M000248566

Cardiac Surgery in the Adult

Cardiac Surgery in the Adult

Second Edition

LAWRENCE H. COHN, M.D.

Virginia and James Hubbard Professor of Cardiac Surgery
Harvard Medical School
Chief, Division of Cardiac Surgery
Brigham and Women's Hospital
Boston, Massachusetts

L. HENRY EDMUNDS, Jr., M.D.

Julian Johnson Professor of Cardiothoracic Surgery
University of Pennsylvania School of Medicine
Philadelphia, Pennsylvania

McGRAW-HILL
Medical Publishing Division

New York Chicago San Francisco Lisbon London Madrid
Mexico City Milan New Delhi San Juan Seoul Singapore Sydney Toronto

Cardiac Surgery in the Adult, Second Edition

1234567890 KGP/KGP 09876543

ISBN 0-07-139129-0

This book was set in Berkley Old Style Medium by TechBooks.
The editors were Marc Strauss and Kitty McCullough.
Project management was provided by Andover Publishing Services.
The production supervisor was Richard Ruzycka.
The cover designer was Aimee Nordin.
The index was prepared by Andover Publishing Services.
Quebecor/Kingsport was printer and binder.

This book is printed on acid-free paper.

Cataloging-in-Publication data is on file for this title at the Library of Congress.

To our patients

Contents

PART III ISCHEMIC HEART DISEASE

PART IVa VALVULAR HEART DISEASE: AORTIC VALVE DISEASE

PART IVb VALVULAR HEART DISEASE: MITRAL VALVE DISEASE

PART IVc VALVULAR HEART DISEASE: OTHER VALVE LESIONS

Contributors

David H. Adams, M.D. [39]
Marie-Josée and Henry R. Kravis Professor of Cardiothoracic Surgery
Mount Sinai School of Medicine
Chairman, Department of Cardiothoracic Surgery
Mount Sinai Medical Center
New York, New York

Arvind K. Agnihotri, M.D. [26]
Instructor in Surgery
Division of Cardiac Surgery
Department of Surgery
Harvard Medical School
Boston, Massachusetts

Cary W. Akins, M.D. [23]
Clinical Professor of Surgery
Harvard Medical School
Cardiac Surgical Unit
Massachusetts General Hospital
Boston, Massachusetts

Michelle A. Albert, M.D. [8]
Instructor in Medicine
Cardiovascular Division
Brigham and Women's Hospital
Department of Medicine
Harvard Medical School
Boston, Massachusetts

Curtis A. Anderson, M.D. [46]
Research Fellow in Cardiac Surgery
Brigham and Women's Hospital
Boston, Massachusetts

Robert H. Anderson, M.D. [2]
Professor
Institute of Child Health and Great Ormond Street Hospital for Children
University College London
London, England

The number(s) in brackets following the contributor's name indicates the chapter(s) authored or coauthored by the contributor.

Mark P. Anstadt, M.D. [16]
Interim Chief and Program Director
Cardiothoracic Surgery
Medical College of Georgia
Augusta, Georgia

Elliott M. Antman, M.D. [8]
Associate Professor of Medicine
Harvard Medical School
Director of the Samuel A. Levine Cardiac Unit
Cardiovascular Division
Brigham and Women's Hospital
Boston, Massachusetts

Sary Aranki, M.D. [38]
Associate Professor of Surgery
Harvard Medical School
Division of Cardiac Surgery
Brigham and Women's Hospital
Boston, Massachusetts

Vinay Badhwar, M.D. [64]
Assistant Professor of Surgery
University of South Florida
Director, Heart Failure Program
Northside Heart Institute
St. Petersburg, Florida

James M. Bailey, M.D., Ph.D. [4]
Associate Professor
Director, Critical Care Service
Department of Anesthesiology
Emory University School of Medicine
Atlanta, Georgia

Leora B. Balsam, M.D. [61]
Research Fellow
Department of Cardiothoracic Surgery
Stanford University School of Medicine
Stanford, California

William A. Baumgartner, M.D. [60]
Cardiac Surgeon-in-Charge
Professor of Surgery
Department of Cardiac Surgery
Johns Hopkins University School of Medicine
Baltimore, Maryland

Joseph E. Bavaria, M.D. [51]
Assistant Professor of Surgery
Division of Cardiothoracic Surgery
Department of Surgery
University of Pennsylvania School of Medicine
Philadelphia, Pennsylvania

Brian T. Bethea, M.D. [60]
Fellow in Cardiothoracic Surgery
Department of Cardiac Surgery
Johns Hopkins University School of Medicine
Baltimore, Maryland

Steven F. Bolling, M.D. [64]
Professor of Surgery
Section of Cardiac Surgery
University of Michigan
Ann Arbor, Michigan

John G. Byrne, M.D. [42]
Associate Professor of Surgery
Harvard Medical School
Division of Cardiac Surgery
Brigham and Women's Hospital
Boston, Massachusetts

Albert T. Cheung, M.D. [9]
Associate Professor of Anesthesia
Department of Anesthesia
University of Pennsylvania School of Medicine
Philadelphia, Pennsylvania

W. Randolph Chitwood, Jr., M.D. [44]
Professor and Chairman
Department of Surgery
Brody School of Medicine
East Carolina University
Greenville, North Carolina

Albert J. Chong, M.D. [34]
Surgical Research Fellow
Division of Cardiothoracic Surgery
Washington University School of Medicine
St. Louis, Missouri

George T. Christakis, M.D. [32]
Associate Professor
Division of Cardiac Surgery
Sunnybrook and Women's College Health Sciences Center
University of Toronto
Toronto, Ontario
Canada

Lawrence H. Cohn, M.D. [30, 38, 42, 46]
Virginia and James Hubbard Professor of Cardiac Surgery
Harvard Medical School
Chief, Division of Cardiac Surgery
Brigham and Women's Hospital
Boston, Massachusetts

Robert W. Colman, M.D. [11]
Professor of Medicine
Temple University School of Medicine
Philadelphia, Pennsylvania

John V. Conte, M.D. [60]
Associate Professor of Surgery
Department of Cardiac Surgery
Johns Hopkins University School of Medicine
Baltimore, Maryland

Joseph S. Coselli, M.D. [48]
Professor and Chief
Division of Cardiothoracic Surgery
Baylor College of Medicine
Houston, Texas

Delos M. Cosgrove, III, M.D.
Chairman
Department of Thoracic and Cardiovascular Surgery
The Cleveland Clinic Foundation
Cleveland, Ohio

James L. Cox, M.D. [53]
Chairman and CEO
The World Heart Foundation
Washington, DC

Willard M. Daggett, Jr., M.D. [26]
Professor of Surgery
Division of Cardiac Surgery
Department of Surgery
Harvard Medical School
Boston, Massachusetts

Tirone E. David, M.D. [31, 33]
Head, Division of Cardiovascular Surgery
Melanie Munk Chair of Cardiovascular Surgery
Professor of Surgery
University of Toronto
Toronto, Ontario
Canada

William J. DeBois, M.B.A., C.C.P. [12]
Chief Perfusionist
Department of Cardiothoracic Surgery
Weill Medical College of Cornell University
New York, New York

Nimesh D. Desai, M.D. [32]
Cardiac Surgery Resident
Division of Cardiac Surgery
Sunnybrook and Women's College Health Sciences Center
University of Toronto
Toronto, Ontario
Canada

Todd M. Dewey, M.D. [22]
Cardiopulmonary Research Science and Technology Institute (CRISTI)
Dallas, Texas

Verdi J. DiSesa, M.D. [43]
Chief, Section of Cardiac Surgery
The Chester County Hospital
West Chester, Pennsylvania

John R. Doty, M.D. [35]
Chief Resident
Division of Cardiac Surgery
The Johns Hopkins Hospital
Baltimore, Maryland

Donald B. Doty, M.D. [35]
Chief, Department of Surgery
LDS Hospital
Salt Lake City, Utah

L. Henry Edmunds, Jr., M.D. [11, 28]
Julian Johnson Professor of Cardiothoracic Surgery
University of Pennsylvania School of Medicine
Philadelphia, Pennsylvania

Laurence M. Epstein, M.D. [52]
Associate Professor of Medicine
Harvard Medical School
Chief, Arrhythmia Service
Director, Electrophysiology and Pacing Laboratory
Division of Cardiology
Brigham and Women's Hospital
Boston, Massachusetts

James I. Fann, M.D. [36]
Assistant Professor
Department of Cardiothoracic Surgery
Stanford University Medical Center
Stanford, California
Cardiac Surgery Section
VA Palo Alto Health Care System
Palo Alto, California

Suellen P. Ferraris, Ph.D. [6]
Research Assistant Professor
Department of Surgery
University of Kentucky Chandler Medical Center
Lexington, Kentucky

Victor A. Ferraris, M.D., Ph.D. [6]
Tyler Gill Professor and Chief
Division of Cardiothoracic Surgery
University of Kentucky Chandler Medical Center
Lexington, Kentucky

Farzan Filsoufi, M.D. [39]
Assistant Professor of Cardiothoracic Surgery
Mount Sinai School of Medicine
Director, Cardiac Valve Center
Mount Sinai Medical Center
New York, New York

Thomas F. Floyd, M.D. [9]
Assistant Professor of Anesthesia
Department of Anesthesia
University of Pennsylvania School of Medicine
Philadelphia, Pennsylvania

Vladimir Formanek, M.D. [10]
Instructor in Anesthesiology
Harvard Medical School
Department of Anesthesiology, Perioperative and Pain Medicine
Brigham and Women's Hospital
Boston, Massachusetts

John A. Fox, M.D. [10]
Instructor in Anesthesiology
Harvard Medical School
Director of Intraoperative Echocardiography
Department of Anesthesiology, Perioperative and Pain Medicine
Brigham and Women's Hospital
Boston, Massachusetts

O. H. Frazier, M.D. [63]
Co-Director
Cardiovascular Research Laboratories
Chief, Cardiopulmonary Transplant Service
Texas Heart Institute at St. Luke's Episcopal Hospital
Houston, Texas

Andrew Friedrich, M.D. [10]
Instructor in Anesthesiology
Harvard Medical School
Department of Anesthesiology, Perioperative and Pain Medicine
Brigham and Women's Hospital
Boston, Massachusetts

James S. Gammie, M.D. [15]
Assistant Professor of Surgery
University of Maryland Medical Center
Baltimore, Maryland

Timothy J. Gardner, M.D. [21]
William Maul Measey Professor and Chief
Division of Cardiothoracic Surgery
Department of Surgery
University of Pennsylvania School of Medicine
Philadelphia, Pennsylvania

Bernard J. Gersh, M.B., Ch.B., D. Phil. [19]
Professor of Medicine
Mayo Medical School
Rochester, Minnesota

A. Marc Gillinov, M.D. [37]
Staff Surgeon
Surgical Director of the Center for Atrial Fibrillation
Department of Thoracic and Cardiovascular Surgery
The Cleveland Clinic Foundation
Cleveland, Ohio

Thomas G. Gleason, M.D. [51]
Cardiac Surgery Fellow
Division of Cardiothoracic Surgery
Department of Surgery
University of Pennsylvania School of Medicine
Philadelphia, Pennsylvania

Donald D. Glower, M.D. [29]
Professor of Surgery
Duke University Medical Center
Durham, North Carolina

Jeffey P. Gold, M.D. [18]
Professor and Chair
Department of Cardiovascular and Thoracic Surgery
Albert Einstein College of Medicine
Montefiore Medical Center
New York, New York

Joseph H. Gorman, III, M.D. [28]
Assistant Professor of Surgery
University of Pennsylvania School of Medicine
Philadelphia, Pennsylvania

Robert C. Gorman, M.D. [28]
Assistant Professor of Surgery
University of Pennsylvania School of Medicine
Philadelphia, Pennsylvania

G. Randall Green, M.D. [45]
Fellow, Department of Thoracic and Cardiovascular Surgery
University of Virginia Health Sciences Center
Charlottesville, Virginia

Randall B. Griepp, M.D. [47]
Professor of Cardiothoracic Surgery
Department of Cardiothoracic Surgery
Mount Sinai School of Medicine
New York, New York

Bartley P. Griffith, M.D. [59]
Professor of Surgery
Chief, Division of Cardiac Surgery
University of Maryland School of Medicine
Baltimore, Maryland

Gary Grunkemeier, Ph.D. [7]
Director, Medical Data Research Center
Providence Health System
Portland, Oregon

Tomas Gudbjartsson, M.D. [38]
Cardiac Surgical Fellow
Department of Cardiac Surgery
Brigham and Women's Hospital
Boston, Massachusetts

Robert A. Guyton, M.D. [3]
Professor and Chief of Cardiothoracic Surgery
Emory University School of Medicine
Atlanta, Georgia

John W. Hammon, Jr., M.D. [11]
Professor of Surgery
Bowman Gray School of Medicine
Wake Forest University
Winston-Salem, North Carolina

Craig R. Hampton, M.D. [34]
Senior Research Fellow
Division of Cardiothoracic Surgery
Department of Surgery
The University of Washington
Seattle, Washington

Eugene A. Hessel II, M.D. [11]
Professor of Anesthesiology and Surgery (Cardiothoracic)
Director, Cardiothoracic Anesthesia
Department of Anesthesiology
University of Kentucky Medical Center
Lexington, Kentucky

Neil B. Ingels, Jr., Ph.D. [36]
Head, Laboratory of Cardiovascular Physiology and Biophysics
Research Institute of the Palo Alto Medical Foundation
Palo Alto, California

O. Wayne Isom, M.D. [12]
Professor and Chairman
Department of Cardiothoracic Surgery
Weill Medical College of Cornell University
New York, New York

M. Salik Jahania, M.D. [14]
Assistant Professor
Division of Cardiothoracic Surgery
University of Kentucky Chandler Medical Center
Lexington, Kentucky

Stuart W. Jamieson, M.B., F.R.C.S. [16]
Professor of Surgery
Chief, Division of Cardiothoracic Surgery
University of San Diego Medical Center
San Diego, California

Ruyun Jin, M.D. [7]
Postdoctoral Fellow, Medical Data Research Center
Providence Health System
Portland, Oregon

Ralph A. Kelly, M.D. [27]
Vice President, Clinical Research
Genzyme Corporation
Framingham, Massachusetts

Karl H. Krieger, M.D. [12]
Professor and Vice-Chairman
Department of Cardiothoracic Surgery
Weill Medical College of Cornell University
New York, New York

Irving L. Kron, M.D. [45]
Professor and Chairman
Department of Thoracic and Cardiovascular Surgery
University of Virginia Health Sciences Center
Charlottesville, Virginia

Eugene L. Kukuy, M.D. [62]
Cardiothoracic Surgery Post-Doctorate Research Fellow
Clinical Pacemaker FellowColumbia University
Division of Cardiothoracic Surgery
Department of Surgery
New York Presbyterian Hospital
New York, New York

Hillel Laks, M.D. [56]
Professor and Chief
Division of Cardiothoracic Surgery
Department of Surgery
David Geffen School of Medicine
University of California, Los Angeles
Los Angeles, California

Robert D. Lasley, Ph.D. [14]
Professor
Division of Cardiothoracic Surgery
University of Kentucky Chandler Medical Center
Lexington, Kentucky

Martin LeBoutillier III, M.D. [43]
Attending Staff
Section of Cardiac Surgery
The Chester County Hospital
West Chester, Pennsylvania

Leonard Y. Lee, M.D. [12]
Assistant Professor
Department of Cardiothoracic Surgery
Weill Medical College of Cornell University
New York, New York

Daniel C. Lee, M.D. [24]
Research Fellow
Division of Cardiothoracic Surgery
Department of Surgery
Columbia University College of Physicans and Surgeons
New York, New York

Jerrold H. Levy, M.D. [4]
Professor and Chairman for Research
Department of Anesthesiology
Emory University School of Medicine
Atlanta, Georgia

James E. Lowe, M.D. [16, 29]
Professor of Surgery
Division of Cardiovascular and Thoracic Surgery
Duke University Medical Center
Durham, North Carolina

Bruce W. Lytle, M.D. [25]
Surgeon
Department of Thoracic and Cardiovascular Surgery
The Cleveland Clinic Foundation
Cleveland, Ohio

Michael J. Mack, M.D. [22]
Cardiopulmonary Research Science and Technology Institute (CRISTI)
Dallas, Texas

Michael M. Madani, M.D. [50]
Assistant Clinical Professor of Surgery
Division of Cardiothoracic Surgery
University of San Diego Medical Center
San Diego, California

Joren C. Madsen, M.D. [26]
Associate Professor of Surgery
Division of Cardiac Surgery
Department of Surgery
Harvard Medical School
Boston, Massachusetts

Abeel A. Mangi, M.D. [57]
Surgical Resident
Department of Surgery
Massachusetts General Hospital
Boston, Massachusetts

Daniel Marelli, M.D. [56]
Assistant Professor
Division of Cardiothoracic Surgery
Department of Surgery
David Geffen School of Medicine
University of California, Los Angeles
Los Angeles, California

Dale H. Marsh, M.D. [41]
Surgical Resident
Mayo Clinic
Rochester, Minnesota

Manu M. Mathur, M.D. [47]
Consultant Cardiothoracic Surgeon
Royal North Shore Hospital
Sydney
Australia

John E. Mayer, Jr., M.D. [65]
Professor of Surgery
Harvard Medical School
Senior Associate in Cardiac Surgery
Children's Hospital
Boston, Massachusetts

Patrick M. McCarthy, M.D. [17]
Surgical Director, Kaufman Center for Heart Failure
Program Director, Heart Transplantation
Department of Cardiothoracic Surgery
The Cleveland Clinic Foundation
Cleveland, Ohio

Philippe Menasche, M.D., Ph.D. [11]
Professor of Cardiac Surgery
Hôpital Européen Georges Pompidou
Assistance Publique- Hôpitaux de Paris and University of Paris
Paris
France

Robert M. Mentzer, Jr., M.D. [14]
Frank C. Spencer Professor and Chairman
Department of Surgery
Professor of Physiology
Director of the UK Transplant Center
University of Kentucky Chandler Medical Center
Lexington, Kentucky

Lynda L. Mickleborough, M.D. [54]
Professor of Cardiac Surgery
University of Toronto
University Health Network
Toronto, Ontario
Canada

Tomislav Mihaljevic, M.D. [30]
Associate Cardiac Surgeon
Assistant Professor of Surgery
Harvard Medical School
Division of Cardiac Surgery
Brigham and Women's Hospital
Boston, Massachusetts

Michael R. Mill, M.D. [2]
Professor of Surgery
Chief, Division of Cardiothoracic Surgery
University of North Carolina School of Medicine
Chapel Hill, North Carolina

D. Craig Miller, M.D. [36]
Thelma and Henry Doelger Professor of Cardiovascular Surgery
Department of Cardiothoracic Surgery
Stanford University Medical School
Stanford, California

R. Scott Mitchell, M.D. [49]
Professor of Cardiovascular Surgery
Department of Cardiothoracic Surgery
Stanford University Medical School
Stanford, California

Nader Moazami, M.D. [17]
Assistant Professor of Surgery
Director of Cardiac Transplantation
Division of Cardiothoracic Surgery
Washington University School of Medicine
St. Louis, Missouri

Susan D. Moffatt, M.D., Ph.D. [49]
Fellow in Cardiovascular Surgery
Department of Cardiothoracic Surgery
Stanford University Medical School
Stanford, California

Ashby C. Moncure, M.D. [23]
Clinical Professor of Surgery
Harvard Medical School
Vascular Surgical Unit
Massachusetts General Hospital
Boston, Massachusetts

Paulo L. Moreno, M.D. [48]
Cardiovascular Surgeon
Instituto de Cardiologia do Rio Grande do Sul
Porto Alegre
Brazil

Jeff Myers, M.D. [56]
Clinical Instructor
Division of Cardiothoracic Surgery
Department of Surgery
David Geffen School of Medicine
University of California, Los Angeles
Los Angeles, California

Timothy J. Myers, B.S. [63]
Manager, Clinical Research and Regulatory Affairs
Cardiovascular Research Laboratories
Texas Heart Institute at St. Luke's Episcopal Hospital
Houston, Texas

Yoshifumi Naka, M.D., Ph.D. [62]
Herbert Irving Assistant Professor of Surgery
Director, Mechanical Circulatory Support
Division of Cardiothoracic Surgery
Department of Surgery
New York Presbyterian Hospital
New York, New York

L. Wiley Nifong, M.D. [44]
Assistant Professor
Department of Surgery
Brody School of Medicine
East Carolina University
Greenville, North Carolina

Jonah Odim, M.D., Ph.D. [56]
Assistant Professor
Division of Cardiothoracic Surgery
Department of Surgery
David Geffen School of Medicine
University of California, Los Angeles
Los Angeles, California

Mehmet C. Oz, M.D. [24]
Professor of Surgery
Director, Cardiovascular Institute
Vice Chairman, Department of Surgery
Columbia University College of Physicans
and Surgeons
New York, New York

Robert F. Padera, Jr., M.D., Ph.D. [5]
Resident in Pathology
Brigham and Women's Hospital
Clinical Fellow in Pathology
Harvard Medical School
Boston, Massachusetts

Subroto Paul, M.D. [30]
Surgical Research Fellow
Brigham and Women's Hospital
Harvard Medical School
Boston, Massachusetts

Bradley J. Phillips, M.D. [42]
Research Fellow
Division of Cardiac Surgery
Brigham and Women's Hospital
Boston, Massachusetts

Mark Plunkett, M.D. [56]
Assistant Professor
Division of Cardiothoracic Surgery
Department of Surgery
David Geffen School of Medicine
University of California, Los Angeles
Los Angeles, California

Robert S. Poston, M.D. [59]
Assistant Professor of Surgery
University of Maryland School of Medicine
Baltimore, Maryland

René Prêtre, M.D. [13]
Professor of Surgery
Department of Cardiovascular Surgery
University Hospital Zürich
Zürich
Switzerland

Michael J. Reardon, M.D. [58]
Professor of Surgery
Baylor College of Medicine
Houston, Texas

Bruce A. Reitz, M.D. [61]
The Norman E. Shumway Professor and Chairman
Department of Cardiothoracic Surgery
Stanford University School of Medicine
Stanford, California

Robert J. Rizzo, M.D. [46]
Assistant Professor of Surgery
Harvard Medical School
Division of Cardiac Surgery
Brigham and Women's Hospital
Boston, Massachusetts

Robert C. Robbins, M.D. [61]
Associate Professor of Cardiothoracic Surgery
Department of Cardiothoracic Surgery
Stanford University School of Medicine
Stanford, California

Marc Ruel, M.D., M.P.H. [27]
Assistant Professor of Surgery
University of Ottawa
Attending Cardiac Surgeon
University of Ottawa Heart Institute
Ottawa, Ontario
Canada

Rawn Salenger, M.D. [15]
Resident
Cardiothoracic Surgery
UMASS Memorial Medical Center
Worcester, Massachusetts

S. Dinakar Satti, M.D. [52]
Instructor in Medicine
Harvard Medical School
Attending Physician, Division of Cardiology
Brigham and Women's Hospital
Boston, Massachusetts

Joseph S. Savino, M.D. [9]
Associate Professor of Anesthesia
Section Chief, Cardiovascular Thoracic Anesthesia and Intensive Care
Department of Anesthesia
University of Pennsylvania School of Medicine
Philadelphia, Pennsylvania

Hartzell V. Schaff, M.D. [41]
Stuart W. Harrington Professor of Surgery
Mayo Clinic
Rochester, Minnesota

Frederick J. Schoen, M.D., Ph.D. [5]
Professor of Pathology
Harvard Medical School
Executive Vice Chairman and Director, Cardiac Pathology
Department of Pathology
Brigham and Women's Hospital
Boston, Massachusetts

Frank W. Sellke, M.D. [27]
Johnson & Johnson Professor of Surgery
Harvard Medical School
Chief, Division of Cardiothoracic Surgery
Beth Israel Deaconess Medical Center
Boston, Massachusetts

Nyma A. Shah, B.S. [63]
Research Coordinator
Cardiovascular Research Laboratories
Texas Heart Institute at St. Luke's Episcopal Hospital
Houston, Texas

Richard J. Shemin, M.D. [40]
Professor and Chairman
Department of Cardiothoracic Surgery
Boston University School of Medicine
Vice Chairman, Division of Surgery
Chief of Cardiothoracic Surgery
Co-director Cardiovascular Center
Boston Medical Center
Boston, Massachusetts

Stanton K. Shernan, M.D. [10]
Assistant Professor of Anesthesiology
Harvard Medical School
Director of Cardiac Anesthesiology
Department of Anesthesiology, Perioperative and Pain Medicine
Brigham and Women's Hospital
Boston, Massachusetts

Hugh C. Smith, M.D. [19]
Professor of Medicine
Mayo Medical School
Rochester, Minnesota

W. Roy Smythe, M.D. [58]
Assistant Professor of Thoracic and Cardiovascular Surgery
The University of Texas M.D. Anderson Cancer Center
Houston, Texas

David Spielvogel, M.D. [47]
Assistant Professor of Cardiothoracic Surgery
Department of Cardiothoracic Surgery
Mount Sinai School of Medicine
New York, New York

Henry M. Spotnitz, M.D. [55]
George H. Humphreys II Professor of Surgery
Vice-Chair, Research and Information Systems
Cardiothoracic Surgery Division
Department of Surgery
Columbia University College of Physicans and Surgeons
New York, New York

Larry W. Stephenson, M.D. [1]
Ford-Webber Professor of Surgery
Chief, Division of Cardiothoracic Surgery
Wayne State University School of Medicine
Detroit, Michigan

Thoralf M. Sundt III, M.D. [19]
Associate Professor of Surgery
Mayo Medical School
Rochester, Minnesota

Fraser W.H. Sutherland, M.A., F.R.C.S. (Eng.) [65]
Research Fellow in Cardiac Surgery
Harvard Medical School and Children's Hospital
Boston, Massachusetts
Specialist Registrar in Cardiothoracic Surgery
The Royal Infirmary of Edinburgh
United Kingdom

Kenichi A. Tanaka, M.D. [4]
Assistant Professor
Department of Anesthesiology
Emory University School of Medicine
Atlanta, Georgia

Windsor Ting, M.D. [24]
Assistant Professor
Division of Cardiothoracic Surgery
Department of Surgery
Columbia University College of Physicans and Surgeons
New York, New York

David F. Torchiana, M.D. [57]
Chief, Division of Cardiac Surgery
Department of Surgery
Massachusetts General Hospital
Boston, Massachusetts

Marko I. Turina, M.D. [13]
Head of Cardiac Surgery and Professor of Surgery
Department of Cardiovascular Surgery
University Hospital Zürich
Zürich
Switzerland

Thomas J. Vander Salm, M.D. [15]
Professor of Surgery
UMASS Memorial Medical Center
Worcester, Massachusetts

Edward D. Verrier, M.D. [34]
Vice Chairman, Department of Surgery
William K. Edmark Professor of Cardiovascular Surgery
Chief, Division of Cardiothoracic Surgery
The University of Washington
Seattle, Washington

Venkataramana Vijay, M.D. [18]
Assistant Professor
Department of Cardiovascular and Thoracic Surgery
Albert Einstein College of Medicine
Montefiore Medical Center
New York, New York

Jakob Vinten-Johansen, Ph.D. [3]
Professor
Division of Cardiothoracic Surgery
Associate Professor
Department of Physiology
Director, Cardiothoracic Research Laboratory
Emory University School of Medicine
Atlanta, Georgia

Andrew Wechsler, M.D. [30]
Stanley K. Brockman Professor and Chairman
Department of Cardiovascular Medicine and Surgery
Drexel University College of Medicine
Philadelphia, Pennsylvania

Benson R. Wilcox, M.D. [2]
Professor of Surgery
Division of Cardiothoracic Surgery
University of North Carolina School of Medicine
Chapel Hill, North Carolina

James T. Willerson, M.D. [20]
President
University of Texas Health Science Center at Houston
Medical Director
Texas Heart Institute
Chief of Cardiology
St. Luke's Episcopal Hospital and Texas Heart Institute
Houston, Texas

Y. Joseph Woo, M.D. [21]
Assistant Professor of Surgery
Division of Cardiothoracic Surgery
Department of Surgery
University of Pennsylvania School of Medicine
Philadelphia, Pennsylvania

David D. Yuh, M.D. [60. 61]
Assistant Professor of Surgery
Department of Cardiac Surgery
Johns Hopkins University School of Medicine
Baltimore, Maryland

Zhi-Qing Zhao, M.D., Ph.D. [3]
Assistant Professor
Division of Cardiothoracic Surgery
Emory University School of Medicine
Atlanta, Georgia

Foreword

It is altogether fitting and proper that this second edition of *Cardiac Surgery in the Adult* reaches publication just in time to celebrate the 50th anniversary of open heart surgery. On September 5, 1952, at the University of Minnesota, F. John Lewis successfully closed an atrial septal defect in a 5-year-old girl using general hypothermia. She remains well to this day. On May 6, 1953, at the Jefferson Hospital in Philadelphia, John H. Gibbon, Jr., successfully closed an atrial septal defect in a 16-year-old woman during 26 minutes of cardiopulmonary bypass. The cork was out of the bottle, but it remained for C. Walton Lillihei and John W. Kirklin of the Mayo Clinic to make open heart surgery a safe and practicable approach, applying it first to congenital heart disease and then to heart disease in the adult. It is interesting that for a brief period in the 1950s only the University of Minnesota and the Mayo Clinic, 90 miles apart, were available to the patient requiring open heart surgery.

Fifty years later, surgery of the heart is a procedure performed many times every day. Another significant change is the emergence of pediatric cardiac surgery as a standalone specialty. This is despite the fact that the arterial switch procedure for transposition had its origin in direct coronary artery surgery. Indeed, many other crossover points exist between pediatric and adult surgery. Hopefully, this interdependence will not disappear as these two disciplines seemingly go their separate ways.

Readers of this volume will be rewarded by finding all they need to know in one well-edited book. There remains, however, a supreme golden rule in heart surgery, which states that, on the morning of postoperative day one, the open heart surgical patient must be awake, alert, and ready for extubation and transfer to regular floor care. It goes without saying that the bleeding, as always, has stopped!

Norman E. Shumway, M.D., Ph.D.
Professor of Cardiothoracic Surgery
Stanford University School of Medicine

Preface

The second edition of *Cardiac Surgery in the Adult* builds on the great success of the first edition, edited by Dr. L. Henry Edmunds. The first edition became the gold standard for adult cardiac surgical textbooks, departing from traditional multi-subspecialty thoracic textbooks involving pediatric, general thoracic, and adult cardiac surgery. Dr. Edmunds' edition blazed a trail by focusing on the information about adult cardiac surgery and provided a tremendous leap forward in our knowledge base.

In the second edition, we have added 19 new chapters in areas related to new technology, and subdivided previous chapters because of the expanded information that is now available in many areas. For example, there are entirely new chapters on minimally invasive valve surgery, coronary angiogenesis, and endovascular stent management of thoracic aortic disease. We have added a new chapter on intraoperative echocardiography for surgeons. The chapter on extracorporeal circulation now contains four major subchapters in order to organize and clearly present the enormous expansion of knowledge about artificial circulation. Other chapters from the first edition have been divided into several new chapters because of the increase in knowledge, particularly in the area of aortic valve surgery. There are now chapters on aortic valve repair and valve-sparing operations, stented bioprosthetic valves, stentless valves (including autograft, homograft, and porcine valves), as well as separate chapters on surgery for endocarditis of the aortic and mitral valves. Because of the continuing evolution of cardiac arrhythmia surgery, we have added a chapter on cardiologic intervention therapy as well as a separate chapter on surgery for ventricular and atrial arrhythmias. Two new chapters involving nontransplant surgical options for heart failure, an increasingly complex field, are also included, as well as one on tissue engineering. What the cardiac surgeon does in the 21st century has changed; perhaps there will be a lesser emphasis on coronary surgery because of interventional techniques, but the cardiac surgeon still has an extremely full and complex array of operations to understand and use on an aging patient population with increasingly complex disease states. We believe that the information in this volume will help to address virtually all the new areas of cardiac surgery that will be employed in the 21st century.

In assuming the editorship of this book, I felt it was important to publish this information as quickly as possible to maximize the effect of the new technology. Thus, the call for chapters was sent out in November 2001 and all chapters were received by the end of September 2002, allowing for publication in early 2003, to commemorate the 50th anniversary of the first successful open heart operation using cardiopulmonary bypass. Textbooks are relevant only to the degree that the information in them is current, and we believe that to be a central part of our mission.

I am indebted to several people for the production of this volume. First and foremost, L. Henry "Hank" Edmunds, M.D., asked me to carry on the legacy of this very important book, and for this I am very grateful. His help has been incredibly important, and his experience, invaluable. His editorial duties with the *Annals of Thoracic Surgery* have made him a superb editor, and he has been of tremendous help to me. I am indebted to Marc Strauss, my editor at McGraw-Hill, who has been extremely supportive and helpful in every way in getting this book organized and completed. I am also very grateful to Ann Maloney, my administrative assistant in the Division of Cardiac Surgery at the Brigham, who was extremely helpful in pointing out ways to improve efficiency and helping to politely cajole chapter authors to get their chapters in on time. Also, Kitty McCullough at McGraw-Hill and Susan Hunter at Andover Publishing Services helped with the technical construction of this book and deserve tremendous credit.

But in the final analysis the most deserving thanks must go to all of the chapter authors, who are among the busiest cardiac surgeons on earth. They took the time and energy to produce superb analysis of their particular areas of expertise on schedule.

I would like to thank Norman Shumway, who was not only my cardiac surgical mentor but who has also been a great supporter of mine throughout my career and who has written a pithy Foreword for this book.

Finally, to my family, who have supported me during the increased amount of time that this project has taken, I give my love and thanks.

Lawrence H. Cohn, M.D.
Boston, Massachusetts
2003

Cardiac Surgery in the Adult

Part **I**

Fundamentals

Chapter 1

History of Cardiac Surgery

Larry W. Stephenson

The development of major surgery was retarded for centuries by a lack of knowledge and technology. Significantly, the general anesthetics, ether and chloroform, were not developed until the middle of the 19th century. These agents made major surgical operations possible, which created an interest in repairing wounds to the heart, leading some investigators in Europe to conduct studies in the animal laboratory on the repair of heart wounds. The first simple operations in humans for heart wounds were soon reported in the medical literature.

HEART WOUNDS

On July 10, 1893, Dr. Daniel Hale Williams (Fig. 1-1), a surgeon from Chicago, successfully operated on a 24-year-old man who had been stabbed in the heart during a fight. The patient was admitted to Chicago's Provident Hospital on July 9 at 7:30 P.M. The stab wound was slightly to the left of the sternum and dead center over the heart. Initially, the wound was thought to be superficial, but during the night the patient experience persistent bleeding, pain, and pronounced symptoms of shock. Williams opened the patient's chest and tied off an artery and vein that had been injured inside the chest wall, likely causing the blood loss. Then he noticed a tear in the pericardium and a puncture wound to the heart, "about one-tenth of an inch in length."[1]

The wound in the right ventricle was not bleeding, so Williams did not place a stitch through the heart wound. He did, however, stitch closed the hole in the pericardium. The patient recovered. Williams reported this case four years later.[1] This operation, which is frequently referred to, is probably the first successful surgery involving a documented stab wound to the heart. At the time, Williams' surgery was considered bold and daring, and although he did not actually place a stitch through the wound in the heart, his treatment seems to have been appropriate. Under the circumstances, he most likely saved the patient's life.

A few years after Williams' case, a couple of other surgeons actually sutured heart wounds, but the patients did not survive. Dr. Ludwig Rehn (Fig. 1-2), a surgeon in Frankfurt, Germany, performed what many consider the first successful heart operation.[2] On September 7, 1896, a 22-year-old man was stabbed in the heart and collapsed. The police found him pale, covered with cold sweat, and extremely short of breath. His pulse was irregular and his clothes were soaked with blood. By September 9, his condition was worsening,

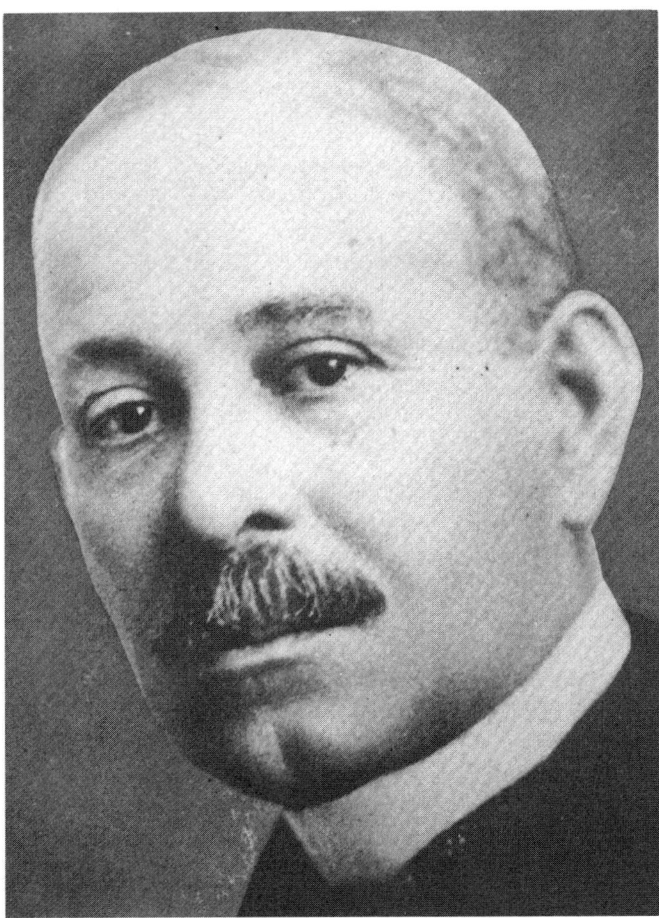

FIGURE 1–1 Dr. Daniel Hale Williams, a surgeon from Chicago who successfully operated on a patient with a wound to the chest involving the pericardium and the heart. *(Reproduced with permission from Organ CH Jr, Kosiba MM: The Century of the Black Surgeons: A USA Experience. Norman, OK, Transcript Press, 1987; p 312.)*

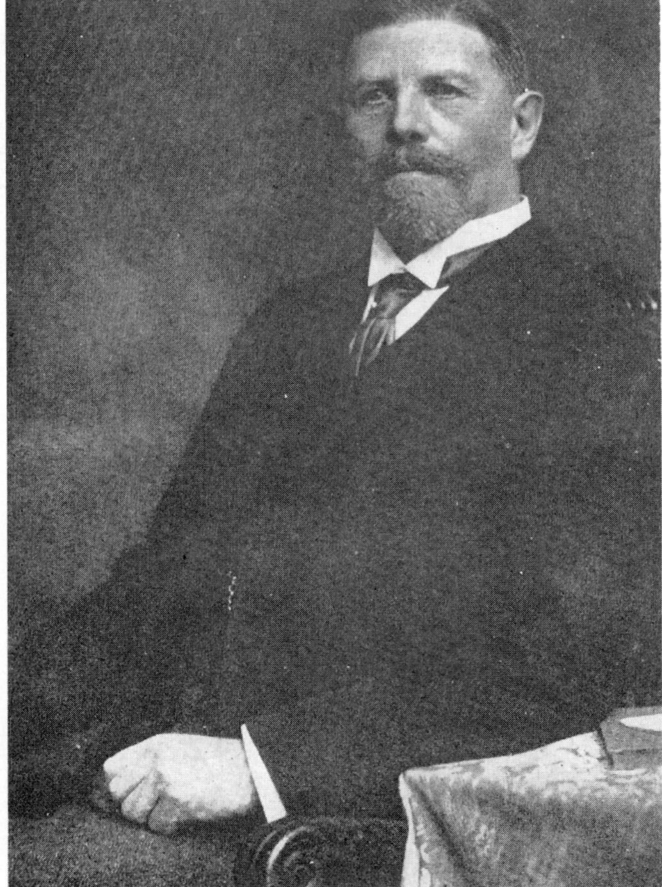

FIGURE 1–2 Dr. Ludwig Rehn, a surgeon from Frankfurt, Germany, who performed the first successful suture of a human heart wound. *(Reproduced with permission from Mead R: A History of Thoracic Surgery. Springfield, IL, Charles C Thomas, 1961; p 887.)*

as shown in Dr. Rehn's case notes:

> Pulse weaker, increasing cardiac dullness on percussion, respiration 76, further deterioration during the day, diagnostic tap reveals dark blood. Patient appears moribund. Diagnosis: increasing hemothorax. I decided to operate entering the chest through the left fourth intercostal space, there is massive blood in the pleural cavity. The mammary artery is not injured. There is continuous bleeding from a hole in the pericardium. This opening is enlarged. The heart is exposed. Old blood and clots are emptied. There is a 1.5 cm gaping right ventricular wound. Bleeding is controlled with finger pressure. . . .
>
> I decided to suture the heart wound. I used a small intestinal needle and silk suture. The suture was tied in diastole. Bleeding diminished remarkably with the third suture, all bleeding was controlled. The pulse improved. The pleural cavity was irrigated. Pleura and pericardium were drained with iodoform gauze. The incision was approximated, heart rate and respiratory rate decreased and pulse improved postoperatively.
>
> . . . Today the patient is cured. He looks very good. His heart action is regular. I have not allowed him to work physically hard. This proves the feasibility of cardiac suture repair without a doubt! *I hope this will lead to more investigation regarding surgery of the heart. This may save many lives.*

Ten years after Rehn's initial repair, he had accumulated a series of 124 cases with a mortality of only 60%, quite a feat at that time.[3]

Dr. Luther Hill was the first American to report the successful repair of a cardiac wound, in a 13-year-old boy who was a victim of multiple stab wounds.[4] When the first doctor arrived, the boy was in profound shock. The doctor remembered that Dr. Luther Hill had spoken on the subject of repair of cardiac wounds at a local medical society meeting in Montgomery, Alabama. With the consent of the boy's parents,

Dr. Hill was sent for. He arrived sometime after midnight with six other physicians. One was his brother. The surgery took place on the patient's kitchen table in a rundown shack. Lighting was provided by two kerosene lamps borrowed from neighbors. One physician administered chloroform anesthesia. The boy was suffering from cardiac tamponade as a result of a stab wound to the left ventricle. The stab wound to the ventricle was repaired with two catgut sutures. Although the early postoperative course was stormy, the boy made a complete recovery. That patient, Henry Myrick, eventually moved to Chicago, where, in 1942, at the age of 53, he got into a heated argument and was stabbed in the heart again, very close to the original stab wound. This time, Henry was not as lucky and died from the wound.

Another milestone in cardiac surgery for trauma occurred during World War II when Dwight Harken, then a U.S. Army surgeon, removed 134 missiles from the mediastinum, including 55 from the pericardium and 13 from cardiac chambers, without a death.[5] It is hard to imagine this type of elective (and semielective) surgery taking place without sophisticated indwelling pulmonary artery catheters, blood banks, and electronic monitoring equipment. Rapid blood infusion consisted of pumping air into glass bottles of blood.

OPERATIVE MANAGEMENT OF PULMONARY EMBOLI

Frederic Trendelenburg was the first to attempt a pulmonary embolectomy. In his classic paper that appeared in 1908,[6] he stated that the clinical picture is characteristic: rapid collapse, frequently accompanied by substernal pain that often causes the patient to suddenly scream wildly. He reported on animal studies in 1907; following rapid exposure of the heart, he quickly incised the conus pulmonalis, inserted a cannula, advanced it into the pulmonary artery, and removed emboli using suction. Further experimentation revealed that a direct incision in the artery with removal of the emboli using forceps (those designed for removal of polyps) was much easier. He describes his first unsuccessful pulmonary embolectomy in a human. That operation became famous and is known as the *Trendelenburg operation*.

Trendelenburg subsequently reported two more cases, both fatal.[7] The first of those two patients died 15 hours postoperatively of cardiac failure, the second 37 hours postoperatively. Kirschner, Trendelenburg's student, reported the first patient who fully recovered after undergoing pulmonary embolectomy in 1924.[8] In 1937, John Gibbon estimated that 9 of 142 patients who had undergone the Trendelenburg procedure worldwide left the hospital alive.[9] These dismal results were a stimulus for Gibbon to start work on a pump oxygenator that could maintain the circulation during pulmonary embolectomy. Sharp was first to perform pulmonary embolectomy using cardiopulmonary bypass, in 1962.[10]

SURGERY OF THE PERICARDIUM

Morgagni reported seven cases of constrictive pericarditis in 1761 and described the dangers of cardiac compression by stating that the heart was "so constricted and confined that it could not receive a proper quantity of blood to pass through it."[11] Pick presented a paper in 1896 in which he described the course of chronic pericarditis under the guise of cirrhosis of the liver.[12] Weill in 1895 and Delorme in 1898 proposed excision of the thickened fibrous pericardium in constrictive pericarditis.[13,14] Pericardial resection was introduced independently by Rehn[15] and Sauerbruch.[16] Since Rehn's report, there have been few advances in the surgical treatment of constrictive pericarditis. Some operations are now performed with the aid of cardiopulmonary bypass. In certain situations, radical pericardiectomy that removes most of the pericardium posterior to the phrenic nerves is done.

CATHETERIZATION OF THE RIGHT SIDE OF THE HEART

Although cardiac catheterization is *not* considered heart surgery, it is an invasive procedure and some catheter procedures have replaced heart operations. Warner Forssmann is credited with the first heart catheterization. He performed the procedure on himself and reported it in *Kleinische Wochenschrift*.[17] In 1956, Forssmann shared the Nobel Prize in Physiology or Medicine with Andre F. Cournand and Dickenson W. Richards, Jr. His 1929 paper states, "These are reasons why one often hesitates to use intercardiac injections. Often, time is wasted with other measures. This is why I kept looking for different, safer access to the cardiac chambers: the catheterization of the right heart via the venous system." He goes on to say,

> I confirmed these facts by studies on a cadaver, catheterizing any vein near the elbow, the catheter would pass easily into the right ventricle. . . .
>
> After these successful preliminary studies, I attempted the first experiment on a living human, performing the experiment on myself. In a preliminary experiment, I had asked a colleague to puncture my right brachial vein with a large-bore needle. Then I advanced a well-lubricated No. 4 ureteral catheter through the cannula into the vein. . . . One week later I tried it again without assistance this time. I proceeded with vena puncture in my left antebrachial vein and introduced the catheter to its full length of 65 cm. . . .
>
> I checked the catheter position radiologically, after having climbed stairs from the OR to the radiology department. A nurse was holding a mirror in front of the x-ray screen for me to observe the catheter advance in position. The length of the catheter did not allow further advancement than into the right atrium. I paid particular attention to the possible effects on the cardiac conduction system, but I could not detect any effect.

In this report by Forssmann, a photograph of the x-ray taken of Forssmann with the catheter in his heart is presented. Forssmann, in that same report, goes on to present the first clinical application of the central venous catheter for a patient in shock with generalized peritonitis. Forssmann concludes his paper by stating, "I also want to mention that this method allows new options for metabolic studies and studies about cardiac physiology."

In a 1951 lecture, Forssmann discussed the tremendous resistance he faced during his initial experiments.[18] "Such methods are good for a circus, but not for a respected hospital," was the answer to his request to pursue physiological studies using cardiac catheterization. His progressive ideas pushed him into the position of an outsider with ideas too crazy to give him a clinical position. Klein applied cardiac catheterization for cardiac output determinations using the Fick method a half year after Forssmann's first report.[19] In 1930 Forssmann described his experiments with catheter cardiac angiography.[20] Further use of this new methodology had to wait until Cournand's work in the 1940s.

HEART VALVE SURGERY BEFORE THE ERA OF CARDIOPULMONARY BYPASS

The first clinical attempt to open a stenotic valve was carried out by Theodore Tuffier on July 13, 1912.[21] Alexis Carrel was present at the operation.[22] Tuffier used his finger to reach the stenotic aortic valve. He was able to dilate the valve by supposedly pushing the invaginated aortic wall through the stenotic valve. The 26-year-old patient recovered and returned to his home in Belgium. One must be skeptical as to what was accomplished. Russell Brock attempted to dilate calcified aortic valves in humans in the late 1940s by passing an instrument through the valve from the innominate or another artery.[23] His results were poor, and he abandoned the approach. During the next several years, Brock[24] and Bailey et al[25] used different dilators and various approaches to dilate stenotic aortic valves in patients. Mortality for these procedures that were often done in conjunction with mitral commissurotomy was high.

Harvey Cushing attempted to create mitral stenosis in dogs but was not successful.[26] He encouraged Elliott Cutler, a young surgeon working with him, to continue. In collaboration with a Boston cardiologist, Samuel Levine, Cutler worked 2 years on a mitral valvulotomy procedure in the laboratory.[27] Their first patient was a desperately ill 12-year-old girl who was confined to bed for 6 months before operation. She underwent successful valvulotomy on May 20, 1923, using a teratomy knife. Unfortunately, most of Cutler's subsequent patients died because he created too much regurgitation with his valvulotome, and he soon gave up the operation. In 1925 Mr. Souttar, an English surgeon, successfully performed a mitral valvulotomy using his finger to fracture the commissures in a young female who had been bedridden for 6 months.[28] His case was successful, but he did not do more operations.

In 1961 Dr. Dwight Harken wrote Henry Suttar a letter and asked him why he did not continue with his mitral valvuloplasty. He replied: "Thank you so much for your very kind letter. I did not repeat the operation because I could not get another case. Although my patient made an uninterrupted recovery, the physicians declared that it was all nonsense and in fact the operation was unjustifiable. In fact, it is of no use to be ahead of one's time. . . ."[29] Two decades passed before there was a resurgence of interest in valvular surgery.

In Charles Bailey's 1949 paper titled "The Surgical Treatment of Mitral Stenosis," he states, "After 1929 no more surgical attempts [on mitral stenosis] were made until 1945. Dr. Dwight Harken, Dr. Horace Smithy, and the author recently made operative attempts to improve mitral stenosis. Our clinical experience with the surgery of the mitral valves has been 5 cases to date. During the past 8 years, the author and his associates have performed operations on the mitral valves of 60 mongrel dogs."[30] Bailey goes on to state several conclusions from their animal research. He then describes his five cases, four of whom died and only one of whom lived a long life.

Bailey's home base, Hahnemann Hospital, refused to allow him to attempt any more mitral commissurotomies after two deaths. He became known as the "butcher of Hahnemann Hospital."[29] However, his cardiologist, Dr. Durant, continued to support him. On June 10, 1948, Bailey scheduled cases 4 and 5. The patient operated on at Philadelphia General Hospital in the morning died (case 4). The surgical team regrouped and rushed to Episcopal Hospital, where the second operation was started promptly before the bad morning news was known and before the hospital administration forbade the procedure. The surgery was completed, and 1 week later Bailey brought the patient by train 1000 miles to Chicago, where he presented the woman to the American College of Chest Physicians.[31] A few days after Bailey's success, on June 16 in Boston, Dr. Dwight Harken successfully performed his first valvulotomy for mitral stenosis. Three months later, Russell Brock in England did his first successful clinical case. He did not report this, however, until 1950, when he described success with six patients.[32]

The first successful pulmonary valvulotomy was performed by Thomas Holmes Sellers on December 4, 1947. A systemic pulmonary artery shunt was planned on the left side, but the attempt was abandoned in this patient with severe tetralogy of Fallot and advanced bilateral pulmonary tuberculosis.[33] The pericardium was opened. Dr. Sellers could feel the stenotic valve each time it pushed through the pulmonary trunk during ventricular systole. Sellers used a tenotomy knife, which he passed through the right ventricle to perform the valvulotomy. The patient made a good recovery and was markedly improved.

Russell Brock also attempted pulmonary valvulotomies in a number of patients during the same period using various techniques. Brock's first three patients died, but he eventually developed a successful procedure similar to Sellers'.[34]

In the early 1950s, Charles Hufnagel, in Washington, DC, and J. M. Campbell, in Oklahoma, independently developed and implanted artificial valves in the descending aorta of dogs. The valves consisted of a mobile ball inside a Lucite case.[35,36] After presenting this first model of a mechanical prosthesis at the American College of Surgeons meeting in 1949, Hufnagel applied this concept clinically for the treatment of aortic valvular insufficiency. In his first clinical paper published in *Surgery* in 1954,[37] Hufnagel reported a series of 23 patients starting September 1952 who had this operation for aortic insufficiency. There were 4 deaths among the first 10 patients and 2 deaths among the next 13. Hufnagel's caged ball valve, which used multiple-point fixation rings to secure the apparatus to the aorta, was the only surgical treatment for aortic valvular incompetence until the advent of cardiopulmonary bypass and the development of heart valves that could be sewn into the aortic annulus position.

The first surgical treatment of multiple valvular disease was by Trace et al.[38] After closed mitral commissurotomy on May 2, 1952, in a 24-year-old woman, the surgeon noted that the right auricular appendage was gravely distended and pointed directly toward the left. Its pulsation was noticed and it was quite blue-purple in color. The purse-string was being placed around the appendage in order to explore it when the patient's heart became arrhythmic. It was deemed advisable to terminate the surgical procedure at this point. The patient did poorly postoperatively. In the 2 weeks after the first operation, a tricuspid commissurotomy was performed. The patient made a good recovery and at 1-year follow-up remained improved.

Combined mitral and tricuspid commissurotomy was performed by Brofman in 1953.[39] Likoff et al[40] reported a series of 74 patients who had combined aortic and mitral valve commissurotomies in 1955 with up to a 2-year follow-up. C. Walton Lillehei was the first to report repair of multiple valvular lesions using cardiopulmonary bypass. On May 23, 1956, he successfully performed an open mitral commissurotomy and aortic valvuloplasty in a 52-year-old man with mitral stenosis and combined aortic stenosis and incompetence.[41] Borman performed a quadruple valve commissurotomy in October 1973 in a 12-year-old Israeli girl with stenosis of all four valves.[42]

CONGENITAL CARDIAC SURGERY BEFORE THE HEART-LUNG MACHINE ERA

Congenital cardiac surgery began when John Streider at the Massachusetts General Hospital first successfully interrupted a ductus on March 6, 1937. The patient was septic and died on the fourth postoperative day. At autopsy, vegetations filled the pulmonary artery down to the valve.[43] On August 16, 1938, Robert Gross, at Boston Children's Hospital,

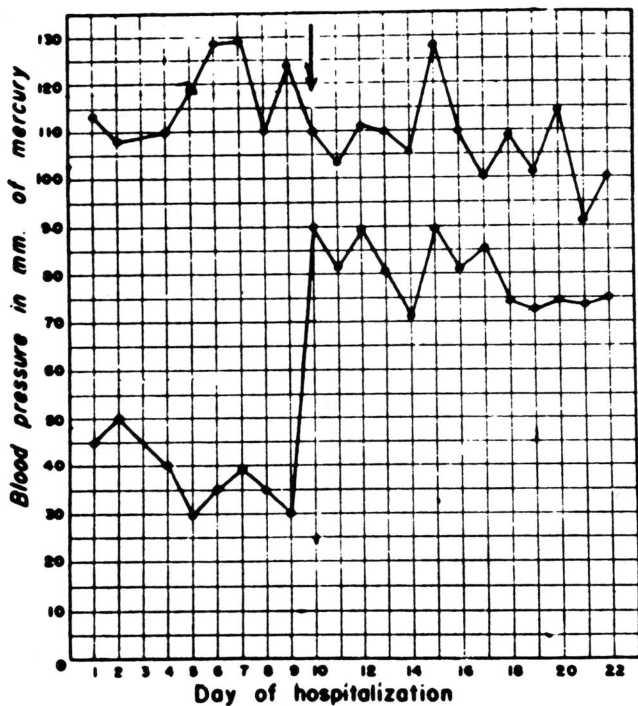

FIGURE 1–3 Ligation of patent ductus arteriosus. Daily blood pressure readings of the patient with a patent ductus arteriosus before and after operation (arrow). *(Reproduced with permission from Gross RE, Hubbard JH: Surgical ligation of a patent ductus arteriosus: report of first successful case. JAMA 1939; 112:729.)*

operated on a 7-year-old girl with dyspnea after moderate exercise.[44] Dr. Gross described the ductus as 7 to 8 mm in diameter and 5 to 6 mm in length. A no. 8 braided silk tie was placed around the ductus with an aneurysm needle, and the vessel was occluded temporarily for a 3-minute observation. During this time, blood pressure rose from 100/35 to 125/90. According to Dr. Gross, "Since there was no embarrassment of the circulation, it was decided to ligate the ductus permanently." The patient made an uneventful recovery (Fig. 1-3).

Modifications of the ductus operation soon followed. In 1944 Dr. Gross reported a technique for successfully dividing the ductus. The next major congenital lesion to be overcome was coarctation of the aorta. Dr. Clarence Crafoord, in Stockholm, Sweden, successfully resected a coarctation of the aorta in a 12-year-old boy on October 19, 1944.[45] Twelve days later he successfully resected the coarctation of a 27-year-old patient. Dr. Gross, in Boston, who had been working on a coarctation model in the laboratory, first operated on a 5-year-old boy with this condition on June 28, 1945.[46] After he excised the coarctation and rejoined the aorta, the patient's heart suddenly stopped. The patient died in the operating room. One week later, however, Dr. Gross operated on a second patient, a 12-year-old girl. This patient's operation was successful (Fig. 1-4). Dr. Gross had been unaware of

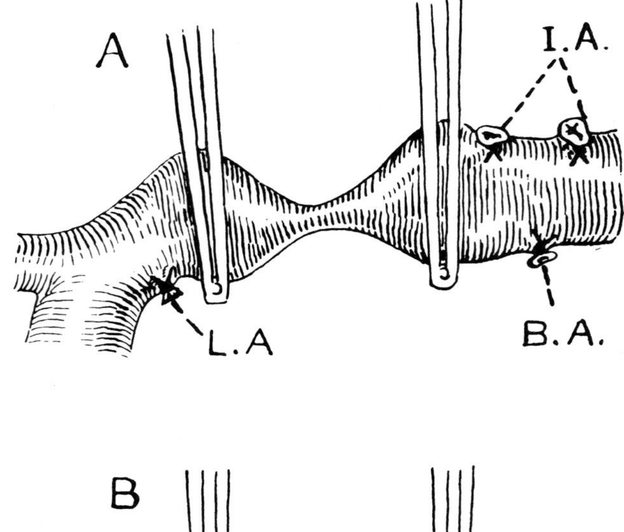

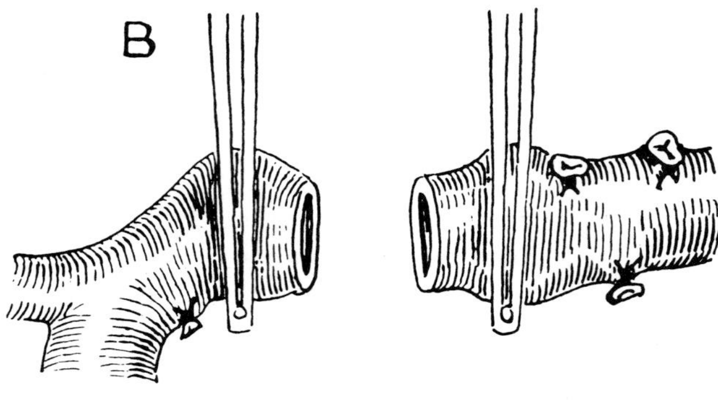

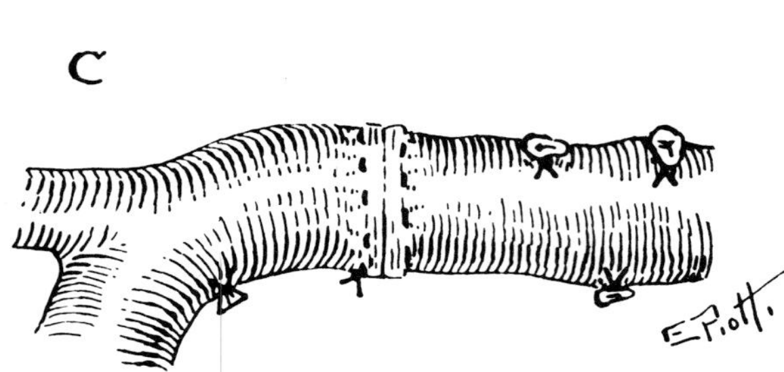

FIGURE 1–4 Resection of aortic coarctation. (A) Section of aorta mobilized by freeing it from its bed and dividing regional intercostal arteries (I.A.), bronchial artery (B.A.), and ligamentum arteriosum (L.A.). Clamps applied to aorta. (B) Segment of aorta excised. (C) Aorta reconstructed by end-to-end anastomosis, with continuous, everting, mattress-type silk suture. *(Reproduced with permission from Gross RE: Surgical correction for coarctation of the aorta. Surgery 1945; 18:673.)*

Dr. Crafoord's successful surgery several months previously, probably because of World War II.

In 1945 Dr. Gross reported the first successful case of surgical relief for tracheal obstruction from a vascular ring.[47] In the 5 years that followed Gross's first successful operation, he reported 40 more cases.[48]

The famous Blalock-Taussig operation also was first reported in 1945. The first patient was a 15-month-old girl with a clinical diagnosis of tetralogy of Fallot with a severe pulmonary stenosis.[49] At age 8 months the baby had her first cyanotic spell, which occurred after eating. Dr. Helen Taussig, the cardiologist, followed the child for 3 months, and during that time cyanosis increased and she failed to gain weight. She was readmitted and during the next 6 weeks refused most of her feedings, lost weight, and weighed only 4 kg at operation. The operation was performed by Dr. Alfred Blalock at Johns Hopkins University on November 29, 1944. The left subclavian artery was anastomosed to the left pulmonary artery in an end-to-side fashion (Fig. 1-5). The postoperative course was described as stormy; she was discharged 2 months postoperatively. Two additional successful cases were done within 3 months of their first patient.

Thus, within a 7-year period, three congenital cardiovascular defects, patent ductus arteriosus, coarctation of the

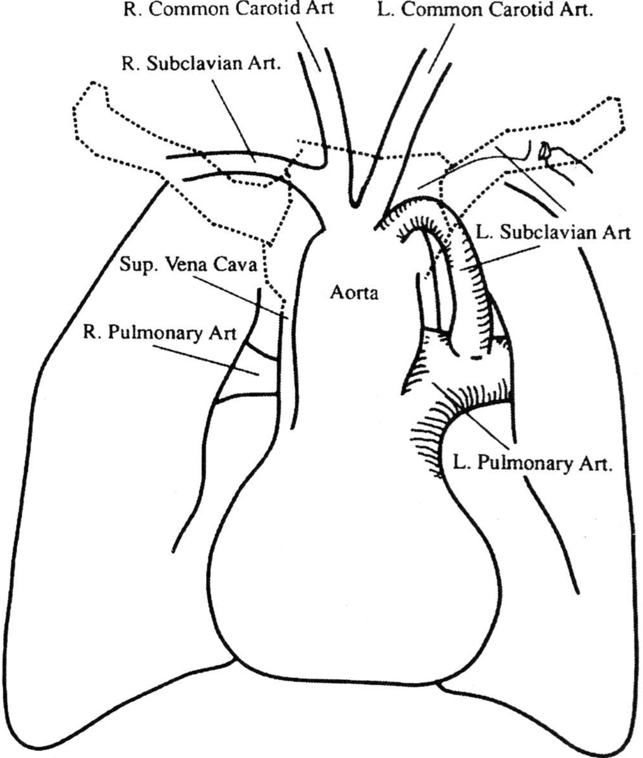

FIGURE 1–5 Diagram of the first Blalock-Taussig anastomosis. *(Reproduced with permission from Blalock A, Taussig HB: The surgical treatment of malformations of the heart in which there is pulmonary stenosis or pulmonary atresia. JAMA 1945; 128:189.)*

aorta, and vascular ring, were attacked surgically and treated successfully. However, the introduction of the Blalock-Taussig shunt was probably the most powerful stimulus to the development of cardiac surgery, because this operation palliated a complex intracardiac lesion and focused attention on the pathophysiology of cardiac disease.

Anomalous coronary artery in which the left coronary artery communicates with the pulmonary artery was the next surgical conquest. The surgery was performed on July 22, 1946, and was reported by Gunnar Biorck and Clarence Crafoord.[50] The patient was a 15-year-old boy who was unable to do gymnastics or play football because of dyspnea shortly after beginning exercise. At operation, the ductus arteriosus was found to be a cord, but there was a thrill over the pericardium. When the pericardium was opened, the anomalous coronary artery was identified and doubly ligated. The patient made an uneventful recovery.

Muller[51] reported successful surgical treatment of transposition of the pulmonary veins in 1951, but the operation addressed a partial form of the anomaly. Later in the 1950s, Gott, Varco, Lillehei, and Cooley reported successful operative variations for anomalous pulmonary veins.

Another of Gross's pioneering surgical procedures was the surgical closure of an aortopulmonary window in a 4-year-old girl who had dyspnea with slight exertion and a cardiac murmur that was consistent with a patent ductus.[52] The operation was carried out on May 22, 1948. After dissecting the posterior aspect of the great vessels, a similar plane was developed between the vessels above the shunt, and an aneurysm needle was passed completely around the shunt.[52] A piece of linen tape 1 cm wide was drawn around the vessel so that it encircled the shunt. At this point, arterial blood began to escape from the depths of the wound so that it was evident that the thin posterior wall of the shunt had been slightly torn. Believing that the one hope of controlling the situation might be to quickly tie the tape that had been placed previously, this was now rapidly and tightly drawn down. Fortunately, all bleeding stopped. All the thrill in the pulmonary artery disappeared. The chest was closed, and the patient made a satisfactory convalescence.

Gross stated, "After successfully treating the child, it is felt that the fortunate outcome had been attended by a high degree of luck and that simple ligature might lead to disaster if attempted in all cases of aortopulmonary artery fenestration. As far as is known, this is the first instance of successful surgical correction of this congenital abnormality." Others were soon to follow using various techniques to interrupt the aortopulmonary window. Cooley et al[53] were the first to report on the use of cardiopulmonary bypass to repair this defect and converted a difficult and hazardous procedure into a relatively straightforward one.

The cavopulmonary anastomosis has had several variations by different designers. Carlon et al[54] are credited with first proposing the anastomosis in 1951. Glenn[55] reported the first successful clinical application in the United States in 1958 for what has been termed the *Glenn shunt*. Similar work was done in Russia during the 1950s by several investigators. On January 3, 1957, Galankin,[56] a Russian surgeon, performed a cavopulmonary anastomosis in a 16-year-old patient with tetralogy of Fallot. The patient made a good recovery with significant improvement in exercise tolerance and cyanosis.

THE DEVELOPMENT OF CARDIOPULMONARY BYPASS

The development of the heart-lung machine made repair of intracardiac lesions possible. To bypass the heart, one needs a basic understanding of physiology of the circulation, a method of preventing the blood from clotting, a mechanism to pump blood, and finally, a method to ventilate the blood.[57]

Before 1900, physiologists were already interested in isolated organ perfusion and therefore needed a method to oxygenate blood. Von Frey and Gruber[58] described a blood pump in 1885 in which gas exchange occurred as blood flowed into a thin film over the inner surface of a slanted rotating cylinder. In 1895 Jacobi passed blood through an excised animal's lung that was aerated by artificial respiration.[59] In 1926, Professors S. S. Brukhonenko and S. Terebinsky[60] in Russia designed a machine that used an excised lung from a donor animal as an oxygenator and two mechanically actuated blood pumps. Their machine was used initially to perfuse isolated organs but later was used to perfuse entire animals.

Alexis Carrel, a Nobel laureate, and Charles Lindbergh, the famous aviator, developed a device that successfully perfused the thyroid gland of a cat for 18 days, beginning April 5, 1935.[61] A picture of the two investigators with their perfusion apparatus appeared on the July 1, 1935, cover of *Time* magazine.[62] At the end of that time, much of the tissue was partially preserved, and pieces grew epithelial cells in tissue culture. According to Edwards and Edwards,[61] many other organs were perfused over the next few years by Carrel and Lindbergh. Hearts were kept beating for several days. Although perfused organs survived surprisingly well, all showed progressive degenerative changes in a few days. Edema fluid filled tissue spaces, arteries became calcified, and connective tissue cells outgrew the more specialized cells.

One of the key requirements of the heart-lung machine was anticoagulation. Heparin was discovered by a medical student, Jay McLean, working in the laboratory of Dr. William Howell, a physiologist at Johns Hopkins.[63] In 1915 Howell gave McLean the task of studying a crude brain extract known to be a powerful thromboplastin. Howell believed that the thromboplastic activity was caused by cephalin contained in the extract. McLean's job was to fractionate the extract and purify the cephalin. McLean also studied extracts prepared from heart and liver. McLean discovered that a substance in the extract was retarding coagulation. McLean wrote[64]:

> I went one morning to the door of Dr. Howell's office, and standing there (he was seated at his desk), I said, Dr. Howell, I have discovered antithrombin. He smiled and said, "Antithrombin is a protein and you are working with phospholipids. Are you sure that salt is not contaminating your substance?"... I told him that I was not sure of that, but it was a powerful anticoagulant. He was most skeptical, so I had the diener, John Schweinhand, bleed a cat. Into a small beaker full of its blood, I stirred all of the proven batch of heparphosphotides, and placed this on Dr. Howell's laboratory table and asked him to tell when it clotted. It never did.

McLean described his finding in February 1916 at a medical society meeting in Philadelphia and later reported it in an article entitled, "The Thromboplastic Action of Cephalin."[64,65] Howell and Holt[66] reported their work on heparin in 1918. In the 1920s, animal experiments confirmed that heparin was an effective anticoagulant.[67]

John Gibbon contributed more to the success of the development of the heart-lung machine than anyone else. His interest began as a young doctor one night in 1930 in Boston "during an all-night vigil by the side of a patient with a massive embolus..."[68]

> My job that night was to take the patient's blood pressure and pulse every 15 minutes and plot it on a chart. During the 17 hours by the patient's side, the thought constantly recurred that the patient's hazardous condition could be improved if some of the blue blood in the patient's distended veins could be continuously withdrawn into an apparatus where the blood could pick up oxygen and discharge carbon dioxide and then pump this blood into the patient's arteries. At 8 A.M. the patient's blood pressure could not be measured. Dr. Edward Churchill, the chief of surgery, immediately opened the chest through an anterior left thoracotomy, then occluded both the pulmonary artery and the aorta as they exited from the heart. He opened the pulmonary artery and removed massive blood clots. The patient did not survive.

Gibbon's work on the heart-lung machine took place over the next 20 years, in laboratories at the Massachusetts General Hospital, the University of Pennsylvania, and Thomas Jefferson University. In 1937, Gibbon reported the first successful demonstration that life could be maintained by an artificial heart and lung and that the native heart and lungs could resume function. Unfortunately, only three animals recovered adequate cardiorespiratory function after total pulmonary artery occlusion and bypass, and even they died a few hours later.[69] Gibbon's work was interrupted by World War II; afterwards, he resumed his work at the Thomas Jefferson Medical College in Philadelphia. Meanwhile, other groups, including Clarence Crafoord in Stockholm, Sweden, J. Jongbloed at the University of Utrecht in Holland, Clarence Dennis at the University of Minnesota, Mario Digliotti and coworkers at the University of Turino in Italy, and Forest Dodrill at Harper Hospital in Detroit, also worked on a heart-lung machine.[70]

Clarence Dennis's first clinical attempt at open heart surgery was in a 6-year-old girl with end-stage cardiac disease.[71] Her heart was already massive, and her only hope was surgical closure of an atrial septal defect. At operation on April 5, 1951, her circulation was supported by a heart-lung machine that Dennis and his coworkers had developed.[72] The atrial septal defect was very difficult to close. Although the heart-lung machine functioned well, the patient did not survive, probably because of a combination of blood loss and surgically induced tricuspid stenosis.

In August of 1951, Mario Digliotti used his heart-lung machine to partially support the circulation at the flow of 1 L/min in a 49-year-old patient during resection of a large mediastinal tumor.[73] During the operation, the patient developed hypotension and cyanosis. He was therefore placed on partial bypass at 1 L/min for 20 minutes. Although the mass was resected successfully, the Italian machine was never used for open heart surgery in humans.

Forest Dodrill and colleagues used the mechanical blood pump they developed with General Motors on a 41-year-old man.[74] The machine was used to substitute for the left ventricle for 50 minutes while a surgical procedure was carried out to repair the mitral valve; the patient's own lungs were used to oxygenate the blood. This, the first clinically successful total left-sided heart bypass in a human, was performed on July 3, 1952, and followed from Dodrill's experimental work with a mechanical pump for univentricular, biventricular, or cardiopulmonary bypass. Although Dodrill et al had used their pump with an oxygenator for total heart bypass in animals,[75] they felt that left-sided heart bypass was the most practical method for their first clinical case. When their patient was interviewed at age 68, he recalled seeing dogs romping on the roof of a nearby building from his hospital room in 1952. Later he learned that they had been used in the final test of the Dodrill-General Motors mechanical heart machine (Fig. 1-6).

Later, on October 21, 1952, Dodrill et al used their machine in a 16-year-old boy with congenital pulmonary stenosis to perform a pulmonary valvuloplasty under direct vision; this was the first successful right-sided heart bypass.[76] Between July 1952 and December 1954, Dodrill performed approximately 13 clinical operations on the heart and thoracic aorta using the Dodrill-General Motors machine, with at least 5 hospital survivors.[77] While he used this machine with an oxygenator in the animal laboratory, he did not start using an oxygenator with the Dodrill-General Motors mechanical heart clinically until early 1955.

Hypothermia was another method to stop the heart and allow it to be opened. In 1950, Bigelow et al[78] reported on 20 dogs that had been cooled to 20°C, with 15 minutes of circulatory arrest; 11 animals also had a cardiotomy. Only

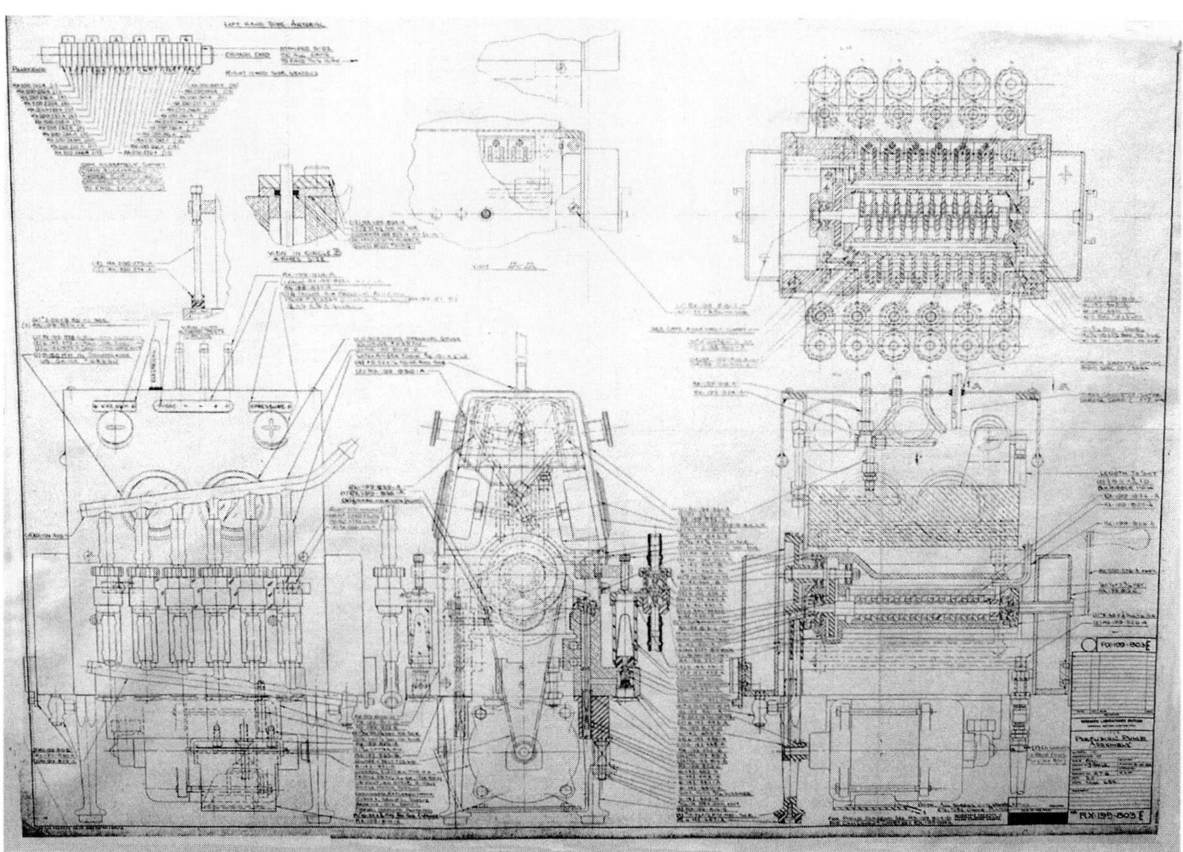

FIGURE 1–6 Blueprints by General Motors engineers of the Dodrill-GMR Mechanical Heart. *(Courtesy of Calvin Hughes, M.D.)*

6 animals survived after rewarming. Bigelow and colleagues continued to study hypothermia.[79–81]

John Lewis closed an atrial septal defect in a 5-year-old girl on September 2, 1952, using a hypothermic technique[82]:

> She was wrapped in refrigerated blankets until after a period of two hours and ten minutes her rectal temperature had fallen to 28°C. At this point the chest was entered through the bed of the right fifth rib. The cardiac inflow was occluded for a total of five and one-half minutes and during this time the septal defect was closed under direct vision. The patient was rewarmed by placing her in hot water kept at 45°C, and after 35 minutes her rectal temperature had risen to 36°C, at which time she was removed from the bath. Recovery from the anesthesia was prompt and her subsequent postoperative convalescence was uneventful.

Shortly thereafter, Swan et al[83] reported successful results in 13 clinical cases using a similar technique. But the use of systemic hypothermia for open intracardiac surgery was relatively short-lived; after the heart-lung machine was introduced clinically, it appeared that deep hypothermia was obsolete. However, during the 1960s it became apparent that operative results in infants under 1 year of age using cardiopulmonary bypass were poor. In 1967, Hikasa et al,[84] from Kyoto, Japan, published an article that reintroduced profound hypothermia for cardiac surgery in infants and used the heart-lung machine for rewarming. Their technique involved surface cooling to 20°C, cardiac surgery during circulatory arrest for 15 to 75 minutes, and rewarming with cardiopulmonary bypass. At the same time, other groups reported using profound hypothermia with circulatory arrest in infants with the heart-lung machine for cooling and rewarming.[85–88] Results were much improved, and subsequently the technique also was applied for resection of aortic arch aneurysms.

After World War II, John Gibbon resumed his research. He eventually met Thomas Watson, chairman of the board of the International Business Machines (IBM) Corporation. Watson was fascinated by Gibbon's research and promised help. Soon afterward, six IBM engineers arrived and built a machine that was similar to Gibbon's earlier machine, which contained a rotating vertical cylinder oxygenator and a modified DeBakey rotary pump (Fig. 1-7). Gibbon successfully used this new machine for intercardiac surgery on small dogs and had several long-term survivors, but the blood oxygenator was too small for human patients. Eventually, the team developed a larger oxygenator that the IBM engineers incorporated into a new machine.[89]

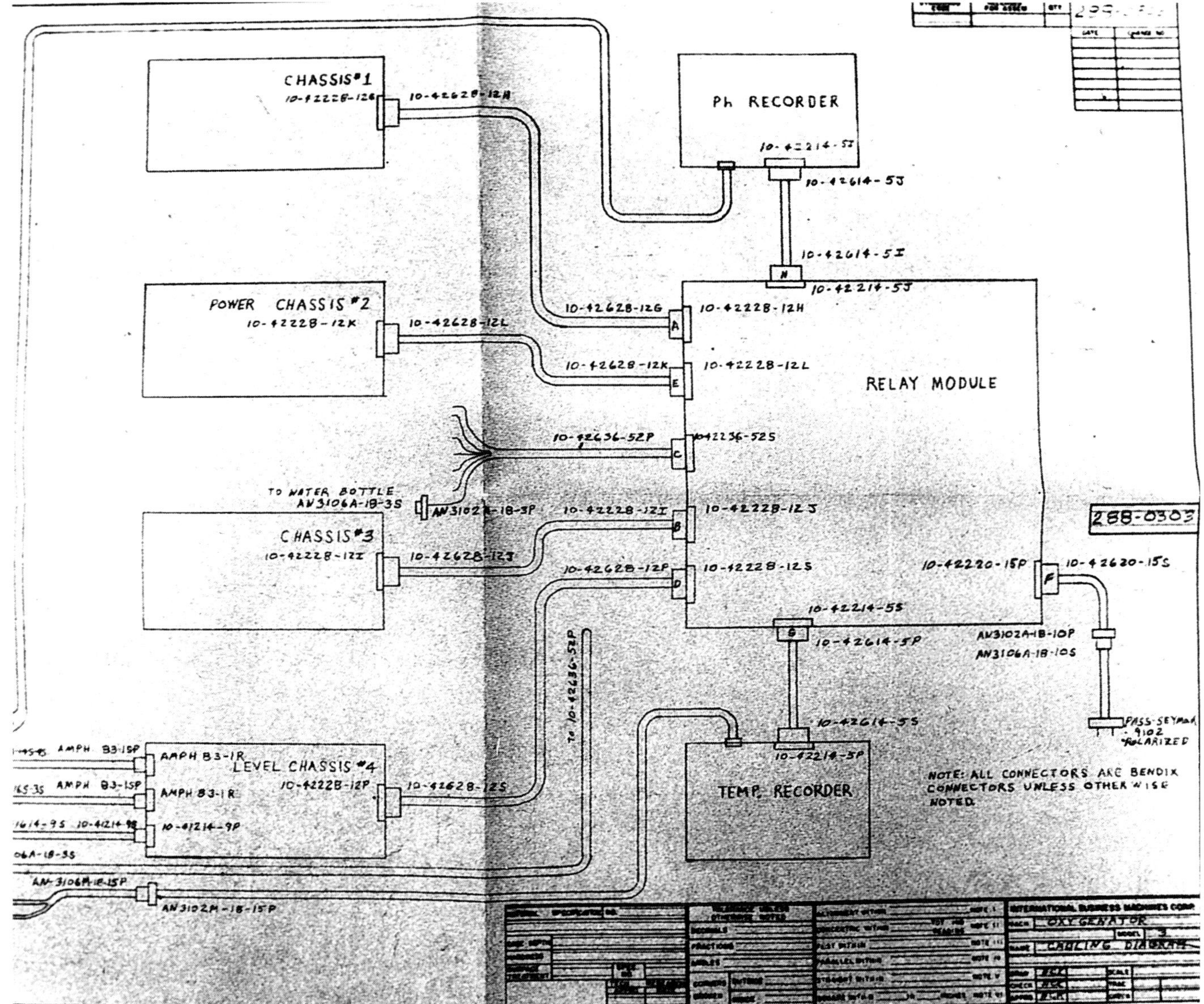

FIGURE 1–7 A schematic drawing by IBM engineers of the pump oxygenator they designed and constructed under Gibbon's direction. (*Courtesy of Thomas Jefferson University Archives, Scott Memorial Library, Philadelphia, PA.*)

In 1949, Gibbon's early mortality in dogs was 80%, but it gradually improved.[90] Gibbon operated on a 15-month-old girl with severe congestive heart failure. The preoperative diagnosis was atrial septal defect, but at operation, none was found. She died, and a huge patent ductus was found at autopsy. The next patient was an 18-year-old girl with congestive heart failure due to an atrial septal defect. This defect was closed successfully on May 6, 1953, with the Gibbon-IBM heart-lung machine. The patient recovered, and several months later the defect was confirmed closed at cardiac catheterization.[90] Unfortunately, Gibbon's next two patients did not survive intracardiac procedures when the heart-lung machine was used. These failures distressed Dr. Gibbon, who declared a one-year moratorium for the heart-lung machine until more work could be done to solve the problems causing the deaths.

During this period, C. Walton Lillehei and colleagues at the University of Minnesota studied a technique called *controlled cross-circulation*.[57] With this technique the circulation of one dog was temporarily used to support that of a second dog while the second dog's heart was temporarily stopped and opened. After a simulated repair in the second dog, the animals were disconnected and allowed to recover.

Lillehei et al[91] used their technique at the University of Minnesota to correct a ventricular septal defect in a 12-month-old infant on March 26, 1954 (Fig. 1-8). Either a parent or a close relative with the same blood type was connected to the child's circulation. In Lillehei's first clinical case,

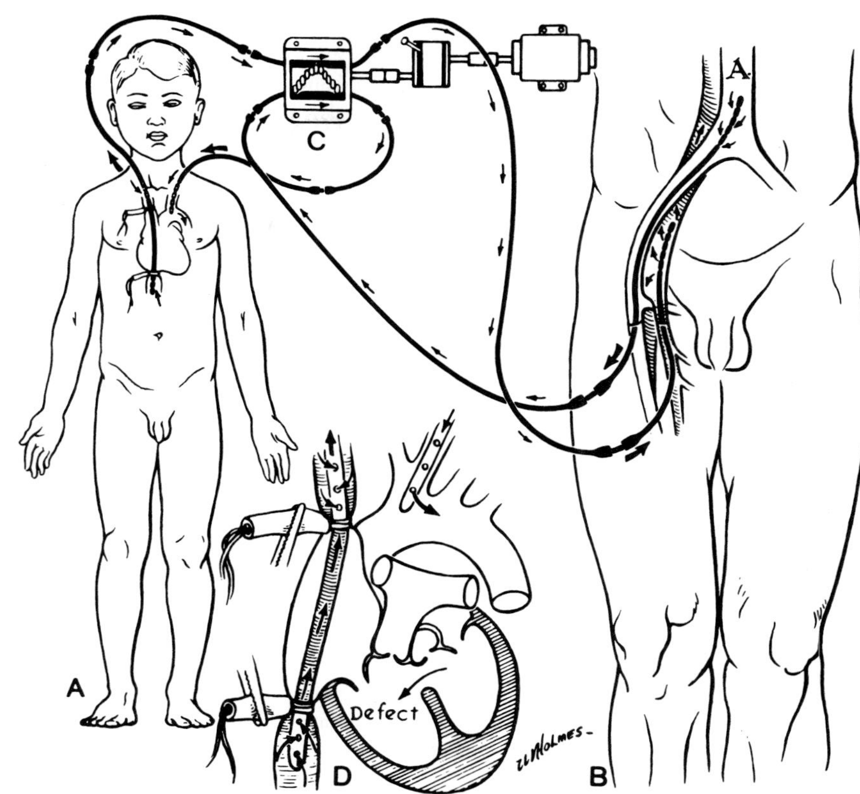

FIGURE 1–8 A depiction of the method of direct vision intracardiac surgery utilizing extracorporeal circulation by means of controlled cross-circulation. (A) The patient, showing sites of arterial and venous cannulations. (B) The donor, showing sites of arterial and venous (superficial femoral and great saphenous) cannulations. (C) The Sigma motor pump controlling precisely the reciprocal exchange of blood between the patient and donor. (D) Close-up of the patient's heart, showing the vena caval catheter positioned to draw venous blood from both the superior and inferior venae cavae during the cardiac bypass interval. The arterial blood from the donor circulated to the patient's body through the catheter that was inserted into the left subclavian artery. *(Reproduced with permission from Lillehei CW, Cohen M, Warden HE, et al: The results of direct vision closure of ventricular septal defects in eight patients by means of controlled cross circulation. Surg Gynecol Obstet 1955; 101:446. Copyright American College of Surgeons.*)

it was the child's father. The patient had been hospitalized 10 months for uncontrollable heart failure and pneumonitis. The patient made an uneventful recovery until death on the 11th postoperative day from a rapidly progressing tracheal bronchitis. At autopsy, the VSD was closed, and the respiratory infection was confirmed as the cause of death. Two weeks later the second and third patients had VSDs closed by the same technique 3 days apart. Both remained long-term survivors with normal hemodynamics confirmed by cardiac catheterization.

In 1955 Lillehei et al[92] published a report of 32 patients that included repairs of ventricular septal defects, tetralogy of Fallot, and atrioventricularis communis defects. By July of 1955, the blood pump used for systemic cross-circulation by Lillehei et al was coupled with a bubble oxygenator developed by Drs. DeWall and Lillehei, and cross-circulation was abandoned after use in 45 patients during 1954 and 1955. Although its clinical use was short-lived, cross-circulation was an important steppingstone in the development of cardiac surgery.[57]

Meanwhile, at the Mayo Clinic only 90 miles away, John W. Kirklin and colleagues launched their open heart program on March 5, 1955.[93] They used a heart-lung machine based on the Gibbon-IBM machine, but with their own modifications. Dr. Kirklin wrote[94]:

> We investigated and visited the groups working intensively with the mechanical pump oxygenators. We visited Dr. Gibbon in his laboratories in Philadelphia, and Dr. Forest Dodrill in Detroit, among others. The Gibbon pump oxygenator had been developed and made by the International Business Machine Corporation and looked quite a bit like a computer. Dr. Dodrill's heart-lung machine had been developed and built for him by General Motors and it looked a great deal like a car engine. We came home, reflected and decided to try to persuade the Mayo Clinic to let us build a pump oxygenator similar to the Gibbon machine, but somewhat different. We already had had about a year's experience in the animal laboratory with David Donald using a simple pump and bubble oxygenator when we set about very early in 1953, the laborious task of building a Mayo-Gibbon pump oxygenator and continuing the laboratory research.
>
> Most people were very discouraged with the laboratory progress. The American Heart Association and the National Institutes of Health had stopped funding any projects for the study of heart-lung machines, because it was felt that the problem was physiologically insurmountable. David Donald and I undertook a series of laboratory experiments lasting about a year and a half during which time the engineering shops at the Mayo Clinic constructed a pump oxygenator based on the Gibbon model.[95]
>
> . . . The electrifying day came in the spring of 1954 when the newspapers carried an account of Walt Lillehei's successful open heart operation on a small child. Of course, I was terribly envious and yet I was terribly admiring at the same moment. That admiration increased exponentially when a short time later, a few of my colleagues and I visited Minneapolis and observed one of what was now a series of successful open heart operations with control cross-circulation.

> ... [I]n the winter of 1954 and 1955 we had 9 surviving dogs out of 10 cardiopulmonary bypass runs. With my wonderful colleague and pediatric cardiologist, Jim DuShane, we had earlier selected 8 patients for intracardiac repair. Two had to be put off because two babies with very serious congenital heart disease came along and we decided to fit them into the schedule. We had determined to do all 8 patients even if the first 7 died. All of this was planned with the knowledge and approval of the governance of the Mayo Clinic. Our plan was then to return to the laboratory and spend the next 6 to 12 months solving the problems that had arisen in the first planned clinical trial of a pump oxygenator.... We did our first open heart operation on a Tuesday in March 1955.

Kirklin continued[94]:

> Four of our first 8 patients survived, but the press of the clinical work prevented our ever being able to return to the laboratory with the force that we had planned. By now, Walt Lillehei and I were on parallel, but intertwined paths. I am extremely grateful to Walt Lillehei and am very proud for the two of us, that during that 12 to 18 months when we were the only surgeons in the world performing open intracardiac operations with cardiopulmonary bypass and surely in intense competition with each other, we shared our gains and losses with each other. We continued to communicate and we argued privately in nightclubs and on airplanes rather than publicly over our differences. Walt was more cheerful and more optimistic than I when we discussed problems. I remember saying to him one day, "Walt, I am so discouraged with complete atrial ventricular canal." "Oh, sure," he said, "that is a tough lesion, but we will learn to do well with it."

By the end of 1956, many university groups around the world had launched into open heart programs. Currently, it is estimated that more than one million cardiac operations are performed each year worldwide with the use of the heart-lung machine. In most cases, the operative mortality is quite low, approaching 1% for some operations. Little thought is given to the courageous pioneers in the 1950s whose monumental contributions made all this possible.

EXTRACORPOREAL LIFE SUPPORT

Extracorporeal life support is an extension of cardiopulmonary bypass. Cardiopulmonary bypass initially was limited to no more than 6 hours. The development of membrane oxygenators in the 1960s permitted longer support. Donald Hill and colleagues, in 1972, treated a 24-year-old man who developed shock lung after blunt trauma.[96] The patient was supported for 75 hours using a heart-lung machine with a membrane oxygenator, cannulated via the femoral vein and artery. The patient was weaned and recovered. Hill's second patient was supported for 5 days and recovered. This led to a randomized trial supported by the National Institutes of Health to determine the efficacy of this therapy for adults with respiratory failure. The study was conducted from 1972 to 1975 and showed no significant difference in survival between patients managed by extracorporeal life support (9.5%) and those who received conventional ventilatory therapy (8.3%).[97] Because of these results, most U.S. centers abandoned efforts to support adult patients using extracorporeal life support (ECLS), also known as *extracorporeal membrane oxygenation* (ECMO).

One participant in the adult trial decided to study neonates. The usual causes of neonatal respiratory failure have in common abnormal postnatal blood shunts known as *persistent fetal circulation* (PFC).[98–101] This is a temporary, reversible phenomenon. In 1976, Bartlett and colleagues, at the University of Michigan, were the first to successfully treat a neonate using extracorporeal life support. Since that time, two prospective studies have shown the efficacy of ECLS for management of neonatal respiratory failure.[102,103] More than 8000 neonatal patients have been treated using ECLS worldwide with a survival rate of 82% (ELSO registry data).

MYOCARDIAL PROTECTION

Alexis Carrel reported in 1914 that "The arresting of the circulation of the heart has already been performed in many ways by various experimenters. We ourselves have used all known methods of stopping the circulation through the heart."[104] He also referred to work of Borrel and others, who had experimented with different forms of myocardial preservation. Carrel goes on to state, "When the above-mentioned precautions were taken, it was possible to clamp the pedicle of the heart (aorta and pulmonary artery) for two and a half or three minutes without any subsequent trouble. As soon as the clamp was removed, the heart resumed its pulsations, and after a very short time, the pulsations were again normal."

Melrose et al[105] in 1955 presented the first experimental study describing induced arrest by potassium-based cardioplegia. Blood cardioplegia was used "to preserve myocardial energy stores at the onset of cardiac ischemia." These authors state, "Ringer drew attention in 1883 to the effect of the differentiations on the heartbeat and Hooker in 1929 suggested that potassium inhibition induced by an excess of potassium chloride could be used to stop the heart when its beat was disorganized by ventricular fibrillation." Melrose goes on to state that "... they have succeeded in evolving a reliable method of stopping and restarting the heart at both normal and reduced body temperatures." Unfortunately, the Melrose solution proved to be toxic to the myocardium, and as a result, cardioplegia was not used widely for several years.

Gay and Ebert[106] and Tyres et al[107] demonstrated that cardioplegia with lower potassium concentrations was safe. Studies by Kirsch et al,[108] Bretschneider et al,[109] and Hearse et al[110] demonstrated the effectiveness of cardioplegia with other constituents and renewed interest in this technique. Gay and Ebert in 1973 demonstrated a significant

TABLE 1–1 First successful intracardiac repairs using cardiopulmonary bypass or cross-circulation

Lesion	Year	Reference	Comment
Atrial septal defect	1953	Gibbon[90]	May 6, 1953
Ventricular septal defect	1953	Lillehei[238]	Cross-circulation
Complete atrioventricular canal	1954	Lillehei[92]	Cross-circulation
Tetralogy of Fallot	1954	Lillehei[91]	Cross-circulation
Tetralogy of Fallot	1955	Kirklin[93]	Cardiopulmonary bypass (CPB)
Total anomalous pulmonary veins	1956	Kirklin[239]	
Congenital aneurysm sinus of Valsalva	1956	Kirklin[240]	
Congenital aortic stenosis	1956	Kirklin[241]	First direct visual correction
Aortopulmonary window	1957	Cooley[242]	First closure using CPB
Double outlet right ventricle	1957	Kirklin[243]	Extemporarily devised correction
Corrected transposition great arteries	1957	Lillehei[244]	
Transposition great arteries: atrial switch	1959	Senning[245]	Physiologic total correction
Coronary arterial-venous fistula	1959	Swan[246]	
Ebstein's anomaly	1964	Hardy[247]	Repair of atrialized tricuspid valve
Tetralogy with pulmonary atresia	1966	Ross[248]	Used aortic allograft
Truncus arteriosus	1967	McGoon[249]	Used aortic allograft
Tricuspid atresia	1968	Fontan[250]	Physiologic correction
Single ventricle	1970	Horiuchi[251]	
Subaortic tunnel stenosis	1975	Konno[252]	
Transposition great arteries: arterial switch	1975	Jatene[253]	Anatomic correction
Hypoplastic left heart syndrome	1983	Norwood[254]	Two-stage operation
Pediatric heart transplantation	1985	Bailey[255]	

reduction in myocardial oxygen consumption during potassium-induced arrest when compared with that of the fibrillating heart.[106] They also showed that the problems in the use of the Melrose solution in the early days of cardiac surgery probably were due to its hyperosmolar properties and perhaps not to the high potassium concentration.

In a 1978 publication by Follette et al,[111] the technique of blood cardioplegia was reintroduced. In experimental and clinical studies, these authors demonstrated that hypothermic, intermittent blood cardioplegia provided better myocardial protection than normothermic, continuous coronary perfusion and/or hypothermic, intermittent blood perfusion without cardioplegia solution. The composition of the best cardioplegia solution remains controversial, and new formulations, methods of delivery, and recommended temperature continue to evolve.

EVOLUTION OF CONGENITAL CARDIAC SURGERY DURING THE ERA OF CARDIOPULMONARY BYPASS

With the advent of cardiopulmonary bypass using either the cross-circulation technique of Lillehei et al or the version of the mechanical heart-lung machine used by Kirklin et al, the two groups led the way for intracardiac repairs for many of the commonly occurring congenital heart defects. Because of the morbidity associated with the heart-lung machine, palliative operations also were developed to improve circulatory physiology without directly addressing the anatomic pathology. These palliative operations included the Blalock-Taussig subclavian-pulmonary arterial shunt[49] with modifications by Potts et al[112] and Waterston et al,[113] the Blalock-Hanlon operation to create an atrial septal defect,[114] and the Galankin-Glenn superior vena cava–right pulmonary arterial shunt.[55]

As the safety of cardiopulmonary bypass steadily improved, surgeons addressed more and more complex abnormalities of the heart in younger and younger patients. Some of the milestones in the development of operations to correct congenital heart defects using cardiopulmonary bypass appear in Table 1-1. These advances coincided with simultaneous advances in the surgery of adult heart disease, and the same surgeons operated on both children and adults. In the 1970s, although dependent on the same technology and basic knowledge, pediatric and adult cardiac surgery began to separate. Operations for more complex congenital lesions in younger and younger patients required new techniques, and likewise the advent of direct operations for ischemic heart disease required new technology and methods to deal with damaged ventricles and acute complications of ischemia. With the exception of sporadic patients who reached adult life with uncorrected or partially corrected congenital heart defects, cardiac surgery in the adult represents the surgery of acquired heart disease. Nevertheless, a close connection continues because the advances in one subspecialty usually are applicable in the other, and this kinship and interdependence probably will remain for the foreseeable future.

VALVULAR SURGERY: CARDIOPULMONARY BYPASS ERA

Cardiac valve repair or replacement under direct vision awaited the development of the heart-lung machine. The first successful aortic valve replacement in the subcoronary position was performed by Dr. Dwight Harken and associates.[115] A caged ball valve was used. Many of the techniques described in Harken's 1960 report are similar to those used today for aortic valve replacement.

That same year, Starr and Edwards[116] successfully replaced the mitral valve using a caged ball valve of their own design. Starr later wrote[117]:

> In 1958, Lowell Edwards presented himself in my office with a proposal to develop an implantable artificial heart. I learned that he was a retired engineer with considerable financial resources. His visit was fortuitous, because just about that time, I had become interested in valvular prostheses. . . . Edwards agreed to begin the project by working on one valve at a time. . . . The obvious direction then was towards the ball valve prosthesis. I drew out for Edwards the general configuration of the Hufnagel valve. He then drew out for me how he thought that particular valve could be adapted for intracardiac use using an open cage. The first animal to have this implant survived for more than a year, but all other subsequent animals died of thrombosis. . . . The big breakthrough came at the end of 1958 when we developed the Silastic shield for the ball valve, which allowed an 80 percent long-term survival. . . . A Silastic shield over the area where thrombus formed on the valve would give us a chance to have long-term survivors.

The first successful operation was done in September of 1960 on a young girl in her mid-twenties. The patient was in pulmonary edema on oxygen prior to operation, and in excellent condition and wide awake on the evening of the day of the surgery.

By 1967, nearly 2000 Starr-Edwards valves had been implanted, and the caged ball valve prosthesis was established as the standard against which all other mechanical prostheses would be compared.

In 1964, Starr et al reported 13 patients who had undergone multiple valve replacement.[118] One patient had the aortic, mitral, and tricuspid valves replaced on February 21, 1963. Cartwright et al, however, on November 1, 1961, were first to successfully replace both the aortic and mitral valves with ball valve prostheses that they had developed.[119] Knott-Craig et al,[120] from the Mayo Clinic, successfully replaced all four heart valves in a patient with carcinoid involvement.

In 1961, Andrew Morrow and Edwin Brockenbrough[121] reported the treatment for idiopathic hypertrophic subaortic stenosis by resecting a portion of the thickened ventricular septum. They referred to this as *subaortic ventriculomyotomy*. They gave credit to William Cleland and H. H. Bentall in London, who had encountered this condition unexpectedly at operation and resected a small portion of the ventricular mass. The patient improved, but no postoperative hemodynamic studies had been reported. The subaortic ventriculomyotomy became the standard surgical treatment for this cardiac anomaly, although in some patients systolic anterior motion (SAM) of the anterior leaflet of the mitral valve necessitates mitral valve replacement with a low-profile mechanical valve.

An aortic homograft valve was used clinically for the first time by Heimbecker et al in Toronto for replacement of the mitral valve in one patient and an aortic valve in another.[122] Survival was short, 1 day in one patient and 1 month in the other. Donald Ross reported on the first successful aortic valve placement with an aortic valve homograft.[123] He used a technique of subcoronary implantation developed in the laboratory by Carlos Duran and Alfred Gunning in Oxford.

The technique of aortic valve replacement with a pulmonary autograft initially described by Ross in 1967 is advocated by some groups for younger patients who require aortic valve replacement.[124,125] An aortic or pulmonary valve homograft is used to replace the pulmonary valve that has been transferred to the aortic position.

Other autogenous materials that have been used to manufacture valve prostheses include pericardium, fasciae latae, and dura mater. In the 1960s, Binet et al[126] began to develop and test tissue valves. In 1964, Duran and Gunning in England replaced an aortic valve in a patient using a xenograft porcine aortic valve. Early results with formaldehyde-fixed xenografts were good,[126] but in a few years these valves began to fail because of tissue degeneration and calcification.[127] Carpentier et al revitalized interest in xenograft valves by fixating porcine valves with gluteraldehyde. Carpentier also mounted his valves on a stent, to produce a bioprosthesis. Carpentier-Edwards porcine valves and Hancock and Angell-Shiley bioprostheses became popular and were implanted in large numbers of patients.[128,129]

Carpentier later wrote, "In 1964 as a young resident in thoracic surgery, I was asked by J. P. Binet, chief of the service, to collect homograft valves from cadavers. Studies of the anatomy of the valves in various animal species showed that the valves from the pigs were the closest to those of humans."[130] Carpentier described the first successful xenograft valve replacement in 1965, followed by 12 other operations, but within 5 years all the heterograft valves had to be replaced. Carpentier goes on to state:

> The use of formalin proposed by O'Brien did not significantly improve the results. I began mounting the valves on a stent in 1966, which permitted the use of heterograft valves in the mitral position. It became obvious that the future of tissue valves would depend upon the development of methods of preparation capable of preventing inflammatory cell reaction, and penetration into the tissue. My background in chemistry is obviously insufficient. I decided to abandon surgery for two days a week to follow the teaching program in chemistry at the Faculty of Sciences and prepare a Ph.D. It is certainly not easy to become a student in chemistry when you are 35 and an associate professor of surgery.
>
> I began to investigate numerous cross-linking inducing factors and found that gluteraldehyde was able to almost eliminate inflammatory reaction. . . .

With the development of cardiopulmonary bypass, valves could be approached under direct vision, and for the first time mitral insufficiency could be attacked by reparative techniques. Techniques for mitral annuloplasty were described by Wooler et al,[131] Reed et al,[132] and Kaye et al.[133] The next step forward was development of annuloplasty rings by Carpentier and Duran. In the 1970s, few groups were involved in valve repairs. Slowly, techniques evolved, were tested clinically, and were followed over the years. Carpentier led the field by establishing the importance of careful analysis of valve pathology, described in detail several techniques of valve repair, and reported good results after early and late follow-up, especially with concomitant use of annuloplasty rings.[134]

From 1966 to 1968, a small epidemic of infective endocarditis in Detroit among heroin addicts broke out. Patients were dying of intractable gram-negative tricuspid valve endocarditis, often due to *Pseudomonas aeruginosa*. Long-term antibiotic administration in combination with tricuspid valve replacement was 100% fatal. These results prompted Agustin Arbulu and colleagues to remove the tricuspid valve entirely without replacing it in seven dogs in 1969. Six survived with satisfactory hemodynamic performance. Starting in 1970, Arbulu operated on 55 patients; in 53, the tricuspid valve was removed without replacing it.[135,136] At 25 years, the actuarial survival is 61%.

CORONARY ARTERY SURGERY

Alexis Carrel remarked in 1910[137]:

> I attempted to perform an indirect anastomosis between descending aorta and the left coronary artery. It was for many reasons a difficult operation. On account of the continuous motion of the heart, it was not easy to dissect and to suture the artery. In one case, I implanted one end of a long carotid artery, preserved in a cold storage, on the descending aorta. The other end was passed through the pericardium and anastomosed to the pericardial end of the coronary near the pulmonary artery. Unfortunately, the operation was too slow. Three minutes after the interruption of the circulation fibrillary contractions appeared, but the anastomosis took five minutes. By massage of the heart, the dog was kept alive, but he died less than two hours afterwards. It shows that the anastomosis must be done in less than three minutes.

In 1930, Claude Beck, a Cleveland surgeon, developed methods to indirectly revascularize the hearts of animals by attaching adjacent tissues in hopes of forming collateral blood flow to ischemic myocardium.[138] These tissues included pericardium, pericardial fat, pectoralis muscle, and omentum. Postmortem examination showed that anastomotic vessels did develop between these tissues and the myocardium. In the first patient, Beck roughened the outer surface of the heart with a burr and then sutured a pedicle graft of pectoralis muscle to the left ventricular wall.[139] The patient made an uneventful recovery and was angina-free after the operation. Beck subsequently performed this operation with modifications on 16 patients.[140]

Arthur Vineberg, a Canadian surgeon, in 1946 reported implanting the internal mammary artery through a tunnel in the myocardium, but he did not actually anastomose the left internal mammary artery to a coronary artery.[141] He showed in animals that communications developed between the internal mammary and the coronary arteries. Contemporary surgeons, however, remained skeptical, but Mason Sones validated Vineberg's concept by demonstrating communications between the graft in the myocardium and the coronary system by angiography in two patients operated on 5 and 6 years earlier. In the middle 1960s the Vineberg operation with many variations was performed at many institutions in the United States and Canada.[142]

At the same time, other surgeons performed coronary arterial endarterectomies. Longmire et al[143] were the first to report endarterectomy of the coronary arteries for the treatment of ischemic coronary disease. In 1958 they reported five patients, with four hospital survivors. Although the operation was used subsequently by other groups, mortality was high, and the procedure was abandoned as an isolated operation.

Selective coronary angiography was developed by Sones and Shirey, at the Cleveland Clinic, and reported in their 1962 classic paper, "Cine Coronary Arteriography."[144] They used a catheter to directly inject contrast material into the coronary artery ostia. This technique gave a major impetus to direct revascularization of obstructed coronary arteries.

From 1960 to 1967, several sporadic instances of coronary grafting were reported. All were isolated cases and, for uncertain reasons, were not reproduced. None had an impact on the development of coronary surgery. Dr. Robert H. Goetz performed what appears to be the first clearly documented coronary artery bypass operation in a human, which was successful. The surgery took place at Van Etten Hospital in New York City on May 2, 1960.[145] He operated on a 38-year-old male who was severely symptomatic and used a nonsuture technique to connect the right internal mammary artery to a right coronary artery. It took him 17 seconds to join the two arteries using a hollow metal tube. The right internal mammary artery–coronary artery connection was confirmed patent by angiography performed on the 14th postoperative day. The patient remained asymptomatic for about a year, then developed recurrent angina and died of a myocardial infarction on June 23, 1961. Goetz was severely criticized by his medical and surgical colleagues for this procedure, although he had performed it successfully many times in the animal laboratory. He never attempted another coronary bypass operation in a human.

Another example involved a case of autogenous saphenous vein bypass grafting performed on November 23, 1964, in a 42-year-old man who was scheduled to have endarterectomy of his left coronary artery.[146] Since the lesion involved the entire bifurcation, endarterectomy with venous patch graft was abandoned as too hazardous. The anterior descending coronary artery was softer distal to the bifurcation. An autogenous saphenous vein graft was therefore placed from the aorta to the left anterior descending. This was probably the first clinical case of successful coronary artery bypass surgery using saphenous vein. The authors, Garrett, Dennis, and DeBakey, however, did not report this case until 1973. The patient was alive at that time, and angiograms showed the vein graft to be patent.

Shumaker[147] credits Longmire with the first internal mammary to coronary artery anastomosis. It was almost surely Longmire, long-time chairman at UCLA, and his associate, Jack Cannon, who first performed an anastomosis between the internal mammary artery and a coronary branch, probably in early 1958. Longmire wrote:

> At that time we were doing the coronary thromboendarterectomy procedure, we also, I think, performed a couple of the earliest internal mammary–coronary anastomoses.... We were forced into it when the coronary artery we were endarterectomizing disintegrated, and in desperation we anastomosed the internal mammary artery to the distal end of the right coronary artery—and later decided it was a good operation.

The reference that Shumaker gives for this quotation from Longmire is a personal communication to Shumaker in 1990, which is 32 years after the fact!

As early as 1952, Vladimir Demikhov, the renowned Soviet surgeon, was anastomosing the internal mammary artery to the left coronary artery in dogs.[148] In 1967, at the height of the Cold War, a Soviet surgeon from Leningrad, V. I. Kolessov, reported his experience with mammary artery–coronary artery anastomoses for treatment of angina pectoris in six patients, in an American surgical journal.[149] The first patient in that series was done in 1964. Operations were performed through a left thoracotomy without extracorporeal circulation or preoperative coronary angiography. The following year, Green et al[150] and Bailey and Hirose[151] separately published reports in which the internal mammary artery was used for coronary artery bypass in patients. Bailey and Hirose carried out the anastomosis on the beating heart and advocated using loupes for magnification. Green et al advocated using cardiopulmonary bypass, fibrillating the vented heart, cross-clamping the aorta, and washing all blood from the coronary system while performing the anastomosis.

Rene Favalaro from the Cleveland Clinic used saphenous vein for bypassing coronary obstructions.[152] Favalaro's 1968 article focused on 15 patients, who were part of a larger series of 180 patients who had undergone the Vineberg procedure. In these 15 patients with occlusion of the proximal right coronary artery, an interpositional graft of saphenous vein also was placed between the ascending aorta and the right coronary artery distal to the blockage. The right coronary was divided, and the vein graft was anastomosed end-to-end. Favalaro states that this procedure was done because of the unfavorable results with pericardial patch reconstruction of the coronary artery. In an addendum to that paper, 55 cases were added, 52 for segmental occlusion of the right coronary and 3 others for circumflex disease.

The contributions by Favalaro, Kolessov, Green et al, and Bailey and Hirose were all important, but arguably the official start of coronary bypass surgery as we know it today happened in 1969 when W. Dudley Johnson and coworkers from Milwaukee reported their series of 301 patients who had undergone various operations for coronary disease since February of 1967.[153] In that report, the authors presented their results with direct coronary surgery during a 19-month period (Fig. 1-9). They state:

> After two initial and successful patch grafts, the vein bypass technique has been used exclusively. Early results were so encouraging that last summer the vein graft technique was expanded and used to all major branches. Vein grafts to the left side of the arteries run from the aorta over the pulmonary artery and down to the appropriate coronary vessel. Right-sided grafts run along the atrio-ventricular groove and also attach directly to the aorta. There is almost no limit of potential (coronary) arteries to use. Veins can be sutured to the distal anterior descending or even to posterior marginal branches. Double vein grafts are now used in over 40 percent of patients and can be used to any combination of arteries.

Johnson goes on to say:

> Our experience indicates that five factors are important to direct surgery. One: Do not limit grafts to proximal portions of large arteries.... Two: Do not work with diseased arteries. Vein grafts can be made as long as necessary and should be inserted into distal normal arteries. Three: Always do end-to-side anastomosis.... Four: Always work on dry, quiet field. Consistently successful fine vessel anastomoses cannot be done on a moving, bloody target.... Five: Do not allow the hematocrit to fall below 35.

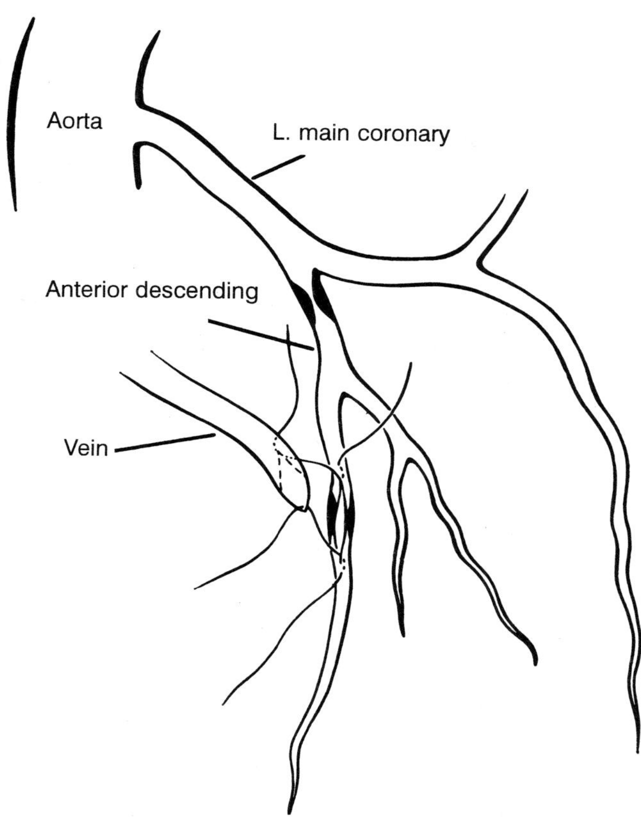

FIGURE 1–9 W. Dudley Johnson method of myocardial revascularization. Veins are usually inserted into an area of normal artery; however, if a second area of atherosclerosis occurs (commonly in the mid-anterior descending artery), the arteriotomy extends across the plaque into normal artery on each end. The vein is sutured as a patch graft always extending the anastomosis to normal artery proximally and distally. With progressive atherosclerosis this maneuver preserves bidirectional flow. (***Reproduced with permission from Johnson WD, Flemma RJ, Lepley D Jr, Ellison EH: Extended treatment of severe coronary artery disease: a total surgical approach. Ann Surg 1969; 171:460.***)

In discussing Dr. Johnson's presentation, Dr. Frank Spencer commented, "I would like to congratulate Dr. Johnson very heartily. We may have heard a milestone in cardiac surgery today. Because for years, pathologists, cardiologists, and many surgeons have repeatedly stated that the pattern of coronary artery disease is so extensive that direct anastomosis can be done in only 5 to 7 percent of patients. If the exciting data by Dr. Johnson remain valid and the grafts remain patent over a long period of time, a total revision of thinking will be required regarding the feasibility of direct arterial surgery for coronary artery disease."[153]

The direct anastomosis between the internal mammary artery and the coronary artery was not initially as popular as the vein graft technique; however, due to the persistence of Drs. Green, Loop, Grondin, and others, internal mammary artery grafts eventually became the conduit of choice when their superior long-term patency became known.[154]

Denton Cooley and colleagues made two important contributions to the surgery for ischemic heart disease.[155] In 1956, with the use of cardiopulmonary bypass, they were the first to repair a ruptured interventricular septum following acute myocardial infarction. The patient initially did well but died 6 weeks after operation of complications. Cooley et al also were the first to report the resection of a left ventricular aneurysm with the use of cardiopulmonary bypass.[156]

Beck[157] in 1944 was the first to successfully excise a left ventricular aneurysm, and Bailey et al[158] in 1951 had five survivors of six attempts with a clamp and oversew technique.

ARRHYTHMIC SURGERY

Sealy et al at Duke University developed the first successful surgical treatment for cardiac arrhythmias.[159,160] A 32-year-old fisherman was referred for symptomatic episodes of atrial tachycardia that caused congestive heart failure. On May 2, 1968, after epicardial mapping, a 5- to 6-cm cut was made extending from the base of the right atrial appendage to the right border of the right atrium during cardiopulmonary bypass. The incision transsected the conduction pathway between the atrium and ventricle. Subsequent epicardial mapping indicated eradication of the pathway. Six weeks after operation heart size had decreased and lung fields had cleared. The patient eventually returned to work.

A year earlier, Dr. Dwight McGoon at the Mayo Clinic closed an atrial septal defect in a patient who also had the Wolf-Parkinson-White syndrome (WPW).[160] At operation, Dr. Birchell mapped the epicardium of the heart and localized the accessory pathway to the right atrioventricular groove. Lidocaine was injected into the site, and the delta wave immediately disappeared. Unfortunately, conduction across the pathway reappeared a few hours later. This was probably the first attempt to treat the WPW syndrome surgically. As a result of knowledge gained from the surgical treatment for WPW syndrome, over 95% of all refractory clinical cases are now treated successfully by nonsurgical means.[160]

Guiraudon et al,[161] from Paris, France, reported their results with an encircling endomyocardial ventriculotomy for the treatment of malignant ventricular arrhythmias. The following year, in 1979, Josephson et al[162] described a more specific procedure for treatment of malignant ventricular arrhythmias. After endocardial mapping, the endocardial source of the arrhythmia was excised. Although the Guiraudon technique usually isolated the source of the arrhythmia, the incision also devascularized healthy myocardium and was associated with high mortality. Endocardial resection was safer and more efficacious, and became the basis of all approaches for the treatment of ischemic ventricular tachycardia.[160]

Ross et al,[163] in Sydney, Australia, and Cox et al,[164] in St. Louis, Missouri, used cryosurgical treatment of atrial ventricular node reentry tachycardia. Subsequently, Cox, after years of laboratory research, developed the Maze operation for atrial fibrillation.[165]

Stimulated by the death of a close personal friend from ventricular arrhythmias, Dr. Mirowski developed a prototype defibrillator over a 3-month period in 1969. In 1980, Mirowski et al described three successful cases using their implantable myocardial stimulator at Johns Hopkins.[166]

PACEMAKERS

Lidwill and Booth in Australia supposedly revived a stillborn infant with electrical pacing in the 1920s.[167] Hyman temporarily paced the heart using two needle electrodes that were passed through the ribs and an electrical device of his own design. In the early 1950s, Bigelow and colleagues reported controlling the heart rate in dogs using external pacemakers.[78]

Paul Zoll is given credit for ushering in the clinical era of pacemaking. In 1952, he reported on two patients suffering from recurring prolonged ventricular standstill whom he treated with an external pacemaker.[168] The first patient was a 75-year-old man with complete heart block who had been revived with 34 intracardiac injections of epinephrine over a 4-hour period. Zoll applied electric shocks 2 milliseconds in duration that were transmitted through the chest wall at frequencies from 25 to 60 per minute and increased the intensity of the shock until ventricular responses were observed. After 25 minutes of intermittent stimulation, however, the patient died. Many subsequent patients, however, recovered.

The next step came when Lillehei et al reported a series of patients who had external pacing after open heart surgery during the 1950s.[169] The field of open heart surgery gave a major impetus to the development of pacemakers, because there was a high incidence of heart block following many intracardiac repairs. The major difference between Zoll's pacing and that of Lillehei et al was that Zoll used external electrodes placed on the chest wall, whereas Lillehei et al attached electrodes directly to the heart at operation. Lillehei et al used a relatively small external pacemaker to stimulate the heart and much less electric current. This form of heart pacing was better tolerated by the patient and was a more efficient way to stimulate the heart. The survival rate of Lillehei's patients with surgically induced heart block was significantly improved.

During this period, progress was made toward a totally implantable pacemaker. Elmquist and Senning[170] developed a pacer battery that was small enough for an epigastric pocket with electrodes connected to the heart. They implanted the unit in a patient with atrioventricular block in 1958. Just before implantation, the patient had 20 to 30 cardiac arrests a day. To avoid publicity, the implantation was done in the evening when the operating rooms were empty. The first pacemaker that was implanted functioned only 8 hours; the second pacemaker implanted in the same patient had better success. The patient survived until January 2002 and had many additional pacemakers. Chardack, Gage, and Greatbatch are perhaps better known for their development of the totally implantable pacemaker.[171] In 1961 they reported a series of 15 patients who had pacemakers implanted that they had developed. The technique for inserting permanent transvenous bipolar pacemaker electrodes was developed in 1962 by Parsonnet et al[172] in the United States and Ekestrom et al[173] in Sweden.

Early implantable pacemakers were fixed-rate, asynchronous devices that delivered an impulse independent of the underlying cardiac rhythm. During the past 35 years, enormous progress has been made in the field of pacing technology. The number of individuals with artificial pacemakers is unknown; however, estimates indicate that approximately 500,000 Americans are living with a pacemaker and that each year another 100,000 or more patients require permanent pacemakers in the United States.

HEART, HEART-LUNG, AND LUNG TRANSPLANTATION

Alexis Carrel and Charles Guthrie reported transplantation of the heart and lungs while at the University of Chicago in 1905.[174] The heart of a small dog was transplanted into the neck of a larger one by anastomosing the caudad ends of the jugular vein and carotid artery to the aorta and pulmonary artery. The animal was not anticoagulated, and the experiment ended about 2 hours after circulation was established because of blood clot in the cavities of the transplanted heart. Carrel also reported in 1906 that he had transplanted the heart and lungs of a 1-week-old cat into the neck of a larger cat.[175] The coronary circulation was immediately reestablished, and the "auricles began to beat. The lungs became red and after a few minutes effective pulsation of the ventricles appeared." Carrel stated that a phlegmon of the neck terminated this observation 2 days later.

Vladimir Demikhov, the great Soviet investigator, described more than 20 different techniques for heart transplantation in 1950.[176] He also published various techniques for heart and lung transplantation. He was even able to perform an orthotopic heart transplant in a dog before the heart-lung machine was developed. This was accomplished by placing the donor heart above the dog's own heart, and then with a series of tubes and connections, he rerouted the blood from one heart to the other until he had the donor heart functioning in the appropriate position and the native heart removed. One of his dogs climbed the steps of the Kremlin on the sixth postoperative day but died shortly afterwards of rejection.

Richard Lower and Norman Shumway established the technique for heart transplantation as it is performed today.[177] Preservation of the cuff of recipient left and right atria with part of the atrial septum was described earlier by Brock[178] in England and Demikhov[148] in the Soviet

Union, but it became popular only after Shumway and Lower reported it in their 1960 paper. Shumway stated[179]:

> In 1958 when I started work at Stanford, the idea [cardiac transplantation] grew out of our local cooling experiments, since we had one hour of aortic cross-clamping during cardiopulmonary bypass. Accordingly we decided to remove the heart at the atrial level and then to suture it back into position. After several of these experiments, we found it would be easier to remove the heart of another dog and to do the actual allotransplant. Something like 20 to 30 experiments were performed before we had a survivor. All of this was done before chemical immune suppression was available.

The first attempt at a human heart transplantation was made by Hardy et al[180] at the University of Mississippi. Since no human donor organ was available at the time, a large chimpanzee's heart was used; however, it was unable to support the circulation because of hyperacute rejection.

The first human-to-human heart transplant occurred December 3, 1967, at the Groote Schuur Hospital in Capetown, South Africa.[181] The surgical team, headed by Christiaan Barnard, transplanted the heart of a donor who had been certified dead after the electrocardiogram showed no activity for 5 minutes into a 54-year-old man whose heart was irreparably damaged by repeated myocardial infarctions. The second human heart transplant using a human donor was performed on a child 3 days after the first on December 6, 1967, by Adrian Kantrowitz in Brooklyn, New York. Dr. Kantrowitz's patient died of a bleeding complication within the first 24 hours.[182] Barnard's patient, Lewis Washkansky, died on the 18th postoperative day. At autopsy, the heart appeared normal, and there was no evidence of chronic liver congestion, but bilateral pneumonia, possibly due to severe myloid depression from immunosuppression, was present.[183]

On January 2, 1968, Barnard performed a second heart transplant on Phillip Blaiberg, 12 days after Washkansky's death.[184] Blaiberg was discharged from the hospital and became a celebrity during the several months he lived after the transplant. Blaiberg's procedure indicated that a heart transplant was an option for humans suffering from end-stage heart disease. Within a year of Barnard's first heart transplant, 99 heart transplants had been performed by cardiac surgeons around the world. However, by the end of 1968, most groups abandoned heart transplantation because of the extremely high mortality related to rejection. Shumway and Lower, Barnard, and a few others persevered both clinically and in the laboratory. Their efforts in discovering better drugs for immunosuppression eventually established heart transplantation as we know it today.

A clinical trial of heart-lung transplantation was commenced at Stanford University in 1981 by Reitz et al.[185] Their first patient was treated with a combination of cyclosporine and azothioprine. The patient was discharged from the hospital in good condition and was well more than 5 years after the transplant. Reitz's clinical success was based on earlier experiments with primates using allografts.[186,187] These primate recipients survived for more than 140 days when cyclosporine A was used for immune suppression. Several of these animals lived for more than 5 years after allotransplantation.[188]

The current success with heart, heart-lung, and lung transplantation is in part related to the discovery of cyclosporine by workers at the Sandoz Laboratory in Basel, Switzerland, in 1970. In December of 1980, cyclosporine was introduced at Stanford for cardiac transplantation. The incidence of rejection was not reduced, nor was the incidence of infection. However, these two major complications of cardiac transplantation were less severe when cyclosporine was used. Availability of cyclosporine stimulated many new programs across the United States in the mid-1980s.

Andre Juvenelle showed that animals could survive autologous lung transplantation for many years.[189] Lung transplantation from dog to dog was fatal when attempted in the early 1950s.[190] Some animals, however, survived with an autotransplant up to 29 days before succumbing to rejection.[191] The first human lung transplant was performed by Hardy et al[192] at the University of Mississippi on June 11, 1964. A pneumonectomy for carcinoma with pleural adhesions had to be performed first. The patient died on the 17th postoperative day. In 1971, a Belgian surgeon, Fritz Derom, achieved a 10-month survival in a patient with pulmonary silicosis.[193]

Much of the credit, however, for the success of lung transplantation belongs to the Toronto group whose efforts were headed by Joel Cooper. Their successes were based on laboratory experimentation and the discovery of cyclosporine. After losing an early patient to bronchial anastomotic dehiscence in 1978, the group substituted cyclosporine for cortisone and wrapped the bronchial suture line with a pedicle of omentum. They also developed a comprehensive preoperative preparation program that increased the strength and nutritional status of the recipients. In 1986, Cooper and associates presented their first two successful patients, who had returned to normal activities and were alive 14 and 26 months after operation.[194] This success was the culmination of more than 40 previous attempts throughout the world made after Derom's case.

HEART ASSIST AND ARTIFICIAL HEARTS

The concept of intraaortic counterpulsation was first described by Harken[195] in 1958 and reported by Clauss et al[196] in 1961. This idea proposed removal of blood via the femoral artery during systole and rapid reinfusion of the same blood during diastole to increase coronary perfusion. Technical difficulties and complications secondary to hemolysis delayed clinical use until 1962, when Moulopoulos et al introduced a balloon catheter placed in the thoracic aorta.[197] In 1963, Kantrowitz et al reported the first use of the intraaortic balloon pump in three patients.[198] All were in cardiogenic shock but improved during balloon pumping. One survived to leave the hospital.

Akutsu and Kolff reported the development and first application of a totally artificial heart in an animal model at the Cleveland Clinic in 1957.[199] The authors implanted a totally artificial heart in a living dog that survived for 90 minutes with the mechanical heart.

In 1963, Liotta et al reported a 42-year-old man who had a stenotic aortic valve replaced but suffered a cardiac arrest the following morning.[200] The patient was resuscitated but developed severe ventricular failure. An artificial intrathoracic circulatory pump was implanted. The patient's pulmonary edema cleared, but he died 4 days later with the pump working continuously. In 1966, the same group used a newer intrathoracic pump to support another patient who could not be weaned from cardiopulmonary bypass. This pump maintained the circulation. The patient eventually died before the pump could be removed.[201] Later that year, the same group used a left ventricular assist device in a woman who could not be weaned from cardiopulmonary bypass after double valve replacement.[202] After 10 days of circulatory assistance, the patient was weaned successfully from the device and recovered. This woman was probably the first patient to be weaned from an assist device and to leave the hospital.

The first human application of a totally artificial heart was by Denton Cooley and colleagues as a "bridge" to transplantation.[203] They implanted a totally artificial heart in a patient who could not be weaned from cardiopulmonary bypass. After 64 hours of artificial heart support, heart transplantation was performed, but the patient died of *Pseudomonas* pneumonia 32 hours after transplantation. The first two patients successfully bridged to transplantation were reported at almost the same time and in the same location by different groups. On September 5, 1984, in San Francisco,[204] Donald Hill implanted a Pierce-Donachy left ventricular assist device in a patient in cardiogenic shock. The patient received a successful transplant 2 days later and was later discharged. The assist device used by Hill was developed at Pennsylvania State University by Pierce and Donachy. Phillip Oyer and associates at Stanford University placed an electrically driven Novacor left ventricular assist device in a patient in cardiogenic shock on September 7, 1984.[205] The patient was transplanted successfully and survived beyond 3 years. The device used by the Stanford group was developed by Peer Portner.

The first implantation of a permanent totally artificial heart (Jarvik-7) was performed by DeVries et al at the University of Utah in 1982.[206] By 1985, they had implanted the Jarvik in four patients, and one survived for 620 days after implantation. This initial clinical experience was heavily based on the work of Kolff and associates.

The effort to use autologous skeletal muscle to assist the failing circulation began in 1959 when Adrian Kantrowitz wrapped diaphragm around the canine aorta to produce diastolic counterpulsation.[207] The problem of muscle fatigue was solved in 1969 when Salmons and Vrbova[208] discovered that fast-twitch fibers found in skeletal muscle could be transformed into slow-twitch fatigue-resistant fibers by chronic electrical stimulation of the motor nerve. That observation led Macoviak et al and Mannion et al to develop electrical conditioning protocols for fiber transformation of large canine muscles[209,210] and Dewar et al[211] to develop the concept of burst stimulation to increase the force of muscle contraction. These advances prompted several surgeons to wrap latissimus dorsi muscle around ventricles of failing hearts and stimulate the muscle to contract during systole. Alain Carpentier first performed this procedure in a patient in 1985.[212] Subsequently, more than 600 patients worldwide have had this procedure, known as *cardiomyoplasty*. Carpentier's group was also first to wrap latissimus dorsi muscle around the human aorta and then stimulate the muscle during cardiac diastole and use this as an aortic diastolic counterpulsator somewhat like the intra-aortic balloon pump. To date, at least 25 of these clinical procedures have been done worldwide.[213] An alternative method to harness skeletal muscle power to the circulation is to wrap a muscle around a pericardial or endothelial cell-lined pouch attached to the thoracic aorta.[214] Canine studies have demonstrated that these skeletal muscle ventricles continue to function for over four years.[215]

THORACIC AORTA SURGERY

Alexis Carrel was responsible for one of the great surgical advances of the 20th century: techniques for suturing and transplanting blood vessels.[216] Although Carrel initially developed his methods of blood vessel anastomosis in Lyon, France, his work with Charles Guthrie in Chicago led to many major advances in vascular, cardiac, and transplantation surgery. In a short period of time, these investigators perfected techniques for blood vessel anastomoses and transposition of arterial and venous segments using both fresh and frozen grafts. After leaving Chicago, Carrel continued to expand his work on blood vessels and organ transplantation and in 1912 received the Nobel Prize. Interestingly, Carrel's work did not receive immediate clinical application.

Rudolph Matas pioneered clinical vascular surgery. Matas's work took place before drugs were available to prevent blood clotting, before antibiotics, and without reliable blood vessel substitutes.[217] Matas performed 620 vascular operations between 1888 and 1940. Only 101 of these were attempts to repair arteries; most involved ligation. Matas developed three variations of his well-known endoaneurysmorrhaphy procedure. The most advanced was to reconstruct the wall of the blood vessel from within while using a rubber tube as a stent.

Vascular surgery advanced tentatively during World War II as traumatic injuries to major blood vessels were repaired in some soldiers with results significantly better than with the standard treatment of ligation.[218] The successful treatment of coarctation of the aorta by Crafoord and Gross added a major boost to the reconstructive surgery of arteries.

Shumaker reported the excision of a small descending thoracic aortic aneurysm with reanastomosis of the aorta in 1948.[219] Swan et al[220] repaired a complex aneurysmal coarctation and used aortic homograft for reconstruction in 1950. Gross[221] reported a series of similar cases using homograft replacement. In 1951, DuBost et al,[222] from Paris, resected an intra-abdominal aortic aneurysm with homograft replacement.

In 1953, Henry Bahnson,[223] from Johns Hopkins, successfully resected six saccular aneurysms of the aorta in eight patients. In the same year, DeBakey and Cooley[224] reported a 46-year-old man who had resection of a huge aneurysm of the descending thoracic aorta that measured approximately 20 cm in length and in greatest diameter. The aneurysm was resected and replaced with an aortic homograft approximately 15 cm in length.

During the Korean War, the arterial homograft and autogenous vein graft were used to reconstruct battlefield arterial injuries and reduce the overall amputation rate to 11.1%,[225] compared to the rate of 49.6 % reported in World War II. Although the vein autograft remains the first-choice peripheral vascular conduit today, the arterial homograft was superseded by the development of synthetic vascular grafts by Arthur Voorhees at Columbia University in 1952. Voorhees et al developed Vinyon-N cloth tubes to substitute for diseased arterial segments,[226] but because of kinking, these smooth-lined tubes could not be used across joints. Development of the crimped graft by Edwards and Tapp[227] and the introduction of Dacron by DeBakey[228] were important milestones. DeBakey's account of his discovery of Dacron reflects the resourcefulness and innovation of these pioneering surgeons[228]:

> We were greatly impressed with the report of Voorhees on the use of a fabric woven of Vinyon-N. On my first trip to obtain some of these fabrics from a department store here, I found that they only had some sheets of Dacron. I purchased several yards and cut them in different sizes to make tubes by sewing on my wife's sewing machine. I had been taught by my mother as a boy to sew and I became an expert not only in the use of the sewing machine, but also on the other aspects of sewing. These tubes proved highly successful in animals, and although we later obtained sheets of Orlon, Teflon, nylon and Ivalon, none of these were as good as the original Dacron fabric. It was rather interesting and an example of serendipity that the first material we obtained (Dacron), the only one available at the store at the time, proved later to be the best. One of these Dacron grafts that I had fabricated as a bifurcation graft was used to replace an aneurysm of the abdominal aorta in September, 1954.

Another advance in aortic surgery appeared in 1955 when DeBakey et al[229] reported six cases of aortic dissection treated by aggressive surgery. This paper included a description of pathologic and hemodynamic factors associated with the dissections and led to a more logical approach to treatment of these lesions. Because mortality of operation for acute dissections remained high, Myron Wheat, Jr., introduced medical therapy for the disease.[230]

During the late 1950s the Houston group, Michael DeBakey, Denton Cooley, Stanley Crawford, and their other associates, systematically developed operations for resection and graft replacement of the ascending aorta,[231] descending aorta, and the thoracoabdominal aorta.[232] Cardiopulmonary bypass was used for the ascending aortic resections. The high risk of paraplegia highlighted a major complication of thoracoabdominal aortic resections. The Houston group was the first to resect an aortic arch with the use of cardiopulmonary bypass in 1957[233] and replace the arch with a reconstituted aortic arch homograph (Fig. 1-10). More interesting is that Cooley et al, using great ingenuity, resected a large aortic arch aneurysm that also involved a portion of the descending aorta in a 49-year-old patient on June 24, 1955. The surgery was done, without the use of cardiopulmonary bypass, by first sewing in a temporary graft from the ascending aorta to the distal descending aorta and sewing in two more temporary limbs off that graft, which were anastomosed to the left and right carotid arteries while the aneurysm was resected and a permanent graft was placed.[234]

In 1968, Bentall and De Bono[235] introduced replacement of the ascending aorta and aortic valve with reanastomoses of the coronary ostia to the replacement graft. They described the composite-graft technique for replacement of the ascending aorta with reimplantation of the coronary arteries into the composite Dacron graft containing the prosthetic aortic valve. As previously mentioned, Cooley and DeBakey were first to replace the supracoronary ascending aorta in 1956. In 1963 Starr et al[236] reported replacing the supracoronary ascending aorta and also the aortic valve at the same sitting. The technique of fashioning buttons of aortic tissue adjacent to the coronary ostia and then incorporating these buttons into the aortic graft along with the aortic valve replacement was described by Wheat et al[237] in 1964. Bentall and De Bono incorporated the aortic prosthesis into the tube graft and used the Wheat technique for implanting the coronary arteries into the composite graft.

SUMMARY

The history of adult cardiac surgery continues to be written and will continue to evolve as long as acquired heart disease shortens lives. In the early days after the introduction of cardiopulmonary bypass, the pace of advance was torrid but, in a way, narrowly focused. Now hundreds of thousands of clinicians, scientists, and engineers are involved in a broad and deep effort to develop new and safer operations and procedures, new valves, new revascularization techniques, new biomaterials, new heart substitutes, new life-support

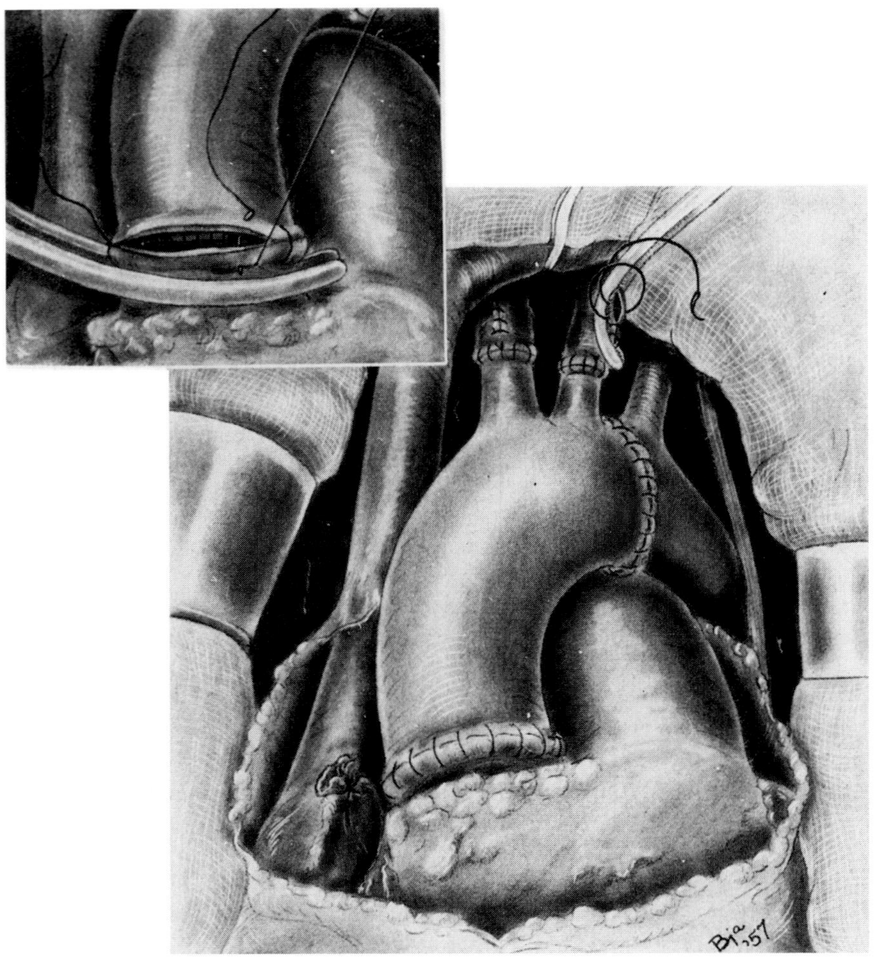

FIGURE 1–10 Homograft replacement of the ascending aorta. Drawings showing final anastomosis of homograft to base of ascending aorta (*inset*) and appearance after completion of all anastomoses to homograft. (*Reproduced with permission from DeBakey ME, Crawford ES, Cooley DA, Morris GC Jr: Successful resection of fusiform aneurysm of aortic arch with replacement by homograft. Surg Gynecol Obstet 1957; 105:657. Copyright American College of Surgeons.*)

systems, and new methods to control cardiac arrhythmias and ventricular remodeling after injury. This research and development are supported by a vigorous infrastructure of basic science in biology and medicine, chemistry and pharmacology, and engineering and computer technology. The history of cardiac surgery is only a prelude; the moving finger writes and having writ moves on to a bright, exciting future.

REFERENCES

1. Williams DH: Stab wound of the heart, pericardium–Suture of the pericardium–Recovery–Patient alive three years afterward. *Med Record* 1897; p 1–8.
2. Rehn L: On penetrating cardiac injuries and cardiac suturing. *Arch Klin Chir* 1897; 55:315.
3. Rehn L: Zur chirurgie des herzens und des herzbeutels. *Arch Klin Chir* 1907; 83:723; quoted from Beck CS: Wounds of the heart: the technic of suture. *Arch Surg* 1926; 13:212.
4. Hill LL: A report of a case of successful suturing of the heart, and table of thirty seven other cases of suturing by different operators with various terminations, and the conclusions drawn. *Med Rec* 1902; 2:846.
5. Harken DE: Foreign bodies in and in relation to the thoracic blood vessels and heart, I: techniques for approaching and removing foreign bodies from the chambers of the heart. *Surg Gynecol Obstet* 1946; 83:117.
6. Trendelenburg F: Operative management of pulmonary emboli. *Verh Dtsch Ges Chir* 1908; 89.
7. Trendelenburg F: Zur operation der embolie der lungenarterie. *Dtsch Med Wochenschr* 1908; 34:1172.
8. Kirschner M: Ein durch die Trendelenburgische operation geheiter fall von embolie der art. pulmonalis. *Arch Klin Chir* 1924; 133:312.
9. Gibbon JH: Artificial maintenance of circulation during experimental occlusion of pulmonary artery. *Arch Surg* 1937; 34:1105.
10. Sharp EH: Pulmonary embolectomy: successful removal of a massive pulmonary embolus with the support of cardiopulmonary bypass. Case report. *Ann Surg* 1962; 156:1.
11. Morgagni GB: De sedibus et causis morborum per anatomen indagatis. Benetiis, typ. Remondiniana, 1761.
12. Pick F: Ueber chronoische, unter dem bilde der lebercirrhose verlautende pericarditis (pericarditsische pseudolebercirrhose) nebst bemerkungen ueber zuckergussleber (Curshmann). *Z Klin Med* 1896; 29:385.
13. Weill E: *Traite clinique des maladies du coeur chez les enfants.* Paris, Doin, 1895.
14. Delorme E: Sur un traitement chirurgical de la symphyse cardopericardique. *Gaz Hop* 1898; 71:1150.

15. Rehn I: Zur experimentellen pathologie des herzbeutels. *Verh Dtsch Ges Chir* 1913; 42:339.
16. Sauerbruch R: *Die Chirurgie der Brustorgane,* vol II. Berlin, 1925.
17. Forssmann W: Catheterization of the right heart. *Klin Wochenshr* 1929; 8:2085.
18. Forssmann W: 21 jahre herzkatheterung, rueckblick and ausschau. *Verh Dtsch Ges Kreislaufforschung* 1951; 17:1.
19. Klein O: Zur bestimmung des zirkulatorischen minutenvoumnens beim menschen nach dem fisckschen prinzip. *Meunsch Med Wochenschr* 1930; 77:1311.
20. Forssmann W: Ueber kontrastdarstellung der hoehlen des lebenden rechten herzens and der lungenschlagader. *Muensch Med Wochenschr* 1931; 78:489.
21. Tuffier T: Etat actuel de la chirurgie intrathoracique. *Trans Int Congr Med* 1913 (London 1914), 7; *Surgery* 1914; 2:249.
22. Shumaker HB Jr: *The Evolution of Cardiac Surgery*. Bloomington, Indiana University Press, 1992; p 116.
23. Brock RC: The arterial route to the aortic and pulmonary valves: the mitral route to the aortic valves. *Guys Hosp Rep* 1950; 99:236.
24. Brock, Sir Russell: Aortic subvalvular stenosis: surgical treatment. *Guys Hosp Rep* 1957; 106:221.
25. Bailey CP, Bolton HE, Nichols HT, et al: Commissurotomy for rheumatic aortic stenosis. *Circulation* 1954; 9:22.
26. Cushing H, Branch JRB: Experimental and clinical notes on chronic valvular lesions in the dog and their possible relation to a future surgery of the cardiac valves. *J Med Res* 1908; 17:471.
27. Cutler EC, Levine SA: Cardiotomy and valvulotomy for mitral stenosis. *Boston Med Surg J* 1923; 188:1023.
28. Suttar HS: Surgical treatment of mitral stenosis. *Br Med J* 1925; 2:603.
29. Acierno LJ: *The History of Cardiology*. New York, Parthenon Publishing Group, 1994; p 633.
30. Bailey CP: The surgical treatment of mitral stenosis. *Dis Chest* 1949; 15:377.
31. Naef AP: *The Story of Thoracic Surgery*. New York, Hogrefe & Huber, 1990; p 94.
32. Baker C, Brock RC, Campbell M: Valvulotomy for mitral stenosis: report of six successful cases. *Br Med J* 1950; 1:1283.
33. Sellors TH: Surgery of pulmonary stenosis: a case in which the pulmonary valve was successfully divided. *Lancet* 1948; 1:988.
34. Shumaker HB Jr: *The Evolution of Cardiac Surgery*. Bloomington, Indiana University Press, 1992; p 98.
35. Hufnagel CA: Aortic plastic valvular prostheses. *Bull Georgetown Med Cent* 1951; 4:128.
36. Campbell JM: Artificial aortic valve. *J Thorac Cardiovasc Surg* 1958; 19:312.
37. Hufnagel CA, Harvey WP, Rabil PJ, et al: Surgical correction of aortic insufficiency. *Surgery* 1954; 35:673.
38. Trace HD, Bailey CP, Wendkos MH: Tricuspid valve commissurotomy with a one year follow-up. *Am Heart J* 1954; 47:613.
39. Brofman BL: Right auriculoventricular pressure gradients with special reference to tricuspid stenosis. *J Lab Clin Med* 1953; 42:789.
40. Likoff W, Berkowitz D, Denton C, et al: A clinical evaluation of surgical treatment of combined mitral and aortic stenosis. *Am Heart J* 1955; 219:394.
41. Lillehei CW, Gott VL, DeWall RA, et al: The surgical treatment of stenotic and regurgitant lesions of the mitral and aortic valves by direct utilization of a pump oxygenator. *J Thorac Surg* 1958; 35:154.
42. Borman JB, Applebaum A, Hirsch M, et al: Quadruple valve commissurotomy. *J Thorac Cardiovasc Surg* 1975; 70:713.
43. Graybiel A, Strieder JW, Boyer NH: An attempt to obliterate the patent ductus in a patient with subacute endarteritis. *Am Heart J* 1938; 15:621.
44. Gross RE, Hubbard JH: Surgical ligation of a patent ductus arteriosus: report of first successful case. *JAMA* 1939; 112:729.
45. Crafoord C, Nylin G: Congenital coarctation of the aorta and its surgical treatment. *J Thorac Cardiovasc Surg* 1945; 14:347.
46. Gross RE: Surgical correction for coarctation of the aorta. *Surgery* 1945; 18:673.
47. Gross RE: Surgical relief for tracheal obstruction from a vascular ring. *N Engl J Med* 1945; 233:586.
48. Gross RE, Neuhauser EBD: Compression of the trachea or esophagus by vascular anomalies: surgical therapy in 40 cases. *Pediatrics* 1951; 7:69.
49. Blalock A, Taussig HB: The surgical treatment of malformations of the heart in which there is pulmonary stenosis or pulmonary atresia. *JAMA* 1945; 128:189.
50. Biorck G, Crafoord C: Arteriovenous aneurysm on the pulmonary artery simulating patent ductus arteriosus botalli. *Thorax* 1947; 2:65.
51. Muller WH Jr: The surgical treatment of the transposition of the pulmonary veins. *Ann Surg* 1951; 134:683.
52. Gross RE: Surgical closure of an aortic septal defect. *Circulation* 1952; 5:858.
53. Cooley DA, McNamara DR, Latson JR: Aorticopulmonary septal defect: diagnosis and surgical treatment. *Surgery* 1957; 42:101.
54. Carlon CA, Mondini PG, de Marchi R: Surgical treatment of some cardiovascular diseases. *J Int Coll Surg* 1951; 16:1.
55. Glenn WWL: Circulatory bypass of the right side of the hearts, IV: Shunt between superior vena cava and distal right pulmonary artery—report of clinical application. *N Engl J Med* 1958; 259:117.
56. Galankin NK: Proposition and technique of cavo-pulmonary anastomosis. *Exp Biol (Russia)* 1957; 5:33.
57. Lillehei CW: Historical development of cardiopulmonary bypass. *Cardiopulmonary Bypass* 1993; 1:26.
58. von Frey M, Gruber M: Untersuchungen uber den stoffwechsel isolierter ograne. Ein respirations-apparat fur isolierte organe. *Virchows Arch Physiol* 1885; 9:519.
59. Jacobi C: Ein betrag zur technik der kunstlichen durchblutung uberlebender organe. *Arch Exp Pathol* (Leipzig) 1895; 31:330.
60. Brukhonenko SS, Terebinsky S: Experience avec la tete isole du chien, I: Techniques et conditions des experiences. *J Physiol Pathol Genet* 1929; 27:31.
61. Edwards WS, Edwards PD: *Alexis Carrel: Visionary Surgeon*. Springfield, IL, Charles C Thomas, 1974; p 93.
62. Edwards WS, Edwards PD: *Alexis Carrel: Visionary Surgeon*. Springfield, IL, Charles C Thomas, 1974; p 95.
63. Johnson SL: *The History of Cardiac Surgery, 1896–1955*. Baltimore, Johns Hopkins Press, 1970; p 121.
64. McLean J: The discovery of heparin. *Circulation* 1959; 19:78.
65. Letter from Jay McLean to Charles H. Best on November 14, 1940; quoted from Best CH: Preparation of heparin and its use in the first clinical case. *Circulation* 1959; 19:79.
66. Howell WH, Holt E: Two new factors in blood coagulation: heparin and pro-antithrombin. *Am J Physiol* 1918; 47:328.
67. Best C: Preparation of heparin and its use in the first clinical cases. *Circulation* 1959; 19:81.
68. Gibbon JH Jr: The gestation and birth of an idea. *Phila Med* 1963; 59:913.
69. Gibbon JH Jr: Artificial maintenance of circulation during experimental occlusion of the pulmonary artery. *Arch Surg* 1937; 34:1105.
70. Johnson SL: *The History of Cardiac Surgery, 1896–1955*. Baltimore, Johns Hopkins Press, 1970; p 145.
71. Johnson SL: *The History of Cardiac Surgery, 1896–1955*. Baltimore, Johns Hopkins Press, 1970; p 148.
72. Dennis C, Spreng DS, Nelson GE, et al: Development of a pump oxygenator to replace the heart and lungs: an apparatus applicable

to human patients, and application to one case. *Ann Surg* 1951; 134:709.
73. Digliotti AM: Clinical use of the artificial circulation with a note on intra-arterial transfusion. *Bull Johns Hopkins Hosp* 1952; 90:131.
74. Dodrill FD, Hill E, Gerisch RA: Temporary mechanical substitute for the left ventricle in man. *JAMA* 1952; 150:642.
75. Dodrill FD, Hill E, Gerisch RA: Some physiologic aspects of the artificial heart problem. *J Thorac Surg* 1952; 24:134.
76. Dodrill FD, Hill E, Gerisch RA, Johnson A: Pulmonary valvuloplasty under direct vision using the mechanical heart for a complete bypass of the right heart in a patient with congenital pulmonary stenosis. *J Thorac Surg* 1953; 25:584.
77. Stephenson LW: Forest Dewey Dodrill—Heart Surgery Pioneer, Part II. *J Cardiac Surg (in press)*.
78. Bigelow WG, Callaghan JC, Hopps JA: General hypothermia for experimental intracardiac surgery. *Am Surg* 1950; 132:531.
79. Bigelow WG, Lindsay WK, Harrison RC, et al: Oxygen transport and utilization in dogs at low body temperatures. *Am J Physiol* 1950; 160:125.
80. Bigelow WG, Hopps JA, Callaghan JA: Radiofrequency rewarming in resuscitation from severe hypothermia. *Can J Med Sci* 1952; 30:185.
81. Bigelow WG: Intellectual humility in medical practice and research. *Surgery* 1969; 132:849.
82. Lewis FJ, Taufic M: Closure of atrial septal defects with the aid of hypothermia: Experimental accomplishments and the report of one successful case. *Surgery* 1953; 33:52.
83. Swan H, Zeavin I, Blount SG Jr, Virtue RW: Surgery by direct vision in the open heart during hypothermia. *JAMA* 1953; 153:1081.
84. Hikasa Y, Shirotani H, Satomura K, et al: Open heart surgery in infants with the aid of hypothermic anesthesia. *Arch Jpn Chir* 1967; 36:495.
85. Horiuchi T, Koyamada K, Matano I, et al: Radical operation for ventricular septal defect in infancy. *J Thorac Cardiovasc Surg* 1963; 46:180.
86. Dillard DH, Mohri H, Hessel EA 2nd, et al: Correction of total anomalous pulmonary venous drainage in infancy utilizing deep hypothermia with total circulatory arrest. *Circulation* 1967; 35(suppl I):I105.
87. Wakusawa R, Shibata S, Saito H, et al: Clinical experience in 52 cases of open heart surgery under simple profound hypothermia. *Jpn J Anesth* 1968; 18:240.
88. Barratt-Boyes BG, Simpson MM, Neutze JM: Intracardiac surgery in neonates and infants using deep hypothermia. *Circulation* 1970; 61(suppl III):III73.
89. Johnson SL: *The History of Cardiac Surgery, 1896–1955*. Baltimore, Johns Hopkins Press, 1970; p 143.
90. Gibbon JH Jr: Application of a mechanical heart and lung apparatus to cardiac surgery. *Minn Med* 1954; 37:171.
91. Lillehei CW, Cohen M, Warden HE, et al: The results of direct vision closure of ventricular septal defects in eight patients by means of controlled cross circulation. *Surg Gynecol Obstet* 1955; 101:446.
92. Lillehei CW, Cohen M, Warden HE, et al: The direct vision intracardiac correction of congenital anomalies by controlled cross circulation. *Surgery* 1955; 38:11.
93. Kirklin JW, DuShane JW, Patrick RT, et al: Intracardiac surgery with the aid of a mechanical pump-oxygenator system (Gibbon type): report of eight cases. *Mayo Clin Proc* 1955; 30:201.
94. Kirklin JW: The middle 1950s and C. Walton Lillehei. *J Thorac Cardiovasc Surg* 1989; 98:822.
95. Spencer FC: Intellectual creativity in thoracic surgeons. *J Thorac Cardiovasc Surg* 1983; 86:167.
96. Hill JD, O'Brien TG, Murray JJ, et al: Prolonged extracorporeal oxygenation for acute post-traumatic respiratory failure (shock-lung syndrome): use of the Bramson membrane lung. *N Engl J Med* 1972; 286:629.
97. Zapol WM, Snider MT, Hill JD, et al: Extracorporeal membrane oxygenation in severe acute respiratory failure: a randomized prospective study. *JAMA* 1979; 242:2193.
98. Bartlett RH, Gazzaniga AB, Jefferies R: Extracorporeal membrane oxygenation (ECMO) cardiopulmonary support in infancy. *ASAIO Trans* 1976; 22:80.
99. Bartlett RH, Andrews AF, Toomasian J: Extracorporeal membrane oxygenation (ECMO) for newborn respiratory failure: 45 cases. *Surgery* 1982; 92:425.
100. Bartlett RH, Gazzaniga AV, Toomasian J, et al: Extracorporeal membrane oxygenation (ECMO) in neonatal respiratory failure: 100 cases. *Ann Surg* 1986; 204:236.
101. Toomasian JM, Snedecor SM, Cornell RG, et al: National experience with extracorporeal membrane oxygenation for newborn respiratory failure: data from 715 cases. *ASAIO Trans* 1988; 34:140.
102. Bartlett RH, Roloff DW, Cornell RG, et al: Extracorporeal circulation in neonatal respiratory failure: a prospective randomized study. *Pediatrics* 1989; 84:957.
103. O'Rourke PP, Crone RK, Vacanti JP, et al: Extracorporeal membrane oxygenation and conventional medical therapy in neonates with persistent pulmonary hypertension of the newborn: a prospective randomized study. *Pediatrics* 1989; 84: 957.
104. Carrel, A: Experimental operations on the orifices of the heart. *Ann Surg* 1914; 40:1.
105. Melrose DG, Dreyer B, Bentall MB, Baker JBE: Elective cardiac arrest. *Lancet* 1955; 2:21.
106. Gay WA Jr, Ebert PA: Functional metabolic, and morphologic effects of potassium-induced cardioplegia. *Surgery* 1973; 74: 284.
107. Tyers GFO, Todd GJ, Niebauer IM, et al: The mechanism of myocardial damage following potassium-induced (Melrose) cardioplegia. *Surgery* 1978; 78:45.
108. Kirsch U, Rodewald G, Kalmar P: Induced ischemic arrest. *J Thorac Cardiovasc Surg* 1972; 63:121.
109. Bretschneider HJ, Hubner G, Knoll D, et al: Myocardial resistance and tolerance to ischemia: physiological and biochemical basis. *J Cardiovasc Surg* 1975; 16:241.
110. Hearse DJ, Stewart DA, Braimbridge MV, et al: Cellular protection during myocardial ischemia. *Circulation* 1976; 16:241.
111. Follette DM, Mulder DG, Maloney JV, Buckberg GD: *J Thorac Cardiovasc Surg* 1978; 78:604.
112. Potts WJ, Smith S, Gibson S: Anastomosis of the aorta to a pulmonary artery. *JAMA* 1946; 132.
113. Waterston DJ: Treatment of Fallot's tetralogy in children under one year of age. *Rozhl Chir* 1962; 41:181.
114. Blalock A, Hanlon CR: The surgical treatment of complete transposition of the aorta and the pulmonary artery. *Surg Gynecol Obstet* 1950; 90:1.
115. Harken DE, Soroff HS, Taylor WJ, et al: Partial and complete prostheses in aortic insufficiency. *J Thorac Cardiovasc Surg* 1960; 40:744.
116. Starr A, Edwards ML: Mitral replacement: clinical experience with a ball-valve prosthesis. *Ann Surg* 1961; 154:726.
117. Spencer FC: Intellectual creativity in thoracic surgeons. *J Thorac Cardiovasc Surg* 1983; 86:168.
118. Starr A, Edwards LM, McCord CW, et al: Multiple valve replacement. *Circulation* 1964; 29:30.
119. Cartwright RS, Giacobine JW, Ratan RS, et al: Combined aortic and mitral valve replacement. *J Thorac Cardiovasc Surg* 1963; 45:35.
120. Knott-Craig CJ, Schaff HV, Mullany CJ, et al: Carcinoid disease of the heart: surgical management of ten patients. *J Thorac Cardiovasc Surg* 1992; 104:475.

121. Morrow AG, Brockenbrough EC: Surgical treatment of idiopathic hypertrophic subaortic stenosis: technic and hemodynamic results of subaortic ventriculomyotomy. *Ann Surg* 1961; 154:181.
122. Heimbecker RO, Baird RJ, Lajos RJ, et al: Homograft replacement of the human valve: a preliminary report. *Can Med Assoc J* 1962; 86:805.
123. Ross DN: Homograft replacement of the aortic valve. *Lancet* 1962; 2:487.
124. Ross DN: Replacement of aortic and mitral valves with a pulmonary autograft. *Lancet* 1967; 2:956.
125. Gerosa G, McKay R, Davies J, et al: Comparison of the aortic homograft and the pulmonary autograft for aortic valve or root replacement in children. *J Thorac Cardiovasc Surg* 1991; 102:51.
126. Binet JP, Carpentier A, Langlois J, et al: Implantation de valves heterogenes dans le traitment des cardiopathies aortiques. *C R Acad Sci Paris* 1965; 261:5733.
127. Binet JP, Planche C, Weiss M: Heterograft replacement of the aortic valve, in Ionescu MI, Ross DN, Wooler GH (eds): *Biological Tissue in Heart Valve Replacement*. London, Butterworth, 1971; p 409.
128. Carpentier A: Principles of tissue valve transplantation, in Ionescu MI, Ross DN, Wooler GH (eds): *Biological Tissue in Heart Valve Replacement*. London, Butterworth, 1971; p 49.
129. Kaiser GA, Hancock WD, Lukban SB, Litwak RS: Clinical use of a new design stented xenograft heart valve prosthesis. *Surg Forum* 1969; 20:137.
130. Spencer FC: Intellectual creativity in thoracic surgeons. *J Thorac Cardiovasc Surg* 1983; 86:168.
131. Wooler GH, Nixon PG, Grimshaw VA, et al: Experiences with the repair of the mitral valve in mitral incompetence. *Thorax* 1962; 17:49.
132. Reed GE, Tice DA, Clause RH: A symmetric, exaggerated mitral annuloplasty: repair of mitral insufficiency with hemodynamic predictability. *J Thorac Cardiovasc Surg* 1965; 49:752.
133. Kay JH, Zubiate T, Mendez MA, et al: Mitral valve repair for significant mitral insufficiency. *Am Heart J* 1978; 96:243.
134. Carpentier A: Cardiac valve surgery: the French correction. *J Thorac Cardiovasc Surg* 1983; 86:23.
135. Arbulu A, Thoms NW, Chiscano A, Wilson RF: Total tricuspid valvulectomy without replacement in the treatment of *Pseudomonas* endocarditis. *Surg Forum* 1971; 22:162.
136. Arbulu A, Holmes RJ, Asfaw I: Surgical treatment of intractable right-sided infective endocarditis in drug addicts: 25 years experience. *J Heart Valve Dis* 1993; 2:129.
137. Carrel A: On the experimental surgery of the thoracic aorta and the heart. *Ann Surg* 1910; 52:83.
138. Beck CS: The development of a new blood supply to the heart by operation, in Levy RL (ed): *Disease of the Coronary Arteries and Cardiac Pain*. New York, Macmillan, 1936; ch 17.
139. Beck CS: The development of a new blood supply to the heart by operation. *Ann Surg* 1935; 102:805.
140. Beck CS: Coronary sclerosis and angina pectoris: treatment by grafting a new blood supply upon the myocardium. *Surg Gynecol Obstet* 1937; 64:270.
141. Vineberg AM: Development of an anastomosis between the coronary vessels and a transplanted internal mammary artery. *Can Med Assoc J* 1946; 55:117.
142. Vineberg AM: Medical news section. *JAMA* 1975; 234:693.
143. Longmire WP Jr, Cannon JA, Kattus AA: Direct-vision coronary endarterectomy for angina pectoris. *N Engl J Med* 1958; 259:993.
144. Sones FM, Shirey EK: Cine coronary arteriography. *Mod Concepts Cardiovasc Dis* 1962; 31:735.
145. Konstantinov IE: Robert H. Goetz: the surgeon who performed the first successful clinical coronary artery bypass operation. *Ann Thorac Surg 2000;* 69:1966.
146. Garrett EH, Dennis EW, DeBakey ME: Aortocoronary bypass with saphenous vein grafts: seven-year follow-up. *JAMA* 1973; 223:792.
147. Shumaker HB Jr: *The Evolution of Cardiac Surgery*. Indianapolis, Indiana University Press, 1992; p 141.
148. Demikhov VP: *Experimental Transplantation of Vital Organs*. Authorized translation from the Russian by Basil Haigh. New York, Consultants Bureau, 1962.
149. Kolessov VI: Mammary artery–coronary artery anastomosis as a method of treatment for angina pectoris. *J Thorac Cardiovasc Surg* 1967; 54:535.
150. Green GE, Stertzer SH, Reppert EH: Coronary arterial bypass grafts. *Ann Thorac Surg* 1968; 5:443.
151. Bailey CP, Hirose T: Successful internal mammary–coronary arterial anastomosis using a minivascular suturing technic. *Int Surg* 1968; 49:416.
152. Favalaro RG: Saphenous vein autograft replacement of severe segmental coronary artery occlusion. *Ann Thorac Surg* 1968; 5:334.
153. Johnson WD, Flemma RJ, Lepley D Jr, Ellison EH: Extended treatment of severe coronary artery disease: a total surgical approach. *Ann Surg* 1969; 171:460.
154. Loop FD, Lytle BW, Cosgrove DM, et al: Influence of the internal-mammary-artery graft on 10-year survival and other cardiac events. *N Engl J Med* 1986; 314:1.
155. Cooley DA, Belmonte BA, Zeis LB, Schnur S: Surgical repair of ruptured interventricular septum following acute myocardial infarction. *Surgery* 1957; 41:930.
156. Cooley DA, Henly WS, Amad KH, Chapman DW: Ventricular aneurysm following myocardial infarction: results of surgical treatment. *Ann Surg* 1959; 150:595.
157. Beck CS: Operation for aneurysm of the heart. *Ann Surg* 1944; 120:34.
158. Bailey CP, Bolton HE, Nichols H, et al: Ventriculoplasty for cardiac aneurysm. *J Thorac Surg* 1958; 35:37.
159. Cobb FR, Blumenshein SD, Sealy WC, et al: Successful surgery interruption of the bundle of Kent in a patient with Wolff-Parkinson-White syndrome. *Circulation* 1968; 38: 1018.
160. Cox JL: Arrhythmia surgery, in Stephenson LW, Ruggiero R (eds): *Heart Surgery Classics*. Boston, Adams Publishing Group, 1994; p 258.
161. Guiraudon G, Fontaine G, Frank R, et al: Encircling endocardial ventriculotomy: a new surgical treatment for life-threatening ventricular tachycardias resistant to medical treatment following myocardial infarction. *Ann Thorac Surg* 1978; 26:438.
162. Josephson ME, Harken AH, Horowitz LN: Endocardial excision: a new surgical technique for the treatment of recurrent ventricular tachycardia. *Circulation* 1979; 60:1430.
163. Ross DL, Johnson DC, Denniss AR, et al: Curative surgery for atrioventricular junctional (AV node) reentrant tachycardia. *J Am Coll Cardiol* 1985; 6:1383.
164. Cox JL, Holman WL, Cain ME: Cryosurgical treatment of atrioventricular node reentrant tachycardia. *Circulation* 1987; 76:1329.
165. Cox JL: The surgical treatment of atrial fibrillation, IV: Surgical technique. *J Thorac Cardiovasc Surg* 1991; 101:584.
166. Mirowski M, Reid PR, Mower MM, et al: Termination of malignant ventricular arrhythmias with an implanted automatic defibrillator in human beings. *N Engl J Med* 1980; 303:322.
167. Bakken EE: Pacemakers and defibrillators, in Stephenson LW, Ruggiero R (eds): *Heart Surgery Classics*. Boston, Adams Publishing Group, 1994; p 298.
168. Zoll PM: Resuscitation of the heart in ventricular standstill by external electrical stimulation. *N Engl J Med* 1952; 247:768.

169. Lillehei CW, Gott VL, Hodges PC Jr, et al: Transistor pacemaker for treatment of complete atrioventricular dissociation. *JAMA* 1960; 172:2006.
170. Elmquist R, Senning A: Implantable pacemaker for the heart, in Smyth, CN (ed): *Medical Electronics: Proceedings of the Second International Conference on Medical Electronics, Paris, June,* 1959. London, Iliffe & Sons, 1960.
171. Chardack WM, Gage AA, Greatbatch W: Correction of complete heart block by a self-contained and subcutaneously implanted pacemaker: clinical experience with 15 patients. *J Thorac Cardiovasc Surg* 1961; 42:814.
172. Parsonnet V, Zucker IR, Gilbert L, et al: An intracardiac bipolar electrode for interim treatment of complete heart block. *Am J Cardiol* 1962; 10:261.
173. Ekestrom S, Johansson L, Lagergren H: Behandling av Adams-Stokes syndrom med en intracardiell pacemaker elektrod. *Opusc Med* 1962; 7:1.
174. Carrel A, Guthrie CC: The transplantation of vein and organs. *Am Med* 1905; 10:101.
175. Shumaker HB Jr: *The Evolution of Cardiac Surgery*. Indianapolis, Indiana University Press, 1992; p 317.
176. Demikhov VP: Experimental transplantation of an additional heart in the dog. *Bull Exp Biol Med* (Russia) 1950; 1:241.
177. Lower RR, Shumway NE: Studies on orthotopic homotransplantation of the canine heart. *Surg Forum* 1960; 11:18.
178. Brock R: Heart excision and replacement. *Guys Hosp Rep* 1959; 108:285.
179. Spencer F: Intellectual creativity in thoracic surgeons. *J Thorac Cardiovasc Surg* 1983; 86:172.
180. Hardy JD, Chavez CM, Hurrus FD, et al: Heart transplantation in man and report of a case. *JAMA* 1964; 188:1132.
181. Barnard CN: A human cardiac transplant: an interim report of a successful operation performed at Groote Schuur Hospital, Cape Town. *S Afr Med J* 1967; 41:1271.
182. Kantrowitz A: Heart, heart-lung and lung transplantation, in Stephenson LW, Ruggiero R (eds): *Heart Surgery Classics*. Boston, Adams Publishing Group, 1994; p 314.
183. Thomson G: Provisional report on the autopsy of LW. *S Afr Med J* 1967; 41:1277.
184. Ruggiero R: Commentary on Barnard CN: A human cardiac transplant: an interim report of a successful operation performed at Groote Schuur Hospital, Cape Town. *S Afr Med J* 1967; 41:1271; in Stephenson LW, Ruggiero R (eds): *Heart Surgery Classics*. Boston, Adams Publishing Group, 1994; p 327.
185. Reitz BA, Wallwork JL, Hunt SA, et al: Heart-lung transplantation: successful therapy for patients with pulmonary vascular disease. *N Engl J Med* 1982; 306:557.
186. Reitz BA, Burton NA, Jamieson SW, et al: Heart and lung transplantation: autotransplantation and allotransplantation in primates with extended survival. *J Thorac Cardiovasc Surg* 1980; 80:360.
187. Castaneda AR, Arnar O, Schmidt-Habelman P, et al: Cardiopulmonary transplantation in primates. *J Cardiovasc Surg* 1972; 37:523.
188. Harjula A, Baldwin J, Henry D, et al: Minimal lung pathology on long-term primate survivors of heart-lung transplantation. *Transplantation* 1987; 44:852.
189. Juvenelle AA, Citret C, Wiles CE Jr, Stewart JD: Pneumonectomy with replantation of the lung in dog for physiologic studies. *J Thorac Surg* 1951; 21:111.
190. Naef AP: *The Story of Thoracic Surgery: Milestones and Pioneers.* Toronto, Hogrefe & Huber, 1990; p 132.
191. Metras H: Note preliminaire sur la greffe du poumon chez le chien. *C R Acad Sci (Paris)* 1950; 231:1176.
192. Hardy JD, Webb WR, Dalton ML Jr, Walker GR Jr: Lung homotransplantation in man: report of the initial case. *JAMA* 1963; 286:1065.
193. Derom F, Barbier F, Ringoir S, et al: Ten-month survival after lung homotransplantation in man. *J Thorac Cardiovasc Surg* 1971; 61:835.
194. Cooper JD, Ginsberg RJ, Goldberg M, et al: Unilateral lung transplantation for pulmonary fibrosis. *N Engl J Med* 1986; 314:1140.
195. Harken DE: Presentation at the meeting of the International College of Cardiology, Brussels, 1958.
196. Clauss RH, Birtwell WC, Altertal G, et al: Assisted circulation, I: The arterial counterpulsator. *J Thorac Cardiovasc Surg* 1961; 41:447.
197. Moulopoulos SD, Topaz S, Kolff WJ: Diastolic balloon pumping in the aorta: mechanical assistance to the failing heart. *Am Heart J* 1962; 63:669.
198. Kantrowitz A, Tjonneland S, Freed PS, et al: Initial clinical experience with intraaortic balloon pumping in cardiogenic shock. *JAMA* 1968; 203:135.
199. Akutsu T, Kolff WJ: Permanent substitutes for valves and hearts. *Trans ASAIO* 1958; 4:230.
200. Liotta D, Hall W, Henly WS, et al: Prolonged assisted circulation during and after cardiac or aortic surgery: Prolonged partial left ventricular bypass by means of intracorporeal circulation. *Am J Cardiol* 1963; 12:399.
201. Shumaker HB Jr: *The Evolution of Cardiac Surgery,* Bloomington, Indiana University Press, 1992.
202. DeBakey ME: Left ventricular heart assist devices, in Stephenson LW, Ruggiero R (eds): *Heart Surgery Classics,* Boston, Adams Publishing Group, 1994.
203. Cooley DA, Liotta D, Hallman GL, et al: Orthotopic cardiac prosthesis for two-staged cardiac replacement. *Am J Cardiol* 1969; 24:723.
204. Hill JD, Farrar DJ, Hershon JJ, et al: Use of a prosthetic ventricle as a bridge to cardiac transplantation for postinfarction cardiogenic shock. *N Engl J Med* 1986; 314:626.
205. Starnes VA, Ayer PE, Portner PM, et al: Isolated left ventricular assist as bridge to cardiac transplantation. *J Thorac Cardiovasc Surg* 1988; 96:62.
206. DeVries WC, Anderson JL, Joyce LD, et al: Clinical use of total artificial heart. *N Engl J Med* 1984; 310:273.
207. Kantrowitz A, McKinnon W: The experimental use of the diaphragm as an auxiliary myocardium. *Surg Forum* 1959; 9:266.
208. Salmons S, Vrbova G: The influence of activity on some contractile characteristics of mammalian fast and slow muscles. *J Physiol* 1960; 150:417.
209. Macoviak JA, Stephenson LW, Armenti F, et al: Electrical conditioning of in situ skeletal muscle for replacement of myocardium. *J Surg Res* 1982; 32:429.
210. Mannion JD, Bitto T, Hammond RL, et al: Histochemical and fatigue-resistant characteristics of conditioned canine latissimus dorsi muscle. *Circ Res* 1986; 58:298.
211. Dewar ML, Drinkwater DC, Wittnich C, Chiu RC-J: Synchronously stimulated skeletal muscle graft for myocardial repair: an experimental study. *J Thorac Cardiovasc Surg* 1984; 87:325.
212. Carpentier A, Chachques JC: Myocardial substitution with a stimulated skeletal muscle: first successful clinical case. *Lancet* 1985; 1:1267.
213. Chachques JC, Radermecker M, Granjean P, et al: Dynamic aortomyoplasty for long-term circulatory support: experimental studies and clinical experience, in Carpentier A, Chachques JC, Grandjean PA (eds): *Cardiac Bioassist,* New York, Futura, 1997; p 481.

214. Thomas GA, Baciewicz FA, Hammond RL, et al: Power output of pericardium-lined skeletal muscle ventricles, left ventricular apex to aorta configuration: up to eight months in circulation. *J Thorac Cardiovasc Surg* 1998; 116:1029.
215. Thomas GA, Hammond RL, Greer K, et al: Functional assessment of skeletal muscle ventricles after pumping for up to four years in circulation. *Ann Thorac Surg* 2000; 70;1281.
216. Edwards WS, Edwards PD: *Alexis Carrel: Visionary Surgeon.* Springfield, IL, Charles C Thomas, 1974; p 26.
217. Acierno LJ: *The History of Cardiology.* New York, Parthenon, 1994; p 603.
218. DeBakey ME, Simeone FA: Battle injuries of the arteries in World War II. *Am J Surg* 1946; 123:534.
219. Shumaker HB: Surgical cure of innominate aneurysm: report of a case with comments on the applicability of surgical measures. *Surgery* 1947; 22:739.
220. Swan HC, Maaske M, Johnson M, Grover R: Arterial homografts, II: resection of thoracic aneurysm using a stored human arterial transplant. *Arch Surg* 1950; 61:732.
221. Gross RE: Treatment of certain aortic coarctations by homologous grafts: a report of nineteen cases. *Ann Surg* 1951; 134:753.
222. DuBost C, Allary M, Oeconomos N: Resection of an aneurysm of the abdominal aorta: reestablishment of the continuity by a preserved human arterial graft, with results after five months. *Arch Surg* 1952; 62:405.
223. Bahnson HT: Definitive treatment of saccular aneurysms of the aorta with excision of sac and aortic suture. *Surg Gynecol Obstet* 1953; 96:383.
224. DeBakey ME, Cooley DA: Successful resection of aneurysm of thoracic aorta and replacement by graft. *JAMA* 1953; 152:673.
225. Hughes CW: Acute vascular trauma in Korean War casualties. *Surg Gynecol Obstet* 1954; 99:91.
226. Voorhees AB Jr, Janetzky A III, Blakemore AH: The use of tubes constructed from Vinyon N cloth in bridging defects. *Ann Surg* 1952; 135:332.
227. Edwards WS, Tapp JS: Chemically treated nylon tubes as arterial grafts. *Surgery* 1995; 38:61.
228. Spencer FC: Intellectual creativity in thoracic surgeons. *J Thorac Cardiovasc Surg* 1983; 86:164.
229. DeBakey ME, Cooley DA, Creech O Jr: Surgical consideration of dissecting aneurysm of the aorta. *Ann Surg* 1955; 142:586.
230. Wheat MW Jr, Palmer RF, Bartley TD, Seelman RC: Treatment of dissecting aneurysms of the aorta without surgery. *J Thorac Cardiovasc Surg* 1965; 50:364.
231. Cooley DA, DeBakey ME: Resection of entire ascending aorta in fusiform aneurysm using cardiac bypass. *JAMA* 1956; 162:1158.
232. DeBakey ME, Creech O Jr, Morris GC Jr: Aneurysm of the thoracoabdominal aorta involving the celiac superior mesenteric, and renal arteries: report of four cases treated by resection and homograft replacement. *Ann Surg* 1956; 144:549.
233. DeBakey ME, Crawford ES, Cooley DA, Morris GC Jr: Successful resection of fusiform aneurysm of aortic arch with replacement by homograft. *Surg Gynecol Obstet* 1957; 105:657.
234. Cooley DA, Mahaffey DE, DeBakey ME. Total excision of the aortic arch for aneurysm. *Surg Gyn Obstet* 1955; 101;667.
235. Bentall H, De Bono A: A technique for complete replacement of the ascending aorta. *Thorax* 1968; 23:338.
236. Starr A, Edwards WL, McCord MD, et al: Aortic replacement. *Circulation* 1963; 27:779.
237. Wheat MW Jr, Wilson JR, Bartley TD: Successful replacement of the entire ascending aorta and aortic valve. *JAMA* 1964; 188:717.
238. Lillehei CW, Cohen M, Warden HE, et al: The results of direct vision closure of ventricular septal defects in eight patients by means of controlled cross circulation. *Surg Gynecol Obstet* 1955; 101:446.
239. Burroughs JT, Kirklin JW: Complete correction of total anomalous pulmonary venous correction: report of three cases. *Mayo Clin Proc* 1956; 31:182.
240. McGoon DC, Edwards JE, Kirklin JW: Surgical treatment of ruptured aneurysm of aortic sinus. *Ann Surg* 1958; 147:387.
241. Ellis FH Jr, Kirklin JW: Congenital valvular aortic stenosis: anatomic findings and surgical techniques. *J Thorac Cardiovasc Surg* 1962; 43:199.
242. Cooley DA, McNamara DG, Jatson JR: Aortico-pulmonary septal defect: diagnosis and surgical treatment. *Surgery* 1957; 42:101.
243. Kirklin JW, Harp RA, McGoon DC: Surgical treatment of origin of both vessels from right ventricle including cases of pulmonary stenosis. *J Thorac Cardiovasc Surg* 1964; 48:1026.
244. Anderson RC, Lillihei CW, Jester RG: Corrected transposition of the great vessels of the heart. *Pediatrics* 1957; 20:626.
245. Senning A: Surgical correction of transposition of the great vessels. *Surgery* 1959; 45:966.
246. Swan H, Wilson JH, Woodwork G, Blount SE: Surgical obliteration of a coronary artery fistula to the right ventricle. *Arch Surg* 1959; 79:820.
247. Hardy KL, May IA, Webster CA, Kimball KG: Ebstein's anomaly: a functional concept and successful definitive repair. *J Thorac Cardiovasc Surg* 1964; 48:927.
248. Ross DN, Somerville J: Correction of pulmonary atresia with a homograft aortic valve. *Lancet* 1966; 2:1446.
249. McGoon DC, Rastelli GC, Ongley PA: An operation for the correction of truncus arteriosus. *JAMA* 1968; 205:59.
250. Fontan F, Baudet E: Surgical repair of tricuspid atresia. *Thorax* 1971; 26:240.
251. Horiuchi T, Abe T, Okada Y, et al: Feasibility of total correction for single ventricle: a report of total correction in a six-year-old girl. *Jpn J Thorac Surg* 1970; 23:434. (In Japanese.)
252. Konno S, Iami Y, Iida Y, et al: A new method for prosthetic valve replacement in congenital aortic stenosis associated with hypoplasia of the aortic valve ring. *J Thorac Cardiovasc Surg* 1975; 70:909.
253. Jatene AD, Fontes VF, Paulista PP, et al: Anatomic correction of transposition of the great vessel. *J Thorac Cardiovasc Surg* 1976; 72:364.
254. Norwood WI, Lang P, Hansen DD: Physiologic repair of aortic atresia-hypoplastic left heart syndrome. *N Engl J Med* 1983; 308:23.
255. Bailey LL, Gundry SR, Razzouk AJ, et al: Bless the babies: one hundred fifteen late survivors of heart transplantation during the first year of life. *J Thorac Cardiovasc Surg* 1993; 105:805.

Chapter 2

Surgical Anatomy of the Heart

Michael R. Mill/Benson R. Wilcox/Robert H. Anderson

A thorough knowledge of the anatomy of the heart is a prerequisite for the successful completion of the myriad procedures performed by the cardiothoracic surgeon. In this chapter, we describe the normal anatomy of the heart, including its position and relationship to other thoracic organs. We describe the incisions used to expose the heart for various operations, and discuss in detail the cardiac chambers and valves, coronary arteries and veins, and the important but surgically invisible conduction tissues.

OVERVIEW

Location of the Heart Relative to Surrounding Structures

The overall shape of the heart is that of a three-sided pyramid located in the middle mediastinum (Fig. 2-1). When viewed from its apex, the three sides of the ventricular mass are readily seen (Fig. 2-2). Two of the edges are named. The acute margin lies inferiorly and describes a sharp angle between the sternocostal and diaphragmatic surfaces. The obtuse margin lies superiorly, and is much more diffuse. The posterior margin is unnamed, but is also diffuse in its transition.

One third of the cardiac mass lies to the right of the midline, and two thirds to the left. The long axis of the heart is oriented from the left epigastrium to the right shoulder. The short axis, which corresponds to the plane of the atrioventricular groove, is oblique and is oriented closer to the vertical than to the horizontal plane (Fig. 2-1).

Anteriorly, the heart is covered by the sternum and the costal cartilages of the third, fourth, and fifth ribs. The lungs

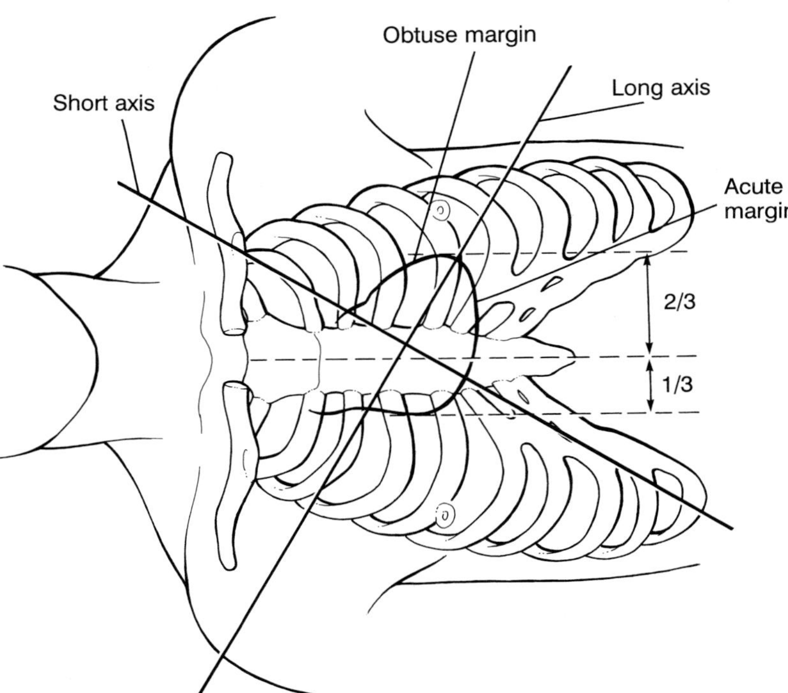

FIGURE 2–1 This diagram shows the heart within the middle mediastinum with the patient supine on the operating table. The long axis lies parallel to the interventricular septum, whereas the short axis is perpendicular to the long axis at the level of the atrioventricular valves.

contact the lateral surfaces of the heart, whereas the heart abuts onto the pulmonary hila posteriorly. The right lung overlies the right surface of the heart and reaches to the midline. In contrast, the left lung retracts from the midline in the area of the cardiac notch. The heart has an extensive diaphragmatic surface inferiorly. Posteriorly, the heart lies on the esophagus and the tracheal bifurcation, and bronchi that extend into the lung. The sternum lies anteriorly and provides rigid protection to the heart during blunt trauma and is aided by the cushioning effects of the lungs.

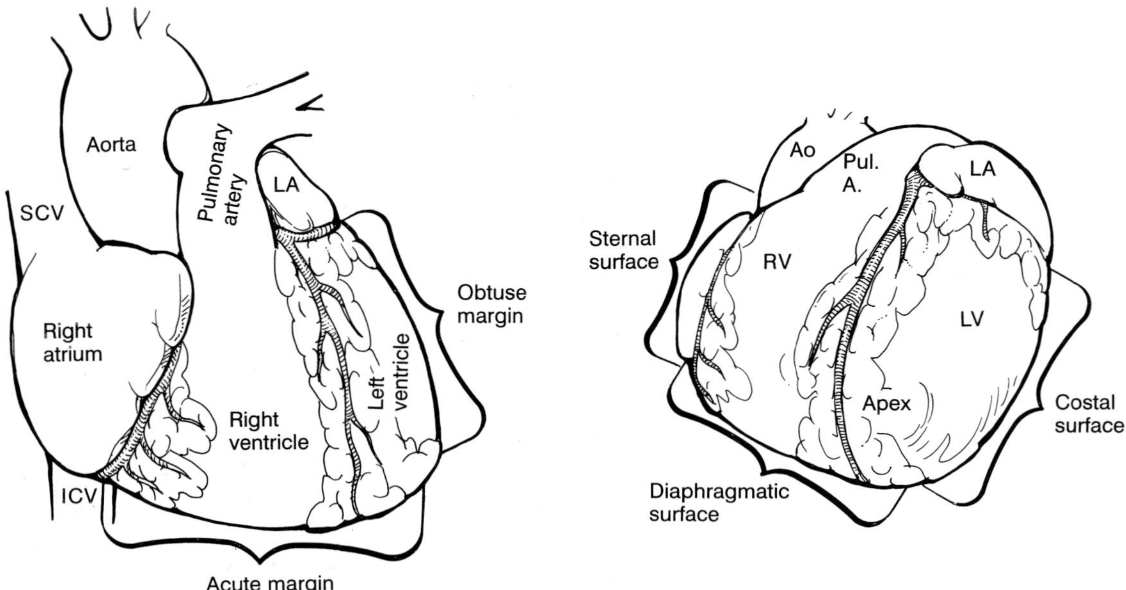

FIGURE 2–2 This diagram shows the surfaces and margins of the heart as viewed anteriorly with the patient supine on the operating table (left), and as viewed from the cardiac apex (right).

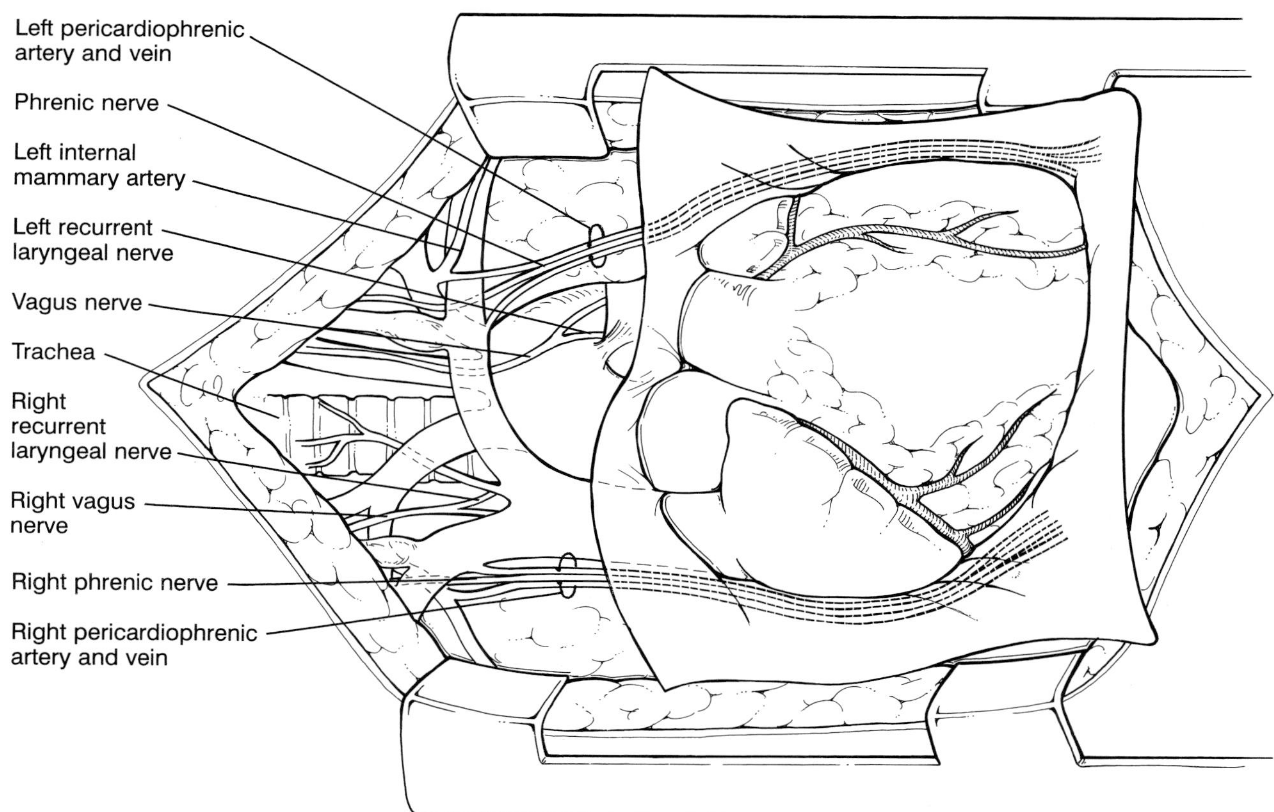

FIGURE 2–3 **Diagram of the heart in relation to the vagus and phrenic nerves as viewed through a median sternotomy.**

The Pericardium and Its Reflections

The heart lies within the pericardium, which is attached to the walls of the great vessels and to the diaphragm. The pericardium can be visualized best as a bag into which the heart has been placed apex first. The inner layer, in direct contact with the heart, is the visceral epicardium, which encases the heart and extends several centimeters back onto the walls of the great vessels. The outer layer forms the parietal pericardium, which lines the inner surface of the tough fibrous pericardial sack. A thin film of lubricating fluid lies within the pericardial cavity between the two serous layers. Two identifiable recesses lie within the pericardium and are lined by the serous layer. The first is the transverse sinus, which is delineated anteriorly by the posterior surface of the aorta and pulmonary trunk and posteriorly by the anterior surface of the interatrial groove. The second is the oblique sinus, a cul-de-sac located behind the left atrium, delineated by serous pericardial reflections from the pulmonary veins and the inferior caval vein.

Mediastinal Nerves and Their Relationships to the Heart

The vagus and phrenic nerves descend through the mediastinum in close relationship to the heart (Fig. 2-3). They enter through the thoracic inlet, with the phrenic nerve located anteriorly on the surface of the anterior scalene muscle and lying just posterior to the internal thoracic artery (internal mammary artery) at the thoracic inlet. In this position, it is vulnerable to injury during dissection and preparation of the internal thoracic artery for use in coronary arterial bypass grafting. On the right side, the phrenic nerve courses on the lateral surface of the superior caval vein, again in harm's way during dissection for venous cannulation for cardiopulmonary bypass. The nerve then descends anterior to the pulmonary hilum before reflecting onto the right diaphragm, where it branches to provide its innervation. In the presence of a left-sided superior caval vein, the left phrenic nerve is directly applied to its lateral surface. The nerve passes anterior to the pulmonary hilum and eventually branches on the surface of the diaphragm. The vagus nerves enter the thorax posterior to the phrenic nerves and course along the carotid arteries. On the right side, the vagus gives off the recurrent laryngeal nerve that passes around the right subclavian artery before ascending out of the thoracic cavity. The right vagus nerve continues posterior to the pulmonary hilum, gives off branches of the right pulmonary plexus, and exits the thorax along the esophagus. On the left, the vagus nerve crosses the aortic arch, where it gives off the recurrent laryngeal branch. The recurrent nerve passes around the arterial ligament before ascending in the tracheoesophageal groove. The vagus nerve continues posterior to the pulmonary hilum, gives rise to the left pulmonary plexus, and then continues inferiorly out of the thorax along the esophagus. A delicate nerve trunk known as the subclavian loop carries fibers from the stellate ganglion to the eye and head. This branch is located adjacent to the subclavian arteries bilaterally. Excessive dissection of the subclavian artery during shunt procedures may injure these nerve roots and cause Horner's syndrome.

SURGICAL INCISIONS

Median Sternotomy

The most common approach for operations on the heart and aortic arch is the median sternotomy. The skin incision is made from the jugular notch to just below the xiphoid process. The subcutaneous tissues and presternal fascia are incised to expose the periostium of the sternum. The sternum is divided longitudinally in the midline. After placement of a sternal spreader, the thymic fat pad is divided up to the level of the brachiocephalic vein. An avascular midline plane is identified easily, but is crossed by a few thymic veins that are divided between fine silk ties or hemoclips. Either the left or right, or occasionally both, lobes of the thymus gland often are removed in infants and young children to improve exposure and to minimize compression on extracardiac conduits. If a portion of the thymus gland is removed, excessive traction may result in injury to the phrenic nerve. The pericardium is opened anteriorly to expose the heart. Through this incision, operations within any chamber of the heart or on the surface of the heart, and operations involving the proximal aorta, pulmonary trunk, and their primary branches can be performed. Extension of the superior extent of the incision into the neck along the anterior border of the right sternocleidomastoid muscle provides further exposure of the aortic arch and its branches for procedures involving these structures. Exposure of the proximal descending thoracic aorta is facilitated by a perpendicular extension of the incision through the third intercostal space.

Bilateral Transverse Thoracosternotomy (Clam Shell Incision)

The bilateral transverse thoracosternotomy (clam shell incision) is an alternative incision for exposure of the pleural spaces and heart. This incision may be made through either the fourth or fifth intercostal space, depending on the intended procedure. After identifying the appropriate interspace, a bilateral submammary incision is made. The incision is extended down through the pectoralis major muscles to enter the hemithoraces through the appropriate intercostal space. The right and left internal thoracic arteries are dissected and ligated proximally and distally prior to transverse division of the sternum. Electrocautery dissection of the pleural reflections behind the sternum allows full exposure to both hemithoraces and the entire mediastinum. Bilateral chest spreaders are placed to maintain exposure. Morse or Haight retractors are particularly suitable with this incision. The pericardium may be opened anteriorly to allow access to the heart for intracardiac procedures. When required, standard cannulation for cardiopulmonary bypass is achieved easily. This incision is popular for bilateral sequential double lung transplants and heart-lung transplants because of enhanced exposure of the apical pleural spaces. When made in the fourth intercostal space, the incision is useful for access to the ascending, arch, and descending thoracic aorta.

Anterolateral Thoracotomy

The right side of the heart can be exposed through a right anterolateral thoracotomy. The patient is positioned supine, with the right chest elevated to approximately 30 degrees by a roll beneath the shoulder. An anterolateral thoracotomy incision can be made that can be extended across the midline by transversely dividing the sternum if necessary. With the lung retracted posteriorly, the pericardium can be opened just anterior to the right phrenic nerve and pulmonary hilum to expose the right and left atria. The incision provides access to both the tricuspid and mitral valves and the right coronary artery. Cannulation may be performed in the ascending aorta and the superior and inferior caval veins. Aortic cross-clamping, administration of cardioplegia, and removal of air from the the heart after cardiotomy are difficult through this approach. This incision is particularly useful, nonetheless, for performance of the Blalock-Hanlon atrial septectomy or for valvar replacement after a previous procedure through a median sternotomy. A left anterolateral thoracotomy performed in a similar fashion to that on the right side may be used for isolated bypass grafting of the circumflex coronary artery, or for left-sided exposure of the mitral valve.

Posterolateral Thoracotomy

A left posterolateral thoracotomy is used for procedures involving the distal aortic arch and descending thoracic aorta. With left thoracotomy, cannulation for cardiopulmonary bypass must be done through the femoral vessels. A number of variations of these incisions have been utilized for minimally invasive cardiac surgical procedures. These include partial sternotomies, parasternal incisions, and limited thoracotomies.

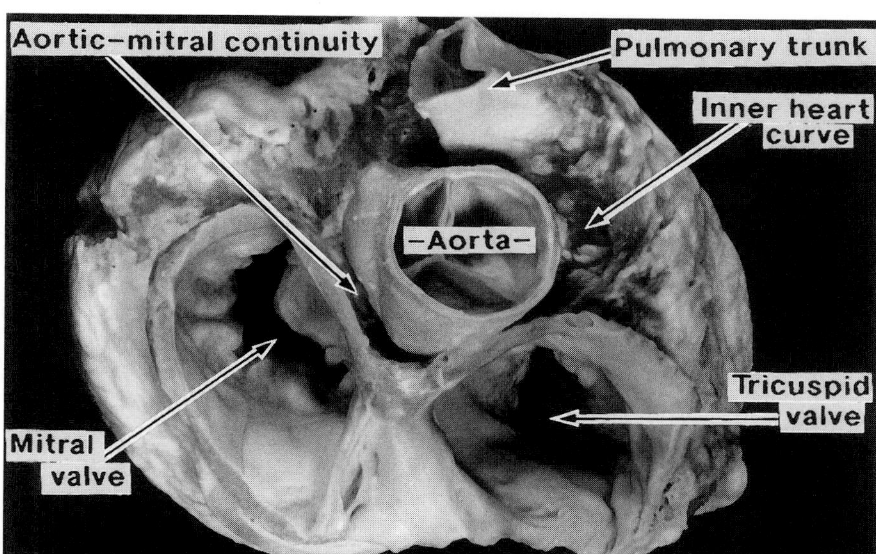

FIGURE 2–4 This dissection of the cardiac short axis, seen from its atrial aspect, reveals the relationships of the cardiac valves.

RELATIONSHIP OF THE CARDIAC CHAMBERS AND GREAT ARTERIES

The surgical anatomy of the heart is best understood when the position of the cardiac chambers and great vessels is known in relation to the cardiac silhouette. The atrioventricular junction is oriented obliquely, lying much closer to the vertical than to the horizontal plane. This plane can be viewed from its atrial aspect (Fig. 2-4) if the atrial mass and great arteries are removed by a parallel cut just above the junction. The tricuspid and pulmonary valves are widely separated by the inner curvature of the heart lined by the transverse sinus. Conversely, the mitral and aortic valves lie adjacent to one another, with fibrous continuity of their leaflets. The aortic valve occupies a central position, wedged between the tricuspid and pulmonary valves. Indeed, there is fibrous continuity between the leaflets of the aortic and tricuspid valves through the central fibrous body.

With careful study of this short axis, several basic rules of cardiac anatomy become apparent. First, the atrial chambers lie to the right of their corresponding ventricles. Second, the right atrium and ventricle lie anterior to their left-sided counterparts. The septal structures between them are obliquely oriented. Third, by virtue of its wedged position, the aortic valve is directly related to all of the cardiac chambers. Several other significant features of cardiac anatomy can be learned from the short axis section. The position of the aortic valve minimizes the area of septum where the mitral and tricuspid valves attach opposite each other. Because the tricuspid valve is attached to the septum further toward the ventricular apex than the mitral valve, a part of the septum is interposed between the right atrium and the left ventricle to produce the muscular atrioventricular septum. The central fibrous body, where the leaflets of the aortic, mitral, and tricuspid valves all converge, lies cephalad and anterior to the muscular atrioventricular septum. The central fibrous body is the main component of the fibrous skeleton of the heart and is made up, in part, by the right fibrous trigone, a thickening of the right side of the area of fibrous continuity between the aortic and mitral valves, and in part by the membranous septum, the fibrous partition between the left ventricular outflow tract and the right heart chambers (Fig. 2-5). The membranous septum itself is divided into two parts by the septal leaflet of the tricuspid valve, which is directly attached across it (Fig. 2-6). Thus, the membranous septum has an atrioventricular component between the right atrium and left ventricle, as well as an interventricular component. Removal of the noncoronary leaflet of the aortic valve demonstrates the significance of the wedged position of the left ventricular outflow tract in relation to the other cardiac chambers. The subaortic region separates the mitral orifice from the ventricular septum; this separation influences the position of the atrioventricular conduction tissues and the position of the leaflets and tension apparatus of the mitral valve (Fig. 2-7).

THE RIGHT ATRIUM AND TRICUSPID VALVE

Appendage, Vestibule, and Venous Component

The right atrium has three basic parts: the appendage, the vestibule, and the venous component (Fig. 2-8). Externally, the right atrium is divided into the appendage and the venous component, which receives the systemic venous return. The junction of the appendage and the venous component is identified by a prominent groove, the terminal groove. This corresponds internally to the location of the terminal crest.

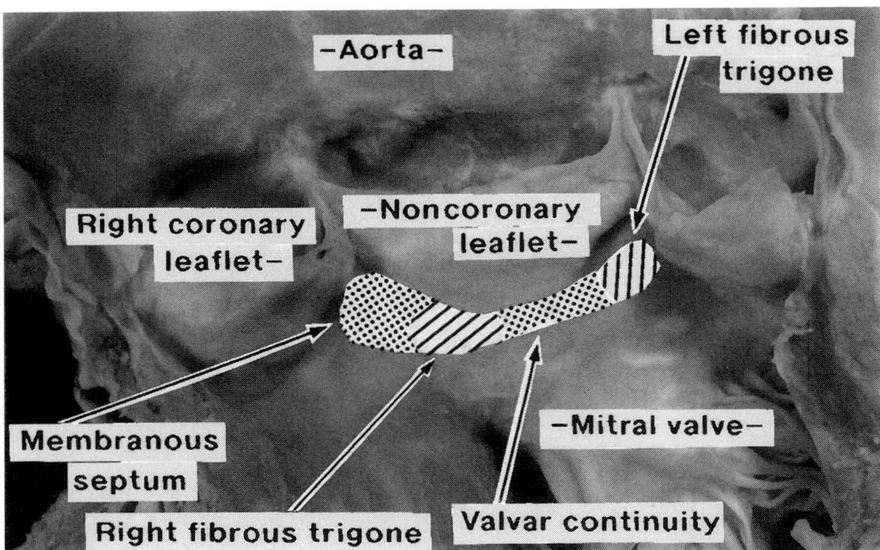

FIGURE 2–5 This view of the left ventricular outflow tract, seen from the front in anatomic orientation, shows the limited extent of the fibrous skeleton of the heart.

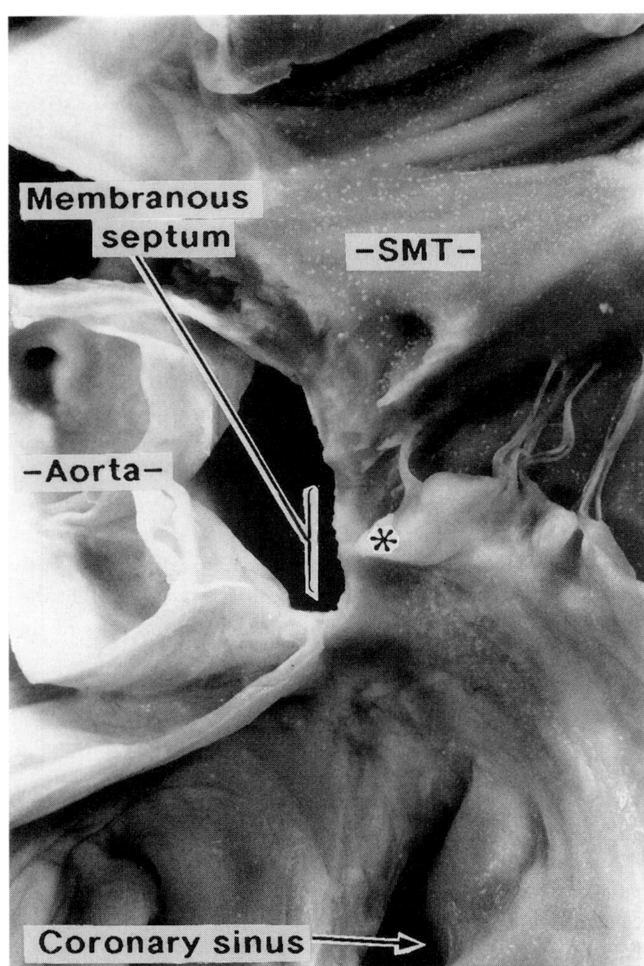

FIGURE 2–6 This dissection, made by removing the right coronary sinus of the aortic valve, shows how the septal leaflet of the tricuspid valve (asterisk) divides the membranous septum into its atrioventricular and interventricular components. SMT = septomarginal trabeculation.

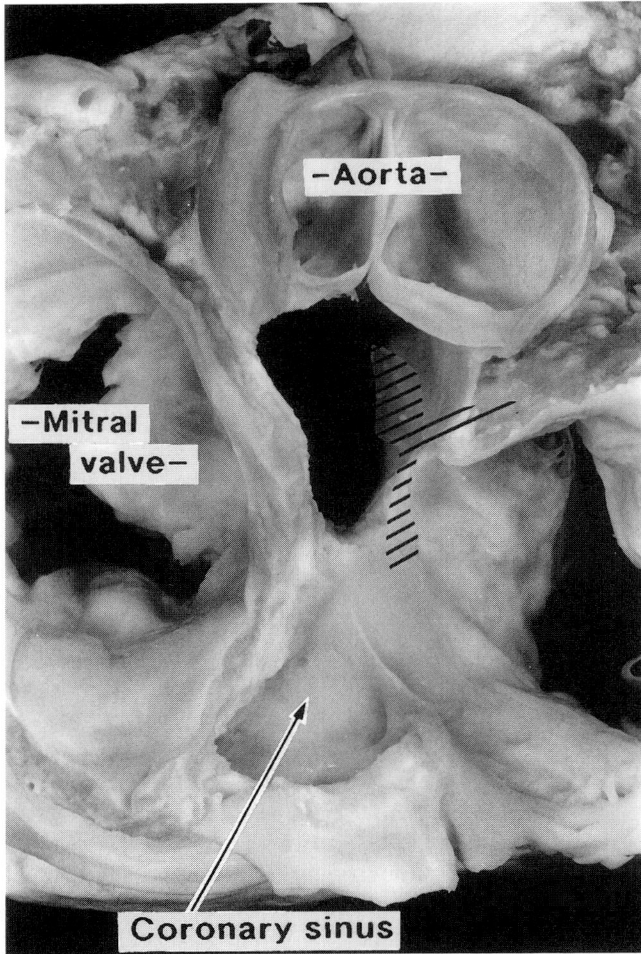

FIGURE 2–7 This dissection, made by removing the noncoronary aortic sinus (compare with Figs. 2-4 and 2-6) shows the approximate location of the atrioventricular conduction axis (hatched area) and the relationship of the mitral valve to the ventricular septum.

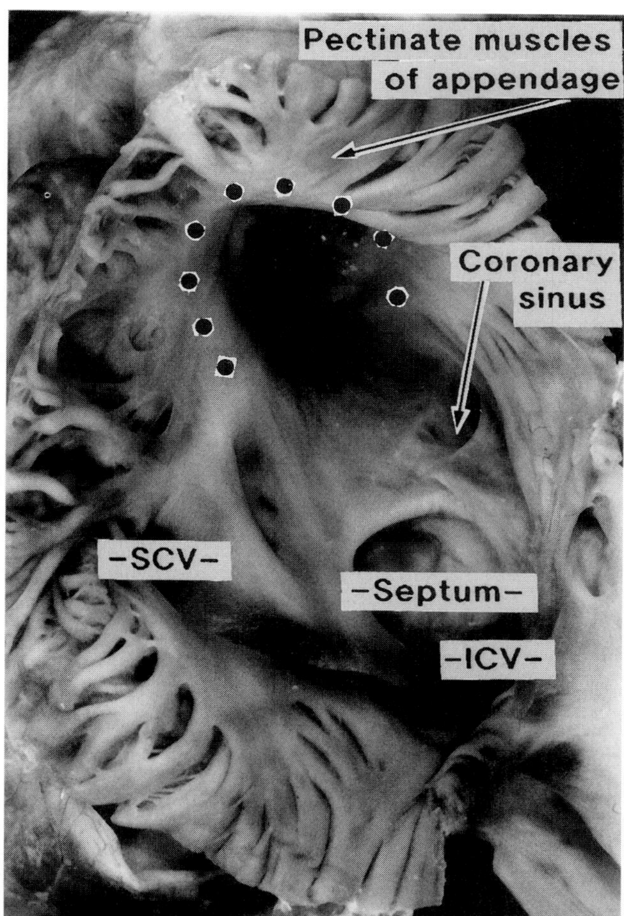

FIGURE 2–8 This view of the right atrium, seen in surgical orientation, shows the pectinate muscles lining the appendage, the smooth vestibule (circles) surrounding the orifice of the tricuspid valve, and the superior caval vein (SCV), inferior caval vein (ICV), and coronary sinus joining the smooth-walled venous component. Note the prominent rim enclosing the oval fossa, which is the true atrial septum (see Fig. 2-11).

The right atrial appendage has the shape of a blunt triangle, with a wide junction to the venous component across the terminal groove. The appendage also has an extensive junction with the vestibule of the right atrium; the latter structure is the smooth-walled atrial myocardium that inserts into the leaflets of the tricuspid valve. The most characteristic and constant feature of the morphology of the right atrium is that the pectinate muscles within the appendage extend around the entire parietal margin of the atrioventricular junction (Fig. 2-9). These muscles originate as parallel fibers that course at right angles from the terminal crest. The venous component of the right atrium extends between the terminal groove and the interatrial groove. It receives the superior and inferior caval veins and the coronary sinus.

Sinus Node

The sinus node lies at the anterior and superior extent of the terminal groove, where the atrial appendage and the superior caval vein are juxtaposed. The node is a spindle-shaped structure that usually lies to the right or lateral to the superior cavoatrial junction (Fig. 2-10). In approximately 10% of cases, the node is draped across the cavoatrial junction in horseshoe fashion.[1]

The blood supply to the sinus node is from a prominent nodal artery that is a branch of the right coronary artery in approximately 55% of individuals, and a branch of the circumflex artery in the remainder. Regardless of its artery of origin, the nodal artery usually courses along the anterior interatrial groove toward the superior cavoatrial junction, frequently within the atrial myocardium. At the cavoatrial junction, its course becomes variable and may circle either anteriorly or posteriorly, or rarely both anteriorly and posteriorly, around the cavoatrial junction to enter the node. Uncommonly, the artery arises more distally from the right coronary artery and courses laterally across the atrial

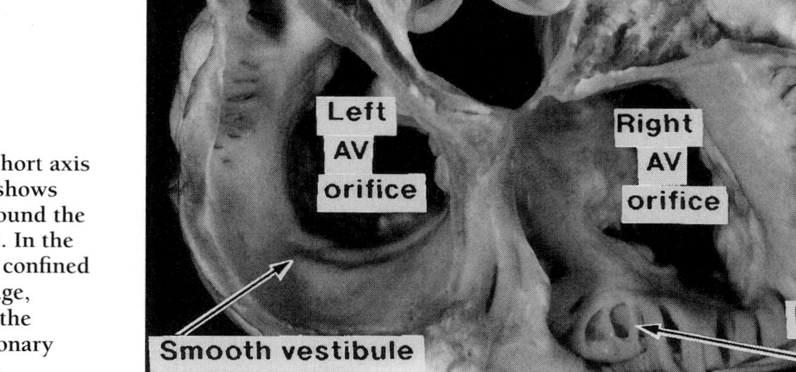

FIGURE 2–9 This dissection of the short axis of the heart (compare with Fig. 2-4) shows how the pectinate muscles extend around the parietal margin of the tricuspid valve. In the left atrium, the pectinate muscles are confined within the tubular left atrial appendage, leaving the smooth vestibule around the mitral valve confluent with the pulmonary venous component of the left atrium.

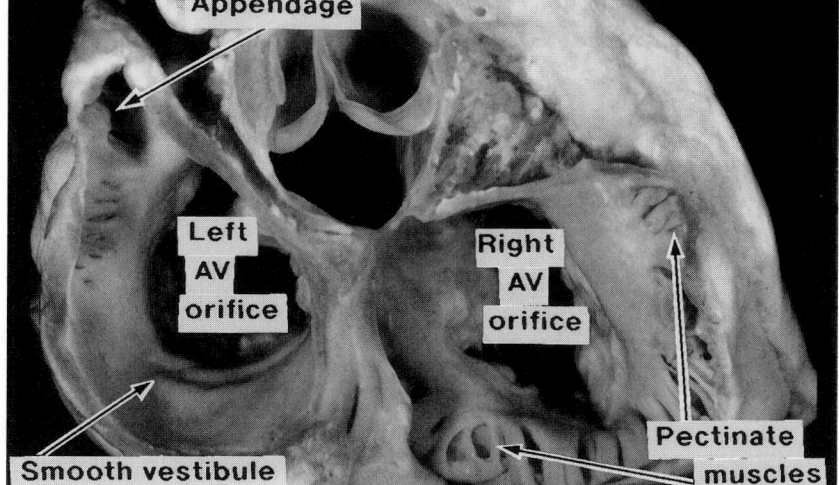

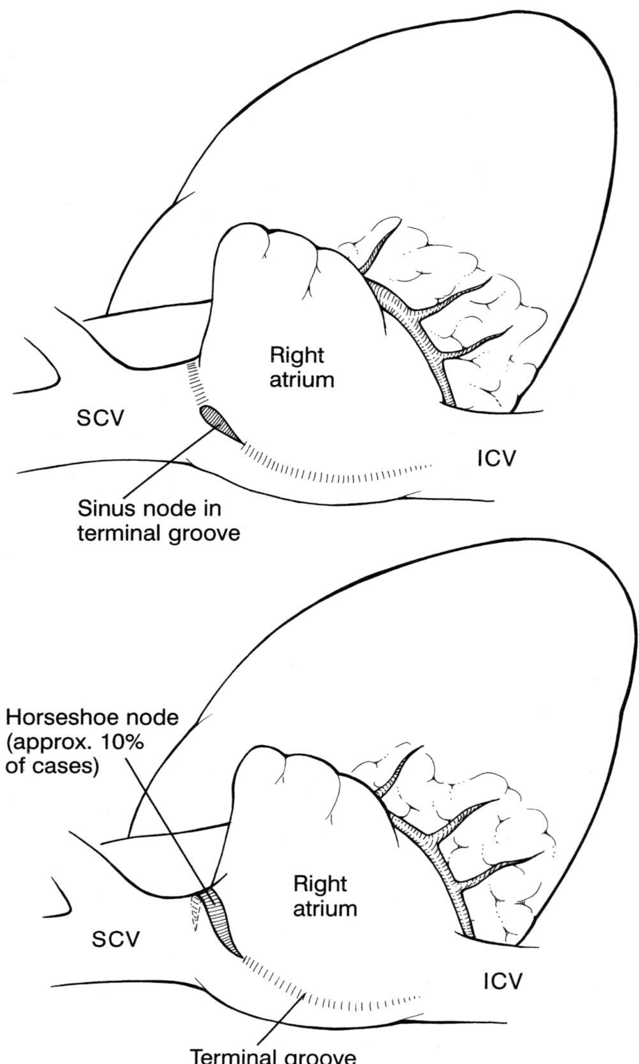

FIGURE 2–10 This diagram shows the location of the sinus node at the superior cavoatrial junction. The node usually lies to the right (lateral) side of the junction, but may be draped in horseshoe fashion across the anterior aspect of the junction. SCV, ICV = superior and inferior caval veins.

appendage. This places it at risk of injury during a standard right atriotomy. The artery also may arise distally from the circumflex artery to cross the dome of the left atrium, where it is at risk of injury when utilizing a superior approach to the mitral valve. Incisions in either the right or left atrial chambers always should be made with this anatomical variability in mind. In our experience, these vessels can be identified by careful gross inspection, and prompt modification of surgical incisions made accordingly.

Atrial Septum

The most common incision into the right atrium is made into the atrial appendage parallel and anterior to the terminal groove. Opening the atrium through this incision confirms that the terminal groove is the external marking of the prominent terminal crest. Anteriorly and superiorly, the crest curves in front of the orifice of the superior caval vein to become continuous with the so-called septum secundum, which, in reality, is the superior rim of the oval fossa. When the right atrium is inspected through this incision, there appears to be an extensive septal surface between the tricuspid valve and the orifices of the caval veins. This septal surface includes the opening of the oval fossa and the orifice of the coronary sinus. The apparent extent of the septum is spurious, as the true septum between the atrial chambers is virtually confined to the oval fossa (Fig. 2-11).[2,3] The superior rim of the fossa, although often referred to as the septum secundum, is an extensive infolding between the venous component of the right atrium and the right pulmonary veins. The inferior rim is directly continuous with the so-called sinus septum that separates the orifices of the inferior caval vein and the coronary sinus (Fig. 2-12).

The region around the coronary sinus is where the right atrial wall overlies the atrioventricular muscular septum. Removing the floor of the coronary sinus reveals the anterior extension of the atrioventricular groove in this region. Only a small part of the anterior rim of the oval fossa is a septal structure. The majority is made up of the anterior atrial wall overlying the aortic root. Thus, dissection outside the limited margins of the oval fossa will penetrate the heart to the outside, rather than provide access to the left atrium via the septum.

Atrioventricular Septum and Node: Triangle of Koch

In addition to the sinus node, another major area of surgical significance is occupied by the atrioventricular node. This structure lies within the triangle of Koch, which is demarcated by the tendon of Todaro, the septal leaflet of the tricuspid valve, and the orifice of the coronary sinus (Fig. 2-13). The tendon of Todaro is a fibrous structure formed by the junction of the eustachian valve and the thebesian valve (the valves of the inferior caval vein and coronary sinus, respectively). The entire atrial component of the atrioventricular conduction tissues is contained within the triangle of Koch, which must be avoided to prevent surgical damage to atrioventricular conduction. The atrioventricular bundle (of His) penetrates directly at the apex of the triangle of Koch before it continues to branch on the crest of the ventricular septum (Fig. 2-14). The key to avoiding atrial arrhythmias is careful preservation of the sinus and atrioventricular nodes and their blood supply. No advantage is gained in attempting to preserve nonexistent tracts of specialized atrial conduction tissue, although it makes sense to avoid prominent muscle bundles where parallel orientation of atrial myocardial fibers favors preferential conduction (Fig. 2-15).

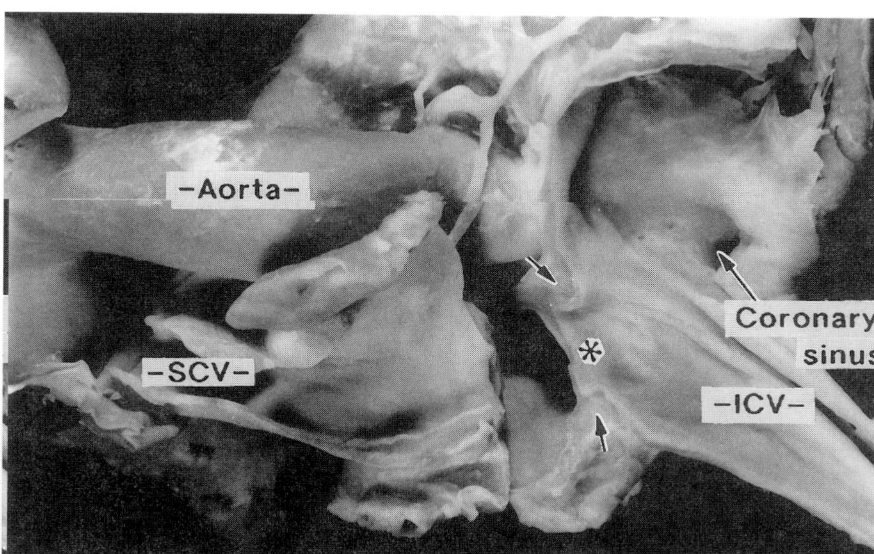

FIGURE 2–11 This transection across the middle of the oval fossa (asterisk) shows how the so-called septum secundum, the rim of the fossa, is made up of the infolded atrial walls (arrows). SCV, ICV = superior and inferior caval veins.

Tricuspid Valve

The vestibule of the right atrium converges into the tricuspid valve. The three leaflets reflect their anatomic location, being septal, anterosuperior, and inferior (or mural). The leaflets join together over three prominent zones of apposition; the peripheral ends of these zones usually are described as commissures. The leaflets are tethered at the commissures by fan-shaped cords arising from prominent papillary muscles. The anteroseptal commissure is supported by the medial papillary muscle. The major leaflets of the valve extend from this position in anterosuperior and septal directions. The third leaflet is less well defined. The anteroinferior commissure is usually supported by the prominent anterior papillary muscle. Often, however, it is not possible to identify a specific inferior papillary muscle supporting the inferoseptal commissure. Thus, the inferior leaflet may seem duplicated. There is no well-formed collagenous annulus for the tricuspid valve. Instead, the atrioventricular groove more or less folds directly into the tricuspid valvar leaflets at the vestibule, and the atrial and ventricular myocardial masses are separated almost exclusively by the fibro-fatty tissue of the groove. The entire parietal attachment of the tricuspid valve usually is encircled by the right coronary artery running within the atrioventricular groove.

THE LEFT ATRIUM AND MITRAL VALVE

Appendage, Vestibule, and Venous Component

Like the right atrium, the left atrium has three basic components: the appendage, vestibule, and venous component (Fig. 2-16). Unlike the right atrium, the venous component is considerably larger than the appendage and has a narrow junction with it that is not marked by a terminal groove or crest. There also is an important difference between the relationship of the appendage and vestibule between the left and right atria. As shown, the pectinate muscles within the right atrial appendage extend all around the parietal margin of the

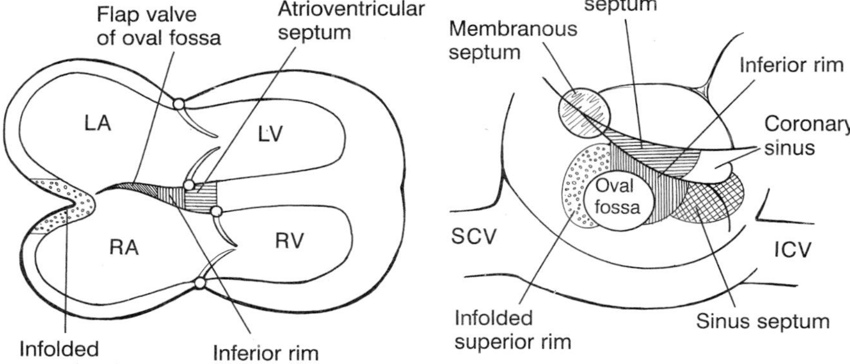

FIGURE 2–12 This diagram demonstrates the components of the atrial septum. The only true septum between the two atria is confined to the area of the oval fossa. SCV, ICV = superior and inferior caval veins.

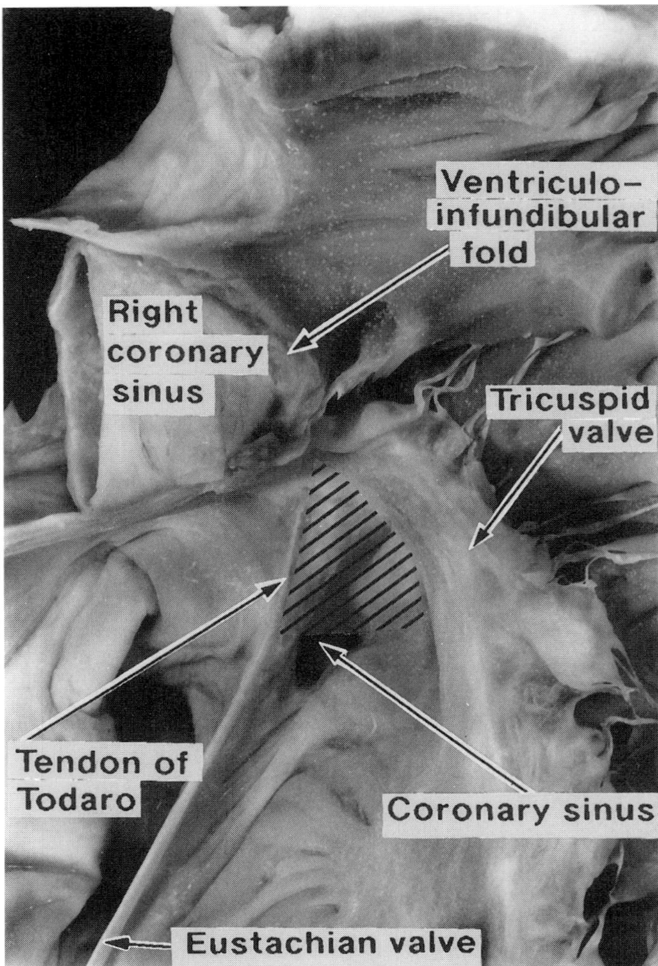

FIGURE 2–13 This dissection, made by removing part of the subpulmonary infundibulum, shows the location of the triangle of Koch (shaded area).

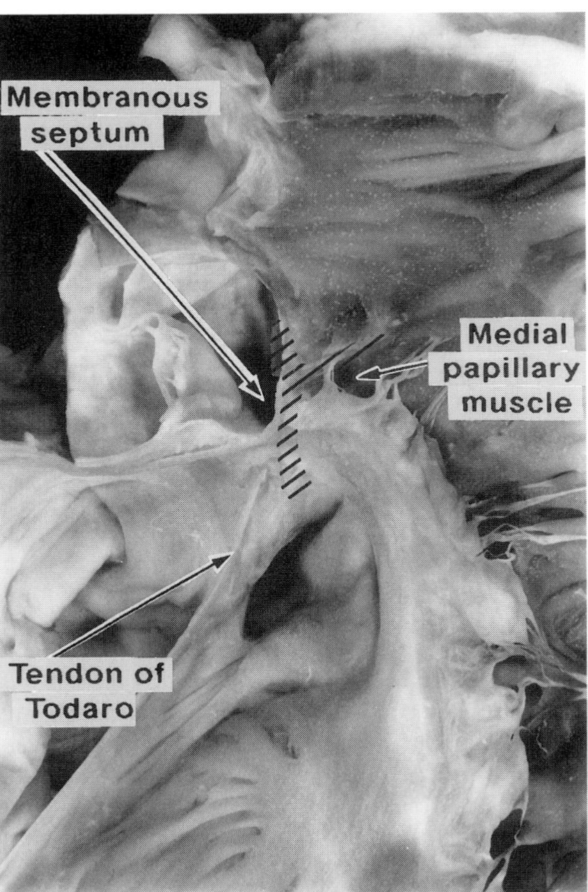

FIGURE 2–14 Further dissection of the heart shown in Fig. 2-13 reveals that a line joining the apex of the triangle of Koch to the medial papillary muscle marks the location of the atrioventricular conduction axis.

vestibule. In contrast, the left atrial appendage has a limited junction with the vestibule, and the pectinate muscles are located almost exclusively within the appendage (Fig. 2-8). The larger part of the vestibule that supports and inserts directly into the mural leaflet of the mitral valve is directly continuous with the smooth atrial wall of the pulmonary venous component.

Because the left atrium is posterior and tethered by the four pulmonary veins, the chamber is relatively inaccessible. Surgeons use several approaches to gain access. The most common is an incision just to the right of and parallel to the interatrial groove, anterior to the right pulmonary veins. This incision can be carried beneath both the superior and inferior caval veins parallel to the interatrial groove, to provide wide access to the left atrium. A second approach is through the dome of the left atrium. If the aorta is pulled anteriorly and to the left, an extensive trough may be seen between the right and left atrial appendages. An incision through this trough, between the pulmonary veins of the upper lobes, provides direct access to the left atrium. When this incision is made, it is important to remember the location of the sinus node artery, which may course along the roof of the left atrium if it arises from the circumflex artery. The left atrium also can be reached via a right atrial incision and an opening in the atrial septum.

When the interior of the left atrium is visualized, the small size of the mouth of the left atrial appendage is apparent. It lies to the left of the mitral orifice as viewed by the surgeon. The majority of the pulmonary venous atrium usually is located inferiorly away from the operative field. The vestibule of the mitral orifice dominates the operative view. The septal surface is located anteriorly, with the true septum relatively inferior (Fig. 2-17).

Mitral Valve

The mitral valve is supported by two prominent papillary muscles located in anterolateral and posteromedial positions. The two leaflets of the mitral valve have markedly

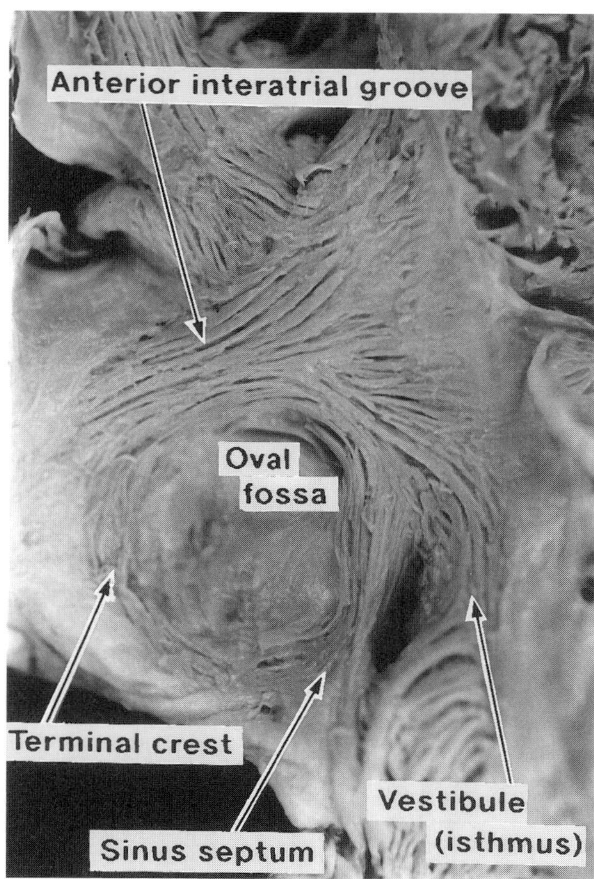

FIGURE 2–15 This dissection, made by careful removal of the right atrial endocardium, shows the ordered arrangement of myocardial fibers in the prominent muscle bundles that underscore preferential conduction. There are *no* insulated tracts running within the internodal atrial myocardium. Dissection made by Prof. Damian Sanchez-Quintana.

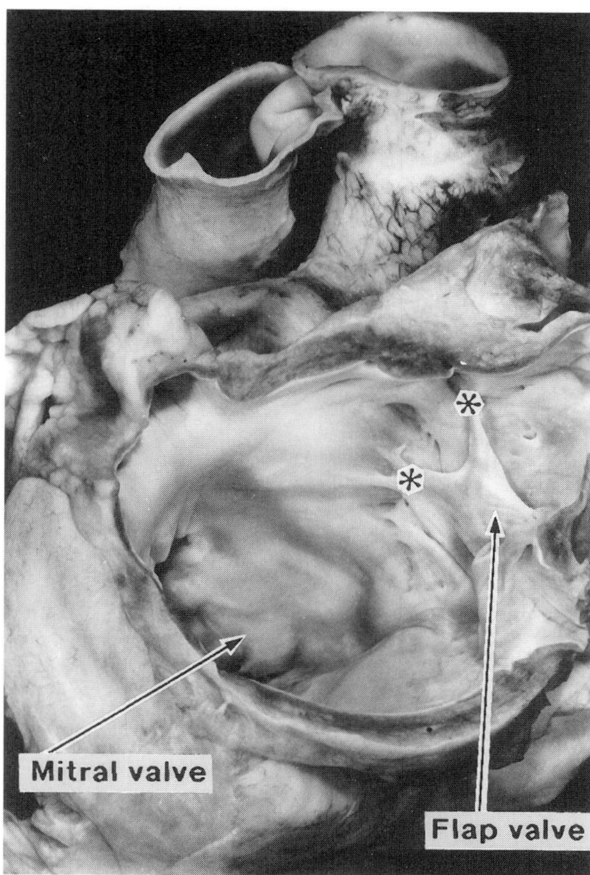

FIGURE 2–17 This view of the opened left atrium shows how the septal aspect is dominated by the flap valve, which is attached by its horns (asterisks) to the infolded atrial groove.

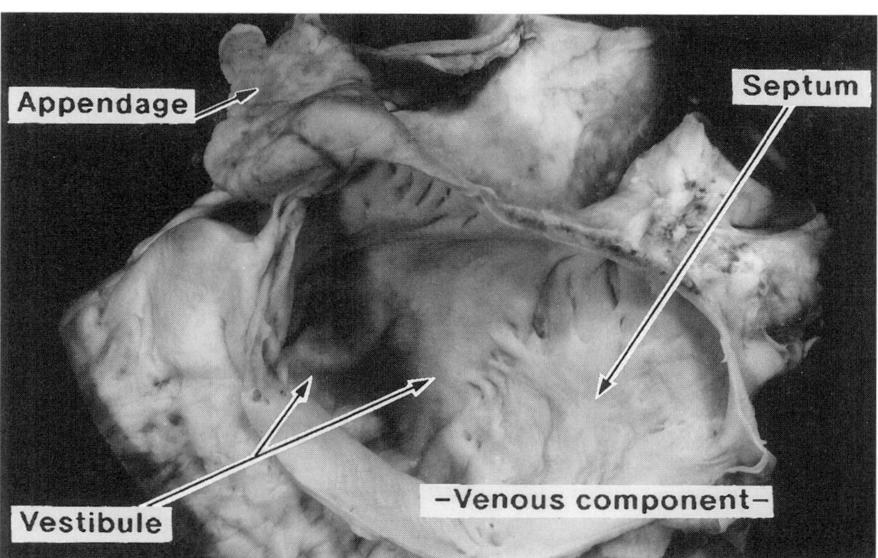

FIGURE 2–16 Like the right atrium, the left atrium (seen here in anatomic orientation) has an appendage, a venous component, and a vestibule. It is separated from the right atrium by the septum.

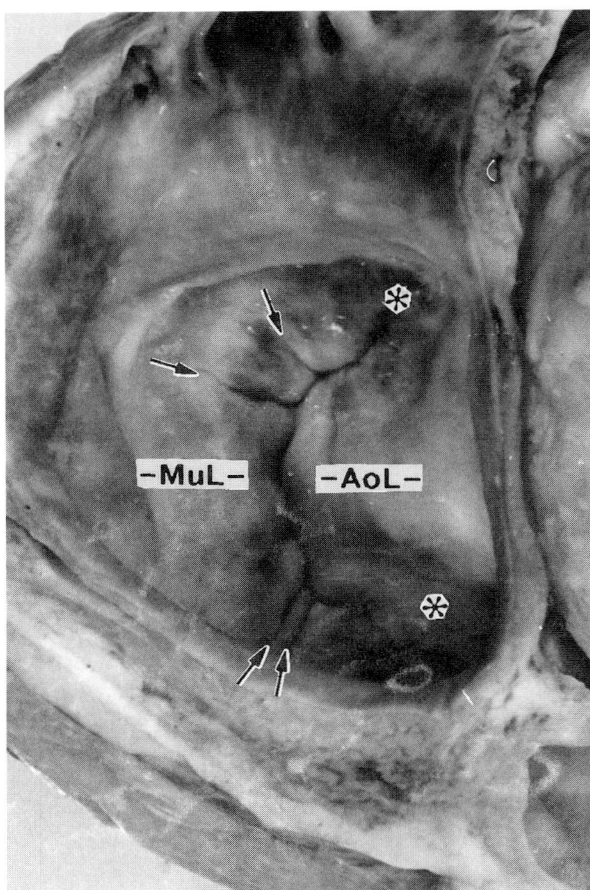

FIGURE 2–18 This view of the opened left atrium shows the leaflets of the mitral valve in closed position. There is a concave zone of apposition between them (between asterisks) with several slits seen in the mural leaflet (MuL). Note the limited extent of the aortic leaflet (AoL) in terms of its circumferential attachments.

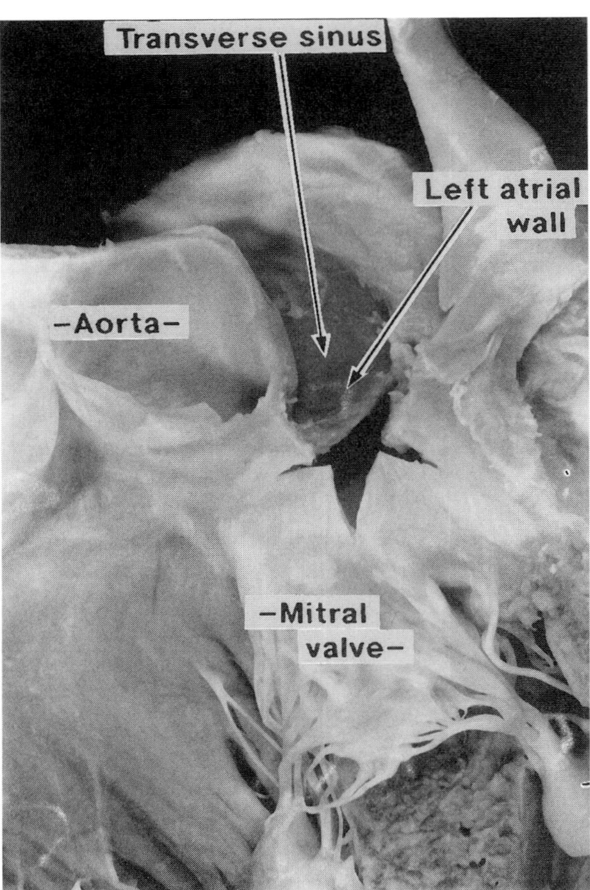

FIGURE 2–19 This dissection simulates the incision made through the aortic-mitral fibrous curtain to enlarge the orificial diameter of the subaortic outflow tract in a normal heart. Dissection made by Dr. Manisha Lal Trapasia.

different appearances (Fig. 2-18). The aortic (or anterior) leaflet is short, relatively square, and guards approximately one third of the circumference of the valvar orifice. This leaflet is in fibrous continuity with the aortic valve and, because of this, is best referred to as the aortic leaflet, since it is neither strictly anterior nor superior in position. The other leaflet is much shallower but guards approximately two thirds of the circumference of the mitral orifice. As it is connected to the parietal part of the atrioventricular junction, it is most accurately termed the mural leaflet, but is often termed the posterior leaflet. It is divided into a number of subunits that fold against the aortic leaflet when the valve is closed. Although generally there are three, there may be as many as five or six scallops in the mural leaflet.

Unlike the tricuspid valve, the mitral valve leaflets are supported by a rather dense collagenous annulus, although it may take the form of a sheet rather than a cord. This annulus usually extends parietally from the fibrous trigones, the greatly thickened areas at either end of the area of fibrous continuity between the leaflets of the aortic and mitral valves (Fig. 2-6). The area of the valvar orifice related to the right fibrous trigone and central fibrous body is most vulnerable with respect to the atrioventricular node and penetrating bundle (Fig. 2-7). The midportion of the aortic leaflet of the mitral valve is related to the commissure between the noncoronary and left coronary cusps of the aortic valve. An incision through the atrial wall in this area may be extended into the subaortic outflow tract, and may be useful for enlarging the aortic annulus during replacement of the aortic valve (Fig. 2-19). The circumflex coronary artery is adjacent to the left half of the mural leaflet, whereas the coronary sinus is adjacent to the right half of the mural leaflet (Fig. 2-20). These structures can be damaged during excessive dissection, or by excessively deep placement of sutures during replacement or repair of the mitral valve. When the circumflex artery is dominant, the entire attachment of the mural leaflet may be intimately related to this artery (Fig. 2-21).

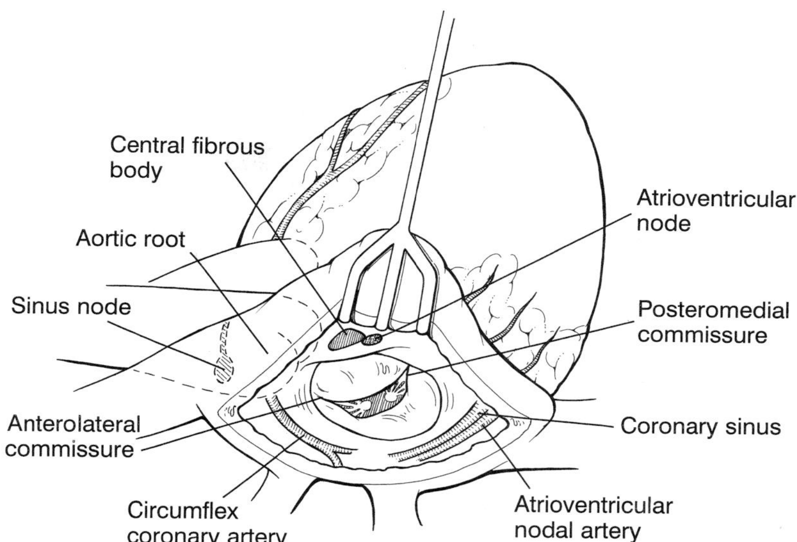

FIGURE 2–20 This diagram depicts the mitral valve in relationship to its surrounding structures as viewed through a left atriotomy.

THE RIGHT VENTRICLE AND PULMONARY VALVE

Inlet and Apical Trabecular Portions

The morphology of both the right and left ventricles can be understood best by subdividing the ventricles into three anatomically distinct components: the inlet, apical trabecular, and outlet portions.[2] This classification is more helpful than the traditional division of the right ventricle into the sinus and conus parts. The inlet portion of the right ventricle surrounds the tricuspid valve and its tension apparatus. A distinguishing feature of the tricuspid valve is the direct attachment of its septal leaflet. The apical trabecular portion of the right ventricle extends out to the apex. Here, the wall of the ventricle is quite thin and vulnerable to perforation by cardiac catheters and pacemaker electrodes.

Outlet Portion and Pulmonary Valve

The outlet portion of the right ventricle consists of the infundibulum, a circumferential muscular structure that supports the leaflets of the pulmonary valve. Because of the semilunar shape of the pulmonary valvar leaflets, this valve does not have an annulus in the traditional sense of a ring-like attachment. The leaflets have semilunar attachments that cross the musculoarterial junction in a corresponding semilunar fashion (Fig. 2-22). Therefore, instead of a single annulus, three rings can be distinguished anatomically

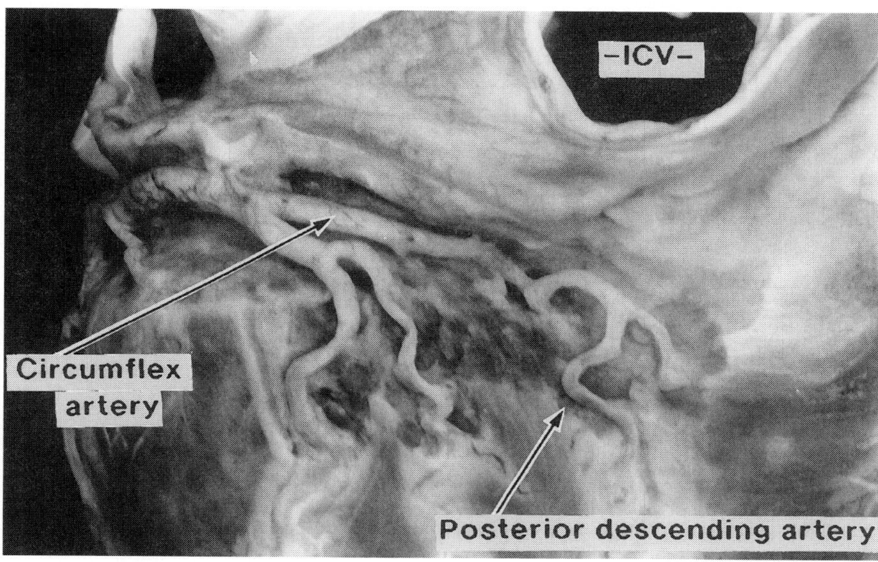

FIGURE 2–21 The extensive course of a dominant circumflex artery within the left atrioventricular groove shown in anatomic orientation. ICV = inferior caval vein.

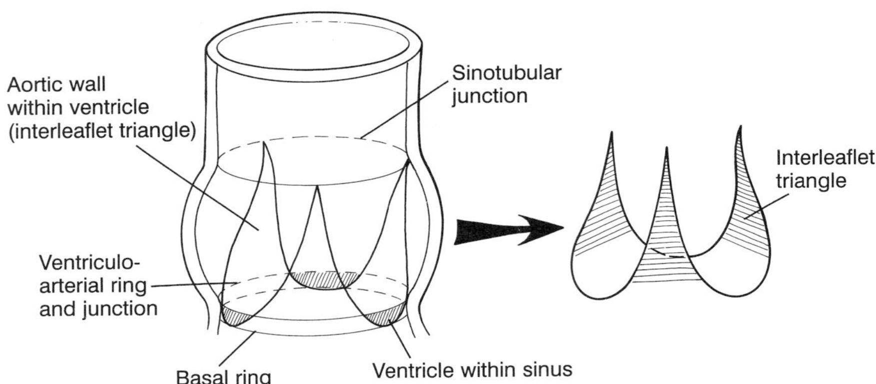

FIGURE 2–22 The semilunar valves do not have an annulus in the traditional sense. Rather, three rings can be identified anatomically: (1) at the sinotubular junction; (2) at the musculoarterial junction; and (3) at the base of the sinuses within the ventricle.

in relation to the pulmonary valve. Superiorly, the sinotubular ridge of the pulmonary trunk marks the level of peripheral apposition of the leaflets (the commissures). A second ring exists at the ventriculoarterial junction. A third ring can be constructed by joining together the basal attachments of the three leaflets to the infundibular muscle. None of these rings, however, corresponds to the attachments of the leaflets, which must be semilunar to permit the valve to competently open and close. In fact, these semilunar attachments, which mark the hemodynamic ventriculoarterial junction, extend from the first ring, across the second, down to the third, and back in each cusp (Fig. 2-23).

Supraventricular Crest and Pulmonary Infundibulum

A distinguishing feature of the right ventricle is a prominent muscular shelf, the supraventricular crest, which separates the tricuspid and pulmonary valves (Fig. 2-24). In reality, this muscular ridge is the posterior part of the subpulmonary muscular infundibulum that supports the leaflets of the pulmonary valve. In other words, it is part of the inner curve of the heart. Incisions through the supraventricular crest run into the transverse septum and may jeopardize the right

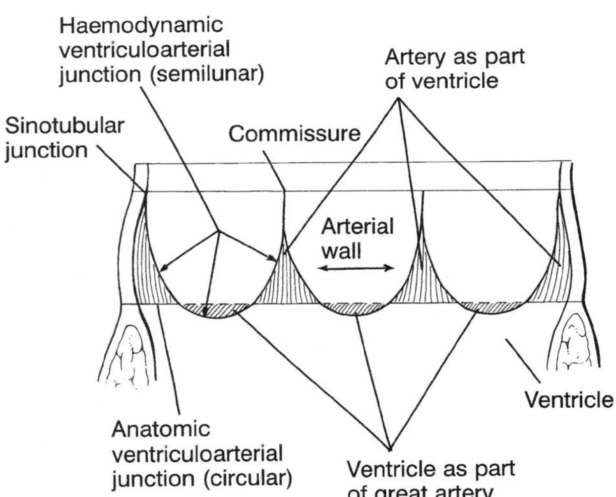

FIGURE 2–23 The hemodynamic ventriculoarterial junction of the semilunar valves extends from the sinotubular junction across the anatomic ventriculoarterial junction to the basal ring and back in each leaflet (see Fig. 2-22). This creates a portion of ventricle as part of the great artery in each sinus, and a triangle of artery as part of the ventricle between each leaflet.

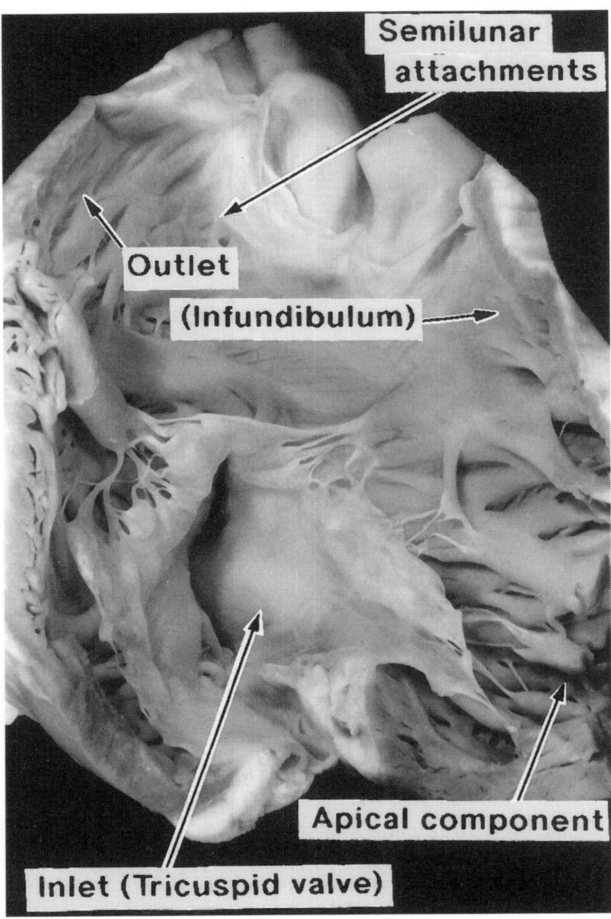

FIGURE 2–24 View of the opened right ventricle, in anatomic orientation, showing its three component parts and the semilunar attachments of the pulmonary valve. These are supported by the supraventricular crest.

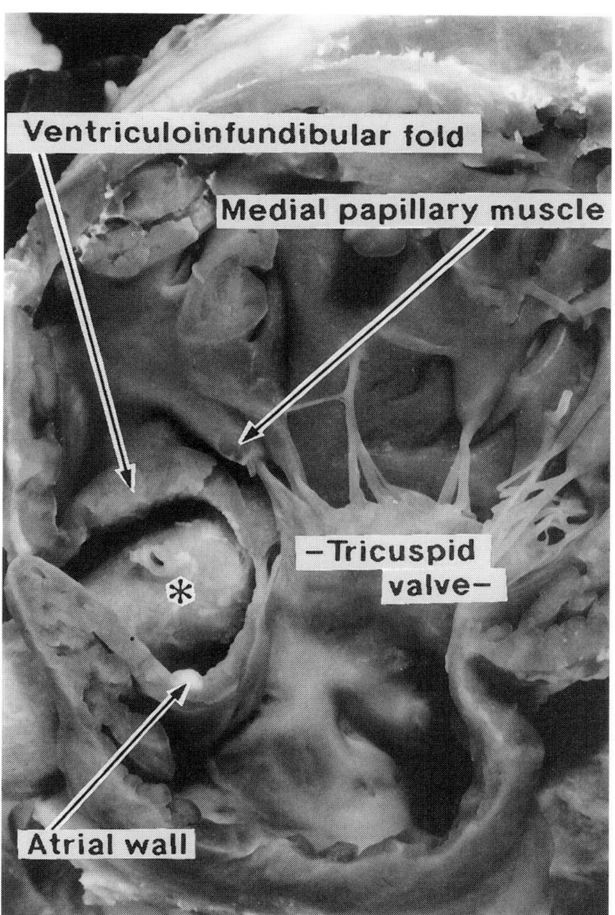

FIGURE 2–25 This dissection, viewed in surgical orientation, shows how the greater part of the supraventricular crest is formed by the freestanding subpulmonary infundibulum in relation to the right coronary aortic sinus (asterisk).

coronary artery. Although this area is often considered the outlet component of the interventricular septum, in fact the entire subpulmonary infundibulum, including the ventriculoinfundibular fold, can be removed without entering the left ventricular cavity. This is possible because the leaflets of the pulmonary and aortic valves are supported on separate sleeves of right and left ventricular outlet muscle. There is an extensive external tissue plane between the walls of the aorta and the pulmonary trunk (Fig. 2-25), and the leaflets of the pulmonary and aortic valves have markedly different levels of attachments within their respective ventricles. This feature enables enucleation of the pulmonary valve, including its basal attachments within the infundibulum, during the Ross procedure without creating a ventricular septal defect. When the infundibulum is removed from the right ventricle, the insertion of the supraventricular crest between the limbs of the septomarginal trabeculation is visible (Fig. 2-26). This trabeculation is a prominent muscle column that divides superiorly into anterior and posterior limbs. The anterior limb runs superiorly into the infundibulum and supports the leaflets of the pulmonary valve. The posterior limb extends backwards beneath the ventricular septum and runs into the inlet portion of the ventricle. The medial papillary muscle arises from this posterior limb. The body of the septomarginal trabeculation runs to the apex of the ventricle, where it divides into smaller trabeculations. Two of these trabeculations may be particularly prominent. One becomes the anterior papillary muscle and the other crosses the ventricular cavity as the moderator band (Fig. 2-27).

THE LEFT VENTRICLE AND AORTIC VALVE

Inlet and Apical Trabecular Portions

The left ventricle can be subdivided into three components, similar to the right ventricle. The inlet component

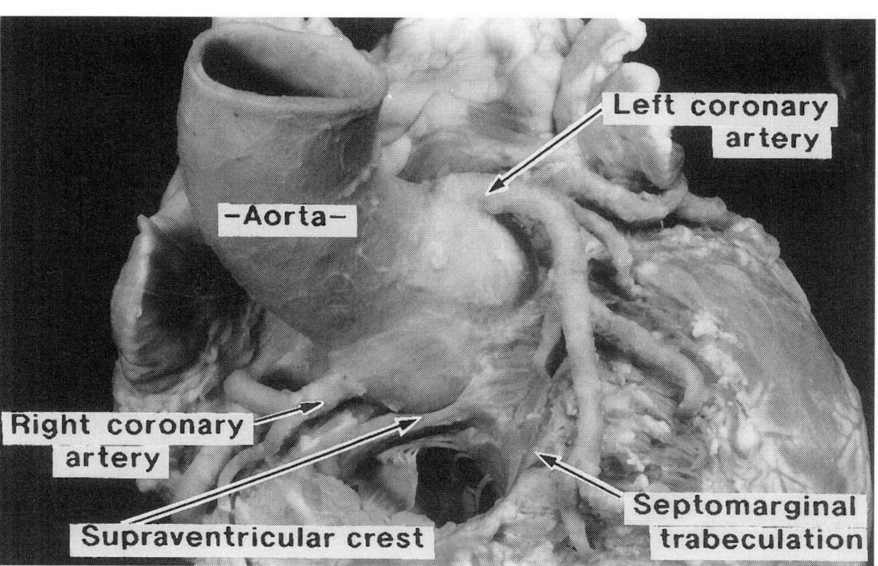

FIGURE 2–26 Removal of the freestanding subpulmonary infundibulum reveals the insertion of the supraventricular crest between the limbs of the septomarginal trabeculation, and shows the aortic origin of the coronary arteries (anatomic orientation).

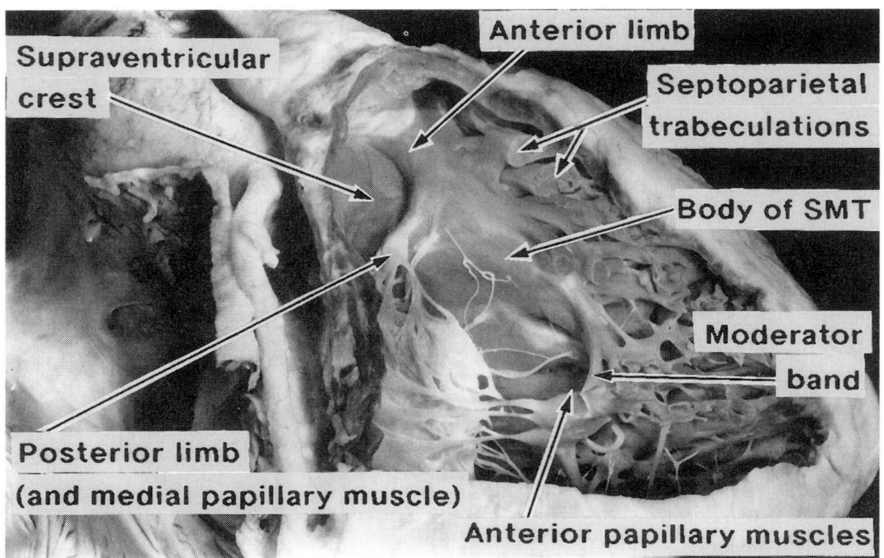

FIGURE 2–27 This dissection of the right ventricle, in anatomic orientation, shows the relations of supraventricular crest and septomarginal (SMT) and septoparietal trabeculations.

surrounds, and is limited by, the mitral valve and its tension apparatus. The two papillary muscles occupy anterolateral and posteromedial positions and are positioned rather close to each other. The leaflets of the mitral valve have no direct septal attachments because the deep posterior diverticulum of the left ventricular outflow tract displaces the aortic leaflet away from the inlet septum. The apical trabecular component of the left ventricle extends to the apex, where the myocardium is surprisingly thin. The trabeculations of the left ventricle are quite fine compared with those of the right ventricle (Fig. 2-28). This characteristic is useful for defining ventricular morphology on diagnostic ventriculograms.

Outlet Portion

The outlet component supports the aortic valve and consists of both muscular and fibrous portions. This is in contrast to the infundibulum of the right ventricle, which is comprised entirely of muscle. The septal portion of the left ventricular outflow tract, although primarily muscular, also includes the membranous portion of the ventricular septum. The posterior quadrant of the outflow tract consists of an extensive fibrous curtain that extends from the fibrous skeleton of the heart across the aortic leaflet of the mitral valve, and supports the leaflets of the aortic valve in the area of aortomitral continuity (Fig. 2-5). The lateral quadrant of the outflow tract is again muscular and consists of the lateral margin of

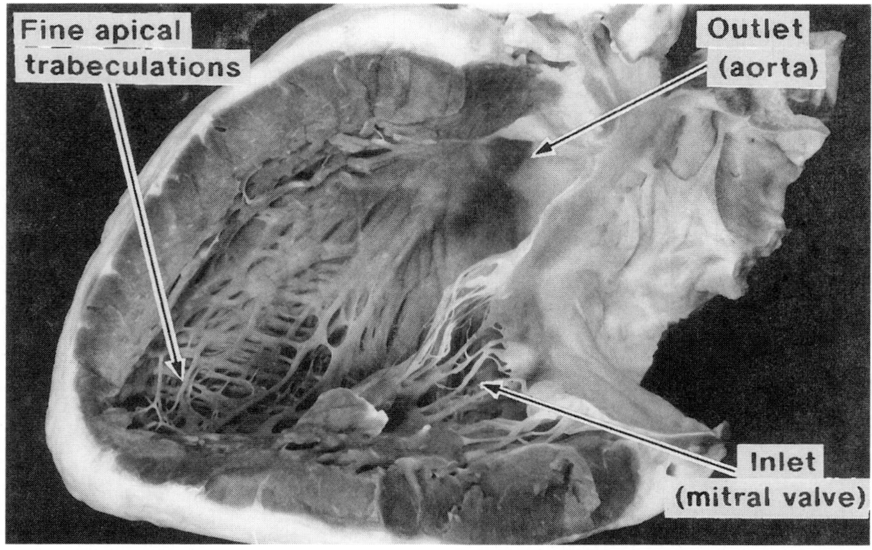

FIGURE 2–28 This dissection of the left ventricle shows its component parts and characteristically fine apical trabeculations (anatomic orientation).

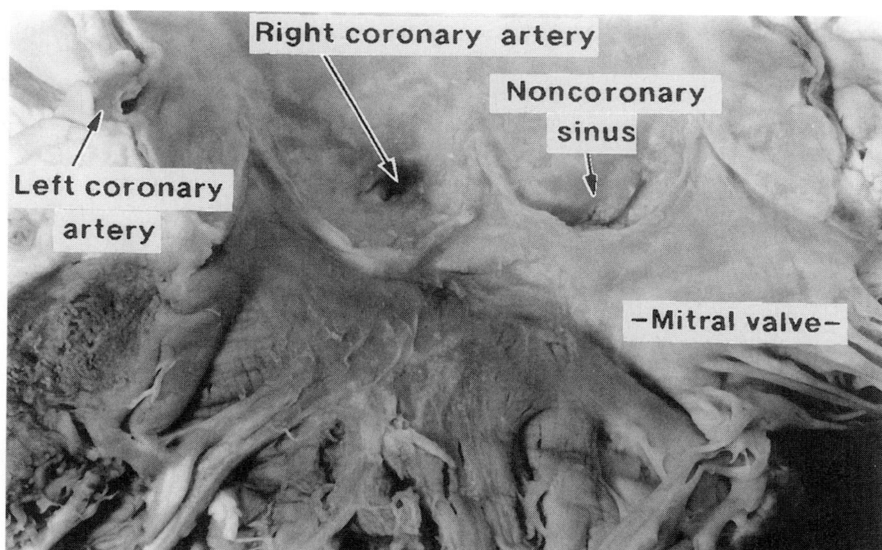

FIGURE 2–29 This dissection in anatomic orientation, made by removing the aortic valvar leaflets, emphasizes the semilunar nature of the hinge points (see Figs. 2-22 and 2-23). Note the relationship to the mitral valve (see Fig. 2-5).

the inner curvature of the heart, delineated externally by the transverse sinus. The left bundle of the cardiac conduction system enters the left ventricular outflow tract posterior to the membranous septum and immediately beneath the commissure between the right and noncoronary leaflets of the aortic valve. After traveling a short distance down the septum, the left bundle divides into anterior, septal, and posterior divisions.

Aortic Valve

The aortic valve is a semilunar valve, morphologically quite similar to the pulmonary valve. Likewise, it does not have a discrete annulus. Because of its central location, the aortic valve is related to each of the cardiac chambers and valves (Fig. 2-4). A thorough knowledge of these relationships is essential to understanding aortic valve pathology and many congenital cardiac malformations.

The aortic valve consists primarily of three semilunar leaflets. As with the pulmonary valve, attachments of the leaflets extend across the ventriculoarterial junction in a curvilinear fashion. Each leaflet, therefore, has attachments to the aorta and within the left ventricle (Fig. 2-29). Behind each leaflet, the aortic wall bulges outward to form the sinuses of Valsalva. The leaflets themselves meet centrally along a line of coaptation, at the center of which is a thickened nodule, called the nodule of Arantius. Peripherally, adjacent to the commissures, the line of coaptation is thinner and normally may contain small perforations. During systole, the leaflets are thrust upward and away from the center of the aortic lumen, whereas, during diastole, they fall passively into the center of the aorta. With normal valvar morphology, all three leaflets meet along lines of coaptation and support the column of blood within the aorta to prevent regurgitation into the ventricle. Two of the three aortic sinuses give rise to coronary arteries, from which arise their designations as right, left, and noncoronary sinuses.

By sequentially following the line of attachment of each leaflet, the relationship of the aortic valve to its surrounding structures can be clearly understood. Beginning posteriorly, the commissure between the noncoronary and left coronary leaflets is positioned along the area of aorto-mitral valvar continuity. The fibrous subaortic curtain is beneath this commissure (Fig. 2-29). To the right of this commissure, the noncoronary leaflet is attached above the posterior diverticulum of the left ventricular outflow tract. Here the valve is related to the right atrial wall. As the attachment of the noncoronary leaflet ascends from its nadir toward the commissure between the noncoronary and right coronary leaflets, the line of attachment is directly above the portion of the atrial septum containing the atrioventricular node. The commissure between the noncoronary and right coronary leaflets is located directly above the penetrating atrioventricular bundle and the membranous ventricular septum (Fig. 2-30). The attachment of the right coronary leaflet then descends across the central fibrous body before ascending to the commissure between the right and left coronary leaflets. Immediately beneath this commissure, the wall of the aorta forms the uppermost part of the subaortic outflow. An incision through this area passes into the space between the facing surfaces of the aorta and pulmonary trunk (Fig. 2-30). As the facing left and right leaflets descend from this commissure, they are attached to the outlet muscular component of the left ventricle. Only a small part of this area in the normal heart is a true outlet septum, since both pulmonary and aortic valves are supported on their own sleeves of myocardium. Thus, although the outlet components of the right and left ventricle face each other, an incision below the aortic valve

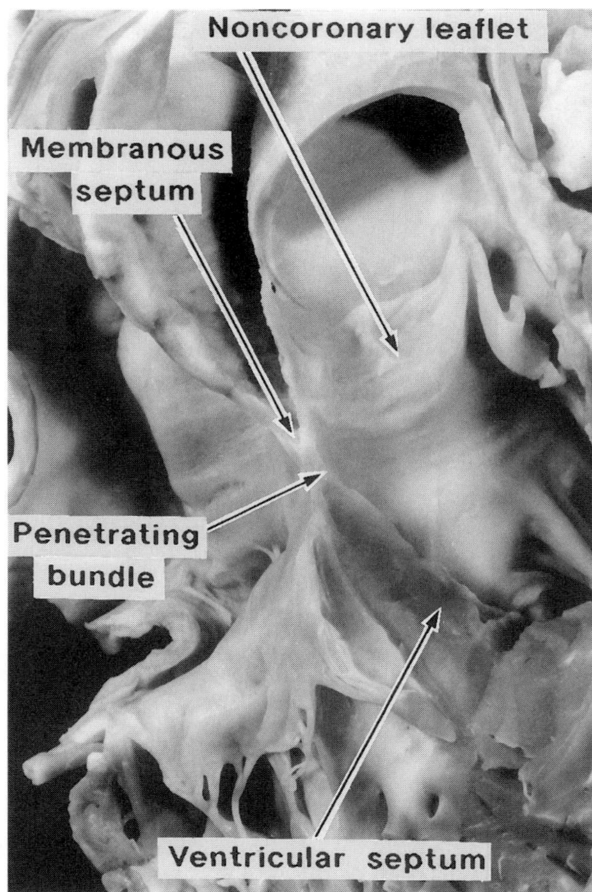

FIGURE 2–30 Dissection made by removing the right and part of the left aortic sinuses to show the relations of the fibrous triangle between the right and noncoronary aortic leaflets (anatomic orientation).

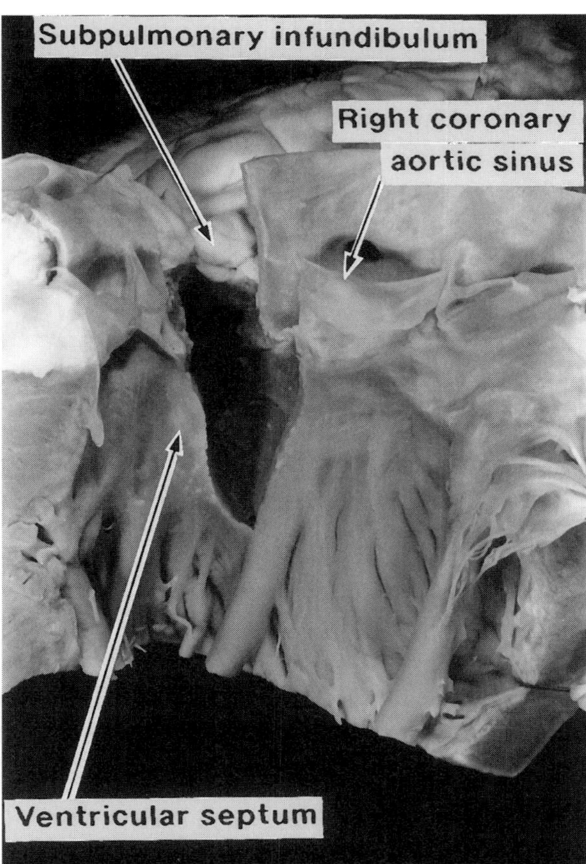

FIGURE 2–31 This incision, made in a normal heart, simulates the Konno-Rastan procedure for enlargement of the aortic root.

enters low into the infundibulum of the right ventricle. As the lateral part of the left coronary leaflet descends from the facing commissure to the base of the sinus, it becomes the only part of the aortic valve that is not intimately related to another cardiac chamber.

The anatomy of the aortic valve and its relationship to surrounding structures is important to successful replacement of the aortic valve, particularly when enlargement of the aortic root is required. The Konno-Rastan aortoventriculoplasty involves opening and enlarging the anterior portion of the subaortic region.[4,5] The incisions for this procedure begin with an anterior longitudinal aortotomy that extends through the commissure between the right and left coronary leaflets. Anteriorly, the incision is extended across the base of the infundibulum. The differential level of attachment of the aortic and pulmonary valve leaflets permits this incision without damage to the pulmonary valve (Fig. 2-31). Posteriorly, the incision extends through the most medial portion of the supraventricular crest into the left ventricular outflow tract. By closing the resulting ventricular septal defect with a patch, the aortic outflow tract is widened to allow implantation of a larger valvar prosthesis. A second patch is used to close the defect in the right ventricular outflow tract.

Alternative methods to enlarge the aortic outflow tract involve incisions in the region of aortomitral continuity. In the Manouguian procedure (Fig. 2-19), a curvilinear aortotomy is extended posteriorly through the commissure between the left and noncoronary leaflets down to, and occasionally into, the aortic leaflet of the mitral valve.[6] A patch is used to augment the incision posteriorly. When the posterior diverticulum of the outflow tract is fully developed, this incision can be made without entering other cardiac chambers, although not uncommonly the roof of the left atrium is opened. The Nicks procedure for enlargement of the aortic root involves an aortotomy that passes through the middle of the noncoronary leaflet into the fibrous subaortic curtain and may be extended into the aortic leaflet of the mitral valve.[7] This incision also may open the roof of the left atrium. When these techniques are used, any resultant defect in the left atrium must be closed carefully.

As discussed previously, the differential level of attachment of aortic and pulmonary valves, as well as the muscular nature of their support, allows the pulmonary valve to be

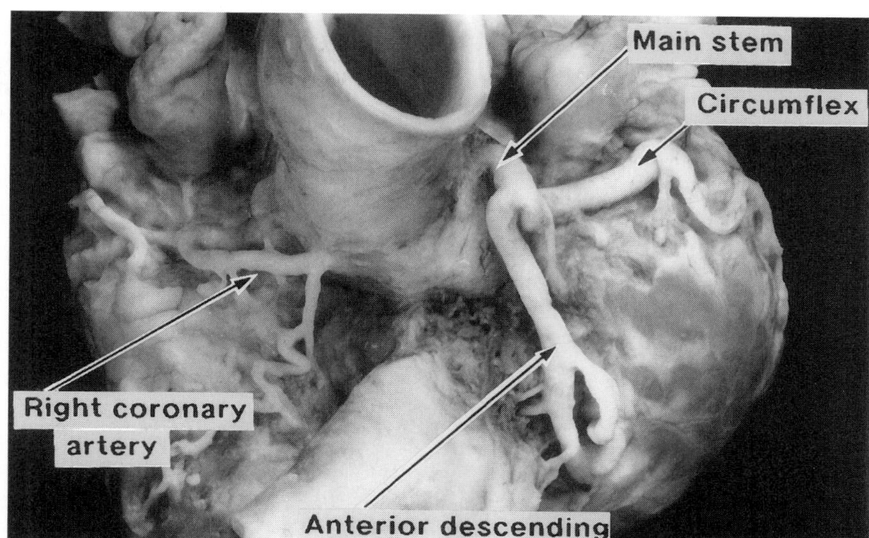

FIGURE 2–32 The short extent of the main stem of the left coronary artery is seen before it branches into the circumflex and anterior descending arteries. Note the small right coronary artery in this heart, in which the circumflex artery was dominant (see Fig. 2-21).

harvested and used as a replacement for the aortic valve in the Ross procedure.[8,9] This procedure can be combined with the incisions of the Konno-Rastan aortoventriculoplasty to repair left ventricular outflow tract obstructions in young children with a viable autograft that has potential for growth and avoids the need for anticoagulation.

Accurate understanding of left ventricular outflow tract anatomy is also important in the treatment of aortic valvar endocarditis.[10,11] Because of the central position of the aortic valve relative to the other valves and cardiac chambers (Fig. 2-4), abscess formation can produce fistulas between the aorta and any of the four chambers of the heart. Patients may, therefore, present with findings of left heart failure, left-to-right shunting, and/or complete heart block in addition to the usual signs of sepsis and systemic embolization.

THE CORONARY ARTERIES[12–14]

The right and left coronary arteries originate behind their respective aortic valvar leaflets (Fig. 2-26). The orifices usually are located in the upper third of the sinuses of Valsalva, although individual hearts may vary markedly. Because of the oblique plane of the aortic valve, the orifice of the left coronary artery is superior and posterior to that of the right coronary artery. The coronary arterial tree is divided into three segments; two (the left anterior descending artery and the circumflex artery) arise from a common stem. The third segment is the right coronary artery. The dominance of the coronary circulation (right versus left) usually refers to the artery from which the posterior descending artery originates, not the absolute mass of myocardium perfused by the left or right coronary artery. Right dominance occurs in 85% to 90% of normal individuals. Left dominance occurs slightly more frequently in males than females.

Main Stem of the Left Coronary Artery

The main stem of the left coronary artery courses from the left sinus of Valsalva anteriorly, inferiorly, and to the left between the pulmonary trunk and the left atrial appendage (Fig. 2-32). Typically it is 10 to 20 mm in length but can extend to a length of 40 mm. The left main stem can be absent, with separate orifices in the sinus of Valsalva for its two primary branches (1% of patients). The main stem divides into two major arteries of nearly equal diameter: the left anterior descending artery and the circumflex artery.

Left Anterior Descending Artery

The left anterior descending (or interventricular) coronary artery continues directly from the bifurcation of the left main stem, coursing anteriorly and inferiorly in the anterior interventricular groove to the apex of the heart (Fig. 2-33). Its branches include the diagonals, the septal perforators, and the right ventricular branches. The diagonals, which may be two to six in number, course along the anterolateral wall of the left ventricle and supply this portion of the myocardium. The first diagonal generally is the largest and may arise from the bifurcation of the left main stem (formerly known as the intermediate artery). The septal perforators branch perpendicularly into the ventricular septum. Typically there are three to five septal perforators; the initial one is the largest and commonly originates just beyond the takeoff of the first diagonal. This perpendicular orientation is a useful marker for identification of the left anterior descending artery on coronary angiograms. The septal perforators supply blood to the anterior two thirds of the ventricular septum. Right ventricular branches, which may not always be present, supply blood to the anterior surface of the right ventricle. In approximately 4% of hearts, the left anterior

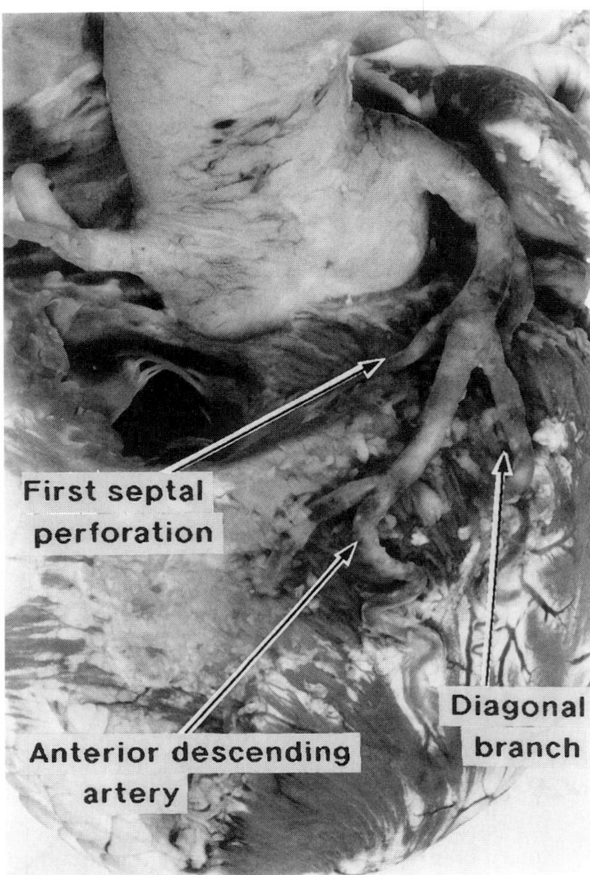

FIGURE 2–33 The important branches of the anterior descending artery are the first septal perforating and diagonal arteries.

descending artery bifurcates proximally and continues as two parallel vessels of approximately equal size down the anterior interventricular groove. Occasionally, the artery wraps around the apex of the left ventricle to feed the distal portion of the posterior interventricular groove. Rarely, it extends along the entire length of the posterior groove to replace the posterior descending artery.

Circumflex Artery

The left circumflex coronary artery arises from the left main coronary artery roughly at a right angle to the anterior interventricular branch. It courses along the left atrioventricular groove and, in 85% to 95% of patients, terminates near the obtuse margin of the left ventricle (Fig. 2-34). In 10% to 15% of patients, it continues around the atrioventricular groove to the crux of the heart to give rise to the posterior descending artery (left dominance; see Fig. 2-21). The primary branches of the left circumflex coronary artery are the obtuse marginals. They supply blood to the lateral aspect of the left ventricular myocardium, including the posteromedial papillary muscle. Additional branches supply blood to the left atrium and, in 40% to 50% of hearts, the sinus node. When the circumflex coronary artery supplies the posterior descending artery, it also supplies the atrioventricular node.

Right Coronary Artery

The right coronary artery courses from the aorta anteriorly and laterally before descending in the right atrioventricular groove and curving posteriorly at the acute margin of the right ventricle (Fig. 2-35). In 85% to 90% of hearts, the right coronary artery crosses the crux, where it makes a characteristic U-turn before bifurcating into the posterior descending artery and the right posterolateral artery. In 50% to 60% of hearts, the artery to the sinus node arises from the proximal portion of the right coronary artery. The blood supply to the atrioventricular node (in patients with right dominant circulation) arises from the midportion of the U-shaped segment. The posterior descending artery runs along the posterior interventricular groove, extending for a variable distance toward the apex of the heart. It gives off perpendicular branches, the posterior septal perforators, that

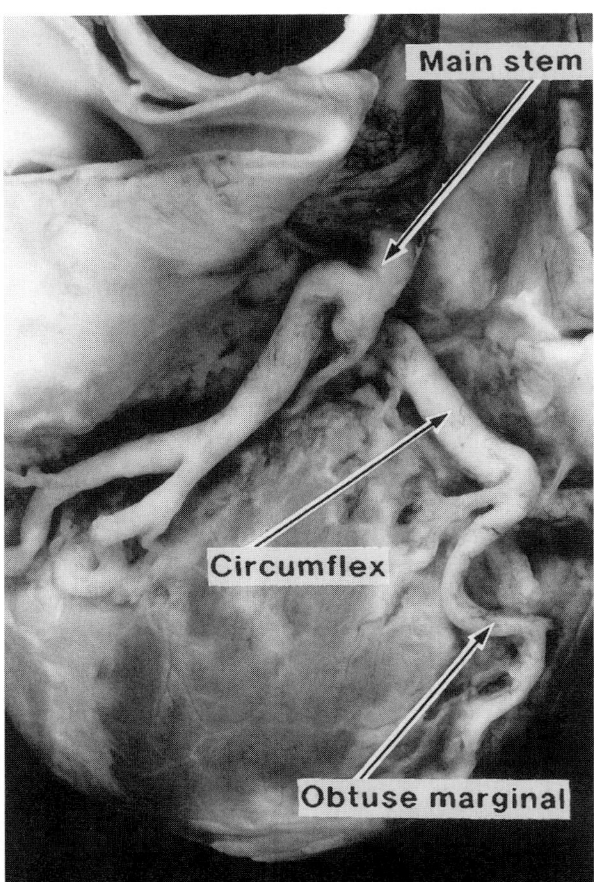

FIGURE 2–34 The important branches of the circumflex artery, seen in anatomic orientation.

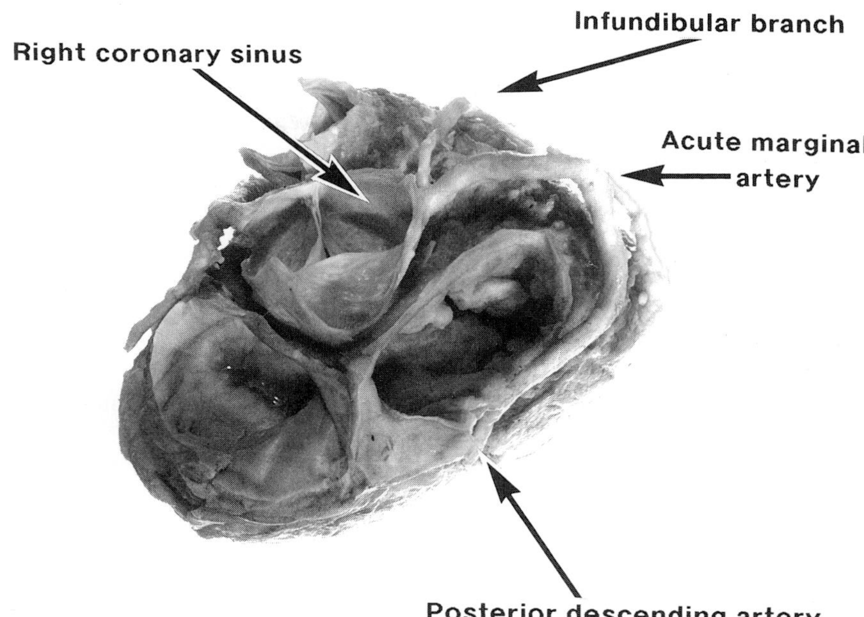

FIGURE 2–35 This dissection shows the relationships and branches of the right coronary artery.

course anteriorly in the ventricular septum. Typically, these perforators supply the posterior one third of the ventricular septal myocardium.

The right posterolateral artery gives rise to a variable number of branches that supply the posterior surface of the left ventricle. The circulation of the posteroinferior portion of the left ventricular myocardium is quite variable. It may consist of branches of the right coronary artery, the circumflex artery, or both. The acute marginal arteries branch from the right coronary artery along the acute margin of the heart, before its bifurcation at the crux. These marginals supply the anterior free wall of the right ventricle. In 10% to 20% of hearts, one of these acute marginal arteries courses across the diaphragmatic surface of the right ventricle to reach the distal ventricular septum. The right coronary artery supplies important collaterals to the left anterior descending artery through its septal perforators. In addition, its infundibular (or conus) branch, which arises from the proximal portion of the right coronary artery, courses anteriorly over the base of the ventricular infundibulum and may serve as a collateral to the anterior descending artery. Kugel's artery is an anastomotic vessel between the proximal right coronary and the circumflex coronary artery that can also provide a branch that runs through the base of the atrial septum to the crux of the heart, where it supplies collateral circulation to the atrioventricular node.[15]

THE CORONARY VEINS[14]

A complex network of veins drains the coronary circulation. An extensive degree of collateralization amongst these veins and the coronary arteries, and the paucity of valves within coronary veins, enables the use of retrograde coronary sinus cardioplegia for intraoperative myocardial protection. The venous circulation can be divided into three systems: the coronary sinus and its tributaries, the anterior right ventricular veins, and the thebesian veins.

Coronary Sinus and Its Tributaries

The coronary sinus predominantly drains the left ventricle and receives approximately 85% of coronary venous blood. It lies within the posterior atrioventricular groove and empties into the right atrium at the lateral border of the triangle of Koch (Fig. 2-36). The orifice of the coronary sinus is guarded by the crescent-shaped thebesian valve. The named tributaries of the coronary sinus include the anterior interventricular vein, which courses parallel to the left anterior descending coronary artery. Adjacent to the bifurcation of the left main stem, the anterior interventricular vein courses leftward in the atrioventricular groove, where it is referred to as the great cardiac vein. It receives blood from the marginal and posterior left ventricular branches before becoming the coronary sinus at the origin of the oblique vein (of Marshall) at the posterior margin of the left atrium. The posterior interventricular vein, or middle cardiac vein, arises at the apex, courses parallel to the posterior descending coronary artery, and extends proximally to the crux. Here, this vein drains either directly into the right atrium or into the coronary sinus just prior to its orifice. The small cardiac vein runs posteriorly through the right atrioventricular groove.

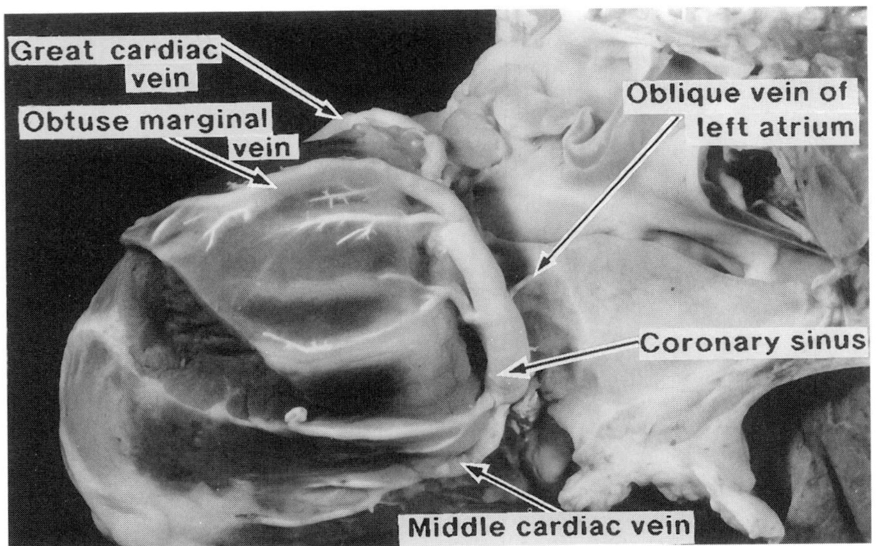

FIGURE 2–36 The coronary veins on the diaphragmatic surface of the heart, seen in anatomic orientation, have been emphasized by filling them with sealant. The tributaries of the coronary sinus are well demonstrated. Note that, strictly speaking, the sinus does not commence until the oblique vein enters the great cardiac vein.

Anterior Right Ventricular Veins

The anterior right ventricular veins travel across the right ventricular surface to the right atrioventricular groove, where they either enter directly into the right atrium or coalesce to form the small cardiac vein. As indicated, this vein travels down the right atrioventricular groove, around the acute margin, and enters into the right atrium directly or joins the coronary sinus just proximal to its orifice.

Thebesian Veins

The thebesian veins are small venous tributaries that drain directly into the cardiac chambers. They exist primarily in the right atrium and right ventricle.

REFERENCES

1. Anderson KR, Ho SY, Anderson RH: The location and vascular supply of the sinus node in the human heart. *Br Heart J* 1979; 41:28.
2. Wilcox BR, Anderson RH: *Surgical Anatomy of the Heart*. New York, Raven Press, 1985.
3. Sweeney LJ, Rosenquist GC: The normal anatomy of the atrial septum in the human heart. *Am Heart J* 1979; 98:194.
4. Konno S, Imai Y, Iida Y, et al: A new method for prosthetic valve replacement in congenital aortic stenosis associated with hypoplasia of the aortic valve ring. *J Thorac Cardiovasc Surg* 1975; 70:909.
5. Rastan H, Koncz J: Aortoventriculoplasty: a new technique for the treatment of left ventricular outflow tract obstruction. *J Thorac Cardiovasc Surg* 1976; 71:920.
6. Manouguian S, Seybold-Epting W: Patch enlargement of the aortic valve ring by extending the aortic incision into the anterior mitral leaflet: new operative technique. *J Thorac Cardiovasc Surg* 1979; 78:402.
7. Nicks R, Cartmill T, Berstein L: Hypoplasia of the aortic root. *Thorax* 1970; 25:339.
8. Ross DN: Replacement of aortic and mitral valve with a pulmonary autograft. *Lancet* 1967; 2:956.
9. Oury JH, Angell WW, Eddy AC, Cleveland JC: Pulmonary autograft—past, present, and future. *J Heart Valve Dis* 1993; 2:365.
10. Wilcox BR, Murray GF, Starek PJK: The long-term outlook for valve replacement in active endocarditis. *J Thorac Cardiovasc Surg* 1977; 74:860.
11. Frantz PT, Murray GF, Wilcox BR: Surgical management of left ventricular-aortic discontinuity complicating bacterial endocarditis. *Ann Thorac Surg* 1980; 29:1.
12. Anderson RH, Becker AE: *Cardiac Anatomy*. London, Churchill Livingstone, 1980.
13. Kirklin JW, Barratt-Boyes BG: Anatomy, dimensions, and terminology, in Kirklin JW, Barratt-Boyes BG (eds): *Cardiac Surgery,* 2nd ed. New York, Churchill Livingstone, 1993; p 3.
14. Schlant RC, Silverman ME: Anatomy of the heart, in Hurst JW, Logue RB, Rachley CE, et al (eds): *The Heart,* 6th ed. New York, McGraw-Hill, 1986; p 16.
15. Kugel, MA: Anatomical studies on the coronary arteries and their branches: 1. Arteria anastomotica auricularis magna. *Am Heart J* 1927; 3:260.

Chapter 3

Cardiac Surgical Physiology

Jakob Vinten-Johansen/Zhi-Qing Zhao/Robert A. Guyton

The cardiac surgeon is a practitioner of the art of medicine, a healer who attempts to understand disease processes with the goal of reversing or assuaging these disease states. Basic to the understanding of cardiac disease is a working knowledge of the normal functioning of the heart and of the specialized cells that comprise the cardiovascular system, for without this understanding of normal function, abnormal physiology escapes recognition. Hence, the cardiac surgeon must also be a practicing physiologist, continuously applying his or her understanding of cardiovascular physiology to the patient with cardiac disease. In addition, the cardiac surgeon must design and implement strategies of myocardial protection that preserve the normal physiology of the heart and constituent cells under conditions of cardiopulmonary bypass and off-pump surgery. The purpose of this chapter is to present a *manageable, working outline of cardiac physiology* that can be used in daily practice by the practitioner as a framework against which pathologic processes can be measured, assessed, and attacked.

The challenge of writing such a chapter of basic cardiovascular physiology is to present complex data, synthesized from numerous sources, that encapsulates our

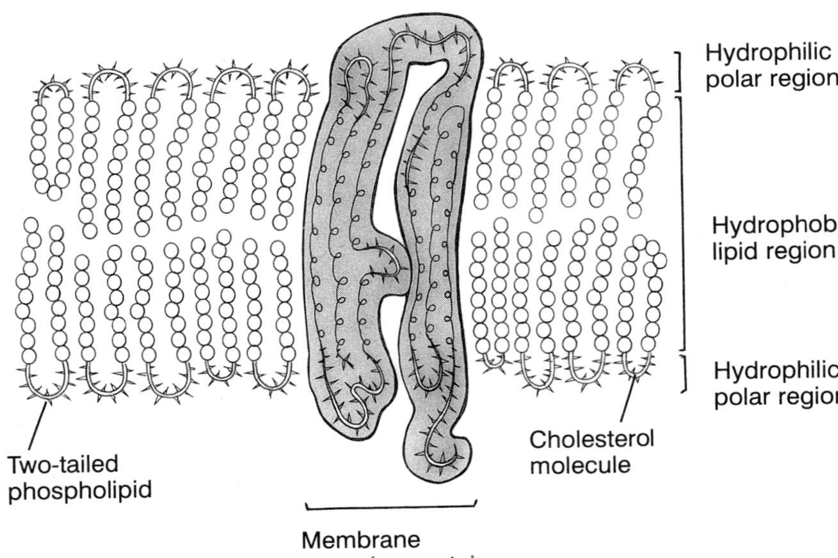

FIGURE 3–1 The sarcolemma is a phospholipid bilayer in which molecules of phospholipids and cholesterol are aligned with both hydrophobic domains of molecules on the interior of the membrane and hydrophilic portions of molecules on the outside. Membrane-spanning proteins are located in this bilayer. The protein shown here is similar to many ion channels, with six hydrophobic alpha-helices spanning the membrane and surrounding a central channel.

understanding at the systems level, at the cellular and subcellular levels, and finally at the molecular level. The latter is important because all the aforementioned levels are a convergence of complex and myriad molecular interactions. The challenge is to maintain simplicity without sacrificing completeness or accuracy, so that the surgeon may apply the fund of knowledge to daily practice and the broad spectrum of patients encountered. Basic, reasonably well established concepts will be presented, with the full understanding that many of these concepts are currently being challenged by our penetration to the molecular level of investigation.[1–3]

SPECIAL ELECTRICAL AND MEMBRANE PROPERTIES OF CARDIAC CELLS

The Cell Membrane or Sarcolemma

The cardiac cell is surrounded by a membrane (*plasmalemma* or *sarcolemma*) with unique properties. These properties allow the *origination* and then the *conduction* of an electrical signal through the heart, leading to near-synchronous depolarization of atrial myocytes and, with an appropriate delay, synchronous depolarization of ventricular myocytes that optimizes ventricular loading conditions. The sarcolemma further possesses properties that lead to the *initiation of the excitation-contraction coupling* process. Finally, the sarcolemma allows *regulation of excitation, contraction, and intracellular metabolism* in response to neuronal and chemical stimulation. Each of these functions will be considered, with emphasis upon those features of the cardiac sarcolemma that differ from the plasmalemma of other cells.

BASIC COMPOSITION OF THE SARCOLEMMA: THE PHOSPHOLIPID BILAYER

A *phospholipid bilayer* provides a barrier between the extracellular compartment and the intracellular compartment or *cytosol*. The sarcolemma, which is only two molecules thick, consists of phospholipids and cholesterol aligned so that the lipid, or hydrophobic, portion of the molecule is on the inside of the membrane, and the hydrophilic portion of the molecule is on the outside (Fig. 3-1). The phospholipid bilayer provides a fluid barrier, like a film of oil on the surface of water, that is particularly *impermeable to diffusion of ions*. Small lipid-soluble molecules such as oxygen and carbon dioxide diffuse easily through the membrane. The water molecule, although insoluble in the membrane, is small enough that it diffuses easily through the membrane (or through pores in the membrane). Other, slightly larger molecules (sodium, chloride, potassium, calcium) cannot easily diffuse through the lipid bilayer and require specialized mechanisms (channels) for transport.[1–4]

The specialized ion transport systems within the sarcolemma consist of *membrane-spanning proteins* that float in and penetrate through the lipid bilayer, with a helical hydrophobic segment spanning the membrane and hydrophilic segments on the outside and inside of the membrane. These proteins, many of which have now been isolated and sequenced, are associated with three different types of ion transport: (1) *diffusion through transmembrane channels* that can be opened or closed (gated) in response to electrical or chemical (ligand) stimuli; (2) *exchange (antiport)* of one ion for another with binding of these ions to portions of the transmembrane protein for exchange in response to an electrochemical gradient; and (3) *active (energy-dependent) transport* of ions against an electrochemical gradient.

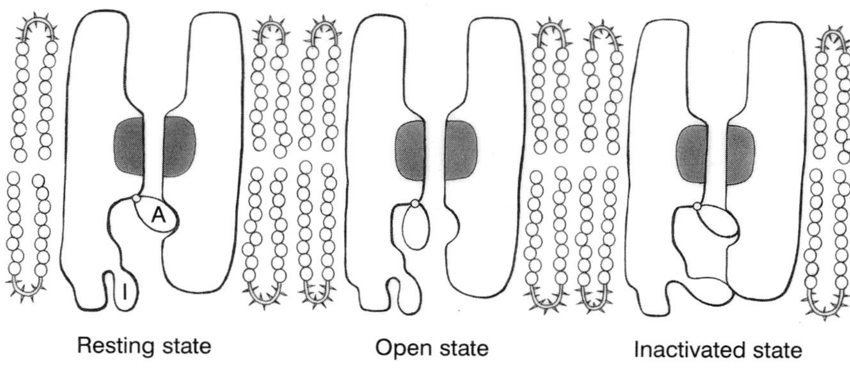

FIGURE 3–2 A sodium ion channel is schematically depicted in this figure. The shaded region within the narrow portion of the pore is the selectivity filter. *A* represents the activation gate, and *I* represents the inactivation gate. In the resting state, the inactivation gate is open and the activation gate is closed. As the transmembrane potential rises from –80 to –60 mV, the activation gate opens, leading to the open state that allows the passage of sodium ions through the channel. Within a few milliseconds, the inactivation gate closes, leading to the inactivated state.

In addition to the proteins that facilitate ion movement, other proteins are located in the sarcolemma that serve as *receptors* for neuronal or chemical control of cellular processes. Familiar examples of this type of protein are beta-adrenergic receptors and muscarinic acetylcholine receptors.

SARCOLEMMAL CHANNELS: VOLTAGE-GATED AND LIGAND-GATED

The protein components of many different ion channels have remarkably similar amino acid sequences, indicating a common evolutionary heritage. Most of the voltage-gated channels consist of tetrameters of four subunits that surround the water-filled pore through which ions cross the membrane. Each subunit has six membrane-spanning alpha helices. A schematic diagram of an ion channel is shown in Figure 3-2. Each channel contains a *selectivity filter* that selectively allows the passage of particular ions based upon pore size and electrical charge, and an *activation gate* that is regulated by conformational changes induced by either a voltage-sensitive or a ligand-binding region of the protein. Many channels also have an *inactivation gate* that is again either voltage or ligand controlled. The function of this gate will be considered in the following discussion of sodium channels.[2,3,5]

Voltage-gated sodium channels The voltage-gated sodium channel is prominent in most electrically excitable muscle and nerve cells. As will be discussed below, the energy-dependent sodium-potassium pump generates a large concentration gradient of sodium from 142 mEq/L outside the cell to 10 mEq/L inside the cell. In addition, the resting electrical membrane potential of −70 to −90 millivolts (mv) acts as a significant magnet drawing the positively charged sodium ion inward. There is, therefore, both a powerful concentration gradient and a strong electrical force favoring the influx of Na^+ from the outside of the cell to the inside; by convention, the flow of a positive ion from outside to inside is termed an *inward current*. As electrical depolarization begins, the activation gate of the sodium channel opens as the resting potential rises to between −70 and −50 mv. As the activation gate opens, Na^+ ions rapidly rush inward, thereby depolarizing the sarcolemmal membrane. The inactivation gate of the sodium channel begins to close at about the same voltage, but with a built-in time delay such that the sodium channel is open for only a few milliseconds. Because these channels open and close so quickly, they have been called *fast channels*. The sodium channel remains closed by the inactivation gate until the resting negative membrane potential of −70 to −90 mv is restored. In cardiac cells, the repolarization phase is delayed by the *plateau* of the action potential.[6–8]

Voltage-gated calcium channels There are two important populations of calcium channels. The *T (transient)-calcium channels* open as the membrane potential rises to −60 to −50 mv, and then close quickly by action of an inactivation gate. These T-calcium channels are important in early depolarization, especially in atrial pacemaker cells, but they contribute little to the sustained depolarization of the plateau of the action potential, and have much less activity in the ventricles.

A second major calcium channel, the slow channel, is especially important in cardiac muscle, since it leads to an inward (depolarizing) current that is slowly inactivated and therefore prolonged. After the initial depolarization phase of the membrane during the action potential, these slow, *L (long-lasting) channels* open at a less negative potential (−30 to −20 mv), and are inactivated slowly, thereby contributing an inward calcium current (Fig. 3-3) that sustains the action potential and provides a *pulse of cytosolic calcium* that also acts as a *trigger of* the excitation-contraction sequence. The activity of this channel is altered by catecholamine stimulation. Beta-receptor stimulation activates a G-protein that, in turn, stimulates a cyclic AMP–dependent protein kinase to phosphorylate a portion of this L-calcium channel. Conformational changes occur that cause an increased influx of calcium ions, an increased calcium accumulation, and an associated increase in the strength of sarcomere contraction. These effects can be attenuated by inhibitory G-proteins, which are activated by stimulation

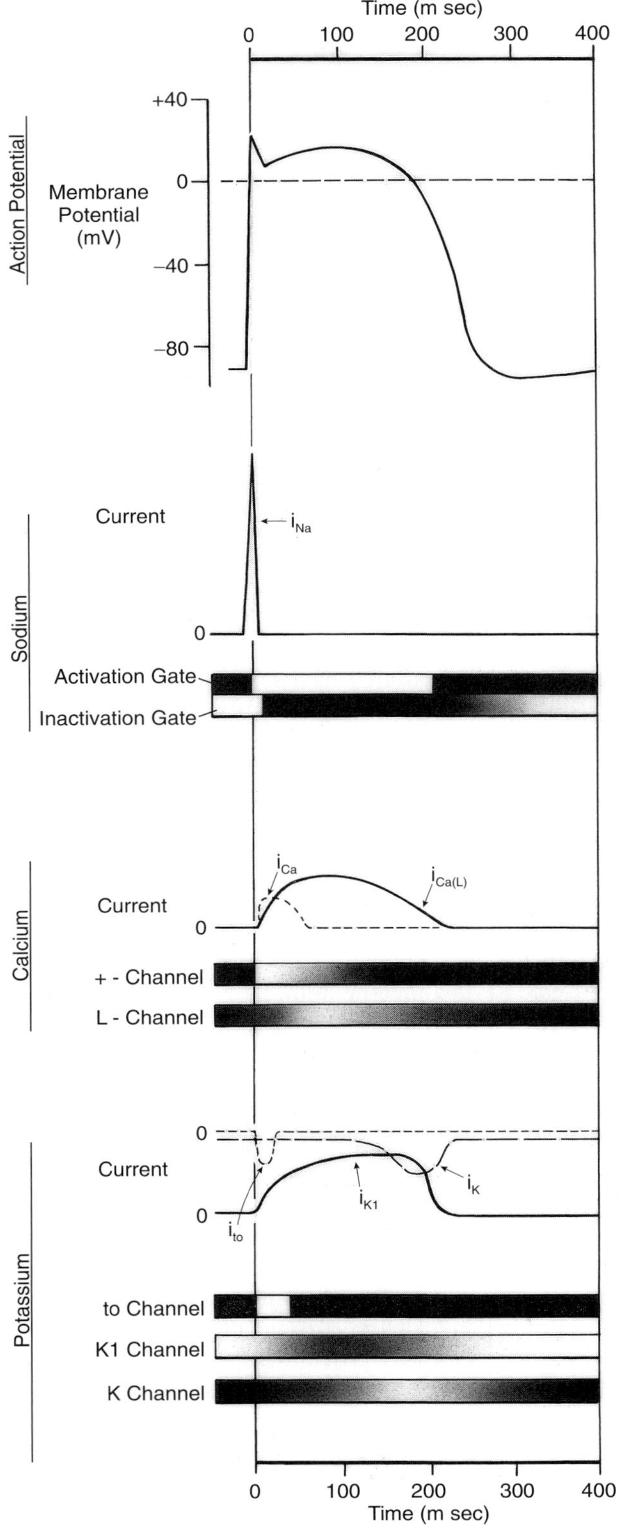

FIGURE 3–3 A typical *ventricular* myocyte action potential and the ion currents contributing to it are schematically represented. Inward (depolarizing) currents are depicted as positive, and outward (repolarizing) currents are depicted as negative. The horizontal filled bars show the state of the gate of the ion channel (white = open; black = closed; shaded = partially open). In the case of the sodium channel, both the activation and inactivation gates are shown (i = current; Na = sodium; Ca = calcium; K = potassium).

of acetylcholine and adenosine receptors. The sarcolemmal L-calcium channels are voltage-gated, but, by the receptor system, they are prominently *regulated* by the neurohumoral control system.[9,10]

Potassium channels Cardiac cells contain a variety of potassium channels, both voltage-regulated and ligand-gated. Three of these voltage-regulated potassium channels are important in the repolarization of the cell membrane.[11,12]

The potassium channel primarily responsible for the bulk of the potassium permeability of the sarcolemma is that channel associated with the *first potassium current,* or i_{K1}. This channel is *open* at negative membrane potentials and tends to close at positive membrane potentials; in fact, this channel tends to favor inward K^+ flow. With time, the channel reopens, strongly favoring repolarization at the end of the plateau (phase 2) of the action potential.

A second potassium channel is *closed* by negative membrane potentials. As the sarcolemma depolarizes, this channel opens in a delayed manner, leading to an outward current at the end of the plateau of the action (phase 2) potential, which helps to repolarize the membrane. This current is called i_K or the *delayed rectifier current*. This channel is highly *regulated,* and signal transduction molecules such as cyclic AMP, protein kinase C, and protein kinase A increase this current.[13]

A third voltage-regulated potassium channel opens briefly with depolarization, allowing a *transient outward* current, i_{to}, which contributes to very early repolarization of the action potential, thereby helping to create the hyperpolarized spike of the Purkinje fiber action potential.

Several ligand-gated potassium channels have been identified. *Acetylcholine-activated and adenosine-activated potassium channels* are time-independent, and lead to hyperpolarization in pacemaker and nodal cells, thereby delaying spontaneous depolarization. A *calcium-activated potassium channel* opens in the presence of high levels of cytosolic calcium and probably enhances the delayed rectifier current leading to early termination of the action potential. An *ATP-sensitive potassium channel* (K_{ATP} channel) is closed in the metabolically normal myocyte, but is opened in the metabolically starved myocyte in which ATP stores have been depleted, leading to hyperpolarization of the cell, thereby retarding depolarization and contraction.

ENERGY-DEPENDENT ION PUMPS AND ION EXCHANGE

Sodium-potassium ATP-dependent pump The sodium-potassium pump utilizes the energy obtained from the hydrolysis of ATP to move three Na^+ ions out of the cell and two K^+ ions into the cell. This process is fueled by the energy provided by the hydrolysis of ATP to ADP and inorganic phosphate. The energy is expended in moving both Na^+ and K^+ against a concentration gradient. Because there is a net outward current (three Na^+ ions for two K^+ ions), the pump is electrogenic, and contributes about 10 mV to the resting membrane potential. The activity of the pump is strongly stimulated by attachment of Na^+ to the Na^+ binding site on the inside of the membrane; activity of the pump increases proportionately to the *third power* of the cytosolic sodium concentration).[1] The Na-K ATPase pump has a very high affinity for ATP, so that the pump continues to function even if ATP levels are moderately reduced. There is, however, a second *regulatory* ATP binding site on the sodium pump with a lower affinity for ATP, which accelerates the turnover of ions when ATP is bound. This regulatory site on the Na^+-K^+ ATPase pump will decrease the activity of the pump during modest reductions in intracellular ATP levels.[3,14]

ATP-dependent calcium pump A second energy-dependent pump is important in regulating the calcium level of the cytosol. This pump functions by binding ATP and calcium, hydrolyzing the ATP, and utilizing the consequent energy to transport calcium out of the cell against a strong concentration gradient. This action represents a net outward current, but the magnitude of this current is quite small since the bulk of calcium transferred out of the cell occurs with sodium-calcium exchange (described below). The c-terminal portion of the protein that makes up the sarcolemmal calcium pump inhibits the pump by interacting with the ATP- and calcium-binding sites of the protein. A cytosolic protein, calmodulin, can complex with calcium and bind to this c-terminal domain, facilitating the action of the pump. The pump is therefore stimulated by increased calcium levels within the cytosol, which teleologically contributes to calcium homeostasis.[3,15,16]

Sodium-calcium exchange Yet another complex protein bridges the sarcolemma and facilitates an exchange of sodium ions for calcium ions. The energy used for this exchange comes from the electrochemical gradient favoring the influx of sodium ions into the cell. In the "forward direction," three extracellular sodium ions are exchanged for one intracellular calcium ion, leading to a net single positive charge transported into the cell with each exchange. The exchange is therefore electrogenic and may contribute a few millivolts to the resting membrane potential. The exchange system is sensitive to the concentration of sodium and calcium on both sides of the membrane, and to the membrane potential. Indeed, when the membrane is depolarized the pump may be temporarily reversed, pumping small amounts of calcium into the cell. If external sodium concentrations decrease, the driving force for removal of calcium from the cell is decreased, leading to an *increase* in cytosolic calcium (and a consequent increase in contraction). This explains an observation made some years ago that hyponatremia can lead to an *increase* in cardiac contractility. As another example, if the intracellular sodium concentration increases, as occurs with ischemia, the gradient for sodium influx is reduced, and the pump slows down or actually reverses, extruding sodium in exchange for an influx (and accumulation) of calcium. This mechanism has been suggested to be central to the accumulation of calcium during ischemia. The sodium-calcium exchange mechanism has a maximum exchange rate that is some 30 times higher than the sarcolemmal ATP-dependent calcium pump described above and is likely the primary mechanism for removal of excess cytosolic calcium.[10]

Sodium-hydrogen exchange The sodium-hydrogen exchange pump located in the sarcolemma normally (in the forward direction) extrudes one intracellular hydrogen ion in exchange for one extracellular sodium ion, and is therefore electroneutral. The energy to drive this exchange comes from the electrochemical gradient favoring sodium influx. This mechanism has been implicated in the maintenance of neutral intracellular pH. During ischemia, the intracellular accumulation of hydrogen ions essentially reverses the direction of the pump, thereby buffering the degree of intracellular acidosis, but at the expense of accumulating high concentrations of sodium ions. The accumulation of sodium ions may then trigger reversal of the sodium-calcium exchange pump to favor the accumulation of calcium intracellularly. This is a purported mechanism underlying injury or cell death during ischemia-reperfusion.

T-tubules and the Sarcoplasmic Reticulum

T-TUBULES

A system of *transverse tubules* (t-tubules) extends the sarcolemma into the interior of the cardiac cell. These tubules are generally perpendicular to the sarcomere at the level of the z-lines. The t-tubules may also run longitudinally along the sarcomere. By extending the extracellular space into the cell, the electrical excitation of the sarcolemma can be brought very close to the contractile proteins, enabling more rapid contraction and relaxation of these contractile elements than would be the case if diffusion of a transmitting chemical were the method for delivery of the contraction signal into the center of the cell. The transverse tubules contain the calcium channels described above, which are in close relationship to the *foot proteins* of the *subsarcolemmal cisternae*.

SUBSARCOLEMMAL CISTERNAE

The bulk of the sarcoplasmic reticulum (SR) in the cardiac cell contains only small amounts of RNA and is not concerned with protein synthesis. Its primary function is *excitation-contraction* coupling by sudden release of calcium to stimulate the contraction proteins and then rapid removal of this calcium to allow relaxation of the contractile elements. The *subsarcolemmal cisternae* and the *sarcotubular network* are the two portions of the sarcoplasmic reticulum concerned with this process. The subsarcolemmal cisternae are beneath the sarcolemma and surround the t-tubules. Specialized bulky proteins are found in the membrane of the sarcoplasmic reticulum with a large protein component extending into the gap between the subsarcolemmal cisternae and the sarcolemma or the t-tubule. These *foot proteins* respond to the release of calcium by the sarcolemma (or t-tubule) by rapid opening of a calcium channel (actually a part of the foot protein), which allows release of a much larger quantity of calcium from the subsarcolemmal cisternae. This is *"calcium-triggered" calcium release* with calcium transported across the sarcolemma leading to calcium release from the subsarcolemmal cisternae. The magnitude of calcium release from the subsarcolemmal cisternae appears to be related to the magnitude of the trigger. The calcium channels appear then to close (perhaps in response to the high concentrations of cytosolic calcium), and calcium uptake can occur by the energy-dependent calcium pump of the sarcoplasmic reticulum, which is located primarily in the *sarcotubular network*.[2,3,16]

THE SARCOTUBULAR NETWORK

The portion of the smooth sarcoplasmic reticulum that is responsible for the uptake of calcium from the cytosol is called the *sarcotubular network*. This network of tubules surrounds the contractile elements of the sarcomere, while the t-tubules and the sarcolemma cisternae are at the level of the z-line. Calcium uptake is accomplished by a high density of ATP-dependent calcium pumps. A large number of these pumps are necessary because calcium ion movement through the pumps is much slower than it is through calcium channels. Calcium concentration in the extracellular fluid or in the sarcoplasmic reticulum is in the millimolar level, whereas cytosolic calcium concentration is about 0.2 micromolar. This huge downhill gradient has been estimated to lead to a calcium channel flow of 3 million ions per second through a single channel. The calcium pump, on the other hand, has been estimated to pump 30 ions per second. It has been estimated that each cardiac cell contains approximately 3000 sarcolemmal calcium channels, 12,000 sarcoplasmic reticulum calcium-release channels, and 150 million sarcoplasmic reticulum calcium pump sites. The pumps appear to work throughout the cardiac cycle but their ability to remove calcium is obviously overwhelmed during the short period of time that the calcium channels are opened by depolarization.[3]

Regulation of calcium transport by the cardiac sarcoplasmic reticulum occurs primarily at the site of the calcium pump. The sarcolemmal calcium pump has a c-terminal portion that inhibits the ATPase- and calcium-binding sites of that protein, as described earlier. This c-terminal portion is not present on the sarcoplasmic reticulum calcium pump; instead, a protein called *phospholamban* in the cytosol has an amino acid sequence very similar to the c-terminal portion of the sarcolemmal calcium pump. Phospholamban inhibits the basal rate of calcium transport by the cardiac sarcoplasmic reticulum calcium pump. This inhibition can be reversed when phospholamban is phosphorylated by a cyclic AMP–dependent or a calcium-calmodulin–dependent protein kinase. This effect appears to be a very important mechanism by which beta-adrenergic stimulation regulates the heart; increased levels of cytosolic cyclic AMP are a consequence of activation of the beta catecholamine receptor. As phospholamban is phosphorylated, there is accelerated calcium turnover and increased sensitivity of the calcium pump, which facilitates uptake of calcium from the cytosol and relaxation of the heart when the heart comes under the influence of beta-adrenergic agonists. It should be noted that phosphorylation of phospholamban does *not* affect the sarcolemmal calcium pump, thereby tending to favor retention of calcium within the cell (increasing the calcium content of the sarcoplasmic reticulum at the expense of calcium removed from the cell through the sarcolemma). This might lead to an increased pulse of calcium within the cell, thereby favoring increased contractility.[10,16]

Electrical Activation of the Heart

THE NEGATIVE RESTING MEMBRANE POTENTIAL

The cardiac cell, in its polarized (diastolic) state, has a *resting electrical transmembrane potential* across the sarcolemma that is determined primarily by the concentration gradient of potassium across the membrane (developed by the sodium-potassium pump described earlier). Since the sarcolemma prevents the diffusion of large anions (e.g., proteins and organic phosphates) and is relatively permeable at rest to potassium ions because of the open state of most potassium channels but less permeable to sodium, potassium ions flow across the membrane in response to the concentration gradient. This leads to an outward flow of positive ions until a *Donnan equilibrium* is established such that the electronegativity of the cell interior retards potassium ion efflux to the same degree that the concentration gradient favors K^+ efflux. For potassium ions, this electronegativity is quantified by the Nernst equation: $Em = 61.5 \log (K_o / K_i)$. With approximate K^+ concentrations inside and outside the cell of 100 mM and 4 mM, respectively, the resting transmembrane potential of cardiac cells is predicted to be −86 mV, which is very close to measured values, suggesting that the transmembrane gradient at rest is largely a potassium current.[1,2]

DEPOLARIZATION OF THE SARCOLEMMA: THE ACTION POTENTIAL

A typical ventricular action potential is depicted in Figure 3-3. An electric current traveling longitudinally along the membrane from another cell, such as an upstream pacemaker cell, depolarizes the membrane. As the transmembrane potential decreases to approximately −60 millivolts, the "fast" sodium channel opens. This channel remains open for only a few milliseconds before the inactivation gate of the sodium channel closes. This inward movement of sodium ions causes the rapid spike of the action potential (*phase 0*); the rapid depolarization completely depolarizes the cell and, in fact, the transmembrane potential becomes slightly positive due to the positively charged amino acids on proteins. A transient potassium current (i_{to}) causes a very early repolarization (*phase 1*) of the action potential, but this fast channel closes quickly. The plateau of the action potential (*phase 2*) is sustained at a neutral or slightly positive level by an inward flowing calcium current, first from the transient calcium channel and second through the long-lasting calcium channel. The plateau is also sustained by a decrease in the outward potassium current (i_{k1}). With time, the long-lasting calcium current begins to close also, and the repolarizing potassium current (i_k, the delayed rectifier current) leads to the initiation of *phase 4* of the action potential. As repolarization progresses, the stronger first potassium current (i_{k1}) dominates, leading to full repolarization of the membrane to the resting negative potential. During the bulk of the depolarized interval (*phase 4*) the first potassium current predominates in myocardial tissue (i.e., myocytes).

Because the sodium channels cannot respond to a second wave of depolarization until the inactivation gates are reopened, the membrane is *refractory* to the propagation of a second impulse during this time interval, referred to as the *absolute refractory period*. As the membrane is repolarized during early phase 3 of the action potential, and some of the sodium channels have been reactivated, a short interval exists during which only very strong impulses can be propagated, which is termed the *relative refractory period*. A drug that acts to speed up the kinetics of the inactivation gate will shorten both the absolute and the relative refractory periods.[1–3,17–19]

SPONTANEOUS DEPOLARIZATION: PACEMAKER ACTIVITY

The action potential of the slow fibers of the nodal tissue (sinoatrial node, or SA node, and atrioventricular node, or AV node) differs from that in the fast fibers of the ventricular myocytes, as shown in Figure 3-4. The rapid upstroke and overshoot of phase 0 are less prominent or even absent due to a lack of fast Na^+ channels. In addition, the plateau phase is abbreviated because of the lack of a sustained active Na^+ inward current, and the lack of a sustained calcium current. Third, the repolarization phase leads to a resting phase that begins to depolarize again, as opposed to the relatively stable resting membrane potential of ventricular myocytes. The slowly depolarizing phase 4 resting potential is called the *diastolic depolarization current,* or the *pacemaker potential.* Continued depolarization of the membrane potential ultimately reduces it to the threshold potential that stimulates another action potential. This diastolic depolarization

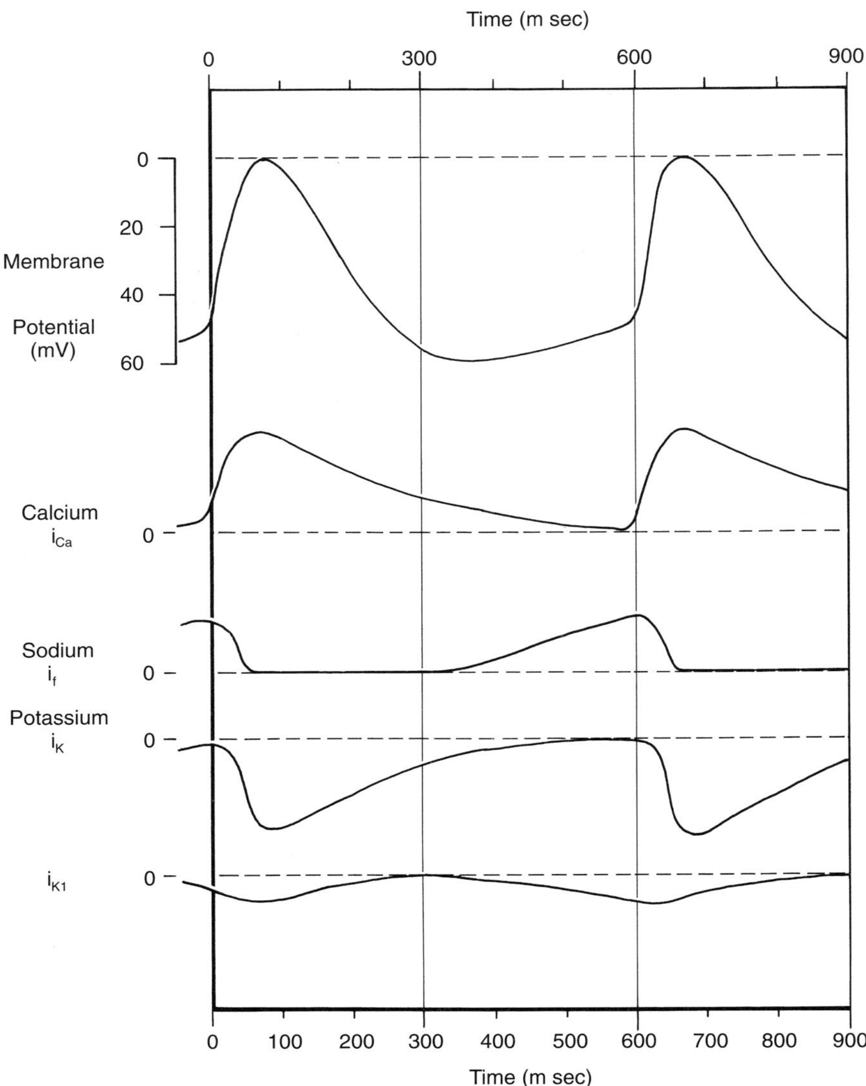

FIGURE 3–4 The membrane potential of a spontaneously depolarizing cell of the SA node, and the ion currents contributing to it. Inward (depolarizing) currents are depicted as positive, and outward (repolarizing) currents are depicted as negative (i = current; Na = sodium; Ca = calcium; K = potassium).

potential is the mechanism underlying the property of *automaticity* in cardiac pacemaker cells. Diastolic depolarization is due to the concerted and net actions of (1) a decrease in the outward K^+ current during early diastole (phase 4), (2) persistence of the slow inward Ca^{2+} current, and (3) an increasing inward Na^+ current over time during diastole. The third current most likely predominates in nodal and conduction tissue. The slope of the diastolic depolarization determines the rate of action potential generation in the pacemaker cells, and hence is a primary mechanism determining heart rate. The slope of the diastolic potential is greatest (faster rate of depolarization) in the SA node, and hence action potentials are generated at a faster rate of 70 to 80 per minute, followed by the AV node with a slightly slower rate of depolarization, and a frequency of action potential generation of 40 to 60 times per minute. The ventricular myocytes have the slowest rate of diastolic depolarization, with a frequency of 30 to 40 times per minute. Once a depolarization is initiated in a pacemaker cell and propagated, it will depolarize the remainder of the heart in a synchronized and well-choreographed manner. Hence, there is a hierarchy of pacemaker activity: the primary site in the SA node generates a heart rate of 70 to 80 beats per minute; the secondary pacemaker is a slower pacemaker site (40 to 60 per minute); and the ventricular myocytes generate 30 to 40 heart beats per minute. If a pacemaker site drops out due to pathology or drug-induced slowing of the diastolic potential, the next pacemaker site in line will take over, with a heart rate typical for that site. The slope of the diastolic depolarization, and hence heart rate, is decreased by acetylcholine (parasympathetic action); hyperpolarization (more negative resting potential) or raising the threshold potential will also increase the time to reach threshold and initiate another pacemaker signal, resulting in a decrease in heart rate. Beta-adrenergic agonists such as epinephrine and norepinephrine will accelerate the rate of depolarization, which will then increase heart rate.

PROPAGATION OF THE ACTION POTENTIAL

Each myocyte is electrically connected to the next myocyte by an intercalated disc at the end of the cell. These discs contain *gap junctions* that allow free permeability of charged molecules from one cell to the next. These pores in the intercalated discs are composed of a protein, *connexin*. Permeability through the cardiac gap junction is increased by both ATP- and cyclic AMP–dependent kinases. This allows the gap junctions to close if ATP levels fall, thereby reducing electrical and presumably mechanical activity, which is essential in limiting cell death when one region of the heart is damaged. It also allows conduction to increase when cyclic AMP increases in response to adrenergic stimulation.

After spontaneous depolarization occurs in the pacemaker cells of the AV node, the action potential is conducted throughout the heart. Special electrical pathways facilitate this conduction. These cells are, in general, large cells that lead to rapid conduction of the action potential. Three internodal paths exist through the atrium between the sinoatrial node and the atrioventricular node. After traversing the AV node, the action potential is propagated rapidly through the bundle of His and into the Purkinje fibers located on the endocardium of the left and right ventricles. Rapid conduction through the atrium causes contraction of most of the atrial muscle synchronously (within 60 to 90 milliseconds). Similarly, the rapid conduction of the signal throughout the ventricle leads to synchronous contraction of the bulk of the ventricular myocardium (within 60 milliseconds). The delay of the propagation of the action potential through the AV node by 120 to 140 milliseconds allows the atria to complete contraction before the ventricles contract (i.e., *sequential* atrioventricular contraction). Slow conduction in the AV node is related to a relatively higher internal resistance because of a small number of gap junctions between cells, and to slowly rising action potentials. In parts of the AV node, functional fast sodium channels are absent and depolarization is dependent upon the "slow" calcium channels.[2,3] The nodal delay allows the atrium to pump an aliquot of blood (up to 10% of left ventricular volume) into the ventricle just prior to ventricular contraction, thereby optimizing preload of the ventricle. The atrial contraction is shown as the "a" wave, also known as the "atrial kick," on a ventricular pressure tracing.

ARRHYTHMIAS

Aberrant pacemaker foci One innocuous type of abnormal cardiac rhythm that frequently occurs is the origin of extracardiac beats from abnormal *aberrant* pacemaker foci. Spontaneously depolarizing areas occur in the heart in the SA node, the AV node, and the His-Purkinje system. Ordinarily, the SA node spontaneously depolarizes first such that the cardiac beat originates from this primary pacemaker site. If the SA node is damaged or slowed by vagal stimulation or drugs (e.g., acetylcholine), pacemakers in the AV node or the His-Purkinje system may take over. Occasionally, aberrant foci in the heart spontaneously depolarize, thereby leading to the insertion of aberrant beats from either the atrium or the ventricle. These beats ordinarily do not interfere with the normal depolarization of the heart and have a very little tendency to degenerate into disorganized electrical activity. Therefore, these beats are generally not clinically threatening.

Reentry arrhythmias, unidirectional block A second type of cardiac rhythm, *reentry arrhythmias* are perhaps the most common dangerous cardiac rhythm. This type of rhythm is caused by propagation of an action potential through the heart in a "circus" movement. In ordinary circumstances, the action potential depolarizes the entire atrium or the entire ventricle in a short enough time interval so that all of the muscle is *refractory* to further stimulation at the same time. However, if a portion of the previously depolarized myocardium has repolarized before the propagation of the action potential is completed throughout the atrium or ventricle, then that action potential can continue its propagation into this repolarized muscle. Such an event generally requires either dramatic slowing of conduction of the action potential, a long conduction pathway, or a shortened refractory period (Fig. 3-5). All of these situations occur clinically. Ischemia leads to slowing of the sodium-potassium pump by the ATP-dependent regulation system described above, which leads to a decreased resting membrane potential and *slowing* of the propagation of the action potential. Hyperkalemia similarly leads to an increase in the extracellular potassium level, a decrease in the resting membrane potential, and a *slowing* of the propagation of the action potential. Progressive atrial dilation, as occurs with mitral valve disease, leads to a *long conduction pathway* around the atrium that can ultimately lead to the development of a reentry or "circus" movement in the atrium. Adrenergic stimulation leads to a shortened refractory period (by mechanisms described below), which increases the likelihood of a reentry arrhythmia. It should be noted that most reentry circuits require *unidirectional propagation of the action potential* along the reentry pathway. The conditions for unidirectional propagation are often created by ischemia or by myocardial damage.[3]

A special type of reentry arrhythmia occurs in the Wolff-Parkinson-White syndrome in which an *accessory pathway* electrically connects the atrium and the ventricle. This accessory pathway can complete a circular electrical pathway between the atrium and the ventricle, which meets the conditions described in the preceding paragraph for a reentry arrhythmia: conduction is unidirectional across the AV node because of the special properties of the AV node, and

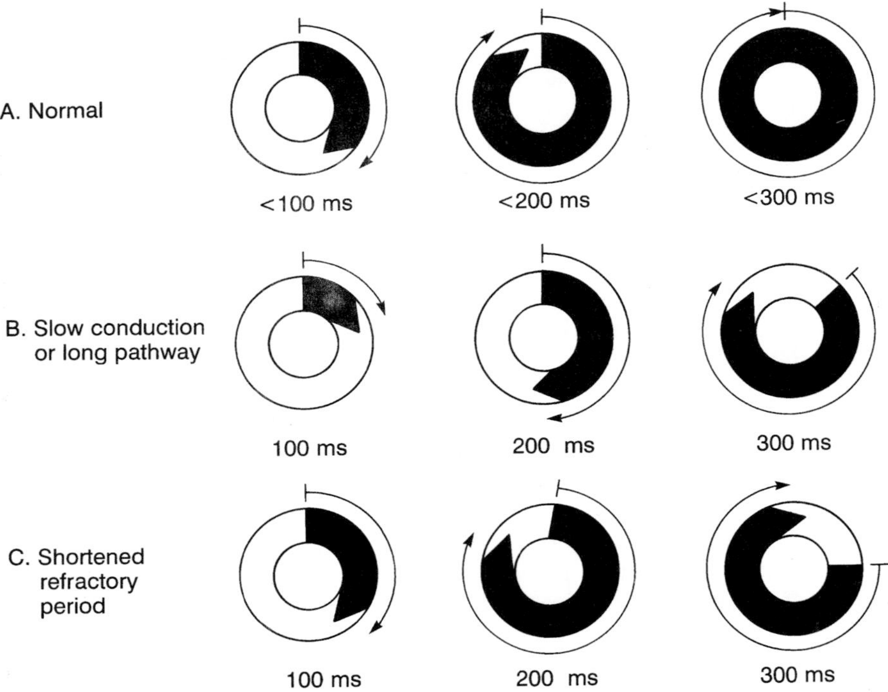

FIGURE 3–5 Three conditions predisposing to reentry or "circus" pathways for action potential propagation are shown. Muscle that is refractory to action potential propagation is shown as black. Normally, as the action potential travels through the atrium or ventricle, all the muscle is depolarized sufficiently that the action potential encounters no more nonrefractory muscle and stops (A). If there is slowed conduction speed or a long pathway (B), the action potential may find repolarized (nonrefractory) muscle and continue in a circular path. Similarly, a shortened refractory period (C) may lead to rapid repolarization and predispose to a reentry continuation of the action potential.

conduction is thereby delayed. The aberrant pathway allows retrograde induction from the ventricle back to the atrium, completing the circle necessary for the reentry circuit. We therefore have a circular pathway with unidirectional, delayed conduction. The accessory pathway of the Wolff-Parkinson-White syndrome is dangerous in another way. Because it does not have the inherent delay and refractory period of the AV node, rapid atrial tachycardias can be conducted in a 1:1 manner across the accessory pathway, leading to ventricular rates as fast as 300 beats per minute, which is a potentially lethal situation in a patient with atrial fibrillation and an accessory pathway.

Afterpotentials or parasystole Most ventricular tachyarrhythmias are reentry arrhythmias. The primary exception to this rule is *parasystole* or *afterpotentials*. Normally, ventricular action potentials have a flat phase 4 during diastole without spontaneous depolarization. If, however, they have elevated levels of cytosolic calcium, there may be a transient diastolic inward (depolarizing) current, probably related to activity of the sodium-calcium exchange pump. Afterpotentials are thought to underline the development of ventricular automaticity during digitalis toxicity. The afterdepolarizations associated with digitalis toxicity appear to be *delayed* afterdepolarizations. Another type of afterdepolarization is an *early* afterdepolarization, which occurs *before* the end of complete repolarization. This early afterdepolarization appears to be the mechanism for the ventricular tachycardia called torsades de pointes, in which varying QRS complexes appear. A prolongation of the QT interval and the varying QRS complexes in torsades de pointes indicate a heterogeneity of the action potential duration within the ventricle, thereby predisposing to ventricular fibrillation.[18]

Antiarrhythmic agents, proarrhythmic agents Antiarrhythmic agents generally act on the two major factors causing arrhythmias, e.g., automaticity and reentry. There are four classes of antiarrhythmic agents.

Class I agents are *sodium channel blockers*. Class IA agents (quinidine, procainamide) inhibit "open" sodium channels, as opposed to class IB agents, which inhibit inactive or closed sodium channels, leading to a slowing of conduction in the heart. The class IA agents have additional effects, perhaps upon the inactivation gate of the sodium channel, that prolong the action potential and thereby increase the refractory period. Class IB agents such as lidocaine and diphenylhydantoin moderately inhibit sodium channels and may shorten the refractory interval. These agents are particularly effective in inhibiting the opening of sodium channels in relatively depolarized cells so that they are especially effective in decreasing spontaneous depolarization (or automaticity), and they are useful when the myocardium is ischemic with many depolarized myocytes. Class IC agents markedly inhibit sodium channel opening, decrease the velocity of the action potential upstroke, and mildly prolong the refractory period. These agents delay conduction and prevent automaticity.

Class II antiarrhythmic drugs are drugs that cause *beta-adrenergic blockade*. These drugs inhibit adrenergic stimulation of calcium channel opening by competitively inhibiting the effect of beta-adrenergic agonists, which are discussed below.

Class III antiarrhythmic agents *prolong the cardiac action potential*. This appears to be primarily an inhibitory effect upon the repolarizing potassium current leading to an increased refractory period without a reduced conduction velocity. Examples of these drugs are amiodarone, bretylium, and sotalol. These agents have a low arrhythmogenic potential.

Class IV agents are *calcium channel blockers*. These drugs are especially important in decreasing the rate of conduction through the AV node.

Many antiarrhythmic drugs have a paradoxical *proarrhythmic* effect. As discussed above, many drugs, particularly the class IA and IC drugs, lead to a decrease in conduction velocity. As illustrated in Figure 3-5, a decrease in conduction velocity increases the likelihood of a reentry arrhythmia. If the refractory period is prolonged, as is the case with class IA drugs, then the tendency of the more rapid conduction may be counterbalanced by a longer refractory period, and reentry arrhythmias may not occur. If, on the other hand, as is the case with the class IC drugs, the conduction velocity is slowed and the refractory period is not sufficiently prolonged, reentry arrhythmias become more likely. Class IC drugs have been shown to have a great clinical risk in prolonged prophylactic use, presumably because of their proarrhythmic effect.[20]

Regulation of Cellular Function by Sarcolemmal Receptors

PARASYMPATHETIC REGULATION

The parasympathetic nervous system is particularly important in control of the pacemaker cells of the SA node. Acetylcholine released by the nerve endings of the parasympathetic system stimulates *muscarinic receptors* in the heart. These activated receptors, in turn, produce an intracellular stimulatory G-protein that opens *acetylcholine gated potassium channels*. An increased outward (repolarizing) flow of potassium leads to *hyperpolarization* of the SA node cells. Stimulation of the muscarinic receptors also inhibits the formation of cyclic AMP; decreased cyclic AMP levels inhibit the opening of calcium channels. A decreased inward flow of calcium, combined with an increased outward flow of potassium, leads to a sometimes dramatic slowing of the spontaneous diastolic depolarization of the sinoatrial nodal cell (see Fig. 3-4). A similar effect in the AV node leads to slowing of conduction through the AV node by the hyperpolarization of cells and inhibition of the slow calcium channel.[2]

ADRENERGIC STIMULATION AND BLOCKADE

Among the most important sarcolemmal receptors are the beta-adrenergic receptors. There are two types of beta-adrenergic receptors: the beta$_1$-adrenergic receptors, which predominate in the heart, and the beta$_2$-adrenergic receptors, which are present in the lungs and the liver. In the human, approximately 15% of the beta receptors in the ventricles are beta$_2$ receptors, but a larger portion of beta$_2$ receptors are present in the atrium. *Cardioselective* beta blockers (metoprolol, atenolol, acebutolol) act predominantly on the heart because there are bound more tightly to beta$_1$ receptors than to beta$_2$ receptors. The number of beta receptors per unit area of the sarcolemma is not fixed, but can increase or decrease in various circumstances. These changes are called *upregulation* or *downregulation* of receptor density, respectively. Beta receptors are downregulated after cardiopulmonary bypass and ischemia. Beta receptors can be internalized during cardiopulmonary bypass, which leads to an attenuated beta-adrenergic response by decreased receptor density. In addition to changes in receptor density, the receptors can be *desensitized* or "*internalized*" by chemical changes such that, although the receptors are still present, they are not as available for signal transmission.[21] Acidemia is associated with a desensitization of beta receptors.

The beta-adrenergic receptor couples with *adenyl cyclase*, another sarcolemmal protein. As diagrammed in Figure 3-6, when the receptor site is occupied by a catecholamine, a *stimulatory G-protein* is formed, which combines with GTP. This activated G-protein–GTP complex then promotes the activity of adenyl cyclase, leading to the formation of *cyclic AMP* from ATP. Cyclic AMP has classically been described as the "*second messenger*" of the beta-adrenergic receptor system, but one should probably consider the stimulatory G-protein to be the second messenger and cyclic AMP to be the third messenger. The stimulatory G-protein directly stimulates *calcium channel opening*. The third messenger, increased cyclic AMP, also actively promotes calcium channel opening. As described earlier in the discussion of the sarcoplasmic reticulum calcium channels, cyclic AMP and increased cytosolic calcium lead to phospholamban activation, which then leads to *increased calcium uptake* by the sarcoplasmic reticulum.

The increased tendency for calcium channels to open during beta-receptor stimulation leads to a number of electrophysiologic effects associated with these drugs. There is *accelerated discharge rate of the SA node* and other spontaneously depolarizing areas of the heart. There is *accelerated conduction* through the AV node, an area of the heart in which depolarization is particularly dependent upon calcium channels. The increased cytosolic levels of calcium lead to a *positive inotropic effect* by mechanisms to be discussed later in the chapter. The increased activity of the sarcoplasmic reticulum calcium pump stimulated by phospholamban leads to a more rapid removal of calcium from the cytoplasm at the termination of systole, thereby leading to a *more rapid relaxation of the cell*. Therefore, beta-adrenergic receptor stimulation leads to a positive *inotropic* effect, a positive *lusitropic* (relaxation) effect, a positive *chronotropic* (heart rate) effect, and a positive *dromotropic* (conduction velocity) effect. These effects are mediated by a series of messengers, the stimulatory G-protein, cyclic AMP, phospholamban, and increased cytosolic calcium levels.[22,23]

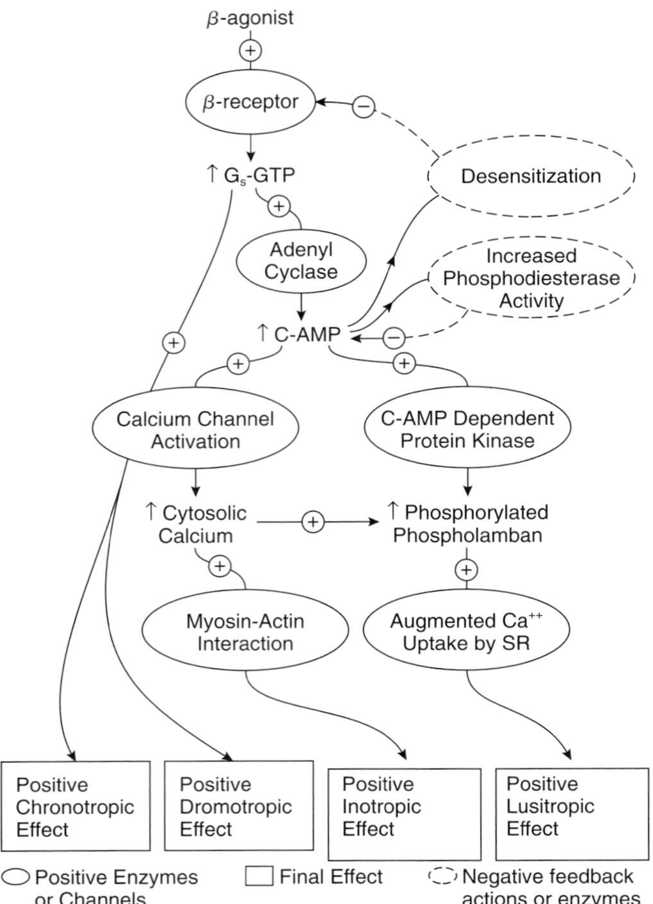

FIGURE 3–6 Adrenergic stimulation via the action of beta agonists on beta receptors leads to a cascade of events in the myocyte, some of which are shown here. Note that an increase in cyclic adenosine monophosphate (cAMP) causes the activation of two inhibitory pathways, retarding excessively sustained adrenergic stimulation (G_s = stimulatory G-protein; GTP = guanosine triphosphate; SR = sarcoplasmic reticulum).

Also shown in Figure 3-6 are two negative feedback systems that contribute to the diminished response (tachyphylaxis) observed when beta-agonist stimulation is repetitive or persistent. Increased cyclic AMP leads to increased phosphorylation of beta receptors which, in turn, leads to *internalization* of the receptor (or downregulation). Increased levels of cyclic AMP lead to increased activity of *phosphodiesterase,* the enzyme that degrades cyclic AMP.

A new class of inotropic drugs, *phosphodiestrase inhibitors* (amrinone, milrinone) inhibit the breakdown of cyclic AMP and thereby increase its level in the cytosol. Because of the site of action of the phosphodiestrase inhibitors, their effect is generally *additive* with that of beta agonists. Also, since they do not stimulate the production of the stimulatory G-protein (G_s) depicted in Figure 3-6, they have a lesser effect on calcium channel activation, and therefore have less of the troublesome positive chronotropic and dromotropic effect of beta-adrenergic stimulation.[23,24]

Cyclic AMP appears to play a central role in the regulation of the cardiac cell. Cytosolic levels of cyclic AMP are increased by activation of receptors other than beta receptors (i.e., for histamine, dopamine, glucagon), and are decreased by inhibitory G-proteins produced by stimulation of muscarinic receptors by acetylcholine and by stimulation of adenosine receptors.

Beta-blocking drugs compete with beta agonists for binding sites on the beta-adrenergic receptor, thereby preventing activation of the receptor. They cause, therefore, according to the scheme shown in Figure 3-6, a negative chronotropic effect, a negative inotropic effect, and a negative lusitropic effect. These drugs are particularly useful in pathologic conditions in which excessive adrenergic stimulation might cause ischemia by an undesirable increase in oxygen consumption. By decreasing cyclic AMP levels (and by other mechanisms) beta blockers lead to *resensitization* of beta receptors in the sarcolemma. If beta-receptor blockers are suddenly stopped, a resensitization occurs, which has led to an increased density of active beta receptors on the cell membrane. This may cause a temporarily enhanced (and potentially dangerous) sensitivity to adrenergic stimulation.

ADENOSINE

Adenosine is an especially useful drug in treating rapid supraventricular tachycardias. The vast majority of adenosine's physiological effects are exerted by interactions with sarcolemmal receptors. There are four types of adenosine receptors. The A_1 receptors are located on cardiomyocytes, and inhibit adenyl cyclase activity via an inhibitory G-protein (G_o, G_i). Activation of adenosine A_1 receptors leads to inhibition of the slow calcium channel and opening of an adenosine-activated ATP-sensitive potassium (K_{ATP}) channel. This leads to hyperpolarization in pacemaker cells, slowing spontaneous depolarization and depressed depolarization in nodal cells (remember that calcium channels are generally responsible for depolarization in these cells rather than sodium channels), and leading to delayed conduction through the AV node and a slowed ventricular response to atrial tachycardia.[2,25] Adenosine has also been used as an arresting agent in cardioplegia solutions, based on its hyperpolarizing effects, with varying degrees of success.[26,27]

CARDIAC GLYCOSIDES

Cardiac glycosides (oubain, digitoxin, digoxin) act, not through a separate receptor protein, but by binding to and inhibiting the ATP-dependent sodium-potassium pump. Inhibition of the pump leads to a slightly increased intracellular concentration of sodium. By the mechanism discussed earlier when considering the sodium-calcium exchange system, the driving force for calcium removal from the cell (the sodium gradient across the sarcolemma) is decreased, and

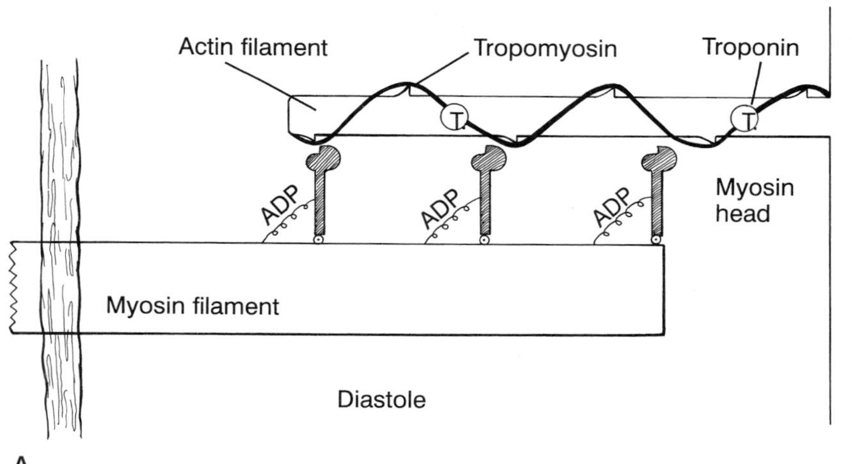

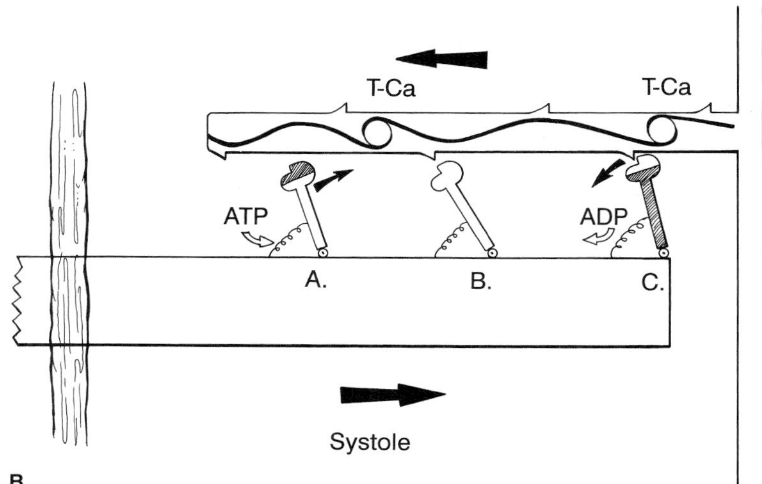

FIGURE 3–7 The interaction of actin and myosin filaments converts chemical energy into mechanical movement. In diastole, the active sites on the actin filament are covered by tropomyosin. When calcium combines with troponin, the tropomyosin is pulled away from the actin active sites, allowing the energized myosin heads (depicted in solid black and cocked at right angles to the filament) to engage and sweep the actin filament along. The myosin heads are deenergized in this process. Myosin ATPase recocks (reenergizes) the head by utilizing the energy derived from the hydrolysis of ATP. In systole, a deenergizing head (C), a deenergized head (B), and a reenergizing head (A) are shown.

the increased intracellular sodium concentration leads to less calcium binding to the intracellular portion of the sodium-calcium exchange protein. These two effects decrease the extrusion of calcium from the cell, which, in turn, leads to an increased strength of myocardial contraction, as will be discussed later. Because increased extracellular levels of potassium may stimulate the sodium-potassium pump, hyperkalemia tends to reverse the effects of digitalis toxicity, while hypokalemia tends to amplify these effects.[2,3,22]

CALCIUM CHANNEL BLOCKERS

Calcium channel blockers bind to the membrane-spanning protein of the L-type calcium channel. There are three chief categories of these drugs, represented by nifedipine, verapamil, and diltiazem. Each category appears to bind in a different site on the calcium channel protein, leading, to different effects upon these voltage-gated and time-dependent channels. Diltiazem and verapamil are particularly useful in slowing AV conduction, thereby decreasing the ventricular response to atrial tachycardias, because AV nodal depolarization is primarily dependent upon a calcium current in the general absence of functional sodium channels.[2]

CONTRACTION OF CARDIAC MUSCLE

The Contractile Element (Sarcomere)

The myocyte is made up of a number of *myofibrils*. Each myofibril is made up of a number of *sarcomeres* connected end-to-end by dense attachments between sarcomeres at the Z-band (the insertion site of the actin filament), which are in turn bundled to form myocytes. A portion of a sarcomere is schematically depicted in Figure 3-7. The sarcomere is considered to be the functional unit of the heart since the entire process of contraction and relaxation occurs within each sarcomeric unit. Each sarcomere is made up of several proteins that are important in generating cardiac contraction, or in regulating contraction. One of the major contractile proteins is *myosin,* found in the "thick filament" of the sarcomere, shown in Figure 3-7A. Myosin consists of a tail of two "heavy" chains intertwined to form a helix, forming in turn a rigid backbone of the thick filament to which a globular head is attached. The globular head of myosin is attached to the heavy chain backbone by a mobile hinge. Two pairs of light chains are associated with the hinged portion of the myosin molecule. In the sarcomere, the heavy myosin tails are connected to each other tail-to-tail, with the globular heads projecting outward. The globular head of myosin has two important biological functions. First, it binds and hydrolyzes the high-energy phosphate ATP by virtue of its ATPase activity. The resultant release of energy fuels contraction. Second, myosin has a binding site for actin, a process that is necessary for contraction to take place. Actin is the protein found in the "thin filament" of the sarcomere (Fig. 3-7A). It is a globular monomeric protein (G-actin) that is polymerized into filaments (F-actin); two filaments intertwine to form a double-stranded helix with a groove running the length of the filament. Actin has two important biological functions: (1) it binds to the myosin globular head to form the actomyosin complex; and (2) it activates the myosin ATPase to hydrolyze ATP to ADP and P_i.

In addition to the major contractile proteins actin and myosin, there are two regulatory proteins that modulate the activity of actin and myosin during the molecular process of contraction. Tropomyosin is a filamentous protein composed of two tightly coiled helical peptide chains; the helical coil of tropomyosin lays in the groove formed by the two intertwined filaments of actin. Tropomyosin binds another complex of regulatory proteins, called *troponin* ("T" in Figure 3-7A). The troponin complex consists of three units. Troponin I is the inhibitory component that covers the binding site on actin and prevents interaction with myosin and formation of the actomyosin cross-bridge. Troponin T is primarily a structural component that anchors the 3-unit troponin complex to tropomyosin. The binding of calcium to troponin C removes the troponin I–induced masking of the myosin binding site on actin, thereby allowing cross-bridge formation between actin and myosin.

During diastole, troponin C remains unbound to Ca^{2+}, and the myosin binding site on actin is inhibited from interacting with myosin. Depolarization of the sarcolemmal membrane and the t-tubule extensions of this membrane into the middle of the myocyte leads to influx of calcium ions via the sarcolemmal L-type calcium channels. This influx occurs in close proximity to the foot protein. These foot proteins are a portion of the subsarcolemmal cisternae in which a large quantity of intracellular calcium is concentrated. The increased intracellular pool of Ca^{2+} may also be contributed by the electrogenic sodium-calcium exchanger, which exchanges intracellular sodium for extracellular Ca^{2+} in a 3 Na^+:1 Ca^{2+} stoichiometry. The T-type Ca^{2+} channel may make small contributions to the "triggering" Ca^{2+} pool. The intracellular accumulation of Ca^{2+} in the proximity of the sarcoplasmic reticulum stimulates a rapid and larger-scale release of calcium from the sarcoplasmic reticulum into the cytoplasm. This mechanism of Ca^{2+} release has a high gain, prompting a cyclic or regenerative release, associated with an abundant release of Ca^{2+} per stimulation. The influx of Ca^{2+} through the sarcolemmal L-type channels and the subsequent "calcium-induced calcium release" from the sarcoplasmic reticulum increases the intracellular Ca^{2+} calcium levels by approximately two orders of magnitude (from 10^{-7} M in diastole to 10^{-5} M in systole). This Ca^{2+}-induced Ca^{2+} release from the sarcoplasmic reticulum provides sufficient calcium to bind to troponin C which, in turn, triggers the contractile sequence: the binding of Ca^{2+} to troponin C causes a conformational change in the troponin molecule, which lifts the inhibitory effect of troponin I, thereby allowing the binding between actin and myosin to form the actomyosin cross-bridge (Fig. 3-7A). Formation of the cross-bridge activates the ATPase on myosin, which then hydrolyzes ATP to ADP and P_i. The hydrolysis products are released from the myosin binding site, prompting a move in the myosin "hinge" at the globular head. This movement of the myosin globular head ratchets the actin filament forward into a contraction, thereby moving the Z-lines closer together (Fig. 3-7B). At the end of the hinge movement, calcium is removed from troponin C, the inhibition of the myosin binding site is restored, and the actin and myosin disengage. ATP reassociates with the myosin head, which then cocks the myosin globular head at the hinge, making it ready for another contraction. This process then repeats itself until the end of muscular contraction is signaled, perhaps by the removal of intracellular calcium by active energy-requiring sequestration into the sarcoplasmic reticulum by action of SERCA2, the protein associated with the sarcoplasmic reticulum responsible for calcium uptake, and by other energy-dependent pump systems. According to this molecular scheme of muscle contraction, both the contraction (systole) phase and the relaxation (diastole) phase are ATP-requiring steps. The transduction of electrical depolarization into a mechanical contraction requires the presence of calcium, making calcium the *excitation-contraction coupler*.

The strength of the myocardial contraction appears to be mediated primarily by the degree of uncovering of the actin active sites as tropomyosin is pulled away from the active sites after calcium has bound to troponin. The magnitude of this effect is dependent upon the affinity of troponin for calcium and the availability of calcium ions, that is, the magnitude of the calcium influx and accumulation during systole. The magnitude of the initial calcium ion influx through the sarcolemmal calcium channels is altered by cyclic AMP levels, by stimulatory G-proteins from beta-adrenergic receptors, and by inhibitory G-proteins from adenosine and acetylcholine receptors. This change in the magnitude of the calcium trigger leads to a change of the magnitude of the cytosolic calcium release from the sarcoplasmic reticulum. The rate of uptake of calcium from the cytosol is altered by cyclic AMP, as depicted in Figure 3-6. In addition to this mechanism, cyclic AMP can phosphorylate a portion of the troponin molecule, thereby facilitating the rapid release of calcium from troponin, and increasing the rate of relaxation of the actin-myosin complex.[10,28]

In addition to regulation of the strength of contraction by the primary mechanism of cytosolic calcium levels, the rate at which binding of ATP reenergizes the myosin heads can alter the speed and strength of the contraction. The rate of this reaction can be altered by phosphorylation of the myosin molecule during beta-adrenergic stimulation, leading to an increased rate of the myosin ATPase activity. Changes in the rate of cross-bridge cycling may also be caused by alterations in the myosin heavy chains, which is a consequence of the synthesis of various isoforms of myosin under regulation by gene expression.[3,18]

Regulation of the Strength of Contraction by Initial Sarcomere Length

In the heart, as in skeletal muscle, a relationship exists between resting sarcomere length and the strength of contraction. In skeletal muscle this relationship is bell-shaped, with maximum contraction occurring at a sarcomere length of approximately 2.2 micrometers. It has been proposed that force declines at a greater sarcomere length, because there is a decreased overlap of actin and myosin and thereby a decreased availability of actin-myosin cross-bridges. In the heart, a decrease in contractility related to decreased overlap of the filaments does not seem to occur clinically, as the resting length of the cardiac sarcomere rarely exceeds 2.2 to 2.4 micrometers. As the heart attempts to dilate beyond this state, a stiff parallel elastic element prevents further dilation. Even if chamber dilation does occur, there appears to be primarily *slippage* of fibers or myofibers rather than stretching of sarcomeres.[2] The increase in contractility that is associated with stretching of the myocardium appears rather to be related to an increased sensitivity of the contractile elements to cytosolic calcium. A calcium influx during excitation-contraction coupling that will cause approximately 50% maximal tension if the initial sarcomere length is 1.95 micrometers will lead to more than 75% maximal tension if the initial sarcomere is 2.4 micrometers.[2] This poorly understood but dramatically increased length-dependent sensitivity to calcium is an important part of the ascending limb of the Starling curve observed in the intact ventricle.

THE PUMP

Mechanics

The heart is a pump whose primary purpose is the conversion of chemical to mechanical energy to the end that blood flow can distribute oxygen and nutrients according to metabolic needs, and wash out carbon dioxide and waste products. In the preceding sections, an understanding of the conversion of ATP to mechanical energy in the form of sarcomere contraction has been developed. The electrical mechanism by which the mechanical activity of the heart is synchronized has also been considered. In this section, we will attempt to describe the function of the heart as an organ, a syncytium of myocytes made up of sarcomeres that contract in near synchrony to deliver external work by ejecting a volume of blood from the right or left ventricular cavity against an aortic or pulmonary artery pressure. The following discussion will center upon the left ventricle.

THE FRANK-STARLING RELATIONSHIP

Almost a century ago, two renowned physiologists (Frank and Starling) simultaneously developed the concept that, within physiologic limits, the heart will function as a sump pump. That is, the greater the heart is filled during diastole, the greater the quantity of blood that will be pumped out of the heart during systole. Under normal circumstances the heart pumps all the blood that comes back to it without excessive elevation of venous pressures. This relationship for the left ventricle is depicted in Figure 3-8. In the normal heart, as ventricular filling is increased, the strength of ventricular contraction increases as sarcomeres are stretched. This axiom is related by unknown mechanisms to increased sensitivity to cytosolic calcium as described earlier. This sarcomere length–dependent force of contraction is know as the Frank-Starling relationship.

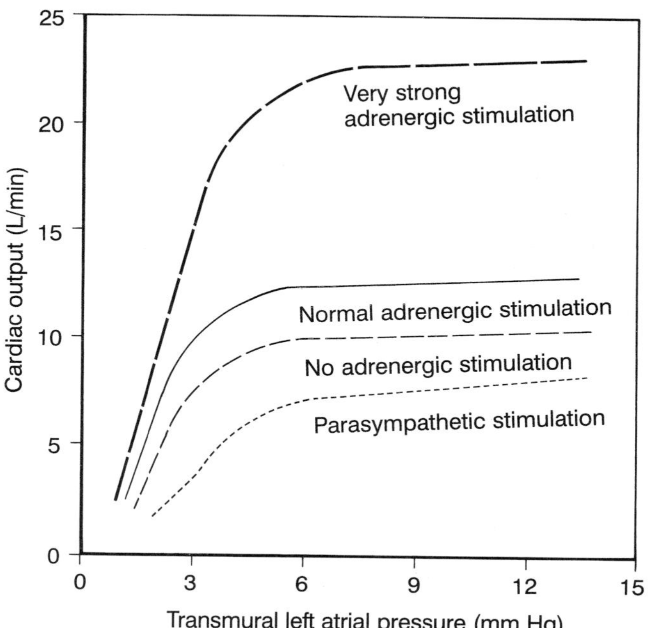

FIGURE 3–8 Starling curves for the left ventricle. The influence of four different states of neurohumoral stimulation on global ventricular performance is shown.

Also depicted in Figure 3-8 are two other states, a condition of normal adrenergic stimulation and a condition of maximal adrenergic stimulation. With sympathetic stimulation, the heart contracts more forcefully with every beat, termed a positive inotropic effect. Equally important, however, are the other stimulatory effects on chronotropic, dromotropic, and lusitropic states. The heart rate increases dramatically, conduction velocity increases, the action potential is shortened, and the velocity of contraction is increased, leading to a shortening of systole with sympathetic stimulation. An increased rate of relaxation (lusitropy) facilitates a greater rate of ventricular filling. This is particularly important with tachycardia. During pacing, the duration of systole remains relatively constant, while it is the duration of diastole that is abbreviated. If the length of systole remains at 300 milliseconds as the heart rate is increased, as it tends to do if the heart rate is increased by pacing, then when the heart rate reaches 120 with a cardiac cycle duration of 500 milliseconds, the time available for the heart to relax and fill is shortened to only 200 milliseconds. This reduction in filling time will lead to a dynamic diastolic failure of the heart with backing up of blood in the systemic and pulmonary veins. With electrical pacing, a heart rate of between 100 and 150 beats per minute will achieve a maximal cardiac output. With sympathetic stimulation, however, the accompanying positive dromotropic and inotropic effects lead to a dramatic shortening of systole relative to diastole. Because of these effects, the optimal heart rate for maximal cardiac output during sympathetic stimulation is approximately 200 beats per minute (with a cardiac cycle length of only 300 milliseconds).[1]

PRELOAD AND DIASTOLIC DISTENSIBILITY AND COMPLIANCE

The preload of the left ventricle describes the intracavitary pressure and volume immediately prior to contraction. From the clinician's point of view, preload has traditionally been considered to be the filling *pressure*. Since physiologists are more concerned with the degree of stretch of the sarcomere, preload to them generally means the initial *volume* of the ventricle. The relationship between the end-diastolic pressure and the end-diastolic volume is complex. Several different diastolic pressure-volume relationships are shown in Figure 3-9. As end-diastolic volume increases, and the heart stretches, the end-diastolic pressure also increases. The *compliance,* or distensibility of the ventricle, is defined as the change in volume divided by the change in pressure. Conversely, the *stiffness* of the ventricle is the reciprocal of compliance, or the change in pressure divided by the change in volume.

A number of factors affect the diastolic pressure-volume relationship. A fibrotic heart, a hypertrophied heart, or an aging heart becomes increasingly stiff (Figs. 3-9C and 3-9E). In the case of fibrosis, this increasing stiffness is related to the development of a greater collagen network. In the case of hypertrophy, this increased stiffness is related both to stiffening of the noncontractile components of the heart and also to impaired relaxation of the heart. Relaxation, as described earlier, is an active, energy-requiring process. This process is accelerated by catecholamine stimulation, but is impaired by ischemia, by hypothyroidism, and by chronic congestive heart failure. Examination of the diastolic pressure-volume curves in Figure 3-9 allows one to appreciate the potential importance of these changes in static (end-diastolic) and dynamic (from mitral valve opening to beginning of systole) diastolic distensibility in pathologic cardiac conditions.[29,30]

AFTERLOAD AND AORTIC IMPEDANCE

The afterload of an isolated muscle is the tension against which it contracts. When considering the heart as an organ, the afterload of the left ventricle is generally considered to be the pressure developed during ventricular systole, which in turn is determined by the aortic pressure against which the ventricle must eject. The greater the afterload, the more mechanical energy that must be imparted to the ejected blood to bring it from atrial pressure to aortic pressure. In addition to the potential energy imparted to the ejected blood by a change in pressure, the contracting left ventricle generates an additional kinetic energy. This additional kinetic energy is utilized to overcome the compliance of the distensible aorta and systemic arterial tree in order to cause the actual flow of blood into the arterial system. The energy necessary for this flow to occur is ordinarily small unless there is some obstruction to flow, such as aortic stenosis. If one considers only the energy used to change the pressure of blood, one relates afterload to *resistance,* which equals the change in pressure divided by cardiac output. If one wishes to more accurately describe the forces resisting ejection of blood from the ventricle, then one must consider compliance, kinetic energy, and potential energy, and one must speak therefore of aortic *impedance* rather than resistance. This distinction becomes important if there is an impediment to aortic flow or if disease processes alter the compliance of the aortic/arterial system.

PRESSURE-VOLUME LOOPS

The function of the heart is to generate a cardiac output and pressure that are sufficient to adequately perfuse all tissues of the body under a very wide range of conditions ranging from total rest (sleep) to strenuous exercise. Accordingly, the function of the heart can be described and quantified in terms of the pressure and volumes generated, i.e., the pressure-volume relationship. As discussed below, the *position* of the loops on the volume axis, the stroke volume (together reflecting the ejection fraction), and the trajectory (slope and x-axis intercept) of the end-systolic pressure-volume point as preload or afterload are varied are used

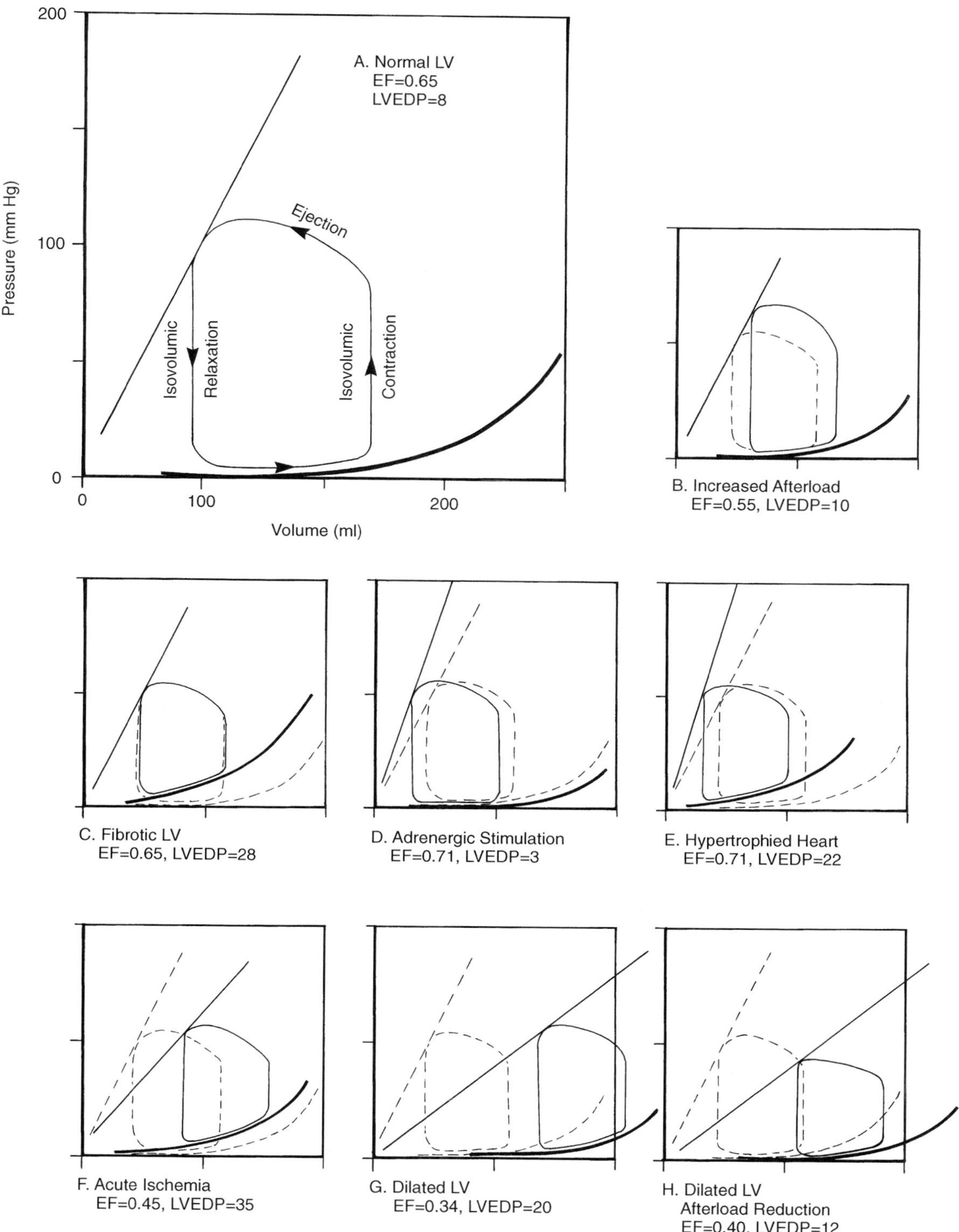

FIGURE 3–9 Left ventricular pressure-volume curves for various physiologic and pathologic conditions. The bold curved line at the bottom of each loop series represents the diastolic pressure-volume relationship. The straight line located on the upper left side of each loop series is the end-systolic pressure-volume relationship. The stroke volume for each curve has been arbitrarily set at 75 mL. Systolic aortic pressure is 115 mm Hg in all curves except B (increased afterload, systolic pressure 140 mm Hg) and H (reduced afterload, systolic pressure 90 mm Hg); LV = left ventricle; EF = ejection fraction; LVEDP = left ventricular end-diastolic pressure, in mm Hg.

to describe the inotropic state and overall performance of the heart, independent of preload or afterload. The basic ventricular pressure-volume "loop" formed by the simultaneous development of pressure and volume in the left ventricle is shown in Figure 3-9A. The basis for the ventricular pressure-volume relationship is the force-length relationship between sarcomere length and peak developed force in cardiac muscle. The Frank-Starling mechanism regulating force and extent of contraction (stroke volume) as a function of end-diastolic length (volume) is consistent with the pressure-volume relationships of the heart. However, the latter perspective of cardiac function has distinct advantages over the Frank-Starling relationship, as will be discussed.

Referring to Figure 3-9A, the end-diastolic point is a conventional starting point to describe the trajectory of the pressure-volume loop. Blood pressure increases after electrical activation of the left ventricle, thereby closing the mitral valve, and intraventricular pressure is generated *isovolumically* without ejection of blood volume (isovolumic contraction in Fig. 3-9A). When left ventricular pressure exceeds that in the aorta, the aortic valve opens, and ejection of blood into the aorta is accompanied by a corresponding decrease in ventricular volume (ejection phase). At the end of systolic ejection, left ventricular pressure decreases rapidly, and pressure differential between ventricle and aorta closes the aortic valve, forming the dichrotic notch, or incisura, in the aortic pressure wave, which is used clinically to mark the end of systole. Relaxation proceeds first isovolumically, since the mitral and aortic valves are both closed, followed by rapid and then slower filling phases of the ventricular chamber after the mitral valve opens (diastolic filling phase). The most important points of the pressure-volume loop from which descriptive data are derived are the *end-systolic pressure-volume* (ESPV) *point* located in the upper left corner of the loop, and *end-diastolic pressure-volume* (EDPV) *point* located in the lower right corner of the loop. The area within the pressure-volume loop represents the *internal work* of the chamber, as opposed to the *external work* determined by the product of stroke volume and aortic pressure measured external to the heart. Pressure-volume loops may be visualized clinically with ventriculography during left heart catheterization, and with echocardiography. However, accurate representation, particularly of left ventricular pressure, requires that high-fidelity measurements be made to avoid artifacts found in simple fluid-filled systems.

The inotropic state (contractility) of the left ventricular chamber relates to the strength of contraction, expressed physiologically in terms of force, velocity, and extent of muscle shortening, and expressed clinically in terms of stroke volume, cardiac output, and end-diastolic pressure and volume. Unfortunately, contractility is influenced by so many different factors, including preload, afterload, and heart rate, that it is difficult to quantify in clinically useful terms. One might compare the attempt to quantify the contractility of the heart to quantifying the vitality of a society. One can easily say that contractility and vitality have improved or diminished, but quantification and describing how and why contractility and vitality have changed are elusive. However, the instantaneous pressure-volume relationship can be used to quantify contractility, or the inotropic state, of the left (and right) ventricle. Contractility can be described physiologically using the end-systolic pressure-volume relationship (ESPVR) by the slope (E_{es}) and volume axis intercept (V_0) of the ESPVR (Fig. 3-10). A series of pressure-volume loops are inscribed during transient preload reduction induced by temporary caval occlusion, during which the loops move from right to left, or conversely during increased preload, during which the loops move from left to right. The end-systolic points in the series of declining loops conform to a linear relationship, forming the linearized end-systolic pressure-volume relationship, or ESPVR. The line connecting end-systolic pressure and volume of all the loops is actually somewhat curvilinear over a wide range of ventricular pressures (from 150 to 30 mm Hg ventricular pressure); it asymptotes horizontally at higher pressures and vertically at lower pressures. However, within a clinical range of systolic pressures (80 to 120 mm Hg), the end-systolic pressure-volume line is largely linear. An increase in inotropic state of the left ventricle is expressed as an increase in slope and sometimes a decrease in V_0. Conversely, a decrease in inotropic state is expressed as a decrease in slope (sometimes together with an increase in V_0; Fig. 3-10). The advantage of using the ESPVR to describe and quantify contractility is that hemodynamic conditions (i.e., preload, afterload) do not affect the slope or intercept descriptors used to quantify inotropic state to the same extent as they do when using the Starling curve concept of describing inotropic state.

Besides quantifying global contractility of the left ventricle, pressure-volume loops can be used to analyze various physiologic and pathophysiologic situations. Figure 3-9B demonstrates the effect of an increase in afterload. Increased afterload moves the end-systolic pressure-volume point slightly upward and to the right, thereby also increasing end-diastolic volume. In the normal heart, stroke volume can be maintained during increased afterload by increasing end-diastolic volume with a minimal rise in end-diastolic pressure, and no change in contractility is required. Note, however, that because the pressure-volume loop is shifted to the right secondary to increased end-diastolic volume, the ejection fraction is slightly decreased if stroke volume remains constant. Figure 3-9C shows the effect of a decrease in ventricular compliance (bold curve) such as may result from hypertrophy, fibrosis, or cardiac tamponade. If systolic function is maintained (same slope and volume axis intercept of the end-systolic pressure-volume line), stroke volume can be maintained without ventricular distention, but at the price of an increased end-diastolic pressure. Note that ejection fraction in this circumstance has not changed, indicating that ejection fraction generally reflects contractility or systolic function rather than diastolic function.

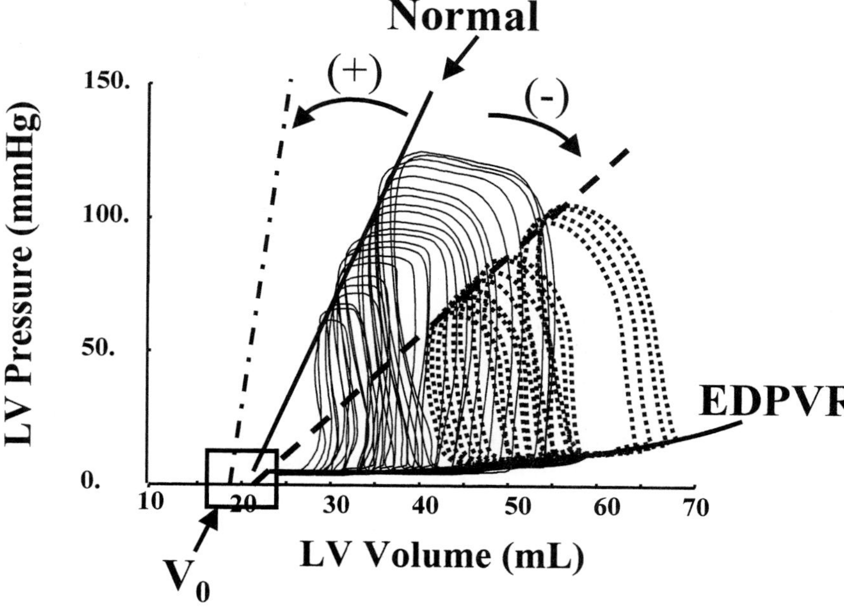

FIGURE 3–10 Two series of declining left ventricular pressure loops generated during transient bicaval occlusion. Loops were generated in normal left ventricles (Normal) and after 30 minutes of global normothermic ischemia and subsequent reperfusion (dashed lines). The end-systolic pressure-volume points from each series are connected the a line generated by linear regression. The end-diastolic pressure-volume relationship indicating chamber stiffness (inverse of compliance) is generated by fitting the end-diastolic point from each loop to an exponential curve. The volume axis intercept (V_0) is shown in the inset. A negative inotropic effect (i.e., ischemia/reperfusion) is characterized by a decrease in the ESPVR slope, while a positive inotropic state is characterized by an increase in ESPVR slope. Notice that the V_0 for these conditions are in close proximity (inset). In some cases, a negative inotropic state is associated with a decrease in slope and an increase in V_0.

Figure 3-9D demonstrates the effect of adrenergic stimulation under the conditions that stroke volume is held constant. A positive inotropic effect combines with the positive lusitropic effect of adrenergic stimulation leading to a decrease in end-diastolic pressure, a shift of the pressure-volume loop to the left, and an increase in the ejection fraction. Figure 3-9E represents the hypertrophied heart with adrenergically mediated compensation. In this situation, as opposed to that in Fig. 3-9C, diastolic compliance is decreased and systolic contractility is increased. A constant stroke volume leads to an increase in end-diastolic filling pressure with a shift of the pressure-volume loop to the left with decreased intropy, and a consequent decrease in ejection fraction. Note that the ability of the hypertrophied heart to increase stroke volume is severely limited because of decreased diastolic compliance. This example illustrates the advantage of the pressure-volume loop approach of analyzing function, in that the separate contributions of inotropic state change and preload changes can be dissected out, in contrast to the Starling curve approach. Figure 3-9F represents an ischemic heart with decreased diastolic compliance and decreased contractility. Ischemia, and subsequent reperfusion, leads to an acute shift in the pressure-volume loop to the right (reflecting loss of contractility) and up (representing a decrease in compliance) if stroke volume is to be maintained. These changes in the position of the loops in the pressure-volume plane are consistent with clinical observations of an acute decrease in ejection fraction and increase in left ventricular filling pressure.

Figure 3-9G shows the right shift of failing hearts that have undergone significant dilatation. Notice that it can be determined that filling pressures are not increased due to compliance changes per se, but rather because the left ventricle has moved upward on the compliance curve reflecting the mechanical properties of the dilated myocardium as opposed to a fibrotic process. Figure 3-9H shows the benefits of afterload reduction in the failing heart. Notice compared to Figure 3-9G that afterload reduction has moved the curve back to the left, thereby decreasing both the degree of chamber dilatation and ejection fraction. However, little benefit is gained in stroke volume unless positive inotropic agents are used, which would shift the ESPVR line to the left (toward the dashed line), and the degree of dilatation would be reduced and both stroke volume and ejection fraction would be increased.

OTHER CLINICAL INDICES OF CONTRACTILITY

For decades clinicians have attempted to assess contractility with an index that was independent of heart rate, preload, and afterload. Contractility, however, is clearly not independent of heart rate, afterload, or preload, and this attempt is futile. However, a number of indices have been described that allow the clinician to determine, in general, whether contractility has increased or decreased in clinical situations. One measure of contractility is represented by the family of Frank-Starling curves depicted in Figure 3-8. If one can determine, for example, that at a constant heart rate, aortic pressure, and cardiac output, the left ventricular preload is higher at time B than it is at time A, then one might conclude that contractility is diminished at time B relative to time A. This conclusion makes, however, the somewhat tenuous assumption that the diastolic pressure-volume relationship of the heart has not changed between time A and time B.

Ejection fraction is a second clinical index of contractility that is commonly utilized. Again ejection fraction gives one a general idea of contractility but, as can be seen by examination of the pressure-volume loops in Figure 3-9, ejection fraction is easily changed by preload and afterload alterations without requiring any change in contractility.

The use of the end-systolic pressure-volume relationship to quantify inotropic state of the left ventricle has been discussed above. The advantages of using this index, rather than the more commonly used ejection fraction and filling pressures, is that the contribution of changes in inotropic state (contributed by pathology such as ischemia, or therapy such as inotropic agents) can be separated from hemodynamic conditions or chronotropic changes. In addition, as has been discussed above, changes in inotropy can be separated from changes in filling dynamics. The disadvantage in using the pressure-volume concept clinically is that volume, or its surrogate measure diameter, is difficult to obtain.

A final index of contractility, which is perhaps a better index with regards to independence from other parameters, is the preload recruitable stroke work (PRSW) relationship. If one plots end-diastolic volume on the abscissa and stroke work on the ordinate from a family of pressure-volume loops obtained by inferior vena cava occlusion, one obtains a quite linear relationship, the slope of which appears to be related to contractility in a manner that is independent (within physiologic ranges) of preload and afterload. Internal stroke work can be determined by integration of the area of the pressure-volume loops as described above.[31] The preload recruitable stroke work can be viewed as complementary to the ESPVR. The advantage of the PRSW relationship is that it gives overall performance of the left ventricle, combining systolic and diastolic components, while the ESPVR allows one to separate these two components of performance. The PRSW shares the same difficulty in obtaining the measurement in the clinical setting.

MYOCARDIAL WALL TENSION

As changes in left ventricular geometry are considered, one must remember that the left ventricle is a pressurized, irregularly shaped chamber. The pressure within the chamber and the geometry of the ventricle determine the circumferential stress or tension in the wall of this chamber. The model of the ventricle as a cylinder can be used to approximate the effects of ventricular dilation on wall tension. In this circumstance, wall tension is proportional to the pressure times the radius of the cylinder, a relationship known as the *law of LaPlace*. Because the cylinder is thick walled, increasing wall thickness leads to decreased tension as a greater number of muscle fibers reduces the tension on each fiber. Tension, therefore, is proportional to pressure times radius divided by wall thickness. This concept has several important implications. If systolic pressure within the ventricle is chronically increased (as it is in aortic stenosis), then compensatory hypertrophy or thickening of the ventricular wall can bring systolic wall tension back close to normal. The price that is paid for this return of systolic wall tension to normal is that end-diastolic pressures must be higher (with increased wall thickness and constant chamber radius) in order to achieve the same diastolic wall tension, and thereby end-diastolic sarcomere length. This is the geometric explanation for the shift in the diastolic pressure-volume curve observed in Figure 3-9E in the hypertrophied heart.

In the heart that has systolic failure, compensation can occur with progressive ventricular dilation. This allows wall tension and diastolic sarcomere stretching to be increased at nearly normal end-diastolic pressures due to the increased diastolic diameter of the heart. Once again, there is a price to be paid. As the heart contracts, it remains dilated throughout the cardiac cycle (Fig. 3-9G). This dilation means that wall tension at end systole is also increased, thereby requiring *excessive energy utilization* from this dilated, failing heart as will be discussed in the following section.

Energetics

CHEMICAL FUELS

The major fuels that serve as an energy supply for the myocardium are carbohydrates (glucose and lactate) and nonesterified free fatty acids. Under ordinary conditions, when sufficient oxygen is present, these fuels are broken down to acetyl coenzyme A, which enters the tricarboxylic acid cycle (Krebs cycle) in the mitochondria to form ATP. The heart is quite flexible in the aerobic state in its use of fuels. In the fasting state when free fatty acid levels are high, lipids may account for 70% of the fuel utilized by the heart. On the other hand, after a high carbohydrate meal or glucose feeding, blood glucose and insulin levels are high and free fatty acids are low. Glucose will then become the major fuel of the heart, accounting for close to 100% of metabolism. During acute exercise, lactate levels rise. These elevated lactate levels inhibit the uptake of free fatty acids. Carbohydrates, mostly lactate, can then account for up to 70% of the cardiac fuel use.[32]

In hypoxic or relatively anaerobic conditions, glycolysis is stimulated, with concomitant increase in glucose uptake from the blood and breakdown of glycogen in the myocyte to glucose. This anaerobic glycolysis can produce two moles of ATP from every mole of glucose metabolized. By-products of this anaerobic system of ATP production are lactate or hydrogen ions, which, when combined with decreased cytosolic ATP levels, lead to a rapid diminution in contractility and a decreased rate of relaxation of the affected sarcomeres. There is a dramatic difference in the quantity of ATP produced by oxidative metabolism; i.e., for 1 mole of glucose, 2 moles of ATP are produced by anaerobic glycolysis, compared to 38 moles of ATP with aerobic metabolism.

Most of the ATP utilized by the heart (60%–70%) is expended in the cyclic contraction of the muscle. An additional 10% to 15% of the ATP is required for maintaining the concentration gradients across the cell membrane (primarily through the sodium-potassium pump). A small portion is wasted in so-called futile cycles, such as the constant uptake and release of calcium by mitochondria, the breakdown and regeneration of glycogen, and the synthesis of triglycerides. In all of these situations a great portion of the actual energy liberated by ATP hydrolysis is converted into heat. Only about 20% to 25% of the total chemical energy of ATP is actually converted into mechanical work.

ATP is compartmentalized in the cell in the mitochondrial and cytosolic compartments. ATP molecules generated within the mitochondria cannot cross the mitochondrial membrane into the cytosol. A mitochondrial *creatine kinase isoenzyme* is situated within the mitochondrial membrane such that intramitochondrial ATP can lead to generation of *creatine phosphate,* which freely traverses the outer myocardial membrane into the cytosol. In the cytosol, the shuttled creatine phosphate reacts with ADP to form ATP. The rapid formation of ATP from creatine phosphate explains the observation that, when the cell becomes acutely hypoxic, creatine phosphate levels fall rapidly to near zero, while ATP levels fall much more slowly. A specific cardiac isoenzyme of creatine kinase (CK-MB) is released into the circulating blood with myocyte necrosis, and is used as a marker for myocardial cell death.[32]

With ischemia and hypoxia, ATP breaks down to ADP and subsequently to AMP, adenosine, and inosine. Adenosine is particularly important because diffusion of this nucleoside to local coronary vessels can lead to coronary vasodilatation, which may increase local coronary flow and reverse the ischemic/hypoxic state (metabolic control mechanism of blood flow, discussed later). Adenosine, inosine, and hypoxanthine are lost from the ischemic myocardium by washout. If an aerobic state is restored, ATP levels can be partially restored by salvage pathways leading to regeneration of adenosine nucleotides from inosine, hypoxanthine, or inosine monophosphate. These salvage pathways operate fairly quickly.

The *de novo* synthesis of ATP also operates in the postischemic recovery period. However, this *de novo* synthesis takes hours or even days to restore significant ATP levels. Considerable controversy has existed concerning the ATP levels found in damaged cells, and the prediction of recovery, viability, or function. Because very low ATP values have been found in cells that subsequently recovered, it is now thought that very low ATP levels are not necessarily a *cause* of cellular necrosis, but cells dying of ischemia *always* contain very low levels of ATP. It may be that the ATP turnover rate, of which the oxygen consumption rate is a surrogate measure, is more indicative of cell viability and function.

DETERMINANTS OF OXYGEN CONSUMPTION

In the normal myocardium with adequate oxygen delivery, nearly all chemical energy used by the heart is generated by oxidative phosphorylation, regardless of the substrate used. The anaerobic metabolism is very limited in the heart since anaerobic enzymes are not present in sufficient concentrations. Therefore, the rate of oxygen consumption ($M\dot{V}O_2$) is largely indicative of the metabolic rate of the heart assuming that oxygen supply is adequate to meet or exceed demands. Therefore, measurement of $M\dot{V}O_2$ has been used to estimate the energy expenditure of the heart. Oxygen consumption is calculated as the product of the arterial-venous oxygen content difference and coronary blood flow, optionally indexed to heart weight in one fashion or another. Therefore, $M\dot{V}O_2 = ((CaO_2 - CvO_2) / CBF) / \text{heart weight}$, where $M\dot{V}O_2$ is myocardial oxygen consumption, CaO_2 is arterial oxygen content in mL O_2/100 mL blood, CvO_2 is coronary venous (i.e., coronary sinus) oxygen content in mL O_2/100 mL blood, and CBF is coronary blood flow in mL/min.

As discussed above, the bulk of the energy utilized by the contracting heart is expended in the contractile cycle. The remainder of the energy is expended in cellular homeostasis (maintaining ionic balance, cell viability) and electrical activation. Changes in the rate of oxygen consumption of the heart are directly related to changes in the contraction cycle and workload. Energy utilization by the heart can be increased by an increase in the workload of the heart, that is, the energy which the heart must impart to the blood as it passes through the left ventricle, or by a decrease in the efficiency with which the heart converts chemical energy to mechanical energy. Since the minute work of the heart is the heart rate times the stroke volume times developed pressure, then the energy imparted by the heart to the blood is related to each of these three factors. An increase in heart rate, an increase in stroke volume, or an increase in left ventricular (or aortic) pressure leads to an increase in oxygen demand. There is a great difference, however, in the change in cardiac efficiency as heart rate, stroke volume, or aortic pressure is altered.

The primary determinant of oxygen demands in the heart is the development of tension or wall stress with each cardiac cycle. This tension or wall stress must first alter series elastic elements and parallel elastic elements and to rearrange the geometry of the ventricle with each cardiac cycle before ejection even occurs. Indeed, during the period of isovolumic contraction, energy is expended by the heart without the delivery of any potential energy to the blood.[33] The energetic cost of actually ejecting blood out of the ventricular chamber is approximately 20% to 30% of that required to generate pressure isovolumically. This may lead to the conclusion that pressure work (generating pressure) is much more costly than is the volume work used to generate increased stroke volume. Studies more recent than those conducted by Sarnoff et al in the mid-1950s have shown that indeed volume work is only slightly less expensive compared to pressure work. Since the increase in stroke volume as a form of volume work is also accompanied by an increase in aortic pressure, some of the energy requirement comes from generating pressure. The concept unifying pressure work and volume work, as codeterminants of oxygen demands, into a single determinant is that wall stress or wall tension is the major determinant of oxygen utilization of the heart.

Cardiac efficiency relates oxygen consumption to cardiac work. Hence, cardiac efficiency = work / $M\dot{V}O_2$. The overall efficiency of the heart ranges from 5% to 40% depending on the type of work (pressure vs. volume vs. velocity) performed.[34–37] The low efficiency of the heart is due to the expenditure of a predominant portion of the oxygen consumed in generating pressure and stretching internal elastic components of the myocardium during isovolumic systole (a form of internal work), which does not contribute to the development of stroke volume and hence to external work. The velocity of shortening, affected in part by inotropic state of the myocardium, also is not factored into the work equation, but contributes significantly to oxygen consumption.

Following cardiac surgery, cardiac efficiency generally decreases due to the increase in $M\dot{V}O_2$ relative to the cardiac work performed. The additional oxygen consumed may be due to an increase in basal metabolism and/or an increase in the cost of the excitation-contraction process, or inefficiencies of ATP production at the mitochondrial level. These changes can only be assessed using the pressure-volume approach, which limits its clinical applicability because of the problems associated with attaining ventricular volume measurements as discussed above.

Because heart rate and aortic pressure are relatively prominent in the determination of myocardial oxygen consumption, two clinical indices based upon heart rate and aortic pressure have been developed for estimation of myocardial oxygen consumption. These are the double product (the heart rate times the blood pressure) and the *tension time index* (the average ejection pressure of the left ventricle multiplied by the duration of ejection). Both of these indices correlate well with cardiac oxygen consumption, but neither takes into account the effect of ventricular dilation or altered contractility.[38] Dilation of the heart during cardiac surgery, i.e., during aortic regurgitation in the absence of left ventricular venting, during the weaning process after removal of the aortic cross-clamp, or with heart failure, is an energetic disaster. Because of the law of LaPlace, the wall tension is much greater in a dilated heart than in a small heart for any given value of developed pressure. Because the inefficiencies of cardiac contraction are associated with the development of tension in the myocardium, these inefficiencies are greatly exaggerated in the dilated heart. In the failing heart, an increase in work output cannot generally be achieved by increased contractility because of receptor downregulation or desensitization, and increased stroke volume can be accomplished only by an increase in end-systolic volume and an increase in heart rate. This leads to an exaggerated increase in oxygen utilization by the dilated heart secondary to both increased wall stress and heart rate. Similar considerations apply to the postsurgical heart, which demonstrates chamber dilatation and a decrease in stroke volume or cardiac index early after weaning from cardiopulmonary bypass.

CORONARY BLOOD FLOW

Normal Coronary Blood Flow

Resting coronary blood flow is slightly less than 1 mL per gram of heart muscle per minute. This blood flow is delivered to the heart through large epicardial conductance vessels and then into the myocardium by penetrating arteries leading to a plexus of capillaries. The bulk of the resistance to coronary flow is in the penetrating arterioles (20–120 μm in size). Because the heart is metabolically very active, there is a high density of capillaries such that there is approximately one capillary for every myocyte, with an intercapillary distance at rest of approximately 17 μm. There is a greater capillary density in subendocardial myocardium compared to subepicardial tissue. When there is an increased myocardial oxygen demand (e.g., with exercise), myocardial blood flow can increase to three or four times normal. This increased blood flow is accomplished by vasodilation of the resistance vessels, and by recruitment of additional capillaries (many of which are closed in the resting state). This capillary recruitment is important in decreasing the intercapillary distance and thereby decreasing the distance that oxygen and nutrients must diffuse through the myocardium.

The blood flow pattern from a coronary artery perfusing the left ventricle, measured by flow probe, is phasic in nature, with greater blood flow occurring in diastole than in systole.[39] The cyclical contraction and relaxation of the left ventricle produces these phases in the blood flow pattern by increasing mechanical resistance forces due to extravascular compression of the arteries and intramyocardial microvessels. There is a gradient in these systolic extravascular compressive forces, being greater or equal to intracavitary pressure in the subendocardial tissue, and decreasing toward the subepicardial tissue. Hence, compression of subendocardial vessels is greater than of subepicardial vessels. Coronary blood flow is less during systole relative to that occurring during diastole. During contraction of the myocardium, the squeezing of the myocardium increases resistance of the arterial vasculature by compressing it, termed extravascular compression. The extravascular compression and resistance to blood flow are greatest in the subendocardial tissue. Measurement of transmural blood flow distribution during systole shows that subepicardial vessels are preferentially perfused, while subendocardial vessels are significantly hypoperfused. During the end of systole, blood flow actually reverses, and becomes retrograde primarily in the epicardial surface vessels due to greater pressure generation in the underlying midmyocardial layers and endocardial layer compared to the overlying epicardial tissue.[40] During diastole, the mural vascular resistance due to extravascular compressive forces releases, and blood flow is distributed to both subepicardial and subendocardial tissue. Hence, the subendocardial myocardium is perfused primarily during diastole, while subepicardial myocardium is perfused during both systole and diastole. A greater capillary density per square millimeter in the subendocardium compared to the subepicardial tissue facilitates the distribution of blood flow to the inner layer of myocardium. In addition, the subendocardial tissue has a greater oxygen demand, requiring a greater oxygen supply from blood flow, since the wall tension generated and the sarcomere shortening is greater in this region. Therefore, the greater blood flow during diastole is due to (1) selective perfusion of the subendocardial myocardium, (2) the higher metabolic demands of the subendocardial myocardium, and (3) continued perfusion of the subepicardial tissue. Myocardial blood flow is normally greater in the subendocardial tissue than in the subepicardial tissue, reflecting the greater oxygen demands in this region.[41] This regional distribution of blood flow during the cardiac cycle has implications regarding the susceptibility of the subendocardium to tissue injury and necrosis during severe coronary artery stenosis and total ischemia.

In contrast to the phasic nature of blood flow in the left coronary artery, blood flow in the right coronary artery is relatively constant during the cardiac cycle. The constancy of blood flow is related to the lower intramural pressures and near absence of extravascular compressive forces in the right ventricle compared to the left ventricle. The lower extravascular compressive forces generated in the myocardial wall of the right ventricle do not impede blood flow to the same degree as in the left ventricle.

Control of Coronary Blood Flow

Nutrient coronary blood flow is ordinarily tightly coupled to the metabolic needs of the heart. Since approximately 70% of the oxygen available in coronary arterial blood is extracted under normal conditions, and blood flow can increase 3- to 5-fold, adjustments in coronary blood flow are the primary mechanism by which increased oxygen demands are met. Because of the aerobic nature of the myocardium, sufficient oxygen is required to meet the ambient demands of the heart. A delicate balance between oxygen needs and oxygen availability requires a precise system for regulating local coronary blood flow. Local coronary blood flow is controlled by a balance of vasodilatory and vasoconstrictor mechanisms. The three components of this delicate system are (1) the *metabolic vasodilatory system,* (2) the *neurogenic control system,* and (3) the *vascular endothelium.*[42] Mechanical factors, such as extravascular compressive forces or myogenic responses, play little part in adjusting coronary blood flow to meet ambient demands under normal circumstances.

The metabolic vasodilatory mechanism causes local vasodilation of resistance vessels whenever local nutrient blood flow is insufficient to meet metabolic demand. Moment-to-moment control of coronary tone is imposed by appropriate adjustment, principally of the resistance vessels, i.e., arterioles and precapillary sphincters. The primary mediator of the metabolic control mechanism appears to be adenosine, which is generated within the myocyte, is freely diffusible across the cell membrane, and is released into the interstitial compartment. In the abluminal compartment, adenosine acts directly upon the smooth muscle cells in the arterioles to cause relaxation by activation of A_2 receptors. Adenosine is the breakdown product of ATP hydrolysis to ADP and AMP. When blood flow is sufficient to meet oxygen demands, ADP is efficiently phosphorylated to ATP, and little adenosine is formed. However, when the oxygen supply falls below the demands even temporarily, the oxygen supply/demand mismatch can not sustain the rapid rephosphorylation of ADP to ATP, and ultimately more adenosine is formed and diffuses into the parenchyma and adjacent microvessels. This increased adenosine then dilates the vessels until sufficient oxygen is supplied to the myocardium to support ADP phosphorylation and less adenosine is formed. Adenosine is therefore the coupling agent between oxygen demands and oxygen supply. This metabolic control mechanism can rapidly adjust blood flow in response to even transient increases or decreases in energy need. Other mediators of local control of coronary blood flow are carbon dioxide, lactic acid, and histamine. Ions may play an important role in regulating coronary blood flow. A buildup of hydrogen ions in myocardium causes vasodilation; recent evidence suggests the role of a chloride channel in regulation of microcirculation.

The sympathetic nervous system acts through *alpha receptors* (which cause vasoconstriction) and *beta receptors* (which cause vasodilation). There appears to be direct innervation of the large conductance vessels and lesser direct innervation of the smaller resistance vessels, although sympathetic receptors on the smooth muscle cells of the resistance vessels certainly can respond to humoral catecholamines. Alpha receptors predominate over beta receptors such that when norepinephrine is released from the sympathetic nerve endings, vasoconstriction ordinarily occurs. A second substance, *neuropeptide-y,* appears to be stored with and released with norepinephrine, and may have a role in coronary vasoconstriction.

The endothelium plays a very important role in the regulation of local coronary blood flow. Endothelium-dependent adjustment of coronary artery blood flow is accomplished by a dynamic balance between vasodilator and vasoconstrictor factors. Vasodilators include endothelial derived relaxing factor (EDRF), identified as nitric oxide (NO•) synthesized from L-arginine by endothelial nitric oxide synthase, or eNOS) and endothelially released adenosine. The vasoconstrictors are principally represented by the endothelially derived constricting peptide endothelin-1. Nitric oxide generation from the endothelium is stimulated by a number of factors including adenosine, acetylcholine, and shear stress secondary to increased intraluminal blood flow. This nitric oxide leads to powerful vasodilation of the resistance vessels. If the endothelium is intact, acetylcholine from the sympathetic nerves or coronary artery shear stress causes vasodilation through generation of NO•. If the endothelium is not functionally intact, acetylcholine causes vasoconstriction by direct stimulation of the vascular smooth muscle to contract. NO• is a potent inhibitor of platelet aggregation and neutrophil function (superoxide generation, adherence, and migration), which has implications in the anti-inflammatory response to ischemia-reperfusion and cardiopulmonary bypass.

Endothelin-1 (ET-1) is a 21-amino-acid peptide derived from preproendothelin-1 in the endothelium by the actions of endothelin-converting enzyme (ECE). Endothelin-1 interacts principally with specific endothelin receptors, ET_A, on vascular smooth muscle, and causes smooth muscle vasoconstriction. Endothelin-1 counteracts the vasodilator effects of endogenous adenosine, NO•, and prostacyclin (PGI_2), and is important in regulating basal coronary artery blood flow in health and disease. This balance between endogenous vasoconstrictors and vasodilators in control of basal coronary artery blood flow was demonstrated in experimental studies in which ET_A receptor antagonists were infused into the coronary circulation, accompanied by an increase in coronary blood flow due to a block of endogenous ET-1–mediated constriction, and an unmasking of endogenous vasodilation (mediated partially by NO•). Endothelin-1 is rapidly synthesized in vascular endothelium, particularly during ischemia, hypoxia, and other stress conditions, where it acts in a paracrine fashion similar to the local effects of adenosine and NO•. ET-1 has a short half-life (4–7 minutes), which exceeds that of adenosine (8–12 seconds) and NO• (microseconds). However, the avid binding of ET-1 to ET_A receptors prolongs its effects beyond the half-life. Human coronary arteries demonstrate abundant endothelin-1 binding sites, suggesting that ET-1 has potentially important consequences in the control of coronary blood flow in humans. Changes in coronary blood flow in ischemia-reperfusion, congestive heart failure, hypertension, and atherosclerosis may be, in part, mediated or exacerbated by an overexpression of endothelin-1, which may overwhelm the vasodilatory effects of local autacoids like adenosine and NO•. Increased age may exacerbate the vasoconstrictor responses to ET-1, which are further exaggerated by a concomitant decrease in tonic NO• production. In addition, the levels of ET-1 have been observed to increase with myocardial ischemia-reperfusion and after cardiac surgery.

Under ordinary circumstances the metabolic vasodilatory system is by far the most powerful force acting on the resistance vessels. For example, the increased metabolic activity caused by sympathetic stimulation leads to vasodilation of the coronary arterioles through the metabolic system, despite a direct vasoconstriction effect of norepinephrine.[43–45]

Autoregulation

Coronary artery blood flow is also determined by perfusion pressure. In a noncompliant and nonreactive conduit such as plastic tubing, the flow is linearly related to pressure, and inversely related to resistance. In the coronary vasculature, however, blood flow can remain constant over a range of perfusion pressures at a constant level of work. This *autoregulation* of blood flow adjusts vascular resistance appropriately to match blood flow needs, likely by the metabolic mechanisms described above. For example, at a given level of cardiac work, a reduction in perfusion pressure is associated with a decrease in vascular resistance, thereby maintaining blood flow. Conversely, if perfusion pressure increases, vascular resistance decreases to maintain relatively constant blood flow. This autoregulatory "plateau" occurs between approximately 60 and 120 mm Hg perfusion pressure. If distal coronary artery perfusion pressure is reduced, for example, by a greater than critical stenosis (see below) or by hypotension, vasodilator capacity will be exhausted and coronary blood flow will decrease, following a linear relationship with perfusion pressure. Because the subendocardial regional of the left ventricle has a lower coronary vascular reserve, maximal dilation is reached in this region before the subepicardial tissue, and a preferential hypoperfusion of the subendocardial tissue results.

Coronary Artery Stenosis

Atherosclerotic coronary artery disease is the most common cause of death in the United States, accounting for approximately one third of all mortality. Atherosclerotic disease primarily affects the large conductance vessels of the heart. The hemodynamic effect that a coronary artery stenosis has upon blood flow may be considered in terms of *Poiseuille's law*, which describes the resistance of a viscous fluid to laminar flow through a cylindrical tube. Resistance is *inversely proportional to the fourth power of the radius and directly proportional to the length of the narrowing*. Therefore, diameter narrowing has a tremendous effect on distal vascular resistance in a diseased coronary artery. Generally, conductance vessels are sufficiently large that a 50% reduction in the diameter of the vessel has minimal hemodynamic effect. A 60% reduction in the diameter of the vessel has only a very small hemodynamic effect. As the stenosis progresses beyond 60%, however, the small decreases in diameter have significant effects on blood flow. By

Poiseuille's law a 1-cm, 80% stenosis has a resistance that is 16 times as high as the resistance of a 1-cm, 60% stenosis. Similarly, if this stenosis progresses to a 90% stenosis, the resistance is 256 times as great as the resistance of a 60% stenosis.[46]

These considerations are especially important when one understands that atherosclerosis may leave partially intact the ability of the conductance vessel to constrict. Indeed, the endothelium is often destroyed or damaged, so that the vasoconstrictor mechanisms are often relatively unopposed by the impaired vasodilatory mechanism, and hence constriction is exaggerated. Suppose an epicardial vessel has an atherosclerotic lesion leading to an 80% diameter reduction in the lumen of that vessel. If the individual should attempt to exercise or should become excited, sympathetic stimulation could lead to vasoconstriction of that epicardial vessel such that the residual lumen is further narrowed to a 90% obstruction. This would lead to a 16-fold increase in coronary vascular resistance.[47]

Another important concept is that of coronary blood flow reserve. Coronary reserve may be defined as the capacity of the coronary vasculature to increase nutrient flow. A short-term occlusion of the coronary artery, or a local infusion of a vasodilator such as adenosine, will maximally dilate the target coronary artery and unmask its coronary reserve. Ordinarily, coronary flow reserve is such that blood flow may be increased to three to four or more times resting levels. As proximal atherosclerotic disease progresses, coronary reserve remains essentially normal until the proximal stenosis exceeds 60%. As the proximal resistance with stenosis increases between 60% and 90%, coronary reserve progressively decreases as the capacity of the distal resistance vessels to dilate is exhausted. At the point where there is no coronary reserve left, but *basal* blood flow is not affected by the stenosis (i.e., is sufficient to meet demands), the stenosis becomes a critical lesion. As the proximal narrowing approaches 90%, the ability of the resistance vessels to dilate is essentially fully utilized, further dilation is not possible, and coronary reserve becomes zero. In this condition, a stimulus that increases myocardial oxygen demand (such a tachycardia, hypertension, or exercise) cannot be met by dilation of the distal vasculature, and myocardial ischemia results.[42] During exercise, turbulence in the coronary artery or sympathetic stimulation may further decrease blood flow below that predicted from the fixed stenosis, so that the degree of stenosis is dynamic.

In the human, coronary arterial vessels are end vessels with little collateral flow between major branches except in pathologic situations. With sudden coronary occlusion in the human heart there usually is very modest collateral flow through very small vessels (20–200 microns in size). Unfortunately, this flow is generally insufficient to maintain cellular viability in the collateralized region. Collateral flow gradually begins to increase over the next 8 to 24 hours, doubling by about the third day after total occlusion. Collateral blood flow development appears to be nearly complete after 1 month, restoring normal or nearly normal resting flow to the surviving myocardium in the ischemic region. Previous ischemic events or gradually developing stenoses can lead to larger preexisting collaterals in the human heart. The presence of these preexisting collaterals has been shown to be important in the prevention of ischemic damage if coronary occlusion should occur.[48]

The development of collateralized regions in the human heart leads to some unusual pathophysiologic possibilities. Presuming that the collateralized region is distal to a totally occluded conductance vessel, flow into the collateralized region is dependent upon a second, nearby conductance vessel. If this second conductance vessel develops a flow-limiting stenosis and there is a sudden sustained increase in myocardial oxygen demand, then the resistance vessels related to that second conductance vessel will dilate, causing an increased pressure gradient across the secondary proximal stenosis, decreased pressure in the collateral vessels, and consequent ischemia of the collateralized region similar to coronary steal. This can cause angina pectoris or even *infarction at a distance* (narrowing of the stenotic left anterior descending by this mechanism could cause infarction of a collateralized region on the inferior surface of the heart).

The subendocardium of the heart is particularly susceptible to reductions in perfusion caused by proximal stenosis or total occlusion. This is related to (1) the greater systolic compressive forces exerted on subendocardial vasculature during systole, (2) the smaller flow reserve in the subendocardial vascular bed due to a greater degree of vasodilation, and (3) the greater degree of wall tension and segmental shortening, and hence regional oxygen demands, compared to the subepicardial region. In addition, if the heart begins to fail acutely and end-diastolic pressure is elevated to 25, 30, or 35mm Hg, then there is diastolic as well as systolic compression of the subendocardial vasculature. Studies have shown that flow to the subepicardium of the heart is effectively autoregulated as long as the pressure in the distal coronary artery is above approximately 40 mm Hg. Flow to the subendocardium, however, is effectively autoregulated only down to a mean distal coronary artery pressure of approximately 60 to 70 mm Hg as alluded to above. Below that level, local coronary flow reserve in the subendocardium is exhausted, and local blood flow decreases linearly with decreases in distal coronary artery pressure. These effects generally lead to more extensive subendocardial ischemia and infarction than subepicardial ischemia in the face of severe coronary stenosis or coronary occlusion. Subendocardial perfusion problems are obviously increased by situations such as chronic hypertension and aortic stenosis, which lead to an increased wall thickness and increased systolic and diastolic wall tension. Aortic regurgitation particularly threatens the subendocardium as diastolic systemic arterial pressures are reduced at the same time that intraventricular systolic and diastolic pressures are elevated.[39,49]

Endothelial Dysfunction

During the last two decades, much has been learned about the active participation of the coronary vascular endothelium in regulating both coronary blood flow and interactions with inflammatory blood cells, notably polymorphonuclear leukocytes (neutrophils, PMNs). The regulation of coronary blood flow and cell-cell interactions involves vasodilator and vasoconstrictor substances released by the coronary artery vascular endothelium. One of the most well-known vasoactive substances is endothelium-derived relaxing factor (EDRF). In 1986, Furchgott first proposed that EDRF is the diffusible free radical gas nitric oxide (NO•). NO• is synthesized from L-arginine by nitric oxide synthase in the presence of molecular oxygen, and with triggering from calcium. Besides endothelium-derived NO•, a number of vasoconstrictor substances are produced by the endothelium, including endothelin-1, angiotensin II, and superoxide free radical. Under normal conditions, endothelium-derived vasodilator substances are in balance with vasoconstrictor substances. This delicate balance can be tipped by numerous diseases, including ischemia-reperfusion, hypertension, diabetes, and hypercholesterolemia, that reduce the tonic generation and release of NO•, and allow an overbalance of vasoconstrictor substance, both effects causing vasoconstriction. This impaired generation of NO• is a major manifestation of endothelial dysfunction caused by all the aforementioned diseases. Endothelial dysfunction contributes to the microvascular blood flow defects and increased inflammatory-like responses mediated principally by neutrophils that occur particularly with ischemia-reperfusion injury.

NO• normally is a major player in local regulation of coronary arterial tone by overwhelming the action of endothelium-derived vasoconstrictor substances, which are also tonically released by the coronary artery endothelium. NO• is released by the coronary vascular endothelium by both soluble factors and mechanical signals. Acetylcholine and ATP stimulate the release of NO•, while shear stress and pulsatile stress also prompt elaboration of NO•. Shear stress in the coronary vasculature is related to perfusion pressure and blood flow velocity. However, in some pathologic states the ability of the endothelium to generate nitric oxide is impaired, and vasoconstriction may predominate, mediated by the relative overexpression of endothelin-1. Reperfusion after temporary myocardial ischemia is one situation in which NO• production may be impaired, leading to a vicious cycle in which the vasodilatory reserve of the resistance vessels is reduced with a consequent and progressive "low-flow" or "no-flow" phenomenon. The coronary vascular NO• system may also be impaired in some cases after coronary artery bypass surgery. As discussed below, the involvement of endothelium-derived NO• has an impact on the pathogenesis of postoperative infarction of a revascularized area, even if that same area was not ischemic preoperatively.[50–52]

In addition to the vasodilatory effects of autacoids such as NO•, the endothelium is important in preventing cell-cell interactions between blood-borne inflammatory cells (i.e., leukocytes and platelets) that initiate a local or systemic inflammatory reaction. Inflammatory cascades occur with sepsis, ischemia-reperfusion, and cardiopulmonary bypass. Under normal conditions, the vascular endothelium repels the interaction of neutrophils and platelets with the vascular endothelium by tonically releasing adenosine and NO•, both of which have potent antineutrophil and platelet inhibitory effects. However, damage to the vascular endothelium caused by adhesion of neutrophils to its surface, and subsequent release of oxygen radicals and proteases, amplifies the inflammatory response and decreases the tonic generation and release of adenosine and NO•, which then permits further interaction with activated inflammatory cells. The activities of activated neutrophils have downstream physiological consequences on other tissues, notably the heart, including increasing vascular permeability, creating blood flow defects (no-reflow phenomenon), and promoting the pathogenesis of necrosis and apoptosis.[53] Triggers of these inflammatory reactions in the heart include cytokines (IL-1, IL-6, IL-8), complement fragments (C3a, C5a, membrane attack complex), oxygen radicals, and thrombin, which upregulate adhesion molecules expressed on both inflammatory cells (CD11a/CD18) and endothelium (P-selectin, E-selectin, and ICAM-1). The release of cytokines and complement fragments during cardiopulmonary bypass activates the vascular endothelium on a systemic basis, which contributes to the inflammatory response to cardiopulmonary bypass.[54] Both adenosine and NO• have been used therapeutically to reduce the inflammatory responses to cardiopulmonary bypass, and to reduce ischemic-reperfusion injury. This treatment has reduced endothelial damage from surgical and nonsurgical ischemia-reperfusion and cardiopulmonary bypass.[55–57]

The Sequelae of Myocardial Hypoperfusion: Infarction, Myocardial Stunning, and Myocardial Hibernation

If local coronary blood flow is acutely reduced to less than 20% of resting levels, a portion of the myocardium in the affected region will die. Cardiac muscle requires approximately 1.3 mL of oxygen per 100 g of muscle per minute for cellular survival, in comparison with approximately 8 mL of oxygen per 100 g per minute in the normally contracting left ventricle. As oxygen delivery is reduced, contraction decreases dramatically (within 8 to 10 heartbeats). If the reduction in regional myocardial blood flow is moderate, regional contraction is prominently diminished, but the metabolic processes of the heart remain intact. Stated another way, the contractile activity of the heart decreases to the point that is sustainable by the oxygen availability. This condition can lead to a chronic hypocontractile state known as *hibernation*.

Hibernation appears to be associated with a decrease in the magnitude of the pulse of calcium involved in the excitation-contraction process such that the calcium levels developed within the cytosol during each heartbeat are inadequate for effective contraction to occur. With reperfusion, hibernating myocardium can very quickly resume normal and effective contraction.[58–60]

If the extent of reduction of coronary blood flow is more severe, mild to moderate abnormalities in cellular homeostasis occur. There is reduction in cellular levels of ATP leading to a loss of adenine nucleotides from the cell. If this reduction in coronary flow is sustained, progressive loss of adenine nucleotides and the elevation of intracellular and intramitochondrial calcium may lead to cellular death and subsequent necrosis. If the myocyte is reperfused prior to irreversible damage to subcellular organelles, the myocyte may slowly recover. A period of days is necessary for full recovery of myocyte ATP levels as adenine nucleotides must be resynthesized. During this time contractile processes are impaired. This impairment seems to be related to reversible damage to the contractile proteins such that their responsiveness to cytosolic levels of calcium is diminished. The magnitude of the cytosolic pulse of calcium with each heartbeat appears to be nearly normal, but the magnitude of the consequent contraction is greatly reduced. Over a period of 1 to 2 weeks this myocardium gradually recovers. This gradually recovering myocardium is called *stunned myocardium*.[59,61]

Reperfusion of ischemic myocardium may lead to a further progression of cellular damage and necrosis rather than to immediate recovery. This *reperfusion injury* is multifactorial. Damaged endothelium in the reperfused region can cause adhesion and activation of leukocytes and platelets as described above. Oxygen free radicals can be released, particularly if reperfusion is accomplished with blood that is excessively oxygenated, causing further damage to subcellular organelles. Membrane leakage often leads to elevation of intracellular calcium levels with uptake of calcium into the mitochondria and subsequent formation of insoluble calcium phosphate crystals. Temporary derangement of the ATP-dependent sodium-potassium pump can lead to loss of cell volume regulation with consequent leakage of water into the cell, explosive cell swelling, and rupture of the cell membrane. Techniques have been developed for modification of reperfusion injury with the goal being to minimize the adverse sequelae of reperfusion, so that the maximum number of myocytes may be salvaged. As might be suspected from the previous discussion, these techniques have included leukocyte depletion or inactivation, prevention of endothelial activation, free radical scavenging, reperfusion with solutions low in calcium content, and reperfusion with hyperosmolar solutions.[62,63] Both adenosine and low-dose $NO^{\bullet}$ are among potent inflammatory agents that have shown benefit in attenuating neutrophil-mediated damage, infarction, and apoptosis.[55,64]

The metabolic changes that occur with ischemia-reperfusion represent a complex system of adaptive mechanisms that allow the myocyte to survive despite a temporary reduction in oxygen delivery. These adaptive mechanisms may be triggered by a very brief coronary occlusion (as short as 5 minutes) such that the negative sequelae of a subsequent prolonged coronary occlusion are greatly minimized. This phenomenon has been called *ischemic preconditioning*. A coronary occlusion that might cause as much as 40% myocyte death in a region subjected to prolonged ischemia may be reduced to only 10% myocyte death if the prolonged period of ischemia is preceded by a 5-minute interval of "preconditioning" coronary occlusion. After more than 13 years of aggressive research, the mechanisms of this intrinsic protective system are still elusive, and are still currently a topic of intense investigation.[62,65,66]

HEART FAILURE

Forms of Heart Failure: Systolic and Diastolic Heart Failure

Heart failure is a progressive and chronic disorder that occurs when the ability of the heart to fill and/or pump is impaired such that the heart is unable, with acceptable filling (venous) pressures, to deliver adequate blood to the tissues to meet metabolic needs at rest or during mild to moderate exercise. The syndrome of heart failure is characterized by low cardiac output, impaired exercise capacity, neurohormonal activation, and enhanced oxidative stress, as well as premature myocardial cell death. Heart failure may be primarily *systolic failure* such that an impairment of contractility leads to low cardiac output and excessive filling pressures (Fig. 3-9F). The early stages of acute myocardial infarction involving a large area of the left ventricle at risk are an example of systolic heart failure. With the loss of contractile function of the area of myocardium undergoing infarction, the ventricular mass is insufficient to maintain a normal stroke volume. Cardiomyopathy is a form of disease that affects the global myocardium, as opposed to a specific region as in myocardial infarction. In both cases, the left ventricle dilates, which causes the pressure-volume relations of the left ventricle to shift to the right (Fig. 3-9F). In this situation, the diastolic portion of the pressure-volume curves is not greatly changed. However, the global systolic performance of the heart (i.e., the ability to pump blood) may be inadequate to meet even resting needs (particularly if there is systolic bulging of a large infarction).[67,68]

Diastolic failure may occur without an impairment of systolic contractility if the myocardium becomes fibrotic or hypertrophied, or if there is an external constraint on filling such as with pericardial tamponade. Increased stiffness of the left ventricular myocardium is associated with an excessive upward shift in the diastolic pressure-volume curve

(Fig. 3-9C and 9E). The most common cause of increased myocardial stiffness is chronic hypertension with consequent left ventricular hypertrophy and diastolic stiffness (related both to myocyte hypertrophy and increased fibrosis of the ventricle).[69,70]

The most common form of heart failure is mixed systolic and diastolic failure. This is the case in chronic cardiac decompensation in which systolic function has been impaired (often by multiple myocardial infarctions) and diastolic stiffness has increased because of proliferation of interstitial cells and collagen, leading to a fibrotic heart.

Early Cardiac and Systemic Sequelae of Heart Failure

The adaptive homeostatic reactions of the body leading to heart failure depend upon the duration of the ongoing pathologic process. When cardiac function acutely deteriorates and cardiac output diminishes, adaptive hemodynamic responses come into play as an early compensatory mechanism. Neurohumoral reflexes attempt to restore both cardiac output and blood pressure. Activation of the sympathetic adrenergic system in the heart and in the peripheral vasculature causes systemic vasoconstriction (via an alpha-adrenergic effect) and increases heart rate and contractility (via a beta-adrenergic effect), responses that are evoked to maintain blood pressure. A variety of mediators formed during this adaptive stage, including norepinephrine, angiotensin II, vasopressin (antidiuretic hormone), and endothelin, not only help in renal retention of salt and water leading to rapid volume expansion but also cause vasoconstriction. Aldosterone output is increased, again helping conserve sodium. The concerted responses of the adrenergic system and the renin-angiotensin system, therefore, recruit changes in the primary determinants of stroke volume and cardiac output—preload, afterload, and contractility. These early compensatory responses to hypotension secondary to heart failure lead to an expansion of blood volume, thereby shifting the pressure-volume loop to the left as shown in Figure 3-9F (dashed line), which in turn restores cardiac output and blood pressure despite diminished contractility.

The heart responds to loss of systolic function by progressively dilating. This dilation leads to preservation of stroke volume by Frank-Starling mechanisms but increased stroke volume is achieved at the expense of ejection fraction, as shown in Figure 3-9G as a right shift in the pressure-volume relations of the left ventricle with an increase in end-diastolic volume (and pressure). In addition to a global dilatation response, acute alterations in cardiac geometry may occur early after a large myocardial infarction, with thinning of the left ventricular wall in the region of the infarct as well as expansion of overall left ventricular cavity size. This is particularly true if the infarct is apical, because of geometric considerations related to the thinness of the left ventricular wall in the region of the apex related to the short radius of curvature of the left ventricular apex. As volume expansion occurs, production of the cardiac atrial naturetic peptide is increased, which tends to prevent excessive sodium retention and inhibit activation of the renin-angiotensin and aldosterone systems.[71–77]

Cardiac and Systemic Maladaptive Consequences of Chronic Heart Failure

During the acute phase of heart failure, the above-described hemodynamic responses are adaptive and help the heart to respond to exercise, blood loss, and acute myocardial ischemia. However, as the pathological process progresses, this response becomes maladaptive and contributes significantly to long-term problems in patients with heart failure (Fig. 3-11). In the late stage of heart failure, the kidney tends to continue to retain sodium and become hyporesponsive to atrial naturetic peptide. The initial response of the heart to sympathetic stimulation is diminished with desensitization of beta-adrenergic receptors as a consequence of sustained stimulation. Circulating catecholamine levels are elevated, but these increased circulating levels are of little benefit because of progressive desensitization of receptors.[21,72]

Left ventricular dilation is accompanied, at least in the early phases, by hypertrophy of the myocytes as well as by lengthening of the myocytes as sarcomeres are added. In addition, there is significant slippage of myofibrils leading to dilation without an increase in the number of myocytes. Angiotensin and aldosterone both appear to stimulate collagen formulation and proliferation of fibroblasts in the heart, leading to an increase in the ratio of interstitial tissue to myocardial tissue in the noninfarcted regions of the heart. The progressive dilation of the heart after chronic heart failure leads to an increase in the wall tension necessary to generate systolic intracavitary pressures by the law of LaPlace. The progressive fibrosis of the heart caused by left ventricular remodeling leads to increased diastolic stiffness and an inability to increase contractility in response to increased filling pressure. Fibrosis and increased ventricular size predispose to reentry ventricular arrhythmias that are a common cause of death in the late stages of heart failure. This rapidly deteriorating clinical cycle explains the result in one clinical study in which the 5-year survival rate was only 25% in men and 38% in women.[74,76–80] Hence, heart failure progresses as a result of a vicious cycle of left ventricular dilatation and remodeling, responses that decrease cardiac performance further.

Evidence has accumulated over the past decade that suggests endothelial dysfunction, release of cytokines (including tumor necrosis factor, interleukins, interferons, and transforming growth factor), and apoptotic cell death may participate in the development of heart failure as a maladaptive reaction (Fig. 3-10). Endothelial dysfunction is evidenced by reduced responses to the endothelium-dependent

External stimuli
Heart attacks (+)
Viral infections (+)
Illicit drugs (+)
Excessive drug intake (+)

Neurohumoral regulators
Catecholamines (+)
Angiotension II (+)
Vasopressin (+)
Endothelin-1 (+)

Inflammatory reactions
Nitric oxide (-)
Free radicals (+)
Cytokines (TNFα) (+)

Growth
Early gene expression (+)
Transcription factors (+)

Acute adaptive responses (short-term)

Maintain cardiac output
Salt and water retention (+)
vasoconstriction
Arrhythmias, sudden death

Attack foreign bodies
Self-defense (+)
Myocardial stunning

Adaptive hypertrophy
Sarcomere number (+)
Maintain cardiac output

Maladaptive responses (long-term)

Cardiac output (-)
Edema
Cardiac energy demand (+)
Pulmonary congestion (+)

Endothelial dysfunction
Necrotic cell death
Apoptotic cell death

Na^+-H^+ exchanger (+)
Maladaptive hypertrophy
Remodeling
Fibrosis

Heart failure (maladaptive responses)
systolic failure
diastolic failure
Combined systolic/diastolic failure

FIGURE 3–11 A flow chart shows the pathophysiology of heart failure from stimulus (etiology) to acute adaptive and chronic maladaptive responses. (+) indicates positive stimulation; (−) indicates negative factors that tend to reduce stimulation of heart failure.

vasodilator acetylcholine, reduced production of the vasodilator autacoids adenosine and nitric oxide, and an overproduction of endothelin-1. In support of this, reduced availability of nitric oxide and increased production of vasoconstrictor agents such as endothelin and angiotensin II have been reported in failing hearts.[81] Heart failure is often accompanied by changes in the endogenous antioxidant defense mechanisms of the heart as well as evidence of oxidative injury to the myocardium. Cytokines, released from systemic and local inflammatory responses in the failing heart, not only directly activate inflammatory cells to release superoxide radicals and cause endothelial dysfunction by augmenting inflammatory cell–endothelial cell interactions as discussed previously, but may also directly induce necrotic and apoptotic myocyte cell death.[82,83] More recent data from experimental studies and clinical observations suggest that cardiomyocyte apoptosis detected in the perinecrotic zone of infarcts may account for the progression of tissue injury towards to development of negative ventricular remodeling and heart failure.[84,85] Compensatory hemodynamic alterations seen at this stage, coupled with ventricular dilation, may continually induce transcription factors and maladaptive hypertrophy. Persistent growth stimulation in terminally differentiated cells may lead paradoxically to apoptotic cell death. Recently, activation of sodium-hydrogen exchange has been linked with the hypertrophic processes and induction of the remodeling at late stage of heart failure.[86]

Therapeutic Strategies for Managing Heart Failure

Treatment of the patient with heart failure is primarily based on diagnosis, identification of causes, and the etiology of failure.[81] The interventions commonly used to treat heart failure include angiotensin-converting enzyme (ACE) inhibitors, angiotensin-receptor blockers, beta-adrenergic receptor blockers, diuretics, and aldosterone blockers. For heart failure with left ventricular systolic dysfunction induced by ischemic heart disease, for example, ACE inhibitors have shown particular clinical benefit in treating peripheral vasoconstriction by reducing afterload and diminishing the direct effect of angiotensin II in promoting fibrosis in the remodeling heart. It has not yet been established that angiotensin-receptor blockers are as effective as the ACE inhibitors, and therefore they are only good for patients who are unable to tolerate ACE inhibitors because of cough or angioedema.[87] Treatment of heart failure with beta-adrenergic receptor blockers often leads to a temporary increase in symptoms followed by a sustained and long-term improvement in cardiovascular function. This appears to be related to a reversal, at least in part, of the desensitization of adrenergic receptors. Diuretics reduce extracellular fluid retention and alleviate symptoms of heart failure, but they also lower preload and consequently decrease cardiac output by Frank-Starling mechanisms. Therefore, they should be used with frequent monitoring in patients with end-stage heart failure.[81] It has been proposed that aldosterone blockers may contribute the beneficial long-term effects in inhibition of growth factor–stimulated response that causes left ventricular dilation, remodeling, and fibrosis.[29,77,88] To date, there are several promising studies that show beneficial effects in the treatment of heart failure with antioxidant therapy, antiapoptotic agents, vasopeptide inhibitors, endothelin antagonists, tumor necrosis factor-alpha inhibitors, and sodium-hydrogen exchange inhibitors.[86,87]

Progress in the treatment of chronic congestive heart failure is a dramatic example of successful therapy based upon an understanding of pathophysiology, which in turn is possible by increasingly accurate concepts of normal cardiac physiology.

REFERENCES

1. Guyton AC: Muscle blood flow and cardiac output during exercise; the coronary circulation; and ischemic heart disease, in Guyton AC (ed): *Textbook of Medical Physiology,* Philadelphia, WB Saunders, 1991; p 234.
2. Opie LH: Fuels: carbohydrates and lipids, in Swynghedauw B, Taegtmeyer H, Ruegg JC, Carmeliet E(eds): *The Heart: Physiology and Metabolism.* New York, Raven Press, 1991; p 208.
3. Katz AM: The cardiac action potential, in Katz AM (ed): *Physiology of the Heart.* New York, Raven Press, 1992; p 438.
4. Katz AM: Regulation of cardiac contraction and relaxation, in Willerson JT, Cohn JN(eds): *Cardiovascular Medicine.* New York, Churchill Livingstone, 1995; p 790.
5. Andersen OS, Koeppe RE: Molecular determinants of channel function. *Physiol Rev* 1992; 72:S89.
6. Catterall WA: Cellular and molecular biology of voltage-gated sodium channels. *Physiol Rev* 1992; 72:S15.
7. Armstrong CM: Voltage-development ion channels and their gating. *Physiol Rev* 1992; 72:S5.
8. Levitan IB: Modulation of ion channels by protein phosphorylation and dephosphorylation. *Annu Rev Physiol* 1994; 56:193.
9. McDonald TF, Pelzer S, Trautwein, et al: Regulation and modulation of calcium channels in cardiac, skeletal, and smooth muscle cells. *Physiol Rev* 1994; 74:365.
10. Barry WH, Bridge JHB: Intracellular calcium homeostasis. *Circulation* 1993; 87:1806.
11. Pongs O: Molecular biology of voltage-dependent potassium channels. *Physiol Rev* 1992; 72:S69.
12. Pallotta BS, Wagoner PK: Voltage-dependent potassium channels since Hodgkin and Huxley. *Physiol Rev* 1992; 72:S49.
13. Agus ZS, Morad M: Modulation of cardiac ion channels by magnesium. *Annu Rev Physiol* 1991; 53:299.
14. Horisberger JD, Lemas V, Kraehenbuhl JP: Structure-function relationship of Na, K-ATPase. *Annu Rev Physiol* 1991; 53:565.
15. Carafoli E: Calcium pump of the plasma membrane. *Physiol Rev* 1991; 71:129.
16. Pozzan T, Rizzuto R, Volpe P, et al: Molecular and cellular physiology of intracellular calcium stores. *Physiol Rev* 1994; 74:595.
17. Coraboeuf E, Nargeot J: Electrophysiology of human cardiac cells. *Cardiovasc Res* 1993; 27:1713.
18. Swynghedauw B: Cardiac hypertrophy and failure, in Willerson JT, Cohn JN(eds): *Cardiovascular Medicine.* New York, Churchill Livingstone, 1995; p 771.

19. Naccarelli GV: Recognition and physiologic treatment of cardiac arrhythmias and conduction disturbances, in Willerson JT, Cohn JN (eds): *Cardiovascular Medicine.* New York, Churchill Livingstone, 1995; p 1282.
20. Naccarelli GV: Anti-arrhythmic drugs, in Willerson JT, Cohn JN (eds): *Cardiovascular Medicine.* New York, Churchill Livingstone, 1995; p 1421.
21. Homcy CJ, Vatner ST, Vatner DE: Beta-adrenergic receptor regulation in the heart in pathophysiologic states: abnormal adrenergic responsiveness in cardiac disease. *Ann Rev Physiol* 1991; 53:137.
22. Feldman AM: Classification of positive inotropic agents. *J Am Coll Cardiol* 1993; 22:1223.
23. Leier CV: Current status of non-digitalis positive inotropic drugs. *Am J Cardiol* 1992; 69:120G.
24. Honerjager P: Pharmacology of bipyridine phosphodiesterase III inhibitors. *Am Heart J* 1991; 1939.
25. Olah ME, Stiles GL: Adenosine receptors. *Annu Rev Physiol* 1992; 54:211.
26. de Jong JW, van der Meer P, Owen P, et al: Prevention and treatment of ischemic injury with nucleosides. *Bratislavske Lekarske Listy* 1991; 92:165.
27. Boehm DH, Human PA, Reichenspurner H, et al: Adenosine and its role in cardioplegia: effects on postischemic recovery in the baboon. *Transplant Proc* 1990; 22:545.
28. Ebashi S: Excitation-contraction coupling and the mechanism of muscle contraction. *Annu Rev Physiol* 1991; 53:1.
29. Klug D, Robert V, Swynghedauw B: Role of mechanical and hormonal factors in cardiac remodeling and the biologic limits of myocardial adaptation. *Am J Cardiol* 1993; 71:46A.
30. Folkow B, Svanborg B: Physiology of cardiovascular aging. *Physiol Rev* 1993; 73:725.
31. Glower DD, Spratt JA, Snow ND, et al: Linearity of the Frank-Starling relationship in the intact heart: the concept of preload recruitable stroke work. *Circulation* 1985; 71:994.
32. Taegtmeyer H: Myocardial metabolism, in Willerson JT, Cohn JN(eds): *Cardiovascular Medicine.* New York, Churchill Livingstone, 1995; p 752.
33. Indolfi C, Ross J: The role of heart rate in myocardial ischemia and infarction: implications of myocardial perfusion-contraction matching. *Prog Cardiovasc Dis* 1993; 36:61.
34. Carden DL, Young JA, Granger DN: Pulmonary microvascular injury after intestinal ischemia-reperfusion: role of P-selectin. *J Appl Physiol* 1993; 75:2529.
35. Luscinskas FW, Brock AF, Arnaout MA, et al: Endothelial-leukocyte adhesion molecule-1-dependent and leukocyte (CD11/CD18)-dependent mechanisms contribute to polymorphonuclear leukocyte adhesion to cytokine-activated human vascular endothelium. *J Immunol* 1989; 142:2257.
36. Li J, Bukoski RD: Endothelium-dependent relaxation of hypertensive resistance arteries is not impaired under all conditions. *Circ Res* 1993; 72:290.
37. Johnston WE, Robertie PG, Dudas LM, et al: Heart rate-right ventricular stroke volume relation with myocardial revascularization. *Ann Thorac Surg* 1991; 52:797.
38. Vinten-Johansen J, Duncan HW, Finkenberg JG, et al: Prediction of myocardial O_2 requirements by indirect indices. *Am J Physiol* 1982; 243:H862.
39. Beyar R: Myocardial mechanics and coronary flow dynamics, in Sideman S, Beyar R(eds): *Interactive Phenomena in the Cardiac System.* New York, Plenum Press, 1993; p 125.
40. Yamada H, Yoneyama F, Satoh K, et al: Comparison of the effects of the novel vasodilator FK409 with those of nitroglycerin in isolated coronary artery of the dog. *Br J Pharmacol* 1991; 103:1713.
41. Vinten-Johansen J, Weiss HR: Regional O_2 consumption in canine left ventricular myocardium in experimental acute aortic valvular insufficiency. *Cardiovasc Res* 1981; 15:305.
42. Bradley AJ, Alpert JS: Coronary flow reserve. *Am Heart J* 1991; 1116.
43. Umans JG, Levi R: Nitric oxide in the regulation of blood flow and arterial pressure. *Annu Rev Physiol* 1995; 57:771.
44. Gross SS, Wolin MS: Nitric oxide: pathophysiological mechanisms [review]. *Annu Rev Physiol* 1995; 57:737.
45. Highsmith RF, Blackburn K, Schmidt DJ: Endothelin and calcium dynamics in vascular smooth muscle. *Ann Rev Physiol* 1992; 54:257.
46. Katritsis D, Choi MJ, Webb-Peploe MM: Assessment of the hemodynamic significance of coronary artery stenosis: theoretical considerations and clinical measurements. *Prog Cardiovasc Dis* 1991; 34:69.
47. Cohn PF: Mechanisms of myocardial ischemia. *Am J Cardiol* 1992; 70:14G.
48. Charney R, Cohen M: The role of the coronary collateral circulation in limiting myocardial ischemia and infarct size. *Am Heart J* 1993; 126:937.
49. Guyton RA, McClenathan JH, Newman GE, et al: Significance of subendocardial ST segment depression, local ischemia and subsequent necrosis. *Am J Cardiol* 1997; 40:373.
50. Treasure CB, Alexander RW: The dysfunctional endothelium in heart failure. *J Am Coll Cardiol* 1993; 22:129A.
51. Meredith IT, Anderson TJ, Uehata A, et al: Role of endothelium in ischemic coronary syndromes. *Am J Cardiol* 1993; 72:27C–32C.
52. Harrison DG: Endothelial dysfunction in the coronary microcirculation: a new clinical entity or an experimental finding? [editorial; comment]. *J Clin Invest* 1993; 91:1.
53. Jordan JE, Zhao Z-Q, Vinten-Johansen J: The role of neutrophils in myocardial ischemia-reperfusion injury. *Cardiovasc Res* 1999; 43:860.
54. Boyle EM, Pohlman TH, Johnson MC, et al: Endothelial cell injury in cardiovascular surgery: the systemic inflammatory response. *Ann Thorac Surg* 1997; 63:277.
55. Vinten-Johansen J: Cardioprotection from ischemic-reperfusion injury by adenosine, in Abd-Elfattah AS, Wechsler AS(eds): *Purines and Myocardial Protection.* Boston, Kluwer Academic Publishers, 1995; p 315.
56. Vinten-Johansen J, Thourani VH, Ronson RS, et al: Broad spectrum cardioprotection with adenosine. *Ann Thorac Surg* 1999; 68:1942.
57. Vinten-Johansen J, Sato H, Zhao Z-Q: The role of nitric oxide and NO-donor agents in myocardial protection from surgical ischemic-reperfusion injury. *Int J Cardiol* 1995; 50:273.
58. Ross J: Myocardial perfusion-contraction matching implications for coronary heart disease and hibernation. *Circulation* 1991; 83:1076.
59. Marban E: Myocardial stunning and hibernation: the physiology behind the colloquialisms [review]. *Circulation* 1991; 83:681.
60. Guth BD, Schulz R, Heusch G: Time course and mechanisms of contractile dysfunction during acute myocardial ischemia. *Circulation* 1993; 87(suppl IV):IV-35.
61. Kusuoka H, Marban E: Cellular mechanisms of myocardial stunning [review]. *Ann Rev Physiol* 1992; 54:243.
62. Granger DN, Korthuis RJ: Physiologic mechanisms of postischemic tissue injury. *Annu Rev Physiol* 1995; 57:311.
63. Vinten-Johansen J, Thourani VH: Myocardial protection: an overview. *J Extracorp Tech* 2000; 32:38.
64. Vinten-Johansen J, Zhao Z-Q, Sato H: Reduction in surgical ischemic-reperfusion injury with adenosine and nitric oxide therapy. *Ann Thorac Surg* 1995; 60:852.
65. Klonger RA, Yellon D: Does ischemic preconditioning occur in patients? *J Am Coll Cardiol* 1994; 24:1133.
66. Carroll R, Yallon DM: Myocardial adaptation to ischemia—the preconditioning phenomenon. *Int J Cardiol* 1999; 68(suppl I): S93.

67. Gaasch WH: Diagnosis and treatment of heart failure based on left ventricular systolic or diastolic dysfunction. *JAMA* 1994; 271:1276.
68. Goldsmith SR, Dick C: Differentiating systolic from diastolic heart failure: pathophysiologic and therapeutic considerations. *Am J Med* 1993; 95:645.
69. Litwin SE, Grossman W: Diastolic dysfunctions a cause of heart failure. *J Am Coll Cardiol* 1993; 22(suppl A):49A.
70. Bonow RO, Udelson JE: Left ventricular diastolic dysfunction as a cause of congestive heart failure. *Ann Intern Med* 1992; 117:502.
71. Brandt RR, Wright RS, Redfield, et al: Atrial natriuretic in heart failure. *J Am Coll Cardiol* 1993; 22(suppl A):86A.
72. Floras JS: Clinical aspects of sympathetic activation and parasympathetic withdrawal in heart failure. *J Am Coll Cardiol* 1993; 22(suppl A):72A.
73. Swan HJC: Left ventricular systolic and diastolic dysfunction in the acute phases of myocardial ischemia and infarction, and in the later phases of recovery: function follows morphology. *Eur Heart J* 1993; 14(suppl A):48.
74. Pfeffer MA: Left ventricular remodeling after acute myocardial infarction. *Annu Rev Med* 1995; 46:455–466.
75. Cohn JN: Heart failure, in Willerson JT, Cohn JN (eds): *Cardiovascular Medicine*. New York, Churchill Livingstone, 1995; p 947.
76. Komuro I, Yazaki I: Control of cardiac gene expression by mechanical stress. *Annu Rev Physiol* 1993; 55:55.
77. Schwartz K, Chassagne C, Boheler K: The molecular biology of heart failure. *J Am Coll Cardiol* 1993; 22(suppl A):30A.
78. Weber KT, Brilla CG: Pathological hypertrophy and cardiac interstitium. *Circulation* 1991; 83:1849.
79. Ross J: Left ventricular function after coronary artery reperfusion. *Am J Cardiol* 1993; 72:91G.
80. Pfeffer JM, Fischer TA, Pfeffer MA: Angiotensin-converting enzyme inhibition and ventricular remodeling after myocardial infarction. *Annu Rev Physiol* 1995; 57:805–826.
81. Katz AM (eds): *Heart Failure: Pathophysiology, Molecular Biology, and Clinical Management*. Philadelphia, Lippincott Williams & Wilkins, 2000.
82. Mak S, Newton GE: The oxidative stress hypothesis of congestive heart failure: radical thoughts [reviews]. *Chest* 2001; 120:2035.
83. Zhao Z-Q, Velez DA, Wang N-P, et al: Progressively developed myocardial apoptotic cell death during late phase of reperfusion. *Apoptosis* 2001; 6:279.
84. Leri A, Liu Y, Malhotra A, et al: Pacing-induced heart failure in dogs enhances the expression of p53 and -53-dependent genes in ventricular myocytes. *Circulation* 1998; 97:194.
85. Elsässer A, Suzuki K, Schaper J: Unresolved issues regarding the role of apoptosis in the pathogenesis of ischemic injury and heart failure. *J Mol Cell Cardiol* 2000; 32:711.
86. Karmazyn M: Role of sodium-hydrogen exchange in cardiac hypertrophy and heart failure: a novel and promising therapeutic target. *Basic Res Cardiol* 2001; 96:325.
87. Kostuk WJ: Congestive heart failure: what can we offer our patients? *CMAJ* 2001; 165:1053.
88. Bristow MR: Changes in myocardial and vascular receptors in heart failure. *J Am Coll Cardiol* 1993; 22(suppl A):61A.

Chapter 4

Cardiac Surgical Pharmacology

James M. Bailey/Kenichi A. Tanaka/Jerrold H. Levy

Clinical pharmacology associated with cardiac surgery is fascinating and challenging. The perioperative period is often characterized by the administration of multiple, potent, rapid-acting drugs with diverse, and sometimes opposing, effects and side effects. In this chapter we summarize the pharmacology of the agents most commonly used for the treatment of the primary physiological disturbances associated with cardiac surgery, hemodynamic instability, respiratory insufficiency, and alterations of hemostasis. Even with this restriction, we must consider a wide variety of chemical classes and mechanisms of action. However, the common theme is that pharmacologic effect is achieved via control of intracellular ion fluxes.

It is worthwhile to briefly review several basic subcellular/molecular pathways. As shown in Figure 4-1, the action potential in myocardial cells is a reflection of ion fluxes across the cell membrane, especially Na^+, K^+, and Ca^{++}.[1,2] Numerous drugs used to control heart rate and rhythm act by altering Na^+ (lidocaine, procainamide), K^+ (amiodarone, bretylium), or Ca^{++} (verapamil) currents. Calcium also has a dominant effect on the inotropic state.[3,4] Myocardial contractility is a manifestation of the interaction of actin and myosin, with the conversion of chemical energy from ATP hydrolysis into mechanical energy. The interaction of actin and myosin in myocytes is inhibited by the associated protein tropomyosin. This inhibition is "disinhibited" by intracellular calcium. A very similar situation occurs in vascular smooth muscle, where the interaction of actin and myosin (leading to vasoconstriction) is modulated by the protein calmodulin, which requires calcium as a cofactor. Thus, intracellular calcium has a "tonic" effect in both the myocardium and in vascular smooth muscle.

Numerous drugs used during or around cardiac surgery act by altering intracellular calcium.[3,4] Catecholamines (epinephrine, dobutamine, etc.) with beta-agonist activity regulate intramyocyte calcium levels via the nucleotide cyclic adenosine monophosphate (cAMP) (Fig. 4-2). Beta agonists bind to receptors on the cell surface that are coupled to the intracellular enzyme adenylate cyclase via the stimulatory transmembrane GTP binding protein. This leads to increased cAMP synthesis, and cAMP in turn acts as a "second messenger" for a series of intracellular reactions culminating in higher levels of intracellular calcium during systole. Less well known is that drugs with only alpha-adrenergic agonist activity may also increase intracellular Ca^{++} levels, although by a different mechanism.[5,6] While under investigation, the probable basis for the inotropic effect of alpha-adrenergic drugs is the stimulation of phospholipase C, which catalyzes hydrolysis of phosphatidyl inositol to diacylglycerol and inositol triphosphate (Fig. 4-2). Both of these compounds increase the sensitivity of the myofilament to calcium, while inositol triphosphate stimulates the release of calcium from its intracellular storage site, the sarcoplasmic reticulum. There is still some debate about the mechanism for the inotropic effect of alpha-adrenergic agonists and its significance for the acute pharmacologic manipulation of contractility, but there is little debate about the importance of this mechanism in vascular smooth muscle, where the increase in intracellular calcium

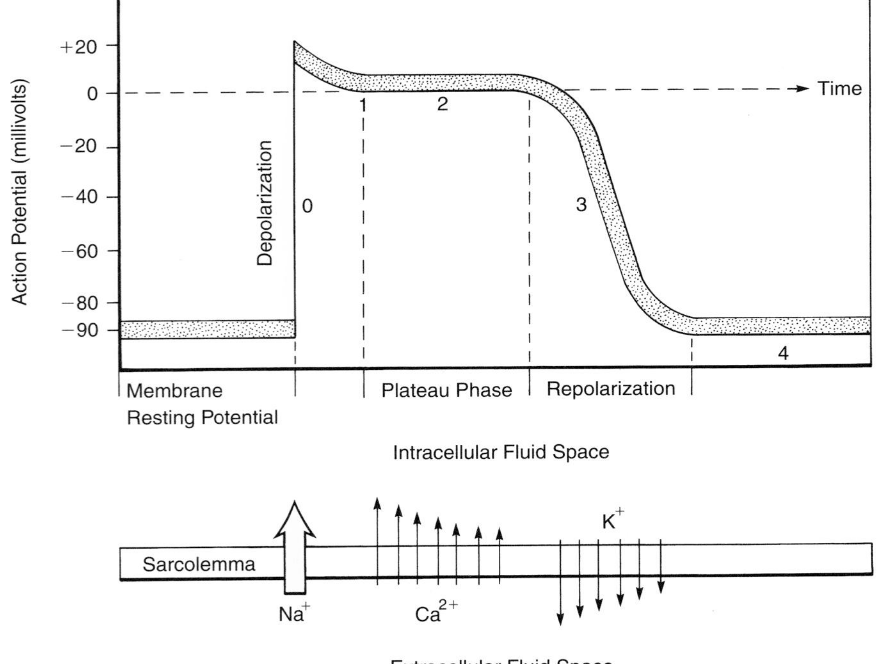

FIGURE 4–1 Cardiac ion fluxes and the action potential. The resting membrane potential is largely a reflection of the intercellular/intracellular potassium gradient. Depolarization of the membrane during phase 4 triggers an initial fast sodium channel with overshoot (phase 0) followed by recovery (phase 1) to a plateau (phase 2) maintained by an inward calcium flux, and then repolarization owing to an outward potassium flux (phase 3).

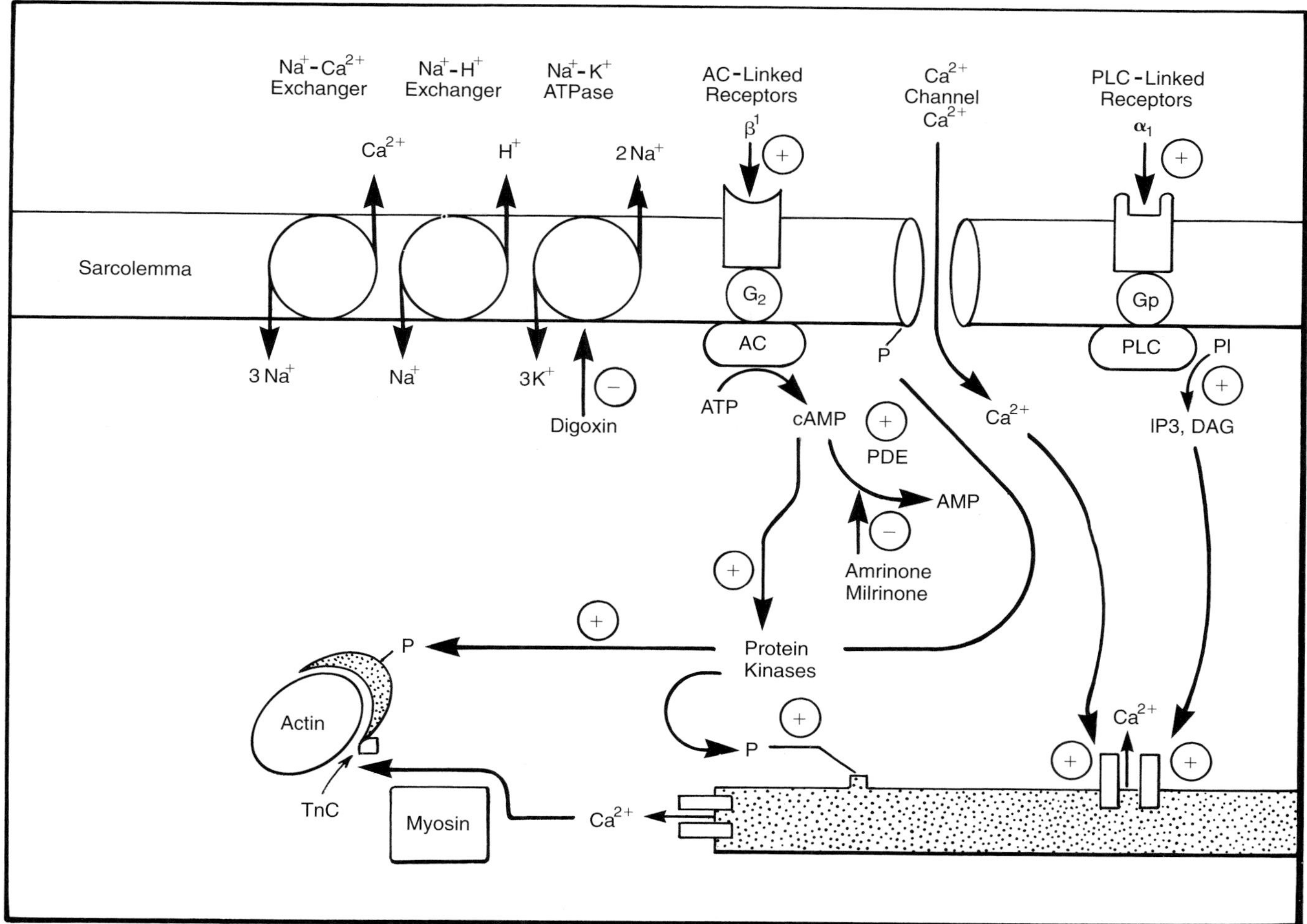

FIGURE 4–2 Mediators of cardiac contractility. Myocardial contractility is a manifestation of the interaction of actin and myosin, which is facilitated by the binding of calcium to troponin C (TnC). Intercellular calcium levels are controlled by direct flux across the membrane, by cyclic AMP, and by inositol triphosphate (IP3) and diacylglycerol (DAG) produced by the action of phospholipase C (PLC). The synthesis of cyclic AMP is catalyzed by adenylate cyclase (AC), which is activated by binding of agonist to the beta-adrenergic receptor, and its breakdown is catalyzed by phosphodiesterase (PDE), which is inhibited by amrinone and milrinone. The action of PLC is activated by binding of agonist to the alpha-adrenergic receptor.

stimulated by alpha-adrenergic agonists can significantly increase smooth muscle tone. However, intracellular calcium in vascular smooth muscle is also controlled by cyclic nucleotides.[7,8] In contrast to the myocyte, in vascular smooth muscle cAMP has a primary effect of stimulating the uptake of calcium into intracellular storage sites, decreasing its availability (Fig. 4-3). Thus, drugs that stimulate cAMP production (beta agonists) or inhibit its breakdown (phosphodiesterase inhibitors) will cause vasodilation. In addition, cyclic guanosine monophosphate (cGMP) (Fig. 4-3) also increases intracellular calcium storage, decreasing its availability for modulating the interaction of actin and myosin. Several commonly used pharmacologic agents act via cGMP. For example, nitric oxide stimulates the enzyme guanylate cyclase, increasing cGMP levels. Drugs such as nitroglycerin and sodium nitroprusside achieve their effect by producing nitric oxide as a metabolic product. Vasodilation is also produced by "cross-talk" between K^+ and Ca^{++} fluxes. Decreased levels of ATP, acidosis, and elevated tissue lactate increase the permeability of the ATP-sensitive K^+ channel. This increased permeability results in hyperpolarization of the cell membrane that inhibits the entry of Ca^{++} into the cell. This results in decreased vascular tone.

The simplistic overview of pathways of cardiac pharmacology summarized in Figures 4-1 through 4-3 also suggests

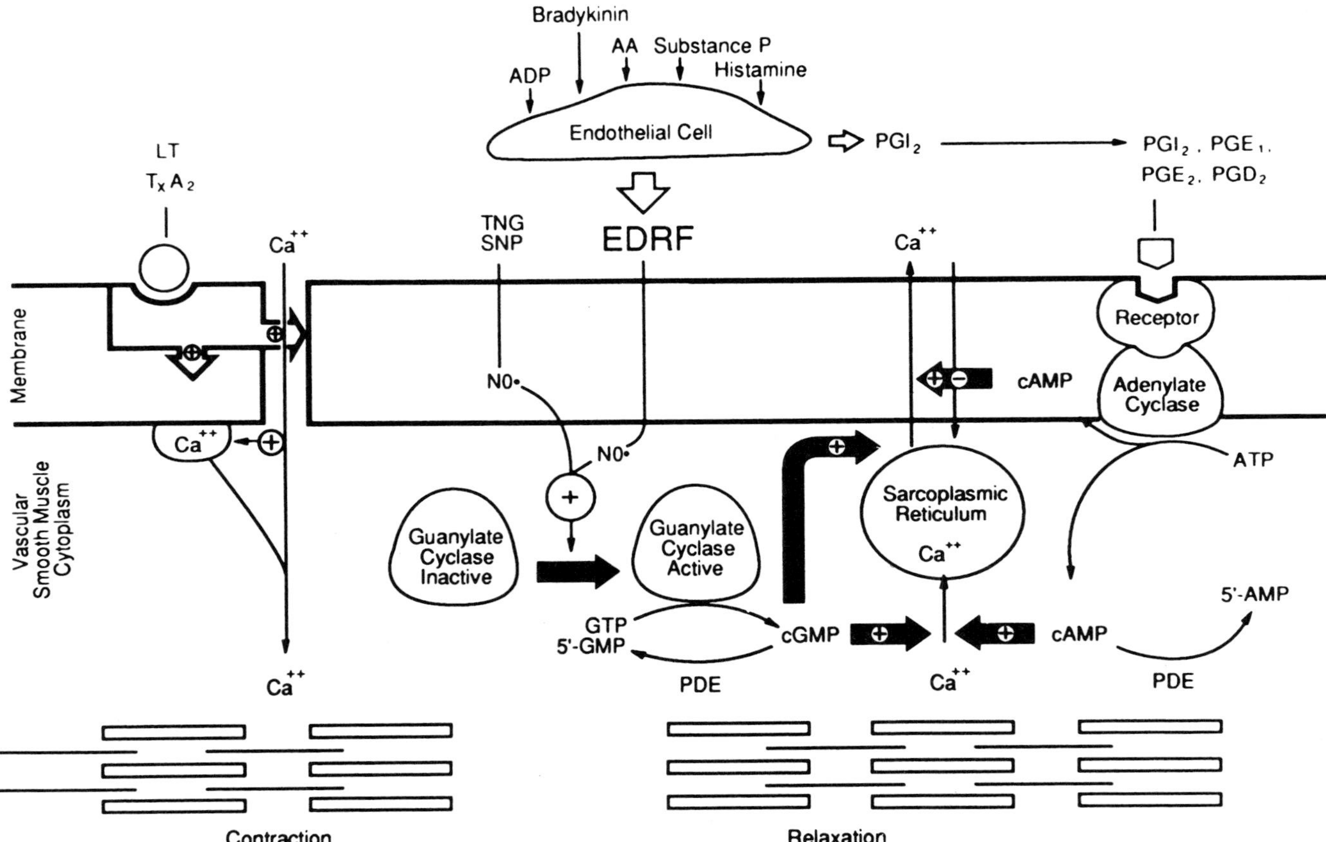

FIGURE 4–3 Mediators of vascular tone. Cyclic AMP and cyclic GMP increase the uptake of calcium into cellular storage sites in vascular smooth muscle, leading to vasodilation. The synthesis of cyclic GMP is catalyzed by guanylate cyclase, which is activated by nitric oxide (NO), which, in turn, is produced by nitroglycerin (NTG) and sodium nitroprusside (SNP). Excessive vasodilation often is a reflection of other endogenous mediators such as prostaglandins (PGI_2, PGE_1, PGE_2, PGD_2) and thromboxane A_2 (TxA_2). Several mediators, such as arachidonic acid (AA), bradykinin, histamine, and substance P, stimulate the release of endothelium-derived relaxing factor (EDRF), which is identified with NO.

the primary cause of difficulty in the clinical use of the drugs discussed in this chapter. The mechanisms of action for control of heart rate and rhythm, contractility, and vascular tone are interrelated. For example, beta-adrenergic agonists not only increase intracellular calcium to increase contractility, but they also alter K^+ currents, leading to tachycardia. Catecholamines not only may have beta-adrenergic agonist activity, with inotropic and chronotropic effects, but they may possess alpha-agonist activity, leading to increased intracellular calcium in vascular smooth muscle and vasoconstriction. Phosphodiesterase inhibitors may increase contractility by increasing cAMP in the myocyte, but may also cause excessive vasodilation by increasing cAMP in the vasculature. The interplay of the various mechanisms means that the clinical art of cardiac surgical pharmacology lies as much in the selection of drugs for their side effects as for their primary therapeutic effects.

ANTIARRHYTHMICS

Arrhythmias are common in the cardiac surgical period. A stable cardiac rhythm requires depolarization and repolarization in a spatially and temporally coordinated manner, and dysrhythmias may occur when this coordination is disturbed. The mechanisms for arrhythmias can be divided into abnormal impulse initiation, abnormal impulse conduction, or combinations of both.[9,10] Abnormal impulse initiation occurs as a result of increased automaticity (spontaneous depolarization of tissue which does not normally have pacemaking activity) or as a result of triggered activity from abnormal conduction after depolarizations during phase 3 or 4 of the action potential. Abnormal conduction often involves reentry phenomena, with recurrent depolarization around a circuit due to unilateral conduction block in ischemic or damaged myocardium and retrograde activation via an alternate pathway through normal tissue. In this simplistic view, it is logical that dysrhythmias could be suppressed by slowing the conduction velocity of ectopic foci, allowing normal pacemaker cells to control heart rate, or by prolonging the action potential duration (and hence refractory period) to block conduction into a limb of a reentry circuit.

Antidysrhythmic agents are often classified by a scheme originally proposed by Vaughan Williams and subsequently modified,[11,12] and although alternative schemes describing specific channel-blocking characteristics have been proposed and may be more logical,[13] we will organize our discussion using the Vaughan Williams system of 4 major drug categories. In this scheme, class I agents are those with local anesthetic properties that block Na^+ channels, class II drugs are beta-blocking agents, class III drugs prolong action potential duration, and class IV are calcium entry blockers. Amiodarone will be discussed in detail due to its expanding role in treating both supraventricular and ventricular arrhythmias, and because its use has replaced many of the previous agents. Because of the efficacy of intravenous amiodarone and its recommendations in ACLS guidelines, many of the older drugs used in cardiac surgery have a historical perspective, and will be briefly considered.

Class I Agents

While each of the class I agents blocks Na^+ channels, they may be subclassified on the basis of electrophysiological differences. These differences can be explained, to some extent, by consideration of the kinetics of the interaction of the drug and the Na^+ channel.[14,15] Class I drugs bind most avidly to open (phase 0 of the action potential—see Figure 4-1) or inactivated (phase 2) Na^+ channels. Dissociation from the channel occurs during the resting (phase 4) state. If the time constant for dissociation is long in comparison to the diastolic interval (corresponding to phase 4), the drug will accumulate in the channel to reach a steady state, slowing conduction in normal tissue. This occurs with class Ia (procainamide, quinidine, disopyramide) and class Ic (encainide, flecainide, lorcainide, propafenone) drugs. In contrast, for the class Ib drugs (lidocaine, tocainide, mexiletine), the time constant for dissociation from the Na^+ channel is short, drug does not accumulate in the channel, and conduction velocity is minimally affected. However, in ischemic tissue the depolarized state is more persistent, leading to greater accumulation of agent in the Na^+ channel, and slowing of conduction in the damaged myocardium.

Procainamide is a class Ia drug that has a variety of electrophysiological effects.[16] Administration may be limited by the side effects of hypotension and decreased cardiac output.[17,18] The loading dose is 20 to 30 mg/min, up to 17 mg/kg, and should be followed by an intravenous infusion of 20 to 80 mg/kg/min. Since procainamide prolongs action potential duration, widening of the QRS complex often heralds a potential overdose. The elimination of procainamide involves hepatic metabolism, acetylation to a metabolite with antiarrhythmic and toxic side effects, and renal elimination of this metabolite. Thus the infusion rate for patients with significant hepatic or renal disease should be at the lower level of this range.

Class Ib drugs include what is probably the best known antiarrhythmic agent, lidocaine. As noted above, lidocaine is a Na^+ channel blocker that has little effect on conduction velocity in normal tissue but slows conduction in ischemic myocardium.[14,15] Other electrophysiological effects include a decrease in action potential duration but a small increase in the ratio of effective refractory period to action potential duration. The exact role of these electrophysiological effects on arrhythmia suppression is unclear. Lidocaine has no significant effects on atrial tissue and it is not recommended for therapy in shock-resistant ventricular tachycardia/fibrillation (VT/VF) in the *Guidelines 2000 for Emergency Cardiovascular Care*.[19] After an initial bolus dose of 1 to 1.5 mg/kg of lidocaine, plasma levels decrease rapidly due to redistribution to muscle, fat, etc. Effective plasma concentrations are maintained only by following the bolus dose with an infusion of 20 to 50 mg/kg/min.[20] Elimination occurs via hepatic metabolism to active metabolites that are cleared by the kidney. Consequently, the dose should be reduced by approximately 50% in patients with liver or kidney disease. The primary toxic effects are associated with the central nervous system, and a lidocaine overdose may cause drowsiness, depressed level of consciousness, or seizures in very high doses. Negative inotropic or hypotensive effects are less pronounced than with most other antiarrhythmics. The other class Ib drugs likely to be encountered in the perioperative period are the oral agents tocainide and mexiletine, which have effects very similar to lidocaine.[15]

The class Ic agents, including flecainide, encainide, and propafenone, markedly decrease conduction velocity.[20,21] The Cardiac Arrhythmia Suppression Trial (CAST) study[20,21] of moricizine found that, while ventricular arrhythmias were suppressed, the incidence of sudden death was greater than placebo with encainide and flecainide, and these drugs are not in wide use. Propafenone is available for oral use. The usual adult dose is 150 to 300 mg every 8 hours. It has beta-blocking (with resultant negative inotropic effects) as well as NA^+ channel-blocking activity, lengthens the PR, QRS, and QT duration, and may be used to treat both atrial and ventricular dysrhythmia.[15]

Class II Agents

Beta-receptor blocking agents are another important group of antiarrhythmic (denoted class II in the Vaughan Williams scheme). However, because of their use as antihypertensive as well as antiarrhythmic agents they are discussed elsewhere in this chapter, and we will move on to consider bretylium, amiodarone, and sotalol, the class III agents in the Vaughan Williams scheme. These drugs have a number of complex ion channel-blocking effects, but possibly the most important activity is K^+ channel blockade.[22] Since the flux of K^+ out of the myocyte is responsible for repolarization, an important electrophysiological effect of Class III drugs is prolongation of the action potential.[23]

Class III Agents

Ibutilide, dofetilide, sotalol, and bretylium are class III agents. Intravenous ibutilide and oral dofetilide are approved for the treatment of atrial fibrillation, but carry the risk of torsades de pointes.[24,25] Sotalol is a nonselective beta blocker that also has K^+ channel-blocking activity.[26] In the United States, it is available only for oral administration and has an approved indication for the treatment of life-threatening ventricular arrhythmias, although it is effective against atrial arrhythmias also. It is not a first-line therapy and should be reserved for arrhythmias refractory to other therapy. Bretylium is not recommended in the *Guidelines 2000 for Emergency Cardiovascular Care.*[19]

Class IV Agents

Calcium entry blockers (class IV in the Vaughan Williams scheme), such as verapamil and diltiazem, are antiarrhythmics. In sinoatrial and atrioventricular nodal tissue, Ca^{++} channels contribute significantly to phase 0 depolarization and the atriovetricular (AV) nodal refractory period is prolonged by Ca^{++} entry blockade.[27,28] This explains the effectiveness of verapamil and diltiazem in the treatment of supraventricular arrhythmias. It is also clear why these drugs are negative inotropes. Both verapamil and diltiazem are effective in slowing the ventricular response to atrial fibrillation, flutter, or paroxysmal supraventricular tachycardia and in converting to sinus rhythm.[29–31] Verapamil has greater negative inotrope effects than diltiazem and, for this reason it is rarely used for supraventricular arrhythmias. The intravenous dose of diltiazem is 0.25 mg/kg with a second dose of 0.35 mg/kg if the response is inadequate after 15 minutes. The loading dose should be followed by an infusion of 5 to 15 mg/hr. Intravenous diltiazem, although useful for rate control, has been replaced by intravenous amiodarone for the most part in clinical therapy of supraventricular tachycardia (SVT) and prophylaxis (see amiodarone, to follow).

Other Drugs

One of the difficulties of classifying antiarrhythmics by the Vaughan Williams classification is that not all drugs can be incorporated into this scheme. Three examples are digoxin, adenosine, and magnesium, each of which has important uses in the perioperative period.

Digoxin inhibits the Na^+/K^+ ATPase, leading to decreased intracellular K^+, a less negative resting membrane potential, increased slope of phase 4 depolarization, and decreased conduction velocity. These direct effects, however, are usually dominated by indirect effects, including inhibition of reflex responses to congestive heart failure and a vagotonic effect.[10,32] The net effect is greatest at the AV node, where conduction is slowed and refractory period is increased, explaining the effectiveness of digoxin in slowing the ventricular response to atrial fibrillation. The major disadvantages of digoxin are the relatively slow onset of action and numerous side effects including proarrhythmia effects, and it is now rarely used for rate control in acute atrial fibrillation because of the advent of IV amiodarone and diltiazem.

Adenosine is an endogenous nucleoside that has an electrophysiological effect very similar to acetylcholine. Adenosine decreases AV node conductivity and its primary antiarrhythmic effect is to break AV nodal reentrant tachycardia.[33] An intravenous dose of 100 to 200 μ/kg is the treatment of choice for paroxysmal supraventricular tachycardia. Adverse effects, such as bronchospasm, are short-lived because its plasma half-life is so short (1–2 seconds). This short half-life makes it ideal for the treatment of reentry dysrhythmia, in which transient interruption can fully suppress the dysrhythmia.

Appropriate acid-base and electrolyte balance is important because electrolyte imbalance can perturb the membrane potential, leading to arrhythmia generation, as can altered acid-base status, via effects on K^+ concentrations and sympathetic tone. Therapy for dysrhythmia should include correction of acid-base and electrolyte imbalance. Magnesium supplementation should be considered.[34] Magnesium deficiency is common in the perioperative period and magnesium administration has been shown to decrease the incidence of postoperative dysrhythmia.[35]

AMIODARONE

Intravenous amiodarone has become one of the most administered intravenous antiarrhythmics used in cardiac surgery because of its broad spectrum of efficacy. Amiodarone was originally developed as an antianginal agent because of its vasodilating effects, including coronary vasodilation.[36] It has a variety of ion channel-blocking activities.[10,29,36] The resultant electrophysiological effects are complex, and there are also differences in the acute intravenous and chronic oral administration. Acute intravenous administration can produce decreases in heart rate and blood pressure, but there are minimal changes in QRS duration or QT interval. After chronic use, there may be significant bradycardia and increases in action potential duration in AV nodal and ventricular tissue, with increased QRS duration and QT interval.[37–39]

Pharmacokinetics

Amiodarone is a complex drug, markedly lipophilic, undergoes variable absorption (35% to 65%) after oral administration, and is extensively taken up by multiple tissues with interindividual variation and complex pharmacokinetics.[38–40] The short initial context-sensitive half-life after intravenous administration represents drug redistribution. The true elimination half-life for amiodarone is extremely long, up to 40 to 60 days. Because of the huge volume of distribution (approximately 60 L/kg) and a very long duration of action, an active metabolite loading period of several months may be required before reaching steady-state tissue concentrations. Further, in life-threatening arrhythmias, intravenous loading is often starting to establish initial plasma levels. Measuring amiodarone plasma concentrations is not useful, due to the complex pharmacokinetics and the metabolites of the parent drug. Plasma concentrations greater than 2.5 mg/L have been associated with increased risk of toxicity. The optimal dose of amiodarone has not been well characterized, and may vary depending on the specific arrhythmias treated. Further, there may be differences in dose requirements for therapy of supraventricular and ventricular arrhythmias.[37–40]

Because of these distinctive pharmacokinetic properties, steady-state plasma levels are slowly achieved. Oral administration for a typical adult consists of a loading regimen of 80 to 1600 mg/day (in 2 or 3 doses) for 10 days, 600 to 800 mg/day for 4 to 6 weeks, and then maintenance doses of 200 to 600 mg/day. For intravenous loading specific studies will be reviewed, but recommended dosing is 150 mg given over 10 minutes for acute therapy in an adult, followed first by a secondary loading infusion of 60 mg/hr for 6 hours and then by a maintenance infusion of 30 mg/hr to achieve a 1000 mg/day dosing.[37–40]

Electrophysiology

The electrophysiological actions of amiodarone are complex and incompletely understood. Amiodarone produces all four effects according to the Vaughan Williams classification. It also has been shown to have use-dependent class I activity, inhibition of the inward sodium currents, and class II activity.[10] The antiadrenergic effect of amiodarone, however, is different from that of beta-blocker drugs because it is noncompetitive and additive to the effect of beta blockers. Amiodarone depresses sinoatrial node automaticity that slows the heart rate and conduction, and increases refractoriness of the AV node, properties useful in the management of supraventricular arrhythmia. Its class III activity results in increases in atrial and ventricular refractoriness and in prolongation of the QTc interval. The effects of oral amiodarone on sinoatrial and AV nodal function are maximal within 2 weeks, whereas the effects on VT and ventricular refractoriness tend to emerge more gradually during oral therapy, becoming maximal after 10 weeks or more.

Indications

The primary indication for amiodarone is ventricular tachycardia or fibrillation refractory to other therapy.[40–48] It is the most efficacious agent for reducing ventricular arrhythmias and suppresses the incidence of post–myocardial infarction sudden death.[37] It is also effective, in doses lower than those used for ventricular dysrhythmia, for the treatment of atrial dysrhythmia and is effective in converting atrial fibrillation to sinus rhythm (see atrial fibrillation).

Side Effects

Although there are numerous adverse reactions to amiodarone, they occur with long-term oral administration and have not been associated with acute intravenous administration. The most serious is pulmonary toxicity, which has not been reported with acute administration in a perioperative setting. Some case series have reported an increased risk of marked bradycardia and hypotension immediately after cardiac surgery in patients already on amiodarone at the time of surgery.[49,50] Other case-control studies, however, have not reproduced this finding.[51] None of the placebo-controlled trials of prophylactic amiodarone for perioperative AF prevention found any adverse cardiovascular effects of the drug.[52–56] Thus, it is relatively unlikely that amiodarone poses a serious cardiovascular risk to the postoperative patient. Case reports and case series of postoperative acute pulmonary toxicity are similarly lacking in the rigor of randomized controlled methodology.

PHARMACOLOGIC THERAPY OF SPECIFIC ARRHYTHMIAS

Ventricular Tachyarrhythmias

Intravenous amiodarone is approved for rapid control of recurrent VT or VF. Three randomized controlled trials of patients with recurrent in-hospital, hemodynamically unstable VT or VF with 2 or more episodes within the past 24 hours who failed to respond to or be intolerant of lidocaine, procainamide, and (in 2 of the trials) bretylium have been reported.[42,44,46] Patients were critically ill with ischemic cardiovascular disease, 25% were on a mechanical ventilator or intra-aortic balloon pump before enrollment, and 10% were undergoing cardiopulmonary resuscitation at the time of enrollment.

One study compared 3 doses of intravenous amiodarone: 525, 1050, and 2100 mg per day.[44] Because of the use of investigator-initiated, intermittent, open-label amiodarone boluses for recurrent VT, the actual mean amiodarone doses received by the 3 groups were 742, 1175, and 1921 mg/d. There was no statistically significant difference in the number of patients without VT/VF recurrence during the 1-day study period: 32 of 86 (41%), 36 of 92 (45%), and 42 of 92 (53%) for the low-, medium-, and high-dose groups, respectively. The number of supplemental amiodarone 150-mg bolus infusions given by blinded investigators was statistically significantly less in those randomized to higher doses of amiodarone.

A wider range of amiodarone doses (125, 500, and 1000 mg/d) was evaluated by Sheinman et al, including a low dose that was expected to be subtherapeutic.[46] This stronger study design, however, was also confounded by open-label bolus amiodarone injections given by study investigators. There was, however, a trend toward a relationship between intended amiodarone dose and VT/VF recurrence rate ($p = .067$). After adjustment for baseline imbalances, the median 24-hour recurrence rates of VT/VF, from lowest to highest doses, were 1.68, 0.96, and 0.48 events per 24 hours.

The third study compared two intravenous amiodarone doses (125 and 1000 mg/d) to bretylium (2500 mg/d).[42] Once again, the target amiodarone dose ratio of 8 to 1 was compressed to 1.8 to 1 as a result of open-label boluses. There was no significant difference in the primary outcome, which was median VT/VF recurrence rate over 24 hours. For low-dose amiodarone, high-dose amiodarone, and bretylium, these rates were 1.68, 0.48, and 0.96 events per 24 hours, respectively ($p = .237$). There was no difference between high-dose amiodarone and bretylium; however, more than 50% of patients had crossed over from bretylium to amiodarone by 16 hours.

The failure of these studies to provide clear evidence of amiodarone efficacy may be related to the "active-control" study design used, a lack of adequate statistical power, high rates of supplemental amiodarone boluses, and high crossover rates. Nonetheless, these studies provide some evidence that IV amiodarone (1 g/d) is moderately effective during a 24-hour period against VT and VF.

SUSTAINED MONOMORPHIC VENTRICULAR TACHYCARDIA AND WIDE QRS TACHYCARDIA

Although the most effective and rapid treatment of any hemodynamically unstable sustained ventricular tachyarrhythmia is electrical cardioversion or defibrillation, intravenous antiarrhythmic drugs can be used for arrhythmia termination if the ventricular tachycardia (VT) is hemodynamically stable. The *Guidelines 2000 for Emergency Cardiovascular Care*[19] removed the former recommendation of lidocaine and adenosine use in stable wide QRS tachycardia, now labeled as "acceptable" but not primarily recommended (lidocaine) or not recommended (adenosine). Intravenous procainamide and sotalol are effective, based on randomized but small studies[10]; amiodarone is also considered acceptable.[19]

SHOCK-RESISTANT VENTRICULAR FIBRILLATION

The *Guidelines 2000 for Emergency Cardiovascular Care* recommend at least three shocks and epinephrine or vasopressin before any antiarrhythmic drug is administered.[10,19] No large-scale controlled randomized studies have demonstrated efficacy for lidocaine, bretylium, or procainamide in shock-resistant VF,[10,19] and lidocaine and bretylium are no longer recommended in this setting.[19] Two pivotal studies have been reported recently studying the efficacy of agents in acute shock-resistant cardiac arrest.

The Amiodarone in the Out-of-Hospital Resuscitation of Refractory Sustained Ventricular Tachycardia (ARREST) study was randomized, double-blind, and placebo-controlled. The ARREST study in 504 patients showed that amiodarone 300 mg administered in a single intravenous bolus significantly improves survival to hospital admission in cardiac arrest still in VT or VF after three direct-current shocks (44% vs. 34%, $p < .03$).[43] Although the highest survival rate to hospital admission (79%) was achieved when the amiodarone was given within 4 to 16 minutes from dispatch, there was no significant difference in the proportional improvement in the amiodarone group compared with the placebo group when the drug administration was delayed (up to 55 minutes). Amiodarone also had the highest efficacy in those patients (21% of all study patients) who had a return of spontaneous circulation before drug administration (survival to hospital admission to 64% from 41% in the placebo group). Among patients with no return of spontaneous circulation, amiodarone only slightly improved outcome (38% vs. 33%).

Dorian performed a randomized trial comparing intravenous lidocaine with intravenous amiodarone as an adjunct to defibrillation in victims of out-of-hospital cardiac arrest.[48] Patients were enrolled if they had out-of-hospital ventricular fibrillation resistant to three shocks, intravenous epinephrine, and a further shock, or if they had recurrent ventricular fibrillation after initially successful defibrillation. They were randomly assigned in a double-blind manner to receive intravenous amiodarone plus lidocaine placebo or intravenous lidocaine plus amiodarone placebo. The primary end point was the proportion of patients who survived to be admitted to the hospital. In total, 347 patients (mean age, 67 ± 14 years) were enrolled. The mean interval between the time at which paramedics were dispatched to the scene of the cardiac arrest and the time of their arrival was 7 ± 3 minutes, and the mean interval from dispatch to drug administration was 25 ± 8 minutes. After treatment with amiodarone, 22.8% of 180 patients survived to hospital admission, as compared with 12.0% percent of 167 patients treated with lidocaine ($p = .009$). Among patients for whom the time from dispatch to the administration of the drug was equal to or less than the median time (24 minutes), 27.7% of those given amiodarone and 15.3% of those given lidocaine survived to hospital admission ($p = .05$). The authors concluded that compared with lidocaine, amiodarone leads to substantially higher rates of survival to hospital admission in patients with shock-resistant out-of-hospital ventricular fibrillation.

Supraventricular Arrhythmias

A supraventricular arrhythmia is any tachyarrhythmia that requires atrial or atrioventricular junctional tissue for initiation and maintenance. It may arise from reentry caused by unidirectional conduction block in one region of the heart and slow conduction in another, from enhanced automaticity akin to that seen in normal pacemaker cells of the sinus node and in latent pacemaker cells elsewhere in the heart, or from triggered activity, a novel type of abnormally enhanced impulse initiation caused by membrane currents that can be activated and inactivated by premature stimulation or rapid pacing.[56–58] Pharmacologic approaches to the treatment of supraventricular arrhythmias, including atrial fibrillation, atrial flutter, atrial tachycardia, AV reentrant tachycardia, and AV nodal reentrant tachycardia, continue to evolve.[56–60] Because atrial fibrillation is perhaps the most common arrhythmia after cardiac surgery, this condition will be emphasized in detail.

Atrial Fibrillation

Atrial fibrillation (AF) is a common complication of cardiac surgery that increases the length of stay in the hospital with resultant increases in health care resource utilization.[56–61] Advanced age, previous AF, and valvular heart operations are the most consistently identified risk factors for this arrhythmia. Because efforts to terminate AF after its initiation are problematic, current interests are directed at therapies to prevent postoperative AF. Most studies suggest that prophylaxis with antiarrhythmic compounds can significantly decrease the incidence of AF, length of hospital stay, and cost. Newer class III antiarrhythmic drugs (i.e., sotalol, ibutilide) may also be effective, but potentially pose the risk of drug-induced polymorphic ventricular tachycardia (torsades de pointes). Defining which subpopulations benefit most from such therapy is particularly important as older and more critically ill patients undergo surgery.

In addition to beta-adrenergic blockers, amiodarone has evolved as an effective approach for prophylactic therapy of AF. However, most clinicians are confused by the different studies that have evaluated oral versus intravenous (IV) amiodarone. IV amiodarone has continue to evolve in clinical practice because acute loading with oral therapy is often not feasible, in part due to time required and due to the complex pharmacokinetics and variable absorption of oral therapy. There may also be additional benefits of prophylactic therapies in high-risk patients, especially those prone to ventricular arrhythmias (i.e., patients with preexisting heart failure).

Two pivotal studies deserve mention regarding prophylaxis with amiodarone. To determine if IV amiodarone would prevent atrial fibrillation and decrease hospital stay after cardiac surgery, Daoud assessed preoperative prophylaxis in 124 patients who were given either oral amiodarone (64 patients) or placebo (60 patients) for a minimum of seven days before elective cardiac surgery.[62] Therapy consisted of 600 mg of amiodarone per day for seven days, then 200 mg per day until the day of discharge from the hospital. The preoperative total dose of amiodarone was 4.8 ± 0.96 g over a period of 13 ± 7 days. Postoperative atrial fibrillation occurred in 16 of the 64 patients in the amiodarone group (25%) and 32 of the 60 patients in the placebo group (53%). Patients in the amiodarone group were hospitalized for significantly fewer days than were patients in the placebo group (6.5 ± 2.6 vs. 7.9 ± 4.3 days, $p = .04$). Total hospitalization costs were significantly less for the amiodarone group than for the placebo group ($18,375 ± $13,863 vs. $26,491 ± $23,837, $p = .03$). Guarnieri evaluated 300 patients randomized in a double-blind fashion to IV amiodarone (1 g/d for 2 days) versus placebo immediately after open-heart surgery.[54] The primary end points of the trial were incidence of atrial fibrillation and length of hospital stay. Atrial fibrillation occurred in 67/142 (47%) patients on placebo versus 56/158 (35%) on amiodarone ($p = .01$). Length of hospital stay for the placebo group was 8.2 ± 6.2 days, and 7.6 ± 5.9 days for the amiodarone group. Low-dose IV amiodarone was safe and effective in reducing the incidence of atrial fibrillation after heart surgery, but did not significantly alter length of hospital stay.

In summary, AF is a frequent complication of cardiac surgery. Many cases can be prevented with appropriate prophylactic therapy. Beta-adrenergic blockers should be administered to most patients without contraindication. Prophylactic amiodarone should be considered in patients at high risk for postoperative AF. The lack of data on cost benefits and cost-efficiency in some studies may reflect the lack of higher risk patients in the study. Patients who are poor candidates for beta blockade may not tolerate sotalol, while amiodarone does not have this limitation. Additional studies need also to be performed to better assess the role of prophylactic therapy in off-pump cardiac surgery.

INOTROPIC AGENTS

Some depression of myocardial function is common after cardiac surgery.[63–65] The etiology is multifactorial—preexisting disease, incomplete repair or revascularization, myocardial edema, postischemic dysfunction, reperfusion injury, etc.—and is usually reversible. Adequate cardiac output can usually be maintained by exploiting the Starling curve with higher preload. But often the cardiac function curve is flattened and it is necessary to utilize inotropic agents to maintain adequate organ perfusion.

The molecular basis for the contractile property of the heart is the interaction of the proteins actin and myosin, in which chemical energy (in the form of ATP) is converted into mechanical energy. In the relaxed state (diastole) the interaction of actin and myosin is inhibited by tropomyosin, a protein associated with the actin-myosin complex. With the onset of systole, Ca^{++} enters the myocyte (during phase 1 of the action potential). This influx of Ca^{++} triggers the release of much larger amounts of Ca^{++} from the sarcoplasmic reticulum. The binding of Ca^{++} to the C subunit of the protein troponin interrupts the inhibition of the actin-myosin interaction by tropomyosin, facilitating the hydrolysis of ATP with the generation of a mechanical force. With repolarization of the myocyte and the completion of systole, Ca^{++} is taken back up into the sarcoplasmic reticulum, allowing tropomyosin to again inhibit the interaction of actin and myosin with consequent relaxation of contractile force. Thus, *inotropic action is mediated by intracellular* Ca^{++}.[66] A novel drug, levosimendan, currently under clinical development in the United States but approved in several countries, increases the sensitivity of the contractile apparatus to Ca^{++},[67] whereas the positive inotropic agents available for clinical use achieve their end by increasing intracellular Ca^{++} levels.

The first drug to be considered is simply Ca^{++} itself. In general, administration of calcium will increase the inotropic state of the myocardium, when measured by load-independent methods, but it will also increase vascular tone (afterload) and impair diastolic function. Also, the effects of calcium on myocardial performance are dependent on the plasma Ca^{++} concentration. Ca^{++} plays important roles in cellular function and the intracellular Ca^{++} concentration is highly regulated by membrane ion channels and intracellular organelles.[68,69] If the extracellular Ca^{++} concentration is normal, administration of Ca^{++} will have little effect on the intracellular level and will have less pronounced hemodynamic effects. On the other hand, if the ionized plasma calcium is low, exogenous calcium administration may increase cardiac output and blood pressure.[70] It should also be realized that even with normal plasma Ca^{++} concentrations, administration of Ca^{++} may increase vascular tone, leading to increased blood pressure but no change in cardiac output. This increased afterload, as well as the deleterious effects on diastolic function, may be the basis of the observation that Ca^{++} administration can blunt the response to epinephrine.[71] Routine use of Ca^{++} at the end of bypass should be tempered by the realization that Ca^{++} may have little effect on cardiac output while increasing systemic vascular resistance, although this in itself may be of importance. If there is evidence of myocardial ischemia, Ca^{++} administration may be deleterious since it may exacerbate both coronary spasm and the pathways leading to cellular injury.[72,73]

Digoxin, while not effective as acute therapy for low cardiac output syndrome in the perioperative period, nevertheless well illustrates the role of intracellular Ca^{++}. Digoxin functions by inhibiting the Na^+/K^+ ATPase, which is responsible for the exchange of intracellular Na^+ with extracellular K^+.[3,4] It is thus responsible for maintaining the intracellular/extracellular K^+ and Na^+ gradients. When it is inhibited, intracellular Na^+ levels increase. The increased intracellular Na^+ is an increased chemical potential for driving the Ca^{++}/Na^+ exchanger, an ion exchange mechanism in which intracellular Na^+ is removed from the cell in exchange for Ca^{++}. The net effect is an increase in intracellular Ca^{++}, with an enhancement of the inotropic state.

By far the most commonly used positive inotropic agents are the beta-adrenergic agonists. The $beta_1$ receptor is part of a complex comprised of the receptor on the outer surface of the cell membrane, coupled with membrane-spanning G-proteins (so named because they bind GTP), which, in turn, stimulate adenylate cyclase on the inner surface of the membrane, catalyzing the formation cyclic adenosine monophosphate (cAMP). The inotropic state is modulated by cAMP via its catalysis of phosphorylation reactions by protein kinase A. These phosphorylation reactions "open" Ca^{++} channels on the cell membrane and lead to greater release and uptake of Ca^{++} from the sarcoplasmic reticulum.[3,4]

There are a large number of drugs that will stimulate $beta_1$ receptors and have a positive inotropic effect, including epinephrine, norepinephrine, dopamine, isoproterenol, and dobutamine, the most commonly used catecholamines in the perioperative period. While there are differences in their binding at the $beta_1$ receptor, the most important differences between the various catecholamines are their relative effects on alpha- and $beta_2$-adrenergic receptors. In general, alpha stimulation of receptors on the peripheral vasculature causes vasoconstriction while $beta_2$ stimulation leads to vasodilation (see the discussion elsewhere in this chapter). For some time it was believed that $beta_2$ and alpha receptors were found only in the peripheral vasculature, as well as a few other organs, but not in the myocardium. However, recent investigation has shown that alpha receptors are found in the myocardium and mediate a positive inotropic effect.[5,6] The mechanism for this positive inotropic effect is probably the stimulation of phospholipase C leading to hydrolysis of phosphatidyl inositol to diacylglycerol and inositol triphosphate, compounds that increase Ca^{++} release from the sarcoplasmic reticulum and increase myofilament sensitivity to Ca^{++}. It is also possible that alpha-adrenergic agents increase intracellular Ca^{++} by prolonging action potential duration via inhibition of outward K^+ currents during repolarization or by activating the Na^+/H^+ exchange mechanism, increasing intracellular pH, and increasing myofilament sensitivity to Ca^{++}. Just as the exact mechanism is uncertain, the exact role of alpha-adrenergic stimulation in control of the inotropic state is unclear, although it is apparent that onset of the effect is slower than that of $beta_1$ stimulation.

In addition to the discovery of alpha receptors in the myocardium, it has also been discovered that $beta_2$ receptors are present in the myocardium.[74] The fraction of $beta_2$ receptors (compared to $beta_1$ receptors) is increased in chronic heart failure, possibly explaining the efficacy of drugs with $beta_2$ activity in this setting. This phenomenon is part of the general observation of $beta_1$-receptor downregulation (decrease in receptor density) and desensitization (uncoupling of effect from receptor binding) that is observed in chronic heart failure.[75] Interestingly, it has been demonstrated in a dog model that this same phenomenon occurs with cardiopulmonary bypass (CPB).[76] In this situation, a newer class of drugs, the phosphodiesterase inhibitors, may be of benefit. These drugs, typified by the agents available in the United States, amrinone and milrinone, increase cAMP levels independently of the beta receptor by selectively inhibiting the myocardial enzyme responsible for the breakdown of cAMP.[3,4]

In clinical use, selection of a particular inotropic agent is usually based more on its side effects than its direct inotropic properties. Of the commonly used catecholamines, norepinephrine has alpha and $beta_1$ but little $beta_2$ activity and is both an inotrope and a vasopressor. Epinephrine and dopamine are mixed agonists with alpha, $beta_1$, and $beta_2$ activity. At lower doses they are primarily inotropes and not vasopressors, although vasopressor effects become more pronounced at higher doses. This is especially true for dopamine, which achieves effects at higher doses by stimulating the release of norepinephrine.[77] Dobutamine is a more selective $beta_1$ agonist, in contrast to isoproterenol, which is a mixed beta agonist. Selection of a drug depends on the particular hemodynamic problem at hand. For example, depressed myocardial function in the presence of profound vasodilation may require a drug with both positive inotropic and vasopressor effects, while a patient who is vasoconstricted may benefit from some other choice. We highly recommend an empirical approach to the selection of inotropic agents with careful monitoring of the response to the drug and selection of the agent that achieves the desired effect.

Clinical experience indicates that phosphodiesterase inhibitors can be very effective when catecholamines do not produce an adequate cardiac output.[78–80] There are few differences in the hemodynamic effects of the two drugs available for use in the United States, amrinone and milrinone. Both agents increase contractility with little effect on heart rate and both are vasodilators. There is significant venodilation, as well as arteriodilating, and maintaining adequate preload is important in avoiding significant hypotension.[81] We prefer milrinone to amrinone because of a less pronounced thrombocytopenia, a problem with both drugs.[82] If amrinone is used, it should be noted that the bolus dose recommended in the product insert, 0.75 mg/mL, is inadequate to maintain therapeutic plasma levels, and a loading dose of 1.5 to 2.0 mg/mL should be used.[83] With either drug, administering the loading dose over 15 to 30 minutes may ameliorate possible hypotension. It should also be realized that despite the fact that both drugs have long half-lives, plasma levels drop quickly after a loading dose due to redistribution and the loading dose should be followed immediately by a continuous infusion.[83,84] Because of their long half-lives, it is relatively difficult to readily titrate plasma levels, in comparison to catecholamines (which have plasma half-lives of a few minutes).

Phosphodiesterase inhibitors, specifically milrinone, are being increasingly used to facilitate separation from CPB and for the treatment of low cardiac output syndrome after cardiac surgery.[82,85–87] A study by Doolan et al also demonstrated that milrinone, in comparison to placebo, significantly facilitated separation of high-risk patients from CPB.[88]

Levosimendan

Levosimendan is one of the first agents of a new class of drugs known as calcium sensitizers. The molecule is a pyridazinone-dinitrile derivative with additional action on adenosine triphosphate (ATP)-sensitive potassium channels.[67,89,90] Levosimendan is used intravenously for the treatment of decompensated cardiac failure, demonstrating enhanced contractility with no increase in oxygen demands, and produces antistunning effects without increasing myocardial intracellular calcium concentrations or prolonging myocardial relaxation. Levosimendan also causes coronary and systemic vasodilation. In patients with decompensated congestive heart failure, IV levosimendan significantly reduced the incidence of worsening CHF or death. IV levosimendan significantly increased cardiac output or cardiac index and decreased filling pressure in the acute treatment of stable or decompensated CHF in large, double-blind, randomized trials and after cardiac surgery in smaller trials. Levosimendan is well tolerated and has not been shown to be arrhythmogenic. In addition to sensitizing troponin to intracellular calcium, levosimendan has been shown to inhibit phosphodiesterase III and open ATP-sensitive potassium channels (K(ATP)), which may produce vasodilation. Unlike currently available intravenous inotropes, levosimendan does not increase myocardial oxygen utilization, has not been shown to be proarrhythmic, and has been used effectively in the presence of beta-blocking medications. Levosimendan also has not been shown to impair ventricular relaxation, which was an initial concern with this class of drugs. Clinical studies of levosimendan have demonstrated short-term hemodynamic benefits of levosimendan over both placebo and dobutamine. While large-scale, long-term morbidity and mortality data are scarce, the Levosimendan Infusion versus Dobutamine in severe low-output heart failure (LIDO) study suggested a mortality benefit of levosimendan over dobutamine up to 180 days after treatment. Clinical studies comparing levosimendan with other positive inotropes, namely milrinone, are lacking. Levosimendan treatment appears to be well tolerated, with the primary adverse events being headache and hypotension.

Clinical Trials

Despite their common use after cardiac surgery, there have been relatively few comparative studies of inotropic agents in the perioperative period. In 1978, Steen et al reported the hemodynamic effects of epinephrine, dobutamine, and epinephrine immediately after separation from CPB.[91] The largest mean increase in cardiac index was achieved with dopamine at 15 μg/kg/min. However, it should be noted that the only epinephrine dose studied was 0.04 μg/kg/min. In a later comparison of dopamine and dobutamine, Salomon et al concluded that dobutamine produced more consistent increases in cardiac index, although the hemodynamic differences were small and all patients had good cardiac indices at the onset of the study.[92] Fowler et al also found insignificant differences in the hemodynamic effects of dobutamine and dopamine, although they reported that coronary flow increased more in proportion to myocardial oxygen consumption with dobutamine.[93] While neither of these groups reported significant increases in heart rate for either dopamine or dobutamine, clinical experience has been otherwise. This is supported by a study by Sethna et al, who found that the increase in cardiac index with dobutamine is simply due to increased heart rate, although they found that myocardial oxygen was maintained.[94] Butterworth et al subsequently demonstrated that the older and much cheaper agent, epinephrine, effectively increased stroke volume without as great an increase in heart rate as dobutamine.[95] More recently, Feneck et al compared dobutamine and milrinone and found them to be equally effective in the treatment of low cardiac output syndrome after cardiac surgery.[96] This study was a comparison of two drugs, and the investigators emphasized that the most efficacious therapy is probably combinations of drugs. In particular, phosphodiesterase inhibitors require the synthesis of cAMP to be effective, and thus use of a combination of a beta$_1$-adrenergic agonist and a phosphodiesterase inhibitor would be predicted to be more effective than either agent alone.

Finally, it must also be realized that while global hemodynamic goals (heart rate, blood pressure, filling pressures, cardiac output) may be achieved, this does not guarantee adequate regional perfusion, in particular renal and mesenteric perfusion. To date, there have been few investigations of regional perfusion after cardiac surgery. There has been more interest in regional (especially mesenteric) perfusion in the critical care medicine literature, and some of the critical care investigations may be relevant to postoperative care of the cardiac surgical patient. Two studies have indicated that epinephrine may impair splanchnic perfusion, especially in comparison to the combination of norepinephrine and dobutamine.[97,98] Norepinephrine alone has variable effects on splanchnic blood flow in septic shock,[99] although the addition of dobutamine can significantly improve splanchnic perfusion when blood pressure is supported with norepinephrine.[98] Low-dose dopamine improves splanchnic blood flow,[100] but there is evidence that dopamine in higher doses impairs gastric perfusion.[101] The relevance of these studies of septic patients for the cardiac surgical patient is unclear, although there are similarities between the inflammatory response to CPB and sepsis.

VASOPRESSORS

Cardiopulmonary bypass is often characterized by derangements of vascular tone. In some cases, CPB induces elevations in endogenous catecholamines as well as other mediators, such as serotonin and arginine vasopressin (AVP), leading to vasoconstriction. However, often CPB is characterized by endothelial injury and a systemic inflammatory response, with a cascade of cytokine and inflammatory mediator release and profound vasodilation. The pathophysiology has a striking resemblance to that of sepsis or an anaphylactic reaction. Furthermore, vasodilation after cardiac surgery may be exacerbated by the preoperative use of angiotensin-converting enzyme inhibitors and post-CPB use of milrinone.

The mechanisms of vasodilatory shock have recently been reviewed.[102] Vascular tone is modulated by intracellular Ca^{++}, which binds calmodulin. The Ca^{++}-calmodulin complex activates myosin light chain kinase, which catalyzes the phosphorylation of myosin to facilitate the interaction with actin. Conversely, intracellular cGMP activates myosin phosphatase (also via a kinase-mediated phosphorylation of myosin phosphatase) that dephosphorylates myosin and inhibits the interaction of actin and myosin. A primary mediator of vasodilatory shock is nitric oxide (NO), which is induced by cytokine cascades. NO activates guanylate cyclase, with resultant loss of vascular tone. Another mechanism of vasodilation that may be particularly relevant to prolonged CPB is the activation of ATP-sensitive potassium (K_{ATP}) channels. These channels are activated by decreases in cellular ATP or increases in hydrogen ion or lactate. All of these could result from the abnormal perfusion associated with CPB and/or hypothermia. Increases in potassium channel conductance result in hyperpolarization of the vascular smooth muscle membrane, which decreases Ca^{++} flux into the cell, leading to decreased vascular tone. A third mechanism of vasodilatory shock that also may be particularly relevant to cardiac surgery is deficiency of vasopressin. As noted above, CPB often induces the release of vasopressin, and this may contribute to the excessive vasoconstriction sometimes seen after CPB. However, it has been observed in several experimental models of shock that the initially high levels of vasopressin decrease as shock persists, leading some investigators to suggest that vasopressin stores are limited and are depleted by the initial response to hypotension.

Excessive vasodilation during shock is usually treated with catecholamines, most typically phenylephrine, dopamine, epinephrine, or norepinephrine.[103] Although catecholamines produce both alpha- and beta-adrenergic effects, $alpha_1$-adrenergic receptor stimulation produces vasoconstriction. As noted earlier, stimulation of these receptors activates membrane phospholipase-C, which in turn hydrolyzes phosphatidylinositol 4,55 diphosphate.[7] This leads to the subsequent generation of two second messengers, including diacyl glycerol and inositol triphosphate. Both of these second messengers increase cytosolic Ca^{++} by different mechanisms, which include facilitating release of calcium from the sarcoplasmic reticulum, and potentially increasing the calcium sensitivity of the contractile proteins in vascular smooth muscle.

Mediator-induced vasodilation is often poorly responsive to catecholamines,[103] and the most potent pressor among catecholamines, norepinephrine, is often required. Some clinicians are concerned about renal, hepatic, and mesenteric function during norepinephrine administration. It should be noted, however, that in septic patients norepinephrine can improve renal function[102–107] and there is evidence it may improve mesenteric perfusion as well.[108] Given the hemodynamic similarities between septic patients and some patients at the end of cardiopulmonary bypass, it would be hoped that these results could be extrapolated to the cardiac surgical patient. However, this has not been confirmed by a systematic study. And in some cases of profound vasodilatory shock, even norepinephrine is inadequate to restore systemic blood pressure. In this situation, low doses of vasopressin may be useful. Argenziano et al[109] studied 40 patients with vasodilatory shock (defined as mean arterial blood pressure less than 70 mm Hg with a cardiac index greater than 2.5 L/min/m^2) after cardiac surgery. Arginine vasopressin levels were inappropriately low in this group of patients, and low-dose vasopressin infusion (0.1 units/min or less) effectively restored blood pressure and reduced norepinephrine requirements without significant change in cardiac index. These observations were very similar to an earlier report of the use of vasopressin in vasodilatory septic shock.[110] Vasopressin has also been reported to be useful in the treatment of milrinone-induced hypotension.[111] In this latter report, vasopressin was reported to increase urine output, presumably via glomerular efferent arteriole constriction. However, the overall effects on renal function are unclear. And there are still important unanswered questions about vasopressin and mesenteric perfusion. While vasopressin may effectively restore blood pressure in vasodilatory shock, it must be remembered that in physiologic concentrations it is a mesenteric vasoconstrictor and mesenteric hypoperfusion may be a factor in the development of sepsis and multiorgan dysfunction syndrome.

TABLE 4–1 Vasodilators used in the treatment of hypertension and heart failure

Angiotensin-converting enzyme inhibitors
Angiotensin II antagonists
$Alpha_1$-adrenergic antagonists: prazosin
$Alpha_2$-adrenergic agonists (clonidine)
Nitrates
Hydralazine
Calcium channel blockers:
Dihydropyridine agents: nifedipine, nicardipine, felodipine, amlodipine
Diltiazem
Verapamil

VASODILATORS

Different pharmacologic approaches are available to produce vasodilation (Table 4-1). Potential therapeutic approaches include: (1) blockade of $alpha_1$-adrenergic receptors, ganglionic transmission, and calcium channel receptors; (2) stimulation of central $alpha_2$-adrenergic receptors or vascular guanylate cyclase and adenylate cyclase; (3) inhibition of phosphodiesterase enzymes and inhibition of angiotensin-converting enzymes.[112] Adenosine in low concentrations is also a potent vasodilator with a short half-life but is used, as noted earlier, for its ability to inhibit atrioventricular conduction. Losartan, a novel angiotensin II antagonist (AII), has just been released for the treatment of hypertension but is not available for intravenous use.

Stimulation of Adenylate Cyclase (Cyclic AMP)

Prostacyclin, prostaglandin E1, and isoproterenol increase cyclic nucleotide formation (adenosine-3′, 5′-monophosphate; cyclic AMP) in vascular smooth muscle to produce calcium mobilization out of vascular smooth muscle. Inhibiting the breakdown of cyclic AMP by phosphodiesterase will also increase cyclic AMP.[112] Increasing cyclic AMP in vascular smooth muscle facilitates calcium uptake by intracellular storage sites, thus decreasing calcium available for contraction. The net effect of increasing calcium uptake is to produce vascular smooth muscle relaxation and, hence, vasodilation. However, most catecholamines with $beta_2$-adrenergic activity (i.e., isoproterenol) and phosphodiesterase inhibitors have positive inotropic and other side effects that include tachycardia, glycogenolysis, and kaluresis.[113] Prostaglandins (prostacyclin and prostaglandin E1) are potent inhibitors of platelet aggregation and activation. Catecholamines with $beta_2$-adrenergic activity, phosphodiesterase inhibitors, and prostaglandin E1 and prostacyclin have been used to vasodilate the pulmonary circulation in patients with pulmonary hypertension and right ventricular failure.[113]

TABLE 4–2 Mechanisms of nitrate tolerance

Classic
Decreased bioconversion to nitric oxide
Desensitization of guanylyl cyclase
Neurohumoral adaptations
Renin-angiotensin system activation
Increased vasopressin, catecholamines
Novel
Increased superoxide anion production
Increased production of endothelin-1 via protein kinase C–mediated mechanisms

Nitrates, Nitrovasodilators, and Stimulation of Guanylyl Cyclase (Cyclic GMP)

The vascular endothelium modulates vascular relaxation by releasing both nitric oxide and prostacyclin.[114–116] Inflammatory mediators can also stimulate the vascular endothelium to release excessive amounts of endothelium-derived relaxing factor (EDRF or nitric oxide), which activates guanylyl cyclase to generate cyclic GMP.[89,90] Nitrates and sodium nitroprusside, however, generate nitric oxide directly, independent of vascular endothelium.[115,116] The active form of any nitrovasodilator is nitric oxide (NO), in which the nitrogen is in a +2 oxidation state. For any nitrovasodilator to be active, it must be first converted to nitric oxide. For nitroprusside, this is easily accomplished because nitrogen is in a +3 oxidation state, with the nitric oxide molecule bound to the charged iron molecule in an unstable manner, allowing nitroprusside to readily donate its nitric oxide moiety. In the case of nitroglycerin, nitrogen molecules exist in a +5 oxidation state, and thus they must undergo significant metabolic transformations before they are converted to an active molecule. Nitroglycerin is a relatively selective coronary vasodilator and does not produce coronary steal as compared to nitroprusside because the small intracoronary resistance vessels, those less than 100 microns, lack whatever metabolic transformation pathway required to convert nitroglycerin into its active form of nitric oxide.[115,116] Chronic nitrate therapy can produce tolerance through different mechanisms, as shown in Table 4-2.[114–118] Sodium nitroprusside and nitroglycerin are effective vasodilators that produce venodilation that contributes significantly to the labile hemodynamic state.[114] Intravenous volume administration is often required with nitroprusside due to the relative intravascular hypovolemia.

Dihydropyridine Calcium Channel Blockers

Dihydropyridine calcium channel blockers are direct arterial vasodilators.[119] Nifedipine was the first dihydropyridine calcium channel blocker, and the newer second-generation water-soluble agents that are available in intravenous form include isradipine and nicardipine. Isradipine and nicardipine produce arterial vasodilation without any effects on the vascular capacitance bed, no effects on atrioventricular nodal conduction, and no depression of ventricular function (i.e., contractility).[120–125] Nicardipine is the first intravenous drug of this class to be available in the United States, and it offers a novel and important therapeutic option to treat perioperative hypertension following cardiac surgery. Because currently available intravenous calcium channel blockers have longer half-lives than nitrovasodilators, rapid loading infusion rates or bolus loading doses need to be administered to obtain therapeutic levels. Bolus nicardipine administration can also be used to treat acute hypertension that occurs during the perioperative period (i.e., intubation, extubation, cardiopulmonary bypass–induced hypertension, and aortic cross-clamping).

Phosphodiesterase Inhibitors

The phosphodiesterase inhibitors currently available for use produce both positive inotropic effects and vasodilation.[126] When administered to patients with ventricular dysfunction, they increase cardiac output, while decreasing pulmonary artery occlusion pressure, systemic vascular resistance, and pulmonary vascular resistance. Because of their unique mechanisms of vasodilation, they are especially useful for patients with acute pulmonary vasoconstriction and right ventricular dysfunction. Multiple forms of the drug are currently under investigation. The bipyridines (amrinone and milrinone), the imidazolones (enoximone), and the methylxanthines (aminophylline) are the ones most widely available. Papaverine, a benzyl isoquinolinium derivative isolated from opium, is a nonspecific phosphodiesterase inhibitor and vasodilator used by cardiac surgeons for its ability to dilate the internal mammary artery.[126]

Angiotensin-Converting Enzyme Inhibitors

The angiotensin-converting enzyme (ACE) inhibitors have growing use in the management of heart failure, and more patients are receiving these drugs. The ACE inhibitors prevent the conversion of angiotensin I to angiotensin II by inhibiting an enzyme called kininase in the pulmonary and systemic vascular endothelium. This enzyme is also important for the metabolism of bradykinin, a potent endogenous vasodilator, and for release of EDRF. Although there is little data in the literature regarding the preoperative management of patients receiving these drugs, withholding them on the day of surgery has been our clinical practice based on their potential to produce excessive vasodilation during CPB. Although Tuman was unable to find any difference in blood pressure during CPB in patients receiving ACE inhibitors, contact activation during CPB has the ability to generate bradykinin and thus amplify the potential for vasodilation.[127] The vasoconstrictor requirements were increased after bypass in his study.

Angiotensin II Receptor Blockers

Angiotensin-converting enzyme (ACE) inhibitors may not be tolerated in some patients due to cough (common) and angioedema (rare). Inhibition of kininase II by ACE inhibitors leads to bradykinin accumulation in the lungs and vasculature, which probably causes cough and vasodilation. Alternative treatment with angiotensin II–receptor blockers (ARBs) may be less frequently associated with these side effects because ARBs do not affect kinin metabolism. Six ARBs are currently available for antihypertensive therapy in the United States: losartan (Cozaar), valsartan (Diovan), irbesartan (Avapro), candesartan (Atacand), eprosartan (Teveten), and telmisartan (Micardis). Mortality in chronic heart failure is related to activation of the autonomic nervous and renin-angiotensin systems, and ACE inhibitor therapy seems to attenuate progression of myocardial dysfunction and remodeling. ACE inhibitors do not completely block angiotensin II (A-II) production,[128] and may even increase circulating A-II levels in patients with heart failure.[129]It was initially thought that ARBs might offer advantages over ACE inhibitors for heart failure therapy in terms of tolerability and more complete A-II blockade. Although ARBs were more tolerated,[130] all-cause mortality and the number of sudden deaths or resuscitated cardiac arrests were not different when losartan (Cozaar) and captopril (Capoten) were compared in patients (>60 years old, NYHA class II-IV, LVEF <40%).[131] Hence, the long-term benefits from ACE inhibitor therapy are, at least in part, attributable to increased bradykinin formation.[132,133] For the treatment of heart failure, combination therapies with ACE inhibitors and ARBs are currently being investigated.[134,135] Perioperative hypotension may be encountered in ARB-treated patients as well as ACE inhibitor–treated patients, and increased inotropic support may be required.[136–138]

PHARMACOLOGIC MANIPULATION OF THE HEMOSTATIC SYSTEM DURING CARDIAC SURGERY

Numerous pharmacologic approaches to manipulate the hemostatic system in cardiac surgery include attenuating hemostatic system activation, preserving platelet function, and decreasing the need for transfusion of allogeneic blood products.[139–141] Different approaches currently available or under investigation are shown in Tables 4-3 and 4-4. Pharmacologic approaches to reduce bleeding and transfusion requirements in cardiac surgical patients are based on either preventing or reversing the defects associated with the CPB-induced coagulopathy.

TABLE 4–3 Novel anticoagulant agents affecting the hemostatic system

Therapeutic class	Agents	Indications
Anti-inflammatory	Adhesion molecule inhibitors Aprotinin complement inhibitors (pexelizumab) Interleukin antagonists P-selection inhibitors	All agents except aprotinin are in clinical development
Antiplatelet inhibitors (intravenous)	Abciximab (ReoPro) Eptifibatide (Integrelin) Tirofiban (Aggrastat)	Percutaneous coronary interventions
Antiplatelet inhibitors (oral)	Clopidogrel (Plavix)	Reduction of atherosclerotic events (myocardial infarction, stroke, and vascular death)
Antithrombotic	Argatroban (Novastan) Bivalirudin (Angiomax) Dermatin sulfate (Orgaran) Pentasaccharide (Fondaparinux) Recombinant hirudin (lepirudin)	Anticoagulation in patients with heparin-induced thrombocytopenia (except for pentacaccharide, which is in phase 3 clinical studies)
Broad-spectrum biologicals	Activated protein C Antithrombin Aprotinin (Trasylol)	In phase 3 studies for sepsis For antithrombin deficiency states Prophylactic use to reduce blood loss and transfusions in patients undergoing CPB

Source: Reproduced with permission from Levy JH: Pharmacologic preservation of the hemostatic system during cardiac surgery. Ann Thorac Surg 2001; 72:1814S.

TABLE 4–4 Agents that improve hemostatic function in the bleeding patient

Therapeutic class	Agents	Indications
Blood components	Fresh frozen plasma	Factor deficiency, reversal of warfarin, increased prothrombin time
	Cryoprecipitate	Von Willebrand's disease, hypofibrinogenemia
	Platelets	Thrombocytopenia, platelet dysfunction
Factor concentrates	Recombinant factor VIII	Hemophilia
	Recombinant factor IX	Hemophilia
	Recombinant factor VIIa (NovoSeven)	Hemophilia with factor inhibitors; use reported with intractable, life-threatening bleeding
Fibrinolytic inhibitors	Aprotinin (Trasylol) Epsilon aminocaproic acid Tranexamic acid	All agents used to decrease bleeding during cardiac surgery, but aprotinin is the only drug FDA-approved to reduce bleeding
Pharmacologic agents	Desmopressin	Hemophilia A with factor VIII coagulant activity levels greater than 5%, used also to improve platelet function in renal failure
Protease inhibitors	Protinin (Trasylol)	Prophylactic use to reduce blood loss and transfusions in patients undergoing CPB
Topical agents	Fibrin glue/fibrin tissue adhesives	Tissue sealant applied for refractory bleeding

Source: Reproduced with permission from Levy JH: Pharmacologic preservation of the hemostatic system during cardiac surgery. Ann Thorac Surg 2001; 72:1814S.

Pharmacology of Anticoagulation

Anticoagulation therapy is based on inhibiting thrombus formation; however, thrombus is due to both thrombin activation and platelet activation (Table 4-5). Because of the complex humoral amplification system linking both hemostatic and inflammatory responses, there are multiple pathways to generate thrombin and platelet activation. During cardiac surgery, multiple aspects of the extracorporeal system can generate thrombin.

Heparin

Heparin is purified from either porcine intestine or from beef lung. Heparin that is used for cardiac surgery includes fragments that range from 3,000 to 30,000 daltons, and is also called unfractionated.[141] Heparin acts as an anticoagulant by binding to antithrombin III (AT III), enhancing the rate of thrombin-AT III complex formation, and also inhibiting other clotting factors.[142] One major advantage of unfractionated heparin is that it can be reversed immediately by protamine. Because heparin also binds to other proteins, it can also produce platelet dysfunction. Heparin dosing for CPB ranges from 300 to 500 units/kg. Despotis reported that the maintenance of patient-specific heparin concentrations during CPB was associated with more effective suppression of hemostatic activation.[143,144] Further, Mochizuki has shown that excess protamine can further alter coagulation and coagulation tests, and the careful exact titrated reversal of heparin avoiding excess protamine may be an important contribution to work by Despotis.[145] Heparin-induced thrombocytopenia (HIT) is an adverse effect of heparin produced by antibodies (IgG) to the composite of heparin-platelet factor 4 (PF4) that leads to the formation of immune complexes.[145] These immune complexes bind to platelets via platelet Fc-receptors (CD 32) producing intravascular platelet activation, thrombocytopenia, and platelet activation with potential thromboembolic complications that can result in limb loss or death.

TABLE 4–5 Preoperative anticoagulants used in cardiac surgical patients

	Heparin	LMWH	Warfarin
Chemistry	Glycosaminoglycan MW = 15.000	MW = 5.000	4-Hydroxy-coumarin
Mechanism of action	Binds to antithrombin lll to inhibit thrombin	Inhibition Ila-Xa	Vitamin K antagonist (factors II, VII, IX, X)
Bioavailability	30%	100%	
Half-life	IV: 45–60 min	SC: 4–7 h	40 h
Laboratory evaluation	ACT - APTT	Anti-Xa	PT/INR
Reversal	Protamine, 1 mg/100 U heparin	Protamine reverses 60%–80%	Vitamin K, FFP (2–4 units)

Low Molecular Weight Heparin

Low molecular weight heparin (LMWH) is manufactured by depolymerizing unfractionated heparin to produce a mean molecular weight of approximately 5000 daltons.[146–148] A pentasaccharide sequence is required for attachment of a heparin fragment to antithrombin, and additional 13-saccharide residues are necessary to allow the heparin fragment to simultaneously attach itself to the heparin-binding domain of thrombin.[146–148] LMWH fragments of less than 18 saccharides retain the critical pentasaccharide sequence required for formation of a Xa-antithrombin complex; LMWH inhibits both factor Xa and thrombin, but the ratio of factor Xa to thrombin is increased.[146–148] LMWH is widely used in cardiovascular medicine but poses a problem for cardiac surgical patients because of its long half-life. PTT and ACT are not affected by LMWH, and LMWH is not readily reversible with protamine.

Antithrombin

Antithrombin (AT) levels are normally present as approximately 100% activity, but decrease approximately 30% in patients receiving heparin. Following initiation of CPB, AT decreases by 40% to 50%, an important consideration that may be critical in determining the extent of thrombin inhibition, especially during CPB.[149] Despotis suggested better anticoagulation during CPB may be associated with less bleeding postprocedure, presumably related to preservation of critical coagulation components. One promising therapy currently under investigation is the use of purified antithrombin III (AT).[150] Supplemental AT, through improved heparin sensitivity and enhanced anticoagulation, may preserve hemostasis during CPB.[151]

New Anticoagulants

The new intravenous antithrombins recombinant hirudin (Refludan), bivalirudin (Hirulog), and argatroban inhibit fibrin-bound thrombin independent of AT.[152–158] The direct thrombin inhibitors do not require AT or access to the heparin binding site of thrombin, and inhibit fibrin-bound as well as fluid-phase thrombin.[41] Recombinant hirudin (lepirudin), a 65-amino-acid polypeptide, is the most potent antithrombin. Although lepirudin has been used for cardiac surgical patients with HIT, it is nonreversible, its effect is difficult to monitor, and it is eliminated by renal mechanisms. Argatroban is a synthetic intravenous direct thrombin inhibitor with a relatively short elimination half-life that is approved for use in patients with HIT. Argatroban requires hepatic elimination, and can be used in patients with renal failure. Bivalirudin (Angiomax) is a short-acting hirudin analogue that requires infusions to be effective, and has been studied in patients with acute coronary syndromes.[159]

When patients with HIT require CPB, danaparoid (Orgaran), ancrod, recombinant hirudin (Refludan), and several other drug combinations have been used with various degrees of success.[160–163] One of the major problems with these drugs is their lack of reversibility and thus potential to produce bleeding. Danaparoid has a long half-life ($t_{\frac{1}{2}}$ of anti–factor Xa activity of 24 hours), and monitoring is complicated by the need to measure anti–factor Xa. Recombinant hirudin, a direct thrombin inhibitor modified from a leech salivary protein, is the most potent and specific thrombin inhibitor currently known. It acts independently of cofactors such as antithrombin. Potzsch et al have reported using lepirudin during cardiopulmonary bypass for patients with HIT using a 0.25-mg/kg bolus and then 5-mg boluses when hirudin concentration was <2500 ng/mL as determined by ecarin clotting time.[157] Koster has reported that the use of tirofiban, a platelet inhibitor, appears to be a better solution to this problem.[164]

Aprotinin

Aprotinin is a naturally occurring polypeptide with a molecular weight of 6512 daltons that reversibly complexes with the active serine site in various proteases in plasma to inhibit the serine proteases, trypsin, kallikrein, plasmin, and elastase, reversibly. Multiple mechanisms are responsible for aprotinin's ability to reduce bleeding after CPB.[163–170] Aprotinin is the most potent antifibrinolytic agent. The propagation of the "intrinsic" fibrinolysis through factor XII–mediated kallikrein activation and the generation of plasmin through "extrinsic" or tPA-mediated activation of plasminogen is effectively inhibited by approximately 4 μmol/L of aprotinin, which is maintained in plasma with the high-dose regimen. Aprotinin also has multiple anti-inflammatory effects, and inflammation and hemostasis are closely linked. Finally, aprotinin has been studied in multiple placebo-controlled studies, and is the only agent approved by the FDA to reduce bleeding in cardiac surgical patients.[167–170]

Antifibrinolytic Agents and Desmopressin

The synthetic lysine analogues epsilon aminocaproic acid (EACA; Amicar) and tranexamic acid inhibit fibrinolysis by attaching to the lysine binding site of the plasmin(ogen) molecule, displacing plasminogen from fibrin. Levi et al reported a meta-analysis of all randomized, controlled trials of the three most frequently used pharmacological strategies to decrease perioperative blood loss (aprotinin, lysine analogues [aminocaproic acid and tranexamic acid], and desmopressin).[170] Studies were included if they reported at least one clinically relevant outcome (mortality, rethoracotomy, proportion of patients receiving a transfusion, or perioperative myocardial infarction) in addition to perioperative blood loss. In addition, a separate meta-analysis was done for studies concerning complicated cardiac surgery. A total of 72 trials (8409 patients) met the inclusion criteria. Treatment with aprotinin decreased mortality almost 2-fold (OR = 0.55; 95% CI, 0.34–0.90) compared with placebo. Treatment with aprotinin and with lysine analogues decreased the frequency of surgical reexploration (OR = 0.37; 95% CI, 0.25–0.55 and OR = 0.44, 95% CI, 0.22–0.90, respectively). These two treatments also significantly decreased the proportion of patients receiving any allogeneic blood transfusion. The use of desmopressin resulted in a small decrease in perioperative blood loss, but was not associated with a beneficial effect on other clinical outcomes. Aprotinin and lysine analogues did not increase the risk of perioperative myocardial infarction; however, desmopressin was associated with a 2.4-fold increase in the risk of this complication. Studies in patients undergoing complicated cardiac surgery showed similar results.

Acquired Platelet Dysfunction

Acquired functional platelet disorders are caused by the multitude of potent antiplatelet agents that patents receive for atherosclerotic vascular disease or during percutaneous interventions.[171–173] Clopidogrel (Plavix), a drug that selectively interferes with ADP-induced platelet aggregation, is commonly used in patients with ischemic heart disease and those undergoing angioplasty.[172] Clopidogrel requires 3 to 5 days for the onset to occur, and a similar length of time for the effect to disappear.[172] Because of the pivotal role of the platelet glycoprotein (GP) IIb/IIIa complex in platelet-mediated thrombus formation, three different GP IIb/IIIa antagonists are currently available, but differ in antagonist affinity, reversibility, and receptor specificity.[171] Glycoprotein (GP) IIb/IIIa (IIbß3) is a receptor on platelets that binds to key hemostatic proteins, including fibrinogen and von Willebrand factor (vWF), to allow cross-linking of platelets and platelet aggregation. By blocking this final common pathway using GP IIb/IIIa antagonists, these drugs function as inhibitors of platelet participation in acute thrombosis. Various antagonists of GP IIb/IIIa are available and include the monoclonal antibody abciximab (ReoPro); tirofiban (Aggrastat), a nonpeptide fiban molecule; and eptifibatide (Integrelin), a cyclic peptide. Tirofiban and eptifibatide are cleared predominantly through renal mechanisms and have a circulating plasma half-life of approximately 2 to 4 hours, and while abciximab has a relatively short plasma half-life, the monoclonal antibody avidly binds to platelets with a relatively longer duration of action.[171]

Antiplatelet agents are used primarily to treat and prevent arterial thrombosis. Ticlopidine and clopidogrel are believed to inhibit the binding of adenosine 5′-diphosphate (ADP) to its platelet receptor; this ADP-receptor blockade leads to direct inhibition of the binding of fibrinogen to the glycoprotein IIb/IIIa complex.[172]Clopidogrel was approved by the FDA for the reduction of ischemic events in patients with recent myocardial infarction, stroke, or peripheral arterial disease with no added risk for neutropenia. The combination of clopidogrel and aspirin, as well as the use of clopidogrel in coronary stenting, is rapidly growing. Many heart centers now administer clopidogrel before anticipated stenting procedures. The variability in bleeding in patients receiving these agents for cardiac surgery may relate to the time and duration of therapy.

TABLE 4–6 Recommendations for managing patients receiving platelet inhibitors for cardiac surgery

Stop therapy
Do not give platelet transfusions prior to surgery, or revasculariztion
Give normal doses of heparin
Platelet transfusions as needed after cardiopulmonary bypass

Previous recommendations for managing patients receiving antiplatelet agents and requiring cardiac surgery are summarized in Table 4-6. The fact that a patient is receiving antiplatelet agents should not preclude urgent revascularization. Platelets may be needed and should be available when operating on abciximab-treated patients. Platelets should not be administered prophylactically. Although recommendations have been made on reducing heparin dosing, we believe there are no data to support reductions in heparin dosing during CPB and for cardiac surgery. Therefore, standard loading doses should be considered and additional heparin doses, based on time and duration of bypass or on actual heparin levels, should be maintained. Further, the heparin is reduced at the end of CPB.

Protamine

One of our most unusual clinical practices is to anticoagulate patients with heparin, an extract from bovine lung or porcine intestine, and reverse the heparin with protamine, which is a histone and a basic arginine-rich polypeptide extracted from salmon sperm. Protamine immediately reverses heparin by nonspecific polyionic-polycationic (acid-base) interactions. There are different methods to determine the amount of protamine to be administered: Use a ratio of 1.3 mg protamine per 100 units heparin administered; determine heparin levels based on heparin-protamine titrations; or use a dose based on the total amount of heparin administered over time.[174]

Protamine, a polypeptide isolated from fish sperm, does have the potential to produce anaphylactic reactions, and other potential adverse drug reactions.[175,176] Although rapid protamine administration has the potential to produce hemodynamic instability, the life-threatening reactions to protamine seen clinically represent immediate hypersensitivity reactions.[175,176] The incidence of anaphylaxis appears to be higher in certain patient groups, including diabetics receiving protamine-containing insulin like NPH. We have reported that the incidence of anaphylaxis to protamine in NPH insulin–dependent diabetics is 0.6% to 2% compared to 0.06% in most other patients.[175,176] Other patient groups may be at an increased risk for adverse reactions to protamine including patients with a prior vasectomy or previous fish allergy; however, data do not support this contention.[175–176]

New methods for reversing anticoagulation were once under investigation but may never come to market and include heparin binding filters, recombinant platelet factor 4, and heparinase.[177]

Antifibrinolytics

As discussed above, patients following fibrinolytic therapy have a complex coagulopathic state. Because of the potential half-lives of the fibrinolytic agents, using drugs that counteract their effects is potentially useful. Epsilon-aminocaproic acid (EACA; Amicar) and its analogue, tranexamic acid, are derivatives of the amino acid lysine. Both of these drugs inhibit the proteolytic activity of plasmin and the conversion of plasminogen to plasmin by plasminogen activators. Although aprotinin in clinically used concentrations is the most potent inhibitor of fibrinolysis and would represent a useful therapy, it is not approved for this use.[169] Additional coagulation factors and platelets may be required in addition to inhibiting fibrinolysis to reverse the coagulopathy.

Blood Products

Blood products are widely administered in cardiac surgical patients and represent a major utilization for hospitals. Once widely administered as part of empirical therapy, specific indications for coagulation factors need to be determined prior to their administration (Table 4-7). In addition to costs, blood products carry significant risks. Although the risk of viral-induced transmission is low, immunosuppressive effects, transfusion-related acute lung injury, and costs need to be considered when administering blood products. The role of fresh frozen plasma administration needs to be considered because it represents an often inappropriately used product. Specific indications for blood products are listed in Table 4-7. Each institution needs to develop its own algorithm for blood product administration in cardiac surgical patients. Using specific therapies, excessive and inappropriate transfusions can be avoided.

TABLE 4–7 Indications for blood product administration in the bleeding cardiac surgical patient

Blood product	Indication	Doses
Red blood cells	Low Hct	
Fresh frozen plasma	Warfarin therapy	2–4 units
	Documented coagulation factor deficiency	
	Abnormal PT	
Platelets	Low platelet count, e.g., <50,000–100,000	1 unit/10 kg
	Platelet dysfunction, e.g., abnormal TEG	
Cryoprecipitate	Low fibrinogen, e.g., <150 mg/dL	
	Fibrin glue	
Bovine thrombin	Fibrin glue	
Antithrombin III	Inadequate ACT (pt on heparin)	500–1000 units

Recombinant Coagulation Products

Coagulation products used to manage bleeding in patients with hemophilia, von Willebrand's disease (vWD), or acquired inhibitors to antihemophilic factor include AHF concentrates, factor IX concentrates, factor VIIa concentrate, factor IX complexes, anti-inhibitor coagulant complexes, and desmopressin acetate. These commercially available products are used to manage acute bleeding or to prevent excessive bleeding during cardiac and noncardiac surgery in patients with hematologic disorders. Recombinant activated factor VIIa (rFVIIa; NovoSeven, Novo Nordisk A/S) has been used as a novel and effective treatment for patients with hemophilia with inhibitors for the treatment of bleeding, and to secure hemostasis in complex clinical situations.[178–181]

The role of rFVIIa in the treatment of bleeding was evaluated in an open pilot study in patients with complicated cardiac surgical procedures. Blood loss and hemostatic effects and safety following rFVIIa administration were evaluated.[181] Five patients undergoing closure of atrial septal defect, De Vega's procedure (mitral valve replacement with tricuspid valve repair), and arterial switch (2.5 years old) were evaluated. Four patients received rFVIIa intraoperatively, while the fifth received it postoperatively. Satisfactory hemostasis was achieved with a single dose (30 μg/kg) of rFVIIa. Four hours after treatment, mean blood loss was 262 mL for adults (220–334 mL) and 85 mL for the child. No significant adverse events were reported. Laboratory parameters indicated a mean 18.5-fold (range 3.7–42) increase in FVII levels at 30 minutes postinjection and a mean reduction of 12 seconds (range 3–39 seconds) in prothrombin time.[182]

The modes of action of rFIIa are multiple, including tissue-factor–dependent mechanisms and generation of factors Xa and IXa on the surface of activated platelets. These studies relate thrombin generation on activated platelets to the high level of recombinant factor VIIa binding to platelet surfaces. Therapeutic doses of recombinant factor VIIa are not established; different doses have been used during surgery in patients with hemophilia and inhibitors, and with refractory bleeding following cardiac surgery. The

TABLE 4–8 Location and actions of beta-adrenergic receptors

Tissue	Receptor	Action	Opposing actions
Heart			
Sinus & AV nodes	1	↑ Automaticity	Cholinergic receptors
Conduction pathways	1	↑ Conduction velocity	Cholinergic receptors
		↑ Automaticity	Cholinergic receptors
Myofibils	1	↑ Contractility	—
		↑ Automaticity	—
Vascular smooth muscle (arterial, venous)	2	Vasodilation	Alpha-adrenergic receptors
Bronchial smooth muscle	2	Bronchodilation	Cholinergic receptors
Kidneys	1	↑ Renin release (juxtaglomerular cells)	$Alpha_1$-adrenergic receptors
Liver	2	↑ Glucose metabolism	$Alpha_1$-adrenergic receptors
		↑ Lipolysis	
Fat/adipose tissue	3	↑ Lipolysis	—
Skeletal muscle	2	↑ Potassium uptake glycogenolysis	—
Eye—ciliary muscle	2	Relaxation	Cholinergic receptors
Gl tract	2	↑ Motility	Cholinergic receptors
Gallbladder	2	Relaxation	Cholinergic receptors
Urinary bladder detrusor muscle	2	Relaxation	Cholinergic receptors
Uterus	2	Relaxation	Oxytocin
Platelets	2	↓ Aggregation	$Alpha_2$-adrenergic receptors (aggregation)

Source: Reproduced with permission from Lefkowitz RH, Hoffman BB, Taylor P: Neurotransmission: the autonomic and somatic motor nervous system, in Hardman JL, Molinoff PB, Ruddon RW, Gilman AG (eds): The Pharmacological Basis of Therapeutics. New York, McGraw-Hill, 1996; p 84.

use of recombinant factor VIIa has been reported to control bleeding in patients with thrombocytopathies, liver disease, and liver transplantation, and patients undergoing cardiac surgery. Recommended dose ranges for rFVIIa usually vary from 60 to 120 μg/kg, although 90 μg/kg is usually the initial starting dose.[180]

Fibrinolytics

Patients may also have received fibrinolytic drugs, including tissue plasminogen activator (TPA), streptokinase, or urokinase. These drugs inactivate fibrinogen and other adhesive proteins, and have the potential to affect platelets as well.[181] Patients receiving these drugs within 24 hours of surgery should be considered to be at a high risk for coagulopathy, and fibrinogen levels should be measured.

BETA-ADRENERGIC RECEPTOR BLOCKERS

Not surprisingly, most of the effects observed after administration of a beta-adrenergic receptor blocker reflect the reduced responsiveness of tissues containing beta-adrenergic receptors to cathecholamines present in the vicinity of those receptors. Hence, the intensity of the effects of beta blockers is dependent on both the dose of the blocker as well as the receptor concentrations of catecholamines, primarily epinephrine and norepinephrine. In fact, a purely competitive interaction of beta blockers and catecholamines can be demonstrated in normal human volunteers as well as in isolated tissues studied in the laboratory. The presence of disease and other types of drugs modifies the responses to beta blockers observed in patients, but the underlying competitive interaction is still operative. The key to successful utilization of beta-adrenergic receptor blockers is to titrate the dose to the desired degree of effect and to remember that excessive effects from larger than necessary doses of beta-adrenergic receptor blockers can be overcome by (1) administering a catecholamine to compete at the blocked receptors, and/or (2) administering other types of drugs to reduce the activity of counterbalancing autonomic mechanisms that are unopposed in the presence of beta-receptor blockade. An example of the latter is propranolol-induced bradycardia, which reflects the increased dominance of the vagal cholinergic mechanism on cardiac nodal tissue. Excessive bradycardia may be relieved by administering atropine to block the cholinergic receptors, which are also located in the sinus and atrioventricular (AV) nodes.

Knowledge of the type, location, and action of beta receptor is fundamental to understanding and predicting effects of beta-adrenergic receptor–blocking drugs (Table 4-8).[183] Beta-adrenergic receptor blockers are competitive inhibitors;

TABLE 4–9 Beta-adrenergic receptor blockers

Generic name	Trade name	Dosage forms	β_1-selective
Acebutolol	Sectral	PO	Yes
Atenolol	Tenormin	IV, PO	Yes
Betaxolol	Kerlone	PO	Yes
Bisoprolol	Zebeta	PO	Yes
Esmolol	Brevibloc	IV	Yes
Metoprolol	Lopressor, Toprol-XL	IV, PO	Yes
Carvedilol*	Coreg	PO	No
Carteolol	Cartrol	PO	No
Labetalol*	Normodyne, Trandate	IV, PO	No
Nadolol	Corgard	PO	No
Penbutolol	Levatol	PO	No
Pindolol	Visken	PO	No
Propranolol	Inderal	IV, PO	No
Sotalol	Betapace	PO	No
Timolol	Blocadren	PO	No

*Alpha$_1$:beta-adrenergic blocking ratio; carvedilol 1:10, labetalol 1:3 (oral)/1:7 (IV).

Source: Reproduced with permission from Hug CJ: Beta-adrenergic blocking drugs, in Drug Evaluations Annual 1994. Chicago, American Medical Association, 1993; p 539.

hence the intensity of blockade is dependent on both the dose of the drug and receptor concentrations of catecholamines, primarily epinephrine and norepinephrine.

Beta-adrenergic receptor antagonists (blockers) include many drugs (Table 4-9) that are typically classified by their relative selectivity for beta$_1$ and beta$_2$ receptors (i.e., cardioselective or nonselective); the presence or absence of agonistic activity; membrane-stabilizing properties; alpha-receptor blocking efficacy; and various pharmacokinetic features (e.g., lipid solubility, oral bioavailability, elimination half-time).[184] The practitioner must realize that the selectivity of individual drugs for beta$_1$ and beta$_2$ receptors is relative, not absolute. For example, the risk of inducing bronchospasm with a beta$_1$-adrenergic (cardioselective) blocker (e.g., esmolol, metoprolol) may be relatively less than with a nonselective blockers (e.g., propranolol); however, the risk is still present.

Acute Myocardial Infarction

Clinical trials of intravenous beta-adrenergic blockers in the early phases of acute myocardial infarction suggest that mortality decreases by 10%. Following myocardial infarction, chronic oral beta-blocking agents reduce the incidence of recurrent myocardial infarction. A randomized, controlled trial of atenolol (Tenormin) in the perioperative period was performed by Mangano and his group. In their study, the incidence of myocardial ischemia was reduced by 50% in patients receiving atenolol. Overall mortality after discharge was lower in the atenolol group compared to the control group over a two-year period (10% vs. 21%).[185] However, atenolol did not result in the reduction of death during hospitalization or of perioperative myocardial infarction. Poldermans and his group performed another randomized, controlled perioperative trial in using bisoprolol (Zebeta) in high-risk vascular surgical patients. Bisoprolol therapy, started one week before a major surgery and continued for 30 days postoperatively, has significantly reduced the rate of death and nonfatal myocardial infarction.[186] The follow-up of their study showed that the reduction of cardiac events persisted over two years in the bisoprolol-treatment group (12 % vs. 32 %).[187]

Supraventricular Tachycardias and Ventricular Dysrhythmias

Beta-adrenergic blocking agents are Vaughan Williams class II antidysrhythmics that primarily block cardiac responses to catecholamines. Propranolol (Inderal), esmolol (Brevibloc), and acebutolol (Sectral) are commonly used for this indication. Beta-blocking agents decrease spontaneous depolarization in the sinus and atrioventricular (AV) nodes, decrease automaticity in Purkinje fibers, increase AV nodal refractoriness, increase threshold for fibrillation (but not for depolarization), and decrease ventricular slow responses that are dependent on catecholamines. Amiodarone, a class III agent, also exerts noncompetitive alpha- and beta-adrenergic blockade, which may contribute its antidysrhythmic and antihypertensive actions.[188] Sotalol is another class III antidysrhythmic with nonselective beta-blocking action. There is evidence that beta-blocking agents also decrease intramyocardial conduction in ischemic tissue and reduce the risks of dysrhythmias, to the extent that they decrease myocardial ischemia. Beta-adrenergic blockers are not particularly effective in controlling dysrhythmias that are not induced or maintained by catecholamines.

Hypertension

Hypertension is a major risk factor for the development of heart failure and other end-organ damage. Beta blockers, along with diuretics, are considered to be the initial drug of choice for uncomplicated hypertension in patients aged less than 65 years.[189]

During the early phases of therapy there is a decrease in cardiac output, a rise in systemic vascular resistance (SVR), and relatively little change in mean arterial blood pressure. Within hours to days, SVR normalizes and blood pressure declines. In addition, the release of renin from the juxtaglomerular apparatus in the kidney is inhibited ($beta_1$ blockade). Beta-blocking agents with intrinsic agonistic activity reduce systemic vascular resistance below pretreatment levels, presumably by activating $beta_2$ receptors in vascular smooth muscle. Most beta-adrenergic blockers are used in conjunction with other agents in the treatment of chronic hypertension. When combined with a vasodilator, beta blockers limit reflex tachycardia. For example, when propranolol is combined with intravenous nitroprusside (a potent arterial dilator), it prevents reflex release of renin and reflex tachycardia induced by nitroprusside.

Acute Dissecting Aortic Aneurysm

The primary goal in the management of dissecting aneurysms is to reduce stress on the dissected aortic wall by reducing the systolic acceleration of blood flow. Beta blockers reduce cardiac inotropy and reduce ventricular ejection fraction. Beta blockers may also limit reflex sympathetic responses to vasodilators that are used to control systemic arterial pressure.

Pheochromocytoma

The presence of catecholamine-secreting tissue is tantamount to the continuous or intermittent infusion of a varying mixture of norepinephrine and epinephrine. It is absolutely essential that virtually complete alpha-adrenergic receptor blockade be established prior to the administration of the beta blocker in order to prevent exacerbation of hypertensive episodes by unopposed alpha-adrenergic receptor activity in vascular smooth muscle.

Chronic Heart Failure

It is now understood that the activation of the autonomic nervous system (ANS) and rennin-angiotensin system (RAS) as a compensatory mechanism to the failing heart may actually contribute to the deterioration of myocardial function. Mortality in chronic heart failure (CHF) seems related to activation of ANS and RAS. Progression of myocardial dysfunction and remodeling may be attenuated by the use of beta-blocking agents and ACE inhibitors. Carvedilol (Coreg) is a beta blocker approved by the FDA to treat patients with heart failure. It has an $alpha_1$- and nonselective beta-blocking activity (alpha:beta = 1:10). It is contraindicated in severe decompensated heart failure and asthma. In patients with atrial fibrillation and left heart failure treated with carvedilol, improved ejection fraction and a trend of decreased incidence of death and CHF hospitalization were observed in a retrospective analysis of a U.S. carvedilol study.[190] There are several on-going clinical trials with carvedilol, metoprolol (Toprol), or bisoprolol (Zebeta). The results of these studies may provide answers as to which beta-blocking agent would most successfully treat specific patient populations.

TABLE 4–10 Clinical applications of beta-adrenergic receptor blockers

Angina pectoris
Acute myocardial infarction (prophylaxis)
Supraventricular tachycardia
Ventricular dysrhythmias
Hypertension (usually in combination with other drugs)
Pheochromocytoma (after alpha-receptor blockade is established)
Acute dissecting aortic aneurysm
Hyperthyroidism
Hypertrophic obstructive cardiomyopathy (IHSS)
Dilated cardiomyopathy (selected patients)
Migraine prophylaxis
Acute panic attack
Alcohol withdrawal syndrome
Glaucoma (topically)

Source: Reproduced with permission from Hug CJ: Beta-adrenergic blocking drugs, in Drug Evaluations Annual 1994. Chicago, American Medical Association, 1993; p 539.

Other Indications

The other clinical applications of beta-adrenergic receptor blockers listed in Table 4-10 are based on largely symptomatic treatment or empiric trials of beta-adrenergic antagonists.

Side Effects and Toxicity

The most obvious and immediate signs of a toxic overdose of a beta-adrenergic receptor blocker are hypotension, bradycardia, congestive heart failure, decreased AV conduction, and a widened QRS complex on the electrocardiogram. Treatment is aimed at blocking the cholinergic receptor responses to vagal nerve activity (e.g., atropine) and administering a sympathomimetic to compete with the beta blockers at adrenergic receptors. In patients with asthma and COPD, beta blockers may cause bronchospasm. Beta blockers may increase levels of plasma triglycerides and reduce levels of HDL cholesterol.[191] Rarely, beta blockers may mask the symptoms of hypoglycemia in diabetic patients. Other side effects include mental depression, physical fatigue, altered sleep patterns, sexual dysfunction, and gastrointestinal symptoms including indigestion, constipation, and diarrhea.

Drug Interactions

Pharmacokinetic drug interactions include reduced gastrointestinal absorption of the beta blocker (aluminum-containing antacids, cholestyramine), increased biotransformation of the beta blocker (phenytoin, phenobarbital, rifampin, smoking), and increased bioavailability due to decreased biotransformation (e.g., cimetidine, hydralazine). Pharmacodynamic interactions include an additive effect with calcium channel blockers to decrease conduction in the heart and a reduced antihypertensive effect of beta blockers when administered with some of the NSAIDs.

DIURETICS

Diuretics are drugs that act directly on the kidneys to increase urine volume and to produce a net loss of solute (principally sodium and other electrolytes) and water. Diuretics and beta blockers are initial drugs of choice for uncomplicated hypertension in patients younger than 65 years.[189] The currently available diuretic drugs have a number of other uses in medicine (e.g., glaucoma, increased intracranial pressure). The principal indications for the use of diuretics by intravenous administration in the perioperative period are (1) to increase urine flow in oliguria, (2) to reduce intravascular volume in patients at risk of acute congestive heart failure from excessive fluid administration or acute heart failure, and (3) to mobilize edema.

Renal function depends on adequate renal perfusion to maintain the integrity of renal cells and to provide the hydrostatic pressure that produces glomerular filtration. There are no drugs that act directly on the renal glomerulus to affect glomerular filtration rate (GFR). In the normal adult human of average size, GFR averages 125 mL/min and urine production approximates 1 mL/min. In other words, 99% of the glomerular filtrate is reabsorbed. Diuretics act primarily on specific segments of the renal tubule to alter reabsorption of electrolytes, principally sodium, and water.

There are two basic mechanisms behind the renal tubular reabsorption of sodium. (1) Sodium is extruded from the tubular cell into peritubular fluid primarily by active transport of the sodium ion, which reflects the action of the Na^+-K^+ ATPase pump and also the bicarbonate reabsorption mechanism (see below). This extrusion of sodium creates an electrochemical gradient causing diffusion of sodium from the tubular lumen into the tubular cell. (2) Sodium moves from the glomerular filtrate in the tubular fluid into the peritubular fluid by several different mechanisms. The most important quantitatively is the sodium electrochemical gradient created by the active extrusion of sodium from the tubular cell into peritubular fluid. In addition, sodium is coupled with organic solutes and phosphate ions, exchanged for hydrogen ions diffusing from the tubular cell into the tubular lumen, and coupled to the transfer of a chloride ion or a combination of a potassium and two chloride ions (Na^+-K^+-$2Cl^-$ cotransport) from tubular fluid into the tubular cell. Diuretics are classified by their principal site of action in the nephron and by the primary mechanism of their naturetic effect (Table 4-11).

TABLE 4–11 Classification of diuretics

Site of action	Mechanism	
Osmotic	Proximal convoluted and late proximal for NA^+ diffusion from tubular fluid into tubular cell	↓ Electrochemical gradient
	Late proximal tubule	↓ Gradient for Cl^- (accompanying Na^+ diffusion)
	Thick ascending loop of Henle	↓ Na^+-K^+-$2Cl^-$ cotransport
Carbonic	Proximal convoluted tubule anhydrase inhibitors	↓ Na^+-H^+ exchange$^+$
Thiazides	Distal convoluted tubule	↓ NA^+-Cl^- cotransport
High ceiling loop diuretics	Thick ascending loop of Henle	↓ NA^+-K^+-$2Cl^-$ cotransport
Potassium-sparing	Late distal tubule and collecting duct	↓ Electrogenic NA^+ entry into cells (driving force for K^+ secretion)

Source: Reproduced with permission from Wener IM: Drugs affecting renal function and electrolyte metabolism, in Gilman AG, Rall TW, Nies AS, Taylor P (eds): The Pharmacological Basis of Therapeutics, 8th ed. New York, Pergamon Press, 1990; p 708.

Osmotic Diuretics

Mannitol is the principal example of this type of diuretic, which is used for two primary indications: (1) prophylaxis and early treatment of acute renal failure which is characterized by a decrease in GFR leading to a decreased urine volume and a increase in the concentration of toxic substances in the renal tubular fluid; (2) to enhance the actions of other diuretics by retaining water and solutes in the tubular lumen, thereby providing the substrate for the action of other types of diuretics. Normally, 80% of the glomerular filtrate is reabsorbed isosmotically in the proximal tubules. By its osmotic effect, mannitol limits the reabsorption of water and dilutes the proximal tubular fluid. This reduces the electrochemical gradient for sodium and limits its reabsorption so that more is delivered to the distal portions of the nephron. Mannitol produces a prostaglandin-mediated increase in renal blood flow that partially washes out the medullary hypertonicity, which is essential for the countercurrent mechanism promoting the reabsorption of water in the late distal tubules and collecting system under the influence of ADH. Mannitol is often used (25–50 g) as a part of the priming solution of cardiopulmonary bypass for the above-mentioned indications. The principal toxicity of mannitol is acute expansion of the extracellular fluid volume leading to congestive heart failure in the patient with compromised cardiac function.

High Ceiling (Loop) Diuretics

Furosemide (Lasix), bumetanide (Bumex), and ethacrynic acid (Edecrin) are three chemically dissimilar compounds that have the same primary diuretic mechanism of action. They act on the tubular epithelial cell in the thick ascending loop of Henle to inhibit the Na^+-K^+-$2Cl^-$ cotransport mechanism. Their peak diuretic effect is far greater than that of the other diuretics currently available. Administered intravenously, they have a rapid onset and relatively short duration of action, the latter reflecting both the pharmacokinetics of the drugs and the body's compensatory mechanisms to the consequences of diuresis. These three diuretics increase renal blood flow without increasing GFR and redistribute blood flow from the medulla to the cortex and within the renal cortex. These changes in renal blood flow are also short-lived, reflecting the reduced extracellular fluid volume resulting from diuresis. Minor actions, including carbonic anhydrase inhibition by furosemide and bumetanide and actions on the proximal tubule and on sites distal to the ascending limb, remain controversial. All three of the loop diuretics increase the release of renin and prostaglandin, and indomethacin blunts the release as well as the augmentation in renal blood flow and naturesis. All three of the loop diuretics produce an acute increase in venous capacitance for a brief period of time after the first intravenous dose is administered, and this effect is also blocked by indomethacin.

Potassium, magnesium, and calcium excretion are increased in proportion to the increase in sodium excretion. In addition, there is augmentation of titratable acid and ammonia excretion by the distal tubules leading to metabolic alkalosis, which is also produced by contraction of the extracellular volume. Hyperuricemia can occur but usually is of little physiological significance. The nephrotoxicity of cephaloridine, and possibly other cephalorsporins, is increased. A rare but serious side effect of the loop diuretics is deafness, which may reflect electrolyte changes in the endolymph.

Because of their high degree of efficacy, prompt onset, and relatively short duration of action, the high ceiling or loop diuretics are favored for intravenous administration in the perioperative period to treat the three principal problems cited above. Dosage requirements vary considerably among patients. Some may only require furosemide 3 to 5 mg IV to produce a good diuresis. And for some patients the less potent benzothiazides may be sufficient.

Benzothiazides

Hydrochlorothiazide (HCTZ) is the prototype of more than a dozen currently available diuretics in this class. Although the drugs differ in potency, they all act by the same mechanism of action and have the same maximum efficacy. All are actively secreted into the tubular lumen by tubular cells and act in the early distal tubules to decrease the electroneutral Na^+-Cl^- cotransport reabsorption of sodium. Their moderate efficacy probably reflects the fact that more than 90% of the filtrated sodium is reabsorbed before reaching the distal tubules. Their action is enhanced by their combined administration with an osmotic diuretic such as mannitol. The benziothiazides increase urine volume and the excretion of sodium, chloride, and potassium. The decreased reabsorption of potassium reflects the higher rate of urine flow through the distal tubule (diminished reabsorption time).

This class of diuretics produces the least disturbance of extracellular fluid composition, reflecting their moderate efficacy as diuretics and perhaps suggesting their usefulness when a moderate degree of diuretic effect is indicated. Their principal side effects include hyperuricemia, decreased calcium excretion, and enhanced magnesium loss. Hyperglycemia can occur and reflects multiple variables. With prolonged use and the development of a contracted extracellular fluid volume, urine formation decreases (i.e., tolerance develops to their diuretic actions). These agents also have a direct action on the renal vasculature to decrease GFR.

Carbonic Anhydrase Inhibitors

Acetazolamide (Diamox) is the only diuretic of this class available for intravenous administration. Its use is primarily directed to alkalinization of urine in the presence of metabolic alkalosis, which is a common consequence of prolonged diuretic therapy. It acts in the proximal convoluted tubule to inhibit carbonic anhydrase in the brush border of the tubular epithelium, thereby reducing the destruction of bicarbonate ions (i.e., conversion to CO_2 that diffuses into the tubular cell). The carbonic anhydrase enzyme in the cytoplasm of the tubular cell is also inhibited, with a consequence that the conversion of CO_2 to carbonic acid is markedly reduced as is the availability of hydrogen ions for the Na-H exchange mechanism. Hence, the reabsorption of both sodium and bicarbonate in the proximal tubules is diminished. However, more than half of the bicarbonate is reabsorbed in more distal segments of the nephron, thereby limiting the overall efficacy of this class of diuretics.

Potassium-Sparing Diuretics

Spironolactone (Aldactone) is a competitive antagonist of aldosterone. Spironolactone binds to the cytoplasmic aldosterone receptor and prevents its conformational change to the active form, thereby aborting the synthesis of active transport proteins in the late distal tubules and collecting system where the reabsorption of sodium and secretion of potassium are reduced.

Triamterene (Dyrenium) and amiloride (Midamor) are potassium-sparing diuretics with a mechanism of action independent of the mineralocorticoids. They have a moderate naturetic effect leading to an increased excretion of sodium and chloride with little change or a slight increase in potassium excretion when the latter is low. When potassium secretion is high, they produce a sharp reduction in the electrogenic entry of sodium ions into the distal tubular cells and thereby reduce the electrical potential that is the driving force for potassium secretion.

Both types of potassium-sparing diuretics are used primarily in combination with other diuretics to reduce potassium loss. Their principal side effect is hyperkalemia. It is appropriate to limit the intake of potassium when using this type of diuretic. It is also appropriate to use this type of diuretic cautiously in patients taking ACE inhibitors, which decrease aldosterone formation and consequently increase serum potassium concentrations.

Other Measures to Enhance Urine Output and Mobilization of Edema Fluid

The infusion of albumin (5%–25% solutions) or other plasma volume expanders (e.g., hetastarch) is often employed in an attempt to draw water and its accompanying electrolytes (i.e., edema fluid) osmotically from the tissues into the circulating blood and thereby enhance their delivery to the kidney for excretion. In the presence of a reduced circulating blood volume, this approach seems to be a logical method to increase the circulating blood volume and renal perfusion. The limiting feature of this approach to enhancing diuresis relates to the fact that the osmotic effect of albumin and plasma expanders is transient because they can diffuse (at a rate slower than water) from blood through capillary membranes into tissue. The albumin or plasma expander then tends to hold water and its accompanying electrolytes in tissue (i.e., rebound edema). The same limiting feature applies to osmotic diuretics such as mannitol, which may transiently draw water and its accompanying electrolytes from tissues into the circulating blood for delivery to the kidney, where the mannitol passes through the glomerulus and delays the reabsorption of water and its accompanying electrolytes from the proximal tubular fluid. While this mechanism may enhance the actions of other diuretics, it is a transient effect limited by the diffusion of mannitol from blood into tissues with the production of rebound edema.

Dopamine (Intropin), at doses 1 to 3 μg/kg/min, has been used conventionally to support mesenteric and renal perfusion. Its vascular action is mediated via vascular dopamine-1 (D_1) receptors in coronary, mesenteric, and renal vascular beds. By activating adenyl cyclase and raising intracellular concentrations of cyclic-AMP, D_1-receptor agonist causes vasodilatation. There are also dopamine-2 (D_2) receptors that antagonize D_1-receptor stimulation. Fenoldopam (Corlopam), a parenteral D_1-receptor-specific agonist, was recently approved by FDA. The JNC VI recommendation includes this drug for hypertensive emergencies.[192,193] Infusion of fenoldopam (0.1–0.3 μg/kg/min) causes an increase in glomerular filtration rate, renal blood flow, and Na^+ excretion.

Clinical trials of dopamine failed to show improvement in renal function, which may probably be due to nonspecificity of dopamine. As a catecholamine and a precursor in the metabolic synthesis of norepinephrine and epinephrine, dopamine has inotropic and chronotropic effects on the heart. The inotropic effect is mediated by $beta_1$-adrenergic receptors and usually requires infusion rates higher than those able to produce enhanced renal perfusion and diuresis. However, there are extremely varied pharmacokinetic responses to dopamine infusion even in healthy subjects[194]; therefore, the use of a "renal dose" dopamine regimen may not always result in the desirable effects. Stimulation of catecholamine receptors and D_2 receptors antagonizes the effects of D_1-receptor stimulation. There are a small number of studies where the improved renal outcome shown with the use of the D_1-receptor-specific agonist fenoldopam.[195–197] A further large-scale study is needed to answer whether prophylactic use of fenoldopam reduces the incidence of perioperative renal insufficiency.

HERBAL MEDICINE

A large number of Americans take herbal remedies for their health. Most of these herbal therapies are not supported by clear scientific evidence, or under rigorous control of

TABLE 4–12 Commonly used herbal remedies

Name	Common uses	Side effects / drug interactions
Cayenne (paprika)	Muscle spasm, Gl disorders	Skin ulcers / blistering Hypothermia
Echinacea	Common cold, antitussive, urinary tract infections	May cause hepatotoxicity May decrease effects of steroids and cyclosporine
Ephedra (ma-huang)	Antitussive, bacteriostatic	Enhanced sympathomimetic effects with guanethedine or monoamine oxidase inhibitor (MAO I) Arrhythmias with halothane or digoxin Hypertension with oxytocin
Feverfew	Migraine, antipyretic	Platelet inhibition, rebound headache, aphthous ulcers, GI irritation
Garlic	Lipid lowering, antihypertensive, antithrombotic	May potentiate warfarin
Ginger	Antinauseant, antispasmodic	May potentiate warfarin
Gingko	Improve circulation	May potentiate aspirin and warfarin
Ginseng	Adaptogenic, enhance energy level, antioxidant	Ginseng abuse syndrome: sleepiness, hypertonia, edema May cause mania in patients on phenelzine May decrease effects of warfarin Postmenopausal bleeding Mastalgia
Goldenseal	Diuretic, anti-inflammatory, laxative, hemostatic	Overdose may cause paralysis; aquaretic (no sodium excretion); may worsen edema / hypertension
Kava-kava	Anxiolytic	Potentiate barbiturates and benzodiazepines Potentiate ethanol May increase suicide risk in depression
Licorice	Antitussive, gastric ulcers	High blood pressure, hypokalemia, and edema
Saw palmetto	Benign prostatic hypertrophy, antiandrogenic	Additive effects with other hormone therapy (e.g., HRT)
St. John's wort	Antidepressant, anxiolytic	Possible interaction with MAO inhibitors Decrease metabolism of fentanyl and ondansetron
Valerian	Mild sedative, anxiolytic	Potentiate barbiturates and benzodiazepines

FDA.[198] Patients who take alternative remedies may not necessarily disclose this information to their physicians.[199] There are increasing concerns regarding serious drug interactions between herbal therapy and prescribed medication. Some of the most common herbal remedies and drug interactions are summarized in Table 4-12.[200]

DRUGS FOR AIRWAY MANAGEMENT

Airway management in cardiovascular surgical patients is very important because these patients often present with coexisting conditions that may complicate endotracheal intubation. For example, a patient with morbid obesity and sleep apnea may require awake intubation with a fiberoptic bronchoscope, or a history of smoking and chronic obstructive pulmonary disease (COPD) may make the patient susceptible to rapid desaturation and/or bronchospasm. Airway management in the perioperative period is a primary responsibility of the anesthesiologist, but the surgeon becomes involved in the absence of the anesthesiologist or in assisting the anesthesiologist in difficult situations. Airway management involves instrumentation and mechanics (not discussed here) and employs drugs to overcome pathophysiological problems that contribute to airway obstruction and to facilitate manipulation and instrumentation of the airway. Most of the drugs utilized for these purposes are taken from drug classes that have other important therapeutic applications (e.g., sympathomimetics).

Five major challenges may be encountered in airway management. Each of these is described succinctly below in order to facilitate understanding of the roles that drugs play in meeting the challenges. For the most part, details of pharmacology such as doses, side effects, and toxicity are left to standard textbooks of pharmacology and drug compendia. The five challenges are: (1) overcoming airway obstruction; (2) preventing pulmonary aspiration; (3) performing endotracheal intubation; (4) maintaining intermittent positive pressure ventilation (IPPV); and (5) reestablishing spontaneous ventilation and airway protective reflexes.

Airway Obstruction

Obstruction to gas flow can occur from the entry of a foreign object (including food) into the airway and as a result of pathophysiological processes involving airway structures (e.g., trauma, edema). In the anesthetized or comatose patient, the loss of muscle tone can allow otherwise normal tissues (e.g., tongue, epiglottis) to collapse into the airway and cause obstruction. The first measure in relieving such obstructions involves manipulation of the head and jaw, insertion of an artificial nasal or oral airway device, and evacuation of obstructing objects and substances (e.g., blood, secretions, food particles). Except for drugs used to facilitate endotracheal intubation (see below), the only drug useful to improve gas flow through a narrowed airway is a mixture of helium and oxygen (heliox), which has a much reduced viscosity resulting in reduced resistance to gas flow.

Aspiration

The upper airway (above the larynx/epiglottis) is a shared porthole to the lungs (gas exchange) and gastrointestinal tract (fluids and nutrition). Passive regurgitation or active vomiting resulting in accumulation of gastric contents in the pharynx places the patient at risk of pulmonary aspiration, especially under circumstances in which airway reflexes (glottic closure, coughing) and voluntary avoidance maneuvers are suppressed (e.g., anesthesia, coma). Particulate matter can obstruct the tracheal bronchial tree and acidic fluid ($pH < 2.5$) can injure the lung parenchyma. The resulting pneumonitis can cause significant morbidity (e.g., ARDS) and has a high mortality rate. Preoperative restriction of fluids and food (NPO status) does not guarantee the absence of aspiration risks. Similarly, the advance placement of a naso/orogastric tube may serve to reduce intragastric pressure but does not guarantee complete removal of gastric contents. Nevertheless, both NPO orders and insertion of a naso/orogastric tube under some circumstances are worthwhile measures to reduce the risks of pulmonary aspiration. In some circumstances, the deliberate induction of vomiting in a conscious patient may be indicated, but is rarely done and almost never involves the use of an emetic drug. In fact, more often antiemetic drugs are employed to reduce the risks of vomiting during airway manipulation and induction of anesthesia.

Drug therapy to reduce the risks of pulmonary aspiration is focused on decreasing the quantity and acidity of gastric contents and on facilitating endotracheal intubation (see below). Nonparticulate antacids (e.g., sodium citrate [Bicitra]) are utilized to neutralize the acidity of gastric fluids. Drugs to reduce gastric acid production include H_2-receptor blockers (e.g., cimetidine [Tagamet], ranitidine [Zantac], famotidine [Pepcid]) and inhibitors of gastric parietal cell hydrogen-potassium ATPase (proton pump inhibitors, e.g., omeprazole [Prilosec], lansoprazole [Prevacid], esomeprazole [Nexium]). Metoclopramide (Reglan) enhances gastric emptying and increases the gastroesophageal sphincter tone. Cisapride (Propulsid) also increases gastrointestinal motility via the release of acetylcholine at the myenteric plexus.

Antiemetic drugs are more commonly used in the postoperative period and include several different drug classes: anticholinergics (scopolamine [Transderm Scop]), antihistamines (hydroxyzine [Vistaril], promethazine [Pherergan]), and antidopaminergics (droperidol [Inapsine], prochlorperazine [Compazine]). Antidopaminergic agents may cause extrapyramidal side effects in elderly patients. More costly, but effective, alternatives are the use of antiserotoninergics (e.g., ondansetron [Zofran], dolasetron [Anzmet]).

Of course, the most widely used measure to minimize the risks of pulmonary aspiration in the anesthetized or comatose patient is endotracheal intubation.

Endotracheal Intubation

Drugs are employed for three purposes in facilitating endotracheal intubation: (1) to improve visualization of the larynx during laryngoscopy; (2) to prevent closure of the larynx; (3) to facilitate manipulation of the head and jaw.

For bronchoscopy, laryngoscopy, or fiberoptic endotracheal intubation, the reflex responses to airway manipulation can be suppressed by several different methods, alone or in combination. Topical anesthesia (2% or 4% lidocaine spray) can be used to anesthetize the mucosal surfaces of the nose, oral cavity, pharynx, and epiglottis. Atomized local anesthetic can be inhaled to anesthetize the mucosa below the vocal cords. The subglottic mucosa can also be topically anesthetized by injecting local anesthetic into the tracheal lumen through the cricothyroid membrane. A bilateral superior laryngeal nerve block eliminates sensory input from mechanical contact or irritation of the larynx above the vocal cords. It must be remembered that anesthesia of the mucosal surfaces to obtund airway reflexes compromises the reflex protective mechanisms of the airway and increases the patient's vulnerability to aspiration of substances from the pharynx. Improvement of visualization of the larynx includes decreasing salivation and tracheal bronchial secretions by administration of an anticholinergic drug (e.g., glycopyrrolate), reducing mucosal swelling by topical administration of a vasoconstrictor (e.g., phenylephrine), and minimizing bleeding due to mucosal erosion by instrumentation, which also is minimized by topical vasconstrictors.

The role of steroids in minimizing acute inflammatory responses in the airway may have some delayed benefit, but they are usually not indicated just prior to intubation.

Systemic drugs, usually administered intravenously, can be used to obtund the cough reflex. Intravenous lidocaine (1–2 mg/kg) transiently obtunds the cough reflex without affecting spontaneous ventilation to any significant degree. The risks of CNS stimulation and seizure-like activity have to be kept in mind and can be reduced by the prior administration of an intravenous barbiturate or benzodiazepine in small doses. Intravenous opioids are effective in suppressing cough reflexes, but the doses required impair spontaneous ventilation to the point of apnea. A combination of an intravenous opioid with a major tranquilizer (e.g., neuroleptanalgesia) allows the patient to tolerate an endotracheal tube with much smaller doses of the opioid and less embarrassment of spontaneous ventilation. Small doses of opioids are also useful in obtunding airway reflexes during general anesthesia provided either by intravenous (e.g., thiopental) or inhaled anesthetics (e.g., isoflurane). Not only do the opioids obtund the cough reflex that results in closure of the larynx, but also they are useful in limiting the autonomic sympathetic response to endotracheal intubation that typically leads to hypertension and tachycardia.

Skeletal muscle relaxants are most commonly used in conjunction with a general anesthetic to allow manipulation of the head and jaw and to prevent reflex closure of the larynx. Of course, they also render the patient apneic, and there are two common procedures utilized to maintain oxygenation of the patient's blood. (1)The patient breathes 100% oxygen by mask while still awake to eliminate nitrogen from the lungs, and then a rapid-sequence administration of an intravenous anesthetic (e.g., thiopental) is immediately followed by a rapid-acting neuromuscular blocker (e.g., succinylcholine, rocuronium [Zemuron]), and cricoid pressure is applied (Sellick maneuver). As soon as the muscle relaxation is apparent (30–90 seconds), laryngoscopy is performed, an endotracheal tube is inserted, the tracheal tube cuff is inflated, and the position of the tube in the trachea is verified. (2) When there is minimal risk of pulmonary aspiration (presumed empty stomach), the patient is anesthetized and paralyzed while ventilation is supported by intermittent positive pressure delivered via a face mask. At the appropriate time, laryngoscopy is performed and the endotracheal tube is inserted.

Normalizing Pulmonary Function During Positive Pressure Ventilation

Once an endotracheal tube is in place, it is common practice in the operating room to maintain general anesthesia and partial muscular paralysis in order to facilitate positive pressure ventilation and continued toleration of the endotracheal tube by the patient. Postoperatively in the PACU and ICU, general anesthesia and partial muscular paralysis may be continued if prolonged positive ventilation is anticipated, or sedatives may be administered by intravenous infusion to allow toleration of the endotracheal tube in anticipation of recovery of spontaneous ventilation and tracheal extubation.

Three other problems are encountered in the patient whose ventilation is supported mechanically by way of an endotracheal tube: (1) poor ventilatory compliance, (2) bronchonstriction, and (3) impaired gas exchange.

Poor ventilatory compliance can reflect limited compliance of the chest wall and diaphragm, limited compliance of the lungs per se, or both. Deepening general anesthesia and administration of a skeletal muscle relaxant can be used to reduce intercostal and diaphragmatic muscle tone, but they obviously cannot improve the chest cavity compliance that is fixed by disease (e.g., scoliosis, emphysema).

Poor lung compliance may reflect pulmonary interstitial edema, consolidation, bronchial obstruction (e.g., mucus plugs), bronchoconstriction, or compression of the lung by intrathoracic substances (e.g., pneumothorax, hemothorax, tumor mass). The treatment of these involves drug therapy of heart failure and infection and procedures such as bronchoscopy, thoracentesis, etc.

Bronchoconstriction may exist chronically (e.g., asthma, reactive airways disease), and these conditions can be exacerbated by the collection of tracheal bronchial secretions in the presence of an endotracheal tube, which reduces the effectiveness of coughing in clearing the airway. Occasionally bronchonstriction can be induced by mechanical stimulation of the airway by an endotracheal tube or other object in an otherwise normal patient. Drug treatment is focused on reducing bronchial smooth muscle tone (beta$_2$ sympathomimetic, anticholinergic), minimizing tracheal bronchial secretions, and decreasing sensory input from the tracheal bronchial tree (e.g., topical anesthetic, deeper general anesthesia, intravenous lidocaine, or an opioid). Acute treatment of bronchonstriction may involve any combination of the following: (1) aerosolized beta$_2$ sympathomimetic and/or anticholinergic, and (2) systemic intravenous administration of a beta$_2$ sympathomimetic, a phosphodiestrerase inhibitor (e.g., theophylline salts [aminophylline]), and/or an anticholinergic.

Intravenous steroids are indicated in severe bronchonstriction, especially in the asthmatic patient for whom they have been effective in the past. With the administration of 100% oxygen, blood oxygenation is not usually the main problem in the patient with bronchonstriction; it is the progressive development of hypercarbia and the trapping of air in lung parenchyma, which reduces ventilatory compliance and increases intrathoracic pressure. This in turn reduces venous return and may cause a tamponade-like impairment of cardiac function.

Impaired alveolar capillary membrane gas exchange can result from alveolar pulmonary edema (treated by diuretics, inotropes, and vasodilators), decreased pulmonary perfusion (treated by inotropes and vasodilators), and lung consolidation (antibiotic therapy for infection).

Restoration of Spontaneous Ventilation and Airway Protective Mechanisms

The anesthesiologist attempts to tailor the anesthetic plan according to postoperative expectations for the patient. In the relatively healthy patient for whom tracheal extubation can be anticipated in the operating room, the goal is to have the patient breathing spontaneously with airway reflexes intact and the patient arousable to command immediately upon completion of the surgical operation. The challenge for the anesthesiologist is to maintain satisfactory general anesthesia through the entire course of the surgical operation and yet have the patient sufficiently recovered from anesthetic drugs, including hypnotics and opioids, shortly after conclusion of the operation. If that is not possible, then the patient is transferred to the PACU to allow additional time for elimination of drugs depressing spontaneous ventilation and cough reflexes. Another possibility is to administer antagonists to opioids (e.g., naloxone) and benzodiazepines (e.g., flumazenil), but this approach risks sudden awakening, pain, and uncontrolled autonomic sympathetic activity leading to undesirable hemodynamic changes. And there is the risk of recurrent ventilatory depression because it is difficult to match the doses of the antagonists to the residual amounts of anesthetic drugs. On the other hand, it is fairly routine for the effects of neuromuscular blockers to be antagonized by administration of an anticholinesterase (e.g., neostigmine) in combination with an anticholinergic (e.g., atropine) to limit the autonomic cholinergic side effects of the anticholinesterase.

When the expectation is for maintenance of mechanical ventilation for some time in the postoperative period, then the patient's toleration of the endotracheal tube is facilitated by the persistent effect of residual anesthetic drugs subsequently supplemented by administration of intravenous hypnotics (e.g., propofol) and opioids (e.g., fentanyl, morphine). These agents can be associated with a number of side effects, including respiratory depression, especially when agents are used concurrently. Dexmedetomidine (Precedex), an alpha$_2$-adrenergic agonist, may offer advantages for sedation during and weaning from mechanical ventilation because it provides sedation, pain relief, anxiety reduction, stable respiratory rates, and predictable cardiovascular responses.[201–203] Dexmedetomidine facilitates patient comfort, compliance, and comprehension by offering sedation with the ability to rouse patients. This "rousability" allows patients to remain sedated yet communicate with health care workers.

When the appropriate time comes to have the patient take over his/her own ventilation completely, these sedative and analgesic drugs are weaned to a level allowing satisfactory maintenance of blood oxygenation and carbon dioxide removal, easy arousal of the patient, and at least partial restoration of airway reflex mechanisms.

REFERENCES

1. Lynch C III: Cellular electrophysiology of the heart, in Lynch C III (ed): *Cellular Cardiac Electrophysiology: Perioperative Considerations.* Philadelphia, JB Lippincott, 1994; p 1.
2. Katz AM: Cardiac ion channels. *N Engl J Med* 1993; 328:1244.
3. Colucci WS, Wright RF, Braunwald E: New positive inotropic agents in the treatment of heart failure: part I. *N Engl J Med* 1986; 314:290.
4. Colucci WS, Wright RF, Braunwald E: New positive inotropic agents in the treatment of heart failure: part II. *N Engl J Med* 1986; 314:349.
5. Terzic A, Puceat M, Vassort G, Vogel SM: Cardiac alpha 1 adreno receptors: an overview. *Pharmacol Rev* 1993; 45:147.
6. Berridge MJ: Inositol lipids and calcium signaling. *Proc R Soc Lond (Biol)* 1988; 234:359.
7. Lucchesi BR: Role of calcium on excitation-coupling in cardiac and vascular smooth muscle. *Circulation* 1978; 8:IV-1.
8. Kukovertz WR, Poch G, Holzmann S: Cyclic nucleotides and relaxation of vascular smooth muscle, in Vanhoutte PM, Leusen I (eds): *Vasodilation.* New York, Raven Press, 1981; p 339.
9. Smith WM: Mechanisms of cardiac arrhythmias and conduction disturbances, in Hurst JW (ed): *The Heart*, 7th ed. New York, McGraw-Hill, 1990; p 473.
10. Pinter A, Dorian P: Intravenous antiarrhythmic agents. *Curr Opin Cardiol* 2001; 16:17.
11. Roden DM: Antiarrhythmic drugs: from mechanisms to clinical practice. *Heart* 2000; 84:339.
12. Vaughan Williams EM: A classification of antiarrhythmic agents reassessed after a decade of new drugs. *J Clin Pharmacol* 1984; 24:129.
13. The Task Force of the Working Group on Arrhythmias of the European Society of Cardiology: The "Sicilian Gambit:"a new approach to the classification of antiarrhythmic drugs based on their actions on arrhythmic mechanisms. *Eur Heart J* 1991; 12:1112.
14. Hondeghem LM: Antiarrhythmic agents: modulated receptor applications. *Circulation* 1987; 75:514.
15. Barber MJ: Class I antiarrhythmic agents, in Lynch C III (ed): *Clinical Cardiac Electrophysiology: Perioperative Considerations.* Philadelphia, JB Lippincott, 1994; p 85.
16. Hoffman BF, Rosen MR, Wit AL: Electrophysiology and pharmacology of cardiac arrhythmias, VII: cardiac effects of quinidine and procainamide. *Am Heart J* 1975; 90:117.
17. Giardenia EG, Heissenbuttel RH, Bigger JT Jr: Intermittent intravenous procaine amide to treat ventricular arrhythmias: correlation of plasma concentration with effect on arrhythmia, electrocardiogram, and blood pressure. *Ann Intern Med* 1973; 78:183.
18. Cummins RO (ed): *Textbook of Advanced Cardiac Life Support.* Dallas, American Heart Association, 1994; p 7–1.
19. The International Guidelines 2000 for CPR and ECC. *Circulation* 2000; 102(8 suppl):I112.
20. Cardiac Arrhythmia Suppression Trial (CAST) Investigators: Preliminary report, effect of encainide and flecainide on mortality in a randomized trial of arrhythmia suppression after myocardial infarction. *N Engl J Med* 1989; 321:406.
21. Echt DS, Liebson PR, Mitchell LB, et al: Mortality and morbidity in patients receiving encainide, flecainide or placebo: the Cardiac Arrhythmia Suppression Trial. *N Engl J Med* 1991; 324:781.

22. Escande D, Henry P: Potassium channels as pharmacologic targets in cardiovascular medicine. *Eur Heart J* 1993; 14 (suppl): 2.
23. Singh BN: Arrhythmia control by prolonging repolarization: the concept and its potential therapeutic impact. *Eur Heart J* 1993; 14(suppl):14.
24. Kudenchuk PJ: Advanced cardiac life support antiarrhythmic drugs. *Cardiol Clin* 2002; 20:79.
25. Balser JR: Perioperative arrhythmias: incidence, risk assessment, evaluation, and management. *Card Electrophysiol Rev* 2002; 6:96.
26. Mahmarian JJ, Verani MS, Pratt CM: Hemodynamic effects of intravenous and oral sotalol. *Am J Cardiol* 1990; 65:28A.
27. Levy JH, Huraux C, Nordlander M: Treatment of perioperative hypertension, in Epstein M (ed): *Calcium Antagonists in Clinical Medicine*. Philadelphia, Hanley and Belfus, 1997; p 345.
28. Conti VR, Ware DL: Cardiac arrhythmias in cardiothoracic surgery. *Chest Surg Clin N Am* 2002; 12:439.
29. Waxman HL, Myerburg RJ, Appel R, Sung RJ: Verapamil for control of ventricular rate in paroxysmal supraventricular tachycardia and atrial fibrillation or flutter: a double-blind randomized crossover study. *Ann Intern Med* 1981; 94:1.
30. Salerno DM, Dias VC, Kleiger RE, et al: Efficacy and safety of intravenous diltiazem for treatment of atrial fibrillation and atrial flutter: the Diltiazem-Atrial Fibrillation/Flutter Study Group. *Am J Cardiol* 1989; 63:1046.
31. Ellenbogen KA, Dias VC, Plumb VJ, et al: A placebo-controlled trial of continuous intravenous diltiazem infusion for 24-hour heart rate control during atrial fibrillation and atrial flutter: a multi-center study. *J Am Coll Cardiol* 1991; 18:891.
32. Smith TW, Antman EM, Friedman PL et al: Digitalis glycosides: mechanisms and manifestations of toxicity: part I. *Prog Cardiovasc Dis* 1984; 26:413.
33. DiMarco JP, Sellers TD, Berne RM, et al: Adenosine: electrophysiological effects and therapeutic use for terminating paroxysmal supraventricular tachycardia. *Circulation* 1983; 68:1254.
34. Hollifield JW: Potassium and magnesium abnormalities: diuretics and arrhythmias in hypertension. *Am J Med* 1984; 77:28.
35. England MR, Gordon G, Salem M, Chernow B: Magnesium administration and dysrhythmia after cardiac surgery: a placebo-controlled, double-blind, randomized trial. *JAMA* 1992; 268:2395.
36. Singh BN, Vaughan Williams EM: The effect of amiodarone, a new antianginal drug, on cardiac muscle. *Br J Pharmacol* 1970; 39:657.
37. Connolly SJ: Evidence-based analysis of amiodarone efficacy and safety. *Circulation* 1999; 100:2025.
38. Chow MS: Intravenous amiodarone: pharmacology, pharmacokinetics, and clinical use. *Ann Pharmacother* 1996; 30:637.
39. Mitchell LB, Wyse G, Gillis AM, Duff HJ: Electropharmacology of amiodarone therapy initiation. *Circulation* 1989; 80:34.
40. Holt DW, Tucker GT, Jackson PR, Storey GCA: Amiodarone pharmacokinetics. *Am Heart J* 1983; 106:840.
41. Fogoros RN, Anderson KP, Winkle RA, et al: Amiodarone: clinical efficacy and toxicity in 96 patients with recurrent, drug-refractory arrhythmias. *Circulation* 1983; 68:88.
42. Kowey PR, Levine JH, Herre JM, et al: Randomized, double-blind comparison of intravenous amiodarone and bretylium in the treatment of patients with recurrent, hemodynamically destabilizing ventricular tachycardia or fibrillation. *Circulation* 1995; 92:3255.
43. Kudenchuk PJ, Cobb LA, Copass MK, et al: Amiodarone for resuscitation after out-of-hospital cardiac arrest due to ventricular fibrillation. *N Engl J Med* 1999; 341:871.
44. Levine JH, Massumi A, Scheinman MM, et al: Intravenous amiodarone for recurrent sustained hypotensive ventricular tachyarrhythmias. Intravenous Amiodarone Multicenter Trial Group. *J Am Coll Cardiol* 1996; 27:67.
45. Morady F, Sauve MJ, Malone P, et al: Long-term efficacy and toxicity of high-dose amiodarone therapy for ventricular tacycardia or ventricular fibrillation. *Am J Cardiol* 1983; 52:975.
46. Scheinman MM, Levine JH, Cannom DS, et al: Dose-ranging study of intravenous amiodarone in patients with life-threatening ventricular tachyarrhythmias. *Circulation* 1995; 92:3264.
47. Scheinman MM, Winkle RA, Platia EV, et al: Intravenous amiodarone for recurrent sustained hypotensive ventricular tachyarrhythmias. *J Am Coll Cardiol* 1996; 27:67.
48. Dorian P, Cass D, Schwartz B, et al: Amiodarone as compared with lidocaine for shock-resistant ventricular fibrillation. *N Engl J Med* 2002; 346:884
49. Kupferschmid JP, Rosengart TK, McIntosh CL, et al: Amiodarone-induced complications after cardiac operation for obstructive hypertrophic cardiomyopathy. *Ann Thorac Surg* 1989; 48:359.
50. Rady MY, Ryan T, Starr NJ: Preoperative therapy with amiodarone and the incidence of acute organ dysfunction after cardiac surgery. *Anesth Analg* 1997; 85:489.
51. Daoud EG, Strickberger SA, Man KC, et al: Preoperative amiodarone as prophylaxis against atrial fibrillation after heart surgery. *N Engl J Med* 1997; 337:1785.
52. Dorge H, Schoendube FA, Schoberer M, et al: Intraoperative amiodarone as prophylaxis against atrial fibrillation after coronary operations. *Ann Thorac Surg* 2000; 69:1358.
53. Giri S, White CM, Dunn AB, et al: Oral amiodarone for prevention of atrial fibrillation after open heart surgery, the Atrial Fibrillation Suppression Trial (AFIST): a randomised placebo-controlled trial. *Lancet* 2001; 357:830.
54. Guarnieri T, Nolan S, Gottlieb SO, et al: Intravenous amiodarone for the prevention of atrial fibrillation after open heart surgery: the Amiodarone Reduction in Coronary Heart (ARCH) trial. *J Am Coll Cardiol* 1999; 34:343.
55. Lee SH, Chang CM, Lu MJ, et al: Intravenous amiodarone for prevention of atrial fibrillation after coronary artery bypass grafting. *Ann Thorac Surg* 2000; 70:157.
56. Carlson MD: How to manage atrial fibrillation: an update on recent clinical trials. *Cardiol Rev* 2001; 9:60.
57. Fuster V, Ryden LE, Asinger RN, et al: ACC/AHA/ESC guidelines for the management of patients with atrial fibrillation: executive summary. *Circulation* 2001; 104:2118.
58. Maisel WH, Rawn JD, Stevenson WG: Atrial fibrillation after cardiac surgery. *Ann Intern Med* 2001; 135:1061.
59. Hogue CW Jr, Hyder ML: Atrial fibrillation after cardiac operation: risks, mechanisms, and treatment. *Ann Thorac Surg* 2000; 69:300.
60. Reddy P, Richerson M, Freeman-Bosco L, et al: Cost-effectiveness of amiodarone for prophylaxis of atrial fibrillation in coronary artery bypass surgery. *Am J Health Syst Pharm* 1999; 56:2211.
61. Reiffel JA: Drug choices in the treatment of atrial fibrillation. *Am J Cardiol* 2000; 85:12D.
62. Daoud EG, Strickberger SA, Man KC, et al: Preoperative amiodarone as prophylaxis against atrial fibrillation after heart surgery. *N Engl J Med* 1997; 337:1785.
63. Gray R, Maddahi J, Berman D, et al: Scintigraphic and hemodynamic demonstration of transient left ventricular dysfunction immediately after uncomplicated coronary artery bypass grafting. *J Thorac Cardiovasc Surg* 1979; 77:504.
64. Mangano DT: Biventricular function after myocardial revascularization in humans: deterioration and recovery patterns during the first 24 hours. *Anesthesiology* 1985; 62:571.
65. Breisblatt WM, Stein K, Wolfe CJ, et al: Acute myocardial dysfunction and recovery: a common occurrence after coronary bypass surgery. *J Am Coll Cardiol* 1990; 15:1261.
66. Fabiato A, Fabiato F: Calcium and cardiac excitation-contraction coupling. *Ann Rev Physiol* 1979; 41:473.

67. Figgitt DP, Gillies PS, Goa KL: Levosimendan. *Drugs* 2001; 61:613.
68. Doggrell SA, Brown L: Present and future pharmacotherapy for heart failure. *Expert Opin Pharmacother* 2002; 3:915.
69. Endoh M: Mechanism of action of $Ca2^+$ sensitizers—update 2001. *Cardiovasc Drugs Ther* 2001; 15:397.
70. Drop LJ, Geffin GA, O'Keefe DD, et al: Relation between ionized calcium concentration and ventricular pump performance in the dog under hemodynamically controlled conditions. *Am J Cardiol* 1981; 47:1041.
71. Zaloga GP, Strickland RA, Butterworth JF, et al: Calcium attenuates epinephrine's β-adrenergic effects in postoperative heart surgery patients. *Circulation* 1990; 81:196.
72. Engelman RM, Hadji-Rousou I, Breyer RH, et al: Rebound vasospasm after coronary revascularization in association with calcium antagonist withdrawal. *Ann Thorac Surg* 1984; 37:469.
73. Cheung JY, Bonventre JV, Malis CD, Leaf A: Calcium and ischemic injury. *N Engl J Med* 1986; 314:1670.
74. Del Monte F, Kaumann AJ, Poole-Wilson PA, et al: Coexistence of functioning $\beta 1$ and $\beta 2$-adrenoreceptors in single myocytes from human ventricle. *Circulation* 1993; 88:854.
75. Bristow MR, Ginsburg R, Minobe W, et al: Decreased catecholamine sensitivity and β-adrenergic receptor density in failing human hearts. *N Engl J Med* 1982; 307:205.
76. Schwinn DA, Leone BJ, Spahn DR, et al: Desensitization of myocardial β-adrenergic receptors during cardiopulmonary bypass: evidence for early uncoupling and late down-regulation. *Circulation* 1991; 84:2559.
77. Port JD, Gilbert EM, Larabee P, et al: Neurotransmitter depletion compromises the ability of indirect acting amines to provide inotropic support in the failing human heart. *Circulation* 1990; 81:929.
78. Goenen M, Pedemonte O, Baele P, Col J: Amrinone in the management of low cardiac output after open heart surgery. *Am J Cardiol* 1985; 56:33B.
79. Robinson RJS, Tchervenkov C: Treatment of low cardiac output after aortocoronary surgery using a combination of norepinephrine and amrinone. *J Cardiothorac Anesth* 1987; 3:229.
80. Prielipp RC, Butterworth JF 4th, Zaloga GP, et al: Effects of amrinone on cardiac index, venous oxygen saturation and venous admixture in patients recovering from cardiac surgery. *Chest* 1991; 99:820.
81. Levy JH, Bailey JM: Amrinone: its effects on vascular resistance and capacitance in human subjects. *Chest* 1994; 105:62.
82. Levy JH, Bailey JM, Deeb GM: Intravenous milrinone in cardiac surgery. *Ann Thorac Surg* 2002; 73:325.
83. Bailey JM, Levy JH, Rogers G, et al: Pharmacokinetics of amrinone during cardiac surgery. *Anesthesiology* 1991; 75:961.
84. Bailey JM, Levy JH, Kikura M, et al: Pharmacokinetics of intravenous milrinone in patients undergoing cardiac surgery. *Anesthesiology* 1994; 81:616.
85. Feneck RO: Effects of variable dose in patients with low cardiac output after cardiac surgery. European Multicenter Trial Group. *Am Heart J* 1991; 121(6 Pt 2):1995.
86. Kikura M, Levy JH, Michelsen LG, et al: The effect of milrinone on hemodynamics and left ventricular function after emergence from cardiopulmonary bypass. *Anesth Analg* 1997; 85:16.
87. Butterworth JF 4th, Hines RL, Royster RL, James RL: A pharmacokinetic and pharmacodynamic evaluation of milrinone in adults undergoing cardiac surgery. *Anesth Analg* 1995; 81:783.
88. Doolan LA, Jones EF, Kalman J, et al: A placebo-controlled trial verifying the efficacy of milrinone in weaning high-risk patients from cardiopulmonary bypass. *J Cardiothorac Vasc Anesth* 1997; 11:37.
89. Follath F, Cleland JG, Just H, et al: Efficacy and safety of intravenous levosimendan compared with dobutamine in severe low-output heart failure (the LIDO study): a randomised double-blind trial. *Lancet* 2002; 360:196.
90. Slawsky MT, Colucci WS, Gottlieb SS, et al: Acute hemodynamic and clinical effects of levosimendan in patients with severe heart failure. *Circulation* 2000; 102:2222.
91. Steen H, Tinker JH, Pluth JR, et al: Efficacy of dopamine, dobutamine, and epinephrine during emergence from cardiopulmonary bypass in man. *Circulation* 1978; 57:378.
92. Salomon NW, Plachetka JR, Copeland JG: Comparison of dopamine and dobutamine following coronary artery bypass grafting. *Ann Thorac Surg* 1981; 3:48.
93. Fowler MB, Alderman EL, Oesterle SN, et al: Dobutamine and dopamine after cardiac surgery: greater augmentation of myocardial blood flow with dobutamine. *Circulation* 1984; 70:1103.
94. Sethna DH, Gray RJ, Moffit EA, et al: Dobutamine and cardiac oxygen balance in patients following myocardial revascularization. *Anesth Analg* 1982; 61:917.
95. Butterworth JF 4th, Prielipp RC, Royster RL, et al: Dobutamine increases heart rate more than epinephrine in patients recovering from aortocoronary bypass surgery. *J Cardiothorac Vasc Anesth* 1992; 6:535.
96. Feneck RO, Sherry KM, Withington S, et al: Comparison of the hemodynamic effects of milrinone with dobutamine in patients after cardiac surgery. *J Cardiothorac Vasc Anesth* 2001; 15:306.
97. Meier-Hellmann A, Reinhart K, Bredle DL, et al: Epinephrine impairs splanchnic perfusion in septic shock. *Crit Care Med* 1997; 25:399.
98. Levy B, Bollaert PE, Charpentier C, et al: Comparison of norepinephrine and dobutamine to epinephrine for hemodynamics, lactate metabolism, and gastric tonometric variables in septic shock: a prospective, randomized study. *Intensive Care Med* 1997; 23:282.
99. Ruokonen E, Takala J, Kari A, et al: Regional blood flow and oxygen transport in septic shock. *Crit Care Med* 1993; 21:1296.
100. Meier-Hellmann A, Bredle DL, Specht M, et al: The effects of low-dose dopamine on splanchnic blood flow and oxygen utilization in patients with septic shock. *Intensive Care Med* 1997; 23:31.
101. Marik PE, Mohedin M: The contrasting effects of dopamine and norepinephrine on systemic and splanchnic oxygen utilization in hyperdynamic sepsis. *JAMA* 1994; 272:1354.
102. Landry DW, Oliver JA: The pathogenesis of vasodilatory shock. *N Engl J Med* 2001; 345:588.
103. Levy JH: *Anaphylactic Reactions in Anesthesia and Intensive Care,* 2d ed. Boston, Butterworth-Heinemann, 1992.
104. Desjars P, Pinaud M, Potel G, et al: A reappraisal of norepinephrine in human septic shock. *Crit Care Med* 1987; 15:134.
105. Meadows D, Edwards JD, Wilkins RG, Nightingale P: Reversal of intractable septic shock with norepinephrine therapy. *Crit Care Med* 1998; 16:663.
106. Hesselvik JF, Broden B: Low dose norepinephrine in patient with septic shock and oliguria: effects on afterload, urine flow, and oxygen transport. *Crit Care Med* 1989; 17:179.
107. Martin C, Eon B, Saux P, et al: Renal effects of norepinephrine used to treat septic shock patients. *Crit Care Med* 1990; 18:282.
108. Marik PE, Mohedin M: The contrasting effects of dopamine and norepinephrine on systemic and splanchnic oxygen utilization in hyperdynamic sepsis. *JAMA* 1994; 272:1354.
109. Argenziano M, Chen JM, Choudhri AF, et al: Management of vasodilatory shock after cardiac surgery: identification of predisposing factors and use of a novel pressor agent. *J Thorac Cardiovasc Surg* 1998; 116:973.
110. Landry DW, Levin HR, Gallant EM, et al: Vasopressin deficiency in vasodilatory septic shock. *Crit Care Med* 1997; 25:1279.

111. Gold JA, Cullinane S, Chen J, et al: Vasopressin as an alternative to norepinephrine in the treatment of milrinone-induced hypotension. *Crit Care Med* 2000; 28:249.
112. Levy JH: The ideal agent for perioperative hypertension. *Acta Anaesth Scand* 1993; 37:20.
113. Huraux C, Makita T, Montes F, Szlam F: A comparative evaluation of the effects of multiple vasodilators on human internal mammary artery. *Anesthesiology* 1998; 88:1654.
114. Harrison DG, Bates JN: The nitrovasodilators: new ideas about old drugs. *Circulation* 1993; 87:1461.
115. Anderson TJ, Meredith IT, Ganz P, et al: Nitric oxide and nitrovasodilators: similarities, differences and potential interactions. *J Am Coll Cardiol* 1994; 24:555.
116. Harrison DG, Kurz MA, Quillen JE, et al: Normal and pathophysiologic considerations of endothelial regulation of vascular tone and their relevance to nitrate therapy. *Am J Cardiol* 1992; 70:11B.
117. Munzel T, Giaid A, Kurz S, Harrison DG: Evidence for a role of endothelin 1 and protein kinase C in nitrate tolerance. *Proc Natl Acad Sci U S A* 1995; 92:5244.
118. Munzel T, Sayegh H, Freeman, Harrison DG: Evidence for enhanced vascular superoxide anion production in tolerance: a novel mechanism underlying tolerance and cross-tolerance. *J Clin Invest* 1995; 95:187.
119. Fleckenstein A: Specific pharmacology of calcium in the myocardium, cardiac pacemakers and vascular smooth muscle. *Ann Rev Pharmacol* 1977; 17:149.
120. Begon C, Dartayet B, Edouard A, et al: Intravenous nicardipine for treatment of intraoperative hypertension during abdominal surgery. *J Cardiothorac Anesth* 1989; 3:707.
121. Cheung DG, Gasster JL, Neutel JM, Weber MA: Acute pharmacokinetic and hemodynamic effects of intravenous bolus dosing of nicardipine. *Am Heart J* 1990; 119:438.
122. David D, Dubois C, Loria Y: Comparison of nicardipine and sodium nitroprusside in the treatment of paroxysmal hypertension following aortocoronary bypass surgery. *J Cardiothorac Vasc Anesth* 1991; 5:357.
123. Lambert CR, Grady T, Hashimi W, et al: Hemodynamic and angiographic comparison of intravenous nitroglycerin and nicardipine mainly in subjects without coronary artery disease. *Am J Cardiol* 1993; 71:420.
124. Singh BN, Josephson MA: Clinical pharmacology, pharmacokinetics, and hemodynamic effects of nicardipine. *Am Heart J* 1990; 119:427A.
125. Leslie J, Brister N, Levy JH, et al: Treatment of postoperative hypertension after coronary artery bypass surgery: double-blind comparison of intravenous isradipine and sodium nitroprusside. *Circulation* 1994; 90:II 256.
126. Huraux C, Makita T, Montes F, et al: A comparative evaluation of the effects of multiple vasodilators on human internal mammary artery. *Anesthesiology* 1998; 88:1654.
127. Tuman K: Angiotensin converting enzyme inhibitors increase vasoconstrictor requirements after cardiopulmonary bvypass. *Anesth Analg* 1995; 80:473.
128. Dzau VJ, Sasamura H, Hein L: Heterogeneity of angiotensin synthetic pathways and receptor subtypes: physiological and pharmacological implications. *J Hypertens* 1993; 11(suppl 3):S13.
129. Bergmeier C, Kilkowski A, Senges J: Chronic heart failure and b-blocker therapy: B-adrenergic blockade in patients with chronic heart failure reduces morbidity and mortality [in German]. *Herzschrittmachertherapie und Elektrophysiologie* 1999; 10 (suppl 2):93.
130. Urata H, Nishimura H, Ganten D, Arakawa K: Angiotensin-converting enzyme-independent pathways of angiotensin II formation in human tissues and cardiovascular diseases. *Blood Press* 1996; 2(suppl):22.
131. Granger CB, Ertl G, Kuch J, et al: Randomized trial of candesartan cilexetil in the treatment of patients with congestive heart failure and a history of intolerance to angiotensin-converting enzyme inhibitors. *Am Heart J* 2000; 139:609.
132. Pitt B, Poole-Wilson PA, Segal R, et al: Effect of losartan compared with captopril on mortality in patients with symptomatic heart failure: randomised trial—The Losartan Heart Failure Survival Study ELITE II. *Lancet* 2000; 355:1582.
133. McDonald KM, Mock J, D'Aloia A, et al: Bradykinin antagonism inhibits the antigrowth effect of converting enzyme inhibition in the dog myocardium after discrete transmural myocardial necrosis. *Circulation* 1995; 91:2043.
134. Wollert KC, Studer R, Doerfer K, et al: Differential effects of kinins on cardiomyocyte hypertrophy and interstitial collagen matrix in the surviving myocardium after myocardial infarction in the rat. *Circulation* 1997; 95:1910.
135. McKelvie RS, Yusuf S, Pericak D, et al: Comparison of candesartan, enalapril, and their combination in congestive heart failure: randomized evaluation of strategies for left ventricular dysfunction (RESOLVD) pilot study. The RESOLVD pilot study investigators. *Circulation* 1999; 100:1056.
136. Cohn JN: Improving outcomes in congestive heart failure: Val-HeFT. *Cardiology* 1999; 91(suppl 1):19.
137. Brabant SM, Bertrand M, Eyraud D, et al: The hemodynamic effects of anesthetic induction in vascular surgical patients chronically treated with angiotensin II receptor antagonists. *Anesth Analg* 1999; 89:1388.
138. Brabant SM, Eyraud D, Bertrand M, Coriat P: Refractory hypotension after induction of anesthesia in a patient chronically treated with angiotensin receptor antagonists. *Anesth Analg* 1999; 89:887.
139. Furie B, Furie BC: Molecular and cellular biology of blood coagulation. *N Engl J Med* 1992; 326:800.
140. Turpie AGG, Weitz JI, Hirsh J: Advances in antithrombotic therapy: novel agents. *Thromb Haemost* 1995; 74:565.
141. Levy JH: review ATS.
142. Hirsh J, Raschke R, Warkentin TE, et al: Heparin: mechanism of action, pharmacokinetics, dosing considerations, monitoring, efficacy and safety. *Chest* 1995; 108(suppl):258S.
143. Despotis GJ, Joist JH, Hogue CW Jr, et al: More effective suppression of hemostatic system activation in patients undergoing cardiac surgery by heparin dosing based on heparin blood concentrations rather than ACT. *Thromb Haemost* 1996; 76:902.
144. Despotis GJ, Summerfield AL, Joist JH, et al: Comparison of activated coagulation time and whole blood heparin measurements with laboratory plasma anti-Xa heparin concentration in patients having cardiac operations. *J Thorac Cardiovasc Surg* 1994; 108:1076.
145. Mochizuki T, Olson PJ, Ramsay JG, Szlam F, Levy JH: Protamine reversal of heparin affects platelet aggregation and activated clotting time after cardiopulmonary bypass. *Anesth Analg* 1998; 87:781.
146. Warkentin TJ: Current agents for the treatment of patients with heparin-induced thrombocytopenia. *Curr Opin Pulm Med* 2002; 8:405.
147. Weitz JI: Low-molecular-weight heparins. *N Engl J Med.* 1997; 337:688.
148. Antman EM, Handin R: Low-molecular-weight heparins: an intriguing new twist with profound implications. *Circulation* 1998; 98:287.
149. Levy JH: Novel intravenous antithrombins. *Am Heart J* 2001; 141:1043.
150. Zaidan JR, Johnson S, Brynes R, et al: Rate of protamine administration: its effect on heparin reversal and antithrombin recovery after coronary atery surgery. *Anesth Analg* 1986; 65:377.

151. Levy JH, Montes F, Szlam F, Hillyer C: In vitro effects of antithrombin III on the activated coagulation time in patients on heparin therapy. *Anesth Analg* 2000; 90:1076.
152. Levy JH, Despotis GJ, Szlam F, et al: Recombinant human transgenic antithrombin in cardiac surgery: a dose finding study. *Anesthesiology* 2002; 96:1095.
153. Lewis BE, Walenga JM, Wallis DE: Anticoagulation with Novastan (argatroban) in patients with heparin-induced thrombocytopenia and heparin-induced thrombocytopenia and thrombosis syndrome. *Semin Thromb Hemost* 1997; 23:197.
154. Matsuo T, Kario K, Chikahira Y, et al: Treatment of heparin-induced thrombocytopenia by use of argatroban, a synthetic thrombin inhibitor. *Br J Haematol* 1992; 82:627.
155. Fareed J, Callas D, Hoppensteadt DA, et al: Antithrombin agents as anticoagulants and antithrombotics: implications in drug development. *Semin Hematol* 1999; 36(suppl 1):42.
156. Greinacher A, Volpel H, Janssens U, et al: Recombinant hirudin (lepirudin) provides safe and effective anticoagulation in patients with heparin-induced thrombocytopenia: a prospective study. *Circulation* 1999; 99:73.
157. Potzsch B, Madlener K, Seelig C, et al: Monitoring of r-hirudin anticoagulation during cardiopulmonary bypass: assessment of the whole blood ecarin clotting time. *Thromb Haemost* 1997; 77:920.
158. Kong DF, Topol EJ, Bittl JA, et al: Clinical outcomes of bivalirudin for ischemic heart disease. *Circulation* 1999; 100:2049.
159. Weitz JI, Huboda M, Massel D, et al: Clot-bound thrombin is protected from inhibition by heparin-antithrombin III but is susceptible to inactivation by antithrombin III-independent inhibitors. *J Clin Invest* 1990; 86:385.
160. Despotis GJ, Filos K, Gravlee G, Levy JH: Anticoagulation monitoring during cardiac surgery: a survey of current practice and review of current and emerging techniques. *Anesthesiology* 1999; 91:1122.
161. Follis F, Schmidt CA: Cardiopulmonary bypass in patients with heparin-induced thrombocytopenia and thrombosis. *Ann Thorac Surg* 2000; 70:2173.
162. Magnani HN: Heparin-induced thrombocytopenia (HIT): an overview of 230 patients treated with orgaran (Org 10172). *Thromb Haemost* 1993; 70:554.
163. Teasdale SJ, Zulys VJ, Mycyk T, et al: Ancrod anticoagulation for cardiopulmonary bypass in heparin-induced thrombocytopenia and thrombosis. *Ann Thorac Surg* 1989; 48:712.
164. Koster A, Kuppe H, Hetzer R, et al: Emergent cardiopulmonary bypass in five patients with heparin-induced thrombocytopenia Type II employing recombinant hirudin. *Anesthesiology* 1999; 89:777.
165. Peters DC, Noble S: Aprotinin: an update of its pharmacology and therapeutic use in open heart surgery and coronary artery bypass surgery. *Drugs* 1999; 57:233.
166. Mannucci PM: Hemostatic drugs. *N Engl J Med* 1998; 339:245.
167. Levy JH, Bailey JM, Salmenperrä M: Pharmacokinetics of aprotinin in preoperative cardiac surgical patients. *Anesthesiology* 1994; 80:1013.
168. Levy JH, Pifarre R, Schaff H, et al: A multicenter, placebo-controlled, double-blind trial of aprotinin to reduce blood loss and the requirement of donor blood transfusion in patients undergoing repeat coronary artery bypass grafting, *Circulation* 1995; 92:2236.
169. Alderman EL, Levy JH, Rich J, et al: International multi-center aprotinin graft patency experience (IMAGE). *J Thorac Cardiovasc Surg* 1998; 116:716.
170. Levi M, Cromheecke ME, de Jonge E, et al: Pharmacological strategies to decrease excessive blood loss in cardiac surgery: a meta-analysis of clinically relevant endpoints. *Lancet* 1999; 354:1940.
171. Mojcik CF, Levy JH: Aprotinin and the systemic inflammatory response after cardiopulmonary bypass. *Ann Thorac Surg* 2001; 71:745.
172. Levy JH, Smith P: Platelet inhibitors and bleeding in cardiac surgical patients. *Ann Thorac Surg* 2000; 70:(suppl): 59.
173. Jarvis B, Simpson K: Clopidogrel: a review of its use in the prevention of atherothrombosis. *Drugs* 2000; 60:347.
174. Despotis GJ, Filos K, Gravlee G, Levy J: Anticoagulation monitoring during cardiac surgery: a survey of current practice and review of current and emerging techniques. *Anesthesiology* 1999; 91:1122.
175. Levy JH, Zaidan JR, Faraj BA: Prospective evaluation of risk of protamine reactions in NPH insulin-dependent diabetics. *Anesth Analg* 1986; 65:739.
176. Levy JH, Schwieger IM, Zaidan JR, et al: Evaluation of patients at risk for protamine reactions. *J Thorac Cardiovasc Surg* 1989; 98:200.
177. Levy JH, Cormack J, Morales A: Heparin neutralization by recombinant platelet factor 4 and protamine. *Anesth Analg* 1995; 81:35.
178. Hedner U: NovoSeven as a universal haemostatic agent. *Blood Coag Fibrinolysis* 2000; 11:(suppl 1):S107.
179. Shapiro AD, Gilchrist GS, Hoots WK, et al: Prospective, randomised trial of two doses of rFVIIa (Novoseven) in haemophilia patients with inhibitors undergoing surgery. *Thromb Haemost* 1998; 80:773.
180. Al Douri M, Shafi T, Al Khudairi D, et al: Effect of the administration of recombinant activated factor VII (rFVIIa; NovoSeven) in the management of severe uncontrolled bleeding in patients undergoing heart valve replacement surgery. *Blood Coag Fibrinolysis* 2000; (suppl 1):S121.
181. Zietkiewicz M, Garlicki M, Domagala J, et al: Successful use of activated recombinant factor VII to control bleeding abnormalities in a patient with a left ventricular assist device. *J Thorac Cardiovasc Surg* 2002; 123:384.
182. Argenziano M, Chen JM, Choudhri AF, et al: Management of vasodilatory shock after cardiac surgery: identification of predisposing factors and use of a novel pressor agent. *J Cardiovasc Thorac Surg* 1998; 116:973.
183. Lefkowitz RH, Hoffman BB, Taylor P: Neurotransmission: the autonomic and somatic motor nervous system, in Hardman JL, Molinoff PB, Ruddon RW, Gilman AG (eds): *The Pharmacological Basis of Therapeutics*. New York, McGraw-Hill, 1996; p 110.
184. Hug CJ: Beta-adrenergic blocking drugs, in *Drug Evaluations Annual* 1994. Chicago, American Medical Association, 1993; p 539.
185. Mangano DT, Layug EL, Wallace A, Tateo I: Effect of atenolol on mortality and cardiovascular morbidity after noncardiac surgery. Multicenter Study of Perioperative Ischemia Research Group. *N Engl J Med* 1996; 335:1713.
186. Poldermans D, Boersma E, Bax JJ, et al: The effect of bisoprolol on perioperative mortality and myocardial infarction in high-risk patients undergoing vascular surgery. Dutch Echocardiographic Cardiac Risk Evaluation Applying Stress Echocardiography Study Group. *N Engl J Med* 1999; 341:1789.
187. Poldermans D, Boersma E, Bax JJ, et al: Bisoprolol reduces cardiac death and myocardial infarction in high-risk patients as long as 2 years after successful major vascular surgery. *Eur Heart J* 2001; 22:1353.
188. Frumin H, Kerin NZ, Rubenfire M: Classification of antiarrhythmic drugs. *J Clin Pharmacol* 1989; 29:387.
189. Joint National Committee: The sixth report of the Joint National Committee on prevention, detection, evaluation, and treatment of high blood pressure. *Arch Intern Med* 1997; 157:2413.
190. Joglar JA, Acusta AP, Shusterman NH, et al: Effect of carvedilol on survival and hemodynamics in patients with atrial

fibrillation and left ventricular dysfunction: retrospective analysis of the U.S. Carvedilol Heart Failure Trials Program. *Am Heart J* 2001; 142:498.

191. Lind L, Pollare T, Berne C, Litheli H: Long-term metabolic effects of antihypertensive drugs. *Am Heart J* 1994; 128:1177.
192. Sheps SG: Overview of JNC VI: new directions in the management of hypertension and cardiovascular risk. *Am J Hypertens* 1999; 12(suppl II): 65S.
193. Tumlin JA, Dunbar LM, Oparil S, et al: Fenoldopam, a dopamine agonist, for hypertensive emergency: a multicenter randomized trial. Fenoldopam Study Group. *Acad Emerg Med* 2000; 7:653.
194. MacGregor DA, Smith TE, Prielipp RC, et al: Pharmacokinetics of dopamine in healthy male subjects. *Anesthesiology* 2000; 92:338.
195. Halpenny M, Lakshmi S, O'Donnell A, et al: Fenoldopam: renal and splanchnic effects in patients undergoing coronary artery bypass grafting. *Anaesthesia* 2001; 56:953.
196. Halpenny M, Markos F, Snow HM, et al: The effects of fenoldopam on renal blood flow and tubular function during aortic cross-clamping in anaesthetized dogs. *Eur J Anaesthiol* 2000; 17:491.
197. Gilbert TB, Hasnain JU, Flinn WR, et al: Fenoldopam infusion associated with preserving renal function after aortic cross-clamping for aneurysm repair. *J Cardiovasc Pharmacol Ther* 2001; 6:31.
198. Eisenberg DM, Davis RB, Ettner SL, et al: Trends in alternative medicine use in the United States, 1990–1997: results of a follow-up national survey. *JAMA* 1998; 280:1569.
199. Ang-Lee MK, Moss J, Yuan CS: Herbal medicines and perioperative care. *JAMA* 2001; 286:208.
200. American Society of Anesthesiologists: What You Should Know About Your Patients' Use of Herbal Medicines. http://www.asahq.org/ProfInfo/herb/herbbro.html.
201. Venn RM, Bryant A, Hall GM, Grounds RM: Effects of dexmedetomidine on adrenocortical function, and the cardiovascular, endocrine and inflammatory responses in post-operative patients needing sedation in the intensive care unit. *Br J Anaesth* 2001; 86:650.
202. Venn RM, Hell J, Grounds RM: Respiratory effects of dexmedetomidine in the surgical patient requiring intensive care. *Crit Care* (Lond) 2000; 4:302.
203. Dutta S, Karol MD, Cohen T, et al: Effect of dexmedetomidine on propofol requirements in healthy subjects. *J Pharm Sci* 2001; 90:172.

Chapter 5

Cardiac Surgical Pathology

Frederick J. Schoen/Robert F. Padera, Jr.

In the past several decades, the virtual explosion in the number and scope of surgical and interventional diagnostic and therapeutic procedures performed on patients with cardiovascular diseases has launched cardiovascular pathology into the forefront of patient care.[1] Pathology-based investigation of the safety and efficacy of diagnostic tests, therapeutic procedures, and devices has contributed to clinical progress. Cardiovascular clinicians benefit from pathologic data that facilitate informed choices among surgical or catheter-based interventional options and optimize short- and long-term patient management, including recognition of complications. Importantly, beyond implicit clinical benefit, studies of cardiac pathology and pathobiology serve as the cornerstone of modern cardiovascular research.

This chapter summarizes pathologic considerations most relevant to surgery in the major forms of acquired cardiovascular disease. Both clinicopathologic correlations and

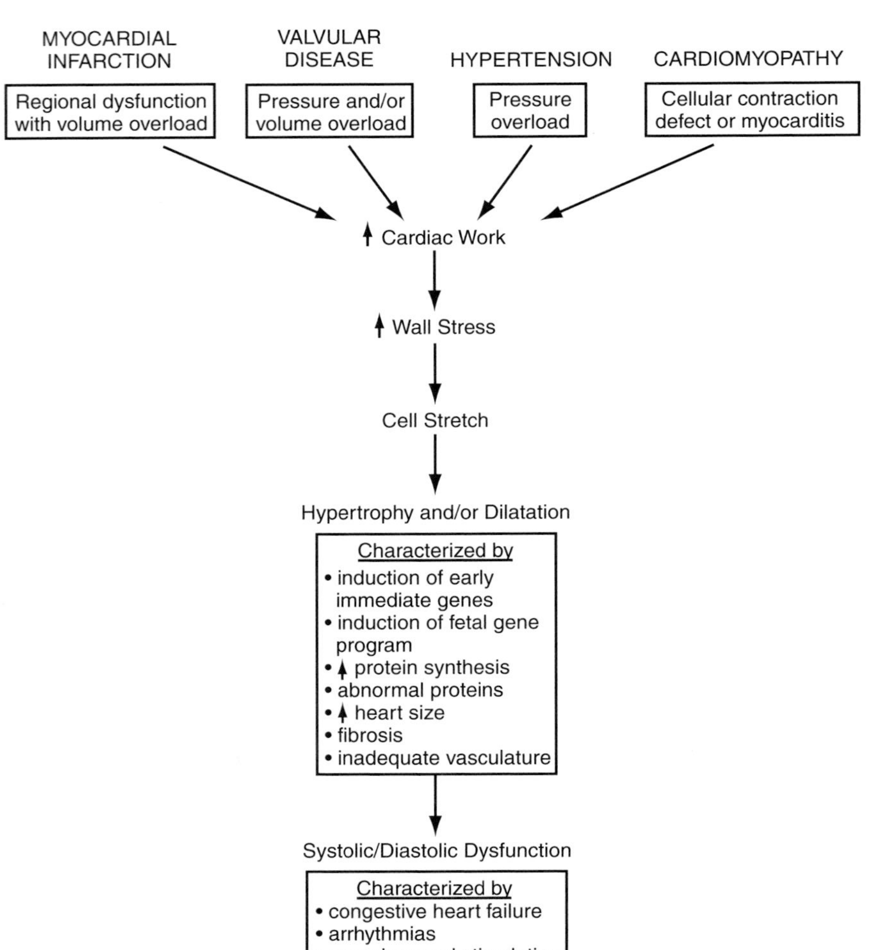

FIGURE 5–1 **Summary of the macroscopic, cellular, and extracellular changes in cardiac hypertrophy and heart failure.** *(Modified with permission from Schoen FJ: The heart, in Cotran RS, Kumar V, Collins T (eds): Robbins Pathologic Basis of Disease, 6th ed. Philadelphia, WB Saunders, 1999; p 543.)*

pathophysiologic mechanisms are emphasized. In view of space limitations, several relevant areas (e.g., aortic disease) are necessarily omitted from discussion and others (e.g., cardiac assist devices) are attenuated as they are discussed in greater detail elsewhere in the text. Moreover, although we have not included the key pathologic considerations herein, we are mindful that the number of adults with congenital heart disease is increasing rapidly and that they have unique and important pathological issues.[2] Many of these considerations have recently been summarized in another venue.[3]

GENERAL CONSIDERATIONS

Myocardial Hypertrophy

Cardiac hypertrophy is the compensatory response of the myocardium to increased work (Fig. 5-1).[4] Myocardial hyperfunction induces an increase in the overall mass and size of the heart that reflects increased size of myocytes through addition of contractile elements (sarcomeres) and mitochondria. Cardiac myocyte diameters, normally approximately 15 μm, can increase to 25 μm or more in hypertrophy.[5] Since cardiac myocytes are terminally differentiated cells that cannot divide, functional augmentation of myocyte number (hyperplasia) does not occur in the adult heart. Since the vasculature does not proliferate commensurate with increased cardiac mass, hypertrophied myocardium is usually relatively deficient in blood vessels. Moreover, myocardial fibrous tissue is often increased.

The pattern of hypertrophy reflects the nature of the stimulus. Pressure-overloaded ventricles (e.g., resulting from hypertension or aortic stenosis) develop concentric hypertrophy with an increased ventricular mass, wall thickness, and ratio of wall thickness to cavity radius without appreciable dilation. In contrast, volume-overloaded ventricles (e.g., resulting from chronic aortic or mitral regurgitation) develop hypertrophy with chamber dilation in which both ventricular radius and wall mass are increased. In this case, dilation may mask the degree of hypertrophy, and despite often markedly increased cardiac muscle mass, wall thickness frequently is not appreciably thickened, and may be near or less than normal. Pressure-overload hypertrophy is accomplished predominantly by augmentation of cell width via parallel addition of sarcomeres; in contrast, volume overload and/or dilation stimulate augmentation of both cell width and length via both parallel and series addition of sarcomeres. In situations such as myocardial infarction where there is local myocyte necrosis, the noninfarcted regions of myocardium not only hypertrophy (termed compensatory hypertrophy) but also may be overwhelmed by mechanical disadvantage and generally accumulate degenerative changes. In contrast to the regional changes resulting from myocardial infarction, the chamber wall is affected globally by the increased chamber pressure of hypertension, the increased pressure or volume workload of valvular heart disease, and in dilated cardiomyopathy.

Molecular changes that initially mediate enhanced function in hypertrophied hearts may subsequently contribute to the development of heart failure.[6–9] Hemodynamic overload alters myocardial gene expression, leading to reexpression of a pattern of protein synthesis similar to that of proliferating cells in general and of fetal cardiac myocytes during development. Proteins comprising contractile elements and those involved in excitation-contraction coupling and energy utilization are altered quantitatively or through production of different isoforms; the variant proteins may be less functional than the normal. Hypertrophied and/or failing myocardium may have additional abnormalities that include reduced adrenergic responsiveness, decreased calcium availability, impaired mitochondrial function, and microcirculatory spasm. Apoptosis of cardiac myocytes, potentially triggered by the same mechanical forces, neurohormonal activation, hypoxia, or cytokines that prompted the adaptive changes, also plays a role in the development of heart failure.[10,11] A further understanding of myocyte apoptosis may lead to novel therapeutic strategies for the treatment of heart failure.

The mechanical changes described above initially enhance function and are thereby adaptive, but they may ultimately become deleterious and contribute to cardiac failure. Thus, cardiac hypertrophy comprises a tenuous balance between adaptive characteristics and potentially deleterious structural, functional, and biochemical/molecular alterations including enlarged muscle mass with enhanced metabolic requirements, synthesis of abnormal proteins, decreased capillary/myocyte ratio, fibrosis, microvascular spasm, and impaired contractile mechanisms. Hypertrophy (with or without chamber dilation) also decreases myocardial compliance and may thereby hinder diastolic filling. In addition, left ventricular hypertrophy is an independent risk factor for cardiac mortality and morbidity, especially for sudden death.[12]

Left ventricular hypertrophy is reversible in many cases following removal of the stimulus,[13] but it is uncertain to what extent hypertrophy is capable of resolution in individual patients. However, the hemodynamic adjustment that occurs following cardiac valve surgery is not always accompanied by reversal of the myocardial changes secondary to the valvular disorder, and progressive cardiac failure may ensue despite valve replacement or repair (Fig. 5-2). Even in ventricles that are well compensated postoperatively, regression of hypertrophy often is incomplete with some degree of hypertrophy persisting for decades. In addition, the increased cardiac muscle mass in many patients requiring cardiac surgery, with its attendant global ischemia, renders intraoperative myocardial preservation difficult to achieve and the heart thereby particularly susceptible to ischemic damage.

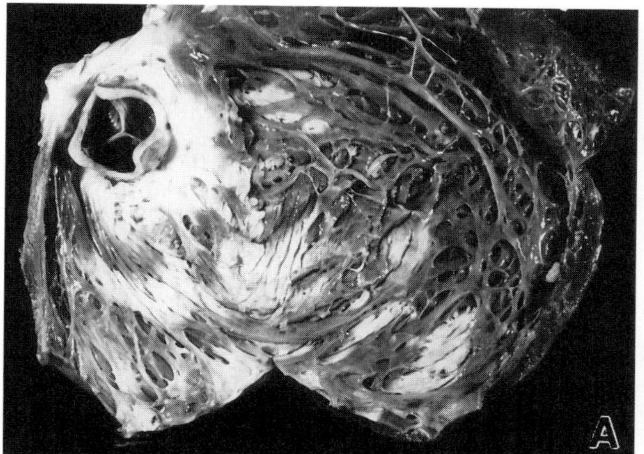

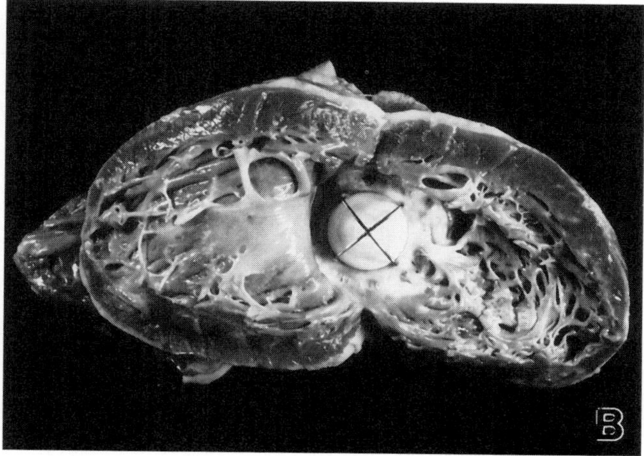

FIGURE 5–2 Late postoperative cardiac failure necessitating heart transplantation. (A) Four years following mitral valve replacement with a porcine bioprosthesis for congenital deformity causing mitral regurgitation. (B) Twenty-eight years following mitral valve replacement with a caged-disk valve for rheumatic mitral stenosis. In both cases the myocardial degradation secondary to the underlying disease progressed despite an intact valve prosthesis.

Atherosclerosis

Atherosclerosis is a chronic, progressive, multifocal disease of the vessel wall intima whose characteristic lesion is the atheroma or plaque that forms through the key processes of intimal thickening (mediated predominantly by smooth muscle cell proliferation) and lipid accumulation (mediated primarily by monocyte phagocytosis).[14–17] Atherosclerosis primarily affects the large elastic arteries and large and medium-sized muscular arteries of the systemic circulation, particularly at points of branches, sharp curvatures, and bifurcations. Atherosclerosis of native coronary arteries generally is limited to the large epicardial vessels, especially the proximal portions of the left anterior descending (LAD) and circumflex, and the right coronary diffusely, and does not involve their intramural branches. In contrast, the arteriosclerosis that affects the coronary arteries of transplanted hearts is a diffuse process that involves distal, intramural vessels as well as the larger epicardial vessels. Venous bypass grafts interposed within branches of the arterial system can develop rapidly progressive intimal thickening and ultimately atherosclerotic obstructions, yet arterial grafts such as the internal mammary artery are largely spared. Atheromas in the coronary arteries may be either concentric (25%-30%) or eccentric (70%-75%), with a plaque-free segment often comprising a substantial fraction of the vessel wall. In early lesions, the plaque bulges outward at the expense of the media with the arterial lumen remaining circular in cross-section at essentially the same original diameter (a process termed vascular remodeling).[18,19]

The prevailing theory of atherogenesis and atherosclerosis (termed the response-to-injury hypothesis) centers around interactions between endothelial cells and smooth muscle cells of the arterial wall, monocytes and platelets in the bloodstream, and plasma lipoproteins (Fig. 5-3).[20–22] Endothelial cell injury from chronic hypercholesterolemia, homocystinemia, chemicals in cigarette smoke, viruses, localized hemodynamic forces, systemic hypertension, hyperglycemia, or the local effects of cytokines causes endothelial activation. Endothelial activation that causes maladaptive processes leading to disease (such as atherosclerosis or hypertension) is called endothelial dysfunction. Endothelial dysfunction is manifested by: (1) vasoconstriction due to decreased production of the vasodilator nitric oxide, (2) increased permeablilty to lipoproteins, (3) expression of tissue factor leading to thrombosis, and (4) expression of certain injury-induced adhesion molecules leading to adherence of platelets and inflammatory cells.[23,24] Progression through an early, subendothelial lesion (often called a fatty streak) to a mature, complex atheromatous plaque results from (1) monocyte adherence to endothelial cells, migration into the subendothelial space, and transformation into tissue macrophages; (2) smooth muscle cell migration from the media into the intima, and proliferation and secretion of collagen and other extracellular matrix constituents; (3) lipid accumulation, both intracellularly (foam cells) in macrophages and smooth muscle cells as well as extracellularly; (4) lipoprotein oxidation in the vessel wall leading to generation of potent biological stimuli such as chemoattractants and cytotoxins; (5) persistent chronic inflammation, especially at the junction with the uninvolved arterial wall (the "shoulder"); and (6) cell death with release of intracellular lipids (mostly cholesterol esters), and subsequent calcification.

Mature atherosclerotic plaques consist of a central core of lipid and cholesterol crystals and cells such as macrophages, smooth muscle cells, and foam cells along with necrotic debris, proteins, and degenerating blood elements.[25,26] This core is separated from the lumen by a fibrous cap rich in collagen. The composition of atheromas can vary considerably among individuals, among arteries in the same individual, or among regions of one artery, especially in regards to the proportion of lipid to connective tissue. The natural history of atheromatous plaque and the efficacy and safety of interventional therapies likely depend on relative plaque composition, the spatial distribution of the constituents, and the integrity of the fibrous cap.[27–30] These features can be evaluated using intravascular ultrasound. The distinction between soft atheromas, consisting primarily of necrotic debris and therefore potentially moldable, and hard, fibrocalcific plaques may be important clinically; plaque mechanical properties can determine the propensity to complications as well as influence the success rate of interventions such as balloon angioplasty. The integrity of the fibrous cap is the principal determinant of plaque stability.

The clinical manifestations of advanced atherosclerosis in the coronary arteries are generally due to their encroachment of the lumen leading to progressive stenosis, or to acute plaque disruption with thrombosis (see later discussion in section on ischemic heart disease) (Fig. 5-4). However, slowly developing occlusions over time may stimulate collateral vessels that protect against distal myocardial ischemia and infarction even with an eventual high-grade stenosis. Aneurysms may form secondary to atherosclerosis as a result of atrophy or necrosis of the media, but this process is more common in the aorta than in the coronary circulation.

Ischemic Myocardial Injury

Cardiac ischemia occurs when there is inadequate perfusion to meet the metabolic needs of the tissue.[31] It is most often caused by inadequate local coronary blood flow resulting from obstruction or narrowing secondary to atherosclerosis, thrombosis, embolism, or spasm. Decreased coronary perfusion also follows systemic hypotension, in shock, and during cardiopulmonary bypass leading to global hypoperfusion. Moreover, ischemia is potentiated when the oxygen supply is decreased secondary to anemia, hypoxia, or cardiac failure. Ischemia can also result from increased cardiac demand

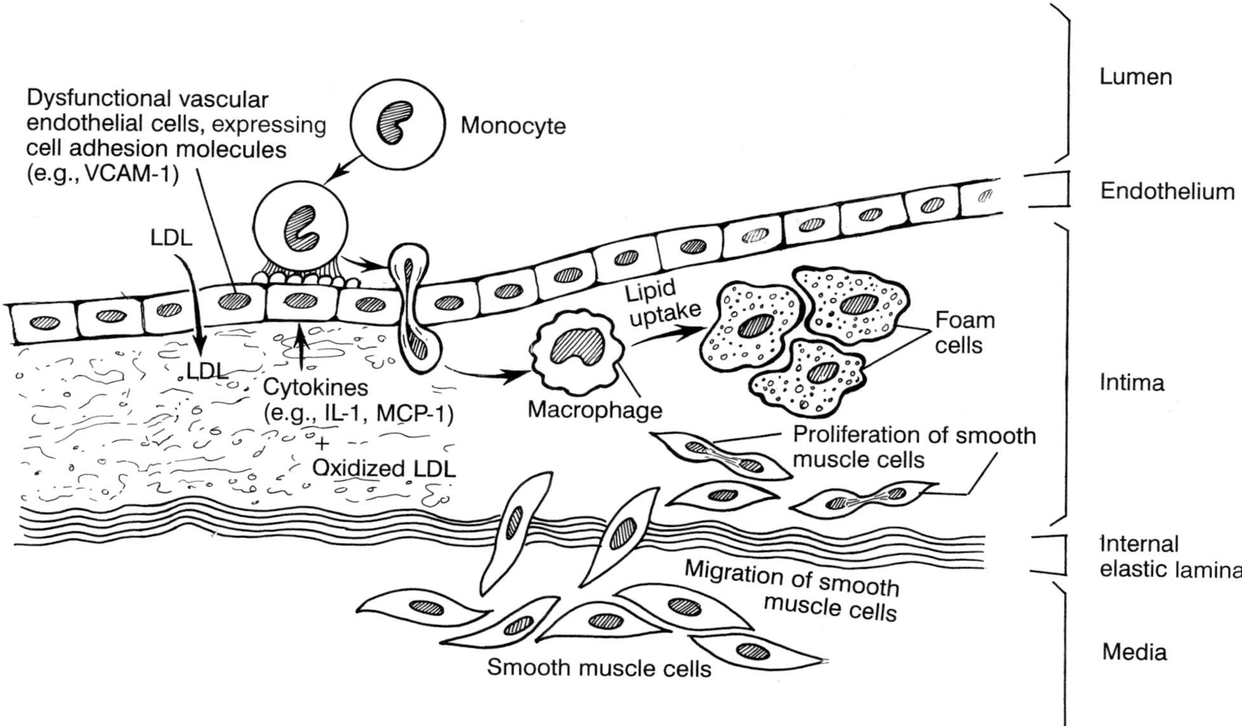

FIGURE 5–3 Schematic diagram of the sequence of cell-level events and cellular interactions in atherosclerosis. Hyperlipidemia and other risk factors cause endothelial injury, resulting in adhesion of platelets and monocytes and release of growth factors, including platelet-derived growth factor (PDGF), which stimulate smooth muscle cell migration and proliferation. Smooth muscle cells produce large amounts of extracellular matrix, including collagen and proteoglycans. Foam cells of atheromatous plaques are derived from both macrophages and smooth muscle cells—from macrophages via the very-low-density lipoprotein (VLDL) receptor and low-density lipoprotein (LDL) modifications recognized by scavenger receptors (e.g., oxidized LDL), and from smooth muscle cells by less certain mechanisms. Extracellular lipid is derived by insudation from the vessel lumen, particularly in the presence of hypercholesterolemia, and also from degenerating foam cells. Cholesterol accumulation in the plaque reflects an imbalance between influx and efflux, and high-density lipoprotein (HDL) likely helps clear cholesterol from these accumulations. *(Reproduced with permission from Schoen FJ, Cotran RS: Blood vessels, in Cotran RS, Kumar V, Collins T (eds): Pathologic Basis of Disease, 6th ed. Philadelphia, WB Saunders, 1999; p 493.)*

secondary to exercise, tachycardia, hyperthyroidism, or ventricular hypertrophy and/or dilation. The consequences of ischemia depend on its severity and duration, and on the preexisting adaptive and nutritional/metabolic state of the affected cells and tissues. Infarction, a loss of cardiac myocytes by necrosis, is caused by severe prolonged ischemia. However, chronic ischemia insufficient to cause infarction may lead to the development of collateral vessels, while brief periods of ischemia followed by reperfusion lead to changes in myocyte metabolism (ischemic preconditioning) that are protective against more severe ischemic events.[32] Ischemic myocardium salvaged by reperfusion may remain viable but suffer transient (hours to days) contractile dysfunction; this condition is termed stunned myocardium or postischemic dysfunction. The progressive effects of ischemia and salvage by reperfusion are discussed below.

PROGRESSION OF DAMAGE

Intracellular changes following the onset of myocardial ischemia are sequential and complex (Table 5-1).[33,34] Cardiac myocyte ischemia induces anaerobic glycolysis within seconds, leading to inadequate production of high-energy phosphates such as ATP and the accumulation of metabolites such as lactic acid leading to intracellular acidosis. Myocardial function is exquisitely sensitive to these biochemical consequences of severe ischemia; following the onset of ischemia, a contractility defect is evident within seconds with total loss of contraction within 2 minutes. Ischemic changes in an individual cell are initially sublethal and potentially reversible if the duration of ischemic injury is short and perfusion is restored prior to the onset of irreversible changes (15-20 min). Irreversible (lethal) injury of cardiac myocytes

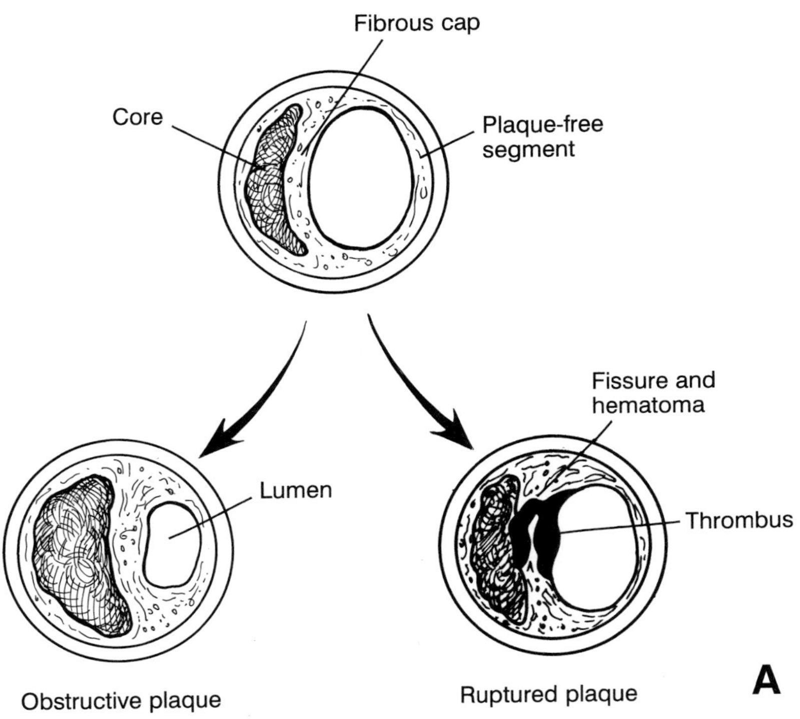

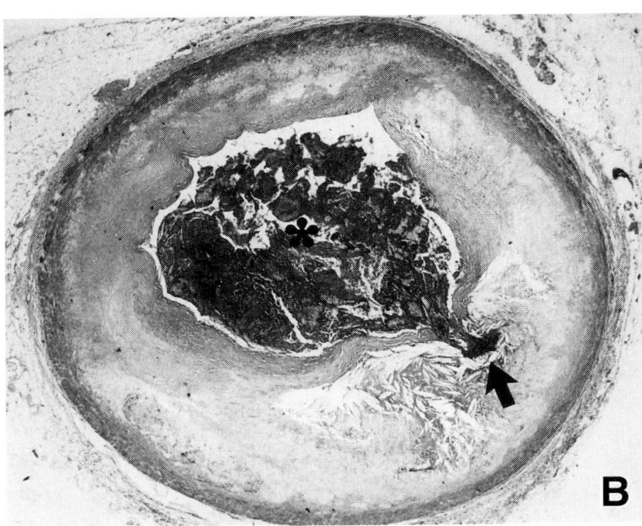

FIGURE 5–4 Consequences of coronary arterial atherosclerosis. (A) Progression of fibrous atheromatous plaque with core of extracellular lipid and necrotic debris covered by intact fibrous cap (top) to either severe chronic stenosis (lower left) or acute plaque fissuring, eventuating in a complicated lesion with a surface defect, hematoma, or mural thrombus (lower right). (B) Coronary thrombosis, superimposed on atherosclerotic plaque, triggering fatal myocardial infarction. A fissure breaching the fibrous cap and extending into the plaque necrotic core (arrow) presumably initiated the occlusive thrombus (asterisk). Hematoxylin and eosin 15X. *(B: Reproduced with permission from Schoen FJ: Interventional and Surgical Cardiovascular Pathology: Clinical Correlations and Basic Principles. Philadelphia, WB Saunders, 1989.)*

TABLE 5–1 Approximate time of onset and recognition of key features of ischemic myocardial injury

Event/process	Time of onset	Pathologic feature	Time of recognition
Onset of anerobic metabolism	Within seconds	Ultrastructural features of reversible injury	5–10 min
Loss of contractility	<2 min	Ultrastructural features of irreversible damage	20–40 min
ATP* reduced		Wavy fibers	1–3 h
to 50% of normal	10 min	Staining defect with tetrazolium dye	2–3 h
to 10% of normal	40 min	Classic histologic features of necrosis	6–12 h
Irreversible cell injury	20-40 min	Gross alterations	12–24 h
Microvascular injury	>1 h		

*ATP = Adenosine triphosphate.

with cell membrane structural defects occurs only after 20 to 40 minutes within the most severely ischemic area. When ischemic injury is of sufficient severity and duration, groups of involved cells die, and myocardial infarction results.

Within the region made vulnerable by loss of perfusion, termed the area at risk, not all cells are equally injured. A gradient of ischemia exists across the myocardium; the most affected regions, and therefore the first to become necrotic, are the subendocardium and papillary muscles in the center of the perfusion defect. However, the myocytes immediately beneath the endocardium to a depth of approximately 1 mm usually are effectively perfused by the well-oxygenated blood in the left ventricular chamber and therefore protected from ischemic damage. As uninterrupted ischemia progresses, there is a wavefront of cell death outward from the mid-subendocardial region toward and eventually encompassing the lateral borders and less ischemic subepicardial and peripheral regions. While the mechanism of cell death in myocardial infarction has traditionally been thought of as coagulation necrosis, recent evidence suggests that apoptosis may also play a role.[35,36] In human myocardial infarction, approximately 50% of the area at risk becomes necrotic in approximately 3 to 4 hours. The final transmural extent of an infarct is generally established within 6 to 12 hours. Restoration of flow via therapeutic intervention can alter the outcome depending on the interval between the onset of ischemia and reperfusion.

Within a few minutes of the onset of ischemia, reversible ultrastructural changes can be observed using transmission electron microscopy, including glycogen depletion, cellular and mitochondrial swelling, myofibrillar relaxation, and margination of nuclear chromatin. This is followed by the development of amorphous mitochondrial densities and sarcolemmal disruption as evidence of necrosis. However, neither reversible ischemia nor necrosis existing less than at least 6 or more hours before patient death can be detected grossly or microscopically. On gross examination at autopsy of a patient who died at least 2 to 3 hours following the onset of infarction, the presence of a necrotic region may often be indicated as a staining defect with triphenyl tetrazolium chloride (TTC), a dye that turns viable myocardium a brick-red color on reaction with intact myocardial dehydrogenases.[37] However, these and other changes occurring less than about 6 hours prior to death are not visible on routine light microscopic evaluation. The earliest light microscopic features include clusters of necrotic myocytes that exhibit intense eosinophilia, nuclear pyknosis and loss, and stretched and wavy myocytes. Inflammatory exudation with polymorphonuclear leukocytes can usually be seen after 6 to 12 hours and peaks within 1 to 3 days. The inflammatory reaction continues with removal of necrotic tissue by macrophages (3-5 days) and is followed by a fibroblastic reparative response accompanied by neovascularization (granulation tissue) beginning after 1 to 2 weeks at the margins of preserved tissue. The infarcted tissue is replaced by scar that reaches maturity by about 6 weeks.

Healing of myocardial ischemic injury may be slowed by anti-inflammatory agents administered following myocardial infarction, as a component of immunosuppressive therapy following transplantation, or in otherwise debilitated or malnourished patients.[38,39] Sublethal but chronic ischemic injury may be revealed by myocyte vacuolization, usually most prevalent in the subendocardium. Overall, the repair sequence following an infarct is similar to that which follows tissue injury of diverse causes and at various noncardiac anatomic sites.

Although cardiac myocytes are not traditionally thought capable of regeneration, mitotic activity has been reported at the viable borders of myocardial infarcts.[40] In addition, myocytes bearing a Y chromosome have been found in the heart of female donors transplanted to male recipients, raising the possibility that endogenous primitive stem cells, either circulating or resident, may play a role in repair of myocardial infarcts.[41]

EFFECTS OF REPERFUSION

The progression of myocardial ischemic injury can be modified by restoration of blood flow (reperfusion) to jeopardized myocardium. Reperfusion occurring before the onset of irreversibility (about 20 minutes in the most severely ischemic regions) may substantially limit infarct size or prevent cell death altogether. Later reperfusion up to 6 to 12 hours does not prevent infarction entirely, but does salvage myocytes located at the leading edge of the "wavefront" that are only reversibly injured. The potential for recovery decreases with increasing severity and duration of ischemia (Fig. 5-5). Late reperfusion beyond the interval at which myocyte salvage continues to be possible may also lead to functional benefits by mechanisms that are yet poorly understood.[42,43]

The gross and microscopic findings of reperfusion of ischemic myocardium are summarized in Figure 5-6. The microscopic pattern of reperfusion includes hemorrhage and necrotic myocytes with contraction bands, which are transverse eosinophilic lines across the cell that represent clusters of hypercontracted sarcomeres. Contraction bands are a manifestation of irreversible injury including cell membrane damage that is followed by a massive influx of calcium from the restored blood flow leading to intense sarcomeric contraction.[44] In cases of reperfusion after global ischemia, the left ventricle may undergo a massive tetanic contraction to a small, hard mass; this is termed the stone heart syndrome.[45]

Restoration of systemic pressure to an artery supplying a healthy microvasculature will often restore adequate blood flow. However, since microvascular damage accompanies severe, prolonged ischemia, the effects of ischemic vascular injury followed by reperfusion may include: (1) hemorrhage, visible grossly and microscopically, due to vascular wall incompetence; or (2) microvascular occlusion due to endothelial or interstitial edema, hypercontracted ischemic myocytes, and/or plugging by platelet or neutrophil aggregates.

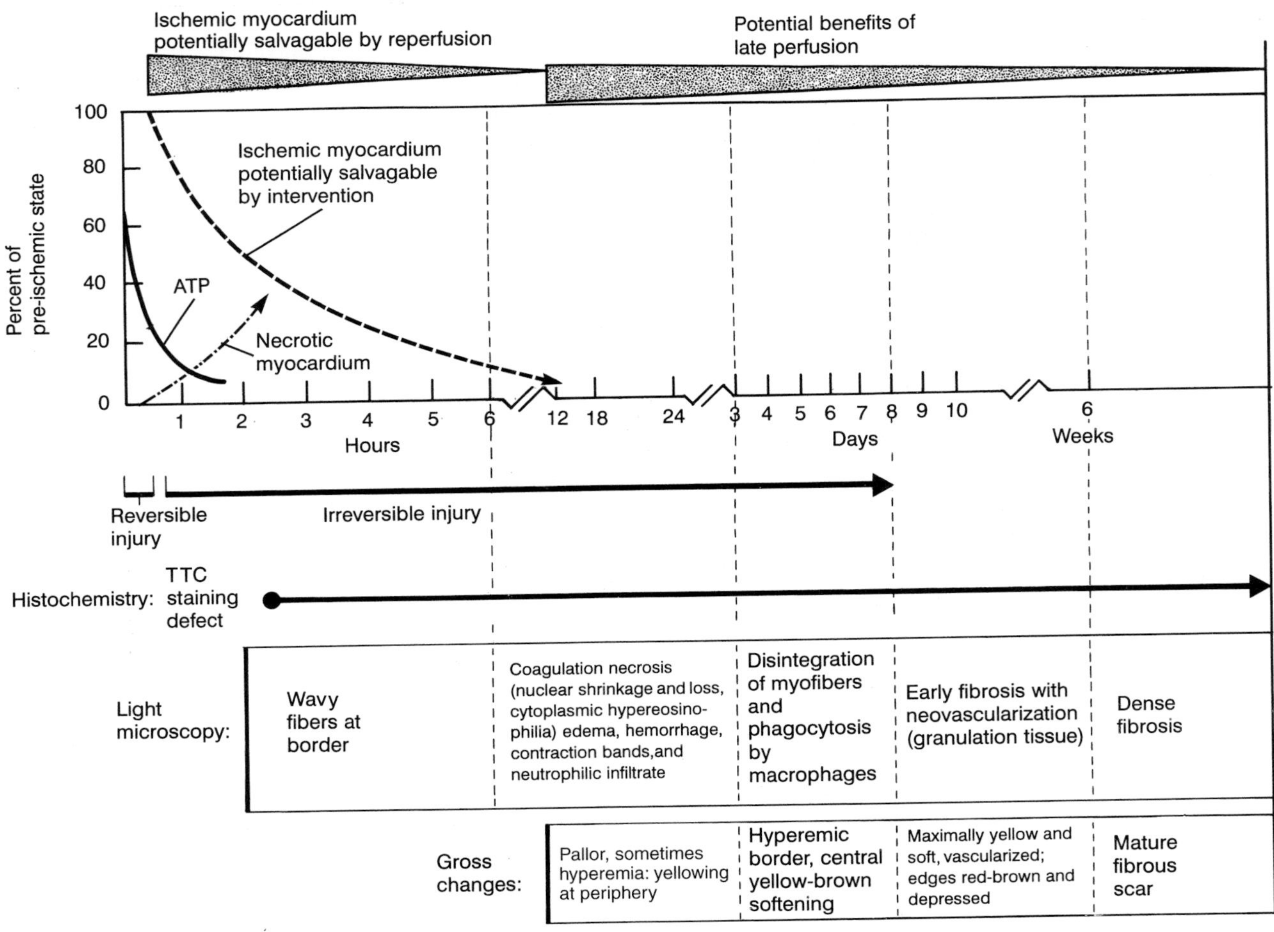

FIGURE 5–5 Temporal sequence of early biochemical, ultrastructural, histochemical, and histologic findings after onset of severe myocardial ischemia. The time frames for early and late reperfusion of the myocardium supplied by an occluded coronary artery are schematically shown at the top of the figure. For approximately one-half hour following the onset of even the most severe ischemia, myocardial injury is potentially reversible. Thereafter, progressive loss of viability occurs to completion by 6 to 12 hours. The benefits of reperfusion are greatest when it is achieved early, with progressively smaller benefit occurring as reperfusion is delayed. *(Modified with permission from Antman E, Braunwald E: Acute myocardial infarction, in Braunwald E, Zipes DP, Libby P (eds): Heart Disease: A Textbook of Cardiovascular Medicine. Philadelphia, WB Saunders, 2001; p 1114.)*

These vascular effects cause the no-reflow phenomenon, which may inhibit the perfusion of damaged regions.

Reperfusion may actually damage some of the ischemic but viable myocytes (reperfusion injury), but the amount of salvaged myocardium usually outweighs the extent of this damage.[46,47] Reperfusion injury is mediated primarily by toxic oxygen species (such as free radicals) that are overproduced by myocytes or polymorphonuclear leukocytes upon restoration of oxygen supply to the tissues, but complement activation may also contribute. Consequently, injury may be reduced by free radical scavengers such as superoxide dismutase and catalase, inhibitors of polymorphonuclear leukocyte endothelial cell adhesion, or drugs that regulate complement.[48–50] Arrhythmias also may occur after reperfusion, possibly secondary to myocyte damage by oxygen free radicals and/or increased intracellular calcium.

Metabolic and functional recovery of successfully reperfused myocardium is not instantaneous, with contractile dysfunction persisting for hours to days following brief periods of ischemia; this dysfunction is termed myocardial stunning.[51,52] Myocardial stunning may occur after angioplasty, thrombolysis, cardiopulmonary bypass, or even ischemia related to unstable angina or stress. The use of cardiac assist devices may allow the stunned myocardium to recover in these situations of reversible cardiac failure.[53–55] The mechanism of myocardial stunning likely involves the generation of oxygen radicals, alterations of calcium metabolism, and changes in the sarcomere.

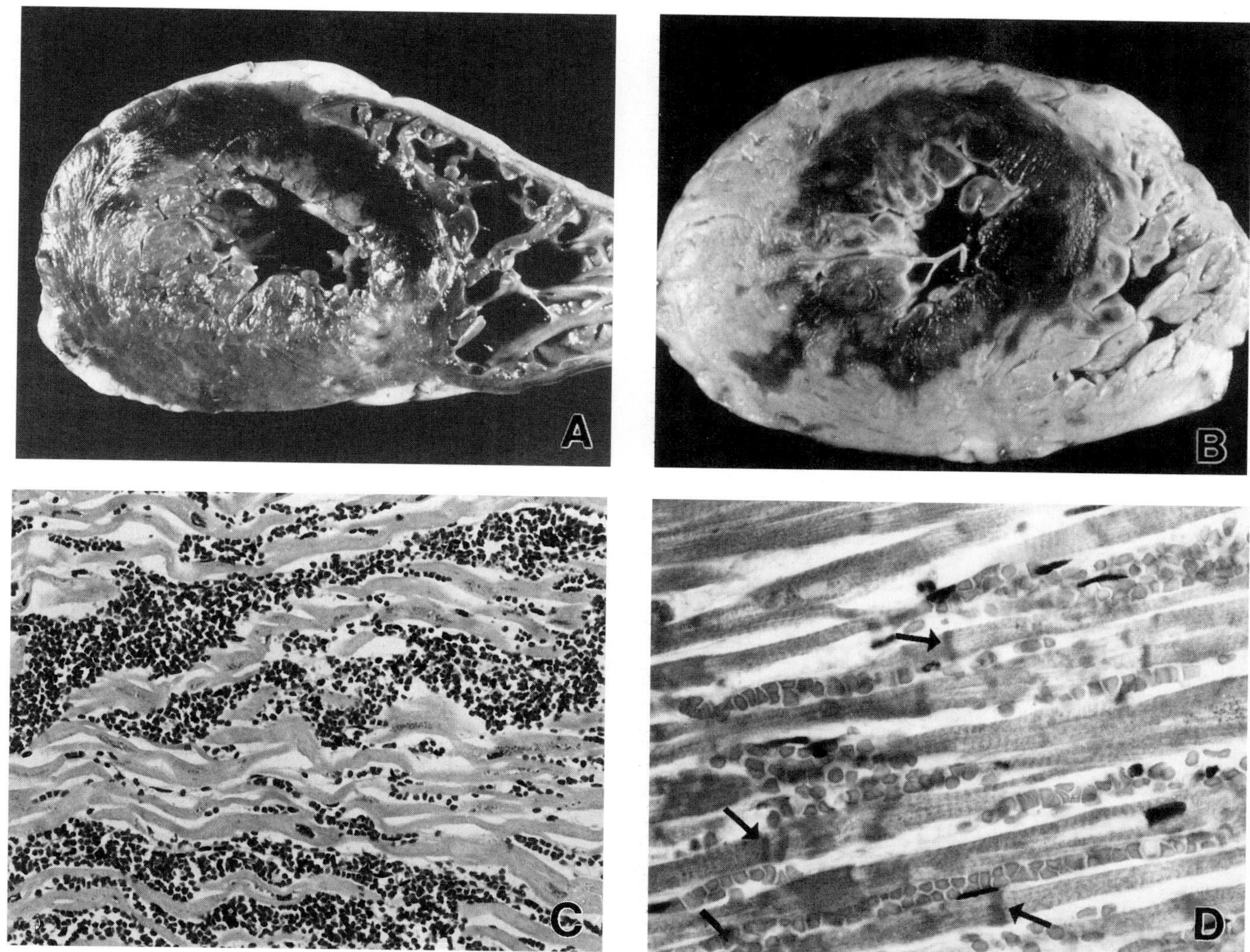

FIGURE 5–6 Morphological effects of reperfusion following severe myocardial ischemia. (A) Large, densely hemorrhagic anteroseptal acute myocardial infarct from patient treated by streptokinase intracoronary thrombolysis for left anterior descending (LAD) artery thrombus, approximately 4 hours following onset of chest pain. (B) Subendocardial circumferential hemorrhagic acute myocardial necrosis in a large hypertrophied heart 2 days postoperative cardiac transplantation. (C) Photomicrograph of myocardial interstitial hemorrhage from heart shown in (A). Hematoxylin and eosin 375X. (D) Photomicrograph of myocardial necrosis with contraction bands (contraction band necrosis). Contraction bands are noted by arrows. Hematoxylin and eosin 375X. *(A, C, and D: Reproduced with permission from Schoen FJ: Interventional and Surgical Cardiovascular Pathology: Clinical Correlations and Basic Principles. Philadelphia, WB Saunders, 1989.)*

Viable regions of myocardium with chronically impaired function in the setting of chronically reduced coronary blood flow are termed hibernating myocardium.[56,57] Myocardial hibernation is characterized by: (1) persistent wall motion abnormality; (2) low myocardial blood flow; and (3) evidence of viability of at least some of the affected areas. Contractile function of hibernating myocardium improves if blood flow returns toward normal or if oxygen demand is reduced. Correction of this abnormality is likely responsible for the reversal of long-standing defects in ventricular wall motion that may be observed following coronary bypass graft surgery or angioplasty. Efforts are underway to image hibernating myocardium and therefore identify those patients who would benefit from restoration of adequate coronary blood flow.[58,59]

Adaptation to short-term transient ischemia may induce tolerance against subsequent, more severe ischemic insults in a process termed ischemic preconditioning.[60] A short (5-min) period of cardiac ischemia followed by reperfusion is capable of protecting the affected myocardium against injury from a more intense period of subsequent ischemia. The mechanism of this protection is uncertain, but stimulation of adenosine receptors when adenosine is released during ischemia, enhanced expression of heat-shock proteins (which makes the heart more resistant to prolonged ischemia), and involvement of protein kinase C and ATP-dependent potassium channels have been suggested.[61,62] Pharmacologic stimulation of these pathways is under investigation to derive the benefits of preconditioning without actually subjecting the myocardium to ischemia.

Biomaterials and Tissue Engineering

Biomaterials are synthetic or modified biologic materials that are used in implanted or extracorporeal medical devices that augment or replace body structures and functions.[63,64] Examples of such biomaterials include polymers, metals, ceramics, carbons, processed collagen, and chemically treated animal or human tissues, the latter exemplified by glutaraldehyde-preserved heart valves, pericardium, and blood vessels. The first generation of biomedical materials (e.g., metals used for early valve substitutes and orthopedic hardware) was generally designed to be inert; the goal was to reduce the host inflammatory responses to the implanted material. By the mid-1980s, a second generation of bioactive biomaterials was emerging that could interact with the host in a beneficial manner (e.g., hydroxyapatite ceramics, biodegradable polymer sutures). With a greater understanding of material-tissue interactions at the cellular and molecular levels, a third generation of materials is being designed to stimulate specific cellular and tissue responses at the molecular level.[65]

Comprising effects of both the implant on the host tissues and the host on the implant, biomaterial-tissue interactions

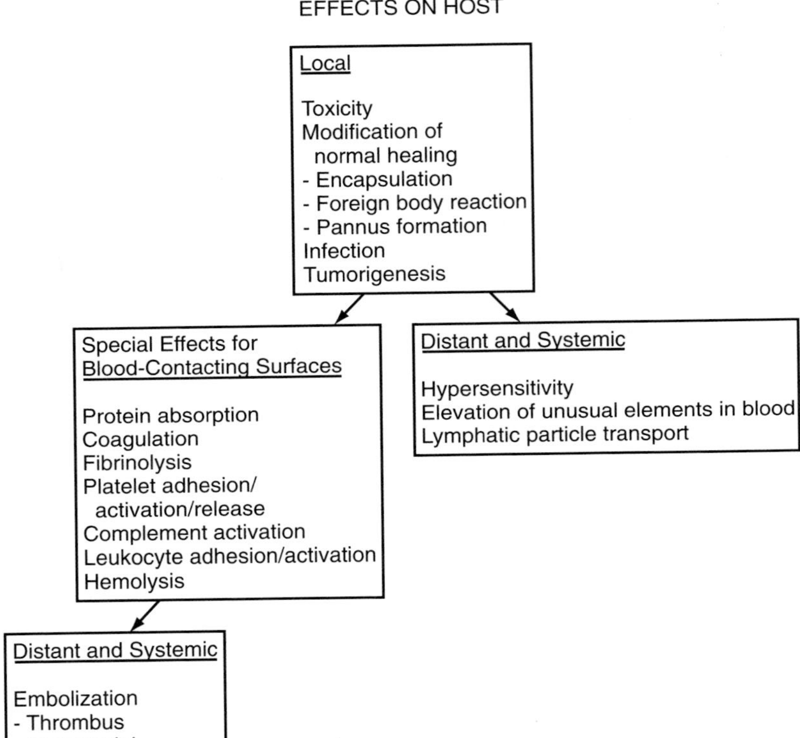

FIGURE 5–7 Overview of potential interactions of biomaterials with tissue, comprising local, distant, and systemic effects of the biomaterial on the host tissue as well as the physical and biological effects of the environment on the materials and the device. These interactions comprise the pathophysiological basis for device complications and failure modes. *(Reproduced with permission from Schoen FJ: Introduction to host reactions to biomaterials and their evaluation, in Ratner BD, Hoffman AS, Lemons JE, Schoen FJ (eds): Biomaterials Science: An Introduction to Materials in Medicine. San Diego, Academic Press, 1996; p 165.)*

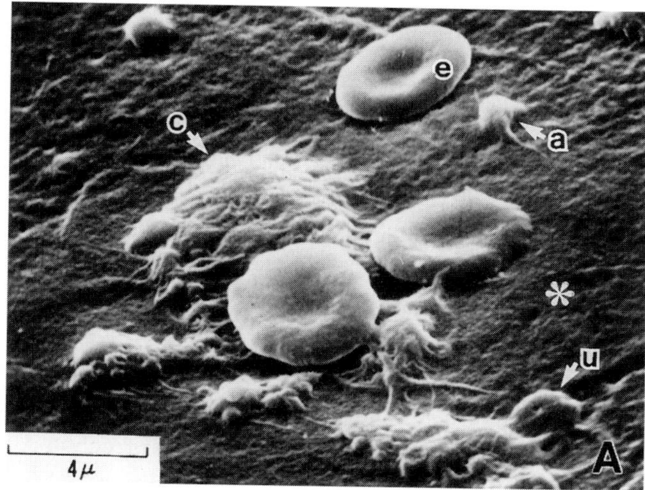

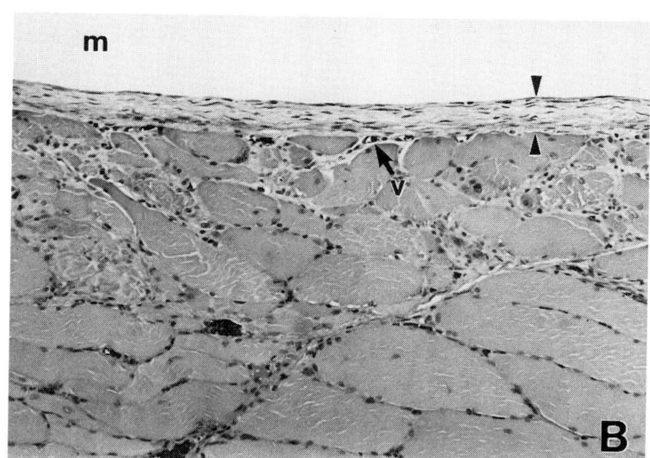

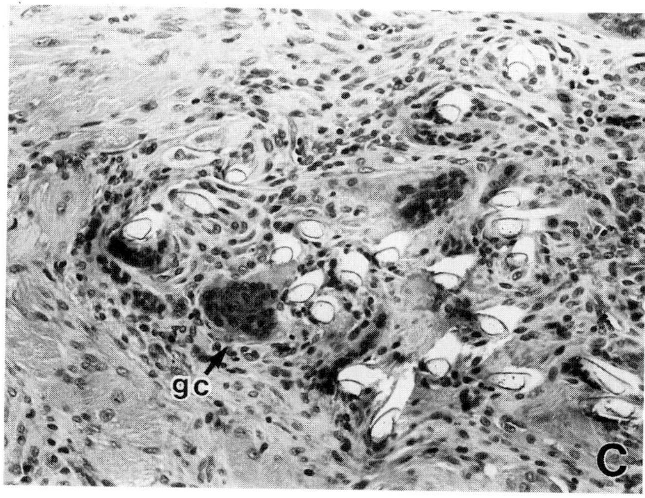

FIGURE 5–8 Morphology of biomaterials-tissue interactions. (A) Scanning electron photomicrograph of early thrombotic deposits on heart valve material exposed to calf blood for a few minutes in an extracorporeal experiment. Numerous platelets in various stages of adhesion ranging from relatively unaffected (u) to adherent to activated (a) forms, some aggregated in clumps (c), are adherent to a background of protein absorption (asterisk). Erythrocytes (e) are probably passively adsorbed in early surface induced thrombus formation. (B) Photomicrograph of experimental tissue reaction to relatively inert biocompatible material (m), implanted into rabbit muscle. A thin discrete fibrous capsule with virtually no inflammatory cell infiltrate is adjacent to the implant (between arrowheads). Fine vascularity (v) is noted at the interface between the fibrous capsule and the surrounding muscle. Hematoxylin and eosin 150X. (C) Granulomatous inflammatory response to surgically implanted Dacron mesh. This is an intense inflammatory response that includes abundant foreign body giant cells (gc). Hematoxylin and eosin 200X. *(A: Reproduced with permission from Schoen FJ: Cardiac valve prostheses: pathological and bioengineering considerations. J Card Surg 1987; 2:265. B and C: Reproduced with permission from Schoen FJ: Interventional and Surgical Cardiovascular Pathology: Clinical Correlations and Basic Principles. Philadelphia, WB Saunders, 1989.)*

are important in mediating prosthetic device complications (Fig. 5-7).[66] Major morphologic effects of biomaterials on tissues are illustrated in Figure 5-8. Complications of cardiovascular medical devices, irrespective of anatomic site of implantation, can be grouped into six major categories: (1) thrombosis and thromboembolism; (2) device-associated infection; (3) exuberant or defective healing; (4) degeneration, fracture, or other biomaterials failure; (5) adverse local tissue interaction, such as toxicity or traumatic hemolysis; and (6) adverse effects distant from the intended site of the device, such as biomaterials migration or systemic hypersensitivity.

No synthetic or modified biological surface is as thromboresistant as the normal, unperturbed endothelium. Like a blood vessel denuded of endothelium, foreign materials on contact with blood spontaneously and rapidly (within seconds) absorb a film of plasma components, primarily protein, followed by platelet adhesion.[67] If conditions of relatively static flow are present, macroscopic thrombus can ensue.

BLOOD-SURFACE INTERACTION

Thromboembolic complications of cardiovascular devices cause significant mortality and morbidity.[68] Thrombotic deposits can impede the function of a prosthetic heart valve, vascular graft, or blood pump, or cause distal emboli. As in the cardiovascular system in general, surface thrombogenicity, hypercoagulability, and locally static blood flow (Virchow's triad), present individually or in combination, determine the relative propensity toward thrombus formation and location of thrombotic deposits with specific devices. Considerable evidence implicates a primary role for blood platelets in the thrombogenic response to artificial surfaces (see Fig. 5-8A).[69] However, the clinical approach to control of thrombosis in cardiovascular devices uses systemic anticoagulants, particularly coumadin (warfarin). This agent inhibits thrombin formation but does not inhibit platelet-mediated thrombosis. The specific physical and chemical characteristics of materials that regulate the outcomes of blood-surface interaction are incompletely understood.

Coagulation proteins, complement products, other proteins, and platelets also are activated, damaged, and consumed by blood-material interactions.For example, blood contact with the large areas of synthetic surfaces during the extracorporeal perfusion of cardiopulmonary bypass (CPB) may have at least four consequences: (1) activation and resultant dysfunction of platelets; (2) progressive denaturation of plasma proteins and lipoproteins; (3) activation of coagulation proteins and the fibrinolytic system and, through interaction with inflammatory pathways, production of various bioactive molecules, including bradykinin, a potent vasodilator; and (4) activation of complement through the alternative pathway, with production of C3a and C5a, inducing polymorphonuclear leukocyte stasis in the pulmonary circulation with the occasional sequelae of acute pulmonary hypertension and inflammatory lung injury.

Hemolysis (damage to red blood cells) in implants and extracorporeal circulatory systems results from both blood-surface interactions and turbulence. Erythrocytes have reduced survival following cardiopulmonary bypass. Also, with earlier model heart valve prostheses, renal tubular hemosiderosis or cholelithiasis occurred in many patients, indicative of chronic hemolysis. With contemporary valves, hemolysis generally is modest and well compensated, but may be accentuated by valve dysfunction.

TISSUE-SURFACE INTERACTION

Synthetic biomaterials typically are not immunogenic, but they elicit a foreign body reaction, a special form of non-immune inflammatory response with an infiltrate predominantly composed of macrophages.[70,71] Although immunologic reactions have been proposed rarely for synthetic biomaterial-tissue interactions, they are theoretically possible with tissue-derived biomaterials, and antibodies can be elicited by implantation of some materials in finely pulverized form.[72,73] Nevertheless, clinical cardiovascular device failure owing to immunologic reactivity is rare. For most biomaterials implanted into solid tissue, encapsulation by a relatively thin fibrous tissue capsule (composed of collagen and fibroblasts) resembling a scar ultimately occurs, often with a fine capillary network at its junction with normal tissue (see Fig. 5-8B). An ongoing inflammatory infiltrate consisting of monocytes/macrophages and multinucleated foreign body giant cells in the vicinity of a foreign body generally suggests persistent tissue irritation (see Fig. 5-8C).

VASCULAR GRAFT HEALING

The healing of fabric prostheses or components within the cardiovascular system can yield exuberant fibrous tissue at the anastomosis as an overactive but physiologic repair response (Fig. 5-9).[74] Synthetic and biological vascular grafts often fail because of generalized or anastomotic narrowing mediated by connective tissue proliferation in the intima, and heart valve prostheses can have excessive pannus that occludes the orifice. Intimal hyperplasia results primarily from smooth muscle cell migration, proliferation, and extracellular matrix elaboration following and possibly mediated by acute or ongoing endothelial cell injury. Contributing factors include: (1) surface thrombogenesis; (2) delayed or incomplete endothelialization of the fabric; (3) disturbed flow across the anastomosis; and (4) mechanical factors at the junction of implant and host tissues.

Tissue lining a vascular graft or coating a heart valve sewing cuff has two principal sources: overgrowth from the host vessel across anastomotic sites, and tissue ingrowth through fabric interstices. In a graft with interstices large enough to permit ingrowth of fibrovascular elements, endothelial cells can arise from capillaries extending from outside to inside the graft and migrate to the luminal surface at a large distance from the anastomosis. However, since most clinical vascular grafts are impervious, in order to obviate hemorrhage, existing grafts (and other fabrics used as cardiovascular implants) heal primarily by ingrowth of endothelium and smooth muscle cells from the cut edges of the adjacent artery or other tissue. A third mechanism, deposition of functional endothelial cells from the circulating blood, is

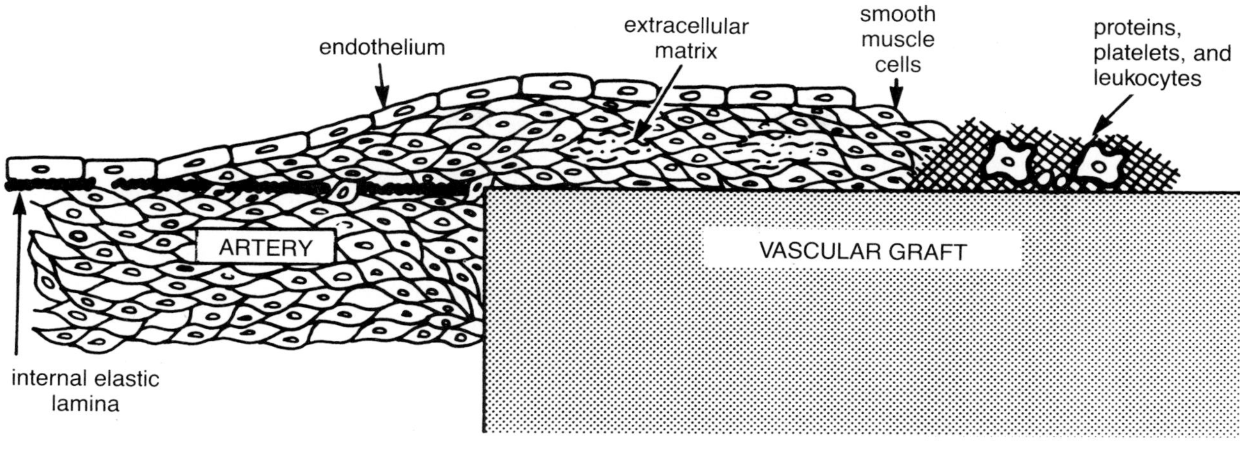

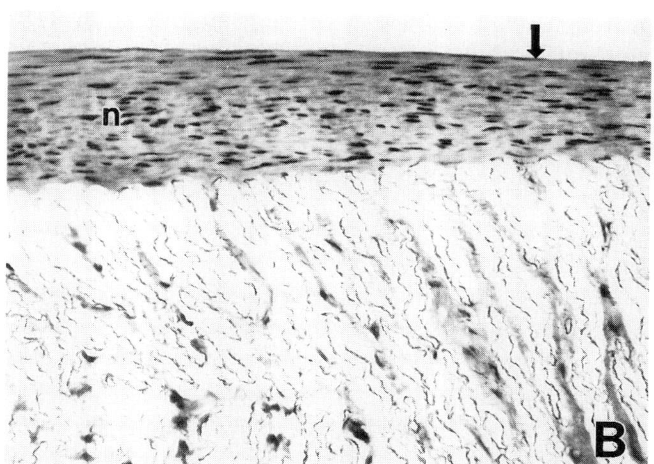

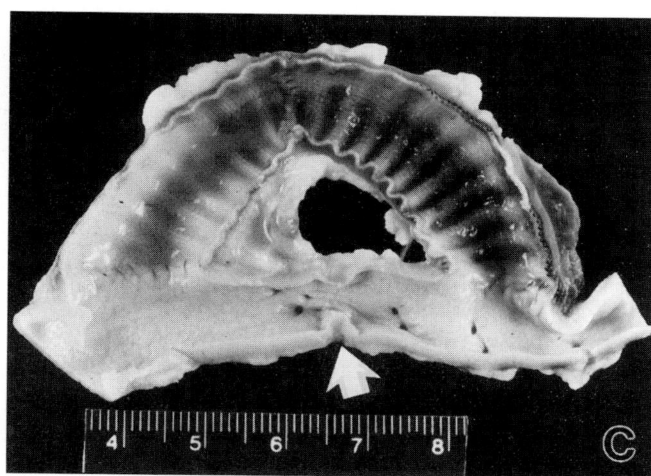

FIGURE 5–9 Vascular graft healing. (A) Schematic diagram of pannus formation, the major mode of graft healing with currently available vascular grafts. Smooth muscle cells migrate from the media to the intima of the adjacent artery and extend over and proliferate on the graft surface. The thin smooth muscle cell layer is covered by a proliferating layer of endothelial cells. (B) Neointima (n), consisting of smooth muscle cells and extracellular matrix covered by endothelium in an experimental ePTFE graft in the rabbit aorta. The blood-contacting surface is indicated by arrow. Hematoxylin and eosin 150X. (C) Experimental composite vascular graft composed of dissimilar grafts anastomosed together, used to bypass a surgically created stenotic segment in the sheep aorta (arrow), from a study of variables in graft healing. The extent of healing is vastly different between the gelatin-coated graft (left) and the albumin-coated graft (right). *(A and B: Reproduced with permission from Schoen FJ: Interventional and Surgical Cardiovascular Pathology: Clinical Correlations and Basic Principles. Philadelphia, WB Saunders, 1989. C: Reproduced by permission from Kadoba K, Schoen FJ, Jonas RA: Experimental comparison of albumin-sealed and gelatin-sealed knitted Dacron conduits. J Thorac Cardiovasc Surg 1992; 103:1059.)*

now believed to exist, but the extent of functional endothelialization via this route is not yet known.[75]

Humans have a limited ability to spontaneously endothelialize cardiovascular prostheses, and full endothelialization of clinical grafts (yielding an intact *neointima*) usually does not occur. Luminal coverage develops relatively slowly and incompletely. For uncertain reasons, endothelial cell coverage generally is restricted to a zone near an anastomosis, typically 10 to 15 mm, thereby allowing healing of intracardiac fabric patches and prosthetic valve sewing rings, but not long vascular grafts. Thus, except adjacent to an anastomosis, a compacted platelet-fibrin aggregate (*pseudointima*) comprises the inner lining of clinical fabric grafts, even after long-term implantation. Because firm adherence of such linings to the underlying graft may be impossible, dislodgment of the lining and formation of a flap-valve can occur and cause acute obstruction.[76] Current research centers on the design of novel vascular graft materials that enhance endothelial cell attachment, grafts preseeded with unmodified or genetically engineered endothelial cells, and attempts to block smooth muscle cell proliferation.[77–81]

INFECTION

Infection occurs in as many as 5% to 10% of patients with implanted prosthetic devices and is a frequent source of morbidity and mortality.[82] Because medical devices usually are coated with platelet-fibrin thrombus and are remote from capillary vessels, associated infections often are difficult to treat with antibiotics and are resistant to host defenses. Consequently, such infections generally persist until the devices are removed.

Early implant infections (less than 1-2 months postoperatively) most likely result from intraoperative contamination or early postoperative wound infection. In contrast, late infections generally occur by a hematogenous route, and can be initiated by bacteremia induced by therapeutic dental or genitourinary procedures.Antibiotics given prophylactically at device implantation and shortly before subsequent diagnostic and therapeutic procedures may protect against implant infection. Infections associated with foreign bodies are characterized microbiologically by a high prevalence of coagulase-negative staphylococci, including *Staphylococcus epidermidis,* an organism with low virulence, and an infrequent cause of non–prosthesis-associated deep infections, as well as other more virulent staphylococci, especially *S. aureus,* and less virulent strains of streptococci.[83,84]

The presence of a foreign body potentiates infection in several ways. Microorganisms may inadvertently be introduced by device contamination, provided access to deeper tissue by damage to natural barriers against infection during implantation or subsequent device function, and permitted to survive adjacent to the implant. Many strains of bacteria, particularly *S. epidermidis,* are adept at adhering to synthetic surfaces and creating a biofilm that protects against the host humoral and cellular immune defenses.[85] Moreover, an implanted foreign body could limit phagocyte migration into infected tissue or interfere with inflammatory cell phagocytic mechanisms, by release of soluble implant components or surface-mediated interactions.

Despite the large numbers of implants used clinically over an extended duration, neoplasms occurring at the site of implanted cardiovascular and other medical devices are exceedingly rare.[86,87]

TISSUE ENGINEERING

A logical future thrust of biomaterials science, *tissue engineering* combines the principles and methods of the life sciences with those of engineering to develop implantable medical devices that use living cells together with extracellular components (either natural or synthetic).[88–91] Tissue engineering utilizes third-generation biomaterials, designed to stimulate specific cellular responses at the molecular level and thereby providing the scientific foundation for molecular design of scaffolds that can be seeded with cells in vitro for subsequent implantation or specifically attract functional cells in vivo.

In implantable medical devices that use cells together with extracellular components, the cells are either transplanted or induced in the recipient by implantation of an appropriate bioresorbable substrate. In the usual approach to engineering tissues, the first step involves the seeding of cells on a synthetic polymer or natural material (such as collagen or chemically treated tissue) scaffold, and a tissue is matured in vitro. A typical scaffold is a bioresorbable polymer in a porous configuration, adhesive for cells in the desired geometry for the engineered tissue. The cells are either differentiated cells, or undifferentiated "stem cells."[92] When placed in a metabolically and mechanically supportive environment with growth media (in a *bioreactor*), the cells proliferate and elaborate extracellular matrix in the form of a "new" tissue (the *construct*). In the second step, the construct is implanted in the appropriate anatomic location. Remodeling of the construct in vivo following implantation is intended to recapitulate normal functional architecture of an organ or tissue. Progress has already been made toward tissue engineered heart valves,[93,94] vascular grafts,[95–97] and segments of myocardium.[98]

Another approach to myocardial tissue engineering is cell transplantation into the myocardium as a means of augmentation. Numerous investigators have injected autologous or allogenic fetal cardiomyocytes, myoblasts, or isolated skeletal muscle satellite, and bone marrow stromal cells or mesenchymal stem cells have been studied.[99] Injection of bone-marrow–derived cells into myocardium following ischemic injury resulted in improved function and replacement of dead myocardial tissue by cells that expressed cardiac muscle-specific proteins.[100]

ISCHEMIC HEART DISEASE

The ischemic heart disease syndromes are primarily caused by atherosclerosis and its complications secondary to a complex dynamic interaction among fixed atherosclerotic narrowing of the epicardial coronary arteries, intraluminal thrombosis overlying a ruptured or fissured atherosclerotic plaque, platelet aggregation, and vasospasm, causing diminished coronary perfusion (Fig. 5-10). Increased myocardial demand, anemia, and systemic hypotension can also contribute acutely to the development of ischemic heart disease.

Pathogenesis

ROLE OF FIXED CORONARY OBSTRUCTIONS

In the absence of significant pathology, coronary arterial flow provides adequate myocardial perfusion at rest, and compensatory vasodilation provides flow reserve that is more than

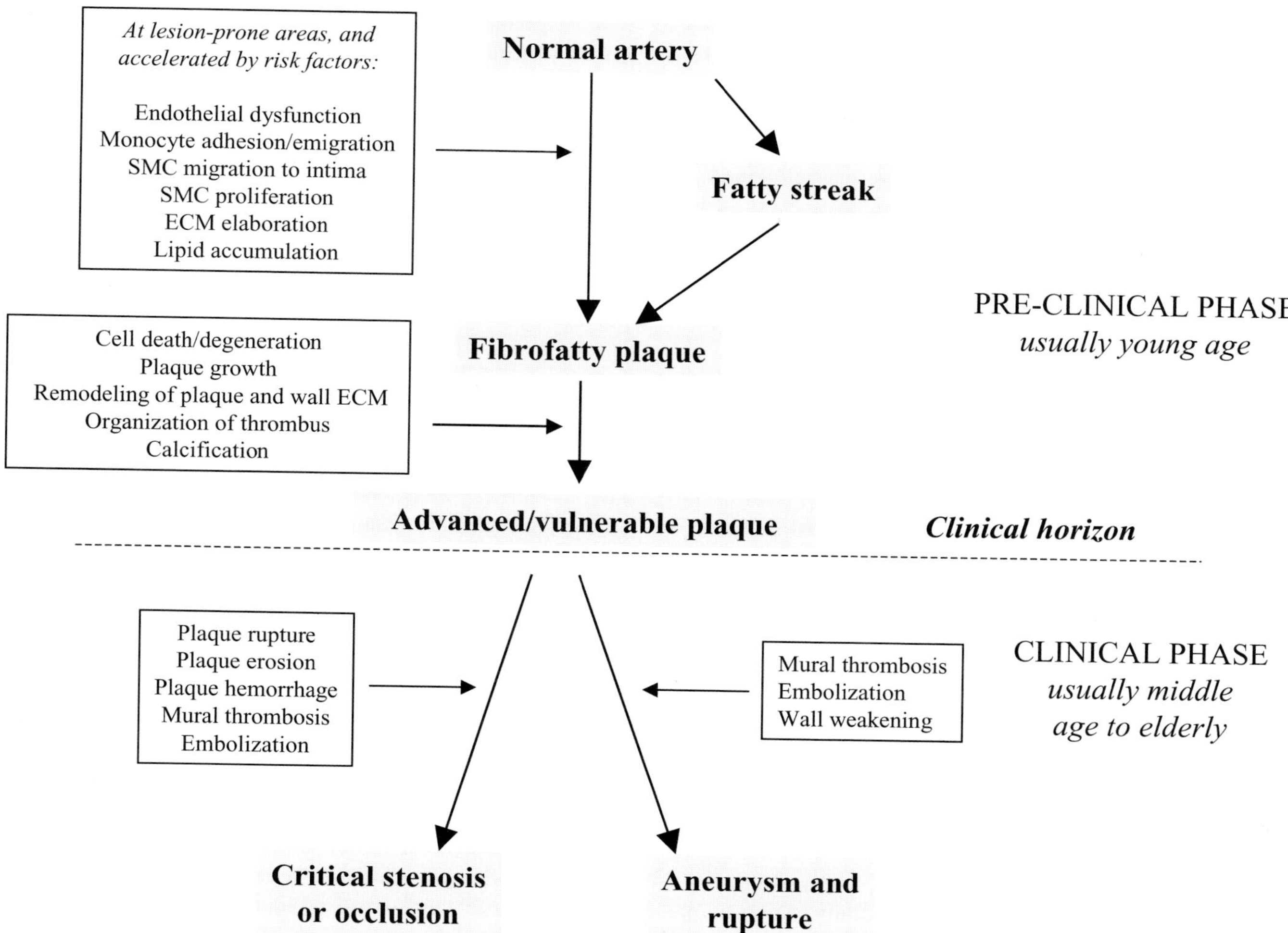

FIGURE 5–10 Summary of the pathology, pathogenesis, complications, and natural history of atherosclerosis. Plaques usually develop slowly and insidiously over many years, beginning in childhood or shortly thereafter and exerting their clinical effect in middle age or later. As described in the text, they may progress from a fatty streak to a fibrous plaque and then to plaque complications that lead to disease. The schematic diagram interrelates the morphology, pathogenesis, and complications of atherosclerosis and provides a unified approach to this serious disease process. SMC = smooth muscle cell; EMC = extracellular matrix. *(Reproduced with permission from Schoen FJ, Cotran RS: Blood vessels, in Kumar V (ed): Basic Pathology, 6th ed. Philadelphia, WB Saunders, 2002, p 325.)*

sufficient to accommodate the increased metabolic demands during vigorous exertion. When the luminal cross-sectional area is decreased by 75% or more, coronary blood flow generally becomes limited with exertion; with 90% or greater reduction, coronary flow may be inadequate even at rest. Over 90% of patients with ischemic heart disease have advanced stenosing coronary atherosclerosis (fixed obstructions), and most myocardial infarcts occur in patients with coronary atherosclerosis.[101] Most have one or more lesions causing at least 75% reduction of the cross-sectional area in one or more of the major epicardial arteries. Thus, the clinical effects of stable advanced atherosclerotic plaques in the coronary arteries are due to their encroachment on the lumen, leading to stenosis.

However, the onset and prognosis of ischemic heart disease and other complications of atherosclerosis are not well predicted by the angiographically determined extent and severity of fixed anatomic disease.[102–105] Dynamic vascular changes are largely responsible for the conversion of chronic stable angina or an asymptomatic state to acute ischemic heart disease. The most common such acute event leading to coronary occlusion is fracture of the fibrous cap leading to hemorrhage into the plaque, followed by platelet aggregation and thrombosis.

Nonatherosclerotic causes of coronary artery obstruction can also occur; the most common causes are infectious disease (e.g., tuberculosis), autoimmune diseases (e.g., SLE and rheumatoid arthritis), vasculitis (e.g., Buergers disease and

Kawasaki disease), fibromuscular dysplasia, and dissection, spasm, embolism. Obstruction of the small intramural coronary arteries is seen in several disease states, including diabetes, deposition diseases such as Fabry disease and amyloidosis, progressive systemic sclerosis (scleroderma), and as a proliferative intimal lesion in the coronary arteries of cardiac allografts.

ROLE OF ACUTE PLAQUE CHANGE

The acute coronary syndromes (unstable angina, acute myocardial infarction, and sudden ischemic death) usually are precipitated by atherosclerotic plaque disruption with hemorrhage, fissuring, and/or ulceration. Fissures and ruptures most frequently occur at the lateral portions of the fibrous cap, with stresses highest at its junction with the adjacent plaque-free segment of the arterial wall.[106] Vasospasm, tachycardia, hypercholesterolemia, and intraplaque hemorrhage are likely contributors, as are stresses induced by blood flow and/or coronary intramural pressure or tone in plaque.

Plaque alterations precipitating the acute coronary syndrome span a broad morphologic range from minimal surface erosions to lacerations that extend deep within the plaque. In some cases, coronary artery thrombosis results from a superficial erosion of the intima without a frank rupture through the plaque fibrous cap. Endothelial cells may undergo apoptosis in response to inflammatory mediators, and this loss of endothelial cells can uncover the thrombogenic subendothelial matrix.[107] Even in the absence of actual sloughing of endothelial cells, an altered balance between prothrombotic and fibrinolytic properties of the endothelium may provoke thrombosis in situ. Regardless of the extent of injury, the result is flow disruption and exposure of the luminal blood to a thrombogenic surface (collagen, lipid, or necrotic debris), thereby setting the stage for mural or total thrombosis (see Fig. 5-4B).

Pathologic and clinical studies show that plaques that undergo abrupt disruption leading to coronary occlusion often are those that previously produced only mild to moderate luminal stenosis.[102–105] Overall, approximately two thirds of plaques that rupture with subsequent occlusive thrombosis cause occlusion of only 50% or less before plaque rupture, and in 85% of patients, stenosis is initially less than 70%. It is presently impossible to reliably predict plaque disruption or subsequent thrombosis in an individual patient.

Coronary artery imaging is an area of current interest and importance.[108,109] Although x-ray coronary angiography remains the gold standard, a noninvasive test that would reduce the procedural risk of this invasive modality is highly desirable. Calcification of the coronary arteries can be detected noninvasively by electron beam computed tomography. Radiographically visible calcium in the epicardial coronary arteries predicts the extent of atherosclerotic disease, but cannot identify features of plaque instability. However, since plaque burden correlates with cardiovascular risk, coronary calcium tends to be a good prognostic indicator of future myocardial ischemic events.[110] In contrast, three-dimensional coronary magnetic resonance angiography may permit reliable detection of coronary artery disease, whether or not calcification is present, as this technique has the potential to visualize both the coronary lumen and the atherosclerotic plaques in the arterial wall.[111] Intravascular ultrasound (IVUS) is an invasive technique that can provide precise information about the degree of stenosis, and the location and nature of atherosclerotic plaque.

The events that trigger abrupt changes in plaque configuration and superimposed thrombosis are complex and poorly understood. Influences both intrinsic (e.g., plaque structure and composition) and extrinsic to the plaque (e.g., blood pressure, platelet reactivity) are likely important. Surface erosions, fissures, and ruptures are more likely to occur in soft and eccentric plaques than in hard and concentric lesions. Similarly, plaques contain large areas of foam cells and extracellular lipid, and those in which the fibrous caps are thin or contain clusters of inflammatory cells are more susceptible to rupture.[112–114] Plaques that are prone to rupture are termed vulnerable plaques. There is evidence that lipid lowering by diet or drugs such as statins can reduce the onset of coronary thrombotic complications by stabilizing plaque through reducing accumulation of macrophages expressing matrix-degrading enzymes and tissue factor, and reducing activation of smooth muscle cells and endothelial cells.[115] The pronounced circadian periodicity for the time of onset of acute myocardial infarction and other acute coronary syndromes, with a peak incidence between 9:00 A.M. and 11:00 A.M., suggests that the physiologic morning surge in blood pressure and heightened platelet reactivity may contribute to plaque disruption.

The fibrous cap is a highly dynamic tissue that can undergo continuous remodeling. The inflammatory process largely controls the balance of collagen synthetic and degradative activity, which determines stability and prognosis. Lesions prone to rupture have a thin collagen layer and few smooth muscle cells. These cells are responsible for the repair and maintenance of the all-important collagenous matrix and are a rich source of extracellular matrix macromolecules in the artery wall.[114] Smooth muscle cells and macrophages can undergo apoptosis within the plaque induced by proinflammatory cytokines and *fas* ligand, factors overexpressed in atherosclerotic plaques. Cytokines induce production of matrix metalloproteinases by macrophages; these enzymes degrade the collagen that lends strength to the fibrous cap. Inflammation may also contribute to coronary thrombosis by altering the balance between prothrombotic and fibrinolytic properties of the endothelium. For example, endothelial cells exposed to proinflammatory cytokines express tissue factor procoagulant, and plaque rupture may expose necrotic and apoptotic cells and cell debris to the circulating blood. It is thus not surprising that several serum markers of inflammation such as C-reactive protein and pregnancy-associated plasma protein A (PAPP-A) have been linked to atherosclerosis and the acute coronary syndromes.[116–118] C-reactive protein has multiple direct atherothrombotic effects and increases risk of acute coronary events, while PAPP-A, a metalloproteinase and prothrombotic inflammatory marker, is expressed in ruptured and eroded but not stable plaque.

Potential outcomes for unstable lesions include thrombotic occlusion, nonocclusive thrombosis, healing at the site of plaque erosion, athero- or thromboembolization, organization of mural thrombus (plaque progression), and organization of the occlusive mass with recanalization. Among these outcomes, the most common fate is plaque progression, owing either to resealing of the plaque fissure or to organization of a nonocclusive mural thrombus. Indeed, asymptomatic plaque rupture and its subsequent healing is likely an important mechanism of stenosis progression.

Pathology of Coronary and Myocardial Interventions

THROMBOLYSIS

Revascularization by thrombolysis in early acute myocardial infarction limits infarct size and improves cardiac function and survival.[119–122] The pathophysiologic basis of thrombolytic therapy is as follows: (1) Untreated thrombotic occlusion of a coronary artery causes transmural infarction; (2) the extent of necrosis during an evolving myocardial infarction progresses as a wavefront and becomes complete only 6 hours or more following coronary occlusion (see Fig. 5-5); (3) both early- and long-term mortality following acute myocardial infarction correlate strongly with the amount of residual functioning myocardium; and (4) early reperfusion rescues some jeopardized myocardium. The benefits of thrombolytic therapy depend on and are assessed by the amount of myocardium salvaged, recovery of left ventricular function, and resultant reduction in mortality. These important clinical end points are largely determined by the time interval between onset of symptoms and a successful intervention, adequacy of early coronary reflow, and the degree of residual stenosis of the infarct vessel. Recanalization rates vary from 60% to 90%, where the best efficacy relates to the earliest time of infusion of thrombolytic agents such as streptokinase, urokinase, or tissue-derived plasminogen activator. The maximal time for substantial myocardial salvage is approximately 4 hours for intracoronary and 3 hours for intravenous administration, but some studies suggest that some benefit can occur following later reperfusion, usually within 12 hours of symptoms. Spontaneous recanalization, presumably owing to inherent thrombolysis, can be beneficial to left ventricular function within 24 hours of infarct initiation. However, spontaneous thrombolysis with reperfusion probably occurs in fewer than 10% of patients within the critical 3 to 4 hours after symptom onset.

Successful thrombolytic therapy often reestablishes antegrade flow in the infarct-related coronary artery but does not reverse factors responsible for initiating the original thrombosis, such as advanced atherosclerotic plaque, intimal rupture, enhanced platelet adhesiveness, or coronary spasm. High-grade residual stenosis and the persistence of the nidus of the original thrombosis are likely to be associated with recurrent ischemic events as evidenced by postinfarction angina or recurrent infarction. Thus, balloon angioplasty and stent placement or surgical revascularization during infarct evolution constitutes a more effective management of the underlying disease process than thrombolysis alone.[123]

The most common complications of thrombolytic reperfusion are failure to achieve clot lysis, reperfusion arrhythmias, coronary rethrombosis, and myocardial and systemic hemorrhage. Failure of thrombolytic therapy occurs in 20% to 30% of patients and is related to the presence of critical and disrupted plaques with complex geometry, plaque rupture with luminal obstruction by thromboatheromatous debris, and old organizing thrombus. Acute reocclusion occurs in 15% to 35% of patients and appears to be related to incomplete thrombolysis and the unstable nature of the underlying atherosclerotic plaque. Other complications include coronary embolism and hemopericardium. The most frequent and potentially the most serious complication of thrombolytic therapy is bleeding, with hemorrhage at sites of vascular punctures the most common (>70%) and intracranial hemorrhage (approximately 1%) the most dreaded.

ANGIOPLASTY, ATHERECTOMY, AND STENTS

Percutaneous transluminal coronary angioplasty (PTCA) is used in patients with stable angina, unstable angina, or acute myocardial infarction.[124] Angioplasty has also been applied to obstructions in saphenous vein grafts, internal mammary artery grafts, and coronary arteries in transplanted hearts. PTCA is successful in 85% to 95% of cases (including vein grafts and internal mammary arteries) and is associated with a mortality rate of 1%.

In PTCA, the progressive and substantial expansile force induced by the inflated balloon causes the plaque to split at its weakest point, a site not necessarily most severely involved with atherosclerosis.[125] Structural/stress analysis based on intravascular ultrasound imaging can predict the location of plaque fracture that accompanies angioplasty. The split extends at least to the intimal-medial border and often into the media, with consequent circumferential and longitudinal dissection of the media (Fig. 5-11). Acute dissection may contribute to the propensity for acute closure that occurs in up to 5% of patients. For example, a dissection that involves a considerable portion of the circumference can generate a flap that may impinge on the lumen. Alternatively, a dissection that involves a substantial proximal-to-distal segment of the vessel, which traverses a large plaque-free

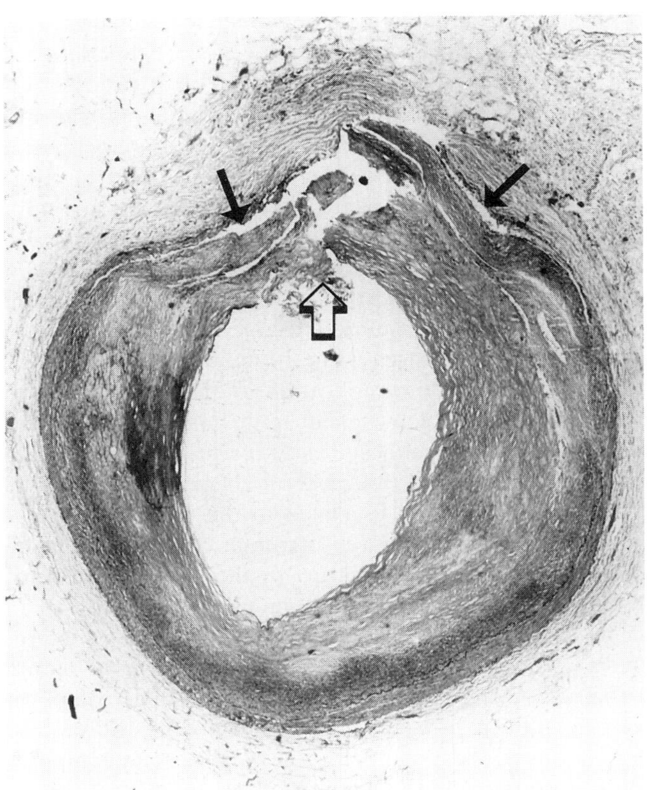

FIGURE 5–11 Acute changes of percutaneous transluminal coronary angioplasty (PTCA) on coronary arterial atherosclerotic plaque. The changes induced by balloon angioplasty consist of fracture of the plaque (open arrow) with deep extension of the wall defect and partial circumferential dissection (closed arrows). Verhoff van Giesen stain (for elastin) 20X. *(Reproduced with permission from Schoen FJ: Blood vessels, in Cotran RS, Kumar V, Collins T: Pathologic Basis of Disease, 6th ed. Philadelphia, WB Saunders, 1999; p 493.)*

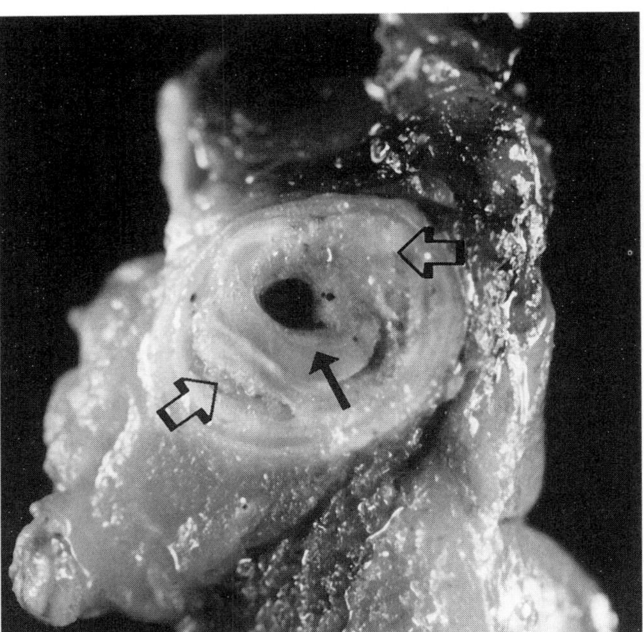

FIGURE 5–12 Proliferative restenosis after percutaneous transluminal coronary angioplasty. This gross cross-section of a coronary artery from a patient who died several months after angioplasty illustrates both the original, previously disrupted atherosclerotic plaque (open arrows) and markedly occlusive concentric fibrous tissue that formed after the procedure (arrow). *(Reproduced with permission from Schoen FJ: Blood vessels, in Cotran RS, Kumar V, Collins T: Pathologic Basis of Disease, 6th ed. Philadelphia, WB Saunders, 1999; p 493.)*

wall segment, can induce compression of the vessel at a point of minimal disease.

Dissimilar plaques respond differently to balloon dilation, and the composition and configuration of the original atherosclerotic lesion play a key role in the outcome of angioplasty. Immediate success probably is enhanced in dilated arteries having eccentric plaques with large lipid-rich necrotic cores and/or calcification, in contrast to concentric fibrotic lesions. For eccentric atheromas, balloon-induced splits most commonly involve the junction between the plaque and the disease-free portion of the arterial wall.

Thus, the key vascular consequences of angioplasty are plaque fracture, medial dissection, and stretching of the media beyond the dissection. These are accompanied by local flow abnormalities and generation of new, thrombogenic blood-contacting surfaces (similar to what is observed with spontaneously disrupted plaque) and can lead to platelet deposition and occlusive thrombosis. The immediate postangioplasty healing process is not well understood, but dissolution of soft atheromatous material, retraction of the split plaque, thrombus formation, and intimal healing with reendothelialization likely occur.

The long-term success of angioplasty is limited by the development of progressive, proliferative restenosis, which occurs in 30% to 40% of patients, most frequently within the first 4 to 6 months (Fig. 5-12). Although vessel wall recoil and organization of thrombus likely contribute, the major process leading to restenosis is excessive medial smooth muscle proliferation as an exaggerated response to angioplasty-induced injury, similar in some respects to the processes of atherosclerosis and vascular graft healing. Medial smooth muscle cells migrate to the intima where, along with existing plaque smooth muscle cells, they proliferate and secrete abundant extracellular matrix. Early lesions have a loose myxoid matrix in which numerous stellate smooth muscle cells are haphazardly arranged. Over weeks to months, the extracellular matrix becomes more densely collagenous, and the neointima becomes less cellular, with scattered spindle-shaped cells in a more laminar arrangement. Moreover, following prominent thrombus formation or in a hyperlipidemic patient, the site of healing may contain foam cells and cholesterol crystals, resembling a mature fibrofatty atheroma. Interest in locally delivered pharmacologic

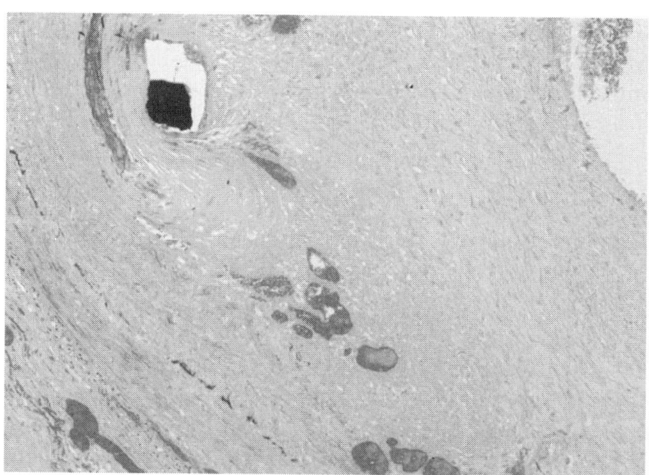

FIGURE 5–13 Metallic coronary artery stent implanted long-term, demonstrating thickened proliferative neointima separating the stent wires (black structure) from the lumen. Movat stain. ***(Reproduced with permission from Schoen FJ, Edwards WD: Pathology of cardiovascular interventions including endovascular therapies, revascularization, vascular replacement, cardiac assist/replacement, arrythmia control, and repaired congenital heart disease, in Silver MD, Gotlieb AI, Schoen FJ (eds): Cardiovascular Pathology, 3d ed. Philadelphia, Churchill Livingstone, 2001; p 678.)***

and molecular therapies to mitigate restenosis has been longstanding; regrettably, success has been limited.[126–130]

Coronary atherectomy of primary or restenosis lesions can be achieved percutaneously with a catheter that mechanically removes obstructive tissue by excision. Deep arterial resection, including medial and even adventitial elements, occurs frequently but has not been associated with acute symptomatic complications. The morphology of arterial vessel healing after directional or rotational atherectomy is similar to that following angioplasty.[131,132]

Metallic balloon-expandable and self-expanding coronary stents have had an immense impact on the outcome of catheter-based therapies. As expandable tubes of metallic mesh that are inserted percutaneously at the time of PTCA to preserve luminal patency in both native coronary arteries and vein grafts, such devices provide a larger and more regular lumen by acting as a scaffold to support the intimal dissections that occur in PTCA. They mechanically prevent vascular spasm and increase blood flow, all of which minimize thrombus formation and reduce the impact of postangioplasty restenosis.[133–135] Stenting has recently been shown to be superior to angioplasty alone in patients with acute myocardial infarction.[136] The complications and limitations of stenting include initial failure, early thrombosis, and late restenosis. Subacute stent thrombosis occurs in 1% to 3% of patients, usually within 7 to 10 days of the procedure; antiplatelet treatment minimizes this risk.

Stent implantation is accompanied by damage to the endothelial lining and stretching of the vessel wall, stimulating early adherence and accumulation of platelets and leukocytes. Covered initially by a variable platelet-fibrin coating, stent wires may eventually become completely covered by an endothelium-lined neointima, with the wires embedded in a layer of intimal thickening consisting of α-actin positive smooth muscle cells in a collagenous matrix.[137–139] Nevertheless, the neointima may thicken, and proliferative restenosis can occur even in the presence of a stent (Fig. 5-13).[140] In-stent restenosis correlates with disruption of the internal elastic lumina, protrusion of struts into lipid-laden portions of the plaque, and intimal neovascularization. Although the clinical paradigm has suggested that a larger lumen after angioplasty diminishes angiographic and clinical restenosis, intimal growth is greater when struts penetrate more deeply into the lipid core of the plaque.[141] Attempts to reduce in-stent restenosis include intracoronary radiotherapy, the delivery of recombinant vascular endothelial growth factor with a balloon catheter to speed endothelialization of a stent, gene therapy, and local drug delivery.[142–146] Antiproliferative agents such as sirolimus and paclitaxel released in a controlled fashion from coated stents have shown impressive promise in reducing the neointimal proliferation that causes stent restenosis.[146,147]

CORONARY ARTERY BYPASS GRAFT SURGERY

Coronary artery bypass graft (CABG) surgery improves survival in patients with significant left main coronary artery disease, with three-vessel disease, or with reduced ventricular function.[148–151] CABG surgery prolongs and improves the quality of life in patients with left main equivalent disease (proximal left anterior descending and proximal left circumflex), but does not protect them from the risk of subsequent myocardial infarction. The main mechanism for these benefits is the reperfusion of hibernating (viable, but poorly functioning owing to low flow) myocardium leading to increased left ventricular function. Over 90% of appropriately selected patients report a reduction in angina pectoris after CABG surgery.

The hospital mortality rate for CABG surgery is approximately 1% in low-risk patients, with less than 3% of patients suffering perioperative myocardial infarction. The most consistent predictors of mortality after CABG are urgency of operation, age, prior cardiac surgery, female sex, low left ventricular ejection fraction, degree of left main stenosis, and number of vessels with significant stenoses. The benefit of CABG is greatest in the highest, risk patients with the most severe disease; it is not surprising, therefore, that a recent increase in morbidity and mortality has accompanied an increase in CABG performed in an older and sicker population. In low- and moderate-risk patients, however, medical therapy and PTCA have results similar to CABG.

The most common mode of death after CABG is acute cardiac failure. The underlying cause of this acute failure leading to low output or arrhythmias is unclear in many cases. Many such patients have no detectable myocardial necrosis either clinically or at autopsy, and in others, the extent of necrosis noted at autopsy seems insufficient to account for the profound ventricular dysfunction encountered clinically. Possible explanations include: (1) evolving myocardial necrosis either undetectable clinically or too recent to detect at autopsy; (2) postischemic dysfunction of viable myocardium, for which no morphologic markers of the dysfunctional state are known; or (3) a metabolic cause, such as hypokalemia, for which there is no morphologic counterpart. Therefore, although established myocardial necrosis causes cardiac dysfunction in some patients with postoperative failure, it may not be the predominant lesion or the cause of death. When such necrosis is detected at autopsy, it may indicate that a potentially larger volume of adjacent morphologically normal myocardium was dysfunctional.

Perioperative infarction usually is caused by either hypotensive episodes during anesthesia induction or inadequate intraoperative regional preservation due to severe obstruction of the feeding artery and poor collaterals. Such necrosis usually predominates in the subendocardium and often has the morphology of necrosis with contraction bands. As in cardiac surgery in general, perioperative myocardial infarction is more likely to occur in patients with cardiomegaly than in those with normal-sized hearts.

Early thrombotic occlusion of the graft vessel may occur, with inadequate distal run-off from extremely small distal native coronaries (often further compromised by atherosclerosis) comprising the major mechanism. Additional factors include acute graft dissection at the anastomotic site, atherosclerosis or arterial branching at the anastomotic site, distortion of a graft that is too short or too long for the intended bypass, as well as patient factors including continued hyperlipidemia or smoking. In some cases, thrombosis occurring early postoperatively involves only the distal portion of the graft, suggesting that early graft thrombosis is frequently initiated at the distal anastomosis. Antiplatelet therapy has resulted in improved patency rates, and graft thromboses account for only a minority of early cardiac deaths; most patients who die early have patent grafts.

The patency of saphenous vein grafts is reported as 60% at 10 years, due to several pathologic mechanisms such as early thrombosis, progressive intimal thickening, and obstructive atherosclerosis.[152,153] Between 1 month and 1 year, graft stenosis is usually caused by intimal hyperplasia with excessive smooth muscle proliferation and extracellular matrix production similar to that seen following angioplasty. Atherosclerosis becomes more the dominant mechanism in graft occlusion 1 to 3 years after CABG. As in the coronary arteries, atherosclerosis in bypass grafts can cause myocardial ischemia through progressive luminal stenosis or plaque rupture with secondary thrombotic obstruction. The potential for disruption and embolization of atherosclerotic lesions in vein grafts exceeds that for native coronary atherosclerotic lesions. Plaques in grafts generally involve dilated segments, often have poorly developed fibrous caps with large necrotic cores, and develop secondary dystrophic calcific deposits that may extend to the lumen (Fig. 5-14). Thus, atheroembolization is a major risk, often with catastrophic results; balloon angioplasty or intraoperative manipulation of grafts may stimulate atheroembolism.[154]

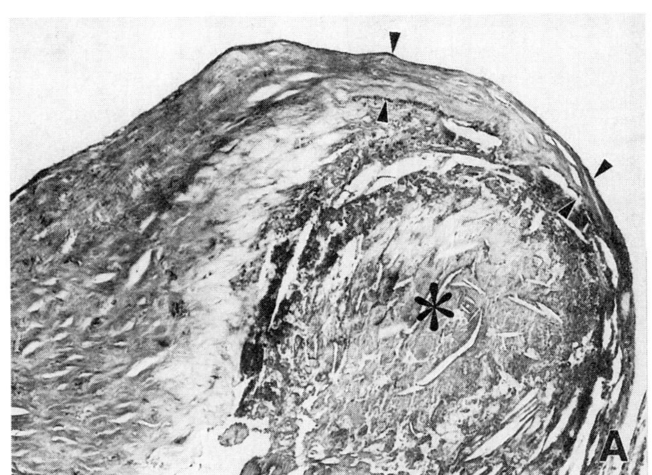

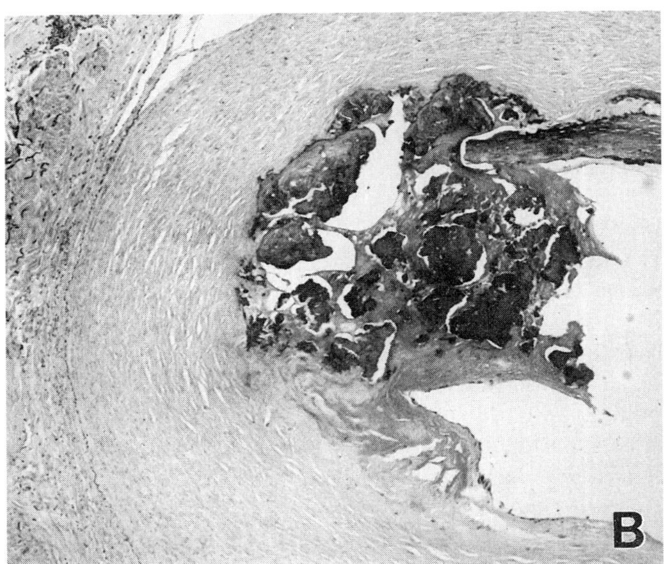

FIGURE 5–14 Atherosclerosis of saphenous vein bypass grafts. (A) Typical fibrous cap (between arrowheads) is attenuated over the necrotic core (asterisk). (B) Prominent calcification at the luminal surface. Hematoxylin and eosin (A) 100X; (B) 60X. *(Reproduced with permission from Schoen FJ: Interventional and Surgical Cardiovascular Pathology: Clinical Correlations and Basic Principles. Philadelphia, WB Saunders, 1989.)*

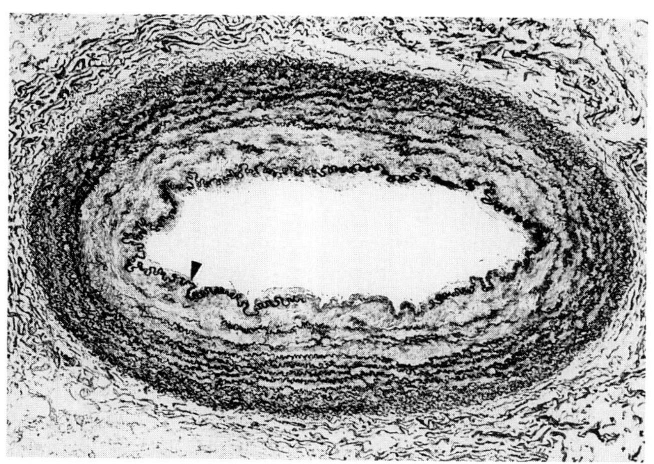

FIGURE 5–15 Internal mammary artery removed 13 years following function as aortocoronary bypass, demonstrating near-normal morphology and with minimal intimal thickening. The internal elastic lamina is indicated by arrowhead. Verhoff von Giesen stain (for elastin) 60X. ***(Reproduced with permission from Schoen FJ: Interventional and Surgical Cardiovascular Pathology: Clinical Correlations and Basic Principles. Philadelphia, WB Saunders, 1989.)***

In contrast to saphenous vein grafts, the internal mammary artery has a greater than 90% patency rate at 10 years (Fig. 5-15).[155] Multiple factors likely contribute to the remarkably higher long-term patency of IMA grafts compared to vein grafts. Free saphenous vein grafts sustain not only disruption of their vasa vasora and nerves but also endothelial damage, medial ischemia, and acutely increased internal pressure. In contrast, the internal mammary artery generally requires minimal surgical manipulation, maintains its nutrient blood supply, is accustomed to arterial pressures, needs no proximal anastomosis, and has an artery-to-artery distal anastomosis, as well as having minimal preexisting atherosclerosis. The sizes of graft and recipient vessel are comparable with the internal mammary artery but disparate (graft substantially larger) with saphenous vein. Radial and gastroepiploic arteries are also used successfully.[156]

TRANSMYOCARDIAL LASER REVASCULARIZATION

Transmyocardial laser revascularization (TMR) is used in selected patients with coronary artery disease that is refractory to conventional revascularization techniques and to maximal medical therapy.[157,158] Performed on a beating heart through a left thoracotomy, the operation employs a high-energy laser to bore transmural channels into the left ventricle. The hypothesis is that blood will flow directly from the left ventricular chamber into the channels and then into the intramyocardial vascular plexus, thereby restoring perfusion to potentially viable myocardium in a manner reminiscent of normal reptilian hearts. Although some clinical trials report a decrease in anginal symptoms after TMR, the morphologic basis for success is yet uncertain.[159–161]

Intramyocardial channels generated by TMR initially have a central region of destroyed myocardium surrounded by a thin rim of necrotic tissue (Fig. 5-16). Over the first 24 hours, the channels fill with blood and fibrin and are surrounded by myocardium with contraction band necrosis (see Fig. 5-16A). After 2 to 3 weeks, the channels are filled with

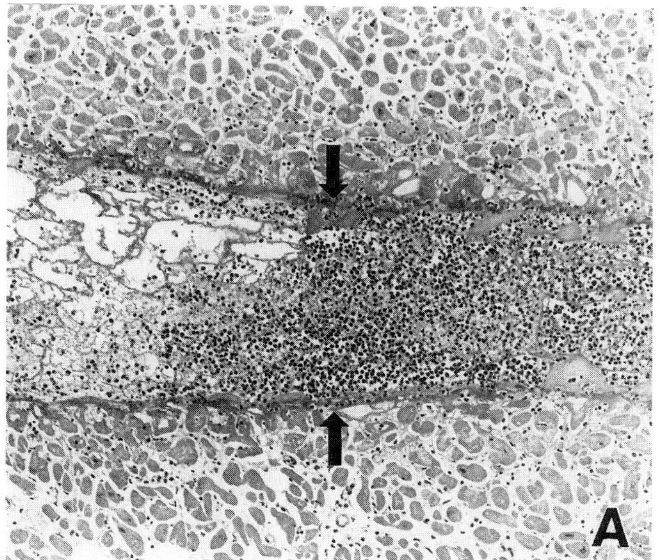

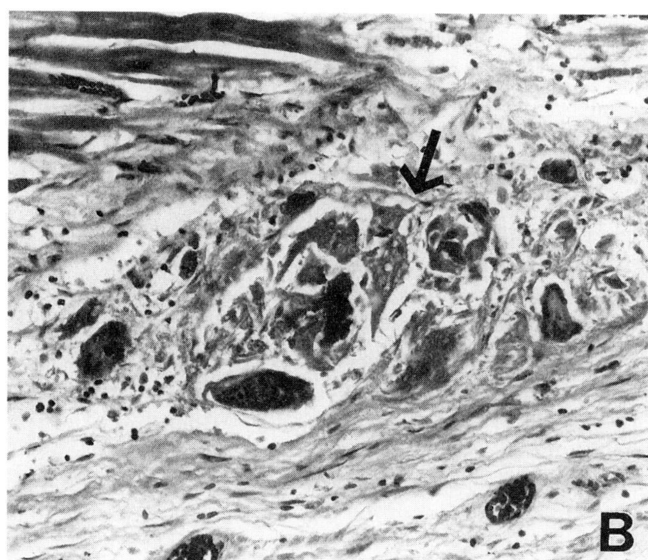

FIGURE 5–16 Myocardial changes following transmyocardial laser revascularization. (A) Transmyocardial channel (between arrows) filled with fibrin and inflammatory cells from patient who died 3 days following the procedure. (B) Transmyocardial channel filled with organizing fibrin (arrow) in patient who died 18 days following the procedure. No patent channels were noted in either case. Hematoxylin and eosin 150X.

vascularized granulation tissue in keeping with the general time course of wound healing (see Fig. 5-16B). Clinical studies and examinations of hearts from patients who have died at various postmortem intervals fail to reveal patent channels.[162,163] The leading hypothesis for the reported efficacy of TMR is the stimulation of neovascularization in the vicinity of the channels[164,165]; denervation of these areas may also play a role in the reduction of symptomatic angina. Ongoing studies are directed at elucidating the mechanisms of action of TMR and clinical indications for its use.

Myocardial Infarction and Its Complications

Coronary atherosclerosis with acute plaque rupture and superimposed thrombosis typically results in a transmural infarct, where ischemic necrosis involves at least half and usually the full or nearly full thickness of the ventricular wall in the distribution of the involved coronary artery. In contrast, a subendocardial (nontransmural) infarct constitutes an area of ischemic necrosis limited to the inner third or at most half of the ventricular wall. This process can be multifocal, often extending laterally beyond the perfusion territory of a single coronary artery. Subendocardial infarcts are commonly associated with diffuse stenosing coronary atherosclerosis without acute plaque rupture or superimposed thrombosis in the setting of episodic hypotension, global ischemia, or hypoxemia. A subendocardial infarct can also result from a coronary thrombus that is nonocclusive or becomes lysed before the progressive myocardial necrosis becomes transmural. In both transmural and subendocardial infarcts, a 1- to 2-mm rim of subendocardium may survive due to diffusion of oxygen and nutrients from the blood in the ventricular cavity.

The electrocardiographic findings of a transmural infarct usually involve ST segment elevations and the development of abnormal Q waves, while subendocardial infarcts have ST segment and T-wave changes without abnormal Q waves. Q-wave infarcts are generally larger both by enzyme elevations and pathologic determination and carry a less favorable short-term prognosis than non–Q-wave infarcts.

The short-term mortality rate from acute myocardial infarction has declined from 30% in the 1960s to 10% to 13% today. The rate is even lower, about 7%, for patients who receive aggressive reperfusion and pharmacologic therapy. However, half of all deaths from myocardial infarction occur within the first hour after the onset of symptoms, often before the individuals reach the hospital. Poor prognostic factors include advanced age, female gender, diabetes mellitus, and a previous myocardial infarction. The most important factors in long-term prognosis are left ventricular function and the extent of obstructive lesions in vessels perfusing viable myocardium. The overall mortality rate following myocardial infarction is 30% in the first year, with survivors having an additional 3% to 4% mortality per year thereafter.

Important and frequent complications of myocardial infarction include ventricular dysfunction, cardiogenic shock, arrhythmias, myocardial rupture, infarct extension and expansion, papillary muscle dysfunction, right ventricular involvement, ventricular aneurysm, pericarditis, and systemic arterial embolism.[166] About one half of patients with myocardial infarction will experience one or more of these complications, with the specific complication and prognosis dependent on infarct size, location, and transmurality. Patients with anterior infarcts are at greatest risk for regional dilation and mural thrombi and have a substantially worse clinical course than those with inferior-posterior infarcts. In contrast, inferior-posterior infarcts are more likely to have serious conduction blocks and right ventricular involvement. Mechanical complications are more frequent and significant in patients with transmural lesions.

Many patients have cardiac rhythm abnormalities following myocardial infarction, even though histologic evidence of direct conduction system involvement is present only in a minority. These abnormalities require aggressive treatment when they impair hemodynamics as can occur with either brady- or tachyarrhythmias, compromise myocardial viability by increasing oxygen requirements, or predispose to malignant ventricular tachycardia or fibrillation. The proposed mechanisms for generation of arrhythmias include the presence of electrically unstable ischemic myocardium at the edge of an infarct causing a micro-reentry phenomenon, and the release of arrhythmogenic metabolites such as lactic acid and potassium from necrotic tissue.[167,168] Autopsy studies of sudden death victims and clinical studies of resuscitated survivors show that only a minority develop a full-blown acute myocardial infarction. Thus, ischemia caused by severe chronic coronary arterial stenosis can lead directly to lethal arrhythmias. Heart block following myocardial infarction usually is transient, but persistent heart block in the proximal atrioventricular conduction system may necessitate pacemaker implantation. Tachyarrhythmias usually originate in areas of severely ischemic or necrotic myocardium. Arrhythmias that develop long after infarction likely originate at the junction between scar tissue and viable myocardium.

Myocardial infarcts produce functional abnormalities approximately proportional to their size. Large infarcts have a higher probability of cardiogenic shock, arrhythmias, and late congestive heart failure. Nonfunctional scar tissue resulting from previous infarctions and areas of stunned or hibernating myocardium may also contribute to overall ventricular dysfunction. Cardiogenic shock occurs in 10% to 15% of patients following myocardial infarction and is generally indicative of a large infarct (often >40% of the left ventricle). The high mortality of myocardial dysfunction and cardiogenic shock has been alleviated somewhat in recent years by the use of intra-aortic balloon pumps and ventricular assist devices to bridge patients through phases of prolonged but reversible functional abnormalities after myocardial infarction.

Frequently catastrophic, cardiac rupture syndromes include three entities: (1) rupture of the ventricular free wall (most common), usually with hemopericardium and cardiac tamponade; (2) rupture of the ventricular septum (less common), leading to an acquired ventricular septal defect with a left-to-right shunt; and (3) papillary muscle rupture (least common), resulting in the acute onset of severe mitral regurgitation. Cardiac rupture is the cause of death in 8% to 10% of patients with fatal acute transmural myocardial infarcts. Ruptures tend to occur relatively early following infarction (mean interval of 4–5 days, range of 1–10 days) with as many as 25% presenting within 24 hours of myocardial infarction. Even though they can be associated with large or small infarcts, free-wall and septal ruptures almost always involve transmural infarcts.[169] Although the lateral wall is the least common site for left ventricular infarction, it is the most common site for postinfarction free-wall rupture. Acute free-wall ruptures usually are rapidly fatal; repair is rarely possible.[170,171]

A fortuitously located pericardial adhesion that arrests the rapidly moving blood front and aborts a rupture may result in the formation of a false aneurysm, defined as a contained rupture with a hematoma communicating with the ventricular cavity.[172] False aneurysms contain no myocardial elements in their walls, consisting only of epicardium and adherent parietal pericardium and thrombus; half eventually rupture.

Acute ventricular septal defects secondary to postinfarction septal rupture complicate 1% to 2% of infarcts. Infarct-related septal defects are of two types: (1) single or multiple sharply localized, jagged, linear passageways that connect the ventricular chambers (simple type), usually involving the anteroapical aspect of the septum; and (2) defects that tunnel serpiginously through the septum to a somewhat distant opening on the right side (complex type), usually involving the basal inferoseptal wall.[173] In simple lesions, neither gross hemorrhage nor peripheral laceration is present. In complex lesions, the tract may extend into regions remote from the site of the infarct. Without surgery, the prognosis following infarct-related septal rupture is poor; 50% of patients die within the first week (half of these within 24 hours), and only 15% to 20% percent survive beyond 2 months.

Mitral regurgitation secondary to either subendocardial or transmural myocardial infarction reflects loss of the structural or functional integrity of the mitral valve apparatus, usually at the level of the papillary muscle. Mitral regurgitation in this setting has an acute onset, and its severity varies depending on the location and extent of papillary muscle disruption. If only part of a papillary muscle group is involved, the degree of regurgitation will be less severe than if the entire muscle group ruptures. Since chordae tendineae arise from the heads of the papillary muscles and provide continuity with each of the valve leaflets, interference with the structure or function of either papillary muscle can result in dysfunction of both mitral valve leaflets.

Papillary muscles are perfused with blood vessels that have traversed the entire transmural extent of the myocardium, and thus are particularly vulnerable to ischemic injury. Since the collateral circulation of the posterior myocardium is not as extensive as it is in the anterolateral segments, the posterior medial papillary muscle is more susceptible to widespread necrosis and is more commonly (85%) the site of rupture.[174,175] Papillary muscle rupture can occur later than other rupture syndromes (as late as 1 month after MI), since local healing can be delayed because of the limited vasculature and resultant inaccessibility of inflammatory cells.

Other mechanisms can produce mitral regurgitation in the setting of chronic ischemic heart disease. These mechanisms include an ischemic papillary muscle that fails to tighten the chordae during systole, and a fibrotic, shortened papillary muscle that fixes the chordae deeply within the ventricle. Ventricular dilation secondary to left ventricular failure can cause stretching of the mitral annulus and malalignment of the papillary muscle axes, leading to functional mitral regurgitation.[176]

Isolated right ventricular infarction is rare. However, involvement of the right ventricle by extension of an inferoseptal infarct occurs in approximately 10% of transmural infarcts and can have important functional consequences, including right ventricular failure with or without tricuspid regurgitation and arrhythmias.[177,178]

Infarct extension is characterized by new or recurrent necrosis in the same distribution as a completed recent infarct, associated with an increase in the amount of necrotic myocardium.[179,180] Extension most often occurs between 2 to 10 days after the original infarction, forms along the lateral and subepicardial borders, and histologically appears younger than the necrotic myocardium of the original infarct.

In contrast, infarct expansion is a disproportionate thinning and dilation of the infarcted region occurring through a combination of (1) slippage between muscle bundles, reducing the number of myocytes across the infarct wall; (2) disruption of the normal myocardial cells; and (3) tissue loss within the necrotic zone.[181] This regional dilation contributes to a significant increase in ventricular volume, increasing the wall stress and workload of noninfarcted myocardium and predisposing to late aneurysm formation. In addition, extension predisposes to intracardiac mural thrombus formation via myocardial contractility abnormalities causing stasis and endocardial damage causing thrombogenicity. Patients with infarct expansion, which can be detected by echocardiography in 30% of transmural infarcts, have increased morbidity and mortality.

Following myocardial infarction, structural changes occur both in the necrotic zone and uninvolved areas of the heart.[182–185] The composite process, called ventricular remodeling, occurs by a combination of left ventricular dilation, wall thinning by infarct expansion, compensatory hypertrophy of noninfarcted myocardium, and potentially late aneurysm formation.[186,187] Ventricular remodeling begins at the time of acute infarction and probably continues for months to years, until either a stable hemodynamic state is achieved or progressively severe cardiac decompensation occurs. Compensatory hypertrophy of noninfarcted myocardium is initially hemodynamically beneficial, but late decreases in ventricular performance with depression of regional and global contractile function may reflect degenerative changes. This congestive heart failure secondary to coronary artery disease occurs when the overall function of nonscarred myocardium can no longer maintain an adequate cardiac output. Moreover, the vulnerability of regions of hyperfunctioning residual myocardium to additional ischemic episodes may be increased.[188]

A ventricular aneurysm most commonly results from a large transmural infarct that undergoes expansion and heals as scar tissue that paradoxically bulges during ventricular systole.[189] In contrast to false aneurysms, and even though their walls are frequently as thin as 1 mm, true ventricular aneurysms rarely rupture because of their tough fibrous or fibrocalcific nature.[190] Markedly hypertrophied myocardial remnants as well as mummified myocardium (necrotic but inadequately healed) often are present in aneurysm walls, indicating incomplete healing of an infarct. Although 50% of patients with chronic fibrous aneurysms have mural thrombus contained within the ventricle, systemic embolization occurs in only approximately 5% of cases. Some pharmacologic approaches to limiting infarct size, such as steroids and other anti-inflammatory agents, could exacerbate infarct expansion and aneurysm formation.

VALVULAR HEART DISEASE

Normal valve function requires integrity and coordinated interactions among all components in the system. For the atrioventricular valves (mitral and tricuspid), these elements include leaflets, commissures, annulus, chordae tendineae (tendinous cords), papillary muscles, and the atrial and ventricular myocardium. For the semilunar valves (aortic and pulmonary), the key structures are the cusps, commissures, and their respective supporting structures in the aortic and pulmonary roots.

Structure-Function Correlations in Normal Valves

The anatomy of the mitral and aortic valves is illustrated in Figure 5-17.

MITRAL VALVE

Of the two leaflets of the mitral valve (see Fig. 5-17A), the anterior (also called septal, or aortic) leaflet is roughly triangular and deep, with the base inserting on approximately one third of the annulus. The posterior (also called mural, or ventricular) leaflet, although more shallow, is attached to about two thirds of the annulus and typically has a scalloped appearance. The mitral leaflets have a combined area approximately twice that of the annulus; they meet during systole with apposition to approximately 50% of the depth of the posterior leaflet and 30% that of the anterior leaflet. Each leaflet receives chordae tendineae from both the anterior and posterior papillary muscles.

The mitral valve orifice is D-shaped, with the flat anteromedial portion comprising the attachment of the anterior mitral leaflet in the subaortic region. This part of the annulus is fibrous and noncontractile; the posterolateral portion of the annulus is muscular and contracts during systole to asymmetrically reduce the area of the orifice. The edges of the mitral leaflets are held in or below the plane of the orifice by the chordae tendineae, which are pulled from below by the contracting papillary muscles during systole. This serves to draw the leaflets to closure and maintain competence. The orifice of the tricuspid valve is larger and less distinct than that of the mitral; its three leaflets (anterior, posterior, and septal) are larger and thinner than those of the mitral valve.

AORTIC VALVE

The three aortic valve cusps (left, right, and noncoronary) attach to the aortic wall in a semilunar fashion, ascending to the commissures and descending to the base of each cusp (see Fig. 5-17B). Commissures are spaced approximately 120 degrees apart and occupy the three points of the annular crown, representing the site of separation between adjacent cusps. Behind the valve cusps are dilated pockets of aortic root, called the sinuses of Valsalva, from which the right and left coronary arteries arise from individual orifices behind the right and left cusps, respectively. At the midpoint of the free edge of each cusp is a fibrous nodule called the nodule of Arantius. A thin, crescent-shaped portion of the cusp on either side of the nodule, termed the lunula, defines the surface of apposition of the cusps when the valve is closed (approximately 40% of the cuspal area). Fenestrations (holes) near the free edges commonly occur as a developmental or degenerative abnormality. They generally are small (less than 2 mm in diameter) and have no functional significance, since the lunular tissue does not contribute to separating aortic from ventricular blood during diastole. In contrast, cuspal defects below the lunula are not only associated with functional incompetence, but also suggest previous or active infection. The pulmonary valve cusps and surrounding tissues have architectural similarity to but are more delicate than those

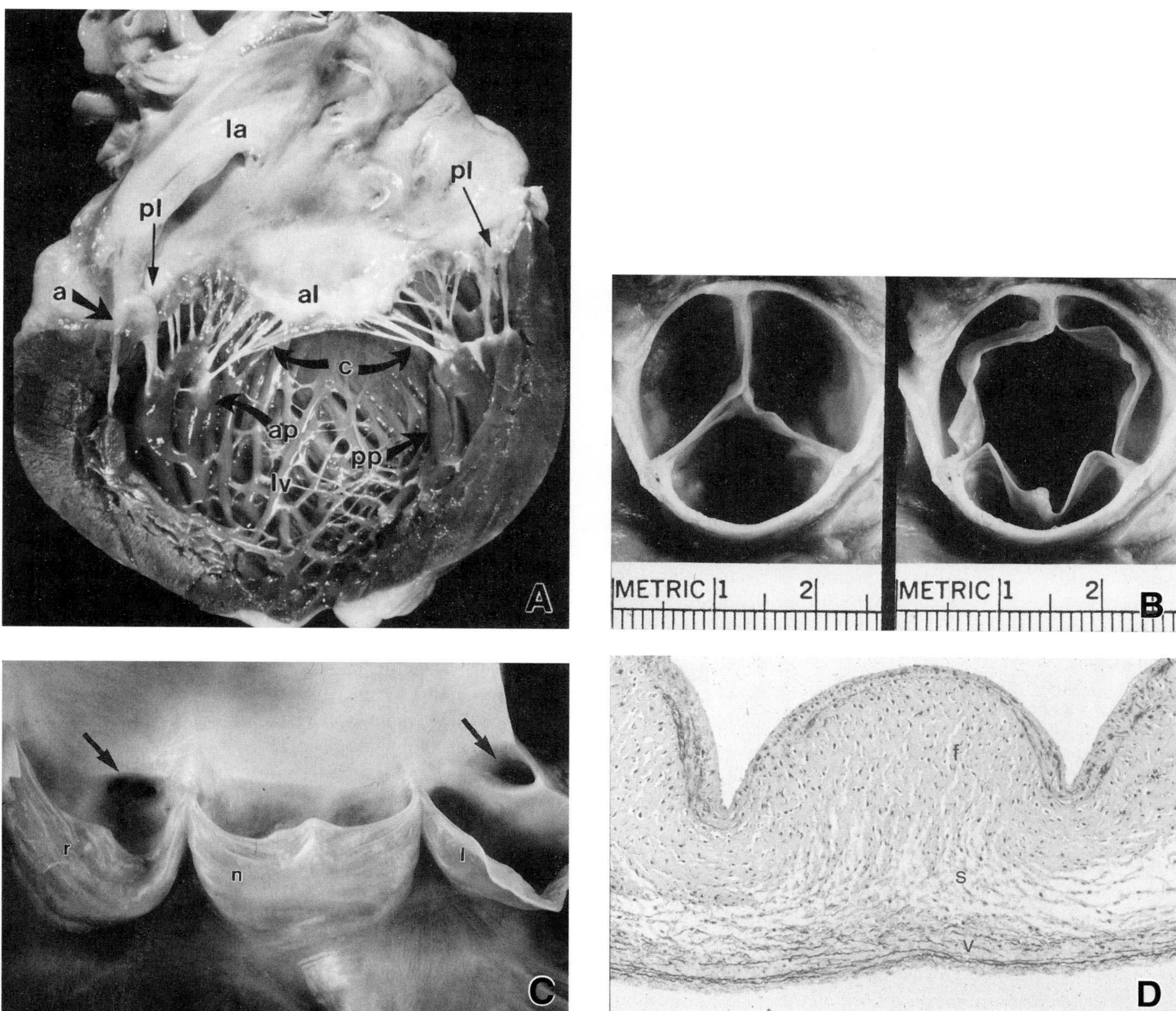

FIGURE 5–17 Normal mitral and aortic valves. In (A), an opened left ventricle of the normal heart, various components of the mitral apparatus are demonstrated. al = anterior leaflet; pl = posterior leaflet; a = annulus; c = chordae tendineae; ap = anterior papillary muscle; pp = posterior papillary muscle; la = left atrium; lv = left ventricle. (B) Aortic valve viewed from distal aspect in closed (left) and open (right) phases. The closed cusps are closely opposed during ventricular diastole and open against the aortic wall during systole. (C) Aortic valve, opened anteriorly to reveal the relationships of the anterior mitral leaflet (lower right) to the aortic valve cusps (lrn = left/right/noncoronary, respectively) and coronary arterial orifices (arrows). (D) Normal aortic valve histology, demonstrating layered structure, including the fibrosa (f) and spongiosa (s), the predominant layers. The inflow surface is at bottom. Verhoeff van Giesen elastic tissue stain 150X. *(A: Reproduced with permission from Schoen FJ: Interventional and Surgical Cardiovascular Pathology: Clinical Correlations and Basic Principles. Philadelphia, WB Saunders, 1989. B, C, and D: Reproduced with permission from Schoen FJ, Edwards WD: Valvular heart disease: general principles and stenosis, in Silver MD, Gotlieb AI, Schoen FJ (eds): Cardiovascular Pathology, 3d ed. New York, Churchill Livingstone, 2001; p 402.)*

of the corresponding aortic components, and lack coronary arterial origins.

VALVE HISTOLOGY

All cardiac valves essentially have the same microscopically inhomogeneous architecture, consisting of four well-defined tissue layers. Using the aortic valve as an example (see Fig. 5-17C), the thin ventricular layer (ventricularis) faces the left ventricular chamber, and is comprised predominantly of collagenous fibers with radially aligned elastic fibers covered by an endothelial lining. The rich elastin of the ventricularis enables the cusps to have minimal surface area when the valve is open but stretch during diastolic back pressure to form a large coaptation area. The spongiosa is centrally located and is composed of loosely arranged collagen and abundant proteoglycan. This layer has negligible structural strength, but accommodates the shape changes of the cusp during the cardiac cycle, lubricates relative movement between layers, and absorbs shock during closure. The fibrosa is a thick fibrous layer that provides structural integrity and mechanical stability and is composed predominantly of circumferentially aligned, densely packed collagen fibers, largely arranged parallel to the cuspal free edge. Finally, the aortalis is a thin layer that consists of a few collagen fibers lined by endothelial cells along the aortic surface of the cusps. Normal human aortic and pulmonary valve cusps have few blood vessels; they are sufficiently thin to be perfused from the surrounding blood. In contrast, the mitral and tricuspid leaflets contain a few capillaries in their most basal thirds.

During valve closure, cusps and leaflets do not touch along only their free edges like closing double doors. Rather, adjacent cusps coapt with a substantial area of surface-to-surface contact. This involves, for example, approximately a third of the atrioventricular valve leaflets. Thus, normal cusp and leaflet areas are substantially greater than are needed to simply close the valve orifice.

The orientation of architectural elements is nonrandom in the plane of the cusp, yielding unequal mechanical properties of the valve cusps in different directions (anisotropic behavior). Consequently, although the pressure differential across the closed aortic valve during the diastolic phase induces a large load on the cusps, the geometry of the whole valve and the fibrous network within the cusps effectively transfers the resultant stresses to the annulus and aortic wall. With specializations that include crimp of collagen fibers along their length, and bundles of collagen in the fibrous layer oriented toward commissures that produce grossly visible corrugations, cusps are extremely soft and pliable when unloaded, but taut and stiff during the closed phase. This minimizes sagging of the cusp centers, preserves maximum coaptation, and prevents regurgitation. For the mitral valve, the subvalvular apparatus including tendinous cords and papillary muscles is critical to maintain valve competency.

Etiology and Pathologic Anatomy of Valvular Heart Disease

Cardiac valve operations usually are undertaken for dysfunction caused by calcification, fibrosis, fusion, retraction, perforation, rupture, stretching, dilation, or congenital malformations of the valve leaflets/cusps or associated struts. Valvular stenosis, defined as inhibition of forward flow secondary to obstruction caused by failure of a valve to open completely, is almost always caused by a primary cuspal abnormality and a chronic disease process. In contrast, valvular insufficiency, defined as reverse flow caused by failure of a valve to close completely, may result from either intrinsic disease of the valve cusps or from damage to or distortion of the supporting structures (e.g., the aorta, mitral annulus, chordae tendineae, papillary muscles, and ventricular free wall) without primary cuspal pathology. Regurgitation may appear either acutely, as with rupture of cords, or chronically, as with leaflet scarring and retraction. Both stenosis and insufficiency can coexist in a single valve, usually with one process predominating. The most commonly encountered morphologies of valvular heart disease are illustrated in Figures 5-18 and 5-19.

Changing disease patterns and an aging U.S. population have altered the relative frequency of the major causes of valve disease in the late 20th century.[191,192] Degenerative (senile) calcific aortic valve disease is the most common cause of aortic stenosis; calcification of congenitally bicuspid aortic valves comprises the second most common cause. Postinflammatory (rheumatic) disease has continued to decline as a cause of aortic valve dysfunction. Indeed, the leading cause of chronic aortic insufficiency is aortic root dilation, causing stretching and outward bowing of the commissures and a lack of cuspal coaptation. Over the age of 40, aortic root dilation is most often due to age-related aortic degeneration or, less commonly, aortitis. Under 40 years, root dilation occurs most frequently in association with Marfan syndrome, other connective tissue disorders, or operated congenital heart disease. Moreover, whereas postrheumatic deformity remains the leading cause of mitral stenosis, its incidence continues to decline. Moreover, myxomatous mitral valve disease and ischemic mitral regurgitation are the leading causes of pure mitral valve regurgitation; indeed, these pathologies are often amenable to and comprise the major indications for mitral valve repair.

DEGENERATIVE CALCIFIC AORTIC VALVE STENOSIS

The most frequent valvular abnormality requiring surgery, acquired aortic stenosis (AS) usually is the consequence of age-related calcium phosphate deposition in either anatomically normal aortic valves or in congenitally bicuspid valves as a result of accelerated wear (see Fig. 5-18A).[193–195] Stenotic, previously normal tricuspid valves come to clinical

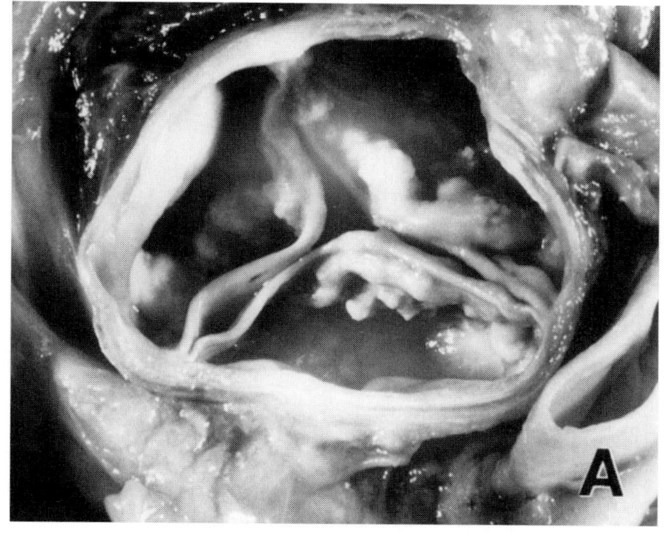

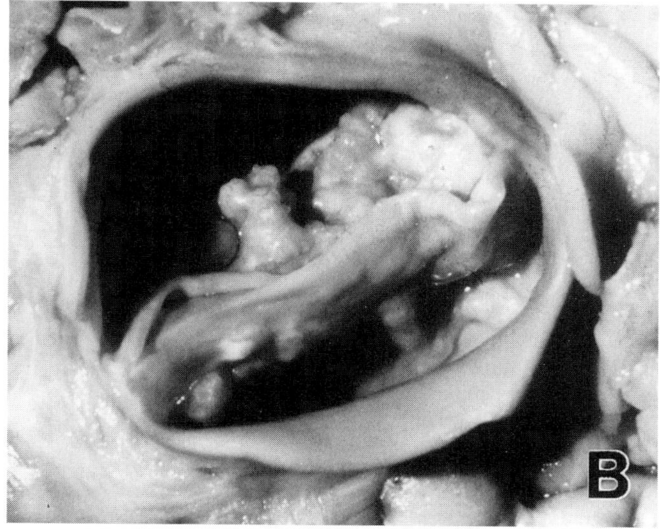

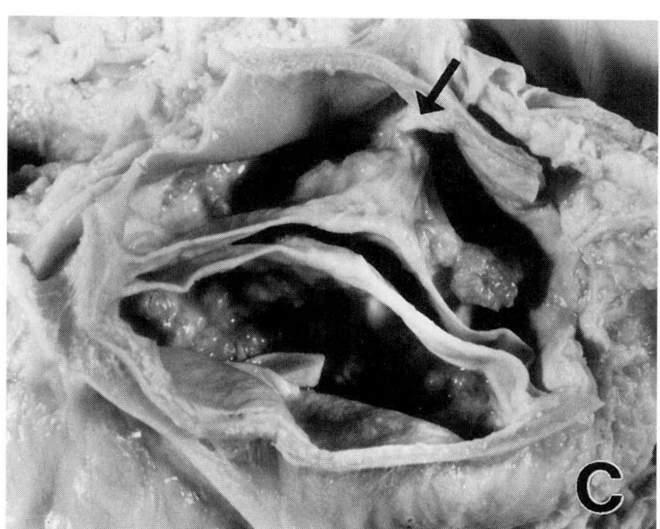

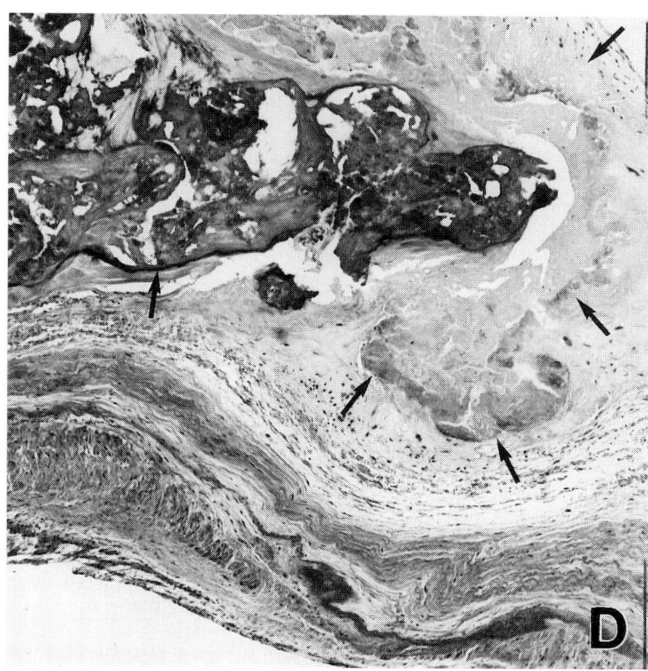

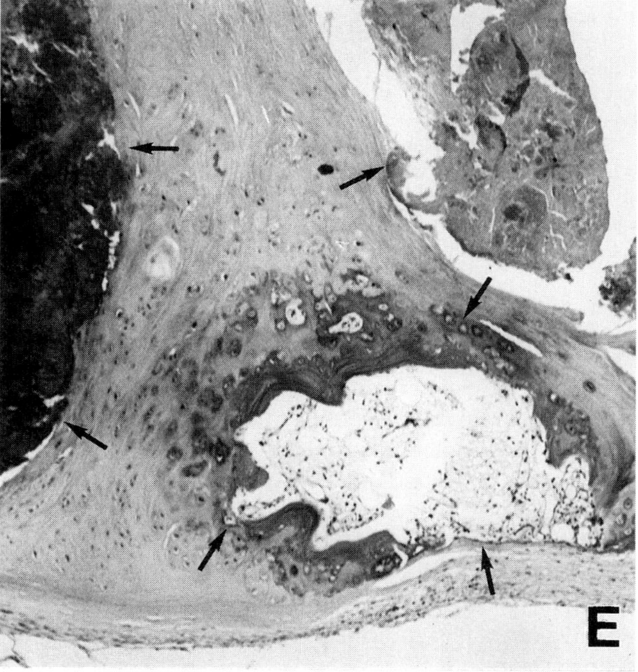

FIGURE 5–18 Calcific aortic stenosis. (A) Calcification of anatomically normal tricuspid aortic valve in an elderly patient, characterized by mineral deposits localized to basal aspect of cusps; cuspal free edges and commissures are not involved. (B) Congenitally bicuspid aortic valve, characterized by two equal cusps with basal mineralization. (C) Congenitally bicuspid aortic valve having two unequal cusps, the larger with a central raphe (arrow). (D) and (E) Photomicrographs of calcific deposits in calcific aortic stenosis; deposits are rimmed by arrows. Hematoxylin and eosin 15X. (D) Shows deposits with underlying cusp largely intact; transmural calcific deposits are shown in (E). (*A and B: Reproduced with permission from Schoen FJ, St. John Sutton M: Contemporary issues in the pathology of valvular heart disease. Hum Pathol 1987; 18:568. Copyright WB Saunders, 1987. C: Reproduced by permission from Schoen FJ: Interventional and Surgical Cardiovascular Pathology: Clinical Correlations and Basic Principles. Philadelphia, WB Saunders, 1989.*)

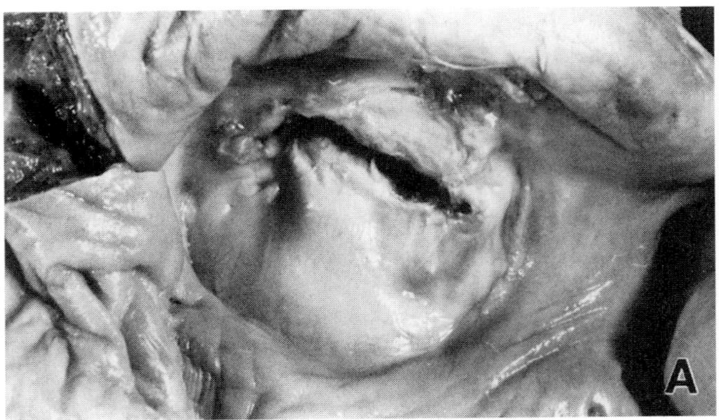

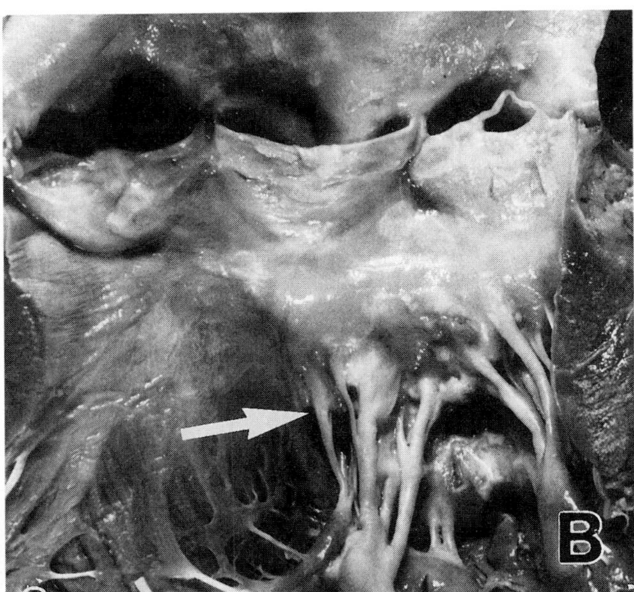

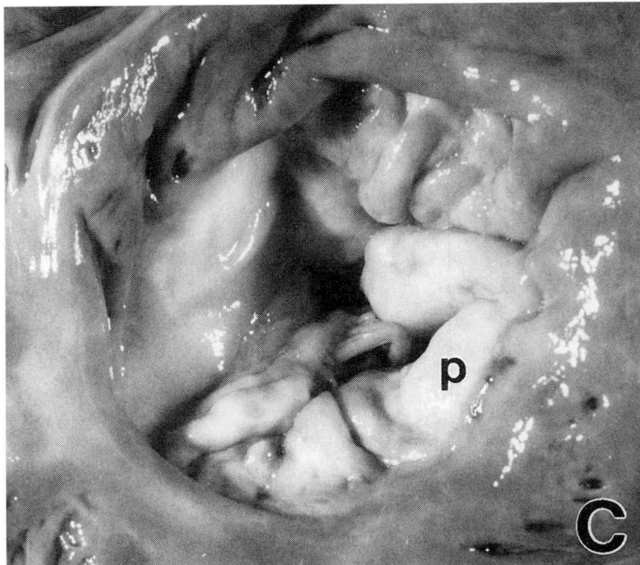

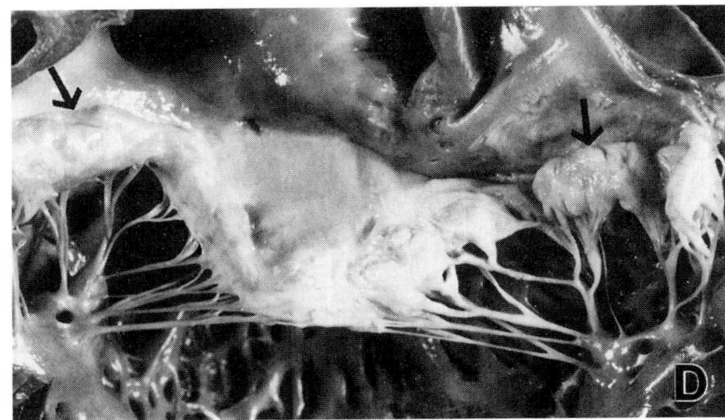

FIGURE 5–19 Major etiologies of mitral valvular disease. (A) Atrial view, and (B) subvalvular and aortic aspect of valve from patient with rheumatic mitral stenosis. There are severe valvular changes, including diffuse leaflet fibrosis and commissural fusion and ulceration of the free edges of the valve, as well as prominent subvalvular involvement with distortion (arrow in [B]). (C) and (D) Myxomatous degeneration of the mitral valve. In (C) (left atrial view), there is prolapse of a redundant posterior leaflet (p), whereas in (D) from another case, the opened annulus reveals a redundant posterior mitral leaflet (arrows), with thin elongated chordae tendineae. The patient with the valve shown in (D) had chronic mitral regurgitation with prolapse noted clinically, and Marfan syndrome. *(Reproduced with permission from Schoen FJ: Interventional and Surgical Cardiovascular Pathology: Clinical Correlations and Basic Principles. Philadelphia, WB Saunders, 1989.)*

attention primarily in the eighth to ninth decades of life, while bicuspid valves with superimposed age-related degenerative calcification generally become symptomatic earlier (usually sixth to seventh decades). Calcific degeneration affects men and women equally.

Nonrheumatic, calcific aortic stenosis is characterized by heaped-up, calcified masses initiated in the cuspal fibrosa at the points of maximal cusp flexion (the margins of attachment); they protrude distally from the aortic aspect into the sinuses of Valsalva, inhibiting cuspal opening. The dystrophic calcification process does not involve the free cuspal edges and largely preserves the microscopic layered architecture. In contrast to rheumatic aortic stenosis, appreciable commissural fusion is absent in calcific aortic stenosis and the mitral valve generally is uninvolved. Aortic valve sclerosis comprises a common, earlier, and hemodynamically less significant stage of the calcification process. Nevertheless, aortic sclerosis is associated with an increase of approximately 50% in the risk of death from cardiovascular causes and the risk of myocardial infarction, even in the absence of hemodynamically significant obstruction of left ventricular outflow.[196]

Aortic valves are congenitally bicuspid in approximately 1% to 2% of the population, with men affected 3 to 4 times more frequently than are women. The two cusps are typically of unequal size, with the larger (conjoined) cusp having a midline raphe, representing an incomplete separation or congenital fusion of two cusps. Less frequently, the cusps are of equal size, and a raphal ridge may or may not be identifiable (see Figs. 5-18B and 5-18C). When a raphe is present, the most commonly fused cusps are the right and left, accounting for about 75% of cases. Neither stenotic nor symptomatic at birth or throughout early life, bicuspid valves are predisposed to accelerated calcification, with about 85% becoming stenotic. About 15% of the time, they become purely incompetent, complicated by infective endocarditis, or associated with acute aortic dissection. Usually, an uncomplicated bicuspid valve is encountered at autopsy.

Aortic stenosis leads to a gradually increasing pressure gradient across the valve, which may reach 75 to 100 mg Hg in severe cases, with a left ventricular pressure of 200 mg Hg or more. Cardiac output is maintained by the development of concentric left ventricular hypertrophy secondary to pressure overload. The onset of symptoms such as angina, syncope, or heart failure in aortic stenosis heralds the exhaustion of compensatory cardiac hyperfunction, and carries a poor prognosis if not treated by aortic valve replacement (>50% mortality within 3-5 years). If cardiac output is low, as may occur in heart failure or in the elderly, then neither the gradient nor the resultant murmur may appear significant and aortic stenosis can be missed clinically. Other complications of calcific aortic stenosis include embolization that may occur spontaneously or during interventional procedures, hemolysis, and extension into the ventricular septum causing conduction abnormalities.

MITRAL ANNULAR CALCIFICATION

Degenerative calcific deposits also can develop in the ring (annulus) of the mitral valve; elderly individuals, especially women, are most commonly affected, although annular calcification can accompany mitral valve myxomatous degeneration. Although generally asymptomatic, the calcific nodules may lead to regurgitation by interference with systolic contraction of the mitral valve ring or, very rarely, stenosis by impairing opening of the mitral leaflets. Occasionally, the calcium deposits may penetrate sufficiently deeply to impinge on the atrioventricular conduction system and produce arrhythmias (and rarely sudden death). Patients with mitral annular calcification have an increased risk of stroke, and the calcific nodules can be the nidus for thrombotic deposits or infective endocarditis.[197]

RHEUMATIC HEART DISEASE

Rheumatic fever is an acute, often recurrent, inflammatory disease that generally follows a pharyngeal infection with group A beta-hemolytic streptococci, principally in children.[198,199] In the past several decades, rheumatic fever and rheumatic heart disease have declined markedly but not disappeared in the United States and other developed countries. Evidence strongly suggests that rheumatic fever is the result of an immune response to streptococcal antigens, inciting either a cross-reaction to tissue antigens, or a streptococcal-induced autoimmune reaction to normal tissue antigens.[200] The cardiac surgical implications of rheumatic fever primarily relate to chronic rheumatic heart disease, characterized by chronic, progressive, deforming valvular disease (particularly mitral stenosis) that produces permanent dysfunction and severe, sometimes fatal, cardiac failure decades later.

Chronic rheumatic heart disease most frequently affects the mitral and to a lesser extent the aortic and/or the tricuspid valves. Chronic rheumatic valve disease is characterized by fibrous or fibrocalcific distortion of leaflets or cusps, valve commissures, and chordae tendineae, with or without annular or papillary muscle deformities (see Figs. 5-19A and 5-19B). Stenosis results from leaflet and chordal fibrous thickening and from commissural and chordal fusion, with or without secondary calcification. Regurgitation entails related mechanisms, including scarring-induced retraction of chordae and leaflets and, less commonly, fusion of a commissure in an opened position. Chordal rupture only very rarely involves a rheumatic valve. Combinations of lesions may yield valves that are both stenotic and regurgitant. Although considered the pathognomonic inflammatory myocardial lesions in acute rheumatic fever, Aschoff nodules are found infrequently in myocardium sampled at autopsy or at valve replacement surgery, most likely reflecting an extended interval from acute disease to critical functional impairment.[201]

MYXOMATOUS DEGENERATION OF THE MITRAL VALVE (MITRAL VALVE PROLAPSE)

Myxomatous mitral valve disease is the most frequent cause of chronic, pure, isolated mitral regurgitation.[202,203] One or both mitral leaflets are enlarged, redundant, or floppy and will prolapse, or balloon back into the left atrium during ventricular systole (see Fig. 5-19C). The three characteristic anatomic changes in mitral valve prolapse are: (1) interchordal ballooning (hooding) of the mitral leaflets or portions thereof (most frequently involving the posterior leaflet), sometimes accompanied by elongated, thinned, or ruptured cords; (2) rubbery diffuse leaflet thickening that hinders adequate coaptation and interdigitation of leaflet tissue during valve closure; and (3) substantial annular dilation, with diameters and circumferences that may exceed 3.5 and 11.0 cm, respectively (see Fig. 5-19D).[204,205] Pathological mitral annular enlargement is usually confined to the posterior leaflet, since the anterior leaflet is firmly anchored by the fibrous tissue at the aortic valve end and is far less distensible. The key microscopic change in myxomatous degeneration is attenuation or focal disruption of the fibrous layer (with loss of collagen) of the valve,[206] on which the structural integrity of the leaflet depends. This is accompanied by focal or diffuse thickening of the spongy layer by proteoglycan deposition. These changes weaken the leaflet. Deposited amorphous extracellular matrix gives the tissue an edematous, blue appearance on routine hematoxylin and eosin staining, an appearance called myxomatous by pathologists. Concomitant involvement of the tricuspid valve is present in 20% to 40% of cases, and the aortic and pulmonary valves also may be affected. Myxomatous tricuspid valve may be associated with primary pulmonary disease owing to altered right-sided hemodynamics.

Secondary changes may occur, including: (1) focal padlike fibrous thickening along both surfaces of the valve leaflets; (2) linear thickening of the subjacent mural endocardium of the left ventricle as a consequence of friction-induced injury by cordal hamstringing of the prolapsing leaflets; (3) thrombi on the atrial surfaces of the leaflets, particularly in the recesses behind the ballooned leaflet segments; (4) calcification along the base of the posterior mitral leaflet; and (5) chordal thickening and fusion with some features that resemble postrheumatic disease. The pathogenesis of myxomatous degeneration is uncertain, but this valvular abnormality is a common feature of Marfan syndrome and occasionally occurs with other hereditary disorders of connective tissues such as Ehlers-Danlos syndrome, suggesting an analogous but localized connective tissue defect. Excessive remodeling of connective tissue marks the disease, but it is yet unknown whether this is causal or secondary.[206]

In a subgroup of affected individuals that is largely unidentifiable beforehand, mitral valve prolapse is associated with infective endocarditis, stroke, or other manifestation of thromboembolism, progressive congestive heart failure, or sudden death. Distinction should be made between the clinical diagnosis of mitral valve prolapse in young people and the pathologic diagnosis of a myxomatous mitral valve in mature individuals. The former generally is associated with a competent and minimally distorted valve and occurs in women more frequently than in men. The latter, in contrast, affects men more often than women and usually is associated with a severely regurgitant valve that is structurally deformed. More important, only a small fraction of young people with clinically detected mitral valve prolapse will develop severely distorted and incompetent mitral valves as they grow older.

INFECTIVE ENDOCARDITIS

Infective endocarditis is characterized by colonization or invasion of the heart valves, mural endocardium, aorta, aneurysmal sacs, or other blood vessels by a microbiologic agent, leading to the formation of friable vegetations laden with organisms.[207] Virtually any type of microbiologic agent can cause infective endocarditis, but most cases are bacterial.

The so-called Duke criteria provide a standardized assessment of patients with suspected infective endocarditis that integrates factors predisposing patients to the development of infective endocarditis, blood-culture evidence of infection, echocardiographic findings, and clinical and laboratory information.[208] The previously important clinical findings of petechiae, subungual hemorrhages, Janeway lesions, Osler's nodes, and Roth's spots in the eyes (secondary to retinal microemboli) have now become uncommon owing to the shortened clinical course of the disease as a result of antibiotic therapy.

The clinical classification into acute and subacute forms is based on the range of severity of the disease and its tempo, on the virulence of the infecting microorganism, and on the presence of underlying cardiac disease. Acute endocarditis is a destructive infection, often involving a previously normal heart valve, with a highly virulent organism, and leads to death within days to weeks in over 50% of patients. In contrast, in a more indolent lesion often called subacute endocarditis, organisms of low virulence cause infection on previously deformed valves; the infection pursues a protracted course of weeks to months and may be undetected and untreated.

Vegetations in both acute and subacute endocarditis are composed of fibrin, inflammatory cells, and organisms. *Staphylococcus aureus* is the leading cause of acute endocarditis and produces necrotizing, ulcerative, invasive, and highly destructive valvular infections. The subacute form is usually caused by *Streptococcus viridans*. Cardiac abnormalities, such as rheumatic heart disease, congenital heart disease (particularly anomalies that have small shunts or tight stenoses creating high-velocity jet streams), myxomatous mitral valves, mildly calcified bicuspid aortic valves, and artificial valves and their sewing rings, predispose to endocarditis. In intravenous drug abusers, left-sided lesions predominate, but right-sided valves are commonly affected; the usual organism is *S. aureus*.[209] In about 5% to 20% of all cases of endocarditis, no organism can be isolated from the blood (culture-negative endocarditis), often because of prior antibiotic therapy.

The complications of endocarditis include valvular insufficiency (or rarely stenosis), abscess of the valve annulus (ring abscess), suppurative pericarditis, and embolization. With appropriate antibiotic therapy, vegetations may undergo healing, with progressive sterilization, organization, fibrosis, and occasionally calcification. Regurgitation generally occurs on the basis of cusp or leaflet perforation, chordal rupture, or fistula formation from a ring abscess into an adjacent cardiac chamber or great vessel. Ring abscesses tend to be associated with virulent organisms, are technically difficult to deal with surgically, and are associated with a relatively high mortality rate.

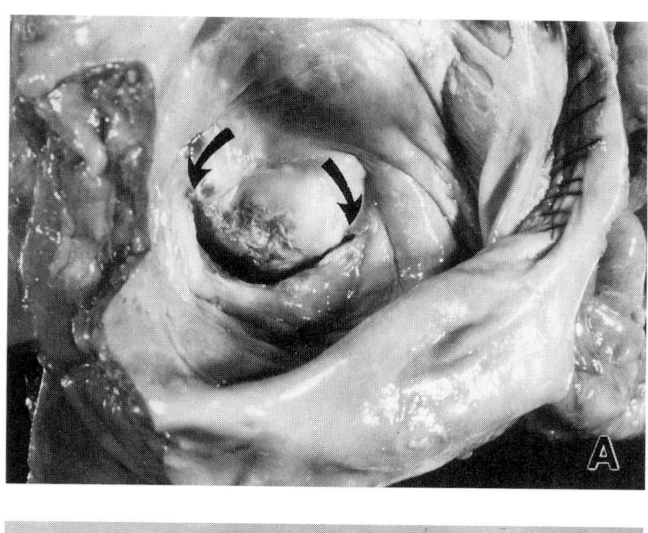

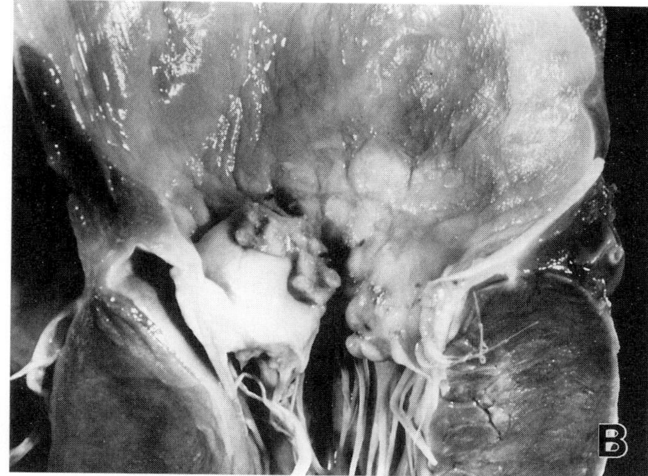

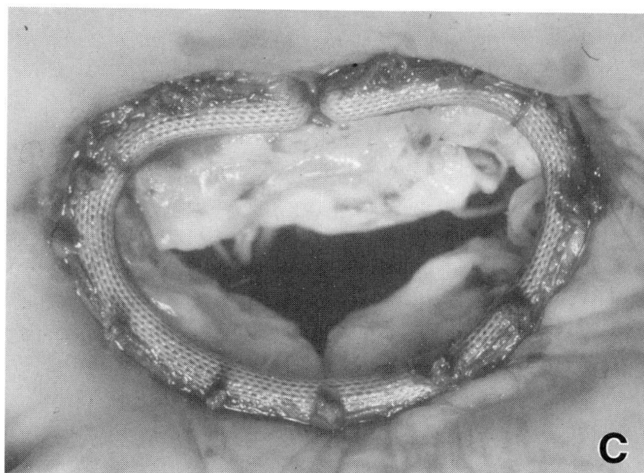

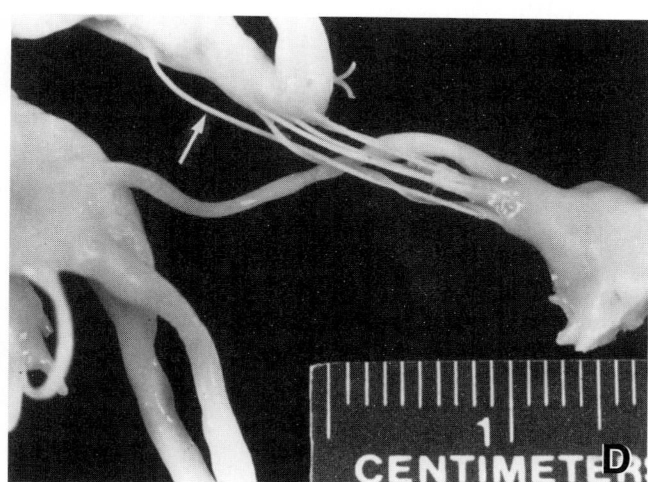

FIGURE 5–20 Valvular reconstructive procedures: mitral valve disease. (A) Open mitral commissurotomy for mitral stenosis. Incised commissures are indicated by arrows. (B) Mitral valve repair with partial leaflet excision. (C) Mitral valve repair with annuloplasty ring. (D) ePTFE suture replacement (arrow) of ruptured cord in myxomatous mitral valve. *(A: Reproduced with permission from Schoen FJ, St. John Sutton M: Contemporary issues in the pathology of valvular heart disease. Hum Pathol 1987; 18:568. Copyright WB Saunders, 1987. D: Reproduced with permission from Schoen FJ, Edwards WD: Valvular heart disease: general principles and stenosis, in Silver MD, Gotlieb AI, Schoen FJ (eds): Cardiovascular Pathology, 3d ed, Churchill Livingstone, 2001; p 402.)*

Valve Reconstruction

Reconstructive procedures to eliminate mitral insufficiency of various etiologies and to minimize the severity of rheumatic mitral stenosis are now highly effective and commonplace, accounting presently for over 70% of mitral valve operations.[210,211] Reconstructive therapy of selected patients with aortic insufficiency and aortic dilation may also be done,[212,213] but repair of aortic stenosis has been notably less successful.[214,215] The major advantages of repair over replacement relate to the elimination of both prosthesis-related complications and the need for chronic anticoagulation. Other reported advantages include a lower hospital mortality, better long-term function, and a lower rate of postoperative endocarditis. Figure 5-20 illustrates the pathologic anatomy of various mitral valve reconstruction procedures, and Figure 5-21 illustrates aortic valve repairs.

MITRAL VALVE REPAIR

The hemodynamic disturbances in most forms of mitral valve disease are the result of structural deformities at different and often multiple levels within the complex mitral

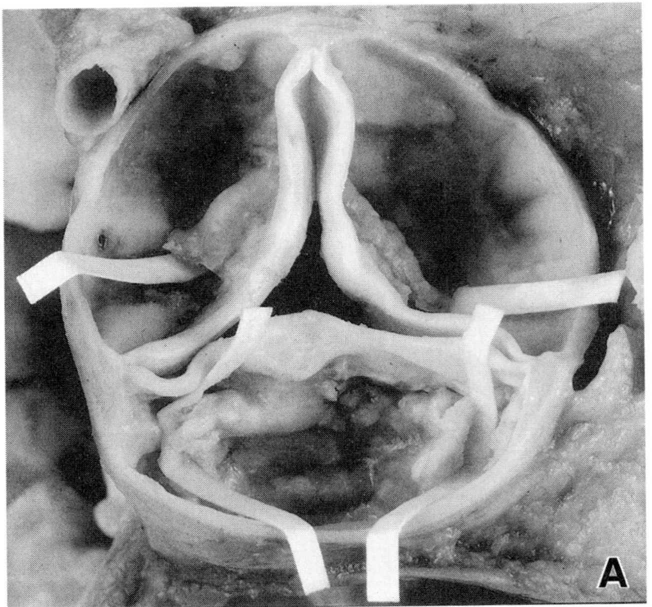

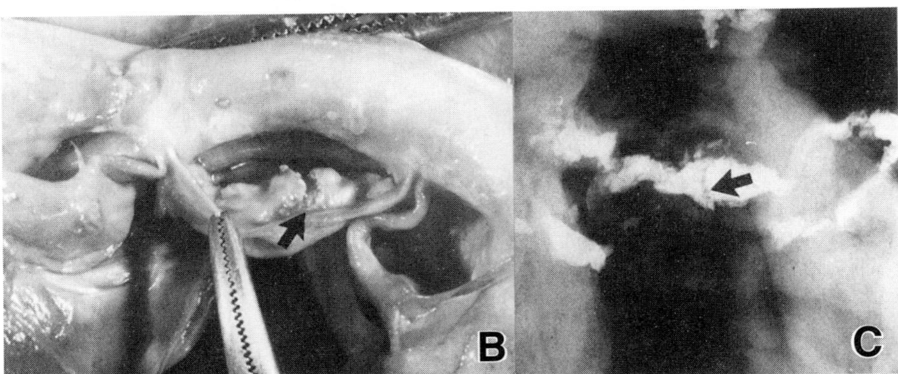

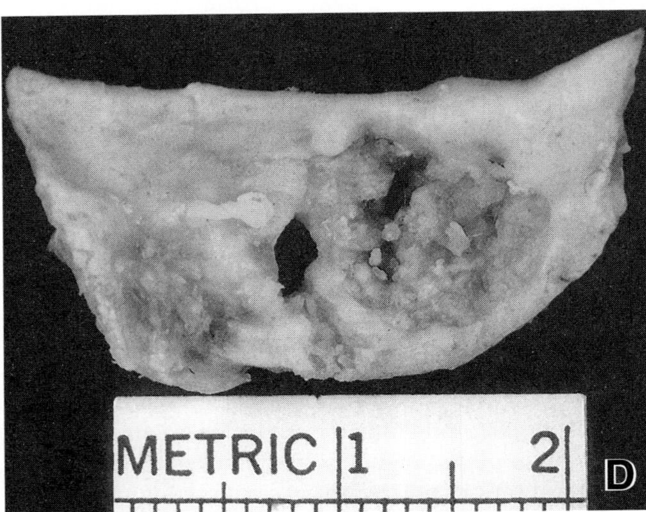

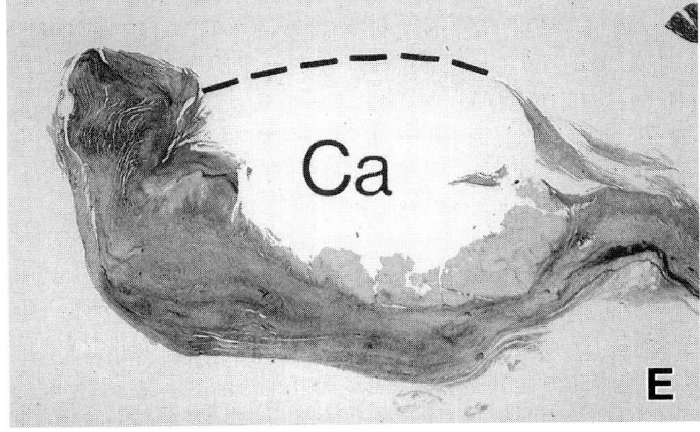

FIGURE 5–21 Valvular reconstructive procedures: aortic stenosis. (A) Aortic valve balloon valvuloplasty for degenerative calcific aortic stenosis, demonstrating fractures of nodular deposits of calcifications highlighted by tapes and (B and C) catheter balloon valvuloplasty–induced fracture of large calcific nodule of noncoronary cusp of aortic valve with calcific stenosis. This patient died during the procedure, owing to wide-open aortic insufficiency with inability of the cusp to close because of slight malposition of the edges of the calcific nodule with impingement of its fracture fascicles. (B) Gross photograph; (C) Specimen radiograph. Fracture site of nodular calcific deposit is demonstrated by arrows in (B) and (C). (D) and (E) Operative decalcification of the aortic valve. (D) Aortic valve after operative mechanical decalcification demonstrating perforated cusp. (E) Histologic cross section of aortic valve cusp after decalcification with lithotripter. Weigert elastic stain. Ca = calcium. *(A, D, and E: Reproduced with permission from Schoen FJ, Edwards WD: Valvular heart disease: general principles and stenosis, in Silver MD, Gotlieb AI, Schoen FJ (eds): Cardiovascular Pathology, 3d ed. New York, Churchill Livingstone, 2001; p 402. B and C: Reproduced with permission from Schoen FJ: Interventional and Surgical Cardiovascular Pathology: Clinical Correlations and Basic Principles. Philadelphia, WB Saunders, 1989.)*

apparatus. Identification of each component of the anatomic lesion and an underlying understanding of normal valve anatomy and function are essential to adequate valve reconstruction (see Fig. 5-20).[216]

In general, reconstructive techniques are more easily applied to mitral valves with nonrheumatic disease than those affected by rheumatic disease. The fibrosis and shortening of both chordae and leaflets that cause mitral stenosis and are the result of an advanced rheumatic process makes gaining adequate mobility and adequate leaflet area difficult. Commissurotomy may be employed in the operative repair of some stenotic mitral valves. Since the annular portions of the leaflet are normally devoid of chordal support, splitting them to 2 to 3 mm from the annulus may avoid the potential complication of a new or residual regurgitant jet. Anterior leaflet mobility often is sufficient to allow an acceptable mitral opening despite posterior leaflet immobility, and pliable leaflets can partially compensate for a rigid subvalvar apparatus. Five factors compromise the late functional results of mitral commissurotomy: (1) left ventricular dysfunction; (2) pulmonary venous hypertension and right-sided cardiac factors, including right ventricular failure, tricuspid regurgitation, or a combination of these; (3) systemic embolization; (4) other coexistent cardiac disorders, such as coronary artery or aortic valve diseases; and (5) residual or progressive mitral valve disease. Late deterioration following mitral commissurotomy may occur owing to restenosis of the valve, residual (unrelieved) stenosis, or regurgitation induced at operation. Leaflet calcification, subvalvar (predominantly chordal) fibrotic changes, and significant regurgitation owing to scar retraction limit the ability to perform reconstructive surgical repair, and thereby necessitate valve replacement of a stenotic mitral valve.

Structural defects seen in mitral regurgitation include: (1) dilation of the mitral annulus; (2) elongation or rupture of chordae tendineae, permitting leaflet prolapse into the atrium; (3) redundancy and deformity of leaflets; (4) leaflet perforations or defects; (5) restricted leaflet motion as a result of commissural fusion in an opened position, and leaflet retraction, chordal shortening or thickening or both. Necrosis without rupture of a papillary muscle following an acute myocardial infarction generally does not itself induce insufficiency. More frequently, mitral regurgitation results from the underlying necrotic and nonfunctional free-wall segment or distortion of the papillary muscle geometry by ventricular dilation, where lateral movement of the papillary muscles alters the axis of their tension on the cords.

Leaflet abnormalities causing mitral regurgitation include retraction, redundancy, and perforation. The posterior leaflet is more delicate, has a shorter annulus-to-free-edge dimension than the anterior, and is therefore more prone to postinflammatory fibrous retraction. Following resection of excess anterior or posterior leaflet tissue in valves with redundancy, annuloplasty with or without a prosthetic ring is used to reduce the annulus dimension to correspond to the amount of leaflet tissue available. Tissue substitutes such as glutaraldehyde-pretreated xenograft or autologous pericardium can be used to repair or enlarge leaflets. Ruptured or elongated chordae may be repaired by shortening or replacement with pericardial tissue or thick suture material.

CATHETER BALLOON VALVULOPLASTY

Percutaneous transluminal balloon dilation of stenotic valves has been used successfully to relieve some congenital and acquired stenoses of native pulmonary, aortic, and mitral valves, and stenotic right-sided porcine bioprosthetic valves.[217–219] Mitral valvuloplasty yields favorable results in elderly patients with mitral stenosis complicated by pulmonary hypertension, a difficult group of patients to manage surgically. For acquired calcific aortic stenosis, individual functional responses to balloon dilation vary considerably and data suggest a modest incremental benefit, high early mortality, and high restenosis rate.[220] Some patients have dramatic improvement in valvular and ventricular function, whereas others show little change. The major complications of balloon valvuloplasty include cerebrovascular accident secondary to embolism, massive regurgitation owing to valve trauma, cardiac perforation with tamponade, and, with mitral valvuloplasty, creation of an atrial septal defect owing to septal dilation.

Improvement following catheter balloon valvuloplasty of aortic stenosis derives from commissural separation, fracture of calcific deposits, and displacing and stretching of the valve cusps (see Fig. 5-21A). Fractured calcific nodules can themselves prove dangerous (see Figs. 5-21B and C).[221] In pediatric cases in which the cusps are generally pliable, cuspal stretching, tearing, or avulsion may also occur. In the relief of mitral stenosis, balloon valvuloplasty largely involves commissural separation; thus, this procedure is unlikely to provide significant alteration in the subvalvular pathology of the chordae and papillary muscles of patients with rheumatic mitral stenosis. Commissural splitting generally is successful only in valves with little or no commissural calcification. Thus, balloon valvuloplasty has been far more applicable in third world countries in which rheumatic mitral stenosis is commonly severe but noncalcific at a young age, rather than in the United States, in which the disease is usually only severe and calcific in middle-aged or elderly adults.

SURGICAL DEBRIDEMENT

Since valvular aortic stenosis in most patients over 60 years of age is characterized by calcific deposits superimposed upon a valve largely free of either congenital or rheumatic deformities, such valves are stenotic simply because the leaflets are immobilized by extensive deposits of calcium. However, because the calcific deposits arise deep in the valve fibrous layer (see Figs. 5-18D and E), their removal by sharp dissection

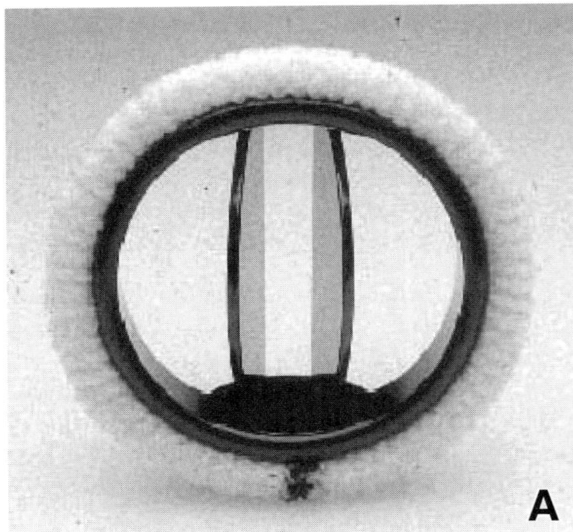

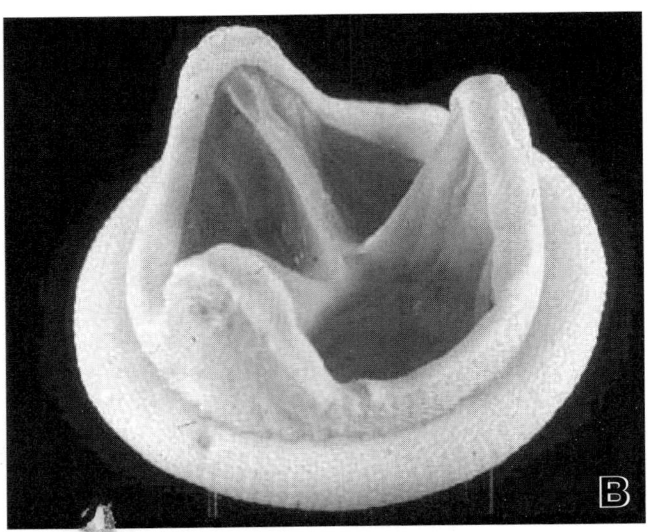

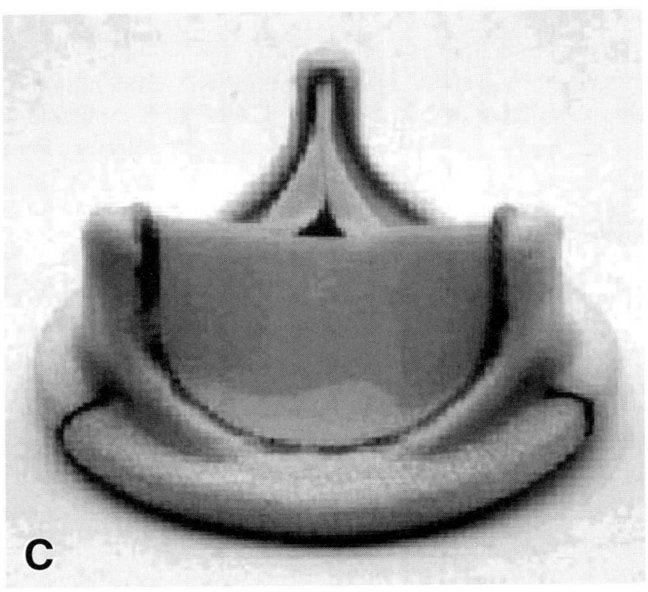

FIGURE 5–22 Photographs of the most widely used valve substitutes. (A) Bileaflet tilting disk mechanical heart valve (St. Jude Medical, St. Jude Medical Inc., St. Paul, MN). (B) Porcine aortic valve bioprosthesis (Hancock, Medtronic Heart Valves, Santa Ana, CA). *(A and B: Reproduced with permission from Schoen FJ: Approach to the analysis of cardiac valve prostheses as surgical pathology or autopsy specimens. Cardiovasc Pathol 1995; 4:241, and Schoen FJ: Pathology of heart valve substitution with mechanical and tissue prostheses, in Silver MD, Gotlieb AI, Schoen FJ (eds): Cardiovascular Pathology, 3rd ed, Churchill Livingstone, 2001.)* (C) Bovine pericardial bioprosthesis (Carpentier-Edwards, Edwards Life Sciences, Santa Ana, CA).

or ultrasonic debridement generally requires surgical dissection that removes the fibrosa and may cause damage to the spongiosa, resulting in severe compromise of cuspal mechanical integrity (see Figs. 4-21D and E).[222] In some cases, vegetations of infective endocarditis may be surgically debrided.

Valve Replacement

Severe symptomatic valvular heart disease other than pure mitral stenosis or incompetence is most frequently treated by excision of the diseased valve(s) and replacement by a functional substitute. Five factors principally determine the results of valve replacement in an individual patient: (1) technical aspects of the procedure; (2) intraoperative myocardial ischemic injury; (3) irreversible and chronic structural alterations in the heart and lungs secondary to the valvular abnormality; (4) coexistent obstructive coronary artery disease; and (5) valve prosthesis reliability and host-tissue interactions.

VALVE TYPES AND PROGNOSTIC CONSIDERATIONS

Cardiac valvular substitutes are of two generic types, mechanical and biological tissue (Fig. 5-22 and Table 5-2).[223–225] Prostheses function passively, responding to pressure and flow changes within the heart. Mechanical valves are usually composed of nonphysiologic biomaterials that employ a rigid, mobile occluder (pyrolytic carbon disk) in a metallic cage (cobalt-chrome or titanium alloy) as in the Bjork-Shiley, Hall-Medtronic, or OmniScience valves, or two carbon hemidisks in a carbon housing as in the

TABLE 5–2 Complications of substitute heart valves

Generic	Specific
Thrombotic limitations	Thrombosis
	Thromboembolism
	Anticoagulation-related hemorrhage
Infection	Prosthetic valve endocarditis
Structural dysfunction (intrinsic)	Wear
	Fracture
	Poppet escape
	Cuspal tear
	Calcification
	Commisural region dehiscence
Nonstructural dysfunction (most extrinsic)	Pannus (tissue overgrowth)
	Entrapment by suture or tissue
	Paravalvular leak
	Disproportion
	Hemolytic anemia
	Noise

Source: Modified with permission from Schoen FJ, Levy RJ, Piehler HR: Pathological considerations in replacement cardiac valves. Cardiovasc Pathol 1992; 1:29.

St. Jude Medical, Edwards-Duromedics, or CarboMedics CPHV prostheses. Pyrolytic carbon has high strength and fatigue and wear resistance, with exceptional biocompatibility including thromboresistance.[227] In contrast, tissue valves are more anatomically similar to natural valves. The major advantages of tissue valves compared to mechanical prostheses are their pseudoanatomic central flow and relative nonthrombogenicity, usually not requiring anticoagulant therapy. It is estimated that slightly more than half of all valves implanted in the present era are mechanical (mostly bileaflet tilting disk); the remainder are bioprosthetic, mostly xenografts fabricated from porcine aortic valve or bovine pericardium, which have been preserved in a dilute glutaraldehyde solution, with a small percentage of cryopreserved allografts. In the past decade, innovations in tissue valve technologies and design have caused this segment of the market to grow disproportionately and expanded indications for their use (Fig. 5-23).[228]

Early mortality after cardiac valve replacement now is generally in the range of 3% to 5%, with the majority of deaths owing to hemorrhage, pulmonary failure, low cardiac

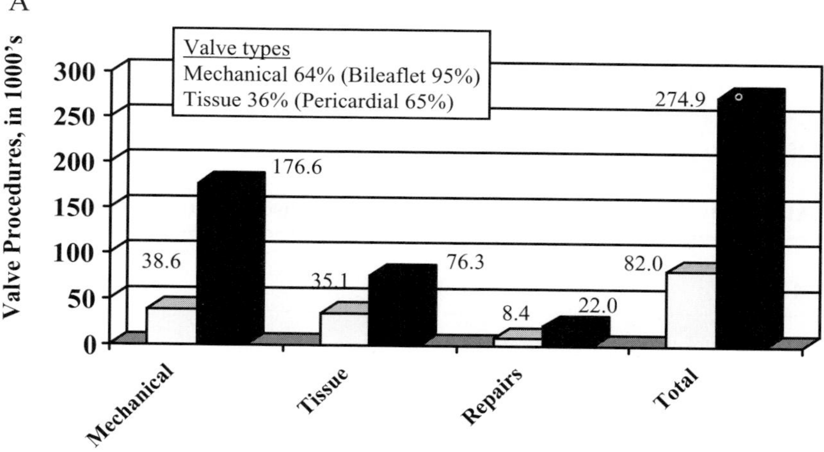

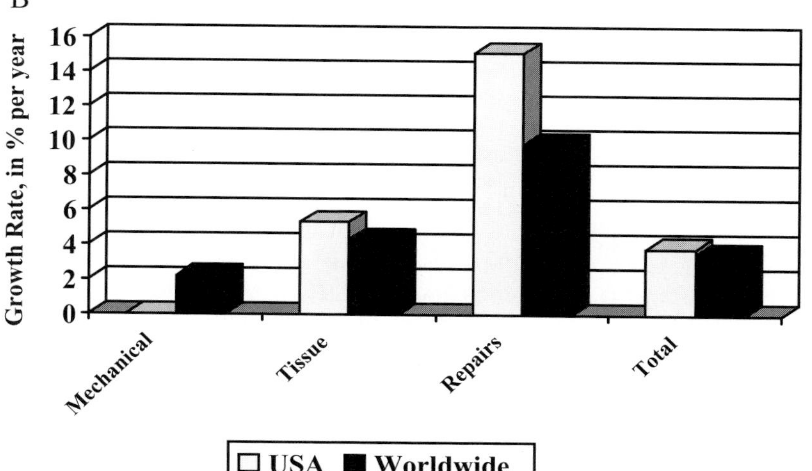

FIGURE 5–23 U.S. and worldwide use of substitute heart valves and heart valve repairs, estimated 2000. (A) Usage. (B) Growth rate. While mechanical valves are implanted more frequently than tissue valves, the growth rate of tissue valves is approximately 4%, much more than that of mechanical valves. Ninety-five percent of mechanical valves are bilateral tilting disk valves; 65% of tissue valves are pericardial bioprostheses. The overall growth rate of repair operations is more than 10%. Approximately 7000 cryopreserved valves are implanted in the United States with a growth rate of approximately 5% per year (worldwide data not available). *(Data courtesy of St. Jude Medical, Inc.)*

output, and sudden death with or without myocardial necrosis or documented arrhythmias. Early prosthetic valve–associated complications are unusual.[229] Potential complications related to valve insertion include hemorrhagic disruption and dissection of the atrioventricular groove, perforation or entrapment of the left circumflex coronary artery by a suture, and pseudoaneurysm or rupture of the left ventricular free wall.

Improvement in late outcome has derived from earlier referral of patients for valve replacement, decreased intraoperative myocardial damage, and improved surgical technique and cardiac valve prostheses. Following valve replacement with currently used devices, the probability of 5-year survival is about 80% and of 10-year survival about 70%, dependent on overall functional state, preoperative left ventricular function, left ventricular and left atrial size, and extent and severity of coronary artery disease. Preservation of the subvalvular apparatus has also been an important advance.[230]

VALVE-RELATED COMPLICATIONS

Prosthetic valve–associated pathology becomes an important consideration beyond the early postoperative period. The few randomized studies available show that with contemporary mechanical prosthetic and bioprosthetic valves, approximately 60% or more patients have an important device-related complication within 10 years postoperatively.[213–215,231,232] However, thrombotic and thromboembolic problems that frequently complicate mechanical valves tend to occur earlier than the structural failures that complicate tissue valve prostheses.[233] Valve-related complications frequently necessitate reoperation, now accounting for approximately 5% to 15% of all valve procedures, and they may cause death. Late death following valve replacement results predominantly from either cardiovascular pathology not related to the substitute valve or prosthesis-associated complications. Moreover, late death is caused by a device-related complication in 25% to 61% of patients.[229,234] As might be expected, autopsy studies generally reveal a higher rate of valve-related pathology than clinical investigations. One fifth or more of valve recipients will ultimately die suddenly; in one autopsy study of a highly selected referral population, 40% of valve recipients who died suddenly had a valve-related cause.[235]

Four categories of valve-related complications are most important: thromboembolism and related problems, infection, structural dysfunction (i.e., failure or degeneration of the biomaterials comprising a prosthesis), and nonstructural dysfunction (i.e., miscellaneous complications and modes of failure not encompassed in the previous groups) (Table 5-2).[226,236–243] The clinicomorphologic features of these problems have been widely described in the literature. The relative performance and risk of complications of various types of widely used substitute heart valve types are summarized in Table 5-3. The risk of some valve-related complications (particularly thromboembolism) is

TABLE 5–3 Types and characteristics of commonly used substitute heart valves*

Valve type	Model(s)	Hemodynamics	Freedom from thrombosis/thromboembolism	Durability
Mechanical				
Caged ball	Starr-Edwards	+§	+	+++
Single tilting disk	Bjork-Shiley Hall-Medtronic Omnicarbon	++	++	+++†
Bileaflet tilting disk	St. Jude Medical CarboMedics Edwards-Duromedics	+++	+++	+++‡
Tissue				
Heterograft/xenograft bioprostheses	Carpentier-Edwards (porcine and bovine pericardial) Hancock (porcine) Ionescu-Shiley (bovine pericardial) Mitroflow (bovine pericardial)	++	+++	++
Homograft/allograft	Cryopreserved human aortic/pulmonic valve	++++	++++	++

*Presently or previously.

† Except Bjork-Shiley 60°/70° convexo-concave valve (see text).

‡ Except previous model of Edwards-Duromedics valve (see text).

§ Performance criteria: + = least favorable to ++++ = most favorable.

Source: Data adapted from Vongpatanasin W, et al: Prosthetic heart valves. N Engl J Med 1996; 335:407.

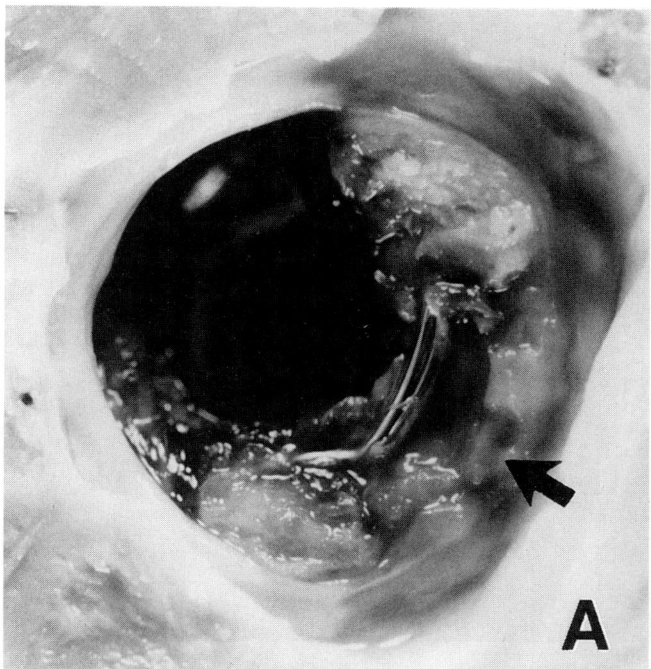

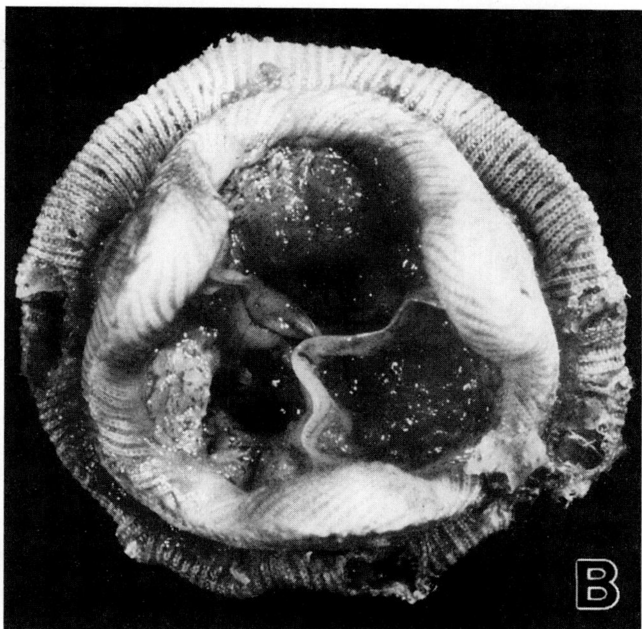

FIGURE 5–24 Thrombotic occlusion of substitute heart valves. (A) Tilting disk prosthesis. Thrombus was likely initiated in the region of stasis immediately distal to the smaller of the two orifices through which blood flows (arrow), causing near-total occluder immobility. (B) Porcine bioprosthesis, with thrombus filling the bioprosthetic sinuses of Valsalva. *(A: Reproduced with permission from Anderson JM, Schoen FJ: Interactions of blood with artificial surfaces, in Buchart EG, Bodnar E (eds): Thrombosis, Embolism, and Bleeding. London, ICR Publishers, 1992; p 160. B: Reproduced with permission from Schoen FJ, Hobson CE: Anatomic analysis of removed prosthetic heart valves: causes of failure of 33 mechanical valves and 58 bioprostheses, 1980 to 1983. Hum Pathol 1985; 16:549.)*

potentiated by preoperative or postoperative functional impairment.

Thromboembolic complications are the major cause of mortality and morbidity after cardiac valve replacement with mechanical valves, and patients with them require chronic therapeutic anticoagulation with warfarin derivatives.[244] Thrombotic deposits can immobilize the occluder or shed emboli (Fig. 5-24). Tissue valves are less thrombogenic than mechanical valves, with most patients not requiring long-term anticoagulation unless they have atrial fibrillation or another specific indication. Nevertheless, the rate of thromboembolism in patients with mechanical valves on anticoagulation is not widely different from that in patients with bioprosthetic valves without anticoagulation (2% to 4% per year). Chronic oral anticoagulation also induces a risk of hemorrhage.[244]

Virchow's triad of factors promoting thrombosis (surface thrombogenicity, hypercoagulability, and locally static blood flow) largely predicts the relative propensity toward and locations of thrombotic deposits. For example, with caged-ball prostheses, thrombi form distal to the poppet at the cage apex. Tilting disk prostheses are particularly susceptible to total thrombotic occlusion or emboli from small thrombi, both generally initiated in a stagnation zone in the minor orifice of the outflow region of the prosthesis; bileaflet tilting disk valves are most vulnerable near the hinges where the leaflets insert into the housing. In contrast, the unusual late thrombosis of a bioprosthetic valve is marked by large thrombotic deposits in one or more of the prosthetic sinuses of Valsalva. Usually, no causal underlying cuspal pathology can be demonstrated by routine microscopic studies. Some valve thromboemboli, especially early postoperatively with any valve type, are thought to be initiated at the valve sewing cuff. Noninvasive visualization of prosthetic valve thrombi is aided by transesophageal endocardiography.[245]

As with other devices in which nonphysiologic artificial surfaces are exposed to blood at high fluid shear stresses, platelet deposition dominates initial blood-surface interaction and prosthetic valve thromboembolism correlates strongly with altered platelet function.[246] Nevertheless, although platelet-suppressive drugs largely normalize indices of platelet formation and partially reduce the frequency of thromboembolic complications in patients with mechanical prosthetic valves, antiplatelet therapy alone is insufficient to adequately prevent thromboembolism. The friability and susceptibility to embolization of thrombi that form on bioprosthetic or mechanical valves are prolonged because lack of adjacent vascular tissue retards their histologic

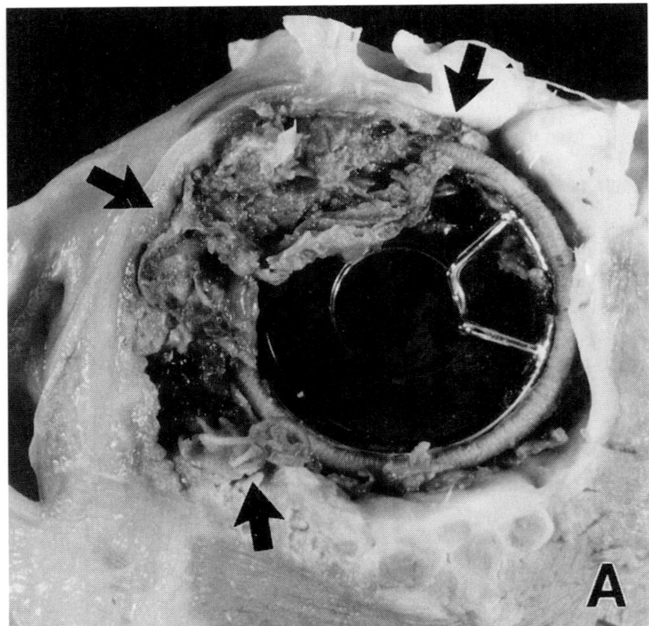

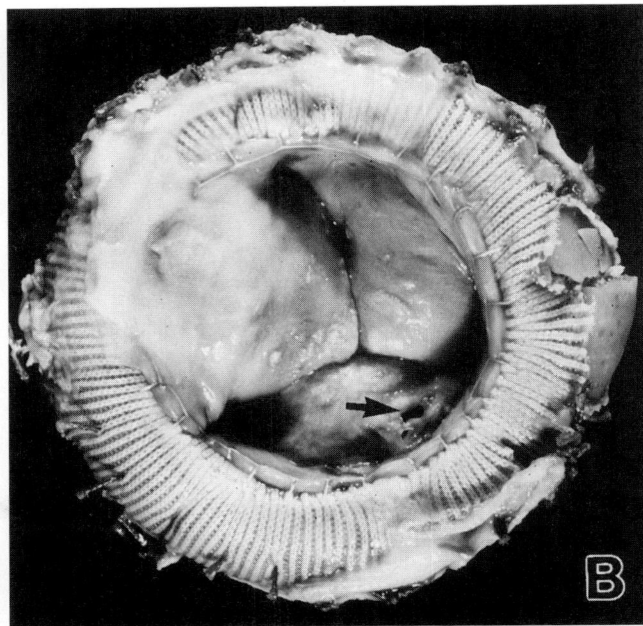

FIGURE 5–25 Prosthetic valve endocarditis. (A) Endocarditis with large ring abscess (arrows) observed from ventricular surface of aortic Bjork-Shiley tilting disk prosthesis in patient who died suddenly. Ring abscess impinges on proximal atrioventricular conduction system. (B) Bioprosthetic valve endocarditis with cuspal perforation by organism-induced necrosis (arrow). *(A: Reproduced by permission from Schoen FJ: Cardiac valve prostheses: pathological and bioengineering considerations. J Cardiac Surg 1987; 2:65. B: Reproduced by permission from Schoen FJ, et al: Long-term failure rate and morphologic correlations in porcine bioprosthetic heart valves. Am J Cardiol 1983; 51:957.)*

organization. For similar reasons, the age of such thrombi is difficult to determine microscopically. Moreover, in selected circumstances, thrombolytic therapy may be a practical nonsurgical option.[247,248]

Prosthetic valve infective endocarditis (Fig. 5-25) occurs in 3% to 6% of recipients of substitute valves.[207,249] Infection is generally categorized into early (usually less than 60 days postoperative) and late.[250–255] The microbial etiology of early prosthetic valve endocarditis is dominated by the staphylococcal species *S. epidermidis* and *S. aureus*, even though prophylactic regimens used today are targeted against these microorganisms. The clinical course of early prosthetic valve endocarditis tends to be fulminant, with rapid deterioration of hemodynamic status due to valvular or annular destruction or persistent bacteremia. In late endocarditis, a probable source of infection can be found in 25% to 80% of patients, the most frequent initiators being dental procedures, urologic infections and interventions, and indwelling catheters. The most common organisms in these late infections are *S. epidermidis, S. aureus, Streptococcus viridans,* and enterococci. Surgical reintervention usually is indicated for large highly mobile vegetations or cerebral thromboembolic episodes. Transesophageal echocardiography enhances diagnosis of prosthetic valve endocarditis and its intracardiac complications.[253] Rates of infection of bioprostheses and mechanical valves are similar, but previous endocarditis as the original indication for valve replacement markedly increases the risk.

Virtually all infections associated with mechanical prosthetic valves and some with bioprosthetic valves are localized to the prosthesis–tissue junction at the sewing ring, and accompanied by tissue destruction around the prosthesis (see Fig. 5-25A). This comprises a ring abscess, with potential paraprosthetic leak, dehiscence, fistula formation, or heart block caused by conduction system damage. In addition, bioprosthetic valve infections may involve, and are occasionally limited to, the cuspal tissue, sometimes causing secondary cuspal tearing or perforation with valve incompetence or obstruction (see Fig. 5-25B). Cases without annular involvement have a better prognosis than those associated with infected annular margins of resection. Additional complications of prosthetic valve endocarditis include embolization of vegetations and congestive heart failure secondary to obstruction or regurgitation.

Prosthetic valve dysfunction owing to materials degradation can necessitate reoperation or cause prosthesis-associated death (Fig. 5-26). Durability considerations vary widely for mechanical valves and bioprostheses, for specific types of each, for different models of a particular prosthesis (utilizing different materials or having different design

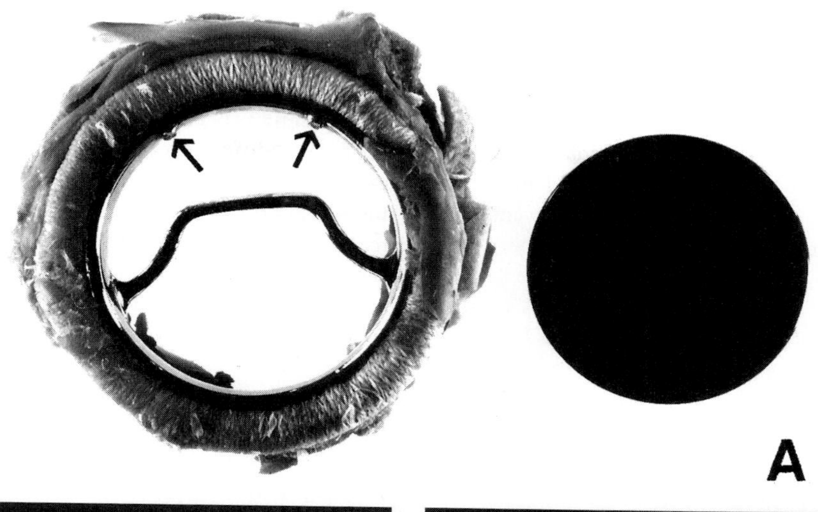

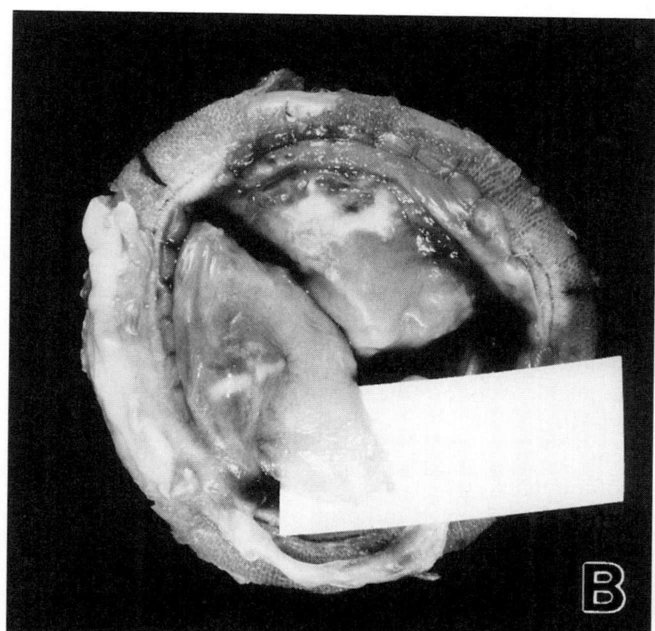

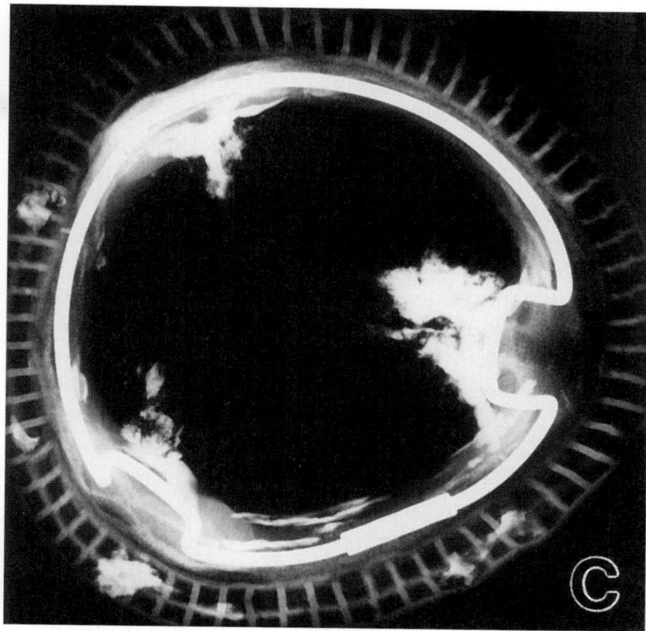

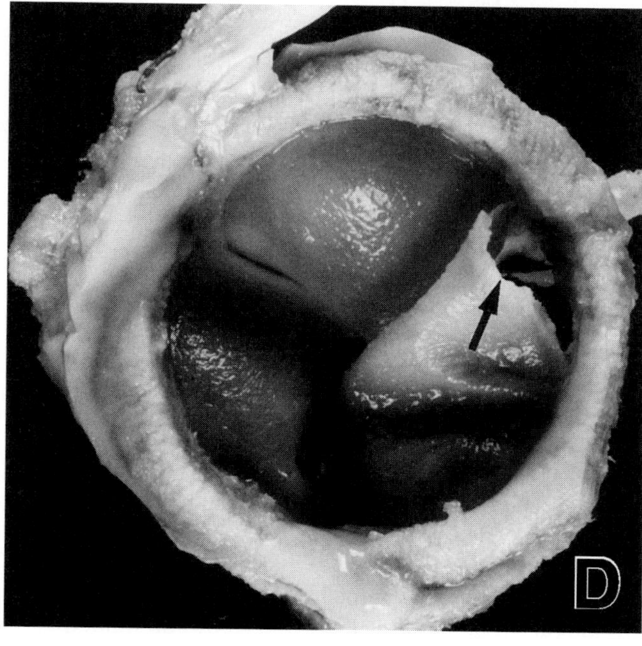

FIGURE 5–26 Structural valve dysfunction. (A) Disk escape owing to fractured lesser strut of a Bjork-Shiley heart valve prosthesis. This model had the strut welded to the metal frame. Both the fractured strut and the disk embolized; the strut was not found at autopsy. The fracture sites are indicated by arrows. (B) and (C) Porcine valve primary tissue failure owing to calcification with secondary cuspal tear leading to severe regurgitation. (B) Gross photograph; (C) specimen radiograph. Dense calcific deposits are apparent in the commissures. (D) Clinical Ionescu-Shiley mitral bovine pericardial bioprostheses with extensive tear of one cusp (arrow) and resultant incompetence.
(A: Reproduced with permission from Schoen FJ, et al: Pathological considerations in substitute heart valves. Cardiovasc Pathol 1992; 1:29. B and C: Reproduced with permission from Schoen FJ, Hobson CE: Anatomic analysis of removed prosthesic heart valves: causes of failure of 33 mechanical valves and 58 bioprostheses 1980 to 1983. Hum Pathol 1985; 16:549. D: Reproduced by permission from Schoen FJ: Cardiac valve prostheses: pathological and bioengineering considerations. J Cardiovasc Surg 1987; 2:65.)

features), and even for the same model prosthesis placed in the aortic rather than the mitral site. Moreover, although mechanical valve failure is often catastrophic and may be life-threatening, bioprosthetic valve failure generally causes slowly progressive symptomatic deterioration, often permitting reoperation.

Fractures of metallic or carbon valve components occur rarely. Of approximately 86,000 Bjork-Shiley 60- and 70-degree Convexo-Concave heart valves implanted, a cluster of over 500 cases has been reported in which the welded outlet strut fractured because of metal fatigue, leading to disk escape (see Fig. 5-26A). Although complete strut fracture is usually fatal, elective removal of structurally intact prostheses has not been recommended. However, a cineangiographic imaging technique may facilitate detection of single leg strut fractures at a presymptomatic stage in some patients, thereby allowing consideration of elective valve removal.[254] In contrast, fractures of carbon components (disks or housing) are unusual in most single leaflet or bileaflet tilting disk valves.[255] However, a group of 37 fractures of an estimated 20,000 Edwards-Duramedics bileaflet tilting valves has occurred, possibly a combined result of carbon coating defects and cavitation bubbles impacting on the carbon surfaces during function.[256,257] Fracture of the St. Jude bileaflet tilting disk valve has been rarely reported.[258]

In contrast, structural dysfunction of tissue valves is the major cause of failure of the most widely used bioprostheses (flexible-stent-mounted, glutaraldehyde-preserved porcine aortic valves, and bovine pericardial valves) (see Figs. 5-26B and 5-26C).[259] Within 15 years following implantation, 30% to 50% of porcine aortic valves implanted as either mitral or aortic valve replacements require replacement because of primary tissue failure.[260] Cuspal mineralization is the major responsible pathologic process with regurgitation through secondary tears the most frequent failure mode.[226,238,243,259] There is increasing recognition that noncalcific structural damage owing to collagen fiber disruption is an important mode of bioprosthetic heart valve failure.[261] Pure stenosis owing to calcific cuspal stiffening and noncalcific cuspal tears or perforations (reflecting direct mechanical destruction of collagen) occurs less frequently. Calcific deposits are usually localized to cuspal tissue (intrinsic calcification), but calcific deposits extrinsic to the cusps may occur in thrombi or endocarditic vegetations. Calcification is markedly accelerated in younger patients, with children and adolescents having an especially accelerated course.

Bovine pericardial valves suffer primarily design-related tearing, with calcification frequent but less limiting.[263,264] Abrasion of the pericardial tissue is an important contributing factor.[265]

The morphology and determinants of calcification of bioprosthetic valve tissue have been widely studied in experimental models. The process is initiated primarily within residual membranes and organelles of the nonviable connective tissue cells that have been devitalized by glutaraldehyde pretreatment procedures.[259,266–269] This dystrophic calcification mechanism involves reaction of calcium-containing extracellular fluid with membrane-associated phosphorus, causing calcification of the collagen. The determinants of accelerated calcification include recipient metabolic factors such as young age, valve factors such as glutaraldehyde fixation, and increased mechanical stress. The function of the native cardiac valve is contingent on a highly adapted, complex, and dynamic architecture in which cells and extracellular matrix elements support substantial repetitive movement and ongoing repair of injury.[270] Substantial changes are induced by the preservation and manufacture of a bioprosthesis, these rendering the tissue different in many respects from that of a native valve. The pathological changes in bioprosthetic valves that occur following implantation are, to a large extent, rationalized on the basis of these differences and the superimposed alterations that occur following implantation,[271] as discussed below. They include:

1. Endothelial cells are lost and the cusp/blood interface is subendothelial connective tissue. This may permit penetration into the cusp of plasma, erythrocytes, and inflammatory cells.
2. Following cross-linking, the interstitial cells are nonviable. Without the synthetic capabilities of viable interstitial cells, bioprostheses have no mechanism to remodel and replace collagen and other matrix components that are progressively degraded by mechanical damage and proteolysis.
3. Cross-linked cellular debris, collagen, and elastin can serve as foci for calcification. Natural inhibitors to mineralization may be diminished or unavailable.
4. The cuspal microstructure is fixed/locked in a static geometry, often characteristic of one phase of the cardiac cycle, with altered mechanical properties. Thus, the normal cyclical rearrangements that occur during valve function cannot occur, leading to loss of tissue compliance and abnormal motion of the cusps.

Commissural region dehiscence of the aortic wall tissue from the inside of porcine bioprosthetic valve stents causing insufficiency has been described in several valve models (Fig. 5-27).[272,273]

Extrinsic (nonstructural) complications of substitute heart valves are illustrated in Figure 5-28. The most common, paravalvular defects may be clinically inconsequential or may aggravate hemolysis or cause heart failure through regurgitation. Early paravalvular leaks may be the result of either suture knot failure, inadequate suture placement, or separation of sutures from a pathologic annulus in endocarditis with ring abscess, myxomatous valvular degeneration, or calcified valvular annulus as in calcific aortic stenosis or mitral annular calcification. Late small paravalvular leaks usually are caused by anomalous tissue retraction from the sewing

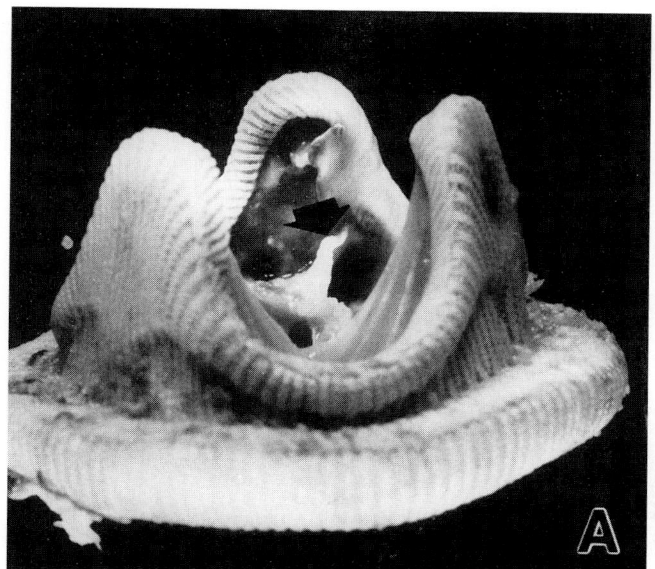

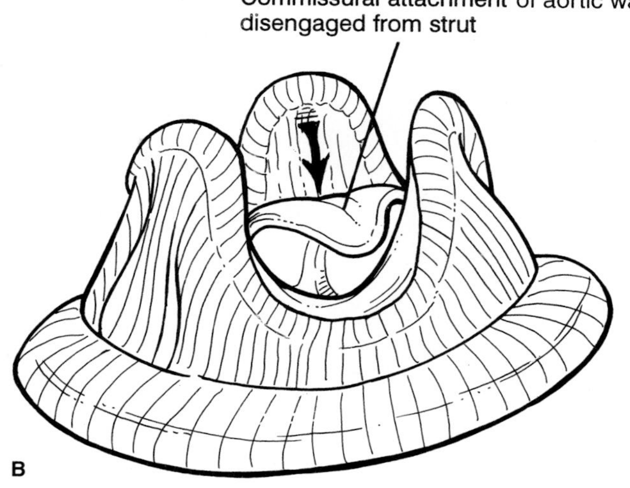

FIGURE 5–27 Dehiscence of commissural region of Hancock Standard porcine bioprosthetic valve. (A) Gross photograph. (B) Schematic diagram (arrow denotes loss of attachment of commissural support). Removed for regurgitation, this valve had prolapse of one cusp, minimal calcification, and no cuspal tears.

ring between sutures during healing and tend to be small and difficult to locate by surgical or pathological examination (see Fig. 5-28A). However, in a particular case, the cause of a paravalvular leak may be obscure. The determinants of sewing ring healing are poorly understood.

Some studies have suggested that the St Jude Medical bileaflet tilting disk valve with a silver coating (Silzone) introduced to prevent bacterial colonization of the valves and consequent prosthetic valve endocarditis has a higher than expected rate of paravalvular leak.[274] This valve has a conventional polyethylene terephthalate (PET) polyester sewing ring coated with metallic silver by an ion beam vapor deposition process. Although it has been theorized that this increased risk of PV leaks is due to an inhibition of normal fibroblast response and incorporation of the fabric of the sewing cuff into host tissues in some patients, this remains unproven.[275]

Hemolysis owing to turbulent flow and blood–material surface interactions is an ever-present risk. It was more common with earlier model heart valve prostheses and resulted in renal tubular hemosiderosis or cholelithiasis in many patients. Although severe hemolytic anemia is unusual with contemporary valves, paravalvular leaks or dysfunction owing to materials degeneration may induce clinically important hemolysis.

Extrinsic factors can mediate late prosthetic valve stenosis or regurgitation, including a large mitral annular calcific nodule, septal hypertrophy, exuberant overgrowth of fibrous tissue (Fig. 5-28B), interference by retained valve remnants (such as a retained posterior mitral leaflet or components of the submitral apparatus; Fig. 5-28C), or unraveled, long, or looped sutures or knots (Figs. 4-28D, E, and F). For bioprosthetic valves, cuspal motion can be restricted by sutures looped around stents, and suture ends cut too long may erode into or perforate a bioprosthetic valve cusp.

VALVULAR ALLOGRAFTS/HOMOGRAFTS

Aortic or pulmonary valves (with or without associated vascular conduits) transplanted from one individual to another have exceptionally good hemodynamic profiles, a low incidence of thromboembolic complications without chronic anticoagulation, and a low reinfection rate following valve replacement for endocarditis.[276,277] Early valvular allografts sterilized and/or preserved with chemicals (using propriolactone or ethylene oxide) or irradiation suffered a high rate of leaflet calcification and rupture, resulting in failure rates of nearly 50% at 10 to 12 years and 50% to 90% at 15 to 20 years.[278] Pathologic examination of such valves revealed variable host fibrous tissue overgrowth and marked structural changes, including loss of architectural elements and cellularity, fibrosis, calcification, and often cuspal ruptures.[279]

Subsequent technical developments have led to cryopreserved allografts, in which freezing is performed with protection from crystallization by dimethyl-sulfoxide; storage until valve use is done at –196°C in liquid nitrogen. Contemporary allograft valves yield freedom from degeneration and have durability equal to or better than those of conventional porcine bioprosthetic valves (approximately 50%-90%

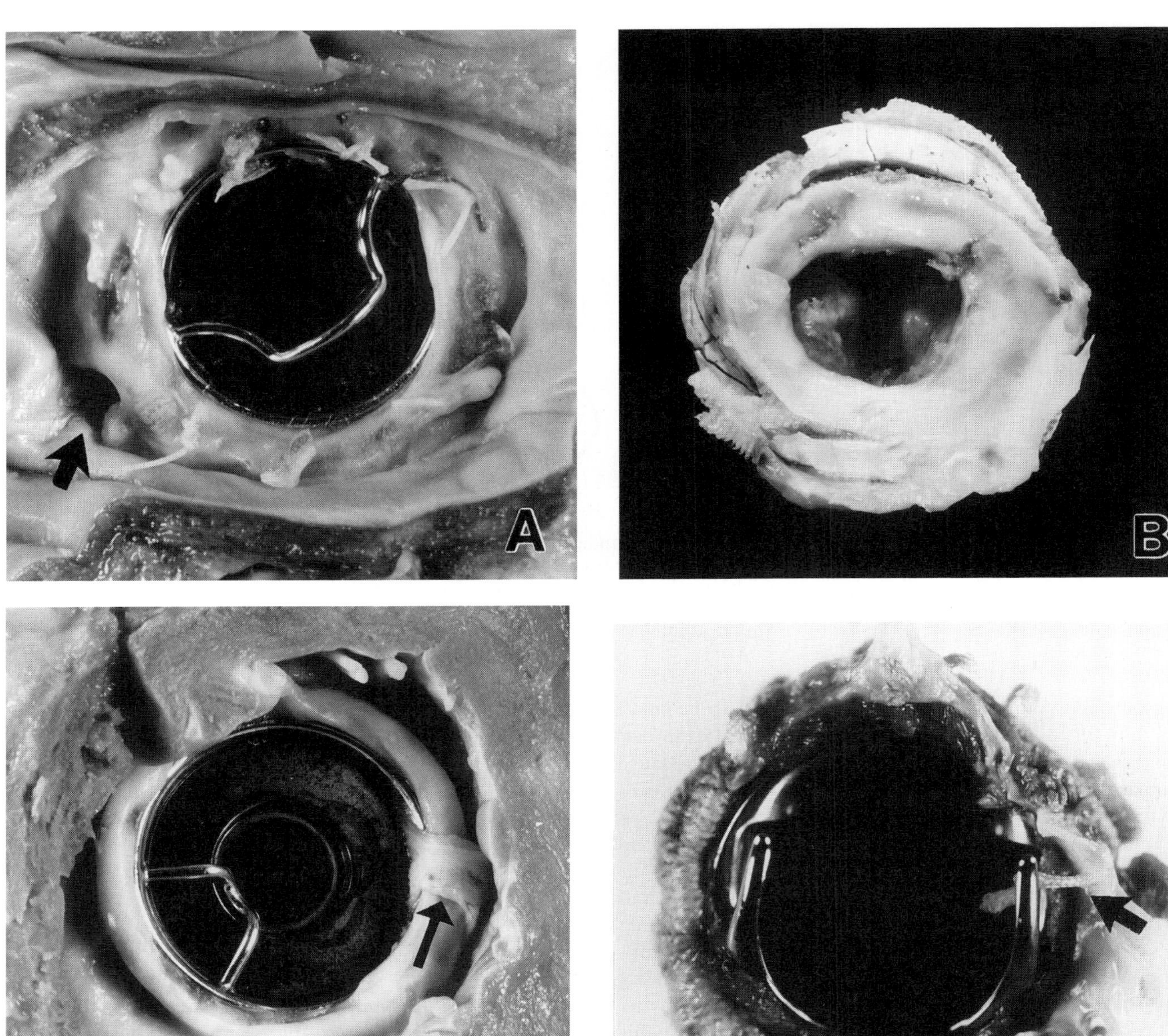

FIGURE 5–28 Nonstructural dysfunction of prosthetic heart valves. (A) Late paravalvular leak adjacent to mitral valve prosthesis (arrow). (B) Tissue overgrowth compromising inflow orifice of porcine bioprosthesis. (C) Immobility of tilting disk leaflet by impingement of retained component of submitral apparatus (arrow) that had moved through orifice late following mitral valve replacement surgery. (D) Suture with long end inhibiting free-disk movement of Lillehei-Kaster tilting disk valve (arrow). *(A and C: Reproduced with permission from Schoen FJ: Histologic considerations in replacement heart valves and other cardiovascular prosthetic devices, in Schoen FJ, Gimbrone MA (eds): Cardiovascular Pathology: Clinicopathologic Correlations and Pathogenetic Mechanisms. Philadelphia, Williams & Wilkins, 1995; p 194. B: Reproduced with permission from Schoen FJ, et al: Pathologic considerations in substitute heart valves. Cardiovasc Pathol 1992; 1:29. D: Reproduced by permission from Schoen FJ: Pathology of cardiac valve replacement, in Morse D, Steiner RM, Fernandez J (eds): Guide to Prosthetic Cardiac Valves. New York, Springer-Verlag, 1985; p 209.)*

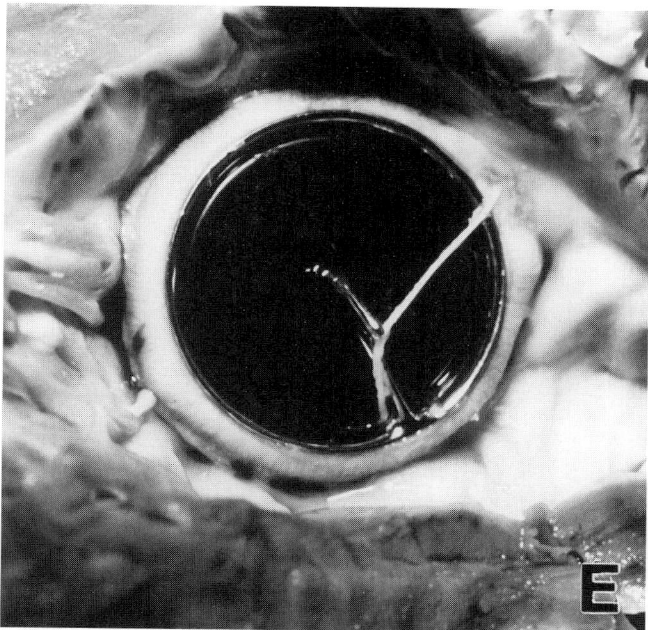

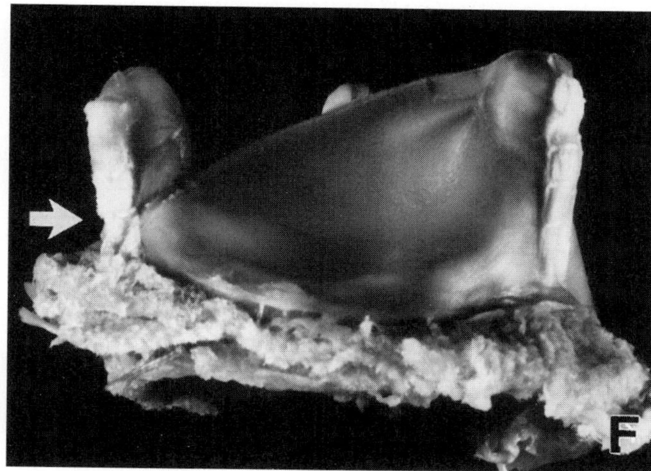

FIGURE 5–28 (*continued*) **Nonstructural dysfunction of prosthetic heart valves. (E) Suture looped around central strut of a Hall-Medtronic tilting disk valve causing disk immobility. (F) Suture looped around stent post of bovine pericardial bioprosthesis causing stenosis (arrow).** *(E: Photo courtesy of Office of the Chief Medical Examiner, New York City. F: Reproduced with permission from Schoen FJ: Cardiac valve prostheses: pathologic and bioengineering considerations. J Cardiac Surg 1987; 2:65.)*

valve survival at 10–15 years compared with 40%-60% for bioprostheses).

Some studies suggest that a fraction of viable cells may remain at the time of implantation of grafts cryopreserved using current technology.[280] However, unknown are the extent of residual cells and their functional activity and whether allograft cell viability at implantation is actually an important determinant of long-term durability. While cellular preservation may enhance both thromboresistance and durability, the presence of viable cells could have deleterious consequences, via immunologic reactivity.

We studied 33 explanted left- and right-sided cryopreserved human allograft heart valves/conduits in place several hours to 9 years in children and adults.[281] Cryopreserved human allograft heart valves/conduits implanted more than 1 day had progressively severe loss of normal structural demarcations. Long-term explants were generally devoid of both surface endothelium and deep connective tissue cells and had hyalinized collagen, laminated elastin, and minimal inflammatory cellularity (Fig. 5-29). No morphological evidence of immunologic rejection was noted. Our studies and most others demonstrate that cryopreserved allograft heart valves/conduits are morphologically nonviable; the structural basis for their favorable function seems primarily related to the largely preserved collagen. Allograft valves do not have the capacity to grow, remodel, or exhibit active metabolic functions, and their degeneration generally is not secondary to immunologic responses.

PULMONARY VALVULAR AUTOGRAFTS

Often called the Ross operation in recognition of its originator, pulmonary autograft replacement of the aortic valve is technically difficult but yields excellent hemodynamic performance, avoids anticoagulation, carries a low risk of thromboembolism, and is purported to permit growth of the autograft proportional to the somatic growth of a child or young adult.[282–285] The risk of late valve failure requiring reoperation for either the autograft valve or the homograft right ventricular outflow tract reconstruction is low. Ross et al have reported freedom from autograft replacement of 85% at 20 years and a freedom from all valve-related events of 70% at 20 years.[282] With the more recently used implantation of the autograft as a root replacement and the cryopreserved pulmonary homograft for right ventricular outflow tract reconstruction, actuarial freedom from reoperation (autograft or homograft) was 89% ± 3% at 5 years, and 92% ± 3% for the autograft alone. Late autograft valve failure was most frequently due to aortic annulus dilation and less frequently to degeneration. Autograft dysfunction can be corrected by autograft repair in patients with central insufficiency and aortic annular dilation.

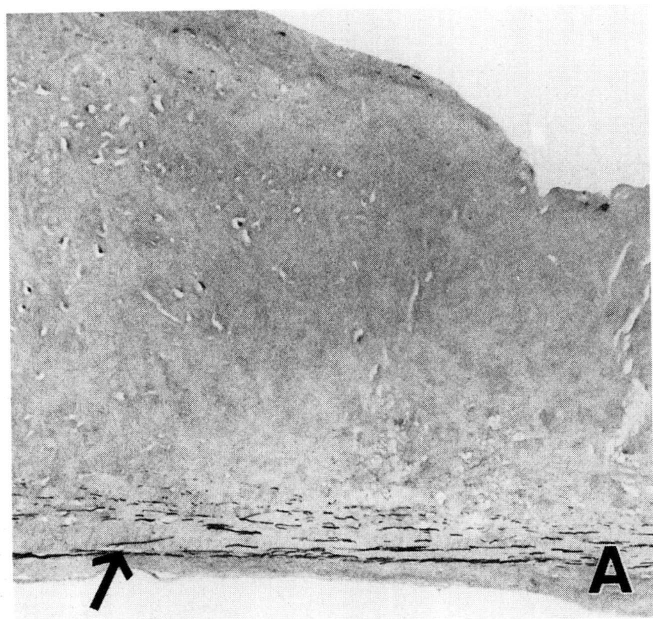

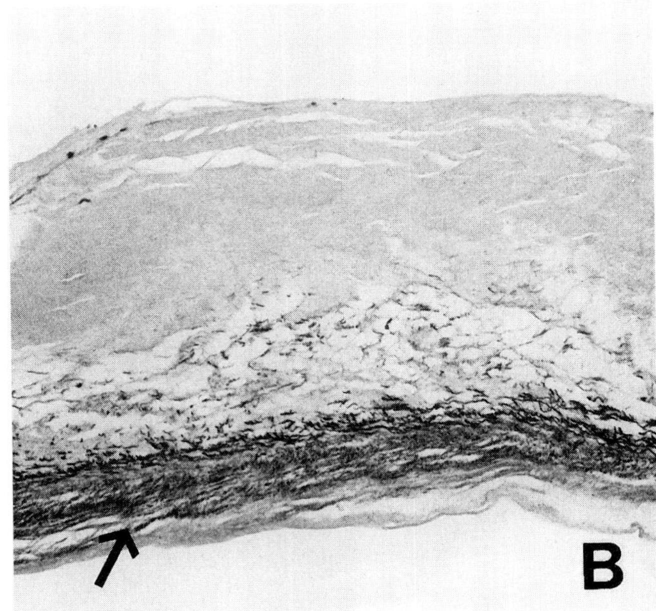

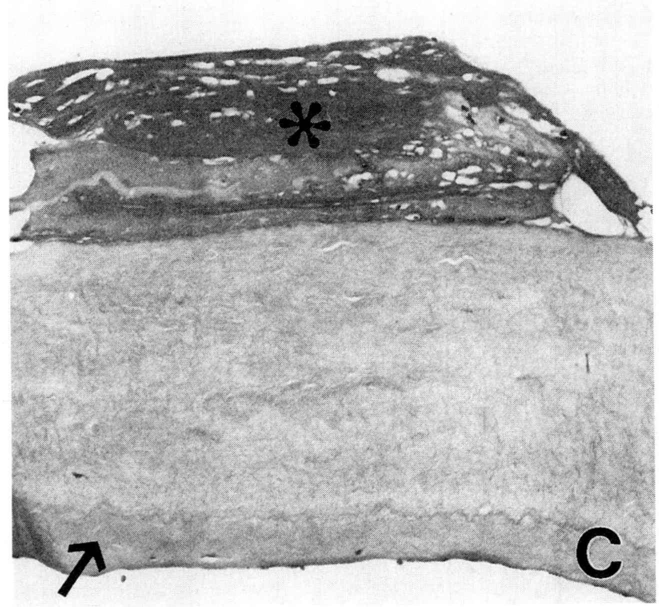

FIGURE 5–29 Late allograft (homograft) valve morphology. (A) Cryopreserved aortic valve allograft removed at 3 years for aortic insufficiency. (B) Cryopreserved aortic valve allograft removed 5 years postoperatively for stenosis. (C) Pulmonic valve allograft removed following 7 years for conduit stenosis in a child. Elastin staining (black), varies from marked in (B) to minimal in (A) to nonexistent in (C) (arrows). In each, there is minimal residual endothelial or deep connective tissue cellularity and host inflammatory cells, and there is a mural thrombus on the outflow surface in (C). All stained with Verhoff van Geisen for elastin, each 100X.

Despite the wide use of the Ross procedure, the structural features, cell viability, and extracellular matrix (ECM) remodeling of pulmonary autograft (PA) valves have not been described. We have studied pulmonary autografts in place for 15 days to 6 years (E Rabkin, FJ Schoen, unpublished data). The pulmonary autograft cusps showed (1) near-normal trilaminar structure, (2) near-normal collagen architecture, (3) viable endothelium and interstitial cells, (4) usual outflow surface corrugations, (5) sparse inflammatory cells, and (6) absence of calcification and thrombus. They often also had an irregular layer of intimal thickening (up to 1 mm), particularly on the ventricular aspect. Long-term explants were markedly hypercellular. Interstitial cells of short-term explants were largely myofibroblasts of vimentin/α-actin phenotype and showed strong metalloproteinase (in the form of MMP-13) activity indicative of active collagen remodeling (likely due to mechanical adaptation). In contrast, long-term explants were stained predominantly for vimentin and had weaker expression of MMP-13, resembling quiescent fibroblast-like cells of normal valves. It remains unknown whether the cuspal changes represent adaptation to the altered mechanical or other conditions of the aortic site or a response to injury engendered by the procedure. The arterial walls showed considerable transmural damage (probably ischemic injury caused by disruption of vasa vasorum) with scaring and loss of medial SMC and elastin. Thus, pulmonary autograft valve cusps undergo early remodeling but maintain remarkably preserved semilunar valve morphology, cell viability, and collagen microstructure up to 6 years. The early necrosis and healing with probable resultant loss of strength/elasticity of the "new" aortic wall may potentiate late dilation.

STENTLESS PORCINE AORTIC VALVE BIOPROSTHESES

Nonstented (stentless) porcine aortic valve bioprostheses comprise glutaraldehyde-pretreated pig aortic root and valve cusps that have no supporting stent. Two such models were approved by the U.S. FDA in 1997 for insertion into the aortic site: St. Jude Medical Toronto SPV (St. Jude Medical Inc., St. Paul, MN) and Medtronic Freestyle (Medtronic Heart Valves, Santa Ana, CA) bioprostheses.[286,287] They differ slightly in overall configuration (particularly the amount of aortic wall included), details of glutaraldehyde pretreatment conditions, and overall fabrication, and whether anticalcification technology is used (the FreeStyle valve is treated with 2-amino-oleic acid [AOA]). Other variants of this concept are also in clinical trials.[288] The principal advantage of a stentless porcine aortic valve is that it allows for the implantation of a larger bioprosthesis (than stented) in any given aortic root, which may enhance hemodynamics and thereby ventricular remodeling and patient survival.[289]

The potential and observed complications with nonstented bioprostheses are comparable to those of stented valves. However, nonstented porcine aortic valves have greater portions of aortic wall exposed to blood than in currently used stented valves, and calcification of the aortic wall is potentially deleterious. Indeed, allograft valved conduits frequently fail because of calcific stenosis, with prominent deposits in the wall.[290] Calcification of the wall portion of a stentless valve could stiffen the root, altering hemodynamic efficiency; cause nodular calcific obstruction or wall rupture; or provide a nidus for emboli. Important in this respect is the observation that some anticalcification agents (see below), including AOA and ethanol, prevent experimental cuspal but not aortic wall calcification. In an initial pathology analysis of nonstented valves, aortic wall calcification was not a problem.[291]

NEW DEVELOPMENTS

Methods are being actively studied and some are being used clinically to prevent calcification in bioprosthetic valves.[292–296] Other approaches to provide improved valves include modifications of bioprosthetic valve stent design and tissue-mounting techniques to reduce cuspal stresses, tissue treatment alternatives to glutaraldehyde to enhance durability and postimplantation biocompatibility, nonstented porcine valves, minimally cross-linked autologous pericardial valves, flexible trileaflet polymeric (polyurethane) prostheses, and mechanical and tissue valves with novel design features to improve hemodynamics, enhance durability, and reduce thromboembolism.

MYOCARDIAL DISEASE

Two broad categories of myocardial disease are distinguished: primary or idiopathic cardiomyopathy, defined as heart muscle disease of unknown cause, and specific cardiomyopathy, defined as heart muscle disease of known cause or associated with disorders of other systems.[297,298] Myocardial dysfunction also frequently occurs as a complication of ischemic, valvular, hypertensive (systemic and pulmonary), and congenital heart disease and some pericardial disease, through hypertrophy and subsequent degenerative changes and/or ischemic damage. Impairment of ventricular performance in the setting of coronary atherosclerosis often is called ischemic cardiomyopathy.

There are three functional/pathophysiologic/anatomic patterns: dilated, hypertrophic, and restrictive. The cause of a specific cardiomyopathy is often revealed by light and/or electron microscopic examination, whereas the morphology is nonspecifically abnormal in idiopathic cardiomyopathy. Moreover, in idiopathic dilated cardiomyopathy, the severity of the morphologic changes does not necessarily correlate with the severity of dysfunction or the patient's prognosis. The understanding and potential treatment of myocardial disease have advanced substantially over the last decade as a result of genetic studies and their correlations with clinical features.[299–302]

Endomyocardial biopsy is used in the diagnosis and management of patients with myocardial disease and in the ongoing surveillance of cardiac transplant recipients.[303] The bioptome, inserted into the right internal jugular or femoral vein and advanced under fluoroscopic or echocardiographic guidance through the tricuspid valve, obtains 1- to 3-mm fragments of endomyocardium, most frequently from the apical half of the right side of the ventricular septum. Interpretation of right-sided biopsy specimens assumes that this location produces representative pathology. Since most myocardial diseases affect both ventricles, correlation between right- and left-sided findings generally is good.

Cardiomyopathy

The most common variants of cardiomyopathy are the dilated and hypertrophic types. Both are illustrated in Figure 5-30.

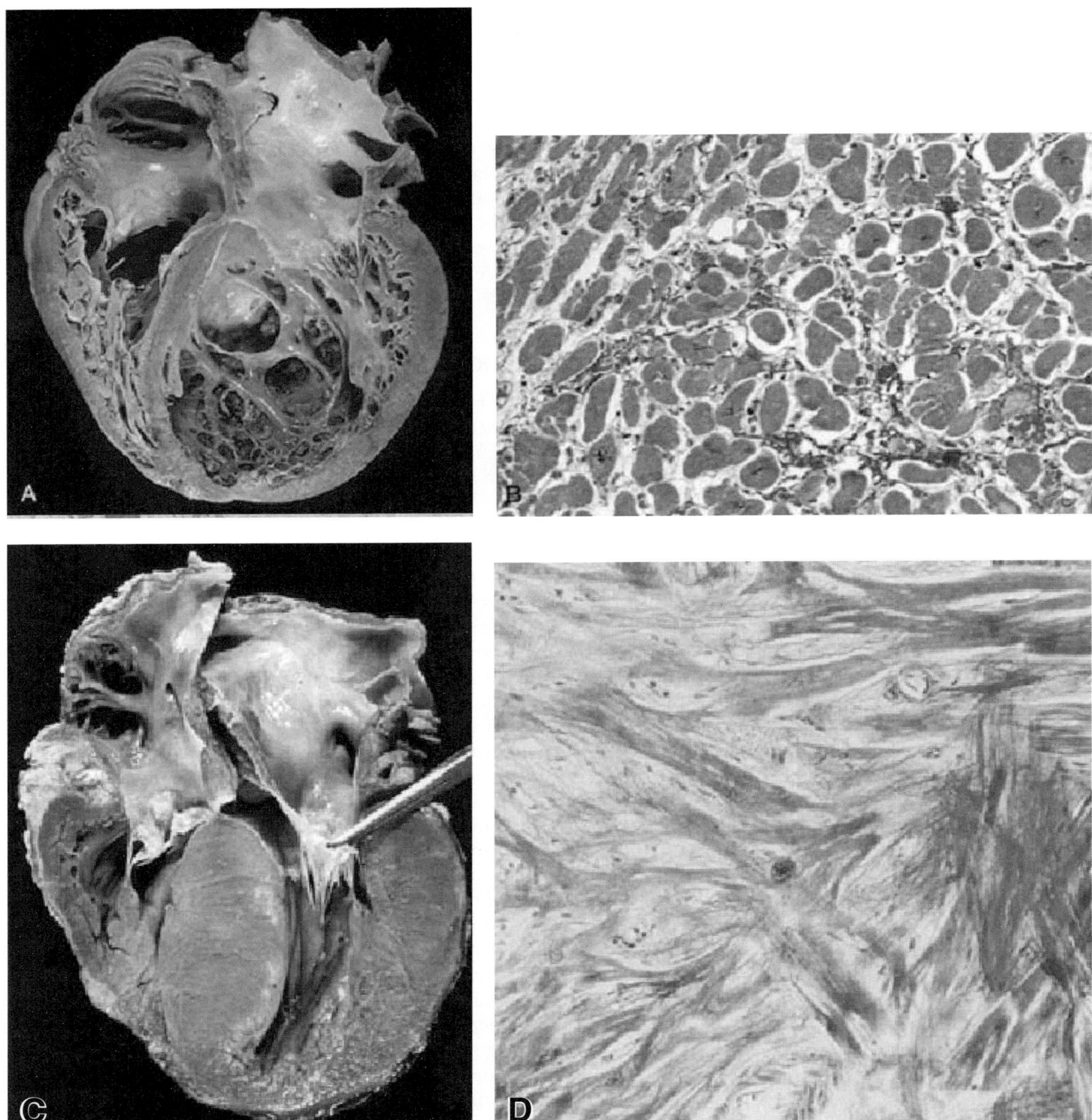

FIGURE 5–30 Cardiomyopathy. (A) and (B) Dilated cardiomyopathy. (A) Gross photo showing four-chamber dilation and hypertrophy. There is granular mural thrombus at the apex of the left ventricle (on the right in this apical four-chamber view). The coronary arteries were unobstructed. (B) Histology, demonstrating irregular hypertrophy and interstitial fibrosis. (C) and (D) Hypertrophic cardiomyopathy with asymmetric septal hypertrophy. (C) Gross photo. The septal muscle bulges into the left ventricular outflow tract, and the left atrium is enlarged. The anterior mitral leaflet has been moved away from the septum to reveal a fibrous endocardial plaque (see text). (D) Histologic appearance demonstrating disarray, extreme hypertrophy, peculiar branching of myocytes, and interstitial fibrosis characteristic of hypertrophic cardiomyopathy. *(Reproduced with permission from Schoen FJ, Interventional and Surgical Cardiovascular Pathology: Clinical Correlations and Basic Principles. Philadelphia, W.B. Saunders, 1989, and Schoen FJ: The heart, in Cotran RS, Kumar V, Collins T (eds): Pathologic Basis of Disease, WB Saunders, 1999; p 543.)*

DILATED CARDIOMYOPATHY

Dilated cardiomyopathy is characterized by hypertrophy, dilation, and systolic ventricular dysfunction. Dilated cardiomyopathy has a familial basis in approximately 30% to 40% of cases, with autosomal dominant (most common), autosomal recessive, and X-linked and mitochondrial inheritance all described.[300,301,304] Mutations in several different genes can cause autosomal dominant dilated cardiomyopathy, including the cytoskeletal protein-encoding genes β- and δ-sarcoglycan, dystrophin, and lamin A/C, as well as the sarcomeric protein-encoding genes actin, β-myosin heavy chain, cardiac troponin T, and α-tropomyosin. These mutations are thought to cause disease through force transmission abnormalities leading to reduced force generation by the cardiac myocytes. A history of chronic alcoholism can be elicited in 20% of patients, and biopsy-proven myocarditis precedes the development of cardiomyopathy in 5% to 10%. Pregnancy-associated nutritional deficiency or immunologic reaction is another possible contributory factor.

The primary functional abnormality in dilated cardiomyopathy is impairment of left ventricular systolic function, as measured by the ejection fraction (<25% in end-stage, normal approximately 50% to 65%). Pathologic findings include cardiomegaly with heart weight two to three times normal and four-chamber dilation (see Fig. 5-30A). Cardiac mural thrombi, a potential source of thromboemboli, are sometimes present and predominate in the left ventricle but may occur in any chamber. The histologic changes comprise myocyte hypertrophy and interstitial and endocardial fibrosis of variable degree, but they do not reflect an etiologic agent (see Fig. 5-20B). Moreover, the myocardial histology in dilated cardiomyopathy is indistinguishable from that in myocardial failure secondary to ischemic or valvular heart disease.

A recently described variant of dilated cardiomyopathy is arrhythmogenic right ventricular cardiomyopathy, characterized by a severely thinned right ventricular wall, with extensive fatty infiltration, loss of myocytes with compensatory myocyte hypertrophy, and interstitial fibrosis.[300,305–307] Sometimes familial, this disorder is most commonly associated with right-sided and sometimes left-sided heart failure and various rhythm disturbances, particularly ventricular tachycardia and sudden death.[308]

HYPERTROPHIC CARDIOMYOPATHY

Hypertrophic cardiomyopathy is characterized by a heavy, muscular, hypercontracting heart, in striking contrast to the flabby, hypocontracting heart of dilated cardiomyopathy. It represents a diastolic, rather than systolic, disorder.

The essential anatomic feature of hypertrophic cardiomyopathy is massive myocardial hypertrophy without dilation (see Fig. 5-30A).[309] The classic pattern is characterized by disproportionate thickening of the ventricular septum relative to the free wall of the left ventricle (ratio >1.5), termed asymmetric septal hypertrophy, and is usually localized to the subaortic region. When the basal septum is markedly thickened at the level of the mitral valve, the outflow of the left ventricle may be narrowed during systole. Endocardial thickening in the left ventricular outflow tract and thickening of the anterior mitral leaflet result from contact between the two during ventricular systole (observed by echocardiography as systolic anterior motion of the mitral valve), correlating with systolic left ventricular outflow tract obstruction. In about 10% of cases, left ventricular hypertrophy is symmetric, and in other cases disproportionate hypertrophy involves the midventricular or apical septum, extends onto the left ventricular free wall anteriorly or inferiorly, or causes right ventricular outflow tract obstruction.

The most important microscopic features in hypertrophic cardiomyopathy include: (1) disarray of myocytes and contractile elements within cells (myofiber disarray) typically involving 10% to 50% of the septum; (2) extreme myocyte hypertrophy, with transverse myocyte diameters frequently more than 40 μm (normal approximately 15–20 μm); and (3) interstitial and replacement fibrosis (see Fig. 5-30D).

Hypertrophic cardiomyopathy has an extremely variable course, with potential complications including atrial fibrillation with mural thrombus formation and embolization, infective endocarditis of the mitral valve, intractable cardiac failure, and sudden death. Sudden death occurs in approximately 2% to 3% of adults and 4% to 6% of children per year, is the most common cause of death from hypertrophic cardiomyopathy, and is particularly common in young males with familial hypertrophic cardiomyopathy or a family history of sudden death. The risk is related to the degree of hypertrophy.[310,311] Cardiac failure from hypertrophic cardiomyopathy results from reduced stroke volume due to decreased diastolic filling of the massively hypertrophied left ventricle. Although symptoms are not solely a result of ventricular septal thickening, some patients benefit from thinning of the septum by surgical myotomy/myectomy.[312,313] More recently, the technique of chemical septal ablation appears to be a safe and effective procedure, with hemodynamic and functional improvement.[314,315] End-stage heart failure can be accompanied by dilation, for which cardiac transplantation may be recommended.

Hypertrophic cardiomyopathy has a genetic basis in most cases.[300–302,309,312,316] In approximately half or more of patients the disease is familial, and the pattern of transmission is autosomal dominant with variable expression; remaining cases appear to be sporadic. Various mutations have been identified in hypertrophic cardiomyopathy; all are genes for sarcomeric proteins including β-myosin heavy chain, troponin T and I, α-tropomyosin, and titin. The mechanism by which defective sarcomeric proteins produce the phenotype of hypertrophic cardiomyopathy is uncertain. Therefore, cardiac hypertrophy in HCM is likely a "compensatory" phenotype due to increased cardiac myocyte stress or altered Ca^{2+} sensitivity of the contractile apparatus imparted by the mutant contractile proteins. Accordingly, increased myocyte stress leads to expression of a variety of cardiac genes that activate the transcription machinery leading to hypertrophy and other phenotypes of HCM. This would suggest that the pathogenesis of hypertrophy, a common programmed response of the myocardium to any form of stress, whether caused by a genetic defect or by an acquired condition, involves common pathways. Interestingly, different responsible gene mutations carry vastly differing prognoses, and certain genetic defects indicate a relatively high likelihood of sudden death.[317]

RESTRICTIVE CARDIOMYOPATHY

Restrictive cardiomyopathy is characterized by impeded diastolic relaxation and left ventricular filling, with systolic function often unaffected. Any disorder that interferes with ventricular filling can cause restrictive cardiomyopathy (including eosinophilic endomyocardial disease, amyloidosis, hemochromatosis, or postirradiation fibrosis) or mimic it (constrictive pericarditis or hypertrophic cardiomyopathy). Morphologically, the ventricles are of approximately normal size or slightly enlarged, but the cavities are not dilated and the myocardium is firm. Biatrial dilation commonly is observed. Distinct morphologic patterns indicative of specific heart muscle disease may be revealed by light or electron microscopy of endomyocardial biopsy specimens, including deposition of amyloid or of products of an inborn error of metabolism such as trihexosylceramide in Fabry disease.[318]

Cardiac Transplantation

Cardiac transplantation provides long-term survival and rehabilitation for many individuals with end-stage cardiac failure.[319] Overall predicted 1-year survival is presently approximately 86% and 5-year survival is about 70%.[320] The most common indications for cardiac transplantation, accounting for 90% of the patients, are idiopathic cardiomyopathy and end-stage ischemic heart disease; other recipients have congenital, other myocardial, or valvular heart disease.[321,322]

Hearts explanted at the time of transplantation typically have the expected pathologic features of the underlying diseases. However, previously undiagnosed conditions and unexpected findings may be encountered. Most frequent is eosinophilic or hypersensitivity myocarditis, seen in approximately 20% of explants and characterized by a focal or diffuse mixed inflammatory infiltrate, rich in eosinophils, and generally associated with minimal associated myocyte necrosis.[323,324] In virtually all cases, the myocarditis represents hypersensitivity to one or more of the many drugs taken by transplant candidates, including dobutamine, and is unrelated to but superimposed on the original disease necessitating transplantation. Several diseases responsible for the original cardiac failure can recur in and cause dysfunction of the allograft, including amyloidosis, sarcoidosis, giant-cell myocarditis, acute rheumatic carditis, and Chagas' disease.[321,322,325]

Recipients of heart transplants undergo surveillance endomyocardial biopsies according to an institution-specific schedule, which typically evolves from weekly during the early postoperative period, to twice weekly until 3 to 6 months, and then approximately two to four times annually following 1 year, or at any time when there is a change in clinical state. Histologic findings of rejection frequently precede clinical signs and symptoms of acute rejection. Optimal biopsy interpretation requires four or more pieces of myocardial tissue; reviews of technical details and artifacts are available.[321,322,326]

The major sources of mortality and morbidity following cardiac transplantation are perioperative ischemic injury, infection, allograft rejection, lymphoproliferative disease, and obstructive graft vasculopathy. A particularly interesting recent finding is that of recipient cells that have migrated (presumably from the bone marrow) to the donor heart.[327] The significance of these cells is yet unknown.

EARLY ISCHEMIC INJURY

Ischemic injury can originate in the unavoidable ischemia that accompanies procurement and implantation of the donor heart. Several time intervals are potentially important: (1) the donor interval between brain death and heart removal, perhaps partially related to terminal administration of pressor agents or the release of norepinephrine and cytokines associated with brain death; (2) the interval of warm ischemia between donor cardiectomy to cold storage; (3) the interval during cold transport; and (4) the interval during warming, trimming, and reimplantation, or some combination of these. Existing hypertrophy and coronary obstructions tend to enhance injury, whereas decreased tissue temperature and cardioplegic arrest slow chemical reactions and thereby protect myocytes from progressive ischemic damage. However, when the heart is not filled with oxygenated blood during transport, the subendocardial myocytes normally perfused from the lumen are especially vulnerable to ischemic injury. As in other situations of transient myocardial ischemia, frank necrosis or prolonged ischemic dysfunction of viable myocardium or both may be present. Massive myocardial injury can cause potentially fatal low cardiac output in the perioperative period.

Perioperative myocardial ischemic injury as diagnosed by conventional histologic criteria is prevalent in endomyocardial biopsies early after heart transplantation.[322,328,329] The histologic progression of healing of myocardial necroses in transplanted hearts, as noted on subsequent endomyocardial

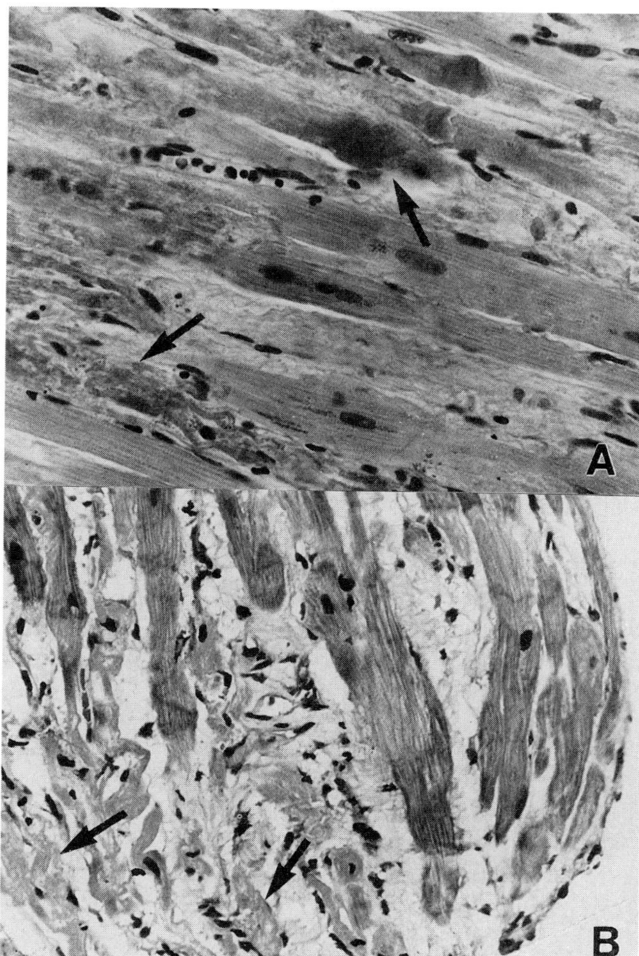

FIGURE 5–31 Perioperative ischemic myocardial injury demonstrated on endomyocardial biopsy. (A) Coagulative myocyte necrosis (arrows). (B) Healing perioperative ischemic injury with predominantly interstitial inflammatory response (arrows), not encroaching on and clearly separated from adjacent viable myocytes. The infiltrate consists of a mixture of polymorphonuclear leukocytes, macrophages, lymphocytes, and plasma cells. Hematoxylin and eosin 200X. (*Reproduced with permission from Schoen FJ: Interventional and Surgical Cardiovascular Pathology: Clinical Correlations and Basic Principles. Philadelphia, WB Saunders, 1989.*)

biopsies, is prolonged and the cellular infiltrate may be distorted owing to the anti-inflammatory effects of immunosuppressive therapy (Fig. 5-31). Therefore, the repair phase of perioperative myocardial necrosis frequently confounds the diagnosis of rejection in the first postoperative month, and in some cases, for as long as 6 weeks. In contrast, ischemic necrosis noted 3 to 6 months postoperatively is usually secondary to occlusive graft vasculopathy. It remains to be determined whether and to what degree early ischemic injury has a late impact on allograft dysfunction, possibly through loss of myocytes, accumulation of fibrosis, potentiation of rejection, or stimulation of graft vasculopathy.

REJECTION

Improved immunosuppressive regimens in heart transplant patients have substantially decreased the incidence of serious rejection episodes. Nonetheless, rejection phenomena still cause cardiac failure or serious arrhythmias in some patients. Hyperacute rejection occurs rarely, most often when a major blood group incompatibility exists between donor and recipient, and acute rejection is unusual earlier than 2 to 4 weeks postoperatively. Acute rejection episodes occur largely but not exclusively in the first several months after transplantation. However, since rejection can occur years postoperatively, many transplant centers continue late surveillance biopsies at widely spaced intervals.[330]

The histologic features of acute rejection are an inflammatory cell infiltrate, with or without damage to cardiac myocytes; in late stages, vascular injury may become prominent (Fig. 5-32). The International Society for Heart and Lung Transplantation (ISHLT) working formulation, illustrated in Figure 5-33, is most widely accepted and used to guide immunosuppressive therapy in heart transplant recipients.[331,332] In this grading system, grade 0 represents no evidence of rejection or healed rejection. Mild rejection (ISHLT grades 1A and 1B) is characterized by a focal or diffuse, respectively, mild perivascular (or interstitial) lymphocytic infiltrate without myocyte damage. Lymphocytic inflammatory infiltrates with associated myocyte encroachment or damage, generally called moderate rejection, can be limited to a single focus (ISHLT grade 2), present in a multifocal pattern (ISHLT grade 3A), or distributed diffusely (ISHLT grade 3B). In severe rejection (ISHLT grade 4), myocyte necrosis is more evident, there is often patchy interstitial hemorrhage owing to vascular damage, and vasculitis (usually arteriolitis) may be prominent. The increased inflammatory infiltrate often also includes neutrophils or eosinophils, presumably in response to myocyte necrosis or vascular damage.

Immunosuppressive protocols and the threshold for treatment of histologic rejection vary greatly among heart transplant centers (Table 5-4); in particular, the clinical significance of mild to moderate rejection is controversial.[333,334] ISHLT grades 1A, 1B, and 2 have been shown to resolve without specific change in management in over 80% of cases and, therefore, these levels of rejection remain untreated in many (but not all) heart transplant centers.[333] Progression of lower rejection grades to advanced rejection on subsequent biopsies becomes less likely with increasing postoperative interval, and is especially unusual beyond 2 years (Fig. 5-34).[333,334]

Other important findings in surveillance endomyocardial biopsies that must be distinguished from rejection, but probably have no independent clinical significance, include lymphoid infiltrates either confined to the endocardium or extending into the underlying myocardium and often accompanied by myocyte damage (Quilty A or B lesions,

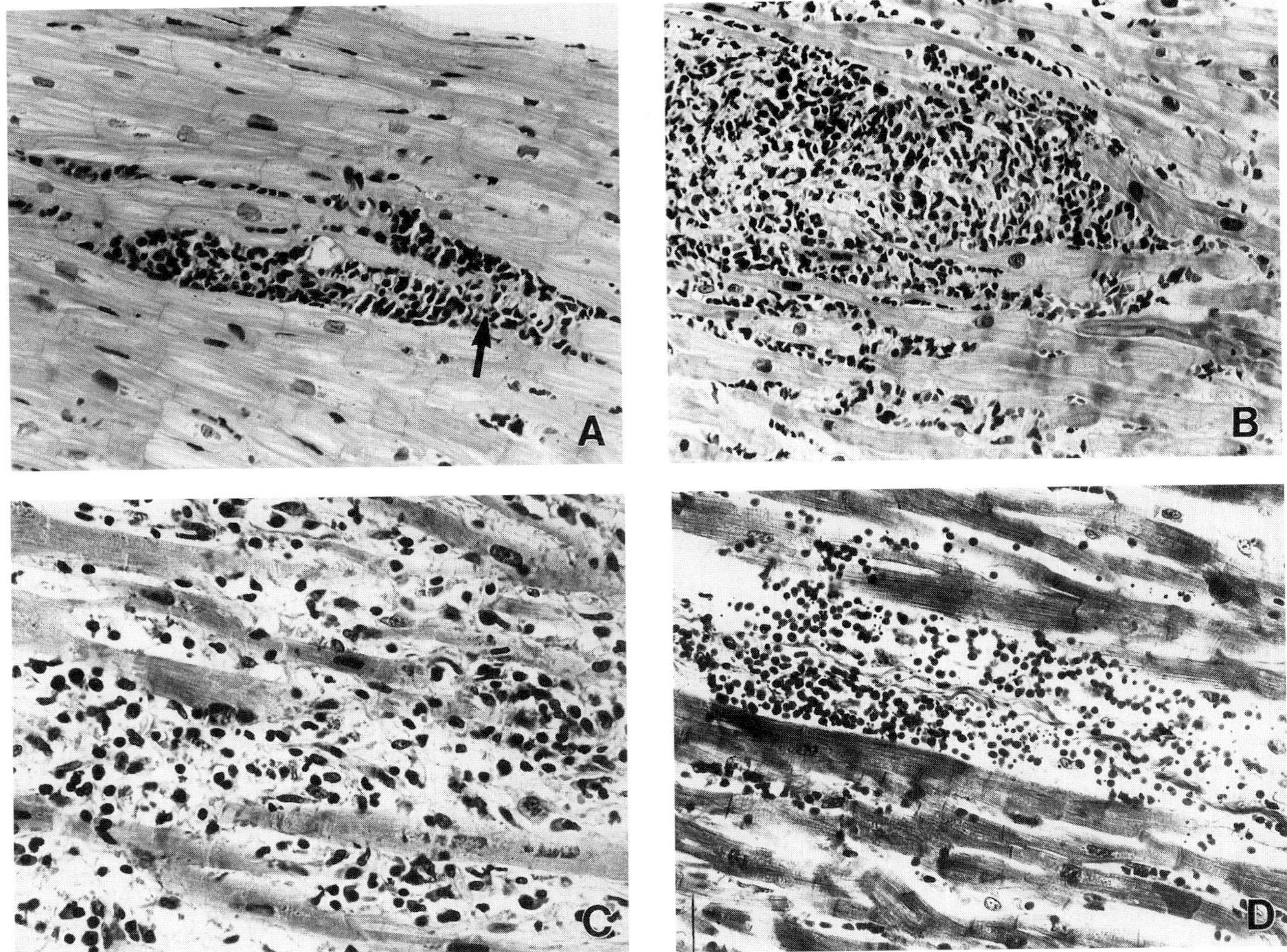

FIGURE 5–32 Histologic features of rejection. (A) Focal moderate rejection with necrosis. The area of myocyte necrosis is indicated by an arrow. (B) More intense focus of inflammatory infiltrate, with large focus of myocyte necrosis. (C) Fatal rejection with extensive infiltrate and myocyte necrosis. (D) Fatal rejection with widespread myocardial hemorrhage and edema. Hematoxylin and eosin 375X. *(Reproduced by permission from Schoen FJ: Interventional and Surgical Cardiovascular Pathology: Clinical Correlations and Basic Principles. Philadelphia, WB Saunders, 1989.)*

respectively), and healing previous biopsy sites. Lymphoproliferative disorders and infections may also be seen in biopsies.

Apoptosis of myocytes occurs during rejection, with its prevalence paralleling the severity of rejection. The intensity of cellular infiltration correlates with the degree of apoptosis, which may be mediated by NO-dependent mechanisms. Apoptosis of other donor cells, including interstitial and endothelial cells, may influence the degree of vascular injury contributing to a deterioration of the transplant.[335]

INFECTION

The immunosuppressive therapy required in all heart transplant recipients confers an increased risk of infection with bacterial, fungal, protozoan, and viral pathogens, with cytomegalovirus (CMV) and *Toxoplasma gondii* remaining the most common opportunistic infections. Prophylaxis in the form of oral gancyclovir is typically given to patients at high risk of primary CMV infection (donor seropositive, recipient seronegative). Viral and parasitic infections can present a challenge in endomyocardial biopsies as the multifocal lymphocytic infiltrates with occasional necrosis seen with these infections can mimic rejection.

GRAFT VASCULOPATHY (GRAFT CORONARY ARTERIOSCLEROSIS)

Graft vasculopathy is the major limitation to long-term graft and recipient survival following heart

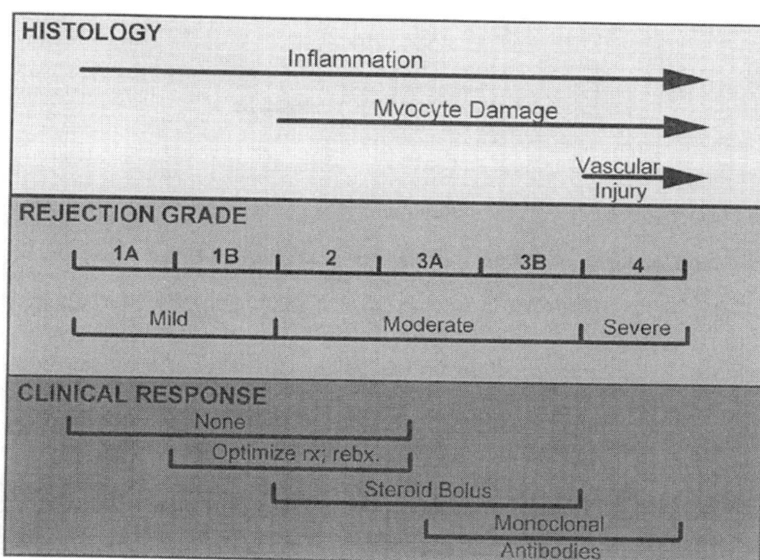

FIGURE 5–33 Comparison of histology with rejection grade and clinical response. In general, increasing grades of rejection represent increasing amounts and severity of inflammation and myocyte damage. There is great variation among transplant centers in the clinical response to rejection grades. That response is most uniform at both ends of the spectrum; i.e., grades 0 and 1A are generally not treated; grades 3B and 4 are treated aggressively with augmented immunosuppression. Variation occurs most frequently in response to intermediate grades such as grade 2. rx = therapy; rebx = rebiopsy. *(Reproduced with permission from Winters GL, Schoen FJ: Pathology of cardiac transplantation, in Silver MD, Gotlieb AI, Schoen FJ (eds): Cardiovascular Pathology, 3d ed. Churchill Livingstone, 2001; p 725.)*

transplantation.[321,322,325,336,337] Up to 50% of recipients have angiographically evident disease 5 years after transplantation.[338,339] However, graft vasculopathy may become significant at any time and can progress at variable rates. Nearly half of our posttransplant deaths owing to graft coronary disease at the Brigham and Women's Hospital have occurred within 6 to 12 months postoperatively.[340]

Graft vasculopathy (Fig. 5-35) represents a diffuse process that begins in small distal vessels and ultimately involves both intramyocardial and epicardial allograft vessels, leading to myocardial infarction, arrhythmias, congestive heart failure, or sudden death.[321,322,326,341] Although this process has been called accelerated atherosclerosis, the morphology of the obstructive lesion of graft vasculopathy is distinctive in comparison to typical atherosclerosis (Table 5-5).[342,343] The vessels involved have concentric occlusions characterized by marked intimal proliferation of myofibroblasts and smooth muscle cells with deposition of collagen, ground substance, and lipid. Lymphocytic infiltration varies from almost none to quite prominent, with the lymphocytes often noted in a subendothelial location. The internal elastic lamina often is almost completely intact, with only focal fragmentation. The resulting myocardial pathology includes subendocardial myocyte vacuolization (indicative of sublethal ischemic injury) and myocardial coagulation necrosis (indicative of infarction).

Although the precise mechanisms of graft vasculopathy are not definitely established, there is mounting evidence that graft vasculopathy is caused by both chronic allogenic immune response to the transplant and nonimmunologic factors that contribute to vascular injury. Endothelial injury, both cell-mediated and humoral, is likely the initiating event; endothelial cell dysfunction precedes the angiographic manifestations of graft vasculopathy. Alloreactive T-cells, activated by MHC class II molecules on donor endothelium, secrete cytokines that amplify the immune

TABLE 5–4 Typical paradigm for clinical response to surveillance endomyocardial biopsy results following cardiac transplantation*

Histologic	Descriptive rejection level	Clinical response
No infiltrate or infiltrate without myocyte damage	No/mild rejection	No response
Infiltrate with myocyte damage (one or few sites)	(Low) moderate rejection	Adjustment of maintenance immunosuppression and early biopsy and/or bolus immunotherapy**
Multifocal infiltrate with myocyte damage	(High) moderate rejection	Bolus immunotherapy**
Widespread inflammation/myocyte injury/vascular injury	Severe rejection	Antibody therapy

*In patients without hemodynamic compromise or clinical change and potentially influenced by postoperative interval, intensity, and extent of rejection activity on previous biopsy; maintenance immunosuppression regimen; nature, duration, and interval since completion of previous treatment; previous biopsy history, treatment regimens, and response; complications of immunosuppression, including toxicity; and cyclosporine serum levels.

**Usually with corticosteroids.

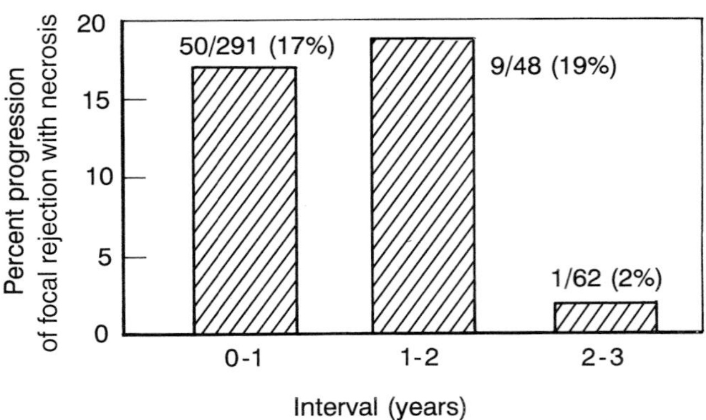

FIGURE 5–34 Relationship between posttransplant interval and outcome as probability of progression of an ISHLT grade 2 rejection diagnosed by endomyocardial biopsy. The probability of progression decreased markedly beyond 2 years postoperatively. *(Data from Winters GL, Loh E, Schoen FJ: Natural history of focal moderate cardiac allograft rejection: is treatment warranted? Circulation 1995;91:1975.)*

TABLE 5–5 Characteristics of graft arteriosclerosis versus typical atherosclerosis

Graft arteriosclerosis	Typical atherosclerosis
Rapid onset (mo-y)	Slow onset (many years)
Risk factors uncertain	Hypertension, lipids, smoking, etc.
Usually silent/congestive heart failure, sudden death	Chest pain, etc.
Diffuse	Focal
Epicardial/intramural	Epicardial
Concentric	Eccentric
Lesions rarely complicated	Lesions often complicated
Smooth muscle cells, macrophages, lymphocytes	Smooth muscle cells, macrophages, foam cells
Primary immunologic mechanism(s)	Complicated stimuli
Difficult to treat; retransplant usually only option	Revascularization by angioplasty, aortocoronary bypass

Source: Reproduced with permission from Schoen FJ, Libby P: Cardiac transplant graft arteriosclerosis. Trends Cardiovasc Med 1991; 1:216.

response and result in upregulation of endothelial cell adhesion molecules, leading to accumulation of macrophages in the vessel wall and a localized, sustained inflammatory response. Activated macrophages, foam cells that have taken up oxidized LDL, and lymphocytes express cytokines and growth factors such as PDGF, FGF, and TGF-β that promote proliferation of smooth muscle and myofibroblast and extracellular matrix synthesis. Hyperlipidemia, specifically high levels of oxidized LDL, can predict the development of graft vasculopathy. Advanced donor age, CMV infection, perioperative graft ischemia, and diabetes have been associated with graft vasculopathy, but their roles in the evolution of the disease remain uncertain. There is no apparent difference in the frequency with which graft vasculopathy

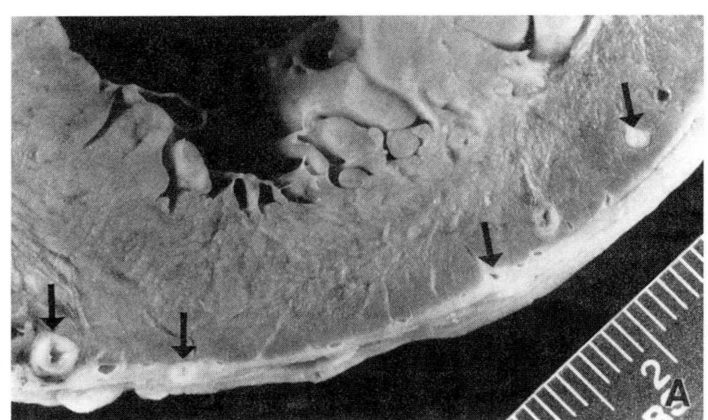

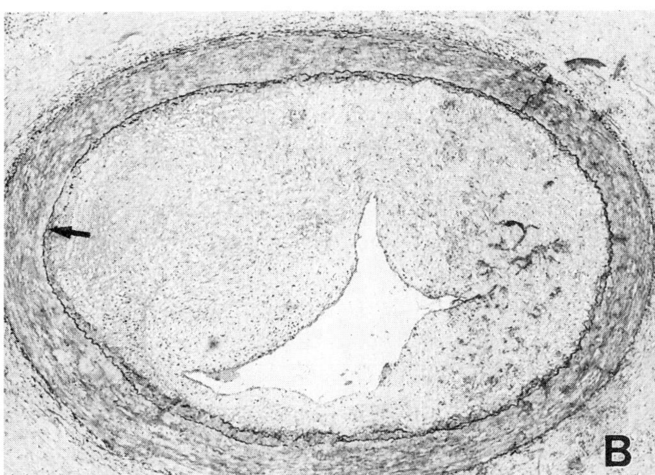

FIGURE 5–35 Gross and microscopic features of graft coronary disease. (A) Gross photograph of transverse cross-section of heart from patient who died of graft arteriosclerosis. Severe concentric stenosis of epicardial and large intramural coronaries is apparent (arrows). (B) Histologic appearance of graft arteriosclerosis as low-power photomicrograph of vessel cross section, demonstrating severe, near-complete, and predominantly concentric intimal proliferation with nearly intact internal elastic lamina (arrow). Verhoff-van Gieson stain (for elastin) 60X. *(A: Reproduced with permission from Schoen FJ, Libby P: Cardiac transplant graft arteriosclerosis. Trends Cardiovasc Med 1991; 1:216. B: Reproduced with permission from Schoen FJ: Interventional and Surgical Cardiovascular Pathology: Clinical Correlations and Basic Principles. Philadelphia, WB Saunders, 1989.)*

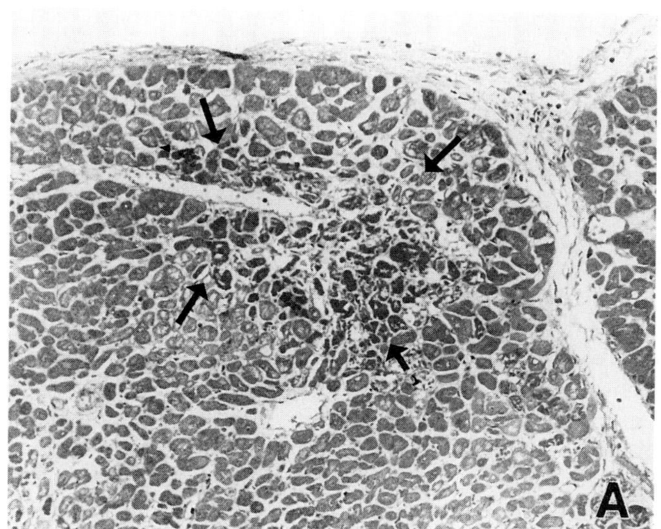

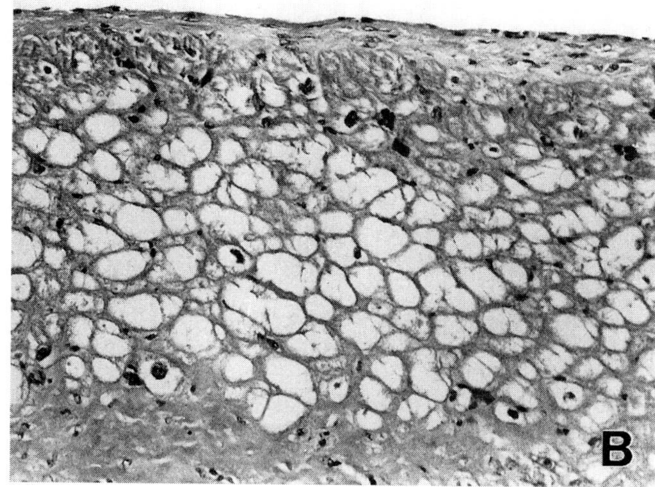

FIGURE 5–36 Graft arteriosclerosis–induced myocardial pathology in heart transplant recipients: (A) Myocardial microinfarct indicative of disease of small intramural arteries (outlined by arrows) and (B) subendocardial myocyte vacuolization indicative of severe chronic ischemia. Hematoxylin and eosin, 375X.

develops in patients who were transplanted for end-stage coronary artery disease and those operated for idiopathic cardiomyopathy. Recent studies suggest that the intimal cells present in the intima in graft arteriosclerosis may be at least partially derived from the bone marrow of the recipient.[344] Interestingly, cells from the donor are also found in the myocardium and resemble cardiac myocytes.

Early diagnosis of graft vasculopathy is limited by the lack of clinical symptoms of ischemia in the denervated allograft, by the relative insensitivity of coronary angiography, which frequently underestimates the extent and severity of this diffuse disease, and by the exclusive or predominant involvement of small intramyocardial vessels. Histologic changes of chronic ischemia such as subendothelial myocyte vacuolization can be seen on surveillance biopsies and may suggest graft vasculopathy (Fig. 5-36). Coronary angiography is nevertheless performed for diagnosis and surveillance purposes and the presence of angiographically detectable disease is of prognostic relevance. Intravascular ultrasound (IVUS) allows exact delineation of vessel wall morphology and quantification of intimal thickness and vascular dimensions. The presence of severe intimal thickening by IVUS predicts cardiac events and early death in transplant recipients.[346] Although not usually amenable to angioplasty, endarterectomy, or coronary artery bypass grafting because of their diffuse distribution, stenoses may be alleviated by these procedures in occasional cases. Pharmacologic therapy aimed at preventing disease progression with calcium antagonists, ACE inhibitors, and HMG-CoA reductase inhibitors has shown some benefit. For most cases, however, retransplantation is the only effective therapy for established graft atherosclerosis.

POSTTRANSPLANT LYMPHOPROLIFERATIVE DISORDERS

Posttransplant lymphoproliferative disorders (PTLDs) are a well-recognized complication of the high-intensity long-term immunosuppressive therapy required to prevent rejection in cardiac allografts. Several factors increase the risk of developing PTLD, including pretransplant Epstein-Barr virus (EBV) seronegativity (10- to 75-fold increase), young recipient age, and cytomegalovirus infection or mismatching (donor-positive, recipient-negative).[347,348] The incidence of PTLD in cardiac transplant recipients is approximately 3%, and the mortality can be as high as 80%.[349]

PTLDs can present as an infectious mononucleosis-like illness or with localized solid tumor masses, especially in extranodal sites (e.g., heart, lungs, gastrointestinal tract). The vast majority (>90%) of PTLDs derive from the B-cell lineage and are associated with EBV infection, although T- or NK-cell origin and late-arising EBV-negative lymphoid malignancies have been described. There is strong evidence that the lesions progress from polyclonal B-cell hyperplasias ("early lesions") to lymphomas ("monomorphic PTLDs") in a short period of time, in association with the appearance of cytogenetic abnormalities.[350] Therapy centers on a stepwise approach of antiviral treatment and reduction of immunosuppression, and then progression to lymphoma chemotherapy. Monoclonal antibodies (rituximab) against the B-cell marker CD20 have yielded impressive initial results and may become an important component of PTLD therapy.[351] As the understanding of the risk factors and pathogenesis of PTLDs has expanded, preemptive or prophylactic therapies may help prevent this complication of transplantation.

CARDIAC ASSIST AND MECHANICAL REPLACEMENT

Continuing and increasing discrepancy between the number of available donor hearts (less than 3000 per year)[352,353] and the number of patients who might benefit from cardiac transplantation (estimated 30,000 to 100,000 per year)[354] has prompted efforts in the development of ventricular assist devices (VADs), total artificial hearts, and cardiomyoplasty techniques.[355,356] These areas are briefly reviewed in the following sections, from the perspective of cardiac pathology.

Cardiac Assist Devices and Total Artificial Hearts

First employed successfully by DeBakey in 1963, mechanical cardiac assist devices and artificial hearts have traditionally been used in two settings: for ventricular augmentation sufficient to permit a patient to survive postcardiotomy or postinfarction cardiogenic shock while ventricular recovery is occurring, and as a bridge to transplantation when ventricular recovery is not expected and the goal is hemodynamic support until a suitable donor organ is located.[357–359] More recently, left ventricular assist devices (LVADs) have been shown to provide long-term cardiac support with survival and quality-of-life improvement over optimal medical therapy in patients with end-stage congestive heart failure who are not candidates for transplantation.[360] LVADs are also being investigated as a "bridge-to-recovery" in patients with congestive heart failure to induce reverse ventricular remodeling leading to an improvement in cardiac function that would eventually allow device removal. The first total artificial heart implants in the United States since the mid-1980s are currently being evaluated (AbioCor, ABIOMED Corp.).[361]

The major complications of cardiac assist devices are hemorrhage, thrombosis/thromboembolism, and infection (Fig. 5-37).[362–367] Hemorrhage continues to be a problem in device recipients, although the risk of major hemorrhage has been decreasing with improved therapies and methods. Many factors predispose to perioperative hemorrhage including: (1) coagulopathy secondary to hepatic dysfunction, poor nutritional status, and antibiotic therapy; (2) platelet dysfunction and thrombocytopenia secondary to cardiopulmonary bypass; and (3) the extensive nature of the required surgery.

Nonthrombogenic blood-contacting surfaces are essential for a clinically useful cardiac assist device or artificial heart. Indeed, thromboembolism occurred in most patients having long-term implantation of the Jarvik-7 artificial heart and is a major design consideration for current devices. Thrombi form primarily in association with crevices and voids, especially in areas of disturbed blood flow such as near connections of conduits and other components to each other and to the natural heart (see Figs. 5-37A and B). Most pumps have used smooth polymeric pumping bladders; these are frequently associated with thromboembolic complications. One approach (HeartMate, Thoratec) to the design of the blood pump is the use of textured polyurethane and titanium surfaces, which accumulate a limited platelet/fibrin pseudointimal membrane that is resistant to thrombosis, allowing only antiplatelet therapy for anticoagulation in most device recipients.[368] The safety of this surface was evident in the Randomized Evaluation of Mechanical Assistance for the Treatment of Congestive Heart Failure (REMATCH) Trial of the HeartMate device.[360]

Infectious complications have been a major limiting factor in the prolonged use of cardiac assist devices. Infection can occur within the device but may also be associated with percutaneous drive lines (see Fig. 5-37C). Susceptibility to infection is not only potentiated by the usual prosthesis-associated factors, but also by the multisystem organ damage from the underlying disease, the periprosthetic culture medium provided by postoperative hemorrhage, and by prolonged hospitalization with the associated risk of nosocomial infections. These infections are a significant cause of morbidity and mortality and are often resistant to antibiotic therapy and host defenses. However, infection is not an absolute contraindication to subsequent cardiac transplantation.[369] In the REMATCH trial, sepsis accounted for 17 of the 41 deaths among the 68 patients receiving LVADs.[360]

Other complications include hemolysis, pannus formation around anastomotic sites, calcification (see Figs. 5-37D and E), and device malfunction. Device failure can occur secondary to fracture or tear of one of the prosthetic valves within the device conduits, as this application provides a particularly severe test of valve durability (see Fig. 5-37F). Device failure can also occur secondary to damage or dehiscence to the pumping bladder (see Fig. 5-37G). These complications can be fatal, or make a patient ineligible for future transplantation.

Many pathophysiologic changes occur during the progression to end-stage heart failure, ranging from the subcellular (e.g., abnormal mitochondrial function and calcium metabolism) to the organ and system level (e.g., ventricular dilation, decreased ejection fraction, and neurohormonal changes), leading to the signs and symptoms of congestive failure. Implantation of an LVAD can reverse many of these changes ("reverse remodeling"), leading to increased cardiac output, decreased ventricular end-diastolic volume, and normalization of neurohormonal status such that a certain fraction of patients can be weaned from the device without the need for subsequent cardiac transplantation. Current research focuses on the mechanisms of cardiac recovery, identification of patients who could achieve recovery, and specifics such as the timing and duration of therapy.[370–372]

Skeletal Muscle Augmentation of Cardiac Function

Autologous skeletal muscle has been used to provide active cardiac assist in the form of both cardiomyoplasty and skeletal muscle ventricles for patients with heart failure.[373–375]

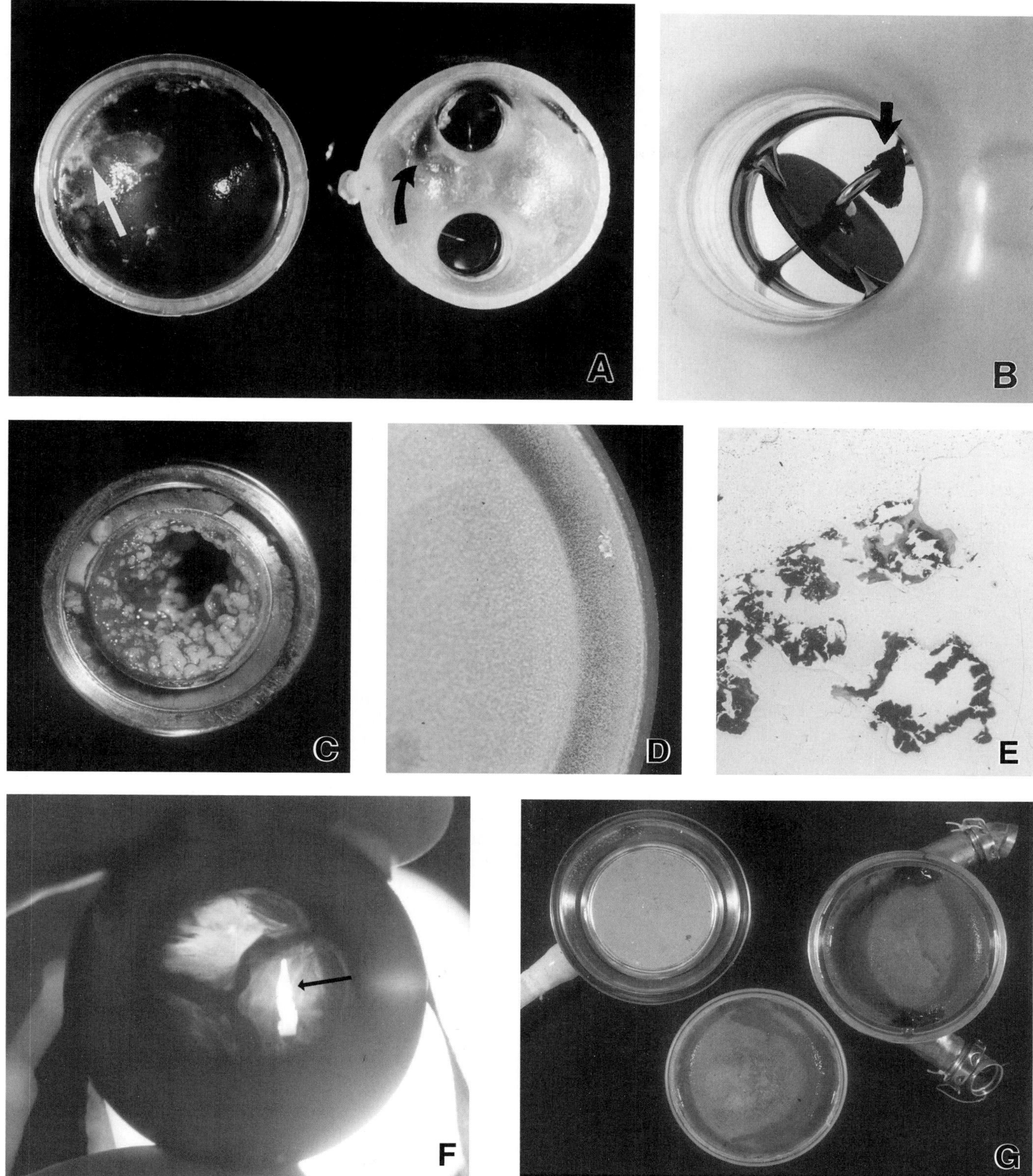

FIGURE 5–37 Complications of left ventricular assist devices (LVADs). (A and B) Thrombotic deposits at the pump outflow and bladder/housing junction, respectively. (C) Fungal infection in LVAD outflow graft. (D and E) Focal calcification of clinical left ventricular assist device. (D) A gross photograph. (E) Histologic section demonstrating calcification (black) (von Kossa stain). (F) Cuspal tear in inflow valve of LVAD. This patient was not a transplant candidate and had been on the LVAD as destination therapy for about 12 months before the tear occurred causing regurgitation. The valve was replaced without incident. (G) Dehiscence of the bladder of a left ventricular assist device. *(A and B: Reproduced with permission from Fyfe B, Schoen FJ: Pathologic analysis of 34 explanted Symbion ventricular assist devices and 10 explanted Jarvik-7 total artificial hearts. Cardiovasc Pathol 1993; 2:187. C, D, E, and G: reproduced with permission from Schoen FJ, Edwards WD: Pathology of cardiovascular interventions, including endovascular therapies, revascularization, vascular replacement, cardiac assist/replacement, arrhythmia control and repaired congenital heart disease, in Silver MD, Gotlieb AI, Schoen FJ (eds): Cardiovascular Pathology, 3d ed. Philadelphia, WB Saunders, 2001; p 678.)*

In cardiomyoplasty, the latissimus dorsi is wrapped around the ventricles, and this has been shown to stabilize left ventricular size and prevent further dilation. Skeletal muscle can adapt its physiological, biochemical, and structural characteristics to overcome fatigue and adjust to a more demanding pattern of use by increases in capillary density, activity of oxidative enzymes, and mitochondrial volume. While these procedures had some promising experimental and clinical results,[373–376] interest in their application has waned due to several factors including the improvement in medical therapy for congestive heart failure, the development of the mechanical cardiac assist devices discussed above, and the hesitancy of clinicians to refer patients for this procedure given the alternative therapies.

NEOPLASTIC HEART DISEASE

Although metastatic tumors to the heart are present in 1% to 3% of patients dying of cancer, primary tumors of the heart are unusual.[377–379] The frequency of primary cardiac neoplasia is about 0.02% based on data from 22 large autopsy series.[380] The most common tumors, in descending order of frequency, are: myxomas, lipomas, papillary fibroelastomas, angiomas, fibromas, and rhabdomyomas, all benign and accounting for approximately 80% of primary tumors of the adult heart. The remaining 20% are malignant tumors, including angiosarcomas and other sarcomas. Many cardiac tumors have a genetic basis.[381]

Myxoma

Myxomas are the most common primary tumor of the heart in adults, accounting for about 50% of all benign cardiac tumors.[382] They typically arise in the left atrium (80%) along the interatrial septum near the fossa ovalis. Occasionally, myxomas arise in the right atrium (15%), the ventricles (3%-4%), or valves. These tumors arise more frequently in women and usually present between the ages of 50 and 70 years. Sporadic cases of myxoma are almost always single, while familial cases can be multiple and present at an earlier age. The Carney complex, a multiple neoplasia syndrome featuring cardiac and cutaneous myxomas, endocrine and neural tumors, as well as pigmented skin and mucosal lesions, is inherited as an autosomal dominant trait.[383,384] A careful history and physical examination in patients with cardiac myxoma is important to identify other signs of the Carney complex as this diagnosis carries implications for family members of the patient.

Myxomas range from small (<1 cm) to large (up to 10 cm) and form sessile or pedunculated masses that vary from globular and hard lesions mottled with hemorrhage to soft, translucent, papillary, or villous lesions having a myxoid and friable appearance (Fig. 5-38). The pedunculated form frequently is sufficiently mobile to move into or sometimes through the ipsilateral atrioventricular valve annulus during ventricular diastole, causing intermittent and often position-dependent obstruction. Sometimes, such mobility exerts a wrecking ball effect, causing damage to and secondary fibrotic thickening of the valve leaflets.

Clinical manifestations are most often determined by tumor size and location; some myxomas are incidentally detected in patients undergoing echocardiography for other indications while others may present with sudden death. Symptoms are generally a consequence of valvular obstruction, embolization, or a syndrome of constitutional symptoms. Intracardiac obstruction may mimic the presentation of mitral or tricuspid stenosis with dyspnea, pulmonary edema, and right-sided heart failure. Fragmentation of a left-sided tumor with embolization may mimic the presentation of infective endocarditis with transient ischemic attacks, strokes, and cutaneous lesions; emboli from right-sided lesions may present as pulmonary hypertension. Constitutional symptoms such as fever, erythematous rash, weight loss, and arthralgias may be due to the release of the acute phase reactant interleukin-6 from the tumor leading to these inflammatory and autoimmune manifestations. Echocardiography, including transesophageal echocardiography, provides a means to noninvasively identify the masses and their location, attachment, and mobility. Surgical removal usually is curative with excellent short- and long-term prognosis. Rarely, the neoplasm recurs months to years later, usually secondary to incomplete removal of the stalk.

Histologically, myxomas are composed of stellate or globular cells, often in formed structures that variably resemble poorly formed glands or vessels, endothelial cells, macrophages, mature or immature smooth muscle cells, and a variety of intermediate forms embedded within an abundant acid mucopolysaccharide matrix and covered by endothelium. Although it has long been questioned whether cardiac myxomas are hamartomas or organized thrombi, the weight of evidence is on the side of benign neoplasia. All the cell types present are thought to derive from differentiation of primitive multipotential mesenchymal cells.

Other Cardiac Tumors and Tumor-Like Conditions

Cardiac lipomas are discrete masses that are typically epicardial, but may occur anywhere within the myocardium or pericardium. Most are clinically silent, but some may cause symptoms such as arrhythmias, pericardial effusion, or intracardiac obstruction. Magnetic resonance imaging is useful in the diagnosis of adipocytic lesions due to its ability to identify fatty tissues. Histologically, these tumors are comprised of mature adipocytes, identical to lipomas elsewhere. A separate, non-neoplastic condition called lipomatous hypertrophy of the interatrial septum is characterized

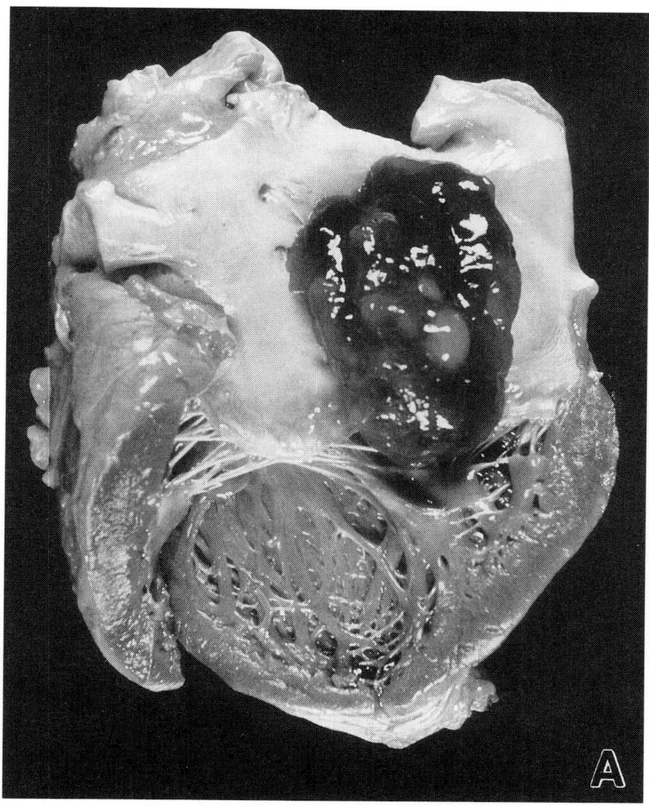

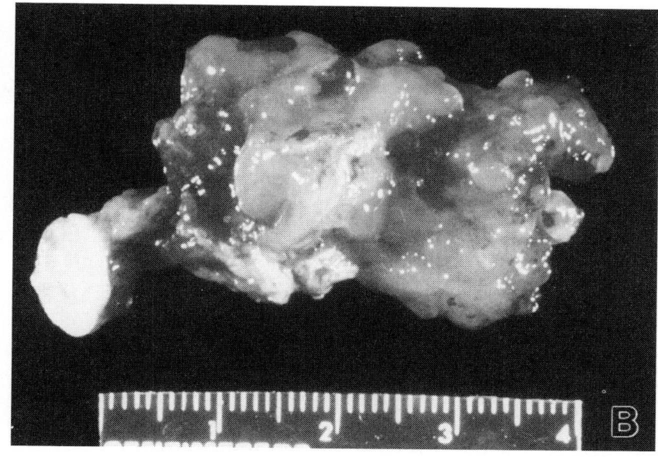

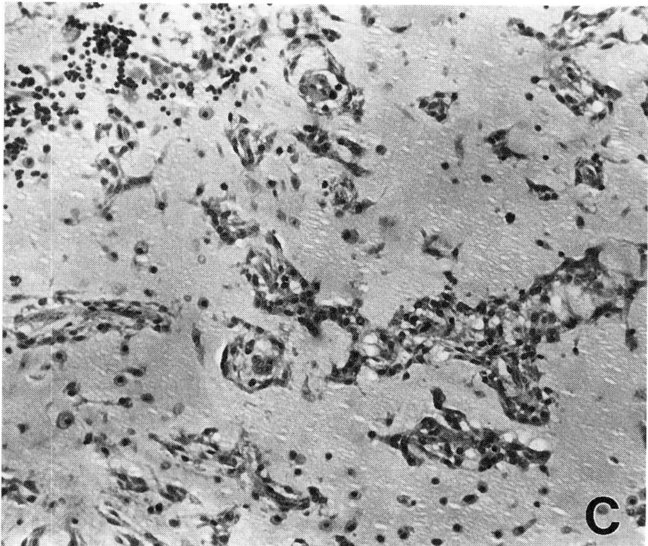

FIGURE 5–38 Gross and histologic features of cardiac myxomas. (A) Smooth, round, hemorrhagic left atrial myxoma, noted at autopsy. The tumor mass nearly fills the left atrium and extends into the mitral valve orifice. (B) Irregular polypoid, gelatinous friable myxoma mass, surgically removed. The resection margin that surrounds the proximal portion of the stalk is at left. (C) Characteristic histologic features of myxoma, including individual tumor cells and clusters and islands scattered throughout the characteristic granular extracellular matrix. Hematoxylin and eosin 50X. *(A: Reproduced with permission from Schoen FJ: The heart, in Cotran RS, Kumar V, Collins T (eds): Pathologic Basis of Disease, 6th ed., Philadelphia, WB Saunders, 1994; p 543. B: Reproduced by permission from Schoen FJ: Interventional and Surgical Cardiovascular Pathology: Clinical Correlations and Basic Principles. Philadelphia, WB Saunders, 1989.)*

by accumulation of unencapsulated adipose tissue in the interatrial septum that can lead to arrhythmias.

Papillary fibroelastomas[385] are usually solitary and located on the valves, particularly the ventricular surfaces of semilunar valves and the atrial surfaces of atrioventricular valves. They constitute a distinctive "sea anemone" cluster of hair-like projections up to 1 cm or more in length, and can mimic valvular vegetations echocardiographically (Fig. 5-39).[386] Histologically, they are composed of a dense core of irregular elastic fibers, coated with myxoid connective tissue, and lined by endothelium. They may contain focal platelet-fibrin thrombus and serve as a source for embolization, commonly to cerebral or coronary arteries. Surgical excision is recommended to eliminate these embolic events. Although classified with neoplasms, fibroelastomas may represent organized thrombi, similar to the much smaller,

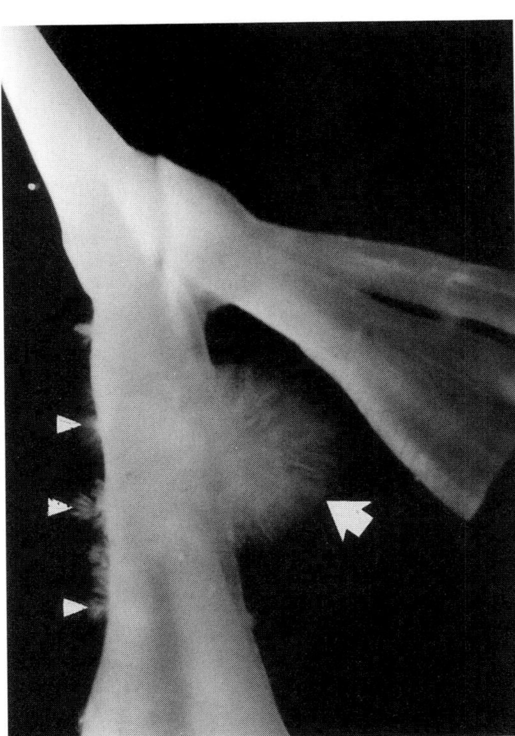

FIGURE 5–39 Papillary fibroelastoma. Gross photograph demonstrating resemblance of this lesion to sea anemone, with papillary fronds, arising from the chordae tendineae and near the mitral leaflet (large arrow). In this case multiple lesions were present, all associated with the mitral valve apparatus (small arrowheads). *(Reproduced with permission from Colucci W, Schoen FJ: Primary tumors of the heart, in Braunwald E, Zipes DP, Libby P (eds): Heart Disease: A Textbook of Cardiovascular Medicine, 6th ed. Philadelphia, WB Saunders, 2001; p 1807.)*

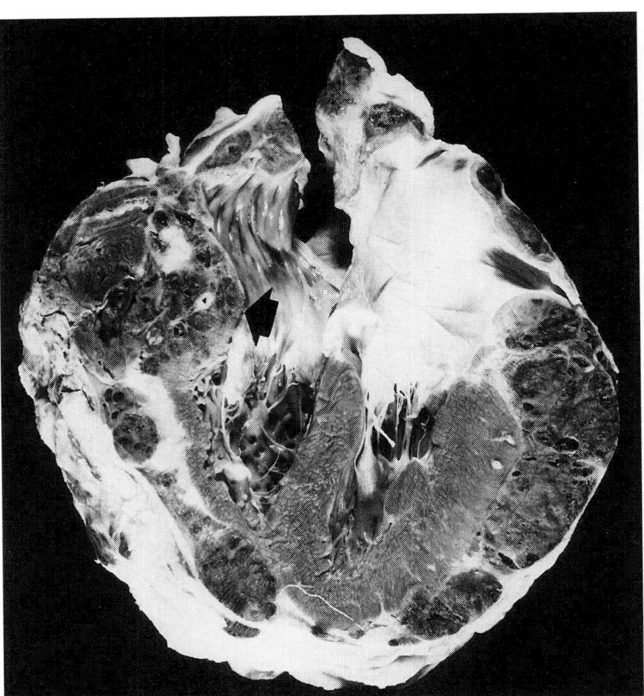

FIGURE 5–40 Massive pericardial angiosarcoma with deep myocardial invasion at multiple sites, particularly at right atrium (arrow). *(Reproduced with permission from Schoen FJ: Interventional and Surgical Cardiovascular Pathology: Clinical Correlations and Basic Principles. Philadelphia, WB Saunders, 1989.)*

usually trivial, whisker-like Lambl's excrescences that are frequently found on the aortic valves of older individuals.

Rhabdomyomas comprise the most frequent primary tumor of the heart in infants and children. They are usually multiple and involve the ventricular myocardium on either side of the heart. They consist of gray-white myocardial masses up to several centimeters in diameter that may protrude into the ventricular or atrial chambers causing functional obstruction. These tumors tend to spontaneously regress, so surgery is usually reserved for patients with severe hemodynamic disturbances or arrhythmias refractory to medical management. Most cardiac rhabdomyomas occur in patients with tuberous sclerosis, the clinical features of which also include infantile spasms, skin lesions (hypopigmentation, shagreen patch, subcutaneous nodules), retinal lesions, and angiomyolipomas. This disease, in its familial form, exhibits autosomal dominant inheritance, but about half the cases are sporadic owing to new mutations. Histologically, rhabdomyomas contain characteristic "spider cells," which are large, myofibril-containing rounded or polygonal cells with numerous glycogen-laden vacuoles separated by strands of cytoplasm running from the plasma membrane to the centrally located nucleus.

Cardiac fibromas, while also occurring predominantly in children and presenting with heart failure or arrhythmias, or incidentally, differ from rhabdomyomas in being solitary lesions that may show calcification on a routine chest radiograph. Fibromas are white, whorled masses that are typically ventricular. There is an increased risk of cardiac fibromas in patients with Gorlin syndrome (nevoid basal cell carcinoma syndrome), an autosomal dominant disorder characterized by skin lesions, odontogenic keratocysts of the jaw, and skeletal abnormalities. Gorlin syndrome is a result of germline mutations in the PTC gene on chromosome 9; the role of this gene product in myocardial growth and development is unknown. Histologically, fibromas consist of fibroblasts showing minimal atypia and collagen with the degree of cellularity decreasing with increasing age of the patient at presentation. While they are grossly well circumscribed, there is usually an infiltrating margin histologically. Calcifications and elastin fibers are not uncommon in these lesions.

Sarcomas, with angiosarcomas and rhabdomyosarcomas being the most common, are not distinctive from their counterparts in other locations. They tend to involve the right side of the heart, especially the right atrioventricular groove

(Fig. 5-40). The clinical course is rapidly progressive as a result of local infiltration with intracavity obstruction and early metastatic events.

Recently described, and of importance only insofar as they need to be distinguished from primary cardiac tumors or metastatic carcinoma, are peculiar microscopic-sized cellular cardiac lesions that have been noted incidentally as part of endomyocardial biopsy or surgically removed tissue specimens or at cardiac surgery, free-floating or loosely attached to a valvular or endocardial mass.[387,388] Termed mesothelial/monocytic incidental cardiac excrescences (MICE), they appear histologically largely as clusters and ribbons of mesothelial cells and entrapped erythrocytes and leukocytes, embedded within a fibrin mesh. Some represent reactive mesothelial and/or monocytic (histiocytic) hyperplasia, whereas others are now considered to be artifacts formed by compaction of mesothelial strips (likely from the pericardium) or other tissue debris and fibrin, which are transported via catheters or around an operative site on a cardiotomy suction tip.

REFERENCES

1. Braunwald E: Shattuck lecture—Cardiovascular medicine at the turn of the millennium: triumphs, concerns and opportunities. *N Engl J Med* 1997; 337:1360.
2. Webb CL, Jenkins KJ, Karpawich PP, et al: Collaborative care for adults with congenital heart disease. *Circulation* 2002; 105:2318.
3. Schoen FJ, Edwards WD: Pathology of cardiovascular interventions, including endovascular therapies, revascularization, vascular replacement, cardiac assist/replacement, arrhythmia control and repaired congenital heart disease, in Silver MD, Gotlieb AI, Schoen FJ (eds): *Cardiovascular Pathology*. Philadelphia, Churchill Livingstone, 2001; p 678.
4. Schoen FJ: The heart, in Cotran RS, Kumar V, Collins T (eds): *Robbins Pathologic Basis of Disease*, 6th ed. Philadelphia, WB Saunders, 1999; p 543.
5. Schoen FJ, Lawrie GM, Titus JL: Left ventricular cellular hypertrophy in pressure- and volume-overload valvular heart disease. *Hum Pathol* 1984; 15:860.
6. Sadoshima J, Izumo S: The cellular and molecular response of cardiac myocytes to mechanical stress. *Annu Rev Physiol* 1997; 59:551.
7. Johnatty SE, Dyck JRB, Michael LH, Olson EN, Abdellatif M: Identification of genes regulated during mechanical load-induced cardiac hypertrophy. *J Mol Cell Cardiol* 2000; 32:805.
8. Swynghedauw B, Baillard C: Biology of hypertensive cardiomyopathy. *Curr Opin Cardiol* 2000; 15:247.
9. Nicol RL, Frey N, Olson EN: From the sarcomere to the nucleus: role of genetics and signaling in structural heart disease. *Annu Rev Genomics Hum Genet* 2000; 1:179.
10. Fortuno MA, Ravassa S, Fortuna A, et al: Cardiomyocyte apoptotic cell death in arterial hypertension: mechanisms and potential management. *Hypertension* 2001; 38:1406.
11. Narula J, Arbustini E, Chandrashekhar Y, et al: Apoptosis and the systolic dysfunction in congestive heart failure: apoptosis interruptus and zombie myocytes. *Cardiol Clin* 2001; 19:113.
12. Levy D, Garrison RJ, Savage DD, et al: Prognostic implications of echocardiographically determined left ventricular mass in the Framingham Heart Study. *N Engl J Med* 1990: 322:1561.
13. Devereux RB: Regression of left ventricular hypertrophy: how and why? [editorial]. *JAMA* 1996; 275:1517.
14. Schoen FJ, Cotran RS: Blood vessels, in Cotran RS, Kumar V, Collins T (eds): *Robbins Pathologic Basis of Disease*, 6th ed. Philadelphia, WB Saunders, 1999; p 493.
15. Gotlieb AI, Silver MD: Atherosclerosis: pathology and pathogenesis, in Silver MD, Gotlieb AI, Schoen FJ (eds.): *Cardiovascular Pathology*, 3d ed. Philadelphia, WB Saunders 2001; p 68.
16. Libby P: The vascular biology of atherosclerosis, in Braunwald E, Libby P, Zipes DP (eds): *Heart Disease: A Textbook of Cardiovascular Medicine*, 6th ed. Philadelphia, WB Saunders, 2001; p 995.
17. Glass CK, Witztum JL: Atherosclerosis: the road ahead. *Cell* 2001; 104:503.
18. Gibbons GH, Dzau VJ: The emerging concept of vascular remodeling. *N Engl J Med* 1994; 330:1431.
19. Schoenhagen P, Ziada KM, Vince DG, et al: Arterial remodeling and coronary artery disease: the concept of "dilated" versus "obstructive" coronary atherosclerosis. *J Am Coll Cardiol* 2001; 38:297.
20. Ross R: Atherosclerosis: an inflammatory disease. *N Engl J Med* 1999; 340:115.
21. Gimbrone MA, Topper JN, Nagel T, et al: Endothelial dysfunction, hemodynamic forces, and atherogenesis. *Ann NY Acad Sci* 2000; 902:230.
22. Fuster V, Gotto AM, Libby P, et al: 27th Bethesda Conference: matching the intensity of risk factor management with the hazard for coronary disease events. Task Force I: Pathogenesis of coronary disease: the biologic role of risk factors. *J Am Coll Cardiol* 1996; 27:964.
23. Herrmann J, Lerman A: The endothelium: dysfunction and beyond. *J Nucl Cardiol* 2001, 8:197.
24. Stevens T, Rosenberg R, Aird W, et al: NHLBI workshop report: endothelial cell phenotypes in heart, lung, and blood disease. *Am J Physiol Cell Physiol* 2001; 281:C1422.
25. Virmani R, Kolodgie FD, Burke AP, et al: Lessons from sudden coronary death: a comprehensive morphological classification scheme for atherosclerotic lesions. *Arterioscler Thromb Vasc Biol* 2000; 20:1262.
26. Libby P: Current concepts of the pathogenesis of the acute coronary syndromes. *Circulation* 2001; 104:365.
27. Richardson PD, Davies MJ, Born GVR: Influence of plaque configuration and stress distribution on fissuring of coronary atherosclerotic plaques. *Lancet* 1989; 941.
28. Kolodgie FD, Burke AP, Farb A: The thin-cap fibroatheroma: a type of vulnerable plaque: the major precursor lesion to acute coronary syndromes. *Curr Opin Cardiol* 2001; 16:285.
29. Huang H, Virmani R, Younis H, et al: The impact of calcification on the biomechanical stability of atherosclerotic plaques. *Circulation* 2001; 103:1051.
30. Nissen SE, Yock P: Intravascular ultrasound: novel pathophysiological insights and current clinical applications. *Circulation* 2001; 103:604.
31. Schoen FJ: *Interventional and Surgical Cardiovascular Pathology: Clinical Correlations and Basic Principles*. Philadelphia, WB Saunders, 1989.
32. Kloner RA, Jennings RB: Consequences of brief ischemia: stunning, preconditioning, and their clinical implications. *Circulation* 2001; 104:2981 and 3158.
33. Jennings RB, Steenbergen C Jr, Reimer KA: Myocardial ischemia and reperfusion, in Schoen FJ, Gimbrone MA (eds): *Cardiovascular Pathology: Clinicopathologic Correlations and Pathogenetic Mechanisms*. Baltimore, Williams & Wilkins, 1995; p 47.
34. Baroldi G: Myocardial cell death, including ischemic heart disease and its complications, in Silver MD, Gotlieb AI, Schoen FJ (eds.): *Cardiovascular Pathology*. Philadelphia, Churchill Livingstone, 2001; p 198.

35. James TN: Apoptosis in cardiac disease. *Am J Med* 1999; 107:606.
36. Anversa P, Cheng W, Liu Y, et al: Apoptosis and myocardial infarction. *Basic Res Cardiol* 1998; 93:8.
37. Vargas SO, Sampson BA, Schoen FJ: Pathologic detection of early myocardial infarction: a critical review of the evolution and usefulness of modern techniques. *Mod Pathol* 1999; 12:635.
38. Hammerman H, Kloner RA, Hale S, et al: Dose-dependent effects of short-term methylprednisolone on myocardial infarct extent, scar formation, and ventricular function. *Circulation* 1983; 68:446.
39. Fyfe B, Loh E, Winters GL, et al: Heart transplantation-associated perioperative ischemic myocardial injury: morphological features and clinical significance. *Circulation* 1996; 93:1133.
40. Beltrami AP, Urbanek K, Kajstura J, et al: Evidence that cardiac myocytes divide after myocardial infarction. *N Engl J Med* 2001; 344:1750.
41. Quaini F, Urbanek K, Beltrami AP, et al: Chimerism of the transplanted heart. *N Engl J Med* 2002; 346:5.
42. Brodie BR, Stuckey TD, Hansen C, et al: Benefit of late coronary reperfusion in patients with acute myocardial infarction and persistent ischemic chest pain. *Am J Cardiol* 1994; 74:538.
43. Richard V, Murry CE, Reimer KA: Healing of myocardial infarcts in dogs: effects of late reperfusion. *Circulation* 1995; 92:1891.
44. Reichenbach DD, Cowan MJ: Healing of myocardial infarction with and without reperfusion. *Maj Probl Pathol* 1991; 23:86.
45. Hutchins GM, Silverman KJ: Pathology of the stone heart syndrome: massive myocardial contraction band necrosis and widely patent coronary arteries. *Am J Pathol* 1979; 95:745.
46. Ambrosio G, Tritto I: Reperfusion injury: experimental evidence and clinical implications. *Am Heart J* 1999; 138:S67.
47. Park JL, Lucchesi BR: Mechanisms of myocardial reperfusion injury. *Ann Thorac Surg* 1999; 68:1905.
48. Dhalla NS, Elmoselhi AB, Hata T, et al: Status of myocardial antioxidants in ischemia-reperfusion injury. *Cardiovasc Res* 2000; 47:446.
49. Rusnak JM, Kopecky SL, Clements IP, et al: An anti-CD11/CD18 monoclonal antibody in patients with acute myocardial infarction having percutaneous transluminal coronary angioplasty (the FESTIVAL study). *Am J Cardiol* 2001; 88:482.
50. Monsinjon T, Richard V, Fontaine M: Complement and its implications in cardiac ischemia/reperfusion: strategies to inhibit complement. *Fundam Clin Pharmacol* 2001; 15:293.
51. Bolli R, Marban E: Molecular and cellular mechanisms of myocardial stunning. *Physiol Rev* 1999; 79:609.
52. Kloner RA, Jennings RB: Consequences of brief ischemia: stunning, preconditioning, and their clinical implications, pts 1 and 2. *Circulation* 2001; 104:2981 and 3158.
53. Leavitt JI, Better N, Tow DE, et al: Demonstration of viable, stunned myocardium with technetium-99m-sestamibi. *J Nucl Med* 1994; 35:1805.
54. Schoen FJ, Palmer DC, Bernhard WF, et al: Clinical temporary ventricular assist. *J Thorac Cardiovasc Surg* 1986; 92: 1071.
55. Kern KB, Hilwig RW, Rhee KH, et al: Myocardial dysfunction after resuscitation from cardiac arrest: an example of global myocardial stunning. *J Am Coll Cardiol* 1996; 28:232.
56. Dispersyn GD, Ramaekers FC, Borgers M: Clinical pathophysiology of hibernating myocardium. *Coron Artery Dis* 2001; 12: 381.
57. Bax JJ, Visser FC, Poldermans D, et al: Time course of functional recovery of stunned and hibernating segments after surgical revascularization. *Circulation* 2001; 104(suppl):I314.
58. Kim RJ, Wu E, Rafael A, et al: The use of contrast-enhanced magnetic resonance imaging to identify reversible myocardial dysfunction. *N Engl J Med* 2000; 343:1445.
59. Perrone-Filardi P, Chiariello M: The identification of myocardial hibernation in patients with ischemic heart failure by echocardiography and radionuclide studies. *Prog Cardiovasc Dis* 2001; 43:419.
60. Miller MJ: Preconditioning for cardioprotection against ischemia reperfusion injury: the roles of nitric oxide, reactive oxygen species, heat shock proteins, reactive hyperemia and antioxidants—a mini review. *Can J Cardiol* 2001; 17: 1075.
61. O'Rourke B: Myocardial K(ATP) channels in preconditioning. *Circ Res* 2000; 87:845.
62. Latchman DS: Heat shock proteins and cardiac protection. *Cardiovasc Res* 2001; 51:637.
63. Peppas N, Langer R: New challenges in biomaterials. *Science* 1994; 263:1715.
64. Ratner BD, Hoffman S, Schoen FJ, et al: *Biomaterials Science: An Introduction to Materials in Medicine*. San Diego, Academic Press, 1996.
65. Hench LL, Polak JM: Third-generation biomedical materials. *Science* 2002; 295:1014.
66. Schoen FJ: Introduction to host reactions to biomaterials and their evaluation, in Ratner BD, Hoffman AS, Schoen FJ, et al (eds): *Biomaterials Science: An Introduction to Materials in Medicine*. San Diego, Academic Press, 1996; p 165.
67. Janvier G, Baquey C, Roth C, et al: Extracorporeal circulation, hemocompatibility and biomaterials. *Ann Thorac Surg* 1996; 62:1926.
68. Harker LA, Ratner BD, Didisheim P: *Cardiovascular Biomaterials and Biocompatibility: A Guide to the Study of Blood-Tissue-Material Interactions*. Supplement to *Cardiovasc Pathol* 1993.
69. Anderson JM, Schoen FJ: Interactions of blood with artificial surfaces, in Butchart EG, Bodnar E (eds): *Current Issues in Heart Valve Disease: Thrombosis, Embolism and Bleeding*. London: ICR Publishers, 1992; p 160.
70. Tang L, Eaton JW: Inflammatory responses to biomaterials. *Am J Clin Pathol* 1995; 103:466.
71. Tang L, Eaton JW: Natural responses to unnatural materials: a molecular mechanism for foreign body reactions. *Mol Med* 1999; 5:351.
72. Kossovsky N, Freiman CJ: Physiochemical and immunological basis of silicone pathophysiology. *J Biomater Sci-Polymer Edn* 1995; 7:101.
73. Love JW: *Autologous Tissue Heart Valves*. Austin TX, RG Landes Co, 1993; p 42.
74. Schoen FJ, Edwards WD: Pathology of cardiovascular interventions, including endovascular therapies, revascularization, vascular replacement, cardiac assist/replacement, arrhythmia control, and repaired congenital heart disease, in Silver MD, Gotlieb AI, Schoen FJ (eds): *Cardiovascular Pathology*, 3rd ed. Philadelphia, Churchill Livingstone, 2001; p 678.
75. Rafii S: Circulating endothelial precursors: mystery, reality, and promise. *J Clin Invest* 2000; 105:17.
76. DiDonato RM, Danielson GK, McGoon DC, et al: Left ventricle-aortic conduits in pediatric patients. *J Thorac Cardiovasc Surg* 1984; 88:82.
77. Mann MJ, Gibbons GH, Kernoff RS, et al: Genetic engineering of vein grafts resistant to atherosclerosis. *Proc Natl Acad Sci USA* 1995; 92:4502.
78. Dunne PF, Newman KD, Jones M, et al: Seeding of vascular grafts with genetically modified endothelial cells. *Circulation* 1996; 93:1439.
79. Consigny PM: Endothelial cell seeding on prosthetic surfaces. *J Long Term Eff Med Implants* 2000; 10:79.
80. Tassiopoulos AK, Greisler HP: Angiogenic mechanisms of endothelialization of cardiovascular implants: a review of recent investigative strategies. *J Biomater Sci Polym Ed* 2000; 11:1275.

81. Salacinski HJ, Tiwari A, Hamilton G, et al: Cellular engineering of vascular bypass grafts: role of chemical coatings for enhancing endothelial cell attachment. *Med Biol Eng Comput* 2001; 39:609.
82. Reid G: Bacterial colonization of prosthetic devices and measures to prevent infection. *New Horiz* 1998; 6(suppl):S58.
83. Rupp ME, Archer GL: Coagulase-negative staphylococci: pathogens associated with medical progress. *Clin Infect Dis* 1994; 19:231.
84. O'Gara JP, Humphreys H: Staphylococcus epidermidis biofilms: importance and implications. *J Med Microbiol* 2001; 50:582.
85. An YH, Friedman RJ: Concise review of mechanisms of bacterial adhesion to biomaterial surfaces. *J Biomed Mater Res (Appl Biomater)* 1998; 43:338.
86. Weinberg DS, Maini BS: Primary sarcoma of the aorta associated with a vascular prosthesis: a case report. *Cancer* 1980; 46:398.
87. Schoen FJ: Tumorigenesis and biomaterials, in Ratner BD, Hoffman S, Schoen FJ, et al (eds): *Biomaterials Science: An Introduction to Materials in Medicine*. San Diego, Academic Press, 1996; p 200.
88. Vacanti JP, Langer R: Tissue engineering: the design and fabrication of living replacement devices for surgical reconstruction and transplantation. *Lancet* 1999; 354:SI32.
89. Fuchs JR, Nasseri BA, Vacanti JP: Tissue engineering: a 21st century solution to surgical reconstruction. *Ann Thorac Surg* 2001; 72:577.
90. Griffith LG, Naughton G: Tissue engineering—current challenges and expanding opportunities. *Science* 2002; 295:1009.
91. Rabkin E, Schoen FJ: Cardiovascular tissue engineering. *Cardiovasc Path (in press)*.
92. Blau HM, Brazelton TR, Weimann JM: The evolving concept of a stem cell: entity or function? *Cell* 2001; 105:829.
93. Hoerstrup SP, Sodian R, Daebritz S, et al: Functional living trileaflet heart valves grown in-vitro. *Circulation* 2000; 102: III-44.
94. Rabkin E, Hoerstrup SP, Aikawa M, et al: Evolution of cell phenotype and extracellular matrix in tissue-engineered heart valves during in-vitro maturation and in-vivo remodeling. *J Heart Valve Dis* 2002;11:1.
95. L'Heureux N, Paquet S, Labbe R, et al: A completely biological tissue-engineered human blood vessel. *FASEB J* 1998; 12:47.
96. Niklason LE, Gao J, Abbott WM, et al: Functional arteries grown in-vitro. *Science* 1999; 284:489.
97. Kaushall S, Amiel GE, Gulesarian KJ, et al: Functional small diameter neovessels using endothelial progenitor cells expanded ex-vivo. *Nature Med* 2001; 7:1035.
98. Carrier RL, Rupnick M, Langer R, et al: Effects of oxygen on engineered cardiac muscle. *Biotech Bioeng* 2002; 78:617.
99. Suzuki K, Murtuza B, Heslop L, et al: Single fibers of skeletal muscle as a novel graft for cell transplantation to the heart. *J Thorac Cardiovasc Surg* 2002;123:984.
100. Orlic D, Kajstura J, Chimenti S, et al: Bone marrow cells regenerate infarcted myocardium. *Nature* 2001; 410:701.
101. Burke AP, Farb A, Malcolm GT, et al: Coronary risk factors and plaque morphology in men with coronary disease who died suddenly. *N Engl J Med* 1997; 336:1276.
102. Fuster V: Mechanisms leading to myocardial infarction: insights from studies of vascular biology. *Circulation* 1994; 90:2126.
103. Muller JE, Abela GS, Nesto RW, et al: Triggers, acute risk factors and vulnerable plaques: The lexicon of a new frontier. *J Am Coll Cardiol* 1994; 23:809.
104. Fayad ZA, Fuster V: Clinical imaging of the high-risk or vulnerable atherosclerotic plaque. *Circ Res* 2001; 89:305.
105. Kern MJ, Meier B: Evaluation of the culprit plaque and the physiological significance of coronary atherosclerotic narrowings. *Circulation* 2001; 103:3142.
106. Lee RT, Loree HM, Cheng GC, et al: Computational structural analysis based on intravascular ultrasound imaging prior to in vitro angioplasty: prediction of plaque fracture locations. *J Am Coll Cardiol* 1993; 21:777.
107. Mallat Z, Tedgui A: Current perspective on the role of apoptosis in atherothrombotic disease. *Circ Res* 2001; 88:998.
108. Kim WY, Danias PG, Stubber M, et al: Coronary magnetic resonance angiography for the detection of coronary stenoses. *N Engl J Med* 2001; 345:1863.
109. Keelan PC, Bielak LF, Ashai K, et al: Long-term prognostic value of coronary calcification detected by electron-beam computed tomography in patients undergoing coronary angiography. *Circulation* 2001; 104:412.
110. Schmermund A, Erbel R: Unstable coronary plaque and its relation to coronary calcium. *Circulation* 2001; 104:1682.
111. Kim WY, Danias PG, Stuber M, et al: Coronary magnetic resonance angiography for the detection of coronary stenoses. *N Engl J Med* 2001; 345:1863.
112. Aikawa M, Rabkin E, Sugiyama S, et al: An HMG-CoA reductase inhibitor, cerivastatin, suppresses growth of macrophages expressing matrix metalloproteinases and tissue factor in-vivo and in-vitro. *Circulation* 2001; 103:276.
113. Rabbani R, Topol EJ: Strategies to achieve coronary arterial plaque stabilization. *Cardiovasc Res* 1999; 41:402.
114. Schwartz SM, Virmani R, Rosenfeld ME: The good smooth muscle cells in atherosclerosis. *Curr Athero Rep* 2000; 2:422.
115. Ambrose JA, Eulogio E, Martinez MD: A new paradigm for plaque stabilization. *Circulation* 2002; 105:2000.
116. Blake GJ, Ridker PM: Novel clinical markers of vascular wall inflammation. *Circ Res* 2001; 89:763.
117. Bayes-Genis A, Conover CA, Overgaard MT, et al: Pregnancy-associated plasma protein A as a marker of acute coronary syndromes. *N Engl J Med* 2001; 345:1022.
118. Libby P, Ridker PM, Maseri A: Inflammation and atherosclerosis. *Circulation* 2002; 105:1135.
119. Antman EM, Braunwald E: Acute myocardial infarction, in Braunwald E, Zipes DD, Libby P (eds): *Heart Disease: A Textbook of Cardiovascular Medicine*, 6th ed. Philadelphia, WB Saunders, 2001: p 1114.
120. Ohman EM, Harrington RA, Cannon CP, et al: Intravenous thrombolysis in acute myocardial infarction. *Chest* 2001; 119:253S.
121. Topol EJ: Acute myocardial infarction: thrombolysis. *Heart* 2000; 83:122.
122. Gensini GF, Comeglio M, Falai M: Advances in antithrombotic therapy of acute myocardial infarction. *Am Heart J* 1999; 138:S171.
123. Zijlstra F, Hoorntje JCA, de Boer MJ, et al: Long-term benefit of primary angioplasty as compared with thrombolytic therapy for acute myocardial infarction. *N Engl J Med* 1999; 341:1413.
124. Landau C, Lange RA, Hillis LD: Percutaneous transluminal coronary angioplasty. *N Engl J Med* 1994; 330:981.
125. Virmani R, Farb A, Burke AP: Coronary angioplasty from the perspective of atherosclerotic plaque: morphologic predictors of immediate success and restenosis. *Am Heart J* 1994; 127:163.
126. Riessen R, Isner JM: Prospects for site-specific delivery of pharmacologic and molecular therapies. *J Am Coll Cardiol* 1994; 23:1234.
127. Lincoff AM, Topol EJ, Ellis SG: Local drug delivery for the prevention of restenosis. *Circulation* 1994; 90:2070.
128. Casscells W: Growth factor therapies for vascular injury and ischemia. *Circulation* 1995; 91:2699.
129. Bennett MR, Schwartz SM: Antisense therapy for angioplasty restenosis. *Circulation* 1995; 92:1981.
130. Kibbe MR, Billiar TR, Tzeng E: Gene therapy for restenosis. *Circ Res* 2000; 86:829.
131. Stertzer SH, Rosenblum J, Shaw RE, et al: Coronary rotational ablation: initial experience in 302 procedures. *J Am Coll Cardiol* 1993; 21:287.

132. Diethrich EB: Classical and endovascular surgery: indications and outcomes. *Surg Today* 1994; 24:949.
133. Serruys PW, de Jaegere P, Kiemeneij F, et al: A comparison of balloon-expandable-stent implantation with balloon angioplasty in patients with coronary artery disease. *N Engl J Med* 1994; 331:489.
134. Eeckhout E, Kappenberger L, Goy J-J: Stents for intracoronary placement: current status and future directions. *J Am Coll Cardiol* 1996; 27:757.
135. Al Suwaidi J, Berger PB, Holmes DR Jr: Coronary artery stents. *JAMA* 2000; 284:1828.
136. Stone GW, Grines CL, Cox DA, et al: Comparison of angioplasty with stenting, with or without abciximab, in acute myocardial infarction. *N Engl J Med* 2002; 346:957.
137. van Beusekom HMM, van der Giessen WJ, van Suylen RJ, et al: Histology after stenting of human saphenous vein bypass grafts: observations from surgically excised grafts 3 to 320 days after stent implantation. *J Am Coll Cardiol* 1993; 21:45.
138. Carter AJ, Laird JR, Kufs WM, et al: Coronary stenting with a novel stainless steel balloon-expandable stent: determinants of neointimal formation and changes in arterial geometry after placement in an atherosclerotic model. *J Am Coll Cardiol* 1996; 27:1270.
139. Farb A, Sangiorgi G, Carter AJ, et al: Pathology of acute and chronic coronary stenting in humans. *Circulation* 1999; 99:44.
140. Virmani R, Farb A: Pathology of in-stent restenosis. *Curr Opin Lipid* 1999; 10:499.
141. Farb A, Weber DK, Kolodgie FD, et al: Morphological predictors of restenosis after coronary stenting in humans. *Circulation* 2002; 105:2974.
142. Tepe G, Dinkelborg LM, Brehme U, et al: Prophylaxis of restenosis with 186Re-labeled stents in a rabbit model. *Circulation* 2001; 104:480.
143. Farb A, Heller PF, Shroff S, et al: Pathological analysis of local delivery of paclitaxel via a polymer-coated stent. *Circulation* 2001; 104:473.
144. Salame MY, Verheye S, Cracker IR, et al: Intracoronary radiation therapy. *Eur Heart J* 2001; 22:629.
145. Williams DO, Sharaf BL: Intracoronary radiation: it keeps on glowing. *Circulation* 2000; 101:350.
146. Sousa JE, Costa MA, Abizaid AC, et al: Sustained suppression of neointimal proliferation by sirolimus-eluting stents: one-year angiographic and intravascular ultrasound follow-up. *Circulation* 2001; 104:1996.
147. Colombo A, Stankovic G, Moses JW: Selection of coronary stents. *J Am Coll Cardiol* 2002; 40:1021.
148. Moustapha A, Anderson HV: Revascularization interventions for ischemic heart disease. *Curr Opin Cardiol* 2000; 15:463.
149. Pretre R, Turina MI: Choice of revascularization strategy for patients with coronary artery disease. *JAMA* 2001; 285:992.
150. Pitt M, Lewis ME, Bonser RS: Coronary artery surgery for ischemic heart failure: risks, benefits and the importance of assessment of myocardial viability. *Prog Cardiovasc Dis* 2001; 43:373.
151. Patil CV, Nikolsky E, Boulos M, et al: Multivessel coronary artery disease: current revascularization strategies. *Eur Heart J* 2001; 22:1183.
152. Bourassa MG: Long-term vein graft patency. *Curr Opin Cardiol* 1994; 9:685.
153. Nwasokwa ON: Coronary artery bypass graft disease. *Ann Intern Med* 1995; 123:528.
154. Saber RS, Edwards WD, Holmes DR Jr, et al: Balloon angioplasty of aortocoronary saphenous vein bypass grafts: a histopathologic study of six grafts from five patients, with emphasis on restenosis and embolic complications. *J Am Coll Cardiol* 1988; 12:1501.
155. Loop FD, Lytle BW, Cosgrove DM, et al: Influence of the internal-mammary-artery graft on 10-year survival and other cardiac events. *N Engl J Med* 1986; 314:1.
156. Barner HB: Remodeling of arterial conduits in coronary grafting. *Ann Thorac Surg* 2002; 73:1341.
157. Bridges CR: Myocardial laser revascularization: the controversy and the data. *Ann Thorac Surg* 2000; 69:655.
158. Nathan M, Aranki S: Transmyocardial laser revascularization. *Curr Opin Cardiol* 2001; 16:310.
159. Cooley DA, Frazier OH, Kadipasaoglu KA, et al.: Transmyocardial laser revascularization: clinical experience with twelve-month follow-up. *J Thorac Cardiovasc Surg* 1996; 111:791.
160. Horvath KA, Mannting F, Cummings N, et al: Transmyocardial laser revascularization: operative techniques and clinical results at two years. *J Thorac Cardiovasc Surg* 1996; 111:1047.
161. Horvath KA: Results of clinical trials of transmyocardial laser revascularization versus medical management for end-stage coronary disease. *J Clin Laser Med Surg* 2000; 18:247.
162. Fleischer KJ, Goldschmidt-Clermont PJ, Fonger JD, et al: One-month histologic response of transmyocardial laser channel with molecular intervention. *Ann Thorac Surg* 1996; 62:1051.
163. Kohmoto T, Fischer PE, Gu A, et al: Physiology, histology and 2-week morphology of acute transmyocardial channels made with a CO_2 laser. *Ann Thorac Surg* 1997; 63:1275.
164. Malekan R, Reynolds C, Narula N, et al: Angiogenesis in transmyocardial laser revascularization: a nonspecific response to injury. *Circulation* 1998; 98:II62.
165. Whittaker P: Transmyocardial revascularization: the fate of myocardial channels. *Ann Thorac Surg* 1999; 68:2376.
166. Prieto A, Eisenberg J, Thakur RK: Nonarrhythmic complications of acute myocardial infarction. *Cardiol Clin North Am* 2001; 19:397.
167. Huikuri HV, Castellanos A, Myerburg RJ: Sudden death due to cardiac arrhythmias. *N Engl J Med* 2001; 345:1473.
168. Virmani R, Burke AP, Farb A: Sudden cardiac death. *Cardiovasc Pathol* 2001; 10:211.
169. Batts KP, Ackermann DM, Edwards WD: Postinfarction rupture of the left ventricular free wall: clinicopathologic correlates in 100 consecutive autopsy cases. *Hum Pathol* 1990; 21:530.
170. Sutherland FWH, Guell FJ, Pathi VL, et al: Postinfarction ventricular free wall rupture: strategies for diagnosis and treatment. *Ann Thorac Surg* 1996; 61:1281.
171. McMullan MH, Maples MD, Kilgore TL Jr., et al: Surgical experience with left ventricular free wall rupture. *Ann Thorac Surg* 2001; 71:1894.
172. Frances C, Romero A, Grady D: Left ventricular pseudoaneurysm. *J Am Coll Cardiol* 1998; 32:557.
173. Birnbaum Y, Fishbein MC, Blanche C, et al: Ventricular septal rupture after acute myocardial infarction. *N Engl J Med* 2002; 347:1426.
174. Barbour DJ, Roberts WC: Rupture of a left ventricular papillary muscle during acute myocardial infarction: analysis of 22 necropsy patients. *J Am Coll Cardiol* 1986; 8:558.
175. Samman B, Korr KS, Katz AS, et al: Pitfalls in the diagnosis and management of papillary muscle rupture: a study of four cases and review of the literature. *Clin Cardiol* 1995; 18: 591.
176. Stanley AW Jr., Athanasuleas CL, Buckberg GD, RESTORE Group: Left ventricular remodeling and functional mitral regurgitation: mechanisms and therapy. *Semin Thorac Cardiovasc Surg* 2001; 13:486–495.
177. Zehender M, Kasper W, Kauder E, et al: Right ventricular infarction as an independent predictor of prognosis after acute inferior myocardial infarction. *N Engl J Med* 1993; 328:981.
178. Kinch JW, Ryan TJ: Right ventricular infarction. *N Engl J Med* 1994; 330:1211.

179. Weissman HF, Healy B: Myocardial infarct expansion, infarct extension, and reinfarction: pathophysiologic concepts. *Prog Cardiovasc Dis* 1987; 30:73.
180. Muller JE, Rude RE, Braunwald E, et al: Myocardial infarct extension: occurrence, outcome, and risk factors in the multicenter investigation of limitation of infarct size. *Ann Intern Med* 1988; 108:1.
181. Weiss JL, Marino PN, Shapiro EP: Myocardial infarct expansion: recognition, significance and pathology. *Am J Cardiol* 1991; 68:35D.
182. Yousef ZR, Redwood SR, Marber MS: Postinfarction left ventricular remodeling: a pathophysiological and therapeutic review. *Cardiovasc Drugs Ther* 2000; 14:243.
183. Cohn JN, Ferrari R, Sharpe N: Cardiac remodeling—concepts and clinical implications: a consensus paper from an international forum on cardiac remodeling. *J Am Coll Cardiol* 2000; 35:569.
184. Francis GS: Pathophysiology of chronic heart failure. *Am J Med* 2001; 7A:37S.
185. Anversa P, Nadal-Ginard B: Myocyte renewal and ventricular remodelling. *Nature* 2002; 415:249.
186. Vaughan DE, Pfeffer MA: Post-myocardial infarction ventricular remodeling: animal and human studies. *Cardiovasc Drugs Ther* 1994; 8:453.
187. Cohn JN: Structural basis for heart failure: ventricular remodeling and its pharmacological inhibition. *Circulation* 1995; 91:2504.
188. Anversa P, Sonnenblick EH: Ischemic cardiomyopathy: pathophysiologic mechanisms. *Prog Cardiovasc Dis* 1990; 33:49.
189. Cabin HS, Roberts WC: True left ventricular aneurysm and healed myocardial infarction: clinical and necropsy observations including quantification of degrees of coronary arterial narrowing. *Am J Cardiol* 1980; 46:754.
190. Brown SL, Gropler RJ, Harris KM: Distinguishing left ventricular aneurysm from pseudoaneurysm: a review of the literature. *Chest* 1997; 111:1403.
191. Dare AJ, Veinot JP, Edwards WD, et al: New observations on the etiology of aortic valve disease: a surgical pathologic study of 236 cases from 1990. *Hum Pathol* 1993; 24:1330.
192. Dare AJ, Harrity PJ, Tazelaar HD, et al: Evaluation of surgically excised mitral valves: revised recommendations based on changing operative procedures in the 1990s. *Hum Pathol* 1993; 24:1286.
193. Sabet HY, Edwards WD, Tazelaar HD, Daley RC: Congenitally bicuspid aortic valves: a surgical pathology study of 542 cases (1991 through 1996) and a literature review of 2,715 additional cases. *Mayo Clin Proc* 1999; 74:14.
194. Carabello BA: Aortic stenosis. *N Engl J Med* 2002; 346:677.
195. Carabello BA: Evaluation and management of patients with aortic stenosis. *Circulation* 2002; 105:1746.
196. Otto CM, Lind BK, Kitzman DW, et al: Association of aortic-valve sclerosis with cardiovascular mortality and morbidity in the elderly. *N Engl J Med* 1999;341:142.
197. Benjamin EJ, Plehn JF, D'Agostino RB, et al: Mitral annular calcification and the risk of stroke in an elderly cohort. *N Engl J Med* 1992; 327:374.
198. Kaplan EL: Global assessment of rheumatic fever and rheumatic heart disease at the close of the century: influences and dynamics of populations and pathogens: a failure to realize prevention? *Circulation* 1993; 88:1964.
199. Stollerman GH: Rheumatic fever in the 21st century. *Clin Infect Dis* 2001; 33:806.
200. Rullan E, Sigal LH: Rheumatic fever. *Curr Rheumatol Rep* 2001; 3:445.
201. Roberts WC, Virmani R: Aschoff bodies at autopsy in valvular heart disease. *Circulation* 1978; 57:803.
202. Hanson EW, Neerhut RK, Lynch C 3rd: Mitral valve prolapse. *Anesthesiology* 1996; 85:178.
203. Jacobs W, Chamoun A, Stouffer GA: Mitral valve prolapse: a review of the literature. *Am J Med Sci* 2001; 321:401.
204. Carabello BA: The pathophysiology of mitral regurgitation. *J Heart Valve Dis* 2000; 9:600.
205. Otto CM: Evaluation and management of chronic mitral regurgitation. *N Engl J Med* 2001; 345:740.
206. Rabkin E, Aikawa M, Stone JR, et al: Activated interstitial myofibroblasts express catabolic enzymes and mediate matrix remodeling in myxomatous heart valves. *Circulation* 2001: 104:2525.
207. Mylonakis E, Calderwood SB: Infective endocarditis in adults. *N Engl J Med* 2001; 345:1318.
208. Durack DT, Lukes AS, Bright DK et al: New criteria for diagnosis of infective endocarditis: utilization of specific echocardiographic findings. *Am J Med* 1994; 96:200.
209. Frontera JA, Gradon JD: Right-sided endocarditis in injection drug users: review of proposed mechanisms of pathogenesis. *Clin Infect Dis* 2000; 102:2842.
210. Reul RM, Cohn LH: Mitral valve reconstruction for mitral insufficiency. *Prog Cardiovasc Dis* 1997; 39:567.
211. Bolling SF: Mitral valve reconstruction in the patient with heart failure. *Heart Fail Rev* 2001; 6:177.
212. Duran C, Kumar N, Gometza B, et al: Indications and limitations of aortic valve reconstruction. *Ann Thorac Surg* 1991; 52:447.
213. David TE, Feindel CM, Bos J: Repair of the aortic valve in patients with aortic insufficiency and aortic root aneurysm. *J Thorac Cardiovasc Surg* 1995; 109:345.
214. Mezzacapo B: Abrasion-debridement of aortic valve calcific stenosis: immediate and mid-term clinical results. *J Cardiovasc Surg* (Torino) 1998; 39:667.
215. Kellner HJ, Pracki P, Hildenbrandt A, et al: Aortic valve debridement by ultrasonic surgical aspirator in degenerative, aortic valve stenosis: follow-up with Doppler echocardiography. *Eur J Cardiothorac Surg* 1996; 10:498.
216. Byrne JG, Aranki SF, Cohn LH: Repair versus replacement of mitral valve for treating severe ischemic mitral regurgitation. *Coron Artery Dis* 2000; 11:31.
217. Vahanian A: Balloon valvuloplasty. *Heart* 2001; 85:223.
218. Iung B, Vahanian A: The long-term outcome of balloon valvuloplasty for mitral stenosis. *Curr Cardiol Rep* 2002; 4:118.
219. Rao PS: Long-term follow-up results after balloon dilation of pulmonic stenosis, aortic stenosis, and coarctation of the aorta: a review. *Prog Cardiovasc Dis* 1999; 42:59.
220. Antunes MJ: Valvuloplasty for acquired aortic valve disease. *Thorac Cardiovasc Surg* 1997; 45:159.
221. Treasure CB, Schoen FJ, Treseler PA, et al: Leaflet entrapment causing acute severe aortic insufficiency during balloon aortic valvuloplasty. *Clin Cardiol* 1989; 12:405.
222. Schoen FJ, Edwards WD: Valvular heart disease: general principles and stenosis, in Silver MD, Gotlieb AI, Schoen FJ (eds): *Cardiovascular Pathology*, 3d ed. Philadelphia, WB Saunders, 2001; p 402.
223. Sapirstein JS, Smith PK: The "ideal" replacement heart valve. *Am Heart J* 2001; 141:856.
224. Turina J, Hess OM, Turina M, et al: Cardiac bioprostheses in the 1990s. *Circulation* 1993; 88:775.
225. Vongpatanasin W, Hillis LD, Lange RA: Prosthetic heart valves. *N Engl J Med* 1996; 335:407.
226. Schoen FJ: Pathology of heart valve substitution with mechanical and tissue prosthesis, in Silver MD, Gotlieb AI, Schoen FJ (eds): *Cardiovascular Pathology*. Philadelphia, Churchill Livingstone, 2001; p 629.
227. Cao H: Mechanical performance of pyrolytic carbon in prosthetic heart valve applications. *J Heart Valve Dis* 1996; 5(suppl I):532.
228. Fann JI, Burdon TA: Are the indications for tissue valves different in 2001 and how do we communicate these changes to our cardiology colleagues? *Curr Opin Cardiol* 2001 16:126.

229. Schoen FJ, Titus JL, Lawrie GM: Autopsy-determined causes of death after cardiac valve replacement. *JAMA* 1983; 249: 899.
230. Reardon MJ, David TE: Mitral valve replacement with preservation of the subvalvular apparatus. *Curr Opin Cardiol* 1999; 14:104-110.
231. Bloomfield P, Wheatley DJ, et al: Twelve-year comparison of a Bjork-Shiley mechanical heart valve with porcine bioprostheses. *N Engl J Med* 1991; 324:573.
232. Hammermeister KE, Sethi GK, Henderson WG, et al: Outcomes 15 years after valve replacement with a mechanical versus a bioprosthetic valve: final report of the Veterans Affairs randomized trial. *J Am Coll Cardiol* 2000; 36:1152.
233. Blackstone EH, Kirklin JW: Death and other time-related events after valve replacement. *Circulation* 1985; 72:753.
234. Rose AG: Autopsy-determined causes of death following heart valve replacement. *Am J Cardiovasc Pathol* 1987; 1:30.
235. Burke AP, Farb A, Sessums L, et al: Causes of sudden cardiac death in patients with replacement valves: an autopsy study. *J Heart Valve Dis* 1994; 3:310.
236. Vaideeswar P, Deshpande JR, Sivaraman A: Cardiac valve prostheses at autopsy: an analysis of 337 cases with clinicopathologic correlation. *Cardivasc Pathol* 1997; 6:279.
237. Schoen FJ: Pathologic considerations in replacement heart valves and other cardiovascular prosthetic devices, in Schoen FJ, Gimbrone MA (eds): *Cardiovascular Pathology: Clinicopathologic Correlations and Pathogenetic Mechanisms*. Baltimore, Williams & Wilkins, 1995; p 194.
238. Ferrans VJ, Hilbert SL, Fujita S, et al: Abnormalities in explanted bioprosthetic cardiac valves, in Virmani R, Atkinson JB, Fenoglio JJ (eds): *Cardiovascular Pathology*. Philadelphia, WB Saunders, 1993; p 373.
239. Hwang MH, Burchfiel CM, Sethi GK, et al: Comparison of the causes of late death following aortic and mitral valve replacement. *J Heart Valve Dis* 1994; 3:17.
240. Edmunds LH, Cohn LH, Weisel RD: Guidelines for reporting morbidity and mortality after cardiac valvular operations. *J Thorac Cardiovasc Surg* 1988; 96:351.
241. Schoen FJ, Levy RJ, Piehler HR: Pathologic considerations in replacement cardiac valves. *Cardiovasc Pathol* 1992; 1:29.
242. Schoen FJ: Surgical pathology of removed natural and prosthetic heart valves. *Hum Pathol* 1987; 18:558.
243. Schoen FJ, Hobson CE: Anatomic analysis of removed prosthetic heart valves: causes of failure of 33 mechanical valves and 58 bioprostheses, 1980 to 1983. *Hum Pathol* 1985; 16:549.
244. Height SE, Smith MP: Strategems for anticoagulant therapy following mechanical heart valve replacement. *J Heart Valve Dis* 1999; 8:662.
245. Koca V, Bozat T, Sarikamis C, et al: The use of transesophageal echocardiography guidance of thrombolytic therapy in prosthetic mitral valve thrombosis. *J Heart Valve Dis* 2000; 9:374.
246. Anderson JM, Kottke-Marchant K: Platelet interactions with biomaterials and artificial devices. *CRC Crit Rev Biocompat* 1985; 1:111.
247. Lengyel M, Vandor L: The role of thrombolysis in the management of left-sided prosthetic valve thrombosis: a study of 85 cases diagnosed by transesophageal echocardiography. *J Heart Valve Dis* 2001; 10:636.
248. Hurrell DG, Schaff HV, Tajik AJ: Thrombolytic therapy for obstruction of mechanical prosthetic valves. *Mayo Clin Proc* 1996; 71:605.
249. Piper C, Korfer R, Horstkotte D: Prosthetic valve endocarditis. *Heart* 2001; 85:590.
250. Chastre J, Trouillet JL: Early infective endocarditis on prosthetic valves. *Eur Heart J* 1995; 16(suppl):32.
251. Horstkotte D, Piper C, Niehues R, et al: Late prosthetic valve endocarditis. *Eur Heart J* 1995; 16(suppl):39.
252. Gordon SM, Serkey JM, Longworth DL, et al: Early onset prosthetic valve endocarditis: the Cleveland Clinic experience 1992–1997. *Ann Thorac Surg* 2000; 69:1388.
253. Lengyel M: The impact of transesophageal echocardiography on the management of prosthetic valve endocarditis: experience of 31 cases and review of the literature. *J Heart Valve Dis* 1997; 6: 204.
254. O'Neill WW, Chandler JG, Gordon RE, et al: Radiographic detection of strut separations in Bjork-Shiley convexo-concave mitral valves. *N Engl J Med* 1995; 333:414.
255. Copeland JG: The CarboMedics prosthetic heart valve: a second generation bileaflet prosthesis. *Semin Thorac Cardiovasc Surg* 1996; 8:237.
256. Klepetko W, et al: Leaflet fracture in Edwards-Duramedics bileaflet valves. *J Thorac Cardiovasc Surg* 1989; 97:90.
257. He Z, Xi B, Zhu K, et al: Mechanisms of mechanical heart valve cavitation: investigation using a tilting disk valve model. *J Heart Valve Dis* 2001; 10:666.
258. Odell JA, Durandt J, Shama DM, Vythilingum S: Spontaneous embolization of a St. Jude prosthetic mitral valve leaflet. *Ann Thorac Surg* 1985; 39:569.
259. Schoen FJ, Levy RJ: Tissue heart valves: current challenges and future research perspectives. *J Biomed Mater Res* 1999; 47: 439.
260. Grunkemeier GL, Jamieson WR, Miller DC, et al: Actuarial versus actual risk of porcine structural valve deterioration. *J Thorac Cardiovasc Surg* 1994; 108:709.
261. Sacks MS, Schoen FJ: Collagen fiber disruption occurs independent of calcification in clinically explanted bioprosthetic heart valves. *J Biomed Mater Res* 2002; 62:359.
262. Vesely I, Barber JE, Ratliff NB: Tissue damage and calcification may be independent mechanisms of bioprosthetic heart valve failure. *J Heart Valve Dis* 2001; 10:471.
263. McGonagle-Wolff K, Schoen FJ: Morphologic findings in explanted Mitroflow pericardial bioprosthetic valves. *Am J Cardiol* 1992; 70:263.
264. Masters RG, Walley VM, Pipe AL, et al: Long-term experience with the Ionescu-Shiley pericardial valve. *Ann Thorac Surg* 1995; 60(suppl):S288.
265. Hilbert SL, Ferrans VJ, McAllister HA, et al: Ionescu-Shiley bovine pericardial bioprostheses: histologic and ultrastructural studies. *Am J Pathol* 1992; 140:1195.
266. Rao KP, Shanthi C: Reduction of calcification by various treatments in cardiac valves. *J Biomater Appl* 1999; 13:238.
267. Valente M, Bortolotti U, Thiene G: Ultrastructural substrates of dystrophic calcification in porcine bioprosthetic valve failure. *Am J Pathol* 1985; 119:12.
268. Schoen FJ, Levy RJ, Nelson AC, et al: Onset and progression of experimental bioprosthetic heart valve calcification. *Lab Invest* 1985; 52:523.
269. Schoen FJ, Tsao JW, Levy RJ: Calcification of bovine pericardium used in cardiac valve bioprostheses: implications for the mechanisms of bioprosthetic tissue mineralization. *Am J Pathol* 1986; 123:134.
270. Schoen FJ: Aortic valve structure-function correlations; role of elastic fibers no longer a stretch of the imagination. *J Heart Valve Dis* 1997; 6:1.
271. Schoen FJ: Future directions in tissue heart valves: impact of recent insights from biology and pathology. *J Heart Valve Dis* 1999; 8:350.
272. Allard MF, Thompson CR, Baldelli RJ, et al: Commissural region dehiscence from the stent post of Carpentier-Edwards bioprosthetic cardiac valves. *Cardiovasc Pathol* 1995; 4:155.

273. Walley VM, Bedard JP: Displacement of a commissure of the Intact porcine bioprosthesis resulting in valvular insufficiency. *Cardiovasc Pathol* 1996; 5:175.
274. Schaff HV, Carrel TP, Jamieson WR, et al: Paravalvular leak and other events in silzone-coated mechanical heart valves: a report from AVERT. *Ann Thorac Surg* 2002; 73:785.
275. Bodnar E: The Silzone dilemma—what did we learn? *J Heart Valve Dis* 2000;9:170.
276. Kirklin JK, Smith D, Novick W, et al: Long-term function of cryopreserved aortic homografts. *J Thorac Cardiovasc Surg* 1993; 106:154.
277. O'Brien MF, Harrocks S, Stafford EG, et al: The homograft aortic valve: a 29-year, 99.3% follow up of 1,022 valve replacements. *J Heart Valve Dis* 2001; 10:334.
278. Grunkemeier GL, Bodnar E: Comparison of structural valve failure among different models of homograft valves. *J Heart Valve Dis* 1994; 3:556.
279. Hudson REB: Pathology of the human aortic valve homograft. *Br Heart J* 1966; 28:291.
280. O'Brien M, Stafford E, Gardner M, et al: A comparison of aortic valve replacement with viable cryopreserved and fresh allograft valves with a note on chromosomal studies. *J Thorac Cardiovasc Surg* 1987; 94:812.
281. Mitchell RN, Jonas RA, Schoen FJ: Structure-function correlations in cryopreserved allograft cardiac valves: viability, durability, and immunogenicity. *Ann Thorac Surg* 1995; 60:S108.
282. Ross D, Jackson M, Davies J: Pulmonary autograft aortic valve replacement: long-term results. *J Cardiac Surg* 1991; 6:529.
283. Dacey LJ: Pulmonary homografts: current status. *Curr Opin Cardiol* 2000; 15:86.
284. Elkins RC, Lane MM, McCue C: Pulmonary autograft reoperation: incidence and management. *Ann Thorac Surg* 1996; 62:450.
285. Oury JH: Clinical aspects of the Ross procedure: indications and contraindications. *Semin Thorac Cardiovasc Surg* 1996; 8:328.
286. David TE, Feindel CM, Scully HE, et al: Aortic valve replacement with stentless porcine aortic valves: a ten-year experience. *J Heart Valve Dis* 1998;7:250.
287. Westaby S, Jin XY, Katsuma T, et al: Valve replacement with a stentless bioprosthesis: versatility of the porcine aortic root. *J Thorac Cardiovasc Surg* 1998; 116:477.
288. Jin XY, Dhital K, Bhattacharya K, et al: Fifty-year hemodynamic performance of the prima stentless aortic valve. *Ann Thorac Surg* 1998; 66:805.
289. David TE, Puschmann R, Ivanov J, et al: Aortic valve replacement with stentless and stented porcine valves: a case-match study. *J Thorac Cardiovasc Surg* 1998; 116:236.
290. Cleveland DC, Williams WG, Razzouk AJ, et al: Failure of cryopreserved homograft valved conduits in the pulmonary circulation. *Circulation* 1992; 86(suppl II):II-150.
291. Fyfe BS, Schoen FJ: Pathologic analysis of non-stented Freestyle™ aortic root bioprostheses treated with amino acid oleic acid (AOA). *Semin Thorac Cardiovasc Surg* 1999; 11:151.
292. Schoen FJ, Levy RJ, Hilbert SL, et al: Antimineralization treatments for bioprosthetic heart valves. *J Thorac Cardiovasc Surg* 1992; 104:1285.
293. Chen W, Schoen FJ, Levy RJ: Mechanism of efficacy of 2-amino oleic acid for inhibition of calcification of glutaraldehyde-pretreated porcine bioprosthetic heart valves. *Circulation* 1994; 90:323.
294. Vyavahare N, Jones PL, Hirsch D, et al: Prevention of glutaraldehyde-fixed bioprosthetic heart valve calcification by alcohol pretreatment: further mechanistic studies. *J Heart Valve Dis* 2000; 9:561.
295. Schoen FJ, Levy RJ: Pathology of substitute heart valves: new concepts and developments. *J Cardiac Surg* 1994; 9(suppl):222.
296. Schoen FJ, Levy RJ: Tissue heart valves: current challenges and future research perspectives. *J Biomed Mater Res* 1999; 47:439.
297. Edwards WD: Cardiomyopathies. *Maj Probl Pathol* 1991; 23:257.
298. Report of the 1995 World Health Organization/International Society and Federation of Cardiology Task Force on the Definition and Classification of Cardiomyopathies. *Circulation* 1996; 93:841.
299. Fatkin D, Graham RM: Molecular mechanisms of inherited cardiomyopathies. *Physiol Rev* 2002; 82:945.
300. Franz WM, Muller OJ, Katus HA: Cardiomyopathies: from genetics to the prospect of treatment. *Lancet* 2001; 358:1627.
301. Towbin JA, Bowles NE: The failing heart. *Nature* 2002; 415:227.
302. Roberts R, Sigwart U: New concepts in hypertrophic cardiomyopathies. *Circulation* 2001;104:2113, 2249.
303. Hauck AJ, Edwards WD: Histopathologic examination of tissues obtained by endomyocardial biopsy, in Fowles RE (ed.): *Cardiac Biopsy*. New York, Futura, 1992; p 95.
304. Grunig E: Frequency and phenotypes of familial dilated cardiomyopathy. *J Am Coll Cardiol* 1998; 31:186.
305. Thiene G, Nava A, Corrado D, et al: Right ventricular cardiomyopathy and sudden death in young people. *N Engl J Med* 1988; 318:129.
306. Thiene G, Basso C: Arrhythmogenic right ventricular cardiomyopathy: an update. *Cardiovasc Path* 2001; 10:109.
307. Gemayel C, Pelliccia A, Thompson PD: Arrhythmogenic right ventricular cardiomyopathy. *J Am Coll Cardiol* 2001; 38:1773.
308. Corrado D, Basso C, Nava A, et al: Arrhythmogenic right ventricular cardiomyopathy: current diagnostic and management strategies. *Cardiol Rev* 2001; 9:259.
309. Maron BJ: Hypertrophic cardiomyopathy: a systematic review. *JAMA* 2002; 287:1308.
310. Spirito P, Bellone P, Harris KM, et al: Magnitude of left ventricular hypertrophy predicts the risk of sudden death in hypertrophic cardiomyopathy. *N Engl J Med* 2000; 342:1778.
311. Elliot PM, Polemiecki J, Dickie S, et al: Sudden death in hypertrophic cardiomyopathy: identification of high risk patients. *J Am Coll Cardiol* 2000; 36:2212.
312. Spirito P, Seidman CE, McKenna WJ, et al: Management of hypertrophic cardiomyopathy. *N Engl J Med* 1997; 30:775.
313. Brunner-La Schonbeck MH, Rocca HP, Vogt PR, et al: Long-term follow-up in hypertrophic obstructive cardiomyopathy after septal myomectomy. *Ann Thorac Surg* 1998; 65:1207.
314. Shamin W, Yousufuddin M, Wang D, et al: Nonsurgical reduction of the interventricular septum in patients with hypertrophic cardiomyopathy. *N Engl J Med* 2002; 347:1326.
315. Nagueh SF, Ommen SR, Lakkis KM, et al: Comparison of ethanol septal reduction therapy with surgical myectomy for the treatment of hypertrophic obstructive cardiomyopathy. *J Am Coll Cardiol* 2001; 38:1706.
316. Towbin JA: Molecular genetics of hypertrophic cardiomyopathy. *Curr Cardiol Rep* 2000; 2:134.
317. Watkins H, Rosenzweig A, Hwang DS, et al: Characteristics and prognostic implications of myosin missense mutations in familial hypertrophic cardiomyopathy. *N Engl J Med* 1992; 326:1108.
318. Hancock EW: Differential diagnosis of restrictive cardiomyopathy and constrictive pericarditis. *Heart* 2001; 86:343.
319. Valente HA, Schroeder JS: Recent advances in cardiac transplantation [editorial]. *N Engl J Med* 1995; 333:660.
320. Deng MC: Cardiac transplantation. *Heart* 2002; 87:177.
321. Winters GL: Heart transplantation: explant, biopsy, and autopsy characteristics, in McManus B (ed): *Atlas of Cardiovascular Pathology for the Clinician*. Philadelphia, Current Medicine, 2001; p 184.
322. Winters GL, Schoen FJ: Pathology of cardiac transplantation, in Silver MD, Gotlieb AI, Schoen FJ (eds.): *Cardiovascular Pathology*. Philadelphia, Churchill Livingstone, 2001; p 725.

323. Gravanis MB, Hertzler GL, Franch RH, et al: Hypersensitivity myocarditis in heart transplant candidates. *J Heart Lung Transplant* 1991; 10:688.
324. Spear G: Eosinophilic explant carditis with eosinophilia: hypersensitivity to dobutamine infusion. *J Heart Lung Transplant* 1995; 14:755.
325. Billingham ME: Pathology of human cardiac transplantation, in Schoen FJ, Gimbrone MA (eds): *Cardiovascular Pathology: Clinicopathologic Correlations and Pathogenetic Mechanisms*. Baltimore, Williams & Wilkins, 1995; p 108.
326. Tazelaar HD, Edwards WD: Pathology of cardiac transplantation: recipient hearts (chronic heart failure) and donor hearts (acute and chronic rejection). *Mayo Clin Proc* 1992; 67:685.
327. Anversa P, Nadal-Ginard B: Myocyte renewal and ventricular remodeling. *Nature* 2002; 415:240.
328. Fyfe B, Loh Evan, Winters GL, et al: Heart transplantation–associated perioperative ischemic myocardial injury. *Circulation* 1996; 93:1133.
329. Day JD, Rayburn BK, Gaudin PB, et al: Cardiac allograft vasculopathy: the central pathogenetic role of ischemia-induced endothelial cell injury. *J Heart Lung Transplant* 1995; 14:S142.
330. Sethi GK, Kosaraju S, Arabia FA, et al: Is it necessary to perform surveillance endomyocardial biopsies in heart transplant recipients? *J Heart Lung Transplant* 1995; 14:1047.
331. Caves PK, Stinson EB, Billingham ME, et al: Serial transvenous biopsy of the transplanted human heart: Improved management of acute rejection episodes. *Lancet* 1974; 1:821.
332. Billingham ME, Cary NRB, Hammond ME, et al: A working formulation for the standardization of nomenclature in the diagnosis of heart and lung rejection: heart rejection study group. *J Heart Transplant* 1990; 9:587.
333. Winters GL, Loh E, Schoen FJ: Natural history of focal moderate cardiac allograft rejection: is treatment warranted? *Circulation* 1995; 91:1975.
334. Brunner-LaRocca HP, Sutsch G, Schneider G, et al: Natural course of moderate cardiac allograft rejection (International Society for Heart Transplantation grade 2) early and late after transplantation. *Circulation* 1996; 94:1334.
335. Miller LW, Granville DJ, Narula J, et al: Apoptosis in cardiac transplant rejection. *Cardiol Clin* 2001; 19:41.
336. Schoen FJ, Libby P: Cardiac transplant graft arteriosclerosis. *Trends Cardiovasc Med* 1991; 1:216.
337. Behrendt D, Ganz P, Fang JC: Cardiac allograft vasculopathy. *Curr Opin Cardiol* 2000; 15:422.
338. Gao SZ, Schroeder JS, Alderman EL, et al: Prevalence of accelerated coronary artery disease in heart transplant survivors: comparison of cyclosporin and azathioprine regimens. *Circulation* 1989; 80(suppl):III-100.
339. Constanzo MR, Naftel DC, Pritzker MR, et al: Heart transplant coronary artery disease detected by coronary angiography: a multiinstitutional study of preoperative donor and recipient risk factors. Cardiac Transplant Research Database. *J Heart Lung Transplant* 1998; 17:744.
340. Winters GL, Schoen FJ: Graft arteriosclerosis-induced myocardial pathology in heart transplant recipients: predictive value of endomyocardial biopsy. *J Heart Lung Transplant* 1997; 16:985.
341. Neish AS, Loh E, Schoen FJ: Myocardial changes in cardiac transplant-associated coronary arteriosclerosis: potential for timely diagnosis. *J Am Coll Cardiol* 1992; 19:586.
342. Johnson DE, Alderman EL, Schroeder JS, et al: Transplant coronary artery disease: histopathologic correlations with angiographic morphology. *J Am Coll Cardiol* 1991; 17:449.
343. Liu G, Butany J: Morphology of graft arteriosclerosis in cardiac transplant recipients. *Hum Pathol* 1992; 23:768.
344. Shimizu K, Sugiyama S, Aikawa M, et al: Host bone marrow cells are a source of donor intimal smooth muscle-like cells in murine aortic transplant arteriopathy. *Nature Med* 2001;7:378.
345. Quaini F, Urbanek K, Beltrami AP, et al: Chimerism of the transplanted heart. *N Engl J Med* 2002; 346:5.
346. Rickenbacher PR, Pinto FJ, Lewis NP, et al: Prognostic importance of intimal thickness as measured by intracoronary ultrasound after cardiac transplantation. *Circulation* 1995; 92:3445.
347. Cockfield SM: Identifying the patient at risk for post-transplant lymphoproliferative disorder. *Transpl Infect Dis* 2001; 3:70.
348. Nalesnik MA: The diverse pathology of post-transplant lymphoproliferative disorders: the importance of a standardized approach. *Transpl Infect Dis* 2001; 3:88.
349. Armatige JM, Kormos RL, Stuart RS, et al: Posttransplant lymphoproliferative disease in thoracic organ transplant patients: ten years of cyclosporin-based immunosuppression. *J Heart Lung Transplant* 1991; 10:877.
350. Cleary ML, Warnke R, Sklar J: Monoclonality of lymphoproliferative lesions in cardiac transplant recipients: clonal analysis based on immunoglobulin-gene rearrangements. *N Engl J Med* 1984; 310:477.
351. Zilz ND, Olson LJ, McGregor CG: Treatment of post-transplant lymphoproliferative disorders with monoclonal CD20 (rituximab) after heart transplantation. *J Heart Lung Transplant* 2001; 20:770.
352. Hosenpud JD, Bennett LE, Keck BM, et al: The registry of the International Society for Heart and Lung Transplantation: seventeenth official report—2000. *J Heart Lung Transplant* 2000; 19:909.
353. *2002 Heart and Stroke Statistical Update*. Dallas, American Heart Association, 2001.
354. McCarthy PM, Smith WA: Mechanical circulatory support—a long and winding road. *Science* 2002; 295:998.
355. Hunt SA, Frazier OH: Mechanical circulatory support and cardiac transplantation. *Circulation* 1998; 97:2079.
356. Goldstein DJ, Oz MC, Rose EA: Implantable left ventricular assist devices. *N Engl J Med* 1998; 339:1523.
357. Mehta SM, Aufiero TX, Pae WE Jr, et al: Combined registry for the clinical use of mechanical ventricular assist pumps and the total artificial heart in conjunction with heart transplantation: sixth official report—1994. *J Heart Lung Transplant* 1995; 14:585.
358. Olsen DB: The history of continuous-flow blood pumps. *Artif Organs* 2000; 24:401.
359. Frazier OH, Myers TJ, Jarvik RK, et al: Research and development of an implantable, axial-flow left ventricular assist device: the Jarvik 2000 heart. *Ann Thorac Surg* 2001; 71:S125.
360. Rose EA, Gelijns AC, Moskowitz AJ, et al: Long-term use of a left ventricular assist device for end-stage heart failure. *N Engl J Med* 2001; 345:1435.
361. Marshall E: A space age vision advances in the clinic. *Science* 2002; 295:1000.
362. Murray KD, Olsen DB: Artificial organs, in Ratner BD, Hoffman AS, Schoen FJ, et al (eds): *Biomaterials Science: An Introduction to Materials in Medicine*. San Diego, Academic Press, 1996; p 389.
363. Schoen FJ, Anderson JM, Didisheim P, et al: Ventricular assist device (VAD) pathology analyses: guidelines for clinical studies. *J Appl Biomat* 1990; 1:45.
364. Borovetz HS, Ramasamy N, Zerbe TR, et al: Evaluation of an implantable ventricular assist system for humans with chronic refractory heart failure. *ASAIO J* 1995; 41:42.
365. Kunin CK, Dobbins JJ, Melo JC: Infectious complications in four long-term recipients of the Jarvik-7 artificial heart. *JAMA* 1988; 259:860.
366. Ward RA, Wellhausen SR, Dobbins JJ, et al: Thromboembolic and infectious complications of total artificial heart implantation. *Ann NY Acad Sci* 1987; 516:638.

367. Fyfe B, Schoen FJ: Pathologic analysis of 34 explanted Symbion ventricular assist devices and 10 explanted Jarvik-7 total artificial hearts. *Cardiovasc Pathol* 1993; 2:187.
368. Long JW: Advanced mechanical circulatory support with the HeartMate left ventricular assist device in the year 2000. *Ann Thorac Surg* 2001; 71:S176.
369. Herrmann M, Weyand M, Greshake B, et al: Left ventricular assist device infection is associated with an increased mortality but is not a contraindication to transplantation. *Circulation* 1997; 95:814.
370. Hetzer R, Muller JH, Weng Y, et al: Bridging-to-recovery. *Ann Thorac Surg* 2001; 71:S109.
371. Young JB: Healing the heart with ventricular assist device therapy: mechanisms of cardiac recovery. *Ann Thorac Surg* 2001; 71: S210.
372. Kumpati GS, McCarthy PM, Hoercher KJ: Left ventricular assist device bridge to recovery: a review of the current status. *Ann Thorac Surg* 2001; 71:S103.
373. Oakley RM, Jarvis JC: Cardiomyoplasty: a critical review of experimental and clinical results. *Circulation* 1994; 90:2085.
374. Magovern GJ Sr, Simpson KA: Clinical cardiomyoplasty: review of the ten-year United States experience. *Ann Thorac Surg* 1996; 61:413.
375. Salmons S: Permanent cardiac assistance from skeletal muscle: a prospect for the new millennium. *Artif Organs* 1999; 23:380.
376. Park SE, Cmolik BL, Lazzara RR, et al: Right latissimus dorsi cardiomyoplasty augments left ventricular systolic performance. *Ann Thorac Surg* 2001; 71:2077.
377. Colucci WS, Schoen FJ: Primary tumors of the heart, in Braunwald E, Zipes DD, Libby P (eds): *Heart Disease: A Textbook of Cardiovascular Medicine*, 6th ed. Philadelphia, WB Saunders, 2001; p 1807.
378. Burke A, Virmani R: *Tumors of the Heart and Great Vessels, Atlas of Tumor Pathology*, 3rd Series. Washington DC, Armed Forces Institute of Pathology, 1996.
379. Shapiro LM: Cardiac tumors: diagnosis and management. *Heart* 2001; 85:218.
380. Reynen K: Frequency of primary tumors of the heart. *Am J Cardiol* 1996; 77:107.
381. Vaughan CJ, Veugelers M, Basson CT: Tumors of the heart: molecular genetic advances. *Curr Opin Cardiol* 2001; 16:195.
382. Reynen K: Cardiac myxomas. *N Engl J Med* 1995; 333: 1610.
383. Stratakis CA, Kirschner LS, Carney JA: Clinical and molecular features of the Carney complex: diagnostic criteria and recommendations for patient evaluation. *J Clin Endocrinol Metab* 2001; 86:4041.
384. Basson CT, Aretz HT: A 27-year-old woman with two intracardiac masses and a history of endocrinopathy. *N Engl J Med* 2002; 346:1152.
385. Shahian DM, Labib SB, Chang G: Cardiac papillary fibroelastoma. *Ann Thorac Surg* 1995; 59:538.
386. Howard RA, Aldea GS, Shapira OM, et al: Papillary fibroelastoma: increasing recognition of a surgical disease. *Ann Thorac Surg* 1999; 68:1881.
387. Courtice RW, Stinson WA, Walley VM: Tissue fragments recovered at cardiac surgery masquerading as tumoral proliferations. *Am J Surg Pathol* 1994; 18:167.
388. Chan JKC: Cardiac MICE: the dust settles. *Adv Anatomic Pathol* 1995; 2:48.

Chapter 6

Risk Stratification and Comorbidity

Victor A. Ferraris/Suellen P. Ferraris

HISTORICAL PERSPECTIVES AND THE PURPOSE OF OUTCOME ASSESSMENT: NIGHTINGALE, CODMAN, AND COCHRANE

> It may seem a strange principle to enunciate as the very first requirement in a Hospital that it should do the sick no harm. It is quite necessary, nevertheless, to lay down such a principle, because the actual mortality in hospitals . . . is very much higher than . . . the mortality of the same class of diseases among patients treated out of hospital. . . .
>
> Florence Nightingale, 1863

The formal assessment of patient care had its beginnings in the mid-1800s. One of the earliest advocates of analyzing outcome data was Florence Nightingale, who was troubled by observations that hospitalized patients died at rates higher than those of patients treated outside of the hospital.[1,2] She also noted a vast difference in mortality rates among different hospitals, with London hospitals having a mortality rate as high as 92%, while smaller rural hospitals had a much lower mortality rate (12%-15%). Although England had tracked hospital mortality rates since the 1600s, the analysis of these rates was in its infancy during Nightingale's era. Yearly mortality statistics were calculated by dividing the number of deaths in a year by the average number of hospitalized patients on a single day of that year. Nightingale made the important observation that raw mortality rates were not an accurate reflection of outcome, since some patients were sicker when they presented to the hospital, and therefore would be expected to have a higher mortality. This was the beginning of risk adjustment based on severity of disease. She was able to carry her observations to the next level by suggesting simple measures, such as improved sanitation, less crowding, and locating hospitals distant from crowded urban areas, that would ultimately result in dramatic improvement in patients' outcomes—an example of a quality improvement project (see below).

Ernest Amory Codman, a Boston surgeon, was one of the most outspoken early advocates of outcome analysis and scrutiny of results. Codman was a classmate of Harvey Cushing, and he became interested in the issues of outcome analysis after a friendly bet with Cushing about who had the lowest complication rate associated with the delivery of anesthesia. In the early 1900s as medical students, they were responsible for administering anesthesia. Since vomiting and aspiration were common upon induction of anesthesia, many operations were over before they started. Cushing and Codman compared their results and kept records concerning the administration of anesthesia while they were medical students. This effort not only represented the first intraoperative patient records, but also served as a foundation for Codman's later interest (almost passion) for the documentation of outcomes. Codman actually paid a publisher to disseminate the results obtained in his privately owned Boston hospital.[3] Codman was perhaps the first advocate of searching for a cause of all complications. He linked specific outcomes to specific interventions (or errors). He believed that most bad outcomes were the result of errors or omissions by physicians, and completely ignored any contribution to outcome from hospital-based and process-related factors. His efforts were not well received by his peers, and eventually his private hospital closed because of lack of referrals.

Both Codman and Nightingale viewed outcome analysis as an intermediate step toward the improvement of patient care. It was not enough to know the rates of a given outcome. While it is axiomatic that any valid comparison of quality of care or patient outcome must account for severity of illness, this is only the initial step toward improving patient outcome.

Further definition of outcome assessment occurred in the mid-1900s. As more and more therapeutic options became available to treat the diseases that predominated in the early 20th century (e.g., tuberculosis), a need arose to determine the best alternative among multiple therapies, leading to the advent of the controlled randomized trial and tests of effectiveness of therapy. One of the earliest randomized trials was conducted to determine whether streptomycin was effective against tuberculosis.[4] Although the trial proved streptomycin's effectiveness, it also stimulated a great deal of controversy. After World War II, several clinicians advocated the use of randomized, controlled trials to better identify the optimal treatment to provide the best outcome. Foremost among these was Archie Cochrane. Every physician should know about Archie Cochrane (Fig. 6-1). He is as close to a true hero as a physician can get, but there may be those who see him as the devil incarnate. As you can see from some of the highlights of his career (see Fig. 6-1), he lived during an exciting time. In the 1930s Professor Cochrane was branded as a "Trotskyite" because he advocated a national health

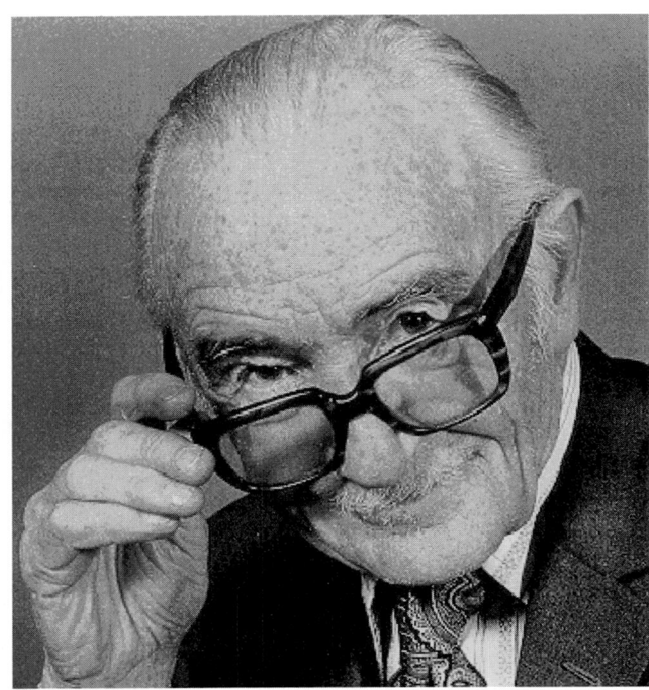

- 1934-6 : Medical student, University College Hospital, London.
- 1936 : International Brigade, Spanish Civil War
- 1939-46 : Captain, Royal Army Medical Corps
- 1941 : Taken prisoner of war in June 1941 in Crete; POW medical officer in Salonica (Greece) and Hildburghausen, Elsterhorst and Wittenberg-am-Elbe (Germany).
- 1947-48 : Studied the epidemiology of tuberculosis at Henry Phipps Institute, Philadelphia, USA.
- 1948-60 : Member, Medical Research Council Pneumoconiosis Research Unit, Penarth, Wales.
- 1960-69 : David Davies Professor of Tuberculosis and Chest Diseases, Welsh National School of Medicine, Cardiff, Wales.
- 1960-74 : Director, Medical Research Council Epidemiology Research Unit, Cardiff, Wales.
- 1972 : Publication by the Nuffield Provincial Hospitals Trust of his book *Effectiveness and Efficiency—Random Reflections on Health Services*.

FIGURE 6–1 Portrait of Archie Cochrane with brief biography.

system for Great Britain. His advocacy was tempered by 4 years as a prisoner of war in multiple German POW camps during World War II. He saw soldiers die from tuberculosis, and he was never sure what the best treatment was. He could choose among collapse therapy, bed rest, supplemental nutrition, or even high-dose vitamin therapy. A quote from his book sums up his frustration:

> I had considerable freedom of clinical choice of therapy: my trouble was that I did not know which to use and when. I would gladly have sacrificed my freedom for a little knowledge.[5]

His experience with the uncertainty about the best treatment for tuberculosis and other chest diseases continued after the war, when he became a researcher in pulmonary disease for the Medical Research Council in Great Britain. His continued interest in tuberculosis was now heightened by the fact that he had contracted the disease. Archie wanted to know the best drug therapy for tuberculosis, since there were now drugs available that could treat this disease, with streptomycin being the first really effective drug against mycobacterium tuberculosis.[4] He was a patron of the randomized controlled trial (or RCTs, as he liked to refer to them) to test important medical hypotheses. He used the evidence gained from these RCTs to make decisions about the best therapy based on available evidence—the beginning of "evidence-based" practice. He felt that RCTs were the best form of evidence to support medical decision making (so-called "class 1" evidence). Initially he was a voice in the wilderness, but this eventually changed. In 1979 he criticized the medical profession for not having a critical summary, organized by specialty and updated periodically, of relevant RCTs. In the 1980s, a database of important RCTs dealing with perinatal medicine was developed at Oxford. In 1987, the year before Cochrane died, he referred to a systematic review of randomized controlled trials (RCTs) of care during pregnancy and childbirth as "a real milestone in the history of randomized trials and in the evaluation of care," and suggested that other specialties should copy the methods used. This led to the opening of the first Cochrane center (in Oxford) in 1992 and the founding of the Cochrane Collaboration in 1993.

The Cochrane Web site (http://www.cochrane.org/) has summaries of all available RCTs on a wide range of medical subjects. Thus it is fair to call Archie Cochrane the "father of evidence-based medicine," Evidence-based medicine has, at its heart, the imperative to improve outcomes by comparing alternative therapies to determine which is the best. Evidence-based studies that involve randomized trials have the advantage of being able to infer cause and effect (i.e., a new therapy or drug *causes* improved outcome). On the other hand, observational studies (or retrospective studies) are able to define only associations between therapies and outcome, not prove cause and effect.

DEFINITIONS

Risk Stratification

Risk stratification means arranging patients according to the severity of their illness. Implicit in this definition is the ability to predict outcomes from a given intervention based on preexisting illness or the severity of intervention. Risk stratification is therefore defined as the ability to predict outcomes from a given intervention by arranging patients according to the severity of their illness. The usefulness of any risk stratification system arises from how the system links severity to a specific outcome.

There have been numerous attempts at describing severity of illness by means of a tangible score or number. Table 6-1 is a partial listing of some of the severity measures commonly used in risk assessment of cardiac surgical patients. This list is not meant to be comprehensive, but it does give an overview of the types of risk stratification schemes that have been used for cardiac patients. The risk stratification systems listed in Table 6-1 are in constant evolution, and the descriptions in the table may not reflect current or future versions of these systems. All of these severity measures share 2 common features. First, they are all linked to a specific outcome. Second, all measures view a period of hospitalization as the episode of illness. The severity indices listed in Table 6-1 define severity predominantly based on clinical measures (e.g., risk of death, clinical instability, treatment difficulty, etc.). Two of the severity measures shown in Table 6-1 (MedisGroups used in the Pennsylvania Cardiac Surgery Reporting System and the Canadian Provincial Adult Cardiac Care Network of Ontario) define severity based on resource use (e.g., hospital length-of-stay, cost, etc.) as well as on clinical measures.[6,7] Of the 9 severity measures listed in Table 6-1, only one, the APACHE III system, computes a risk score independent of patient diagnosis.[8] All of the others in the table are diagnosis-specific systems that use only patients with particular diagnoses in computing severity scores.

Each of the risk stratification measures shown in Table 6-1 has been tested against a validation set of patients and found to be an adequate measure of the risk of operative mortality or of other outcome. However, assessing the validity and performance of various risk-adjustment methods entails more than simple cross-validation. No severity tool will ever perfectly describe patients' risks for death, complications, or increased resource use. The most important reason that risk-adjustment methods fail to completely predict outcomes is that the data set used to derive the risk score comes from retrospective, observational data that contain inherent selection bias; i.e., patients were given a certain treatment that resulted in a particular outcome because a clinician had a certain selection bias about what treatment that particular patient should receive. In observational data sets, patients are not allocated to a given treatment in a randomized manner. In addition, clinician bias is not always

TABLE 6–1 Examples of risk stratification systems used for patients undergoing cardiac surgical procedures

Severity system	Data source	Classification approach	Outcomes measured
APACHE III[8]	Values of 17 physiologic parameters and other clinical information	Integer scores from 0 to 299 measured within 24 hours of ICU admission	In-hospital death
Pennsylvania[6]	Clinical findings collected at time of admission	Probability of in-hospital death ranging from 0 to 1 based on logistic regression model and MediQual's Atlas admission severity score	In-hospital death and cost of procedure
NY[175,189,266]	Condition-specific clinical variables from discharge record	Probability of in-hospital death ranging from 0 to 1 based on logistic regression model	In-hospital death
STS[103,105,267]	Condition-specific clinical variables from discharge record	Bayesian algorithm used to assign patient to risk interval (percent mortality interval); more recently converted to logistic regression model	In-hospital death and morbidity
VA[181,268,269]	Condition-specific clinical variables measured 30 days after operation	Logistic regression model used to assign patient to risk interval (percent mortality interval)	In-hospital death and morbidity
Parsonnet[270–273]	Condition-specific clinical variables from discharge record	Additive multiple regression model with scores between 0 and 158 based on 14 weighted risk factors	Death within 30 days of operation
Canadian[7,274]	Condition-specific clinical variables entered at time of referral for cardiac surgery	Range of scores from 0 to 16 based on logistic regression odds ratio for 6 key risk factors	In-hospital mortality, ICU stay, and postoperative length of stay
New England[138,193,275]	Condition-specific clinical variables and comorbidity index entered from discharge record	Scoring system based on logistic regression coefficients used to calculate probability of operative mortality from 7 clinical variables and 1 comorbidity index	In-hospital mortality
Cleveland[276]	Condition-specific clinical variables from discharge record	Range of scores from 0 to 33 based on univariate odds ratio for each of 13 risk factors	In-hospital death or death within 30 days of operation

Penn = Pennsylvania Cost Containment Committee for Cardiac Surgery; NY = New York State Department of Health Cardiac Surgery Reporting System; STS = Society of Thoracic Surgeons Risk Stratification System; VA = Veteran's Administration Cardiac Surgery Risk Assessment Program; Parsonnet = Parsonnet Risk Stratification Model; Canadian = Ontario Ministry of Health Provincial Adult Cardiac Care Network: New England = Northern New England Cardiovascular Disease Study Group; Cleveland = Cleveland Clinic Foundation Risk Stratification System.

founded in evidence-based data. An excellent review of the subtleties of evaluating the performance of risk-adjustment methods is given in the book by Iezzoni, and this reference is recommended to the interested reader.[9] More attention is paid to the quality of risk-adjustment systems in subsequent sections.

Outcomes and Risk Stratification

There are at least 4 outcomes of interest to surgeons dealing with cardiac surgical patients: mortality, serious nonfatal morbidity, resource utilization, and patient satisfaction. Which patient characteristics constitute important risk factors may depend largely on the outcome of interest. For example, Table 6-2 lists the multivariate factors and odds ratios associated with various outcomes of interest for our patients having cardiac operations.[10–12] The clinical variables associated with increased resource utilization after operation are different than those associated with increased mortality risk. As a generalization, the risk factors associated with in-hospital death are likely to reflect concurrent, disease-specific variables, while factors associated with increased resource utilization reflect serious comorbid illness.[10,11,13] For example, mortality risk after coronary artery bypass graft (CABG) is associated with disease-specific factors such as ventricular ejection fraction, recent myocardial infarction, and hemodynamic instability at the time of operation. Risk factors for increased resource utilization (as measured by length of stay and hospital cost) include comorbid illnesses such as peripheral vascular disease, renal

TABLE 6–2 Multivariate factors associated with various outcomes of cardiac surgery[10,11]

	Relative risk of outcome			
Variable	**Serious morbidity (95% CI)**	**Mortality (95% CI)**	**Decreased cost (95% CI)**	**Decreased LOS (95% CI)**
Congestive heart failure	4.81 (2.16-5.98)	9.20 (6.02-14.0)	0.56 (0.51-0.63)	0.79 (0.73-0.85)
NYS predicted mortality risk		1.28 (1.16-1.41)	0.93 (0.89-0.97)	0.78 (0.76-0.80)
Type of operation		6.04 (3.48-10.5)	0.43 (0.40-0.47)	0.53 (0.48-0.59)
Creatinine > 2.5 mg/100 cc			0.40 (0.33-0.49)	0.47 (0.38-0.58)
Priority		18.6 (7.42-46.6)	0.53 (0.50-0.56)	
Age/RBC volume (per 0.01 unit increase)	6.93 (3.21-11.5)		0.61 (0.55-0.67)	0.32 (0.30-0.36)
Reoperative procedure			0.68 (0.62-0.76)	
Preoperative IABP			0.65 (0.56-0.75)	
Hypertension	5.62 (2.11-15.2)		0.86 (0.81-0.92)	0.83 (0.78-0.89)
More than one prior MI			0.83 (0.75-0.91)	
Dialysis-dependent renal failure			0.61 (0.47-0.78)	
Peripheral vascular disease				0.85 (0.71-0.94)
Prior CNS disease	3.41 (2.99-4.91)			0.81 (0.72-0.92)
COPD				0.87 (0.79-0.94)

COPD = chronic obstructive pulmonary disease; IABP = intra-aortic balloon counterpulsation; RBC = red blood cell.

dysfunction, hypertension, and chronic lung disease. It is not surprising that comorbid conditions are important predictors of hospital charges, since patients with multiple comorbidities often require prolonged hospitalization, not only for treatment of the primary surgical illness but also for treatment of the comorbid conditions.

Operative mortality is an easily defined, readily measured outcome. Most studies that have attempted to define effective care have focused on mortality as an outcome. However, outcomes such as resource utilization or quality of life indicators may be more relevant postoperative factors in many instances. Outcome measures other than operative mortality are particularly important when deciding how to spend health care dollars.[14,15]

Measures of Comorbidity

Comorbidities are coexisting diagnoses that are indirectly related to the principal surgical diagnosis but may alter the outcome of an operation. Physicians or hospitals that care for patients with a higher prevalence of serious comorbid conditions are clearly at a significant disadvantage in unadjusted comparisons. The prevalence of comorbid illness in patients with cardiac disease has been well demonstrated. In one series of patients with myocardial infarction, 26% also had diabetes, 30% had arthritis, 6% had chronic lung problems, and 12% had gastrointestinal disorders.[16]

Several indices of comorbidity are available. Table 6-3 compares 5 commonly used comorbidity measures: the Charlson index, the RAND Corporation index, the Greenfield index, the Goldman index, and the APACHE III scoring system.[16–23] There are many limitations of comorbidity indices, and they are not applied widely in studies of efficacy or medical effectiveness. Perhaps the most serious drawback of comorbidity scoring systems is the imprecision of the databases used to form the indices. Most of the data used to construct the indices come from two sources: (1) administrative databases in the form of computerized discharge abstract data, and (2) out-of-hospital follow-up reports. Discharge abstracts include clinical diagnoses that are often assigned by nonphysicians who were not involved in the care of the patient. Comprehensive entry of correct diagnoses is not a high priority for most clinicians, and problems with discharge coding have been identified by Iezzoni and others.[24–26] These authors found that many conditions that are expected to increase the risk of death are actually associated with a lower mortality. The presumed explanation for this paradoxical finding is that less serious diagnoses are unlikely to be coded and entered in the records of the most seriously ill patients. Likewise, the accuracy of out-of-hospital follow-up studies is hard to validate, and they may contain significant inaccuracies. Because of these shortcomings, analyses that compare physician or hospital outcomes and that do not provide adequate adjustment for patient comorbidity are likely to discriminate against providers or hospitals that treat disproportionate numbers of elderly patients with multiple comorbid conditions.

A vivid example of failure to adjust for severity of illness occurred when the leaders of the Health Care Financing Administration (HCFA) released hospital mortality figures in

TABLE 6–3 Five comorbidity indices

Comorbidity index	Data source and purpose	Classification approach	Most significant comorbidities
Charlson[17]	Abstract of medical records and follow-up data used to predict death at 1 year	Weighted relative risks from Cox proportional hazards model used to create comorbidity index	AIDS, metastatic tumor, and moderate to severe liver disease
APACHE III[19]	Inpatient ICU records used to develop chronic health evaluation as part of overall index	Scores ranging from 0 to 299 created from logistic regression model with in-hospital mortality as outcome	AIDS, severe liver failure, lymphoma/leukemia, metastatic tumor
Keeler/RAND[20]	Medicare administrative database used to evaluate 30-day mortality risk	Weights assigned based on regression coefficients of significant logistic regression variables	Cancer, chronic renal failure, hypoalbuminemia, disease of the thorax, and use of nasogastric tube
Goldman[23]	Preoperative examination of patients undergoing noncardiac operations	Weights assigned for comorbidities based on discriminant analysis	Third heart sound, MI within 6 months, non–sinus rhythm, aortic stenosis, type of operation
Greenfield/ICED[16,21,22]	Abstracts of medical records and outpatient follow-up to assess functional status 1 year after acute event	Combines measures of physiologic derangement and impairment related to comorbidity; variables derived from clinical experience	Functional status, acute exacerbation of comorbid condition, and baseline comorbidities including metastatic cancer, liver disease, renal failure, and cardiac disease

March of 1986. Significantly higher death rates than predicted were reported for 142 hospitals. At the facility with the most aberrant death rate, 87.6% of Medicare patients died compared to a Medicare average of 22.5%. What was not taken into account was that this particular facility was a hospice caring for terminally ill patients.[27] The HCFA model had not adequately accounted for patient risks and comorbidities.

Risk adjustment for severity of illness and comorbidity is equally important for patients about to undergo stressful interventions such as surgical operations or chemotherapy. For example, Goldman et al reported that preexisting heart conditions and other comorbid diseases were important predictors of postoperative cardiac complications for patients undergoing noncardiac procedures.[23] The Goldman scoring system is commonly used by anesthesiologists in assessing patients preoperatively, especially prior to noncardiac procedures.

USES OF OUTCOMES ANALYSIS AND RISK STRATIFICATION

The tools of risk stratification and outcome analysis can be used to judge effectiveness of care and to aid providers in quality improvement in a number of areas, including the following: (1) cost containment, (2) patient education, (3) effectiveness-of-care studies, and (4) improving provider practices. Table 6-4 provides an idealized list of some of the potentially beneficial uses and goals of risk stratification.

Improving the Quality of Care

The ultimate goal of risk stratification and outcome assessment is to account for differences in patient risk factors so that patient outcomes can be used as an indicator of quality of care. A major problem arises in attaining this goal because uniform definitions of quality of care are not available. This is particularly true of cardiovascular disease. For example, there are substantial geographic differences in the rates at which patients with cardiovascular diseases undergo diagnostic procedures and, incidentally, there is little, if any, evidence that these variations are related to survival or improved outcome.[28–31] In one study, coronary angiography was performed after acute myocardial infarction in 45% of patients in Texas compared to 30% of patients in New York State ($p<.001$).[29] In these patient populations the differences in the rates of coronary revascularization were not as dramatic, and the survival in these patients was not related to the type of treatment or diagnostic procedures. Regional variations of this sort suggest that a rigorous definition of the "correct" treatment of acute myocardial infarction, and

TABLE 6–4 Uses of risk stratification and outcome assessment

Risk stratification goal	Example of methodology	Potential benefit
Cost containment	Risk-adjusted patient care costs determined and tracked over time	Cost-efficient institutions or physicians benefit from savings and patients benefit from decreased cost
Improve physician practices	Physician-specific risk-adjusted outcomes determined and made available to practitioners in a nonpunitive way	Physicians improve practice patterns by careful analysis of risk-adjusted data
Improve patient education	Risk-adjusted provider profiles (both hospital and physician specific) made available to the public in a nonthreatening, nonpunitive manner	Patients understand the risks of a given procedure and have more accurate expectations about given intervention; patients have better understanding of "high-risk"
Evaluate effectiveness of care	Risk stratification of population-based retrospective studies used to identify high-risk subsets	Efficacy trials devised and implemented to test benefit in high-risk subsets; with refinements, may allow comparison among providers with goal of improving outliers

other cardiovascular diseases, is elusive, and the definition of quality of care for such patients is imperfect. Similar imperfections exist for nearly all outcomes in patients with cardiothoracic disorders.

Recognizing the difficulties in defining "best practices" for a given illness, professional organizations have opted to promote practice guidelines or "suggested therapy" for given diseases.[32] These guidelines represent a compilation of available published evidence, including randomized trials and risk-adjusted observational studies, as well as consensus among panels of experts proficient at treating the given disease.[33] For example, the practice guideline for coronary artery bypass grafting is available for both practitioners and the lay public on the Internet (http://www.acc.org/clinical/guidelines/bypass/execIndex.htm). Table 6-5 summarizes the 1999 AHA/ACC guidelines for coronary artery bypass grafting in patients with acute (Q-wave) myocardial infarction. These guidelines were developed using available randomized controlled trials, risk-adjusted observational studies, and expert consensus. They are meant to provide clinicians with accepted standards of care that most would agree upon, with an ultimate goal of limiting deviations from accepted standards.

The methodology for developing guidelines for disease treatment is evolving. Many published guidelines do not adhere to accepted standards for developing guidelines.[34] The

TABLE 6–5 1999 AHA/ACC guidelines for CABG in ST-segment elevation (Q-wave) MI

Indication and clinical condition	Definition of level of evidence
Class I None.	*Class I* Conditions for which there is evidence and/or general agreement that a given procedure or treatment is useful and effective.
Class IIa 1. Ongoing ischemia/infarction not responsive to maximal nonsurgical therapy.	*Class II* Conditions for which there is conflicting evidence and/or a divergence of opinion about the usefulness or efficacy of a procedure.
Class IIb 1. Progressive LV pump failure with coronary stenosis compromising viable myocardium outside the initial infarct area. 2. Primary reperfusion in the early hours ($\leq$ 6 to 12 hours) of an evolving ST-segment elevation MI.	*Class IIa* Weight of evidence/opinion is in favor of usefulness/efficacy. *Class IIb* Usefulness/efficacy is less well established by evidence/opinion.
Class III 1. Primary reperfusion late ($\geq$12 hours) in evolving ST-segment elevation MI without ongoing ischemia.	*Class III* Conditions for which there is evidence and/or general agreement that the procedure/treatment is not useful/effective and in some cases may be harmful.

AHA = American Heart Association; ACC = American College of Cardiology; MI = myocardial infarction; LV = left ventricle.

greatest improvement is needed in the identification, evaluation, and synthesis of the scientific evidence.

EFFICACY STUDIES VERSUS EFFECTIVENESS STUDIES

There have been many efficacy studies relating to cardiothoracic surgery. These studies attempt to isolate one procedure or device and evaluate its effect on patient outcomes. The study population in efficacy studies is specifically chosen to contain as uniform a group as possible. Typical examples of efficacy studies include randomized, prospective, clinical trials (RCTs) comparing use of a procedure or device in a well-defined treatment population compared to an equally well-defined control population.

Efficacy studies are different from effectiveness studies.[5] The latter deal with whole populations and attempt to determine the treatment option that provides optimal outcome in a population that would typically be treated by a practicing surgeon. An example of an effectiveness study is a retrospective study of outcome in a large population treated with a particular heart valve. Risk stratification is capable of isolating associations between outcome and risk factors. Methodological enhancements in risk adjustment are capable of reducing biases inherent in population-based, retrospective studies,[35] but they can never eliminate all confounding biases in observational studies.

One reasonable strategy for using risk stratification to improve patient care is to isolate high-risk subsets from population-based, retrospective studies (i.e., effectiveness studies), and then to test interventions to improve outcome in high-risk subsets using RCTs. This is a strategy that should ultimately lead to the desired goal of improved patient care. For example, a population-based study on postoperative blood transfusion revealed that the following factors were significantly associated with excessive blood transfusion (defined as more than 4 units of blood products after CABG): (1) template bleeding time, (2) red blood cell volume, (3) cardiopulmonary bypass time, and (4) age.[36] Cross-validation of these results was carried out on a similar population of patients undergoing CABG at another institution. Based on these retrospective studies, it was reasonable to hypothesize that interventions aimed at reducing blood transfusion after CABG were most likely to benefit patients with prolonged bleeding time and low red blood cell volume. A prospective clinical trial was then performed to test this hypothesis using two blood conservation techniques, platelet-rich plasma saving and whole blood sequestration, in patients undergoing CABG. The results of this stratified, prospective clinical trial showed that blood conservation interventions were beneficial in the high-risk subset of patients.[37] The implications of these studies are that more costly interventions such as platelet-rich plasma saving are only justified in high-risk patients, with the high-risk subset being defined by risk stratification methodologies. Other strategies have been developed that use risk-adjustment methods to improve quality of care, and these methods will be discussed below.

Other Goals of Outcomes Analysis

Financial factors are a major force behind health care reform. America's health care costs amount to 15% to 20% of the gross national product, and this figure is rising at a rate of 6% annually. Institutions who pay for health care are demanding change, and these demands are fueled by studies that suggest that 20% to 30% of care is inappropriate.[38] Charges of inappropriate care stem largely from the observation that there are wide regional variations in the use of expensive procedures.[39,40] This has resulted in a shift in emphasis, with health care costs being emphasized on equal footing with clinical outcomes of care. Relman suggested that clinical outcomes will be used by patients, payors, and providers as a basis for distribution of future funding of health care.[41] While wide differences in use of cardiac interventions initially fueled charges of overuse in certain areas,[42] recent evaluations suggest that underuse of indicated cardiac interventions (either PTCA or CABG) may be a cause of this variation.[42–47] Whether caused by underuse or overuse of cardiovascular services, regional variations in resource utilization make it difficult to use outcomes as an indicator of quality of care.

If the causes of regional variations in the use of cardiac interventions seem puzzling, then physician practice behavior might seem bizarre. One study showed that there were unbelievably large variations in care delivered to patients having cardiac surgery.[48] Among 6 institutions that treated very similar patients (Veteran's Administration medical centers), there were large differences in the percentage of elective, urgent, and emergent cases at each institution, ranging from 58% to 96% elective, 3% to 31% urgent, and 1% to 8% emergent.[48] There was also a 10-fold difference in the preoperative use of intra-aortic balloon counterpulsation for control of unstable angina, varying from 0.8% to 10.6%.[48] Similar variations in physician-specific transfusion practices,[49] ordering of blood chemistry tests,[50] anesthetic practices,[51] treatment of chronic renal failure,[52] and use of antibiotics[53–55] have been observed. This variation in clinical practice may reflect uncertainty about the efficacy of available interventions, or differences in practitioners' clinical judgment. Some therapies with proven benefit are underused.[51,52] Whatever the causes of variations in physician practice, they distort the allocation of health care funds in an inappropriate way. Solutions to this problem involve altering physician practice patterns, something that has been extremely difficult to do.[56] How can physician practice patterns be changed in order to improve outcome? Evidence suggests that the principal process of outcome assessment—the case-by-case review (traditionally done in the morbidity and mortality conference format)—may not be cost-effective and may not improve quality[57] and should be replaced by profiles of practice patterns at institutional, regional, or national levels. One proposed model for quality improvement involves oversight that emphasizes the appropriate balance between internal mechanisms of quality improvement (risk-adjusted outcome analysis) and external accountability.[57]

TOOLS FOR RISK STRATIFICATION AND OUTCOMES ANALYSIS

Databases

Perhaps the most important tool of any outcome assessment endeavor is a database that is made up of a representative sample of the study group of interest. The accuracy of the data elements in any such database cannot be overemphasized.[58–60] Factors such as the source of data, the outcome of interest, the methods used for data collection, standardized definitions of the data elements, data reliability checking, and the time frame of data collection are essential features that must be considered when either constructing a new database or deciding how to use an existing database.[59,60] The quality of the database of interest must be evaluated.

Data obtained from claims databases have been criticized. Because these data are generated for the collection of bills, their clinical accuracy is inadequate, and it is likely that these databases overestimate complications for billing purposes.[61,62] Furthermore, claims data were found to underestimate the effects of comorbid illness and to have major deficiencies in important prognostic variables for CABG, namely left ventricular function and number of diseased vessels.[63] The Duke Databank for Cardiovascular Disease found major discrepancies between clinical and claims databases, with claims data failing to identify more than half of the patients with important comorbid conditions such as congestive heart failure, cerebrovascular disease, and angina.[64] The Health Care Financing Administration (HCFA) uses claims data to evaluate variations in the mortality rates in hospitals treating Medicare patients. After an initially disastrous effort at risk adjustment from claims data,[65,66] new algorithms were developed. Despite these advances, the HCFA administration halted release of the 1993 Medicare hospital mortality report because of concerns about the database and fears that the figures would unfairly punish inner-city public facilities.[67] The importance of the quality of databases used to generate comparisons cannot be overemphasized.

Analytic Tools of Risk Stratification

Implicit in risk adjustment is the use of some analytic technique to determine the significant risk factors that are predictive of the outcome of interest. Some physicians take the "ostrich" approach when it comes to any statistical concept more sophisticated than the *t* test. This approach is both unscientific and potentially harmful to patient care. The current shift to outcomes analysis carries with it a more intensive reliance on statistical techniques that are capable of evaluating large populations with multiple variables of interest in an interdependent manner—i.e., multivariate analyses. A modicum of statistical knowledge helps unravel the intricacies of risk adjustment and provides confidence in the results of risk-adjustment methodologies. The following sections are not intended to provide the reader with exhaustive knowledge of the statistics of outcome analysis, but rather to provide a resource for critical assessment of these methods and to stimulate the interest of readers to learn more about this important field. Perhaps the biggest single benefit of risk adjustment for outcome analysis will come from physicians increasing their knowledge base about these analytic techniques and gaining confidence in the methodology.

Regression Analysis

The starting point for understanding multivariate statistical methods is a firm grasp of elementary statistics. Several basic texts on statistics are available that are enjoyable reading for the interested health care professional.[68–70] These texts are a painless way to become familiar with the basic terminology regarding variable description, simple parametric (normally distributed) univariate statistics, linear regression, analysis of variance, nonparametric (not normally distributed) statistical techniques, and ultimately multivariate statistical methods.

A statistical technique that is commonly used to describe how one variable (the dependent or outcome variable) depends on or varies with a set of independent (or predictor) variables is *regression analysis*. The dependent or outcome variable of interest can be either continuous (e.g., hospital cost or length of stay) or discrete (e.g., mortality). Discrete outcome variables can be either dichotomous (two discrete values, such as alive or dead) or nominal (multiple discrete values, such as improved, unimproved, or worse). The relationship between the outcome variable and the set of descriptor variables can be any type of mathematical relationship. The books by Glantz and Slinker and by Harrell provide an enjoyable primer on regression analysis and are geared to the biomedical sciences.[70,71]

Regression analysis means determining the relationship that describes how an outcome variable depends on (or is associated with) a set of independent predictor variables. Put in simple terms, multivariate regression analysis is "model building." The resultant model is useful only if it accurately predicts outcomes for patients by determining significant risk factors associated with the outcome of interest—i.e., risk adjustment of outcome. When the outcome variable of interest is a continuous variable such as hospital cost, linear multivariate regression is often used to construct a model to predict outcome. A multivariate linear regression model contains a set of independent variables that are linearly related to, and can be used to predict, an outcome variable. These significant independent variables are termed risk factors, and knowledge of these risk factors allows separation of patients according to their degree of risk—i.e., risk stratification. The linear regression model has two important features. First, the model allows one to estimate the expected risk of a patient based on his/her risk characteristics. Second, various health care providers can be compared by comparing their observed outcomes to the outcomes that would be predicted from consideration of the risk factors of the patients that they treat (so-called observed to expected ratio or "O/E" ratio).

Statistical terminology used to describe variables and variable distribution patterns is particularly important in understanding linear regression statistical modeling. An important concept is statistical variance (R^2). R^2 is a summary measure of performance of the statistical model. R^2 is often described by saying that it is the fraction of the total variability of the dependent variable explained by the statistical model. Most investigators routinely report R^2 as a measure of the performance of linear regression risk-adjustment models.[72] For example, the APACHE III risk-adjustment scoring system described in Table 6-1 can be used to predict ICU length of stay. When this is done, the model is associated with an R^2 value of 0.15.[19,72] This implies that 15% of the variability in ICU length of stay can be explained by the variables encompassed in the APACHE III score. Another way of saying this is that 85% of the variability in ICU length of stay is *not* explained by the APACHE III scoring system. This R^2 value does not rate the APACHE III scoring system very highly for predicting ICU length of stay. The APACHE III scoring system uses patient data obtained within 24 hours of admission to the ICU to predict outcome and was developed to predict in-hospital mortality, not hospital costs or length of stay. We have found that the outcome of patients admitted to the ICU depends on events that happen after admission (especially iatrogenic events occurring in the ICU) more so than patient characteristics present on admission to the ICU.[73] Hence, it is not surprising that the APACHE III score does not account for all of the variability in ICU length of stay. In addition, it is not clear what level of R^2 can be expected when the APACHE III system is used in a very different context than the one for which it was designed. Shwartz and Ash give an excellent review of evaluating the performance of risk-adjustment methods using R^2 as a measure of model performance, and their work provides an enlightening insight into the tools of risk adjustment.[74] Hartz et al point out that it is unlikely that any large multivariate regression model will completely account for all of the variability of any complex outcome.[75] When the outcome variable of interest is a discrete variable (e.g., mortality), then nonlinear regression analysis is used. Logistic regression is the nonlinear method most widely used to model dichotomous outcomes in the health sciences. Logistic regression makes use of the mathematical fact that the expression, $e^x/(1-e^x)$, assumes values between 0 and 1 for all positive values of x. The value x in the expression can be a linear sum of predictor variables (either continuous or discrete) and the value of $e^x/(1-e^x)$ is the probability of outcome between 0 (e.g., survival) and 1 (e.g., death) for any value of predictor variables. Computer iteration techniques can be used to produce a model consisting of a set of independent variables that best predict the occurrence of a dichotomous outcome variable. The significant independent variables identified by the logistic regression model are risk factors that allow risk stratification of patients according to their risk of experiencing the dichotomous outcome (e.g., survival versus death).

TABLE 6–6 Formulas for analysis of risk-adjusted dichotomous outcomes

Statistical term	Formula*
Prevalence	(A + C) / (A + B + C + D)
Positive predictive value (PPV)	A / (A + B)
Negative predictive value (NPV)	D / (C + D)
Sensitivity (rate of correct positive predictions)	A / (A + C)
Specificity (rate of correct negative predictions)	D / (B + D)

*A = true positive cases; B = false positive cases; C = true negative cases; D = false negative cases.

The performance of logistic regression models can be assessed in several ways. However, there is less agreement about how best to measure performance for models that predict binary outcomes than there is about the use of R^2 to evaluate linear regression models. One commonly used parameter to evaluate the performance of logistic regression models is the c-statistic.[76] The c-statistic is equal to the area under the receiver operator characteristic (ROC) curve and can be generated from the sensitivity and specificity of measurements of any dichotomous outcomes. Table 6-6 describes the formulas for the statistical terms commonly used to describe dichotomous outcomes.

Figure 6-2 depicts the ability of a logistic regression model to predict patients who will receive a blood transfusion after CABG based on preoperative variables including preoperative aspirin use.[77] This figure is an ROC curve derived from a plot of the sensitivity versus 1 minus the specificity (same as a plot of the true positive rate on the Y-axis versus the false positive rate on the X-axis). The ROC curve in Figure 6-2 is produced by assuming a particular cutoff point for a predicted probability of one outcome (e.g., patients with a predicted probability greater than 0.5 of receiving any transfusion after CABG are considered to be positive for receiving a blood transfusion). The c-statistic for the prediction model is 0.738, suggesting only fair ability of the model to predict postoperative blood transfusion. To put this in perspective, a c-statistic of 1.0 indicates perfect discrimination of the

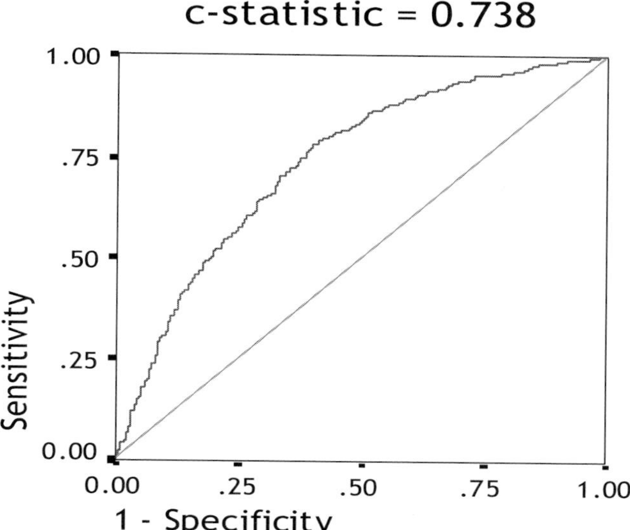

FIGURE 6–2 Receiver operating characteristic (ROC) curve demonstrating association of preoperative aspirin use in 2606 patients before CABG with postoperative blood transfusion. For this analysis, postoperative transfusion was considered a dichotomous variable (patients either received a transfusion or they did not). The area between the diagonal line and the upper curve represents the c-statistic.[77]

model, and a c-statistic of 0.5 indicates no discrimination. So a c-statistic of 0.738 is about halfway between perfect and worthless. An excellent critique of the various methods used to assess performance of regression models of dichotomous outcomes is given by Ash and Shwartz in the book by Iezzoni.[78]

Hierarchical Models and Logistic Regression

Logistic regression models have been used to develop risk profiles for providers (both hospitals and individual surgeons), or so-called report cards.[79–86] This has caused anguish on the part of providers,[87] and concern on the part of statisticians and epidemiologists.[79,80] The typical approach that report cards take is to grade surgeons by their operative mortality for CABG. In order to grade a provider, the expected number of deaths (E or expected rate) calculated from deaths observed in the entire provider group is compared to the observed number of risk-adjusted deaths for the provider (O or observed rate). This gives an O/E ratio, which is a ratio of the risk-adjusted observed mortality rate to the expected mortality rate based on the group logistic model. In order to make comparisons between providers, a confidence interval (usually a 95% confidence interval) is assigned to the observed mortality rates, and the between-provider mortality rates are presented as a range of values for each provider (Fig. 6-3A). The expected mortality rates are assumed to be independent of the observed mortality rates—an incorrect assumption. Furthermore, no sampling error is attached to the expected values—another incorrect assumption. The effect of making these two assumptions is to identify too many outliers (in either direction).

Statistical methodology to account for these incorrect assumptions has been available for many years. The methodology involves construction of hierarchical regression models. Hierarchy means nesting, and the name of these models implies that they incorporate (or nest) other levels of analysis within the analysis of provider mortality. For example, patients are nested within provider groups (patients treated by a given provider), but then patients are also nested within hospital groups (patients treated at a given hospital). The most important feature of hierarchical models is that the model recognizes that the nested observations may be correlated (e.g., mortality may depend on the surgeon, the hospital where care is provided, and other unspecified variables such as referral patterns, academic status, hospital size and location, etc.) and that different sources of variation can occur at each level (or nest). Computer-intensive methods are available to produce hierarchical models for risk-adjusted surgeon mortality. Most statisticians recognize hierarchical models as the preferred method to perform this type of provider analysis, but the methods are complex, labor-intensive, and not included in most commercially available computer software.

Traditional logistic regression modeling to rank surgeons according to their risk-adjusted mortality rates results in exaggerated (incorrect) provider profiles.[28,79,80,88–90] Goldstein and Spiegelhalter reexamined the 1994 New York State publicly disseminated mortality data using hierarchical logistic regression.[88] Figure 6-3 summarizes their findings. The hierarchical analysis dampens the surgeon mortality rates towards the mean of all providers. More importantly, the New York State report identified three outliers (2 low and 1 high) based on simple logistic regression, while hierarchical analysis identified only one outlier (1 high). Similar results have been obtained by Grunkemeier et al when they applied the principles of hierarchical regression analysis to the Providence Health System logistic regression model for CABG operative mortality.[80]

The use of simplistic models, as in the case of the New York State or the Providence Health System logistic regression models, is incorrect, and probably unethical, given the potential impact that outlier status might have on a surgeon's practice. Two impediments to widespread use of hierarchical models are the absence of the necessary large data sets and the lack of readily available easy-to-use software packages. There are statistical "workarounds" that adjust data sets to obtain similar results to those obtained from hierarchical models,[28,91] but it is unclear if such adjustment produces a result that is qualitatively different from that produced by standard hierarchical analysis. At present, hierarchical regression is the "gold standard" for risk adjustment of dichotomous outcomes and producing provider report cards. Unfortunately, this gold standard is rarely used.

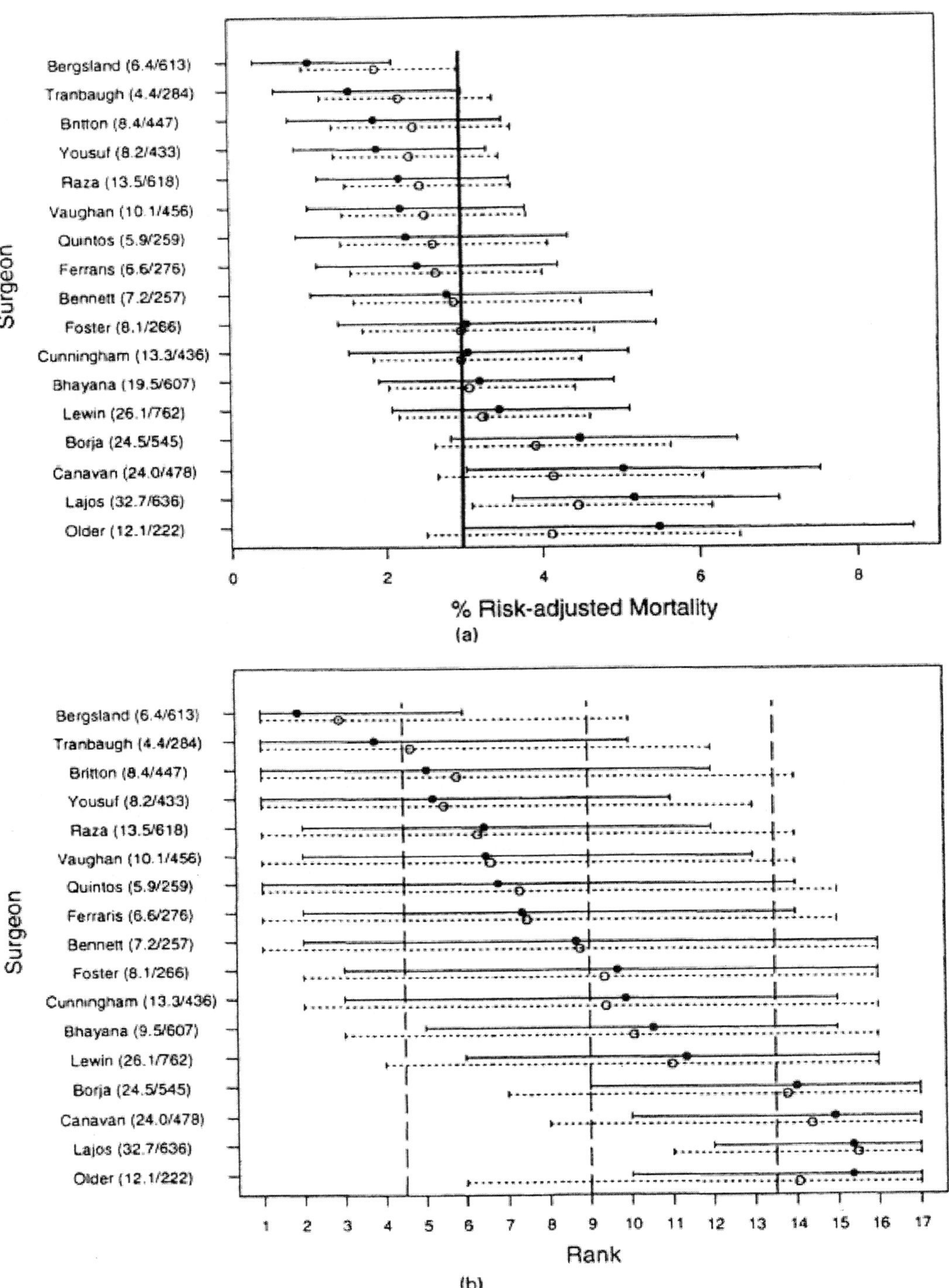

FIGURE 6–3 Comparison of classical statistical point and interval estimates to estimates from hierarchical models for a sample of New York surgeons performing coronary artery bypass grafting. (A) Estimates and 95% intervals for risk-adjusted mortality rates, classical approach (black circle) and estimates from hierachical models (open circle). The state average of 2.99% is shown with the vertical line. (B) Mean and 95% intervals for rank of surgeon, classical approach (solid circle) and estimates from hierachical models (open circle). *(Reproduced with permission from Goldstein H, Spiegelhalter DJ: League tables and their limitations: statistical issues in comparisons of institutional performance (with discussion). J R Stat Soc 1996; 159:385.)*

Statistics of Survival

When the outcome of interest is a time-dependent variable (e.g., hospital length of stay or survival after valve implantation), then regression modeling may be a more complex but still manageable process. Regression models for time-dependent outcome variables can be developed using computer iteration methods. Several excellent texts are available that cover the gamut of technical information from the relatively simple[92,93] to the complex.[94–96] One model that has been used extensively in the biomedical sciences is the Cox proportional hazards regression model.[94] In some regression models, such as logistic regression, the dependent or outcome variable is known with precision. With time-dependent outcome variables, the possibility exists that only a portion of the survival time is observed for some patients. Thus the data available for analysis will consist of some outcomes that are incomplete or "censored." Some regression models, such as logistic regression, do not easily adapt to censored data. Cox's model overcomes these technical problems by assuming that the independent variables are related to survival time by a multiplicative effect on the hazard function—thus it is a "proportional hazards" model. The hazard function is defined as the slope of the survival curve (or the time decay curve) for a series of time-dependent observations. In the Cox model, one assumes that the hazard functions are proportional, a reasonable assumption when comparing survival in two or more similar groups. Hence, it is not necessary to know the underlying survival function in order to determine the relative importance of independent variables that contribute to the overall survival curve. Table 6-7 shows an example of the use of Cox regression to evaluate the independent variables that are predictive of hospital length of stay (a time-dependent outcome variable) for patients undergoing CABG.[11] For the purposes of this analysis, hospital deaths were considered censored observations. The independent variables shown in Table 6-7 are considered risk factors for increased length-of-stay, and can be used to stratify patients into groups with varying risk of prolonged hospitalization.

Measures of the performance of Cox regression models are less well developed than those for logistic regression or for multivariate linear regression. Simple methods of checking the predictive value of Cox models are usually reported in the medical literature. One of the most commonly used methods is called cross-validation, or jackknife analysis. This consists of using Cox regression to determine significant independent variables predictive of outcome in a "training" set of data. The significant variables and their coefficients from the Cox model are then used to compute values of the outcome variables in a different data set (called the validation set, or the jackknife set). The agreement between the predicted values and the observed values in the validation set is used as an index of the performance of the Cox model. Figure 6-4 shows a cross-validation set of data used to check the results of the Cox regression described in Table 6-7. This figure shows fair "validation" of the Cox model using a relatively small data set (1200 patients operated upon during 1994 at a single institution). Performance of Cox models can also be expressed in terms of ROC curves and the c-statistic as for logistic regression models.

Bayesian Analysis: Models Based on Experience

Thomas Bayes was a nonconformist minister and mathematician who is given credit for describing the probability of an event based on knowledge of prior probabilities that the same event has already occurred.[97] Using the Bayesian approach, three sets of probabilities are defined: (1) the probability

TABLE 6–7 Cox proportional hazards regression model for significant predictor variables associated with increased hospital length of stay in 938 patients undergoing CABG during 1993[11]

Risk factor (patients with risk factor)	Observed LOS	95% Cl	Odds ratio	Chi^2 improvement
None (40 patients)*	5.9 days	0.7 days	1.00	
Age/RBCVOL (385 patients with ≥ mean value of 0.0390)	10.0 days	0.98 days	1.83 per 0.01 unit of Age/RBCVOL	72.907
CHF (91 patients)	11.6 days	2.3 days	4.34	17.729
Hypertension (646 patients)	9.0 days	0.6 days	2.31	12.296
Peripheral vascular disease (74 patients)	10.1 days	1.4 days	3.01	8.053
Renal dysfunction (17 patients)**	12.8 days	3.8 days	5.64	6.904
COPD (213 patients)	9.4 days	0.9 days	2.23	7.259
Previous stroke (51 patients)	11.1 days	2.2 days	3.20	5.017

Age/RBCVOL = age in years divided by red blood cell volume obtained from nomogram of patient height, weight, gender, and preoperative hematocrit; CHF = congestive heart failure immediately preceding CABG; COPD = chronic obstructive pulmonary disease.

*For purposes of calculating zero risk factor scores, age/RBCVOL was assumed to be less than 0.0250 (one standard deviation below the mean).

**Serum creatinine ≥2.5 mg/% but not dialysis-dependent.

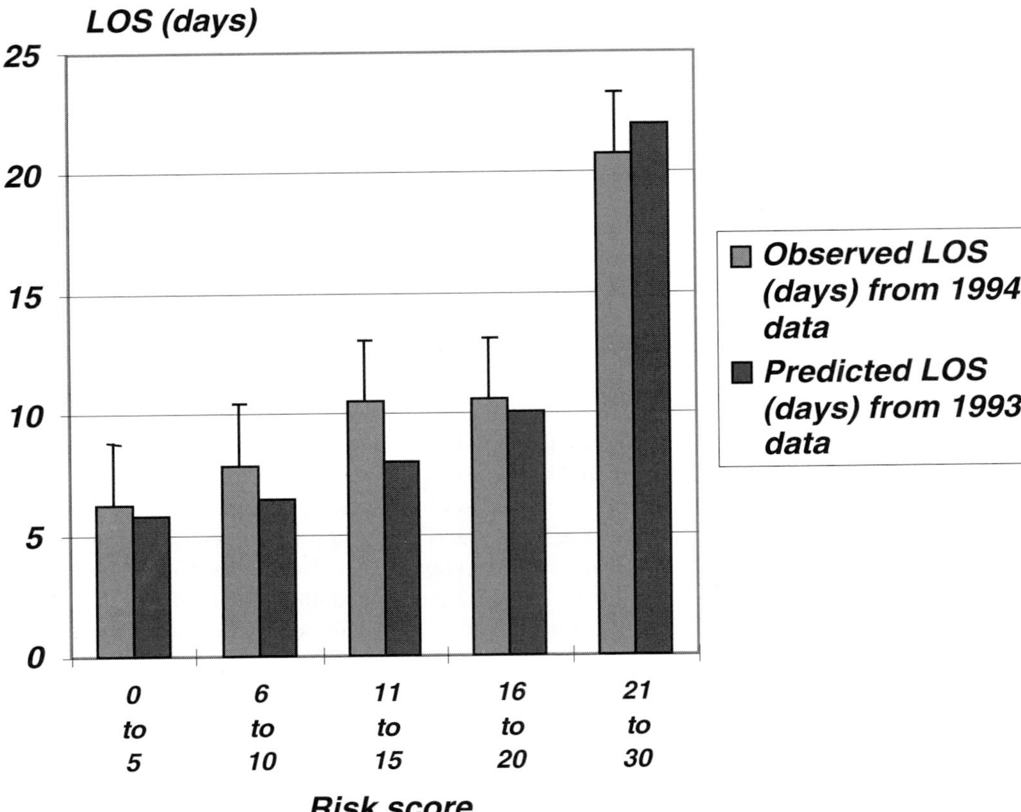

FIGURE 6–4 Cross-validation of Cox regression model used to predict hospital length of stay after CABG. Data from patients operated upon in 1993 were used as the "training" data set to predict values for LOS in patients undergoing operation in 1994 ("validation set"). Risk scores were generated by assigning numerical weights to significant variables in the Cox model based on regression coefficients shown in Table 6-7. The methods used to derive the patient risk scores are described in the references.[11,287] *(Reproduced with permission from Ferraris VA, Ferraris SP: Risk factors for postoperative morbidity. J Thorac Cardiovasc Surg 1996; 111:731.)*

of an event before the presence of a new finding is revealed (prior probability); (2) the probability that an event is observed given that an independent variable is positive (conditional probability); and (3) the probability of an event occurring after the presence of a new finding is revealed (posterior probability). The mathematical relationship between the three probabilities is Bayes' theorem. The prior and posterior probabilities are defined with respect to a given set of independent variables. In the sequential process common to all Bayesian analyses, the posterior probabilities for one finding become the prior probabilities for the next, and a mathematical combination of prior and conditional probabilities produces posterior probabilities. Bayes' theorem can be expressed in terms of the nomenclature of Table 6-6 as:

$$P_{\text{Bayes}} = \text{Sensitivity} \times \text{prior probability} / (\text{sensitivity} \times \text{prior probability}) + [\text{False positive rate} \times (1 - \text{prior probability})]$$

where P_{Bayes} is defined as the probability of a given outcome if prior probabilities are known. The principles of Bayesian statistics have been used widely in decision analysis[98] and can also be used to generate multivariate regression models based on historical data about independent variables.[99–102] Bayesian multivariate regression models are generated using computer-based iterative techniques[99,102–104] and have been used in the past, but not at present, to develop the risk stratification analysis for the Society of Thoracic Surgeons National Cardiac Database.[103,105] Evaluation of the performance of the Bayesian statistical regression models is usually done by cross-validation studies similar to those used to validate the Cox survival regression model in Figure 6-4. Performance of Bayesian models can also be expressed in terms of ROC curves and the c-statistic as for logistic regression models. Marshall et al have shown that Bayesian models of risk adjustment give comparable results and produce ROC curves similar to those generated from logistic regression analysis using conventional models.[106]

Meta-analysis

An implicit part of assessing outcome is the development of a best standard of care for a given illness or disease process. Once the most efficacious treatment is known, then comparisons with, or deviations from, the standard can be assessed—a process called "benchmarking." As mentioned above, the "best standard" is not always known. Meta-analysis is a quantitative approach for systematically assessing the results of multiple previous studies to determine the best or preferred outcome. The overall goal of meta-analysis is to combine the results of previous studies to arrive at a consensus conclusion about the best outcome. Stated in a different way, meta-analysis is a tool used to summarize efficacy studies (preferably RCTs) of an intervention in a defined population with a disease in order to determine which intervention is likely to be effective in a large population with a similar disorder. Meta-analysis is a tool that can relate efficacy studies to effectiveness of an intervention by summarizing available medical evidence.

In summarizing available medical evidence on a given subject, information retrieval is king. Nowhere is this more evident than in the Cochrane Collection of available randomized trials on various medical subjects. For example, a recent Cochrane review found 17 trials that evaluated postoperative neurological deficit in patients having hypothermic cardiopulmonary bypass (CPB) compared to normothermic CPB.[107] This compares to a recently published meta-analysis on a similar topic that found only 11 trials with which to perform a similar analysis.[108] The Cochrane reviewers perform an exhaustive search of all available literature, using not only MEDLINE but also unpublished trials, and so-called "fugitive literature" (government reports, proceedings of conferences, published Ph.D. theses, etc.). The average thoracic surgeon has not heard of "publication bias," but the Cochrane reviewers are acutely aware of it. They realize that RCTs that have a negative result are less likely to pass the peer-review editorial process into publication than RCTs with a significant treatment effect—so called "publication bias" in favor of positive clinical trials.[109] So for each of the Cochrane reviews, attempts are made to find unpublished and/or negative trials to add to the body of evidence about a given subject.

All trials or observational studies that address the same outcomes of a given intervention are not the same. There are almost always subtle differences in study design, sample size, analysis of results, and inclusion/exclusion criteria. The object of comparing multiple observational studies and RCTs on the same treatment outcome is to come up with a single summary estimate of the effect of the intervention. Calculating a single estimate in the face of such diversity may give a misleading picture of the truth. There are no statistical tricks that account for bias and confounding in the original studies. Heterogeneity of the various RCTs and observational studies on the same or similar treatment outcome is the issue. This heterogeneity makes comparison of RCTs a daunting task, about which volumes have been written.[15]

There are at least two types of heterogeneity that confound summary estimates of multiple RCTs—clinical heterogeneity and statistical heterogeneity. Statistical heterogeneity is present when the between-study variance is large; i.e., similar treatments result in widely varying outcomes in different trials. This form of heterogeneity is easiest to measure. For example, Berlin et al evaluated 22 separate meta-analyses and found that only 14 of 22 had no evidence of statistical heterogeneity.[110] Three of the remaining 8 comparative studies gave different results depending on the type of statistical methods used for the analysis—the more statistical heterogeneity, the less certain the statistical inferences from the analysis.

Clinical heterogeneity of groups of RCTs that assess similar outcomes is much more difficult to assess. Measurement of treatment outcomes has plagued reviewers who try to summarize RCTs. Many RCTs address similar treatment options (e.g., hypothermic CPB versus normothermic CPB) but measure slightly different outcomes (e.g., stroke or neuropsychological dysfunction). For example, the Cochrane Heart Group found 17 RCTs that addressed the effect of CPB temperature on postoperative stroke.[107] Only 4 of these 17 RCTs measured neuropsychological function, while all 17 measured neurological deficit associated with CPB. In summarizing the results of multiple RCTs comparing a given treatment, it is necessary to match "apples with apples" when looking at outcomes. In this analysis by the Cochrane Heart Group, there was a trend towards a reduction in the incidence of nonfatal strokes in the hypothermic group (OR = 0.68; 95% CI, 0.43-1.05). Conversely, the number of non–stroke-related perioperative deaths tended to be higher in the hypothermic group (OR = 1.46; 95% CI, 0.9-2.37). When all "bad" outcomes (stroke, perioperative death, myocardial infarction, low-output syndrome, intra-aortic balloon pump use) were pooled, neither hypothermia nor normothermia had a significant advantage (OR = 1.07; 95% CI, 0.92-1.24). This suggests that there is clinical heterogeneity among the various RCTs evaluated. There are statistical "tricks," such as stratification or regression, that can investigate and explore the differences among studies, but it is unlikely that clinical heterogeneity can be completely removed from the meta-analysis. Importantly, the Cochrane Group concludes from these data that there is no definite advantage of hypothermia over normothermia in the incidence of clinical events following CPB. This constitutes good evidence (multiple well-done RCTs) to support the notion that normothermic and hypothermic CPB have equal efficacy for most outcomes. An expert panel reviewing the Cochrane evidence might suggest that there is class I evidence (according to the ACC/AHA guideline nomenclature) that neither normothermic nor hypothermic CPB results in increased incidence of perioperative complications. This is an entirely different conclusion than Bartels et al made in their meta-analysis about the same interventions. These authors suggest that there is little evidence to support the usefulness/efficacy of hypothermia in CPB.[108] No one can say which meta-analysis is closer to the truth. Much depends on the details of the meta-analyses, but logic suggests that the higher quality study including more available RCTs and statistically rigorous analysis comes closer to the scientific truth.

There is some concern about the findings of meta-analysis.[111–113] LeLorier et al found significant discrepancies between the conclusions of meta-analyses and subsequent large RCTs.[112,113] On review of selected meta-analyses, Bailar found that "problems were so frequent and so serious, including bias on the part of the meta-analyst, that it was difficult to trust the overall 'best estimates' that the method often produces."[114,115] Great caution must be used in the interpretation of meta-analyses, but the technique has gained a strong following among clinicians since it may be applied even when the summarized studies are small and there is substantial variation in many of the factors that may have an important bearing on the findings.

"Breakthrough Statistics"

The use of complex statistics is becoming more common in assessing medical data. Arguably, the understanding of this complex material on the part of clinicians has not advanced at a similar rate. In an attempt to address this knowledge gap, Blackstone coined the term "breakthrough statistics" to denote newer methods that are available to handle complex, but clinically important, research questions.[35] His goal was to acquaint clinicians with the methods in a nontechnical fashion "so that you may read reports more knowledgeably, interact with your statistical collaborators more closely, or encourage your statistician to consider these methods if they are applicable to your clinical research."[35] These worthy goals have direct relevance to outcomes assessment and risk stratification.

BALANCING SCORES

One of Blackstone's breakthrough statistical methods deals with a very common problem: the assessment of nonrandomized comparisons. Observational studies, or nonrandomized comparisons, can detect associations between risk and outcome but cannot, strictly speaking, determine which risks *cause* the particular outcome. Traditionally only RCTs have been able to determine cause and effect. A so-called breakthrough technique to allow nonrandomized comparisons to come closer to inferring cause and effect is the use of balancing scores.

Simple comparison of two nonrandomized treatments is confounded by selection factors. That means that a clinician decided to treat a particular patient with a given treatment for some reason that was not obvious and was not necessarily evidence-based. The selection factors used in this nonrandomized situation are difficult to control, and RCTs eliminate this type of bias. However, RCTs are often not applicable to the general population of interest since they are very narrowly defined.[116]

Use of nonrandomized comparisons is more versatile and less costly. One of the earliest methods used to account for selection bias was patient matching. Two groups who received different treatment were matched as closely as possible for all factors except the variable of interest. Balancing scores were developed as an extension of patient matching. In the early 1980s, Rosenbaum and Rubin introduced the idea of balancing scores to analyze observational studies.[117] They called the simplest form of a balancing score a *propensity score*. Their techniques were aimed at drawing causal inference from nonrandomized comparisons. The propensity score is a probability of group membership. For example, in a large group of patients having CABG, some receive aspirin before operation and others do not. One might ask whether preoperative aspirin causes increased postoperative blood transfusion. The propensity score is a probability between 0 and 1 that can be calculated for each patient, and this score represents their probability of getting an aspirin before operation. If the aspirin and nonaspirin patients are matched by their propensity scores, the patients will be as nearly matched as possible for every preoperative characteristic excluding the outcome of interest. Not all the patients may be included in the analysis because some aspirin users may have a propensity score that is not closely matched to a nonaspirin user. But those aspirin users who have a matching propensity score to a nonaspirin user will be very closely matched for every variable except for the outcome variable of interest. This is as close to a randomized trial comparison as you can get without actually doing a randomized trial.

How is the propensity score calculated? The relevant question asked to construct the propensity score is which factors predict group membership (e.g., who will receive aspirin and who will not). The probability of receiving an aspirin is a dichotomous variable that can be modeled like any other binary variable. For example, logistic regression can be used to identify factors associated with aspirin use. In the logistic regression analysis to develop the propensity score, as many risk factors as possible are included in the model, and the logistic equation is solved (or modeled) for the probability of being in the aspirin group. This probability is the propensity score. An example of the results obtained from this type of analysis is shown in Table 6-8.[77] In this analysis, 2606 patients (1900 preoperative aspirin users and 606 nonusers) were "balanced" by being divided into 5 equal quintiles according to their propensity scores. Quintile 1 had the least chance of receiving aspirin while quintile 5 had the greatest chance of receiving aspirin before operation. Within each quintile, the patients were matched as closely as possible for all variables except for the outcome variable of interest, i.e., receiving any blood transfusion after CABG, almost like a randomized trial. Notice that within each quintile, aspirin users and nonusers were

TABLE 6–8 Effect of aspirin (ASA) on postoperative blood transfusion using propensity score-matched quintiles

	Quintile									
	1 (n = 521)		2 (n = 521)		3 (n = 521)		4 (n = 521)		5 (n = 521)	
	ASA	No ASA	ASA	No ASA	ASA	No ASA	ASA	No ASA	ASA	No ASA
Total patients	267	254	335	166	381	141	423	98	444	77
Received blood transfusion (%)	**31***	**14**	27	25	18	22	21	16	21	19
Women (%)	43	43	34	34	25	23	23	25	19	16
Renal insufficiency (%)	5.2	5.1	3.6	3.1	1.9	2.5	2.5	2.6	1.7	0
Age, y (SD)	64 (11)	65 (10)	63 (11)	62 (11)	63 (10)	62 (10)	62 (10)	63 (11)	63 (10)	64 (10)
Weight, kg (SD)	79 (15)	78 (16)	84 (19)	84 (17)	84 (17)	86 (17)	86 (18)	85 (17)	88 (21)	90 (21)
CPB time, min (SD)	162 (81)	162 (63)	144 (51)	148 (51)	144 (62)	141 (51)	135 (52)	143 (43)	137 (47)	136 (41)

*$p < .001$, Chi-square, compared to no ASA in quintile 1.

closely matched for other variables, such as preoperative renal function, gender, and cardiopulmonary bypass time. This indicates that the propensity score matching did what it was intended to do: match the patients for all variables except for the outcome variable of interest (i.e., postoperative transfusion). The results show that the propensity scored quintiles are asymmetric—i.e., there is not a consistent association between aspirin and blood transfusion across all quintiles. In the strata that are least likely to receive preoperative aspirin, there are patients who are more likely to receive postoperative transfusion (i.e., patients in quintile 1 have the longest cardiopulmonary bypass time, the greatest number of women, and the largest number of patients with preoperative renal dysfunction). This implies that some patients may have been recognized as high risk preoperatively and were not given aspirin—i.e., selection bias exists in the data set. There is some evidence that well-done observational studies give comparable results to RCTs dealing with the similar outcomes,[118,119] and balancing scores provide optimal means of analyzing nonrandomized studies.

BOOTSTRAPPING

The importance of risk factor identification for comparing outcomes has already been stressed. Risk factor identification for a given outcome has become commonplace in medicine. A problem arises from this dependence on risk factor analysis, especially logistic regression. Different observers analyzing the same risk factors to predict outcome get different results. Table 6-9 is an example of the variability in risk factor identification that can result. In this table, Grunkemeier et al compared 13 published multivariate risk models for mortality following CABG.[80] The number of independent risk factors cited by any one model varied from 5 to 29! Naftel described 9 different factors that contribute to different investigators obtaining different models to predict outcome (i.e., different sets of risk factors associated with the same outcome).[120] Some or all of these factors may affect the risk models listed in Table 6-9. One of Naftel's factors that is important in differentiating various models of CABG mortality is variable selection. In Table 6-9, 13 different groups found 13 different variable patterns that apparently adequately predicted operative mortality. How can this be? Recent breakthrough statistical methods have surfaced that address variable selection in statistical modeling.

In the early 1980s, the ready availability of computers began to surface to the consciousness of investigators. Efron et al popularized computer-intensive computational techniques that were not readily available until computers were on every investigator's desk.[121–124] They coined the term "bootstrap" to describe these computer-intensive methods. Bootstrap analysis is a data-based simulation method for statistical inference. Efron's group and others found that by taking repeated random samples from a data set (1000 random samples is typical) and determining risk factors for an outcome from each of the new data sets using statistical modeling, the predictor variables obtained from all the 1000 random samples were usually different. However, some variables were never selected in the model and others were selected consistently. The frequency of occurrence of risk factors among the 1000 or more models provides variables that have a high degree of reproducibility and reliability as independent risk factors of the given outcome. This process is called "bootstrap bagging,"[125] and it has formalized the development of model building, which had previously been more of an art than a science. As a result of this work with bootstrap analysis, model building and risk adjustment will be held to a more rigorous scientific standard.

TOTAL QUALITY MANAGEMENT AND RISK ANALYSIS

Cardiac surgeons now treat patients that were considered inoperable as recently as a decade ago. Yet almost no one is happy with the health care system. It costs too much, excludes many, is inefficient, and is ignorant about its own

TABLE 6–9 Risk models for operative mortality for CABG

Risk model	NYS[189]	Canada[277]	Mass[190]	Emory[278]	VA[279]	Australia[280]	Toronto[281]	CCF[282]	Israel[283]	Alabama[284]	NNE[138]	NYC[285]	Parsonnett[286]	Sum
Patients (no.)	174,210	57,187	50,357	17,128	13,368	12,712	12,003	7,491	4,918	4,835	3,654	3,055	2,152	
Risk factors (no.)	29	16	13	7	6	9	5	9	7	9	9	10	8	
Age	x	x		x	x	x	x	x	x	x	x	x	x	12
Gender	x	x	x	x	x		x	x		x		x		9
Urgency	x		x		x	x		x		x	x	x		8
EF	x	x			x		x	x		x	x	x		8
Renal dysfunction	x	x	x	x						x	x		x	7
Previous CABG	x		x	x				x			x	x		6
NYHA class	x	x	x	x		x				x				6
Left main CAD	x	x						x		x	x	x		6
# diseased vessels	x	x			x			x		x		x		6
PVD	x		x			x		x	x					5
Diabetes	x	x			x					x			x	5
Prior stroke	x		x	x		x								4
Intraop/postop variables			x				x		x				x	4
Prior MI	x	x	x	x										4
Body size	x	x										x		3
Preop IABP	x	x				x								3
Shock	x	x									x			3
COPD	x	x												2
Prior PTCA	x		x											2
Angina		x					x							2
IV NTG	x					x								2
Arrhythmias	x								x					2
Hx of heart operation		x				x								2
Hemodynamic instability	x												x	2
Charison comorbidity											x	x		2
Dialysis dependence	x	x												2
Pulmonary hypertension	x												x	2
Diuretics	x					x								2
HTCVD								x						1
Serum albumin									x					1
Race	x													1
Previous CHF											x			1
MI timing	x													1

Cardiac index			x			1
LVEDP				x		1
CVA timing	x					1
Liver disease		x				1
Neoplasia		x				1
Ventricular aneurysm		x				1
Steroids	x					1
Digitalis	x					1
Thrombolytic therapy					x	1
Arterial bicarbonate			x			1
Calcified aorta					x	1

NYS = New York State; Mass = Massachusetts; VA = Veterans' Administration; CCF = Cleveland Clinic Foundation; NNE = Northern New England; NYC = New York City; EF = ejection fraction; NYHA = New York Heart Association; CAD = coronary artery disease; PVD = peripheral vascular disease; MI = myocardial infarction; IABP = intra-aortic balloon pump; COPD = chronic obstructive pulmonary disease; PTCA = percutaneous transluminal coronary angioplasty ± stent; NTG = nitroglycerin; Hx = history; HTCVD = hypertensive cardiovascular disease; LVEDP = left ventricular end-diastolic pressure; CVA = cerebrovascular accident.

Source: Reproduced with permission from Grunkemeier GL, Zerr KJ, Jin R: Cardiac surgery report cards: making the grade. Ann Thorac Surg 2001; 72:1845.

effectiveness. This state of confusion has been likened to the conditions that existed with Japanese industry after World War II. Out of the confusion and crisis of post–World War II, Japan became a monolith of efficiency. Two major architects of this transformation were an American statistician, W. Edwards Deming, and a Romanian-American theoretician, J.M. Juran. They led the way in establishing and implementing certain principles of management and efficiency based on quality.

Deming's and Juran's principles[126–129] have been given the acronym of "total quality management," or TQM. The amazing turnaround in Japanese industry has led many organizations to embrace the principles of TQM, including organizations involved in the delivery and assessment of health care.[130] Using this approach, health care is viewed as a process requiring raw materials (e.g., sick patients), manufacturing steps (e.g., delivery of care to the sick), and finished products (e.g., outcomes of care). Managerial interventions are important at each step of the process to insure high-quality product. Table 6-10 outlines the key features of TQM.

An important component of the TQM process is the use and availability of statistical methods to provide the necessary information to managers and workers who must make decisions about the health care process.[131–133] Although the statistical methods of TQM have a slightly different focus than those outlined above for risk adjustment, the goal is the same—i.e., improving the quality of health care. Hence, it is reasonable to include a description of the methods of TQM, since those methods will inevitably come up in discussions about health care outcomes and assessing risks for these patient outcomes.

Table 6-11 provides an outline of the sequential steps involved in solving a problem using TQM. Risk stratification plays an important role in the TQM process. One of the most important applications of risk stratification in TQM is in the early stages of the project, when the definition of the problems that affect quality is being considered. Usually a problem is identified from critical observations—e.g., excessive blood transfusion after operation may result in increased morbidity, including disease transmission, increased infection risk, and increased cost. Tools such as flow diagrams

TABLE 6–10 Principles of total quality management (TQM) applied to health care

Principle	Explanation
Health care delivery is a process.	The purpose of a process is to add value to the input of the process. Each person in an organization is part of one or more processes.
Quality defects arise from problems with the process.	Former reliance on quotas, numerical goals, and discipline of workers is unlikely to improve quality, since these measures imply that workers are at fault and that quality will get better if workers do better. The problem is with the process, not with the worker. Quality improvement involves "driving out fear" on the part of the worker, and breaking down barriers between departments so that everyone may work effectively as a team for the organization.
Customer-supplier relationships are the most important aspect of quality.	A customer is anyone who depends on the organization. The goal of quality improvement is to improve constantly and to establish a long-term relationship of loyalty and trust between the customer (patient) and supplier (health care organization) and, thereby, meet the needs of the patient. The competitive advantage for an organization that can better meet the needs of the customer is obvious. The organization will gain market share, reduce costs, and waste less effort in activities that do not add value for patients.
Understand the causes of variability.	Failure to understand variation in critical processes within the organization is the cause of many serious quality problems. Unpredictable processes are flawed and are difficult to study and assess. Managers must understand the difference between random (or common-cause) variation and special variation in a given outcome.
Develop new organizational structures.	Managers are leaders, not enforcers. Eliminate management by objective numerical goals. Remove barriers that rob workers of their right to pride of workmanship. Empower everybody in the organization to achieve the transformation to a quality product.
Focus on the most "vital few" processes.	This is known as the Pareto principle (first devised by Juran), which states that whenever a number of individual factors contribute to an outcome, relatively few of those items account for the bulk of the effect. By focusing on the "vital few," the greatest reward for effort will occur.
Quality reduces cost.	Poor quality is costly. Malpractice suits, excessive use of costly laboratory tests, and unnecessarily long hospital stays are examples of costly poor quality. The premise that it is too costly to implement quality control is incorrect.
Statistics and scientific thinking are the foundation of quality.	Managers must make decisions based on accurate data, using scientific methods. Not only managers, but all members of the organization utilize the scientific method for improving processes as part of their normal daily activity.

TABLE 6–11 Steps in a TQM project

Step	Goal	Tools
1. Definition of problem	List and prioritize problems that effect quality. Define project and identify team to solve problem.	Flow process diagram Pareto chart Customer surveys Risk stratification to identify high-risk subsets
2. Diagnosis of problem	Formulate and test hypotheses about the cause of the problem.	Process flow diagram Experimental design methods Statistics to test hypotheses
3. Remedy for problem	Managers and workers participate in training and implementing new or revised process.	Managerial skills in initiating training, implementing solutions, designing controls, and dealing with resistance
4. Check performance of new process	Monitor process for effectiveness and develop new TQM projects based on results of modifications to the old process.	Sampling methods to get representative sample of outcome Control charts used at every level of the organization—graphs, histograms, stem-and-leaf displays, CUSUM methods, regression analysis, etc.

that document all of the steps in the process (e.g., steps involved in the blood transfusion process after CABG) are helpful in this phase of the analysis. A logical starting point for efforts to improve the quality of the blood transfusion process would be to focus on a high-risk subset of patients who consume a disproportionate amount of resources. An Italian economist, named Pareto, made the observation that a few factors account for the majority of the outcomes of a complex process, and this has been termed the "Pareto principle."

The Pareto principle has proven to be a valuable tool in improving quality. A graphical method of identifying the spectrum of outcomes in a process is included in most statistics programs, and is termed a Pareto diagram. Figure 6-5 is an example of a Pareto diagram for blood product transfusion. The data are arranged in histogram format, and the population distribution of patients receiving transfusion is plotted simultaneously. The Pareto diagram is an example of a graphical method of risk identification. By looking at the diagram, it is possible to identify a subset of patients who

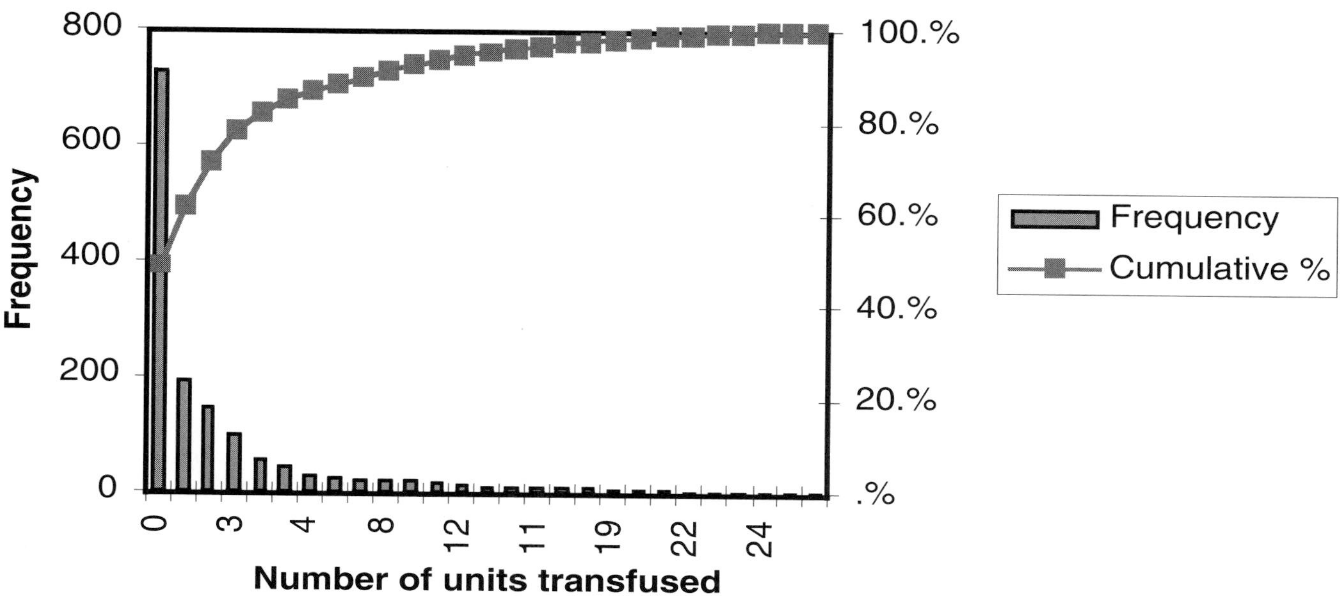

FIGURE 6–5 Pareto diagram of blood transfusion in 1489 patients undergoing cardiac procedures at Albany Medical Center Hospital during 1994.

consume more than a certain threshold of blood products. For example, it can be estimated that 20% of the patients consume 80% of the blood products transfused. Substantial savings in cost and possibly other morbidity will result by decreasing the amount of blood transfusion in these "high-end" users. Strategies can be devised and tested to decrease blood product consumption in the high-risk subset, and ultimately monitors must be set up to test the effectiveness of the new strategies.

Application of the Pareto principle is a valuable tool in risk stratification and TQM, but some of the risk stratification analytic tools previously discussed can be equally useful in the TQM process. For example, linear regression analysis might be used to identify which of several factors are most important in predicting improved blood transfusion profiles after CABG, or Cox analysis might be used to identify risk factors for increased hospital length of stay in patients at high risk for excessive blood transfusion. Other tools of TQM such as data sampling strategies and use of control charts play an important role in the process.

Several tools that are typically used in industrial quality improvement and process control[134] have been applied to medicine and, in particular, cardiothoracic surgery.[135–137] Shahian et al used control charts to evaluate special and usual variability of outcomes in patients having average-risk CABG.[135] Again, for this type of analysis, CABG is viewed as a process with raw materials (patients with coronary artery disease), manufacturing steps (CABG), and output (operative outcomes). The outcomes are tracked over time using control charts, a well-known quality improvement tool. Control charts are plots of data over time. The data points are usually plotted in conjunction with overlying lines that represent upper and lower control limits. The control limits are established by considering historical data (e.g., rate of blood transfusion or the operative mortality rate). When a data point falls outside of the control limits, it is said to be "out of control." Causes of a process being out of control include either usual causes (random) or special (nonrandom) causes. Shahian et al found that certain postoperative complications (e.g., postoperative bleeding, leg wound infections, and total major complications) were out of control in the early part of their study. After implementing quality improvement measures, these complication rates showed progressive improvement, with the net effect being improvement in the length of hospital stay.

A variation on the control chart methodology, called the cumulative sum analysis, or CUSUM, was used by Novick et al to analyze the effect of changing from on-pump CABG to off-pump CABG as a primary means of operative coronary revascularization.[136] These authors found that the CUSUM methodology was more sensitive than standard statistical techniques in detecting a cluster of surgical failures or successes.

Another example of a TQM project that has been carried out in clinical cardiothoracic surgery is the study reported by de Levalet al.[137] In this study, surgeons identified an increase in the mortality rate of infants undergoing total repair of D-transposition of the great vessels; the authors applied the principles of TQM to the process of care of these infants. They were able to identify risk factors for poor outcome and to separate the sources of variation in mortality rate into either random (common cause) variation or nonrandom (special cause) variation. By identifying and altering nonrandom causes of increased mortality, which were presumably related to the surgeon or to the process of care, they were able to make a positive impact on patient outcome. Examples like this go far beyond simple risk analysis and begin to get at the true value of these techniques, i.e., improving patient outcomes.

Another set of innovative TQM studies has been carried out by the Northern New England Cardiovascular Disease Study Group.[138–141] These investigators used a risk-adjustment scheme (Tables 6-1 and 6-9) to predict mortality in patients undergoing CABG at 5 different institutions. After risk stratification, significant variability was found among the different institutions and providers. Statistical methods suggested that the variation in mortality rate was nonrandom ("special variability" in the TQM vernacular). A peer-based, confidential TQM project was initiated to address this variability and to improve outcomes in the region. In order to study this nonrandom variability, representatives from each institution visited all institutions and reviewed the processes involved in performing CABG. Surgical technique, communication among providers, leadership, decision making, training levels, and environment were assessed at each institution. Significant variation among many of the processes was observed, and attempts to correct deficiencies were undertaken at each institution. Subsequent publications from these authors suggest that this approach improves outcomes for all providers at all institutions.[141]

RISKS OF OPERATION FOR ISCHEMIC HEART DISEASE

Risks Factors for Operative Mortality

By far, the bulk of available experience with risk stratification and outcome analysis in cardiothoracic surgery deals with risk factors associated with operative mortality, particularly in patients undergoing coronary revascularization. Most of the risk stratification analyses shown in Table 6-1 and Table 6-9 have been used to evaluate life or death outcomes in surgical patients with ischemic heart disease, in part because mortality is such an easy end point to measure and track. As previously mentioned, each of the risk stratification systems shown in Table 6-1 and Table 6-9, with the exception of the APACHE III system, computes a risk score based on risk factors that are dependent on patient diagnosis. The definition of operative mortality varies among the different systems (either 30-day mortality or in-hospital mortality), but the risk factors identified by each of the stratification schemes in Table 6-9 show many similarities. Some variables are risk factors in almost all stratification systems; some variables are never significant risk factors. Each of the models has been validated using separate data sets; hence, there is some justification in using any of the risk stratification methods both in preoperative assessment of patients undergoing coronary artery bypass grafting (CABG) and in making comparisons among providers (either physicians or hospitals), but certain caveats exist about the validity and reliability of these models (see below). At present it is not possible to recommend one risk stratification method over another. In general, the larger the sample size, the more risk factors can be found.

A large number of patient variables other than those shown in Table 6-9 have been proposed as risk factors for operative mortality following coronary revascularization. Such variables as serum BUN,[142] cachexia,[143] oxygen delivery,[144] HIV,[145] case volume,[146–149] low hematocrit on bypass,[150] use of the internal mammary artery,[151] the diameter of the coronary artery,[152] and resident involvement in the operation[153,154] fit this description. On the surface, the clinical relevance of these variables may seem undeniable in published reports, but very few of these putative risk factors have been tested with the rigor of the variables shown in Table 6-9. The regression diagnostics (e.g., ROC curves and cross-validation studies) performed on the models included in Tables 6-1 and 6-9 suggest that the models are good, but not perfect, at predicting outcomes. In statistical terms this means that all of the variability in operative mortality is not explained by the set of risk factors included in the regression models. Hence, it is possible that inclusion of new putative risk factors in the regression equations may improve the validity and precision of the models. New regression models, and new risk factors, must be scrutinized and tested using cross-validation methods and other regression diagnostics before acceptance. It is uncertain whether inclusion of many more risk factors will significantly improve the quality and predictive ability of regression models. For example, the STS risk stratification model described in Tables 6-1 and 6-9 includes many predictor variables, while the Toronto risk-adjustment scheme includes only 5 predictor variables. Yet the regression diagnostics for these two models are similar, suggesting that both models have equal precision and predictive capabilities. This suggests that the models are effective at predicting population behavior but not necessarily suited for predicting individual outcomes. Further work needs to be done, both to explain the differences in risk factors seen between the various risk stratification models and to determine which models are best suited for studies of quality improvement.

Many critical features of any risk-adjustment outcome program must be considered when determining quality of the risk stratification method or when comparing one to another (see below). Daley provides a summary of the key features that are necessary to validate any risk-adjustment model.[59,155] She makes the point that no clear-cut evidence exists that differences in risk-adjusted mortalities across providers reflect differences in the process and structure of care.[156] This issue needs further study.

Risk Factors for Postoperative Morbidity and Resource Utilization

Patients with nonfatal outcomes following operations for ischemic heart disease make up more than 95% of the pool of patients undergoing operation. Of approximately 500,000 patients having CABG yearly, between 50% and 75% have what is characterized by both the patient and provider as an uncomplicated course following operation. The complications occurring in surviving patients range from serious organ system dysfunction to minor limitation or dissatisfaction with lifestyle, and account for a significant fraction of the cost of the procedures. We estimate that as much as 40% of the yearly hospital costs for CABG are consumed by 10% to 15% of the patients who have serious complications after operation.[11] This is an example of the Pareto principle described above, and also suggests that reducing morbidity in CABG patients would have significant impact on cost reduction.

A great deal of information has been accumulated on nonfatal complications after operation for ischemic heart disease. Several large databases have been used to identify risk factors for both nonfatal morbidity and increased resource utilization. Table 6-12 is a summary of some of the risk factors that have been identified by available risk stratification models using either serious postoperative morbidity or increased resource utilization as measures of undesirable outcomes.

Occasionally studies appear that suggest that a particular patient variable is *not* a risk factor for a particular patient outcome. Care must be exercised in interpreting negative results. Many putative risk factors labeled as "no different from control" in studies using inadequate samples have not received a fair test. For example, Burns et al studied preoperative template bleeding times in 43 patients undergoing elective CABG.[157] They found no increased postoperative blood loss in patients with prolonged bleeding times. In this small sample size, there was a trend toward more units of blood transfused, but differences between high and low bleeding time groups were "not significant" at the $\alpha = 5\%$ ($p = .05$). Using the author's data, it is possible to compute a β error for this negative observation of less than 0.5. This means that there is as much as a 50% chance that the negative finding is really a false-negative result. We have found elevated bleeding time (> 10 minutes) to be a significant multivariate risk factor for excessive blood transfusion after CABG in two different studies.[36,37] Although there is controversy about the

TABLE 6–12 Risk factors associated with either increased length of stay (L) or increased incidence of organ failure morbidity (M) or both (L/M) following coronary revascularization

Risk factor	Boston[287]	Albany[11]	VA[179–181]	Canada[7]
Demographics				
Advanced age	L		M	L
Increased ratio of age/red blood cell volume		L/M		
Female gender				L
Disease-specific diagnoses				
CHF or cardiomegaly	L	L/M	M	
Concomitant valve disease			M	L
Reoperation			M	L
LV dysfunction (ejection fraction)				L
Surgical priority			M	L
IABP preop	L			
Active endocarditis			M	
Comorbid conditions				
Obesity	L			
Renal dysfunction	L	L	M	
Peripheral vascular disease		L	M	
Chronic obstructive lung disease		L		
Cerebrovascular disease		L/M		
Hypertension		L/M		

CHF = congestive heart failure; LV = left ventricular; IABP = intra-aortic balloon counterpulsation.

value of bleeding time as a screening test,[158,159] it is possible that discarding the bleeding time after an inconclusive negative trial, such as that of Burns et al, may ignore a potentially important risk factor.[160]

Patient Satisfaction as an Outcome

Other post-CABG outcomes, such as patient satisfaction and sense of well-being, have been less well studied. The increasing importance of patient-reported outcomes reflects the increasing prevalence of chronic disease in our aging population. The goals of therapeutic interventions are often to relieve symptoms and improve quality of life, rather than cure a disease and prolong survival. This is especially important in selecting elderly patients for operation. One report from the United Kingdom suggests that as many as one third of patients over the age of 70 did not have improvement in their disability and overall sense of well-being after cardiac operation.[161] Risk stratification methodology may prove to be important in identifying elderly patients who are optimal candidates for revascularization based on quality of life considerations.

Surprisingly little published information is available regarding long-term functional status or patient satisfaction following CABG. One comparative study found no difference between patients older than 65 years and those 65 or younger with regard to quality of life outcomes (symptoms, cardiac functional class, activities of daily living, and emotional and social functioning).[162] This study also found a direct relationship between clinical severity and quality of life indicators, since patients with less comorbid conditions and better preoperative functional status had better quality of life indicators 6 months after operation. Rumsfeld et al found that improvement in the self-reported quality of life (from Form SF-36) was more likely in patients who had relatively poor health status before CABG compared to those who had relatively good preoperative health status.[163] Interestingly, these same authors found that the poor self-reported quality of life indicator, as measured by SF-36 questionnaire, was an independent predictor of operative mortality following CABG.[164] These findings suggest that the risks of patient dissatisfaction after CABG are dependent on preoperative comorbid factors as well as on the indications for, and technical complexities of, the operation itself. At present no risk stratification scheme has been devised to identify patients who are likely to report dissatisfaction with operative intervention following CABG.

There are several difficulties with measurement of patient-reported outcomes, and consequently cardiothoracic surgeons have not been deeply involved with systematic measurements of patient satisfaction after operation. One problem is that patient-reported outcomes may be dependent on the type of patient who is reporting them and not on the type of care received. For example, younger Caucasian patients with better education and higher income are more likely to give less favorable ratings of physician care.[165] However, considerable research has been done dealing with instruments to measure patient satisfaction. At least two of these measures, the Short-Form Health Survey (SF-36)[166] and the San Jose Medical Group's Patient Satisfaction Measure,[167] have been used to monitor patient satisfaction over time. The current status of these and other measures of patient satisfaction does not allow comparisons among providers, because the quality of the data generated by these measures is poor. These instruments are characterized by low response rates, inadequate sampling, infrequent use, and unavailability of satisfactory benchmarks. Nonetheless, available evidence indicates that patient-reported outcomes can be measured reliably[168,169] and that feedback on patient satisfaction data to physicians can significantly improve physician practices.[170] It is likely that managed care organizations and hospitals will use patient-reported outcome measures to make comparisons between institutions and between individual providers. Risk-adjustment methods for patient-reported outcomes will be required to provide valid comparisons of this type.

VALIDITY AND RELIABILITY OF RISK STRATIFICATION METHODS

There is little or no consensus about how to assess the validity of risk-adjustment methodology. As pointed out by Daley, the concept of validity is something that everyone understands but for which no single meaning exists.[156] The concept of validity is made up of many parts. According to Daley, 5 of these parts are as follows:

1. Face validity: Will whoever uses the risk model accept it as valid?
2. Content validity: Does the model include risk factors that should have been included based on known risks?
3. Construct validity: How well does the model compare to other measures of the same outcome?
4. Predictive validity: How well does the model predict outcome in patients not used to construct the model?
5. Attributional validity: Does the model measure the attribute of effectiveness of care, not patient variability?

Of these components, face and content validity are arguably the most important. Clinicians can readily accept the results of risk stratification efforts if the model uses variables that are familiar and includes risk factors that the clinician recognizes as important in determining outcome. All of the risk models shown in Table 6-9 satisfy some or all of these criteria of validity. There is no objective measure that defines validity, but most clinicians would agree that the risk models have relevance to clinical practice and contain many of the features that one would expect to be predictive of morbidity and mortality for CABG.

The reliability of a risk stratification model is more easily measured than validity. Reliability of a risk-adjustment method refers to the statistical term of "precision," or the ability to repeat the observations using similar input variables and similar statistical techniques with resultant similar outcome findings. There are literally hundreds of sources of variability in any risk stratification model. Some of these include errors in data input, inconsistencies in coding or physician diagnosis, variations in use of therapeutic intervention, data fragility (final model may be very dependent on a few influential outliers), and the type of rater (physician, nurse, or coding technician), to name a few.[171] The most common measure of reliability is Cohen's kappa coefficient, which measures the level of agreement between two or more observations compared to agreement due to chance alone.[172] The kappa coefficient is defined as:

$$\kappa = (P_o - P_c)/(1 - P_c)$$

where P_c is the fraction representing the agreement that would have occurred by chance, and P_o is the observed agreement between two observers. If two observations agree 70% of the time for an observation where agreement by chance alone would occur 54% of the time (i.e., $P_o = 0.7$ and $P_c = 0.54$), then kappa = 0.35. Landis and Koch have offered a performance estimate of kappa[173] as follows:

0 to 0.2: slight agreement
0.2 to 0.4: fair agreement
0.4 to 0.6: good agreement
0.6 to 0.8: substantial agreement
0.8 to 1.0: near perfect agreement

Other methods of measuring the agreement between two models include weighted kappa, interclass correlation coefficient, the tau statistic, and the gamma statistic. These methods are discussed in the work of Hughes and Ash,[171] and any of these methods offer an objective means of assessing the reliability of a risk-adjustment model.

Surprisingly little work has been done in assessing the reliability and validity of the risk-adjustment methods used with large cardiac surgical databases. It is absolutely essential that validity and reliability be tested in these models, both in order for clinicians to feel comfortable with the comparisons generated by the risk stratification models, and for policy makers (either government or managed care organizations) to feel confident in making decisions based on risk-adjusted outcomes.

Risk Stratification to Measure the Effectiveness of Care

The biggest single shortcoming of risk-adjustment methodology is its lack of proven effectiveness in delineating quality of care. Even though it may seem obvious that differences in risk-adjusted outcomes reflect differences in quality of care, this is far from proven. What little information there is available on this subject is inconsistent. Hartz et al compared hospital mortality rates for patients undergoing CABG.[174] They found that differences in hospital mortality rates were correlated with differences in quality of care between hospitals. Hannan et al attempted to evaluate the quality of care in outlier hospitals in the New York State risk-adjusted mortality cohort.[175] They concluded, as did Hartz et al, that risk-adjusted mortality rates for CABG were a reflection of quality of care. The measures of quality used in these studies were somewhat arbitrary and did not reflect a complete array of factors that might be expected to influence outcomes after CABG. In TQM jargon, the entire clinical process of surgical intervention for coronary revascularization was not assessed. Other studies have not found a correlation between global hospital mortality rates and quality of care indicators.[83,176–178] Indeed, one study suggested that nearly all of the variation in mortality among hospitals reflects variation in patient characteristics rather than in hospital characteristics,[178] while another study found that identifying poor-quality hospitals on the basis of mortality rate performance, even with perfect risk adjustment, resulted in less than 20% sensitivity and greater than 50% predictive error.[83] These studies suggest that reports that measure quality using risk-adjusted mortality rates misinform the public about hospital (or physician) performance.

Two ongoing quality improvement studies are using risk-adjusted outcome measurements to assess and influence the clinical process of coronary artery bypass grafting: the Northern New England Cardiovascular Disease Study[138–141] and the Veteran's Administration Cardiac Surgery Risk Assessment Program.[179–181] Results from these studies suggest that using risk-adjusted outcomes (e.g., mortality and cost) as internal reference levels tracked over time (similar to the control charts of TQM described above) can produce meaningful improvements in outcomes. Whether these risk-adjusted outcomes can be used to indicate quality of care or cost-effectiveness of providers across all institutions is another question that remains unanswered. At present, equating risk-adjusted outcome measurements with effective care is not justified.[176–178,182–188]

Controversy exists as to whether changes in a physician's report card over time reflect changes in care or whether these changes are due to other factors not related to the care delivery of individual provider's. Hannan et al suggested that the public release of surgeon-specific, risk-adjusted mortality rates led to a decline in overall mortality in the state of New York from 4.17% in 1989 to 2.45% in 1992 and hence to an improvement in the quality of care.[189] The cause of this decline in operative mortality is uncertain, but probably represents a combination of improvement in the process of care (especially in the outlier hospitals), the retirement of low-volume surgeons, and an overall national trend toward decreased CABG mortality. Ghali et al found that states adjacent to New York that did not have report cards had comparable decreased CABG operative mortality during the same time period.[190] Without any formal quality improvement initiative or report card, the operative morality rate in Massachusetts decreased from 4.7% in 1990 to 3.3% in 1994. This occurred while the expected operative mortality of patients increased from 4.7% to 5.7%.

The decline in New York State operative mortality over time associated with the publication of surgeon-specific mortality rates was greater than the overall national decrease in CABG death rates. Peterson et al found that the reduction in observed CABG mortality was 22% in New York versus 9% in the rest of the nation, a highly significant difference.[191] An interesting finding in this study is that the only other area in the United States with a comparable decline in CABG mortality to that of New York was northern New England. The Northern New England Cooperative Group established a confidential TQM approach to improve CABG outcomes[139,140,192–194] at about the same time that New York State report cards were published in the lay press.

Ethical Implications of Risk Stratification: The Dilemma of Managed Care

An important component of new proposals for health care reform is mandated reports on quality of care.[195] While reporting on quality of care sounds appealing, there are many problems associated with this effort, some of which present the clinician with an ethical dilemma.[187,196–198] There is general agreement that quality indicators should be risk-adjusted to allow fair comparisons among providers. Risk adjustment in this setting is extremely difficult and may be misleading, and, what is worse, may not reflect quality of care at all. The release of risk-adjusted data may alienate providers and result in the sickest patients having less accessibility to care. This may have already happened in New York State[87,188,199] and in other regions where risk-adjusted mortality and cost data have been released to the public. Of even more concern is the selection bias that seems to exist in managed care HMO enrollment. Morgan et al suggest that Medicare HMOs benefit from the selective enrollment of healthier Medicare recipients and the disenrollment or outright rejection of sicker beneficiaries.[200] This form of separation of patients into unfavorable or favorable risk categories undermines the effectiveness of the Medicare managed care system and highlights the subtle selection bias that can result when financial incentives overcome medical standards. Careful population-based

TABLE 6–13 (*Continued*)

New Jersey State Department of Health	Health care consumers in the state of New Jersey	By mail (New Jersey Department of Health and Senior Services, Office of Research and Development, P.O. Box 360, Trenton, NJ 08625)	Risk-adjusted hospital mortality rates for CABG
New York State Department of Health	Patients having cardiac procedures in New York State	Internet (http://www.health.state.ny.us/nysdoh/consumer/heart/1996-98cabg.pdf)	Surgeon-specific and hospital-specific in-hospital mortality rates for CABG
Pennsylvania Health Care Cost Containment Council	Patients who require CABG in the state of Pennsylvania	Internet (http://www.phc4.org/reports/cardiaccare.htm)	Hospital- and surgeon-specific CABG mortality rates
Rand Corporation	Provide the public with summary data about health care outcomes for cardiac surgery	Internet (http://www.rand.org/publications/MR/MR1255/MR1255.app4.pdf)	Summary of publicly available CABG mortality rates with critical appraisal of methods and some estimation of appropriateness of care
Society of Thoracic Surgeons	Provide the public with results of cardiac surgery over as broad of a population as possible (including VA, Northern New England Consortium, and Great Britain)	Internet (http://www.ctsnet.org/section/outcomes/)	Mortality and other outcomes data for a variety of thoracic procedures; some of the data is presented as raw mortality data without risk adjustment; one of the only databases that includes noncardiac surgery
Solucient Corp., Inc. (Top 100 Heart Hospitals)	Provide the public with rather arbitrary rating of overall quality of cardiac care at hospitals	Internet (http://www.100tophospitals.com/Media/releases/nr010702_cardio.htm)	Rates all hospitals in the U.S. that do cardiac surgery and lists the top 100 heart hospitals
WebMD, Inc.	Provide information to consumers and physicians about a broad spectrum of health care issues	Internet (http://my.webmd.com/content/dmk/dmk_article_53203)	Information about CABG and expected outcomes
Women's Heart Foundation	Provide health-related information for women	Internet (http://www.womensheart-foundation.org/content/HeartSurgery/state_report_cards_on_ohs.asp)	Links to Internet-available report cards on cardiac surgery

discussion) will become more important as refinements in risk-adjustment methodology progress.

Information Management: Electronic Medical Records

As already mentioned, accurate patient data are essential in order to apply the principles of risk stratification and quality improvement outlined in this chapter. The quality and accuracy of administrative (or claims) databases have been questioned.[24,61,63–66] Therefore, risk-adjustment methodology has placed greater reliance on data extracted from the medical record. The American College of Surgeons was among the earliest advocates of the utility of medical records for quality review.[252] In the 1960s, Weed advocated standardization and computerization of medical records.[253–255]

Little substantive progress had been made as far as the computerization of medical records until the need arose for management of large amounts of data of the sort required for risk adjustment and outcomes assessment. Medical records are an invaluable source of information about patient risk factors and outcomes. With these facts in mind, more and more pilot studies are being undertaken to computerize and standardize the medical record in a variety of clinical situations.[245,256–264] Iezzoni has pointed out the difficulties with computerized medical records and suggests that they may not adequately reflect the importance of chronic disability and decreased functional status.[265] Nevertheless, it is apparent that the need for data about large groups of patients exists, especially for managed care and capitation initiatives. It is reasonable to expect that efforts to computerize medical records will expand. Applications of electronic medical records that may be available in the future for cardiothoracic surgeons include monitoring of patient outcomes,[256] supporting clinical decision making with real-time analysis of the electronic medical record,[257,259,262] and real-time tracking of resource utilization using computerized hospital records.[260]

CONCLUSIONS

Risk stratification and outcomes analysis will have an increasing role in cardiac surgery. The methods of risk analysis are straightforward but are in their early stages. The goal of risk adjustment in the analysis of outcomes is to account for the contribution of patient-related risk factors, in order that patient outcomes can be used as an indicator of the quality of care rendered by physicians and hospitals. The future will undoubtedly see refinements in risk-adjustment methods and increasing use of these techniques at all levels of health care delivery, including the distribution of health care dollars. Thoracic surgeons have been at the forefront of these methodologies (sometimes unwillingly), but much work remains to be done in the area of education about the use of risk stratification and application of risk-adjusted outcome analysis toward improving quality of care. We are obliged to have an understanding of the techniques, with the ultimate goal being to improve patient outcomes and maintain high professional quality.

REFERENCES

1. Nightingale F: *Notes on Hospitals*. London, Longman, Green, Longman, Roberts, and Green, 1863.
2. Cohen IB: Florence Nightingale. *Sci Am* 1984; 250:128.
3. Codman E: *A Study in Hospital Efficiency as Demonstrated by the Case Report of the First Five Years of a Private Hospital*. Boston, Thomas Todd Company, 1917.
4. Daniels M, Hill A: Chemotherapy of pulmonary tuberculosis in young adults: an analysis of the combined results of three Medical Research Council trials. *BMJ* 1952; 1:1162.
5. Cochrane A: *Effectiveness & Efficiency: Random Reflections on Health Services*. London, Royal Society of Medicine Press Limited, 1971; p. 1.
6. Steen PM, Brewster AC, Bradbury RC, et al: Predicted probabilities of hospital death as a measure of admission severity of illness. *Inquiry* 1993; 30:128.
7. Tu JV, Jaglal SB, Naylor CD: Multicenter validation of a risk index for mortality, intensive care unit stay, and overall hospital length of stay after cardiac surgery. Steering Committee of the Provincial Adult Cardiac Care Network of Ontario. *Circulation* 1995; 91:677.
8. Knaus WA, Wagner DP, Zimmerman JE, Draper EA: Variations in mortality and length of stay in intensive care units. *Ann Intern Med* 1993; 118:753.
9. Iezzoni LI: *Risk Adjustment for Measuring Healthcare Outcomes*. Chicago, Health Administration Press, 1997.
10. Ferraris VA, Ferraris SP, Singh A: Operative outcome and hospital cost. *J Thorac Cardiovasc Surg* 1998; 115:593.
11. Ferraris VA, Ferraris SP: Risk factors for postoperative morbidity. *J Thorac Cardiovasc Surg* 1996; 111:731.
12. Iezzoni LI: Risk adjustment for medical effectiveness research: an overview of conceptual and methodological considerations. *J Invest Med* 1995; 43:136.
13. Riordan CJ, Engoren M, Zacharias A, et al: Resource utilization in coronary artery bypass operation: does surgical risk predict cost? *Ann Thorac Surg* 2000; 69:1092.
14. Gold MR, Siegel JE, Russell LB, Weinstein MC: *Cost-effectiveness in Health and Medicine*. Oxford, Oxford University Press, 1996.
15. Petitti D: Meta-analysis, decision analysis, and cost-effectiveness analysis, in Kelsey JL MM, Stolley PD, Vessey MP (eds): *Monographs in Epidemiology and Biostatistics*, Vol. 31. New York, Oxford University Press, 2000.
16. Stewart AL, Greenfield S, Hays RD, et al: Functional status and well-being of patients with chronic conditions: results from the Medical Outcomes Study. *JAMA* 1989; 262:907.
17. Charlson ME, Pompei P, Ales KL, MacKenzie CR: A new method of classifying prognostic comorbidity in longitudinal studies: development and validation. *J Chron Dis* 1987; 40:373.
18. Charlson ME, Sax FL, MacKenzie CR, et al: Morbidity during hospitalization: can we predict it? *J Chron Dis* 1987; 40:705.
19. Knaus WA, Wagner DP, Draper EA, et al: The APACHE III prognostic system: risk prediction of hospital mortality for critically ill hospitalized adults. *Chest* 1991; 100:1619.
20. Keeler EB, Kahn KL, Draper D, et al: Changes in sickness at admission following the introduction of the prospective payment system. *JAMA* 1990; 264:1962.
21. Greenfield S, Apolone G, McNeil BJ, Cleary PD: The importance of co-existent disease in the occurrence of postoperative complications and one-year recovery in patients undergoing total hip replacement: comorbidity and outcomes after hip replacement. *Med Care* 1993; 31:141.
22. Greenfield S, Aronow HU, Elashoff RM, Watanabe D: Flaws in mortality data: the hazards of ignoring comorbid disease. *JAMA* 1988; 260:2253.
23. Goldman L, Caldera DL, Nussbaum SR, et al: Multifactorial index of cardiac risk in noncardiac surgical procedures. *N Engl J Med* 1977; 297:845.
24. Iezzoni LI, Foley SM, Daley J, et al: Comorbidities, complications, and coding bias: does the number of diagnosis codes matter in predicting in-hospital mortality? *JAMA* 1992; 267:2197.
25. Iezzoni LI, Daley J, Heeren T, et al: Using administrative data to screen hospitals for high complication rates. *Inquiry* 2000; 31:40.
26. McCarthy EP, Iezzoni LI, Davis RB, et al: Does clinical evidence support ICD-9-CM diagnosis coding of complications? *Med Care* 2000; 38:868.
27. Brinkley J: U.S. releasing lists of hospitals with abnormal mortality rates. *New York Times*, March 12, 1986; p 1.
28. Gatsonis CA, Epstein AM, Newhouse JP, et al: Variations in the utilization of coronary angiography for elderly patients with an acute myocardial infarction: an analysis using hierarchical logistic regression. *Med Care* 1995; 33:625.
29. Guadagnoli E, Hauptman PJ, Ayanian JZ, et al: Variation in the use of cardiac procedures after acute myocardial infarction. *N Engl J Med* 1995; 333:573.
30. Mark DB, Naylor CD, Hlatky MA, et al: Use of medical resources and quality of life after acute myocardial infarction in Canada and the United States. *N Engl J Med* 1994; 331:1130.
31. Anderson GM, Grumbach K, Luft HS, et al: Use of coronary artery bypass surgery in the United States and Canada: influence of age and income. *JAMA* 1993; 269:1661.
32. Chassin MR: Improving quality of care with practice guidelines. *Front Health Serv Manage* 1993; 10:40.

33. Eagle KA, Guyton RA, Davidoff R, et al: ACC/AHA Guidelines for Coronary Artery Bypass Graft Surgery: a report of the American College of Cardiology/American Heart Association Task Force on Practice Guidelines (Committee to Revise the 1991 Guidelines for Coronary Artery Bypass Graft Surgery). *J Am Coll Cardiol* 1999; 34:1262.
34. Shaneyfelt TM, Mayo-Smith MF, Rothwangl J: Are guidelines following guidelines? The methodological quality of clinical practice guidelines in the peer-reviewed medical literature. *JAMA* 1999; 281:1900.
35. Blackstone EH: Breaking down barriers: helpful breakthrough statistical methods you need to understand better. *J Thorac Cardiovasc Surg* 2001; 122:430.
36. Ferraris VA, Gildengorin V: Predictors of excessive blood use after coronary artery bypass grafting: a multivariate analysis. *J Thorac Cardiovasc Surg* 1989; 98:492.
37. Ferraris VA, Berry WR, Klingman RR: Comparison of blood reinfusion techniques used during coronary artery bypass grafting. *Ann Thorac Surg* 1993; 56:433.
38. Barbour G: The role of outcomes data in health care reform. *Ann Thorac Surg* 1994; 58:1881.
39. Chassin MR: Explaining geographic variations: the enthusiasm hypothesis. *Med Care* 1993; 31:YS37.
40. Wennberg JE, Freeman JL, Shelton RM, Bubolz TA: Hospital use and mortality among Medicare beneficiaries in Boston and New Haven. *N Engl J Med* 1989; 321:1168.
41. Relman AS: Assessment and accountability: the third revolution in medical care. *N Engl J Med* 1988; 319:1220.
42. Schneider EC, Leape LL, Weissman JS, et al: Racial differences in cardiac revascularization rates: does "overuse" explain higher rates among white patients? *Ann Int Med* 2001; 135:328.
43. Philbin EF, McCullough PA, DiSalvo TG, et al: Underuse of invasive procedures among Medicaid patients with acute myocardial infarction. *Am J Public Health* 2001; 91:1082.
44. Filardo G, Maggioni AP, Mura G, et al: The consequences of underuse of coronary revascularization; results of a cohort study in Northern Italy. *Eur Heart J* 2001; 22:654.
45. Kravitz RL, Laouri M: Measuring and averting underuse of necessary cardiac procedures: a summary of results and future directions. *Jt Comm J Qual Improv* 1997; 23:268.
46. Peterson ED, Shaw LK, DeLong ER, et al: Racial variation in the use of coronary-revascularization procedures: are the differences real? Do they matter? *N Engl J Med* 1997; 336:480.
47. Asch SM, Sloss EM, Hogan C, et al: Measuring underuse of necessary care among elderly Medicare beneficiaries using inpatient and outpatient claims. *JAMA* 2000; 284:2325.
48. Tobler HG, Sethi GK, Grover FL, et al: Variations in processes and structures of cardiac surgery practice. *Med Care* 1995; 33:OS43.
49. Stover EP, Siegel LC, Parks R, et al: Variability in transfusion practice for coronary artery bypass surgery persists despite national consensus guidelines: a 24-institution study. Institutions of the Multicenter Study of Perioperative Ischemia Research Group. *Anesthesiology* 1998; 88:327.
50. Lyon AW, Greenway DC, Hindmarsh JT: A strategy to promote rational clinical chemistry test utilization. *Am J Clin Pathol* 1995; 103:718.
51. Macario A, Chung A, Weinger MB: Variation in practice patterns of anesthesiologists in California for prophylaxis of postoperative nausea and vomiting. *J Clin Anesth* 2001; 13:353.
52. Nissenson AR, Collins AJ, Hurley J, et al: Opportunities for improving the care of patients with chronic renal insufficiency: current practice patterns. *J Am Soc Nephrol* 2001; 12:1713.
53. Nourse C, Byrne C, Leonard L, Butler K: Glycopeptide prescribing in a tertiary referral paediatric hospital and applicability of hospital infection control practices advisory committee (HICPAC) guidelines to children. *Eur J Pediatr* 2000; 159:193.
54. Gonzales R, Malone DC, Maselli JH, Sande MA: Excessive antibiotic use for acute respiratory infections in the United States. *Clin Infect Dis* 2001; 33:757.
55. Jones MI, Greenfield SM, Bradley CP: Prescribing new drugs: qualitative study of influences on consultants and general practitioners. *BMJ* 2001; 323:378.
56. Schneider EC, Eisenberg JM: Strategies and methods for aligning current and best medical practices: the role of information technologies. *West J Med* 1998; 168:311.
57. American College of Physicians. The oversight of medical care: a proposal for reform. *Ann Intern Med* 1994; 120:423.
58. Ebert PA: The importance of data in improving practice: effective clinical use of outcomes data. *Ann Thorac Surg* 1994; 58:1812.
59. Daley J: Criteria by which to evaluate risk-adjusted outcomes programs in cardiac surgery. *Ann Thorac Surg* 1994; 58:1827.
60. Edwards FH, Clark RE, Schwartz M: Practical considerations in the management of large multiinstitutional databases. *Ann Thorac Surg* 1994; 58:1841.
61. Jollis JG, Ancukiewicz M, DeLong ER, et al: Discordance of databases designed for claims payment versus clinical information systems: implications for outcomes research. *Ann Intern Med* 1993; 119:844.
62. Hannan EL, Racz MJ, Jollis JG, Peterson ED: Using Medicare claims data to assess provider quality for CABG surgery: does it work well enough? *Health Serv Res* 1997; 31:659.
63. Green J, Wintfeld N: How accurate are hospital discharge data for evaluating effectiveness of care? *Med Care* 1993; 31:719.
64. Lee TH: *Evaluating the Quality of Cardiovascular Care: A Primer*. Bethesda, MD, American College of Cardiology Press, 1995; p 35.
65. Blumberg MS: Comments on HCFA hospital death rate statistical outliers. *Health Serv Res* 1987; 21:715.
66. Dubois RW: Hospital mortality as an indicator of quality, in Goldfield N, Nash DB (eds): *Providing Quality Care*. Philadelphia, American College of Physicians, 1989; p 107.
67. Podolsky D, Beddingfield KT: America's best hospitals. *U.S. News and World Report* 1993; 115:66.
68. Glantz SA: *Primer of Biostatistics*. New York, McGraw-Hill, 2002.
69. Motulsky H: *Intuitive Biostatistics*. New York, Oxford University Press, 1995.
70. Harrell FE: *Regression Modeling Strategies: With Applications to Linear Models, Logistic Regression, and Survival Analysis*. New York, Springer, 2001.
71. Glantz SA, Slinker BK: *Primer of Applied Regression and Analysis of Variance*. New York, McGraw-Hill, 2001.
72. Thomas JW, Ashcraft ML: Measuring severity of illness: six severity systems and their ability to explain cost variations. *Inquiry* 1991; 28:39.
73. Ferraris VA, Propp ME: Outcome in critical care patients: a multivariate study. *Crit Care Med* 1992; 20:967.
74. Shwartz M, Ash AS: Evaluating the performance of risk-adjustment methods: continuous measures, in Iezzoni LI (ed): *Risk Adjustment for Measuring Health Care Outcomes*. Ann Arbor, MI, Health Administration Press, 1994; p 287.
75. Hartz AJ, Kuhn EM, Kayser KL: Report cards on cardiac surgeons. *N Engl J Med* 1995; 333:939.
76. Harrell FE, Lee KL, Califf RM, et al: Regression modelling strategies for improved prognostic prediction. *Stat Med* 1984; 3:143.
77. Ferraris VA, Ferraris SP, Joseph O, et al: Aspirin and postoperative bleeding after coronary artery bypass grafting. *Ann Surg* 2002; 235:820.
78. Ash RS, Shwartz M: Evaluating the performance of risk-adjustment methods: dichotomous measures, in Iezzoni L (ed):

Risk Adjustment for Measuring Health Care Outcomes. Ann Arbor, MI, Health Administration Press, 1997; p 427.

79. Shahian DM, Normand SL, Torchiana DF, et al: Cardiac surgery report cards: comprehensive review and statistical critique. *Ann Thorac Surg* 2001; 72:2155.
80. Grunkemeier GL, Zerr KJ, Jin R: Cardiac surgery report cards: making the grade. *Ann Thorac Surg* 2001; 72:1845.
81. Schneider EC, Epstein AM: Use of public performance reports: a survey of patients undergoing cardiac surgery. *JAMA* 1998; 279:1638.
82. Hofer TP, Hayward RA, Greenfield S, et al: The unreliability of individual physician "report cards" for assessing the costs and quality of care of a chronic disease. *JAMA* 1999; 281:2098.
83. Thomas JW, Hofer TP: Accuracy of risk-adjusted mortality rate as a measure of hospital quality of care. *Med Care* 1999; 37:83.
84. Bindman AB: Can physician profiles be trusted? *JAMA* 1999; 281:2142.
85. Marshall MN, Shekelle PG, Leatherman S, Brook RH: The public release of performance data: what do we expect to gain? A review of the evidence. *JAMA* 2000; 283:1866.
86. Marshall MN: Accountability and quality improvement: the role of report cards. *Qual Health Care* 2001; 10:67.
87. Ferraris VA: The dangers of gathering data. *J Thorac Cardiovasc Surg* 1992; 104:212.
88. Goldstein H, Spiegelhalter DJ: League tables and their limitations: statistical issues in comparisons of institutional performance (with discussion). *J R Stat Soc* 1996; 159:385.
89. Thomas N, Longford NT, Rolph JE: Empirical Bayes methods for estimating hospital-specific mortality rates. *Stat Med* 1994; 13:889.
90. Shwartz M, Ash AS, Iezzoni LI: Comparing outcomes across providers, in Iezzoni LI (ed): *Risk Adjustment for Measuring Healthcare Outcomes*. Chicago, Health Administration Press, 1997; p 471.
91. Hartz AJ, Kuhn EM, Kayser KL, et al: Assessing providers of coronary revascularization: a method for peer review organizations. *Am J Public Health* 1992; 82:1631.
92. Lagakos SW: Statistical analysis of survival data, in Bailar JC, Mosteller F (eds): *Medical Uses of Statistics*. Boston, NEJM Books, 1992; p 281.
93. Marubini E, Valsecchi MG: *Analyzing Survival Data from Clinical Trials and Observational Studies*. New York, Wiley, 1995.
94. Cox DR, Oakes D: *Analysis of Survival Data*. London, Chapman and Hall, 1984.
95. Kalbfleisch JD, Prentice RL: *The Statistical Analysis of Failure Time Data*. New York, Wiley, 1980.
96. Lee E: *Statistical Methods for Survival Data Analysis*. New York, Wiley, 1992.
97. Bayes T: An essay towards solving a problem in the doctrine of chances, in Press SJ (ed): *Bayesian Statistics: Principles, Models, and Applications*. New York, Wiley, 1989; p 189.
98. Pauker SG, Kassirer JP: Decision analysis, in Bailar JC, Mosteller F (eds): *Medical Uses of Statistics*. Boston, NEJM Books, 1992; p 159.
99. Edwards FH, Graeber GM: The theorem of Bayes as a clinical research tool. *Surg Gynecol Obstet* 1987; 165:127.
100. Press SJ: *Bayesian Statistics: Principles, Models, and Applications*. New York, Wiley, 1989.
101. Bernardo JM: *Bayesian Theory*. New York, Wiley, 1994.
102. Spiegelhalter DJ, Myles JP, Jones DR, Abrams KR: Bayesian methods in health technology assessment: a review. *Health Technol Assess* 2000; 4:1.
103. Edwards FH, Clark RE, Schwartz M: Coronary artery bypass grafting: the Society of Thoracic Surgeons National Database experience. *Ann Thorac Surg* 1994; 57:12.
104. Casella G: An introduction to empirical Bayes data-analysis. *Am Statistician* 1985; 39:83.
105. Hattler BG, Madia C, Johnson C, et al: Risk stratification using the Society of Thoracic Surgeons Program. *Ann Thorac Surg* 1994; 58:1348.
106. Marshall G, Shroyer AL, Grover FL, Hammermeister KE: Bayesian-logit model for risk assessment in coronary artery bypass grafting. *Ann Thorac Surg* 1994; 57:1492.
107. Rees K, Beranek-Stanley M, Burke M, Ebrahim S: Hypothermia to reduce neurological damage following coronary artery bypass surgery. *Cochrane Database Syst Rev* 2001; 1:CD002138.
108. Bartels C, Gerdes A, Babin-Ebell J, et al: Cardiopulmonary bypass—"evidence- or experience-based." *J Thorac Cardiovasc Surg* 2002; 124:20.
109. Begg CB, Berlin JA: Publication bias and dissemination of clinical research. *J Natl Cancer Inst* 1989; 81:107.
110. Berlin JA, Laird NM, Sacks HS, Chalmers TC: A comparison of statistical methods for combining event rates from clinical trials. *Stat Med* 1989; 8:141.
111. Tierney WM: Meta-analysis and bouillabaisse. *Ann Intern Med* 1996; 125:519.
112. LeLorier J, Gregoire G, Benhaddad A, et al: Discrepancies between meta-analyses and subsequent large randomized, controlled trials. *N Engl J Med* 1997; 337:536.
113. LeLorier J, Gregoire G: Comparing results from meta-analyses vs large trials. *JAMA* 1998; 280:518.
114. Bailar JC: The promise and problems of meta-analysis. *N Engl J Med* 1997; 337:559.
115. Bailar JC: The practice of meta-analysis. *J Clin Epidemiol* 1995; 48:149.
116. Longford NT: Selection bias and treatment heterogeneity in clinical trials. *Stat Med* 1999; 18:1467.
117. Rosenbaum PR, Rubin DB: The central role of the propensity score in observational studies for causal effects. *Biometrika* 1983; 70:41.
118. Benson K, Hartz AJ: A comparison of observational studies and randomized, controlled trials. *N Engl J Med* 2000; 342:1878.
119. Concato J, Shah N, Horwitz RI: Randomized, controlled trials, observational studies, and the hierarchy of research designs. *N Engl J Med* 2000; 342:1887.
120. Naftel DC: Do different investigators sometimes produce different multivariable equations from the same data? *J Thorac Cardiovasc Surg* 1994; 107:1528.
121. Efron B, Tibshirani R: *An Introduction to the Bootstrap*. New York, Chapman & Hall, 1993.
122. Diaconis P, Efron B: Computer-intensive methods in statistics. *Sci Amer* 1983; 248:116.
123. Efron B: Model selection and the bootstrap. *Math Soc Sci* 1983; 5:236.
124. Efron B: The bootstrap and modern statistics. *J Am Stat Assoc* 2000; 95:1293.
125. Breiman L: Bagging predictors. *Machine Learning* 1996; 26:123.
126. Deming WE: *Out of the Crisis*. Cambridge, MA, Massachusetts Institute of Technology Center for Advanced Engineering Study, 1986.
127. Juran JM, Gryna FM: *Juran's Quality Control Handbook*. New York, McGraw-Hill, 1988.
128. Juran JM: *Juran on Leadership for Quality: An Executive Handbook*. New York, Free Press, 1989.
129. Juran JM: *A History of Managing for Quality: The Evolution, Trends, and Future Directions of Managing for Quality*. Milwaukee, WI, ASQC Quality Press, 1995.
130. Berwick DM, Godfrey AB, Roessner J, National Demonstration Project on Quality Improvement in Health Care (eds): *Curing Health Care: New Strategies for Quality Improvement*. San Francisco, Jossey-Bass, 1990.

131. Plsek PE: Resource B: A primer on quality improvement tools, in Berwick DM, Godfrey AB, Roessner J, National Demonstration Project on Quality Improvement in Health Care (eds): *Curing Health Care: New Strategies for Quality Improvement.* San Francisco, Jossey-Bass, 1990; p 177.
132. Ryan T: *Statistical Methods for Quality Improvement.* New York, Wiley, 1989.
133. Walton M: *The Deming Management Method.* New York, Putnam, 1986.
134. Ryan TP: *Statistical Methods for Quality Improvement.* New York, Wiley, 2000.
135. Shahian DM, Williamson WA, Svensson LG, Restuccia JD, Dagostino RS: Applications of statistical quality control to cardiac surgery. *Ann Thorac Surg* 1996; 62:1351.
136. Novick RJ, Fox SA, Stitt LW, et al: Cumulative sum failure analysis of a policy change from on-pump to off-pump coronary artery bypass grafting. *Ann Thorac Surg* 2001; 72:S1016.
137. de Leval MR, Francois K, Bull C, Brawn W, Spiegelhalter D: Analysis of a cluster of surgical failures: application to a series of neonatal arterial switch operations. *J Thorac Cardiovasc Surg* 1994; 107:914.
138. O'Connor GT, Plume SK, Olmstead EM, et al: Multivariate prediction of in-hospital mortality associated with coronary artery bypass graft surgery. Northern New England Cardiovascular Disease Study Group. *Circulation* 1992; 85:2110.
139. O'Connor GT, Plume SK, Olmstead EM, et al: A regional prospective study of in-hospital mortality associated with coronary artery bypass grafting. The Northern New England Cardiovascular Disease Study Group. *JAMA* 1991; 266:803.
140. Kasper JF, Plume SK, O'Connor GT: A methodology for QI in the coronary artery bypass grafting procedure involving comparative process analysis. *Qual Rev Bull* 1992; 18:129.
141. Nugent WC, Schults WC: Playing by the numbers: how collecting outcomes data changed by life. *Ann Thorac Surg* 1994; 58:1866.
142. Hartz AJ, Kuhn EM, Kayser KL, Johnson WD: BUN as a risk factor for mortality after coronary-artery bypass-grafting. *Ann Thorac Surg* 1995; 60:398.
143. Otaki M: Surgical treatment of patients with cardiac cachexia: an analysis of factors affecting operative mortality. *Chest* 1994; 105:1347.
144. Boyd O, Grounds RM, Bennett ED: A randomized clinical-trial of the effect of deliberate perioperative increase of oxygen delivery on mortality in high-risk surgical patients. *JAMA* 1993; 270:2699.
145. Frater RW, Sisto D, Condit D: Cardiac surgery in human immunodeficiency virus (HIV) carriers. *Eur J Cardiothorac Surg* 1989; 3:146.
146. Mandal AK, Kaushik VS, Oparah SS: Risk of aortocoronary bypass-surgery in a low-volume inner-city hospital. *J Natl Med Assoc* 1991; 83:519.
147. Nallamothu BK, Saint S, Ramsey SD, Hofer TP, Vijan S, Eagle KA: The role of hospital volume in coronary artery bypass grafting: is more always better? *J Am Coll Cardiol* 2001; 38:1923.
148. Hannan EL, Kilburn H, Bernard H, Odonnell JF, Lukacik G, Shields EP: Coronary-artery bypass-surgery: the relationship between inhospital mortality-rate and surgical volume after controlling for clinical risk-factors. *Med Care* 1991; 29:1094.
149. Sowden AJ, Deeks JJ, Sheldon TA: Volume and outcome in coronary-artery bypass graft-surgery: true association or artifact? *BMJ* 1995; 311:151.
150. DeFoe GR, Ross CS, Olmstead EM, et al: Lowest hematocrit on bypass and adverse outcomes associated with coronary artery bypass grafting. Northern New England Cardiovascular Disease Study Group. *Ann Thorac Surg* 2001; 71:7696.
151. Leavitt BJ, O'Connor GT, Olmstead EM, et al: Use of the internal mammary artery graft and in-hospital mortality and other adverse outcomes associated with coronary artery bypass surgery. *Circulation* 2001; 103:507.
152. O'Connor NJ, Morton JR, Birkmeyer JD, et al: Effect of coronary artery diameter in patients undergoing coronary bypass surgery. Northern New England Cardiovascular Disease Study Group. *Circulation* 1996; 93:652.
153. Sethi GK, Hammermeister KE, Oprian C, Henderson W: Impact of resident training on postoperative morbidity in patients undergoing single valve-replacement. *J Thorac Cardiovasc Surg* 1991; 101:1053.
154. Kress DC, Kroncke GM, Chopra PS, et al: Comparison of survival in cardiac surgery at a Veterans Administration-hospital and its affiliated university hospital. *Arch Surg* 1988; 123:439.
155. Hammermeister KE, Daley J, Grover FL: Using outcomes data to improve clinical practice: what we have learned. *Ann Thorac Surg* 1994; 58:1809.
156. Daley J: Validity of risk-adjustment methods, in Iezzoni LI (ed): *Risk Adjustment for Measuring Healthcare Outcomes.* Chicago, Health Administration Press, 1997; p 331.
157. Burns ER, Billett HH, Frater RW, Sisto DA: The preoperative bleeding time as a predictor of postoperative hemorrhage after cardiopulmonary bypass. *J Thorac Cardiovasc Surg* 1986; 92:3102.
158. Gewirtz AS, Miller ML, Keys TF: The clinical usefulness of the preoperative bleeding time. *Arch Pathol Lab Med* 1996; 120:353.
159. De Caterina R, Lanza M, Manca G, et al: Bleeding time and bleeding: an analysis of the relationship of the bleeding time test with parameters of surgical bleeding. *Blood* 1994; 84:3363.
160. Freiman JA, Chalmers TC, Smith HJ, Kuebler RR: The importance of beta, the type II error, and sample size in the design and interpretation of the randomized controlled trial, in Bailar JC, Mosteller F (eds): *Medical Uses of Statistics.* Boston, NEJM Books, 1992; p 357.
161. Kallis P, Unsworth-White J, Munsch C, et al: Disability and distress following cardiac surgery in patients over 70 years of age. *Eur J Cardiothorac Surg* 1993; 7:306.
162. Guadagnoli E, Ayanian JZ, Cleary PD: Comparison of patient-reported outcomes after elective coronary artery bypass grafting in patients aged greater than or equal to and less than 65 years. *Am J Cardiol* 1992; 70:60.
163. Rumsfeld JS, Magid DJ, O'Brien M, et al: Changes in health-related quality of life following coronary artery bypass graft surgery. *Ann Thorac Surg* 2001; 72:2026.
164. Rumsfeld JS, MaWhinney S, McCarthy M, et al: Health-related quality of life as a predictor of mortality following coronary artery bypass graft surgery. Participants of the Department of Veterans Affairs Cooperative Study Group on Processes, Structures, and Outcomes of Care in Cardiac Surgery. *JAMA* 1999; 281:1298.
165. Lee TH, Shammash JB, Ribeiro JP, et al: Estimation of maximum oxygen uptake from clinical data: performance of the Specific Activity Scale. *Am Heart J* 1988; 115:203.
166. Ware JE, Sherbourne CD: The MOS 36–item short-form health survey (SF-36): I, conceptual framework and item selection. *Med Care* 1992; 30:473.
167. Lee TH, American College of Cardiology: Private Sector Relations Committee: *Evaluating the Quality of Cardiovascular Care: A Primer.* Bethesda, MD, American College of Cardiology, 1995; p 53.
168. Ware JE Jr, Davies AR, Rubin HR: Patients' assessment of their care, in U.S. Congress Office of Technology Assessment (ed): *The Quality of Medical Care: Information for Consumers.* Washington, DC, U.S. Government Printing Office, Vol. (OTA-H-386), June, 1988.
169. Kaplan SH, Ware JE Jr: The patient's role in health care and quality assessment, in Goldfield N, Nash DB (eds): *Providing Quality Care:*

The Challenge to Clinicians. Philadelphia, American College of Physicians, 1989.
170. Cope DW, Linn LS, Leake BD, Barrett PA: Modification of residents' behavior by preceptor feedback of patient satisfaction. *J Gen Intern Med* 1986; 1:394.
171. Hughes JS, Ash AS: Reliability of risk-adjustment methods, in Iezzoni LI (ed): *Risk Adjustment for Measuring Healthcare Outcomes*. Chicago, Health Administration Press, 1997; p 365.
172. Fleiss JL: *Statistical Methods for Rates and Proportions*. New York, Wiley, 1981.
173. Landis JR, Koch GG: The measurement of observer agreement for categorical data. *Biometrics* 1977; 33:159.
174. Hartz AJ, Kuhn EM, Green R, Rimm AA: The use of risk-adjusted complication rates to compare hospitals performing coronary artery bypass surgery or angioplasty. *Int J Technol Assess Health Care* 1992; 8:524.
175. Hannan EL, Kilburn H, O'Donnell JF, et al: Adult open heart surgery in New York State: an analysis of risk factors and hospital mortality rates. *JAMA* 1990; 264:2768.
176. Park RE, Brook RH, Kosecoff J, et al: Explaining variations in hospital death rates: randomness, severity of illness, quality of care. *JAMA* 1990; 264:484.
177. Thomas JW, Holloway JJ, Guire KE: Validating risk-adjusted mortality as an indicator for quality of care. *Inquiry* 1993; 30:6.
178. Silber JH, Rosenbaum PR, Ross RN: Comparing the contributions of groups of predictors—which outcomes vary with hospital rather than patient characteristics. *J Am Stat Assoc* 1995; 90:7.
179. Hammermeister KE, Burchfiel C, Johnson R, Grover FL: Identification of patients at greatest risk for developing major complications at cardiac surgery. *Circulation* 1990; 82(5 suppl):IV380.
180. Grover FL, Hammermeister KE, Burchfiel C: Initial report of the Veterans Administration Preoperative Risk Assessment Study for Cardiac Surgery. *Ann Thorac Surg* 1990; 50:12.
181. Hammermeister KE, Johnson R, Marshall G, Grover FL: Continuous assessment and improvement in quality of care: a model from the Department of Veterans Affairs Cardiac Surgery. *Ann Surg* 1994; 219:281.
182. Koska MT: Are severity data an effective consumer tool? *Hospitals* 1989; 63:24.
183. Iezzoni LI: Using risk-adjusted outcomes to assess clinical practice: an overview of issues pertaining to risk adjustment. *Ann Thorac Surg* 1994; 58:1822.
184. Wu AW: The measure and mismeasure of hospital quality: appropriate risk-adjustment methods in comparing hospitals. *Ann Intern Med* 1995; 122:149.
185. Daley J, Henderson WG, Khuri SF: Risk-adjusted surgical outcomes. *Ann Rev Med* 2001; 52:275.
186. Iezzoni LI, Greenberg LG: Widespread assessment of risk-adjusted outcomes: lessons from local initiatives. *Jt Comm J Qual Improv* 1994; 20:305.
187. Kassirer JP: The use and abuse of practice profiles. *N Engl J Med* 1994; 330:634.
188. Green J, Wintfeld N: Report cards on cardiac surgeons: assessing New York State's approach. *N Engl J Med* 1995; 332:1229.
189. Hannan EL, Kilburn H, Racz M, Shields E, Chassin MR: Improving the outcomes of coronary artery bypass surgery in New York State. *JAMA* 1994; 271:761.
190. Ghali WA, Ash AS, Hall RE, Moskowitz MA: Statewide quality improvement initiatives and mortality after cardiac surgery. *JAMA* 1997; 277:379.
191. Peterson ED, DeLong ER, et al: The effects of New York's bypass surgery provider profiling on access to care and patient outcomes in the elderly. *J Am Coll Cardiol* 1998; 32:993.
192. Malenka DJ, O'Connor GT: A regional collaborative effort for CQI in cardiovascular disease. Northern New England Cardiovascular Study Group. *Jt Comm J Qual Improv* 1995; 21:627.
193. O'Connor GT, Plume SK, Wennberg JE: Regional organization for outcomes research. *Ann N Y Acad Sci* 1993; 703:44.
194. Borer A, Gilad J, Meydan N, et al: Impact of active monitoring of infection control practices on deep sternal infection after open-heart surgery. *Ann Thorac Surg* 2001; 72:515.
195. Epstein AM: Changes in the delivery of care under comprehensive health-care reform. *N Engl J Med* 1993; 329:1672.
196. McNeil BJ, Pedersen SH, Gatsonis C: Current issues in profiling quality of care. *Inquiry* 1992; 29:298.
197. Kassirer JP: Managed care and the morality of the marketplace. *N Engl J Med* 1995; 333:50.
198. Epstein A: Sounding board: performance reports on quality—prototypes, problems, and prospects. *N Engl J Med* 1995; 333:57.
199. Omoigui N, Annan K, Brown K, et al: Potential explanation for decreased CABG-related mortality in New York State: outmigration to Ohio. *Circulation* 1994; 90:93.
200. Morgan RO, Virnig BA, DeVito CA, Persily NA: The Medicare-HMO revolving door—the healthy go in and the sick go out. *N Engl J Med* 1997; 337:169.
201. Van de Ven WP, Van Vliet RC, Van Barneveld EM, Lamers LM: Risk-adjusted capitation: recent experiences in The Netherlands. *Health Aff (Millwood)* 1994; 13:120.
202. Gauthier AK, Lamphere JA, Barrand NL: Risk selection in the health care market: a workshop overview. *Inquiry* 1995; 32:14.
203. Kronick R, Zhou Z, Dreyfus T: Making risk adjustment work for everyone. *Inquiry* 1995; 32:41.
204. Bowen B: The practice of risk adjustment. *Inquiry* 1995; 32:33.
205. Newhouse JP: Patients at risk: health reform and risk adjustment. *Health Aff (Millwood)* 1994; 13:132.
206. Rodwin MA: Conflicts in managed care. *N Engl J Med* 1995; 332:604.
207. Walker LM: Managed care 1995: turn capitation into a money-maker. *Medical Economics* 1995; 72:58.
208. Morain C: When managed care takes over, watch out! *Med Economics* 1995; 72:38.
209. Himmelstein DU, Woolhandler S, Hellander I, Wolfe SM: Quality of care in investor-owned vs not-for-profit HMOs. *JAMA* 1999; 282:159.
210. Woolhandler S, Himmelstein DU: Costs of care and administration at for-profit and other hospitals in the United States. *N Engl J Med* 1997; 336:769.
211. Anonymous: Iowa: classic test of a future concept. *Med Outcomes & Guidelines Alert* 1995: 3:8.
212. Gardner E: Florida hospitals plan quality-indicator project. *Mod Healthcare* 1993; 6:36.
213. Petitti DB: *Meta-Analysis, Decision Analysis, and Cost-Effectiveness Analysis: Methods for Quantitative Synthesis in Medicine*. New York, Oxford University Press, 2000; p 140.
214. Hunink MG: In search of tools to aid logical thinking and communicating about medical decision making. *Med Decis Making* 2001; 21:267.
215. Eddy DM, Hasselblad V, Shachter R: A Bayesian method for synthesizing evidence: the confidence profile method. *Int J Technol Assess Health Care* 1990; 6:31.
216. Eddy DM: Clinical decision making: from theory to practice: resolving conflicts in practice policies. *JAMA* 1990; 264:389.
217. Gage BF, Cardinalli AB, Albers GW, Owens DK: Cost-effectiveness of warfarin and aspirin for prophylaxis of stroke in patients with nonvalvular atrial fibrillation. *JAMA* 1995; 274:1839.
218. Riley G, Lubitz J: Outcomes of surgery among the Medicare aged: surgical volume and mortality. *Health Care Financing Rev* 1985; 7:37.
219. Showstack JA, Rosenfeld KE, Garnick DW, et al: Association of volume with outcome of coronary artery bypass graft surgery: scheduled vs nonscheduled operations. *JAMA* 1987; 257:785.

220. Hannan EL, O'Donnell JF, Kilburn H, et al: Investigation of the relationship between volume and mortality for surgical procedures performed in New York State hospitals. *JAMA* 1989; 262:503.
221. Farley DE, Ozminkowski RJ: Volume-outcome relationships and in-hospital mortality: the effect of changes in volume over time. *Med Care* 1992; 30:77.
222. Grumbach K, Anderson GM, Luft HS, et al: Regionalization of cardiac surgery in the United States and Canada: geographic access, choice, and outcomes. *JAMA* 1995; 274:1282.
223. Hannan EL, Siu AL, Kumar D, et al: The decline in coronary artery bypass graft surgery mortality in New York State: the role of surgeon volume. *JAMA* 1995; 273:209.
224. Shroyer ALW, Marshall G, Warner BA, et al: No continuous relationship between Veterans Affairs hospital coronary artery bypass grafting surgical volume and operative mortality. *Ann Thorac Surg* 1996; 61:17.
225. Sollano JA, Gelijns AC, Moskowitz AJ, et al: Volume-outcome relationships in cardiovascular operations: New York State, 1990–1995. *J Thorac Cardiovasc Surg* 1999; 117:419.
226. Hewitt M, for the Committee on Quality of Health Care in America and the National Cancer Policy Board: *Interpreting the Volume-Outcome Relationship in the Context of Health Care Quality*. Workshop summary. Washington, DC, Institute of Medicine, 2000.
227. Luft HS, Bunker JP, Enthoven AC: Should operations be regionalized? The empirical relation between surgical volume and mortality. *N Engl J Med* 1979; 301:1364.
228. Tu JV, Naylor CD: Coronary artery bypass mortality rates in Ontario: a Canadian approach to quality assurance in cardiac surgery. Steering Committee of the Provincial Adult Cardiac Care Network of Ontario. *Circulation* 1996; 94:2429.
229. Crawford FA, Anderson RP, Clark RE, et al: Volume requirements for cardiac surgery credentialing: a critical examination. The Ad Hoc Committee on Cardiac Surgery Credentialing of The Society of Thoracic Surgeons. *Ann Thorac Surg* 1996; 61:12.
230. Brennan TA, Leape LL, Laird NM, et al: Incidence of adverse events and negligence in hospitalized patients. Results of the Harvard Medical Practice Study I. *N Engl J Med* 1991; 324:370.
231. Thomas EJ, Studdert DM, Burstin HR, et al: Incidence and types of adverse events and negligent care in Utah and Colorado. *Med Care* 2000; 38:261.
232. Kohn LT, Corrigan J, Donaldson MS, Institute of Medicine (U.S.), Committee on Quality of Health Care in America: *To Err Is Human: Building a Safer Health System*. Washington, DC, National Academy Press, 2000.
233. Runciman WB, Webb RK, Helps SC, et al: A comparison of iatrogenic injury studies in Australia and the USA, II: reviewer behaviour and quality of care. *Int J Qual Health Care* 2000; 12:379.
234. Vincent CA: Research into medical accidents: a case of negligence? *BMJ* 1989; 299:1150.
235. Donchin Y, Gopher D, Olin M, et al: A look into the nature and causes of human errors in the intensive care unit. *Crit Care Med* 1995; 23:294.
236. Brennan TA: The Institute of Medicine report on medical errors: could it do harm? *N Engl J Med* 2000; 342:1123.
237. Richardson WC, Berwick DM, Bisgard JC, et al: The Institute of Medicine Report on Medical Errors: misunderstanding can do harm. Quality of Health Care in America Committee. *MedGenMed* 2000; Sep 19:E42.
238. Hayward RA, Hofer TP: Estimating hospital deaths due to medical errors: preventability is in the eye of the reviewer. *JAMA* 2001; 286:415.
239. Wears RL, Janiak B, Moorhead JC, et al: Human error in medicine: promise and pitfalls, part 2. *Ann Intern Med* 2000; 36:142.
240. Berwick DM, Leape LL: Reducing errors in medicine. *Qual Health Care* 1999; 8:145.
241. de Leval MR, Carthey J, Wright DJ, et al: Human factors and cardiac surgery: a multicenter study. *J Thorac Cardiovasc Surg* 2000; 119:661.
242. Langdorf MI, Fox JC, Marwah RS, et al: Physician versus computer knowledge of potential drug interactions in the emergency department. *Acad Emerg Med* 2000; 7:1321.
243. Soza H: Reducing medical errors through technology. *Cost Qual* 2000; 6:24.
244. Tierney WM, Overhage JM, Takesue BY, et al: Computerizing guidelines to improve care and patient outcomes: the example of heart failure. *J Am Med Inform Assoc* 1995; 2:316.
245. Overhage JM, Tierney WM, McDonald CJ: Computer reminders to implement preventive care guidelines for hospitalized patients. *Arch Intern Med* 1996; 156:1551.
246. Litzelman DK, Tierney WM: Physicians' reasons for failing to comply with computerized preventive care guidelines. *J Gen Intern Med* 1996; 11:497.
247. Orr RK: Use of an artificial neural network to quantitate risk of malignancy for abnormal mammograms. *Surgery* 2001; 129:459.
248. Katz S, Katz AS, Lowe N, Quijano RC: Neural net-bootstrap hybrid methods for prediction of complications in patients implanted with artificial heart valves. *J Heart Valve Dis* 1994; 3:49.
249. Tu JV, Guerriere MR: Use of a neural network as a predictive instrument for length of stay in the intensive care unit following cardiac surgery. *Comput Biomed Res* 1993; 26:220.
250. Steen PM: Approaches to predictive modeling. *Ann Thorac Surg* 1994; 58:1836.
251. Freeman RV, Eagle KA, Bates ER, et al: Comparison of artificial neural networks with logistic regression in prediction of in-hospital death after percutaneous transluminal coronary angioplasty. *Am Heart J* 2000; 140:511.
252. American College of Surgeons: Standard of efficiency for the first hospital survey by the College. *Bull Am Coll Surg* 1918; 3:1.
253. Weed LL: Medical records that guide and teach. *N Engl J Med* 1968; 278:652 concl.
254. Weed LL: Medical records that guide and teach. *N Engl J Med* 1968; 278:593.
255. Weed LL: What physicians worry about: how to organize care of multiple-problem patients. *Mod Hospital* 1968; 110:90.
256. Henzler C, Harper JJ: Implementing a computer-assisted appropriateness review using DRG 182/183. *Jt Comm J Qual Improv* 1995; 21:239.
257. Safran C, Rind DM, Davis RB, et al: Guidelines for management of HIV infection with computer-based patient's record. *Lancet* 1995; 346:341.
258. Rector AL, Nowlan WA, Kay S, Goble CA, Howkins TJ: A framework for modelling the electronic medical record. *Methods Inf Med* 1993; 32:109.
259. Tierney WM: Improving clinical decisions and outcomes with information: a review. *Int J Med Inform* 2001; 62:1.
260. Tierney WM, Miller ME, Overhage JM, McDonald CJ: Physician inpatient order writing on microcomputer workstations: effects on resource utilization. *JAMA* 1993; 269:379.
261. Overhage JM, Tierney WM, Zhou XH, McDonald CJ: A randomized trial of "corollary orders" to prevent errors of omission. *J Am Med Inform Assoc* 1997; 4:364.
262. McConnell T: Safer, cheaper, smarter: Computerized physician order entry promises to streamline and improve healthcare delivery. *Health Manage Technol* 2001; 22:16.
263. Dexter PR, Perkins S, Overhage JM, et al: A computerized reminder system to increase the use of preventive care for hospitalized patients. *N Engl J Med* 2001; 345:965.
264. Kuperman GJ, Teich JM, Gandhi TK, Bates DW: Patient safety and computerized medication ordering at Brigham and Women's Hospital. *Jt Comm J Qual Improv* 2001; 27:509.

265. Iezzoni L: Measuring the severity of illness and case mix, in Goldfield ND (ed): *Providing Quality Care: The Challenge to Clinicians*. Philadelphia, American College of Physicians, 1989; p 70.
266. Hannan EL, Kumar D, Racz M, Siu AL, Chassin MR: New York State's Cardiac Surgery Reporting System: four years later. *Ann Thorac Surg* 1994; 58:1852.
267. Edwards FH, Grover FL, Shroyer AL, et al: The Society of Thoracic Surgeons National Cardiac Surgery Database: current risk assessment. *Ann Thorac Surg* 1997; 63:903.
268. Grover FL, Johnson RR, Shroyer AL, et al: The Veterans Affairs Continuous Improvement in Cardiac Surgery Study. *Ann Thorac Surg* 1994; 58:1845.
269. Grover FL, Shroyer AL, Hammermeister KE: Calculating risk and outcome: the Veterans Affairs database. *Ann Thorac Surg* 1996; 62:S6.
270. Parsonnet V, Dean D, Bernstein AD: A method of uniform stratification of risk for evaluating the results of surgery in acquired adult heart disease. *Circulation* 1989; 79:I3.
271. Nashef SA, Carey F, Silcock MM, et al: Risk stratification for open heart surgery: trial of the Parsonnet system in a British hospital. *BMJ* 1992; 305:1066.
272. Martinez-Alario J, Tuesta ID, Plasencia E, et al: Mortality prediction in cardiac surgery patients: comparative performance of Parsonnet and general severity systems. *Circulation* 1999; 99:2378.
273. Parsonnet V, Bernstein AD, Gera M: Clinical usefulness of risk-stratified outcome analysis in cardiac surgery in New Jersey. *Ann Thorac Surg* 1996; 61:S8.
274. Tu JV, Wu K: The improving outcomes of coronary artery bypass graft surgery in Ontario, 1981 to 1995. *CMAJ* 1998; 159:221.
275. O'Connor GT, Plume SK, Olmstead EM, et al: A regional intervention to improve the hospital mortality associated with coronary artery bypass graft surgery. The Northern New England Cardiovascular Disease Study Group. *JAMA* 1996; 275:841.
276. Higgins TL, Estafanous FG, Loop FD, et al: Stratification of morbidity and mortality outcome by preoperative risk factors in coronary artery bypass patients: a clinical severity score. *JAMA* 1992; 267:2344.
277. Ghali WA, Quan H, Brant R: Coronary artery bypass grafting in Canada: national and provincial mortality trends, 1992–1995. *CMAJ* 1998; 159:25.
278. Weintraub WS, Wenger NK, Jones EL, et al: Changing clinical characteristics of coronary surgery patients: differences between men and women. *Circulation* 1993; 88:II79.
279. Grover FL, Johnson RR, Marshall G, Hammermeister KE: Factors predictive of operative mortality among coronary artery bypass subsets. *Ann Thorac Surg* 1993; 56:1296.
280. Iyer VS, Russell WJ, Leppard P, Craddock D: Mortality and myocardial infarction after coronary artery surgery: a review of 12,003 patients. *Med J Aust* 1993; 159:166.0
281. Ivanov J, Tu JV, Naylor CD: Ready-made, recalibrated, or remodeled? Issues in the use of risk indexes for assessing mortality after coronary artery bypass graft surgery. *Circulation* 1999; 99: 2098.
282. Higgins TL, Estafanous FG, Loop FD, et al: ICU admission score for predicting morbidity and mortality risk after coronary artery bypass grafting. *Ann Thorac Surg* 1997; 64:1050.
283. Mozes B, Olmer L, Galai N, Simchen E: A national study of postoperative mortality associated with coronary artery bypass grafting in Israel. ISCAB Consortium. Israel Coronary Artery Bypass Study. *Ann Thorac Surg* 1998; 66:1254.
284. DeLong ER, Peterson ED, DeLong DM, et al: Comparing risk-adjustment methods for provider profiling. *Stat Med* 1997; 16:2645.
285. Reich DL, Bodian CA, Krol M, et al: Intraoperative hemodynamic predictors of mortality, stroke, and myocardial infarction after coronary artery bypass surgery. *Anesth Analg* 1999; 89:814.
286. Bernstein AD, Parsonnet V: Bedside estimation of risk as an aid for decision-making in cardiac surgery. *Ann Thorac Surg* 2000; 69:823.
287. Lahey SJ, Borlase BC, Lavin PT, Levitsky S: Preoperative risk factors that predict hospital length of stay in coronary artery bypass patients >60 years old. *Circulation* 1992; 86:II181.

Chapter 7

Statistical Treatment of Outcome Data

Gary Grunkemeier/Ruyun Jin

The results (outcomes) of cardiac surgery can be measured in several ways. The type of variable used as the measure of a particular outcome determines the statistical methods that should be used for its analysis. For example, some administrative outcomes are captured by *continuous* variables, such as hospital charges (in dollars) or length of stay (in days). Other outcomes are collected as *categorical* variables, such as discharge destination (acute care facility, specialized nursing facility, home). But the major outcomes of interest to clinicians are described by variables that indicate the occurrence of (usually adverse) *events,* such as death, stroke, infection, or reoperation. Therefore, in this relatively short overview, we will concentrate on the statistical methods commonly used for analyzing outcome *events*.

For statistical purposes, we must differentiate between two different types of events, based on their timing: *early* (one-time) events and *late* (time-related) events. We somewhat arbitrarily divide the areas of statistical inquiry into three major categories, based on the goals of the analysis: *summarize, compare,* and *model*. This chapter will describe and illustrate the *statistical methods* most often used in each situation.

EVENT TYPES

There are two fundamentally different types of events: (1) *early* or "operative" events, which occur within a short period of time (usually within the first 30 days following surgery), so that it is possible to say definitely whether each patient did or did not suffer the event; (2) *late,* or time-related events, which occur any time from 30 days after surgery up until the death of the patient. In the usual ongoing analysis, some patients will have experienced a late event, while others have not but are still alive and at risk for the event and may have it in the future. Different types of analysis must be used for these two types of events.

One-time Events

In cardiac surgery, early events are defined as occurring within 30 days of surgery or before hospital discharge, whichever is sooner. By the time of the analysis, the early outcome of every patient is presumably known. Thus every patient has a "yes" or "no" value for the event being studied, and an estimate of the prevalence of the event can be given as the ratio of patients with the event to total patients, usually multiplied by 100 and expressed as a percentage.

Time-related Events

Late events are those that occur after 30 days. The analysis of these events is complicated by the fact that: (1) the time of occurrence must be taken into account since, for example, a death at 6 months will have a different effect on the analysis than a death at 6 years, and (2) at the time of analysis the outcome of many or most of the patients will not yet be known. Their event status is termed *censored,* which means only that it is known not to have occurred by the time of the current follow-up. For example, a patient in the study who had surgery 5 years ago and is still alive has a time of death that is not yet known. But we have partial information about his or her survival time, namely that it exceeds, or is *censored at,* 5 years. When dealing with censored data it is necessary to use special statistical methods. It is not appropriate, for example, to summarize late mortality by a simple percentage such as the number of late deaths divided by the number of patients. Mortality varies over, and must be related to, postoperative time.

ANALYSIS GOALS

Statistics are used for many tasks of varying complexity. The most common ones used for evaluating cardiac surgery outcome events are to: (1) *summarize* the results from a single series; (2) *compare* the results between two series or two subgroups of the same series based on a single discriminating variable or risk factor; and (3) construct a multivariable *model,* which provides the simultaneous effect of many risk factors.

Summarize

A study usually includes many patients and, rather than enumerating the outcome of interest for each individual, the first use of statistics is to summarize the outcome for the entire group with a single, representative number (statistic). Most common is the sample average or *mean* value. A single-valued estimate such as this is called a *point estimate;* but, acknowledging the imprecision of a single estimated value, a range of values should also be given. The *standard error* (SE) is a measure of the precision of this estimate, and a *confidence interval* (CI), a range of values for the estimate which are consistent with the observed data, can be constructed using the standard error and in other, often better, ways.

Compare

A study often consists of evaluating subgroups of patients who received different treatments in order to determine the best one. Thus, in addition to summarizing the outcomes from the subgroups, we are interested in comparing their summary statistics. To do so, we typically compute another statistic that combines data from both groups and that approximately follows some known statistical reference distribution, such as a normal (bell-shaped) or other (chi-square, *t,* etc.) distribution. We then see how extreme or improbable the value computed from our data is in that reference distribution, if there were in fact no difference between the two groups we are comparing. This probability is called the *p*-value, and when it is smaller than .05 (5%), the difference we have observed is said to be *statistically significant.*

A completely different method of making comparisons and of constructing CIs that has gained much prominence recently with the availability of computing power and specific software is the *bootstrap* method. Instead of basing these statistics on an assumed distribution, it uses many repeated random samples from the data itself to produce this distribution.

Model: Multivariable Regression

Comparing the outcomes between two groups based on a single factor, as described in the previous section, is called *univariable analysis,* to distinguish it from *multivariable* analysis, in which several characteristics of each subgroup are considered simultaneously. Most clinical studies are based on observational data collected in the normal delivery of care, and the patient subgroups possibly differ with regard to several influential characteristics. A *multiple regression* analysis can determine the influence of the treatment under study on the outcome variable after simultaneously adjusting for these potential differences. The result is a *statistical model,* which consists of the group of factors which significantly affect the outcome, and which may or may not ultimately include the treatment being studied. Each factor is assigned a coefficient that indicates the amount of weight given to that factor in the model. The model hopefully gives us a fuller understanding of the interrelationship among the treatment being studied, the outcome variable, and other important risk factors. One can compute the expected outcome for any patient using these weights applied to the values of the patient's particular set of risk factors.

A way of contrasting this technique with that described in the previous section is that the univariate comparison provides a raw or *unadjusted* comparison, while the regression model provides a comparison of *adjusted* outcomes. The comparison between treatments has been adjusted for the other risk factors by which the treatment groups may differ.

CLINICAL MATERIAL

To describe and illustrate the statistical methods most frequently used in the cardiac surgical literature for the two types of events, we will use data collected on isolated mitral valve

TABLE 7–1 Heart valve summary data by valve model

	Previous	Current
Patients (no.)	565	691
Mean age ± S.E. (y)	52.4 ± 11.4	59.3 ± 12.8
Female (%)	62.1	61.9
REDO (%)	5.0	16.5
CABG (%)	9.4	19.4

REDO = re-replacement valve surgery; CABG = coronary artery bypass surgery.

replacement using Starr-Edwards valves. Dr. Albert Starr and his group at the Oregon Health Sciences University and Providence St. Vincent Medical Center in Portland, Oregon, implanted these valves from 1965 to 1994. Table 7-1 contains a summary of selected variables used to illustrate the statistical methods. Several valve models are represented in this group: "Current" refers to the Model 6120 introduced in 1965, which is still in current use; "Previous" refers to all the other, mostly cloth-covered, models which have been discontinued. Patients with the Current model valve have a higher mean age, more valve re-replacement surgery (REDO), and more concomitant coronary bypass surgery (CABG).

EARLY (ONE-TIME) EVENTS

We will use operative mortality to illustrate the statistical treatment of early events.

Summarize

The mean (point estimate) for operative mortality is computed as the number of operative deaths divided by the number of patients. Multiplying by 100 converts this decimal to a percentage. The standard error of a proportion (P) based on a sample of size N equals the square root of P(1 – P) / N. Thus, the percentages of patients with early death (SE) are 4.8% (0.9%) and 9.0% (1.1%) for the Previous and Current valve models, respectively. Table 7-2 shows these values, with 95% confidence intervals computed by two popular methods. The first method is based on the fact that the binomial distribution, which governs proportions, can be approximated by the normal (bell-shaped) distribution as the sample size increases. This CI is easily computed as the point estimate plus and minus twice the SE. The second CI method uses the binomial distribution directly.[1]

Compare

To demonstrate a univariate comparison, we will use operative mortality between the two valve models. This does not

TABLE 7–2 Summary and univariate comparison of early mortality by valve model

	Previous	Current
Patients (no.)	565	691
Operative deaths (no.)	27	62
Operative mortality		
Point estimate (%)	4.8	9.0
Standard error (%)	0.9	1.1
95% confidence interval (%)		
Normal approximation	(3.0, 6.5)	(6.8, 11.1)
Exact binomial	(3.2, 6.9)	(6.9, 11.4)

Comparison statistics	***p*-value (2-sided)**
Pearson chi-square	.004
With continuity correction	.006
Fisher's exact test	.004

seem very interesting clinically, since model of valve would seem to have little to do with operative mortality; nevertheless, many valve comparison papers attempt to draw clinical conclusions from just such questionable comparisons. The Current model has a higher operative mortality and, since the 95% confidence intervals do not overlap (Table 7-2), one can surmise that the difference will be significant.[2] Comparing two proportions gives rise to a matrix with two rows and two columns, called a two-by-two *contingency table*. The most common method for extracting a *p*-value from such a matrix is the *(Pearson) chi-square* test. This test has an alternative, more conservative form, using a *continuity correction*. Validity of the chi-square test depends on having an adequate sample size (technically, each cell of the table should have an *expected* size of at least 5), and when this is not the case then *Fisher's exact test* is often used. All three tests find the difference in operative mortality to be highly significant; that is, the *p*-values are much less than the required .05 (Table 7-2).

Model: Logistic Regression

The univariate comparison above showed that operative mortality with the Current valve was significantly higher than for with the Previous valve. But patients with the Current valve were older, with more CABG and REDO operations (Table 7-1). Could the apparent difference in operative mortality between valve models be due to these patient characteristics? A multivariable analysis may answer this question.

For binary outcomes like operative mortality, the most common method for developing a multivariable model is *logistic regression*.[3] A logistic regression was done, with operative death as the outcome (dependent variable) and the patient characteristics plus valve model as potential risk factors (independent variables). A stepwise regression program

TABLE 7–3 Multivariate modeling of early mortality using logistic regression

Variable	Univariate p-value	Multivariate				
		Coefficient	SE	p-value	Odds ratio	95% Confidence interval
Age	.000	.034	.011	.002	1.04	(1.01, 1.06)
CABG	.000	.976	.251	.000	2.65	(1.62, 4.34)
Valve	.004			.169		
Female	.472			.934		
REDO	.738			.416		

CABG = coronary artery bypass surgery; REDO = re-replacement valve surgery.

begins by doing a univariate test of each potential risk factor (using a different method than those used in Table 7-2), as shown in Table 7-3. In addition to valve model, age and CABG are also significantly different (their p-values are less than .05). After the stepwise procedure, only age and CABG are still significant, and they are *risk factors,* since their coefficients are positive numbers (meaning they add to the risk). After the effect of age and CABG is accounted for in the model, however, the effect due to type of valve is no longer significant ($p = .169$). Thus, according to this analysis, the apparent increase in operative mortality with the Current valve is an artifact; Current valve type is a surrogate for older age and more bypass surgery, which themselves are responsible for the increased mortality.

For technical reasons, logistic regression does not use the *probability* (P) of death directly as the dependent variable in the model. Instead, it uses the logarithm of the *odds,* $P/(1-P)$, of death. To facilitate interpretation of a regression coefficient B, it should be converted into an *odds ratio* (OR) by using the *exponential* function. Most statistical programs do this automatically, and the odds ratios are often labeled exp(B). The 95% CI for the odds ratio is computed as the exponential of the normal approximation CI (mean plus and minus twice the SE) for the coefficient itself.

The OR of a binary variable like CABG (2.65 in Table 7-3) means that the odds of mortality for a patient having concomitant CABG are 2.65 times that of a patient not undergoing CABG. This is the point estimate; the interval estimate (Table 7-3) ranges from 1.62 to 4.34. When the coefficient is significantly greater than zero (as it is for CABG, $p < .001$), the OR will be significantly greater than 1, and the lower limit of the 95% confidence interval (Table 7-3) will be greater than 1 (as it is for CABG, 1.62). For a continuous variable such as age, the OR of 1.04 means that for each year of age, the odds of dying are multiplied by 1.04.

TIME-RELATED EVENTS

We use both death and thromboembolism (TE) to illustrate methods for the analysis of time-related events.

Summarize

SURVIVAL CURVE

A single percentage is adequate to summarize mortality at a single point in time, such as the operative period (above). But to express the pattern over time of late survival requires a different estimate at virtually every postoperative interval, a *survivorship function,* whose plot is the familiar *survival curve.* The most common way of estimating a survival curve is the Kaplan-Meier (KM) method,[4] called *nonparametric* or *distribution-free* because it does not presuppose any particular statistical distribution. If all the patients in a given series were dead, the survival curve would be very simple to construct, as the percentage that had lived until each point in time. The KM method allows these percentages to be estimated before all the patients have died in an ongoing series, using the assumption that patients who are still alive (and have a *censored* survival time) will have the same risk of future death as those who have already died. Figure 7-1 shows the KM survival curve for the mitral valve patients.

LINEARIZED RATE

Besides survival curves, there are several other statistical functions that characterize the distribution of a time-related event. Survival curves are the easiest to interpret and apply to a patient or a population, since they summarize the possibly varying risks over time to produce the probability of being alive at each point in time. But another function, the hazard function or hazard rate, which measures the instantaneous risk at each point in time, is useful for deciding whether a risk is constant or changing (increasing or decreasing) over time. In general, the hazard function is difficult to draw without smoothing the points; but in the special situation in which the hazard function is constant over time, it is called a linearized rate.[5] The linearized rate is estimated as the number of events divided by the total follow-up years. Multiplying this by 100 converts it to "events per 100 patient-years," often abbreviated as "percent per patient-year" or "percent per year." Early events are usually not included in the calculation,

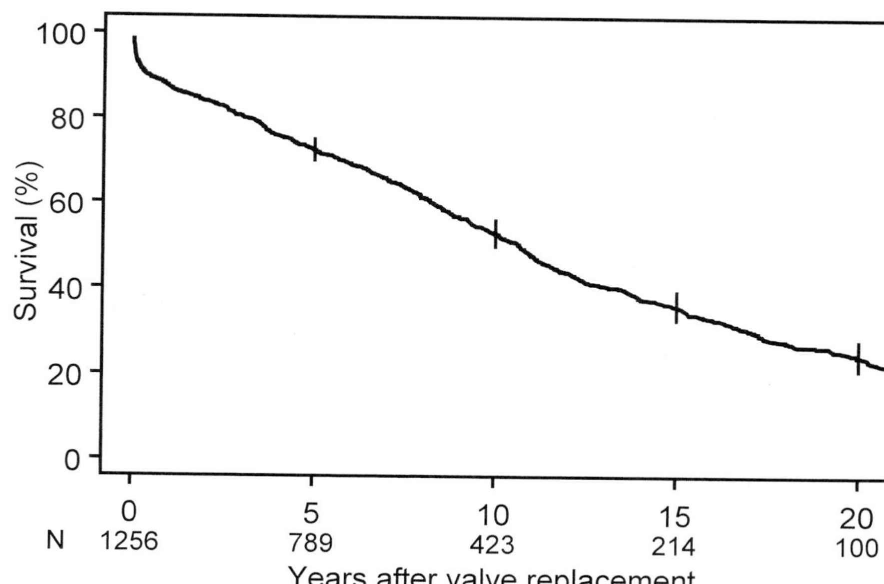

FIGURE 7–1 Kaplan-Meier survival curve. Vertical lines at selected intervals indicate the 95% confidence intervals of the event-free percentages. Numbers below the horizontal axis indicate the number of patients remaining at risk.

because the risk of most events is higher for a time after operation, so the assumption of a constant hazard would not hold.

Table 7-4 shows the linearized death rates by valve model, based on late deaths and late follow-up (patient-years beyond 30 days). Confidence intervals are given by two methods: using the normal approximation (point estimate plus and minus two SEs) and a method suggested by Cox,[6] which was recommended after a comparison of several methods.[7] Cox's method also agrees with the *probability interval* produced by Bayesian analysis using a noninformative prior.[8] The CIs given by the two methods in Table 7-4 agree very well, differing from each other only in the second decimal place.

TABLE 7–4 Summary and univariate comparison of linearized rates of late mortality by valve model

	Previous	Current
Late deaths (no.)	324	302
Late follow-up (patient-years)	5,377	4,818
Linearized death rate		
Point estimate (%/y)	6.0	6.3
Standard error (%/y)	0.3	0.3
95% confidence interval (%/year)		
Normal approximation	(5.37, 6.68)	(5.56, 6.98)
Cox's method	(5.40, 6.71)	(5.59, 7.01)

Comparison statistics	*p*-value (2-sided)
Normal approximation	.621
Cox's method	.621
Linearized rate method	.622

"ACTUAL" ANALYSIS

The KM method is often used for events other than death. Figure 7-2 contains a KM thromboembolism-free curve for the mitral valve patients. When used for events such as thromboembolism that are not necessarily fatal, KM estimates the probability of being event-free given the unrealistic condition that death does not occur. But patients do, in fact, die before such an event has happened to them, so the KM event-free estimate is lower than the real (actual) event-free percentage. Another method, called cumulative incidence in the statistical literature and "actual" analysis in the cardiac literature, provides a mortality-adjusted event-free percentage.[9,10] The actual TE-free curve for this mitral valve series is indeed higher than the KM TE-free curve (Figure 7-2).

Compare

The statistic most often chosen to compare KM curves is called the *logrank* statistic.[11] Figure 7-3 shows the survival curves for the Previous and Current valve models including all events, early and late. The Previous model has significantly better survival according to this univariate comparison.

Univariate analysis using linearized rates, for late events only, shows no significant difference between late survival using three different methods: a normal approximation method, a method recommended by Cox,[6] and a likelihood ratio test (Table 7-4).

Model: Cox Regression

Analogous to logistic regression, which provides multivariable analysis of the simple percentages associated with

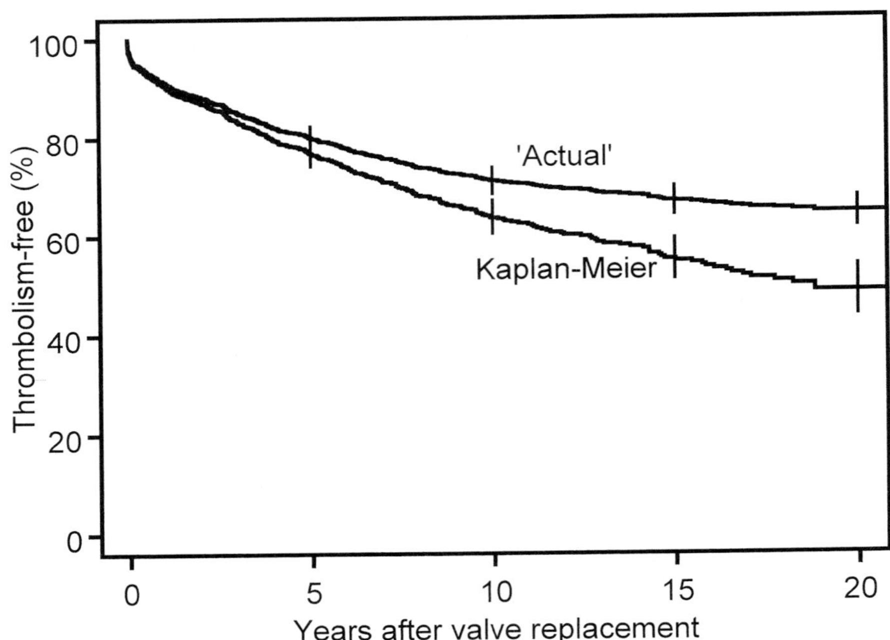

FIGURE 7–2 Thromboembolism-free curves constructed by the Kaplan-Meier method and the "actual" (cumulative incidence) method. Vertical lines at selected intervals indicate the 95% confidence intervals of the event-free percentages.

operative mortality, there is a widely used method for assessing multivariable influences on late survival: *Cox regression* or *proportional hazards regression*.[12] This analysis is usually applied to all events, early and late. Table 7-5 shows the result of this regression as applied to the valve data set. The univariate comparisons done by the stepwise regression program show all of the factors except REDO to be significant. The final model includes REDO, but valve type, which was significant by univariate analysis, is no longer significant after the other four risk factors are included in the model. There is a similarity between Table 7-5 and Table 7-3, in that taking the exponential function of the coefficients provides more useful statistics. Here exp(B) gives a *hazard ratio* (HR) instead of an odds ratio. The 95% CI for the HR is computed as the exponential of the normal approximation CI (mean plus and minus twice the SE) for the coefficient. Female has a negative coefficient, which results in an HR less than 1; this means female gender is a protective factor rather than a

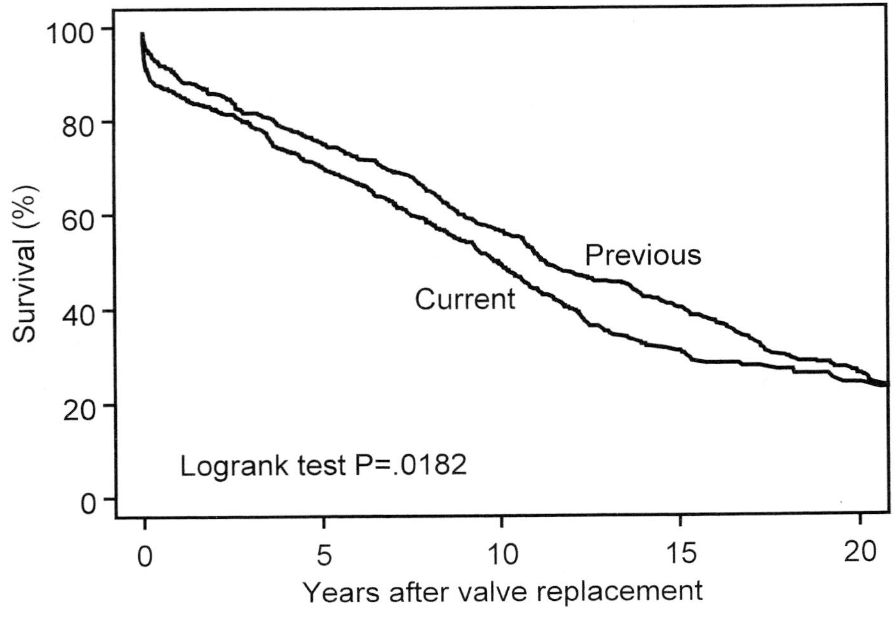

FIGURE 7–3 Survival by valve model. Overall survival significantly favors the Previous valve model, according to this misleading univariate analysis that ignores the higher mortality risk of the patients with the Current valve model.

TABLE 7–5 Multivariate modeling of late survival by Cox regression

Variable	Univariate *p*-value	Multivariate Coefficient	SE	*p*-value	Hazard ratio	95% Confidence interval
Age	.000	.045	.004	.000	1.05	(1.04, 1.05)
CABG	.000	.331	.109	.002	1.39	(1.12, 1.72)
Female	.016	−.181	.080	.024	0.84	(0.71, 0.98)
REDO	.125	.253	.126	.045	1.29	(1.01, 1.65)
Valve	.028			.266		

CABG = coronary artery bypass surgery; REDO = re-replacement valve surgery.

risk factor. Since the upper limit of the 95% CI is less than 1, female gender is a significant protective factor.

CONCLUSIONS

1. Different analytical methods must be used for outcome events after surgery depending on whether they are one-time (operative) or time-related (late).
2. Factors found significant on univariate analysis are often overturned by multivariate analysis, because they are surrogates for other more clinically fundamental variables. This was the case with valve model, in both the early and overall analysis of mortality. The converse can also happen; REDO was not significant for overall mortality by itself, but became so in concert with other risk factors.
3. Linearized rates provide a convenient single-parameter summary of late event rates, but should not be used unless the hazard function is approximately constant.
4. Kaplan-Meier analysis estimates survival probabilities as a function of time after surgery. When used for events that are not necessarily fatal, KM estimates probabilities as if death were eliminated, while "actual" analysis gives a true mortality-adjusted estimate of the event probabilities.

REFERENCES

1. Ling RF: Just say no to binomial (and other discrete distributions) tables. *Am Statistician* 1992; 46:53.
2. Browne RH: On visual assessment of the significance of a mean difference. *Biometrics* 1979; 35:657.
3. Hosmer DW, Lemeshow S: *Applied Logistic Regression*. New York, Wiley, 2000; p 307.
4. Kaplan EL, Meier P: Nonparametric estimation from incomplete observations. *J Amer Stat Assn* 1958; 53:457.
5. Lachin JM: *Biostatistical Methods*. New York, Wiley, 2000.
6. Cox DR: Some simple approximate tests for Poisson variates. *Biometrika* 1953; 40:354.
7. Grunkemeier GL, Anderson WN Jr: Clinical evaluation and analysis of heart valve substitutes. *J Heart Valve Dis* 1998; 7:163.
8. Martz HF, Waller RA: *Bayesian Reliability Analysis*. New York, Wiley, 1982; p 745.
9. Grunkemeier GL, Jamieson WR, Miller DC, et al: Actuarial versus actual risk of porcine structural valve deterioration. *J Thorac Cardiovasc Surg* 1994; 108:709.
10. Grunkemeier GL, Anderson RP, Miller DC, et al: Time-related analysis of nonfatal heart valve complications: cumulative incidence (actual) versus Kaplan-Meier (actuarial). *Circulation* 1997; 96: II70.
11. Peto R, Pike MC, Armitage P, et al: Design and analysis of randomized clinical trials requiring prolonged observation of each patient, II: Analysis and examples. *Br J Cancer* 1997; 35:1.
12. Cox DR: Regression methods and life table. *J Royal Stat Soc, Series B* 1972; 34:187.

Part II

Perioperative/ Intraoperative Care

Chapter 8

Preoperative Evaluation for Cardiac Surgery

Michelle A. Albert/Elliott M. Antman

Cardiac surgery, including coronary artery bypass grafting and surgery for valvular disease, represents one of the most common classes of surgical procedures performed worldwide. Advances in the percutaneous management of coronary artery disease as well as in cardiac surgical techniques have led to improved outcomes with consequent longer life expectancy for patients. Developments relating to antiplatelet drug therapy, rapamycin-coated stents to minimize restenosis risk, and advanced catheter-guided techniques allow more patients to be treated via percutaneous means, thereby channeling older and sicker patients to coronary bypass grafting surgery.[1–6] Greater numbers of patients with depressed left ventricular function, multiple comorbidities, failed interventional procedures, and prior revascularization operations are now referred for cardiac surgery.[7–9] As a result, preoperative risk assessment is even more critical to ensure the safe performance of cardiac surgical procedures and the achievement of low mortality rates. Furthermore, advances in cardiac surgery utilizing novel approaches such as robotically assisted surgery, off-pump coronary artery bypass graft (CABG) procedures, and minimally invasive valve surgery with robotics extend the operative options for patients.[8–12] Along with the implementation of proper quality surveillance mechanisms, these improvements translate into an improved risk-adjusted mortality for CABG of less than 2% for the general population and 3% to 4% for the Medicare population.[13–15] This chapter reviews the information essential to the cardiologist and surgeon in the evaluation and management of patients prior to cardiac surgery.

THE PHYSICAL EXAMINATION

The preoperative physical examination is a critical aspect of a patient's evaluation for CABG since the findings can greatly influence perioperative management. During the physical examination, particular attention should be paid to the patient's risk for endocarditis, the presence of aortic insufficiency, the presence of vascular disease, and the neurologic status. Examination of the head, eyes, ears, throat, and teeth for infection is helpful in the assessment of an individual's risk of endocarditis in valvular surgery. Inspection of the patient's skin is helpful in detecting and preventing infection (e.g., the presence of tinea pedis on the lower extremities increases the risk of lower extremity cellulitis). Identifying the presence of an aortic regurgitation murmur is important because regurgitation can worsen during cardiopulmonary bypass and acute left ventricular distention may develop.

The physical examination also helps to identify potential contraindications to the use of an intra-aortic balloon pump, which include aortic insufficiency, severe peripheral vascular insufficiency, abdominal aortic aneurysm, or significant atherosclerosis. Attention should also be paid to the patency of the venous system in the lower extremities since extensive varicosities may necessitate the use of arm veins as conduits; if the latter are needed, then avoidance of intravenous line placement in the arm from which veins will be harvested is necessary. In the event of reoperation, noninvasive imaging of the lower extremities as well as imaging of the left internal mammary artery during cardiac catheterization may be desirable to assess patency of potential conduits.

Since neurologic status may be compromised perioperatively and/or postoperatively, carotid ultrasound should be performed on all patients, and combined endarterectomy/CABG should be considered in those individuals with a history of prior stroke, severe bilateral stenoses, or contralateral occlusion and in patients with a history of neurologic symptoms that could represent cerebral ischemia.[16,17] In addition, perioperative identification of any baseline neurologic deficits provides an important reference in the event of neurofunctional deterioration postoperatively.

Additionally, since women who have had left radical mastectomy can have alterations in thoracic blood flow, patency of the left internal mammary artery may be compromised; the left anterior descending artery then becomes ineffective as a conduit.[18]

Minimally invasive direct access (MIDA) cardiac surgical procedures are becoming more frequent as innovative surgical techniques evolve. Advantages of MIDA procedures include improvement in morbidity, shorter hospital stay, and less neurologic complications. Table 8-1 outlines the most frequently performed novel cardiac procedures and lists the preoperative considerations for each.

TABLE 8–1 Novel cardiac surgical techniques

Technique	Reason/advantage	Preoperative considerations
MIDA-AVR	Reduce chest trauma; minimize blood loss; accelerate patient recovery	Body habitus; elderly patients; CXR; defibrillator pads; TEE guidance
MIDA-MVR	Reduce chest trauma; minimize blood loss; accelerate patient recovery	Body habitus; elderly patients; CXR; defibrillator pads; TEE guidance
MIDA-CABG	Reduce chest trauma; accelerate patient recovery	Body habitus; elderly patients; CXR; defibrillator pads; TEE guidance
Robotic-assisted CABG	Can perform on beating heart	
Off-pump CABG	Elderly patients; reduces oxidative stress and inflammation; comorbidities; less need for blood transfusions; shorter hospital stay; decrease in deep sternal wound infections; possibility of reduced cerebral dysfunction	Body habitus; elderly patients; CXR; defibrillator pads; TEE guidance
TMR	Refractory angina despite maximal medical therapy ± revascularization procedures	Anginal class III/IV; left ventricular free wall ischemia; poor-quality target vessels

MIDA = minimally invasive direct access; AVR = aortic valve replacement; MVR = mitral valve replacement; TMR = transmyocardial laser revascularization.

Source: Adapted from refs. 11, 101-104.

PREOPERATIVE LABORATORY EVALUATION

Basic laboratory testing prior to cardiac surgery should include a complete blood count, coagulation screen, chemistry profile, stool hematest, evaluation of ventricular function, and assessment of coronary anatomy via cardiac catheterization (Table 8-2). Because heparinization and hemodilution will occur on cardiopulmonary bypass, anemia should be avoided preoperatively and maintenance of a hematocrit above 35% is preferable. The causes of occult bleeding should also be sought and treated. For example, preoperative correction of occult gastrointestinal bleeding detected via hemocult stool testing limits the risk of GI bleeding during heparinization and may also influence the type of prosthetic valve inserted. Additionally, patients with conditions that potentially increase myocardial oxygen demand, such as congestive heart failure, aortic stenosis, and left main coronary artery disease, should be advised against autologous blood donation preoperatively. Evidence of increased risk for bleeding can be assessed via a coagulation screen. Prolonged bleeding time, thrombocytopenia, or increased INR or aPTT may necessitate corrective transfusions preoperatively or even lead to postponement of surgery. Also, a white blood cell count higher than 10,000/μL or white cells in the urine may generate the search for and treatment of potential occult infection.

Electrolyte abnormalities increase the risk of arrhythmias, and should be corrected prior to anesthesia induction. Similarly, attention must be given to abnormal renal and liver function, which can worsen perioperatively and thereby compromise drug clearance. This is particularly true of anesthetics. Furthermore, patients with renal dysfunction may require temporary or even permanent hemodialysis.

TABLE 8–2 Preoperative tests for cardiac surgery

Preoperative laboratory test	Abnormal finding	Comment
Complete blood count	1. Anemia, especially Hct <35%	1. Anticipate that hemodilution will occur on cardiopulmonary bypass and blood loss will occur intraoperatively. In stable patients, preoperative iron supplementation (weeks) or erythropoietin therapy (days) should be considered. Patients with unstable angina, congestive heart failure, aortic stenosis, and left main coronary artery disease should be advised against autologous donation of blood in the preoperative period.
	2. WBC >10,000	2. Search for possible infection.
Coagulation screen	1. Prolonged bleeding time 2. Elevated PT and/or PTT 3. Thrombocytopenia	All these laboratory abnormalities suggest that the patient is at risk for bleeding postoperatively and may have excessive chest tube drainage. Corrective measures (e.g., vitamin K, fresh frozen plasma, platelet transfusions) should be considered preoperatively, and surgery may need to be postponed. Hematological consultation may be required if an inherited defect in coagulation (e.g., von Willebrand factor deficiency) is suspected.
Chemistry profile	1. Elevated BUN/creatinine	1. Abnormal renal function that may worsen in the perioperative period (caused by nonpulsatile flow on cardiopulmonary bypass and potential low flow postoperatively); may necessitate temporary or even permanent hemodialysis.
	2. Potassium <4.0 mEq/ liter and/or magnesium <2.0 mEq/liter	2. Electrolyte deficits may place the patient at risk of arrhythmias perioperatively and should be corrected before induction of anesthesia.
	3. Abnormal liver function tests	3. Patient may clear anesthetic agents as well as other cardioactive drugs more slowly. Low albumin level may indicate a state of relative malnutrition that may need to be corrected with nutritional support perioperatively.
Stool hematest	Positive for occult blood	Because heparinization will take place while on the cardiopulmonary bypass apparatus, the patient may be at risk for GI bleeding perioperatively. The source of GI heme loss should be investigated preoperatively if clinical circumstances permit. The potential for bleeding in the future may influence the choice of prosthetic valve inserted.
Pulmonary function	Reduced VC or prolonged FEV_1	Anticipate longer than usual process of weaning from ventilator postoperatively if FEV_1 <65% of VC or FEV_1 <1.5-2.0 liters. Obtain baseline arterial blood gas analysis on room air to help guide respiratory management postoperatively.
Thyroid function	These tests are not ordered routinely but should be performed in cases of suspected hypothyroidism or hyperthyroidism, known thyroid dysfunction during replacement therapy, and atrial fibrillation in patients who have not undergone evaluation of thyroid function	Hypothyroid patients require prolonged period of ventilatory support postoperatively because of slower clearance of anesthetic agents. Hyperthyroid patients have a hypermetabolic state that places them at increased risk of myocardial ischemia, vasomotor instability, and poorly controlled ventricular rate in atrial fibrillation.
Echocardiography	1. Decreased LV ejection fraction	1. Patients with decreased LV function are at higher perioperative risk for surgery. Selected patients should undergo viability assessment.
	2. Decreased RV function	2. RV dysfunction increases perioperative risk and identification may lead to preoperative assessment of reversibility of pulmonary hypertension.
	3. Aortic stenosis	3. Mild to moderate aortic stenosis (gradient <25 mm Hg) may be treated by prophylactic valve replacement in selected low-risk patients.
	4. Aortic insufficiency	4. Ventricular dimension will help guide decisions to perform valve replacement in addition to revascularization in patients with combined aortic regurgitation and coronary disease.

(*Continued*)

TABLE 8–2 (*Continued*)

Preoperative laboratory test	Abnormal finding	Comment
	5. Mitral insufficiency	5. Moderate or severe mitral regurgitation may warrant valve exploration in patients undergoing coronary revascularization.
	6. LV aneurysm	6. May alert surgeons to the need of aneurysmectomy in selected patients.
	7. Ventricular septal defect	7. Identification will suggest the need for early surgical intervention.
Cardiac catheterization	1. Elevated LV end-diastolic pressure and pulmonary capillary wedge pressure	1. May remain elevated in the early postoperative period and indicate a need for careful attention to maintenance of adequate preload postoperatively.
	2. Elevated right atrial pressure	2. May reflect tricuspid regurgitation or RV dysfunction from prior infarction. Such patients require vigorous volume expansion postoperatively to maintain adequate cardiac output.
	3. Elevated pulmonary artery pressure (and pulmonary vascular resistance)	3. Fixed pulmonary vascular resistance should be suspected when the pulmonary artery diastolic pressure exceeds the mean pulmonary capillary wedge pressure. Vigorous oxygenation and pharmacological support with a pulmonary vasodilator (isoproterenol, prostaglandin E_1) are important in such cases. Patients with a pulmonary artery diastolic pressure equal to the pulmonary capillary wedge pressure usually have more rapid resolution of pulmonary hypertension postoperatively.
	4. LV mural thrombus	4. Increased risk of stroke perioperatively.
	5. Status of internal mammary arteries	5. Highly desirable arterial conduits for planned revascularization surgery. Particular care required during reoperation if patent internal mammary artery bypass is in place from previous surgery.
	6. Status of saphenous vein grafts	6. "Pseudoextravasation" of dye outside the lumen in a patent graft with slow flow probably represents thrombus-filled atherosclerotic aneurysm of the graft.

BUN = blood urea nitrogen; FEV_1 = volume of air expired at 1 second; GI = gastrointestinal; Hct = hematocrit; LV = left ventricular; PT = prothrombin time; PTT = partial thromboplastin time; RV = right ventricular; VC = vital capacity; WBC = white blood cell count.

Source: Reproduced with permission from Adams DH, Antman EM: Medical management of the patient undergoing cardiac surgery, in Braunwald E, Zipes D, Libby P (eds): Heart Disease. Philadelphia, WB Saunders, 2001; p 2059.

Additionally, patients with relative malnutrition as evidenced by a low serum albumin (<2.5g/dL) are at greater risk of sepsis and respiratory failure and may need nutritional correction for at least 1 to 2 weeks prior to elective cardiac surgery.

Finally, although thyroid function tests should not be ordered routinely, they are necessary in patients with suspected or confirmed thyroid dysfunction (on replacement therapy) and in individuals who have known arrhythmias, such as atrial fibrillation, who have not undergone thyroid function evaluation. Hyperthyroidism places patients at increased risk of myocardial ischemia, heart failure, vasomotor instability, and poorly controlled ventricular rate during atrial fibrillation. In contrast, hypothyroidism produces a hypometabolic state with resultant slower clearance of anesthetic agents and consequent prolonged ventilatory requirement.

Heparin-induced Thrombocytopenia

Heparin-induced thrombocytopenia (HIT) or "white clot syndrome" is an immune-mediated, potentially life-threatening thrombotic complication of heparin therapy that occurs in 3% to 5% of individuals approximately 5 to 14 days after heparin exposure.[19,20] HIT should be suspected in any patient who experiences a 50% or greater decrease in platelet count from baseline or a 30% or greater decrease in platelet count and associated thrombotic complication while on unfractionated heparin for at least 5 days. HIT can occur earlier in patients who are within 3 months of previous exposure to heparin. Thrombocytopenia usually resolves within one week of heparin discontinuation, but thrombotic tendency can persist for up to one month. Though HIT can occur with the use of low molecular weight heparin (LMWH), the incidence and development of thrombosis is much less frequent.[21]

Antibodies to heparin-platelet factor 4 cause platelet activation and aggregation as well as thrombin formation, resulting most commonly in deep venous thrombosis, pulmonary embolism, or cerebral sinus thrombosis.[22] Following CABG, HIT may present as graft occlusion, left atrial thrombus, valvular thrombosis, or pulmonary embolism.[23] On average, 25% to 50% of cardiopulmonary bypass patients who receive heparin acquire HIT-IgG, but only approximately 7% develop HIT.[24,25]

Many surgeons still prefer to use unfractionated heparin (UFH) during cardiopulmonary bypass because of familiarity, the need to employ specialized monitoring when using alternative agents, and the lack of antidotes for alternative agents. Besides the use of lepirudin, an irreversible antithrombin, or argatroban, a reversible direct thrombin inhibitor, reduction of thrombosis during cardiopulmonary bypass in patients with known HIT can be achieved by limiting UFH exposure time or by delaying surgery until 3 months after the patient's UFH exposure.[26] Otherwise, after receiving UFH, platelet counts should be monitored every 3 days from day 3 to day 14 of UFH exposure. In patients with HIT, warfarin initiation should be done in the presence of lepirudin or argatroban due to warfarin's association with limb gangrene when used as the sole agent.[27]

Hypercoaguable Disorders

Management of patients with hypercoaguable syndromes can be especially challenging in the setting of cardiac surgery where the need to control postoperative bleeding is crucial in preventing potentially life-threatening complications such as pericardial tamponade. Common (factor V Leiden, G20210A prothrombin gene) and relatively uncommon (antithrombin deficiency, protein C and protein S deficiency) causes of thrombosis have different risk associations. For example, the relative risk of venous thrombosis in the Caucasian population can range from 2.5 for the prothrombin gene mutation to 25 in the presence of antithrombin deficiency.[28] Furthermore, approximately 50% of cases of venous thrombosis associated with these hereditary disorders are provoked by known risk factors such as surgery. Therefore, aggressive prophylaxis with subcutaneous UFH or LMWH is warranted prior to surgery for patients who are not taking long-term anticoagulation.[29] In contrast, for those on long-term anticoagulation, the decision to continue treatment for thrombosis in the cardiac surgery setting should be individualized. In general, warfarin therapy can be switched to LMWH 3 to 5 days prior to cardiac surgery. Anticoagulation using UFH as a bridge should be resumed as soon as the bleeding risks associated with cardiac surgery have been stabilized, usually within 2 to 3 days postoperatively. The patients at highest risk for venous thrombosis are those within 3 months of an episode of thrombosis and those with conditions that predispose to the highest risk of thrombosis, such as antithrombin deficiency.[28]

Patients with antiphospholipid antibody syndrome (lupus anticoagulant/anticardiolipin antibodies, history of arterial or venous thrombosis, and/or recurrent fetal loss) deserve special mention because this syndrome can be associated with valvular heart disease (32% to 36% requiring replacement).[30–32] Perioperative management, including the choice of prosthetic valve, is challenging and requires a multidisciplinary approach due to the risk of thrombophilia, abnormal prolongation in clotting times, and the presence of thrombocytopenia. During cardiopulmonary bypass, anticoagulation monitoring is difficult using standard means. Therefore, preoperative in vitro testing to identify the most reliable assay for heparin monitoring during cardiopulmonary bypass may be necessary.[33] Potential heparin assays include protamine titration, kaolin, and the anti-Xa methods that measure heparin's in vitro effects differently.[32]

Multiple Anticoagulants in the Setting of Failed Percutaneous Intervention

Advances in cardiology have resulted in the almost standard use of glycoprotein IIb/IIIa inhibitors, aspirin, and intravenous heparin UFH or subcutaneous LMWH in patients with non–ST and ST-elevation myocardial infarction (STEMI) who undergo early percutaneous intervention (PCI).[1,2] However, prospective, randomized evidence involving patients who have received multiple anticoagulants for PCI who subsequently required urgent or semi-urgent cardiac surgery is lacking. Clinical decisions should therefore be based on the known bleeding risks and pharmacology associated with individual agents, available subgroup analyses, and surgical urgency.

In the PURSUIT trial, patients who received the glycoprotein IIb/IIIa inhibitor eptifibatide within 30 days of CABG did not experience higher rates of bleeding, probably due to the short half-life of the drug.[1] However, the CURE trial showed that the antiplatelet agent clopidogrel was beneficial in patients with acute coronary syndromes undergoing PCI but was associated with a concomitant increased risk of major bleeding.[34] Though clopidogrel can decrease mortality, it may potentially pose serious problems with major perioperative bleeding (clopidogrel vs. placebo groups: 3.7% vs. 2.7%; relative risk [RR] = 1.38; 95% CI, 1.13-1.67; $p = .001$). In further subgroup analysis, there was no significant increase in bleeding after CABG (1.3% vs. 1.1%; RR = 1.26; 95% CI, 0.93-1.71). The median time between discontinuation of clopidogrel and CABG was 5 days. For those patients who stopped taking clopidogrel within 5 days prior to CABG, the rate of major bleeding was 9.6% in the clopidogrel-treated patients and 6.3% in the placebo group (RR = 1.53, $p = .06$). However, these studies were not designed to address bleeding complications with CABG, and the surgeon often relies on experience with the respective agents to dictate the timing of cardiac surgery.

Yende et al investigated the effect of clopidogrel on bleeding complications after CABG, and noted that clopidogrel use increased the need for reexploration and blood product transfusion after CABG.[35] By contrast, Grubitzsch et al found no significant increase in reexploration rate or transfusion requirement after CABG in patients who had received excessive preoperative anticoagulation.[36] Overall, it is presumably safer to have patients wait at least a week after discontinuing these agents before undergoing elective cardiac surgery. One exception may be when clopidogrel is being taken in the context of new stent implantation for coronary artery restenosis. In this instance, the risk of stent thrombosis may outweigh the risk of bleeding complications.

Limited data are available regarding the use of fibrinolytic agents prior to CABG. However, in a subgroup analysis of the Global Utilization of Streptokinase and Tissue Plasminogen Activator for Occluded Coronary Arteries trial (GUSTO I), patients who underwent PCI or CABG after receiving fibrinolytics had a lower rate (0%) of intracranial hemorrhage than those treated with repeat fibrinolysis (1.3%) or medical therapy (0.5%) ($p = .046$).[37] By contrast, in the Assessment of the Safety of a New Thrombolytic Study (ASSENT 2), no difference in the rate of intracranial hemorrhage was observed among the revascularization, repeat fibrinolysis, and conservative treatment groups.[37]

PREOPERATIVE ESTIMATION OF MORBIDITY AND MORTALITY RISK

Preoperative risk assessment has important implications for patient well-being, containment of hospital costs, and provision of data to identify perioperative issues in need of improvement. Several scoring systems have been developed to assess perioperative risk, particularly in the setting of isolated CABG. Figure 8-1 shows the most commonly used clinical severity scoring system from the Northern New England Cardiovascular Disease Study Group. The major risk factors for adverse outcome during CABG include advanced age, emergency surgery, history of prior CABG, dialysis dependency, and creatinine of 2 mg/dL or higher.

Due to the changing profile of patients undergoing cardiac surgery, accurate preoperative risk stratification has become increasingly difficult. Factors affecting outcome data include surgery type, follow-up time, and medical therapy after hospitalization, as well as geographic, cultural, social, and economic issues.[38,39] Immer et al compared three different scores (Parsonnet, French, and Higgins scores) used for preoperative risk stratification of postoperative morbidity, mortality, and hospital length of stay for 1299 consecutive patients undergoing CABG and/or heart valve surgery.[40] All three scoring systems performed well, with c-statistics between 0.76 and 0.79. The Higgins and French scores were especially useful in predicting postoperative outcome. Both of these scoring systems showed a progressive increase in cardiac risk class with increasing cardiac risk score. Rumsfeld et al examined a nontraditional approach to cardiac surgical risk stratification that involved assessment of a patient's self-perceived health status using the physical component summary (PCS) scores from the preoperative short-form 36 (SF-36) health status survey.[41] After adjustment for known clinical risk factors of mortality following CABG, the PCS from the preoperative SF-36 was found to be an independent predictor of mortality such that a 10 point or 1 SD decrement in baseline PCS was associated with a 39% increase in 6-month mortality (95% CI, 1.11-1.77; $p = .006$). As noted by the authors, this study may have had a selection bias towards lower risk elective cases and did not determine the predictors of the baseline PCS. While the role of these data in the preoperative evaluation of cardiac surgery patients remains unclear, they illustrate that in addition to physician-determined components of risk stratification, patient self-report may provide a complementary, noninvasive, cost-effective measurement of mortality prediction.

RISK FACTORS FOR MORBIDITY AND MORTALITY

Atrial Fibrillation

Commonly encountered after cardiac surgery, atrial fibrillation occurs in as many as 10% to 40% of patients after CABG and in up to 65% of patients undergoing combined CABG and valve surgery.[42–45] Atrial fibrillation occurs most frequently within 24 to 48 hours after surgery, and, although usually considered benign and self-limited, it is associated with prolonged hospitalization, hemodynamic instability, and thromboembolization.[46–49] For example, the risk of stroke increases 3-fold in patients with postoperative atrial fibrillation. Many patients (25% to 80%) spontaneously convert to sinus rhythm within 24 hours.[50]

The mechanism of atrial fibrillation following cardiac surgery is not well understood, but possible etiologies include multiple wavelet reentry in the atria, rapid firing of an atrial focus, and less likely atrial ischemia.[45,51] Preoperative clinical predictors of atrial fibrillation after cardiac surgery include increased age, history of hypertension, male sex, and a previous history of atrial fibrillation and congestive heart failure.[43,45,46,52] Less well characterized predictors of postoperative atrial fibrillation include aortic cross-clamp time, pulmonary vein venting, respiratory disease, and prolonged ventilation.[45]

The prophylactic use of beta-blocker therapy decreases the incidence of post–CABG atrial fibrillation by as much as 70% to 80%.[53] Preoperative initiation of beta-blocker therapy probably attenuates the high sympathetic tone associated with cardiac surgery. Prophylactic use of calcium channel blockers and digoxin does not reduce the incidence of atrial fibrillation.[45] Several studies have demonstrated the efficacy of amiodarone in decreasing the incidence of postoperative atrial fibrillation when started one week prior to surgery and continued until hospital discharge.[54,55] Sotalol, a class III antiarrhythmic drug, also reduces the incidence of postoperative atrial fibrillation compared to placebo and half-dose beta blockade.[56,57] Additionally, prophylactic continuous atrial overdrive pacing via temporary epicardial wires or from the right atrium also shows promise in decreasing the incidence of atrial fibrillation post–CABG.[58,59]

PREOPERATIVE ESTIMATION OF RISK OF MORTALITY, CEREBROVASCULAR ACCIDENT, AND MEDIASTINITIS			
For use *only* in isolated CABG surgery			
Directions: Locate outcome of interest, e.g., mortality. Use the score in that column for each relevant preoperative variable, and then sum these scores to get the total score. Take the total score and look up the approximate preoperative risk in the table below			
PATIENT OR DISEASE CHARACTERISTICS	**MORTALITY SCORE**	**CVA SCORE**	**MEDIASTINITIS SCORE**
Age 60–69	2	3.5	
Age 70–79	3	5	
Age ≥80	5	6	
Female sex	1.5		
EF <40%	1.5	1.5	2
Urgent surgery	2	1.5	1.5
Emergency surgery	5	2	3.5
Prior CABG	5	1.5	
PVD	2	2	
Diabetes			1.5
Dialysis or creatinine ≥2	4	2	2.5
COPD	1.5		3.5
Obesity (BMI 31–36)			2.5
Severe obesity (BMI ≥37)			3.5
Total score			

PERIOPERATIVE RISK			
TOTAL SCORE	**MORTALITY (%)**	**CVA (%)**	**MEDIASTINITIS (%)**
0	0.4	0.3	0.4
1	0.5	0.4	0.5
2	0.7	0.7	0.6
3	0.9	0.9	0.7
4	1.3	1.1	1.1
5	1.7	1.5	1.5
6	2.2	1.9	1.9
7	3.3	2.8	3.0
8	3.9	3.5	3.5
9	6.1	4.5	5.8
10	7.7	≥6.5	≥6.5
11	10.6		
12	13.7		
13	17.7		
14	≥28.3		

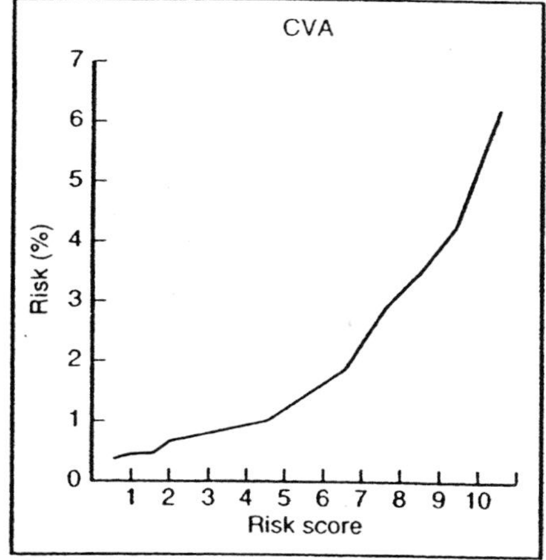

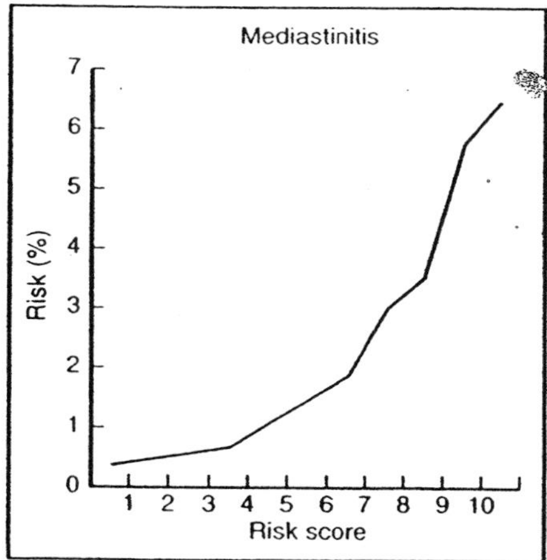

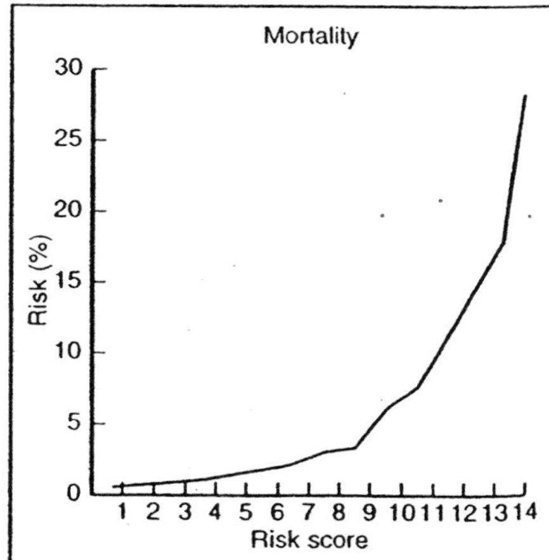

FIGURE 8–1 Preoperative estimation of risk of mortality, cerebrovascular accident, and mediastinitis, developed by the Northern New England Cardiovascular Disease Study Group. *(Adapted with permission from Eagle KA, Guyton RA, Davidoff R, et al: ACC/AHA guidelines for CABG. J Am Coll Cardiol 1999; 34:1262.)*

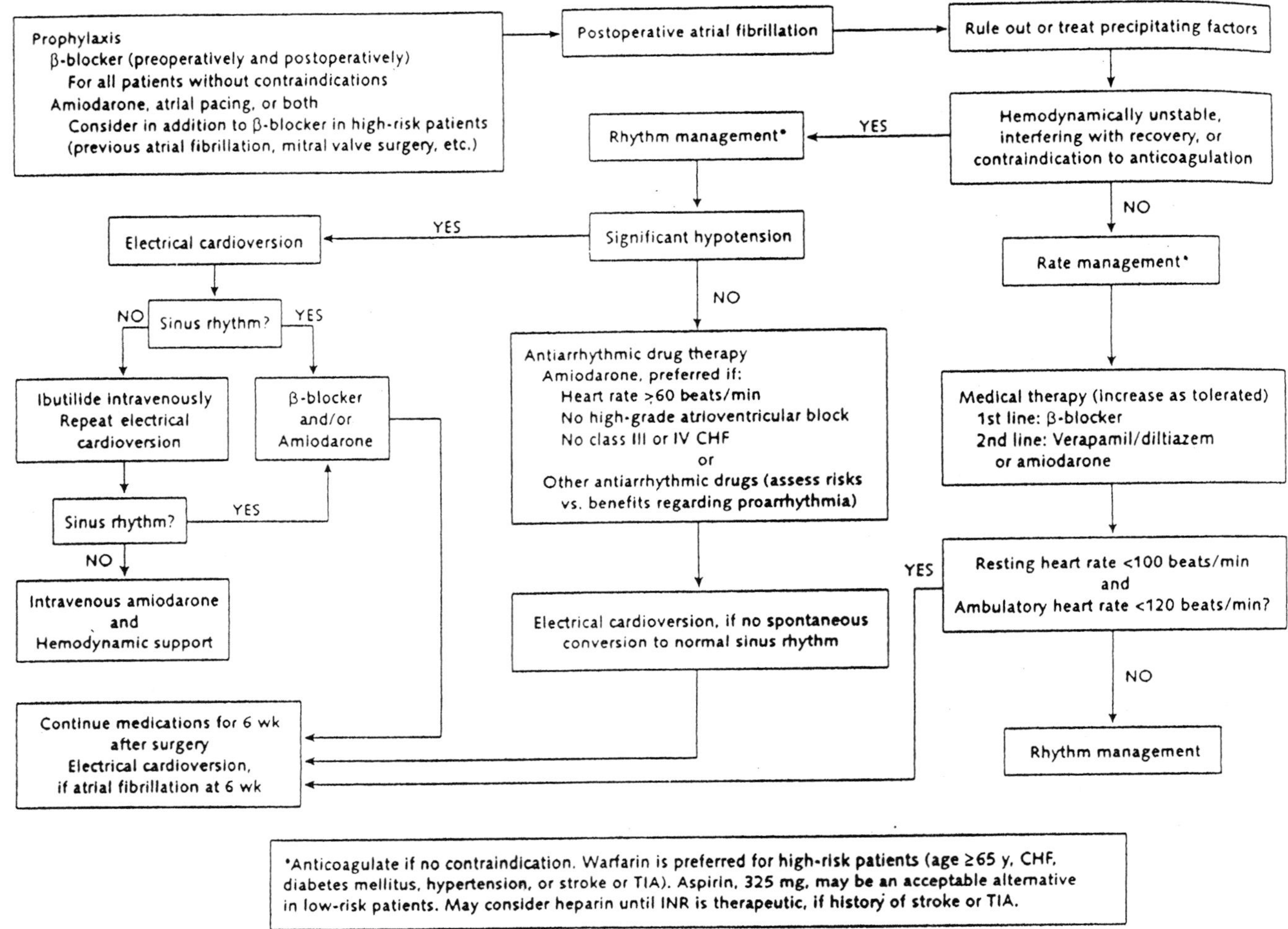

FIGURE 8–2 Algorithm for the prevention and management of atrial fibrillation after cardiac surgery. *(Adapted with permission from Maisel WH, Rawn JD, Stevenson WG: Atrial fibrillation after cardiac surgery. Ann Intern Med 2001; 135:1061.)*

For patients with persistent atrial fibrillation after cardiac surgery, priority should be given to electrolyte repletion and rate control. While beta blockers are considered first-line therapy, calcium channel blockers such as verapamil and diltiazem are also useful in controlling ventricular rate. Amiodarone is also useful in the provision of rate control, particularly in those individuals who are unable to tolerate beta blockers or calcium channel blockers because of hypotension. Antiarrhythmic therapy is usually reserved for those individuals who have persistent or recurrent atrial fibrillation. Class IA (disopyramide, quinidine, procainamide), IC (propafenone, flecainide), and III agents (sotalol, amiodarone, ibutilide, dofetilide) all have varying degrees of efficacy for conversion of post–CABG atrial fibrillation.[45] Cardiology consultation is prudent prior to using any of these agents since they are contraindicated in select patient populations and the risk for drug-induced proarrhythmia is high. Electrical cardioversion should be performed if the patient demonstrates hemodynamic instability and in those patients with persistent symptoms or rapid ventricular rate despite optimal drug therapy. Figure 8-2 outlines an algorithm for the prevention and management of atrial fibrillation after cardiac surgery.

Anticoagulation in patients with postoperative atrial fibrillation for 48 hours or more should be individualized. Heparin therapy as a bridge to a therapeutic INR (2 to 3) with warfarin is troublesome because it is associated with higher rates of large pericardial effusion and cardiac tamponade compared to aspirin or placebo.[45] Generally, most patients with persistent atrial fibrillation at discharge will spontaneously convert to sinus rhythm within 6 weeks.[60]

Renal Disease

Acute renal failure develops in approximately 1% to 5% patients after cardiac surgery.[61] Morbidity and mortality related to renal disease after cardiac surgery are heavily dependent on comorbid disease. Risk factors for acute renal failure

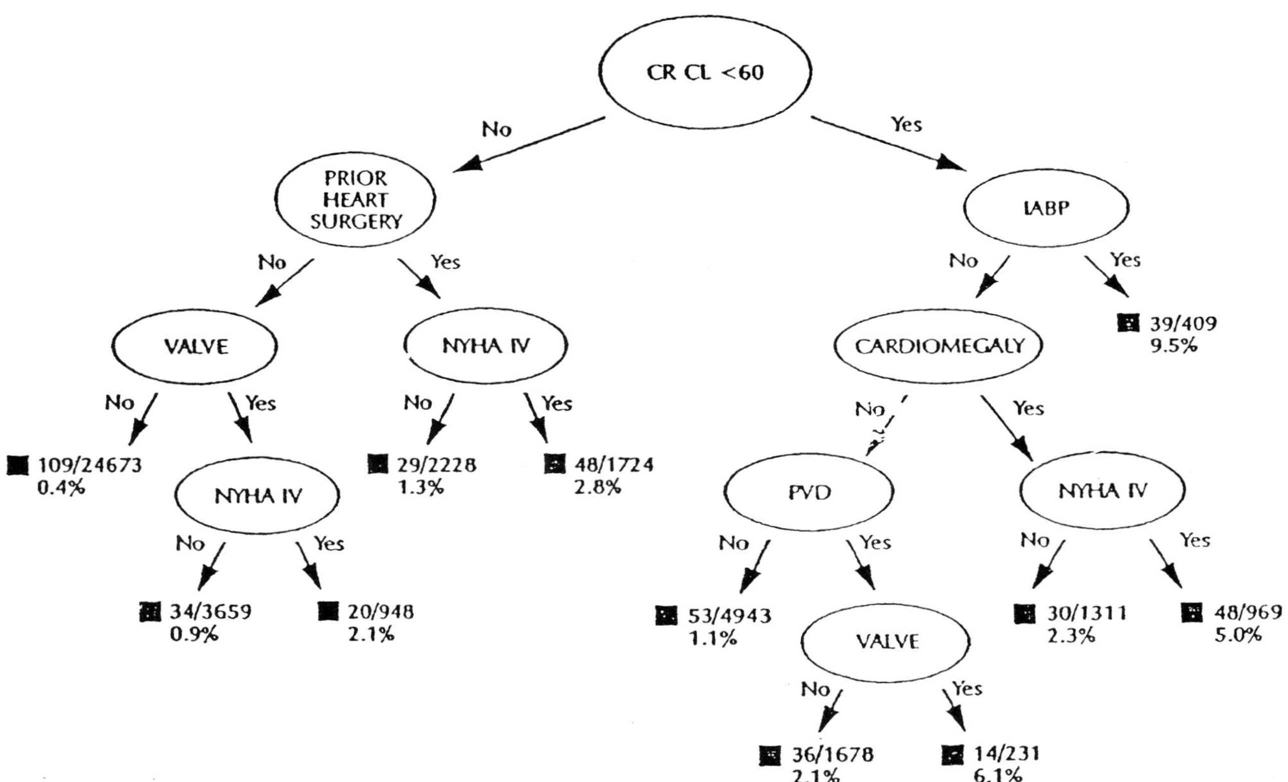

FIGURE 8–3 Recursive partitioning analysis of the risk of renal failure after CABG. CrCl = estimated creatinine clearance; LVEF = left ventricular ejection fraction; IABP = intra-aortic balloon pump; PVD = peripheral vascular disease. *(Adapted and modified with permission from Fortescue EB, Bates DW, Chertow GM: Predicting acute renal failure after coronary bypass surgery: cross-validation of two risk-stratification algorithms. Kidney Int 2000; 57:294.)*

include advanced age, baseline renal dysfunction, left ventricular dysfunction, peripheral vascular disease, clinical signs of poor cardiac function such as pulmonary rales, and the use of an intra-aortic balloon pump.[61–63] Dialysis is necessary in 1% of patients who develop acute renal failure; the 30-day mortality is almost 64% for those patients with acute renal failure compared to 4.3% for those with normal renal function.[61] The VA Continuous Improvement in Cardiac Surgery Program developed a recursive partitioning clinical risk algorithm that performs well across different patient populations.[64] It helps to identify individuals who are at high risk of developing acute renal failure (Fig. 8-3).

Age

The prevalence of cardiac surgical procedures in the elderly continues to increase as life expectancy improves and procedural benefits outweigh the risks. Moreover, the outcome of surgical coronary revascularization has progressively improved despite increased numbers of elderly patients and worsened preoperative risk profiles over the past several decades. Operative mortality in patients more than 70 years old still remains higher than in younger patients, with octogenarians having the highest operative risk (Table 8-3).[6] Identified risk factors for poor operative outcome include lower BMI, advanced NYHA class, and higher prevalence of diabetes, renal dysfunction, peripheral vascular disease, and previous CABG. Mortality statistics may also vary based on multiple socioeconomic and demographic factors. For example, whereas a study by Zacek et al reported higher mortality in patients who were aged 70 years and older versus those younger than 70 (7.3% vs. 2.3%; $p < .005$), a Canadian study reported operative mortality declining from 7.2% in 1982–1986 to 4.4% in 1987–1991 in the elderly.[5,8] The latter study also stratified patients by risk and demonstrated that while the prevalence of high-risk elderly patients increased significantly over time, operative mortality decreased for medium- and high-risk patients. Possible reasons for better outcomes include improved myocardial protection and anesthetic techniques perioperatively, as well as greater use of arterial grafts. However, patients aged 75 years and older tend to have a higher incidence of mental confusion and reduced quality of life compared to their younger counterparts.[65]

By contrast, younger women have a higher mortality after CABG compared with their male counterparts. Vaccarino

TABLE 8–3 Operative mortality by age group

Reference	Year of publ.	30-day mortality (%)			
		Patients aged under 70	Over 70	Over 75	Over 80
Gann	1977		6.7		
Knapp	1981	1.1	1.6		
Gersh	1983	4.6	6.6	9.5	
Hibler	1983	4.6	5.0	20.0	
Hochberg	1984	4.0	12.0		
Horneffer	1987	2.2	9.3		
Goldman	1988	2.9	6.2		
Horvath	1990			10.8	
Freeman	1991				12.9
Ko	1991				12.0
Tsai	1991				7.0
Hannan	1994				
Curtis	1994		5.2		
He	1994		8.9		
Katz	1995		6.4		
Morris	1996				7.8
MEDICARE	1995				11.5
KCH - unit HK	2000		5.9		

Source: Reproduced with permission from Zacek P, Dominik J, Harrer J, et al: Morbidity and mortality in patients 70 years of age and over undergoing isolated coronary artery bypass surgery. Acta Medica (Hradec Kralove) 2001; 44:109.

et al reported that despite having higher ejection fractions and fewer diseased coronary arteries, women less than 50 years old had in-hospital mortality rates that were 3 times higher than men (3.4% vs. 1.1%).[66] Although the reason for this difference is uncertain, the women had more comorbidities compared with men.

Ventricular Dysfunction

Viable myocardium that has not been revascularized in persons with ischemic heart disease and congestive heart failure promotes the development of further functional and myocardial disability.[67–69] Though poor left ventricular function is considered a major risk factor for cardiac surgery, surgical revascularization improves ventricular function in those individuals with hibernating myocardium.[67] For individuals with ejection fractions less than 30%, low cardiac output syndrome and supraventricular arrhythmias are the most common complications, and in this group mortality rates approach 10%.[70] However, CABG improves both ventricular function and the 3-year survival rate, making adequate assessment of myocardial viability via thallium reperfusion imaging, positron-emission tomography, or stress echocardiography necessary prior to surgery.[67,68,71]

Despite advances in surgical techniques, 1% of cardiac surgery patients develop postoperative ventricular dysfunction.[72] In these individuals, implantation of ventricular assist devices as either a bridge to recovery or to transplantation can be beneficial, particularly in the bridge to transplant subgroup, often resulting in successful discharge from the hospital.[72]

Patients with left ventricular dysfunction and valvular disease such as mitral regurgitation or aortic stenosis require special preoperative management. Individuals with mitral regurgitation and heart failure should receive preoperative afterload reduction with angiotensin-converting enzyme (ACE) inhibitors or intravenous sodium nitroprusside to maintain systolic blood pressures in the 90 to 100 mm Hg range. While patients with aortic stenosis and hemodynamically significant cerebral or renovascular disease should not receive the latter therapies, intra-aortic balloon counterpulsation (IABP) may be useful in such subgroups. Intra-aortic balloon support can also be used in the setting of acute mitral regurgitation due to papillary muscle rupture as well as in infarct-related ventricular septal defect. Preoperative IABP use in high-risk patients decreases mortality and shortens ICU stay due to enhanced hemodynamic performance.[73]

Right ventricular dysfunction also increases perioperative risk and patients should be assessed for pulmonary hypertension (pulmonary artery systolic pressure >60 mm Hg), documentation of a history of inferior myocardial infarction, or chronic tricuspid regurgitation. Right ventricular dysfunction caused by increased pulmonary vascular resistance should be treated with inotropes that have vasodilator properties such as dobutamine (5 μg/kg/min) and milronone (5 μg/kg/min). Intravenous nitrates, prostacyclin

(0.5-2.0 ng/kg/min), and nitric oxide (10-20 ppm) are also effective agents for lowering pulmonary vascular resistance with resultant improvement in right ventricular function.[74]

Pulmonary Disease

In patients with chronic obstructive pulmonary disease (COPD), prolonged weaning from mechanical ventilation postoperatively is common if FEV_1 is less than 65% of VC or if FEV_1 is less than 1.5 L. CABG patients with severe COPD are more likely to develop ventilatory failure and have higher mortality rates than those with mild-to-moderate or no COPD (death: 19% vs. 4% vs. 2%, $p = .02$).[75] Preoperative screening of arterial oxygen concentration on room air can provide guidance in respiratory management postoperatively. The role of preoperative spirometry and perioperative bronchodilators remains unclear in stable patients and cannot be recommended on a routine basis.

Reoperation

Approximately 3% to 20% of patients who undergo CABG will require reoperation within a decade; reoperations represent roughly 20% of CABG operations performed yearly.[76] With aging of the population, the number of reoperations is expected to increase. Operative mortality for reintervention is almost two times higher than for the initial procedure, hovering between 1% and 6% in most case series.[77,78] Furthermore, emergency reoperations increase the baseline operative mortality rate 4-fold.[76] One study demonstrated that reoperations in patients over 70 years old were associated with a 7% operative mortality and 90% survival rate at approximately 2.8 years, suggesting that reintervention in this subset of patients has an acceptable morbidity and mortality profile.[79] Preoperative risk factors for reoperation include female sex, a history of diabetes, hypertension, renal insufficiency, hyperlipidemia, smoking, and reduced ventricular function.

Nutrition and BMI

The postoperative hypermetabolic state requires increased nutrition in order to facilitate wound healing and to meet corporal metabolic demands. Consequently, patients who are malnourished preoperatively should receive at least 2 to 4 weeks of intensive nutritional bolstering prior to elective surgery, and all patients should resume an oral diet within 24 hours after uncomplicated surgery. Since perioperative stroke may limit the ability of some patients to protect their airway, a swallowing evaluation is mandatory in this subset of patients. Early enteral feeding is warranted in those individuals who have no contraindications to feeding. Low body mass index (<20 kg/m^2) and hypoalbuminemia (<2.5 g/dL) are independently associated with increased risk of morbidity and mortality after cardiac surgery.[80] Patients with decreased albumin levels are at increased risk for bleeding, renal failure, prolonged ventilatory support, and reoperation. While obesity is not associated with increased mortality, patients with high percent body fat and poor aerobic capacity are at higher risk for sternal wound infection (OR = 2.3; $p < .001$), saphenous vein harvest site infection, and atrial arrhythmias.[80–82]

Diabetes

Diabetes is an important independent risk factor for atherosclerotic heart disease. Although the BARI trial did not evaluate stented patients, it demonstrated that diabetic patients with multivessel disease have greater survival with CABG compared to those who receive PCI.[83] Furthermore, Morricone et al showed that although diabetic CABG patients did not have higher mortality rates compared to nondiabetics, diabetics tended to have more renal and neurologic complications, experienced longer ICU stays, required more blood transfusions, and had higher reopening rates.[84] Diabetics who underwent valve operations had a 5-fold increased risk of having a major pulmonary complication.

Carotid Artery Disease

Approximately 1% to 6% of persons develop neurologic complications after cardiac surgery.[85–87] Stroke is the most debilitating of these complications, with an estimated 15,000 victims yearly.[87] Carotid artery disease is present in up to as many as 30% of patients who have postoperative strokes. Cerebral microembolization from the arterial tree during CABG is likely the most common culprit. In fact, atherosclerosis of the ascending aorta is an independent predictor of long-term neurologic insult and mortality.[88] For patients undergoing CABG, the incidence of carotid artery disease can be as high as 22% (3% in unselected populations), depending on multiple factors including screening method, age, diabetic status, the presence of left main disease or left ventricular dysfunction, female sex, and a history of smoking or prior cerebrovascular attacks.[89]

Indeed, patients with concomitant carotid and coronary disease often present a management challenge to physicians because they have decreased long-term survival compared to their counterparts who have only coronary disease.[89] Generally, perioperative stroke risk is believed to be highest (>5%) in patients with more than 80% unilateral stenosis, bilateral stenoses of at least 50%, and unilateral occlusion with at least a 50% carotid artery lesion on the contralateral side.[89] Consequently, all patients who fall into one of these categories should be considered for combined carotid endarterectomy (CEA) and CABG. Several authors report operative mortalities between 0% and 5%, and perioperative neurologic and myocardial events of approximately 3%.[89–93] At 5 years, over 85% of these patients are stroke-free.[9] In selected patients with asymptomatic significant carotid artery disease, CEA results in a lower incidence of subsequent long-term neurologic events.[94] Hence, screening of cardiac surgical candidates via carotid artery ultrasound is advisable to enable detection of significant carotid stenoses prior to surgery in those individuals at increased risk of perioperative stroke.

Though the treatment of patients with asymptomatic severe carotid artery stenoses undergoing CABG remains controversial, combined CABG/CEA is recommended in symptomatic patients with carotid artery stenosis. Although perioperative myocardial infarction and mortality are generally higher with combined CABG/CEA than with CABG alone, the former is still preferred in this group.[95,96] Similarly, selected asymptomatic patients with unilateral or bilateral high-grade stenoses benefit from combined CABG/CEA due to long-term neurologic protection.[96–98]

The timing of CEA in relation to CABG is institution-dependent; however, there appears to be no demonstrated difference in mortality or morbidity whether CEA is done before or during CABG.[99] Carotid artery stenting can also be performed in close proximity to CABG. Potential advantages of carotid artery stenting include minimizing the need for systemic heparinization prior to CABG. At present, stenting can be safely performed 4 weeks prior to CABG. Thus carotid artery stenting might be advantageous in patients with stable carotid and coronary disease, in elderly patients who are at high risk for thoracotomy, and in patients who have concomitant carotid artery disease and single-vessel left anterior descending artery disease for which minimally invasive surgery is planned. Babatasi et al reported 97% procedural success with coronary artery stenting in a series of 36 patients treated with carotid stenting and CABG.[100] In this study, CABG was performed within a mean of 24.3 days after carotid artery stenting with no embolizations or deaths and a minor stroke rate of 3.6%; 2 patients developed restenosis at 23 $\pm$ 2 months. However, the data regarding CABG/CEA continue to evolve.

Bradyarrhythmias and Atrioventricular and Intraventricular Block

Preoperative temporary transvenous pacemaker wire insertion is recommended in patients with hemodynamic instability and high-grade heart block (third degree or Mobitz II). Permanent epicardial pacing lead implantation should be done intraoperatively for patients undergoing tricuspid valve replacement with a mechanical prosthesis, due to the contraindication of passing a transvenous lead through the latter. For individuals with permanent pacemakers, information regarding patient pacemaker dependency as well as the make, model, and settings of the device should be clearly documented in the medical record. Previously implanted automatic cardioverter-defibrillator devices should be disabled before surgery to minimize inappropriate shocks caused by electrocautery signal sensing intraoperatively. Bedside external defibrillation equipment must therefore be readily available.

REFERENCES

1. PURSUIT Trial Investigators: Inhibition of platelet glycoprotein IIb/IIIa with eptifibatide in patients with acute coronary syndromes. *N Engl J Med* 1998; 339:436.
2. Platelet Receptor Inhibition in Ischemic Syndrome Management (PRISM) Study Investigators: a comparison of aspirin plus tirofiban with aspirin plus heparin for unstable angina. *N Engl J Med* 1998; 338:1498.
3. Hofma SH, van Beusekom HM, Serruys PW, van Der Giessen WJ: Recent developments in coated stents. *Curr Interv Cardiol Rep* 2001; 3:28.
4. Suzuki T, Kopia G, Hayashi S, et al: Stent-based delivery of sirolimus reduces neointimal formation in a porcine coronary model. *Circulation* 2001; 104:1188.
5. Zacek P, Dominik J, Harrer J, et al: Morbidity and mortality in patients 70 years of age and over undergoing isolated coronary artery bypass surgery. *Acta Medica* (Hradec Kralove) 2001; 44:109.
6. Deiwick M, Tandler R, Mollhoff T, et al: Heart surgery in patients aged eighty years and above: determinants of morbidity and mortality. *Thorac Cardiovasc Surg* 1997; 45:119.
7. Trachiotis GD, Weintraub WS, Johnston TS, et al: Coronary artery bypass grafting in patients with advanced left ventricular dysfunction. *Ann Thorac Surg* 1998; 66:1632.
8. Ivanov J, Weisel RD, David TE, Naylor CD: Fifteen-year trends in risk severity and operative mortality in elderly patients undergoing coronary artery bypass graft surgery. *Circulation* 1998; 97:673.
9. Eagle KA, Guyton RA, Davidoff R, et al: ACC/AHA guidelines for coronary artery bypass graft surgery: executive summary and recommendations: a report of the American College of Cardiology/American Heart Association Task Force on Practice Guidelines (Committee to revise the 1991 guidelines for coronary artery bypass graft surgery). *Circulation* 1999; 100:1464.
10. Filsoufi F, Aklog L, Adams DH: Minimally invasive CABG. *Curr Opin Cardiol* 2001; 16:306.
11. Byrne JG, Hsin MK, Adams DH, et al: Minimally invasive direct access heart valve surgery. *J Card Surg* 2000; 15:21.
12. Grossi EA, Galloway AC, Ribakove GH, et al: Impact of minimally invasive valvular heart surgery: a case-control study. *Ann Thorac Surg* 2001; 71:807.
13. Katz NM, Gersh BJ, Cox JL: Changing practice of coronary bypass surgery and its impact on early risk and long-term survival. *Curr Opin Cardiol* 1998; 13:465.
14. Aldea GS, Gaudiani JM, Shapira OM, et al: Effect of gender on postoperative outcomes and hospital stays after coronary artery bypass grafting. *Ann Thorac Surg* 1999; 67:1097.
15. Mullany CJ, Mock MB, Brooks MM, et al: Effect of age in the Bypass Angioplasty Revascularization Investigation (BARI) randomized trial. *Ann Thorac Surg* 1999; 67:396.
16. Rizzo RJ, Whittemore AD, Couper GS, et al: Combined carotid and coronary revascularization: the preferred approach to the severe vasculopath. *Ann Thorac Surg* 1992; 54:1099.
17. Vassilidze TV, Cernaianu AC, Gaprindashvili T, et al: Simultaneous coronary artery bypass and carotid endarterectomy: determinants of outcome. *Tex Heart Inst J* 1994; 21:119.
18. Hanet C, Marchand E, Keyeux A: Left internal mammary artery occlusion after mastectomy and radiotherapy. *Am J Cardiol* 1990; 65:1044.
19. King DJ, Kelton JG: Heparin-associated thrombocytopenia. *Ann Intern Med* 1984; 100:535.
20. Warkentin TE, Kelton JG: Heparin-induced thrombocytopenia. *Prog Hemost Thromb* 1991; 10:1.
21. Warkentin TE, Levine MN, Hirsh J, et al: Heparin-induced thrombocytopenia in patients treated with low-molecular-weight heparin or unfractionated heparin. *N Engl J Med* 1995; 332:1330.

22. Chong BH: Heparin-induced thrombocytopenia. *Br J Haematol* 1995; 89:431.
23. Singer RL, Mannion JD, Bauer TL, et al: Complications from heparin-induced thrombocytopenia in patients undergoing cardiopulmonary bypass. *Chest* 1993; 104:1436.
24. Visentin GP, Malik M, Cyganiak KA, Aster RH: Patients treated with unfractionated heparin during open heart surgery are at high risk to form antibodies reactive with heparin:platelet factor 4 complexes. *J Lab Clin Med* 1996; 128:376.
25. Trossaert M, Gaillard A, Commin PL, et al: High incidence of anti-heparin/platelet factor 4 antibodies after cardiopulmonary bypass surgery. *Br J Haematol* 1998; 101:653.
26. Deitcher SR, Carman TL: Heparin-induced thrombocytopenia: natural history, diagnosis, and management. *Vasc Med* 2001; 6: 113.
27. Warkentin TE, Russett JI, Hohnston M, Kelton JG: Warfarin treatment of deep venous thrombosis complicating heparin-induced thrombocytopenia is a risk factor for initiation of venous limb gangrene: report of nine patients implicating the interacting procoagulant effects of two anticoagulant agents. *Thromb Haemost* 1995; 73:1110.
28. Kearon C, Crowther M, Hirsh J: Management of patients with hereditary hypercoagulable disorders. *Annu Rev Med* 2000; 51:169.
29. Clagett GP, Anderson FA Jr, Geerts W, et al: Prevention of venous thromboembolism. *Chest* 1998; 114:531S.
30. Garcia-Torres R, Amigo MC, de la Rosa A, et al: Valvular heart disease in primary antiphospholipid syndrome (PAPS): clinical and morphological findings. *Lupus* 1996; 5:56.
31. Brenner B, Blumenfeld Z, Markiewicz W, Reisner SA: Cardiac involvement in patients with primary antiphospholipid syndrome. *J Am Coll Cardiol* 1991; 18:931.
32. Levine JS, Branch DW, Rauch J: The antiphospholipid syndrome. *N Engl J Med* 2002; 346:752.
33. Hogan WJ, McBane RD, Santrach PJ, et al: Antiphospholipid syndrome and perioperative hemostatic management of cardiac valvular surgery. *Mayo Clin Proc* 2000; 75:971.
34. The CURE Investigators: Effects of clopidogrel in addition to aspirin in patients with acute coronary syndromes without ST-segment elevation. *N Engl J Med* 2001; 345:494.
35. Yende S, Wunderink RG: Effect of clopidogrel on bleeding after coronary artery bypass surgery. *Crit Care Med* 2001; 12:2271.
36. Grubitzsch H, Wollert HG, Eckel L: Emergency coronary artery bypass grafting: does excessive preoperative anticoagulation increase bleeding complications and transfusion requirements? *Cardiovasc Surg* 2001; 9:510.
37. Barbash GI, Birnbaum Y, Bogaerts K, et al: Treatment of reinfarction after thrombolytic therapy acute myocardial infarction: an analysis of outcome and treatment choices in the Global Utility of Streptokinase and Tissue Plasminogen Activators for Occluded Coronary Arteries (GUSTO I) and Assessment of the Safety of a New Thrombolytic (ASSENT 2) studies. *Circulation* 2001; 103:954.
38. Jones RH, Hannan EL, Hammermeister KE, et al: Identification of preoperative variables needed for risk adjustment of short-term mortality after coronary artery bypass graft surgery. The Working Group Panel on the Cooperative CABG Database Project. *J Am Coll Cardiol* 1996; 28:1478.
39. Pinna-Pintor P, Bobbio M, Sandrelli L, et al: Risk stratification for open heart operations: comparison of centers regardless of the influence of the surgical team. *Ann Thorac Surg* 1997; 64:410.
40. Immer F, Habicht J, Nessensohn K, et al: Prospective evaluation of 3 risk stratification scores in cardiac surgery. *Thorac Cardiovasc Surg* 2000; 48:134.
41. Rumsfeld JS, MaWhinney S, McCarthy M Jr, et al: Health-related quality of life as a predictor of mortality following coronary artery bypass graft surgery. Participants of the Department of Veterans Affairs Cooperative Study Group on Processes, Structures, and Outcomes of Care in Cardiac Surgery. *JAMA* 1999; 281:1298.
42. Lauer MS, Eagle KA, Buckley MJ, DeSanctis RW: Atrial fibrillation following coronary artery bypass surgery. *Prog Cardiovasc Dis* 1989; 31:367.
43. Aranki SF, Shaw DP, Adams DH, et al: Predictors of atrial fibrillation after coronary artery surgery: current trends and impact on hospital resources. *Circulation* 1996; 94:390.
44. Mathew JP, Parks R, Savino JS, et al: Atrial fibrillation following coronary artery bypass graft surgery: predictors, outcomes, and resource utilization. MultiCenter Study of Perioperative Ischemia Research Group. *JAMA* 1996; 276:300.
45. Maisel WH, Rawn JD, Stevenson WG: Atrial fibrillation after cardiac surgery. *Ann Intern Med* 2001; 135:1061.
46. Almassi GH, Schowalter T, Nicolosi AC, et al: Atrial fibrillation after cardiac surgery: a major morbid event? *Ann Surg* 1997; 226:501.
47. Creswell LL, Schuessler RB, Rosenbloom M, Cox JL: Hazards of postoperative atrial arrhythmias. *Ann Thorac Surg* 1993; 56:539.
48. Yousif H, Davies G, Oakley CM: Peri-operative supraventricular arrhythmias in coronary bypass surgery. *Int J Cardiol* 1990; 26:313.
49. Taylor GJ, Malik SA, Colliver JA, et al: Usefulness of atrial fibrillation as a predictor of stroke after isolated coronary artery bypass grafting. *Am J Cardiol* 1987; 60:905.
50. Cochrane AD, Siddins M, Rosenfeldt FL, et al: A comparison of amiodarone and digoxin for treatment of supraventricular arrhythmias after cardiac surgery. *Eur J Cardiothorac Surg* 1994; 8:194.
51. Haissaguerre M, Jais P, Shah DC, et al: Spontaneous initiation of atrial fibrillation by ectopic beats originating in the pulmonary veins. *N Engl J Med* 1998; 339:659.
52. Svedjeholm R, Hakanson E: Predictors of atrial fibrillation in patients undergoing surgery for ischemic heart disease. *Scand Cardiovasc J* 2000; 34:516.
53. Andrews TC, Reimold SC, Berlin JA, Antman EM: Prevention of supraventricular arrhythmias after coronary artery bypass surgery: a meta-analysis of randomized control trials. *Circulation* 1991; 84:III236.
54. Daoud EG, Strickberger SA, Man KC, et al: Preoperative amiodarone as prophylaxis against atrial fibrillation after heart surgery. *N Engl J Med* 1997; 337:1785.
55. Butler J, Harriss DR, Sinclair M, Westaby S: Amiodarone prophylaxis for tachycardias after coronary artery surgery: a randomised, double blind, placebo controlled trial. *Br Heart J* 1993; 70:56.
56. Nystrom U, Edvardsson N, Berggren H, et al: Oral sotalol reduces the incidence of atrial fibrillation after coronary artery bypass surgery. *Thorac Cardiovasc Surg* 1993; 41:34.
57. Suttorp MJ, Kingma JH, Peels HO, et al: Effectiveness of sotalol in preventing supraventricular tachyarrhythmias shortly after coronary artery bypass grafting. *Am J Cardiol* 1991; 68:1163.
58. Blommaert D, Gonzalez M, Mucumbitsi J, et al: Effective prevention of atrial fibrillation by continuous atrial overdrive pacing after coronary artery bypass surgery. *J Am Coll Cardiol* 2000; 35: 1411.
59. Greenberg MD, Katz NM, Iuliano S, et al: Atrial pacing for the prevention of atrial fibrillation after cardiovascular surgery. *J Am Coll Cardiol* 2000; 35:1416.
60. Landymore RW, Howell F: Recurrent atrial arrhythmias following treatment for postoperative atrial fibrillation after coronary bypass operations. *Eur J Cardiothorac Surg* 1991; 5:436.
61. Chertow GM, Lazarus JM, Christiansen CL, et al: Preoperative renal risk stratification. *Circulation* 1997; 95:878.
62. Gailiunas P Jr, Chawla R, Lazarus JM, et al: Acute renal failure following cardiac operations. *J Thorac Cardiovasc Surg* 1980; 79:241.

63. Abrahamov D, Tamariz M, Fremes S, et al: Renal dysfunction after cardiac surgery. *Can J Cardiol* 2001; 17:565.
64. Fortescue EB, Bates DW, Chertow GM: Predicting acute renal failure after coronary bypass surgery: cross-validation of two risk-stratification algorithms. *Kidney Int* 2000; 57:2594.
65. Heijmeriks JA, Dassen W, Prenger K, Wellens HJ: The incidence and consequences of mental disturbances in elderly patients post cardiac surgery— comparison with younger patients. *Clin Cardiol* 2000; 23:540.
66. Vaccarino V, Abramson JL, Veledar E, Weintraub WS: Sex differences in hospital mortality after coronary artery bypass surgery: evidence for a higher mortality in younger women. *Circulation* 2002; 105:1176.
67. Palazzo RS, Barner HB: Surgery for ischemic heart disease. *Curr Opin Cardiol* 1994; 9:216.
68. Vanoverschelde JL, Gerber BL, D'Hondt AM, et al: Preoperative selection of patients with severely impaired left ventricular function for coronary revascularization: role of low-dose dobutamine echocardiography and exercise-redistribution-reinjection thallium SPECT. *Circulation* 1995; 92:II37.
69. Salati M, Lemma M, Di Mattia DG, et al: Myocardial revascularization in patients with ischemic cardiomyopathy: functional observations. *Ann Thorac Surg* 1997; 64:1728.
70. Nemec P, Bedanova H, Necas J, et al: Coronary artery bypass grafting in patients with left ventricular ejection fraction of 30% or less. *Bratisl Lek Listy* 2001; 102:15.
71. Pasquet A, Lauer MS, Williams MJ, et al: Prediction of global left ventricular function after bypass surgery in patients with severe left ventricular dysfunction: impact of pre-operative myocardial function, perfusion, and metabolism. *Eur Heart J* 2000; 21:125.
72. Dekkers RJ, FitzGerald DJ, Couper GS: Five-year clinical experience with Abiomed BVS 5000 as a ventricular assist device for cardiac failure. *Perfusion* 2001; 16:13.
73. Christenson JT, Simonet F, Badel P, Schmuziger M: Evaluation of preoperative intra-aortic balloon pump support in high risk coronary patients. *Eur J Cardiothorac Surg* 1997; 11:1097.
74. Fullerton DA, Jones SD, Jaggers J, et al: Effective control of pulmonary vascular resistance with inhaled nitric oxide after cardiac operation. *J Thorac Cardiovasc Surg* 1996; 111:753.
75. Kroenke K, Lawrence VA, Theroux JF, et al: Postoperative complications after thoracic and major abdominal surgery in patients with and without obstructive lung disease. *Chest* 1993; 104:1445.
76. Merlo C, Aidala E, La Scala E, et al: Mortality and morbidity in reoperation comparing to first intervention in coronary revascularization. *J Cardiovasc Surg* (Torino) 2001; 42:713.
77. Horton DA, Hicks RG: Reoperation for recurrent coronary artery disease–a ten year experience. *Aust N Z J Med* 1992; 22:364.
78. Lytle BW, McElroy D, McCarthy P, et al: Influence of arterial coronary bypass grafts on the mortality in coronary reoperations. *J Thorac Cardiovasc Surg* 1994; 107:675.
79. Awad WI, De Souza AC, Magee PG, et al: Re-do cardiac surgery in patients over 70 years old. *Eur J Cardiothorac Surg* 1997; 12:40.
80. Engelman DT, Adams DH, Byrne JG, et al: Impact of body mass index and albumin on morbidity and mortality after cardiac surgery. *J Thorac Cardiovasc Surg* 1999; 118:866.
81. Cook JW, Pierson LM, Herbert WG, et al: The influence of patient strength, aerobic capacity and body composition upon outcomes after coronary artery bypass grafting. *Thorac Cardiovasc Surg* 2001; 49:89.
82. Moulton MJ, Creswell LL, Mackey ME, et al: Obesity is not a risk factor for significant adverse outcomes after cardiac surgery. *Circulation* 1996; 94:II87.
83. Berger PB, Velianou JL, Aslanidou Vlachos H, et al: Survival following coronary angioplasty versus coronary artery bypass surgery in anatomic subsets in which coronary artery bypass surgery improves survival compared with medical therapy: results from the Bypass Angioplasty Revascularization Investigation (BARI). *J Am Coll Cardiol* 2001; 38:1440.
84. Morricone L, Ranucci M, Denti S, et al: Diabetes and complications after cardiac surgery: comparison with a non-diabetic population. *Acta Diabetol* 1999; 36:77.
85. Gardner TJ, Horneffer PJ, Manolio TA, et al: Major stroke after coronary artery bypass surgery: changing magnitude of the problem. *J Vasc Surg* 1986; 3:684.
86. Bull DA, Neumayer LA, Hunter GC, et al: Risk factors for stroke in patients undergoing coronary artery bypass grafting. *Cardiovasc Surg* 1993; 1:182.
87. Furlan AJ, Sila CA, Chimowitz MI, Jones SC: Neurologic complications related to cardiac surgery. *Neurol Clin* 1992; 10:145.
88. Davila-Roman VG, Murphy SF, Nickerson NJ, et al: Atherosclerosis of the ascending aorta is an independent predictor of long-term neurologic events and mortality. *J Am Coll Cardiol* 1999; 33:1308.
89. Lazar HL, Menzoian JO: Coronary artery bypass grafting in patients with cerebrovascular disease. *Ann Thorac Surg* 1998; 66:968.
90. Schwartz LB, Bridgman AH, Kieffer RW, et al: Asymptomatic carotid artery stenosis and stroke in patients undergoing cardiopulmonary bypass. *J Vasc Surg* 1995; 21:146.
91. Brenner BJ, Brief DK, Alpert JS: The risk of stroke in patients with asymptomatic carotid stenosis undergoing cardiac surgery: a follow-up study. *J Vasc Surg* 1987; 1:269.
92. Rice PL, Pifarre R, Sullivan HJ, et al: Experience with simultaneous myocardial revascularization and carotid endarterectomy. *J Thorac Cardiovasc Surg* 1980; 79:922.
93. Babu SC, Shah PM, Singh BM, et al: Coexisting carotid stenosis in patients undergoing cardiac surgery: indications and guidelines for simultaneous operations. *Am J Surg* 1985; 150:207.
94. Executive Committee for the Asymptomatic Carotid Atherosclerosis Study: Endarterectomy for asymptomatic carotid artery stenosis. *JAMA* 1995; 273:1421.
95. Hamulu A, Yagdi T, Atay Y, et al: Coronary artery bypass and carotid endarterectomy: combined approach. *Jpn Heart J* 2001; 42:539.
96. Estes JM, Khabbaz KR, Barnatan M, et al: Outcome after combined carotid endarterectomy and coronary artery bypass is related to patient selection. *J Vasc Surg* 2001; 33:1179.
97. Dylewski M, Canver CC, Chanda J, et al: Coronary artery bypass combined with bilateral carotid endarterectomy. *Ann Thorac Surg* 2001; 71:777.
98. Gaudino M, Glieca F, Luciani N, et al: Should severe monolateral asymptomatic carotid artery stenosis be treated at the time of coronary artery bypass operation? *Eur J Cardiothorac Surg* 2001; 19:619.
99. Lord RS, Graham AR, Shanahan MX, et al: Combined carotid coronary reconstructions–synchronous or sequential? *Aust N Z J Surg* 1985; 55:329.
100. Babatasi G, Massetti M, Theron J: Coexistent coronary and cerebrovascular disease: a place for carotid stenting. *Ann Thorac Surg* 1999; 68:297.
101. Nathan M, Aranki S: Transmyocardial laser revascularization. *Curr Opin Cardiol* 2001; 16:310.
102. Adams DH, Antman EM: Medical management of the patient undergoing cardiac surgery, in Braunwald E, Zipes D, Libby P (eds): *Heart Disease*. Philadelphia, WB Saunders, 2001; p 2059.
103. Cremer JT, Wittwer T, Boning A, et al: Minimally invasive coronary artery revascularization on the beating heart. *Ann Thor Surg* 2000; 67:1787.
104. Cartier R, Brann S, Dagenais F, et al: Systematic off-pump coronary artery revascularization in multivessel disease. *J Thorac Cardiovasc Surg* 2000; 119:221.

Chapter 9

Cardiac Anesthesia

Joseph S. Savino/Thomas F. Floyd/Albert T. Cheung

The objectives of a general anesthetic are to provide the patient with analgesia, amnesia, and unconsciousness while supporting vital physiologic function and creating satisfactory operating conditions. An effective general anesthetic prevents patient movement and blunts the physiologic responses to surgical trauma, nociception, and hemodynamic perturbations and permits recovery at a predictable time after operation. To accomplish this, the anesthesiologist must act as the patient's medical intensivist: support life with mechanical ventilation, control the circulation, and diagnose and treat acute emergencies during surgical incision, rapid changes in body temperature, extracorporeal circulation, and acute shifts in intravascular volume. The task in cardiac surgery is unique because of the nature of the operations and the narrow tolerance for hemodynamic alterations in patients with critical cardiac disease. Furthermore, anesthetic management of the cardiac surgical patient is intimately related to the planned operative procedure and the anticipated timing of intraoperative events.

The choice of general anesthetics is often dictated by the patient's preoperative cardiovascular function, drug pharmacokinetics, and the dose-dependent pharmacologic actions of the anesthetics. Surgical incision in the presence of inadequate concentrations of a volatile anesthetic produces hypertension, tachycardia, tachypnea, and movement. In the absence of stimulation, the same anesthetic produces cardiovascular depression, hypotension, and apnea. The anesthesiologist titrates the anesthetic to a measurable end point by monitoring cardiovascular effects. There is no direct method for assessing or monitoring adequacy of analgesia or state of awareness in a paralyzed patient, although the BIS monitor offers some insight. The BIS monitor is an integrated EEG system that relates a bispectral index to depth of general anesthesia.[1,2]

PREOPERATIVE EVALUATION

The preoperative visit by the anesthesiologist is aimed at formulation of an anesthetic plan based on the patient's surgical illness, scheduled operation, and concomitant medical problems. The anesthesiologist is responsible for informing the patient of the conduct of the planned anesthetic and associated risks and obtaining consent for the anesthesia and related procedures. The medical history is elicited by questioning the patient and reviewing the medical records. The nature and severity of the surgical illness and related cardiovascular and pulmonary disease often dictate the choice of anesthetic drugs and monitors. All anesthetic drugs have a direct effect on cardiac function, vascular tone, or the autonomic nervous system. The anesthesiologist must know the status of the cardiovascular system, related morbidity, and concurrent medications to safely design the anesthetic for a patient undergoing heart surgery.

The exchange of information between patient and physician is often a balance between providing sufficient insight regarding possible complications and producing harmful anxiety. An outline of upcoming events accompanied by an informative discussion of risks and options usually leads to informed consent. Laboratory tests are ordered to complement findings of the medical history and physical examination. Routine preoperative tests for patients scheduled for a cardiac operation include a complete blood and platelet count, electrolyte battery, determination of blood glucose, serum creatinine, and blood urea nitrogen levels, prothrombin time and partial thromboplastin time, chest radiograph, electrocardiogram (ECG), and urinalysis.

The American Society of Anesthesiologists (ASA) has developed a physical status classification as a general measure of the patient's severity of illness (Table 9-1).[3] Concurrent medical illness often defines an acceptable range for monitored parameters that are controlled during cardiac surgery, contributes to postoperative morbidity, or influences the response to a specific drug. Acceptable intraoperative blood pressure is defined by the range of blood pressure before surgery. A severely hypertensive patient may inadequately perfuse vital organs if the blood pressure during surgery is maintained within a "normal" range rather than within the patient's usual range. A previous stroke with apparent recovery may become manifest after general anesthesia without evidence of a new neurologic injury. Chronic obstructive pulmonary disease and its response to bronchodilators permit guided management of perioperative bronchospasm and inadequate respiration. Prior surgical and anesthetic procedures are investigated by reviewing medical records. A history of a difficult intubation or adverse response to a specific drug is highly relevant to the anesthesia plan.

TABLE 9–1 American Society of Anesthesiologists' physical status classification

Class 1: Normal healthy patient
Class 2: Systemic disease without end-organ dysfunction
Class 3: Systemic disease with end-organ dysfunction that is not incapacitating (e.g., diabetes mellitus with abnormal renal function)
Class 4: Systemic disease with end-organ dysfunction that is incapacitating (e.g., diabetes mellitus with renal failure and ketoacidosis)
Class 5: Moribund patient unexpected to survive beyond 24 hours (e.g., diabetes mellitus with renal failure, ketoacidosis, and infarcted bowel requiring vasopressor support)
E*: Emergency surgery

*The E is added to the classification number.

Concurrent medications usually are continued until the operation, although the dose may be altered or a shorter-acting preparation substituted. Oral medications are administered according to schedule on the day of surgery with a small sip of water. Intravenous heparin given for unstable angina pectoris is not discontinued before surgical incision. For patients scheduled for late afternoon surgery and not receiving maintenance intravenous fluids, preoperative diuretics may be withheld to avoid dehydration. The physical examination includes measurement of vital signs and height and weight and a comprehensive assessment of the heart, lungs, peripheral vasculature, nervous system, and airway. Samsoon's modification of the Mallampati classification to predict a difficult airway is based on the examiner's ability to view intraoral structures[4,5]:

Class 1: Soft palate, tonsillar fauces, tonsillar pillars, and uvula
Class 2: Soft palate, tonsillar fauces, and uvula
Class 3: Soft palate and base of uvula
Class 4: Soft palate not visualized

Classes 1 and 2 represent airway anatomy associated with minimal difficulty with tracheal intubation. Classes 3 and 4 are more likely associated with an inability to intubate the trachea using conventional direct laryngoscopy. Other features associated with difficult intubations include a recessed chin, small mouth, large tongue, and inability to sublux the mandible.

Before the patient enters the operating room, the anesthesiologist formulates a plan to control the circulatory response to anesthesia, secure the airway, and maintain body homeostasis. Emergency operation frequently is incompatible with leisurely preparation but is dictated by a sense of urgency. Rarely is there no opportunity to provide reassurance or to meticulously prepare for anesthesia and operation.

MONITORING PHYSIOLOGICAL FUNCTIONS DURING ANESTHESIA

Extensive physiological monitoring is employed during cardiac operations because virtually every major physiological system required for life is affected. The reasons for physiological monitoring are: (1) to ensure patient safety in the absence of protective reflexes made ineffective by anesthetic drugs; (2) to enable pharmacological and mechanical control of vital function; and (3) to diagnose acute emergencies that require immediate treatment. For example, morbidity as a consequence of breathing circuit disconnects, loss of oxygen from the hospital's central supply, or unrecognized esophageal or main-stem intubations can be prevented by capnography, pulse oximetry, airway pressure monitors, oxygen analyzers, and a stethoscope.

The senses of touch, hearing, and sight are the basic monitors. Electronic monitors are vigilance aids that supplement the anesthesiologist's perceptions. In setting up a monitoring and diagnostic system, it is important to establish the sensitivity and specificity for detecting physiological changes and disease. Sensitivity is a measure of the ability of a monitor to detect change in whatever is measured (measurand). Specificity is the degree that a change in the measurand is peculiar to a singular condition or disease. Sensitivity and specificity of a monitor depend on sensor calibration, accuracy, and precision. A sensor is an instrument that detects change in the measurand and provides a corresponding output signal. Calibration is the relationship between the measurand and the output signal, such that the magnitude of the output signal reflects the magnitude of the parameter being measured. Pressure transducers, light detectors, flowmeters, thermistors, and gas analyzers are examples of sensors commonly used in the operating room. The ideal sensor is accurate during static and dynamic conditions, precise, reliable, safe, practical, and inexpensive. Accuracy is defined by how well the output signal agrees with the true value or a calibration quality standard. Precision is a measure of repeatability. A sensor is precise if it provides little variability between repeated measures. A pulse oximeter is an accurate monitor of percentage of oxyhemoglobin because it agrees with in vitro measures (between values of 80% to 100%). Thermodilution is an imprecise method of determining cardiac output because successive measurements vary by 20% or more. All monitors are properly calibrated prior to clinical use, and specifications for accuracy and precision must be established to maximize sensitivity and specificity for detecting diagnosing change.

The selection of monitors is dictated by the utility of the generated data, expense, and risk. Routine or essential monitors that have been deemed cost-effective with low risk-benefit ratios include pulse oximetry, noninvasive blood pressure, capnography, temperature, ECG, precordial or esophageal stethoscope, and oxygen analyzers. These have been defined by the American Society of Anesthesiologists (House of Delegates, 1989) as essential monitors to be used in all surgical patients requiring anesthesia unless there are contraindications (e.g., esophageal stethoscope during esophageal surgery) (Table 9-2). Other noninvasive and invasive monitors are used only with clear indication.

The growth in monitoring technology and sophistication is paralleled by an equal growth in cost. The balance between cost and enhancement of patient safety must be considered when additional monitoring is selected. It is difficult to justify a monitor that provides data that do not influence medical or surgical management. Improved safety decreases patient morbidity and mortality, decreases the direct costs of health care providers, and reduces legal costs, insurance premiums, and possibly the risk of early retirement by physicians. However, monitors do not interpret data and must themselves be monitored by a human being.

TABLE 9–2 Physiological monitors

Organ system	ASA standard operating room monitors	Additional monitoring for cardiac surgery
Cardiovascular	ECG Noninvasive blood pressure	Invasive blood pressure CVP PAP/PAOP Cardiac output Svo_2 TEE
Pulmonary	Capnography Pulse oximeter Airway pressures Stethoscope Oxygen analyzer	Arterial blood gases
Nervous system		EEG SSEP Transcranial Doppler CSF pressure
Metabolic	Temperature Urine output	Serum electrolytes Acid-base Glucose Serum osmolarity Hematocrit

Measurement of Blood Pressure

Blood pressure changes abruptly during anesthesia and surgery and is the most commonly measured index of cardiovascular stability in the perioperative period. Anesthetics and surgery cause changes in blood pressure that may be great enough to cause harm unless anticipated and treated. A change in blood pressure alters perfusion pressure but may not change organ blood flow. Most vital organs have autoregulation of blood flow in response to changes in mean arterial blood pressure, permitting a constant blood flow over a range of perfusion pressures.[6] In hypertensive patients, the boundaries for autoregulation are shifted so that significant decreases in organ perfusion may occur with blood pressures in the "normal" range. Both the type and dose of anesthetic medications affect the relationship between vital organ perfusion and blood pressure. Volatile anesthetics are potent vasodilators that tend to disrupt autoregulation in a dose-dependent manner to render blood flow more linearly dependent on blood pressure (Fig. 9-1).

Although noninvasive blood pressure monitoring suffices for most patients during routine noncardiac surgery, direct measure of arterial blood pressure with an indwelling

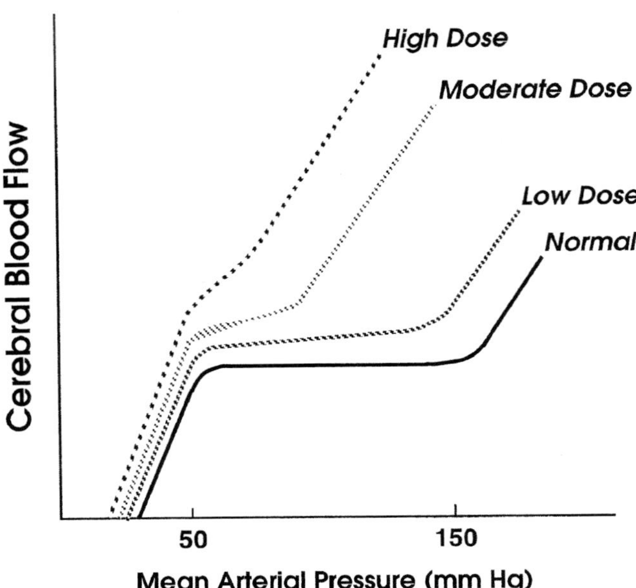

FIGURE 9–1 Autoregulation maintains a constant cerebral blood flow between mean arterial blood pressures of 50 to 150 mm Hg in the conscious, unanesthetized state. Increasing doses of potent inhalation anesthetics produce a dose-dependent disruption of autoregulation due to cerebral vasodilatation. *(Modified with permission from Shapiro H: Anesthesia effects upon cerebral blood flow, cerebral metabolism, electroencephalogram and evoked potentials, in Miller RD (ed): Anesthesia, 2d ed. New York, Churchill-Livingstone, 1986; p 1249.)*

catheter is necessary for cardiac surgery in order to detect changes rapidly, to measure nonpulsatile blood pressure during cardiopulmonary bypass, and to facilitate blood sampling for laboratory analysis. The measuring system includes an intra-arterial catheter and low-compliance saline-filled tubing connected to a transducer with a pressure-sensing diaphragm. The transducer has a strain gauge that converts the mechanical energy (displacement of the diaphragm by a change in pressure) into an electric signal that is typically displayed as a pressure waveform with numeric outputs for systolic, diastolic, and mean pressures. The mean blood pressure is determined by calculating the area under several pulse waveforms and averaging over time. This represents a more accurate measure of mean arterial blood pressure than weighted averages of systolic and diastolic pressures.

The transducer requires a zero reference at the level of the right atrium. Any movement of the patient or the transducer that changes the vertical distance between the transducer and the right atrium affects the value of the blood pressure measured. If the transducer is lowered, the pressure diaphragm senses arterial blood pressure plus hydrostatic pressure generated from the vertical column of fluid contained in the tubing and displays a falsely high blood pressure. A transducer elevated above the zero reference level decreases the displayed blood pressure. A 1-cm column of water (blood) exerts a hydrostatic pressure equal to 0.74 mm Hg. Small changes in patient or transducer position have a relatively insignificant effect on arterial blood pressure measurements but have a more important effect on lower amplitude pressure measurements, such as central venous, pulmonary artery, and pulmonary artery occlusion pressures.

The intra-arterial cannula, tubing, and transducer assembly are prepared prior to surgery and flushed with heparinized saline. All air bubbles must be cleared from the system to prevent damping and air embolism. The radial artery is the most common site for the insertion of an intra-arterial catheter. The increased use of arterial conduits for coronary grafts limits the possible sites for monitoring. Twenty-gauge catheters are preferred because larger catheters are more likely to cause thrombosis. Thrombosis of the radial artery does not produce ischemia of the hand and fingers in the presence of intact ulnar blood flow and a patent palmar arch although distal emboli remain a risk. The Allen test was designed to assess ulnar and palmar arch blood flow during abrupt occlusion of the radial artery, but its value to predict morbidity with radial artery cannulation is equivocal.[7] Other sites selected for the insertion of an intra-arterial catheter include the brachial, axillary, and femoral arteries.

The contour of the arterial pressure waveform is different in central and peripheral arteries. The propagating pressure waveform loses energy and momentum with a corresponding delay in transmission, loss of high-frequency components such as anacrotic and dicrotic notches, lower systolic and pulse pressures, and decreased mean pressure.[8] The changes in the pulse waveform can be attributed to damping, blood viscosity, vessel diameter, vessel elastance, and the effects of reflectance of the incident arterial waveform by the artery-arteriolar junction.[9,10] The blood pressure waveform measured in the ascending aorta is minimally affected by reflected waves in contrast to the measurement of blood pressure in the dorsalis pedis or radial artery. Vasodilators decrease terminal impedance at the artery-arteriolar junction and decrease the resonant frequency of the arterial waveform.

The contour of the pressure waveform is affected by the physical construction of the monitoring system. A hyperresonant response to a change in pressure, or *ringing*, occurs when the frequency response of the monitoring system (extension tubing, catheter, stopcocks) is close to the frequency of the pressure waveform.[8] The natural or *resonant frequency* fn of a monitoring system is defined by

$$fn = \frac{1}{2\pi}\sqrt{\frac{\pi D^2}{4pL \cdot C}}$$

where C = compliance of the measuring system, L = length of the tubing, D = diameter of the catheter extension tubing, and p = density of the solution.

To prevent ringing, the natural frequency of the monitoring system, fn, must be greater than the frequencies of the pulse waveform. Any process that decreases *fn*, such as narrow, long, compliant tubing, may cause ringing.[11] Ringing increases the value of the systolic blood pressure and decreases the value of the diastolic blood pressure but generally does not affect the value of the mean arterial pressure.

Damping is the tendency of the measuring system, through frictional losses, to blunt the peaks and troughs in a signal.[12] Kinks in the pressure tubing or catheter, stopcocks, and air bubbles contribute to damping. Overdamped systems underestimate systolic blood pressure and overestimate diastolic blood pressure. When long lengths of tubing are necessary, deliberate damping may improve the fidelity of the arterial waveform.

Testing a measuring system for ringing and damping ensures that an arterial contour is faithfully reproduced. A simple test is the brief flush of a high-pressure heparinized saline-filled catheter-extension assembly. Flush and release should produce a rapid return of the pressure waveform to baseline with minimal oscillations. A gradual return to baseline and loss of higher-frequency components of the waveform suggest overdamping. A rapid return to baseline followed by sustained oscillations suggests ringing.

Electrocardiogram

The intraoperative electrocardiogram (ECG) monitor has evolved from the fading ball oscilloscope to a sophisticated microprocessor analog display. ECG signals are digitally filtered to eliminate electrical artifact produced by high-frequency (60-Hz) electrical power lines, electrocautery, patient movement, and baseline drift. The bandwidth filter modes are diagnostic, monitor, and filter. The diagnostic mode has the widest bandwidths (least filtered signal) and is preferred for detecting ST-segment changes caused by myocardial ischemia. Monitor and filter modes have progressively narrower bandwidths that effectively eliminate high-frequency interference and baseline drift but decrease the sensitivity of detecting ST-segment changes and decrease the specificity of ST-segment change to diagnose myocardial ischemia. Abnormal ST-segment depression (>1 mV) can occur from excessive low-frequency filtering and result in the misdiagnosis of myocardial ischemia. Filter modes are useful for detecting P waves and changes in cardiac rhythm in the presence of high-frequency interference.

The ECG is the most sensitive and practical monitor for the detection and diagnosis of disorders of cardiac rhythm and conduction and myocardial ischemia and infarction. Continuous monitoring of leads II and V_5 is common (Fig. 9-2). Together, these leads detect greater than 90% of ischemic episodes in patients with coronary artery disease who have noncardiac surgery.[13] The ECG leads selected for monitoring of myocardial ischemia can be guided by preoperative testing. Myocardium at risk, identified by exercise testing or coronary angiograms, can be monitored by selecting the lead with the appropriate vector. A reversible perfusion defect of

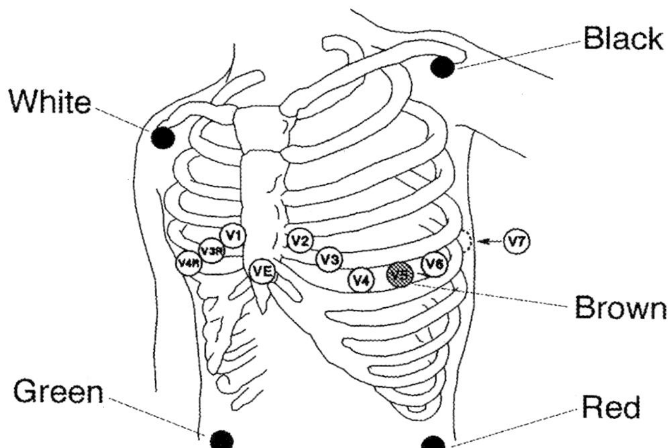

FIGURE 9–2 Standard intraoperative electrocardiogram (ECG) lead placement. Typically, leads II and V_5 are continuously monitored.

the inferior wall of the left ventricle during an exercise thallium reperfusion scan may encourage the anesthesiologist to specifically monitor leads II, III, and AVF.

Diagnostic criteria for myocardial ischemia based on the ECG are (1) acute ST-segment depression greater than 0.1 mV 60 msec beyond the J point or (2) acute ST-segment elevation greater than 0.2 mV 60 msec beyond the J point (see Fig. 9-3).[14] The normal ST-segment curves smoothly into the T wave. Flat ST segments that form an acute angle with the T wave or downsloping ST segments are worrisome for subendocardial ischemia. ST-segment elevation occurs with transmural myocardial injury but also may occur after direct-current (DC) cardioversion and in normal adults. The lack of specificity of ST-T wave changes for myocardial ischemia is a major limitation of intraoperative ECG monitoring. Pericarditis, myocarditis, mitral valve prolapse, stroke, and digitalis therapy may produce changes in the ST segment that mimic myocardial ischemia.

Digital signal processing handles much larger quantities of information compared to the unaided eye and may increase the ability to detect ischemic episodes. ST-segment position analyzers automatically measure the displacement of the ST segment from a predetermined reference and enhance the ability to quantify changes in ST-segment position. Appropriate application requires accurate identification of the various loci in the P-QRS-T wave complex. The operator defines the baseline and the J point of a reference QRS complex by movement of a cursor. New QRS-T wave complexes are superimposed onto a predefined mean reference complex. Vertical ST-segment displacement is measured in millivolts and displayed graphically in 1-mV increments (see Fig. 9-3). Because the accuracy of automated ST-segment monitoring is vulnerable to baseline drift and dependent on the appropriate identification of the PR and ST segments, the diagnosis of myocardial ischemia is always verified by inspecting the actual ECG tracing.

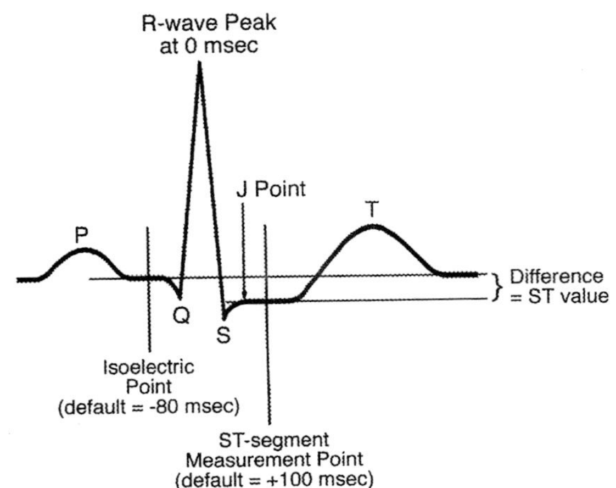

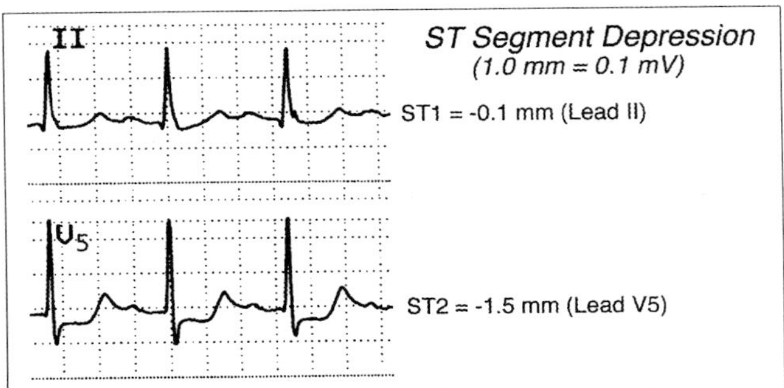

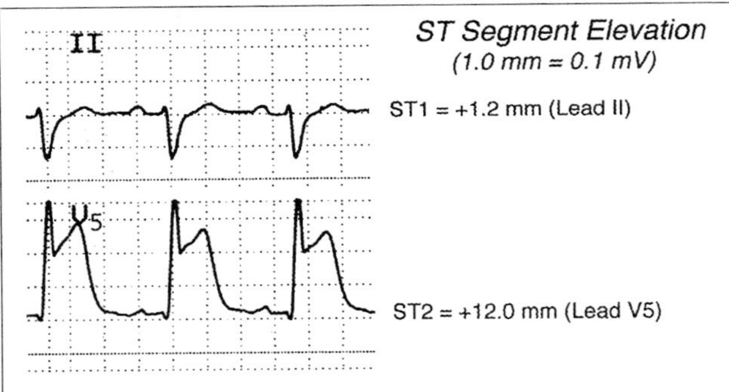

FIGURE 9–3 Automated ST-segment monitoring of the ECG can be used to detect intraoperative myocardial ischemia. General criteria for myocardial ischemia are ST-segment depression greater than 0.1 mV or ST-segment elevation greater than 0.4 mV that persists for longer than 1 minute. At fast heart rates, the ST-segment measurement point may occur on the upslope of the T wave, causing erroneous indication of ST-segment elevation.

Disturbances of rhythm and conduction are common during anesthesia and especially during cardiac surgery. Instrumentation of the heart, hypothermia, electrolyte abnormalities, myocardial reperfusion, myocardial ischemia, and mechanical factors such as surgical manipulation of the heart affect the normal propagation of the cardiac action potential. Heart rate is measured by averaging several RR intervals of the ECG. The ECG may not sense the R wave of the selected lead if the electrical vector is isoelectric. A prominent T wave or pacemaker spike may be miscounted as an R wave by the ECG and artifactually double the rate. Usually, heart rate is best monitored by selecting the lead with an upright R wave and adjusting the sensitivity.

The QT interval can only be measured on hard copy. A normal QT interval is less than half the RR interval, but the QT interval must be corrected for heart rates higher than 90 or lower than 65 beats per minute. A prolonged QT interval increases the risk of reentrant ventricular tachydysrhythmias and may occur from hypokalemia, hypothermia, and toxic drug effect (quinidine or procainamide). The electrically dormant heart during aortic cross-clamping and perfusion with cold cardioplegia is monitored by the ECG. Hypothermia decreases action potential conduction velocity and high-dose potassium decreases the transcell membrane potassium concentration gradient to prevent depolarization of cardiac muscle. During cardiopulmonary bypass and aortic cross-clamping, the loss and persistent absence of electromechanical activity suggest that myocardial oxygen consumption is maintained at a minimum.

Monitoring the ECG is most valuable when it begins before induction of general anesthesia. A hard copy of the pertinent leads permits comparison should a change be detected. An abnormal or marginal finding is less worrisome if it was present in the preoperative ECG and remains unchanged during the perioperative period. However, new-onset ST-T wave changes or disturbances in rhythm and conduction suggest an ongoing active process that usually requires immediate attention.

Capnography

Capnometry is the measure of carbon dioxide (CO_2) concentration in a gas. The capnogram is the continuous graphic display of airway carbon dioxide partial pressure (Fig. 9-4). Changes in its contour reflect disorders of ventilation, carbon dioxide production, or carbon dioxide transport to the lungs. The capnogram is the single most effective monitor for detecting esophageal intubation, apnea, breathing circuit disconnects, accidental extubation of the trachea, and airway obstruction. Tracheal intubation is verified by detection of

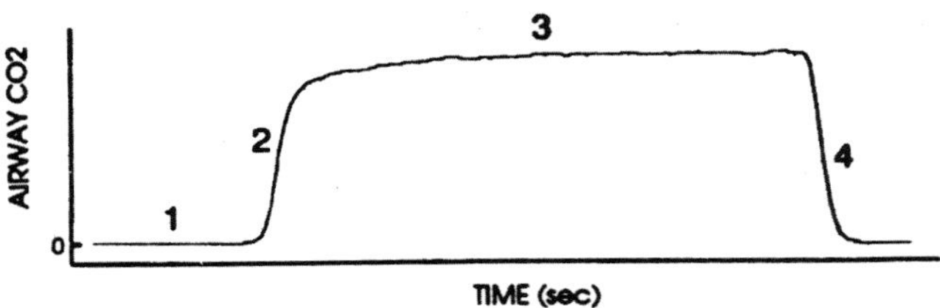

FIGURE 9–4 The normal capnogram: (1) inspired CO_2 concentration = zero, (2) washout of anatomic dead space, (3) plateau represents alveolar gas CO_2 content, and (4) beginning of inhalation.

physiologic carbon dioxide concentrations in the exhaled gas. A steep increase in the phase 3 slope in the exhaled CO_2 concentration suggests partial airway obstruction, either mechanical (tube kinking) or physiologic (bronchospasm). A progressive decrease in exhaled carbon dioxide concentration occurs with decreased CO_2 production (hypothermia), increased minute ventilation, increase in physiologic dead space ventilation (e.g., pulmonary embolus), or low cardiac output. A progressive increase in exhaled carbon dioxide concentration occurs with hypoventilation, increased CO_2 production (malignant hyperthermia), or increased delivery of CO_2 to the lungs, such as occurs during weaning off bypass. The contour of the capnogram is also affected by the expiratory flow rate, distribution of pulmonary blood flow, distribution of ventilation, and the use of sidestream or mainstream carbon dioxide analyzers. Despite the interplay of mechanical and physiologic factors that affect the shape of the capnogram, any abrupt change in contour always signifies an acute change in the patient's cardiovascular, pulmonary, or metabolic state.

Pulse Oximetry

Pulse oximeters were universally adopted into the practice of anesthesia almost immediately after their introduction despite lack of data demonstrating improved outcome with their use. Oxyhemoglobin saturation and arterial oxygen tension are measured routinely during cardiac surgery by intermittent arterial blood sampling. Arterial blood gas analysis does not replace the pulse oximeter, which continuously measures arterial hemoglobin saturation and pulse rate. The pulse oximeter detects decreasing percentages of oxyhemoglobin before changes in the color of the patient's skin or blood are evident.[15] The pulse oximeter is reusable, inexpensive, and noninvasive, and provides continuous online data. Its major limitations include electrical interference, motion artifact, high failure rate during periods of low flow or inadequate perfusion, and the need for pulsatile flow for proper operation.[16]

Pulse oximetry measures the percentage of oxyhemoglobin in arterial blood by transillumination and detection of differences in the optical absorption properties of oxy- and deoxyhemoglobin. Transmission oximetry at wavelengths of 660 and 940 nm and photoplethysmography and rapid signal processing permit reliable and rapid determination of the relative proportion of oxy- and deoxyhemoglobin. Oxyhemoglobin has a higher optical absorption in the infrared spectrum (940 nm), whereas reduced hemoglobin absorbs more light in the red band (660 nm). The ratio R of light absorbance at the two wavelengths is a function of the relative proportions of the two forms of hemoglobin.

Photoplethysmography permits the measure of arterial hemoglobin saturation by isolating the pulsatile component of the absorbed signal. The peaks and troughs in the blood volume of the finger or ear being transilluminated produce a corresponding pulsatile effect on light absorption, rendering the calculated oxyhemoglobin saturation independent of nonpulsatile venous blood and soft tissue. Calculation of arterial hemoglobin saturation is based on calibration algorithms derived from healthy volunteers. The R values were determined by in vitro measures of oxyhemoglobin saturation and are less accurate at oxyhemoglobin saturations below 70%. Motion artifact produces a high absorption of light at both wavelengths and an R value of approximately 1 that corresponds to an oxyhemoglobin saturation of approximately 85%.

The pulse oximeter is unable to distinguish other hemoglobin species that absorb light at the emitted wavelengths. Methemoglobin (ferric instead of ferrous hemoglobin) has similar absorption at both 660 and 940 nm with an R value of 1 and a corresponding displayed saturation of 85% regardless of the true value. Carbon monoxide poisoning produces carboxyhemoglobin that has significant absorption at 660 nm and is erroneously interpreted by the pulse oximeter as oxyhemoglobin.

Measurement of Temperature

Profound changes in body temperature during cardiac surgery are common, often deliberate, and affect vital organ function (Fig. 9-5). Anesthetized patients are poikilothermic. Intrinsic temperature regulation normally controlled by the hypothalamus fails during general anesthesia. Hypothermia occurs by passive and active heat loss. Passive mechanisms of cooling include radiation, evaporation, convection, and conduction. Active cooling usually occurs with extracorporeal circulation and with the use of cold or iced solutions poured into the chest cavity. Deliberate hypothermia during cardiac surgery is designed to arrest and cool the heart and decrease systemic oxygen consumption. Hyperthermia may result from preexisting fever, bacteremia, malignant hyperthermia, or overzealous rewarming during cardiopulmonary bypass.

Malignant hyperthermia is a rare inherited disorder of muscle and is potentially fatal.[17] It is an autosomal dominant trait with variable penetrance that is almost always quiescent until the patient is exposed to a triggering agent, such as volatile anesthetics or succinylcholine. Malignant hyperthermia is associated with derangements in calcium metabolism. Ineffective uptake of calcium by sarcoplasmic reticulum and abnormal release of calcium from intracellular storage sites occurs with massive skeletal muscle depolarization in response to triggering agents. Clinical manifestations of malignant hyperthermia include increased production of carbon dioxide, tachycardia, and increased cardiac output, followed by fever, metabolic and respiratory acidosis, hyperkalemia, cellular hypoxia, rhabdomyolysis, myoglobinuria, renal failure, and cardiovascular collapse. Serum creatine kinase is increased and may be of diagnostic value. The fever may reach 43°C but may be masked by deliberate

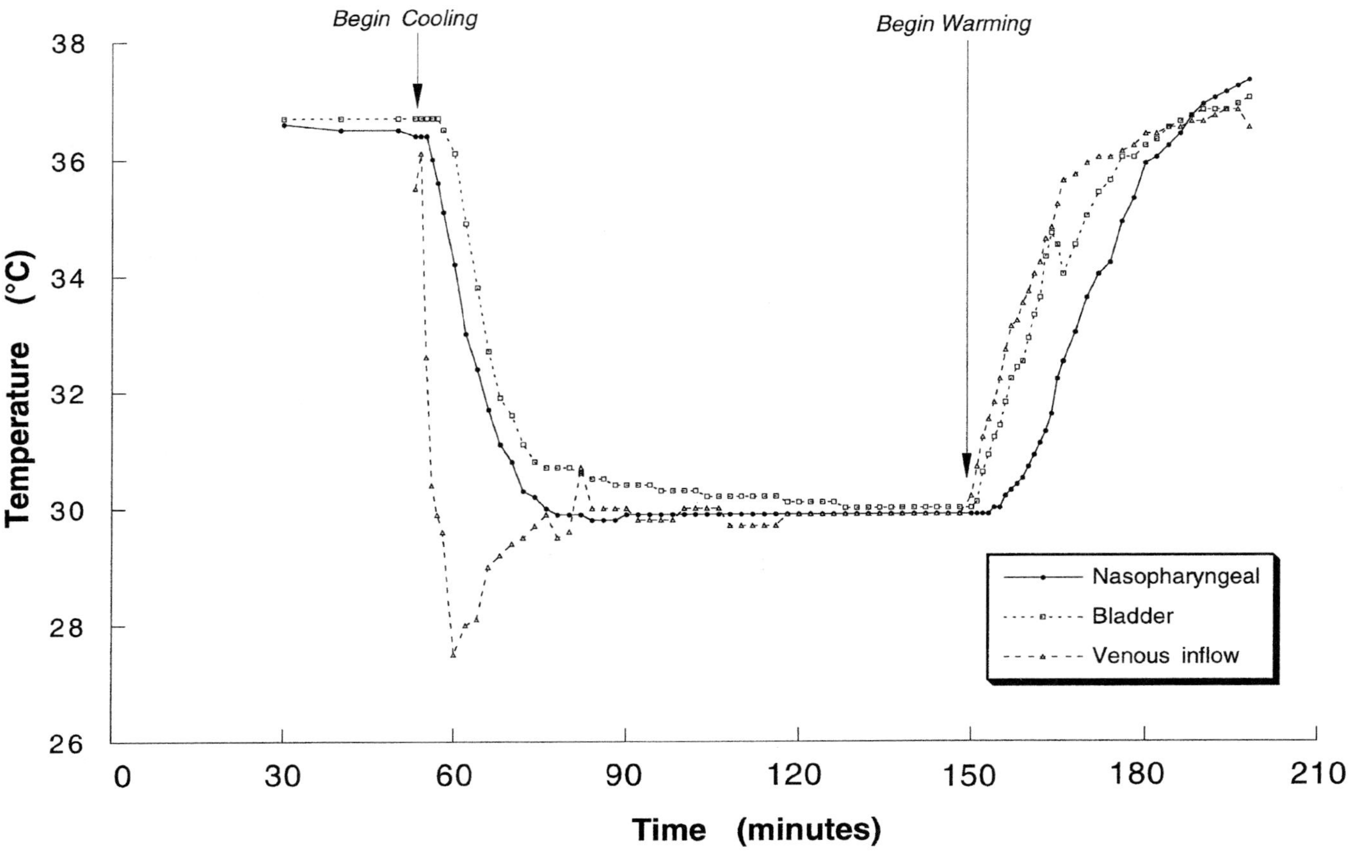

FIGURE 9–5 Changes in body temperature during hypothermic cardiopulmonary bypass. A brisk diuresis accompanied rewarming, rendering the urine an ultrafiltrate of blood and resulting in the urine (bladder) temperature closely tracking temperature measured in the venous blood in the cardiopulmonary bypass machine.

hypothermia during cardiopulmonary bypass. Despite increased awareness, improved monitors, and the advent of established treatment algorithms with dantrolene, mortality rates remain high. Treatment is aimed at discontinuing the trigger agent and controlling body temperature through active cooling. Oxygen, hyperventilation, and correction of metabolic acidosis and electrolyte abnormalities are the cornerstone of therapy.

Dantrolene blocks calcium release and is administered at a dose of 2 mg/kg intravenously every 5 minutes for a total dose of 10 mg/kg.[18] Intravenous dantrolene is generally continued at 12-hour intervals for a minimum of 24 hours because episodes of malignant hyperthermia may recur even after the trigger agent has been discontinued. The incidence of malignant hyperthermia is approximately 1 in 62,000 anesthetics. Patients with a history of malignant hyperthermia and those with most types of muscular dystrophies are at increased risk. Not all episodes of malignant hyperthermia lead to progressive metabolic and cardiovascular collapse. Unexplained fever after an anesthetic or in the recovery room may identify a patient at increased risk. Testing by in vitro skeletal muscle responses to halothane and/or caffeine is recommended for the preoperative diagnosis of patients suspected to be at increased risk. High-risk patients can be anesthetized safely by using anesthetic drugs such as narcotics, barbiturates, nitrous oxide, local anesthetics, and nondepolarizing muscle relaxants that are not believed to trigger malignant hyperthermia.

Hypothermia after cardiopulmonary bypass is the result of ineffective rewarming, cold operating rooms, cold wet surgical drapes, a large surgical incision, and the administration of cold intravenous fluids. Hypothermia exacerbates dysrhythmias and coagulopathy, potentiates the effects of anesthetic drugs and neuromuscular blockers, increases vascular resistance, decreases the availability of oxygen, and contributes to postoperative shivering. The elderly are especially susceptible because of limited compensatory reserve.

Temperature is typically monitored from several sites during cardiac surgery. Blood temperature is measured from the tip of the pulmonary artery catheter and within the cardiopulmonary bypass circuit (typically venous and arterial lines). Blood temperature is the first to change in response to deliberate hypothermia or active rewarming during cardiopulmonary bypass. Nasopharyngeal and tympanic

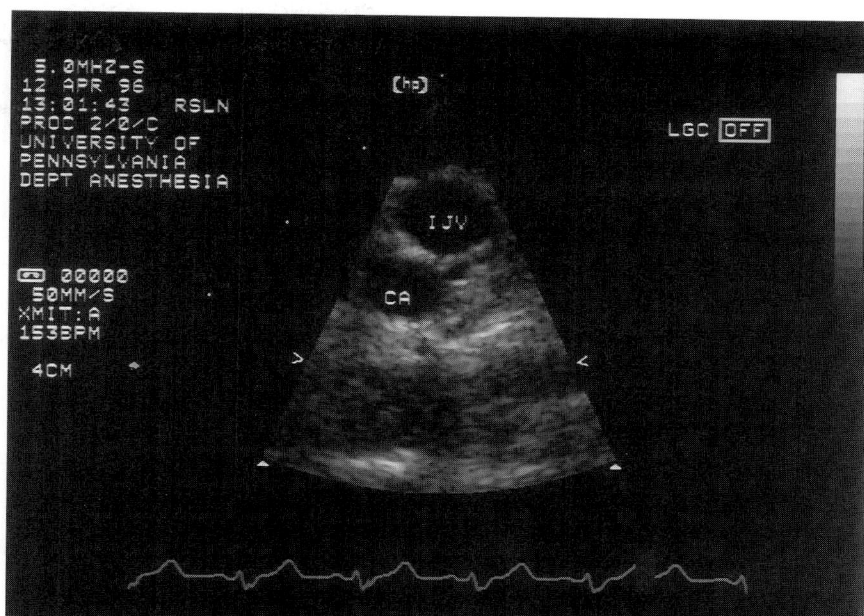

FIGURE 9–6 A two-dimensional short-axis image of the internal jugular vein (IJV) and carotid artery (CA) using a handheld ultrasound transducer.

temperatures reflect the temperature of the brain and closely track blood temperature because these sites are highly perfused. Rectal and bladder temperatures provide a measure of core temperature only at equilibrium. Esophageal temperature often underestimates core temperature because of the cooling effects of ventilation in the adjacent trachea. Axillary and inguinal temperature are shell measurements and are impractical.

The degree and site of temperature change are important indicators of an intact circulatory system. A persistent discrepancy in temperature between two sites may be a sign of malperfusion. Rewarming during cardiopulmonary bypass is normally associated with an increase in nasopharyngeal or tympanic temperature accompanied by a more gradual increase in temperature in organs with low perfusion. A persistently cold nasopharynx with a normal rate of increase in rectal temperature may be due to aortic dissection and hypoperfusion of the head.

Measurement of Cardiac Output and Central Venous and Pulmonary Artery Pressures

Cannulation of the central venous circulation permits central administration of drugs, passage of catheters and pacing electrodes into the heart, rapid administration of fluids through short, large-bore cannulas, and the measure of central venous pressure. The most commonly used site for central venous access is the internal jugular vein because of easy, reliable insertion, easy access from the head of the table, decreased risk of pneumothorax, and decreased risk of catheter kinking during sternal retraction. The subclavian vein is the preferred site for the insertion of a central venous catheter for long-term intravenous total parenteral nutrition because of a decreased risk of blood-borne infection.[19] The most important complication of internal jugular vein cannulation is inadvertent puncture or cannulation of the carotid or subclavian artery. Cannulation of the central venous circulation is confirmed by transducing the pressure waveform prior to the insertion of a large-bore catheter. Ultrasound-guided cannulation of the internal jugular vein renders the procedure less dependent on anatomic landmarks and is associated with a decrease in the number of unsuccessful cannulation attempts (Fig. 9-6).[20]

Central venous pressure (CVP) is an index of right ventricular preload. The pulsatile a, c, and v pulse waveforms are a function of uninterrupted return of venous blood to the right atrium, right atrial contraction and right atrial size and compliance, intrathoracic pressure, and mechanical properties of the tricuspid valve and right ventricle. The normal CVP is 6 to 10 mm Hg and is measured at end-exhalation. A decrease in CVP suggests hypovolemia or vasodilation. An increased CVP with normal cardiac function occurs with hypervolemia, vasoconstriction, and increased intrathoracic pressure. CVP is increased by positive pressure ventilation and positive end-expiratory pressure. Systemic hypotension accompanied by an increased CVP suggests cardiac dysfunction. The most common cause of venous hypertension is left-sided heart failure, although acute left ventricular dysfunction may cause an increase in left atrial and pulmonary artery occlusion pressure without significant change in CVP.

Pulmonary artery catheters are inserted via the central venous circulation through the right side of the heart with the catheter tip positioned just downstream to the pulmonic valve. The pulmonary artery catheter measures pulmonary

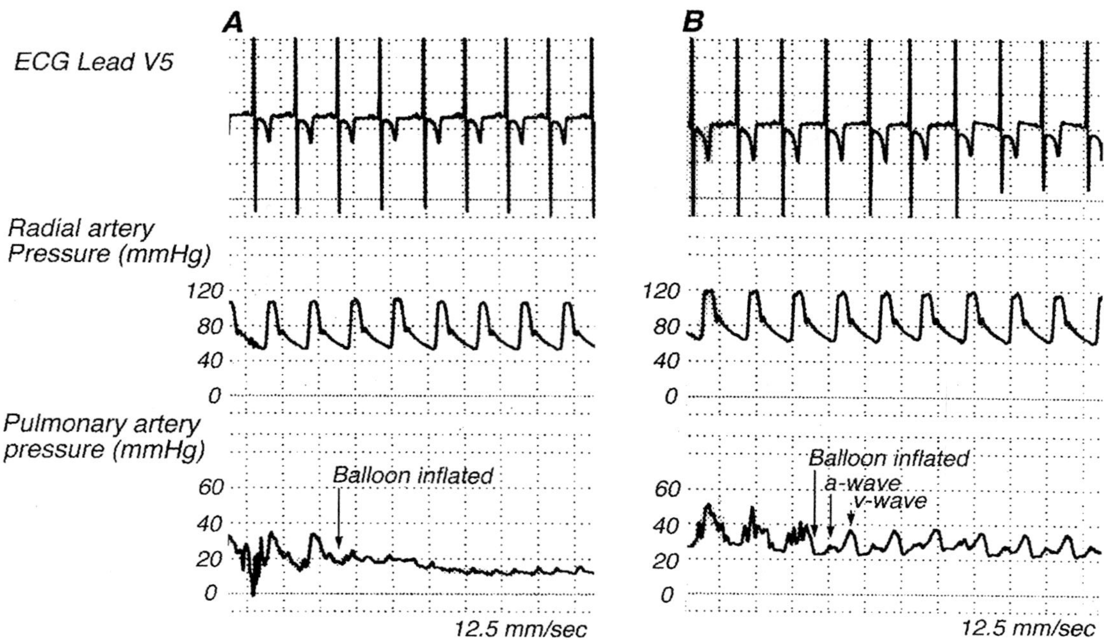

FIGURE 9–7 Pulmonary artery occlusion pressure tracing at two time points. The acute onset of myocardial ischemia (B) was associated with ST-segment depression in ECG lead V_5, increased pulmonary artery pressures, and a prominent v wave.

artery pressure, pulmonary artery occlusion pressure, cardiac output, and mixed venous oxygen saturation and permits calculation of the derived values of systemic and pulmonary vascular resistance. The pulmonary artery occlusion pressure is an index of left ventricular preload in the absence of mitral stenosis. However, the use of a pressure measurement to estimate preload is limited because of variability in left ventricular size and compliance. The hemodynamic parameters derived from the pulmonary artery catheter may be used to detect myocardial ischemia if ischemia produces ventricular dysfunction that is associated with a decrease in cardiac output, increase in left ventricular end-diastolic pressure, or pulmonary hypertension (Fig. 9-7). However, hemodynamic parameters derived from the pulmonary artery catheter are not as sensitive or as specific for detecting myocardial ischemia as the ECG.[21] Pulmonary artery occlusion pressure is affected by volume status, myocardial compliance, mode of ventilation, and ventricular afterload.

Complications associated with the insertion of a pulmonary artery catheter include dislodgment of pacemaker wires or right atrial or ventricular clot or tumor, atrial and ventricular arrhythmias, pulmonary infarction, pulmonary artery rupture, catheter entrapment, and heart block. The incidence of right bundle branch block (RBBB) is approximately 3% and may cause complete heart block in patients with a preexisting left bundle branch block (LBBB).[22] A mechanism to treat complete heart block (e.g., external pacer) should be available for these patients. The passage of the pulmonary artery catheter can be delayed for most patients until after sternotomy, when heart block can be treated with epicardial pacing wires. Chronic indwelling pulmonary artery catheters are associated with a progressive thrombocytopenia.[23] Heparin-bonded catheters decrease the incidence of thrombus formation,[24] but high-dose aprotinin may increase the risk of early thrombus formation.[25]

Multiport pulmonary artery catheters equipped with a tip thermistor permit the measure of pulmonary blood flow or cardiac output by thermodilution. Thermodilution cardiac output is an indicator-dilution technique. The indicator, a known volume of cold saline, is injected rapidly into the right atrium. Cardiac output is calculated from the rate of change in blood temperature in the pulmonary artery over time using the Stewart Hamilton equation[26,27]:

$$\mathrm{CO} = \frac{V(T_B - T_I)K_1K_2}{\int_0^{\infty} \Delta T_B(t)\,dt}$$

where CO = cardiac output, V = volume of injectate, T_B = blood temperature at time = 0, T_I = injectate temperature at time = 0, $\Delta T_B(t)$ is the change in blood temperature at time = t, K_1 = density factor, and K_2 = computation factor.

Thermodilution measures the degree of mixing that occurs between the cold injectate and blood. More mixing implies increased flow. Complete mixing of 10 mL of cold injectate with a circulating blood volume produces a small decrease in temperature at the catheter tip. Poor mixing, suggestive of slow, sluggish flow, produces a large decrease in temperature as the injectate bolus passes the thermistor.

The derived value for cardiac output is inversely proportional to the area under the thermodilution curve. Rapid infusion of cold intravenous fluids at the time of measurement may falsely increase the derived cardiac output. Thermodilution measures right-sided cardiac output, which does not equal left-sided cardiac output in patients with intracardiac shunts. There are no outcome data to support the routine use of a pulmonary artery catheter in cardiac surgery.

Cardiac output may be monitored continuously using a specialized pulmonary artery catheter. The continuous cardiac output catheter intermittently heats blood adjacent to a proximal portion of the catheter and senses changes in blood temperature at the catheter tip using a fast-response thermistor. The method requires no manual injections, and values are acquired, averaged, and updated automatically every several minutes. Disadvantages include increased cost and a cardiac output display that is not instantaneous but is an average value over the prior 2 to 10 minutes. Other methods of measuring cardiac output that do not depend on an indwelling pulmonary artery catheter include transthoracic bioimpedance, echocardiography, and analysis of the aortic pressure pulse contour. These have proven cumbersome, impractical, or unreliable for routine use.[28]

Mixed venous oxygen saturation (Svo_2) can be measured intermittently by manual blood sampling from the pulmonary artery or continuously using a modified pulmonary artery catheter equipped with an oximeter. The Svo_2 provides a continuous monitor of cardiovascular well-being. Assuming normal oxygen consumption, a normal Svo_2 generally denotes adequate oxygen delivery but does not provide information about the adequacy of perfusion to specific organs. A normal Svo_2 may not reflect adequate tissue perfusion in patients with intracardiac shunts, sepsis, or liver failure. A decrease in Svo_2 is rarely caused by an increase in oxygen consumption during cardiac surgery but is more likely a sign of decreasing oxygen delivery due to decreased cardiac output, anemia, or hypoxia.

Svo_2 provides an alternative method to calculate cardiac output if oxygen consumption is assumed to be constant. By the Fick equation, cardiac output is equal to the rate of systemic oxygen consumption divided by the arterial-venous oxygen content difference:

$$O_2\ \text{delivery} = CO \times Cao_2$$

$$O_2\ \text{delivery} = \dot{V}o_2 + (CO \times Cvo_2)$$

$$CO \times Cao_2 = \dot{V}o_2 + (CO \times Cvo_2)$$

$$CO(Cao_2 - Cvo_2) = \dot{V}o_2$$

$$CO = \frac{\dot{V}o_2}{Cao_2 - Cvo_2}$$

where $\dot{V}o_2$ = oxygen consumption, CO = cardiac output, Cao_2 = oxygen content in arterial blood, and Cvo_2 = oxygen content in mixed venous blood.

Although routine use of a pulmonary artery catheter for monitoring patients during cardiac operation is debated, it does provide clinical information that is used to direct therapy in high-risk patients (Fig. 9-8). Hypotension associated with increased cardiac output with a normal pulmonary artery occlusion pressure is likely caused by vasodilation and is effectively treated by a vasoconstrictor such as phenylephrine, vasopressin, or norepinephrine. Hypotension associated with a low cardiac output and a low pulmonary artery occlusion pressure indicates hypovolemia and is treated with volume expansion (Fig. 9-9). Hypotension associated with a low cardiac output and increased pulmonary artery and pulmonary artery occlusion pressure indicates cardiac dysfunction and may require treatment with an inotropic or anti-ischemic medication. An insidious decrease in Svo_2 may be an early warning of impending circulatory insufficiency due to a decrease in arterial oxygen tension, ventricular dysfunction, bleeding, or tamponade. Svo_2 pulmonary artery catheters serve as diagnostic tools and vigilance monitors, especially in the intensive care unit, where early deterioration in cardiac function can be detected and treated before an adverse event occurs.

Anesthetic Gas Monitors

Inhaled volatile anesthetics are different from other parenteral medications. The dose of the drug administered is dictated by its concentration in the blood rather than by a set standard. The concentration of an anesthetic in the exhaled gas at end-exhalation reflects the alveolar gas concentration that is in direct equilibrium with the blood. Monitoring the concentration of anesthetic in the end-tidal gas mixture adds precision to the administration of inhaled anesthetics and guards against inadvertent overdose.

The concentration of anesthetic gases is measured clinically by mass spectroscopy. A gas sample retrieved from the breathing circuit is analyzed off-line by measuring the dispersion of the ionized sample as it is accelerated and deflected by a magnetic field. The site of impact on a collecting plate is specific for a gas species, and the number of impacts represents the relative concentration of the gas species in the sample. The end-tidal concentration is determined by gating the measure of the anesthetic gas to the carbon dioxide expirogram (capnogram). Other methods of measuring anesthetic and respiratory gases include infrared spectroscopy, Raman spectroscopy, electrochemical and polarographic sensors, and piezoelectric absorption.[29]

Measurement of Electrolyte Concentration

Electrolyte abnormalities occur commonly during and after cardiopulmonary bypass and are monitored intermittently using routine laboratory tests that are promptly reported to the operating room.[30] Reliable on-line measurements of electrolytes are not yet available. The capability to detect and

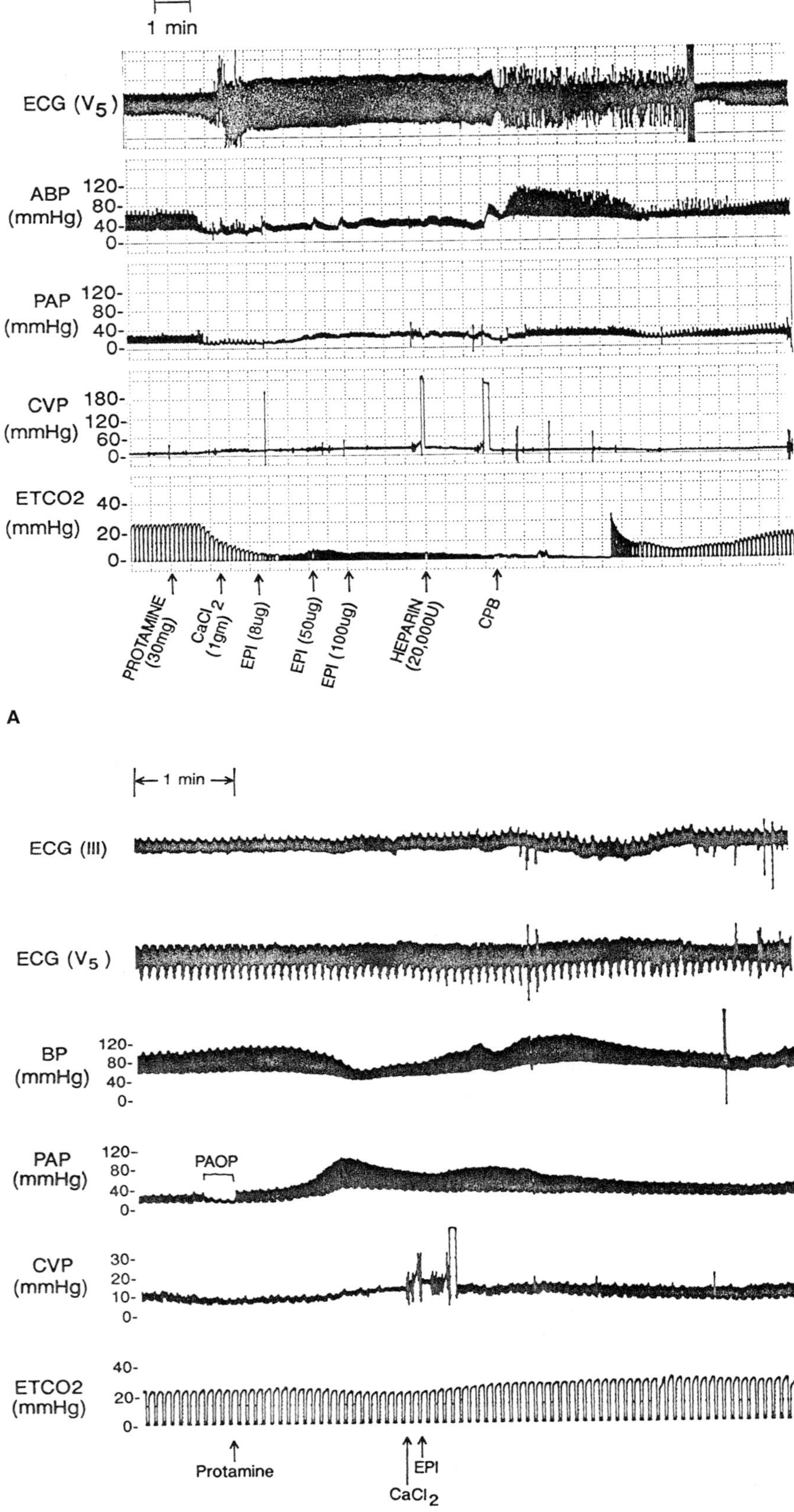

FIGURE 9–8 Intraoperative hemodynamic recordings showing the time sequence of systemic severe vasodilation (panel A) and catastrophic pulmonary vasoconstriction–type (panel B) protamine reactions during the reversal of heparin anticoagulation in patients undergoing heart operation. Arterial blood pressure (ABP) and pulmonary artery pressure (PAP) decrease in parallel during systemic vasodilation. In contrast, an increase in PAP and central venous pressure (CVP) precedes the decrease in ABP during the pulmonary vasoconstriction–type reaction. The decreases in end-tidal carbon dioxide concentration ($ETCO_2$) during the protamine reactions reflect the decrease in blood flow through the lungs.

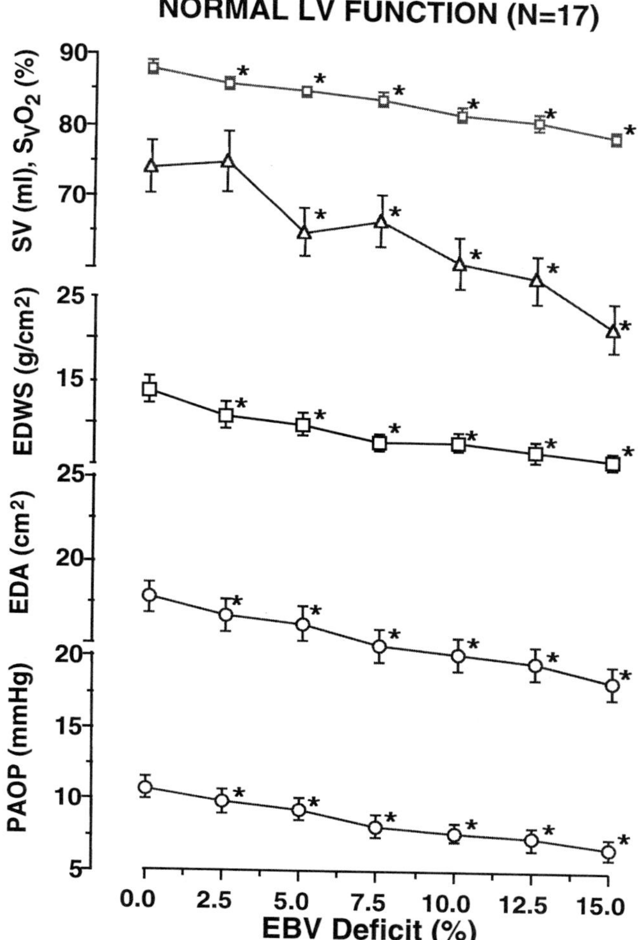

FIGURE 9–9 Decreased left ventricular preload produced by graded estimated blood volume deficits (EBV) was associated with serial decreases in the mixed venous oxygen saturation (Svo_2), cardiac stroke volume (SV), left ventricular end-diastolic meridional wall stress (EDWS), left ventricular end-diastolic cavity cross-sectional area (EDA), and pulmonary artery occlusion pressure (PAOP). Patients with dilated cardiomyopathy displayed less change in SV and Svo_2 in response to equivalent EBV deficits. *$p < .05$ versus baseline value (ANOVA for repeated measures). *(Modified with permission from Cheung AT, Weiss SJ, Savino JS: Protamine-induced right-to-left intracardiac shunting. Anesthesiology 1991; 75:904.)*

correct electrolyte disturbances is an important aspect of intraoperative care.

Abnormalities in sodium and water homeostasis are caused primarily by hemodilution with solutions used to prime the cardiopulmonary bypass circuit. Nonosmotic secretion of arginine vasopressin provoked by surgical stress, pain, hypotension, or nonpulsatile perfusion contributes to the development of hyponatremia by stimulating renal retention of free water. A 2- to 5-mEq/L decrease in the plasma sodium concentration is expected after beginning cardiopulmonary bypass and does not normally require treatment. Hyperglycemia or excessive mannitol administration causes pseudohyponatremia by decreasing the plasma sodium concentration. Hypernatremia is usually caused by excessive diuresis without free water repletion or by the administration of hypertonic sodium bicarbonate solutions. Hyperkalemia is common because high-potassium cardioplegic solutions are distributed into the systemic circulation. Hyperkalemia during cardiac surgery also may be caused by hemolysis, acidosis, massive depolarization of muscle, and tissue cell death. Increasing serum potassium concentration is manifested by peaked T waves, a widened QRS complex, disappearance of the P wave, heart block, and conduction abnormalities that may be life-threatening. Very high concentrations of potassium used to provide cardioplegia inhibit spontaneous depolarization and produce asystole. Patients with diabetes mellitus are at increased risk for hyperkalemia because cellular uptake of potassium is mediated by insulin. Impaired renal excretion of potassium enhances hyperkalemia in patients with renal insufficiency. The initial treatment of hyperkalemia is aimed at redistributing extracellular potassium into cells, but the elimination of potassium from the body requires excretion by the kidneys or gastrointestinal tract. Insulin and glucose administration rapidly decrease extracellular potassium by redistributing the ion into cells. Alkalosis, hyperventilation, and beta-adrenergic agonists also favor redistribution of potassium into cells, but the response is less predictable. Calcium carbonate and calcium chloride antagonize the effects of hyperkalemia at the cell membrane. A typical intravenous dose of glucose and insulin for the acute treatment of hyperkalemia is 1 g/kg of glucose and 1 unit of regular insulin per 4 g of glucose administered.

Hypokalemia is also common during cardiac surgery and may be caused by hemodilution with nonpotassium priming solutions, diuresis, or increased sympathetic tone during nonpulsatile perfusion. Intraoperative hypokalemia is exacerbated by preoperative potassium depletion due to chronic diuretic therapy. $Beta_2$-adrenergic agonists acutely decrease the plasma potassium concentration by directly stimulating cellular uptake of potassium. Hypokalemia predisposes to atrial arrhythmias, ventricular ectopy, digitalis toxicity, and prolonged response to neuromuscular blocking drugs. Hypokalemia is treated by slow administration of KCl in increments of 10 mEq, with potassium concentrations measured between doses.

Hypocalcemia decreases myocardial contractility and peripheral vascular tone and is associated with tachycardia.[31,32] Hypocalcemia produces prolongation of the QT interval and T-wave inversions, but significant arrhythmias due to disturbances in ionized calcium concentration are not common. Hypocalcemia occurs soon after the onset of cardiopulmonary bypass but may resolve without treatment. Increasing serum concentrations of parathyroid hormone during cardiopulmonary bypass may, in part, explain the gradual increase in ionized calcium concentration to pre–cardiopulmonary bypass levels.[33] The etiology of cardiopulmonary bypass–induced hypocalcemia is probably multifactorial, but hemodilution and decreased metabolism of citrate after rapid blood transfusion are contributing factors. The routine administration of calcium salts without prior measurement of ionized calcium concentration poses the risk of hypercalcemia. Excessive calcium administration may increase the risk of postoperative pancreatitis and myocardial reperfusion injury.[34]

Magnesium deficiency is common in cardiac surgical patients, and acute magnesium supplementation decreases the incidence of postoperative cardiac dysrhythmias and overall morbidity after cardiac operations.[35,36] However, measuring total plasma magnesium concentration has questionable clinical significance because the value primarily reflects the concentration of protein-bound magnesium and not physiologically active, ionized magnesium.[37]

Perioperative glucose control effects outcome after heart surgery. Aggressive protocols aimed at maintaining normoglycemia with the use of insulin infusions during cardiac surgery and into the early postoperative period lead to a decrease in morbidity (e.g., sternal wound infection) and possibly mortality.[37,38] However, aggressive control of blood glucose in diabetes increases the incidence of hypoglycemia, which can have severe consequences if not detected early and treated.[39]

Monitoring the Nervous System

Anesthetics produce characteristic changes in the electrical activity of the brain. The cellular mechanism of general anesthetics is controversial. Unconsciousness and general anesthesia are not achieved by producing energy failure in the brain. The central nervous system cellular concentrations of ATP, ADP, phosphocreatine, glucose, and glycogen are increased and lactate concentrations are decreased during general anesthesia. Most general anesthetics, and especially the extensively studied barbiturates, decrease cerebral metabolic rate and oxygen consumption.

A myriad of neurologic complications may be associated with cardiac surgery,[40] including stroke, paralysis, cognitive dysfunction, blindness, and peripheral nerve injury.

STROKE

Stroke associated with cardiac surgery occurs in 3% to 8%[41,42] of cases, but the incidence may alarmingly approach 35% to 70% in those with multiple risk factors such as previous stroke, carotid disease, advanced age, hypertension, and diabetes mellitus.[41] The majority of strokes are not identified immediately after cardiac surgery, but occur in the first several days postoperatively. The cause of these strokes and their causal relationship to cardiopulmonary bypass remain unclear.

Strokes may be related to micro- or macroemboli but may also be secondary to regional hypoperfusion. The combination of preexisting regional hypoperfusion and embolic phenomenon may be particularly deleterious.[43] The existence of a heavily calcified aorta increases the risk of stroke secondary to macroemboli.[44] Efforts to reduce the incidence of stroke in this patient group include the use of "off-pump" coronary artery bypass grafting, epiaortic ultrasound to identify "safe" areas for cannulation, and single clamping techniques for proximal anastamoses.[45] Previous work in animal models has demonstrated that in regions of the brain with compromised blood flow, acute anemia may not be well tolerated.[46] Acute anemia in individuals at risk for cerebrovascular disease may be exacerbated by an imbalance in oxygen supply and demand.[47]

The possibility exists to intervene to alter the course of perioperative stroke in individuals at high risk. For example, the application of intra-arterial thrombolytics in a highly selective fashion to the affected cerebral arteries can be done with acceptable morbidity even early after cardiac surgery.[48,49]

PARALYSIS

Paralysis, a devastating complication, is associated with dissection of the thoracic aorta, with repair of descending thoracic and thoracoabdominal aneurysm, and most recently after placement of endovascular stents.[50] The incidence in repair of a descending thoracic or thoracoabdominal aneurysm is 5% to 10%[51,52] and may exceed 25% in certain high-risk groups.[53] The likely cause is hypoperfusion of the spinal cord during aortic cross-clamping and ligation of intercostal and lumbar arteries.[54] Risk factors for paralysis include extent of the aneurysm and acuteness of disease. Those subjects without demonstrated flow in intercostals within the aneurysm may be at lower risk for paralysis after resection,[55] presumably because collateral blood supply to the cord in the involved region has been allowed to slowly occur, while subjects experiencing acute dissection, which does not permit time for collateralization, may experience a high rate of paralysis.

Intraoperative monitoring including motor evoked potentials and somatosensory potentials may be of some benefit to detect early spinal cord ischemia[56,57] yet may lack the sensitivity and specificity necessary to reliably guide intervention.[58] Preemptive measures to limit the degree of spinal cord ischemia have included identification and reimplantation of the artery of Adamkiewicz as well as intercostal vessels,[59,60] placement of cerebrospinal fluid (CSF) drainage catheters to increase the mean arterial pressure to CSF pressure gradient, epidural cooling of the spinal cord,[61,62] and distal perfusion techniques such as left atrial-femoral artery (LA-FA) bypass to enhance cord perfusion from below the inferior clamp site.[63,64] All of the above techniques have met with potentially important but limited success and controlled studies demonstrating a difference in outcome do not exist.[65] Recent work has emphasized the importance of addressing spinal cord ischemia in a similar fashion to the management of coronary or cerebral ischemia.[66] A continuum of injury exists from infarcted to ischemic tissue. Signs of spinal cord ischemia may improve or deteriorate with time and there may be, at the very least, an opportunity to ameliorate the extent of the injury through early intervention, such as increasing perfusion pressure and decreasing CSF pressure through drainage.[67] Most treatments are fraught with risk (e.g., the placement of CSF drainage catheters).[68]

COGNITIVE DYSFUNCTION

Postoperative alterations in cognitive function include disturbances of memory, attention, and intellectual function. Cognitive dysfunction occurs after cardiac operations at a rate estimated as high as 80% in the acute phase after surgery and may persist in 20% to 40% of cases depending on length of follow-up.[69] More than any other factor, advanced age has been consistently identified as the greatest risk factor for cognitive dysfunction after cardiac surgery with cardiopulmonary bypass. Early and late mortality may be markedly increased, quality of life is diminished, and costs of care are increased in the short and long run.[70]

Etiology has focused upon a myriad of potential causes[71] that predominantly include the effects of cardiopulmonary bypass such as hypotension,[72] microemboli,[73] open versus closed cardiac procedures,[74] acute anemia,[75] changes in brain water content,[76] hypoxemia, rewarming strategies,[77] cold versus warm cardiopulmonary bypass,[78] pH management strategy (alpha-stat vs. pH-stat),[79] pulsatile versus nonpulsatile perfusion,[80] bypass duration,[81] flow rates,[82] hypo- and hyperglycemia,[83] presence of the apolipoprotein E $\in -4$ allele,[84] and immunologic mechanisms.[85] Lastly, although cognitive dysfunction in the general population has been associated with chronic hypotension[86] and congestive heart failure,[87] the role of left ventricular function in cognition surrounding cardiac surgery is not known.

Research outside the arena of cardiac surgery into neurologic injury in cerebrovascular disease has focused upon the immune system as the generator of mediators and modulators of the cerebral endothelium[88,89] and of blood-brain barrier permeability.[90] One theory of immunologic mediated neuronal injury postulates a cascade of events initiated by complement- and neutrophil-mediated vascular endothelial damage and disruption of the blood-brain barrier, thus allowing neutrophil access to the parenchyma with resultant neural destruction.[88,90]

NEUROLOGIC SEQUELAE IN NONCARDIAC SURGERY

It would be irresponsible not to mention that stroke and cognitive dysfunction occur in patients after noncardiac surgery at a rate that is significantly less than that which is seen in the cardiac surgery group, yet the incidence is not negligible,[91–93] and may also be associated with prolonged deficits.[94,95] There may be similar risk factors and similar pathophysiologic mechanisms in this group of patients, especially in the origins of delayed stroke in the perioperative period. Investigations may ultimately even implicate the anesthetic agents themselves,[96] irrespective of issues of intraoperative hemodynamic management.

Neurophysiological monitoring techniques permit assessment of nervous system function during and early after operation because clinical evaluation is not possible. Techniques to monitor neurophysiological function during general anesthesia include electroencephalography (EEG) and somatosensory evoked potentials (SSEP). The EEG is a recording of the spontaneous electrical activity of the cerebral cortex and is defined by frequency, amplitude, and spatial distribution.[97] The amplitude of electrical activity decreases by more than 80% when the recording electrode is displaced only 2 cm from the site of maximum amplitude. This necessitates multiple electrodes and channel recordings to obtain a spatial representation of the EEG rhythm.[98] A change in EEG amplitude or frequency may be produced by cerebral ischemia, anesthetics, or hypothermia. Barbiturates produce a flat EEG, whereas enflurane may cause seizure-like activity. EEG burst suppression is not uncommon after induction of general anesthesia but does not exclude an impending neurologic catastrophe if induced by changes in cerebral blood flow. While continuous EEG monitoring may detect cerebral ischemia during carotid operations, its application during cardiac operations is problematic because the decrease in EEG frequency and amplitude due to anesthesia and hypothermia during operation cannot be distinguished from changes caused by cerebral ischemia.[99,100] Electrical artifacts from the heart-lung machine also interfere with the ability to continuously monitor the EEG during operation. Intraoperative monitoring of SSEP to detect cerebral ischemia overcomes some of the problems inherent to EEG monitoring because the temperature dependency of SSEP is well established.[101] Embolic stroke and brachial plexus injury[65,66] can be detected using intraoperative SSEP monitoring, but the utility, sensitivity, and specificity of this technique for detecting, preventing, and guiding the treatment of neurologic complications remain to be established (Fig. 9-10).[102,103]

Alternatively, intraoperative transesophageal echocardiography (TEE) and transcranial Doppler (TCD) may be used to detect arterial embolic events (Fig. 9-11). The embolic burden to the cerebral circulation measured by quantitative TCD correlates with the incidence of intraoperative surgical manipulation and postoperative neurologic deficits.[104] Intraoperative TEE can be applied to detect right-to-left intracardiac shunting through an atrial septal defect,[105,106] intracardiac masses,[107,108] or residual air within the cardiac chambers.[109] Routine epiaortic ultrasonography to assess the degree of aortic atherosclerosis and guide the insertion of the aortic cannula and application of the aortic cross-clamp

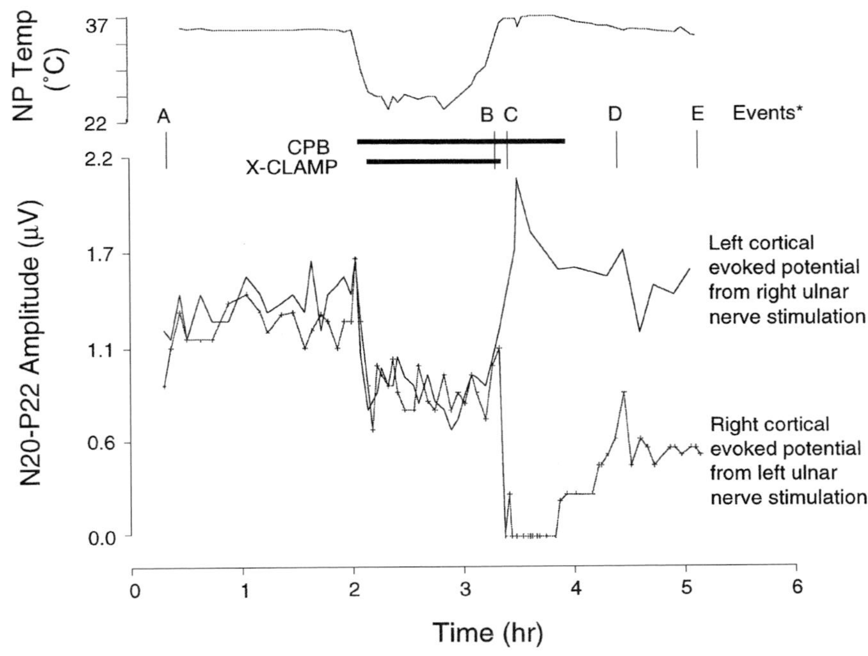

FIGURE 9–10 Intraoperative monitoring of somatosensory evoked potentials (SEPs) was used for the acute detection of embolic stroke during mitral valve replacement. The symmetric changes in the peak-to-peak amplitudes of N20-P22 SEPs before removal of the aortic cross-clamp were caused by the decrease in body temperature during deliberate hypothermia. The asymmetric decrease in the right cortical SEPs after removal of the aortic cross-clamp was associated with an acute embolic stroke to the right thalamus or right somatosensory cortex. CPB = cardiopulmonary bypass; NP = nasopharyngeal temperature; X-clamp = ascending aorta cross-clamp. *(Reproduced with permission from Cheung AT, Savino JS, Weiss SJ, et al: Detection of acute embolic stroke during mitral valve replacement using somatosensory evoked potential monitoring. Anesthesiology 1995; 83:201.)*

may decrease the risk of embolic stroke, but outcome data to suggest efficacy are sparse.[110]

ANESTHESIA

Anesthetic techniques presently employed for patients undergoing cardiac operations have been selected after extensive testing and clinical experience. Current clinical practice techniques have minimal organ toxicity, predictable cardiovascular and physiological effects, well-established pharmacokinetic behavior, and excellent safety profiles. No benchmark anesthetic technique has been defined for all patients undergoing cardiac operations.[111–114] Combining drugs that selectively provide hypnosis, amnesia, analgesia, and muscle relaxation permits control of the anesthetic state and minimizes side effects of a single anesthetic drug used in high concentrations. Achieving the desired anesthetic state while preserving or improving vital organ function during operation requires an understanding of the physiological actions of anesthetics, individually and in combination, in patients with a wide range of medical conditions.

Anesthesia drug management is dictated, in part, by the underlying cardiovascular disorder. Coronary artery disease renders the ventricle susceptible to myocardial ischemia, and management is designed to support coronary perfusion pressure while decreasing myocardial oxygen demands. Tachycardia, hypertension, and increased inotropic state caused by nociception during operation are prevented by anticipating the inciting events and providing effective anesthesia. In contrast, patients with heart failure due to valvular disease, dilated cardiomyopathy, or cardiac tamponade may be dependent on underlying sympathetic tone to support the circulation. In these patients, the anesthetist must be prepared to pharmacologically replace endogenous catecholamines while the patient is anesthetized.

Anesthetic-induced hemodynamic perturbations must be considered when assessing valve function intraoperatively using TEE (Fig. 9-12). Patients with regurgitant valve lesions frequently exhibit acute hemodynamic improvement during anesthesia because systemic oxygen demand and ventricular afterload decrease with anesthetic agents. Potent volatile anesthetics produce varying degrees of dose-dependent vasodilation and afterload reduction: isoflurane > enflurane > halothane. Assessment of mitral regurgitant grade during general anesthesia is not necessarily predictive of regurgitant grade in the awake state and may lead to mismanagement.[115,116] Provocative pharmacological testing may be required to mimic circulatory conditions in the awake, exercising patient. Stress-testing the mitral valve may be achieved with incremental doses of phenylephrine to increase the transmitral systolic pressure gradient; however, the determinants of regurgitant volume are many, and it is unlikely that phenylephrine reliably reproduces the cardiovascular conditions that occur when a patient is exercising.

Maintenance of cardiovascular stability during general anesthesia for patients with aortic stenosis is based on avoiding systemic vasodilation and tachycardia and preserving sinus rhythm. Systemic vasodilation provides no significant decrease in left ventricular afterload because of the stenotic aortic valve. Tachycardia is poorly tolerated due to shortened diastole and decreased filling of the noncompliant left

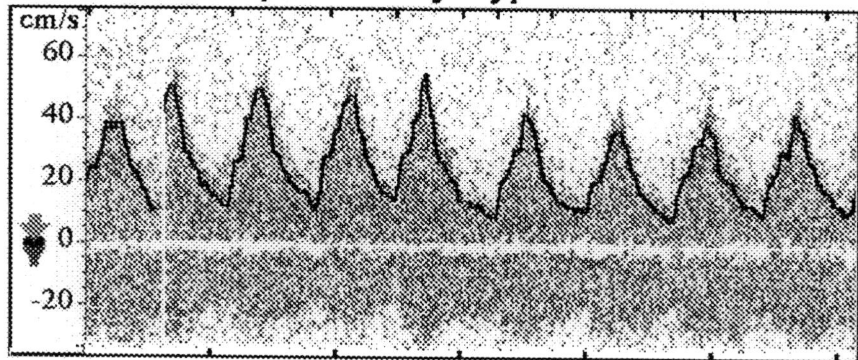

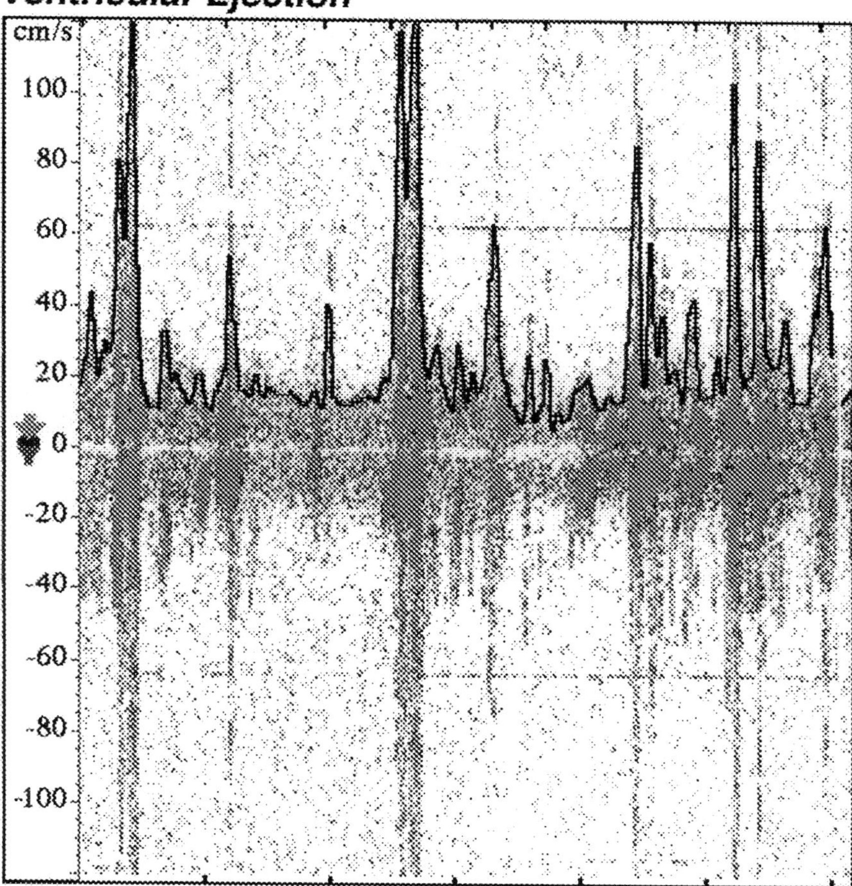

FIGURE 9–11 Middle cerebral artery blood flow velocity measured intraoperatively using a 2-MHz transcranial Doppler ultrasound transducer. The phasic velocity profile in the top panel was recorded before cardiopulmonary bypass. The irregular high-velocity, high-amplitude signals recorded in the lower panel indicate microemboli traveling through the middle cerebral artery immediately after ventricular ejection.

ventricle. Nonsynchronous atrial contraction, a common occurrence during induction of general anesthesia, may produce significant hypotension and rapid deterioration in stroke volume. Narcotic-based anesthetics possess many desired hemodynamic attributes for patients with aortic stenosis. Synthetic narcotics are potent vagotonic drugs that decrease heart rate with minimal vasodilating effects and provide profound analgesia.

Anesthetics and Neuromuscular Blockers

INHALED ANESTHETICS

Inhaled anesthetics alone produce all the conditions necessary for operation.[117] All inhaled anesthetics cause circulatory depression at concentrations necessary to produce general anesthesia. When ventilation is controlled, circulatory actions of the inhaled anesthetics usually limit the anesthetic

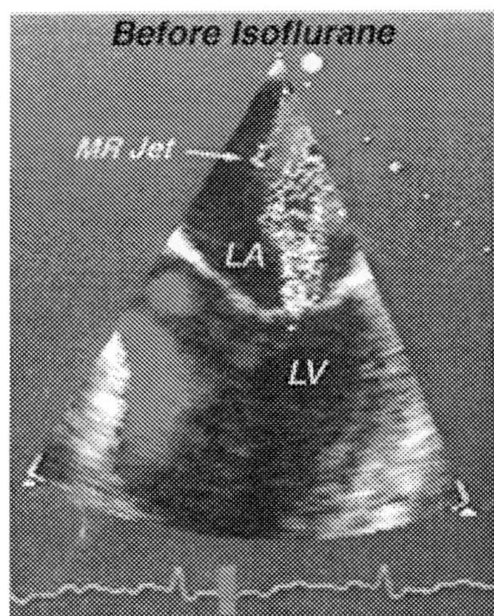

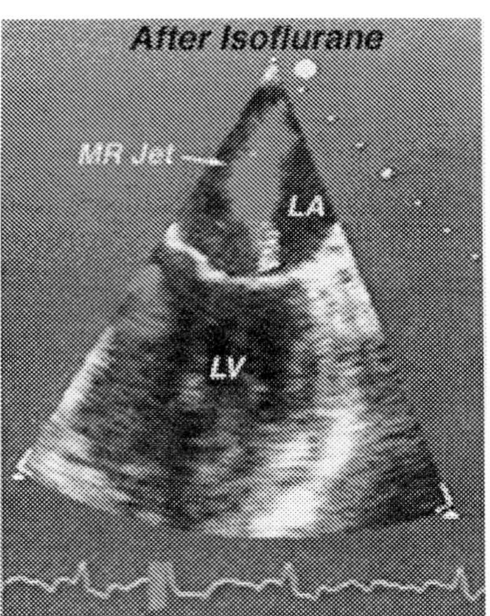

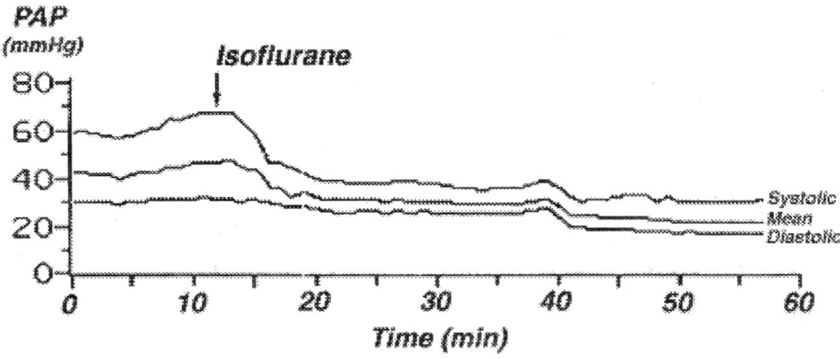

FIGURE 9–12 The relationship of increasing doses of isoflurane to the magnitude of mitral regurgitation and pulmonary artery pressures. The systemic unloading effects of isoflurane decreased mitral regurgitation from moderate to mild and decreased pulmonary artery pressures almost to normal.

dose that can be tolerated, especially in patients with cardiovascular disease. For this reason, lower doses of inhaled anesthetics are usually combined with other anesthetics to produce general anesthesia for cardiac operations.

The decrease in blood pressure caused by volatile anesthetics is a direct result of vasodilation and depression of myocardial contractility and an indirect result of attenuation of sympathetic nervous system activity. The decrease in blood pressure is so predictable that it is often used as a sign for assessing the depth of anesthesia. Overdose with inhaled anesthetics is manifested by hypotension, arrhythmias, and bradycardia that, if unrecognized, may lead to circulatory shock.

The inhaled anesthetics decrease myocardial contractility based on both experimental and clinical studies (Fig. 9-13).[118–120] Inhalation anesthetics produce a dose-dependent decrease in mean maximal velocity of circumferential shortening, mean maximal developed force, and dP/dt.[121–123] The effects of each individual inhaled anesthetic on cardiovascular function depend on selective dose-dependent effects of the drug on myocyte contraction and relaxation, vascular smooth muscle tone, and sympathetic nervous system reflexes, as well as the underlying disease state, intravascular volume status, surgical stimulation, temperature, mode of ventilation, and acid-base status. The decrease in blood pressure in response to 1.0 minimum alveolar concentration (MAC) of halothane is primarily the result of decreased cardiac output caused by direct myocardial depression. Despite a decrease in myocardial contractility, cardiac output is generally unchanged at 1.0 MAC of isoflurane because of direct arterial vasodilation and preservation of baroceptor reflexes, with a resulting decrease in ventricular afterload and increase in heart rate and stroke volume (Fig. 9-14).[124] Halothane, enflurane, isoflurane, desflurane, and sevoflurane decrease global left ventricular systolic function at any given left ventricular loading condition or at any given degree of underlying sympathetic tone (Fig. 9-15). Experimental studies suggest these agents cause minimal changes in left ventricular diastolic compliance but impair left ventricular diastolic relaxation in a dose-dependent manner.[125] These agents have minimal direct effects on left ventricular preload. Left and right ventricular end-diastolic pressures may increase during anesthesia because of impaired diastolic filling and decreased cardiac output. Halothane and enflurane are the most potent direct myocardial depressants, followed by isoflurane, desflurane, and sevoflurane.

Patients in shock or with profound ventricular dysfunction may not tolerate the cardiovascular depressant effects of

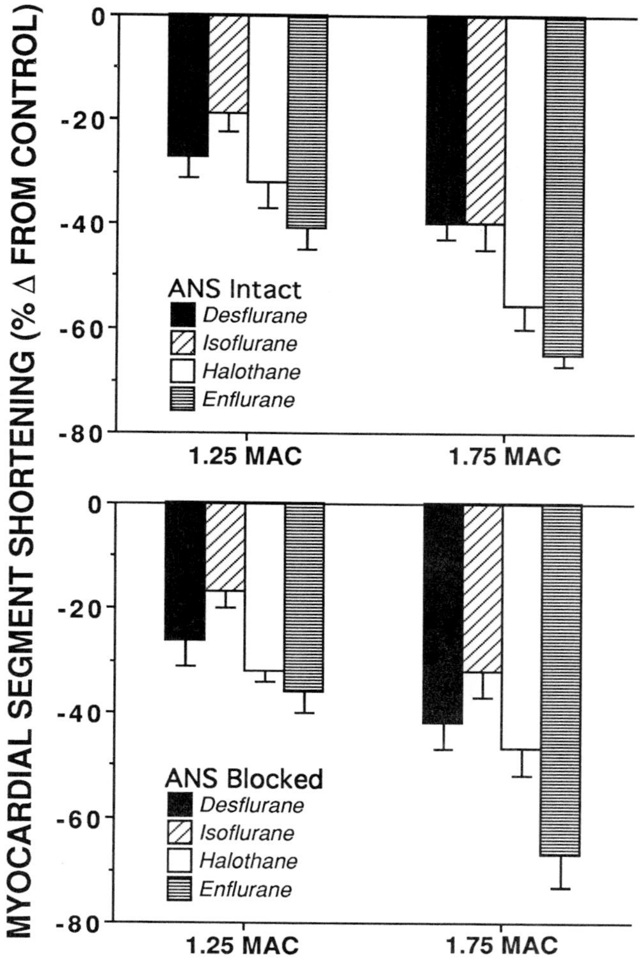

FIGURE 9–13 The actions of inhaled anesthetics on left ventricular myocardial segment shortening as measured in chronically instrumented dogs with an intact and blocked autonomic nervous system (ANS). All inhaled anesthetics caused a significant decrease in segment shortening at both 1.25 and 1.75 MAC in comparison with awake animals. *(Reproduced with permission from Pagel PS, Kampine JP, Schmeling WT, Warltier DC: Comparison of the systemic and coronary hemodynamic actions of desflurane, isoflurane, and enflurane in the chronically instrumented dog. Anesthesiology 1991; 74:539.)*

inhaled anesthetics given in concentrations that are needed to produce anesthesia. Volatile anesthetics have a proportionally greater negative inotropic effect on diseased myocardium compared with normal myocardium. In contrast, sympathetic nervous system activation due to nociception may mask clinical signs of circulatory depression caused by inhaled anesthetics. Cardiodepressants and adrenergic antagonists potentiate the cardiovascular depressant actions of inhaled anesthetics.

The administration of inhaled anesthetics in patients with preexisting cardiovascular diseases has potential advantages. The myocardial depressant and arterial vasodilating actions of anesthetics benefit patients with coronary insufficiency if perfusion pressure is maintained. The negative inotropic properties of inhalation anesthetics decrease myocardial oxygen demand and may create a more favorable myocardial oxygen balance. The vasodilating and antihypertensive actions of anesthetics effectively control an increase in blood pressure in response to surgical pain, but anesthetic-induced hypotension may reduce coronary perfusion pressure and coronary blood flow.

Enflurane is a mild coronary vasodilator, while halothane has little effect on coronary vascular tone. Regional wall motion abnormalities and ECG evidence of myocardial ischemia associated with enflurane or halothane are due to decreases in coronary perfusion pressure rather than to a redistribution of myocardial blood flow.[126,127] Isoflurane causes endothelium-dependent inhibition of the contractile response of canine coronary arteries.[128] The direct coronary artery vasodilating action of isoflurane may increase coronary blood flow but also may increase the risk of myocardial ischemia in patients with steal-prone coronary anatomy by attenuating autoregulation of coronary blood flow. Coronary anatomy associated with isoflurane-induced coronary steal is a total occlusion of a major coronary branch and a hemodynamically significant (greater than 50%) stenosis in the artery that supplies the collateral-dependent myocardium. The proposed mechanism is vasodilation and a decrease in coronary perfusion pressure downstream to the stenosis that decreases blood flow through the high-resistance, less-responsive collateral network.[129] However, there is no convincing clinical evidence that isoflurane should be avoided in patients with coronary artery disease any more than other nonselective coronary vasodilators (e.g., nitroprusside).[130] The increase in heart rate and sympathetic tone associated with isoflurane and desflurane increases oxygen demand by producing tachycardia and may cause myocardial ischemia in susceptible patients. This is more important than the theoretical risk of coronary steal.[131–133]

Volatile anesthetics have anti-ischemic, preconditioning properties resulting in cardioprotection against myocardial infarction via K_{ATP} channels.[134] Isoflurane, desflurane, and sevoflurane have cardioprotective properties independent from anesthetic improvement of myocardial oxygen supply demand balance.[135] However, there are no clinical outcome data to suggest that anesthetized patients with coronary artery disease fare better with the use of volatile anesthetics compared to intravenous agents.

Halothane sensitizes the myocardium to epinephrine-induced ventricular dysrhythmias and may be problematic in patients at risk for ventricular tachycardia, especially if sympathomimetics are given concurrently. The subcutaneous dose of epinephrine required to cause ventricular premature contractions during anesthesia with isoflurane, enflurane, or desflurane is approximately 4-fold greater than the dose required during halothane anesthesia.[136,137] The susceptibility to catecholamine-induced dysrhythmias is exacerbated by hypercarbia.

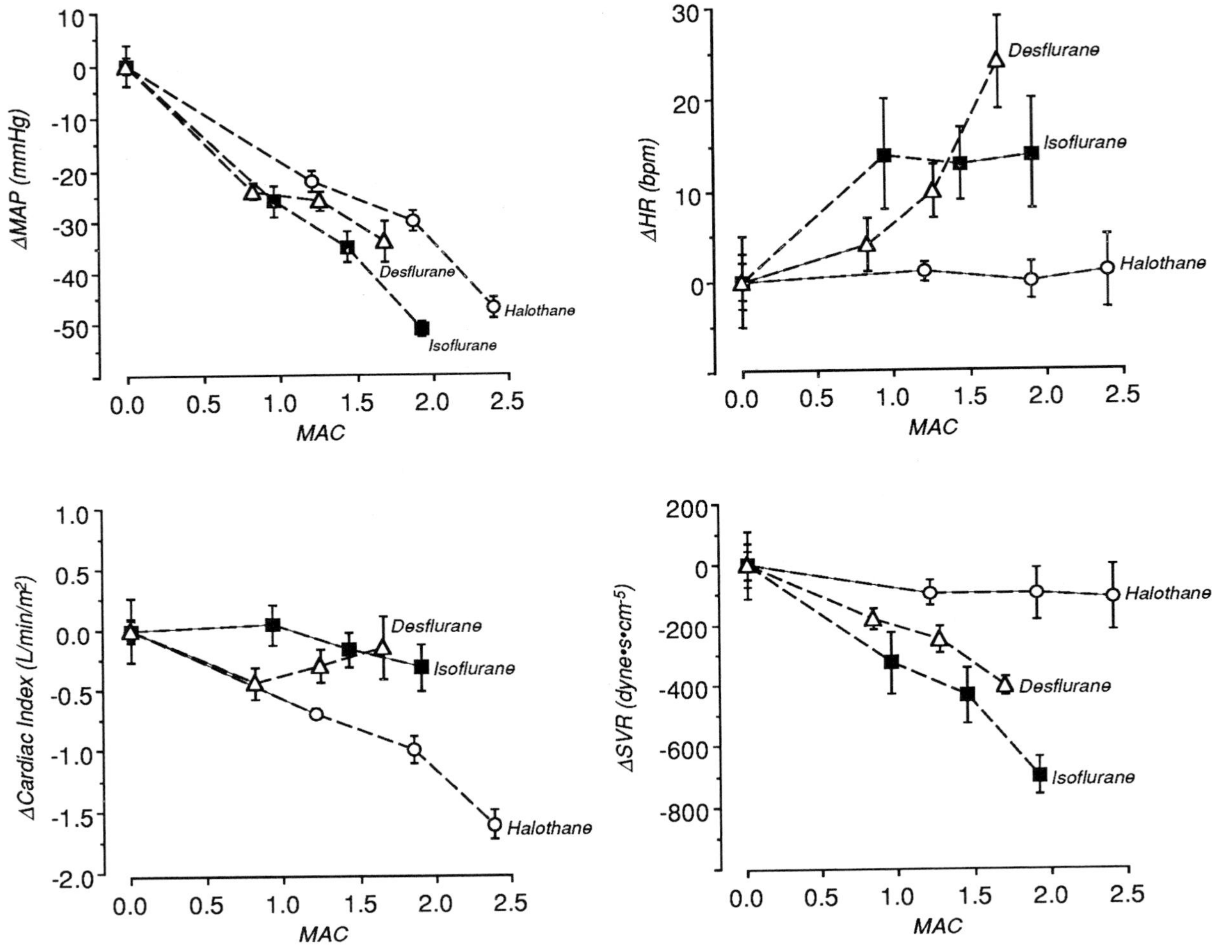

FIGURE 9–14 Dose-dependent changes in mean arterial pressure, heart rate, cardiac index, and systemic vascular resistance produced by halothane, isoflurane, and desflurane in normocarbic adults. Despite the myocardial depressant effects of isoflurane and desflurane, cardiac output is maintained during anesthesia with these agents in part because of a decrease in left ventricular afterload and increase in heart rate. *(Data from Weiskopf RB, Cahalan MK, Eger EI 2nd, et al: Cardiovascular actions of desflurane in normocarbic volunteers. Anesth Analg 1991; 73:143. Used with permission.)*

Junctional rhythms are observed often with all inhaled anesthetics but most commonly with enflurane. The loss of atrial augmentation of ventricular preload with a junctional rhythm contributes to a decrease in blood pressure during inhalation anesthesia. Junctional rhythms are frequently problematic in patients with aortic stenosis and left ventricular hypertrophy who have poor ventricular diastolic compliance. Junctional rhythms can be treated with transesophageal, transvenous, or direct atrial pacing, decreasing the dose of inhalation anesthetic, or administering an anticholinergic drug such as glycopyrrolate or atropine.

Regional blood flow to other vital organs may be modified by inhaled anesthetics because of their effects on metabolic demands and autoregulation. The normal circulatory response to hypotension and low cardiac output is redistribution of blood flow to vital organs (brain, heart, kidneys) and a decrease in blood flow to skin, muscle, and the gastrointestinal system. Volatile inhalation anesthetics impair this protective response and compromise vital organ perfusion if administered in high doses during periods of circulatory shock.

Nitrous oxide (N_2O) is also an inhaled anesthetic but not potent enough to be used alone for general anesthesia. It is often used with other anesthetics because it decreases the MAC of halothane and isoflurane. N_2O is rarely used during cardiac operations because it diffuses into and expands the volume of gas-containing cavities and may increase the size of arterial gas emboli.

Rare cases of acute postoperative hepatic necrosis have been attributed to halothane administration.[138] Although the epidemiologic evidence implicating halothane as the cause of this syndrome remains controversial, the incidence

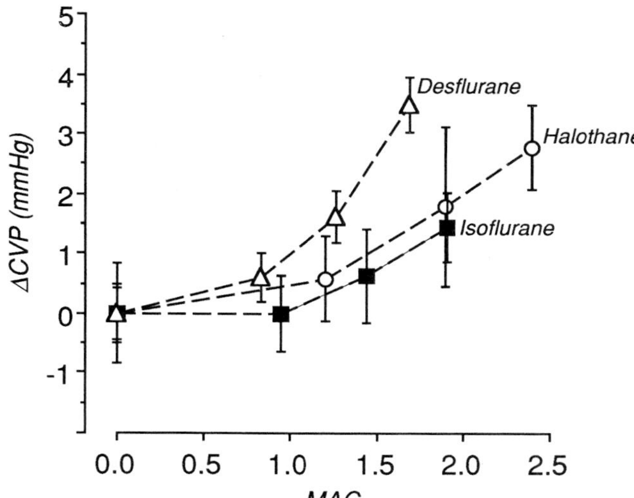

FIGURE 9–15 Dose-dependent changes in central venous pressure produced by halothane, isoflurane, and desflurane in normocarbic adults. *(Data from Weiskopf RB, Cahalan MK, Eger EI 2nd, et al: Cardiovascular actions of desflurane in normocarbic volunteers. Anesth Analg 1991; 73:143. Used with permission.)*

of this idiosyncratic reaction is estimated in the range of 1 in 10,000 to 1 in 35,000 halothane anesthetics. Repeated exposures to halothane, reduced splanchnic blood flow, obesity, hypoxemia, enhanced reductive metabolism of the drug, and increased levels of hepatic enzymes induced by chronic drug use, malnutrition, and underlying liver disease appear to be risk factors for postoperative hepatitis. The perceived risk of halothane-induced hepatitis has favored increased use of newer anesthetic agents such as enflurane, isoflurane, and desflurane. Sevoflurane, a newer generation ether volatile agent, offers lack of airway reactivity, nonpungent odor, low flammability, rapid induction and emergence, and minimal cardiovascular and respiratory side effects.[139,140] The accumulation of Compound A, a potential renal toxin and byproduct of sevoflurane use, has been associated only with low fresh gas flow (<1 L/min). These newer agents undergo minimal hepatic metabolism, do not decrease hepatic blood flow, and have not been implicated in anesthetic-induced liver dysfunction.

In general, carefully conducted clinical trials suggest that almost any inhaled anesthetic can be administered safely to patients with cardiovascular disease if the hemodynamic condition of the patient is closely controlled.[113,137]

SEDATIVE-HYPNOTICS

Sedative-hypnotics are a broad class of anesthetic drugs that includes barbiturates, benzodiazepines, etomidate, propofol, and ketamine. They are used for preoperative sedation, produce immediate loss of consciousness during intravenous induction of general anesthesia, supplement the actions of the inhaled anesthetics, and provide sedation in the immediate postoperative period. The circulatory effects of individual agents are an important consideration for patients with cardiovascular disease. The sedative-hypnotics have direct effects on cardiac contractility and vascular tone in addition to indirect effects on autonomic tone.

The barbiturates, such as thiopental or methohexital, are negative inotropic agents. They produce dose-dependent decreases in ventricular dP/dt and the force-velocity relationship of ventricular muscle.[141] Induction of general anesthesia with a barbiturate is associated with a decrease in blood pressure and cardiac output. In comparison with barbiturates, propofol appears to cause less myocardial depression.[142,143] The decrease in arterial pressure after propofol administration is attributed primarily to arterial and venous dilatation.[144,145] Propofol is well suited for continuous intravenous infusion for sedation because it has a short duration of action and can be titrated to effect. Propofol given intravenously for sedation in an nonintubated patient requires the presence of an anesthesiologist because respiratory depression is common. Etomidate and ketamine are administrated for rapid induction of general anesthesia in patients with preexisting hemodynamic compromise because they generally cause little or no change in circulatory parameters.[146] These agents are useful for unstable patients undergoing emergency operation, reexploration for bleeding, or cardioversion. Etomidate has virtually no effect on myocardial contractility even in diseased ventricular muscle.[147,148] However, etomidate inhibits adrenal synthesis of cortisol by blocking beta hydroxylase and therefore is limited to short-term use as an intravenous anesthetic induction agent. Ketamine often increases heart rate and blood pressure after anesthetic induction because it maintains sympathetic tone.[149] The direct negative inotropic and vasodilating effects of ketamine can be unmasked when it is administered to critically ill patients with catecholamine depletion.[150] Ketamine is not used routinely because it may cause postoperative delirium, especially if it is administered in the absence of other sedative-hypnotics.

Centrally acting $alpha_2$-adrenergic agonists such as clonidine possess sedative and analgesic actions but do not produce anesthesia. Preoperative administration of clonidine to cardiac surgical patients decreases narcotic requirements and improves hemodynamic stability during operation.[151] $Alpha_2$ agonists are potent sympatholytic agents and also may be effective at attenuating sympathetically mediated myocardial ischemia.[152] Dexmedetomidine is a highly selective intravenous $alpha_2$-adrenergic agonist with sedative actions.[153] Dexmedetomidine administered at a rate of 0.2 to 0.7 μg/kg/h intravenously provides effective postoperative sedation for intubated cardiac surgical patients and decreases the need for narcotic analgesics by approximately 50%. Because $alpha_2$-adrenergic agonists have little or no respiratory depressant actions, weaning from mechanical ventilatory support and tracheal extubation can be accomplished without interruption of the dexmedetomidine infusion. The most common adverse effects of dexmedetomidine are hypotension and bradycardia. At dexmedetomidine doses greater than 1.0 μg/kg/h, arterial pressure may increase due to direct activation of the alpha$_{2B}$ receptor subtype, which produces peripheral vasoconstriction. Dexmedetomine-induced vasoconstriction causes an increase in systemic vascular resistance, an increase in pulmonary vascular resistance, and a decrease in cardiac output.

NARCOTIC ANESTHETICS

Narcotics remain an important adjunct for cardiac anesthesia. Analgesic actions are mediated by direct activation of opioid receptors in the central nervous system, spinal cord, and periphery. The three types of opioid receptors most studied are the mu, delta, and kappa receptors. Mu receptors are densely concentrated in the neocortex, brainstem, and regions of the central nervous system associated with nociception and sensorimotor integration.[154] Two different mu receptor subtypes produce analgesia and respiratory depression, leading to the possible development of selective agonist or antagonist compounds.

Narcotic-based anesthetics offer the advantages of profound analgesia, attenuation of sympathetically mediated cardiovascular reflexes in response to pain, and virtually no direct effects on myocardial contractility or vasomotor tone. Narcotics may be administered intravenously, intrathecally, or into the lumbar or thoracic epidural space. Even though narcotics have little direct action on the cardiovascular system, they may cause profound hemodynamic changes indirectly by attenuating sympathetic tone. Narcotics decrease serum catecholamine levels and produce cardiovascular depression indirectly, especially in a patient who is critically ill and dependent on endogenous catecholamines (e.g., those with hypovolemia or cardiac tamponade). Morphine sulfate may decrease blood pressure by provoking the release of histamine.

Problems encountered with narcotic-based anesthetics include difficulty estimating the dose required because of patient variability, predicting the duration of postoperative narcotic-induced respiratory depression, and ensuring hypnosis during operation. Rapid administration of narcotics is associated with muscle rigidity that may impede the ability to ventilate the patient immediately after the induction of general anesthesia.[156] The rigidity usually affects the thoracic and abdominal musculature and is commonly observed with doses of narcotic used in cardiac anesthesia. Myoclonic activity often associated with muscle rigidity can easily be mistaken for grand mal seizures. There is no evidence that opioids induce seizures when there is adequate oxygenation and ventilation.[157] Opioid-induced muscle rigidity is immediately reversed by the administration of neuromuscular blockers.

The nonselective opioid antagonist naloxone reverses narcotic-induced respiratory depression. Narcotic antagonists must be titrated carefully to effect. Sudden reversal of opioid-mediated analgesia may produce systemic and pulmonary hypertension and tachycardia and is potentially life-threatening for patients with coronary artery disease.[158] The reversing effect of naloxone on narcotic-induced respiratory depression is significantly shorter than the respiratory depressant effects of most opioids, except for ultrashort-acting synthetic narcotics (e.g., alfentanil, remifentanil). A patient who receives a single intravenous dose of naloxone is susceptible to renarcotization after initial reversal of respiratory depression. For this reason, the initial bolus dose of naloxone is typically followed by an intramuscular injection or intravenous infusion, and patients are monitored closely. Longer acting opioid antagonists include nalmefene, which has an elimination half-life ($t_{1/2B}$)of 8.5 hours, in contrast with the $t_{1/2B}$ of 1.5 hours for naloxone.[159] Mixed opioid agonists-antagonists (e.g., nalbuphine) may decrease the risk of hypertension, tachycardia, and dysrhythmias but do not reverse respiratory depression as reliably as naloxone.[160]

Opioid tolerance is a decrease in response (both analgesia and respiratory depression) to a narcotic due to prior exposure. Tachyphylaxis is the rapid development of drug tolerance. Drug dependence is a patient condition or disorder that occurs as a consequence of sustained exposure to a drug such that withdrawal or antagonism of the drug prohibits normal function.[155] Perioperative exposure to morphine and synthetic narcotics is unlikely to produce the downregulation and desensitization of opioid receptors believed necessary for narcotic dependence.[161] Acute tolerance to fentanyl in humans is likely to occur only after prolonged infusion and to a lesser extent in the perioperative period. Cardiac surgical patients receiving narcotic infusions in the intensive care unit develop tolerance and require increasing doses to sustain the desired effect.[162]

The synthetic narcotics such as fentanyl, sufentanil, and alfentanil overcome some of the problems of morphine-based anesthetics because of increased lipid solubility, more rapid onset of action, increased anesthetic potency, absence of histamine release, and independence of renal function for drug clearance. Development of short-acting narcotic anesthetics also may improve the ability to control anesthetic depth without prolonging recovery time. Ultrashort-acting narcotics (e.g., remifentanil) may have a unique niche in cardiac anesthesia because their effect is terminated almost immediately on stopping the drug infusion due to rapid in vivo ester hydrolysis.[163] Other side effects of narcotics include pruritus, nausea, constipation, and urinary retention.

NEUROMUSCULAR BLOCKING DRUGS

Neuromuscular blocking drugs are administered to facilitate intubation of the trachea, prevent patient movement during operation, improve surgical exposure of the operating field, and attenuate metabolic demands caused by shivering during hypothermia. Except for succinylcholine, the

TABLE 9–3 Neuromuscular blocking drugs

Drug	ED_{95} (mg/kg)	Dose (mg/kg)	Onset (min)	Duration (min)	Effects of drug on: HR	BP	CO	Histamine release	Renal elimination
Succinylcholine	0.25	1.5	1-1.5	12-15	(+)	(+)	(0)	(+)	0%
D-Tubocurarine	0.51	0.6	3-5	180-240	(+)	(−)	(−)	(+ + +)	60%
Pancuronium	0.07	0.1	3-5	180-240	(++)	(+)	(+)	(0)	70%
Metocurine	0.28	0.4	3-5	240	(+)	(−)	(0)	(++)	90%
Gallamine	3.0	3.5	3-5	180	(+ + +)	(++)	(++)	(0)	100%
Vecuronium	0.06	0.1	2-3	75-120	(0)	(0)	(0)	(0)	15%
Atracurium	0.25	0.5	2-3	60-90	(0)	(−)	(0)	(+)	<5%
Doxicurium	0.04	0.06	3-5	180-240	(0)	(0)	(0)	(0)	75%
Rocuronium	0.3	0.6	1-2	45-90	(0)	(0)	(0)	(0)	0%
Mivacurium	0.1	0.2	2-3	40-60	(0)	(0)	(0)	(+)	<5%

ED_{95} = dose required to produce 95% suppression of muscle twitch in response to nerve stimulation; dose = initial dose required for intubation of the trachea; onset = time required to achieve conditions required for tracheal intubation; duration = time after injection required for recovery to 95% of baseline function; (+) = increase; (−) = decrease; (0) = no effect; HR = heart rate; BP = arterial pressure; CO = cardiac output; histamine release = drug-induced histamine release; renal elimination = percentage of injected dose that is dependent on renal function for excretion.

neuromuscular blocking drugs used in clinical practice are typically nondepolarizing, competitive antagonists of acetylcholine at the nicotinic acetylcholine receptor at the motor end plate. Succinylcholine is an acetycholine agonist that produces rapid, short-acting muscle paralysis by depolarizing the motor end plate.

Muscle relaxants are chosen based on the desired speed of onset, duration of action, route of elimination, spectrum of cardiovascular side effects, and cost (Table 9-3). The newer neuromuscular blocking drugs such as vecuronium, cis-atracurium, doxacurium, and rocuronium have virtually no cardiovascular side effects and are not dependent on renal function for elimination. Metocurine and gallamine are completely dependent on renal function for elimination and are infrequently used in clinical practice. Succinylcholine has the most rapid onset of action (90 seconds) but produces unpredictable changes in heart rate, increases serum potassium concentration by approximately 0.5 mEq/L, may cause life-threatening hyperkalemia in patients with denervation, burn, or compression injuries, and can trigger malignant hyperthermia in susceptible individuals. Pancuronium increases blood pressure and heart rate by blocking muscarinic acetylcholine receptors in the sinoatrial node, increases sympathetic activity via antimuscarinic actions, and inhibits reuptake of catecholamines. The neuromuscular blockers D-tubocurarine, metocurine, mivacurium, and atracurium may decrease blood pressure and increase heart rate indirectly by mediating release of histamine. The cardiovascular effects of these neuromuscular blockers may be attenuated by pretreatment with H_1- and H_2-receptor antagonists. Long-term administration of vecuronium is associated with development of myopathy in patients on glucocorticoid therapy.[164]

Discontinuing general anesthesia or sedation before complete recovery from neuromuscular blockade is very distressing for a patient because the awake, alert, and paralyzed patient has no means to communicate discomfort. Discontinuing mechanical ventilatory support in patients with residual neuromuscular blockade may cause acute or delayed respiratory failure. Even mild residual neuromuscular blockade contributes to pulmonary insufficiency by compromising mechanics of breathing and decreasing negative inspiratory force, vital capacity, tidal volume, and the ability to generate an effective cough. Muscle fatigue may produce airway obstruction by decreasing muscle tone in the oropharynx. Recovery from nondepolarizing neuromuscular blockade may be hastened by administering an acetylcholine-esterase inhibitor, such as neostigmine or edrophonium, that decreases degradation of acetylcholine at the neuromuscular junction and thereby increases the concentration of the neurotransmitter at the motor end plate. The undesirable systemic effects of acetylcholine-esterase inhibitors are bronchospasm, bradycardia, and hypersalivation, which can be minimized by simultaneous administration of anticholinergic agents such as atropine or glycopyrrolate. Severe bradycardia has been described in heart transplant patients after reversal of neuromuscular blockade, possibly due to the non-antagonized parasympathetic activity associated with acetylcholinesterase inhibitors in the denervated heart.[165] Reliable reversal of neuromuscular blockade with cholinesterase inhibitors is usually achieved only after muscle strength has recovered spontaneously to approximately 25% of baseline levels. Recovery of neuromuscular function is measured by a train-of-four twitch monitor applied to the ulnar nerve.

LOCAL ANESTHETICS

Local anesthetic drugs block the propagation of action potentials in electrically excitable tissue. Local anesthetics can be delivered by topical application to mucosa, infiltration into tissues, injection into the region of a peripheral nerve, infusion into the epidural space, or injection intrathecally into cerebrospinal fluid. Regional nerve blocks can be used to supplement a general anesthetic or to provide postoperative analgesia. Epinephrine is often added to local anesthetic solutions to prolong the anesthetic duration, but may cause tachycardia or cardiac arrhythmias when absorbed into the systemic circulation. Inadvertent intravascular injection of a local anesthetic may cause seizures, myocardial depression, hypotension, bradycardia, ventricular arrhythmias, or even cardiac arrest. Among the local anesthetics, bupivacaine has the greatest potential for cardiac toxicity. Ropivacaine is less cardiotoxic than bupivacaine.[166,167]

Special Anesthetic Techniques

EMERGENCY AIRWAY MANAGEMENT

Establishing a patent and secure airway is essential for the conduct of general anesthesia and is the first step in emergency life support for cardiovascular resuscitation. Tracheal intubation for airway protection and mechanical ventilation can be challenging in a patient with cardiovascular disease. Anesthesia is often necessary to facilitate tracheal intubation; however, the effects of general anesthetics on respiratory and circulatory function typically produce respiratory depression and may cause apnea, instability of the patient's airway, aspiration pneumonitis, hypoxia, hypercarbia, and cardiovascular collapse. Inadequate anesthesia during tracheal intubation may provoke myocardial ischemia or tachyarrhythmias in susceptible patients. The American Society of Anesthesiologists has established practice guidelines for the emergency management of the difficult airway.[168] The difficult airway (e.g., Mallampati class 4) often can be intubated with the patient in a sedated state using fiberoptic bronchoscopy. This technique requires time and special equipment. The risk of hypertension, tachycardia, and discomfort during tracheal intubation in an awake patient can be offset partially by topical anesthesia. Other techniques include mask ventilation, laryngeal mask ventilation, esophageal-tracheal combitube ventilation, blind oral or nasal intubation, direct laryngoscopy, rigid ventilating bronchoscopy, light wand intubation, retrograde intubation, transtracheal jet ventilation, cricothyroidotomy, and tracheostomy.

SINGLE-LUNG VENTILATION

Single-lung ventilation, or the ability to collapse one lung and selectively ventilate the contralateral lung, is necessary for operative exposure when the heart or great vessels are approached through a lateral thoracotomy incision. Selective lung ventilation is integral in the intraoperative management of patients undergoing minimally invasive direct coronary artery bypass (MIDCAB) procedures. Adequate surgical exposure with minithoracotomy for coronary revascularization without cardiopulmonary bypass requires deflation of the left lung. Single-lung ventilation is also used in patients undergoing thoracoscopic procedures, lung transplantation, thoracic aortic operations, mitral valve surgery through a right thoracotomy, closure of large bronchopleural fistulas, intrathoracic robotic surgery, or life-threatening hemoptysis. Single-lung ventilation may be achieved using double-lumen endobronchial tubes (Fig. 9-16) or bronchial blockers (Fig. 9-17).

Wire-guided bronchial blocker kits often contain an adapter for a standard endotracheal tube with ports for the bronchial blocker and fiberoptic bronchoscope. A central lumen for the blocker contains a monofilament loop that passes out the end of the catheter. Placement of the loop over a fiberoptic bronchoscope permits the bronchial blocker to be guided directly into position using the bronchoscope. Removal of the monofilament loop from the central lumen provides a port for venting the nonventilated lung. Bronchial blockers for lung isolation are preferred when the larynx is too small to accommodate a double lumen endobronchial tube (rare in the adult patient), when it is difficult or dangerous to change an existing endotracheal tube, or when the tracheal or mainstem bronchus is distorted by a mediastinal mass or aortic aneurysm.

The routine use of fiberoptic bronchoscopy has decreased the complication rates and eliminated uncertainty regarding positioning of these devices in the airway. Hypoxemia caused by transpulmonary shunt through the nonventilated lung during single-lung ventilation often requires modification of the anesthetic technique to preserve hypoxic pulmonary vasoconstriction.

REGIONAL ANESTHESIA AND ANALGESIA

Epidural or intrathecal administration of local anesthetics and narcotics can provide profound postoperative analgesia after thoracic and major abdominal operations with less sedation or respiratory depression compared to parenteral narcotic analgesia.[169–171] However, the risk of hematoma in the spinal canal during or after cardiopulmonary bypass and heparinization has limited the use of epidurals for cardiac surgery. Patient-controlled epidural analgesia using infusion pumps can be triggered by patient demand with a predetermined maximum lockout dose to prevent overdose. Patient-controlled epidural analgesia is an effective method to titrate the dose of epidural local anesthetic and narcotic based on clinical need. The potential clinical advantages of epidural or intrathecal analgesia are less postoperative pain, decreased duration of postoperative ventilatory support, attenuation of the surgical stress responses, and improved pulmonary function.[172]

The epidural catheter is most often inserted prior to operation before systemic anticoagulation. Instrumentation of

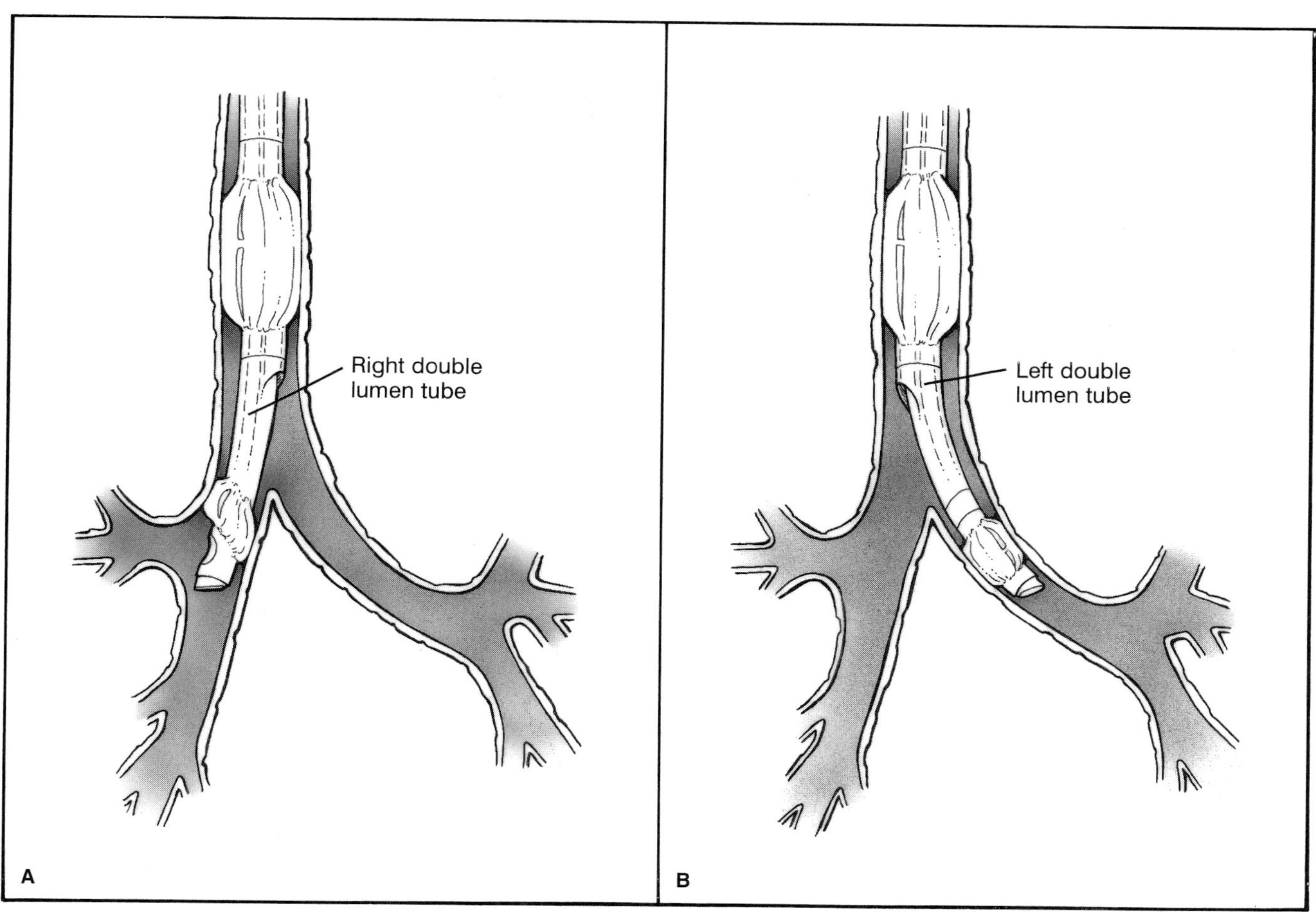

FIGURE 9–16 (A) Right-sided double-lumen endobronchial tube positioned such that Murphy's eye is aligned with the orifice of the right upper lobe bronchus. Indications for a right-sided tube are surgery involving the left main-stem bronchus, patients with a prior left pneumonectomy, stenosis, compression, or mass in the left main bronchus, and circumstances in which the trachea needs to be protected from soilage from contents in the right lung (e.g., abscess). (B) Left-sided double-lumen endobronchial tube.

the epidural space for insertion of the catheter or removal of the epidural catheter is contraindicated in anticoagulated patients and in patients with coagulopathy because of the risk of epidural hematoma formation.[173,174] Epidural analgesia is provided by administering a continuous infusion of dilute solution of local anesthetic or narcotic, or a combination of the two, into the epidural catheter (e.g., bupivacaine 0.05% and fentanyl 2 μg/mL at a rate of 4 to 8 mL per hour).

The most common side effect of epidural analgesia is hypotension caused by local anesthetic blockade of the preganglionic vasomotor efferents of the sympathetic nervous system and loss of compensatory vasoconstriction. This side effect can be decreased by decreasing the concentration of the local anesthetic relative to the narcotic analgesic used in the epidural infusion. Respiratory depression can also occur with systemic absorption of the narcotic. The onset of respiratory depression is sometimes delayed or unpredictable. Nausea and pruritis are also common side effects of epidural or intrathecal narcotics. Epidural hematoma formation causing spinal cord compression is a rare, but potentially catastrophic complication of epidural and intrathecal analgesia, with an estimated frequency of 1 in 150,000 cases.[175]

Thoracic epidural anesthesia has been employed successfully for treatment of refractory angina.[176,177] Selective anesthesia of T1 to T5 thoracic dermatomes with epidural local anesthetic inhibits sympathetic innervation of the heart and regional vasculature. Thoracic epidural anesthesia decreases left ventricular contractility and heart rate while prolonging phase IV of the cardiac action potential.[178] The decrease in myocardial oxygen consumption, reduced arrhythmogenicity, and increase in diameter of the stenotic coronary arteries are the proposed mechanisms for the abolition of chest pain in unstable angina patients who receive thoracic epidural local anesthetic.[179–183] With exercise testing, these patients have a smaller ischemic burden (less ST-segment depression) for a given workload with epidural anesthesia compared with

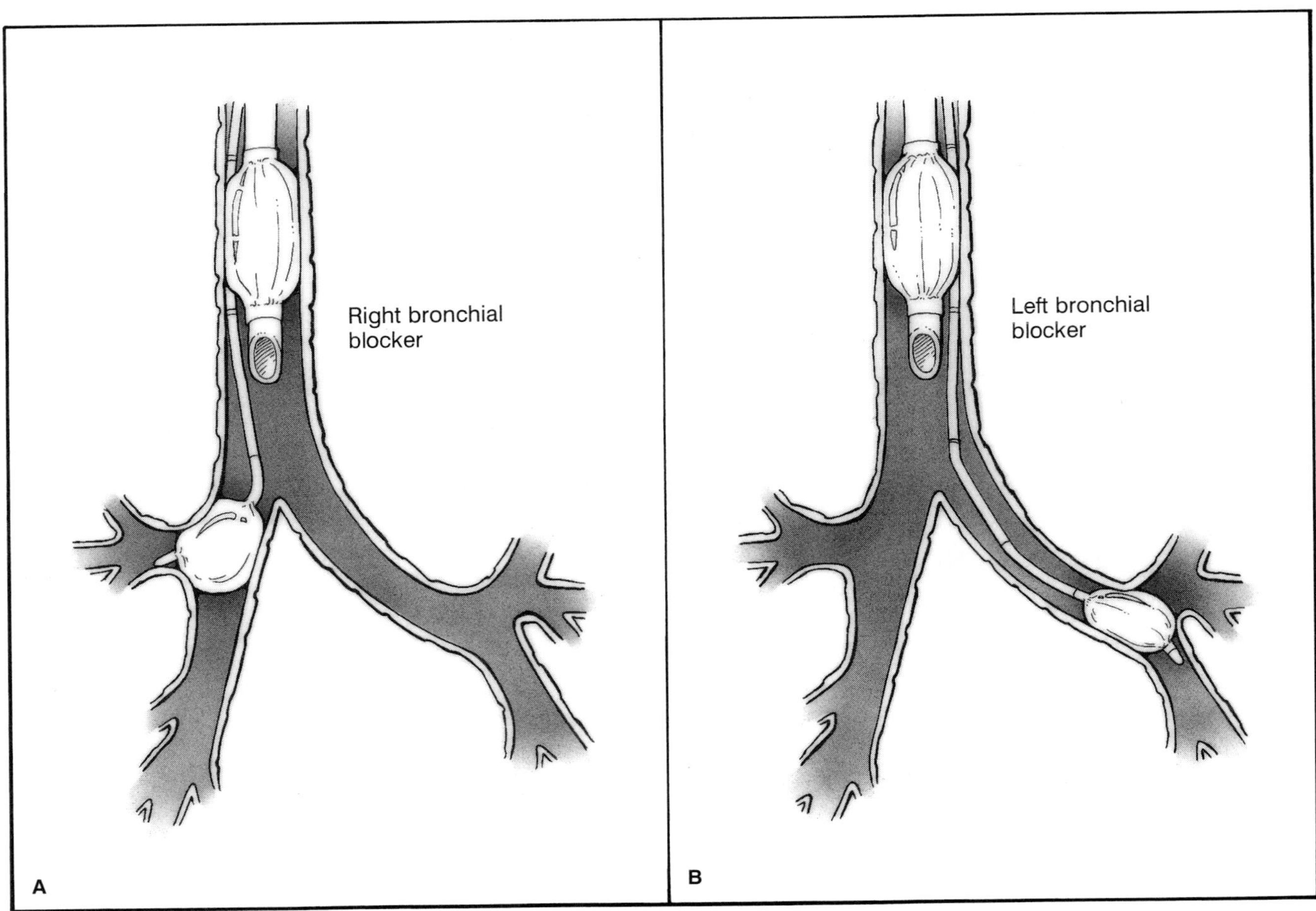

FIGURE 9–17 Bronchial blockers permit single-lung ventilation but do not permit suctioning or rapid deflation of the nonventilated lung. Position of the bronchial blocker is less stable compared with a double-lumen endobronchial tube.

control exercise without epidural anesthesia. Treatment of myocardial ischemia with an infusion of local anesthetics or opioids into the epidural space is not without risk in patients who are likely to receive anticoagulants and/or thrombolytics and who may have significant preexisting left ventricular dysfunction.

CONTROLLING LUMBAR CEREBROSPINAL FLUID PRESSURE

Several studies and clinical experience suggest that spinal fluid drainage may improve neurologic outcome from spinal cord ischemia during thoracoabdominal aortic operations.[183–186] Although the clinical efficacy of lumbar CSF drainage remains controversial, the technique is routine at some institutions.[187–188] CSF drainage and a decrease in the lumbar CSF pressure can be achieved by aseptically inserting a subarachnoid catheter through a Tuohy needle positioned in a lower lumbar vertebral interspace. The catheter is typically inserted 1 to 2 hours before systemic anticoagulation with the patient in a lateral decubitus position. CSF is passively drained to reduce lumbar CSF pressure to approximately 10 to 12 mm Hg during operation. Reducing CSF pressure further may cause an abducens nerve palsy and postoperative diplopia. The catheter is secured and CSF drainage continued typically for 24 hours after operation. In the absence of spinal cord ischemia, the catheter is capped at 24 hours after operation and removed at 48 hours after operation. Emergent implementation of lumbar CSF drainage to a target lumbar CSF pressure of 10 mm Hg combined with augmentation of the mean arterial pressure to 100 mm Hg has been reported to successfully reverse delayed-onset paraplegia or paraparesis in some patients after thoracic aortic reconstruction.[189] Complications associated with lumbar CSF catheters include meningitis, persistent CSF leak, breakage and retention of a catheter fragments, and epidural hematoma. The risk of epidural hematoma is increased when the CSF catheter is inserted or removed in anticoagulated patients.

THE CONDUCT OF ANESTHESIA, SURGERY, NURSING, AND PERFUSION

Cardiac surgery is conducted in an interdisciplinary environment among surgeon, anesthesiologist, perfusionist, and nursing staff. The operating room requires a minimum of 800 sq ft to comfortably accommodate the patient, health care providers, standard operating room equipment, cell saver, heart-lung machine, and assist devices, if needed.[190] The required square footage may be greater for the higher technology procedures such as robotic surgery.

The anesthetic begins before the patient arrives in the operating room. Patients are premedicated with a sedative-hypnotic (e.g., scopolamine, benzodiazepine) and analgesic (e.g., morphine) unless the associated mild degree of respiratory depression is unwarranted. The patient's identification and scheduled procedure are verified immediately on arrival in the operating room. The patient is escorted into the operating room and placed onto the operating table, and routine noninvasive monitors are applied. The physical condition of the patient is assessed clinically, and medical events that occurred over the previous 12 to 24 hours are reviewed. For elective surgery, the patient should have fasted for a minimum of 6 hours prior to induction of general anesthesia. Prophylactic antibiotics are administered after insertion of an intravenous catheter. A catheter is inserted in the radial artery. A blood sample is acquired for laboratory analysis, and a blood type and crossmatch are requested if not done already. A central venous catheter is always indicated, although in many patients it can be inserted after the induction of general anesthesia. A pulmonary artery catheter is commonly used to provide measures of cardiac output and estimate ventricular filling pressures.[191] Large-bore intravenous catheters are inserted for patients who are undergoing reoperation because of the possibility of rapid blood loss during sternotomy. The immediate availability of typed and crossmatched blood is verified before skin incision. Patients undergoing reoperations are more likely to have a positive antibody screen that delays the availability of blood products. External defibrillation pads are always applied to patients undergoing reoperation or in procedures in which access to the heart with internal paddles is not readily available.

Anesthesia care begins in the preinduction period, documents significant events of surgery, and becomes part of the patient's medical record. Prior to induction of general anesthesia, a baseline set of hemodynamic measurements is obtained and recorded. These measures often guide the choice of anesthetic drugs and technique, provide a baseline for comparison later, and confirm hemodynamic data acquired during cardiac catheterization. Automated record keepers eventually may relieve the anesthetist of recording this data.

Induction of general anesthesia is achieved by inhalation of volatile potent anesthetics, the intravenous administration of sedative-hypnotics, or both. Inhalation inductions permit maintenance of spontaneous ventilation and a controlled titration of anesthetic dose but prolong the excitatory phase of anesthesia when the patient is prone to cough, move, develop laryngospasm, or vomit and aspirate. Inhalation inductions are not used commonly in adults. Intravenous induction produces rapid apnea that requires immediate ventilatory support. Administration of neuromuscular blocking drugs produces profound muscle paralysis and facilitates laryngoscopy and tracheal intubation. Vasoactive drugs are titrated, if necessary, to counteract the cardiovascular effects of anesthetics. Laryngoscopy is extremely stimulating (painful) and, if the patient is inadequately anesthetized, causes severe hypertension and tachycardia and stimulates vasovagal reflexes. The inability to ventilate or intubate the trachea in a patient after the induction of general anesthesia is a medical crisis and may require transtracheal jet ventilation, cricothyroidotomy, or tracheostomy. Patients with a history of a technically difficult tracheal intubation, poor dentition, large tongue, limited mouth opening, inability to sublux the mandible, or a recessed chin are at increased risk of airway complications, and it may be prudent to secure the airway while they are still awake. Successful intubation of the trachea is verified by the appearance of a carbon dioxide expirogram. Most adult patients can be intubated with an 8.0-mm-internal-diameter polyvinyl chloride endotracheal tube that accommodates an adult flexible bronchoscope. The tip of the tracheal tube is secured above the carina by documenting breath sounds bilaterally. The patient is positioned prior to surgical preparation and draping. Regions susceptible to pressure injuries are protected and padded.

Maintenance of general anesthesia is achieved by continuous or intermittent administration of anesthetic drugs titrated to effect while monitoring the conduct of operation and vital physiological functions. Short-acting vasoactive agents with rapid onset of action are usually preferred for controlling the circulation because conditions constantly change. The cardiovascular actions of inhaled anesthetics are often utilized for short-term blood pressure control because effective concentrations can be reached quickly and monitored in real time by expired gases. Direct-acting vasodilators may be required for blood pressure control if the patient cannot tolerate the myocardial depressant effects of an inhaled anesthetic. Vasopressors and inotropic agents sometimes are required to support the circulation in response to anesthetic-induced vasodilation and cardiac depression. Utilizing nitroglycerin to modify venous capacitance permits buffering acute changes in intravascular volume. Heart rate can be controlled by short-acting cardioselective beta-adrenergic agonists and antagonists, vagolytic agents, or chronotropic drugs or, alternatively, by direct cardiac pacing. The urgency to control hemodynamic parameters with pharmacologic therapy must be tempered

TABLE 9–4 Checklist for preparation to separate from cardiopulmonary bypass

1. Stable rhythm, preferably with a synchronized atrial contraction
2. Pacemaker and cables available
3. Positive inotropes available (e.g., epinephrine, dopamine)
4. Vasodilators available (e.g., nitroglycerine, nitroprusside)
5. Vasopressors available (e.g., phenylephrine, norepinephrine)
6. Adequate levels of anesthesia and paralysis
7. Normothermia: nasopharyngeal temperature = 37°C, rectal or bladder temperature = 35°C
8. Normal serum electrolyte concentrations: K^+, Ca^{+2}
9. Normal serum glucose
10. Normal blood acid-base status
11. No systemic oxygen debt: oxygen saturation in cardiopulmonary bypass venous inflow >70%
12. Acceptable O_2-carrying capacity: hemoglobin concentration
13. Normal systemic vascular resistance
14. Recalibration of pressure transducers
15. ECG in diagnostic mode
16. Clearance of air by TEE
17. Hemothorax evacuated
18. Ventilation with 100% oxygen and atelectatic lungs reexpanded

by recognizing the risk of drug overdose from overzealous treatment. Intraoperative events associated with acute increases in anesthetic requirements are sternotomy, chest wall retraction, manipulations and cannulation of the aorta, rewarming during cardiopulmonary bypass, and sternal wiring. Intraoperative awareness from insufficient anesthesia may occur during cardiac surgery, especially if the anesthetist places a greater emphasis on avoiding cardiovascular actions of anesthetic agents than on providing sufficient anesthesia.

Initiation of cardiopulmonary bypass acutely changes circulating drug concentrations. The addition of 2 L of pump prime has a negligible effect on plasma concentrations of lipophilic drugs with a large volume of distribution but significantly decreases the concentration of drugs distributed primarily in the intravascular space. Despite measurable decreases in blood anesthetic concentrations during cardiopulmonary bypass, the anesthetic level may not change because systemic hypothermia decreases anesthetic requirements, potentiates the effects of neuromuscular blocking drugs, and increases the solubility of volatile anesthetics in blood. Rewarming returns anesthetic requirements to baseline levels and predisposes to inadequate anesthesia if therapeutic drug concentrations are not maintained. The judicious use of sedative-hypnotics, analgesics, and amnestic agents during rewarming decreases the incidence of recall but does not guarantee unconsciousness. Volatile inhalation anesthetics can be given during cardiopulmonary bypass by adding them to the oxygen-rich gas mixture ventilating the pump oxygenator. This use of volatile anesthetics requires an effective scavenging system to prevent accumulation of anesthetic gases in ambient air.

Separation from cardiopulmonary bypass requires effective communication among members of the intraoperative team. Similar to an airline pilot preparing to land, the cardiac anesthesiologist has a checklist that ensures that all systems are in working order (Table 9-4).

ANESTHESIA IN THE IMMEDIATE POSTOPERATIVE PERIOD

Continuous monitoring of physiological functions during transport to the postoperative intensive care unit is paramount because of the possibility of hemodynamic instability. Cardiac output, blood pressure, and vascular tone decrease acutely in the immediate postoperative period because surgical stimulation no longer increases sympathetic tone. Vasodilation also occurs from increases in cutaneous blood flow during active rewarming. Reducing positive pressure ventilatory support during weaning from mechanical ventilation may alter hemodynamic function by increasing venous return and decreasing pulmonary vascular resistance. Sedative-hypnotic or analgesic drugs administered in the immediate postoperative period contribute to changes in the circulatory state.

Anesthesia is required in the early postoperative period because of mechanical ventilatory support, hypothermia, and the possibility of hypertension and tachycardia from pain and tracheal intubation if abrupt emergence occurs. Several hours may be needed to achieve criteria for tracheal extubation (e.g., minimal bleeding, cardiovascular stability, systemic rewarming). Arrival in the intensive care unit triggers a battery of laboratory tests designed to assess rapid changes in vital organ function and prompt corrective therapy. These tests include a chest radiograph, complete blood and platelet count, chemistry battery with blood urea nitrogen and serum creatinine, serum glucose, ECG, prothrombin time and partial thromboplastin time, and arterial blood gases.

Preemptive patient management during operation and in the early postoperative period can decrease intensive care unit and hospital length of stay after cardiac surgery.[192] Traditionally, high-dose narcotic anesthesia provided profound analgesia, sympathetic blockade, and a gradual emergence that was managed over a time course of 8 to 12 hours. With high-dose narcotic anesthesia, patient recovery often was determined by the duration of action of the anesthetic given in the operating room. The time required for recovery from general anesthesia may be decreased by short-acting sedative-hypnotics (e.g., propofol) or analgesics administered by infusion that continues into the postoperative period and permits recovery according to the patient's condition rather than the anesthetic. Implementation of protocol-based care plans, designed to expedite patient recovery after cardiac operations, requires a coordinated effort and mutual understanding between the anesthesiologist, surgeon, and critical care team.

Hemodynamic management of cardiac surgical patients is integrated with anesthetic management. The ability to rapidly establish a diagnosis and circulation during anesthesia is essential for safe conduct of cardiac operations. The challenge to maintain control of the cardiovascular system during the course of a typical operation is complicated by actions of the anesthetic drugs on the circulation, autonomic nervous system reflexes, variability in individual responses to vasoactive drug therapy, continuous fluctuations in the intensity of painful stimuli, rapid intravascular volume shifts, the patient's underlying medical condition, and the urgency of operation.

REFERENCES

1. O'Connor MF, Daves SM, Tung A, et al: BIS monitoring to prevent awareness during general anesthesia. *Anesthesiology* 2001; 94:520.
2. Szekely B, Saint-Marc T, Degremont AC, et al: Value of bispectral index monitoring during cardiopulmonary resuscitation. *Br J Anaesth* 2002; 88:443.
3. Owens WD, Felts JA, Spitznagel EL: ASA Physical Status Classifications: a study of consistency of ratings. *Anesthesiology* 1978; 49:239.
4. Samsoon GLT, Young JRB: Difficult tracheal intubation: a retrospective study. *Anaesthesia* 1987; 42:487.
5. Mallampati SR, Gatt SP, Gugino LD, et al: A clinical sign to predict difficult tracheal intubation: a prospective study. *Can Anaesth Soc J* 1985; 32:429.
6. Strandgaard S, Olesen J, Skinhoj E, Lassen NA: Autoregulation of brain circulation in severe arterial hypertension. *BMJ* 1973; 1:507.
7. Cheng EY, Lauer KK, Stommel KA, Guenther NR: Evaluation of the palmar circulation by pulse oximetry. *J Clin Monit* 1989; 5:1.
8. Bedford RF, Shah NK: Blood pressure monitoring: invasive and noninvasive, in Blitt CD, Hines RL (eds): *Monitoring in Anesthesia and Critical Care Medicine*, 3d ed. New York, Churchill Livingstone, 1995; p 95.
9. O'Rourke MF: Pressure and flow waves in systemic arteries and the anatomical design of the arterial system. *J Appl Physiol* 1967; 23:139.
10. Brunner JMR, Krenis LJ, Kunsman JM, et al: Comparison of direct and indirect methods of measuring arterial blood pressure, part I. *Med Instrum* 1981; 15:11.
11. Boutros A, Albert S: Effect of the dynamic response of transducer-tubing system on accuracy of direct blood pressure measurement in patients. *Crit Care Med* 1983; 11:124.
12. Prys-Roberts C: Measurement of intravascular pressure, in Saidman LJ, Smith NT (eds): *Monitoring in Anesthesia*. New York, Churchill Livingstone, 1978.
13. London M, Hollenberg M, Wong M, et al: Intraoperative myocardial ischemia: localization by continuous 12-lead electrocardiography. *Anesthesiology* 1988; 69:232.
14. Mangano DT, Browner WS, Hollenberg M, et al: Association of perioperative myocardial ischemia with cardiac morbidity and mortality in men undergoing noncardiac surgery. *N Engl J Med* 1990; 323:1781.
15. Moller JT, Johannessen NW, Espersen K, et al: Randomized evaluation of pulse oximetry in 20,802 patients, II: perioperative events and postoperative complications. *Anesthesiology* 1993; 78:445.
16. Pan PH, Gravenstein N: Intraoperative pulse oximetry: frequency and distribution of discrepant data. *J Clin Anesth* 1994; 6:491.
17. Strazis KP, Fox AW: Malignant hyperthermia: a review of published cases. *Anesth Analg* 1993; 77:297.
18. Murphy FL: Hazards of anesthesia, in Longnecker DE, Murphy FL (eds): *Dripps Introduction to Anesthesia*, 9th ed. Philadelphia, WB Saunders, 1996.
19. Reed CR, Sessler CN, Glauser FL, Phelan BA: Central venous catheter infections: concepts and controversies. *Intensive Care Med* 1995; 21:177.
20. Troianos CA, Jobes DR, Ellison N: Ultrasound-guided cannulation of the internal jugular vein: a prospective, randomized study. *Anesth Analg* 1991; 72:823.
21. Van Daele ME, Sutherland GR, Mitchell MM, et al: Do changes in pulmonary capillary wedge pressure adequately reflect myocardial ischemia during anesthesia? A correlative preoperative hemodynamic, electrocardiographic and transesophageal echocardiographic study. *Circulation* 1990; 81:865.
22. Sprung CL, Elser B, Schein RMH, et al: Risk of right bundle branch block and complete heart block during pulmonary artery catheterization. *Crit Care Med* 1989; 17:1.
23. Kim YL, Richman KA, Marshall BE: Thrombocytopenia associated with Swan Ganz catheterization in patients. *Anesthesiology* 1980; 53:261.
24. Mangano DT: Heparin bonding and long-term protection against thrombogenesis. *N Engl J Med* 1982; 307:894.
25. Bohrer H, Fleischer F, Lang J, Vahl C: Early formation of thrombi on pulmonary artery catheters in cardiac surgical patients receiving high-dose aprotonin. *J Cardiothorac Anesth* 1990; 4:222.
26. Swan HJC, Ganz W, Forrester J, et al: Catheterization of the heart in man with use of a flow directed balloon tipped catheter. *N Engl J Med* 1970; 283:447.
27. Reich DL, Kaplan JA: Hemodynamic monitoring, in Kaplan JA (ed): *Cardiac Anesthesia*. Philadelphia, WB Saunders, 1993; p 261.
28. Savino JS, Troianos CA, Aukburg, et al: Measurement of pulmonary blood flow with transesophageal two-dimensional and Doppler echocardiography. *Anesthesiology* 1991; 75:445.
29. Philip JH, Feinstein DM, Raemer DB: Monitoring anesthetic and respiratory gases, in Blitt CD, Hines RL (eds): *Monitoring in Anesthesia and Critical Care Medicine*, 3d ed. New York, Churchill Livingstone, 1995; p 363.
30. Cheung A, Chernow B: Perioperative electrolyte disorders, in Benumof JL, Saidman LJ (eds): *Anesthesia and Perioperative Complications*. St Louis, Mosby-Year Book, 1991; p 466.
31. Drop LJ: Ionized calcium, the heart, and hemodynamic function. *Anesth Analg* 1985; 64:432.
32. Bronsky B, Dubin A, Waldstein SS, et al: Calcium and the electrocardiogram, 1: electrocardiographic manifestations of hypoparathyroidism. *Am J Cardiol* 1961; 7:823.
33. Robertie PG, Butterworth JF, Royster RL, et al: Normal parathyroid hormone responses to hypocalcemia during cardiopulmonary bypass. *Anesthesiology* 1991; 75:43.
34. Fernandez-del Castillo C, Harringer W, Warshaw AL, et al: Risk factors for pancreatic cellular injury after cardiopulmonary bypass. *N Engl J Med* 1991; 325:382.
35. Algio LS, Stanford GG, Maddi R, et al: Hypomagnesemia is common following cardiac surgery. *J Cardiothorac Vasc Anesth* 1991; 5:201.
36. England MR, Gordon G, Salem M, Chernow B: Magnesium administration and dysrhythmias after cardiac surgery: a placebo-controlled, double-blind, randomized trail. *JAMA* 1992; 268: 2395.
37. Vyvyan HA, Mayne PN, Cutfield GR: Magnesium flux and cardiac surgery: a study of the relationship between magnesium exchange, serum magnesium levels and postoperative arrhythmias. *Anaesthesia* 1994; 49:245.

38. Furnary AP, Zerr KJ, Grunkemeier GL, Starr A: Continuous intravenous insulin infusion reduces the incidence of deep sternal wound infection in diabetic patients after cardiac surgical procedures. *Ann Thorac Surg* 1999; 67:352.
39. van den Berghe G, Wouters P, Weekers F, et al: Intensive insulin therapy in the surgical intensive care unit. *N Eng J Med* 2001; 345:1359.
40. Floyd TF, Cheung AT, Stecker MM: Postoperative neurologic assessment and management of the cardiac surgical patient. *Semin Thorac Cardiovasc Surg* 2000; 12:337.
41. McKhann GM, Goldsborough MA, Borowicz LM Jr, et al: Predictors of stroke risk in coronary artery bypass patients. *Ann Thorac Surg* 1997; 63:516.
42. Newman MF, Wolman R, Kanchuger M, et al: Multicenter preoperative stroke risk index for patients undergoing coronary artery bypass graft surgery. Multicenter Study of Perioperative Ischemia (McSPI) Research Group. *Circulation* 1996; 94:II74.
43. Caplan LR, Hennerici M: Impaired clearance of emboli (washout) is an important link between hypoperfusion, embolism, and ischemic stroke. *Arch Neurol* 1998; 55:1475.
44. van der Linden J, Hadjinikolaou L, Bergman P, Lindblom D: Postoperative stroke in cardiac surgery is related to the location and extent of atherosclerotic disease in the ascending aorta. *J Am Coll Cardiol* 2001; 38:131.
45. Rokkas CK, Kouchoukos NT: Surgical management of the severely atherosclerotic ascending aorta during cardiac operations. *Semin Thorac Cardiovasc Surg* 1998; 10:240.
46. Dexter F, Hindman BJ: Effect of haemoglobin concentration on brain oxygenation in focal stroke: a mathematical modelling study. *Br J Anaesth* 1997; 79:346.
47. Goto T, Yoshitake A, Baba T, et al: Cerebral ischemic disorders and cerebral oxygen balance during cardiopulmonary bypass surgery: preoperative evaluation using magnetic resonance imaging and angiography. *Anesth Analg* 1997; 84:5.
48. Chalela JA, Katzan I, Liebeskind DS, et al: Safety of intra-arterial thrombolysis in the postoperative period. *Stroke* 2001; 32:1365.
49. Moazami N, Smedira NG, McCarthy PM, et al: Safety and efficacy of intraarterial thrombolysis for perioperative stroke after cardiac operation. *Ann Thorac Surg* 2001; 72:1933.
50. Gravereaux EC, Faries PL, Burks JA, et al: Risk of spinal cord ischemia after endograft repair of thoracic aortic aneurysms. *J Vasc Surg* 2001; 34:997.
51. Coselli JS, LeMaire SA, Miller CC 3rd, et al: Mortality and paraplegia after thoracoabdominal aortic aneurysm repair: a risk factor analysis. *Ann Thorac Surg* 2000; 69:409.
52. Safi HJ, Miller CC 3rd: Spinal cord protection in descending thoracic and thoracoabdominal aortic repair. *Ann Thorac Surg* 1999; 67:1937.
53. Grabitz K, Sandmann W, Stuhmeier K, et al: The risk of ischemic spinal cord injury in patients undergoing graft replacement for thoracoabdominal aortic aneurysms. *J Vasc Surg* 1996; 23:230.
54. Griepp RB, Ergin MA, Galla JD, et al: Looking for the artery of Adamkiewicz: a quest to minimize paraplegia after operations for aneurysms of the descending thoracic and thoracoabdominal aorta. *J Thorac Cardiovasc Surg* 1996; 112:1202.
55. Svensson LG, Hess KR, Coselli JS, Safi HJ: Influence of segmental arteries, extent, and atriofemoral bypass on postoperative paraplegia after thoracoabdominal aortic operations. *J Vasc Surg* 1994; 20:255.
56. van Dongen EP, Schepens MA, Morshuis WJ, et al: Thoracic and thoracoabdominal aortic aneurysm repair: use of evoked potential monitoring in 118 patients. *J Vasc Surg* 2001; 34:1035.
57. Jacobs M, Meylaerts SA, de Haan P, et al: Strategies to prevent neurologic deficit based on motor-evoked potentials in type I and II thoracoabdominal aortic aneurysm repair. *J Vasc Surg* 1999; 29:48.
58. Shiiya N, Yasuda K, Matsui Y, et al: Spinal cord protection during thoracoabdominal aortic aneurysm repair: results of selective reconstruction of the critical segmental arteries guided by evoked spinal cord potential monitoring. *J Vasc Surg* 1995; 21:970.
59. Svensson LG: Management of segmental intercostal and lumbar arteries during descending and thoracoabdominal aneurysm repairs. *Semin Thorac Cardiovasc Surg* 1998; 10:45.
60. Ross SD, Kron IL, Parrino PE, et al: Preservation of intercostal arteries during thoracoabdominal aortic aneurysm surgery: a retrospective study. *J Thorac Cardiovasc Surg* 1999; 118:17.
61. Albin MS, White RJ, Locke GE, Kretchmer HE: Spinal cord hypothermia by localized perfusion cooling. *Nature* 1966; 210: 1059.
62. Cambria RP, Davison JK: Regional hypothermia for prevention of spinal cord ischemic complications after thoracoabdominal aortic surgery: experience with epidural cooling. *Semin Thorac Cardiovasc Surg* 1998; 10:61.
63. Bonatti J, Watzka S, Antretter H, et al: Spinal cord protection in descending and thoracoabdominal aortic surgery–the role of distal perfusion. *Thorac Cardiovasc Surg* 1996; 44:136.
64. Robertazzi RR, Acinapura AJ: The efficacy of left atrial to femoral artery bypass in the prevention of spinal cord ischemia during aortic surgery. *Semin Thorac Cardiovasc Surg* 1998; 10: 67.
65. Ling E, Arellano R: Systematic overview of the evidence supporting the use of cerebrospinal fluid drainage in thoracoabdominal aneurysm surgery for prevention of paraplegia. *Anesthesiology* 2000; 93:1115.
66. Azizzadeh A, Huynh TT, Miller CC 3rd, Safi HJ: Reversal of twice-delayed neurologic deficits with cerebrospinal fluid drainage after thoracoabdominal aneurysm repair: a case report and plea for a national database collection. *J Vasc Surg* 2000; 31:592.
67. Ortiz-Gomez JR, Gonzalez-Solis FJ, Fernandez-Alonso L, Bilbao JI: Reversal of acute paraplegia with cerebrospinal fluid drainage after endovascular thoracic aortic aneurysm repair. *Anesthesiology* 2001; 95:1288.
68. Weaver KD, Wiseman DB, Farber M, et al: Complications of lumbar drainage after thoracoabdominal aortic aneurysm repair. *J Vasc Surg* 2001; 34:623.
69. Newman MF, et al: Longitudinal assessment of neurocognitive function after coronary-artery bypass surgery. *N Engl J Med* 2001; 344:395.
70. Vingerhoets G, Van Nooten G, Vermassen F, et al: Short-term and long-term neuropsychological consequences of cardiac surgery with extracorporeal circulation. *Eur J Cardiothorac Surg* 1997; 11:424.
71. Selnes OA, Goldsborough MA, Borowicz LM Jr, et al: Determinants of cognitive change after coronary artery bypass surgery: a multifactorial problem. *Ann Thorac Surg* 1999; 67:1669.
72. Mutch WA, Sutton IR, Teskey JM, et al: Cerebral pressure-flow relationship during cardiopulmonary bypass in the dog at normothermia and moderate hypothermia. *J Cereb Blood Flow Metab* 1994; 14:510.
73. Braekken SK, Russell D, Brucher R, et al: Cerebral microembolic signals during cardiopulmonary bypass surgery: frequency, time of occurrence, and association with patient and surgical characteristics. *Stroke* 1997; 28:1988.
74. Heyer EJ, Delphin E, Adams DC, et al: Cerebral dysfunction after cardiac operations in elderly patients. *Ann Thorac Surg* 1995; 60:1716.
75. Jonas RA: Optimal hematocrit for adult cardiopulmonary bypass. *J Cardiothorac Vasc Anesth* 2001; 15:672.
76. Harris DN, Oatridge A, Dob D, et al: Cerebral swelling after normothermic cardiopulmonary bypass. *Anesthesiology* 1998; 88:340.

77. Grigore AM, Grocott HP, Mathew JP, et al: The rewarming rate and increased peak temperature alter neurocognitive outcome after cardiac surgery. *Anesth Analg* 2002; 94:4.
78. Cook DJ, Oliver WC Jr, Orszulak TA, Daly RC: A prospective, randomized comparison of cerebral venous oxygen saturation during normothermic and hypothermic cardiopulmonary bypass. *J Thorac Cardiovasc Surg* 1994; 107:1020.
79. Patel RL, Turtle MR, Chambers DJ, et al: Alpha-stat acid-base regulation during cardiopulmonary bypass improves neuropsychologic outcome in patients undergoing coronary artery bypass grafting. *J Thorac Cardiovasc Surg* 1996; 111:1267.
80. Undar A, Calhoon JH, Cossman RM, Johnson SB: The effects of pulsatile cardiopulmonary bypass on cerebral and renal blood flow in dogs [letter; comment]. *J Cardiothorac Vasc Anesth* 1998; 12:126.
81. Croughwell ND, Reves JG, White WD, et al: Cardiopulmonary bypass time does not affect cerebral blood flow. *Ann Thorac Surg* 1998; 65:1226.
82. Sungurtekin H, Plochl W, Cook DJ: Relationship between cardiopulmonary bypass flow rate and cerebral embolization in dogs. *Anesthesiology* 1999; 91:1387.
83. Jacobs A, Neveling M, Horst M, et al: Alterations of neuropsychological function and cerebral glucose metabolism after cardiac surgery are not related only to intraoperative microembolic events. *Stroke* 1998; 29:660.
84. Tardiff BE, Newman MF, Saunders AM, et al: Preliminary report of a genetic basis for cognitive decline after cardiac operations. The Neurologic Outcome Research Group of the Duke Heart Center. *Ann Thorac Surg* 1997; 64:715.
85. Boyle EM Jr, Pohlman TH, Johnson MC, Verrier ED: Endothelial cell injury in cardiovascular surgery: the systemic inflammatory response. *Ann Thorac Surg* 1997; 63:277.
86. Zuccala G, Onder G, Pedone C, et al: Cognitive dysfunction as a major determinant of disability in patients with heart failure: results from a multicentre survey. On behalf of the GIFA (SIGG-ONLUS) Investigators. *J Neurol Neurosurg Psychiatry* 2001; 70:109.
87. Almeida OP, Flicker L: The mind of a failing heart: a systematic review of the association between congestive heart failure and cognitive functioning. *Intern Med J* 2001; 31:290.
88. Stanimirovic D, Satoh K: Inflammatory mediators of cerebral endothelium: a role in ischemic brain inflammation. *Brain Pathol* 2000; 10:113.
89. Starzyk RM, Rosenow C, Frye J, et al: Cerebral cell adhesion molecule: a novel leukocyte adhesion determinant on blood-brain barrier capillary endothelium. *J Infect Dis* 2000; 181: 181.
90. Abbott NJ: Inflammatory mediators and modulation of blood-brain barrier permeability. *Cell Mol Neurobiol* 2000; 20: 131.
91. Riis J, Lomholt B, Haxholdt O, et al: Immediate and long-term mental recovery from general versus epidural anesthesia in elderly patients. *Acta Anaesthesiol Scand* 1983; 27:44.
92. Turnipseed WD, Berkoff HA, Belzer FO: Postoperative stroke in cardiac and peripheral vascular disease. *Ann Surg* 1980; 192:365.
93. Bedford PD: Adverse cerebral effects of anaesthesia in old people. *Lancet* 1955; 2:259.
94. Moller JT, Cluitmans P, Rasmussen LS, et al: Long-term postoperative cognitive dysfunction in the elderly ISPOCD1 study. ISPOCD investigators. International Study of Post-Operative Cognitive Dysfunction [see comments] [published erratum appears in *Lancet* 1998; 351:1742]. *Lancet* 1998; 351:857.
95. Abildstrom H, Rasmussen LS, Rentowl P, et al: Cognitive dysfunction 1–2 years after non-cardiac surgery in the elderly. ISPOCD group. International Study of Post-Operative Cognitive Dysfunction. *Acta Anaesthesiol Scand* 2000; 44:1246.
96. Kofke WA, Garman RH, Garman R, Rose ME et al: Opioid neurotoxicity: fentanyl-induced exacerbation of cerebral ischemia in rats. *Brain Res* 1999; 818:326.
97. Personnet F, Sindon M, Laviron A, et al: Human cortical electrogenesis: stratigraphy and spectral analysis, in Petsche H, Brazier MAB (eds): *Synchronization of EEG Activity in Epilepsies*. New York, Springer-Verlag, 1972; p 235.
98. Allison T: Calculated and empirical evoked-potential distribution in human recordings, in Otto DA (ed): *Multidisciplinary Perspectives in Event-Related Brain Potential Research*. Washington, DC, US Environmental Protection Agency, 1978.
99. Bashein G, Nessly ML, Bledsoe SW, et al: Electroencephalography during surgery with cardiopulmonary bypass and hypothermia. *Anesthesiology* 1992; 76:878.
100. Levy WJ: Monitoring of the electroencephalogram during cardiopulmonary bypass. *Anesthesiology* 1992; 76:876.
101. Markand ON, Warren C, Mallik GS, et al: Temperature-dependent hysteresis in somatosensory and auditory evoked potentials. *Electroencephalogr Clin Neurophysiol* 1990; 77:425.
102. Cheung AT, Savino JS, Weiss SJ, et al: Detection of acute embolic stroke during mitral valve replacement using somatosensory evoked potential monitoring. *Anesthesiology* 1995; 83: 208.
103. Hickey C, Gugino LD, Aglio LS: Intraoperative somatosensory evoked potential monitoring predicts peripheral nerve injury during cardiac surgery. *Anesthesiology* 1993; 78:29.
104. Clark RE, Brillman J, Davis DA, et al: Microemboli during coronary artery bypass grafting. *J Thorac Cardiovasc Surg* 1995; 109:249.
105. Cheung AT, Weiss SJ, Savino JS: Protamine-induced right-to-left intracardiac shunting. *Anesthesiology* 1991; 75:904.
106. Weiss SJ, Cheung AT, Stecker MM, et al: Fatal paradoxical cerebral embolization during bilateral knee arthroplasty. *Anesthesiology* 1996; 84:721.
107. Pearson AC, Labovitz AJ, Tatineni S, Gomez CR: Superiority of transesophageal echocardiography in detecting cardiac source of embolism in patients with cerebral ischemia of uncertain etiology. *J Am Coll Cardiol* 1991; 17:66.
108. Cheung AT, Levin SK, Weiss SJ, et al: Intracardiac thrombus: a risk of incomplete anticoagulation for cardiac operations. *Ann Thorac Surg* 1994; 58:541.
109. Savino JS, Weiss SJ: Images in clinical medicine: right atrial tumor. *N Engl J Med* 1995; 333:1608.
110. Davila-Roman VG, Barzilai B, Wareing TH, et al: Intraoperative ultrasonographic evaluation of the ascending aorta in 100 consecutive patients undergoing cardiac surgery. *Circulation* 1991; 84 (suppl III):III47.
111. Tuman KJ, McCarthy RJ, Spiess BD, Ivankovich AD: Comparison of anesthetic techniques in patients undergoing heart valve replacement. *J Cardiothorac Anesth* 1990; 4:159.
112. Tuman KJ, McCarthy RJ, Spiess BD, et al: Does choice of anesthetic agent significantly affect outcome after coronary artery surgery? *Anesthesiology* 1989; 70:189.
113. Slogoff S, Keats AS: Randomized trial of primary anesthetic agents on outcome of coronary artery bypass operations. *Anesthesiology* 1989; 70:179.
114. Mora CT, Dudek C, Torjman MC, White PF: The effects of anesthetic technique on the hemodynamic response and recovery profile in coronary revascularization patients. *Anesth Analg* 1995; 81:900.
115. James KB, Marwick T, Cosgrove DML: Underestimation of mitral regurgitation under general anesthesia. *J Thorac Cardiovasc Surg* 1992; 104:534.
116. Konstadt SN, Louie EK, Shore-Lesserson L, et al: The effects of loading changes on intraoperative Doppler assessment of mitral regurgitation. *J Cardiothorac Vasc Anesth* 1994; 8:19.

117. Longnecker DE, Cheung AT: Pharmacology of inhalational anesthetics, in Longnecker DE, Tinker JH, Morgan GE (eds): *Principles and Practice of Anesthesiology*, 2d ed. St Louis, Mosby, 1998; p 1123.
118. Kikura M, Ikeda K: Comparison of effects of sevoflurane/nitrous oxide and enflurane/nitrous oxide on myocardial contractility in humans. *Anesthesiology* 1992; 79:235.
119. Pagel PS, Kampine JP, Schmeling WT, Warltier DC: Comparison of the systemic and coronary hemodynamic actions of desflurane, isoflurane, halothane, and enflurane in the chronically instrumented dog. *Anesthesiology* 1991; 74:539.
120. Stowe DF, Monroe SM, Marijic J, et al: Comparison of halothane, enflurane, and isoflurane with nitrous oxide on contractility and oxygen supply and demand in isolated hearts. *Anesthesiology* 1991; 75:1062.
121. Kemmotsu S, Hasimoto Y, Sheimosato S: Inotropic effects of isoflurane on mechanics of contraction in isolated cat papillary muscles from normal and failing hearts. *Anesthesiology* 1973; 39:470.
122. Brown BR, Richard J: A comparative study of the effects of five general anesthetics on myocardial contractility: isometric conditions. *Anesthesiology* 1971; 34:236.
123. Van Tright P, Christian CC, Fagraeus L, et al: Myocardial depression by anesthetic agents: quantitation based on end-systolic pressure-dimension relations. *Am J Cardiol* 1984; 53:243.
124. Kotrly KJ, Ebert TH, Vucins E, et al: Baroreflex reflex control of heart rate during isoflurane anesthesia in humans. *Anesthesiology* 1984; 60:173.
125. Pagel PS, Kampine JP, Schmeling WT, Warltier DC: Alteration of left ventricular diastolic function by desflurane, isoflurane, and halothane in the chronically instrumented dog with autonomic nervous system blockade. *Anesthesiology* 1991; 74:1103.
126. Buffington CW: Impaired systolic thickening associated with halothane in the presence of a coronary stenosis is mediated by changes in hemodynamics. *Anesthesiology* 1986; 64:632.
127. Gelman S, Fowler KC, Smith LR: Regional blood flow during isoflurane and halothane anesthesia. *Anesth Analg* 1984; 63:557.
128. Blaise G, Sill JC, Nugent M, et al: Isoflurane causes endothelium-dependent inhibition of contractile responses of canine coronary arteries. *Anesthesiology* 1987; 67:513.
129. Becker LC: Conditions for vasodilator-induced coronary steal in experimental myocardial ischemia. *Circulation* 1978; 57: 1103.
130. Hogue CW Jr, Lerbst TJ, Pond C, et al: Perioperative myocardial ischemia. *Anesthesiology* 1993; 79:514.
131. Helman JD, Leung JM, Bellows WH, et al: The risk of myocardial ischemia in patients receiving desflurane versus sufentanil anesthesia for coronary artery bypass graft surgery. *Anesthesiology* 1992; 77:47.
132. Inoue K, Reichelt W, el-Banayosy A, et al: Does isoflurane lead to a higher incidence of myocardial infarction and perioperative death than enflurane in coronary artery surgery? A clinical study of 1178 patients. *Anesth Analg* 1990; 71:469.
133. Ebert TJ, Muzi M: Sympathetic hyperactivity during desflurane anesthesia in healthy volunteers. *Anesthesiology* 1993; 79: 444.
134. Zaugg M, Lucchinetti E, Spahn D, Pasch T, Schaub M: Volatile anesthetics mimic cardiac preconditioning by priming the activation of mito K_{ATP} channels via multiple signaling pathways. *Anesthesiology* 2002: 97:4.
135. Zaugg M, Lucchinetti E, Spahn D, et al: Differential effects of anesthetics on mitochondrial K_{ATP} channel activity and cardiomyocyte protection. *Anesthesiology* 2002; 97:15.
136. Siemikawa K, Ishizseka N, Suzaki M: Arrhythmogenic plasma levels of epinephrine with halothane, enflurane, and pentobarbital anesthesia in the dog. *Anesthesiology* 1983; 58:322.
137. Thomson IR, Bowering JB, Hudson RJ, et al: A comparison of desflurane and isoflurane in patients undergoing coronary artery surgery. *Anesthesiology* 1991; 75:776.
138. Cheung AT, Marshall BE: The inhaled anesthetics, in Longnecker DE, Murphy FL (eds): *Dripps Introduction to Anesthesia*, 9th ed. Philadelphia, WB Saunders, 1996.
139. Varadarajan SG, An J, Novalija E, Stowe DF. Sevoflurane before or after ischemia improves contractile and metabolic function while reducing myoplasmic Ca(2+) loading in intact hearts. *Anesthesiology* 2002; 96:125.
140. Loeckinger A, Keller C, Lindner KH, Kleinsasser A: Pulmonary gas exchange in coronary artery surgery patients during sevoflurane and isoflurane anesthesia. *Anesth Analg* 2002; 94:1107
141. Stowe DF, Bosnjak ZJ, Kampine JP: Comparison of etomidate, ketamine, midazolam, propofol, and thiopental on function and metabolism of isolated hearts. *Anesth Analg* 1992; 74:547.
142. Park WK, Lynch C III: Propofol and thiopental depression of myocardial contractility: a comparative study of mechanical and electrophysiologic effects in isolated guinea pig ventricular muscle. *Anesth Analg* 1992; 74:395.
143. Lepage J-YM, Pinaud ML, Helias JH, et al: Left ventricular performance during propofol and methohexital anesthesia: isotopic and invasive cardiac monitoring. *Anesth Analg* 1991; 73:3.
144. Muzi M, Berens RA, Kampine JP, Ebert TJ: Ventilation contributes to propofol-mediated hypotension in humans. *Anesth Analg* 1992; 74:877.
145. Rouby JJ, Andreev A, Leger P, et al: Peripheral vascular effects of thiopental and propofol in humans with artificial hearts. *Anesthesiology* 1991; 75:32.
146. Gooding JM, Corssen G: Effect of etomidate on the cardiovascular system. *Anesth Analg* 1977; 56:717.
147. Riou B, Lecarpentier Y, Chemla D, Viars P: In vitro effects of etomidate on intrinsic myocardial contractility in the rat. *Anesthesiology* 1990; 72:330.
148. Riou B, Lecarpentier Y, Viars P: Effects of etomidate on the cardiac papillary muscle of normal hamsters and those with cardiomyopathy. *Anesthesiology* 1993; 78:83.
149. White PF, Way WL, Trevor AJ: Ketamine-Mits pharmacology and therapeutic uses. *Anesthesiology* 1982; 56:119.
150. Waxman K, Shoemaker WC, Lippmann M: Cardiovascular effects of anesthetic induction with ketamine. *Anesth Analg* 1980; 59:355.
151. Flacke JW, Bloor BC, Flacke WE, et al: Reduced narcotic requirement by clonidine with improved hemodynamic and adrenergic stability in patients undergoing coronary bypass surgery. *Anesthesiology* 1987; 67:11.
152. Schulz R, Guth BD, Heusch G: Pharmacological mechanisms to attenuate sympathetically induced myocardial ischemia. *Cardiovasc Drugs Ther* 1989; 3:L43.
153. Talke P, Li J, Jjain U, et al: Effects of perioperative dexmedetomidine infusion in patients undergoing vascular surgery: the study of perioperative ischemia research group. *Anesthesiology* 1995; 82:620.
154. Mansour A., Khachaturian H, Lewis ME, et al: Anatomy of CNS opioid receptors. *Trends Neurosci* 1988; 11:308.
155. Bovill JG, Boer F: Opioids in cardiac anesthesia, in Kaplan J (ed): *Cardiac Anesthesia*, 3d ed. Philadelphia, WB Saunders, 1993; p 467.
156. Benthuysen JL, Smith NT, Sanford TJ, et al: Physiology of alfentanil-induced rigidity. *Anesthesiology* 1986; 64:440.
157. Smith NT, Benthuysen JL, Bickford RG, et al: Seizures during opioid anesthetic induction: are they opioid induced rigidity? *Anesthesiology* 1989; 71:852.
158. Azar I, Turndorf H: Severe hypertension and multiple atrial premature contractions following naloxone administration. *Anesth Analg* 1979; 58:524.

159. Gal TJ, DiFazio CA: Prolonged antagonism of opioid action with intravenous nalmefene in man. *Anesthesiology* 1986; 64:175.
160. Bailey PL, Clark NJ, Pace NL, et al: Failure of nalbuphine to antagonize morphine: a double-blind comparison with naloxone. *Anesth Analg* 1986; 65:605.
161. Puttfarcken PS, Cox BM: Morphine induced desensitizations and down-regulation at mu receptors in 7315c pituitary tumor cells. *Life Sci* 1989; 45:1937.
162. Shafer A, White PF, Schuttlrt J, Rosenthal MH: Use of fentanyl infusion in the intensive care unit: tolerance to its anesthetic effects? *Anesthesiology* 1983;59:245.
163. Egan TD, Lemmens HJ, Fiset P, et al: The pharmacokinetics of the new short-acting opioid remifentanil (GI87084B) in healthy adult male volunteers. *Anesthesiology* 1993; 79:881.
164. Douglas JA, Tuxen DV, Horne M, et al: Myopathy in severe asthma. *Am Rev Respir Dis* 1992; 146:517.
165. Backman SB, Stein RD, Ralley FE, Fox GS: Neostigmine-induced bradycardia following recent vs remote cardiac transplantation in the same patient. *Can J Anaesth* 1996; 43(4): 394.
166. Santos AC, DeArmas PI: Systemic toxicity of levobupivacaine, bupivacaine, and ropivacaine during continuous intravenous infusion to nonpregnant and pregnant ewes. *Anesthesiology* 2001; 95:1256.
167. Ohmura S, Kawada M, Ohta T, et al: Systemic toxicity and resuscitation in bupivacaine-, levobupivacaine-, or ropivacaine-infused rats. *Anesth Analg* 2001; 93:743.
168. American Society of Anesthesiologists Task Force on Management of the Difficult Airway: Practice guidelines for management of the difficult airway. *Anesthesiology* 1993; 78:597.
169. Swenson JD, Hullander RM, Wingler K, Leivers D: Early extubation after cardiac surgery using combined intrathecal sufentanil and morphine. *J Cardiothorac Vasc Anesth* 1994; 8:509.
170. Fitzpatrick GJ, Moriarty DC: Intrathecal morphine in the management of pain following cardiac surgery: a comparison with morphine IV. *Br J Anaesth* 1988; 60:639.
171. Aun C, Thomas D, St. John-Jones L, et al: Intrathecal morphine in cardiac surgery. *Eur J Anaesth* 1985; 2:419.
172. Scott NB, Turfrey DJ, Ray AA, et al: A prospective randomized study of the potential benefits of thoracic epidural anesthesia and analgesia in patients undergoing coronary artery bypass grafting. *Anesth Analg* 2001; 93:528.
173. Moore R, Follette DM, Berkoff HA: Poststernotomy fractures and pain management in open cardiac surgery. *Chest* 1994; 106: 1339.
174. Robinson RJ, Brister S, Jones E, Quigly M: Epidural meperidine analgesia after cardiac surgery. *Can Anaesth Soc J* 1986; 33: 550.
175. Vandermeulen EP, Van Aken H, Vermylen J: Anticoagulants and spinal-epidural anesthesia. *Anesth Analg* 1994; 79:1165.
176. Blomberg S, Curelaru I, Emanuelsson H, et al: Thoracic epidural anaesthesia in patients with unstable angina pectoris. *Eur Heart J* 1989; 10:437.
177. Blomberg SG: Long-term home self-treatment with high thoracic epidural anesthesia in patients with severe coronary artery disease. *Anesth Analg* 1994; 79:413.
178. Goertz AW, Seeling W, Heinrich H, et al: Influence of high thoracic epidural anesthesia on left ventricular contractility assessed using the end-systolic pressure-length relationship. *Acta Anaesthesiol Scand* 1993; 37:38.
179. Blomberg S, Curelaru I, Emanuelsson H, et al: Thoracic epidural anaesthesia in patients with unstable angina pectoris. *Eur Heart J* 1989; 10:437.
180. Reiz S, Nath S, Rais O: Effects of thoracic epidural block and prenalterol on coronary vascular resistance and myocardial metabolism in patients with coronary artery disease. *Acta Anaesthesiol Scand* 1980; 24:11.
181. Blomberg S, Emanuelsson H, Ricksten SE: Thoracic epidural anesthesia and central hemodynamics in patients with unstable angina pectoris. *Anesth Analg* 1989; 65:558.
182. Kock M, Blomberg S, Emanuelsson H, et al: Thoracic epidural anesthesia improves global and regional left ventricular function during stress-induced myocardial ischemia in patients with coronary artery disease. *Anesth Analg* 1990; 71:625.
183. Acher CW, Wynn MM, Archibald J: Naloxone and spinal fluid drainage as adjuncts in the surgical treatment of thoracoabdominal and thoracic aneurysms. *Surgery* 1990; 108:755.
184. Blaisdell FW, Cooley DA: The mechanism of paraplegia after temporary thoracic aortic occlusion and its relationship to spinal fluid pressure. *Surgery* 1962; 51:1351.
185. Svensson MB, Von Ritter CM, Groeneveld HT, et al: Cross-clamping of the thoracic aorta: influence of aortic shunts, laminectomy, papaverine, calcium channel blocker, allopurinol and superoxide dismutase on spinal cord blood flow and paraplegia in baboons. *Ann Surg* 1986; 204:388.
186. Bower TC, Murray MJ, Gloviczki P, et al: Effects of thoracic aortic occlusion and cerebrospinal fluid drainage on regional spinal cord blood flow in dogs: correlation with neurologic outcome. *J Vasc Surg* 1988; 9:135.
187. Murray MJ, Werner E, Oliver WC, et al: Anesthetic management of descending thoracic and thoracoabdominal aortic aneurysm repair: effects of CSF drainage and mild hypothermia. *J Cardiothorac Vasc Anesth* 1993; 7:266.
188. Crawford ES, Svensson LG, Hess KR, et al: A prospective randomized study of cerebrospinal fluid drainage to prevent paraplegia after high risk surgery on the thoracoabdominal aorta. *J Vasc Surg* 1991; 13:36.
189. Cheung AT, Weiss SJ, McGarvey M, et al: Interventions for reversing delayed-onset postoperative paraplegia after thoracic aortic reconstruction. *Ann Thorac Surg* 2002; 74:413.
190. ACC/AHA guidelines and indications for coronary artery bypass graft surgery: a report of the American College of Cardiology/American Heart Association Task Force on cardiovascular procedures. *Circulation* 1991; 83:1125.
191. Practice guidelines for pulmonary artery catheterization: a report by the American Society of Anesthesiologists Task Force on Pulmonary Artery Catheterization. *Anesthesiology* 1993; 78:380.
192. Ramsay JG, DeLima LGR, Wynands JE, et al: Pure opioid vs opioid-volatile anesthesia for coronary artery bypass graft surgery: a prospective randomized double-blinded study. *Anesth Analg* 1994; 78:867.

Chapter **10**

Intraoperative Echocardiography

John A. Fox/Vladimir Formanek/Andrew Friedrich/ Stanton K. Shernan

Since its introduction into clinical practice in the 1980s, the utility of intraoperative echocardiography has becoming increasingly more evident as anesthesiologists, cardiologists, and surgeons continue to appreciate its potential applications. The recent publications of guidelines describing the indications for performing intraoperative echocardiography and technique for acquiring a comprehensive transesophageal echocardiographic (TEE) examination (Fig. 10-1) have facilitated the growth of this important diagnostic tool.[1,2] TEE provides real-time, noninvasive imaging of the heart and great vessels while simultaneously permitting quantification of blood flow and overall cardiac performance without interrupting the surgical procedure. Consequently, the information provided by a comprehensive TEE examination can significantly contribute to the perioperative management of cardiac surgical patients.[3–7] This chapter provides an introductory overview of the utility of intraoperative TEE and its impact on cardiac surgical and anesthetic decision making.

VALVULAR DISEASE

Mitral Valve

Over the last several years, the impact of TEE's influence on perioperative cardiac surgical decision making has become increasingly more appreciated. TEE, however, has been particularly useful in the perioperative evaluation of mitral valve (MV) disease. Early studies commented on the use of MV scanning on the field by the surgeon[8]; however, because of the MV's orientation in relation to the esophagus,

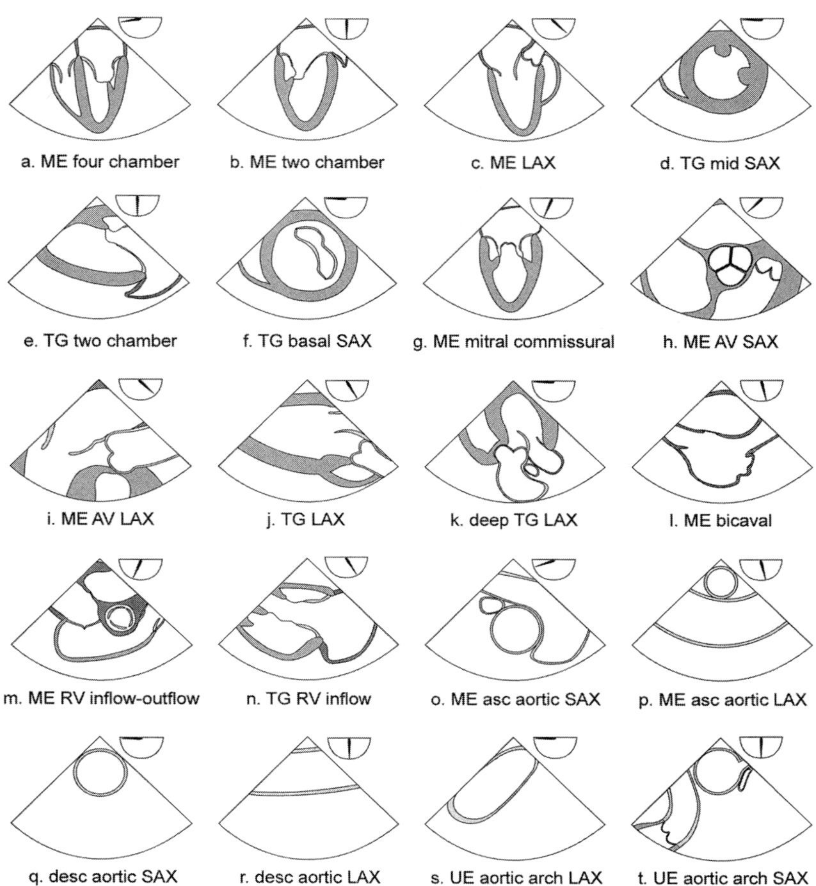

FIGURE 10–1 The 20 multiplane views of a comprehensive intraoperative multiplane transesophageal examination. *(Reproduced with permission from Shanewise JS, Cheung AT, Aronson S, et al: ASE/SCA Guidelines for Performing a Comprehensive Intraoperative Multiplane Transesophageal Echocardiography Examination: Recommendations of the American Society of Echocardiography Council for Intraoperative Echocardiography and the Society of Cardiovascular Anesthesiologists Task Force for Certification in Perioperative Transesophageal Echocardiography. Anesth Analg 1999; 89:870.)*

excellent intraoperative echocardiographic windows for two-dimensional (2-D) and both qualitative and quantitative Doppler evaluation can easily be obtained. Accordingly, TEE has supplanted surgeon-guided epicardial scanning for evaluation of the MV.[9]

A thorough TEE examination of the MV requires the utilization of all echocardiographic modalities. In the initial pre–cardiopulmonary bypass (CPB) period, 2-D echocardiography defines the extent and etiology of MV pathology. The severity and location of MV disease, including subvalvular involvement, annular calcification and dilation, bileaflet prolapse, and anterior mitral leaflet (AML) disease, along with the degree of left ventricular (LV) function, should be assessed. This information, when integrated and evaluated, can be helpful in determining whether MV replacement (MVR), repair, or neither is indicated. It is also important to diagnose if existing severe mitral regurgitation (MR) is primarily associated with ischemia as opposed to rheumatic or myxomatous disease, since the extent of surgical treatment for ischemic MR remains controversial. Although the 2-D anatomic images and the color flow Doppler (CFD) modalities are used most often during interrogation of the MV in the operating suite, a complete echocardiographic evaluation using pulse wave (PWD) and continuous wave Doppler (CWD) can assist in determining the severity of blood flow disturbances associated not only with MR, but also with mitral stenosis (MS).[1]

Clinical studies have suggested that the *pre–CPB* TEE exam prompts changes in surgery in 9% to 14%[8–11] of patients undergoing MV surgery. The population of patients influenced by the pre–CPB TEE exam includes those initially scheduled only for coronary bypass grafting (CABG) who also require an MV procedure. In addition, the pre–CPB exam also influences surgical decision-making in those patients scheduled for an MV procedure based upon the *preoperative* transthoracic echocardiographic (TTE) or TEE exam, who actually only require a CABG due to "improvement" in the severity of MV disease as determined by the *pre–CPB* TEE examination in the operating room. The influence of changes in hemodynamic loading conditions during general anesthesia on transmitral flow and pressure, the potential changes in the patient's overall medical condition since the time of the preoperative echocardiographic exam, the technical limitations of TTE in comparison to TEE, and the general subjectivity of the assessment among different echocardiographers must all be taken into consideration when making the final surgical decision regarding the most appropriate MV procedure.

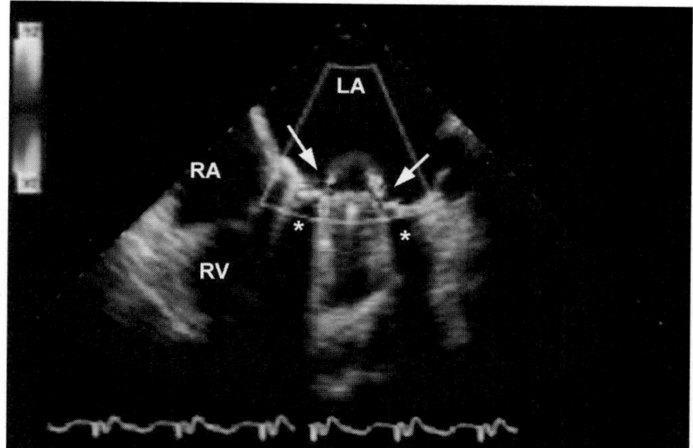

FIGURE 10–2 Normal prosthetic mitral valve regurgitation. All prosthetic valves demonstrate some degree of transvalvular regurgitation. In this color flow Doppler examination of a St. Jude mitral valve prosthesis (St. Jude Medical Inc., St. Paul, MN), two jets of mitral regurgitation are demonstrated (arrows). These regurgitant jets are normal for this valve and originate from the hinge points of the dual tilting disks. The valve sewing ring prevents ultrasound propagation, thus producing "drop out" beyond the ring (asterisks). Left ventricular cavity visualization is also obscured by the valve disks. LA = left atrium; RA = right atrium; RV = right ventricle.

The initial *post–CPB* TEE exam is essential in helping to determine the competency of the replaced or repaired MV, and to evaluate persistent MR and/or systolic anterior motion (SAM). It is especially important for the echocardiographer to fully understand the normal flow patterns and acceptable transvalvular pressure gradients following various types of MV repairs and replacements. Almost all MV replacements will exhibit physiologic, regurgitant transvalvular flow patterns that are acceptable and anticipated, although they vary significantly depending upon the specific prosthetic (Fig. 10-2). Most small perivalvular jets detected by CFD are insignificant, although larger "leaks" may become associated with hemolysis, hemodynamic instability, or valvular dehiscence. Hemodynamic loading conditions and LV function must also be taken into consideration in the assessment of residual MR. Following MV procedures, several studies have suggested that, in approximately 5% to 11% of cases,[3,8–11] the post–CPB TEE exam may identify persistent lesions that require additional, immediate surgical intervention.

GENERAL IMPACT OF INTRAOPERATIVE ECHOCARDIOGRAPHY ON MITRAL SURGERY

In an early study of the utility of epicardial scanning in 100 patients undergoing MV repair, Stewart et al[8] noted that 6 patients required an immediate return to CPB for further MV evaluation and repair. Three of these patients had SAM, 2 patients had residual 2+ or higher MR, and 1 patient had a flail leaflet. In this study, 2 patients with 3+ MR were not reoperated on immediately, but required a second procedure within 5 days due to hemodynamic compromise.

Another series employing TEE reported outcomes in 586 cardiac valve procedures[9] included 92 patients undergoing MV procedures. In these 92 MV patients, the pre–CPB TEE impacted surgical decision-making in a "minor" way in 14% of the cases. Minor changes included discovering an unknown LV thrombus, repairing an unknown ruptured chord, and identification of a valvular vegetation. Pre–CPB TEE had a "major" impact on an additional 11% of the mitral patients in this series including discovery of unknown lesions on the aortic (AV), tricuspid (TV), or MV (n = 7), existence of an ASD (n = 2), or unknown asymmetric septal hypertrophy (n = 1). The post–CPB TEE in 10 mitral patients (11%) determined the need for further MV surgery because the repairs were not judged to be adequate.

In a large series of 3245 adult patients undergoing a wide variety of cardiac surgical procedures, new information resulting in a modification of the surgical procedure was identified during the pre–CPB intraoperative TEE examination in 12% of 1265 patients undergoing MV surgery. Of note, 96 patients scheduled for MV surgery and a concomitant procedure were found to have a "normal" valve, and consequently did not require an MV procedure. Post–CPB, 6% of the MV surgical patients were noted to have a "new echocardiographic finding."[10] A smaller study, which prospectively followed 203 cardiac surgical patients who underwent intraoperative TEE, found a similar incidence of 17% unknown pre–CPB findings in 8 of 46 patients requiring MV procedures, and a return to CPB in 4.7% (2 of 46) mitral surgical patients.[11] Another large series, reporting on 6340 patients who had intraoperative echocardiographic examinations over a 10-year period, noted that return to CPB was required in 7% of 2226 MV repair procedures.[3] Despite the experience in MV repairs in this surgical group, the incidence of returning to bypass because of an unsatisfactory initial repair did not decrease over the 10 years, suggesting that more difficult repairs were being attempted.

To date, there are no prospective, large-scale, *randomized* trials that have specifically identified a consistent, independent advantage for intraoperative TEE. The wide-scale acceptance of intraoperative TEE during MV procedures has made it difficult if not impossible to conduct such a study. Data from several clinical investigations, however, have implicated an important, clinically significant and cost-effective role for TEE as a safe and valuable hemodynamic monitor in identifying high-risk patients, in assisting in the determination of the definitive surgical approach, and in providing a timely post–CPB evaluation of the procedure, thereby allowing for immediate intervention or at least the opportunity to triage patients appropriately. In the near future, the role of intraoperative TEE in patients undergoing MV procedures will most certainly become even more important with the development of three-dimensional (3-D) TEE and the further introduction of newer, minimally

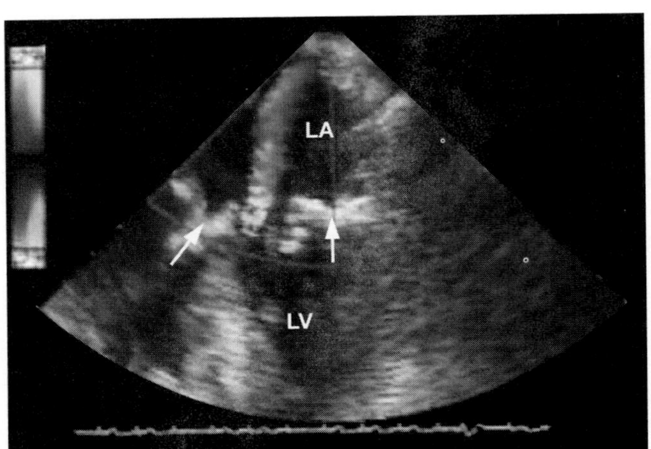

FIGURE 10–3 Moderate mitral regurgitation is demonstrated in this color flow Doppler image following mitral valve repair. The regurgitation jet extends to the back of the left atrium (LA) and is broad-based. The arrows indicate the borders of the ring placed during the repair. LV = left ventricle.

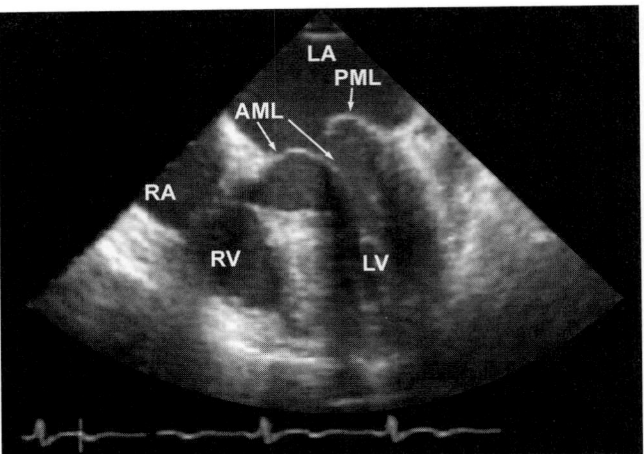

FIGURE 10–4 Elongated, redundant mitral valve leaflets are potential risk factors for systolic anterior motion following mitral valve repair. In the example shown, a redundant posterior mitral leaflet (PML) has prolapsed into the left atrium (LA), and the elongated anterior mitral leaflet (AML) extends deep into the left ventricle (LV) during systole. RA = right atrium; RV = right ventricle.

invasive approaches in which direct surgical visualization and inspection may be more limited.

PERSISTENT MITRAL REGURGITATION FOLLOWING MITRAL VALVE REPAIR

It is clear from the studies cited that intraoperative echocardiography can provide the surgeon with an immediate evaluation of MV function after repair. Moderate to severe residual MR (Fig. 10-3) will usually necessitate a return to CPB for further evaluation and definitive surgery. One main question arises regarding MV repairs and the utility of intraoperative echo: What is the outcome of patients who have trace to mild residual MR after repair?

One study attempting to address this topic included 76 patients with residual 1+ or 2+ MR following MV repair, in whom the surgical team decided not to return to CPB.[12] These patients were compared to a control group matched for preoperative risk who also underwent MV repair without evidence of residual MR. Follow-up data were available for an average of 3 years for each group. There was no difference in morbidity (congestive heart failure, embolic events, or surgical mortality) between the two groups; however, reoperation for a second MV procedure was required in only 3 of the "no MR" group compared to 9 patients in whom persistent MR was initially demonstrated. The authors concluded that insignificant residual MR should not raise excessive concern but expressed caution about the trend toward reoperation.

SYSTOLIC ANTERIOR MOTION FOLLOWING MITRAL VALVE REPAIR

Following MV repair, the presence of left ventricular outflow tract (LVOT)obstruction has typically been associated with SAM. Risk factors for SAM include *preoperative* evidence of excessive or redundant posterior (PML) and/or AML tissue (Fig. 10-4), nondilated LV, and a narrow mitroaortic angle. Postoperative risk factors for SAM include persistent AML redundancy, excessive PML resection, the selection of an annuloplasty ring that is either too small or incorrectly oriented, and an hypertrophied/hyperdynamic LV. All of those factors contribute to a Venturi effect that "pulls" the AML and coaptation point toward the ventricular septum during systole.

The mechanism of SAM following MV repair may not be as simple as a "Venturi" effect on the AML, but instead may involve a more complex relationship between the MV leaflets and adjacent ventricular structures. Maslow et al studied the intraoperative TEE in 11 patients who developed SAM following MV repair in an attempt to determine if there were any common echocardiographic findings.[13] Off-line measurements included mitral annular diameter, PML and AML lengths, and distance from the coaptation point of the MV to the ventricular septum. These measurements were compared to 22 matched control patients who underwent MV repair without evidence of SAM. Before repair, patients who displayed SAM following MV repair had a shorter anterior leaflet (2.13 ± 0.34 cm vs. 2.68 ± 0.39 cm), a longer posterior leaflet (2.18 ± 0.37 cm vs. 1.42 ± 0.27 cm), a shorter AML/PML ratio (0.99 ± 0.14 vs. 1.95 ± 0.27), and a shorter distance from coaptation point to the ventricular septum (2.53 ± 0.34 cm vs. 3.01 ± 0.56 cm). Surprisingly, the mitral annular diameters were not different in each group. In an illustration of the complexity of the mechanism of SAM following repair, the lower AML/PML ratio implied a relatively greater contribution of the PML to the coaptation of the MV, which may predispose to SAM following repair. Additionally, a shorter distance between the valvular coaptation point and the ventricular septum may also predict SAM following MV repair.

Another echocardiographic study comparing 8 patients who developed SAM[14] with a control population who did not develop SAM following repair found that the AML was significantly longer than the PML (3.5 ± 0.40 cm vs. 2.8 ± 0.32 cm) and the ratio of the AML/PML to be almost identical. In this investigation, however, measurements of the mitral leaflet lengths were performed in mid-diastole, whereas in the previous study the mitral leaflet lengths were measured at the start of ventricular systole, making a comparison between the studies somewhat difficult.

Several studies have identified SAM as a contribution to the requirement for early and late MV reoperation.[15,16] Freeman et al[16] reported on 143 MV procedures for MR associated with myxomatous degeneration. Over 9% of these patients demonstrated echocardiographic evidence of SAM following MV repair. Although all of these patients had PML prolapse, 7 also had AML prolapse. The majority underwent PML resection (n = 10), and 12 underwent ring annuloplasty (Duran = 10, Carpentier = 2). In this investigation, reinstitution of CPB was required in 5 patients due to persistent 3+ to 4+ MR, which resolved following the second procedure. In the remaining 8 patients, SAM and concurrent MR were associated with hypovolemia and a relative hyperdynamic heart. Resolution of hemodynamic instability and pathology was achieved with volume resuscitation and by reducing the administration of inotropic therapy. Marwick et al[15] reported that 10 of 309 mitral patients were observed to have LVOT obstruction and all 10 required reinstitution of CPB for either removal of the MV ring (n = 5) or MVR (n = 5).

In the absence of an echocardiographic evaluation, the diagnosis of and treatment of SAM following MV repair can be challenging, since commonly employed post–CPB therapeutic interventions (such as the use of inotropic agents) may actually be relatively contraindicated and lead to further hemodynamic compromise. Thus, it is essential to include a comprehensive evaluation for the presence of SAM in the post–CPB TEE examination following MV repair. The echocardiographic evaluation of SAM following MV repair includes a 2-D assessment of the mitral apparatus (Fig. 10-5A), a qualitative and quantitative CFD analysis of the MR jet (Fig. 10-5B), and a quantification of the pressure gradient across the LVOT obstruction. The CFD jet is typically directed toward the left pulmonary vein and away from the atrial septum as the AML is pulled toward the LVOT. Obstruction in the LVOT can produce pressure gradients as high as 100 mm Hg. Typically the Doppler flow velocity profile associated with dynamic LVOT obstruction can be differentiated from the profile associated with aortic stenosis (AS) by its "dagger" shape and mid-systolic acceleration. It would seem reasonable to assume that in the presence of echocardiographic confirmation of SAM and a hypovolemic and/or hyperdynamic LV, a trial of volume resuscitation and reduction of intropic therapy as suggested by Freeman et al[16] is initially warranted, followed by a reevaluation of any persistent MR and LVOT obstruction before returning to CPB. Maslow et al[13] reported that SAM resolved completely in 4 patients with this treatment and, in another 4 patients, SAM was still present but without CFD evidence of LVOT obstruction or MR. The authors do not comment on whether the 3 remaining patients required further surgery.

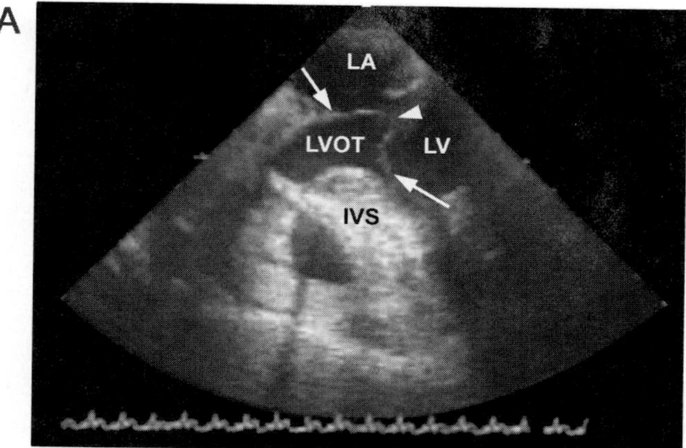

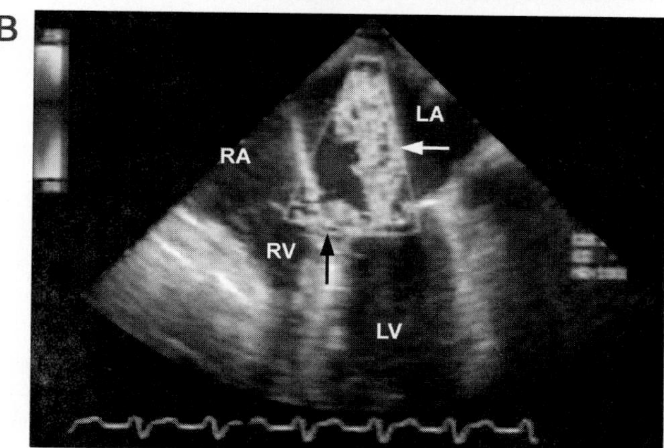

FIGURE 10–5 Systolic anterior motion following mitral valve repair. (A) The anterior mitral leaflet (arrows) is hinged toward the left ventricular outflow tract (LVOT) and intraventricular septum (IVS), thereby obstructing flow during systole. The hinge point of the leaflet is indicated by the arrowhead. (B) Color flow Doppler demonstrates high-velocity flow in the left ventricular outflow tract (black arrow) and severe mitral regurgitation (white arrow) associated with systolic anterior motion. RA = right atrium; RV = right ventricle; LA = left atrium; LV = left ventricle.

ISCHEMIC MITRAL REGURGITATION

By definition, ischemic MR presents in patients who have significant coronary artery disease with relatively normal mitral leaflet morphology. Mitral regurgitation associated with ischemia may be caused by annular dilatation in the presence

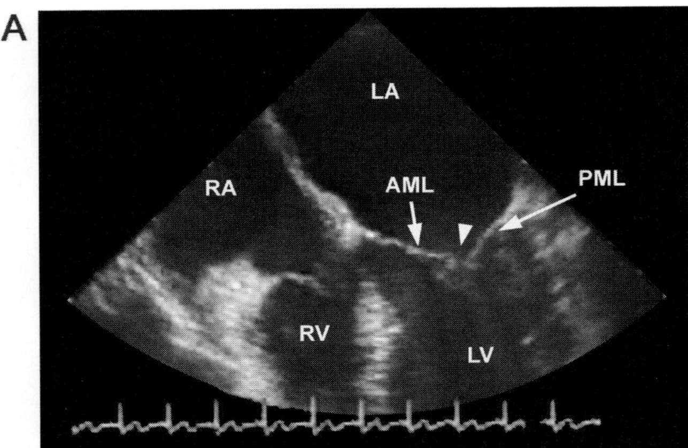

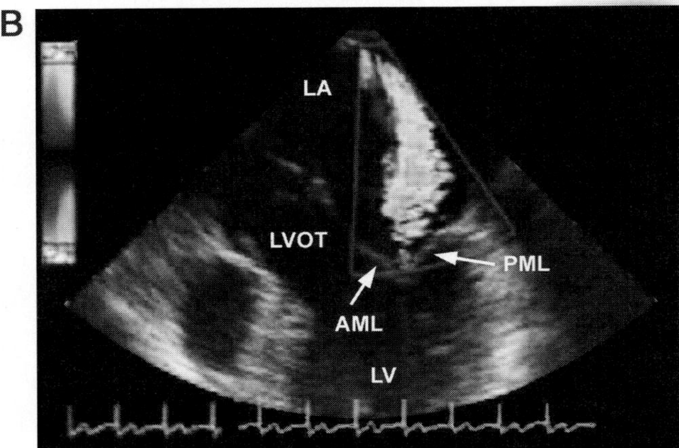

FIGURE 10–6 Ischemic mitral regurgitation. (A) Mid-esophageal, four-chamber transesophageal echocardiographic view demonstrating impaired anterior and posterior mitral leaflet coaptation (arrowhead) and tethering of the posterior mitral leaflet in a patient with ischemic mitral regurgitation. (B) Color flow Doppler demonstrating central and slight posterolateral eccentricity of a severe ischemic mitral regurgitation jet. LA = left atrium; LVOT = left ventricular outflow tract; RA = right atrium; RV = right ventricle.

of normal mitral leaflet motion or by restricted systolic leaflet motion with or without annular dilatation (Fig. 10-6).[17] Echocardiography is an essential diagnostic technique for evaluating the mechanism of ischemic MR and quantifying valvular dysfunction.

Several studies have attempted to investigate the utility of intraoperative echocardiography in patients who present with ischemic MR. One study looked at the impact of intraoperative TEE in this group of patients.[18] Over a 2-year period, 246 patients with ischemic heart disease who underwent surgery with TEE monitoring were evaluated. Each of these patients had cardiac catheterization results within 3 months of surgery that graded the degree of MR. The degree of MR present intraoperatively was compared to the degree of MR obtained at catheterization. In 134 patients, the degree of MR at catheterization agreed with the degree of MR found by TEE. However, in 53 patients, MR was graded higher by TEE, and in 59 patients MR was graded less by TEE compared to the results obtained during cardiac catheterization. As a result of the intraoperative TEE data, only a CABG procedure was performed in 22 patients in whom a CABG/MVR was originally scheduled, and in 5 other patients scheduled for only CABG, an MV procedure was also performed. From this data, intraoperative TEE impacted the surgical procedure in a major way in 27 of 246 (10.9%) of the patients with ischemic MR.

A retrospective review of 269 patients referred for surgery with the diagnosis of moderate ischemic MR (determined by catheterization, preoperative echocardiogram, or both) yielded 136 patients who underwent CABG only.[17] The remaining 133 underwent an MV repair along with the CABG and were consequently excluded from the analysis. In the group of 136 patients who underwent CABG alone, the authors compared the pre- and postoperative TTE evaluation with the intraoperative TEE assessment. Because these patients were scheduled only for CABG and intraoperative echocardiography was left to the discretion of the surgical and anesthesia team, intraoperative TEE was performed in only 38 of these patients. Similarly, only 68 patients underwent a postoperative TTE within 6 weeks of the hospitalization. By definition, all patients arrived in the operating room with 3+ MR, but the 38 patients who had intraoperative TEE had a decrease in average grade of MR to 1.4+. In addition, the postoperative TTE assessment of persistent MR revealed an increase in grade to an average of 2.2+. These results suggested that, under general anesthesia, intraoperative TEE may underestimate the degree of ischemic MR.

Bach et al[19] studied MR jet area and diameter in 46 patients who underwent MR surgery and noted that in the 12 patients who had ischemic heart disease, both these measures decreased under general anesthesia. Jet area decreased from 10.0 ± 3.8 cm^2 to 5.7 ± 3.5 cm^2 and jet diameter decreased from 1.10 ± 0.29 cm to 0.79 ± 0.33 cm, lending further credence to a cautionary note on interpretation of intraoperative TEE results in patients with ischemic MR.

In patients with ischemic MR, intraoperative echo results should be interpreted with the following considerations in mind. First, changes in loading conditions have been shown to dramatically affect the degree of MR evaluated intraoperatively in the pre–CPB period.[20] Consequently, it is important to evaluate the degree of MR intraoperatively (while a patient is under general anesthesia and receiving positive pressure ventilation) only after hemodynamics have been optimized with volume infusions and/or vasconstriction to reflect preoperative values. Second, the assessment of MR jet size by CFD is a relatively subjective assessment. Consequently, interobserver variability and differences between TTE and TEE techniques must also be considered when there is a discrepancy between grades of MR severity. Thus, other factors including clinical signs and symptoms of congestive heart failure as well as further supportive evidence of a significant regurgitant lesion such as elevated pulmonary artery pressures and Doppler echocardiographic evidence of jet eccentricity, increased LA size, and abnormal pulmonary venous flow patterns should also be considered.[21]

PROSTHETIC MITRAL VALVE REPLACEMENT

All prosthetic valves have characteristic regurgitant CFD jets that must be recognized and distinguished from pathologic transvalvular and paravalvular lesions.[22] For example, the St. Jude prosthetic valve (St. Jude Medical, Inc., St. Paul, MN) is manufactured to permit 3 to 5 small, transvalvular, washout jets along the leaflet hinge points, which serve to prevent thrombus formation. Pathologic transvalvular regurgitant jets are often associated with leaflets that are torn or stented open with clot, abscesses, or excessive subvalvular tissue.

Small paravalvular jets are not uncommon and frequently resolve spontaneously (Fig. 10-7A). Meloni et al studied 27 cardiac surgical patients undergoing MVR to assess regurgitant characteristics of MV biologic and mechanical prostheses immediately after implantation.[22] Physiologic transvalvular regurgitant jets were observed in both biologic and mechanical prostheses. Trivial periprosthetic jets were observed in 14 patients (maximum jet area 0.46 cm^2; range 0.1-1.5 cm^2). Cardiopulmonary bypass was reinitiated in 2 patients with MV regurgitant jet areas of 3.6 cm^2 and 5.5 cm^2; however, prosthetic dehiscence was discovered by direct inspection in only the latter case. Morehead et al also studied 27 cardiac surgical patients undergoing aortic valve replacement (AVR) (n = 11), MVR (n = 15), or AVR/MVR (n = 1), and hypothesized that although paravalvular jets visualized by intraoperative TEE immediately post–CPB are common, they tend to improve with restoration of normal coagulation parameters.[23] In this patient population, only 29 of the original 55 jets were still identified following protamine administration, and jet areas decreased from 2.0 cm^2 ± 2.2 cm^2 to 0.86 ± 1.7cm^2. None of the patients required immediate reexploration. Thus the results from these trials would suggest that most residual regurgitant jets visualized by intraoperative echocardiography following MVR are trivial. Alternatively, large paravalvular jets usually have to be repaired immediately to prevent excessive hemolysis, hemodynamic instability, and possible valve dehiscence (Fig. 10-7B).

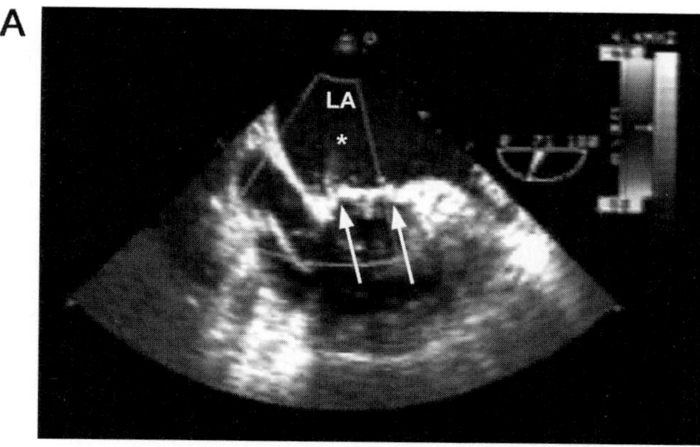

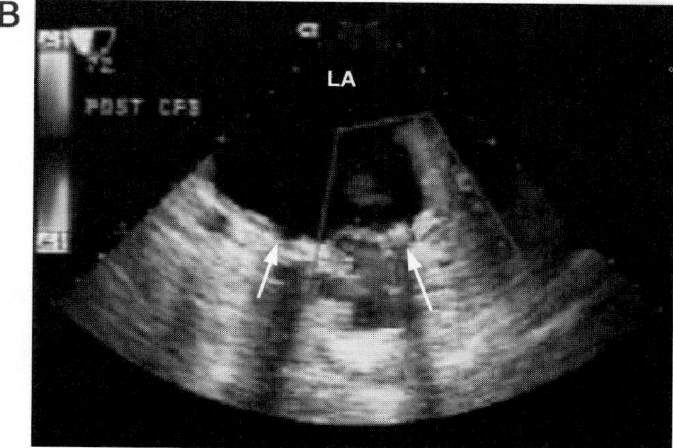

FIGURE 10–7 Perivalvular leaks following mitral valve replacement. (A) Small perivalvular leaks (asterisk) visualized around the mitral valve sewing ring often close following heparin reversal. (B) More widely based perivalvular leaks usually require surgical intervention. LA = left atrium; arrows = sewing rings.

Aortic Valve

For most cases in which the AV is replaced, the pathology has been well delineated by preoperative echocardiography and angiography (Fig. 10-8). Consequently, the likelihood of the intraoperative TEE exam impacting directly on the surgical management of the AV per se is low. In a retrospective study by Nowrangi et al, none of the 383 patients in their series who underwent aortic valve replacement (AVR) for AS required aortic prosthesis modification post–CPB, based on the intraoperative TEE examination.[24] However, in that same study, intraoperative TEE altered the planned operation in 13% of the patients. The changes in surgical plan based solely on new data from the intraoperative pre–CPB TEE exam included performance or cancellation of an MV procedure, PFO closure, and removal of LAA thrombi and other intracardiac masses. In addition, intraoperative TEE measurement of aortic annular size, which the investigators were able to do reliably, allowed homografts to be thawed and prepared prior to aortotomy, potentially decreasing the duration of CPB.

The question of whether to replace a regurgitant MV at the time of AVR for AS has also been addressed specifically in several recent studies.[25–27] Although all of the studies are retrospective, have limited follow-up periods, and use echocardiographic indices of MR as clinical end points, the weight of the available evidence suggests that, in the absence of significant intrinsic disease of the MV and chordal apparatus, MR is improved by AVR alone in the majority of cases.

A

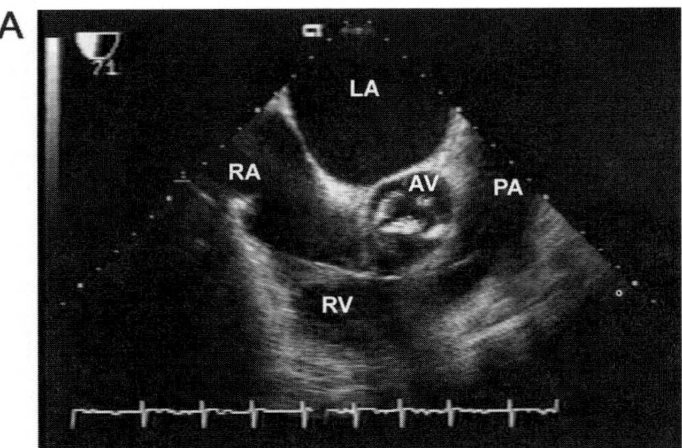

B

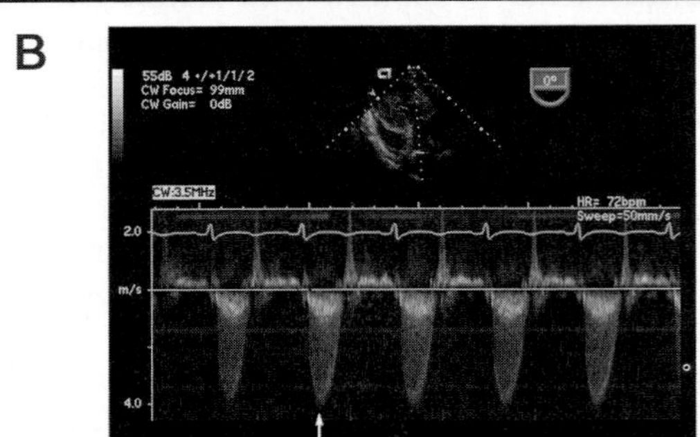

FIGURE 10–8 Aortic stenosis. (A) This two-dimensional transesophageal echocardiographic image demonstrates a calcified and stenotic aortic valve. (B) A continuous wave Doppler flow velocity profile is used to measure the velocity (arrow) across the stenotic aortic valve. The velocity across the aortic valve is nearly 4 m/s, which is consistent with a transvalvular pressure gradient (ΔP) of 64 mm Hg according to the modified Bernoulli equation: $\Delta P = 4(v)^2$. LA = left atrium; RA = right atrium;AV = aortic valve; PA = pulmonary artery; RV = right ventricle.

Suggested mechanisms for this improvement are reduction of the transmitral pressure gradient and favorable changes in ventricular morphology that occur as a result of the AVR.[28]

Because of its ability to provide detailed information about the structure and function of the entire valvular apparatus, TEE assessment of the AV has a growing impact upon surgical decision-making in cases of aortic insufficiency (AI), especially those due to aortic dissection. Moskowitz et al studied 50 consecutive patients with acute type A aortic dissection, and defined the severity and mechanism of AI in each case.[29] They identified three mechanisms of AI which were amenable to surgical repair: (1) incomplete closure of intrinsically normal leaflets due to leaflet tethering by a dilated sinotubular junction; (2) leaflet prolapse due to disruption of leaflet attachments by a dissection flap that extends into the aortic root; and (3) prolapse of the dissection flap through intrinsically normal leaflets, which disrupts leaflet coaptation. Generally, accepted echocardiographic criteria for a normal aortic root include a valvular annular diameter of 19 to 23 mm and symmetrical sinuses, with a sinotubular junction diameter at most 3 mm larger than the valve annulus. In the presence of an anatomically abnormal AV (i.e., bicuspid AV, Marfan's syndrome, leaflet thickening, or aortitis), AVR was determined to be necessary. Of the 16 patients with AI and intrinsically normal leaflets, 15 underwent successful AVR, and did not require subsequent surgery at a median follow-up of 23 months. The lone patient who did not undergo a valve-sparing procedure was excluded at the surgeon's discretion after a complicated intraoperative course unrelated to the AV. The authors concluded that TEE can successfully define the severity and mechanisms of AI in cases of type A aortic dissection, and assist the surgeon in distinguishing repairable valves from those requiring replacement.

Pulmonic Valve

Pulmonic stenosis is rare in the adult patient and is usually associated with a congenital syndrome such as tetraology of Fallot, or a primary etiology including unicuspid, bicuspid, or quadricuspid forms of the valve. Severe pulmonary regurgitation is most usually seen in patients with signs of pulmonary hypertension due to congenital defects (i.e., intracardiac shunts) or due to MV disease. However, mild degrees of pulmonary regurgitation occur in 40% to 70% of the normal adult patient population.[30]

Pulmonic valve (PV) replacement associated with primary pathology is usually limited to procedures involving congenital heart disease. However, the introduction of the Ross procedure, in which a diseased AV is replaced with the native PV, has promoted interest in the intraoperative echocardiographic evaluation of this structure. Elkins et al reported on 206 patients who underwent Ross procedures.[31] Eleven patients required autograft reoperations for valve insufficiency (Fig. 10-9). Three patients required a procedure

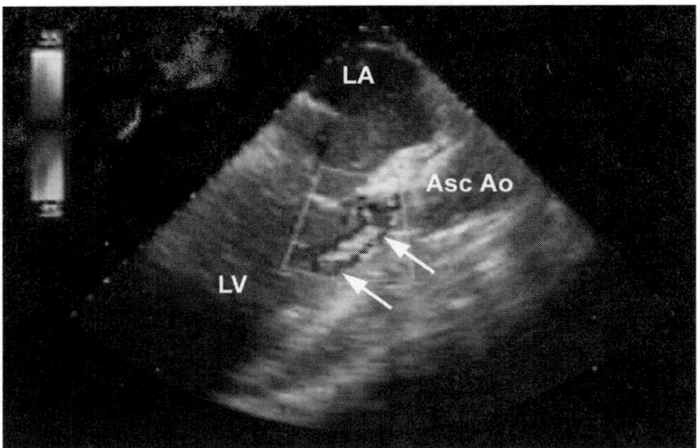

FIGURE 10–9 Moderate to severe aortic insufficiency (arrows) following a Ross procedure. Patients with significant aortic valve dilatation are at risk for postoperative aortic insufficiency unless the surgical procedure is altered to downsize the aortic annulus. LA = left atrium; LV = left ventricle; Asc Ao = ascending aorta.

within 6 months and the remaining 8 required reoperation from 1 to 6.2 years later. Intraoperative echocardiography demonstrated 1+ to 2+ AI in 2 of the 3 early reoperation patients. Autograft mismatch was most likely responsible for the AI in 1 patient with a dilated aorta. The second patient had "malalignment of the autograft valve commissures in a scalloped subcoronary implant." In 5 of the 8 patients in whom reoperation was required over a postoperative period of 1 to 6.2 years, the intraoperative TEE evaluation demonstrated abnormal findings. Three of the patients who had significant aortic dilation and left the operating room with 1+ to 2+ AI required reoperation at 2.1, 4.4, and 5.4 years. Two of these 3 patients underwent successful reduction annuloplasty while the third patient required valve replacement after an initial failed attempt at repair. The 2 remaining patients, who had bicuspid AV disease and mild AI preoperatively and only trace or mild AI after autograft replacement, developed progressive AI and aortic annular dilatation by the time reoperation was required.

The same authors reported on 20 patients (median age: 27 years) with significant annular dilatation who underwent Ross procedures.[32] Sixteen had more than a 4-mm discrepancy between the aortic and pulmonary valvular annulae according to preoperative echocardiographic examination, which was confirmed by intraoperative TEE. A modification of the Ross procedure was performed in this subpopulation, in which a proximal suture line of the autograft was reinforced with a Dacron strip and the annulus downsized to fit the PV annulus. In these cases, perioperative grading of 0 to 1+ AI in 18 of 20 patients and 2+ AI in the remaining 2 patients was confirmed at the time of the 1-year postoperative echocardiographic examination. None of these patients required reoperation during a follow-up period from 1 month to 5.6 years. Thus intraoperative evaluation of PV anatomy and function prior to resection, calculation of the AV/PV annular ratio (Fig. 10-10), and the post–CPB assessment of autograft function are all important components of a comprehensive intraoperative TEE examination during the Ross procedure.

Several studies report on perioperative echocardiographic measures of reconstructed right ventricular outflow tract (RVOT) hemodynamic profiles. In 109 consecutive patients who underwent reconstruction of the RVOT with a homograft, 105 had subsequent follow-up TTE at 39 ± 20 months.[33] Although the authors do not comment on the results of the intraoperative echocardiographic examination, none of the patients had a transvalvular pressure gradient greater than 20 mm Hg measured 1 week postoperatively by TTE. At 39 months, 30 patients had pulmonary gradients between 20 and 40 mm Hg and 4 patients had a gradient greater than 40 mm Hg. In another study of 60 patients undergoing the same procedure, implantation of an oversized homograft in the RVOT led to an increase in gradient in across the PV from 3.0 ± 0.3 to 6.8 ± 0.5 mm Hg.[34] At 1-year follow-up of 54 patients, the peak gradient across the valve was 14.0 ± 1.1 mm Hg. Thus it would seem that an increase in the trans-PV gradient following placement of the homograft is inevitable, and independent of the intraoperative echocardiographic measurement.

A
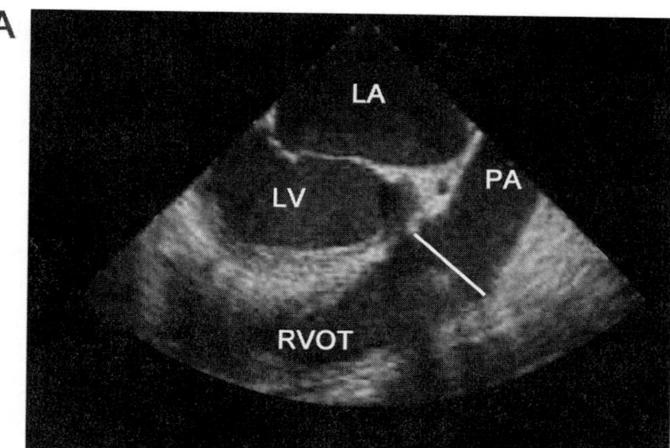

B
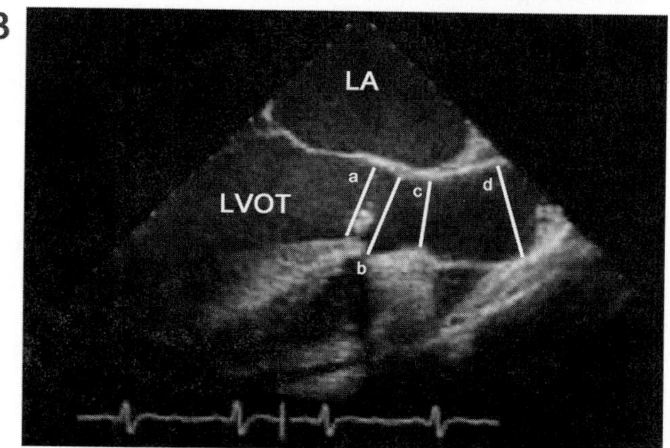

FIGURE 10–10 Pulmonary artery and aortic measurements prior to Ross procedure. (A) Measurement of the pulmonic valve (PV) annular diameter (straight line). (B) Aortic valve and ascending aortic diameters measured in a mid-esophageal, aortic valve long axis transesophageal echocardiographic view. Line a = aortic valve annulus; line b = sinus of Valsalva; line c = sinotubular junction; line d = ascending aorta; RVOT = right ventricular outflow tract; PA = pulmonary artery; LV = left ventricle; LA = left atrium; LVOT = left ventricular outflow tract.

Tricuspid Valve

A comprehensive echocardiographic examination of the tricuspid valve (TV) includes 2-D evaluation for leaflet pathology (i.e., prolapse, calcification, chordal rupture) and annular dimensions. Utilization of Doppler echocardiography is essential for the evaluation of severity of tricuspid regurgitation (TR) and tricuspid stenosis (TS). In one series of patients undergoing TV replacement (TVR), TR was the primary pathology in 75% compared to only 2% of the patients who had pure TS.[35] Although a variety of congenital and acquired disorders of the TV are responsible for valve pathology,[36] TR is most commonly associated with normal leaflet morphology in the presence of RV and/or LV failure with concurrent pulmonary hypertension.

Early studies using epicardial echocardiography intraoperatively were able to establish the utility of CFD in the evaluation of TV disease.[37,38] In 18 patients undergoing TVR, the immediate post–CPB measurement of TR correlated with echocardiographic evaluation several weeks postoperatively.[38] Interestingly, there was poor correlation in this study with RA V wave and degree of TR. Grading of TR, however, is not as standardized at grading of MR. Early studies measured the degree of TR according to CFD jet extension into the RA. A jet that extended just beyond the TV was graded as 1+. A step-up in grade was assigned for each one-third extension into the RA up to 4+ for a jet that extended to the back of the RA.

A study of 66 patients in a database with "moderate or severe" TR by TTE compared 19 echocardiographic findings in an attempt to develop a TR severity score.[39] Severe TR was defined by the presence of at least two of the following three clinical findings: (1) V waves in the jugular venous pulsations, (2) pulsatile liver, and (3) seesaw movement in the parasternal area. In this case series, 38 patients had clinical evidence of TR. Four of the 19 echocardiographic signs had a greater than 80% positive predictive value of detecting clinical TR. Hepatic vein systolic flow reversal, paradoxical atrial septal movement, TR jet area greater than 9 cm^2, and RA area greater than 30 cm^2 had predictive values of severe TR of 91.2%, 82.8%, 81.4%, and 80.6%, respectively (Fig. 10-11).

The post–CPB intraoperative TEE examination has been instrumental in evaluating TV integrity following repair.[40–42] One case series of 389 patients undergoing TVR revealed a 5.1% incidence of immediate reoperation. Other studies have reported a similar incidence of echocardiography-documented TV repair failure in the range of 5% to 10%.[40,42] The post–CPB results following TV repair have not been studied in a randomized population of cardiac surgical patients. It is reasonable to assume, however, that the identification of persistent TR by echocardiography permits early surgical reintervention, and therefore reduces the potential for postoperative morbidity.

A

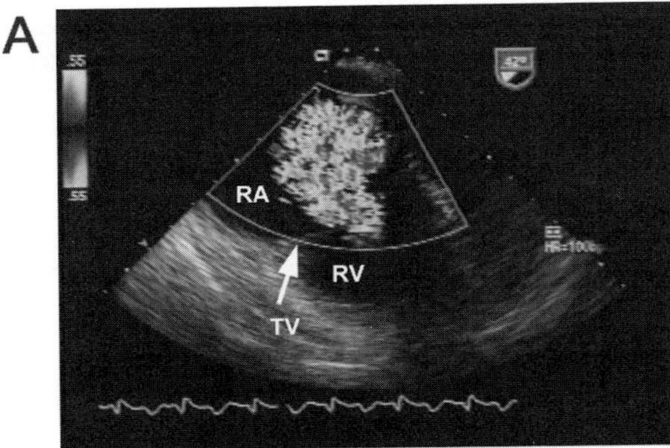

B

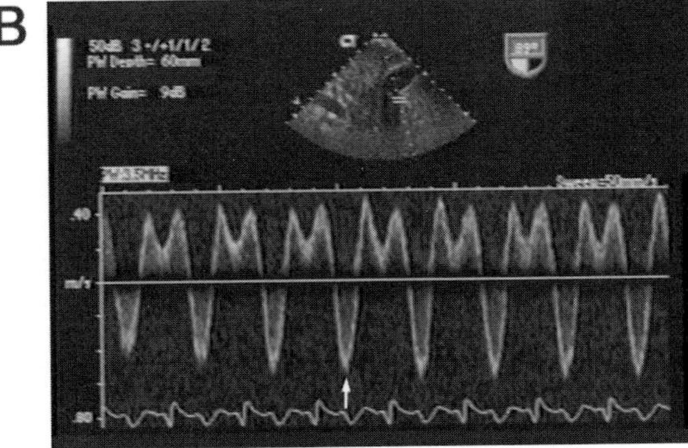

FIGURE 10–11 Severe tricuspid regurgitation. (A) Enlarged right atrium and color flow Doppler evidence of severe tricuspid regurgitation. (B) Hepatic vein Doppler flow velocity profile demonstrating systolic flow reversal (arrow) consistent with severe tricuspic regurgitation. RV = right ventricle; TV = tricuspid valve.

VENTRICULAR FUNCTION: REGIONAL AND GLOBAL

The primary purposes for any cardiac surgical preoperative risk stratification scheme are to identify patients for whom the risk/benefit ratio of coronary revascularization is most advantageous, to facilitate consultations with other medical specialists, to delineate appropriate postoperative triaging, and to assist in containing hospital expenses. There are several variables describing cardiac surgical patient demographics and comorbidity that have been studied extensively as potential predictors of postoperative adverse events.[43–48] The preoperative estimate of ventricular systolic function is considered one of the more important risk factors and predictors of postoperative outcome in patients undergoing surgical coronary revascularization.[49,50] The beneficial effect of revascularization of dysfunctional myocardium in chronic ischemic heart disease has traditionally been measured by its effect on improvement of resting regional and global LV function.[51–53] Although several studies have described the prognostic value of preoperative echocardiographic evaluation of ventricular function for predicting survival after revascularization, many of these studies have been limited by relatively small sample sizes, lack of serial echocardiographic measurements, and only short-term follow-up.[54–58] In addition, there is still some controversy regarding the independent value of preoperative ejection fraction (EF),[59] the relative value of global versus regional measures of LV function,[60] and the role of RV dysfunction[61] as predictors of morbidity and mortality following CABG. Thus, further investigation of the relationship between perioperative echocardiographic measures of global and regional ventricular systolic function and postoperative adverse events is warranted.

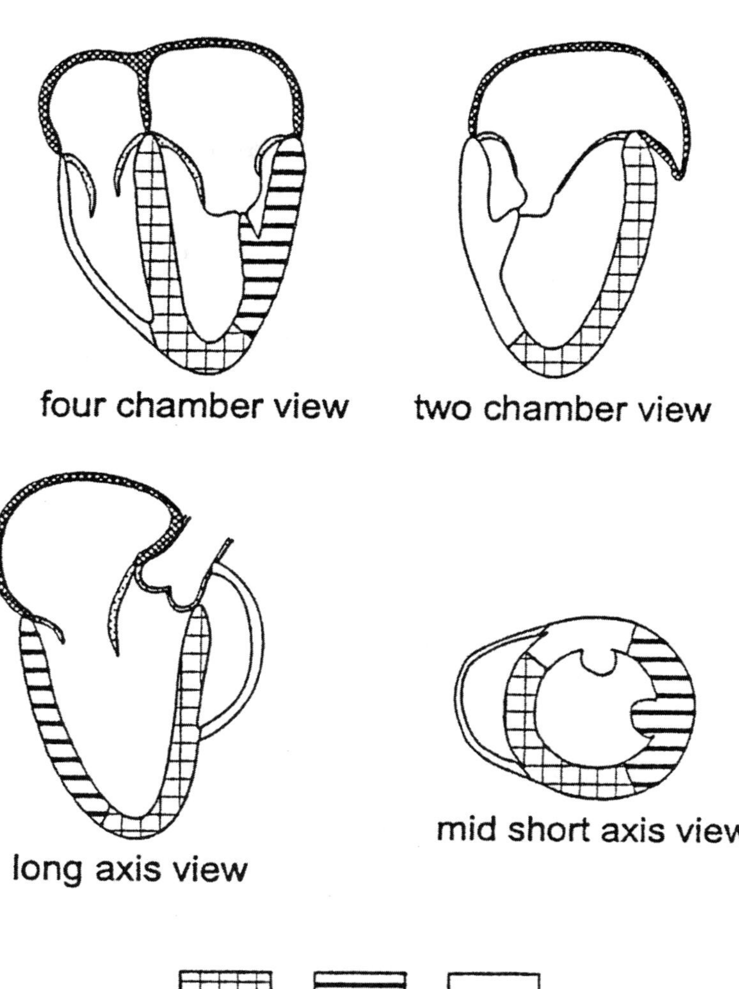

FIGURE 10–12 Regional coronary artery distribution relative to standard transesophageal echocardiographic views. LAD = left anterior descending coronary artery; Cx = left circumflex coronary artery; RCA = right coronary artery. *(Reproduced with permission from Shanewise JS, Cheung AT, Aronson S, et al: ASE/SCA Guidelines for Performing a Comprehensive Intraoperative Multiplane Transesophageal Echocardiography Examination: Recommendations of the American Society of Echocardiography Council for Intraoperative Echocardiography and the Society of Cardiovascular Anesthesiologists Task Force for Certification in Perioperative Transesophageal Echocardiography. Anesth Analg 1999; 89:870.)*

Regional Left Ventricular Function

Segmental wall motion abnormalities (SWMA) of the LV develop within seconds of regional myocardial oxygen deprivation, often preceding or even occurring in the absence of ECG changes.[62–64] Although segmental shortening may decline with as little as a 10% to 20% reduction in coronary blood flow, akinesis and dyskinesis require a greater than 90% and greater than 95% reduction, respectively. The echocardiographic evaluation of SWMA includes an assessment of both inward endocardial border excursion and wall thickening during systole, which can be determined by both qualitative visual assessment or quantitative linear measurements.[65,66] Abnormalities in wall thickening tend to occur before changes in endocardial excursion and better define the boundaries of an ischemic area, but both techniques are often used. Normally, endocardial excursion is greater than 30% and myocardial wall thickness increases by 40% to 50% during systole.[67] Ideally a significant difference in visual SWMA requires a change of at least two grades (e.g., normal to severe hypokinesis or severe hypokinesis to dyskinesis) since intra- and interobserver variability has been demonstrated with this technique.[68] Acute changes in loading conditions, afterload, and rhythm can also interfere with the interpretation of SWMA.[69] Furthermore, the appearance of SWMA in the absence of ischemia can be seen with tangential views or with translational and rotational movement of the heart especially in the septal region after pericardiotomy.[70] Finally, tethering of infarcted or stunned segments may present as SWMA, although a sudden, severe decrease or cessation of LV segmental contraction is almost certainly due to myocardial ischemia. Despite these limitations, the diagnosis of new SWMA by TEE remains an important influence in guiding anti-ischemia therapy in CABG patients.[71]

The TEE visual evaluation of regional LV function is often confined to the transgastric, short axis view at the mid-papillary level (TG mid SAX; see Fig. 10-1D) since all four LV walls corresponding to the territorial distribution of the three respective epicardial coronary arteries may be visualized simultaneously (Fig. 10-12). Split screens or multiple

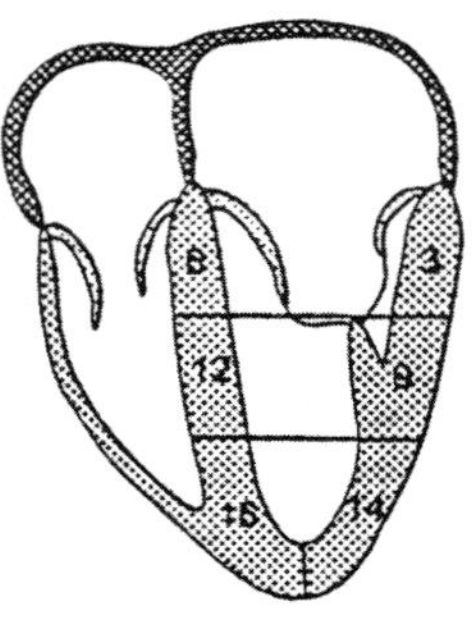

a. four chamber view

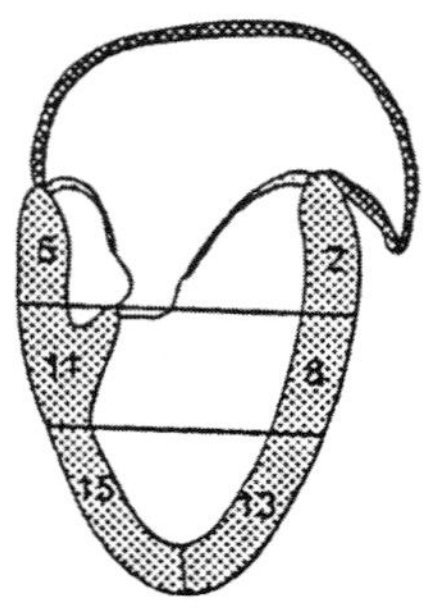

b. two chamber view

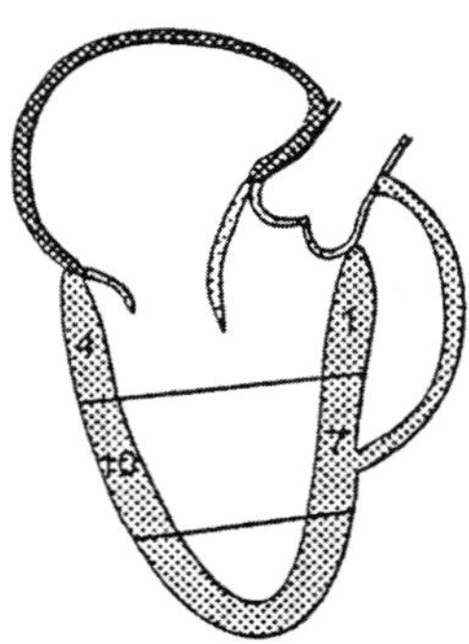

c. long axis view

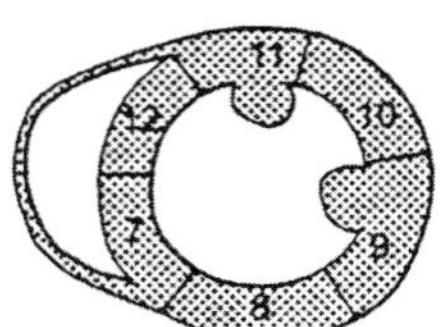

d. mid short axis view

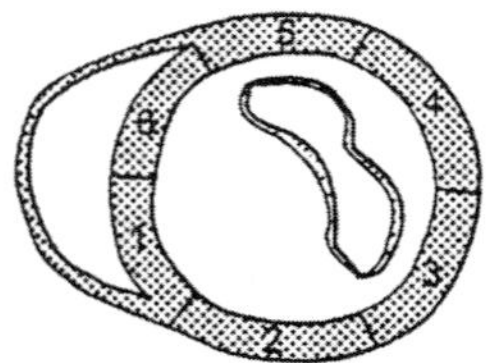

e. basal short axis view

Basal Segments	Mid Segments	Apical Segments
1= Basal Anteroseptal	7= Mid Anteroseptal	13= Apical Anterior
2= Basal Anterior	8= Mid Anterior	14= Apical Lateral
3= Basal Lateral	9= Mid Lateral	15= Apical Inferior
4= Basal Posterior	10= Mid Posterior	16= Apical Septal
5= Basal Inferior	11= Mid Inferior	
6= Basal Septal	12= Mid Septal	

FIGURE 10–13 Regional left ventricular wall segments according to standard transesophageal echocardiographic views. *(Reproduced with permission from Shanewise JS, Cheung AT, Aronson S, et al: ASE/SCA Guidelines for Performing a Comprehensive Intraoperative Multiplane Transesophageal Echocardiography Examination: Recommendations of the American Society of Echocardiography Council for Intraoperative Echocardiography and the Society of Cardiovascular Anesthesiologists Task Force for Certification in Perioperative Transesophageal Echocardiography. Anesth Analg 1999; 89:870.)*

saved images can be helpful for making comparisons and determining changes in SWMA over time (i.e., pre– versus post–CPB). The use of the TG mid SAX view as a single plane is practical for continuous long-term evaluation; however, this view does not include apical and basal levels. In addition, evaluation of the lateral and septal walls, which are parallel to the ultrasound beam, may be limited by echocardiographic "drop-out" in this short axis view. A more complete assessment can be performed using the 16-segment model and scoring system established by the American Society of Echocardiography (Fig. 10-13).[1] The use of additional TEE viewing planes has been shown to improve SWMA detection. In one recent study, only 17% of SWMA were detected in the TG-mid SAX view.[72] Although the introduction of other short axis views increased the detection of SWMA to 65%, the introduction of multiplane views was required to capture the remaining 35%.

Myocardial contrast echocardiography can also be used to enhance endocardial borders and improve the qualitative assessment of SWMA.[73] In addition, contrast echocardiography can be employed intraoperatively to evaluate myocardial perfusion and to assess the quality of coronary artery bypass grafts and the adequacy of cardioplegia delivery. Myocardial contrast echocardiography is performed by injecting nontoxic solutions containing gaseous microbubbles, which circulate with blood flow and reflect ultrasonic signals. In one study of 15 patients undergoing CABG surgery, at least one LV segment could not be adequately seen by at least one observer during the examination. However, 60% of the segments could be seen after contrast injection (OPTISON; Amersham Health, Princeton, NJ).[74] In addition, 16% of the segments were graded differently after the contrast agent injection, although 2.2% differed more than one grade or changed from "not seen" to "seen." Thus, the use of contrast agents may facilitate the detection of LV SWMA.

Intraoperative administration of low-dose dobutamine combined with TEE has also been proposed to be a valuable technique for predicting functional recovery in regional LV function following CABG surgery. It is extremely important to distinguish dysfunctional myocardial regions that are viable from those that are irreversibly injured in patients undergoing coronary revascularization procedures. Experimental and clinical evidence have confirmed that low-dose dobutamine increases coronary blood flow and contractility without an associated increase in regional myocardial oxygen demand. Aronson et al analyzed 560 LV segments in 40 patients scheduled for elective CABG surgery for SWMA at four stages in the procedure: baseline (after general anesthesia induction and endotracheal intubation), with administration of low-dose dobutamine (5 μg/kg/min) before CPB, after separation from CPB (early), and after protamine administration (late).[75] Changes in regional myocardial function after low-dose dobutamine were highly predictive of early and late changes in regional myocardial function compared to baseline regional scores. Thus, intraoperative low-dose dobutamine stress testing may be considered a reliable method for predicting regional myocardial reserve and determining anticipated functional recovery after coronary revascularization.

Endocardial motion can also be displayed in color, using Color Kinesis technology (CK; Philips, Andover, MA) or color Doppler tissue imaging (DTI). CK automatically detects endocardial motion in real time using integrated backscatter data to identify pixel transitions between blood-tissue interfaces throughout the cardiac cycle. The speed and direction of endocardial motion are displayed as a composite of different, user-selected, frame-specific colors superimposed upon the 2-D gray scale at end systole and at end diastole. Although CK facilitates the detection of endocardial border excursion, wall thickening is not further optimized. In comparison to conventional 2-D analysis of endocardial motion, CK is a sensitive but not particularly specific method for evaluating SWMA.[76–78] In addition, CK technology may be limited by interference from ultrasound "drop-out," image clutter, and translational motion of the heart. Regional LV function may also be evaluated using DTI, which uses Doppler frequency shift signals to continuously display the velocity and direction of myocardial wall motion either in color or as a spectral waveform analysis of velocities over time.

The use of TEE for evaluating perioperative ischemic myocardial injury is considered a class II indication according to the guidelines published by the SCA/ASE.[2] In several studies, the echocardiographic demonstration of new SWMA in the perioperative period has been shown to be a more reliable sign of myocardial ischemia and infarction compared to ST-segment changes.[79,80] For example, in a study of 50 patients undergoing cardiovascular surgery, new significant SWMA occurred in 24 patients whereas ischemic ST-segment changes only occurred in 6 patients.[81] Three patients who sustained intraoperative myocardial infarction (MI) developed significant SWMA in the corresponding area of myocardium, which persisted until the end of surgery, but only 1 of these 3 patients had ischemic ST-segment changes intraoperatively.

In another study, investigators diagnosed new SWMA in 19 of 179 (10.6%) patients undergoing CABG surgery, and 14 of 71 patients (19.7%) undergoing other cardiac surgical procedures (combined CABG/valve, valve, and aortic surgery).[82] Intraoperative TEE directed the management of 18 of 33 (54%) of these patients who developed new SWMA. Finally, in another study, TEE was compared to Holter ECG in a series of 351 patients undergoing CABG surgery, to determine if either technique had clinical value in identifying those patients in whom MI (creatine kinase-MB $\geq$100 ng/mL) was likely to develop.[83] Electrocardiographic or TEE evidence of intraoperative ischemia was present in 126 (36%) of the patients; however, the concordance between the two techniques was poor (positive concordance = 17%; Kappa statistic = 0.13). Myocardial infarction occurred in 62 (17%) of the patients, and 32 (52%) of them had previous intraoperative ischemia of which 28 (88%) were identified by TEE, yet only 13 (41%) were identified by ECG. In this study, SWMA were more commonly observed compared to ECG changes and concordance between the two modalities was low. Logistic regression analysis revealed that TEE was twice as predictive as ECG in identifying patients who develop a perioperative MI. Thus perioperative identification of SWMA remains an important technique for diagnosing myocardial ischemic events and identifying patients at risk for MI following cardiac surgery.

Global Left Ventricular Function

Global LV function is an important predictor of outcome in patients undergoing major surgery. In patients undergoing CABG surgery, global ventricular function, as assessed by EF, is more important in determining survival than the number of diseased vessels.[84,85] The ASE Guidelines for Quantification of the Left Ventricle recommend that, following optimization of image quality (assuring the best resolution of endocardial border definition by using the proper transducer frequency, dynamic range, depth, and transmit zone), LV dimensions, areas, and volume can be acquired to facilitate quantification of contractile function and cardiac performance.[69] Therefore, a comprehensive evaluation of LV function involves an integration of different ventricular performance constituents (i.e., preload, afterload, and contractility) in addition to an evaluation of global measures. Furthermore, echocardiographic evaluation of trans-MV (LV filling) and pulmonary venous (LA filling) Doppler flow velocity profiles can be useful in the assessment of LV diastolic function.

FRACTIONAL SHORTENING AND FRACTIONAL AREA CHANGE

The simplest echocardiographic method for evaluating global LV function involves indirect measures of EF. Fractional shortening (FS) is derived from the difference between end-diastolic internal diameter (EDID) and end-systolic

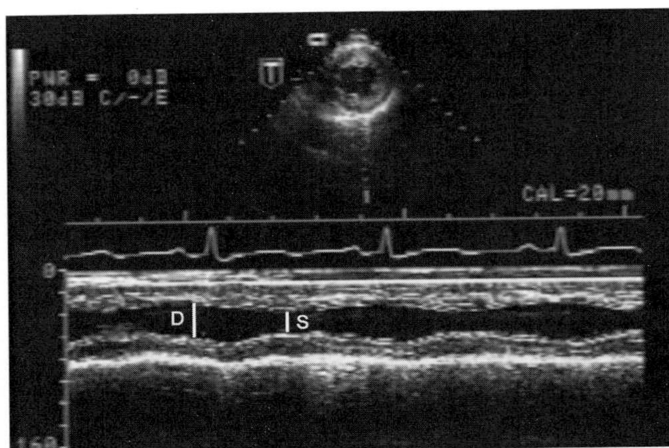

FIGURE 10–14 Fractional shortening of the left ventricle is derived from an M-mode view of a transgastric mid short axis echocardiogram. The internal diameters of the LV are measured during diastole (D) and systole (S).

internal diameter (ESID) divided by the EDID as imaged in the TGSA-MP view (mean: 33%; range: 28%-41%):

$$FS = \frac{EDID - ESID}{EDID} \times 100\%$$

FS is usually measured in the TG-mid SAX view and evaluated using M-mode echocardiography with the ultrasound beam oriented through the center of the LV (Fig. 10-14).

Fractional area change (FAC) uses 2-D echocardiography to derive the difference between end-diastolic area (EDA) and end-systolic area (ESA) divided by the EDA (mean: 57%; range: 37%-76%):

$$FAC = \frac{EDA - ESA}{EDA} \times 100\%$$

Circumferential areas are obtained by tracing around the LV endocardial borders (planimetry) during the corresponding phase of the cardiac cycle in the TG-mid SAX view since 85% of cardiac contractility occurs along this axis (Fig. 10-15). FAC is limited by the ability to obtain optimal cardiac images, errors in tracing or dimensional measurements, and the inherent limitations of equating 2-D measurements with 3-D physiological data. Although FAC correlates reasonably well with other approximations of the global EF, significant limitations apply. For example, FAC like other measures of EF is load-dependent and thus markedly affected by acute changes in preload and afterload without changing the intrinsic systolic function of the LV. Despite these limitations, FAC has been shown to significantly correlate with radionucleotide EF (r = 0.85; SEE = 9.6%).[86]

A

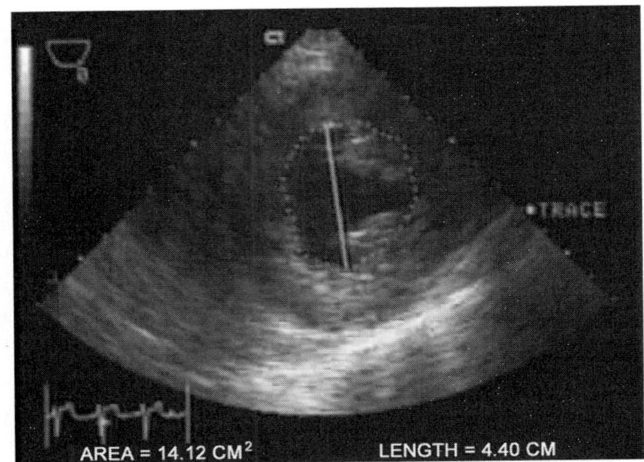

B

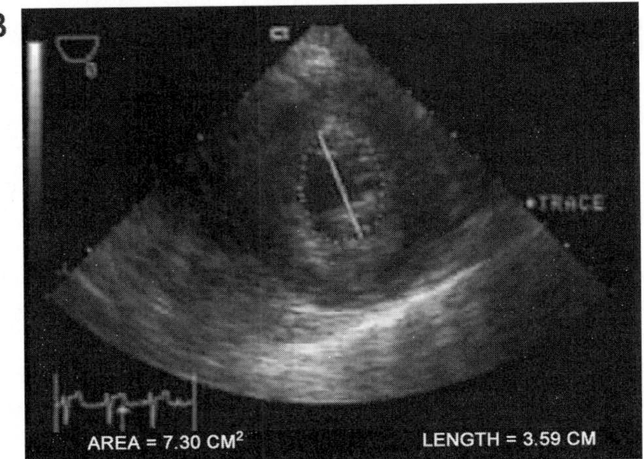

FIGURE 10–15 Fractional area of change of the left ventricle is derived by planimetering the area of the left ventricular cavity in the transgastric mid short axis echocardiogram during (A) diastole and (B) systole.

EJECTION FRACTION

Since TEE is primarily a 2-D technology and volume is a 3-D property, one must accept certain assumptions about ventricular geometry and use mathematical formulae to calculate volume from internal dimensions by "summing areas" or disks along one or more ventricular axes. Measurement of EF requires that LV volumes be measured in the TG-mid SAX view and one or more long axis views (i.e., mid-esophageal 4-chamber and mid-esophageal 2-chamber views) (Fig. 10-16). Acoustic quantification and automated border detection (AQ and ABD: Philips Medical Systems; Andover, MA) utilize unprocessed radio frequency data to discriminate blood from myocardial tissue to provide continuous, real-time, on-line estimates of EF and stroke volume. These estimates correlate favorably with radionucleotide-derived and thermodilution-acquired estimates.[87]

STROKE VOLUME AND CARDIAC OUTPUT

Cardiac output and its individual components can also be evaluated echocardiographically. Blood velocity can be measured using PWD or CWD. Stroke volume is calculated from the product of velocity-time integral (VTI: integrated area within the Doppler flow velocity profile) and the measured

A

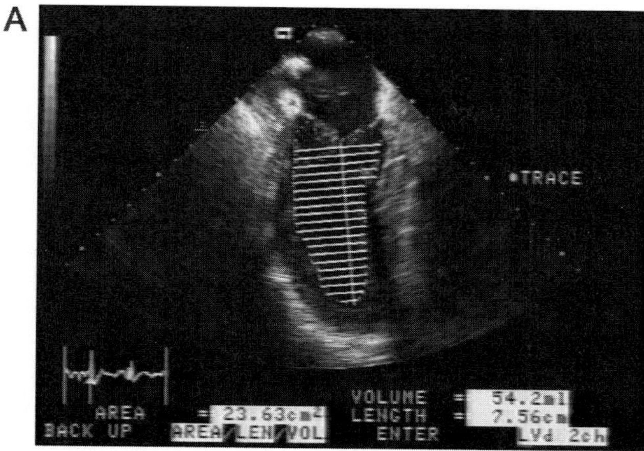

B

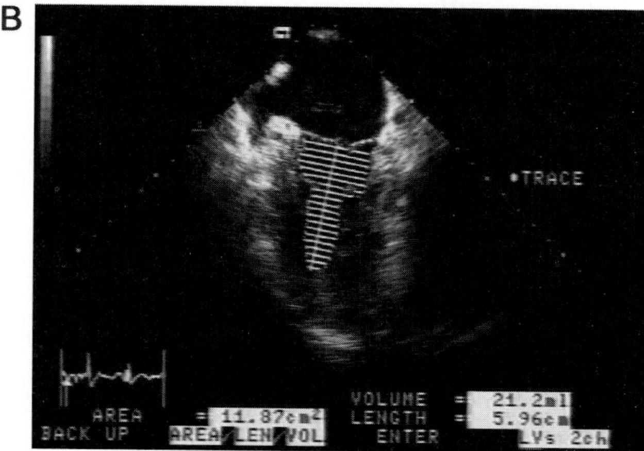

FIGURE 10–16 According to Simpson's rule, the LV end-diastolic volume and LV end-systolic volume can be determined by assuming that the LV is composed of a series of disk-shaped slices, which can each be measured and summed. (A) LV end-diastolic volume. (B) LV end-systolic volume.

area through which blood is flowing. Furthermore, cardiac output (CO) can be obtained according to the following formula:

$$CO = VTI \times area \times heart\ rate$$

Cardiac output measurement using Doppler echocardiography assumes laminar blood flow, a uniform Doppler flow velocity profile, parallel alignment of the Doppler beam with blood flow, and visualization of a circular and unchanging measured area. Despite these limiting factors, CO measurement using echocardiography has been performed in several different intracardiac locations (MV, AV, pulmonary artery/RVOT) and has been validated against classical techniques such as thermodilution.[88–90]

Left Ventricular Diastolic Function

Diastolic dysfunction describes a limitation of the ventricle to fill to an adequate end-diastolic volume without an abnormal increase in end-diastolic pressure. The main determinants of diastolic filling include myocardial relaxation, passive LV filling characteristics (LV compliance), LA function, heart rate, and MV integrity. Doppler echocardiographic evaluation of the trans-MV (LV-filling) and pulmonary venous (LA-filling) flow velocity profiles can provide information pertaining to LV diastolic function (Fig. 10-17).[91] The normal trans-MV Doppler flow velocity profile is characterized by an early E-wave velocity, which reflects LV relaxation and compliance as well as a later diastolic A-wave, which is more dependent upon the contractile state of the LA and the balance between LA and LV compliance. The normal pulmonary venous Doppler flow velocity profile is characterized by a systolic forward velocity reflecting LA relaxation and atrioventricular interactions, an early diastolic velocity reflecting LA filling while the MV is open, and a small late diastolic flow reversal during atrial contraction.

In early diastolic dysfunction, the ratio of the early-to-late trans-MV velocity (E/A ratio), which is normally larger than 1, decreases to less than 1 in response to impaired LV relaxation (E-to-A reversal).[91] Similarly, the diastolic component of the pulmonary venous Doppler flow velocity profile becomes significantly diminished compared to the systolic component. As diastolic dysfunction progresses, LV compliance becomes compromised resulting in an increased LVEDP and LAP. When the elevated LAP becomes the driving force for trans-MV flow, a restrictive pattern develops characterized by a supranormal trans-MV E/A ratio and a significantly blunted pulmonary venous systolic velocity compared to the diastolic velocity. Complementary changes occur in the pulmonary venous flow pattern over the spectrum of diastolic dysfunction (see Fig. 10-17). Perioperative LV diastolic function evaluation using trans-MV and pulmonary venous Doppler flow velocity profiles is limited due to the significant influence of acute changes in loading conditions, heart rate, and rhythm on these echocardiographic measurements. Newer echocardiographic techniques for assessing LV diastolic function, including Doppler tissue imaging of mitral annular motion and transmitral color M-mode propagation velocity, reportedly are less vulnerable to the effects of acute changes in loading conditions and therefore may be particularly useful in the perioperative period.[92]

Preoperative diastolic dysfunction has been reported in 30% to 70% of cardiac surgical patients and has been associated with difficult weaning from CPB, the need for more frequent inotropic and vasoactive pharmacological support, and increased morbidity.[93,94] Following CPB, acute or worsening diastolic dysfunction of varying degrees associated with ischemia-reperfusion injury, hypothermia, metabolic disturbances, or myocardial edema occurs in many patients and may persist for several minutes to days.[95,96] Therefore the availability and feasibility of echocardiography for diagnosing the presence and progression of perioperative diastolic function should assist in the identification of high-risk cardiac surgical patients who may benefit from appropriate triage and therapeutic intervention.

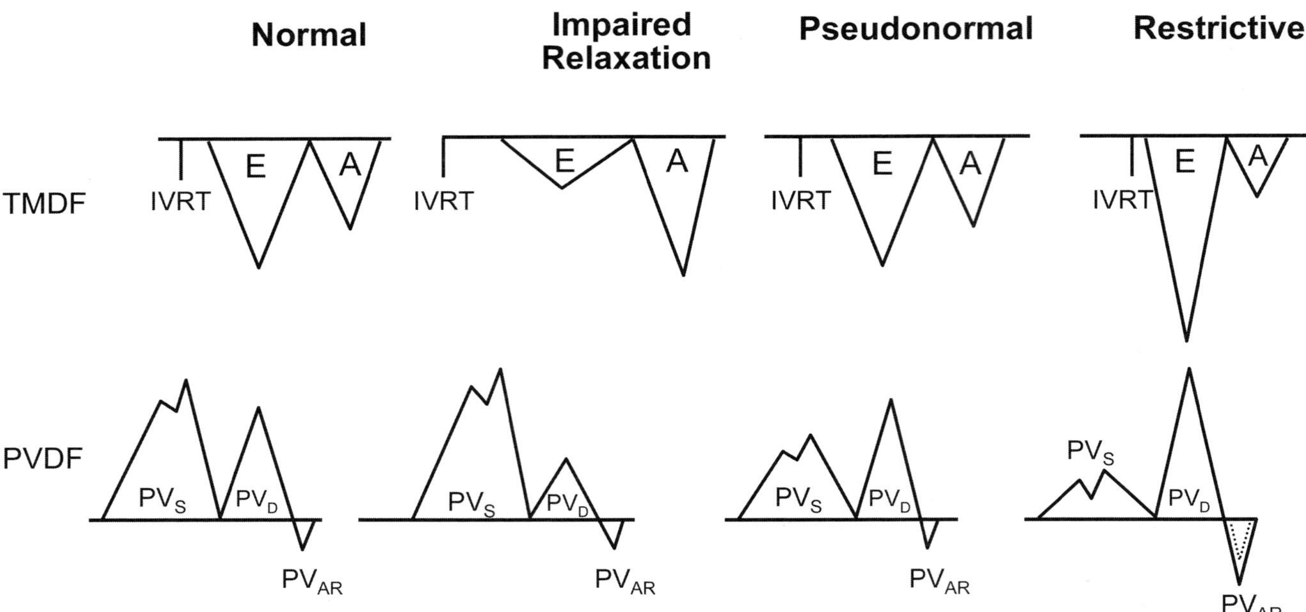

FIGURE 10–17 Transmitral and pulmonary venous Doppler flow velocity profiles. The impact of progressive left ventricular diastolic dysfunction on transmitral (TMDF; top) and pulmonary venous Doppler flow (PVDF; bottom) velocity profiles. E = E-wave; A = A-wave; IVRT = LV isovolumic relaxation time; PV_{AR}= late diastolic retrograde velocity; PV_{S1}= first systolic component; PV_{S2}= second systolic component; PV_D = diastolic component.

Right Ventricular Function

The ASE/SCA guidelines divide the RV into the free wall (with basal, apical, anterior, and inferior segments), the septal wall, and RV outflow.[1] The four conventional TEE views for evaluating RV function include the ME 4-chamber (see Fig. 10-1A), TG mid SAX (see Fig. 10-1D), ME RV inflow-outflow (see Fig. 10-1M), and TG RV inflow (see Fig. 10-1N). Compared to the evaluation of LV function, objective quantification of RV function is more difficult by both TTE and TEE.[97,98] The RV free wall is extremely thin, with an end-diastolic thickness of less than 5 mm. Consequently, evaluation of wall thickening and evaluation of RWMA may be difficult except in the presence frank akinesis or dyskinesis. In addition, the asymmetrical and crescent-shaped RV does not lend itself to volumetric measurement by ultrasound. Furthermore, the RV contains multiple trabeculations making endocardial border detection and accurate volume tracing difficult. Standard geometric formulas for volume calculations have only limited applicability given the shape of the RV. Attempts at modeling the RV in the TTE literature according to complex geometric shapes (i.e., ellipse, half cylinder, half conical structure, prism, a pyramid with a triangular base, or a three-dimensional parallelogram) have met with varying degrees of success when compared to volumetric methods (angiography, nuclear magnetic resonance, or formalin casting).[3] Few studies have attempted to evaluate geometric models of the RV in a varying number of patients with a wide spectrum of RV pathology, and they have no immediate intraoperative application.[102,103]

Despite these limitations, RV dysfunction is conventionally diagnosed echocardiographically by evaluating measures of both RV dimensions and RWMA. Because of its thin wall, the RV will dilate in response to volume overload. A comparison of RV to LV area is often used as a subjective measure of RV dilation, being described as mild (RV area smaller than LV area), moderate, (RV equals LV area), or severe (RV larger than LV area).[2] Because of its highly unusual geometry, it is essential to scan the RV in multiple planes in order to diagnose pathological RV dilation.

Regional dysfunction of the RV can also be evaluated by diagnosing the presence of hypokinetic, akinetic, or dyskinetic systolic RWMA. Additional echocardiographic features including RV free wall hypokinesis, systolic and diastolic septal flattening,[99] and dilation of the RA, IVC, and pulmonary artery in the presence of TR may support a diagnosis of RV failure.[100–102] However, in an intraoperative clinical setting, semiquantification of the RV area compared to the LV area is usually sufficient.

Although objective echocardiographic signs of RV systolic dysfunction may be difficult to determine,subjective signs of RV dysfunction have been used to demonstrate its incidence in the perioperative period.[103] In one retrospective study involving 66 emergent intraoperative TEE exams in 46 cardiac surgical patients, 2 of the 66 had a main TEE finding of “severe right heart dysfunction.”[103] In this study the main diagnoses were aortic dissection (n = 14) and severe LV dysfunction (n = 17). Another similar case series looked at urgently requested TEE exams in the cardiac surgical intensive care unit, and found, out of 130 emergent TEEs, 18 resulted in a diagnosis of RV dysfunction.[104] The incidence of RV dysfunction was surpassed only by LV dysfunction (n = 39).

Nonetheless, there are few studies that systematically investigate the utility of intraoperative echocardiography in evaluating RV function. In a study involving 16 patients undergoing CABG, Rafferty et al attempted to correlate RV EF (as measured by a rapid-response thermodilution pulmonary artery catheter) with an echocardiographic calculation using an off-line analysis of planimetered RV systolic and diastolic volumes in the ME 4-chamber and the TG mid SAX views, as well as systolic and diastolic length changes along a major axis and minor axis in the ME 4-chamber view.[105] Measurements were taken after general anesthesia induction, following sternotomy/pericardotomy, and after CPB. Although thermodilution RVEF did not change after CPB (EF PRE = 41%; EF POST = 37%), planimetered EF changed from 50% before CPB to 37% after CPB, indicating how difficult it is to correlate echocardiographic images of the RV.

A more recent study[106] demonstrated the utility of echocardiography for evaluating RV function postoperatively in cardiac surgical patients by administering incremental doses of dobutamine and obtaining RV pressure-area measurements using automated endocardial border detection. In addition, the echocardiographic measurement of RV cross-sectional area was validated intraoperatively as a surrogate for RV volume. Echocardiographic measurements were obtained from the difference between RV systolic and diastolic cross-sectional areas. Stroke volume was also measured directly by the investigators by placing an electromagnetic flow probe around the main pulmonary artery. Snares were placed around the IVC and then slowly tightened until a systolic radial artery pressure reached 70 mm Hg before being released to vary loading conditions. RV cross-sectional area as determined by automated border detection was shown to correlate with changing flow rate. The authors emphasized, however, that the utility of echocardiography for measuring RV stroke volume should be interpreted with caution since maintaining the image of the RV in a ME 4-chamber view required strict vigilance on behalf of the ultrasonographer, and had not been verified in previous studies.

Intraoperative RV systolic and diastolic function have also been evaluated echocardiographically by assessing Doppler hepatic venous flow velocity (HVF) patterns before and after CPB. The normal HVF pattern is characterized by forward flow in systole that exceeds the forward flow velocity in early diastole. The systolic component is produced by RV contraction with a combination of atrial relaxation and descent of the TV annulus. Alternatively, the diastolic component is a result of TV opening and RV relaxation and compliance. In addition, reversed flow associated with atrial contraction and late systole may also be observed. The results from two studies that evaluated changes in HVF patterns in cardiac surgical patients implicated that the development of post–CPB diastolic predominance suggested the presence of a reduction in RA compliance or relaxation associated with impaired RV relaxation and contraction. In addition, the demonstration of increased end-systolic reversal supports a diagnosis of RV stunning and dysfunction.[107,108]

Ventricular Dysfunction Associated with Pulmonary Embolism

Pulmonary embolism (PE) is a relatively rare but important cause of acute RV heart failure. The sensitivity (58%-97%) and specificity (88%-100%) of TEE for directly visualizing a pulmonary embolus in situ is somewhat variable especially for peripheral pulmonary emboli.[109] Consequently, indirect echocardiographic signs including the presence of mobile thrombus in the RA, RV, vena cavae, and/or main pulmonary artery are often considered highly suggestive of an acute PE, especially when visualized concurrently with evidence of acute RV failure in a high-risk patient. Initial RV dilation accompanied by tricuspid regurgitation is associated with an inability to compensate for sudden increases in resistance to flow in the pulmonary artery that occur following a clinically significant PE. An end-diastolic ratio of RV/LV diameter of 0.6 correlates with a significant RV pressure overload, whereas a ratio of 0.8 indicates a PE.[110] RV systolic dysfunction follows acute dilation, often manifesting with a paradoxical shift and flattening of the interventricular septum and echocardiographic evidence of an underfilled LV.[111]

A characteristic abnormal motion of the RV free wall relative to the apex has been demonstrated in patients with documented PE.[112] Normally, the RV contracts with a spiral motion that pulls the TV toward the apex. The RV free wall subsequently contracts inward toward the septum, creating the bellows-like effect. Finally, the RV is pulled by the contracting LV near the site of mutual attachment. In contrast, patients who have a PE demonstrate a bulging or akinesis of the middle portion of the RV free wall, while the apex continues to contract normally. In the study by McConnell et al, this unique pattern of RV motion was initially described in 14 patients with documented PE, and was validated retrospectively by viewing the TTE of 85 patients who had RV dysfunction from a variety of etiologies and sources.[112] The echocardiographic finding of RV free wall akinesis with normal apical contraction had a 77% sensitivity and a 94% specificity for the diagnosis of PE. The authors speculated that the mechanism for this abnormal RV motion could be due to localized RV ischemia or RV apical tethering to a normal or hyperdynamic contracting left ventricle. Despite the apparent importance of this "pathognomonic" finding, the use of TEE may still be limited by difficulty in routinely visualizing the RV apex.

PERICARDIAL EFFUSIONS AND CARDIAC TAMPONADE

Pericardial Effusions

Two-dimensional echocardiographic visualization of the pericardial cavity as an "echo-free space" depends upon the volume and pattern of fluid distribution around the heart. Small pericardial effusions (<100 mL; <10 mm in width) tend to be localized behind the posterior LV wall.[113] Moderate sized effusions (100-500 mL; 10-15 mm in width) expand laterally, apically, and anteriorly and can be visualized throughout the entire cardiac cycle. Large pericardial effusions (>500 mL; >15 mm in width) tend to be more evenly distributed around the heart, although preferential posterior accumulation is still common.[114] Large, chronically accumulating pericardial fluid effusions are often associated with excessive anteroposterior heart motion, and counterclockwise rotation in the horizontal plane.

Pericardial effusions can be identified postoperatively in approximately 85% of cardiac surgical patients although their size may vary, usually peaking by the 10th postoperative day.[115] The clinical presentation of postoperative effusions may also vary from a spurious finding in an asymptomatic patient to hemodynamic instability associated with local or circumferential cardiac chamber compression. The absolute size of the effusion, however, does not necessarily correlate with clinical signs since even relatively small, rapidly accumulating effusions may produce symptoms. Although postoperative effusions may present as an isolated anterior effusion, they are often located posteriorly and loculated by restraint from adhesions within the pericardial space.[116] Postoperative hemopericardium can present with thrombus usually along the anterolateral RA free wall, and may also cause compression and hemodynamic compromise.[117] Moderate or large pericardial effusions requiring surgical intervention also develop in patients with renal failure and following pericardial infiltration from lung and breast carcinoma.[118]

Pericardial Tamponade

Cardiac tamponade is a clinical syndrome defined as the decompensated phase of cardiac compression resulting from increased intrapericardial compression. Severe cardiac tamponade causing significant impairment of ventricular filling often requires surgical intervention to prevent circulatory collapse. Patients with severe cardiac tamponade usually become symptomatic when an excessively large or rapidly accumulating pericardial effusion develops (i.e., perioperative coagulopathy, vascular incisional or anastomotic dehiscence, ascending aortic dissection, coronary artery dissection following angioplasty, cardiac trauma, etc.). Postoperative pericardial tamponade has been reported in up to 2% of cardiac surgical patients.[119]

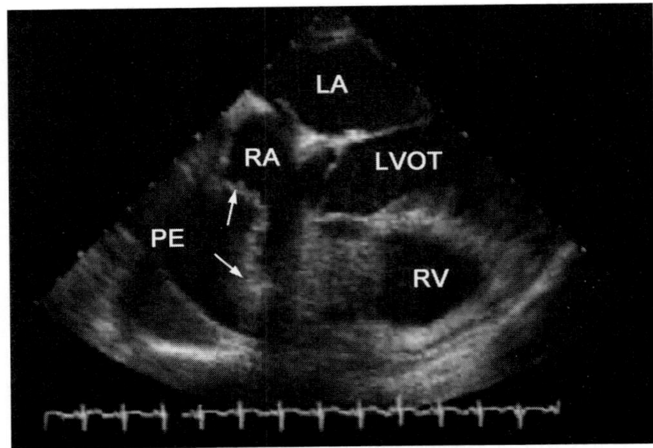

FIGURE 10–18 Two-dimensional transesophageal echocardiogram reveals the classic echocardiographic finding of diastolic right atrial (RA) collapse (arrows) and a large pericardial effusion (PE). LA = left atrium; RV = right ventricle; LVOT = left ventricular outflow tract.

TWO-DIMENSIONAL ECHOCARDIOGRAPHY

Although a variety of 2-D echocardiographic signs have been reported in patients with symptomatic pericardial tamponade, the most important include evidence of RA and RV diastolic collapse (Fig. 10-18).[120] Many of the described classic echocardiographic features of cardiac tamponade may not be present when small increases in intrapericardial volume are associated with rapid rises in pericardial pressure (i.e., cardiac trauma) or when effusions are loculated.[121] Following pericardiocentesis, cardiac pressure and volume corrections are more likely to reflect the presence and degree of cardiac compression rather than the amount of fluid removed. After drainage, the more compliant RV may dilate significantly and develop abnormal septal motion consistent with volume overload and congestive heart failure.[122] LV dilation ("pericardial shock") and pulmonary edema may also develop following pericardiocentesis in patients with underlying myocardial disease, due to the acute increase in venous return in the presence of persistent compensatory increases in peripheral resistance.[122]

DOPPLER ECHOCARDIOGRAPHY

In comparison to 2-D echocardiography, Doppler echocardiographic features of pericardial tamponade are more sensitive measures of clinical severity.[123] Doppler findings of pericardial tamponade are based upon alterations of intrathoracic and intracardiac pressures that occur during respiration and an exaggeration of ventricular interdependence. Normally during spontaneous respiration, changes in intrathoracic pressures are almost equally transmitted to the pericardial space and intracardiac chambers. Significant pericardial effusions often blunt the transmission of intrathoracic pressure. Consequently, LA and LV filling pressure gradients are decreased during spontaneous *inspiration*, resulting in diminished pulmonary venous forward diastolic velocities, delayed MV opening, prolonged isovolumic relaxation time, and decreased mitral E-wave velocity.[124] Similarly, relative increases in LA and LV filling pressure gradients during spontaneous *expiration* are responsible for corresponding increases in LA and LV Doppler inflow velocities. Exaggeration of ventricular interdependence with pericardial tamponade is responsible for reciprocal changes in right-sided intracardiac flows, resulting in increased tricuspid early E-wave filling velocities during spontaneous inspiration. These transvalvular Doppler flow velocities tend to normalize following therapeutic pericardiocentesis.[125] Alterations in the respiratory variation of RA inflow velocities (i.e., vena cavae and hepatic veins) are also altered by cardiac tamponade pathophysiology. For example, hepatic vein forward velocities decrease and reverse flows increase during spontaneous expiration.[123]

The identification of a significant pericardial effusion in a hemodynamically unstable, symptomatic patient can provide sufficient evidence to warrant prompt surgical intervention, thus avoiding a delay in diagnosis and further morbidity or mortality. In patients who require surgical intervention, perioperative echocardiography including 2-D and Doppler can provide important information related to the determination of postoperative functional status. Understanding the utility of perioperative echocardiography in evaluating patients with significant pericardial effusions is therefore an important component of the ultrasonographer's knowledge base.

AORTIC DISSECTION AND ATHEROMATOUS DISEASE

Ascending Aortic Dissection

The sensitivity of TEE in the diagnosis of thoracic aortic dissections has been well documented in the literature. For example, in the previously cited study by Moskowitz et al,[29] an intimal dissection flap was identified in all 50 patients studied, highlighting the high sensitivity of TEE for diagnosis of aortic dissection (Fig. 10-19). This has been a consistent finding in other studies of multiplane TEE in the setting of aortic dissection.[126] With reported sensitivities of 98% to 100%, TEE is comparable to MRI and superior to CT or aortography as a screening test. Characteristic echocardiographic findings in cases of aortic dissection include the intimal flap, which appears as an undulating, intralumenal density; the presence of two separate echoes in the aortic wall, one representing the intima and inner media, the other the outer media and adventia; and the presence of two lumens with different CFD patterns.[127] The limitation of TEE as a diagnostic modality for aortic dissection is its tendency to produce false-positive results, as a consequence of reverberation

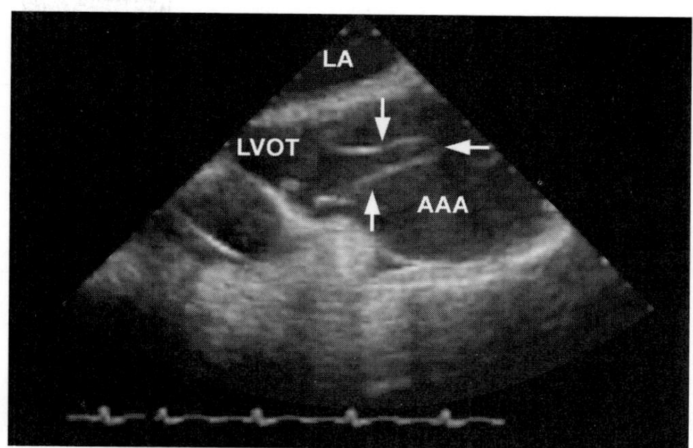

FIGURE 10–19 Mid-esophageal long axis ascending aortic transesophageal echocardiographic view of an ascending aortic aneurysm (AAA) and dissection. Arrows point toward the intimal flap. LA = left atrium; LVOT = left ventricular outflow tract.

artifacts, in dilated ascending aortas. The specificity of multiplane TEE in these cases is 94% to 95%, which is inferior to the specificity of 98% to 100% quoted for MRI and the basis of the recommendation by one group that MRI should be the initial diagnostic test on hemodynamically stable patients.[128] This limitation can be minimized with utilization of M-mode technology, which in one study improved the specificity of TEE to 100%.[129]

Although there has yet to be a randomized, prospective trial comparing initial diagnostic tests and their effect on outcome in acute aortic dissection, TEE is emerging as the technique of choice for this disease process because of its efficiency and high level of accuracy. In addition, because of its aforementioned utility in predicting suitability of valve-sparing surgical techniques and its ability to assess the adequacy of surgical intervention immediately after CPB, TEE has been used as the sole diagnostic modality for management of these patients, with favorable results.[130,131]

Echocardiographic Evaluation of Aortic Atheromatous Disease

Postoperative neurologic dysfunction in the cardiac surgical population continues to be a significant cause of mortality, morbidity, and increased cost. In 1996, a prospective multicenter study of 2108 patients undergoing CABG showed an incidence of adverse cerebral outcome of 6.1%.[132] This figure is of particular concern in view of the fact that the patients who suffered postoperative neurologic dysfunction in this study had a significantly higher mortality rate (16% vs. 2%, $p < .001$), had a longer length of hospital stay (22 days vs. 9.5 days, $p < .001$), and were less likely to be discharged home (46% vs. 90%, $p < .001$) than patients who did not sustain neurologic injury. The risk factor most predictive of poor neurologic outcome in this study was the presence of

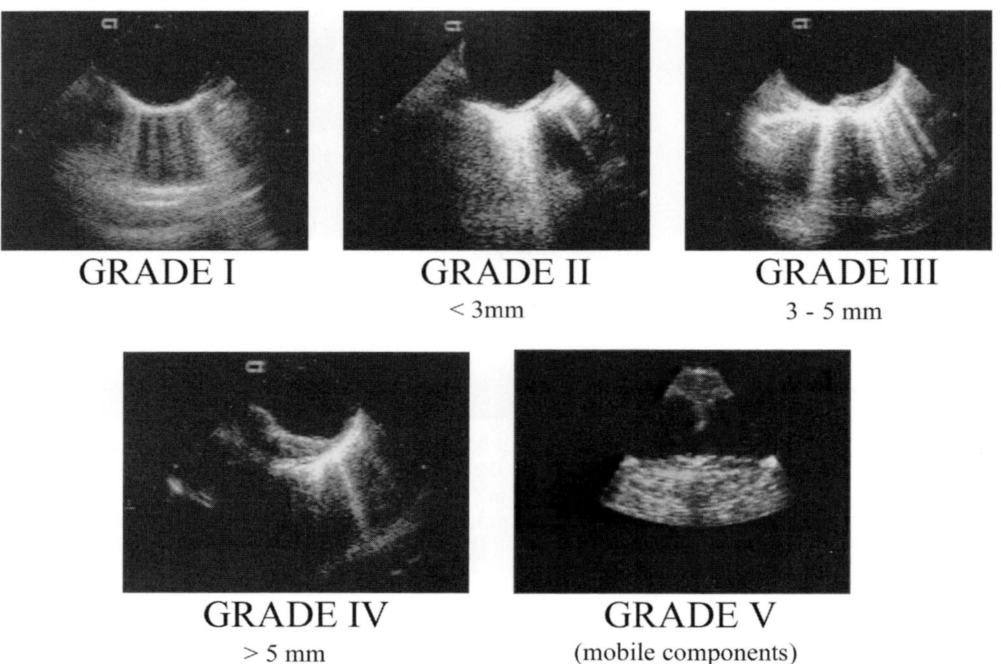

FIGURE 10–20 Grading of descending aortic atheromatous disease by transesophageal echocardiography.

ascending aortic atheroma, which increased the incidence of adverse neurologic outcome more than 4-fold over that seen in patients without aortic disease. These authors concluded that this finding supported "the theory that most strokes are caused by large atherosclerotic emboli liberated by surgical manipulation of the aorta."[132]

The association between ascending aortic atheroma and postoperative neurologic dysfunction was originally hypothesized in case reports from the surgical literature in the 1970s,[133,134] and was further advanced by autopsy studies[135] and several retrospective series that examined the link between aortic atheromas, as diagnosed by intraoperative TEE, and postoperative embolic stroke. Most notable among these investigations was a study by Davila-Roman,[136] which observed a significantly higher occurrence of intraoperative stroke (15%) in patients with aortic arch atheromas than in those without aortic arch disease (2%). In addition, a study by Stern[137] similarly reported an intraoperative stroke incidence of 11.6%, versus a general institutional intraoperative stroke incidence of 2.2%, in patients with aortic arch atheromas larger than 5 mm in diameter. Aortic atheromatous disease is generally classified according to plaque thickness and mobility (Fig. 10-20).[138] The causal relationship of aortic atheromas to embolic stroke was ultimately demonstrated in prospective studies[139–141] of nonsurgical patients during the 1990s. These studies showed an approximately 4-fold increase in the risk of future embolic stroke for patients with significant aortic atheromatous disease, as diagnosed by echocardiographic imaging.

Although there are currently no prospective, randomized studies on the impact of surgical technique upon neurologic outcome in patients with aortic atheromatous disease, the above data have made the prevention of embolization of aortic atheroma one of the goals of modern cardiac surgical practice. Several uncontrolled studies have suggested the possibility of improved neurologic outcomes in this patient subgroup through utilization of surgical techniques that minimize manipulation of the diseased aorta, such as alteration of the aortic cannulation or cross-clamp site,[142] replacement of the ascending aorta,[143] or off-pump coronary artery bypass graft surgery.[144] If and when the efficacy of such techniques is proven definitively, the identification of high-risk patients will be an essential component of the therapeutic plan.

Historically, the preoperative chest x-ray, cardiac catheterization, and manual palpation of the aorta constituted the predominant diagnostic regimen for identification of aortic atheroma. Unfortunately, although each of these modalities has reasonable specificity for the presence of atheromatous disease, none is sensitive enough to be particularly useful as a screening tool. Chest radiography, which has a predictive value of 84% for identifying atheroma if aortic knob calcification is seen, has a sensitivity of only 52%; cardiac catheterization provides no additional information beyond that obtained from the chest x-ray alone.[145] The diagnostic utility of manual palpation of the aorta has been studied more extensively, but with equally unimpressive results. For example, Ohteki et al[146] found that palpation detected only

25% of atherosclerotic plaques seen echocardiographically, and Sylviris found that palpation undergraded the severity of ascending aortic atheromas, compared with ultrasound imaging, in up to 69% of patients.[147]

Newer imaging modalities such as CT, magnetic resonance imaging (MRI), and ultrasound have improved the clinician's ability to diagnose thoracic aortic atheromatous disease. Several studies have investigated the sensitivity and specificity of these tests for the detection of this entity. CT scanning, when compared with TEE, has been shown to have a sensitivity of 87% and a specificity of 82% for the detection of protruding aortic atheromas.[148] Better results have been observed with MRI, which has a sensitivity and specificity equivalent to TEE for detection of the presence of atheroma, but its tendency to undergrade the thickness of the plaques represents a diagnostic limitation.[149]

As a result of these and similar studies, echocardiography has emerged as the gold standard for detection of atheromatous disease of the thoracic aorta. In the cardiac surgical patient, however, the opportunity to place an ultrasound transducer directly upon the ascending aorta has generated an additional debate as to the optimal mode of echocardiographic scanning. This debate has arisen because of the fact that ultrasound is unable to adequately penetrate air-filled structures, such as the trachea and proximal bronchi. This gives epiaortic scanning a physical advantage over TEE for the assessment of the distal ascending aorta and proximal arch, which lie above the trachea and bronchi; these aortic segments represent a "blind spot" in the TEE field of vision. Several recent studies investigated whether the theoretical advantages of epiaortic scanning resulted in improved sensitivity for the diagnosis of aortic atheromas in cardiac surgical patients. Konstadt et al[150] showed that TEE failed to visualize as much as 42% of the ascending aorta, and as a result failed to diagnose severe plaques, as seen by epiaortic scanning, in 36% of patients. Davila-Roman et al[151] compared biplane TEE with epiaortic ultrasound and found that TEE underdiagnosed atheromatous disease in 39% of proximal ascending aortic segments and 66% of distal ascending aortic segments. Similarly, Sylviris et al[147] reported that TEE undergraded atheromas in 50% of patients in both mid and distal ascending aortic segments, but only in 9% of patients in the proximal segments. Thus, for the detection of atheroma in the areas of the aorta most frequently manipulated during cardiac surgery, it can be concluded that epiaortic scanning is superior to TEE.

However, not every patient undergoing cardiac surgery requires epiaortic scanning prior to aortic manipulation.[152] In the absence of significant risk factors for aortic atheromatous disease, such as age older than 65 years, diabetes mellitus, smoking, and peripheral vascular disease, the incidence of ascending aortic disease is very low, and epiaortic scanning is unlikely to provide useful information. Furthermore, the negative predictive value of TEE examination of the thoracic aorta for atheromatous disease of the ascending aorta has been shown to be 100%[153] so that an intraoperative TEE exam that is negative for atheroma effectively obviates the need for epiaortic scanning. The optimal approach for detection of ascending aortic disease in cardiac surgical patients should incorporate consideration of risk factors and results of the TEE exam before time is spent on the epiaortic examination.

INTRACARDIAC MASSES

One of the major indications for the use of perioperative TEE in cardiac surgical patients is to assess and evaluate intracardiac masses prior to resection. Since the ultrasound beam is not traveling through the chest cavity as in transthoracic echocardiography (TTE), the images of cardiac masses obtained by TEE are usually clearer, more defined, and often quite dramatic.[154] In a series of 93 nonsurgical patients, TEE identified intracardiac and paracardiac masses in all but 89 (96%) of the cases, whereas TTE identified only 54 (58%).[155] In addition, TTE was not able to visualize thrombi in the left atrial appendage (LAA) (n =12), LA (n = 6), superior vena cava (SVC) (n = 3), or right pericardial space (n = 5). LV thrombi detected in 5 patients by TTE, however, were not visualized by TEE.

If TEE is not performed prior to surgery, the intraoperative echocardiographic examination must reconfirm the diagnosis from other preoperative imaging modalities and assure the surgical team that the intracardiac mass does not have any extracardiac extension. Proper determination of the size, shape, and mobility of the intracardiac mass can assist the surgical team in determining the CPB cannulation technique and sites if it appears that the attachment of the structure is tenuous, suggesting the possibility of embolism from surgical manipulation. In addition, knowledge of potential obstructive effects of the mass on transvalvular flow patterns may be helpful in diagnosing the etiology of pre–CPB hemodynamic instability and supports the potential benefits of changing patient positioning, administering fluid resuscitation or vasoactive medications, and/or determining the urgency of initiating CPB.

Intracardiac Thrombus

Transesophageal echocardiography is a particularly useful technique for diagnosing the presence and location of thrombus in all cardiac chambers with the exception of the LV. In particular, thrombus in the LV apex may be difficult to visualize via a TEE approach compared to TTE.[155] TEE is particularly useful for identifying thrombus in the LAA. In a study by Click et al, unexpected thrombi were identified by TEE in 37 out of 3245 patients (1.1%), thus altering the surgical procedure in 36 patients.[10]

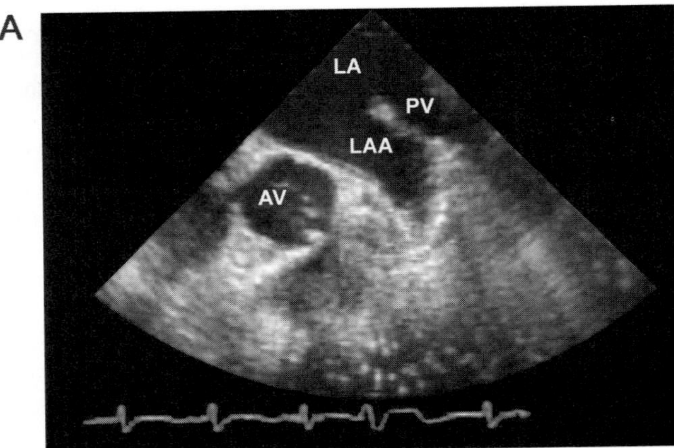

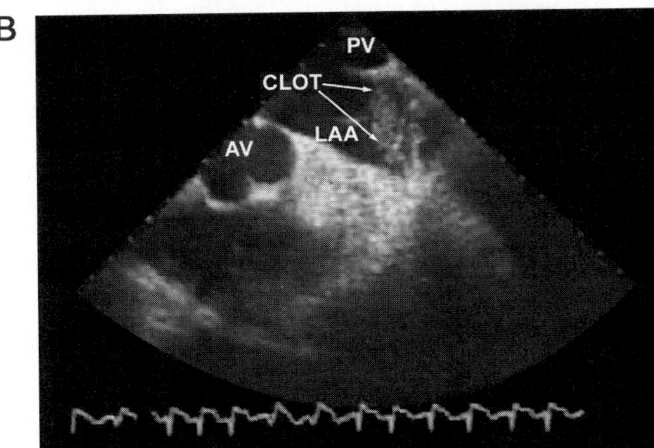

FIGURE 10–21 Transesophageal echocardiographic image of the left atrial appendage (LAA). (A) Normal LAA. (B) LAA with clot. PV = pulmonary vein; AV = aortic valve.

Patients at risk for intracardiac thrombus formation include those with stasis of blood flow associated with atrial fibrillation, LA enlargement, isolated MS, or decreased CO. Echocardiographic spontaneous contrast indicating relative stasis often appears as a smoky texture within the LA and alerts the ultrasonographer to interrogate the LAA for thrombus.[156] The echocardiographic characteristics of an atrial thrombus include layering, an area of central echolucency, and broad-based attachment to the atrial wall or septum. In addition, the absence of contraction can be used to distinguish thrombus from endocardium especially in the presence of protruding trabeculations and atrial ridges, which can often be confused with isolated clots (Fig. 10-21).

Cardiac Tumors

Primary malignant cardiac tumors are fortunately rare in the adult. However, malignant tumors that originate in the thorax may extend directly to the heart, compressing cardiac chambers or compromising the integrity of adjacent great vessels.[158] Echocardiographic delineation of the extension and origination of intra- and pericardial tumors can have major impact in determining the extent of the surgery.

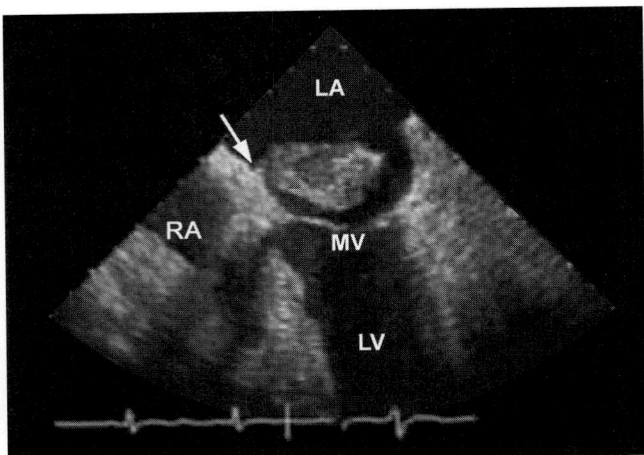

FIGURE 10–22 Left atrial myxoma attached by stalk (arrow) to atrial septum. LV = left ventricle; MV = mitral valve; LA = left atrium; RA = right atrium.

The majority of benign primary cardiac tumors are atrial myxomas. Almost 80% of these solitary tumors originate in the LA, but they have been known to occur in the RA and RV. Rarely, myxomas have been reported simultaneously in multiple locations. Typical echocardiographic characteristics of myxomas include a rounded shape, smooth margins, lack of laminated appearance, and a definitive site of attachment (stalk) most frequently from the fossa ovalis of the interatrial septum (Fig. 10-22). The tumor's site of origin may have particularly important implications for involvement of adjacent, indirectly involved structures including the MV. In addition, identifying the location and extent of RA myxomas may be important for guiding the appropriate positioning of inferior vena cava (IVC) and SVC cannulae.[158] Finally, following resection of a myxoma, intraoperative post–CPB TEE is necessary to determine the completion of resection and to assure that the atrial septum is intact.

Normal Intracardiac Structures

The accurate diagnosis of abnormal cardiac masses requires a fundamental appreciation for variants of normal anatomy. Intracardiac structures that may be confused with pathologic masses include the eustachian valve (EV),[159] Chiari network,[160] RV trabeculations,[161] moderator band, the LAA, and lipomatous infiltrations of the atrial septum.[162,163]

The EV and Chiari network are remnants of an embryologic membrane in the RA that directs flow from the IVC to the foramen ovale. The EV, located at the junction of the IVC and RA, is a mobile, thin structure that can often be confused with thrombus (Fig. 10-23).[159,160] The Chiari network, found in 1.0% to 1.5% of patients studied by TTE,

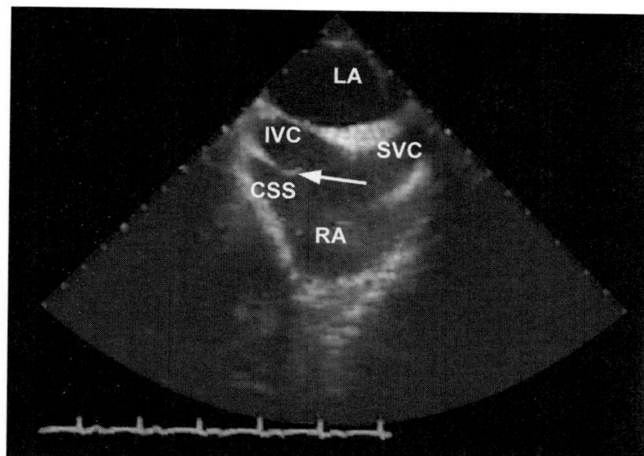

FIGURE 10–23 A mid-esophageal bicaval transesophageal echocardiographic view of a prominent eustachian valve (arrow). LA = left atrium; RA = right atrium; SVC = superior vena cava; IVC = inferior vena cava; CSS = coronary sinus.

is located near the coronary sinus and also appears as a highly mobile, thin filamentous structure.[161] The Chiari network is usually much longer than the EV and may be distinguished from thrombus by the presence of a broader base of attachment.

The RV also has many prominent trabeculations and a thickened muscular moderator band extending from the ventricular septum to one of the papillary muscles (Fig. 10-24). In the presence of RV hypertrophy, both of these normal structures may erroneously be diagnosed as pathology. In some patients, the LAA may be very prominent and possess trabeculations in its walls.[163] In addition, LAA inversion during CPB may give the appearance of an intra-atrial thrombus.[164]

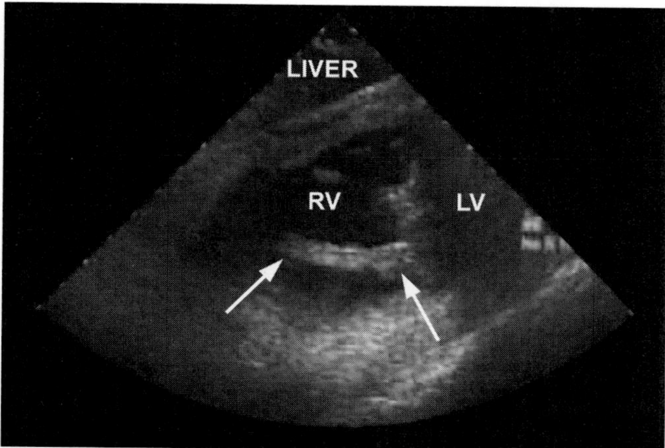

FIGURE 10–24 A transgastric mid short axis transesophageal echocardiographic view of a large moderator band in the right ventricle (arrows). RV = right ventricle; LV = left ventricle.

CONGENITAL CARDIAC DISEASE

Transesophageal echocardiography has proven itself to be a major diagnostic modality in the evaluation of patients of all ages with congenital heart disease. In one study comparing TEE with magnetic resonance imaging (MRI) in the preoperative evaluation of 85 adult patients (mean age: 29.6 years; range: 12-57 years), TEE was more helpful for the diagnosis of intracardiac anatomy than MRI. Alternatively, MRI was better as a technique for diagnosing extracardiac anatomy.[165] Several studies surveyed the impact of intraoperative TEE on congenital heart surgery in the pediatric population[166,167] and found the technique to be comparable to current imaging modalities.

Muhiudeen et al compared the pre- and postoperative diagnostic utility of TEE with epicardial scanning in 90 pediatric patients (mean age: 4.1 years) with congenital heart disease.[166] In the pre–CPB evaluation of 130 different congenital lesions (shunts and regurgitant and obstructive lesions), TEE failed to diagnosis correctly only 7 anomalies. Epicardial scanning missed 2 anomalies and was superior only in the pre–CPB diagnosis of obstructive lesions of the RVOT. Given that epicardial scanning requires interrupting the surgical procedure and raises the potential for breaking sterility, the conclusion from this study was that TEE was comparable to epicardial scanning for the perioperative evaluation of most congenital lesions.

Post–CPB findings in another study of children undergoing open heart surgery for congenital defects demonstrated that TEE had a major impact in reinitiating CPB.[167] Successful TEE exams performed in 227 out of 230 pediatric patients (mean age: 4.4 years) demonstrated an incomplete repair in 17 (7.5%) of the cases. The initial diagnoses in these patients were VSD (n = 5), subaortic stenosis (n = 9), and 1 each of transposition, aortic valve (AV) disease, and double outlet RV. Although these data represent a pediatric population, inferences can be made pertaining to the overall utility of perioperative echocardiography in the evaluation of congenital heart lesions.

The importance of performing a comprehensive intraoperative TEE exam and understanding anomalies associated with the primary diagnosis are essential in the evaluation of the adult patient undergoing surgery for congenital heart disease. Both are needed to avoid overlooking unsuspected lesions that would warrant surgical repair. In adult patients with extremely complex congenital heart disease, close collaboration with an expert ultrasonographer who specializes in complex congenital adult heart disease may be necessary to assure the highest standard of care. Discussion of the ultrasound characteristics of complex congenital lesions is beyond the scope of this chapter; however, the impact of intraoperative ultrasound on common lesions of the atrial septum provides an example of the utility of intraoperative echocardiography in adult congenital heart surgery.

Atrial Septal Defects

Atrial septal defects (ASD) including ostium secundum, ostium primum, sinus venosus, and coronary sinus defects are among the most common congenital heart defects found in adults. Although many of these lesions may be well defined preoperatively, a comprehensive TEE examination must confirm not only the presence of the known congenital lesion but also the direction and quantification of shunting. In addition, it is imperative for the ultrasonographer to rule out the presence of collateral pathology (e.g., cleft anterior MV leaflet associated with ostium primum defects) and any additional concurrent congenital lesions that may have a direct impact on the surgical procedure. Immediately following CPB, a thorough intraoperative TEE exam including 2-D and CFD must also be performed to ensure anatomic integrity of the surgical repair. The intravenous injection of saline contrast may be particularly useful for detecting trans-septal flow.[166]

A sinus venosus ASD may be difficult to thoroughly evaluate preoperatively by TTE. Consequently, a comprehensive intraoperative pre–CPB TEE examination focusing on the location and size of the lesion as well as the presence of any concurrent congenital pathology (e.g., anomalous pulmonary venous return) is of critical importance (Fig. 10-25). The post–CPB TEE examination may also be particularly important since repair of these defects, using a patch or a baffle, may involve the pulmonary veins, may obstruct the IVC, or may not completely close the defect. In each of these instances, the diagnosis may be made immediately by the intraoperative TEE.

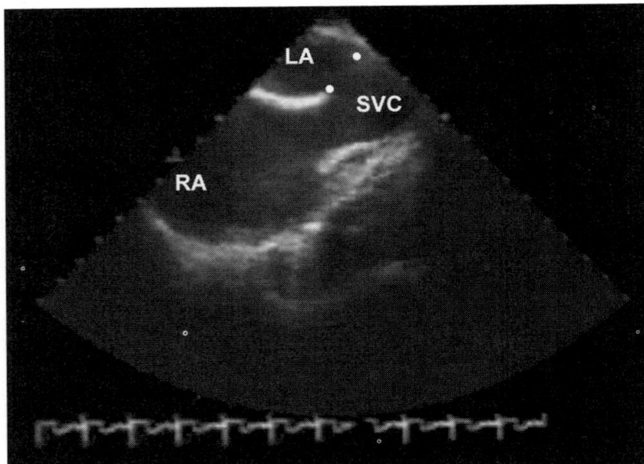

FIGURE 10–25 The close proximity of the transesophageal echo probe to the left atrium (LA) permits accurate visualization of atrial septal defects. A sinus venosus defect (white dots) is clearly evident in this mid-esophageal bicaval view. SVC = superior vena cava; RA = right atrium; LA = left atrium.

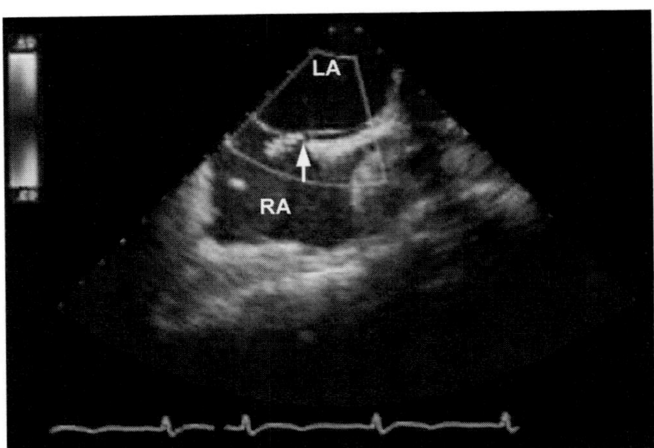

FIGURE 10–26 Color flow Doppler demonstrating patent foramen ovale (arrow). LA = left atrium; RA = right atrium.

Patent Foramen Ovale

A patent foramen ovale (PFO) at least 0.2 to 0.6 cm in diameter can be found in more than 25% of surgical patients (Fig. 10-26).[168] In comparison to TTE, TEE with its clear views of the of the atrial septum has been shown in numerous studies to permit a more thorough evaluation of PFO anatomy and the presence of trans-septal shunting.[169,170]

The importance of confirming the presence of a PFO using TEE is supported by the inherent risk of paradoxical embolization.[171] Nonsurgical data suggest that serious consideration must be made for intervening in a patient who presents for cardiac surgery and show a constellation of echocardiographic findings of a PFO and an atrial septal aneurysm,[172,173] defined as an atrial septum larger than 1.5 cm with a 1.1-cm extrusion into either the RA or LA with contraction.[174] In a multicenter, 4-year study involving 581 young patients (mean age: 44.5) who had an ischemic stroke with no significant risk factors (i.e., no source of emboli or significant atherosclerosis), patients who presented with a PFO and an atrial septal aneurysm diagnosed by TEE had a recurrent stroke rate of 15.2% compared to rates of 2.3% in patients with a PFO alone and 4.3% in patients with neither.[172] All patients in this study who had an atrial septal aneurysm also had a PFO (100%), whereas others have demonstrated the incidence of PFO in atrial aneurysm patients to be closer to 70%.[174]

HEART TRANSPLANTS AND VENTRICULAR ASSIST DEVICES

Heart Transplantation

In the heart transplant recipient, the value of the pre–CPB echocardiographic examination is usually limited to its utility as a monitor of ventricular performance. In addition, since most transplant recipients present with a history of severe, chronic cardiomyopathy and cardiomegaly, the potential for the stasis of blood flow is significant. Consequently, a comprehensive echocardiographic investigation for the presence of intracardiac thrombus is warranted prior to excessive manipulation and cannulation.

Once the donor heart is placed, a thorough post–CPB echocardiographic examination of RV and LV regional and global function is essential to guide appropriate pharmacologic or surgical intervention. Depending on the duration of donor ischemia time, the adequacy of myocardial protection during CPB, the duration of CPB, and the presence of recipient pulmonary hypertension, the incidence of RV and/or LV dysfunction is variable. Interestingly, interventricular septal hypokinesis persisting through 12 postoperative months has been demonstrated in the majority of cardiac transplant recipients in at least two investigations.[175,176] Explanations for this echocardiographic finding included perioperative septal ischemia, development of RV dysfunction in the presence of pulmonary hypertension, or the development of posttransplantation subendocardial coronary artery disease. Consequently, the presence of isolated interventricular septal hypokinesis in an otherwise hemodynamically stable cardiac transplant recipient should not necessarily cause concern.

The atrial suture lines between the donor and recipient cuffs may have a distinctive "hour-glass" echocardiographic appearance.[177–180] Stenosis of the suture line that impedes intracardiac flow has been reported. In one study of 64 transplant recipients who underwent echocardiographic examination at an average of 31 months postoperatively, spontaneous echo contrast was seen in 35 of the patients by TEE, and 18 patients had evidence of LA thrombus (38%).[179] Another study demonstrated only a 25% incidence of spontaneous LA echo contrast by TEE, but a 50% incidence of suspicious LA or RA masses suggestive of intra-atrial thrombus.[177] Therefore, a comprehensive intraoperative echocardiographic examination should include confirmation of atrial size and geometry, which may correlate with the potential for intra-atrial thrombus formation.

Postoperative MR and TR following cardiac transplantation have been well documented in the literature.[177–179,181] In these TEE studies acquired from 5 to 31 months postoperatively, an incidence of 73% to 100% of mild to moderate TR and 53% to 77% of mild to moderate MR has been reported. The etiology of posttransplant MR includes the development of an enlarged LA with mitral annular dilatation and resultant annuloventricular disproportion,[182,183] cardiac edema,[184] SAM,[185] and subacute bacterial endocarditis.[186] Posttransplant TR has been attributed to annular dilatation secondary to alterations in RV geometry associated with subclinical rejection or adaptation to higher pulmonary pressures.[181] In addition, direct and indirect injury to the TV during endomyocardial biopsy has also been reported.[187–189] Consequently, the documentation of valve function by intraoperative echocardiography in the immediate post–CPB period should be an essential component of a routine examination in a heart transplant recipient.

Ventricular Assist Devices

Several important principles should be incorporated into a comprehensive intraoperative echocardiographic examination of patients receiving ventricular assist devices (VAD). Before implantation, it is important to document the extent of ventricular regional and global dysfunction. Patients undergoing VAD placement are also susceptible to preoperative intracardiac thrombus formation, which has been demonstrated in 12% of this high-risk patient population.[177] Interrogating the extent and location of significant concurrent valvular disease is also important. The demonstration of significant AI in 4 patients undergoing the placement of a HeartMate (Thermocardiosystems Inc, Woburn, MA) resulted in the requirement for an additional AV procedure to assure appropriate VAD function via the ascending aortic outflow cannula.[177] TR, diagnosed by intraoperative echocardiography in 23 of the patients, did not require a concurrent repair. Finally, the documentation of a PFO may have important consequences in patients scheduled for a VAD. Following left VAD (LVAD) placement, the subsequent decrease in LA and LV pressures could promote predominant right to left shunting via a PFO.[175,177] In the 91 HeartMate patients discussed above, 8 were found to have a PFO that was closed during surgery and another patient was subsequently discovered to have a PFO after implantation, which was subsequently closed after reinitiating CPB.

Immediately following the placement of a single VAD, it is imperative to monitor function of both the recipient and nonassisted ventricle. In the HeartMate series, 11 patients undergoing LVAD placement required a subsequent right VAD upon the confirmation of RV failure by intraoperative TEE.[177] It is also important to document that the assisted chamber is being effectively unloaded and that the inflow cannula is properly positioned (Fig. 10-27). Of the 91 patients in this series, 3.3% of the cases required cannula repositioning based on TEE evidence. Finally, it is important to document the presence of intracavitary air following any open cardiac procedure because of the inherent risk of embolization. Significant "microair" was found in 91% of patients, which required halting of VAD flow until the air could be vented for several minutes.[177]

Echocardiography has also been utilized in the postoperative period during weaning from a VAD. In one case series, a SWMA scoring system for the RV and LV acquired by TEE[181] was used to predict successful weaning from centrifugal or pneumatic pump systems in 16 ICU patients. In each patient, the device flows were decreased and inotropic support was increased while the ventricular walls were scored. This study emphasizes the potential perioperative utility of TEE

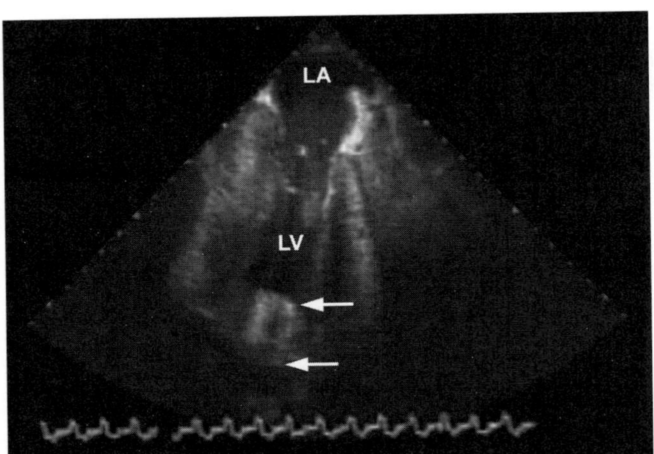

FIGURE 10–27 A mid-esophageal two-chamber transesophageal echocardiographic view demonstrating appropriate positioning of the left ventricular (LV) inflow cannula (arrows) of a HeartMate ventricular assist device. The cannula inlet (top arrow) is aligned with transmitral inflow and not obstructed by the left ventricular walls. LA = left atrium.

in this high-risk population. This same series reported that 3 patients developed extracardiac thrombus that compressed the cannula. In addition, intraventricular thrombus was visualized in 2 patients by TEE near the cannula inlet, which required subsequent surgical removal.

SAFETY AND COMPLICATIONS OF INTRAOPERATIVE TRANSESOPHAGEAL ECHOCARDIOGRAPHY

A discussion on the impact of a new technology on outcome is not complete without consideration for safety and potential complications. The evidence that TEE is a relatively safe procedure comes mainly from the cardiology literature, but there are several case series focusing on intraoperative complications. Initial safety data were reported in 1991 from a survey of 15 European centers, which included 10,419 TEE examinations performed from 1982–89.[190] In 201 patients (1.9%), the probe could not be placed in the esophagus due to operator inexperience (n = 198) and/or the presence of a tracheostomy (n = 1) or esophageal diverticulum (n = 2). In 88 awake patients (0.6%), the exam could not be completed due to either probe intolerance (n = 65) or non–life-threatening pulmonary (n = 8), cardiac (n = 8), or bleeding (n = 1) complications. The echocardiography exam had to be terminated prematurely due to vomiting in 5 patients. Finally, 1 patient who had an undiagnosed esophageal tumor died from a bleeding complication. Comparable complication rates have been reported in a large series of patients undergoing TEE examinations from the Mayo Clinic.[191,192] Among 15,381 patients in this series, 2 deaths, 3 esophageal tears, and 18 cases of hematemesis were reported. In addition, the incidence of hypoxia/laryngospasm (0.7%) and minor cardiovascular problems including superventricular tachycardia, hypotension, and hypertension (1%) was also noted.

Several case series have reported specifically on the low rate of significant complications associated with intraoperative TEE.[193–195] A 1993 study involving 846 intraoperative TEE examinations reported no deaths or esophageal perforations but did include 1 incidence of a chipped tooth, 3 pharyngeal abrasions, and 1 unilateral vocal cord paralysis.[195] A large case series retrospectively studied 7200 patients who underwent TEE in the operating room and reported no deaths that were directly attributed to the TEE and an overall 0.2% incidence of morbidity.[193] In 2 patients, the endotracheal tube was advanced into the left mainstem bronchus during the intraoperative study, resulting in transient hypoxia until the endotracheal tube was repositioned. No hemodynamic perturbations were reported in these anesthetized patients associated specifically with the TEE placement or examination. Swallowing abnormalities were reported in 7 patients postoperatively. Finally, 1 patient suffered an esophageal perforation that required surgical repair on the second postoperative day. Although esophageal perforation remains a relatively infrequent complication associated with TEE, at least 12 cases of perioperative TEE-associated pharyngeal or esophageal perforations have been reported in neonates and adult surgical patients with the vast majority of these cases involving patients undergoing cardiac surgical procedures.[193,196–204] The high morbidity and mortality associated with this potential complication suggests that the placement of a TEE probe should be avoided in patients with esophageal or gastric pathology and in those patients in whom probe insertion or advancement within the esophagus is difficult.

The most frequent controversy in the cardiac surgical literature regarding intraoperative TEE complications focuses on a perceived association with postoperative dysphagia. An initial study in 1991, retrospectively reviewed 1245 cardiac surgical patients and reported a 1.8% incidence of dysphagia in the 217 patients who had a TEE placed compared to a 1.6% incidence in the 1028 patients in whom TEE was not performed.[205] Although there was no statistical difference between the two populations, the authors concluded that the number of patients was insufficient to completely exclude the possibility of a very weak association between TEE and dysphagia. Hogue et al also investigated the association between intraoperative TEE and dysphagia in 879 cardiac surgical patients.[206] Barium swallows demonstrating esophageal dysfunction were obtained in 34 patients who experienced dysphagia or coughing while drinking water following extubation. In comparison to the rest of the population, those patients with dysphagia were older, had lower CO, were more likely to require an intra-aortic balloon counterpulsation, had longer intubation times, and had a higher incidence of TEE probe placement (68% to 48%).

Even though age, duration of tracheal intubation, and intraoperative TEE were independent predictors of swallowing dysfunction, the authors noted that confounding variables may have accounted for this relationship.

A retrospective chart review of 838 consecutive cardiac surgical patients also found 10 of 126 TEE-studied patients had postoperative dysphagia compared to 13 of 712 with dysphagia who did not have an intraoperative TEE.[195] Again, the patients who underwent TEE examination had longer intubation times (34.1 hours vs. 17.5 hours) and more frequently underwent valve or combined valve/coronary artery bypass graft procedures (60.3% vs. 20.7%) than the non-TEE cohort. In addition, the need for TEE was not assigned randomly but was determined at the discretion of the surgeon and/or anesthesiologist. Other smaller studies of 57 and 41 patients have not demonstrated this correlation between TEE and dysphagia or any esophageal injury.[194,207]

Many studies may underestimate the true incidence of TEE-associated complications due to conservative definitions of clinically significant adverse events, limitations in standardizing the evaluation of patient's subjective complaints, and ascribing truly related complications to other etiologies. In addition, it is difficult to assess consequences associated with the "distraction factor" of intraoperative multitasking and patient care while performing intraoperative TEE. Morbidity associated with intraoperative TEE may be minimized by avoiding its use in patients with obvious contraindications to gastroesophageal manipulation, adhering to conservative judgment in abandoning probe insertion when significant resistance is encountered, and maintaining strict vigilance while continuing to observe and care for patients during the examination. The relatively low reported incidence of morbidity suggests that intraoperative TEE is a relatively safe diagnostic monitor that continues to serve as an invaluable tool in the perioperative management of cardiac surgical patients.

REFERENCES

1. Shanewise JS, Cheung AT, Aronson S, et al: ASE/SCA Guidelines for Performing a Comprehensive Intraoperative Multiplane Transesophageal Echocardiography Examination: Recommendations of the American Society of Echocardiography Council for Intraoperative Echocardiography and the Society of Cardiovascular Anesthesiologists Task Force for Certification in Perioperative Transesophageal Echocardiography. *Anesth Analg* 1999; 89:870.
2. Thys DA (chair): Practice Guidelines for Perioperative Transesophageal Echocardiography: A Report by the American Society of Anesthesiologists and the Society of Cardiovascular Anesthesiologists Task Force on Transesophageal Echocardiography. *Anesth Analg* 1996; 84:986.
3. Stewart WJ, Thomas JD, Klein AL, et al: Ten year trends in utilization of 6340 intraoperative echos. *Circulation* 1995; 92(suppl I): 2453.
4. Chaliki HP, Click RL, Abel MD: Comparison of intraoperative transesophageal echocardiographic examinations with the operative findings: prospective review of 1918 cases. *J Am Soc Echocardiogr* 1999; 12; 237.
5. Brandt RR, Oh JK, Abel MD, et al: Role of emergency intraoperative transesophageal echocardiography. *J Am Soc Echocardiogr* 1998; 11:972.
6. Wake PJ, Ali M, Carroll J, et al: Clinical and echocardiographic diagnoses disagree in patients with unexplained hemodynamic instability after cardiac surgery. *Can J Anaesth* 2001; 48:778.
7. Mishra M, Chauhan R, Sharma KK, et al: Real-time intraoperative echocardiography—how useful? Experience of 5,016 cases. *J Cardiothorac Vasc Anesth* 1998; 12:625.
8. Stewart WL, Currie PJ, Salcedo EE, et al: Intraoperative Doppler color flow mapping for decision-making in valve repair for mitral regurgitation: technique and results in 100 patients. *Circulation* 1990; 81:556.
9. Sheikh KH, deBruijn NP, Rankin JS, et al: The utility of transesophageal echocardiography and Doppler color flow imaging in patients undergoing cardiac valve surgery. *J Am Coll Cardiol* 1990; 15:363.
10. Click RL, Abel, MD, Schaff HV: Intraoperative transesophageal echocardiography: 5–year prospective review of impact on surgical management. *Mayo Clin Proc* 2000; 75:241.
11. Michel-Cherqui M, Ceddaha A, Liu N, et al: Assessment of systematic use of intraoperative transesophageal echocardiography during cardiac surgery in adults: a prospective study of 203 patients. *J Cardiothorac Vasc Anesth* 2000; 14:45.
12. Fix J, Isada L, Cosgrove D, et al: Do patients with less than "echo-perfect" results from mitral valve repair by intraoperative echocardiography have a different outcome? *Circulation* 1993; 88:39.
13. Maslow AD, Regan AMM, Haering JM, et al: Echocardiographic predictors of left ventricular outflow tract obstruction and systolic anterior motion of the mitral valve after mitral valve reconstruction for myxomatous valve disease. *J Am Coll Cardiol* 1999; 34:2096.
14. Shah PM, Raney AA: Echocardiographic correlates of left ventricular outflow obstruction and systolic anterior motion following mitral valve repair. *J Heart Valve Dis* 2001; 10:302.
15. Marwick TH, Stewart WJ, Currie PH, Cosgrove DM: Mechanisms of failure of mitral valve repair: an echocardiographic study. *Am Heart J* 1991; 122:149.
16. Freeman WK, Schaff HV, Khandheria BK, et al: Intraoperative evaluation of mitral valve regurgitation and repair by transesophageal echocardiography: incidence and significance of systolic anterior motion. *J Am Coll Cardiol* 1992; 20:599.
17. Aklog L, Filsoufi F, Flores KQ, et al: Does coronary artery bypass grafting alone correct moderate ischemic mitral regurgitation? *Circulation* 2001; 104(suppl I):I-68.
18. Sheikh KH, Bengtson JR, Rankin JS, et al: Intraoperative transesophageal Doppler color flow imaging used to guide patient selection and operative treatment of ischemic mitral regurgitation. *Circulation* 1991; 84:594.
19. Bach DS, Deeb GM, Bolling SF: Accuracy of intraoperative transesophageal echocardiography for estimating the severity of functional mitral regurgitation. *Am J Cardiol* 1995; 76:508.
20. Konstadt SN, Louie EK, Shore-Lesserson L, et al: The effects of loading changes on intraoperative Doppler assessment of mitral regurgitation. *J Cardiothorac Vasc Anesth* 1994; 8:19.
21. Thomas L, Foster E, Hoffman JIE, Schiller NB: The mitral regurgitation index: an echocardiographic guide to severity. *J Am Coll Cardiol* 1999; 33:2016.
22. Meloni L, Aru G, Abbruzzese PA, et al: Regurgitant flow of mitral valve prosthesis: an intraoperative transesophageal echocardiographic study. *J Am Soc Echocardiogr* 1994; 7:36.

23. Morehead AJ, Firstenberg MS, Takahiro S, et al: Intraoperative echocardiographic detection of regurgitant jets after valve replacement. *Ann Thorac Surg* 2000; 69:135.
24. Nowrangi SK, Connolly HM, Freeman WK, Click RL: Impact of intraoperative transesophageal echocardiography among patients undergoing aortic valve replacement for aortic stenosis. *J Am Soc Echocardiogr* 2001; 14:863.
25. Christenson JT, Jordan B, Bloch A, et al: Should a regurgitant mitral valve be replaced simultaneously with a stenotic aortic valve? *Tex Heart Inst J* 2000; 27:350.
26. Tunick PA, Gindea A, Kronzon I: Effect of aortic valve replacement for aortic stenosis on severity of mitral regurgitation. *Am J Cardiol* 1990; 65:1219.
27. Brasch AV, Khan SS, DeRobertis MA, et al: Change in mitral regurgitation severity after aortic valve replacement for aortic stenosis. *Am J Cardiol* 2000; 85:1271.
28. Harris KM, Malenka DJ, Haney MF, et al: Improvement in mitral regurgitation after aortic valve replacement. *Am J Cardiol* 1997; 80:741.
29. Moskowitz HD, Levine RA, Hilgenberg AD, Isselbacher EM: Transesophageal echocardiographic description of the mechanisms of aortic regurgitation in acute type a aortic dissection: implications for aortic valve repair. *J Am Coll Cardiol* 2000; 36:884.
30. Weyman AE: Right ventricular outflow tract, in Weyman AE (ed): *Principles and Practice of Echocardiography,* 2d ed. Philadelphia, Lea and Febiger, 1994.
31. Elkins RC, Lane MM, McCue C: Pulmonary autograft reoperation: incidence and management. *Ann Thorac Surg* 1996; 62:450.
32. Elkins RC, Knott-Craig CJ, Howell CE: Pulmonary autografts in patients with aortic annulus dysplasia. *Ann Thorac Surg* 1996; 61:1141.
33. Raanani E, Yau TM, David TE, et al: Risk factors for late pulmonary homograft stenosis after the Ross procedure. *Ann Thorac Surg* 2000; 70:1953.
34. Moidl R, Simon P, Kupilik N, et al: Increased pulmonary flow velocities in oversized homografts in patients after the Ross procedure. *Eur J Cardiothorac Surg* 1997; 12:569.
35. Pearlman AS: Role of echocardiography in the diagnosis and evaluation of severity of mitral and tricuspid stenosis. *Circulation* 1991; 84(suppl I):I-193.
36. Blaustein AS, Ramanathan A: Tricuspid valve disease: clinical evaluation, physiopathology, and management. *Cardiol Clin* 1998; 16:551.
37. Czer LSC, Maurer G, Bolger A, et al: Tricuspid valve repair: operative and follow-up evaluation by Doppler color flow mapping. *J Thorac Cardiovasc Surg* 1989; 98:101.
38. Goldman ME, Guarino T, Fuster V: The necessity for tricuspid valve repair can be determined intraoperatively by two-dimensional echocardiography. *J Thorac Cardiovasc Surg* 1987; 94:542.
39. Shapira Y, Porter A, Wurzel M, et al: Evaluation of tricuspid regurgitation severity: echocardiographic and clinical correlation. *J Am Soc Echocardiogr* 1998; 11:652.
40. Grimm RA, Stewart WJ: The role of intraoperative echocardiography in valve surgery. *Cardiol Clin* 1998; 16:477.
41. DeSimone R, Lange R, Saggau W, et al: Intraoperative transesophageal echocardiography for the evaluation of mitral, aortic, tricuspid valve repair: a tool to optimize surgical outcome. *Eur J Cardiothorac Surg* 1992; 6:665.
42. Johnston SR, Freeman WK, Schaff HV, et al: Severe tricuspid regurgitation after mitral valve repair: diagnosis by intraoperative transesophageal echocardiography. *J Am Soc Echocardiogr* 1990; 3:416.
43. Higgins T, Estafanous F, Lloyd F, et al: Stratification of morbidity and mortality outcome by preoperative risk factors in coronary artery bypass patients: a clinical severity score. *JAMA* 1992; 207:2344.
44. Edwards F, Carey J, Grover F, et al: Impact of gender on coronary bypass operative mortality. *Ann Thorac Surg* 1998; 66:125.
45. Ferraris V, Ferraris S: Risk factors for postoperative morbidity. *J Thorac Cardiovasc Surg* 1996; 111:731.
46. Tu J, Jagal S, Naylor S: Steering Committee of the Provincial Adult Cardiac Care Network of Ontario: multicenter validation of a risk index for mortality, intensive care unit stay, and overall hospital length of stay after cardiac surgery. *Circulation* 1995; 91:677.
47. Brooks M, Jones R, Bach R, et al: Predictors of morbidity and mortality from cardiac causes in the bypass angioplasty revascularization investigation (BARI) randomized trial and registry. *Circulation* 2000; 101:2682.
48. Vogt A, Grube E, Glunz H, et al: Determinants of mortality after cardiac surgery: results of the Registry of the Arbeitsgemeinschaft Leitender Kardiologischer Krankenhausarzte (ALKK) on 10,525 patients. *Eur Heart J* 2000; 21:28.
49. Eagle K, Guyton R, Davidoff R, et al: ACC/AHA guidelines for coronary artery bypass surgery. *J Am Coll Cardiol* 1999; 34:1262.
50. Cohn P, Gorlin R, Cohn L, et al: Left ventricular ejection fraction as a prognostic guide in surgical treatment of coronary and valvular heart disease. *Am J Cardiol* 1979; 34:136.
51. Senior R, Glenville B, Basu S, et al: Dobutamine echocardiography and thallium-201 imaging predict functional improvement after revascularization in severe ischemic left ventricular dysfunction. *Br Heart J* 1995; 74:358.
52. La Canna G, Alfieri O, Giubbibi R, et al: Echocardiography during infusion of dobutamine for identification of reversible dysfunction in patients with chronic coronary artery disease. *J Am Coll Cardiol* 1994; 23:617.
53. Cigarroa C, de Fillipi C, Brickner E, et al: Dobutamine stress echocardiography identifies hibernating myocardium and predicts recovery of left ventricular function after coronary revascularization. *Circulation* 1993; 88:430.
54. Meluzin J, Cerny J, Frelich M, et al: Prognostic value of the amount of dysfunctional but viable myocardium in revascularized patients with coronary artery disease and left ventricular dysfunction. *J Am Coll Cardiol* 1998; 32:912.
55. Olsen P, Kassis E, Niebuhr-Jorgensen U: Coronary artery bypass surgery in patients with severe left ventricular dysfunction. *Thorac Cardiovasc Surg* 1993; 41:118.
56. Luciani G, Montalbano G, Casali G, et al: A functional outcome after myocardial revascularization in ischemic ventricular failure. *G Ital Cardiol* 1998; 28:859.
57. Pasquet A, Lauer M, Williams M, et al: Prediction of global left ventricular function after bypass surgery in patients with severe left ventricular dysfunction: impact of preoperative myocardial function, perfusion, and metabolism. *Eur Heart J* 2000; 21:125.
58. Bax J, Poldermans D, Elhendy A, et al: Improvement of left ventricular ejection fraction, heart failure symptoms and prognosis after revascularization in patients with chronic coronary artery disease and viable myocardium detected by dobutamine stress echocardiography. *J Am Coll Cardiol* 1999; 34:163.
59. Zaroff J, Aronson S, Lee B, et al: The relationship between immediate outcome after cardiac surgery, homogeneous cardioplegia delivery, and ejection fraction. *Chest* 1994; 106:38.
60. Rocchi G, Poldermans D, Bax J: Usefulness of the ejection fraction response to dobutamine infusion in predicting functional recovery after coronary artery bypass grafting in patients with left ventricular dysfunction. *Am J Cardiol* 2000; 15:1440.
61. Mangano D: Biventricular function after myocardial revascularization in humans: deterioration and recovery patterns during the first 24 hours. *Anesthesiology* 1985; 62:571.

62. Battler A, Froelicher VF, Gallagher K, et al: Dissociation between regional myocardial dysfunction and ECG changes during ischemia in the conscious dog. *Circulation* 1980; 62:735.
63. Hauser AM, Gangadharan F, Ramos R, et al: Sequence of mechanical, electrocardiographic and clinical effects of repeated coronary artery occlusion in human beings: echocardiographic observations during coronary angioplasty. *J Am Coll Cardiol* 1985; 5:193.
64. Wohlgelernter D, Jaffe C, Cabin H, et al: Silent ischemia during coronary occlusion produced by balloon inflation: relation to regional myocardial dysfunction. *J Am Coll Cardiol* 1987; 10:491.
65. Smith J, Cahalan M, Benefield D, et al: Intraoperative detection of myocardial ischemia in high-risk patients: electrocardiography versus two-dimensional echocardiography. *Circulation* 1985; 72:1015.
66. Koolen JJ, van Visser C, Wezel H, et al: Influence of coronary artery bypass surgery on regional left ventricular wall motion: an intraoperative two-dimensional transesophageal echocardiographic study. *J Cardiothorac Anesth* 1987; 1:276.
67. Schiller N, Shah P, Crawford M, et al: Recommendations for quantitation of the left ventricle by two-dimensional echocardiography: American Society of Echocardiography Committee on Standards, Subcommittee on Quantitation of Two-Dimensional Echocardiograms. *J Am Soc Echocardiogr* 1989; 2:358.
68. Deutsch H, Curtis J, Leischik R, et al: Reproducibility of assessment of left ventricular function using intraoperative transesophageal echocardiography. *Thorac Cardiovasc Surg* 1993; 41:54.
69. Seeberger M, Cahalan M, Rouine-Rapp K, et al: Acute hypovolemia may cause segmental wall motion abnormalities in the absence of myocardial ischemia. *Anesth Analg* 1997; 86:1252.
70. Okada R: Relationship between septal perfusion, viability and motion before and after coronary artery bypass surgery. *Am Heart J* 1992; 124:1190.
71. Bergquist B, Wayne H, Leung J: Transesophageal echocardiography in myocardial revascularization, II: influence on intraoperative decision making. *Anesth Analg* 1996; 82:1139.
72. Rouine-Rapp K, Ionescu P, Balea M, et al: Detection of intraoperative segemental wall-motion abnormalities by transesophageal echocardiography: the incremental value of additional cross sections in the transverse and longitudinal planes. *Anesth Analg* 1996; 83:1141.
73. Cohen JL, Cheirif J, Segar DS, et al: Improved left ventricular endocardial border delineation and opacification with OPTISON (FS069), a new echocardiographic contrast agent: results of a phase III multicenter trial. *J Am Coll Cardiol* 1998; 32:746.
74. Erb JM, Shanewise JS, Michelsen LG, Aronson S: Changes in intraoperative regional wall motion assessment using contrast echocardiography during cardiac surgery. *Anesth Analg* 1999; 88:SCA102.
75. Aronson S, Dupont F, Savage R, et al: Changes in regional myocardial function after coronary artery bypass graft surgery are predicted by intraoperative low-dose dobutamine echocardiography. *Anesthesiology* 2000; 93:685.
76. Mor-avi V, Vignon P, Koch R, et al: Segemental analysis of color kinesis images: new method for quantification of the magnitude and timing of endocardial motion during left ventricular systole and diastole. *Circulation* 1996; 93:1877.
77. Lau Y, Puryear J, Gan S, et al: Assessment of left ventricular wall motion abnormalities with the use of color kinesis: a valuable visual and training aid. *J Am Soc Echocardiogr* 1997; 10:665.
78. Hartmann T, Kolev N, Blaichar A, et al: Validity of acoustic quantification colour kinesis for detection of left ventricular regional wall motion abnormalities: a transesophageal echocardiographic study. *Br J Anaesth* 1997; 79:482.
79. Leung J, Okelly B, Browner W, et al: Prognostic importance of post bypass regional wall-motion abnormalities in patients undergoing coronary artery bypass graft surgery. *Anesthesiology* 1989; 71:16.
80. Van Daele M, Sutherland G, Mitchell M, et al: Do changes in pulmonary capillary wedge pressure adequately reflect myocardial ischemia during anesthesia? A correlative preoperative hemodynamic, electrocardiographic and transesophageal echocardiographic study. *Circulation* 1990; 81:865.
81. Smith J, Cahalan M, Benefiel D, et al: Intraoperative detection of myocardial ischemia in high-risk patients: electrocardiography versus two-dimensional transesophageal echocardiography. *Circulation* 1985; 72:1015.
82. Afifi S, Podgoreanu M, Davis E, et al: Is the routine use of intraoperative transesophageal echocardiography (TEE) justified? *Anesth Analg* 2000; 90:SCA82.
83. Communale M, Body S, Ley C, et al: The concordance of intraoperative left ventricular wall-motion abnormalities and electrocardiographic S-T segment changes: association with outcome after coronary revascularization. *Anesthesiology* 1998; 88:945.
84. Poortmans G, Schupfer G, Roosens C, Poelaert J: Transesophageal echocardiographic evaluation of left ventricular function. *J Cardiothorac Vasc Anesth* 2000; 14:588.
85. Mock M, Ringqvist I, Fisher L, et al: Survival of medically treated patients in the coronary artery surgery study (CASS) registry. *Circulation* 1982; 66:562.
86. Liu N, Darmon P, Saada M, et al: Comparison between radionucleotide ejection fraction and fractional area changes derived from transesophageal echocardiography using automated border detection. *Anesthesiology* 1996; 85:468.
87. Gorscan J 3rd, Lazar J, Schulman D, Follansbee W: Comparison of left ventricular function by echocardiographic automated border detection and by radionucleotide ejection fraction. *Am J Cardiol* 1993; 72:810.
88. Perrino A, Harris S, Luther M: Intraoperative determination of cardiac output using multiplane transesophageal echocardiography: a comparison to thermodilution. *Anesthesiology* 1998; 89:350.
89. Maslow A, Communale M, Haering J, Watkins J: Pulsed wave Doppler measurement of cardiac output from the right ventricular outflow tract. *Anesth Analg* 1996; 83:466.
90. Darmon P, Hillel Z, Mogtader A, et al: Cardiac output by transesophageal echocardiography using continuous wave Doppler across the aortic valve. *Anesthesiology* 1994; 80:796.
91. Appleton C, Hatle L: The natural history of left ventricular filling abnormalities: assessment by two-dimensional and Doppler echocardiography. *Echocardiography* 1992; 9:437.
92. Garcia M, Thomas J, Klein A: New Doppler echocardiographic applications for the study of diastolic function. *J Am Coll Cardiol* 1998; 32:865.
93. Djaiani G, McCreath B, Ti L, et al: Mitral flow propagation velocity identifies patients with abnormal diastolic function during coronary bypass surgery. *Anesth Analg* 2002; 95:524.
94. Bernard F, Denault A, Babin D, et al: Diastolic dysfunction is predictive of difficult weaning from cardiopulmonary bypass. *Anesth Analg* 2001; 92:291.
95. De Hert S, Rodrigus I, Haenen L, et al: Recovery of systolic and diastolic left ventricular function early after cardiopulmonary bypass. *Anesthesiology* 1996; 85:1063.
96. McKenney P, Apstein C, Mendes L, et al: Increased left ventricular diastolic chamber stiffness immediately after coronary artery bypass surgery. *J Am Coll Cardiol* 1994; 5:1189.
97. Jiang L, Wiegers SE, Weyman AE: Right ventricle, in Weyman AE (ed): *Principles and Practice of Echocardiography,* 2d ed. Philadelphia, Lea and Febiger, 1994.
98. Otto C: Echocardiographic evaluation of left and right ventricular systolic function, in Otto C (ed): *Textbook of Clinical Echocardiography,* 2d ed. Philadelphia, WB Saunders, 2000.

99. Jardin F, Dubourg O, Gueret P, et al: Quantitative two-dimensional echocardiography in massive pulmonary embolism: emphasis on ventricular interdependence and leftward septal displacement. *J Am Coll Cardiol* 1987; 10:1201.
100. Ryan T, Petrovic O, Dillon JC, et al: An echocardiographic index for separation of right ventricular volume and pressure overload. *J Am Coll Cardiol* 1985; 5: 918.
101. King ME, Braun H, Goldblatt A, et al: Interventricular septal configuration as a predictor of right ventricular systolic hypertension in children: a cross-sectional echocardiographic study. *Circulation* 1983; 68:68.
102. Fenely M, Garagham T: Paradoxical and pseudo paradoxical interventricular septal motion in patients with right ventricular volume overload. *Circulation* 1986; 74:230.
103. Hamel E, Pacouret G, Vincentelli D, et al: Thrombolysis or heparin therapy in massive pulmonary embolism with right ventricular dilation (results from a 128-patient monocenter registry). *Chest* 2001; 120:120.
104. Wake PJ, Ali M, Carroll J, et al: Clinical and echocardiographic diagnoses disagree in patients with unexplained hemodynamic instability after cardiac surgery. *Can J Anaesth* 2001; 48:778.
105. Rafferty T, Durkin M, Harris S, et al: Transesophageal two-dimensional echocardiographic analysis of right ventricular systolic performance indices during coronary artery bypass grafting. *J Cardiothorac Vasc Anesth* 1993; 7:160.
106. Ochai Y, Morita S, Tanoue Y, et al: Use of transesophageal echocardiography for postoperative evaluation of right ventricular function. *Ann Thorac Surg* 1999; 67:146.
107. Nomura T, Lebowitz L, Koide Y: Evaluation of hepatic venous flow using transesophageal echocardiography in coronary artery bypass surgery: an index of right ventricular function. *J Cardiothorac Vasc Anesth* 1995; 1:9.
108. Gardeback M, Settergren G, Brodin L: Hepatic blood flow and right ventricular function during cardiac surgery assessed by transesophageal echocardiography. *J Cardiothorac Vasc Anesth* 1996; 10:318.
109. Leibowitz D: Role of echocardiography in the diagnosis and treatment of acute pulmonary embolus. *J Am Soc Echocardiogr* 2001; 14:921.
110. Wake PJ, Ali M, Carroll J, et al: Clinical and echocardiographic diagnoses disagree in patients with unexplained hemodynamic instability after cardiac surgery. *Can J Anaesth* 2001; 48:778.
111. Come PC: Echocardiographic evaluation of pulmonary embolism and its response to therapeutic interventions. *Chest* 1992; 101:151S.
112. McConnell M, Solomon SD, Rayan ME, et al: Regional right ventricular dysfunction detected by echocardiography in acute pulmonary embolism. *Am J Cardiol* 1996; 78:469.
113. Feigenbaum H: Pericardial disease, in Feigenbaum H (ed): *Echocardiography,* 5th ed. Baltimore, Williams & Wilkins, 1994; p 556.
114. Martin R, Rakowski H, French J, Popp R: Localization of pericardial effusion with wide-angle phased array echocardiography. *Am J Cardiol* 1978; 42:904.
115. Weitzman L: The incidence and natural history of pericardial effusion after cardiac surgery: an echocardiographic study. *Circulation* 1984; 69:506.
116. Douglas P: Pericardial disease, in Sutton M, Oldershaw P (eds): *Textbook of Adult and Pediatric Echocardiography and Doppler.* Boston, Blackwell Scientific Publications, 1989; p 381.
117. Fyke F 3rd: Detection of intrapericardial hematoma after open-heart surgery: the role of echocardiography and computer tomography. *J Am Coll Cardiol* 1985; 5:1496.
118. Friedberg C: *Diseases of the Heart.* Philadelphia, WB Saunders, 1966.
119. Pepi M, Muratori M, Barbieri P, et al: Pericardial effusion after cardiac surgery: incidence, site, size and hemodynamic consequences. *Br Heart J* 1994; 72:327.
120. Oh J: Pericardial disease, in Oh J, Seward J, Tajik A (eds): *The Echo Manual,* 2d ed. Philadelphia, Lippincott Williams & Wilkins, 1999; p 181.
121. Russo A, O'Connor W, Waxman H: Atypical presentation and echocardiographic findings in patients with cardiac tamponade occurring early and late after cardiac surgery. *Chest* 1993; 104:71.
122. Spodick D: Pericardial diseases, in Braunwald E, Zipes D, Libby P (eds): *Heart Disease,* 6th ed. Philadelphia, WB Saunders, 2001; p 1823.
123. Burstow D, Oh J, Bailey K, et al: Cardiac tamponade: characteristic Doppler observations. *Mayo Clin Proc* 1989; 64:312.
124. Klein A, Cohen G, Petrolungo J, et al: Differentiation of constrictive pericarditis from restrictive cardiomyopathy by Doppler transesophageal echocardiographic measurements of respiratory variations in pulmonary venous flow. *J Am Coll Cardiol* 1993; 2:1935.
125. Appleton C, Hatle L, Pop R: Cardiac tamponade and pericardial effusion: respiratory variation in transvalvular flow velocities studied by Doppler echocardiography. *J Am Coll Cardiol* 1988; 11:1020.
126. Keren A, Kim CB, Hu BS, et al: Accuracy of biplane and multiplane transesophageal echocardiography in diagnosis of typical acute aortic dissection and intramural hematoma. *J Am Coll Cardiol* 1996; 28:627.
127. Willens HJ, Kessler KM: Transesophageal echocardiography in the diagnosis of diseases of the thoracic aorta, part 1. *Chest* 1999; 116:1772.
128. Nienaber CA, Kodolitsch YV, Nicholas V, et al: The diagnosis of thoracic aortic dissection by noninvasive imaging procedures. *N Engl J Med* 1993; 328:1.
129. Evangelista A, Garcia del Castillo H, Gonzalez-Alujas T, et al: Diagnosis of ascending aortic dissection by transesophageal echocardiography: utility of M-mode in recognizing artifacts. *J Am Coll Cardiol* 1996; 27:102.
130. Adachi H, Omoto R, Kyo S, et al: Emergency surgical intervention of acute aortic dissection with rapid diagnosis by transesophageal echocardiography. *Circulation* 1991; 84(suppl III):14.
131. Banning AB, Masani ND, Ikram S, et al: Transesophageal echocardiography as the sole diagnostic investigation in patients with suspected thoracic aortic dissection. *Br Heart J* 1994; 72:461.
132. Roach GW, Kanchuger M, Mangano C, et al: Adverse cerebral outcomes after coronary bypass surgery. *N Engl J Med* 1996; 335: 1857.
133. Stoney WS, Mulherin JL Jr, Alford WC Jr, et al: Unexpected death following aorto coronary bypass. *Ann Thorac Surg* 1976; 21: 528.
134. McKibbin DW, Gott VL, Hutchins GM, et al: Fatal cerebral atheromatous embolization after cardiopulmonary bypass. *J Thorac Cardiovasc Surg* 1976; 71:741.
135. Amarenco P, Cohen A, Tzourio C, et al: The prevalence of ulcerated plaques in the aortic arch in patients with stroke. *N Engl J Med* 1992; 326:221.
136. Davila-Roman VG, Barzilai B, Wareing TH, et al: Atherosclerosis of the ascending aorta: prevalence and role as an independent predictor of cerebrovascular events in cardiac patients. *Stroke* 1994; 25:2010.
137. Stern A, Tunick PA, Culliford AT, et al: Protruding aortic arch atheromas: risk of stroke during heart surgery with and without aortic arch endarterectomy. *Am Heart J* 1999; 138:746.
138. Ribakove G, Katz E, Gallaway A, et al: Surgical implications of transesophageal echocardiography to grade the atheromatous aortic arch. *Ann Thorac Surg* 1992; 53:758.

139. Tunick PA, Rosenzweig BP, Katz ES, et al: High risk for vascular events in patients with protruding aortic atheromas: a prospective study. *J Am Coll Cardiol* 1994; 23:1085.
140. The French Study of Aortic Plaques in Stroke Group: Atherosclerotic disease of the aortic arch as a risk factor for recurrent ischemic stroke. *N Engl J Med* 1996; 334:1216.
141. Mitusch R, Dorothy C, Wucherpfennig H, et al: Vascular events during follow-up in patients with aortic arch atherosclerosis. *Stroke* 1997; 28:36.
142. Wareing TH, Davila-Roman VG, Barzilai B, et al: Management of the severely atherosclerotic aorta during cardiac operations. *J Thorac Cardiovasc Surg* 1992; 103:453.
143. Kouchoukos NT, Wareing TH, Daily BB, Murphy SF: Management of the severely atherosclerotic aorta during cardiac operations. *J Card Surg* 1994; 9:490.
144. Trehan N, Mishra M, Bapna R, et al: Significantly reduced incidence of stroke during coronary artery bypass grafting using transesophageal echocardiography. *Eur J Cardiothorac Surg* 1997; 11:234.
145. Marschall K, Kanchuger M, Kessler K, et al: Superiority of transesophageal echocardiography in detecting aortic arch atheromatous disease: identification of patients at increased risk of stroke during cardiac surgery. *J Cardiothorac Vasc Anesth* 1994; 8:5.
146. Ohteki H, Itoh T, Natswaki M, et al: Intraoperative ultrasonic imaging of the ascending aorta in ischemic heart disease. *Ann Thorac Surg* 1990; 539.
147. Sylivris S, Calafiore P, Mataloanis G, et al: The intraoperative assessment of ascending aortic atheroma: epiaortic imaging is superior to both transesophageal echocardiography and direct palpation. *J Cardiothorac Vasc Anesth* 1997; 11:704.
148. Tennenbaum A, Garniek A, Shemesh J, et al: Dual-helical CT for detecting aortic atheromas as a source of stroke: comparison with transesophageal echocardiography. *Radiology* 1998; 208:153.
149. Kurz SM, Lee VS, Tunick PA, et al: Atheromas of the thoracic aorta: comparison of TEE and MRA [abstract]. *J Am Coll Cardiol* 1999; 33(suppl A):414A.
150. Konstadt SN, Reich DL, Stanley TE 3rd, et al: The ascending aorta: how much does transesophageal echocardiography see? *Anesth Analg* 1994; 78:240.
151. Davila-Roman VG, Phillips KJ, Daily BB, et al: Intraoperative transesophageal echocardiography and epiaortic ultrasound for assessment of atherosclerosis of the thoracic aorta. *J Am Coll Cardiol* 1996; 28:942.
152. Ostrowski JW, Kanchuger MS: Epiaortic scanning is not routinely necessary for cardiac surgery. *J Cardiothorac Vasc Anesth* 2000; 14:91.
153. Konstadt SN, Reich DL, Stanley TE 3rd, et al: Transesophageal echocardiography can be used to screen for ascending aortic atherosclerosis. *Anesth Analg* 1995; 81:225.
154. Matsuzaki M, Toma Y, Kusukawa R: Clinical applications of transesophageal echocardiography. *Circulation* 1990; 82:709.
155. Mugge A, Daniel WG, Haverich A, Lichtlen PR: Diagnosis of noninfective cardiac mass lesions by two-dimensional echocardiography: comparison of the transthoracic and transesophageal approaches. *Circulation* 1991; 83:70.
156. Black, IW, Hopkins AP, Lee LCL, et al: Left atrial spontaneous contrast: a clinical and echocardiographic analysis. *J Am Coll Cardiol* 1991; 18:398.
157. Feigenbaum H: Cardiac masses, in Feigenbaum H (ed): *Echocardiography,* 5th ed. Baltimore, Williams & Wilkins, 1994; p 589.
158. Raichlen J: Cardiac masses, tumors and thrombi, in St John Sutter M, Oldershaw PJ, Kotler MN (eds): *Textbook of Echocardiography and Doppler in Adults and Children,* 2d ed. Boston, Blackwell Science, 1996; p 437.
159. Seward JB, Khanderia BK, Oh JK, et al: Critical appraisal of transesophageal echocardiography: limitations, pitfalls and complications. *J Am Soc Echocardiogr* 1992; 5:288.
160. Stoddard MF, Liddell N.E, Longacker RA, Dawkins PR: Transesophageal echocardiography: normal variants and mimickers. *Am Heart J* 1992; 124:1587.
161. Cujec B, Mycyk T, Khouri M: Identification of Chiari's network with transesophageal echocardiography. *J Am Soc Echocardiogr* 1992; 5:96.
162. Pochis WT, Saeian K, Sagar K: Usefulness of transesophageal echocardiography in diagnosing lipomatous hypertrophy of the atrial septum with comparison to transthoracic echocardiography. *Am J Cardiol* 1992; 70:396.
163. Alam M, Sun I: Transesophageal echocardiographic evaluation of left atrial mass lesions. *J Am Soc Echocardiogr* 1992; 4:323.
164. Aronson S, Ruo W, Sand M: Invert left atrial appendage appearing as a left atrial mass with transesophageal echocardiography during cardiac surgery. *Anesthesiology* 1992; 76:1054.
165. Hirsch R, Kilner PJ, Connelly MS, et al: Congenital heart disease: diagnosis in adolescents and adults with congenital heart disease: prospective assessment of individual and combined roles of magnetic resonance imaging and transesophageal echocardiography. *Circulation* 1994; 90:2937.
166. Muhiudeen IA, Roberson DA, Silverman NH, et al: Intraoperative echocardiography for evaluation of congenital heart defects in infants and children. *Anesthesiology* 1992; 76:165.
167. Stevenson JG, Sorensen GK, Gartman DM, et al: Transesophageal echocardiography during repair of congenital cardiac defects: identification of residual problems necessitating reoperation. *J Am Soc Echocardiogr* 1993; 6:356.
168. Sukernik MR, Mets B, Bennett-Guerrero E: Patent foramen ovale and its significance in the perioperative period. *Anesth Analg* 2001; 93:1137.
169. Schneider B, Zienkiewicz T, Jansen V, et al: Diagnosis of patent foramen ovale by transesophageal echocardiography and correlation with autopsy findings. *Am J Cardiol* 1996; 77:1202.
170. Konstadt SN, Louie EK, Black S, et al: Intraoperative detection of patent foramen ovale by transesophageal echocardiography. *Anesthesiology* 1991; 74:212.
171. Stone DA, Godard J, Corretti MC, et al: Patent foramen ovale: association between the degree of shunt by contrast transesophageal echocardiography and the risk of future ischemic neurologic events. *Am Heart J* 1996; 131:158.
172. Mas JL, Arquizian C, Lamy C: Recurrent cerebrovascular events associated with patent foramen ovale, atrial septal aneurysm or both. *N Engl J Med* 2001; 345:1740.
173. Mugge A, Daniel WG, Angermann C, et al: Atrial septal aneurysm in adult patients: a multicenter study using transthoracic and transesophageal echocardiography. *Circulation* 1995; 91:2785.
174. Pearson AC, Nagelhout D, Castello R: Atrial septal aneurysm and stroke: a transesophageal echocardiographic study. *J Am Coll Cardiol* 1991; 18:1223.
175. Gorcsan J 3rd, Snow FR, Paulsen W, et al: Echocardiographic profile of the transplanted human heart in clinically well recipients. *J Heart Lung Transplant* 1992; 11:80.
176. Rees AP, Milani RV, Lavine CJ: Valvular regurgitation and right-sided cardiac pressures in heart transplant recipients by complete Doppler and color flow evaluation. *Chest* 1993; 104:82.
177. Angermann CE, Spes CH, Tammen A, et al: Anatomic characteristics and valvular function of the transplanted heart: transthoracic versus transesophageal echocardiographic findings. *J Heart Transplant* 1990; 9:331.
178. Polanco G, Jafri SM, Alam M, Levine BT: Transesophageal echocardiographic findings in patients with orthotopic heart transplantation. *Chest* 1992; 101;599.

179. Derumeaux G, Mouton-Schleifer D, Soyer R, et al: High incidence of left atrial thrombus detected by transoesophageal echocardiography in heart transplant recipients. *Eur Heart J* 1995; 16:120.
180. Goldstein DJ, Garfein ES, Aaronson K, et al: Mitral valve replacement and tricuspid valve repair after cardiac transplantation. *Ann Thorac Surg* 1997; 63:1463.
181. Rees AP, Milani RV, Lavine CJ, et al: Valvular regurgitation and right-sided cardiac pressures in heart transplant recipients by complete Doppler and color flow evaluation. *Chest* 1993; 104:82.
182. Stevenson L, Dadourian B, Kobashigawa J, et al: Mitral regurgitation after cardiac transplantation. *Am J Cardiol* 1987; 60:119.
183. Deleuze P, Benvenuti C, Mazzucotelli J, et al: Orthotopic cardiac tranplantation with direct caval anastomosis: is it the optimal procedure? *J Thorac Cardiovasc Surg* 1995; 109:731.
184. Cladellas M, Abadal M, Pons-Llado G, et al: Early transient multivalvular regurgitation detected by pulsed Doppler in cardiac transplantation. *Am J Cardiol* 1986; 58:1122.
185. Chatel D, Paquin S, Oroudji M, et al: Systolic anterior motion of the anterior mitral leaflet after heart transplantation. *Anesthesiology* 1999; 91:1535.
186. Copeland JG, Rosado LJ, Sethi G, et al: Mitral valve replacement six years after cardiac transplantation. *Ann Thorac Surg* 1991; 51:1014.
187. Stahl RD, Karwande SV, Olsen SL, et al: Tricuspid valve dysfunction in the transplanted heart. *Ann Thorac Surg* 1995; 59:477.
188. Huddleston CB, Rosenbloom M, Goldstein JA, Pasque MK: Biopsy-induced tricuspid regurgitation after cardiac transplantation. *Ann Thorac Surg* 1994; 57:832.
189. Weston MW, Vijayanagar R, Sastry N: Closure of a patent foramen ovale and tricuspid valve replacement after heart transplantation. *Ann Thorac Surg* 1996; 61:717.
190. Daniel WG, Erbel R, Kasper W, et al: Safety of transesophageal echocardiography: a multicenter survey of 10,419 examinations. *Circulation* 1991; 83:817.
191. Transesophageal echocardiography, in Oh J, Seward JB, Tajik AJ (eds):*The Echo Manual,* 2d ed. Philadelphia, Lippincott Williams & Wilkins, 1999.
192. Khandheria BK: The transesophageal echocardiographic examination: is it safe? *Echocardiography* 1994; 7:55.
193. Kallmeyer JI, Collard CD, Fox JA, et al: The safety of intraoperative transesophageal echocardiography: a case series of 7200 cardiac surgical patients. *Anesth Analg* 2001; 92:1126.
194. Hulyalkar AR, Ayd JD: Low risk of gastroesophageal injury associated with transesophageal echocardiography during cardiac surgery. *J Cardiothorac Vasc Anesth* 1992; 2:175.
195. Rafferty T, LaMantina KR, Davis E, et al: Quality assurance for intraoperative transesophageal echocardiography monitoring: a report of 846 procedures. *Anesth Analg* 1993; 76:228.
196. Kharasch ED, Sivarajan M: Gastroesophageal perforation after intraoperative transesophageal echocardiography. *Anesthesiology* 1996; 85:426.
197. Massey SR, Pitis A, Mehta D, et al: Oesophageal perforation following perioperative transesophageal echocardiography. *Br J Anaesth* 2000; 84:643.
198. Muhiudeen-Russell IA, Miller-Hance WC, Silverman NH: Unrecognized esophageal perforation in a neonate during transesophageal echocardiography. *J Am Soc Echocardiogr* 2001; 14:747.
199. Spahn DR, Schmid S, Carrell T, et al: Hypopharynx perforation by a transesophageal echocardiography probe. *Anesthesiology* 1995; 82:581.
200. Badaoui R, Choufane S, Riboulot M, et al: Esophageal perforation after transesophageal echocardiography. *Ann Fr Anesth Reanim* 1994; 13:850.
201. Brinkman WT, Shanewise JS, Clenments SD, et al: Transesophageal echocardiography: not an innocuous procedure. *Ann Thorac Surg* 2001; 72:1725.
202. Lecharny JB, Philip I, Depoix JP: Oesophageal perforation after intraoperative transesophageal echocardiography in cardiac surgery. *Br J Anaesth* 2002; 88:592.
203. Zalunardo MP, Bimmler D, Grob UC, et al: Late oesophageal perforation after intraopoerative transoesophageal echocardiography. *Br J Anaesth* 2002; 88:595.
204. Shapira MY, Hirshberg B, Agid R, et al: Esophageal perforation by a transesophageal echocardiogram. *Echocardiography* 1999; 65:151.
205. Messina AG, Paranicas M, Fiamengo S, et al: Risk of dysphagia after transesophageal echocardiography. *Am J Cardiol* 1991; 67:313.
206. Hogue, CW, Lappas, DG, Creswell LL, et al: Swallowing dysfunction after cardiac operations. *J Thorac Cardiovasc Surg* 1995; 110:512.
207. Owall A, Stahl L, Settergren G: Incidence of sore throat and patient complaints after intraoperative transesophageal echocardiography during cardiac surgery. *J Cardiothorac Vasc Anesth* 1992; 6:15.

Chapter 11

Extracorporeal Circulation

L. Henry Edmunds, Jr./Eugene A. Hessel II/ Robert W. Colman/ Philippe Menasche/John W. Hammon, Jr.

Introduction

L. Henry Edmunds, Jr.

Cardiac surgery is unique because blood exposed to nonendothelial cell surfaces is collected and continuously recirculated throughout the entire body. This contact with synthetic surfaces in the perfusion circuit and multiple tissues within the wound triggers a massive defense reaction that involves at least five plasma protein systems and five blood cells. This reaction—the inflammatory response to cardiopulmonary bypass—initiates a powerful thrombotic stimulus and the production, release, and circulation of a host of microemboli and vasoactive and cytotoxic substances that affect every organ and tissue within the body. Cardiopulmonary bypass and open heart surgery are simply not possible without heparin; thus the inflammatory response to cardiopulmonary bypass describes the consequences of exposing *heparinized* blood to nonendothelial cell–covered surfaces.

Much has been learned about the inflammatory response since early pioneers first described hemolysis, thrombocytopenia, and production of emboli during and after open heart surgery. Still much remains to be learned and the nirvana of a truly nonthrombogenic synthetic surface remains far beyond the horizon. This chapter summarizes applications of extracorporeal circulation as used in adult cardiac surgery. The presentation is divided into four sections. Section 11A describes the components and operation of perfusion systems and related special topics. The inflammatory response is separated into two middle sections (11B and 11C) for simplification and clarity; in reality the reactions of blood elements with each other are extensively intertwined and overlapping during cardiopulmonary bypass. The consequences of extracorporeal perfusion in terms of organ damage are summarized in section 11D.

11A: Perfusion Systems

Eugene A. Hessel II/L. Henry Edmunds, Jr.

COMPONENTS

During cardiopulmonary bypass (CPB) for clinical cardiac surgery, blood is typically drained by gravity into the venous reservoir of the heart-lung machine via cannulas placed in the superior and inferior vena cavae or a single cannula placed in the right atrium. Blood from this reservoir is pumped through a membrane oxygenator into the systemic arterial system, usually through a cannula placed in the distal ascending aorta (Fig. 11-1). This basic extracorporeal perfusion system can be adapted to provide partial or total circulatory and respiratory support or partial support for the left or right heart or for the lungs separately.

The complete heart-lung machine includes many additional components (Fig. 11-2).[1] Most manufacturers consolidate a *membrane oxygenator, venous reservoir,* and *heat exchanger* into one unit. A *microfilter-bubble trap* is added to the arterial line. Depending on the operation various suction systems are used to return blood from the surgical field, cardiac chambers, and/or the aorta. Aspirated blood passes through a *cardiotomy reservoir* and *microfilter* before returning to the venous reservoir. Optionally, but increasingly recommended, field blood is washed in a *cell saver system* and returned to the perfusate as packed red cells. In addition to adjusting pump flow, partial and occluding *clamps* on venous and arterial lines are used to direct and regulate flow. *Sites* for obtaining blood samples and *sensors* for monitoring pressures, temperatures, oxygen saturation, blood gases, and pH are included, as are various safety devices.

A separate circuit for administering *cardioplegic* solutions at controlled composition, rate, and temperature is usually included in the system. Less often a *hemoconcentrator* (for removal of water and small molecules) is added to the primary circuit.

Venous Cannulation and Drainage

PRINCIPLES OF VENOUS DRAINAGE

Venous blood usually enters the circuit by gravity or siphonage into a venous reservoir placed 40 to 70 cm below the level of the heart. The amount of drainage is determined by central venous pressure; the height differential; resistance in cannulas, tubing, and connectors; and absence of air within the system. Central venous pressure is determined by intravascular volume and venous compliance, which is influenced by medications, sympathetic tone, and anesthesia. Inadequate blood volume or excessive siphon pressure may cause compliant venous or atrial walls to collapse against cannular intake openings to produce "chattering" or "fluttering." This phenomenon is corrected by adding volume to the patient.

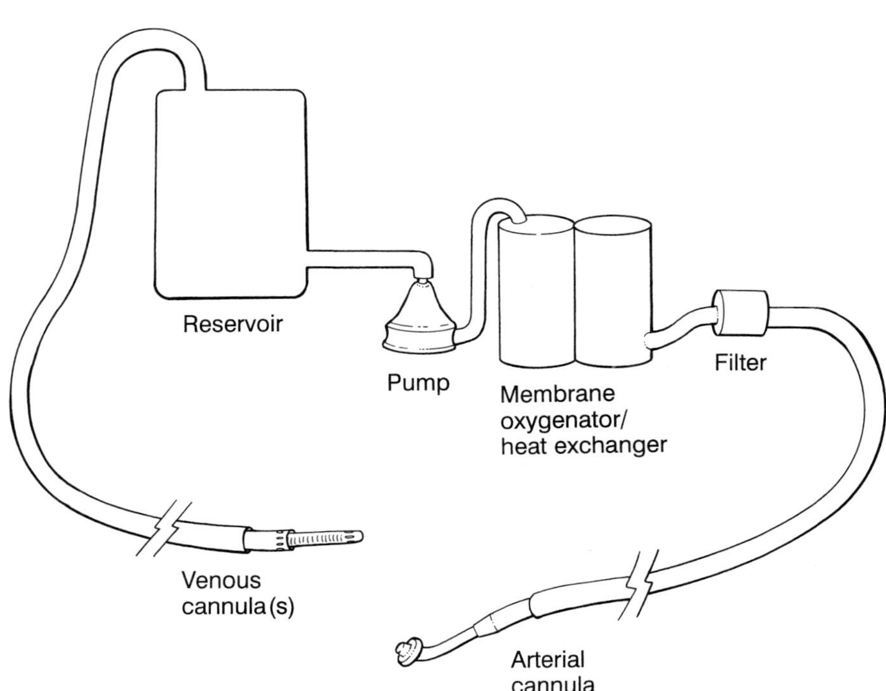

FIGURE 11–1 Basic cardiopulmonary bypass circuit with membrane oxygenator and centrifugal pump.

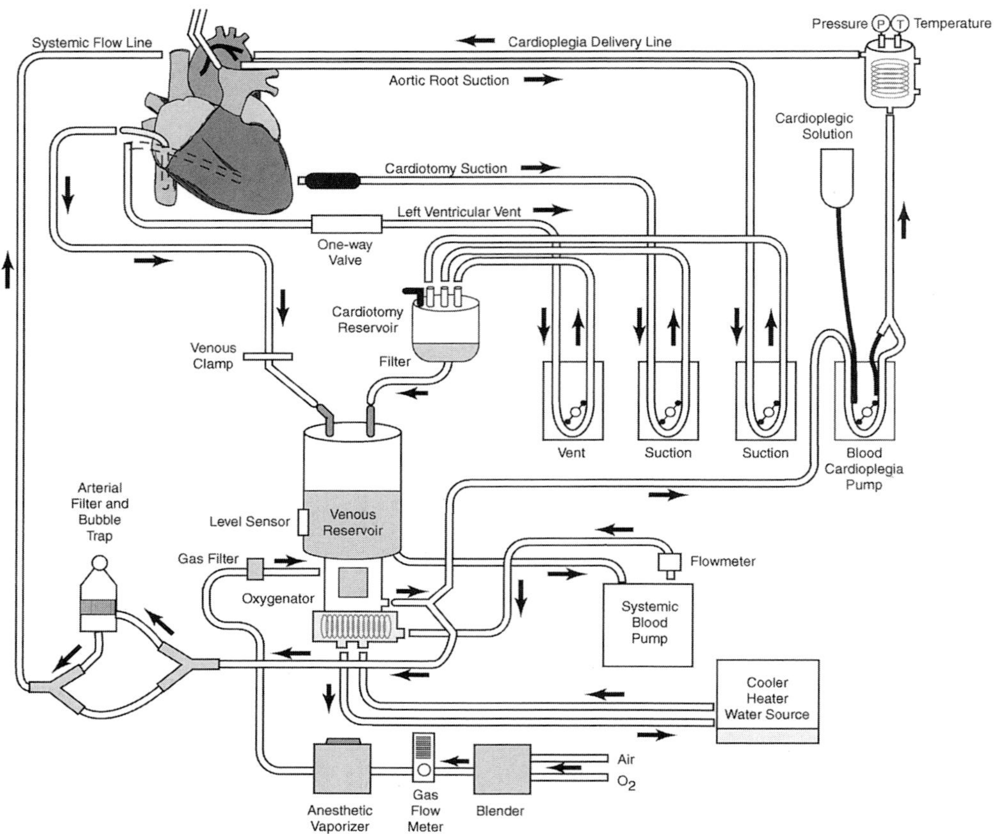

FIGURE 11–2 Diagram of a typical cardiopulmonary bypass circuit with vent, field suction, aortic root suction, and cardioplegic system. Blood is drained from a single "two-stage" catheter into the venous reservoir, which is part of the membrane oxygenator/heat exchanger unit. Venous blood exits the unit and is pumped through the heat exchanger and then the oxygenator. Arterialized blood exits the oxygenator and passes through a filter/bubble trap to the aortic cannula, which is usually placed in the ascending aorta. Blood aspirated from vents and suction systems enters a separate cardiotomy reservoir, which contains a microfilter, before entering the venous reservoir. The cardioplegic system is fed by a spur from the arterial line to which the cardioplegic solution is added and is pumped through a separate heat exchanger into the antegrade or retrograde catheters. Oxygenator gases and water for the heat exchanger are supplied by independent sources.

VENOUS CANNULAS AND CANNULATION

Venous cannulas are usually made out of flexible plastic, which may be stiffened against kinking by wire reinforcement. Tips are straight or angled and often are constructed of thin, rigid plastic or metal. Size is determined by patient size, anticipated flow rate, and an index of catheter flow characteristics and resistance (provided by the manufacturer). For an average adult with 60-cm negative siphon pressure, a 30F cannula in the superior vena cava (SVC) and 34F in the IVC or a single 42F cavoatrial catheter suffices. Catheters are typically inserted through purse-string guarded incisions in the right atrial appendage, lateral atrial wall, or directly in the SVC and IVC.

Three basic approaches for central venous cannulation are used: bicaval, single atrial, or cavoatrial ("two stage") (Fig. 11-3). *Bicaval cannulation* and caval tourniquets are necessary to prevent bleeding and air entry into the system when the right heart is entered during CPB. Because of coronary sinus return, caval tourniquets should not be tightened without decompressing the right atrium. Bicaval cannulation without caval tapes is often preferred to facilitate venous return during exposure of the left atrium and mitral valve.

Single venous cannulation is adequate for most aortic valve and coronary artery surgery; however, usually a cavoatrial cannula ("two-stage") is employed (Fig. 11-3B). This catheter is typically introduced via the right atrial appendage. Its narrowed distal end is threaded into the IVC while the wider proximal portion has side holes designed to rest within the right atrium. It tends to be more stable and provide better drainage than a single cannula, but proper positioning is critical.[2] With single cannulas, elevation of the heart may

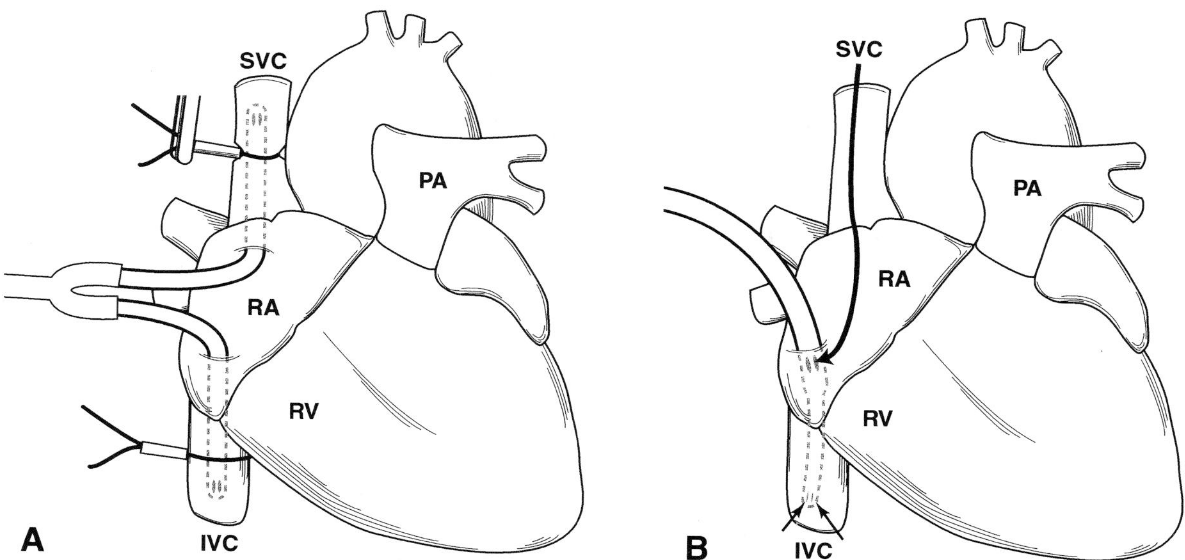

FIGURE 11–3 Placement of venous cannulas. (A) Cannulation of both cavae from incisions in the right atrium. (B) Cannulation using the "two-stage cannula." Blood in the right atrium is captured by vents in the expanded shoulder several inches from the narrower IVC catheter tip.

kink the junction of the SVC with the atrium and partially obstruct venous drainage.

At times, venous cannulation is accomplished via the femoral or iliac vein. This either open or percutaneous cannulation is used for emergency closed cardiopulmonary assist, for support of particularly ill patients before induction of anesthesia, for prevention or management of bleeding complications during sternotomy, for reoperations,[3] for certain types of aortic and thoracic surgery, and for applications of CPB that do not require thoracotomy. Adequate flow rates require using a cannula that is as large as possible and advancing the catheter into the right atrium guided by transesophageal echocardiography (TEE). Specially designed commercially manufactured long, ultrathin, wire-reinforced catheters are available for this purpose.

PERSISTENT LEFT SUPERIOR VENA CAVA

A persistent left superior vena cava (PLSVC) is present in 0.3% to 0.5% of the general population and usually drains into the coronary sinus; however, in about 10% of cases it drains into the left atrium.[4–6] The presence of a PLSVC should be suspected when the (left) innominate vein is small or absent and when a large coronary sinus or the PLSVC itself is seen on baseline TEE.[7,8]

A PLSVC may complicate retrograde cardioplegia or entry into the right heart.[9] If an adequate-sized innominate vein is present (30% of patients), the PLSVC can simply be occluded during CPB, if the ostium of the coronary sinus is present.[10] If the right SVC is not present (approximately 20% of patients with PLSVC), the left cava cannot be occluded. If the innominate vein is absent (40% of patients) or small (about 33%), occlusion of the PLSVC may cause venous hypertension and possible cerebral injury. In these patients a cannula is passed retrograde into the PLSVC through the coronary sinus ostium and secured. Alternatively, a cuffed endotracheal tube may be used as a cannula.[11]

AUGMENTED OR ASSISTED VENOUS RETURN

Negative pressure is sometimes applied to the venous lines to provide assisted venous drainage using a roller pump or centrifugal pump,[12] or by applying a regulated vacuum to a closed hard-shell venous reservoir (vacuum-assisted venous drainage, VAVD).[13] This may permit use of smaller diameter catheters[14] and may be helpful when long, peripheral catheters are used. Augmented negative pressure in the venous line increases the risk of aspirating gross or microscopic air and causing cerebral injury,[15–18] hemolysis, or aspiration of air into the blood compartment of membrane oxygenators. Positive pressure in the venous reservoir can cause air to enter the venous lines and right heart.[19] These potential complications require special safety monitors and devices and adherence to detailed protocols.[19,20]

COMPLICATIONS ASSOCIATED WITH VENOUS CANNULATION AND DRAINAGE

These include atrial arrhythmias, atrial or caval tears and bleeding, air embolization, injury or obstruction due to catheter malposition, reversing arterial and venous lines, and unexpected decannulation. Placing tapes around the cavae may lacerate branches, nearby vessels (e.g., right pulmonary artery), or the cava itself. Before or after CPB, catheters may compromise venous return to the right atrium from the body. Venous catheters and/or caval tapes may displace or compromise central venous or pulmonary arterial monitoring catheters; conversely, monitoring catheters may compromise the function of caval tapes.

Any intracardiac catheter may be trapped by sutures, which may impede removal before or after the wound is closed. Any connection between the atmosphere and cannula intake ports may entrain air to produce an air lock or gaseous microembolism. Assisted venous drainage (AVD) increases the risk of air entrainment.[21,22] Finally, improperly placed purse-string sutures may obstruct a cava when tied.[23]

CAUSES OF LOW VENOUS RETURN

Low venous pressure, hypovolemia, drug- or anesthetic-induced venous dilatation, inadequate differential height between heart and reservoir, too small cannula size, cannula obstruction from any cause, air locks, or excessive flow resistance in the drainage system are possible causes of reduced venous return. Partial obstruction of the venous line may distend the right ventricle and impair later contractility.

Arterial Cannulation

ARTERIAL CANNULAS

The tip of the arterial cannula is usually the narrowest part of the perfusion system and at required flows small aortic and arterial catheters produce high pressure differentials, jets, turbulence, and cavitation. Most arterial catheters are rated by a performance index, which relates external diameter, flow, and pressure differential.[24] High-velocity jets may damage the aortic wall, dislodge atheroemboli, produce dissections, disturb flow to nearby vessels, and cause cavitation and hemolysis. Pressure differences that exceed 100 mm Hg cause excessive hemolysis and protein denaturation.[25] Weinstein[26] attributed a predominance of left-sided stroke following cardiac surgery to the sand-blasting effect of end-hole aortic cannulas directing debris into the left carotid artery. Aortic catheters with only side ports[27] are designed to minimize jet effects and better distribute arch vessel perfusion and pressure[28] and may be associated with fewer strokes.[26]

Recently a dual-stream aortic perfusion catheter has been developed that features an inflatable horizontal streaming baffle that is designed to protect the arch vessels from atherosclerotic and other emboli and permits selective cerebral hypothermia.[29,30] Another novel aortic cannula features a side port that deploys a 120-μm mesh filter to remove particulate emboli beyond the ascending aorta.[31] Although this catheter increased the pressure gradient by 50%,[32] it removed an average of 8 emboli in 99% of 243 patients and cerebral injuries were less than expected.[33]

CONNECTION TO THE PATIENT

Anatomic sites available for arterial inflow include the proximal aorta, innominate artery and distal arch, and femoral, external iliac, axillary, and subclavian arteries. The choice is influenced by the planned operation[34] and distribution of atherosclerotic disease.[35]

ATHEROSCLEROSIS OF THE ASCENDING AORTA

Dislodgement of atheromatous debris from the aortic wall from manipulation,[36] cross-clamping, or the sand-blasting effect of the cannula jet is a major cause of perioperative stroke[37,38] and a risk factor for aortic dissection[39] and postoperative renal dysfunction.[40] Simple palpation during transient hypotension or transesophageal echocardiography (TEE) is less sensitive and accurate for detecting severe atherosclerosis than epiaortic ultrasonic scanning.[36,41,42] TEE views of the middle and distal ascending aorta are often inadequate,[41–44] but some recommend this method for screening.[44,45] Epiaortic scanning is preferred for all patients who have a history of transient ischemic attack, stroke, severe peripheral vascular disease, palpable calcification in the ascending aorta, calcified aortic knob on chest radiograph, age older than 50 to 60 years, or TEE findings of moderate aortic atherosclerosis.[36] Calcified aorta ("porcelain aorta"), which occurs in 1.2% to 4.3% of patients,[46,47] is another indication for changing the location of the aortic cannula.[48,49] Alternative sites include the distal aortic arch[46,50] and innominate, axillary-subclavian, or femoral arteries.

ASCENDING AORTIC CANNULATION

The distal ascending aorta is the preferred cannulation site because of ease and fewest complications. Most surgeons place two purse-string sutures (1.0-1.3 cm diameter) partially through the aortic wall, followed by a 4- to 5-mm, full-thickness stab wound, and insert the cannula under a finger while the mean arterial pressure is approximately 60 to 80 mm Hg. Usually the cannula is inserted 1 to 2 cm with a whiff of back bleeding, rotated to ensure that the tip is completely within the lumen, and positioned to direct flow to the mid transverse aorta. A few surgeons prefer a long catheter with the tip placed beyond the left subclavian artery.[51] Proper cannula placement is critical[28] and is confirmed by noting pulsatile pressure in the aortic line monitor and equivalent pressure in the radial artery. Once inserted the cannula must be adequately secured in place.

Complications of ascending aorta cannulation Complications include difficult insertion; bleeding; tear in the aortic wall; intramural or malposition of the cannula tip (in or against the aortic wall, toward the valve, or in an arch vessel)[52]; atheromatous emboli; failure to remove all air from the arterial line after connection; injury to the aortic back wall; high line pressure indicating obstruction to flow; inadequate or excessive cerebral perfusion[53]; inadvertent decannulation; and aortic dissection.[54,55] It is essential to monitor aortic line and radial artery pressures and to carefully observe the aorta for possible cannula-related complications during onset of CPB and during placement of aortic clamps. Asymmetric cooling of the face or neck may suggest a problem with cerebral perfusion. Late bleeding and infected or noninfected false aneurysms are delayed complications of aortic cannulation.

Aortic dissection occurs in 0.01% to 0.09% of aortic cannulations[39,55–58] and is more common in patients with aortic root disease. The first clues may be discoloration beneath the adventia near the cannula site, an increase in arterial line pressure, or a sharp reduction in return to the venous reservoir. TEE may be helpful in confirming the diagnosis,[59] but prompt action is necessary to limit the dissection and maintain perfusion. The cannula must be promptly transferred to a peripheral artery or uninvolved distal aorta. Blood pressure should be controlled pharmacologically and perfusion cooling to temperatures less than 20°C initiated. During hypothermic circulatory arrest, the aorta is opened at the original site of cannulation and repaired by direct suture, patch, or circumferential graft.[57,58] When recognized early, survival rates range from 66% to 85%, but when discovered after operation survival is approximately 50%.

CANNULATION OF THE FEMORAL OR ILIAC ARTERY

These vessels are usually the first alternative to aortic cannulation, but are also indicated for initiating cardiopulmonary bypass quickly for severe bleeding, cardiac arrest, acute intraoperative dissection or severe shock, limited access cardiac surgery, and selected reoperative patients.[3] Femoral or iliac cannulation limits cannula size but the retrograde distribution of blood flow is similar to antegrade flow.[60]

Femoral cannulation is associated with many complications[3,61] that include tears, dissection, late stenosis or thrombosis, bleeding, lymph fistula, infection in the groin, or cerebral and coronary atheroembolism. In patients with prior aortic dissections femoral perfusion may cause malperfusion; thus some surgeons recommend alternative cannulation sites for these patients.[62,63] Ischemic complications of the distal leg may occur during prolonged (3-6 hours) retrograde perfusions[64,65] unless perfusion is provided to the distal vessel. This may be provided by a small Y catheter in the distal vessel[65] or a side graft sutured to the artery.[66]

Retrograde arterial dissection is the most serious complication of femoral or iliac arterial cannulation and may extend to the aortic root and/or cause retroperitoneal hemorrhage. The incidence is between 0.2% and 1.3%[67–70] and is associated with a mortality of about 50%. This complication is more likely in diseased arteries and in patients over 40 years old. The diagnosis is similar for an aortic cannula dissection and may be confirmed by TEE of the descending thoracic aorta.[59] Antegrade perfusion in the true lumen must be immediately resumed by either the heart itself or by cannulation in the distal aorta or axillary-subclavian artery. It is not always necessary to repair the dissected ascending aorta unless it affects the aortic root.[67–69]

OTHER SITES FOR ARTERIAL CANNULATION

The axillary-subclavian artery is increasingly used for cannulation.[71–75] Advantages include freedom from atherosclerosis, antegrade flow into the arch vessels, and protection of the arm and hand by collateral flow. Because of these advantages and the dangers of retrograde perfusion in patients with aortic dissection, some surgeons prefer this cannulation site for these patients.[63,75,76] Brachial plexus injury and axillary artery thrombosis are reported complications.[71] The axillary artery is approached through a subclavicular incision; the intrathoracic subclavian artery may be cannulated through a left thoracotomy.[77]

Occasionally the innominate artery may be cannulated through a purse-string suture without obstructing flow around a 7F to 8F cannula to the right carotid artery.[34,49] The ascending aorta can also be cannulated by passing a cannula through the aortic valve from the left ventricular apex.[78,79] Coselli and Crawford[80] also describe retrograde perfusion through a graft sewn to the abdominal aorta.

Venous Reservoir

The venous reservoir serves as volume reservoir and is placed immediately before the arterial pump when a membrane oxygenator is used (see Fig. 11-1). This reservoir serves as a high-capacitance (i.e., low-pressure) receiving chamber for venous return, facilitates gravity drainage, is a venous bubble trap, provides a convenient place to add drugs, fluids, or blood, and adds storage capacity for the perfusion system. As much as 1 to 3 L of blood may be translocated from patient to circuit when full CPB is initiated. The venous reservoir also provides several seconds of reaction time if venous return is suddenly decreased or stopped during perfusion.

Reservoirs may be rigid (hard) plastic canisters ("open" types) or soft, collapsible plastic bags ("closed" types). The rigid canisters facilitate volume measurements and management of venous air, often have larger capacity, are easier to prime, permit suction for vacuum-assisted venous drainage, and may be less expensive. Some hard-shell venous reservoirs incorporate macrofilters and microfilters and can serve as cardiotomy reservoirs and to receive vented blood.

Disadvantages include the use of silicon antifoam compounds, which may produce microemboli,[81,82] risk of microembolism, and increased activation of blood elements.[83] Soft bag reservoirs eliminate the blood-gas interface and by collapsing reduce the risk of pumping massive air emboli.

Oxygenators

Membrane oxygenators imitate the natural lung by interspersing a thin membrane of either microporous polypropylene (0.3- to 0.8-μm pores) or silicone rubber between the gas and blood phases. Compared to bubble oxygenators, membrane oxygenators are safer, produce less particulate and gaseous microemboli,[84,85] are less reactive to blood elements, and allow superior control of blood gases.[86,87] With microporous membranes, plasma-filled pores prevent gas entering blood but facilitate transfer of both oxygen and CO_2. Because oxygen is poorly diffusible in plasma, blood must be spread as a thin film (approximately 100 μm) over a large area with high differential gas pressures between compartments to achieve oxygenation. Areas of turbulence and secondary flow enhance diffusion of oxygen within blood and thereby improve oxyhemoglobin saturation.[88] Carbon dioxide is highly diffusible in plasma and easily exits the blood compartment despite small differential pressures across the membrane.

The most popular design uses sheaves of hollow fibers (120-200 μm) connected to inlet and outlet manifolds within a hard-shell jacket (Fig. 11-4). The most efficient configuration creates turbulence by passing blood between fibers and oxygen within fibers. Arterial P_{CO_2} is controlled by gas flow, and P_{O_2} is controlled by the fraction of inspired oxygen (F_{IO_2}) produced by an air-oxygen blender. Modern membrane oxygenators add up to 470 mL of O_2 and remove up to 350 mL CO_2 per minute at 1 to 7 liters of flow with priming volumes of 220 to 560 mL and resistances of 12 to 15 mm Hg per liter blood flow. Most units combine a venous reservoir, heat exchanger, and hollow fiber membrane oxygenator into one compact unit.

Oxygen and CO_2 diffuse across thin silicone membranes, which are made into envelopes and wound around a spool to produce a spiral coil oxygenator. Gas passes through the envelope and blood passes between the coil windings. Because of protein leakage, which degrades membrane function, these spiral coil oxygenators are preferred over hollow fiber microporous oxygenators for the prolonged perfusions (days) used in respiratory support.

A new membrane oxygenator features a very thin (0.05 μm), solid membrane on the blood side of a highly porous support matrix. This membrane reduces the risk of gas emboli and plasma leakage during prolonged CPB, but may impair transfer of volatile anesthetics.[89]

Flow regulators, flow meters, gas blender, oxygen analyzer, gas filter, and moisture trap are parts of the oxygenator gas supply system used to control the ventilating gases within membrane oxygenators. Often an anesthetic vaporizer is added, but care must be taken to prevent volatile anesthetic liquids from destroying plastic components of the perfusion circuit.

Bubble oxygenators are obsolete in the United States, but are used elsewhere for short-term CPB because of cost and efficiency. Because each bubble presents a new foreign surface to which blood elements react, bubble oxygenators cause progressive injury to blood elements and entrain more gaseous microemboli.[90,91] In bubble oxygenators, venous

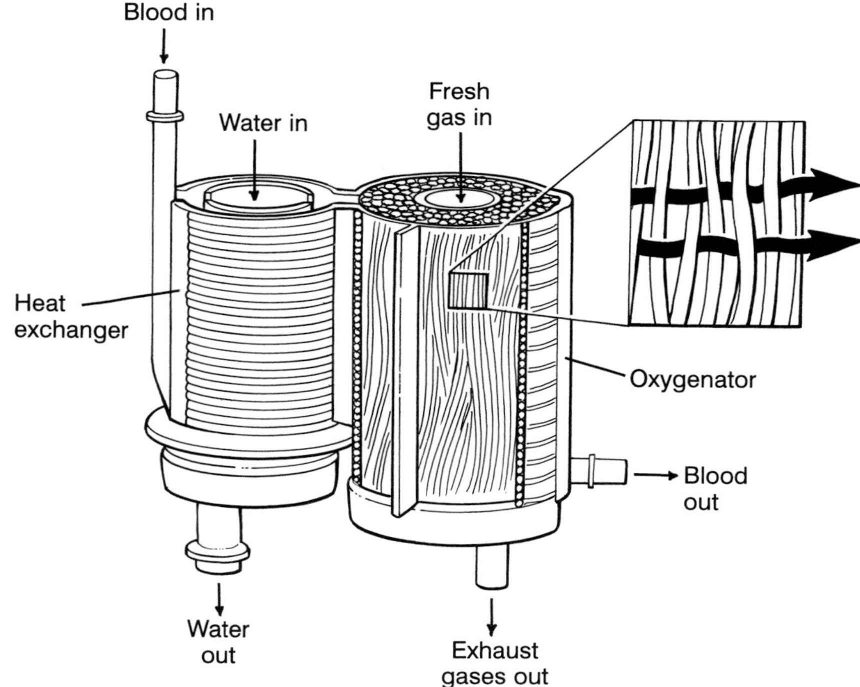

FIGURE 11–4 Diagram of a hollow fiber membrane oxygenator and heat exchanger unit. Blood enters the heat exchanger first and flows over water-cooled or -warmed coils and then enters the oxygenator to pass between woven strands of hollow fibers. Oxygen enters one end of the bundles of hollow fibers and exits at the opposite end. The hollow fiber bundles are potted at each end to separate the blood and gas compartments. Oxygen and carbon dioxide diffuse in opposite directions across the aggregate large surface of the hollow fibers.

TABLE 11–1 Roller versus centrifugal pump

	Roller pump	Centrifugal pump
Description	Nearly occlusive Afterload independent	Nonocclusive Afterload sensitive
Advantages	Low prime volume Low cost No potential for backflow Shallow sine-wave pulse	Portable, position insensitive Safe positive and negative pressure Adapts to venous return Superior for right or left heart bypass Preferred for long-term bypass Protects against massive air embolism
Disadvantages	Excessive positive and negative pressure Spallation Tubing rupture Potential for massive air embolism Necessary occlusion adjustments Requires close supervision	Large priming volume Requires flowmeter Potential passive backward flow Higher cost

blood drains directly into a chamber into which oxygen is infused through a diffusion plate (sparger). The sparger produces thousands of small (approximately 36 μm) oxygen bubbles within blood. Gas exchange occurs across a thin film at the blood-gas interface around each bubble. Carbon dioxide diffuses into the bubble and oxygen diffuses outward into blood. Small bubbles improve oxygen exchange by effectively increasing the surface area of the gas-blood interface,[92] but are difficult to remove. Large bubbles facilitate CO_2 removal. Bubbles and blood are separated by settling, filtration, and defoaming surfactants in a reservoir. Bubble oxygenators add 350 to 400 mL oxygen to blood and remove 300 to 330 mL CO_2 per minute at flow rates from 1 to 7 L/min.[86,93] Priming volumes are less than 500 mL. Commercial bubble oxygenators incorporate a reservoir and heat exchanger within the same unit and are placed upstream to the arterial pump.

Oxygenator malfunction requiring change during CPB occurs in 0.02% to 0.26% of cases,[94–96] but the incidence varies between membrane oxygenator designs.[97] Development of abnormal resistant areas in the blood path is the most common cause,[96] but other problems include leaks, loss of gas supply, rupture of connections, failure of the blender, and deteriorating gas exchange. Blood gases need to be monitored to ensure adequate CO_2 removal and oxygenation. Heparin coating may reduce development of abnormally high resistance areas.[95]

Heat Exchangers

Heat exchangers control body temperature by heating or cooling blood passing through the perfusion circuit. Hypothermia is frequently used during cardiac surgery to reduce oxygen demand or to facilitate operative exposure by temporary circulatory arrest. Gases are more soluble in cold than in warm blood; therefore, rapid rewarming of cold blood in the circuit or body may cause formation of bubble emboli.[98] Most membrane oxygenator units incorporate a heat exchanger upstream to the oxygenator to minimize bubble emboli. Blood is not heated above 40°C to prevent denaturation of plasma proteins, and temperature differences within the body and perfusion circuit are limited to 5°C to 10°C to prevent bubble emboli. The heat exchanger may be supplied by hot and cold tap water, but separate heater/cooler units with convenient temperature-regulating controls are preferred. Leakage of water into the blood path can cause hemolysis and malfunction of heater/cooler units may occur.[94]

Separate heat exchangers are needed for cardioplegia. The simplest system is to use bags of precooled cardioplegia solution. More often cardioplegia fluid is circulated through through a dedicated heat exchanger or tubing coils placed in an ice or warm water bath.

Pumps

Most heart-lung machines use two types of pumps, although roller pumps can be used exclusively (Table 11-1). Centrifugal pumps are usually used for the primary perfusion circuit for safety reasons and for a possible reduction in injury to blood elements. However, this latter reason remains highly controversial and unproven.[99–104]

Centrifugal pumps (Fig. 11-5) consist of a vaned impeller or nested, smooth plastic cones, which when rotated rapidly, propel blood by centrifugal force.[105] An arterial flowmeter is required to determine forward blood flow, which varies with the speed of rotation and the afterload of the arterial line. Unless a check valve is used,[106] the arterial line must be clamped to prevent backward flow when the pump is off. Centrifugal blood pumps generate up to 900 mm Hg of forward pressure, but only 400 to 500 mm Hg of negative pressure and, therefore, less cavitation and fewer gaseous microemboli. They can pump small amounts of air, but become

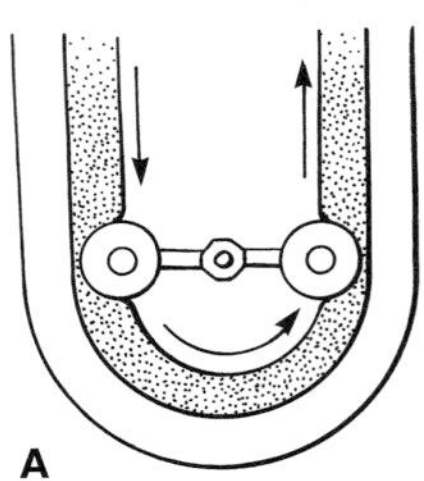

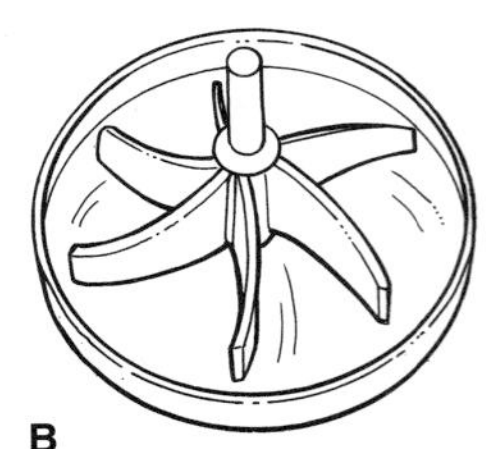

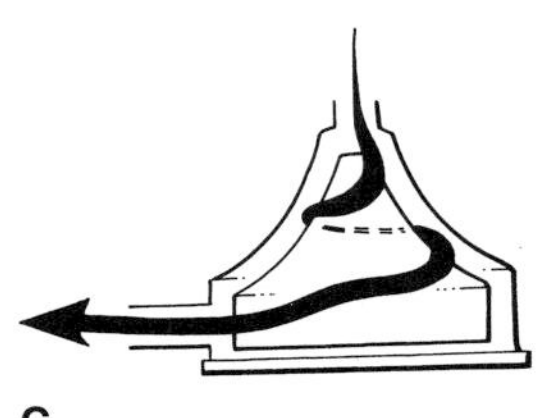

FIGURE 11–5 Diagrams of blood pumps. (A) Roller pump with two rollers, 180 degrees apart. The compression of the rollers against the raceway is adjustable and is set to be barely nonocclusive. Blood is propelled in the direction of rotation. (B) The impeller pump uses vanes mounted on a rotating central shaft. (C) The centrifugal pump uses three rapidly rotated, concentric cones to propel blood forward by centrifugal force.

"deprimed" if over 30 to 50 mL of air enters the blood chamber. Centrifugal pumps are probably superior for temporary extracorporeal assist devices and left heart bypass, and for generating pump-augmented venous return.

Roller pumps consist of a length of 1/4- to 5/8-inch (internal diameter) polyvinyl, silicone, or latex tubing, which is compressed by two rollers 180° apart, inside a curved raceway. Forward flow is generated by roller compression and flow rate depends upon the diameter of the tubing, rate of rotation, the length of the compression raceway, and completeness of compression. Compression is adjusted before use to be barely nonocclusive against a standing column of fluid that produces 45 to 75 mm Hg back pressure.[107–110] Hemolysis and tubing wear are minimal at this degree of compression.[107] Flow rate is determined from calibration curves for each pump for different tubing sizes and rates of rotation. Roller pumps are inexpensive, reliable, safe, insensitive to afterload, and have small priming volumes, but can produce high negative pressures and microparticles shed from compressed tubing (spallation).[111] Roller pumps are vulnerable to careless operation that results in: propelling air; inaccurate flow calibration; backflow when not in use if rollers are not sufficiently occlusive; excessive pressure with rupture of connections if arterial inflow is obstructed; tears in tubing; and changing roller compression settings during operation. Roller pumps, but not centrifugal pumps, are used for sucker systems and for delivering cardioplegic solutions.

Centrifugal pumps produce pulseless blood flow and standard roller pumps produce a sine wave pulse around 5 mm Hg. The arterial cannula dampens the pulse of pulsatile pumps, and it is difficult to generate pulse pressures above 20 mm Hg within the body during full CPB.[112,113] To date no one has conclusively demonstrated the need for pulsatile perfusion during short-term or long-term CPB or circulatory assistance.[114–117]

Complications that may occur during operation of either type of pump include loss of electricity; loss of the ability to control pump speed, which produces "runaway pump" or "pump creep" when turned off; loss of the flow meter or RPM indicator; rupture of tubing in the roller pump raceway; and reversal of flow by improper tubing in the raceway. A means to manually provide pumping in case of electrical failure should always be available.

Filters and Bubble Traps

MICROEMBOLI

During clinical cardiac surgery with CPB the wound and the perfusion circuit generate gaseous and biologic and nonbiologic particulate microemboli (<500 μM diameter).[31,118–123] Microemboli produce much of the morbidity associated with cardiac operations using CPB (see section 11D). Gaseous emboli contain oxygen or nitrogen and may enter the perfusate from multiple sources and pass through other components of the system.[18,21] Potential sources of gas entry include stopcocks, sampling and injection sites,[122] priming solutions, priming procedures, intravenous fluids, vents, the cardiotomy reservoir, tears or breaks in the perfusion circuit, loose purse-string sutures (especially during augmented venous return),[18] rapid warming of cold blood,[98] cavitation, oxygenators, venous reservoirs with low perfusate levels,[21,82] and the heart and great vessels. Bubble oxygenators produce many gaseous emboli; membrane oxygenators produce very few.[84–86] Aside from mistakes (open stopcocks, empty venous reservoir, air in the heart) the cardiotomy reservoir is the largest source of gaseous emboli in membrane oxygenator perfusion systems.

Blood produces a large number of particulate emboli related to thrombus formation (clots), fibrin, platelet and platelet-leukocyte aggregation, hemolyzed red cells, cellular debris, and generation of chylomicrons, fat particles, and denatured proteins.[124] Stored donor blood is also an important source of blood-generated particles.[125] Other biologic emboli include atherosclerotic debris and cholesterol crystals and calcium particles dislodged by cannulation, manipulation for exposure, or the surgery itself. Both biologic and nonbiologic particulate emboli are aspirated from the wound. Bits of muscle, bone, and fat are mixed with suture material, talc, glue, and dust and aspirated into the cardiotomy reservoir.[125,126] Materials used in manufacture, spallated material, and dust may also enter the perfusate from the perfusion circuit[125] if it is not first rinsed by recirculating saline through a prebypass microfilter, which is discarded.

In vivo microemboli are detected by transcranial Doppler ultrasound,[127] fluorescein angiography,[84] TEE, and retinal inspection. In the circuit, microemboli are monitored by arterial line ultrasound[128] or monitoring screen filtration

TABLE 11–2 Minimizing microemboli

Membrane oxygenator, centrifugal arterial pump
Cardiotomy reservoir filter ($\leq 40\mu m$)
Arterial line filter/bubble trap ($\leq 40\mu m$)
Keep temperature differentials <8°C-10°C
Prime with CO_2 flush; recirculate with saline and filter ($5\mu m$)
Prevent air entry into circuit
Snug purse-string sutures
Three-way stopcocks on all sampling ports
Meticulous syringe management
Adequate cardiotomy reservoir volume (for debubbling)
Avoid excessive suction on vents
One-way valved purge lines for bubble traps
Use TEE to locate trapped intracardiac air; de-air thoroughly
Wash blood aspirated from the surgical field
Prevent thrombus formation with adequate anticoagulation
Assess inflow cannulation site by epiaortic ultrasound imaging
Cannulate distal aorta or axillary artery
Consider use of special aortic cannulas

pressure. Microfilter weights and examination, histology of autopsy tissues, and electron particle size counters of blood samples[125] verify microemboli beyond the circuit.

Prevention and control of microemboli Table 11-2 outlines methods to reduce microembolism. Major methods include using a membrane oxygenator and cardiotomy reservoir filter; minimizing and washing blood aspirated from the field[129]; and preventing air entry into the circuit and using left ventricular vents when the heart is opened.[130,131]

The brain receives 14% of the cardiac output and is the most sensitive organ for microembolic injury.[132] Strategies to selectively reduce microembolism to the brain include reducing Pa_{CO_2} to cause cerebral vasoconstriction[133]; hypothermia[134]; placing aortic cannulas downstream to the cerebral vessels[50,51,122]; and using special aortic cannulas with[29–31,33] or without[26] special baffles or screens designed to prevent cannula-produced cerebral atherosclerotic emboli.

Two types of blood microfilters are available for use within the perfusion circuit: depth and screen.[135–137] Depth filters consist of packed fibers or porous foam, have no defined pore size, present a large, tortuous, wetted surface, and remove microemboli by impaction and absorption. Screen filters are usually made of woven polyester or nylon thread, have a defined pore size, and filter by interception. Screen filters vary in pore size and configuration and block most air emboli; however, as pore size decreases, resistance increases. As compared to no filter, studies indicate that all commercial filters effectively remove gaseous and particulate emboli.[138–141] Most investigations find that the Dacron wool depth filter is most effective, particularly in removing micro- and macroscopic air. Pressure differences across filters vary between 24 and 36 mm Hg at 5 L/min flow. Filters cause slight hemolysis and tend to trap some platelets; nylon filters may activate complement.[135,136]

The need for microfilters in the cardiotomy suction reservoir is universally accepted,[126] and most commercial units contain an integrated micropore filter. The need for a filter in the cardioplegia delivery system, however, is questionable,[142] and the need for an arterial line filter is unsettled.[137] In vitro studies demonstrate that an arterial filter reduces circulating microemboli[139–141] and clinical studies are confirmatory.[140,141] However, these filters do not remove all microemboli generated by the extracorporeal circuit.[18,122,126,143] When bubble oxygenators are used, studies show equivocal or modest reductions in microemboli[84,144–146] and neurologic outcome markers.[146–150] In contrast, membrane oxygenators produce far fewer microemboli and when used without an arterial filter, the numbers of microemboli are similar to those found with bubble oxygenators plus arterial line filters.[85,137]

Although efficacy of arterial line microfilters remains unsettled, use is almost universal.[151] Filters are effective bubble traps, but increase costs, occasionally obstruct during use, are difficult to de-air during priming, and should be used with a bypass line and valved purge line to remove air.

Other sources of biologic microemboli may be more important. Cerebral microemboli are most numerous during aortic cannulation,[152–154] application and release of aortic clamps,[153,154] and at the beginning of cardiac ejection after open heart procedures.[155] Furthermore, as compared to perfusion microemboli, surgically induced emboli are more likely to cause postoperative neurologic deficits.[156]

LEUKOCYTE-DEPLETING FILTERS

Leukocyte-depleting filters are discussed in section 11C and have been recently reviewed.[157–160] These filters reduce circulating leukocyte counts in most studies,[161–163] but fail to produce convincing evidence of clinical benefit.[164–166]

Tubing and Connectors

The various components of the heart-lung machine are connected by polyvinyl tubing and fluted polycarbonate connectors. Medical grade polyvinyl chloride (PVC) tubing is universally used because it is flexible, compatible with blood, inert, nontoxic, smooth, nonwettable, tough, transparent, resistant to kinking and collapse, and can be heat sterilized. To reduce priming volume, tubing connections should be short; to reduce turbulence, cavitation, and stagnant areas, the flow path should be smooth and uniform without areas of constriction or expansion. Wide tubing improves flow rheology, but also increases priming volume. In practice 1/2- to 5/8-inch (internal diameter) tubing is used for most adults, but until a compact, integrated, complete heart-lung machine can be designed and produced as a unit, the flow path produces some turbulence. Careless tubing connections are sources of air intake or blood leakage and all connections must be secure. For convenience and safety, most tubing and connectors are prepackaged and disposable.

Heparin-Coated Circuits

Heparin can be attached to blood surfaces of all components of the extracorporeal circuit by ionic or covalent bonds. The Duraflo II heparin coating ionically attaches heparin to a quaternary ammonium carrier (alkylbenzyl dimethyl-ammonium chloride), which binds to plastic surfaces (Edwards Lifesciences, Irvine, CA). Covalent attachment is produced by first depositing a polyethylenimine polymer spacer onto the plastic surface, to which heparin fragments bind (Carmeda Bioactive Surface, Medtronic Inc., Minneapolis, MN). Ionic-bound heparin slowly leaches, but this is irrelevant in clinical cardiac surgery. The use of heparin-coated circuits during CPB has spawned an enormous literature[167–172] and remains controversial largely because studies are contaminated by patient selection, reduced doses of systemic heparin, and washing or discarding field-aspirated blood.[172] There is no credible evidence that heparin-coated perfusion circuits reduce the need for systemic heparin or reduce bleeding or thrombotic problems associated with CPB (see section 11B). Although the majority of studies indicate that heparin coatings reduce concentrations of C3a and C5b-9,[173] the inflammatory response to CPB is not reduced (see section 11C) and the evidence for clinical benefit is not convincing.[174,175]

Other surface modifications and coatings in development[168] include a phosphorylcholine coating,[176] surface-modifying additives,[179] a trillium biopassive surface,[177,178] and a synthetic protein coating[180] (see also section 11C).

Cardiotomy Reservoir and Field Suction

Blood aspirated from the surgical wound may be directed to the cardiotomy reservoir for defoaming, filtration, and storage before it is added directly to the perfusate. A sponge impregnated with a surfactant removes bubbles by reducing surface tension at the blood interface and macro, micro, or combined filters remove particulate emboli. Negative pressure is generated by either a roller pump or by vacuum applied to the rigid outer shell of the reservoir. The degree of negative pressure and blood level must be monitored to avoid excessive suction or introducing air into the perfusate.

The cardiotomy suction and reservoir are major sources of hemolysis, particulate and gaseous microemboli, fat globules, cellular aggregates, platelet injury and loss, thrombin generation, and fibrinolysis.[82,118,126,181,182] Air aspirated with wound blood contributes to blood activation and destruction and is difficult to remove because of the high proportion of nitrogen, which is poorly soluble in blood. High suction volumes and admixture of air are particularly destructive of platelets and red cells.[181,183] Commercial reservoirs are designed to minimize air entrainment and excessive injury to blood elements. Air and microemboli removal are also facilitated by allowing aspirated blood to settle within the reservoir before it is added to the perfusate.

An alternative method for recovering field-aspirated blood is to dilute the blood with saline and then remove the saline to return only packed red cells to the perfusate. Centrifugal cell washers (e.g., Haemonetics Cell Saver, Meomonetics Corp., Braintree, MA) automate this process, which has the advantage of removing air, thrombin, and nearly all biologic and nonbiologic microemboli from the aspirate at the cost of discarding plasma. A third alternative is to discard all field-aspirated blood.[184] Increasingly, field-aspirated blood is recognized as a major contributor to the thrombotic, bleeding, and inflammatory complications of CPB (see sections 11B and 11C).

Venting the Heart

If the heart is unable to contract, distention of either ventricle is detrimental to subsequent contractility.[185] Right ventricular distention during cardiac arrest or ventricular fibrillation is rarely a problem, but left ventricular distention can be insidious in that blood can enter the flaccid, thick-walled chamber from multiple sources during this period. During CPB blood escaping atrial or venous cannulas and from the coronary sinus and thebesian veins may pass through the unopened right heart into the pulmonary circulation. This blood plus bronchial venous blood, blood regurgitating through the aortic valve, and blood from undiagnosed abnormal sources (patent foramen ovale, patent ductus, etc.) may distend the left ventricle unless a vent catheter is used (Fig. 11-6). During CPB bronchial venous blood and noncoronary collateral flow average approximately 140 $\pm$ 182 and 48 $\pm$ 74 mL/min, respectively.[186]

There are several methods for venting the left heart during cardiac arrest. Few surgeons vent the left ventricular apex directly because of inconvenience and myocardial injury. Most often a multihole, soft-tip catheter (8-10F) is inserted into the junction of the right superior pulmonary vein and left atrium (see Fig. 11-6) or left atrial appendage and may or may not be passed into the left ventricle. Others prefer to place a small suction catheter into the pulmonary artery.[187] The ventricle can also be vented by passing a catheter retrograde across the aortic valve when working on the mitral valve. Vent catheters are drained to the cardiotomy reservoir by a roller pump, vacuum source, or gravity drainage,[188,189] but must be carefully monitored for malfunction. Although inspection and palpation may detect ventricular distention, TEE monitoring or direct measurements of left atrial or pulmonary arterial pressures are more reliable. The heart is no longer vented for most myocardial

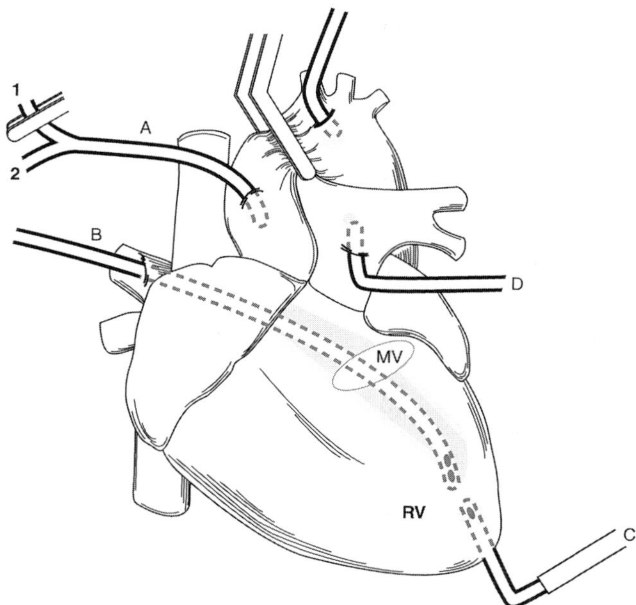

FIGURE 11–6 Diagram shows locations used to vent (decompress the heart). (A) Aortic root vent, which can also be used to administer cardioplegic solution after the ascending aorta is clamped. (B) A catheter placed in the right superior pulmonary vein/left atrial junction can be passed through the mitral valve into the left ventricle. (C) Direct venting of the left ventricle at the apex. (D) Venting the main pulmonary artery, which decompresses the left atrium because pulmonary veins lack valves.

revascularization operations, but the ventricle must be protected from distention.[190–192] If the heart cannot remain decompressed during distal anastomoses, a vent should be inserted. Often the cardioplegia line inserted into the aortic root is used for venting when not used for cardioplegia.[193]

The most common and serious complication of left heart venting is residual air when the heart is filled and begins to contract. De-airing maneuvers and TEE are important methods for ensuring removal of all residual air. In addition, many surgeons aspirate the ascending aorta via a small metal or plastic cannula to detect and remove any escaping air as the heart begins to eject.[194,195] Bleeding problems or direct injury to the myocardium are other complications associated with left ventricular vents.

Cardioplegia Delivery Systems

Cardioplegic solutions contain 8 to 20 mEq/L potassium, magnesium, and often other components and are infused into the aortic root proximal to the aortic cross clamp or retrograde into the coronary sinus to arrest the heart in diastole. The carrier may be crystalloid or preferably blood and is infused at temperatures around 4°C or 37°C, depending upon surgeon's preference. Normothermic cardioplegia must be delivered almost continuously to keep the heart arrested; cold cardioplegia is infused intermittently. Cardioplegic solutions are delivered through a separate perfusion system that includes a reservoir, heat exchanger, roller pump, bubble trap, and perhaps microfilter (see Fig. 11-2). Temperature and infusion pressure are monitored. The system may be completely independent of the main perfusion circuit or branch from the arterial line. The system also may be configured to vent the aortic root when between infusions.

Antegrade cardioplegia is delivered through a small cannula in the aortic root or via handheld cannulas directly into the coronary ostia when the aortic valve is exposed. Retrograde cardioplegia is delivered through a cuffed catheter inserted blindly into the coronary sinus.[196] Proper placement of the retrograde catheter is critical, but not difficult, and is verified by palpation, TEE, color of the aspirated blood, or pressure waveform of a catheter pressure sensor.[197] Complications of retrograde cardioplegia include rupture or perforation of the sinus, hematoma, and rupture of the catheter cuff.[198,199]

Hemoconcentrators (Hemofiltration/Ultrafiltration)

Hemoconcentrators, like oxygenators, contain one of several available semipermeable membranes (typically hollow fibers) that transfer water, electrolytes (e.g., potassium), and molecules up to 20 kD out of the blood compartment.[200] Hemoconcentrators may be connected to either venous or arterial lines or a reservoir in the main perfusion circuit, but require high pressure in the blood compartment to effect fluid removal. Thus a roller pump is needed unless connected to the arterial line. Suction may or may not be applied to the air side of the membrane to facilitate filtration. Up to 180mL/min of fluid can be removed at flows of 500 mL/min.[201] Hemoconcentrators conserve platelets and most plasma proteins as compared to centrifugal cell washers and may allow greater control of potassium concentrations than diuretics.[202] Aside from cost, disadvantages are few and adverse effects are rare.[201]

Perfusion Monitors and Safety Devices

Table 11-3 lists monitors and safety devices that are commonly used during CPB. *Pressure in the arterial line* between pump and arterial line filter is monitored continuously to instantly detect any increased resistance to arterial inflow into the patient. This pressure should be higher than radial arterial pressure because of resistance of the filter (if used) and cannula. The arterial pressure monitor may be connected to an audible alarm or the pump switch to alert the perfusionist of abrupt increases.

An *arterial line flowmeter* is essential for centrifugal pumps and may be desirable to confirm flow calculations with roller pumps.

TABLE 11–3 Safety devices and procedures

Device or procedure	Usage (%)*
Low venous blood level alarm	60-100
With pump cut-off	34-80
High arterial line pressure alarm	84-94
With pump cut-off	35-75
Macrobubble detector	42-88
With pump cut-off	62-63
Arterial line filter	44-99
Pre-bypass recirculation/filtration	75-81
Oxygen supply filter	81-95
In-line venous oxygen saturation	75-76
In-line arterial oxygen saturation	12-13
Oxygenator gas supply oxygen analyzer	43-53
One-way valved intracardiac vent lines	18-73
Batteries in heart-lung machine	29-85
Alternate dedicated power supply	36
Electrical generator	28
Backup arterial pump head	80
Backup heater-cooler	97
Backup oxygen supply	88-91
Emergency lighting	62-91
Pre-bypass activated clotting time	74-99
Activated clotting time during CPB	83
Pre-bypass check list	74-95
Written protocols	49-75
Log of perfusion incidents	46
Log of device failures	52

*Usage data represent ranges from various surveys: references 94, 151, 354, 363, and 364.

Flow-through devices are available to continuously measure *blood gases, hemoglobin/hematocrit, and some electrolytes*.[203] These devices in the venous line permit rapid assessment of oxygen supply and demand.[204–206] In the arterial line the devices offer better control of blood gases.[207] The need for these devices is unproven and because reliability is still uncertain, use may distract operative personnel and spawn unnecessary laboratory measurements.[208–211] The use of automated analyzers by the perfusion team in the operating room is an alternative if frequent measurement of blood gases, hematocrit, and electrolytes is desirable.[203]

The *flow and concentration of oxygen* entering the oxygenator should be monitored.[212] Some teams also monitor exit gases to indirectly estimate metabolic activity and depth of anesthesia.[212] Some manufacturers recommend monitoring the *pressure gradient across membrane oxygenators,* which may be an early indication of oxygenator failure.[95–97]

Temperatures of the water entering heat exchangers must be monitored and carefully controlled to prevent blood protein denaturation and gaseous microemboli.[98] During operations using deep hypothermia changes in venous line temperatures reflect rates of temperature change in the patient and arterial line temperatures help protect against brain hyperthermia during rewarming.

A *low-level sensor* with alarms on the venous reservoir and a bubble detector on the arterial line are desirable safety devices. A *one-way valve* is recommended in the purge line between an arterial filter/bubble trap and cardiotomy reservoir to prevent air embolism. Some perfusionists also use these valves in the venous and vent lines to protect against retrograde air entry into the circulation or in the arterial line to prevent inadvertent exsanguination.[106]

Automatic data collection systems are available for preoperative calculations and to process and store data during CPB.[213,214] Computer systems for operating CPB are in development.[215]

CONDUCT OF CARDIOPULMONARY BYPASS

The Perfusion Team

Although the surgeon is directly responsible to the patient for the outcome of the operation, he or she needs a close working relationship with the anesthesiologist and perfusionist. These three principals must communicate freely, often, and candidly. Their overlapping and independent responsibilities relevant to CPB are best defined by written policies that include protocols for various types of operations and emergencies and by periodic multidisciplinary conferences.

The surgeon determines the planned operation, target perfusion temperatures, methods of cardioplegia, cannulations, and anticipated special procedures. During operation the surgeon communicates the procedural steps involved in connecting and disconnecting the patient to CPB and interacts with the other principals to coordinate perfusion management with surgical exposure and working conditions. The perfusionist is responsible for setting up and priming the heart-lung machine, performing safety checks, operating the heart-lung machine, monitoring the conduct of bypass, monitoring anticoagulation, adding prescribed drugs, and maintaining a written perfusion record.

The anesthesiologist monitors the operative field, anesthetic state and ventilation of the patient, the patient's physiology, and conduct of perfusion. A vigilant anesthesiologist is the safety officer and often "troubleshooter" of these complex procedures and is in the best position to anticipate, detect, and correct deviations from desired conditions. In addition the anesthesiologist provides TEE observations before, during, and immediately after bypass. While the surgeon corrects the anatomic pathology, the anesthesiologist and perfusionist maintain the patient's life and expectation of recovery

Assembly of Heart-Lung Machine

The perfusionist is responsible for setting up and preparing the heart-lung machine and all components necessary for the proposed operation. Most perfusionists use commercial, sterile, pre-prepared customized tubing packs that are connected to the various components that constitute the heart-lung machine. This dry assembly takes about 10 to 15 minutes, and the system can be kept in standby for up to 7 days. Once the system is primed with fluid, which takes about 15 minutes, it should be used within 8 hours. After assembly the perfusionist conducts a safety inspection and completes a written prebypass checklist.

PRIMING

Adult extracorporeal perfusion circuits require 1.5 to 2.0 L of balanced electrolyte solution (lactated Ringer's solution, Normosol-A, Plasma-Lyte). Before connections are made to the patient, the prime is recirculated through a micropore filter to remove particulate and air emboli. The priming volume represents approximately 30% to 35% of the patient's blood volume and reduces the hematocrit to about two-thirds of the preoperative value. The addition of crystalloid cardioplegia causes further dilution. Thus sometimes a unit of banked blood is added to raise the perfusate hematocrit to a predetermined minimum (e.g., 25% or more). Porcine heparin (2000 units) is added to each unit of banked whole blood to ensure anticoagulation. There is no consensus regarding the optimal hematocrit during CPB; most perfusates have hematocrits between 20% and 25% when used with moderate hypothermia (25°C-32°C). Dilution reduces perfusate viscosity, which is not a problem during clinical CPB, but also reduces oxygen-carrying capacity; mixed venous oxygen saturations below 60% usually prompt either transfusion or increased pump flow.[204,205] Sometimes 12.5 to 50 g of mannitol is added to stimulate diuresis and possibly minimize postoperative renal dysfunction.

Efforts to avoid the use of autologous blood include reducing the priming requirement of the machine by using smaller-diameter and shorter tubing lengths and operating the machine with minimal perfusate in the venous and cardiotomy reservoirs. This latter practice increases the risk of air embolism, the risk of which can be reduced by using collapsible reservoirs and reservoir level sensors that stop the pump. Autologous blood prime is another method, which displaces and then removes crystalloid prime by bleeding the patient into the circuit just before beginning CPB.[216,217] This method reduces perfusate volume, but phenylephrine may be required to maintain stable hemodynamics.[216,217] The method reduces transfusions and does not affect clinical outcome.

The use of colloids (albumin, gelatins, dextrans, and hetastarches) in the priming volume is controversial.[218] Colloids reduce the fall in colloid osmotic pressure[219,220] and may reduce the amount of fluid entering the extracellular space. The question is whether or not clinical outcome is improved. Prospective clinical studies have failed to document significant clinical benefits with albumin,[219–224] which is expensive and may have adverse effects.[225,226] Hetastarch may contribute to postoperative bleeding.[227] McKnight et al found no influence of prime composition on postoperative nitrogen balance.[228] Because of possible adverse effects, including neurologic deficits, the addition of glucose and/or lactate to the prime is avoided.[229,230]

Anticoagulation and Reversal

Porcine heparin (300-400 units/kg IV) is given before arterial or venous cannulas are inserted. CPB is not started until anticoagulation is confirmed by either an activated clotting time (ACT) or the Hepcon test. Although widely used, bovine heparin is more antigenic in inducing antiplatelet IgG antibodies than is porcine heparin.[231] The anticoagulation effect is measured about 3 minutes after heparin administration. However, groups differ in the minimum ACT that is considered safe for CPB. The minimum ACT is 400 seconds; many groups recommend 480 seconds[232] because heparin only partially inhibits thrombin formation during CPB (see section 11B). In patients who have received aprotinin, ACT should be measured using kaolin as opposed to celite, because celite artifactually and erroneously increases ACT. Failure to achieve a satisfactory ACT may be due to inadequate heparin or to low concentrations of antithrombin. If a total of 500 units/kg of heparin fails to adequately prolong ACT, fresh frozen plasma (or recombinant antithrombin when available[233]) is needed to increase antithrombin concentrations to overcome "heparin resistance." Antithrombin is a necessary cofactor that binds circulating thrombin; heparin accelerates this reaction a thousandfold. See section 11B for mangagement of patients with suspected or proven heparin-induced antiplatelet IgG antibodies and alternative anticoagulants to heparin.

During CPB, ACT or the Hepcon test is measured every 30 minutes. If ACT goes below the target level, more heparin is given. Usually one third of the initial heparin bolus is given every hour even when the ACT is within the normal range. The Hepcon test titrates the heparin concentration and is more reproducible than ACT, but ACT provides satisfactory monitoring of anticoagulation. Although excessively high concentrations of heparin (ACT >1000 sec) may cause remote bleeding away from operative sites, low concentrations increase circulating thrombin concentrations and risk clotting within the extracorporeal perfusion circuit.

One mg of protamine (not to exceed 3 mg/kg) is given for each 100 units of heparin injected in the initial bolus dose. The heparin-protamine complex activates complement and often causes acute hypotension, which may be attenuated by adding calcium (2 mg/1 mg protamine). After a third of the planned protamine dose, blood must not be returned to the cardiotomy reservoir from the surgical field. Rarely, protamine may cause an anaphylactic reaction in patients with antibodies to protamine insulin.[234] Neutralization of heparin is usually confirmed by an ACT or Hepcon test and more protamine (50 mg) is given if either test remains prolonged and bleeding is a problem. Heparin rebound is the term used to describe a delayed heparin effect due to release of tissue heparin after protamine is cleared from the circulation. Although protamine is a mild anticoagulant, one or two supplemental 25- to 50-mg doses can be given empirically if heparin rebound is suspected. In most instances the heart-lung machine should be available for immediate use until the patient leaves the operating room.

Starting Cardiopulmonary Bypass

CPB is started at the surgeon's request with concurrence of the anesthesiologist and perfusionist. As venous return enters the machine, the perfusionist progressively increases arterial flow while monitoring the patient's blood pressure and volume levels in all reservoirs. Six observations are critical:

1. Is venous drainage adequate for the desired flow?
2. Is pressure in the arterial line acceptable?
3. Is arterial blood adequately oxygenated?
4. Is systemic arterial pressure acceptable?
5. Is systemic venous pressure acceptable?
6. Is the heart adequately decompressed?

Once full stable cardiopulmonary bypass is established for at least 2 minutes, lung ventilation is discontinued, perfusion cooling may begin, and the aorta may be clamped for arresting the heart.

Cardioplegia

Antegrade blood or crystalloid cardioplegia is administered directly into the aortic root at 60 to 100 mm Hg pressure proximal to the aortic cross-clamp by a dedicated cardioplegia roller pump (see Fig. 11-2). Blood entering the coronary sinus is captured by the right atrial or unsnared caval catheters; right ventricular distention is prevented. Usually the heart is cooled to a prespecified myocardial temperature range. The heart usually arrests within 30 to 60 seconds; delay indicates problems with delivery of the solution or unrecognized aortic regurgitation. Some surgeons monitor myocardial temperature or pH via direct needle sensors.[235]

The usual flow of retrograde cardioplegia is 200 to 400 mL/min at coronary sinus pressures between 30 and 50 mm Hg.[236] Higher pressures may injure the coronary venous system[198]; low pressures usually indicate inadequate delivery due to malposition of the catheter or leakage around the catheter cuff, but may indicate a tear in the coronary sinus.[199] Induction of electrical arrest is slower (2 to 4 minutes) than with antegrade, and retrograde cardioplegia may provide incomplete protection of the right ventricle.[196,237]

Key Determinants of Safe Perfusion

The following offers rational guidelines for management of CPB, which uses manipulation of temperature, hematocrit, pressure, and flow rate to adequately support cellular metabolism during nonphysiologic conditions.

BLOOD FLOW RATE

Normally, basal cardiac output is determined by oxygen consumption, which is approximately 250 mL/min. It is impractical to measure oxygen consumption during cardiac surgery; therefore, the generally accepted flow rate at 35° to 37°C and hematocrit of 25% is approximately 2.4 L/min/m^2 in deeply anesthetized and muscle-relaxed patients. Hemodilution reduces blood oxygen content from approximately 20 mL/dL to 10 to 12 mL/dL; consequently flow rate must increase over resting normal cardiac output or oxygen demand must decrease. The resistance of venous catheters, turbulence, and loss of physiologic controls of the vasculature are reasons venous return and maximum pump flows are limited.

Hypothermia reduces oxygen consumption by a factor of 0.5 for every 10°C decrease in temperature. However, at both normothermia and hypothermia maximal oxygen consumption falls with decreasing flow as described in the following equation:

$$V\text{O}_2 = 0.44(\text{Q} - 62.7) + 71.6$$

This relationship at various temperatures is depicted in Figure 11-7. For this reason Kirklin and Barratt-Boyes[238] recommend that flows be reduced only to levels which permit at least 85% of maximal an oxygen consumption. At 30°C this flow rate is approximately 1.8 L/min/m^2; at 25°C, 1.6 L/min/m^2; and at 18°C, 1.0 L/min/m^2.

As long as mean arterial pressure remains above 50 to 60 mm Hg (i.e., above the autoregulatory range), cerebral blood flow is preserved even if systemic flow is less than normal. However, there is a hierarchal reduction of flow to other organs as total systemic flow is progressively reduced. First skeletal muscle flow falls, then abdominal viscera and bowel, and finally kidneys.

PULSATILE FLOW

Theoretical benefits of pulsatile blood flow include transmission of more energy to the microcirculation, which reduces critical capillary closing pressure, augments lymph flow, and improves tissue perfusion and cellular metabolism. Pulsatile flow, theoretically, also reduces vasocontrictive reflexes and neuroendocrine responses and may increase oxygen consumption, reduce acidosis, and improve organ perfusion. However, despite extensive investigation no one has convincingly demonstrated a benefit of pulsatile blood

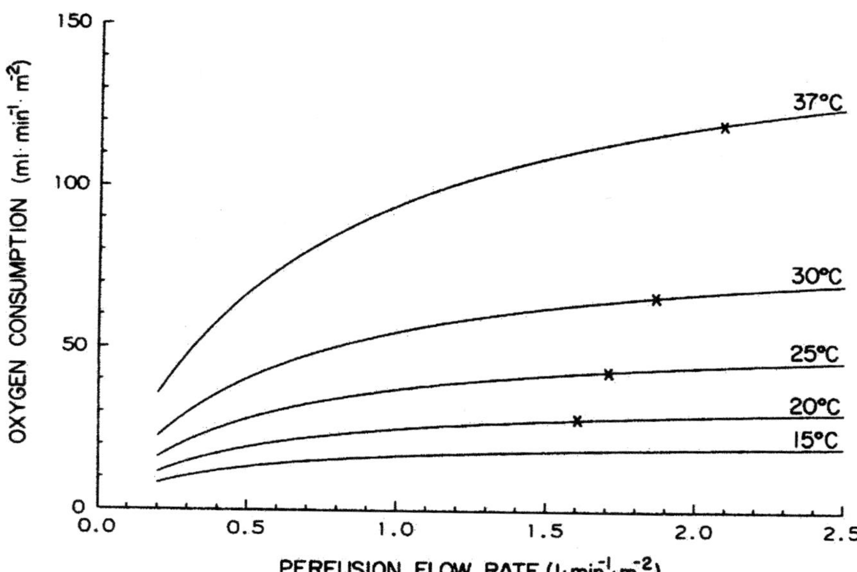

FIGURE 11–7 Nomogram relating oxygen consumption to perfusion flow rate and temperature. The small x's indicate clinical flow rates used by Kirklin and Barratt-Boyes. (*Reproduced with permission from Kirklin JW, Barratt-Boyes BG: Hypothermia, circulatory arrest, and cardiopulmonary bypass, in Kirklin JW, Barratt-Boyes BG (eds): Cardiac Surgery, 2d ed. New York, Churchill Livingstone, 1993; p 91.*)

flow over nonpulsatile blood flow for short- or long-term CPB.[112,115,116,239–243] Two studies reported the association of pulsatile flow with lower rates of mortality, myocardial infarction, and low cardiac output syndrome,[244,245] but others failed to detect clinical benefits.[246–251]

Pulsatile CPB, which actually reproduces the normal pulse pressure within the body, is expensive, complicated, and requires a large-diameter aortic cannula. Higher nozzle velocities increase trauma to blood elements,[252] and pulsations may damage micromembrane oxygenators.[253] Thus for clinical CPB, nonpulsatile blood flow is an acceptable, nonphysiologic compromise with few disadvantages.

ARTERIAL PRESSURE

Systemic arterial blood pressure is a function of flow rate, blood viscosity (hematocrit), and vascular tone. Perfusion of the brain is normally protected by autoregulation, but autoregulation appears to be lost somewhere between 55 and 60 mm Hg during CPB at moderate hypothermia and a hematocrit of 24%.[133,254–256] Cerebral blood flow may still be adequate at lower arterial pressures,[257,258] but the only prospective randomized study found a lower combined major morbidity/mortality rate when mean arterial pressure was maintained near 70 mm Hg (average 69 ± 7) rather than below 60 (average 52).[259] In older patients, who may have vascular disease[260] and/or hypertension, mean arterial blood pressure is generally maintained between 70 and 80 mm Hg at 37°C. Higher pressures are undesirable because collateral blood flow to the heart and lungs increases blood in the operative field.

Hypotension during CPB may be due to low pump flow, aortic dissection, measurement error, or vasodilatation. Phenylephrine is most often used to elevate blood pressure, but arginine vasopressin (0.05-0.1 unit/min) has recently been introduced. If anesthesia is adequate, hypertension is preferably treated with nitroprusside instead of nitroglycerin, which predominately dilates veins.

HEMATOCRIT

The ideal hematocrit during CPB remains controversial because of competing advantages and disadvantages. Low hematocrits reduce blood viscosity and hemolysis, reduce oxygen-carrying capacity, and reduce the need for autologous blood transfusion. In general, viscosity remains stable when percent hematocrit and blood temperature (in °C) are equal (i.e., viscosity is constant at hematocrit 37%, temperature 37°C, or at hematocrit 20%, temperature 20°C). Hypothermia reduces oxygen consumption and permits perfusion at 26°C to 28°C with hematocrits between 18% and 22%, but at higher temperatures limits on pump flow may not satisfy oxygen demand.[261–263] Hill[264] found that hematocrit during CPB did not affect either hospital mortality or neurologic outcome, but DeFoe observed[265] increasing hospital mortality with hematocrits below 23% during CPB; thus the issue remains unresolved.[266] However, higher hematocrits (25%-30%) during CPB appear justified[263] in view of the increasing safety of autologous blood transfusion, improved neurologic outcomes with higher hematocrits in infant cardiac surgery,[267] and more frequent operations near normothermia in older sicker patients.

TEMPERATURE

The ideal temperature for uncomplicated adult cardiac surgery is also an unsettled question.[263] Until recently nearly all operations reduced body temperature to 25° to 30°C during CPB to protect the brain, support hypothermic cardioplegia, permit perfusion at lower flows and hematocrits, and increase the safe duration of circulatory arrest in case of emergency. Hypothermia, however, interferes with enzyme and organ function, aggravates bleeding, increases systemic vascular resistance, delays cardiac recovery, lengthens duration of bypass, increases the risk of cerebral hyperthermia, and is associated with higher levels of depression and anxiety postoperatively.[268] Since the embolic risk of cerebral injury often is greater than perfusion risk, perfusion at higher temperatures (33°C-35°C), or "tepid" CPB, is recommended, in part because detrimental high blood temperatures are avoided during rewarming.[269] Increasingly, efforts are made to avoid cerebral hyperthermia during and after operation, and one study suggests improved neuropsychometric outcomes if patients are rewarmed to only 34°C.[270]

pH/P_{CO_2} MANAGEMENT

There are two strategies for managing pH/P_{CO_2} during hypothermia: pH stat and alpha stat. During deep hypothermia and circulatory arrest (see below) there is increasing evidence that pH-stat management may produce better neurologic outcomes during pediatric cardiac surgery.[267] Alpha stat may be better in adults.[248,271,272] pH stat maintains temperature-corrected pH 7.40 at all temperatures and requires the addition of CO_2 as the patient is cooled. Alpha stat allows the pH to increase during cooling so that blood becomes alkalotic. Cerebral blood flow is higher, and pressure is passive and uncoupled from cerebral oxygen demand with pH stat. With alpha stat, cerebral blood flow is lower, autoregulated, and coupled to cerebral oxygen demand.[273]

ARTERIAL Pa_{O_2}

Pa_{O_2} should probably be kept above 150 mm Hg to assure complete arterial saturation. Whether or not high levels (i.e., >200 mm Hg) are detrimental has not been determined.

GLUCOSE

Although Hill[264] found no relationship between blood glucose concentrations during CPB and adverse neurologic outcome, others are concerned that hyperglycemia (>180 mg/dL) aggravates neurologic injury[230] and other morbidity/mortality.[274]

Patient Monitors

Systemic arterial pressure is typically monitored by radial, brachial, or femoral arterial catheter; central venous pressure is routinely monitored by a jugular venous catheter. Routine use of a Swan-Ganz pulmonary arterial catheter is controversial and not necessary for uncomplicated operations in low-risk patients.[275] During CPB the pulmonary artery catheter should be withdrawn into the main pulmonary artery to prevent lung perforation and suture ensnarement.

TRANSESOPHAGEAL ECHOCARDIOGRAPHY

A comprehensive transesophageal echocardiography (TEE) examination[276] is an important monitor during most applications of CPB[277] to assess catheter and vent insertion and location[196,278,279]; severity of regional atherosclerosis[43,44]; myocardial injury, infarction, dilatation, contractility, thrombi, and residual air; undiagnosed anatomic abnormalities[276]; valve function after repair or replacement; diagnosis of dissection[59,280]; and adequacy of de-airing at the end of CPB.[281]

TEMPERATURE

Bladder or rectal temperature is usually used to estimate temperature of the main body mass, but does not reflect brain temperature.[282] Esophageal and pulmonary artery temperatures may be affected by local cooling associated with cardioplegia. The jugular venous bulb temperature is considered the best surrogate for brain temperature, but is difficult to obtain.[283] Nasopharyngeal or tympanic membrane temperatures are more commonly used, but tend to underestimate jugular venous bulb temperature during rewarming by 3° to 5°C.[284] During rewarming, arterial line temperature correlates best with jugular venous bulb temperature.[285]

NEUROPHYSIOLOGIC MONITORING

The efficacy of neurophysiologic monitoring during CPB is under investigation and not yet established as necessary. Techniques being investigated include jugular venous bulb temperature and saturation, transcranial Doppler ultrasound, near-infrared transcranial reflectance spectroscopy (NIRS), and the raw or processed electroencephalogram (EEG).[286,287]

ADEQUACY OF PERFUSION

During CPB oxygen consumption (V_{O_2}) equals pump flow rate times the difference in arterial (Ca_{O_2}) and venous oxygen content (Cv_{O_2}). For a given temperature, maintaining V_{O_2} at 85% predicted maximum during CPB assures adequate oxygen delivery (see Fig. 11-7).[238] Oxygen delivery (D_{O_2}) equals pump flow times Ca_{O_2} and should be above 250 mL/min/m^2 during normothermic perfusion.[261] Mixed venous oxygen saturation (Sv_{O_2}) assesses the relationship between D_{O_2} and V_{O_2}; values below 60% indicate inadequate oxygen delivery. Because of differences in regional vascular tone, higher Sv_{O_2} does not assure adequate oxygen delivery to all vascular beds.[210,288] Metabolic acidosis (base deficit) or elevated lactic acid levels also indicate inadequate perfusion.

URINE OUTPUT

Urine output is usually monitored but varies with renal perfusion, temperature, composition of the pump prime, diuretics, absent pulsatility, and hemoconcentration. Urine production is reassuring during CPB and oliguria requires investigation.

GASTRIC TONOMETRY AND MUCOSAL FLOW

These Doppler and laser measurements gauge splanchnic perfusion but are rarely used clinically.

Stopping Cardiopulmonary Bypass

Prior to stopping CPB the patient is rewarmed to 34°C to 36°C, the heart is defibrillated, and the lungs are reexpanded (40 cm H_2O pressure) and ventilated. Cardiac rhythm is monitored, and hematocrit, blood gases, acid-base status, and plasma electrolytes are reviewed. If the heart has been opened, TEE is recommended for detection and removal of trapped air before ejection begins. Caval catheters are adjusted to ensure unobstructed venous return to the heart. If inotropic drugs are anticipated, these are started at low flow rates. Vent catheters are removed, although sometimes an aortic root vent is placed on gentle suction to remove undiscovered air.

Once preparations are completed, the surgeon, anesthesiologist, and perfusionist begin to wean the patient off CPB. The perfusionist gradually occludes the venous line and simultaneously reduces pump input as cardiac rate and rhythm, arterial pressure and pulse, and central venous pressure are monitored and adjusted. Initially blood volume within the pump is kept constant, but as pump flow approaches zero, volume is added or removed from the patient to produce arterial and venous pressures within the physiologic ranges. During weaning, cardiac filling and contractility is often monitored by TEE, and intracardiac repairs and regional myocardial contractility are assessed. Pulse oximetry saturation near 100%, end-tidal CO_2 greather than 25 mm Hg, and mixed venous oxygen saturation higher than 65% confirm satisfactory ventilation and circulation. When cardiac performance is satisfactory and stable, all catheters and cannulas are removed, protamine is given to reverse heparin, and blood return from the surgical field is discontinued.

Once the patient is hemodynamically stable, as determined by surgeon and anesthesiologist, and after starting wound closure, the perfusate may be returned to the patient in several ways. The entire perfusate may be washed and returned as packed cells. Excess fluid may be removed by a hemoconcentrator. More often the perfusate, which still contains heparin, is gradually pumped into the patient for hemoconcentration by the kidneys. Occasionally some of the perfusate must be bagged and given later. The heart-lung machine should not be completely disassembled until the chest is closed and the patient is ready for transfer.

SPECIAL TOPICS

Special Applications of Extracorporeal Perfusion

Reoperations, surgery of the descending thoracic aorta, and minimally invasive procedures may be facilitated by surgical incisions other than midline sternotomy. These alternative incisions often require alternative methods for connecting the patient to the heart-lung machine. Some alternative applications of CPB are presented below.

RIGHT THORACOTOMY

Anterolateral incisions through the 4th or 5th interspaces provide easy access to the cavae and right atrium, adequate access to the ascending aorta, and no direct access to the left ventricle. Adequate exposure of the ascending aorta is available for cross-clamping, aortotomy, and administration of cardioplegia by retracting the right atrial appendage. Deairing the left ventricle (e.g., after mitral valve repair) is more difficult. External pads facilitate defibrillation.

LEFT THORACOTOMY

Lateral or posterolateral incisions in the left chest are used for a variety of operations. Venous return may be captured by cannulating the pulmonary artery via a stab wound in the right ventricle, or by retrograde cannulation of the left pulmonary artery or cannulation of the left iliac or femoral vein. With iliac or femoral cannulation, venous return is augmented by threading the cannula into the right atrium using TEE guidance.[289] The descending thoracic aorta or left subclavian, iliac, or femoral arteries are accessible for arterial cannulation.

LEFT HEART BYPASS

Left heart bypass utilizes the beating right heart to pump blood through the lungs to provide gas exchange.[290] An oxygenator is not used and intake cannulation sites are exposed through a left thoracotomy. The left superior pulmonary vein–left atrial junction is an excellent cannulation site for capturing blood. The left atrial appendage can also be used, but is more friable and difficult. The apex of the left ventricle is infrequently used because of myocardial injury. The tip of the intake catheter must be free in the left atrium and careful technique is required to avoid air entry during cannulation and perfusion. The extracorporeal circuit typically consists only of tubing and a centrifugal pump and does not include a reservoir, heat exchanger, or bubble trap. This reduces the thrombin burden (see section 11B) and may permit reduced or no heparin, if anticoagulation poses an additional risk (e.g., in acute head injury). Otherwise, full heparin doses are recommended. The reduced perfusion circuit precludes the ability to add or sequester fluid, adjust temperature, or intercept systemic air emboli. Intravenous volume expanders may be needed to maintain adequate flows; temperature can usually be maintained without a heat exchanger.[291]

Full left heart bypass may be employed for left-sided coronary artery surgery by draining all of the pulmonary venous return out of the left atrium and leaving no blood for left ventricular ejection. If the heart fibrillates, blood can still passively pass through the right heart and lungs, but often an elevated central venous pressure is required.[292]

Partial left heart bypass is identical in configuration and cannulation to full left heart bypass and is used to facilitate surgery on the descending thoracic aorta. The patient's left ventricle supplies blood to the aorta proximal to aortic clamps, and the circuit supplies blood to the distal body. Typically about two-thirds normal basal cardiac output (i.e., 1.6 L/min/m^2) is pumped to the lower body. Arterial pressure is monitored proximal (radial or brachial) and distal (right femoral, pedal) to the aortic clamps. Blood volume in the body and circuit is assessed by central venous pressure and TEE monitoring of chamber dimensions. Management is more complicated because of the single venous circulation and separated arterial circulations.[290,293]

PARTIAL CARDIOPULMONARY BYPASS

Partial CPB with an oxygenator is also used to facilitate surgery of the descending thoracic aorta. After left thoracotomy, systemic venous and arterial cannulas are placed as described above. The perfusion circuit includes a reservoir, pump, oxygenator, heat exchanger, and bubble trap. The beating left ventricle supplies the upper body and heart, so lungs must be ventilated and upper body oxygen saturation should be independently monitored. Blood flow to the separate upper and lower circulations must be balanced as described for partial left heart bypass above.

FULL CARDIOPULMONARY BYPASS

Full CPB with peripheral cannulation is used when access to the chest is dangerous because of proximity of the heart, vital vessels (e.g., mammary arterial graft), or pathologic condition (e.g., ascending aortic mycotic aneurysm) abutting the anterior chest wall.[3] The patient is supine and a complete extracorporeal perfusion circuit is prepared and primed. Venous cannulas may be inserted into the right atrium via the iliac or femoral vessels and/or the right jugular vein. The iliac, femoral, or axillary-subclavian arteries may be used for arterial cannulation. Initiation of CPB decompresses the heart, but cooling is usually deferred to keep the heart beating and decompressed until the surgeon can insert a vent catheter.

FEMORAL VEIN TO FEMORAL ARTERY BYPASS

Femoral vein to femoral artery bypass with full CPB is used to initiate bypass outside the operating room for emergency circulatory assistance,[3] supportive angioplasty,[294] or accidental hypothermia. Femoral vessel cannulation is occasionally used during other operations to facilitate control of bleeding (e.g., cranial aneurysm, tumor invading the inferior vena cava) or ensure oxygenation (e.g., lung transplantation, upper airway reconstruction).

CANNULATION FOR MINIMALLY INVASIVE (LIMITED ACCESS) SURGERY

Off-pump coronary artery bypass (OP-CAB) describes construction of coronary arterial bypass grafts on the beating heart without CPB. Minimally invasive direct coronary artery bypass (MID-CAB) refers to coronary arterial bypass grafting with or without CPB through small, strategically placed incisions. Peripheral cannulation sites, described above, may be used, but often central cannulation of the aorta, atrium, or central veins is accomplished using specially designed or smaller cannulas placed through the operative incision or through a separate small incisions in the chest wall.[295,296] Venous return may be augmented by applying negative pressure (see discussion of venous cannulation above); often soft tipped arterial catheters are used to minimize arterial wall trauma.[27]

The Port-Access System provides a means for full CPB, cardioplegia administration, and aortic cross-clamping without exposing the heart and can be used for both valvular and coronary arterial operations.[70,279] Through the right internal jugular vein separate transcutaneous catheters are inserted into the coronary sinus for retrograde cardioplegia and the pulmonary artery for left heart venting. A multilumen catheter is inserted through the femoral artery and using TEE and/or fluoroscopy is positioned in the ascending aorta for arterial pump inflow, for balloon occlusion of the ascending aorta, and for administration of antegrade cardioplegia into the aortic root. Venous return is captured by a femoral venous catheter advanced into the right atrium. The system allows placement of small skin incisions directly over the parts of the heart that require surgical attention.

Minimally invasive surgery using CPB is associated with potential complications that include perforation of vessels or

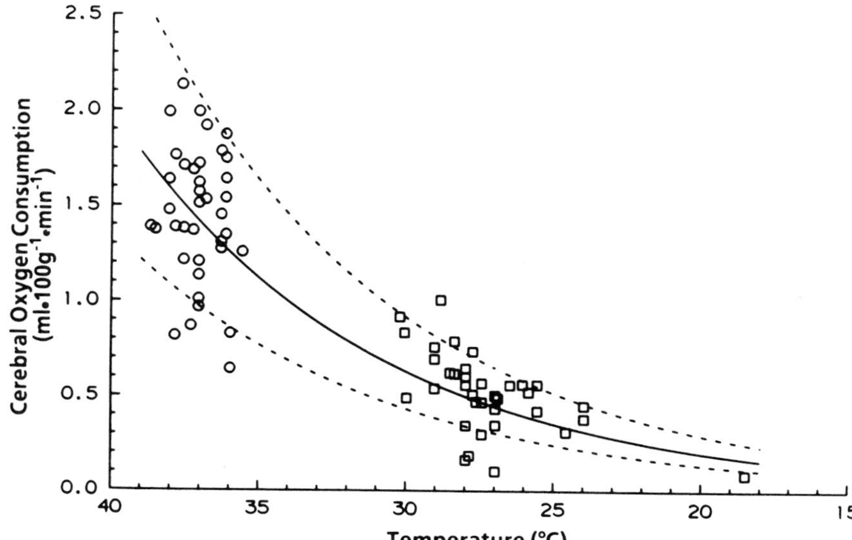

FIGURE 11–8 Relation between cerebral oxygen consumption and nasopharyngeal temperature during CPB at 2 L/min/m^2. *(Reproduced with permission from Kirklin JW, Barratt-Boyes BG: Hypothermia, circulatory arrest, and cardiopulmonary bypass, in Kirklin JW, Barratt-Boyes BG (eds): Cardiac Surgery, 2d ed. New York, Churchill Livingstone, 1993; p 91.)*

cardiac chambers, aortic dissection, incomplete de-airing, systemic air embolism, and failure of the balloon aortic clamp. Because CO_2 is heavier than air and more soluble in blood, the surgical field is sometimes flooded with CO_2 at 5- to 10-L/min flow to displace air when the heart is open. The balloon aortic clamp can leak, prolapse through the aortic valve, or move distally to occlude arch vessels. For safety the position of the occluding balloon is closely monitored by TEE, bilateral radial arterial pressures, and one of the following: transcranial Doppler ultrasound, cerebral near-infrared spectroscopy, or electroencephalogram.[296a]

Deep Hypothermic Circulatory Arrest

Deep hypothermic circulatory arrest (DHCA) is used for operations involving the aortic arch, porcelain aorta, thoracoabdominal aneurysms, pulmonary thromboendarterectomy, selected uncommon cardiovascular and neurologic procedures,[297,298] and certain complex congenital heart procedures. The technology involves reducing body temperature to less than 20°C, arresting the circulation for a short period, and then rewarming to 37°C. Deep hypothermia reduces cerebral oxygen consumption (Fig. 11-8), and attenuates release of toxic neurotransmitters and reactive oxidants during ischemia and reperfusion.[299]

Because perfusion cooling produces differential temperatures within both the body and brain,[282] more than one temperature is customarily monitored. Bladder, pulmonary artery, esophageal, or rectal temperatures are used to estimate body temperature. Nasopharyngeal and tympanic membrane temperatures are imperfect surrogates for mean brain temperature. Most surgical teams cool to either EEG silence, jugular venous saturation above 95%, or for at least 30 minutes before stopping circulation at nasopharyngeal or tympanic membrane temperatures below 20°C. Caloric exchange is proportional to body mass, rate of perfusion, and temperature differences between patient and perfusate; however, rates of perfusion cooling and rewarming are restricted (see the section on heat exchangers above). Perfusion cooling is usually supplemented by surface cooling using hypothermia blankets and/or packing the head in ice. Hyperthermia is avoided by keeping arterial inflow temperature below 37°C during rewarming.

Changes in temperature affect acid-base balance, which must be monitored and managed during deep hypothermia. The pH-stat protocol (CO_2 is added to maintain temperature corrected blood pH at 7.4) may be preferred over the alpha-stat protocol, which allows cold blood to become alkalotic. Compared to alpha-stat, pH-stat increases the rate and uniformity of brain cooling,[300,301] slows the rate of brain oxygen consumption by 30% to 40% at 17°C,[301–303] and improves neurologic outcomes in animal models[267,304,305] and perhaps in infants,[306–308] but not necessarily in adults.[309] Hyperglycemia appears to increase brain injury and is avoided during deep hypothermia.[310] The value of high-dose corticosteroids or barbiturates remains unproven.

The safe duration of circulatory arrest during deep hypothermia is unknown. In adults arrest times as short as 25 minutes are associated with poor performance on neuropsychologic tests of fine motor function and memory.[311] Ergin[312] found duration of arrest was a predictor of temporary neurologic dysfunction, which correlated with long-term neuropsychologic deficits.[313] At 18°C, cerebral metabolism and oxygen consumption are 17% to 40% of normothermia[314–316] and abnormal encephalographic patterns and cerebrovascular responses can be detected after 30 minutes of circulatory arrest.[314,317] Most investigators,[318–322] but not all[323] report increased mortality and adverse neurologic outcomes after 40 to 65 minutes of circulatory arrest. Most surgeons try to keep the period of arrest at less than 45 minutes and, if the operation allows, many perfuse for 10 to 15 minutes between serial arrest periods of 10 to 20 minutes.

Antegrade and Retrograde Cerebral Perfusion

Antegrade cerebral perfusion is used in lieu of DHCA or as a supplement. The cerebral vessels can be cannulated separately and perfused together by a single pump[324] or perfused collectively after a graft with a side branch is sewn to the top of the aortic arch from which the innominate, left carotid, and left subclavian arteries originate. Separate perfusion of separately cannulated vessels is rarely done. Perfusion is usually provided by a separate roller pump that receives blood from the arterial line. Line pressure is monitored and a microfilter may or may not be used. The cerebral vessels are collectively perfused with cold blood between 10° and 18°C and at approximate flows of 10 mL/kg/min; perfusion pressures are restricted to 30 to 70 mm Hg. At the present time each individual surgeon seems to have a preferred protocol between these broad ranges.[325–332] The adequacy of cerebral perfusion can be assessed by monitoring jugular venous saturation or near-infrared spectroscopy. Selective antegrade cerebral perfusion risks dislodging atheromatous emboli or causing air embolism, cerebral edema, or injury from excessive perfusion pressure.

Retrograde cerebral perfusion (RCP) was introduced in 1980 as emergency treatment for massive air embolism.[333] Ueda introduced continuous RCP for cerebral protection as an adjunct to deep hypothermic circulatory arrest during aortic surgery.[334] During RCP and DHCA the superior vena cava is perfused at blood pressures usually between 25 and 40 mm Hg, temperatures between 8°C and 18°C, and flows between 250 and 400 mL/min from a spur off the arterial line, which is clamped downstream to the spur. Some surgeons advocate much higher pressures and flows to compensate for runoff and have not shown detrimental effects.[335] A snare is usually placed around the superior caval catheter cephalad to the azygous vein to reduce runoff. The IVC may or may not be occluded.[322,336–339]

Retrograde cerebral perfusion has been widely and safely used,[321,335,339–347] but its effectiveness in protecting the brain is not clear.[322,328,348] The method can wash out some particulate emboli entering from arteries, which is a major cause of brain injury after aortic surgery.[337,349] However, it is not clear how adequately and completely all regions of the brain are perfused.[322,339,348,350] Lin[342] found cortical flows to be only 10% of control values. RCP slows but does not arrest the decrease in cerebral oxygen saturation[324,335] and the decay in amplitude of somatosensory evoked potentials.[351] Others from clinical comparisons and animal studies believe RCP provides some cerebral protection over DHCA alone.[321,335,339,341,342,344,345,347,352] A few studies report that antegrade cerebral perfusion provides better protection than retrograde.[324,338,353]

Complications and Risk Management

Life-threatening incidents occur in 0.4% to 2.7% of operations with CPB and the incidence of serious injury or death is between 0.06% and 0.08% (Table 11-4).[94,151,354] Massive air embolism, aortic dissection, dislodgement of cannulas, and clotting within the circuit during perfusion are the principal causes of serious injury or death. Malfunctions of the heater-cooler, oxygenator, pumps, and electrical supply are the most common threatening incidents related to equipment. Other threatening incidents include premature takedown or clotting within the perfusion circuit.

TABLE 11–4 Adverse incidents involving cardiopulmonary bypass

	Incidence (events/1000)	Death or serious injury(%)*
Protamine reaction	1.3	10.5
Thrombosis during cardiopulmonary bypass	0.3-0.4	2.6-5.2
Aortic dissection	0.4-0.8	14.3-33.1
Dislodgement of cannula	0.2-1.6	4.2-7.1
Rupture of arterial connection	0.2-0.6	0-3.1
Gas embolism	0.2-1.3	0.2-8.7
Massive systemic gas embolism	0.03-0.07	50-52
Electrical power failure	0.2-1.8	0-0.6
Pump failure	0.4-0.9	0-3.5
Heater-cooler problems	0.5-3	0
Replace oxygenator during CPB	0.2-1.3	0-0.7
Other oxygenator problems	0.2-0.9	0
Urgent re-setup after takedown	2.9	13
Early unplanned cessation of CPB	0.2	0-0.7

*Percentage of incidents that resulted in death or serious injury. Data derived from references 94, and 151.

Complications related to connections to and from the heart-lung machine and perfusion during operation are described above with descriptions of the various components of the perfusion circuit.

MASSIVE AIR EMBOLISM

The incidence of massive air embolism is between 0.003% to 0.007% with 50% of outcomes adverse.[94,151] Air can enter any component of the perfusion circuit at anytime during operation if the integrity of the circuit is broken.[355] Stopcocks, connections, vent catheters, empty reservoirs, purse-string sutures, cardioplegia infusion catheters, and unremoved air in opened cardiac chambers are the most common sources of air emboli. Uncommon sources include oxygenator membrane leaks, residual air in the circuit after priming, reversal of flow in venous or arterial lines, and unexpected inspiration by the patient during cannula removal.

Massive air embolism during perfusion is a catastrophe and management guidelines are evolving.[20,333,355–358] Perfusion should stop immediately and clamps should be placed on both venous and arterial lines. Air in the circuit should be rapidly removed by recirculation and entrapment of all air in a reservoir or bubble trap. The patient should be immediately placed in steep Trendelenburg position and blood and air at the site of entry should be aspirated until no air is retrieved. TEE should be rapidly employed to search for air, but perfusion must resume promptly depending upon body temperature to prevent ischemic brain damage. Cooling to deep hypothermia should be considered to protect the brain and other organs while air is located and removed. As soon as possible, retrograde perfusion of the brain should be undertaken while the aortic arch is simultaneously aspirated with the patient in steep Trendelenburg position. Corticosteroids and/or barbiturates may be considered. Depending upon circumstances and availability, hyperbaric oxygen therapy may be helpful if patients can be treated within 5 hours of operation.[357,359]

RISK MANAGEMENT

Minimizing risks of extracorporeal perfusion requires strict attention to personnel training, preparation and training for emergencies, equipment function, and record keeping.[20] All members of the operative team must be trained, certified, and recertified in their respective roles and participate in continuing education programs. A policy manual for the perfusion team and written protocols should be developed and continuously updated for various types of operations and emergencies. Emergency kits are prepared for out-of-operating-room crises. Adequate supplies are stocked in designated locations with sufficient inventory to support any operation or emergency for a specified period. An inventory of supplies is taken and recorded at regular intervals. Checklists are prepared and used for setting up the perfusion system and connecting to the patient. Equipment is inspected at regular intervals; worn, loose, or outdated parts are replaced; and preventive maintenance is provided and documented. New equipment is thoroughly checked before use and instructions are thoroughly digested by all user personnel. Safety alarms are optional; none replace the vigilance and attention of all OR personnel during an operation. Complete, signed written records are required for every perfusion; adverse events are recorded in a separate log and reviewed by the entire OR team. A continuous quality assurance program is desirable.[360]

During the procedure communication must be open between the surgeon, anesthetist, and perfusionist to coordinate activites. Statements are verbally acknowledged. Distractive conversations are discouraged. The entire OR team is committed to a zero-error policy, which can only be achieved by discipline and attention to details.[354,361,362]

11B: Thrombosis and Bleeding

L. Henry Edmunds, Jr./Robert W. Colman

Within the body the endothelial cell, the only surface in contact with circulating blood, simultaneously maintains the fluidity of blood and the integrity of the vascular system. This remarkable cell maintains a dynamic equilibrium by producing anticoagulants to maintain blood in a fluid state and by generating procoagulant substances to enhance gel formation when perturbed. Coagulation proteins circulate as inert zymogens, which convert to active enzymes when stimulated. Likewise, blood cells remain quiescent until activated to express surface receptors and release proteins and enzymes involved in the coagulation equilibrium. The continuous exposure of heparinized blood to the perfusion circuit and to nonendothelial cell tissues of the wound during clinical cardiac surgery produces an intense thrombotic stimulus that involves both the tissue factor pathway (extrinsic coagulation pathway) in the wound and the contact and intrinsic coagulation pathways in the perfusion circuit. Heparin does not block thrombin formation; during extracorporeal perfusion (ECP) heparin partially inhibits thrombin after it is produced. Thrombin is continuously generated and circulated despite massive doses of heparin in all applications of extracorporeal perfusion.[365–369]

INITIAL REACTIONS IN THE PERFUSION CIRCUIT

When heparinized blood contacts any biomaterial, plasma proteins are instantly adsorbed (<1 second) onto the surface to form a *monolayer* of selected proteins.[370–372] For each protein the amount adsorbed depends upon its bulk concentration in plasma and the *intrinsic surface activity* of the biomaterial. Different biomaterials have different intrinsic surface activities for each plasma protein. The physical and chemical composition of the *biomaterial surface* determine the intrinsic surface activity of the biomaterial, but intrinsic surface activity is not predictable from knowledge of chemical and physical characteristics. Thus intrinsic surface activity differs among biomaterial surfaces, among plasma proteins, and among different bulk concentrations of plasma proteins. Concentrations of plasma proteins on a given biomaterial differ from concentrations in bulk plasma. Similarly, concentrations of surface-adsorbed proteins from the same plasma differ on different biomaterials. The composition of the protein monolayer is specific for the biomaterial and for various concentrations of proteins in the plasma, but the topography of the adsorbed protein layer may not be uniform across the surface of the biomaterial.[373] Thus it is not possible to predict the "thrombogenicity" of any biomaterial except by trial and error.

On most biomaterial surfaces fibrinogen is selectively adsorbed, but the adsorbed concentration of fibrinogen and other proteins may change over time.[372] Surface-adsorbed proteins "compete" for space on the biomaterial surface, but are tightly packed, irreversibly bound, and immobile. The density of surface-adsorbed proteins is 100 to 1000 times greater than the density of proteins in bulk plasma.[373] The complexity of blood-biomaterial interactions is further compounded by the fact that adsorbed proteins often undergo limited conformational changes[374,375] that may expose "receptor" amino acid sequences that are recognized by specific blood cells or bulk plasma proteins. Conformational changes of adsorbed factor XII and fibrinogen initiate activation of the contact pathway and platelet surface adhesion, respectively; similar changes in complement protein 3 participate in activation of the complement system.[375] For a given adsorbed protein these conformational changes may vary between biomaterial surfaces and in turn vary the reactivity of the adsorbed protein with cells and blood proteins in the bulk phase.

Thus heparinized blood does not directly contact biomaterial surfaces in extracorporeal perfusion circuits, but contacts monolayers of densely packed, immobile plasma proteins arranged in undefined mosaics that differ between locations and possibly across time. All biomaterial surfaces, including heparin-coated surfaces, are *procoagulant*[367,376]; only the endothelial cell is truly nonthrombogenic (Fig. 11-9).

ANTICOAGULATION

ECP and cardiopulmonary bypass (CPB) are not possible without anticoagulation; the large procoagulant surface quickly overwhelms natural circulating anticoagulants—antithrombin, proteins C and S, tissue factor pathway inhibitor, and plasmin—to produce thrombin and thrombosis within the circuit. Thrombin is produced in extracorporeal perfusion systems with small surface areas and high-velocity flow,[368,377,378] but thrombosis may not be apparent if other procoagulants (e.g., addition of blood from wounds) are absent. Generation of thrombin varies widely between applications of extracorporeal technology (see below), but this powerful and potentially dangerous enzyme is produced whenever blood contacts a nonendothelial cell surface (Fig. 11-10).

During CPB and open heart surgery (OHS) high concentrations of heparin (3-4 mg/kg, initial dose) are needed to maintain the fluidity of blood. Heparin has both advantages and disadvantages; the most notable advantages are parenteral use, immediate onset of action, and rapid reversal by protamine or recombinant platelet factor 4.[379] Heparin does not directly inhibit coagulation, but acts by accelerating the actions of the natural protease, antithrombin.[380]

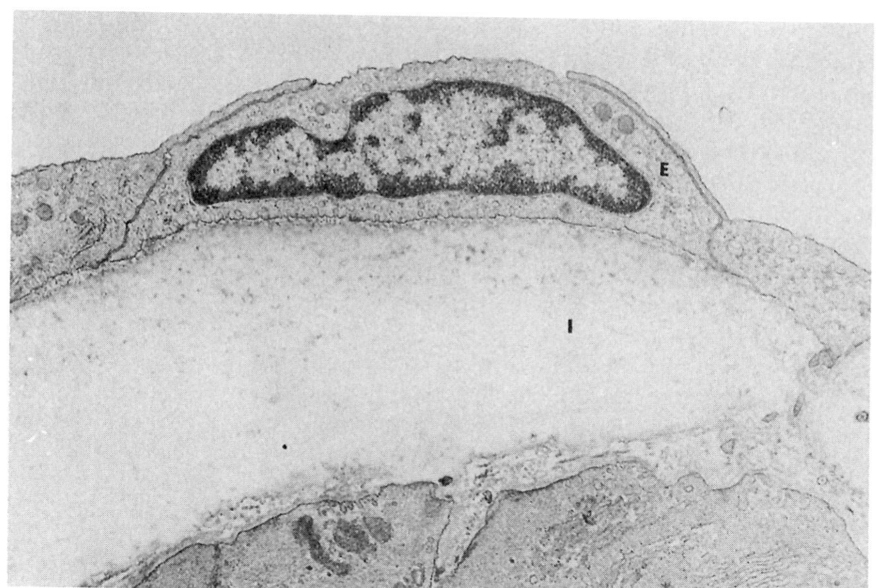

FIGURE 11–9 Electron micrograph of a rabbit endothelial cell (E), the only known nonthrombogenic surface. Note the overlapping junctions with neighboring endothelial cells. Endothelial cells rest on the internal elastic lamina (I), which abut medial smooth muscle cells. The vessel lumen is at the top. (*Reproduced with permission from Stemerman MB: Anatomy of the blood vessel wall, in Colman RW, Hirsh J, Marder VJ, Salzman E (eds): Hemostasis and Thrombosis: Basic Principles and Clinical Practice, 2d ed. Philadelphia, JB Lippincott, 1987; p 775.*)

Heparin-catalyzed antithrombin, however, does not inhibit thrombin bound to fibrin[381] or factor Xa bound to platelets within clots[382]; thus heparin only partially inhibits thrombin in vivo. Antithrombin primarily binds thrombin; its action on factors Xa and IXa is much slower. Heparin inhibits coagulation at the end of the cascade after nearly all other coagulation proteins have been converted to active enzymes. In addition, heparin to varying degrees activates several blood constituents: platelets,[383–385] factor XII,[386] complement, neutrophils, and monocytes.[387–389] Heparin increases the sensitivity of platelets to soluble agonists,[385] inhibits binding to von Willebrand factor,[390] and modestly increases template bleeding times.[384] Thrombin concentrations cannot be measured in real time and only insensitive, indirect methods are available to regulate heparin anticoagulation in the operating room.[391–393]

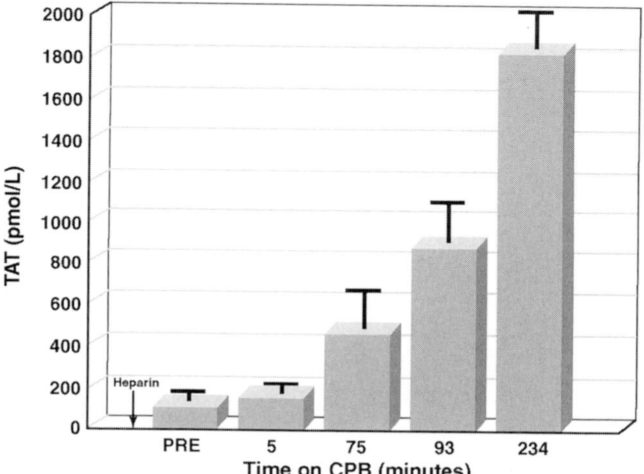

FIGURE 11–10 Plasma thrombin-antithrombin (TAT) measurements of thrombin generation during CPB and clinical cardiac surgery of varying duration. (*Data from Brister SJ, Ofosu FA, Buchanan MR: Thrombin generation during cardiac surgery: is heparin the ideal anticoagulant? Thromb Haemost 1993; 70:259.*)

Heparin is also associated with some clinical idiosyncrasies. In some patients recent, prolonged parenteral heparin may reduce antithrombin concentrations and produce *heparin resistance*.[380,394,395] Insufficient antithrombin may also occur due to insufficient synthesis or increased consumption in some cyanotic infants, premature babies, cachectic patients, and patients with advanced liver or renal disease. The deficiency in antithrombin prevents heparin from prolonging activated clotting times to therapeutic levels. In these patients fresh frozen plasma is needed to increase plasma antithrombin concentrations to inhibit thrombin. *Heparin rebound* is a delayed anticoagulant effect after protamine neutralization due to the rapid metabolism of protamine and delayed seepage of heparin into the circulation from lymphatic tissues and other deposits. Heparin is also associated with an allergic response in some patients that produces heparin-induced thrombocytopenia (HIT) with or without thrombosis (see below). Lastly, heparin only partially suppresses thrombin formation during CPB and all applications of extracorporeal perfusion and mechanical circulatory and respiratory assistance despite doses 2 to 3 times those used for other indications (see Fig. 11-10).[365–368] Thus heparin is far from an ideal anticoagulant.

Potential alternatives for heparin during ECP include low molecular weight heparin, danaparoid (Organan), recombinant hirudin (Lepirudin), and the organic chemical, argatroban (Texas Biotechnology Corp.). All have important drawbacks and are approved for use in heparin-induced thrombocytopenia and in patients with circulating IgG anti-heparin-PF4 complex antibodies (see below). Low molecular weight heparins have long half-lives in plasma

(4-8 hours), require antithrombin as a cofactor, primarily inhibit factor Xa, and are not reversible by protamine.[396,397] Although less antigenic than standard heparin, low molecular weight heparins can stimulate production of IgG anti-heparin-PF4 complex antibodies.[397] Danaparoid is a mixture of heparin sulfate, dermatan sulfate, and chrondroitin sulfate that catalyzes antithrombin to inhibit thrombin and factor Xa. To a lesser extent, Danaparoid also catalyzes inhibition of thrombin by heparin cofactor II. The anticoagulant effect is long lasting (plasma half-life 4.3 hours)[398] and is not reversed by protamine.

Recombinant hirudin (Lepirudin) is a direct inhibitor of thrombin, is effective rapidly, does not have an effective antidote, is monitored by the partial thromboplastin time, is cleared by the kidney, and has a relatively short half-life in plasma (40 minutes).[399] This drug has been successfully used during CPB and open heart surgery, but in many instances bleeding after bypass has been troublesome and substantial. A newer drug is a semisynthetic bivalent thrombin inhibitor composed of 12 amino acids from hirudin, which binds to exosite 1 of thrombin linked to an active site-directed moiety, D Phe Pro Arg Pro, by four glycines.[400] This drug, bivalirudin (Angiomax), has a shorter half-life than hirudin and therefore may be safer. In addition, only a small amount is excreted by the kidney. In coronary angioplasty, bivalirudin was as effective as heparin but there was less bleeding. Argatroban is also a direct thrombin inhibitor[401] with rapid onset of action and short plasma half-life (40-50 minutes).[402] Argatroban is metabolized in the liver and is without an antidote, but can be monitored with partial thromboplastin times or activated clotting times. At present there is little clinical experience with argatroban or bivalirudin in cardiac surgical patients.

HEPARIN-ASSOCIATED THROMBOCYTOPENIA, HEPARIN-INDUCED THROMBOCYTOPENIA, AND HEPARIN-INDUCED THROMBOCYTOPENIA AND THROMBOSIS

Heparin-associated thrombocytopenia (HAT) is a benign, nonimmune, 5% to 15% decrease in platelet count that occurs within a few hours to 3 days after heparin exposure. The etiology is due to mild platelet stimulation from multifactorial causes; bleeding does not occur; and the condition is clinically inconsequential.[403]

Heparin-induced thrombocytopenia (HIT) and heparin-induced thrombocytopenia and thrombosis (HITT) are different manifestations of the same immune disease. Heparin binds to platelets in the absence of an antibody and releases small amounts of platelet factor 4 (as occurs in HAT). PF4 avidly binds heparin to form a heparin-PF4 (H-PF4) complex, which is antigenic in some people. In these individuals IgG antibodies to the *H-PF4 complex* are produced within 5 to 15 days after exposure to heparin and continue to circulate in the absence of more heparin for approximately 3 to 6 months.[404] *IgG-anti-H-PF4 antibodies* plus *H-PF4 complexes* form *HIT complexes,* which unite IgG Fc terminals to platelet Fc receptors (Fig. 11-11). This binding strongly stimulates platelets to release more PF4.[405] A self-perpetuating, accelerating cascade of platelet activation, release, and aggregation ensues. Since platelet granules contain several procoagulatory proteins (e.g., thrombin, fibronectin, factor V, fibrinogen, von Willebrand factor), release also activates coagulation proteins to generate thrombin.

The intensity of the immune reaction varies between patients, but also varies by the indications for heparin use. Both heparin and PF4 must be available to form the antigenic H-PF4 complex. Patients who do not have conditions that activate platelets have a low incidence of HIT following administration of heparin, because few PF4 molecules are available to form H-PF4 complexes. In medical patients the incidence of thrombocytopenia after heparin is about 0.5%; the incidence of HITT is approximately 0.25%; and only 3% have IgG anti-H-PF4 antibodies by enzyme immunoassay.[406] Large doses of heparin are given and huge numbers of platelets are activated during CPB. Thus after CPB, 50% of patients have IgG anti-H-PF4 antibodies; 2% have immune heparin-induced thrombocytopenia; and approximately 1% develop HITT.[406] A combination of three ingredients is necessary to produce HIT or HITT: heparin, platelet factor 4, and IgG anti-H-PF4 antibodies. Since IgG antibodies are transient, a second heparin exposure 6 months after HIT is not likely to produce HIT or HITT,[404] but will stimulate production of new IgG antibodies to the H-PF4 complex. The danger is a second heparin exposure when IgG anti-H-PF4 antibodies are still circulating.

IgG anti-H-PF4 antibodies are detected in two ways. The serotonin release test detects the release of radioactive serotonin from normal platelets washed by the patient's serum.[407] An enzyme immunoassay measures IgG anti-H-PF4 antibodies directly. Both assays are equally sensitive in patients with clinical HIT, but the enzyme immunoassay is more sensitive in detecting IgG anti-H-PF4 antibodies in patients without other evidence of the disease.[407]

The clinical presentation of HIT may be insidious. If the platelet count was originally normal, the earliest sign is an abrupt decrease of at least 50% in platelet count (to less than 150,000/μL) in a patient who has had exposure to heparin within the past 5 to 15 days.[404] This event is a preoperative stop sign for elective cardiac operations. After CPB, platelet counts below 80,000/μL should trigger an order to stop all heparin, including heparin flushes, and to obtain daily platelet counts. The patient should be thoroughly examined for deep vein thrombosis, extremity ischemia, stroke, myocardial infarction, or any evidence of intravascular thrombosis using ultrasound and appropriate radiographic technology. Any evidence of vascular thrombosis should prompt a plasma sample for IgG anti-H-PF4 antibodies. A positive antibody test confirms the diagnosis of HIT in patients with

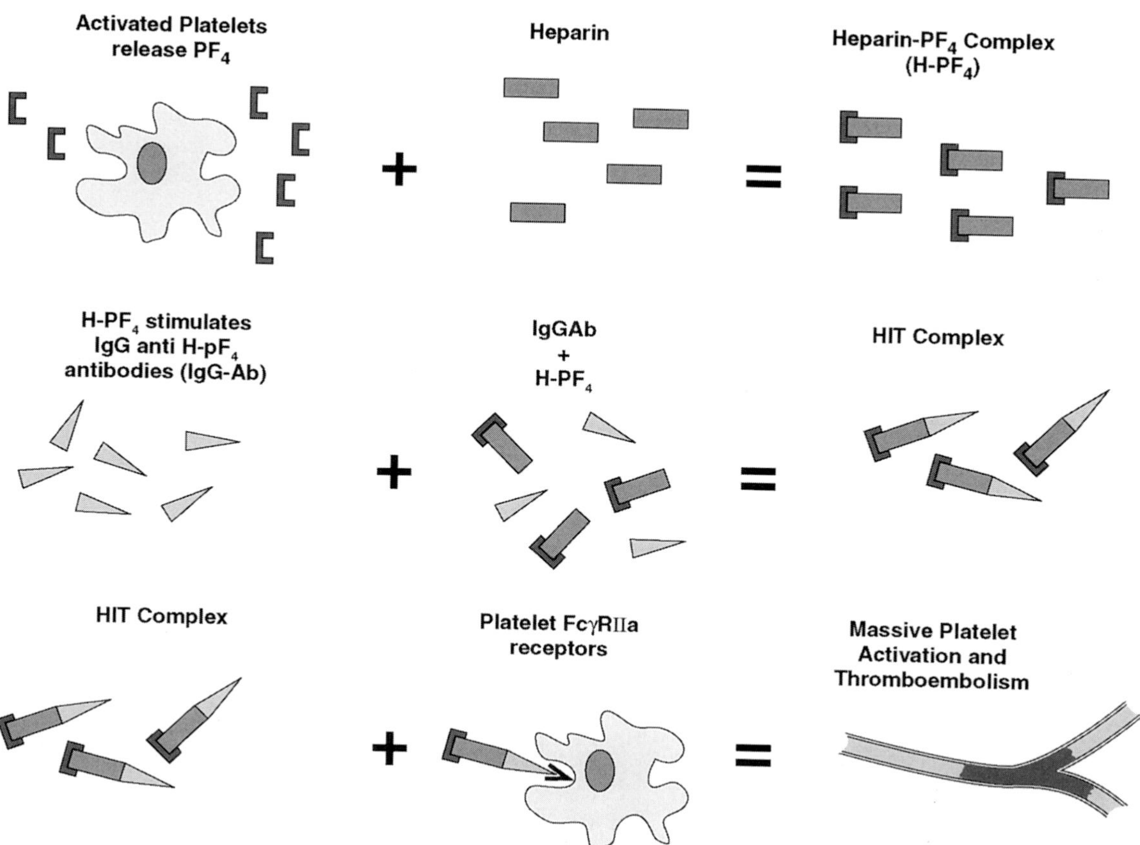

FIGURE 11–11 The generation of HIT complexes. Read each horizontal group of three left to right beginning at top left. See text for full explanation.

thrombocytopenia and HITT in those with either venous or arterial thrombosis or both. It is important to stress that HIT or HITT is a clinical diagnosis and that a positive antibody test is not required before stopping heparin.

Once the diagnosis of HIT or HITT is suspected, management must focus on prevention of further intravascular thrombosis. Bleeding is rarely the problem; intravascular thrombosis is. Neither heparin nor platelet transfusions should be given; platelet transfusions only add more PF4 if heparin and IgG anti-H-PF4 antibodies are still circulating. If heparin is proven absent from the circulation, platelet transfusions may be used very cautiously if the patient has significant nonsurgical bleeding. Surgical measures to reopen thrombosed large arteries are usually futile because the platelet-rich thrombus (white clot) often extends into small arteries and arterioles. An inferior vena cava filter is recommended if pulmonary embolism is likely or has occurred.

Modern management also includes full anticoagulation with recombinant hirudin (Lepirudin), argatroban, or possibly bivalirudin to prevent further extension of thrombosis or development of clinical intravascular thrombosis. This may occur in 40% to 50% of patients with HIT who are treated only with heparin cessation.[408] At present there is little experience with argatroban in cardiac surgical patients with HITT, but the drug is a direct thrombin inhibitor, has attractive pharmokinetics, and is approved for patients with HITT. Full anticoagulation with hirudin in fresh postoperative cardiac surgical patients is recommended, but the safety zone between bleeding and thrombosis is narrow. The patient must be carefully monitored for pericardial tamponade and signs of hidden bleeding. Hirudin is monitored by aPTT and the range used is similar to that with intravenous heparin. The effective blood concentration of hirudin for thrombin inhibition is 0.5 to 1.5 μg/mL.[409] To achieve this, 0.2 mg/kg/h infusions are recommended.[409] Dose must be reduced in patients with renal failure because the kidney clears the drug. Argatroban is sometimes a better choice, but it should be remembered that it is difficult to manage in the presence of liver disease since it is metabolized in that organ. In most patients oral anticoagulation with warfarin is started at the same time as intravenous hirudin, but warfarin should not be started prior to hirudin.

Emergency or urgent open heart surgery with CPB using hirudin is possible in patients with circulating IgG anti-HPF4 antibodies. The therapeutic level of drug should be between 3.5 and 4.5 μg/mL during CPB.[409] Greinacher recommends bolus doses of 0.25 mg/kg IV and 0.2 mg/kg in the priming volume followed by an infusion of 0.5 mg/min until 15 minutes before stopping CPB.[409] At that time 5 mg of hirudin is added to the perfusate to prevent clotting within the heart-lung machine.

Patients who require elective cardiac surgery are best deferred until circulating IgG anti-H-PF4 antibodies are absent by enzyme immunoassay. Patients with a history of HIT who require elective cardiac surgery with CPB should have IgG anti-H-PF4 antibodies measured in their serum before surgery is scheduled. If antibodies are absent, elective surgery can be safely carried out using heparin anticoagulation, *if the first reexposure to heparin is the bolus dose given just before starting CPB*. Since HIT requires the presence of the H-PF4 complex plus IgG anti-H-PF4 antibodies to form the HIT complex, and since it takes about 5 days to produce these antibodies, HIT or HITT will not occur if no further heparin is given after operation.

GENERATION OF THROMBIN

Generation of thrombin during cardiopulmonary bypass and other applications of extracorporeal circulatory technology is the cause of the thrombotic and bleeding complications associated with ECP. Theoretically, if thrombin formation could be completely inhibited during ECP, the consumptive coagulopathy, which consumes coagulation proteins and platelets and causes bleeding complications, would not occur.

Thrombin generation and the fibrinolytic response primarily involve the extrinsic and intrinsic coagulation pathways, the contact and fibrinolytic plasma protein systems, and platelets, monocytes, and endothelial cells.

Contact System

The contact system includes four primary plasma proteins—factor XII, prekallikrein, high molecular weight kininogen (HMWK), and C-1 inhibitor[410]—and is activated during CPB and clinical cardiac surgery.[411] This system is involved in complement and neutrophil activation and the inflammatory response to ECP, but is not involved in thrombin formation in vivo. However, when blood contacts a negatively charged surface (protein surfaces contain both positive and negative charges) in ECP, small amounts of factor XII are adsorbed and undergo a conformational change to factor XIIa.[373,412] Factor XIIa in the presence of HMWK activates factor XI and initiates the intrinsic coagulation pathway (Fig. 11-12). Thrombin also activates factor XI, and is the predominating agonist in vivo in pathologic states.[413]

Intrinsic Coagulation Pathway

The intrinsic coagulation pathway probably does not generate thrombin in vivo, but does initiate thrombin formation when blood contacts nonendothelial cell surfaces such as perfusion circuits.[414,415] Factor XIa, produced by activation of the contact system and subsequently thrombin generation, activates factor IX, which forms part of the intrinsic tenase complex.[416,417] Factor XI is primarily activated by thrombin (see Fig. 11-12).

Extrinsic (Tissue Factor) Coagulation Pathway

The extrinsic coagulation pathway is the major coagulation pathway in vivo and is a major source of thrombin generation during CPB and clinical cardiac surgery.[418,419] Exposure of blood to tissue factor initiates the extrinsic coagulation pathway.[417] Tissue factor (TF) is a cell-bound glycoprotein that is constitutively expressed on the cellular surfaces of fat, muscle, bone, epicardium, adventia, injured endothelial cells, and many other cells except pericardium.[419–421] Plasma TF associated with wound monocytes is a second source of TF and may be an important source during CPB and clinical cardiac surgery (authors' unpublished data; ref. 422). Tissue factor is the cofactor for the activation of factor VII to factor VIIa, which is part of extrinsic tenase (see Fig. 11-12).

Tenase Complexes

Intrinsic and extrinsic tenase catalyze the activation of factor X to factor Xa (see Fig. 11-12). Extrinsic tenase is formed by the combination of tissue factor, factor VIIa, calcium, and a phospholipid surface to cleave a small peptide from factor X to form factor Xa.[417] Extrinsic tenase also generates small amounts of factor IXa,[423] which greatly accelerates formation of intrinsic tenase and is the major pathway for the formation of factor Xa. Intrinsic tenase is produced by the combination of factor IXa, factor VIIIa, and calcium on the surface of an activated platelet,[424] and catalyzes production of factor Xa 50 times faster than extrinsic tenase.[417] Factor Xa activates factors V and VII in feedback loops.

Common Coagulation Pathway

Factor Xa is the gateway protein of the common coagulation pathway. Factor Xa slowly cleaves prothrombin to α-thrombin, the active enzyme, and a fragment, F1.2, but the reaction is 300,000 times faster if catalyzed by the *prothrombinase complex*.[417] The prothrombinase complex is produced when factor Xa, in the presence of Ca^{2+}, is anchored by factor Va onto a phospholipid surface provided by platelets, monocytes, or endothelial cells.[417] Either factor Xa or thrombin activates factor V to factor Va. The prothrombinase complex cleaves prothrombin to α-thrombin and a fragment, F1.2,

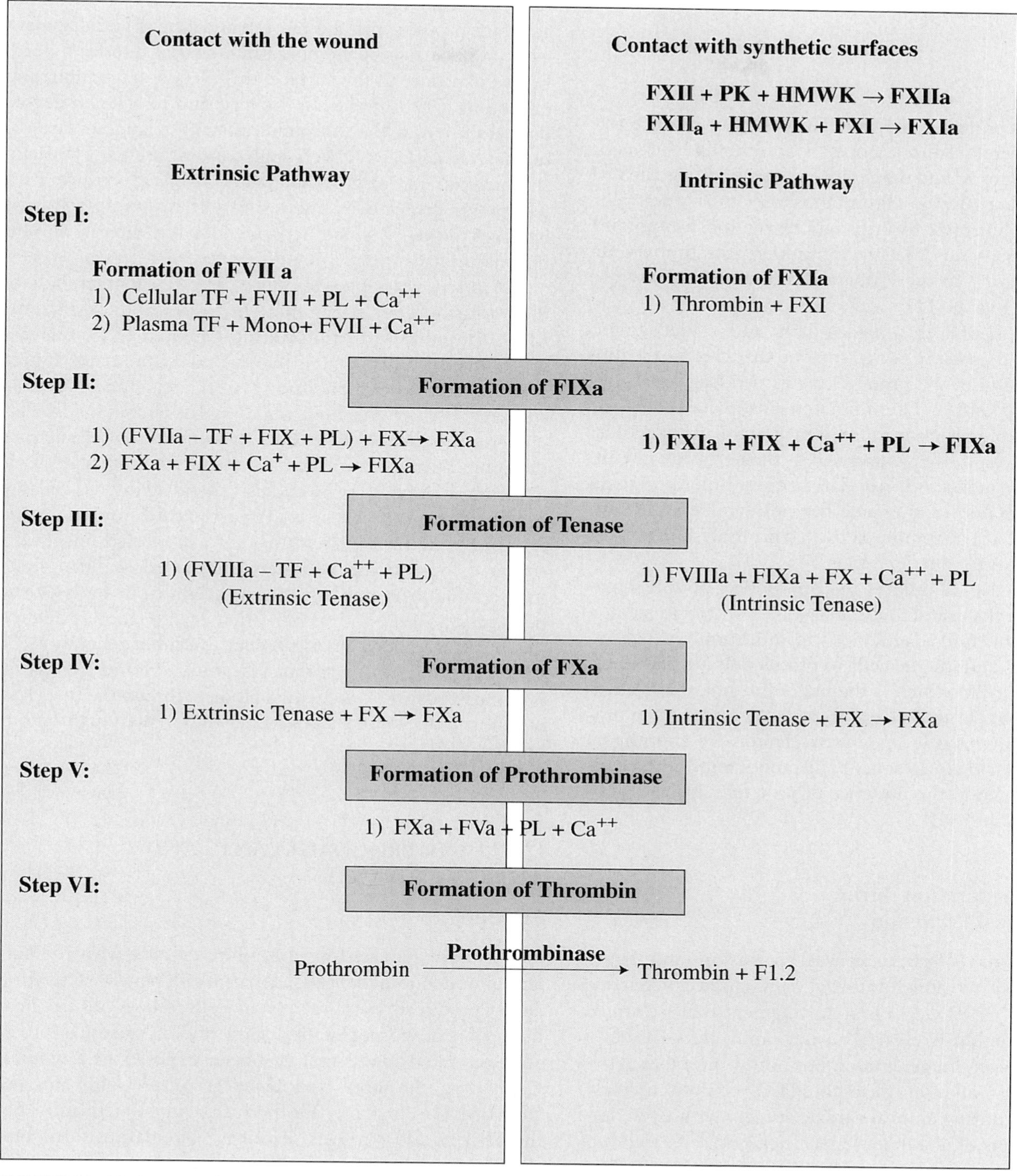

FIGURE 11–12 Steps in the generation of thrombin in the wound and in the perfusion circuit via the extrinsic, intrinsic, and common coagulation pathways. PK, prekallikrein; HMWK, high molecular weight kininogen; Ca++, calcium ion; PL, cellular phospholipid surface; TF, tissue factor; mono, monocyte. Activated coagulation proteins are indicated by the suffix "a."

and is the major pathway producing thrombin.[417] F1.2 is a useful marker of the reaction.

Thrombin

Thrombin is a powerful enzyme that accelerates its own formation by several feedback loops.[425] Thrombin is the major activator of factor XI and the exclusive activator of factor VIII in the intrinsic pathway. Thrombin is a secondary activator of factor VII, but once formed may be the most important activator in the wound. Lastly, thrombin is the primary activator of factor V in the formation of the prothrombinase complex (see Fig. 11-12).

Thrombin has both procoagulant and anticoagulant properties.[425] Thrombin is the enzyme that cleaves fibrinogen to fibrin and in the process creates two fragments, fibrinopeptides A and B. Thrombin activates platelets via the platelet thrombin receptor and thus may be the major agonist for platelets both in the wound and in the perfusion circuit. Thrombin also activates factor XIII to cross-link fibrin to an insoluble form and to attenuate fibrinolysis. Lastly, thrombin activates TAFI, thrombin-activated fibrinolysis inhibitor, which alters fibrin to reduce lysis.[425]

Thrombin also stimulates the production of anticoagulants. Surface glycosaminoglycans, such as heparan sulfate, inhibit thrombin and coagulation via antithrombin. Thrombin stimulates endothelial cells to produce tissue plasminogen activator, t-PA, which is the major enzyme that cleaves plasminogen to plasmin. Thrombin also stimulates the production of nitric oxide and prostaglandin by endothelial cells. Thrombin in the presence of thrombomodulin activates protein C, which in the presence of protein S destroys activated factor V and VIII.

Thrombin Generation during Extracorporeal Perfusion

All applications of extracorporeal perfusion and exposure of blood to nonendothelial cell surfaces generate thrombin.[365–367] F1.2 is a protein fragment that is formed when prothrombin is cleaved to thrombin; thus F1.2 is a measure of thrombin generation but not of thrombin activity. F1.2 and thrombin-antithrombin (TAT) complex increase progressively during clinical cardiac surgery with CPB, during applications of circulatory assist devices[368,379] and during extracorporeal life support (ECLS) (see Fig. 11-10). The amount of thrombin produced seems to vary with the intensity of the stimuli for thrombin production and may vary with age, comorbid disease, and clinical health of the patient. The cytokines, IL-1β and TNF-α, are procoagulant and inhibit the thrombomodulin/protein C anticoagulant pathway and stimulate production of type I plasminogen activator inhibitor.[426] Complex cardiac surgery that requires several hours of CPB produces more F1.2[366] than short procedures with minimal exposure of circulating blood to the wound (e.g., first-time myocardial revascularization).[427] Thrombin generation varies with the amount and type of anticoagulant used; surface area of the blood-biomaterial interface; duration of exposure to the surface; turbulence, stagnation, and cavitation within perfusion circuits; and to a lesser degree temperature and the "thromboresistant" characteristics of biomaterial surfaces.[428] Very high concentrations of heparin, sufficient to increase spontaneous bleeding, reduce F1.2 production probably by interfering with thrombin-activated feedback loops,[429] since heparin does not directly inhibit thrombin formation.

For many years blood contact with the biomaterials of the perfusion circuit was thought to be the major stimulus to thrombin formation during CPB and OHS. Increasing evidence indicates that the wound is the major source of thrombin generation during CPB and clinical cardiac surgery.[365,366,430] This understanding has encouraged development of strategies to reduce the amounts of circulating thrombin during clinical cardiac surgery by either discarding wound blood[431] or by exclusively salvaging red cells by centrifugation in a cell saver. The reduced thrombin formation in the perfusion circuit has also supported misguided strategies for reducing the systemic heparin dose during first-time coronary revascularization procedures using heparin-bonded circuits.[427,432] While there is no good evidence that heparin-bonded circuits reduce thrombin generation,[367] there is strong evidence that discarding wound plasma or limiting exposure of circulating blood to the wound (e.g., less bleeding in the wound) does reduce the circulating thrombin burden.[376,432]

CELLULAR PROCOAGULANTS AND ANTICOAGULANTS

Platelets

Platelets are activated by thrombin, contact with the surface of nonendothelial cells, heparin, and platelet-activating factor produced by a variety of cells during all applications of extracorporeal perfusion and/or recirculation of anticoagulated blood that has been exposed to a wound. Circulating thrombin and platelet contact with surface-adsorbed fibrinogen in the perfusion circuit are probably the earliest and strongest agonists. Circulating thrombin, although rapidly inhibited by antithrombin, is a powerful agonist and binds avidly to two specific thrombin receptors on platelets: PAR-1 and GPIbα.[433] As CPB continues, C5a, C5b-9,[434,435] plasmin,[436] hypothermia,[437] platelet-activating factor (PAF), interleukin-6,[438] cathepsin G, serotonin, epinephrine, eicosanoids, and other agonists also activate platelets and contribute to their loss and dysfunction.

The initial platelet reaction to agonists is shape change. Circulating discoid platelets extend pseudopods, centralize

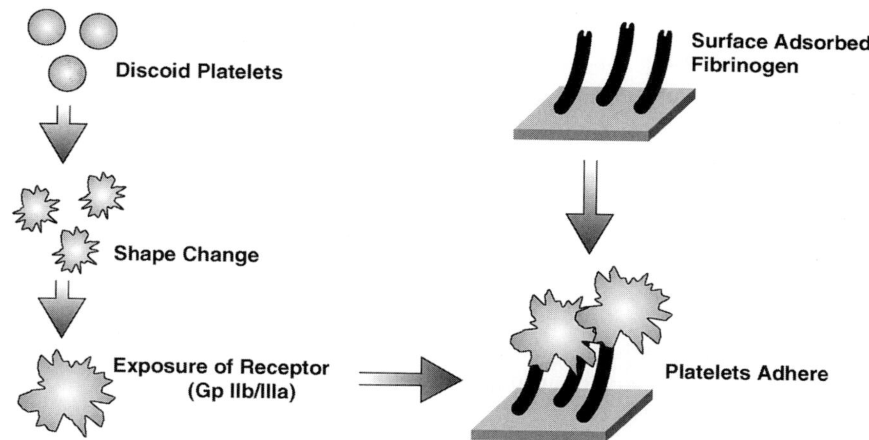

FIGURE 11–13 Adhesion of activated platelets binding to surface-adsorbed fibrinogen via GPIIb/IIIa ($\alpha_{IIb}\beta3$) receptors. The same receptors bind plasma fibrinogen molecules to form platelet aggregates.

granules, express GPIb and GPIIb/IIIa receptors,[439] and secrete soluble and bound P selectin receptors from alpha granules.[440] GPIIb/IIIa ($\alpha_{IIb}\beta3$) receptors almost instantaneously bind platelets to exposed binding sites on the α- and γ-chains on surface-adsorbed fibrinogen (Fig. 11-13).[441] The number of adherent platelets is proportional to the amount of surface-adsorbed fibrinogen recognized by fibrinogen antibody,[442] but the density of adherent platelets also varies with the chemical and physical composition of the surface biomaterial.[443,444] Rough surfaces accumulate more platelets than smooth surfaces.[445] Fewer platelets adhere to polyurethane, cuprophane, and PMEA (poly 2-methoxyethylacrylate) than to silicone rubber.[374,428] Platelet adhesion and aggregate formation reduce the circulating platelet count, which is already reduced by dilution with pump priming solutions.

Plasma fibrinogen forms bridges between platelets expressing GPIIb/IIIa receptors to produce circulating platelet aggregates. Platelet bound P-selectin binds platelets to monocytes and neutrophils to form aggregates.[446] During ECP some adherent platelets detach, leaving membrane fragments behind,[447] to produce platelet microparticles and partially fragmented platelets.[448,449] Some of these platelet membrane fragments also detach and circulate.[448,449]

A small percentage of activated platelets synthesize and release a variety of chemicals and proteins from granules that include thromboxane A2,[450] platelet factor 4, β-thromboglobulin,[451] P-selectin, and serotonin. Platelet lysosomes release neutral proteases and acid hydrolases.[452]

During ECP the circulating platelet pool is reduced by dilution, adhesion, aggregation, destruction, and consumption. The platelet mass consists of a reduced number of morphologically normal platelets, platelets with pseudopod formation, new and larger platelets released from megakaryocytes,[453] partially and completely degranulated platelets, platelet membrane fragments, platelet microparticles, and resealed platelets that have lost some of their membrane receptors.[446,447,452,453] Most of the circulating platelets appear structurally normal,[453] but bleeding times increase and remain prolonged for several hours after protamine.[454] The functional state of the circulating intact platelet during and early after CPB is reduced, but it is not clear whether this functional defect is intrinsic or extrinsic to the platelet. Flow cytometry studies of circulating intact platelets show little change in platelet membrane receptors.[455] In prolonged applications of ECP, platelets are consumed and may or may not be adequately replaced by new platelets from the bone marrow.[456]

Monocytes

During CPB and clinical cardiac surgery the concentration of plasma tissue factor, which normally is 0.26 to 1.1 pM,[422,457] doubles to 2.0 pM.[422] During cardiac surgery wound plasma contains 6 to 11 pM.[422] In the wound with calcium present, monocytes associate with plasma tissue factor to rapidly accelerate the conversion of factor VII to factor VIIa (authors' unpublished data). This association is specific for monocytes—the reaction is essentially nil for platelets, neutrophils, and lymphocytes—and does not occur if monocytes, plasma tissue factor, or factor VII is not present. Monocytes also synthesize and express tissue factor, but this process, which peaks 3 to 4 hours after monocytes are activated,[458] is not a major source of tissue factor during CPB and clinical heart surgery but does occur during prolonged perfusions.[459] Plasma microparticles, also present in wound plasma, are procoagulant[460] and monocytes may express the procoagulant CD 11b receptor,[461] but the clinical importance of these pathways in thrombin generation is not clear and probably minor. The major sources of tissue factor in the wound are the combination of monocytes, plasma tissue factor, and cell-bound tissue factor.

Agonists for activating monocytes during CPB and clinical cardiac surgery include C5a,[462] endotoxin, IL-6, IL-1β, tumor necrosis factor (TNF-α), and monocyte chemotactic protein-1 (MCP-1). Monocytes and macrophages produce

MCP-1, IL-1β, IL-6, and TNF-α[463,464]; express tissue factor,[458] Mac-1,[461] L-selectin, and monocyte chemotactic protein –1 (MCP-1)[465]; and form aggregates with platelets.[440] For the most part, monocyte reactions are slow and peak concentrations of cytokines occur several hours after CPB ends.[466–468]

Endothelial Cells

Endothelial cells, charged with maintaining the fluidity of circulating blood and the integrity of the vascular system, are activated during CPB and clinical cardiac surgery by thrombin, C5a,[469] IL-1, and TNF-α.[470] Endothelial cells produce both procoagulants and anticoagulants. Procoagulant activities of endothelial cells include expression of tissue factor and production of a host of procoagulant proteins, including collagen, elastin, microfibillar protein, laminin, fibronectin, thrombospondin, von Willebrand factor, factor V, platelet-activating factor, and plasminogen activator inhibitor 1, and the vasoconstrictors, endothelin-1 and renin. Endothelial cells also bind von Willebrand factor, vibronectin, and factors IXa and Xa. Anticoagulant activities of endothelial cells include the production of tissue plasminogen activator (t-PA), heparin sulfate, dermatan sulfate, protein S (which accelerates the activation of protein C), tissue factor inhibitor protein, thrombomodulin and protease nexin 1 (which both bind thrombin), prostacyclin,[471] nitric oxide, and adenosine. Prostacyclin concentrations increase rapidly at the beginning of CPB and then begin to decrease.[472] During clinical cardiac surgery endothelin-1 peaks several hours after CPB ends.[473]

Except for expression of tissue factor and expression of CD11b/CD18 (Mac-1), which is weakly procoagulant, endothelial cell receptors do not participate heavily in thrombin generation during ECP.

Neutrophils

During ECP neutrophils express Mac-1 receptors,[474] which bind factor X and fibrinogen and weakly facilitate thrombin formation. Neutrophils secrete elastase, which can destroy protease inhibitors such as antithrombin and coagulation factors such as factor V and may contribute significantly to the equilibrium between the fluid and gel forms of blood.

EMBOLI

A vast number of particulate emboli are produced during all applications of ECP and most of these emboli originate from blood constituents (see sections 11A and 11D). These macro- and microemboli contribute to temporary and permanent organ damage and impairment of neurocognitive function. Emboli directly produced by activation of the coagulation system during ECP include fibrin; platelet microparticles, fragments, and aggregates; and platelet-leukocyte aggregates.

FIBRINOLYSIS

Circulating thrombin activates endothelial cells to produce tissue plasminogen activator (t-PA), which binds avidly to fibrin.[475–477] Endothelial cells are the principal source of t-PA.[476] The combination of t-PA, fibrin, and plasminogen cleaves plasminogen to plasmin; plasmin cleaves fibrin.[476] This reaction produces the protein fragment, D-dimer, which is a useful marker of fibrinolysis, and a marker of thrombin activity because fibrin is cleaved from fibrinogen by thrombin. Kallikrein, produced by the contact system, cleaves pro-urokinase to urokinase; however, this enzyme is less important in fibrinolysis than t-PA because urokinase binds poorly to fibrin.[476] F1.2, D-dimer, and fibrinopeptide A (produced by the conversion of fibrinogen to fibrin) increase during extracorporeal perfusion, indicating ongoing thrombin production, fibrin formation, and fibrinolysis.[366,367,478,479] D-dimer and other fibrin degradation products are themselves anticoagulants inhibiting fibrin polymerization.[476]

Fibrinolysis is controlled by native protease inhibitors, α2-antiplasmin, α2-macroglobulin, and plasminogen activator inhibitor-1.[477] Plasminogen activator inhibitor-1, produced by endothelial cells, directly inhibits t-PA and urokinase, but little is produced during CPB and open cardiac surgery.[480] Alpha 2-antiplasmin rapidly inhibits unbound plasmin, preventing the enzyme from circulating, but poorly inhibits plasmin bound to fibrin. Alpha 2-macroglobulin is a slow inhibitor of plasmin.

Plasmin is both a stimulator and inhibitor of platelets depending upon concentration and temperature.[481] High concentrations of plasmin at normothermia and low concentrations during hypothermia cause conformational changes in platelets, centralization of platelet granules, and internalization of platelet GPIb receptors but not GPIIb/IIIa receptors.[482]

CONSUMPTIVE COAGULOPATHY

Simultaneous and ongoing thrombin formation and fibrinolysis is by definition a consumptive coagulopathy[483] and is present in all applications of ECP. In the normal state the fluidity of blood and the integrity of the vascular system are established and maintained by an equilibrium between procoagulants favoring clot and anticoagulants favoring liquidity (Fig. 11-14A). Blood contact with ECP systems and the wound disrupts this equilibrium to produce a massive procoagulant stimulus that overwhelms natural

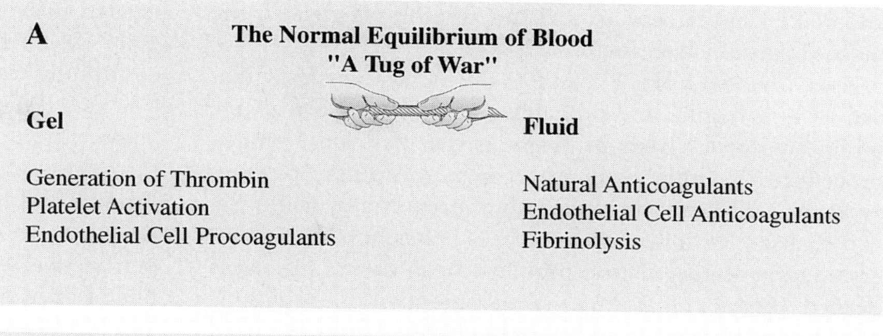

B

A New Equilibrium
CPB and OHS

Thrombosis

Wound and Circuit
Generator of Thrombin
Platelet Activation
Soluble Tissue Factor

Bleeding

Heparin
Fibrinolysis
Platelet Dysfunction

FIGURE 11–14 (A) The balance between procoagulant and anticoagulant forces that produces an equilibrium allows blood to circulate. (B) During CPB and OHS (open heart surgery) the normal equilibrium is disturbed by changes in both procoagulants and anticoagulants. Imbalance of procoagulants risks thrombosis; an imbalance of anticoagulants risks bleeding.

anticoagulants; therefore, an exogenous anticoagulant, heparin, is required for nearly all applications of ECP (Fig. 11-14B). Exceptions are only possible in applications that produce a relatively weak procoagulant stimulus and a minimal thrombin burden that can be contained by natural anticoagulants. Surgeons must realize that any blood exposure to nonendothelial cell surfaces, including prosthetic heart valves, produces a procoagulant stimulus whether or not clot is produced. Except for the healthy endothelial cell, no nonthrombogenic surface exists.

This concept of an equilibrium between procoagulants and anticoagulants is helpful in managing the thrombotic and bleeding complications associated with all applications of ECP. During ECP procoagulant stimuli, manifested by thrombin formation that is not measurable in real time, must be balanced by *either* increased anticoagulation or a reduction in the thrombin burden to maintain equilibrium. After ECP, anticoagulants must be inhibited to avoid excessive bleeding. During consumptive coagulopathy, coagulation proteins and platelets are consumed and may become too deficient to generate thrombin and fibrin-platelet clots. In cardiac surgical patients many additional variables affect the coagulation equilibrium and impact the availability of coagulation proteins and functional platelets. These variables include the quantity of blood in contact with the wound; surface area of the perfusion system; duration of perfusion; circulating anticoagulants; and to lesser degrees temperature and the rheology and biomaterials of the perfusion system. Patient factors also affect the coagulation equilibrium; these include age, infection, history or presence of cardiogenic shock, massive blood losses and transfusions, platelet coagulation deficiencies, fibrinolysis, liver disease, cachexia, reoperation, and hypothermia.

MANAGEMENT OF BLEEDING

The cornerstone of bleeding management is meticulous surgical hemostasis during all phases of an operation. The surgical techniques, topical agents, and customary drugs used do not need reiteration for trained surgeons. Most cardiac surgical operations involving CPB are accompanied by net blood losses between 200 to 600 mL. Reoperations; complex procedures; prolonged (>3 hours) cardiopulmonary bypass; and patient factors listed above may be associated with excessive and ongoing blood losses. Most surgeons use an antifibrinolytic, such as aprotonin or epsilon amino caproic acid, to reduce fibrinolysis in prolonged or complex operations. Problem patients who bleed excessively after heparin neutralization require an attempt to rebalance pro- and anticoagulants to near normal, pre–CPB concentrations.

The most useful tests in the operating room are an activated clotting time or a protamine titration test to assess the presence of heparin; prothrombin time to uncover deficiency in the extrinsic coagulation pathway; and platelet count. If heparin is neutralized, the partial thromboplastin time may be measured to assess possible deficiency of coagulation proteins. Other tests such as measurements of fibrinogen, template bleeding time, and the thromboelastograph are controversial and/or difficult to obtain. Platelet counts below 80,000 to 100,000/μL should initiate platelet transfusions in bleeding patients, except those with IgG anti-H-PF4 antibodies, to add functioning platelets to the mass of partially dysfunctional platelets.

Measurements of F1.2 and D-dimer are two tests that can be very helpful and probably should be made available on an emergency basis in hospitals that perform complex procedures and offer mechanical circulatory and respiratory assistance. F1.2 measures thrombin formation by factor Xa, and if absent or low, there may be a deficiency in the concentrations of coagulation proteins; fresh frozen plasma is needed. If F1.2 and D-dimer (a measurement of fibrinolytic activity) are both elevated, thrombin is being formed and an antifibrinolytic (aprotinin or epsilon amino caproic acid) is needed to neutralize plasmin. If both markers or F1.2 remain elevated after the antifibrinolytic drug, this indicates continuing thrombin generation and the cause (e.g., infection usually) should be aggressively treated with antibiotics. Some thrombin is needed to stop bleeding, but excessive thrombin production feeds the consumptive coagulopathy. As with diffuse intravascular coagulopathy,[483] no guaranteed therapeutic recipe is known; success requires patience, persistence, and judicious use of platelets, antifibrinolytics, fresh frozen plasma, and replacement transfusions to rebalance the coagulation equilibrium at near normal concentrations of the constituents.

11C: The Inflammatory Response

Philippe Menasche/L. Henry Edmunds, Jr.

The inflammatory response to cardiopulmonary bypass (CPB) is initiated by contact between heparinized blood and nonendothelial cell surfaces.[484–486] Blood contact with nonendothelial cell surfaces in the wound and in the perfusion circuit activates plasma zymogens and cellular blood elements that constitute part of the body's defense reaction to all noxious substances including infectious agents, toxins, foreign antigens, allergens, and also injuries. All surgery, like accidental trauma, triggers an acute inflammatory response, but the continuous exposure of heparinized blood to nonendothelial cell surfaces followed by reinfusion and circulation within the body greatly magnifies this response in operations in which CPB is used. Although far from fully described and understood, this primarily "blood injury" produces a unique response, which is different in detail from that caused by other threats to homeostasis.

The principal blood elements involved in this acute defense reaction are contact and complement plasma protein systems, neutrophils, monocytes, endothelial cells, and to a lesser extent platelets. Lymphocytes are also altered by CPB,[487,488] but are more involved in the immune response to foreign proteins and acute rejection and do not materially contribute to the acute response to CPB. Likewise, eosinophils and basophil/mast cells are primarily activated by IL-5 and IgE antibodies, respectively, and have prominent roles in allergy, parasitic diseases, and histamine production. When activated during CPB, the principal blood elements release vasoactive and cytotoxic substances; produce cell signaling inflammatory and inhibitory cytokines; express complementary cellular receptors that interact with specific cell signaling substances and other cells; and generate a host of vasoactive and cytotoxic substances that circulate.[489] Normally these reactive blood elements mediate and regulate the defense reaction,[490–492] but during CPB an orderly, targeted response is overwhelmed by the massive activation and circulation of these reactive blood elements.

Admittedly there is considerable overlap between the plasma and blood cellular responses involved in bleeding and thrombosis, ischemia/reperfusion,[493] acute rejection, and acute and chronic inflammation, but these responses are separated in this book in the interests of simplification. This section offers a simplified overview of the acute inflammatory response to cardiopulmonary bypass; the detailed interactions of the body's defense system against hurtful stimuli are under active and intense investigation and are far beyond the authors' expertise.

PRIMARY BLOOD CONSTITUENTS

Complement

The complement system constitutes a group of more than 30 plasma proteins that interact to produce powerful vasoactive anaphylatoxins, C3a, C4a, and C5a, and the terminal complement cytotoxic complex, C5b-9.[494] Complement is activated by three pathways, but only the classical and alternative pathways are involved in cardiopulmonary bypass,[495,496] although a role for the manose-lectin pathway has not been excluded. Direct contact between heparinized blood and the synthetic surfaces of the extracorporeal perfusion circuit activates the contact plasma proteins and the classical complement pathway.[495] Activation of C1, possibly by activated factor XIIa, sequentially activates C2 and C4 to form C4b2a (classical C3 convertase) that cleaves C3 to form C3a and C3b (Fig. 11-15).[494]

Generation of C3b activates the alternative pathway, which involves factors B and D in the formation of C3bBb, which is the alternative pathway C3 convertase that cleaves C3 to form C3a and C3b (see Fig. 11-15). Whereas the classical pathway proceeds in sequential steps, the alternative pathway contains a feedback loop that greatly amplifies cleavage of C3 by membrane-bound C3 convertase to membrane-bound C3b and C3a. During CPB complement is largely activated by the alternative pathway.[496–498]

The complement system is activated at three different times during CPB and cardiac surgery: during blood contact with nonendothelial cell surfaces[495,499]; after protamine administration and formation of the protamine-heparin complex[495,500]; and after reperfusion of the ischemic, arrested heart.[485] CPB and myocardial reperfusion activate complement by both the classical and alternative pathways; the heparin-protamine complex activates complement by the classical pathway.[495] Other agonists that activate the classical pathway during CPB include endotoxin,[496] apoptotic cells, and C-reactive protein.[494]

The two C3 convertases effectively merge the two complement pathways by producing C3b, which activates C5 to C5a and C5b (see Fig. 11-15). C3a and C5a are potent vasoactive anaphylatoxins. C5a, which avidly binds to neutrophils and therefore is difficult to detect in plasma, is the major agonist. C3b acts as an opsonin, which binds target cell hydroxyl groups and renders them susceptible to phagocytic cells expressing specific receptors for C3b.[494,497] C5b is the first component of the terminal pathway that ultimately

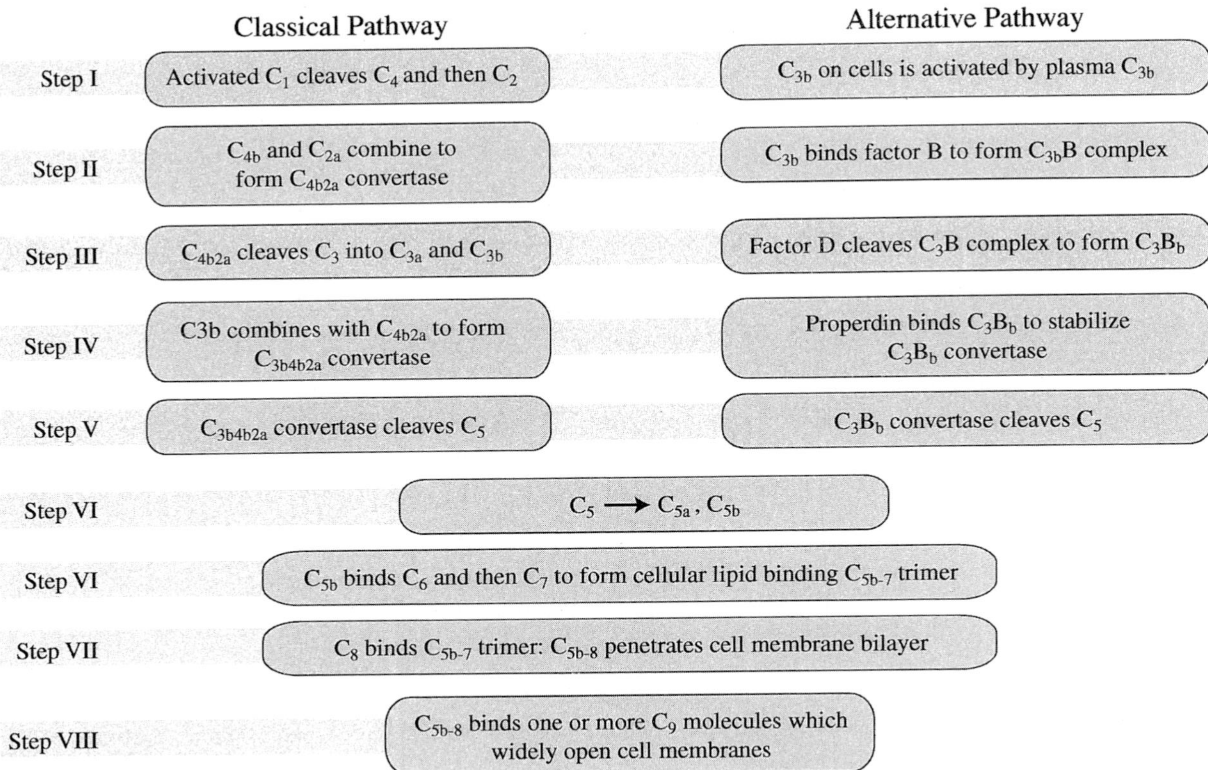

FIGURE 11–15 Steps in activation of the classical and alternative complement pathways and formation of the membrane attack complex, C5b-9. *(Adapted with permission from Walport MJ: Complement. N Engl J Med 2001; 344:1058; and Plumb ME, Sadetz JM: Proteins of the membrane attack complex, in Volkankis JE, Frank ME (eds): The Human Complement System in Health and Disease. New York, Marcel Dekker, 1998; p 119.)*

leads to formation of the membrane attack complex, C5b-9. In prokaryotic cells like erythrocytes, C5b-9 creates transmembrane pores, which cause death by intracellular swelling following loss of the intracellular/interstitial osmotic gradient. In eukaryotic cells, deposits of C5b-9 may not be immediately lethal but may eventually cause injury mediated by release of arachidonic acid metabolites (thromboxane A2, leukotrienes) and oxygen free radicals by macrophages and neutrophils, respectively.[497]

Together, C5a and C5b-9 play major roles in promoting neutrophil–endothelial cell interactions through upregulation of specific adhesion molecules (see below). Importantly, C5b-9 may also activate platelets and promote platelet-monocyte aggregates.[501] As such, these complement proteins contribute to neutrophil loss from the circulation by adhesion to surface-bound platelets,[501] but more importantly to endothelial cells. The interaction between complement proteins and neutrophils contributes to postoperative organ damage in both adults[502] and in children.[503]

Normally, several regulatory proteins modulate the inflammatory actions of C5a and C5b-9 by inactivating convertases, which cleave C3 and C5,[504] but these inhibitors are usually overwhelmed during CPB. Two proteins, factors H and I, are soluble; three others, complement receptor 1 (CD35), decay accelerating factor, and membrane cofactor protein (CD46), are membrane bound.[494] Factor I cleaves C3 into inactive iC3b, which cannot form C3 convertase, but can be an opsonin.[505] Factor H is the dominant complement regulatory protein and competes with factor B in binding to C3.[494] CD59 and homologous restriction factor are direct inhibitors of the membrane attack complex.[497,506]

Neutrophils

Leukocyte counts decrease in response to hemodilution during CPB and increase moderately after operation.[486,507] Only a few neutrophils attach to synthetic surfaces, to each other, or to platelets and monocytes.[507,508] Nevertheless, neutrophils are strongly activated during cardiopulmonary bypass (Fig. 11-16).[486,509] The principal agonists are kallikrein[510] and C5a[511,512] produced by the contact and complement systems, respectively.[511,513,514] C5a, generated early during CPB and clinical cardiac surgery, is a particularly potent chemotactic protein that induces neutrophil

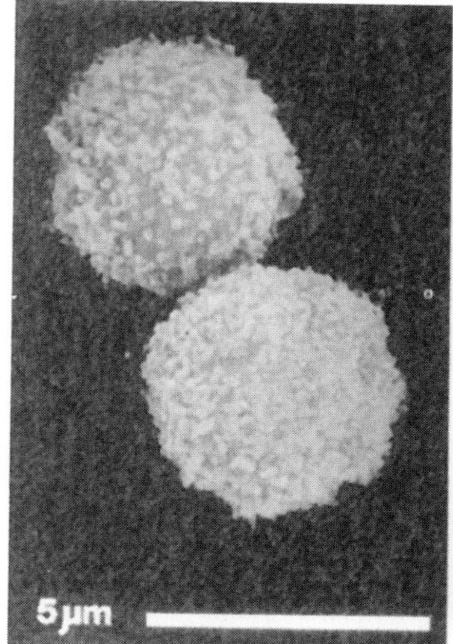

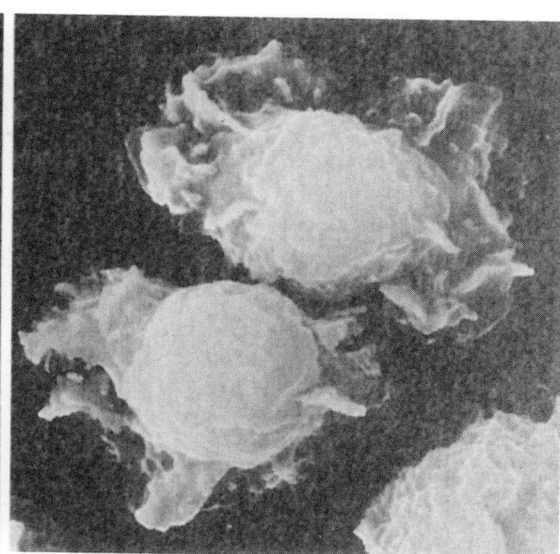

FIGURE 11–16 Scanning electron micrographs of resting neutrophils (left) and 5 seconds after exposure to a chemoattractant. (*Reproduced with permission from Baggiolini M: Chemokines and leukocyte traffic. Nature 1998; 392:565.*)

chemotaxis, degranulation, and superoxide generation.[515] Other agonists involved during CPB include IL1-β,[516] TNF-α,[492,517] IL-8,[518] C5b-9,[512] factor XIIa,[519] heparin, histamine, hypochlorous acids, and products of arachidonate metabolism: B4 (LTB4),[492] platelet activating factor (PAF), and thromboxane A2.[515] Lastly, CPB, perhaps mediated by IL-6 and IL-8,[520] partially inhibits neutrophil apoptosis and prolongs the period of neutrophil activity.[521]

Neutrophils are recruited to localized areas of injury or inflammation by chemokines, complement proteins (C5a), IL-1β, TNF-α, and adhesion molecules. Neutrophils respond to the CXC (α) family of chemokines that includes IL-8, platelet factor 4 (PF4), neutrophil activating factor-2 (NAF-2), and granulocyte chemotactic protein 2.[522–524] During CPB thrombin stimulates endothelial cell production of PAF (platelet activating factor).[492] Thrombin and PAF cause rapid expression of P-selectin by endothelial cells[490] and circulating IL-1β and TNF-α stimulate endothelial cells to synthesize and express E-selectin.[490,525] Regional vasoconstriction reduces blood flow rates within local vascular beds to allow neutrophils to marginate near endothelial cell surfaces. L-selectins are constitutively expressed by all types of activated leukocytes and lightly bind to endothelial cell mucin-like glycoproteins before being shed with the onset of transmigration.[490] P-selectin weakly binds to PSGL-1 (P-selectin glycoprotein-1) on neutrophils[526]; E-selectin binds to a different sialyl Lewis antigen (CD62E). Selectin binding causes the slowly passing neutrophils to roll and eventually stop (Fig. 11-17).[527] Stronger adherence is produced by intracellular adhesion molecule-1 (ICAM-1) expressed on endothelial cells, which binds β2 neutrophil integrins, principally CD11b/CD18 (Mac-1) and to some extent CD11a/CD18.[490,528] These adhesion molecules from the immunoglobulin superfamily completely stop neutrophils[529] and the process of transmigration begins in response to chemoattractants and cytotoxins produced in the extravascular space.[530,531] PECAM-1 expressed on leukocytes and endothelial cells mediates transmigration of leukocytes.[532] This trafficking is strongly regulated by IL-8 produced by neutrophils, macrophages, and other cells. During CPB neutrophils express the Mac-1 (CD11b/CD18) receptor[533,534] and CD11c/CD18, which binds to fibrinogen and a complement fragment,[528] and VLA-4 (α1β4) receptors that are involved in cellular adhesion.[528] Neutrophil receptor CXCR1 is not affected by CPB, but CXCR2 is downregulated.[535]

Using pseudopods and following the scent of complement proteins (C5a, C3b, and iC3b),[536] IL-8,[492,518,537,538] hypochlorous acids, leukotriene B4,[539] and locally produced IL-1 and TNF-α,[492,537] neutrophils arrive at the scene of inflammation to begin the process of phagocytosis and release of cytotoxins. Organs and tissues experience periods of ischemia followed by reperfusion (lung, heart, brain) during CPB, and as a result express adhesion receptors[540] and reactive oxidants,[541] and are sources of neutrophil chemoattractants.[520,542]

Neutrophils vary considerably between individuals in expression of adhesive receptors[543] and responsiveness to chemoattractants during CPB. There also is substantial variation in measurements of soluble and cellular adhesion receptors.[534] The presence of diabetes,[544] oxidative stress,[545] and perhaps genetic factors (see below) influences expression of cellular and soluble adhesive receptors and cytokines, which affect neutrophil adhesion and release of granule contents. It is difficult to show a correlation between markers of neutrophil activation and measurements of organ dysfunction.[546]

Neutrophils contain a potent arsenal of proteolytic and cytotoxic substances. Azurophilic granules contain lysozyme, myeloperoxidase, cationic proteins, elastase,

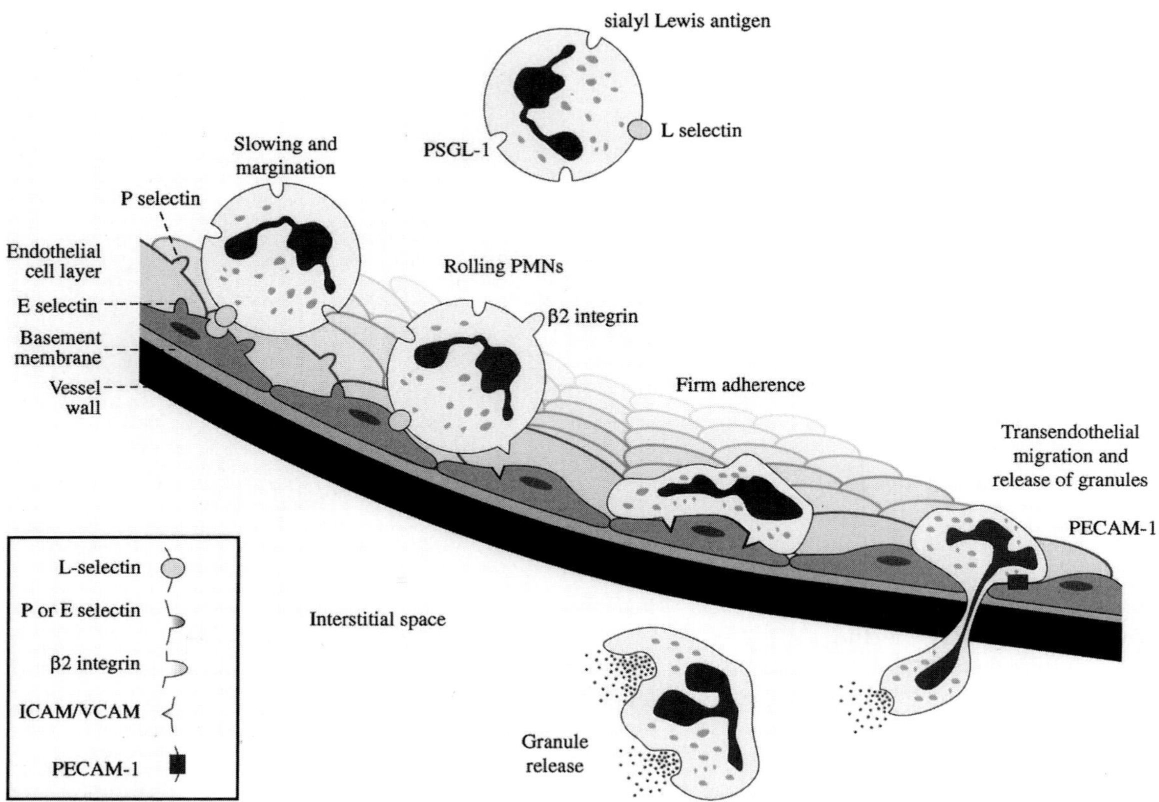

FIGURE 11–17 Mechanism of arrest and transmigration of neutrophils into the interstitial space. Neutrophils constitutively express L-selectin, which binds to endothelial cell glycoprotein ligands. Simultaneously, early response cytokines stimulate endothelial cells to rapidly express P-selectin and later E-selectin receptors, which weakly bind neutrophil PSGL-1 ligands. Marginated neutrophils, which are slowed by local vasoconstriction and reduced blood flow, lightly adhere to endothelial cells via selectin expression and begin to roll. Neutrophils activated by C5a, kallikrein, and early response cytokines express $\beta 2$ CD11b and c receptors, which bind firmly to cytokine-activated endothelial cell intergrins, ICAM-1 and VCAM-1. Once arrested, L-selectins are shed and PECAM receptors on endothelial cell surfaces mediate neutrophil transmigration through endothelial cell junctions, led by chemoattractants into the interstitial space.

collagenases, proteinase 3, acid hydrolases, defensins, and phospholipase.[547] Specific granules contain $\beta 2$ integrins, lactoferrin, lysozyme, type IV collagenase, histaminase, heparanase, complement activator, alkaline phosphatase, and membrane-associated NADPH (nicotinamide adenine dinucleotide) phosphate oxidase.[515] Activated neutrophils, in a "respiratory burst," also produce cytotoxic reactive oxygen and nitrogen intermediates including superoxide anion, hydrogen peroxide, hydroxyl radicals, singlet oxygen molecules, N-chloramines, hypochlorous acids, and peroxynitrite.[490,548] Finally, neutrophils produce arachidonate metabolites, prostaglandins, leukotrienes, and platelet-activating factor. During CPB these vasoactive and cytotoxic substances are produced and released into the extracellular environment and circulation.[486,489] Circulation of these substances mediates many of the manifestations of the "whole body inflammatory response" or "systemic inflammatory response syndrome" (SIRS) associated with CPB and clinical cardiac surgery.[549]

Monocytes

Monocytes and macrophages (tissue monocytes) are relatively large, long-lived cells that are involved in both acute and chronic inflammation. Monocytes respond to chemical signals, are mobile, phagocytize microorganisms and cell fragments, produce and secrete chemical mediators, participate in the immune response, and generate cytotoxins.[550] Monocytes are activated during CPB[551] and have a major role in thrombin formation[552] (see section 11B). Monocytes also produce and release many inflammatory mediators during acute inflammation including proinflammatory cytokines (principally TNF-α, IL-1β, IL-6, IL-8, and MCP-1), reactive oxygen and nitrogen intermediates, and prostaglandins.[524]

The mechanism by which monocytes are initially activated during CPB is not known, but the most likely candidates are C5a,[550] thrombin,[553] platelet factor 4 (PF-4), and bradykinin,[554] which are four potent agonists rapidly generated from blood contact with nonendothelial cell surfaces. Monocytes possess a huge list of surface receptors,[550] but those apt to be involved in the inflammatory response to CPB are C5a and three other complement proteins; IL-1, CD11b/CD18, and CD 11c/CD18; LTB4; and the C-C family of chemokine receptors.[550] Monocytes also possess C-reactive protein receptors, which, when activated, strongly upgrade proinflammatory cytokine production.[491]

C-C chemokines, MCP-1-4 (monocyte chemotactic protein), MIP-α, MIP-β (monocyte inhibitor protein), and RANTES (regulated upon activation, normal T cell expressed and presumably secreted), are produced by a variety of cells including monocytes and are potent activators of monocytes.[550] LTB4, cathepsin G, and azurodidin from neutrophils[538]; C5a; PF-4, platelet-derived growth factor, and platelet-activating factor (PAF); thrombin[553]; and the C-C family of chemokines are chemotactic for monocytes. Monocytes express $\beta 1$, $\beta 2$, and VLA-4 ($\alpha 1 \beta 4$) integrins, which adhere to the immunoglobulin endothelial cell receptors ICAM-1, 2, and VCAM-1 to enable monocyte trafficking in response to chemotactic stimuli.[490]

Monocytes are the major source of the early response cytokines IL-1β and TNF-α,[491,554] which play an important role in directing both neutrophils and monocytes to local sites of inflammation. Monocytes are also the major producer of IL-8,[491] which also is produced by neutrophils[492] and induces neutrophil chemotaxis.[490] Other cytokines produced by monocytes include IL-1α, IL-6, and IL-10.[491] Monocytes also produce important growth factors, matrix proteins, interferons, and a variety of enzymes, including elastase, collagenases, acid hydrolases, prostaglandins, and lipooxygenase products,[524] and contain myeloperoxidase, which converts H_2O_2 into more powerful oxidants. Most of the cytotoxic substances—both oxygen-dependent (superoxide anion, hydroxyl radical, singlet oxygen, N-chloramines, and hypochlorous acids) and oxygen-independent (prostaglandins, leukotrienes, platelet activating factor, lysosomal proteases, lactoferrin, lysozyme, and defensins)—are released into phagosomes, and the amount of monocyte-derived cytotoxins that circulate is difficult to differentiate from cytotoxins produced by activated neutrophils. Lastly, monocytes generate nitric oxide (NO), which can react with reactive oxygen intermediates to produce reactive nitrogen compounds.

Endothelial Cells

Endothelial cells are activated during CPB and OHS by a variety of agonists. The principal agonists for endothelial cell activation during CPB are thrombin, C5a,[555] and the cytokines IL-1β and TNF-α.[537,556] Other agonists, such as endotoxin, histamine, and INF-γ (from lymphocytes), are less important during CPB, and endothelial cells are largely unresponsive to chemokines.[525]

IL-1β and TNF-α induce the early expression of P-selectin and the later synthesis and expression of E-selectin, which are involved in the initial stages of neutrophil and monocyte adhesion.[490] The two cytokines also induce expression of ICAM-1 and VCAM-1, which firmly bind neutrophils and monocytes to the endothelium and initiate leukocyte trafficking to the extravascular space (see Fig. 11-17).[492,525,537] Experimentally ICAM-1 is upregulated during CPB in pulmonary vessels[557] and there is evidence that P- and E-selectins are upregulated during CPB and in myocardial ischemia-reperfusion sequences. IL-1β and TNF-α induce endothelial cell production of the chemotactic proteins IL-8 and MCP-1, and induce production of PGI2 (prostacyclin) by the cyclooxygenase pathway[532,558] and NO by NO synthase.[532,559] These two vasodilators reduce shear stress and increase vascular permeability and therefore enhance leukocyte adhesion and transmigration. Lastly, IL-1β and TNF-α stimulate endothelial cell production of proinflammatory cytokines, IL-1, IL-6, IL-8, MCP-1, and PAF.[525]

In addition to NO and PGI2, endothelial cells produce the vasoconstrictor endothelin-1[489,560] and inactivate other vasoactive mediators, including histamine, norepinephrine, and bradykinin.[561] Prostacyclin concentrations increase rapidly at the beginning of CPB and then begin to decrease.[562] Endothelin-1 peaks several hours after CPB ends.[563]

Platelets

Platelets are probably initially activated during CPB by thrombin, which is the most potent platelet agonist, but plasma epinephrine, PAF, vasopressin,[564] cathepsin G[565] from other cells, serotonin and ADP secreted by platelets, and internally generated thromboxane A2[566] contribute to activation as CPB continues.[489] Platelets possess several protease-activated receptors[564] to most of these agonists and to collagen, which has an important role in adhesion and thrombus formation. Collagen binding causes release of thromboxane A2 and ADP, which help recruit platelets.[564] Platelets contribute to the inflammatory response by synthesis and release of eicosanoids[566]; serotonin from dense granules; IL-1β[567]; CXC chemokines, PF4, NAP-2 (neutrophil activating protein), IL-8, and ENA-78 (endothelial cell neutrophil attractant); and C-C chemokines, MIP-1a, MCP-3, and RANTES[568] from alpha granules. Platelets also produce and release acid hydrolases from membrane-bound lysozymes. Platelet-secreted cytokines, NAP-2, RANTES, PF4, IL-1β, IL-8, and ENA-78 may be particularly involved in the inflammatory response to CPB because of strong activation of platelets in both the wound and perfusion circuit.

Circulating monocytes and neutrophils constitutively express PSGL-1, which interacts with aggregated platelets via P-selectin expressed on activated platelets.[526] Platelets aggregate using platelet GPIIb/IIIa ($\alpha 2b\beta 3$) receptors attached to symmetrical fibrinogen molecules to form bridges between platelets. During CPB platelets aggregate with each other and also to monocytes and neutrophils.[507,561]

OTHER MEDIATORS OF INFLAMMATION

Anaphylatoxins

The anaphylatoxins C3a, C4a, and C5a are bioactive protein fragments released by cleavage of complement proteins C3, C4, and C5. These fragments have potent proinflammatory and immunoregulatory functions and contract smooth muscle cells, increase vascular permaeability, serve as chemoattractants, and in the case of C5a, activate neutrophils and monocytes.[514] Anaphylatoxins contribute to increased pulmonary vascular resistance, edema, and neutrophil sequestration and an increase in extravascular water during CPB. The duration of postoperative ventilation directly correlates with plasma C3a concentrations.[502] C3a and C5a are important mediators in ischemia/reperfusion injuries. All three anaphylatoxins are produced during CPB, but the amount of C4a is small until protamine is given[569,570] and nearly all C5a is bound to neutrophils.[492] C3a is the principal circulating anaphylatoxin.[485,569,570]

Cytokines

Cytokines are small, cell-signaling peptides produced and released into blood or the extravascular environment by both blood and tissue cells. Cytokines stimulate specific receptors on other cells to initiate a response in that cell. All blood leukocytes and endothelium produce cytokines, but many tissue cells including fibroblasts, smooth muscle cells, cardiac myocytes, keratinocytes, chrondrocytes, hepatocytes, microglial cells, astrocytes, endometrial cells, and epithelial cells also produce cytokines.[537,554,571] IL-1β and TNF-α are early response cytokines that are promptly produced at the site of injury by resident macrophages.[537] These cytokines stimulate surrounding stromal and parenchymal cells to produce more IL-1β and TNF-α and chemokines, particularly IL-8 and MCP-1, which are powerful chemoattractants for neutrophils and macrophages, respectively. Together with IL-6, the cytokine that regulates production of acute-phase proteins (e.g., C-reactive protein, α2-macroglobulin) by the liver,[572] these five cytokines are the major proinflammatory cytokines involved in the acute inflammatory response to CPB.

The major anti-inflammatory cytokine involved during CPB is IL-10.[573] IL-10 inhibits synthesis of proinflammatory cytokines by monocytes and macrophages[574] and induces production of IL-1 receptor antagonist IL-1ra, which downgrades the response to IL-1.[554,575] IL-13 downregulates production of IL-1, IL-8, and Il-10 and reduces monocyte production of reactive oxidants[576]; its role during CPB is undetermined.

Proinflammatory cytokines increase during and after clinical cardiac surgery using CPB, but peak concentrations usually occur 12-24 hours after CPB ends (Fig. 11-18).[570,577–581] Measured amounts differ greatly in timing and within and between studies, probably because of differences in the duration of CPB, perfusion temperatures,[582] perfusion equipment, and aortic cross-clamp times; differences in methods of myocardial protection; possibly variable concentrations of inhibitory cytokines[583,584]; and perhaps exogenous factors such as priming solutions, anesthesia, and intravascular drugs.[570,577–581] Plasma concentrations of proinflammatory cytokines are significantly higher during normothermic (37°C) versus tepid (32°C-34°C) CPB.[582] The ischemic/reperfused heart is a major source of inflammatory cytokines and reactive oxidants.[541,542,585]

Some of the variation in measurements between studies also may be due to patient factors such as age, left ventricular function, and genetic factors.[586] The presence of the APOE4 allele (one of the common human polymorphisms of the gene encoding apolipoprotein E) is associated with increased TNF-α and IL-8.[586] Patients who are homozygous for TNF-β2 have elevated levels of TNF-α and IL-8 during both on- and off-pump cardiac surgery.[587] Carriers of APOE4 have reduced concentrations of IL-1ra, the inhibitory peptide of IL-1.[588] Additional hints of a genetic role in the acute inflammatory response are the association between postoperative serum creatinine and different APOε alleles[589] and the association between length of stay after coronary artery surgery and 174GG polymorphism of the IL-6 gene.[590]

α_2-Macroglobulin (α_2-M) is a ubiquitous plasma protein that inhibits all four classes of proteases and has been shown to specifically bind to TNF-α, ILl-β, IL-6, and IL-8.[591] The precise role of α_2-M in the regulation of cytokines is unknown, but the inhibitor may be involved in clearance of plasma and extravascular cytokines.[591]

Reactive Oxidants

Neutrophils, monocytes, and macrophages produce reactive oxidants, which are cytotoxic inside the phagosome, but act as cytotoxic mediators of acute inflammation outside. Four enzymes generate a large menu of reactive oxidants: NADPH (nicotinamide adenine dinucleotide phosphate) oxidase, superoxide dismutase, nitric oxide synthase, and myeloperoxidase.[548] The enzyme NADPH oxidase adds a free electron to molecular oxygen to create superoxide (O_2^-) and two hydrogen ions, H^+. Superoxide dismutase catalyzes the conversion of superoxide to hydrogen peroxide, H_2O_2, and molecular oxygen. Nitric oxide synthase produces

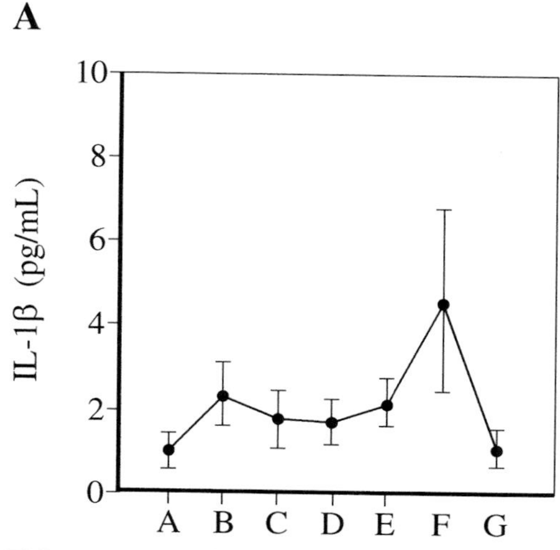

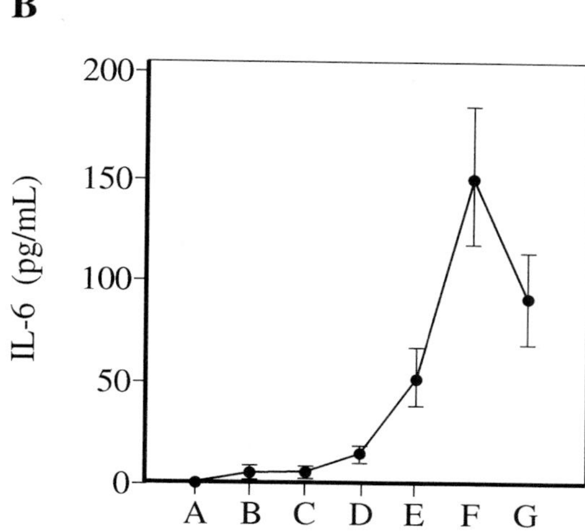

FIGURE 11–18 Changes in IL-1β (A) and IL-6 (B) in 30 patients who had elective first-time myocardial revascularization. Letters on x-axis represent the following events: A, induction of anesthesia; B, 5 minutes after heparin; C, 10 minutes after starting CPB; D, end of CPB; E, 20 minutes after protamine; F, 3 hours after CPB; G, 24 hours after CPB. *(Redrawn from Steinberg JB, Kapelanski DP, Olson JD, Weiler JM: Cytokine and complement levels in patients undergoing cardiopulmonary bypass. J Thorac Cardiovasc Surg 1993; 106:1008.)*

nitric oxide (NO) from NADPH, arginine, and oxygen, and myeloperoxidase uses $H_2O_2$to oxidize halide ions to hypochlorous acids.[592] The four products produced by these enzymes, O_2^-, H_2O_2, NO, and HOCl, generate all reactive oxidants from nonenzymatic reactions with other molecules or ions.[548]

Free radicals have one or more unpaired electrons and are highly reactive in scavenging hydrogen ions from other molecules. OH· is produced from H_2O_2 by low-valence iron or copper ions, which are reduced to the original low valence after the reaction by various reducing agents, such as ascorbic acid. Secondary free radicals, containing carbon, oxygen, nitrogen, or sulfur, are formed when a free radical reacts with molecules that lack unpaired electrons[548]; this self-perpetuating sequence produces a chain reaction of highly cytotoxic substances.

HOCl reacts with amines and amino acids, which are widely distributed in biological systems, to form chloramines and aldehydes, respectively. The products of HOCl reactions are often more toxic than the parent molecule. To varying degrees, some chloramines are lipid soluble.[548] Singlet oxygen ($^1O_2$) is a very reactive form of oxygen that is produced by neutrophils by an oxidized halogen and hydrogen peroxide. Peroxynitrite is formed by NO and superoxide (O_2^-), which produces an unknown nitrating agent that catalyzes nitration in neutrophils and macrophages.[548]

Endotoxins

Endotoxins, including lipopolysaccharides, are fragments of bacteria that are powerful agonists for complement,[593] neutrophils, monocytes, and other leukocytes. Endotoxins have been detected during CPB[593–596] and after aortic cross-clamping using a very sensitive bioassay.[597,598] Sources include contaminants within sterilized infusion solutions, the bypass circuit, and possibly the gastrointestinal tract due to changes in microvascular intestinal perfusion, which may translocate bacteria.[599] Intestinal microvascular blood flow is sensitive to both flow rate and duration of CPB. In some instances leakage of endotoxin into the systemic circulation occurs if clearance by the hepatic Kupffer cells fails. The quantitative significance of the role of endotoxin in the acute inflammatory response to CPB is unknown.

Metalloproteinases

CPB induces the synthesis and release of matrix metalloproteinases,[600] which are one of the four major classes of mammalian proteinases. These proteolytic enzymes have a major role in degradation of collagens and proteins in the extracellular matrix and vascular basement membrane and in the pathogenesis of atherosclerosis and postinfarction left ventricular remodeling. The interstitial collagenases, MMP-8 and MMP-13, increase approximately 4-fold, peak at the end of CPB and 30 minutes later, respectively, and soon return to normal plasma concentrations. The gelatinase pro-MMP-9 increases 3-fold with release of the aortic cross-clamp and remains elevated 24 hours after CPB ends. The increase in pro-MMP-2 is modest, but it remains elevated at 24 hours. The significance and possible injury produced by activation of these interstitial degradation enzymes over the long term remain to be determined.

Angry Blood

Blood circulating during clinical cardiac surgery with cardiopulmonary bypass is a stew of vasoactive and cytotoxic substances, activated blood cells, and microemboli. Shear stress, turbulence, cavitation, and other rheologic forces and C5b-9 cause hemolysis of some red cells. Complement anaphylatoxins,[514] bradykinin formed by activation of the contact proteins,[490,513] and proinflammatory cytokines stimulate endothelial cells to contract, allowing extravasation of intravascular fluid into the extravascular space.[601] Numerous circulating vasoactive substances cause vasoconstriction or vasodilatation of heterogeneous regional vascular networks.[489] As neutrophils and monocytes migrate across the endothelial cell barrier, stromal and parenchymal cells are exposed to a cytotoxic environment mediated by neutral proteases, collagenases, and gelatinases, reactive oxidants, lipid peroxides, C5b-9, and other cytotoxins.[486,545,602,603] This injury is magnified by microemboli produced from platelet-leukocyte aggregates, lipids, and other blood elements and emboli from other sources (see sections 11B and 11D). The manifestations of the inflammatory response include systemic symptoms such as malaise, fever, increased heart rate, mild hypotension,[582] interstitial fluid accumulation,[604] and temporary organ dysfunction, particularly of the brain, heart, lungs, and kidneys.

The magnitude of this defense reaction during and after CPB is influenced by many exogenous factors that include the surface area of the perfusion circuit, the duration of blood contact with extravascular surfaces, general health and preoperative organ function of the patient, blood loss and replacement, organ ischemia and reperfusion injury, sepsis, different degrees of hypothermia, periods of circulatory arrest, genetic profiles, corticosteroids, and other pharmacologic agents.

CONTROL OF THE ACUTE INFLAMMATORY RESPONSE TO CARDIOPULMONARY BYPASS

Off-Pump Cardiac Surgery

Myocardial revascularization without either CPB or cardioplegia reduces the acute inflammatory response but does not prevent it.[605–607] The response to surgical trauma, manipulation of the heart, pericardial suction, heparin, protamine, other drugs, and anesthesia produces an increase in the markers of acute inflammation, C3a, C5b-9, proinflammatory cytokines (TNF-α, IL-6, IL-8), neutrophil elastase, and reactive oxidants,[545] but the magnitude of the response is significantly less than that observed with CPB.[606–608] Although it has not been shown that the attenuated acute inflammatory response directly reduces organ dysfunction,[605,608] elderly patients and those with reduced renal and pulmonary function tolerate off-pump surgery with less morbidity and mortality than patients treated with CPB.[608–611]

Cardiopulmonary Bypass without an Oxygenator: The Drew-Anderson Technique

In 1959 Drew and Anderson introduced deep hypothermia and the use of the patient's own lungs for gas exchange during open cardiac surgery using separate right and left perfusion systems.[612] Richter et al reintroduced this method for coronary revascularization at 30°C to 32°C and demonstrated that absence of an oxygenator significantly reduced peak concentrations of IL-6 and IL-8 without changing the anti-inflammatory cytokines IL-1ra and IL-10.[613] These cytokine changes correlated with better postoperative blood gases and pulmonary function, smaller blood losses, and shorter times to extubation. A later study confirmed attenuation of the pulmonary inflammatory response by demonstrating lower levels of cytokines and fewer platelet-monocyte microaggregates in blood exiting from the lung, as compared with conventional bypass.[614] This method is not likely to achieve wide acceptance because of the need for multiple cannulations and a cluttered operative field. Miniaturization of perfusion circuits, however, may be feasible and preliminary data suggest that this approach attenuates the inflammatory response.[615]

Perfusion Temperature

Release of mediators of inflammation is temperature sensitive. Normothermic CPB increases the release of cytokines and other cellular and soluble mediators of inflammation,[582] whereas hypothermia reduces production and release of these mediators until rewarming begins.[616] Perfusion at tepid temperatures between 32°C and 34°C is a reasonable compromise for many operations requiring 1 to 2 hours of CPB.[580,602]

Perfusion Circuit Coatings

Ionic- or covalent-bonded heparin perfusion circuits are the most widely used surface coatings and are often combined with reduced doses of systemic heparin in first-time myocardial revascularization patients.[617] It is well established that heparin is an agonist for platelets, complement, factor XII, and leukocytes (see section 11B), but there is no reproducible evidence that heparin coating either produces a nonthrombogenic surface or reduces activation of the clotting cascade.[618–622] A review of a large portion of this literature concluded that heparin-bonded circuits reduced concentrations of the terminal complement complex, C5b-9 (Fig. 11-19),[623] but for nearly every study showing a beneficial anti-inflammatory or anti-thrombotic effect another study shows no effect.[621] Clinical trials that have combined

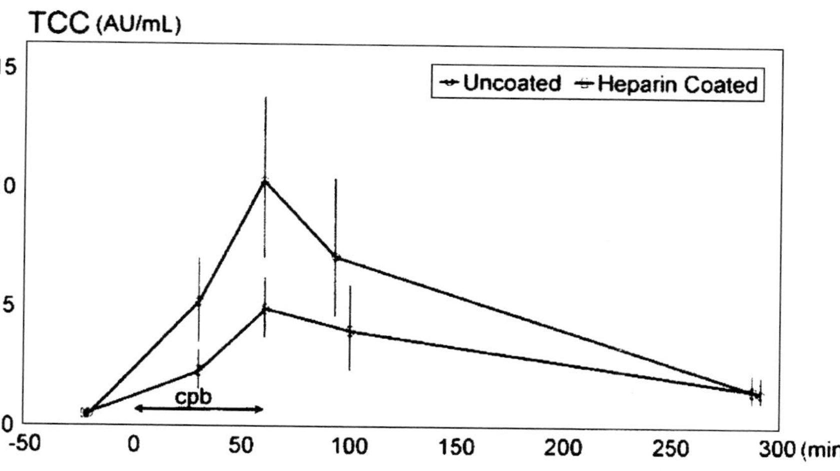

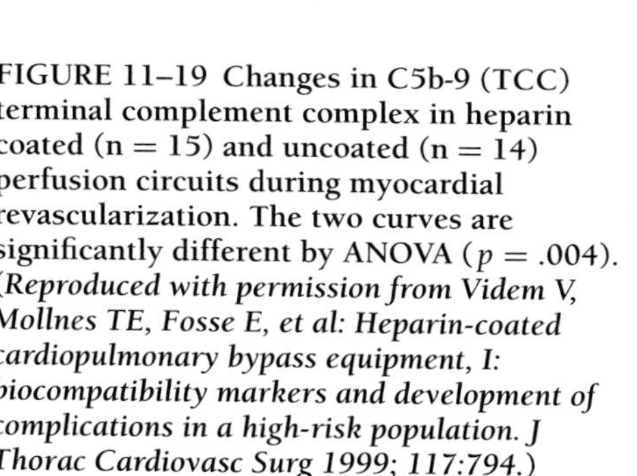
FIGURE 11–19 Changes in C5b-9 (TCC) terminal complement complex in heparin coated (n = 15) and uncoated (n = 14) perfusion circuits during myocardial revascularization. The two curves are significantly different by ANOVA ($p = .004$). *(Reproduced with permission from Videm V, Mollnes TE, Fosse E, et al: Heparin-coated cardiopulmonary bypass equipment, I: biocompatibility markers and development of complications in a high-risk population. J Thorac Cardiovasc Surg 1999; 117:794.)*

heparin-coated circuits with reduced systemic heparin and exclusion of field-aspirated blood from the perfusion circuit have demonstrated modest clinical benefits.[624] However, most trials, including a large European trial of 805 patients, have not observed clinical benefits except in certain subsets of patients that are not the same between studies[617,625–629] and which report sporadic differences that barely reach statistical significance.[628,629] Excluding unwashed field blood from the perfusion circuit reduces admixture of high concentrations of thrombin,[552] fibrinolysins,[630] cytokines, and activated complement (authors' unpublished data) and leukocytes to the perfusate. Exclusion of these inflammatory mediators may be more important in reducing the amounts of vasoactive and cytotoxic substances circulating within the body than the heparin surface coating.

New surface coatings are being developed or undergoing clinical trials.[631] Surface-modifiying additives (SMA) are chemicals used in low concentrations to reduce interfacial energy and modify the mosaic of adsorbed surface plasma proteins. One commercially available SMA uses a triblock copolymer containing polar and nonpolar chains of polycaprolactone-polydimethylsiloxane-polycaprolactone.[632] In clinical trials this surface significantly reduced platelet loss and granule release, and reduced markers of thrombin generation.[632,633] PMEA (poly-2-methylethylacrylate) is another manufactured surface coating designed to reduce surface adsorption of plasma proteins. Laboratory studies show reduced surface adsorption of fibrinogen and reduced bradykinin and thrombin generation in pigs.[634] Early clinical studies show significant reductions in C3a, C4D, and neutrophil elastase, but ambivalent effects on IL-6 and platelets.[635,636]

Modified Ultrafiltration

Although effective in pediatric cardiac surgery,[637,638] ultrafiltration to remove intravascular (and extravascular) water and inflammatory substances has produced mixed results in adults.[639,640] Dialysis during CPB in adults may be beneficial in removing water, potassium, and protein wastes in patients with renal insufficiency.

Leukocyte Filtration

The role of neutrophils in the acute inflammatory response has led to development of leukocyte-depleting filters for the CPB circuit. Multiple groups have investigated these filters in clinical trials, but consistent efficacy in reducing markers of neutrophil activation and improvement in respiratory or renal function are lacking. Most clinical studies fail to document significant leukocyte depletion or clinical benefits.[641–643] Active sequestration of leukocytes and platelets using a separate cell separator during CPB may have beneficial clinical effects,[644,645] but requires a separate inflow cannula and separator system.

Complement Inhibitors

The central role of complement in the acute inflammatory response to CPB provides ample rationale for inhibition. The anaphylatoxins and C5b-9 are direct mediators of the inflammatory response, and C5a is the principal agonist for activating neutrophils and is a potent chemoattractant for neutrophils, monocytes, macrophages, eosinophils, basophils, and microglial cells.[514] C1-inhibitor (C1-Inh) is a natural inhibitor of complement C1 components C1s and C1r, factor XIIa, kallikrein, and factor XIa.[504] Factor H and C4BP inhibit C3 and C5 convertase subunits, but are poor inhibitors of induced activation of the complement system.[504] None of these inhibitors are attractive candidates for inhibiting complement activation during CPB.

The sequential activation cascade with convergence of the classical and alternative pathways at C3 offers many opportunities for inhibition by recombinant proteins. Using

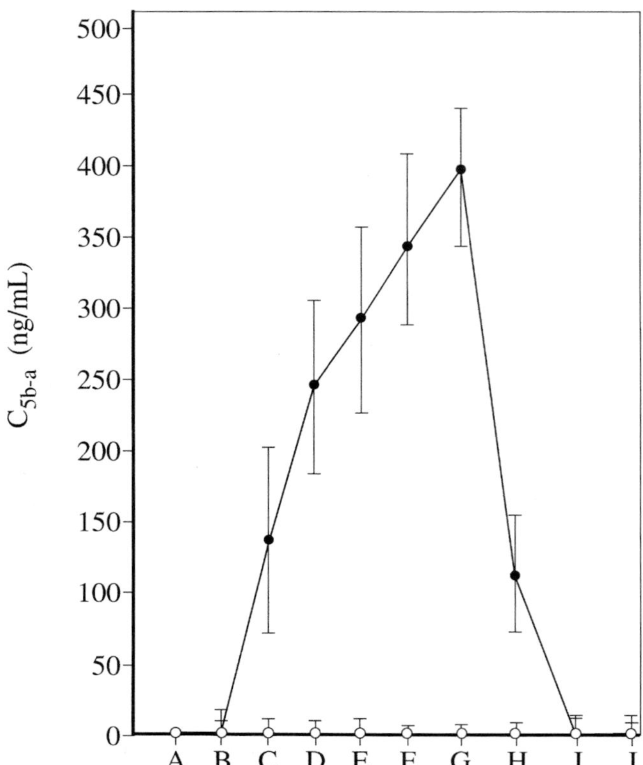

FIGURE 11–20 Inhibition of C5b-9, complement terminal attack complex, with placebo (solid circles) and 2 μg/kg of h5G1.1-scFv (open circles) during clinical cardiac surgery with CPB. Letters on x-axis represent the following events: A, before heparin; B, 5 minutes after drug; C, 5 minutes after cooling to 28°C; D, after beginning rewarming; E, 5 minutes after reaching 32°C; F, 5 minutes after reaching 37°C; G, 5 minutes after CPB; H, 2 hours after CPB; I, 12 hours after CPB; J, 24 hours after CPB. HcG1.1-scFv completely inhibited formation of the C5b-9 terminal attack complex. (*Data redrawn from Fitch JCK, Rollins S, Matis L, et al: Pharmacology and biological efficacy of a recombinant, humanized, single-chain antibody C5 complement inhibitor in patients undergoing coronary artery bypass graft surgery with cardiopulmonary bypass. Circulation 1999; 100:2499.*)

a humanized, recombinant antibody to C5 (h5G1.1-scFv), Fitch et al demonstrated that generation of C5b-9 was completely blocked in a dose-response manner (Fig. 11-20) and that neutrophil and monocyte CD11b/CD18 expression was attenuated in patients during and for several hours after clinical cardiac surgery using CPB.[646] In addition they observed reduction in markers of myocardial and cognitive functional injury.[646]

Fung et al[496] used an anti-factor D monoclonal antibody to inhibit production of complement proteins, Bb, C3a, sC5b-9, and C5a, via the alternate pathway and attenuate upregulation of neutrophil and platelet adhesive receptors during CPB in vitro.[496] Undar confirmed these results during CPB in baboons and additionally found inhibition of complement C4d, attenuation of IL-6 concentrations, and reduced markers of cardiac injury.[647] Compstatin, a very small (1593-Da) synthetic peptide, binds C3 and therefore inhibits both the classical and alternative pathways.[494] This peptide inhibits generation of C3a and sC5b-9 and neutrophil binding during in vitro CPB.[648] In baboons, after activation of complement by the heparin-protamine complex, compstatin completely inhibits C3 cleavage without causing any change in hemodynamic measurements or side effects.[649]

Other complement recombinant protein inhibitors have been developed and are under active investigation and in clinical trials because of the importance of this plasma protein system in CPB, ischemia/reperfusion, and injuries that summon the acute inflammatory response.[504,650–652] Experimentally, recombinant soluble complement inhibitor 1 (sCR1) improves cardiac and pulmonary function after CPB in pigs.[653] Recombinant soluble complement receptor I and CAB-2, a chimeric protein constructed from the genes encoding the complement regulatory proteins, human membrane cofactor protein, and human decay-accelerating factor target C3/C5 convertases, have been developed and are under investigation.[501,504,651,654] Although any effective and safe inhibitor is welcome, C3 may be a better target for inhibition because both activation pathways are blocked at the point of convergence and because C3 concentrations in plasma are 15 times greater than C5.[504,649,655]

Glucocorticoids

Many investigators have used glucocorticoids to suppress the acute inflammatory response to CPB and clinical cardiac surgery, but beneficial effects in adult patients have been inconsistent.[656–658] Steroids reduce release of rapid-response cytokines, TNF-α, and IL-1β from macrophages,[659] enhance release of IL-10,[660,661] and suppress expression of endothelial cell selectins and neutrophil integrins.[662] Clinically, glucocorticoids decrease endotoxin release,[663] shift the cytokine balance towards the anti-inflammatory side,[659,663–666] and decrease expression of neutrophil integrins.[656] Clinical results from a few randomized trials are conflicting: one study observed earlier extubation and reduced shivering,[667] but another found increased blood glucose levels and delayed extubation.[668] Differences in specific steroids, dosing, and timing may explain some of these discrepancies.

Recent observations regarding the inhibitory effect of glucocorticoids on transcription factor nuclear factor κB (NF kappa B) may provide a rationale for using glucocorticoids to suppress the acute inflammatory response to CPB.[669] This inducible transcription factor controls the expression of genes encoding a wide array of proinflammatory mediators, including cytokines, inducible NO synthase (iNOS), and adhesion molecules, and is activated by IL-1β, TNF-α, reactive oxidants, and other noxious stimuli.[658,670] Given the multiplicity and redundancy of pathways involved in the inflammatory response to bypass, inhibition of a common "upstream" control point in transcriptional regulation of inflammatory genes is an attractive strategy. Kovacich et al showed that inhibiting NF-kappa B prevents IL-1-mediated hypotension.[671] Thus the use of glucocorticoids for controlling the inflammatory response to CPB is conceptually attractive.[672]

Protease Inhibitors

Aprotinin is a natural serine protease inhibitor in the kunin superfamily that strongly inhibits plasmin and weakly inhibits kallikrein.[673] Plasma concentrations of 4-10 KIU (kallikrein inhibitory units) of aprotinin completely inhibit plasmin, but 250 to 400 KIU are required to fully inhibit kallikrein.[673] Clinical doses of aprotinin totally inhibit plasmin, but are not sufficient to completely inhibit kallikrein.[674] The antifibrinolytic and platelet-sparing effects of the drug are well known and significantly reduce blood losses during and after complex cardiac surgery.[675–677] The anti-inflammatory effects of aprotinin are more difficult to quantitate and may reflect multiple mechanisms including partial kallikrein inhibition, direct effects, and inhibition of NF-kappa B.

In vitro aprotinin inhibits kallikrein formation, and attenuates complement activation and release of platelet beta thromboglobulin and neutrophil elastase.[678] Aprotinin also reduces neutrophil transmigration and expression of ICAM-1 and VCAM-1 by endothelial cells.[679,680] Clinically, aprotinin reduces circulating TNF-α, IL-6, IL-8, and neutrophil CD11b expression,[657,681,682] and synergistically increases IL-10 synthesis.[661,682] The drug may also attenuate neutrophil activation and myocardial damage during aortic cross-clamping[683] and reduce overall mortality.[676] Nevertheless, low- or high-dose aprotinin used in large, randomized controlled clinical trials fails to show a reduction in proinflammatory cytokines, activated complement, neutrophil elastase, and myeloperoxidase.[633,684] Thus the efficacy of aprotinin as an anti-inflammatory agent remains unresolved.

Nafamostat mesilate is a trypsin-like protease inhibitor that inhibits platelet aggregation and release, formation of kallikrein, and factor XIIa and neutrophil elastase release during in vitro extracorporeal recirculation.[685] Early clinical trials show that nafamostat mesilate inhibits fibrinolysis, preserves platelet numbers and function, reduces blood loss, and attenuates the acute inflammatory response by suppressing IL-6, IL-8, and malondialdehyde formation and neutrophil integrin expression.[686,687]

Other Inhibitors

Sodium nitroprusside is a vasodilator and potent activator of nitric oxide synthase (NOS), which catalyzes the production of nitric oxide (NO) from arginine, oxygen, and NADPH.[548] During clinical cardiac surgery sodium nitroprusside attenuates complement activation in children[688] and production of proinflammatory cytokines and retention of platelet-leukocyte coaggregates in reperfused hearts of adults.[689] NO, however, reacts with superoxide (O_2^-) to form reactive nitrogen molecules, which are cytotoxic[548]; thus, its clinical benefit is unclear.

Generation of reactive oxidants, initially from C5a activation of neutrophils,[690] oxidizes membrane phospholipids to form lipid peroxidases, conjugated dienes, and malondialdehyde and other reactive species during cardiopulmonary bypass.[690,691] Ischemia/reperfusion injuries produce the greatest concentrations of reactive oxidants and lipid peroxidases[691,692] and have stimulated studies using antioxidants to counteract these cytotoxins.[692–695] Although exogenous vitamin E prevents depletion of circulating α-tocopherol during clinical cardiac surgery,[693] beneficial effects in terms of reduced myocardial or pulmonary injury are inconclusive.[692,693,695]

Platelets, endothelial cells, neutrophils, and monocytes are regulated by two cyclic nucleotides: cyclic adenine monophosphate (cAMP) or cyclic guanosine monophosphate (cGMP). Increased cAMP inhibits NF-κB transcription in monocytes and endothelial cells.[696] A multitude of phosphodiesterases (9 families) control intracellular concentrations of the two cyclic nucleotides and provide a mechanism for controlling regional groups of cells.[697] A variety of drugs have been developed to inhibit specific PDE families; some have been studied for their effects on the acute inflammatory response to CPB. One study in patients who had clinical cardiac surgery with CPB shows no change in hemodynamics or oxygen transport and metabolism but does show improved splanchnic circulation and reduced absorbtion of endotoxin and production of IL-6.[698]

Comment

As summarized above, CPB and clinical cardiac surgery unleash a broad and intense acute inflammatory response that varies in degree between patients. The cause is the continuous recirculation of blood that is sequentially in contact with the wound, perfusion circuit, and intravascular compartment to which is added the washout of reperfused ischemic organs and tissues. The acute inflammatory response together with microembolization is responsible for most of the morbidity of CPB and clinical cardiac surgery. Given the magnitude and diversity of the acute inflammatory response, it appears unlikely that drug cocktails or indirect measures directed against specific mediators of this response will prove more than mildly effective. Efforts to temporarily inhibit the more important mediators, specifically complement[699] and neutrophils, during the perioperative period are more attractive and achievable targets that could produce more immediate clinical benefits. Because our patients are vulnerable to infection and other forms of injury during and immediately after operation and because the acute inflammatory response is an important first step in healing, the clinician must remember that temporary, reversible inhibitors are probably safer than permanent inhibitors.

11D: Organ Damage

John W. Hammon, Jr./L. Henry Edmunds, Jr.

Cardiopulmonary bypass preempts normal reflex and chemoreceptor control of the circulation, initiates coagulation, activates blood cells, releases circulating cell-signaling proteins, generates vasoactive and cytotoxic substances, and produces a variety of microemboli. Venous pressure is elevated, plasma colloid osmotic pressure is reduced, flow is nonpulsatile, and temperature is manipulated. Tissues and organs suffer from regional malperfusion of blood flow that is independent of physiologic controls, and is caused by bombardment of microemboli, increased interstitial water, and perfusion with an enzymatic stew of cytotoxic substances. Reversible and irreversible cell injury occur, but damage is diffusely distributed throughout the entire body as individual cells or small groups of cells are affected. Ischemia-reperfusion injury augments damage to the heart and on occasion to other organs. Amazingly, the body is able to withstand and for the most part repair this physiologic chaos and massive assault of angry blood. This section summarizes the reversible and permanent organ damage produced by cardiopulmonary bypass (CPB) and complements the preceding three sections of this chapter and the chapter on ischemia and reperfusion (see Ch. 3).

MECHANISMS

Cardiac output during CPB is carefully monitored and synchronized with temperature and hemoglobin concentration to ensure that the entire body is adequately supplied with oxygen (see earlier section on extracorporeal perfusion systems). Excessive hemodilution reduces oxygen delivery,[700] and hemoglobin concentrations below 8 g/L cause organ dysfunction at temperatures above 30°C.[701] However, regional hypoperfusion is not monitored[702]; is independent of reflex and chemoreceptor controls; and is influenced by the inflammatory response, which produces circulating vasoactive substances,[703,704] defined as substances that cause vascular smooth muscle cells and/or endothelial cells to contract or relax (see earlier section on inflammatory response). Regional perfusion is also influenced by acid-base relationships during cooling and may affect postoperative organ function.[705,706] Alpha-stat management (pH increases during cooling) decreases cerebral perfusion during hypothermia; pH stat (pH 7.40 is maintained by adding CO_2) improves organ perfusion but may increase embolic injury.[707] Temperature differences within the body and within organs produce regional temperature-perfusion mismatch,[708] which can precipitate regional hypoperfusion and acidosis due to inadequate oxygen delivery. There is no method to monitor regional perfusion during cardiopulmonary bypass, and even direct temperature surveillance of vital organs may fail to detect temperature differences within the organ.

The inflammatory response produces the terminal complement attack complex, anaphylatoxins, cytotoxic proteases,[709] collagenases, gelatinases, metalloproteinases,[710] reactive oxidants, free radicals, lipid peroxide, endotoxin, inflammatory cytokines, and activated neutrophils and monocytes that can and do destroy organ and tissue cells (see section 11C). These agents directly access the specialized cells of every organ by passing between endothelial cell junctions to reach the interstitial compartment. Reduced plasma colloid osmotic pressure, elevated venous pressure, and widened endothelial cell junctions[711] increase the volume of the interstitial space during CPB in proportion to the duration of bypass, magnitude of the dissection, transfusions, and other factors. In prolonged complicated perfusions the interstitial compartment may increase 18% to 33%,[712] but intracellular water does not increase during CPB.

Microemboli are defined as particles less than 500 microns in diameter. They enter the circulation during CPB from a variety of sources.[713] Table 11-5 summarizes sources of gas, foreign, and blood-generated microemboli, which are more fully discussed in section 11A. Air entry into the perfusion circuit produces the most dangerous gas emboli because nitrogen is poorly soluble in blood and is not a metabolite. Carbon dioxide is rapidly soluble in blood and is sometimes used to flood the surgical field to displace air.[714] Foreign emboli, largely generated in the surgical wound, reach the circulation from the surgical field via the cardiotomy reservoir. The cardiotomy reservoir is the primary source of foreign emboli and the major source of blood-generated emboli, particularly fat emboli.[715] Extensive activation and physical damage to blood elements produce a wide variety of emboli, which tend to increase with the duration of perfusion.[716,717]

STRATEGIES FOR REDUCING MICROEMBOLI

Although discussed in earlier sections, the principal methods for reducing circulating microemboli deserve emphasis and include the following: adequate anticoagulation; membrane oxygenator; washing blood aspirated from the surgical wound[718]; filter in the cardiotomy reservoir; secure purse-string sutures around cannulas; strict control of all air entry sites within the perfusion circuit; removal of residual air from the heart and great vessels; avoidance of atherosclerotic emboli; and selective filtration of cerebral vessels.[719,720]

Many intraoperative strategies are available to reduce cerebral atherosclerotic embolization. These include routine epicardial echocardiography of the ascending aorta to detect both anterior and posterior atherosclerotic plaques

TABLE 11–5 Major sources of microemboli

Gas	Foreign	Blood
Bubble oxygenators	Atherosclerotic debris	Fibrin
Air entry into the circuit	Fat, fat droplets	Free fat
Residual air in the heart	Fibrin clot	Aggregated chylomicrons
Loose purse-string sutures	Cholesterol crystals	Denatured proteins
Cardiotomy reservoir	Calcium particles	Platelet aggregates
Rapid rewarming	Muscle fragments	Platelet-leukocyte aggregates
Cavitation	Tubing debris, dust	Hemolyzed red cells
	Bone wax, talc	Transfused blood
	Silicone antifoam	
	Glue, Surgicel	
	Cotton sponge fibers	

and to find sites free of atherosclerosis for placing the aortic cannula.[721] Recently, special catheters with or without baffles or screens have been developed to reduce the number of atherosclerotic emboli that reach the cerebral circulation.[719–724] In patients with moderate or severe ascending aortic atherosclerosis a single application of the aortic clamp as opposed to partial or multiple applications is strongly recommended and has been shown to reduce postoperative neuronal and neurocognitive deficits in a large clinical series.[725] Retrograde cardioplegia is preferred over antegrade cardioplegia in these patients to avoid a sandblasting effect of the cardioplegic solution.[726] No aortic clamp may be safe or even possible in some patients with severe atherosclerosis or porcelain aorta. If intracardiac surgery is required in these patients, deep hypothermia may be used with or without graft replacement of the ascending aorta. If only revascularization is needed, pedicled single or sequential arterial grafts,[727] T or Y grafts from a pedicled mammary artery,[728] or vein grafts anastomosed to arch vessels can be used.

In-depth or screen filters (see section 11A) are essential for cardiotomy reservoirs and are usually used in arterial lines. The efficacy of arterial line filters is controversial since screen filters with a pore size less than 25 to 40 microns cannot be used because of flow resistance across the filter. Moreover, air and fat emboli can pass through filters and air and atherosclerotic emboli may enter the circulation downstream to the filter.

CARDIAC INJURY

It is difficult to separate postoperative cardiac dysfunction from injury due to CPB, ischemia/reperfusion, direct surgical trauma, the disease being treated, and maladjustment of preload and afterload to myocardial contractile function. The heart, like all organs and tissues, is subject to microemboli, protease and chemical cytotoxins, activated neutrophils and monocytes, and regional hypoperfusion during CPB before and after cardioplegia or fibrillatory arrest. Some degree of myocardial "stunning" during the period coronary blood flow is interrupted is inevitable,[729] as is some degree of reperfusion injury after ischemia. Both myocardial edema and distention of the flaccid cardioplegic heart during aortic cross-clamping[730] reduce myocardial contractility. Lastly, if myocardial contractility is weak, excessive preload or high afterload during weaning from CPB increases ventricular end-diastolic volume, myocardial wall stress, and oxygen consumption. Thus postoperative performance of the heart depends upon many variables and not just the injuries produced by CPB.

NEUROLOGIC INJURY

Because the brain controls all body activity, even small injuries to it may produce detectable, functional losses that are not detectable or important in other organs. Regional hypoperfusion, edema, microemboli, and circulating cytotoxins may cause subtle losses in cognitive function, behavioral patterns, and physiologic and physical function that can pass unnoticed, be accepted and dismissed, or profoundly compromise the patient's quality of life. Thus the brain is the most sensitive organ exposed to damage by CPB and also the organ that it is most important to protect.

Assessment

Routine assessment of neurologic injury due to cardiopulmonary bypass is not done for most patients because of the priority of the cardiac lesion and because of costs in time and money. General neurologic examinations by untrained individuals or by members of the surgical team are not adequate to rule out subtle neurologic injuries, and this is the principal reason that the incidence of post–CPB, nonstroke, neurologic injury varies widely in the surgical literature.[731–733]

For studies designed to assess or reduce neurologic injury caused by CPB, nonroutine preoperative and postoperative tests are required. These special tests include a complete neurologic examination by a trained neurologist. To improve accuracy, a single neurologist should conduct all serial examinations. A standardized protocol of examination should be followed, with uniform reporting of results. The basic, structured examination includes a mental state examination; cranial nerve, motor, sensory, and cerebellar examinations; and examination of gait, station, deep tendon, and primitive reflexes.

The most obvious neuropsychologic abnormalities are coma, delirium, and confusion, but transitory episodes of delirium and confusion are often dismissed as due to anesthesia or medications. More subtle losses are determined by comparison of preoperative and postoperative performances using a standard battery of neuropsychologic tests prepared by a group of neuropsychologists.[734] A 20% decline in two or more of these tests suggests a neuropsychologic deficit that should be followed until resolved or not resolved.[735]

Computed axial tomograms (CAT) or magnetic resonance imaging (MRI) scans are essential for the definitive diagnosis of stroke, delirium, or coma. Preoperative imaging is usually not necessary when new techniques such as diffusion-weighted MRI imaging, MRI spectroscopy, or MRI angiography are used to assess possible new lesions after operation.[736–738]

Biochemical markers of neurologic injury after cardiac surgery are relatively nonspecific and inconclusive. Neuron-specific enolase (NSE) is an intracellular enzyme found in neurons, normal neuroendocrine cells, platelets, and erythrocytes.[739] S-100 is an acidic calcium-binding protein found in the brain.[740,741] The beta dimer resides in glial and Schwann cells. Both S-100 and NSE increase in spinal fluid with neuronal death[740,742] and may correlate with neurologic injury after CPB,[742] but the tests are contaminated by red cell and platelet destruction and are often elevated following prolonged CPB in patients without otherwise detectable neurologic injury.[743]

Populations at Risk

Advancing age increases the risk of stroke or cognitive impairment in the general population, and surgery, regardless of type, increases the risk still higher.[744] A European study compared 321 elderly patients without surgery to 1218 patients who had noncardiac surgery and found a 26% incidence of cognitive dysfunction 1 week after operation and a 10% incidence at 3 months.[745] Between 1974 and 1990 the number of patients undergoing cardiac surgery over age 60 and over age 70 increased 2-fold and 7-fold, respectively.[746] Figure 11-21 illustrates the relationship between age and cognitive dysfunction after CABG and demonstrates a steep increase after the age of 60. Genetic factors also influence the incidence of cognitive dysfunction following cardiac surgery.[747] The incidence of cognitive dysfunction at 1 week following cardiac surgery is approximately double that of noncardiac surgery.

As the age of cardiac surgical patients increases, the number with multiple risk factors for neurologic injury also increases. Risk factors for adverse cerebral outcomes are listed in Table 11-6.[748] These factors are divided into stroke with a permanent fixed neurologic deficit (type 1) and coma or delirium (type 2). Hypertension and diabetes occur in approximately 55% and 25% of cardiac surgical patients, respectively.[749] Fifteen percent have carotid stenosis of 50% or greater, and up to 13% have had a transient ischemic attack or prior stroke.[749] The total number of atherosclerotic stenoses in the brachiocephalic vessels adds to the risk of stroke or cognitive dysfunction,[750] as does the severity of atherosclerosis in the ascending aorta as detected by

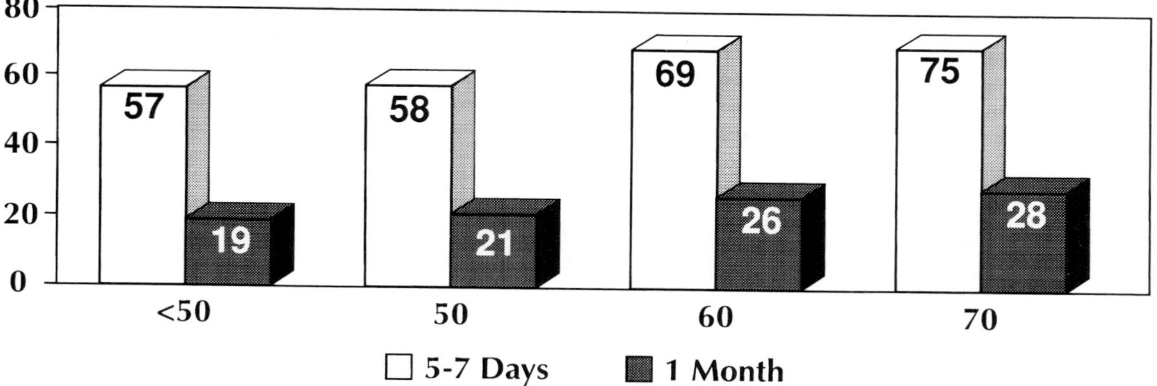

FIGURE 11–21 Effect of age by decade on neuropsychologic outcome after CABG. Abnormal neuropsychologic outcomes at 1 week and 1 month postoperative are more common with advancing age. Percentages of patients with deficits on two or more tests are shown (N = 374). (*Reproduced with permission from Hammon JW, Stump DA, Kon ND, et al: Risk factors and solutions for the development of neurobehavioral changes after coronary artery bypass grafting. Ann Thorac Surg 1998: 63:1613.*)

TABLE 11–6 Adjusted odds ratios for type I and type II cerebral outcomes associated with selected risk factors

Factor	Model for type I cerebral outcome	Model for type II cerebral outcome
Significant factors, $p < .05$		
Proximal aortic atherosclerosis	4.52	
History of neurologic disease	3.19	
Use of intra-aortic balloon pump	2.60	
Diabetes mellitus	2.59	
History of hypertension	2.31	
History of pulmonary disease	2.09	2.37
History of unstable angina	1.83	
Age (per additional decade)	1.75	2.20
Systolic blood pressure >180 mm Hg at admission		3.47
History of excessive alcohol consumption		2.64
History of CABG		2.18
Dysrhythmia on day of surgery		1.97
Antihypertensive therapy		1.78
Other factors (p not significant)		
Perioperative hypotension	1.92	1.88
Ventricular venting	1.83	
Congestive heart failure on day of surgery		2.46
History of peripheral vascular disease		1.64

Source: Adapted with permission from Roach GW, Kanchugar M, Mangano CM, et al: Adverse cerebral outcomes after coronary bypass surgery: multicenter study of perioperative ischemia research groups and the ischemia research and education foundation investigators. N Engl J Med 1996; 335: 1857.

epiaortic ultrasound scanning.[751] Palpable ascending aortic atherosclerotic plaques markedly increase the risk of right carotid arterial emboli as detected by Doppler ultrasound.[752] The incidence of severe aortic atherosclerosis is 1% in cardiac surgical patients less than 50 years old and is 10% in those aged 75 to 80.[753]

Mechanisms of Injury

The two major causes of organ dysfunction and injury during CPB are microemboli and hypoperfusion, which are to some extent mutually exclusive. Microemboli are distributed in proportion to blood flow[754]; thus reduced cerebral blood flow reduces microembolic injury but increases the risk of hypoperfusion.[754] During CPB both alpha-stat acid-base management and phenylepherine reduce cerebral injury in adults, probably by causing cerebral vessel vasoconstriction and reducing the number of microemboli.[755,756] Air,[757] atherosclerotic debris,[758] and fat are the major types of microemboli causing brain injury in clinical practice, and all cause neuronal necrosis by blocking small cerebral vessels.[707,759] Massive air embolism causes a large ischemic injury, but gaseous cerebral microemboli may directly damage endothelium in addition to blocking blood flow.[759] The recent identification of unique small capillary arteriolar dilatations (SCADs) in the brain associated with fat emboli (Fig. 11-22)[760] raises the possibility that these emboli not only block small vessels but also release cytotoxic free radicals, which may significantly increase the damage to lipid-rich neurons.

Anemia and elevated cerebral temperature increase cerebral blood flow but may cause inadequate oxygen delivery to the brain[761]; however, these conditions are easily avoided during clinical cardiac surgery. Although some investigators speculate that normothermic and/or hyperthermic CPB cause cerebral hypoperfusion,[762] experimental studies indicate that cerebral blood flow increases with temperature.[754] Brain injuries associated with this practice are more likely due to increased cerebral microemboli, which produce larger lesions at higher cerebral temperatures.[754] Reduced brain temperature is protective against neural cell necrosis and remains an important neuroprotective strategy.

Additional Neuroprotective Strategies

Primary strategies for avoiding air, atherosclerotic particulates, and blood-generated microembolism are presented above and in section 11A. Recommended conditions for protecting the brain during CPB include mild hypothermia (32°C-34°C) and hematocrit above 25%.[763] Temporary increases in cerebral venous pressure caused by superior vena cava obstruction and excessive rewarming above blood temperatures of 37°C should be avoided.[764–766] Either jugular venous bulb oxygen saturation or near-infrared cerebral oximetry are recommended for monitoring cerebral perfusion in patients who may be at high risk for cerebral injury.[767]

Barbiturates reduce cerebral metabolism by decreasing spontaneous synaptic activity[768] and provide a definite neuroprotective effect during clinical cardiac surgery using CPB.[769] Unfortunately, these agents delay emergence from

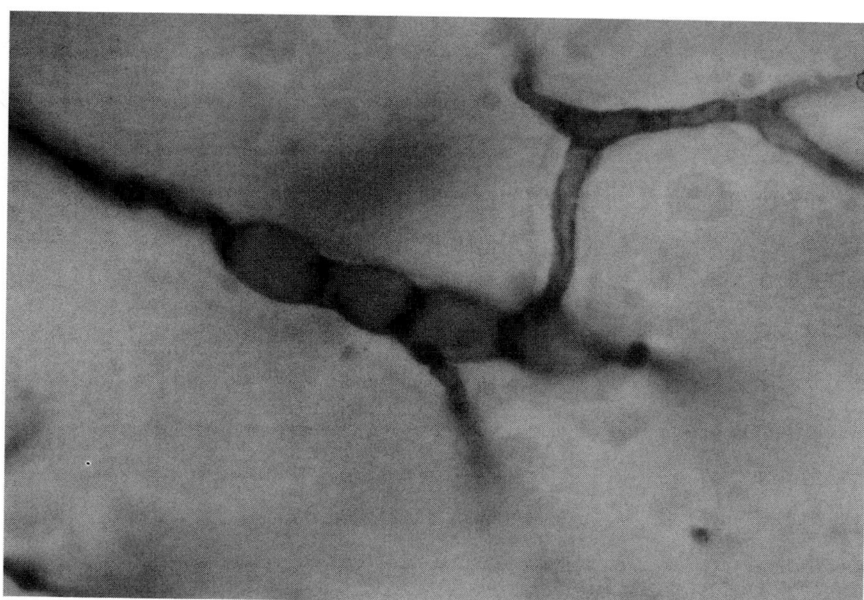

FIGURE 11–22 Small capillary and arterial dilatations (SCADs) in cerebral vessels in a patient who expired 48 hours after CABG using cardiopulmonary bypass. (Alkaline phosphatase-stained celloidin section, 100 μm thick: X100.)

anesthesia and prolong intensive care unit stays. NMDA (N-methyl-D asparate) antagonists, which are effective in animals, provide mild protection compared to control patients, but have a high incidence of neurologic side effects.[770] A small study demonstrated a neuroprotective effect of lidocaine.[771] Currently no agent is recommended for protection of the central nervous system during CPB.

Off-pump myocardial revascularization theoretically avoids many of the causes of cerebral injury due to CPB, but, as noted above, many causes of neuronal injury are independent of CPB and related to atherosclerosis and air entry sites into the circulation. Measurements of carotid emboli by Doppler ultrasound indicate fewer emboli and improved neurocognitive outcomes in patients who have off-pump surgery as compared to those with on-pump revascularization[772,773]; however, a definitive, randomized trial, which is necessary to neutralize patient-related causes of injury, has not been done.

Prognosis

Neuropsychologic deficits that are present after 3 months are almost always permanent.[774] Assessments after that time are confounded by development of new deficits, particularly in aged patients.[775]

LUNG INJURY

Patient factors and the separate effects of operation and CPB combine to compromise lung function early after operation. Chronic smoking and emphysema are the most common patient factors, but muscular weakness, chronic bronchitis, occult pneumonia, preoperative pulmonary edema, and unrelated respiratory disease are other contributors to postoperative pulmonary dysfunction. Incisional pain, lack of movement, shallow respiratory sighs, increased work of breathing, reduced pulmonary compliance, weak cough, increased pulmonary arterial-venous shunting, and interstitial edema, to some degree, are consequences of anesthesia and any operation. CPB significantly adds to this injury.

During CPB the lungs are supplied by the bronchial arteries and pulmonary arterial blood flow may be absent or minimal. Whether or not alveolar cells suffer an ischemic/reperfusion injury is unclear, but the lungs are subject to many insults that combine to increase pulmonary capillary permeability and interstitial lung water. Hemodilution, reduced plasma oncotic pressure, and temporary elevation of left atrial or pulmonary venous pressure during CPB or during weaning from CPB increase extravascular lung water.[776,777] Microemboli[778] and circulating cellular, vasoactive, and cytotoxic mediators of the inflammatory response[779–783] reach the lung via bronchial arteries during CPB and with resumption of the pulmonary circulation during weaning. These agents increase pulmonary capillary permeability, perivascular edema, and bronchial secretions, and perhaps cause observed changes in alveolar surfactant.[784] The combination of increased interstitial lung water and bronchial secretions, altered surfactant, patient factors, and the consequences of operation reduces pulmonary compliance and functional residual capacity and increases the work of breathing.[785] All of these changes combine to enhance regional atelectasis, increase susceptibility to infection, and increase the physiologic arterial-venous shunt, which reduces systemic arterial Pa_{O_2}.

Postoperative respiratory care is based upon restoring normal pulmonary capillary permeability and interstitial lung volume; preventing atelectasis; reinflating atelectatic segments; maintaining normal arterial blood gases; and preventing infection and facilitating removal of bronchial mucus. Improved postoperative respiratory care, an understanding of the mechanisms of lung injury during CPB, and efforts to prevent or control the causes of injury[786,787] have markedly reduced the incidence of pulmonary complications in recent years.[785] (See Ch. 15 for a more detailed discussion of postoperative care.)

Acute respiratory distress syndrome (ARDS) is a rare complication of lung injury during cardiopulmonary bypass and is usually caused by intrabronchial bleeding from traumatic injury by the endotracheal tube or pulmonary artery catheter[788] or to extravasation of blood into alveoli from acute increases in pulmonary venous pressure or severe pulmonary capillary toxic injury.

RENAL INJURY

As with other organs, the preoperative health of the kidneys is a major factor in the ability of that organ to withstand the microembolic, cellular,[789] and regional malperfusion injuries caused by CPB. Risk factors for postoperative renal dysfunction include age over 70 years, diabetes mellitus, previous cardiac surgery, congestive heart failure, and a complex, prolonged operation.[790] The incidence of acute renal failure requiring dialysis after CPB is remarkably low, averaging 1%; however, the incidence increases to 5% with complex operations.[791]

Some degree of renal injury is inevitable during CPB[792] and postperfusion proteinuria occurs in all patients.[793] Increased expression of neutrophil CD 11b receptors and elevated neutrophil count are significantly related to postoperative acute renal failure, defined as a 150% increase in plasma creatinine over baseline.[789] Renal blood and plasma flow, creatinine clearance, free water clearance, and urine volume decrease without hemodilution.[794] Hemodilution attenuates most of these functional changes and also reduces the risk of hemoglobin precipitation in renal tubules if plasma-binding proteins become saturated with free hemoglobin during extracorporeal perfusion. Hemoglobin is toxic to renal tubules and precipitation can block both blood and urine flow to the tubules.[795] Hemodilution dilutes plasma hemoglobin; improves flow to the outer renal cortex; improves total renal blood flow; increases creatinine, electrolyte, and water clearance; and increases glomerular filtration and urine volume.[794]

Perioperative periods of low cardiac output and/or hypotension added to the microembolic, cellular, and cytotoxic injuries of CPB and to any preoperative renal disease are the major cause of postoperative renal failure.[789,796] Low cardiac output reduces renal perfusion pressure and causes angiotensin II production and renin release, which further decrease renal blood flow. Kidneys, already compromised by preoperative disease and the CPB injury, are particularly sensitive to ischemic injury secondary to low cardiac output and hypotension. Thus perioperative management includes efforts to maximize cardiac output using dopamine or dobutamine if necessary,[797] avoiding renal arterial vasoconstrictive drugs, providing adequate crystalloid infusions to maintain urine volume, and alkalinizing urine to minimize precipitation of tubular hemoglobin if excessive hemolysis has occurred. Preliminary studies with a natruetic peptide found in human urine, urodilantin, indicate the possibility of attenuating postoperative oliguria.[798]

If perioperative low cardiac output and hypotension do not occur,[796] the normal kidney has sufficient functional reserve to provide adequate renal function during and after operation. The appearance of oliguric renal failure is ominous and usually requires dialysis, which is generally permanent if required for more than 2 weeks.[799] Oliguric renal failure markedly increases morbidity and mortality by approximately 8-fold.[800]

INJURY TO THE LIVER AND GASTROINTESTINAL ORGANS

Although subjected to microemboli, cytotoxins, and regional malperfusion during CPB, the enormous functional reserve and reparative processes of the normal liver nearly always overcome the injury without consequences. Often liver enzymes are mildly elevated,[801] and 10% to 20% of patients are mildly jaundiced.[802] Extensive red cell hemolysis increases the likelihood of mild jaundice. Persistent and rising jaundice 2 or more days after CPB may precede development of liver failure and is associated with increased morbidity and mortality.[803] Catastrophic liver failure, however, occurs in patients with overwhelming sepsis, oliguric renal failure, anesthetic or drug toxicity, or after a prolonged period of low cardiac output or an episode of hemorrhagic shock and multiple blood transfusions and is uniformly fatal.[804] The liver usually is involved in patients who develop multiorgan failure.

PANCREATIC INJURY

Less then 1% of patients develop clinical pancreatitis after CPB, but approximately 30% develop a transitory, asymptomatic increase in plasma amylase and/or lipase.[805–807] Autopsy studies of the pancreas soon after CPB indicate occasional evidence of histologic pancreatitis.[808] A history of recurrent pancreatitis, perioperative circulatory shock or hypotension, excessively prolonged CPB, and continuous, high doses of inotropic agents are risk factors for developing postoperative pancreatitis.[809] Experimentally and clinically, high doses of calcium increase intracellular trypsinogen activation and histologic evidence of pancreatitis.[810–812] Fulminant pancreatits is very rare, but is often fatal.[813]

STOMACH AND GUT INJURY

CPB at adequate flow rates does not decrease splanchnic blood flow.[814] Risk factors for gastrointestinal complications include advanced age, emergency surgery, prolonged CPB, postoperative low cardiac output or shock, prolonged vasopressor therapy, and elevated preoperative systemic venous pressure.[815]

CPB decreases gastric pH, which declines further after operation.[816] Prior to the advent of H2 blockers and regular use of antacids, duodenal and/or gastric erosion, ulcer, and bleeding were frequent complications following clinical cardiac surgery[817] and were associated with mortality that approached 33% to 50%.[818] These complications are now uncommon.

Several days to 1 week after operation very elderly patients rarely may develop mesenteric vasculitis or severe mesenteric vasoconstriction in response to vasopressors that proceeds to small bowel ischemia and/or infarction. New onset abdominal pain with a silent, rigid abdomen and abrupt rise in white count may be the only signs of this catastrophic complication, which is frequently fatal. If suspected before infarction, infusion of papaverine or alternative vasodilators directly into the mesenteric arteries may prevent or limit subsequent infarction.[819,820] The role of CPB in the etiology of this complication is not known.

REFERENCES

11A: Perfusion Systems

1. Gravlee GP, Davis RF, Kurusz M, Utley JR: *Cardiopulmonary Bypass: Principles and Practice,* 2d ed. Philadelphia, Lippincott Williams & Wilkins, 2000.
2. Arom KV, Ellestad C, Grover FL, Trinkle JK: Objective evaluation of the efficacy of various venous cannulas. *J Thorac Cardiovasc Surg* 1981; 81:464.
3. Merin O, Silberman S, Brauner R, et al: Femoro-femoral bypass for repeat open-heart surgery. *Perfusion* 1998; 13:455.
4. Winter FS: Persistent left superior vena cava: survey of world literature and report of thirty additional cases. *Angiology* 1954; 5:90.
5. Choudhry AK, Conacher ID, Hilton CJ, et al: Persistent left superior vena cava. *J Cardiothorac Anesth* 1989; 3:616.
6. Horrow JC, Lingaraju N: Unexpected persistent left superior vena cava: diagnostic clues during monitoring. *J Cardiothorac Anesth* 1989; 3:611.
7. Hasel R, Barash PG: Dilated coronary sinus on pre-bypass echocardiography. *J Cardiothorac Vasc Anesth* 1996; 10:430.
8. Gardino C, Chew S, Forbess J, et al: Persistent left superior vena cava and partial anomalous pulmonary venous connection: incidental diagnosis by transesophageal echocardiography during coronary artery bypass surgery. *J Am Soc Echocard* 1999; 12:682.
9. Shahian DM: Retrograde coronary sinus cardioplegia in the presence of persistent left superior vena cava. *Ann Thorac Surg* 1992; 54:1214.
10. Yokota M, Kyoku I, Kitano M, et al: Atresia of the coronary sinus orifice: fatal outcome after intraoperative division of the drainage left superior vena cava. *J Thorac Cardiovasc Surg* 1989; 98:30.
11. Harris AM, Shawkat S, Bailey JS: The use of an endotracheal tube for cannulation of left superior vena cava via coronary sinus for repair of a sinus venosus atrial septal defect. *Br Heart J* 1987; 58:676.
12. Toomasian JM, McCarthy JP: Total extrathoracic cardiopulmonary support with kinetic assisted venous drainage: experience in 50 patients. *Perfusion* 1998; 13:137.
13. Taketani S, Sawa Y, Massai T, et al: A novel technique for cardiopulmonary bypass using vacuum system for venous drainage with pressure relief valve: an experimental study. *Artif Organs* 1998; 22:337.
14. Humphries K, Sistino JJ: Laboratory evaluation of the pressure flow characteristics of venous cannulas during vaccum-assisted venous drainage. *J Extracorp Tech* 2002; 34:111.
15. Willcox TW, Mitchell SJ, Gorman DF: Venous air in the bypass circuit: a source of arterial line emboli exacerbated by vacuum-assisted venous drainage. *Ann Thorac Surg* 1999; 68:1285.
16. La Pietra A, Groggi EA, Pua BB, et al: Assisted venous drainage presents the risk of undetected air microembolism. *J Thorac Cardiovasc Surg* 2000; 120:856.
17. Jahangiri M, Rayner A, Keogh B, Lincoln C: Cerebrovascular accident after vacuum-assisted venous drainage in a Fontan patient: a cautionary tale. *Ann Thorac Surg* 2001; 72:1727.
18. Willcox TW: Vacuum-assisted venous drainage: to air or not to air, that is the question: has the bubble burst? *J Extracorp Tech* 2002; 34:24.
19. Davila RM, Rawles T, Mack MJ: Venoarterial air embolus: a complication of vacuum-assisted venous drainage. *Ann Thorac Surg* 2001; 71:1369.
20. Hessel EA II: Cardiopulmonary bypass equipment, in Estafanous FG, Barash PG, Reves JG (eds): *Cardiac Anesthesia: Principles and Clinical Practice,* 2d ed. Philadelphia, Lippincott Williams & Wilkins, 2001; p 335.
21. Jones TJ, Deal DD, Vernon JC, et al: How effective are cardiopulmonary bypass circuits at removing gaseous microemboli? *J Extracorp Tech* 2002; 34:34.
22. Jahangiri M, Rayner A, Keogh B, Lincoln C: Cerebrovascular accident after vacuum-assisted venous drainage in a Fontan patient: a cautionary tale. *Ann Thorac Surg* 2001; 72: 1727.
23. Ambesh SP, Singh SK, Dubey DK, Kaushik S: Inadvertent closure of the superior vena cava after decannulation: a potentially catastrophic complication after termination of bypass [letter]. *J Cardiothorac Vasc Anesth* 1998; 12:723.
24. Brodman R, Siegel H, Lesser M, Frater R: A comparison of flow gradients across disposable arterial perfusion cannulas. *Ann Thorac Surg* 1985; 39:225.
25. Galletti PM, Brecher GA: *Heart-lung Bypass.* New York: Grune & Stratton, 1962.
26. Weinstein GS: Left hemispheric strokes in coronary surgery: implication for end-hole aortic cannulas. *Ann Thorac Surg* 2001; 71:128.
27. Muehrcke DD, Cornhill JF, Thomas JD, Cosgrove DM: Flow characteristics of aortic cannulae. *J Card Surg* 1995; 10:514.
28. Joubert-Hubner E, Gerdes A, Klarproth P, et al: An in-vitro evaluation of aortic arch vessel perfusion characteristics comparing single versus multiple stream aortic cannulae. *Eur J Cardiothorac Surg* 1999; 15:359.
29. Cook DJ, Zehr KJ, Orszulak TA, Slater JM: Profound reduction in brain embolization using an endoaortic baffle during bypass in swine. *Ann Thorac Surg* 2002; 73:198.
30. Macoviak JA, Hwang J, Boerjan KL, Deal DD: Comparing dual-stream and standard cardiopulmonary bypass in pigs. *Ann Thorac Surg* 2002; 73:203.
31. Reichenspurner H, Navia JA, Benny G, et al: Particulate embolic capture by an intra-aortic filter device during cardiac surgery. *J Thorac Cardiovasc Surg* 2000; 119:233.

32. Gerdes A, Hanke T, Sievers H-H: In vivo hydrodynamics of the Embol-X cannula. *Perfusion* 2002; 17:153.
33. Harringer W: Capture of a particulate embolic during cardiac procedures in which aortic cross-clamp is used. *Ann Thorac Surg* 2000; 70:1119.
34. Banbury MK, Cosgrove DM 3rd: Arterial cannulation of the innominate artery. *Ann Thorac Surg* 2000; 69:957.
35. Mills NL, Everson CT: Atherosclerosis of the ascending aorta and coronary artery bypass: pathology, clinical correlates, and operative management. *J Thorac Cardiovasc Surg* 1991; 102:546.
36. Beique FA, Joffe D, Tousignant G, Konstadt S: Echocardiographic-based assessment and management of atherosclerotic disease of the thoracic aorta. *J Cardiothorac Vasc Anesth* 1998; 12:206.
37. Blauth CI, Cosgrove DM, Webb BW, et al: Atheroembolism from the ascending aorta. *J Thorac Cardiovasc Surg* 1992; 103:1104.
38. Barbut D, Grassineau D, Lis E, et al: Posterior distribution of infarcts in strokes related to cardiac operation. *Ann Thorac Surg* 1998; 65:1656.
39. Murphy DA, Craver JM, Jones EL, et al: Recognition and management of ascending aortic dissection complicating cardiac surgical operations. *J Thorac Cardiovasc Surg* 1983; 85:247.
40. Davila-Roman VG, Kouchoukos NT, Schechtman KB, Barzilai B: Atherosclerosis of the ascending aorta is a predictor of renal dysfunction after cardiac operations. *J Thorac Cardiovasc Surg* 1999; 117:111.
41. Davila-Roman V, Phillips K, Davila R, et al: Intraoperative transesophageal echocardiography and epiaortic ultrasound for assessment of atherosclerosis of the thoracic aorta. *J Am Coll Cardiol* 1996; 28:942.
42. Sylivris S, Calafiore P, Matalanis G, et al: The intraoperative assessment of ascending aortic atheroma: epiaortic imaging is superior to both transesophageal and direct palpation. *J Cardiothorac Vasc Anesth* 1997; 11:704.
43. Konstadt SN, Reich DL, Quintana C, Levy M: The ascending aorta: how much does transesophageal echocardiography see? *Anesth Analg* 1994; 78:240.
44. Wilson MJ, Boyd SYN, Lisagor PG, et al: Ascending aorta atheroma assessed intra-operatively by epiaortic and transesophageal echocardiography. *Ann Thorac Surg* 2000; 70:35.
45. Konstadt SN, Reich DL, Kahn R, Viggiani RF: Transesophageal echocardiography can be used to screen for ascending aortic atherosclerosis. *Anesth Analg* 1995; 81:225.
46. Gaudino M, Glieca F, Alessandrini F, et al: The unclampable ascending aorta in coronary artery bypass patients: a surgical challenge of increasing frequency. *Circulation* 2000; 102:1497.
47. Gillinov AM, Lytle BW, Hoang V, et al: The atherosclerotic aorta at aortic valve replacement: surgical strategies and results. *J Thorac Cardiovasc Surg* 2000; 120:957.
48. Byrne JG, Aranki SF, Cohn LH: Aortic valve operations under deep hypothermic circulatory arrest for the porcelain aorta: "no-touch" technique. *Ann Thorac Surg* 1998; 65:1313.
49. Prifti E, Frati G: Innominate artery cannulation in patients with severe porcelain aorta. *Ann Thorac Surg* 2001; 71:399.
50. Borger MA, Taylor RL, Weisel RD, et al: Decrease cerebral emboli during distal aortic arch cannulation: a randomized clinical trial. *J Thorac Cardiovasc Surg* 1999; 118:740.
51. Grossi EA, Kanchuger MS, Schwartz DS, et al: Effect of cannula length on aortic arch flow: protection of the atheromatous aortic arch. *Ann Thorac Surg* 1995; 59:710.
52. McLeskey CH, Cheney FW: A correctable complication of cardiopulmonary bypass. *Anesthesiology* 1982; 56:214.
53. Watson BG: Unilateral cold neck. *Anaesthesia* 1983; 38:659.
54. Magner JB: Complications of aortic cannulation for open-heart surgery. *Thorax* 1971; 26:172.
55. Salama FD, Blesovsky A: Complications of cannulation of the ascending aorta for open heart surgery. *Thorax* 1970; 25:604.
56. Taylor PC, Groves LK, Loop FD, Effler DB: Cannulation of the ascending aorta for cardiopulmonary bypass. *J Thorac Cardiovasc Surg* 1976; 71:255.
57. Gott JP, Cohen CL, Jones EL: Management of ascending aortic dissections and aneurysms early and late following cardiac operations. *J Card Surg* 1990; 5:2.
58. Still RJ, Hilgenberg AD, Akins CW, et al: Intraoperative aortic dissection. *Ann Thorac Surg* 1992; 53:374.
59. Troianos CA, Savino JS, Weiss RL: Transesophageal echocardiographic diagnosis of aortic dissection during cardiac surgery. *Anesthesiology* 1991; 75:149.
60. Lees MH, Herr RH, Hill JD, et al: Distribution of systemic blood flow of the rhesus monkey during cardiopulmonary bypass. *J Thorac Cardiovasc Surg* 1971; 61:570.
61. Salerno TA, Lince DP, White DN, et al: Arch versus femoral artery perfusion during cardiopulmonary bypass. *J Thorac Cardiovasc Surg* 1978; 78:681.
62. Svensson LG: Editorial comment: autopsies in acute Type A aortic dissection, surgical implications. *Circulation* 1998; 98:II-302.
63. Van Arsdell GS, David TE, Butany J: Autopsies in aortic Type A aortic dissection. Surgical implications. *Circulation* 1998; 98: II-299.
64. Hendrickson SC, Glower DD: A method for perfusion of the leg during cardiopulmonary bypass via femoral cannulation. *Ann Thorac Surg* 1998; 65:1807.
65. Gates JD, Bichell DP, Rizzu RJ, et al: Thigh ischemia complicating femoral vessel cannulation for cardiopulmonary bypass. *Ann Thorac Surg* 1996; 61:730.
66. Van derSalm TJ: Prevention of lower extremity ischemia during cardiopulmonary bypass via femoral cannulation. *Ann Thorac Surg* 1997; 63:251.
67. Biegutay AM, Garamella JJ, Danyluk M, Remucal HC: Retrograde aortic dissection occurring during cardiopulmonary bypass. *JAMA* 1976; 236:465.
68. Benedict JS, Buhl TL, Henney RP: Acute aortic dissection during cardiopulmonary bypass. *Arch Surg* 1974; 108:810.
69. Carey JS, Skow JR, Scott C: Retrograde aortic dissection during cardiopulmonary bypass: "nonoperative" management. *Ann Thorac Surg* 1977; 24:44.
70. Galloway AC, Shemin RJ, Glower DD, et al: First report of the Port-Access International Registry. *Ann Thorac Surg* 1999; 67:51.
71. Sabik JF, Lytle BW, McCarthy PM, Cosgrove DM: Axillary artery: an alternative site of arterial cannulation for patients with extensive and peripheral vascular disease. *J Thorac Cardiovasc Surg* 1995; 109:885.
72. Bichell DP, Balaguer JM, Aranki SF, et al: Axilloaxillary cardiopulmonary bypass: a practical alternative to femorofemoral bypass. *Ann Thorac Surg* 1997; 64:702.
73. Baribeau YR, Westerbrook BM, Charlesworth DC, Maloney CT: Arterial inflow via an axillary artery graft for the severely atherosclerotic aorta. *Ann Thorac Surg* 1998; 66:33.
74. Gerdes A, Joubert-Hubner E, Esders K, Sievers H-H: Hydrodynamics of aortic arch vessel during perfusion through the right subclavian artery. *Ann Thorac Surg* 2000; 69:1425.
75. Neri E, Massetti M, Capannini G, et al: Axillary artery cannulation in type A aortic dissection operations. *J Thorac Cardiovasc Surg* 1999; 118:324.
76. Svensson LG: Editorial comment: autopsies in acute Type A aortic dissection, surgical implications. *Circulation* 1998; 98:II-302.
77. Whitlark JD, Sutter FP: Intrathoracic subclavian artery cannulation as an alternative to the femoral or axillary artery cannulation [letter]. *Ann Thorac Surg* 1998; 66:296.

78. Golding LAR: New cannulation technique for the severely calcified ascending aorta. *J Thorac Cardiovasc Surg* 1985; 90:626.
79. Fukuda I, Aikawa S, Imazuru T, Osaka M: Transapical aortic cannulation for acute aortic dissection with diffuse atherosclerosis. *J Thorac Cardiovasc Surg* 2002; 123:369.
80. Coselli JS, Crawford ES: Femoral artery perfusion for cardiopulmonary bypass in patients with aortoiliac artery obstruction. *Ann Thorac Surg* 1987; 43:437.
81. Orenstein JM, Sato N, Arron B, et al: Microemboli observed in deaths following cardiopulmonary bypass surgery: silicone antifoam agents and polyvinyl chloride tubing as source of emboli. *Hum Pathol* 1982; 13:1082.
82. Mitchell SJ, Wilcox T, Gorman DF: Bubble generation and venous air filtration by hard-shell venous reservoirs: a comparative study. *Perfusion* 1997; 12:325.
83. Schonberger JPAM, Everts PAM, Hoffman JJ: Systemic blood activation with open and closed venous reservoirs. *Ann Thorac Surg* 1995; 59:1549.
84. Blauth CI, Smith PL, Arnold JV, et al: Influence of oxygenator type on the prevalence and extent of micro-emboli retinal ischemia during cardiopulmonary bypass: assessment by digital image analysis. *J Thorac Cardiovasc Surg* 1990; 99:61.
85. Griffin S, Pugsley W, Treasure T: Microembolism during cardiopulmonary bypass: a comparison of bubble oxygenator with arterial line filter and membrane oxygenator alone. *Perfusion* 1991; 6:99.
86. Pearson DT: Gas exchange; bubble and membrane oxygenators. *Semin Thorac Cardiovasc Surg* 1990; 2:313.
87. Masters RG, Bethune DW: Pro and con: bubble oxygenators are outdated and no longer appropriate for cardiopulmonary bypass. *J Cardiothorac Anesth* 1989; 3:235.
88. Drinker PA, Bartlett RH, Bialer RM, Noyes BS Jr: Augmentation of membrane gas transfer by induced secondary flows. *Surgery* 1969; 66:775.
89. Wiesenack C, Wiesner G, Keyl C, et al: In vivo uptake and elimination of isoflurane by different membrane oxygenators during cardiopulmonary bypass. *Anesthesiology* 2002; 97:133.
90. Clark RE, Beauchamp RA, Magrath RA, et al: Comparison of bubble and membrane oxygenators in short and long term perfusions. *J Thorac Cardiovasc Surg* 1979; 78:655.
91. Edmunds LH Jr, Ellison, N, Colman, RW, et al: Platelet function during open heart surgery: comparison of the membrane and bubble oxygenators. *J Thorac Cardiovasc Surg* 1982; 83:805
92. Hammond GL, Bowley WW: Bubble mechanics and oxygen transfer. *J Thorac Cardiovasc Surg* 1976; 71:422.
93. High KM, Snider MT, Bashein G: Principles of oxygenator function: gas exchange, heat transfer, and blood-artificial surface interaction, in Gravlee GP, Davis RF, Utley JR (eds): *Cardiopulmonary Bypass: Principles and Practice*. Baltimore, Williams & Wilkins, 1993; p 28.
94. Jenkins OF, Morris R, Simpson JM: Australasian perfusion incident survey. *Perfusion* 1997; 12:279.
95. Wahba A, Philipp A, Behr R, Birnbaum DE: Heparin-coated equipment reduces the risk of oxygenator failure. *Ann Thorac Surg* 1998; 65:1310.
96. Fisher AR: The incidence and cause of emergency oxygenator changeovers. *Perfusion* 1999; 14:207.
97. Svenmarker S, Haggmark S, Jansson E, et al: The relative safety of an oxygenator. *Perfusion* 1997; 12:289.
98. Geissler HJ, Allen JS, Mehlhorn U, et al: Cooling gradients and formation of gaseous microemboli with cardiopulmonary bypass: an echocardiographic study. *Ann Thorac Surg* 1997; 64:100.
99. Moen O, Fosse E, Broten J, et al: Difference in blood activation related to roller/centrifugal pumps and heparin coated/uncoated surfaces in a cardiopulmonary bypass model circuit. *Perfusion* 1996; 11:113.
100. Tamari Y, Lee-Sensiba K, Leonard EF, et al: The effects of pressure and flow on hemolysis caused by Bio-Medics centrifugal pumps and roller pumps: guidelines for choosing a blood pump. *J Thorac Cardiovasc Surg* 1993; 106:997.
101. Driessen JJ, Fransen G, Rondelez L, et al: Comparison of the standard roller pump and a pulsatile centrifugal pump for extracorporeal circulation during routine coronary artery bypass grafting. *Perfusion* 1991; 6:303.
102. Wahba A, Philip A, Bauer MF, et al: The blood saving potential of vortex versus roller pump with and without aprotinin. *Perfusion* 1995; 10:333.
103. Ashraf S, Bhattacharya K, Zachanias S, et al: Serum S100B release after coronary artery bypass grafting: roller versus centrifugal pump. *Ann Thorac Surg* 1998; 66:1958.
104. Baufreton C, Intractor L, Jansen PGM, et al: Inflammatory response to cardiopulmonary bypass using roller or centrifugal pumps. *Ann Thorac Surg* 1999; 67:972.
105. Leschinsky BM, Zimin NK: Centrifugal blood pumps–a brief analysis: development of new designs. *Perfusion* 1991; 6:115.
106. Kolff J, McClurken JB, Alpern JB: Beware centrifugal pumps: not a one-way street, but a dangerous siphon! *Perfusion* 1990; 5:225.
107. Bernstein EF, Gleason LR: Factors influencing hemolysis with roller pumps. *Surgery* 1967; 61:432.
108. Reed CC, Kurusz M, Lawrence AE: *Safety Techniques in Perfusion*. Stafford, TX, Quali-Med, Inc, 1988.
109. Stammers AH: Extracorporeal devices and related technologies, in Kaplan JA (ed.): *Cardiac Anesthesia,* 4th ed. Philadelphia, WB Saunders, 1999; p 1018.
110. Mongero LB, Beck JR, Orr TR, et al: Clinical evaluation of setting pump occlusion by the dynamic method: effect on flow. *Perfusion* 1998; 13:360.
111. Uretzky G, Landsburg G, Cohn D, et al: Analysis of microembolic particles originating in extracorporeal circuits. *Perfusion* 1987; 2:9.
112. Wright G: Hemodynamic analysis could resolve the pulsatile blood flow controversy [current review]. *Ann Thorac Surg* 1994; 58:1199.
113. Wright G: Mechanical simulation of cardiac function by means of pulsatile blood pumps. *J Cardiothorac Vasc Anesth* 1997; 11:299.
114. Edmunds LH Jr: Pulseless cardiopulmonary bypass. *J Thorac Cardiovasc Surg* 1982; 84:800.
115. Boucher JK, Rudy LW, Edmunds LH Jr: Organ blood flow during pulsatile cardiopulmonary bypass. *J Appl Physiol* 1974; 36:86.
116. Tominaga R, Smith WA, Massiello A, et al: Chronic nonpulsatile blood flow, I: cerebral autoregulation in chronic nonpulsatile biventricular bypass: carotid blood flow response to hypercapnia. *J Thorac Cardiovasc Surg* 1994; 108:907.
117. Rudy LW Jr, Heymann MA, Edmunds LH Jr: Distribution of systemic blood flow during cardiopulmonary bypass. *J Appl Physiol* 1973; 34:194.
118. Pearson DT: Micro-emboli: gaseous and particulate, in Taylor KM (ed.): *Cardiopulmonary Bypass: Principles and Management*. Baltimore, Williams & Wilkins, 1986; p 313.
119. Butler BD, Kurusz M: Gaseous microemboli: a review. *Perfusion* 1990; 5:81.
120. Blauth CI: Macroemboli and microemboli during cardiopulmonary bypass. *Ann Thorac Surg* 1995; 598:300.
121. Moody DM, Brown WR, Challa VR: Brain micro embolic associated with cardiopulmonary bypass: a histologic and magnetic resonance imaging study. *Ann Thorac Surg* 1995; 59:1304.
122. Borger MA, Feindel CM: Cerebral emboli during cardiopulmonary bypass: effect of perfusionist interventions and aortic cannulas. *J Extracorp Tech* 2002; 34:29.

123. Barbut D, Yao F-S, Lo Y-W, et al: Determination of size of aortic emboli and embolic load during coronary artery bypass grafting. *Ann Thorac Surg* 1997; 63:1262.
124. Lee WH Jr, Krumhaar D, Fonkalsrud EW, et al: Denaturation of plasma proteins as a cause of morbidity and death after intracardiac operations. *Surgery* 1961; 50:1025.
125. Liu J-F, Su Z-F, Ding W-X: Quantitation of particle microemboli during cardiopulmonary bypass: experimental and clinical studies. *Ann Thorac Surg* 1992; 54:1196.
126. Brooker RF, Brown WR, Moody DM, et al: Cardiotomy suction: a major source of brain lipid emboli during cardiopulmonary bypass. *Ann Thorac Surg* 1998; 65:1651.
127. Ringelstein EB, Droste DW, Babikian VL, et al: Consensus on microembolus detection by TCD. *Stroke* 1998; 29:725.
128. Wright G, Furness A, Haigh S: Integral pulse frequency modulated ultrasound for the detection and quantification of gas microbubbles in flowing blood. *Perfusion* 1987; 2:131.
129. Kincaid E, Jones T, Stump D, et al: Processing scavenged blood with a cell saver reduces cerebral lipid microembolization. *Ann Thorac Surg* 2000; 70:1296.
130. Hammon JW, Stump DA, Hines M, et al: Prevention of embolic events during coronary artery bypass graft surgery. *Perfusion* 1994; 9:412.
131. Hammon JW, Stump DA, Kon ND, et al: Risk factors and solutions for the development of neurobehavioral changes after coronary artery bypass grafting. *Ann Thorac Surg* 1997; 63: 1613.
132. Edmunds LH Jr: Thromboembolic complications of current cardiac valvular prostheses. *Ann Thorac Surg* 1982; 34: 96.
133. Plochl W, Cook DJ: Quantification and distribution of cerebral emboli during cardiopulmonary bypass in the swine: the impact of Pa_{CO_2}. *Anesthesiology* 1999; 90:183.
134. Cook DJ, Plochl W, Orszulak TA: Effect of temperature and PaCO2 on cerebral embolization during cardiopulmonary bypass in swine. *Ann Thorac Surg* 2000; 69:415.
135. Berman L, Marin F: Micropore filtration during cardiopulmonary bypass, in Taylor KM (ed.): *Cardiopulmonary Bypass: Principles and Management*. Baltimore, Williams & Wilkins, 1986; p 355.
136. Marshall L: Filtration in cardiopulmonary bypass: past, present and future. *Perfusion* 1988; 3:135.
137. Joffe D, Silvay G. The use of microfilters in cardiopulmonary bypass. *J Cardiothorac Vasc Anesth* 1994; 8:685.
138. Ware JA, Scott MA, Horak JK, Solis RT: Platelet aggregation during and after cardiopulmonary bypass: effect of two different cardiotomy filters. *Ann Thorac Surg* 1982; 34:204.
139. Gourlay T, Gibbons TG, Fleming J, Taylor KM: Evaluation of a range of arterial line filters: part I. *Perfusion* 1987; 2:297.
140. Gourlay T, Gibbons M, Taylor KM: Evaluation of a range of arterial line filters: part II. *Perfusion* 1988; 3:29.
141. Gourlay T: The role of arterial line filters in perfusion safety. *Perfusion* 1988; 3:195.
142. Munsch C, Rosenfeldt F, Chang V: Absence of particle-induced coronary vasoconstriction during cardioplegic infusion: is it desirable to use a microfilter in the infusion line? *J Thorac Cardiovasc Surg* 1991; 101:473.
143. Clark RE, Brillman J, Davis DA, et al: Microemboli during coronary artery bypass grafting: genesis and effect on outcome. *J Thorac Cardiovasc Surg* 1995; 109:249.
144. Muraoka R, Yokota M, Aoshima M, et al: Subclinical changes in brain morphology following cardiac operations as reflected by computed tomographic scans of the brain. *J Thorac Cardiovasc Surg* 1981; 81:364.
145. Henriksen L, Hjelms E: Cerebral blood flow during cardiopulmonary bypass in man: effect of arterial filtration. *Thorax* 1986; 41:386.
146. Pugsley W, Klinger L, Paschalie C, et al: The impact of microemboli during cardiopulmonary bypass on neurological functioning. *Stroke* 1994; 25:1393.
147. Garvey JW, Willner A, Wolpowitz A, et al: The effect of arterial filtration during open heart surgery on cerebral function. *Circulation* 1983; 64(suppl 2):2.
148. Nussmeier NA, Fish KJ: Neuropsychologic dysfunction after cardiopulmonary bypass: a comparison of two institutions. *J Cardiothorac Vasc Anesth* 1991; 5:584.
149. Aris A, Solanes H, Camara ML, et al: Arterial line filtration during cardiopulmonary bypass. *J Thorac Cardiovasc Surg* 1986; 91:526.
150. Mossing KA: Post cardiotomy delirium and microfiltration [Master of Arts dissertation]. University of Washington, 1975.
151. Mejak BL, Stammers A, Raush E, et al: A retrospective study of perfusion incidents and safety devices. *Perfusion* 2000; 15:51.
152. Sylivris S, Levi C, Matalanis G, et al: Pattern and significance of cerebral microemboli during coronary artery bypass grafting. *Ann Thorac Surg* 1998; 66:1674.
153. Grocott HP, Croughwell ND, Amory DW, et al: Cerebral emboli and serum S-100-B during cardiac operation. *Ann Thorac Surg* 1998; 65:1645.
154. Aldea GS, O'Gara P, Shapira OM, et al: Effects of anticoagulation protocol on outcome in patients undergoing CABG with heparin-bonded cardiopulmonary bypass circuits. *Ann Thorac Surg* 1998; 65:425.
155. Milsom FP, Mitchell SJ. A dual-vent left heart de-airing technique markedly reduces carotid artery microemboli. *Ann Thorac Surg* 1998; 66:785.
156. Clark RE, Brillman J, Davis DA, et al: Microemboli during coronary artery bypass grafting: genesis and effects on outcome. *J Thorac Cardiovasc Surg* 1995; 109:249.
157. Morris SJ: Leucocyte reduction in cardiovascular surgery. *Perfusion* 2001; 11:371.
158. Matheis G, Scholz M, Simon A, et al: Leukocyte filtration in cardiac surgery: a review. *Perfusion* 2001; 16:361.
159. Ortolana G, Aldea GS, Lilly K, et al: A review of leukofiltration in cardiac surgery: the time course of reperfusion injury may facilitate study design of anti-inflammatory effects. *Perfusion* 2002; 17(suppl):53.
160. Taylor KM (ed): Perfusion workshop 2001: therapeutic filtration perfusion. *Perfusion* 2002; 17(suppl):1.
161. Gu YJ, deVries AJ, Voa P, et al: Leukocyte depletion during cardiac operations: a new approach through the venous bypass circuit. *Ann Thorac Surg* 1999; 67:604.
162. Lazar HL, Zhang X, Hamasaki T, et al: Role of leukocyte depletion during cardiopulmonary bypass and cardioplegic arrest. *Ann Thorac Surg* 1995; 60:1745.
163. Gott JP, Cooper, WA, Schmidt FE, et al: Modifying risk for extracorporeal circulation: Trial of four anti-inflammatory strategies. *Ann Thorac Surg* 1998; 66:747.
164. Hurst T, Johnson D, Cujec B, et al: Depletion of activated neutrophils by a filter during cardiac valve surgery. *Can J Anaesth* 1997; 44:131.
165. Baksaas ST, Videm V, Mollnes TE, et al: Leukocyte filtration during cardiopulmonary bypass hardly changed leukocyte counts and did not influence myeloperoxidase, complement, cytokines or platelets. *Perfusion* 1998; 13:429.
166. Chen Y-F, Tsai W-C, Lin C-C, et al: Leukocyte depletion attenuates expression of neutrophil adhesion molecules during cardiopulmonary bypass in human beings. *J Thorac Cardiovasc Surg* 2001; 123:218.
167. Mahoney CB: Heparin-bonded circuits: clinical outcome and costs. *Perfusion* 1998; 13:1892.
168. Hsu L-C: Heparin-coated CPB circuits: current status. *Perfusion* 2001; 16:417.

169. Ovrum E, Mollnes TE, Fosse E, et al: High and low heparin dose with heparin-coated cardiopulmonary bypass: activation of complement and granulocytes. *Ann Thorac Surg* 1995; 60:1755.
170. Aldea GS, Soltow LO, Chandler WL, et al: Limitation of thrombin generation, platelet activation, and inflammation by elimination of cardiotomy suction in patients undergoing coronary artery bypass grafting treated with heparin-bonded circuits. *J Thorac Cardiovasc Surg* 2002; 123:742.
171. Heyer EJ, Lee KS, Manspeizer HE, et al: Heparin-bonded CPB circuits reduce cognitive dysfunction. *J Cardiothorac Vasc Anesth* 2001; 16:37.
172. Edmunds LH Jr, Stenach N: The blood-surface interface, in Gravlee GP, Davis RF, Kurusz M, Utley JR (eds): *Cardiopulmonary Bypass: Principles and Practice,* 2d ed. Media, PA, Williams & Wilkins, 2000; p 149.
173. Videm V, Mollnes TE, Fosse E, et al: Heparin-coated cardiopulmonary bypass equipment, I: biocompatibility markers and development of complications in a high-risk population. *J Thorac Cardiovasc Surg* 1999; 117:794.
174. Wildevuur CRH, Jansen DGM, Bezemer PD, et al: Clinical evaluation of Duraflo II heparin treated extracorporeal circuits. *Eur J Cardiothorac Surg* 1997; 11:616.
175. Ranucci M, Mozzucco A, Pessotto R, et al: Heparin-coated circuits for high-risk patients: a multi-center prospective randomized trial. *Ann Thorac Surg* 1999; 67:994.
176. DeSomer F, VanBelleghem Y, Cases F, et al: Phosphorylcholine coating offers natural platelet preservation during CPB. *Perfusion* 2002; 17:39.
177. Ereth MH, Nuttall GA, Clarke SH, et al: Biocompatibility of trillium biopassive surface-coated oxygenator versus un-coated oxygenator during CPB. *J Cardiothorac Vasc Anesth* 2001; 15:545.
178. Stammers AH: Biocompatibilty of trillium biopassive surface-coated oxygenator during CPB [editorial]. *J Cardiothorac Vasc Anesth* 2001; 15:539.
179. Gu YJ, Boonstra PW, Rijnsburger AA, et al: Cardiopulmonary bypass circuit treated with surface-modifying additives: a clinical evaluation of blood compatibility. *Ann Thorac Surg* 1998; 65: 1343.
180. Wimmer-Greinecker G, Matheis G, Martens S, et al: Synthetic protein treated versus heparin coated cardiopulmonary surfaces: similar clinical results and minor biochemical differences. *Eur J Cardiothorac Surg* 1999; 16:211.
181. Edmunds LH Jr, Saxena NH, Hillyer P, Wilson TJ: Relationship between platelet count and cardiotomy suction return. *Ann Thorac Surg* 1978; 25:306.
182. Wright G, Sanderson JM: Cellular aggregation and trauma in cardiotomy suction systems. *Thorax* 1979; 34:621.
183. Boonstra PW, van Imhoff GW, Eysman L, et al: Reduced platelet activation and improved hemostasis after controlled cardiotomy suction during clinical membrane oxygenator perfusions. *J Thorac Cardiovasc Surg* 1985; 89:900.
184. Tabuchi N, Haan J, Boonstra PW, van Oeveren W: Activation of fibrinolysis in the pericardial cavity during cardiopulmonary bypass. *J Thorac Cardiovasc Surg* 1993; 106:828.
185. Downing SW, Edmunds LH Jr: Release of vasoactive substances during cardiopulmonary bypass. *Ann Thor Surg* 1992; 54:1236.
186. Baile EM, Ling IT, Heyworth JR, et al: Bronchopulmonary anastomotic and noncoronary collateral blood flow in humans during cardiopulmonary bypass. *Chest* 1985; 87:749.
187. Little AG, Lin CY, Wernley JA, et al: Use of the pulmonary artery for left ventricular venting during cardiac operations. *J Thorac Cardiovasc Surg* 1984; 87:532.
188. Casha AR: A simple method of aortic root venting for CABG [letter]. *Ann Thorac Surg* 1998; 66:608.
189. Victor S, Kobeer M: Venting and de-airing without a roller pump [letter]. *Ann Thorac Surg* 1993; 55:807.
190. Olinger GM, Bonchek LI: Ventricular venting during coronary revascularization: assessment of benefit by intraoperative ventricular function curves. *Ann Thorac Surg* 1978; 26:525.
191. Kanter KR, Schaff HV, Gott VL: Reduced oxygen consumption with effective left ventricular venting during postischemic reperfusion. *Circulation* 1982; 66(suppl 1):1.
192. Breyer RN, Meredith JW, Mills SA, et al: Is a left ventricular vent necessary for coronary artery bypass procedures performed with cardioplegia arrest? *J Thorac Cardiovasc Surg* 1983; 86:338.
193. Salomon NW, Copeland JG: Single catheter technique for cardioplegia and venting during coronary artery bypass grafting. *Ann Thorac Surg* 1980; 29:88.
194. Marco JD, Barner HB: Aortic venting: comparison of vent effectiveness. *J Thorac Cardiovasc Surg* 1977; 73:287.
195. Brenner WI, Wallsh E, Spencer FC: Aortic vent efficiency: a quantitative evaluation. *J Thorac Cardiovasc Surg* 1971; 61:258.
196. Clements F, Wright SJ, deBruijn N: Coronary sinus catheterization made easy for port-access minimally invasive cardiac surgery. *J Cardiothorac Vasc Anesth* 1998; 12:96.
197. Aldea GS, Connelly G, Fonger JD, et al: Directed atraumatic coronary sinus cannulation for retrograde cardioplegia administration. *Ann Thorac Surg* 1992; 54:789.
198. Panos AL, Ali IS, Birnbaum PL, et al: Coronary sinus injuries during retrograde continuous normothermic blood cardioplegia. *Ann Thorac Surg* 1992; 54:1132.
199. Kurusz M, Girouard MK, Brown PS Jr: Coronary sinus rupture with retrograde cardioplegia. *Perfusion* 2002; 17:77.
200. Journois D, Israel-Biet E, Pouard P, et al: High volume, zero-balance hemofiltration to reduce delayed inflammatory response to cardiopulmonary bypass in children. *Anesthesiology* 1996; 85:965.
201. Boldt J, Zickmann B, Fedderson B, et al: Six different hemofiltration devices for blood conservation in cardiac surgery. *Ann Thorac Surg* 1991; 51:747.
202. High KM, Williams DR, Kurusz M: Cardiopulmonary bypass circuits and design, in Hensley FA Jr, Martin DE (eds): *A Practical Approach to Cardiac Anesthesia,* 2d ed. Boston, Little, Brown, 1995; p 465.
203. Stammers AH: Monitoring controversies during cardiopulmonary bypass: how far have we come? *Perfusion* 1998; 13:35.
204. Baraka A, Barody M, Harous S, et al: Continuous venous oximetry during cardiopulmonary bypass: influence of temperature changes, perfusion flow and hematocrit level. *J Cardiothorac Anesth* 1990; 4:35.
205. Swan H, Sanchez M, Tyndall M, Koch C: Quality control of perfusion: monitoring venous blood oxygen tension to prevent hypoxic acidosis. *J Thorac Cardiovasc Surg* 1990; 99:868.
206. Rubsamen DS: Continuous blood gas monitoring during cardiopulmonary bypass—how soon will it be the standard of care? [editorial]. *J Cardiothorac Anesth* 1990; 4:1.
207. Pearson DT: Blood gas control during cardiopulmonary bypass. *Perfusion* 1988; 31:113.
208. Mark JB, Fitzgerald D, Fenton T, et al: Continuous arterial and venous blood gas monitoring during cardiopulmonary bypass. *J Thorac Cardiovasc Surg* 1991; 102:431.
209. McDaniel LB, Zwischenberger JM, Vertrees RA, et al: Mixed venous oxygen saturation during cardiopulmonary bypass poorly predicts regional venous saturation. *Anesth Analg* 1994; 80:466.
210. Lindholm L, Hansdottir V, Lundqvist M, Jeppsson A: The relationship between mixed venous and regional venous oxygen saturation during cardiopulmonary bypass. *Perfusion* 2002; 17:133.
211. Nicolson SC, Jobes DR, Steven JM, et al: Evaluation of a user-operative patient-site blood gas and chemistry monitor in children undergoing cardiac surgery. *J Cardiothorac Anesth* 1989; 3:741.

212. Kirson LE, Goldman JM: A system for monitoring the delivery of ventilating gas to the oxygenator during cardiopulmonary bypass. *J Cardiothorac Vasc Anesth* 1994; 8:51.
213. Berg E, Knudsen N: Automatic data collection for cardiopulmonary bypass. *Perfusion* 1988; 3:263.
214. Gourlay T: Computers in perfusion practice. *Perfusion* 1987; 2:79.
215. Beppu T, Imai Y, Fukui Y: A computerized control system for cardiopulmonary bypass. *J Thorac Cardiovasc Surg* 1995; 109:428.
216. Rosengart T, DeBois W, O'Hara M, et al: Retrograde autologous priming for cardiopulmonary bypass: a safe and effective means of decreasing hemodilution and transfusion requirements. *J Thorac Cardiovasc Surg* 1998; 115:426.
217. Shapira O, Aldea G, Treanor P, et al: Reduction of allogeneic blood transfusions after open heart operations by lowering cardiopulmonary bypass prime volume. *Ann Thorac Surg* 1998; 65:724.
218. Boldt J: Volume therapy in cardiac surgery: does the kind of fluid matter? *J Cardiothorac Vasc Anesth* 1999; 13:752.
219. Hoeft A, Korb H, Mehlhorn U, et al: Priming of CPB with human albumin or ringer lactate: effect on colloid osmotic pressure and extravascular lung water. *Br J Anaesth* 1991; 66:77.
220. London MJ, Franks M, Verrier ED, et al: The safety and efficacy of ten percent penta starch as a CPB priming solution: a randomized clinical trial. *J Thorac Cardiovasc Surg* 1992; 104:284.
221. Marelli D, Paul A, Samson R, et al: Does the addition of albumin to the prime solution in cardiopulmonary bypass affect clinical outcome? *J Thorac Cardiovasc Surg* 1989; 98:751.
222. Scott DA, Hore PJ, Cannata J, et al: A comparison of albumin, polygeline and crystalloid priming solutions for CPB in patients having coronary artery bypass surgery. *Perfusion* 1995; 10:415.
223. Jenkins IR, Curtis AP: The combination of mannitol and albumin in the priming solution reduces positive intraoperative fluid balance during CPB. *Perfusion* 1995; 10:301.
224. Buhre W, Hoeft A, Schorn B, et al: Acute effects of mitral valve replacement on extravascular lung water in patients receiving colloid or crystalloid priming of CPB. *Br J Anaesth* 1997; 79:311.
225. Cochrane Injuries Group Albumin Reviews: Human albumin administration in critically ill patients: systemic review of randomized controlled trials. *BMJ* 1998; 317:235.
226. Wilkes MM, Navicks RJ: Patient survival after human albumin administration: a meta-analysis of randomized, controlled trials. *Ann Intern Med* 2001; 135:149.
227. Wilkes MM, Navickis RJ, Sibbald WJ: Albumin versus hydroxyethyl starch in CPB surgery: a meta-analysis of post-operative bleeding. *Ann Thorac Surg* 2001; 72:527.
228. McKnight CK, Elliott MJ, et al: The cardiopulmonary bypass pump priming fluid and nitrogen balance after open heart surgery in adults. *Perfusion* 1986; 1:47.
229. McKnight CK, Elliott MJ, Pearson DT, et al: The effect of four different crystalloid bypass pump priming fluids upon the metabolic response to cardiac operations. *J Thorac Cardiovasc Surg* 1985; 90:97.
230. Lanier WL: Glucose management during cardiopulmonary bypass: cardiovascular and neurologic implications. *Anesth Analg* 1991; 72:423.
231. Francis JL, Palmer GJ III, Moroose R, Drexler A: Comparative effects of bovine and porcine heparin on heparin antibody formation following cardiovascular surgery. *Ann Thorac Surg (in press)*.
232. Bull BS, Huse WM, Brauer FS, et al: Heparin therapy during extracorporeal circulation: the use of a drug response curve to individualize heparin and protamine dosage. *J Thorac Cardiovasc Surg* 1975; 69:685.
233. Levy JH, Despotis GJ, Szlam F, et al: Recombinant human transgenic antithrombin in cardiac surgery: a dose finding study. *Anesthesiology* 2002; 96:1095.
234. Weiss ME, Nyhan D, Peng Z, et al: Association of protamine IgE and IgG antibodies with life-threatening reactions to intravenous protamine. *N Engl J Med* 1989; 320:886.
235. Khabbaz KR, Zankoul F, Warner KG: Intraoperative metabolic monitoring of the heart, II: online measurement of myocardial tissue pH. *Ann Thorac Surg* 2001; 72:S2227.
236. Ikonomidis JS, Yau IM, Weisel RD, et al: Optimal flow rates for retrograde warm cardioplegia. *J Thorac Cardiovasc Surg* 1994; 107:510.
237. Honkonen EL, Kaukinen L, Pehkoneu EJ, Kaukinen S: Myocardial cooling and right ventricular function in patients with right coronary artery disease: antegrade vs. retrograde cardioplegia. *Acta Anaesthesiol Scand* 1997; 41:287.
238. Kirklin JW, Barrett-Boyes BE: *Cardiac Surgery,* 2d ed. New York, Wiley, 1993; Ch. 2.
239. Taylor KM, Bain WH, Maxted KJ, et al: Comparative studies of pulsatile and nonpulsatile bypass, I: pulsatile system employed and its hematologic effects. *J Thorac Cardiovasc Surg* 1978; 75:569.
240. Shevde K, Finlayson DC: Pro and con: pulsatile flow in preferable to non-pulsatile flow during cardiopulmonary bypass. *J Cardiothorac Anesth* 1987; 2:165.
241. Munoz HR, Sacco CM: Cardiac mechanical energy and effects on the arterial tree. *J Cardiothorac Vasc Anesth* 1997; 11:289.
242. Hornick P, Taylor K: Pulsatile and nonpulsatile perfusion: the continuing controversy. *J Cardiothorac Vasc Anesth* 1997; 11:310.
243. Mangano CM, Hill L, Cartwright CR, Hindman BJ: Nonpulsatile versus pulatile perfusion, in Kaplan JA (ed): *Cardiac Anesthesia,* 4th ed. Philadelphia, WB Saunders, 1999; p 1065.
244. Taylor KM, Bain WH, Davidson KG, Turner MA: Comparative clinical study of pulsatile and non-pulsatile perfusion in 350 consecutive patients. *Thorax* 1982; 37:324.
245. Murkin JM, Martzke JS, Buchan AM, et al: A randomized study of the influence of perfusion technique and pH management in 316 patients undergoing coronary artery bypass surgery, I: mortality and cardiovascular morbidity. *J Thorac Cardiovasc Surg* 1995; 110:340.
246. Shaw PJ, Bates D, Cartlige NEF: Analysis of factors predisposing to neurological injury in patients undergoing coronary bypass operations. *QJM* 1989; 72:633.
247. Henze T, Stephen H, Sonntag H: Cerebral dysfunction following extracorporeal circulation for aorta coronary bypass surgery: no difference in neuropsychological outcomes after pulsatile versus non pulsatile flow. *J Thorac Cardiovasc Surg* 1990; 38:65.
248. Murkin JM, Martzke JS, Buchan AM, et al: A randomized study of the influence of perfusion technique and pH management strategy in 316 patients undergoing coronary artery bypass surgery, II: neurological and cognitive outcomes. *J Thorac Cardiovasc Surg* 1995; 110:349.
249. Ohri SK, Desai JB, Gaer JAR, et al: Intra-abdominal complications after cardiopulmonary bypass. *Ann Thorac Surg* 1991; 52:826.
250. Badner NH, Murkin JM, Lok P: Differences in pH management and pulsatile/nonpulsatile perfusion during cardiopulmonary bypass do not influence renal function. *Anesth Analg* 1992; 75:696.
251. Louagie YA, Gonzalez M, Collard E, et al: Does flow character of cardiopulmonary bypass make a difference? *J Thorac Cardiovasc Surg* 1992; 104:1628.
252. Rees W, Schiessler A, Schulz F, et al: Pulsatile extra-corporeal circulation: fluid-mechanic considerations. *Perfusion* 1993; 8:459.
253. Gourlay T, Taylor KM: Pulsatile flow and membrane oxygenators. *Perfusion* 1994; 9:189.
254. Sugurtekin H, Boston US, Cook DJ: Bypass flow, mean arterial pressure, and cerebral perfusion during cardiopulmonary bypass in dogs. *J Cardiothorac Vasc Anesth* 2000; 14:25.

255. Sadahiro M, Haneda K, Mohri H: Experimental study of cerebral autoregulation during cardiopulmonary bypass with or without pulsatile perfusion. *J Thorac Cardiovasc Surg* 1994; 108:446.
256. Schwartz AE, Sandhu AA, Kaplan RJ et al: Cerebral blood flow is determined by cardiopulmonary bypass arterial pressure and not cardiopulmonary bypass flow rate. *Ann Thorac Surg* 1995; 60:165.
257. Hill SE, van Wermeskerken GK, Lardenoye J-WH, et al: Intraoperative physiologic variables and outcome in cardiac surgery, part I: in-hospital mortality. *Ann Thorac Surg* 2000; 69:1070.
258. Slogoff S, Reul GL, Keats AS, et al: Role of perfusion pressure and flow in major organ dysfunction after cardiopulmonary bypass. *Ann Thorac Surg* 1990; 50:511.
259. Gold JP, Charlson MR, Williams-Russa P, et al: Improvements of outcomes after coronary artery bypass: a randomized trial comparing intraoperative high versus low mean arterial pressure. *J Thorac Cardiovasc Surg* 1995; 110:1302.
260. Hartman GS, Yao F-S, Bruefach M, et al: Severity of aortic atheromatous disease diagnosed by transesophageal echocardiography predicts stroke and other outcomes associated with coronary artery surgery: a prospective study. *Analg Anesth* 1996; 83:701.
261. Liam B-L, Plöchl W, Cook DJ, et al: Hemodilution and whole body oxygen balance during normothermic cardiopulmonary bypass in dogs. *J Thorac Cardiovasc Surg* 1998; 115:1203.
262. Cook DJ, Orszulak TA, Daly RC: Minimum hematocrit at differing cardiopulmonary bypass temperatures in dogs. *Circulation* 1998; 98(suppl II):II-170.
263. Cook DJ: Optimal conditions for cardiopulmonary bypass. *Semin Cardiothorac Vasc Anesth* 2001; 5:265.
264. Hill SE, VanWermesker, Ken GK, et al: Intraoperative physiologic variables and outcome in cardiac surgery, part I: in-hospital mortality. *Ann Thorac Surg* 2000; 69:1070.
265. DeFoe GR, Ross CS, Olmstead EM, et al: Lowest hematocrit on bypass and adverse outcomes associated with coronary artery bypass grafting. *Ann Thorac Surg* 2001; 71:769.
266. Groom RC: High or low hematocrits during cardiopulmonary bypass for patients undergoing coronary artery bypass graft surgery? An evidence-based approach to the question. *Perfusion* 2002; 17:99.
267. Jonas RA. Optimal pH strategy for hypothermic circulatory arrest [editorial]. *J Thorac Cardiovasc Surg* 2001; 121:204.
268. Khatri P, Babyak M, Croughwell ND, et al: Temperature during coronary artery bypass surgery affects quality of life. *Ann Thorac Surg* 2001; 71:110.
269. Engleman RM, Pleet AB, Hicks R, et al: Is there a relationship between systemic perfusion temperature during coronary artery bypass grafting and extent of intraoperative ischemic central nervous system injury? *J Thorac Cardiovasc Surg* 2000; 119:230.
270. Nathan HJ, Wells GA, Munson JL, Wozny D: Neuroprotective effect of mild hypothermia in patients undergoing coronary artery surgery with cardiopulmonary bypass. A randomized trial. *Circulation* 2001; 104(suppl I):I-85.
271. Stephan H, Weyland A, Kazmaier S, et al: Acid-base management during hypothermic cardiopulmonary bypass does not affect cerebral metabolism but does affect blood flow and neurologic outcome. *Br J Anaesth* 1992; 69:51.
272. Patel RL, Turtle MR, Chambers DJ, et al: Alpha-stat acid base regulation during cardiopulmonary bypass improves neuropsychologic outcome in patients undergoing coronary artery bypass grafting. *J Thorac Cardiovasc Surg* 1996; 111:1267.
273. Murkin JM, Farrar JK, Tweed WA, et al: Cerebral autoregulation and flow/metabolism coupling during cardiopulmonary bypass: rhe influence of $PaCO_2$. *Anesth Analg* 1987; 66:825.
274. Van den Berghe G, Wouters P, Weekers, et al: Intensive insulin therapy in critically ill patients. *N Engl J Med* 2001; 345:1359.
275. Bernard GR, Sopko G, Cerra F, et al: National Heart Lung and Blood Institute and Food and Drug Administration Workshop Report: Pulmonary Artery Catheterization and Clinical Outcomes (PACC). *JAMA* 2000; 283:2568.
276. Shanewise JS, Cheung AT, Aronson S, et al: ASE/SCA guidelines for performing a comprehensive intraoperative multiplane transesophageal echocardiography examination: recommendation of the American Society of Echocardiography council for intraoperative echocardiography and the Society of Cardiovascular Anesthesiologists task force for certification in perioperative echocardiography. *Anesth Analg* 1999; 99:870.
277. Lucina MG, Savage RM, Hearm C, Kraenzler EJ: The role of transesophageal echocardiography on perfusion management. *Semin Cardiothorac Vasc Anesth* 2001; 5:321.
278. Paul D, Hartman GS: Foley balloon occlusion of the atheromatous ascending aorta: the role of transesophageal echocardiography. *J Cardiothorac Vasc Anesth* 1998; 12:61.
279. Siegel LC, St Goar FG, Stevens JH, et al: Monitoring considerations for Port-Access cardiac surgery. *Circulation* 1997; 96:562.
280. Yamada E, Matsumura M, Kimura S, et al: Usefulness of transesophageal echocardiography in detecting changes in flow dynamics responsible for malperfusion phenomena observed during surgery of aortic dissection. *Am J Cardiol* 1997; 79:1149.
281. Tingleff J, Joyce FS, Pettersson G: Intraoperative echocardiographic study of air embolism during cardiac operations. *Ann Thorac Surg* 1995; 60:673.
282. Stone JG, Young WL, Smith CR, et al: Do standard monitoring sites reflect true brain temperature when profound hypothermia is rapidly induced and reversed? *Anesthesiology* 1995; 82:344.
283. Rumana CS, Gopinath SP, Uzura M, et al: Brain temperature exceeds systemic temperature in head-injured patients. *Crit Care Med* 1998; 26:562.
284. Johnson RZ, Fox MA, Grayson A, et al: Should we rely on nasopharyngeal temperature during cardiopulmonary bypass? *Perfusion* 2002; 17:145.
285. Nussmeier NA, personal communication, 2002.
286. Stump DA, Jones JJ, Rorie KD: Neurophysiologic monitoring and outcomes in cardiovascular surgery [review article]. *J Cardiothorac Vasc Anesth* 1999; 13:600.
287. Edmunds HL: Advances in neuromonitoring for cardiothoracic and vascular surgery. *J Cardiothorac Vasc Anesth* 2001; 15:241.
288. McDaniel LB, Zwischenberger JM, Vertrees RA, et al: Mixed venous oxygen saturation during cardiopulmonary bypass poorly predicts regional venous saturation. *Anesth Analg* 1994; 80:466.
289. Wenger R, Bavaria JE, Ratcliffe M, Edmunds LH Jr: Flow dynamics of peripheral venous catheters during extracorporeal membrane oxygenator (ECMO) with a centrifugal pump. *J Thorac Cardiovasc Surg* 1988; 96:478.
290. Hessel EA II: Bypass techniques for descending thoracic aortic surgery. *Semin Cardiothorac Vasc Anesth* 2001; 5:293.
291. Ireland KW, Follette DM, Iguidbashian J, et al: Use of a heat exchanger to prevent hypothermia during thoracic and thoracoabdominal aneurysm repairs. *Ann Thorac Surg* 1993; 55:534.
292. Edmunds LH Jr, Austen WG, Shaw RS, Kosminski S: Clinical and physiologic considerations of left heart bypass during cardiac arrest. *J Thorac Cardiovasc Surg* 1961; 41:356.
293. O'Connor CJ, Rothenberg DM: Anesthetic considerations for descending thoracic aortic surgery: part II. *J Cardiothorac Vasc Anesth* 1995; 9:734.
294. Hedlund KD, Dattilo R: Supportive angioplasty [letter]. *Perfusion* 1990; 5:297.
295. Toomasian JM: Cardiopulmonary bypass for less invasive procedures. *Perfusion* 1999; 14:279.

296. Taylor KM (ed): 1997 Hammersmith perfusion workshop: perfusion techniques for minimally invasive cardiac surgery. *Perfusion* 1998; 13:225.
296a. Grocott HP, Smith MS, Glower DC, Clements FM: Endovascular aortic balloon clamp malposition during minimally invasive cardiac surgery. *Anesthesiology* 1998; 88:1396.
297. Young WL, Lawton MT, Gupta DF, Hashimoto T: Anesthetic management of deep hypothermic circulatory arrest for cerebral aneurysm surgery. *Anesthesiology* 2002; 96:497.
298. Lawton MT, Roudzens PA, Zabramski JM, Spetzler RF: Hypothermic circulatory arrest in neurovascular surgery: evolving indications and predictions of patient outcome. *Neurosurgery* 1998; 43:10.
299. Soong WAL, Uysal S, Reich DL: Cerebral protection during surgery of the aortic arch. *Semin Cardiothorac Vasc Anesth* 2001; 5:286.
300. Hiramatsu T, Miura T, Forbess JM, et al: pH strategies and cerebral energetics before and after circulatory arrest. *J Thorac Cardiovasc Surg* 1995; 109:948.
301. Kurth CD, O'Rourke MM, O'Hara IB: Comparison of pH-stat and alpha stat cardiopulmonary bypass on cerebral oxygenation and blood flow in relation to hypothermic circulatory arrest in piglets. *Anesthesiology* 1998; 98:110.
302. Hindman BJ, Dexter F, Cutkomp J, Smith T: pH-stat management reduces cerebral metabolic rate for oxygen during profound hypothermia (17°C): a study during cardiopulmonary bypass in rabbits. *Anesthesiology* 1995; 82:983.
303. Sharyak LA, Chai PJ, Kern FH, et al: Blood gas management and degree of cooling: effects on cerebral metabolism before and after circulatory arrest. *J Thorac Cardiovasc Surg* 1995; 110: 1649.
304. Sakamoto T, Zurakowski D, Duebener LF, et al: Combination of alpha-stat strategy and hemodilution exacerbates neurologic injury in a survival piglet model with deep hypothermic circulatory arrest. *Ann Thorac Surg* 2002; 73:180.
305. Priestley MA, Golden JA, O'Hara IB, et al: Comparison of neurologic outcome after deep hypothermic circulatory arrest with alpha-stat and pH-stat cardiopulmonary bypass in newborn pigs. *J Thorac Cardiovasc Surg* 2001; 121:336.
306. Jonas RA, Bellinger DC, Rappaport LA et al: Relation of pH-strategy and development outcome after hypothermic circulatory arrest. *J Thorac Cardiovasc Surg* 1993; 106:362.
307. du Plessis AJ, Jonas RA, Wypij J, et al: Perioperative effects of alpha-stat versus pH-stat strategies for deep hypothermic cardiopulmonary bypass in infants. *J Thorac Cardiovasc Surg* 1997; 114:991.
308. Bellinger DC, Wypij D, du Plessis AJ, et al: Developmental and neurologic effects of alpha-stat versus pH-stat strategies for deep hypothermic cardiopulmonary bypass in infants. *J Thorac Cardiovasc Surg* 2001; 121:374.
309. Hindman BJ: Choice of α-stat or ph-stat management and neurologic outcomes after cardiac surgery: it depends. *Anesthesiology* 1998; 98:5.
310. Ekroth R, Thompson RJ, Lincoln C, et al: Elective deep hypothermia with total circulatory arrest: changes in plasma creatine kinase BB, blood glucose, and clinical variables. *J Thorac Cardiovasc Surg* 1989; 97:30.
311. Reich DL, Uysal S, Sliwinski M, et al: Neuropsychological outcome following deep hypothermia circulatory arrest in adults. *J Thorac Cardiovasc Surg* 1999; 117:156.
312. Ergin MA, Galla JD, Lansman SL, et al: Hypothermic circulatory arrest in operations on the thoracic aorta. *J Thorac Cardiovasc Surg* 1994; 107:788.
313. Ergin MA, Uysal S, Reich DL, et al: Temporary neurological dysfunction after deep hypothermic circulatory arrest: a clinical marker of long term functional deficit. *Ann Thorac Surg* 1999; 67:1886.
314. Mezrow CK, Midulla PS, Sadeghi AM, et al: Quantitative electroencephalography: a method to assess cerebral injury after hypothermic circulatory arrest. *J Thorac Cardiovasc Surg* 1995; 109:925.
315. McCullough JN, Zhang N, Reich DL, et al: Cerebral metabolic suppression during hypothermic circulatory arrest in humans. *Ann Thorac Surg* 1999; 67:1895.
316. Ehrlich MP, McCullough JN, Zhang N, et al. Effect of hypothermia on cerebral blood flow and metabolism in the pig. *Ann Thorac Surg* 2002; 73:191.
317. Mezrow CK, Gandsas A, Sadeghi AM, et al. Metabolic correlates of neurologic and behavioral injury after prolonged hypothermic circulatory arrest. *J Thorac Cardiovasc Surg* 1995; 109:959.
318. Newberger JW, Jonas RA, Wernovsky G, et al: A comparison on the perioperative neurologic defect of hypothermic circulatory arrest versus low flow cardiopulmonary in infant heart surgery. *N Engl J Med* 1993; 329:1057.
319. Svensson LG, Crawford ES, Hess KR, et al: Deep hypothermia with circulatory arrest: determinants of stroke and early mortality in 656 patients. *J Thorac Cardiovasc Surg* 1993; 106:19.
320. Bellinger DC, Jonas RA, Rappaport LA, et al: Developmental and neurologic status of children after heart surgery with hypothermic circulatory arrest or low-flow cardiopulmonary bypass. *N Engl J Med* 1995; 332:549.
321. Deeb GM, Jenkins E, Bolling SF, et al: Retrograde cerebral perfusion during hypothermic circulatory arrest reduces neurologic morbidity. *J Thorac Cardiovasc Surg* 1995; 109:259.
322. Wong CH, Bonser RS: Does retrograde cerebral perfusion affect risk factors for stroke and mortality after hypothermic circulatory arrest? *Ann Thorac Surg* 1999; 67:1900.
323. Grabenwoger M, Ehrlich M, Cartes-Zumelzu F, et al: Surgical treatment of aortic arch aneurysms in profound hypothermia and circulatory arrest. *Ann Thorac Surg* 1997; 64:1067.
324. Higami T, Kozawa S, Asada T, et al: Retrograde cerebral perfusion versus selective cerebral perfusion as evaluated by cerebral oxygen saturation during aortic arch reconstruction. *Ann Thorac Surg* 1999; 67:1091.
325. Kazui T, Kimura N, Yamada O, Komatsu S: Surgical outcome of aortic arch aneurysms using selective cerebral perfusion. *Ann Thorac Surg* 1994; 57:904.
326. Tanaka H, Kazui T, Sato H, et al: Experimental study on the optimal flow rate and pressure for selective cerebral perfusion. *Ann Thorac Surg* 1995; 59:651.
327. Ohmi M, Tabayashi K, Hata M, et al: Brain damage after aortic arch repair using selective cerebral perfusion. *Ann Thorac Surg* 1998; 66:1250.
328. Griepp RB: Strategies for cerebral protection during aortic aneurysm surgery, in Kawashima Y and Takamoto S (eds): *Brain Protection in Aortic Surgery*. New York, Elsevier Science, 1997; p 127.
329. Bachet J, Guilmet D, Goudot B, et al: Cold cerebroplegia: a new technique of cerebral protection during operations on the transverse aortic arch. *J Thorac Cardiovasc Surg* 1991; 102:85.
330. Bachet J, Guilmet D, Banfi C, et al: Surgery of aortic arch aneurysm with cold blood antegrade cerebroplegia, in Kawashima Y, Takamoto S (eds): *Brain Protection in Aortic Surgery*. New York, Elsevier Science, 1997; p 139.
331. Alamanni F, Agrifoglio M, Pompilio G, et al: Aortic arch surgery: pros and cons of selective cerebral perfusion: a multivariable analysis for cerebral injury during hypothermic circulatory arrest. *J Cardiovasc Surg* 1995; 36:31.

332. Dossche KM, Schepens MAAM, Morshuis WJ, et al: Antegrade selective cerebral perfusion in operations on the proximal thoracic aorta. *Ann Thorac Surg* 1999; 67:1904.
333. Mills NL, Ochsner JL: Massive air embolism during cardiopulmonary bypass: causes, prevention, and management. *J Thorac Cardiovasc Surg* 1980; 80:708.
334. Ueda Y, Miki S, Kusuhara K, et al: Surgical treatment of aneurysm or dissection involving the ascending aorta and aortic arch, utilizing circulatory arrest and retrograde cerebral perfusion. *J Cardiovasc Surg* 1990; 31:553.
335. Ganzel BL, Edmonds HL Jr, Pank JR, Goldsmith LJ: Neurophysiologic monitoring to assure delivery of retrograde cerebral perfusion. *J Thorac Cardiovasc Surg* 1997; 113:748.
336. DeBrux J-L, Subayi J-B, Pegis J-D, Dillet J: Retrograde cerebral perfusion: anatomic study of the distribution of blood to the brain. *Ann Thorac Surg* 1995; 60:1294.
337. Juvonen T, Weisz DJ, Wolfe D, et al: Can retrograde perfusion mitigate cerebral injury after particulate embolization? A study in a chronic porcine model. *J Thorac Cardiovasc Surg* 1998; 115:1142.
338. Juvonen T, Zhang N, Wolfe D, et al: Retrograde cerebral perfusion enhances cerebral protection during prolonged hypothermic circulatory arrest: a study in a chronic porcine model. *Ann Thorac Surg* 1998; 66:38.
339. Dong P, Guan Y, He M, et al: Clinical application of retrograde cerebral perfusion for brain protection during surgery of ascending aortic aneurysm—a report of 50 cases. *J Extracorp Tech* 2002; 34:101.
340. Lytle BW, McCarthy PM, Meaneu KM, et al: Systemic hypothermia and circulatory arrest combined with arterial perfusion of the superior vena cava. *J Thorac Cardiovasc Surg* 1995; 109:738.
341. Usui A, Abe T, Murase M: Early clinical results of retrograde cerebral perfusion for aortic arch operations in Japan. *Ann Thorac Surg* 1996; 62:94.
342. Lin PJ, Chang GH, Tan PPC, et al: Prolonged circulatory arrest in moderate hypothermia with retrograde cerebral perfusion: is brain ischemic? *Circulation* 1996; 95 (suppl II):II-166.
343. Raskin SA, Fuselier VW, Reeves-Viets JL, Coselli JS: Deep hypothermic circulatory arrest with and without retrograde cerebral perfusion. *Int Anesth Clinics* 1996; 34:177.
344. Coselli JS, LeMaire SA: Experience with retrograde cerebral perfusion during proximal aortic surgery in 290 patients. *J Card Surg* 1997; 12:322.
345. Safi HJ, Letson GV, Illiopoulous DC, et al: Impact of retrograde cerebral perfusion on ascending aorta and arch aneurysm repair. *Ann Thorac Surg* 1997; 63:1601.
346. Moshkovitz Y, David TE, Caleb M, et al: Circulatory arrest under moderate systemic hypothermia and cold retrograde cerebral perfusion. *Ann Thorac Surg* 1998; 66:1179.
347. Okita Y, Takamota S, Ando M, et al: Mortality and cerebral outcome in patients who underwent aortic arch operations using deep hypothermic circulatory arrest with retrograde cerebral perfusion: no relation of early death, stroke, delirium to the duration of circulatory arrest. *J Thorac Cardiovasc Surg* 1998; 115:129.
348. Murkin JM: Retrograde cerebral perfusion: is the brain really being perfused? [editorial]. *J Cardiothorac Vasc Anesth* 1998; 12:249.
349. Kouchoukos NT: Adjuncts to reduce the incidence of embolic brain injury during operations on the aortic arch. *Ann Thorac Surg* 1994; 57:243.
350. Katz MG, Khazin V, Steinmetz A, et al: Distribution of cerebral flow using retrograde versus antegrade cerebral perfusion. *Ann Thorac Surg* 1999; 97:1065.
351. Cheung AT, Bavaria JE, Weiss SJ, et al: Neurophysiologic effects of retrograde cerebral perfusion used for aortic reconstruction. *J Cardiothorac Vasc Anesth* 1998; 12:252.
352. Safi HT, Illiopoulos DC, Gopinath SP, et al: Retrograde cerebral perfusion during profound hypothermia and circulatory arrest in pigs. *Ann Thorac Surg* 1995; 59:1107.
353. Ye J, Ryner LN, Kozlowski P, et al: Retrograde cerebral perfusion results in flow distribution abnormalities and neuronal damage. *Circulation* 1998; 98:II-313.
354. Kurusz M: Lessons from perfusion surveys. *Perfusion* 1997; 12:221.
355. Kurusz M, Butler BD, Katz J, Conti VR: Air embolism during cardiopulmonary bypass. *Perfusion* 1995; 10:361.
356. Bayindir O, Paker T, Akpinar B, et al: Case conference: a 58–year-old man had a massive air embolism during cardiopulmonary bypass. *J Cardiothorac Vasc Anesth* 1991; 5:627.
357. Kols A, Ammar R, Weisz G, Melamed Y: Hyperbaric oxygenation for arterial air embolism during cardiopulmonary bypass. *Ann Thorac Surg* 1993; 55:401.
358. Larach DR, Gibbs NM: Anesthetic management during cardiopulmonary bypass, in Hensley FA Jr, Martin DE, Gravlee GP (eds): *A Practical Approach to Cardiac Anesthesia*, 3rd ed. Philadelphia: Lippincott Williams & Wilkins, 2003.
359. Ziser A, Adir Y, Lavon H, Shupof A: Hyperbaric oxygen therapy for massive arterial air embolism during cardiac operations. *J Thorac Cardiovasc Surg* 1999; 117:818.
360. Pedersen T, Kaargen AL, Benze S: An approach toward total quality assurance in cardiopulmonary bypass: which data to register and how to assess perfusion quality. *Perfusion* 1996; 11:39.
361. Palanzo DA: Perfusion safety: past present and future. *J Cardiothorac Vasc Anesth* 1997; 11:383.
362. Taylor KM (ed): Proceedings of 1996 Hammersmith Perfusion Workshop: safety, standards and education. *Perfusion* 1997; 12:217.
363. Cecere G, Groom R, Forest R, et al: A 10–year review of pediatric perfusion practice in North America. *Perfusion* 2002; 17:83.
364. Silvay G, Ammar T, Reich DL, et al: Cardiopulmonary bypass for adult patients: a survey of equipment and techniques. *J Cardiothorac Vasc Anesth* 1995; 9:420.

11B: Thrombosis and Bleeding

365. Boisclair MD, Lane DA, Philippou H, et al: Thrombin production, inactivation and expression during open heart surgery measured by assays for activation fragments including a new ELISA for prothrombin Fragment F1+2. *Thromb Haemost* 1993; 70:253.
366. Brister SJ, Ofosu FA, Buchanan MR: Thrombin generation during cardiac surgery: is heparin the ideal anticoagulant? *Thromb Haemost* 1993; 70:259.
367. Gorman RC, Ziats NP, Gikakis N, et al: Surface-bound heparin fails to reduce thrombin formation during clinical cardiopulmonary bypass. *J Thorac Cardiovasc Surg* 1996; 111:1.
368. Spanier T, Oz M, Levin H, Weinberg A, et al: Activation of coagulation and fibrinolytic pathways in patients with left ventricular assist devices. *J Thorac Cardiovasc Surg* 1996; 112:1090.
369. Bowen FW, Edmunds LH Jr: Coagulation, anticoagulation, and the interaction of blood and artificical surfaces, in Zwischenberger JB, Steinhorn RH, Bartlett RH (eds): *ECMO Extracorporeal Cardiopulmonary Support in Critical Care*. Extracorporeal Life Support Organization Publication, 2000.
370. Uniyal S, Brash JL: Patterns of adsorption of proteins from human plasma onto foreign surfaces. *Thromb Haemost* 1982; 47:285.
371. Ziats NP, Pankowsky DA, Tierney BP, et al: Adsorption of Hageman factor (factor XII) and other plasma proteins to biomedical polymers. *J Lab Clin Med* 1990; 116:687.

372. Horbett TA: Principles underlying the role of adsorbed plsma proteins in blood interactions with foreign materials. *Cardiovasc Pathol* 1993; 2:137S.
373. Horbett TA: Proteins: structure, properties, and adsorption to surfaces, in Ratner BD, Hoffman AS, Schoen FJ, and Lemons JE (eds): *Biomaterials Science: An Introduction to Materials in Medicine*. San Diego, Academic Press, 1996; p 133.
374. Brash JL, Scott CF, ten Hove P, et al: Mechansim of transient adsorption of fibrinogen from plasma to solid surfaces: role of the contact and fibrinolytic systems. *Blood* 1988; 71:932.
375. Lindon JN, McManama G, Kushner L, et al: Does the conformation of adsorbed fibrinogen dictate platelet interactions with artificial surfaces? *Blood* 1986; 68:355.
376. Edmunds LH Jr, Stenach N: The blood-surface interface, in Gravlee GP, Davis RF, Kurusz M, Utley JR (eds): *Cardiopulmonary Bypass: Principles and Practice,* 2d ed. Media, PA, Williams & Wilkins, 2000; p 149.
377. Muehrcke DD, McCarthy PM, Stewart RW, et al: Complications of extracorporeal life support systems using heparin-bound surfaces. *J Thorac Cardiovasc Surg* 1995; 110:843.
378. Edmunds LH Jr: Blood activation in mechanical circulatory assist devices. *J Congestive Heart Failure Circ* 2000; 1(suppl):141.
379. Bernabei AF, Gikakis N, Maione T, et al: Reversal of heparin anticoagulation by recombinant platelet factor 4 and protamine sulfate in baboons during cardiopulmonary bypass. *J Thorac Cardiovasc Surg* 1995; 109:765.
380. Rosenberg RD, Edelberg M, Zhang L: The heparin-antithrombin system: a natural anticoagulant mechanism, in Colman RW, Hirsh J, Marder VJ, et al (eds): *Hemostasis and Thrombosis: Basic Principles and Clinical Practice*. Philadelphia, JB Lippincott, 2001; p 711.
381. Weitz JI, Hudoba M, Massel D, et al: Clot-bound thrombin is protected from inhibition by heparin- antithrombin III-independent inhibitors. *J Clin Invest* 1990; 86:385.
382. Eisenberg PR, Siegel JE, Abendschein DR, Miletich JP: Importance of factor Xa in determining the procoagulant activity of whole-blood clots. *J Clin Invest* 1993; 91:1877.
383. Ellison N, Edmunds LH Jr, Colman RW: Platelet aggregation following heparin and protamine administration. *Anesthesiology* 1978; 48:65.
384. Khuri S, Valeri CR, Loscalzo J, et al: Heparin causes platelet dysfunction and increases fibrinolysis before the institution of cardiopulmonary bypass. *Ann Thorac Surg* 1995; 60:1008.
385. Salzman EW, Rosenberg RD, Smith MH, et al: Effect of heparin and heparin fractions on platelet aggregation. *J Clin Invest* 1980; 65:64.
386. Sobel M, McNeill PM, Carlson PL, et al: Heparin inhibition of von Willebrand factor-dependent platelet function in vitro and in vivo. *J Clin Invest* 1991; 87:1878.
387. Pixley RA, Cassello A, De La Cadena RA, et al: Effect of heparin on the activation of factor XII and the contact system in plasma. *Thromb Haemost* 1991; 66:540.
388. Wachtfogel YT, Harpel PC, Edmunds LH Jr, Colman RW: Formation of C1s-C1-inhibitor, kallikrien-C1-inhibitor and plasmin-alpha 2–plasmin inhibitor complexes during cardiopulmonary bypass. *Blood* 1989; 73:468.
389. Cavarocchi NC, Schaff HV, Orszulak TA, et al: Evidence for complement activation by protamine-heparin interaction after CPB. *Surgery* 1985; 98:525.
390. Kirklin JK, Chenoweth DE, Naftel DC, et al: Effects of protamine administration after cardiopulmonary bypass on complement, blood elements, and the hemodynamic state. *Ann Thorac Surg* 1986; 41:193.
391. Despotis GJ, Summerfield MD, Joist JH, et al: Comparison of activated coagulation time and whole blood heparin measurements with laboratory plasma anti-Xa heparin concentration in patients having cardiac operations. *J Thorac Cardiovasc Surg* 1994; 108:1076.
392. Hardy J-F, Belisle S, Robitaille D, et al: Measurement of heparin concentration in whole blood with the Hepcon/HMS device does not agree with laboratory determination of plasma heparin concentration using a chromogenic substrate for activated factor X. *J Thorac Cardiovasc Surg* 1996; 112:154.
393. Shore-Lesserson L, Gravlee GP: Anticoagulation for cardiopulmonary bypass, in Gravlee GP, Davis RF, Kurusz M, Utley JR (eds): *Cardiopulmonary Bypass: Principles and Practice*. Philadelphia, Lippincott Williams & Wilkins, 2000; p 435.
394. Dietrich W, Spannagl M, Schramm W, et al. The influence of preoperative anticoagulation on heparin response during cardiopulmonary bypass. *J Thorac Cardiovasc Surg* 1991; 102:505.
395. Tait R, Walker I, Perry D, et al. Prevalence of antithrombin III deficiency subtypes in 4000 healthy blood donors. *Thromb Haemost* 1992; 65:839.
396. Gikakis N, Rao AK, Miyamoto S, Gorman et al: Enoxaparin suppresses thrombin formation and activity during cardiopulmonary bypass in baboons. *J Thorac Cardiovasc Surg* 1998; 116:1043.
397. Hirsh J, Levine MN: Low molecular weight heparin. *Blood* 1992; 79:1.
398. Danhof M, de Boer A, Magnani HN, Stiekema JC: Pharmacokinetic considerations on Orgaran (Org 10172) therapy. *Haemostasis* 1992; 22:73.
399. Stringer KA, Lindenfeld J: Hirudins: antithrombin anticoagulants. *Ann Pharmacother* 1992; 26:1535.
400. Gladwell TD: Bivalirudin: a direct thrombin inhibitor. *Clin Ther* 2002; 1:38.
401. Fitzgerald D, Murphy N: Argatroban: a synthetic thrombin inhibitor of low relative molecular mass. *Coron Artery Dis* 1996; 7:455.
402. Swan SK, St Perer JV, Lanbrecht LJ, Hursting MJ: Comparison of anticoagulant effects and safety of argatroban and heparin in healthy subjects. *Pharmacotherapy* 2000; 20:756.
403. Horne DK 3rd: Nonimmune heparin-platelet interactions: implications for the pathogenesis of heparin-induced thrombocytopenia, in Warkentin TE, Greinacher A (eds): *Heparin-Induced Thrombocytopenia*. New York, Marcel Dekker, 2001; p 123.
404. Warkentin TE, Kelton JG: Temporal aspects of heparin-induced thrombocytopenia. *N Engl J Med* 2001; 344:1286.
405. Amiral J, Meyer D: Heparin-dependent antigens in heparin-induced thrombocytopenia, in Warkentin TE, Greinacher A (eds): *Heparin-Induced Thrombocytopenia*. New York, Marcel Dekker, 2001; p 137.
406. Lee DH, Warkentin TE: Frequency of heparin-induced thrombocytopenia, in Warkentin TE, Greinacher A (eds): *Heparin-Induced Thrombocytopenia*. New York, Marcel Dekker, 2001; p 87.
407. Warkentin TE, Greinacher A: Laboratory testing for heparin-induced thrombocytopenia, in Warkentin TE, Greinacher A (eds): *Heparin-Induced Thrombocytopenia*. New York, Marcel Dekker, 2001; p 231.
408. Wallis DE, Workman KL, Lewis BE, et al: Failure of early heparin cessation as treatment for heparin-induced thrombocytopenia. *Am J Med* 1999; 106:629.
409. Greinacher A: Recombinant hirudin for the treatment of heparin-induced thrombocytopenia, in Warkentin TE, Greinacher A (eds): *Heparin-Induced Thrombocytopenia*. New York, Marcel Dekker, 2001; p 349.
410. Colman RW: Contact activation pathway: inflammatory, fibrinolytic, anticoagulant, antiadhesive and antiangiogenic activities, in Colman RW, Hirsh J, Marder VJ, et al (eds):

Hemostasis and Thrombosis: Basic Principles and Practice. Philadelphia, Lippincott Williams & Wilkins, 2001; p 103.
411. Wachtfogel YT, Harpel PC, Edmunds LH Jr, Colman RW: Formation of C1s-C1-inhibitor, kallikrein-C1 inhibitor and plasmin-alpha 2-plasmin-inhibitor complexes during cardiopulmonary bypass. *Blood* 1989; 73:468.
412. Samuel M, Pixley RA, Villanueva MA, et al: Human factor XII (Hageman factor) autoactivation by dextran sulfate: circular dichroism, fluorescence and ultraviolet difference spectroscopic studies. *J Biol Chem* 1992; 267:19691.
413. Butenas S, van't Veer C, Mann KG: Evaluation of the initiation phase of blood coagulation using ultra sensitive assays for serine proteases. *J Biol Chem* 1997; 272:21527.
414. Gikakis N, Khan MMH, Hiramatsu Y, et al: Effect of factor Xa inhibitors on thrombin formation and complement and neutrophil activation during in-vitro extracorporeal circulation. *Circulation* 1996; 94(suppl II):341.
415. Sundaram S, Gikakis N, Hack CE, et al: Nafamostat mesilate, a broad spectrum protease inhibitor, modulates cellular and humoral activation in simulated extracorporeal circulation. *Thromb Haemost* 1996; 75:76.
416. Walsh PN: Factor XI, in Colman RW, Hirsh J, Marder VJ, et al (eds): *Hemostasis and Thrombosis: Basic Principles and Practice.* Philadelphia, Lippincott Williams & Wilkins, 2001; p 191.
417. Jenny NS, Mann KG: Thrombin, in Colman RW, Hirsh J, Marder VJ, et al (eds): *Hemostasis and Thrombosis: Basic Principles and Practice.* Philadelphia, Lippincott Williams & Wilkins, 2001; p 171.
418. Boisclair MD, Lane DA, Philippou H, et al: Mechanisms of thrombin generation during surgery and cardiopulmonary bypass. *Blood* 1993; 82:3350.
419. Chung JH, Gikakis N, Rao AK, et al: Pericardial blood activates the extrinsic coagulation pathway during clinical cardiopulmonary bypass. *Circulation* 1996; 93:2014.
420. Drake TA, Morrissey JH, Edgington TS: Selective cellular expression of tissue factor in human tissues. *Am J Pathol* 1989; 134:1087.
421. Drake TA, Ruf W, Morrissey JH, Edgington TS: Functional tissue factor is entirely cell surface expressed on lipopolysaccharide-stimulated human blood monocytes and a constitutively tissue factor-producing neoplastic cell line. *J Cell Biol* 1989; 109:389.
422. Philippou H, Adami A, Davidson SJ, et al: Tissue factor is rapidly elevated in plasma collected from the pericardial cavity during cardiopulmonary bypass. *Thromb Haemost* 2000; 84:124.
423. Bauer KA, Kass BL, ten Cate H, et al: Factor IX is activated in vivo by the tissue factor mechanism. *Blood* 1990; 76:731.
424. Scandura JM, Walsh PN: Factor X bound to the surface of activated human platelets is preferentially activated by platelet-bound factor IXa. *Biochemistry* 1996; 35:8890.
425. Hirsh J, Colman RW, Marder VJ, et al: Overview of thrombosis and its treatment, in Colman RW, Hirsh J, Marder VJ, et al (eds): *Hemostasis and Thrombosis: Basic Principles and Practice.* Philadelphia, Lippincott Williams & Wilkins, 2001; p 1071.
426. Mantovani A, Dejana E, Introna M, Bussolino F: Cytokines and endothelial cells, in Remick DG, Friedland JS (eds): *Cytokines in Health and Disease,* 2d ed. New York, Marcel Dekker, 1997; p 323.
427. Ovrum E, Holen EA, Tangen G, et al: Completely heparinized cardiopulmonary bypass and reduced systemic heparin: clinical and hemostatic effects. *Ann Thorac Surg* 1995; 60:365.
428. Rubens FD, Labow RS, Lavallee GR, et al: Hematologic evaluation of cardiopulmonary bypass circuits prepared with a novel block copolymer. *Ann Thorac Surg* 1999; 67:696.
429. Despotis GJ, Joist JH, Hogue CW, et al: More effective suppression of hemostatic system activation in patients undergoing cardiac surgery by heparin dosing based on heparin blood concentrations rather than ACT. *Thromb Haemost* 1996; 76:902.
430. Philippou H, Adami A, Boisclair MD, Lane DA: An ELISA for factor X activation peptide: application to the investigation of thrombogenesis in cardiopulmonary bypass. *Br J Haematol* 1995; 90:432.
431. Tabuchi N, Haan J, Boonstra PW, van Oeveren W: Activation of fibrinolysis in the pericardial cavity during cardiopulmonary bypass. *J Thorac Cardiovasc Surg* 1993; 106:828.
432. Aldea GS, O'Gara P, Shapira OM, et al: Effect of anticoagulation protocol on outcome in patients undergoing CABG with heparin-bonded cardiopulmonary bypass circuits. *Ann Thorac Surg* 1998; 65:425.
433. Coughlin SR, Vu T-K H, Hung DT, Wheaton VI: Characterization of a functional thrombin receptor. *J Clin Invest* 1992; 89:351.
434. Wiedmer T, Esmon CT, Sims PJ: Complement proteins C5b-9 stimulate procoagulant activity through the platelet prothrombinase. *Blood* 1986; 68:875.
435. Rinder CS, Rinder HM, Johnson K, et al: Blockade of C5a and C5b-9 generation inhibits leukocytes and platelet activation during extracorporeal circulation. *J Clin Invest* 1995; 96:1564.
436. Niewiarowski S, Senyi AF, Gilles P: Plasmin-induced platelet aggregation and platelet release reaction. *J Clin Invest* 1973; 52:1647.
437. Michelson AD, MacGregor H, Barnard MR, et al: Reversible inhibition of human platelet activation by hypothermia in vivo and in vitro. *Thromb Haemost* 1994; 71:633.
438. Weerasinghe A, Taylor KM: The platelet in cardiopulmonary bypass. *Ann Thorac Surg* 1998; 66:2145.
439. Lefkovits J, Plow EF, Topol EJ: Platelet glycoprotein Iib/IIIa receptors in cardiovascular medicine. *N Engl J Med* 1995; 332:1553.
440. Rinder CS, Bonnert J, Rinder HM, et al: Platelet activation and aggregation during cardiopulmonary bypass. *Anesthesiology* 1991; 74:388.
441. Gluszko P, Rucinski B, Musial J, et al: Fibrinogen receptors in platelet adhesion to surfaces of extracorporeal circuit. *Am J Physiol* 1987; 252:H615.
442. Lindon JN, McManama G, Kushner L, et al: Does the conformation of adsorbed fibrinogen dictate platelet interactions with artificial surfaces? *Blood* 1986; 68:355.
443. Salzman EW, Lindon J, Brier D: Surface-induced platelet adhesion, aggregation and release, in Vroman L, Leonard E (eds): *The Behavior of Blood and Its Components in Interfaces.* New York: New York Academy of Science, 1977; p 114.
444. Didisheim P, Tirrell MV, Lyons CS, et al: Relative role of surface chemistry and surface texture in blood-material interactions. *Trans Am Soc Artif Intern Org* 1983; 29:169.
445. Rinder HM, Bonan JL, Rinder CS, et al: Activated and unactivated platelet adhesion to monocytes and neutrophils. *Blood* 1991; 78:1760.
446. George JN, Pickett EB, Saucerman S, et al: Platelet surface glycoproteins; studies on resting and activated platelets and platelet membrane microparticles in normal subjects, and observations in patients during adult respiratory distress syndrome and cardiac surgery. *J Clin Invest* 1986; 78:340.
447. Miyamoto S, Marcinkiewicz C, Edmunds LH Jr, Niewiarowski S: Measurement of platelet microparticles during cardiopulmonary bypass by means of captured ELISA for GPIIb/IIIa. *Thromb Haemost* 1998; 80:225.
448. Addonizio VP Jr, Smith JB, Strauss JF 3rd, et al: Thromboxane synthesis and platelet secretion during cardiopulmonary bypass with bubble oxygenator. *J Thorac Cardiovasc Surg* 1980; 79:91.
449. Hennessy VL Jr, Hicks RE, Niewiarowski S, et al: Effects of surface area and composition on the function of human platelets during extracorporeal circulation. *Am J Physiol* 1977; 232:H622.

450. Addonizio VP Jr, Strauss JF 3rd, Li-Feng C, et al: Release of lysosomal hydrolases during extracorporeal circulation. *J Thorac Cardiovasc Surg* 1982; 84:28.
451. Laufer N, Merin G, Grover NB, et al: The influence of cardiopulmonary bypass on the size of human platelets. *J Thorac Cardiovasc Surg* 1975; 70:727.
452. Wenger RK, Lukasiewicz H, Mikuta BS, et al: Loss of platelet fibrinogen receptors during clinical cardiopulmonary bypass. *J Thorac Cardiovasc Surg* 1989; 97:235.
453. Zilla P, Fasol R, Groscurth P, et al: Blood platelets in cardiopulmonary bypass operations. *J Thorac Cardiovasc Surg* 1989; 97:379.
454. Edmunds LH Jr, Ellison N, Colman RW, et al: Platelet function during open heart surgery: comparison of the membrane and bubble oxygenators. *J Thorac Cardiovasc Surg* 1982; 83:805.
455. Kestin AS, Valeri CR, Khuri SF, et al: The platelet function defect of cardiopulmonary bypass. *Blood* 1993; 82:107.
456. Anderson HL 3rd, Cilley RE, Zwischenberger JB, et al: Thrombocytopenia in neonates after extracorporeal membrane oxygenation. *Trans Am Soc Artif Intern Organs* 1986; 32:534.
457. Giesen PLA, Rauch U, Bohrmann B, et al: Blood-borne tissue factor: another view of thrombosis. *Proc Natl Acad Sci U S A* 1999; 96:2311.
458. Gregory SA, Morrissey JH, Edgington TS: Regulation of tissue factor gene expression in the monocyte procoagulant response to endotoxin. *Mol Cell Biol* 1989; 9:2752.
459. Kappelmayer J, Bernabei A, Edmunds LH Jr, et al: Tissue factor is expressed on monocytes during simulated extracorporeal circulation. *Circ Res* 1993; 72:1075.
460. Nieuwland R, Berckmans RJ, Rotteveel-Eijkman RC, et al: Cell-derived microparticles generated in patients during cardiopulmonary bypass are highly procoagulant. *Circulation* 1997; 96:3534.
461. Parratt R, Hunt BJ: Direct activation of factor X by monocytes occurs during cardiopulmonary bypass. *Br J Haemat* 1998; 101:40.
462. Ember JA, Jagels MA, Hugli TE: Characterization of complement anaphylatoxins and their biological responses, in Volankis JE, Frank MM (eds): *The Human Complement System in Health and Disease*. New York: Marcel Dekker, 1998; p 241.
463. Fingerle-Rowson G, Auers J, Kreuzer E, et al: Down-regulation of surface monocyte lipopolysaccharide-receptor CD14 in patients on cardiopulmonary bypass undergoing aorta-coronary bypass operation. *J Thorac Cardiovasc Surg* 1998; 115:1172.
464. Haeffner-Cavaillon N, Roussellier N, Ponzio O, et al: Induction of interleukin-1 production in patients undergoing cardiopulmonary bypass. *J Thorac Cardiovasc Surg* 1989; 98:1100.
465. Enofsson M, Thelin S, Siegbahn A: Monocyte tissue factor expression, cell activation, and thrombin formation during cardiopulmonary bypass: a clinical study. *J Thorac Cardiovasc Surg* 1997; 113:576.
466. Steinberg JB, Kapelanski DP, Olson JD, Weiler JM: Cytokine and complement levels in patients undergoing cardiopulmonary bypass. *J Thorac Cardiovasc Surg* 1993; 106:1008.
467. Fering B, Philip I, Dehoux M, et al: Circulating cytokines in patients undergoing normothermic cardiopulmonary bypass. *J Thorac Cardiovasc Surg* 1994; 108:636.
468. Kawahito K, Kawakami M, Fujiwara T, et al: Interleukin-8 and monocyte chemotactic activating factor responses to cardiopulmonary bypass. *J Thorac Cardiovasc Surg* 1995; 110:99.
469. Saadi S, Platt JL: Endothelial cell responses to complement activation, in Volankis JE, Frank MM (eds): *The Human Complement System in Health and Disease*. New York: Marcel Dekker, 1998; p 335.
470. Asimakopoulos G, Taylor KM: Effects of cardiopulmonary bypass on leukocyte and endothelial adhesion molecules. *Ann Thorac Surg* 1998; 66:2135.
471. Vane JR, Anggard EE, Botting RM: Regulatory functions of the vascular endothelium. *N Engl J Med* 1990; 323:27.
472. Faymonville ME, Deby-Dupont G, Larbuisson R, et al: Prostaglandin E2, prostacyclin, and thromboxane changes during nonpulsatile cardiopulmonary bypass in humans. *J Thorac Cardiovasc Surg* 1986; 91:858.
473. Hashimoto K, Horikoshi H, Miyamoto H, et al: Mechanisms of organ failure following cardiopulmonary bypass: the role of elastase and vasoactive mediators. *J Thorac Cardiovasc Surg* 1992; 104:666.
474. Kappelmeyer J, Bernabei A, Gikakis N, et al: Upregulation of Mac-1 surface expression on neutrophils during simulated extracorporeal circulation. *J Lab Clin Med* 1993; 121:118.
475. Levin EG, Marzec U, Anderson J, et al: Thrombin stimulates tissue plasminogen activator from cultured human endothelial cells. *J Clin Invest* 1984; 74:1988.
476. Francis CW, Marder VJ: Physiologic regulation and pathologic disorders of fibrinolysis, in Colman RW, Hirsh J, Marder VJ, et al: *Hemostasis and Thrombosis: Basic Principles and Practice*. Philadelphia, Lippincott Williams & Wilkins, 2001; p 975.
477. Bachmann F. Plasminogen-plasmin enzyme system, in Colman RW, Hirsh J, Marder VJ, et al: *Hemostasis and Thrombosis: Basic Principles and Practice*. Philadelphia, Lippincott Williams & Wilkins, 2001; p 275.
478. Stibbe J, Kluft C, Brommer EJP, et al: Enhanced fibrinoytic activity during cardiopulmonary bypass in open-heart surgery in man is caused by extrinsic (tissue-type) plasminogen activator. *Eur J Clin Invest* 1984; 14:375.
479. Gram J, Janetzko T, Jespersen J, Bruhn HD: Enhanced effective fibrinolysis following the neutralization of herparin in open heart surgery increases the risk of post-surgical bleeding. *Thromb Haemost* 1990; 63:241.
480. Lu H, Du-Bruit C, Soria J, et al. Postoperative hemostasis and fibrinolysis in patients undergoing cardiopulmonary bypass with or without aprotinin therapy. *Thromb Haemost* 1994; 72:438.
481. Lu H, Soria C, Cramer EM, et al: Temperature dependence of plasmin-induced activation or inhibition of human platelets. *Blood* 1991; 77:996.
482. Cramer EM, Lu H, Caen JP, et al: Differential redistribution of platelet glycoproteins Ib and IIb/IIIa after plasmin stimulation. *Blood* 1991; 77:894.
483. Feinstein DI, Marder VJ, Colman RW: Consumptive thrombohemorrhagic disorders, in Colman RW, Hirsh J, Marder VJ, et al: *Hemostasis and Thrombosis: Basic Principles and Practice*. Philadelphia, Lippincott Williams & Wilkins, 2001; p 1197.

11C: The Inflammatory Response

484. Lee WH Jr, Krumhaar D, Fonkalsrud EW, et al: Denaturation of plasma proteins as a cause of morbidity and death after intracardiac operations. *Surgery* 1961; 50:1025.
485. Chenoweth DE, Cooper SW, Hugli TE, et al: Complement activation during cardiopulmonary bypass: evidence for generation of C3a and C5a anaphylactoxins. *N Engl J Med* 1981; 304:497.
486. Wachtfogel YT, Kucich U, Greenplate J, et al: Human neutrophil degranulation during extracorporeal circulation. *Blood* 1987; 69:324.
487. Roth J, Golub S, Cuckingnan R, et al: Cell-mediated immunity is depressed following cardiopulmonary bypass. *Ann Thorac Surg* 1981; 31:350.
488. DePalma L, Yu M, McIntosh CL, et al: Changes in lymphocyte subpopulations as a result of cardiopulmonary bypass. *J Thorac Cardiovasc Surg* 1991; 101:240.
489. Downing SW, Edmunds LH Jr: Release of vasoactive substances during cardiopulmonary bypass. *Ann Thorac Surg* 1992; 54:1236.

490. Warren JS, Ward PA: The inflammatory response, in Beutler E, Coller BS, Lichtman MA, et al: *Williams Hematology,* 6th ed. New York, McGraw-Hill, 2001; p 67.
491. Wewers MD: Cytokines and macrophages, in Remick DG, Friedland JS (eds): *Cytokines in Health and Disease,* 2d ed. New York, Marcel Dekker, 1997; p 339.
492. Fantone JC: Cytokines and neutrophils: neutrophil-derived cytokines and the inflammatory response, in Remick DG, Friedland JS (eds): *Cytokines in Health and Disease,* 2d ed. New York, Marcel Dekker, 1997; p 373.
493. Weisman HF, Bartow T, Leppo MK, et al: Recombinant soluble CR1usppressed complement activation, inflammation, and necrosis associated with reperfusion of ischemic myocardium. *Trans Assoc Am Physicians* 1990; 103:64.
494. Walport MJ: Complement. *N Engl J Med* 2001; 344:1058.
495. Wachtfogel YT, Harpel PC, Edmunds LH Jr, Colman RW: Formation of C1s-C1-inhibitor, kallikrien-C1-inhibitor and plasmin-alpha 2-plasmin inhibitor complexes during cardiopulmonary bypass. *Blood* 1989; 73:468.
496. Fung M, Loubser PG, Ündar A, et al: Inhibition of complement, neutrophil, and platelet activation by an anti-factor D monoclonal antibody in simulated cardiopulmonary bypass circuits. *J Thorac Cardiovasc Surg* 2001; 122:113.
497. Moat NE, Shore DF, Evans TW: Organ dysfunction and cardiopulmonary bypass: the role of complement and complement regulatory proteins. *Eur J Cardiothorac Surg* 1993; 7:563.
498. Kirklin JK, Chenoweth DE, Naftel DC, et al: Effects of protamine administration after cardiopulmonary bypass on complement, blood elements, and the hemodynamic state. *Ann Thorac Surg* 1986; 41:193.
499. van Oeveren W, Kazatchkine MD, Descamps-Latscha B, et al: Deleterious effects of cardiopulmonary bypass: a prospective study of bubble versus membrane oxygenation. *J Thorac Cardiovasc Surg* 1985; 89:888.
500. Cavarocchi NC, Schaff HV, Orszulak TA, et al: Evidence for complement activation by protamine-heparin interaction after cardiopulmonary bypass. *Surgery* 1985; 98:525.
501. Rinder CS, Rinder HM, Smith MJ, et al: Selective blockade of membrane attack complex formation during simulated extracorporeal circulation inhibits platelet but not leukocyte activation. *J Thorac Cardiovasc Surg* 1999; 118:460.
502. Kirklin JK, Westaby S, Blackstone EH, et al: Complement and the damaging effects of cardiopulmonary bypass. *J Thorac Cardiovasc Surg* 1983; 86:845.
503. Seghaye MC, Duchateau J, Grabitz RG, et al: Complement activation during cardiopulmonary bypass in infants and children: relation to postoperative multiple system organ failure. *J Thorac Cardiovasc Surg* 1993; 106:978.
504. Sahu A, Lambris JD: Complement inhibitors: a resurgent concept in anti-inflammatory therapeutics. *Immunopharmacology* 2000; 49:133.
505. Lambris JD, Sahu A, Wetsel RA: The chemistry and biology of C3, C4 and C5, in Volanakis JE, Frank MM (eds): *The Human Complement System in Health and Disease.* New York, Marcel Dekker, 1998; p 83.
506. Gralinski MR, Park JL, Lucchesi BR: Complement in myocardial tissue injury, in Haunsø S, Aldershville J, Svendsen JH (eds): *Coronary Microcirculation During Ischemia and Reperfusion.* Copenhagen, Munksgaard, 1997; p 211.
507. Rinder CS, Bonan JL, Rinder HM, et al: Cardiopulmonary bypass induces leukocyte-platelet adhesion. *Blood* 1992; 79:1201.
508. Stahl RF, Fisher CA, Kucich U: Effects of simulated extracorporeal circulation on human leukocyte elastase release, superoxide generation, and procoagulant activity. *J Thorac Cardiovasc Surg* 1991; 101:230.
509. Dreyer WJ, Smith CW, Entman ML: Neutrophil activation during cardiopulmonary bypass. *J Thorac Cardiovasc Surg* 1993; 105:763.
510. Schapira M, Despland E, Scott CF, et al: Purified human plasma kallikrein aggregates human blood neutrophils. *J Clin Invest* 1982; 69:1199.
511. Chenoweth DE, Hugli TE: Demonstration of specific C5a receptor on intact human polymorphonuclear leukocytes. *Proc Natl Acad Sci U S A* 1978; 75:3943.
512. Rinder CS, Rinder HM, Smith BR, et al: Blockade of C5a and C5b-9 generation inhibits leukocyte and platelet activation during extracorporeal circulation. *J Clin Invest* 1995; 96:1564.
513. Colman RW: Surface-mediated defense reactions: the plasma contact activation system. *J Clin Invest* 1984; 73:1249.
514. Ember JA, Jagels MA, Hugli TE: Characterization of complement anaphylatoxins and their biological responses, in Volankis JE, Frank MM (eds): *The Human Complement System in Health and Disease.* New York, Marcel Dekker, 1998; p 241.
515. Smolen JE, Boxer LA: Functions of neutrophils, in Beutler E, Coller BS, Lichtman MA, et al: *Williams Hematology,* 6th ed. New York, McGraw-Hill, 2001; p 761.
516. Klempner MS, Dinarello CA, Gallin JI: Human leukocyte pyrogen induces release of specific granule contents from human neutrophils. *J Clin Invest* 1978; 61:1330.
517. Insel PA: Analgesic-antipyretic and antiinflammatory agents and drugs employed in the treatment of gout, in Hardman JG, Limbird LE (eds): *Goodman and Gilman's The Pharmacological Basis of Therapeutics.* New York, McGraw-Hill, 1996; p 618.
518. Kawahito K, Kawahami M, Fujiwara T, et al: Interleukin-8 and monocyte chemotactic activating factor responses to cardiopulmonary bypass. *J Thorac Cardiovasc Surg* 1995; 110:99.
519. Wachtfogel YT, Pixley RA, Kucich U, et al: Purified plasma factor XIIa aggregates human neutrophils and causes degranulation. *Blood* 1986; 67:1731.
520. Elgebaly SA, Hashmi FH, Houser SL, et al: Cardiac-derived neutrophil chemotactic factors: detection in coronary sinus effluents of patients undergoing myocardial revascularization. *J Thorac Cardiovasc Surg* 1992; 103:952.
521. Chello M, Mastroroberto P, Quirino A, et al: Inhibition of neutrophil apoptosis after coronary bypass operation with cardiopulmonary bypass. *Ann Thorac Surg* 2002; 73:123.
522. Abboud CN, Lichtman MA: Structure of the marrow and the hematopoietic microenvironment, in Beutler E, Coller BS, Lichtman MA, et al: *Williams Hematology,* 6th ed. New York, McGraw-Hill, 2001; p 29.
523. Baggiolini M, Dewald B, Moser B: Interleukin-8 and related chemotactic cytokines—CXC and CC chemokines. *Adv Immunol* 1994; 55:97.
524. Lehrer RI, Ganz T: Biochemistry and function of monocytes and macrophages, in Beutler E, Coller BS, Lichtman MA, et al: *Williams Hematology,* 6th ed. New York, McGraw-Hill, 2001; p 865.
525. Mantovani A, Dejana E, Introna M, Bussolino F: Cytokines and endothelial cells, in Remick DG, Friedland JS (eds): *Cytokines in Health and Disease,* 2d ed. New York, Marcel Dekker, 1997; p 323.
526. Yang J, Furie BC, Furie B: The biology of P-selectin glycoprotein ligand-1: its role as a selectin counterreceptor in leukocyte-endothelial and leukocyte-platelet interaction. *Thromb Haemost* 1999; 81:1.
527. Springer TA: Traffic signals for lymphocyte circulation and leukocyte migration: the multistep paradigm. *Cell* 1994; 76:301.
528. Asimakopoulos G, Taylor KM: Effects of cardiopulmonary bypass on leukocyte and endothelial adhesion molecules. *Ann Thorac Surg* 1998; 66:2135.

529. Babior BM, Golde DW: Production, distribution and fate of neutrophils, in Beutler E, Coller BS, Lichtman MA, et al: *Williams Hematology,* 6th ed. New York, McGraw-Hill, 2001; p 755.
530. Smith WB, Gamble JR, Clarklewis I, Vadas MA: Chemotactic desensitization of neutrophils demonstrates interleukin-8 (IL-8)-dependent and IL-8-independent mechanisms of transmigration through cytokine-activated endothelium. *Immunology* 1993; 78:491.
531. Cotran RS, Briscoe DM: Endothelial cells in inflammation, in Kelly W, et al (eds): *Textbook of Rheumatology,* 5th ed. Philadelphia, WB Saunders, 1997; p 183.
532. Hajjar KA, Esmon NL, Marcus AJ, Muller WA: Vascular function in hemostasis, in Beutler E, Coller BS, Lichtman MA, et al: *Williams Hematology,* 6th ed. New York, McGraw-Hill, 2001; p 1451.
533. Kappelmeyer J, Bernabei A, Gikakis N, et al: Upregulation of Mac-1 surface expression on neutrophils during simulated extracorporeal circulation. *J Lab Clin Med* 1993; 121:118.
534. Asimakopoulos G, Kohn A, Stefanou DC, et al: Leukocyte integrin expression in patients undergoing cardiopulmonary bypass. *Ann Thorac Surg* 2000; 69:1192.
535. Chishti AD, Dark JH, Kesteven P, et al: Expression of chemokine receptors CXCR1 and CXCR2 during cardiopulmonary bypass. *J Thorac Cardiovasc Surg* 2001; 122:1162.
536. Asghar SS, Pasch MC: Complement as a promiscuous signal transduction device. *Lab Invest* 1998; 78:1203.
537. Kunkel SL, Lukasc NW, Chensue SW, Strieter RM: Chemokines and the inflammatory response, in Remick DG, Friedland JS (eds): *Cytokines in Health and Disease,* 2d ed. New York, Marcel Dekker, 1997; p 121.
538. Baggiolini M, Dewald B, Moser B: Interleukin-8 and related chemotactic cytokines—CXC and CC chemokines. *Adv Immunol* 1994; 55:97.
539. Gadaleta D, Fahey AL, Verma M, et al: Neutrophil leuktriene generation increases after cardiopulmonary bypass. *J Thorac Cardiovasc Surg* 1994; 108:642.
540. Kilbridge PM, Mayer JE, Newburger JW, et al: Induction of intercellular adhesion molecule-1 and E-selectin mRNA in heart and skeletal muscle of pediatric patients undergoing cardiopulmonary bypass. *J Thorac Cardiovasc Surg* 1994; 107:1183.
541. Hayashi Y, Sawa Y, Ohtake S, et al: Peroxynitrite formation from human myocardium after ischemia-reperfusion during open heart operation. *Ann Thorac Surg* 2001; 72:571.
542. Liebold A, Keyl C, Birnbaum DE: The heart produces but the lungs consume pro-inflammatory cytokines following cardiopulmonary bypass. *Eur J Cardiothorac Surg* 1999; 15:340.
543. Ilton MK, Langton PE, Taylor ML, et al: Differential expression of neutrophil adhesion molecules during coronary artery surgery with cardiopulmonary bypass. *J Thorac Cardiovasc Surg* 1999; 118:930.
544. Chello M, Mastroroberto P, Cirillo F, et al: Neutrophil-endothelial cells modulation in diabetic patients undergoing coronary artery bypass grafting. *Eur J Cardiothorac Surg* 1998; 14:373.
545. Matata BM, Galiñanes M: Cardiopulmonary bypass exacerbates oxidative stress but does not increase proinflammatory cytokine release in patients with diabetes compared with patients without diabetes: regulatory effects of exogenous nitric oxide. *J Thorac Cardiovasc Surg* 2000; 120:1.
546. Mair P, Mair J, Seibt I, et al: Plasma elastase concentrations and pulmonary function after cardiopulmonary bypass. *J Thorac Cardiovasc Surg* 1994; 108:184.
547. Borregaard N, Cowland JB: Granules of the human neutrophilic polymorphonuclear leukocyte. *Blood* 1997; 89:3503.
548. Babior BM: Phagocytes and oxidative stress. *Am J Med* 2000; 109:33.
549. Blackstone EH, Kirklin JW, Stewart RW, et al: The damaging effects of cardiopulmonary bypass, in Wu KK, Roxy EC (eds): *Prostaglandins in Clinical Medicine: Cardiovascular and Thrombotic Disorders.* Chicago, Yearbook Medical Publishers, 1982, p 355.
550. Douglas SD, Ho W-Z: Morphology of monocytes and macrophages, in Beutler E, Coller BS, Lichtman MA, et al: *Williams Hematology,* 6th ed. New York, McGraw-Hill, 2001; p 855.
551. Kappelmayer J, Bernabei A, Edmunds LH Jr, et al: Tissue factor is expressed on monocytes during simulated extracorporeal circulation. *Circ Res* 1993; 72:1075.
552. Chung JH, Gikakis N, Drake TA, et al: Pericardial blood activates the extrinsic coagulation pathway during clinical cardiopulmonary bypass. *Circulation* 1996; 93:2014.
553. Naldini A, Sower L, Bocci V, et al: Thrombin receptor expression and responsiveness of human monocytic cells to thrombin is linked to interferon-induced cellular differentiation. *J Cell Physiol* 1998; 77:76.
554. Tocci MJ, Schmidt JA: Interleukin-1: structure and function, in Remick DG, Friedland JS (eds): *Cytokines in Health and Disease,* 2d ed. New York, Marcel Dekker, 1997; p 1.
555. Saadi S, Platt JL: Endothelial cell responses to complement activation, in Volankis JE, Frank MM (eds): *The Human Complement System in Health and Disease.* New York, Marcel Dekker, 1998; p 335.
556. Francis CW, Marder VJ: Physiologic regulation and pathologic disorders of fibrinolysis, in Colman RW, Hirsh J, Marder VJ, et al (eds): *Hemostasis and Thrombosis: Basic Principles and Practice.* Philadelphia, Lippincott Williams & Wilkins, 2001; p 975.
557. Dreyer WJ, Burns AR, Phillips SC, et al: Intercellular adhesion molecule-1 regulation in the canine lung after cardiopulmonary bypass. *J Thorac Cardiovasc Surg* 1998; 115:689.
558. Rosenkranz WP, Sessa WC, Milstien S, et al: Regulation of nitric oxide synthesis by proinflammatory cytokines in human umbilical vein endothelial cells: elevations in tetrahydrobiopterin levels endhance endothelial nitric oxide synthase specific activity. *J Clin Invest* 1994; 93:2236.
559. Habib A, Creminon C, Frobert Y, et al: Demonstration of an inducible cyclooxygenase in human endothelial cells using antibodies raised against the carboxyl-terminal region of the cyclooxygenase-2. *J Biol Chem* 1993; 268:23448.
560. Vane JR, Anggard EE, Botting RM: Regulatory functions of the vascular endothelium. *N Engl J Med* 1990; 323:27.
561. Jaffe EA: Endothelial cell structure and function, in Hoffman R, Benz EJ Jr, Shattil SJ, et al (eds): *Hematology.* New York, Churchill Livingstone, 1991; p 1198.
562. Faymonville ME, Deby-Dupont G, Larbuisson R, et al: Prostaglandin E2, prostacyclin, and thromboxane changes during nonpulsatile cardiopulmonary bypass in humans. *J Thorac Cardiovasc Surg* 1986; 91:858.
563. Hashimoto K, Horikoshi H, Miyamoto H, et al: Mechanisms of organ failure following cardiopulmonary bypass: the role of elastase and vasoactive mediators. *J Thorac Cardiovasc Surg* 1992; 104:666.
564. Abrams CS, Brass LF: Platelet signal transduction, in Colman RW, Hirsh J, Marder VJ, et al (eds): *Hemostasis and Thrombosis: Basic Principles and Practice.* Philadelphia, Lippincott Williams & Wilkins, 2001; p 541.
565. Selak MA, Chignard M, Smith JB: Cathepsin G is a strong platelet agonist released by neutrophils. *Biochem J* 1988; 251;293.
566. Funk CD: Platelet eicosanoids, in Colman RW, Hirsh J, Marder VJ, et al (eds): *Hemostasis and Thrombosis: Basic Principles and Practice.* Philadelphia, Lippincott Williams & Wilkins, 2001; p 533.

567. Hawrylowicz CM, Santoro AS, Platt FM, Unanue ER: Activated platelets express IL-1 activity. *J Immunol* 1989; 143:4015.
568. Fukami MH, Holmsen H, Kowalska A, Niewiarowski S: Platelet secretion, in Colman RW, Hirsh J, Marder VJ, et al (eds): *Hemostasis and Thrombosis: Basic Principles and Practice.* Philadelphia, Lippincott Williams & Wilkins, 2001; p 559.
569. Tamiya T, Yamasaki M, Maeo Y, et al: Complement activation in cardiopulmonary bypass with special reference to anaphylatoxin production in membrane and bubble oxygenators. *Ann Thorac Surg* 1988; 46:47.
570. Steinberg JB, Kapelanski DP, Olson JD, Weiler JM: Cytokine and complement levels in patients undergoing cardiopulmonary bypass. *J Thorac Cardiovasc Surg* 1993; 106:1008.
571. Tracey KJ: Tumor necrosis factor, in Remick DG, Friedland JS (eds): *Cytokines in Health and Disease,* 2d ed. New York, Marcel Dekker, 1997; p 223.
572. Cox G, Gauldie J. Interleukin-6, in Remick DG, Friedland JS (eds): *Cytokines in Health and Disease,* 2d ed. New York, Marcel Dekker, 1997; p 81.
573. Seghaye M-C, Duchateau J, Bruniaux J, et al: Interleukin-10 release related to cardiopulmonary bypass in infants undergoing cardiac operations. *J Thorac Cardiovasc Surg* 1996; 111:545.
574. de Waal Malefyt R, Abrams J, Bennett B, et al: Interleukin-10 (IL-10) inhibits cytokine synthesis by human monocytes: an autoregulatory role of IL-10 produced by monocytes. *J Exp Med* 1991; 174:1209.
575. Powrie F, Bean A, Moore KW: Interleukin-10, in Remick DG, Friedland JS (eds): *Cytokines in Health and Disease,* 2d ed. New York, Marcel Dekker, 1997; p 143.
576. Minty AJ: Interleukin-13, in Remick DG, Friedland JS (eds): *Cytokines in Health and Disease,* 2d ed. New York, Marcel Dekker, 1997; p 185.
577. Hennein HA, Ebba H, Rodriguez JL, et al: Relationship of the proinflammatory cytokines to myocardial ischemia and dysfunction after uncomplicated coronary revascularization. *J Thorac Cardiovasc Surg* 1994; 108:626
578. Frering B, Philip I, Dehoux M, et al: Circulating cytokines in patients undergoing normothermic cardiopulmonary bypass. *J Thorac Cardiovasc Surg* 1994; 108:636.
579. Haeffner-Cavaillon N, Roussellier N, Ponzio O, et al: Induction of interleukin-1 production in patients undergoing cardiopulmonary bypass. *J Thorac Cardiovasc Surg* 1989; 98:1100.
580. Menasché P: The inflammatory response to cardiopulmonary bypass and its impact on postoperative myocardial function. *Curr Opin Cardiol* 1995; 10:597.
581. Enofsson M, Thelin S, Siegbahn A: Monocyte tissue factor expression, cell activation, and thrombin formation during cardiopulmonary bypass: a clinical study. *J Thorac Cardiovasc Surg* 1997; 113:576.
582. Menasché PH, Haydar S, Peynet J, et al: A potential mechanism of vasodilatation after warm heart surgery: the temperature-dependent release of cytokines. *J Thorac Cardiovasc Surg* 1994; 107:293.
583. Deng MC, Dasch B, Erren M, Möllhoff T, Scheld HH: Impact of left ventricular dysfunction on cytokines, hemodynamics, and outcome in bypass grafting. *Ann Thorac Surg* 1996; 62:184.
584. Sablotzki A, Welters I, Lehmann N, et al: Plasma levels of immunoinhibitory cytokines interleukin-10 and transforming growth factor-b in patients undergoing coronary artery bypass grafting. *Eur J Cardiothorac Surg* 1997; 11:763.
585. Wan S, DeSmet JM, Barvais L, et al: Myocardium is a major source of proinflammatory cytokines in patients undergoing cardiopulmonary bypass. *J Thorac Cardiovasc Surg* 1996; 112:806.
586. Drabe N, Zünd G, Grünenfelder J, et al: Genetic predisposition in patients undergoing cardiopulmonary bypass surgery is associated with an increase of inflammatory cytokines. *Eur J Cardiothorac Surg* 2001; 20:609.
587. Schroeder S, Borger N, Wrigge H, et al: A tumor necrosis factor gene polymorphism influences the inflammatory response following cardiac surgery. *Ann Thorac Surg (in press).*
588. Grocott HP, Newman MF, El-Moalem H, et al: Apolipoprotein E genotype differentially influences the proinflammatory and anti-inflammatory response to cardiopulmonary bypass. *J Thorac Cardiovasc Surg* 2001; 122:622.
589. Chew ST, Newman MF, White WD, et al: Preliminary report on the association or apolipoprotein E polymorphisms with post-operative peak serum creatinine serum concentrations in cardiac surgical patients. *Anesthesiology* 2000; 93:325.
590. Burzotta F, Iacoviello L, DiCastelnuovo A, et al: Relationship of the –174G/C polymorphism of interleukin-6 to interleukin-6 plasma levels and to length of hospitalization after surgical coronary revascularization. *Am J Cardiol* 2001; 88:1125.
591. Pizzo SV, Wu SM: a-Macroglobulins and kunins, in Colman RW, Hirsh J, Marder VJ, et al (eds): *Hemostasis and Thrombosis: Basic Principles and Practice.* Philadelphia, Lippincott Williams & Wilkins, 2001; p 367.
592. Hampton MB, Kettle AJ, Winterbourn DD: Inside the neutrophil phagosome: oxidants, myiloperoxidase and bacterial killing. *Blood* 1998; 92:3007.
593. Taggart DP, Sundaram S, McCartney C, et al: Endotoxemia, complement, and white blood cell activation in cardiac surgery: a randomized trial of laxatives and pulsatile perfusion. *Ann Thorac Surg* 1994; 57:376.
594. Andersen LW, Baek L, Degn H, et al: Presence of circulating endotoxins during cardiac operations. *J Thorac Cardiovasc Surg* 1987; 93:115.
595. Kharazmi A, Andersen LW, Baek L, et al: Endotoxemia and enhanced generation of oxygen radicals by neutrophils from patients undergoing cardiopulmonary bypass. *J Thorac Cardiovasc Surg* 1989; 98:381.
596. Nilsson L, Kulander L, Nystrom S-O, Eriksson O: Endotoxins in cardiopulmonary bypass. *J Thorac Cardiovasc Surg* 1990; 100:777.
597. Rocke DA, Gaffin SL, Wells MT, et al: Endotoxemia associated with cardiopulmonary bypass. *J Thorac Cardiovasc Surg* 1987; 93:832.
598. Jansen NJG, van Oeveren W, Gu YJ, et al: Endotoxin release and tumor necrosis factor formation during cardiopulmonary bypass. *Ann Thorac Surg* 1992; 54:744.
599. Neuhof C, Wendling J, Friedhelm D, et al: Endotoxemia and cytokine generation in cardiac surgery in relation to flow mode and duration of cardiopulmonary bypass. *Shock* 2001; 16:39.
600. Joffs C, Gunasinghe HR, Multani MM, et al: Cardiopulmonary bypass induces the synthesis and release of matrix metalloproteinases. *Ann Thorac Surg* 2001; 71:1518.
601. Smith EEJ, Naftel DC, Blackstone EH, Kirklin JW: Microvascular permeability after cardiopulmonary bypass. *J Thorac Cardiovasc Surg* 1987; 94:225.
602. Ohata T, Sawa Y, Kadoba K, et al: Role of nitric oxide in a temperature dependent regulation of systemic vascular resistance in cardiopulmonary bypass. *Eur J Cardiothorac Surg* 2000; 18:342.
603. Faymonville ME, Pincemail J, Duchateau MD, et al: Myeloperoxidase and elastase as markers of leukocyte activation during cardiopulmonary bypass in humans. *J Thorac Cardiovasc Surg* 1991; 102:309.
604. Pacifico AD, Digerness S, Kirklin JW: Acute alterations of body composition after open intracardiac operations. *Circulation* 1970; 41:331.
605. Menasché PH: The systemic factor: The comparative roles of cardiopulmonary bypass and off-pump surgery in the genesis of

patient injury during and following cardiac surgery. *Ann Thorac Surg* 2001; 72: S2260.

606. Struber M, Cremer JT, Gohrbandt B, et al: Human cytokine responses to coronary artery bypass grafting with and without cardiopulmonary bypass. *Ann Thorac Surg* 1999; 68:1330.
607. Ascione R, Lloyd CT, Underwood MJ: Inflammatory response after coronary revascularization with and without cardiopulmonary bypass. *Ann Thorac Surg* 2000; 69:1198.
608. Ascione R, Caputo M, Angelini GD: Off-pump coronary artery bypass grafting: not a "flash in the pan." *Ann Thorac Surg (in press)*.
609. Hirose H, Amano A, Takahashi A: Off-pump coronary artery bypass grafting for elderly patients. *Ann Thorac Surg* 2001; 72:2013.
610. Ascione R, Lloyd CT, Underwood MJ, et al: On-pump versus off-pump coronary revascularization: evaluation of renal function. *Ann Thorac Surg* 1999; 68:493.
611. Cleveland JC Jr, Shroyer LW, Chen AY, et al: Off-pump coronary artery bypass grafting decreases risk-adjusted mortality and morbidity. *Ann Thorac Surg* 2001;72:1282.
612. Drew CE, Anderson IM: Profound hypothermia in cardiac surgery. *Lancet* 1959; 1:748.
613. Richter JA, Meisner H, Tassani P, et al: Drew-Anderson technique attenuates systemic inflammatory response syndrome and improves respiratory function after coronary artery bypass grafting. *Ann Thorac Surg* 1999; 69:77.
614. Massoudy P, Zahler S, Tassani P, et al: Reduction of pro-inflammatory cytokine levels and cellular adhesion in CABG procedures with separated pulmonary and systemic extracorporeal circulation without an oxygenator. *Eur J Cardiothorac Surg* 2000; 17: 729.
615. Fromes Y, Gaillard D, Ponzio O, et al: Reduction of the inflammatory response following coronary bypass grafting with total minimal extracorporeal circulation. Proceedings of the Joint Meeting of the European Association for Cardiothoracic Surgery & the European Society of Thoracic Surgeons. Lisbon, Portugal, September 16–19, 2001; p 556.
616. Menasché P, Peynet J, Heffner-Cavaillon N, et al: Influence of temperature on neutrophil trafficking during clinical cardiopulmonary bypass. *Circulation* 1995; 92(suppl II): II-334.
617. Øvrum E, Tangen G, Øystese R, et al: Comparison of two heparin-coated extracorporeal circuits with reduced systemic anticoagulation in routine coronary artery bypass operations. *J Thorac Cardiovasc Surg* 2001; 121:324.
618. Wagner WR, Johnson PC, Thompson KA, Marrone GC: Heparin-coated cardiopulmonary bypass circuits: hemostatic alterations and postoperative blood loss. *Ann Thorac Surg* 1994; 58:734.
619. Gorman RC, Ziats NP, Gikakis N, et al: Surface-bound heparin fails to reduce thrombin formation during clinical cardiopulmonary bypass. *J Thorac Cardiovasc Surg* 1996; 111:1.
620. Muehrcke DD, McCarthy PM, Stewart RW, et al: Complications of extracorporeal life support systems using heparin-bound surfaces. *J Thorac Cardiovasc Surg* 1995; 110:843.
621. Edmunds LH Jr, Stenach N: The blood-surface interface, in Gravlee GP, Davis RF, Kurusz M, Utley JR (eds): *Cardiopulmonary Bypass: Principles and Practice,* 2d ed. Media, PA, Williams & Wilkins, 2000; p 149.
622. Butler J, Murithi EW, Pathi VL, et al: Duroflo II heparin bonding does not attenuate cytokine release or improve pulmonary function. *Ann Thorac Surg* 2002; 74:139.
623. Videm V, Mollnes TE, Fosse E, et al: Heparin-coated cardiopulmonary bypass equipment, I: biocompatibility markers and development of complications in a high-risk population. *J Thorac Cardiovasc Surg* 1999; 117:794.
624. Aldea GS, O'Gara P, Shapira OM, et al: Effect of anticoagulation protocol on outcome in patients undergoing CABG with heparin-bonded cardiopulmonary bypass circuits. *Ann Thorac Surg* 1998; 65:425.
625. Fosse E, Thelin S, Svennevig JL, et al: Duraflo II coating of cardiopulmonary bypass circuits reduces complement activation, but does not affect the release of granulocyte enzymes in fully heparinized patients: a European multicenter study. *Eur J Cardiothorac Surg* 1997; 11:320.
626. Muehrcke DD, McCarthy PM, Kottke-Marchant K, et al: Biocompatibility of heparin-coated extracorporeal bypass circuits: a randomized masked clinical trial. *J Thorac Cardiovasc Surg* 1996; 112:472.
627. McCarthy PM, Yared JP, Foster RC, et al: A prospective randomized trial of Duraflo II heparin-coated circuits in cardiac reoperations. *Ann Thorac Surg* 1999; 67:1268.
628. Wildevuur ChRH, Jansen PGM, Bezemer PD, et al: Clinical evaluation of Duraflo II heparin treated extracorporeal circulation circuits (2nd version). The European Working Group on Heparin Coated Extracorporeal Circulation Circuits. *Eur J Cardiothorac Surg* 1997; 11: 616.
629. Ranucci M, Mazzucco A, Pessotto R, et al: Heparin-coated circuits for high-risk patients: a multicenter, prospective, randomized trial. *Ann Thorac Surg* 1999; 67: 994.
630. Tabuchi N, Haan J, Boonstra PW, van Oeveren W: Activation of fibrinolysis in the pericardial cavity during cardiopulmonary bypass. *J Thorac Cardiovasc Surg* 1993; 106:828.
631. Wendel HP, Ziemer G: Coating-techniques to improve the hemocompatibility of artificial devices used for extracorporeal circulation. *Eur J Cardiothorac Surg* 1999; 16: 342.
632. Rubens FD, Labow RS, Lavallee GR, et al: Hematologic evaluation of cardiopulmonary bypass circuits prepared with a novel block copolymer. *Ann Thorac Surg* 1999; 67:689.
633. Defraigne J-O, Pincemail J, Dekoster G, et al: SMA circuits reduce platelet consumption and platelet factor release during cardiac surgery. *Ann Thorac Surg* 2000; 70:2075.
634. Suhara H, Sawa Y, Nishimure M, et al: Efficacy of a new coating material, PMEA, for cardiopulmonary bypass circuits in a porcine model. *Ann Thorac Surg* 2001; 71:1603.
635. Gunaydin S, Farsak B, Kocakulak M, et al: Clinical performance and biocompatibility of poly (2-methoxyethylacrylate) coated extracorporeal circuits. *Ann Thorac Surg* 2002; 74:819.
636. Ninomiya M, Miyaji K, Takamoto S: Poly (2-methoxyethylacrylate)-coated bypass circuits reduce perioperative inflammatory response. *Ann Thorac Surg (in press)*.
637. Naik SK, Knight A, Elliot M: A prospective randomized study of a modified technique of ultrafiltration during pediatric open-heart surgery. *Circulation* 1991; 84(suppl III): III-422.
638. Wang MJ, Chiu IS, Hsu CM, et al: Efficacy of ultrafiltration in removing inflammatory mediators during pediatric cardiac operations. *Ann Thorac Surg* 1996; 61:651.
639. Luciani GB, Menon T, Vecchi B, et al: Modified ultrafiltration reduces morbidity after adult cardiac operations: a prospective, randomized clinical trial. *Circulation* 2001; 104(suppl I): I-253.
640. Grunefelder J, Zund G, Schoeberlein A, et al: Modified ultrafiltration lowers adhesion molecules and cytokine levels after cardiopulmonary bypass without clinical relevance in adults. *Eur J Cardiothorac Surg* 2000; 17:77.
641. Gu JY, de Vries AJ, Vos P, et al: Leukocyte depletion during cardiac operation: a new approach through the venous bypass circuit. *Ann Thorac Surg* 1999; 67:604.
642. Hurst T, Johnson D, Cujec B, et al: Depletion of activated neutrophils by a filter during cardiac valve surgery. *Can J Anaesth* 1997; 44:131.
643. Baksaas ST, Videm V, Mollnes TE, et al: Leukocyte filtration during cardiopulmonary bypass hardly changed leukocyte counts

and did not influence myeloperoxidase, complement, cytokinin or platelets. *Perfusion* 1998; 13:429.
644. Chiba Y, Morioka K, Muraoka R, et al: Effects of depletion of leukocytes and platelets on cardiac dysfunction after cardiopulmonary bypass. *Ann Thorac Surg* 1998; 65:107.
645. Morioka K, Muraoka R, Chiba Y, et al: Leukocyte and platelet depletion with a blood cell separator: effects on lung injury after cardiac surgery with cardiopulmonary bypass. *J Thorac Cardiovasc Surg* 1996; 111:45.
646. Fitch JCK, Rollins S, Matis L, et al: Pharmacology and biological efficacy of a recombinant, humanized, single-chain antibody C5 complement inhibitor in patients undergoing coronary artery bypass graft surgery with cardiopulmonary bypass. *Circulation* 1999; 100:2499.
647. Undar A, Eichstaedt, Clubb FJ Jr, et al: Novel anti-factor D monoclonal antibody inhibits complementand leukocyte activation in a baboon model of cardiopulmonary bypass. *Ann Thorac Surg* 2002; 74;355.
648. Nilsson B, Larsson R, Hong J, et al: Compstatin inhibits complement and cellular activation in whole blood in two models of extracorporeal circulation. *Blood* 1998; 92:1661.
649. Soulika AM, Khan MM, Hattori T, et al: Inhibition of heparin/protamine complex-induced complement activation by compstatin in baboons. *Clin Immunol* 2000; 96:212.
650. Larsson R, Elgue G, Larsson A, et al: Inhibition of complement activation by soluble recombinant CR1 under conditions resembling those in a cardio-pulmonary circuit: reduced up-regulation of CD11b and complete abrogation of binding of PMNs to the biomaterial surface. *Immunopharmacology* 1997; 38:119.
651. Moran P, Beasley H, Gorrell A, et al: Human recombinant soluble decay accelerating factor inhibits complement activation in vitro and in vivo. *J Immunol* 1992; 149:1736.
652. Christiansen D, Milland J, Thorley BR, et al: A functional analysis or recombinant soluble CD46 in vivo and a comparison with recombinant soluble forms of CD55 and CD35 in vitro. *Eur J Immunol* 1996; 26:578.
653. Chai PJ, Nassar R, Oakeley AE, et al: Soluble complement receptor-1 protects heart, lung, and cardiac myofilament function from cardiopulmonary bypass damage. *Circulation* 2000; 101:541.
654. Finn A, Morgan BP, Rebuck N, et al: Effect of inhibition of complement activation using recombinant soluble complement receptor 1 on neutrophil CD11b/CD18 and L-selectin expression and release of interleukin-8 and elastase in simulated cardiopulmonary bypass. *J Thorac Cardiovasc Surg* 1996; 111:451.
655. Rinder CS, Rinder HM, Johnson K, et al: Role of C3 cleavage in monocyte activation during extracorporeal circulation. *Circulation* 1999; 100: 553.
656. Hill GE, Alonso A, Thiele GM, Robbins RA: Glucocorticoids blunt neutrophil CD11b surface glycoprotein upregulation during cardiopulmonary bypass in humans. *Anesth Analg* 1994; 79:23.
657. Hill GE, Alonso A, Spurzem JR, et al: Aprotinin and methylprednisolone equally blunt cardiopulmonary bypass-induced inflammation in humans. *J Thorac Cardiovasc Surg* 1995; 110:1658.
658. Paparella D, Yau TM, Young E: Cardiopulmonary bypass induced inflammaion: pathophysiology and treatment update. *Eur J Cardiothorac Surg* 2002; 21:232.
659. Hall RI, Smith MS, Rocker G: The systemic inflammatory response to cardiopulmonary bypass: pathophysiological, therapeutic and pharmacological considerations. *Anesth Analg* 1997; 85:766.
660. Tabardel Y, Duchateau J, Schmartz D, et al: Corticosteroids increase blood interleukin-10 levels during cardiopulmonary bypass in men. *Surgery* 1996; 119:76.
661. Hill GE, Diego RP, Stammers AH, et al: Aprotinin enhances the endogenous release of interleukin-10 after cardiac operations. *Ann Thorac Surg* 1998; 65:66.
662. Cronstein BN, Kimmel SC, Levin RI, et al: A mechanism for the antiinflammatory effects of corticosteroids: the glucocorticoid receptor regulates leukocyte adhesion to endothelial cells and expression of endothelial-leukocyte adhesion molecule 1 and intercellular adhesion molecule 1. *Proc Natl Acad Sci U S A* 1992; 89:9991.
663. Wan S, LeClerc JL, Huynh C-H, et al: Does steroid pretreatment increase endotoxin release during clinical cardiopulmonary bypass? *J Thorac Cardiovasc Surg* 1999; 117:1004.
664. Teoh KH, Bradley CA, Gauldie J, Burrows H: Steroid inhibition of cytokine-mediated vasodilation after warm heart surgery. *Circulation* 1995; 92(suppl II): II-347.
665. Kawamura T, Inada K, Nara N, et al: Influence of methylprednisolone on cytokine balance during cardiac surgery. *Crit Care Med* 1999; 27:545.
666. Harig F, Hohenstein B, von der Emde J, Weyand M: Modulating IL-6 and IL-10 levels by pharmacologic strategies and the impact of different extracorporeal circulation parameters during cardiac surgery. *Shock* 2001; 16:33.
667. Yared JP, Starr NJ, Torres FK, et al: Effects of single dose, postinduction dexamethasone on recovery after cardiac surgery. *Ann Thorac Surg* 2000; 69:1420.
668. Chaney MA, Durazo-Arvizu RA, et al: Methylprednisolone does not benefit patients undergoing coronary artery bypass grafting and early tracheal extubation. *J Thorac Cardiovasc Surg* 2001; 121:561.
669. Steer JH, Kroeger KM, Abraham LJ, Joyce DA: Glucocorticoids suppress tumor necrosis factor-alpha expression by human monocytic THP-1 cells by suppressing transactivation through adjacent NF-kappaB and c-Jun-activating transcription factor-2 binding sites in the promoter. *J Biol Chem* 2000; 275:18432.
670. Florens E, Salvi S, Peynet J, et al: Can statins reduce the inflammatory response to cardiopulmonary bypass? A clinical study. *J Card Surg* 2001; 16:232.
671. Kovacich JG, Boyle EM, Morgan EN, et al: Inhibition of the transcriptional activator protein nuclear factor kB prevents hemodynamic instability associated with the whole-body inflammatory response syndrome. *J Thorac Cardiovasc Surg* 1999; 118:154.
672. Christman JW, Lancaster LH, Blackwell TS: Nuclear factor kappa B: a pivotal role in the systemic inflammatory response syndrome and new target for therapy. *Intensive Care Med* 1998; 24:1131.
673. Gallimore MJ, Fuhrer G, Heller W, Hoffmeister HE: Augmentation of kallikrein and plasmin inhibition capacity by aprotinin using a new assay to monitor therapy. *Adv Exp Med Biol* 1989; 247B:55.
674. Levy JH, Bailey, JM, Salmenpera M: Pharmacokinetics of aprotinin in preoperative cardiac surgical patients. *Anesthesiology* 1994; 80:1013.
675. Lu H, DuBuit C, Soria J, et al: Postoperative hemostasis and fibrinolysis in patients undergoing cardiopulmonary bypass with or without aprotinin therapy. *Thromb Haemost* 1994; 72:438.
676. Levi M, Cromheecke ME, de Jonge E, et al: Pharmacological strategies to decrease excessive blood loss in cardiac surgery: a meta-analysis of clinically relevant endpoints. *Lancet* 2000; 354:1940.
677. Gott JP, Cooper WA, Schmidt FE, et al: Modifying risk for extracorporeal circulation: trial of four anti-inflammatory strategies. *Ann Thorac Surg* 1998; 66:747.
678. Wachtfogel YT, Kucich U, Hack CE, et al: Aprotinin inhibits the contact, neutrophil, and platelet activation systems during

simulated extracorporeal perfusion. *J Thorac Cardiovasc Surg* 1993; 106:1.
679. Asimakopoulos G, Thompson R, Nourshargh S, et al: An anti-inflammatory property of aprotinin detected at the level of leukocyte extravasation. *J Thorac Cardiovasc Surg* 2000; 120:361.
680. Asimakopoulos G, Lidington EA, Mason J, et al: Effect of aprotinin on endothelial cell activation. *J Thorac Cardiovasc Surg* 2001; 122:123.
681. Hill GE, Pohorecki R, Alonso A, et al: Aprotinin reduces interleukin-8 production and lung neutrophil accumulation after cardiopulmonary bypass. *Anesth Analg* 1996; 83:696.
682. Greilich PE, Okada K, Latham P, et al: Aprotinin but not Î-aminocaproic acid decreases interleukin-10 after cardiac surgery with extracorporeal circulation. Randomized, double-blind, placebo-controlled study in patients recieving aprotinin and Î-aminocaproic acid. *Circulation* 2001; 104(suppl I): I-265.
683. Wendel HP, Heller W, Michel J, et al: Lower cardiac troponin T levels in patients undergoing cardiopulmonary bypass and receiving high-dose aprotinin therapy indicate reduction of perioperative myocardial damage. *J Thorac Cardiovasc Surg* 1995; 109:1164.
684. Ashraf S, Tian Y, Cowan D, et al: "Low-dose" aprotinin modifies hemostasis but not proinflammatory cytokine release. *Ann Thorac Surg* 1997; 63:68.
685. Sundaram S, Gikakis N, Hack CE, et al: Nafamostat mesilate, a broad spectrum protease inhibitor, modulates platelet, neutrophil and contact activation in simulated extracorporeal circulation. *Thromb Haemost* 1996; 75:76.
686. Murase M, Usui A, Tomita Y, et al: Nafamostat mesilate reduces blood loss during open heart surgery. *Circulation* 1993; 88(suppl II): II-432.
687. Sawa Y, Shimazaki Y, Kadoba K, et al: Attenuation of cardiopulmonary bypass-derived inflammatory reactions reduces myocardial reperfusion injury in cardiac operations. *J Thorac Cardiovasc Surg* 1996; 111:29.
688. Seghaye M-C, Duchateau J, Grabitz RG, et al: Effect of sodium nitroprusside on complement activation induced by cardiopulmonary bypass: a clinical and experimental study. *J Thorac Cardiovasc Surg* 1996; 111:882.
689. Massoudy P, Zahler S, Freyholdt T, et al: Sodium nitroprusside in patients with compromised left ventricular function undergoing coronary bypass: reduction of cardiac proinflammatory substances. *J Thorac Cardiovasc Surg* 2000; 119:566.
690. Cavarocchi NC, England MD, Schaff HV, et al: Oxygen free radical generation during cardiopulmonary bypass: correlation with complement activation. *Circulation* 1986; 74(suppl III): III-130.
691. England MD, Cavarocchi NC, O'Brien JF, et al: Influence of antioxidants (mannitol and allopuringol) on oxygen free radical generation during and after cardiopulmonary bypass. *Circulation* 1986; 74(suppl III):III-134.
692. Menasche P, Piwnica A: Free radicals and myocardial protection: a surgical viewpoint. *Ann Thorac Surg* 1989; 47:939.
693. Royston D, Fleming MI, Desai JB, et al: Increased production of peroxidation products associated with cardiac operations. *J Thorac Cardiovasc Surg* 1986; 91:759.
694. Westhuyzen J, Cochrane AD, Tesar PJ, et al: Effect of preoperative supplementation with a-tocopherol and ascorbic acid on myocardial injury in patients undergoing cardiac operations. *J Thorac Cardiovasc Surg* 1997; 113:942.
695. Wagner FM, Wever AT, Ploetze K, et al: Do vitamins C and E attenuate the effects of reactive oxygen species during pulmonary reperfusion and thereby prevent injury? *Ann Thorac Surg* 2002; 74:811.
696. Ollivier V, Parry GCN, Cobb RR, et al: Elevated cyclic AMP inhibits NF-kappa B-mediated transcription in human monocytic cells and endothelial cells. *J Biol Chem* 1996; 271:20828.
697. Beavo JA, Conti M, Heaslip RJ: Multiple cyclic nucleotide phospodiestereases. *Mol Pharmacol* 1994; 46:399.
698. Mollhoff T, Loick HM, Van Aken H, et al: Milrinone modulates endotoxemia, systemic inflammation and subsequent acute phase response after cardiopulmonary bypass (CPB). *Anesthesiology* 1999; 90:72.
699. Plumb ME, Sadetz JM: Proteins of the membrane attack complex, in Volkankis JE, Frank ME (eds): *The Human Complement System in Health and Disease*. New York, Marcel Dekker, 1998; p 119.

11D: Organ Damage

700. Levy JH, Hug CC: Use of cardiopulmonary bypass in studies of the circulation. *Br J Anaesth* 1988; 60:35S.
701. Carson JL, Poses RM, Spence RK, et al: Severity of anaemia and operative mortality and morbidity. *Lancet* 1988; 1:727.
702. Kolkka R, Hilberman M: Neurologic dysfunction following cardiac operation with low-flow, low-pressure cardiopulmonary bypass. *J Thorac Cardiovasc Surg* 1980; 79:432.
703. Downing SW, Edmunds LH Jr: Release of vasoactive substances during cardiopulmonary bypass. *Ann Thorac Surg* 1992; 54:1236.
704. Robicsek F, Masters TN, Niesluchowski W, et al: Vasomotor activity during cardiopulmonary bypass, in Utley JR (ed): *Pathophysiology and Techniques of Cardiopulmonary Bypass*, vol II. Baltimore, Williams & Wilkins, 1983; p 1.
705. Murkin JM, Martzke JS, Buchan AM, et al: A randomized study of the influence of perfusion technique and pH management strategy in 316 patients undergoing coronary artery bypass surgery, II: neurologic and cognitive outcomes. *J Thorac Cardiovasc Surg* 1995; 110: 349.
706. Patel RL, Turtle MR, Chambers DJ, et al: Alpha-stat acid-base regulation during cardiopulmonary bypass improves neuropsychologic outcome in patients undergoing coronary artery bypass grafting. *J Thorac Cardiovasc Surg* 1996; 111:1267.
707. Stump DA, Brown WR, Moody DM, et al: Microemboli and neurologic dysfunction after cardiovascular surgery. *Semin Cardiothorac Vascular Anesth* 1999; 3:47.
708. Stone JG, Young WL, Smith CR, et al: Do standard monitoring sites reflect true brain temperature when profound hypothermia is rapidly induced and reversed? *Anesthesiology* 1995; 82:344.
709. Faymonville ME, Pincemail J, Duchateau MD, et al: Myeloperoxidase and elastase as markers of leukocyte activation during cardiopulmonary bypass in humans. *J Thorac Cardiovasc Surg* 1991; 102:309.
710. Joffs C, Gunasinghe HR, Multani MM, et al: Cardiopulmonary bypass induces the synthesis and release of matrix metalloproteinases. *Ann Thorac Surg* 2001; 71:1518.
711. Smith EEJ, Naftel DC, Blackstone EH, Kirklin JW: Microvascular permeability after cardiopulmonary bypass. *J Thorac Cardiovasc Surg* 1987; 94:225.
712. Pacifico AD, Digerness S, Kirklin JW: Acute alterations of body composition after open intracardiac operations. *Circulation* l970;41:331.
713. Edmunds LH Jr, Williams W: Microemboli and the use of filters during cardiopulmonary bypass, in Utley JR (ed): *Pathophysiology and Techniques of Cardiopulmonary Bypass,* vol II. Baltimore, Williams & Wilkins, 1983; p. 101.
714. Webb WR, Harrison LH, Helmcke FR, et al: Carbon dioxide field flooding minimizes residual intracardiac air after open-heart operations. *Ann Thorac Surg* 1997; 64:1489.
715. Brooker RF, Brown WR, Moody DM, et al: Cardiotomy suction: a major source of brain lipid emboli during cardiopulmonary bypass. *Ann Thorac Surg* 1998; 65:1651.

716. Lee WH Jr, Krumhaar D, Fonkalsrud EW, et al: Denaturation of plasma proteins as a cause of morbidity and death after intracardiac operations. *Surgery* 1961; 50:1025.
717. Slogoff S, Girgis KZ, Keats AS: Etiologic factors in neuropsychiatric complications associated with cardiopulmonary bypass. *Anesth Analg* 1982; 61:903.
718. Kincaid EH, Jones TJ, Stump DA, et al: Processing scavenged blood with a cell saver reduces cerebral lipid microembolization. *Ann Thorac Surg* 2000; 70:1296.
719. Reichenspurner H, Navia JA, Benny G et al: Particulate embolic capture by an intra-aortic filter device during cardiac surgery. *J Thorac Cardiovasc Surg* 2000; 119:233.
720. Cook DJ, Zehr KJ, Orszulak TA, Slater JM: Profound reduction in brain embolization using an endoaortic baffle during bypass in swine. *Ann Thorac Surg* 2002; 73: 198.
721. Barzilai B, Marshall WG Jr, Saffitz Je, et al: Avoidance of embolic complications by ultrasonic characterization of the ascending aorta. *Circulation* 1989; 80:1275.
722. Weinstein GS: Left hemispheric strokes in coronary surgery: implication for end-hole aortic cannulas. *Ann Thorac Surg* 2001; 71:128.
723. Macoviak JA, Hwang J, Boerjan KL, Deal DD: Comparing dual-stream and standard cardiopulmonary bypass in pigs. *Ann Thorac Surg* 2002; 73:203.
724. Harringer W: Capture of a particulate embolic during cardiac procedures in which aortic cross-clamp is used. *Ann Thorac Surg* 2000; 70:1119.
725. Hammon JW, Stump DA, Kon ND, et al: Risk factors and solutions for the development of neurobehavioral changes after coronary artery bypass grafting. *Ann Thorac Surg* 1998; 63:1613.
726. Loop FD, Higgins TL, Panda R, et al: Myocardial protection during cardiac operations: decreased morbidity and lower cost with blood cardioplegia and coronary sinus perfusion. *J Cardiovasc Surg* 1992; 104:608.
727. Sundt TM, Barner HB, Camillo CJ, et al: Total arterial revascularization with an internal thoracic artery and radial artery T graft. *Ann Thorac Surg* 1999; 68:399.
728. Tector AJ, Amundsen S, Schmahl TM, et al: Total revascularization with T Grafts. *Ann Thorac Surg* 1994; 57:33.
729. Menninger FJ 3rd, Rosenkranz ER, Utley JR, et al: Interstitial hydrostatic pressure in patients undergoing CABG and valve replacement. *J Thorac Cardiovasc Surg* 1980; 79:181.
730. Downing SW, Savage EB, Streicher JS, et al: The stretched ventricle: myocardial creep and contractile dysfunction after acute nonischemic ventricular distention. *J Thorac Cardiovasc Surg* 1992; 104:996.
731. Shaw PJ: The incidence and nature of neurological morbidity following cardiac surgery: a review. *Perfusion* 1989; 4:83.
732. Newman S: The incidence and nature of neuropsychological morbidity following cardiac surgery. *Perfusion* 1989; 4:93.
733. Svensson LG, Nadolny EM, Kimmel WA: Multimodal protocol influence on stroke and neurocognitive deficit prevention after ascending/arch aortic operations. *Ann Thorac Surg (in press)*.
734. Newman S, Smith P, Treasure T, et al: Acute neuropsychological consequences of coronary artery bypass surgery. *Curr Psychol Res Rev* 1987; 6:115.
735. Murkin JM, Stump DA, Blumenthal JA, et al: Defining dysfunction: group means versus incidence analysis-a statement of consensus. *Ann Thorac Surg* 1997; 64:904.
736. Baird A, Benfield A, Schlaug G, et al: Enlargement of human cerebral ischemic lesion volumes measured by diffusion-weighted magnetic resonance imaging. *Ann Neurol* 1997; 41:581.
737. Bendszus M, Reents W, Franke D, et al: Brain damage after coronary artery bypass grafting. *Arch Neurol* 2002; 59:1090.
738. Rosen B, Belliveau J, Vevea J, et al: Perfusion imaging with NMR contrast agents. *Magn Reson Med* 1990; 14:249.
739. Maragos PJ, Schmechel DE: Neuro-specific enolase, a clinically useful marker for neurons and neuroendocrine cells. *Annu Rev Neuro Sci* 1987; 10:269.
740. Persson L, Hardemark HG, Gustafsson J, et al: S-100 protein and neuro-specific enolase in cerebrospinal fluid and serum: markers of cell damage in human central nervous system. *Stroke* 1987; 18:911.
741. Zimmer DB, Cornwall EH, Landar A, Song W: The S-100 protein family: history, function, and expression. *Brain Res Bull* 1995; 37: 417.
742. Johnsson P, Blomquist S, Luhrs C, et al: Neuron-specific enolase increases in plasma during and immediately after extracorporeal circulation. *Ann Thorac Surg* 2000; 69:750.
743. Anderson RE, Hansson LO, Liska J, et al: The effect of cardiotomy suction on the brain injury marker S100 b after cardiopulmonary bypass. *Ann Thorac Surg* 2000; 69:847.
744. Shaw PJ, Bates D, Cartlidge NE, et al: Neurologic and neuropsychological morbidity following major surgery: comparison of coronary artery bypass and peripheral vascular surgery. *Stroke* 1987; 18:700.
745. Moller JT, Cluitmans P, Rasmussen LS, et al: Long-term postoperative cognitive dysfunction in the elderly ISPOCD1 study. ISPOCD investigators, International Study of Post-Operative Cognitive Dysfunction. *Lancet* 1998; 351:857.
746. Jones EL, Weintraub WS, Craver JM, et al: Coronary bypass surgery: is the operation different today? *J Thorac Cardiovasc Surg* 1991; 101:108.
747. Tardiff BE, Newman MF, Saunders AM, et al: Preliminary report of a genetic basis for cognitive decline after cardiac operations. *Ann Thorac Surg* 1997; 64:715.
748. Roach GW, Kanchugar M, Mangano CM, et al: Adverse cerebral outcomes after coronary bypass surgery: multicenter study of perioperative ischemia research groups and the ischemia research and education foundation investigators. *N Engl J Med* 1996; 335:1857.
749. Weintraub WS, Wenger NK, Jones EL, et al: Changing clinical characteristics of coronary surgery patients: differences between men and women. *Circulation* 1993; 88:79.
750. Goto T, Baba T, Yoshitake A, et al: Craniocervical and aortic atherosclerosis as neurologic risk factors in coronary surgery. *Ann Thorac Surg* 2000; 69:834.
751. Wareing TH, Davila-Roman VG, Daily BB, et al: Strategy for the reduction of stroke incidence in cardiac surgical patients. *Ann Thorac Surg* 1993; 55:1400.
752. Stump DA, Brown WR, Moody DM, et al: Microemboli and neurologic dysfunction after cardiovascular surgery. *Semin Cardiothorac Vasc Anesth* 1999; 3:47.
753. Tuman KJ, McCarthy RJ, Najafi H, et al: Differential effects of advanced age on neurologic and cardiac risks of coronary operations. *J Thorac Cardiovasc Surg* 1992; 104:1510.
754. Jones TJ, Stump DA, Deal D, et al: Hypothermia protects the brain from embolization by reducing and redirecting the embolic load. *Ann Thorac Surg* 1999; 68:1465.
755. Gold JP, Charlson ME, Williams-Russo P: Improvement of outcomes after coronary artery bypass; a randomized trial comparing high verus low mean arterial pressure. *J Thorac Cardiovasc Surg* 1995; 110:1302.
756. Murkin JM, Farrar JK, Tweed WA, et al: Cerebral autoregulation and flow/metabolism coupling during cardiopulmonary bypass: the role of $PaCO_2$. *Anesth Analg* 1987; 66:665.
757. Hill AG, Groom RC, Tewksbury L, et al: Sources of gaseous microemboli during cardiopulmonary bypass. *Proc Am Acad Cardiovasc Perfus* 1988; 9:122.

758. Blauth CI: Macroemboli and microemboli during cardiopulmonary bypass. *Ann Thorac Surg* 1995; 59:1300.
759. Helps SC, Parsons DW, Reilly PL, et al: The effect of gas emboli on rabbit cerebral blood flow. *Stroke* 1990; 21:94.
760. Moody DM, Brown WR, Challa VR, et al: Efforts to characterize the nature and chronicle the occurrence of brain emboli during cardiopulmonary bypass. *Perfusion* 1995; 9:316.
761. Cook DJ, Oliver WC, Orsulak TA, et al: Cardiopulmonary bypass temperature, hematocrit, and cerebral oxygen delivery in humans. *Ann Thorac Surg* 1995; 60:1671.
762. Martin TC, Craver JM, Gott MP, et al: Prospective, randomized trial of retrograde warm-blood cardioplegia: myocardial benefit and neurological threat. *Ann Thorac Surg* 1994; 59:298.
763. Engelman RM, Pleet AB, Rouson JA, et al: What is the best perfusion temperature for coronary revascularization? *J Thorac Cardiovasc Surg* 1996; 112:1622.
764. Avraamides EJ, Murkin JM: The effect of surgical dislocation of the heart on cerebral blood flow in the presence of a single, two-stage venous cannula during cardiopulmonary bypass. *Can J Anaesth* 1996; 43:A36.
765. Nathan HJ, Wells GA, Munson JL, Wozny D: Neuroprotective effect of mild hypothermia in patients undergoing coronary artery surgery with cardiopulmonary bypass. *Circulation* 2001; 104(suppl I): I-85.
766. Jones T, Roy RC: Should patients be normothermic in the immediate postoperative period? *Ann Thorac Surg* 1999; 68:1454.
767. Brown R, Wright G, Royston D: A comparison of two systems for assessing cerebral venous oxyhaemoglobin saturation during cardiopulmonary bypass in humans. *Anaethesia* 1993; 48:697.
768. Michenfelder JD: The interdependency of cerebral functional and metabolic effects following massive doses of thiopental in the dog. *Anesthesiology* 1974; 41:231.
769. Nussmeier N, Arlund C, Slogoff S: Neuropsychiatric complications after cardiopulmonary bypass: cerebral protection by a barbiturate. *Anesthesiology* 1986; 64:165.
770. Arrowsmith JE, Harrison MJG, Newman SP, et al: Neuroprotection of the brain during cardiopulmonary bypass: a randomized trial of remacemide during coronary artery bypass in 171 patients. *Stroke* 1998; 29:2357.
771. Mitchell SJ, Pellet O, Gorman DF: Cerebral protection by lidocaine during cardiac operations. *Ann Thorac Surg* 1999; 67:1117.
772. Diegeler A, Hirsch R. Schneider F, et al: Neuromonitoring and neurocognitive outcome in off-pump versus conventional coronary bypass operation. *Ann Thorac Surg* 2000; 69:1162.
773. Dijk DV, Jansen EWL, Hijman R, et al: Cognitive outcome after off-pump and on-pump coronary artery bypass graft surgery. *JAMA* 2002; 287:1405.
774. Newman MF, Kirchner JL, Phillips-Bute B, et al: Longitudinal assessment of neurocognitive function after coronary artery bypass grafting. *N Engl J Med* 2001; 344:395.
775. Sotaniemi KA: Cerebral outcome after extracorporeal circulation: comparison between prospective and retrospective evaluations. *Arch Neurol* 1983; 40:75.
776. Maggart M, Stewart S: The mechanisms and management of noncardiogenic pulmonary edema following cardiopulmonary bypass. *Ann Thorac Surg* 1987; 43:231.
777. Lloyd J, Newman J, Brigham K: Permeability pulmonary edema: diagnosis and management. *Arch Intern Med* 1984; 144:143.
778. Allardyce D, Yoshida S, Ashmore P: The importance of microembolism in the pathogenesis of organ dysfunction caused by prolonged use of the pump oxygenator. *J Thorac Cardiovasc Surg* 1966; 52:706.
779. Tonz M, Mihaljevic T, von Segesser LK, et al: Acute lung injury during cardiopulmonary bypas: are the neutrophils responsible? *Chest* 1995; 108:1551.
780. Chenoweth DE, Cooper SW, Hugli TE, et al: Complement activation during cardiopulmonary bypass: evidence for generation of C3a and C5a anaphylatoxins. *N Engl J Med* 1981; 304:497.
781. Royston D, Fleming JS, Desai JB, et al: Increased production of peroxidation products associated with cardiac operations. *J Thorac Cardiovasc Surg* 1986; 91:759.
782. Craddock PR, Fehr J, Brigham KL, et al: Complement and leukocyte-mediated pulmonary dysfunction in hemodialysis. *N Engl J Med* 1977; 296:769.
783. Hammerschmidt DE, Stroncek DF, Bowers TK, et al: Complement activation and neutropenia during cardiopulmonary bypass. *J Thorac Cardiovasc Surg* 1981; 81:370.
784. McGowan FX, del Nido PJ, Kurland G, et al: Cardiopulmonary bypass significantly impairs surfactant activity in children. *J Thorac Cardiovasc Surg* 1993; 106:968.
785. Oster JB, Sladen RN, Berkowitz DE: Cardiopulmonary bypass and the lung, in Gravlee GP, Davis RF, Kurusz M, Utley JR (eds): *Cardiopulmonary Bypass: Principles and Practice*. Philadelphia, Lippincott Williams & Wilkins, 2000; p 367.
786. Magnusson L, Zemgulis V, Tenling A, et al: Use of a vital capacity maneuver to prevent atelectasis after cardiopulmonary bypass: an experimental study. *Anesthesiology* 1998; 88:134.
787. Cogliati AA, Menichetti A, Tritapepe L, et al: Effects of three techniques of lung management on pulmonary function during cardiopulmonary bypass. *Acta Anaesth Belg* 1996; 47:73.
788. Sirivella A, Gielchinsky I, Parsonnet V: Management of catheter-induced pulmonary artery perforation: a rare complication in cardiovascular operations. *Ann Thorac Surg* 2001; 72:2056.
789. Rinder CS, Fontes M, Mathew JP, et al: Neutrophil CD11b upregulation during cardiopulmonary bypass is associated with postoperative renal injury. *Ann Thorac Surg (in press)*.
790. Chertow G, Mazarus J, Christiansen C, et al: Preoperative renal risk stratification. *Circulation* 1997; 95:878.
791. Zanardo G, et al: Acute renal failure in the patient undergoing cardiac operation: prevalence, mortality rate, and main risk factors. *J Thorac Cardiovasc Surg* 1994; 107:1489.
792. Settergren G, Ohqvist G. Renal dysfunction during cardiac surgery. *Curr Opin Anesthesiol* 1994; 7:59.
793. Feindt PR, Walcher S, Volkmer I, et al: Effects of high-dose aprotinin on renal function in aortocoronary bypass grafting. *Ann Thorac Surg* 1995; 60:1076.
794. Utley JR: Renal function and fluid balance with cardiopulmonary bypass, in Gravlee GP, Davis RF, Utley JR (eds): *Cardiopulmonary Bypass: Principles and Practice*. Baltimore, Williams & Wilkins, 1993; p 488.
795. Clyne DH, Kant KS, Pesce AJ, et al: Nephrotoxicity of low molecular weight serum proteins: physicochemical interactions between myoglobin, hemoglobin, Bence Jones proteins and Tamm-Horsfall mucoprotein. *Curr Prob Clin Biochem* 1979; 9:299.
796. Abel, RM, Buckley, MJ, Austen, WG, et al: Etiology, incidence and prognosis of renal failure following cardiac operations: results of a prospective analysis of 500 consecutive patients. *J Thorac Cardiovasc Surg* 1976; 71:32.
797. Conger J: Interventions in clinical acute renal failure: what are the data? *Am J Kidney Dis* 1995; 26:565.
798. Wiebe K, Meyer M, Wahlers T, et al: Acute renal failure following cardiac surgery is reverted by administration of urodilatin (INN: ularitide). *Eur J Med Res* 1996; 1:259.
799. Blachey JD, Henrich WL: The diagnosis and management of acute renal failure. *Semin Nephrol* 1981; 1:11.
800. Mangano C, et al: Renal dysfunction after myocardial revascularization: risk factors, adverse outcomes and hospital resource utilization. The Multicenter Study of Perioperative Ischemia Research Group. *Anesth Analg* 1998; 1:3.

801. Welbourn N, Melrose DG, Moss DW: Changes in serum enzyme levels accompanying cardiac surgery with extracorporeal circulation. *J Clin Pathol* 1966; 19:220.
802. Collins JD, Ferner R, Murray A, et al: Incidence and prognostic importance of jaundice after cardiopulmonary bypass surgery. *Lancet* 1983; 1:1119.
803. Ryan TA, Rady MY, Bashour CA, et al: Predictors of outcome in cardiac surgical patients with prolonged intensive care stay. *Chest* 1997; 112:1035.
804. Krasna MJ, Flancbaum L, Trooskin SZ, et al: Gastrointestinal complications after cardiac surgery. *Surgery* 1988; 104:773.
805. Rattner DW, Gu Z-Y, Vlahakes GJ, et al: Hyperamylasemia after cardiac surgery. *Ann Surg* 1989; 209:279.
806. Fernandez-del Castillo C, Harringer W, Warshaw AL, et al: Risk factors for pancreatic celular injury after cardiopulmonary bypass. *N Engl J Med* 1991; 325:382.
807. Haas GS, Warshaw AL, Daggett WM, et al: Acute pancreatitis after cardiopulmonary bypass. *Am J Surg* 1985; 149:508.
808. Feiner H: Pancreatitis after cardiac surgery: a morphologic study. *Am J Surg* 1976; 131:684.
809. Lefor AT, Vuocolo P, Parker FB Jr, et al: Pancreatic complications following cardiopulmonary bypass: factors influencing mortality. *Arch Surg* 1992; 127:1225.
810. Izsak EM, Shike M, Roulet M, et al: Pancreatitis in association with hypercalcemia in patients receiving total parenteral nutrition. *Gastroenterology* 1980; 79:555.
811. Mithofer K, Fernandes-del Castillo C, Frick TW, et al: Acute hypercalcemia causes acute pancreatitis and ectopic trypsinogen activation in the rat. *Gastroenterology* 1995; 109:239.
812. Waele BD, Smitz J, Willems G: Recurrent pancreatitis secondary to hypercalcemia following vitamin D poisoning. *Pancreas* 1989; 4:378.
813. Rose DM, Ranson JHC, Cunningham JN, et al: Patterns of severe pancreatic injury following cardiopulmonary bypass. *Ann Surg* 1984; 199:168.
814. Mori A, Watanabe K, Onoe M, et al: Regional blood flow in the liver, pancreas and kidney during pulsatile and nonpulsatile perfusion under profound hypothermia. *Jpn Circ J* 1988; 52:219.
815. Decker GAG, Josselsohn E, Svensson L, et al: Acute gastroduodenal complications after cardiopulmonary bypass surgery. *S Afr J Surg* 1984; 22:261.
816. Fiddian-Green RG, Baker S: Predictive valve of the stomach wall pH for complications after cardiac operations: comparison with other monitoring. *Crit Care Med* 1987; 15:153.
817. Shangraw RE: Splanchnic, hepatic and visceral effects, in Gravlee GP, Davis RF, Utley JR (eds): *Cardiopulmonary Bypass: Principles and Practice*. Baltimore, Williams & Wilkins, 1993; p 391.
818. Heikkinen LO, Ala-Kulju KV: Abdominal complications following cardiopulmonary bypass in open-heart surgery. *Scand J Thorac Cardiovasc Surg* 1987; 21:1.
819. Hanks JB, Curtis SE, Hanks BB, et al: Gastrointestinal complications after cardiopulmonary bypass. *Surgery* 1982; 92:394.
820. Moneta GL, Misbach GA, Ivey TD: Hypoperfusion as a possible factor in the development of gastrointestinal complications after cardiac surgery. *Am J Surg* 1985; 149:648.

Chapter **12**

Transfusion Therapy and Blood Conservation

Leonard Y. Lee/William J. DeBois/Karl H. Krieger/O. Wayne Isom

With the development of cardiac surgery in the 1950s to correct congenital heart defects came the need for large-volume blood transfusions. In the 1960s and 1970s, the introduction of valve prostheses and direct grafting of coronary arteries made the correction of acquired heart disease a possibility. These landmarks, along with the liberal use of homologous blood transfusion therapy, led to the rapid growth of the field. Commensurate with the growth of cardiac surgery as a field was an increasing incidence of transfusion-transmitted hepatitis in the 1970s, ultimately alerting the public and treating physicians to the concept of blood conservation. The emergence of infection by HIV greater heightened the interest in this area, leading to the current practices of blood conservation therapy in cardiac surgery.

Historically, open heart surgery has been associated with a high usage of blood transfusion. Some reports suggest that up to 70% of this patient population require blood transfusions, resulting in an average of 2 to 4 donor exposures per patient.[1,2] It has been reported that 10% of all red blood cell units transfused in the United States are administered during coronary bypass surgery.[3] Almost all patients received blood transfusion in the early days of cardiac surgery. However, with an increased awareness of blood-borne infectious diseases, lack of donors, great cost to both the patient and the institution, allergic reaction, blood-type mismatch, and the needs of special populations such as Jehovah's Witnesses, a greater effort has been made to perform open heart procedures without blood transfusions even in high-risk patients. Advances in perioperative medications minimizing blood loss, greater tolerance of lower hematocrits especially on bypass, and improvements in surgical techniques resulting in shorter operative times have allowed for these extensive procedures to be performed without significant blood loss.

The high transfusion rates associated with cardiac surgery have been well characterized and are likely due to the coagulopathy, platelet dysfunction, and red cell hemolysis that occur as a result of the cardiopulmonary bypass circuit.[4–6] The introduction of hemodilution using crystalloid pump-priming solution rather than whole blood dramatically reduced the transfusion requirements seen during coronary artery bypass graft (CABG) procedures.[7] While this technique has reduced the amount of blood transfused during cardiopulmonary bypass (CPB), the resulting hemodilution contributes to the risk of low intraoperative and postoperative hematocrit, especially in patients who weigh less than 70 kg, thereby posing a new risk for transfusion.

Efforts at reducing the use of homologous blood in cardiac surgery began almost 40 years ago. The efforts to decrease allogeneic blood exposures have been a topic of constant review and attention because of the desires of both patients and their physicians to conserve blood during the perioperative

TABLE 12–1 Literature review of blood conservation techniques in patients undergoing combined procedures

Year	Reference	Patients (no.)	Preop. donation	Intraop. donation	Trigger CPB	Trigger postop.	Med. shed	Drugs	Transfused (%)	Units/ patient
1967	Beall[44]	1818	No	1180	NS	NS	No	No	8.6	NS
1975	Cohn[45]	400	No	50C-1000	15	NS	No	No	96.5	3.9
1976	Cove[46]	44	Yes	No	NS	NS	No	No	75	2.0
1977	Kaplan[47]	60	No	750	NS	NS	No	No	100	5.5
1977	Lilleaasen[48]	30	No	855	NS	NS	No	No	100	3.85
1978	Schaff[49]	63	NS	NS	NS	35	Yes	No	NS	2.4
1979	Thurer[50]	54	No	NS	NS	30	Yes	No	59	1.6
1979	Lambert[51]	774	NS	NS	NS	NS	No	Ami	67	5.5
1983	Johnson[52]	168	NS	No	NS	NS	Yes	No	NS	1.0
1987	Love[53]	58	Yes	No	NS	NS	Yes	No	36	1.1
1988	Giordano[54]	65	No	500	NS	25	No	No	NS	6.32
1988	Giordano[55]	50	No	No	NS	NS	NS	No	NS	13.7
1989	Page[56]	50	No	Yes	17	30	Yes	No	88	3.15
1989	Lepore[57]	67	No	NS	NS	NS	Yes	No	74.6	2.7
1989	DelRossi[26]	170	NS	No	NS	30	No	Ami	NS	2.8
1989	Britton[58]	104	Yes	1000	NS	NS	No	No	34	0.7
1990	Horrow[27]	18	No	No	NS	NS	Yes	Trax	NS	0.6
1991	Horrow[59]	77	NS	NS	NS	24	Yes	Trax	32	NS
1991	Carey[60]	222	Yes	No	21	24	Yes	No	53	2.2
1992	Scott[61]	60	Yes	575	18	24	Yes	No	58	4.0
1992	Ikeda[62]	3022	No	Yes	21	NS	Yes	No	72	9
1992	Dzik[63]	79	Yes	NS	NS	NS	NS	NS	32	NS
1993	Helm[64]	35	No	1562	15	22	Yes	No	17	1.0
1994	Rosengart[65]	15	No	1180	15	NS	Yes	Ap	0	0
1994	Wong[66]	20	No	1200	18	24	No	No	30	0.45
1994	Murkin[67]	29	No	No	NS	20	No	Ap	58.6	4.1
1994	Axford[68]	16	No	No	NS	25	Yes	No	62	8.6
1995	Shinfield[69]	20	No	No	NS	NS	NS	Ap	50	1.1
1995	Spiess[70]	591	NS	NS	NS	NS	No	No	78.5	6
1995	Parolari[71]	1310	Yes	Yes	NS	24	No	Ap	21.1	0.84
1995	Sandrelli[22]	348	Yes	Yes	18	24	Yes	Ap	12.6	0.34
1998	Shapira[72]	114	No	No	20	25	No	Ami	35	0.7
2001	Tempe[73]	60	No	Yes	NS	24	No	Ap	60	0.75
2001	Van der Linden[74]	636	No	Yes	20	21	No	Ap	18	0.51

NS = not stated.

period. These joint efforts have affected virtually every aspect of the manner in which heart surgery and cardiopulmonary bypass are performed. Our experience combined with the experiences of others has led to the development of an integrated, comprehensive blood conservation program that makes the goal of bloodless heart surgery possible.

PAST EXPERIENCES: A REVIEW OF THE LITERATURE

Since the earlier days of cardiac surgery, there have been several reports of minimizing the use of blood and blood products both intraoperatively as well as postoperatively. While most of these studies have focused on the use of one particular modality or pharmacologic agent, these techniques were applied in the context of an entire set of blood conservation measures. Collectively the results of these reports provide an important body of information that can be used as an aid to evaluating the relative effectiveness of various combinations of the presently available blood conservation techniques.

Table 12-1 summarizes the findings of 34 studies of patients undergoing non–CABG or combined procedures requiring cardiopulmonary bypass. Table 12-2 similarly summarizes the findings of 39 studies of patients undergoing CABG only. These studies provide information about the techniques applied as well as outcome measures of patients receiving homologous transfusions. Although preoperative autologous donation was only sporadically applied (12/73 studies), nonblood prime was almost universally applied (65/73 studies). The majority of studies achieving very low transfusion rates used low to low-moderate transfusion triggers both during and following CPB. Conversely,

TABLE 12–2 Literature review of blood conservation techniques in patients undergoing CABG

Year	Reference	Patients (no.)	Preop. donation	Intraop. donation	Trigger CPB	Trigger postop.	Med. shed	Drugs	Transfused (%)	Units/ patient
1974	Zubiate[75]	477	Yes	1800	15	22	No	No	29	1.1
1978	Yeh[76]	240	NS	NS	NS	33	No	No	77.8	1.45
1979	Schaff[77]	135	No	NS	NS	NS	Yes	No	100	2.4
1979	Cosgrove[8]	50	No	675	15	NS	Yes	No	6	0.06
1980	Bayer[78]	1246	NS	NS	NS	NS	NS	No	NS	2.6
1984	Weisel[79]	13	No	NS	21	21	No	No	50	1.4
1985	Cosgrove[19]	441	No	NS	15	22	Yes	No	10	0.3
1986	Belcher[80]	90	No	550	NS	25	No	No	10	0.18
1987	Breyer[81]	43	No	No	18	25	Yes	No	42	2.23
1988	Hartz[82]	21	NS	NS	NS	NS	NS	NS	30	NS
1989	Dietrich[83]	25	No	739	15	30	Yes	No	68	1.6
1989	Tyson[84]	52	No	Yes	NS	25	Yes	No	74.5	4.5
1989	Owings[85]	107	Yes	250–500	NS	NS	Yes	No	27	0.8
1990	LoCicero[86]	100	No	No	NS	NS	Yes	No	31	0.7
1990	Jones[87]	50	NS	1000	21	23	Yes	No	34	0.67
1991	Jones[88]	100	No	1000	15	21	Yes	No	18	0.31
1991	Ovrum[10]	121	No	815	15	25	Yes	No	4.1	0.06
1991	Ovrum[9]	500	No	799	15	25	Yes	No	2.4	NS
1992	Davies[89]	32	No	857	20	24	No	No	NS	1.6
1992	Watanabe[90]	26	Yes	NS	18	21	NS	Epo	0	0
1992	Johnson[91]	18	Yes	750	NS	25	Yes	No	0	0
1993	Kulier[92]	12	Yes	No	NS	NS	NS	Epo	0.08	0.33
1993	Karski[93]	75	NS	NS	18	20	Yes	Trax	28	NS
1993	Sutton[94]	60	No	No	NS	NS	No	No	NS	1.7
1993	Ward[95]	17	No	No	24	24	Yes	No	89	NS
1993	Tobe[96]	24	No	750	NS	NS	Yes	No	71	4.1
1993	Schoenberger[97]	50	No	799	18	25	Yes	No	35	0.8
1994	Paone[98]	314	No	No	18	20	No	No	31.5	2.34
1994	Lemmer[99]	151	No	No	18	21	Yes	Trax	40	2.2
1994	Petry[100]	45	No	500–1000	20	30	No	No	66	1.3
1994	Arom[101]	100	NS	NS	NS	NS	No	Ami	NS	1.4
1995	Helm[42]	45	No	1607	15	22	Yes	No	28	1.2
1996	Helm[102]	100	No	1450	15	22	Yes	Ap/Epo	0	0
1997	Rosengart[103]	30	No	1300	15	22	Yes	Ap/Epo	0	0
1999	Rousou[104]	175	NS	No	20	20	No	Ami	4	NS
2001	Karkouti[105]	1007	No	Yes	18	20	Yes	TA	29.4	0.5

NS = not stated.

the studies reporting high rates of transfusion either used higher transfusion triggers, or the triggers were not stated, indicating that the investigators likely did not recognize, or place enough emphasis on, this essential blood conservation measure. Finally, the studies that achieved overall transfusion rates of less than 30% used the cornerstones of blood conservation, namely pre- or intraoperative autologous blood donation, nonblood priming, return of residual circuit blood to the patient, low or moderately low intra- and postoperative transfusion triggers, and reinfusion of shed mediastinal blood. Several of these studies bear special attention.

The first program to report less than 10% transfusion rates in non–Jehovah's Witness CABG patients was that of Cosgrove et al at the Cleveland Clinic in 1978.[8] This report of 50 patients undergoing elective CABG demonstrated transfusion rates of only 6% with a mean of 0.06 units per patient receiving blood. Included in Cosgrove's study were the 6 principal techniques of blood conservation stated earlier, many of which are still used today in blood conservation programs throughout the world, namely:

1. Intraoperative autologous donation
2. Nonblood prime
3. Return of all residual CPB circuit blood
4. Intraoperative salvage
5. Use of the lowest safe level of anemia during CPB as well as in the postoperative period
6. Reinfusion of shed mediastinal blood

Later studies took advantage of pharmacologic developments such as serine protease inhibitors, antifibrinolytics, and erythropoietin. By the early 1990s, these pharmacologic adjuncts to blood conservation had become readily available and could be categorized as those agents useful in perioperative stimulation of bone marrow for red blood cell production (erythropoietin) and those agents useful in reducing postoperative bleeding (serine protease inhibitors and antifibrinolytics).

In 1990, Ovrum et al confirmed the effectiveness of the simple "core" approach to blood conservation.[9] In 121 consecutive elective CABG patients, the authors achieved a transfusion rate of 4.1% and 0.06 unit per patient. In 1991 Ovrum applied these same principles to 500 elective CABG patients and obtained similar low rates of transfusion (2.4% of patients).[10] The authors found this 6-step blood conservation program to be simple, safe, and cost-effective.

By the 1990s, there were also some technical advances in cardiopulmonary bypass designed to minimize the need for transfusions as well as for hemodilution. With better oxygenators came a reduction in the volume of the CPB circuit, accompanied by a reduction in the amount of hemodilution that occurred.[11] Circuit volume could be further reduced by replacing as much of the crystalloid circuit prime as possible with autologous blood drained from the arterial cannula into the circuit immediately prior to CPB, called retrograde autologous priming (RAP), as well as displacing the venous side of the crystalloid prime when first initiating CPB.[12] These relatively simple maneuvers can reduce the crystalloid prime to a volume of roughly 200 mL. In addition, technical advances such as leukocyte filters and heparin-bonded circuits reduced the inflammatory response of the body to the blood interface with the CPB circuit, which can ultimately lead to less homologous blood requirement.[13,14]

The addition of newer pharmacologic and technologic advances to the proven "core" conservation measures as established by Cosgrove and Ovrum had the potential to markedly reduce and even eliminate the need for transfusion even in the face of the more difficult patient characteristics increasingly being encountered. This then became the goal of blood conservation programs.

PREOPERATIVE MANAGEMENT

Identification of Patients at Risk

The coagulopathy associated with CPB is primarily related to the interaction of blood components with the artificial surfaces of the CPB circuit, which results in derangements in platelet function, abnormal functioning of the coagulation cascades, and excessive fibrinolysis. The administration of high-dose heparin to prevent coagulation within the CPB circuit and hypothermia achieved during bypass further contribute to hemostatic derangements. Finally, while the use of asanguinous crystalloid prime rather than the whole-blood pump prime utilized historically has dramatically reduced the amount of blood transfused during CPB, the resulting hemodilution contributes to the risk of low intraoperative and postoperative hematocrit, which can be independent risk factors for transfusion in the postoperative period. Other risk factors can be assessed in the preoperative state, which can identify those patients that may be at high risk of bleeding, or with low red cell mass, both of which may require autologous blood transfusions.

One of the most important predictors of postoperative bleeding in the surgical patient is a personal or family history of any excessive bleeding or documented bleeding disorders. Many disorders can be confirmed with simple laboratory tests demonstrating some level of coagulation derangement. However, in the cardiothoracic patient population, medications and acquired medical diseases and their associated hemostatic defects are likely to be the most common risk for bleeding. Some of the most commonly seen problems are summarized in Tables 12-3 and 12-4. Notably, the use of aspirin alone, or included in other medications intended for pain relief or treatment of other ailments, is very common. The prevalence among patients undergoing unplanned surgery may be as high as 50% and even higher among patients with previously diagnosed coronary artery disease.[15,16] The currently published data would suggest that this does not represent a significant bleeding risk, and there is little evidence to suggest that bleeding times correlate with operative blood loss in these patients.[17,18]

One of the primary concerns in blood conservation is the patient's size and preoperative red cell volume. Two early reports by Cosgrove and Utley demonstrated these factors in addition to preoperative anemia as independent risk factors for blood transfusion.[19,20] As will be discussed later in the chapter, there are several relatively simple manipulations to the cardiopulmonary bypass circuit that can be made to reduce the amount of hemodilution that the patient

TABLE 12–3 Medications associated with an increased risk of bleeding

Drugs	Effect on hemostasis
Aspirin	Irreversible platelet inhibition by blocking platelet cyclooxygenase
Heparin	Inhibition of factors II and X, both direct and indirect thrombycytopenia Mostly antibody mediated (HIT)
Coumadin	Multiple factor deficiency by blocking gamma-carboxylation Vitamin K-dependent factors
Antibiotics	Multiple factor deficiency due to vitamin K malabsorption
Multiple drugs	Thrombocytopenia due to bone marrow inhibition of platelet production

TABLE 12–4 Acquired diseases associated with an increased risk of bleeding

Condition	Effect on hemostasis
ESRD/uremia	Irreversible platelet dysfunction by platelet inhibitory metabolites
Liver disease	Multiple factor deficiency due to defective synthesis
	Thrombocytopenia due to hypersplenism
Malabsorption	Multiple factor deficiency from vitamin K deficiency
SLE	Thrombocytopenia and thrombocytopathy due to platelet autoantibodies
	Factor deficiency due to prothrombin deficiency occasionally associated with lupus-type inhibitor
Amyloid	Capillary fragility due to vascular amyloid infiltration
	Factor X deficiency due to absorption by amyloid
Malignancy	Thrombocytopenia and anemia due to chemotherapy
	Thrombocytopenia due to marrow infiltration of tumor
	Factor deficiency due to DIC (advanced stages of cancer) as well as some chemotherapeutic agents

experiences while on bypass to reduce the overall risk of transfusions.

Autologous Blood Donation

Preoperative autologous donation (PAD) is a recognized strategy to reduce the risk of homologous blood transfusion in the perioperative period. Although this technique has been in practice since the 1960s, its use in cardiac surgery did not achieve widespread acceptance until the 1980s, with the advent of HIV, as an effort to reduce homologous blood exposures. Unfortunately, in cardiac surgery, the acuteness of the operations and dealing with an older and sicker patient population often precludes PAD, since there must be enough preoperative time for autologous collection as well as for red cell mass regeneration prior to arriving in the operating room. However, for that select, elective, cardiac surgical patient for whom PAD is possible, it is a good option to reduce homologous blood exposures.

Several preoperative characteristics can identify the cardiac patient who is eligible for PAD. The first criterion is that the patient be able to wait the required time for donation and red cell regeneration. This length of time typically varies depending upon the type of surgical procedure planned (larger operative procedures likely requiring a larger amount of blood) and the patient characteristics (body size, blood volume, and hematocrit). In general, this time is a minimum of 2 weeks per unit of blood donated to allow for red blood cell regeneration. The second criterion is that the patient be healthy enough to undergo donation. This criterion would preclude patients with severe left main stem stenosis, critical aortic stenosis, congestive heart failure, or idiopathic hypertrophic subaortic stenosis, as well as patients with severe coronary artery disease and ongoing ischemia, given that many of these patients would have been screening failures for criterion 1. The third criterion is that the patient not have active endocarditis. The time between donation and receiving the PAD unit is ample time for bacteria to replicate in the donated unit with resulting bacteremia which is potentially life-threatening. The fourth criterion is that the patient has an adequate hematocrit and red cell mass. A preoperative hematocrit of less than 33% regardless of red cell mass is a contraindication to PAD according to the American Association of Blood Bank (AABB) guidelines. A patient with a hematocrit greater than 33% may be eligible provided that other criteria are met.

Several options exist for these patients who were historically not eligible for PAD. Recombinant erythropoietin can be used to accelerate red cell production in anemic patients; this strategy is commonly used in Jehovah's Witness patients to increase their red cell mass prior to surgery.[21] However, this can be quite costly; as a result, it is usually reserved for those patients who are unable to tolerate homologous blood transfusions whether for religious reasons or because they have a rare blood type. An alternative strategy is to stimulate the body to increase the release of endogenous erythropoietin by allowing patients with hematocrits below the traditional cutoff to undergo PAD. The resultant anemia experienced by the patient in the post-donation period is a strong stimulant for endogenous erythropoietin production, ultimately leading to an increase in red cell mass.[22]

Red cell mass is related to patient body size.[23] A traditional cutoff of 110 pounds had been used for PAD. The AABB does, however, make specific allowances for PAD in smaller patients. The current recommendation is that no more than 15% of the patient's effective blood volume be removed at any given time, which takes into account smaller patient body size. PAD should be aggressively pursued for these small patients with low red cell mass and hematocrit because they are at highest risk of receiving a blood transfusion at sometime during their hospital stay. The mean rate of red cell generation of the studies that provided adequate data is 0.46 units per week, or slightly less than 1 unit every 2 weeks.[24] In conjunction with PAD, oral iron therapy should be initiated at the time of first donation to ensure adequate iron stores for red cell regeneration.

Due to the relatively acute illness of the population, rarely is there sufficient time for PAD in the cardiothoracic surgical patient. In addition, PAD has been largely supplanted by intraoperative blood salvage techniques, for reasons of cost-effectiveness (blood withdrawal, preparation, storage, and potential erythropoietin therapy add to costs) and because of advances in intraoperative blood salvage techniques such as intraoperative autologous donation (IAD; discussed later in this chapter), retrograde autologous prime of the CPB circuit, use of cell saver, and regular use of cardiotomy suction.

PHARMACOLOGIC STRATEGIES FOR BLOOD CONSERVATION

A number of drugs have been used to decrease blood loss and the use of blood transfusion associated with cardiac surgery (Table 12-5). Interest has been recently renewed in antifibrinolytics, a relatively old class of drug. Currently, three such medications are used clinically; two are synthetic antifibrinolytics (epsilon-aminocaproic acid and tranexamic acid) and one is naturally occurring (aprotinin derived from bovine lung). Linked with the resurgence of interest in these drugs is interest in diminishing homologous blood transfusions related to cardiac surgery.

Epsilon-Aminocaproic Acid

Epsilon-aminocaproic acid (EACA) is a synthetic antifibrinolytic agent first described in 1959, which derives its effect by forming reversible complexes with either plasminogen or plasmin, saturating the lysine binding sites and thus displacing plasminogen and therefore plasmin from the surface of fibrin. This blockage of plasminogen binding to fibrin blocks plasminogen activation and therefore fibrinolysis. The overall effect is to block the dissolution of the fibrin clot.

Several studies have demonstrated the efficacy of EACA in reducing bleeding following open heart surgery. First utilized in situations in which excessive bleeding was encountered, Lambert et al used EACA in 1979 to successfully treat patients with coagulation disorders, who comprise 20% of total primary coronary bypass patients.[25] DelRossi used EACA in 1989 as a prophylactic tool to reduce blood loss in 350 patients undergoing CPB, having an impact on both blood loss and transfusion of autologous blood and blood products.[26]

TABLE 12–5 Antifibrinolytics used in cardiac surgery and their mechanism of action

Antifibrinolytic	Mechanism of action
Epsilon-aminocaproic acid (Amicar)	Forms a complex with plasminogen through lysine-binding sites, thus blocking their adhesion to fibrin
Tranexamic acid (Cyklokapron)	Forms a complex with plasminogen through lysine-binding sites, thus blocking their adhesion to fibrin
Aprotinin (Trasylol)	Serine protease inhibitor with an antifibrinolytic effect carried by the inhibition of plasmin and kallikrein Protection of platelet GpIb, reducing thrombin-mediated consumption of the platelets

Tranexamic Acid

The mechanism of action of tranexamic acid (TA) is similar to EACA. The significant difference between EACA and TA is that TA is roughly 10 times more potent than EACA. As with EACA, postoperative bleeding and homologous blood requirements were similarly decreased with the use of TA, as shown by Horrow in 1990 in 38 patients undergoing CPB.[27]

Aprotinin

Aprotinin is a low molecular weight serine-protease inhibitor, with a lysine residue occupying its active center. It is a naturally occurring polypeptide isolated from bovine lung. Reversible enzyme-inhibitor complexes with various proteases are formed, displaying activity against trypsin, plasmin, streptokinase-plasma complex, tissue kallikrein, and plasma kallikrein. Because aprotinin is a nonspecific serine antiprotease, it intervenes in the coagulation cascade in multiple loci, working to decrease bleeding in CPB patients by its antiplasmin and antikallikrein effects.

Aprotinin was first used in cardiac surgery by Tice et al, who described the administration of 10,000 to 20,000 kallikrein inhibitory units (KIU) resulting in rapid establishment of hemostasis in 5 patients that had undergone CPB; they also demonstrated increased bleeding and increased fibrinolytic activity.[28] The currently accepted regimen of high-dose aprotinin (5-6 million unit average total dose) is reflective of the experiences of the Hammersmith group, which serendipitously saw a reduction in bleeding in patients receiving aprotinin to reduce kallikrein-mediated lung inflammation during CPB.[29] Since this report, multiple reports have emerged citing the efficacy of aprotinin as compared to other antifibrinolytics and controls in reducing bleeding complications, homologous blood transfusions, and inflammation primarily in the reoperative setting.[30–32]

TOPICAL HEMOSTATIC AGENTS

The limited efficacy of topical agents such as oxidized cellulose and microfibrillar collagen has led to the development of new products with novel applicator systems that are direct activators of the clotting cascade. Additionally, pericardial lavage with aprotinin or EACA has been shown to be ineffective at reducing transfusion requirements and may enhance mediastinal adhesion formation.[33–35] As a result of the limitations of more traditional agents, the new generation topical agents have gained appeal due to their inherent effectiveness as well as their ease of use.

Bioglue (Cryolife, Inc., Kennesaw, GA) is a biological glue initially approved for use in the repair of aortic dissection. This product is composed of purified bovine serum, albumin, and gluteraldehyde. The action is almost instantaneous because gluteraldehyde exposure leads to the tenuous binding of lysine molecules, proteins, and tissue surfaces. Raanani described the use of Bioglue as an aid in aortic reconstructive surgery, avoiding the use of stiff Teflon felt strips.[36]

Tisseel VH (Baxter Healthcare Corp., Glendale, CA) is a topical protein solution sealer which is sprayed onto hemorrhagic surfaces. This fibrin sealant contains fibrinogen, thrombin, calcium chloride, and aprotinin. When the protein and thrombin solutions are mixed and topically sprayed, a viscous solution that rapidly sets into an elastic coagulum is produced. A study by Rousou demonstrated that fibrin sealant was safe in regard to viral transmission and highly effective in controlling localized bleeding in cardiac operations.[37]

The gelatin-based hemostatic sealant FloSeal (Fusion Medical Technologies, Inc., Mountain View, CA) activates the clotting cascade and simultaneously forms a nondisplacing hemostatic plug. A FloSeal kit contains a bovine-derived gelatin matrix, a bovine-derived thrombin component, and a syringe applicator. The gelatinous matrix is biocompatible and reabsorbed in 6 to 8 weeks. In a series of patients undergoing open heart procedures, the Fusion Matrix Group studied FloSeal versus Gelfoam-Thrombin in procedures in which standard surgical means were ineffective at controlling bleeding.[38] FloSeal stopped bleeding in a significantly higher number of patients than did standard therapy with no differences in adverse events; however, there was no mention of each product's effect on transfusion rates.

PLATELET INHIBITORS AND THEIR EFFECT ON BLOOD USAGE

Platelet inhibition with the relatively new drug class glycoprotein (GP) IIb/IIIa receptor antagonists has greatly reduced the need for emergent CABG in those patients undergoing angioplasty or coronary stenting procedures. However, these agents pose a new challenge for the cardiac surgical team for those patients referred for surgery in terms of bleeding risk (Table 12-6).

The final common pathway of platelet aggregation leading to coronary artery occlusion is the cross-linking of receptor GP IIb/IIIa on adjacent platelets by adhesive plasma proteins (fibrinogen). As a result, receptor blockade of GP IIb/IIIa results in blocking platelet aggregation and subsequent thrombus formation. A population of patients with ischemic heart disease who may be expected to require CABG despite maximal therapy with GP IIb/IIIa inhibitors still remains. Currently, there are no controlled studies of GP IIb/IIIa inhibitors' effect on patients undergoing CABG. However, the use of these inhibitors may enhance the risk of bleeding compared to elective procedures in patients not receiving these agents. The currently utilized agents are summarized in Table 12-6. Current guidelines for patients requiring coronary artery bypass surgery include:

TABLE 12–6 Antiplatelet agents

Drug	Binding	Mechanism	Half-life
Clopidogrel (Plavix)	Irreversible	ADP-mediated platelet aggregation	8 h
Abciximab (ReoPro)	Noncompetitive	GP IIb/IIIa inhibition	30 min
Tirofiban (Aggrastat)	Reversible	GP IIb/IIIa inhibition	2.2 h
Eptifibatide (Integrillin)	Reversible	GP IIb/IIIa inhibition	2.5 h

1. Stop the GP IIb/IIIa inhibitor.
2. Delay surgery for up to 12 hours if abciximab, tirofiban, or eptafibitide is used and delay up to 7 days if clopidogrel is used.
3. Maintain standard heparin dosing despite elevated bleeding times.
4. Utilize ultrafiltration via zero balance technique while on CPB.
5. Transfuse platelets as needed as opposed to prophylactically, preferably once off CPB and after protamine administration.[39]

INTRAOPERATIVE AND POSTOPERATIVE MANAGEMENT

Intraoperative Period

Intraoperative autologous donation (IAD) of whole blood has many advantages over PAD. IAD does not require a delay in surgery; it can be performed efficiently and with minimal additional cost. In addition, the blood product obtained by IAD is whole blood, which is transfused within 2 to 3 hours of collection and therefore contains active platelets and factors. The resultant advantages are the avoidance of coagulopathy frequently seen after CPB, and the addition of red cell mass capable of oxygen transport. The storage process limits the amount of blood loss during surgery via lap pads and discard suction, and spares the damaging effects of the heart-lung machine, which include contact activation of platelets and complement as well as red blood cell hemolysis. Because IAD serves to decrease red cell requirements in a volume-dependent manner, the maximum amount of blood should be removed from each individual patient in order to optimize blood conservation efforts. The amount of blood that an individual patient is capable of donating via IAD is strictly dependent upon the patient's own physiologic parameters, estimated blood volume (based on height-weight normogram), pre–IAD hematocrit, and pre–CPB hematocrit.[40]

Minimal hemodilution by red cell priming of the CPB circuit is a useful technique in avoiding transfusions. These techniques include low-prime circuitry and retrograde autologous prime (RAP).[41] Up to 90% of the crystalloid prime of the CPB circuit can be displaced with autologous blood utilizing RAP. This technique involves partial priming of the bypass circuit with the patient's own blood from the arterial cannula just prior to instituting CPB. In addition, the venous loop can also be primed in a similar manner when first instituting CPB, displacing the crystalloid prime in the venous loop. The result is the replacement of virtually all of the crystalloid prime with autologous blood, thereby reducing the amount of hemodilution the patient experiences on CPB.

TRANSFUSION TRIGGERS

The literature indicates that the anesthetized patient on full cardiopulmonary bypass at moderate hypothermia can safely tolerate a hematocrit as low as 15%, with the exception of those patients at risk for decreased cerebral oxygen delivery, namely those with a history of CVA, diabetes, cerebrovascular disease.[42] These latter patients can tolerate a hematocrit as low as 18% when utilizing moderate hypothermia.[43] Once the patient is warm and being weaned from CPB, these percentage points are raised by 2% each (17% and 20%, respectively) since the relative protective effects of the hypothermia are no longer present. In our institution, once off CPB, our practice has been to retransfuse all or as much as possible remaining blood in the CPB circuit to the patient, then give all available cell saver blood including any blood remaining in the CPB circuit that was not initially given back to the patient, then any IAD, and then finally PAD if available. Then and only then, if the hematocrit remains unsatisfactorily low, does the patient receive homologous blood.

Once the patient leaves the operating room, we use a transfusion trigger corresponding with a hematocrit of 22% in the asymptomatic patient. In patients greater than 80 years of age, a trigger of 24% is utilized. These numbers are meant to serve as guidelines; if a patient is at all symptomatic (tachycardic, hypotensive, ischemic, or with any evidence of end organ hypoperfusion), the patient will receive homologous blood transfusion therapy. To safely and appropriately apply minimum safe transfusion standards, the cardiac surgeon or anesthesiologist must have an understanding of the lowest safe level of anemia under the variety of conditions encountered by the cardiac surgical patient. This understanding can then be combined with an assessment of the patient's clinical status to determine the true need for red cell transfusion.

TABLE 12–7 Relative costs of blood conservation agents used in a single institution

Agents	Approximate cost
EACA (Amicar)	$30.00 per case
Tranexemic acid	$25.00 per case
Aprotinin (Trasylol)	$1200.00 per case
Erythropoietin (Procrit)	$130.00 per 20,000-unit dose
Homologous banked PRBC	$210.00 per unit
PAD	$340.00 per unit
Platelets (pheresed only)	$600.00 per 6 units
FFP	$55.00 per unit
Cryoprecipitate	$53.00 per 10 units
Blood irradiation	$16.00 per bag
Blood CMV testing	$25.00 per bag

COST OF BLOOD CONSERVATION

In today's economic environment, it is important to discuss patient treatment modalities in terms of cost. There is no question that some aspects of the blood conservation approach are more costly than others (Table 12-7). However, when taken in the context of the cost of blood products, their usage, the potential reduction in the risk of reexplorations, as well as the reduction or elimination of the risks of homologous blood exposures, these costs may seem a little more reasonable.

CONCLUSION

Historically, cardiac surgery has been associated with a high incidence of blood transfusion, with up to 70% of these patients receiving homologous blood transfusions at some point during their hospital stay. However, with improving technology, awareness of blood conservation techniques, and better pharmacologic agents, a multidisciplinary approach to blood conservation can make "bloodless heart surgery" entirely possible. For the purely elective case, these techniques are initiated preoperatively with PAD, while other patients are eligible for one or all of the remainder of the in-hospital techniques described. Using a team approach that both optimizes and integrates the use of each of these measures, the use of homologous blood can be markedly reduced in a majority of cardiac surgical patients.

REFERENCES

1. Belisle S, Hardy JF: Hemorrhage and the use of blood products after adult cardiac operations: myths and realities. *Ann Thorac Surg* 1996; 62:1908.
2. Goodnough LT, Despostis GJ, Hohue CW, et al: On the need for improved transfusion indicators in cardiac surgery. *Ann Thorac Surg* 1995; 60:473.

3. Surgenor DM, Wallace EL, Churchill WH, et al: Red cell transfusion in coronary artery bypass surgery. *Transfusion* 1992; 32:458.
4. Boyle EM, Verrier VD Spiess BD: The procoagulant response to injury. *Ann Thorac Surg* 1997; 64:S16.
5. Hunt BJ, Parratt RN, Segal HC, et al: Activation of coagulation and fibrinolysis during cardiothoracic operations. *Ann Thorac Surg* 1998; 65:712.
6. Woodman RC, Harker LA: Bleeding complications associated with cardiopulmonary bypass. *Blood* 1990; 76:1680.
7. Cooley DA, Beall AC, Grondin P: Open-heart operations with disposable oxygenators, 5 percent dextrose prime, and normothermia. *Surgery* 1962; 52:713.
8. Cosgrove DM, Thurer RL, Lytle BW, et al: Blood conservation during myocardial revascularization. *Ann Thorac Surg* 1979; 28:184.
9. Ovrum E, Holen EA, Linstein MA: Elective coronary artery bypass without homologous blood transfusion. *Scand J Thorac Cardiovasc Surg* 1991; 25:13.
10. Ovrum E, Holen EA, Abdelnoor M, et al: Conventional blood conservation techniques in 500 consecutive coronary artery bypass operations. *Ann Thorac Surg* 1991; 51:500.
11. DeBois WJ, Sukhram Y, McVey, J, et al: Reduction in homologous transfusion using a low prime circuit. *J Extracorp Tech* 1996; 28:58.
12. Rosengart TR, DeBois WJ, O'Hara M, et al: Retrograde autologous priming for cardiopulmonary bypass: a safe and effective means of decreasing hemodilution and transfusion requirements. *J Thorac Cardiovasc Surg* 1998; 115:426.
13. Lilly KJ, O'Gara PJ, Treanor PR, et al: Heparin-bonded circuits without a cardiotomy: a description of a minimally invasive technique of cardiopulmonary bypass. *Perfusion* 2002; 7:95.
14. Hamada Y, Kawachi K, Nakata T, et al: Antiinflammatory effect of heparin-coated circuits with leukocyte-depleting filters in coronary bypass surgery. *Artif Organs* 2001; 25:1004.
15. Ferraris VA, Swanson E: Aspirin usage and perioperative blood loss in patients undergoing unexpected operations. *Surg Gynecol Obstet* 1983; 156:439.
16. Ferraris VA, Gildengorin VJ: Predictors of excessive blood use after coronary artery bypass grafting: a multivariate analysis. *Thorac Cardiovasc Surg* 1989; 98:492.
17. Bashein G, Nessly ML, Rice AL, et al: Preoperative aspirin therapy and reoperation for bleeding after coronary artery bypass surgery. *Arch Intern Med* 1991; 151:89.
18. Rodgers RP, Levin J: A critical reappraisal of the bleeding time. *Semin Thromb Hemost* 1990; 16:1.
19. Cosgrove DM, Loop FD, Lytle BW, et al: Determinants of blood utilization during myocardial revascularization. *Ann Thorac Surg* 1985; 40:380.
20. Utley JR, Wallace DJ, Thomason ME, et al: Correlates of preoperative hematocrit value in patients undergoing coronary artery bypass. *J Thorac Cardiovasc Surg* 1989; 98:451.
21. Rosengart TK, Helm RE, DeBois WJ, et al: Open heart operations without transfusion using a multimodality blood conservation strategy in 50 Jehovah's Witness patients: implications for a "bloodless" surgical technique. *J Am Coll Surg* 1997; 184:618.
22. Sandrelli L, Pardini A, Lorusso R, et al: Impact of autologous blood predonation on a comprehensive blood conservation program. *Ann Thorac Surg* 1995; 59:730.
23. Goodnough LT, Verbrugge D, Marcus RE, et al: The effect of patient size and dose of recombinant human erythropoietin therapy on red blood cell volume expansion in autologous blood donors for elective orthopedic operation. *J Am Coll Surg* 1994; 179:171.
24. Owings DV, Kruskall MS, Thurer RL, et al: Autologous blood donations prior to elective cardiac surgery: safety and effect on subsequent blood use. *JAMA* 1989; 262:1963.
25. Lambert CJ, Marengo-Rowe AJ, Leveson JE, et al: The treatment of postperfusion bleeding using epsilon-aminocaproic acid, cryoprecipitate, fresh-frozen plasma, and protamine sulfate. *Ann Thorac Surg* 1979; 28:440.
26. DelRossi AJ, Cernaianu AC, Botros S, et al: Prophylactic treatment of postperfusion bleeding using EACA. *Chest* 1989; 96:27.
27. Horrow JC, Hlavacek J, Strong MD, et al: Prophylactic tranexamic acid decreases bleeding after cardiac operations. *J Thorac Cardiovasc Surg* 1990; 99:70.
28. Tice DA, Worth MH Jr: Recognition and treatment of postoperative bleeding associated with open-heart surgery. *Ann N Y Acad Sci* 1968; 146:745.
29. Royston D: The serine antiprotease aprotinin (Trasylol): a novel approach to reducing postoperative bleeding. *Blood Coagul Fibrinolysis* 1990; 1:55.
30. Barrons RW, Jahr JS: A review of post–cardiopulmonary bypass bleeding, aminocaproic acid, tranexamic acid, and aprotinin. *Am J Ther* 1996; 3:821.
31. Casati V, Guzzon D, Oppizzi M, et al: Hemostatic effects of aprotinin, tranexamic acid and epsilon-aminocaproic acid in primary cardiac surgery. *Ann Thorac Surg* 1999; 68:2252.
32. Laupacis A, Fergusson D: Drugs to minimize perioperative blood loss in cardiac surgery: meta-analyses using perioperative blood transfusion as the outcome. The International Study of Perioperative Transfusion (ISPOT) Investigators. *Anesth Analg* 1997; 85:1258.
33. De Bonis M, Cavaliere F, Alessandrini F, et al: Topical use of tranexamic acid in coronary artery bypass operations: a double-blind, prospective, randomized, placebo-controlled study. *Thorac Cardiovasc Surg* 2000; 119:575.
34. Cicek S, Theodoro DA: Topical aprotinin in cardiac operations: a note of caution. *Ann Thorac Surg* 1996; 61:1039.
35. O'Regan DJ, Giannopoulos N, Mediratta N, et al: Topical aprotinin in cardiac operations. *Ann Thorac Surg* 1994; 58:778.
36. Raanani E, Latter DA, Errett LE, et al: Use of "BioGlue" in aortic surgical repair. *Ann Thorac Surg* 2001; 72:638.
37. Rousou J, Levitsky S, Gonzalez-Lavin L, et al: Randomized clinical trial of fibrin sealant in patients undergoing resternotomy or reoperation after cardiac operations: a multicenter study. *J Thorac Cardiovasc Surg* 1989; 97:194.
38. Oz MC, Cosgrove DM III, Badduke BR, et al: Controlled clinical trial of a novel hemostatic agent in cardiac surgery. The Fusion Matrix Study Group. *Ann Thorac Surg* 2000; 69:1376.
39. Lee LY, DeBois W, Krieger KH, et al: The effects of platelet inhibitors on blood use in cardiac surgery. *Perfusion* 2002; 17:33,
40. Helm RE, Klemperer JD, Rosengart TK, et al: Intraoperative autologous blood donation preserves red cell mass but does not decrease postoperative bleeding. *Ann Thorac Surg* 1996; 62:1431.
41. Rosengart TK, DeBois W, O'Hara M, et al: Retrograde autologous priming for cardiopulmonary bypass: a safe and effective means of decreasing hemodilution and transfusion requirements. *J Thorac Cardiovasc Surg* 1998; 115:426.
42. Helm RE, Klemperer JD, Rosengart TK, et al: Intraoperative autologous blood donation preserves red cell mass but does not decrease postoperative bleeding. *Ann Thorac Surg* 1996; 62:1431.
43. Fang WC, Helm RE, Krieger KH, et al: Impact of minimum hematocrit during cardiopulmonary bypass on mortality in patients undergoing coronary artery surgery. *Circulation* 1997; 96 (9 suppl):II194.
44. Beall AC Jr, Yow EM Jr, Bloodwell RD, et al: Open heart surgery without blood transfusion. *Arch Surg* 1967; 94:567.
45. Cohn LH, Fosberg AM, Anderson WP, Collins JJ Jr: The effects of phlebotomy, hemodilution and autologous transfusion on systemic oxygenation and whole blood utilization in open heart surgery. *Chest* 1975; 68:283.
46. Cove H, Matloff J, Sacks HJ, et al: Autologous blood transfusion in coronary artery bypass surgery. *Transfusion* 1976; 16:245.

47. Kaplan JA, Cannarella C, Jones EL, et al: Autologous blood transfusion during cardiac surgery: a re-evaluation of three methods. *J Thorac Cardiovasc Surg* 1977; 74:4.
48. Lilleaasen P: Moderate and extreme haemodilution in open-heart surgery: blood requirements, bleeding and platelet counts. *Scand J Thorac Cardiovasc Surg* 1977; 11:97.
49. Schaff HV, Hauer JM, Bell WR, et al: Autotransfusion of shed mediastinal blood after cardiac surgery: a prospective study. *J Thorac Cardiovasc Surg* 1978; 75:632.
50. Thurer RL, Lytle BW, Cosgrove DM, Loop FD: Autotransfusion following cardiac operations: a randomized, prospective study. *Ann Thorac Surg* 1979; 27:500.
51. Lambert CJ, Marengo-Rowe AJ, Leveson JE, et al: The treatment of postperfusion bleeding using epsilon-aminocaproic acid, cryoprecipitate, fresh-frozen plasma, and protamine sulfate. *Ann Thorac Surg* 1979; 28:440.
52. Johnson RG, Rosenkrantz KR, Preston RA, et al: The efficacy of postoperative autotransfusion in patients undergoing cardiac operations. *Ann Thorac Surg* 1983; 36:173.
53. Love TR, Hendren WG, O'Keefe DD, Daggett WM: Transfusion of predonated autologous blood in elective cardiac surgery. *Ann Thorac Surg* 1987; 43:508.
54. Giordano GF, Rivers SL, Chung GK, et al: Autologous platelet-rich plasma in cardiac surgery: effect on intraoperative and postoperative transfusion requirements. *Ann Thorac Surg* 1988; 46:416.
55. Giordano GF, Goldman DS, Mammana RB, et al: Intraoperative autotransfusion in cardiac operations: effect on intraoperative and postoperative transfusion requirements. *J Thorac Cardiovasc Surg* 1988; 96:382.
56. Page R, Russell GN, Fox MA, et al: Hard-shell cardiotomy reservoir for reinfusion of shed mediastinal blood. *Ann Thorac Surg* 1989; 48:514.
57. Lepore V, Radegran K: Autotransfusion of mediastinal blood in cardiac surgery. *Scand J Thorac Cardiovasc Surg* 1989; 23:47.
58. Britton LW, Eastlund DT, Dziuban SW, et al: Predonated autologous blood use in elective cardiac surgery. *Ann Thorac Surg* 1989; 47:529.
59. Horrow JC, Van Riper DF, Strong MD, et al: Hemostatic effects of tranexamic acid and desmopressin during cardiac surgery. *Circulation* 1991; 84:2063.
60. Carey JS, Cukingnan RA, Carson E: Transfusion therapy in cardiac surgery: impact of the Paul Gann Blood Safety Act in California. *Am Surg* 1991; 57:830.
61. Scott EP, Quinley ED: Is the deferred-donor notification process effective? *Transfusion* 1992; 32:696.
62. Ikeda S, Johnston MF, Yagi K, et al: Intraoperative autologous blood salvage with cardiac surgery: an analysis of five years' experience in more than 3,000 patients. *J Clin Anesth* 1992; 4:359.
63. Dzik WH, Fleisher AG, Ciavarella D, et al: Safety and efficacy of autologous blood donation before elective aortic valve operation. *Ann Thorac Surg* 54(6):1177, 1992.
64. Helm RE, Klemperer JD, Rosengart TK, et al: Intraoperative autologous blood donation preserves red cell mass but does not decrease postoperative bleeding. *Ann Thorac Surg* 1996; 62:1431.
65. Rosengart TK, Helm RE, Klemperer J, et al: Combined aprotinin and erythropoietin use for blood conservation: results with Jehovah's Witnesses. *Ann Thorac Surg* 1994; 58:1397.
66. Wong CA, Franklin ML, Wade LD: Coagulation tests, blood loss, and transfusion requirements in platelet-rich plasmapheresed versus nonpheresed cardiac surgery patients. *Anesth Analg* 1994; 78:29.
67. Murkin JM, Lux J, Shannon NA, et al: Aprotinin significantly decreases bleeding and transfusion requirements in patients receiving aspirin and undergoing cardiac operations. *J Thorac Cardiovasc Surg* 1994; 107:554.
68. Axford TC, Dearani JA, Ragno G, et al: Safety and therapeutic effectiveness of reinfused shed blood after open heart surgery. *Ann Thorac Surg* 1994; 57:615.
69. Shinfeld A, Zippel D, Lavee J, et al: Aprotinin improves hemostasis after cardiopulmonary bypass better than single-donor platelet concentrate. *Ann Thorac Surg* 1995; 59:872.
70. Spiess BD, Gillies BS, Chandler W, Verrier E: Changes in transfusion therapy and reexploration rate after institution of a blood management program in cardiac surgical patients. *J Cardiothorac Vasc Anesth* 1995; 9:168.
71. Parolari A, Antona C, Rona P, et al: The effect of multiple blood conservation techniques on donor blood exposure in adult coronary and valve surgery performed with a membrane oxygenator: a multivariate analysis on 1310 patients. *J Card Surg* 1995; 10:227.
72. Shapira OM, Aldea GS, Treanor PR, et al: Reduction of allogeneic blood transfusions after open heart operations by lowering cardiopulmonary bypass prime volume. *Ann Thorac Surg* 1998; 65:724.
73. Tempe DK, Banerjee A, Virmani S, et al: Comparison of the effects of a cell saver and low-dose aprotinin on blood loss and homologous blood usage in patients undergoing valve surgery. *J Cardiothorac Vasc Anesth* 2001; 15:326.
74. Van der Linden P, De Hert S, Daper A, et al: A standardized multidisciplinary approach reduces the use of allogeneic blood products in patients undergoing cardiac surgery. *Can J Anaesth* 2001; 48:894.
75. Zubiate P, Kay JH, Mendez AM, et al: Coronary artery surgery: a new technique with use of little blood, if any. *J Thorac Cardiovasc Surg* 1974; 68:263.
76. Yeh T Jr, Shelton L, Yeh TJ: Blood loss and bank blood requirement in coronary bypass surgery. *Ann Thorac Surg* 1978; 26:11.
77. Schaff HV, Hauer J, Gardner TJ, et al: Routine use of autotransfusion following cardiac surgery: experience in 700 patients. *Ann Thorac Surg* 1979; 27:493.
78. Bayer WL, Coenen WM, Jenkins DC, Zucker ML: The use of blood and blood components in 1,769 patients undergoing open-heart surgery. *Ann Thorac Surg* 1980; 29:117.
79. Weisel RD, Charlesworth DC, Mickleborough LL, et al: Limitations of blood conservation. *J Thorac Cardiovasc Surg* 1984; 88:26.
80. Belcher P, Lennox SC: Reduction of blood use in surgery for coronary artery disease. *J Cardiovasc Surg (Torino)* 1986; 27:657.
81. Breyer RH, Engelman RM, Rousou JA, Lemeshow S: Blood conservation for myocardial revascularization: is it cost effective? *J Thorac Cardiovasc Surg* 1987; 93:512.
82. Hartz RS, Smith JA, Green D: Autotransfusion after cardiac operation: assessment of hemostatic factors. *J Thorac Cardiovasc Surg* 1988; 96:178.
83. Dietrich W, Barankay A, Dilthey G, et al: Reduction of blood utilization during myocardial revascularization. *J Thorac Cardiovasc Surg* 1989; 97:213.
84. Tyson GS, Sladen RN, Spainhour V, et al: Blood conservation in cardiac surgery: preliminary results with an institutional commitment. *Ann Surg* 1989; 209:736.
85. Owings DV, Kruskall MS, Thurer RL, Donovan LM: Autologous blood donations prior to elective cardiac surgery: safety and effect on subsequent blood use. *JAMA* 1989; 262:1963.
86. LoCicero J 3rd, Massad M, Gandy K, et al: Aggressive blood conservation in coronary artery surgery: impact on patient care. *J Cardiovasc Surg (Torino)* 1990; 31:559.
87. Jones JW, McCoy TA, Rawitscher RE, Lindsley DA: Effects of intraoperative plasmapheresis on blood loss in cardiac surgery. *Ann Thorac Surg* 1990; 49:585.
88. Jones JW, Rawitscher RE, McLean TR, et al: Benefit from combining blood conservation measures in cardiac operations. *Ann Thorac Surg* 1991; 51:541.

89. Davies GG, Wells DG, Sadler R, et al: Plateletpheresis and transfusion practice in heart operations. *Ann Thorac Surg* 1992; 54:1020.
90. Watanabe Y, Fuse K, Naruse Y, et al: Subcutaneous use of erythropoietin in heart surgery. *Ann Thorac Surg* 1992; 54:479.
91. Johnson RG, Thurer RL, Kruskall MS, et al: Comparison of two transfusion strategies after elective operations for myocardial revascularization. *J Thorac Cardiovasc Surg* 1992; 104:307.
92. Kulier AH, Gombotz H, Fuchs G, et al: Subcutaneous recombinant human erythropoietin and autologous blood donation before coronary artery bypass surgery. *Anesth Analg* 1993; 76:102.
93. Karski JM, Teasdale SJ, Norman PH, et al: Prevention of postbypass bleeding with tranexamic acid and epsilon-aminocaproic acid. *J Cardiothorac Vasc Anesth* 1993; 7:431.
94. Sutton RG, Kratz JM, Spinale FG, Crawford FA Jr: Comparison of three blood- processing techniques during and after cardiopulmonary bypass. *Ann Thorac Surg* 1993; 56:938.
95. Ward HB, Smith RR, Landis KP, et al: Prospective, randomized trial of autotransfusion after routine cardiac operations. *Ann Thorac Surg* 1993; 56:137.
96. Tobe CE, Vocelka C, Sepulvada R, et al: Infusion of autologous platelet rich plasma does not reduce blood loss and product use after coronary artery bypass: a prospective, randomized, blinded study. *J Thorac Cardiovasc Surg* 1993; 105:1007.
97. Schonberger JP, Bredee JJ, Tjian D, et al: Intraoperative predonation contributes to blood saving. *Ann Thorac Surg* 1993; 56:893.
98. Paone G, Spencer T, Silverman NA: Blood conservation in coronary artery surgery. *Surgery* 1994; 116:672.
99. Lemmer JH Jr, Stanford W, Bonney SL, et al: Aprotinin for coronary bypass operations: efficacy, safety, and influence on early saphenous vein graft patency: a multicenter, randomized, double-blind, placebo-controlled study. *J Thorac Cardiovasc Surg* 1994; 107:543.
100. Petry AF, Jost J, Sievers H: Reduction of homologous blood requirements by blood-pooling at the onset of cardiopulmonary bypass. *J Thorac Cardiovasc Surg* 1994; 107:1210.
101. Arom KV, Emery RW: Decreased postoperative drainage with addition of epsilon-aminocaproic acid before cardiopulmonary bypass. *Ann Thorac Surg* 1994; 57:1108.
102. Helm RE, Rosengart TK, Gomez M, et al: Comprehensive multimodality blood conservation: 100 consecutive CABG operations without transfusion. *Ann Thorac Surg* 1998; 65:125.
103. Rosengart TK, Helm RE, DeBois WJ, et al: Open heart operations without transfusion using a multimodality blood conservation strategy in 50 Jehovah's Witness patients: implications for a "bloodless" surgical technique. *J Am Coll Surg* 1997; 184:618.
104. Rousou JA, Engelman RM, Flack JE 3rd, et al: The "primeless pump": a novel technique for intraoperative blood conservation. *Cardiovasc Surg* 1999; 7:228.
105. Karkouti K, Cohen MM, McCluskey SA, Sher GD: A multivariable model for predicting the need for blood transfusion in patients undergoing first-time elective coronary bypass graft surgery. *Transfusion* 2001; 41:1193.

Chapter 13

Deep Hypothermic Circulatory Arrest

René Prêtre/Marko I. Turina

Hypothermia is the most efficient measure to prevent or reduce ischemic damage to the central nervous system when blood circulation is reduced. The central nervous system has a high metabolic rate and limited energy stores, which make it extremely vulnerable to ischemia. Because the central nervous system is the organ that is most sensitive to ischemia, attention has been mainly centered on neurologic outcome when perfusion was reduced, with the indirect assumption that, if the brain or the spinal cord could tolerate undamaged the reduced perfusion, the other organs would too. With the introduction of regional cerebral perfusion, many surgeons have shifted their practice from a deep to a moderate systemic hypothermia during repair of the thoracic aorta. Consideration (which will not be discussed here) should then be given to a specific protection of the abdominal viscera when a long period of reduced perfusion is anticipated.

CEREBRAL METABOLIC RATE

Reduction of Metabolism

Hypothermia reduces the metabolic rate of the central nervous system and lengthens the period of tolerated ischemia. The central nervous system almost exclusively extracts its energy through the aerobic process of glycolysis. The uptake of oxygen or glucose is consequently a reliable parameter of the cerebral metabolic rate. Using oxygen and glucose consumption, animal studies showed a drop of the brain metabolic rate of 50% at 28°C, 19% at 18°C, and 11% at 8°C.[1,2] Comparable results, using less precise methods of measurement, were obtained in humans (Table 13-1).[3] The reduction of metabolic rate in relation to temperature espouses an exponential curve, with a greater drop at high temperatures (about 6% for 1°C around 37°C) than at low temperatures (about 1% at 15°C).[1,3,4] A luxurious perfusion of the brain is rapidly set when the metabolic rate is reduced and perfusion flow rate maintained. The arteriovenous difference of oxygen, glucose, and brain-produced metabolites decreases. The luxurious perfusion is, however, of limited help in view of an ischemic period because additional energetic reserve cannot be stored in neurons. The obvious clinical implication of these findings is that, although reduced, the metabolism of the brain is not suppressed by hypothermia, and actually remains relatively high at 18°C, a common target temperature in surgical practice. Assuming an ischemic tolerance of 5 minutes at normothermia, the calculated safe period of circulatory arrest for the central nervous system would not exceed 25 minutes at 18°C and 38 minutes at 13°C (see Table 13-1).[3]

Cellular activity, be it mechanical, biochemical, or electrical, is an important determinant of energetic requirement superimposed on basal metabolism.[5] Obtaining a complete suppression of cerebral electrical activity should consequently be an important goal in the strategy of brain

TABLE 13–1 Effect of temperature on cerebral metabolic rate

Temperature (°C)	CMR (% baseline)	Duration of safe CA (min)	$CMRO_2$ (mL/100g/min)	pMPFR (mL/kg/min)
37	100	5	1.48	100
32	70 (66-74)	7.5 (6.5-8)	0.82	56
30	56 (52-60)	9 (8-10)	0.65	44
28	48 (44-52)	10.5 (9.5-11.5)	0.51	34
25	37 (33-42)	14 (12-15)	0.36	24
20	24 (21-29)	21 (17-24)	0.20	14
18	17 (20-25)	25 (21-30)	0.16	11
15	14 (11-18)	31 (25-38)	0.11	8

CMR: cerebral metabolic rate; CA: circulatory arrest; $CMRO_2$: cerebral metabolism rate for oxygen; pMPFR: predicted minimal perfusion flow rate.

Data derived from McCullough JN, Zhang N, Reich DL, et al: Cerebral metabolic suppression during hypothermic circulatory arrest in humans. Ann Thorac Surg 1999; 67:1895; and Kern FH, Ungerleider RV, Reves JG, et al: Effect of altering pump flow rate on cerebral blood flow and metabolism in infants and children. Ann Thorac Surg 1993; 56:1366.

protection when a significant period of cerebral ischemia is anticipated. In the clinical setting, electrocerebral silence (as assessed by electroencephalography) is obtained at a mean nasopharyngeal temperature of 17.5°C.[6] Wide variations in the temperature inducing silence, however, exist between individuals and methods of cooling. The variations are also amplified by the fact that the brain temperature is not measured directly. In one large study, the minimal nasopharyngeal temperature to obtain electrocerebral silence in all patients was 12.5°C; at the classical 18°C, 40% of patients still exhibited electrical activity.[6]

Duration of Circulatory Arrest

The duration of safe circulatory arrest at a given temperature should not be seen as a clear-cut time period, but as a broad one during which successive biochemical alterations, followed by ultrastructural and then structural changes, arise (Fig. 13-1). The potential for recovery exists during the initial phase of biochemical alteration, but decreases as ischemia persists and becomes more dependent on reperfusion conditions. The cerebral metabolic rates of oxygen and glucose have often been used as surrogates for adequate energetic metabolism of the brain and consequently adequate maintenance of cellular homeostasis.[7,8] The recovery of oxygen consumption is already impaired after 15 minutes of ischemia at 18°C,[2] and cerebral-produced lactate (a marker of anaerobic metabolism) is detectable in the effluent blood after 20 minutes of ischemia.[9] Definitive damage to the brain, however, is unlikely if perfusion is adequately reinstituted after this time period.

Monitoring the evolution of intracellular high-energy molecules and pH specifies more precisely the moment when the exhaustion of energetic substrates may trigger the cascade of deleterious biochemical reactions. Nuclear magnetic resonance can provide continuous measurements

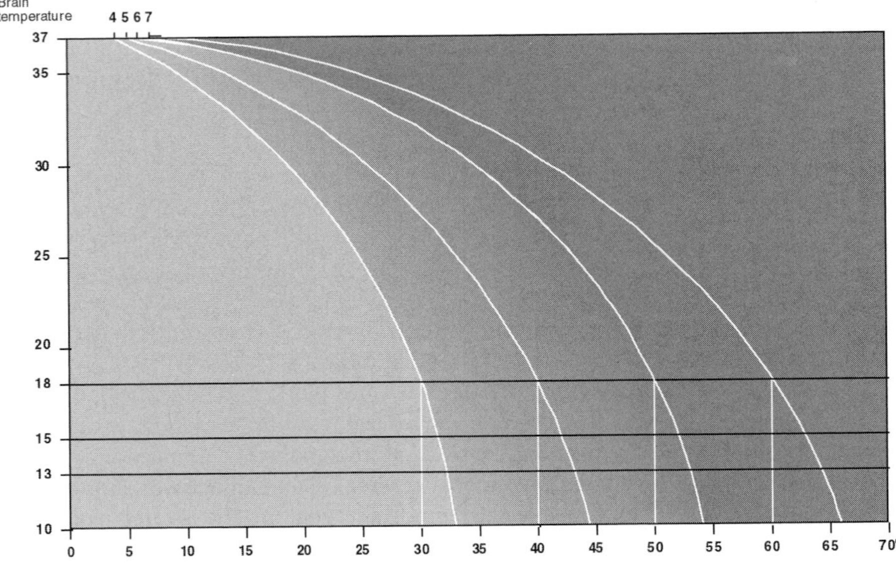

FIGURE 13–1 Consequences of circulatory arrest in relation to temperature and duration of cerebral ischemia. The light color depicts the periods of safe circulatory arrest. The dark color depicts the periods of obligatory harmful circulatory arrest. The transitional area depicts the periods where the risk and extent of brain damage are dependent on the conduct of surgery and pharmacological intervention. The light gray area is compatible with reversible deficits, while the dark gray area is associated with irreversible injuries.

of the relative concentration of phosphocreatine and adenosine triphosphate, the principal energetic molecules of the brain, as well as that of inorganic phosphate (the split product of these molecules) and intracellular pH. The electromagnetic signal of phosphocreatine decreases rapidly, followed by that of adenosine triphosphate, after institution of circulatory arrest.[5] These signals become hardly detectable after 32 to 36 minutes of ischemia at 15°C in animals.[10–12] Parallel to their disappearance, the signals of inorganic phosphate and pH progressively rise within the cells.

DIRECT AND SECONDARY ISCHEMIC INJURY

Direct Injuries

Cessation of blood delivery to neurons leads to an immediate reduction in the production of energetic molecules and sets a state of progressive energy failure. Cellular injury occurs because of a rapidly occurring intracellular acidosis and a more progressive dissipation of ionic gradient across membranes. The dissipation of ionic gradient initiates a cascade of destructive events that rapidly escape regulatory control.[5] At this stage, accumulation of calcium within cells (which interferes with many fundamental biochemical reactions) and attraction of osmotically obligated water are striking.[13]

The endothelial cells are also extremely sensitive to ischemia. The continuous activation and production of vasoactive factors (among which nitric oxide plays a central role) are impaired after endothelial ischemia. The endothelial dysfunction results in an increase in cerebral vascular resistance.[11,14] This is clinically exemplified by the loss of the diastolic perfusion of the brain in Doppler analysis of the middle cerebral artery after circulatory arrest.[15] Nitric oxide is a potent short-acting vasodilatator that regulates on-line the local vascular tone. The molecule further inhibits the aggregation of platelets and adherence of neutrophils to the endothelium, two critical steps in the initiation of reperfusion injuries.[16,17] The stimulation of nitric oxide production after circulatory arrest improves cerebral perfusion and accelerates recovery of high-energy phosphate and cerebral metabolism.[11,14]

Secondary Injuries

Secondary injuries occur upon and after restitution of perfusion. Reperfusion injuries operate at a cellular and at a vascular level. At the cellular level, the restitution of oxygen provokes the formation of highly reactive free radicals, able to disintegrate the membrane structure. At the vascular level, the recirculation of blood in ischemic territories induces a tight aggregation and adhesion of thrombocytes and neutrophils to the endothelium. These cellular complexes release potent inflammatory mediators and vasoconstrictor agents. Movement of blood elements becomes sluggish in small capillaries and can shut the microcirculation down and reestablish ischemia. Although a strong theoretical background supports the mechanisms of reperfusion injuries, their real contribution after deep hypothermic circulatory arrest (DHCA) remains uncertain.[13] At the vascular level, the risk of blood slugging seems greatly attenuated by the hemodilution induced by cardiopulmonary bypass.

Electrical hyperactivity of the brain after ischemia can produce extensive damage, because the condition recreates a cellular energetic mismatch and induces the release of toxic neurotransmitters. The mammalian brain is paradoxically extraordinarily vulnerable to its own neurotransmitters when released in the extracellular space.[18] Glutamate is the principal excitatory neurotransmitter of the brain and is found in extremely high concentration within neurons and astrocytes. The death of one cell liberates the neurotransmitter into the extracellular space, and puts all the surrounding neurons in danger, especially in the context of reduced defense capacity. A series of events, starting with the overexcitation of a neuron and ending in its death, rapidly propagates and exponentially expands the brain damage. It is unknown if premature resumption of brain activity (before replenishment of energy stores) can trigger the cascade of harmful events. It is, however, evident that hyperactivity of the brain during the rewarming period results in the extracellular release of glutamate.[18] Administration of glutamate antagonists after ischemic injury to the brain has shown a protective effect in animals and humans, already in the absence of cerebral hyperactivity.[19,20] These antagonists could prove valuable in circumscribing brain damage once significant neuronal injury has occurred, especially in case of electrical hyperactivity.

Protracted cellular dysfunction and apoptosis lead to a delayed (after a few days) neuronal death. The prolonged inability of the neuron to restore calcium homeostasis and ensure the turnover of cytostructure proteins is responsible for a progressive loss of cellular function and eventual death.[5,21,22] Apoptosis (programmed cellular death) is an active, energy-dependent process characterized by the silent breakdown and phagocytosis of a cell. A profound or long-lasting ischemia results in cellular necrosis, while a less severe ischemia results in apoptosis. The importance of apoptotic cell clearance is not well established but certainly underestimated, because of the swiftness of the process and the fact that it leaves no inflammatory traces. Apoptosis has often been documented in zones of borderline ischemia—in zones with moderate energy depletion—like the penumbra surrounding a focal ischemia.[21,23]

CEREBRAL BLOOD FLOW

Low-flow and Intermittent Perfusion

Low-flow and intermittent perfusion of the brain are able to maintain and respectively restore intracellular stores of high-energy substrates, prevent anaerobic glycolysis and intracellular acidosis, and consequently prolong cerebral tolerance to ischemia. Continuous monitoring of high-energy molecules established that the minimal perfusion flow able to maintain metabolic homeostasis in animals at 15°C was 10 mL/kg/min (a flow corresponding to 10% of full flow).[12] The minimal flow rate in humans, extrapolated from the slope of metabolic rate reduction, is 11 mL/kg/min at 18°C (Table 13-1).[24,25] In clinical practice, however, wide ranges of minimal flow rates (ranging from 5 to 30 mL/kg/min at 18°C) have been determined at a given temperature.[25] The wide variation is probably a consequence of blood (hematocrit, management of carbon dioxide) and hemodynamic (pulsatility, evolution of the "noncerebral" systemic resistance) factors. These facts argue for the use of a significant residual flow (a flow 50% greater than the predicted minimal perfusion flow rate of Table 13-1 for temperatures above 25°C, and 100% greater for temperatures under 25°C), when a low-flow perfusion strategy is adopted. Lower flow rates should not be used without a close monitoring of the jugular venous saturation or cerebral oxygenated state.[26] A continuous drop in venous saturation or a reduction in cerebral oxyhemoglobin detected by near infrared spectroscopy is an absolute sign of insufficient brain perfusion.

Intermittent perfusion of the brain also results in the absence of lactate production and rapid resumption of normal cerebral metabolism and perfusion after circulatory arrest.[27,28] Oxygen saturation in the sagittal sinus falls precipitously (to 16%) after 60 minutes of noninterrupted circulatory arrest, while it remains around 55% with intermittent perfusion.[27] This higher oxygen saturation, in combination with the higher blood pH and lower lactate production, acknowledges the nutritive role of intermittent perfusion at low temperatures. Metabolic homeostasis is maintained throughout when intermittent perfusion was established after a relatively short period of ischemia (after every 20 minutes at 18°C). Extending the ischemic period to 30 minutes results in a moderate production of lactate and subsequent impaired oxygen extraction in the brain.[2,28] Concerns that repetitive episodes of reperfusion may result in neuronal damage (as has been documented at normothermia[29,30]) have not been validated in the model of deep hypothermic circulatory arrest. One may at least speculate that reperfusion injuries do not happen if recirculation is established before the occurrence of anaerobic glycolysis.

Pulsatile Flow

Pulsatile perfusion provides hemodynamic advantages over nonpulsatile perfusion that become significant with borderline pressure and perfusion flow.[31,32] Once the perfusion pressure falls under the closing pressure of the precapillary arterioles, the vascular bed shuts down and is no longer perfused. The peak pressure in pulsatile perfusion is able to maintain the microcirculation open with a lower mean perfusion pressure and, consequently, a lower flow rate. The phenomenon is amplified after circulatory arrest.[32] A high perfusion pressure (higher than the pressure necessary to maintain a capillary bed open) is necessary to reopen closed vascular beds. The postischemic dysfunction of the endothelial cells (with the loss of the vasodilatation dominance[33]) further increases the critical reopening pressure of the capillaries. The peak pressure in a pulsatile perfusion overcomes more quickly this critical pressure. This results in a swifter and more homogenous restitution of brain perfusion. Cerebral vascular resistance is reduced and recovery of cerebral metabolic rate improves with pulsatile perfusion after circulatory arrest.[31,32]

MANAGEMENT OF TEMPERATURE

pH Strategy

Two strategies for blood gas management are possible during hypothermia. Alpha-stat management (the mechanism prevailing in reptiles) aims at maintaining normal acidemia and blood gases (a pH of 7.40 and a Pa_{CO_2} of 40 mm Hg) in the rewarmed (to 37°C) blood. In vivo, the hypothermic blood is alkalemic and hypocapnic. pH-stat management (the mechanism prevailing in hibernating animals) aims at maintaining normal values in vivo, in the hypothermic blood. When rewarmed to 37°C, the blood becomes acidemic and hypercapnic.

Alpha-stat management preserves autoregulation of brain perfusion and optimizes cellular enzyme activity. Because of blood alkalemia, the curve of oxyhemoglobin dissociation is shifted toward the right, corresponding to an increased affinity of oxygen for hemoglobin. With the further shift of oxyhemoglobin to the right due to hypothermia, the availability of oxygen carried by the hemoglobin molecule becomes tremendously reduced. At deep temperature reductions, oxygen diluted in blood represents the major source of oxygen to tissues.

The pH-stat strategy results in a powerful and sustained dilatation of the cerebral vessels because of the high level of carbon dioxide. Autoregulation of brain perfusion is lost and cerebral blood flow greatly increased. The time for temperature equilibration between blood and brain is shortened, resulting in a quick and homogenous cooling of the brain. Hypercapnia shifts the oxyhemoglobin dissociation curve toward the left and results in an increased availability of oxygen to tissues.

A comparison between the two strategies has been performed mainly in neonates or small animals. In piglets, a pH-stat strategy resulted in improved recovery of cerebral metabolism, and better histologic and behavioral scores.[34] In neonates, the same strategy provided superior psychometric scores at midterm evaluation.[35] The superiority of the pH strategy has not been confirmed in adults, however.

Prospective studies found no differences[36] or even worse neuropsychologic outcome.[37–39] Because it maintains a physiological coupling between cerebral blood flow and metabolism, the alpha-stat strategy appears advantageous in adults, in whom the risk of under- or overperfusion within the brain is substantial. Cerebral edema, which can be a consequence of cerebral overperfusion, is less likely to occur. Finally, the preservation of cerebral autoregulation may attenuate the uneven distribution of blood, which is prone to occur in patients with an underlying vasculopathy like atherosclerosis, hypertension, and diabetes.

Cooling and Rewarming

The time required to obtain equilibration of temperature between blood and tissues depends on the temperature gradient on one hand, and on the blood flow in the tissue and a tissue-specific coefficient of temperature exchange on the other hand. Cooling or rewarming over a short period of time results in wide variations of temperature between organs, and also within an organ itself. A slow rate of cooling or rewarming and a high blood flow are the two factors ensuring homogenous changes of the body temperature. Occlusive vascular disease and altered vascular reactivity may significantly reduce cerebral perfusion and delay temperature equilibration. Enhancement of cerebral cooling can be achieved by local cooling. Ice packed around the head efficiently reduces the temperature of the brain cortex and subcortical area by heat conduction across the skull.

Oxygen availability is reduced during hypothermia because of the shift to the right of the oxyhemoglobin curve. The parallel decrease in metabolic rate is likely to preserve an appropriate balance between availability and requirement of oxygen. During rapid cooling, however, the affinity of oxygen to hemoglobin rises sharply during the period that the tissue temperature is not equilibrated with that of blood. This effect, combined with the dilution of blood by the priming volume of cardiopulmonary bypass, may temporarily create a state of insufficient oxygen availability. Studies in animals confirm that expedited cooling associated with excessive hemodilution resulted in an uncompensated consumption of energetic molecules and in the development of cellular acidosis before institution of circulatory arrest. In one study, it was demonstrated that an increased concentration of hemoglobin was able to compensate for the decreased oxygen availability related to hypothermia. Intracellular acidosis was not present with a hematocrit of 30%, mild with a hematocrit of 20%, and severe with a hematocrit of 10%.[40,41] Using intravital microscopy, these investigators further established that the cerebral capillary flow was maintained despite increased blood viscosity (which is associated with high hematocrit values).[41,42] These findings support the consensus that cooling should be performed slowly and with an adequate hematocrit.

Rewarming represents a critical time period—perhaps the most decisive one—during which any additional harm to cerebral cells might induce permanent injury or precipitate their death. It seems logical to strive to obtain rapidly a stable energetic and biochemical homeostasis to prevent the occurrence of secondary injuries. Once initiated, the pathological processes are difficult to stop. Moreover, the final impact of a specific therapeutic action is often uncertain, owing to the complexity of interrelated biochemical derangements.

Providing a favorable hematologic environment, ensuring optimal hemodynamic conditions, and avoiding cerebral hyperactivity should set the best conditions for optimal recovery of the energy-depleted brain. It is, therefore, important to restart perfusion slowly after circulatory arrest. An initial period of "cold blood–low-pressure reperfusion" washes out accumulated metabolites, buffers free radicals, and provides substrates for regeneration of high-energy molecules before the resumption of cerebral electrical activity. A sufficient hematocrit during this reperfusion period is theoretically attractive because of its buffer, redox, and free radical scavenging capacity.[43] Glycemia should be monitored closely and hyperglycemia treated aggressively. Hyperglycemia, stimulated by the release of endogenous catecholamines, increases intracellular acidosis and can prevent or delay the restitution of metabolic homeostasis.[43] During rewarming, cerebral vascular resistance and energetic metabolism are impaired in proportion to the severity of ischemia.[44,45] Cerebral perfusion is reduced, glucose is in part diverted to the less efficient anaerobic pathway, and oxygen coupling with the oxidative phosphorylation is disturbed.[21] This vulnerable period can last for 6 to 8 hours after initiation of reperfusion.[45,46] During this time, an abnormally high extraction of oxygen and glucose is necessary to sustain the cerebral metabolic rate.[45] Jugular venous oxygen saturation is often below 40% during this recovering period.[45] Cerebral autoregulation may become unable to compensate for another reduction in oxygen delivery, which could occur with postoperative events like acute hypotension, hypoxemia, or anemia.

The temperature of the perfusate at the end the rewarming phase should be managed carefully. Hyperthermia exacerbates cerebral activity and disturbs cellular metabolism after circulatory arrest.[47] The perfusate temperature should not be allowed to exceed 37°C, keeping in mind that a relative hypothermia might actually be beneficial for optimal brain recovery.[48] Electrical hyperactivity of the brain can trigger overwhelmingly destructive reactions.[18] The disorder is not uncommon after prolonged circulatory arrest and is actually considered a sign of ischemic injury.[49] Detection of increased cerebral activity should prompt immediate therapeutic action, which includes deep anesthesia, appropriate sedation, and reduction of temperature. Monitoring the electrical activity of the brain during the rewarming phase (and thereafter if circulatory arrest has exceeded the safe ischemic period or if signs of abnormal electrical activity are present) could help limit the extent of secondary damage to the brain.

NEUROLOGIC INJURY AFTER DHCA IN CLINICAL PRACTICE

Neurologic deficit after DHCA encompasses a wide scale of disorders ranging from deep coma to subtle, hardly perceptible alterations in cognitive functions or behavior. In the immediate postoperative period, the return of sophisticated neurologic functions is often obscured by the administration of sedative and analgesic agents. Neurologic injury presents at that time mostly as a focal or diffuse deficit. A focal deficit is due to interruption of blood in a terminal vascular territory, usually following embolism of material or gas bubbles. Less frequently, a prolonged subliminar perfusion of the brain can result in a localized necrosis in the transition area between two vascular territories (the so-called watershed lesion). The clinical expression is typically motor-sensory deficit, aphasia, or cortical blindness. Computed tomography and magnetic resonance imaging are usually able to detect a sharply demarcated area of necrosis in the brain (Fig. 13-2). The prevalence of a focal deficit in clinical series ranges from 5% to 10% after aortic surgery with the use of deep hypothermic circulatory arrest. Age, atherosclerosis, and manipulation of the aorta are risk factors, but not the duration of circulatory arrest.[50] Retrograde perfusion of the aorta during cardiopulmonary bypass (with the arterial cannula inserted in a femoral or iliacal artery) has also been associated with an increased risk of focal cerebral deficit. The retrograde flow of blood in the aorta can dislodge floating atheromatous plaques and thrombi loosely attached to the wall of thoracic aortic aneurysms.

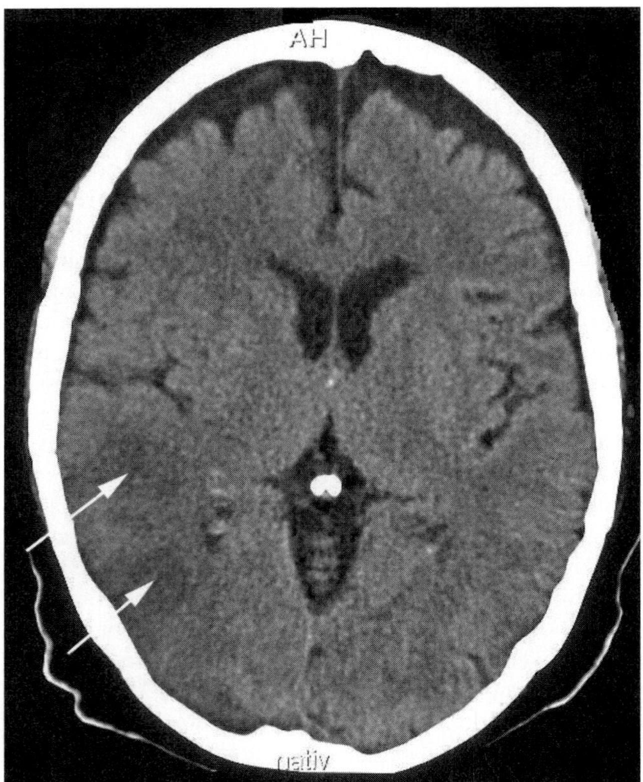

FIGURE 13–2 Computed tomography, performed two days after surgery, showing multiple focal ischemic lesions of the brain. Areas of demarcated necrosis can be seen (arrows) in the temporo-occipital junction of the right hemispheres. The damage was attributed to a retrograde perfusion of the aorta leading to dislodgment and embolization to the brain of mural thrombi.

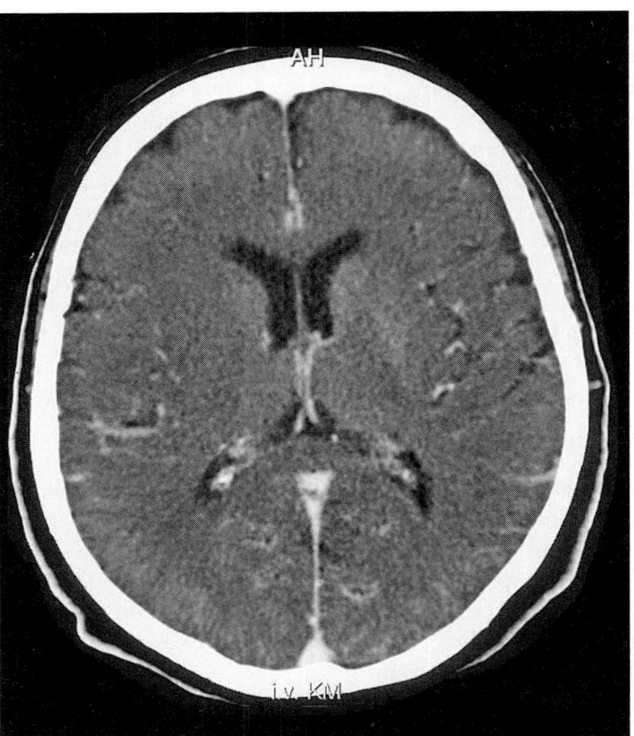

FIGURE 13–3 Computed tomography with contrast enhancement showing signs of diffuse anoxic lesions of the brain. Of note is the blurred delineation of the cerebral cortex and basal ganglia on the right side.

Diffuse neurologic deficits are due to a global cerebral ischemia that induces various levels of cellular dysfunction. In the mild forms, the cerebral cells are viable but temporarily unable to function properly. Cerebral areas with reduced perfusion (due to atherosclerosis) or with increased metabolic activity (like the hippocampus, which is responsible for the acquisition and treatment of new information) are most vulnerable and affected first by ischemia. The spectrum of neuropsychologic disorders ranges from benign and reversible conditions like transient confusion, stupor, delirium, and agitation to more serious and debilitating ones like seizures, parkinsonism, and coma. Imaging techniques are usually normal, although, in the most severe forms, scattered areas of necrosis may progressively appear (Fig. 13-3). The wide range (from 3% to 30%) of prevalence of diffuse deficit after circulatory arrest quoted in the literature reflects the subtle

TABLE 13–2 Adjunctive methods to improve brain protection

	Clearly documented	Possible	Hypothetical
Slow systemic cooling and rewarming	x		
Ice-packing of the head	x		
Waiting for electrocerebral silence	x		
Continuous antegrade perfusion of the brain	x		
Intermittent antegrade perfusion of the brain	x		
Continuous retrograde perfusion of the brain		x	
High hematocrit (~20%)		x	
Pharmacologic blockade of excitatory neurotransmitters		x	
Pharmacologic enhancement of vascular function			x
Pharmacologic prevention of reperfusion injuries			x

and often unrecognized nature of most deficits. Scrupulous postoperative evaluation of neurologic function discloses a frequency between 10% and 20%.[51,52] Age, improper conduct of cardiopulmonary bypass, and prolonged duration of circulatory arrest are common risk factors for diffuse deficit. Disorders that impair vascular reactivity and cerebral autoregulation, like diabetes and hypertension, have sporadically been associated with an increased incidence of diffuse deficit.[53]

For a long time, only relatively coarse and persistent neurologic deficits were accounted for in clinical series. The harm of circulatory arrest was underestimated, and, more worrying, the duration of safe circulatory arrest was erroneously inferred. With refinement in neurologic evaluation including behavioral and cognitive testing, it appears that subtle deficits occur in a much larger proportion of patients after shorter ischemic times. Transient neurologic dysfunction, a condition once not considered as a deficit, appears now as a definitive marker of long-lasting cerebral injury. One quarter of patients with transient deficit perform poorly in postoperative neuropsychologic testing and the deficit, affecting mainly memory and fine motor function, persists in many of them after hospital discharge.[51,52] The risk of transient neurologic deficit starts when deep hypothermic circulatory arrest exceeds 25 minutes.[51,52] The risk is initially linearly related to the duration of circulatory arrest and rises more steeply after 50 minutes of ischemia.[50] Transient neurologic dysfunction might represent the subtlest clinical derangement of the brain that appears first during circulatory arrest.

Based upon these findings and accumulated experience, it appears that the great majority of patients can support unharmed a circulatory arrest of 30 minutes at 18°C, provided that electrocerebral silence has been obtained. No deficit or only a transient neurologic dysfunction is expected when the ischemic period extends to 40 minutes, provided that rewarming is correctly performed and hemodynamic stability maintained postoperatively. With an arrest time superior to 40 minutes, neurologic deficit is prone to occur particularly in high-risk patients, such as older patients and those presenting with diabetes or hypertension. Further cooling of the brain to 13°C to 15°C reduces the risk and makes a deficit again unlikely if the arrest time does not exceed 40 minutes or makes it no more severe than a transient dysfunction if it lasts 50 minutes. In these cases, careful rewarming with close monitoring of cerebral activity, deep anesthesia, and hemodynamic stability are decisive for a favorable outcome.

PREVENTION OF ISCHEMIC NEUROLOGIC DAMAGE

Reduction of cerebral metabolism and swift surgery are the two fundamental measures that should be taken to prevent or reduce brain damage during circulatory arrest. Adjunctive protective measures are summarized in Tables 13-2 and 13-3. Selective perfusion of the brain has emerged as an important adjunctive measure (Figs. 13-4 and 13-5). The efficacy and safety of selective perfusion have progressively

TABLE 13–3 Methods to prevent particulate embolism to the brain

	Clearly documented	Hypothetical
No manipulation of the aorta and arch arteries before CA	x	
Avoidance of retrograde perfusion of the aorta	x	
Continuous perfusion of the brain through the right subclavian artery	x	
Continuous retrograde perfusion of the brain	x	
PH alpha-stat strategy during hypothermia		x

CA = circulatory arrest.

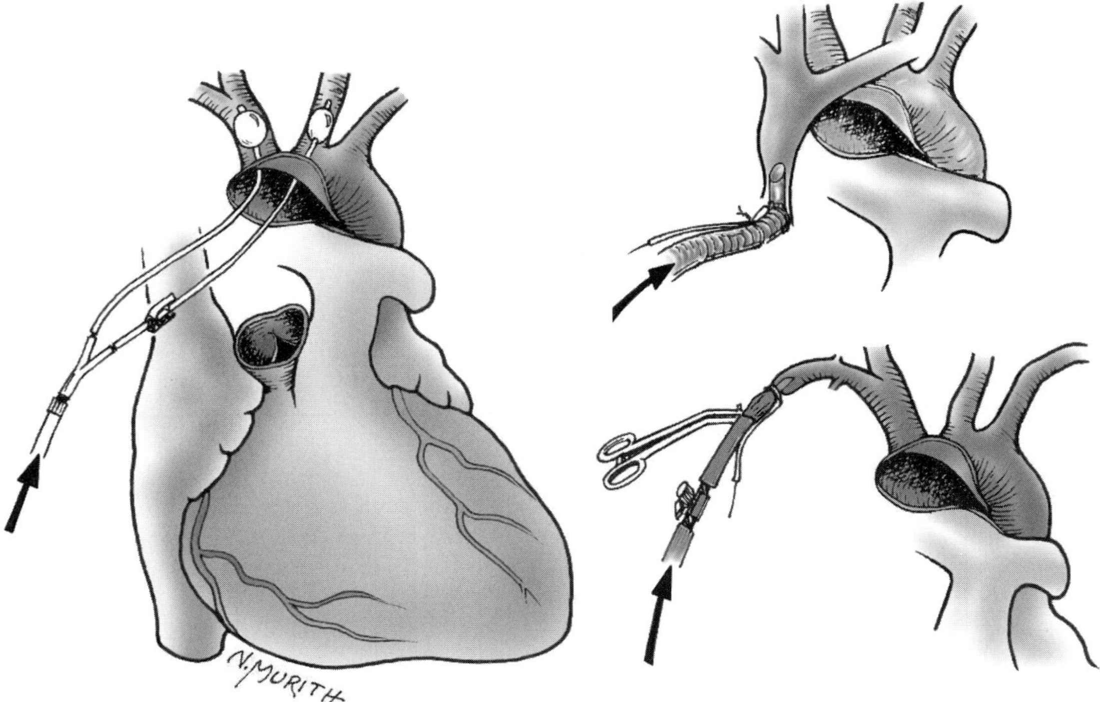

FIGURE 13–4 Bilateral antegrade cerebral perfusion obtained by selective cannulation of the innominate and left common carotid artery. Upper right: retrograde cerebral perfusion via the superior vena cava. Lower right: regional cerebral perfusion (unilateral antegrade perfusion) via cannulation of the right subclavian artery.

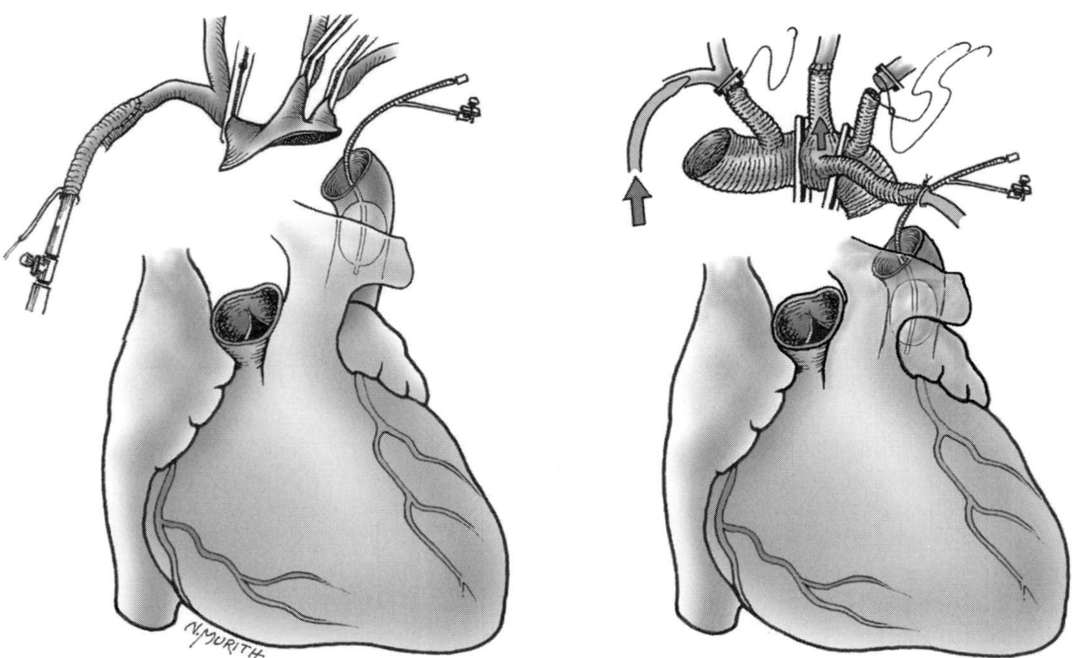

FIGURE 13–5 Sequential bilateral antegrade perfusion of the brain. The branch of a multiple-arms graft is initially connected to the left common carotid artery allowing rapid establishment of a bilateral perfusion of the brain. The other anastomoses are performed thereafter. Perfusion of the right subclavian artery through a graft allows monitoring of the perfusion pressure via the right radial artery.

allowed modulation of the level of systemic cooling. When the anticipated ischemic period does not exceed 20 minutes (for instance, as illustrated in Figure 13-4, for a hemiarch replacement), systemic cooling could be set at 25°C. The duration of cardiopulmonary bypass to equilibrate temperature during cooling and rewarming is greatly reduced. Homeostasis of the blood is in turn less disturbed, particularly regarding platelet function and coagulation. When the anticipated ischemic time exceeds 40 minutes (for instance, as illustrated in Figure 13-5, for a complete resection of the aortic arch), deep systemic hypothermia to 18°C or lower remains the safest measure to protect not only the brain but also the spinal cord and abdominal organs.

Antegrade Cerebral Perfusion

Antegrade perfusion of the brain through cannulae inserted in the innominate (or more distally in the right common carotid artery) and left common carotid artery provides the most physiologic and efficient perfusion of the brain. Perfusate temperature is usually set at 18°C and flow is set between 10 and 20 mL/kg/min or adjusted to maintain a pressure between 40 and 50 mm Hg in the right radial artery. Clinical results, especially regarding swift recovery of cerebral function, have been outstanding with this method of perfusion.[54–58] The necessity to cannulate relatively small and often diseased arch arteries and the presence of additional cannulae in the operating field constitute the main drawbacks of the technique. Cannulation of the common carotid arteries can result in dissection of the arterial wall and embolism of atheromatous plaque material or air. Furthermore, the flow in the artery is dependent on proper positioning of the tip of the cannula within the vessel. For these reasons, many surgeons rely on a unilateral perfusion of the brain, with the sole cannulation and perfusion of the right subclavian artery. The right vertebral and right common carotid artery territories are perfused in an antegrade fashion. The blood reaches the left cerebral hemisphere through the circle of Willis and, to a lesser extent, through cervicofacial connections. It is, therefore, important that the left common carotid and left subclavian arteries be occluded to avoid a steal of blood down these arteries. Occlusion (usually with an inflatable balloon) of the descending aorta is also a useful maneuver to improve overall body perfusion. Effective somatic perfusion (including the abdominal organs, spinal cord, and lower limb musculature) has been documented with this maneuver.[59]

The presence of an aberrant right subclavian artery (also called arteria lusoria) is obviously a contraindication to the use of this perfusion method. The aberrant origin of the artery is usually readily identified by computed tomography or magnetic resonance. The burst of blood from the descending aorta during the opening of the aortic arch should alert the surgeon to this anatomic variation, and prompt a direct cannulation of the ostium of the right and left common carotid arteries.

Sequential perfusion of the cerebral arteries provides additional safety to unilateral cerebral perfusion, and avoids cannulation of small or diseased arch arteries. The right subclavian artery remains perfused during the whole procedure. A vascular graft is immediately sewn on a common patch of aortic wall including all the arch vessels,[60] or the second branch of a multiple-arm prosthesis is anastomosed to the left common carotid artery. Perfusion is then instituted through this additional graft and enhances, after a short period of time, cerebral perfusion.

Retrograde Cerebral Perfusion

The value of retrograde cerebral perfusion in protecting the human brain has still not been clearly elucidated. No animal model truly replicates the complex anatomy and physiology of the human brain, and none allows a fine neuropsychologic evaluation. Conflicting results and conclusions in clinical and experimental studies have, therefore, been reported. Accepted facts include a deep and homogenous cooling of the brain hemispheres (the cooling scalp effect) and the expulsion of solid particles or gaseous bubbles from the arch arteries. Controversies surround the possible nutritive value of retrograde perfusion. The nutritive value has been demonstrated in rabbits but not in dogs, pigs, or baboons.[61–63] In humans, signs of cerebral perfusion and oxygen uptake have been documented,[64] but the amount of perfusate providing cerebral nutrition is low, corresponding to about 5% of total retrograde flow.[62,65] The blood delivered in the superior vena cava flows preferentially in the low-pressure inferior vena cava, via the azygos system, the perivertebral venous plexus, and the thoracic wall veins.[66] Even within the brain, the distribution of retrograde flow is uneven, with a preferential distribution in the sagittal sinus and hemispheric veins.[67] The large steal of blood to the inferior venous territory is corroborated by the clinical finding of an extremely small proportion of perfused blood flowing out of the arch arteries. Occlusion of the inferior vena cava to decrease the pressure gradient between the two venous territories effectively reduces the amount of stolen blood, but increases the sequestration of fluid in the interstitial tissue.[68] Interstitial edema is another potential problem of retrograde perfusion, which can lead to cerebral edema and hypertension, particularly when the perfusion pressure exceeds 25 mm Hg. Finally, the finding that the human jugular system may contain competent valves[69] casts definitive doubts regarding the reliability of retrograde cerebral perfusion.

Clinical series, however, have reported encouraging results. A reduction in both mortality and incidence of neurologic damage has been regularly documented with the adjunctive use of retrograde cerebral perfusion to classical hypothermia.[58,70–73] Some studies confirmed the limited capacity of retrograde perfusion to sustain cerebral metabolism, and stressed the fact that the occurrence of neurologic damage was only delayed.[62,74] Indeed, the risk rises sharply after 60 minutes of deep hypothermic circulatory arrest, perhaps at the extinction of intracellular energy substrates. If most surgeons acknowledge the capacity of retrograde cerebral perfusion to prolong the period of safe circulatory arrest, they consider the method a valuable but not an alternative adjunct to conventional methods when long periods of circulatory arrest are contemplated.[58,70–73]

Integrated Perfusion

Probably the safest approach to a patient requiring a long period of circulatory arrest resides in the integration of complementary methods of perfusion and monitoring.[50] Retrograde perfusion of the aorta through the femoral artery should be avoided in the presence of a thoracic aortic aneurysm in order to reduce the risk of particulate dislodgment with embolization in the brain and myocardium. Antegrade perfusion of the aorta is performed with cannulation of the ascending aorta or right subclavian artery. The body is cooled to 18°C. Electroencephalogram and venous jugular saturation are monitored to ensure adequate reduction of cerebral metabolism. Circulatory arrest is established only after electrocerebral silence is obtained and jugular venous saturation is superior to 95%. During the 10 to 20 minutes preceding circulatory arrest, the temperature of the perfusate can be lowered to 13°C to further reduce brain temperature and metabolism. The arch arteries are connected to a graft (either with the use of a patch of aortic wall or separately), and antegrade perfusion of the brain is resumed before more extensive resection and repair of the aorta is performed. When the risk of particle embolization to the brain is substantial (old age, severe atherosclerosis of the aorta, arch aneurysm with thrombotic material), a short period of retrograde cerebral perfusion can be performed to wash out the arch arteries before antegrade perfusion is definitively reestablished.[50]

REFERENCES

1. Michenfelder JD, Milde JH: The effect of profound levels of hypothermia (below 14 degrees C) on canine cerebral metabolism. *J Cereb Blood Flow Metab* 1992; 12:877.
2. Mault JR, Ohtake S, Klingensmith ME, et al: Cerebral metabolism and circulatory arrest: effects of duration and strategies for protection. *Ann Thorac Surg* 1993; 55:57.
3. McCullough JN, Zhang N, Reich DL, et al: Cerebral metabolic suppression during hypothermic circulatory arrest in humans. *Ann Thorac Surg* 1999; 67:1895.
4. Greeley WJ, Ungerleider RM, Kern FH, et al: Effects of cardiopulmonary bypass on cerebral blood flow in neonates, infants, and children. *Circulation* 1989; 80:I209.
5. Siesjo BK, Katsura K, Zhao Q, et al: Mechanisms of secondary brain damage in global and focal ischemia: a speculative synthesis. *J Neurotrauma* 1995; 12:943.
6. Stecker MM, Cheung AT, Pochettino A, et al: Deep hypothermic circulatory arrest, I: effects of cooling on electroencephalogram and evoked potentials. *Ann Thorac Surg* 2001; 71:14.
7. Greeley WJ, Kern FH, Meliones JN, Ungerleider RM: Effect of deep hypothermia and circulatory arrest on cerebral blood flow and metabolism. *Ann Thorac Surg* 1993; 56:1464.
8. Mault JR, Whitaker EG, Heinle JS, et al: Cerebral metabolic effects of sequential periods of hypothermic circulatory arrest. *Ann Thorac Surg* 1994; 57:96.
9. Kimura T, Muraoka R, Chiba Y, et al: Effect of deep hypothermic circulatory arrest on cerebral anaerobic metabolisms: preliminary report. *Nippon Geka Gakkai Zasshi* 1994; 95:480.
10. Kawata H, Fackler JC, Aoki M, et al: Recovery of cerebral blood flow and energy state in piglets after hypothermic circulatory arrest versus recovery after low-flow bypass. *J Thorac Cardiovasc Surg* 1993; 106:671.
11. Hiramatsu T, Jonas RA, Miura T, et al: Cerebral metabolic recovery from deep hypothermic circulatory arrest after treatment with arginine and nitro-arginine methyl ester. *J Thorac Cardiovasc Surg* 1996; 112:698.
12. Swain JA, McDonald TJ Jr, Griffith PK, et al: Low-flow hypothermic cardiopulmonary bypass protects the brain. *J Thorac Cardiovasc Surg* 1991; 102:76.
13. Siesjo BK, Zhao Q, Pahlmark K, et al: Glutamate, calcium, and free radicals as mediators of ischemic brain damage. *Ann Thorac Surg* 1995; 59:1316.
14. Tsui SS, Kirshbom PM, Davies MJ, et al: Nitric oxide production affects cerebral perfusion and metabolism after deep hypothermic circulatory arrest. *Ann Thorac Surg* 1996; 61:1699.
15. Astudillo R, van der Linden J, Ekroth R, et al: Absent diastolic cerebral blood flow velocity after circulatory arrest but not after low flow in infants. *Ann Thorac Surg* 1993; 56:515.
16. Kubes P, Suzuki M, Granger DN: Nitric oxide: an endogenous modulator of leukocyte adhesion. *Proc Natl Acad Sci U S A* 1991; 88:4651.
17. Nakanishi K, Vinten Johansen J, Lefer DJ, et al: Intracoronary L-arginine during reperfusion improves endothelial function and reduces infarct size. *Am J Physiol* 1992; 263:H1650.
18. Lipton SA, Rosenberg PA: Excitatory amino acids as a final common pathway for neurologic disorders. *N Engl J Med* 1994; 330:613.
19. Erdo SL, Schafer M: Memantine is highly potent in protecting cortical cultures against excitotoxic cell death evoked by glutamate and N-methyl-D-aspartate. *Eur J Pharmacol* 1991; 198:215.
20. Seif el Nasr M, Peruche B, Rossberg C, et al: Neuroprotective effect of memantine demonstrated in vivo and in vitro. *Eur J Pharmacol* 1990; 185:19.
21. Siesjo BK, Siesjo P: Mechanisms of secondary brain injury. *Eur J Anaesthesiol* 1996; 13:247.
22. Fujie W, Kirino T, Tomukai N, et al: Progressive shrinkage of the thalamus following middle cerebral artery occlusion in rats. *Stroke* 1990; 21:1485.
23. Hartley A, Stone JM, Heron C, et al: Complex I inhibitors induce dose-dependent apoptosis in PC12 cells: relevance to Parkinson's disease. *J Neurochem* 1994; 63:1987.
24. Croughwell N, Smith LR, Quill T, et al: The effect of temperature on cerebral metabolism and blood flow in adults during cardiopulmonary bypass. *J Thorac Cardiovasc Surg* 1992; 103:549.
25. Kern FH, Ungerleider RM, Reves JG, et al: Effect of altering pump flow rate on cerebral blood flow and metabolism in infants and children. *Ann Thorac Surg* 1993; 56:1366.
26. Shin'oka T, Nollert G, Shum Tim D, et al: Utility of near-infrared spectroscopic measurements during deep hypothermic circulatory arrest. *Ann Thorac Surg* 2000; 69:578.
27. Langley SM, Chai PJ, Miller SE, et al: Intermittent perfusion protects the brain during deep hypothermic circulatory arrest. *Ann Thorac Surg* 1999; 68:4.

28. Kimura T, Muraoka R, Chiba Y, et al: Effect of intermittent deep hypothermic circulatory arrest on brain metabolism. *J Thorac Cardiovasc Surg* 1994; 108:658.
29. Nakano S, Kato H, Kogure K: Neuronal damage in the rat hippocampus in a new model of repeated reversible transient cerebral ischemia. *Brain Res* 1989; 490:178.
30. Shuaib A, Ijaz S, Kalra J, Code W: Repetitive transient forebrain ischemia in gerbils: delayed neuronal damage in the substantia nigra reticulata. *Brain Res* 1992; 574:120.
31. Watanabe T, Washio M: Pulsatile low-flow perfusion for enhanced cerebral protection. *Ann Thorac Surg* 1993; 56:1478.
32. Onoe M, Mori A, Watarida S, et al: The effect of pulsatile perfusion on cerebral blood flow during profound hypothermia with total circulatory arrest. *J Thorac Cardiovasc Surg* 1994; 108: 119.
33. Cooper WA, Duarte IG, Thourani VH, et al: Hypothermic circulatory arrest causes multisystem vascular endothelial dysfunction and apoptosis. *Ann Thorac Surg* 2000; 69:696.
34. Priestley MA, Golden JA, O'Hara IB, et al: Comparison of neurologic outcome after deep hypothermic circulatory arrest with alpha-stat and pH-stat cardiopulmonary bypass in newborn pigs. *J Thorac Cardiovasc Surg* 2001; 121:336.
35. Jonas RA, Bellinger DC, Rappaport LA, et al: Relation of pH strategy and developmental outcome after hypothermic circulatory arrest. *J Thorac Cardiovasc Surg* 1993; 106:362.
36. Bashein G, Townes BD, Nessly ML, et al: A randomized study of carbon dioxide management during hypothermic cardiopulmonary bypass. *Anesthesiology* 1990; 72:7.
37. Murkin JM, Martzke JS, Buchan AM, et al: A randomized study of the influence of perfusion technique and pH management strategy in 316 patients undergoing coronary artery bypass surgery, II: neurologic and cognitive outcomes. *J Thorac Cardiovasc Surg* 1995; 110:349.
38. Patel RL, Turtle MR, Chambers DJ, et al: Alpha-stat acid-base regulation during cardiopulmonary bypass improves neuropsychologic outcome in patients undergoing coronary artery bypass grafting. *J Thorac Cardiovasc Surg* 1996; 111:1267.
39. Tanaka J, Shiki K, Asou T, et al: Cerebral autoregulation during deep hypothermic nonpulsatile cardiopulmonary bypass with selective cerebral perfusion in dogs. *J Thorac Cardiovasc Surg* 1988; 95: 124.
40. Duebener LF, Sakamoto T, Hatsuoka S, et al: Effects of hematocrit on cerebral microcirculation and tissue oxygenation during deep hypothermic bypass. *Circulation* 2001; 104:I260.
41. Shin'oka T, Shum Tim D, Jonas RA, et al: Higher hematocrit improves cerebral outcome after deep hypothermic circulatory arrest. *J Thorac Cardiovasc Surg* 1996; 112:1610.
42. Shin'oka T, Shum Tim D, Laussen PC, et al: Effects of oncotic pressure and hematocrit on outcome after hypothermic circulatory arrest. *Ann Thorac Surg* 1998; 65:155.
43. Anderson RV, Siegman MG, Balaban RS, et al: Hyperglycemia increases cerebral intracellular acidosis during circulatory arrest. *Ann Thorac Surg* 1992; 54:1126.
44. Greeley WJ, Kern FH, Ungerleider RM, et al: The effect of hypothermic cardiopulmonary bypass and total circulatory arrest on cerebral metabolism in neonates, infants, and children. *J Thorac Cardiovasc Surg* 1991; 101:783.
45. van der Linden J, Astudillo R, Ekroth R, et al: Cerebral lactate release after circulatory arrest but not after low flow in pediatric heart operations. *Ann Thorac Surg* 1993; 56:1485.
46. Mezrow CK, Sadeghi AM, Gandsas A, et al: Cerebral effects of low-flow cardiopulmonary bypass and hypothermic circulatory arrest. *Ann Thorac Surg* 1994; 57:532.
47. Shum Tim D, Nagashima M, Shinoka T, et al: Postischemic hyperthermia exacerbates neurologic injury after deep hypothermic circulatory arrest. *J Thorac Cardiovasc Surg* 1998; 116: 780.
48. The Hypothermia after Cardiac Arrest Study Group: Mild therapeutic hypothermia to improve the neurologic outcome after cardiac arrest. *N Engl J Med* 2002; 346:549.
49. Newburger JW, Jonas RA, Wernovsky G, et al: A comparison of the perioperative neurologic effects of hypothermic circulatory arrest versus low-flow cardiopulmonary bypass in infant heart surgery. *N Engl J Med* 1993; 329:1057.
50. Ergin MA, Griepp EB, Lansman SL, et al: Hypothermic circulatory arrest and other methods of cerebral protection during operations on the thoracic aorta. *J Card Surg* 1994; 9:525.
51. Reich DL, Uysal S, Sliwinski M, et al: Neuropsychologic outcome after deep hypothermic circulatory arrest in adults. *J Thorac Cardiovasc Surg* 1999; 117:156.
52. Ergin MA, Uysal S, Reich DL, et al: Temporary neurological dysfunction after deep hypothermic circulatory arrest: a clinical marker of long-term functional deficit. *Ann Thorac Surg* 1999; 67:1887.
53. Kumral E, Yuksel M, Buket S, et al: Neurologic complications after deep hypothermic circulatory arrest: types, predictors, and timing. *Tex Heart Inst J* 2001; 28:83.
54. Bachet J, Guilmet D, Goudot B, et al: Antegrade cerebral perfusion with cold blood: a 13-year experience. *Ann Thorac Surg* 1999; 67:1874.
55. Dossche KM, Morshuis WJ, Schepens MA, Waanders FG: Bilateral antegrade selective cerebral perfusion during surgery on the proximal thoracic aorta. *Eur J Cardiothorac Surg* 2000; 17: 462.
56. Di Bartolomeo R, Di Eusanio M, Pacini D, et al: Antegrade selective cerebral perfusion during surgery of the thoracic aorta: risk analysis. *Eur J Cardiothorac Surg* 2001; 19:765.
57. Kazui T, Washiyama N, Muhammad BA, et al: Total arch replacement using aortic arch branched grafts with the aid of antegrade selective cerebral perfusion. *Ann Thorac Surg* 2000; 70:3.
58. Okita Y, Minatoya K, Tagusari O, et al: Prospective comparative study of brain protection in total aortic arch replacement: deep hypothermic circulatory arrest with retrograde cerebral perfusion or selective antegrade cerebral perfusion. *Ann Thorac Surg* 2001; 72:72.
59. Pigula FA, Gandhi SK, Siewers RD, et al: Regional low-flow perfusion provides somatic circulatory support during neonatal aortic arch surgery. *Ann Thorac Surg* 2001; 72:401.
60. Hagl C, Ergin MA, Galla JD, et al: Neurologic outcome after ascending aorta-aortic arch operations: effect of brain protection technique in high-risk patients. *J Thorac Cardiovasc Surg* 2001; 121:1107.
61. Midulla PS, Gandsas A, Sadeghi AM, et al: Comparison of retrograde cerebral perfusion to antegrade cerebral perfusion and hypothermic circulatory arrest in a chronic porcine model. *J Card Surg* 1994; 9:560.
62. Ye J, Yang L, Del Bigio MR, et al: Retrograde cerebral perfusion provides limited distribution of blood to the brain: a study in pigs. *J Thorac Cardiovasc Surg* 1997; 114:660.
63. Boeckxstaens CJ, Flameng WJ: Retrograde cerebral perfusion does not perfuse the brain in nonhuman primates. *Ann Thorac Surg* 1995; 60:319.
64. Pagano D, Boivin CM, Faroqui MH, Bonser RS: Retrograde perfusion through the superior vena cava perfuses the brain in human beings. *J Thorac Cardiovasc Surg* 1996; 111:270.
65. Ye J, Yang L, Del Bigio MR, et al: Neuronal damage after hypothermic circulatory arrest and retrograde cerebral perfusion in the pig. *Ann Thorac Surg* 1996; 61:1316.
66. de Brux JL, Subayi JB, Pegis JD, Pillet J: Retrograde cerebral perfusion: anatomic study of the distribution of blood to the brain. *Ann Thorac Surg* 1995; 60:1294.
67. Ye J, Ryner LN, Kozlowski P, et al: Retrograde cerebral perfusion results in flow distribution abnormalities and neuronal damage: a

magnetic resonance imaging and histopathological study in pigs. *Circulation* 1998; 98:1313.

68. Juvonen T, Zhang N, Wolfe D, et al: Retrograde cerebral perfusion enhances cerebral protection during prolonged hypothermic circulatory arrest: a study in a chronic porcine model. *Ann Thorac Surg* 1998; 66:38.
69. Dresser LP, McKinney WM: Anatomic and pathophysiologic studies of the human internal jugular valve. *Am J Surg* 1987; 154:220.
70. Coselli JS, LeMaire SA: Experience with retrograde cerebral perfusion during proximal aortic surgery in 290 patients. *J Card Surg* 1997; 12(2 suppl):322.
71. Bavaria JE, Pochettino A: Retrograde cerebral perfusion (RCP) in aortic arch surgery: efficacy and possible mechanisms of brain protection. *Semin Thorac Cardiovasc Surg* 1997; 9:222.
72. Kitamura M, Hashimoto A, Aomi S, et al: Medium-term results after surgery for aortic arch aneurysm with hypothermic cerebral perfusion. *Eur J Cardiothorac Surg* 1995; 9:697.
73. Safi HJ, Letsou GV, Iliopoulos DC, et al: Impact of retrograde cerebral perfusion on ascending aortic and arch aneurysm repair. *Ann Thorac Surg* 1997; 63:1601.
74. Reich DL, Uysal S, Ergin MA, et al: Retrograde cerebral perfusion during thoracic aortic surgery and late neuropsychological dysfunction. *Eur J Cardiothorac Surg* 2001; 19:594.

Chapter 14

Myocardial Protection

Robert M. Mentzer, Jr./M. Salik Jahania/Robert D. Lasley

The term "myocardial protection" refers to strategies and methodologies used either to attenuate or to prevent postischemic myocardial dysfunction that occurs during and after heart surgery. Postischemic myocardial dysfunction is attributable, in part, to a phenomenon known as ischemia/reperfusion-induced injury. Clinically, it is manifest by low cardiac output and hypotension, and may be subdivided into two subgroups: reversible injury and irreversible injury. The two are typically differentiated by the presence of ECG abnormalities, elevations in the levels of specific plasma enzymes or proteins such as creatine kinase and troponin I or T, and/or the presence of regional or global echocardiographic wall motion abnormalities. With respect to coronary artery bypass surgery alone, 10% of patients may experience myocardial infarction, severe ventricular dysfunction, heart failure, and/or death, despite advances in surgical technique. The impact from these complications both on families and on society is enormous. From an economic standpoint alone, such dysfunctions consume an estimated additional $2 billion in U.S. health care resources each year.[1] The purpose of this chapter is to review the history of myocardial protection, to update the reader regarding the current protective techniques, to examine the mechanisms underlying ischemia/reperfusion injury, and to discuss several new strategies currently under investigation.

HISTORY

Over the past 50 years, many therapeutic strategies have been developed to protect the heart during surgery (Table 14-1). This concept of shielding the heart from perioperative insult originated in 1950 with the review article by Bigelow et al in which hypothermia was reported "as a form of anesthetic" that could be used to expand the scope of surgery.[2] It was proposed that hypothermia could be used as "a technique that might permit surgeons to operate on the bloodless heart without recourse to extracorporeal pumps and perhaps allotransplantation of organs."[2] Five years later, Melrose et al reported another way to reliably stop and restart the heart by injecting potassium citrate into the root of the aorta at both normal and reduced body temperatures.[3] Soon thereafter, the clinical application of potassium citrate arrest was adopted by many centers. Interest in using the "Melrose technique" waned, however, with subsequent reports that potassium citrate arrest was associated with myocardial injury and necrosis. Within a short time, many cardiac surgeons shifted from using potassium-induced arrest to normothermic cardiac ischemia (normothermic heart surgery performed with the aorta occluded while the patient was on cardiopulmonary bypass), intermittent aortic occlusion, or coronary artery perfusion. Experimental and clinical evidence showed, however, that normothermic cardiac

TABLE 14–1 Therapeutic innovations for myocardial protection

Reference	Year	Innovation
Bigelow WG[2]	1950	Studied the application of hypothermia to cardiac surgery in canines
Swan H[250]	1953	Showed that hypothermic arrest (26°C) in humans provided a bloodless field for operating
Melrose DG, Bentall HH[3]	1955	Introduced the concept of reversible chemical cardiac arrest in canines
Lillehei CW[94]	1956	Detailed a method for delivering hypothermic crystalloid cardioplegia by cannulating coronary arteries
Lam CR[251]	1957	One of the earliest known uses of the term "cardioplegia"
Gerbode F, Melrose DG[252]	1958	Used potassium citrate to induce cardiac arrest in humans
McFarland JA[253]	1960	Challenged the safety of the Melrose technique; changed from potassium arrest to intermittent aortic occlusion or coronary artery perfusion for myocardial protection
Bretschneider HJ[7]	1964	Developed a sodium-poor, calcium-free, procaine-containing solution to arrest the heart
Sondergaard KT[254,255]	1964	Adopted Bretschneider's cardioplegic solution and was one of the first to routinely use it for myocardial protection in clinical practice
Gay WA, Ebert PA[13]	1973	Credited with revival of potassium-induced cardioplegia; demonstrated that potassium solution could arrest a canine heart for 60 minutes without cellular damage
Roe BB[14]	1973	Demonstrated that "the modalities of cardioplegia, hypothermia, and capillary washout" provided effective myocardial protection
Tyers WA[4]	1974	Demonstrated that an infusion of cold blood to keep the myocardial tissue below 4° provided 90 minutes of ischemia in animals
Hearse DJ[8]	1975	Emphasized preischemic infusions to negate ischemic injuries in rats; this formula became known as St. Thomas solution no. 1
Braimbridge MV[9]	1975	One of the first to use St. Thomas solution no. 1 clinically
Effler DB[256]	1976	Recommended simple aortic clamping at operating room temperatures
Buckberg GD[16]	1979	Introduced the use of blood as the vehicle for infusing potassium into coronary arteries
Akins CW[83]	1984	Utilized technique of hypothermic fibrillatory arrest for coronary revascularization without cardioplegia
Murray CE[257]	1986	Noted that brief periods of ischemia and reperfusion enable the heart to withstand longer periods of ischemia
Lichtenstein SV[88] and Salerno TA[89]	1991	Reported clinically beneficial results using continuous, warm blood cardioplegia

ischemia was associated with metabolic acidosis, hypotension, and low cardiac output.[4–6]

As a consequence, there was a renewed interest in discovering ways to arrest the heart. Bretschneider published the principle of arresting the heart with a low-sodium, calcium-free solution.[7] It was Hearse and colleagues, however, who studied the various components of cardioplegic solutions, which led to the development and use of St. Thomas solution.[8] The components of this crystalloid solution were based on Ringer's solution with its normal concentrations of sodium and calcium, with the addition of potassium chloride (16 mmol/L) and 16 mmol/L of magnesium chloride to arrest the heart instantly. The latter component was shown by Hearse to provide an additional cardioprotective benefit. In 1975, Braimbridge et al introduced this crystalloid solution into clinical practice at St. Thomas Hospital.[9]

Gay and Ebert showed experimentally that lower concentrations of potassium chloride could achieve the same degree of chemical arrest and myocardial protection afforded by the Melrose solution without the associated myocardial necrosis reported earlier.[10–13] Shortly thereafter, Roe et al reported an operative mortality of 5.4% for patients who underwent cardiac surgery with potassium-induced arrest as the primary form of myocardial protection.[14] In 1977, Tyers et al reported that potassium cardioplegia provided satisfactory protection in over 100 consecutive cardiac patients.[15]

By the 1980s, the use of normothermic aortic occlusion had been replaced for the most part with the use of cardioplegia to protect the heart during cardiac surgery. The major controversy at the time (and one that persists today) was not whether cardioplegic solutions should be used, but what the ideal components of those solutions were. The chief variants consisted of: (1) the Bretschneider solution, consisting primarily of sodium, magnesium, and procaine; (2) the St. Thomas solution, consisting of potassium, magnesium, and procaine added to Ringer's solution; and (3) potassium-enriched solutions, containing no magnesium or procaine (Table 14-2). Coincident to this controversy, another variant

TABLE 14–2 **Components of various cardioplegic solutions**

Solution	Usual components*							Other components
	Sodium	Potassium	Magnesium	Calcium	Bicarbonate	pH	Osmolarity (mOsm/L)	
Bretschneider's no. 3	12.0	10.0	2.0	–	–	5.5–7.0	320	Procaine; mannitol
Lactated Ringer's	130.0	24.0	–	1.5	–	7.14	–	Lactate; chlorine
Tyer's	138.0	25.0	1.5	0.5	20.0	7.8	275	Acetate; gluconate; chloride
St. Thomas no. 2	110.0	16.0	16.0	1.2	10.0	7.8	324	Lidocaine
Roe's	27.0	20.0	1.5	–	–	7.6	347	Glucose; tris buffer
Gay/Ebert	38.5	40.0	–	–	10.0	7.8	365	Glucose
Birmingham	100.0	30.0	–	0.7	28.0	7.5	300–385	Glucose; chloride; albumin; mannitol
Craver's	154.0	25.0	–	–	11.0	–	391	Dextrose
Lolley's	–	20.0	–	–	4.4	7.78	350	Dextrose; mannitol; insulin

*Values are expressed in millimoles per liter unless otherwise noted.

of cardioplegia was introduced, that of using potassium-enriched blood cardioplegia.[16,17] The theory was that blood would be a superior delivery vehicle based on its oxygenating and buffering capacity. Ironically, Melrose et al initially used blood as the vehicle to deliver high concentrations of potassium citrate more than 20 years earlier.

While hypothermia and potassium infusions remain the cornerstone of myocardial protection during on-pump heart surgery, there are many other cardioprotective techniques and methodologies available.[3,18] While many of these techniques have been reported to confer superior protection and improve patient outcomes, the ideal cardioprotective technique, solution, and/or method of administration has yet to be found. Fortunately, the majority of cardioprotective strategies now available do allow patients to undergo conventional and complex heart operations with an operative mortality rate ranging from less than 2% to 4%.

ISCHEMIA/REPERFUSION INJURY

While the etiology of postischemic myocardial dysfunction after cardiac surgery is multifactorial, three basic types of injury occur during heart surgery: myocardial stunning, apoptosis, and myocardial infarction. Myocardial stunning is an injury that may last for only a few hours or persist for several days despite the restoration of normal blood flow. Cells that have been reversibly injured (stunned) exhibit no sign of ultrastructural damage. Apoptosis is "suicidal" programmed cell death, characterized by retention of an intact cell membrane, cell shrinkage, chromatin condensation, and phagocytosis without inflammation.[19–21] There is increasing evidence that apoptotic death of cardiomyocytes caused by ischemia/reperfusion contributes significantly to the development of infarction as well as the loss of cells surrounding the infarct area. A large fraction of dying cells may exhibit features of both apoptosis and necrosis, i.e., both nuclear condensation and plasma membrane damage. Ultimately, however, after more prolonged ischemia, the heart begins to sustain irreversible injury in the form of infarction and necrosis. This is manifest as membrane destruction, cell swelling, DNA degradation, cytolysis, and the induction of an inflammatory response.

While the consequences of inadequate myocardial protection are usually apparent in the immediate postoperative period, the full impact may not be fully appreciated for months. Klatte et al reported that patients with increased peak creatine kinase-myocardial band (CK-MB) enzyme ratios after CABG surgery exhibited a greater 6-month mortality.[22] Specifically, the 6-month mortality rates for patients with peak CK-MB ratios of <5, ≥ 5 to <10, ≥ 10 to <20, and ≥ 20 upper limits of normal were 3.4%, 5.8%, 7.8%, and 20.2%, respectively. Conversely, the cumulative 6-month survival was inversely related to the peak CK-MB ratio. These observations support the concept that myocardial injury occurring as a result of inadequate myocardial protection intraoperatively is associated with subsequent death.

In order to appreciate the strategies that have evolved to protect the myocardium during heart surgery it is important to understand the mechanisms implicated in the etiology of the various types of myocardial ischemia/reperfusion injury. Significant evidence now exists that the primary mediators of reversible and irreversible myocardial ischemia/reperfusion injury include intracellular Ca^{2+} overload during ischemia and reperfusion, and oxidative stress induced by reactive oxygen species (ROS) generated at the onset of reperfusion (Fig. 14-1).[23–25] The molecule nitric oxide (NO) can also interact with ROS to generate various reactive nitrogen species that appear capable of both contributing to and reducing injury.[26,27] In addition, metabolic alterations occurring

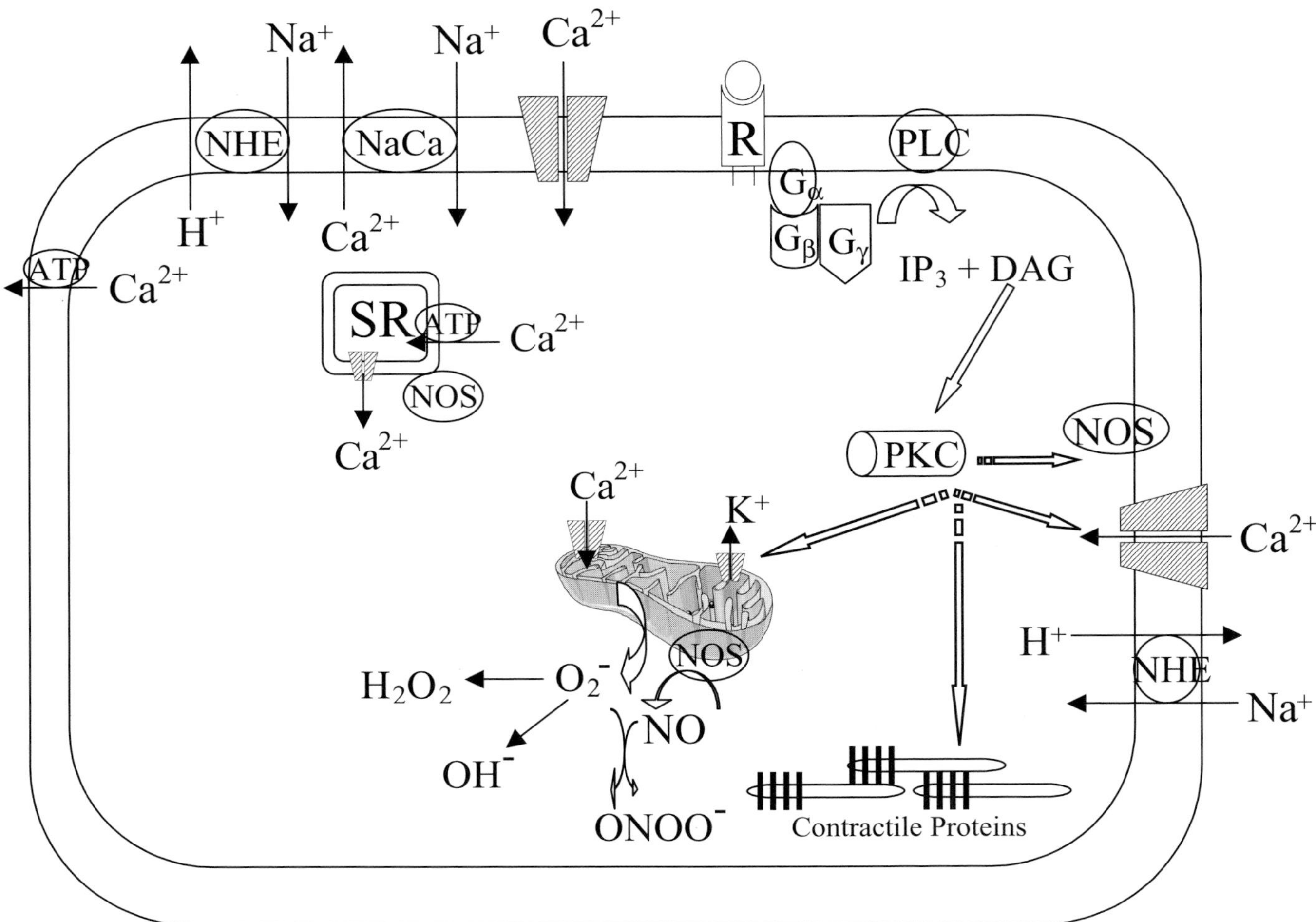

FIGURE 14–1 Intracellular mechanisms regulate cardiomyocyte Ca^{2+} homeostasis and reactive oxygen species formation, the two primary mediators of myocyte ischemia/reperfusion injury. During ischemia, intracellular Ca^{2+} increases via the inability of energy-dependent Ca^{2+} pumps in the sarcolemma and sarcoplasmic reticulum (SR) to maintain normal low resting cytosolic Ca^{2+} concentrations. Activation of various G protein–coupled receptors (R, alpha- and beta-adrenergic, angiotensin, endothelin, etc.) initiates signaling mechanisms (stimulatory G proteins [G_s] and PLC [phospholipase C]) and also increases Ca^{2+}. The generation of inositol triphosphate (IP3) from this latter pathway increases Ca^{2+} release from intracellular stores, including SR. Diacylglycerol (DAG) formation via the PLC pathway leads to the activation of Ca^{2+} dependent and independent isoforms of protein kinase C (PKC). PKC phosphorylation of various proteins and enzymes further modulates Ca^{2+} concentration, metabolism, and contractile protein Ca^{2+} sensitivity. The sodium-hydrogen exchanger (NHE) exchanges intracellular H^+ for extracellular Na^+, and the resulting increase in intracellular Na^+ may result in reverse Na^+-Ca^{2+} exchange via the sodium-calcium exchanger (NaCa). During reperfusion, the generation of reactive oxygen species (superoxide anion [O_2^-], hydroxyl anion [OH^-], and hydrogen peroxide [H_2O_2]) oxidizes various proteins (Ca^{2+} pumps, SR Ca^{2+} release channels, contractile proteins, etc.) that contribute to both reversible and irreversible injury. Superoxide may combine with nitric oxide (NO) generated from sarcolemmal NOS and possibly mitochondrial NOS to form peroxynitrite ($ONOO^-$) and other reactive nitrogen species to modulate ischemia/reperfusion injury. Early reperfusion is also associated with increased NHE activity, further exacerbating Ca^{2+} overload via reverse Na^+-Ca^{2+} exchange. Preischemic activation of some myocyte inhibitory G protein (G_i)–coupled receptors, such as adenosine A_1 and opioid receptors, reduces these deleterious effects of ischemia/reperfusion. It has also been proposed that PKC may phosphorylate an ATP-dependent K^+ channel in the mitochondrial membrane and/or membrane-bound nitric oxide synthase (NOS) that protects the myocyte against ischemia/reperfusion injury.

during ischemia can contribute directly and indirectly to Ca^{2+} overload and ROS formation. For example, decreased cytosolic phosphorylation potential ([ATP] / ([ADP] × [Pi]) results in less free energy from ATP hydrolysis than is necessary to drive the energy-dependent pumps (SR Ca^{2+}-ATPase, the sarcolemmal Ca^{2+}-ATPase) that maintain intracellular calcium homeostasis.[28] Restoration of intracellular pH at the onset of reperfusion via Na^+-H^+ exchange contributes to intracellular Ca^{2+} overload via reversed Na^+-Ca^{2+} exchange.[29,30]

The metabolic changes that occur during ischemia also reduce the endogenous antioxidant defense systems of cardiac myocytes. The first line of defense against mitochondrial ROS formation and its deleterious effects is the GSH (reduced glutathione)/GSSG (oxidized glutathione) system, which is directly linked to the NADPH/$NADP^+$ ratio via the enzyme glutathione reductase. The depletion of glutathione levels increases ROS formation, oxidative stress, and $[Ca^{2+}]_i$.[31–34] Since NADPH is not formed during ischemia, the normal metabolic mechanism for regenerating the reduced glutathione does not function. Thus, the formation of ROS during reperfusion occurs at a time when the myocyte's endogenous defense mechanisms are depressed. The NADPH/$NADP^+$ ratio is a primary determinant of the redox state of the cell, and there is evidence that redox state plays a key role in determining the bioactivity and redox state of NO.[27,35,36] In addition, there are several reports that, in the absence of normal levels of its cofactors, nitric oxide synthase (NOS) itself can generate superoxide anion.[37,38] Although systolic calcium $[Ca^{2+}]_i$ may return to normal levels early in reperfused stunned myocardium, the transient increases in intracellular $[Ca^{2+}]_i$ can activate Ca^{2+}-dependent protein kinase (PKC); proteases, such as calpain; and endonucleases.[39–41] Calpain activation and subsequent action on contractile proteins has been implicated in the reduction in myofilament Ca^{2+} sensitivity observed in stunned myocardium.[42,43]

Similarly, there is significant evidence that ROS are involved in mediating myocardial stunning. Various spin trap agents and chemical probes have demonstrated the rapid release of ROS into the vascular space during reperfusion after brief ischemia in vivo.[44–47] It is also now recognized that mitochondria are a primary source of intracellular ROS in cardiac myocytes.[48,49] Scavengers of ROS and antioxidants attenuate myocardial stunning in vitro and in vivo, and these interventions are effective when administered prior to or at the onset of reperfusion.[23,50,51] It has been shown that ROS can attack thiol residues of numerous proteins such as the SR Ca^{2+}-ATPase, the ryanodine receptor, and contractile proteins.[52–54] This may explain why myofibrils isolated from in vivo reperfused stunned, but not ischemic, myocardium exhibit reduced Ca^{2+} sensitivity.[55]

More prolonged ischemia, which produces irreversible injury, is associated with more severe intracellular Ca^{2+} overload and further depletion of endogenous antioxidants, conditions which both contribute to and are exacerbated during reperfusion by the production of ROS. The production of ROS during reperfusion appears to contribute to Ca^{2+} overload, as exposure of normal myocytes to exogenous ROS is associated with increased L-type Ca^{2+} channel current and increased $[Ca^{2+}]_i$.[34,56–57] Conversely, increases in $[Ca^{2+}]_i$ during ischemia/reperfusion may adversely affect mitochondrial function, leading to further ROS production.[58–59] Mitochondria can buffer small increases in intracellular Ca^{2+} via the Ca-uniporter, a process that is energetically favorable due to the $[Ca^{2+}]$ gradient and the mitochondrial membrane potential. During reperfusion, the increase in cytosolic Ca^{2+} enhances mitochondrial Ca^{2+} uptake. Since excess cytosolic Ca^{2+} has been associated with the loss of myocyte viability, mitochondrial Ca^{2+} buffering is initially cardioprotective.[60] However, continued mitochondrial Ca^{2+} buffering in the face of decreased antioxidant reserves and excess ROS formation sets up a cycle which may ultimately lead to the total collapse of mitochondrial membrane potential and cell death.[58] The synergistic interactions between Ca^{2+} overload and ROS formation during conditions of decreased antioxidant reserves may also provide an explanation of why ROS scavengers are not very effective at reducing irreversible injury when administered at reperfusion.[61,62]

Historically, myocardial ischemia/reperfusion injury has been characterized as either reversible or irreversible (based on staining techniques, enzyme release, and histology). There is now increasing evidence that this injury represents a transition from reversible to irreversible injury, and that it occurs as a continuum and not as an all-or-none phenomenon. For example, apoptosis occurs prior to severe depletion in ATP and loss of membrane integrity, but ultimately leads to cell death.[20,21] The phenomenon of apoptosis appears to commence during reperfusion with the formation of intracellular ROS and/or intracellular calcium overload (Fig. 14-2).[63–65] This process is initiated by the translocation of the proapoptotic proteins Bad and Bax from the cytosol to the mitochondrial membrane. Heterodimerization of Bad or Bax with the anti-apoptotic Bcl-2 or Bcl-xl can lead to the release of the mitochondrially localized cytochrome c into the cytosol.[66–68] Formation of a cytosolic complex consisting of cytochrome c, apoptosis activating factor-1 (APAF-1), and caspase-9 leads to activation of caspase 3 and the cleavage of poly (ADP)-ribosylating (PARP) protein. Activation of PARP is the final step in apoptosis, leading to DNA fragmentation.[69] As described above, the increased intracellular ROS and/or intracellular calcium overload collapse the mitochondrial membrane potential, leading to mitochondrial permeability transition pore (MPTP) opening, which if not reversed can result in the loss of mitochondrial proteins, such as cytochrome c.[58]

The physiological relevance of apoptosis during myocardial ischemia/reperfusion has yet to be determined. This is due to the fact that the majority of reports on apoptosis in this setting have been based on measurements of DNA

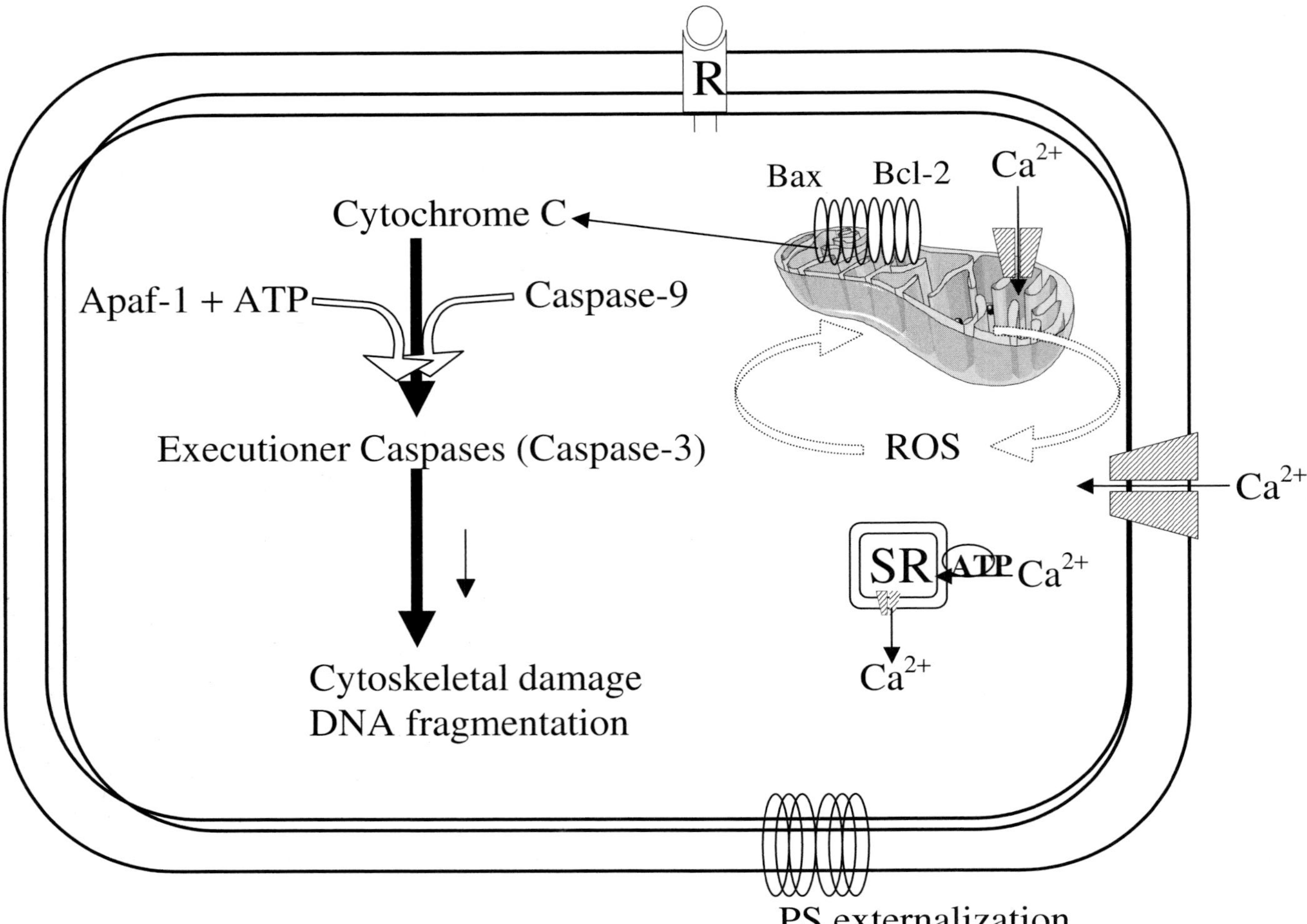

FIGURE 14–2 Proposed mechanisms of cardiomyocyte apoptosis following ischemia/reperfusion injury. Intracellular Ca^{2+} overload during ischemia and reperfusion and reactive oxygen species (ROS) formation during reperfusion are thought to be the primary mediators of the intrinsic pathway of apoptosis. The mechanisms of Ca^{2+} overload and ROS formation are described in detail in the text. Ischemia/reperfusion-associated effects on metabolism and decreased levels of the endogenous antioxidant glutathione lead to excess electron leak from the mitochondrial electron transport chain generating mitochondrial ROS. The mitochondrial Ca^{2+} uniporter can buffer increases in cytosolic Ca^{2+}, but increased mitochondrial Ca^{2+} can induce excess ROS formation. Likewise, ROS formation can induce intracellular Ca^{2+} overload. Through mechanisms that are not well defined, two families of closely related proteins (Bcl-2 and Bax) modulate the cell's response to apoptotic stimuli. Bcl-2 is an antiapoptotic protein that appears to be capable of inhibiting cytochrome c release either directly or by forming a complex with and inhibiting the proapoptotic family of proteins (Bax). Bax is thought to translocate from the cytosol to the mitochondrial membrane during the apoptotic process. Two early events in apoptosis are the externalization of phosphatidylserine (PS) residues in the sarcolemma and the release of cytochrome c from the mitochondria. The significance of PS externalization is not clear; however, its occurrence can be detected with fluorescently tagged annexin-5, thus permitting the detection of the early stages of apoptosis. Cytochrome c released from the mitochondria complexes with an apoptotic protease-activating factor-1 (Apaf-1) and procaspase 9. In the presence of near normal ATP levels, procaspase 9 is cleaved into the active caspase 9 with the resulting activation of the cytosolic protease caspase 3, often referred to as the executioner caspase. Caspase 3 protease activity leads to irreversible damage to cell morphology and DNA fragmentation and laddering.

fragmentation and laddering, the final steps in apoptotic cell death. Once DNA is fragmented, the cell's ability to synthesize new proteins to repair itself is severely compromised, and these cells, even if they survive a first ischemic episode, may die at an accelerated rate during subsequent stress or ischemia. However, studies conducted in other tissues and in isolated cells (including cardiomyocytes) indicate that the apoptotic program can be detected much earlier than these late stages. One of the earliest signs of apoptosis is the translocation of phosphatidylserine from the inner face of the plasma membrane to the cell surface, a process that can be detected by annexin V, which has a strong affinity for phosphatidylserine.[70,71] Apoptosis in cardiac myocytes can be demonstrated with (FITC)-conjugated annexin V staining of the plasma membrane much earlier than DNA fragmentation (via the TUNEL assay and DNA laddering).[72–75] There are also reports that this early stage of apoptosis does not irreversibly commit cells to programmed cell death in noncardiac tissue, and that a significant proportion of myocytes, when submitted to simulated ischemia/reperfusion, exhibit signs of early apoptosis (positive annexin-FITC staining, intact membrane cell death, decreased cell width, and increased mitochondrial [Ca^{2+}]).[75–77]

Thus, it appears that ischemia/reperfusion injury (myocardial stunning, apoptosis, infarction) is manifest in a variety of interrelated ways. For example, apoptosis may proceed to necrosis when mitochondria are no longer able to withstand the intracellular Ca^{2+} overload and oxidative stress induced by ROS, and when oxidative phosphorylation is unable to keep pace with energy demands. Due to the resulting decrease in the myocardial phosphorylation potential, energy-dependent ion pumps cannot maintain normal ion gradients. This results in cell swelling and, ultimately, loss of membrane integrity. These disturbances can be further exacerbated by the influx of macrophages and leukocytes, complement activation, and endothelial plugging by platelets and neutrophils. If cell death in ischemic/reperfused myocardium progresses from apoptosis to necrosis, and if early apoptosis is indeed reversible, then one therapeutic approach for the treatment or prevention of ischemia/reperfusion injury would be to target the early events in apoptosis. Regardless of which stage is being addressed, current cardioprotection strategies are designed to reduce cellular and subcellular ROS formation and oxidative stress, to enhance the heart's endogenous antioxidant defense mechanisms, and to prevent intracellular Ca^{2+} overload.

NONCARDIOPLEGIC TECHNIQUES

Intermittent Cross-clamping with Fibrillation

One of the earliest forms of cardioprotection, still used at some centers today, is known as intermittent aortic cross-clamping with fibrillation and moderate hypothermic perfusion (30°C to 32°C). Using this approach, coronary artery bypass surgery can be performed on the unarrested heart with ascending aorta cannulation and generally a two-stage single venous cannula. This technique allows the surgeon to operate in a relatively quiet field (during ventricular fibrillation) and to avoid the consequences of profound metabolic changes that occur with more prolonged periods of ischemia. The duration of fibrillation is determined by how long it takes to complete the distal anastomoses. After completion of the last distal graft, the heart can be defibrillated and the proximal aortic-based graft anastomoses performed on the beating heart, using an aortic partial occlusion clamp.

As a result of increasing pressures to reduce costs, and yet maintain acceptable levels of myocardial protection, there has been a renewed interest in this approach. There are, in fact, a number of reports that indicate that satisfactory protection can be conferred using this technique. In 1992, Bonchek et al reported a large clinical series in which the advantages and safety of using this technique were meticulously analyzed.[78] In this study, the authors reviewed the outcomes of the first 3000 patients at their institution who underwent primary coronary bypass surgery utilizing the intermittent aortic cross-clamping technique. Preoperative risk factors (age, gender, left ventricular dysfunction, preoperative intra-aortic balloon pumping, and urgency of operation) and operative deaths were analyzed as well. In this series, 29% of the patients were more than 70 years of age; 27% were females; 9.7% had an ejection fraction less than 0.30; 13% had a myocardial infarction less than one week preoperatively; and 31% had preinfarction angina in the hospital. Only 26% underwent purely elective operations. Using the noncardioplegic cardioprotective technique, the authors reported an elective operative mortality of rate 0.5%, an urgent mortality rate of 1.7%, and an emergency rate of 2.3%. Postoperatively, inotropic support was needed in only 6.6% of the patients and only 1% required intra-aortic balloon pumping. It is important to note, however, that this was a retrospective, single-center institutional experience. The findings would have been more enlightening if the analysis had included a similarly matched group of patients at the same institution in which cardioplegic arrest had been employed. Nevertheless, the findings do suggest that noncardioplegic strategies can provide a satisfactory means of myocardial protection even in high-risk patients.

As a result, a minority of surgeons continue to use this technique.[79–81] In 2002, Raco et al[82] reported the results of 800 consecutive coronary artery bypass grafting operations performed by a single surgeon using aortic cross-clamping in both elective and nonelective procedures. The patients were divided into three cohorts: (1) elective, (2) urgent, and (3) emergent. The mean age, number of distal grafts, and mortality in the elective group were 61.5 years, 3.2, and 0.6%, respectively. For the urgent group, they were 63.1 years, 3.2, and 3.1 %. In the emergent group they were 63.8 years, 2.9, and 5.6%. These findings support the contention that intermittent aortic cross-clamping is a safe technique both in elective and nonelective patients when performed by an experienced surgeon.

SYSTEMIC HYPOTHERMIA AND ELECTIVE FIBRILLATORY ARREST

Although infrequently used, this technique appears to be a safe approach to protecting the heart during coronary artery bypass surgery. In 1984, Atkins et al reported a low incidence of perioperative infarction and a low hospital mortality rate in 500 consecutive patients using this technique.[83] With this method, systemic hypothermia (28°C), elective fibrillatory arrest, and maintenance of systemic perfusion pressure between 80 mm Hg and 100 mm Hg are the key elements. Upon fibrillatory arrest, the local vessel can be isolated and myocardial revascularization performed. The limitations of this technique include: (1) the surgical field may be obscured by blood during revascularization; (2) ventricular fibrillation is associated with increased muscular tone, which can limit the surgeon's ability to position the heart for optimal exposure; and (3) it is generally not applicable for intracardiac procedures.

CARDIOPLEGIC TECHNIQUES

Cardioplegic solutions contain a variety of chemical agents that are designed to arrest the heart rapidly in diastole, create a quiescent operating field, and provide reliable protection against ischemia/reperfusion injury. In general, there are two types of cardioplegic solutions: crystalloid cardioplegia and blood cardioplegia. These solutions are administered most frequently under hypothermic conditions.

Cold Crystalloid Cardioplegia

There are basically two types of crystalloid cardioplegic solutions: the intracellular type and the extracellular type. The intracellular types are characterized by absent or low concentrations of sodium and calcium. The extracellular types contain relatively higher concentrations of sodium, calcium, and magnesium. Both groups avoid concentrations of potassium greater than 40 mmol/L, contain bicarbonate for buffering, and are osmotically balanced. In both types the concentration of potassium used ranges between 10 mmol/L and 40 mmol/L (for potassium 1 mmol/L = 1 mEq/L). Examples of some of the various crystalloid cardioplegic solutions used are shown in Table 14-2.

OPERATIVE PROCEDURE

While the degree of core cooling varies from center to center, patients undergoing cardiac surgery are placed on cardiopulmonary bypass and often cooled to between 33°C and 28°C. To initiate immediate chemical arrest, the solution is infused after cross-clamping the aorta through a cardioplegic catheter inserted into the aorta proximal to the cross-clamp. The catheter may or may not be accompanied by a separate vent cannula. The cold hyperkalemic crystalloid solution is then infused (antegrade) at a volume that generally does not exceed 1000 mL. One or more infusions of 300 to 500 mL of the cardioplegic solution may be administered if there is evidence of electrical heart activity resumption, or if a prolonged ischemic time is anticipated. If myocardial revascularization is being performed, the aortic cross-clamp can be removed after completing the distal anastomoses, and the heart reperfused while the proximal anatomoses are completed, using a partial occlusion clamp. Alternatively, the proximal grafts can be performed after the distal grafts have been completed with the cross-clamp still in place (the single-clamp technique). Another approach is to perform the proximal aortic grafts first, then cross-clamp the aorta and infuse the cardioplegic solution. When valve repair or replacement is being performed, the crystalloid cardioplegia can be administered directly into the coronary arteries via cannulation of the coronary ostia. Crystalloid cardioplegia can also be administered retrograde via a coronary sinus catheter, with or without a self-inflating silicone cuff.

RESULTS

Numerous studies have been performed to determine the efficacy of using cold crystalloid cardioplegic solutions to protect the heart during cardiac surgery. While there is considerable controversy regarding the "ideal" solution and its components, there is evidence that in those centers in which crystalloid cardioplegia is used almost exclusively, excellent myocardial protection can be achieved. In many reports the perioperative myocardial infarction rate is less than 4%, and the operative mortality rate is less than 2%.

Cold Blood Cardioplegia

Cold blood cardioplegia, widely employed throughout the world, is the cardioplegic technique most commonly used in the United States today. Although there are a variety of formulations, it is usually prepared by combining autologous blood obtained from the extracorporeal circuit while the patient is on cardiopulmonary bypass with a crystalloid solution consisting of citrate-phosphate-dextrose (CPD), tris-hydroxymethyl-aminomethane (tham) or bicarbonate (buffers), and potassium chloride. The CPD is used to lower the ionic calcium, the buffer is used to maintain an alkaline pH of approximately 7.8, and the final concentration of potassium is used to arrest the heart (approximately 30 mmol/L).

Prior to administering blood cardioplegia, the temperature of the solution is usually lowered with a heat exchanging coil to between 12°C and 4°C. The ratio of blood to crystalloid varies among centers, with the most common ratios being 8:1, 4:1, and 2:1. This in turn affects the final hematocrit of the blood cardioplegia infused. For example, if the hematocrit of the autologous blood obtained from the extracorporeal circuit is 30, these ratios would result in a blood cardioplegia with a hematocrit of approximately 27, 24, and 20, respectively.

The use of undiluted blood cardioplegia or "miniplegia" (using a minimum amount of crystalloid additives) has also been reported to be effective. In an acute ischemia/reperfusion canine preparation, Velez and colleagues tested the hypothesis that an all-blood cardioplegia (66:1 blood to crystalloid ratio) would provide superior protection compared to a 4:1 blood cardioplegia delivered in a continuous retrograde fashion.[84] They found very little difference between the animal groups with respect to infarct size or postischemic recovery of function. This is consistent with the findings by Rousou et al years earlier that it is the level of hypothermia that is important in blood cardioplegia, not necessarily the hematocrit.[85]

The rationales for using blood as a vehicle for hypothermic potassium-induced cardiac arrest include:

1. It can provide an oxygenated environment.
2. It can provide a method for intermittent reoxygenation of the heart during arrest.
3. It can limit hemodilution when large volumes of cardioplegia are used.
4. It has an excellent buffering capacity.
5. It has excellent osmotic properties.
6. The electrolyte composition and pH are physiologic.
7. It contains a number of endogenous antioxidants and free radical scavengers.
8. It can be less complex than other solutions to prepare.

With respect to efficacy, there are numerous preclinical studies as well as nonrandomized and randomized clinical trials that demonstrate that cold blood cardioplegia is an effective way to provide excellent myocardial protection. While many of these same studies have also suggested that cold blood cardioplegia is superior to cold crystalloid cardioplegia, it is important to note that other investigators have shown crystalloid cardioplegia to be just as cardioprotective as well as cost-effective, if not more so, and that crystalloid cardioplegia more reliably ensures a quiet, bloodless operative field. Unfortunately, many of the clinical trials that have compared the efficacy of blood and crystalloid cardioplegia have been single-center studies, involved a limited number of patients, focused on a specific subset of patients, and/or omitted details of the clinical management of the two techniques.

Warm Blood Cardioplegia

The concept of using warm (normothermic) blood cardioplegia as a cardioprotective strategy in humans dates back to the 1980s. In 1982, Rosenkranz et al reported that warm induction with normothermic blood cardioplegia, with a multidose cold blood cardioplegia maintenance of arrest, resulted in better recovery of function in canines than a similar protocol using cold blood induction.[86] In 1986, Teoh et al reported an experimental study demonstrating that a terminal infusion of warm blood cardioplegia before removing the cross-clamp (a "hot shot") accelerated myocardial metabolic recovery.[87] This was followed by reports in 1991 by Lichtenstein et al that normothermic blood cardioplegia in humans is an effective cardioprotective approach.[88] They compared the results of 121 consecutive patients who received antegrade normothermic blood cardioplegia during myocardial revascularization operations with a historical group of 133 patients who received antegrade hypothermic blood cardioplegia. The operative mortality in the warm cardioplegic group was 0.9% compared to 2.2% for the historical controls. At about the same time, Salerno et al reported a series of 113 consecutive patients in which continuous warm blood cardioplegia was administered via the coronary sinus.[89] In this series, 96% had spontaneous return of rhythm upon reperfusion, 7% needed transient intra-aortic balloon pump circulatory support, 6% had evidence of a perioperative myocardial infarction, and 3% did not recover. A control cohort was not provided for comparison.

Despite these encouraging reports, there are still concerns with this approach. For example, for any given patient it is not known just how long the warm heart can tolerate an ischemic event, which may occur when the infusion is interrupted, flow rates are reduced due to an obscured surgical field, or a maldistribution of the cardioplegic solution occurs. Another concern is the report by Martin et al which suggested that the use of warm cardioplegia is associated with increased incidence of neurological deficits.[90] In their prospective, randomized study (conducted on more than 1000 patients), the efficacy of warm blood cardioplegia and cold oxygenated crystalloid cardioplegia was analyzed. While operative mortalities were similar between the warm blood group and the cold oxygenated crystalloid cardioplegia cohort (1.0% vs.1.6%, respectively), the incidence of permanent neurologic deficits was threefold greater in the warm blood group (3.1% vs.1.0%). Thus, it appears that warm blood cardioplegia offers no distinct advantage over cold blood or cold crystalloid cardioplegia, and it may be less than ideal if its delivery is interrupted for any reason.

Tepid Blood Cardioplegia

Both cold blood (4°C to10°C) and warm blood cardioplegic solutions (37°C) have temperature-related advantages and disadvantages. As a consequence, a number of studies were performed in the 1990s to determine the optimal temperature.

Hayashida et al were one of the first groups to study specifically the efficacy of tepid (29°C) blood cardioplegia.[91] In this study, 72 patients undergoing coronary artery bypass grafting were randomized to receive cold (8°C) antegrade or retrograde, tepid (29°C) antegrade or retrograde, or warm (37°C) antegrade or retrograde blood cardioplegia. While protection was adequate for all three, the tepid antegrade cardioplegia was the most effective in reducing anaerobic lactate acid release during the arrest period. These authors reported similar findings when the tepid solution was delivered continuously retrograde and intermittently antegrade.[92] Since then, other studies have also demonstrated that tepid blood cardioplegia is safe and effective. The majority of these studies, however, have been single-center studies and/or conducted in a relatively small cohort of patients. Whether tepid cardioplegia confers better protection over other current methodologies remains to be determined.

Methods of Delivery

In addition to a variety of solutions and temperatures, there are also many different ways of administering the solutions (Fig. 14-3). As one might expect with so many options, the optimal delivery method of a cardioplegic solution also remains controversial. These include: intermittent antegrade, antegrade via the graft, continuous antegrade, continuous retrograde, intermittent retrograde, antegrade followed by retrograde, and simultaneous antegrade and retrograde infusions. While all methods are generally good, comparisons are difficult because there are numerous confounding factors such as the: (1) composition of the solution, (2) temperature of the solution, (3) duration of the infusion, (4) infusion pressure, (5) type and complexity of the operation, (6) need for surgical exposure, and (7) expected versus actual cross-clamp time. One method that is being used more frequently is the retrograde technique. This approach originated with a concept developed by Pratt in 1898, who suggested that oxygenated blood could be supplied to the ischemic heart via the coronary venous system.[93] Sixty years later, Lillehei et al used retrograde coronary sinus perfusion to protect the heart during aortic valve surgery.[94] Today, it is an accepted method for delivering a cardioplegic solution and is used frequently as an adjunct to antegrade cardioplegia.

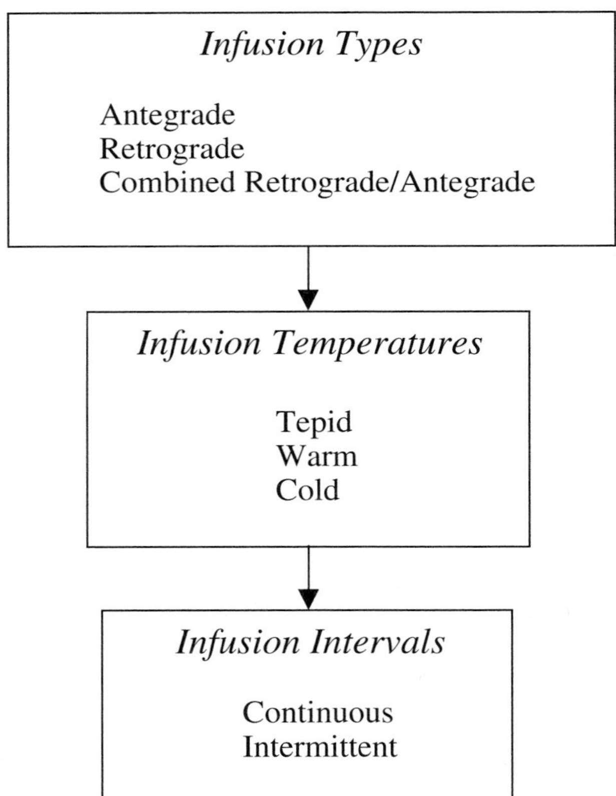

FIGURE 14–3 Methods and delivery of cardioplegic solutions.

In favor of the retrograde approach is the theoretical advantage of ensuring a more homogeneous distribution of the cardioplegic solution to regions of the heart that are poorly collateralized. It is also effective in: (1) the setting of aortic regurgitation and valve surgery; (2) reducing the risk of embolization from saphenous vein grafts that could occur during antegrade perfusion during reoperative coronary artery surgery; and (3) delivering cardioplegia in a continuous manner.

Despite these advantages, retrograde cardioplegia is not without its limitations. Numerous experimental and clinical studies have shown that cardioplegia administered via the coronary sinus can result in a poor distribution of the solution to the right ventricle. This may be related to the variable venous anatomy of the heart. Because the anterior region of the right ventricle is not drained by the coronary sinus, and it is not uncommon for the heart to have a number of coronary sinus anomalies, these factors may result in the heterogeneous distribution of cardioplegic solutions and thus limit myocardial protection.

As a consequence, a technique for simultaneously delivering cardioplegia both antegrade and retrograde is available. The feasibility and safety of this approach was reported in 1984 by Ihnken et al.[95] In a more recent study, Cohen et al used sonicated albumen and transesophageal echocardiography intraoperatively to assess the effects of delivering a cardioplegic solution antegrade and retrograde simultaneously.[96] Compared to the antegrade or retrograde routes, the best and most consistent perfusion of the anterior left and right ventricles was achieved using the simultaneous technique. These investigators also reported that antegrade infusion resulted in superior perfusion of the left ventricle when compared to retrograde delivery alone, and that right ventricular perfusion was inconsistent with both antegrade and retrograde delivery. Thus, it remains to be determined in which setting the simultaneous use of both methods is most appropriate.

With respect to intermittent cardioplegic infusions versus continuous infusions, the major advantage of the former is the ability to achieve and to sustain a dry quiescent operative field. While a continuous infusion, especially if it

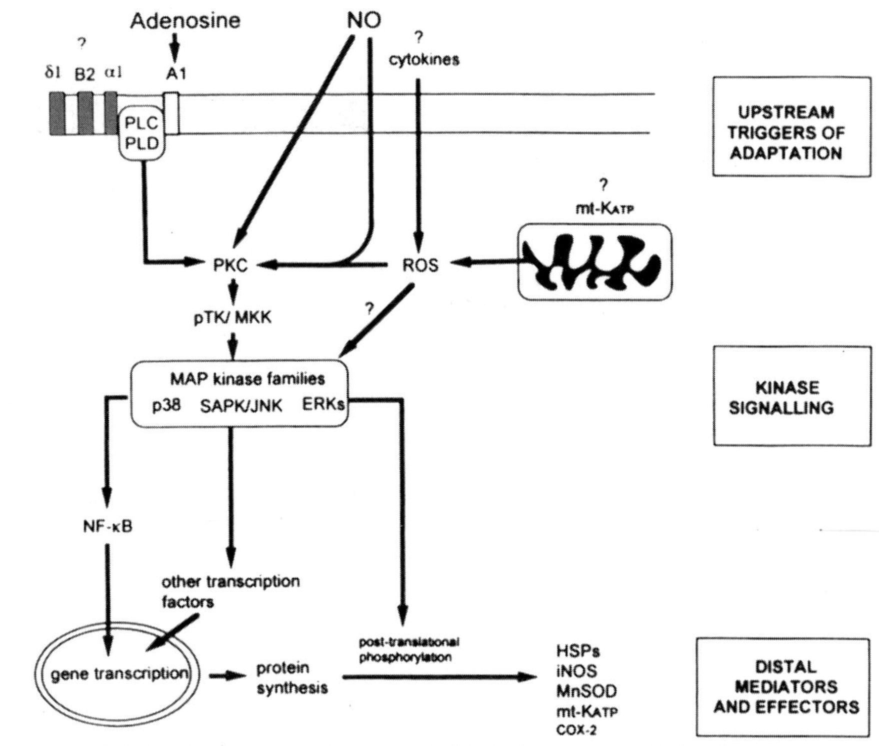

FIGURE 14–4 Proposed mechanisms of late-phase preconditioning. Important upstream triggers of adaptation include adenosine, nitric oxide (NO), and reactive oxygen species (ROS). It is also possible that other ligands binding with 7 transmembrane domain receptors such as bradykinin, opioids, and noradrenaline may act as triggers of delayed preconditioning, but there is only indirect evidence for this at present. Mitochondrial K_{ATP} channel (MT-K_{ATP}) opening may initiate delayed protection, speculatively through the generation of superoxide anion. The rapid release of cytokines may also trigger delayed protection. The activation of a complex kinase signaling cascade is proposed, and experimental evidence suggests the activation of protein kinase C-ε and $-\mu$ isoforms (PKC); tyrosine phosphorylation by protein tyrosine kinases (pTK) and MAP kinases (MKK); and involvement of some MAP kinase familes. Activation of NF-κB occurs rapidly and may be a key transciptional mechanism, although other transcription factors are activated also by preconditioning. De novo protein synthesis is proposed to be central to the mechanism of delayed preconditioning, but it is likely that posttranslational modifications of constituitively expressed proteins may also be involved. The identities of distal mediators and the effectors of protection are not established. Possible candidates include members of the heat shock protein family (HSPs), inducible nitric oxide synthase (iNOS), and manganese-dependent superoxide dismutase (Mn-SOD). The regulation of proteins associated with mt-K_{AT}P function may be involved. Cyclo-oxygenase-2 (COX-2) may be upregulated in delayed preconditioning. The final common pathway leading to cell survival during index ischemia is unknown, but it is highly likely that several distal proteins cooperate to confer protection. (*Reproduced with permission from Springer-Verlag from Baxter GF, Ferdinandy P: Delayed preconditioning of myocardium: current perspectives. Basic Res Cardiol 2001; 96:338.*)

is oxygenated, has the theoretical advantage of minimizing ischemia, from a practical aspect it is unlikely that this can be achieved reliably. There is also the theoretical potential for an excessive infusion of cardioplegic solution.

PROTECTION STRATEGIES UNDER INVESTIGATION

Ischemic Preconditioning

Ischemic preconditioning is an adaptive biological phenomenon in which the heart (and numerous other tissues) becomes more tolerant to a period of prolonged ischemia if first exposed to a prior episode of brief ischemia and reperfusion. This adaptation to ischemia was first described by Murry et al, and is referred to as classic or early phase preconditioning.[97] This increased tolerance to ischemia is associated with a reduction in infarct size, apoptosis, and reperfusion-associated arrhythmias.[98–102] It has been demonstrated in every animal species studied and appears to persist as long as 1 to 2 hours after the ischemic preconditioning stimulus.[103,104] It becomes ineffective when the sustained ischemic insult exceeds 3 hours.[105] This suggests that the protection is conferred only when prolonged ischemia is followed by timely reperfusion.[106]

Further characterization of this phenomenon has also revealed a second phase of protection that requires 24 hours to appear and is sustained for up to 72 hours. This has been referred to as the second window of protection (SWOP), late phase preconditioning, or delayed preconditioning. Unlike classical preconditioning, which protects only against infarction, the late phase protects against both infarction and myocardial stunning.[99,107] This observation, coupled with a longer interval of protection, has resulted in major investigative efforts to elucidate the intracellular mechanism(s) that underlie both phenomena. The assumption is that a better understanding of these mechanism(s) could lead to the development of potent new therapeutic modalities that are more effective in treating or preventing the deleterious consequences of ischemia/reperfusion injury.

To elucidate the trigger(s) and mediator(s) of this powerful endogenous defense mechanism, numerous in vivo and in vitro studies have been performed. One of the earliest hypotheses was that the adenosine receptor (the A_1 receptor) was the primary mediator of this phenomenon (Fig. 14-4).[104,108] Subsequent studies have shown, however, that in addition to adenosine, there are multiple guanine nucleotide binding (G) protein coupled receptors that, once activated, can mimic protection against infarction (e.g., bradykinin, endothelin, alpha$_1$-adrenergic, muscarinic, angiotensin II, and delta-opioid receptors).[104,108] Transient infusion of exogenous agents that mimic ischemic preconditioning is referred to as pharmacologic preconditioning. Exactly which of these receptors is the most important in mediating endogenous preconditioning is unknown, since there appear to be species differences and redundant pathways. Regardless, it is now thought that these triggers of ischemic preconditioning result in alterations in certain enzymes, such as tyrosine kinases, protein kinase C (PKC), and mitogen-activated protein kinases or c- jun-N-terminal kinases, which in turn confer protection against irreversible injury prior to the onset of prolonged ischemia.[104,108] While the actual effector(s) of the protection has yet to be determined, one hypothesis is that the activation of these signaling pathways ultimately leads to the activation of an ATP-sensitive K^+ (K_{ATP}) channel in the mitochondria.[104,108]

While early-phase preconditioning shares many of the same signaling mechanisms with late-phase preconditioning, the most obvious difference between the two is the apparent requirement for protein synthesis in the latter. Both late-phase ischemic and pharmacologic preconditioning have been shown to be associated with the upregulation of various proteins, such as heat shock proteins, inducible NOS (iNOS), cyclo-oxygenase 2, and manganese superoxide dismutase.[109–111]

To date, the evidence that ischemic preconditioning exists in the human heart is circumstantial. A number of investigators have reported that patients experiencing angina prior to a myocardial infarct have better in-hospital prognoses and a reduced incidence of cardiogenic shock, fewer and less severe episodes of congestive heart failure, and smaller infarcts as assessed by cardiac enzyme release.[112–115] There are also follow-up studies that suggest patients who have had preinfarction angina prior to an infarct have better long-term survival rates.[116–118] There are also a myriad of reports that patients who undergo percutaneous transluminal coronary angioplasty (PTCA) have an enhanced tolerance to ischemia after the first balloon inflation, providing that the first balloon inflation exceeds 60 to 90 seconds.[106] Chest pain severity, regional wall motion abnormalities, ST-segment elevation, QT dispersion, lactate production, and CK-MB release have all been reported to be attenuated in this setting as well.[119–124]

In patients undergoing PTCA, a preconditioning-like effect has also been mimicked by the administration of a variety of pharmacologic agents that are known to induce preconditioning in animal studies. For example, the administration of adenosine prior to PTCA has been reported to attenuate myocardial ischemic indices during the first balloon inflation. Conversely, the administration of bamiphylline or aminophylline (nonselective adenosine receptor antagonists) reportedly abolishes markers of myocardial ischemia during the second balloon inflation.[125] Tomai et al reported that the administration of oral glibenclamide (a K_{ATP} channel blocker) before angioplasty abolishes the reduction in ischemic indices observed after subsequent balloon inflations.[126] This finding is consistent with the observation that nicorandil (a potassium channel opener) administration is associated with a reduction in ECG evidence of ischemia during PTCA.[127] Opioid and bradykinin receptor activation have also been implicated in mediating the myocardial protection induced by the first balloon inflation.[128] Thus, there are many observational studies that support the hypothesis that myocardial protection conferred by ischemic preconditioning and its possible mediators in animal studies is translatable to humans. It is important to note, however, that classic or early ischemic preconditioning observed in animals is associated with a reduction in infarct size, not stunning, and that many of the clinical studies are either retrospective in nature or have used surrogate markers of injury as end points.

With respect to cardiac surgery, one of the first studies indicating that preconditioning may exist in humans was conducted by Yellon et al in 1993.[129] In this study, patients undergoing cardiac surgery were subjected to a protocol that involved 2 cycles of 3 minutes of global ischemia. Cross-clamping the aorta intermittently and pacing the heart at 90 beats per minute were used to induce ischemia. This was followed by 2 minutes of reperfusion before a 10-minute period of global ischemia and ventricular fibrillation. Myocardial biopsies were obtained during a 10-minute period of global ischemia, and ATP tissue content was measured. The results showed that the ATP levels in the biopsies obtained from patients subjected to the preconditioning-like protocol were higher. However, since ATP content is not a marker of necrosis, a follow-up study was performed and troponin T serum levels were used. In this study the investigators reported that the release of this marker of necrosis was also less in patients subjected to the preconditioning protocol.[130]

Whether the phenomenon of ischemic preconditioning plays any role in conferring protection when the intermittent cross-clamp technique is used perioperatively is unknown. It is important to note, however, that Teoh et al reported that ischemic preconditioning might confer additional myocardial protection beyond that provided by intermittent cross-clamp fibrillation in patients undergoing coronary artery bypass surgery.[131] The fact that other human studies have not shown additional protection when ischemic preconditioning was added to a myocardial protection protocol makes the use of this procedure less likely.[132,133] For the immediate future, the most promising strategy for developing new methods to protect the heart against ischemia/reperfusion injury lies with the elucidation of the intracellular events underlying the phenomenon of late-phase ischemic preconditioning (Fig. 14-4).

TABLE 14–3 Cardiac adenosine receptor subtypes

Receptor subtype	G protein coupling	Location	Effect
A_1	G_i	Myocyte	Negative chronotropic and dromotropic; antiadrenergic; extracardiac: CNS depression, antilipolytic effects
A_{2a}	G_s	Myocyte, EC, VSM	Coronary vasodilation
A_{2b}	G_s	VSM, EC	Mast cell degranulation, angiogenesis
A_3	G_i, G_q?	Lungs and liver?	Hemopoiesis

EC = endothelial cell; VSM = vascular smooth muscle. Question marks indicate that specific effects have not been definitively determined. See text for more detailed descriptions.

Adenosine

There is considerable experimental evidence that the preischemic administration of the nucleoside adenosine retards the rate of ischemia-induced ATP depletion, prolongs the time to onset of ischemic contracture, attenuates myocardial stunning, enhances postischemic myocardial energetics, and reduces infarct size.[134] As mentioned earlier, there is also evidence that adenosine may play a role in mediating the infarct size–limiting effects of ischemic preconditioning.[104,135] A transient infusion of adenosine or certain adenosine receptor agonists prior to ischemia is associated with infarct size reduction similar to that of ischemic preconditioning.[135–137] There are, however, conflicting reports regarding the ability of adenosine receptor antagonists to block ischemic preconditioning.[138,139] When analyzing these studies, it is important to recognize a small but important difference between adenosine preconditioning and adenosine pretreatment. The former involves a brief infusion of adenosine that is terminated prior to the onset of ischemia, whereas the latter involves the continuous infusion of adenosine until the onset of ischemia. The significance of this difference lies with the observation that adenosine pretreatment, not adenosine preconditioning, attenuates myocardial stunning.[140,141] Myocardial stunning is the most common form of injury in patients after heart surgery. The beneficial effects of adenosine infusions prior to ischemia appear to be due to the direct effects of adenosine on the cardiac myocyte since: (1) adenosine must be infused at a dose that reaches the interstitial fluid (ISF) space that surrounds the cardiac myocyte; and (2) adenosine reduction of ischemic and hypoxic injury can be demonstrated in isolated myocyte preparations.[142–144]

Although the cardioprotective effects of adenosine have been recognized for some time, there are still many questions regarding its mechanism of action. Genetic, biochemical, and pharmacologic studies indicate that there are at least four distinct sarcolemmal adenosine receptor subtypes, designated A_1, A_{2a}, A_{2b}, and A_3(Table 14-3), that couple to a variety of guanine nucleotide binding (G) proteins, G_o, $G_{i\alpha 2}$, $G_{i\alpha 3}$, G_q, and Gs, depending upon the receptor subtype and tissue studied. Currently, there is direct evidence that two, possibly three, of these receptors are expressed in the adult heart. Radioligand binding studies have documented the presence of A_1 and A_{2a} adenosine receptors in mammalian myocardium, and numerous studies since have reported the physiological roles of these receptors.[145] The results of recent studies suggest that adenosine A_{2b} receptors may be expressed in the coronary vasculature.[146,147] Although there are some reports of A_3 receptor mRNA expression in cardiac tissue, presently there is no definitive evidence for the expression of this receptor in the normal mammalian heart.[148,149]

In normal myocardium, activation of A_1 receptors on atrial myocytes exerts negative chronotropic, dromotropic, and inotropic effects via modulation of K^+ and Ca^{2+} channel conductances. Activation of the same receptor exerts few, if any, direct effects in ventricular myocardium. However, A_1 receptor activation significantly blunts the metabolic and contractile effects of beta-adrenergic receptor stimulation.[150] Adenosine cardioprotection appears to be another physiologically relevant indirect effect of A_1 receptor activation. The administration of various A_1 receptor agonists prior to ischemia in multiple species and preparations, including human papillary muscle strips and atrial myocytes, has also been shown to mimic the cardioprotective effects of adenosine.[134,151] Likewise, there are reports that the beneficial effects of adenosine pretreatment are blocked by the A_1 receptor antagonist 1,3-dipropyl-8-cyclopentylxanthine (DPCPX).[134] Like the A_1 antiadrenergic effect, the A_1 receptor cardioprotective effect is blocked by pertussis toxin pretreatment, which ADP ribosylates and blocks G_i protein activation.[152] Preischemic adenosine A_1 receptor activation appears more effective in modulating the deleterious effects of ischemia, since A_1 receptor agonist infusion during reperfusion appears to exert little or no beneficial effect afterwards.[153]

With respect to the A_{2a} receptor, recent studies indicate that selective adenosine A_{2a} receptor activation can be beneficial to the reperfused myocardium. Reperfusion infusions of the relatively selective A_{2a} agonist 2-[4-[(2-carboxyethyl)-phenyl]-ethylamino]-5′-N-ethylcarboxamidoadenosine (CGS21680), at doses that exert minimal effects on systemic blood pressure and heart rate, have been shown to decrease infarct size in intact canine and porcine myocardium.[154–157] There is now evidence that adenosine A_{2a} receptor activation during reperfusion in stunned porcine myocardium is associated with a flow-independent increase in myocardial contractility (assessed by load-insensitive measurements of preload recruitable stroke work index). This effect appears to occur only in the stunned myocardium. This is in contrast to earlier studies that showed adenosine infusion upon reperfusion had little or no effect on infarct size. These negative findings were probably due to the rapid rate of degradation of adenosine in blood and the use of high-dose adenosine which may have masked or offset any potential beneficial effects of selective A_{2a} receptor activation. In addition to vascular smooth muscle and endothelial cells, adenosine A_{2a} receptors have been shown to be expressed in porcine, human, and rat ventricular myocytes.[158,159] This suggests that the beneficial effect of A_{2a} agonists may be due to a direct effect on the cardiac myocytes.

More recent studies have suggested that the A_3 receptor plays an important role in conferring protection.[160,161] This hypothesis has been supported by studies with novel adenosine agonists, such as N^6-(3-iodobenzyl)-adenosine-5′-N-methyluronamide (IBMECA) and 2-chloro-N^6-(3-iodobenzyl)-adenosine-5′-N-methyluronamide (Cl-IBMECA). These agents exhibit selectivity for cloned A_3 receptors.[162–164] However, there have been no reports verifying the expression of A_3 receptors on mammalian adult cardiomyocytes. Moreover, the effects of these agents can be blocked by A_1 and A_{2a} receptor antagonists.[165–167] It is also important to note that A_3 receptor agonists have been reported to simulate apoptosis in several cell types, including neonatal rat ventricular myocytes, an undesirable effect if applicable to adult myocytes.[168,169]

As noted earlier, the specific subcellular events and signaling pathways that are involved after the adenosine receptor has been activated have yet to be clearly defined. There is no known direct signaling mechanism activated by adenosine in normal ventricular myocardium. The mechanisms that have received the most interest and study are the stimulation of protein kinase C (PKC) isoforms and/or ATP-dependent K^+ (K_{ATP}) channels.[104,135] It has been proposed that A_1 receptor activation results in the cytosol-to-membrane translocation of one or more PKC isoforms, which phosphorylate the K_{ATP} channels, leading to increased channel activity.[104] Another possibility is that the A_1 receptor can activate a protein tyrosine kinase and p38 mitogen activated protein (MAP) kinase, processes that occur distal to PKC.[170] The evidence that supports this hypothesis is based on pharmacologic studies designed to explore the effects of specific agents on infarct size. However, other studies indicate that adenosine A_1 receptor activation blunts the PKC-dependent negative inotropic effects in intact myocardium and isolated myocytes, and may, in fact, activate a serine-threonine protein phosphatase.[171–174] With respect to the K_{ATP} channel mechanism, there is evidence that adenosine activates sarcolemmal K_{ATP} channels in neonatal rat ventricular myocytes (although there is no direct evidence that this occurs in adult myocytes).[175] This latter observation and recent results with the agent diazoxide (a mitochondrial K_{ATP} channel activator) have led to the hypothesis that adenosine A_1 cardioprotection is mediated via the activation of mitochondrial K_{ATP} channels.[104] It is possible that the A_1 receptor activates a PKC isoform that translocates to mitochondria to phosphorylate the K_{ATP} channel, and (in a yet-to-be-determined manner) confers myocardial protection.

Another possibility is that activation of the A_1 receptor results in an attenuation of oxidative stress. Both adenosine and A_1 receptor agonists have been shown to attenuate the deleterious contractile and metabolic effects of hydrogen peroxide.[176,177] They have also been reported to decrease lipid peroxidation and increase the activity of superoxide dismutase, catalase, glutathione peroxidase, and glutathione reductase in various cell types.[178] This suggests that adenosine may play an important role in counteracting the deleterious effects of the formation of reactive oxygen species (a major component of ischemia/reperfusion injury) and in this manner attenuate stunning, apoptosis, and myocardial infarction.

Adenosine A_1 receptor agonists, in addition to their acute cardioprotective effects, have been shown to induce a second window of protection (SWOP) or delayed preconditioning. The injection of various species with the A_1 receptor agonist 2-chloro-N^6-cyclopentyladenosine (CCPA) has been shown to reduce myocardial infarct size 24 hours later, an effect that has been shown to persist for 72 hours in the rabbit.[179–185] This is similar to the second window of protection induced by a transient ischemic episode. If A_1receptor–mediated delayed and ischemia-induced late-phase preconditioning share some of the same signaling pathways, this would implicate a trigger role for the upregulation of inducible nitric oxide synthase (iNOS).[186]Although 24-hour CCPA protection is associated with the upregulation of iNOS in murine myocardium, a loss of protection in iNOS knockout mice has not been a consistent finding, and NOS inhibitors do not block the A_1 SWOP in rabbit myocardium.[181,183] Thus much work needs to be done to fully understand the mechanism underlying A_1 delayed preconditioning and ischemia-induced late-phase preconditioning. A better understanding of both phenomena could lead to new therapies designed to protect the heart during cardiac surgery.

Although there have been fewer studies on adenosine A_{2a} receptor–mediated attenuation of myocardial reperfusion injury, there appears to be more definitive evidence regarding its mechanism of action. Adenosine- and A_{2a} agonist–induced reduction in infarct size are associated with decreased neutrophil infiltration and adherence to coronary endothelium.[155,156,187] Although this effect could simply be the result, rather than the cause, of myocardial protection, it is known that adenosine A_{2a} receptors are expressed on neutrophils, and that their activation leads to decreased superoxide radical production.[188] As described earlier, adenosine A_{2a} receptors are also expressed on coronary endothelial cells, and there is evidence that their activation may result in nitric oxide (NO) release.[189] The platelet antiaggregatory effects of adenosine may also play a role in A_{2a}-mediated reduction of reperfusion injury.

With respect to clinical studies, Lee et al pretreated 7 patients undergoing coronary artery bypass surgery with adenosine and compared their postoperative course to a similar group of untreated patients.[190] Adenosine was infused incrementally before the initiation of cardiopulmonary bypass at a rate of 50 μg/kg/min every minute until a dose of 350 μg/kg/min was reached. The total duration of the adenosine infusion lasted for 10 minutes, or until the patient developed systemic arterial pressures less than 70 mm Hg, at which time the infusion was discontinued. Five minutes after completion of the adenosine or the saline control infusion, patients were placed on cardiopulmonary bypass and underwent coronary artery bypass grafting. Cold blood cardioplegia was used to facilitate the arrest. The investigators reported that adenosine pretreatment was associated with improved postoperative myocardial function. Major limitations of this study were the small number of patients studied and limited number of parameters used to assess ventricular function. In contrast, Fremes et al reported the results of an open label, nonrandomized adenosine study in which no effect was observed.[191] In this study, the patients also underwent coronary artery bypass surgery. Antegrade warm blood cardioplegia was used, with adenosine added to the initial 1-L dose and the final 500-mL dose of cardioplegia. The adenosine concentrations studied were 15, 20, and 25 μmol/L. These investigators found that adenosine could be safely added as a supplement to cardioplegic solutions, but the agent had no effect on myocardial function at the doses studied.

A similar lack of efficacy in humans was reported by Cohen et al in a phase II double-blind, placebo-controlled trial performed in patients also undergoing coronary artery bypass surgery.[192] Patients were treated with placebo (saline) or warm blood cardioplegia supplemented with 15 μM, 50 μM, or 100 μM adenosine. These investigators also reported that the adenosine additive had no effect on survival, on the incidence of myocardial infarction (as determined by CK-MB levels), or on the incidence of low cardiac output syndrome. A major limitation of this study was the use of low concentrations of adenosine in the setting of warm blood cardioplegia. The nucleoside is rapidly metabolized to inosine and hypoxanthine, and the half-life in blood is measured in seconds.

In contrast, Mentzer et al reported a beneficial effect in an open label, single-center study in which the safety, tolerance, and efficacy of high doses of adenosine were assessed.[193] Like the previous studies, adenosine was added to cold blood cardioplegia in patients undergoing coronary artery bypass surgery. In this study, 61 patients were randomized to receive standard cold blood cardioplegia or cold blood cardioplegia containing 1 of 5 adenosine doses (100 μM, 500 μM, 1 mM, 2 mM, and 2 mM with a preischemic infusion of 140 μg/kg/min). Invasive and noninvasive studies of myocardial function were obtained at 1, 2, 4, 8, 16, and 24 hours postbypass. This included the recording of inotropic utilization rates for the postoperative treatment of low cardiac output. Blood samples were collected before and after the first, second, and last dose of cardioplegia, as well as at 1 hour and 24 hours after cessation of cardiopulmonary bypass, for the measurement of nucleoside levels. These investigators found that high-dose adenosine treatment was associated with a 249-fold increase in the plasma adenosine concentration and a 69-fold increase in the combined levels of adenosine and its degradation products, inosine and hypoxanthine. The high-dose adenosine and associated high plasma levels of adenosine were associated with a reduction in postbypass inotropic drug utilization and improved regional wall motion and global function measured by transthoracic echocardiography.

Using a similar protocol, Mentzer et al examined the effects of high-dose adenosine treatment in 253 patients randomized to one of three treatment arms.[194] This was a double-blind, placebo-controlled multicenter trial. The three cohorts consisted of those patients who were administered intraoperative cold blood cardioplegia, those administered cold blood cardioplegia containing 500 μM adenosine, and those receiving cold blood cardioplegia containing 2 mM adenosine. Patients receiving the adenosine cardioplegia were also given an infusion of adenosine (200 μg/kg/min) 10 minutes before and 15 minutes after removal of the aortic cross-clamp. Invasive and noninvasive measurements of ventricular performance were obtained before, during, and after surgery. The results of this study revealed a trend toward a decrease in high-dose inotropic agent utilization rates and a lower incidence of myocardial infarction. A composite outcome analysis showed that patients who received the high-dose adenosine were less likely to experience one of five adverse events: high-dose dopamine use, epinephrine use, insertion of an intra-aortic balloon pump, myocardial infarction, or death. A major limitation of this study was the failure to demonstrate a reduction in dopamine use or overall inotropic use, the two primary end points of the study. Another factor was the relatively low adverse event rates of myocardial infarction and death, namely 5.1% and 3.6%.

In summary, there is preclinical and clinical evidence that adenosine is a cardioprotective agent. Its clinical use, however, is somewhat limited since large doses are associated with marked hypotension. Although this can be easily managed while the patient is on cardiopulmonary bypass, it would be preferable to use a more selective A_1 receptor agonist that would confer protection without peripheral vasodilation. The administration of such an agent prior to surgery (much in the same way that late-phase preconditioning has a salutary effect in limiting myocardial stunning, apoptosis, and infarction 24 hours later) could result in a reduction in the current rates of postoperative stunning and infarction, and represent a significant advance in the field of myocardial protection.

Sodium/Hydrogen Exchange Inhibition

The sodium hydrogen exchangers (NHEs) are a family of membrane proteins that are involved in the transport of hydrogen ions in exchange for sodium ions. The driving force behind the exchange is the transmembrane Na^+ gradient, the Ca^{2+} gradient, and the membrane potential.[195,196] The gradient is regulated by the intracellular pH through interaction of H^+, with a sensor site on the exchanger protein (Fig. 14-5). To date, seven NHEs have been identified and are designated as NHE-1 through NHE-7.[197–200] In contrast to the NHE-1 and NHE-6 isoforms, which are ubiquitously distributed, the NHE-2 and NHE-5 isoforms have a much more limited expression. All isoforms except NHE-6 and NHE-7, which are located intracellularly, are localized primarily in the sarcolemmal membrane. In the mammalian heart the NHE-1 is the predominant isoform, although NHE-6 has been identified in the heart as well.[197–199] While the exact role the exchanger plays in the normal excitation-contraction coupling process has yet to be determined, there is increasing evidence that these proteins perform an important role in many pathophysiological conditions. They have been implicated in the etiology of arrhythmias, stunning, apoptosis, necrosis associated with acute myocardial ischemia/reperfusion injury, and postinfarction ventricular remodeling and heart failure.[201,202]

One of the primary mechanisms of injury that all these conditions have in common is the deleterious effect of an excess accumulation of intracellular calcium.[203] Normally, sodium-hydrogen (Na^+/H^+) exchange plays an important role in regulating cardiac myocyte physiology. The influx of extracellular Na^+ via its concentration gradient is coupled to the efflux of H^+, helping to maintain the intracellular pH. The Na^+/Ca^{2+} exchanger uses the normal Na^+ gradient to extrude Ca^{2+} in order to maintain normal intracellular Ca^{2+} homeostasis. However, during ischemia intracellular Na^+ accumulates due to decreased activity of the Na^+/K^+ ATPase, and increased production of H^+ due to anaerobic glycolysis. During the initial phase of reperfusion, the Na^+/H^+ exchanger is accelerated in an attempt to restore intracellular pH. This results in even more sodium and ultimately more Ca^{2+} accumulating intracellularly. As a consequence of increased intracellular sodium, the Na^+/Ca^{2+} exchanger operates in the reverse direction, resulting in a marked increase in the intracellular Ca^{2+} concentration (Ca^{2+} overload).

This Ca^{2+} overload can result in the activation of various enzyme systems and signaling pathways that over time can lead to cell contracture, membrane rupture, gap junction dysfunction, and cell death.[204] As a consequence of this deleterious process, numerous preclinical

A. non-ischemic

3Na+ 2K+ out NCX NHE Na+ pump in Ca2+ 3Na+ pHi ≈ 7.2

B. ischemic

Ca2+ Na+ out NCX NHE Na+ pump in Ca2+ Ca2+ 3Na+ Na+ Na+ H+ H+ Ca2+ Ca2+ Na+ Na+ H+ H+ H+ Ca2+ Ca2+ Ca2+ Na+ Na+ Na+ H+ H+ pHi ≈ 6.4

C. ischemic + NHE inhibitor

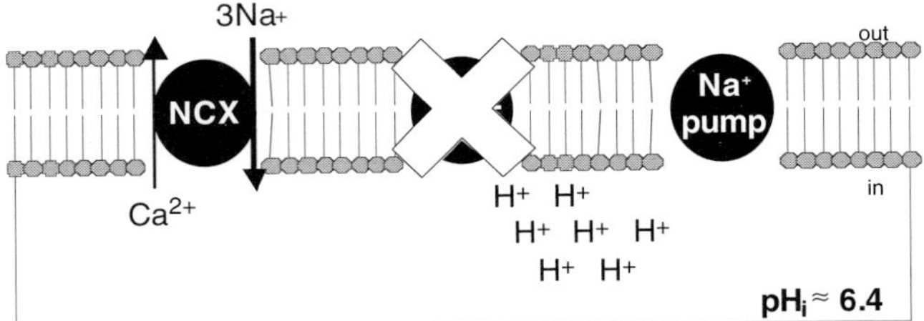

FIGURE 14–5 Potential mechanism through which Na^+/H^+ exchanger (NHE) inhibition preserves intracellular ion homeostasis and thereby myocardial integrity and function after ischemia and reperfusion. (A) Under basal conditions, NHE is relatively quiescent, the Na^+/K^+ ATPase (Na^+ pump) utilizes ATP to extrude Na^+, and the bidirectional Na^+/Ca^{2+} exchanger (NCX) works predominantly in forward (Ca^{2+} efflux) mode. (B) During ischemia, NHE becomes activated in response to intracellular acidosis and possibly by other NHE-stimulatory factors. The resulting influx of Na^+, occurring in the presence of ischemia-induced attenuation of Na^+ pump activity, causes the intracellular accumulation of Na^+. Such a rise in the intracellular Na^+ concentration during ischemia alters the reversal potential of the NCX in a manner that inhibits its operation in forward mode but favors its operation in reverse (Ca^{2+} influx) mode, thus producing intracellular Ca^{2+} accumulation (Ca^{2+} overload) during both ischemia and subsequent reperfusion. (C) NHE inhibitors are likely to afford a cardioprotective effect during ischemia and reperfusion by inhibiting this sequence at an early stage, through the limitation of Na^+ influx during ischemia. Note that the illustration has been simplified for clarity, and that mechanisms other than NHE activity are also likely to contribute to the intracellular accumulation of Na^+ and consequently Ca^{2+} during ischemia and reperfusion. *(Reproduced with permission from the American College of Cardiology Foundation, from Avkiran M, Marber MS: Na^+/H^+ exchange inhibitors for cardioprotective therapy: progress, problems and prospects. J Am Coll Cardiol 2002; 39:749.)*

studies have been performed to determine whether interruption of the process that leads to calcium overload can prevent ischemia/reperfusion injury. This has involved the use of agents with NHE inhibitor properties such as amiloride and its 5-amino-substituted derivatives, and the more novel benzoylguanidine derivatives: cariporide (HOE-642), eniporide (EMD-96785), and zoniporide (CP-597, 396).[197,202,205,206]

One of the first studies to suggest that inhibition of the Na^+-H^+ exchange mechanism might exert a beneficial effect on postischemic recovery of ventricular function was reported by Karmazyn in 1988.[207] Using the isolated rat heart subjected to low-flow ischemia, this investigator reported that the compound amiloride improved contractile recovery and decreased creatine kinase and 6-ketoprostaglandin $F_{1\alpha}$ release. In addition to NHE inhibition, however, the compound was known to exhibit numerous other pharmacologic properties. Using the more selective NHI inhibitor HOE-694, du Toit and Opie[208] found that this agent, given either prior to global ischemia or at the onset of reperfusion, attenuated myocardial stunning in the ejecting isolated perfused rat heart. Amiloride, at a 100-fold higher dose, was also protective, although only when administered prior to ischemia. When given at the time of reperfusion, both agents were reported to reduce the incidence of reperfusion arrhythmias. Likewise, Sack et al reported that HOE-694 given prior to ischemia and throughout reperfusion improved regional ventricular function and decreased the incidence of arrhythmias following brief coronary occlusion in the intact pig.[209] Using a chronic porcine preparation, Klein et al demonstrated that pigs treated with HOE-694 10 minutes prior to 45 minutes of regional ischemia showed a significant decrease in infarct size and an improved regional systolic shortening after 24 hours of reperfusion.[210] When the drug was administered 10 minutes prior to reperfusion, less infarct size reduction and no improvement in function were observed. This is consistent with the report by Rohmann et al, who found that HOE-694 pretreatment reduced infarct size to a much greater extent when administered prior to reperfusion.[211] Over time, the beneficial effects of NHE inhibition have been corroborated by numerous other investigators in a variety of experimental animals and under numerous conditions (Fig. 14-6).[212–216] Thus, it is not surprising that there has been considerable interest in exploring the use of these agents in the clinical setting.

One of the first trials to examine the efficacy of using an NHE inhibitor was reported by Rupprecht et al.[217] In this study, the NHE inhibitor cariporide was administered to patients within 6 hours after the onset of symptoms of an anterior myocardial infarction. One hundred patients were randomized to receive placebo or cariporide prior to reperfusion therapy. Cardiac enzymes were determined in blood samples obtained at predetermined times after reperfusion. Left ventricular function was ascertained by contrast ventriculography before treatment and 3 weeks after treatment.

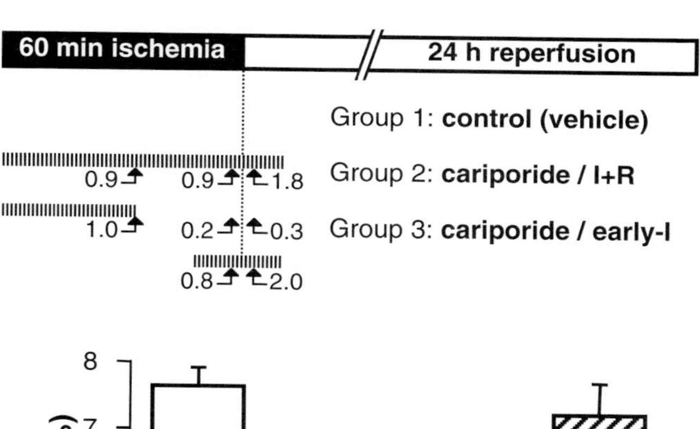

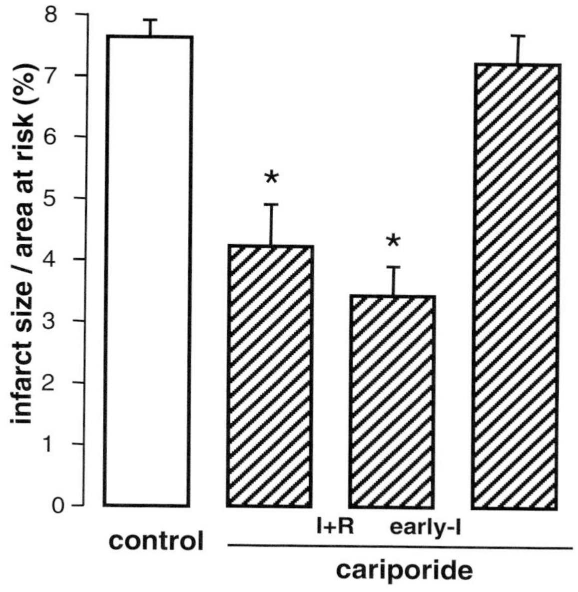

FIGURE 14–6 Effects on infarct size of intracoronary infusion of the Na^+/H^+ exchanger (NHE) inhibitor cariporide during various periods, in pig hearts subjected to 60 min of regional low-flow ischemia and 24 h of reperfusion. Infarct size was measured at the end of 24 h of reperfusion by both histochemical and histologic methods. The top panel illustrates the experimental protocol, with the vertically hatched bars indicating the periods of cariporide infusion and the arrows showing the coronary sinus cariporide concentrations (in μmol/L) after 30 min of ischemia, immediately before reperfusion and immediately after reperfusion, in the various study groups. Note that a minimum concentration of approximately 1 μmol/L cariporide is required for effective inhibition of sarcolemmal NHE activity in cardiac ventricular myocytes. As shown, infarct size was significantly limited by the intracoronary infusion of cariporide during the first 30 min of ischemia or throughout the entire 60 min of ischemia plus the first 10 min of reperfusion. In contrast, infusion of cariporide during the last 15 min of ischemia plus the first 10 min of reperfusion provided no benefit, even though the coronary sinus cariporide concentrations at the end of ischemia and the beginning of reperfusion were sufficient to inhibit NHE activity. Thus, NHE activity during early ischemia, rather than that during late ischemia and early reperfusion, appears to be the principal determinant of the extent of myocardial infarction. I = ischemia; R = reperfusion, $^*p < .05$ versus control. The figure is based on data from Klein et al[210] (*Reproduced with permission from the American College of Cardiology Foundation, from Avkiran M, Marber MS: Na^+/H^+ exchange inhibitors for cardioprotective therapy: progress, problems and prospects. J Am Coll Cardiol 2002; 39:750.*)

In the cariporide group of patients, the ejection fraction was greater, the resolution of regional left ventricular wall motion abnormalities tended to occur earlier, and the cumulative release of CK-MB was less. These findings supported the contention that NHE inhibition is beneficial to patients at risk of sustaining a reperfusion injury.

In a subsequent study performed by Zeymer et al, the salutary effects of NHE inhibitor therapy were not confirmed.[218] In the ESCAMI (Evaluation of the Safety and Cardioprotective Effects of Eniporide in Acute Myocardial Infarction) trial, 433 patients with either an anterior or inferior myocardial infarction were studied. Patients were randomized to receive placebo or three different doses (low, intermediate, or high) of eniporide. Treatment was initiated in the form of a 10-minute infusion prior to the start of coronary angioplasty or within 15 minutes after the start of thrombolytic therapy. The initial findings indicated a reduction in cumulative cardiac enzyme release of approximately 15% and 30% with the low- and intermediate-dose eniporide therapies, respectively. There was, however, no observable effect at the highest dose studied. Consequently, 978 additional patients were recruited to the placebo, low-dose, and intermediate-dose eniporide groups. The results of this second phase (the extended study), however, failed to substantiate the positive findings of the first stage of the trial; i.e., there was no significant reduction in cardiac enzyme release by eniporide.[218] This led to the conclusion that NHE inhibition was not effective in attenuating reperfusion injury.

Curiously, both of these studies were undertaken with the assumption that the beneficial effect of NHE inhibition would be realized during late ischemia or early reperfusion, despite considerable preclinical data that indicated that the salutary effect was realized during early ischemia. Despite these observations, a third clinical trial (GUARDIAN) was initiated to determine effective dosing and clinical efficacy in the heterogeneous group of patients experiencing variable degrees of ischemia.[203] Specifically, 11,590 patients with unstable angina and non–ST elevation myocardial infarction who were undergoing high-risk percutaneous and surgical revascularization were randomized to receive a placebo, and one of three doses of cariporide for the period of risk. The results of this study also indicate that NHE inhibition failed to reduce the incidence of myocardial infarction and death. In a subgroup analysis, however, there did appear to be a salutary effect among patients undergoing coronary artery bypass surgery. In this cohort, there was a 25% risk reduction for myocardial infarction or death for 6 months after surgery. Thus, while the GUARDIAN trial failed to show a clinical benefit of NHE inhibition in all patients studied, the findings suggested that NHE inhibition was beneficial when administered to patients undergoing cardiac surgery. Whether NHE inhibition is an effective form of protection against myocardial stunning, apoptosis, infarction, ventricular remodeling, and heart failure in humans during heart surgery awaits further study.

Nitric Oxide

There is increasing evidence that the signaling molecule nitric oxide (NO) plays an important role in modulating the heart's tolerance to ischemia. However, the combination of the short half-life of NO, the multiple redox states in which it can exist, the subcellular compartmentalization of NOS isoforms, and the multiple targets of its actions has hindered the determination of the specific role this molecule plays in modulating ischemia/reperfusion injury. This explains, in part, why NO and related reactive nitrogen species have been reported to both exacerbate injury and exert a cardioprotective effect.[219] For the most part, however, studies performed using in vivo preparations indicate that the administration of NO donors reduces infarct size.[219] There are also reports that the infusion of NOS inhibitors during reperfusion exacerbates ischemia/reperfusion injury.[220,221] These reports are consistent with evidence that NO modulates coronary blood flow, and that the molecule can reduce neutrophil adherence to endothelium and inhibit platelet aggregation. There is also evidence that NO produced during reperfusion may scavenge the oxygen free radical superoxide (O_2^-), an effect observed in oxidant stressed cells exposed to constant low levels (1-2 μM) of NO. [222,223]

Additional support for the beneficial effects of NO is derived from studies of late-phase ischemic preconditioning. Several reports (in multiple species) indicate that delayed protection against infarction induced by ischemic and pharmacologic preconditioning is blocked by various NOS inhibitors.[224–229] Conversely, delayed preconditioning can be induced by NO donors.[226,230] There are also reports of increased iNOS upregulation following delayed ischemic and pharmacologic preconditioning, and that this protection is ablated in iNOS knockout mice.[181,185,186,231,232] Late-phase preconditioning against myocardial stunning has also been reported to be induced by nitroglycerin and the NO donor SNAP.[233] If NO does play a role in mediating late-phase preconditioning, it is still not known whether this protection is a direct result of increased NO production during prolonged ischemia/reperfusion or whether a transient increase in NO production during the preconditioning period triggers the upregulation of one or more endogenous protective proteins.

Although acute ischemic preconditioning has cardioprotective effects similar to delayed preconditioning and may have some common signal transduction mechanisms, there is much less evidence supporting NO as a trigger or mediator of this form of preconditioning. While there are reports that transient infusions of NO donors mimic acute ischemic preconditioning, there are also reports in multiple species that NOS inhibitors do not block early-phase conditioning.[233–238] Moreover, as in the studies on late-phase preconditioning, there have been very few, if any, studies in which NO levels have actually been measured.

With respect to clinical studies, there is only a modest amount of evidence that the NO mechanism can be manipulated to confer myocardial protection in humans. Leesar et al reported that the infusion of nitroglycerin (an NO donor) 24 hours prior to angioplasty mimicked the protection associated with the first balloon inflation in the control group in terms of ST-segment shifts, regional wall motion abnormalities, and chest pain scores.[239] Zhang and Galinanes studied the effects of arginine (a precursor to NO) on human myocardial specimens obtained from right atrial appendages of patients undergoing elective coronary artery bypass graft surgery.[240] The tissues were subjected to 120 minutes of simulated ischemia followed by 120 minutes of reoxygenation. Ischemic injury was assessed by measuring the leakage of lactate dehydrogenase into the incubation medium and the capacity of the tissue to reduce MTT [3-(4-dimethylthiazol-yl)-2,5-diphenyltetrazolium bromide] to a formazan product. In this study, L-arginine (a precursor of NO) decreased LDH leakage but had no effect on MTT reduction or oxygen consumption. However, the effect of arginine was not reversed by L-NAME (an NO synthase inhibitor), nor was it mimicked by S-nitroso-N-acetylpenicillamine (an NO donor). These data suggested that L-arginine was effective, but provided only a modest degree of protection against simulated ischemia/reperfusion injury in human myocardial atria tissue.

In a more relevant setting, Carrier et al reported that an L-arginine-enriched blood cardioplegia solution provided superior protection in 200 patients undergoing coronary artery bypass surgery.[241] This was a prospective, randomized, double-blind clinical trial that compared standard blood cardioplegia to an L-arginine-enriched solution. The results indicated that the use of the arginine-supplemented blood cardioplegic solution was associated with a reduction in the release of a biochemical marker (troponin T) of myocardial damage.

All of these studies are limited, however, because the demonstration of efficacy was dependent on the measurement of surrogate markers of injury and sample sizes were small. Additional preclinical studies and clinical trials are needed to demonstrate whether NO plays an important role in protecting the ischemic heart. As noted by Wang and colleagues, the potential cytoprotective role of iNOS-derived NO needs to be reconciled with the known detrimental actions associated with iNOS in the setting of septic shock, organ rejection, inflammation, autoimmune diseases, and ischemic brain injury.[186]

MYOCARDIAL PROTECTION DURING BEATING HEART SURGERY

As many as 10% to 15% of the patients in the United States who undergo coronary artery bypass surgery have the operation performed on the beating heart. The acceptance of this technique is due, in part, to the development and availability of better shunt appliances and mechanical stabilization devices, as well as the demonstration of satisfactory outcomes.[242] The infarction rate among patients undergoing beating heart coronary artery surgery (OPCAB) has been reported to range between 0% and 5%, while on-pump surgery ranges between 2% and 6%.[243–245] If sensitive myocardial marker proteins are used to detect myocardial necrosis, it is possible that cell necrosis may be less in OPCAB patients. The fact that any necrosis occurs suggests that even OPCAB patients may be susceptible to ischemia/reperfusion injury. For the most part, however, little is known about the indications for and long-term outcomes of beating heart surgery. Likewise, there is a paucity of data regarding the extent to which the myocardium is reversibly or irreversibly damaged after OPCAB surgery. This is due, in part, to the fact that the primary focus among beating heart advocates has been the demonstration of feasibility, safety, and cost-effectiveness.

In an effort to elucidate the impact of regional myocardial ischemia/reperfusion injury on regional myocardial function and metabolism during OPCAB surgery, Dapunt et al studied the effects of performing a left internal mammary artery to left anterior coronary artery (LAD) anastomosis on the beating heart in an in vivo juvenile porcine heart preparation.[246] The anastomosis was performed during either a 15-minute LAD occlusion or 15-minute intra–LAD shunt insertion to maintain blood supply to the myocardium distal to the anastomosis. Functional and biochemical data were obtained at baseline, 15 minutes after LAD occlusion or shunt insertion, and after 30 minutes of reperfusion. In both groups, the regional left ventricular wall motion score index (WMSI) (using epimyocardial echocardiography) was similar at 15 minutes after occlusion or shunt insertion. After 30 minutes of reperfusion, however, both global and regional WMSI were markedly better in the shunt insertion group compared to the occlusion group. Myocardial adenine nucleotide glycogen contents were significantly lower in the occlusion group, while HSP 70 expression was greater. The major limitations of this study include the following: (1) only healthy pig hearts were used, (2) only one anastomosis was performed, (3) the investigators did not assess the impact of the surgery on cardiac enzyme release, and (4) the duration of reperfusion was limited. While the salutary effect of shunting is noteworthy, equally important were the findings that the hearts in the nonshunted animals were susceptible to ischemia/reperfusion injury. This suggests that patients with multivessel disease and poor ventricular function who undergo OPCABG might benefit from additional forms of myocardial protection.

In an effort to clarify the incidence of perioperative myocardial injury as determined by myocardial marker protein release, Bonatti et al studied 15 consecutive patients undergoing beating heart surgery.[247] A stabilizing device was used along with the short-acting beta blocker esmolol to reduce heart rate and myocardial contractility. Target vessels were snared using silicone tube–armed prolene sutures placed around a bolster of epicardial and myocardial tissue. Prior to performing each anastomosis, the vessel was occluded for 5 minutes and reperfused for another 5 minutes. Intraoperative and postoperative assessments included echocardiography, ECG monitoring, and the measurement of creatine kinase and cardiac troponin I. The results of this study revealed that 9 of 14 surviving patients showed signs of transient myocardial ischemia on ECG, echocardiography, or both. This was observed only intraoperatively during target vessel occlusion in 3 patients, and postoperatively in 3 patients. Three other patients exhibited reversible signs of ischemia both intraoperatively and postoperatively. The Tn I level was elevated in 4 of the 9 patients showing ischemia, and the CK-MB mass concentration was elevated in 5. There was one death related to severe myocardial ischemia with infarction confirmed on autopsy. The overall conclusion was that despite the use of an agent to reduce heart rate and contractility, subclinical myocardial injury is a common event in coronary artery surgery on the beating heart.

In contrast, Koh et al reported their findings in a prospective observational study that compared 18 patients undergoing coronary grafting on the beating heart with 8 patients undergoing grafting with cardiopulmonary bypass.[248] In the beating heart surgery cohort, pharmacologic agents were not used to slow the heart rate. These investigators found that the intraoperative and serial venous cardiac troponin T concentrations were lower in the beating heart surgery group. Neither group required inotropic support or pacing, and none of the patients sustained a perioperative myocardial infarct as determined by ECG. The conclusion of these investigators was that their results provided strong evidence that a lower degree of myocardial injury is associated with beating heart coronary surgery. Again, it is important to note that some degree of myocyte injury was observed regardless of whether the surgery was performed on or off pump.

To determine if the reversible injury that occurs during OPCAB surgery can be reduced using pharmacologic agents, Hendrikx et al studied the phenomenon in an in vivo, stunning only, sheep preparation.[249] Animals were randomized to one of four groups. Group I received no treatment, Group II was administered the NHE inhibitor cariporide, Group III was given aprotinin, and Group IV was treated with a combination of cariporide and aprotinin. Each animal was then subjected to 20 minutes of regional ischemia by temporarily occluding the first lateral branch of the circumflex artery. This was followed by 1 hour of reperfusion. These investigators found that compared to the control group, both cariporide and aprotinin treatments, and especially the combination of the two, were associated with a marked attenuation of stunning. Thus, there is some preclinical evidence that patients undergoing beating heart surgery could benefit from pharmacologic pretreatment with selected cardioprotective agents.

SUMMARY

While considerable progress has been made in the field of myocardial protection, the ideal solution, technique, or delivery method has yet to be identified. This is due, in part, to our increasing awareness of the complexity of ischemia/reperfusion injury, and the recognition that the definition of ideal protection is no longer limited to the time that the patient is in the operating room. As long as the incidence of myocardial stunning ranges from 20% to 80%, postischemic ventricular dysfunction from 3% to 7%, severe dysfunction in high-risk patients from 15% to 20%, and non-Q-wave infarction and Q-wave infarction from 5% to 7%, there is clearly a need to develop new therapeutic strategies to protect the heart during heart surgery. This need is even greater when one considers that long-term survival after heart operations is determined, in part, by adequate myocardial protection during the operation itself.

REFERENCES

1. Mangano DT: Cardiovascular morbidity and CABG surgery—a perspective: epidemiology, costs, and potential therapeutic solutions. *J Card Surg* 1995; 10:366.
2. Bigelow WG, Lindsay WK, Greenwood WF: Hypothermia: its possible role in cardiac surgery: an investigation of factors governing survival in dogs at low body temperatures. *Ann Surg* 1950; 132:849.
3. Melrose DG, Dreyer B, Bentall HH, et al: Preliminary communication: elective cardiac arrest. *Lancet* 1955; 2:21.
4. Tyers GF, Hughes HC, Todd GJ, et al: Protection from ischemic cardiac arrest by coronary perfusion with cold Ringer's lactate solution. *J Thorac Cardiovasc Surg* 1974; 67:411.
5. Colapinto ND, Silver MD: Prosthetic heart valve replacement: causes of early postoperative death. *J Thorac Cardiovasc Surg* 1971; 61:938.
6. Iyengar SR, Ramchand S, Charrette EJ, et al: An experimental study of subendocardial hemorrhagic necrosis after anoxic cardiac arrest. *Ann Thorac Surg* 1972; 13:214.
7. Bretschneider HJ, Hübner G, Knoll D, et al: Myocardial resistance and tolerance to ischemia: physiological and biochemical basis. *J Cardiovasc Surg* 1975; 16:241.
8. Hearse DJ, Stewart DA, Braimbridge MV: Cellular protection during myocardial ischemia: the development and characterization of a procedure for the induction of reversible ischemic arrest. *Circulation* 1976; 54:193.
9. Braimbridge MV, Chayen J, Bitensky L, et al: Cold cardioplegia or continuous coronary perfusion? *J Thorac Cardiovasc Surg* 1977; 74:900.
10. Greenburg JJ, Edmunds LH, Brown RB: Myocardial metabolism and post arrest function in the cold and chemically arrested heart. *Surgery* 1960; 48:31.
11. Webb WR, Dodds RP, Unal MO, et al: Suspended animation of the heart with metabolic inhibitors. *Ann Surg* 1966; 164:343.
12. Mundth ED, Sokol DM, Levine FH, et al: Evaluation of methods for myocardial protection during extended periods of aortic cross-clamping and hypoxic cardiac arrest. *Bull Soc Intern Chir* 1970; 29:227.
13. Gay WA, Ebert PA: Functional, metabolic and morphologic effects of potassium-induced cardioplegia. *Surgery* 1973; 74:284.

14. Roe BB, Hutchinson JC, Fishman NH, et al: Myocardial protection with cold, ischemic, potassium-induced cardioplegia. *J Thorac Cardiovasc Surg* 1977; 73:366.
15. Tyers GF, Manley NJ, Williams EH, et al: Preliminary clinical experience with isotonic hypothermic potassium-induced arrest. *J Thorac Cardiovasc Surg* 1977; 74:674.
16. Buckberg GD: A proposed "solution" to the cardioplegia controversy. *J Thorac Cardiovasc Surg* 1979; 77:803.
17. Follette DM, Mulder DG, Maloney JV, et al: Advantages of blood cardioplegia over continuous coronary perfusion or intermittent ischemia. *J Thorac Cardiovasc Surg* 1978; 76:604.
18. Abd-Elfattah AS, Ding M, Wechsler AS: Intermittent aortic crossclamping prevents cumulative adenosine triphosphate depletion, ventricular fibrillation, and dysfunction (stunning): is it preconditioning? *J Thorac Cardiovasc Surg* 1994; 110:328.
19. Anversa P, Cheng W, Liu Y, et al: Apoptosis and myocardial infarction. *Basic Res Cardiol* 1998; 93(suppl 3):8.
20. Gill C, Mestril R, Samali A: Losing heart: the role of apoptosis in heart disease—a novel therapeutic target? *FASEB J* 2002; 16:135.
21. Elsasser A, Suzuki K, Lorenz-Meyer S, et al: The role of apoptosis in myocardial ischemia: a critical appraisal. *Basic Res Cardiol* 2001; 96:219.
22. Klatte K, Chaitman BR, Theroux P, et al: Increased mortality after coronary artery bypass graft surgery is associated with increased levels of postoperative creatine kinase-myocardial band isoenzyme release. *J Am Coll Cardiol* 2001; 38:1070.
23. Bolli R, Marban E: Molecular and cellular mechanisms of myocardial stunning. *Physiol Rev* 1999; 79:609.
24. Park JL, Lucchesi BR: Mechanisms of myocardial reperfusion injury. *Ann Thorac Surg* 1999; 68:1905.
25. Piper HM, Garcia-Dorado D: Prime causes of rapid cardiomyocyte death during reperfusion. *Ann Thorac Surg* 1999; 68:1913.
26. Beckman JS, Koppenol WH: Nitric oxide, superoxide, and peroxynitrite: the good, the bad, and ugly. *Am J Physiol* 1996; 271:C1424.
27. Droge W: Free radicals in the physiological control of cell function. *Physiol Rev* 2002; 82:47.
28. Mallet RT, Bunger R: Energetic modulation of cardiac inotropism and sarcoplasmic reticular Ca^{2+} uptake. *Biochim Biophys Acta* 1994; 1224:22.
29. Lemasters JJ, Bond JM, Chacon E, et al: The pH paradox in ischemia-reperfusion injury to cardiac myocytes. *EXS* 1996; 76:99.
30. Eigel BN, Hadley RW: Antisense inhibition of Na+/Ca2+ exchange during anoxia/reoxygenation in ventricular myocytes. *Am J Physiol* 2001; 281:H2184.
31. Verbunt RJ, Van der Laarse A: Glutathione metabolism in nonischemic and postischemic rat hearts in response to an exogenous prooxidant. *Mol Cell Biochem* 1997; 167:127.
32. Vaage J, Antonelli M, Bufi M, et al: Exogenous reactive oxygen species deplete the isolated rat heart of antioxidants. *Free Radic Biol Med* 1997; 22:85.
33. Palace V, Kumar D, Hill MF, et al: Regional differences in nonenzymatic antioxidants in the heart under control and oxidative stress conditions. *J Mol Cell Cardiol* 1999; 31:193.
34. Sharikabad MN, Hagelin EM, Hagberg IA, et al: Effect of calcium on reactive oxygen species in isolated rat cardiomyocytes during hypoxia and reoxygenation. *J Mol Cell Cardiol* 2000; 32:441.
35. Gow AJ, Ischiropoulos H: Nitric oxide chemistry and cellular signaling. *J Cell Physiol* 2001; 187:277.
36. Espey MG, Miranda KM, Feelisch M, et al: Mechanisms of cell death governed by the balance between nitrosative and oxidative stress. *Ann N Y Acad Sci* 2000; 899:209.
37. Xia Y, Tsai AL, Berka V, et al: Superoxide generation from endothelial nitric-oxide synthase: a Ca^{2+}/calmodulin-dependent and tetrahyrobiopterin regulatory process. *J Biol Chem* 1998; 273:25804.
38. Gao WD, Atar D, Backx PH, et al: Relationship between intracellular calcium and contractile force in stunned myocardium: direct evidence for decreased myofilament Ca^{2+} responsiveness and altered diastolic function in intact ventricular muscle. *Circ Res* 1995; 76:1036.
39. Vasquez-Vivar J, Kalyanaraman B, Martasek P, et al: Superoxide generation by endothelial nitric oxide synthase: the influence of cofactors. *Proc Nat Acad Sci* 1998; 95:9220.
40. Kositprapa C, Zhang B, Berger S, et al: Calpain-mediated proteolytic cleavage of troponin I induced by hypoxia or metabolic inhibition in cultured neonatal cardiomyocytes. *Mol Cell Biochem* 2000; 214:47.
41. Matsumura Y, Saeki E, Otsu K, et al: Intracellular calcium level required for calpain activation in a single myocardial cell. *J Mol Cell Cardiol* 2001; 33:1133.
42. Urthaler F, Wolkowicz PE, Digerness SB, et al: MDL-28170, a membrane-permeant calpain inhibitor, attenuates stunning and PKC epsilon proteolysis in reperfused ferret hearts. *Cardiovasc Res* 1997; 35:60.
43. Tsuji T, Ohga Y, Yoshikawa Y, et al: Rat cardiac contractile dysfunction induced by Ca2+ overload: possible link to the proteolysis of alpha-fodrin. *Am J Physiol* 2001; 281:H1286.
44. Sekili S, McCay PB, Li XY, et al: Direct evidence that the hydroxyl radical plays a pathogenetic role in myocardial "stunning" in the conscious dog and demonstration that stunning can be markedly attenuated without subsequent adverse effects. *Circ Res* 1993; 73:705.
45. Obata T, Hosokawa H, Yamanaka Y: In vivo monitoring of norepinephrine and ·OH generation on myocardial ischemic injury by dialysis technique. *Am J Physiol* 1994; 266:H903.
46. Tang XL, Kaur H, Sun JZ, et al: Effect of the hydrophilic alphatocopherol analog MDL 74,405 on detection of hydroxyl radicals in stunned myocardium in dogs. *Am Heart J* 1995; 130:940.
47. Gorodetskaya EA, Kalenikova EI: Formation of hydroxyl radicals during myocardial reperfusion after experimental ischemia of different duration. *Bull Exp Biol Med* 2001; 131:533.
48. Vanden Hoek TL, Shao Z, Li C, et al: Mitochondrial electron transport can become a significant source of oxidative injury in cardiomyocytes. *J Mol Cell Cardiol* 1997; 29:2441.
49. Narayan P, Kilpatrick EL, Mentzer RM, et al: Adenosine A_1 receptor activation reduces reactive oxygen species and attenuates stunning in ventricular myocytes. *J Mol Cell Cardiol* 2001; 33:121.
50. Li Q, Bolli R, Qiu Y, et al: Gene therapy with extracellular superoxide dismutase attenuates myocardial stunning in conscious rabbits. *Circulation* 1998; 98:1438.
51. Sun JZ, Tang XL, Park SW, et al: Evidence for an essential role of reactive oxygen species in the genesis of late preconditioning against myocardial stunning in conscious pigs. *J Clin Invest* 1996; 97:562.
52. Xu KY, Zweier JL, Becker LC: Hydroxyl radical inhibits sarcoplasmic reticulum $Ca^{(2+)}$-ATPase function by direct attack on the ATP binding site. *Circ Res* 1997; 80:76.
53. Sulakhe PV, Vo XT, Phan TD, et al: Phosphorylation of inhibitory subunit of troponin and phospholamban in rat cardiomyocytes: modulation by exposure of cardiomyocytes to hydroxyl radicals and sulfhydryl group reagents. *Mol Cell Biochem* 1997; 175:98.
54. Kawakami M, Okabe E: Superoxide anion radical-triggered Ca2+ release from cardiac sarcoplasmic reticulum through ryanodine receptor Ca2+ channel. *Mol Pharmacol* 1998; 53:497.
55. Miller WP, McDonald KS, Moss RL: Onset of reduced Ca^{2+} sensitivity of tension during stunning in porcine myocardium. *J Mol Cell Cardiol* 1996; 28:689.
56. Josephson RA, Silverman HS, Lakatta EG, et al: Study of the mechanisms of hydrogen peroxide and hydroxyl free radical-induced

cellular injury and calcium overload in cardiac myocytes. *J Biol Chem* 1991; 266:2354.

57. Thomas GP, Sims SM, Cook MA, et al: Hydrogen peroxide-induced stimulation of L-type calcium current in guinea pig ventricular myocytes and its inhibition by adenosine A_1 receptor activation. *J Pharmacol Exp Ther* 1998; 286:1208.
58. Halestrap AP, Kerr PM, Javadov S, et al: Elucidating the molecular mechanism of the permeability transition pore and its role in reperfusion injury of the heart. *Biochim Biophys Acta* 1998; 1366:79.
59. Delcamp TJ, Dales C, Ralenkotter L, et al: Intramitochondrial [Ca^{2+}] and membrane potential in ventricular myocytes exposed to anoxia-reoxygenation. *Am J Physiol* 1998; 275:H484.
60. Miyata H, Lakatta EG, Stern MD, et al: Relation of mitochondrial and cytosolic free calcium to cardiac myocyte recovery after exposure to anoxia. *Circ Res* 1992; 71:605.
61. Tanaka M, Richard VJ, Murry CE, et al: Superoxide dismutase plus catalase therapy delays neither cell death nor the loss of the TTC reaction in experimental myocardial infarction in dogs. *J Mol Cell Cardiol* 1993; 25:367.
62. Watanabe BI, Premaratne S, Limm W, et al: High- and low-dose superoxide dismutase plus catalase does not reduce myocardial infarct size in a subhuman primate model. *Am Heart J* 1993; 126:840.
63. Gottlieb RA, Burleson KO, Kloner RA, et al: Reperfusion injury induces apoptosis in rabbit cardiomyocytes. *J Clin Invest* 1994; 94:1621.
64. Maulik N, Yoshida T, Das DK: Oxidative stress developed during the reperfusion of ischemic myocardium induces apoptosis. *Free Radic Biol Med* 1998; 24:869.
65. Freude B, Masters TN, Robicsek F, et al: Apoptosis is initiated by myocardial ischemia and executed during reperfusion. *J Mol Cell Cardiol* 2000; 32:197.
66. Kirshenbaum LA, de Moissac D: The bcl-2 gene product prevents programmed cell death of ventricular myocytes. *Circulation* 1997; 96:1580.
67. Kluck RM, Bossy-Wetzel E, Green DR, et al: The release of cytochrome c from mitochondria: a primary site for BCL-2 regulation of apoptosis. *Science* 1997; 275:1132.
68. Yang J, Liu X, Bhalla K, et al: Prevention of apoptosis by BCL-2: release of cytochrome c from mitochondria blocked. *Science* 1997; 275:1129.
69. Haunstetter A, Izumo S: Apoptosis: basic mechanisms and implications for cardiovascular disease. *Circ Res* 1998; 82:1111.
70. Martin SJ, Reutelingsperger CP, McGahon AJ, et al: Early redistribution of plasma membrane phosphatidylserine is a general feature of apoptosis regardless of the initiating stimulus: inhibition by over expression of Bcl-2 and Abl. *J Exp Med* 1995; 182:1545.
71. van Engeland M, Nieland LJ, Ramaekers FC, et al: Annexin V–affinity assay: a review on an apoptosis detection system based on phosphatidylserine exposure. *Cytometry* 1998; 31:1.
72. Maulik N, Kagan VE, Tyurin VA, et al: Redistribution of phosphatidylethanolamine and phosphatidylserine precedes reperfusion-induced apoptosis. *Am J Physiol* 1998; 274:H242.
73. Rucker-Martin C, Henaff M, Hatem SN, et al: Early redistribution of plasma membrane phosphatidylserine during apoptosis of adult rat ventricular myocytes *in vitro*. *Basic Res Cardiol* 1999; 94:171.
74. van Heerde WL, Robert-Offerman S, Dumont E, et al: Markers of apoptosis in cardiovascular tissues: focus on Annexin V. *Cardiovasc Res* 2000; 45:549.
75. Narayan P, Mentzer RM, Lasley RD: Annexin V staining following reperfusion detects cardiomyocytes with unique properties. *Am J Physiol* 2001; 281:H1931.
76. Hammill AK, Uhr JW, Scheuermann RH: Annexin V staining due to loss of membrane asymmetry can be reversible and precede commitment to apoptotic death. *Exp Cell Res* 1999; 251:16.
77. Maiese K, Vincent AM: Membrane asymmetry and DNA degradation: functionally distinct determinants of neuronal programmed cell death. *J Neurosci Res* 2000; 59:568.
78. Bonchek LI, Burlingame MW, Vazales BE, et al: Applicability of non-cardioplegic coronary bypass to high-risk patients: selection of patients, technique, and clinical experience in 3000 patients. *J Thorac Cardiovasc Surg* 1992; 103:230.
79. Taggart DP, Bhusari S, Hooper J, et al: Intermittent ischemic arrest in coronary artery surgery: coming full circle? *Br Heart J* 1994; 72:136.
80. Casthely PA, Shah C, Mekhijian H, et al: Left ventricular diastolic function after coronary bypass grafting: a correlative study with three different myocardial protection techniques. *J Thorac Cardiovasc Surg* 1997; 114:254.
81. Cohen AS, Hadjinikolaou L, McColl A, et al: Lipid peroxidation antioxidant status and troponin-T following cardiopulmonary bypass: a comparison between intermittent crossclamp with fibrillation and crystalloid cardioplegia. *Eur J Cardiothorac Surg* 1997; 12:248.
82. Raco L, Mills E, Millner RJ: Isolated myocardial revascularization with intermittent aortic cross-clamping: experience with 800 cases. *Ann Thorac Surg* 2002;73:1436.
83. Akins CW: Noncardioplegic myocardial preservation for coronary revascularization. *J Thorac Cardiovasc Surg* 1984; 88:174.
84. Velez DA, Morris CD, Budde JM, et al: All-blood (miniplegia) versus dilute cardioplegia in experimental surgical revascularization of evolving infarction. *Circulation* 2001; 104:I296.
85. Rousou JA, Engelman RM, Breyer RH, et al: The effect of temperature and hematocrit level of oxygenated cardioplegic solutions on myocardial preservation. *J Thorac Cardiovasc Surg* 1988; 95:625.
86. Rosenkranz ER, Vinten-Johansen J, Buckberg GD, et al: Benefits of normothermic induction of blood cardioplegia in energy-depleted hearts, with maintenance of arrest by multidose cold blood cardioplegic infusions. *J Thorac Cardiovasc Surg* 1982; 84:667.
87. Teoh KH, Christakis GT, Weisel RD, et al: Accelerated myocardial metabolic recovery with terminal warm blood cardioplegia. *J Thorac Cardiovasc Surg* 1986; 91:888.
88. Lichtenstein SV, Ashe KA, EL Dalati H, et al: Warm heart surgery. *J Thorac Cardiovasc Surg* 1991; 101:269.
89. Salerno TA, Houck JP, Barrozo CA, et al: Retrograde continuous warm blood cardioplegia: a new concept in myocardial protection. *Ann Thorac Surg* 1991; 51:245.
90. Martin TD, Craver JM, Gott JP, et al: Prospective, randomized trial of retrograde warm blood cardioplegia: myocardial benefit and neurologic threat. *Ann Thorac Surg* 1994; 57:298.
91. Hayashida N, Ikonomides JS, Weisel RD, et al: The optimal cardioplegic temperature. *Ann Thorac Surg* 1994; 58:961.
92. Hayashida N, Isomura T, Sato T, et al: Minimally diluted tepid blood cardioplegia. *Ann Thorac Surg* 1998; 65:615.
93. Pratt FH. The nutrition of the heart through the vessels of Thebesius and the coronary veins. *Am J Physiol* 1898; 1:86.
94. Lillehei CW, Dewall RA, Gott VL, et al: The direct vision correction of calcification of calcific aortic stenosis by means of pump-oxygenator and retrograde coronary sinus perfusion. *Dis Chest* 1965; 30:123.
95. Ihnken K, Morita K, Buckberg GD, et al: The safety of simultaneous arterial and coronary sinus perfusion: experimental background and initial clinical results. *J Card Surg* 1994; 9:15.
96. Cohen G, Borger MA, Weisel RD, et al: Intraoperative myocardial protection: current trends and future perspectives. *Ann Thorac Surg* 1999; 68:1995.
97. Murry CE, Jennings RB, Reimer KA: Preconditioning with ischemia: a delay of lethal cell injury in ischemic myocardium. *Circulation* 1986; 74:1124.
98. Sun JZ, Tang XL, Knowlton AA, et al: Late preconditioning against myocardial stunning: an endogenous protective mechanism that

confers resistance to postischemic dysfunction 24 h after brief ischemia in conscious pigs. *J Clin Invest* 1995; 95:388.

99. Bolli R: The early and late phases of preconditioning against myocardial stunning and the essential role of oxyradicals in the late phase: an overview. *Basic Res Cardiol* 91:57, 1996.
100. Shiki K, Hearse DJ: Preconditioning of the ischemic myocardium: reperfusion-induced arrhythmias. *Am J Physiol* 1987; 253:H1470.
101. Lasley RD, Konyn PJ, Hegge JO, et al: The effects of ischemic and adenosine preconditioning on interstitial fluid adenosine and myocardial infarct size. *Am J Physiol* 1995; 269:H1460.
102. Jahania MS, Lasley RD, Mentzer RM: Ischemic preconditioning does not acutely improve load-insensitive parameters of contractility in in vivo stunned porcine myocardium. *J Thorac Cardiovasc Surg* 1999; 117:810.
103. Kloner RA, Jennings RB: Consequences of brief ischemia: stunning, preconditioning, and their clinical implications, part 2. *Circulation* 2001; 104:3158.
104. Cohen MV, Baines CP, Downey JM: Ischemic preconditioning: from adenosine receptor of KATP channel. *Ann Rev Physiol* 2000; 62:79.
105. Yellon DM, Baxter GF, Garcia-Dorado D, et al: Ischaemic preconditioning: present position and future directions. *Cardiovasc Res* 1998; 37:21.
106. Yellon DM, Dana A: The preconditioning phenomenon: a tool for the scientist or a clinical reality? *Circ Res* 2000; 87:543.
107. Bolli R: The late phase of preconditioning. *Circ Res* 2000; 87:972.
108. Schulz R, Cohen MV, Behrends M, et al: Signal transduction of ischemic preconditioning. *Cardiovasc Res* 2001; 52:181.
109. Guo Y, Bao W, Wu WJ, et al: Evidence for an essential role of cyclooxygenase-2 as a mediator of the late phase of ischemic preconditioning in mice. *Basic Res Cardiol* 2000; 95:479.
110. Dana A, Skarli M, Papakrivopoulou J, et al: Adenosine A(1) receptor induced delayed preconditioning in rabbits: induction of p 38 mitogen-activated protein kinase activation and Hsp27 phosphorylation via a tyrosine kinase- and protein kinase C-dependent mechanism. *Circ Res* 2000; 86:989.
111. Wang Y, Guo Y, Zhang SX, et al: Ischemic preconditioning upregulates inducible nitric oxide synthase in cardiac myocyte. *J Mol Cell Cardiol* 2002; 34:5.
112. Kloner RA, Shook T, Przyklenk K, et al: Previous angina alters in-hospital outcome in TIMI 4: a clinical correlate to preconditioning? *Circulation* 1995; 91:37.
113. Anzai T, Yoshikawa T, Asakura Y, et al: Preinfarction angina as a major predictor of left ventricular function and long-term prognosis after a first Q wave myocardial infarction. *J Am Coll Cardiol* 1995; 26:319.
114. Ottani F, Galvani M, Ferrini D, et al: Prodromal angina limits infarct size: a role for ischemic preconditioning. *Circulation* 1995; 91:291.
115. Tamura K, Tsuji H, Nishiue T, et al: Association of preceding angina with in-hospital life-threatening ventricular tachyarrhythmias and late potentials in patients with a first acute myocardial infarction. *Am Heart J* 1997; 133:297.
116. Ishihara M, Sato H, Tateishi H, et al: Implications of prodromal angina pectoris in anterior wall acute myocardial infarction: acute angiographic findings and long-term prognosis. *J Am Coll Cardiol* 1997; 30:970.
117. Kloner RA, Shook T, Antman EM, et al: Prospective temporal analysis of the onset of preinfarction angina versus outcome: an ancillary study in TIMI-9B. *Circulation* 1998; 97:1042.
118. Dana A, Yellon DM: Cardioprotection by pre-infarct angina: is it ischaemic preconditioning? *Eur Heart J* 1998; 19:367.
119. Deutsch E, Berger M, Kussmaul WG, et al: Adaptation to ischemia during percutaneous transluminal coronary angioplasty: clinical, hemodynamic, and metabolic features. *Circulation* 1990; 82:2044.
120. Cribier B, Korsatz L, Koning R, et al: Improved myocardial ischemic response and enhanced collateral circulation with long repetitive coronary occlusion during angioplasty: a prospective study. *J Am Coll Cardiol* 1992; 20:578.
121. Eltchaninoff H, Cribier B, Tron C, et al: Adaptation to myocardial ischemia during coronary angioplasty demonstrated by clinical, electrocardiographic, echocardiographic, and metabolic parameters. *Am Heart J* 1997; 133:490.
122. Okishige K, Yamashita K, Yoshinaga H, et al: Electrophysiologic effects of ischemic preconditioning on QT dispersion during coronary angioplasty. *J Am Coll Cardiol* 1996; 28:70.
123. Airaksinen KE, Huikuri HV: Antiarrhythmic effect of repeated coronary occlusion during balloon angioplasty. *J Am Coll Cardiol* 1997; 29;1035.
124. Laskey WK: Beneficial impact of preconditioning during PTCA on creatine kinase release. *Circulation* 1999; 99:2085.
125. Tomai F, Crea F, Gaspardone A, et al: Effects of A1 adenosine receptor blockade by bamiphylline on ischaemic preconditioning during coronary angioplasty. *Eur Heart J* 1996; 17:846.
126. Tomai F, Crea F, Gaspardone A, et al: Ischemic preconditioning during coronary angioplasty is prevented by glibenclamide, a selective ATP-sensitive K+ channel blocker. *Circulation* 1994; 90:700.
127. Saito S, Mizumura T, Takayama T, et al: Antiischemic effects of nicorandil during coronary angioplasty in humans. *Cardiovasc Drugs Ther* 1995; 9:257.
128. Tomai F, Crea F, Gaspardone A, et al: Effects of naloxone on myocardial ischemic preconditioning in humans. *J Am Coll Cardiol* 1999; 33:1863.
129. Yellon DM, Alkjulaifi AM, Puglesy WB: Preconditioning the human myocardium. *Lancet* 1993; 342:276.
130. Jenkins DP, Puglesy WB, Alkjulaifi AM, et al: Ischaemic preconditioning reduces troponin T release in patients undergoing coronary artery bypass surgery. *Heart* 1997; 77:314.
131. Teoh LK, Grant R, Huff JA, et al: The effect of preconditioning (ischemic and pharmacological) on myocardial necrosis following coronary artery bypass graft surgery. *Cardiovasc Res* 2002; 53:174.
132. Perrault LP, Menasche P: Preconditioning: can nature's shield be raised against surgical ischemic-reperfusion injury? *Ann Thorac Surg* 1999; 68:1988.
133. Ghosh S, Standen NB, Galinianes M: Failure to precondition pathological human myocardium. *J Am Coll Cardiol* 2001; 37:711.
134. Lasley RD: The protective effects of adenosine in reversibly and irreversibly injured ischemic myocardium, in Pelleg A, Belardinelli L (eds): *Effects of Extracellular Adenosine and ATP on Cardiomyocytes*. Austin, TX, R.G. Landes Company, 1998; p 133.
135. Downey JM, Cohen MV, Ytrehus K, et al: Cellular mechanisms in ischemic preconditioning: the role of adenosine and protein kinase C. *Ann N Y Acad Sci* 1994; 723:82.
136. Thornton JD, Liu GS, Olsson RA, et al: Intravenous pretreatment with A_1-selective adenosine analogues protects the heart against infarction. *Circulation* 1992; 85:659.
137. Lasley RD, Konyn PJ, Hegge JO, et al: The effects of ischemic and adenosine preconditioning on interstitial fluid adenosine and myocardial infarct size. *Am J Physiol* 1995; 269:H1460.
138. Armstrong S, Downey JM, Ganote CE: Preconditioning of isolated rabbit cardiomyocytes: induction by metabolic stress and blockade by the adenosine antagonist SPT and calphostin C, a protein kinase C inhibitor. *Cardiovasc Res* 1994; 28:72.
139. Lasley RD, Noble MA, Konyn PJ: Different effects of an adenosine A_1 analogue and ischemic preconditioning in isolated rabbit hearts. *Ann Thorac Surg* 1995; 60:1698.
140. Sekili S, Jeroudi MO, Tang XL, et al: Effect of adenosine on myocardial "stunning" in the dog. *Circ Res* 1995; 76:82.

141. Randhawa MPS, Lasley RD, Mentzer RM: Salutary effects of exogenous adenosine on canine myocardial stunning *in vivo*. *J Thorac Cardiovasc Surg* 1995; 110:63.
142. Lasley RD, Mentzer RM: Dose dependent effects of adenosine on interstitial fluid adenosine and postischemic function in the isolated rat heart. *J Pharmacol Exper Ther* 1998; 286:806, 1998.
143. Rice PJ, Armstrong SC, Ganote CE: Concentration-response relationships for adenosine agonists during preconditioning of rabbit cardiomyocytes. *J Mol Cell Cardiol* 1996; 28:1355.
144. Narayan P, Kilpatrick EL, Mentzer RM, et al: Adenosine A_1 receptor activation reduces reactive oxygen species and attenuates stunning in ventricular myocytes. *J Mol Cell Cardiol* 2001; 33:121.
145. Olah ME, Stiles GL: Adenosine receptor-mediated signal transduction, in Pelleg A, Belardinelli L (eds): *Effects of Extracellular Adenosine and ATP on Cardiomyocytes*. Austin, TX, R.G. Landes Company, 1998; p 7.
146. Olanrewaju HA, Mustafa SJ: Adenosine A(2A) and A(2B) receptors mediated nitric oxide production in coronary artery endothelial cells. *Gen Pharmacol* 2000; 35:171.
147. Morrison RR, Talukder MA, Ledent C, et al: Cardiac effects of adenosine in A(2A) receptor knockout hearts: uncovering A(2B) receptors. *Am J Physiol* 2002; 282:H437.
148. Zhou QY, Li C, Olah ME, et al: Molecular cloning and characterization of an adenosine receptor: the A_3 adenosine receptor. *Proc Natl Acad Sci U S A* 1992; 189:7432.
149. Wang JL, Drake F, Sajjadi GS, et al: Dual activation of adenosine A_1 and A_3 receptors mediates preconditioning of isolated cardiac myocytes. *Eur J Pharm* 1997; 320:241.
150. Dobson JG, Fenton RA, Romano FD: The antiadrenergic actions of adenosine in the heart, in Gerlach E, Becker BF (eds): *Topics and Perspectives in Adenosine Research*. Berlin, Springer-Verlag, 1987; p 356.
151. Lasley RD, Narayan P, Mentzer RM: New insights into adenosine receptor modulation of myocardial ischemia-reperfusion injury. *Drug Develop Res* 2001; 52:357.
152. Lasley RD, Mentzer RM: Pertussis toxin blocks adenosine A_1 receptor mediated protection of the ischemic rat heart. *J Mol Cell Cardiol* 1993; 25:815.
153. Baxter GF, Hale SL, Miki T, et al: Adenosine A_1 agonist at reperfusion trial (AART): results of a three-center, blinded, randomized, controlled experimental infarct study. *Cardiovasc Drugs Ther* 2000; 14:607.
154. Shlack W, Schafer M, Uebing A, et al: Adenosine A_2-receptor activation at reperfusion reduces infarct size and improves myocardial wall function in dog heart. *J Cardiovasc Pharmacol* 1993; 22:89.
155. Zhao ZQ, Sato H, Williams MW, et al: Adenosine A_2-receptor activation inhibits neutrophil-mediated injury to coronary endothelium. *Am J Physiol* 1996; 271:H1456.
156. Jordan JE, Zhao ZQ, Sato H, et al: Adenosine A2 receptor activation attenuates reperfusion injury by inhibiting neutrophil accumulation, superoxide generation and coronary endothelial adherence. *J Pharmacol Exp Ther* 1997; 280:301.
157. Lasley RD, Jahania MS, Mentzer RM: Beneficial effects of the adenosine A_{2a} agonist CGS 21680 in infarcted and stunned porcine myocardium. *Am J Physiol* 2001; 280:H1660.
158. Marala RB, Mustafa SJ: Immunological characterization of adenosine A_{2A} receptors in human and porcine cardiovascular tissues. *J Pharmacol Exp Ther* 1998; 286:1051.
159. Kilpatrick EL, Narayan P, Mentzer RM, et al: Rat ventricular myocyte adenosine A_{2a} receptor activation fails to alter cAMP or contractility: role of receptor localization. *Am J Physiol* 2002; 282:H1035.
160. Liu GS, Richards SC, Olsson RA, et al: Evidence that the adenosine A_3 receptor may mediate the protection afforded by preconditioning in the isolated rabbit heart. *Cardiovasc Res* 1994; 28:1057.
161. Armstrong S, Ganote CE: Adenosine receptor specificity in preconditioning of isolated rabbit cardiomyocytes: evidence of A_3 receptor involvement. *Cardiovasc Res* 1994; 28:1049.
162. Tracey WR, Magee W, Masamune H, et al: Selective adenosine A_3 receptor stimulation reduces ischemic myocardial injury in the rabbit heart. *Cardiovasc Res* 1997; 33:410.
163. Tracey WR, Magee W, Masamune H, et al: Selective activation of adenosine A_3 receptors with N^6-(3–chlorobenzyl)-5′-N-methylcarboxamidoadenosine (CB-MECA) provides cardioprotection via K_{ATP} channel activation. *Cardiovasc Res* 1998; 40:138.
164. Auchampach JA, Rizvi A, Qiu Y, et al: Selective activation of A_3 adenosine receptors with N^6-(3–iodobenzyl)adenosine-5′-N-methyluronamide protects against myocardial stunning and infarction without hemodynamic changes in conscious rabbits. *Circ Res* 1997; 80:800.
165. Lasley RD, Narayan P, Jahania MS, et al: Species-dependent hemodynamic effects of adenosine A_3 receptor agonists IBMECA and Cl-IBMECA. *Am J Physiol* 1999; 45:H2076.
166. Visser SS, Theron AJ, Ramafi G, et al: Apparent involvement of the A(2A) subtype adenosine receptor in the anti-inflammatory interactions of CGS 21680, cyclopentyladenosine, and IB-MECA with human neutrophils. *Biochem Pharmacol* 2000; 60:993.
167. Kilpatrick EL, Narayan P, Mentzer RM, et al: Adenosine A_3 agonist cardioprotection in isolated rat and rabbit hearts is blocked by the A_1 antagonist DPCPX. *Am J Physiol* 2001; 281:H47.
168. Abbracchio MP, Rainaldi G, Giammarioli AM, et al: The A_3 adenosine receptor mediates cell spreading, reorganization of actin cytoskeleton, and distribution of Bcl-XL: studies in human astroglioma cells. *Biochem Biophys Res Commun* 1997; 241:297.
169. Shneyvays V, Nawrath H, Jacobson KA, et al: Induction of apoptosis in cardiac myocytes by an A_3 adenosine receptor agonist. *Exp Cell Res* 1998; 243:383.
170. Nakano A, Baines CP, Kim SO, et al: Ischemic preconditioning activates MAPKAPK2 in the isolated rabbit heart: evidence for involvement of p38 MAPK. *Circ Res* 2000; 86:144.
171. Lasley RD, Noble MA, Paulsen KL, et al: Adenosine attenuates phorbol ester-induced negative inotropic and vasoconstrictive effects in the isolated rat heart. *Am J Physiol* 1994; 266:H2159.
172. Narayan P, Valdivia HH, Mentzer RM, et al: Adenosine A_1 receptor stimulation antagonizes the negative inotropic effects of the PKC activator dioctanoylglycerol. *J Mol Cell Cardiol* 1998; 30: 913.
173. Gupta RC, Neumann J, Watanabe AM: Comparison of adenosine and muscarinic receptor-mediated effects on protein phosphatase inhibitor-1 activity in the heart. *J Pharmacol Exp Ther* 1993; 266:16.
174. Narayan P, Mentzer RM, Lasley RD: The phosphate inhibitor cantharidin blocks the adenosine A_1 receptor anti-adrenergic effect in rat cardiac myocytes. *Am J Physiol* 2000; 278:H1.
175. Kirsch GE, Codina J, Birnbaumer L, et al: Coupling of ATP-sensitive K+ channels to A1 receptors by G proteins in rat ventricular myocytes. *Am J Physiol* 2000; 259:H820.
176. Karmazyn M, Cook MA: Adenosine A_1 receptor activation attenuates cardiac injury produced by hydrogen peroxide. *Circ Res* 1992; 71:1101.
177. Thomas GP, Sims SM, Cook MA, et al: Hydrogen peroxide-induced stimulation of L-type calcium current in guinea pig ventricular myocytes and its inhibition by adenosine A1 receptor activation. *J Pharmacol Exp Ther* 1998; 286:1208.
178. Maggirwar SB, Dhanraj DN, Somani SM, et al: Adenosine acts as an endogenous activator of the cellular antioxidant defense system. *Biochem Biophys Res Commun* 1994; 201:508.

179. Baxter GF, Marber MS, Patel VC, et al: Adenosine receptor involvement in a delayed phase of myocardial protection 24 hours after ischemic preconditioning. *Circulation* 1994; 90:2993.
180. Baxter GF, Yellon DM. Time course of delayed myocardial protection after transient adenosine A1-receptor activation in the rabbit. *J Cardiovasc Pharmacol* 1997; 29:631.
181. Zhao T, Xi L, Chelliah J, et al: Inducible nitric oxide synthase mediates delayed myocardial protection induced by activation of adenosine A(1) receptors: evidence from gene-knockout mice. *Circulation* 2000; 102:902.
182. Dana A, Jonassen AK, Yamashita N, et al: Adenosine A(1) receptor activation induces delayed preconditioning in rats mediated by manganese superoxide dismutase. *Circulation* 2000; 101:2841.
183. Dana A, Baxter GF, Yellon DM: Delayed or second window preconditioning induced by adenosine A1 receptor activation is independent of early generation of nitric oxide or late induction of inducible nitric oxide synthase. *J Cardiovasc Pharmacol* 2001; 38:278.
184. Takano H, Bolli R, Black RG, et al: A(1) or A(3) adenosine receptors induce late preconditioning against infarction in conscious rabbits by different mechanisms. *Circ Res* 2001; 88:520.
185. Bell RM, Smith CC, Yellon DM: Nitric oxide as a mediator of delayed pharmacological (A(1) receptor triggered) preconditioning: is eNOS masquerading as iNOS? *Cardiovasc Res* 2002; 53:405.
186. Wang Y, Guo Y, Zhang SX, et al: Ischemic preconditioning upregulates inducible nitric oxide synthase in cardiac myocyte. *J Mol Cell Cardiol* 2002; 34:5.
187. Olafsson B, Forman MB, Puett DW, et al: Reduction of reperfusion injury in the canine preparation by intracoronary adenosine: importance of the endothelium and the no-reflow phenomenon. *Circulation* 1987; 76:1135.
188. Cronstein BN, Rosenstein ED, Kramer SB, et al: Adenosine; a physiologic modulator of superoxide anion generation by human neutrophils: adenosine acts via an A2 receptor on human neutrophils. *J Immunol* 1985; 135:1366.
189. Abebe W, Hussain T, Olanrewaju H, et al: Role of nitric oxide in adenosine receptor-mediated relaxation of porcine coronary artery. *Am J Physiol* 1995; 269:H1672.
190. Lee HT, LaFaro RJ, Reed GE: Pretreatment of human myocardium with adenosine during open heart surgery. *J Card Surg* 1995; 10:665.
191. Fremes SE, Levy SL, Christakis GT, et al: Phase 1 human trial of adenosine-potassium cardioplegia. *Circulation* 1995; 94:II370.
192. Cohen G, Feder-Elituv R, Iazetta J, et al: Phase 2 studies of adenosine cardioplegia. *Circulation* 1998; 98:II225.
193. Mentzer RM, Rahko PS, Molina-Viamonte V, et al: Safety, tolerance and efficacy of adenosine as an additive to blood cardioplegia in humans during coronary artery bypass surgery. *Amer J Cardiol* 1997; 79:38.
194. Mentzer RM, Birjiniuk V, Khuri S, et al: Adenosine myocardial protection: preliminary results of a phase II clinical trial. *Ann Surg* 1999; 229:643.
195. Phillipson KD: Na(+)-Ca(2+) exchange: three new tools. *Circ Res* 2002; 90:118.
196. Forlich O, Karmazyn M: The Na-H exchanger revisited: an update on Na-H exchange regulation and the role of the exchanger in hypertension and cardiac function in health and disease. *Cardiovasc Res* 1997; 36:138.
197. Karmazyn M, Sostaric JV, Gan XT: The myocardial Na+/H+ exchanger: a potential therapeutic target for the prevention of myocardial ischaemic and reperfusion injury and attenuation of postinfarction heart failure. *Drugs* 2001; 61:375.
198. Yokoyama H, Gunasegaram S, Harding SE, et al: Sarcolemmal Na+/H+ exchanger activity and expression in human ventricular myocardium. *J Am Coll Cardiol* 2000; 36:534.
199. Orlowski J. Na+/H+ exchangers. Molecular diversity and relevance to heart. *Ann N Y Acad Sci* 1999; 874:346.
200. Karmazyn M. Sodium-hydrogen exchange in heart disease. *Science & Medicine* 2002; 8:18.
201. Karmazyn M, Gan XT, Humphreys RA, et al: The myocardial Na(+)-H(+) exchange: structure, regulation, and its role in heart disease. *Circ Res* 1999; 85:777.
202. Avkiran M, Marber MS: Na(+)/H(+) exchange inhibitors for cardioprotective therapy: progress, problems and prospects. *J Am Coll Cardiol* 2002; 39:747.
203. Theroux P, Chaitman BR, Danchin N, et al: Inhibition of the sodium-hydrogen exchanger with cariporide to prevent myocardial infarction in high-risk ischemic situations: main results of the GUARDIAN trial. Guard During Ischemia Against Necrosis (GUARDIAN) investigators. *Circulation* 2000; 102:3032.
204. Kloner RA, Bolli R, Marban E, et al: Medical and cellular implications of stunning, hibernation, and preconditioning: an NHLBI workshop. *Circulation* 1999; 97:1848.
205. Pierce GN, Czubryt MP: The contribution of ionic imbalance to ischemia/reperfusion-induced injury. *J Mol Cell Cardiol* 1995; 27:53.
206. Avkiran M: Sodium-hydrogen exchange in myocardial ischemia and reperfusion: a critical determinant of injury?, in Karmazyn M (ed): *Myocardial Ischemia: Mechanisms, Reperfusion, Protection*, Vol. 76. Boston, Birkhauser Verlag, 1996; p 299.
207. Karmazyn M: Amiloride enhances postischemic ventricular recovery: possible role of Na+-H+ exchange. *Am J Physiol* 1988; 255:H608.
208. du Toit EF, Opie LH: Role for the Na+/H+ exchanger in reperfusion stunning in isolated perfused rat heart. *J Cardiovasc Pharmacol* 1993; 22:877.
209. Sack S, Mohri M, Schwarz ER, et al: Effects of a new Na+/H+ antiporter inhibitor on postischemic reperfusion in pig heart. *J Cardiovasc Pharmacol* 1994; 23:72.
210. Klein HH, Pich S, Bohle RM, et al: Myocardial protection by Na(+)-H+ exchange inhibition in ischemic, reperfused porcine hearts. *Circulation* 1995; 92:912.
211. Rohmann S, Weygandt H, Minck KO. Preischaemic as well as postischaemic application of a Na+/H+ exchange inhibitor reduces infarct size in pigs. *Cardiovasc Res* 1995; 30:945.
212. Gumina RJ, Mizumura T, Beier N, et al: A new sodium/hydrogen exchange inhibitor, EMD 85131, limits infarct size in dogs when administered before or after coronary artery occlusion. *J Pharmacol Exp Ther* 1998; 286:175.
213. Garcia-Dorado D, Gonzalez MA, Barrabes JA, et al: Prevention of ischemic rigor contracture during coronary occlusion by inhibition of Na(+)-H+ exchange. *Cardiovasc Res* 1997; 35:80.
214. Miura T, Ogawa T, Suzuki K, et al: Infarct size limitation by a new Na(+)-H+ exchange inhibitor, Hoe 642: difference from preconditioning in the role of protein kinase C. *J Am Coll Cardiol* 1997; 29:693.
215. Linz W, Albus U, Crause P, et al: Dose-dependent reduction of myocardial infarct mass in rabbits by the NHE-1 inhibitor cariporide (HOE 642). *Clin Exp Hypertens* 1998; 20:733.
216. Klein HH, Bohle RM, Pich S, et al: Time-dependent protection by Na+/H+ exchange inhibition in a regionally ischemic, reperfused porcine heart preparation with low residual blood flow. *J Mol Cell Cardiol* 1998; 30:795.
217. Rupprecht H, Dahl J, Terres W, et al: Cardioprotective effects of the Na+/H+ exchange inhibitor cariporide in patients with acute anterior myocardial infarction undergoing direct PTCA. *Circulation* 2000; 101:2902.
218. Zeymer U, Suryapranata H, Monassier JP, et al: The Na+/H+ exchange inhibitor eniporide as an adjunct to early reperfusion

therapy for acute myocardial infarction: results of the Evaluation of the Safety and Cardioprotective Effects of Eniporide in Acute Myocardial Infarction (ESCAMI) trial. *J Am Coll Cardiol* 38:1644, 2001.

219. Bolli R: Cardioprotective function of inducible nitric oxide synthase and role of nitric oxide in myocardial ischemia and preconditioning: an overview of a decade of research. *J Mol Cell Cardiol* 2001; 33:1897.
220. Weyrich AS, Lefer DJ, Lefer AM: Diminished basal nitric oxide release after myocardial ischemia and reperfusion promotes neutrophil adherence to coronary endothelium. *Circ Res* 1993; 72:403.
221. Williams MW, Taft CS, Ramnauh S, et al: Endogenous nitric oxide (NO) protects against ischaemia-reperfusion injury in rabbits. *Cardiovasc Res* 1995; 10:79.
222. Wink DA, Hanbauer I, Krishna MC, et al: Nitric oxide protects against cellular damage and cytotoxicity from reactive oxygen species. *Proc Nat Acad Sci U S A* 1993; 90:9813.
223. Xia Y, Tsai A-L, Berka V, et al: Superoxide generation from endothelial nitric-oxide synthase: a Ca^{2+}/calmodulin-dependent and tetrahydrobiopterin regulatory process. *J Biol Chem* 1998; 273:25804.
224. Qiu Y, Rizvi A, Tang XL, et al: Nitric oxide triggers late preconditioning against myocardial infarction in conscious rabbits. *Am J Physiol* 1997; 273:H2931.
225. Zhao L, Weber PA, Smith JR, et al: Role of inducible nitric oxide synthase in pharmacological "preconditioning" with monophosphoryl lipid A. *J Mol Cell Cardiol* 1997; 29:1567.
226. Bolli R, Manchikalapudi S, Tang XL, et al: The protective effect of late preconditioning against myocardial stunning in conscious rabbits is mediated by nitric oxide synthase: evidence that nitric oxide acts both as a trigger and as a mediator of the late phase of ischemic preconditioning. *Circ Res* 1997; 81:1094.
227. Takano H, Manchikalapudi S, Tang XL, et al: Nitric oxide synthase is the mediator of late preconditioning against myocardial infarction in conscious rabbits. *Circulation* 1998; 98:441.
228. Imagawa J, Yellon DM, Baxter GF. Pharmacological evidence that inducible nitric oxide synthase is a mediator of delayed preconditioning. *Br J Pharmacol* 1999; 126:701.
229. Xuan YT, Tang XL, Qiu Y, et al: Biphasic response of cardiac NO synthase isoforms to ischemic preconditioning in conscious rabbits. *Am J Physiol* 2000; 279:H2360.
230. Takano H, Tang XL, Qiu Y, et al: Nitric oxide donors induce late preconditioning against myocardial stunning and infarction in conscious rabbits via an antioxidant-sensitive mechanism. *Circ Res* 1998; 83:73.
231. Kim SJ, Kim YK, Takagi G, et al: Enhanced iNOS function in myocytes one day after brief ischemic episode. *Am J Physiol* 2002; 282:H423.
232. Guo Y, Jones WK, Xuan YT, et al: The late phase of ischemic preconditioning is abrogated by targeted disruption of the inducible NO synthase gene. *Proc Natl Acad Sci U S A* 1999; 96:11507.
233. Shinmura K, Tang XL, Takano H, et al: Nitric oxide donors attenuate myocardial stunning in conscious rabbits. *Am J Physiol* 1998; 277(6 Pt 2):H2495.
234. Lochner A, Marais E, Genade S, et al: Nitric oxide: a trigger for classic preconditioning? *Am J Physiol* 2000; 279:H2752.
235. Bell RM, Yellon DM: The contribution of endothelial nitric oxide synthase to early ischaemic preconditioning: the lowering of the preconditioning threshold: an investigation in eNOS knockout mice. *Cardiovasc Res* 2001; 52:274.
236. Nakano A, Liu GS, Heusch G, et al: Exogenous nitric oxide can trigger a preconditioned state through a free radical mechanism, but endogenous nitric oxide is not a trigger of classical ischemic preconditioning. *J Mol Cell Cardiol* 2000; 32:1159.
237. Weselcouch EO, Baird AJ, Sleph P, et al: Inhibition of nitric oxide synthesis does not affect ischemic preconditioning in isolated perfused rat hearts. *Am J Physiol* 1995; 268:H242.
238. Post H, Schulz R, Behrends M, et al: No involvement of endogenous nitric oxide in classical ischemic preconditioning in swine. *J Mol Cell Cardiol* 2000; 32:725.
239. Leesar MA, Stoddard MF, Dawn B, et al: Delayed preconditioning-mimetic action of nitroglycerin in patients undergoing coronary angioplasty. *Circulation* 2001; 103:2935.
240. Zhang JG, Galinanes M: Role of the L-arginine/nitric oxide pathway in ischaemic/reoxygenation injury of the human myocardium. *Clin Sci* (Lond) 2000; 99:497.
241. Carrier M, Pellerin M, Perrault LP, et al: Cardioplegic arrest with L-arginine improves myocardial protection: results of a prospective randomized clinical trial. *Ann Thorac Surg* 2002; 3;837.
242. Menon AK, Albes JM, Oberhoff M,et al: Occlusion versus shunting during MIDCAB: effects on left ventricular function and quality of anastomosis. *Ann Thorac Surg* 2002; 73:1418.
243. Cremer J, Strüber M, Wittwer T, et al: Morbidity of cardiopulmonary bypass and potential benefits of minimally invasive coronary surgery off pump. *Cor Europaeum* 1997; 6:164.
244. Benetti F, Mariani MA, Sani G, et al: Video-assisted minimally invasive coronary operations without cardiopulmonary bypass: a multicenter study. *J Thorac Cardiovasc Surg* 1996; 112:1478.
245. Subramanian VA: Clinical experience with minimally invasive reoperative coronary bypass surgery. *Eur J Cardiothorac Surg* 1997; 10:1058.
246. Dapunt OE, Raji MR, Jeschkeit S, et al: Intracoronary shunt insertion prevents myocardial stunning in a juvenile porcine MIDCAB model absent of coronary artery disease. *Eur J Cardiothorac Surg* 1999; 15:173.
247. Bonatti J, Hangler H, Hormann C, et al: Myocardial damage after minimally invasive coronary artery bypass grafting on the beating heart. *Ann Thorac Surg* 1998; 66:1093.
248. Koh TW, Carr-White GS, DeSouza AC, et al: Intraoperative cardiac troponin release and lactate metabolism during coronary artery surgery: comparison of beating heart with conventional coronary artery surgery with cardiopulmonary bypass. *Heart* 1999; 81:495.
249. Hendrikx M, Rega F, Jamaer L, et al: Na(+)/H(+)-exchange inhibition and aprotinin administration: promising tools for myocardial protection during minimally invasive CABG. *Eur J Cardiothorac Surg* 2001; 19:633.
250. Swan H, Virtue RW, Blount SG Jr, et al: Hypothermia in surgery: analysis of 100 clinical cases. *Ann Surg* 1955; 142:382.
251. Lam CR, Cahagan T, Sergeant C, et al: Clinical experiences with induced cardiac arrest during intracardiac surgical procedures. *Ann Surg* 1957; 146:439.
252. Gerbode F, Melrose DG: The use of potassium arrest in open cardiac surgery. *Am J Surg* 1958; 96:221.
253. McFarland JA, Thomas LB, Gilbert JW, et al: Myocardial necrosis following elective cardiac arrest induced with potassium citrate. *J Thorac Cardiovasc Surg* 1960; 40:200.
254. Søndergaard T, Senn A: Klinische Erfahrungen mit der Kardioplegie nach Bretschneider. *Langenbecks Arch Chir* 1967; 319:661.
255. Søndergaard T, Berg E, Staffeldt I, et al: Cardioplegic cardiac arrest in aortic surgery. *J. Cardiovasc Surg* (Torino) 1975; 16:288.
256. Effler DB: The mystique of myocardial preservation. *J Thorac Cardiovasc Surg* 1976; 72:468.
257. Murry CE, Jennings RB, Reimer KA: Preconditioning with ischemia: a delay of lethal cell injury in ischemic myocardium. *Circulation* 1986; 74:1124.

Chapter 15

Postoperative Care of Cardiac Surgical Patients

Rawn Salenger/James S. Gammie/Thomas J. Vander Salm

OVERVIEW OF MAJOR DERANGEMENTS

Major physiological derangements must be treated in patients recovering from a cardiac surgical operation. These fall into two types: those existing preoperatively and those that occur as a consequence of the operation and cardiopulmonary bypass (CPB). The goal is to restore normal homeostasis. The most important factor contributing to this restoration, of course, is the proper conduct of a well-conceived operation.

Because so many systems may be deranged, a systems-oriented approach is necessary to deal with problems in an orderly fashion.[1] The cardiac system, usually the most perturbed, is the primary determinant of recovery, and consequently requires the greatest effort to restore normal function. Measured cardiac output, clinical signs of cardiac adequacy, and blood pressure must be maintained, and cardiac distension and ischemia must be avoided. A low cardiac index during the early postoperative period markedly increases the probability of death.[2,3] With the physiological trauma of recent cardiopulmonary bypass, hearts are susceptible to ventricular arrhythmias early after operation and to atrial arrhythmias later.

Fluid accumulation in the perioperative period and interstitial edema cause pulmonary dysfunction. The goal is to wean the patient from mechanical ventilation and high oxygen concentrations as quickly as is commensurate with adequate spontaneous ventilation, ability to protect the airway, and satisfactory oxygenation.

High urine output usually results from operations performed on cardiopulmonary bypass; anything less raises the alarm of renal insufficiency and requires immediate evaluation and treatment. Renal dysfunction occurs commonly after heart operations, and early and aggressive treatment reduces the otherwise high mortality accompanying this complication.[4]

Neurologic complications occur more commonly after heart operations than after most other types of surgery. Early, careful assessment and documentation of the return of mental and central and peripheral neurologic function are required. Although many central deficits occurring in the perioperative period cannot be treated, others can be, and early diagnosis allows treatment before changes become irreversible.

Excessive bleeding complicates heart operations more often than other operations. Consistent, systematic intraoperative control of bleeding contributes more than any other factor to tolerable postoperative blood loss. Even then, excessive bleeding occurs with a frequency higher than with most other operations. Bleeding may be from surgical bleeding sites or caused by the temporary coagulation disorder that accompanies nearly all heart surgery.

INFLAMMATORY RESPONSE TO CARDIOPULMONARY BYPASS

CPB harms patients, even while it enables life-preserving operations. In a time-dependent fashion, CPB activates plasma proteins and blood and endothelial cells.[5–12] These complex reactions activate the complement, clotting, and fibrinolytic cascades and cause a bleeding tendency, microemboli, fluid retention, and perturbation of the hormonal milieu.[13–16] A detailed description of these events is provided in Chapter 11.

COMPLICATIONS: ANTICIPATION AND TREATMENT

A protocol for postoperative care is useful if it anticipates and prevents complications while minimizing utilization of hospital resources. Many complications that occur from cardiac operations, such as renal failure, pulmonary dysfunction, and bleeding, may be anticipated. Accordingly, early and aggressive treatment mitigates morbidity and shortens convalescence.

Hemodynamic malfunction may be caused by the underlying heart disease, but to assume so precludes correcting mechanical complications of the operation at a time when damage may be minimized. Postcardiac surgical units routinely monitor the electrocardiogram (ECG), arterial blood pressure, and filling pressures (right atrial, left atrial, and/or pulmonary artery pressure) and also utilize continuous displays of arterial and mixed venous oxygen saturations (via pulse oximetry and oxymetric pulmonary artery catheters, respectively). These indices allow minute-to-minute assessment of cardiopulmonary physiology. Deviations from expected normal ranges prompt immediate reevaluation of heart and lung function (Table 15-1). As a working policy, therefore, all hemodynamic malfunctions—low cardiac output, low blood pressure, elevated left or right atrial pressures—are first considered a direct mechanical complication of the operation performed or a result of mechanical ventilation or drug administration. Reparable maladies such as coronary artery graft occlusion or spasm, prosthetic paravalvular leak, mechanical valve leaflet immobility, pericardial tamponade, pneumothorax, hemothorax, endotracheal tube malposition, and incorrect doses of intravenous infusions are considered first.

Commonly used medications are listed in Table 15-2. Examples of standard postoperative orders are included in Table 15-3. Details of patient care are included in the following sections.

TABLE 15–1 Expected values following cardiac surgery

Mean arterial pressure (MAP)	70-95 mm Hg
Systolic blood pressure (SBP)	90-140 mm Hg
Right atrial pressure (RAP)	5-15 mm Hg
Left atrial pressure (LAP)	5-15 mm Hg
Cardiac index (CI) = CO/BSA	2.0-4.4 L/min
Systemic vascular resistance (SVR)	SVR = (MAP − RAP / CO) × 80
SVRI = (MAP − RAP / CI) × 80	1400-2800 dyn · s · cm^5/m^2

TABLE 15–2 Commonly Used Postoperative Medications

Medication	Clinical effect	Adverse effect	Dosing(IV)
Epinephrine	Positive inotrope Positive chronotrope At low doses, causes vasodilation from $beta_2$ activity $>2\mu g/min$ raises BP via increasing alpha activity	Increases myocardial O_2 consumption Tachycardia Arrhythmogenic High doses can exacerbate metabolic acidosis from alpha effect	0.008-0.06 $\mu g/kg/min$ (0.5-4.0 $\mu g/min$)
Norepinephrine	Raises BP and SVR Less positive inotropy	Increases myocardial O_2 consumption Intense vasoconstriction can lead to visceral and renal ischemia Exacerbates metabolic acidosis by increasing anaerobic glycolysis and lactate production Exacerbates hyperglycemia	0.03-0.3 $\mu g/kg/min$ (2.0-20 $\mu g/min$)
Phenylephrine	Raises BP and SVR Often reflex decrease in HR Useful in patients with high cardiac index and severely vasodilated	Increases myocardial O_2 consumption Tolerance develops Can cause visceral and renal ischemia Can exacerbate metabolic acidosis	0.15-3.0 $\mu g/kg/min$ (10-200 $\mu g/min$)
Dopamine	At 2-3 $\mu g/kg/min$, mainly renal vasodilation via dopaminergic receptors At 4-10 $\mu g/kg/min$, mainly positive inotropic and chronotropic effects via $beta_1$ receptors At >10 $\mu g/kg/min$, mainly raises BP and SVR via alpha receptors Receptor stimulation overlap occurs	Raises myocardial O_2 consumption Arrhythmogenic	2.0-20 $\mu g/kg/min$
Dobutamine	Positive inotrope Positive chronotrope May decrease SVR	Hypertension (alpha effect) Hypotension ($beta_2$ effect) Arrhythmogenic May raise myocardial O_2 consumption	2.0-20 $\mu g/kg/min$
Milrinone	Positive inotrope Decreases SVR Decreases pulmonary vascular resistance (ideal for RV failure) Decreases coronary vascular resistance Most favorable effect on myocardial O_2 consumption	Hypotension	Loading dose: 50-75 $\mu g/kg$ Maintenance: 0.25-0.75 $\mu g/kg/min$
Nitroprusside	Arterial vasodilatation Increases venous capacitance Decreases SVR and PVR Rapid onset Short half-life	Reflex tachycardia Inhibition of hypoxic pulmonary vasoconstriction leading to increased V/Q mismatch Tachyphylaxis Cyanide toxicity[a] Metabolic acidosis Methemoglobinemia Thiocyanate toxicity[b] Seizures Psychosis	0.3-10 $\mu g/kg/min$ Usual dose: 0.3-4.0 $\mu g/kg/min$
Nitroglycerin	Increases venous capacitance (major effect) Coronary vasodilatation Decreases SVR and PVR (less than nitroprusside)	Tolerance can occur with continuous dosing Methemoglobinemia[c]	0.1-10 $\mu g/kg/min$ (10-700 $\mu g/min$)

(*Continued*)

TABLE 15–2 (*Continued*) Commonly Used Postoperative Medications

Medication	Clinical effect	Adverse effect	Dosing(IV)
Calcium	Positive inotrope Stabilizes myocardial membranes in setting of hyperkalemia	Temporary effect	1g CaCl
Triiodothyronine	Positive inotrope Decreases SVR	Tachycardia May be arrhythmogenic	Loading dose: 0.4-0.8 μg/kg in OR after x-clamp removed Maintenance: 0.1-0.12 μg/kg/h over 6 h

[a]Higher risk with hepatic dysfunction.
[b]Higher risk with renal dysfunction.
[c]Higher risk with renal or hepatic dysfunction.

TABLE 15–3 Routine Postoperative Orders

ALL OTHER ORDERS
Admission Date:
Time:
Allergies:
Diet: NPO
VS and I&O's q15 min until stable then q30min ×2, then q 1h.
Neurovascular checks of leg & calf swelling/tenseness q 1h.
Activity: bed rest only; HOB up 30° if BP stable.
Wrist restraints as per ICU life support equipment removal prevention protocol.
Mediastinal tubes to ____ cm water suction.
Pleural chest tube to ____ cm water suction.
Blake drains to bulb suction.
Do not milk tubes or drains.
NGT to low continuous suction.
Foley to bedside drainage.
Vent @___FIO^2, ____PEEP, ____VT, ____IMV, wean per protocol.
Continuous pulse oximetry.
Pacemaker: ____ if NSR and HR >80, set pacer at VD 50 bpm.
Portable AP CXR on arrival to ICU, POD #1 & # 2.
EKG on arrival to ICU; then AM POD #1 & #3; obtain q d if pt. on procainamide, quinidine, sotalol, or amiodarone
Weight q d starting POD #1.
ADM Labs: chem 7, Hct, PTT, ABG.
Subsequent Labs: Hct, K^+, @ 3h and 6h.
Labs in AM: CBC, chem 7, ABG.
Daily: PT/INR for warfarin pts., and PTT if on heparin.
POD #2 Labs: CBC, chem 7.

FOR RADIAL ARTERY GRAFT PATIENTS:
Wound care: neurovascular & dressing checks q 1h × 24h, then q 4h.
Sign over bed stating, "No IV's or venipuncture in arm of harvest."

MEDICATION ORDERS
IV infusions mixed per standard:
1. ____________ @ ____________
Wean to keep ________ > ________
2. ____________ @ ____________
Wean to keep ________ > ________
3. ____________ @ ____________
Wean to keep ________ > ________
4. ____________ @ ____________
Wean to keep ________ > ________
5. Magnesium sulfate 4g. IV in 250 cc NS over 4 hours; omit in renal failure.
6. KCI 10 mEq via central vein for K^+ 4.0-4.5
KCI 20 mEq via central vein for K^+ 3.5-3.9
KCI 30 mEq via central vein for K^+ <3.5
7. Antibiotic: ________ g IV on admission and q ___ h D/C in 24 h.
8. Morphine ________ mg IV q 1-2h prn pain, or codeine 30 mg po q 3h prn.
9. Acetaminophen 650 mg PR q 4hrs prn temp >38.5°C and notify H.O.
10. Carafate 1g NGT/po q 6hrs. while in ICU.
11. Colace 100 mg po BID.
12. Digoxin (as per afib prophylaxis protocol).
13. Metoprolol ___ mg po q 12h, start POD# 1 (as pre afib prophylaxis protocol).

FOR CABG PATIENTS:
ASA 325 mg per NGT qd (start POD# 1)
Change to enteric coated ASA when taking po.
Omit ASA if pt. has hx of peptic ulcer disease or is on warfarin/heparin.

FOR LIMA PATIENTS:
Nifedipine 10 mg po/NGT q 6h × 36h.
Hold for SBP <90 mm Hg (and call H.O.)
Hold if pt. is on isordil
Clamp NGT for 1.5 h after po meds

TABLE 15–3 (*Continued*) Routine Postoperative Orders

FOR IABP PATIENTS: IABP ratio __: __ Check ABI's and pulses on arrival to ICU, then as per protocol. Signature: ________ Beeper: ________	FOR RADIAL ARTERY GRAFT PATIENTS: NTG qtt @ ________ Once taking po, start imdur 30 mg po qd. D/C NTG qtt 60 minutes after 1st dose imdur. FOR IABP PATIENTS: Dextran 10% in D5W @ 25 cc/hr IV. Begin when coags are within normal limits.

HEART

Minimal Requirements

Adequate cardiac function is an absolute requirement for successful recovery from any operation, including one on the heart itself. During the immediate postoperative period, minimum requirements of systemic and pulmonary blood flow must be met to avoid organ dysfunction. Normal renal, gastrointestinal, and neurologic functions are the best indices of adequate systemic circulation, but other parameters, including measurements of cardiac output and oxygen utilization (VO_2), are also useful.

Under basal conditions, oxygen consumption can be measured directly; taken from tables that correct for age, sex, and size; or estimated utilizing calculations based on the patient's size (125 mL O_2 per minute per m^2).[17] A value for oxygen consumption provides a means of estimating cardiac output from measurements of mixed venous and arterial oxygen content using the Fick equation (Table 15-4). Frequently, measurements of mixed venous oxygen saturation (SvO_2) are used to determine whether the cardiac output meets systemic demands. An SvO_2 greater than 60% is acceptable for an awake normothermic patient. Following cardiac surgery, a number of factors may affect the oxygen content of blood, the ability of blood to release oxygen where it is needed, and the body's demand for oxygen (Table 15-5). The essence of postoperative critical care is to ensure the adequacy of systemic oxygen supply relative to demand.[18,19]

TABLE 15–4 Fick equation of cardiac output*

CI (cardiac index) = O_2 consumption (mL/min/m^2) / arteriovenous O_2 difference (mL/L)

Requires	Assumptions
Estimate of body O_2 consumption Measurement of arterial and mixed venous (pulmonary arterial) O_2 saturation	No significant intracardiac shunt Inconsequential bronchial and thebesian venous drainage
Arteriovenous O_2 difference = ($SaO_2 - SvO_2$) × 1.39(Hgb) × 10	A static level of O_2 consumption

*According to the Fick principle, if O_2 consumption and arterial O_2 saturation are constant, then changes in cardiac output would be directly reflected by changes in the SvO_2. SvO_2 is easily measured and can be used as a surrogate for cardiac output. An adequate SvO_2, however, does not ensure a normal cardiac output if all of the above assumptions are not true. A further assumption regarding tissue perfusion is that the measured cardiac output is available uniformly to peripheral organs. Local vasodilatation and shunting can lead to tissue ischemia/acidosis despite normal or elevated measured cardiac output.

Determinants of Cardiac Output

The cardiac output, expressed as liters per minute per square meter (cardiac index; CI), is the most commonly used measure of cardiac performance in the immediate postoperative period. Although other methods are possible, the thermodilution technique using a pulmonary artery catheter and room temperature injectate is simple and sufficiently precise.[20] A normal value for CI after surgery is between 2.0 and 4.4 L/min/m^2.[21]

Dietzman et al[3] first reported the association between low cardiac output and mortality after cardiac surgery, and this observation was confirmed subsequently by others.[22–26] A normal recovery from cardiac surgery can be expected when the CI is maintained above 2.0 to 2.2 L/min/m^2.[27] Treatment of low cardiac output is predicated on manipulation of its primary determinants (Table 15-6).

The determinants of cardiac output are heart rate and stroke volume. The latter is influenced by the cardiac rhythm, ventricular preload and afterload, and myocardial contractility. Although the *heart rate* is usually slightly increased immediately after surgery, patients using large

TABLE 15–5 Factors affecting systemic oxygen supply and demand after cardiac surgery

	Supply	Demand
INCREASE	Hyperoxygenation Augmented CO Mild peripheral acidosis	Fever Pain Agitation Shivering Hyperdynamic state
DECREASE	Hypothermia Anemia Profound alkalosis	Hypothermia Anesthesia/analgesia

TABLE 15–6 Treatment of low cardiac output (CI <2.0-2.2 L/min/m²)

1. Consider surgical complications, including coronary graft occlusion, valve malfunction, tamponade, bleeding, coronary spasm
2. Optimize heart rate and rhythm
   Increase rate to 90-100 beats per minute
   Atrial pacing if no heart block
   A-V pacing if heart block exists

3. Low blood pressure (SBP <100 mm Hg or MAP <70 mm Hg)
   - If LAP * <15 mm Hg and HCT ≥25, administer Ringer's lactate or hetastarch
   - If LAP <15 mm Hg and HCT <25, administer PRBCs
   - If LAP ≥15 mm Hg, start dopamine or other inotropic agent, then add nipride when MAP >70 mm Hg

4. Normal or high blood pressure (SBP >100 mm Hg or MAP >70 mm Hg)
   - If LAP <15 mm Hg and HCT ≥25, administer Ringer's lactate or hetastarch, plus nipride or other vasodilator
   - If LAP <15 mm Hg and HCT <25, administer PRBCs, plus nipride or other vasodilator
   - If LAP ≥15 mm Hg, administer nipride/other vasodilator and consider diuretic

5. If CI and BP still low, place IABP

*PA diastolic pressure can be used in place of LAP.

amounts of beta blockers preoperatively or with an intrinsic rhythm disturbance may have a slow heart rate. Conversely, some patients, particularly younger ones or those with profound left ventricular dysfunction, may be tachycardic. The optimal heart rate balances coronary blood flow (which takes place mainly during diastole) with cardiac output and is usually between 80 and 100 beats per minute.[28] Normal sinus *rhythm* ensures atrioventricular synchrony and maximizes cardiac efficiency.[29] Loss of sinus rhythm (junctional rhythm or atrial fibrillation) usually reduces cardiac output by 10% to 25%.[30] Patients with slow sinus rhythm (less than 70 beats per minute) or junctional (AV nodal) rhythm usually can be paced via atrial pacing wires placed at the time of surgery to improve cardiac output.[31] Slowing a rapid rhythm (>110 bpm) is important to reduce the likelihood of developing myocardial ischemia in the immediate postoperative period when coronary flow reserve is limited. Reduction of exogenous catecholamines; administration of narcotics, sedatives, antipyretics, or intravenous fluids; and the use of antiadrenergics such as beta blockers are employed to slow a rapid heart rate.

Ventricular *preload* refers to sarcomere length at end-diastole when both passive filling and the contribution of atrial contraction are complete. Sarcomere length cannot be measured directly, and therefore, a number of surrogate measurements are used. These include left ventricular end-diastolic volume (LVEDV), which is related to left ventricular end-diastolic pressure (LVEDP). The relationship LVEDV/LVEDP is referred to as *ventricular compliance*, a combination of active relaxation of the actin-myosin complex and the passive viscoelastic properties of the myocardium.[32,33] Hearts with reduced ventricular compliance (a frequent finding after heart surgery[34]) exhibit diastolic dysfunction and therefore require a higher LVEDP to achieve a given preload. For example, patients with left ventricular hypertrophy secondary to aortic stenosis have poor left ventricular compliance. Left atrial pressure closely approximates LVEDP and its direct measurement is especially helpful in patients undergoing complex operations or with preexisting left ventricular dysfunction. Pulmonary capillary wedge pressure or pulmonary artery diastolic pressure provide good estimates of the left atrial pressure when pulmonary congestion, edema, and inflammation are absent—conditions rarely met immediately after cardiac surgery.[35]

To maintain adequate preload, volume replacement frequently is necessary immediately after heart surgery due to loss of arterial and venous vasomotor tone, increased capillary permeability, bleeding, and high volumes of urine.[36] Often, judicious fluid administration is all that is required to maintain hemodynamic stability or to treat low cardiac output accompanied by vasoconstriction. Lactated Ringer's solution is appropriate initially, but infusion of hydroxyethyl starch (hetastarch) or blood products may be indicated. Limited animal and retrospective data have raised concern regarding coagulation abnormalities associated with the use of hetastarch after cardiac surgery.[37–39] The preponderance of evidence, however, suggests that when administered in quantities under 20cc/kg/24h hetastarch does not cause increased bleeding, and is at least as effective as albumin solutions for volume expansion,[37,39–50] at half the cost. Transfusion of packed red blood cells should be governed by logical protocols and good clinical judgment with regard to the rate of blood loss. In general, blood is not necessary unless the hematocrit is less than 25%. Strategy based on recent data suggests that the mortality rate rises sharply if the *intraoperative* hematocrit is allowed to drop below 23%.[51]

Ventricular *afterload* refers to systolic wall stress, which is determined by intraventricular systolic pressure and ventricular wall thickness.[52] Ventricular wall thickness changes minimally during heart surgery, and therefore changes in ventricular systolic pressure have the most impact on afterload. In the absence of left ventricular outflow obstruction, systolic blood pressure determines afterload and thereby influences both stroke volume and myocardial oxygen demand.[53,54] Manipulations of systemic vascular resistance can improve cardiac output and the adequacy of coronary blood flow.[55,56]

Hypertension, or at least systemic vasoconstriction, is common after cardiac surgery.[57] Increased arterial resistance has been associated with low Po_2 in skeletal muscle and secondary metabolic acidosis despite adequate cardiac output and oxygen content of arterial blood.[58] The microcirculatory changes that produce inadequate tissue perfusion appear to resolve after a period of 6 to 8 hours, but this interval does not correlate with rewarming following moderately hypothermic cardiopulmonary bypass.[59] Humoral factors may play a role, since a number of circulating mediators are present and produce the whole-body inflammatory response to CPB.[8,60] Regardless of etiology, sodium nitroprusside is an effective means to reduce afterload during and after cardiac surgery.[57,61,62] The administration of this and other drugs via computer-controlled systems offers several advantages[63–65] but cannot substitute for a competent bedside clinician.

Some patients have a lowered systemic vascular resistance (SVR) during and immediately after cardiopulmonary bypass. The accompanying hypotension sometimes requires treatment with vasoconstrictors that are usually agents with pronounced alpha-adrenergic effects such as phenylephrine or norepinephrine. Christakis et al[66] reported the incidence of low SVR to be more common in patients undergoing normothermic perfusion and in those with longer cardiopulmonary bypass times.[66] Diabetics, patients with peripheral vascular disease, and those with a left ventricular ejection fraction of less than 0.40 are less likely to develop low systemic vascular resistance and associated hypotension. Phenylephrine has been shown to decrease flow in internal mammary grafts but not in saphenous vein grafts, whereas norepinephrine does not change and epinephrine increases flow in the internal mammary artery.[67]

Most surgeons assess *myocardial contractility* before, during, and after a cardiac operation by indirect methods. Measurements of ejection fraction, ventricular wall motion, and cardiac output all depend on loading conditions present at the time, as well as intrinsic myocardial contractility. In the research laboratory, changes in the ventricular pressure/volume relationship during a cardiac cycle can be used to generate a load-independent assessment of contractility,[68] but this methodology is impractical for routine clinical use. Thus appropriate assumptions regarding contractility are made when changes in cardiac output are not explained by the other determinants.

Following heart surgery, dysfunction of either ventricle may limit overall cardiac performance. Measurement and comparison of right and left atrial pressures (reflective of respective ventricular end-diastolic pressures) provide important information.[69] When the atrioventricular valves are normal, the ventricle with the highest corresponding atrial pressure is the one limiting cardiac performance. Therapeutic interventions, including but not limited to the use of inotropes, are aimed at supporting that ventricle.

PERIOPERATIVE VENTRICULAR DYSFUNCTION

Causes

The factor that contributes the most to depressed postoperative cardiac function is the pathology that existed immediately prior to operation. Even when reconstructive surgery is successful, it is unusual to see an immediate improvement in contractile function (without the administration of inotropes). Thus adequate cardiac reserve must be present to withstand the demands of heart surgery. Preoperative cardiac abnormalities are not limited to systolic function but may involve diastolic, valvular, electrophysiologic, and vascular function. Optimal perioperative care is aimed at compensating for this impaired preoperative function.

The operation itself may cause left ventricular dysfunction and low cardiac output. Contributors to cardiac dysfunction include inadequate protection of the myocardium during periods of aortic cross-clamping, myocardial and pulmonary edema, acute left ventricular distension or other trauma, uncorrected valvular lesions, and reduced coronary blood flow. The investigation as to whether the operation has been adequate to correct preexisting pathology begins as soon as the aortic cross-clamp is removed. Search for graft occlusion, valvular incompetence, cardiac compression, or intracardiac shunting continues throughout the postoperative period. Useful tools include assessment of wall motion abnormalities by direct visualization or echocardiography (usually transesophageal), the electrocardiogram, cardiac enzymes, blood gases obtained from the pulmonary and systemic vasculature, and right and left atrial pressure measurements. Discovery of an inadequate operation usually demands immediate reoperation.

PERICARDIAL TAMPONADE

Pericardial tamponade can occur either when the heart is too large for the available space (after sternum closure) because of the myocardial, lung, and mediastinal edema resulting from a long operation or when postoperative fluid collection compresses a heart that previously fit comfortably in the pericardial space. Compression of the heart, especially of the right atrium and ventricle, can reduce overall cardiac function dramatically. Increased right-sided heart pressures impair venous return and consequently diminish left ventricular preload.

Sternal closure tamponade This will be evident as soon as sternal closure is attempted. Delayed sternal closure is an accepted technique for avoiding compression of the seriously impaired or markedly edematous heart in the immediate postoperative period.[70–72] Infectious complications are minimized by covering the wound with an occlusive watertight dressing[70] and instituting continuous irrigation of the mediastinum with a diluted povidone-iodine solution.[73,74] Because of the concern for possible iodine toxicity, antibiotic solutions may also be used. Closure of the sternum is usually possible in 2 to 4 days after achieving a negative fluid balance of several liters.[71]

Fluid accumulation tamponade This occurs in the early postoperative period from an accumulation of undrained blood and clot in patients who initially demonstrate adequate ventricular performance but have copious bleeding in the initial hours after surgery. Coagulopathy correction results in formation of a pericardial clot, with consequent inability of the mediastinal tubes to evacuate the accumulating blood. Tamponade results. Acute tamponade is usually associated with a rapid increase in right and left atrial pressures, which tend to equalize. Tamponade is almost invariably associated with widening of the mediastinal silhouette on the chest radiograph. The association of rising atrial pressures, diminished cardiac output, and a widening mediastinum is sufficient to prompt surgical exploration.

Although the majority of patients develop some degree of pericardial effusion in the days following heart surgery, only a minority develop signs and symptoms of tamponade.[75] Delayed pericardial tamponade may develop insidiously. It can occur as late as several weeks after operation and is more common in patients receiving anticoagulants.[76,77] Delayed tamponade is not associated with the postpericardiotomy syndrome (fever, pain, friction rub)[78] but rarely may be caused by chylopericardium.[79,80] Prolonged drainage of the pericardial space does not prevent subsequent development of delayed tamponade.[81]

The use of echocardiography to diagnose early or delayed tamponade has been well described,[82–84] and this test is indicated in patients with unexplained poor cardiac performance following heart surgery.[85] Measurement of an exaggerated pulsus paradoxus (a decrease in systolic blood pressure during inspiration) remains a reliable clinical indicator and, together with adequate radiologic examination, indicates the need for drainage. Although percutaneous catheter drainage is useful for effusions unassociated with heart surgery, the safest treatment for delayed tamponade after median sternotomy is surgical, usually by a simple subxyphoid approach.[86]

SUPPORT OF CARDIAC PERFORMANCE

Pharmacologic Support

If ventricular function is depressed following a cardiac operation, treatment with vasodilators and volume loading may not be sufficient to ensure adequate circulation. Ventricular contractility should be augmented, usually with inotropic agents. There are excellent reviews on this subject,[87–89] and a thorough understanding of the pharmacology involved is required to care for postoperative cardiac patients. Inotropic agents may be divided into catecholamines and noncatecholamines. The former include natural or synthetic adrenergic agents that stimulate alpha and beta receptors in the heart, lungs, and peripheral vasculature (Table 15-7). Noncatecholamines include calcium, digoxin, amrinone, and milrinone.

Patients likely to benefit from catecholamine support are those with low cardiac output (CI <2.0 L/min/m^2), with optimized heart rate, rhythm, ventricular preload, and afterload, and without evidence of acute cardiac tamponade. Dopamine and dobutamine enhance heart rate and cardiac output equally, but dobutamine produces greater reductions in left ventricular preload and afterload.[90] Dobutamine augments myocardial coronary blood flow more than dopamine.[91] Dopamine works well in conjunction with vasodilators for low cardiac output after heart surgery.[92,93] As with all adrenergic agents, the hemodynamic effects of these

TABLE 15–7 Adrenergic receptor activity of commonly used catecholamines*

Drug	α Peripheral	β_1 Cardiac	β_2 Peripheral	DA_1 Peripheral	DA_2 Peripheral
Epinephrine	++++	++++	++++	0	0
Norepinephrine	+++	++++	+	0	0
Phenylephrine	++++	0	0	0	0
Dopamine	++++	++++	++	++++	++++
Dobutamine	+	++++	++	0	0

*Peripheral alpha receptors (α) cause vasoconstriction. $Beta_1$ receptors mainly have a positive inotropic and chronotropic effect. $Beta_2$ receptors also have positive inotropic and chronotropic action on the heart, and peripherally cause vasodilatation (particularly in skeletal muscle vasculature).

DA_1, dopamine 1, or postsynaptic receptor causing direct vasodilation; DA_2, dopamine 2, or presynaptic receptor causing vasodilation by inhibition of norepinephrine release.

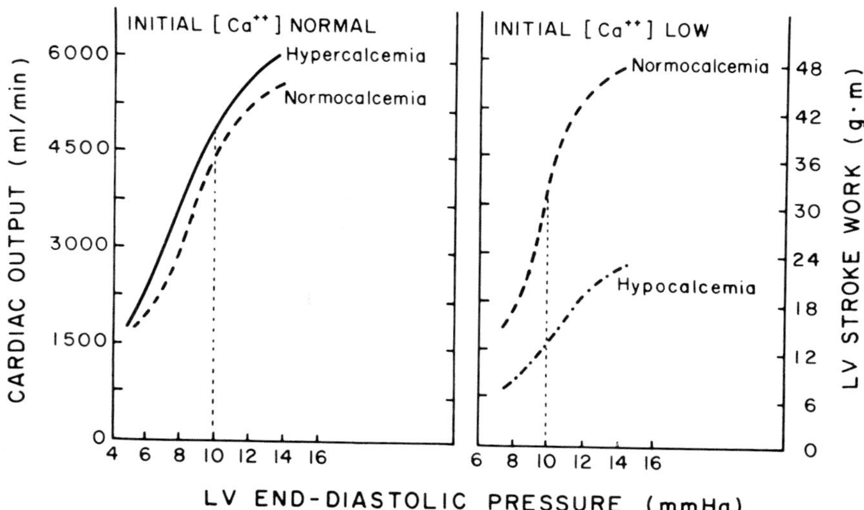

FIGURE 15–1 Influence of initial calcium concentration on left ventricular response to calcium administration. *(Reproduced with permission from Drop LJ: Ionized calcium, the heart, and hemodynamic function. Anesth Analg 1985; 64:432.)*

drugs depend on dosage. When dopamine is administered at less than 8 μg/kg per minute, beta and dopaminergic receptor stimulation predominates and enhances cardiac output and renal blood flow.[94] At doses greater than 10 μg/kg per minute, alpha vasoconstrictor effects predominate, and tachycardia may ensue. The underlying pathophysiology and age of the patient may alter the expected response.

The effect of epinephrine on both alpha- and beta-adrenergic receptors makes it a useful agent following cardiac surgery. The effects of epinephrine vary by dosage. At low doses (<0.02 μg/kg/min), epinephrine stimulates peripheral $beta_2$ receptors and causes vasodilation. Higher doses cause increasing cardiac effects, and the highest doses can cause vasoconstriction via peripheral alpha receptor stimulation. The response of an individual patient's peripheral and pulmonary hemodynamics is somewhat unpredictable, especially after cardiopulmonary bypass. Steen et al[95] investigated the effects of epinephrine after cardiac surgery and discovered a consistent increase in cardiac output but variable changes in mean arterial pressure. Stephenson et al[96] demonstrated similar increases in cardiac output with epinephrine infusions after heart surgery and showed that hypertension and tachycardia occurred when higher doses were used.

Norepinephrine, another naturally occurring catecholamine, is used after heart surgery when blood pressure is low. In addition to pronounced effects on peripheral alpha receptors, norepinephrine is a potent $beta_1$ agonist and therefore increases myocardial inotropy. The increased blood pressure that these two effects provide must be balanced against increased myocardial oxygen consumption and reduced renal, mesenteric, and peripheral perfusion that may ensue, especially at higher doses.

Isoproterenol stimulates $beta_1$- and $beta_2$-adrenergic receptors but has little alpha action. Isoproterenol increases heart rate and contractility and decreases systemic vascular resistance. Isoproterenol is potentially useful when reactive pulmonary hypertension and right-sided heart failure contribute to postoperative low cardiac output, as may occur following mitral valve surgery or cardiac transplantation. Its nonselective beta-adrenergic stimulation, which may cause tachyarrhythmias and systemic vasodilation, limits its utility in other situations.

Calcium, in its ionized form, is critical for excitation-contraction coupling in cardiac muscle.[97] Low calcium ion concentrations depress ventricular function and peripheral resistance and contribute to hypotension and low cardiac output. In addition, adequate calcium is necessary for the action of many cardiovascular drugs, including catecholamines. Drop and Scheidegger[98] demonstrated that a calcium bolus injection is associated with increased myocardial contractility, an effect that is directly related to the initial calcium level (Fig. 15-1). Shapira et al[99] also showed that a bolus of calcium can cause transient hemodynamic improvement in patients after cardiopulmonary bypass but that a continuous infusion of calcium does not sustain the beneficial effect. Because of these and similar[100,101] observations, many surgeons administer a bolus of calcium (500 to 1000 mg) immediately before weaning from cardiopulmonary bypass when serum ionized calcium levels are generally low.

Inamrinone (initially named amrinone) is a noncatecholamine bypyridine derivative that inhibits phosphodiesterase to slow the hydrolysis of adenosine 3', 5'-cyclic monophosphate (cAMP).[102] Because its congener, milrinone, causes less thrombocytopenia, milrinone has largely replaced inamrinone in clinical use.[103–106] Increased vascular (systemic and pulmonary) and myocardial cAMP augments cardiac output through pulmonary and systemic vasodilation and inotropic effects.[107–110] Milrinone also partially reverses the reduction in ventricular compliance induced by cardiopulmonary bypass.[111] It is useful in cases of right ventricular and biventricular failure due to its ability to reduce right ventricular afterload. Milrinone clearly improves separation from cardiopulmonary bypass in patients who have preexisting left ventricular dysfunction.[112] Since the mechanism of action complements that of catecholamines, which stimulate production of cAMP, these drugs can be used in combination with milrinone to achieve a synergistic effect.

Phosphodiesterase inhibitors appear to improve myocardial relaxation[113] as well as coronary,[114] skeletal muscle,[115] and mesenteric blood flow.[116] Their use is not associated with an increase in myocardial oxygen consumption,[110,117] a finding that contrasts with all the catecholamines. Unfortunately, these agents cost substantially more than do traditional inotropes. They have a slight proarrhythmic effect.[118]

Once acute problems have subsided, some patients in sinus rhythm require chronic augmentation of contractile function. The use of digitalis in this setting has long been argued, but there is evidence that it increases contractility.[119] Newer agents such as enoximone, another type III phosphodiesterase inhibitor, and vesnarinone, a quinalone with immunomodulatory properties, may be available for treatment of chronic heart failure, perhaps used in combination with beta-blocking agents.[120–122] Their role in the immediate postoperative period is not defined.

THYROID HORMONE

Several studies have demonstrated that cardiopulmonary bypass and hypothermic cardiac arrest result in low serum levels of thyroid hormone.[13,123–125] The pattern of thyroid hormone depletion after cardiopulmonary bypass is similar to that seen in other acute nonthyroid illnesses and the euthyroid sick syndrome. Traditionally, triiodothyronine replacement has not been administered to this group of patients. Several studies have challenged this view by demonstrating improved recovery of ischemic myocardium in animals[126–129] and improved hemodynamics with a lower incidence of atrial fibrillation in a small number of patients after cardiopulmonary bypass.[125,130–134] Thyroid supplementation to unstable organ donors may improve outcomes in cardiac transplantation.[135–138]

Triiodothyronine (T3) augments cardiac output via nucleus-mediated mechanisms and direct stimulation of calcium-ATPase in the sarcolemma and sarcoplasmic reticulum.[139] Enhancement of calcium transport reduces the cytoplasmic calcium concentration, which aids in myocardial relaxation. This action improves myocardial compliance and diastolic function in postischemic stunned myocardium.[13,123,124,139] Triiodothyronine also decreases cardiac work postoperatively by acutely decreasing systemic vascular resistance.[132,140,141]

A number of studies, however, including a trial of over 200 patients, have failed to demonstrate any significant hemodynamic benefit from administering triiodothyronine to patients after cardiopulmonary bypass.[141–143] This may be related to intramyocardial T3 levels. Although serum levels of thyroid hormone are decreased for up to one week after cardiopulmonary bypass,[13,124] the myocyte may not be depleted of thyroid hormone.[144] Concerns regarding enhanced myocardial oxygen demand and conflicting data about atrial arrhythmias have further limited widespread use of this hormone.[145,146] Further investigation will help elucidate the multiple cardiovascular effects of triiodothyronine and possibly define the subset of patients who will benefit from this therapy.

Mechanical Circulatory Support

Pharmacologic inotropic support is the first line of therapy for the patient who fails to separate from cardiopulmonary bypass or who experiences pump failure in the early postoperative period. The decision to add mechanical support (IABP or a ventricular assist device) to chemical support is frequently based on the presence of low cardiac output (CI <2.0 L/min/m^2) despite maximal inotropic support. Examination of levels of inotropic support at the time of separation from cardiopulmonary bypass in a group of adult patients undergoing cardiac surgery demonstrated a linear correlation between the level of pharmacologic inotropic support administered and hospital mortality. Patients requiring three high-dose inotropes at the time of weaning from cardiopulmonary bypass had a mortality of 80%.[147] This series also showed greatly improved hospital discharge rates for patients who underwent ventricular assist device (VAD) insertion based on a defined formula (cardiogenic shock despite administration of two high-dose inotropes) that emphasized early insertion. It is clear that high-dose pharmacologic inotropic support alone may stabilize a patient's hemodynamics and permit transfer to the intensive care unit, but that a significant proportion of these patients will ultimately succumb to multisystem organ failure.

INTRA-AORTIC BALLOON COUNTERPULSATION

Intra-aortic balloon pumping (IABP) was first performed clinically by Kantrowitz et al in 1968.[148] IABP uses the principle of diastolic counterpulsation, in which the balloon inflates in synchrony and out of phase with the cardiac cycle. Benefits of this technique include augmentation of diastolic coronary perfusion pressure, reduced systolic afterload, and increased cardiac output with an improvement in the myocardial oxygen supply/demand ratio. Major contraindications to IABP use include severe atherosclerotic disease of the aorta or iliofemoral arteries, descending aortic dissection, and aortic insufficiency. If indicated, insertion of the IABP can be accomplished bedside in the ICU. IABPs are used perioperatively in 8% to 12% of cardiac surgical operations.

There are significant practice pattern variations in regards to timing of insertion, with the percentage of IABPs inserted preoperatively ranging from 20% to 70%.[149–151] Complications of femoral IABP placement include lower extremity ischemia and thrombocytopenia.[152–156]

VENTRICULAR ASSIST DEVICES

The intra-aortic balloon pump is an attractive form of circulatory support for the patient undergoing cardiac surgery because of its ease of insertion and removal. However, the IABP only yields a modest increase in cardiac output and does not displace a significant volume. Failure of the IABP to improve hemodynamic performance of the failing heart should prompt consideration of rapid institution of mechanical circulatory support. An ideal circulatory support device would be rapidly and easily implanted and explanted, permit uni- or biventricular assist, have minimal anticoagulation requirements, provide maximal LV unloading, reliably provide intermediate length support (7-14 days), permit ambulation, have a low infection rate, and be easy to convert to a long-term device. Such a device does not exist. Currently available options include the centrifugal pump, extracorporeal life support (ECLS), the Abiomed BVS-5000, and the Thoratec system.

BLEEDING

Causes

PREDISPOSITION TO BLEEDING

Although infrequent, preoperative disorders may cause postoperative bleeding. Acute myocardial infarction treated with thrombolytic therapy within hours before surgical revascularization causes a profound bleeding diathesis that can be controlled with fibrinogen replacement and/or aprotinin.[157,158] Aspirin taken within 1 week before operation may increase the bleeding time but infrequently increases postoperative blood loss.[159,160] A heart operation may be necessary after patients have had percutaneous coronary angioplasty or stent insertion. These patients will often be under the influence of platelet inhibitors such as the glycoprotein IIb/IIIa inhibitors eptifibatide, tirofiban, or abciximab; or the ADP binding inhibitor, clopidogrel. Platelet transfusion to counteract all these antiplatelet drugs and fresh frozen plasma or cryoprecipitate for the GP IIb/IIIa inhibitors will attenuate resultant coagulopathy.[161]

Other intrinsic clotting abnormalities are encountered occasionally; however, almost all can be ruled out in the absence of a history of unusual bleeding with lacerations, operations, or dental procedures. We do not recommend a routine preoperative bleeding time but do obtain a careful bleeding history.

MECHANICAL, ANATOMIC, OR SURGICAL CAUSES

In the presence of excessive bleeding (over 500 mL in the first hour), the first question is whether or not bleeding is coming from an anatomic source. Such sources include vascular anastomoses, side branches of saphenous veins or internal mammary arteries, cannulation sites, aortotomies or cardiotomies, left ventricular aneurysm resection lines, the distal transected end of an internal mammary artery, edges of pericardium, the coronary sinus and great coronary vein, sternal wire sites, and pleural or pericardial fat. If bleeding is exceptionally brisk or an anatomic source is suspected, the remedy is immediate operation.

BLEEDING DIATHESIS

Cardiac surgery causes a postoperative bleeding tendency.[162–167] The primary cause appears to be fibrinolysis caused by blood contact with the biomaterial components of the heart-lung machine and by blood suctioned from pericardial and pleural wells. (See Chapter 11 for a detailed discussion of the pathogenesis.) The degree of fibrinolysis correlates with the duration of cardiopulmonary bypass.[163] Platelet dysfunction and heparin[168] also contribute to postoperative bleeding. Hemodilution decreases platelet numbers. Most cardiac operations use moderate hypothermia, and persistent or recurrent hypothermia commonly occurs early after operation. Hypothermia-induced dysfunction of platelets and coagulation enzymes also causes a bleeding diathesis. Heparin rebound—the recurrence of measurable heparin activity after complete neutralization with protamine—occurs frequently and is probably caused by elution of heparin from plasma proteins.[169] This problem is easily managed by protamine administration.[170]

Diagnosis

We define excessive bleeding as a chest tube effluent exceeding 500 mL/h in the first hour, 400 mL/h during the first 2 hours, 300 mL/h during the first 3 hours, or 200 mL/h during the first 6 hours. In addition, sudden increases in bleeding rate signify excessive bleeding and suggest a new arterial or intracardiac source. Massive bleeding is considerably in excess of these parameters and usually is accompanied by hemodynamic compromise.

At times, blood accumulates in the pericardial space but does not drain because clots fill the chest tubes. In these instances, the clot fills not only the chest tube but also the pericardium. Vigorous chest tube stripping can create high negative pressures but rarely succeeds in clearing clot from the tube. The clot cannot be removed in this manner because the tube is surrounded by a mediastinal clot that has the consistency of Jello. The high vacuum created by stripping can suck a saphenous vein graft into the chest tube and kink

TABLE 15–8 Postoperative coagulopathy

	Tests							
Cause	PT	PTT	TT	Platelet count	RT	FIB	FSP	Treatment
Heparin excess	N-↑	↑	↑↑	N	N	N	N	Protamine sulfate titrated with ACT or heparin assay
Fibrinolysis	↑	↑	↑	N	↑	N-↓	↑	EACA 4-8 g IV over 10 min followed by 1gm/h infusion for 5-8 h (or until clotting factors N); FFP
Excessive consumption*	↑	↑	↑	↓	↑	↓↓	↑	Treat cause, FFP, cryoprecipitate, platelets
Thrombocytopenia or platelet dysfunction	N	N	N	N↓**	N	N	N	Platelets

*Rare excessive consumption [also known as diffuse intravascular coagulation (DIC)] always has associated fibrinolysis.

**Platelets may be reduced in number as well as function.

PT = prothrombin time; PTT = partial thromboplastin time; TT = thrombin time; RT = reptilase time; FIB = fibrinogen; FSP = fibrin split products; ACT = activated clotting time; EACA = epsilon-aminocaproic acid; FFP = fresh-frozen plasma; N = normal; sl = slightly;↑ = elevated; ↑↑ = very elevated; ↓ = low; ↓↓ = very low.

or occlude the graft. Chest tubes should not be stripped! Reexploration of the wound and manual removal of the clot are required.

Our routine postoperative laboratory test to screen for clotting disorders is an activated partial thromboplastin time (PTT). For patients with excessive bleeding or a markedly elevated PTT, other tests are performed. These include a prothrombin time (PT), thrombin time (TT), fibrinogen determination, and platelet count. Elevated fibrin degradation products (FDP) or d-dimer indicates fibrinolysis, but a low plasma fibrinogen concentration is sufficient to initiate antifibrinolytic therapy. If inadequate heparin neutralization exists, it may be identified by an elevated PTT or TT, and a normal reptilase test. An analysis of the causes of bleeding and recommended treatments are given in Table 15-8. In addition to these tests, a comparison of the blood hematocrit with one from a freshly drawn sample from the chest tube differentiates fresh bleeding and excessive serum reflux or lymphatic drainage. Finally, if pericardial tamponade is suspected, the chest x-ray taken immediately after operation should be compared with that taken several hours later; tamponade in the absence of widened mediastinum is rare.

Treatment

INTRAOPERATIVE PREVENTION

The vast majority of excessive postoperative bleeding episodes can be prevented by a meticulous, systematic operation and sternal closure. At the completion of an orderly, carefully performed operation, and after neutralization of heparin with protamine, a compulsively thorough search for bleeding should be done. Beginning superficially, the skin and suprasternal tissues are inspected, followed by the sternum and periosteum. The internal mammary bed comes next, followed by reinsertion of the sternal retractor and examination of the pericardial and pleural fat and the veins in the region of the left innominate vein. Finally, all anastomoses, aortotomies, and cardiotomies and the lengths of all grafts are examined. Excessive bleeding during this inspection often precludes finding specific bleeding sites. Patience must be called upon to continue a systematic search for bleeding. Because some patients do not tolerate lifting the heart, the surgeon must be assured that the posterior surface is not bleeding before bypass is terminated. This routine was clearly advocated by Najafi, who stated, "The surgeon's determination to gain reliable hemostasis is the prerequisite for preventing reoperation for bleeding after cardiac operations."[171]

PHARMACOLOGIC PREVENTION

Regardless of efforts to prevent bleeding, a bleeding diathesis may still produce excessive blood loss after complex and long operations. Pharmacologic therapy of this nonsurgical clotting disorder is often helpful. Antifibrinolytic agents such as epsilon-aminocaproic acid and tranexamic acid and the protease inhibitor aprotinin reduce postoperative blood loss after heart operations.[172–176] However, aprotinin, the most effective of these agents, may contribute to renal dysfunction and early coronary artery graft thrombosis.[177–179] For this reason, and because of its considerable cost (about $1000 per patient), we reserve aprotinin for long operations with predictable excessive bleeding. We recommend, and routinely administer, epsilon-aminocaproic acid: 10 g with the skin incision, 10 g during the operation, and the final 10 g immediately before heparin reversal with protamine for other operations.

Desmopressin acetate (DDAVP) also has been given to reduce postoperative bleeding, but its effectiveness is unclear.[180–182] However, the drug appears to be effective in reducing postoperative bleeding in patients who receive preoperative aspirin.[183–185]

REINFUSION OF SHED BLOOD

During cardiac operations, blood in the pericardium or pleural spaces is routinely aspirated back into the perfusion circuit. This admixture of circulating and shed blood probably contributes to some of the clotting disorders that occur after heart operations.[186] Before heparin and after protamine, many centers reinfuse packed cells separated from washed blood aspirated from the field. After operation, chest tube effluent may be reinfused. This blood has already clotted in the mediastinum and hence contains high levels of fibrin degradation products and low levels of fibrinogen. Accordingly, fibrinolysis is detectable after reinfusion of shed blood, but this does not lead to a significant clotting disorder.[187–192] Nevertheless, we find that reinfusion is neither necessary nor cost-effective in most patients (in whom average postoperative blood loss over the first 24 hours is between 500 and 750 mL).

VOLUME REPLACEMENT

Volume replacement should satisfy two seemingly opposing goals: (1) maintenance of adequate intravascular volume for adequate blood circulation, (2) without increasing diffuse organ edema that accompanies heart operations. Blood oxygen-carrying capacity also must be adequate. If oxygenation and mixed venous O_2 saturation are adequate, we do not transfuse patients unless the hematocrit falls below 25%.

BLOOD FACTOR REPLACEMENT

Component factor replacement is unnecessary unless bleeding is excessive and tests (Table 15-8) indicate a bleeding diathesis. For patients who require replacement, the usual clotting disorder demonstrates an elevated PT, PTT, and TT and a depressed fibrinogen concentration and platelet count. If the reptilase time is normal, heparin excess is present, and extra protamine should be given. If the reptilase test is elevated, fibrinogen deficiency and fibrinolysis are present in most cases. Continued bleeding and continued red cell replacement exacerbate this deficiency. Fibrinogen must be replaced after calculating the deficit. Although normal serum fibrinogen levels are between 200 and 400 mg/dL, a fibrinogen concentration of above 100 mg/dL should be sufficient to prevent bleeding due to hypofibrinogenemia. The deficit is calculated by subtracting the patient's serum fibrinogen concentration from 100 mg/dL and multiplying this by the patient's serum volume in deciliters. Volume replacement is calculated by dividing the deficit by the amount of fibrinogen in 1 unit of replacement. Fresh-frozen plasma contains about 500 mg per unit, and cryoprecipitate contains about 150 mg per unit. After replacing the deficit amount, serum fibrinogen should be remeasured. Continued bleeding further reduces the fibrinogen and must be treated with additional replacement.

In patients with excessive bleeding and a bleeding diathesis or a low platelet count, we replace platelets empirically and usually administer 6 to 10 units before assessing the response.

OTHER METHODS OF CONTROLLING BLEEDING

Increasing positive end-expiratory pressure (PEEP) may control excessive bleeding, but pressures approaching 20 cm H_2O may cause hypotension and reduced cardiac output.[193–195]

Other mechanical methods include placing a tamponading pack in the mediastinum, either with the chest closed or open. Sometimes the pack is covered with a rubber glove to reduce the possibility that bleeding will restart when the pack is removed. Lastly, high vacuum applied through a catheter to a specific bleeding area that cannot be controlled with sutures may cause local tamponade of the bleeding area.[196,197]

Reexploration for Bleeding

Excessive bleeding, as defined above, requires reexploration if clotting studies are normal. Delays in reexploration only increase morbidity by requiring more blood transfusions that further increase the bleeding tendency, increase organ edema, and exacerbate heart, lung, and renal dysfunction.

The decision to reexplore is more difficult if clotting studies are abnormal. If the bleeding rate does not produce hemodynamic compromise, and if pericardial tamponade is absent, replacement of clotting factors and protamine administration may be pursued aggressively. When clotting studies have returned to normal, or nearly so, the bleeding rate may be reassessed by criteria listed above to determine the need for reexploration.

When the clotting abnormality persists despite treatment, and if bleeding persists, reexploration should be performed. The likelihood of finding nonsurgical bleeding is high, but the likelihood of stopping the bleeding even without an anatomic source is also high. Evacuation of mediastinal clots seems to facilitate cessation of bleeding, even when no anatomically correctable site can be found.[198]

Massive bleeding demands immediate reexploration, as does pericardial tamponade.

ICU Emergency Sternotomy

Massive, sudden hemorrhage, and impending or actual cardiac arrest unresponsive to standard therapy usually require reopening the sternotomy in the ICU. The goals of reopening the chest are to release tamponade, prevent exsanguination, and facilitate better cardiac function. If the heart is still contracting, the act of releasing the sternum alone may result in hemodynamic improvement. Blood is aspirated while searching for sites of bleeding or kinked grafts. Massive bleeding can be controlled on the way to the operating room. Either pleura is opened if a pneumothorax is present. While this is being accomplished, an assistant should perform open heart massage. After these simple maneuvers are complete, the patient is transported to the operating room. Survival after emergently reopening the chest in the ICU varies from 20% to 70%.[199–204]

LUNG

The goal of pulmonary management after heart surgery is a rapid transition from a patient who is anesthetized, intubated, and ventilated to one who is awake, extubated, and breathing spontaneously with adequate oxygenation.

Initial Assessment

In postcardiotomy patients who have extensive and invasive monitoring, there is a tendency to observe and treat the numbers rather than to rely on clinical assessment. On arrival to the ICU, most patients will be intubated and still asleep. Skin color and feel give early warning of poor cardiac output and poor oxygenation. Chest auscultation confirms adequate air exchange in both lungs.

Arterial blood gases (ABGs) should be obtained on admission to the ICU even though subsequent ventilator weaning may be monitored by pulse oximetry. A chest x-ray confirms proper endotracheal tube position and reveals pleural effusions, pulmonary edema, and atelectasis. The film also serves as a baseline for comparison of mediastinal width should a question of pericardial tamponade subsequently be raised.

Pulmonary Dysfunction

PULMONARY EFFECTS OF CARDIOPULMONARY BYPASS

Cardiopulmonary bypass (CPB) injures most organs, including the lung. Extracorporeal perfusion produces multiple emboli of gas, fibrin, fat, cells, and other biologic debris. Bypass activates coagulation, contact, complement and fibrinolytic systems, and leukocytes, monocytes, platelets, and endothelial cells (see Ch. 11).

The combination of microemboli and activated blood enzymes leads to increased functional residual capacity (FRC), pulmonary shunting with an increased alveolar-arterial oxygen gradient, ventilation/perfusion mismatch, microatelectasis, endothelial cell swelling, and increased total-body and lung fluid.[205,206] The degree of damage increases with the time on CPB and is worse with bubble oxygenators than with membrane oxygenators.[207,208] The pulmonary damage also correlates with the amount of pulmonary extracellular water and the degree of complement activation (as measured by C3a), and both these changes correlate with the duration of CPB.[7,207,209]

If patients sustain pulmonary insult from CPB, then performing coronary artery surgery off-pump would be expected to improve postoperative pulmonary function. Although some trials demonstrate that patients who undergo off-pump coronary artery bypass require less time on the ventilator,[210–212] numerous other trials demonstrate no difference in pulmonary function or time to extubation.[213–217] More investigation will be needed to understand if a pulmonary benefit exists with off-pump surgery.

Several methods to minimize this lung injury have been proposed. Intraoperative leukocyte depletion (by filtration) has produced inconsistent results.[218–220] Prostaglandin E1 (PGE1) or a synthetic analogue reduces the duration of ventilation and improves oxygenation postoperatively.[221,222] Pharmacologic inhibition of platelet-activating factor decreases pulmonary vascular resistance, increases oxygenation, and decreases histologic lung damage.[223]

The use of PEEP postoperatively increases FRC but may not reduce intrapulmonary shunting.[224] However, in our experience, increasing levels of PEEP usually improve oxygenation in patients with excessive shunting. Very high levels, above 10 to 15 cm H_2O, may impair cardiac function.

PHRENIC NERVE PALSY

Left lower lobe atelectasis or infiltrates are quite common after heart operations.[225] Reasons for this include wound pain, sedation, the supine position, hesitancy to cough, and general weakness of the patient. Partial palsy of one or both phrenic nerves may contribute.[225–227] More severe or complete phrenic palsy can be caused by topical cold or iced slush in the pericardium. Phrenic nerve palsy, particularly if bilateral, can lead to severe or even fatal pulmonary dysfunction.[228–230]

OTHER CAUSES

Preoperative pulmonary dysfunction contributes to postoperative dysfunction.[231] In patients with poor pulmonary function, both the incidence of pulmonary complications and the duration of intensive care increase. Patients with obstructive pulmonary disease fare less well than those with restrictive disease.

Persistent left ventricular failure after cardiac operations increases end-capillary hydrostatic pressure and favors fluid extravasation into alveoli. Interstitial and alveolar fluid inhibits oxygen transfer, increases shunting, decreases compliance, increases secretions, and facilitates atelectasis and pneumonia. Excessive pain, by inhibiting deep breathing, also leads to atelectasis and pneumonia. Epidural anesthesia effectively relieves severe pain and may be helpful in the uncommon patient who develops sternal fractures during operation.[232]

Ventilation

INITIAL MANAGEMENT: VENTILATOR SETTINGS

The ventilator is adjusted to achieve adequate oxygenation (PO_2 of 80 to 100 mm Hg), carbon dioxide elimination (PCO_2 of 35 to 45 mm Hg), and normal pH (7.3 to 7.5). Higher tidal volumes with lower rates help reduce atelectasis without hyperventilation. PEEP also helps to maintain lung volumes and prevent atelectasis. Low amounts of PEEP are tolerated well by all patients except those with emphysematous air trapping; in these patients, PEEP may be contraindicated. Typical initial ventilator settings are: minute volume, 120 mL/kg/min; tidal volume, 15 mL/kg; rate, 8 breaths per minute; and PEEP, 5 cm H_2O. The inspired initial oxygen concentration (FIO_2) is usually 0.9 but is quickly lowered to 0.5 or less as permitted by an initial ABG measurement. Subsequently, FIO_2 is progressively reduced and monitored by transcutaneous O_2 saturation.

MAINTENANCE

Intermittent mandatory ventilation (IMV) with PEEP of 5 mm Hg maintains alveolar expansion and facilitates weaning by gradual reduction in the ventilatory rate, but may not always prevent postoperative atelectasis.[233] FIO_2 is rapidly reduced as tolerated. Excessive secretions are removed by suction. An in-line suction catheter reduces airway contamination that may occur with repeated insertions of an independent suction catheter into the endotracheal tube. When the secretions are due to pulmonary edema, however, PEEP and addressing the cause constitute the best method of controlling them.

Shivering following hypothermic CPB increases systemic oxygen consumption and predisposes to respiratory and metabolic acidosis.[234] Shivering is best treated by rewarming with radiant heat but may be arrested temporarily with narcotics or muscle relaxants.[235,236]

VENTILATOR WEANING

Whereas we once deferred extubation until the day after the operation, we now wean patients from the ventilator and extubate them as quickly as possible after (and occasionally before) leaving the operating room. This requires modification of the high-dose narcotic anesthesia protocol that is often used to blunt the sympathetic response in patients with ischemic heart disease.[237,238] Perioperative myocardial infarctions increase if anesthesia is insufficient to prevent sympathetic discharge.[237,238] However, other factors besides anesthesia also must be considered in a decision for early extubation. These include duration of cardiopulmonary bypass, extent of rewarming, preoperative pulmonary status, age, comorbidity, and adequacy of hemodynamics and hemostasis. The efficacy of the operation itself is a major factor in the decision for early extubation. Early extubation is safe and improves cardiac function by increasing preload as capacitance blood volume shifts into the chest.[239–241] Early extubation allows shorter stays in the ICU and decreased costs.

WEANING CRITERIA

If the initial ABGs are adequate, weaning the FIO_2 to 0.5 or less may be performed by monitoring arterial O_2 saturation (SaO_2) by pulse oximetry. Weaning from controlled ventilation to spontaneous unassisted ventilation may be monitored similarly. However, adequate O_2 saturation does not ensure absence of CO_2 retention. Careful clinical assessment usually indicates satisfactory CO_2 elimination. Rising blood pressure, rapid or shallow ventilation, and agitation suggest inadequate CO_2 elimination; ABGs must be measured if there is any question of the adequacy of alveolar ventilation or CO_2 removal. Even if ventilator weaning proceeds smoothly, ABGs should be remeasured prior to extubation to confirm the absence of CO_2 retention and acidosis. Contraindications to extubation include inadequate ABG values, inadequate ventilatory mechanics, early pneumonia, unstable hemodynamics, and systemic complications.

For extubation, ABG criteria are:
- PO_2 >80 mm Hg with $FIO_2 \leq 0.5$
- pH (on CPAP) $\geq$7.35 (no respiratory acidosis)
- $PCO_2 \leq$ 45 mm Hg

Ventilatory criteria are:
- Vital capacity (VC) $\geq$15 mL/kg
- Negative inspiratory force (NIF) $\geq$20 cm H_2O

Clinical requirements are:
- Alert, awake
- Absence of excessive bleeding, hemodynamic instability, or dangerous arrhythmia

When an intubated patient is breathing without assistance other than a positive airway pressure of 8 cm H_2O or less, certain clinical parameters predict failure to extubate or the need for reinstitution of mechanical ventilatory support. These include tachycardia, tachypnea, excessive ventilatory effort, and sweating. The physiologic index most predictive of failure to wean and extubate is the minute frequency of spontaneous ventilation (f) divided by the tidal volume (Vt) in liters. When high, this index reflects a clinical picture of a patient with rapid, shallow breathing. When *f*/Vt is less than 105, 78% of patients can be weaned and extubated successfully.[242] When greater than 105, 95% of patients cannot be weaned and extubated successfully. A Vt of 0.325 L is a good threshold value for predicting weaning success or failure.

Ventilator weaning, in uncomplicated cases, is quite simple. When the patient is fully awake and without excessive bleeding or hemodynamic instability, the ventilator is switched to spontaneous ventilation with CPAP of 5 mm Hg and F_{IO_2} less than 0.5. If, after 30 minutes, the patient is comfortable, and without tachycardia, tachypnea, or dyspnea, the endotracheal tube is removed and replaced with humidified mask oxygen.

POSTEXTUBATION SUPPORT

Immediately after extubation, administer humidified oxygen at 10 L/min and at a concentration 10% greater than the patient received while intubated. Oxygen delivery may be decreased safely if the O_2 saturation remains above 97% to 98%. Usually by the second postoperative day supplemental oxygen may be given via nasal prongs at progressively decreasing rates as long as the O_2 saturation remains above 90%. Sa_{O_2} is maintained over 95% during the first 2 to 3 days after extubation and over 90% thereafter. Incentive spirometry helps the patient to visually assess and improve his or her ventilatory effort. Lobar collapse either before or after extubation may be treated by tracheal suctioning but usually requires bronchoscopy. Chest physiotherapy is particularly helpful in raising secretions and encouraging cough. During these first few postextubation days, several pulmonary complications may occur; anticipating problems allows earlier treatment and preempts an extended convalescence.

REINTUBATION

A few patients are too weak to sustain adequate ventilatory efforts despite having satisfied extubation criteria. They develop retained secretions and atelectasis and may progress to pneumonia. Treatment consists of chest physical therapy, nasotracheal suctioning, and occasionally bronchoscopy. Should these measures not restore adequate ventilatory mechanics, or should excessive weakness persist, reintubation is necessary.

This step must not be delayed to the point that more severe pulmonary complications ensue. The same clinical factors that predict failure to wean also predict the need for reintubation. Air hunger, feeble ventilatory effort, tachypnea, shallow breathing, or gross inability to clear secretions requires reintubation and mechanical ventilation. Other reintubation criteria include a rising Pa_{CO_2} from a normal value to 50 mm Hg over a few hours, hypoxia despite an increasing F_{IO_2}, and a falling cardiac output.[243] A venous P_{CO_2} can be measured in lieu of an arterial sample. Venous P_{CO_2} is invariably 6 or 7 mm Hg higher than the simultaneous Pa_{CO_2}.

COMPLICATIONS

Prolonged mechanical ventilation predisposes to pneumonia. The endotracheal tube not only bypasses defenses of the upper airway and tracheal cilia but also allows direct ingress of bacteria. The importance of strict asepsis during ventilator maintenance and endotracheal suctioning cannot be overemphasized. The drawbacks of endotracheal intubation and predisposition to pneumonia strengthen the argument for early extubation.

Noncardiogenic pulmonary edema develops from an allergic reaction, probably to blood or its products or to protamine.[244,245] The edema presents as fulminating pulmonary edema with normal left atrial or pulmonary capillary wedge pressures and usually occurs either in the operating room or in the immediate postoperative period. The copious fluid bubbling from the endotracheal tube has a high protein content. When this edema occurs after cardiopulmonary bypass, the turgid, edematous lungs develop such severe air trapping that ventilation may cause the lungs to tamponade the heart, especially if sternal closure is attempted. Effective treatment consists of bronchodilators, corticosteroids, isoproterenol, and positive-pressure ventilation with high levels of PEEP. Because of tissue edema, sternal closure may effectively tamponade the heart and may need to be deferred. An intra-aortic balloon may be required to support cardiac function despite the absence of intrinsic cardiac abnormalities.

Barotrauma occurs most commonly in patients who require high levels of PEEP or high peak inspiratory pressure during mechanical ventilation. Sudden hypoxia suggests pneumothorax, either simple or tension, and demands immediate investigation. If present, prompt chest tube insertion is required. This complication is most common early after operation in elderly patients who cannot be extubated early and usually is due to rupture of apical blebs.

With an open pleural space, as often occurs from harvesting the internal mammary artery, postoperative bleeding may produce hemothorax rather than excessive blood drainage. An unexplained fall in hematocrit or hemodynamic instability suggests this possibility, and requires a chest x-ray for evaluation. Hemothorax requires chest tube insertion.

Late pleural effusions occur more commonly on the left than on the right, as does left lower lobe atelectasis. This predilection remains even without harvesting the left internal mammary artery. Effusions may require thoracentesis or occasionally a chest tube.

Pulmonary embolism occurs infrequently after heart operations (incidence 0.56%) but carries a high mortality of 34%.[246] Risk factors include preoperative bed rest or hospitalization of more than 1 day, groin cardiac catheterization within 15 days of operation, and postoperative congestive heart failure or bed rest of more than 3 days.

Long-Term Ventilator Support

CAUSES OF FAILURE TO WEAN FROM MECHANICAL VENTILATION

Infrequently, a postoperative patient may require prolonged ventilator support for more than several days. Failure to wean has two causes: failure of gas exchange at the alveolar level and failure to ventilate adequately. The two most common reasons for deficiency in gas exchange are left-sided heart failure with pulmonary congestion and the adult respiratory distress syndrome (ARDS).

Predictable failure of ventilator weaning occurs in several circumstances. These include chronic illness with poor nutrition (cachexia) and ventilatory (diaphragm and chest wall) muscle weakness, central nervous system dysfunction, pain, mechanical disruption of the bony chest wall, chronic lung disease with stiff lung parenchyma, and sepsis. Muscle weakness also may be caused by hypothyroidism and deficiencies of magnesium, potassium, calcium, and phosphate.[247,248]

WEANING AFTER PROLONGED MECHANICAL VENTILATION

In patients who need prolonged ventilator support, weaning attempts must be preceded by elimination of the causes of ventilator dependence. When excessive lung water impedes weaning, negative fluid balance is required. In the patient with renal dysfunction, a compromise must be struck between the pulmonary and renal systems, usually in the favor of the lungs. During mild dehydration, the blood urea nitrogen (BUN) level may rise temporarily. Likewise, pneumonia must be resolved by appropriate antibiotics and airway toilet. When the disorders promoting ventilator dependence are corrected, the same weaning criteria as for the acute postoperative patient are used.

WEANING TECHNIQUES

The process of weaning from long-term ventilator support may be considered endurance training for the chest wall muscles and diaphragm. This consists of progressively increasing ventilatory load until mechanical ventilation can be discontinued. Spontaneous breathing trials (SBT) are performed once per day for durations of 30 to 120 minutes, or to the point of failure. Success criteria are stable arterial blood gases, stable hemodynamics, and a stable ventilatory pattern. Failure criteria consist of failing the above, or deterioration of mental status, worsening discomfort, diaphoresis, or signs of increased work of breathing.[249] The SBT can be performed using a T-piece (giving no positive airway pressure), continuous positive airway pressure (CPAP) at a low pressure (5 cm H_2O), or with low levels (5 to 7 cm H_2O of pressure support ventilation (PSV). No convincing evidence suggests the superiority of one method over another. Using one method in a consistent protocol-driven fashion yields the most expeditious weaning, although in difficult weaning cases, it may be helpful to use an alternative method if the primary method continues to be unsuccessful. With all methods, weaning in an upright or sitting position optimizes the likelihood of success.

Tracheostomy

If, after 7 to 10 days of ventilation, weaning does not seem imminent, a tracheostomy should be performed. Tracheostomy offers several advantages over an endotracheal tube. The concern over possible laryngeal damage caused by an endotracheal tube may encourage premature weaning. With a tracheostomy, weaning can be managed independently of extubation. Tracheal toilet is more easily performed via tracheostomy. The dead space of a tracheostomy is less than that of an endotracheal tube, and this may facilitate weaning in a patient with marginal ventilation. A tracheostomy is more comfortable. Once established for a week or more, a tracheostomy offers greater security than an endotracheal tube in case of accidental extubation, because a tracheostomy tube is more easily inserted.

One serious complication of tracheostomy, whether performed by standard or percutaneous techniques, is accidental extubation during the first several days after initial placement. Hasty attempts to replace the tube easily lead to insertion outside the trachea; early accidental tracheostomy decannulation requires endotracheal intubation with subsequent elective reestablishment of the tracheostomy. Because of the possibility of contamination and infection of the median sternotomy incision from the proximity of a tracheostomy incision, the tracheal stoma should be established no lower than the second tracheal ring. With either a tracheostomy or endotracheal tube, obstruction of the tracheal end of the tube may occur from inspissated secretions. Adequate humidification helps prevent this complication. Difficulty passing a suction catheter through the tube suggests the problem, which may require changing the tube.

Percutaneous tracheostomies have replaced open (surgical) tracheostomies for many patients, although questions have been raised about the incidence of complications from the procedure with studies demonstrating both more and fewer complications with the percutaneous method.[250–253] Almost all of our elective tracheostomies are performed percutaneously and at the bedside. In 400 patients (not limited to cardiac surgical patients), there have been no procedure-related deaths, no false passages of dilators or tracheostomy tube, and two conversions to an open technique for bleeding (personal communication, Dr. Alan A. Conlan, May 22, 2002).

General Care

Multiple problems may develop in the patient who requires long-term ventilation, and these are best prevented by prophylaxis.

In an immobile patient, skin breakdown may occur over pressure points. A mattress designed to eliminate constant pressure focused over these pressure points should be used. Pooling of body fluids may cause skin maceration and breakdown. Assiduous nursing care must be employed to prevent pooling of urine, stool, or other fluids.

Inadequate nutrition impairs the ability to wean from the ventilator. Nutritional maintenance is started if the patient has not been extubated by the second postoperative day. Most cardiac patients have an intact gut; enteral feeding has many advantages over parenteral feeding. In these patients, and especially in those receiving narcotics, stool impaction may easily occur. This possibility should be assessed frequently by rectal examination if necessary. Stool softeners are used routinely.

Physical therapy is started to maintain joint mobility through range-of-motion exercises and muscle mass through resistance exercises. Contractures in patients with neurologic dysfunction are prevented with stretching exercises and splinting.

Infection constantly threatens these patients. Assiduous, aseptic care must be given to intravenous lines and all catheters. Intravenous catheters are changed on a regular schedule, usually every 5 days, or immediately if abrupt fever develops. Pulmonary toilet is maintained with strict asepsis.

KIDNEY

Postoperative Renal Function

Urine volume, blood urea nitrogen (BUN) level, and plasma creatinine level are the primary measures of adequate renal function following cardiac surgery. Urine output in the early postoperative course is usually copious as the kidneys excrete the extra volume acquired during cardiopulmonary bypass, and should be a minimum of 0.5 to 1.0 mL/kg/h. When urine volume is less, the cause must be sought.

Causes of Oliguria

The causes of oliguria can be divided into three categories: pre-renal, renal, and postrenal. Following cardiac surgery, postrenal obstruction is usually the result of a kinked or otherwise blocked Foley catheter. This can be diagnosed and usually treated by repositioning and flushing the catheter. If the bladder is obstructed secondary to hematuria and clot formation, this will also often respond to flushing. Ongoing hematuria with obstruction, however, requires continuous bladder irrigation and urology consultation.

With postrenal oliguria ruled out, the task is to differentiate a pre-renal cause from intrinsic renal failure. Pre-renal causes of oliguria are common and include low cardiac output, bleeding, hypovolemia, hypothermia, and intense vasoconstriction. Pre-renal oliguria is a result of decreased renal blood flow, and is often the first sign of generalized inadequate tissue perfusion. An example is the patient with falling urine output secondary to cardiac tamponade. If allowed to persist, inadequate renal perfusion will eventually lead to renal failure from ischemia. When diagnosed early, most causes of pre-renal oliguria can be corrected.

Pre-renal Oliguria

If a pre-renal cause for oliguria exists, and remains untreated, renal parenchymal ischemia will cause acute tubular necrosis (ATN). Obversely, assuming oliguria to be established renal failure becomes self-fulfilling: if renal failure was not present, lack of treatment will cause it. That treatment starts with the elimination of causes of diminished renal perfusion as discussed above.

If, despite this treatment, oliguria persists, early pharmacologic treatment should be used. Many centers use mannitol in the priming solution for cardiopulmonary bypass, and it is the agent of choice for prevention of renal dysfunction when periods of decreased glomerular filtration are anticipated. Pretreatment with intravenous mannitol, continued throughout any ischemic episode, improves subsequent renal blood flow and glomerular filtration.[254] A strong solute diuresis relieves tubular obstruction and reduces tubular cellular swelling.[254,255] Mannitol increases renal blood flow in both dogs and humans during CPB.[256,257]

The renovascular and functional effects of loop diuretics are similar to those of mannitol. Furosemide increases renal blood flow and promotes solute excretion.[258] The theoretical benefit of furosemide in the patient with incipient acute renal failure is to convert oliguric to nonoliguric renal failure. Although this may not improve chances of recovery,[259,260] it avoids some of the complications associated with complete renal shutdown. Furosemide early in renal dysfunction, when only abnormalities in free water clearance are apparent, improves medullary blood flow and free water clearance and identifies patients who are likely to require dialysis by their failure to respond.[261,262]

Dopamine at low doses (3-5 mg/kg/min) enhances renal blood flow. Dopamine and furosemide act synergistically and are more effective than either drug alone.[263] This drug combination prompts a brisk diuresis and reduces serum creatinine levels, possibly by enhancing vasodilatation to allow increased delivery of furosemide to the distal tubule.[264] A continuous infusion of dopamine, furosemide, and mannitol immediately upon the appearance of oliguria is particularly effective in restoring renal function and decreasing the need for dialysis.[265]

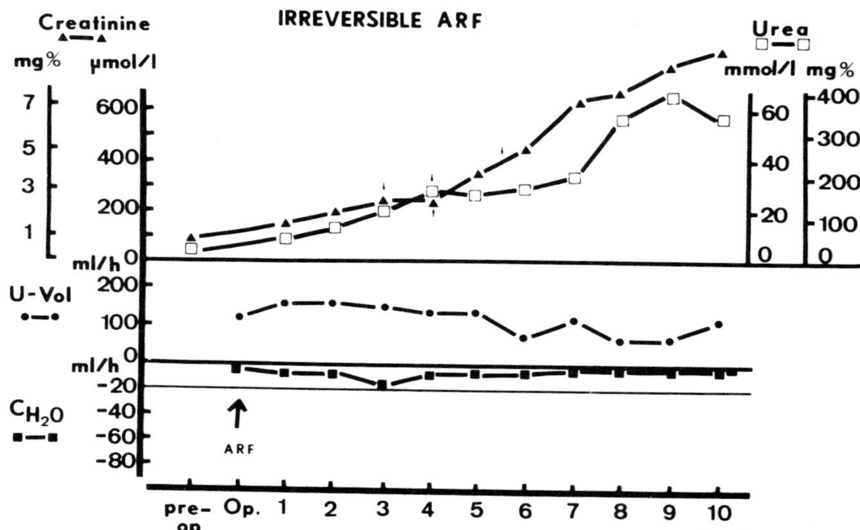

FIGURE 15–2 Representative profiles of serum urea, creatinine, urine volume, and free water clearance (C_{H_2O}) in a patient who developed irreversible acute renal failure following heart surgery. Note that changes in free water clearance preceded significant alterations in seurm urea nitrogen or creatinine.

Other drugs that have some protective effect in experimental models include calcium channel blockers[266,267] and PGE_1.[268,269] None of these agents has found clinical application. The mainstay of early support is improvement in renal blood flow and maintenance of tubular patency by ensuring adequate cardiac output and blood pressure while promoting renal vasodilatation and glomerular filtration with dopamine, mannitol, and furosemide.

Renal Failure

DIAGNOSIS

Because of the frequent difficulty of distinguishing pre-renal and renal causes of oliguria in the early postoperative period, the first responsibility must be to treat *as if* pre-renal causes exist: optimize cardiac output, eliminate vasoconstrictors and hypothermia that cause splanchnic vasoconstriction, and assure adequate blood volume and the absence of significant bleeding.

In the early hours after surgery, BUN and creatinine elevation are neither sensitive nor specific for renal failure. Mild elevations of BUN and creatinine are common after cardiac surgery and may be associated with an adequate or even large urine volume.[270] These changes are nearly always transient, with complete return of normal renal function. In cardiac surgical patients with normal preoperative renal function, 15% have an increase in serum creatinine above 1.5 mg/dL postoperatively. Only a fraction of these patients develop acute renal failure (oliguria, creatinine >2.5 mg/dL), a complication associated with a high mortality rate. New azotemia reflects hypoperfusion of the kidney, and its degree depends on the severity and duration of decreased glomerular filtration.

The insensitivity of BUN and plasma creatinine levels for predicting the onset of acute renal failure has led to other analyses of renal function that are related primarily to renal concentrating capacity.[271,272] Free water clearance is a simple and accurate method of identifying early, subclinical renal dysfunction.[261,262] Free water clearance (C_{H_2O}) can be determined according to the method of Smith[273]:

$$C_{H_2O} = V(1 - U_{osm}/P_{osm})$$

where U_{osm} and P_{osm} are urine and plasma osmolality in mmoles per liter, and V is urine volume (mL/h). Free water clearance values range from –100 (or more negative) to –20 mL/h; pathologic values range from –20 to 0 mL/h or more positive. Abnormal free water clearance is a constant finding that precedes elevations of BUN or creatinine in patients who develop renal failure[271] (Fig. 15-2). However, abnormal free water clearance is also detectable in patients with mild reversible renal insufficiency and therefore is not predictive of renal shutdown. Baek et al[261] and Brown[262] used free water clearance measurements and the response to furosemide to prospectively determine which patients would experience frank renal failure. A response to furosemide correlated with a better prognosis. Thus free water clearance measurements allow earlier detection and treatment of incipient renal failure.

Other tests for renal dysfunction lag behind the free water clearance. These tests include the BUN/creatinine ratio, urine osmolality, and fractional excretion of sodium (Fe_{Na}) (see Table 15-9).

TREATMENT

In the absence of a pre-renal cause for oliguria, acute renal failure exists. Patients at highest risk for acute renal failure are those with preoperative renal dysfunction, diabetes, congestive heart failure, renal artery stenosis, long bypass

TABLE 15–9 Distinguishing pre-renal from renal oliguria

	Pre-renal	Renal
FE^{*}_{Na}	<1	>1
Urinary [Na]	<20 mEq/dL	>20 mEq/dL
Urinary sediment	Bland	Casts
BUN/creatinine	>15:1	<15:1
Urine osmolality	>500 mosm/kg	<400 mosm/kg

*FE_{Na} is calculated using the equation $FE_{Na} = (U_{Na}/S_{Na}) / (U_{cr}/S_{cr}) \times 100$.

runs, advanced age, and emergency operations.[270,274–278] Other contributory factors are hemolysis with the liberation of free hemoglobin during prolonged cardiopulmonary bypass,[279,280] circulatory arrest,[281,282] and perioperative sepsis.

Once renal failure is established, early and aggressive dialysis decreases mortality in surgical patients.[283,284] The goals of dialysis include removal of excess fluid, reduction of serum potassium level, removal of toxic metabolites including nephrotoxins, and correction of metabolic acidosis. Intermittent hemodialysis has been largely replaced by either continuous hemofiltration or hemodialysis.[285] The former refers to ultrafiltration of blood plasma driven across a semipermeable membrane by a pressure gradient, whereas the latter refers to ultrafiltration via osmotic differences between the blood and solute sides of the membrane. The former is primarily used to remove volume, and the latter to reduce levels of specific solutes.

Hemofiltration was first described as continuous arteriovenous hemofiltration (CAVH) and employed to correct the hemodilution following cardiopulmonary bypass.[286–288] The simpler method of continuous venovenous hemofiltration (CVVH) has replaced CAVH and is mainly used, in conjunction with continuous venovenous hemodialysis (CVVHD), in the treatment of acute renal failure.[285,289,290] Arterial catheters are no longer required because CVVHD is performed via a double lumen dialysis catheter placed in a large vein. CVVH machines include a roller pump that allows hypotensive patients to continue therapy. This is in contrast to CAVH, which required a mean arterial pressure of 70 mm Hg to drive the hemofiltration.[285]

The benefit of early hemofiltration/hemodialysis of patients with postoperative renal failure and volume overload is noted above. This slow continuous process has a low risk of inducing hemodynamic instability when compared to conventional intermittent hemodialysis. Other advantages include improved filtration of middle-sized molecules and inflammatory mediators, virtually unlimited potential for fluid removal, and no requirement for a specialized dialysis nurse at the bedside.[285] There is evidence that CVVH provides benefit to patients independent of fluid removal by filtering tumor necrosis factor, complement, and interleukin-6.[289,291–293] Instituting such therapy for patients with renal failure after cardiac surgery may also decrease time on the ventilator, shorten ICU stay, and possibly improve the rate of renal recovery.[289,293]

PROGNOSIS

Despite all supportive measures available today, the prognosis for patients with established acute renal failure after CPB remains poor. Survival is 90% in patients who maintain nonoliguric renal insufficiency,[294] but those who progress to oliguric renal failure have a mortality over 50%.[278,294–296] Most patients who develop acute renal failure have sustained hypotension during the perioperative period and develop failure of several organ systems. Infection becomes a common terminal event in patients who die with renal failure. Age is a significant prognostic factor in determining survival from acute renal failure after heart surgery,[294] although Lange et al[296] did not find age, sex, preoperative renal dysfunction, severity of underlying heart disease, cardiopulmonary bypass time, or oliguria to be significant influences in a univariate analysis of patients who required hemodialysis after heart surgery. They did find that the number and types of complications were significant predictors of outcome; the highest mortality rate was associated with respiratory failure, central nervous system dysfunction, persistent hypotension, and infection. Bhat et al[295] noted a marked increase in mortality in patients whose serum creatinine rose higher than 6 mg/dL.

The best survival occurs in patients who can be maintained in nonoliguric renal failure. Early dialysis and nutritional support in patients with oliguric failure minimize metabolic complications, but the prognosis remains poor because of late septic complications. Although many recover renal function after a brief period (days to weeks) of oliguria, the incidence of chronic dialysis dependency in these patients is significant.

NERVOUS SYSTEM

Postoperative neurologic dysfunction occurs with disturbing frequency. This group of complications can be divided into three categories: central neurologic, neuropsychologic, and peripheral neurologic. Because of differences in definitions, in tests to measure deficits, and in the diligence of postoperative examinations and testing, the medical literature is confusing, especially with respect to the incidence of these complications.

Central Neurologic Complications

Cerebrovascular accidents (CVAs) that result in lasting deficits occur after heart operations in 2% to 5% of patients.[297–300] These may appear after recovery from anesthesia but usually are obvious when the patient awakens. Perioperative strokes kill one-eighth of all patients afflicted.[301]

After a CVA, a computed tomographic (CT) scan demonstrates the cerebral infarction within a day or two. Insofar as no treatment exists, there is little need to document cerebral damage early if the patient is too hemodynamically unstable to travel. However, in the comatose patient, treatable causes may exist and therefore a CT scan should be performed as soon as possible.

Carotid artery stenosis may be a risk factor for stroke in patients without *preoperative neurologic symptoms* only when the stenosis is greater than 80%, although the evidence is contradictory.[298,299,302–306] We are wary of performing cardiac operations in the presence of critical (>80%) stenosis on one or both sides without prior or concomitant carotid endarterectomy. *Symptomatic* carotid stenoses increase the risk of stroke and usually require prophylactic or concomitant carotid endarterectomy.

Perioperative strokes have multiple causes. Operations performed at normothermia have a higher incidence of CVA than those performed at moderate (28 to 32°C) hypothermia.[307] Open heart operations may cause embolic cerebral infarction from air boluses, intracardiac clot, calcified debris, or foreign material (such as felt pledgets). However, the most probable cause of most strokes is atheromatous emboli from the ascending aorta and aortic arch. Increasing age, incidence of aortic atheroma, incidence of peripheral embolization (in autopsy series), and incidence of CVA are closely correlated.[297,299,301,308] If aortic atheromas are documented by echocardiography in older patients, operation is tailored to reduce aortic manipulation and embolization.[299] Some authors find a correlation between low perfusion pressure (50 to 60 mm Hg) during CPB and CVA and recommend higher perfusion pressures (between 80 and 100 mm Hg).[309]

Neuropsychologic Complications

A large number of symptoms fall into this category and range from alterations of mood to bizarre behavior to quantifiable deficits in intellectual function. Postoperative depression occurs commonly, may last 2 to 3 months, and may be sufficiently severe to disrupt families and, rarely, cause patients to become suicidal. Usually, mild symptoms of depression disappear spontaneously and require no treatment other than reassurance. Early postoperative delirium follows a lucid period and presents as paranoia or hallucinations. Together with depression, these disorders occur in about 40% of patients.[310] The reported incidence of delirium varies widely from 7% to 57% of cardiac surgical patients.[311,312] Delirium usually disappears within a week; patient management is facilitated by small doses of haloperidol.

In some studies, deficits in intellectual function such as memory and cognition occur in as many as 75% of patients in the early postoperative period, decline to half that number by 8 weeks, and decline minimally over the next year.[313–316] Others, however, report little change between preoperative and postoperative assessments of intellectual function.[317,318] The changes seem to be caused by cerebral microemboli and correlate with the duration of CPB.[298,313,316,318] Membrane oxygenators as compared with bubble oxygenators reduce the production of microemboli.[319] The incidence of transcranially detected microemboli correlates with both stroke and behavioral change, as well as with cardiac and pulmonary complications and mortality.[320] These neurologic changes also correlate with new cerebral abnormalities detected by magnetic resonance imaging.[321] Increasing age also predicts neuropsychologic deficits.[314,318]

Debate continues regarding decreased neurologic morbidity for patients receiving coronary bypass without cardiopulmonary bypass. Despite the claims of a few investigators,[322,323] off-pump surgery has failed to demonstrate a significant decrease in stroke rate or incidence of neurocognitive dysfunction after heart surgery.[210,212,217,322,324–330]

Peripheral Deficits

Intraoperative femoral arterial bleeding (usually from a recent cardiac catheterization) can compress the femoral nerve. Foot drop can occur from pressure on the peroneal nerve as it wraps around the fibula. This complication of leg positioning for saphenous vein harvesting can be prevented by proper padding or use of a cushion designed to protect the nerve.

Upper extremity deficits are more common and are related to the median sternotomy.[331–334] The incidence increases with wide retraction or placement of the retractor.[331,332] Upper extremity deficits produce sensory deficits in the fourth and fifth fingers and usually disappear within 2 to 3 months. In severe cases, deficits involve a wider area, result in permanent sensory and motor deficits, and can lead to sympathetic dystrophy. These injuries are not completely preventable. In mild forms, sensory deficits occur in as many as 24% of patients[332] and are caused by brachial plexus injury from a first rib fracture or from the plexus stretching over an intact first rib. Nerves C8 and T1 are damaged most commonly.

Injuries of the nerves around the elbow, especially the ulnar nerve, may be confused with brachial plexus injuries. Proper padding prevents these cubital nerve injuries.

GASTROINTESTINAL SYSTEM

Major gastrointestinal complications occur more frequently after cardiac operations than after noncardiac, nonintestinal surgery. The incidence reported is from 0.5% to 3%.[335–341] Decreased visceral blood flow occurring during episodes of hypotension contributes to such complications.[342–344] Pancreatitis, mesenteric ischemia, gastroduodenal ulceration and inflammation, cholecystitis, and hepatic failure have all been attributed to hypotension, shock, or cardiopulmonary bypass.[342,345–350]

The most common major complications are upper gastrointestinal (GI) bleeding from gastritis or ulcer disease, pancreatitis, hollow viscus perforation, mesenteric ischemia, and cholecystitis.[336–338,342,350–352] In aggregate, these complications have a frighteningly high mortality between 20% and 80%; mesenteric ischemia is nearly always fatal.[338–341,346,353–355]

Risk factors for these complications include older age, perioperative hypoperfusion, emergency operation, longer CPB times, need for high-dose vasopressors and intra-aortic balloons, and valve operations.[335,338,342,350,354,355] More than 800 mg of calcium chloride per square meter of body surface area is an independent risk factor for pancreatitis.[349]

Treatment and diagnosis must be pursued vigorously for all these complications, without regard to the recent heart operation. Delayed diagnosis and therapy may initiate a chain reaction that culminates in multiorgan failure. An unexplained, persistent metabolic acidosis should raise the spectre of an intra-abdominal catastrophe.

Mesenteric ischemia can occur secondary to a superior mesenteric artery embolus or low mesenteric flow. An elevated lactate level supports the diagnosis but is nonspecific. Initial treatment for mesenteric ischemia secondary to low flow includes volume resuscitation and minimizing vasopressor therapy. An arteriogram can diagnose mesenteric vasospasm, low flow, or embolic occlusion, but is often impractical in an unstable post–cardiac surgery patient. If the suspicion for mesenteric ischemia is high in an unstable patient, early laparotomy can be life saving. Necrotic bowel is resected and marginal bowel is reassessed at a second look operation in 24 hours. When an embolic cause is likely, a superior mesenteric artery embolectomy can restore mesenteric flow.[353]

An elevated amylase level postoperatively occurs far more often than does clinical pancreatitis. About 30% of patients develop an elevated amylase level postoperatively, but only 10% have an increased lipase or pancreatic amylase level; 20% have a nonpancreatic source for the increased amylase.[356] The clinical setting of abdominal pain and tenderness usually helps distinguish those patients with true pancreatitis. CT scan can serve as an adjunct for the diagnosis. Only 0.04% to 1% of patients develop severe pancreatitis.[349,351] Treatment includes withholding oral intake, nasogastric tube decompression, and possibly, antibiotics. Development of pancreatic abscess requires laparotomy and drainage.

Hollow viscus perforation usually produces free peritoneal air (which should not be confused with air introduced during a median sternotomy incision that extended too far caudally). This usually mandates laparotomy.

Calculous or acalculous cholecystitis can occur in the post–cardiopulmonary bypass patient. Ultrasound or radionuclide scan with hepatobiliary iminodiacetic acid (HIDA) supports this diagnosis. Cholecystectomy is the treatment of choice. In the rare patient that cannot withstand cholecystectomy, cholecystostomy is a reasonable second choice.

Upper gastrointestinal bleeding in the postoperative patient is usually secondary to hemorrhagic stress gastritis or ulceration. Routine stress ulcer prophylaxis after cardiac surgery is widely practiced, but the benefit has not been studied in a randomized trial.[357] Patients at highest risk for upper GI bleeding include those who require prolonged mechanical ventilation, anticoagulation, or steroid therapy.[42,358] Long cardiopulmonary bypass and aortic cross-clamp times have also been associated with an increased risk of postoperative GI bleeding.[358] When considering stress ulcer prophylaxis for high-risk patients, sucralfate may be preferable to ranitidine, which has been linked to increased infectious complications in ICU patients.[359–363] Infections in patients treated with H_2 blockers are theoretically due to loss of gastric acidity and subsequent bacterial colonization of the stomach. Although gastric colonization does occur, it has not been demonstrated conclusively to cause higher rates of pneumonia or other infections in patients treated with H_2 blockers.[364–369] *Helicobacter pylori* has not been shown to be a factor in postoperative stress ulceration for cardiac surgery patients.[358,370]

Endoscopy is used to evaluate and often treat upper GI bleeding. Anticoagulants are stopped temporarily. The severity of bleeding must be weighed against the danger of discontinuing anticoagulation. When the danger of prolonged stoppage is unacceptable, early operation is performed to arrest the bleeding. Tissue valves are preferred for patients at high risk for postoperative upper GI bleeding.

Minor GI complications are more frequent than major complications. Mild postoperative ileus is common and is best treated by extending the duration of nasogastric tube suction. Forcing oral intake while ileus persists only lengthens hospitalization. Diarrhea suggests *Clostridium difficile* enteritis. A stool swab for fecal leukocytes and enterotoxin secures the diagnosis. Treatment requires specific antibiotics (metronidazole or oral vancomycin) and, when necessary, nutritional support.

PROPHYLACTIC ANTIBIOTICS

Operations performed using cardiopulmonary bypass cause major derangements of multiple body systems and of the mediators of inflammation. Immunocompromise seems to be one of the derangements; the incidence of infection without prophylactic antibiotics is as high as 50%. Prophylactic antibiotics reduce this rate substantially.[371] To be effective, antibiotics must be circulating at the start of the operation and must be maintained in an adequate concentration during the entire operation.[372–375] In the immediate postoperative period, antibiotic treatment should be continued for 24 to 48 hours. Administration for longer periods of time affords no better protection against infection.[372–374,376] The choice of antibiotic generally varies with recommendations of hospital epidemiologists or infectious disease committees and varies among institutions.

REFERENCES

1. Kirklin JW: Systems analysis in surgical patients with particular attention to the cardiac and pulmonary subsystems. *The Macewen Memorial Lectures*, no.155. Glasgow, University of Glasgow, 1970.
2. Appelbaum A, Kouchoukos NT, Blackstone EH, Kirklin JW: Early risks of open heart surgery for mitral valve disease. *Am J Cardiol* 1976; 37:201.
3. Dietzman RH, Ersek RA, Lillehei CW, et al: Low output syndrome: recognition and treatment. *J Thorac Cardiovasc Surg* 1969; 57:138.
4. Gailiunas P, Chawla R, Lazarus JM, et al: Acute renal failure following cardiac operations. *J Thorac Cardiovasc Surg* 1980; 79:241.
5. Edmunds LH Jr: Blood-surface interactions during cardiopulmonary bypass. *J Card Surg* 1993; 8:404.
6. Edmunds LH Jr: Inflammatory response to cardiopulmonary bypass. *Ann Thorac Surg* 1998; 66 (5 suppl):S12.
7. Kirklin JK, Westaby S, Blackstone EH, et al: Complement and the damaging effects of cardiopulmonary bypass. *J Thorac Cardiovasc Surg* 1983; 86:845.
8. Downing SW, Edmunds LH Jr: Release of vasoactive substances during cardiopulmonary bypass. *Ann Thorac Surg* 1992; 54:1236.
9. Markewitz A, Faist E, Lang S, et al: Regulation of acute phase response after cardiopulmonary bypass by immunomodulation. *Ann Thorac Surg* 1993; 55:389.
10. Kappelmayer J, Bernabli A, Gikakis N, et al: Upregulation of Mac-1 surface expression on neutrophils during simulated extracorporeal circulation. *J Thorac Cardiovasc Surg* 1993; 121:118.
11. Chenoweth DE, Cooper SW, Hugli TE, et al: Complement activation during cardiopulmonary bypass. *N Engl J Med* 1981; 304:497.
12. Aslan R, Tunerir B, Dernek S, et al: The factors effecting complement activation in open heart surgery. *J Cardiovasc Surg (Torino)* 1992; 33:754.
13. Chu SH, Huang TS, Hsu RB, et al: Thyroid hormone changes after cardiovascular surgery and clinical implications. *Ann Thorac Surg* 1991; 52:791.
14. Tulla H, Takala J, Alhava E, et al: Hypermetabolism after coronary artery bypass. *J Thorac Cardiovasc Surg* 1991; 101:598.
15. Chiara O, Giomarelli PP, Biagioli B, et al: Hypermetabolic response after hypothermic cardiopulmonary bypass. *Crit Care Med* 1987; 15:995.
16. Crock PA, Ley CJ, Martin IK, et al: Hormonal and metabolic changes during hypothermic coronary artery bypass surgery in diabetic and non-diabetic subjects. *Diabet Med* 1988; 5:47.
17. Braunwald AG: Cardiac catheterization, in Grossman W (ed): *Heart Disease*. Philadelphia, WB Saunders, 1992; p 180.
18. Boyd O, Grounds RM, Bennett ED: A randomized clinical trial of the effect of deliberate perioperative increase of oxygen delivery on mortality in high-risk surgical patients. *JAMA* 1993; 270: 2699.
19. Finch CA, Lenfant C: Oxygen transport in man. *N Engl J Med* 1972; 286:407.
20. Chiolero R, Mavrocordatos P, Bracco D, Schutz Y, Cayeux C, Revelly JP: O_2 consumption by the fick method: methodologic factors. *Am J Respir Crit Care Med* 1994; 149:1118.
21. Kumon K, Tanaka K, Hirata T, et al: Organ failures due to low cardiac output syndrome following open heart surgery. *Jpn Circ J* 1986; 50:329.
22. Parr GV, Blackstone EH, Kirklin JW: Cardiac performance and mortality early after intracardiac surgery in infants and young children. *Circulation* 1975; 51:867.
23. Sadeghi N, Sadeghi S, Mood ZA, Karimi A: Determinants of operative mortality following primary coronary artery bypass surgery. *Eur J Cardiothorac Surg* 2002; 21:187.
24. Yau TM, Fedak PW, Weisel RD, et al: Predictors of operative risk for coronary bypass operations in patients with left ventricular dysfunction. *J Thorac Cardiovasc Surg* 1999; 118:1006.
25. Nemec P, Bedanova H, Necas J, et al: Coronary artery bypass grafting in patients with left ventricular ejection fraction of 30% or less. *Bratisl Lek Listy* 2001; 102:15.
26. Bech-Hanssen O, Caidahl K, Wall B, et al: Influence of aortic valve replacement, prosthesis type, and size on functional outcome and ventricular mass in patients with aortic stenosis. *J Thorac Cardiovasc Surg* 1999; 118:57.
27. Kirklin JK, Kirklin JW: Management of the cardiovascular subsystem after cardiac surgery. *Ann Thorac Surg* 1981; 32:311.
28. Kotter GS, Kotrly KJ, Kalbfleisch JH, et al: Myocardial ischemia during cardiovascular surgery as detected by an ST segment trend monitoring system. *J Cardiothorac Anesth* 1987; 1:190.
29. Gosselink AT, Crijns HJ, van den Berg MP, et al: Functional capacity before and after cardioversion of atrial fibrillation: a controlled study. *Br Heart J* 1994; 72:161.
30. Creswell LL, Schuessler RB, Rosenbloom M, Cox JL: Hazards of postoperative atrial arrhythmias. *Ann Thorac Surg* 1993; 56:539.
31. Friesen WG, Woodson RD, Ames AW, et al: A hemodynamic comparison of atrial and ventricular pacing in postoperative cardiac surgical patients. *J Thorac Cardiovasc Surg* 1968; 55:271.
32. Fozzard HA: Relaxation and diastolic properties of the heart, in Smith VE, Weisfeldt ML, Katz AM (eds): *The Heart and Cardiovascular System*. New York, Raven Press, 1986; p 803.
33. Rankin JS, Arentzen CE, McHale PA, et al: Viscoelastic properties of the diastolic left ventricle in the conscious dog. *Circ Res* 1977; 41:37.
34. McKenney PA, Apstein CS, Mendes LA, et al: Increased left ventricular diastolic chamber stiffness immediately after coronary artery bypass surgery. *J Am Coll Cardiol* 1994; 24:1189.
35. Mammana RB, Hiro S, Levitsky S, et al: Inaccuracy of pulmonary capillary wedge pressure when compared to left atrial pressure in the early postsurgical period. *J Thorac Cardiovasc Surg* 1982; 84:420.
36. Norris SO: Managing low cardiac output states: maintaining volume after cardiac surgery. *AACN Clin Issues Crit Care Nurs* 1993; 4:309.
37. Canver CC, Nichols RD: Use of intraoperative hetastarch priming during coronary bypass. *Chest* 2000; 118:1616.
38. Cope JT, Banks D, Mauney MC, et al: Intraoperative hetastarch infusion impairs hemostasis after cardiac operations. *Ann Thorac Surg* 1997; 63:78.
39. Strauss RG: Review of the effects of hydroxyethyl starch on the blood coagulation system. *Transfusion* 1981; 21:299.
40. Mastroianni L, Low HB, Rollman J, et al: A comparison of 10% pentastarch and 5% albumin in patients undergoing open-heart surgery. *J Clin Pharmacol* 1994; 34:34.
41. Lacy JH, Wright CB: Use of plasma volume expanders in myocardial revascularisation. *Drugs* 1992; 44:720.
42. Moggio RA, Rha CC, Somberg ED, et al: Hemodynamic comparison of albumin and hydroxyethyl starch in postoperative cardiac surgery patients. *Crit Care Med* 1983; 11:943.
43. Shatney CH, Deepika K, Militello PR, et al: Efficacy of hetastarch in the resuscitation of patients with multisystem trauma and shock. *Arch Surg* 1983; 118:804.
44. Rackow EC, Falk JL, Fein IA, et al: Fluid resuscitation in circulatory shock: a comparison of the cardiorespiratory effects of albumin, hetastarch, and saline solutions in patients with hypovolemic and septic shock. *Crit Care Med* 1983; 11:839.

45. Eising GP, Niemeyer M, Gunther T, et al: Does a hyperoncotic cardiopulmonary bypass prime affect extravascular lung water and cardiopulmonary function in patients undergoing coronary artery bypass surgery? *Eur J Cardiothorac Surg* 2001; 20:282.
46. Kasper SM, Giesecke T, Limpers P, et al: Failure of autologous fresh frozen plasma to reduce blood loss and transfusion requirements in coronary artery bypass surgery. *Anesthesiology* 2001; 95:81.
47. Diehl JT, Lester JL 3rd, Cosgrove DM: Clinical comparison of hetastarch and albumin in postoperative cardiac patients. *Ann Thorac Surg* 1982; 34:674.
48. Kirklin JK, Lell WA, Kouchoukos NT: Hydroxyethyl starch versus albumin for colloid infusion following cardiopulmonary bypass in patients undergoing myocardial revascularization. *Ann Thorac Surg* 1984; 37:40.
49. Palanzo DA, Parr GV, Bull AP, et al: Hetastarch as a prime for cardiopulmonary bypass. *Ann Thorac Surg* 1982; 34:680.
50. Sade RM, Stroud MR, Crawford FA Jr, et al: A prospective randomized study of hydroxyethyl starch, albumin, and lactated Ringer's solution as priming fluid for cardiopulmonary bypass. *J Thorac Cardiovasc Surg* 1985; 89:713.
51. DeFoe GR, Ross CS, Olmstead EM, et al: Lowest hematocrit on bypass and adverse outcomes associated with coronary artery bypass grafting. Northern New England Cardiovascular Disease Study Group. *Ann Thorac Surg* 2001; 71:769.
52. Yin FC: Ventricular wall stress. *Circ Res* 1981; 49:829.
53. Buckberg GD, Archie JP, Fixler DE, Hoffman JI: Experimental subendocardial ischemia during left ventricular hypertension. *Surg Forum* 1971; 22:124.
54. Franciosa JA, Guiha NH, Limas CJ, et al: Arterial pressure as a determinant of left ventricular filling pressure after acute myocardial infarction. *Am J Cardiol* 1974; 34:506.
55. Fremes SE, Weisel RD, Baird RJ, et al: Effects of postoperative hypertension and its treatment. *J Thorac Cardiovasc Surg* 1983; 86:47.
56. Roberts AJ, Niarchos AP, Subramanian VA, et al: Systemic hypertension associated with coronary artery bypass surgery: predisposing factors, hemodynamic characteristics, humoral profile, and treatment. *J Thorac Cardiovasc Surg* 1977; 74:846.
57. Estafanous FG, Tarazi RC: Systemic arterial hypertension associated with cardiac surgery. *Am J Cardiol* 1980; 46:685.
58. Beerthuizen GI, Goris RJ, Bredee JJ, et al: Muscle oxygen tension, hemodynamics, and oxygen transport after extracorporeal circulation. *Crit Care Med* 1988; 16:748.
59. Kuttila K, Niinikoski J: Peripheral perfusion after cardiac surgery. *Crit Care Med* 1989; 17:217.
60. Bailey DR, Miller ED Jr, Kaplan JA, Rogers PW: The renin-angiotensin-aldosterone system during cardiac surgery with morphine–nitrous oxide anesthesia. *Anesthesiology* 1975; 42:538.
61. Lappas DG, Lowenstein E, Waller J, et al: Hemodynamic effects of nitroprusside infusion during coronary artery operation in man. *Circulation* 1976; 54:III4.
62. Stinson EB, Holloway EL, Derby G, et al: Comparative hemodynamic responses to chlorpromazine, nitroprusside, nitroglycerin, and trimethaphan immediately after open-heart operations. *Circulation* 1975; 52:126.
63. Chitwood WR Jr, Cosgrove DM 3rd, Lust RM: Multicenter trial of automated nitroprusside infusion for postoperative hypertension. Titrator Multicenter Study Group. *Ann Thorac Surg* 1992; 54:517.
64. Cosgrove DM 3rd, Petre JH, Waller JL, et al: Automated control of postoperative hypertension: a prospective, randomized multicenter study. *Ann Thorac Surg* 1989; 47:678.
65. Ferrari HA, Robicsek F: Coronary surgery and computerized monitoring-patient care. *Coll Works Cardiopulm Dis* 1979; 22:98.
66. Christakis GT, Fremes SE, Koch JP, et al: Determinants of low systemic vascular resistance during cardiopulmonary bypass. *Ann Thorac Surg* 1994; 58:1040.
67. DiNardo JA, Bert A, Schwartz MJ, et al: Effects of vasoactive drugs on flows through left internal mammary artery and saphenous vein grafts in man. *J Thorac Cardiovasc Surg* 1991; 102:730.
68. Sagawa K: The ventricular pressure-volume diagram revisited. *Circ Res* 1978; 43:677.
69. Berglund E: Ventricular function, VI: Balance of left and right ventricular output: relation between left and right atrial pressures. *Am J Physiol* 1954; 178:381.
70. Josa M, Khuri SF, Braunwald NS, et al: Delayed sternal closure: an improved method of dealing with complications after cardiopulmonary bypass. *J Thorac Cardiovasc Surg* 1986; 91:598.
71. Furnary AP, Magovern JA, Simpson KA, Magovern GJ: Prolonged open sternotomy and delayed sternal closure after cardiac operations. *Ann Thorac Surg* 1992; 54:233.
72. Fanning WJ, Vasko JS, Kilman JW: Delayed sternal closure after cardiac surgery. *Ann Thorac Surg* 1987; 44:169.
73. Durandy Y, Batisse A, Bourel P, et al: Mediastinal infection after cardiac operation: a simple closed technique. *J Thorac Cardiovasc Surg* 1989; 97:282.
74. Serry C, Bleck PC, Javid H, et al: Sternal wound complications: management and results. *J Thorac Cardiovasc Surg* 1983; 80:861.
75. Weitzman LB, Tinker WP, Kronzon I, et al: The incidence and natural history of pericardial effusion after cardiac surgery—an echocardiographic study. *Circulation* 1984; 69:506.
76. Wickstrom PH, Monson BK, Helseth HK: Delayed postoperative bloody pericardial effusion. *Minn Med* 1985; 68:19.
77. Ofori-Krakye SK, Tyberg TI, Geha AS, et al: Late cardiac tamponade after open heart surgery: incidence, role of anticoagulants in its pathogenesis and its relationship to the postpericardiotomy syndrome. *Circulation* 1981; 63:1323.
78. Nishimura RA, Fuster V, Burgert SL, Puga FJ: Clinical features and long-term natural history of the postpericardiotomy syndrome. *Int J Cardiol* 1983; 4:443.
79. Pereira WM, Kalil RA, Prates PR, Nesralla IA: Cardiac tamponade due to chylopericardium after cardiac surgery. *Ann Thorac Surg* 1988; 46:572.
80. Rose DM, Colvin SB, Danilowicz D, Isom OW: Cardiac tamponade secondary to chylopericardium following cardiac surgery: case report and review of the literature. *Ann Thorac Surg* 1982; 34:333.
81. Smulders YM, Wiepking ME, Moulijn AC, et al: How soon should drainage tubes be removed after cardiac operations? *Ann Thorac Surg* 1989; 48:540.
82. Hochberg MS, Merrill WH, Gruber M, et al: Delayed cardiac tamponade associated with prophylactic anticoagulation in patients undergoing coronary bypass grafting: early diagnosis with two-dimensional echocardiography. *J Thorac Cardiovasc Surg* 1978; 75:777.
83. Spodick DH, Paladino D, Flessas AP: Respiratory effects on systolic time intervals during pericardial effusion. *Am J Cardiol* 1983; 51:1033.
84. Louie EK, Hariman RJ, Wang Y, et al: Effect of acute pericardial tamponade on the relative contributions of systolic and diastolic pulmonary venous return: a transesophageal pulsed Doppler study. *Am Heart J* 1995; 129:124.
85. Reichert CL, Visser CA, Koolen JJ, et al: Transesophageal echocardiography in hypotensive patients after cardiac operations: comparison with hemodynamic parameters. *J Thorac Cardiovasc Surg* 1992; 104:321.
86. Borkon AM, Schaff HV, Gardner TJ, et al: Diagnosis and management of postoperative pericardial effusions and late cardiac tamponade following open-heart surgery. *Ann Thorac Surg* 1981; 31:512.

87. DiSesa VJ: The rational selection of inotropic drugs in cardiac surgery. *J Card Surg* 1987; 2:385.
88. DiSesa VJ: Pharmacologic support for postoperative low cardiac output. *Semin Thorac Cardiovasc Surg* 1991; 3:13.
89. Lollgen H, Drexler H: Use of inotropes in the critical care setting. *Crit Care Med* 1990; 18:S56.
90. DiSesa VJ, Brown E, Mudge GH Jr, et al: Hemodynamic comparison of dopamine and dobutamine in the postoperative volume-loaded, pressure-loaded, and normal ventricle. *J Thorac Cardiovasc Surg* 1982; 83:256.
91. Fowler MB, Alderman EL, Oesterle SN, et al: Dobutamine and dopamine after cardiac surgery: greater augmentation of myocardial blood flow with dobutamine. *Circulation* 1984; 70: I103.
92. Sturm JT, Fuhrman TM, Sterling R, et al: Combined use of dopamine and nitroprusside therapy in conjunction with intra-aortic balloon pumping for the treatment of postcardiotomy low-output syndrome. *J Thorac Cardiovasc Surg* 1981; 82:13.
93. Loeb HS, Ostrenga JP, Gaul W, et al: Beneficial effects of dopamine combined with intravenous nitroglycerin on hemodynamics in patients with severe left ventricular failure. *Circulation* 1983; 68:813.
94. Goldberg LI, Rajfer SI: Dopamine receptors: applications in clinical cardiology. *Circulation* 1985; 72:245.
95. Steen PA, Tinker JH, Pluth JR, et al: Efficacy of dopamine, dobutamine, and epinephrine during emergence from cardiopulmonary bypass in man. *Circulation* 1978; 57:378.
96. Stephenson LW, Blackstone EH, Kouchoukos NT: Dopamine vs epinephrine in patients following cardiac surgery: randomized study. *Surg Forum* 1976; 27:272.
97. Drop LJ: Ionized calcium, the heart, and hemodynamic function. *Anesth Analg* 1985; 64:432.
98. Drop LJ, Scheidegger D: Plasma ionized calcium concentration: important determinant of the hemodynamic response to calcium infusion. *J Thorac Cardiovasc Surg* 1980; 79:425.
99. Shapira N, Schaff HV, White RD, Pluth JR: Hemodynamic effects of calcium chloride injection following cardiopulmonary bypass: response to bolus injection and continuous infusion. *Ann Thorac Surg* 1984; 37:133.
100. Auffant RA, Downs JB, Amick R: Ionized calcium concentration and cardiovascular function after cardiopulmonary bypass. *Arch Surg* 1981; 116:1072.
101. Gallagher JD, Geller EA, Moore RA, et al: Hemodynamic effects of calcium chloride in adults with regurgitant valve lesions. *Anesth Analg* 1984; 63:723.
102. Alousi AA, Johnson DC: Pharmacology of the bipyridines: amrinone and milrinone. *Circulation* 1986; 73:III10.
103. Kikura M, Lee MK, Safon RA, et al: The effects of milrinone on platelets in patients undergoing cardiac surgery. *Anesth Analg* 1995; 81:44.
104. Ansell J, Tiarks C, McCue J, et al: Amrinone-induced thrombocytopenia. *Arch Intern Med* 1994; 144:949
105. Ross MP, Allen-Webb EM, Pappas JB, McGough EC: Amrinone-associated thrombocytopenia: pharmacokinetic analysis. *Clin Pharmacol Ther* 1993; 53:661.
106. Kikura M, Lee MK, Safon RA, et al: The effects of milrinone on platelets in patients undergoing cardiac surgery. *Anesth Analg* 1995; 81:44.
107. Levy JH, Bailey JM, Deeb GM: Intravenous milrinone in cardiac surgery. *Ann Thorac Surg* 2002; 73:325.
108. Baim DS, McDowell AV, Cherniles J, et al: Evaluation of a new bipyridine inotropic agent—milrinone—in patients with severe congestive heart failure. *N Engl J Med* 1983; 309:748.
109. Borow KM, Come PC, Neumann A, et al: Physiologic assessment of the inotropic, vasodilator and afterload reducing effects of milrinone in subjects without cardiac disease. *Am J Cardiol* 1985; 55:1204.
110. Monrad ES, McKay RG, Baim DS, et al: Improvement in indexes of diastolic performance in patients with congestive heart failure treated with milrinone. *Circulation* 1984; 70:1030.
111. Lobato EB, Gravenstein N, Martin TD: Milrinone, not epinephrine, improves left ventricular compliance after cardiopulmonary bypass. *J Cardiothorac Vasc Anesth* 2000; 14:374.
112. Lobato EB, Florete O Jr, Bingham HL: A single dose of milrinone facilitates separation from cardiopulmonary bypass in patients with pre-existing left ventricular dysfunction. *Br J Anaesth* 1998; 81:782.
113. Monrad ES, McKay RG, Baim DS, et al: Improvement in indexes of diastolic performance in patients with congestive heart failure treated with milrinone. *Circulation* 1984; 70:1030.
114. Monrad ES, Baim DS, Smith HS, et al: Effects of milrinone on coronary hemodynamics and myocardial energetics in patients with congestive heart failure. *Circulation* 1985; 71:972.
115. Drexler H, Faude F, Winterer H, et al: [Central and regional vascular hemodynamics of milrinone in experimental heart failure: comparison with captopril and dobutamine]. *Z Kardiol* 1987; 76:507.
116. Drexler H, Faude F, Hoing S, Just H: Blood flow distribution within skeletal muscle during exercise in the presence of chronic heart failure: effect of milrinone. *Circulation* 1987; 76:1344.
117. Martin JL, Likoff MJ, Janicki JS, et al: Myocardial energetics and clinical response to the cardiotonic agent MDL 17043 in advanced heart failure. *J Am Coll Cardiol* 1984; 4:875.
118. Tisdale JE, Patel R, Webb CR, et al: Electrophysiologic and proarrhythmic effects of intravenous inotropic agents. *Prog Cardiovasc Dis* 1995; 38:167.
119. Cook LS, Toal KW, Elkins RC: Cardiovascular time course in patients with postoperative myocardial dysfunction requiring catecholamine administration. *Curr Surg* 1987; 44:124.
120. Gottlieb SS: New approaches to managing congestive heart failure. *Curr Opin Cardiol* 1995; 10:282.
121. Feldman AM, Bristow MR, Parmley WW, et al: Effects of vesnarinone on morbidity and mortality in patients with heart failure. Vesnarinone Study Group. *N Engl J Med* 1993; 329: 149.
122. Shakar SF, Abraham WT, Gilbert EM, et al: Combined oral positive inotropic and beta-blocker therapy for treatment of refractory class IV heart failure. *J Am Coll Cardiol* 1998; 31:1336.
123. Holland FW, Brown PS Jr, Weintraub BD, Clark RE: Cardiopulmonary bypass and thyroid function: a "euthyroid sick syndrome." *Ann Thorac Surg* 1991; 52:46.
124. Murzi B, Iervasi G, Masini S, et al: Thyroid hormones homeostasis in pediatric patients during and after cardiopulmonary bypass. *Ann Thorac Surg* 1995; 59:481.
125. Klemperer JD, Klein I, Gomez M, et al: Thyroid hormone treatment after coronary-artery bypass surgery. *N Engl J Med* 1995; 333:1522.
126. Dyke CM, Yeh T Jr, Lehman JD, et al: Triiodothyronine-enhanced left ventricular function after ischemic injury. *Ann Thorac Surg* 1991; 52:14.
127. Dyke CM, Ding M, Abd-Elfattah AS, et al: Effects of triiodothyronine supplementation after myocardial ischemia. *Ann Thorac Surg* 1993; 56:215.
128. Holland FW, Brown PS Jr, Clark RE: Acute severe postischemic myocardial depression reversed by triiodothyronine. *Ann Thorac Surg* 1992; 54:301.
129. Novitzky D, Matthews N, Shawley D, et al: Triiodothyronine in the recovery of stunned myocardium in dogs. *Ann Thorac Surg* 1991; 51:10.
130. Novitzky D, Cooper DK, Swanepoel A: Inotropic effect of triiodothyronine (T3) in low cardiac output following cardioplegic

arrest and cardiopulmonary bypass: an initial experience in patients undergoing open heart surgery. *Eur J Cardiothorac Surg* 1989; 3:140.

131. Novitzky D, Cooper DK, Barton CI, et al: Triiodothyronine as an inotropic agent after open heart surgery. *J Thorac Cardiovasc Surg* 1989; 98:972.
132. Novitzky D, Fontanet H, Snyder M, et al: Impact of triiodothyronine on the survival of high-risk patients undergoing open heart surgery. *Cardiology* 1996; 87:509.
133. Mullis-Jansson SL, Argenziano M, Corwin S, et al: A randomized double-blind study of the effect of triiodothyronine on cardiac function and morbidity after coronary bypass surgery. *J Thorac Cardiovasc Surg* 1999; 117:1128.
134. Klemperer JD, Klein IL, Ojamaa K, et al: Triiodothyronine therapy lowers the incidence of atrial fibrillation after cardiac operations. *Ann Thorac Surg* 1996; 61:1323.
135. Taniguchi S, Kitamura S, Kawachi K, et al: Effects of hormonal supplements on the maintenance of cardiac function in potential donor patients after cerebral death. *Eur J Cardiothorac Surg* 1992; 6:96.
136. Orlowski JP, Spees EK: Improved cardiac transplant survival with thyroxine treatment of hemodynamically unstable donors: 95.2% graft survival at 6 and 30 months. *Transplant Proc* 1993; 25: 1535.
137. Novitzky D, Wicomb WN, Cooper DK, Tjaalgard MA: Improved cardiac function following hormonal therapy in brain dead pigs: relevance to organ donation. *Cryobiology* 1987; 24:1.
138. Novitzky D, Cooper DK, Chaffin JS, et al: Improved cardiac allograft function following triiodothyronine therapy to both donor and recipient. *Transplantation* 1990; 49:311.
139. Davis PJ, Davis FB: Acute cellular actions of thyroid hormone and myocardial function. *Ann Thorac Surg* 1993; 56:S16–S23.
140. Ojamaa K, Balkman C, Klein IL: Acute effects of triiodothyronine on arterial smooth muscle cells. *Ann Thorac Surg* 1993; 56: S61.
141. Vavouranakis I, Sanoudos G, Manios A, et al: Triiodothyronine administration in coronary artery bypass surgery: effect on hemodynamics. *J Cardiovasc Surg (Torino)* 1994; 35:383.
142. Bennett-Guerrero E, Jimenez JL, White WD, et al: Cardiovascular effects of intravenous triiodothyronine in patients undergoing coronary artery bypass graft surgery: a randomized, double-blind, placebo-controlled trial. Duke T3 study group. *JAMA* 1996; 275:687.
143. Teiger E, Menasche P, Mansier P, et al: Triiodothyronine therapy in open-heart surgery: from hope to disappointment. *Eur Heart J* 1993; 14:629.
144. Gotzsche LS, Weeke J: Changes in plasma free thyroid hormones during cardiopulmonary bypass do not indicate triiodothyronine substitution. *J Thorac Cardiovasc Surg* 1992; 104:273.
145. Lowenstein E: Implications of triiodothyronine administration before cardiac and noncardiac operations. *Ann Thorac Surg* 1993; 56:S43.
146. Clark RE: Triiodothyronine: to be or not to be, that is the question. *Ann Thorac Surg* 1991; 51:5.
147. Samuels LE, Kaufman MS, Thomas MP, et al: Pharmacological criteria for ventricular assist device insertion following postcardiotomy shock: experience with the Abiomed BVS system. *J Card Surg* 1999; 14:288.
148. Kantrowitz A, Tjonneland S, Freed PS, et al: Initial clinical experience with intraaortic balloon pumping in cardiogenic shock. *JAMA* 1968; 203:113.
149. Torchiana DF, Hirsch G, Buckley MJ, et al: Intraaortic balloon pumping for cardiac support: trends in practice and outcome, 1968 to 1995. *J Thorac Cardiovasc Surg* 1997; 113:758.
150. Creswell LL, Rosenbloom M, Cox JL, et al: Intraaortic balloon counterpulsation: patterns of usage and outcome in cardiac surgery patients. *Ann Thorac Surg* 1992; 54:11.
151. Naunheim KS, Swartz MT, Pennington DG, et al: Intraaortic balloon pumping in patients requiring cardiac operations: risk analysis and long-term follow-up. *J Thorac Cardiovasc Surg* 1992; 104:1654.
152. Gol MK, Bayazit M, Emir M, et al: Vascular complications related to percutaneous insertion of intraaortic balloon pumps. *Ann Thorac Surg* 1994; 58:1476.
153. Perler BA, McCabe CJ, Abbott WM, Buckley MJ: Vascular complications of intra-aortic balloon counterpulsation. *Arch Surg* 1983; 118:957.
154. Iverson LI, Herfindahl G, Ecker RR, et al: Vascular complications of intraaortic balloon counterpulsation. *Am J Surg* 1987; 154:99.
155. McCabe JC, Abel RM, Subramanian VA, Guy WA Jr: Complications of intra-aortic balloon insertion and counterpulsation. *Circulation* 1978; 57:769.
156. Vonderheide RH, Thadhani R, Kuter DJ: Association of thrombocytopenia with the use of intra-aortic balloon pumps. *Am J Med* 1998; 105:27.
157. Alajmo F, Calamai G: High-dose aprotinin in emergency coronary artery bypass after thrombolysis. *Ann Thorac Surg* 1992; 54:1022.
158. Skinner JR, Phillips SJ, Zeff RH, Kongtahworn C: Immediate coronary bypass following failed streptokinase infusion in evolving myocardial infarction. *J Thorac Cardiovasc Surg* 1984; 87:567.
159. Rawitscher RE, Jones JW, McCoy TA, Lindsley DA: A prospective study of aspirin's effect on red blood cell loss in cardiac surgery. *J Cardiovasc Surg (Torino)* 1991; 32:1.
160. Reich DL, Patel GC, Vela-Cantos F, et al: Aspirin does not increase homologous blood requirements in elective coronary bypass surgery. *Anesth Analg* 1994; 79:4.
161. Becker RM, Fintel DJ, Green D: *Antithrombotic Therapy,* 2d ed. West Islip, NY, Professional Communications, 2002.
162. Kestin AS, Valeri CR, Khuri SF, et al: The platelet function defect of cardiopulmonary bypass. *Blood* 1993; 82:107.
163. Khuri SF, Wolfe JA, Josa M, et al: Hematologic changes during and after cardiopulmonary bypass and their relationship to the bleeding time and nonsurgical blood loss. *J Thorac Cardiovasc Surg* 1992; 104:94.
164. Edmunds LH Jr: Why cardiopulmonary bypass makes patients sick: strategies to control the blood-synthetic surface interface. *Adv Card Surg* 1995; 6:131.
165. Taylor KM: Perioperative approaches to coagulation defects. *Ann Thorac Surg* 1993; 56:S78.
166. John LC, Rees GM, Kovacs IB: Inhibition of platelet function by heparin: an etiologic factor in postbypass hemorrhage. *J Thorac Cardiovasc Surg* 1993; 105:816.
167. Michelson AD: Bleeding associated with cardiopulmonary bypass in children. *Int J Pediatr Hematol Oncol* 1994; 1:147.
168. Walls JT, Curtis JJ, Silver D, et al: Heparin-induced thrombocytopenia in open heart surgical patients: sequelae of late recognition. *Ann Thorac Surg* 1992; 53:787.
169. Teoh KH, Young E, Bradley CA, Hirsh J: Heparin binding proteins: contribution to heparin rebound after cardiopulmonary bypass. *Circulation* 1993; 88:II420.
170. Martin P, Horkay F, Gupta NK, et al: Heparin rebound phenomenon—much ado about nothing? *Blood Coagul Fibrinolysis* 1992; 3:187.
171. Najafi H: Reoperation for excessive bleeding after cardiac operations. *J Thorac Cardiovasc Surg* 1992; 103:814.
172. Vander Salm TJ, Ansell JE, Okike ON, et al: The role of epsilon-aminocaproic acid in reducing bleeding after cardiac operation: a double-blind randomized study. *J Thorac Cardiovasc Surg* 1988; 95:538.
173. Daily PO, Lamphere JA, Dembitsky WP, et al: Effect of prophylactic epsilon-aminocaproic acid on blood loss and transfusion

requirements in patients undergoing first-time coronary artery bypass grafting: a randomized, prospective, double-blind study. *J Thorac Cardiovasc Surg* 1994; 108:99.
174. Arom KV, Emery RW: Decreased postoperative drainage with addition of epsilon-aminocaproic acid before cardiopulmonary bypass. *Ann Thorac Surg* 1994; 57:1108.
175. Royston D: High-dose aprotinin therapy: a review of the first five years' experience. *J Cardiothorac Vasc Anesth* 1992; 6:76.
176. Royston D: The serine antiprotease aprotinin (Trasylol): a novel approach to reducing postoperative bleeding. *Blood Coagul Fibrinolysis* 1990; 1:55.
177. Cosgrove DM 3rd, Heric B, Lytle BW, et al: Aprotinin therapy for reoperative myocardial revascularization: a placebo-controlled study. *Ann Thorac Surg* 1992; 54:1031.
178. Sundt TM 3rd, Kouchoukos NT, Saffitz JE, et al: Renal dysfunction and intravascular coagulation with aprotinin and hypothermic circulatory arrest. *Ann Thorac Surg* 1993; 55:1418.
179. Laub GW, Riebman JB, Chen C, et al: The impact of aprotinin on coronary artery bypass graft patency. *Chest* 1994; 106:1370.
180. Salzman EW, Weinstein MJ, Reilly D, Ware JA: Adventures in hemostasis: desmopressin in cardiac surgery. *Arch Surg* 1993; 128:212.
181. Temeck BK, Bachenheimer LC, Katz NM, et al: Desmopressin acetate in cardiac surgery: a double-blind, randomized study. *South Med J* 1994; 87:611.
182. Ansell J, Klassen V, Lew R, et al: Does desmopressin acetate prophylaxis reduce blood loss after valvular heart operations? A randomized, double-blind study. *J Thorac Cardiovasc Surg* 1992; 104:117.
183. Dilthey G, Dietrich W, Spannal M, Richter JA: Influence of desmopressin acetate on homologous blood requirements in cardiac surgical patients pretreated with aspirin. *Anesthesiology* 1993; 7:425.
184. Sheridan DP, Card RT, Pinilla JC, et al: Use of desmopressin acetate to reduce blood transfusion requirements during cardiac surgery in patients with acetylsalicylic-acid-induced platelet dysfunction. *Can J Surg* 1994; 37:33.
185. Shirvani R: An evaluation of clinical aspects of post-operative autotransfusion, either alone or in conjunction with pre-operative aspirin, in cardiac surgery. *Br J Clin Pract* 1991; 45:105.
186. de Haan J, Boonstra PW, Monnink SH, et al: Retransfusion of suctioned blood during cardiopulmonary bypass impairs hemostasis. *Ann Thorac Surg* 1995; 59:901.
187. Ovrum E, Holen EA, Lindstein Ringdal MA: Elective coronary artery bypass surgery without homologous blood transfusion: early results with an inexpensive blood conservation program. *Scand J Thorac Cardiovasc Surg* 1991; 25:13.
188. Schaff HV, Hauer JM, Bell WR, et al: Autotransfusion of shed mediastinal blood after cardiac surgery: a prospective study. *J Thorac Cardiovasc Surg* 1978; 75:632.
189. Hartz RS, Smith JA, Green D: Autotransfusion after cardiac operation: assessment of hemostatic factors. *J Thorac Cardiovasc Surg* 1988; 96:178.
190. Breyer RH, Engelman RM, Rousou JA, Lemeshow S: Blood conservation for myocardial revascularization: is it cost effective? *J Thorac Cardiovasc Surg* 1987; 93:512.
191. Griffith LD, Billman GF, Daily PO, Lane TA: Apparent coagulopathy caused by infusion of shed mediastinal blood and its prevention by washing of the infusate. *Ann Thorac Surg* 1989; 47:400.
192. Axford TC, Dearani JA, Ragno G, et al: Safety and therapeutic effectiveness of reinfused shed blood after open heart surgery. *Ann Thorac Surg* 1994; 57:615.
193. Hoffman WS, Tomasello DN, MacVaugh H: Control of postcardiotomy bleeding with PEEP. *Ann Thorac Surg* 1982; 34:71.
194. Ilabaca PA, Ochsner JL, Mills NL: Positive end-expiratory pressure in the management of the patient with a postoperative bleeding heart. *Ann Thorac Surg* 1980; 30:281.
195. Zurick AM, Urzua J, Ghattas M, et al: Failure of positive end-expiratory pressure to decrease postoperative bleeding after cardiac surgery. *Ann Thorac Surg* 1982; 34:608.
196. Bouboulis N, Rivas LF, Kuo J, et al: Packing the chest: a useful technique for intractable bleeding after open heart operation. *Ann Thorac Surg* 1994; 57:856.
197. Vander Salm TJ: Two techniques for the control of cardiac bleeding. *Ann Thorac Surg* 1994; 57:762.
198. Pelletier MP, Solymoss S, Lee A, Chiu RC: Negative reexploration for cardiac postoperative bleeding: can it be therapeutic? *Ann Thorac Surg* 1998; 65:999.
199. Fairman RM, Edmunds LH Jr: Emergency thoracotomy in the surgical intensive care unit after open cardiac operation. *Ann Thorac Surg* 1981; 32:386.
200. Anthi A, Tzelepis GE, Alivizatos P, et al: Unexpected cardiac arrest after cardiac surgery: incidence, predisposing causes, and outcome of open chest cardiopulmonary resuscitation. *Chest* 1998; 113:15.
201. Feng WC, Bert AA, Browning RA, Singh AK: Open cardiac massage and periresuscitative cardiopulmonary bypass for cardiac arrest following cardiac surgery. *J Cardiovasc Surg (Torino)* 1995; 36:319.
202. Hill RC: Open-chest resuscitation and postcardiac surgery arrest. *Chest* 1998; 113:3.
203. Pottle A, Bullock I, Thomas J, Scott L: Survival to discharge following open chest cardiac compression (OCCC): a 4–year retrospective audit in a cardiothoracic specialist center—Royal Brompton and Harefield NHS Trust, United Kingdom. *Resuscitation* 2002; 52:269.
204. Wahba A, Gotz W, Birnbaum DE: Outcome of cardiopulmonary resuscitation following open heart surgery. *Scand Cardiovasc J* 1997; 31:147.
205. Ratliff NB, Young WG Jr, Hackel DB, et al: Pulmonary injury secondary to extracorporeal circulation: an ultrastructural study. *J Thorac Cardiovasc Surg* 1973; 65:425.
206. Gillespie DJ, Didier EP, Rehder K: Ventilation-perfusion distribution after aortic valve replacement. *Crit Care Med* 1990; 18:136.
207. Pacifico AD, Digerness S, Kirklin JW: Acute alterations of body composition after open intracardiac operations. *Circulation* 1970; 41:331.
208. Hill DG, de Lanerolle P, Kosek JC, et al: The pulomary pathophysiology of membrane and bubble oxygenators. *Trans Am Soc Artif Intern Organs* 1975; 21:165.
209. Cohn LH, Angell WW, Shumway NE: Body fluid shifts after cardiopulmonary bypass, I: effects of congestive heart failure and hemodilution. *J Thorac Cardiovasc Surg* 1971; 62:423.
210. Lancey RA SBVT: Off-pump versus on-pump coronary artery bypass surgery: a case-matched comparison of clinical outcomes and costs. *Heart Surg Forum* 2000; 4:277.
211. Magee MJ, Dewey TM, Acuff T, et al: Influence of diabetes on mortality and morbidity: off-pump coronary artery bypass grafting versus coronary artery bypass grafting with cardiopulmonary bypass. *Ann Thorac Surg* 2001; 72:776.
212. Arom KV, Flavin TF, Emery RW, et al: Safety and efficacy of off-pump coronary artery bypass grafting. *Ann Thorac Surg* 2000; 69:704.
213. Yokoyama T, Baumgartner FJ, Gheissari A, et al: Off-pump versus on-pump coronary bypass in high-risk subgroups. *Ann Thorac Surg* 2000; 70:1546.
214. Bowles BJ, Lee JD, Dang CR, et al: Coronary artery bypass performed without the use of cardiopulmonary bypass is associated

with reduced cerebral microemboli and improved clinical results. *Chest* 2001; 119:25.

215. Hernandez F, Clough RA, Klemperer JD, Blum JM: Off-pump coronary artery bypass grafting: initial experience at one community hospital. *Ann Thorac Surg* 2000; 70:1070.
216. Kshettry VR, Flavin TF, Emery RW, et al: Does multivessel, off-pump coronary artery bypass reduce postoperative morbidity? *Ann Thorac Surg* 2000; 69:1725.
217. van Dijk D, Nierich AP, Jansen EW, et al: Early outcome after off-pump versus on-pump coronary bypass surgery: results from a randomized study. *Circulation* 2001; 104:1761.
218. Coleman SM, Demastrice L: Leukocyte depletion reduces postoperative oxygen requirements. *Ann Thorac Surg* 1994; 58:1567.
219. Mihaljevic T, Tonz M, von Segesser LK, et al: The influence of leukocyte filtration during cardiopulmonary bypass on postoperative lung function: a clinical study. *J Thorac Cardiovasc Surg* 1995; 109:1138.
220. Connell RS, Page US, Bartley TD, et al: The effect on pulmonary ultrastructure of dacron-wool filtration during cardiopulmonary bypass. *Ann Thorac Surg* 1973; 15:217.
221. el Gatit A, al Khaja N, Belboul A, et al: Influence of alprostadil on pulmonary dysfunction after a cardiac operation. *Ann Thorac Surg* 1992; 53:1018.
222. Mayumi H, Tokunaga K: Prostaglandin E1 for patients who have both heart and lung failure after cardiotomy. *J Thorac Cardiovasc Surg* 1993; 105:1120.
223. Zehr KJ, Poston RS, Lee PC, et al: Platelet activating factor inhibition reduces lung injury after cardiopulmonary bypass. *Ann Thorac Surg* 1995; 59:328.
224. Downs JB, Mitchell LA: Pulmonary effects of ventilatory pattern following cardiopulmonary bypass. *Crit Care Med* 1976; 4:295.
225. Markand ON, Moorthy SS, Mahomed Y, et al: Postoperative phrenic nerve palsy in patients with open-heart surgery. *Ann Thorac Surg* 1985; 39:68.
226. Large SR, Heywood LJ, Flower CD, et al: Incidence and aetiology of a raised hemidiaphragm after cardiopulmonary bypass. *Thorax* 1985; 40:444.
227. Estenne M, Yernault JC, De Smet JM, De Troyer A: Phrenic and diaphragm function after coronary artery bypass grafting. *Thorax* 1985; 40:293.
228. Benjamin JJ, Cascade PN, Rubenfire M, et al: Left lower lobe atelectasis and consolidation following cardiac surgery: the effect of topical cooling on the phrenic nerve. *Radiology* 1982; 142:11.
229. Dajee A, Pellegrini J, Cooper G, Karlson K: Phrenic nerve palsy after topical cardiac hypothermia. *Int Surg* 1983; 68:345.
230. Diehl JL, Lofaso F, Deleuze P, et al: Clinically relevant diaphragmatic dysfunction after cardiac operations. *J Thorac Cardiovasc Surg* 1994; 107:487.
231. Bevelaqua F, Garritan S, Haas F, et al: Complications after cardiac operations in patients with severe pulmonary impairment. *Ann Thorac Surg* 1990; 50:602.
232. Moore R, Follette DM, Berkoff HA: Poststernotomy fractures and pain management in open cardiac surgery. *Chest* 1994; 106:1339.
233. Good JT Jr, Wolz JF, Anderson JT, et al: The routine use of positive end-expiratory pressure after open heart surgery. *Chest* 1979; 76:397.
234. Zwischenberger JB, Kirsh MM, Dechert RE, et al: Suppression of shivering decreases oxygen consumption and improves hemodynamic stability during postoperative rewarming. *Ann Thorac Surg* 1987; 43:428.
235. Sharkey A, Lipton JM, Murphy MT, Giesecke AH: Inhibition of postanesthetic shivering with radiant heat. *Anesthesiology* 1987; 66:249.
236. Rodriguez JL, Weissman C, Damask MC, et al: Physiologic requirements during rewarming: suppression of the shivering response. *Crit Care Med* 1983; 11:490.
237. Slogoff S, Keats AS: Does perioperative myocardial ischemia lead to postoperative myocardial infarction? *Anesthesiology* 1985; 62:107.
238. Hall RI: Anaesthesia for coronary artery surgery—a plea for a goal-directed approach. *Can J Anaesth* 1993; 40:1178.
239. Gall SA Jr, Olsen CO, Reves JG, et al: Beneficial effects of endotracheal extubation on ventricular performance: implications for early extubation after cardiac operations. *J Thorac Cardiovasc Surg* 1988; 95:819.
240. Chong JL, Grebenik C, Sinclair M, et al: The effect of a cardiac surgical recovery area on the timing of extubation. *J Cardiothorac Vasc Anesth* 1993; 7:137.
241. Butler J, Chong GL, Pillai R, et al: Early extubation after coronary artery bypass surgery: effects on oxygen flux and haemodynamic variables. *J Cardiovasc Surg* (Torino) 1992; 33:276.
242. Yang KL, Tobin MJ: A prospective study of indexes predicting the outcome of trials of weaning from mechanical ventilation. *N Engl J Med* 1991; 324:1445.
243. Postoperative care, in Kirklin JW, Barratt-Boyes BG (eds): *Cardiac Surgery*. New York, Churchill-Livingston, 1993; p 195.
244. Culliford AT, Thomas S, Spencer FC: Fulminating noncardiogenic pulmonary edema: a newly recognized hazard during cardiac operations. *J Thorac Cardiovasc Surg* 1980; 80:868.
245. Olinger GN, Becker RM, Bonchek LI: Noncardiogenic pulmonary edema and peripheral vascular collapse following cardiopulmonary bypass: rare protamine reaction? *Ann Thorac Surg* 1980; 29:20.
246. Gillinov AM, Davis EA, Alberg AJ, et al: Pulmonary embolism in the cardiac surgical patient. *Ann Thorac Surg* 1992; 53:988.
247. Dhingra S, Solven F, Wilson A, McCarthy DS: Hypomagnesemia and respiratory muscle power. *Am Rev Respir Dis* 1984; 129:497.
248. Martinez FJ, Bermudez-Gomez M, Celli BR: Hypothyroidism: a reversible cause of diaphragmatic dysfunction. *Chest* 1989; 96:1059.
249. MacIntyre NR, Cook DJ, Ely EW Jr, et al: Evidence-based guidelines for weaning and discontinuing ventilatory support: a collective task force facilitated by the American College of Chest Physicians; the American Association for Respiratory Care; and the American College of Critical Care Medicine. *Chest* 2001; 120:375S.
250. Massick DD, Yao S, Powell DM, et al: Bedside tracheostomy in the intensive care unit: a prospective randomized trial comparing open surgical tracheostomy with endoscopically guided percutaneous dilational tracheotomy. *Laryngoscope* 2001; 111:494.
251. Dulguerov P, Gysin C, Perneger TV, Chevrolet JC: Percutaneous or surgical tracheostomy: a meta-analysis. *Crit Care Med* 1999; 27:1617.
252. Cheng E, Fee WE Jr: Dilatational versus standard tracheostomy: a meta-analysis. *Ann Otol Rhinol Laryngol* 2000; 109:803.
253. Freeman BD, Isabella K, Lin N, Buchman TG: A meta-analysis of prospective trials comparing percutaneous and surgical tracheostomy in critically ill patients. *Chest* 2000; 118:1412.
254. Frega NS, Dibona DR, Guertler B, Leaf A: Ischemic renal injury. *Kidney Int Suppl* 1976; 10:525.
255. Levinsky NG, Bernard DB, Johnston PA: Mannitol and loop diuretics in acute renal failure, in Brenner BM, Lazarus JM (eds): *Acute Renal Failure*. Philadelphia, WB Saunders, 1983; p 712.
256. Kahn DR, Cerny JC, Lee RS, Sloan H: The effect of mannitol on renal function during open-heart surgery. *Surgery* 1965; 57:676.
257. Schuster SR, Kak M van, Vawter GF, Narter N: An experimental study of the effect of mannitol during cardiopulmonary bypass. *Circulation* 1964; 29:72.
258. Patak RV, Fadem SZ, Lifschitz MD, Stein JH: Study of factors which modify the development of norepinephrine-induced acute renal failure in the dog. *Kidney Int* 1979; 15:227.

259. Kleinknecht D, Ganeval D, Gonzalez-Duque LA, Fermanian J: Furosemide in acute oliguric renal failure: a controlled trial. *Nephron* 1976; 17:51.
260. Nierenberg DW: Furosemide and ethacrynic acid in acute tubular necrosis. *West J Med* 1980; 133:163.
261. Baek SM, Brown RS, Shoemaker WC: Early prediction of acute renal failure and recovery, II: renal function response to furosemide. *Ann Surg* 1973; 178:605.
262. Brown RS: Renal dysfunction in the surgical patient: maintenance of high output state with furosemide. *Crit Care Med* 1979; 7:63.
263. Lindner A, Cutler RE, Goodman G: Synergism of dopamine plus furosemide in preventing acute renal failure in the dog. *Kidney Int* 1979; 16:158.
264. Lindner A: Synergism of dopamine and furosemide in diuretic-resistant, oliguric acute renal failure. *Nephron* 1983; 33:121.
265. Sirivella S, Gielchinsky I, Parsonnet V: Mannitol, furosemide, and dopamine infusion in postoperative renal failure complicating cardiac surgery. *Ann Thorac Surg* 2000; 69:501.
266. Hashimoto K, Nomura K, Nakano M, et al: Pharmacological intervention for renal protection during cardiopulmonary bypass. *Heart Vessels* 1993; 8:203.
267. Zanardo G, Michielon P, Rosi P, et al: Effects of a continuous diltiazem infusion on renal function during cardiac surgery. *J Cardiothorac Vasc Anesth* 1993; 7:711.
268. Abe K, Fujino Y, Sakakibara T: The effect of prostaglandin E1 during cardiopulmonary bypass on renal function after cardiac surgery. *Eur J Clin Pharmacol* 1993; 45:217.
269. Mauk RH, Patak RV, Fadem SZ, et al: Effect of prostaglandin E administration in a nephrotoxic and a vasoconstrictor model of acute renal failure. *Kidney Int* 1977; 12:122.
270. Zanardo G, Michielon P, Paccagnella A, et al: Acute renal failure in the patient undergoing cardiac operation: prevalence, mortality rate, and main risk factors. *J Thorac Cardiovasc Surg* 1994; 107:1489.
271. Holper K, Struck E, Sebening F: The diagnosis of acute renal failure (ARF) following cardiac surgery with cardio-pulmonary bypass. *Thorac Cardiovasc Surg* 1979; 27:231.
272. Kron IL, Joob AW, Van Meter C: Acute renal failure in the cardiovascular surgical patient. *Ann Thorac Surg* 1985; 39:590.
273. Smith HW: *Principles of Renal Physiology*. Baltimore, University Park Press, 1956.
274. Abel RM, Buckley MJ, Austen WG, et al: Etiology, incidence, and prognosis of renal failure following cardiac operations: results of a prospective analysis of 500 consecutive patients. *J Thorac Cardiovasc Surg* 1976; 71:323.
275. Corwin HL, Sprague SM, DeLaria GA, Norusis MJ: Acute renal failure associated with cardiac operations: a case-control study. *J Thorac Cardiovasc Surg* 1989; 98:1107.
276. Andersson LG, Ekroth R, Bratteby LE, et al: Acute renal failure after coronary surgery—a study of incidence and risk factors in 2009 consecutive patients. *Thorac Cardiovasc Surg* 1993; 41:237.
277. Corwin HL, Sprague SM, DeLaria GA, Norusis MJ: Acute renal failure associated with cardiac operations: a case-control study. *J Thorac Cardiovasc Surg* 1989; 98:1107.
278. Zanardo G, Michielon P, Paccagnella A, et al: Acute renal failure in the patient undergoing cardiac operation: prevalence, mortality rate, and main risk factors. *J Thorac Cardiovasc Surg* 1994; 107:1489.
279. Osborn JJ, Cohn K, Hart M: Hemolysis during perfusion. *J Thorac Cardiovasc Surg* 1962; 43:459.
280. Savitsky JP, Doczi J, Black J, Arnold JD: A clinical safety trial of stroma-free hemoglobin. *Clin Pharmacol Ther* 1978; 23:73.
281. Carlson DE, Karp RB, Kouchoukos NT: Surgical treatment of aneurysms of the descending thoracic aorta: an analysis of 85 patients. *Ann Thorac Surg* 1983; 35:58.
282. Roberts AJ, Nora JD, Hughes WA, et al: Cardiac and renal responses to cross-clamping of the descending thoracic aorta. *J Thorac Cardiovasc Surg* 1983; 86:732.
283. Kleinknecht D, Jungers P, Chanard J, et al: Uremic and non-uremic complications in acute renal failure: evaluation of early and frequent dialysis on prognosis. *Kidney Int* 1972; 1:190.
284. Norman JC, McDonald HP, Sloan H: The early and aggressive treatment of acute renal failure following cardiopulmonary bypass with continuous peritoneal dialysis. *Surgery* 1964; 56:240.
285. Meyer MM: Renal replacement therapies. *Crit Care Clin* 2000; 16:29.
286. Walpoth B, Geroulanos S, Turina M, Senning A: [Reducing hemodilution through ultrafiltration following cardiopulmonary bypass]. *Helv Chir Acta* 1980; 47:231.
287. Darup J, Bleese N, Kalmar P, et al: Hemofiltration during extracorporeal circulation (ECC). *Thorac Cardiovasc Surg* 1979; 27:227.
288. Walpoth BH, Amport T, Schmid R, et al: Hemofiltration during cardiopulmonary bypass: quality assessment of hemoconcentrated blood. *Thorac Cardiovasc Surg* 1994; 42:162.
289. Lamer C, Valleaux T, Plaisance P, et al: Continuous arteriovenous hemodialysis for acute renal failure after cardiac operations. *J Thorac Cardiovasc Surg* 1990; 99:175.
290. Morgan JM, Morgan C, Evans TW: Clinical experience of pumped arteriovenous haemofiltration in the management of patients in oliguric renal failure following cardiothoracic surgery. *Int J Cardiol* 1988; 21:259.
291. Baudouin SV, Wiggins J, Keogh BF, et al: Continuous veno-venous haemofiltration following cardio-pulmonary bypass: indications and outcome in 35 patients. *Intensive Care Med* 1993; 19:290.
292. Cole L, Bellomo R, Journois D, et al: High-volume haemofiltration in human septic shock. *Intensive Care Med* 2001; 27:978.
293. Journois D, Israel-Biet D, Pouard P, et al: High-volume, zero-balanced hemofiltration to reduce delayed inflammatory response to cardiopulmonary bypass in children. *Anesthesiology* 1996; 85:965.
294. McLeish KR, Luft FC, Kleit SA: Factors affecting prognosis in acute renal failure following cardiac operations. *Surg Gynecol Obstet* 1977; 145:28.
295. Bhat JG, Gluck MC, Lowenstein J, Baldwin DS: Renal failure after open heart surgery. *Ann Intern Med* 1976; 84:677.
296. Lange HW, Aeppli DM, Brown DC: Survival of patients with acute renal failure requiring dialysis after open heart surgery: early prognostic indicators. *Am Heart J* 1987; 113:1138.
297. Katz ES, Tunick PA, Rusinek H, et al: Protruding aortic atheromas predict stroke in elderly patients undergoing cardiopulmonary bypass: experience with intraoperative transesophageal echocardiography. *J Am Coll Cardiol* 1992; 20:70.
298. Smith PL, Treasure T, Newman SP, et al: Cerebral consequences of cardiopulmonary bypass. *Lancet* 1986; 1:823.
299. Wareing TH, Davila-Roman VG, Daily BB, et al: Strategy for the reduction of stroke incidence in cardiac surgical patients. *Ann Thorac Surg* 1993; 55:1400.
300. Roach GW, Kanchuger M, Mangano CM, et al: Adverse cerebral outcomes after coronary bypass surgery. Multicenter Study of Perioperative Ischemia Research Group and the Ischemia Research and Education Foundation Investigators. *N Engl J Med* 1996; 335:1857.
301. Gardner TJ, Horneffer PJ, Manolio TA, et al: Stroke following coronary artery bypass grafting: a ten-year study. *Ann Thorac Surg* 1985; 40:574.
302. Furlan AJ, Sila CA, Chimowitz MI, Jones SC: Neurologic complications related to cardiac surgery. *Neurol Clin* 1992; 10:145.
303. Harrison MJ, Schneidau A, Ho R, et al: Cerebrovascular disease and functional outcome after coronary artery bypass surgery. *Stroke* 1989; 20:235.

304. Hogue CW Jr, Murphy SF, Schechtman KB, Davila-Roman VG: Risk factors for early or delayed stroke after cardiac surgery. *Circulation* 1999; 100:642.
305. Ali IM, Cummings B, Sullivan J, Francis S: The risk of cerebrovascular accident in patients with asymptomatic critical carotid artery stenosis who undergo open-heart surgery. *Can J Surg* 1998; 41:374.
306. Yoon BW, Bae HJ, Kang DW, et al: Intracranial cerebral artery disease as a risk factor for central nervous system complications of coronary artery bypass graft surgery. *Stroke* 2001; 32:94.
307. Martin TD, Craver JM, Gott JP, et al: Prospective, randomized trial of retrograde warm blood cardioplegia: myocardial benefit and neurologic threat. *Ann Thorac Surg* 1994; 57:298.
308. Blauth CI, Cosgrove DM, Webb BW, et al: Atheroembolism from the ascending aorta: an emerging problem in cardiac surgery. *J Thorac Cardiovasc Surg* 1992; 103:1104.
309. Gold JP, Charlson ME, Williams-Russo P, et al: Improvement of outcomes after coronary artery bypass: a randomized trial comparing intraoperative high versus low mean arterial pressure. *J Thorac Cardiovasc Surg* 1995; 110:1302.
310. Huse-Kleinstoll G, Dahme B, Flemming B, et al: Open-heart surgery: somatic predictors of postoperative psychopathology. *Thorac Cardiovasc Surg* 19779; 27:271.
311. Calabrese JR, Skwerer RG, Gulledge AD, et al: Incidence of postoperative delirium following myocardial revascularization: a prospective study. *Cleve Clin J Med* 1987; 54:29.
312. Dubin WR, Field HL, Gastfriend DR: Postcardiotomy delirium: a critical review. *J Thorac Cardiovasc Surg* 1979; 77:586.
313. Blauth C, Griffin S, Harrison M, et al: Neuropsychologic alterations after cardiac operation. *J Thorac Cardiovasc Surg* 1989; 98:454.
314. Newman S, Smith P, Treasure T: Acute neuropsychological consequences of coronary artery bypass surgery. *Cur Psychiatr Res Rev* 1987; 6:115.
315. Sotaniemi KA, Mononen H, Hokkanen TE: Long-term cerebral outcome after open-heart surgery: a five-year neuropsychological follow-up study. *Stroke* 1986; 17:410.
316. Shaw PJ, Bates D, Cartlidge NE, et al: Neurologic and neuropsychological morbidity following major surgery: comparison of coronary artery bypass and peripheral vascular surgery. *Stroke* 1987; 18:700.
317. O'Brien DJ, Bauer RM, Yarandi H, et al: Patient memory before and after cardiac operations. *J Thorac Cardiovasc Surg* 1992; 104:1116.
318. Townes BD, Bashein G, Hornbein TF, et al: Neurobehavioral outcomes in cardiac operations: a prospective controlled study. *J Thorac Cardiovasc Surg* 1989; 98:774.
319. Johnston WE, Stump DA, DeWitt DS, et al: Significance of gaseous microemboli in the cerebral circulation during cardiopulmonary bypass in dogs. *Circulation* 1993; 88:II319.
320. Clark RE, Brillman J, Davis DA, et al: Microemboli during coronary artery bypass grafting: genesis and effect on outcome. *J Thorac Cardiovasc Surg* 1995; 109:249.
321. Toner I, Peden CJ, Hamid SK, et al: Magnetic resonance imaging and neuropsychological changes after coronary artery bypass graft surgery: preliminary findings. *J Neurosurg Anesthesiol* 1994; 6:163.
322. Diegeler A, Hirsch R, Schneider F, et al: Neuromonitoring and neurocognitive outcome in off-pump versus conventional coronary bypass operation. *Ann Thorac Surg* 2000; 69:1162.
323. Ricci M, Karamanoukian HL, Abraham R, et al: Stroke in octogenarians undergoing coronary artery surgery with and without cardiopulmonary bypass. *Ann Thorac Surg* 2000; 69:1471.
324. Koutlas TC, Elbeery JR, Williams JM, et al: Myocardial revascularization in the elderly using beating heart coronary artery bypass surgery. *Ann Thorac Surg* 2000; 69:1042.
325. Hernandez F, Cohn WE, Baribeau YR, et al: In-hospital outcomes of off-pump versus on-pump coronary artery bypass procedures: a multicenter experience. *Ann Thorac Surg* 2001; 72:1528.
326. Puskas JD, Thourani VH, Marshall JJ, et al: Clinical outcomes, angiographic patency, and resource utilization in 200 consecutive off-pump coronary bypass patients. *Ann Thorac Surg* 2001; 71:1477.
327. Taggart DP, Browne SM, Halligan PW, Wade DT: Is cardiopulmonary bypass still the cause of cognitive dysfunction after cardiac operations? *J Thorac Cardiovasc Surg* 1999; 118:414.
328. Murkin JM: Neurological outcomes after OPCAB: how much better is it? *Heart Surg Forum* 2000; 3:207.
329. Angelini GD, Taylor FC, Reeves BC, Ascione R: Early and midterm outcome after off-pump and on-pump surgery in Beating Heart Against Cardioplegic Arrest Studies (BHACAS 1 and 2): a pooled analysis of two randomised controlled trials. *Lancet* 2002; 359:1194.
330. van Dijk D, Jansen EW, Hijman R, et al: Cognitive outcome after off-pump and on-pump coronary artery bypass graft surgery: a randomized trial. *JAMA* 2002; 287:1405.
331. Vander Salm TJ, Cutler BS, Okike ON: Brachial plexus injury following median sternotomy: part II. *J Thorac Cardiovasc Surg* 1982; 83:914.
332. Vander Salm TJ, Cereda JM, Cutler BS: Brachial plexus injury following median sternotomy. *J Thorac Cardiovasc Surg* 1980; 80:447.
333. Kirsh MM, Magee KR, Gago O, et al: Brachial plexus injury following median sternotomy incision. *Ann Thorac Surg* 1971; 11:315.
334. Treasure T, Garnett R, O'Connor J, Treasure JL: Injury of the lower trunk of the brachial plexus as a complication of median sternotomy for cardiac surgery. *Ann R Coll Surg Engl* 1980; 62:37.
335. Leitman IM, Paull DE, Barie PS, et al: Intra-abdominal complications of cardiopulmonary bypass operations. *Surg Gynecol Obstet* 1987; 165:251.
336. Eustace S, Connolly B, Egleston C, O'Connell D: Imaging of abdominal complications following cardiac surgery. *Abdom Imaging* 1994; 19:405.
337. Tsiotos GG, Mullany CJ, Zietlow S, van Heerden JA: Abdominal complications following cardiac surgery. *Am J Surg* 1994; 167:553.
338. Johnston G, Vitikainen K, Knight R, et al: Changing perspective on gastrointestinal complications in patients undergoing cardiac surgery. *Am J Surg* 1992; 163:525.
339. Zacharias A, Schwann TA, Parenteau GL, et al: Predictors of gastrointestinal complications in cardiac surgery. *Tex Heart Inst J* 2000; 27:93.
340. Sakorafas GH, Tsiotos GG: Intra-abdominal complications after cardiac surgery. *Eur J Surg* 1999; 165:820.
341. Mierdl S, Meininger D, Dogan S, et al: Abdominal complications after cardiac surgery. *Ann Acad Med Singapore* 2001; 30:245.
342. Christenson JT, Schmuziger M, Maurice J, et al: Postoperative visceral hypotension the common cause for gastrointestinal complications after cardiac surgery. *Thorac Cardiovasc Surg* 1994; 42:152.
343. Fiddian-Green RG: Studies in splanchnic ischemia and multiple organ failure, in Marston A, Buckley GB, Fiddian-Green RG: Splanchnic Ischemia and Multiple Organ Failure. London, Edward Arnold, 1989; p 349.
344. Bailey RW, Bulkley GB, Hamilton SR, et al: The fundamental hemodynamic mechanism underlying gastric "stress ulceration" in cardiogenic shock. *Ann Surg* 1987; 205:597.
345. Albes JM, Schistek R, Baier R, Unger F: Intestinal ischemia associated with cardio-pulmonary-bypass surgery: a life threatening complication. *J Cardiovasc Surg (Torino)* 1991; 32:527.
346. Allen KB, Salam AA, Lumsden AB: Acute mesenteric ischemia after cardiopulmonary bypass. *J Vasc Surg* 1992; 16:391.
347. Chu CM, Chang CH, Liaw YF, Hsieh MJ: Jaundice after open heart surgery: a prospective study. *Thorax* 1984; 39:52.
348. Svensson LG, Decker G, Kinsley RB: A prospective study of hyperamylasemia and pancreatitis after cardiopulmonary bypass. *Ann Thorac Surg* 1985; 39:409

349. Fernandez-del Castillo C, Harringer W, et al: Risk factors for pancreatic cellular injury after cardiopulmonary bypass. *N Engl J Med* 1991; 325:382.
350. Rosen HR, Vlahakes GJ, Rattner DW: Fulminant peptic ulcer disease in cardiac surgical patients: pathogenesis, prevention, and management. *Crit Care Med* 1992; 20:354.
351. Egleston CV, Wood AE, Gorey TF, McGovern EM: Gastrointestinal complications after cardiac surgery. *Ann R Coll Surg Engl* 1993; 75:52.
352. Krasna MJ, Flancbaum L, Trooskin SZ, et al: Gastrointestinal complications after cardiac surgery. *Surgery* 1988; 104:773.
353. Mansour MA: Management of acute mesenteric ischemia. *Arch Surg* 1999; 134:328.
354. DePriest JL: Stress ulcer prophylaxis: do critically ill patients need it? *Postgrad Med* 1995; 98:159.
355. Simic O, Strathausen S, Hess W, Ostermeyer J: Incidence and prognosis of abdominal complications after cardiopulmonary bypass. *Cardiovasc Surg* 1999; 7:419.
356. Rattner DW, Gu ZY, Vlahakes GJ, Warshaw AL: Hyperamylasemia after cardiac surgery: incidence, significance, and management. *Ann Surg* 1989; 209:279.
357. van der Voort PH, Zandstra DF: Pathogenesis, risk factors, and incidence of upper gastrointestinal bleeding after cardiac surgery: is specific prophylaxis in routine bypass procedures needed? *J Cardiothorac Vasc Anesth* 2000; 14:293.
358. Halm U, Halm F, Thein D, et al: Helicobacter pylori infection: a risk factor for upper gastrointestinal bleeding after cardiac surgery? *Crit Care Med* 2000; 28:110.
359. O'Keefe GE, Gentilello LM, Maier RV: Incidence of infectious complications associated with the use of histamine2–receptor antagonists in critically ill trauma patients. *Ann Surg* 1998; 227:120.
360. Messori A, Trippoli S, Vaiani M, et al: Bleeding and pneumonia in intensive care patients given ranitidine and sucralfate for prevention of stress ulcer: meta-analysis of randomised controlled trials. *BMJ* 2000; 321:1103.
361. O'Keefe GE, Gentilello LM, Maier RV: Incidence of infectious complications associated with the use of histamine2–receptor antagonists in critically ill trauma patients. *Ann Surg* 1998; 227:120.
362. Maier RV, Mitchell D, Gentilello L: Optimal therapy for stress gastritis. *Ann Surg* 1994; 220:353.
363. Prod'hom G, Leuenberger P, Koerfer J, et al: Nosocomial pneumonia in mechanically ventilated patients receiving antacid, ranitidine, or sucralfate as prophylaxis for stress ulcer: a randomized controlled trial. *Ann Intern Med* 1994; 120:653.
364. Hanisch EW, Encke A, Naujoks F, Windolf J: A randomized, double-blind trial for stress ulcer prophylaxis shows no evidence of increased pneumonia. *Am J Surg* 1998; 176:453.
365. Cook D, Guyatt G, Marshall J, et al: A comparison of sucralfate and ranitidine for the prevention of upper gastrointestinal bleeding in patients requiring mechanical ventilation. Canadian Critical Care Trials Group. *N Engl J Med* 1998; 338:791.
366. Moesgaard F, Jensen LS, Christiansen PM, et al: The effect of ranitidine on postoperative infectious complications following emergency colorectal surgery: a randomized, placebo-controlled, double-blind trial. *Inflamm Res* 1998; 47:12.
367. Thomason MH, Payseur ES, Hakenewerth AM, et al: Nosocomial pneumonia in ventilated trauma patients during stress ulcer prophylaxis with sucralfate, antacid, and ranitidine. *J Trauma* 1996; 41:503.
368. Sirvent JM, Verdaguer R, Ferrer MJ, et al: [Mechanical ventilation-associated pneumonia and the prevention of stress ulcer: a randomized clinical trial of antacids and ranitidine versus sucralfate]. *Med Clin (Barc)* 1994; 102:407.
369. Pickworth KK, Falcone RE, Hoogeboom JE, Santanello SA: Occurrence of nosocomial pneumonia in mechanically ventilated trauma patients: a comparison of sucralfate and ranitidine. *Crit Care Med* 1993; 21:1856.
370. Schilling D, Haisch G, Sloot N, et al: Low seroprevalence of Helicobacter pylori infection in patients with stress ulcer bleeding—a prospective evaluation of patients on a cardiosurgical intensive care unit. *Intensive Care Med* 2000; 26:1832.
371. Fong IW, Baker CB, McKee DC: The value of prophylactic antibiotics in aorat-coronary bypass operations: a double-blind randomized trial. *J Thorac Cardiovasc Surg* 1979; 78:908.
372. Burke JF: Use of preventive antibiotics in clinical surgery. *Am Surg* 1973; 39:6.
373. Burke JF: The effective period of preventive antibiotic action in experimental incisions and dermal lesions. *Surgery* 1961; 50:161.
374. Goldmann DA, Hopkins CC, Karchmer AW, et al: Cephalothin prophylaxis in cardiac valve surgery: a prospective, double-blind comparison of two-day and six-day regimens. *J Thorac Cardiovasc Surg* 1977; 73:470.
375. Stone HH, Haney BB, Kolb LD, et al: Prophylactic and preventive antibiotic therapy: timing, duration and economics. *Ann Surg* 1979; 189:691.
376. Nelson CL, Green TG, Porter RA, Warren RD: One day versus seven days of preventive antibiotic therapy in orthopedic surgery. *Clin Orthop* 1983; 176:258.

Chapter 16

Cardiopulmonary Resuscitation

Mark P. Anstadt/James E. Lowe

Cardiovascular disease remains the leading cause of death in the United States. Over 6 million people in the United States have significant coronary artery disease (CAD).[1] In 1991 an estimated 478,000 deaths were due to coronary artery disease.[1] Nearly a third occurred in persons less than 65 years of age.[1] While death rates from cardiovascular disease decreased 25.7% between 1981 and 1991, the actual number of deaths decreased only 6% due to the aging population.[1,2] More recently it has been estimated that 900,000 acute myocardial infarctions occur annually in the United States.[3] Of the 225,000 deaths, 125,000 occur in the field, which accounts for the majority of sudden cardiac deaths in the United States.[3]

Sudden cardiac death is the unexpected, nontraumatic, abrupt cessation of effective cardiac function in a patient with either no symptoms or acute symptoms for less than 1 hour.[4,5] Prodromal symptoms such as chest pain, palpitations, and fatigue may be present within the preceding 24 hours.[4] One half to two thirds of deaths secondary to coronary artery disease (CAD) occur suddenly, usually within 2 hours of the onset of symptoms.[1,6–8] Most victims of sudden cardiac death die before reaching a hospital.[1] Although the vast majority of sudden deaths in this country are secondary to CAD, other etiologies may be responsible.

Cardiopulmonary resuscitation (CPR) is utilized to sustain cardiovascular and respiratory function. Related clinical investigations have been analyzed to formulate advanced cardiac life support (ACLS) guidelines for the treatment of sudden death. Until recently, ACLS guidelines have reflected somewhat dogmatic approaches for what has become "standard of care." More recent recommendations were based on available scientific data[9] and established by the American Heart Association (AHA) in collaboration with the International Liaison Committee on Resuscitation (ILCOR). ACLS guidelines are now considered *recommendations* formulated from available scientific data, not mandates for a "standard of care."

It has been estimated that CPR is performed on 1% to 2% of all patients admitted to teaching hospitals (including approximately 30% of patients who die in teaching hospitals).[10,11] CPR's underlying goal is to restore spontaneous circulation. Early defibrillation is currently the single most effective means for restoring spontaneous cardiac function and improving survival. When initial attempts fail, restoration of spontaneous circulation (ROSC) is dependent on improving myocardial perfusion combined with treatment of underlying disorders. Novel methods of CPR, circulatory support devices, and new antiarrhythmics may aid in these critical challenges. To date, the survival rates remain disappointingly low,[12–14] and many patients who are successfully resuscitated suffer severe neurologic impairment.[15–17]

TECHNIQUES IN CARDIOPULMONARY RESUSCITATION

Basic life support (BLS) encompasses the techniques utilized to sustain ventilation and blood flow. BLS measures are recommended until advanced cardiac life support (ACLS) measures are available to restore spontaneous circulation. An ABCD algorithm (airway, breathing, circulation, defibrillation) describes the standardized approach to patients in cardiac arrest (Fig. 16-1).[18]

Airway Management

Unresponsive patients mandate activation of the emergency medical system (EMS). Initial steps are then directed toward ensuring a patent airway.[19] The airway can usually be opened using the head-tilt–chin-lift maneuver. The jaw-thrust technique is an alternative for suspected neck trauma; however, it is more difficult to perform.[20] Both relieve posterior displacement of the tongue, which is the most common cause of airway obstruction.[20–22] If no signs of respiration are present, rescue breathing is initiated. Difficult ventilation should be addressed by repositioning and addressing airway foreign bodies. The Heimlich maneuver, or *subdiaphragmatic abdominal thrust*, is recommended for relief of airway obstruction secondary to foreign bodies.[23] Rapid thrusts to the subxiphoid region produce high airway pressures, which may dislodge a foreign body.[24] This should be repeated until ventilation is established. Alternatively, chest thrusts are recommended for obese patients and women in late stages of pregnancy. Magill forceps can be used to retrieve foreign bodies when these techniques fail. Back blows are recommended only for pediatric patients.[24]

Masks and oral and nasal airways may be used for mouth-to-mask ventilation or with bag-valve devices. Mouth-to-mask breathing is more reliable in providing adequate tidal

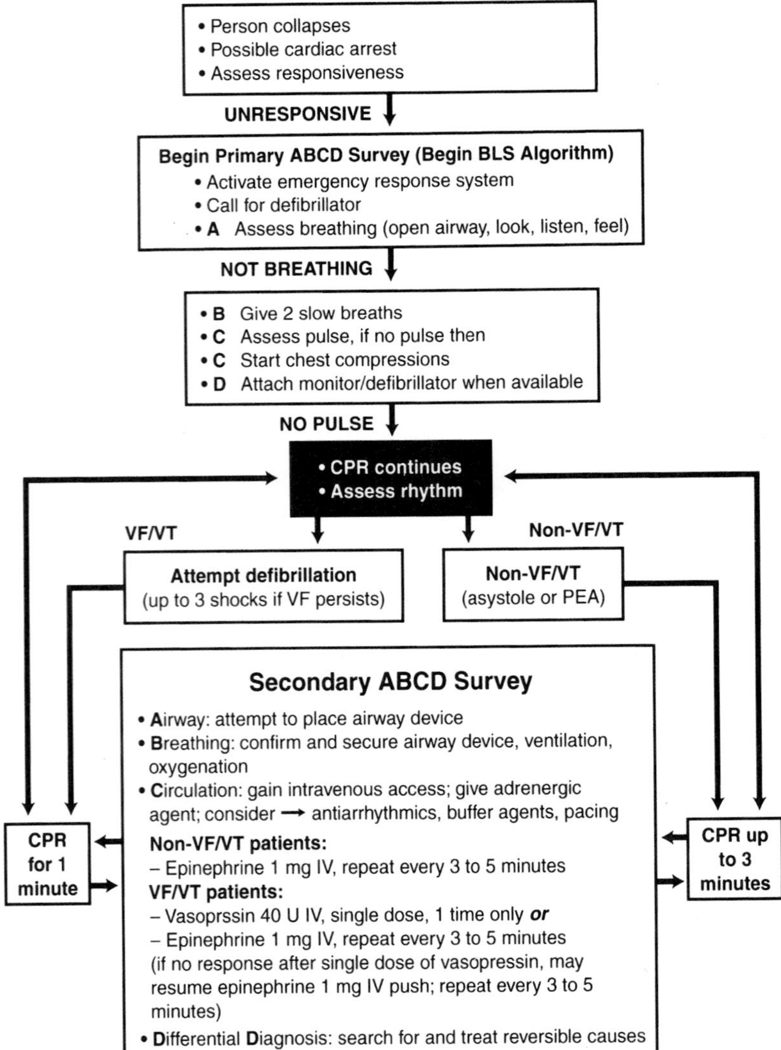

FIGURE 16–1 Universal treatment algorithm for adult emergency cardiac care.

volumes than bag-valve-to-mask respiration.[25–27] Bag-valve devices reduce exposure to potential infection, but require two or more rescuers.[9] Oropharyngeal or nasopharyngeal airways should be used in nonintubated patients. Oropharyngeal airways are not used in conscious patients because of the risk of laryngospasm and regurgitation.[9]

Endotracheal intubation (ETT) is the preferred method of airway management. In addition to maintaining an open airway, the risk of gastric distension and aspiration is decreased, and an alternative route for drug administration is provided.[28] Orotracheal intubation is optimal for resuscitation unless a neck injury is suspected, in which case nasotracheal intubation is recommended. End-tidal CO_2 monitors may be used as an adjunct to confirm tube placement. Esophageal intubation is likely in the absence of elevated end-tidal CO_2.[29,30] Complications of ETT include esophageal intubation, oral trauma, pharyngeal laceration, vocal cord injury, pharyngeal-esophageal perforation, mainstem bronchus intubation, and aspiration.[31–33]

Transtracheal catheter ventilation (TTC) is a temporizing method when other modes of ventilation are not possible. A catheter passed through the cricothyroid membrane is attached to a pressurized oxygen tank (30 to 60 lb/in^2), and inspiratory flow is regulated by a triggered valve. TTC provides limited ventilation and can lead to a respiratory acidosis.[34] Other problems may include pneumothorax, hemorrhage, and esophageal perforation.[35] Cricothyroidotomy is another consideration when endotracheal intubation is not possible.[36] Complications of cricothyroidotomy may include hemorrhage, esophageal perforation, and mediastinal and subcutaneous emphysema.[37] Tracheostomy is rarely indicated for managing cardiac arrest but should be considered when ventilation cannot be otherwise achieved.

Mouth-to-mouth ventilation is recommended in the absence of airway devices. It is effective[38] and generally results in an alveolar PO_2 of approximately 80 mm Hg. Chest movement is observed to assess the adequacy of ventilation at a recommended respiratory rate of 10 to 12 per minute.[9] Cricoid pressure (Sellick maneuver), maintaining a patent airway, and administering slow breaths may decrease the risk of gastric distension, regurgitation, and aspiration.[27,37,39,40] Mouth-to-nose breathing is performed when the mouth cannot be opened or a tight seal is not possible.

There has been great concern about contracting transmissible diseases from cardiac arrest victims during mouth-to-mouth resuscitation, and this fear has reduced enthusiasm for CPR. Barrier devices, such as face shields and mask devices, have been developed to protect EMS personnel from such exposure. Studies indicate minimal risk of the transmission hepatitis B virus (HBV), hepatitis C virus (HCV), or the human immunodeficiency virus (HIV) from CPR procedures.[41,42] However, there is a risk of transmission if blood is inadvertently exchanged with an infected victim.[43] Therefore, rescuers should always observe universal precautions.[41] Herpes[44] and tuberculosis[19,45] have been transmitted to emergency personnel on rare occasions. When mouth to mouth ventilation is not performed, chest compressions alone are better than no resuscitation attempt. A recent randomized trial found patients who received chest compressions alone experienced no significant difference in survival to hospital admission or discharge compared to CPR including mouth-to-mouth ventilation.[46]

Closed Chest Cardiac Massage

Closed chest cardiac massage (CCM) remains the principal means of maintaining the circulation during cardiac arrest. CCM is performed with the victim supine on a flat, firm surface (Fig. 16-2). Compressions over the lower half of the sternum are recommended at a rate of 100/min. Compression depth should be 4 to 6 cm and occupy 50% of the cycle.[47] Complete release after each downstroke allows ventricular filling, and maintaining hand contact with the chest avoids repositioning between compressions.[9] CCM can generate up to 25% to 30% of normal cardiac output.[48–51] Systolic blood pressures usually range from 60 to 80 mm Hg, while diastolic pressures are typically less than 20 mm Hg.[52] Organ perfusion is poor. Cerebral blood flow is reduced to 10% to 15%[52] and coronary perfusion 1 to 5% of normal.[53–55] Clearly, CCM is only a tempory means for providing some blood flow to vital organs. In the absence of definitive interventions (e.g., defibrillation), CCM is unable to sustain life. As the delay to such therapy increases, survival becomes significantly less likely. The possibility of successful ROSC and survival is exceedingly low when CCM is required for more than 30 minutes. However, CCM is the only widely available means of sustaining the circulation while awaiting definitive therapy.

Discontinuation of CPR

Unfortunately, there are no good criteria for discontinuing CPR efforts. Even determining the adequacy of CCM is quite subjective. Palpable pulses only signify the difference between systolic and diastolic pressures,[56] not forward flow. Venous pulse pressures may, in fact, be similar.[57] The presence of reactive pupils and/or spontaneous respirations does indicate some cerebral perfusion, but these findings are frequently absent and poorly correlate with outcome.[58] Aortic diastolic pressure is a measure of CPR effectiveness.[59] Diastolic pressures correlate best with coronary perfusion during CPR.[18] Unfortunately, this measurement is usually not available in the clinical setting.

End-tidal CO_2 ($ETCO_2$) is a noninvasive alternative for assessing CPR. $ETCO_2$ correlates with flows generated during CPR and provides information regarding proper endotracheal tube placement[30,60,61] A low $ETCO_2$ indicates either low blood flow (inadequate CCM), esophageal intubation, airway obstruction, massive pulmonary embolus, or

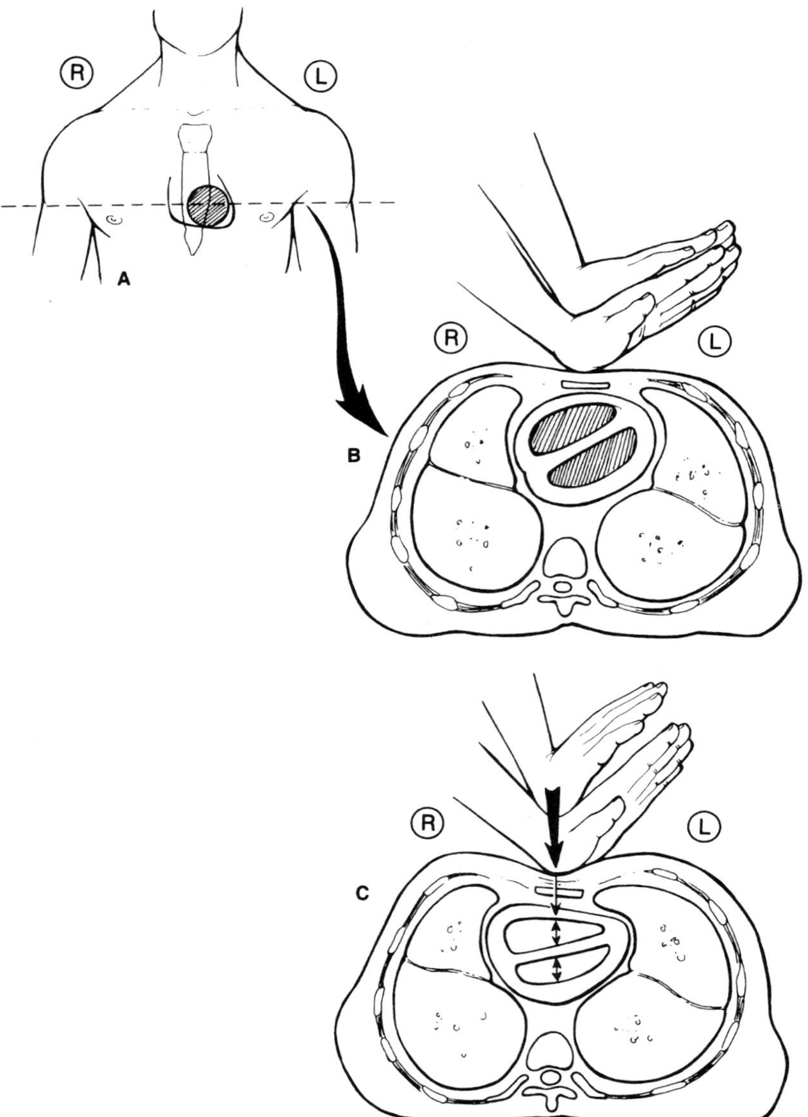

FIGURE 16–2 Cross-sectional view of closed cardiac massage. Compressions are delivered with high velocity and moderate force, resulting in cardiac compression.

hypothermia.[62] Studies have shown that $ETCO_2$ may be predictive of survival in patients suffering from sudden cardiac arrest.[63,64]

Complications of CPR

Common complications of CCM are rib and sternal fractures.[65] Others include aspiration, gastric dilatation, anterior mediastinal hemorrhage, epicardial hematoma, hemopericardium, myocardial contusion, pneumothorax, coronary air embolus, hemothorax, lung contusion, and oral and dental injuries.[65–67] The liver and spleen are the most commonly injured intraabdominal organs, reportedly in 1% to 2% of cases.[65] Rarely, significant injury can involve the trachea, esophagus, stomach, cervical spine, vena cava, retroperitoneum, and myocardium.[65]

SUDDEN DEATH TREATMENT CONSIDERATIONS

Sudden death generally presents as one of three different pathophysiologic conditions: ventricular fibrillation/tachycardia (VF/VT), asystole, or electromechanical dissociation (EMD), also called *pulseless electrical activity* (PEA). VF may persist after initial defibrillation attempts ("*shock-resistant*") or may persist despite multiple therapeutic interventions ("*persistent*" or "*refractory*"). Furthermore, VF may be successfully treated by initial ACLS measures and subsequently recur ("*recurrent*"). These patterns of dysrhythmias are felt to have different etiologies, priorities of treatment, and prognoses. Early identification of the underlying rhythm is important for selecting the recommended treatment algorithm (Fig. 16-1).

Ventricular Tachycardia

Ventricular tachycardia (VT) is a reentrant arrhythmia characterized by premature ventricular depolarizations at a rate greater than 100 beats per minute. Cardiac arrest can occur with rapid, sustained VT. Ventricular fibrillation (VF) is characterized by uncoordinated, continuous contraction of the ventricles. Holter monitors have shown that 80% to 90% of nontraumatic cardiac arrests originate with VF/VT.[68] Over 90% of survivors in most series have VF/VT as the initial rhythm.[69,70] Rapid defibrillation is the most important determinant of survival after cardiac arrest.[71–74] Therefore, defibrillation should precede all other CPR therapy if a device is immediately available.[9] Even minimal delays impact negatively on the success of defibrillation.[75,76] Mortality from sudden death increases 4% to 10% for every minute preceeding initial defibrillation attempts.[73,75,77] Countershocks delivered more than 10 to 12 minutes after the onset of the arrest result in survival rates that approach zero.[78] The current ECC guidelines strongly emphasize early defibrillation and wider use of automated external defibrillation systems.[9]

Treatment of VF and/or pulseless VT, therefore, begins with immediate defibrillation or CPR until one arrives. Recommended energy for the initial defibrillation is 200 J. The electrodes should remain in place on the chest between defibrillation attempts. If monitored VF continues, a second shock of 200 to 300 J is given immediately. A third countershock of 360 J is likewise delivered if the second is without success. It is vital that the three shocks be given consecutively and without delay for ventilations, chest compressions, or other interventions. CPR is performed whenever the three initial defibrillation attempts fail. The patient is intubated and intravenous (IV) access obtained. Figure 16-3 outlines the subsequent treatment algorithm for persistent VF/VT. Epinephrine or vasopressin is given IV or via the endotracheal tube. Vasopressin has recently been added to the ECC guidelines but should only be given once with no subsequent doses. Defibrillation is attempted again with 360 J. The provider may choose to use three stacked shocks at this point. Epinephrine is given every 3 to 5 minutes throughout the resuscitation. Refractory VF is treated with antiarrhythmic agents (Fig. 16-3). There is growing evidence that amiodarone may be the most efficacious drug in this setting.[12,79–81] Lidocaine is still acceptable therapy for recurrent VF and pulseless VT; however, there are insufficient clinical data to recommend it over amiodarone.[82] Magnesium sulfate, particularly if hypomagnesemia is suspected, and procainamide are recommended for intermittent and/or recurrent VF/VT. Bretylium is no longer recommended. The patient should be given a 360-J shock within 30 to 60 seconds of each drug.[9]

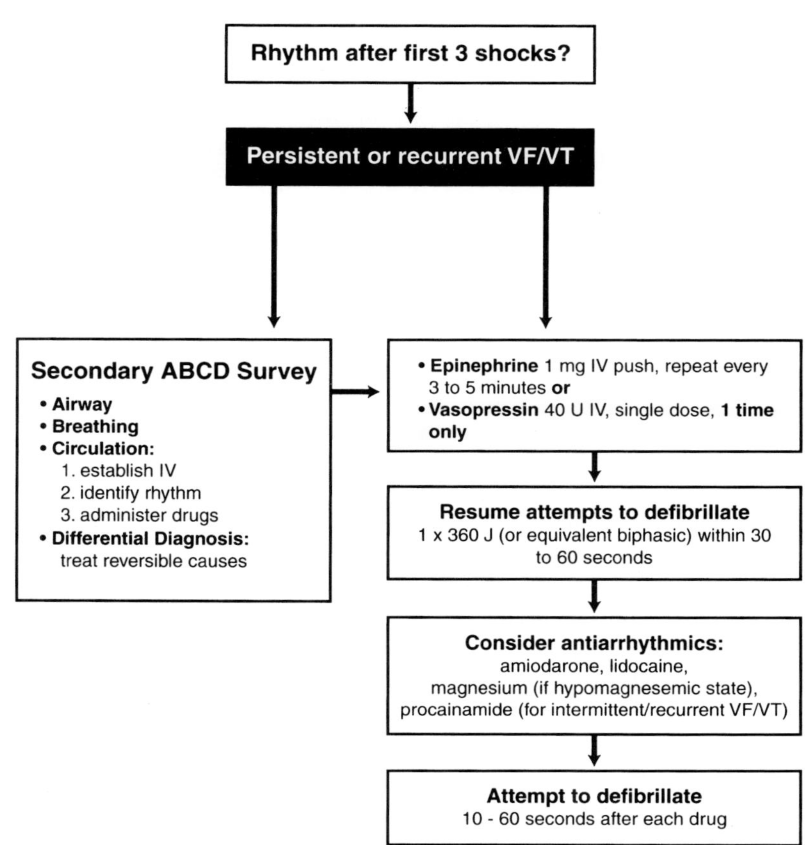

FIGURE 16–3 Treatment algorithm for persistent ventricular fibrillation and pulseless ventricular tachycardia (VF/VT).

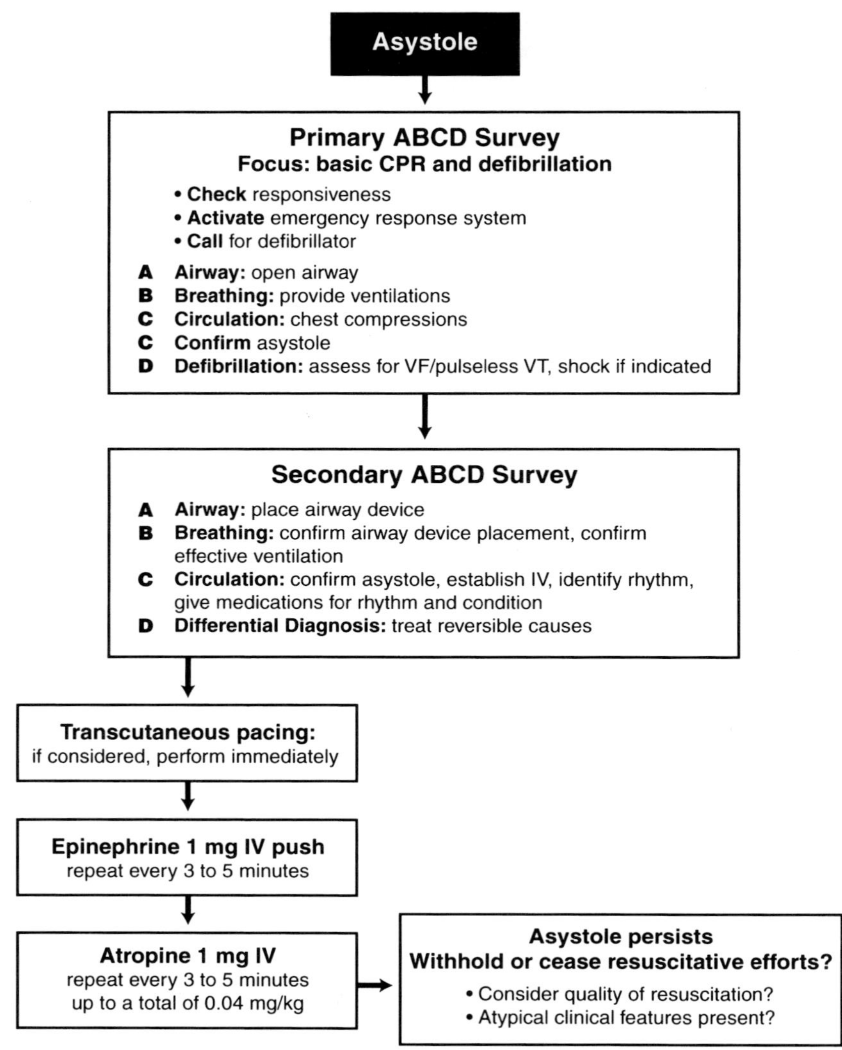

FIGURE 16–4 Algorithm for asystole.

The prognosis of patients found in VF/pulseless VT is better than that for asystole or pulseless electrical activity (PEA). Up to 30% of patients who suffer witnessed VF/VT arrests are successfully resuscitated.[83,84] Early defibrillation has been shown conclusively to improve survival in out-of-hospital arrest.[71,72] Eisenberg et al[71] reported survival increased from 7% to 26% when defibrillation was provided in the field. Stults et al[72] reported similar findings. Failure of initial defibrillation attempts is a poor prognostic sign. Attention should be focused on correcting underlying disorders including metabolic derangements. Emphasis should also be directed toward ensuring effective CPR, antiarrhythmic therapy, and further attempts to defibrillate before discontinuing resuscitative efforts.[9]

Asystole

Asystole is complete absence of electrical and mechanical cardiac activity, which frequently indicates a terminal event. However, CPR efforts can result in survival. Attention must be given to a continued search for treatable causes. Other priorities (Fig. 16-4) include establishing effective CPR and rhythm confirmation.[85] Fine, low-amplitude VF may masquerade as asystole in certain electrocardiographic (ECG) leads.[86] This scenario is thought to be rare, occurring in merely 2.5% of patients diagnosed with asystole in one report.[87] More likely, erroneous diagnoses result from incorrect lead placement and equipment malfunction.[87] Verifying lead placement and connections while confirming asystole in other leads is important. There is no benefit to countershocks in *true* asystole[88,89]; they can only induce a parasympathetic discharge and diminish subsequent chances of restoring circulation.[90,91] If fine VF is strongly suspected, defibrillation should be considered.

Once confirmed, asystole is approached with basic ABCD guidelines (Fig. 16-4). Epinephrine is the only recommended vassopressor and is administered to raise perfusion pressures.[9,92] Vasopressin is not recommended for asystole. Epinephrine is repeated every 3 to 5 minutes during the resuscitation. Atropine is administered every 3 to 5 minutes for

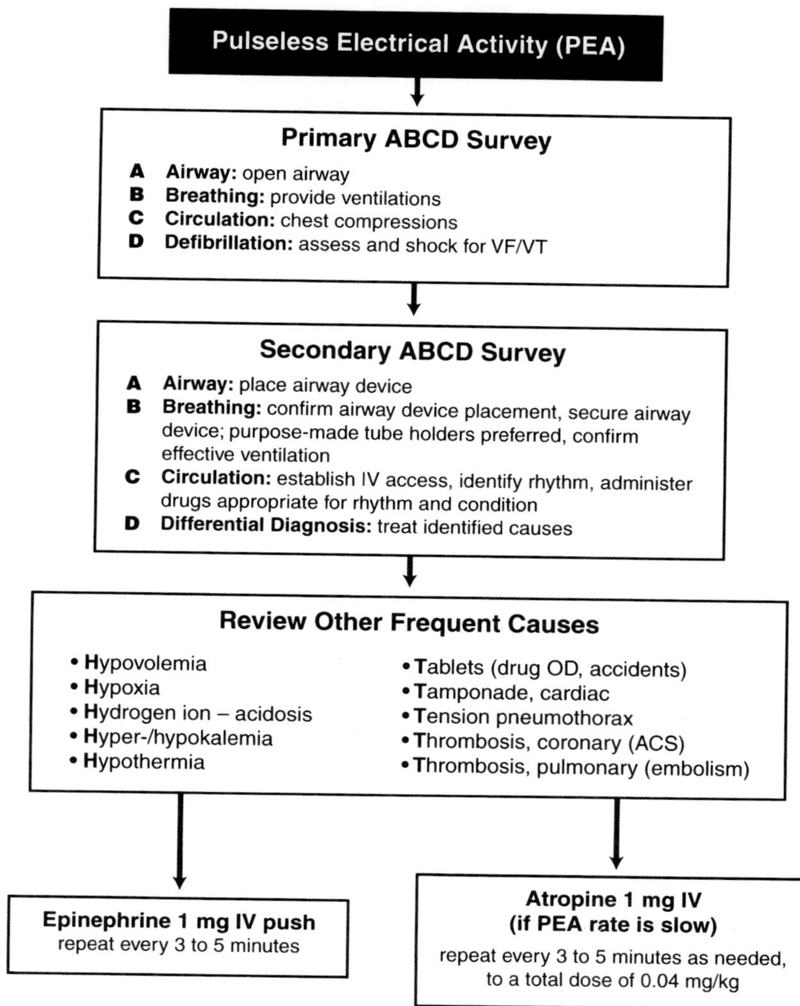

FIGURE 16–5 Treatment algorithm for pulseless electrical activity (PEA)

a total dose of 0.03 to 0.04 mg/kg. Atropine can treat the high parasympathetic tone that underlies severe bradyasystolic arrests.[90,91,93] Transcutaneous or transvenous pacing therapy may also be effective if applied early.[94] Pacing should be applied immediately whenever it is considered, otherwise depleted high-energy phosphates will negate effective cardiac contraction despite successful electrical capture.[95] Unfortunately, the prognosis of asystole remains grim. Less than 2% of these patients survive to discharge.[96] Asystole following countershocks for VF has a better prognosis than asystole occurring after prolonged CPR.[97]

Pulseless Electrical Activity

Pulseless electrical activity (PEA) also carries a poor prognosis and is characterized by organized electrical activity without effective cardiac contractions. PEA is synonymous with electromechanical dissociation (EMD) and includes conditions such as pulseless idioventricular, bradycardiac, and ventricular escape rhythms.[9] These later three dysrhythms have an extremely poor prognosis.[98,99] Overall, PEA is the most common proximate cause of death in delayed or difficult resuscitations.[85] As recommended for asystole, PEA mandates a careful assessment for reversible causes (Fig. 16-5). Rapid, narrow-complex activity increases the probability for treatable conditions.[85,100] Successful resuscitation is otherwise very unlikely. Effective CPR and epinephrine to augment perfusion pressures remain important.[99,101–103] Atropine is indicated for bradycardia.[9] Patients with chest trauma should undergo emergency left anterolateral thoracotomy[104] to address potentially reversible disorders, including cardiac tamponade and cardiovascular injuries. Thoractomy also provides exposure for direct cardiac massage and occlusion of the descending thoracic aorta, which may be lifesaving in the trauma setting.

Cardioversion

Electrical cardioversion is the *only* effective treatment for ventricular fibrillation (VF). Defibrillation depolarizes the entire heart, resulting in temporary asystole.[91,105] Pacemaker cells are then able to restore rhythmic myocardial activation. Myocardial contraction can resume if high-energy phosphate (HEP) stores, depleted rapidly during CPR,[106] are sufficient.[107,108] Although CPR can provide some organ perfusion, early defibrillation remains paramount. The probability of successful defibrillation approaches 90% immediately following a witnessed arrest.[106,109,110] Success rates then decline rapidly. The likelihood of restoring spontaneous circulation decreases 7% to 10% every minute.[78] At best, current CPR can only slow the already deteriorating state. Once a defibrillator is available, it should be attached immediately. When positioned on the chest, quick-look paddles allow rhythm evaluation and VF or pulseless VT treated immediately. Blind defibrillation is rarely indicated due to the wide availability of quick-look paddles. Countershocks for VF or pulseless ventricular tachycardia are delivered asynchronously. Shocks should be synchronized for relatively stable rhythms such as atrial fibrillation/flutter and monomorphic VT.[9] Otherwise, asynchronous countershocks may impinge on the relative refractory period, which risks inducing VF.[111]

Energy levels used for cardioversion are important for successful defibrillation. Low currents may be ineffective, while excessive energy levels can result in myocardial injury.[112,113] Generally, the lowest energy level for reliable defibrillation is preferred. A prospective study demonstrated that 175 J and 320 J were equally effective during the first defibrillation attempt.[114] Based on these data, 200 J is recommended for initial defibrillation attempts.[9] Up to 90% of adults can be successfully defibrillated when 200 J is delivered sufficiently early.[115,116] The range for a second countershock is 200 to 300 J. Decreased transthoracic impedance following repetitive shocks explains the consideration for 200 J during second attempts,[117,118] as subsequent countershocks would be expected to deliver greater energy to the heart. However, increasing energy levels to 300 J may provide more reliable increases in current delivery.[117]

Body size, which is not considered in current guidelines, also impacts on defibrillation energy requirements.[9] The optimal *current* for defibrillation is 30 to 40 A.[119–121] Adults have an average transthoracic impedance of 70 to 80 gV, requiring a 200-J countershock to produce a 30-A current.[122] However, the range of impedance varies significantly[117–121] and depends on many factors, including the energy, chest size, electrode size, interelectrode distance, paddle-skin coupling, phase of respiration, and antecedent countershocks.[117,118,123,124] Therefore, the defibrillation technique is important. Electrodes are positioned to maximize current flow using three paddle arrangements. Most commonly, one electrode is placed on the right parasternal border below the clavicle and the other is positioned in the left midaxillary line, level with the nipple. Alternatives are anteroposterior and apical-posterior positioning.[9] Electrodes must not touch directly or via conductive gels to ensure that current passes through the heart. During open chest resuscitation, one internal paddle is placed over the right ventricle, and the other is placed behind the apex. Larger paddles result in lower resistance.[117,124] Most adult paddles are 8 to 12 cm in diameter. Smaller paddles have high impedance and should be used only if standard adult paddles do not fit in the chest.[125]

Defibrillation threshold (DFT) describes the amount of current required to defibrillate the heart. DFT increases with CPR time. The most important factor affecting the DFT is coronary perfusion pressure. Catecholamines decrease the DFT.[126–128] It was once thought that epinephrine decreased the DFT through its beta-adrenergic effects. However, epinephrine's beneficial effect on DFT is due primarily to increased coronary perfusion pressure (alpha-adrenergic receptor stimulation).[129] The underlying mechanism of the time-dependent increase in DFT during VF is not completely understood. The DFT is not affected by metabolic or respiratory acidosis.[130,131] Recent work implicates adenosine, via adenosine A_1 receptor antiadrenergic effects, as a possible mediator of the increase in DFT with time.[132] Cardiac compression has been shown to reduce defibrillation thresholds during open chest defibrillation.[133] Aminophylline, an adenosine receptor antagonist, decreases the defibrillation threshold.[134–136]

Patients with pacemakers and automatic internal cardiodefibrillators (AICDs) deserve careful consideration. Patients with pacemakers should not have the paddles placed directly over the generator,[137] and must be interrogated to determine pacing thresholds after defibrillation. Patients with AICDs who present with VF or pulseless VT should have external defibrillation performed immediately.[138] AICDs are shielded to withstand external countershocks. AICD patches may increase transthoracic resistance.[139] Therefore, the electrode position should be changed if initial countershocks fail. After successful external defibrillation, the AICD unit should be tested.

New automated external defibrillators (AEDs) are being increasingly utilized. The AED analyzes the ECG pattern, and then sounds an alarm and discharges when VF is detected. AEDs require less training than conventional defibrillators, and there is less delay in administering the countershock.[78,140,141] Several studies with AEDs have shown equivalent or improved survival compared with early defibrillation using manual defibrillators.[142–144] AEDs are endorsed by the AHA for use in out-of-hospital arrest.[145]

Current-based defibrillators have been developed in an effort to improve defibrillation.[119,120,146] These devices should significantly enhance the delivery of *appropriate* energy to the myocardium and increase the likelihood of successful cardioversion while reducing the risk of myocardial trauma. Other areas of investigation include delivery of biphasic (bidirectional) or multipulse, multipathway shocks.[122] These methods are in use for internal defibrillators, but their efficacy for external defibrillation has not been established.[147,148]

A precordial thump is an alternative means of attempting defibrillation and may be used for witnessed arrests when a defibrillator is not immediately available. It has been reported to convert VT to sinus rhythm in 11% to 25% of cases.[149,150] Unfortunately, precordial thumps may convert VT to VF, asystole, or EMD,[150,151] and are very unlikely to convert VF. A precordial thump is not indicated for unwitnessed or out-of-hospital arrests.[9]

PHYSIOLOGY OF CARDIOPULMONARY RESUSCITATION

The mechanism(s) generating forward blood flow during CPR has been a subject of significant controversy. Kouwenhoven postulated that chest compressions are translated directly to the heart through the sternum and spine.[152,153] This mechanism became known as the *cardiac pump*. Multiple laboratory and clinical investigations have verified this as an operative mechanism during closed chest compression.[154–157] However, other operative mechanisms have also been demonstrated during CPR.

Investigations have identified at least two other important mechanisms responsible for blood flow during CPR. The thoracic pump was discovered by the observation that coughing during cardiac arrest generated forward flow. Laboratory[51] work has demonstrated chest compressions cause a general rise in intrathoracic pressures capable of forcing blood into the systemic circulation. The heart in this circumstance merely functions as a conduit. Many studies have validated the thoracic pump mechanism during CPR.[48,158–160]

A third means for generating blood flow during CPR is the abdominal pump. This describes the effects of abdominal compressions, which are now advocated for CPR.[161–164] The abdominal pump operates through arterial and venous components. The arterial component reflects compression of the abdominal aorta, which forces blood into the peripheral circulation. The aortic valve remains closed during abdominal compression and resists retrograde arterial flow. Simultaneously, the venous component pushes blood from the inferior vena cava into the right heart. Both contribute added hemodynamic benefits during recommended techniques for abdominal compressions in CPR.

It is clear that the cardiac, thoracic, and abdominal pump mechanisms are all important means for generating forward flow during CPR. Technique dictates to what extent these three mechanisms contribute. Other factors that can influence the effectiveness of these pumping mechanisms include: cycle rates, compression durations, body habitus, cardiac size, chest wall stiffness, and the presence of pulmonary disease, as well as the duration of the resuscitation effort. The pump mechanism that contributes most toward effective CPR is widely variable. Better understanding of these variables should guide recommendations and improvements in CPR techniques and adjunctive devices.

CPR TECHNIQUES AND MECHANICAL ADJUNCTS

The high mortality rates associated with cardiac arrest have led to increased enthusiasm for several techniques and devices. Combining chest and abdominal pumping techniques within the same compression cycle is termed interposed abdominal compression CPR (IAC-CPR). The technique employs chest compressions with abdominal compression during the relaxation phase of chest compression (Fig. 16-6). The simplest and most studied applications involve compressing the chest and abdomen at equal durations. The method has not been associated with increased intra-abdominal injuries or aspiration. Human studies of IAC-CPR have yielded encouraging results with statistically significant improvement in outcome measures.[165–177] Return of spontaneous circulation and survival to discharge were both improved using IAC-CPR when examining inpatient cardiac arrests.[166,168,169] Therefore, the method is now considered an acceptable alternative to standard CPR for in-hospital arrests. A device that will allow IAC-CPR by a single rescuer is currently under evaluation (Fig. 16-7).

Noninvasive Mechanical Devices

Noninvasive mechanical devices have recently been developed for improving CPR. A pneumatic vest optimizes the thoracic pump mechanism by alternating pressures around

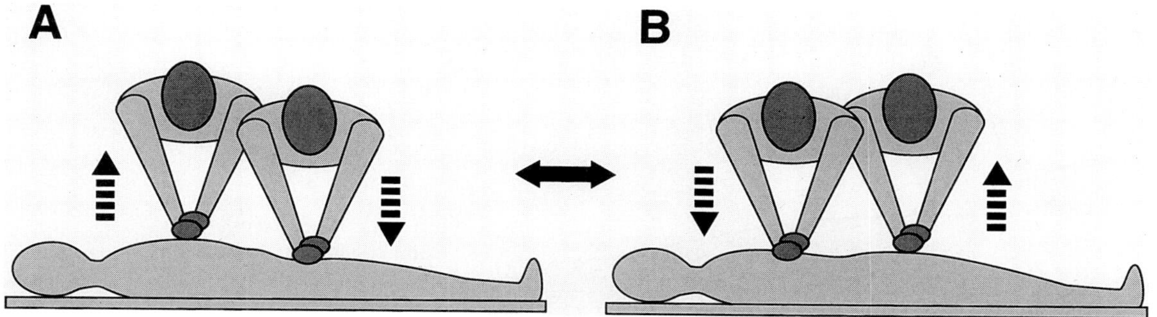

FIGURE 16–6 Interposed abdominal compression (IAC) cardiopulmonary resuscitation (CPR), or IAC-CPR.

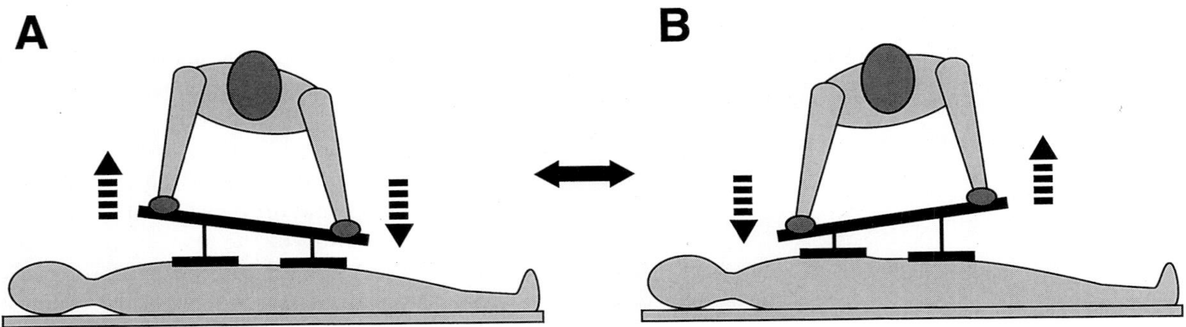

FIGURE 16–7 Device proposed for abdominal compression cardiopulmonary resuscitation (IAC-CPR).

the thoracic cage (Vest-CPR). Vest-CPR utilizes a pneumatic bladder tailored to fit the chest. Air is forced into and out of the vest by a pneumatic drive. Two clinical trials demonstrated improved outcomes with an increased rate of return of spontaneous circulation.[170,171] However, no patients survived to discharge and complete results have not yet been published. The vest is considered an acceptable alternative to standard CPR for ambulance transport or for in-hospital use.

Active Compression-Decompression

Active compression-decompression (ACD) is a promising means for improving CPR. The concept originated from successful resuscitations using a plunger.[172] A device that consists of a hand-held suction cup with a central piston and handle is required (Fig. 16-8). ACD-CPR can increase aortic pressures resulting in improved cerebral, coronary, and renal blood flow.[173–176] Ventricular filling and venous return are augmented by negative intrathoracic pressure during the active decompression phase.[177] Two initial studies reported increased return of spontaneous circulation and 24-hour survival with the ACD device. Survival to discharge was higher with ACD in both studies but did not reach statistical significance.[178,179] Data from 2866 patients using the ACD device were subsequently combined.[180] ACD improved 1-hour survival but long-term outcome was not significantly different from standard CPR. More recently, a randomized clinical trial demonstrated significantly improved 1-year survival following ACD compared to standard CPR.[181] ACD-CPR is considered an acceptable alternative to standard CPR.

Open Chest Cardiac Massage

Several invasive means of supporting the circulation are also advocated for resuscitation. Open chest cardiac massage (OCM) was relatively common prior to 1960.[182] The role for OCM is currently limited to specific circumstances. OCM is indicated for cardiac arrest associated with penetrating thoracic trauma. Other situations in which OCM should be considered include cardiac arrest due to hypothermia, massive pulmonary embolism, pericardial tamponade, or intra-abdominal hemorrhage, and when chest deformity precludes effective CPR. The recommended approach is via a left lateral thoracotomy except following recent cardiac surgery where the prior sternotomy can be reentered. Thoracotomy is carried through the fifth intercostal space and the pericardium opened anterior and parallel to the phrenic nerve. The heart is compressed with two hands or, alternatively, with one hand while the other is used to occlude the thoracic aorta (Fig. 16-9).

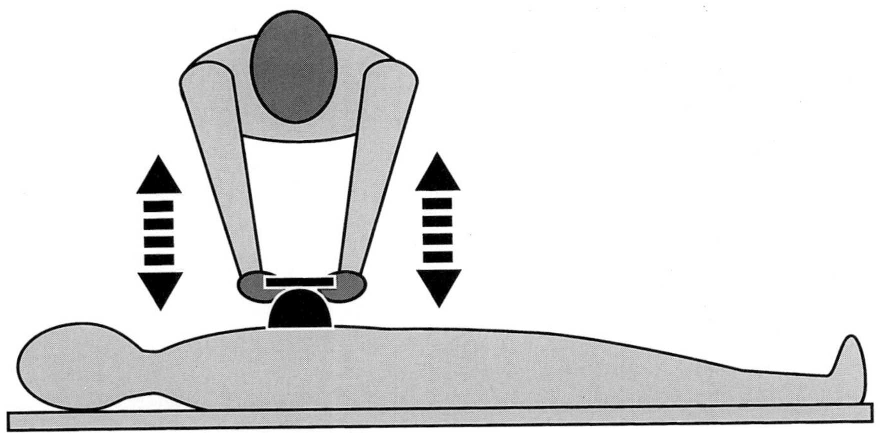

FIGURE 16–8 Active compression-decompression cardiopulmonary bypass (ACD-CPR) using a suction cup device attached to chest wall.

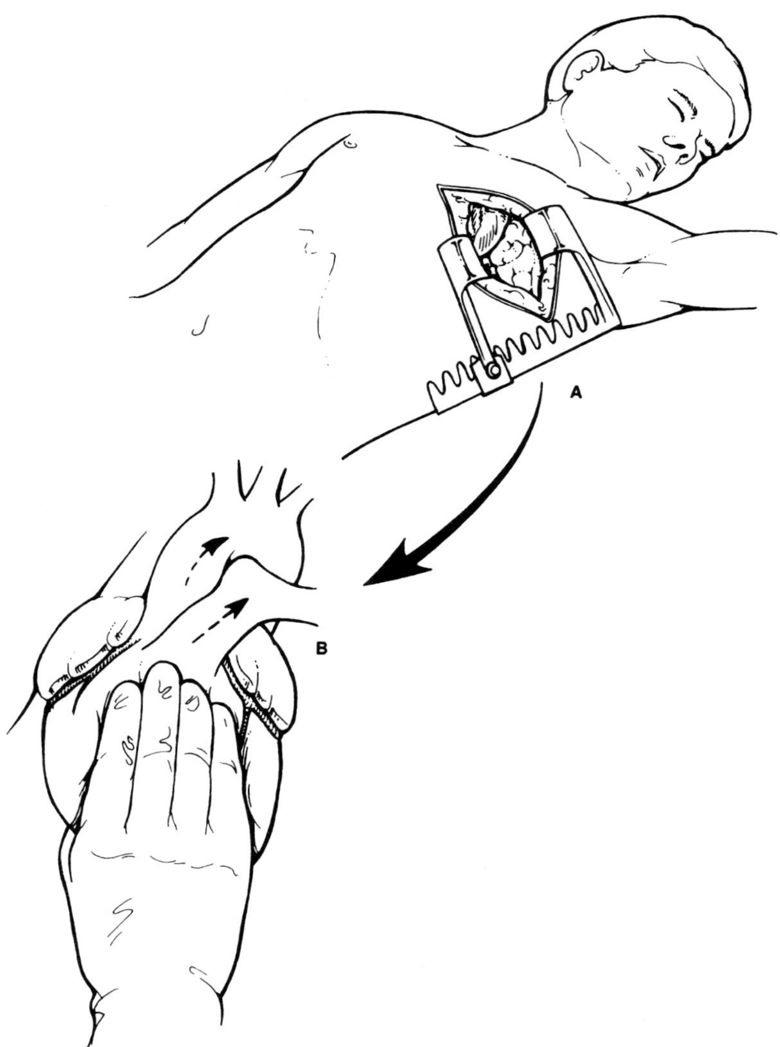

FIGURE 16–9 Technique of open chest cardiac massage. The heart is exposed via an anterolateral thoracotomy through the fifth intercostal space. The pericardium is opened if there is evidence of pericardial tamponade; otherwise, it is left intact. The heart is massaged at a rate of 60 to 80 beats per minute.

Numerous studies have demonstrated superior hemodynamics results during open massage compared to CCM.[56,183–188] Most notable are increased diastolic pressures and reduced central venous pressures,[56,185,188] which demonstrated the favorable effects on coronary perfusion during OCM versus CCM. Cardiac output and cerebral blood flow are also higher during OCM,[186,187,189] and OCM has resulted in successful resuscitation following failed attempts during CCM.[189–191] However, clinical results are not improved when OCM is used following prolonged CPR efforts.[192] Animal studies have suggested that OCM may improve results if applied early after a short period of ineffective CCM.[193] And a recent prospective, nonrandomized clinical trial emphasized the importance of instituting OCM earlier to improve outcome.[194] Patients receiving OCM had improved outcome compared to CCM; however, improvements declined as the period of CCM increased.

Early application of OCM may improve survival. For results to be meaningful, this needs to be determined in a prospective clinical trial. Downtimes prior to thoracotomy must also be minimized to reduce neurologic impairment in survivors. Potential complications of OCM include right ventricular perforation, hemorrhage, lung laceration, phrenic nerve injury, esophageal and aortic injury, cardiac lacerations, and empyema.[191] However, the rate of infection is relatively low, approximately 5%, given the emergent nature of the procedure on an unprepped chest.[195]

Blood Pumps

Blood pumps can also improve resuscitation results. Hemodynamics, survival, and neurologic function are improved in animals treated with early CPB versus those treated with standard CCM.[196–198] However, these devices are generally limited to tertiary care centers. A number of institutions have utilized CPB to selectively bridge patients to transplantation following cardiac arrest.[199–201] The development of portable CPB systems has made the technology more available and CPB has been used successfully in a growing number of centers for select cases of cardiac arrest.[202–208] Growing clinical experience has demonstrated improvements in outcome when CPB is applied within 20 to 30 minutes following cardiac arrest, with long-term survival ranging from 17% to 57%. A registry has reported a 27% survival rate when CPB systems were used for the treatment of 386 patients in cardiac arrest.[209] The possibility of survival appears limited to patients who receive CPB within 30 minutes of a witnessed *normothermic* arrest. *Hypothermic* cardiac arrests represent a unique category in which survival is possible following relatively prolonged arrests. In this setting, CPB has been advocated as the resuscitation method of choice because of its unique ability to rewarm the patient while providing total circulatory support.[165,166] Although treatment protocols have not been well defined, CPB support should be continued until the patient is adequately rewarmed before resuscitative efforts are abandoned.

The intra-aortic balloon pump IABP can improve hemodynamic parameters during CPR.[210,211] However, the value of IABP augmentation during CPR appears very limited. Alternatively, there has been growing interest in using *aortic balloon occlusion catheters*.[212–214] Selective aortic arch perfusion utilizes a catheter inserted via the femoral artery and advanced to the descending thoracic aorta. Balloon occlusion allows selective, retrograde perfusion of the heart and brain. One proposed advantage is that therapeutic agents could be selectively delivered to the heart and brain by this technique.

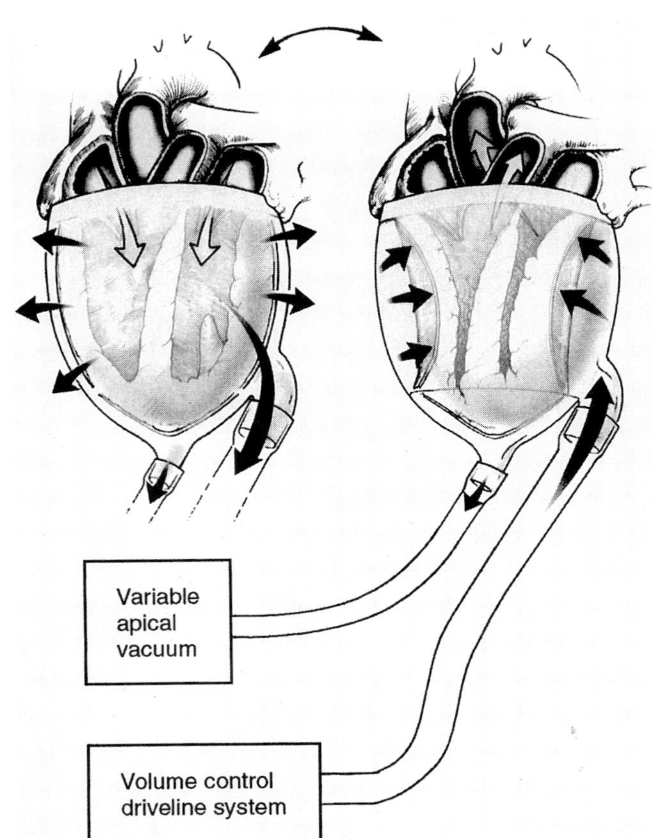

FIGURE 16–10 Direct mechanical ventricular actuation (DMVA). The ventricles are encompassed by a pneumatically regulated heart cup and the arrested heart is compressed (right) and dilated (left).

Direct Mechanical Ventricular Actuation

Direct mechanical ventricular actuation (DMVA) is a unique non–blood contacting method of circulatory support that transfers systolic and diastolic forces directly to the ventricular myocardium (Fig. 16-10). DMVA employs a pneumatically regulated heart cup constructed with a flexible inner membrane and semirigid shell. The device is vacuum attached to the heart via a left anterior thoracotomy. Ventricular compression results in physiologic forward blood flow while active decompression enhances diastolic filling.[215] DMVA can provide hemodynamic support far superior to any other CPR method. Its capability to provide physiologic pulsatile flow may best explain improved neurologic outcome when compared with CPB in animal models.[216–218] DMVA is uniquely capable for resuscitation because it can be applied rapidly. One disadvantage is the requirement for a thoracotomy; however, DMVA's value as an adjunct in resuscitation is complemented by its versatility and lack of blood contact. Clinical experience with DMVA has resulted in successful bridge to transplantation, postcardiotomy support, and long-term recovery from severe myocarditis.[219,220]

PHARMACOLOGIC THERAPY DURING CPR

Peripheral venous access is preferred for purposes of speed and safety and for avoiding CPR interruption. Drugs take 1 to 2 minutes to reach the central circulation during CPR[221] and should be administered as boluses followed by a 20-mL saline flush with extremity elevation.[222] Peak drug concentrations are lower with peripheral than central venous injection.[223] Central access should be considered if the response to peripherally administered drugs is absent. The internal jugular and supraclavicular sites are preferred to the femoral vein because return from the infradiaphragmatic IVC is impaired during CPR.[224] A long femoral line that extends above the diaphragm overcomes this problem. Intravenous fluids are not indicated for routine cardiac arrest without hypovolemia. Fluid administration may adversely affect coronary perfusion pressure and myocardial blood flow by raising right atrial pressure.[225] Fluids can benefit in certain cases of PEA, such as hypovolemia and cardiac tamponade.

When venous access is not possible, drugs may be administered via an endotracheal tube. The medications are given via a catheter passed beyond the tip of the ETT. The dose is 2 to 2.5 times the recommended intravenous dose, diluted in 10 mL of saline or distilled water.[226] Water provides better absorption but has a greater adverse effect on PaO_2 than saline.[227] Several rapid insufflations are given after the bolus to disperse the drug. Intracardiac injection is not recommended for routine use during CPR. It may be used for epinephrine during OCM or when no other access can be obtained during CCM. Disadvantages of intracardiac injection are the need to stop CPR and the high rate of complications. Complications include coronary artery laceration, cardiac tamponade, and pneumothorax.

The principal pharmacologic agents recommended for ACLS have been adrenergic agonists, antiarrhythmics, and buffers. Until recently, alpha-adrenergic agonists have been the only class of drugs that have been shown to improve outcome definitively in CPR.[228–230] The primary benefit is vasoconstriction. Increases in peripheral resistance result in elevated aortic pressure, which improves coronary perfusion. Epinephrine is given for this purpose during cardiac arrest.[129,229–232] Epinephrine's beta-adrenergic effects have not been clearly shown to benefit the treatment of cardiac arrest. The recommended dose of epinephrine for resuscitation is 1.0 mg IV every 3 to 5 minutes throughout the resuscitation attempt.[9] Epinephrine has improved the return of spontaneous circulation and survival rate in animal models of cardiac arrest.[228–230] The minimum coronary perfusion pressure and myocardial blood flow needed to achieve successful defibrillation are 15 mm Hg and 15 to 20 mL/min per 100 g, respectively.[52,85] Standard CPR techniques rarely achieve these requirements in the absence of pressor agents. Anecdotal reports of using higher doses of epinephrine generated enthusiasm.[233–235] Subsequent clinical trials reported higher rates of ROSC, but no significant survival benefit.[236–240] One trial found high-dose epinephrine had more adverse effects,[237] which may be partly explained by increases in oxygen demand.[241]

A number of other nonadrenergic vasocontrictive agents have been studied in an effort to find a more effective drug then epinephrine. Vasopressin has recently emerged as an alternative to epinephrine for treating cardiac arrest. Comparative laboratory and clinical data indicate that vasopressin may be preferable to epinephrine.[242,243] Although further clinical trials are needed, vasopressin is now considered an acceptable alternative to epinephrine for initial treatment of the arrested patient.

The effectiveness of antiarrhythmic agents in the treatment of sudden death has not been well substantiated in previous clinical investigations. Recently, randomized clinical trials have demonstrated amiodarone to be effective in the treatment of cardiac arrest.[12,80,81,244] Amiodarone significantly improved survival to hospital admission compared to placebo for VF/pulseless VT.[244] It was found to be as effective as bretylium for treating VF or unstable VT in another randomized trial. Most recently, amiodarone significantly increased survival to hospital admission compared to lidocaine in a randomized clinical trial for the treatment of sudden death.[12] There was a trend toward increased survival at hospital discharge with amiodarone that did not reach statistical significance. Amiodarone is now recommended for the treatment of persistent VT and/or VF after defibrillation and epinephrine. Currently, lidocaine has more evidence opposing than supporting its use in cardiac arrest.[82] However, it is considered an acceptable alternative to amiodarone.

Procainamide is a ganglionic blocker that slows phase-4 depolarization and intraventricular conduction. It is recommended for recurrent VF/VT and should be administered as an infusion over 30 minutes. Rapid infusion rates are associated with hypotension.[245] Procainamide may be of little benefit *during* cardiac arrest and also may worsen ventricular arrhythmias in the presence of hypokalemia and hypomagnesemia.

Magnesium sulfate should be administered for suspected hypomagnesemia or torsades de pointes. It is recommended for treatment of refractory VF/VT. Hypomagnesemia is associated with ventricular arrhythmias and sudden cardiac death[246] and may hinder potassium replenishment in hypokalemic patients. Common side effects of magnesium sulfate include flushing, mild bradycardia, and hypotension with rapid infusions. Hypermagnesemia can cause flaccid paralysis and cardiorespiratory arrest.

Atropine is a parasympatholytic agent that enhances atrioventricular node conduction and sinus node automaticity. It is indicated for symptomatic bradycardia and asystolic arrest.[90,91,93,247] Asystole secondary to prolonged ischemia is almost uniformly fatal, and although atropine is unlikely to be of real benefit, there is no evidence that it is harmful under these dire circumstances.[97] The dose of atropine in cardiac arrest is 1 mg as an IV bolus, repeated every 3 to 5 minutes to a total dose of 3 mg. For symptomatic bradycardia, the dose is 0.5 to 1 mg (maximum of 2 to 3 mg). Doses lower than 0.5 mg are avoided because they may cause paradoxical bradycardia.[248,249] Adverse effects of atropine include tachycardia and anticholinergic effects.

Sodium bicarbonate is recommended for acidosis during cardiac arrest. It binds hydrogen ions to form carbonic acid, which is converted to CO_2 and eliminated by the lungs. During CPR, CO_2 may accumulate rapidly, leading to a hypercarbic venous acidemia.[250,251] Since CO_2 is diffusible across membranes, paradoxical intracellular acidosis[252] may result and decrease the likelihood of successful resuscitation. Additionally, hypocarbic arterial alkalemia[251] or the so-called venoarterial paradox may develop. Sodium bicarbonate may increase CO_2 levels, worsen the venoarterial paradox, and exacerbate intracellular acidosis.[253,254] Other potential adverse effects of $NaHCO_3$ include alkalemia with a leftward shift of the oxyhemoglobin desaturation curve (less O_2 release to tissues), hyperosmolality, hypernatremia, and decreased coronary perfusion pressure.[255–258] Bicarbonate has not been shown to improve results in cardiac arrest[256,257,259] and is only recommended for patients with preexisting acidosis, hyperkalemia, or tricyclic antidepressant overdose. Otherwise, bicarbonate should be considered for prolonged resuscitations.

CEREBRAL PROTECTION/RESUSCITATION

The objective of CPR is to restore circulation in a neurologically intact individual. The main priority during CPR is to provide sufficient myocardial and cerebral blood flow to prevent irreversible damage prior to definitive intervention. Unfortunately, this goal often is not achieved. *Less than 10% of CPR attempts result in survival without neurologic damage, whether in or out of a hospital.*[260]

Following cardiac arrest, consciousness is lost within 10 seconds.[261] High-energy phosphates and glycogen stores are depleted within 5 minutes.[262] Lactic acid accumulates in neurons and has a direct cytotoxic effect.[263] The limited cerebral blood flow generated by CPR may exacerbate intracellular acidosis by allowing anaerobic metabolism.[264,265] Survival with normal neurologic function becomes unlikely as irreversible brain damage can occur within 4 to 5 minutes of cardiac arrest.[266,267] Restoring circulation within 5 to 20 minutes of sudden death is associated with variable degrees of neurologic damage.[266,268,269]

During CPR, venous valves at the thoracic inlet prevent the transmission of high intrathoracic pressures to the jugular venous system.[270] Cerebral blood flow is usually kept at about 50 mL/min per 100 g by autoregulation when cerebral perfusion pressures are within the normal physiologic range.[260] CPR results in much lower cerebral perfusion pressures, which seldom exceeded 40 mm Hg.[18,52] Cerebral blood flow is only 10% to 15% of normal,[185] which may be more harmful than no flow at all.[265]

Irreversible neuronal injury begins after 5 minutes of ischemia.[266] Because neurons can function in vitro for up to 60 minutes of ischemia,[271] reperfusion may be as important to neurologic outcome as ischemia itself. Reperfusion injury following successful resuscitation has been termed the *postresuscitation syndrome* and appears to be multifactorial. Calcium overload in the mitochondria, free-radical injury, and the no-reflow phenomenon may all contribute to reperfusion injury.[260] The no-reflow phenomenon describes continued hypoperfusion that may last up to 3 hours.[272] Platelet aggregation, altered calcium flux, vasoconstriction, and pericapillary edema are all presumed causative factors.[273] Intracranial pressure may not be an important factor as it usually returns to normal soon after cardiac arrest.[274,275] Cerebral blood flow remains depressed for 18 to 24 hours following a severe ischemic insult.[276] Subsequent periods of hypoperfusion are believed secondary to calcium-induced precapillary vasoconstriction.[277]

Cerebral blood flow is abnormal following ischemic injury.[278] Perfusion is more dependent on arterial pressure and moderate hypotension may lead to further cerebral injury.[279] Patients should be kept normotensive and/or mildly hypertensive in the postresuscitation period.[280,281] Moderate hyperoxia ($Po_2 = 100$ mm Hg) and mild hyperventilation ($Paco_2 = 30$ to 35 mm Hg) are desirable. Arterial pH is kept in the normal range. Anticonvulsants should be given as needed for seizures, which can be subtle and occur in up to 30% of patients.[282,283] Body temperature is kept low to normal to reduce cerebral metabolic demand.[283]

Mild hypothermia has exhibited increasing promise in the prevention of brain damage following cardiac arrest. Earlier experiments using canine models demonstrated improved neurologic function when active cooling followed arrest.[284,285] Clinical trials have subsequently shown cooling shortly following resuscitation from cardiac arrests improves neurologic outcome.[286] Benefits of hypothermia may be greatest when rapid postresuscitation cooling is achieved and maintained for an extended period.[287,288]

Although not well proven, there are other considerations for treating patients in the immediate postresuscitation period. The patient should be monitored closely. Supplemental oxygen and intravenous fluids are given, and urine output is monitored. Patients revived using antiarrhythmic agents should have these agents continued as an infusion. Tachyarrhythmias are the most commonly encountered postresuscitation arrhythmias and are likely secondary to increased circulating catecholamines. Increasing emphasis has been placed on the use of beta-adrenergic blockade in the postresuscitation period.[289] These agents should be considered unless bradycardia is a significant problem. Bradycardia following CPR frequently requires the airway and ventilatory status to be carefully assessed, followed by adminstration of atropine, epinephrine, and/or pacing if the patient becomes hypotensive.

Possibly the greatest impact on survival has been the use of automatic internal cardiodefibrillators and antiarrhythmics in patients who are at increased risk for sudden death. Multiple clinical studies have now shown that survival can be significantly improved with these devices.[146,290–294] Amiodarone has also been shown to be effective in this regard.[295–300] More attention is being directed toward identifying patients who should be considered for such therapy.[295,301–306] To date, many of these treatments have been directed towards patients who have been successfully resuscitated from sudden death.

Predicting which patients are likely to survive *during* resuscitation efforts remains an elusive problem. Patients presenting in VF/VT have a better prognosis compared with those in asystole or PEA.[10,307–311] Advanced age was a negative prognostic indicator in several early series[312,313] but has no independent predictive value when comorbidities are considered.[10,11] Location of the arrest (ICU versus non-ICU) may be an important consideration.[10,11,310,313,314] Patients with noncardiac disorders are more likely to survive if their clinical status was stable prior to cardiac arrest compared

TABLE 16–1 Long-term survival following CPR

Reference	No. cases	No. surviving to discharge	Long-term survival		
			1 y	2 y	4 y
Lund[347]	1263 arrests	97 (10%)	—	80%	—
Rockswald[342]	514 arrests	47 (9%)	85%	50%	—
Goldstein[338]	2171 arrests	142 (7%)	80%	65%	45%
Cobb[348]	VF only	406	74%	64%	50%
Eisenburg[349]	1567 arrests	276 (19%)	76%	66%	49%
Baum[339]	886 VF	146 (16%)	74%	62%	—
Litherthson[329]	301 VF	42 (14%)	Mean survival: 13 months		

to those who were deteriorating.[315] Comorbid conditions associated with more than 95% of mortalities after cardiac arrest include renal failure, metastatic cancer, pneumonia, sepsis, hypotension, stroke, and homebound lifestyle.[10,307–310] Survival is clearly more likely for witnessed arrests and for CPR initiated within 5 minutes, with CPR durations of 15 minutes or less. Mortality increases from 44% for resuscitations less than 15 minutes in duration versus 95% for those that are longer.[10] Survival is rare after 30 minutes of CPR.[10,316,317]

In contrast to inpatient arrest, in which comorbid diseases play a major role in outcome, delayed therapy outweighs all other factors for out-of-hospital arrest. Key determinants of survival include the initial rhythm, witnessed arrest, downtime prior to CPR, and delays in definitive treatment. Survival rates are highly variable among reported series. Becker et al[318] found a 2% overall survival to discharge in metropolitan Chicago. In New York City, Lombardi et al[319] found a 1.4% survival rate, which improved to 5.3% in patients with witnessed VF arrest. Eisenberg et al[320] reported a 22% survival in patients with witnessed arrests; however, downtimes were much shorter. The last study emphasized the importance of early intervention as only 4% of patients suffering unwitnessed arrests survived. CPR initiated within 4 minutes improved survival rates from 12% to 28%. Early definitive care was also associated with improved outcome.[320] As with in-hospital arrest, presenting rhythm was a major determinant for survival, with VF/VT having the best prognosis.[321] Bystander CPR has repeatedly been associated with improved survival rates for victims of cardiac arrest.[322–330] In addition, several studies found less neurologic morbidity in cardiac arrest victims who received bystander CPR.[327,328,331,332] The decrease in hospital mortality from bystander CPR is primarily due to fewer deaths from anoxic encephalopathy during postresuscitation hospitalization.[328,332] Return of consciousness within

TABLE 16–2 Studies reporting morbidity of patients from out-of-hospital cardiac arrest after resuscitation and discharge

Reference	No. cases	No. surviving to discharge	Type of arrest	Morbidity
Lund[347]	1263	94	All	21% impaired
Litherthson[337]	301	42	VF	60% normal 28% partial deficit 12% severe deficit
Rockswald[342]	514	83	All	60% normal 40% severe deficit
Wernberg[350]	1686	72	All	22% partial deficit 6% severe deficit
Snyder[351]	63	25	All	64% excellent 32% good recovery 4% poor recovery
Earnest[16]	117	38	All	53% independent 24% severe deficit
Bergner[352]	—	426	VF	91% independent 9% severe deficit
Abramson[343]	—	100	All	25% prearrest 36% good recovery

24 to 48 hours of arrest is a positive neurologic prognostic sign.[10,333,334]

Long-term survival of those patients discharged after out-of-hospital arrest is reasonably good. The reported 1-year survival rate ranges from 75% to 85%, and approximately 50% are still alive at 4 years[335] (Table 16-1). The majority of these patients ultimately die of cardiac causes.[16,336,337] Positive predictors for long-term survival are cardiac arrest associated with acute MI, no prior history of MI, and short time intervals between arrest, CPR, and definitive care.[338–340] Patients with primary antiarrhythmic events, congestive heart failure, impaired LV function, extensive CAD, and complex premature ventricular depolarizations are less likely to survive long term after discharge.[341]

Unfortunately, only a small proportion of patients who suffer sudden death survive and have a subsequent good quality of life.[335] Depression is a common problem following discharge but usually resolves within a few months.[10] The rate of significant mental impairment in those who survive is variable. Significant neurologic impairment usually results in death prior to hospital discharge. Of those who survived to discharge, a significant proportion have neurologic deficits (Table 16-2).[342] For patients who did not receive early intervention, the outlook is more dismal.[16,343]

ETHICAL CONSIDERATIONS

Resuscitation efforts should be discontinued when continued ACLS efforts do not result in a perfusing rhythm.[344] Discontinuation is generally based on clinical judgement.[345] Unilateral determination of medical futility is made when the patient's underlying medical condition precludes successful resuscitation. Metastatic cancer and sepsis are examples of such conditions.[346] Although several studies show that resuscitation for longer than 30 minutes is unlikely to result in long-term survival, there are many anecdotal reports of neurologically intact survival following prolonged resuscitations.[10,316,317]

CONCLUSION

Until recently, the only factors that have proven to impact CPR favorably are early defibrillation, effective BLS, and epinephrine. Yet overall survival rates remain dismally low. There is a growing pool of evidence that novel methods of CPR and new antiarrhythmics may significantly improve survival in this challenging field. The combination of improved response times, automatic defibrillators, more effective circulatory support methods, and new antiarrhythmic agents has exciting implications. Major improvements in survival and neurologic outcome of out-of-hospital cardiac arrest victims will require continued focus on rapid response and the availability of definitive treatments in the field. Heightened community awareness and organized medical efforts can have a positive impact on these factors.

Future improvements in the field of cardiopulmonary circulation will depend on the timely implementation of promising therapies. Efforts to identify patients at risk for sudden death may provide increasing opportunity for preventative strategies such as AICDs and antiarrhythmics. Most important will be the continued use of well-designed clinical trials to better direct treatment strategies based on valid scientific data.

REFERENCES

1. *Heart and Stroke Facts: 1994 Statistical Supplement*. Dallas, American Heart Association, 1994.
2. Goldman L, Cook EF: The decline in ischemic heart disease mortality rates: an analysis of the comparative effects of medical interventions and changes in lifestyle. *Ann Intern Med* 1984; 101:825.
3. Ryan TJ, Anderson JL, Antman EM, et al: ACC/AHA guidelines for the management of patients with acute myocardial infaraction: a report of the American College of Cardiology/American Heart Association Task Force in Practice Guidelines (Committee on Management of Acute Myocardial infarction). *J Am Coll Cardiol* 1996:28:1328.
4. Myerburg RJ, Castellanos A: Cardiac arrest and sudden death, in Braunwald E (ed): *Heart Disease*. Philadelphia, WB Saunders, 1992; p 756.
5. Eisenberg MS, Bergner L, Hallstrom A: Survivors of out-of-hospital cardiac arrest: morbidity and long-term survival. *Am J Emerg Med* 1984;2:189.
6. Kannel WB, Doyle JT, McNamara PM, et al: Precursors of sudden coronary death: factors related to the incidence of sudden death. *Circulation* 1975; 51:606.
7. Kuller L, Lilienfeld A, Fisher R: Epidemiologic study of sudden and unexpected deaths due to arteriosclerotic heart disease. *Circulation* 1966; 34:1056.
8. Girdon T, Kannel WB: Premature mortality from coronary heart disease: the Framingham study. *JAMA* 1971; 215:1617.
9. The American Heart Association in collaboration with the International Liaison Committee on Resuscitation (ILCOR): Guidelines 2000 for cardiopulmonary resuscitation and emergency cardiovascular care. *Circulation* 2000; 102:1-1.
10. Bedell SE, Delbanco TL, Cook EF, Epstein FH: Survival after cardiopulmonary resuscitation in the hospital. *N Engl J Med* 1983; 309:569.
11. DeBard ML: Cardiopulmonary resuscitation: analysis of six years' experience and review of the literature. *Ann Emerg Med* 1981; 10:408.
12. Dorian P: ALIVE. Presentation at the Amercian Heart Association Scientific Sessions 2001, Anaheim, CA, Nov. 11–14, 2001.
13. Hallstrom A, Cobb L, Johnson E, Copass M: Cardiopulmonary resuscitation by chest compression alone or with mouth to mouth ventilation. *N Engl J Med* 2000; 342:1546.
14. Kudenchuk PJ, Cobb LA, Copass MK, et al: Amiodarone for resuscitation after out-of-hospital cardiac arrest due to ventricular fibrillation. *N Engl J Med* 1993; 341:871.
15. Longstreth WT Jr, Inui TS, Cobb LA, et al: Neurologic recovery after out-of-hospital cardiac arrest. *Ann Intern Med* 1983; 98:588.
16. Earnest MP, Yarnell PR, Merrill SL, et al: Long-term survival and neurologic status after resuscitation from out-of-hospital cardiac arrest. *Neurology* 1980; 30:1298.
17. Plaisance P, Lurie KG, Vicaut E, et al: A comparison of standard cardiopulmonary resuscitation and active compression-decompression resuscitation for out-of-hospital cardiac arrest. *N Engl J Med* 1999; 341:1569.

18. Brown CB, Schlifer J, Jenkins J, et al: Effect of direct mechanical ventricular assistance on myocardial hemodynamics during ventricular fibrillation. *Crit Care Med* 1989; 17:1175.
19. Emergency Cardiac Care Committee and Subcommittees, American Heart Association: Guidelines for cardiopulmonary resuscitation and emergency cardiac care. II: adult basic life support. *JAMA* 1992; 268:2184.
20. Guildner CW: Resuscitation—opening the airway: a comparative study of techniques for opening an airway obstructed by the tongue. *J Am Coll Emerg Phys* 1976; 5:588.
21. Safar P, Escarraga LA, Chang F: Upper airway obstruction in the unconscious patient. *J Appl Physiol* 1959; 14:760.
22. Ruben HM, Elam JO, Ruben AM, et al: Investigation of upper airway problems in resuscitation: studies of pharyngeal X-rays and performance by laymen. *Anesthesiology* 1961; 22:271.
23. Heimlich HJ: A life-saving maneuver to prevent food choking. *JAMA* 1975; 234:398.
24. Day RL, Crelin ES, DuBois AB: Choking: the Heimlich abdominal thrust vs back blows: an approach to measurement of inertial and aerodynamic forces. *Pediatrics* 1982; 70:113.
25. Elling R, Politis J: An evaluation of emergency medical technicians' ability to use manual ventilation devices. *Ann Emerg Med* 1983; 12:765.
26. Hess D, Baran C: Ventilatory volumes using mouth-to-mouth, mouth-to-mask, and bag-valve-mask techniques. *Am J Emerg* Med 1985; 12:765.
27. Melker RJ: Alternative methods of ventilation during respiratory and cardiac arrest. *Circulation* 1986; 74 (suppl IV):IV-63.
28. Pepe PE, Copass MK, Joyce TH: Prehospital endotracheal intubation: rationale for training emergency medical personnel. *Ann Emerg Med* 1985; 14:1085.
29. Sayah AJ, Peacock WF, Overton DT: End-tidal CO_2 measurement in the detection of esophageal intubation during cardiac arrest. *Ann Emerg Med* 1990; 19:857.
30. Falk JL, Rackow EC, Weil MH: End-tidal carbon dioxide concentration during cardiopulmonary resuscitation. *N Engl J* Med 1988; 318:607.
31. Blanc VF, Tremblay NA: The complications of tracheal intubation: a new classification with a review of the literature. *Anesth Analg* 1974; 53:202.
32. Jones GO, Hale DE, Wasmuth CE, et al: A survey of acute complications associated with endotracheal intubation. *Cleve Clin Q* 1968; 204:995.
33. Taryle DA, Chandler JE, Good JT Jr: Emergency room intubations: complications and survival. *Chest* 1979; 75:541.
34. Smith RB, Babinski M, Klain M, et al: Percutaneous transtracheal ventilation. *J Am Coll Emerg Phys* 1976; 5:765.
35. Poon YK: Case history number 89: a life-threatening complication of cricothyroid membrane puncture. *Anesth Analg* 1976; 55:298.
36. McGill J, Clinton JE, Ruiz E: Cricothyroidotomy in the emergency department. *Ann Emerg Med* 1982; 11:361.
37. Ruben H, Knudsen EJ, Carguti G: Gastric inflation in relation to airway pressure. *Acta Anaesthesiol Scand* 1961; 5:107.
38. Elam JO, Greene DG: Mission accomplished: successful mouth-to-mouth resuscitation. *Anesth Analg* 1961; 40:578.
39. Melker RJ: Recommendations for ventilation during cardiopulmonary resuscitation: time for change? *Crit Care Med* 1985; 13:882.
40. Sellick BA: Cricoid pressure to control regurgitation of stomach contents during the induction of anesthesia. *Lancet* 1961; 2:404.
41. Centers for Disease Control: Guidelines for the prevention of transmission of human immunodeficiency virus and hepatitis B virus to health-care and public safety workers. *MMWR* 1989; 38 (suppl 6):1.
42. Sande MA: Transmission of AIDS: the case against casual contagion. *N Engl J Med* 1986; 314:380.
43. Marcus R: Surveillance of health care workers exposed to blood from patients infected with human immunodeficiency virus. *N Engl J Med* 1988; 319:1118.
44. Hendricks AA, Shapiro EP: Primary herpes simplex infection following mouth-to-mouth resuscitation. *JAMA* 1980; 243:257.
45. Haley CE, McDonald RC, Rossi L, et al: Tuberculosis epidemic among hospital personnel. *Infect Control Hosp Epidemiol* 1989; 10:204.
46. Hullston A: Cardiopulmonary resuscitation by chest compression alone or with mouth-to-mouth ventilation. *N Engl J Med* 2000; 342:1546.
47. Taylor GJ, Tucker WM, Green HL, et al: Importance of prolonged compression during cardiopulmonary resuscitation in man. *N Engl J Med* 1977; 296:1515.
48. Del Guercio LMR, Coomaraswany R, State D: Cardiac output and other hemodynamic variables during external massage in man. *N Engl J Med* 1963; 269:1398.
49. Jackson RE, Freeman SB: Hemodynamics of cardiac massage. *Emerg Med Clin North Am* 1983; 1:501.
50. Luce JM, Ross BK, O'Quinn, et al: Regional blood flow during cardiopulmonary resuscitation in dogs using simultaneous and nonsimultaneous compression and ventilation. *Circulation* 1983; 67:258.
51. Maier GW, Tyson GS, Olsen CO, et al: The physiology of external cardiac massage: high-impulse cardiopulmonary resuscitation. *Circulation* 1984; 70:86.
52. Paradis NA, Martin GB, Goetting MG, et al: Simultaneous aortic, jugular bulb, and right atrial pressures during cardiopulmonary resuscitation in humans: insight into mechanisms. *Circulation* 1989; 80:361.
53. Ditchey RV, Winkler JV, Rhodes CA: Relative lack of coronary blood flow during closed chest resuscitation in dogs. *Circulation* 1982; 66:297.
54. Niemann J, Rosborough J, Ung S, et al: Coronary perfusion pressure during experimental cardiopulmonary resuscitation. *Ann Emerg Med* 1982; 11:127.
55. Sanders AB, Ogle M, Ewy GA: Coronary perfusion pressure during cardiopulmonary resuscitation. *Am J Emerg Med* 1985; 3:11.
56. Weale FE, Rothwell-Jackson RL: The efficiency of cardiac massage. *Lancet* 1962; I:990.
57. Coletti RH, Hartjen B, Gozdeziewski S, et al: Origin of canine femoral pulses during standard CPR [abstract]. *Crit Care Med* 1983; 11:218.
58. Kern KB, Sanders AB, Ewy GA: Open-chest cardiac massage after closed-chest compression in a canine model: when to intervene? *Resuscitation* 1987; 15:51.
59. Niemann JT, Criley JM, Rosborough JP, et al: Predictive indices of successful cardiac resuscitation after prolonged arrest and experimental cardiopulmonary resuscitation. *Ann Emerg Med* 1985; 14:521.
60. Weil MH, Bisera J, Trevino RP: Cardiac output and end tidal carbon dioxide. *Crit Care Med* 1985; 13:907.
61. Garnett AR, Ornato JP, Gonzalez ER, et al: End-tidal carbon dioxide measurement during cardiopulmonary resuscitation. *JAMA* 1987; 257:512.
62. Ornato JP: Hemodynamic monitoring during CPR. *Ann Emerg Med* 1993; 22:289.
63. Sanders AB, Ewy GA, Bragg S, et al: Expired P_{CO_2} as a prognostic indicator of successful resuscitation from cardiac arrest. *Ann Emerg Med* 1985; 14:948.
64. Sanders AB, Kern KB, Otto CW, et al: End-tidal carbon dioxide monitoring during cardiopulmonary resuscitation: a prognostic indicator for survival. *JAMA* 1989; 262:1347.
65. Krischer JP, Fine EG, Davis JH, Nagel EL: Complications of cardiac resuscitation. *Chest* 1987; 92:287.
66. Bedell SE, Fulton EJ: Unexpected findings and complications at autopsy after cardiopulmonary resuscitation (CPR). *Arch Intern Med* 1986; 146:1725.

67. Powner DJ, Holcombe PA, Mello LA: Cardiopulmonary resuscitation-related injuries. *Crit Care Med* 1984; 12:54.
68. DeLuna AB, Coumel P, Leclerq JF: Ambulatory sudden cardiac death: mechanism of production of fatal arrhythmia on the basis of data from 157 cases. *Am Heart J* 1989; 117:151.
69. Cobb LA, Werner JA, Trobaugh GB: Sudden cardiac death, I: a decade's experiences with out-of-hospital resuscitation. *Mod Concepts Cardiovasc Dis* 1980; 49:31.
70. Eisenberg MS, Hallstrom AP, Copass MK, et al: Treatment of ventricular fibrillation: emergency medical technician defibrillation and paramedic services. *JAMA* 1984; 251:1723.
71. Eisenberg MS, Copass MK, Hallstrom A: Treatment of out-of-hospital cardiac arrests with rapid defibrillation by emergency medical technicians. *N Engl J Med* 1980; 302:1379.
72. Stults KR, Brown DD, Schug VL, Bean JA: Prehospital defibrillation performed by emergency medical technicians in rural communities. *N Engl J Med* 1984; 310:219.
73. Weaver WD, Cobb LA, Hallstrom AP, et al: Factors influencing survival after out-of-hospital cardiac arrest. *J Am Coll Cardiol* 1986; 7:752.
74. Stiell IG, Wells GA, Field BJ, et al. Improve out-of-hospital cardiac arrest survival through the inexpensive optimization of an existing defibrillation program. OPALS Study Phase II. *JAMA* 1999; 281:1175.
75. Yakatis RW, Ewy GA, Otto CW, et al: Influence of time and therapy on ventricular defibrillation in dogs. *Crit Care Med* 1980; 8:157.
76. Winkle RA, Mead RH, Ruder MA, et al: Effect of duration of ventricular fibrillation on defibrillation efficacy in humans. *Circulation* 1990; 81:1477.
77. Weaver WD, Cobb LA, Hallstrom AP, et al: Considerations for improving survival from out-of-hospital cardiac arrest. *Ann Emerg Med* 1986; 15:1181.
78. Cummins RO: From concept to standard of care? Review of the clinical experience with automated external defibrillators. *Ann Emerg Med* 1989; 18:1270.
79. Levine JH, Massumi A, Scheinman MM, et al: Intravenous amiodarone for recurrent sustained hypotensive ventricular tachyarrhythmias. *J Am Coll Cardiol* 1996; 27:67.
80. Sceinman MM, Levine JH, Cannom DS, et al, for the Intravenous Amiodarone Muilticenter Investigators Group: Dose-ranging study of intravenous amiodarone in patients with life-threatening ventricular tachyarrhythmias. *Circulation* 1995:92:3264.
81. Kowey PR, Levine JH, Herre JM, et al, for the Intravenous Amiodarone Mulitcenter Investigators Group. Randomized, double-blind comparison of intravenous amiodarone and bretylium in the treatment of patients with recurrent, hemodynamically destabilizing ventricular tachycardia or fibrillation. *Circulation.* 1995; 92:3255.
82. Herlitz J, Ekstrom L, Wennerbolom B, et al: Lidocaine in out-of-hospital ventricular fibrillation: does it improve survival? *Resuscitation* 1997; 33:199.
83. Eisenberg M, Bergner L, Hearne T: Out-of-hospital cardiac arrest: a review of major studies and a proposed uniform reporting system. *Am J Public Health* 1980; 79:236.
84. Marwick TH, Case CC, Siskind V, Woodhouse SP: Prediction of survival from resuscitation: a prognostic index derived from multivariate logistic model analysis. *Resuscitation* 1991; 22:129.
85. Lowenstein SR: Cardiopulmonary resuscitation in noninjured patients, in Wilmore DW, Brennan MF, Harken AH, et al (eds): *Care of the Surgical Patient.* New York, Scientific American, 1989; p 1.
86. Ewy GA, Dahl CF, Zimmerman M, Otto C: Ventricular fibrillation masquerading as ventricular standstill. *Crit Care Med* 1981; 9:841.
87. Cummins RO, Austin D: The frequency of "occult" ventricular fibrillation masquerading as a flat line in prehospital cardiac arrest. *Ann Emerg Med* 1988; 17:813.
88. Thompson BM, Brooks RC, Pionkowski RS, et al: Immediate countershock in the treatment of asystole. *Ann Emerg Med* 1984; 13:827.
89. Stults K, Brown D, Kerber R: Should asystole be cardioverted? [abstract]. *Circulation* 1987; 76 (suppl IV):IV-12.
90. Brown DC, Lewis AJ, Criley JM: Asystole and its treatment: the possible role of the parasympathetic nervous system in cardiac arrest. *J Am Coll Emerg Phys* 1979; 8:448.
91. Vassalle M: On the mechanisms underlying cardiac standstill: factors determining success or failure of escape pacemakers in the heart. *J Am Coll Cardiol* 1985; 5:35B.
92. Ralston SH: Alpha agonist drug usage during CPR. *Ann Emerg Med* 1984; 13:786.
93. Daly MD, Angell-James JE, Elsner R: Role of the carotid-body chemoreceptors and their reflex interactions in bradycardia and cardiac arrest. *Lancet* 1979; 1:764.
94. Bocka JJ: External transcutaneous pacemakers. *Ann Emerg Med* 1989; 18:1280.
95. Cummins R, Graves J, Horan S, et al: Prehospital transcutaneous pacing for asystolic arrest [abstract]. *Ann Emerg Med* 1190; 19:239.
96. Niemann JT: Cardiopulmonary resuscitation. *N Engl J Med* 1992; 327:1075.
97. Warner LL, Hoffman JR, Baraff LJ: Prognostic significance of field response in out-of-hospital ventricular fibrillation. *Chest* 1985; 87:22.
98. Steuven HA, Aufderheide TP, Waite EM, Mateer JR: Electromechanical dissociation: six years prehospital experience. *Resuscitation* 1989; 17:173.
99. Charlap S, Kaplan S, Lichstein E, Frishman W: Electromechanical dissociation: diagnosis, pathophysiology, and management. *Am Heart J* 1989; 118:355.
100. Sutton-Tyrell K, Abramson NS, Safar P, et al: Predictors of electromechanical dissociation during cardiac arrest. *Ann Emerg Med* 1988; 17:572.
101. Otto CW: Cardiovascular pharmacology,II: the use of catecholamines, pressor agents, digitalis, and corticosteroids in CPR and emergency cardiac care. *Circulation* 1986; 74(suppl IV):IV-80.
102. Vincent JL, Thijs L, Weil MH, et al: Clinical and experimental studies on electromechanical dissociation. *Circulation* 1981; 64:18.
103. Niemann JT, Haynes KS, Garner D, et al: Postcountershock pulseless rhythms: response to CPR, artificial cardiac pacing and adrenergic agonists. *Ann Emerg Med* 1986; 15:112.
104. Ivatury RR, Rohman M: Emergency department thoracotomy for trauma: a collective review. *Resuscitation* 1987; 15:23.
105. Eysmann SB, Marchlinski FE, Buxton A, Josephson ME: Electrocardiographic changes after cardioversion of ventricular arrhythmias. *Circulation* 1986; 73:73.
106. Hossack KF, Hartwig R: Cardiac arrest associated with supervised cardiac rehabilitation. *J Cardiac Rehab* 1982; 2:402.
107. Neumar RW, Brown CG, Robitaille PM, Altschuld RA: Myocardial high energy phosphate metabolism during ventricular fibrillation with total circulatory arrest. *Resuscitation* 1990; 19:199.
108. Kern KB, Garewal HS, Sanders AB, et al: Depletion of myocardial adenosine triphosphate during prolonged untreated ventricular fibrillation: effect on defibrillation success. *Resuscitation* 1990; 20:221.
109. Fletcher GF, Cantwell JD: Ventricular fibrillation in a medically supervised cardiac exercise program: clinical, angiographic, and surgical correlations. *JAMA* 1977; 238:2627.
110. Van Camp SP, Peterson RA: Cardiovascular complications of outpatient cardiac rehabilitation programs. *JAMA* 1986; 256:1160.
111. Lown B: Electrical reversion of cardiac arrhythmias. *Br Heart J* 1967: 29:469.
112. Ewy GA, Taren D, Banert J, et al: Comparison of myocardial damage from defibrillator discharge at various dosages. *Med Instrum* 1980; 14:9.

113. Warner ED, Dahl AAJ, Webb SW, et al: Myocardial injury from transthoracic countershock. *Arch Pathol Lab Med* 1975; 99:55.
114. Weaver WD, Cobb LA, Copass MK, et al: Ventricular fibrillation: a comparative trial using 175-J and 320-J shocks. *N Engl J Med* 1982; 307:1101.
115. Adgey AAJ, Patton JN, Campbell NPS, Webb SW: Ventricular defibrillation: appropriate energy levels. *Circulation* 1979; 60:219.
116. Gascho JA, Crampton RS, Cherwek ML, et al: Determinants of ventricular defibrillation in adults. *Circulation* 1979; 60:231.
117. Kerber RE, Grayzel J, Hoyt R, et al: Transthoracic resistance in human defibrillation: influence of body weight, chest size, serial shocks, paddle size, and paddle contact pressure. *Circulation* 1981; 63:676.
118. Sirna SJ, Ferguson DW, Charbonnier F, et al: Factors affecting transthoracic impedance during electrical cardioversion. *Am J Cardiol* 1988; 62:1048.
119. Lerman BB, DiMarco JP, Haines DE: Current-based versus energy-based ventricular defibrillation: a prospective study. *J Am Coll Cardiol* 1988; 12:1259.
120. Dalzell GW, Cunningham SR, Anderson J, Adgey AA: Initial experience with a microprocessor controlled current-based defibrillator. *Br Heart J* 1989; 61:502.
121. Kerber RE, Martins JB, Kienzle MG, et al: Energy, current, and success in defibrillation and cardioversion: clinical studies using an automated impedance-based method of energy adjustment. *Circulation* 1988; 77:1038.
122. Kerber RE: Electrical treatment of cardiac arrhythmias: defibrillation and cardioversion. *Ann Emerg Med* 1993; 22:296.
123. Dahl CF, Ewy GA, Ewy MD, Thomas ED: Transthoracic impedance to direct current discharge: Effect of repeated countershocks. *Med Instrum* 1976; 10:151.
124. Connell PN, Ewy GA, Dahl CF, Ewy MD: Transthoracic impedance to defibrillator discharge: effect of electrode size and electrode-chest wall interface. *J Electrocardiol* 1973; 6:313-M.
125. Atkins DL, Sirna S, Kieso R, et al: Pediatric defibrillation: importance of paddle size in determining transthoracic impedance. *Pediatrics* 1988; 82:914.
126. Ruffy R, Schechtman K, Monje E: Beta-adrenergic modulation of direct defibrillation energy in anesthetized dog heart. *Am J Physiol* 1985; 248:H674.
127. Ruffy R, Schechtman K, Monje E: Adrenergically mediated variations in the energy required to defibrillate the heart: observations in closed-chest, nonanesthetized dogs. *Circulation* 1986; 73:374.
128. Rattes MF, Sharma AD, Klein GJ, et al: Adrenergic effects on internal cardiac defibrillation threshold. *Am J Physiol* 1987; 253:H500.
129. Yakaitis RW, Otto CW, Blitt CD: Relative importance of alpha- and beta-adrenergic receptors during resuscitation. *Crit Care Med* 1979; 7:293.
130. Kerber RE, Pandian NG, Hoyt R, et al: Effect of ischemia, hypertrophy, hypoxia, acidosis, and alkalosis on canine defibrillation. *Am J Physiol* 1983; 244:H825.
131. Echt DS, Cato EL, Coxe DR: pH-dependent effects of lidocaine on defibrillation energy requirements in dogs. *Circulation* 1989; 80:1003.
132. Lerman BB, Engelstein ED: Metabolic determinants of defibrillation: role of adenosine. *Circulation* 1995; 91:838.
133. Idriss SF, Anstadt M, Anstadt GL, Ideker R: The effect of cardiac compression on defibrillaton efficacy and the upper limit of vulnerability. *J Cardiovasc Electrophysiol* 1995; 6:368.
134. Viskin S, Belhassewn B, Roth A, et al: Aminophylline for bradyasystolic cardiac arrest refractory to atropine and epinephrine. *Ann Intern Med* 1993; 118:279.
135. Ruffy R, Monje E, Schechtman K: Facilitation of cardiac defibrillation by aminophylline in the conscious, closed-chest dog. *J Electrophysiol* 1988; 2:450.
136. Fredholm BB: Are methylxanthine effects due to antagonism of endogenous adenosine? *Trends Pharmacol Sci* 1980; 1:129.
137. Levine PA, Barold SS, Fletcher RD, Talbot P: Adverse acute and chronic effects of electrical defibrillation on implanted unipolar cardiac pacing systems. *J Am Coll Cardiol* 1983; 1:1413.
138. Cummins RO: *Textbook of Advanced Cardiac Life Support*. Dallas, American Heart Association, 1994.
139. Walls JT, Schuder JC, Curtis JJ, et al: Adverse effects of permanent cardiac internal defibrillator patches on external defibrillation. *Am J Cardiol* 1989; 64:1144.
140. Newman MM: The survival advantage: early defibrillation programs in the fire service. *J Emerg Med Serv* 1987; 12:40.
141. Newman MM: National EMT-D study. *J Emerg Med Serv* 1986; 11:70.
142. Jaggarao NS, Grainger R, Heber M, et al: Use of an automated external defibrillator-pacemaker by emergency medical technicians. *Lancet* 1982; 2:73.
143. Stults KR, Brown DD, Kerber RE: Efficacy of an automated external defibrillator in the management of out-of-hospital cardiac arrest: validation of the diagnostic algorithm and initial clinical experience in a rural environment. *Circulation* 1986; 73:701.
144. Cummins RO, Eisenberg MS, Litwin PE, et al: Automatic external defibrillators used by emergency medical technicians: a controlled clinical trial. *JAMA* 1987; 257:1605.
145. Kerber RE: Statement on early defibrillation. *Circulation* 1991; 84:2233.
146. Bigger JT, Whang W, Rottman JN, et al: Mechanisms of death in the CABG Patch Trial: a randomized trial of implantable cardic defibrillator prophylaxis in patients at high risk of death after coronary artery bypass graft surgery. *Circulation* 1999; 99:1419.
147. Jones DL, Klein JG, Guiraudon GM, et al: Internal cardiac defibrillation in man: pronounced improvement with sequential pulse delivery to two different lead orientations. *Circulation* 1986; 73:484.
148. Kerber RE, Bourland JD, Kallok MJ, et al: Transthoracic defibrillation using sequential and simultaneous dual shock pathways: experimental studies. *PACE* 1990; 13:207.
149. Caldwell G, Millar G, Quinn E, et al: Simple mechanical methods for cardioversion: defence of the precordial thump and cough version. *BMJ* 1985; 291:627.
150. Miller J, Tresch D, Horwitz L, et al: The precordial thump. *Ann Emerg Med* 1984; 13:791.
151. Yakaitis RW, Redding JS: Precordial thumping during cardiac resuscitation. *Crit Care Med* 1973; 1:22.
152. Sabiston DC, Jude JR, Knickerbocker GS, Kouwenhoven WD: Cardiac resuscitation: comparison of the open and closed approach, in *Advances in Cardiopulmonary Diseases*. Chicago, Year Book, 1964; p 305.
153. Kouwenhoven WG, Jude JR, Knickerbocker GG: Closed-chest cardiac massage. *JAMA* 1960; 173:1064.
154. Newton JR, Glower DD, Wolfe JA, et al: A physiologic comparison of external cardiac massage techniques. *J Thorac Cardiovasc Surg* 1988; 95:892.
155. Feneley MP, Maier GW, Gaynor JW, et al: Sequence of mitral valve motion and transmitral blood flow during manual cardiopulmonary resuscitation in dogs. *Circulation* 1987; 76:363.
156. Hackl W, Simon P, Mauritz W, Steinbereithner K: Echocardiographic assessment of mitral valve function during mechanical cardiopulmonary resuscitation in pigs. *Anesth Analg* 1990; 70:350.
157. Deshmukh GH, Weil MH, Rackow EC, et al: Echocardiographic observations during cardiopulmonary resuscitation: a preliminary report. *Crit Care Med* 1985; 13:904.
158. Niemann JT, Rosborough J, Hausknecht M, et al: Cough-CPR: documentation of systemic perfusion in man and in an experimental model: a window to the mechanism of blood flow in external CPR. *Crit Care Med* 1980; 8:141.

159. Rudikoff MT, Maughan WL, Effron M, et al: Mechanism of flow during cardiopulmonary resuscitation. *Circulation* 1980; 61:345.
160. Niemann JT, Rosborough JP, Hausknecht M, et al: Pressure synchronized cineangiography during experimental cardiopulmonary resuscitation. *Circulation* 1981; 64:985.
161. Beyar R, Kishon Y, Kimmel E, et al: Intrathoracic and abdominal pressure variations as an efficient method for cardiopulmonary resuscitation: studies in dogs compared with computer model results. *Cardiovasc Res* 1985; 19:335.
162. Babbs CF, Geddes LA: Effects of abdominal counterpulsation in CPR as demonstrated in a simple electrical model of the circulation. *Ann Emerg Med* 12:247, 1983.
163. Coletti RH, Kasel PS, Cohen SR, et al: Abdominal counterpulsation (AC): a new concept in circulatory assistance. *Trans Am Soc Artif Intern Organs* 1985: 28:563.
164. Ralston SH, Babbs CF, Niebauer MJ: Cardiopulmonary resuscitation with interposed abdominal compression in dogs. *Anesth Analg* 1982; 61:645.
165. Wollenek G, Honarwar N, Golej J, Marx M: Cold water submersion and cardiac arrest in treatment of severe hypothermia with cardiopulmonary bypass. *Resuscitation* 2002; 52:255.
166. Mateer JR, Stueven HA, Thompson BM, et al: Prehospital IAC-CPR versus standard CPR: paramedic resuscitation of cardiac arrest. *Am J Emerg Med* 1985; 3:143.
167. Farstad M, Andersen KS, Koller ME, et al: Rewarming from accidental hypothermia by extracorporeal circulation: a retrospective study. *Eur J Cardiothorac Surg* 2001; 20:58.
168. Sack JB, Kesselbrenner MB, Bergman D: Survival from in-hospital cardiac arrest with interposed abdominal compression during cardiopulmonary resuscitation. *JAMA* 1992; 267:379.
169. Sack JB, Kesselbrenner MB, Jarrad A: Interposed abdominal compression-cardiopulmonary resuscitation and resuscitation outcome during asystole and electromechanical dissociation. *Circulation* 1992; 86:192.
170. Weston CFM, de Latorre FJ, Dick W, et al. VEST-CPR system: results of a multicenter randomized pilot study [abstract]. *J Am Coll Cardiol* 1998; 31(suppl A):403.
171. Halperin HR, Tsitlik JE, Gefland M, et al: A preliminary study of cardiopulmonary resuscitation by circumferential compression of the chest with the use of a pneumatic vest. *N Engl J Med* 1993; 329:762.
172. Lurie KG, Lindo C, Chin J: CPR: The P stands for plumber's helper. *JAMA* 1990; 264:1661.
173. Cohen TJ, Tucker KJ, Redberg RF, et al: Active compression-decompression resuscitation: novel method of cardiopulmonary resuscitation. *Am Heart J* 1992; 124:1145.
174. Lindner KH, Pfenninger EG, Lurie KG, et al: Effects of active compression-decompression resuscitation on myocardial and cerebral blood flow in pigs. *Circulation* 1993; 88:154.
175. Chang MW, Cullen P, Lurie KG, et al: Tissue perfusion during standard versus active compression decompression CPR in the dog [abstract]. *Circulation* 1992; 86:I-233.
176. Schultz JJ, Coffeen P, Sweeney M, et al: Evaluation of standard and active compression-decompression CPR in an acute human model of ventricular fibrillation. *Circulation* 1994; 89:684.
177. Tucker KJ, Idris A: Clinical and laboratory investigations of active compression-decompression cardiopulmonary resuscitation. *Resuscitation* 1994; 28:1.
178. Cohen TJ, Goldner BG, Maccaro PC, et al: A comparison of active compression-decompression cardiopulmonary resuscitation with standard cardiopulmonary resuscitation for cardiac arrests occurring in the hospital. *N Engl J Med* 1993; 329:1918.
179. Tucker KJ, Galli F, Savitt MA, et al: Active compression-decompression resuscitation: effects on initial return of circulation and survival after in-hospital cardiac arrest. *Circulation* 1993; 88:I-10.
180. Mauer DK, Nolan J, Plaisance P, et al. Effect of active compression-decompression resuscitation (ACD-CPR) on survival: a combined analysis of individual patient data [abstract]. *Resuscitation* 1999; 41:249.
181. Plaisance P, and the French Active Compression-Decompression Cardiopulmonary Resuscitation Study Group (Lariboisiere University, Paris, France): A comparison of standard cardiopulmonary resuscitation and active compression-decompression resuscitation for out-of hospital cardiac arrest. *Ann Emerg Med* 2000; 341:569.
182. DeBard ML: The history of cardiopulmonary resuscitation. *Ann Emerg Med* 1980; 9:273.
183. Barnett WM, Alifimoff JK, Paris PM: Comparison of open-chest cardiac massage techniques in dogs. *Ann Emerg Med* 1986; 15:408.
184. Alifimoff JK: Open versus closed chest cardiac massage in non-traumatic cardiac arrest. *Resuscitation* 1987; 15:13.
185. Bircher N, Safar P, Stewart R: A comparison of standard, MAST-augmented, and open-chest CPR in dogs. *Crit Care Med* 1980; 8:147.
186. Bircher N, Safar P: Cerebral preservation during cardiopulmonary resuscitation in dogs. *Crit Care Med* 1985; 13:135.
187. Byrne D, Pass HI, Neeley, et al: External versus internal cardiac massage in normal and chronically ischemic dogs. *Am Surg* 1980; 46:657.
188. Weiser FM, Adler AN, Kuhn LA: Hemodynamic effects of closed and open chest cardiac resuscitation in normal dogs and those with acute myocardial infarction. *Am J Cardiol* 1962; 10:555.
189. Del Guercio LRM, Feins NR, Cohn JD, et al: A comparison of blood flow during external and internal cardiac massage in man. *Circulation* 1965; 31 (suppl I):I–171.
190. Briggs BD, Sheldon DB, Beecher HK: Cardiac arrest: study of a thirty year period of operating room deaths at Massachusetts General Hospital. *JAMA* 1956; 160:1439.
191. Stephenson HE Jr, Reid LC, Hinton JW: Some common denominators in 1200 cases of cardiac arrest. *Ann Surg* 1953; 137:731.
192. Geehr EC, Lewis FR, Auerbach PS: Failure of open-chest massage to improve survival after prehospital nontraumatic cardiac arrest [letter]. *N Engl J Med* 1986; 314:1189.
193. Kern KB, Sanders AB, Badylak SF, et al: Long-term survival with open-chest cardiac massage after ineffective closed-chest compression in a canine model. *Circulation* 1987; 75:498.
194. Takino M, Okada Y: Optimum timing of resuscitation thoracotomy for non-traumatic out-of- hospital cardiac arrest. *Resuscitation* 1993; 26:69.
195. Altemeier WA, Todd J: Studies on the incidence of infection following open-chest cardiac massage for cardiac arrest. *Ann Surg* 1963; 158:596.
196. Martin GB, Nowak RM, Carden DL, et al: Cardiopulmonary bypass versus CPR as treatment for prolonged canine cardiopulmonary arrest. *Ann Emerg Med* 1987; 16:628.
197. Levine R, Gorayeb M, Safar P, et al: Cardiopulmonary bypass after cardiac arrest and prolonged closed-chest CPR in dogs. *Ann Emerg Med* 1980; 16:620.
198. Angelos M, Safar P, Reich H: A comparison of cardiopulmonary resuscitation with cardiopulmonary bypass after prolonged cardiac arrest in dogs: reperfusion pressures and neurologic recovery. *Resuscitation* 1991; 21:121.
199. Bowen FW, Carboni AF, O'Hara ML, et al: Application of "double bridge mechanical" resuscitation for profound cardiogenic shock leading to cardiac transplantation. *Ann Thorac Surg* 2001; 72:86.
200. Pagani FD, Aaronson KD, Swaniker F, Bartlett RH: The use of extracorporeal life support in adult patients with primary cardiac failure as a bridge to implantable left ventricular assist device. *Ann Thorac Surg* 2001; 71:S77.
201. Pagani FD, Aaronson KD, Dyke DB, et al: Assessment of an

extracorporeal life support LAVD bridge to heart transplant strategy. *Ann Thorac Surg* 2000; 70:1977.

202. Younger JG, Schreiner RJ, Swaniker F, et al: Extracorporeal resuscitation of cardiac arrest. *Acad Emerg Med* 1999; 6:700.
203. Tisherman SA, Safar P, Abramsom NS, et al: Feasibility of emergency cardiopulmonary bypass for resuscitation from CPR-resistant cardiac arrest: a preliminary report [abstract]. *Ann Emerg Med* 1991; 20:491.
204. Martin GB, Paradis NA, Rivers EP, et al: Cardiopulmonary bypass in the treatment of cardiac arrest in humans [abstract]. *Crit Care* Med 1990; 18:S247.
205. Hartz R, LoCicero J 3rd, Sanders JH Jr, et al: Clinical experience with portable cardiopulmonary bypass in cardiac arrest patients. *Ann Thorac Surg* 1990; 50:437.
206. Phillps SJ, Zeff RH, Kongtahworn C, et al: Percutaneous cardiopulmonary bypass: application and indication for use. *Ann Thorac Surg* 1989; 47:121.
207. Reichman RT, Joyo CI, Dembitsky WP, et al: Improved patient survival after cardiac arrest using a cardiopulmonary support system. *Ann Thorac Surg* 1990; 49:101.
208. Shawl FA, Domanski MJ, Wish MH, et al: Emergency cardiopulmonary bypass support in paitents with cardic arrest in the catheterization laboratory. *Catheter Cardiovasc Diag* 1990; 19:8.
209. Barlett RH: Extracorporeal life support registry 1995. *ASAIO J* 1997; 43:107.
210. Emerman CL, Pinchak AC, Hagen JF, Hancock D: Hemodynamic effects of the intra-aortic balloon pump during experimental cardiac arrest. *Am J Emerg Med* 1989; 7:378.
211. Wesley RC Jr, Morgan DB: Effect of continuous intra-aortic balloon inflation in canine open-chest cardiopulmonary resuscitation. *Crit Care Med* 1990; 18:630.
212. Manning JE, Baston DN, Payne FB, et al: Selective aortic perfusion during cardiac arrest: enhanced resuscitation using oxygenated perflubron emulsion with or without aortic epinephrine. *Ann Emerg Med* 1997; 29:580.
213. Manning JE, Murphy CA, Baston DN, et al: Aortic arch versus central venous epinephrine during CPR. *Ann Emerg Med* 1993; 22:709.
214. Paradis NA, Rose MI, Gawryl MS: Selective aortic perfusion and oxygenation: an effective adjunct to external chest compression-based cardiopulmonary resuscitation. *J Am Coll Cardiol* 1994; 23:497.
215. Feagins LA, Guil CK, Malon JP, et al: Myocardial dynamics during direct mechanical ventricular actuation of the fibrillating heart. *ASAIO J* 2000; 46:168.
216. Anstadt MP, Hendry PJ, Plunkett MD, et al: Mechanical cardiac actuation achieves hemodynamics similar to cardiopulmonary bypass. *Surgery* 1990; 108:442.
217. Anstadt MP, Taber JE, Hendry PJ, et al: Myocardial tolerance to ischemia after resuscitation: direct mechanical ventricular actuation versus cardiopulmonary bypass. *ASAIO Trans* 1991; 37:M518.
218. Anstadt MP, Stonnington MJ, Tedder M, et al: Pulsatile reperfusion after cardiac arrest improves neurologic outcome. *Ann Surg* 1991; 214:478.
219. Lowe JE, Anstadt MP, VanTright P, et al: First successful bridge to cardiac transplantation using direct mechanical ventricular actuation. *Ann Thorac Surg* 1991; 52:1237.
220. Lowe JE, Hughes C, Biswass SS: Non-blood contacting biventricular support: direct mechanical ventricular actuation. *Operative Tech Thorac Cardiovasc Surg* 1999; 4:345.
221. Kuhn GJ, White BC, Swetman RE, et al: Peripheral vs. central circulation times during CPR: a pilot study. *Ann Emerg Med* 1981; 10:417.
222. Emerman CL, Pinchak AC, Hancock D, Hagen JF: The effect of bolus injection on circulation times during cardiac arrest. *Am J Emerg Med* 1990; 8:190.
223. Barsan WG, Levy RC, Weir H: Lidocaine levels during CPR: differences after peripheral venous, central venous, and intracardiac injections. *Ann Emerg Med* 1981; 10:73.
224. Emerman CL, Bellon EM, Lukens TW, et al: A prospective study of femoral versus subclavian vein catheterization during cardiac arrest. *Ann Emerg Med* 1990; 19:26.
225. Ditchey RV, Lindenfield JA: Potential adverse effects of volume loading on perfusion of vital organs during closed-chest resuscitation. *Circulation* 1984; 69:181.
226. Aitkenhead AR: Drug administration during CPR: what route? *Resuscitation* 1991; 22:191.
227. Hahnel JH, Lindner KH, Schurmann C, et al: Plasma lidocaine levels and PaO_2 with endobronchial administration: dilution with normal saline or distilled water? *Ann Emerg Med* 1990; 19:1314.
228. Redding JS, Pearson JW: Resuscitation from ventricular fibrillation. *JAMA* 1969; 203:255.
229. Pearson JW, Redding JS: Influence of peripheral vascular tone on cardiac resuscitation. *Anesth Analg* 1967; 46:746.
230. Pearson JW, Redding JS: The role of epinephrine in cardiac resuscitation. *Anesth Analg* 1963; 42:599.
231. Michael JR, Guerci AD, Koehler RC, et al: Mechanism by which epinephrine augments cerebral and myocardial perfusion during cardiopulmonary resuscitation. *Circulation* 1984; 69:822.
232. Schleien CL, Dean JM, Koehler RC, et al: Effect of epinephrine on cerebral and myocardial perfusion in an infant animal preparation of cardiopulmonary resuscitation. *Circulation* 1986; 73:809.
233. Koscove EM, Paradis NA: Successful resuscitation from cardiac arrest using high-dose epinephrine therapy: report of two cases. *JAMA* 1988; 259:3031.
234. Martin D, Werman HA, Brown CG: Four case studies: high-dose epinephrine in cardiac arrest. *Ann Emerg Med* 1990; 19:322.
235. Gonzalez ER, Ornato JP, Garnett AR, et al: Dose-dependent vasopressor response to epinephrine during cardiopulmonary resuscitation in humans. *Ann Emerg Med* 1989; 18:920.
236. Lindner KH, Ahnefeld FW, Prengel AW: Comparison of standard and high-dose adrenaline in the resuscitation of asystole and electromechanical dissociation. *Acta Anaesthesiol Scand* 1991; 35:253.
237. Stiell IG, Hebert PC, Weitzman BN, et al: A study of high-dose epinephrine in human CPR. *N Engl J Med* 1992; 327:1047.
238. Callaham M, Madsen CD, Barton CW, et al: A randomized clinical trial of high-dose epinephrine and norepinephrine versus standard dose epinephrine in prehospital cardiac arrest. *JAMA* 1992; 268:2667.
239. Brown CG, Martin DR, Pepe PE, et al: A comparison of standard dose and high dose epinephrine in cardiac arrest outside the hospital. The Multicenter High-Dose Epinephrine Study Group. *N Engl J Med* 1992; 327:1051.
240. Marwick TH, Case C, Siskind V, et al: Adverse effect of early high-dose adrenaline on outcome of ventricular fibrillation. *Lancet* 1988; 2:66.
241. Ditchey RV, Lindenfield J: Failure of epinephrine to improve the balance between myocardial oxygen supply and demand during closed-chest resuscitation in dogs. *Circulation* 1988; 78:382.
242. Lindner KH, Prengel AW, Pfenninger EG, et al: Vasopressin improves vital organ blood flow during closed-chest CPR in pigs. *Circulation* 91:215,1995.
243. Lindner KH, Dirks B, Strohmenger HU, et al: Randomised comparison of epinephrine and vasopression in patients with out-of-hospital ventricular fibrillation. *Lancet* 1997; 349:535.
244. Kudenchuk PJ, Cobb LA, Copass MK, et al: Amiodarone for resuscitation after out-of-hospital cardiac arrest due to ventricular fibrillation. *N Engl J Med* 1999; 341:871.
245. Harrison DC, Sprouse JH, Morrow AG: The antiarrhythmic properties of lidocaine and procainamide: clinical and electrophysiologic studies of their cardiovascular effects in man. *Circulation* 1963; 28:486.

246. Iseri LT: Magnesium and cardiac arrhythmias. *Magnesium* 1986; 5:111.
247. Coon GA, Clinton JE, Ruiz E: Use of atropine for brady-asystolic prehospital cardiac arrest. *Ann Emerg Med* 1981; 10:462.
248. Dauchot P, Gravenstein JS: Bradycardia after myocardial ischemia and its treatment with atropine. *Anesthesiology* 1968; 29:1125.
249. Kotmeier CA, Gravenstein JS: The parasympathomimetic activity of atropine and atropine methylbromide. *Anesthesiology* 1968; 29:1125.
250. Grundler WG, Weil MH, Rackow EC: Arteriovenous carbon dioxide and pH gradients during cardiac arrest. *Circulation* 1986; 74:1071.
251. Weil MH, Rackow EC, Trevino R, et al: Difference in acid-base state between venous and arterial blood during cardiopulmonary resuscitation. *N Engl J Med* 1986; 315:153.
252. Ritter JM, Doktor HS, Benjamin N: Paradoxical effect of bicarbonate on cytoplasmic pH. *Lancet* 1990; 335:1243.
253. Graf H, Leach W, Arieff AI: Evidence for a detrimental effect of bicarbonate therapy in hypoxic lactic acidosis. *Science* 1985; 227:754.
254. von Planta I, Weil MH, von Planta M: Hypercarbic acidosis reduces cardiac resuscitability. *Crit Care Med* 1991; 19:1177.
255. Kette F, Weil MH, Gazmuri RJ: Buffer solutions may compromise cardiac resuscitation by reducing coronary perfusion pressure. *JAMA* 1991; 266:2121.
256. Kette F, Weil MH, von Planta I, et al: Buffer agents do not reverse intramyocardial acidosis during cardiac resuscitation. *Circulation* 1990; 81:1660.
257. Bishop RL, Weisfeldt ML: Sodium bicarbonate administration during cardiac arrest: effect on arterial pH, P_{CO_2}, and osmolality. *JAMA* 1976; 235:506.
258. Douglas ME, Downs JB, Mantini El, Ruis BC: Alteration of oxygen tension and oxyhemoglobin saturation: a hazard of sodium bicarbonate administration. *Arch Surg* 1979; 114:326.
259. Guerci AD, Chandra N, Johnson E, et al: Failure of sodium bicarbonate to improve resuscitation from ventricular fibrillation in dogs. *Circulation* 1986; 74 (suppl IV):IV-75.
260. Safar P: Cerebral resuscitation after cardiac arrest: research initiatives and future directions. *Ann Emerg Med* 1993; 22:324.
261. Rossen R, Kabat H, Anderson JP: Acute arrest of cerebral circulation in man. *Arch Neurol Psychiatry* 1943; 50:510.
262. Nemoto EM: Pathogenesis of cerebral ischemia-anoxia. *Crit Care Med* 1978; 6:203.
263. Rehncrona S, Rosen I, Siesjo BK: Excessive cellular acidosis: an important mechanism of neuronal damage in the brain? *Arch Physiol Scand* 1980; 110:425.
264. Rehncrona S, Mela L, Siesjo BK: Recovery of brain mitochondrial function in the rat after complete and incomplete cerebral ischemia. *Stroke* 1979; 10:437.
265. Siejso BK: Mechanism of ischemic brain damage. *Crit Care Med* 1988; 16:954.
266. Weinberger LM, Gibbon MH, Gibbon JH Jr: Temporary arrest of the circulation to central nervous system: physiologic effects. *Arch Neurol Psychiatry* 1940; 43:615.
267. Cole SL, Corday E: Four minute limit for cardiac resuscitation. *JAMA* 1956; 161:1454.
268. Brierly JB, Meldrum BS, Brown AW: The threshold and neuropathology of anoxic-ischemic cell change. *Arch Neurol* 1973; 29:367.
269. Graham DI: The pathology of brain ischemia and possibilities for therapeutic intervention. *Br J Anaesth* 1985; 57:3.
270. Fischer J, Vaghaiwalla F, Tsitlik J, et al: Determinants and clinical significance of venous valve competence. *Circulation* 1982; 65:188.
271. Kleihues P, Hossmann KA, Pegg AE, et al: Resuscitation of the monkey brain after one hour complete ischemia, III: indications of metabolic recovery. *Brain Res* 1975; 95:61.
272. Ames A 3rd, Wright RL, Kowada M, et al: Cerebral ischemia, III: the no-reflow phenomenon. *Am J Pathol* 1986; 52:437.
273. Kirsch JR, Dean JM, Rogers MC: Current concepts in brain resuscitation. *Arch Intern Med* 1986; 146:1413.
274. Lind B, Snyder J, Safar P: Total brain ischemia in dogs: cerebral physiologic and metabolic changes after 15 minutes of circulatory arrest. *Resuscitation* 1975; 4:97.
275. Snyder JV, Nemoto EM, Carroll RG, et al: Global ischemia in dogs: intracranial pressures, brain blood flow and metabolism. *Stroke* 1975; 6:21.
276. Gadzinski DS, White JD, Hoehner PJ, et al: Canine cerebral cortical blood flow and vascular resistance post cardiac arrest. *Ann Emerg Med* 1982; 11:58.
277. Kagstrom E, Smith ML, Siesjo BK: Cerebral circulatory responses to hypercapnia and hypoxia in the recovery period following complete and incomplete cerebral ischemia in the rat. *Acta Physiol Scand* 1983; 118:281.
278. Siesjo BK: Cerebral circulation and metabolism. *J Neurosurg* 1984; 60:883.
279. Cantu RC, Ames A 3rd, DiGiacinto G, Dixon J: Hypotension: a major factor limiting recovery from cerebral ischemia. *J Surg Res* 1969; 9:525.
280. Wise G, Sutter R, Burkholder J: The treatment of brain ischemia with vasopressor drugs. *Stroke* 1972; 3:135.
281. Sterz F, Leonov Y, Safar P, et al: Hypertension with or without hemodilution after cardiac arrest in dogs. *Stroke* 1990; 21:1178.
282. Snyder BD, Hauser WA, Loewenson RB, et al: Neurologic prognosis after cardiopulmonary arrest, III: seizure activity. *Neurology* 1980; 30:1292.
283. Siesjo BK: *Brain Energy Metabolism*. New York, Wiley, 1978.
284. Weinrach V, Safar P, Tisherman S, et al: Beneficial effect of mild hypothermia and detrimental effect of deep hypothermia after cardiac arrest in dogs. *Stroke* 1992; 23:1454.
285. Sterz F, Safar P, Tisherman S, et al: Mild hypothermic cardiopulmonary resuscitation improves outcome after prolonged cardiac arrest in dogs. *Crit Care Med* 1991; 19:379.
286. Bernard S, Jones B, Horne M: Clinical trail of induced hypothermia in comatose survivors of out-of-hospital cardiac arrest. *Ann Emerg Med* 1997; 30:146.
287. Colbourne F, Corbertt D: Delayed postischemic hypothermia: a six-month survival study using behavioral and histological assessment of neuroprotection. *J Neurosci* 1995; 15:7250.
288. Kuboyama K, Safar P, Radovsky A, er al: Delay in cooling negates the beneficial effect of mild resuscitative cerebral hypothermia after cardiac arrest in dogs: a prospective randomized study. *Crit Care Med* 1993; 21:1348.
289. Exner DV, Reiffel JA, Epstein AE, et al: Beta-blocker use and survival in patients with ventricular fibrillation or symptomatic ventricular tachycardia. The AVID Trial. *J Am Coll Cardiol* 1993; 34:325.
290. Moss AJ, Hall WJ, Cannom DS, et al: Improved survival with an implanted defibrillator in patients with coronary disease at high risk for ventricular arrhythmia. *N Engl J Med* 1996; 335:1933.
291. Mushlin AI, Hall J, Zwanziger J, et al: The cost effectiveness of automatic implanted cardiac defilbrillators: results from MADIT. *Circulation* 1998; 97:2129.
292. The Antiarrhythmics vs Implantable Defibrillator (AVID) Investigators: A comparison of antiarrhythmic drug therapy with implantable defibrillators in patients resuscitated from near fatal ventricular arrhythmias. *N Engl J Med* 1997; 337:1576.
293. Bigger JT, for the CABG Patch Trial Investigators: Prophylactic use of implanted cardiac defibrillators in patients at high risk for ventricular arrhythmias after coronary artery bypass graft surgery. *N Engl J Med* 1997; 337:1569.
294. Buxton AE, Lee KL, Fisher JD, et al: A randomized study of the

prevention of sudden death in patients with coronary artery disease. *N Engl J Med* 1999; 341:1882.

295. Cairns JA, Connolly SJ, Roberts R, et al: Randomized trail of outcome after myocardial infarction in patients with frequent or repetitive ventricular premature depolarisations: CAMIAT. *Lancet* 1997; 349:675.
296. Burkart F, Pfisterer M, Kiowski E, et al: Effect of antiarrhythmic therapy on mortality in survivors of myocardial infarction with asymptomatic complex ventricular arrhythmias. Basel Antiarrhymic Study of Infarct Survival (BASIS). *J Am Coll Cardiol* 1990; 16:1711.
297. Pfisterer ME, Kiowski W, Brunner H, et al: Long term benefit of 1 year amiodarone treatment for persistent complex ventricular arrhythmias after myocardial infarction. *Circulation* 1993; 87:309.
298. The CASCADE Investigators: Cardiac Arrest in Seattle: Conventional vs Amiodarone Drug Evaluation (the CASCADE study). *Am J Cardiol* 1991; 67:578.
299. Greene HL, for the CASCADE Investigators. The CASCADE study: randomized antiarrythmic drug therapy in survivors of cardiac arrest in Seattle. *Am J Cardiol* 1993; 72:70F.
300. Connolly SJ, Gent M, Roberts RS, et al: A randomized trail of the implantable cardioverter defibrillator against amiodarone. *Circulation* 2000; 101:1297.
301. The ESVEM Investigators: The ESVEM Trial: Electrophysiologic study vs electrocardiographic monitoring for selection of antiarrhythmic therapy of ventricular tachyarrhythmias. *Circulation* 1989; 79:1354.
302. The ESVEM Investigators: Determinants of predicted efficacy of antiarrhythmic drugs in the electrophysiologic study vs electrocardiographic monitoring trial. *Circulation* 1993; 87:329.
303. Mason JW, for the ESVEM Investigators: A comparison of electrophysiologic testing with holter monitoring to predict antiarrhythmic drug efficacy for ventricular tachyarrhythmias. *N Engl J Med* 1993; 329:445.
304. Mason JW, for the ESVEM Investigators: A comparison of 7 antiarrhythmic drugs in patients with ventricular tachyarrhythmias. *N Engl J Med* 1993; 329:452.
305. Omioigui NA, Marcus FI, Mason JW, et al: Cost of initial therapy in the electrophysiological study vs ECG monitoring trial (ESVEM). *Circulation* 1995; 91:1070.
306. Reiter MJ, Mann DE, Reiffel JE, et al: Significance and incidence of concordance of drug efficacy predictions by holter monitoring and electrophysiological study in the ESVEM Trial. *Circulation*. 1995; 91:1988.
307. Timerman A, Piegas LS, Sousa EMR: Results of cardiopulmonary resuscitation in a cardiology hospital. *Resuscitation* 1989; 18:75.
308. Urberg M, Ways C: Survival after cardiopulmonary resuscitation for an in-hospital arrest. *J Fam Pract* 1987; 25:41.
309. Rozenbaum EA, Shenkman L: Predicting outcome of in-hospital cardiopulmonary resuscitation. *Crit Care Med* 1988; 16:583.
310. Tortolani AJ, Risucci DA, Rosati RJ, et al: In-hospital cardiopulmonary resuscitation: patient arrest and resuscitation factors associated with survival. *Resuscitation* 1990; 20:115.
311. Castagna J, Weil MH, Shubin H: Factors determining survival in cardiac arrest. *Chest* 1974; 65:527.
312. Camarata SJ, Weil MH, Hanashira PK, Shubin H: Cardiac arrest in the critically ill. I: a study of predisposing causes in 132 patients. *Circulation* 1971; 44:688.
313. McGrath RB: In-hospital cardiopulmonary resuscitation after a quarter of a century. *Ann Emerg Med* 1987; 16:1365.
314. Tweed WA, Bristow G, Donen N, et al: Evaluation of hospital-based cardiac resuscitation, 1973–1977. *Can Med Assoc* J 1980; 122:301.
315. Smith DL, Kim K, Cairns BA, et al: Prospective analysis of outcome after cardiopulmonary resuscitation in critically ill surgical patients. *J Am Coll Surg* 1995; 180:488.
316. Hendrick JM, Pijls NHJ, vander Werf T, et al: Cardiopulmonary resuscitation on the general ward: no category of patients can be excluded in advance. *Resuscitation* 1990; 20:163.
317. Brain Resuscitation Clinical Trial I Study Group: Neurologic recovery after cardiac arrest: effect of duration of ischemia. *Crit Care Med* 1985; 13:930.
318. Becker LB, Ostrander MP, Barrett J, Kondos GT: Outcome of CPR in a large metropolitan area: where are the survivors? *Ann Emerg Med* 1991; 20:355.
319. Lombardi G, Gallagher EJ, Gennis P: Outcome of out-of-hospital cardiac arrest in New York City: the Pre-Hospital Arrest Survival Evaluation (PHASE) study. *JAMA* 1994; 271:678.
320. Eisenberg MS, Bergner L, Hallstrom A: Cardiac resuscitation in the community: importance of rapid provision and implications for program planning. *JAMA* 1979; 241:1905.
321. Cummins RO, Eisenberg MS: Prehospital cardiopulmonary resuscitation: is it effective? *JAMA* 1985; 253:2408.
322. Guzy PM, Pearce ML, Greenfield S: The survival benefit of bystander cardiopulmonary resuscitation in a paramedic-served metropolitan area. *Am J Public Health* 1983; 73:766.
323. Roth R, Stewart RD, Rogers K, et al: Out-of-hospital cardiac arrest: factors associated with survival. *Ann Emerg Med* 1984; 13:237.
324. Jakobsson J, Rehnquist N, Nyquist O: One year's experience of early defibrillation in Stockholm: Department of Anaesthesia, Karolinska Institute, Danderd Hospital, Stockholm, Sweden. *J Intern Med* 1989; 225:297.
325. Tweed WA, Bristow G, Donen N: Resuscitation from cardiac arrest: assessment of a system only basic life support outside of hospital. *Can Med Assoc* J 1980; 122:297.
326. Lund I, Skullberg A: Cardiopulmonary resuscitation by lay people. *Lancet* 1976; 2:702.
327. Copley DP, John AM, Rogers WJ, et al: Improved outcome for prehospital cardiopulmonary collapse with resuscitation by bystanders. *Circulation* 1974; 56:901.
328. Thompson RG, Hallstrom AP, Cobb LA: Bystander-initiated cardiopulmonary resuscitation in the management of ventricular fibrillation. *Ann Intern Med* 1979; 90:737.
329. Gudjonsson H, Baldvinsson E, Oddsson G, et al: Results of attempted cardiopulmonary resuscitation of patients dying suddenly outside the hospital in Reykjavik and the surrounding area 1976–1979. *Acta Med Scand* 1982; 212:247.
330. Eisenberg M, Bergner L, Hallstrom A: Paramedic programs and out-of-hospital cardiac arrest, I: factors associated with successful resuscitation. *Am J Public Health* 1979; 69:30.
331. Luce JM, Cary JM, Ross BK, et al: New developments in CPR. JAMA 1980; 244:1366.
332. Herlitz J, Ekstrom L, Wennerblom, et al: Effect of bystander-initiated cardiopulmonary resuscitation on ventricular fibrillation and survival after witnessed cardiac arrest. *Br Heart J* 1994; 72:408.
333. Levy DE, Bates D, Caronna JJ, et al: Prognosis in nontraumatic coma. *Ann Intern Med* 1981; 94:293.
334. Caronna JJ, Finklestein S: Neurologic syndromes after cardiac arrest. *Stroke* 1978; 9:517.
335. Eisenberg MS, Bergner L, Hallstrom A: Survivors of out-of-hospital cardiac arrest: morbidity and long-term survival. *Am J Emerg Med* 1984; 2:189.
336. Robinson GR, Hess D: Postdischarge survival and functional status following in-hospital cardiopulmonary resuscitation. *Chest* 1994; 105:991.
337. Liberthson RR, Nagel EL, Hirschman JC, Nussenfeld SR: Prehospital ventricular fibrillation: prognosis and follow-up course. *N Engl J Med* 1974; 291:317.
338. Goldstein S, Landis JR, Leighton R, et al: Characteristics of the resuscitated out-of-hospital cardiac arrest victim with coronary artery disease. *Circulation* 1981; 64:977.

339. Baum RS, Alvarez H, Cobb LA: Survival after resuscitation from out-of-hospital ventricular fibrillation. *Circulation* 1974; 50:1231.
340. Cobb LA, Baum RS, Alvarez HA, Schaffer WA: Resuscitation from out-of-hospital ventricular fibrillation: 4 years follow-up. *Circulation* 1975; 51 (suppl III):III-223.
341. Cobb L, Werner J: Predictors and prevention of sudden cardiac death, in Hurst JW, et al (eds): *The Heart*. New York, McGraw-Hill, 1982; p 599.
342. Rockswald G, Sharma B, Ruiz E, et al: Follow-up of 514 consecutive patients with cardiac arrest outside the hospital. *J Am Coll Emerg Phys* 1979; 8:216.
343. Abramson NS, Safar P, Detre K: Brain Resuscitation Clinical Trial II Study Group: Factors influencing neurologic recovery after cardiac arrest [abstract]. *Ann Emerg Med* 1989; 18:477.
344. Emergency Cardiac Care Committee and Subcommittees, American Heart Association: Guidelines for cardiopulmonary resuscitation and emergency cardiac care, VIII: ethical considerations in resuscitation. *JAMA* 1992; 268:2282.
345. Schneiderman LJ, Jecker NS, Jonsen AR: Medical futility: its meaning and ethical implications. *Ann Intern Med* 1990; 112:949.
346. Faber-Langendorff K: Resuscitation of patients with metastatic cancer: is a transient benefit still futile? *Arch Intern Med* 1991; 151:235.
347. Lund I, Skulberg A: Resuscitation of cardiac arrest outside hospitals: experiences with a mobile intensive care unit in Oslo. *Acta Anaesthesiol Scand* 1973; 53 (suppl):13.
348. Cobb L, Hallstrom A, Weaver D, et al: Prognostic factors in patients resuscitated from sudden cardiac death, in Wilhelmsen L, Hjalmarson A (eds): *Acute and Long-Term Management of Myocardial Ischemia*. Molndal, Sweden, Lindgren and Soner, 1978; p 106.
349. Eisenberg MS, Hallstrom A, Bergner L: Long-term survival after out-of-hospital cardiac arrest. *N Engl J Med* 1982; 306:1340.
350. Wernberg M, Thomassen A: Prognosis after cardiac arrest occurring outside intensive care and coronary units. *Acta Anaesthesiol Scand* 1979; 23:69.
351. Snyder B, Loewenson R, Gumnit R, et al: Neurologic prognosis after cardiopulmonary arrest, II: level of consciousness. *Neurology* 1980; 30:52.
352. Bergner L, Eisenberg MS, Hallstrom AP, et al: Health status of survivors of out-of-hospital cardiac arrest. *Circulation* 1982; 66 (suppl II):1401.

Chapter 17

Temporary Circulatory Support

Nader Moazami/Patrick M. McCarthy

Over the past several years, an increasing number of devices have been developed and approved for acute circulatory support. Compared with the devices that are intended for prolonged use as a bridge to transplantation, this group of support devices is more applicable to the acute resuscitative phase of cardiogenic shock. Despite maximal inotropic drugs, intubation, and control of cardiac rhythm, some patients remain hemodynamically unstable and require some type of mechanical circulatory support.[1,2] The need for circulatory support in the postcardiotomy period is relatively low and has been estimated to be in the range of 0.2% to 0.6%,[3] while cardiogenic shock occurs in 2.4% to 12% of patients with acute myocardial infarction,[4] with a mortality as high as 75%.[5]

The expansion of indications for circulatory support, development of better support devices, and improved results mandate that all surgeons acquire an understanding of the circulatory support devices currently available. Studies show that even smaller facilities that do not have cardiac transplantation may have improved patient survival if a device can be rapidly implemented and the patient transferred to a tertiary facility with expanded capabilities.[6] In this chapter we describe the devices currently available, and discuss indications for use, patient management considerations, and the overall morbidity and mortality associated with temporary mechanical support. The goal of the use of temporary assist devices is to achieve improved function of the native heart allowing for removal of the device. If recovery is unlikely, then transition to heart transplantation (Ch. 60) or a chronic assist device (Chs. 62 and 63) may be the only solution for achieving long-term survival.

COUNTERPULSATION

Historical Notes

The concept of increasing coronary blood flow by retarding the systolic pressure pulse was demonstrated by Kantrowitz and Kantrowitz in 1953 in a canine preparation and again by Kantrowitz and McKinnon in 1958 using an electrically stimulated muscle wrap around the descending thoracic aorta to increase diastolic aortic pressure.[7–9] In 1961 Clauss et al used an external counterpulsation system synchronized to the heart beat to withdraw blood from the femoral artery during systole and reinject it during diastole.[10] One year later Moulopoulos, Topaz, and Kolff produced an inflatable latex balloon that was inserted into the descending thoracic aorta through the femoral artery and inflated with carbon dioxide.[11] Inflation and deflation were synchronized to the electrocardiogram to produce counterpulsation that reduced end-systolic arterial pressure and increased diastolic pressure. In 1968 Kantrowitz reported survival of one of three patients with postinfarction cardiogenic shock refractory to medical therapy using an intra-aortic balloon pump.[12] These pioneering studies introduced the concept of supporting the failing circulation by mechanical means. Currently intra-aortic balloon counterpulsation is used in an estimated 70,000 patients annually.[8]

Physiology

The major physiologic effects of the intra-aortic balloon pump (IABP) are reduction of left ventricular afterload and an increase in aortic root and coronary perfusion pressure.[13–15] Important related effects include reduction of left ventricular systolic wall tension and oxygen consumption, reduction of left ventricular end-systolic and diastolic volumes, reduced preload, and an increase in coronary and

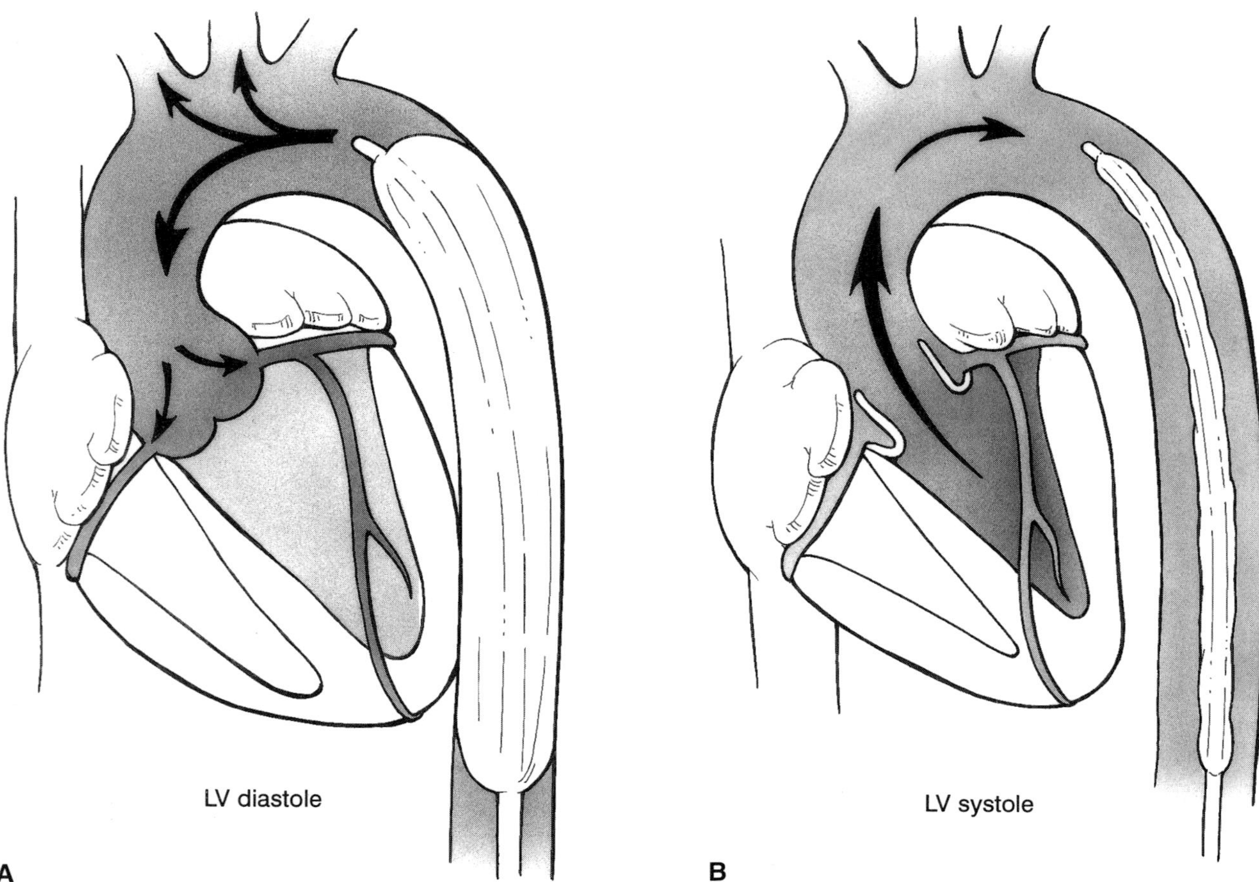

FIGURE 17–1 (A) Balloon inflation during left ventricular (LV) diastole occludes the descending thoracic aorta, closes the aortic valve, and increases proximal coronary and cerebral perfusion. (B) Balloon deflation during LV systole decreases LV afterload and myocardial oxygen demand.

collateral vessel blood flow.[16–19] Cardiac output increases because of improved myocardial contractility owing to increased coronary blood flow and the reduced afterload and preload, but the IABP does not directly move or significantly redistribute blood flow.[20,21] IABP reduces peak systolic wall stress (afterload) by 14% to 19% and left ventricular systolic pressure by approximately 15%.[16,20,22,23] Since peak systolic wall stress is related directly to myocardial oxygen consumption, myocardial oxygen requirements are reduced proportionately.[24–26] Coronary blood flow is subject to autoregulation, and in experimental animals the IABP does not increase flow until hypotension reduces flow to less than 50 mL/100 g ventricle/min.[14] However, as measured by echocardiography and color flow Doppler mapping, peak diastolic flow velocity increases by 117% and the coronary flow velocity integral increases 87% with counterpulsation.[27] Experimentally, collateral blood flow to ischemic areas increases up to 21% at mean arterial pressures higher than 190 mm Hg.[28]

Several variables affect the physiologic performance of the IABP. The position of the balloon should be just downstream to the left subclavian artery (Fig. 17-1). Diastolic augmentation of coronary blood flow increases with proximity to the aortic valve.[29,30] The balloon should fit the aorta so that inflation nearly occludes the vessel. Experimental work indicates that for adults balloon volumes of 30 or 40 mL significantly improve both left ventricular unloading and diastolic coronary perfusion pressure over smaller volumes. Inflation should be timed to coincide with closure of the aortic valve, which for clinical purposes is the dicrotic notch of the aortic blood pressure trace (Fig. 17-2). Early inflation reduces stroke volume, increases ventricular end-systolic and diastolic volumes, and increases both afterload and preload. Diastolic counterpulsation is visualized easily as a pressure curve in the arterial waveform and indicates increased diastolic perfusion of the coronary vessels (and/or bypass grafts).[31,32] Deflation should occur as late as possible to maintain the duration of the augmented diastolic blood pressure, but it must happen before the aortic valve opens and the ventricle ejects. For practical purposes deflation is timed to occur with the onset of the electrocardiographic R-wave. Active deflation of the balloon creates a suction effect that acts to decrease left ventricular afterload (and therefore myocardial oxygen consumption).

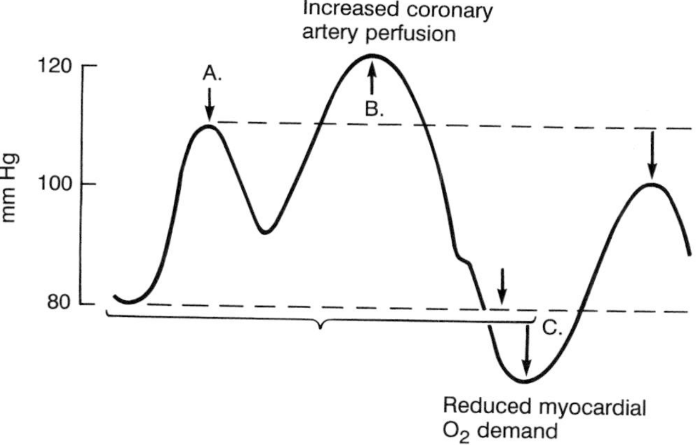

FIGURE 17–2 Illustration showing the effect of the intra-aortic balloon on aortic pressure. After ejection produces the pulse (A), inflation of the balloon increases aortic diastolic pressure (B). At end diastole, sudden deflation reduces aortic end-diastolic pressure (C) below that of an unassisted beat and reduces afterload and myocardial oxygen demand.

Biological factors that influence the in situ hemodynamic performance of the IABP include heart rate and rhythm, mean arterial diastolic pressure, competence of the aortic valve, and the compliance of the aortic wall. Severe aortic regurgitation is a contraindication to the use of the IABP; very low mean aortic diastolic pressures reduce aortic root pressure augmentation and coronary blood flow. A calcified, noncompliant aorta increases diastolic pressure augmentation, but risks injury to the aortic wall.

By far the most important biological variables are heart rate and rhythm. Optimal performance requires a regular heart rate with an easily identified R-wave or a good arterial pulse tracing with a discrete aortic dicrotic notch. Current balloon pumps trigger off the electrocardiographic R-wave or from the arterial pressure tracing. Both inflation and deflation are adjustable, and operators attempt to time inflation to coincide with closure of the aortic valve and descent of the R-wave. During tachycardia the IABP usually is timed to inflate every other beat; during chaotic rhythms the device is timed to inflate in an asynchronous fixed mode that may or may not produce a mean decrease in afterload and an increase in preload. In unstable patients every effort is made to establish a regular rhythm, including a paced rhythm, so that the IABP can be timed properly.

Indications

The traditional indications for insertion of the intra-aortic balloon pump are cardiogenic shock, uncontrolled myocardial ischemic pain, and postcardiotomy low cardiac output.[33–36] In recent years indications for IABP have broadened to include patients with high-grade left main coronary artery stenosis, high-risk or failed percutaneous transluminal coronary angioplasty, atherectomy, or stents; poorly controlled ventricular arrhythmias before or after operation; and patients with postinfarction ventricular septal defect or acute mitral insufficiency after myocardial infarction.[37–40] In addition, the IABP occasionally is used prophylactically in high-risk patients with poor left ventricular function with either mitral regurgitation or preoperative low cardiac output owing to hibernating or stunned myocardium. Patients with these conditions benefit from temporary afterload reduction during weaning from cardiopulmonary bypass, particularly if myocardial contractility is not immediately improved by revascularization. In some institutions a femoral arterial catheter is inserted in anticipation of IABP use in patients undergoing complex procedures who have myocardial dysfunction.[41] In exceptional patients, IABP is used with extracorporeal membrane oxygenation (ECMO) to unload the left ventricle and generate pulsatility while providing circulatory assistance for postcardiotomy patients.[42–44]

Nearly 90% of patients who receive intra-aortic balloon counterpulsation have various manifestations of ischemic heart disease, with or without associated valvular heart disease.[45–47] Patients with valvular heart disease without coronary disease who receive an intraoperative IABP generally have mitral valve disease. A few patients have IABP for end-stage cardiomyopathy, acute endocarditis, or before or after heart transplantation.[48]

Of 231 patients who had IABP insertions at the Cleveland Clinic, Eltchaninoff reports that 83 (34.6%) were for complications of acute myocardial infarction, 44 (18.3%) were owing to failed angioplasty, 48 (20%) were for high-risk angioplasty, and 31 (12.9%) were for stabilization before cardiac surgery.[35] Only 13 (5.4%) were for end-stage cardiomyopathy.

The timing of IABP insertion varies widely between reports. The percentage of IABPs inserted before cardiac surgery varies between 18% at St. Louis University Medical Center and 57% in a group of community hospitals that do cardiac catheterization.[49,50] The percentage of IABPs inserted intraoperatively varies from 42% to 72%, with a smaller number inserted early after operation (3% to 14%).

The overwhelming reason for intraoperative use of the IABP is failure to wean from cardiopulmonary bypass. Approximately 75% of intraoperative balloon insertions are for this reason. Preoperative low cardiac output and postinfarction angina are additional indications for intraoperative insertion of the IABP.

Techniques of Insertion

The intra-aortic balloon pump is usually inserted into the common femoral artery percutaneously.[51] A cutdown is most often used during cardiopulmonary bypass when the pulse is absent. The superficial femoral artery is avoided because of its smaller size and increased possibility of leg ischemia. For patients with small vessels an 8.5F catheter is recommended; otherwise, the 9.5F catheter is used. The iliac and axillary arteries and, very rarely, the abdominal aorta are infrequently used alternative sites.[52,53] Direct insertion into the ascending aorta is used for intraoperative insertions in patients with severe aortoiliac or femoral occlusive disease that prevents passage of the balloon catheter.[54–56]

Approximately two thirds to three quarters of all femoral arterial insertions utilize the percutaneous method.[57] Although percutaneous insertion was associated with a higher incidence of leg ischemia in the past, this is no longer true.[58,59] In the catheterization laboratory both the guidewire and balloon are monitored by fluoroscopy, but this is not essential if not available. The cutdown technique may be done with local anesthesia outside of the operating room, but preferably is done in the operating room with local or general anesthesia. After the femoral artery is exposed, a guidewire is introduced followed by dilating catheters and the balloon. The catheter can be inserted without the sheath in some instances.[60] The balloon catheter usually fits snugly in the arterial wound, so a pursestring suture is not needed. If bleeding is present around the entrance site, sutures are used for control. The wound is closed completely. Regardless of the method of insertion, whenever possible the tip of the balloon is visualized by fluoroscopy or transesophageal echocardiography to place the balloon just downstream to the left subclavian artery.[61]

The timing of inflation and deflation of the balloon must be monitored closely during counterpulsation. This is done by observing the continuously displayed arterial pressure tracing; a second systolic pulse should appear with every heartbeat and begin just after the smaller first pulse begins to decay. Timing the balloon for irregular rhythms is difficult and the circulatory support provided by the balloon is compromised; in these patients attempts are made to convert the patient to a sinus or paced rhythm or to slow (80-90 bpm) atrial fibrillation using appropriate drugs or cardioversion. For tachycardias over 110 to 120 bpm the balloon is timed to provide inflation on alternate beats if the machine is not able to reliably follow each beat. Generally patients are not given heparin for the IABP. The exit site of the catheter must be kept clean with antiseptics and covered in an effort to prevent local infection or septicemia.

A percutaneous IABP can be removed without exposing the femoral puncture site. The balloon catheter is disconnected from the pump and completely deflated using a 50-mL syringe. Using steady pressure over the femoral puncture site, the balloon catheter is withdrawn smoothly and removed, and pressure is maintained over the puncture site for 30 minutes. If the balloon is inserted via a cutdown, the balloon is preferably removed in the operating room. The puncture site is closed with sutures. If blood flow to the lower limb is impaired after removal, a local thromboembolectomy using Fogarty catheters and an angioplasty procedure using a vein patch is performed.

If the percutaneous needle punctures the iliac artery above the inguinal ligament intentionally or inadvertently in obese individuals, removal should be done through a surgical incision in the operating room, because the backward slope of the pelvis makes pressure difficult to maintain after withdrawal and substantial occult retroperitoneal bleeding may occur.

If the common femoral or iliac arteries cannot be used because of occlusive disease or inability to advance the guidewire, the axillary artery usually is exposed below the middle third of the clavicle for insertion.[52,53] This vessel is smaller than the femoral artery, but generally more compliant. Fluoroscopy or transesophageal (not transthoracic) echocardiography is recommended to ensure that the guidewire does not go down the ascending thoracic aorta into the heart.

Transaortic insertion of IABP may be done through an 8- or 10-mm woven Dacron or polyfluorotetraethylene graft that is beveled and sutured end-to-side to the ascending aorta using a side-biting clamp on the aorta.[56] The opposite end of the graft is passed through a stab incision in the chest wall below but near the xiphoid. The balloon is passed through this sleeve into the aorta and guided into the proximal descending thoracic aorta so that the balloon does not occlude the left subclavian orifice when inflated. The suture cuff of the balloon catheter is trimmed so that it can be inserted into the graft and tied tightly to achieve secure hemostasis. This connection is placed just beneath the skin so that none of the graft protrudes. The catheter is secured in place.

A simpler method uses two aortic pursestring sutures to secure the aorta around the balloon catheter. No graft is used, yet bleeding complications are minimal.[54,55] Regardless of the technique of insertion, balloon catheters inserted through the ascending aorta are removed in the operating room to secure closure of the aorta.

Pulmonary arterial counterpulsation is recommended for right heart failure but has not achieved wide use.[62,63] Because of the short length of the pulmonary artery either a prosthetic graft (20-25 mm) is sewn end-to-side to the main pulmonary artery and tied around the balloon catheter placed inside. There are little data regarding the amount of afterload reduction of the right ventricle.

Complications

Reported complication rates of the intra-aortic balloon pump vary between 12.9% and 29% and average approximately 20%.[36,57,64] Life-threatening complications are rare.[65] Leg ischemia is by far the most common complication (incidence 9% to 25%); other complications include balloon rupture, thrombosis within the balloon, septicemia, infection at the insertion site, bleeding, false aneurysm formation, lymph fistula, lymphocele, and femoral neuropathy.[66,67] There is no significant difference in limb ischemia in the five different types of IABPs clinically available.[64,68]

Balloon rupture occurs in approximately 1.7% of patients and usually is indicated by the appearance of blood within the balloon catheter and only occasionally by the pump alarm. Rupture may be slightly more common with transaortic insertion. Although helium usually is used to inflate the balloon, gas embolism has not been a problem. If rupture occurs, the balloon should be deflated forcibly to minimize thrombus formation within the balloon and promptly removed. If the patient is IABP-dependent, a guidewire is introduced through the ruptured balloon, the original balloon is removed, and a second balloon catheter is inserted over the wire. If the ruptured balloon is not removed easily, a second balloon is inserted via the opposite femoral or iliac artery or through the axillary artery to maintain circulatory support.[69]

Removal of a kinked or thrombosed ruptured balloon that cannot be withdrawn by firm traction requires operation. A thrombosed balloon can severely lacerate the femoral artery. The catheter should be withdrawn as far as possible with firm traction. The location of the tip should be determined by x-ray or ultrasound and an incision planned to expose that segment of the vascular system. In the operating room thrombolytic drugs may be considered if these drugs are not contraindicated by recent surgery.[70] The trapped balloon is removed through an arterotomy after control of the vascular segment is obtained.

Although the incidence of clinically significant lower leg ischemia varies from 9% to 25% of patients, up to 47% have evidence of ischemia during the time the IABP is used.[66,67] Thus the preinsertion status of the pedal pulses should be determined and recorded in every patient before the IABP is inserted. After insertion, the circulation of the foot is followed hourly by palpating pulses or by Doppler ultrasound. Foot color, mottling, temperature, and capillary refill are observed; the appearance of pain, dullness to sensation, and minimal circulation indicate severe ischemia that requires restoration of the circulation to the extremity as soon as possible.

There are three alternatives. If the patient is not balloon-dependent, it is removed immediately. In the majority of patients this relieves the distal ischemia; a few patients require surgical exploration of the puncture site, removal of thrombus and/or emboli, and reconstruction of the femoral artery. If the patient is balloon-dependent, a second balloon catheter can be introduced into the opposite femoral or iliac artery and the first removed. If this alternative is not available or attractive, circulation to the ischemic extremity is restored using a cross-leg vascular graft or, less commonly, an axillofemoral graft.[70,71] Prompt revascularization preempts development of the compartment syndrome (incidence 1% to 3%) and the need for fasciotomy. Prompt and aggressive treatment of leg ischemia has reduced the incidence of amputation to 0.5% to 1.5%, but if amputation is necessary the level often is above the knee. Several risk factors for development of leg ischemia have emerged. Female gender, peripheral vascular disease, diabetes, cigarette smoking, advanced age, obesity, and cardiogenic shock are reported to increase the risk of ischemic complications after IABP. Since the IABP is inserted for compelling indications, identification of risk factors does not influence management, except to encourage removal of the device as soon as the cardiac status of the patients allows. In some series longer duration of IABP counterpulsation is associated with an increased risk of complications.[66]

Although most ischemic complications are owing to impairment of arterial inflow, severe atherosclerotic diseases of the descending thoracic aorta may produce embolization of atherosclerotic material that can cause toe ischemia and eventually require amputation. Emboli may also reach the renal and visceral arteries to produce ischemia of these organs. The presence of aortic atherosclerosis can be determined by echocardiography and if present, insertion through the axillary artery considered.[72] The ischemic rate of axillary insertions is not known because of the low number of cases reported.

Approximately 1% of patients develop false aneurysms at the femoral puncture site either in the hospital or shortly after discharge, and rare patients develop an arterial-venous fistula. Both conditions are confirmed readily by duplex scanning and require elective operative repair; neglected false aneurysms can rupture. The rare complication of lymphocele or lymph fistula preferably is treated surgically by local exploration and suture control.

Bleeding produces a local hematoma that is not evacuated unless skin necrosis is likely. If bleeding occurs in the wound, the wound is explored, bleeding is stopped, part of the hematoma is evacuated without extending the dissection, and the wound is reclosed. Bleeding from transaortic insertion is uncommon (3% to 4%). Retroperitoneal bleeding from an iliac artery puncture may not be obvious, but may cause death.

Septicemia occurs in up to 1% of patients, but the risk increases with the duration of IABP. Septicemia is an indication for IABP removal, but if the patient is balloon-dependent, a replacement balloon catheter is inserted in a new site. Septicemia is treated aggressively after blood cultures are obtained with broad-spectrum antibiotics, which are switched to one or more specific antibiotics when the organism is known. Local infections occur in 2% to 3% of patients and usually are treated by drainage, packing, antibiotics, and secondary closure.

Acute aortic dissection from the catheter tip piercing the intima has been reported.[36] This problem is prevented preferably by not advancing the catheter against resistance and monitoring with fluoroscopy or transesophageal echocardiography. Occasional femoral neuropathies resolve over time, but can be disabling. Transaortic IABP is associated with a 2% to 3% incidence of cerebral vascular accidents.[55]

Results

Very few complications of IABP cause death. Rare instances of bleeding (retroperitoneal or aortic), septicemia, central nervous system injury, or aortic dissection may cause or contribute to a patient's death. Mortality is higher in patients with leg ischemic complications than in those without.

Counterpulsation increases coronary arterial flow, reduces afterload and myocardial oxygen consumption, and experimentally reduces infarct size early after infarction.[73] Without revascularization IABP produces a marginal increase in survival, but with revascularization both short-term and long-term survival as well as quality of life are substantially improved.[74–76]

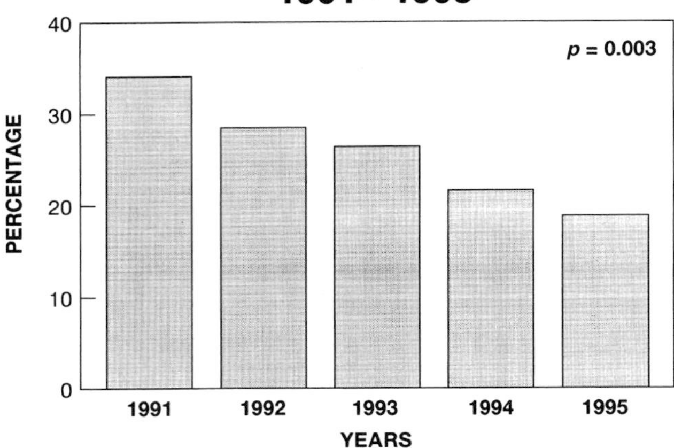

FIGURE 17–3 Hospital mortality for this 5-year period was 26%.

However, mortality is high in patients who receive IABP because of the cardiac problems that led to the need for the device. Overall reported hospital mortality ranges from 26% to 50%, although it has been decreasing. (Fig. 17-3).[77–79] Risk factors for hospital mortality include advanced age, female gender, high NYHA class, preoperative nitroglycerin, operative or postoperative insertion, and transaortic insertion in one study and age and diabetes mellitus in another. A third study correlates hospital death with acute myocardial infarction, ejection fraction less than 3%, NYHA class IV, and prolonged aortic cross-clamp and bypass times.[78] Time of insertion affects hospital mortality: preoperative insertion is associated with a mortality of 18.8% to 19.6%;[48] intraoperative insertion, 27.6% to 32.3%;[48] and postoperative insertion, 39% to 40.5%. Mortality is highest at 68% for patients with pump failure; lowest at 34% for patients with coronary ischemia; and 48% for patients who had a cardiac operation.[33] Risk factors at the time of weaning from cardiopulmonary bypass associated with the likelihood of hospital death are heart block, advanced age, female gender, and elevated preoperative blood urea concentration.[72]

Long-term survival varies with the type of operation and is highest in patients who had cardiac transplantation or myocardial revascularization.[48] Patients who received an IABP and who required valve surgery with or without revascularization have a poorer prognosis. Creswell et al found 58.8% of all patients alive at 1 year and 47.2% alive at 5 years. Nauheim et al found that nearly all survivors are in NYHA class I or II.[45] Approximately 18% of hospital survivors have some symptoms of lower extremity ischemia.[79]Although the literature supports a significant complication rate and mortality with IABP use, the more recent data suggest a trend toward continued improvement of results. The most recent report from the IABP registry from 1996–2000 reports the same trends in terms of IABP usage: hemodynamic support during cardiac catheterization (20.6%), cardiogenic shock (18.8%), weaning from cardiopulmonary bypass (16.1%), preoperative use in high-risk patients (13%), and refractory unstable angina (12.3%).[80] Major complications (including major limb ischemia, severe bleeding, balloon leak, death directly due to IABP insertion or failure) occurred in only 2.6% of cases, with an in-hospital mortality of 21.2%.[80]

Given the overall ease of IABP insertion, excellent physiologic augmentation of coronary blood flow, and LV unloading, this form of therapy should be considered as the first line of mechanical support in patients who do not have significant peripheral vascular disease. There is some suggestion that preoperative prophylactic IABP insertion in high-risk patients (left ventricular EF <40%, unstable angina, left main stenosis >70%, redo CABG) can improve cardiac index, reduce length of ICU stay, and decrease mortality.[81,82]

DIRECT CIRCULATORY SUPPORT

Background

The need for acute cardiac support beyond cardiopulmonary bypass was clear from the early days of cardiac surgery. Spencer et al reported the first successful clinical use of a temporary device in 1965 after four patients were placed on femoral–femoral cardiopulmonary bypass. Only one patient survived to discharge. Subsequently, in 1966 the first successful use of a left ventricular assist device was reported after a double valve operation.[83] Debakey used an assist device that was implanted in an extracorporeal location between the left atrium and the axillary artery, marking the first use of an extracorporeal temporary device support system. The patient survived for 10 days on the pump and was eventually discharged home.

The excitement surrounding these events prompted the formation of the Artificial Heart Program in 1964, sponsored by the National Heart Institute, which encouraged the development of mechanical circulatory support systems.[84] One of the objectives of this program was to promote the development of support systems that would be used in cases of acute hemodynamic collapse.

Ideal Device

Despite recent advances in biotechnology, recognition of many of the problems and complications associated with extracorporeal circulation have delineated the limitations of these devices. The components of an ideal device must overcome some of the existing problems.

An ideal device should support adequate flow, maximize hemodynamics, and unload the ventricle for patients of all sizes. Although using different cannulation approaches can address some of these issues (see below), even under ideal conditions the currently available pumps are only able to support flows up to a maximum of 6 L/min, a limitation in obese patients.

At the other extreme is the need to support patients with small body surface areas. Current devices have addressed the problem associated with variations in patient size by being designed as extracorporeal systems. Therefore, by virtue of having small-diameter cannulas transversing the chest, the pumps can support patients with varying body surface area. The disadvantage of such a system is the potential for driveline and mediastinal infections. In addition, the length of the cannula between the heart and the device, particularly the inflow cannula, predisposes to areas of stasis and potential thrombus generation. Thromboemboli, which occur despite adequate anticoagulation, are one of the leading etiologies of death in patients supported on devices.

All current pumps require anticoagulation that increases the ever-present threat of early postoperative bleeding. In addition, requirements for transfusion of large amounts of coagulation factors and platelets enhance the inflammatory response that is induced by surgery and is further aggravated by the artificial circuit. Activation of the contact and complement systems, as well as release of cytokines by leukocytes, endothelial cells, and macrophages, further increases the potential negative and detrimental effects of use of temporary assist devices.[85,86] The ensuing inflammatory cascade and volume overloading can have detrimental effect on the pulmonary vascular resistance and right ventricular overload, often necessitating addition of a right ventricular assist device.

Current temporary assist devices all have the capability of biventricular support, provided that the lungs can support oxygenation and ventilation. In cases of acute lung injury superimposed on circulatory failure, ECLS (ECMO) is the only device currently approved that can support an in-line oxygenator.

The multitude of clinical scenarios that often lead to the need for mechanical support all require that support be instituted expeditiously. All current devices must therefore be easily implantable. In the postcardiotomy setting with access to the great vessels, the cannulas should allow the versatility of choosing any inflow or outflow site that is clinically indicated (see below). In an active resuscitative setting, such as cardiac arrest in the catheterization laboratory, in which time is critical and transport to the operating room often impractical, percutaneous cannulation must be an option.

Table 17-1 summarizes some of the components of an ideal temporary support device. At present, no single device is inclusive of all the components.

Indications for Support and Patient Selection

A wide range of indications exist for acute mechanical support, but the primary goal is rapid restoration of the circulation and stabilization of hemodynamics. The routine

TABLE 17–1 Characteristics of an ideal temporary support device

1. Accommodates patients of all sizes, regardless of body surface area
2. Easy to insert
3. Maximizes hemodynamics while unloading the heart to allow for myocardial recovery
4. Is adaptable for patients who require biventricular support
5. Supports the use of an oxygenator as needed, particularly in the group of patients with acute lung injury
6. Requires minimal anticoagulation
7. Has a biocompatible surface that does not promote thrombus generation
8. Causes minimal destruction of blood or plasma components
9. Allows for ambulation and physical rehabilitation
10. Converts easily to a long-term implantable device

use of transesophageal echocardiography (TEE) has greatly helped in assessing the etiology of cardiogenic shock by allowing evaluation of ventricular function, regional wall motion abnormalities, and valvular mechanics. In a patient with mechanical complications secondary to myocardial infarction, such as acute rupture with tamponade, acute papillary muscle rupture, or postinfarction ventricular septal defect, emergent surgical correction may obviate the need for device support. Similarly in the postcardiotomy setting with failure to separate from cardiopulmonary bypass, TEE may direct the surgeon to the need for additional revascularization and reparative valve surgery and successful weaning from bypass.

If echocardiography fails to reveal a surgically correctable cause for cardiogenic shock, most surgeons use hemodynamic data to consider the need for mechanical assistance. These criteria include a cardiac index less than 2.2 L/min/ m^2, systolic blood pressure lower than 90 mm Hg, mean pulmonary capillary wedge pressure or central venous pressure higher than 20 mm Hg, and concomitant use of high doses of least two inotropic agents.[87] These situations may be clinically associated with arrhythmias, pulmonary edema, and oliguria. In such circumstances, use of an intra-aortic balloon pump may be considered as the first step. In the postcardiotomy shock setting, without mechanical support, the mortality is greater than 50%.[88] In this setting, some believe that early implantation of an assist device capable of supporting high flows and allowing the heart to rest may improve results and allow for recovery of stunned myocardium.[89] Furthermore, new pharmacologic agents such as the phosphodiesterase inhibitor milrinone, nitric oxide, and vasopressin have helped to optimize hemodynamics during this critical initial period, reducing the need for concomitant right ventricular support.[90,91]

Once mechanical assistance has been instituted, the stabilized patient can undergo periodic evaluation to assess native heart recovery, end-organ function, and neurologic status. We initiate evaluation for cardiac transplantation concomitantly. Patients who do not have occult malignancy, severe untreated infection, or neurologic deficit are selected for cardiac transplantation if all other criteria are met and there is no sign of cardiac recovery. In this subgroup we generally transition to a chronic ventricular assist device until an organ becomes available. In those patients with gradual improvement in myocardial pump function, the devices may be weaned and removed (see below).

CONTINUOUS FLOW PUMPS

There are two types of commercially available pumps for extracorporeal circulation: roller pumps and centrifugal pumps. Roller pumps are used rarely, if ever, for temporary circulatory support beyond routine cardiopulmonary bypass applications because of important disadvantages. Although inexpensive, roller pumps are insensitive to line pressure if the outflow line becomes obstructed, and also require unobstructed inflow. Additionally, they may cause spallation of tubing particles and are subject to tubing failure at unpredictable times. These systems require constant vigilance and are difficult to operate for extended periods. Use of roller pumps beyond 4 to 5 hours is associated with hemolysis, and for this reason roller pumps are inappropriate for mechanical assistance that may involve several days to weeks of support.[92]

Centrifugal Pumps

Centrifugal pumps are familiar assist systems because of their routine use in cardiopulmonary bypass. Although many different pumphead designs are available, they all work on the principle of generating a rotatory motion by virtue of moving blades, impellers, or concentric cones. These pumps can generally provide high flow rates with relatively modest increases in pressure. They require priming and de-airing prior to use in the circuit, and the amount of flow generated is sensitive to outflow resistance and filling pressures. The differences in design of the various commercially available pumpheads are in the numbers of impellers, the shape and angle of the blades, and the priming volume. The only exception is the Medtronic BioPump (Medtronic Bio-Medicus, Eden Prairie, MN), which is based on two concentric cones generating the rotatory motion. The pumpheads are disposable, relatively cheap to manufacture, and are mounted on a magnetic motorized unit that generates the power. Despite design differences, in vitro and in vivo testing has shown no clear superiority of one pump over the other.[93–95] Although earlier designs caused mechanical trauma to the blood elements, leading to excessive hemolysis, the newly engineered pumps are less traumatic and can be used for longer periods. Studies have documented that centrifugal pumps have a superior performance with regards to mechanical injury to red blood cells when compared to roller pumps.[96]

TABLE 17–2 Significance of differences between prevalence of complications among circulatory assist devices

Complication	Centrifugal devices (%)	Pneumatic devices (%)	p-Value
Bleeding/DIC	48.3	38.2	.002
BV failure/low CO	33.1	29.1	NS
Renal failure	30.7	37.2	.030
Infection	11.3	24.3	<.001
Neurologic	11.9	11.7	NS
Thrombus/emboli	9.6	12.9	NS
Hemolysis	5.1	10.4	<.001
Technical problems	3.6	7.4	.003

DIC = disseminated intravascular coagulopathy; BV = biventricular; CO = cardiac output; NS = no significance demonstrated.

COMPLICATIONS

Complications with temporary mechanical assistance are high and very similar for patient on centrifugal pump support or ECLS (see below). The major complications reported by a voluntary registry for temporary circulatory assistance using primarily left ventricular assist devices (LVAD), right ventricular assist devices (RVAD), and biventricular assist devices (BVAD) are bleeding, low cardiac output with BVAD, renal failure, infection, neurologic deficits, thrombosis, and emboli, hemolysis, and technical problems (Table 17-2). The incidence of these complications in 1279 reported patients differed significantly between continuous perfusion systems and pneumatically driven systems (see the following section) with respect to bleeding, renal failure, infection, and hemolysis. Neurologic deficits occurred in approximately 12% of patients, and in Golding's experience noncerebral emboli occurred equally often.[97] Golding also found that 13% of patients also developed hepatic failure. An autopsy study found anatomic evidence of embolization in 63% of patients even though none had emboli detected clinically.[98]

Complications reported from the University of Missouri[99] on 91 patients who had undergone centrifugal mechanical support for postcardiotomy failure are also very similar, with 45% incidence of bleeding, 35% renal failure, 21% infection, and 4.4% thromboembolism. In addition, seal disruption between the pumphead and magnet is a common problem with prolonged support and will cause fluid accumulation in the magnet chamber. Therefore, frequent inspection of the pumps every 12 hours is mandatory.

RESULTS

Although a meaningful comparison of results of centrifugal support from different institutions is not possible, in general overall survival has been in the range of 21% to 41% (Table 17-3). The voluntary registry reported the experience with 604 LVAD, 168 RVAD, and 507 BVAD experiences; approximately 70% were with continuous flow pumps and the remainder with pulsatile pumps.[1] There were no significant differences in the percentage of patients weaned from circulatory assistance or the percentage discharged from the hospital according to the type of perfusion circuitry. Overall 45.7% of patients were weaned and 25.3% were discharged from the hospital.[1] The registry also reports that long-term survival of patients weaned from circulatory support is 46% at 5 years.[1] Most of the mortality occurs in the hospital before discharge or within 5 months of discharge.

Golding reported an identical hospital survival rate for 91 patients in 1992 using only centrifugal pumps, and Noon reported that 21% of 129 patients were discharged.[97,100] Patients who received pulsatile circulatory assistance were supported significantly longer than those supported by centrifugal pumps, but there were no differences in the percentage of patients weaned or discharged.[1] Survivors were supported an average of 3.1 days using continuous flow pumps. Patients supported for acute myocardial infarction did poorly; only 11.5% were discharged.

Data from the University of Missouri Hospital are also very similar.[99] From the 91 patients with postcardiotomy heart failure, 46% were weaned from the device and 21% survived to hospital discharge. Although weaning was more successful with RVAD support alone compared to LVAD or biVAD support (100% for RVAD vs. 48.5% for LVAD, vs. 44.9% for biVAD), survivals were not significantly different (RVAD, 22%; LVAD, 24.3%; biVAD, 18.4%). Joyce reports that 42% of patients supported by Sarn impeller pumps were eventually discharged.[101] This is the highest reported survival and probably reflects the fact that some of these

TABLE 17–3 Review of large series in the literature reporting outcomes of centrifugal mechanical assistance in the setting of postcardiotomy cardiac failure

Reference	Patients (no.)	Biventricular (%)	Mean duration of support, d (range)	Weaned (%)	Survived (%)
Noon[156]	141	16.3	3.8 (1-22)	54	22
Magovern[157]	77	46.8	2.2 (<1-7.7)	56	35
Joyce[158]	34	NR	NR	62	41
Curtis[99]	91	54.0	2.2 (<1-18)	46	21
Combined registry*	559	NR	NR	45	26

*Volunteer registry established by the American Society for Artificial Organs ISHLT.

NR = not reported.

patients received transplants, which is known to improve overall survival.

Extracorporeal Life Support

By the 1960s it was clear that CPB was not suitable for patients requiring circulatory support for several days to weeks. The development of extracorporeal life support (ECLS) as a temporary assist device (also referred to as extracorporeal membrane oxygenation, or ECMO) is a direct extension of the principles of cardiopulmonary bypass and follows the pioneering efforts of Bartlett et al in demonstrating the efficacy of this technology in neonatal respiratory distress syndrome.[102]

There are a number of key differences between CPB and ECLS. The most obvious difference is the duration of required support. Whereas CPB is typically employed for several hours during cardiac surgery, ECLS is designed for longer duration of support. With ECLS a lower dose of heparin is used, and reversal of heparin is not an issue because a continuous circuit is used and areas of stasis have been minimized (such as cardiotomy suction or venous reservoir). In addition, the membrane oxygenator allows for longer duration of support. These differences are thought to reduce the inflammatory response and the more pronounced coagulopathy that can be seen with CPB.[86]

A typical ECLS circuit is demonstrated in Figure 17-4. The system is comprised of the following:

(1) *Hollow-fiber membrane oxygenator with an integrated heat-exchange system*: The microporous membrane provides the necessary gas transfer capability via the micropores where there is direct blood-gas interface with minimal resistance to diffusion. By virtue of the membranes being close to each other, the diffusion distance has been reduced without a significant pressure drop across the system.[103] Control of oxygenation and ventilation is relatively easy. Increasing the total gas flow rate increases CO_2 removal (increasing the "sweep") by reducing the gas phase CO_2 partial pressure and promoting diffusion. Blood oxygenation is simply controlled by changing the fraction of O_2 in the gas supplied to the oxygenator.[103]

(2) *Centrifugal pump*: These pumps are totally nonocclusive and afterload-dependent. An increase in downstream resistance, such as significant hypertension, will decrease forward flow to the body. Therefore, flow is not determined by rotational flow alone, and a flow meter needs to be incorporated in the arterial outflow to quantitate the actual pump output. If the pump outflow should become occluded, the pump will not generate excessive pressure and will not rupture the arterial line. Similarly, the pump will not generate significant negative pressure if the inflow becomes occluded. This protects against cavitation and microembolus formation.

(3) *Heat exchanger*: The heat exchanger allows for control of blood temperature as it passes through the extracorporeal circuit. Generally the transfer of energy occurs by circulating nonsterile water in a countercurrent fashion against the circulating blood. Use of water as the heat exchange medium provides an even temperature across the surface of the heat exchanger without localized hot spots.[103]

(4) *Circuitry interfaced between the patient and the system*: The need for systemic anticoagulation on ECLS and

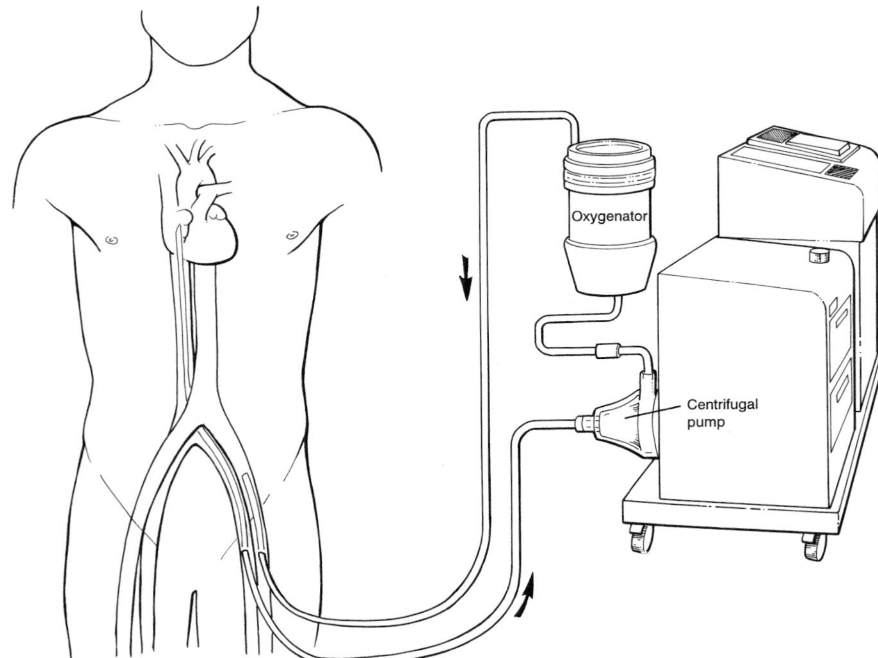

FIGURE 17–4 Percutaneous ECMO support is attained via femoral vessel access. Right atrial blood is drained via a catheter inserted into the femoral vein and advanced into the right atrium. Oxygenated blood is perfused retrograde via the femoral artery. Distal femoral artery perfusion is not illustrated.

the complications associated with massive coagulopathy and persistent bleeding during the postcardiotomy period led to the development of biocompatible heparin-bonded bypass circuits. In 1991, the Carmeda Corporation in Stockholm, Sweden, released a heparin-coating process that could be used to produce an antithrombotic surface.[104] This process was applied to extracorporeal tubing and the hollow-fiber microporous oxygenator surface.[105] Initial experience suggested that the need for systemic anticoagulation had been eliminated. In addition, heparin coating has been associated with a decrease in the inflammatory response with reduced granulocyte activation[106] and complement activation.[107] Bindsler[108] and Mottaghy[109] reported excellent hemodynamic support with minimal postoperative blood loss in experimental animals for up to 5 days. Magovern and Aranki reported similar excellent results with clinical application.[110,111] Although these heparin-bonded circuits were initially thought to completely eliminate the need for heparinization, thrombus formation without anticoagulation remains a persistent problem. In a study of 30 adult patients with cardiogenic shock who underwent ECLS using the heparin-bonded circuits and no systemic anticoagulation, 20% of patients developed left ventricular thrombus shown by transesophageal echocardiography and an additional 6% had visible clot in the pumphead.[112] Protamine administration after starting ECLS can precipitate intracardiac clot. If the left ventricle does not eject and blood remains static within the ventricle, clot formation is more likely. Intracavity clot is more likely in patients with myocardial infarction due to expression of tissue factor by the injured cells. Protamine may bind to the heparinized coating of the new circuit and negate an anticoagulant effect.[113]

CANNULATION

A key difference between the centrifugal pump and ECLS is the presence of an in-line oxygenator. As a result, ECLS can be used for biventricular support by using central cannulation of the right atrium and aorta or by peripheral cannulation. Intraoperatively, the most common application of ECLS has been for patients who cannot be weaned from cardiopulmonary bypass after heart surgery. In these cases, the existing right atrial and aortic cannulas can be used. An alternative strategy, and one that we prefer, is to convert the system to peripheral cannulas and to cannulate both the proximal and distal femoral artery. Conversion permits chest closure and removal of perfusion catheters at the bedside in intensive care.

The cannulation is done by surgical cutdown in the groin for exposure of the common femoral artery and vein. The entire vessel does not need to be mobilized and exposure of the anterior surface of the vessels is sufficient. A purse-string suture is placed over the anterior surface of the vessel. The largest cannula that the vessel can accommodate is selected. Typically arterial cannulas are 16F to 20F and venous

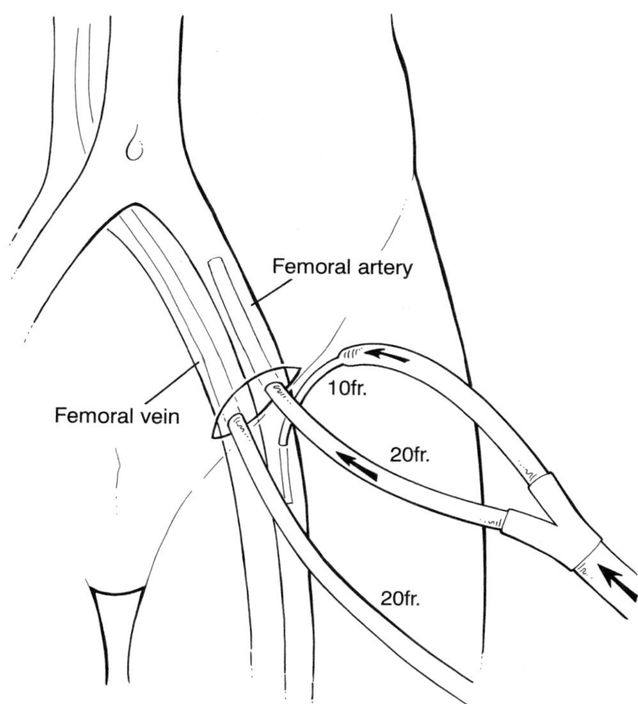

FIGURE 17–5 Surgical exposure of the femoral vessels facilitates cannulation for ECMO. A small 10F cannula is used to perfuse the distal femoral artery.

cannulas are 18F to 28F in size. The cannulation is performed under direct vison using Seldinger's technique. A stab incision is made in the skin with a #11 blade knife, a needle is inserted through the stab incision into the vessel, and a guidewire is gently advanced. Dilators are then sequentially passed to gently dilate the tract and the insertion point in the vessel. The cannulas are then inserted, the guidewire is removed, and a clamp is applied. For venous drainage we typically employ a long 2-stage cannula (Fem-Flex II; Research Medical, Midvale, UT) and direct it to the level of the right atrium under TEE guidance.

To minimize limb complication from ischemia, one strategy is to place a 10F perfusion cannula in the superficial femoral artery downstream to the primary arterial inflow cannula to perfuse the leg (Fig. 17-5). This cannula is connected to a tubing circuit that is spliced into the arterial circuit with a Y-connector.[114] The distal cannula directs continuous flow into the leg and significantly reduces problems with leg ischemia. An alternative strategy is to completely mobilize the common femoral artery and sew a 6- or 8-mm short Dacron graft to its anterior surface as a "chimney." The graft serves as the conduit for the arterial cannula and no obstruction to distal flow exists. This strategy also allows for a more secure connection and avoids problems with inadvertent dislodgement of the cannulas because of loosening of the purse strings. In general, complete percutaneous placement of arterial cannulas is avoided to prevent iatrogenic injury during insertion and ensure proper positioning of the cannulas. However, when venovenous bypass is the only mode of support needed, percutaneous cannulation is performed. Surgical exposure is not necessary and bleeding is less with this technique. Although traditionally the perfusion circuit involves atrial drainage and femoral reinfusion (atriofemoral flow), a recent prospective study has shown the reverse circuit (femoroatrial flow) to provide higher maximal extracorporeal flow, and higher pulmonary arterial mixed venous oxygenation.[115]

Central cannulation is sometimes indicated either because of severe peripheral vascular disease or the desire to deliver the highly oxygenated blood directly to the coronaries and the cerebral circulation. In patients with an open chest, aortic and right atrial cannulas are used. Reinforcing purse-string sutures are placed and tied over rubber chokers and buttons for later tying at decannulation. The catheters are brought through the chest wall through separate stab wounds, and after bleeding is secured, the chest is covered, but not closed, over mediastinal drainage tubes.[92]

An alternative central cannulation site is the axillary artery. Direct cannulation of this artery has been associated with progressive edema of the arm.[116] Therefore, the best strategy to maintain arm perfusion is to expose the axillary artery and sew a 6- or 8-mm graft to the vessel as a "chimney." The cannula is then placed in the graft and tied securely with several circumferential umbilical tapes.

Once instituted, the system can be monitored by trained ICU nurses and maintained by a perfusionist. Evidence of thrombus in the pumphead requires a change. Leakage of plasma across the membrane from the blood phase to the gas phase continues to be a problem, gradually decreasing the efficiency of the oxygenator and increasing resistance to flow, necessitating oxygenator exchanges. Using this system, ECLS flows of 4 to 6 L/min are possible at pump speeds of 3000 to 3200 rpm. Higher pump speeds are avoided to minimize mechanical trauma to blood cells. Other means of improving flow include transfusion of blood, crystalloid, or other colloid solutions to increase the overall circulating volume. Physiologically, ECLS will unload the right ventricle, but will not unload the ejecting left ventricle, even though left ventricular preload is reduced.[117] If the heart is dilated and poorly contracting, the marked increase in afterload provided by the ECLS system offsets any change in end-diastolic left ventricular volume produced by bypassing the heart. The heart remains dilated because the left ventricle cannot eject sufficient volume against the increased afterload to reduce either end-diastolic or end-systolic volume. ECLS, therefore, may theoretically increase left ventricular wall stress and myocardial oxygen consumption unless an intra-aortic balloon pump or other means is used to mechanically unload the left ventricle and reduce left ventricular wall stress.[118] We routinely use IABP in the majority of patients to decrease the increased afterload imposed by ECLS, and add pulsatility to the continuous flow generated by the centrifugal pump. Kolobow has devised a spring-loaded catheter introduced through the femoral vein to render the pulmonary valve incompetent to decompress the left ventricle during ECLS, but this has not been used clinically.[118] Others use atrial septostomy to decompress the left ventricle if the pulmonary artery pressures remain elevated.[119]

An RVAD is rarely indicated in the postcardiotomy setting because in general these patients have global biventricular dysfunction. ECLS as an RVAD (with outflow to the pulmonary artery via the right ventricular outflow tract) may be only used in patients with good function of the left ventricle. Exclusive right ventricular dysfunction is rare but may occur if retrograde cardioplegia is used and fails to protect the right ventricle, in cases of pulmonary thromboendarterectomy, or in patients with right ventricular infarction. Note that if significant pulmonary hypertension is present, this configuration may not adequately load the left ventricle.

COMPLICATIONS

The experience in adults with ECMO for postoperative cardiogenic shock is more limited because of nearly universal bleeding problems associated with the chest wound in combination with heparin anticoagulation with the ECMO circuit.[120] Pennington reported massive bleeding in six of six adults supported by ECMO following cardiac surgery. Even without the chest wound, bleeding was the major complication in a large study of long-term ECMO for acute respiratory insufficiency.[121] Muehrcke reported experience with ECMO using heparin-coated circuitry with no or minimal heparin.[117,122] The incidence of reexpoloration was 52% in the Cleveland Clinic experience; transfusions averaged 43 units of packed cells, 59 units of platelets, 51 units of cryoprecipitate, and 10 units of fresh frozen plasma. Magovern reported somewhat fewer uses of blood products, but treated persistent bleeding by replacement therapy and did not observe evidence of intravascular clots; two patients developed stroke after perfusion stopped. Other important complications associated with ECMO using heparin-coated circuits included renal failure requiring dialysis (47%), bacteremia or mediastinitis (23%), stroke (10%), leg ischemia (70%), oxygenator failure requiring change (43%), and pump change (13%).[117] Nine of 21 patients with leg ischemia required thrombectomy and one amputation. Half of the patients developed marked left ventricular dilatation and six patients developed intracardiac clot detected by transesophageal echocardiography.[90] Intracardiac thrombus may form within a poorly contracting, nonejecting left ventricle or atrium because little blood reaches the left atrium with good right atrial drainage.[40,82,89,108] We have observed intracardiac thrombus in heparinized patients and those perfused with pulsatile devices and a left atrial drainage cannula. The problem, therefore, is not unique to ECMO or the location of the left-sided drainage catheter, but is related to left ventricular function. In patients on ECMO with a left ventricular thrombus, we

TABLE 17–4 Representative clinical trials evaluating extracorporeal membrane oxygenation for the treatment of postcardiotomy cardiogenic shock

Reference	Patients (no.)	Duration of support (range)	Weaned from device, no. (%)	Survived to hospital discharge, no. (%)
Magovern[117]	21	9-92 h	16 (76)	1 (52)
Wang[159]	18	7-456 h	10 (55)	6 (33)
Muehrcke[122]	23	0.5-144 h	9 (39)	7 (30)
Magovern[125]	55	8-137 h	36 (65)	20 (36)

have removed the thrombus at the time a HeartMate LVAD was implanted for a bridge to transplantation.[122]

More recent reports documenting the high incidence of complications with ECLS have continued to plague temporary support mechanisms based on continous flow. Kasirajan reported an 18.9% incidence of intracranial hemorrhage with female gender, heparin use, elevated creatinine, need for dialysis, and thrombocytopenia as important associated risk factors.[123] Smedira recently reported on 107 postcardiotomy patients supported on ECLS with a 48% rate of infection, 39% need for dialysis, 29% neurologic events, 5% pump thrombus formation, and 27% limb complications.[124]

RESULTS

Table 17-4 summarizes some of the reported results with ECLS for postcardiotomy circulatory support. Magovern reported improved results in 14 patients supported by a heparin-coated ECMO circuit after operations for myocardial revascularization.[117] Eleven of 14 patients (79%) with revascularization survived, but none of three patients with mitral valve surgery and none of four patients who underwent elective circulatory arrest survived. Overall, 52% of the whole group survived, but two developed postperfusion strokes that were probably from thrombi produced during perfusion. Although the Cleveland Clinic experience with heparin-coated ECLS circuits produced a survival rate of 30%, the patient population was more diversified and represented only 0.38% of cardiac operations done during the same time period.[112] In a recent report on 82 adult patients supported with ECMO for a variety of indications, survival for postcardiotomy was 36%, whereas none of the patients who had acute cardiac resuscitation survived, and survival for cardiac allograft failure was 50%.[125]

More recently the Cleveland Clinic reported their results looking at 202 adults with cardiac failure treated with ECMD.[85] With an extended follow-up up to 7.5 years (mean 3.8 years), survival was reported to be 76% at 3 days, 38% at 30 days, and 24% at 5 years. Patients surviving 30 days had a 63% chance of being alive at 5 years. Interestingly, patients who were weaned or bridged to transplantation had a higher overall survival (40% and 45%, respectively). Failure to wean or bridge was secondary to end-organ dysfunction and included renal and hepatic failure and occurrence of neurologic events while on support.[85] Another report from the Cleveland Clinic looking at 19,985 patients undergoing cardiac operations found that 107 (0.5%) required ECLS for postcardiotomy failure. Younger age, number of reoperations, emergency operations, higher creatinine, greater left ventricular dysfunction, and history of myocardial infarction were significant predictors of the need for mechanical support.[124] Although overall survival was 35%, survival was 72% in the subgroup bridged to a chronic implantable device system (see below for bridge to bridge experience.)

PULSATILE PUMPS

ABIOMED BVS 5000

In 1992, the ABIOMED device became the first extracorporeal pump designed to provide pulsatile univentricular or biventricular support that was approved by the Food and Drug Administration. It has been used in Europe and the United States for the purpose of postcardiotomy pump failure with more than 850 patients currently reported to the registry. The system is a simple, user-friendly, extracorporeal pulsatile pump that is available in over 450 centers in United States, with the majority being utilized in nontransplant centers. The pump is configured as a dual chamber device containing an atrial chamber that fills passively by gravity and a ventricular chamber that pneumatically pumps the blood to the outflow cannula (Fig. 17-6). The two chambers and the outflow tract are divided by trileaflet polyurethane valves, which allows for unidirectional blood flow.

The pump chamber itself consists of a collapsible polyurethane bladder with a capacity of 100 mL. Passive flow of blood into the atrial chamber is dependent on gravity (the height of the chamber relative to the patients' atrium), the central venous pressure (preload), and the central venous capacitance. The atrial bladder operates in a fill to empty mode and therefore can be affected by changes of the height of the pump relative to the patient or the volume status of the patient. The pump is usually set approximately 25 cm below the bed. The adequacy of filling can be visually assessed because the pump is transparent. The passive filling (absence of a negative pressure generation) is designed to prevent atrial collapse with each pump cycle and also to prevent suctioning of air into the circuitry.

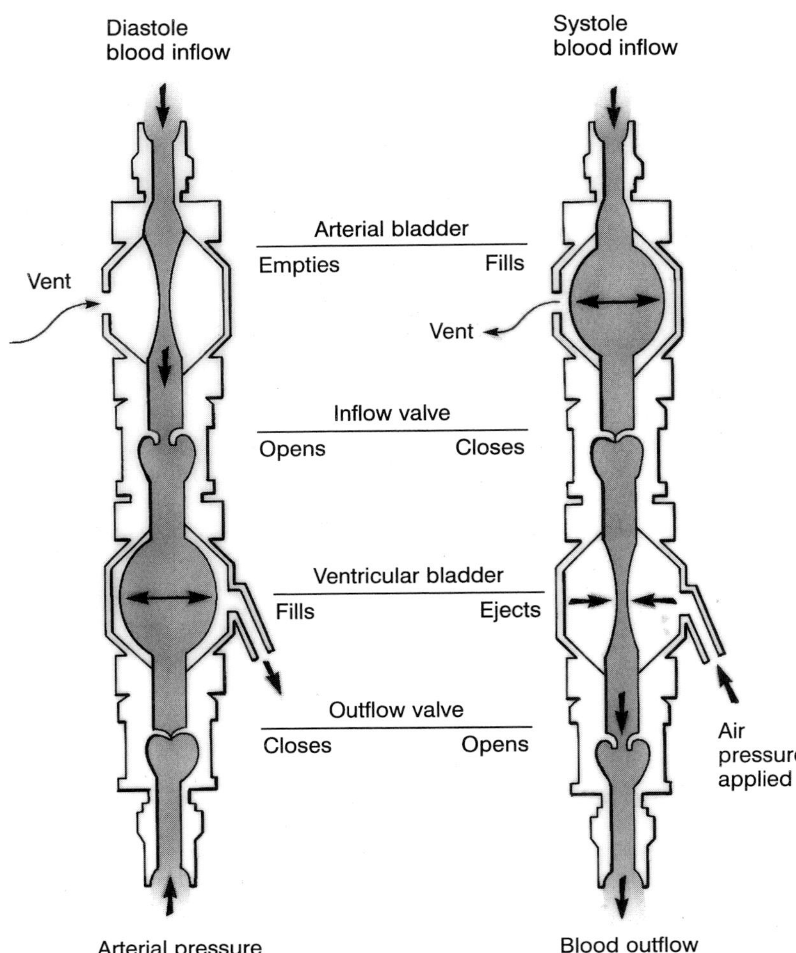

FIGURE 17–6 The ABIOMED BVS 5000. (Left panel) The atrial chamber empties through a one-way valve into the ventricular chamber (diastole). (Right panel) The pneumatically driven pump compresses the ventricular chamber and blood flows through a one-way valve into the patient (systole). The atrial chamber fills by gravity during pump systole.

The ventricular chamber, on the other hand, requires active pulsatile pumping by a pneumatic driveline. Compressed air is delivered to the chamber, causing bladder collapse and forcing blood out of the pump to the patient. During diastole the air is vented to the atmosphere, allowing refilling of the chamber during the next cycle. The rate of pumping and the duration of pump systole and diastole are adjusted by the pump microprocessor that operates asynchronously to the native heart rate. The pump automatically makes adjustments to account for preload and afterload changes and delivers a constant stroke volume of approximately 80 mL. The maximum output is approximately 5 to 6 L/min with the newer BVS 5000*i* console. This design requires minimal input by personnel except during periods of weaning. Medical management should include optimizing patients' hydration status and outflow resistance as the pump's performance depends on these parameters.

The main advantage of the device is the ability to provide independent univentricular or biventricular support as needed. The device has not demonstrated any significant hemolysis and the pulsatile flow may have some degree of physiological benefit. As opposed to the centrifugal pump and ECLS, patients can be extubated and can have limited mobility, such as transfer from bed to chair or dangling of the legs from the bed.

CANNULATION

The cannulas are constructed from polyvinyl chloride and have a velour body sleeve that is tunneled subcutaneously and is designed to promote hemostasis and tissue ingrowth at the exit sites. Three sizes of wire-reinforced inflow cannulas are commercially available (Fig. 17-7). These include a 32F right-angle light-house tip, a 36F malleable cannula with an adjustable backbone, and a 42F right-angle light-house tip cannula.

Arterial cannulas are made of same material but have a precoated Dacron graft attached to the end (Fig. 17-7). They are available in two sizes and are sewn in an end-to-side fashion: a 10-mm graft for anastomosis to the smaller and lower-resistance pulmonary artery and a 12-mm graft for anastomosis to the ascending aorta.

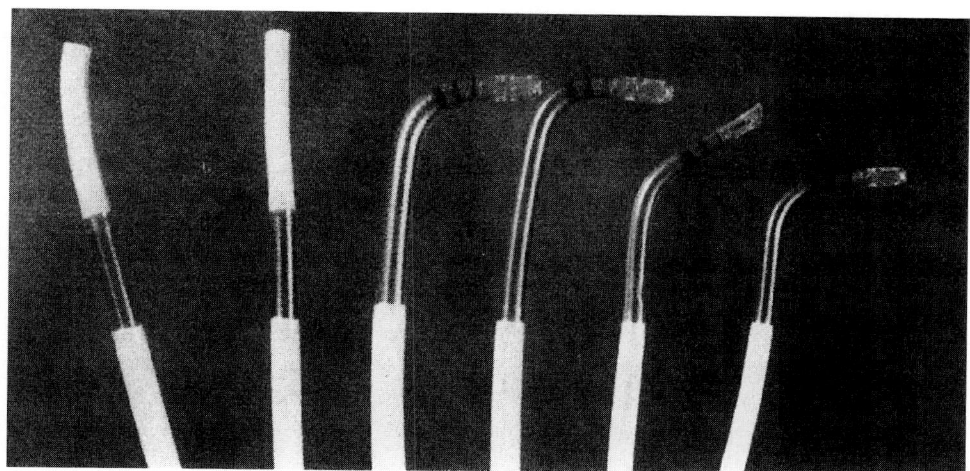

FIGURE 17–7 Inflow and outflow cannulas for the ABIOMED system. The arterial grafts have a Dacron graft at the end for direct end-to-side anastomosis to the aorta or pulmonary artery. The inflow cannulas are either in a right-angle configuration or with a malleable backbone that can be adjusted to the desired angle.

Careful cannula insertion is important for optimal performance. Venous inflow must be unimpeded and outflow grafts must not be kinked. In addition, careful consideration must be given to cannula position when bypass grafts are crossing the epicardial surface of the heart. Depending on the location of these grafts, these cannulas must be placed such that graft compression does not occur. The three-dimensional layout of this geometry needs to be visualized and thought out in advance, particularly if chest closure is planned. Any graft compression will make recovery unlikely if at all possible.

It is technically much easier to use cardiopulmonary bypass for placement of these cannulas, although off-pump insertion is possible and may be preferable in certain clinical situations, particularly for isolated right-sided support.[126] A side-biting clamp is typically used on the aorta to perform the outflow anastomosis. If the patient is on cardiopulmonary bypass, the pulmonary artery anastomosis can be done without the need of a partial cross-clamp. The length of the graft is measured from the anticipated skin exit site to the site of anastomosis, and the Dacron graft is cut to the appropriate length so that there is no excessive tension or any kinking. The cutaneous exit site is planned so that approximately 2 cm of the velour cuff is extending from the skin and the remainder is in the subcutaneous tunnel. The cannula is not tunneled subcutaneously until after completion of the anastomosis. For the aortic anastomosis, incorporation of a Teflon or pericardial strip will help control suture-line bleeding.

Although cannulation for right ventricular outflow is most commonly constructed so that the cannula with the 10-mm Dacron graft is sewn to the pulmonary artery, we prefer an alternative quicker technique that has been recently reported.[127] Two concentric pledgeted purse-string sutures are placed along the right ventricular outflow tract anteriorly. The 36F straight atrial cannula is then introduced in the right ventricular outflow tract through a cruciate incision and directed through the pulmonary valve into the main pulmonary artery. Cannula position is confirmed by palpation and purse strings are tightened and secured with snares. This is an easy, reproducible, and quick technique for RVAD outflow placement and is a useful technique in situations where access to the pulmonary artery is difficult because of scarring or poor visualization. In addition, RVAD placement can be performed without the need for CPB. If this technique is used, the cannula must be externalized from the skin prior to insertion into the pulmonary artery.

For inflow cannulation, a double-pledgeted purse-string suture using 3-0 polypropylene is placed concentrically for cannula placement. Tourniquets must be firmly secured to prevent inadvertent loosening of the purse string and bleeding from the insertion sites. In addition, the heart is generally volume loaded to prevent air embolism during insertion.

For right-sided support, we usually use the 42F right-angle cannula for drainage from the midatrial wall with the cannula directed to the IVC. For left-sided drainage, several options are available. The 36F malleable cannula is used because it provides the versatility to accomodate variations in anatomy and clinical conditions. Left atrial cannulation can be achieved via the interatrial groove, the dome of the left atrium, or the left atrial appendage. Alternatively the body of the right ventricle or the left ventricular apex may be cannulated.[128] There is no need to excise a core of the ventricular apical muscle as is common with other VADs.[129] Ventricular cannulation offers the advantages of excellent ventricular decompression, which may improve ventricular recovery,[130] but bleeding from around the cannula may also become a problem, particularly in the setting of recent myocardial infarction.

TABLE 17–5 Clinical experience with ABIOMED support for postcardiotomy cardiogenic shock

Reference	Patients (no.)	Biventricular support (%)	Mean duration of support (d)	Weaned, no. (%)	Discharged, no. (%)
Guyton[131]	31	52	4.7	17 (55)	9 (29)
Minami[160]	26	31	NR	16 (62)	3 (50)
Körfer[133]	55	NR	5.7 ± 6.9	33 (60)	27 (49)
ABIOMED post–market surveillance study registry*	876	50	5	NR	271 (31)

*Voluntary ABIOMED Registry.

NR = not reported.

Source: ABIOMED post–market surveillance study data courtesy of Diane Walsh, ABIOMED Inc, Danvers, MA.

One of the advantages of the ABIOMED is that the perfusionist can prepare and de-air the circuit while the cannulas are being placed. Connecting the cannulas to the externalized circuit is easy and can be done expeditiously.

The drive console for the ABIOMED BVS 5000 is simple to operate. The control system automatically adjusts the duration of pump diastole and systole, primarily in response to changes in preload. Pump rate and flow are visible on the display monitor. During automated operation, the device can be managed by the bedside nurse and almost never needs additional adjustments.

COMPLICATIONS

As with all patients who require postcardiotomy mechanical support, complications are frequent. Guyton[131] reported 75% bleeding complications, 54% respiratory failure, 52% renal failure, and 26% permanent neurologic deficit. Infection occurred in 13 patients (28%) while on the device, but only 3 cases were considered device-related. Other complications included embolism in 13%, hemolysis in 17%, and mechanical problems related to the atrial cannula site in 13% of patients.[124] No major changes in platelet count or blood chemistries occurred during the period of circulatory support.

Jett et al[128] reported on 55 patients supported on the ABIOMED for a variety of indications including postcardiotomy failure (28), failed transplant allograft (8), acute myocardial infarction (2), and myocarditis (1). They reported a 40% incidence of bleeding, 50% respiratory complications, and 25% neurologic complications. Marelli[126] also reported a similar incidence of complications in 19 status I patients with 6 developing renal failure, 9 reexplored for bleeding, and 3 dying of sepsis and multisystem organ failure. As with all acute mechanical support systems, these relatively high complication rates are a reflection of the significant preexisting hemodynamic insult that occurs, necessitating implementation of mechanical support. Early device insertion should be considered and may improve overall outcome.[87]

RESULTS

The ABIOMED system is available in over 550 U.S centers, with over 5000 patients supported to date. Results from several reports are summarized in Table 17-5. In a multicenter study, Guyton[131] reported 55% of postcardiotomy patients were weaned from support and 29% were discharged from the hospital. However, 47% of patients who had not experienced cardiac arrest before being placed on circulatory support were discharged. Of 14 patients who had presupport cardiac arrest, only 1 (7%) was discharged. In another report of 500 patients treated with the BVS 5000 system, which included 265 (53%) who could not be weaned from cardiopulmonary bypass, 27% of patients were discharged from the hospital.[132] Recent data utilizing this device in a wide range of clinical situations, including postcardiotomy failure, have reported successful weaning in 83% and discharge to home for 45% of patients.[129] These excellent results are also repoted by Marelli[126] in 14 of 19 patients who were weaned or transplanted with a 1-year survival of 79%. Korfer[133] also recently reported 50% hospital discharge in 50 postcardiotomy patients supported with the ABIOMED, and 7 of 14 patients transplanted with a 1-year survival of 86%. The ABIOMED Worldwide registry experience suggests that that better results can be expected from experienced heart transplant programs.[134] In fact, early transfer of patients from smaller facilities (the "spokes") to transplant centers (the "hub") has been shown to result in improved overall survival.[6]

Thoratec Ventricular Assist Device

The Thoratec VAD (Thoratec Laboratories Corp., Berkeley, CA) was introduced clinically in 1976 under an investigational device exemption (IDE) and was approved as a bridge to heart transplantation in 1996. Although it was first used clinically in 1982 for postcardiotomy support, only recently has it been approved for use as a temporary cardiac assist device. As such, it is the only device currently available that bridges the gap between short- and long-term devices. The advantage of this concept is that it allows the device to be

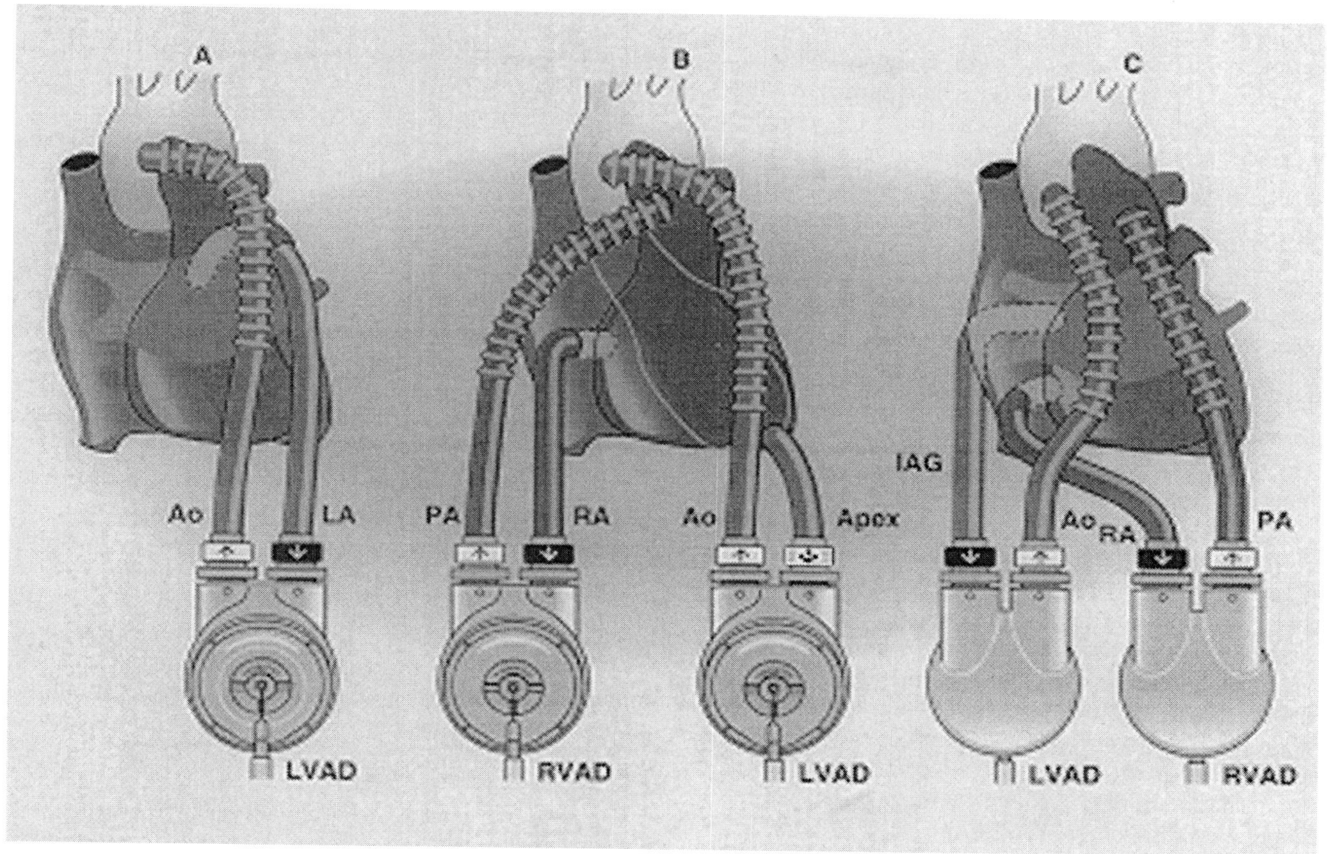

FIGURE 17–8 The Thoratec device shown here can be placed in a variety of positions for support of one or both ventricles. (A) Cannulation of the left atrial appendage. (B) Cannulation of the left ventricular apex. (C) Cannulation of the interatrial groove. (*Courtesy of Nancy E. Olson, Thoratec Corporation.*)

implanted initially with the intent of myocardial recovery, particularly in the postcardiotomy heart failure setting. If myocardial recovery does not occur, then the device can be used long term until a suitable heart becomes available for transplantation. Although this concept is desirable and offers the advantage of avoiding a second operation for transitioning from a temporary support device (bridge to bridge) to a more chronic device (see below), it comes at increased expense (because of the higher price of the pumps) and can also create ethical dilemmas if the patient recovers but is not a transplant candidate.

The device is a pneumatically driven pulsatile pump that contains two polyurethane, seamless bladders within a rigid housing.[135] The inlet and outlet ports contain Bjork-Shiley convexo-concave tilting disc valves to provide unidirectional flow. The effective stroke volume of each prosthetic ventricle is 65 mL. The pneumatic drive console applies alternating negative and positive pressures to fill and empty each prosthetic bladder. Driveline vacuum and positive pressures can be adjusted to improve filling and to improve systemic arterial pressure. The pump eject time (equivalent of ventricular systole) also can be adjusted depending on preload and afterload conditions. One or both pumps may be used to provide univentricular (LVAD or RVAD) or biventricular support (BVAD).

The prosthetic ventricles are placed on the upper abdomen (Fig. 17-8) and are connected to the heart and great vessels by large bore, wire-wrapped, polyurethane cannulas that traverse the chest wall.[136,137] The cannulas are connected to a large console via pneumatic drivelines. The pumps can be operated in three control modes. The fixed rate mode operates independently of the patient's heart, and the operator sets the rate. In the external synchronous mode, the pump empties when triggered by the patient's R-wave on the electrocardiogram. The usual mode for most patients is the full to empty mode in which ejection occurs when the device senses that the prosthetic ventricle is filled. In this volume mode, heart rate is determined by the rate of prosthetic ventricular filling.

Unlike the ABIOMED BVS 5000, the Thoratec pump resides on the upper abdominal wall and is connected to a large, wheeled console containing compressed air tanks. Patients may be ambulatory, but the large console and external configuration of the drive tubes and cannulas make ambulation more difficult, but unlike continuous flow pumps, possible. A smaller portable console is also available for outpatient management in patients that are bridged to recovery.

CANNULATION

The device implantation is typically performed on cardiopulmonary bypass. Recently, a method has been described for off-pump insertion as a right ventricular assist device.[138] As with the ABIOMED, it is important to carefully select the cannula position and cutaneous exit sites. The pump should be planned to rest on the anterior abdominal wall. Lateral placement may lead to excessive tension at the skin exit sites and prevent a seal from being formed. Approximately 1.5 to 2 cm of the felt covering of the cannulas must extend beyond the skin exit site with the remainder in the subcutaneous tunnel to promote ingrowth of tissue and create a seal. The length of the cannulas extending out must be adjusted based on the length of the atrial cannula (if one is used). The end of the atrial cannula widens out to connect to the inflow port of the device and therefore cannot be trimmed. On the other hand, ventricular or outflow cannulas can be trimmed to adjust the length.

The outflow cannula is generally attached first. The arterial cannulas are available with a 14-mm Dacron graft (for the pulmonary artery) or an 18-mm Dacron graft (for the aorta), and must be cut to length after the appropriate exit site has been selected. They come in two lengths, 15 cm and 18 cm, which are again selected based on the patient's anatomy and the planned exit site. The graft is generally sewn on the aorta or pulmonary artery after applying a partial occluding clamp, and sewn with 4-0 polypropylene suture with or without a strip of pericardium or Teflon felt for reinforcement. An alternative technique for pulmonary outflow has been described.[138] This technique involves placement of pledget-reinforced 3-0 polypropylene suture anteriorly over the right ventricular outflow. The right-angle atrial inflow cannula is then immersed in hot water and straightened. This cannula is inserted through a stab incision in the right ventricular outflow tract and directed through the pulmonary valve into the main pulmonary artery. This method of cannula insertion has not been widely reported.

Inflow can be accomplished by cannulation of the atria or the ventricles.[139] All cannulations are generally reinforced with a double layer of pledgeted concentric purse strings. For atrial cannulation, a 51F right-angle cannula is available in two lengths, 25 cm and 30 cm. For the left atrium, the cannula is inserted throught the atrial appendage, the interatrial groove, or the superior dome of the left atrium. For right atrial cannulation, the cannula is inserted into the middle right atrial wall and directed towards the inferior vena cava. If this cannula is inserted towards the tricuspid valve, the leaflets may interfere with proper inflow as they get sucked into the cannula during negative pressure. In addition, if the tip is not advanced to reside properly in the right atrium, negative pressure can intermittently cause the compliant right atrial wall to collapse around the cannula and interfere with proper filling of the pump.

An alternative approach can use the ventricles for inflow cannulation.[138,139] This provides better drainage, higher flows, and perhaps improves the chance of myocardial recovery. This is achieved by placing a concentric layer of pledgeted horizontal mattress sutures at the apex of the left ventricle or the acute margin of the right ventricle (superior to the posterior descending artery). The cannulas used for this purpose can be either the blunt-tip 27-cm straight ventricular tube or the smooth-tipped, beveled 20-cm ventricular tube. The previously placed sutures are sequentially passed through the cuff, the apex of the heart is elevated, and the mean arterial pressure at the aorta is maintained over 70 mm Hg to prevent air embolization during cannula insertion. Either a core of tissue is removed or a cruciate incision is made with care not to cut any of the mattress sutures. The cannula is then inserted and secured by tying the sutures. The free end can then be directed out through the previously planned cutaneous exit site and a tubing clamp is placed on it.

INITIATION OF SUPPORT

Connecting the cannulas to the pump is difficult and must be done with care. The connections to the pump have a sharp beveled edge that should be carefully directed under gentle pressure to fit the cannulas without damaging the inner surface of the tube. In addition, if this tip bends, it may provide a nidus for thrombus formation. The inflow cannula is typically connected first. Prior to connecting the outflow cannula, a purse string is placed on the outflow Dacron graft and a 5F to 7F vascular catheter with an aspiration port is introduced through it and directed into the pump chamber through the outflow valve. This maneuver is critical because de-airing can be difficult as a result of the way the pump sits on the abdomen. The outflow cannula is then connected. Prior to releasing the tubing clamps and flooding the chamber with blood, the air in the chamber is aspirated. Once all the air is evacuated, the de-airing catheter and the inflow tubing clamp are removed, allowing the chamber to fill with blood. Then gentle hand pumping can be performed to ensure complete air evacuation through the opening in the Dacron graft prior to removing the outflow tubing clamp.

We slowly come off cardiopulmonary bypass before starting the pump. This ensures complete filling of the chambers to minimize the possibility of air being introduced into the circuit by the negative pressure of the pump. If a BVAD is in place, we start the LVAD first and then the RVAD. The pump

TABLE 17–6 Pre-market approval experience with Thoratec support for the management of postcardiotomy cardiogenic shock

Variable	Primary cohort*	Posttransplant†	Delayed‡
Demographics:			
Patients (no.)	29	9	15
Men (%)	79	89	80
Age (y):			
Mean	52	49	51
Range	38-66	25-66	23-68
Configuration, no. (%)			
LVAD	14 (48)	0 (0)	3 (20)
RVAD	9 (0)	3 (33)	4 (27)
BVAD	15 (52)	6 (67)	8 (53)
Length of support (d):			
Mean	12	10.3	14.5
Range	0-80	2-26	0-42
Outcome, no. (%)			
Weaned and discharged	10/29 (35)	4 (44)	1 (7)
Alive with device	0 (0)	0 (0)	0 (0)
Dead	19 (65)	5 (56)	14 (93)

*Met all the study inclusion and exclusion criteria for weaning from bypass.

†An additional group of transplant recipients who needed a ventricular assist device immediately after cardiopulmonary bypass.

‡Delayed use (patients left the operating room and came back later because of postcardiotomy cardiogenic shock; they did not meet the study criteria).

BVAD = biventricular assist device; LVAD = left ventricular assist device; RVAD = right ventricular assist device.

Source: Data courtesy of Nancy Olson, Thoratec Inc.

is begun in the fixed rate mode and negative pressure is set low at –5 to –10 mm Hg. The inflow sites should also be covered with saline. Driveline pressure and and systolic duration can be adjusted to optimize pump flows. Additional refinements can be done once the chest is closed.

COMPLICATIONS

The complications reported for the bridge to transplantation are similar to those reported for postcardiotomy patients. In a multicenter trial the most common complications were bleeding in 42%, renal failure in 36%, infection in 36%, neurologic events in 22%, and multisystem organ failure in 16% of patients.[135] Similar complications have been reported from other centers.[135,140,141]

RESULTS

Most temporary use of the Thoratec VAD is for postcardiotomy patients, but the device has also been used for patients after myocardial infarction and during cardiac transplant rejection.[135,142,143] The Thoratec pump has also been used to support a patient with myocarditis who eventually recovered adequate native heart function.[144] After cardiotomy, results are similar to those obtained with continuous flow devices and the ABIOMED BVS 5000. In a review of 145 patients with nonbridge use of the Thoratec device, 37% of patients were weaned and 21% were discharged.[71] More experienced centers have achieved hospital survival rates over 40%.[142,143] Renal failure and myocardial infarction are poor prognostic events for survival.[131]

The Thoratec pre–market approval experience (Table 17-6) for the treatment of 53 patients with postcardiotomy heart failure had an in-hospital survival of 28%. The majority of these patients were supported with a BVAD. The Bad Oeynhausen group, however, has reported a 60% survival for postcardiotomy patients supported with the Thoratec device.[133,145] Clearly the greatest advantage that the Thoratec device offers is that it can be applied for longer duration of support than any other temporary device mentioned previously. This feature may be uniquely advantageous particularly because the duration of support necessary is usually unclear in advance. All other devices mentioned have an increasing complication rate with a longer duration of support. Furthermore, the Thoratec device allows for physical rehabilitation and ambulation of the patients during the recovery period.

BRIDGE TO BRIDGE OR BRIDGE TO HEART TRANSPLANTATION

ECLS is a unique system with many advantages that allow for rapid establishment of circulatory support by peripheral cannulation. The system is simple, relatively cheap, easy to assemble rapidly, and very portable. In addition, there is no need for operating room sternotomy because of the capability for both cardiac and respiratory support through peripheral cannulation. As a result, ECLS is used as a lifesaving option in patients with hemodynamic collapse who initially are not known to be candidates for cardiac transplantation and therefore have a need for more chronic VAD support.[119,146] The patients who are candidates for ECLS include those who present with massive myocardial infarction who remain in cardiogenic shock despite inotropic support and IABP counterpulsation, those with chronic heart failure with acute decompensation, and those in cardiac arrest. Improved results with implantable ventricular assist devices has prompted the implementation of strategies using ECLS as a means to rapidly establish circulatory support to maintain hemodynamics as transplant evaluation is initiated and neurologic status is determined. This strategy is aimed at maximizing patient survival, and limiting the duration of support with temporary assist devices by early transition to a chronic VAD (bridge to bridge) that would allow patient rehabilitation and eventual transplantation. Furthermore, implantation of expensive LVADs is avoided in patients who may have already suffered from the sequelae of multisystem organ failure and are known to have a poor outcome.[147] Pagani recently reported the results of 33 patients with primary cardiac failure who were placed on ECLS.[146] The etiology was ischemic in 58%, nonischemic in 30%, and postcardiotomy in 12%. Overall, 73% of their patients were in cardiac arrest or had experienced a cardiac arrest within 15 to 30 min of initiation of ECLS. Ten patients who were transplant candidates and could not be weaned from ECLS were bridged to an LVAD. Six patients were transplanted and discharged, 2 were alive on the LVAD awaiting transplantation, and 2 died. Overall, ECLS was discontinued in 27% of patients because of absolute contraindication to transplantation, primarily because of neurologic injury. However, 80% of patients transitioned to an LVAD survived. This aggressive strategy and remarkable survival is secondary to selection of patients who are most likely to survive at the expense of more initial deaths on ECLS. If the entire group of patients in this study are considered, only 36% survived to discharge. Interestingly, the need for RVAD support in the group of patients with ECLS as a bridge strategy was 40%, significantly higher than the 10% reported for patients who receive LVADS as the initial device. This may be secondary to the inflammatory response to ECLS and associated increase in pulmonary vascular resistance.[148,149] On the other hand, an increased frequency of multisystem organ failure may lead to a greater need for perioperative biventricular support.[150–152]

Similar improved results have been reported from the Cleveland Clinic, in which 18 of 107 postcardiotomy patients who were appropriate transplant candidates were converted to an LVAD.[124] Of these, 72% survived to transplantation and 92% were alive at 1 year. The successful use of LVADs for postcardiotomy support has also been reported by DeRose in a group of 12 patients.[153] LVAD support was converted to a HeartMate Assist device at a mean of 3.5 days. Of these 8 were transplanted, and 1 was explanted with an overall survival of 75%.

Korfer et al also reported on 68 patients supported with the ABIOMED BVS 5000 system.[133] The majority of these patients were postcardiotomy, with 32 being weaned, and 13 transplanted. Overall survival was 47%. More recently, Korfer reported on 17 patients with postcardiotomy shock who received the Thoratec device. In this group 7 were transplanted and 1 successfully weaned for an overall survival of 47.[145]

Device Selection

To date, insufficient data exist to recommend one device over the other for patients who require temporary mechanical support. The particular device used is often based on availability rather than science. Currently, the majority of heart centers use the ABIOMED BVS 5000 as their primary means of short-term cardiac support.

For centers with multiple devices, patient presentation and cardiopulmonary status will determine the device selected. Patients undergoing cardiopulmonary resuscitation are best serviced by urgent femoral cannulation. This avoids the time delay of transportation and sternotomy. Patients with severe hypoxia and lung injury either from aspiration or pulmonary edema benefit from the oxygenation and lung rest provided with ECMO. Oxygenators have been added to the ABIOMED system but they add substantial afterload to the system and reduce the flow.

For postcardiotomy support all devices have been used with similar success. The Thoratec system is the most versatile, providing both short- and long-term support. If a bridge to bridge strategy is utilized, we prefer ECLS followed by implantation of the TCI HeartMate. Typically, patients are supported on ECLS for 48 to 72 hours while transplant evaluation is completed. They are then transitioned to the HeartMate if myocardial recovery has failed. This approach avoids the high-risk emergency heart transplantation and provides the time necessary for improved organ function.

The best device for acute myocardial infarctions or myocarditis remains uncertain. For fulminant myocarditis the device least traumatic to the heart is advisable, as recovery is likely. Transplantation is more likely for more indolent myocarditis or for giant cell myocarditis, and a chronic implantable system or the Thoratec device may be the best choice. Whether earlier support or direct LV drainage will improve recovery in the setting of an acute MI is unknown.

Patient Management

The ultimate goal is to maintain optimal perfusion of all end-organs, to allow time for recovery from an acute hemodynamic insult, and to prevent further deterioration of organ function. Ideally, pump flow would achieve mixed venous saturation greater than 70%. Low-flow states can often be corrected by intravascular volume expansion. With centrifugal pumps and ECMO, pump speed can be adjusted to control flow and allow some degree of cardiac ejection to decrease the likelihood of stasis and intracardiac thrombus formation. Increasing flow rates by using excessive pump speeds can also cause significant hemolysis. Fluid administration to expand intravascular volume is the best way to increase flow. However, right heart failure may also manifest as a low-flow state in presence of low pulmonary artery pressures. This condition usually requires the institution of right-sided circulatory support and is associated with a lower overall survival.

VENTILATORY SUPPORT

We use pressure-controlled ventilation to maintain peak inspiratory pressures below 35 cm H_2O at tidal volumes of

8 to 10 mL/kg. Inspired oxygen is set initially at 100% with a positive end-expiratory pressure of 5 cm H_2O. Fractional inspired oxygen is then gradually decreased to less than 50% with partial pressure of oxygen maintained between 85 and 100 mm Hg. These measures are instituted to diminish the deleterious effect of barotrauma and oxygen toxicity in the setting of lung injury.

ANTICOAGULATION

Anticoagulation should be done judiciously to balance excessive risk of bleeding against clot formation in the pump. Platelet counts decrease within the first 24 hours of support; therefore, counts are monitored every 8 hours and we routinely transfuse platelets to maintain counts over 50,000/mm^3 during routine support and above 100,000/mm^3 if bleeding is present. Fresh frozen plasma and cryoprecipitate are given to control coagulopathy and maintain fibrinogen greater than 250 mg/dL and also replace other coagulation factors consumed by the circuit. Although other institutions have reported on the use of plasminogen inhibitors such as aminocaproic acid and aprotinin to decrease fibrinolysis,[154] we have not routinely used these drugs because of concern for thrombus formation. In most cases heparin infusion is started soon after adequate hemostasis is present. Anticoagulation is achieved by systemic heparinization with a continuous infusion starting at 8 to 10 U/kg/h and titrated to maintain PTT between 45 and 55 seconds. For ECMO, in most cases heparin infusion is started within 24 hours if used in the postcardiotomy setting but sooner in patients without a sternotomy.

FLUID MANAGEMENT

Patients are aggressively diuresed while on support to minimize third space fluid accumulations. If response to diuretic therapy is suboptimal because of renal insufficiency, we use a hemofilter/dialyzer spliced into the arterial or venous limb of the circuit if feasible. Otherwise, we use continuous venovenous hemodialysis (CVVHD). This system permits control over fluid balance by continuous ultrafiltration that can be adjusted for volume removal and also allows for dialysis as needed.

NEUROLOGIC MONITORING

Patients are sedated with fentanyl or propofol infusion to maintain comfort. Muscle paralysis is utilized as needed to decrease the energy expenditure and to decrease chest wall stiffness to allow for optimal adjustment of the ventilation parameters. All patients are periodically assessed off sedation to establish neurologic function. Response to simple commands, ability to move all extremities, and spontaneous eye movements are used as gross indications of intact sensorium. A low threshold of obtaining CT scans of the head is exercised if any change is noted or index of suspicion is high.

WEANING

A weaning trial is usually attempted after 48 to 72 hours of support. It is critical not to rush weaning and to allow time for myocardial as well as end-organ recovery. The principle of weaning is common to all devices and all have various controls available that allow reduction of flow, thereby enabling more work to be performed by the heart. Flow is gradually reduced at increments of 0.5 to 1 L/min. Adequate anticoagulation is critical during this low-flow phase to prevent pump thrombosis, and in general it is not recommended to reduce flow to less than 2.0 L/min for a prolonged period. We add additional heparin during this period to maintain ACT above 300 seconds. With optimal pharmacologic support, and continuous TEE evaluation of ventricular function, flows are reduced while monitoring systemic blood pressure, cardiac index, pulmonary pressures, and ventricular size. Maintenance of cardiac index and low pulmonary pressures with preserved LV function by echo suggests weaning is likely. A failed attempt at weaning results in resumption of full flow. Absence of ventricular recovery after several wean attempts is a poor prognostic sign. Patients who are transplant candidates undergo a full evaluation and subsequently are staged to a long-term ventricular assist device as a bridge to cardiac transplantation. We and others have found that early conversion to chronic ventricular support is beneficial and improves the low survival that is associated with cardiogenic shock, particularly in the postcardiotomy setting.[119,124,133,153]

SUMMARY OF COMPLICATIONS AND RESULTS

Duration of Support

Complications tend to increase with increasing length of support. Therefore, in general, these devices are used for less than 2 weeks but longer durations have been reported (Table 17-7). An exception to this general rule is the Thoratec device, which can be used for a longer period until cardiac transplantation. The longest reported duration of support with this device is 365 days. Table 17-8 summarizes the indications for which temporary support has been implemented.

TABLE 17–7 Duration of support with temporary assist devices

Device	Median support (d)	Range (d)
Centrifugal pump	2.3	1-14
ECMO	2.5	1-9
ABIOMED	5.6	1-81
Thoratec	42.0	6-365

TABLE 17–8 Indications that temporary device support has been used for acute cardiogenic shock

Postcardiotomy pump failure
Acute myocardial infarction
Decompensated heart failure
Post–cardiac transplantation allograft dysfunction
Acute myocarditis
Deterioration during cardiac catheterization procedures
Right ventricular failure after LVAD placement
Cardiac arrest
Massive pulmonary embolism

Complications

At present all current devices are thrombogenic and require anticoagulation. The delicate balance between overanticoagulation resulting in bleeding versus inadequate anticoagulation and thromboembolism is a major determinant of morbidity.

BLEEDING

During the acute phase, bleeding remains a significant problem, occurring at suture lines and cannulation sites, or often consists of a diffuse coagulopathy that becomes difficult to localize. The high incidence is partly because of the hemostatic disarray associated with the operation, the low-flow physiologic state that necessitates pump placement, and the need for anticoagulation early in the course of support. In general, this translates into a large transfusion requirement that can be detrimental in terms of problems with transfusion reactions, increases in pulmonary vascular resistance, and importantly increased sensitization of patients who may later require transplantation. The need for rapid transfusion often prohibits the use of filters that generally slow the rate of infusion. Golding has reported severe bleeding in 87% of patients supported with centrifugal pumps with a mean transfusion requirement of 53 units of blood.[97] We have seen a median transfusion requirement of 14 units (range 1 to 99) using ECMO.[85]

The use of heparin-coated circuits has failed to reduce the coagulopathy and bleeding associated with ECMO effectively. However, peripheral cannulation with ECMO for acute support is associated with less bleeding than transthoracic approaches in the postcardiotomy setting. Similarly, with the ABIOMED and Thoratec devices, the incidence of bleeding has been as high as 27%.[89,131]

THROMBOEMBOLISM

Despite the development of heparin-coated systems, the incidence of thromboembolism remains a constant threat. Thrombin deposition in centrifugal pumps with increasing duration of support is a well-known phenomenon. Golding reported thromboembolism in 12.7% of 91 patients supported with centrifugal pump for postcardiotomy pump failure.[97] In 202 adult patients supported with ECMO, pumphead thrombus was noted in 5% and neurologic complications occurred in 29%.[85] Both factors were found to have a profound negative impact on survival or ability to be weaned from support. Similarly, thromboembolic incidence of 8% and 13% has been reported for the Thoratec and ABIOMED, respectively. These numbers may underestimate the actual number of thromboembolic episodes. Curtis et al reported autopsy results in 8 patients who had no clinical evidence of thromboembolism. In this group, 5 (63%) were found to have evidence of acute thromboembolic infarction in the cerebral, pulmonary, and system territories.[155]

Weaning and Survival

There are currently no data to indicate that one device is superior over another in terms of weaning and survival. Published reports suggest that weaning can be accomplished in approximately 45% to 60% of patients; however, survival overall is less than 30% with only 50% of weaned patients discharged alive from the hospital. Reports on long-term follow-up in this group are unavailable. The Cleveland Clinic recently demonstrated in a cohort of patients supported on ECMO that the high early attrition rate diminishes rapidly within 6 months of ECMO removal, and 65% of patients discharged are alive at 5 years.[85] Risk factors associated with increased mortality have included age older than 60 years, emergency operations, reoperations, renal insufficiency, and preexisting left ventricular dysfunction. In all series, sepsis, multisystem organ failure, and neurologic complications stand out as the causes of death.

This overall static survival rate in reported series over the last decade has seen significant improvement at transplant and assist centers where appropriate transplant candidates are bridged to transplantation after a period of support. In the Cleveland Clinic experience, ECMO support has been converted to an implantable LVAD in 18 patients.[85] Of these, 72% survived to transplant with 92% 1-year survival. DeRose et al have described the successful use of an implantable LVAD for postcardiotomy support in a group of 12 patients after elective or emergency coronary artery grafting requiring IABP, Bio-Medicus, or ABIOMED LVAD support.[153] All were converted to the TCI HeartMate at a mean of 3.5 days. Of these, 9 were transplanted, 1 was explanted, and all discharged for an overall survival of 75%. Similar results have been described by Korfer.[133] In their experience with 68 patients supported with the ABIOMED BVS 5000, the majority with postcardiotomy failure, 32 were weaned and 13 patients transplanted with an overall survival of 47%. Thoratec VADS was used in another 17 patients at their institution for postcardiotomy support with 8 survivors (47%), 7 patients transplanted, and 1 successfully weaned.

CONCLUSION

Currently a number of options exist for temporary circulatory support, and with advances in technology the number of devices will expand. Each device has advantages and disadvantages and to date none satisfy all the requirements of an ideal device. We have clearly learned many lessons that should direct the development of systems and strategies that maximize survival and reduce complications. In this arena, better understanding of the host inflammatory response, appreciation of the induced derangement in the coagulation cascade, and development of systems that do not require anticoagulation should improve overall outcomes. In addition, development of therapies that alter the reperfusion injury and preserve organ function is important. Agents that affect the inflammatory response in general, such as steroids, aprotinin, and plasmapheresis, or more specific blockades such as leukocyte depletion or direct cytokine inhibition, will need evaluation.

Risk analysis has also taught us that patients requiring postcardiotomy support generally fit into a particular profile. Specifically, these are patients who require emergency operations, have poor ventricular reserve, are older, and have extensive atherosclerotic coronary disease and preexisting renal dysfunction. Preoperative awareness should prompt maximization of medical pharmacologic support and the readiness to implement mechanical devices early in the face of cardiac pump failure.

REFERENCES

1. Mehta SM, Aufiero TX, Pae WE, et al: Results of mechanical ventricular assistance for the treatment of postcardiotomy cardiogenic shock. *ASAIO J* 1996; 42:211.
2. Pae WE Jr, Miller CA, Matthews Y, et al: Ventricular assist devices for postcardiotomy cardiogenic shock: a combined registry experience. *J Thorac Cardiovasc Surg* 1992; 104:541.
3. Torchiana DF, Hirsch G, Buckley MJ, et al: Intraaortic balloon pumping for cardiac support: trends in practice and outcome, 1968 to 1995. *J Thorac Cardiovasc Surg* 1997; 113:758.
4. Goldberg RJ, Gore JM, Alpert JS, et al: Cardiogenic shock after acute myocardial infarction. *N Engl J Med* 1991; 325:1117.
5. Hochman JS, Sleeper LA, Webb JG, et al: Early revascularization in acute myocardial infarction complicated by cardiogenic shock. *N Engl J Med* 1999; 341:625.
6. Helman DN, Morales DL, Edwards NM, et al: Left ventricular assist device bridge to transplant network improves survival after failed cardiotomy. *Circulation* 1999; 68:1187.
7. Kantrowitz A, Kantrowitz A: Experimental augmentation of coronary flow by retardation of arterial pressure pulse. *Surgery* 1953; 34:678.
8. Kantrowitz A: Origins of intraaortic balloon pumping. *Ann Thorac Surg* 1990; 50:672.
9. Kantrowitz A, McKinnon WMP: Experimental use of diaphragm as auxiliary myocardium. *Surg Forum* 1958; 9:266.
10. Clauss RH, Birtwell WC, Albertal G, et al: Assisted circulation, I: the arterial counterpulsator. *J Thorac Cardiovas Surg* 1961; 41:447.
11. Moulopoulos SD, Topaz S, Kolff WJ: Diastolic balloon pumping (with carbon dioxide) in the aorta—a mechanical assistance to the failing circulation. *Am Heart J* 1962; 63:669.
12. Kantrowitz A, Tjonneland S, Freed PS, et al: Initial clinical experience with intraaortic balloon pumping in cardiogenic shock. *JAMA* 1968; 203:135.
13. Weber KT, Janicki JS: Intraaortic balloon counterpulsation. *Ann Thorac Surg* 1974; 17:602.
14. Powell WJ Jr, Daggett WM, Magro AE, et al: Effects of intraaortic balloon counterpulsation on cardiac performance, oxygen consumption, and coronary blood flow in dogs. *Circ Res* 1970; 26:753.
15. Bolooki H: The effects of counterpulsation with an intra-aortic balloon on cardiovascular dynamics and metabolism, in Bolooki H (ed): *Clinical Application of Intra-aortic Balloon Pump*. New York, Futura, 1977; p 13.
16. Urschel CW, Eber L, Forrester J, et al: Alteration of mechanical performance of the ventricle by intraaortic balloon counterpulsation. *Am J Cardiol* 1970; 25:546.
17. Dunkman WB, Leinbach RC, Buckley MJ, et al: Clinical and hemodynamic results of intraaortic balloon pumping and surgery for cardiogenic shock. *Circulation* 1972; 42:465.
18. Fuchs RM, Brin KP, Brinker JA, et al: Augmentation of regional coronary blood flow by intra-aortic balloon counterpulsation in patients with unstable angina. *Circulation* 1983; 68:117.
19. Gundel WD, Brown BG, Gott VL: Coronary collateral flow studies during variable aortic root pressure waveforms. *J Appl Physiol* 1970; 29:579.
20. Buckley MJ, Leinbach RC, Kastor JA, et al: Hemodynamic evaluation of intra-aortic balloon pumping in man. *Circulation* 1970; 42 (suppl II):II130.
21. Scheidt S, Wilner G, Mueller H, et al: Intra-aortic balloon counterpulsation in cardiogenic shock. *New Engl J Med* 1973; 288:979.
22. Rose EA, Marrin CAS, Bregman D, et al: Left ventricular mechanics of counterpulsation and left heart bypass, individually and in combination. *J Thorac Cardiovasc Surg* 1979; 77:127.
23. Mueller H, Ayres SA, Giannelli S, et al: Effect of isoproterenol, l-norepinephrine and intraaortic counterpulsation on hemodynamics and myocardial metabolism in shock following acute myocardial infarction. *Circulation* 1972; 45:335.
24. Graham TP Jr, Covell JW, Sonnenblick EH, et al: Control of myocardial oxygen consumption: relative influence of contractile state and tension development. *J Clin Invest* 1968; 47:375.
25. Weber KT, Janicki JS: Myocardial oxygen consumption: the role of wall force and shortening. *Am J Physiol* 1977; 233:H421.
26. Suga J, Hisano R, Hirata S, et al: Mechanism of higher oxygen consumption rate: pressure-loaded vs. volume-loaded heart. *Am J Physiol* 1982; 242:H942.
27. Katz ES, Tunick PA, Kronzon I: Observations of coronary flow augmentation and balloon function during intraaortic balloon counterpulsation using transesophageal echocardiography. *Am J Cardiol* 1992; 69:1635.
28. Weber KT, Janicki JS: Coronary collateral flow and intraaortic balloon counterpulsation. *Trans Am Soc Artif Intern Organs* 1973; 19:395.
29. Feola M, Adachi M, Akers WW, et al: Intraaortic balloon pumping in the experimantal animal. *Am J Cardiol* 1971; 27:129.
30. Weber KT, Janicki JS, Walker AA: Intra-aortic balloon pumping: an analysis of several variables affecting balloon performance. *Trans Am Soc Artif Org* 1972; 17:486.
31. Kern MJ, Aguirre FV, Tatineni S, et al: Enhanced coronary blood flow velocity during intraaortic balloon counterpulsation in critically ill patients. *J Am Coll Cardiol* 1993; 21:359.
32. Tedoriya T, Akemoto K, Imai T, et al: The effects of blood flows of coronary artery bypass grafts during intra-aortic balloon pumping. *J Cardiovasc Surg* 1994; 35 (suppl 1):99.
33. Sanfelippo PM, Baker NH, Ewy HG, et al: Experience with intraaortic balloon counterpulsation. *Ann Thorac Surg* 1986; 441:36.

34. Creswell LL, Rosenbloom R, Cox JL, et al: Intraaortic balloon counterpulsation: patterns of usage and outcome in cardiac surgery patients. *Ann Thorac Surg* 1992; 54:11.
35. Eltchaninoff H, Dimas AP, Whitlow PL: Complications associated with percutaneous placement and use of intraaortic balloon counterpulsation. *Am J Cardiol* 1993; 71:328.
36. Miller JS, Dodson TF, Sala AA, et al: Vascular complications following intra-aortic balloon pump insertion. *Am Surg* 1992; 58:232.
37. Aguirre FV, Kern MN, Back R, et al: Intraaortic balloon pump support during high-risk coronary angioplasty [review]. *Cardiology* 1994; 84:175.
38. O'Murchu B, Foreman RD, Shaw RE, et al: Role of intraaortic balloon pump counterpulsation in high risk coronary rotational atherectomy. *J Am Coll Cardiol* 1995; 26:1270.
39. Cowell RP, Paul VE, Ilsley CD: The use of intra-aortic balloon counterpulsation in malignant ventricular arrhythmias. *Int J Cardiol* 1993; 39:219.
40. Hansen EC, Levine FH, Kay HR, et al: Control of postinfarction ventricular irritability with the intra-aortic balloon pump. *Circulation* 1980; 62 (suppl I):I130.
41. Pae WE Jr, Pierce WS, Sapirstein JS: Intra-aortic balloon counterpulsation, ventricular assist pumping, and the artificial heart, in Baue AE, Geha AS, Hammond GL, et al (eds): *Glenn's Thoracic and Cardiovascular Surgery,* 6th ed. Stamford, CT, Appleton & Lange, 1995; p 1825.
42. Bavaria JE, Ratcliffe MB, Gupta KB, et al: Changes in left ventricular systolic wall stress during biventricular circulatory assistance. *Ann Thorac Surg* 1988; 45:526.
43. Bavaria JE, Furukawa S, Kreiner G: Effect of circulatory assist devices on stunned myocardium. *Ann Thorac Surg* 1990; 49:123.
44. Phillips SJ, Zeff RH, Kongtahworn C, et al: Benefits of combined balloon pumping and percutaneous cardiopulmonary bypass. *Ann Thorac Surg* 1992; 54:908.
45. Naunheim KS, Swartz MT, Pennington DG, et al: Intraaortic balloon pumping in patients requiring cardiac operations. Risk analysis and long-term follow-up. *J Thorac Cardiovasc Surg* 1992; 104:1654.
46. Waksman R, Weiss AT, Gotsman MS, et al: Intra-aortic balloon counterpulsation improves survival in cardiogenic shock complicating acute myocardial infarction. *Eur Heart J* 1993; 14:71.
47. Mueller HS: Role of intra-aortic counterpulsation in cardiogenic shock and acute myocardial infarction [review]. *Cardiology* 1994; 84:168.
48. Creswell LL, Moulton MJ, Cox JL, et al: Revascularization after acute myocardial infarction. *Ann Thorac Surg* 1995; 60:19.
49. Iverson LIG, Herfindahl, G, Ecker RR, et al: Vascular complications of intraaortic balloon counterpulsation. *Am J Surg* 1987; 154:99.
50. Makhoul RG, Cole CW, McCann RL: Vascular complications of the intra-aortic balloon pump. *Am Surg* 1993; 59:564.
51. Bolooki H: Methods of insertion of intra-aortic balloon, in Bolooki H (ed): *Clinical Application of Intra-aortic Balloon Pump.* New York, Futura 1977; p 55.
52. McBride LR, Miller LW, Naunheim KS, et al: Axillary artery insertion of an intraaortic balloon pump. *Ann Thorac Surg* 1989; 48:874.
53. Blythe D: Percutaneous axillary artery insertion of an intra-aortic balloon pump [letter]. *Anesth Intensive Care* 1995; 23:406.
54. Hazelrigg SR, Auer JE, Seifert PE: Experience in 100 transthoracic balloon pumps. *Ann Thorac Surg* 1992; 54:528.
55. Pinkard J, Utley JR, Leyland SA, et al: Relative risk of aortic and femoral insertion of intraaortic balloon pump after coronary artery bypass grafting procedures. *J Thorac Cardiovasc Surg* 1993; 105:721.
56. Macoviak J, Stephenson LW, Edmunds LH Jr, et al: The intra-aortic balloon pump: an analysis of five years' experience. *Ann Thorac Surg* 1980; 29:451.
57. Mackenzie DJ, Wagner WH, Julber DA, et al: Vascular complications of the intra-aortic balloon pump. *Am J Surg* 1992; 164:517.
58. Goldberg MJ, Rubenfire M, Kantrowitz A, et al: Intraaortic balloon pump insertion: a randomized study comparing percutaneous and surgical techniques. *J Am Coll Cardiol* 1987; 9:515.
59. Gottlieb SO, Brinker JA, Borkon AM, et al: Identification of patients at high risk for complications of intraaortic balloon counterpulsation: a multivariate risk factor analysis. *Am J Cardiol* 1984; 53:1135.
60. Phillips SJ, Tannenbaum M, Zeff RH, et al: Sheathless insertion of the percutaneous intraaortic balloon pump: an alternate method. *Ann Thorac Surg* 1992; 53:162.
61. Tatar H, Cicek S, Demirkilic U, et al: Exact positioning of intraaortic balloon catheter. *Eur J Cardiothorac Surg* 1993; 7:52.
62. Symbas PN, McKeown PP, Santora AH: Pulmonary artery balloon counterpulsation for treatment of intraoperative right ventricular failure. *Ann Thorac Surg* 1985; 39:437.
63. Moran JM, Opravil M, Gorman AJ, et al: Pulmonary artery balloon counterpulsation for right ventricular failure, II: clinical experience. *Ann Thorac Surg* 1984; 38:254.
64. Patel JJ, Kopisyansky C, Boston B, et al: Prospective evaluation of complications associated with percutaneous intraaortic balloon counterpulsation. *Am J Cardiol* 1995; 76:1205.
65. Bolooki H: Clinical and hemodynamic criteria for utilization of the intra-aortic balloon pump (IABP), in Bolooki H (ed): *Clinical Application of Intra-aortic Balloon Pump.* New York, Futura, 1977; p 47.
66. Alle KM, White GH, Harris JP, et al: Iatrogenic vascular trauma associated with intra-aortic balloon pumping: identification of risk factors. *Am Surg* 1993; 59:13.
67. Funk M, Gleason J, Foell D: Lower limb ischemia related to use of the intraaortic balloon pump. *Heart Lung* 1989; 18:542.
68. Nishida H, Koyanagi H, Abe T, et al: Comparative study of five types of IABP balloons in terms of incidence of balloon rupture and other complications: a multi-institutional study. *Artif Organs* 1994; 18:746.
69. Horowitz MD, Otero M, de Marchena EJ, et al: Intraaortic balloon entrapment. *Ann Thorac Surg* 1993; 56:368.
70. Gold JP, Cohen J, Shemin RJ, et al: Femorofemoral bypass to relieve acute leg ischemia during intra-aortic balloon pump cardiac support. *J Vasc Surg* 1986; 3:351.
71. Friedell ML, Alpert J, Parsonnet V, et al: Femorofemoral grafts for lower limb ischemia caused by intra-aortic balloon pump. *J Vasc Surg* 1987; 5:180.
72. Karalis DG, Krishnaswamy C, Victor MF, et al: Recognition and embolic potential of intraaortic atherosclerotic debris. *J Am Coll Cardiol* 1991; 17:73.
73. Maroko PR, Bernstein EF, Libby P, et al: Effects of intraaortic balloon counterpulsation on the severity of myocardial ischemic injury following acute coronary occlusion. *Circulation* 1972; 45:1150.
74. O'Rourke MF, Norris RM, Campbell TJ, et al: Randomized controlled trial of intraaortic balloon counterpulsation in early myocardial infarction with acute heart failure. *Am J Cardiol* 1981; 47:815.
75. DeWood MA, Notske RN, Hensley GR, et al: Intraaortic balloon counterpulsation with and without reperfusion for myocardial infarction shock. *Circulation* 1980; 61:1105.
76. Pierri MK, Zema M, Kligfield P, et al: Exercise tolerance in late survivors of balloon pumping and surgery for cardiogenic shock. *Circulation* 1980; 62:(suppl I):I138.
77. Baldwin RT, Slogoff S, Noon GP, et al: A model to predict survival at time of postcardiotomy intraaortic balloon pump insertion. *Ann Thorac Surg* 1993; 55:908.

78. Pi K, Block PC, Warner MG, et al: Major determinants of survival and nonsurvival of intraaortic balloon pumping. *Am Heart J* 1995; 130:849.
79. Funk M, Ford CF, Foell DW, et al: Frequency of long-term lower limb ischemia associated with intraaortic balloon pump use. *Am J Cardiol* 1992; 70:1195.
80. Ferguson JJ 3rd, Cohen M, Freedman RJ Jr, et al: The current practice of intra-aortic balloon counterpulsation: results from the Benchmark Registry. *J Am Coll Cardiol* 2001; 38:1246.
81. Christenson JT, Badel P, Simonet F, Schmuziger M: Preoperative intraaortic balloon pump enhances cardiac performance and improves the outcome of redo CABG. *Ann Thorac Surg* 1997; 64:1237.
82. Christenson JT, Schmuziger M, Simonet F: Effective surgical management of high-risk coronary patients using preoperative intraaortic balloon counterpulsation therapy. *Cardiovasc Surg* 2001; 9:383.
83. DeBakey ME: Left ventricular bypass pump for cardiac assistance: clinical experience. *Am J Cardiol* 1971; 27:3.
84. Department of Health and Human Services, National Institutes of Health, National Heart, Lung, and Blood Institute: Left heart assist blood pumps (request for proposal). Bethesda, MD, 1977.
85. Smedira NG, Moazami N, Golding CM, McCarthy PM, et al: Clinical experience with 202 adults receiving extracorporeal membrane oxygenation for cardiac failure: survival at five years. *J Thorac Cardiovasc Surg* 2001; 122:92.
86. Peek GJ, Firmin RK: The inflammatory and coagulative response to prolonged extracorporeal membrane oxygenation. *ASAIO J* 1999; 45:250.
87. Samuels LE, Kaufman MS, Thomas MP, et al: Pharmacological criteria for ventricular assist device insertion following postcardiotomy shock: experience with the ABIOMED BVS system. *J Card Surg* 1999; 14:288.
88. Baldwin RT, Slogoff S, Noon GP, et al: A model to predict survival at the time of postcardiotomy intraaortic balloon pumping. *J Thorac Cardiovasc Surg* 1997; 74:709.
89. Jett GK: ABIOMED BVS 5000: experience and potential advantages. *Ann Thorac Surg* 1996; 61:301.
90. Argenziano M, Choudhri AF, Moazami N, et al: A prospective randomized trial of arginine vasopressin in the treatment of vasodilatory shock after left ventricular assist device placement. *Circulation* 1997; 96 (suppl):286.
91. Argenziano M, Choudhri AF, Moazami N, et al: Randomized, double-blind trial of inhaled nitric oxide in LVAD recipients with pulmonary hypertension. *Ann Thorac Surg* 1998; 65:340.
92. Curtis JJ: Centrifugal mechanical assist for postcardiotomy ventricular failure. *Semin Thorac Cardiovasc Surg* 1994; 6:140.
93. Curtis JJ, Wagner-Mann CC, Turpin TA, et al: In vitro evaluation of five commercially available perfusion systems. *Int J Angiol* 1994; 3:128.
94. Magovern GJ Jr: The biopump and postoperative circulatory support. *Ann Thorac Surg* 1993; 55:245.
95. Curtis JJ, Walls JT, Schmaltz RA, et al: Use of centrifugal pumps for postcardiotomy ventricular failure: technique and anticoagulation. *Ann Thorac Surg* 1996; 61:296.
96. Hoerr HR, Kraemer MF, Williams JL, et al: In vitro comparison of the blood handling by the constrained vortex and twin roller blood pumps. *J Extracorpor Technol* 1987; 19:316.
97. Golding LAR, Crouch RD, Stewart RW, et al: Postcardiotomy centrifugal mechanical ventricular support. *Ann Thorac Surg* 1992; 54:1059.
98. Curtis JJ, Walls JT, Boley TM, et al: Autopsy findings in patients on postcardiotomy centrifugal ventricular assist. *ASAIO J* 1992; 38:M688.
99. Curtis JJ, Wagner-Mann C: Extracorporeal support: centrifugal pumps, in Goldstein DJ, Oz MC (eds): *Cardiac Assist Devices.* New York, Futura, 2000; p 215.
100. Noon GP, Ball JW Jr, Short HD: Bio-Medicus centrifugal ventricular support for postcardiotomy cardiac failure: a review of 129 cases. *Ann Thorac Surg* 1996; 61:291.
101. Joyce LD, Kiser JC, Eales F, et al: Experience with generally accepted centrifugal pumps: personal and collective experience. *Ann Thorac Surg* 1996; 61:287.
102. Bartlett RH, Roloff DW, Custer JR, et al: Extracorporeal life support: the University of Michigan experience. *JAMA* 2000; 283:904.
103. High KM, Snider MT, Bashein G: Principles of oxygenator function: gas exchange, heat transfer, and blood-artificial surface interaction, in Gravlee GP, Davis RF, Utley JR (eds): *Cardiopulmonary Bypass Principles and Practice.* Baltimore, Williams & Wilkins, 1993; p 28.
104. Larm O, Larsson R, Olsson P: A new non-thrombogenic surface prepared by selective covalent binding of heparin via a reducing terminal residue. *Biomater Med Devices Artif Organs* 1983; 11:161.
105. Videm V, Mollnes TE, Garred P, Svennevig JL: Biocompatibility of extracorporeal circulation: in vitro comparison of heparin-coated and uncoated oxygenator circuits. *J Thorac Cardiovasc Surg* 1991; 101:654.
106. Redmond JM, Gillinov AM, Stuart RS, et al: Heparin-coated bypass circuits reduce pulmonary injury. *Ann Thorac Surg* 1993; 56:474.
107. Videm V, Svennevig JL, Fosse E, Semb G, et al: Reduced complement activation with heparin-coated oxygenator and tubings in coronary bypass operations. *J Thorac Cardiovasc Surg* 1992; 103:806.
108. Bindsler L, Gouda I, Inacio J, et al: Extracorporeal elimination of carbon dioxide using surface-heparinized veno-venous bypass system. *ASAIO Trans* 1986; 32:530.
109. Mottaghy K, Oedekoven B, Poppei K, et al: Heparin free long-term extracorporeal circulation using bioactive surfaces. *ASAIO Trans* 1989; 35:635.
110. Magovern GJ, Magovern JA, Benckart DH, et al: Extracorporeal membrane oxygenation versus the biopump: preliminary results in patients with postcardiotomy cardiogenic shock. *Ann Thorac Surg* 1994; 57:1462.
111. Aranki SF, Adams DH, Rizzo RJ, et al: Femoral veno-arterial extracorporeal life support with minimal or no heparin. *Ann Thorac Surg* 1993; 56:149.
112. Muehrcke DD, McCarthy PM, Stewart RW, et al: Complications of extracorporeal life support systems using heparin-bound surfaces. *J Thorac Cardiovasc Surg* 1995; 110:843.
113. Von Segessor LK, Gyurech DD, Schilling JJ, et al: Can protamine be used during perfusion with heparin surface coated equipment? *ASAIO Trans* 1993; 39:M190.
114. Pennington DG, Hahn CJ: Discussion of ECMO for cardiac support. *Ann Thorac Surg* 1996; 61:340.
115. Rich PB, Awad SS, Crotti SC, Hirschl RB, et al: A prospective comparison of atrio-femoral and femoro-atrial flow in adult venovenous extracorporeal life support. *J Thorac Cardiovasc Surg* 1998; 116: 628.
116. Edmunds LH Jr, Herrmann HC, DiSesa VJ, et al: Left ventricular assist without thoracotomy: clinical experience with the Dennis method. *Ann Thorac Surg* 1994; 57:880.
117. Magovern GJ Jr, Magovern JA, Benckart DH, et al: Extracorporeal membrane oxygenation: preliminary results in patients with postcardiotomy cardiogenic shock. *Ann Thorac Surg* 1994; 57:1462.
118. Kolobow T, Rossi F, Borelli M, Foti G: Long-term closed chest partial and total cardiopulmonary bypass by peripheral cannulation for severe right and/or left ventricular failure, including ventricular fibrillation. *ASAIO Trans* 1988; 34:485.

119. Pagani FD, Lynch W, Swaniker F, et al: Extracorporeal life support to left ventricular assist device bridge to heart transplant: a strategy to optimize survival and resource utilization. *Circulation* 1999, 100 (19 suppl.):II206.
120. Pennington DG, Merjavy JP, Codd JE, et al: Extracorporeal membrane oxygenation for patients with cardiogenic shock. *Circulation* 1984; 70 (suppl I):I130.
121. Zapol WM, Snider MT, Hill JD, et al: Extracorporeal membrane oygenation in severe acute respiratory failure: a randomized prospective study. *JAMA* 1979; 242:2193.
122. Muehrcke DD, McCarthy PM, Stewart RW, et al: Extracorporeal membrane oxygenation for postcardiotomy cardiogenic shock. *Ann Thorac Surg* 1996; 61:684.
123. Kasirajan V, Smedira NG, McCarthy JF, Casselman F, et al: Risk factors for intracranial hemorrhage in adults on extracorporeal membrane oxygenation. *Eur J Cardiothorac Surg* 1999; 15: 508.
124. Smedira NG, Blackstone EH: Postcardiotomy mechanical support: risk factors and outcomes. *Ann Thorac Surg* 2001; 71:S60.
125. Magovern GJ Jr., Simpson KA: Extracorporeal membrane oxygenation for adult cardiac support: the Allegheny experience. *Ann Thorac Surg* 1999; 68:655.
126. Marelli D, Laks H, Fazio D, et al: Mechanical assist strategy using the BVS 5000i for patients with heart failure. *Ann Thorac Surg* 2000; 70:59.
127. Dewey TM, Chen JM, Spanier TB, Oz MC: Alternative technique of right-sided outflow cannula insertion for right ventricular support. *Ann Thorac Surg* 1998; 66:1829.
128. Jett GK, Lazzara RR: Extracorporeral support: the ABIOMED BVS 5000, in Goldstein DJ, Oz MC (eds): *Cardiac Assist Devices*. New York, Futura, 2000.
129. Arabia FA, Paramesh V, Toporoff B, et al: Biventricular cannulation for the Thoratec ventricular assist device. *Ann Thorac Surg* 1998; 66:2119.
130. Lohmann BP, Swartz RC, Pendelton DJ, et al: Left ventricular versus left atrial cannulation for the Thoratec ventricular assist device. *ASAIO J* 1990; 36:M545.
131. Guyton RA, Schonberger J, Everts P, et al: Postcardiotomy shock clinical evaluation of the BVS 5000 Biventricular System. *Ann Thorac Surg* 1993; 56:346.
132. Jett GK: ABIOMED BVS 5000: Experience and potential advantages. *Ann Thorac Surg* 1996; 61:301.
133. Körfer R, El-Banayosy A, Arusogul L, et al: Temporary pulsatile ventricular assist devices and biventricular assist devices. *Ann Thorac Surg* 1999; 68:678.
134. Jett GK: Postcardiotomy support with ventricular assist devices: selection of recipients. *Semin Thorac Cardiovasc Surg* 1994; 6:136.
135. Farrar DJ, Hill JD: Univentricular and biventricular Thoratec VAD support as a bridge to transplantation. *Ann Thorac Surg* 1993; 55:276.
136. Ganzel BL, Gray LA, Slater AD, et al: Surgical techniques for the implantation of heterotopic prosthetic ventricles. *Ann Thorac Surg* 1989; 47:113.
137. Lohmann DP, Swarta MT, Pennington DG, et al: Left ventricular versus left atrial cannulation for the Thoratec ventricular assist device. *ASAIO Trans* 1990; 36:M545.
138. Rao V, Oz MC, Edwards NM, Naka Y: A new off-pump technique for Thoratec right ventricular assist device insertion. *Ann Thorac Surg* 2001; 71:1719.
139. Arabia FA, Paramesh V, Toporoff B, Arzouman DA, et al: Biventricular cannulation for the Thoratec ventricular assist device. *Ann Thorac Surg* 1998; 66:2119.
140. McBride LR, Naunheim KS, Fiore AC, et al: Clinical experience with 111 Thoratec ventricular assist devices. *Ann Thorac Surg* 1999; 67:1233.
141. Goldstein DJ, Oz MC: Mechanical support for postcardiotomy cardiogenic shock. *Semin Thorac Cardiovasc Surg* 2000; 12:220.
142. Korfer R, El-Banayosy A, Posival H, et al: Mechanical circulatory support with the Thoratec assist device in patients with postcardiotomy cardiogenic shock. *Ann Thorac Surg* 1996; 61:314.
143. Pennington DG, McBride LR, Swartz MT, et al: Use of the Pierce-Donachy ventricular assist device in patients with cardiogenic shock after cardiac operations. *Ann Thorac Surg* 1989; 47:130.
144. Holman WL, Bourge RC, Kirklin JK: Case report: circulatory support for seventy days with resolution of acute heart failure [letter]. *J Thorac Cardiovasc Surg* 1991; 102:932.
145. Körfer R, El-Banayosy A, Arusoglu L, Minami K, et al: Single-center experience with the Thoratec ventricular assist device. *J Thorac Cardiovasc Surg* 2000; 119:596.
146. Pagani FD, Aaronson KD, Swaniker F, Bartlett RH: The use of extracorporeal life support in adult patients with primary cardiac failure as a bridge to implantable left ventricular assist device. *Ann Thorac Surg* 2001; 71:S77.
147. Oz MC, Goldstein DJ, Pepino P, et al: Screening scale predicts patients successfully receiving long term implantable left ventricular assist devices. *Circulation* 1995; 92 (suppl II):II169.
148. Plotz FB, van Oeveren W, Bartlett RH, et al: Blood activation during neonatal extracorporeal life support. *J Thorac Cardiovasc Surg* 1993; 105:823.
149. Jamadar DA, Kazerooni EA, Cascade PN, et al: Extracorporeal membrane oxygenation in adults: radiographic findings and correlation of lung opacity with patient mortality. *Radiology* 1996; 198:693.
150. Reinhartz O, Farrar DJ, Hershon JH, et al: Importance of preoperative liver function as a predictor of survival in patients supported with Thoratec ventricular assist device. *J Thorac Cardiovasc Surg* 1998; 116:633.
151. Farrar DJ, Hill JD, Pennington DG, et al: Preoperative and postoperative comparison of patients with univentricular and biventricular support with the Thoratec ventricular assist device as a bridge to cardiac transplantation. *J Thorac Cardiovasc Surg* 1997; 113:202.
152. Kormos RL, Gasior TA, Kawai A, et al: Transplant candidate's clinical status rather than right ventricular function defines the need for univentricular versus biventricular support. *J Thorac Cardiovasc Surg* 1996; 111:773.
153. DeRose JJ, Umana JP, Argenziano M, et al: Improved results for postcardiotomy cardiogenic shock with the use of implantable left ventricular assist devices. *Ann Thorac Surg* 1997; 64: 1757.
154. Horwitz JR, Cofer BR, Warner BW, et al: A multicenter trial of 6-aminocaproic acid (Amicar) in the prevention of bleeding in infants on ECMO. *J Pediatr Surg* 1998; 33:1610.
155. Curtis JJ, Walls JT, Boley TM, et al: Autopsy findings in patients on postcardiotomy centrifugal ventricular assist. *ASAIO J* 1992; 38:M688.
156. Noon GP, Lafuente JA, Irwin S: Acute and temporary ventricular support with BioMedicus Centrifugal Pump. *Ann Thorac Surg* 1999; 68:650.
157. Magovern GJ Jr: The Biopump and post-operative cirulatory support. *Ann Thorac Surg* 1991; 52:230.
158. Joyce LD, Kiser JC, Eales F, et al: Experience with generally accepted centrifugal pumps: personal and collective experience. *Ann Thorac Surg* 1996; 61:287.
159. Wang SS, Chen YS, Ko WJ, et al: Extracorporeal membrane oxygenation: support for postcardiotomy cardiogenic shock. *Artif Organs* 1996; 20:1287.
160. Minami K, Posival H, el-Banayosi A, et al: Mechanical ventricular support using pulsatile ABIOMED BVS 5000 and centrifugal biomedics pump in postcardiotomy shock. *Int J Artif Organs* 1994; 17:492.

Chapter **18**

Late Complications of Cardiac Surgery

Venkataramana Vijay/Jeffrey P. Gold

The science and art of cardiac surgery continue to evolve at an unprecedented rate. Rapid and diverse developments in technology and pharmacology as well as a better understanding of cardiac pathophysiology have led to this continued expansion of procedures available to patients of all ages suffering from cardiac diseases. In spite of being able to offer a wider spectrum of procedures to older and sicker patients, to patients with more advanced stages of cardiac disease, and to patients with a wider spectrum of noncardiac multisystem comorbidity, the morbidity and mortality after cardiac surgery continue to remain at a stable level or to fall.

Changes in technology have produced a myriad of new devices and exposure techniques, and have redefined our concepts of the role for cardiopulmonary bypass, the very technology around which much of our specialty has been built. Parallel to these new procedures and advanced technologies has been an expansion of the knowledge of the early and late complications following these procedures.

The development and maintenance of large institutional, regional, national, and international databases have allowed surgeons to better understand the outcomes of many of the commonly performed procedures and at the same time to identify the risk factors which are predictive of improved or unsatisfactory outcomes. Both preoperative patient-specific risk factors as well as perioperative process-related factors have been studied extensively, profiling the spectrum of morbidity and mortality of patients undergoing cardiac surgery.

Postoperative complications can be classified in many ways, but the timing of onset or recognition is among the most useful classification systems. Short-term complications are those that are recognized almost immediately following the procedure, occurring within hours to up to thirty days following the procedure. Many data sets categorize short-term complications as those recognized during the initial or primary hospitalization or within the first thirty days following the procedure. Long-term complications, those occurring after the short-term period has elapsed, have also been well studied for many of the procedures that cardiac surgeons commonly employ.

Although typically framed in terms of six months, one year, many years, and extending up to decades after the procedure originally performed, any related cardiac event after the initial period of recovery can be considered within this important category of late surgical sequelae. The patient-related risk factors and the procedural or process-related factors predicting improved or deteriorated outcomes may be similar to those predicting the short-term sequelae for many of the procedures, but in most cases there is an additional set of factors predicting long-term outcomes. The levels of significance of the short-term predictive factors and their associated odds ratios have been different in all instances when long- and short-term outcomes have been compared.

This chapter addresses the long-term outcomes, also known as the late complications, of cardiac surgical procedures. In each instance, the differences and similarities when compared to the immediate or short-term complications will be explored in the context of an understanding of the predictive risk factors attributable to the patient, to the techniques involved with the procedures, and to the postoperative care whenever possible.

Given the long-term nature of the development of these late complications, the completeness of the follow-up, the nature of the follow-up system, and the ability to track large cohorts of patients are extremely important. It is clearly important for surgeons to have access to precise and complete long-term procedure-related data to fully understand current and evolving procedures, as well as to continually modify indications and surgical technique. By design, the long-term specific procedure-related outcomes and complications for valvular heart surgery, coronary heart disease, transplantation, and ventricular replacement devices are extensively covered in other chapters, and as such are not addressed in this chapter.

The recognition of long-term complications may depend upon the development of clinical symptoms and signs or upon routine scheduled provocative testing. Objective tests of cardiac function at rest and with exercise enhance the quantification of long-term outcomes of virtually all procedures we now commonly offer. Stratifying the outcomes of this objective noninvasive or invasive testing forms the basis of much of what we now use to determine indications for almost all aspects of preprocedural selection, intraoperative technique, and postoperative care. Medicine, based upon the pedestal of solid evidence, continues to support much of the decision making within our specialty.

This chapter will attempt to define the scientific basis of the late complications of cardiac surgery procedures. It is organized by the organ systems involved, and whenever possible the discussion is related directly to technical and perioperative considerations. Special attention is focused on neurologic, cognitive, and psychiatric complications, since those have been the focus of much interest and the basis of much procedurally driven decision making. Quality of life, months and years following all cardiac interventions, whatever the basis, underlies the ultimate goal of all of medicine. The closer we can come to understanding the relationships between patient and procedural factors and long-term complications that relate to quality of life, the better care our patients will receive.

MYOCARDIAL ISCHEMIC COMPLICATIONS

Myocardial infarction and ischemia have been reported to complicate most types of surgical procedures, but are particularly important in the setting of major cardiac, vascular, and pulmonary procedures. Recognition and early diagnosis are essential. With improvements in myocardial protection and better perfusion during cardiopulmonary bypass, the incidence of postoperative myocardial infarction has steadily fallen over the course of the past two decades.

The diagnosis of postoperative myocardial infarction has traditionally been based on electrocardiography (EKG). Presence of Q waves has been deemed sufficient to diagnose a perioperative infarction. However, Svedjeholm et al compared accuracy of Q-wave–based postoperative myocardial infarction diagnosis with biochemical markers in 302 consecutive patients. EKG-positive criteria for myocardial infarction were present in 8.1%, but when correlated with CPK-MB and troponin-T levels, only 1% of these cases qualified as positive for myocardial infarction. More than 25% of Q waves were associated with plasma levels of troponin-T below the reference level.[1] Troponin-T is the most reliable marker for postoperative myocardial infarction according to Hake et al, who studied EKG, CPK-MB, and troponin-T in patients suffering myocardial infarctions following coronary surgery.[2]

Iyer studied 12,003 coronary artery bypass graft patients treated over a 12-year period and calculated an overall mortality rate of 0.99% with a postoperative myocardial infarction rate of 1.34%. Bypass time of greater than 100 minutes and presence of unstable angina were the two most important predictors for postoperative myocardial infarction.[3]

COMPLICATIONS OF ARRHYTHMIA AND PACING PROCEDURES

Atrial Arrhythmias

With the advent of various techniques for approach (standard or minimally invasive, epicardial or endocardial) and methods of energy delivery for ablation procedures (cryo, radiofrequency, or microwave), the resultant increase in the number of these operations performed has produced a reasonable database of outcomes.

Guang et al compared freedom from atrial fibrillation at 3 years in two groups of patients requiring mitral valve surgery. Ninety-six patients with mitral valve replacement and radiofrequency ablation (modified Maze III) of the left atrium were contrasted with 87 undergoing mitral valve replacement alone. At three years, 77% of the first cohort were free of atrial fibrillation versus 25% of group II.[4]

Mohr et al evaluated a series of 234 patients undergoing radiofrequency ablation with 31.6% having radiofrequency ablation alone, 24.4% with concomitant mitral repair, 16.2% with mitral valve replacement, 5.1% with aortic valve replacement, and 5.0% with coronary artery bypass grafting. Median sternotomy was used in 43.2% and right video-assisted limited thoracotomy in 56.8%. Of the total group, 83.9% were discharged in sinus rhythm, 7.6% had atrial fibrillation, and 8.5% had atypical flutter. Pacemakers were needed in 9.8%, with 1.3% developing an aortoesophageal fistula with a 4.2% hospital and 2.1% 30-day mortality. At 6 months, 81% of patients were in sinus rhythm; at 12 months, the proportion was 72.5%.[5] Combined endocardial and epicardial approaches have also been tried with similar good success.[6] These studies have documented the efficacy of these procedures in alleviating atrial arrhythmias and in maintaining sinus rhythm at reasonable durations of follow-up.

Circumferential radiofrequency ablation around the pulmonary vein ostia alone, producing atrial electroanatomic remodeling, has been described by Pappone et al. In that study, 251 patients (179 with paroxysmal atrial fibrillation and 72 in permanent atrial fibrillation) were treated with radiofrequency for lesions surrounding the pulmonary veins with intraoperative evidence of pulmonary vein electrical isolation. At 10.4 months follow-up, 85% of the patients with paroxysmal atrial fibrillation and 68% of those with permanent atrial fibrillation were in sinus rhythm. Age, atrial fibrillation duration, and ejection fraction were not predictors for failure to convert. Left atrial diameter, however, was noted to be significantly higher in permanent atrial fibrillation patients with recurrence.[7] Chen et al performed atrial size reduction with ablation in a group of 119 patients, and noted that in patients who converted to sinus rhythm, the right and left atrial sizes were smaller than in those who did not convert.[8] Lim et al studied the influence of atrial fibrillation on outcome following mitral valve repair in 400 patients, and noted that atrial fibrillation did not affect early outcome or durability of mitral repair, but patients in atrial fibrillation had lower survival at 3 years of 82% (vs. 93% in controls) and 73% versus 88% at 5 years. Age older than 70 years, poor left ventricular function, and atrial fibrillation were negative predictors in univariate analysis.[9]

Repetitive atrial flutter following left atrial Maze procedures was noted by Usui et al to be associated with a right atrial isthmus. In their series of 41 patients, 9.8% developed atrial flutter, and it was inducible in all of them through the right atrial isthmus, which was treated subsequently by linear ablation.[10]

Albage et al studied hormonal activation in the perioperative phase and noted that weight gain from fluid retention was higher after the Maze procedure due to elevated antidiuretic hormone and aldosterone levels.[11] Bauer et al, in their study of 72 patients, found that atrial transport function (ATF) return to normal in 87% (echocardiography) and 78% (magnetic resonance imaging) at 12 months. Independent predictors of return of ATF were smaller preoperative left atrial diameter and better preoperative left ventricular ejection fraction.[12]

Ventricular Arrhythmias

Preoperative risk factor analysis for new onset tachyarrhythmias after cardiac surgery by Mayr et al revealed older age, history of congestive heart failure, sepsis, systemic inflammatory response, and multiorgan dysfunction as highly predictive.[13] In a study of 382 coronary artery bypass grafting patients by Steinberg et al, 3.1% experienced one episode of sustained ventricular tachycardia at a mean of 4.1 days after surgery, with an in-hospital mortality rate of 25%. Previous myocardial infarction, severe congestive heart failure, low ejection fraction, noncollateralized occluded vessels on angiogram, and bypass grafting to an infarcted zone were the most predictive of risk for ventricular tachycardia following coronary surgery.[14]

Levine's study of 218 patients with automatic implantable cardioverter-defibrillator (AICD) placed for tachyarrhythmias found that nearly 50% of patients had their first AICD fire (discharge) for syncope, presyncope, or sustained ventricular tachycardia/ventricular fibrillation. Ejection fraction of less than 25% was noted to have an earlier first fire and shortened survival after AICD discharge. Beta blockers and coronary artery bypass grafting were associated with longer interval to first fire, but only coronary artery bypass grafting bestowed prolonged survival.[15]

Pacing Complications

Malpositioned leads in various positions (into the left ventricle through a patent foramen ovale or displaced lead into coronary artery sinus, etc.) have been reported and can be fairly easily diagnosed by x-ray or EKG tracings. Some patients may also present with cerebral embolism from inadvertently placed left ventricular leads.[16] Echocardiography is useful in the diagnosis of such malpositioned leads. Infected transvenous permanent pacemakers can be diagnosed by transthoracic or transesophageal echocardiography. However, transesophageal echocardiography detected lead and valve vegetations in 7 out of 10 patients, compared to only 2 out of 10 by transthoracic echocardiography.[17]

Management in the large majority of these situations involves replacement of the leads. Pacing lead extractions become necessary for dysfunction or incompatibility in 12% of patients, lead endocarditis in 32%, Accufix lead in 14%, pulse generator pocket infection in 22%, or lead erosions in 19%. Jarwe, in his study of 128 lead extractions, noted that 95% of the leads could be completely extracted, 2% partially, and 4% could not be removed. Four complications of two tricuspid leaflet tears, lead migration, and femoral hemorrhage were seen.[18] Femoral lead extraction has now become safe and efficient.

Infections of the pacing systems are infrequent, with *Staphylococcus* being the predominant organism in generator pocket infections. Endocarditis induced by pacemaker leads can arise de novo or as an extension of generator pocket infection. Primary treatment option includes removal of the entire pacing system under antibiotic cover.[19] Explantation, sterilization, and reimplantation have also been successfully employed. New leads are placed, old leads removed, and the sterilized generator reimplanted, producing excellent results in 17 patients over 14 years.[20] Runaway pacemakers have been reported, which usually indicates battery end-of-life and requires generator replacement.[21]

PERICARDIAL COMPLICATIONS

Postpericardiotomy syndrome, pericardial effusions, tamponade, and constrictive pericarditis are some of the well-known late pericardial complications after cardiac surgery.

Postpericardotomy Syndrome

Postpericardiotomy syndrome and post–myocardial infarction pericardial syndrome (Dressler's space syndrome) are characterized by fever with a pleural/pericardial pain component associated with eosinophilia and atypical lymphocytosis. The usual treatment algorithm is nonsteroidal anti-inflammatory agents followed by steroids for persistent effusions. Colchicine has been used in some resistant cases of postpericardiotomy effusions with success. Postperfusion pericardial syndrome is caused by cytomegalovirus inflammation of the pericardium and is characterized by sore throat without pleural/pericardial or eosinophilic accompaniment. Elevated cytomegalovirus titers (Ig M) are usually present.[22]

Pericardial Effusions

Postpericardiotomy effusions have an incidence of 58% to 64% following coronary grafting and valvular surgery. In one study, loculated effusions (57%) were more frequent than diffuse (42%), with tamponade in 1.5%; however, aortic root surgery predisposed to a 6-fold increase in effusions to 31.6%.[23] This certainly warrants surveillance echocardiography every 6 months for 2 years postoperatively, to exclude tamponade physiology, especially for those on anticoagulant therapy. Postpericardiotomy effusions are frequently seen 1 to 2 weeks postoperatively in patients receiving aspirin or warfarin and contribute to 35% of late effusions. Symptoms of postpericardiotomy syndrome, pericardial rub, atrial arrhythmias, cardiac enlargement, and pleural effusions are the most commonly noted. A higher incidence of pericardial and pleural effusions is associated with the use of internal mammary as a conduit.[23–25] Use of anticoagulation contributed to 86% of early and 65% of late pericardial effusions. Diagnosis and treatment by echocardiography is safe and effective. Echo-guided pericardiocentesis is successful in draining 89% to 97% of all effusions and nearly 96% of loculated effusions with a major complication rate of 2% (chamber laceration and pneumothorax). With use of a flexible catheter for extended drainage, incidence of recurrent effusion can be decreased by 50%.[26,27] The subxiphoid approach has a higher recurrence rate while the transthoracic approach is more invasive. These more invasive methods may be reserved for situations in which pericardiocentesis is not feasible.

Refractory supraventricular tachyarrhythmias and chylopericardium (due to operative trauma during mammary artery harvesting) are two unusual presentations of postpericardiotomy effusion.[28,29] A higher incidence of pericardial effusion causing tamponade (8.9%) is seen in heart transplant patients. A weight mismatch (recipient weight greater than donor weight), lack of previous sternotomy, rejection, and cyclosporine use have been implicated. Forty-four percent were treated successfully by pericardiocentesis and 28% required pericardiectomy in one series.[30]

Constrictive Pericarditis

Constrictive pericarditis as a late complication of cardiac surgery has an incidence of 0.2% to 2.0%. The interval between surgery and presentation is an average of 82 days (14 to 186). Risk factor analysis reveals normal left ventricular function, warfarin administration, and inadequate drainage of early postoperative pericardial effusions as the significant causes.[31,32] Diagnosis is established by echocardiography, tomography, and catheterization showing pericardial thickening, constrictive physiology, and characteristic early diastolic dip and late plateau pattern (square root sign). Leaving the pericardium open at initial surgery does not influence the incidence of constrictive pericarditis.[33]

Other rare causes such as tuberculosis, viral, chlamydial, and fungal infections, and autoimmune reactions have also been reported. Treatment by pericardiectomy is the most durable. Use of 0.1% dilute sodium, hyaluronic acid (NaHA), and 0.1% carboxymethylcellulose (CMC) or tissue protective bioabsorbable polymer membrane solutions has been shown experimentally to decrease pericardial and pleural adhesions to 20% while control groups had an 80% incidence.[34,35]

RESPIRATORY COMPLICATIONS

Chest Wall Complications

Sternal or chest wall pain and its inadequate control have a debilitating effect on a patient's recovery and long-term functional status. Mueller et al studied prospectively the location, distribution, and intensity of pain after cardiac surgery in 200 patients. The pain intensity was at its maximum on postoperative days 1 and 2 and decreased to a minimum by day 7; however, the location of pain shifted from midsternal early postoperatively to shoulder pain by day 7. Age had an impact on pain, with patients less than 60 years having a higher intensity.[36] Long-term pain (beyond four weeks) tended to be more osteoarthritic and musculoskeletal with a small percentage developing paresthesias at the costochondral junctions of the left anterior chest, at the site of internal mammary artery harvest.

In a series of 288 patients, a 9% incidence of sternal fractures with a higher association with mammary artery harvest was noted. Of the patients with sternal fracture, 10% had major respiratory compromise from pain, and epidural anesthesia was the most effective in managing these patients.[37] In another study, 13% patients had rib fractures, with 60% involving the first rib (following mammary harvest) and the remaining comprised of costotransverse disarticulations. Rib fractures negatively influence postoperative rehabilitation and overall postsurgical satisfaction with quality of life.[38]

Gust et al performed a randomized trial comparing patient-controlled anesthesia (PCA) with nurse-controlled anesthesia and the effect on atelectasis, rehabilitation, mobility, and overall satisfaction. The study concluded that PCA significantly decreases postoperative pulmonary atelectasis and respiratory complications, and increases return to functional status.[39] Please see the later section on quality of life for further return to work, functional status, and overall satisfaction details.

Sternal Wound Complications

Serious sternal wound infection and dehiscence occurred in 1.86% of a study group of 2579 consecutive cardiac surgical procedures reported by Ottino et al. In univariate analysis for risk factors, age, sex, type of surgical procedure, antibiotic prophylaxis, duration of ventilation, reoperation duration of CBV, blood transfusions, reexploration, rewiring, and ICU length of stay were significant. Multiple regression analysis showed that hospital environment, interval between admission and surgery, reoperation, reexploration, rewiring, and blood transfusions were important in predicting sternal instability, infection, and dehiscence.[40] Stahle et al studied 13,285 cardiac procedures and noted a 1.5% incidence of sternal infection, mediastinitis, and dehiscence. The CABG group had a 1.7% and the valve group a 0.7% incidence. Risk factors in their study were female sex, diabetes, bilateral IMA use, postoperative dialysis, reexploration, and transfusions. Patients with sternal wound complications showed no significant increase in early mortality but had worse long-term survival even after risk adjustments.[41]

Coagulase-negative staphylococcus is the most common organism involved. In the Cleveland Clinic study of 22,180 cardiac procedures, 23% of wound infections were from coagulase-negative staphylococci. Coagulase-negative staphylococcal sternal wound infections were superficial in 56% of the cases, 27% were deep, and 70% had mediastinitis, with 14% having simultaneous blood stream infection. Ninety-two percent of these infections were methicillin resistant. Management included reexploration (39%), flap operation (12%), and sternectomy (5%). Mean interval from operation to onset of sternal infection was 24 days with a mean parenteral antibiotic requirement of 22 days, resulting in an additional direct cost per patient of $20,000 for the entire admission.[42] *Streptococcus, Klebsiella, Enterobacter, Enterococcus, Pseudomonas,* and rarely *Candida albicans* are the other organisms cultured. Obesity and use of ACE inhibitors (the side effect of dry cough with ACE I inhibitors caused sternal instability and dehiscence) have also been implicated.[43] Use of ACE type II receptor inhibitors decreased the incidence.

Symptoms, physical examination, and culture of wound drainage are sufficient to confirm the diagnosis. Computed tomography has a 67% sensitivity and 83% specificity and is not the most accurate diagnostic modality.[44] Management involves several approaches of reinforced sternal wiring, prosthesis insertion for strength of closure, various flap operations, etc. Reinforced sternal closure produces a statistically significant lower rate of dehiscence.[45] Pericostal sutures decreases incidence of dehiscence to 0.38%.[46]

Use of cannulated screws with wire passed through the screw cannula seems to reduce stresses in the sternum.[47] The Ley prosthesis (a 0.5-mm-thick titanium alloy plate for stabilizing the sternum), when compared to controls, significantly reduced the incidence of reexploration and rewiring, thus reducing cardiac surgery ward length of stay and decreasing overall cost.[48] Open chest and delayed sternal closure are required in situations of cardiac edema, intractable bleeding, and arrhythmias.

The incidence of superficial wound infections (1.6%), mediastinitis (1%), and dehiscence (2.4%) following the use of these modalities was similar to controls, indicating that they may be safely used as adjuncts to drainage, debridement, and refixation of the sternum.[49]

Spontaneous right ventricular rupture following sternal dehiscence is a catastrophic complication that occurs between sternal debridement and a flap procedure, with an incidence of 0.07% of all cardiac procedures. Mortality from this complication can be decreased by freeing the right ventricle from the underside of the sternum at the initial sternal debridement followed by flap closure at first instance when primary closure is not feasible.[50]

Muscle flap reconstruction for major sternal infection comprises pectoralis (unilateral or bilateral), rectus abdominis, and/or greater omental flaps. Pectoralis flap advancement provides bulk but causes unsightly deformity and limits functional status. Rectus abdominis flaps are superior functionally but are limited by use of mammary arteries for coronary grafting, since the IMA forms a major part of the rectus blood supply. A delay period after mammary harvest has been suggested to improve collateral blood supply. Omental flaps have been used when rectal flaps are not feasible and have provided bulk and cosmesis. Reinfection rates after muscle flap reconstructions are very low. Freedom from reinfection and reintervention after muscle flap is 72% to 74%, compared to 12% after rewiring alone.[51–54]

Airway and Pulmonary Complications

Durand et al studied pulmonary function tests as predictors of pulmonary outcomes after cardiac surgery, and showed that decreased preoperative vital capacity (less than 2.5 liters) and FeV1 less than 1.5 liters were the most reliable predictors of unfavorable long-term pulmonary outcomes.[55] Bevelaqua et al studied complications after cardiac surgery in patients with severe preoperative pulmonary impairment. Over 65% of these patients had obstructive disease and the remaining restrictive disease. Compared to controls, this entire group had a significantly higher incidence of atelectasis, effusion, bronchospasm, pneumonia, and pneumothorax. It was also found that in these patients, although pulmonary morbidity was higher, overall hospital mortality was comparable to controls. Restrictive disease patients fared better than obstructive. Valve replacement carried a higher morbidity compared to isolated coronary surgery. Perioperative pulmonary function tests can be used to accurately predict postoperative risk for pulmonary complications.[56]

Several studies on ARDS after cardiac surgery place its incidence at 0.4% to 2.5% with a mortality of 15% to 34%. Redo surgery, poor preoperative pulmonary function, transfusions, emergent surgery (shock), smoking, diabetes, poor left ventricular function, and renal failure were predictors of ARDS following cardiac surgery.[57–59]

Morbidity from prolonged ventilatory support (greater than 14 days) was studied by Lo Cicero et al in 581 open heart surgery patients, showing an incidence of 9.9%. Overall mortality was 43% in those who required prolonged ventilation. Of the survivors, 55% required only an endotracheal tube and were extubated within 14 days, while 45% needed tracheostomy. Of the tracheostomy patients, 26% were extubated, 37% died, and 37% remained on mechanical ventilation. Complication rate for patients with endotracheal tubes was 65% compared to 37% for those with tracheostomy.[60] Common tracheostomy complications included sternal infection, stomal infection, minor hemorrhage, tracheal stenosis, tube displacement, delayed wound healing, and soft tissue hemorrhage.[61] Early tracheostomy (14 days) conferred better pulmonary toilet and outcomes.

Vocal cord dysfunction is an overlooked complication after respiratory support for cardiac surgery. Its incidence is about 1.9% of all cardiac surgery. It is usually self-limiting and masquerades as respiratory insufficiency. A small percentage of patients with more permanent vocal cord dysfunction require tracheostomy.[62]

GENITOURINARY COMPLICATIONS

Renal Dysfunction

Several studies have defined by multivariate analysis specific pre-, intra-, and postoperative risk factors that increase chances of acute and long-term renal dysfunction after cardiac surgery. These studies found that 10% to 20% of patients developed transient oliguria and elevation in serum creatinine, with 75% of these spontaneously returning to normal renal function. However, 1% to 5% progressed to renal failure requiring dialysis. Mortality in this group ranged from 38% to 52%.

Preoperative risk factors include age greater than 65 years, diabetes, poor left ventricular function (ejection fraction less than 35%), class III and class IV heart failure, emergent surgery, and preoperative renal dysfunction. Intraoperative causes include prolonged bypass time (greater than 140 minutes), transfusions, reexplorations for bleeding, hypothermic circulatory arrest, use of full-dose aprotinin, low perfusion pressure, low flow rates during bypass, and high on-bypass hematocrits (greater than 35%).

Postoperative renal dysfunction, defined as a decrease by 25% in creatinine clearance from baseline or a value of less than 40 mL/min, results from postoperative hypovolemia, anemia, hypotension, low output syndrome, redo cardiac surgery, excessive use of vasoconstrictor therapy, myoglobinuria, jaundice, sepsis, and pericardial tamponade.[63,64] Off-pump cardiac surgery has in at least one study been shown to attenuate transient renal injury compared to traditional on-pump grafting.[65]

Use of full-dose aprotinin has anecdotally been reported to cause postoperative renal dysfunction from an exaggerated adverse reaction. However, at least two well-known large studies, from Lemmer et al and Mora Mangano et al, evaluated the effect of full-dose aprotinin in coronary grafting on-pump and in other cardiac surgery requiring hypothermic circulatory arrest, and neither study showed any significant renal toxicity or dysfunction, even though a transient postoperative rise in serum creatinine was noted.[66,67]

A concerted effort on the part of the surgeon, anesthesiologist, and perfusionist in addressing each of the listed risk factors is essential to significantly decrease the incidence of postoperative renal dysfunction. If a high likelihood of renal dysfunction is suspected despite the above precautions, intraoperative conventional hemofiltration or modified ultrafiltration can be undertaken. A few studies randomizing conventional hemofiltration (continuous veno-venous hemofiltration or continuous arterio-venous hemofiltration) to modified ultrafiltration have shown that a significant rise in postoperative hematocrit, mean blood pressure, and cardiac index occurred with modified ultrafiltration.[68–70] This improved hemodynamics and resulted in better clinical outcomes and mortality rates in that group of patients. Modified ultrafiltration is known to attenuate systemic inflammatory response by removing serum interleukin-8 plasma.[71]

Cardiac surgery requiring cardiopulmonary bypass has been performed in patients with prior kidney transplantation. The majority of these patients retained full function of the renal graft when measures were taken to ensure that hypotension, fluid overloading, and prolonged bypass were avoided. Some patients may need their immunosuppression to be reinstituted with a bolus dose because CPB dilutes their plasma levels. Less than 2% of these patients experience graft rejection. Perioperative incidence of renal failure requiring dialysis is less than 12%, although a transient rise in serum creatinine may be noted.[72]

Urethral Complications

Urethral complications are seen mainly in those older than 60 years, with an incidence of 4% per year. Factors implicated in development of urethral stricture following cardiac surgery are a combination of urethral hypersensitivity and bulbar and penile urethral ischemia during cardiopulmonary bypass. Pressure necrosis at the urethral orifice of the urinary bladder also occurs from traction on the balloon of the urinary catheter exerted by its weight (collection bag) or from manner of anchoring.

A randomized trial of urethral catheterization to suprapubic catheterization showed a 4-fold increase of stricture with urethral catheterization. Avoiding overinflation of the catheter balloon and traction on the catheter may decrease incidence of this complication.[73]

GASTROINTESTINAL COMPLICATIONS

Due to the absence of early specific clinical signs, gastrointestinal complications after cardiac surgery are often diagnosed late with resultant high mortality. Incidence of all intra-abdominal side effects after cardiopulmonary bypass is about 1% to 2%, but mortality ranges from 12.5% to greater than 90% depending upon the specific complication[74–76] and the surgical intervention needed.

Common in-hospital late complications (beyond 7 to 10 days postoperatively) include bowel ischemia from embolization or low flow, upper or lower gastrointestinal bleeding from gastritis, peptic ulceration and diverticular disease, and diarrhea from pseudomembranous colitis, pancreatitis, cholecystitis, and septic rupture of spleen. In a study of 4923 patients in which 1.3% had GI complications, the most frequent were GI bleeding (40%), pancreatitis (34%), acute cholecystitis (11%), perforated duodenal ulcer (8%), ischemic bowel (5%), and diverticulitis 2%.[77] In another study of 4473 patients in which 0.78% had GI complications, mortality rate by complication was GI bleeding 45%, intestinal infarction 67%, and pancreatitis 100%.[78]

A third study of 6281 patients, evaluating mortality from GI complications requiring intervention based on type of cardiac surgery, showed that CABG had an incidence of 0.4% to 1% mortality from GI complications, valvular surgery 0.8%, cardiac transplantation 6%, acute aortic dissection 9%, and reoperative surgery 6% to 10%. Major associated risk factors were sepsis (odds ratio 38.7), renal failure (odds ratio 3.5), and prolonged ventilatory support (odds ratio 2.7).[79] A retrospective analysis of 4463 patients with a 1.9% incidence of GI complications noted a mortality rate of 70% for medical management of the GI complication versus 50% for surgical management.[80]

Risk factors and predictors of intestinal ischemia and GI complications identified by multivariate analysis in two large series include age older than 70 years, duration of bypass, reoperation, need for transfusion of more than 2 units of blood, heart failure class IV, triple-vessel coronary disease associated with significant peripheral vascular disease, use of intra-aortic balloon counterpulsation, aortic athero emboli, reexploration for bleeding, postoperative low cardiac output, and significant inotropic support. In all patients with GI complications, a combination of at least four of the above predictors was present.[81]

Studies on gut barrier and mucosal function during anesthesia and cardiopulmonary bypass evaluated time sequence between intraoperative and postoperative endotoxemia, intramucosal pH changes, mediator and intestinal permeability, and acute phase proteins and their relationship to postoperative GI complications such as cholecystitis, hepatic, pseudomembranous colitis, and postoperative infections. Intraluminal pH of the stomach dropped significantly (6.98), plasma levels of endotoxin (greater than 0.2 endotoxin units/mL) increased (14-fold), interleukin-6 (IL-6) increased on the second postoperative day (2-fold), and C-reactive protein increased (4-fold) in patients who developed GI and infective complications. Ischemia in splanchnic circulation either intraoperatively (CBV) or postoperatively (low cardiac output) seemed to be the most likely stimuli.[82,83]

Intestinal Complications

Mesenteric ischemia is a rare but catastrophic complication (0.1% of all cardiac surgery) with mortality rates of as high as 91%. Nonocclusive ischemia (45% to 60%) and embolic events are the common causes. Physical examination findings of ileus or acute abdomen with elevated lactate and amylase levels should usually arouse suspicion.

Radiologic and angiographic studies are used to confirm diagnosis. Interventions include intra-arterial papavarine injection, embolectomy (9%), bowel resection (36%), and exploratory laparotomy by itself in 55%. Average in-hospital mortality is 80% to 90% for bowel resection.[84–86] Acute diverticulitis is a rare complication with an incidence of 2% to 5% of all GI complications and conservative management is advocated, usually with good outcomes.[87]

Hepatic Complications

Synthetic and secretory dysfunction of liver, icterus, and hepatic encephalopathy are rare complications of cardiac surgery utilizing cardiopulmonary bypass. Risk factors predicting hepatic dysfunction and adverse outcome include preoperative hepatic dysfunction evidenced by elevated SGOT, SGPT, prothrombin time, conjugated and unconjugated bilirubin, thrombocytopenia, right heart failure with severe hepatic congestion, portal hypertension, cardiac cirrhosis, hypotension, hypoxemia, and amount of transfusions. Age, sex, underlying cardiac lesions, and the presence or absence of hepatitis B are not predictive of postoperative jaundice. Classes B and C of Child's classification of liver dysfunction are the strongest predictors of mortality following cardiac surgery. Elective surgery with Child's class A including CABG and valve replacements survived the surgery, but succumbed late to GI complication such as bleeding or hepatic encephalopathy, etc. Histology shows central necrosis of hepatocytes with sinusoidal dilation. Good pre-, intra-, and postoperative management of systemic perfusion (with high flow rates), optimization of heart and liver function, and pharmacologic/mechanical circulatory support helps to produce better outcomes in patients with liver dysfunction.

Onset of fulminant hepatic dysfunction postoperatively invariably leads to multiorgan failure and is uniformly fatal.[88–91] Conventional tests of hepatic function do not offer precise evaluation of functional liver reserve. The two most common pharmacologic means of assessing hepatic reserve in patients undergoing cardiac surgery are the antipyrine plasma clearance test and the indocyanine green clearance test. Drop in antipyrine clearance (0.4 N mL/min/kg) closely correlated (coefficient $r = 0.699$) with ability to predict postoperative hyperbilirubinemia, while indocyanine green (coefficient $r = 0.477$) was slightly less sensitive and changes depended on cardiac index. These tests can be used to identify patients at risk for postoperative hyperbilirubinemia and hepatic dysfunction.[92,93]

Pancreatic Complications

A study of 5621 cardiac surgery patients showed an incidence of 0.44% of pancreatic complications.[94] Hyperamylasemia is common after cardiac procedures (up to 32% of patients). About 20% of patients with hyperamylasemia (less than 1000 IU/L) had no serum lipase elevations and the elevated amylase was predominantly the salivary isoenzyme. Of the patients with elevated amylase, 10% had subclinical pancreatitis with mild elevations in serum lipase but had a self-limiting GI course. About 3% of patients with elevated amylase and lipase had overt clinical and diagnostic (tomography) signs of severe pancreatitis.[95] Patients with hyperamylasemia had a higher mortality of 9% compared to controls. Acute pancreatitis was by far the common complication (60%) with pancreatic necrosis next. Mortality increased up to 44% with these complications. The risk factors include pre-/postoperative hypotension, excessive use of inotropic support, renal failure, prolonged ventilatory support, intra-aortic balloon usage, and administration of calcium in doses of 800 mg or more/cm^2 of body surface area in the perioperative period.[96] Hyperamylasemia was more commonly seen with nonpulsatile perfusion (in 70% of patients) versus 32% of patients with pulsatile perfusion.[97] Modifying the above risk factors in the perioperative period can result in better outcomes. A 30-fold increase in incidence of pancreatitis is noted in heart/lung transplant recipients due to the combined effects of CPB and immunosuppression.[98]

Splenic Complications

Splenic injury and rupture following cardiac surgery are very rare complications, sometimes noted in patients with myeloid dyscrasias and enlarged spleen or in those with erosion from fulminant pancreatitis or operative trauma exacerbated by full heparinization.[99]

Biliary Complications

Acalculous and calculous cholecystitis have both been described following cardiac surgery and cardiothoracic organ transplantation. In a study of 645 cardiothoracic organ transplantation patients, 5.7% had symptomatic cholecystitis with all of them containing gallstones. Close to 45% of these patients required emergent cholecystectomy, with one mortality. All patients were female with a higher body mass index and a significant proportion had common bile duct stones also.[100] In posttransplant patients, early diagnosis and cholecystectomy with screening for choledocholithiasis produce the best results.

In nontransplant cardiac surgery, acalculous cholecystitis (biliary-based dyskinesia) is as frequent as calculous cholecystitis. Sepsis appears to be a major associated risk with acalculous cholecystitis. Conservative medical management with interval cholecystectomy appears a reasonable approach in nondiabetics. Acalculous cholecystitis also is a frequently associated GI complication in HIV-positive and AIDS patients undergoing cardiac surgery. Aggressive management in this immunosuppressed group produces the best outcomes.

VASCULAR COMPLICATIONS

Monitoring and Access Complications

Catheter access for monitoring and therapeutic reasons is well established. The placement and maintenance of these devices are also associated with a set of late complications. Arterial and venous monitoring and indwelling catheter complications have been described in several studies pertaining to surgical and medical intensive care patients. A brief review of long-term complications is presented here.

ARTERIAL CATHETERS

Frezza et al studied 2119 patients in medical and surgical critical care units with femoral and radial artery monitoring catheters in situ. Site of catheter insertion, intervals to the catheter change, number of changes, bleeding, infection, and ischemia were among the complications studied. Arterial catheters were present in 48% of MICU patients and 33% of SICU patients; 45% of MICU versus 11.5% of SICU patients had femoral catheters; and 78% of SICU and 52% of MICU patients had radial catheters. Catheters were changed in 9.5% of MICU versus 13% of SICU patients. The most common complication was vascular insufficiency (3.4% in MICU and 4.6% in SICU) followed by bleeding (1.8% in MICU and 2.6% in SICU). The catheter infection rates were 0.4% and 0.7%, respectively, with radial and femoral arterial sites having similar infection rates of 43% and 50%. The study concluded that catheter infection rates, timing, number of catheters, and site changes made no significant difference in complication rates.[101–103]

PULMONARY ARTERY CATHETERS

Catheter colonizations and bacteremia with pulmonary artery catheters were studied by Singh et al in 51 critically ill patients having 52 arterial and 37 pulmonary catheterizations. Daily cultures of blood and catheter sites showed a colonization rate of 10% with a 45% bacteremia risk. Presence of concurrent infection and use of antibiotics did not change catheter colonization. Femoral catheters had more colonization than pulmonary or radial.[104,105]

Thrombosis rates of arterial and pulmonary catheters were compared with heparinized and nonheparinized solutions by Zevola et al. Thrombosis rates of pulmonary catheters were no different in the two subgroups; however, arterial catheters failed less often when maintained with heparinized solutions.[106]

CENTRAL VENOUS CATHETERS

Central venous line infections in the SICU were studied by Charalambous et al in 232 consecutive catheter insertions. Their analysis showed that 49% had no microbial growth, 17% were colonized, and 34% were infected. Univariate analysis showed catheter site, placement in operating room versus SICU, and catheter used for monitoring versus fluid and nutrition were all significant factors. Internal jugular insertion site was the single most important predictor of infection in the multivariate analysis. Of the catheter infections, 68% were monomicrobial and 32% were polymicrobial. A concurrent bacteremia was present in 45% of the patients with infected catheters, and death from catheter-related sepsis occurred in 7%. Gram-positive bacteria were found in 86% while others had gram-negative bacteria or *Candida albicans*.[107]

Conduit Harvesting

INTERNAL MAMMARY ARTERY

El-Ansary et al compared the musculoskeletal and neurologic complications of internal mammary artery and saphenous vein harvests and noted an incidence of 78.5% and 45%, respectively, in patients at 3 to 6 weeks following cardiac surgery. The musculoskeletal effects relate to use of retraction and the neurologic side effects pertaining to anterior chest wall relate to internal mammary artery takedown with electrocautery causing injury to intercostal nerve branches.[108]

A higher incidence of pleural changes including thickening occurred in internal mammary artery harvest compared to saphenous vein graft, although incidence and size of left-sided pleural effusions were similar in both groups.[109] Incidental malignancy in internal mammary artery lymph nodes is found very rarely. Undiagnosed lymphomas or carcinoma of the breast or lung are the usual causes. Abnormally enlarged internal thoracic artery lymph nodes should be histopathologically examined.[110]

Chylothorax following median sternotomy and internal mammary artery harvest has an incidence of less than 0.25%. It occurs from injury to lymphatic drainage from the thymus following median sternotomy or from injury to the thoracic duct during internal mammary artery harvest. Conservative management is sufficient in the majority; however, minimally invasive procedures such as video-assisted thoracic surgery (VATS) have provided good results.[111–113]

Phrenic nerve dysfunction is not uncommon after coronary surgery, and a study of risk factors revealed that the use of pericardial ice slush for myocardial protection was the most important predictor followed by mammary artery harvest.[114] An elevated hemidiaphragm with atelectasis is diagnostic. Phrenic nerve dysfunction is usually transient and resolves in less than 3 to 6 weeks. However, in phrenic transsection, diaphragmatic plication may in rare instances become necessary to overcome respiratory failure.

Steal phenomenon from side branches after use of internal mammary artery as conduit has been described, and various forms of therapy have been attempted. Its occurrence is rare and the pathogenesis is controversial. Several studies have used modalities such as Doppler echo and thallium scintiscan to determine the predisposing factors and the extent of steal from the side branches. Selective muscular vasodilation is known to be the most important factor that evokes the steal phenomenon when the first intercostal and/or certain large-caliber pericardial side branches are left in situ during mammary artery harvest. Approximately 25% of patients with a patent internal mammary artery with ischemia in its distribution are noted to have significant side branch collaterals. Marked decrease in distal mammary graft flow with large side branches on arteriography is diagnostic. Percutaneous intervention with transcatheter coil embolization has been successful in management of the unligated side branches. VATS ligation is another safe and minimally invasive option.[115–119]

GASTROEPIPLOIC ARTERY

This artery has been used as an in situ and as a free graft. Short- and mid-term patency rates have been approximately 95% and 92%, respectively. In 104 patients, complications of the following types occurred, requiring catheter-based interventions: 3 occlusions, 5 stenoses, 3 competitive flow, and 8 instances of exercise-induced ischemia.[120] Intraoperative Doppler flow assessment of flow before artery harvest of 25 mL per minute or less suggests unsuitability for grafting.[121]

RADIAL ARTERY

Sensation abnormalities or thumb weakness reflect median nerve and radial nerve injury during radial artery harvest. In a study of 615 patients, Denton et al reported thumb weakness in 5.5% and sensation abnormality in 18.1%. Over a period of 8 to 9 months postoperatively, only 12.1% of patients reported symptoms without improvement. Statistical association was noted with diabetes, peripheral vascular disease, smoking, and elevated creatinine level.[122] Both clinical and laboratory studies have shown that a calcium antagonist in combination with nitroglycerin is more potent than either calcium antagonist or nitroglycerin alone in prevention of radial artery vasospasm in the long term.[123]

Aortic Complications

Postoperative aortic complications of dissection or enlargement have been reported in patients undergoing aortic valve replacement or ascending aortic surgery. Patients with an aortic diameter of 4.0 cm or greater with hypertension were most at risk. The incidence was approximately 0.25% in 8 patients out of 2205 in a study by Milano et al. They concluded with recommendations for aortic root replacement along with other planned aortic surgery in patients with a preoperative aortic diameter greater than 5.0 cm. Congenital bicuspid aortic valve, young age at aortic valve replacement, aortic regurgitation, and fragility or thinning of the aortic valve were strong multivariate analysis predictors for aortic dissection and enlargement.[124–126]

Aneurysms and pseudoaneurysms of the saphenous vein graft–aortic anastomosis site are rare, but may present as paracardiac, hilar, or mediastinal masses on chest radiographs. Fistulous connections with chambers of the heart and cardiac compression are also reported. Mediastinitis appears to be one of the most commonly associated predisposing factors. Rupture of pseudoaneurysms at aortic cannulation sites secondary to mediastinitis has also been documented.[127–129]

HEMATOLOGIC COMPLICATIONS

Hemolysis

Chronic hemolysis from a well-functioning bioprosthesis or mechanical valve is rare. Paravalvular leak is the most common cause for clinically significant hemolysis. A patient-prosthesis mismatch (for example, a 19-mm mechanical valve in a body surface area greater than 1.8 cm^2) or an underlying hemolytic blood dyscrasia such as spherocytosis or thalassemia is another rare cause for hemolysis. Reconstructive patches (Dacron or Hemashield), when subjected to turbulent blood flow in and out of cardiac chambers, pledgets in the blood stream, or other stresses, are other flow-related causes for hemolysis.[130] Ventricular assist devices, pulsatile pumps, and centrifugal or axial flow pumps produce hemolysis enough to elevate bilirubin levels significantly for up to three weeks after implantation, after which there is a gradual downtrend. Intra-aortic balloon usage has also been reported to produce significant hemolysis based on the duration of usage.

Diagnosis is usually made by serial hemoglobin, serum LDH, haptoglobin, and serum and urine bilirubin levels. Patients with hemolysis can be treated conservatively until there is a drop in hemoglobin level to 5 or 6 g/dL (hematocrit of 20%), if the increase in reticulocyte count is over 10%, reflecting adequate bone marrow compensation. Onset of significant bilirubinemia (greater than 4 g/dL) and a packed cell transfusion requirement of 1 to 2 units per week are usually indications for surgical reintervention. A red cell fragility test can be used to detect underlying hemolytic anemia disorder.

Heparin-Induced Thrombocytopenia and Thrombosis

Heparin-induced thrombocytopenia (HIT) and thrombosis (HITT) are the result of autoantibodies directed against heparin-platelet factor 4 complexes that cause platelet activation and aggregation. Based on the platelet count, HIT type I is a milder form, with counts greater than 100,000/dL, and type 2 is the more clinically significant form, with counts less than 100,000/dL. Incidence of type 2 HIT is approximately 5% in patients undergoing cardiac surgery. HITT has been reported to cause stroke, myocardial infarction, graft closure, aortoiliac thrombosis with leg ischemia, mesenteric and deep vein thrombosis, and prosthetic valve thrombosis.[131–136]

Management options may be based on urgency of surgery. A 6- to 8-week observation period decreases the antibody titer significantly, allowing surgery to be performed at full-dose heparin. Serial platelet counts and platelet aggregation tests are mandatory during this period. If surgery cannot be postponed, low molecular weight heparin (LMWH) can be used; however, a cross-reaction risk is then present. Danaparoid (Organon), a mixture of dermatans and heparins that has anticoagulant activity but minimal cross-reaction, is a third option. However, anticoagulation with danaparoid is excessive and difficult to control and reverse. The final option is plasmapheresis. Autoantibodies to heparin can be reduced or eliminated by a series of plasmapheresis treatments.

Neoplastic Hematologic Disorders

Patients with malignant hematologic disorders suffer from an increased risk in undergoing cardiac surgery. Non-Hodgkin's and Hodgkin's lymphoma, multiple myeloma, polycythemia, Waldenström's macroglobulinemia, myelodysplasia, chronic lymphocytic leukemia, and aplastic anemia are some disorders encountered in cardiac surgical practice. Elective cardiac surgery in these patients is complicated by a bleeding diathesis that requires several units of packed cell platelets and FFP concentrate. This predisposes to postoperative multiorgan failure, respiratory insufficiency, and long-term infections. Therefore, risk for morbidity must be carefully weighed against indications for surgery in this group.[137]

Immunologic Alterations

Cardiopulmonary bypass is known to produce a transient immunosuppressive phase immediately postoperatively due to its effect on circulating lymphocytes and monocytes. Total lymphocyte count on bypass drops dramatically. T-cell numbers are significantly decreased, particularly CD4 cells (to as low as 251 cells/dL), while the ratio of CD3 and CD8 cells is retained. Only B cells and natural killer (NK) cells are increased. Expression of class II major histocompatibility antigens from monocytes is also decreased.[138,139] This results in a transient immunosuppression that peaks at postoperative day 1 and gradually returns to normal by day 3.

The outcome of human immunodeficiency virus (HIV) infection after CPB is still unclear. Conflicting reports, mostly anecdotal, claim that a small percentage of HIV patients progress to AIDS after CPB, but there is no conclusive evidence so far. In fact, in one study of a 74-month follow up, no such progression was noted.[140,141] Vijay et al evaluated outcomes in HIV patients undergoing cardiac surgery based on preoperative CD4 count. Elective surgery for noninfective indications in patients with a CD4 count greater than 200 had immediate postoperative outcomes similar to those of the non-HIV population. However, emergent surgery for infective etiology with a CD4 count of less than 200 was uniformly fatal.[142]

NEUROLOGIC COMPLICATIONS

Neurologic complications after cardiac surgery fall into the categories of neurologic deficits, cognitive dysfunction, or encephalopathy. Neurologic deficits include hemiparesis, hemiplegia, and visual defects. The prevalence of stroke is far less than that of neurocognitive dysfunction. In young patients, the risk of stroke after cardiac surgery is 0.5% but gradually increases to 5% at 65 years and to 8% in those over 75 years of age for coronary surgery, and averages about 8% for valvular surgery. Reoperations and combined CABG plus valve replacement can have an incidence of up to 18%.[143–145]

Neurologic Deficits

Aortic atheroma and prior history of stroke are the two most important predictors of stroke following cardiac surgery. Patients who have limited or no atheroma have a less than 2% incidence while those with a grade 4 or grade 5 atheroma have a 40% stroke rate.[146] Patients with carotid stenosis of less than 50% have a 1% or less incidence, while those with 90% stenosis or greater have a 6.5% stroke rate.[147] Other important risk factors for stroke include age, diabetes, peripheral vascular disease, renal failure, aneurysmal disease of the abdominal aorta, left main coronary stenosis, emergent operation, heart failure class, duration of bypass, number of aortic anastomoses, LV venting, intra-aortic balloon pump (IABP), reexplorations, and intraoperative detection of aortic atheroma. Use of a nonmembrane oxygenator and an arterial filter of greater than 40-micron porosity have also been implicated as risk factors.[148,149]

Abraham et al reported the incidence of stroke in off-pump and on-pump groups as 1.2% and 3.6 %, respectively. But the off-pump group had a significantly higher percentage of redos and calcified aortas (26.4% redos in the off-pump group versus 8.7% in on-pump, and 79% versus 2.9% for calcified aortas, respectively), reiterating that the 3-fold reduction of stroke in off-pump may be significant.[150] Other studies have shown no significant difference in perioperative stroke rate between off-pump and on-pump coronary surgery. Use of low-dose heparin combined with lack of the protective effect of CPB (platelet destruction) on coagulation and blood pressure changes during off-pump surgery contribute to cerebral no-reflow phenomenon accounting for some delayed postoperative TIA and stroke incidence. This may account for the lack of significant stroke rate differences between off-pump and on-pump in the long term.

Several therapeutic measures can be adopted during surgery to reduce the risk of nonembolic stroke and neurocognitive dysfunction. EEG and transcranial Doppler (TCD) have been used to monitor adequacy of CPB physiology and cerebral perfusion; however, cumbersomeness of EEG and lack of specificity with TCD have decreased their utility in the operating room.

INVOS-cerebral oximetry (Somanetics Corporation, Troy, MI) is a device that monitors cerebral venous oxygen saturation and has been utilized at several centers as an adjunct to detect cerebral hypoperfusion. This allows certain intraoperative measures to be taken, such as increasing flow rates, increasing mean arterial pressure and hematocrit, increasing Pa_{CO_2}, and deepening the level of anesthesia to augment cerebral oxygenation, which decrease cerebral oxygen demand and thus eliminate nonembolic causes of stroke and cognitive dysfunction. Use of cerebral oximetry in off-pump surgery to decide on timing of conversion to on-pump surgery is recommended based on a decrease in cerebral saturation (less than 50% saturation correlates with postoperative neurocognitive dysfunction) during off-pump cardiac manipulation for graft placement.[151,152]

Certain mechanical devices such as various cannula tips, aortic nets combined with aortic cannulas (EMBOL-X, Mountain View, CA), have shown that a significant embolic load can be removed during the critical portions of surgery that are notorious for showering emboli.[153] A holistic approach to addressing and optimizing all risk factors provides the best chance for a favorable neurologic outcome.

Neurocognitive Function

Evaluation of neurocognitive function consists of eight tests consolidated into five domains: attention, cognitive speed, memory, executive function, and fine motor function. Disturbances in these areas are more pronounced after deep hypothermia and circulatory arrest than after other types of cardiac operations with significantly shorter bypass times. Cognitive defects are subtle and transient in most patients; however, significant defects persist long term and primarily affect functional recovery and overall patient satisfaction, although it is a rare patient who does not return to work because of cognitive deficits. Nevertheless, a 50% or greater negative change in memory, fine motor function, and attention at 1 week after surgery, as determined by a battery of commonly used tests, was a strong predictor of poor performance at 6 weeks and these disabilities persisted up to 6 months to 5 years in some patients.[154]

Newman found that cognitive deficits are evident in approximately 53% of patients at discharge, decreasing to 36% at 6 weeks, and 24% at 6 months. Linguistic function is the best preserved of all cognitive functions. Such neurocognitive decline has been shown to be dramatically reduced in off-pump surgery, compared to a 90% incidence immediately postoperatively in on-pump surgery.[155,156]

Encephalopathy

Encephalopathy (delirium) is seen in 30% to 35% of patients, with confusion being the most common presentation in the absence of focal neurologic deficits. Most episodes peak within 24 hours after surgery and only 10% of patients have symptoms by the 10th day. Encephalopathy is associated with preoperative substance abuse syndromes, metabolic conditions, and dementia, but not with age, alcoholism, narcotics, or sedatives.[157,158] Please refer to the next section for further details on return to work, productive life, and overall satisfaction following neuropsychological disturbances.

QUALITY OF LIFE AFTER CARDIAC SURGERY

Functional benefits are a group of three subsets of quality of life instruments used to assess patients before and after cardiac surgery. They are physical functioning (fewer incapacitated days per month and fewer activity restrictions), sexual functioning (through increased energy, decreased pain and worry), and role functioning (ability to return to work, participate in social activities, resume pursuit of hobby, and so forth).[159]

Coping and emotional response in cardiac surgery patients can be assessed by a coping checklist and a profile of mood state. There is a significant postoperative decrease in dependent coping strategies such as blaming oneself, wishful thinking, and seeking social support. Preoperative emotional state is the single most important predictor of postoperative coping and emotion.[160]

In a study of gender-matched and procedure-matched patients of two groups (one younger than 50 years and the other older than 75 years), incidence and consequences of mental disturbances in elderly patients following cardiac surgery were compared to younger patients. Mental confusion was more prevalent in the older group, 22.6% versus 11.8% in the younger group. Late mortality was significantly worse and the quality of life diminished in the elderly who were confused in the perioperative period.[161]

Another study of 241 patients correlated perioperative neurocognitive function with the quality of life 5 years after surgery. Lower 5-year overall quality of life correlated well with lower general health and less productive working status and neurocognitive decline postoperatively.[162] Patients who suffered from posttraumatic stress disorder in the postoperative phase consistently rated their life satisfaction lower than the controls in the long term.[163]

Several studies have assessed general quality of life and level of satisfaction in the elderly using the Barthel mobility index and the Duke activity index, and found that 99.1% were satisfied with their operation, and 96.5% were in heart failure class I and II with dramatic improvement in functional status following cardiac surgery, thus justifying surgery in this age group.[164,165] A study of survival and functional status after cardiac surgery and long-term intensive care stay showed that the geriatric depression scale assessment put 91% as normal with only 8% in a severely depressed state. Although in-hospital mortality was high at 34%, all survivors had above average functional state and quality of life, justifying the surgery.[166]

With multiple regression analysis, it has become clear that the strongest predictors of return to work are preoperative employment, educational level, higher family income, early surgery, and less postoperative angina and fatigue.

The overall reemployment rate after surgery was 78% in patients who had the above favorable predictors. These results suggest that the determinants of return to work are largely present before surgery, and that a patient's attitude and expectations along with early surgery play an important role.[167,168]

SUMMARY

Over time, the spectrum of surgical procedures available to patients with cardiac and great vessel disease continues to diversify and to mature. In parallel, our ability to match a widening range of surgical procedures with the individual needs of the patient has evolved as well. The relationships among preoperative patient-related risk factors and procedure-related perioperative care form the basis of the ongoing process of surgical care. Through a precise understanding of the long- and short-term benefits of a given surgical procedure, the risks for early and late complications can be evaluated to ensure that responsible clinical decision making occurs.

The close relationships among our nonsurgical colleagues, patients, and families as well as with the other members of the surgical care team facilitate the prevention of many of the above-described late complications of cardiac surgery. In addition, this teamwork also supports the early detection and successful treatment of many late surgical sequelae.

REFERENCES

1. Svedjeholm R, Dahlin LG, Lundberg C, et al: Are electrocardiographic Q-wave criteria reliable for diagnosis of perioperative myocardial infarction after coronary surgery? *Eur J Cardiothorac Surg* 1998; 13:655.
2. Hake U, Schmid FX, Iversen S, et al: Troponin T: a reliable marker of perioperative myocardial infarction? *Eur J Cardiothorac Surg* 1993; 7:628.
3. Iyer VS, Russell WJ, Leppard P, et al: Mortality and myocardial infarction after coronary surgery: a review of 12,003 patients. *Med J Aust* 1993; 159:166.
4. Guang Y, Zhen-jie C, Yong LW, et al: Evaluation of clinical treatment of atrial fibrillation associated with rheumatic mitral valve disease by radiofrequency ablation. *Eur J Cardiothorac Surg* 2002; 21:249.
5. Mohr FW, Fabricius AM, Falk V, et al: Curative treatment of atrial fibrillation with intraoperative radiofrequency ablation: short-term and midterm results. *J Thorac Cardiovasc Surg* 2002; 123:919.
6. Raman JS, Seevanayagam S, Storer M, et al: Combined endocardial and epicardial radiofrequency ablation of right and left atria in the treatment of atrial fibrillation. *Ann Thorac Surg* 2001; 72:S1096.
7. Pappone C, Oreto G, Rosanio S, et al: Atrial electroanatomic remodeling after circumferential radiofrequency pulmonary vein ablation: efficacy of an anatomic approach in a large cohort of patients with atrial fibrillation. *Circulation* 2001; 104:2539.
8. Chen MC, Chang JP, Guo GB, et al: Atrial size reduction as a predictor of the success of radiofrequency maze procedure for chronic atrial fibrillation in patients undergoing concomitant valvular surgery. *J Cardiovasc Electrophysiol* 2001; 12:867.
9. Lim E, Barlow CW, Hosseinpour AR, et al: Influence of late atrial fibrillation on outcome following mitral valve repair. *Circulation* 2001; 104 (suppl I):59.
10. Usui A, Inden Y, Mizutani S, et al: Repetitive atrial flutter as a complication of the left-sided simple maze procedure. *Ann Thorac Surg* 2002; 73:1457.
11. Albage A, van der Linden J, Bengtsson L, et al: Elevations in antidiuretic hormone and aldosterone as possible causes of fluid retention in the Maze procedure. *Ann Thorac Surg* 2001; 72:58.
12. Bauer EP, Szalay ZA, Brandt RR, et al: Predictors for atrial transport function after mini-maze operation. *Ann Thorac Surg* 2001; 72:1251.
13. Mayr A, Knotzer H, Pajk W, et al: Risk factors associated with new-onset tachyarrhythmias after cardiac surgery–a retrospective analysis. *Acta Anaesthesiol Scand* 2001; 45:543.
14. Steinberg JS, Gaur A, Sciacca R, et al: New-onset sustained ventricular tachycardia after cardiac surgery. *Circulation* 1999; 99:903.
15. Levine JH, Mellits ED, Baumgardner RA, et al: Predictors of first discharge and subsequent survival in patients with automatic implantable cardioverter-defibrillators. *Circulation* 1991; 84:558.
16. Arnar DO, Kerber RE: Cerebral embolism resulting from a transvenous pacemaker catheter inadvertently placed in the left ventricle: a report of two cases confirmed by echocardiography. *Echocardiography* 2001; 18:681.
17. Vilacosta I, Sarria C, San Roman JA, et al: Usefulness of transesophageal echocardiography for diagnosis of infected transvenous permanent pacemakers. *Circulation* 1994; 89:2684.
18. Jarwe M, Klug D, Beregi JP, et al: Single center experience with femoral extraction of permanent endocardial pacing leads. *Pacing Clin Electrophysiol* 1999; 22:1202.
19. Choo MH, Holmes DR Jr, Gersh BJ, et al: Permanent pacemaker infections: characterization and management. *Am J Cardiol* 1981; 48:559.
20. Mansour KA, Kauten JR, Hatcher CR Jr: Management of the infected pacemaker: explantation, sterilization, and reimplantation. *Ann Thorac Surg* 1985; 40:617.
21. Bohm A, Hajdu L, Pinter A, et al: Runaway pacemaker syndrome and intermittent non-output as manifestations of end of life of a VVI pacemaker. *Pacing Clin Electrophysiol* 2000; 23:2143.
22. Prince SE, Cunha BA: Postpericardiotomy syndrome. *Heart Lung* 1997: 26:165.

23. Alkhulaifi AM, Speechly-Dick ME, Swanton RH, et al: The incidence of significant pericardial effusion and tamponade following major aortic root surgery. *J Cardiovasc Surg* 1996: 37:385.
24. Ikaheimo MJ, Huikuri HV, Airaksinen KE, et al: Pericardial effusion after cardiac surgery: incidence, relation to the type of surgery, anti-thrombolytic therapy, and early coronary bypass graft patency. *Am Heart J* 1998: 116:97.
25. Pepi M, Muratori M, Barbier B, et al: Pericardial effusion after cardiac surgery: incidence, site, size, and hemodynamic consequences. *Br Heart J* 1994; 72:327.
26. Tsang TS, Barnes ME, Hayes SN, et al: Clinical and echocardiographic characteristics of significant pericardial effusions following cardiothoracic surgery and outcomes of echo-guided pericardiocentesis for management: Mayo Clinic experience 1979–1998. *Chest* 1999; 116:322.
27. Susini G, Pepi M, Sisillo E, et al: Percutaneous pericardiocentesis versus subxiphoid pericardiotomy in cardiac tamponade due to post-operative pericardial effusion. *J Cardiothorac Vasc Anesth* 1993; 7:178.
28. Schactman M, Scott C, Glibbery-Fiesel DR: Chylopericardium following aortic valve replacement and coronary artery bypass surgery: a case report and discussion. *Am J Crit Care* 1994; 3:313.
29. Angelini GD, Bryan AJ, Lamarra M: Refractory supraventricular tachyarrhythmias due to early posterior pericardial effusion following open heart surgery. *Thorac Cardiovasc Surg* 1988; 36:162.
30. Hauptman PJ, Couper GS, Aranki S, et al: Pericardial effusion after cardiac transplantation. *J Am Coll Cardiol* 1994; 23:1625.
31. Kutcher MA, King SB, Alimurung BN, et al: Constrictive pericarditis as a complication of cardiac surgery: recognition of an entity. *Am J Cardiol* 1982; 50:742.
32. Matsuyama K, Matsumoto M, Sugita T: Clinical characteristics of patients with constrictive pericarditis after coronary bypass surgery. *Jpn Circulation J* 2001; 65:480.
33. Duvernoy O, Malm T, Thuomas KA, et al: CT- and MR-based evaluation of pericardial and retrosternal adhesions after cardiac surgery. *J Comput Assist Tomogr* 1991; 15:555.
34. Seeger JM, Kaelin LD, Staples EM, et al: Prevention of postoperative pericardial adhesions using tissue-protective solutions. *J Surg Res* 1997; 68:63.
35. Mitchell JD, Lee R, Neya K, et al: reduction in experimental pericardial adhesions using a hyaluronic acid bioabsorbable membrane. *Eur J Cardiothorac Surg* 1994: 8:149.
36. Mueller XM, Tinguely F, Tevaearai HT: Pain location, distribution, and intensity after cardiac surgery. *Chest* 2000; 118:391.
37. Moore R, Follette DM, Berkoff HA: Poststernotomy fractures and pain management in open cardiac surgery. *Chest* 1994; 106:1339.
38. Gumbs RV, Peniston RL, Nabhani HA, et al: Rib fractures complicating median sternotomy. *Ann Thorac Surg* 1991; 51:952.
39. Gust R, Becher S, Gust A, et al: Effect of patient-controlled analgesia on pulmonary complications after coronary artery bypass grafting. *Crit Care Med* 1999; 27:2218.
40. Ottino G, De Paulis R, Pansini S, et al: Major sternal wound infection after open-heart surgery: a multivariate analysis of risk factors in 2579 consecutive operative procedures. *Ann Thorac Surg* 1987; 44:173.
41. Stahle E, Tammelin A, Bergstrom R, et al: Sternal wound complications—incidence, microbiology and risk factors. *Eur J Cardiothorac Surg* 1997; 11:1146.
42. Mossad SV, Serkey JM, Longworth DL, et al: Coagulase-negative staphylococcal sternal wound infections after open heart operations. *Ann Thorac Surg* 1997; 63:395.
43. Abid Q, Podila SR, Kendall S: Sternal dehiscence after cardiac surgery and ACE type 1 inhibition. *Eur J Cardiothorac Surg* 2001; 20:203.
44. Yamaguchi H, Yamauchi H, Yamada T, et al: Diagnostic validity of computed tomography for mediastinitis after cardiac surgery. *Ann Thorac Cardiovasc Surg* 2001; 7:94.
45. Totaro P, Lorusso R, Zogno M: Reinforced sternal closures for prevention of sternal dehiscence in high-risk patients. *J Cardiovasc Surg* 2001; 42:601.
46. Katz NM: Pericostal sutures to reinforce sternal closure after cardiac surgery. *J Card Surg* 1997; 12:277.
47. Jutley RS, Shepherd DE, Hukins DW, et al: Sternum screw: analysis of a novel approach to the closure of the chest after surgery. *Heart Surg Forum* 2002; 5:69.
48. Astudillo R, Vaage J, Myhre U, et al: Fewer re-operations and shorter age in the cardiac surgical ward when stabilizing the sternum with the Ley prosthesis in postoperative mediastinitis. *Eur J Cardiothorac Surg* 2001; 20:133.
49. Christenson JT, Maurice J, Simonet F, et al: Open chest and delayed sternal closure after cardiac surgery. *Eur J Cardiothorac Surg* 1996; 10:305.
50. Arbulu A, Gursel E, Camaro LG: Spontaneous right ventricular rupture after sternal dehiscence: a preventable complication? *Eur J Cardiothorac Surg* 1996; 10:110.
51. Castello JR, Centella T, Garro L, et al: Muscle flap reconstruction for the treatment of major sternal wound infections after cardiac surgery: a 10-year analysis. *Scand J Plast Reconstr Hand Surg* 1999; 33:17.
52. El Gamel A, Yonan NA, Hassan R, et al: Treatment of mediastinitis: early modified Robicsek closure and pectoralis major advancement flap. *Ann Thorac Surg* 1998; 65:41.
53. De Varennes V, Tchervenkov CI, Kerrigan C, et al: Sternotomy after muscle flap repair of sternal osteomyelitis and mediastinitis. *J Card Surg* 1990; 5:190.
54. Moor EV, Neuman RA, Weinberg A, et al: Transposition of the grade momentum for infected sternotomy wounds in cardiac surgery: report of 16 cases and review of published reports. *Scand J Plast Reconstr Surg Hand Surg* 1999; 33:25.
55. Durand M, Combes B, Eisele JH, et al: Pulmonary function test predict outcome after cardiac surgery. *Acta Anaesthesiol Belg* 1993; 44:17.
56. Bevelaqua F, Garritan S, Haas F, et al: Complications after cardiac operations in patients with severe pulmonary impairment. *Ann Thorac Surg* 1990; 50:602.
57. Milot J, Perron J, Lapasse Y, et al: Incident and predictors of ARDS after cardiac surgery. *Chest* 2001; 119:884.
58. Messent M, Sullivan K, Keogh BF, et al: Adult respiratory distress syndrome following cardiopulmonary bypass: incidence and prediction. *Anesthesia* 1992; 47:267.
59. Kaul TK, Fields DL, Riggins LS, et al: Adult respiratory distress syndrome following cardiopulmonary bypass: incidence, prophylaxis, and management. *J Cardiovasc Surg* 1998; 39:777.
60. Lo Cicero J, McCann B, Massad M, et al: Prolonged ventilatory support after open heart surgery. *Crit Care Med* 1992; 20:990.
61. Wagner F, Nasseri R, Laucke U, et al: Percutaneous dilatational tracheostomy: results on long-term outcome of critically ill patients following cardiac surgery. *Thorac Cardiovasc Surg* 1998; 46: 352.
62. Shafei H, El-Kholy A, Azmy S, et al: Vocal cord dysfunction after cardiac surgery: an overlooked complication. *Eur J Cardiothorac Surg* 1997; 11:564.
63. Abrahamov D, Tamariz M, Fremes S, et al: Renal dysfunction after cardiac surgery. *Can J Cardiol* 2001; 17:565.
64. Suen WS, Mok CK, Chiu SW, et al: Risk factors for development of acute renal failure (ARF) requiring dialysis in patients undergoing cardiac surgery. *Angiology* 1998; 49:789.
65. Loef BG, Epema AH, Navis G, et al: Off-pump coronary revascularization attenuates transient renal damage compared with on-pump coronary revascularization. *Chest* 2002; 121:1190.

66. Lemmer JH Jr, Stanford W, Bonney SL, et al: Aprotinin for coronary artery bypass grafting: effect on postoperative renal function. *Ann Thorac Surg* 1995; 59:132.
67. Mora Mangano CT, Neville MJ, Hsu PH, et al: Aprotinin, blood loss, and renal dysfunction in deep hypothermic circulatory arrest. *Circulation* 2001; 104:I276.
68. Kiziltepe U, Uysalel A, Corapcioglu T, et al: Effects of combined conventional and modified ultrafiltration in adult patients. *Ann Thorac Surg* 2001; 71:684.
69. Alarabi A, Nystrom SO, Stahle E, et al: Acute renal failure and outcome of continuous arteriovenous hemodialysis (CAVHD) and continuous hemofiltration (CAVH) in elderly patients following cardiovascular surgery. *Geriatr Nephrol Urol* 1997; 7:45.
70. Bent P, Tan HK, Bellomo R, et al: Early and intensive continuous hemofiltration for severe renal failure after cardiac surgery. *Ann Thorac Surg* 2001; 71:832.
71. Onoe M, Magara T, Yamamoto Y, et al: Modified ultrafiltration removed serum interleukin-8 faced in adult cardiac surgery. *Perfusion* 2001; 16:37.
72. Reddy VS, Chen AC, Johnson HK, et al: Cardiac surgery after renal transplantation. *Am Surg* 2002; 68:154.
73. Bernstein J, Peijeira J, Elhilala MM: Urethral stenosis following cardiac surgery. *J Urol* 1983; 89:101.
74. Byhahn C, Strouhal U, Martens S, et al: Incidence of gastrointestinal complications in cardiopulmonary bypass patients. *World J Surg* 2001; 25:1140.
75. Egleston CV, Wood AE, Gorey TF, et al: Gastrointestinal complications after cardiac surgery. *Ann R Coll Surg Engl* 1993; 75:52.
76. Aranha GV, Pickleman J, Pifarre R, et al: The reasons for gastrointestinal consultation after cardiac surgery. *Am Surg* 1984; 50:301.
77. Mercado PD, Farid H, O'Connell TX, et al: Gastrointestinal complications associated with cardiopulmonary bypass procedures. *Am Surg* 1994; 60:789.
78. Huddy SP, Joyce WP, Tepper JR. Gastrointestinal complications in 4,476 patients who underwent cardiopulmonary bypass surgery. *Br J Surg* 1991; 78:293.
79. Aouifi A, Piriou V, Bastien O, et al: Severe digestive complications after heart surgery using extracorporeal technologies. *Can J Anesth* 1999; 46:114.
80. Zacharias A, Schwann TA, Parenteau GL, et al: Predictors of gastrointestinal complications and cardiac surgery. *Tex Heart Inst J* 2000; 27:93.
81. Ghosh F, Roberts N, Firmin RK, et al: Risk factors for intestinal ischemia in cardiac surgical patients. *Eur J Cardiothorac Surg* 2002; 21:411.
82. Bolke E, Jehle PM, Orth K, et al: Changes of gut barrier function during anesthesia and cardiac surgery. *Angiology* 2001; 52:477.
83. Riddington DW, Venkatesh B, Boivin CM, et al: Intestinal permeability, gastric intramucosal pH, and systemic endotoxemia in patients undergoing cardiopulmonary bypass. *JAMA* 1996; 275:1007.
84. Klotz S, Vestring T, Rotker J, et al: Diagnosis and treatment of nonocclusive mesenteric ischemia after open heart surgery. *Ann Thorac Surg* 2001; 72:1583.
85. Klempnauer J, Grothues F, Bektas H, et al: Acute mesenteric ischemia following cardiac surgery. *J Cardiovasc Surg* 1997; 38:639.
86. Allen KB, Salam AA, Lumsden AB: Acute mesenteric ischemia after cardiopulmonary bypass. *J Vasc Surg* 1992; 16:391.
87. Burton NA, Albus RA, Grapver GM, et al: Acute diverticulitis following cardiac surgery. *Chest* 1986; 89:756.
88. Chu CM, Chang HC, Liaw YF, et al: Jaundice after open heart surgery: a prospective study. *Thorax* 1984; 39:52.
89. Hill DM, Warren SE, Mitas JA, et al: Hepatic coma after open heart surgery. *South Med J* 1980; 73:906.
90. Ninomiya M, Takamoto S, Kotsuka Y, et al: Indication and perioperative management for cardiac surgery in patients with liver cirrhosis: our experience with three patients. *Jpn J Thorac Cardiovasc Surg* 2001; 49:391.
91. Bizouarn P, Ausseur A, Desseigne P, et al: Early and late outcome after elective cardiac surgery in patients with cirrhosis. *Ann Thorac Surg* 1999; 67:1334.
92. Takeda M, Furuse A, Kawauchi M, et al: Estimation of functional liver reserve in patients before cardiac surgery using antipyrine plasma clearance test. *J Cardiovasc Surg* 1999; 40:817.
93. Watanabe Y, Kumon K: Assessment by pulse dye densitometry indocyanine green (ICG) clearance test of hepatic function of patients before cardiac surgery: its value as a predictor of serious postoperative liver dysfunction. *J Cardiothorac Vasc Anesth* 1999; 13:299.
94. Lefor AT, Vuocolo P, Parker FB Jr, et al: Pancreatic complications following cardiopulmonary bypass: factors influencing mortality. *Arch Surg* 1992; 127:1225.
95. Ihaya A, Nuraoka R, Chiba Y: Hyperamylasemia and subclinical pancreatitis after cardiac surgery. *World J Surg* 2001; 25:862.
96. Rattner DW, Gu ZY, Vlahakes GJ, et al: Hyperamylasemia after cardiac surgery: incidence, significance, and management. *Ann Surg* 1989; 209:279.
97. Moores WY, Gago O, Morris JD, et al: Serum and urinary amylase levels following pulsatile and continuous cardiopulmonary bypass. *J Thorac Cardiovasc Surg* 1977; 74:73.
98. Herline AJ, Binson CW, Wright JK, et al: Acute pancreatitis after cardiac transplantation and other cardiac procedures: case control analysis in 24,631 patients. *Am Surg* 1999; 65:819.
99. Pilkey RM, Lawrence MD, Wolfshon AL, et al: Splenic rupture resulting from acute pancreatitis after cardiac surgery with intra-aortic balloon pumping: case report. *Can J Surg* 1994; 37:428.
100. Lord RV, Ho S, Coleman MJ, Spratt PM: Cholecystectomy in cardiothoracic organ transplant recipients. *Arch Surg* 1998; 133:73.
101. Frezza EE, Mezghebe H: Indications and complications of arterial catheter use in surgical or medical intensive care units: analysis of 4932 patients. *Am Surg* 1998; 64:127.
102. Thomas F, Burke JP, Parker J, et al: The risk of infection related to radial versus femoral sites for arterial catheterization. *Crit Care Med* 1983; 11:807.
103. Martin C, Saux P, Papazian L, et al: Long-term arterial cannulation in ICU patients using the radial artery or dorsalis pedis artery. *Chest* 2001;119:901.
104. Singh S, Nelson N, Acosta I, et al: Catheter colonization and bacteremia with pulmonary and arterial catheters. *Crit Care Med* 1982; 10:736.
105. Michel L, Marsh HM, McMichan JC, et al: Infection of pulmonary artery catheters in critically ill patients. *JAMA* 1981; 245:1032.
106. Zevola DR, Dioso J, Moggio R: Comparison of heparinized and non-heparinized solutions for maintaining patency of arterial and pulmonary artery catheters. *Am J Crit Care* 1997; 6:52.
107. Charalambous C, Swoboda SM, Dick J, et al: Risk factors and clinical impact of central line infection in the surgical intensive care unit. *Arch Surg* 1998; 133:1241.
108. El-Ansary D, Adams R, Gandhi A: Musculoskeletal and neurological complications following coronary artery bypass graft surgery: a comparison between saphenous vein and internal mammary artery grafting. *Aust J Physiother* 2000; 46:19.
109. Peng MJ, Vargas FS, Cukier A, et al: Postoperative pleural changes after coronary revascularization: comparison between saphenous vein and internal mammary artery grafting. *Chest* 1992; 101:327.
110. Guo LR, Myers ML, Kirk ME: Incidental malignancy in internal thoracic artery lymph nodes. *Ann Thorac Surg* 2001; 72:625.
111. Bogers AJ, Pardijs WH, van Herwerden LA, et al: Chylothorax as a complication of harvesting the left internal thoracic artery in coronary bypass grafting. *Eur J Cardiothorac Surg* 1993; 7:555.

112. Joyce LD, Lindsay WG, Nicoloff DM: Chylothorax after median sternotomy for intrapericardial cardiac surgery. *J Thorac Cardiovasc Surg* 1976; 71:476.
113. Jansen JP, Joosten HJ, Postmus BE, et al: Thoracoscopic treatment of postoperative chylothorax after coronary bypass surgery. *Thorax* 1994; 49:1273.
114. Dimopoulou I, Daganou M, Dafni U, et al: Phrenic nerve dysfunction after cardiac operations: electrophysiologic evaluation of risk factors. *Chest* 1998; 113:8.
115. Singh RN, Sosa JA: Internal mammary artery-coronary artery anastomosis: influence of the side branches on surgical results. *J Thorac Cardiovasc Surg* 1981; 82:909.
116. Gaudino M, Serricchio M, Glieca F, et al: Steal phenomenon from mammary side branches: when does it occur? *Ann Thorac Surg* 1998; 66:2056.
117. Gaudino M, Serricchio M, Tondi P, et al: Do internal mammary artery side branches have the potential for hemodynamically significant flow steal? *Eur J Cardiothorac Surg* 1999; 15:251.
118. Chavan A, Mugge A, Hohmann C, et al: Recurrent angina pectoris in patients with internal mammary artery to coronary artery bypass: treatment with coil embolization of unligated side branches. *Radiology* 1996; 200:433.
119. Pagni S, Bousamra M II, Shirley MW, et al: Successful VATS ligation of a large anomalous branch producing IMA steal syndrome after MIDCAB. *Ann Thorac Surg* 2001; 71:1681.
120. Jegaden O, Eker A, Montagna P, et al: Technical aspect and late functional results of gastroepiploic bypass grafting (400 cases). *Eur J Cardiothorac Surg* 1995; 9:575.
121. Tavilla G, Jackimovicz J, Berreklouw E: Intraoperative blood flow measurement of the right gastroepiploic artery using pulsed Doppler echocardiography. *Ann Thorac Surg* 1997; 64: 426.
122. Denton TA, Trento L, Cohen M, et al: Radial artery harvesting for coronary artery bypass operations: neurologic complications and their potential mechanisms. *J Thorac Cardiovasc Surg* 2001; 121:951.
123. Chanda J, Brichkov I, Canver DC: Prevention of radial artery graft vasospasm after coronary bypass. *Ann Thorac Surg* 2000; 70:2070.
124. Natsuaki M, Itoh T, Rikidake K, et al: Aortic complications after aortic valve replacement in patients with dilated ascending aorta and aortic regurgitation. *J Heart Valve Dis* 1998; 7:504.
125. Milano A, Pratali S, De Carlo M, et al: Ascending aorta dissection after aortic valve replacement. *J Heart Valve Dis* 1998; 7:75.
126. von Kodolitsch Y, Simic O, Schwartz A, et al: Predictors of proximal aortic dissection at the time of aortic valve replacement. *Circulation* 1999; 100(19 suppl):II287.
127. Doyle MD, Spizarny DL, Baker DE: Saphenous vein graft aneurysm after coronary bypass grafting surgery. *AJR Am J Roentgenol* 1997; 168:747.
128. Le Breton H, Pavin D, Langanay T, et al: Aneurysms and pseudoaneurysm of saphenous vein coronary artery bypass grafts. *Heart* 1998; 79:505.
129. Smith JA, Goldstein J: Saphenous vein graft pseudoaneurysm formation after postoperative mediastinitis. *Ann Thorac Surg* 1992; 54:766.
130. Ahmad R, Manohit Harajah FM, Deverall PB, et al: Chronic hemolysis following mitral valve replacement. *J Thorac Cardiovasc Surg* 1976; 1:212.
131. Walls JT, Curtis JJ, Silver D, et al: Heparin-induced thrombocytopenia in open heart surgical patients: sequelae of late recognition. *Ann Thorac Surg* 1992; 53:787.
132. Aouifi A, Blanc P, Piriou V, et al: Cardiac surgery with cardiopulmonary bypass in patients with type 2 heparin-induced thrombocytopenia. *Ann Thorac Surg* 2001; 71:678.
133. Glock Y, Szmil E, Boudjema E, et al: Cardiovascular surgery and heparin-induced thrombocytopenia. *Int Angiol* 1988; 7:238.
134. Gillis S, Merin G, Zahger D: Danaparoid for cardiopulmonary bypass in patients with patient with previous heparin-induced thrombocytopenia. *Br J Haematol* 1997; 98:657.
135. Fernandes P, Mayer R, MacDonald JL, et al: Use of danaparoid sodium (Orgaran) as an alternative to heparin sodium during cardiopulmonary bypass: a clinical evaluation of six cases. *Perfusion* 2000; 15:531.
136. Kalangos A, Relland JY, Massonet-Pastel S, et al: Heparin-induced thrombocytopenia and thrombosis following open heart surgery. *Eur J Cardiothorac Surg* 1994; 8:199.
137. Christiansen S, Schmid C, Loher A, et al: Impact of malignant hematological disorders on cardiac surgery. *Cardiovasc Surg* 2000; 8:149.
138. Rinder CS, Mathew JP, Rinder HM, et al: Lymphocyte and monocyte subset changes during cardiopulmonary bypass: effects of aging and gender. *J Lab Clin Med* 1997; 129:592.
139. Misoph M, Babin-Ebell J, Schwendner S, et al: Response of the cellular immune system to cardiopulmonary bypass in vivo. *Thorac Cardiovasc Surg* 1997; 45:217.
140. Everson, Zeigler R, Sabbaga Amato M, et al: Significance of the human immunodeficiency virus infection in patients admitted to cardiac surgery. *J Cardiovasc Surg* 1999; 40:477.
141. Lemma M, Vanelli P, Beretta L, et al: Cardiac surgery in HIV-positive intravenous drug addicts: influence of cardiopulmonary bypass on the progression to AIDS. *Thorac Cardiovasc Surg* 1992; 40:279.
142. Vijay V, Bocker J, Furlong P, et al: Short-term outcomes of cardiac surgery in the HIV positive. *Chest* 2001; 120:306S.
143. Cernaianu AC, Vassilidze TV, Flum DR, et al: Predictors of stroke after cardiac surgery. *J Card Surg* 1995; 4:334.
144. Cheng RT: Neurological complications in heart disease. *Baillieres Clin Neurol* 1997; 2:337.
145. Kuroda Y, Uchimoto R, Karieda R, et al: Central nervous system complications after cardiac surgery: a comparison between coronary artery bypass grafting and valve surgery. *Anesth Analg* 1993; 76:222.
146. Barbut D, Lo Y, Hartman GS, et al: Aortic atheroma is related to outcome but not numbers of emboli during coronary bypass. *Ann Thorac Surg* 1997; 64:454.
147. Babu FC, Shah TM, Singh VM, et al: Coexisting carotid stenosis in patients undergoing cardiac surgery: indications and guidelines for simultaneous operations. *Am J Surg* 1985; 150:207.
148. Van Der Linden J, Hadjinikolaou L, Bergman P, et al: Postoperative stroke in cardiac surgery is related to the location and extent of atherosclerotic disease in the ascending aorta. *J Am Coll Cardiol* 2001; 38:131.
149. Saimanen EI: Perioperative stroke with coronary artery bypass surgery: analysis of risk factors. *Scand Cardiovasc J* 2000: 34:41.
150. Abraham R, Karamanoukian HL, Jajkowski MR, et al: Does avoidance of cardiopulmonary bypass decrease the incidence of stroke in diabetics undergoing coronary surgery? *Heart Surg Forum* 2001; 4:135.
151. Edmonds HL, Rodriguez RA, Audenaert SM, et al: Role of neuromonitoring in cardiovascular surgery. *J Cardiothorac Vasc Anesth* 1996; 10:15.
152. Edmonds HL: Advances in neuromonitoring for cardiothoracic and vascular Surgery. *J Cardiothorac Vasc Anesth* 2001; 15:241.
153. Barbut D, Hinton RB, Szatrowski TP, et al: Cerebral emboli detected during bypass surgery or associated with clamp removal. *Stroke* 1994; 25:2398.
154. Ergin MA, Uysal S, Reich DL, et al: Temporary neurological dysfunction after deep hypothermic circulatory arrest: a clinical

marker of long-term functional deficit. *Ann Thorac Surg* 1999; 67:1887.
155. Newman MF, Reves JG: Towards a new frontier in cardiac surgery. *Ann Thorac Surg* 1997; 632:322.
156. Diegeler A, Hirsch R, Schneider F, et al: Neuromonitoring and neurocognitive outcome in off-pump versus conventional coronary bypass operation. *Ann Thorac Surg* 2000; 69:1162.
157. Barbut D, Caplan LR. Brain complications of cardiac surgery. *Curr Probl Cardiol* 1997; 22:449.
158. Taylor KM. Brain damage during cardiopulmonary bypass. *Ann Thorac Surg* 1994; 42:212.
159. Stanton BA, Jenkins CD, Savageau JA, et al: Functional benefits following coronary artery bypass graft surgery. *Ann Thorac Surg* 1984; 37:286.
160. Crumlish CM: Coping: an emotional response in cardiac surgery patients. *West J Nurs Res* 1994; 16:57.
161. Heijmeriks JA, Dassen W, Prenger K, et al: The incidence and consequences of mental disturbances in elderly patient post cardiac surgery-a comparison with younger patients. *Clin Cardiol* 2000; 23:540.
162. Newman MF, Grocott HV, Mathew JP, et al: Report of the substudy assessing the impact of neurocognitive function on quality of life 5 years after cardiac surgery. *Stroke* 2001; 32: 2874.
163. Stoll C, Schelling G, Goetz AE, et al: Health-related quality of life and post-traumatic stress disorder in patients after cardiac surgery and intensive care treatment. *J Thorac Cardiovasc Surg* 2000; 120:505.
164. Mittermair RP, Muller LC: Quality of life after cardiac surgery in the elderly. *J Cardiovasc Surg* (Torino) 2002; 43:43.
165. Jaejer-AA, Hlatky MA, Paul SM, et al: Functional capacity after cardiac surgery in elderly patients. *J Am Coll Cardiol* 1994; 24:104.
166. Isgro F, Skuras JA, Kiessling AH, et al: Survival and quality of life after a long-term intensive care stay. *Thorac Cardiovasc Surg* 2002; 50:95.
167. Stanton BA, Jenkins CD, Denlinger P, et al: Predictors of employment status after cardiac surgery. *JAMA* 1983; 249:907.
168. Shigenobu M, Senoo Y, Teramoto S: Return to work after heart valve replacement. *Acta Med Okayama* 1989; 43:185.

Part **III**

Ischemic Heart Disease

Chapter 19

Indications for Coronary Revascularization

Thoralf M. Sundt, III/Bernard J. Gersh/Hugh C. Smith

Coronary artery disease remains the most common condition suffered by the patients who consult cardiologists and cardiac surgeons, and the practicing cardiac surgeon is confronted with no clinical question more often than "Is coronary bypass indicated in this patient?" It is our aim to provide a practical overview of the current indications for myocardial revascularization, with sufficient reference to the relevant studies on which they are based to afford the reader an appreciation for the validity of their conclusions as well as their vulnerability to modification as the results of medical and surgical treatments of ischemic heart disease evolve.

In the three and a half decades since coronary artery bypass (CABG) surgery was popularized[1] and the 25 years since the introduction of coronary angioplasty,[2] an enormous volume of data has been collected concerning the results of invasive revascularization. Remarkably, from the outset, many of these studies have been prospectively randomized. Equally remarkable is the dearth of data concerning pharmacologic therapies for chronic coronary artery disease despite remarkable progress in the area. For example, although nitrates are unquestionably effective in relieving symptoms, the impact of long-acting nitrates on clinical outcomes has never been rigorously tested. Furthermore, there has been only one trial of beta-blocker therapy in the treatment of angina, the Atenolol Silent Ischemia Study (ASIST) study, which demonstrated benefit for patients with mild effort-induced angina or silent ischemia.[3] A handful of studies of combination therapy with beta blockers and calcium channel blockers have also demonstrated antianginal benefit.[4–6] Most recently randomized trials of two new drugs, Nicorandil and Ranolazine, have been reported.[7,8] Beyond these, however, few studies of medical therapy alone have been performed.

CLINICAL AND LABORATORY ASSESSMENT OF CORONARY ARTERY DISEASE

A surgeon's first introduction to a patient with coronary artery disease is frequently an angiogram. In addition to the coronary anatomy, however, the clinical presentation as well as the results of noninvasive studies of myocardial perfusion and function are necessary to characterize the pathophysiologic implications of the angiographic disease and its impact on prognosis.

The system proposed by the Canadian Cardiovascular Society for grading the clinical severity of angina pectoris is widely accepted (Table 19-1).[9] Unfortunately, angina is a highly subjective phenomenon for both patient and physician, and prospective evaluation of the assessment of functional classification by the CCS criteria has demonstrated a reproducibility of only 73%.[10] Furthermore, there may be

TABLE 19–1 Canadian Cardiovascular Society angina classification

0 = no angina
1 = angina only with strenuous or prolonged exertion
2 = angina with walking at a rapid pace on the level, on a grade, or up stairs (slight limitation of normal activities)
3 = angina with walking at a normal pace less than 2 blocks or one flight of stairs (marked limitation)
4 = angina with even mild activity

strikingly poor correlation between symptoms and ischemia, as is notoriously the case among diabetic patients with asymptomatic "silent ischemia."

Electrocardiography (ECG) is helpful in assessing ischemic burden if abnormal, but demonstrates no pathognomonic signs in half of patients with chronic stable angina.[11] Conversely, a normal ECG is a strong indicator of normal left ventricular function.[12] Stress ECG is simple and inexpensive, however, and is therefore useful as a screening examination. Among patients with anatomically defined disease, it provides additional information about the severity of ischemia and the prognosis of the disease.[13–15] The sensitivity of the test increases with age, with the severity of disease, and with the magnitude of observed ST-segment shift.[13] If ST-segment depression is greater than 1 mm, stress ECG has a predictive value of 90%, while a 2-mm shift with accompanying angina is virtually diagnostic.[16] Early onset of ST-segment depression and prolonged depression after the discontinuation of exercise are strongly associated with significant multivessel disease. Unfortunately, many patients cannot achieve their target heart rates due to beta blockade, or their exercise tolerance is limited because of coexisting disease. This limits the usefulness of this test in these often high-risk patients. Resting abnormalities in the ECG may also limit the predictive accuracy of the test.

Perfusion imaging with thallium-201 or a technetium-99m tracer may be particularly useful in patients with abnormalities on their baseline ECG. A demonstration of reversible defects by comparison of images obtained after injection of the tracer at peak stress with rest images is indicative of ischemia, and hence viability. An irreversible defect indicates nonviable scar.[17,18] The results obtained with both tracers are similar, with the average sensitivity around 90% and specificity of approximately 75%.[13] For patients unable to exercise, pharmacologic vasodilators such as adenosine or dipyridamole may be used with similar sensitivity.[19–23]

Echocardiographic imaging during exercise or during pharmacologic stress has gained increasing popularity among cardiologists. Comparative studies have demonstrated accuracy similar to nuclear studies[12,24,25] with sensitivity and specificity both around 85%.[13] Patients unable to exercise may be stressed with high-dose dipyridamole[26,27] or more commonly dobutamine at doses from 5 to 40 μg/kg/min.[13,26,27] An initial augmentation of contractility followed by loss or "drop out" is diagnostic of ischemia (and accordingly viability), while failure to augment contractility at low dose suggests scar.[18,28,29]

GUIDELINES FOR REVASCULARIZATION

The guidelines for surgical revascularization have been established by the American College of Cardiology and American Heart Association as shown in Table 19-2.[30] The basis for these guidelines resides in the large body of literature comparing medical therapy with surgical revascularization and, more recently, percutaneous transluminal coronary angioplasty (PTCA).

Before reviewing the results of the seminal trials of CABG versus medical therapy performed in the 1970s, and those of newer prospectively randomized trials comparing the results of surgery with PTCA and medical therapy, some limitations of these trials must be recognized. First, it is difficult to ensure comparable patient populations by virtue of the extraordinary anatomic and physiologic complexity of coronary artery disease as well as the heterogeneity of the patient substrate. Differences in ventricular function and comorbidities such as age, diabetes, peripheral vascular disease, and pulmonary disease may have a profound impact on outcomes such as survival or quality of life. For example, caution must be exercised in interpreting the results of nonrandomized and registry reports of PTCA versus surgery because the patients subjected to the former more often have single- or double-vessel disease,[31,32] whereas the latter commonly have triple-vessel or left main disease.[32] Most prospectively randomized trials are subject to similar limitations as they typically include predominantly low-risk patients. For example, the only currently published prospective study comparing all three options of medical therapy, CABG, and PTCA involves patients with single-vessel disease (left anterior descending). Such patients typically compose a small fraction of the population seen in practice. Therefore, although the studies do provide objective data that are directly applicable to the patient subset represented in the study, extrapolation of the results to the more heterogeneous populations seen clinically can only be made if the implicit caveats are clearly understood. The impact of socioeconomic status on prognosis is an important but less tangible variable as well.

Secondly, as a consequence of the overrepresentation of patients at lowest risk of death in randomized trials, most are statistically underpowered with respect to survival analysis. They therefore frequently employ softer end points such as angina or quality of life, or composite end points of death and myocardial infarction (MI). This is further complicated by relatively short-term follow-up in most studies. Since events such as the need for subsequent revascularization characteristically occur at different time intervals after these

TABLE 19–2 AHA/ACC guidelines for CABG

Asymptomatic/mild angina

Class I

(1) left main stenosis
(2) left main equivalent (proximal LAD and proximal circumflex)
(3) triple-vessel disease

Class IIa

(1) proximal LAD stenosis and one or two vessel disease

Class IIb

(1) one or two vessel disease not involving proximal LAD

Stable angina

Class I

(1) left main stenosis
(2) left main equivalent (proximal LAD and proximal circumflex)
(3) triple vessel disease
(4) two vessel disease with proximal LAD stenosis and EF <50% or demonstrable ischemia
(5) one or two vessel disease without proximal LAD stenosis but with a large territory at risk and high risk criteria on noninvasive testing
(6) disabling angina refractory to medical therapy

Class IIa

(1) proximal LAD stenosis with one vessel disease
(2) one or two vessel disease without proximal LAD stenosis, but with a moderate territory at risk and demonstrable ischemia

Unstable angina

Class I

(1) proximal LAD stenosis with one vessel disease
(2) one or two vessel disease without proximal LAD stenosis, but with a moderate territory at risk and demonstrable ischemia
(3) ongoing ischemia despite medical therapy

Class IIa

(1)proximal LAD stenosis and one or two vessel disease

Class IIb

(1) one or two vessel disease not involving the LAD

ST segment elevation (Q-wave) MI

Class I

None

Class IIa

(1) ongoing ischemia despite medical therapy

Class IIb

(1) progressive heart failure with remote territory at risk
(2) primary reperfusion within 6-12 hours

Poor LV function

Class I

(1) left main stenosis
(2) left main equivalent
(3) proximal LAD stenosis and one to two vessel disease

Class IIa

(1) significant viable territory and noncontractile myocardium

Life-threatening ventricular arrhythmias

Class I

(1) left main disease
(2) three vessel disease

Class IIa

(1) bypassable one or two vessel disease
(2) proximal LAD disease and one or two vessel disease

Failed PTCA

Class I

(1) ongoing ischemia with significant territory at risk
(2) shock

(*Continued*)

TABLE 19–2 (*Continued*) AHA/ACC guidelines for CABG

Class IIa
(1) foreign body in critical position
(2) shock with coagulopathy and no previous sternotomy
Class IIb
(1) shock with coagulopathy and previous sternotomy
Previous CABG
Class I
(1) disabling angina refractory to medical therapy
Class IIa
(1) large territory at risk
Class IIb
(1) ischemic in non-LAD distribution with a functioning LITA graft to LAD without aggressive medical or percutaneous treatment

Definitions:
Class I: Conditions for which there is evidence and/or general agreement that a given procedure or treatment is useful and effective.
Class II: Conditions for which there is conflicting evidence and/or a divergence of opinion about the usefulness or efficacy of a procedure.
Class IIa: Weight of evidence/opinion is in favor of usefulness/efficacy.
Class IIb: Usefulness/efficacy is less well established by evidence/opinion.
Class III: Conditions for which there is evidence and/or general agreement that the procedure/treatment is not useful/effective and in some cases may be harmful.
ACC = American College of Cardiology; AHA = American Heart Association; CABG = coronary artery bypass grafting; EF = ejection fraction; LAD = left anterior descending; LITA = left internal thoracic artery; LVE = left ventricular function.

therapies (restenosis after PTCA vs. graft occlusion after CABG), an 8- to 10-year follow-up period is needed to adequately compare long-term results.

Finally, significant improvements in each of these treatment strategies are occurring constantly. Examples include the use of antiplatelet agents,[33] angiotensin-converting enzyme inhibitors, intravascular stents,[34] internal thoracic aortic grafts, and most recently the impressive beneficial effect of lipid-lowering therapy on the subsequent incidence of coronary events.[35,36] These advances along with aggressive risk factor modifications have steadily reduced the morbidity and mortality of coronary artery disease, making differences in the hard end points of survival difficult to demonstrate for any therapy.[37]

COMPARATIVE TRIALS OF REVASCULARIZATION VS. MEDICAL THERAPY IN STABLE ANGINA

Surgical vs. Medical Therapy

Three major randomized studies, Coronary Artery Surgery Study (CASS),[38] the Veterans Administration Cooperative Study Group (VA),[39,40] and the European Coronary Surgery Study (ECSS),[41,42]as well as several other smaller randomized trials conducted between 1972 and 1984[43–45] provide the most reliable outcome data comparing medical and surgical therapy. Despite the limitations noted above, these studies are remarkably consistent in their major findings and the qualitative conclusions drawn from them can continue to be generalized to our current practice.

The central message from all of these studies is that the relative benefits of bypass surgery over medical therapy on survival are greatest in those patients at highest risk as defined by the severity of angina and/or ischemia, the number of diseased vessels, and the presence of left ventricular dysfunction (Figure 19-1).[39,46,47] For example, thus far no study has shown survival benefit for CABG over medical therapy for patients with single-vessel disease.[47–49] It should be emphasized, however, that these trials involved primarily patients with moderate chronic stable angina. These conclusions may, therefore, not necessarily apply to patients with unstable angina or to patients with more severe degrees of chronic stable angina.

A meta-analysis of the seven randomized trials cited above demonstrated a statistically enhanced survival at 5, 7, and 10 years, for surgically treated patients at highest risk (4.8% annual mortality) and moderate risk (2.5% annual mortality), but no evidence of a survival benefit for those patients at lowest risk.[46] The overall survival benefit at 12 years for the three large and four smaller randomized studies is shown in Figure 19-2. Nonrandomized studies have also demonstrated a beneficial effect of surgery on survival of patients with multivessel disease and severe ischemia regardless of left ventricular function.[50–53]

There have been only two randomized controlled trials of surgery versus medical therapy in the 1990s. Their results make an even stronger case for revascularization. In the Trial of Invasive versus Medical Therapy in Elderly Patients with Chronic Symptomatic Coronary-Artery Disease (TIME) study, the incidence of major adverse events (death, nonfatal MI, or hospitalization) was lower and angina relief and

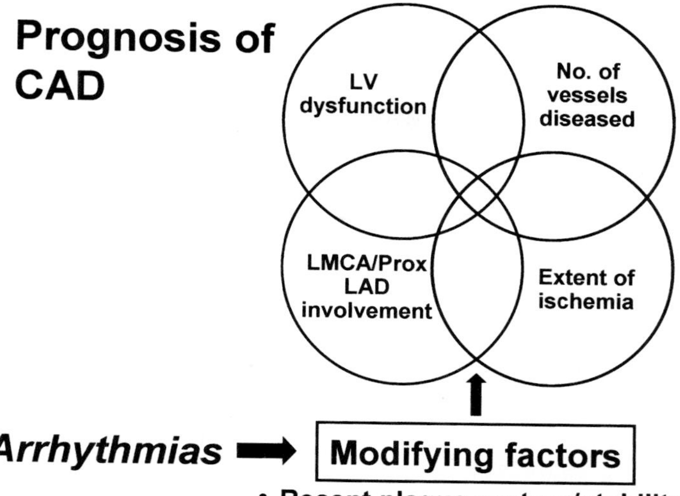

FIGURE 19–1 The decision regarding mode of therapy for coronary artery disease depends upon the individual patient's prognosis as determined by both cardiac and noncardiac conditions.

quality of life superior for those undergoing coronary angiography and surgical revascularization than in those randomized to an initial trial of medical therapy without angiography (19% vs. 49%, $p < .0001$).[54] In the Asymptomatic Cardiac Ischemia Pilot (ACIP) trial, patients with anatomy amenable to CABG were randomized to angina-directed anti-ischemic therapy, drug therapy guided by noninvasive measures of ischemia, or revascularization by CABG or PTCA.[55] At 2 years, mortality was 6.6% in the angina-guided group, 4.4% in the ischemia-guided group, and 1.1% in the revascularization group. The rates of death or MI were 12.1%, 8.8%, and 4.7%, respectively. By pairwise testing, the differences between revascularization and angina-guided therapy were statistically significant.

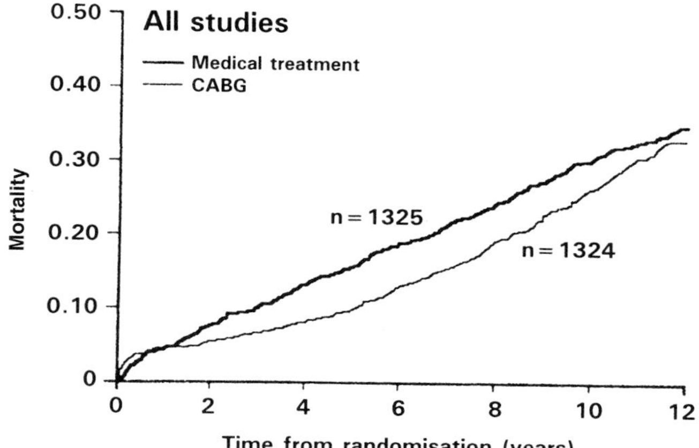

FIGURE 19–2 Survival (mortality) curves for all medically and surgically treated patients with chronic stable angina enrolled in seven prospective, randomized, controlled trials. *(Reproduced with permission from Yusuf S, Zucker D, Peduzzi P, et al: Effect of coronary artery bypass graft surgery on survival: overview of ten-year results from randomized trials by the Coronary Artery Bypass Graft Surgery Trialist Collaboration. Lancet 344:563, 1994.)*

Early concern over a prohibitive operative mortality among patients with impaired ventricular function has been superseded by the recognition that the survival of these patients on medical therapy was much worse than their survival with revascularization. This, coupled with ever improving surgical techniques, such as advances in myocardial preservation and perioperative support, has made this specific subgroup the one in which the relative survival benefit of surgical therapy is the greatest. Accordingly, left ventricular dysfunction in patients with documented ischemia is now considered an important indication—rather than a contraindication—for surgical revascularization.[38,46,50,56,57] Recent evidence that ischemic, viable, hypokinetic myocardium (hibernating or stunned) regains stronger contractile function following effective revascularization has prompted expansion of the indications for surgical revascularization among patients with severe left ventricular dysfunction to include patients who would otherwise be considered candidates for cardiac transplantation. This subject is discussed in more detail below.

In summary, a survival advantage is demonstrable for surgical revascularization over medical therapy in patients with left main disease,[58] those with triple-vessel disease and left ventricular dysfunction,[59,60] those with two-vessel disease and proximal LAD disease,[61] and in patients with severe ischemia and multivessel disease (Figure 19-3).[62,63] Those survival advantages have not been demonstrable among patients with single-vessel disease.[64–66]

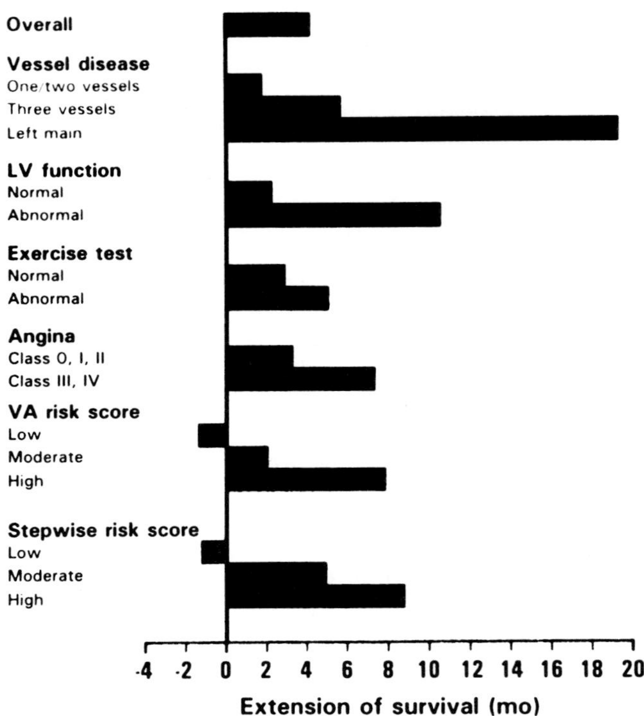

FIGURE 19–3 Extension of survival in months for various subgroups of patients with chronic stable angina treated by surgery as compared with those treated by medicine in seven prospective, randomized, controlled trials. *(Reproduced with permission from Yusuf S, Zucker D, Peduzzi P, et al: Effect of coronary artery bypass graft surgery on survival: overview of ten-year results from randomized trials by the Coronary Artery Bypass Graft Surgery Trialist Collaboration. Lancet 344:563, 1994.)*

Apart from affording a survival benefit, CABG is indicated for the relief of angina pectoris and improvement in the quality of life. Between 80% and 90% of patients who are symptomatic on medical therapy become symptom-free following CABG. This benefit extends to low-risk patients for whom survival benefit from surgery is not likely.[46] Relief of symptoms appears to relate to both the completeness of revascularization and maintenance of graft patency, with the benefit of CABG diminishing with time. Recurrence of angina following CABG surgery occurs at rates of 3% to 20% per year. Although enhanced survival is reported when an internal thoracic artery graft is used to the LAD, there is no significant difference in postoperative freedom from angina.[66] This may be due to vein graft occlusion or progression of native disease in grafted or ungrafted vessels.[39]

Unfortunately, few patients experience an advantage in work rehabilitation with surgery as compared with medical management. Generally, employment declines in both groups and is determined nearly as much by socioeconomic factors as age, preoperative unemployment, and type of job as by type of therapy or clinical factors such as postoperative angina. Notably, surgical revascularization has not been shown to reduce the incidence of nonfatal events such as myocardial infarction (MI) although this may be due to perioperative infarctions that offset the lower incidence of infarction in each study follow-up.[51,67]

PTCA vs. Medical Therapy

Despite the increasing application of catheter-based technology to multivessel disease, the majority of interventions have been historically in single-vessel disease.[32] Accordingly, most of the data comparing angioplasty with medical therapy are derived from studies comprised principally or exclusively of patients with a limited extent of obstructive disease, although most people with angiographically detectable stenosis in one vessel have more extensive atherosclerotic changes throughout most of their coronary vessels. Also, many of these trials antedate the use of IIb/IIIa inhibitors, clopidegrel, and stents. Although angiographic success rates of 85% to 90% are commonplace, no study to date has ever shown a benefit in survival or subsequent MI for PTCA over medical therapy in patients with stable angina pectoris. The results of several recent studies have, however, demonstrated improvement in symptoms and exercise tolerance.

In the Angioplasty Compared with Medical Therapy-I (ACME-I) study, 212 patients with documented ischemia and a single coronary artery stenosis greater than 70% were randomly assigned to medical therapy or angioplasty.[68] After six months, there was no mortality difference in either treatment group; however, PTCA provided more complete angina relief with fewer medications and better quality of life scores as well as longer exercise duration on stress testing than medical therapy.[68] This benefit came at some cost, however; among the 100 angioplasty patients, 19 underwent repeat PTCA and 7 needed CABG surgery during the first six months, compared with 11 angioplasty procedures and no CABG surgery in the patients randomized to medical therapy.[68] Moreover, nearly half of all patients assigned to initial medical therapy were asymptomatic at six months. Because this modest symptomatic benefit was achieved at such a large procedural and financial cost, patients who are either asymptomatic or have mild symptoms should have objective evidence of ischemia prior to PTCA.[69] In a follow-up study by the same investigators, 101 patients with stable angina and two-vessel disease were randomized to PTCA or medical therapy.[70] At six months, both groups had similar improvement in exercise duration, freedom from angina, and overall quality of life. These studies together suggest that, in many patients, an initial trial of medical therapy is appropriate.

Several more recent studies have included patients with multivessel disease. In the Randomized Intervention Treatment of Angina-2 (RITA-2) trial, of 1018 patients with stable angina randomized to medicine or PTCA one third had two-vessel disease and 7% had three-vessel disease. At a median follow-up of 2.7 years, the primary end points of death or MI had occurred twice as often in the PTCA group (6.3 vs. 3.3%, $p < .02$). Surgical revascularization was required during the follow-up interval in 7.9% of the PTCA group, and repeat angioplasty was required in 11%. In the medical group, 23% of patients required revascularization. Angina relief and exercise tolerance were improved to a greater degree in the angioplasty group early, but this difference disappeared by three years.[71] Again, this supports an initial strategy of medical therapy.

Finally, PTCA and medicine as initial strategy were compared among patients with hyperlipidemia in the Atorvastatin vs. Revascularization Trial (AVERT).[72] Among 341 patients with single- or double-vessel disease, ischemic events were actually less common in the medical than in the PTCA groups (13% vs. 21%, $p < .05$). Although criticized for employing outdated angioplasty technology and other issues, the results of this study are consonant with the recent demonstration that lipid-lowering agents may have a powerful impact on ischemic events.[73–75]

PTCA vs. CABG

RANDOMIZED STUDIES

A number of studies comparing an initial strategy of angioplasty versus early surgery have been carried out, all with similar results. It is important to recognize that these studies are comparisons of treatment strategies and not head-to-head comparisons of revascularization techniques. Accordingly, crossover is permitted and end points are selected to determine adverse consequences of the algorithm.

A single-center Swiss study of 134 patients with isolated LAD disease was reported in 1994.[49] At 2.5 years of follow-up there was no significant difference in combined outcomes of MI and cardiac death between treatment groups. There was, however, a greater need for surgical revascularization in the initial PTCA treatment group with 25% requiring a second revascularization procedure compared with only 4.4% in the initial CABG group. Although the PTCA patients were taking significantly more antianginal medication, clinical impairment level, stress test performance, and quality of life indices did not differ at 2 years. These findings held up at 5 years[76] with no difference between groups with respect to mortality or functional outcome but more repeat procedures in the PTCA group.

The Medicine, Angioplasty or Surgery Study (MASS) from Brazil compared medical therapy, PTCA, and CABG using an internal thoracic artery bypass at a single center in 214 patients with stable angina, normal left ventricular function, and proximal stenosis of the left anterior descending coronary artery.[48] In this relatively small but nonetheless important randomized trial, the combined end point of cardiac death, MI, or refractory angina requiring revascularization was statistically significantly less in surgically treated patients. Moreover, there was no significant difference between patients treated medically or with PTCA. In comparison with medical therapy, however, both PTCA and CABG surgery were shown to provide improved relief of severe symptoms of angina pectoris and a lower frequency of inducible ischemia on treadmill exercise testing. There was no difference among the three strategies at the end with respect to mortality or late MI. Similar findings were obtained at 5-year follow-up.[77]

The results of the second MASS trial, which enrolled 611 patients with multivessel disease, have been reported in abstract form.[78] Although technology is a moving target, this trial has the advantage that approximately 70% of PTCA patients had stents placed. Despite this, at one year the medical treatment group had a lower incidence of adverse events and actually had superior angina relief to the PTCA group. Surgical therapy provided the best angina relief and lowest incidence of adverse events.

A number of larger prospectively randomized studies comparing PTCA with CABG have been reported in recent years. All share the limitation that, in general, only a very small minority of patients undergoing revascularization at any center were entered into these trials.[79,80] Accordingly the populations included in the trials may not be generally reflective of clinical practice. For instance, few patients in these studies had significant LV dysfunction, and most randomized patients had only one- or two-vessel disease. In the RITA trial, approximately one third of patients had single-vessel disease.[81] Among clinically eligible patients in the Bypass Angioplasty Revascularization Investigation (BARI)[64] trial and Emory Angioplasty versus Surgery Trial (EAST),[65] approximately two thirds of patients were excluded on angiographic grounds that included chronic total occlusion, left main coronary artery stenosis, diffuse disease, or other anatomic factors making PTCA potentially dangerous.[64,65] Consequently these randomized trials contain only a portion of the spectrum of patients with coronary artery disease encountered clinically.

This has an obvious impact on the likelihood of observing an outcome difference between therapies. As a high proportion of the randomized patients are in the low-risk group, in whom no survival advantage could be demonstrated when CABG surgery was compared with medical therapy in the earlier CAST, ECSS, and VA surgery randomized trials,[38–41] it is possible that any potential survival benefit of CABG surgery over PTCA in high- and moderate-risk groups may be masked.[80]

A second consideration in evaluating these studies is that the success of revascularization procedures depends not only on the criteria employed to define success, but also on the interpretation of those criteria by both patient and physician. In the 1985–1986 National Heart, Lung and Blood Institute PTCA Registry, 99% of patients were discharged alive from hospital and 92% did not sustain a MI or require CABG surgery.[31] In the most recent BARI trial, 99% of patients survived hospitalization and 88.6% of PTCA-treated patients did not have MI or require repeat revascularization by

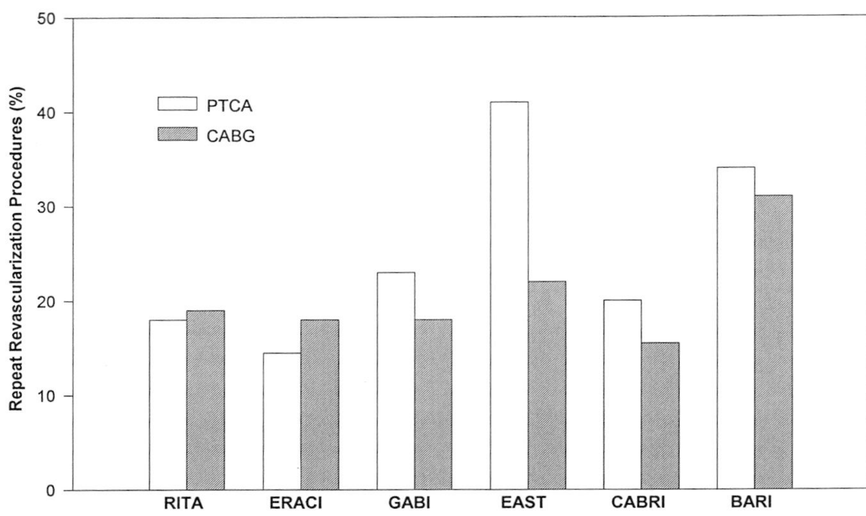

FIGURE 19–4 Risk of repeat revascularization in six randomized trials of PTCA versus CABG surgery. (See refs. 64, 81, 65, 82, and 83 for explanation of acronyms.)

angioplasty or surgery during the initial hospitalization.[64] Employing event-free criteria (death, MI, CABG) for the initial hospitalization, PTCA can be judged successful. However, if a repeat revascularization procedure within five years is regarded as a negative outcome, then only 45.5% of PTCA treated patients are treated successfully.[64] Regardless, the lack of differences in mortality or MI rates permits individuals to select one or the other procedure as initial therapy without the likelihood that they will pay a serious price.

In the BARI, EAST, Coronary Artery Bypass Revascularization Investigation (CABRI), German Angioplasty Bypass Surgery Investigation (GABI), and RITA multivessel PTCA versus CABG surgery trials,[64,65,81,82] mortality and recurrent MI were generally low and similar between 1 and 5 years of follow-up in both the PTCA and CABG treatment groups. Mortality ranged from 3% in the CABRI trial at 1-year follow-up[65] and 3.4% in the RITA trial at 2.5 years[81] to 13% in the BARI trial at 5 years.[64] A similar but slightly higher incidence for MI was noted in some of these trials.

The incidence of repeat revascularization is higher among patients treated with angioplasty than with surgery in all trials carried out to date (Fig. 19-4). The incidence of repeat revascularization in the PTCA-treated patients ranged from 36.5% in the CABRI trial at 1-year follow-up to 62% in the EAST trial at 3 years. The repeat revascularization rate in the EAST trial for angioplasty-treated patients was much higher than that noted in the BARI, CABRI, and RITA trials. There was a concentration of repeat revascularization procedures in trials that required a stress thallium and angiography studies at 1 year; thus some of these procedures may have occurred in the EAST trial as a consequence of protocol-mandated tests rather than clinical indications.[20] In contrast to PTCA, repeat revascularization is less common after CABG in these same studies. The incidence of repeat revascularization procedures in multivessel patients randomized to CABG surgery ranged from 3.5% in the CABRI trial to 13.5% in the EAST trial. Generally, repeat revascularization procedures were required 5 to 8 times more often in patients with multivessel disease initially treated with angioplasty as compared with those randomized to initial CABG surgery. The incidence of angina at follow-up also was generally greater in the PTCA-treated patients than in those randomized to CABG surgery.

In the BARI trial at 5 years, 54.5% of patients initially assigned to PTCA had undergone a repeat revascularization procedure.[64] Of these 23.2% had repeat PTCA, 20.5% underwent CABG surgery, and 10.8% had both PTCA and CABG.[64] Sixty-nine percent of PTCA treated patients who are angina-free at 5 years had not required CABG surgery. Among angina-free patients at 5 years, only 48% of the angioplasty-treated patients compared with 94% of the CABG surgery patients had not had an additional revascularization procedure after their initial procedure.

Several more recent studies of PTCA versus surgery have confirmed these findings. The Argentine Randomized Trial of Coronary Angioplasty vs. Bypass Surgery in Multivessel Disease (ERACI) trial conducted between 1998 and 1990 demonstrated no difference in death or MI, but superior event-free survival in the CABG group at 1 and 3 years.[83,84] In the French Monocentric Study, 152 patients with multivessel disease underwent PTCA or CABG.[85] Again superior event-free survival was seen in the surgical group, driven predominantly by a lesser need for subsequent revascularization.

The impact of stent technology on the comparative results of PTCA and CABG has been recently investigated. In the Arterial Revascularization Therapy Study (ARTS), 1205 patients with multivessel disease underwent CABG or PTCA with stents.[86] No significant differences in the primary end point of freedom from death, stroke, or MI at one year were observed, although the need for revascularization remained higher in the angioplasty than surgery groups. A similar study was performed by the ERACI-2 study group[87]; however, in this study, 30-day mortality was higher in the CABG than in the PTCA group, as was the incidence of Q-wave MI. Repeat revascularization rates were not compared. A concern about the study was the relatively high operative mortality rate (5.7%) in the surgery group as compared with the angioplasty group. The findings of the Surgery or Stent (SOS) study, which compared outcomes in 900 patients with multivessel disease, demonstrated lower all-cause mortality among surgical than angioplasty patients and confirmed higher rates of repeat revascularization after angioplasty.[88] Of particular interest in this study was the reintervention rate, which while still higher than after surgery, was far below that previously reported for angioplasty at only 17%.

It is important to recognize that recent progress in stent technology promises to further reduce the incidence of restenosis, narrowing the gap in late outcome between PTCA and CABG. It is possible that we are on the cusp of a revolution in catheter-based technologies. The use of stents has certainly reduced adverse remodeling,[89] and recent antimitotic drug-eluting stents appear to reduce the restenosis rates even further. The early results with rapamycin suggest that restenosis can be virtually eradicated.[90] Other antimitotic drugs are being tested as well, but results are only preliminary.

In conclusion, the randomized trials of PTCA versus CABG are useful, but only if results are interpreted in the context of the types of patients entering or eligible to enter these trials.[79,80] PTCA is a reasonable alternative to CABG surgery, and for many patients is the preferred initial approach, provided the patient understands that there is a higher incidence of recurrent angina and need for repeat revascularization procedures. This applies to patients with multivessel disease and preserved left ventricular function in the main. For most patients similar to those included in these published trials, it is reassuring that a nonsurgical revascularization procedure does not place them at increased risk of MI or death in comparison with the outcomes of surgical therapy. Extrapolating these results to patients who are not eligible for entry is intellectually flawed and potentially misleading, however.

NONRANDOMIZED DATABASE COMPARISONS

Additional information on the long-term outcome of coronary angioplasty and CABG surgery in patients may be obtained from large, prospectively managed, unrandomized database studies. In the Duke Cardiovascular Disease Databank, 9263 patients undergoing clinically indicated coronary angiography between 1984 and 1990 were followed a mean of 5 years after nonrandomized treatment by CABG, PTCA, or medical therapy.[32] Patients with valvular disease, prior revascularization, significant (more than 75%) left main disease, and congenital and nonischemic cardiomyopathy were excluded. Overall, 39% of the patients had single-vessel disease, 31% two-vessel disease, and 30% three-vessel disease. Initial therapy was medical in 3053 patients, PTCA in 2788 patients, and CABG in 3422 patients. To correct for baseline differences among treatment groups, a standard covariate adjustment was performed that included all identified prognostic factors in a multivariate survival model. Complete follow-up was obtained in 97% of patients. The 5-year survival was 91%, remarkably similar to that reported from Emory, which showed an overall adjusted 5-year survival rate of 93% in both groups.[57] The mortality hazard ratios derived from the Cox regression model to evaluate relative survival differences in this database study are shown for medicine versus CABG surgery in Figure 19-5, PTCA versus medicine in Figure 19-6, and PTCA versus CABG in Figure 19-7.[32]

From a practical standpoint, in this database study as in the randomized trials, the effect of revascularization on survival depended largely on the extent of the coronary artery disease and is an example of the concept of benefit in relationship to a “gradient of risk.” For the least severe (one-vessel) disease, there were no survival advantages of revascularization over medical therapy in up to 5 years of follow-up.[32] For intermediate levels of coronary artery disease severity (i.e., two-vessel disease), there was a higher 5-year survival rate for patients undergoing revascularization than for those treated medically. For patients with the most severe coronary artery disease (i.e., three-vessel disease), CABG surgery provided a significant and consistent survival advantage over medical therapy. PTCA appeared prognostically equivalent to medical therapy in these patients, but only a small number of patients in this subgroup underwent angioplasty. In comparing PTCA with CABG surgery, PTCA demonstrated a small survival advantage over CABG surgery for patients with less severe two-vessel disease, whereas CABG surgery was superior for more severe two-vessel disease (i.e., proximal left anterior descending artery involvement).

SPECIAL CIRCUMSTANCES

Acute Coronary Syndromes

The acute coronary syndromes (ACS) cover a wide spectrum from ST-segment elevation MI with underlying coronary obstruction or Prinzmetal's to variant angina in patients with coronary vasospasm in the absence of significant underlying obstruction. The rubric of the non–ST-segment elevation ACS encompasses the entities of unstable angina, non–Q-wave MI, and postinfarction angina. They denote acute, symptomatic changes in the myocardial oxygen supply demand ratio over a short time span. Prinzmetal's angina, or coronary vasospasm, is diagnosed definitively by electrocardiograms obtained during the episode of pain and is treated medically. Unstable angina is not a uniform clinical entity but describes the spectrum of myocardial ischemia

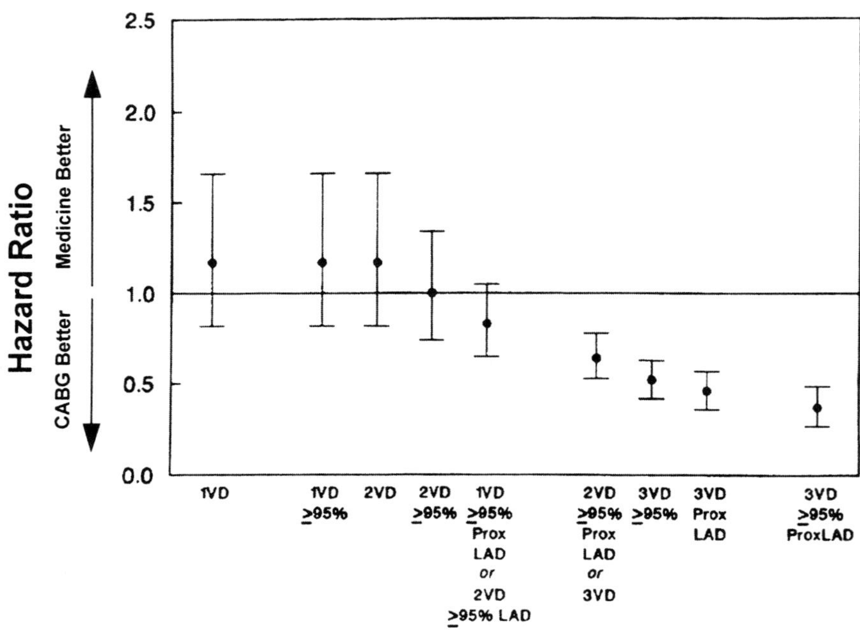

FIGURE 19–5 Hazard (mortality) ratios for CABG surgery versus medicine calculated from the Cox regression model to evaluate relative survival differences. Points indicate hazard ratios for each level of a weighted (0 to 100), hierarchical, prognostic coronary artery disease index. Bars indicate 99% confidence intervals. Horizontal line at 1.0 indicates point of prognostic equivalence between treatments. Hazard ratios below this line favor CABG; those above the line favor medicine. VD, vessel disease; Prox LAD, proximal left anterior descending coronary artery. *(Reproduced with permission from Mark DB, Nelson CL, Califf RM, et al: Continuing evolution of therapy for coronary artery disease; initial results from the era of coronary angioplasty. Circulation 89:2015, 1994.)*

between chronic stable angina and MI. Unstable angina implies a recent change in the severity, character, or trigger threshold of chronic stable angina or new onset angina. Approximately 5.6 million Americans have chronic angina, and about 350,000 develop new angina each year.[91] Unstable angina develops in approximately 750,000 Americans each year and is associated with subsequent MI in approximately 10%. Postinfarction angina is defined as the presence of angina or other evidence of myocardial ischemia in a patient with a recent (one to two weeks) Q-wave or non–Q-wave MI.

Unstable and postinfarction angina are classified into subsets according to the triggering stimulus (A-C) and frequency of pain (I-III).[92] Class A indicates angina precipitated by an extracardiac or indirect stimulus such as an arrhythmia or hypotension that can be reversed by medical management. Class B indicates angina without an extracardiac or indirect stimulus, and class C indicates angina in the presence of acute MI. Class I is new or accelerated angina without pain at rest. Class II is angina at rest within one month but not within 48 hours. Class III is angina at rest within 48 hours.

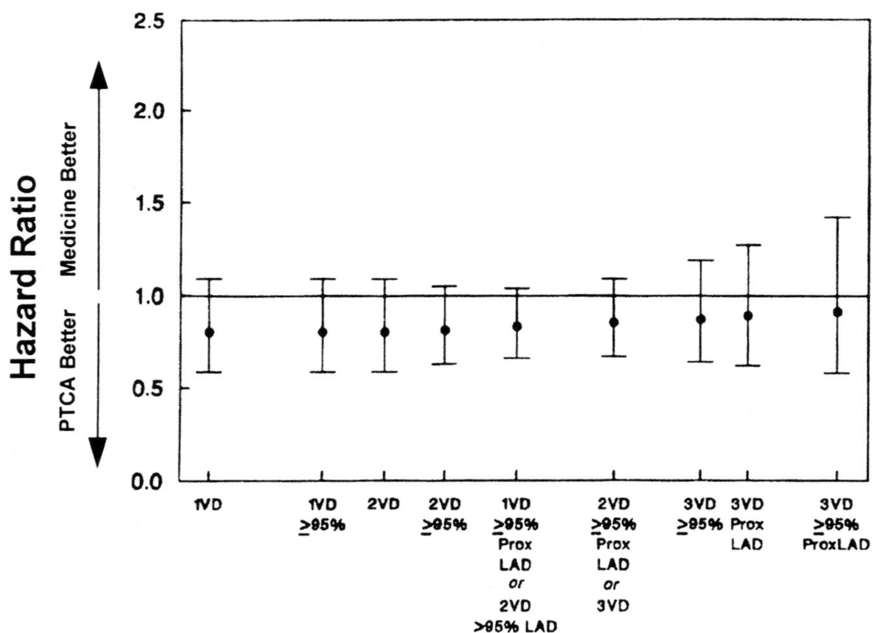

FIGURE 19–6 Hazard ratios for PTCA versus medicine. See Fig. 19-5 for explanation. Points below the horizontal line favor PTCA. *(Reproduced with permission from Mark DB, Nelson CL, Califf RM, et al: Continuing evolution of therapy for coronary artery disease; initial results from the era of coronary angioplasty. Circulation 89:2015, 1994.)*

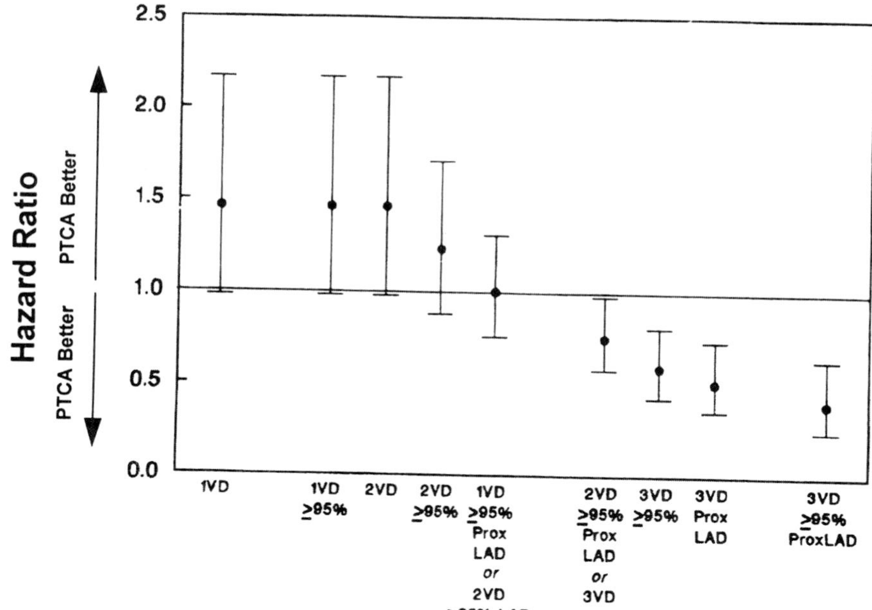

FIGURE 19–7 Hazard ratios for CABG surgery versus PTCA. See Fig. 19-5 for explanation. Points below the horizontal line favor CABG (not PTCA as mislabeled). *(Reproduced with permission from Mark DB, Nelson CL, Califf RM, et al: Continuing evolution of therapy for coronary artery disease; initial results from the era of coronary angioplasty. Circulation 89:2015, 1994.)*

The initial approach to the patient with non–ST-segment elevation ACS is pharmacologic stabilization followed by risk stratification. The latter is based upon multiple clinical, demographic, and ECG variables in addition to the use of serum biomarkers. In institutions with facilities for early angiography, patients at intermediate or high risk (the majority) undergo early angiography with a view to revascularization. In many parts of the world, however, angiographic facilities are limited and an alternative approach based upon pharmacologic stabilization followed by mobilization and risk stratification utilizing stress testing is employed.

The most recent randomized controlled trials of aggressive versus conservative approaches to non–ST-segment elevation ACS are the second Fragmin and Fast Revascularization During Instability in Coronary Artery Disease (FRISC II), Treat Angina with Aggrastat and Determine Cost of Therapy with an Invasive or Conservative Strategy (TACTICS), and Value of First Day Angiography/Angioplasty in Evolving Non-ST Segment Elevation Myocardial Infarction: Open Multicenter Randomized Trial (VINO) trials.[93–95] Despite differences between these trials, the results favor an aggressive strategy with a view towards revascularization in the majority of the patients shown to be at high risk (e.g., older patients, diabetics, those with ST-segment depression on ECG, and those with elevated CPK-MB or serum troponins).

CABG VS. MEDICAL THERAPY

The technical advances in PTCA in the setting of ACS have relegated CABG largely to a secondary position in most acute cases. The special circumstances of postinfarction mechanical complications of papillary muscle rupture, ventricular septal defect, and shock are specifically treated in other chapters of this text. It should be noted, however, that two multicenter trials and one single-center randomized trial involving a total of 823 patients have evaluated the relative merits of CABG surgery and medical therapy in unstable angina between 1972 and 1982.[96–98] Patients with left main disease, poor left ventricular function (ejection fraction less than 30%), and those over age 70 were not included. In the VA cooperative study, improved survival and a lower rate of recurrent angina were shown with surgery, and at both 5 and 8 years there were fewer subsequent hospitalizations in the surgical group for cardiac reasons.[96] Interestingly, there was no difference in progression to Q-wave MI between medical and surgical groups.[96] Like the VA study, the National Cooperative Study Group Trial[97] showed no difference in progression to Q-wave MI and less severe subsequent angina with operation. Unlike the VA trial, however, there was no survival difference at two years (90% in both groups). Of note, 32% of the medical group crossed over to surgery by 24 months. As current medical therapy was not available to these patients, there is significant difficulty in extrapolating the results of these trials to current clinical practice. Finally, Bertolasi et al reported a single-center study of 113 patients, which demonstrated less subsequent angina, fewer infarctions, and a survival benefit for surgery in short-term follow-up.[98]

Among patients with unstable angina or non–Q-wave MI, medical management followed by earlier delayed PTCA or CABG resulted in 6-week mortality and nonfatal MI rates of 2.1% and 6.1% in the Thrombolysis in Myocardial Ischemia (TIMI)-IIIB trial involving 1473 patients.[99] This study compared the results of a strategy of initial stabilization and an aggressive arm involving routine angiography followed by revascularization in the presence of suitable anatomy with a conservative arm reserving angiography for those with recurrent angina or a positive stress test. At 42-day and 1-year follow-up there was no difference in death or MI between the two groups. Subsequent subset analyses have demonstrated a trend in favor of an aggressive approach to revascularization over medical therapy in patients at higher risk as characterized by an elevated CPK-MB fraction (non–Q-wave MI).[99] Somewhat surprisingly, revascularization rates were similar, with only the timing of that revascularization event being different. The addition of thrombolytic therapy in these patients is not beneficial and may be harmful.

The Veterans Affairs Non-Q-Wave Infarcts and Strategies in Hospitals (VANQWISH) trial[100] had a similar design to TIMI-IIIB. In this study, however, a higher early mortality rate was observed in the invasive group than in the medical group, possibly due to the extraordinarily high perioperative mortality rate of 7.7% in the CABG group. The opposite result was found in the FRISC II.[93] These investigators found a benefit with early revascularization, particularly among patients with elevated troponin. The reasons for such different results among these studies is likely due to differences in patient populations studied. It is likely that the higher-risk patients benefit from an aggressive approach, while lower-risk patients have less to gain and so are more likely to suffer adverse consequences.

PTCA FOR ACUTE MYOCARDIAL INFARCTION

Because of the rapidity with which vessel patency can be restored using percutaneous techniques, PTCA has all but replaced CABG in the setting of acute MI. Both thrombolytic therapy and direct or primary angioplasty can restore coronary artery patency and flow during acute MI, but multiple randomized controlled trials have demonstrated the superiority of PTCA when performed promptly. In the absence of hemorrhagic concerns, however, thrombolytic therapy is more widely available and is standard early therapy for acute transmural MI when immediate angioplasty is unavailable.

Several early myocardial reperfusion trials have assessed the role of routine adjunctive angioplasty, given that not all arteries can be reopened by thrombolysis, that reocclusion occurs in some arteries initially opened, and that reocclusion is associated with increased morbidity and mortality.[101,102] In these studies the addition of routine angioplasty to thrombolytic therapy did not enhance patency, improve left ventricular function, or reduce early mortality in comparison with a more conservative approach of ischemia-driven angiography, but did increase expense and vascular bleeding problems.[103–105] A meta-analysis of adjunctive PTCA and thrombolysis versus thrombolysis showed no early benefit of PTCA except in patients who have clinical indications for early revascularization (e.g., postinfarction angina).[106] These studies were performed in an early phase of PTCA, however, and the addition of stents as well as IIb/IIIa inhibitors and new lytics have more recently renewed interest in a combined strategy.

Asymptomatic Coronary Artery Disease

The role of revascularization, either by PTCA or CABG, versus medical therapy in the setting of asymptomatic coronary artery disease has been studied in the ACIP trial.[107] Of 558 patients with coronary artery disease and medically controlled angina, treatment was randomized to revascularization or medical therapy directed toward eliminating angina or eliminating ischemia during ambulatory ECG. Revascularization was more effective than medical therapy in relieving ischemia, and CABG was superior to PTCA (70% freedom from ischemia vs. 46%, $p < .002$). Mortality at one and two years was superior for revascularization as compared with angina-directed medical therapy, but not superior to ischemia-directed medical therapy.[55,108] The greatest benefit was among those patients with the most severe disease.

The documentation of ischemia, however, is critical. Several studies emphasize the flaws in the assumption that one can identify future culprit lesions in the absence of symptoms or documentation of ischemia.[109] Among patients undergoing serial coronary arteriography who subsequently developed acute MI or unstable angina, the severity of stenosis at the time of initial angiogram is poorly predictive of the culprit lesion causing the acute ischemic syndrome.[109–112] In most cases the severity of the lesion responsible for subsequent ischemia was less than 50%, and in many patients it was not present at all on the initial angiogram. The lack of benefit of prophylactic revascularization incidentally raises concern regarding the number of patients undergoing angioplasty who have not undergone stress testing to document objective evidence of ischemia when severe symptoms at the time of presentation were absent.[113] Bech et al have demonstrated that fractional flow reserve exceeded 0.75 in 91 of 325 patients planned for PTCA without noninvasive evaluation of ischemia, and that among those patients angioplasty had no impact on event-free survival or angina.[114]

The Elderly

Age is a predictor of operative risk in most models, but is also a predictor of poor outcome with medical therapy in the presence of coronary artery disease. The Swiss TIME trial was recently reported.[54] In this study, 301 patients over the age of 75 were randomized to medical therapy with or without invasive evaluation. Of those undergoing angiography, two thirds had revascularization. Among those not initially assigned to invasive evaluation, one third had revascularization at some time during the study interval. Approximately two thirds of revascularizations were PTCA. During the 6-month follow-up interval, adverse events (death, MI, rehospitalization) occurred in one half of those assigned to initial therapy without invasive evaluation and in one fifth of the other group. These data suggest that invasive evaluation should be offered to the elderly who are symptomatic on adequate medical therapy.

The choice of mode of revascularization will be particularly impacted in this group of patients by the presence of comorbidities that may increase the risk of surgical intervention, such as cerebrovascular disease, renal dysfunction, and pulmonary disease. The impact of a reduction in operative morbidity through "off-pump" coronary bypass on this choice is as yet unclear. There are an increasing number of studies to suggest that "off-pump" surgery offers its greatest advantage over conventional surgery in just this group of patients with comorbid conditions (see Ch. 22). The majority of these studies are not randomized, however, making their results less conclusive than one would hope. A recently published randomized trial from the Netherlands demonstrated slightly improved neurocognitive outcomes among off-pump patients at 3 months, but this difference became negligible at one year.[115] The Beating Heart Against Cardioplegic Arrest Studies (BHACAS 1 and 2) demonstrated a reduction in morbidity as assessed by atrial fibrillation, sternal wound infection, inotropic requirement, transfusion, and hospital stay, but did not assess neurocognitive outcomes.[116] The impact, therefore, of newer technologies on broadening the indications for CABG in the elderly is as yet unclear.

Severe Left Ventricular Dysfunction

Left ventricular dysfunction is a predictor of increased operative risk for most cardiac surgical procedures, and in the early days of coronary revascularization these patients were not offered CABG. Like age, however, it is also a strong predictor of poor outcome with medical therapy. Accordingly, more recently significant LV dysfunction has been considered an indication rather than contraindication to surgical revascularization. In some patients, LV function has been shown to improve—sometimes dramatically so—after revascularization, leading to the concept of "hibernating" or "stunned" myocardium.[117–120] The diagnosis of viable myocardium that is potentially recoverable depends upon the identification of preserved metabolic activity by positron emission tomography (PET), cell membrane integrity by thallium-201 or technetium-99m SPECT, or dobutamine stress echocardiography.[18,120,121]

Thus far, no prospective randomized trials of medical versus surgical therapy in patients with severe LV dysfunction have been reported, although the NIH-sponsored Surgical Treatment for Ischemic Heart Failure (STICH) trial has just begun. A number of retrospective analyses of the impact of revascularization on outcome in patients with LV dysfunction with or without demonstrable viability have been reported. Recently Allman et al reported the results of a meta-analysis of these studies.[122] Their analysis demonstrated a 79.6% reduction in annual mortality (16% vs. 3.2%, $p < .0001$) when patients with severe three-vessel disease and severely depressed LV function with evidence of viability underwent surgery versus medical therapy. Among those patients without demonstrable viability, the mortality rates were similar (7.7% vs. 6.2%, $p =$ NS). This study is subject to all of the limitations of a retrospective surgical series, including perhaps most importantly the unaccountable effect of the clinical judgment employed in selecting patients for one therapy versus another. The results have been remarkably consistent over the years among virtually all studies, with the greatest benefit of surgical revascularization being sustained by the patients with the worst ventricular function.

The relative roles of CABG and PTCA in this population are not clearly defined despite the number of trials of angioplasty versus surgery. Patients with left ventricular dysfunction may be at higher mortality risk following revascularization by PTCA than by CABG surgery, but the potential survival benefits of CABG surgery have not been demonstrated, perhaps because these patients are underrepresented in these prospective, randomized studies. In a multicenter study of patients with left ventricular dysfunction (ejection fraction less than 40%), slightly more than one quarter of the patients were dead in the 2 years following multivessel angioplasty.[123] Similar results have been reported from other studies of PTCA in patients with multivessel disease and left ventricular dysfunction. Overall, the outcome with PTCA appears less favorable than that obtained after CABG surgery,[57] possibly as a function of more complete revascularization in surgical patients.[124]

Completeness of revascularization may be particularly important in patients with left ventricular dysfunction. An analysis of data from the CASS registry demonstrated that, among patients with triple-vessel disease, 4-year survival was dependent upon the number of vessels bypassed, particularly among those with more severe angina and those with worse ventricular function.[124] For PTCA, complete revascularization of target arteries ranged from 57% to 61% in the prospective, randomized trials in which complete revascularization was not a protocol requirement (BARI, EAST, CABRI). In the GABI and RITA trials, complete revascularization by PTCA was targeted and was achieved in 86% in GABI and in 81% and 63% of patients with two- or three-vessel disease in RITA.[81,82]

Total Occlusion

Revascularization is not possible in most patients with chronic, totally occluded coronary arteries, although the advent of stent technology has offered some improvement in this area. In the randomized trials of multivessel PTCA versus CABG, 35% to 37% of the patients excluded were excluded because of the presence of a chronic total occlusion of a coronary artery serving viable myocardium. Thus the high proportion of trial patients with less than three-vessel disease, well-preserved ventricular function, and absence of chronically occluded arteries produces a study population that favors a higher incidence of complete revascularization by PTCA and attenuated consequences of incomplete revascularization than would be expected in community practices. Among patients with severe angina, triple-vessel disease, and ventricular dysfunction, survival is greater in those with three or more coronary arteries bypassed than in those with only two vessels bypassed.[46,124] CABG surgery improves survival in patients with three- and two-vessel disease with left ventricular dysfunction compared with medical therapy. Although angioplasty may have a similar survival benefit, its influence on this high-risk subgroup has not been fully tested or reported.

Diabetes Mellitus

It has been recognized for many years that patients with diabetes mellitus are at higher risk following percutaneous[125] or surgical[125–128] revascularization. The BARI trial was the first trial large enough to identify significant differences in outcome between diabetic and nondiabetic patients. In this study, which included 353 diabetic patients, a survival benefit was observed among patients undergoing CABG as compared with those undergoing PTCA. The explanation for this is not entirely clear, although an intriguing observation is that while the incidence of subsequent MI is similar between groups, survival following MI is superior among those who have undergone surgical revascularization.[129] In fact, diabetics suffering spontaneous Q-wave MI were more than 10 times as likely to die with their infarction if they had been treated with PTCA as compared with CABG. No such protective effect was seen among nondiabetic patients either with or without Q-wave MI. This survival difference was even more pronounced at 7 years, with 76.4% of diabetics in the surgical arm alive as compared with 55.7% in the angioplasty arm.[130]

The physiologic basis for this difference remains a matter of speculation, although the completeness of revascularization may be a factor. Because of the significant incidence of restenosis after PTCA in diabetics, Van Belle et al analyzed ejection fraction at 6 months and long-term cardiac mortality and morbidity among 513 diabetic patients stratified according to the presence of occlusive restenosis (n = 94), nonocclusive restenosis (n = 257), and no restenosis (n = 162).[131] The mortality rose with restenosis (24% without restenosis, 35% with nonocclusive restenosis, and 59% with occlusion), and ejection fraction fell with occlusion (decrease of 4.8% ± 12.6%). Coronary occlusion was strongly predicted by coronary occlusion by multivariate analysis.

The results of the BARI trial prompted retrospective post hoc analyses of several earlier trials. The results have been variable. An analysis of diabetic patients from the CABRI trial at 8 years demonstrated a mortality rate of 3.5% for CABG patients versus 15.6% for PTCA.[132] There was also a nonsignificant trend for better survival among diabetic patients in the EAST trial.[133] A meta-analysis of pooled data pertaining to diabetic patients from CABRI, EAST, and RITA, however, found similar 5-year mortality rates following CABG or PTCA.[134] Several other data bank studies have also been conducted. The Northern New England Cardiovascular Disease Study Group evaluated survival 5 years after treatment among 7159 diabetic patients with multivessel disease who were treated with CABG or PTCA between 1992 and 1996.[135] Of this group, 38.6% of patients were clinically and angiographically similar to those randomized in BARI. Patients were treated according to physician preference. Those undergoing CABG were more likely to have three-vessel disease and tended to be older with greater degrees of ventricular impairment and obstructive lung disease. There were more women and more urgent interventions in the PTCA group. After adjusting for these variables, PTCA was associated with a significantly greater mortality rate at 5 years (risk ratio = 1.49; 95% CI, 1.02 to 2.17; $p = .037$) and particularly among diabetics with three-vessel disease (hazard ratio 2.01; CI, 1.04 to 3.91; $p = .038$).

Diabetes is a condition characterized biologically by an inflammatory, proliferative, and prothrombotic state. This may account in part for the increased risk of restenosis and occlusion. Since diabetics tend to have more diffuse disease, the importance of complete revascularization—which is more often achieved surgically than percutaneously—may be enhanced. Another explanation may have more to do with patient selection than vascular biology. It has long been recognized from the previously cited studies that the survival advantage of CABG over medical therapy is greater the more extensive the coronary disease, and more recent studies of PTCA versus CABG have demonstrated similar trends. Diabetic patients tend to have more extensive disease, and in the BARI trial diabetics had a higher frequency of three-vessel disease, diffuse disease, proximal LAD disease, and left ventricular dysfunction.

In this respect it is interesting to note that in community studies[136] and the BARI registry,[137] there were no significant differences in outcomes between these therapies in the diabetic subgroup, although diabetics have a poorer outcome with both PTCA and CABG in comparison with nondiabetics. It must be emphasized that in these nonrandomized trials in which the selection of therapy was at the discretion of the physician and the patient, a very clear trend was noted. The "sicker" patients with left ventricular dysfunction and triple-vessel disease were far more likely to undergo CABG in contrast to patients with double-vessel disease and preserved left ventricular function. Therefore, these registry studies suggest that although the differences between bypass surgery and PTCA in diabetics may be due to altered vascular biology, these differences are magnified by the process of randomization in which patients who probably would have been treated with CABG in clinical practice were randomized to PTCA.

From a clinical standpoint in regard to patient selection for coronary revascularization and the method of revascularization, the assessment of diabetics should be based upon standard principles: the severity and extent of coronary disease, the potential for complete revascularization, the presence or absence of left ventricular dysfunction, and the technical suitability of the lesions for PTCA. The results of the aforementioned studies suggest that a preference for surgical over percutaneous revascularization is, at this time, appropriate among diabetics—at least those with extensive disease and/or ventricular dysfunction, although this recommendation may change if new technologies such as coated stents and antiplatelet agents are successful in reducing the risk of restenosis and occlusion. Furthermore, the potential impact of risk factor reduction and the use of insulin providers rather than insulin sensitizers on long-term survival may alter the risk/benefit balance in the future in this important and increasing subset of patients presenting with coronary artery disease. Irrespective of the mode of therapy, an aggressive approach to risk factor modification is required.

REFERENCES

1. Favaloro RG: Saphenous vein autograft replacement of severe segmental coronary artery occlusion: operative technique. *Ann Thorac Surg* 1968; 5:334.
2. Gruentzig AR, Senning A, Siegenthaler WE: Nonoperative dilation of coronary artery stenosis: percutaneous transluminal coronary angioplasty. *N Engl J Med* 1979; 301:62.
3. Pepine C, Cohn PF, Deedwania C, et al: Effects of treatment on outcome in mildly asymptomatic patients with ishemia during daily life. The Atenolol Silent Ischemia Study (ASIST). *Circulation* 1994; 90;762.
4. Detry JM, Lichtlen PR, Magnani B, et al: Amlodipine reduces transient myocardial ischemia in patients with coronary artery disease: double-blind Circadian Anti-Ischemia Program in Europe (CAPE trial). *J Am Coll Cardiol* 1994; 24:1460.
5. Savonitto S, Ardissiono D, Egstrup K, et al: Combination therapy with metoprolol and nifedipine versus monotherapy in patients with stable angina pectoris. Results of the International Multiceneter Angina Exercise (IMAGE) study. *J Am Coll Cardiol* 1996; 27: 311.
6. Von Arnim T, for the TIBBS Investigators: Prognostic significance of transientischemic episodes: response to treatment shows improved prognosis. Results of the Total Ischemic Burden Bisoprolol Study (TIBBs) follow-up. *J Am Coll Cardiol* 1996; 28: 20.
7. The IONA Study Group: Effect of Nicorandil on coronary events in patients with stable angina: the Impact Of Nicorandil in Angina (IONA) randomized trial. *Lancet* 359: 2002; 1269.
8. Late breaking clinical trial abstracts. *Circulation* 2001; 104: 1B.
9. Campeau L: Grading of angina pectoris [letter]. *Circulation* 1976; 54:522.
10. Goldman L, Hashimoto B, Cook EF, et al: Comparative reproducibly and validity of systems for assessing cardiovascular functional class: advantage of a new activity scale. *Circulation* 1976; 54:522.
11. Christian TF, Millder TD, Chareonthaitawee P, et al: Prevalence of normal resting left ventricular function with normal rest electrocardiograms. *Am J Cardiol* 1977; 79:1295.
12. Rihal CS, Eagle KA, Gersh BJ: The utility of clinical, electrocardiographic, and roentgenographic criteria in the estimation of left ventricular function. *Am J Cardiol* 1995; 75:220.
13. Gibbons RJ, Chatterjee K, Daley J, et al: ACC/AHA/ACP-ASIM guidelines for the management of patients with chronic stable angina: a report for the American College of Cardiology/American Heart Association Task Force on Practice Guidelines. *J Am Coll Cardiol* 1999; 33:2092.
14. Gibbons RJ, Balady GJ, Beasley JW, et al: ACC/AHA Guidelines for Exercise Testing: a report of the American College of Cardiology/American Heart Association Task Force on Practice Guidelines (Committee on Exercise Testing). *J Am Coll Cardiol* 1997; 30:260.
15. Chang JA, Froelicher VF: Clinical and exercise test markers of prognosis in patients with stable coronary artery disease. *Curr Probl Cardiol* 1994; 19:533.
16. Ribisl PM, Morris CK, Kawaguchi T, et al: Angiographic patterns and severe coronary artery disease: exercise test correlates. *Arch Intern Med* 1992; 152:1618.
17. Pagley PR, Beller GA, Watson DD, et al: Improved outcome after coronary bypass surgery in patients with ischemic cardiomyopathy and residual myocardial viability. *Circulation* 1997; 96:793.
18. Bonow RO: Identification of viable myocardium [editorial]. *Circulation* 1996; 94:2674.
19. Ritchie JL, Bateman TM, Bonow RO, et al: Guidelines for clinical use of cardiac radionuclide imaging. Report of the American College of Cardiology/American Heart Association Task Force on Assessment of Diagnostic and Therapeutic Cardiovascular Procedures (Committee on Radionuclide Imaging), developed in collaboration with the American Society of Nuclear Cardiology. *J Am Coll Cardiol* 1995; 25:521.
20. Iskandrian AS, Heo J, Lemlek J, et al: Identification of high-risk patients with left main and three-vessel coronary artery disease by adenosine-single photon emission computed tomographic thallium imaging. *Am Heart J* 1993; 125:1130.
21. Taillefer R, Amyot R, Turpin S, et al: Comparison between dipyridamole and adenosine as pharmacologic coronary vasodilators in detection of coronary artery disease with thallium 201 imaging. *J Nucl Cardiol* 1996; 3:204.
22. Pennell DJ, Underwood SR, Ell PJ: Safety of dobutamine stress for thallium-201 myocardial perfusion tomography in patients with asthma. *Am J Cardiol* 1993; 71:1346.
23. Calnon DA, Glover DK, Beller GA, et al: Effects of dobutamine stress on myocardial blood flow, ^{99m}Tc sestamibi uptake, and systolic wall thickening in the presence of coronary artery stenoses: implications for dobutamine stress testing. *Circulation* 1997; 96:2353.
24. Cheitlin MD, Alpert JS, Armstrong WF, et al: ACC/AHA Guidelines for the Clinical Application of Echocardiography. A report of the American College of Cardiology/American Heart Association Task Force on Practice Guidelines (Committee on Clinical Application of Echocardiography). Developed in collaboration with the American Society of Echocardiography. *Circulation* 1997; 95:1686.
25. Fleischmann KE, Hunink MG, Kuntz KM, et al: Exercise echocardiography or exercise SPECT imaging? A meta-analysis of diagnostic test performance. *JAMA* 1998; 280:913.
26. Dagianti A, Penco M, Agati L, et al: Stress echocardiography: comparison of exercise, dipyridamole and dobutamine in detecting and predicting the extent of coronary artery disease. *J Am Coll Cardiol* 1995; 26:18.
27. Beleslin BD, Ostojic M, Stephanovic J, et al: Stress echocardiography in the detection of myocardial ischemia: head-to-head

comparison of exercise, dobutamine, and dipyridamole tests. *Circulation* 1994; 90:1168.
28. Perrone-Filardi P, Pace L, Prastaro M, et al: Assessment of myocardial 24-hour ^{201}T1 tomography versus dobutamine echocardiography. *Circulation* 1996; 94:2712.
29. Bax JJ, Poldermans D, Elhendy A, et al: Improvement of left ventricular ejection fraction, heart failure symptoms and prognosis after revascularization in patients with chronic coronary artery disease: rest-4-hour-24-hour ^{201}T1 tomography versus dobutamine echocardiography. *Circulation* 1994; 94:2712.
30. Eagle KA, Guyton RA, Davidoff R, et al: ACC/AHA guidelines for coronary artery bypass graft surgery: executive summary and recommendations: a report of the American College of Cardiology/American Heart Association Task Force on Practice Guidelines (Committee to Revise the 1991 Guidelines for Coronary Artery Bypass Graft Surgery). *Circulation* 1999; 100:1464.
31. Detre K, Holubkov R, Kelsey S, et al: Percutaneous transluminal coronary angioplasty in 1985–1986 and 1977–1981: The National Heart, Lung and Blood Institute Registry. *N Engl J Med* 1988; 318:265.
32. Mark DB, Nelson CL, Califf RM, et al: Continuing evolution of therapy for coronary artery disease; initial results from the era of coronary angioplasty. *Circulation* 1994; 89:2015.
33. Goldman S, Copeland J, Moritz T, et al: Starting aspirin therapy after operation: effects on early graft patency. *Circulation* 1991; 84:520.
34. Serruys PW, de Jaegere P, Kiemenei F, et al, for the Benestent Study Group: A comparison of balloon expandable stent implantation with balloon angioplasty in patients with coronary artery disease. *N Engl J Med* 1994; 331:489.
35. Shepherd J, Cobbe SM, Ford I, et al, for the West of Scotland Coronary Prevention Study Group: Prevention of coronary heart disease with pravastatin in men with hypercholesterolemia. *N Engl J Med* 1995; 333:1301.
36. Scandinavian Simvastatin Survival Study Group: Randomized trial of cholesterol lowering in 4444 patients with coronary heart disease: the Scandinavian Simvastatin Survival Study (4S). *Lancet* 1994; 344:1383.
37. Pearson T, Rapaport E, Criqui M, et al: Optimal risk factor management in the patient after coronary revascularization: a statement for healthcare professions; from an American Heart Association Writing Group. *Circulation* 1994; 90:3125.
38. CASS Principal Investigators and Their Associates: Coronary Artery Surgery Study (CASS): a randomized trial of coronary artery bypass surgery; survival data. *Circulation* 1983; 68:939.
39. Veterans Administration Coronary Artery Bypass Surgery Cooperative Study Group: Eleven-year survival in the Veterans Administration Randomized Trial of Coronary Bypass Surgery for Stable Angina. *N Engl J Med* 1948; 311:1333.
40. Murphy ML, Hultgren HN, Detre K, et al: Treatment of chronic stable angina: a preliminary report of survival data of the randomized Veterans Administration Cooperative Study. *N Engl J Med* 1977; 1297:621.
41. Varnauskas E: European Coronary Surgery Study Group: Twelve-year follow-up of survival in the randomized European Coronary Surgery Study. *N Engl J Med* 1988; 319:332.
42. European Coronary Surgery Study Group: Prospective randomized study of coronary artery bypass surgery in stable angina pectoris: second interim report. *Lancet* 1980; 2:491.
43. Norris RM, Agnew TM, Brandt PWT, et al: Coronary surgery after recurrent myocardial infarction: progress of a trial comparing surgical and nonsurgical management for asymptomatic patients with advanced coronary disease. *Circulation* 1981; 63:788.
44. Mathur VS, Guinn GA: Prospective randomized study of the surgical therapy of stable angina. *Cardiovasc Clin* 1977; 8:131.
45. Kloster FE, Kremkau EL, Ritzman LW, et al: Coronary bypass for stable angina. *N Engl J Med* 1979; 300:149.
46. Yusuf S, Zucker D, Peduzzi P, et al: Effect of coronary artery bypass graft surgery on survival: overview of ten-year results from randomized trials by the Coronary Artery Bypass Graft Surgery Trialist Collaboration. *Lancet* 1994; 344:563.
47. Alderman EL, Bourassa MG, Cohen LS, et al: Ten-year follow-up of survival and myocardial infarction in the randomized Coronary Artery Surgery Study. *Circulation* 1990; 82:1629.
48. Hueb WA, Bellotti G, de Oliveira SA, et al: The Medicine, Angioplasty, or Surgery Study (MASS): A prospective, randomized trial of medical therapy, balloon angioplasty, or bypass surgery for single proximal left anterior descending artery stenoses. *J Am Coll Cardiol* 1995; 26:1600.
49. Goy JJ, Eeckhout E, Burnand B, et al: Coronary angioplasty versus left internal mammary artery grafting for isolated proximal left anterior descending artery stenosis. *Lancet* 1994; 343:1449.
50. Kaiser GC, Davis KB, Fisher LD, et al: Survival following coronary artery bypass grafting in patients with severe angina pectoris (CASS): an observational study. *J Thorac Cardiovasc Surg* 1985; 89:513.
51. Myers WO, Schaff HV, Fisher LD, et al: Time to first new myocardial infarction in patients with severe angina and three-vessel disease comparing medical and early surgical therapy: a CASS Registry study of survival. *J Thorac Cardiovasc Surg* 1988; 95:382.
52. Mock MB, Ringqvist I, Fisher LD, et al: Survival of medically treated patients in the Coronary Artery Surgery Study (CASS) registry. *Circulation* 1982; 66:562.
53. Harris PJ, Harrell FE Jr, Lee KL, et al: Survival in medically treated coronary artery disease. *Circulation* 1979; 60:1259.
54. The TIME investigators: Trial of Invasive versus Medical Therapy in Elderly Patients with Chronic Symptomatic Coronary-Artery Disease (TIME): a randomized trial. *Lancet* 2001; 358:951.
55. Davies RF, Goldberg AD, Forman S, et al: Asymptomatic Cardiac Ischemia Pilot (ACIP) study two-year follow-up: outcomes of patients randomized to initial strategies of medical therapy versus revascularization. *Circulation* 1997; 95:2037.
56. Kirklin JW, Naftel DC, Blackstone EH, et al: Summary of a consensus concerning death and ischemic events after coronary artery bypass grafting. *Circulation* 1989; 79 (suppl I):I-81.
57. Weintraub WS, Jones EL, King SB III, et al: Changing use of coronary angioplasty in coronary bypass surgery in the treatment of chronic coronary artery disease. *Am J Cardiol* 1990; 65:183.
58. Takaro T, Hultgren HN, Lipton MJ, et al: The VA Cooperative Randomized Study of Surgery for Coronary Arterial Occlusive Disease, II: subgroup with significant left main lesions. *Circulation* 1976; 51(suppl III):III-107.
59. Passamani E, Davis KB, Gillespie MJ, et al: A randomized trial of coronary artery bypass surgery: survival of patients with a low ejection fraction. *N Engl J Med* 1985; 312:1665.
60. Peduzzi P, Hultgren HN: Effect of medical vs surgical treatment on symptoms in stable angina pectoris: the Veterans Administration Cooperative Study of Surgery for Coronary Arterial Occlusive Disease. *Circulation* 1979; 60:888.
61. European Coronary Surgery Study Group: Long-term results of prospective randomized study of coronary artery bypass surgery in stable angina pectoris. *Lancet* 1982; 2:1173.
62. Mock MB, Fisher LD, Holmes DR Jr, et al: Comparison of effects of medical and surgical therapy on survival in severe angina pectoris and two-vessel coronary artery disease with and without left ventricular dysfunction: a Coronary Artery Surgery Study Registry study. *Am J Cardiol* 1988; 61:1198.
63. Weiner DA, Ryan TJ, McCabe CH, et al: The role of exercise testing in identifying patients with improved survival after coronary artery bypass surgery. *J Am Coll Cardiol* 1986; 8:741.

64. The Bypass Angioplasty Revascularization Investigation (BARI) Investigators: A clinical trial comparing coronary bypass surgery with angioplasty in patients with multivessel disease. *N Engl J Med* 1966; 335:217.
65. King SB 3rd, Barnhart HX, Kosinski AS, et al: Angioplasty or surgery for multivessel coronary artery disease: comparison of eligible registry and randomized patients in the EAST trial and influence of treatment selections on outcomes. Emory Angioplasty versus Surgery Trial Investigators. *Am J Cardiol* 1997; 79:1453.
66. Loop FD, Lytle BW, Cosgrove DM, et al: Influence of the internal-mammary-artery graft on 10-year survival and other cardiac events. *N Engl J Med* 1986; 314:1.
67. The VA Coronary Artery Bypass Surgery Cooperative Study Group: Eighteen-year follow-up in the Veterans Affairs Cooperative Study of Coronary Artery Bypass Surgery for stable angina. *Circulation* 1992; 86:121.
68. Parisi AF, Folland ED, Hartigan P (on behalf of the Veterans Affairs ACME Investigators): A comparison of angioplasty with medical therapy in the treatment of single-vessel coronary artery disease. *N Engl J Med* 1992; 326:10.
69. Ryan TJ, Bauman WB, Kennedy J, et al: ACC/AHA task force report: guidelines for percutaneous transluminal coronary angioplasty. A report of the American College of Cardiology/American Heart Association Task Force on Assessment of Diagnostic and Therapeutic Cardiovascular Procedures (Committee on Percutaneous Transluminal Angioplasty). *J Am Coll Cardiol* 1993; 22:2033.
70. Folland ED, Hartigan PM, Parisi AF, for the Veterans Affairs ACME Investigators: Percutaneous transluminal coronary angioplasty versus medical therapy for stable angina pectoris: outcomes for patients with double-vessel versus single-vessel coronary artery disease in a Veterans Affairs cooperative randomized trial. *J Am Coll Cardiol* 1997; 29:1505.
71. Pocock SJ, Henderson RA, Clayton T, et al: Quality of life after coronary angioplasty or continued medical treatment for angina: three-year follow-up in the RITA-2 trial. Randomized Intervention Treatment of Angina. *J Am Coll Cardiol* 2000; 35:907.
72. Scandinavian Simvastatin Survival Study Group: Randomized trial of cholesterol lowering in 4444 patients with coronary heart disease: the Scandinavian Simvastatin Survival Study (4S). *Lancet* 1994; 344:1383.
73. Sacks FM, Pfeffer MA, Moye LA, et al: The effect of pravastatin on coronary events after myocardial infarction in patients with average cholesterol levels. *N Engl J Med* 1996; 335:1001.
74. McCormick LS, Black DM, Waters D, et al: Rationale, design, and baseline characteristics of a trial comparing aggressive lipid lowering with Atorvastatin Versus Revascularization Treatments (AVERT). *Am J Cardiol* 1997; 80:1130.
75. Pitt B, Waters D, Brown WV, et al: Aggressive lipid-lowering therapy compared with angioplasty in stable coronary artery disease. Atorvastatin versus Revascularization Treatment Investigators. *N Eng J Med* 1999; 341:70.
76. Goy JJ, Eeckhout E, Moret C, et al: Five-year outcome in patients with isolated proximal left anterior descending coronary artery stenosis treated by angioplasty or left internal mammary artery grafting: a prospective trial. *Circulation* 1999; 99:3255.
77. Hueb WA, Soares PR, Almeida De Oliveira S, et al: Five-year follow-up of the Medicine, Angioplasty, or Surgery Study (MASS): a prospective, randomized trial of medical therapy, balloon angioplasty, or bypass surgery for single proximal left anterior descending coronary artery stenosis. *Circulation* 1999; 100(19 suppl):II107.
78. The Second Medicine, Angioplasty, or Surgery Study has been completed and the preliminary outcome results were presented in abstract form at the American College of Cardiology, 50th Annual Meeting, Scientific Sessions, Orlando, FL, March, 2001.
79. Pocock SJ, Henderson RA, Rickards AF, et al: Meta-analysis of randomized trials comparing coronary angioplasty with bypass surgery. *Lancet* 1995; 346:1184.
80. Sim I, Gupta M, McDonald K, et al: A meta-analysis of randomized trials comparing coronary artery bypass grafting with percutaneous transluminal coronary angioplasty in multivessel coronary artery disease. *Am J Cardiol* 1995; 76:1025.
81. RITA Trial Participants: Coronary angioplasty versus coronary artery bypass surgery: the Randomized Intervention Treatment of Angina (RITA) trial. *Lancet* 1993; 341:573.
82. Hamm CW, Reimers J, Ischinger T, et al, for the German Angioplasty Bypass Surgery Investigation: A randomized study of coronary angioplasty compared with bypass surgery in patients with symptomatic multivessel coronary disease. *N Engl J Med* 1994; 331:1037.
83. Rodriguez A, Boullon F, Perez-Balino N, et al, on behalf of the ERACI Group: Argentine randomized trial of percutaneous transluminal coronary angioplasty versus coronary artery bypass surgery in multivessel disease (ERACI): in-hospital results and 1-year follow-up. *J Am Coll Cardiol* 1993; 22:1060.
84. Rodriguez A, Mele E, Peyregne E, et al: Three-year follow-up of the Argentine Randomized Trial of Percutaneous Transluminal Coronary Angioplasty Versus Coronary Artery Bypass Surgery in Multivessel Disease (ERACI). *J Am Coll Cardiol* 1996; 27:1178.
85. Carrie DM, Elbaz M, Puel J, et al: Five-year outcome after coronary angioplasty versus bypass surgery in multivessel coronary artery disease: results from the French Monocentric Study. *Circulation* 1997; 96(9 suppl):II-1.
86. Serruys PW, Unger F, Sousa JE, et al, for the Arterial Revascularization Therapies Study Group: Comparison of coronary-artery bypass surgery and stenting for the treatment of multivessel disease. *N Engl J Med* 2001; 344:1117.
87. Rodriguez A, Bernardi V, Navia J, et al: Argentine Randomized Study: Coronary Angioplasty with Stenting versus Coronary Bypass Surgery in patients with Multiple-Vessel Disease (ERACI II): 30-day and one-year follow-up results. ERACI II Investigators. *J Am Coll Cardiol* 2001; 37:51.
88. Preliminary results of SoS were released at the American College of Cardiology 50th Annual Meeting, Scientific Sessions, Orlando, FL, March 2001.
89. Mintz GS, Kent KM, Pichard AD, et al: Intravascular ultrasound insights into mechanisms of stenosis formation and restenosis. *Cardiol Clin* 1997; 15:17.
90. Morice MC, Serruys PW, Sousa JE et al: A randomized comparison of a sirolinus-eluting stent with a standard stent for coronary revascularization. *N Engl J Med* 2002; 346:1773.
91. American Heart Association: *Heart and Stroke Facts: 1995 Statistical Supplement*. Dallas, Texas, American Heart Association, 1996.
92. Braunwald E: Unstable angina: a classification. *Circulation* 1989; 80:410.
93. Wallentin L, Lagerqvist B, Husted S, et al: Outcome at 1 year after an invasive compared with a non-invasive strategy in unstable coronary-artery disease: the FRISC II invasive randomised trial. FRISC II Investigators. *Lancet* 2000; 356:9.
94. Cannon CP, Wientraub WS, Demopoous LA, et al: Comparison of early invasive and conservative strategies in patients with unstable coronary syndromes treated with the glycoprotein Iib/IIIa inhibitor tirofiban. *N Engl J Med* 2001; 344:1879.
95. Spacek R, Widimsky P, Straka Z, et al: Value of first day angiography/angioplasty in evolving non-ST segment elevation myocardial infarction: an open multicenter randomized trial. The VINO study. *Eur Heart J* 2002; 23:230.

96. Luchi RJ, Scott SM, Deupree RH, et al: Comparison of medical and surgical treatment for unstable angina pectoris: results of a Veterans Administration cooperative study. *N Engl J Med* 1987; 316:977.
97. National Cooperative Study Group: Unstable angina pectoris: national cooperative study group to compare surgical and medical therapy, II: in-hospital experience and initial follow-up results in patients with one, two and three vessel disease. *Am J Cardiol* 1978; 42:839.
98. Bertolasi CA, Tronge JE, Riccitelli MA, et al: Natural history of unstable angina with medical or surgical therapy. *Chest* 1976; 70:596.
99. Anderson HV, Cannon CP, Stone PH, et al: One-year results of the Thrombolysis in Myocardial Ischemia (TIMI) IIIB clinical trial: a randomized comparison of tissue-type plasminogen activator versus placebo and early invasive versus early conservative strategies in unstable angina and non–Q wave myocardial infarction. *J Am Coll Cardiol* 1995; 26:1643.
100. Boden WE, O'Rourke RA, Crawford MH, et al: Outcomes in patients with acute non-Q-wave myocardial infarction randomly assigned to an invasive as compared with a conservative management strategy. Veterans Affairs Non-Q-Wave Infarction Strategies in Hospital (VANQWISH) Trial Investigators. *N Engl J Med* 1998; 338:1785.
101. Grines CL, Browne KF, Marco J, et al: A comparison of immediate angioplasty with thrombolytic therapy in acute myocardial infarction. *N Engl J Med* 1993; 328:673.
102. Gibbons RJ, Holmes DR, Reeder GS, et al: Immediate angioplasty compared with the administration of a thrombolytic agent followed by conservative treatment for myocardial infarction. *N Engl J Med* 1993; 328:685.
103. Simoons ML, Betriu A, Col J, et al: Thrombolysis with tissue plasminogen activator in acute myocardial infarction: no additional benefit from immediate percutaneous coronary angioplasty. *Lancet* 1988; 1:197.
104. Topol EJ, Califf RM, George BS, et al: A randomized trial of immediate versus delayed elective angioplasty after intravenous tissue plasminogen activator in acute myocardial infarction. *N Engl J Med* 1987; 317:581.
105. Rogers WJ, Baim DS, Gore JM, et al: Comparison of immediate invasive, delayed invasive, and conservative strategies after tissue-type plasminogen activator: results of the thrombolysis in myocardial infarction (TIMI) phase II-A trial. *Circulation* 1990; 81:1457.
106. Michels KB, Yusuf S: Does PTCA in acute myocardial infarction affect mortality and reinfarction rates? *Circulation* 1995; 91:476.
107. Pepine CJ, Geller NL, Knatterud GL, et al: The Asymptomatic Cardiac Ischemia Pilot (ACIP) Study: Design of a randomized clinical trial, baseline data and implications for a long-term outcome trial. *J Am Coll Cardiol* 1994; 24:1.
108. Rogers WJ, Bourassa MG, Andrews TC, et al: Asymptomatic Cardiac Ischemia Pilot (ACIP) Study: Outcome at 1 year for patients with asymptomatic cardiac ischemia randomized to medical therapy or revascularization. *J Am Coll Cardiol* 1995; 26:594.
109. Little WC, Downes TR, Applegate RJ: The underlying coronary lesion in myocardial infarction: implications for coronary angiography. *Clin Cardiol* 1991; 14:668.
110. Giroud D, Li JM, Urban P, et al: Relation of the site of acute myocardial infarction to the most severe coronary arterial stenosis at prior angiography. *Am J Cardiol* 1992; 69:729.
111. Little WC, Constantinescu M, Applegate RJ, et al: Can coronary angiography predict the site of a subsequent myocardial infarction in patients with mild to moderate coronary artery disease? *Circulation* 1988; 78:1157.
112. Ambrose JA, Winters SL, Arora RR, et al: Coronary angiographic morphology in myocardial infarction: a link between the pathogenesis of unstable angina and myocardial infarction. *J Am Coll Cardiol* 1985; 6:1233.
113. Topol EJ, Ellis SG, Cosgrove DM, et al: Analysis of coronary angioplasty practice in the United States with an insurance-claims data base. *Circulation* 1993; 87:1489.
114. Bech GJ, De Bruyne B, Pijls NH, et al: Fractional flow reserve to determine the appropriateness of angioplasty in moderate coronary stenosis: a randomized trial. *Circulation* 2001; 103:2928.
115. Van Dijk D, Jansen EW, Hijman R, et al, for the Octopus Study Group: Cognitive outcome after off-pump and on-pump coronary artery bypass graft surgery: a randomized trial. [See comments.] *JAMA* 2002; 287:1405.
116. Angelini GD, Taylor FC, Reeves BC, et al: Early and mid-term outcome after off-pump and on-pump surgery in Beating Heart Against Cardioplegic Arrest Studies (BHACAS 1 and 2): a pooled analysis of two randomized controlled trials. *Lancet* 2002; 359:1194.
117. Rahimtoola SH: Coronary bypass surgery for chronic angina, 1981: a perspective. *Circulation* 1982; 65:225.
118. Braunwald E, Rutherford JD: Reversible ishemic left ventricular dysfunction: evidence for "hibernating" myocardium. *J Am Coll Cardiol* 1986; 8:1467.
119. Ross J Jr: Myocardial perfusion-contraction matching: implications for coronary artery disease and hybernation. *Circulation* 1991; 83:1076.
120. Dilsizian V, Bonow RO: Current diagnostic techniques of assessing myocardial viability in hybernating and stunned myocardium. *Circulation* 1993; 87:1.
121. Bax JJ, Wijns W, Cornel JH, et al: Accuracy of currently available techniques for prediction of functional recovery after revascularization on patients with left ventricular dysfunction due to coronary artery disease: comparison of pooled data. *J Am Coll Cardiol* 1997; 30:1451.
122. Allman KC, Shaw LJ, Hachamovitch R, et al: Myocardial viability testing and impact of revascularization on prognosis in patients with coronary artery disease and left ventricular dysfunction: a meta-analysis. *J Am Coll Cardiol* 2002; 39:1151.
123. Ellis SG, Cowley MJ, DiSciascio G, et al: Determinants of 2-year outcome after coronary angioplasty in patients with multivessel disease on the basis of comprehensive procedural evaluation: implications for patient selection. *Circulation* 1991; 83: 1905.
124. Bell MR, Gersh BJ, Schaff HV, et al: Effect of completeness of revascularization on long-term outcome of patients with three-vessel disease undergoing coronary artery bypass surgery: a report from the Coronary Artery Surgery Study (CASS) Registry. *Circulation* 1992; 86:446.
125. Kip KE, Faxon DP, Detre RM, et al: Coronary angioplasty in diabetic patients: the National Heart, Lung and Blood Institute Percutaneous Transluminal Coronary Angioplasty Registry. *Circulation* 1996; 94:1818.
126. Salomon NW, Page US, Okies JE, et al: Diabetes mellitus and coronary artery bypass: short-term risk and long-term prognosis. *J Thorac Cardiovasc Surg* 1983; 85:264.
127. Stein B, Weintraub WS, Gebhart SSP, et al: Influence of diabetes mellitus on early and late outcome after percutaneous transluminal coronary angioplasty. *Circulation* 1995; 91:979.
128. Kornowski R, Mintz GS, Kent KM, et al: Increased restenosis in diabetes mellitus after coronary interventions is due to exaggerated intimal hyperplasia: a serial intravascular ultrasound study. *Circulation* 1997; 95:1366.
129. Detre KM, Lombardero MS, Brooks MM, et al: The effect of previous coronary-artery bypass surgery on the prognosis of patients

with diabetes who have acute myocardial infarction. Bypass Angioplasty Revascularization Investigation Investigators. *N Engl J Med* 2000; 342:989.

130. BARI Investigators: Seven-year outcome in the Bypass Angioplasty Revascularization Investigation (BARI) by treatment and diabetic status. *J Am Coll Cardiol* 2000; 35:1122.
131. Van Belle E, Ketelers R, Bauters C, et al: Patency of percutaneous transluminal angiographic follow-up: the key determinant of survival in diabetics after coronary balloon angioplasty. *Circulation* 2001; 103:1185.
132. Bertrand M: Long-term follow-up of European revascularization trials. Presentation at the 68th Scientific Sessions, Plenary Session XII, American Heart Association, Anaheim, CA, November, 1995.
133. King SB 3rd, Kosinski AS, Guyton RA, et al : Eight-year mortality in the Emory Angioplasty versus Surgery Trial (EAST). *J Am Coll Cardiol* 2002; 35:1116.
134. Ellis SG, Nairns CR: Problem of angioplasty in diabetics. *Circulation* 1997; 96:1707.
135. Niles NW, McGrath PD, Malenka D, et al: Survival of patients with diabetes and multivessel coronary artery disease after surgical or percutaneous coronary revascularization: results of a large regional prospective study. *J Am Coll Cardiol* 2001; 37:1008.
136. Barsness GW, Peterson ED, Ohman EM, et al: Relationhsip between diabetes mellitus and long-term survival after coronary bypass and angioplasty. *Circulation* 1997; 96:2551.
137. Detre KM, Guo P, Holubkov R, Califff RM et al: Coronary revascularization in diabetic patients: a comparison of the randomized and observational components of the Bypass Angioplasty Revascularization Investigation (BARI). *Circulation* 1999; 99:633.

Chapter 20

Myocardial Revascularization with Cardiologic Interventional Devices

James T. Willerson

The incidence of coronary artery disease and stroke has declined during the past three decades, yet acute myocardial infarction (MI) remains the most important cause of death in the United States.[1] It is estimated that today more than 6 million people in this country have a history of heart attack, angina pectoris, or both.[2] Today, many physicians devote their clinical practices solely to the diagnosis and management of patients with obstructive disease of the coronary or peripheral arteries. The approach for treatment of such patients is multifaceted, as new catheter technologies have emerged and operator techniques have improved. The field of interventional cardiology has been evolving since the early 1970s, when Gruentzig[3] introduced the technique of percutaneous transluminal angioplasty. The percutaneous transluminal dilatation technique was used first in the peripheral arteries,[3] and it was applied in the human coronary arteries in 1977,[4,5] opening the way for many new coronary artery interventions.

The decision to perform a revascularization procedure is based on careful evaluation of several factors, including the patient's history, the extent of vascular involvement, anatomical considerations, and risks involved with the procedure itself. It is important for the interventionalist to have a broad knowledge of the literature and to understand the trends in interventional therapy—how techniques are developing, how they are best utilized, and how they compare with other strategies. In the following pages, a summary of current and alternative approaches used in interventional cardiology for the patient with coronary artery disease will be discussed.

THROMBOLYSIS FOR ACUTE MYOCARDIAL INFARCTION

Thrombolytic therapy for acute MI evolved from early attempts in the 1970s to treat patients with MI on an emergent surgical basis.[6] Because cardiac catheterization was required to delineate the coronary anatomy before undertaking coronary bypass, it soon became apparent that thrombotic coronary occlusion was present in most of these patients. Still, many investigators remained unconvinced that total thrombotic occlusion was a significant factor in acute MI. Although thrombolytic therapy was widely tested in Europe throughout the 1970s, it was not uniformly accepted. Interventional studies during that period provided further evidence that thrombotic occlusion was the cause of acute MI and opened the way for the study of both intracoronary and intravenous thrombolytic therapy.

The modern era of thrombolytic therapy began in the late 1970s with the observation by Rentrop[7] that intracoronary streptokinase provided effective thrombolysis for the infarct-related coronary artery and when, in the early and mid-1980s, intravenous streptokinase therapy was shown to reduce mortality in patients with myocardial infarction in the Gruppo Italiano per lo Studio della Streptochinasi nell'Infarcto Miocardio (GISSI) clinical trial.[8] Since that time, numerous clinical trials have been undertaken to test the efficacy of various thrombolytic agents in the treatment of acute myocardial infarction. The results have shown definitively that timely administration of thrombolytic agents reduces infarct size, preserves left ventricular function, and improves short- and long-term survival in patients with acute MI. Despite the irrefutable evidence that thrombolytic therapy is beneficial, controversial issues regarding this therapy remain, such as the choices of the specific drug to be used and the need for adjunctive therapy, including platelet glycoprotein IIb/IIIa receptor antagonists or other platelet antagonists in addition to heparin or low molecular weight heparin.

Thrombolytic Agents

Complete thrombotic coronary occlusion usually results from ulceration or fissuring of vascular endothelium at the site of an atherosclerotic plaque. As a response to vessel injury, platelets adhere to the damaged endothelium and release and/or activate factors that promote thrombosis, vasoconstriction, and fibroproliferation. This results in fibrin formation and thrombotic coronary occlusion. Thrombolytic drugs work by activation of plasminogen to the active enzyme plasmin, which digests the fibrin component of the clot.

Thrombolytic agents may be divided into two general groups—the relatively fibrin-specific and non–fibrin-specific activators. The relatively specific group consists of tissue-type plasminogen activator (t-PA) and its mutants (r-PA and others) and, to a lesser extent, single-chain urokinase plasminogen activator (scu-PA); the relatively nonspecific proteases include streptokinase (SK), urokinase (UK), and anistreplase (APSAC).[9] Four of these drugs, SK, t-PA, urokinase, and APSAC, are commercially available, and two (t-PA and its mutants and SK) are widely used in the treatment of acute MI. The drugs vary according to their clearance, fibrin selectivity, and plasminogen binding, in their potential to induce allergic reactions, and in costs.[10,11]

STREPTOKINASE

Streptokinase was the first thrombolytic protein discovered, and it has been studied more extensively than any other thrombolytic agent. It works by joining to plasminogen in a complex that converts neighboring plasminogen to plasmin.[12] As a product of beta-hemolytic streptococci, streptokinase is antigenic and may produce allergic reactions in patients with recent streptococcal infections. The recommended dose of streptokinase (1.5 million units) is usually sufficient to overcome the neutralizing effect of antibodies; therefore, most patients will develop systemic fibrinolysis. The pharmacologic half-life of streptokinase is 30 minutes; depletion of fibrinogen usually lasts for 24 hours. Antibodies develop approximately 4 days after streptokinase therapy and persist for 6 months to 1 year; therefore, it is recommended that patients not be retreated with streptokinase (or APSAC) during that time.

Streptokinase has been tested in thousands of patients and has shown the ability to improve left ventricular function and save lives. It is less costly than other agents, but it does have the potential for allergic reactions[13] and hypotension.[14]

TISSUE PLASMINOGEN ACTIVATOR

Tissue plasminogen activator (t-PA) is a naturally occurring serine protease that is nonantigenic and may be readministered immediately in the event of reinfarction.[12] Unlike SK and APSAC, t-PA is relatively fibrin-specific and clot-selective, producing more local thrombolysis. One disadvantage of t-PA is that its short half-life (5 minutes) may contribute to infarct vessel reocclusion. This limitation has led to the development of t-PA mutants with glycosylation and other defects that delay the clearance of t-PA and, in experimental animal models, result in more rapid thrombolysis and reduction in the risk of reocclusion.[15–17] Originally, the recommended dose of t-PA was 100 mg over a 3-hour period (60, 20, and 20 mg over hours 1, 2, and 3, respectively). In 1989, Neuhaus et al[18,19] initiated front-loaded or accelerated t-PA dosing by demonstrating that higher patency could be achieved with a regimen of a 15-mg bolus, another 50 mg given in the first 30 minutes, and the remainder (35 mg) infused over the next 60 minutes. More recently, an initial 20-mg bolus is administered, with the remainder of the t-PA being given over 1 hour. With the doses at which t-PA is usually given, the decline in fibrinogen is approximately 50%; therefore, there is less generation of fibrinogen split products.

Even though t-PA is clot-selective, it does not cause fewer bleeding complications than the other drugs. Increased bleeding complications have been noted particularly in patients of smaller body size (less than 165 kg). Therefore, in these patients, the recommended dosage is lowered to 1.25 mg/kg over 3 hours, with 10% as a bolus, 50% for the first hour, and 40% for the last 2 hours. Although acute

TABLE 20–1 GUSTO trial: treatment given and infarct-related artery perfusion status*

	SK + SQH	SK + IVH	Accelerated t-PA + IVH	Combined limb
TIMI perfusion grade 2 or 3 (percent)				
90 min	54	60	81	73
180 min	73	74	76	85
24 h	77	80	86	94
5–7 d	72	84	84	80
TIMI perfusion grade 3 (percent)				
90 min	29	32	54	38
180 min	35	41	43	53
24 h	51	41	45	60
5–7 d	51	58	58	55

*GUSTO = Global Utilization of Streptokinase and Tissue Plasminogen Activator for Occluded Coronary Arteries; TIMI = Thrombolysis in Myocardial Infarction; SK = streptokinase; SQH = subcutaneous heparin; IVH = intravenous heparin; t-PA = tissue-type plasminogen activator.

Source: The GUSTO Investigators: An international randomized trial comparing four thrombolytic strategies for acute myocardial infarction. N Engl J Med 1993; 321:673.

Reproduced with permission from Holmes DR, Califf RM, Topol EJ: Lessons we have learned from the GUSTO trial. J Am Coll Cardiol 1995; 25:7S.

reperfusion rates have been shown to be higher with t-PA than with streptokinase (Tables 20-1 and 20-2),[20] reocclusion also may be higher. In addition, because of its higher fibrinolytic potency, t-PA may induce hemorrhagic stroke at a higher rate than streptokinase. It is also more costly than other thrombolytic drugs—about 5 to 10 times more costly than streptokinase.[21,22]

TABLE 20–2 Definitions of perfusion in the TIMI trial

Grade 0 (no perfusion): There is no antegrade flow beyond the point of occlusion.

Grade 1 (penetration with minimal perfusion): The contrast material passes beyond the area of obstruction, but "hangs up" and fails to opacify the entire coronary bed distal to the obstruction for duration of the cine run.

Grade 2 (partial perfusion): The contrast material passes across the obstruction and opacifies the coronary bed distal to the obstruction. However, the rate of entry of contrast material into the vessel distal to the obstruction or its rate of clearance from the distal bed (or both) are perceptibly slower than its entry into or clearance from comparable areas not perfused by the previously occluded vessel, e.g., the opposite coronary artery or the coronary bed proximal to the obstruction.

Grade 3 (complete perfusion): Antegrade flow into the bed distal to the obstruction occurs as promptly as antegrade flow into the bed proximal to the obstruction, and clearance of contrast material from the involved bed is as rapid as clearance from an uninvolved bed in the same vessel or the opposite artery.

Source: Sheehan FH, Braunwald E, Canner P, et al, and Co-Investigators of the TIMI trial: The effect of intravenous thrombolytic therapy on left ventricular function: a report on tissue-type plasminogen activator and streptokinase from the Thrombolysis in Myocardial Infarction (TIMI Phase 1) Trial. Circulation 1987; 75:817–829. Reproduced with permission from the American Heart Association.

ANISOYLATED PLASMINOGEN STREPTOKINASE ACTIVATOR COMPLEX

Anisoylated plasminogen streptokinase activator complex (APSAC) is a new second-generation thrombolytic agent that was developed to overcome some of the limitations of streptokinase therapy.[12] With APSAC, the active enzymatic site of the plasminogen streptokinase complex is temporarily protected by acylation, therefore allowing rapid intravenous injection of the drug. This results in prolonged fibrinolytic action. Compared with streptokinase, APSAC has greater fibrin binding and a longer duration of action (half-life of 90 minutes). This simplifies intravenous administration of the drug, with improved coronary reperfusion and reduced reocclusion rates. The entire bolus of the drug can be administered over a period of 2 to 5 minutes, and its expense is moderate compared with the other fibrinolytic agents. APSAC is not superior to other drugs, however, in improving ventricular function or reducing mortality.

UROKINASE

Another thrombolytic agent, urokinase, has been approved by the FDA for intravenous administration but is not available for intracoronary use. Urokinase is a proteolytic enzyme produced from human fetal kidney tissue cultures.[12] The usual dosage is 3 million units, which usually is sufficient for depletion of fibrinogen. The dosage consists of 1.5 million units as a bolus, with 1.5 million additional units given over a 1-hour period.

Clinical trials have shown that after intravenous urokinase, the rate of coronary patency is approximately 50% to 70%; reocclusion is 5% to 10%.[23–25] Compared with streptokinase, urokinase has much less antigenicity, can be given in a bolus dose, and has a relatively low rate of reocclusion. There are fewer allergic reactions and less hypotension associated with this drug. The disadvantages include its relative expense compared with other agents and the relative lack of experience with it in the United States. It has been more widely used in Europe.

Indications

The current consensus is that thrombolytic therapy is underutilized in patients with acute MI, despite a broader application of the therapy.[26] The criteria for appropriate patient selection for thrombolytic intervention have evolved as more knowledge is gained through clinical trials. All patients presenting with MI should be considered candidates for intravenous thrombolytic therapy if they are seen less than 6 hours after the onset of symptoms and have no potential bleeding problems. Patients with systemic arterial hypertension are not candidates for thrombolytic therapy as they have an increased risk of intracranial hemorrhage. Because the extent of myocardial damage occurring during acute MI is time-dependent, mortality reduction is greatest in those patients treated early with thrombolytic agents, although beneficial effects have been shown with treatment initiated up to 12 hours after the onset of symptoms.[27–29] It is agreed generally that patients presenting with symptoms of acute myocardial infarction and ST-segment elevation or left bundle-branch block will benefit by thrombolytic therapy. Those with only ST depression should be excluded because thrombolytic therapy is not helpful in these patients and may actually be harmful.

Contraindications

Late presentation after symptom onset, systemic arterial hypertension, and older patient age are the most common contraindications to thrombolytic therapy. Within the past several years, elderly patients with MI have been treated more routinely, however.[30] In a meta-analysis of eight large clinical trials, with regard to older patients, thrombolytic therapy was shown to have the greatest margin of benefit in patients aged 65 to 74 years.[31] In patients older than 75 years, only 18 lives were saved per 1,000 patients; this is owing, in part, to an increase in bleeding complications in this patient subset.

In 1990, Muller and Topol[32] critically reviewed the recommendations regarding patient eligibility for thrombolytic therapy after acute MI by examining studies published during a 10-year period. They examined only randomized, controlled trials of intravenous thrombolysis in acute MI and unstable angina. This study revealed that relatively few patients with MI were considered eligible for the therapy. Those excluded from thrombolysis, however, had a high early mortality. The findings suggested that selected, high-risk subgroups might benefit from thrombolytic therapy. Such groups would include otherwise healthy elderly patients, certain patients presenting more than 6 hours after the onset of symptoms, and those with a history of controlled systolic hypertension or brief nontraumatic cardiopulmonary resuscitation. Their data did not support the use of fibrinolytic therapy as the primary treatment for patients with unstable angina or suspected myocardial infarction in the absence of confirmatory electrocardiographic changes.

Investigators from the Global Utilization of Streptokinase and Tissue Plasminogen Activator for Occluded Coronary Arteries (GUSTO-I) trial developed a multivariable statistical model for risk assessment in candidates for thrombolytic therapy.[33] They used criteria from the large population of 41,021 patients in this trial to analyze the relationship between baseline clinical data and 30-day mortality. They concluded that multiple characteristics of the patient must be considered for an accurate prognosis to be determined. These characteristics include age, medical history, physiological significance of the infarction, and medical treatment.

Specifically, multivariable analysis identified age as the most significant factor influencing 30-day mortality, with rates of 1.1% in the youngest decile (younger than 45 years) and 20.5% in patients older than 75 years. Other factors most significantly associated with increased mortality were lower systolic blood pressure, higher Killip class, elevated heart rate, and anterior infarction. These five factors comprised 90% of the prognostic information in the baseline clinical data. Other less significant factors included previous myocardial infarction, height, time to treatment, diabetes, weight, smoking status, type of thrombolytic, previous bypass surgery, hypertension, and prior cerebrovascular disease.

Choice of Thrombolytic Agent

Information regarding drug selection has become available from three large-scale randomized trials directly comparing the risks and benefits of various thrombolytic agents in acute MI.[34–36] These include the Gruppo Italiano per lo Studio della Sopravvivenze nell'Infarcto Miocardico (GISSI-2) trial and its international extension, the Third International Study of Infarct Survival (ISIS-3), and the GUSTO-I trial (mentioned earlier). In the interpretation of results from these trials, it is agreed generally that the agents most commonly used in the United States—t-PA, SK, and APSAC—all reduce mortality when given to patients with acute evolving MI.

In addition, when the therapy is given to patients presenting up to 12 hours after onset of symptoms, the mortality rate is reduced by approximately 20%. When aspirin therapy is used in patients presenting up to 24 hours after symptoms begin, there is a 23% reduction in mortality. The combination with aspirin enhances the thrombolytic efficacy of streptokinase and, probably, of all thrombolytic interventions.

Heparin (or another thrombin inhibitor) given intravenously in adequate dosage is required to allow t-PA to exert a maximal thrombolytic effect. Aspirin is a cyclooxygenase inhibitor and reduces the availability of thromboxane A_2, a potent promoter of platelet aggregation. Thrombin is formed at sites of vascular injury and constriction and promotes platelet aggregation and vasoconstriction. Thrombolytic therapy activates platelets and the addition of aspirin and thrombin inhibitors counteracts the platelet activation and local effects of thrombin.

The most important finding in the analysis of randomized trials is that earlier administration, as well as more widespread use of thrombolytic therapy and aspirin, would save more lives. In several studies, patients who received streptokinase had slightly fewer strokes than those who received t-PA or APSAC, but the biological difference is very small.

One important contribution of the GUSTO trial, according to Habib,[11] is that it provided compelling evidence for the open artery theory.[37] Regardless of which thrombolytic drug was used, 30-day mortality was substantially higher (8.9% vs. 4.4%, $p = .009$) in patients with a nonperfused infarct-related artery. According to the theory, rapid and complete coronary reperfusion is associated with improved clinical outcome (improved survival and improved ventricular function).[37]

Thrombolysis with Other Treatment Strategies

Thrombolytic therapy has been compared with other treatment strategies in recent years in several clinical trials. The Thrombolysis in Myocardial Ischemia (TIMI)-IIIB clinical trial, which included 1,473 patients, was designed to compare the efficacy of t-PA with early invasive versus early conservative strategies in patients with unstable angina and non–Q-wave myocardial infarction.[38] In this large study of patients with unstable angina and non–Q-wave MI, the incidence of death and nonfatal infarction or reinfarction was low but not trivial after 1 year (4.3% mortality, 8.8% nonfatal infarction). An early invasive management strategy was associated with slightly more coronary angioplasty procedures but equivalent numbers of bypass surgery procedures than was a more conservative early strategy of catheterization, in which revascularization was performed only when there were signs of recurrent ischemia. No difference was seen in death or nonfatal infarction, or both, after 1 year, according to strategy assignment, but fewer patients in the early invasive strategy group underwent later repeat hospital admission (26% vs. 33%, $p = .001$). According to these results, either strategy appears to be acceptable for treatment of patients with unstable angina and non–Q-wave MI; in this regard, physicians have latitude in individualizing care for such patients. In the patients with unstable angina and non–Q-wave infarction, thrombolytic therapy did not reduce mortality or morbidity.

Very recently, however, the Treat Angina with Aggrastat and Determine Cost of Therapy with an Invasive or Conservative Strategy (TACTICS) trial done in a very similar patient population has provided different conclusions.[39] In this trial in patients with unstable angina and non–Q-wave myocardial infarcts, invasive strategy proved superior to conservative therapy in patients with elevations in their serum troponin I or T or C-reactive protein.[39] In patients without elevations in their serum C-reactive protein or troponin I or T, the results were similar between invasive and conservative therapies. This suggests the ability to select patients at highest risk for more aggressive therapy.[39]

Angioplasty and Thrombolytic Therapy

Percutaneous transluminal coronary angioplasty (PTCA) often is performed in patients with acute ST-segment elevation (Q-wave) MIs after thrombolytic therapy or in lieu of thrombolysis. An early trial by Ribeiro et al[40] compared the benefit of thrombolytic therapy utilizing streptokinase with that of direct coronary angioplasty in 100 patients who presented with acute MI at a single interventional center. They excluded patients who were older than 75 years or had prior bypass surgery, Q-wave infarction in the region of ischemia, or excessive risk of bleeding. There were no major differences in the baseline characteristics of the two treatment groups in this study. Results showed no difference in 48-hour infarct-related artery patency or LV-ejection fraction. Also, there were no major bleeding events, and mortality was similar. The investigators concluded that intravenous therapy might be preferred over coronary angioplasty because of the shorter time to treatment.

Several prospective clinical trials in the United States and Europe have been undertaken to test the role and timing of angioplasty after intravenous thrombolytic therapy—the Thrombolysis and Angioplasty in Myocardial Infarction (TAMI) study,[41] the European Co-operative Study,[42] and the Thrombolysis in Myocardial Infarction (TIMI) II-B study.[43,44] These early trials revealed some detrimental effects of aggressive treatment for MI patients. Invasive therapy after intravenous thrombolytic therapy with recombinant tissue-type plasminogen activator (rt-PA) resulted in no additional preservation of ventricular function and no improvement in survival probability. Furthermore, this aggressive approach was associated with greater morbidity and a trend toward higher mortality.

A meta-analysis of randomized clinical trials examining the benefits of PTCA alone and PTCA after thrombolysis revealed less convincing evidence for the superiority of one therapy over another for treatment of acute ST-segment elevation MI.[45] The analyses of the various categories of trials have suggested, however, that primary PTCA may be more beneficial than thrombolytic therapy in the treatment of these acute MIs.[10] According to Ross, the current overall impression is that direct PTCA for acute infarction is an effective method of reperfusion so long as it can be accomplished in the same time frame as can pharmacologic reperfusion.[10] Based on several large-scale trials, however, there has been failure to confirm a lower reocclusion rate for PTCA as compared with plasminogen activator therapy.[10]

Very recently, Stone et al have shown that, at experienced centers, stent implantation with or without the platelet glycoprotein inhibitor abciximab appears to be superior to PTCA in the treatment of acute ST-segment elevation myocardial infarctions.[46] They randomly assigned 2,082 patients with acute ST-segment elevation myocardial infarcts to undergo PTCA (518 patients), PTCA plus abciximab therapy (528 patients), stenting alone with the Multi-Link stent (512 patients), or stenting plus abciximab therapy (524 patients). At 6 months, the primary end point—a composite of death, reinfarction, disabling stroke, and ischemic-driven revascularization of the target vessel—had occurred in 20% of patients after PTCA, 16.5% after PTCA and abciximab, 11.5% after stenting, and 10% after stenting and abciximab ($p < .001$). Rates of angiographically established restenosis were 40.8% after PTCA and 22% after stenting ($p < .001$).

EFFECTS OF GENDER

Stone et al[47] compared in-hospital outcomes in men versus women who were treated by either thrombolytic therapy or primary coronary angioplasty for acute MI. Their study comprised 395 patients (288 men, 107 women) in 12 centers who were prospectively randomized to treatment with t-PA or primary PTCA. The in-hospital mortality in women was 3.3-fold higher than in men (9.3% vs. 2.8%, $p = .005$). Women were older, more often had diabetes mellitus, systemic hypertension, or prior congestive heart failure, and presented later after symptom onset. In contrast, after primary PTCA, women and men had similar in-hospital mortality (4.0% vs. 2.1%, respectively, $p = .46$). Multiple logistic regression analysis of 15 clinical variables showed that treatment with PTCA, as well as younger age, was independently predictive of in-hospital survival in women.

COST

As greater numbers of clinical trials have been undertaken to compare the efficacy of thrombolysis versus primary angioplasty for acute MI, comparisons regarding cost-effectiveness of these separate strategies have been made by several investigators.

According to a study by Goldman,[21] the incremental cost for thrombolysis with streptokinase in patients with acute myocardial infarction ranges from approximately $3,500 to approximately $21,000 per year of life saved. The incremental cost-effectiveness of tissue-type plasminogen activator (t-PA) compared with streptokinase ranges from approximately $16,000 to $60,000 per year of life saved. Combined data from three randomized trials suggest that primary angioplasty can reduce mortality by as much as 63% without any increase in cost. This reduction is much greater than that shown by early administration of thrombolytic therapy or by accelerated t-PA versus streptokinase. The recent study by Stone et al has now established the clinical superiority of stenting over PTCA alone in the treatment of patients with acute ST elevation myocardial infarcts at experienced centers where these patients can be treated relatively acutely.[46]

PERCUTANEOUS TRANSLUMINAL CORONARY ANGIOPLASTY

Indications

The role of PTCA and now stenting in the treatment of coronary artery disease continues to evolve.[48] The original indication for PTCA was the presence of angina pectoris with failure of maximal medical therapy in a patient with an anatomically appropriate lesion (de novo, type A) of a single diseased coronary artery.[49]

Today, PTCA is used in selected patients with multivessel disease, calcified and/or eccentric lesions, distal coronary stenosis, complex or multiple lesions within the same vessel, or saphenous or internal mammary bypass grafts.[50] PTCA also is used as primary therapy for patients with acute ST-segment elevation myocardial infarction (Fig. 20-1),[10,51] and as reviewed above, is even better with stenting.[46] In patients with stable angina and single-vessel disease, PTCA alleviates symptoms more completely than medical therapy alone. It may also reduce the development of unstable angina and result in fewer hospitalizations.

In acute MI, PTCA applied sequentially, that is, after early administration of thrombolytic agents, is not yet considered a preferred treatment since poor results have been shown in some clinical trials. In selected patients, however, PTCA/stenting as an adjunctive therapy (several hours after the occurrence of acute MI) is a common choice and is probably applied in up to one third of patients first treated with a plasminogen activator.[10]

Deciding to utilize PTCA/stenting is dependent on several criteria: lesion classification, the number of lesions or diseased vessels involved, and the patient's history and clinical status. The American College of Cardiology (ACC) and the American Heart Association (AHA) have developed a classification system for patients undergoing PTCA, based on the likelihood of a successful procedure (Table 20-3), and this has been recently updated.[52]

Contraindications

The Task Force also has outlined contraindications to coronary angioplasty (Tables 20-4 and 20-5).

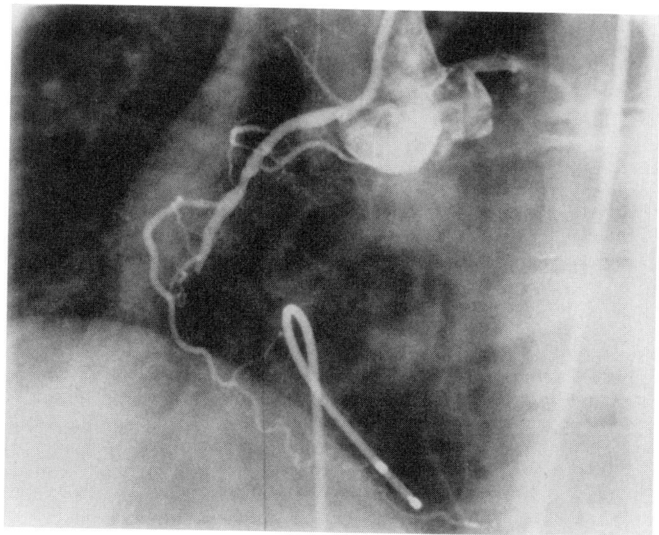
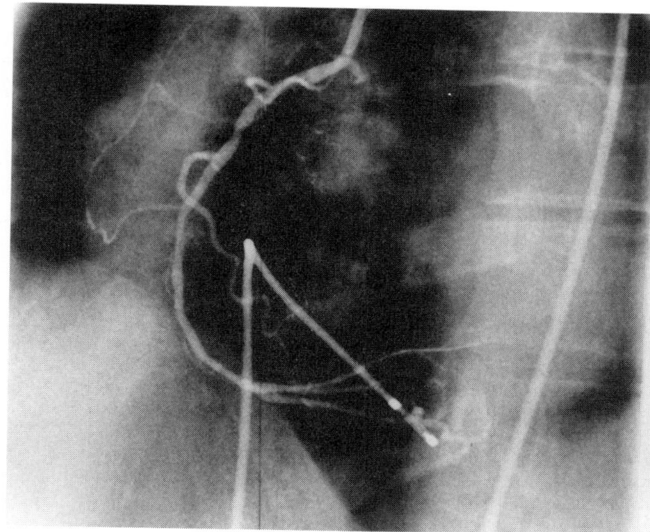

FIGURE 20–1 Acute inferior myocardial infarction, with demonstration of total mid right coronary artery occlusion (left). Angiographic result after direct PTCA (right).

TABLE 20–3 Characteristics of type A, B, and C lesions

Type A lesions (minimally complex)
Discrete (length <10 mm)
Concentric
Readily accessible
Nonangulated segment (<45°)
Smooth contour
Little or no calcification
Less than totally occlusive
Not ostial in location
No major side branch involvement. Absence of thrombus
Type B lesions (moderately complex)*
Tubular (length 10-20 mm)
Eccentric
Moderate tortuosity of proximal segment.
Moderately angulated segment (>45°, <90°).
Irregular contour
Moderate or heavy calcification
Total occlusions <3 mo old
Ostial in location
Bifurcation lesions requiring double guide wires
Some thrombus present
Type C lesions (severely complex)
Diffuse (length >2 cm)
Excessive tortuosity of proximal segment. Extremely angulated segments >90°
Total occlusions >3 mo old and/or bridging collaterals. Inability to protect major side branches
Degenerated vein grafts with friable lesions

*Although the risk of abrupt vessel closure may be moderately high with Type B lesions, the likelihood of a major complication may be low in certain instances such as in the dilation of total occlusions <3 mo old or when abundant collateral channels supply the distal vessel.

Source: Ryan TJ, and the Committee on Percutaneous Transluminal Angioplasty. Guidelines for Percutaneous Transluminal Angioplasty. Circulation 1993; 88:2987–3007. Reproduced with permission from the American Heart Association.

Surgical Backup for PTCA

Early trials showed that angioplasty during the first hours after onset of MI is associated with a lower incidence of reinfarction, intracranial hemorrhage, and death than thrombolysis.[53] For this reason, the procedure has been approved in hospitals that do not have coronary bypass backup programs. However, according to the current Task Force guidelines, the national standard of accepted medical practice for coronary angioplasty requires that an experienced cardiovascular surgical team be available within the institution to perform emergency coronary bypass surgery should the clinical need arise.[52] Surgical consultation is advisable in cases in which the extent of disease indicates that surgery may be a more effective means of therapy than angioplasty.[54]

Single-Vessel Coronary Artery Disease

Patients with single-vessel coronary artery disease with significant symptoms are still one of the largest groups undergoing angioplasty. In this group of patients, a 90% to 95% success rate can be expected.[55,56]

Several studies have been undertaken in recent years to compare the outcome of PTCA with other therapeutic measures in patients with single-vessel disease. The Department of Veterans Affairs Angioplasty Compared with Medical Therapy (ACME) Study addressed 212 patients who had single-vessel lesions of 70% to 99% diameter stenosis and myocardial ischemia by treadmill testing for whom continued medical therapy was still an option.[57] This study showed that PTCA offers earlier and more complete relief of angina than medical therapy and is associated with better performance on the exercise test. The drawbacks of PTCA are its initial higher costs and an association with a higher

TABLE 20–4 Factors predictive of abrupt vessel closure

Preprocedure	Postprocedure
Clinical factors	Intimal dissection >10 mm
Female gender	Residual stenosis >50%
Unstable angina	Transient in-lab closure
Insulin-dependent diabetes mellitus	Residual transstenotic gradient ≥20 mm Hg
Inadequate antiplatelet therapy	
Angiographic factors	
Intracoronary thrombus	
>90% stenosis	
Stenosis length 2 or more luminal diameters	
Stenosis at branch point	
Stenosis on bend (≥45°)	
Right coronary artery stenosis	

Source: Ryan TJ, and the Committee on Percutaneous Transluminal Angioplasty. Guidelines for Percutaneous Transluminal Angioplasty. Circulation 1993; 88:2987–3007. Reproduced with permission from the American Heart Association.

frequency of need for a second procedure. The addition of stenting has further improved the efficacy of angioplasty, reducing the occurrence of restenosis problems requiring a second intervention to the 15% to 20% range. Even more recently, the use of "coated" stents, specifically with rapamycin (Sirolimus), appears to reduce the risk of restenosis to less than 5%.[58]

Angioplasty vs. Surgery

The role of angioplasty in the treatment for multivessel disease has become increasingly common, yet the benefits of this approach versus bypass surgery have not been determined. Coronary bypass surgery offers the advantage of more complete revascularization regardless of the coronary anatomy at the time of the procedure, yet it carries the risks of general anesthesia, mechanical ventilation, midline sternotomy, extracorporeal circulation, and a prolonged recovery time. Coronary angioplasty carries the risks of abrupt vessel closure and early restenosis, and it does not guarantee complete revascularization at the time of the procedure.[51] As noted above, the use of stents, and most likely "coated" stents in the future (most especially rapamycin-coated stents), should make interventional therapy even more attractive. Randomized trials of surgical therapy have shown that the benefits of surgical revascularization are proportional to the amount of myocardium affected by, or at risk for, ischemic injury. Comparisons between angioplasty and bypass surgery in select populations with single- and multivessel coronary artery disease have shown that PTCA is not as effective as surgery for long-term symptomatic control, and that it often requires repeat PTCA or crossover to bypass surgery; however, long-term outcomes (i.e., death and myocardial infarction) are similar.[59] The best "coated" stent may further enhance the effectiveness of PTCA, allowing it to be used successfully and with better long-term results in more patients with two- and three-vessel coronary heart disease. The critical outcome measures of these procedures will be functional status, quality of life, employment, and health care costs.[60]

TABLE 20–5 Factors associated with increased mortality for angioplasty

Clinical Factors	Angiographic Factors
Female gender	Left main coronary disease
Age >65 years	Three-vessel disease
Unstable angina	Left ventricular ejection fraction <0.30
Congestive heart failure	Risk index*
Chronic renal failure	Myocardial jeopardy score
	Proximal right coronary stenosis
	Collaterals originate from dilated vessel

*See also Bergelson BA, Jacobs AK, Cupples LA, et al: Prediction of risk for hemodynamic compromise during percutaneous transluminal coronary angioplasty. *Am J Cardiol* 1992; 70:1540–1545.

Source: Ryan TJ, and the Committee on Percutaneous Transluminal Angioplasty. Guidelines for Percutaneous Transluminal Angioplasty. Circulation 1993; 88:2987–3007. Reproduced with permission from the American Heart Association.

The Coronary Artery Surgery Study (CASS) showed no survival benefits for revascularization among patients who received PTCA without having failed medical therapy. The advantages of PTCA are measured by symptom relief, functional improvement, or reduced cost in this patient subset.[61]

The Emory Angioplasty versus Surgery Trial (EAST)[62] recently assessed the 5-year outcome in 392 patients randomized to coronary surgery (n = 194) or coronary angioplasty (n = 198). Each group had an in-hospital mortality of 1%. Survival was 91% in the CABG group versus 87.9% in the PTCA group ($p = .29$). Whereas there was no difference in mortality at 3 years, by 5 years there was a slight but not significant separation of the curves favoring surgery. Most of the additional revascularization procedures occurred in the first year, and there were more additional revascularization procedures in the PTCA group.

In a similar trial, the Bypass Angioplasty Revascularization Investigation (BARI), 1,800 patients from 16 centers across the United States were enrolled for a 5-year study period.[63,64] This trial was designed to evaluate whether the strategy of PTCA is as safe (regarding mortality) as the strategy of starting with bypass surgery. The surgical cohort of this trial represents the largest group of patients with multivessel coronary artery disease who have been randomly assigned to surgical treatment. Patients were eligible for BARI if they had multivessel coronary artery disease, had a clinical indication for revascularization, and were suitable for both coronary angioplasty and bypass surgery. The results from this study were very similar to those from the EAST trial. One problem patient group that has emerged from these studies are the patients with diabetes, especially insulin-dependent diabetes. They do not have as favorable results from PTCA/stenting as do the nondiabetics. They have higher restenosis rates and greater morbidity, and current data favor surgical revascularization in this group of patients, especially those with two- and three-vessel disease. It has been shown, however, that the combined use of PTCA/stenting with a platelet IIb/IIIa receptor inhibitor, such as Reopro, enhances the effectiveness of PTCA/stenting in the diabetic patient.[65,66]

The Randomized Intervention Treatment of Angina (RITA) trial was established to compare angioplasty with surgical therapy in stable and unstable angina.[67] This trial differed from BARI and EAST in that the lesions in each patient had to be suitable for both angioplasty and surgery. The goal for both strategies is to achieve complete revascularization. At the second year follow-up in RITA, there was no difference between PTCA and bypass surgery for survival following myocardial infarction.[67] Additional revascularization procedures, myocardial infarction, and death were more common among PTCA patients (38%) than among bypass surgery patients (11%) within 2 years of randomization. Repeat coronary angiography was four times more common among PTCA patients (31% vs. 7%).

Other clinical trials that are in progress will include angiography and myocardial perfusion stress testing in their follow-up evaluations.[68,69] In the German Angioplasty Bypass Surgery Investigation (GABI),[68] PTCA and CABG showed equivalent improvement in angina at the end of one year. The patients treated with PTCA were more likely to require further interventions and antianginal drugs, whereas the patients treated with bypass surgery were more likely to sustain an acute MI at the time of the procedure.

In the Coronary Artery Bypass Revascularization Investigation (CABRI), 183 Dutch patients with multivessel disease were randomized to treatment with PTCA or coronary artery bypass surgery between 1988 and 1992.[69] The CABG group consisted of 88 patients with a total of 255 vascular obstructions; the PTCA group comprised 95 patients with 294 vascular lesions. Within 30 days after intervention, the clinical results of the two treatments were the same. The differences in death rate and myocardial infarctions were not significant, in contrast to the difference in the numbers of reinterventions. The death rates were 1.1% and 2.1% for CABG and PTCA, respectively. The proportion of transmural, nonfatal myocardial infarctions was 2.3% in the CABG group versus 3.1% in the PTCA group. The proportion of reinterventions was higher in the PTCA group, 11.4% versus 1.1%. Early results with CABRI indicate that PTCA is a reasonable alternative to coronary surgery in patients with multiple-vessel coronary disease.

In a review of surgery versus angioplasty for coronary artery disease, Wilson and Ferguson[59] concluded that surgical bypass remains the mainstay of therapy for patients with severe disease and a poor prognosis for survival, and it is warranted in patients in whom PTCA/stenting has failed repeatedly. Revascularization should be offered on the basis of symptom severity (in the presence of medical therapy) in accordance with the prognosis for survival, as judged by the extent and severity of disease.

Complications of Angioplasty

Procedural success in angioplasty relates to certain patient characteristics, such as younger age and male gender, and to clinical variables, such as diabetes, prior myocardial infarction, prior bypass surgery, and impairment of left ventricular function.[51] Of major importance in predicting the success of the procedure are the angiographic characteristics of the lesion (or lesions) to be dilated.[70] Long, calcified, or ostial lesions; tortuosity of the vessels; and degenerative vein grafts are particularly challenging for the interventionalist. The risk of abrupt vessel closure and early restenosis must be carefully weighed when determining which patients will most benefit from angioplasty. Other risks associated with the procedure include stroke, myocardial infarction, arrhythmias, and vascular complications at the catheter entry site.

ABRUPT VESSEL CLOSURE

It is estimated that an acute ischemic complication will develop in approximately 7% of patients undergoing coronary angioplasty.[71] In more than half of these patients, thrombus, dissection, or both can be identified angiographically as the underlying cause of abrupt closure.[71] Predictors of dissection-mediated closure include degenerated vein graft, de novo stenosis, proximal tortuosity, high lesion grade, eccentricity, longer lesion length, and angulation.[71] Yellow plaque identified by angioscopy confers a heightened risk of major complications. Lesions containing areas of calcium adjacent to areas of soft plaque have been identified by ultrasound as a powerful predictor of major dissection. The presence of thrombus in the artery to be dilated is associated with a higher risk of postprocedural thrombotic occlusion.

Tan et al[72] examined the determinants of coronary angioplasty success and complications by evaluating the American College of Cardiology/American Heart Association ABC lesions classification scheme and its modifications. They assessed the lesion morphologic determinants of immediate angioplasty outcome in 729 consecutive patients who underwent coronary angioplasty of 994 vessels and 1248 lesions. Angioplasty success was achieved in 91% of lesions, and abrupt closure occurred in 3%. They found that longer lesions, calcified lesions, diameter stenosis of 80% to 99%, and presence of thrombus were predictive of a lower success rate. Longer lesions, angulated lesions, diameter stenosis of 80% to 99%, and calcified lesions were predictive of an abrupt closure.

Despite the various interventions used to prevent abrupt closure, it remains a highly unpredictable occurrence, with a substantial incidence of myocardial infarction and angioplasty-related morbidity and mortality.[73] Intracoronary visualization by intravascular ultrasound can help to identify important characteristics that identify lesions at risk for abrupt closure.[73] Repeat dilatation is often successful in the treatment of abrupt closure.[74]

In one study examining the impact of new devices on the incidence and reversal rate of abrupt closure,[75] abrupt closure occurred in 80 (4.2%) of 1919 consecutive coronary angioplasty procedures; 389 procedures (20%) were performed with the use of stents, coronary atherectomy, or laser balloon angioplasty. Abrupt closure was less frequent following newer coronary interventions (1.8%) compared with standard balloon angioplasty (4.9%, $p = .01$). Although this may have reflected case selection, the results indicated that new interventional devices were associated with a lower incidence of abrupt closure. Most catheterization laboratories administer heparin for 12 to 24 hours after angioplasty to reduce the risk of abrupt closure,[76] and in some cases, such as diabetics and others deemed to be at increased risk, an inhibitor of the platelet glycoprotein IIb/IIIa receptors may be used.

RESTENOSIS

Restenosis has been deemed the Achilles' heel of angioplasty.[77] Despite many innovations in interventional techniques for coronary disease in recent years, restenosis remains the most common complication following PTCA. Restenosis may be described simply as the chronic renarrowing of the dilated vessel in response to the balloon (or other interventional device) injury that typically occurs over 3 to 6 months after the procedure. In other words, coronary arteries that have been subjected to balloon angioplasty or other interventions will be traumatized and undergo wound healing, which culminates in the formation of stenotic lesions.

In 1992, the average restenosis rate reported in the literature was 30%,[77,78] but recent reports have estimated a range of 20% to 55% occurrence of restenosis in arteries subjected to percutaneous interventions.[79,80] Studies of serial longitudinal angiographic evaluations[81] after successful PTCA have shown that 11% of patients will have restenosis within the first month; 39% will have restenosis at the end of the first 3 months; and an additional 6% will have restenosis 3 to 6 months after PTCA. A small number of patients will have angiographic evidence of restenosis at the end of 1 year.

Renarrowing within the first few days after an angioplasty procedure usually represents abrupt closure rather than restenosis. This is often caused by thrombosis superimposed on a vessel wall dissection or intimal flap. Asymptomatic angiographic renarrowing (50% or greater diameter stenosis) has been shown to occur in as many as 7.8% of lesions treated.[82] Some researchers[83] have noted that although anginal symptom recurrence is the hallmark of restenosis, approximately 25% of patients are asymptomatic. Also noteworthy is the fact that among those with recurring angina, up to 44% are not found to have restenosis.[83,84] After the first several days, further renarrowing probably reflects chronic recoil, vessel remodeling, and neointimal proliferation.[80]

Although restenosis does not result in increased mortality (because patients with restenosis develop angina rather than myocardial infarction or sudden death), restenosis does lead to repeat PTCA or coronary artery bypass grafting; thus, it increases morbidity and costs.[85] There is, however, considerable enthusiasm for the use of coated stents, especially rapamycin-coated stents, as a means to reduce the restenosis risk. Stents have reduced the risk of restenosis from 30% to 50% with PTCA alone to 15% to 20% with stents following PTCA. The use of rapamycin-coated stents has reduced the risk of restenosis to less than 5% in the first several hundred patients that have been treated.[58]

Mechanisms of Restenosis Findings from angioscopic, intravascular ultrasound, atherectomy, and autopsy studies have supported the hypothesis that early restenosis is a local vascular manifestation of the general response to injury and wound healing. Restenosis early after angioplasty usually consists of immediate elastic recoil, platelet deposition, and thrombus formation, followed by smooth muscle cell proliferation and matrix formation.[86,87]

The time course of restenosis can be determined from studies of injury in animal models and autopsy studies.[88–95] Within seconds of injury, endothelial removal and endothelial death, as well as some smooth muscle death, smooth muscle separation, and smooth muscle stretch, occur. For the next several minutes, there is platelet attachment, release, aggregation, and coagulation. Within a few days after injury, endothelial and smooth cells and macrophages proliferate and migrate. Over several weeks, synthesis, maturation, and contraction of the extracellular matrix occur, in addition to the remodeling process, during which the vessel may enlarge or decrease in size.

Prevention of Restenosis Angiographic results have shown that arteries undergoing any type of intervention—balloon angioplasty, atherectomy, or laser balloon angioplasty—show a similar extent of restenosis at 6 months.[96] Use of angiography to predict the long-term success or failure of PTCA is of limited value, however, because these images provide only a circumscribed view of the arterial lumen and offer little insight into the morphologic characteristics of the underlying plaque.[97] Intravascular ultrasound has been used with more success to identify patients in whom restenosis is likely to develop, because it provides information about the morphologic features of the atheroma and its composition.[98,99] With ultrasound, the interventional strategy may be modified to optimize lumen size and possibly reduce the risk of restenosis.[99] Restenosis after stent placement is a somewhat different process and one that reflects primarily the proliferative process of smooth muscle cells without vessel recoil.

The process of wound healing after balloon angioplasty begins within minutes or up to 2 hours after the procedure and may continue for weeks or months. This process is dependent not only on the release and complex interaction of thrombosis, cytokines, and growth factors, but also on the extent of healing and the type of injury.[97] Therefore, therapies have to be targeted at processes that occur early after balloon injury to combat the early release of growth factors and cytokines and for processes that occur late (2 to 4 weeks) when factors that induce substance deposition are at their peak.[97] Although a variety of agents designed to reduce the risk of restenosis have been successful in animal studies, no pharmacologic agent has clearly proved to be successful in reducing restenosis in humans, even after more than 50 published major clinical trials randomizing greater than 20,000 patients with the goal of limiting restenosis by pharmacologic means.[100] In addition, few risk factors for restenosis have stood the test of time, and their predictive power is relatively weak,[101] including such factors as lipoprotein (a), low high-density lipoprotein (HDL), prior restenosis, total occlusion, diabetes, or location of the left anterior descending coronary artery.[85,102–109]

Stents have markedly reduced the risk of restenosis, except in diabetic patients as noted earlier, and that may be improved in the diabetic patient by using the platelet glycoprotein IIb/IIIa receptor inhibitor, Reopro, before, during, and following stent placement so the results look similar to those in nondiabetics.[65] Early studies have found that the rapamycin-coated stents may reduce the risk of restenosis to less than 5%, and if this is confirmed in future studies, this will have a major effect on interventional procedures generally. Inhibitors of platelet glycoprotein IIb/IIIa receptors and new therapies are still being sought based on the role of smooth muscle cell proliferation, inflammatory cells, and humoral factors in the restenotic process.[109–117]

Arterial Remodeling One avenue of research in prevention of restenosis involves arterial remodeling. According to Currier and Faxon,[86] restenosis can be thought of not merely as neointimal formation in response to balloon injury, but as arterial remodeling in response to balloon injury and neointimal formation. This remodeling may consist of actual constriction of the artery, as has been described in some animal models and in preliminary fashion in humans, or of compensatory enlargement, as has been described in de novo atherosclerosis and in the hypercholesterolemic rabbit iliac artery model. Compensatory enlargement and chronic constriction may represent two ends of the spectrum of arterial remodeling in response to balloon angioplasty. Thus, therapeutic strategies to alter arterial remodeling in conjunction with altering neointimal formation may be required to reduce restenosis after coronary interventions.

Lipid-lowering Agents Omega-3 fatty acids, in addition to lowering triglyceride level, also affect platelet aggregation and coagulation, which are important in restenosis. Conflicting results have been found in five clinical trials addressing the effect of omega-3 fatty acid supplementation on the risk of restenosis.[118–123] The weight of the evidence suggests, however, that they do not generally reduce the risk of restenosis after PTCA. In one early trial, a beneficial effect on restenosis was shown with the lipid-lowering agent lovastatin[124]; however, subsequent trials were unable to confirm this observation.[125,126] The Lovastatin Restenosis Trial after PTCA[127] also failed to show the efficacy of hypocholesterolemic therapy for reducing the risk of restenosis.

Platelet Inhibitors After coronary angioplasty, patients usually are treated with aspirin, nitrates, calcium channel antagonists, and heparin. Such medications are given specifically to interfere with coronary artery vasoreactivity and platelet function. These drugs are useful in treating coronary vasospasm and preventing abrupt closure. Platelet inhibitors have shown promise for prevention of restenosis in recent clinical studies. One large-scale trial, Evaluation of c7E3 for the Prevention of Ischemia Complications (EPIC), was designed to examine the role of thrombosis, angiotensin II, and oxidation in restenosis. The platelet glycoprotein IIb/IIIa integrin is the receptor that mediates the final common pathway of platelet aggregation. According to the EPIC investigators, agents that block this platelet receptor represent a promising new approach to preventing cardiovascular ischemic complications and late restenosis after PTCA.[128,129] In the trial, which included high-risk patients undergoing coronary intervention procedures, a monoclonal antibody Fab fragment (c7E3) directed against glycoprotein IIb/IIIa integrin was administered as a bolus dose and through infusion (Fig. 20-2). In early results of the trial, c7E3 significantly reduced the 30-day incidence of major ischemic events relative to aspirin and heparin, as well as decreased the need for repeat revascularization during the 6-month follow-up period. However, this finding was not confirmed in later studies

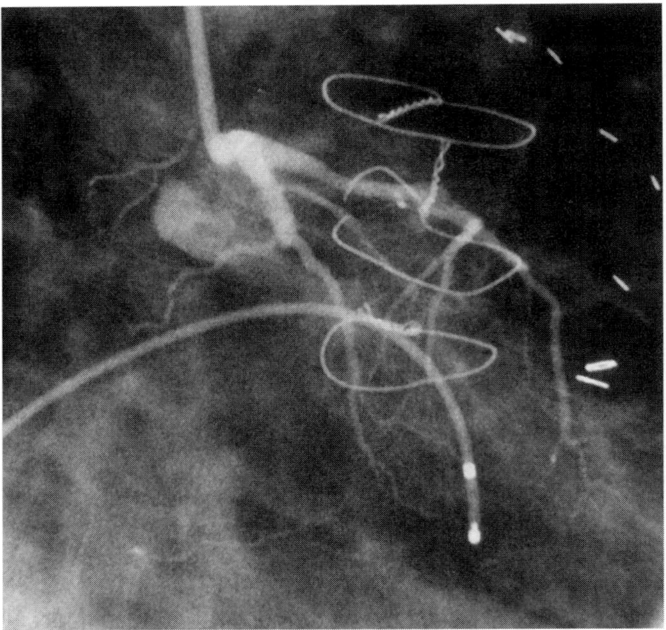

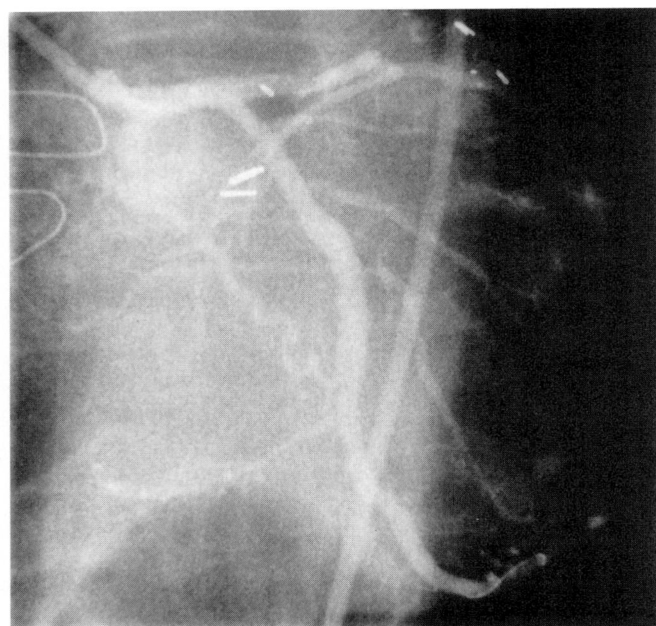

FIGURE 20–2 Acute lateral myocardial infarction (left). Final result after direct PTCA and tandem stenting, with use of c7E3 (Reopro) platelet inhibitor (right).

by these same investigators, and so it is difficult to use this finding from the EPIC trial in the treatment of patients at the current time. The major complication in the EPIC trial was bleeding,[130] the risk of which appeared to be inversely related to body weight.[131]

At The University of Texas Health Science Center and the Texas Heart Institute, we have tested the hypothesis that c7E3 can abolish or attenuate cyclic flow variations in coronary blood flow after angioplasty procedures.[132] After angioplasty, flow variations occur as a result of repetitive accumulation and dislodgment of platelet aggregates at sites of coronary stenosis with endothelial injury.[133] In animal models of coronary thrombosis, cyclic alterations in flow have often preceded thrombotic occlusion or reocclusion.[134] Reopro was shown to eliminate cyclic alterations in coronary blood flow in 4 of 5 patients who developed cyclic flow variations in our observations of 27 patients undergoing angioplasty procedures.[132] Studies are still needed to elucidate the role of the c7E3 antibody in the prevention of restenosis.

ALTERNATIVE APPROACHES TO CONVENTIONAL BALLOON ANGIOPLASTY

Since balloon angioplasty was developed, improvements in the procedure have kept it the primary interventional therapy for patients with ischemic heart disease.[135] However, research has indicated that certain lesion types and patient populations may be treated more effectively with other newer technologies, such as intracoronary stents as already discussed, coronary atherectomy and ablation, and cutting devices. These devices appear to be more effective than conventional angioplasty in treating calcified, eccentric, or ulcerated lesions; ostial stenosis or stenosis of the left anterior descending (LAD) artery; disease in older saphenous vein grafts; restenotic lesions after prior interventions; and dissected vessels with actual or threatened abrupt closure.[136] The challenge for the clinician is deciding the optimal application for these technologies in specific clinical settings.

Stents

The use of vascular endoprostheses or stents developed as a result of complications seen in percutaneous transluminal angioplasty. Appropriate indications for stent placement include restenosis, dissection, abrupt closure, residual stenosis, or reopened total occlusion (Fig. 20-3). Intracoronary stenting has proved to be a successful method of circumventing emergency bypass surgery after acute vessel closure in angioplasty procedures.

The problem of thrombosis associated with angioplasty is not resolved by stent placement. Stents are themselves thrombogenic,[137] and their use requires some form of anticoagulation therapy; recent data suggest that aspirin or aspirin and ticlopidine, or more recently aspirin and clopidogrel (Plavix), is adequate.[138,139] In addition, a clinical trial involving a heparin-coated Palmaz Schatz stent was conducted in Europe (BENESTENT II),[140] and studies involving larger numbers of patients receiving rapamycin-coated stents (RAVEL study) are underway. Additional oral

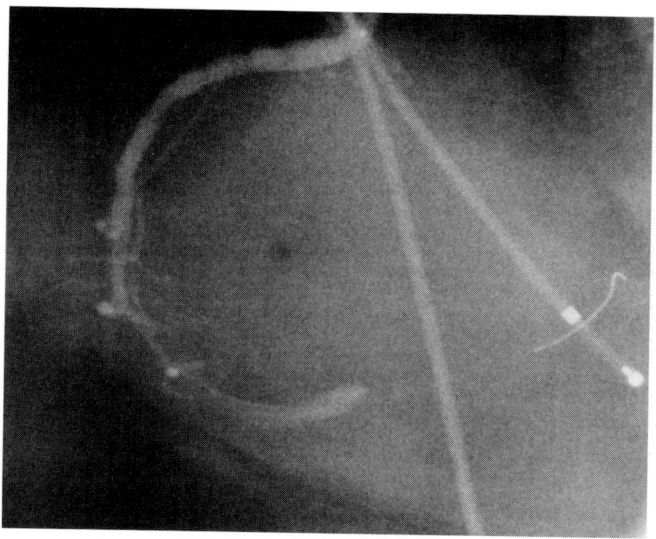

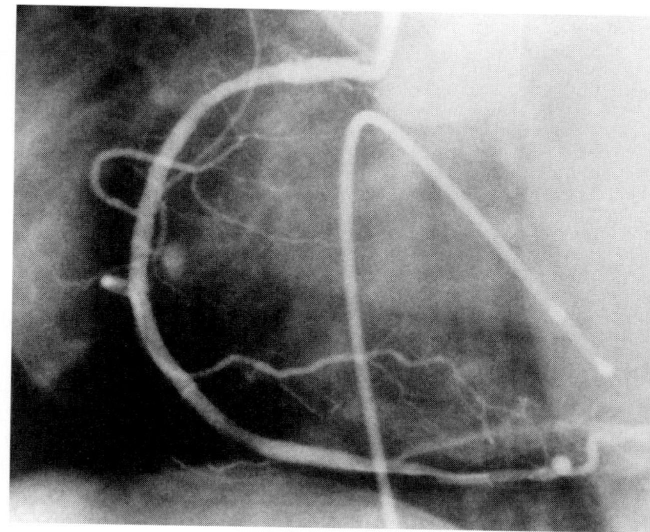

FIGURE 20–3 Severe spiral dissection of the right coronary artery following routine angioplasty (left). Excellent angiographic result after repair of dissection with tandem stenting (right).

anticoagulation will most likely always be needed when stents are placed in human arteries, and recent evidence suggests that Plavix should probably be continued long term after stent placement. The BENESTENT II trial data suggest that a heparin-coated stent reduces the risk of restenosis to approximately 13%. An earlier trial, BENESTENT I, suggested that stents themselves reduce the risk of restenosis from the anticipated 30% to 40% to 22%.[141]

Though it is a rare occurrence, loss of the stent from its delivery system into the peripheral circulation is another possible complication of the stent procedure. In such cases, magnetic resonance imaging may be useful for locating the misplaced device.[142]

There are now reports of stent implantation after myocardial infarction.[143–146] Recent evidence suggests that PTCA/stenting may be the preferred therapy for acute ST-segment elevation MI,[46] and perhaps the preferred therapy for patients with unstable angina/non–ST-segment elevation MIs with elevated serum CRP or troponin I or T concentrations (unstable angina, as reviewed earlier in this chapter).[39]

One disadvantage of coronary stenting is cost. Elective coronary stenting, as performed in the randomized Stent Re-Stenosis Study (STRESS) trial, increased total 1-year medical care costs by approximately $800 per patient, compared with conventional angioplasty. Ongoing refinements in stent design, implantation techniques, and anticoagulation regimens may narrow this cost difference by reducing stent-related vascular complications or length of stay.

Directional Coronary Atherectomy

Directional coronary atherectomy (DCA) has been proposed as an alternative to balloon dilatation for treatment of coronary artery disease, but the long-term efficacy of this procedure is not known. DCA was introduced in 1986 and approved by the FDA for clinical use in 1990. The goal of DCA is for debulking rather than dilating a coronary artery lesion (Fig. 20-4).

In directional atherectomy, a metal cylinder with a lateral window is positioned on the end of a catheter. When introduced into the lesion, the atherectomy catheter's rotating knife cuts into the atheromatous material and traps it inside the metallic reservoir. Although its potential role is not clearly defined, it is believed that, with DCA, selective removal of plaque potentially may minimize the vessel wall damage and lead to subsequent better late outcome. One important advantage of DCA is its usefulness for the in vivo study of coronary artery plaques.[147]

In a study of the clinical and angiographic outcome after directional coronary atherectomy, the procedure was associated with a high procedural success rate (94.8%) and infrequent complications in selected lesion subsets.[148] Late clinical events (death, Q-wave myocardial infarction, coronary bypass surgery, coronary angioplasty) occurred in 69 patients (28%). Independent predictors of late clinical events included diabetes mellitus, unstable angina, and a prior history of restenosis.

DCA for saphenous vein graft lesions was performed at 21 centers during a 2-year period; 318 procedures were performed in 363 vein graft lesions.[149] Angiographic success was achieved in 86% of lesions and clinical success was achieved in 85%. Restenosis was significantly lower in primary vein graft lesions than in vein grafts with prior intervention. This initial multicenter investigation indicates that DCA is safe and effective in selected cases of degenerative vein grafts.

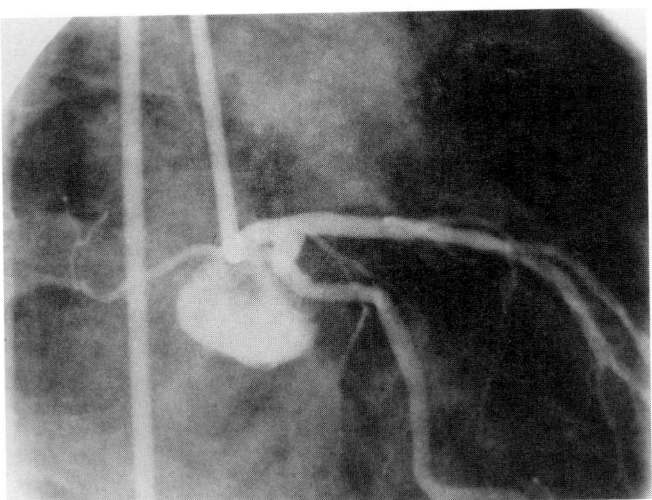

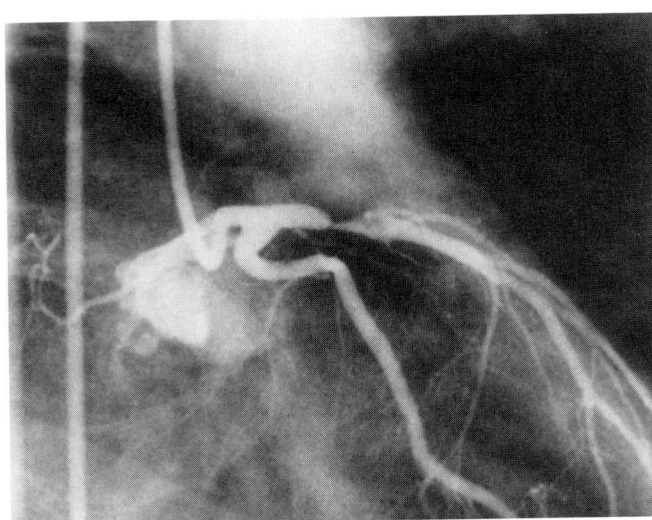

FIGURE 20–4 Stenosis of the proximal left anterior descending coronary artery (left). Angiogram showing result of directional coronary atherectomy procedure following suboptimal balloon angioplasty (right).

Several studies have been undertaken to compare the results of angioplasty with DCA for treatment of coronary lesions. One recent study involving complex lesions showed that DCA is limited by a modest degree of lumen enlargement, frequent need for adjunctive angioplasty, and a high restenosis rate, and appears to offer no advantage over conventional balloon angioplasty for such lesions.[150]

Investigators in the Coronary Angioplasty Versus Excisional Atherectomy Trial (CAVEAT I) examined the efficacy of DCA for ostial coronary lesions.[151] For ostial left anterior descending (LAD) coronary artery stenosis, procedures yielded similar rates of initial success and restenosis, but atherectomy was associated with a higher incidence of non–Q-wave-MI. The predominant angiographic benefit in this study was shown in proximal nonostial lesions of the LAD. At 1-year follow-up in CAVEAT I, of 1012 patients randomized to either angioplasty or DCA, a statistically significant excess of deaths after DCA was revealed that was not evident at 6-month follow-up.[152]

A review of acute and long-term results of coronary stenting and atherectomy in women and the elderly has shown that both techniques can be performed safely and effectively in these patient subsets, despite a somewhat lower success rate and higher rates of acute complications.[153]

Rotablator

The Rotablator, which encompasses an olive-shaped high-speed burr coated with diamond chips, is used primarily for debulking lesions (Fig. 20-5). When introduced into the

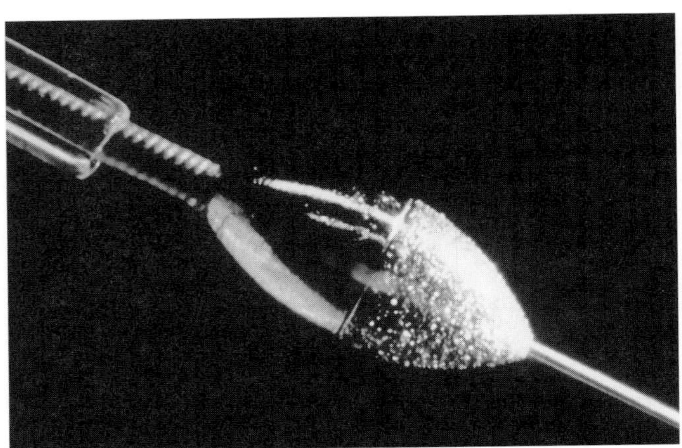

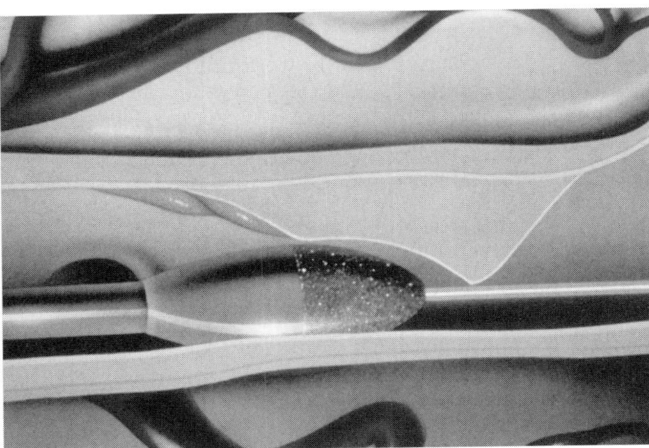

FIGURE 20–5 Rotablator system (left). Artist's depiction of ablation of atherosclerotic plaque using the Rotablator (right). (*Courtesy of Heart Technology, Inc., Redmond, WA.*)

stenosed area of the vessel, the Rotablator attacks preferentially hard resistant material and is thus indicated for calcified lesions. Its fine elliptoid tip rotates at 180,000 rpm, grinding atheroma into millions of tiny fragments. Whereas DCA is used to physically remove plaque from the vessels, the Rotablator is used to ablate the plaque in situ. Its use is contraindicated in irregular or thrombus-containing stenoses, highly angulated stenoses (and possibly right coronary artery stenoses), or in those associated with impaired distal runoff caused by a recent MI or manifest by a fixed thallium defect.[154] The primary success rate with this device is 95%.[155] In most Rotablator procedures, concomitant balloon angioplasty is necessary, however, for creation of a suitable lumen.

Data from the Multicenter Rotablator Registry of two[155] rotational atherectomy procedures in single lesions were analyzed to determine the efficacy of rotational atherectomy for 1078 calcified and 1083 noncalcified lesions.[156] Adjunctive coronary angioplasty was used in 82.9% of calcified and 66.9% of noncalcified lesions. Procedural success (defined as less than 50% residual stenosis without major complications) was achieved in 94.3% of calcified and 95.2% of noncalcified lesions. In this large study, the success rate of rotational atherectomy was not reduced by calcification despite the more frequently complex nature of the calcified lesions. These results underscore the potential for the Rotablator as the interventional device of choice for complex, calcified lesions.

THE FUTURE IN ALTERNATIVE CORONARY INTERVENTIONS

Other new technologies undergoing evaluation for treatment of coronary artery disease include various types of stents, low-speed rotators, and transluminal extraction catheters. Although laser angioplasty initially was greeted with enthusiasm, the current consensus is that its use will be limited.

The adjunctive therapies in use today have made it possible for interventionalists to treat long, calcified, ulcerated, and distal lesions that would not have been possible to treat with balloon angioplasty alone. A lesion-specific approach is commonplace now. The restenosis rate has not been significantly reduced with these adjunctive strategies, although refinements in stent placement are promising.

Coronary angioplasty, now along with stenting, remains the cornerstone of interventional cardiology, currently accounting for more than 90% of all coronary interventions. If selected stent coatings prove as successful as they appear presently, especially rapamycin-coated stents, the future impact of interventional cardiology in patient care will be even greater. It is likely to remain the primary procedure for coronary interventions and the standard against which we measure new therapies in the future. The impact of any new device will depend to a great extent on the technical experience and clinical judgment of the cardiology team. To aid in evaluating the safety and efficacy of new percutaneous transluminal interventional devices, the New Approaches to Coronary Intervention (NACI) voluntary registry was founded in the early 1990s.[157] Reports from this registry should be useful to all physicians interested in keeping abreast of evolving technologies.

Brachytherapy

Local radiotherapy with both beta and gamma emitters has been shown to markedly reduce the risk of restenosis following stent placement in human coronary arteries.[159] This form of therapy has already had a major beneficial impact in preventing restenosis when it has occurred with the original stent placement. General estimates of the risk of restenosis following brachytherapy suggest that in the first year, the incidence is approximately 5% to 15%.[158] Iridium 192 and strontium 90/yttrium 90 have been used for gamma and beta radiation, respectively. Longer term follow-up problems have been identified, including edge restenosis at the distal ends of the radiated segment, the later development of thrombosis, occasional coronary aneurysms, and a rare pseudoaneurysm.[158] Thus, longer term antiplatelet therapy has been recommended in the treatment of these patients, including aspirin and clopidogrel given for at least 1 year following radiation therapy; some physicians give this therapy for even longer periods of time. Clearly, the local radiotherapy has reduced the restenosis rate in patients with in-stent restenosis when a second procedure is needed. Whether this form of therapy will continue to be used if the drug-coated stents, such as rapamycin-coated stents, prove to be as successful in the future as they appear to be presently is uncertain. However, it is the author's belief that localized radiotherapy will be a useful adjunct therapy even in an era where coated stents are the preferred therapy.

ACKNOWLEDGMENTS

The excellent and dedicated assistance of Rebecca Teaff and Linda Spangler in preparing this manuscript is gratefully acknowledged. Case illustrations were generously provided by Emerson Perin, M.D.

REFERENCES

1. Sutherland JE, Persky VW, Brody JA: Proportionate mortality trends: 1950 through 1986. *JAMA* 1990; 264:3178.
2. American Heart Association: *Heart and Stroke Facts*. 1994 Statistical Supplement. Dallas, American Heart Association, 1993.
3. Gruentzig AR, Kumpe DA: Techniques of percutaneous transluminal angioplasty with the Gruentzig balloon catheter. *AJR* 1979; 132:547.

4. Gruentzig A: Transluminal dilatation of coronary artery stenosis. *Lancet* 1978; 1:263.
5. Gruentzig A, Senning A, Siegenthaler WE: Nonoperative dilatation of coronary artery stenosis: percutaneous transluminal coronary angioplasty. *N Engl J Med* 1979; 61:303.
6. O'Neill WW: Angioplasty therapy for acute myocardial infarction: current status and future directions, in Vogel JHK, King SB III (eds): *The Practice of Interventional Cardiology*. St. Louis, Mosby-Yearbook, 1993; p 359.
7. Rentrop P, Blanke H, Kostering H, Karsch KR: Intracoronary application of streptokinase in acute myocardial infarction and non-stable angina pectoris [author's translation; article in German]. *Deutsche Medizinische Wochenschrift* 1980; 105:221.
8. Gruppo Italiano per lo Studio della Streptochinasi nell'Infarcto Miocardio (GISSI): Effectiveness of intravenous thrombolytic therapy in acute myocardial infarction. *Lancet* 1986; 1:397.
9. Topol EJ: Thrombolytic intervention, in Topol EJ (ed): *Textbook of Interventional Cardiology,* 2d ed. Philadelphia, WB Saunders, 1993; p 68.
10. Ross AM: The role of angioplasty in the treatment of acute myocardial infarction, in Vogel JHK, King SB III (eds): *The Practice of Interventional Cardiology*, 2d ed. St. Louis, Mosby-Yearbook, 1993; p 378.
11. Habib GB: Current status of thrombolysis in acute myocardial infarction, I: optimal selection and delivery of a thrombolytic drug. *Chest* 1995; 107:225.
12. Sherry S: Appraisal of various thrombolytic agents in the treatment of acute myocardial infarction. *Am J Med* 1987; 83 (suppl 2A):31.
13. ISIS-2 (Second International Study of Infarct Survival) Collaborative Group: Randomized trial of intravenous streptokinase, oral aspirin, both, or neither among 17,187 cases of suspected acute myocardial infarction; ISIS-2. *Lancet* 1988; ii:349.
14. Lew AS, Laramee P, Cercek B, et al: The hypotensive effect of intravenous streptokinase in patients with acute myocardial infarction. *Circulation* 1985; 72:1321.
15. Willerson JT, Golino P, McNatt J, et al: Thrombolytic therapy: enhancement by platelet and platelet-derived mediator antagonists [review]. *Mol Biol Med* 1991; 8:235.
16. Nicolini FA, Nichols WW, Mehta JL, et al: Sustained reflow in dogs with coronary thrombosis with k2P, a novel mutant of tissue-plasminogen activator. *J Am Coll Cardiol* 1992; 20:228.
17. Rudd PM, Woods RJ, Wormald MR, et al: The effects of variable glycosylation on the functional activities of ribonuclease, plasminogen and tissue plasminogen activator [review]. *Biochimica et Biophysica Acta* 1995; 1248:1.
18. Neuhaus KL, Feuerer W, Jeep-Tebbe S: Improved thrombolysis with a modified dose regimen of recombinant tissue-type plasminogen activator. *J Am Coll Cardiol* 1989; 14:1566.
19. Tebbe U, Tanswell P, Seifried E, et al: Single-bolus injection of recombinant tissue-type plasminogen activator in acute myocardial infarction. *Circulation* 1989; 64:448.
20. Holmes DR Jr, Califf RM, Topol EJ: Lessons we have learned from the GUSTO Trial. *J Am Coll Cardiol* 1995; 25(suppl):10S.
21. Goldman L: Cost and quality of life: thrombolysis and primary angioplasty. *J Am Coll Cardiol* 1995; 25:38S.
22. Mark DB, Hlatky MA, Califf RM, et al: Cost effectiveness of thrombolytic therapy with tissue plasminogen activator as compared with streptokinase for acute myocardial infarction. *N Engl J Med* 1995; 332:1418. [Published erratum in *N Engl J Med* 1995; 334:267; comment in *N Engl J Med* 1995; 332:1443.]
23. O'Rourke M, Baron D, Keogh A, et al: Limitation of myocardial infarction by early infusion of recombinant tissue-type plasminogen activation. *Circulation* 1988; 77:1311.
24. Guerci AD, Gerstenblith G, Brinker JA, et al: A randomized trial of intravenous tissue plasminogen activator for acute myocardial infarction with subsequent randomization to elective coronary angioplasty. *N Engl J Med* 1987; 317:1613.
25. TIMI Research Group: Immediate vs delayed catheterization and angioplasty following thrombolytic therapy for acute myocardial infarction: TIMI A results. *JAMA* 1988; 260:2849.
26. Habib GB: Current status of thrombolysis in acute myocardial infarction, II: optimal utilization of thrombolysis in clinical subsets. *Chest* 1995; 107:528.
27. Schroder R, Biamino G, Leitner EF: Intravenous short-term thrombolysis in acute myocardial infarction. *Circulation* 1981; 64:10.
28. Schroder R, Biamino G, Leitner ER, et al: Intravenous short-term infusion of streptokinase in acute myocardial infarction. *Circulation* 1983; 67:536.
29. Vogel JHK, Coughlin BJ, Setty RK, et al: Thrombolysis in acute myocardial infarction in the community hospital, in Vogel JHK, King SB 3rd (eds): *The Practice of Interventional Cardiology*, 2d ed. St. Louis, Mosby-Yearbook, 1993; p 387.
30. Weaver WD, Litwin PE, Martin JS, et al: Effect of age on use of thrombolytic therapy and mortality in acute myocardial infarction. *J Am Coll Cardiol* 1991; 18:657.
31. Fibrinolytic Therapy Trialists' (FTT) Collaborative Group: Indications for fibrinolytic therapy in suspected acute myocardial infarction: collaborative overview of early mortality and major morbidity results from all randomized trials of more than 1000 patients. *Lancet* 1994; 343:311. [Published erratum appears in *Lancet* 1994; 343:742.]
32. Muller DW, Topol EJ: Selection of patients with acute myocardial infarction for thrombolytic therapy. *Ann Intern Med* 1990; 113:949.
33. Lee KL, Woodlief LH, Topol EJ, et al: Predictors of 30-day mortality in the era of reperfusion for acute myocardial infarction. Results from an international trial of 41,021 patients. GUSTO-I Investigators. *Circulation* 1995; 91:1659.
34. GISSI-2: A factorial randomized trial of alteplase versus streptokinase and heparin versus no heparin among 12,490 patients with acute myocardial infarction. *Lancet* 1990; 336:65.
35. Third International Study of Infarct Survival Collaborative Group: ISIS-3. A randomized comparison of streptokinase vs. tissue plasminogen activator vs. anistreplase and of aspirin plus heparin vs. aspirin alone among 41,229 cases of suspected acute myocardial infarction. *Lancet* 1992; 339:753.
36. The GUSTO Investigators: An international randomized trial comparing four thrombolytic strategies for acute myocardial infarction. *N Engl J Med* 1993; 329:673.
37. Braunwald E: The open artery theory is alive and well—again. *N Engl J Med* 1993; 329:1650.
38. Anderson HV, Cannon CP, Stone PH, et al, for the TIMI IIIB Investigators: One-year results of the Thrombolysis in Myocardial Infarction (TIMI) IIIB Clinical Trial: a randomized comparison of tissue-type plasminogen activator versus placebo and early invasive versus early conservative strategies in unstable angina and non–Q-wave myocardial infarction. *J Am Coll Cardiol* 1995; 26:1643.
39. Cannon, CP, Weintraub, WS, Demopoulos, LA, et al, for the TACTICS—Thrombosis in Myocardial Infarction 18 Investigators: Comparison of early invasive and conservative strategies in patients with unstable coronary syndromes treated with the glycoprotein IIb/IIIa inhibitor tirofiban. *N Engl J Med* 2001; 344 (25):1879.
40. Ribeiro EE, Silva LA, Carneiro R, et al: Randomized trial of direct coronary angioplasty versus intravenous streptokinase in acute myocardial infarction. *J Am Coll Cardiol* 1993; 22:376.
41. Topol EJ, Califf RM, George BS, et al: A randomized trial of immediate versus delayed elective angioplasty after intravenous tissue plasminogen activator in acute myocardial infarction. *N Engl J Med* 1989; 317:581.

42. Simoons ML, Arnold AER, Betriu A, et al: Thrombolysis with tissue plasminogen activator in acute myocardial infarction: no additional benefit from immediate percutaneous coronary angioplasty. *Lancet* 1988; 1:197.
43. The TIMI Research Group: Immediate vs. delayed catheterization and angioplasty following thrombolytic therapy for acute myocardial infarction. *JAMA* 1988; 260:2849.
44. The TIMI Study Group: Comparison of invasive and conservative strategies after treatment with intravenous tissue plasminogen activator in acute myocardial infarction. *N Engl J Med* 1989; 320:618.
45. Michels KB, Yusuf S: Does PTCA in acute myocardial infarction affect mortality and reinfarction rates? A quantitative overview (meta-analysis) of the randomized clinical trials. *Circulation* 1995; 91:476.
46. Stone GW, Grines CL, Cox DA, et al: Comparison of angioplasty with stenting, with or without abciximab, in acute myocardial infarction. *N Engl J Med* 2002; 34613:957.
47. Stone GW, Grines CL, Browne KF, et al: Comparison of in-hospital outcome in men versus women treated by either thrombolytic therapy or primary coronary angioplasty for acute myocardial infarction. *Am J Cardiol* 1995; 75:987.
48. Vaitkus PT: The continuing evolution of percutaneous transluminal coronary angioplasty in the treatment of coronary artery disease. *Coron Artery Dis* 1995; 6:429.
49. Folland ED: Balloon angioplasty, in Topol EJ, Serruys PW (eds): *Interventional Cardiology*. Philadelphia, Current Medicine, 1994.
50. Ryan TJ, Skolnick AE: Indications for coronary angioplasty. *Heart Disease and Stroke,* Jan–Feb 1994; p 29.
51. Ryan TJ, Bauman WB, Kennedy JW, et al: Guidelines for percutaneous transluminal coronary angioplasty: a report of the American Heart Association/American College of Cardiology Task Force on Assessment of Diagnostic and Therapeutic Cardiovascular Procedures (Committee on Percutaneous Transluminal Coronary Angioplasty). *Circulation* 1993; 88:2987.
52. Smith, SC, Dove JT, Jacobs, AK, et al: ACC/AHA Guidelines for percutaneous coronary intervention (Revision of the 1993 PTCA Guidelines)—executive summary: a report of the American College of Cardiology/American Heart Association task force on practice guidelines. Committee to Revise the 1993 Guidelines for Percutaneous Transluminal Coronary Angioplasty; endorsed by the Society for Cardiac Angiography and Interventions. *Circulation* 2001; 103:3019.
53. Ryan TJ: Angioplasty in acute myocardial infarction. *Hosp Pract* 1995; 30:33.
54. Jones R: A symposium: complex angioplasty. *Am J Cardiol* 1992; 69:22F.
55. Segal J, Kern MJ, Scott NA, et al: Alterations of phasic coronary artery flow velocity in humans during percutaneous coronary angioplasty. *J Am Coll Cardiol* 1992; 20:276.
56. Stammen F, Piessens J, Vrolix M, et al: Immediate and short-term results of a 1988–1989 coronary angioplasty registry. *Am J Cardiol* 1991; 67:253.
57. Sousa JE, Marco AC, Alexandre A, et al: Loci of neointimal proliferation after implantation of sirolimus-coated stents in human coronary arteries: a quantitative coronary angiography and three-dimensional intravascular ultrasound study. *Circulation* 2000.
58. Parisi AF, Folland ED, Hartigan P, on behalf of the Veterans Affairs ACME Investigators: A comparison of angioplasty with medical therapy in the treatment of single-vessel coronary artery disease. *N Engl J Med* 1992; 326:10.
59. Wilson JM, Ferguson JJ: Revascularization therapy for coronary artery disease: coronary artery bypass grafting versus percutaneous transluminal coronary angioplasty. *Tex Heart Inst J* 1995; 22:145.
60. Hlatky MA, Charles ED, Nobrega F, et al: Initial functional and economic status of patients with multivessel coronary artery disease randomized in the Bypass Angioplasty Revascularization Investigation (BARI). *Am J Cardiol* 1995; 75:34C.
61. CASS Principal Investigators and their associates: Myocardial infarction and mortality in the Coronary Artery Surgery Study (CASS) randomized trial. *N Engl J Med* 1984; 310:750.
62. Kosinski AS, Barnhart HX, Weintraub WS, et al, and the EAST investigators: Five-year outcome after coronary surgery or coronary angioplasty: results from the Emory Angioplasty vs Surgery Trial (EAST). *Circulation* 1995; 92(suppl):I-543.
63. Schaff HV, Rosen AD, Shemin RJ, et al: Clinical and operative characteristics of patients randomized to coronary artery bypass surgery in the Bypass Angioplasty Revascularization Investigation (BARI). *Am J Cardiol* 1995; 75:18c.
64. Rogers WJ, Alderman EL, Chaitman BR, et al: Bypass Angioplasty Revascularization Investigation (BARI): baseline, clinical and angiographic data. *Am J Cardiol* 1995; 75:9C.
65. Topol EJ, Mark DB, Lincoff AM, et al: Outcomes at 1 year and economic implications of platelet glycoprotein IIb/IIIa blockade in patients undergoing coronary stenting: results from a multicentre randomised trial. EPISTENT Investigators. Evaluation of Platelet IIb/IIIa Inhibitor for Stenting. *Lancet* 1999; 354:2019.
66. King SB, Mahmud E: Will blocking the platelet save the diabetic? *Circulation* 1999; 100:2466.
67. RITA Trial Participants: Coronary angioplasty versus coronary artery bypass surgery: the Randomized Intervention Treatment of Angina (RITA) trial. *Lancet* 1993; 341:573.
68. Hamm CW, Reimers J, Ischinger T, et al: A randomized study of coronary angioplasty compared with bypass surgery in patients with symptomatic multivessel coronary disease. German Angioplasty Bypass Surgery Investigation (GABI). *N Engl J Med* 1994; 331:1037.
69. Breeman A, Serruys PW, van den Brand MJ, et al: Complications shortly after transluminal angioplasty or following coronary surgery in 183 comparable patients with multi-vessel coronary disease. *Nederlands Tijdschrift voor Geneeskunde* 1994; 138:1074.
70. Rozenman Y, Gilon D, Welber S, et al: Clinical and angiographic predictors of immediate recoil after successful coronary angioplasty and relation to late restenosis. *Am J Cardiol* 1993; 72:1020.
71. Ellis SG: Coronary lesions at increased risk. *Am Heart J* 1995; 130:643.
72. Tan K, Sulke N, Taub N, Sowton E: Clinical and lesion morphologic determinants of coronary angioplasty success and complications: current experience. *J Am Coll Cardiol* 1995; 25:855.
73. Sassower MA, Abela GS, Koch JM, et al: Angioscopic evaluation of periprocedural and postprocedural abrupt closure after percutaneous coronary angioplasty. *Am Heart J* 1993; 126:444.
74. Tenaglia AN, Fortin DR, Frid DJ, et al: Long-term outcome following successful reopening of abrupt closure after coronary angioplasty. *Am J Cardiol* 1993; 72:21.
75. Kuntz RE, Piana R, Pomerantz RM, et al: Changing incidence and management of abrupt closure following coronary intervention in the new device era. *Cathet Cardiovasc Diagn* 1992; 27:183.
76. Fail PS, Maniet AR, Banka VS: Subcutaneous heparin in postangioplasty management: comparative trial with intravenous heparin. *Am Heart J* 1993; 126:1059.
77. Swan HJC: Introduction: the practice of interventional cardiology, in Vogel JHK, King SB 3rd (eds): *The Practice of Interventional Cardiology*. St. Louis, Mosby-Yearbook, 1993.
78. Bevans M, Mclimore E: Intracoronary stents: a new approach to coronary artery dilatation. *J Cardiovasc Nursing* 1992; 7:34.
79. Califf RM: Restenosis: the cost to society. *Am Heart J* 1995; 130:680.
80. Fortin DE, Tcheng JE, Hillegass WB, Phillips HR 3rd: Clinical management of restenosis, in Roubin GS, O'Neill WW, Stack RS, et al (eds): *Interventional Cardiovascular Medicine: Principles and Practice*. New York, Churchill Livingstone, 1994; p 555.

81. Nobuyoshi M, Kimura T, Noksaka H, et al: Restenosis after successful coronary angioplasty: serial angiographic follow-up of 229 patients. *J Am Coll Cardiol* 1988; 12:616.
82. Corcos T, Favereau X, Tamburino C, et al: Early restenosis at 24 hours following successful coronary angioplasty: a prospective study in 1000 patients, abstracted. *J Am Coll Cardiol* 1993; 21:322A.
83. Assali A, Beigel Y: Restenosis after PTCA. *Isr J Med Sci* 1995; 31:377.
84. Holmes DR Jr, Vlietstra RE, Smith HC, et al: Restenosis after percutaneous transluminal coronary angioplasty (PTCA): a report from the PTCA registry of National Heart, Lung and Blood Institute. *Am J Cardiol* 1984; 53:77C.
85. Weintraub WS, Ghazzal ZMB, Douglas JS Jr, et al: Long-term clinical follow-up in patients with angiographic restudy after successful angioplasty. *Circulation* 1993; 87:831.
86. Currier JW, Faxon DP: Restenosis after percutaneous transluminal coronary angioplasty: have we been aiming at the wrong target? *J Am Coll Cardiol* 1995; 25:516.
87. Haudenschild CC: Pathogenesis of restenosis. *Z Kardiol* 1989; 78:28.
88. Schwartz SM, Heimark RL, Majesky MW: Developmental mechanisms underlying pathology of arteries. *Physiol Rev* 1990; 70:1177.
89. Casscells W: Migration of smooth muscle cells and endothelial cells: critical events in restenosis. *Circulation* 1992; 86:723.
90. Farb A, Virmani R, Atkinson JB, Kolodgie FD: Plaque morphology and pathologic changes in arteries from patients dying after coronary balloon angioplasty. *J Am Coll Cardiol* 1990; 16:1421.
91. Waller BF, Pinkerton CA, Orr CM, et al: Restenosis 1 to 24 months after clinically successful coronary balloon angioplasty: a necropsy study of 20 patients. *J Am Coll Cardiol* 1991; 17:58B.
92. Gordon D, Reidy MA, Benditt EP, Schwartz SM: Cell proliferation in human coronary arteries. *Proc Natl Acad Sci U S A* 1990; 87:4600.
93. Potkin BN, Roberts WC: Effects of percutaneous transluminal coronary angioplasty on atherosclerotic plaques and relation of plaque composition and arterial size to outcome. *Am J Cardiol* 1988; 62:41.
94. Correa R, Yu Z-X, Flugelman MY, et al: Evidence of FGF receptor expression in smooth muscle cells and macrophages of atherosclerotic and restenotic human arteries [abstract]. *Circulation* 1991; 84(suppl II):II-460.
95. Nobuyoshi M, Kimura T, Ohishi H, et al: Restenosis after percutaneous transluminal coronary angioplasty: pathologic observations in 20 patients. *J Am Coll Cardiol* 1991; 17:433.
96. Kuntz RE, Safian RD, Levine MJ, et al: Novel approach to the analysis of restenosis after the use of three new coronary devices. *J Am Coll Cardiol* 1992; 19:1493.
97. Virmani R, Farb A, Burke AP: Coronary angioplasty from the perspective of atherosclerotic plaque: morphologic predictors of immediate success and restenosis. *Am Heart J* 1994; 127:163.
98. Coy KM, Park JC, Fishbein MC, et al: In vitro validation of three-dimensional intravascular ultrasound for the evaluation of arterial injury after balloon angioplasty. *J Am Coll Cardiol* 1992; 20:692. [Comment appears in *J Am Coll Cardiol* 1992; 20:701.]
99. Jain SP, Jain A, Collins TJ, et al: Predictors of restenosis: a morphometric and quantitative evaluation by intravascular ultrasound. *Am Heart J* 1994; 128:664.
100. Franklin SM, Faxon DP: Pharmacologic prevention of restenosis after coronary angioplasty: review of the randomized clinical trials. *Coron Artery Dis* 1993; 4:232.
101. Casscells W, Engler D, Willerson JT: Mechanisms of restenosis. *Tex Heart Inst J* 1994; 21:68.
102. Popma JJ, Califf RM, Topol EJ: Clinical trials of restenosis after coronary angioplasty [editorial]. *Circulation* 1991; 84:1426.
103. Kuntz RE, Gibson CM, Nobuyoshi M, Baim DS: Generalized model of restenosis after conventional balloon angioplasty, stenting, and directional atherectomy. *J Am Coll Cardiol* 1993; 21:15.
104. Bobbio M, Detrano R, Colombo A, et al: Restenosis rate after percutaneous transluminal coronary angioplasty: a literature overview. *J Invasive Cardiol* 1991; 3:214.
105. Shah PK, Amin J: Low high density lipoprotein level is associated with increased restenosis rate after coronary angioplasty. *Circulation* 1992; 85:1279.
106. Califf RM, Willerson JT: Percutaneous transluminal coronary angioplasty: prevention of occlusion and restenosis, in Fuster V, Verstraete M (eds): *Thrombosis in Cardiovascular Disorders*. Philadelphia, WB Saunders, 1992; p 389.
107. Berger PB, Bell MR, Holmes DR Jr, et al: Effect of restenosis after an earlier angioplasty at another coronary site on the frequency of restenosis after a subsequent coronary angioplasty. *Am J Cardiol* 1992; 69:1096.
108. Gibson CM, Kuntz RE, Nobuyoshi M, et al: Lesion-to-lesion independence of restenosis after treatment by conventional angioplasty, stenting, or directional atherectomy: validation of lesion-based restenosis analysis. *Circulation* 1993; 87:1123.
109. Hermans WR, Rensing BJ, Strauss BH, Serruys PW: Prevention of restenosis after percutaneous transluminal coronary angioplasty: the search for a magic bullet. *Am Heart J* 1991; 122:171.
110. Ferns GA, Raines EW, Sprugel KH, et al: Inhibition of neointimal smooth muscle accumulation after angioplasty by an antibody to PDGF. *Science* 1991; 253:1129.
111. Repine CJ, Hirschfeld JW, MacDonald RG, et al: A controlled trial of corticosteroid to prevent restenosis after angioplasty. *Circulation* 1990; 81:1752.
112. Jonasson L, Holm J, Hannsson GK: Cyclosporin A inhibits smooth muscle proliferation in the vascular response to injury. *Proc Natl Acad Sci U S A* 1988; 85:2303.
113. Epstein SE, Speir E, Ungar EF, et al: The basis of molecular strategies for treating coronary restenosis after angioplasty. *J Am Coll Cardiol* 1994; 23:1278.
114. Speir E, Epstein SG: Inhibition of smooth muscle cell proliferation by an antisense oligodeoxynucleotide targeting the messenger RNA encoding proliferating cell nuclear antigen. *Circulation* 1992; 86:538.
115. Simons M, Edelman ER, DeKeyser JL, et al: Antisense C-myb oligonucleotides inhibit intimal arterial smooth muscle cell accumulation in vivo. *Nature* 1992; 359:67.
116. Zhu N, Liggitt D, Liu Y, et al: Systemic gene expression after intravenous DNA delivery into adult mice. *Science* 1993; 261:209.
117. Geary RL, Lynch CM, Vergel S, et al: Human gene expression in baboons using vascular grafts seeded with retrovirally transduced smooth muscle cell [abstract]. *Circulation* 1993; 88 (suppl I):I-81.
118. Ohman EM, Califf RM, Lee KL, et al: Restenosis after angioplasty: overview of clinical trials using aspirin and omega-3 fatty acids [abstract]. *J Am Coll Cardiol* 1990; 15(suppl A):88A.
119. Stack JD, Pinkerton CA, Van Tassel J, et al: Can oral fish oil supplement minimize restenosis after percutaneous transluminal coronary angioplasty? [abstract]. *J Am Coll Cardiol* 1989; 9: (suppl 2):69A.
120. Reis GJ, Boucher TM, Sipperly ME, et al: Randomised trial of fish oil for prevention of restenosis after coronary angioplasty. *Lancet* 1989; ii:177.
121. Milner MR, Gallino RA, Leffingwell A, et al: Usefulness of fish oil supplements in preventing clinical evidence of restenosis after percutaneous transluminal coronary angioplasty. *Am J Cardiol* 1989; 64:394.
122. Dehmer GJ, Popma JJ, Van den Berg EK, et al: Reduction in the rate of early restenosis after coronary angioplasty by a diet supplemented with N-3 fatty acid. *N Engl J Med* 1988; 319:733.

123. Grigg LE, Kay TWA, Valentine PA, et al: Determinants of restenosis and lack of effect of dietary supplementation with eicosapentanoic acid on the incidence of coronary artery restenosis after angioplasty. *J Am Coll Cardiol* 1989; 13:665.
124. Sahni R, Maniet AR, Voci G, Banba VS: Prevention of restenosis by lovastatin after successful coronary angioplasty. *Am Heart J* 1991; 121:1600.
125. Beigel J, Zafrir N, Teplitsky M, et al: The effect of lovastatin on early restenosis. *J Clin Pharmacol* 1995; 36:599.
126. Hollman J, Konrad K, Raymond R, et al: Lipid lowering for prevention of recurrent stenosis following coronary angioplasty [abstract]. *Circulation* 1989; 80(suppl II):II-65.
127. Weintraub WB, Boccuzzi SJ, Brown CL, et al: Background and method for the lovastatin-restenosis trial after percutaneous transluminal coronary angioplasty. *Am J Cardiol* 1992; 70:293.
128. Topol EJ: Prevention of cardiovascular ischemic complications with new platelet glycoprotein IIb/IIIa inhibitors. *Am Heart J* 1995; 130:666.
129. The EPIC Investigators: Use of a monoclonal antibody directed against the platelet glycoprotein IIb/IIIa receptor in high-risk coronary angioplasty. *N Engl J Med* 1994; 330:956.
130. Aguirre FV, Topol EJ, Ferguson JJ, et al, and the EPIC investigators: Bleeding complications with the chimeric antibody to platelet glycoprotein IIb/IIIa integrin in patients undergoing percutaneous coronary intervention. *Circulation* 1995; 91:2882.
131. Moliterno DJ, Califf RM, Aguirre FV, et al: Effect of platelet glycoprotein IIb/IIIa integrin blockade on activated clotting time during percutaneous transluminal coronary angioplasty or directional atherectomy. Evaluation of c7E3 Fab in the Prevention of Ischemic Complications (EPIC) Trial. *Am J Cardiol* 1995; 75:559.
132. Anderson HV, Kirkeeide RL, Krishnaswami A, et al: Cyclic flow variations after coronary angioplasty in humans: clinical and angiographic characteristics and elimination with 7E3 monoclonal antiplatelet antibody. *J Am Coll Cardiol* 1994; 23:1031.
133. Eidt JR, Ashton J, Golino P, et al: Thromboxane A_2 and serotonin mediate coronary blood flow reductions in unsedated dogs. *Am J Physiol* 1989; 257:H873.
134. Anderson HV, Yao SK, Murphree SS, et al: Cyclic coronary artery flow in dogs after coronary angioplasty. *Coron Artery Dis* 1990; 1:717.
135. Smith JF, Hanley HG, Sheridan FM: Percutaneous interventions for ischemic heart disease. *J La State Med Soc* 1995; 147:223.
136. Baim DS: Assessing new techniques in coronary angioplasty. *Cleve Clin J Med* 1992; 59:142.
137. Nath FC, Muller DW, Ellis SG, et al: Thrombosis of a flexible coil coronary stent: frequency, predictors and clinical outcome. *J Am Coll Cardiol* 1993; 21:622.
138. Van Belle E, McFadden EP, Lablanche JM, et al: Two-pronged antiplatelet therapy with aspirin and ticlopidine without systemic anticoagulation: an alternative therapeutic strategy after bailout stent implantation. *Coron Artery Dis* 1995; 6:341.
139. Colombo A, Hall P, Nakamura S, et al: Intracoronary stenting without anticoagulation accomplished with intravascular ultrasound guidance *Circulation* 1995; 91:1676. [Comments in *Circulation* 1995; 91:1891.]
140. Stratienko AA, Zhu D, Lambert CR, et al: Improved thromboresistance of heparin coated Palmaz-Schatz coronary stents in an animal model [abstract]. *Circulation* 1993; 88:I–596.
141. Serruys PW, de Jaegere P, Kiemeneij F, and the BENESTENT Study Group: A comparison of balloon expandable stent implantation with balloon angioplasty in patients with coronary artery disease. *N Engl J Med* 1994; 331:489.
142. Mohiaddin RH, Roberts RH, Underwood R, Rothman M: Localization of a misplaced coronary artery stent by magnetic resonance imaging. *Clin Cardiol* 1995; 18:175.
143. Wong SC, Franklin MD, Teirstein PS, et al: Stenting in acute myocardial infarction secondary to delayed vessel closure following balloon angioplasty. *J Invasive Cardiol* 1992; 4:331.
144. Wong PHC, Wong CM: Intracoronary stenting in acute myocardial infarction. *Cathet Cardiovasc Diagn* 1994; 33:39.
145. Cannon AD, Roubin GS, Macander PR, Agarwal SK: Intracoronary stenting as an adjunct to angioplasty in acute myocardial infarction. *J Invasive Cardiol* 1991; 3:255.
146. Ahmad T, Webb JG, Carere RR, Dodek A: Coronary stenting for acute myocardial infarction. *Am J Cardiol* 1995; 76:77.
147. Arbustini E, De Servi S, Boscarini M, et al: Diagnostic and research potential of directional atherectomy [in Italian]. *Cardiologia* 1994; 39:65.
148. Popma JJ, Mintz GS, Satler LF, et al: Clinical and angiographic outcome after directional coronary atherectomy: a qualitative and quantitative analysis using coronary arteriography and intravascular ultrasound. *Am J Cardiol* 1993; 72:55E.
149. Cowley MJ, Whitlow PL, Baim DS, et al: Directional coronary atherectomy of saphenous vein graft narrowings: multicenter investigational experience. *Am J Cardiol* 1993; 72:30E.
150. Safian RD, May MA, Lichtenberg A, Schreiber TL, et al: Detailed clinical and angiographic analysis of transluminal extraction coronary atherectomy for complex lesions in native coronary arteries. *J Am Coll Cardiol* 1995; 25:848.
151. Boehrer JD, Ellis SG, Pieper K, et al: Directional atherectomy versus balloon angioplasty for coronary ostial and nonostial left anterior descending coronary artery lesions: results from a randomized multicenter trial. The CAVEAT-I investigators. Coronary Angioplasty Versus Excisional Atherectomy Trial. *J Am Coll Cardiol* 1995; 25:1380.
152. Elliott JM, Berdan LG, Holmes DR, et al: One-year follow-up in the Coronary Angioplasty Versus Excisional Atherectomy Trial (CAVEAT I). *Circulation* 1995; 91:2158.
153. Fishman RF, Kuntz RE, Carrozza JP Jr, et al: Acute and long-term results of coronary stents and atherectomy in women and the elderly. *Coron Artery Dis* 1995; 6:159.
154. Ellis SG, Popma JJ, Buchbinder M, et al: Relation of clinical presentation, stenosis morphology, and operator technique to the procedural results of rotational atherectomy and rotational atherectomy-facilitated angioplasty. *Circulation* 1994; 89:882.
155. Metzger JP, LeFeuvre C, Batisse JP, Vacheron A: New techniques of interventional cardiology. *Press Medicale* 1995; 24:537.
156. MacIsaac AI, Bass TA, Buchbinder M, et al: High speed rotational atherectomy: outcome in calcified and noncalcified coronary artery lesions. *J Am Coll Cardiol* 1995; 26:731.
157. Detre KM, Baim D, Buchbinder M, et al: Baseline characteristics and therapeutic goals, in the New Approaches to Coronary Interventional registry. *Coron Artery Dis* 1993; 4:1013.
158. Teirstein PS: Radiation therapy, in Willerson JT, Cohn JN (eds): *Cardiovascular Medicine,* 2d ed. New York, Churchill Livingstone, 2000; p 827.

Chapter 21

Myocardial Revascularization with Cardiopulmonary Bypass

Y. Joseph Woo/Timothy J. Gardner

HISTORY

Surgery for human atherosclerotic coronary arterial disease began in 1935, when Beck attached a pedicled graft of pectoralis muscle to the heart in an attempt to provide a new blood supply.[1] In 1941, Beck reported constricting the coronary sinus, mechanically abrading the pericardium and epicardium, instilling asbestos and trichloracidic acid into the pericardium, and placing mediastinal fat onto the epicardial surface. In 1951, Vineberg described the implantation of the internal thoracic artery directly into the myocardium.[2] Although long-term patency of the graft was demonstrated later, the amount of blood flow and region of distribution were insignificant with this approach. In the mid-1950s, Murray reported experimental studies of internal thoracic artery–coronary artery anastomoses.[3] In 1953, Gibbon successfully used cardiopulmonary bypass clinically for intracardiac surgery.[4] In the late 1950s, Bailey described direct coronary endarterectomies.[5] In 1961, Senning described a patch angioplasty of a stenotic coronary artery.[6] In 1962, Sohns and Shirey reported the development of coronary angiography, which would subsequently permit guided interventions for distinct coronary stenoses.[7]

Credit for performing the first coronary artery bypass procedure in humans is given to several different surgeons. In 1958, Longmire described a patient in which a coronary endarterectomy was attempted, but the coronary artery disintegrated. In a desperate attempt to reconstruct the coronary, the internal thoracic artery was harvested and anastomosed to the coronary artery.[8] In 1962, Sabiston reported the first aortocoronary bypass, but this patient died in the early postoperative period of a cerebrovascular accident.[9] Garrett and DeBakey are credited by some with performing the first successful aortocoronary bypass in 1964, although this was not reported until 1973.[10] In 1964, Kolesov in Leningrad performed the first planned anastomosis between the left internal thoracic artery and the left anterior descending artery.[11] In 1968, Favolaro reported the first large series of coronary artery bypass graft patients.[12] From the late 1960s and early 1970s, aortocoronary venous bypass grafting, together with internal thoracic artery to coronary artery bypass grafting, grew rapidly in popularity to become one of the most commonly performed major operations today. Likewise, alternative strategies for myocardial revascularization have propagated and exist across a wide spectrum of approaches ranging from variations on the standard operation with elimination of cardiopulmonary bypass, to extensive catheter-based angioplasty and stenting, and finally to laser and genetic endogenous revascularization.[13]

OPERATIVE INDICATIONS

The specific indications for coronary revascularization are covered in Chapter 19, and methods of percutaneous coronary interventions are described in Chapter 20. Globally, the indications for operative myocardial revascularization have been well delineated and can be viewed as specific anatomic criteria such as left main coronary artery disease, multivessel coronary disease, and double-vessel coronary disease with proximal left anterior descending artery involvement, and with or without physiological sequelae such as myocardial ischemia, myocardial infarction, and left ventricular dysfunction.[14–21] Furthermore, an additional subset includes patients undergoing other cardiovascular surgery with coronary artery disease that would otherwise not indicate operative revascularization. In general, only coronary arteries with significant (greater than 70%) stenoses are bypassed, because graft patency is otherwise severely limited by competitive native coronary flow.

PATIENT EVALUATION

A patient referred for myocardial revascularization should undergo a complete history and physical examination with particular attention focused upon identifying coexisting cardiovascular diseases, comorbid processes, and specific issues that may impact the technical aspects of surgery. Standard laboratory data evaluating chemistry, hematologic, and coagulation profiles should be reviewed. Blood bank studies are performed. Diagnostic studies, which consist primarily of coronary angiography, perfusion ischemia-viability studies, electrocardiograms, and echocardiography, are reviewed. Coronary arterial targets are identified and vascular conduits are chosen and assessed by appropriate studies. The timing of surgery is determined and the patient is pharmacologically and hemodynamically optimized. Once all data are obtained, risk stratification can be performed and the patient can provide fully informed consent.[22] The patient can then undergo standard preoperative preparation, which will vary by institution, surgeon, and anesthesiologist.

Specific Comorbidities

Although potential comorbid conditions for coronary artery bypass grafting abound, several specific disease processes should be excluded by history and physical examination and, if present, should be appropriately addressed in an attempt to facilitate safer myocardial revascularization. These conditions include advanced age, cerebrovascular disease, chronic obstructive pulmonary disease, diabetes mellitus, renal insufficiency, hepatic insufficiency, gastrointestinal hemorrhage, a hematologic or pharmacologically induced bleeding disorder, malignancy, HIV infection, prior surgery, radiation/chemotherapy, and likely postoperative debilitation that would require rehabilitation.[23,24]

In 1989, the Society of Thoracic Surgeons initiated a national database to evaluate coronary artery bypass graft and valvular surgery. To date, approximately 1.7 million patients have been registered, and the STS Database is now the largest cardiothoracic surgery outcome and quality improvement program in the world. A particularly useful feature is the ability to obtain immediate risk stratification for a given patient by simple online entry of clinical data. This database can be accessed at http://www.sts.org. Analysis of trends in preoperative risk factors reveals progressively increased severity of risk over the past decade.[25]

ANESTHESIA

The anesthetic management for cardiac surgical patients is detailed in Chapter 9. There exists an ongoing controversy regarding the extent of monitoring required or deemed appropriate for myocardial revascularization procedures performed with cardiopulmonary bypass. Centers vary in their use of pulmonary artery monitoring catheters, oximetric continuous cardiac output monitors, and transesophageal echocardiography. Perioperative antibiotic administration should be designed to prevent primarily gram-positive but also gram-negative infections.[26]

BLOOD CONSERVATION

Although homologous blood products are multiply screened and considered extremely safe in the current era, the remote risk of infection still exists. Blood product administration does increase the risk of multiorgan dysfunction, particularly that of the lungs, and transfusion is costly. Thus, strategies for the conservation of blood abound. These will often include autologous as well as donor-directed blood donation.[27] However, these strategies tend to be less utilized among cardiac surgical patients, particularly autologous donation, where compromised oxygen carrying capacity may exacerbate myocardial ischemia or hemodynamic instability. Preoperative multivitamins, iron, and erythropoietin have been used among patients in an effort to increase red cell mass.[28,29]Intraoperative prebypass hemodilution and blood storage as well as platelet harvest devices have been utilized. Complicated formulas for heparin and protamine dosing have also been used in an attempt to reduce blood loss.[30] Pharmacologic measures with antifibrinolytics such as epsilon-aminocaproic acid and aprotinin are utilized.[31,32] Although of some theoretical concern, aprotinin does not appear to increase the risk of early thrombosis in patients who have primary coronary artery bypass grafts.[33] Also of some potential value are DDAVP and vitamin K.[34] During surgery, the use of a cell saver and a cardiotomy suction device helps to conserve blood, and autotransfusion systems can be utilized postoperatively. Total creatine kinase and lactate dehydrogenase enzyme levels may be elevated because of the hemolysis associated with the use of such systems, and care must be taken in the interpretation of these values.[35] There is also ongoing active research in artificial blood substitute development. These tend to be categorized into two types: liquid compounds with increased oxygen solubility and mammalian hemoglobin derivatives. All of the above issues become particularly relevant when choosing to operate on patients who, for religious or other reasons, refuse the administration of blood products.

INCISIONS

The standard operative approach for coronary revascularization is the median sternotomy, which provides the greatest access to the heart and great vessels. Alternative incisions include partial sternotomy as well as a right or left thoracotomy approach, which can be used to address coronary targets on specific sides. Incisions other than the median sternotomy often require femoral arterial and/or venous access for cardiopulmonary bypass.

CONDUITS

The choice of conduit for coronary artery bypass grafting is influenced by patient age, medical history, target vessels, conduit availability, and surgeon preference. Of particular note, a pedicled arterial graft to a high-outflow system has been clearly shown to significantly improve early and late postoperative survival, and thus should be utilized whenever possible.[36,37] Specific conduits, their evaluation, and their preparation are described in the following sections.

Internal Thoracic Artery

CHARACTERISTICS

The internal thoracic artery possesses distinct molecular and cellular characteristics that contribute to its unique resistance to atherosclerosis and extremely high long-term patency rates. Structurally, there is no vaso vasorum. There is a dense, nonfenestrated, intact internal elastic lamina that inhibits cellular migration and subsequent initiation of hyperplasia. The ITA possesses a thin medial layer with few smooth muscle cells, which provides little vasoreactivity. Even among these few smooth muscle cells, there exist distinct populations with varying biochemical functions and ultrastructural features.[38,39] Saphenous vein smooth muscle cells exhibit markedly enhanced proliferation in response to platelet-derived growth factor as compared with internal thoracic artery smooth muscle cells.[40] Pulsatile mechanical stretch is also a potent mitogen for saphenous vein but not for internal thoracic artery smooth muscle cells.[41] The vasoactivity of the internal thoracic artery has also been well characterized. The internal thoracic artery produces significantly more prostacyclin, a vasodilator and platelet inhibitor, than does the saphenous vein.[42] The potent vasodilator nitric oxide is produced in markedly higher quantities by internal thoracic artery endothelium compared to that of saphenous vein.[41,43] In studies of the human internal thoracic artery, nitric oxide also antagonizes the potent vasocontrictive effects of endogenous endothelin-1.[44] The internal thoracic artery vasodilates in response to milrinone and does not vasoconstrict in response to norepinephrine.[45] Nitroglycerin causes vasodilation in the internal thoracic artery but not in saphenous vein.[46] Conduit resistance to harvest injury may also vary. Scanning electron microscopy of representative sections of internal thoracic artery and saphenous vein conduits at the time of anastomosis revealed large thrombogenic intimal defects with exposed collagen fibrils in veins and essentially no endothelial injury in arteries.[47] Lipid and glycosaminoglycan composition of internal thoracic artery compared to saphenous vein suggests greater atherogenecity

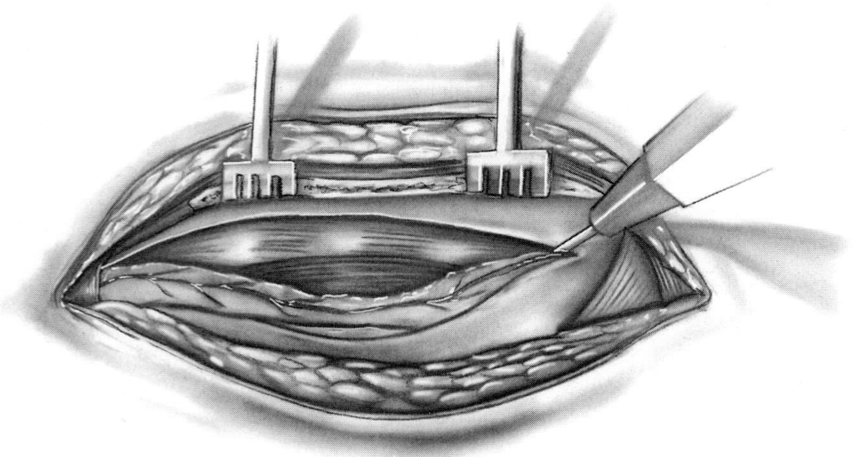

FIGURE 21–1 Left internal thoracic artery harvest. An asymmetric retractor is used to elevate the left hemisternum. The parietal pleura and endothoracic fascia medial and lateral to the internal thoracic artery and accompanying veins are incised with the electrocautery and then, using a combination of blunt and electrocautery dissection, the internal thoracic artery pedicle is separated from the chest wall. Metal clips are used to secure the larger branches. The pedicle can be harvested from the level of the subclavian vein down to the bifurcation of the superior epigastric and musculophrenic arteries. After systemic heparinization, the pedicle is divided distally and flow is assessed.

in saphenous vein.[48] Finally, the pedicled internal thoracic artery can exhibit flow adaptation over time and is often observed to be larger when visualized on late postoperative angiograms.

HARVEST TECHNIQUE

Because the internal thoracic artery is almost always of adequate caliber and provides adequate flow, it is rarely evaluated preoperatively. Occasionally, an internal thoracic artery is imaged at the time of cardiac catheterization. The incidence of subclavian artery or internal thoracic artery ostial stenosis is estimated to be well under 5% in patients undergoing revascularization. The preparation of the internal thoracic artery begins immediately after median sternotomy (Fig. 21-1). A RULTract device or asymmetric sternal retractor is placed to elevate the hemisternum. Care should be taken not to exert excessive traction on the hemisternum as this may cause brachial plexus injury, although this is more commonly a result of overly wide distraction with the sternal retractor.[49] The table is turned away from the surgeon and raised to an appropriate level. The tidal volume on the mechanical ventilator is decreased and the pleural space is opened widely. A moistened laparotomy pad can be placed onto the surface of the lung to keep the lung away from the field of dissection. Alternatively, some surgeons prefer not to enter the pleural space and simply push the parietal pleura away from the endothoracic fascia, utilizing the pleura itself to retract the lung away from the operative field.

Dissection can be initiated at any point along the course of the internal thoracic artery. One technique is to incise the fascia with electrocautery at the most superior aspect of the artery near the level of the subclavian vein. Downward traction on the edge of the fascia together with a combination of cold dissection and electrocautery permits separation of the arterial-venous pedicle from the anterior chest wall. Depending upon size, arterial and venous branches to the chest wall are electrocauterized or secured with metal clips. Dissection is carried out in this manner along the entire course of the artery. Care must be taken not to grasp the artery. Gentle retraction against the artery is safe, but grasping the edge of the pedicle fascia, or even the internal thoracic vein, is preferable. Pulsations within the artery can often be observed visually or manually palpated. The absence of these pulsations does not necessarily correlate with poor internal thoracic artery flow at the time of division. When the majority of the internal thoracic artery is freely dissected, the patient is systemically heparinized. Dissection can then be completed and the distal internal thoracic artery can be divided. At this time, flow can also be evaluated. What may appear to be suboptimal flow in an internal thoracic artery at the time of division is often due to spasm from manipulation and usually improves in a period of time with the topical administration of papaverine solution. The pedicle is examined for hemostasis and is usually wrapped in a papaverine sponge or sprayed with a papaverine solution. Some surgeons directly infuse the distal internal thoracic artery with papaverine solution, but this may cause a frank dissection and studies suggest endothelial and medial injury may result from direct luminal exposure to concentrated papaverine.[50–52]

Preparation of the internal thoracic artery for distal anastomosis can be performed at any convenient time. Options include preparation (1) immediately after harvest, (2) upon identification of likely distal target site, (3) during cardioplegia administration, or (4) after target arteriotomy. The primary advantage of earlier preparation is a small decrement in bypass and cross-clamp time. The advantage of later preparation is the ability to comfortably shorten the conduit and thus utilize a region of larger diameter. To prepare the internal thoracic artery for anastomosis, the adjacent veins and soft tissue are gently dissected away from the artery at the level of planned division. The artery is divided, flow is assessed, and the distal end is spatulated with a fine scissor (Fig. 21-2).

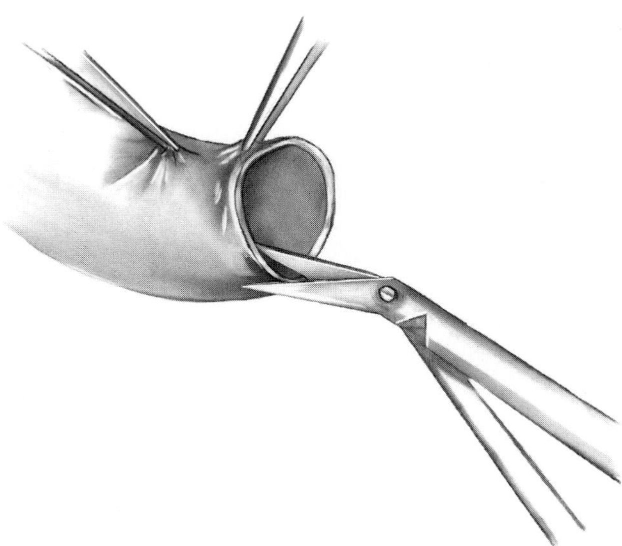

FIGURE 21–2 Preparation of the distal internal thoracic artery for anastomosis. The internal thoracic artery is freed of its adjacent venous structures and areolar tissue and incised with fine scissors along the fascial aspect of the artery for a distance of approximately 5 to 10 mm to create a hood for distal anastomosis. The artery is carefully inspected for any evidence of injury.

When an internal thoracic artery intended for use as a pedicled graft is injured during harvesting, it can often be used as a free graft, depending upon the location of the injury and the location of the intended anastomotic target. Care must be taken with dissection of internal thoracic artery grafts at the superior aspect as the phrenic nerve comes in close proximity to the ITA bilaterally. When a pedicled internal thoracic artery graft is found to be of insufficient length to provide a tension-free anastomosis, the conduit can be lengthened significantly by skeletonizing short segments of the artery, dividing the fascia, muscle, and accompanying veins. One to 1.5 cm of additional length can often be obtained with each region of skeletonization. Harvest of the internal thoracic artery by complete skeletonization is now less commonly practiced. Conflicting data exist regarding whether this technique results in decreased rates of long-term patency.[53] Advantages include increased length, improved ability to identify spasm, facilitation of sequential anastomoses, and increased preservation of sternal blood supply. Clear disadvantages are increased harvest time, spasm, and likelihood of injury.

BILATERAL ITA

A moderate increase in long-term survival and decrease in ischemic events after coronary artery bypass grafting with the use of two versus one pedicled internal thoracic artery grafts have been demonstrated.[54–59] This benefit may not exist in all populations[60] and may not be present in females.[61] The use of bilateral internal thoracic arteries in nondiabetics has been shown to minimally increase the risk of sternal wound complications, particularly in obese patients.[62,63] In diabetics, the risk is significantly increased with the use of bilateral internal thoracic arteries.[64–66] Harvest of the internal thoracic artery results in subtle transient changes in chest wall mechanics that resemble restrictive lung disease, possibly due to pain from asymmetric retraction.[67] Bilateral internal thoracic artery utilization is not recommended in patients with chronic obstructive pulmonary disease. [68]

When bilateral internal thoracic arteries are being harvested, a common practice is to dissect the majority of the left internal thoracic artery, leaving several terminal branches intact along the distal artery. The right internal thoracic artery is then dissected completely and after the administration of systemic heparin, the right internal thoracic artery is divided, followed by completion of the dissection of the left internal thoracic artery and division.

By far the most common scenario of the internal thoracic artery as a conduit is that of a pedicled LITA anastomosed to the left anterior descending artery. Other scenarios include a pedicled right internal thoracic artery to the right coronary artery or branch thereof, a pedicled RITA brought anterior to the aorta or posteriorly through the transverse sinus to anastomose to a circumflex marginal, a pedicled RITA brought anteriorly to supply the LAD with the pedicled LITA used to supply the circumflex marginal, and finally, the RITA used as a free graft.[68–70] It appears that the choice of the target vessel, in regards to outflow, has greater influence on long-term patency than the choice of which internal thoracic artery is used.[71] Graft placement through the transverse sinus may subject the conduit to unrecognized tension and distortion and also obscure bleeding along the pedicle. Scenarios that place a pedicled RITA anteriorly across the mediastinum impose an extremely high risk of conduit injury during future reoperative surgery.

Radial Artery

CHARACTERISTICS

The use of a radial artery as a conduit for coronary artery bypass grafting was first described by Carpentier in 1973.[72] Early patency rates were poor and interest in the use of this conduit faded. The radial artery possesses a pronounced medial layer and is highly vasoreactive.[73,74] Cosmetic concerns have also been cited as a deterrent for radial artery usage. There has been a resurgence in the popularity of the use of the radial artery graft.[75] This has been attributed to enhanced short- to mid-term radial artery patency rates, the observation of improved outcomes with use of two arterial grafts, and interest in total arterial revascularization.[76,77] Bilateral radial artery grafting has been utilized as an effective means of facilitating all arterial revascularization.[78] Improved patency rates may be due to a variety of factors, which include greater utilization of harvesting techniques that do not skeletonize the radial artery but rather harvest essentially an arteriovenous island of tissue, widespread application of calcium channel blockade or nitrates to counter spasm, and other pharmacologic manipulation such as the use lipid-lowering agents to retard graft atherosclerosis.[79,80] Selection of left-sided target vessels with high-grade proximal stenoses and generous outflow improves radial graft patency rates.[81,82] The evaluation of the suitability of the radial artery as a conduit for grafting consists usually of noninvasive duplex ultrasonography, and/or clinical examination with the Allen's test or a variant thereof utilizing a pulse oximeter.[83] The radial artery from the nondominant arm is used unless proven unsatisfactory by the above tests, in which case the dominant arm radial artery can be used.

HARVEST TECHNIQUE

In the operating room, the arm is prepped circumferentially, the hand is wrapped sterilely, and the arm is placed on an arm board at 90° from the long axis of the table. In approximately 90% of the population, harvesting radial artery from the nondominant arm means harvesting from the left arm, which will not interfere with simultaneous left internal thoracic artery harvesting. When radial artery harvesting contralateral to the internal thoracic artery harvest is required, this can often be accomplished with the radial artery harvest surgeon working next to the patient's head and approaching the artery from the superior aspect of the arm. A longitudinal, slightly curved skin incision is made over the course of the radial artery with particular attention to avoiding the lateral antebrachial cutaneous nerve. Injury to this nerve results in forearm numbness. The location of initiation of radial artery dissection varies among surgeons. The artery is usually dissected with adjacent tissue similar to that of internal thoracic artery harvest.[84] Particular attention is paid to avoiding injury to the superficial radial nerve, which is in close lateral proximity to the middle third of the radial artery (Fig. 21-3). Injury to this nerve results in dorsal thenar numbness. Paraesthesias and numbness occur transiently in 25% to 50% of patients undergoing radial artery harvest and persist in 5% to 10%.[85–87] After systemic heparinization, the radial artery is divided proximally and distally and removed with its adjoining venous and soft tissue island. It is usually stored in dilute heparin papaverine solution and can be flushed, depending upon surgeon preference. Hemostasis within the operative field is obtained and the arm is closed in multiple layers, and then abducted and secured to the table. The distal aspect of the excised radial artery is usually marked with a suture for proper identification. Very recently, endoscopic techniques of harvesting radial artery conduits have been reported.[88] Early short-term data suggest no decrement in graft patency.

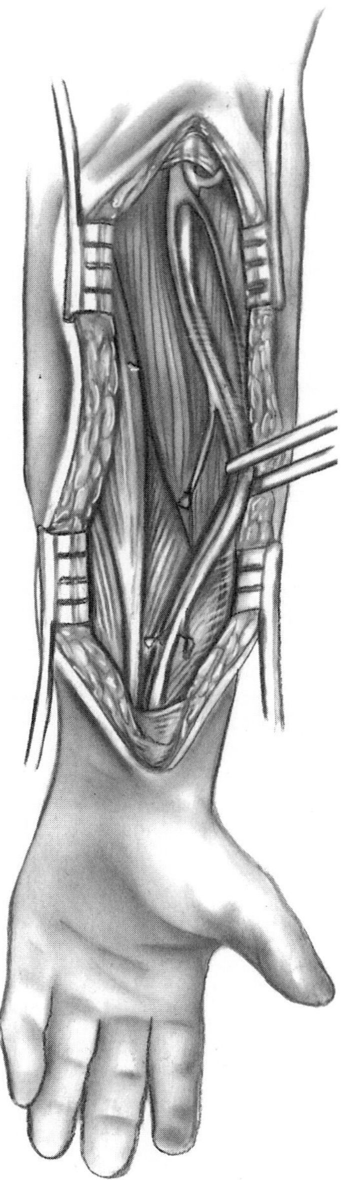

FIGURE 21–3 Left radial artery harvest. The radial artery is harvested with adjacent venous structures. Care is taken to avoid injury to the nearby superficial radial nerve. Dissection is carried from 1 cm below the ulnar radial bifurcation to the level of the wrist crease.

Gastroepiploic Artery

CHARACTERISTICS

The gastroepiploic artery was first described as a coronary artery bypass conduit in 1984 by Pym.[89] This pedicled conduit has primarily been used in reoperative scenarios in the absence of other suitable conduits.[90,91] It is now used more frequently as a secondary, tertiary, or quaternary arterial conduit in an attempt to provide all-arterial revascularization.[92–95] At present, the unclear benefits of third and fourth arterial grafts, the additional operative time required to harvest a gastroepiploic artery, and the involvement of an additional body cavity with potential abdominal complications limit the widespread use of this conduit. However, cellular and physiological studies of the gastroepiploic artery suggest near equivalent biological characteristics to the internal thoracic artery.[96–100]

Guidelines for preoperative assessment of the right gastroepiploic artery are not well delineated. Suspicion of preoperative mesenteric vascular insufficiency may warrant angiographic evaluation. Noninvasive duplex measurement of intra-abdominal vasculature is not always reliable and the role of other noninvasive imaging modalities, such as magnetic resonance imaging, has simply not been studied. Previous abdominal surgery may complicate conduit harvest. Prior gastric surgery, interventional radiology therapies directed towards this vessel, or documented mesenteric vascular insufficiency contraindicate the use of this vessel as a conduit.

HARVEST TECHNIQUE

The harvest technique entails nasogastric decompression and extension of the median sternotomy incision for a few centimeters to perform a limited upper midline laparotomy. The stomach is retracted into the field and the gastroepiploic artery is palpated to evaluate patency. The artery is dissected with its associated veins away from the surrounding gastrocolic omentum (Fig. 21-4). The thin-walled nature of this artery and the tendency for mesenteric vessels to retract into fat and bleed persistently warrant the extensive use of surgical clips to control branches. Alternately, the use of a harmonic scalpel has been advocated. Distally, the dissection is carried for the extent of the artery, which is usually two-thirds along the greater curvature of the stomach. Proximally, the dissection is carried to the duodenum, close to the origin of the gastroepiploic artery from the gastroduodenal artery.[101]

There are several options for the route of entry of the gastroepiploic artery from the abdomen into the pericardium.[102] The pedicle can be placed anterior or posterior to the stomach and duodenum. It can be placed anterior or posterior to the left lateral segment of the liver, and can traverse the peritoneal pericardial junction in a variety of locations. A route posterior to the stomach and duodenum decreases risk of conduit injury on future laparotomy, but increases the possibility of tension on the pedicle resulting from gastric distention. Placement anterior to the stomach and duodenum provides the opposite trade-off. The coronary target and size of the left lateral segment of the liver usually determine the route, with respect to the liver. Entry into the pericardium should be close to the target, yet still allow several

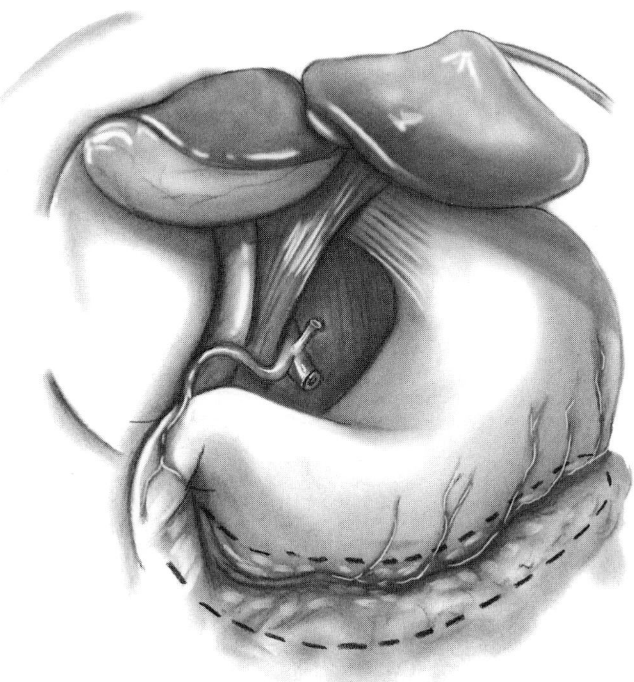

FIGURE 21–4 Right gastroepiploic artery harvest. Via upper midline laparotomy, the left lateral hepatic segment is retracted cephalad and the stomach is exposed. The right gastroepiploic artery is harvested from the stomach and greater omentum with the generous use of surgical clips. The artery is harvested from its most distal extent along the greater curvature of the stomach to the level of the pylorus. The artery can then be brought anterior or posterior to the stomach as well as anterior or posterior to the liver and subsequently through the diaphragm and into the pericardium.

centimeters of conduit to be placed inside the pericardium and loosely draped to provide a tension-free anastomosis and allow cardiac mobility.

Although the gastroepiploic artery is most commonly used to supply the right coronary artery system, it can be used for the left anterior descending and distal circumflex system, depending upon length of conduit. Although primarily used as a pedicled graft, the gastroepiploic artery can be used as a free graft in the setting of inability to reach a target vessel and lack of conduit or desire to use an additional arterial conduit.

Inferior Epigastric Artery

An infrequently used free arterial conduit is the inferior epigastric artery.[103,104] This artery exhibits favorable physiological vasoreactivity characteristics.[105,106] It is rather variable in its diameter, length, and location relative to the rectus muscle, and in ease of harvesting. A paramedian incision beginning below the umbilicus is used to approach the conduit. A midline incision can be used to harvest both inferior

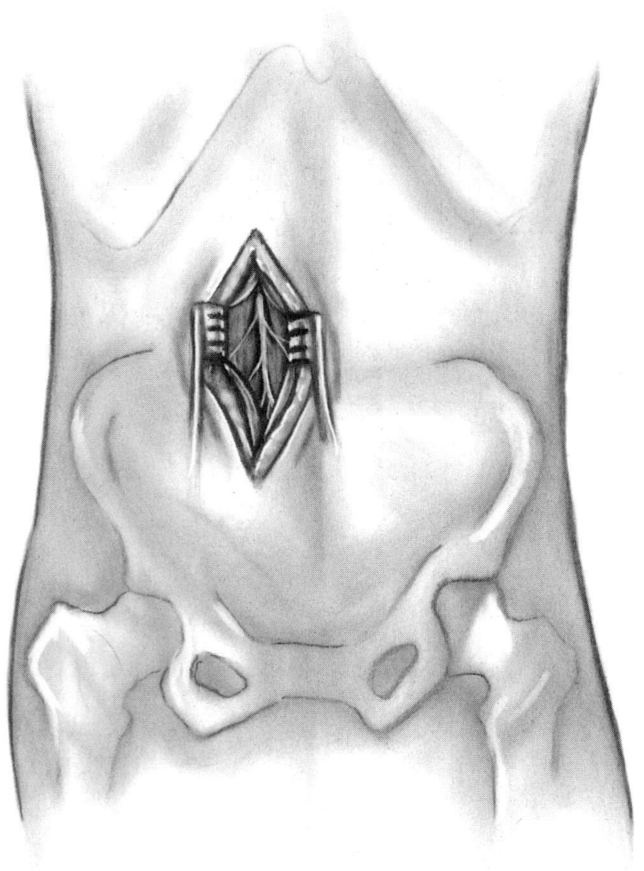

FIGURE 21–5 Epigastric artery harvest. The artery can be approached via a midline or paramedian skin incision with appropriate lateral or medial retraction of the rectus abdominus muscle, respectively. In a majority of cases, the inferior epigastric artery lies deep to the body of the rectus muscle. The dissection can be carried as cephalad as the costal margin and as caudad as the external iliac artery.

epigastric arteries. The rectus sheath is entered and the rectus abdominus muscle is carefully dissected and retracted medially, avoiding avulsion of small vascular branches off the inferior epigastric vessels. The artery, together with its accompanying veins and a small amount of soft tissue, is dissected away from the rectus anteriorly and the peritoneum and pre-peritoneal fat posteriorly (Fig. 21-5). The artery is usually transected just distal to its takeoff from the external iliac artery and divided as far superiorly as technically feasible. It is then treated like a radial artery conduit, in terms of preparation.

Alternative Arterial Conduits

Various other arterial conduits have been anecdotally reported. These include the ulnar, left gastric, splenic, thoracodorsal, and lateral femoral circumflex arteries.[107–111]

Greater Saphenous Vein

CHARACTERISTICS

Greater saphenous vein continues to be the primary conduit for coronary artery bypass grafting in conjunction with a pedicled left internal thoracic artery. Greater saphenous vein has many advantages as a conduit, including availability, accessibility, ease of harvest, reliability, resistance to spasm, and versatility. There are limitations to the greater saphenous vein, including patency rates, size mismatch in either direction, inadequate length, varicosity, sclerosis, and leg healing issues, particularly in patients with peripheral vascular disease. Venous conduit also exhibits poor compliance after arterialization and is prone to progressive atherosclerosis. Ultrasonographic localization and evaluation can be employed when the presence or adequacy of greater saphenous venous conduit is uncertain given specific findings in the history or physical examination.

HARVEST TECHNIQUE

Methods of harvesting the greater saphenous vein vary depending upon the length of segment required. In general, anterior coronary targets require 10 to 15 cm of conduit, lateral targets require 15 cm, and posterior targets require 20 cm. The initiation of vein harvest begins with a skin incision to localize and identify the vein. Then, depending upon whether a completely open, bridged, or endoscopic technique is utilized, the initial skin incision is either extended or additional skin incisions are made (Fig. 21-6). Dissection can be started either in the upper thigh, above the knee, or at the ankle. Identification of the greater saphenous vein is easiest in the ankle, just above the medial malleolus. Patients with peripheral vascular disease and compromised distal arterial blood flow should undergo vein harvest initiated in the thigh. In the lower leg, the saphenous nerve lies in close proximity to the greater saphenous vein and should be preserved. Injury can result in localized numbness or hyperesthesia. When using a totally open technique, the tissue surrounding the vein is dissected away from the vein. All branches are directly ligated in situ and the vein is divided proximally and distally. When using bridged or endoscopic techniques, branches are divided in situ and ligated once the vein is explanted. Once harvested, the vein is cannulated, gently pressurized to identify and ligate additional previously unidentified branches, marked, and stored in heparin solution. Patency rates may be related to endothelial damage induced during harvest and preparation.[112–114] Procurement techniques with minimal vein contact or harvest of adjacent tissue have been advocated.[115,116]

Increasingly popular techniques of endoscopic vein harvest are currently being clinically employed. Initial studies suggest that vein graft patency is equal to that of open techniques and wound complication rates are significantly

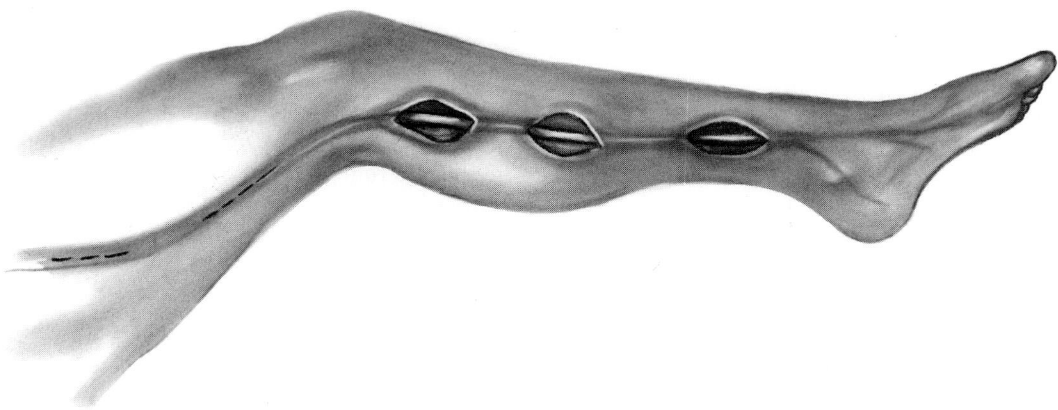

FIGURE 21–6 Left greater saphenous vein harvest. The figure demonstrates a technique of multiple skin bridges between which the left greater saphenous vein has been identified and dissected free of surrounding tissue. With proper retraction and the saphenous vein within the tunnels beneath the skin, bridges can be easily dissected free.

decreased.[117–122] Scanning electron microscopy reveals no difference in degree of endothelial injury.[123]

Lesser Saphenous Vein

This alternative venous conduit can be harvested in a supine position, either by flexing the hip and medially rotating the thigh and knee, thus providing a lateral approach, or by flexing the hip and lifting the leg straight up and providing an inferior approach. A skin incision is usually started midway between the Achilles tendon and the lateral malleolus (Fig. 21-7). Dissection is carried proximally along the leg. Attention should be paid to avoid injuring the sural nerve. The vein is otherwise managed similarly to the greater saphenous vein.

Cephalic Vein

The patency rate of cephalic vein used for aortocoronary bypass is significantly lower than that of other venous and arterial conduits, and thus should be considered essentially a conduit of last resort.[124,125] Vein from the arm and forearm can be used. The arm is prepared and positioned as during radial artery harvest. Incisions are placed along the superior aspect of the either the arm or forearm. The vein is identified and harvested similarly to the greater saphenous

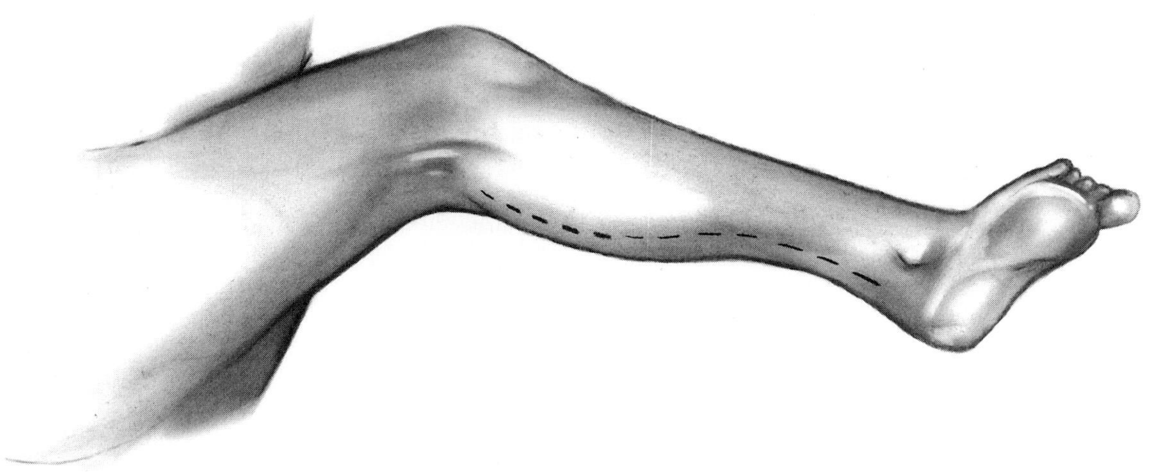

FIGURE 21–7 Right lesser saphenous vein harvest. The figure demonstrates the location of the skin incision for harvest of the right lesser saphenous vein. The lesser saphenous vein can be found posterior to the lateral maleolus and followed cephalad into the popliteal fossa.

vein. Notably, the cephalic vein is relatively thin-walled in comparison to the greater saphenous vein and extra care should be taken during harvest. The cephalic vein is also predisposed to aneurysmal dilatation.

Nonautogenous Conduits

Alternative nonautogenous vascular conduits have been used for coronary artery bypass grafting. These include cryopreserved human saphenous vein allograft, autologous endothelialized vein allograft, processed bovine sacral artery, and various synthetic conduits, such as polytetrafluoroethylene (PTFE).[126–129] Such conduits exhibit extremely low short-term patency rates, and are generally not considered acceptable coronary conduits. Research in tissue engineering approaches such as endothelializing synthetic conduits is being actively pursued.

CARDIOPULMONARY BYPASS

Myocardial revascularization without cardiopulmonary bypass is detailed in Chapter 22. In patients undergoing myocardial revascularization with cardiopulmonary bypass, systemic anticoagulation is initiated prior to cannulation, usually prior to division of the internal thoracic artery conduit. Direct epiaortic ultrasound can be utilized to augment the accuracy of manual palpation of the aorta in identification of suitable cannulation and cross-clamping sites.[130,131] In highly diseased aortas, alternative cannulation sites include femoral and subclavian arteries. Ideally, a cross-clamp site should still be identified.[132,133] Otherwise one can employ techniques such as cold fibrillatory, vented arrest or ascending aortic graft replacement with deep hypothermic circulatory arrest. These methods have essentially been supplanted by off-pump coronary artery bypass grafting using only pedicled arterial conduits, basing proximal inflow off pedicled conduits, brachiocephalic vessels, or (rarely) an uninvolved proximal native coronary artery, or, as will be described later, sutureless, clampless proximal connector devices.[134]

The distal ascending aorta is usually chosen as the site of cannulation. This is usually around the level of the superior pericardial reflection. Two partial-thickness concentric purse-string sutures using 3-0 Tevdek suture are placed in the aorta. Arterial blood pressure should be well controlled during aortic cannulation to avoid the risk of aortic dissection. The aortic adventitia within the purse strings just superior to the aortotomy is grasped with a forceps and using a #11 blade, an aortotomy is created. Bleeding is easily controlled with slight inferior traction of the forceps on the adventitia. An appropriately sized aortic cannula is then inserted into the ascending aorta. If this is not easily accomplished, an aortotomy dilator will facilitate cannulation. Once the aortic cannula is inserted and properly positioned, the purse strings are tightened and the cannula is secured to the skin at an appropriate level. The cannula is then de-aired and connected to the pump tubing.

Attention is then directed to venous cannulation. For standard coronary artery bypass grafting, a two-stage venous cannula inserted in the right atrial appendage is sufficient. A 2-0 Tevdek purse-string suture is placed around the right atrial appendage. A partial occlusion clamp is placed on the right atrial appendage at the level of the purse-string suture. An atriotomy is made with scissors at the tip of the appendage. This incision can then be extended superiorly and inferiorly to a size appropriate for the venous cannula. Small bridging fibers of muscle are divided with scissors to permit easy entry of the cannula. Both edges of the atrial appendage are grasped, the clamp is removed, and the venous cannula is inserted to an appropriate level with the tip in the inferior vena cava. A retrograde coronary sinus cardioplegia catheter is not routinely used, although use in patients with left main disease or severe proximal multivessel disease may be helpful. An aortic root cardioplegia and venting cannula can then be placed, usually at the site of a planned proximal anastomosis. A mattress 4-0 polypropylene pledgeted suture is placed in the ascending aorta and a needle-bearing catheter is placed in the ascending aorta and connected to the cardioplegia line and vent line. The heart is now properly cannulated for cardiopulmonary bypass. All conduits are reinspected and the distal portions can be appropriately prepared for anastomoses.

Prior to initiating bypass, it is helpful to attempt to localize the target vessels, which are often easier to identify when fully distended in their native state. After communication with the anesthesiologist and perfusionist, cardiopulmonary bypass is initiated.

Patients with known mild-to-moderate aortic insufficiency that is not to be surgically addressed may benefit from the placement of a left ventricular venting catheter via the right superior pulmonary vein. This is usually performed immediately after the initiation of cardiopulmonary bypass on a full heart to avoid air entrainment. Systemic cooling can now be initiated, the exact temperature of which is highly variable and surgeon dependent. A systemic temperature of 32 to 34°C is usually sufficient for a standard coronary artery bypass graft procedure. A myocardial temperature probe can now be placed into the interventricular septum, if desired.[135] The ascending aorta is then cross-clamped at the appropriate time, usually upon initiation of ventricular fibrillation or significant bradycardia. Antegrade cardioplegia is then delivered via the aortic root cannula, taking care to confirm an adequate root pressure by palpation and a soft, nondistended left ventricle. Cessation of surface mechanical activity, an isoelectric EKG, and a septal temperature less than 10°C confirm an adequate arrest. There are significant differences on specific cardioplegic composition, quantities, regimens, and delivery techniques. Despite different perioperative outcome parameters attributable to cardioplegia strategy, overall

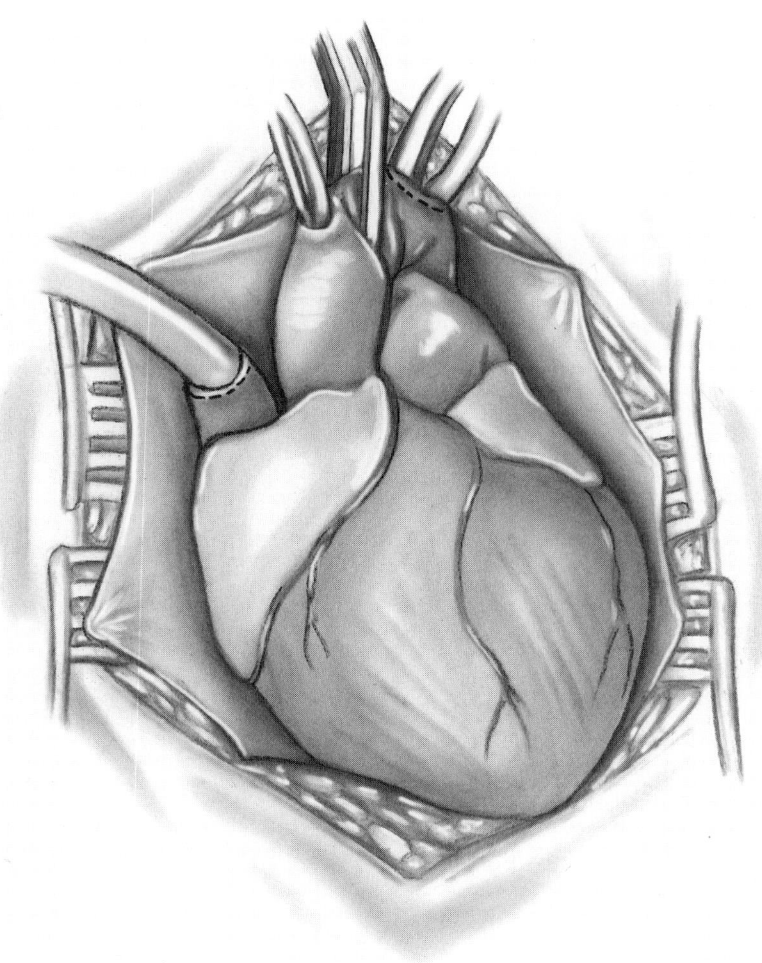

FIGURE 21–8 Cardiopulmonary bypass. The heart is shown here in a pericardial cradle with a venous cannula in the right atrial appendage, an aortic cannula in the distal ascending aorta, an aortic cross-clamp, and a cardioplegia cannula.

survival is not influenced.[136] Readministration of antegrade partial-dose cardioplegia at the completion of distal anastomoses is a common practice (Fig. 21-8).

DISTAL ANASTOMOSES

Sequence of Anastomoses

A sequence of completing distal anastomoses usually entails grafting the most ischemic region first to permit antegrade delivery of cardioplegia via the new graft. Using this strategy, grafts can be placed from most ischemic to least ischemic territories, with, however, the pedicled left internal thoracic artery to left anterior descending artery anastomosis performed last to avoid tension and potential injury. Occasionally, in the setting of severe left main or proximal multivessel coronary artery stenosis, or concomitant valvular surgery, retrograde cardioplegia may be used to augment antegrade delivery. When relying upon retrograde cardioplegia, it is important to recognize that the right ventricle is not well protected and that the grafting sequence should be appropriately adjusted.[137] If cardioplegia delivery is not a concern, completion of posterior anastomoses followed by right-sided anastomoses followed by anterior anastomoses forms a convenient grafting sequence.

Distal Target Selection

Angiographically identified distal target locations are usually confirmed by visual inspection and epicardial examination. Arteriotomy sites should be chosen proximal enough to provide the largest-sized target coronary and distal enough to avoid the region of disease. Regions of branching and bifurcation should be avoided if possible. Targets with intramyocardial location first require dissection of overlying tissue. This can usually be accomplished with sharp knife dissection or electrocautery on a low setting. Localization of intramyocardial vessels can often be accomplished by noting epicardial indentation, accompanying epicardial venous structures, or a faint discoloration or a whitish streak within the reddish brown myocardium. When extreme difficulty is encountered in identifying a left anterior descending artery, one controversial technique that has been described is that of locating

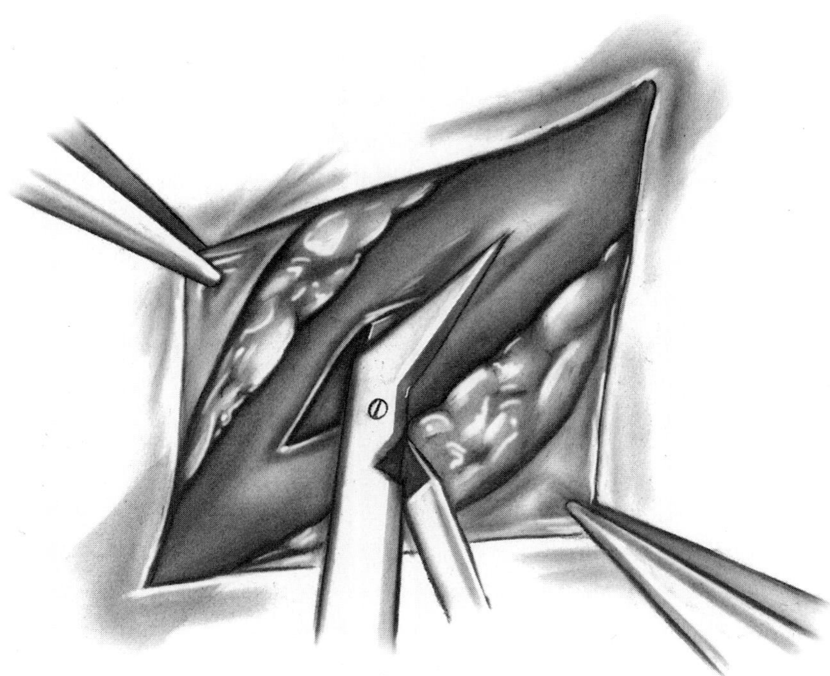

FIGURE 21–9 Coronary arteriotomy. The epicardium overlying the coronary artery has been incised and dissected free of the anterior surface of the coronary artery. An initial arteriotomy is created with a knife, being careful not to injure the posterior intima. The arteriotomy is then extended in both directions with angled fine scissors.

the LAD near the apex of the heart, which is commonly very superficial in this location. A small transverse arteriotomy is then created in this very distal location and a metal probe can be passed retrograde into the LAD and manually palpated more proximally. This arteriotomy can be closed transversely with 8-0 polypropylene suture. Silastic tapes placed through the epicardium, around the proximal coronary artery, or other retracting and positioning techniques can be used to help with visualization and stabilization of the planned arteriotomy site.

Arteriotomy

The target coronary artery, once dissected free of overlying tissue, often displays a thin purplish stripe down the center. This usually correlates with the absence of anterior atheromatous disease and a suitable region of arteriotomy. Either a rounded tip blade or a pointed blade with the sharp side up is used to enter the coronary artery. This arteriotomy is then extended with fine scissors proximally and distally to generate an arteriotomy of approximately 5 mm in size (Fig. 21-9). Depending much upon the size of the native coronary artery and conduit, some surgeons will now probe the distal and/or proximal coronary artery from this arteriotomy prior to performing the anastomosis.

Anastomotic Technique

The previously prepared and beveled or notched conduit is brought to the field. Multiple anastomotic techniques exist and differ in various aspects: continuous versus interrupted versus combined, intiation at the heel versus the toe, and parachute versus anchored. The authors prefer a continuous, parachuting technique initiated at the heel for virtually all distal and proximal anastomoses. Starting slightly to the far side of the heel, a 7-0 polypropylene suture is passed outside-in on the conduit and then inside-out at the corresponding location near the heel of the arteriotomy. Four or five such suture throws are then placed with the conduit in the air, coming around the heel towards the near side. The conduit is then parachuted down onto the arteriotomy, and the suture is continued along the near side towards the toe, around the toe, and then back up the far side until the other end of the suture is met (Fig. 21-10). Precise endothelial approximation is critical. When conduits are notched, the two flanges can potentially be inadvertently included within the anastomosis and must be sutured out of the anastomosis. Bevelling the conduit instead of notching avoids this potential obstruction. Care should be taken to apply a proper amount of tension on the follow-through to avoid both leakage and a purse-string effect, both of which may also be avoided with an increased number of throws. Prior to tying down the suture, the heel and toe can be probed to confirm patency and a venous conduit is usually flushed free of air. The use of an intraluminal coronary occcluder during anastomotic construction may protect against back wall suturing at a minimal risk of endothelial injury. Anastomotic hemostasis can now be confirmed. With nonpedicled conduits, cardioplegia can be administered to the supplied territory. To prevent anastomotic tension and torsion, pedicled conduits can be suture fixated to the adjacent epicardium. This is particularly relevant when further manipulation of the heart for

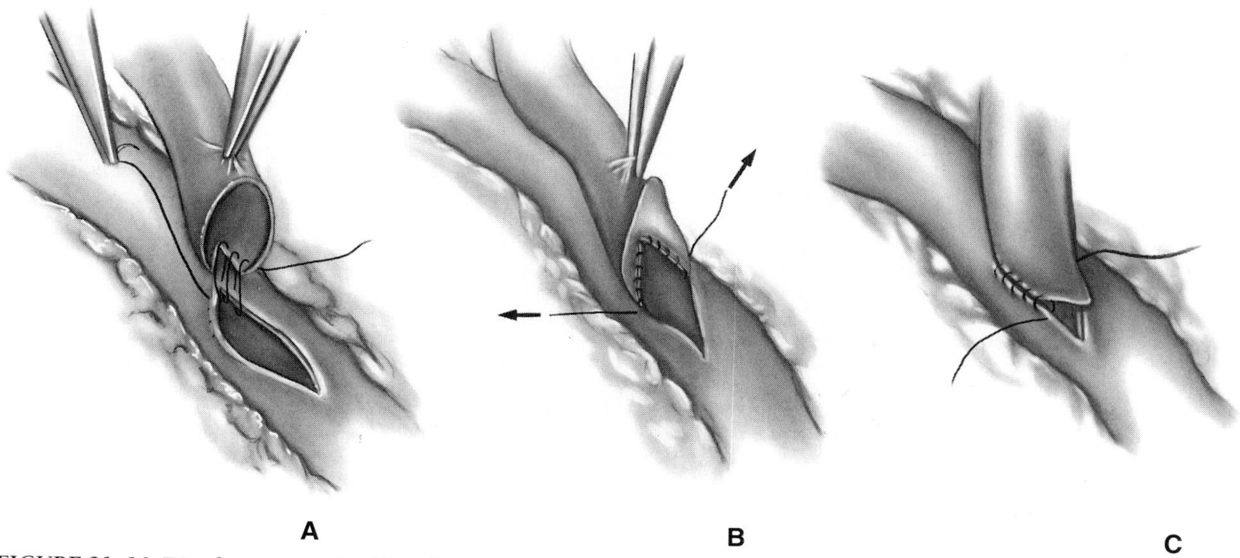

FIGURE 21–10 Distal anastomosis. (A) A fine polypropylene suture is passed through the conduit and coronary artery in a running fashion towards and around the anastomotic heel. (B) After several throws, the conduit is gently parachuted down to the coronary artery. (C) A suture is continued towards and around the anastomotic toe until the other end of the suture is reached.

grafting or concomitant procedures is anticipated. A minority of surgeons advocate the use of interrupted anastomoses to avoid a purse-string effect on the anastomosis. Nitinol clips have been recently introduced to facilitate interrupted distal anastomoses by avoiding the need for tying of multiple sutures. When using a long segment of greater saphenous vein for multiple grafts, the heart should be placed in native position and filled with blood, and the conduit should be filled and cut to an appropriate length for later proximal anastomosis.

Sequential Grafting

Sequential grafting permits the performance of additional distal anastomoses while sparing conduit and additional proximal anastomoses. A purported advantage is the effective augmentation of outflow and, in venous grafts, an increase in patency rates compared to single distal anastomoses.[138–140] Sequential grafting with the internal thoracic artery is occasionally performed, usually to a stenotic diagonal coronary artery, although specific anatomic concerns exist.[141–143] Potential additional advantages with ITA sequential grafting include an arterial revascularization of the second target, and significant coronary flow reserve in the ITA.[144] Routine use of the LITA for multiple sequential anastomoses of the circumflex system and the RITA for the LAD has also been described.[145] The gastroepiploic artery has also been used to sequentially graft multiple inferoposterior targets.[146] A clear disadvantage of sequential grafting is the reliance of two or more distal targets upon a single conduit and proximal anastomosis. A potentially larger region of myocardium may be jeopardized. In general, most surgeons avoid using the left internal thoracic artery for sequential grafting or as a donor for composite Y-grafting of other conduits because of valid concerns of compromising critical LITA to LAD flow.

When planning sequential anastomoses, the most distal anastomosis should be to the largest target vessel with the greatest outflow potential.[147,148] If the reverse situation is created, the most distal anastomosis is at high risk for failure given the likelihood of preferential flow to the more proximal distal anastomosis. Although sequential anastomoses can be performed in any order, completing the distal anastomosis first and moving proximally subsequently is often easier from the spacing and positioning perspective. One exception to this may be the use of a pedicled left internal thoracic artery graft to the left anterior descending artery with a sequenced anastomosis to a diagonal branch more proximally. In this setting, performing the diagonal anastomosis first may be spatially more feasible. Sequential anastomoses are performed in side-to-side fashion. These are usually performed with a longitudinal native coronary arteriotomy and a longitudinal conduit venotomy or arteriotomy. An excessively long arteriotomy and venotomy are avoided to prevent flattening of the conduit. The two incisions can then be aligned in parallel, perpendicular to one another to create a diamond-shaped anastomosis, or at any angle in between depending upon the spatial geometry. When aligned in parallel, the anastomosis can be performed in running fashion heel-to-heel, similar to that described previously for standard distal anastomosis. When aligned at 90°, one can start the anastomosis in the heel of the conduit and match

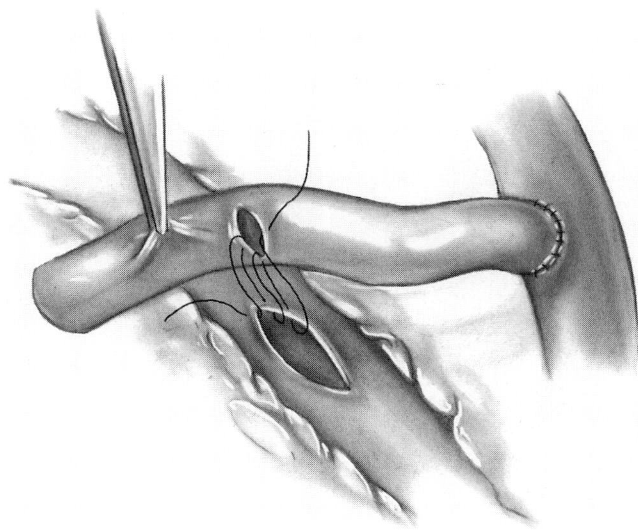

FIGURE 21–11 Sequential distal anastomosis. After determination of the appropriate geometric alignment of the conduit and coronary artery, a coronary arteriotomy and conduit venotomy or arteriotomy are created and, in a manner similar to that described for distal anastomosis, a polypropylene suture is used in continuous fashion beginning near the heel.

this region to the corresponding midportion of either the near or far side of the coronary artery, but subsequently perform the running anastomosis around the arteriotomy in a fashion similar to that described above for a standard distal anastomosis (Fig. 21-11). When aligned at any other angle, the suture placement is modified accordingly. Hemostasis is then confirmed and cardioplegia can be delivered as indicated. In the rare circumstance in which a coronary stenosis occurs at the bifurcation of two graftable vessels, conduit is limited, and a sequential graft is anatomically difficult to align, an alternative is a bifid anastomosis over the coronary bifurcation.

Distal Anastomotic Devices

Several sutureless devices that facilitate distal anastomosis are under active clinical investigation.[149] In general, these are based upon variations of stent technology utilized in an intra- or extraluminal manner.

CORONARY ENDARTERECTOMY

Coronary endarterectomy is a relatively infrequently utilized procedure for creating a distal target from an otherwise unsuitable site. Endarterectomy is considered only for diffusely diseased coronary arteries or occluded coronary arteries that supply a large distribution.[150,151] In general, the larger the size of the distal vessel, the greater the chance of success with endarterectomy.[152] Thus, this technique is utilized more commonly in the right coronary artery than any other distribution. The primary disadvantages of this technique are technical difficulty, increased thrombogenicity in the region of endarterectomy, and the risk of vessel occlusion from an intimal flap. The patency of grafts to endarterectomized vessels is clearly lower than that of grafts to nonendarterectomized vessels.[153] Contemporary endarterectomy series demonstrate improvements in long-term patency.[154,155]

The closed technique for endarterectomy, usually of the right coronary system, entails a slightly longer than standard arteriotomy, followed by elevating the plaque and encircling it with an instrument such as a spatula or an endarterectomy knife. With traction on the plaque and countertraction on the artery, the plaque is extracted (Fig. 21-12). An open endarterectomy, usually of the left anterior descending coronary artery, begins with an arteriotomy along the entire length of the plaque. The plaque is dissected free of the native coronary vessel along its entire length and then removed (Fig 21-13). This technique is particularly useful in the left anterior descending artery because it permits extraction of plaque branches from septal perforators. The native artery is not closed primarily, but rather covered by a long side-to-side anastomosis with a bypass conduit, usually saphenous vein.[156] There are limited reports of long internal thoracic artery anastomoses to endarterectomized left anterior descending arteries.

PROXIMAL ANASTOMOSES

Great variation exists in the technique of performing proximal anastomoses. These differences relate to timing with respect to distal anastomoses, timing with respect to aortic cross-clamp removal, sequence, location, and technical considerations.

Prior to Distal Anastomosis

A minority of surgeons prefer to perform venous and free arterial conduit proximal anastomoses prior to performing the distal anastomoses. There are several primary advantages cited by advocates of this technique. The first advantage is that the performance of the proximal anastomoses can be done with the use of a partial occlusion clamp prior to the initiation of cardiopulmonary bypass, thus decreasing the overall bypass period. The second advantage is that upon completion of the distal anastomoses and removal of the aortic cross-clamp, all regions of the myocardium are immediately revascularized. The third advantage, which is at the same time a disadvantage, is that conduits need to be measured peripherally on a full, beating heart prior to initiation of cardiopulmonary bypass and cut to an appropriate length. This technique, which is somewhat difficult and may occasionally result in undersizing

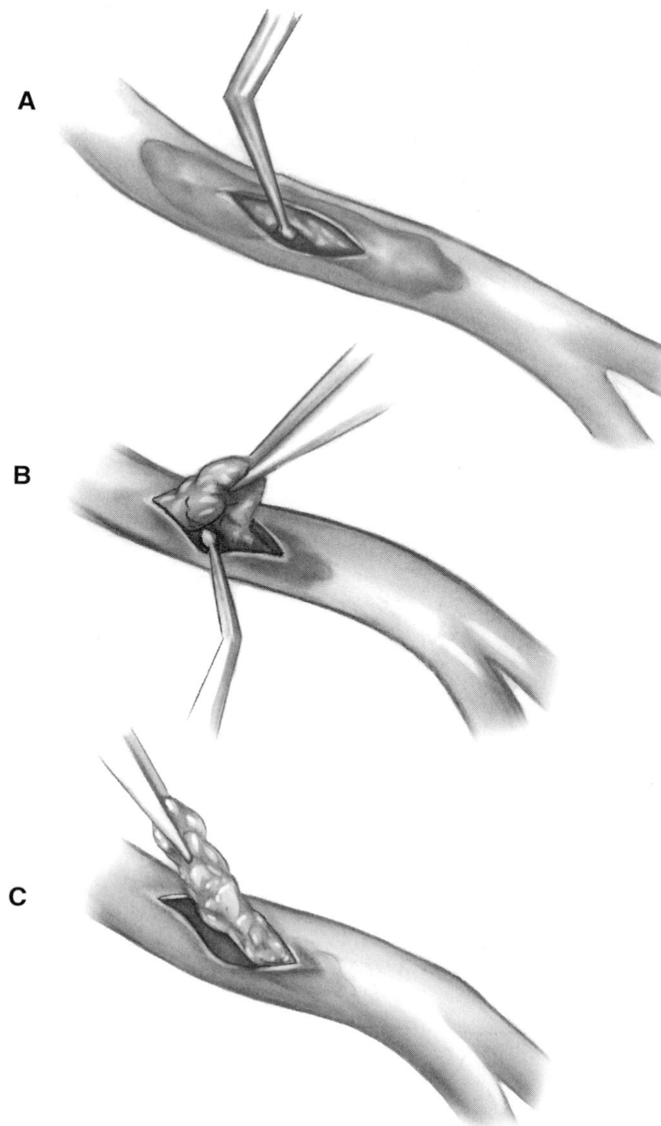

FIGURE 21–12 Closed coronary endarterectomy. (A) A coronary arteriotomy is created and an appropriate dissection plane is initiated between the plaque and the arterial wall. (B) This plane is continued circumferentially around the plaque and extended proximally. The plaque is then extracted from the proximal coronary artery. (C) The dissection plane is carried as far distally as possible from the arteriotomy and the plaque is extracted.

or oversizing of the conduit, does utilize conduit very efficiently. There are many disadvantages to performing proximal anastomoses first. The use of a partial occlusion clamp on the aorta during normal myocardial function increases the risk of traumatizing the aorta and potentially causing a dissection. As mentioned, the grafts need to be measured very carefully to avoid creating too long or too short of a conduit. The technique of measuring conduit first assumes the adequacy of a distal target site for anastomosis. Occasionally, identification of and careful inspection of a planned distal anastomosis site reveals an unsuspected plaque necessitating a more distal anastomosis. This would increase the risk of a precut graft being too short. Many surgeons test the adequacy of a distal anastomosis from a flow and hemostasis standpoint by the manual administration of cardioplegia or heparinized saline via a cannulated graft. This option is eliminated when proximal anastomoses are completed first. Cardioplegia can still be given through the graft, via aortic root administration; however, this requires the heart being returned to native position and the presence of a competent aortic valve. Thus, a leaking distal anastomosis, which requires repair, would potentially necessitate multiple awkward repositionings of the heart.

Single Cross-clamp

This technique entails performance of distal anastomoses followed by proximal anastomoses just prior to the removal of the aortic cross-clamp. This technique is commonly used when coronary artery bypass grafting is performed in conjunction with valvular procedures, but some surgeons advocate this technique in performing coronary bypass grafting by itself. The advantages, when compared to other techniques, include the ability to perform distal anastomoses first, and the ability to place proximal anastomoses onto areas of the aorta that may be otherwise more difficult to access with a partial occlusion clamp, such as the proximal or lateral ascending aorta. The primary purported advantage is the avoidance of additional aortic manipulation and risk of neurologic injury.[157] Disadvantages include longer cross-clamp time and a need to de-air the heart. One can see, in the setting of, for example, an aortic valve replacement with concomitant coronary artery bypass grafting, that the heart needs to be de-aired anyway, and the retrograde coronary sinus cardioplegia catheter can be used to minimize the effects of the additional cross-clamp time required for proximal anastomoses. One also avoids the potential need to place a partial occlusion clamp across an aortotomy suture line.

Partial Occlusion Clamp

This technique is probably still the most common method of completing proximal anastomoses. When performing coronary artery bypass grafting alone, this technique permits the advantages of performing the distal anastomoses first, without increasing the ischemic cross-clamp time. Only the vein graft, and not the heart itself, requires de-airing. The aorta does need to be manipulated during placement of the partial occlusion clamp; however, the risk of initiating dissection is lower, while the patient is still on full bypass and the heart has yet to recover vigorous activity. The locations of proximal anastomoses are somewhat limited to the anterior aspect of the ascending aorta.

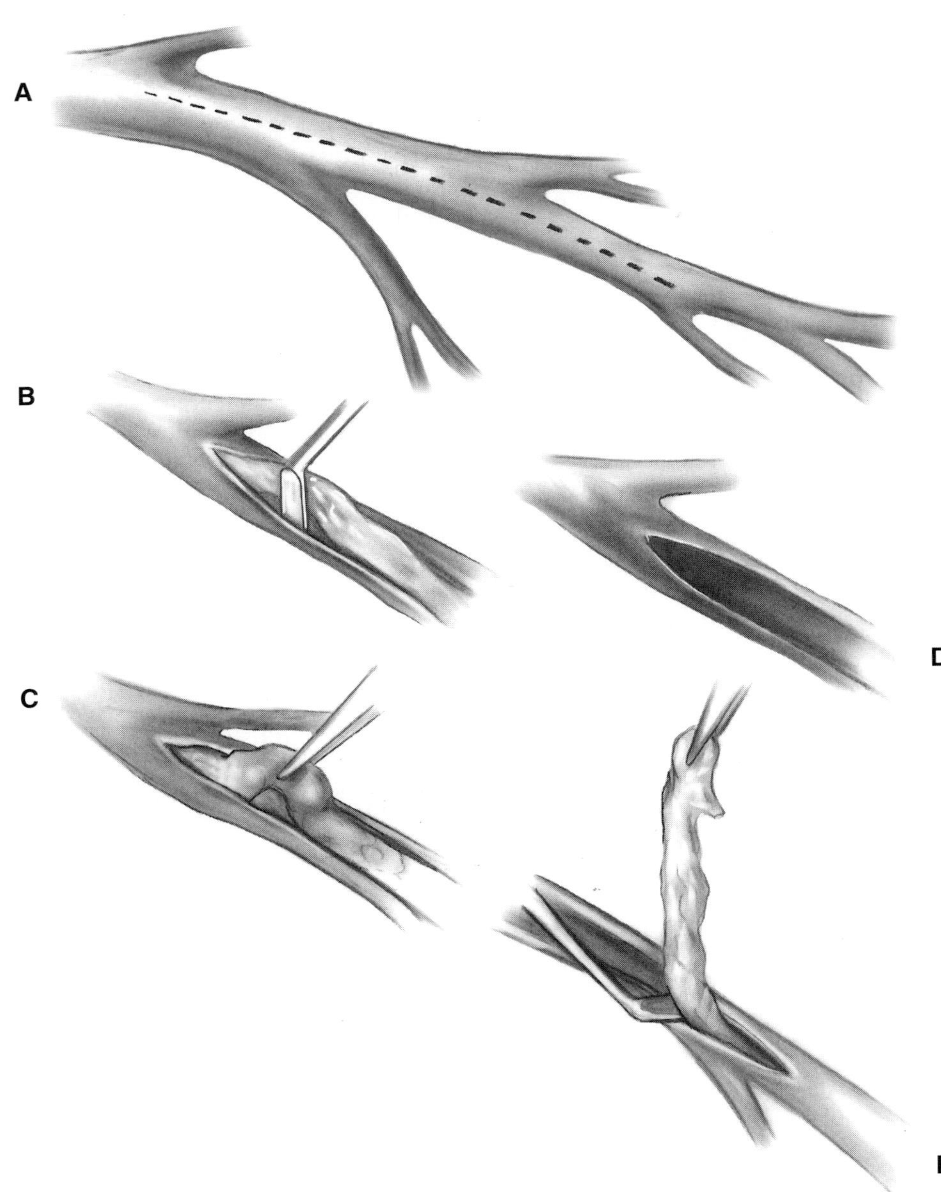

FIGURE 21–13 Open coronary endarterectomy. (A) A long coronary arteriotomy is created. (B) A dissection plane is initiated between the plaque and arterial wall and extended proximally and distally. (C) The proximal extent of the plaque is extracted, if possible, or flushly divided with a sharp knife. (D) The proximal portion of the endarterectomized coronary artery is shown. (E) The endarterectomy dissection plane is continued down to the distal extent of the arteriotomy and the extensive plaque is extracted.

Anastomotic Technique

An appropriate site for aortotomy is identified. The fatty tissue overlying the aorta is removed, an arteriotomy is created with a #11 blade, and a 4.8 punch is used to create a circular aortotomy. When the venous conduit is somewhat smaller in diameter or when using arterial conduits, a 4.0 punch may be preferable. The proximal aspect of the conduit is cut to an appropriate bevel and an additional notch is usually made in the heel. For a venous conduit, a running 5-0 or 6-0 polypropylene suture can be used. For an arterial conduit, a 6-0 or 7-0 polypropylene suture can be used. The long axis of the graft should be aligned at an appropriate angle from the long axis of the ascending aorta in such a way as to provide a gentle curvature with the conduit either around the right atrium for a right-sided graft or over the pulmonary artery for a left-sided graft. Occasionally, left-sided grafts can be taken off the right side of the ascending aorta and routed posteriorly behind the aorta and through the transverse sinus. A running suture is then started outside-in on the conduit, two bites counterclockwise from the heel. The needle is then passed inside-out on the aorta at an appropriate location along the circumference of the arteriotomy such as to generate the appropriate angle of approach of the conduit

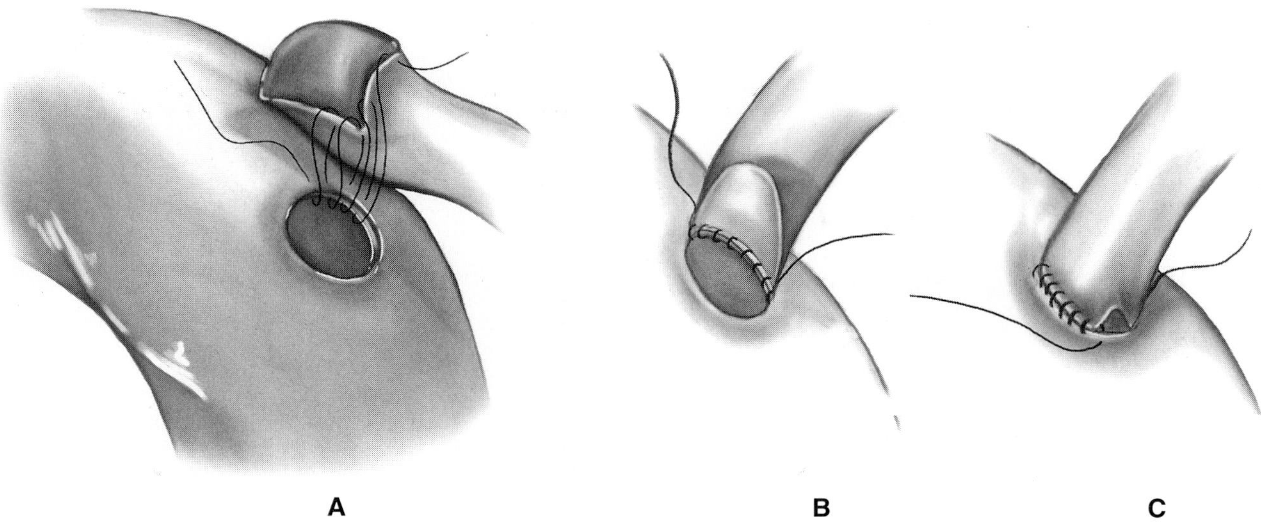

FIGURE 21–14 Proximal anastomosis. (A) The technique of single cross-clamp is demonstrated. An aortotomy is created with a knife and punch. Appropriate conduit length and orientation are established and a fine polypropylene suture is used in a running fashion towards and around the anastomotic heel. (B) The conduit is then carefully parachuted down onto the aorta. (C) The suture is continued towards and around the anastomotic toe.

relative to the long axis of the aorta. As mentioned above, four or five passes are then made in similar fashion moving clockwise along the conduit, coming around the heel. The conduit is then parachuted down onto the aorta and the suture is then continued around over the toe of the anastomosis until completed (Fig. 21-14). Alternatively, once the toe of the anastomosis has been reached, the other needle can be used outside-in on the aorta and used to complete the other half of the anastomosis and meet the other suture essentially at the toe. The site of anastomosis can be marked with a surgical clip or wire of some sort to facilitate future cardiac catheterization, if necessary. To de-air a vein graft, a soft bulldog is placed distally along the graft before the aortic cross-clamp or partial occlusion clamp is removed. A 27-gauge needle is used to pierce the vein graft in its most elevated portion, from which air will usually extrude. The bulldog can then be removed. Hemostasis can be evaluated proximally and distally, as indicated. Generally, arterial conduits are not de-aired in this fashion for fear of conduit needle injury. Conduits such as the free RIMA and radial artery that are harvested with surrounding venous and soft tissue structures should be carefully inspected along the entire length for hemostasis.

Composite Grafts

Various configurations of Y- and T-grafts can be devised to accommodate multiple issues such as limited conduit length and limited aortotomy sites, as well as to minimize aortic proximal anastomoses on single cross-clamp and intentionally base proximal sites on locations other than the ascending aorta (Fig. 21-15). An additional stimulus for creating composite grafts is the concern about long-term arterial conduit patency with direct aortic anastomosis in which there is marked mismatch between aortic wall thickness and conduit size. In such a setting, it may be advantageous to base an arterial conduit proximal on a vein graft, a pedicled arterial graft, or the right subclavian or innominate artery.[158–160] An example is that of basing a radial artery graft off the proximal left internal thoracic artery pedicle.[161] This configuration takes advantage of ITA flow reserve.[162] Disadvantages include technical difficulties and reliance upon a single inflow source for two or more distal targets. The critical LITA to LAD graft may be in jeopardy should there be a technical problem with the composite graft. Delicate all-arterial Y-grafts are usually planned in advance and constructed prior to the initiation of cardiopulmonary bypass. Y-grafting can also be performed more distally along a conduit and used in lieu of sequential grafting. Compared to sequential grafting, this technique requires an additional anastomosis, but may facilitate distal grafting of targets that, because of anatomic alignment, may not be ideally suited for sequential grafting. This technique may also facilitate complete myocardial revascularization with only internal thoracic arteries.[163] Other creative variations such as an inverted "T " comprised of a single radial artery anastomosed to all distal coronary targets in an end-to-side or side-to-side manner and subsequent LITA end-to-side anastomosis into the radial artery have been constructed.[164] As with sequential grafting, a disadvantage of composite grafting is reliance of multiple

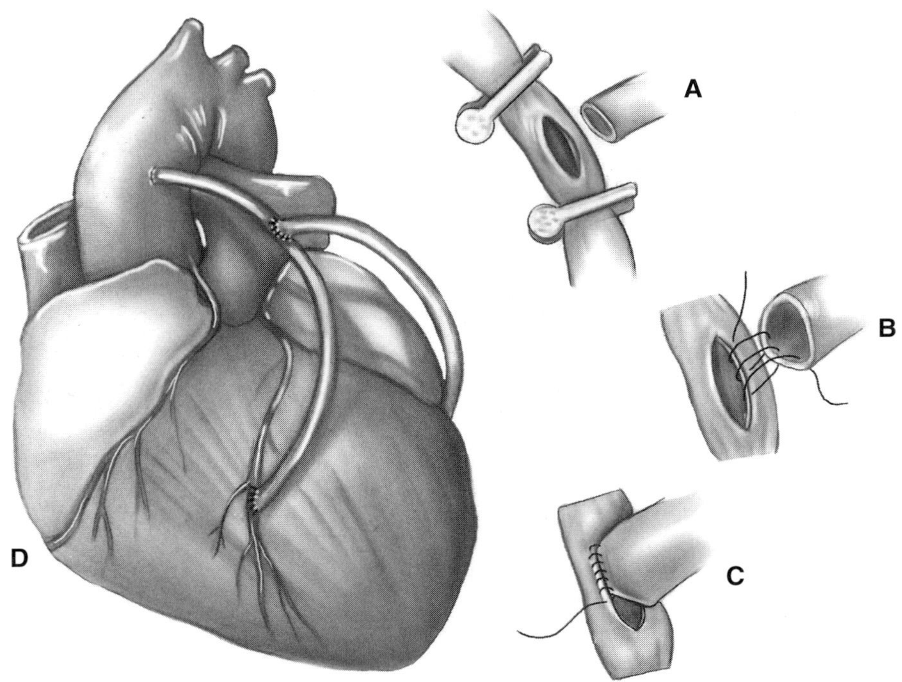

FIGURE 21–15 Y-graft. (A) In the example shown, a completed coronary artery bypass graft is used as a proximal donor site for another conduit. A venotomy or arteriotomy is created in the donor conduit. (B) The recipient conduit is then anastomosed in an end-to-side fashion using a fine polypropylene suture in running fashion, beginning near the heel. (C) The recipient conduit is then gently parachuted down onto the donor conduit. (D) A representative example of a completed Y-graft in a relatively less common configuration of an aortocoronary saphenous vein graft to the LAD with a composite vein graft to an obtuse marginal.

myocardial regions on a single proximal graft. Particular care must also be taken during construction of composite grafts to avoid tension, rotational torsion, or narrowing of either segment.

Proximal Anastomotic Devices

Currently, sutureless proximal anastomotic devices are in various stages of clinical evaluation and commercial availability. These devices are used for creating an aortotomy and subsequently attaching a vein graft to the aorta with a circular wire appliance (Fig. 21-16).[165] These devices obviate the need for application of a partial occlusion clamp. Reportedly, these devices will soon be able to anastomose free arterial conduits as well.

WEANING FROM CARDIOPULMONARY BYPASS

Upon completion of all anastomoses, the patient is extensively prepared for separation from cardiopulmonary bypass (Table 21-1). Critical aspects include the establishment of a stable intrinsic or paced cardiac rhythm, metabolic optimization, appropriate pharmacologic support, and the initiation of effective mechanical ventilation. While closely monitoring the hemodynamic profile, the patient is weaned from cardiopulmonary bypass (Table 21-2). In rare instances, mechanical circulatory support in the form of an intra-aortic balloon counterpulsation or ventricular assist device may be required; these are detailed in Chapter 17.

Once separated from cardiopulmonary bypass, all cannulae are removed with the exception of the aortic cannula. The state of anticoagulation is reversed with a calculated dose of protamine. Systemic hypotension may develop with rapid infusion of protamine, primarily from a vasodilatory effect. This can be treated by slowing the protamine infusion, providing pharmacologic support, and administering volume rapidly via the aortic cannula. With normalization of the activated clotting time, the aortic cannula is removed. All surgical sites are appropriately reinforced and adequate hemostasis is confirmed.

CHEST CLOSURE

Thoracostomy drainage tubes are carefully placed, usually in any opened pleural space, the inferior mediastinum, and the superior mediastinum. Direct contact with conduits is generally avoided.[166] A minority of surgeons will attempt to reapproximate the pericardium in an effort to decrease the risk of cardiovascular injury during reoperation. Thymic and mediastinal tissues in the superior mediastinum can usually be easily reapproximated without undue tension on the heart, great vessels, or grafts.[167] The sternum is usually reapproximated with interrupted stainless steel wire, although heavy suture, bands, and plates have also been utilized. The fascial, subdermal, and skin layers are reapproximated.

In rare instances, prolonged cardiopulmonary bypass and cross-clamp may result in significant myocardial edema and subsequent hemodynamic intolerance of chest closure.

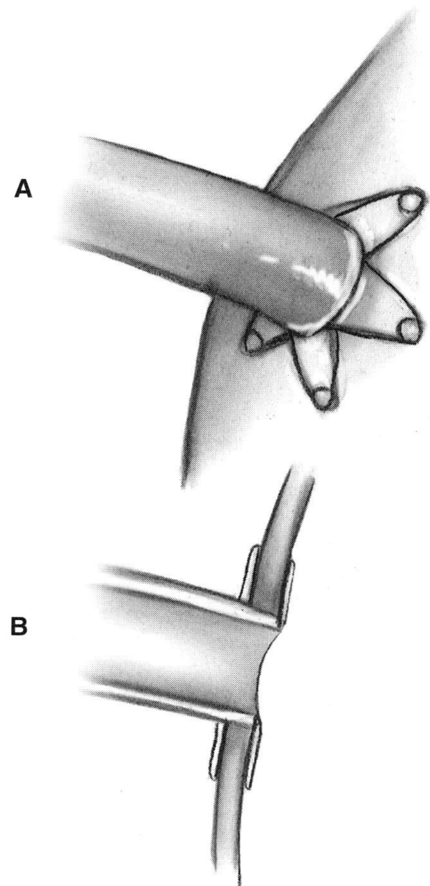

FIGURE 21–16 Sutureless proximal connector. (A) A venous conduit is shown anastomosed in end-to-side fashion to the aorta with a multipronged wire connecting device. (B) The anastomosis is shown in cross-section with two layers of opposing wire connection devices and the venous conduit within the aortic wall.

TABLE 21–1 Preparation of the patient for separation from cardiopulmonary bypass

Overall physiologic
Rewarm patient to 37°C
Correct hemoglobin to 8-10 g/dL
Correct metabolic parameters: acid-base, potassium, calcium, magnesium
Titrate level of anesthetic
Confirm drug and volume infusions
Check appropriate blood products
Level table, zero transducers, and check monitors
Pulmonary
Suction endotracheal tube, fiberoptic bronchoscopy if necessary
Mechanically ventilate with 100% O_2
Treat hydro-hemo-pneumothorax, atelectasis, and bronchospasm
Consider the need for alternate ventilation with PEEP, nitric oxide, or inhaled prostacyclin
Cardiovascular
General
Remove retrograde catheter, intracardiac vent, and caval tapes if present
Establish hemostasis
Evacuate intracardiac air
Confirm conduit patency and alignment
Rhythm
Establish stable rhythm with appropriate rate 80-100 bpm
Rhythm preference SR>AP>AVP>AF>JR>VP>VT>VF>Asystole
Cardioversion, antiarrythmics, and rate controlling agents
Confirm absence of EKG evidence of ischemia
Hemodynamics
Adjust preload with cardiopulmonary bypass machine volume
Augment contractility as needed
Pharmacologically adjust afterload balancing myocardial work versus coronary perfusion pressure (IABP if necessary)

In addition to appropriate pharmacologic and mechanical support, prolonged open sternotomy may be required. Delayed sternal closure should only be attempted after significant diuresis.[168]

POSTOPERATIVE MANAGEMENT

In a carefully coordinated and monitored manner, the patient is transferred to the surgical intensive care unit. The enormous complexities of postoperative care are detailed in Chapter 15.

OUTCOMES

Outcomes can be broadly categorized into perioperative results and long-term results. The perioperative results that are most commonly measured include mortality, major morbidity such as myocardial infarction and cerebrovascular accident, other major organ system failures, reoperation for hemorrhage, and mediastinitis. Other parameters such as length of stay and costs are now being evaluated more commonly. Long-term outcomes most commonly measured include graft patency, recurrence of symptoms such as angina, myocardial infarction, need for reoperation, and overall survival.

Perioperative Mortality

Hospital mortality or 30-day mortality after primary coronary artery bypass grafting has been evaluated extensively and has been reported in the range of 1% to 5% overall for a heterogeneous population. The rate has remained at approximately 3% overall for the past decade despite an increase in preoperative risk.[25,169] The majority of these deaths are related to primary cardiac failure with or without associated myocardial infarction. Risk factors for perioperative mortality can be viewed in two categories. The first category

TABLE 21–2 Primary considerations when unable to separate patient from cardiopulmonary bypass

Metabolic disturbance
Failure to deliver pharmacologic agents
Inadequate ventilation
Hydro-hemo-pneumothorax
Inappropriate rhythm or rate
Significant preload or afterload alteration
Contractile dysfunction
Myocardial ischemia, air/particulate embolism, graft failure, nonrevascularization
Valvular dysfunction
Intracardiac shunt
Occult hemorrhage
Venous inflow or arterial outflow obstruction
Aortic dissection

consists of preoperative factors, such as age, comorbidities, degree of myocardial ischemia and function, and anatomy. The other category of risk factors relates to operative factors such as year of operation, surgeon, cardiopulmonary bypass time, myocardial ischemic time, extent of revascularization, failure to use the internal thoracic artery to the left anterior descending artery, and the need for pharmacologic and mechanical cardiac support.[170]

Perioperative Morbidity

Perioperative myocardial infarction, as defined by elevation of creatine kinase MB fraction and/or troponin I with the development of new electrocardiographic Q-waves, occurs at a rate of approximately 2% to 5% during primary coronary artery bypass grafting procedures. Causes of perioperative myocardial infarction include inadequate myocardial protection, incomplete revascularization, technical issues with bypass grafts, embolism, and hemodynamic instability, among others.

Perioperative neurologic injury can manifest in a wide range of clinical sequelae. These will include anything from subtle neuropsychological changes detected only with intensive testing, to severe gross neurologic deficits of either a transient or permanent nature.[171] These gross deficits occur at rates highly dependent upon patient age. Approximately 0.5% of young patients and 5% of patients older than age 70 will experience gross neurologic deficits after primary coronary artery bypass grafting. The preoperative risk factors of age, hypertension, prior neurologic event, and diabetes repeatedly correlate most highly with the development of stroke after coronary revascularization.[172–175]

The rate of injury to other major organ systems is highly dependent upon multiple variables, particularly preoperative organ status. For example, patients with underlying chronic renal insufficiency are at significantly higher risk of developing post–coronary artery bypass acute tubular necrosis, which will often require temporary or permanent hemodialysis.[176]

Other Perioperative Parameters

Current medical, economic, and environmental factors emphasize the evaluation of additional parameters of outcome, such as time to extubation, time in the intensive care unit, length of stay, and various other costs.[177–182]

Long-Term Graft Patency

The combination of the unique biology of the pedicled internal thoracic artery and the extensive diagonal and septal outflow of the left anterior descending artery provides an extremely durable coronary artery bypass graft. The LITA anastomosed end-to-side to the LAD has a 10-year patency of over 90%, and there are reports of continued patency 15, 20, 25, and 30 years postoperatively.[183] The patency of the pedicled left internal thoracic artery when anastomosed to a target vessel other than the LAD is approximately 90% at 5 years and 80% at 10 years. The pedicled right internal thoracic artery, when anastomosed to the right coronary distribution, results in a 5-year patency rate of approximately 90% and a 10-year patency of approximately 80%. In rare instances, when the pedicled right internal thoracic artery is anastomosed to the left anterior descending artery, the patency rates appear to approach that of the pedicled LITA to LAD anastomosis, thus further supporting the notion that a large vascular runoff bed contributes significantly to long-term patency rates. Free internal thoracic artery grafts yield excellent patency rates of approximately 90% at 5 years.[184,185]

The patency rates of a radial artery graft off the aorta are approximately 80% at 5 years,[82,186] although significantly higher patency rates have been reported.[187,188] Placement of the radial artery graft onto a left-sided target vessel with a high-grade proximal stenosis and good runoff may result in higher patency rates. Basing the radial artery proximally off a vein graft hood or another arterial graft, such as a pedicled internal thoracic artery, also may increase the long-term patency rates.

Pedicled, in situ right gastroepiploic artery grafts have been reported to yield patency rates of approximately 85% to 90% at 5 years.[92,189] Experience is limited and large-scale data are unavailable. Free gastroepiploic grafts based off the aorta yield patency rates similar to that of the radial artery. Patency data for inferior epigastric arterial grafts are very limited and suggest short-term patency rates similar to that of the radial artery.[91,103]

Greater saphenous vein and, to a similar extent, lesser saphenous vein fail in two general modalities. Early graft failure occurs during the first year in approximately 20% to 25% of all venous conduits.[190] This is due to anastomotic problems, graft kinking, conduit harvesting trauma, aortic disease, poor runoff, or progression of native coronary

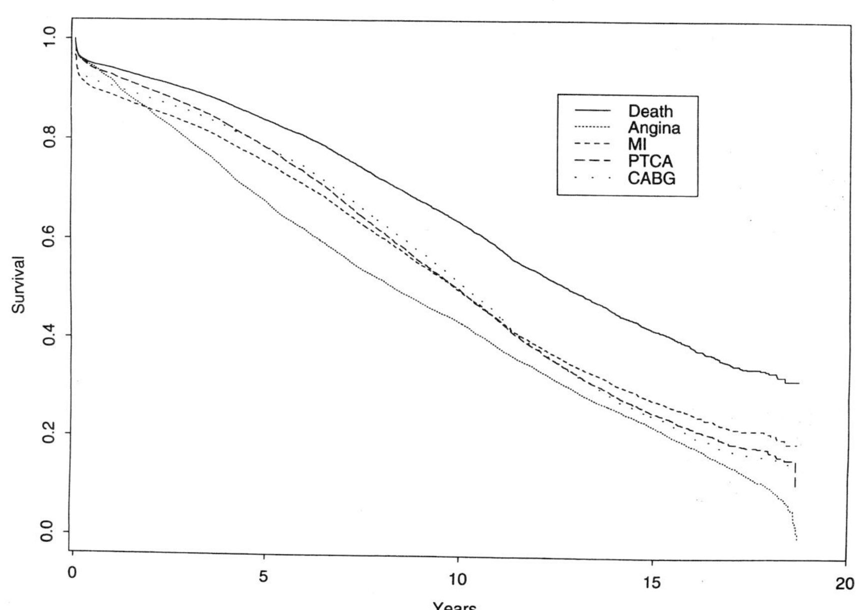

FIGURE 21–17 Kaplan-Meier event-free survival curves for death, angina, myocardial infarction, percutaneous transluminal coronary angioplasty, or repeat coronary artery bypass grafting. Data collected from Emory University Cardiac Surgical Databank, January 1977 to December 1995. N = 23,960.

disease. Late venous conduit failure is due to progression of graft atherosclerosis.[191] Reported 5- and 10-year patency rates for saphenous vein grafts are 60% and 40%, respectively. Improvements in these patency rates may be possible with aspirin administration and aggressive antiatherosclerotic strategies such as the use of lipid-lowering agents.[192–194] Intraoperative gene therapy of saphenous vein conduit with novel antiproliferative agents is under clinical investigation and has yielded encouraging results.[195]

Long-Term Survival

Primary long-term outcomes can be expressed as freedom from the following events: angina, myocardial infarction,

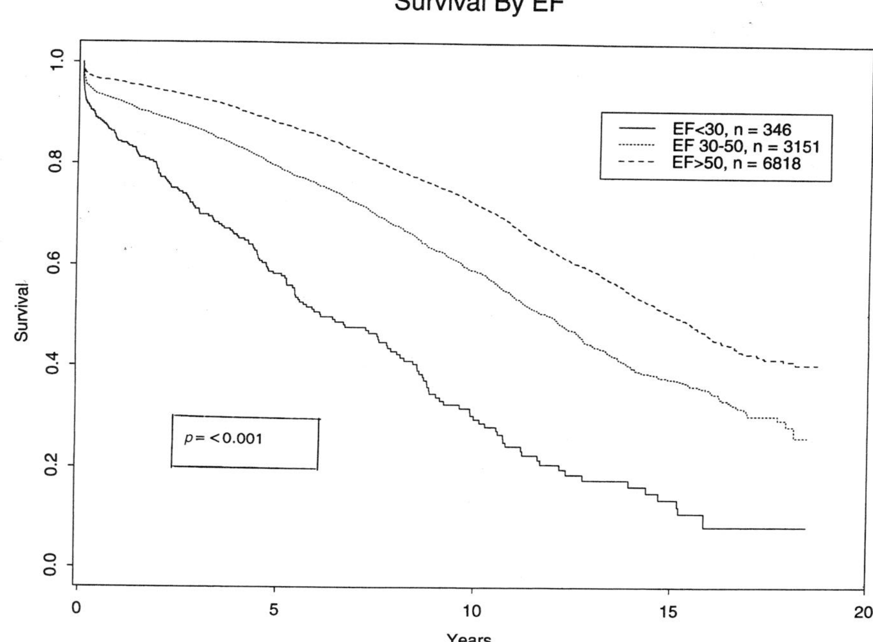

FIGURE 21–18 Kaplan-Meier survival curve for survival in primary coronary artery bypass grafting patients stratified by ejection fraction (EF). Data collected from Emory University Cardiac Surgical Databank, January 1977 to December 1995. N = 23,960, $p < .0001$ for effect of EF on survival.

percutaneous coronary intervention, reoperation, and death. For heterogenous postoperative populations, overall rates of freedom from the above events are excellent.[196–200] A representative event-free survival curve is shown in Figure 21-17. Each of these events, particularly death, can be further stratified based upon preoperative, intraoperative, and postoperative variables. The most striking example would be survival estimates based on preoperative ejection fraction.[201] A representative survival curve by preoperative ejection fraction is displayed in Figure 21-18. Another striking example is the completeness of revascularization and the use of the LITA to LAD.[202–204] Interestingly, very recent data challenge the importance of complete revascularization in long-term outcomes and, in fact, suggest that more than one graft to any non-LAD system may actually be detrimental.[205] Increased utilization of arterial conduits may improve long-term survival.[206] In terms of quality of life, coronary artery bypass grafting provides the greatest improvement to patients with preoperative functional impairment.[207]

SUMMARY

Coronary artery disease is the most prevalent disease condition in industrialized civilization. Operative myocardial revascularization, the most commonly performed major operation overall in the United States, is still considered the gold standard for treatment of most patients with multivessel coronary disease. Cardiopulmonary bypass is currently utilized in approximately 80% of primary coronary artery bypass grafting procedures in the United States today. A pedicled left internal thoracic artery anastomosed to the left anterior descending coronary artery with saphenous vein grafts to the right coronary and left circumflex distributions is the most common combination, although additional pedicled and free arterial grafts are being utilized more commonly. Perioperative major morbidity and mortality rates are very low and long-term outcomes are excellent. Emerging technologic advancements in anastomotic devices, beating heart surgery, and robotics will greatly influence multiple aspects of this operation.[208–212]

REFERENCES

1. Beck C: The development of a new blood supply to the heart by operation. *Ann Surg* 1935; 102:801.
2. Vineberg AM, Miller G: Internal mammary coronary anastomosis in the surgical treatment of coronary artery insufficiency. *Can Med Assoc J* 1951; 64:204.
3. Murray G, Porcheron R, Hilario J, Roschlau W: Anastomosis of a systemic artery to the coronary. *Can Med Assoc J* 1954; 71:594.
4. Gibbon JH: Application of a mechanical heart and lung apparatus to cardiac surgery. *Minn Med* 1954; 37:171.
5. Bailey CP, May A, Lemmon WM: Survival after coronary endarterectomy in man. *JAMA* 1957; 164:641.
6. Senning A: Strip grafting in coronary arteries: report of a case. *J Thorac Cardiovasc Surg* 1961; 41:542.
7. Sones FM Jr, Shirey EK: Cine coronary arteriography. *Mod Concepts Cardiovasc Dis* 1962; 31:735.
8. Longmire WP, Cannon JA, Kattus AA: Direct vision coronary endarterectomy for angina pectoris. *N Engl J Med* 1958; 259:993.
9. Sabiston DC Jr: Direct surgical management of congenital and acquired lesions of the coronary artery. *Prog Cardiovasc Dis* 1963; 6:229.
10. Garrett EH, Dennis EW, DeBakey ME: Aortocoronary bypass with saphenous vein grafts: seven-year follow-up. *JAMA* 1973; 223:792.
11. Kolesov VI: Mammary artery-coronary artery anastomosis as a method of treatment for angina pectoris. *J Thorac Cardiovasc Surg* 1967; 54:535.
12. Favaloro RG: Saphenous vein autograft replacement of severe segmental coronary artery occlusion: operative technique. *Ann Thorac Surg* 1968; 5:334.
13. Rosengart TK, Lee LY, Patel SR, et al: Angiogenesis gene therapy: phase I assessment of direct intramyocardial administration of an adenovirus vector expressing VEGF121 cDNA to individuals with clinically significant severe coronary artery disease. *Circulation* 1999; 100:468.
14. The Bypass Angioplasty Revascularization Investigation (BARI) Investigators: Comparison of coronary bypass surgery with angioplasty in patients with multivessel disease. *N Engl J Med* 1996; 335:217.
15. Cashin WL, Sanmarco ME, Nessim SA, Blankenhorn DH: Accelerated progression of atherosclerosis in coronary vessels with minimal lesions that are bypassed. *N Engl J Med* 1984; 311:824.
16. CASS Principal Investigators and their associates: Coronary Artery Surgery Study (CASS): a randomized trial of coronary artery bypass surgery; survival data. *Circulation* 1983; 68:939.
17. Cosgrove DM, Loop FD, Saunders CL, et al: Should coronary arteries with less than fifty percent stenosis be bypassed? *J Thorac Cardiovasc Surg* 1981; 82:520.
18. Eagle KA, Guyton RA, Davidoff R, et al: ACC/AHA Guidelines for Coronary Artery Bypass Graft Surgery: a Report of the American College of Cardiology/American Heart Association Task Force on Practice Guidelines (Committee to Revise the 1991 Guidelines for Coronary Artery Bypass Graft Surgery). American College of Cardiology/American Heart Association. *J Am Coll Cardiol* 1999; 34:1262.
19. Varnauskas E: European Coronary Surgery Study Group: twelve-year follow-up of survival in the randomized European Coronary Surgery Study. *N Engl J Med* 1988; 319:332.
20. The Veterans Administration Coronary Artery Bypass Surgery Cooperative Study Group: Eleven-year survival in the Veterans Administration randomized trial of coronary bypass surgery for stable angina. *N Engl J Med* 1984; 311:1333.
21. Niles NW, McGrath PD, Malenka D, et al: Survival of patients with diabetes and multivessel coronary artery disease after surgical or percutaneous coronary revascularization: results of a large regional prospective study. *J Am Coll Cardiol* 2001; 37:1008.
22. Fortescue EB, Kahn K, Bates DW: Development and validation of a clinical prediction rule for major adverse outcomes in coronary bypass grafting. *Am J Cardiol* 2001; 88:1251.
23. Craver JM, Puskas JD, Weintraub WW, et al: 601 octogenarians undergoing cardiac surgery and comparison with younger age groups. *Ann Thorac Surg* 1999; 67:1104.
24. Thourani VH, Weintraub WS, Stein B, et al: Influence of diabetes mellitus on early and late outcome after coronary artery bypass grafting. *Ann Thorac Surg* 1999; 67:1045.
25. Ferguson TB Jr, Hammill BG, Peterson ED, et al: A decade of change–risk profiles and outcomes for isolated coronary artery

bypass grafting procedures, 1990–1999: a report from the STS National Database Committee and the Duke Clinical Research Institute. Society of Thoracic Surgeons. *Ann Thorac Surg* 2002; 73:480.

26. Kreter B, Woods M: Antibiotic prophylaxis for cardiothoracic operations: meta-analysis of thirty years of clinical trials. *J Thorac Cardiovasc Surg* 1992; 104:590.
27. Sandrelli L, Pardini A, Lorusso R, et al: Impact of autologous blood predonation on a comprehensive blood conservation program. *Ann Thorac Surg* 1995; 59:730.
28. Yazicioglu L, Eryilmaz S, Sirlak M, et al: Recombinant human erythropoietin administration in cardiac surgery. *J Thorac Cardiovasc Surg* 2001; 122:741.
29. Hayashi J, Kumon K, Takanashi S, et al: Subcutaneous administration of recombinant human erythropoietin before cardiac surgery: a double-blind, multicenter trial in Japan. *Transfusion* 1994; 34:142.
30. Jobes DR, Aitken GL, Shaffer GW: Increased accuracy and precision of heparin and protamine dosing reduces blood loss and transfusion in patients undergoing primary cardiac operations. *J Thorac Cardiovasc Surg* 1995; 110:36.
31. Arom KV, Emery RW: Decreased postoperative drainage with addition of epsilon-aminocaproic acid before cardiopulmonary bypass. *Ann Thorac Surg* 1994; 57:1108.
32. Ray MJ, Hales MM, Brown L, et al: Postoperatively administered aprotinin or epsilon aminocaproic acid after cardiopulmonary bypass has limited benefit. *Ann Thorac Surg* 2001; 72:521.
33. Kalangos A, Tayyareci G, Pretre R, et al: Influence of aprotinin on early graft thrombosis in patients undergoing myocardial revascularization. *Eur J Cardiothorac Surg* 1994; 8:651.
34. Owen CH, Cummings RG, Sell TL, et al: Coronary artery bypass grafting in patients with dialysis-dependent renal failure. *Ann Thorac Surg* 1994; 58:1729.
35. Nguyen DM, Gilfix BM, Dennis F, et al: Impact of transfusion of mediastinal shed blood on serum levels of cardiac enzymes. *Ann Thorac Surg* 1996; 62:109.
36. Loop FD, Lytle BW, Cosgrove DM, et al: Influence of the internal-mammary-artery graft on 10-year survival and other cardiac events. *N Engl J Med* 1986; 314:1.
37. Cameron A, Davis KB, Green G, Schaff HV: Coronary bypass surgery with internal-thoracic-artery grafts—effects on survival over a 15-year period. *N Engl J Med* 1996; 334:216.
38. Li S, Fan YS, Chow LH, van Den Diepstraten C, et al: Innate diversity of adult human arterial smooth muscle cells: cloning of distinct subtypes from the internal thoracic artery. *Circ Res* 2001; 89:517.
39. Ko YS, Yeh HI, Haw M, et al: Differential expression of connexin43 and desmin defines two subpopulations of medial smooth muscle cells in the human internal mammary artery. *Arterioscler Thromb Vasc Biol* 1999; 19:1669.
40. Yang Z, Oemar BS, Carrel T, et al: Differential proliferative properties of smooth muscle cells of human arterial and venous bypass vessels: role of PDGF receptors, mitogen-activated protein kinase, and cyclin-dependent kinase inhibitors. *Circulation* 1998; 97:181.
41. Yang Z, Luscher TF: Basic cellular mechanisms of coronary bypass graft disease. *Eur Heart J* 1993; 14(suppl I):193.
42. Chaikhouni A, Crawford FA, Kochel PJ, et al: Human internal mammary artery produces more prostacyclin than saphenous vein. *J Thorac Cardiovasc Surg* 1986; 92:88.
43. Broeders MA, Doevendans PA, Maessen JG, et al: The human internal thoracic artery releases more nitric oxide in response to vascular endothelial growth factor than the human saphenous vein. *J Thorac Cardiovasc Surg* 2001; 122:305.
44. Wiley KE, Davenport AP: Nitric oxide-mediated modulation of the endothelin-1 signalling pathway in the human cardiovascular system. *Br J Pharm* 2001; 132:213.
45. Gitter R, Anderson JM Jr., Jett GK: Influence of milrinone and norepinephrine on blood flow in canine internal mammary artery grafts. *Ann Thorac Surg* 1996; 61:1367.
46. Jett GK, Arcici JM Jr, Hatcher CR Jr, et al: Vasodilator drug effects on internal mammary artery and saphenous vein grafts. *J Am Coll Cardiol* 1988; 11:1317.
47. Lehmann KH, von Segesser L, Muller-Glauser W, et al: Internal-mammary coronary artery grafts: is their superiority also due to a basically intact endothelium? *Thorac Cardiovasc Surg* 1989; 37:187.
48. Sisto T, Yla-Herttuala S, Luoma J, et al: Biochemical composition of human internal mammary artery and saphenous vein. *J Vasc Surg* 1990; 11:418.
49. Vahl CF, Carl I, Müller-Vahl H: Brachial plexus injury after cardiac surgery. *J Thorac Cardiovasc Surg* 1991; 102:724.
50. Cooper GJ, Gillot T, Parry EA, et al: Papaverine injures the endothelium of the internal mammary artery. *Cardiovasc Surg* 1995; 3:553.
51. Cooper GJ, Gillot T, Francis SE, Angelini GD: Distension produces medial but not endothelial damage in porcine internal mammary artery. *Cardiovasc Surg* 1995; 3:171.
52. Mills NL: Preparation of the internal mammary artery graft with intraluminal papaverine. *J Card Surg* 1991; 6:318.
53. Deja MA, Wos S, Golba KS, et al: Intraoperative and laboratory evaluation of skeletonized versus pedicled internal thoracic artery. *Ann Thorac Surg* 1999; 68:2164.
54. Hirotani T, Shirota S, Cho Y, Takeuchi S: Feasibility and suitability of the routine use of bilateral internal thoracic arteries. *Ann Thorac Surg* 2002; 73:511.
55. Galbut DL, Traad EA, Dorman MJ, et al: Seventeen-year experience with bilateral internal mammary artery grafts. *Ann Thorac Surg* 1990; 49:195.
56. Dion R, Etienne PY, Verhelst R, et al: Bilateral mammary grafting: clinical, functional, and angiographic assessment in 400 consecutive patients. *Eur J Cardiothorac Surg* 1993; 7:287.
57. Taggart DP, D'Amico R, Altman DG: Effect of arterial revascularisation on survival: a systematic review of studies comparing bilateral and single internal mammary arteries. *Lancet* 2001; 358: 870.
58. Endo M, Nishida H, Tomizawa Y, Kasanuki H: Benefit of bilateral over single internal mammary artery grafts for multiple coronary artery bypass grafting. *Circulation* 2001; 104:2164.
59. Berreklouw E, Rademakers PP, Koster JM, et al: Better ischemic event-free survival after two internal thoracic artery grafts: 13 years of follow-up. *Ann Thorac Surg* 2001; 72:1535.
60. Sergeant P, Blackstone E, Meyns B: Validation and interdependence with patient-variables of the influence of procedural variables on early and late survival after CABG. *Eur J Cardiothorac Surg* 1997; 12:1.
61. Kurlansky PA, Traad EA, Glanut DL, et al: Efficacy of single versus bilateral internal mammary artery grafting in women: a long-term study. *Ann Thorac Surg* 2001; 71:1949.
62. He GW, Ryan WH, Acuff TE, et al: Risk factors for operative mortality and sternal wound infection in bilateral internal mammary artery grafting. *J Thorac Cardiovasc Surg* 1994; 107: 196.
63. Kouchoukos NT, Wareing TH, Murphy SF, et al: Risks of bilateral internal mammary artery bypass grafting. *Ann Thorac Surg* 1990; 49:210.
64. Grossi EA, Esposito R, Harris LJ, et al: Sternal wound infections and use of internal mammary artery grafts [see comments]. *J Thorac Cardiovasc Surg* 1991; 102:342.
65. Cosgrove DM, Lytle BW, Loop FD, et al: Does bilateral internal mammary artery grafting increase surgical risk? *J Thorac Cardiovasc Surg* 1988; 95:850.

66. Accola KD, Jones EL, Craver JM, et al: Bilateral mammary artery grafting: avoidance of complications with extended use. *Ann Thorac Surg* 1993; 56:872.
67. Cohen AJ, Moore P, Jones C: Effect of internal mammary harvest on postoperative pain and pulmonary function. *Ann Thorac Surg* 1993; 56:1107.
68. Lev-Ran O, Pevni D, Matsa M, et al: Arterial myocardial revascularization with in situ crossover right internal thoracic artery to left anterior descending artery. *Ann Thorac Surg* 2001; 72:798.
69. Ura M, Sakata R, Nakayama Y, et al: Technical aspects and outcome of in situ right internal thoracic artery grafting to the major branches of the circumflex artery via the transverse sinus. *Ann Thorac Surg* 2001; 71:1485.
70. Tatoulis J, Buxton BF, Fuller JA: Results of 1,454 free right internal thoracic artery-to-coronary artery grafts. *Ann Thorac Surg* 1997; 64:1263.
71. Chow MS, Sim E, Orszulak TA, Schaaf HV: Patency of internal thoracic artery grafts: comparison of right versus left in importance of vessel grafted. *Circulation* 1994; 90(part 2):II129.
72. Carpentier A, Guermonprez JL, Deloche A, et al: The aorta-to-coronary radial artery bypass graft. *Ann Thorac Surg* 1973; 16:111.
73. Chardigny C, Jebara VA, Acar C, et al: Vasoreactivity of the radial artery: comparison with the internal mammary and gastroepiploic arteries with implications for coronary artery surgery. *N Engl J Med* 1993; 88:II115.
74. He GW, Yang CQ: Vasorelaxant effect of phosphodiesterase-inhibitor milrinone in the human radial artery used as coronary bypass graft. *J Thorac Cardiovasc Surg* 2000; 119:1039.
75. Acar C, Jebara VA, Portoghese M, et al: Revival of the radial artery for coronary artery bypass grafting. *Ann Thorac Surg* 1992; 54:652.
76. Tatoulis J, Buxton BF, Fuller JA: Bilateral radial artery grafts in coronary reconstruction: technique and early results in 261 patients. *Ann Thorac Surg* 1998; 66:714.
77. Cohen G, Tamariz MG, Sever JY, et al: The radial artery versus the saphenous vein graft in contemporary CABG: a case-matched study. *Ann Thorac Surg* 2001; 71:180.
78. Tatoulis J, Buxton BF, Fuller JA: Bilateral radial artery grafts in coronary reconstruction: technique and early results in 261 patients. *Ann Thorac Surg* 1998; 66:714.
79. Shapira OM, Alkon JD, Macron DS, et al: Nitroglycerin is preferable to diltiazem for prevention of coronary bypass conduit spasm. *Ann Thorac Surg* 2000; 70:883.
80. Dietl CA, Benoit CH: Radial artery graft for coronary revascularization: technical considerations. *Ann Thorac Surg* 1995; 60:102.
81. Maniar HS, Sundt TM, Barner HB, et al: Effect of target stenosis and location on radial artery graft patency. *J Thorac Cardiovasc Surg* 2002; 123:45.
82. Moran SV, Baeza R, Guarda E, et al: Predictors of radial artery patency for coronary bypass operations. *Ann Thorac Surg* 2001; 72:1552.
83. Ruengsakulrach P, Brooks M, Hare DL, et al: Preoperative assessment of hand circulation by means of Doppler ultrasonography and the modified Allen test. *J Thorac Cardiovasc Surg* 2001; 121:526.
84. Reyes AT, Frame R, Brodman RF: Technique for harvesting a radial artery as a coronary bypass graft. *Ann Thorac Surg* 1995; 59:118.
85. Anyanwu AC, Saeed I, Bustami M, et al: Does routine use of the radial artery increase complexity or morbidity of coronary bypass surgery? *Ann Thorac Surg* 2001; 71:555.
86. Meharwal ZS, Trehan N: Functional status of the hand after radial artery harvesting: results in 3,977 cases. *Ann Thorac Surg* 2001; 72:1557.
87. Denton TA, Trento L, Cohen M, et al: Radial artery harvesting for coronary bypass operations: neurologic complications and their potential mechanisms. *J Thorac Cardiovasc Surg* 2001; 121:951.
88. Genovesi MH, Torrillo L, Fonger J, et al: Endoscopic radial artery harvest: a new approach. *Heart Surg Forum* 2001; 4:223.
89. Pym J, Brown PM, Charrette EJ, et al: Gastroepiploic-coronary anastomosis: a viable alternative bypass graft. *J Thorac Cardiovasc Surg* 1987; 94:256.
90. Mills NL, Everson CT: Right gastroepiploic artery: a third arterial conduit for coronary artery bypass. *Ann Thorac Surg* 1989; 47:706.
91. Manapat AE, McCarthy PM, Lytle BW, et al: Gastroepiploic and inferior epigastric arteries for coronary artery bypass: early results and evolving applications. *N Engl J Med* 1994; 90:II-144.
92. Grandjean JG, Voors AA, Boonstra PW, et al: Exclusive use of arterial grafts in coronary artery bypass operations for three-vessel disease: use of both thoracic arteries and the gastroepiploic artery in 256 consecutive patients. *J Thorac Cardiovasc Surg* 1996; 112:935.
93. Nishida H, Tomizawa Y, Endo M, et al: Coronary artery bypass with only in situ bilateral internal thoracic arteries and right gastroepiploic artery. *Circulation* 2001; 104(suppl 1):I76.
94. Jegaden O, Eker A, Monthena P, et al: Risk and results of bypass grafting using bilateral internal mammary and right gastroepiploic arteries. *Ann Thorac Surg* 1995; 59:955.
95. Grandjean JG, Boonstra PW, den Heyer P, Ebels T: Arterial revascularization with the right gastroepiploic artery and internal mammary arteries in 300 patients. *J Thorac Cardiovasc Surg* 1994; 107:1309.
96. Yang Z, Siebenmann R, Studer M, et al: Similar endothelium-dependent relaxation, but enhanced contractility, of the right gastroepiploic artery as compared with the internal mammary artery. *J Thorac Cardiovasc Surg* 1992; 104:459.
97. Oku T, Yamane S, Suma H, et al: Comparison of prostacyclin production of human gastroepoploic artery and saphenous vein. *Ann Thorac Surg* 1990; 49:767.
98. Kennedy JH: The gastroepiploic artery compared with the internal mammary artery in aortocoronary bypass. *Annales de Chirurgie* 1994; 48:814.
99. Koike R, Suma H, Kondo K, et al: Pharmacological response of internal mammary artery and gastroepiploic artery. *Ann Thorac Surg* 1990; 50:384.
100. Mills NL, Hockmuth DR, Everson CT, et al: Right gastroepiploic artery used for coronary artery bypass grafting: evaluation of flow characteristics and size. *J Thorac Cardiovasc Surg* 1993; 106:579.
101. Mills NL, Everson CT: Technical considerations for use of the gastroepiploic artery for coronary artery surgery. *J Card Surg* 1989; 4:1.
102. Tavilla G, van Son JAM, Verhagen AF, et al: Retrogastric versus antegastric routing and histology of the right gastroepiploic artery. *Ann Thorac Surg* 1992; 53:1057.
103. Buche M, Schroeder E, Gurné O, et al: Coronary artery bypass grafting with the inferior epigastric artery: midterm clinical and angiographic results. *J Thorac Cardiovasc Surg* 1995; 109:553.
104. Barner HB, Naunheim KS, Fiore AC, et al: Use of the inferior epigastric artery as a free graft for myocardial revascularization. *Ann Thorac Surg* 1991; 52:429.
105. Cremer J, Mugge A, Schulze M, et al: The inferior epigastric artery for coronary bypass grafting: functional assessment and clinical results. *Eur J Cardiothorac Surg* 1993; 7:423.
106. Tadjkarimi S, O'Neil GS, Schyns CJ, et al: Vasoconstrictor profile of the inferior epigastric artery. *Ann Thorac Surg* 1993; 56:1090.
107. Buxton BF, Chan AT, Dixit AS, et al Ulnar artery as a coronary bypass graft. *Ann Thorac Surg* 1998; 65:1020.
108. van Aarnhem EE, Schreur JH, Firouzi M, Jansen EW: The left gastric artery as an in-situ conduit in coronary artery bypass grafting. *Ann Thorac Surg* 2001; 71:1013.
109. Edwards WS, Lewis CE, Blakeley WR, et al: Coronary artery bypass with internal mammary and splenic artery grafts. *Ann Thorac Surg* 1973; 15:35.

110. Yaginuma G, Sakurai M, Meguro T, Ota K: Thoracodorsal artery as a free arterial graft for myocardial revascularization. *Ann Thorac Surg* 2001; 72:915.
111. Schamun CM, Duran JC, Rodriguez JM, et al: Coronary revascularization with the descending branch of the lateral femoral circumflex artery as a composite arterial graft. *J Thorac Cardiovasc Surg* 1998; 116:870.
112. Soyombo AA, Angelini GD, Bryan AJ, Newby AC: Surgical preparation induces injury and promotes smooth muscle cell proliferation in a culture of human saphenous vein. *Cardiovasc Res* 1993; 27:1961.
113. Bonchek LI: Prevention of endothelial damage during preparation of saphenous veins for bypass grafting. *J Thorac Cardiovasc Surg* 1980; 79:911.
114. Angelini GD, Passani SL, Breckenridge IM, Newby AC: Nature and pressure dependence of damage induced by distension of human saphenous vein coronary artery bypass grafts. *Cardiovasc Res* 1987; 21:902.
115. Souza DS, Bomfim V, Skoglund H, et al: High early patency of saphenous vein graft for coronary artery bypass harvested with surrounding tissue. *Ann Thorac Surg* 2001; 71:797.
116. Tsui JC, Souza DS, Filbey D, et al: Preserved endothelial integrity and nitric oxide synthase in saphenous vein grafts harvested by a "no-touch" technique. *Br J Surg* 2001; 88:1209.
117. Bitondo JM, Daggett WM, Torchiana DF, et al: Endoscopic versus open saphenous vein harvest: a comparison of postoperative wound complications. *Ann Thorac Surg* 2002; 73:523.
118. Dusterhoft V, Bauer M, Buz S, et al: Wound-healing disturbances after vein harvesting for CABG: a randomized trial to compare the minimally invasive direct vision and traditional approaches. *Ann Thorac Surg* 2001; 72:2038.
119. Meyer DM, Rogers TE, Jessen ME, et al: Histologic evidence of the safety of endoscopic saphenous vein graft preparation. *Ann Thorac Surg* 2000; 70:487.
120. Paletta CE, Huang DB, Fiore AC, et al: Major leg wound complications after saphenous vein harvest for coronary revascularization. *Ann Thorac Surg* 2000; 70:492.
121. Kiaii B, Moon BC, Massel D, et al: A prospective randomized trial of endoscopic versus conventional harvesting of the saphenous vein in coronary artery bypass surgery. *J Thorac Cardiovasc Surg* 2002; 123:204.
122. Crouch JD, O'Hair DP, Keuler JP, et al: Open versus endoscopic saphenous vein harvesting: wound complications and vein quality. *Ann Thorac Surg* 1999; 68:1513.
123. Lancey RA, Cuenoud H, Nunnari JJ: Scanning electron microscopic analysis of endoscopic versus open vein harvesting techniques. *J Cardiovasc Surg* 2001; 42:297.
124. Stoney WS, Alford WC Jr, Burrus GR, et al: The fate of arm veins used for aorta-coronary bypass grafts. *J Thorac Cardiovasc Surg* 1984; 88:522.
125. Wijnberg DS, Boeve WJ, Ebels T, et al: Patency of arm vein grafts used in aorto-coronary bypass surgery. *Cardiothorac Surg* 1990; 4:510.
126. Lamm P, Juchem G, Milz S, et al: Autologous endothelialized vein allograft: a solution in the search for small-caliber grafts in coronary artery bypass graft operations. *Circulation* 2001; 104(suppl 1):I108.
127. Laub GW, Muralidharan S, Clancy R, et al: Cryopreserved allograft veins as alternative coronary artery bypass conduits: early phase results [see comments]. *Ann Thorac Surg* 1992; 54:826.
128. Kruse J, Borsow J, Buntrock P, et al: Aortocoronary vascular prosthesis made of siliconized homologous vein or bovine sacral artery. *Thorac Cardiovasc Surg* 1991; 39(suppl 3):233.
129. Okoshi T, Soldani G, Goddard M, Galletti PM: Very small-diameter polyurethane vascular prostheses with rapid endothelialization for coronary artery bypass grafting. *J Thorac Cardiovasc Surg* 1993; 105:791.
130. Marshall WG Jr, Barzilai B, Kouchoukos NT: Intraoperative ultrasonic imaging of the ascending aorta. *Ann Thorac Surg* 1989; 48:339.
131. Ohteki H, Tsuyoshi I, Natsuaki M, et al: Intraoperative ultrasonic imaging of the ascending aorta in ischemic heart disease. *Ann Thorac Surg* 1990; 50:539.
132. Mills NL, Everson CT: Atherosclerosis of the ascending aorta and coronary artery bypass. *J Thorac Cardiovasc Surg* 1991; 102:546.
133. Wareing TH, Davila-Roman VG, Barzilai B, et al: Management of the severely atherosclerotic ascending aorta during cardiac operations: a strategy for detection and treatment. *J Thorac Cardiovasc Surg* 1992; 103:453.
134. Rowland PE, Grooters RK: Coronary-coronary artery bypass: an alternative. *Ann Thorac Surg* 1987; 43:326.
135. Dearani JA, Axford TC, Patel MA, et al: Role of myocardial temperature measurement in monitoring the adequacy of myocardial protection during cardiac surgery. *Ann Thorac Surg* 2001; 72:S2235.
136. Flack JE, Cook JR, May SJ, et al: Does cardioplegia type affect outcome and survival in patients with advanced left ventricular dysfunction? *Circulation* 2000; 102(suppl III):III84.
137. Allen BS, Winkelmann JW, Hanafy H, et al: Retrograde cardioplegia does not adequately perfuse the right ventricle. *J Thorac Cardiovasc Surg* 1995; 109:1116.
138. Vural KM, Sener E, Tasdemir O: Long-term patency of sequential and individual saphenous vein coronary bypass grafts. *Eur J Cardiothorac Surg* 2001; 19:140.
139. Yamaguchi A, Kitamura N, Miki T, et al: Comparative study in graft patency of individual and sequential grafting as coronary bypass. *Circulation* 1993; 41:577.
140. Kieser TM, Fitzgibbons JM, Keon WJ: Sequential coronary bypass grafts: long-term follow-up. *J Thorac Cardiovasc Surg* 1986; 91:767.
141. Bessone LN, Pupello DF, Hiro SP, et al: Sequential internal mammary artery grafting: a viable alternative in myocardial revascularization. *Cardiovasc Surg* 1995; 3:155.
142. Kesler KA, Sharp TG, Turrentine MW, Brown JW: Technical considerations and early results of sequential left internal mammary artery bypass grafting to the left anterior descending coronary artery system. *J Card Surg* 1990; 5:134.
143. Tashiro T, Todo K, Haruta Y, et al: Sequential internal mammary artery grafts: clinical and angiographic assessment. *Cardiovasc Surg* 1993; 1:720.
144. Hartman JM, Kelder JC, Ackerstaff RG, et al: Different behavior of sequential versus single left internal mammary artery to left anterior descending area grafts (1). *Cardiovasc Surg* 2001; 9: 586.
145. Kootstra GJ, Pragliola C, Lanzillo G: Technique of sequential grafting the left internal mammary artery (LIMA) to the circumflex coronary system. *J Cardiovasc Surg* 1993; 34:523.
146. Ochi M, Bessho R, Saji Y, et al: Sequential grafting of the right gastroepiploic artery in coronary artery bypass surgery. *Ann Thorac Surg* 2001; 71:1205.
147. Christenson JT, Schmuziger M: Sequential venous bypass grafts: results 10 years later. *Ann Thorac Surg* 1997; 63:371.
148. Christenson JT, Simonet F, Schmuziger M: Sequential vein bypass grafting: tactics and long-term results. *Cardiovasc Surg* 1998; 6:389.
149. Eckstein FS, Bonilla LF, Meyer B, et al: Sutureless mechanical anastomosis of a saphenous vein graft to a coronary artery with a new connector device. *Lancet* 2001; 357:931.
150. Brenowitz JB, Kayser KL, Johnson WD: Results of coronary endarterectomy in reconstruction. *J Thorac Cardiovasc Surg* 1988; 95:1.

151. Goldstein J, Cooper E, Saltups A, Boxall J: Angiographic assessment of graft patency after coronary endarterectomy. *J Thorac Cardiovasc Surg* 1991; 102:539.
152. Ferraris VA, Harrah JD, Moritz DM, et al: Long-term angiographic results of coronary endarterectomy. *Ann Thorac Surg* 2000; 69:1737.
153. Qureshi SA, Halim MA, Pillai R, et al: Endarterectomy of the left coronary system: analysis of a ten year experience. *J Thorac Cardiovasc Surg* 1985; 89:852.
154. Asimakopoulos G, Taylor KM, Ratnatunga CP: Outcome of coronary endarterectomy: a case-control study. *Ann Thorac Surg* 1999; 67:989.
155. Shapira OM, Akopian G, Hussain A, et al: Improved clinical outcomes in patients undergoing coronary artery bypass grafting with coronary endarterectomy. *Ann Thorac Surg* 1999; 68:2273.
156. Goldman BS, Christakis GT: Endarterectomy of the left anterior descending coronary artery [review]. *J Cardiac Surg* 1994; 9:89.
157. Dar MI, Gillott T, Ciulli F, Cooper GJ: Single aortic cross-clamp technique reduces S-100 release after coronary artery surgery. *Ann Thorac Surg* 2001; 71:794.
158. Suma H: Innominate and subclavian arteries as an inflow of free arterial graft. *Ann Thorac Surg* 1996; 62:1865.
159. Tector AJ, Amundsen S, Schmal TM, et al: Total revascularization with T-grafts. *Ann Thorac Surg* 1994; 57:33.
160. Calafiore AM, Di Giammarco G, Teodori G, et al: Radial artery and inferior epigastric artery in composite grafts: improved mid-term angiographic results. *Ann Thorac Surg* 1995; 60:517.
161. Barner HB, Sundt TM 3rd, Bailey M, Zang Y: Midterm results of complete arterial revascularization in more than 1,000 patients using an internal thoracic artery/radial artery T graft. *Ann Surg* 2001; 234:447.
162. Royse AG, Royse CF, Groves KL, et al: Blood flow in composite arterial grafts and effect of native coronary flow. *Ann Thorac Surg* 1999; 68:1619.
163. Tector AJ, McDonald ML, Kress DC, et al: Purely internal thoracic artery grafts: outcomes. *Ann Thorac Surg* 2001; 72:450.
164. Tashiro T, Nakamura K, Iwakuma A, et al: Inverted T graft: novel technique using composite radial and internal thoracic arteries. *Ann Thorac Surg* 1999; 67:629.
165. Eckstein FS, Bonilla LF, Englberger L, et al: Minimizing aortic manipulation during OPCAB using the Symmetry aortic connector system for proximal vein graft anastomoses. *Ann Thorac Surg* 2001; 72:S995.
166. Svedjeholm R, Hakanson E: Postoperative myocardial ischemia caused by chest tube compression of vein graft. *Ann Thorac Surg* 1997; 64:1806.
167. Rao V, Komeda M, Weisel RD, et al: Should the pericardium be closed routinely after heart operations? *Ann Thorac Surg* 1999; 67:484.
168. Furnary AP, Magovern JA, Simpson KA, Magovern GJ: Prolonged open sternotomy and delayed sternal closure after cardiac operations. *Ann Thorac Surg* 1992; 54:233.
169. Estafanous FG, Loop FD, Higgins TL, et al: Increased risk and decreased morbidity of coronary artery bypass grafting between 1986 and 1994. *Ann Thorac Surg* 1998; 65:383.
170. Leavitt BJ, O'Connor GT, Olmstead EM, et al:. Use of the internal mammary artery graft and in-hospital mortality and other adverse outcomes associated with coronary artery bypass surgery. *Circulation* 2001; 103:507.
171. McKhann GM, Goldsborough MA, Borowicz LM Jr, et al: Cognitive outcome after coronary artery bypass: a one-year prospective study. *Ann Thorac Surg* 1997; 62:510.
172. Puskas JD, Winston AD, Wright CE, et al: Stroke after coronary artery operation: incidence, correlates, outcome, and cost. *Ann Thorac Surg* 2000; 69:1053.
173. Gardner TJ, Horneffer PJ, Manolio TA, et al: Stroke following coronary artery bypass grafting: a ten-year study. *Ann Thorac Surg* 1985; 40:574.
174. Rao V, Christakis GT, Weisel RD, et al: Risk factors for stroke following coronary bypass surgery. *J Card Surg* 1995; 10:468.
175. McKhann GM, Goldsborough MA, Borowicz LM Jr, et al: Predictors of stroke risk in coronary artery bypass patients. *Ann Thorac Surg* 1997; 62:516.
176. Szczech LA, Best PJ, Crowley E, et al: Outcomes of patients with chronic renal insufficiency in the bypass angioplasty revascularization investigation. *Circulation* 2002; 105:2253.
177. Weintraub WS, Jones EL, Craver J, et al: Determinants of prolonged length of hospital stay after coronary bypass surgery. *N Engl J Med* 1989; 80:276.
178. Weintraub WS, Craver JM, Jones EL, et al: Improving cost and outcome of coronary surgery. *Circulation* 1998; 98(19 suppl):II23.
179. Cowper PA, DeLong ER, Peterson ED, et al: Variability in cost of coronary bypass surgery in New York State: potential for cost savings. *Am Heart J* 2002; 143:130.
180. Mauldin PD, Weintraub WS, Becker ER: Predicting hospital costs for first-time coronary artery bypass grafting from preoperative and postoperative variables. *Am J Cardiol* 1994; 74:772.
181. Engelman RM, Rousou JA, Flack JE 3d, et al: Fast-track recovery of the coronary bypass patient. *Ann Thorac Surg* 1994; 58: 1742.
182. Mounsey JP, Griffith MJ, Heaviside DW, et al: Determinants of the length of stay in intensive care and in hospital after coronary artery surgery. *Br Heart J* 1995; 73:92.
183. Barner HB, Barnett M: Fifteen to 21 year angiographic assessment of internal thoracic artery as a bypass conduit. *Ann Thorac Surg* 1994; 57:1526.
184. Tatoulis J, Buxton BF, Fuller JA, Royse AG: Total arterial coronary revascularization: techniques and results in 3,220 patients. *Ann Thorac Surg* 1999; 68:2093.
185. Loop FD, Lytle BW, Cosgrove DM, et al: Free (aorta-coronary) internal mammary artery graft: late results. *J Thorac Cardiovasc Surg* 1986; 92:827.
186. Acar C, Ramsheyi A, Pagny JY, et al: The radial artery for coronary artery bypass grafting: clinical and angiographic results at five years. *J Thorac Cardiovasc Surg* 1998; 116:981.
187. Calafiore AM, Di Mauro M, D'Alessandro S, et al: Revascularization of the lateral wall: long-term angiographic and clinical results of radial artery versus right internal thoracic artery grafting. *J Thorac Cardiovasc Surg* 2002; 123:225.
188. Iaco AL, Teodori G, Di Giammarco G, et al: Radial artery for myocardial revascularization: long-term clinical and angiographic results. *Ann Thorac Surg* 2001; 72:464.
189. Suma H, Wanibuchi Y, Terada Y, et al: The right gastroepiploic artery graft: clinical and angiographic midterm results in 200 patients. *J Thorac Cardiovasc Surg* 1993; 105:615.
190. Campeau L, Enjalbert M, Lesperance J, et al: Atherosclerosis and late closure of aortocoronary saphenous vein grafts: sequential angiographic studies at 2 weeks, 1 year, 5 to 7 years and 10 to 12 years after surgery. *Circulation* 1983; 68 (suppl II):II-1.
191. Campeau L, Enjalbert M, Lesperance J, et al: The relation of risk factors to the development of atherosclerosis in saphenous-vein bypass grafts and the progression of disease in the native circulation: a study 10 years after aortocoronary bypass surgery. *N Engl J Med* 1984; 311:1329.
192. Blankenhorn DH, Nessim SA, Johnson RL: Beneficial effects of combined colestipol-niacin therapy on coronary atherosclerosis and coronary venous bypass grafts. *JAMA* 1987; 257:323.
193. Goldman S, Copeland J, Moritz T, et al: Starting aspirin therapy after operation: affects on early graft patency. *Circulation* 1991; 84:520.

194. Domanski MJ, Borkowf CB, Campeau L, et al: Prognostic factors for atherosclerosis progression in saphenous vein grafts: the post-coronary artery bypass graft (Post-CABG) trial. Post-CABG Trial Investigators. *J Am Coll Cardiol* 2000; 36:1877.
195. Mann MJ, Dzau VJ: Therapeutic applications of transcription factor decoy oligonucleotides. *J Clin Invest* 2000; 106:1071.
196. Myers WO, Blackstone EH, Davis K, et al: CASS Registry long term surgical survival. Coronary Artery Surgery Study. *J Am Coll Cardiol* 1999; 33:488.
197. Gardner SC, Grunwald GK, Rumsfeld JS, et al: Risk factors for intermediate-term survival after coronary artery bypass grafting. *Ann Thorac Surg* 2001; 72:2033.
198. Dzavik V, Ghali WA, Norris C, et al: Long-term survival in 11,661 patients with multivessel coronary artery disease in the era of stenting: a report from the Alberta Provincial Project for Outcome Assessment in Coronary Heart Disease (APPROACH) Investigators. *Am Heart J* 2001; 142:119.
199. Pell JP, MacIntyre K, Walsh D, et al: Time trends in survival and readmission following coronary artery bypass grafting in Scotland, 1981–96: retrospective observational study. *BMJ* 2002; 324: 201.
200. Graham MM, Ghali WA, Faris PD, et al: Survival after coronary revascularization in the elderly. *Circulation* 2002; 105: 2378.
201. Trachiotis GD, Weintraub WS, Johnston TS, et al: Coronary artery bypass grafting in patients with advanced left ventricular dysfunction. *Ann Thorac Surg* 1998; 66:1632.
202. Van den Brand MJBM, Rensing BJWM, Morel MM, et al: The effect of completeness of revascularization in event-free survival at one year in the ARTS trial. *J Am Coll Cardiol* 2002; 39:559.
203. Scott R, Blackstone EH, McCarthy PM, et al: Isolated bypass grating of the left internal thoracic artery to the left anterior descending coronary artery: late consequences of incomplete revascularization. *J Thorac Cardiovasc Surg* 2000; 120:173.
204. Moon MR, Sundt TM 3rd, Pasque MK, et al: Influence of internal mammary artery grafting and completeness of revascularization on long-term outcome in octogenarians. *Ann Thorac Surg* 2001; 72:2003.
205. VanderSalm TJV, Kip KE, Jones RH, et al: What constitutes optimal surgical revascularization? Answers from the bypass angioplasty revascularization investigation (BARI). *J Am Coll Cardiol* 2002; 39:565.
206. Taggart DP, D'Amico R, Altman DG: Effect of arterial revascularisation on survival: a systematic review of studies comparing bilateral and single internal mammary arteries. *Lancet* 2001; 358:870.
207. Rumsfeld JS, Magid DJ, O'Brien M, et al: Changes in health-related quality of life following coronary artery bypass graft surgery. *Ann Thorac Surg* 2001; 72:2026.
208. Mohr FW, Falk V, Diegeler A, et al: Computer-enhanced "robotic" cardiac surgery: experience in 148 patients. *J Thorac Cardiovasc Surg* 2001; 121:842.
209. Loulmet D, Carpentier A, d'Attellis N, et al: Endoscopic coronary artery bypass grafting with the aid of robotic assisted instruments. *J Thorac Cardiovasc Surg* 1999; 118:4.
210. Boyd WD, Rayman R, Desai ND, et al: Closed-chest coronary artery bypass grafting on the beating heart with the use of a computer-enhanced surgical robotic system. *J Thorac Cardiovasc Surg* 2000; 120:807.
211. Damiano RJ Jr, Tabaie HA, Mack MJ, et al: Initial prospective multicenter clinical trial of robotically-assisted coronary artery bypass grafting. *Ann Thorac Surg* 2001; 72:1263.
212. Kappert U, Schneider J, Cichon R, et al: Development of robotic enhanced endoscopic surgery for the treatment of coronary artery disease. *Circulation* 2001; 104(suppl 1):I102.

Chapter 22

Myocardial Revascularization Without Cardiopulmonary Bypass

Todd M. Dewey/Michael J. Mack

Surgical revascularization of the coronary arterial system remains the foundation of cardiothoracic surgical practice. Coronary artery bypass grafting comprises the majority of open heart procedures performed on a yearly basis by surgeons in this country.[1] Remarkably, with the exception of new techniques of myocardial protection, the technical aspects of the procedure have remained unchanged for decades. While many of the bedrock procedures in other specialties have undergone change and redefinition due to the introduction of facilitating technology, standard bypass grafting has resisted change to a large degree. The enduring nature of coronary artery bypass grafting bespeaks of its proven history of safety and efficacy.[2–7] Additionally, it has been a technique that can be reproducibly performed by a wide variety of operators with varying degrees of technical skill and acumen with generally good results. However, conventional bypass grafting utilizing cardioplegic arrest continues to be associated with singular complications that may negate an otherwise successful procedure.

The success of catheter-based techniques for treating ischemic coronary syndromes, combined with the shift towards less invasive approaches by other surgical specialties, has renewed interest in minimally invasive approaches for cardiac surgery, including beating heart surgery. Initial attempts at reducing insult to the cardiac patient focused mainly on incision size and location. Revascularization was conducted either on an arrested heart using peripheral cannulation (Port Access, Heartport, Redwood City, CA), or on a beating heart with a minimally invasive direct coronary artery bypass (MIDCAB) approach. Lack of demonstrated benefits and technical challenges have since relegated Port Access approaches to primarily intracardiac procedures rather than coronary revascularization.[8] Likewise, the technical challenges associated with the MIDCAB procedure, the rarity of surgical single-vessel disease, and the questionable benefit of thoracotomy over sternotomy have served to limit this approach to less than 2% of all grafting currently performed.[9] Recognition of improved outcomes in selected patients with the elimination of cardiopulmonary bypass serves as the impetus to develop off-pump coronary artery bypass (OPCAB) as a treatment option for multivessel coronary artery disease.[10–14] A recent review of all isolated coronary artery bypass operations performed in the 76 hospitals of the HCA National Hospital System revealed that 3672 (21.6%) were performed without cardiopulmonary bypass.[15] As experience grows, aspects crucial to the success of the operation continue to be refined, thereby enabling the majority if not all coronary revascularization procedures to be performed on the beating heart. Ultimately, the transformation of this technique from compelling idea to central belief relies upon scientifically demonstrating the following: (1) graft patency rates that are superior or equivalent to conventional techniques; (2) reduced morbidity and mortality, especially in high-risk groups; (3) a rapid return to usual functional capacity; and (4) an economic benefit.

PATIENT SELECTION

Currently there are few absolute and only relative contraindications to off-pump surgery. The selection of patients should stem in large part on the operating surgeon's beating heart experience and comfort level. Programs early in their off-pump experience should concentrate on patients with less demanding revascularization requirements (Table 22-1). Optimal candidates for surgeons with limited experience typically include patients who are hemodynamically stable and require a limited number of bypasses (1 to 3) located in easily accessible areas. The left anterior descending (LAD), diagonal artery, right coronary artery (RCA), and posterior descending artery (PDA) are the easiest for inexperienced surgeons to access and graft. Patients should have large target vessels free of diffuse calcific disease, normal ventricular function, and be hemodynamically stable. Furthermore, these procedures should be primary bypasses, not reoperations.

With experience, higher risk and technically more challenging procedures can be undertaken. These include elderly patients, patients with significant comorbidities, and those requiring multiple grafts to the posterior and lateral walls (Table 22-2).[16–21] Difficult patients likely to benefit from off-pump surgery include those with severe left ventricular dysfunction, ischemic mitral insufficiency, or those grafted emergently after an acute myocardial infarction.[21–23] Patients presenting the most significant challenge include those undergoing reoperations or those with small and diffusely diseased vessels.[24,25]

Patients who are either hemodynamically or electrically unstable may not tolerate the manipulation required for off-pump bypass grafting, and therefore represent a population generally not considered candidates for OPCAB. However, this subset of patients may be safely revascularized by performing pump-supported beating heart surgery. Patients are supported by the extracorporeal circuit to maintain hemodynamic stability, but global ischemia is avoided by performing the anastomosis utilizing beating heart techniques. The ability to apply these techniques when needed augments the armamentarium of the practicing surgeon.

TABLE 22–1 OPCAB patient selection in early experience

Anterior vessels
Limited number of bypasses (1-3)
Normal LV function
Epicardial location of targets
Large vessels not diffusely diseased
Hemodynamically stable
Primary revascularization
First case of the day

LV = left ventricular; OPCAB = off-pump coronary artery bypass.

TABLE 22–2 Patients most likely to benefit from OPCAB

Age >70 years
Low ejection fraction
Reoperative surgery
Patients with significant comorbidities
Cerebral vascular disease
Peripheral vascular disease
Hepatic disease
Bleeding disorders
COPD
Renal dysfunction
Atheromatous or calcified aorta
Patients who refuse blood products

COPD = chronic obstructive pulmonary disease; OPCAB = off-pump coronary artery bypass.

ANESTHESIA FOR OFF-PUMP BYPASS GRAFTING

Close collaboration with a familiar and involved anesthesiologist is vital to the performance of off-pump bypass grafting. Lines of communication between the surgeon and the anesthesiologist should be clearly established in order to provide appropriate responses to rapidly changing clinical situations.

Anesthetic techniques for off-pump surgeries are tailored to provide stable hemodynamics, reduce the sequelae of regional myocardial ischemia, and allow early recovery of consciousness and extubation (Table 22-3). These techniques are predicated upon the avoidance of high-dose narcotics and the use of short- and intermediate-acting anesthetic agents.

Without the heat exchanger of the bypass circuit to control the patient's body temperature, maintenance of body heat by ancillary methods becomes necessary. The patient's temperature is maintained by using warming mattresses, infusing warmed fluids, warmed oxygen, and anesthetic gases,

TABLE 22–3 Essentials of anesthetic management in OPCAB

Use intermediate- or short-acting agents
Warming mattresses, warmed fluids and gases
Elevated room temperature
Oximetric pulmonary artery catheters
Transesophageal echocardiography
Trendelenberg's position to increase preload
Volume loading
Nitroglycerine for ischemia prophylaxis
Judicious use of positive inotropes
Avoidance of negative inotropes

OPCAB = off-pump coronary artery bypass.

and keeping the room temperature elevated. The authors' approach is to extubate patients not intubated prior to surgery or in cardiogenic shock in the operating room at the end of the procedure. In 150 consecutive cases, reintubation was required in only 2.6% of patients.

All patients receive continuous oximetric pulmonary artery catheters and transesophageal echocardiography probes. This provides continuous hemodynamic monitoring, and allows treatment to be directed towards specific alterations in the patient's cardiac function. Additionally, undiagnosed intracardiac abnormalities that require treatment and alteration of the operative plan are intermittently identified. Nitroglycerine infusion for ischemic prophylaxis and volume loading are instituted at the beginning of the case. Patients are preload sensitive during the manipulation that occurs when setting up the anastomosis, especially of the posterior circulation vessels. Cardiac displacement leads to right ventricular deformation and decreased pump function without valvular incompetence; this occurs secondary to inflow occlusion or outflow obstruction.[26–31] Volume loading and use of Trendelenburg positioning increases preload, thereby augmenting RV filling pressures and allowing patients to tolerate the distortion in anatomy and maintain adequate cardiac output. Antiarrthymics are instituted as needed but are seldom required. Pacing wires and intraluminal shunts are often placed when grafting poorly collateralized large right coronary arteries because hypotension and bradycardic events are frequently seen with occlusion of these vessels.

Most surgeons believe that negative inotropic or chronotropic agents are to be avoided in off-pump surgery. They provide little assistance in facilitating the construction of the anastomosis, and they reduce cardiac performance enough to make some areas of the heart ungraftable. Utilization of positive inotropes can increase the force of myocardial contraction, thereby accentuating cardiac motion and making target stabilization problematic. During manipulation and positioning of the heart, volume infusion and small aliquots of pressor agents are used to support blood pressure and optimize cardiac output.

Anticoagulation is produced using 1.5 to 2.0 mg/kg of heparin in order to maintain an activated clotting time greater than 300 seconds. At the end of the procedure, the anticoagulation is reversed with protamine sulfate. A bypass circuit is routinely available in the operative suite in the event that conversion to cardiopulmonary support is indicated. Conversion rates vary with surgeon experience, but are generally less than 4%.[32]

SURGICAL TECHNIQUE

Incision

Median sternotomy is the most frequently used route for cardiac access when performing multivessel grafting. Isolated grafting of specific individual vessels can be performed using a variation of thoracotomy, anterior for the left anterior descending artery or lateral for access to the marginal vessels. Median sternotomy allows the surgeon to visualize the operative field from an orientation that is familiar and similar to on-pump procedures. This facilitates target vessel identification as well as harvesting of the internal mammary arteries for use as conduit. Partial sternotomies or parasternal incisions have not proven to be particularly advantageous in terms of postoperative pain or morbidity as compared to full sternotomies. Additionally, should conversion to conventional bypass become necessary, a median sternotomy allows easy access for cannulation of the heart.

Once the conduit is obtained, the retractor is positioned inferiorly in the sternal incision. This placement reduces traction on the brachial plexus and allows easier subluxation of the heart for positioning. Dedicated retractors are now available for beating heart surgery; these tools provide suture holders as well as the ability to attach suction exposure devices and stabilizers (Fig. 22-1). The pericardium is opened in an inverted T-shaped incision. The lateral extensions are exaggerated in order to facilitate mobilization of the apex of the heart, and to create increased space for the right ventricle during positioning. When dealing with hypertrophic hearts it is often helpful to displace the heart into the right chest to aid in exposure of the lateral wall vessels. This is accomplished by incising the right pleura parallel to and along the entire length of the sternotomy. Additionally the pericardial incision is extended posteriorly towards the inferior vena cava along the right diaphragm (Fig. 22-2). This incision is stopped anterior to the phrenic nerve in order to avoid injury. Graft preparation is performed prior to manipulating the heart in order to reduce the amount of time spent with the heart in a nonanatomic position. All varieties of conduit used in conventional bypass grafting can likewise be used in beating heart surgery.[33]

Patient Positioning

Standard positioning for off-pump bypass grafting is to place the patient in Trendelenburg's position and rotated towards the operating surgeon. This position helps maintain hemodynamic stability by augmenting cardiac output by increasing venous return to the heart. Additionally, rightward rotation enlists gravity to facilitate subluxation of the heart, thereby simplifying visualization of the coronary arteries of the lateral, posterior, and inferior walls. Extreme degrees of rotation may be necessary to obtain hemodynamically tolerable positions for some difficult anastomoses.

Target Exposure and Stabilization

Optimal target vessel exposure and three-dimensional stabilization are essential for successful off-pump bypass surgery. Two approaches used to manipulate the heart and expose the

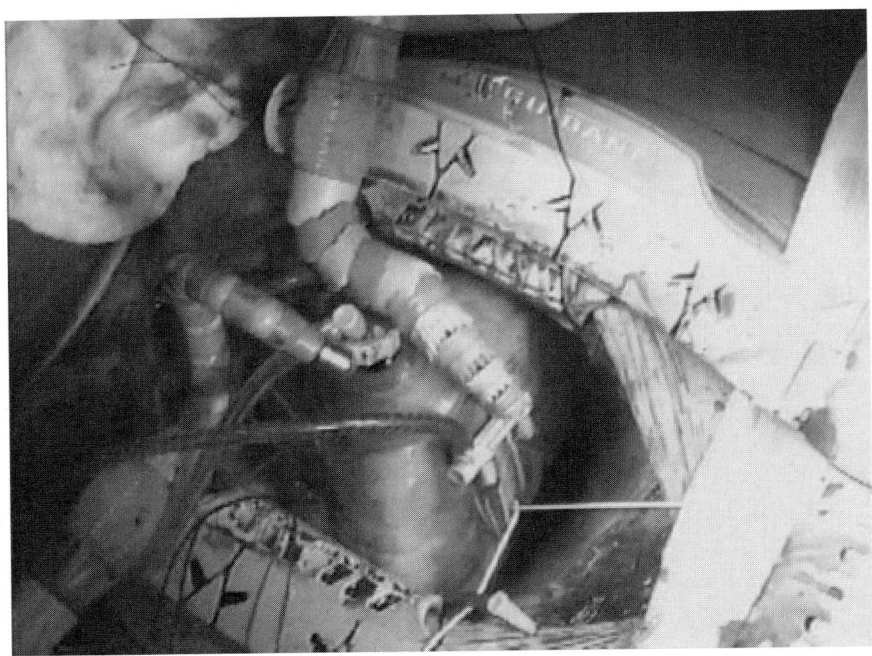

FIGURE 22–1 Custom off-pump sternotomy retractor. Note suture holders and tracts for attachment of stabilizer and suction exposure device.

coronary arteries involve the use of deep pericardial traction sutures or apical suction devices.[34] Deep pericardial traction sutures elevate and rotate the heart by placing tension on and distorting the pericardial well. Typically, three or four sutures are utilized with this technique (Fig. 22-3). The first suture is placed deep in the pericardium just anterior to the left superior pulmonary vein, the second just anterior to the left inferior pulmonary vein, and the third midway between the inferior pulmonary vein and the inferior vena cava. A fourth suture can be placed anterior to the inferior vena cava to expose the diaphragmatic surface of the right ventricle. Differential tension on these sutures rotates the heart and exposes the anterior, lateral, posterolateral, and inferior arteries. Care must be taken to avoid injury to the phrenic nerve, underlying lung, or the pulmonary veins when using this technique.

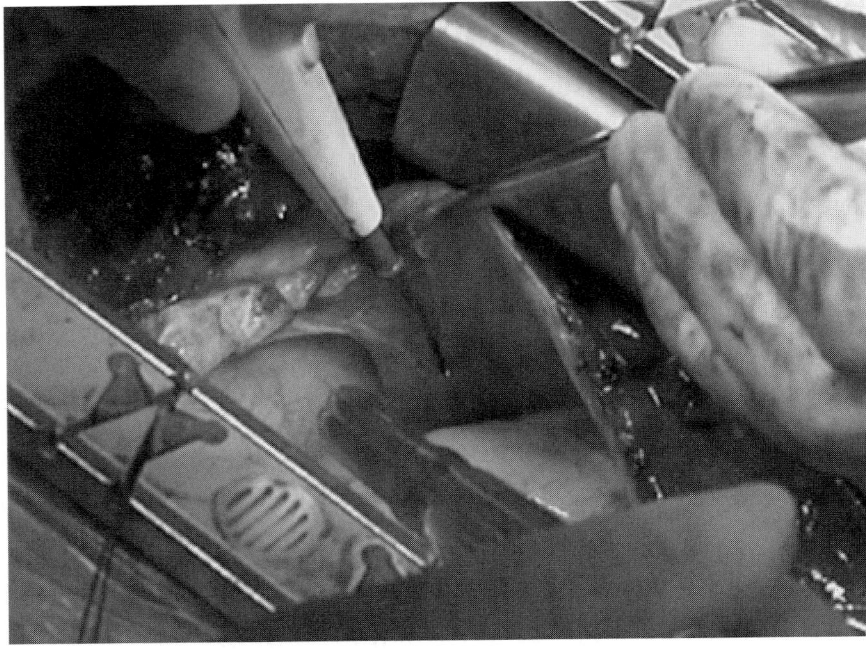

FIGURE 22–2 Extension of the pericardial incision along the right diaphragmatic reflection to create room for the right ventricle during displacement.

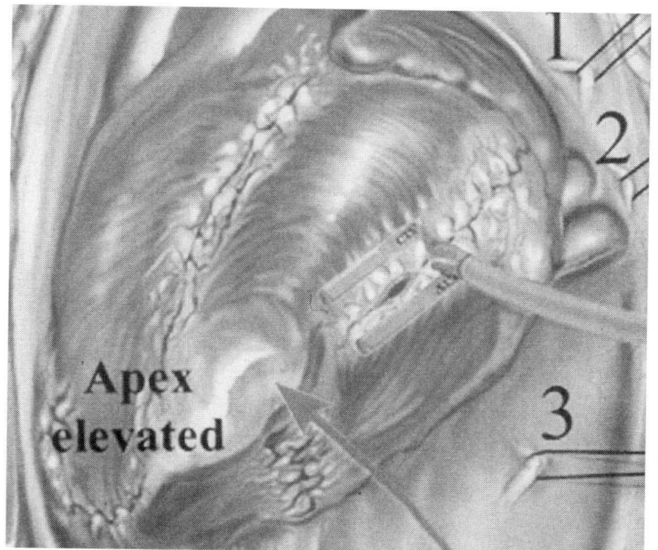

FIGURE 22–3 Placement of deep pericardial sutures for cardiac displacement during exposure of the posterior circulation.

Apical suction devices allow distraction and manipulation of the heart by creating a vacuum-type seal to the epicardial surface (Fig. 22-4). These devices extend from reticulating arms that attach to the sternal retractor and allow the heart to be positioned for optimal vessel exposure. The anterior descending, diagonal, and obtuse marginal vessels are presented by applying suction and moving the apex of the heart towards the right sternum. Suction applied to the acute margin of the heart with retraction towards the left shoulder exposes the distal right coronary artery and its branch vessels. A significant advantage to these devices is that they maintain the normal geometry of the heart and avoid compression to the right ventricle. This improves hemodynamic stability when grafting difficult arteries, especially in patients with reduced ejection fractions.

Stabilization of the target vessel for the anastomosis can be obtained either by using a compression-type stabilizer or a suction stabilizer.[35] Both types are shaped like two-pronged forks. With compression type, immobility of the target is achieved by placing the stabilizer straddling and parallel to the artery and using pressure to stabilize the area. These devices typically have a textured surface to prevent slippage when applied to the epicardium. Suction-type stabilizers consist of pods of suction cups within the prongs of the stabilizer that immobilize the target area by creating a vacuum between the epicardium surface and the stabilizer arm (Fig. 22-5). These tools allow for construction of the anastomosis to take place in a motionless field.

Grafting Strategy

The sequence of graft construction is crucial to the success of the procedure (Table 22-4). In general, collateralized vessels should be grafted before collateralizing vessels. Additionally, a bloodless field is necessary in order to perform a precise distal anastomosis. Proximal control of the vessel selected for grafting is obtained with a soft silastic tape mounted on a blunt needle (Fig. 22-5). This suture is placed circumferentially just proximal to the site of the anastomosis. Tension applied to the suture restricts blood flow by inflow occlusion

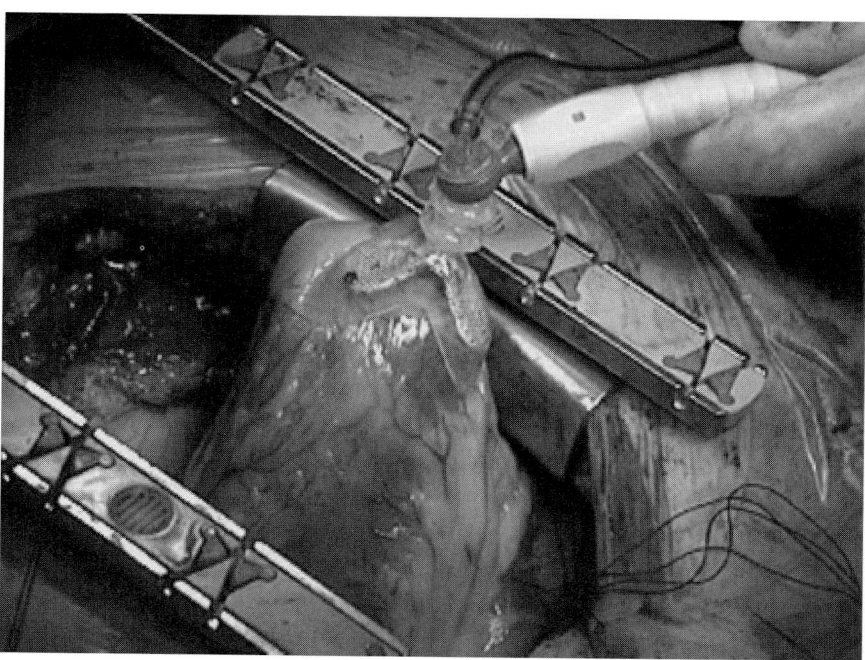

FIGURE 22–4 Attachment of an apical suction device to the epicardial surface to facilitate exposure of the posterior circulation without compression or distortion of the right ventricle.

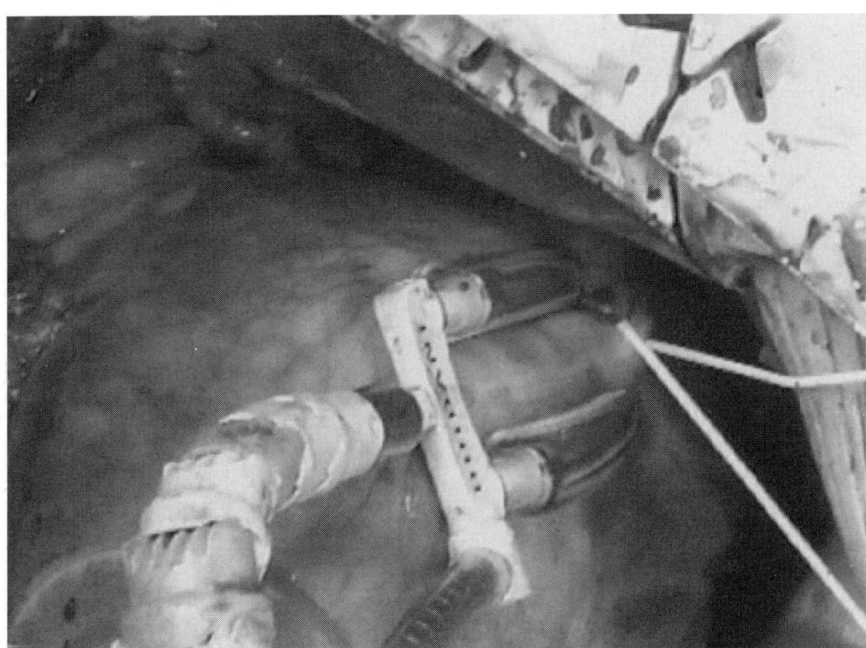

FIGURE 22–5 Suction stabilizer device placed adjacent to the obtuse marginal circumflex branch for local immobilization. Note Silastic snare around the proximal vessel.

and facilitates the anastomosis. A distal snare can be placed if back bleeding from collateralizing vessels is problematic. However, most surgeons avoid distal loops because of potential damage to the intima of the outflow portion of the grafted artery.[36] A misted carbon dioxide blower is also employed to clear blood from the field and open the arteriotomy during the anastomosis (Fig. 22-6). A heparinized, pH-balanced solution should be used in the blower.[37] The flow rate of the carbon dioxide from the blower should be limited to the minimal level needed to perform the anastomosis because excessive gas jet velocity can injure the target coronary endothelium or the conduits.[37] Intracoronary shunts may be employed to provide distal vessel perfusion during the construction of the anastomosis if ischemia is a concern. Patience is rewarded when positioning the heart to expose the target vessels. Small changes in positioning can have profound hemodynamic effects. Avoidance of overreacting to pressure changes and close collaboration with the anesthesiologist generally allow the heart to be positioned with acceptable hemodynamics and exposure for the anastomosis.

TABLE 22–4 Grafting strategy for OPCAB—easiest to hardest

Collateralized vessels before collateralizing
Left anterior descending with LIMA
Proximal anastomosis before distals
Diagonal artery
Main right coronary artery
Posterior descending artery
Distal circumflex, second, third obtuse marginal vessels
Posterior lateral artery
Proximal obtuse marginal artery
Ramus intermedius artery

OPCAB = off-pump coronary artery bypass; LIMA = left internal mammary artery.

The left anterior descending artery (LAD) is typically the first anastomosis performed using the internal mammary artery. This vessel is the easiest to expose and access, and allows revascularization of the septum and anterior wall prior to other provocative maneuvers. Exposure is usually obtained by placing a moist laparotomy pad behind the heart to bring the vessel to the midline. An exception to this strategy is if the anterior descending artery collateralizes a completely occluded right coronary artery (RCA), thereby providing the sole blood supply to the septum, anterior, and inferior walls. This circumstance dictates initial grafting of the right coronary artery in order to limit the amount of myocardium made ischemic during occlusion of the left anterior descending artery. A stabilizing foot is then placed straddling the target area and the vessel exposed. An intramyocardially located LAD can be particularly challenging. This situation can be successfully addressed by careful attention to the details of exposure. The dissection is not initiated until the stabilizing foot is in place. A misted carbon dioxide blower is utilized to maintain a bloodless field. Exposure of the LAD begins distally where it emerges onto the epicardial surface near the apex of the heart. Dissection then proceeds proximally by relocating the stabilizer until a segment of artery suitable for grafting is identified. Shed blood is scavenged using a cell saver. Intracoronary shunts can be used if the arteriotomy is centered over a septal perforator in order to reduce blood loss and aid in visualization. After completion of the LAD anastomosis, a tacking suture is placed to secure

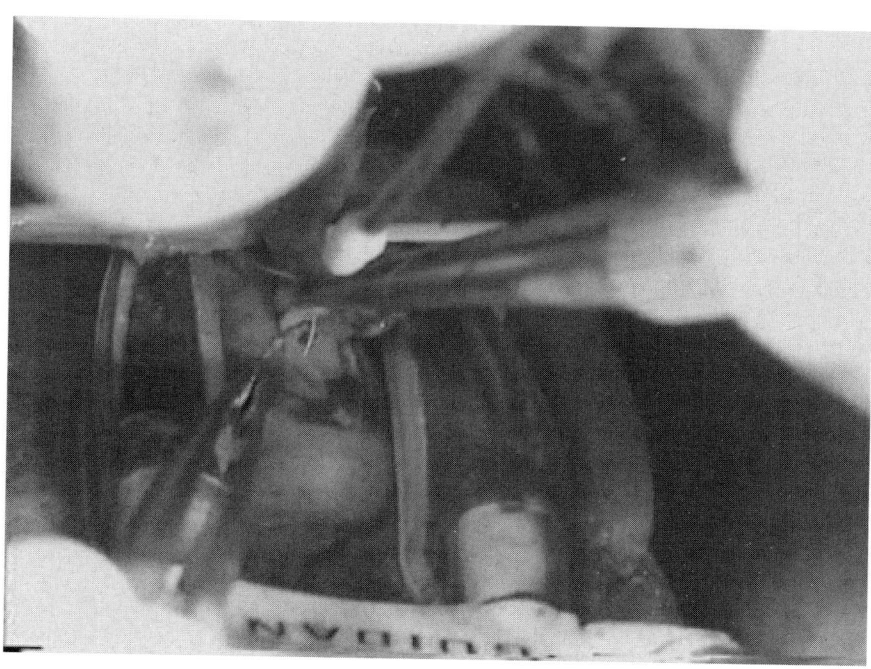

FIGURE 22–6 Creation of a motionless, bloodless operative field for a distal anastomosis to the left anterior descending coronary artery by use of a suction exposure device, a proximal Silastic snare, and a misted CO_2 blower.

the pedicle to the epicardium to eliminate torsion on the anastomosis.

Grafting is then continued by performing the easier anastomoses prior to the more difficult ones. The diagonal arteries on the anterior surface of the heart are relatively straightforward to graft, and can be exposed by either using the laparotomy pad or placing a suction device on the apex of the heart and moving the vessel to the midline. This position is hemodynamically well tolerated in most patients. Grafting then commences in standard fashion by placing the silastic suture for inflow occlusion and stabilizing the target site.

The main right coronary artery, while generally easy to demonstrate, can be problematic to graft. Problems most frequently occur when a large dominant, moderately stenotic right coronary is to be bypassed proximal to the crux. Proximal occlusion causes ischemia to the atrioventricular node; this manifests as bradycardia and heart block that can lead to ventricular distension and cardiovascular collapse. Helpful maneuvers as previously noted include placing atrial and ventricular pacing wires prior to making the arteriotomy, as well as placing an intracoronary shunt to provide perfusion to the atrioventricular node. Trendelenburg positioning and suction distraction on the acute margin of the heart cephalad provide excellent exposure of the mid to distal right coronary artery.

The posterior descending artery follows in degree of difficulty to expose and graft. A similar approach is used to that of exposing the distal right coronary artery but with the angle of distraction oriented more towards the left shoulder of the patient. This positioning simplifies the anastomosis by placing the posterior descending artery on a level plane thereby maintaining a consistent focal length for the surgeon. Bradyarrythmias and hemodynamic problems are rarely seen with occlusion of this vessel, as opposed to the right coronary artery.

The next most accessible vessels would include the mid to distal obtuse marginal branches and the posterior ventricular artery. The heart is positioned with the apex pointing towards the right mid sternum utilizing a suction device. The patient is also rotated to the right towards the surgeon as far as necessary to achieve adequate visualization of the target vessel. Release of right-sided pericardial stay sutures and/or opening of the pleura on the right side avoids compression of the right ventricle and maintains acceptable hemodynamics during the anastomosis.

The ramus intermedius artery presents the most challenge to expose due to compression on the right ventricular outflow tract and pulmonary artery. The introduction of suction devices to position the heart has decreased the hemodynamic alterations associated with exposing this difficult part of the heart. The apex of the heart is retracted towards the patient's right hip, and the table is rotated towards the surgeon. This area of the heart tends to be tethered by the nearby pericardial reflection, reducing its mobility and making exposure difficult.

Debate exists regarding whether the proximal anastomoses should be constructed prior to performance of the distal anastomosis or after. Proponents of constructing the proximal anastomoses first do so in order to provide immediate perfusion to the grafted artery at the conclusion of each distal anastomosis. However, for some surgeons estimating the appropriate graft length can be difficult, and they prefer doing all distal anastomoses first to avoid short or redundant

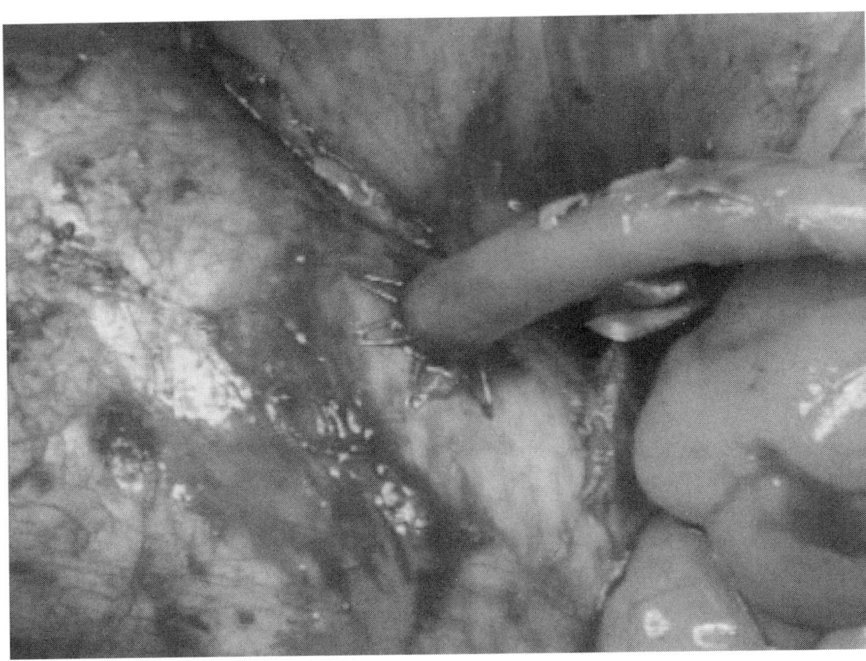

FIGURE 22–7 Aorto–saphenous vein anastomosis performed in a "clampless" fashion with an anastomotic connector.

grafts. With experience, most surgeons can reliably master the skill of estimating graft length. To avoid underestimating the length required, the exact target location should be determined prior to preparing the end of the graft for anastomosis. Additionally, the graft should be sized to the location where the anastomosis will rest with the heart in anatomic position, and not where the anastomosis is performed.

The proximal anastomoses are constructed using a partial occlusion clamp on a depressurized aorta. Many surgeons routinely use epiaortic scanning to survey the aorta for atheromatous disease that can escape even careful palpation.[38] Recent introduction of proximal anastomotic connectors obviates the need for a partial occlusion clamp, thereby reducing the risk of atheromatous embolization or aortic dissection with placement of the clamp (Fig. 22-7).[39]

Upon completion of the grafts, an assessment of the hemodynamic stability, the electrocardiogram (ECG), and the ventricular function of the patient is performed. Many surgeons do not routinely measure intraoperative graft flows, but rely instead on ECG changes or wall motion abnormalities detected by transesophageal echo. Small drainage tubes (19F Blake or Jackson-Pratt) are placed to facilitate immediate extubation. Pacing wires are placed according to the surgeon's discretion. The sternotomy is closed in standard fashion, and cell saver blood is returned to the patient.

PUMP-SUPPORTED BEATING HEART SURGERY

Patients taken to the operating suite who are hemodynamically unstable secondary to an acute myocardial infarction, acute coronary artery closure or dissection, or other catheterization lab misadventure represent a difficult population for traditional beating heart surgery. In these situations, the risk of global myocardial ischemia overshadows the use of extracorporeal circulation. One approach is to initiate cardiopulmonary bypass with standard aortic and venous cannulas, and perform the grafts with the heart beating but supported.[40] The patients are moderately cooled during the procedure, and perfusion pressures are maintained in the range of 60 to 80 mm Hg. Grafting then proceeds in similar fashion to off-pump beating heart surgery. This technique not only supplies hemodynamic stability, but also avoids ischemic cardioplegic arrest. Aortic clamping and manipulation can also be avoided by using anastomotic devices to perform the proximal anastomosis while on bypass.

THORACOTOMY FOR BEATING HEART BYPASS

Access to the heart via thoracotomy has been utilized for valvular procedures, repair of atrial septal defects, aortic arch and descending aortic aneurysm repair, aortic valve replacement, and minimally invasive and reoperative coronary artery bypass grafting.[41,42] Coronary reoperations continue to increase as patients experience progression of native vessel disease or attrition of previous bypass grafts. Patients undergoing reoperative coronary artery bypass grafting have an increased operative mortality and morbidity compared to patients undergoing primary revascularization.[7,43] Various strategies have evolved to minimize the risks of reoperative revascularization. These include avoiding repeat sternotomy when the potential exists to injure patent grafts, reducing the manipulation of the aorta or previous grafts to decrease the potential for embolization, and changing the approach to myocardial protection. Revascularization by minithoracotomy remains an alternative to standard grafting in a population at increased risk for morbidity and mortality.

After induction of general anesthesia and insertion of a double-lumen endotracheal tube, patients are placed in the right lateral decubitus position. Harvesting of bypass conduit (radial artery or saphenous vein) occurs prior to positioning. A left posterolateral thoracotomy incision is performed in the sixth or seventh intercostal space depending upon the target vessel selected for revascularization. The left lung is collapsed and the inferior pulmonary ligament divided. This allows mobilization of the lung superior to the level of the inferior pulmonary vein. Patients with previous LIMA grafts generally have adhesions between the lung and the mammary bed that must be taken down in order to fully mobilize the lung and expose the pericardium. The pericardium is opened longitudinally posterior to the phrenic nerve. Lysis of existing adhesions and target vessel identification are then performed. A Silastic suture is placed proximally around the target vessel to achieve vascular control. A stabilizer is positioned straddling the anastomotic area, and a misted CO_2 blower is used to keep the anastomotic site clear of blood and the edges of the artery separated. Senile grafts can be used as markers to identify the target vessels. The anastomosis is performed in a continuous fashion with a 7-0 prolene suture. The proximal anastomosis is then performed by means of a side-biting clamp on the descending aorta with a running 6-0 prolene suture. Proximal anastomotic connectors greatly facilitate the conduct of the operation and reduce the technical obstacles associated with operating deep within the chest. The graft is then positioned inferiorly to the hilum of the lung in a gentle curve (Fig. 22-8). An initial experience in revascularizing the circumflex distribution utilizing off-pump techniques via left minithoracotomy involving 32 patients was recently published.[44] There was no observed mortality. There was one reoperation for bleeding and one patient with a postoperative neurologic deficit. Off-pump bypass via thoracotomy provides a safe and effective alternative approach for patients requiring limited revascularization.

RESULTS

The argument supporting the efficacy of off-pump bypass surgery has been hindered by the observational nature of the majority of the studies reported in the literature. In designing research protocols, randomized controlled trials are accorded significantly more weight than are observational studies, primarily due to evidence of overestimation of treatment effects.[45–47] Randomized clinical trials also benefit by an absence of selection bias and adherence to an experimental method. Disadvantages to this model revolve around the expense in time and resources to complete trials of sufficient statistical power as to be meaningful within the scope of clinical practice. This is especially true in the investigation of variables with a low incidence of occurrence. In fact, many early studies have been limited by small sample sizes (statistical type II error), thus diminishing the strength of their conclusions. As larger studies, many randomized and controlled, are published, persuasive evidence in support of off-pump surgery continues to be generated.

Mortality

Multiple variables are known to affect patient mortality and morbidity after coronary artery bypass grafting. Opinion as to the safety of OPCAB has been based primarily on retrospective reviews of single and multi-institutional databases comparing large numbers of patients. Unfortunately, equally sized prospective randomized trials have yet to be reported. Two preliminary prospective randomized controlled studies comparing 30-day mortality between OPCAB and conventional bypass grafting have recently been published.[48,49] While no mortality benefit for OPCAB was identified, both studies were small and relatively underpowered to draw meaningful conclusions. A reduction in postoperative morbidity was observed in both reports.

To minimize the role of selection bias in retrospective observational studies, computer matching has been utilized to critically evaluate differences between off-pump and on-pump patients in regard to clinical outcomes. A recently published two-institution retrospective study of 1983 patients operated on from 1998 through 2000 utilized computer matching to compare patients revascularized with either conventional techniques or OPCAB.[50] In an effort to identify and control for selection bias, preoperative risk factors found by logistic regression analysis to be associated with off-pump selection were weighted by odds ratio, and a propensity score calculated for each patient. Off-pump and conventional surgery patients were then computer matched by propensity score, institution, and number of bypasses performed in a 1:2 ratio. These investigators found significant reductions in mortality, the incidence of perioperative myocardial infarction, reoperation for bleeding, transfusion of blood products, prolonged ventilation, and renal failure in the off-pump group (Table 22-5). Additionally, multivariate logistic regression analysis demonstrated that the use of cardiopulmonary bypass was independently associated with a 1.9 (95% CI, 1.2-3.1) times increased risk of death. A similar report compared 200 consecutive off-pump patients with a computer-matched contemporary cohort of 1000 patients.[51] Notable findings in the off-pump group include a mortality rate of 1%, a stroke rate of 1.5%, and a myocardial infarction rate of 1%. These outcomes, however, were not significantly different from the matched on-pump patients.

Several other institutions have also reported their beating heart experience, which correspondingly shows a decrease in

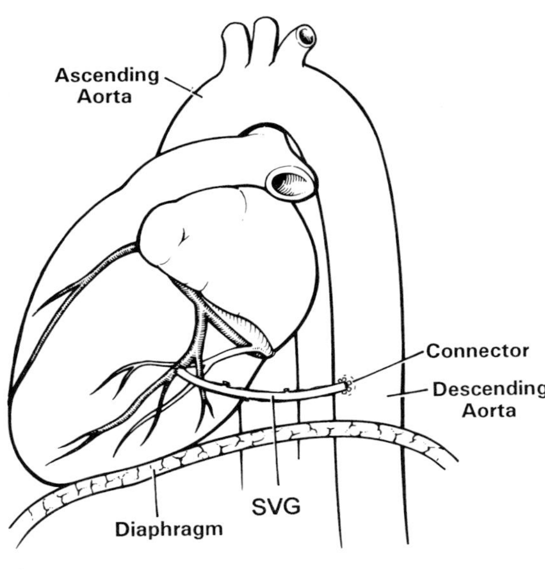

A.

FIGURE 22–8 Saphenous vein graft between descending aorta and an obtuse marginal branch of the circumflex coronary artery with a gentle curve beneath the inferior pulmonary vein.

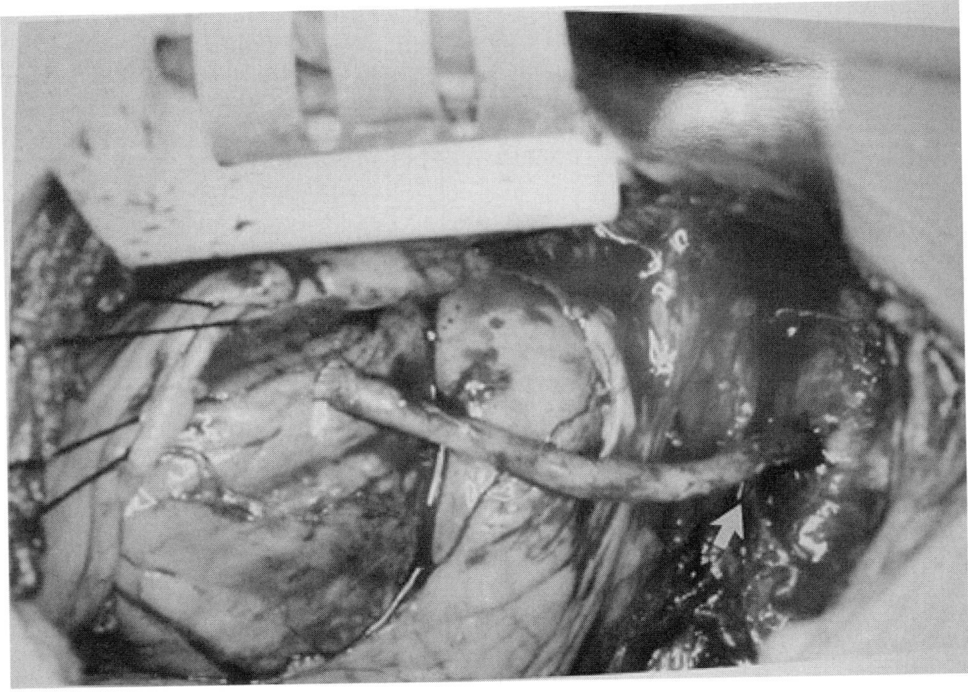

B.

mortality and complication rate in nonrandomized groups. One study recently reported 680 off-pump cases from 34 Department of Veterans Affairs medical centers.[52] Off-pump mortality and overall complication rates were lower (8.8% vs. 14%, $p = .001$) when compared to conventional bypass patients. Several nonrandomized studies examining mortality and risk-adjusted mortality between OPCAB and conventional bypass surgery have also been reported. The two largest studies demonstrate a significant mortality benefit for OPCAB in comparison to the on-pump patients.[53,54] While the other reports did not show significantly improved survival in off-pump patients, their small sample sizes may not have been powered to demonstrate significance (Table 22-5).[55–57]

A review of 17,000 isolated coronary bypass operations performed in 2001 in the 76 hospitals of the HCA National Hospital System demonstrated that 21.6% (3672) were performed off-pump.[15] There was significantly reduced mortality in the off-pump as compared to the on-pump population; 1.98% versus 2.38%, respectively ($p < .05$). Likewise, there

TABLE 22–5 Mortality for OPCAB versus CABG

Reference	OPCAB observed (%)	CABG observed (%)	*p*-value
Cleveland[54]	2.32	2.94	.001
Calafiore[60]	1.40	3.00	.016
Magee[50]	1.82	3.12	.002
Plomondon[52]	2.70	4.00	NS
Kshettry[56]	0.74	2.13	NS
Puskas[51]	1.00	2.20	NS
Pfister[57]	1.40	2.40	NS
Hernandez[55]	2.54	2.57	NS

OPCAB = off-pump coronary artery bypass; CABG = conventional coronary artery bypass grafting; NS = not significant.

was a statistically significant decrease in stroke, renal failure, reoperation for bleeding, length of stay, and hospital cost in the off-pump cohort. Interestingly, these results held true for both high- and low-volume centers.

Finally, two small observational reviews of OPCAB mortality in high-risk cohorts—reoperations and those with predicted mortality greater than 5%—have also been published.[58,59] Both reports demonstrated improved survival in the OPCAB group as compared to conventional bypass cohort. One can infer from the recent literature that OPCAB mortality is no worse than conventional bypass surgery, and probably significantly better in high-risk groups of patients.

Graft Patency

Reliable graft patency has been the foundation of surgical therapy for coronary artery disease. The goal of off-pump bypass grafting is to minimize procedural complications and patient trauma without compromising the outcomes traditionally demonstrated by surgical revascularization. To date no prospective randomized studies comparing the patency of grafts performed off-pump to those performed using conventional techniques have been published. OPCAB graft patency has been presumed equivalent to traditional patency based on several prospective nonrandomized studies (Table 22-6). The largest of these reports was from the group at Emory, who performed angiography on 167 patients out of a consecutive cohort of 200 patients undergoing OPCAB.[51] Angiographic assessment of 421 grafts was performed prior to hospital discharge. Overall graft patency was 98.8%, with 93.2% graded as Fitzgibbon A, 5.5% Fitzgibbon B, and 1.2% graded as Fitzgibbon O. All 163 left internal mammary artery grafts to the left anterior descending artery were patent. Among the grafts to other areas of the heart, 73 out of 74 grafts to the obtuse marginal vessels, 67 out of 68 grafts to the posterior descending artery, and 26 out of 26 right coronary grafts were also patent. This study corroborates the results of several smaller reports published previously that suggest an early patency comparable to the historic patency for conventional patients.

Excellent patency rates for conduits other than saphenous vein and the left internal mammary artery have also been described. A study from the group in Chieti, Italy, reported patency results for 122 OPCAB patients who had primary revascularization using two or more arterial conduits. Angiographic assessment was performed on 67 patients (55%) at an average of 33 ± 3.5 days after surgery. The patency rate was 98.8% overall, and 98.2% for the obtuse marginal branches.[60]

While conclusive evidence of equivalent patency awaits the reporting of large prospective randomized series, extrapolation of current results suggests that OPCAB may provide early patency similar to conventional surgery.

Morbidity

NEUROLOGIC

Of particular interest to off-pump practitioners is the effect of beating heart surgery on the neurologic and neurocognitive outcomes of their patients. Patients with atherosclerosis of the ascending aorta, who are at increased risk for atheromatous embolization from cannulation or aortic manipulation,

TABLE 22–6 Angiographic patency rates after OPCAB

Reference	Year	Patients (no.)	% Angiography	Timing	Grafts (no.)	Patency %
Calafiore[60]	1999	122	55	33-35 days	185	98
Izzat[89]	1999	24	100	intraop	42	95
Akpinar[90]	2000	126	56	P.T.DC	150	95
Omeroglu[91]	2000	696	10	24-61 mo	172	86
Zehr[92]	2000	50	100	<48 h	144	93
Bull[93]	2001	40	100	<48 h	108	97
Kim[94]	2001	122	92	<96 h	355	87*
Puskas[51]	2001	200	84	P.T.DC	399	93*

intraop = intraoperative; P.T.DC = prior to discharge; OPCAB = off-pump coronary artery bypass.
*Fitzgibbon grade A.

may benefit from off-pump CABG.[61,62] These atheromatous plaques have been recognized as sources of macroemboli that may result in postoperative stroke or neurocognitive dysfunction.[63] Early studies reported a reduced rate of release of S100B protein (a marker of cerebral injury) and a lower incidence of high-intensity transient signals by transcranial Doppler ultrasound after off-pump versus on-pump CABG.[64,65] Recent reports, however, call into question the validity of utilizing S100B as a marker because extracerebral sources have been identified. Blood from the surgical field as well as shed postoperative mediastinal blood have been found to contain significant amounts of S100B. Infusion of this blood back into the patient's circulation results in artificially elevated systemic S100B levels and inaccurate interpretation of results.[66] Ultimately, this question will only be resolved with a prospective randomized study.

Attention to the neurologic outcomes after bypass grafting has intensified since the reporting by the Perioperative Ischemia Research Group of a 6.1% incidence of adverse neurologic outcomes in coronary artery bypass patients, equally divided between focal deficits (stroke) (3.1%) and diffuse neurocognitive dysfunction (3%).[67] Patient age was a significant risk factor for the occurrence of a neurologic complication, with patients older than 80 years having a 16% incidence of neurologic problems after coronary artery bypass. Additionally, adverse neurologic events were associated with a 5- to 10-fold increase in observed mortality and a doubling of hospital length of stay. Furthermore, patients suffering neurologic complications were 30% to 47% more likely to be discharged to intermediate or long-term care facilities. In this study, the most significant predictor of stroke was the presence of atherosclerotic disease of the ascending aorta.

These findings were corroborated in a study reporting longitudinally assessed neurocognitive function after bypass grafting.[68] This article demonstrated that cognitive function could be adversely effected for up to five years after bypass grafting. In a randomized series comparing off-pump patients to conventional patients for neurological outcomes, researchers found that adverse changes were present in 90% of the on-bypass patients.[69] Conversely, they identified no neurocognitive changes in the off-pump cohort. These findings correlated with the number of cerebral emboli that were recorded in each group by transcranial Doppler and defined as high-intensive transient signals (HITS). The mean number of HITS were 394 (range 0 to 2217) in the conventional surgery group versus 11 in the off-pump cohort (range 0 to 50).

Neurologic injury remains the predominant complication in the elderly due to an increased incidence of atherosclerotic disease of the ascending aorta and cerebrovascular tree. In a series reported by the group in Buffalo, patients 80 years of age and older undergoing off-pump revascularization experienced significantly lower rates of perioperative stroke and overall complications compared to those undergoing similar procedures with CPB.[70]

TABLE 22–7 OPCAB neurologic events—postoperative stroke

Reference	OPCAB (%)	CABG (%)	*p*-value
Cleveland[54]	1.25	1.99	<.001
Iaco[71]	0.80	6.90	<.05
Van Dijk[48]	0.70	1.40	NS
Sabik[81]	0.70	1.30	NS
Puskas[51]	1.50	2.30	NS
Magee[50]	1.06	1.35	NS
Hernandez[55]	1.30	1.80	NS

OPCAB = off-pump coronary artery bypass; CABG = conventional coronary artery bypass grafting; NS = not significant.

Two recent large nonrandomized studies also report significant reduction in the rates of perioperative stroke in OPCAB patients versus conventional bypass patients (Table 22-7).[54,71] The largest of these reports utilizing the STS National Database documented a stroke rate of 1.25% (n = 11,717) in the OPCAB group versus 1.99% (n = 106,423; $p < .001$) in the bypass cohort. In contrast, two other observational and one prospective randomized trial failed to detect a significant difference in stroke rate between the OPCAB and conventional surgery groups (Table 22-7).

One can hypothesize that improved results should stem from eliminating the source of gaseous and particulate emboli, namely, the extracorporeal circuit. Additionally, neurologic outcomes may be improved by avoiding clamping a diseased ascending aorta, using anastomotic connectors, or placing filters in the aorta to catch particulate matter. A recent report involving 4823 patients compared neurologic outcomes after bypass grafting in which the proximal anastomoses were performed either with or without partial occlusion of the ascending aorta.[72] The patients were distributed into an on-pump cohort of 2830 patients and an OPCAB group of 1993 patients. Aortic manipulation using a side-biting clamp was an independent predictor of neurologic injury regardless of whether the procedure was performed off or on bypass. The variability of neurologic outcomes with OPCAB published in the literature only serves to underscore the difficulty of making meaningful inferences in regard to an event with infrequent incidence. Definitive conclusions regarding the improvement in neurologic and neurocognitive outcomes with off-pump revascularization await the result of a large prospective randomized series.

INFLAMMATORY RESPONSE

Conventional coronary revascularization employs cardiopulmonary bypass to maximally support the patient and provide optimal surgical conditions. However, the motionless and bloodless field obtained comes at a price. Numerous reports in the surgical literature detail the profound systemic effects produced by the exposure of the blood to foreign surfaces and shear stress. Cardiopulmonary bypass is associated with an intense systemic inflammatory response manifested by a systemic and pulmonary capillary leak, as well as pulmonary, renal, and neurocognitive dysfunction. A recent study demonstrated a rapid elevation of complement C3a and elastase upon institution of CPB, which was subsequently followed by increases in interleukin-8, tumor necrosis factor-α, and E-selectin.[73] Elevation of these factors was curtailed in patients having off-pump bypass.

MYOCARDIAL ISCHEMIA

The use of ischemic cardioplegic arrest to provide a flaccid heart has been associated with global myocardial ischemia and myocardial dysfunction.[74] Recent studies demonstrate a reduction in myocardial injury after off-pump versus on-pump CABG.[75,76] Specifically, levels of troponin T and I and creatine kinase MB isoenzymes were lower in the off-pump cohort, implying greater myocardial injury with conventional revascularization. Additionally, investigators have noted a reduced incidence of perioperative myocardial infarction in off-pump patients when compared to on-pump patients with multivessel grafting and complete revascularization.[77]

TRANSFUSION REQUIREMENTS

Two large randomized trials in the literature demonstrate that OPCAB patients require significantly fewer blood transfusions than do conventional bypass patients.[48,78] Additionally, several observational studies have investigated perioperative bleeding, and all confirm significantly less blood loss after OPCAB.

One particular patient subgroup felt to markedly benefit from off-pump surgery is the elderly. It is acknowledged that perioperative morbidity and mortality rates rise with increasing patient age. Additionally, it has been noted that an increasing number of octogenarians are presenting for coronary revascularization. Surgeons from the Washington Hospital Center reported a contemporary series of octogenarians in which off-pump bypass was associated with a substantially reduced rate of intraoperative transfusion, a marked reduction in the postoperative ventilatory time, and a reduced hospital length of stay when compared to conventional surgery.[79]

RENAL DYSFUNCTION

The etiology of renal dysfunction after conventional bypass grafting can be attributed to several factors, such as perioperative cardiovascular compromise with decreased renal perfusion, toxic insult to the kidneys, and the use of extracorporeal circulation. Free plasma hemoglobin, elastase, endothelin, and free radicals including superoxide, hydrogen peroxide, and the hydroxyl radicals can be generated during bypass and induce injury to the renal brush-border membrane. Additionally, nonpulsatile flow, renal hypoperfusion, hypothermia, and duration of bypass are felt to adversely effect renal function. In a prospective randomized study from the Bristol Heart Institute, renal function in 50 patients undergoing OPCAB and conventional bypass grafting was examined by following renal glomerular filtration rates using creatinine clearance and the urinary microalbumin/creatinine ratio.[80] Additionally, renal tubular function was tracked by measuring urinary N-acetyl-ß-glucosamine. While biochemical markers of glomerular filtration rate and renal tubular function were significantly improved in the OPCAB cohort, clinically relevant renal dysfunction was not different. Failure to identify a clinically significant end point can be attributed to the small number of patients randomized and the low incidence of acute renal failure in this population. Three retrospective studies comparing renal function between OPCAB and conventional surgery patients did, however, identify clinically significant acute renal dysfunction as defined by a greater than 50% increase in baseline creatinine or requiring dialysis (Table 22-8).[50,54,81] The large number of patients studied lends support to the conclusions reached in these observational investigations that OPCAB provides improved renal protection when compared to conventional bypass grafting.

TABLE 22–8 **Acute renal dysfunction in OPCAB**

Reference	OPCAB (%)	CABG (%)	*p*-value
Magee[13]	0.87	2.75	.036
Sabik[81]	0	1.50	.03
Cleveland[54]	3.85	4.26	.036

OPCAB = off-pump coronary artery bypass; CABG = conventional coronary artery bypass grafting.

Hospital Length of Stay/Economic Benefits

Current emphasis on cost containment in health care has initiated interest on the economics of surgical procedures. An important component of the cost of providing coronary artery bypass grafting is the length of time patients spend in the hospital after the procedure. The length of hospital stay after coronary artery bypass surgery is a function of multiple variables primarily related to a patient's premorbid condition and morbidity from the surgery. OPCAB has been demonstrated in numerous reports to facilitate earlier discharge for patients having surgical revascularization (Table 22-9). A recent prospective study of 281 patients randomized to OPCAB and conventional surgery demonstrated a significant reduction in length of stay, from 7 days to 6 days.[48] Furthermore, several retrospective studies have also shown significant differences in the length of time spent in the hospital after OPCAB compared to on-pump bypass.[50–53,58,71]

TABLE 22–9 Hospital length of stay

Reference	OPCAB (d)	CABG (d)	*p*-value
Puskas[51]	3.9	5.7	<.001
Iaco[71]	4	4.7	<.001
Calafiore[60]	4.1	5.4	<.001
Arom[58]	6.1	7.1	<.001
Magee[50]	5	6	<.0001
Plomondon[52]	6	7	.0005
Van Dijk[48]*	6	7	<.01

OPCAB = off-pump coronary artery bypass; CABG = conventional coronary artery bypass grafting.
*Randomized controlled trial.

In a prospective randomized study of 200 patients undergoing primary coronary artery bypass grafting from the United Kingdom, OPCAB was shown to be significantly less expensive than conventional surgery.[82] These savings were a result of an increased rate of complications, intubation time, ICU length of stay, and overall hospital length of stay in the on-pump cohort. By reducing the morbidity of the procedure as well as decreasing the incidence of complications, OPCAB has decreased hospital length of stay. This reduction in complications and morbidity translates into a more cost-effective operation.

COMPLICATIONS ASSOCIATED WITH OPCAB

Experience with beating heart surgery has uncovered unique complications associated with the procedure that separate it from conventional techniques. With the elimination of cardiopulmonary bypass, the platelet activation and defunctionalization that occur with exposure of blood to the foreign surface of the extracorporeal circuit are avoided. Comparison of platelet counts before and after bypass shows a striking reduction in absolute numbers[83,84]; furthermore, bleeding times as a measure of impaired hemostasis demonstrate a strong linear correlation with the length of time on bypass.[85] The significance of these changes appears to be increased thromboembolic complications and the introduction of a hypercoagulable state similar to that of any other major surgical procedure.[86] The consequences of this hypercoagulable state include an increased incidence of deep vein thrombosis, pulmonary embolism, and early graft occlusion.[87] Likewise, there have been reports in the literature detailing ascending aortic dissections related to placement of the partial occluding clamp on a distended pulsatile aorta.[88] Early graft occlusion as a result of increased thrombogenicity remains a theoretical concern. One approach has been to institute aggressive antiplatelet therapy in the early postoperative period by the administration of 325 mg of enteric-coated aspirin daily as well as loading patients with 150 mg to 300 mg of clopidrogrel. The patients are maintained on the clopidrogrel for approximately 30 to 90 days. The aspirin is continued indefinitely. An increase in early postoperative bleeding or delayed tamponade with this aggressive approach has not been observed.

Concerns also exist as to the risks and outcomes after a forced conversion from an off-pump approach to cardiopulmonary bypass, either due to unfavorable anatomy or patient deterioration. A review of the authors' experience from January 2000 to July 2001 identified 40 patients out of 1040 (3.8%) undergoing multivessel grafting that had conversion from an off-pump procedure to cardiopulmonary bypass.[85] Patients were classified as emergent, urgent, and elective in regard to the clinical situation surrounding the conversion. Operative mortality in the 40 converted patients was 15%, all of which occurred in the patients having urgent or emergent conversion. Risk factors predisposing to conversion included preoperative placement of an intra-aortic balloon pump, patients having redo bypass grafting, and early surgeon experience. This review demonstrates that delayed conversion to CPB when difficulties arise, especially early in a surgeon's beating heart experience, is associated with increased mortality. Persistence in the face of unfavorable anatomy or hemodynamic deterioration is potentially hazardous.

CONCLUSION

It is anticipated that the number of coronary artery bypass procedures performed without the aid of cardiopulmonary bypass will continue to increase in the near future. The impetus to change established practice patterns rests upon the scientific validation of the clinical benefits of off-pump surgery. Large multicenter studies are needed to produce confirmation of the clinical benefits seen in smaller observational reports. However, performance of these studies can be problematic given the inherent prejudice either for or against the technique by participating surgeons. It is notable that other techniques considered standards of care were introduced and adopted without validation by randomized studies, including the use of the left internal mammary artery as a conduit and mitral valve repair.

Other factors that will encourage the implementation of beating heart surgery include the introduction of new enabling technology and improvements in technique that simplify the procedure. Recent progress in stabilizer technology as well as the introduction of suction exposure and positioning devices further serve to make off-pump bypass increasingly applicable to a broad range of surgeons. Likewise, technologic advances such as anastomotic connectors can reduce operating time and compensate for the somewhat more challenging operative setting.

Coronary artery bypass surgery must continue to evolve in order contend with the success of catheter-based intervention. Surgical revascularization now comprises less than 30% of all coronary revascularization procedures. The anticipated erosion of the surgical patient base with the introduction of drug-eluting stents compels surgeons to identify and implement new techniques that reduce invasiveness while maintaining exceptional long-term results.

REFERENCES

1. Society of Thoracic Surgeons National Database Chicago, IL.
2. The Veterans Administration Coronary Artery Bypass Surgery Cooperative Study Group, 1984: Eleven-year survival in the Veterans Administration Randomized Trial of Coronary Bypass Surgery for stable angina. *N Engl J Med* 1984; 311:133.
3. European Coronary Surgery Study Group: Long-term results of prospective randomized study of coronary artery bypass surgery in stable angina pectoris. *Lancet* 1982; 2:1173.
4. CASS Principal Investigators and their associates: Coronary Artery Surgery Study (CASS): a randomized trial of coronary artery bypass surgery, survival data. *Circulation* 1983; 68:939.
5. Loop FD, Lytle BW, Cosgrove DM, et al: Influence of the internal mammary artery on 10-year survival and other cardiac events. *N Engl J Med* 1986; 316:1.
6. Lytle BW, Loop FD, Cosgrove DM, et al: Long-term (5 to 12 years) serial studies of internal mammary and saphenous coronary bypass grafts. *J Thorac Cardiovasc Surg* 1985; 89:35.
7. Lytle BW, Loop FD, Cosgrove DM, et al: Fifteen hundred coronary reoperations: results and determinants of early and late survival. *J Thorac Cardiovasc Surg* 1987; 93:47.
8. Reichenspurner H, Boehm DH, Welz A, et al: Minimally invasive coronary artery bypass grafting: port-access approach versus off-pump techniques. *Ann Thorac Surg* 1999; 66:1036.
9. Diegler A, Spyrantis N, Matin M, et al: The revival of surgical treatment for isolated proximal high-grade LAD lesions by minimally invasive coronary artery bypass grafting. *Eur J Cardiothorac Surg* 2000; 17:501.
10. Puskas JD, Wright CE, Ronson RS, et al: Off-pump multivessel coronary bypass via sternotomy is safe and effective. *Ann Thorac Surg* 1998; 66:1068.
11. Trehan N, Mishra M, Sharma OM, et al: Further reduction in stroke after off-pump coronary artery bypass grafting: a 10-year experience. *Ann Thorac Surg* 2001; 72:S1026.
12. Guler M, Kirali K, Toker ME, et al: Different CABG methods in patients with chronic obstructive pulmonary disease. *Ann Thorac Surg* 2001; 71:152.
13. Magee NJ, Dewey TM, Acuff TA, et al: Influence of diabetes on mortality and morbidity: off-pump coronary artery bypass grafting versus coronary artery bypass grafting with cardiopulmonary bypass. *Ann Thorac Surg* 2001; 71:776.
14. Dewey TM, Magee MJ, Edgerton JR, et al: Off-pump bypass grafting is safe in patients with left main coronary disease. *Ann Thorac Surg* 2001; 72:788.
15. HCA Case Mix Database, HCA Hospital Company, Nashville, TN.
16. Ricci M, Karamanoukian HL, Abraham R, et al: Stroke in octogenarians undergoing coronary artery surgery with and without cardiopulmonary bypass. *Ann Thorac Surg* 2000; 69:1471A.
17. Stamou SC, Dangas G, Dullum MKC, et al: Beating heart surgery in octogenarians: perioperative outcomes and comparison with younger age groups. *Ann Thorac Surg* 2000; 69:1140.
18. Koutlas TC, Elbeery JR, Williams JM, et al: Myocardial revascularization in the elderly using beating heart coronary artery bypass surgery. *Ann Thorac Surg* 2000; 69:1042.
19. Trehan N, Mishra M, Kasliwal RR, et al: Surgical strategies in patients at high risk for stroke undergoing coronary artery bypass grafting. *Ann Thorac Surg* 2000; 70:1037.
20. Stamou SC, Corso PJ: Coronary revascularization without cardiopulmonary bypass in high-risk patients: a route to the future. *Ann Thorac Surg* 2001; 71:1056.
21. Pasini E, Ferrari G, Cremona G, et al: Revascularization of severe hibernating myocardium in the beating heart: early hemodynamic and metabolic features. *Ann Thorac Surg* 2001; 71:176.
22. Locker C, Shapira I, Paz Y, et al: Emergency myocardial revascularization for acute myocardial infarction: survival benefit of avoiding cardiopulmonary bypass. *Eur J Cardiothorac Surg* 2000; 17:234.
23. Mohr R, Moshkovitch Y, Shapira I, et al: Coronary artery bypass without cardiopulmonary bypass with acute myocardial infarction. *J Thorac Cardiovasc Surg* 1999; 118:50.
24. Yokoyama T, Baumgartner FJ, Gheissari A, et al: Off-pump versus on-pump coronary bypass in high-risk subgroups. *Ann Thorac Surg* 2001; 72:1630.
25. Trehan N, Mishra YK, Malhotra R, et al: Off-pump redo coronary artery bypass grafting. *Ann Thorac Surg* 2000; 70:1026.
26. Watters MPR, Ascione R, Ryder IG, et al: Hemodynamic changes during beating heart coronary surgery with the "Bristol Technique." *Eur J Cardiothorac Surg* 2001; 19:3440.
27. Mathison M, Edgerton JR, Horswell JL, et al: Analysis of hemodynamic changes during beating heart surgical procedures. *Ann Thorac Surg* 2000; 70:1355.
28. Grundeman PF, Borst C Verlaan CWJ, et al: Exposure of circumflex branches in the tilted, beating porcine heart: echocardiographic evidence of right ventricular deformation and the effect of right or left heart bypass. *J Thorac Cardiovasc Surg* 1999; 118:316.
29. Porat E, Sharony R, Ivry S, et al: Hemodynamic changes and right heart support during vertical displacement of the beating heart. *Ann Thorac Surg* 2000; 69:1188.
30. Grundeman PF, Borst C, Van Herwaarden JA, et al: Vertical displacement of the beating heart by the Octopus tissue stabilizer: influence on coronary flow. *Ann Thorac Surg* 1998; 65:1348.
31. Nierich AP, Diephuis J, Jansen EWL, et al: Heart displacement during off pump CABG: how well is it tolerated? *Ann Thorac Surg* 2000; 70:466.
32. Edgerton JR, Dewey TM, Magee MJ, et al: Conversions in off-pump coronary artery bypass grafting (CABG): an analysis of predictors and outcomes. *Ann Thorac Surg (in press)*.
33. Quigley RL, Weiss SJ, Pym J, et al: Creative arterial bypass grafting can be performed on the beating heart. *Ann Thorac Surg* 2001; 72:793.
34. Baumgartner FJ, Gheissari A, Capouya ER, et al: Technical aspects of total revascularization in off-pump coronary bypass via sternotomy approach. *Ann Thorac Surg* 1999; 67:1653.
35. Scott NA, Knight JL, Bidstrup BP, et al: Systematic review of beating heart surgery with the Octopus® tissue stabilizer. *Eur J Cardiothorac Surg* 2002; 21:804.
36. Hangler HB, Pfaller K, Antretter H, et al: Coronary endothelial injury after local occlusion on the human beating heart. *Ann Thorac Surg* 2001; 71:122.
37. Burfiend WR, Duhaylongsod FG, Annex BH, et al: High-flow gas insufflation to facilitate MICABG: effects on coronary endothelium. *Ann Thorac Surg* 1998; 69:1246.
38. Ura M, Sakata R, Nakayama Y, et al: Extracorporeal circulation before and after ultrasonographic evaluation of the ascending aorta. *Ann Thorac Surg* 1999; 67:478.
39. Eckstein FS, Bonilla LF, Englberger L, et al: Minimizing aortic manipulation during OPCAB using the Symmetry connector system for proximal vein graft anastomosis. *Ann Thorac Surg* 2001; 72:S993.
40. Perrault LP, Menasche P, Peynet J, et al: On-pump, beating heart coronary operations in high-risk patients: an acceptable trade-off? *Ann Thorac Surg* 19997; 64:1368.
41. Bolton JWR: Left thoracotomy for reoperative revascularization of the posterior coronary circulation. *J Cardiovasc Surg* 1997; 38:407.

42. Coulson AS, Bakhshay SA, Sloan TJ: Minimally invasive reoperation through lateral thoracotomy for circumflex coronary artery bypass. *Tex Heart Inst J* 1998; 25:170.
43. Edwards FH, Clark RE, Schwartz M: Coronary artery bypass grafting: the Society of Thoracic Surgery national database experience. *Ann Thorac Surg* 1994; 57:12.
44. Dewey TM, Magee MJ, Edgerton J, et al: Left mini-thoracotomy for beating heart bypass grafting: a safe alternative to high-risk intervention for selected grafting of the circumflex artery distribution. *Circulation* 2001; 104(suppl I):I-99.
45. Benson K, Hartz AJ: A comparison of observational studies and randomized, controlled trials. *N Engl J Med* 2000; 342:1878.
46. Concato J, Shah N, Horwitz RI: Randomized, controlled trials, observational studies, and the hierarchy of research designs. *N Engl J Med* 2000; 342:1887.
47. Pocock SJ, Elbourne DR: Randomized trials or observational tribulations? *N Engl J Med* 2000; 342:1907.
48. Van Dijk D, Nierich AP, Jansen EWL, et al: Early outcome after off-pump versus on-pump coronary bypass surgery. *Circulation* 2001; 104:1761.
49. Angelini GD, Taylor FC, Reeves BC, et al: Early and midterm outcome after off-pump and on-pump surgery in beating heart against cardioplegic arrest studies (BHACAS 1 and 2): a pooled analysis of two randomized controlled trials. *Lancet* 2002; 359:1194.
50. Magee MJ, Jablonski KA, Stamou SC, et al: Elimination of cardiopulmonary bypass improves early survival for multivessel coronary artery bypass patients. *Ann Thorac Surg* 2002; 73:1196.
51. Puskas JD, Thourani VH, Marshall JJ, et al: Clinical outcomes, angiographic patency, and resource utilization in 200 consecutive off pump coronary bypass patients. *Ann Thorac Surg* 2001; 71:1477.
52. Plomondon ME, Cleveland JC, Ludwig ST, et al: Off pump coronary artery bypass is associated with improved risk-adjusted outcomes. *Ann Thorac Surg* 2001; 72:14.
53. Calafiore AM, Di Mauro M, Contini M, et al: Myocardial revascularization with and without cardiopulmonary bypass in multivessel disease: impact of the strategy on early outcome. *Ann Thorac Surg* 2001; 72:456.
54. Cleveland JC, Shroyer AL, Chen AY, et al: Off-pump coronary artery bypass grafting decreases risk-adjusted mortality and morbidity. *Ann Thorac Surg* 2001; 72:1282.
55. Hernandez F, Cohn WE, Baribeau YR, et al: In hospital outcomes of off-pump versus on-pump coronary artery bypass procedures: a multicenter experience. *Ann Thorac Surg* 2001; 72:1528.
56. Kshettry VR, Flavin TF, Emery RW, et al: Does multivessel off-pump coronary artery bypass reduce postoperative morbidity. *Ann Thorac Surg* 2000; 69:1725.
57. Pfister AJ, Zaki MS, Garcia JM, et al: Coronary artery bypass without cardiopulmonary bypass. *Ann Thorac Surg* 1992; 54:1085.
58. Arom KV, Flavin TF, Emery RW, et al: Safety and efficacy of off-pump bypass grafting. *Ann Thorac Surg* 2000; 69:704.
59. Stamou SC, Pfister AJ, Dangas G, et al: Beating heart versus conventional single-vessel reoperative coronary artery bypass. *Ann Thorac Surg* 2000; 69:1383.
60. Calafiore AM, Teodori G, Di Giammarco G, et al: Multiple arterial conduits without cardiopulmonary bypass: early angiographic results. *Ann Thorac Surg* 1999; 67:450.
61. Murkin JM, Boyd WD, Ganapathy S, et al: Beating heart surgery: why expect less central nervous system morbidity? *Ann Thorac Surg* 1999; 68:1498.
62. Cernaianu AC, Vassilidze TV, Flum DR, et al: Predictors of stroke after cardiac surgery. *J Card Surg* 1995; 10:334.
63. Trehan N, Mishra M, Kasliwal RR, et al: Reduced neurological injury during CABG in patients with mobile aortic atheromas: a five year follow-up study. *Ann Thorac Surg* 2000; 70:1558.
64. Anderson RE, Hansson LO, Vaage J: Release of S100B during coronary artery bypass grafting is reduced by off-pump surgery. *Ann Thorac Surg* 1999; 67:1721.
65. Watters MPR, Cohen AM, Monk CR, et al: Reduced cerebral embolic signals in beating heart surgery detected by transcranial doppler ultrasound. *Br J Anaesth* 2000; 84:629.
66. Jonsson H, Johnsson P, Alling C, et al: S100beta after coronary artery surgery: release pattern, source of contamination, and relation to neuropsychological outcome. *Ann Thorac Surg* 1999; 68:2202.
67. Roach GW, Kanchuger M, Mangano CM, et al: Adverse cerebral outcomes after coronary bypass surgery. *N Engl J Med* 1996; 335:1857.
68. Newman MF, Croughwell ND, Blumenthal JA, et al: Effect of aging on cerebral autoregulation during cardiopulmonary bypass: association with postoperative cognitive dysfunction. *Circulation* 1994; 90(5 pt 2): II243.
69. Diegeler A, Hirsch R, Schneider F, et al: Neuromonitoring and neurocognitive outcome in off-pump versus conventional coronary bypass operation. *Ann Thorac Surg* 2000; 69:1162.
70. Ricci M, Karamanoukian HL, Abraham R, et al: Stroke in octogenarians undergoing coronary artery surgery with and without cardiopulmonary bypass. *Ann Thorac Surg* 2000; 69:1471.
71. Iaco AL, Contini M, Teodori G, et al: Off or on-pump bypass: what is the safety threshold. *Ann Thorac Surg* 1999; 68:1486.
72. Calafiore AM, Di Mauro M, Teodori G, et al: Impact of aortic manipulation on incidence of cerebrovascular accidents after surgical myocardial revascularization. *Ann Thorac Surg* 2002; 73:1387.
73. Matata BM, Sosnowski AW, Galinanes M: Off-pump bypass graft operation significantly reduces oxidative stress and inflammation. *Ann Thorac Surg* 2000; 69:785.
74. Dailey PO, Pfeffer TA, Wisniewski JB, et al: Clinical comparisons of methods of myocardial protection. *J Thorac Cardiovasc Surg* 1987; 93:324.
75. Koh TW, Carr-White GS, DeSouza AC, et al: Intraoperative cardiac troponin T release and lactate metabolism during coronary artery surgery: comparison of beating heart with conventional coronary artery surgery with cardiopulmonary bypass. *Heart* 1999; 81:495.
76. Krejca M, Skiba J, Szmagala P, et al: Cardiac troponin T release during coronary surgery using intermittent cross-clamp with fibrillation, on-pump and off-pump beating heart. *Eur J Cardiothorac Surg* 1999; 16:337.
77. Bouchard D, Cartier R: Off-pump revascularization of multivessel coronary artery disease has a decreased myocardial infarction rate. *Eur J Cardiothorac Surg* 1998; 14(suppl 1):S20.
78. Ascione R, Williams S, Lloyd CT, et al: Reduced postoperative blood loss and transfusion requirement after beating heart coronary operations: a prospective randomized study. *J Thorac Cardiovasc Surg* 2001; 121:689.
79. Stamou SC, Pfister AJ, Dullum MKC, et al: Beating heart versus conventional coronary artery bypass grafting in octogenarians: early clinical outcomes. *J Am Coll Cardiol* 2000; 35(suppl A):341.
80. Ascione R, Lloyd CT, Underwood MJ, et al: On-pump versus off-pump coronary revascularization: evaluation of renal function. *Ann Thorac Surg* 1999; 68:49.
81. Sabik JF, Gillinov AM, Blackstone EH, et al: Does off-pump coronary surgery reduce morbidity and mortality. *J Thorac Cardiovasc Surg* 2002; 124:698.
82. Ascione R, Lloyd CT, Underwood MJ, et al: Economic outcome of off-pump coronary artery bypass surgery: a prospective randomized study. *Ann Thorac Surg* 1999; 68:2237.
83. Jung G, Razafindranaibe F, Elkouby A, et al: Modification in platelet shape and change in ATP release during CPB. *Haemostasis* 1995; 25:149.
84. Wahba A, Rothe G, Schmitz G, et al: Heparin effect on platelets and fibrinolysis. *Ann Thorac Surg* 1996; 61:1590.

85. Bertolino G, Locatelli A, Noris P, et al: Platelet composition and function in patients undergoing CPB for heart surgery. *Haemotologica* 1996; 81:116.
86. Mariani MA, Gu YJ, Boonstra PW, et al: Procoagulant activity after off pump coronary operation: is the current anticoagulation adequate? *Ann Thorac Surg* 1999; 67:1370.
87. Cartier R, Robitaille D: Thrombotic complications in beating heart operations. *J Thorac Cardiovasc Surg* 2001; 121:920.
88. Chavanon O, Carrier M, Cartier R, et al: Increased incidence of acute ascending aortic dissection with off pump aortocoronary bypass surgery? *Ann Thorac Surg* 2001; 71:117.
89. Izzat MB, Khaw KS, Atassi W, et al: Routine intraoperative angiography improves the early patency of coronary artery grafts performed on the beating heart. *Chest* 1999; 155:987.
90. Akpinar B, Guden M, Sagbas E, et al: Off-pump coronary artery bypass grafting with use of the Octopus 2 stabilization system. *Heart Surg Forum* 2000; 3:282.
91. Omeroglu SN, Kirahi K, Guler M, et al: Midterm angiographic assessment of coronary artery bypass grafting without cardiopulmonary bypass. *Ann Thorac Surg* 2000; 70:844.
92. Zehr K, Harda N, Bonilla LF, et al: Pitfalls and results of immediate angiography after off-pump coronary artery bypass grafting. *Heart Surg Forum* 2000; 3:293.
93. Bull DA, Nuemayer LA, Stringham JC, et al: Coronary artery bypass grafting with cardiopulmonary bypass versus off-pump cardiopulmonary bypass grafting: does eliminating the pump reduce morbidity and cost? *Ann Thorac Surg* 2001; 71:170.
94. Kim KB, Lim C, Lee C, et al: Off-pump coronary artery bypass may decrease the patency of saphenous vein grafts. *Ann Thorac Surg* 2001; 72:S1033.

Chapter 23

Myocardial Revascularization with Carotid Artery Disease

Cary W. Akins/Ashby C. Moncure

Next to operative mortality, an irreversible perioperative cerebrovascular accident is the most dreaded perioperative complication of myocardial revascularization, primarily because of the devastating consequences to the patient, but also because of the significantly increased cost of hospitalization and posthospital care. Perioperative stroke following coronary artery bypass grafting increasingly concerns the cardiac surgeon, because the average age of coronary bypass patients continues to rise and with it the risk of stroke. This chapter will investigate the relationship of carotid artery disease to perioperative neurologic complications following myocardial revascularization and evaluate treatment options for dealing with severe carotid artery stenosis that may occur in patients presenting for coronary artery bypass grafting (CABG).

PERIOPERATIVE STROKE

Incidence of Perioperative Stroke

To better understand the magnitude of the problem of perioperative cerebrovascular accidents after CABG, one need only review the literature on the rising incidence of stroke. In 1986 Gardner et al[1] reported the risk of stroke in their coronary bypass patients to be a direct function of patient age. For patients younger than 45 years the risk of perioperative stroke was 0.2%, rising to 3.0% for patients in their 60s, and to 8.0% for patients older than 75. The risk factors associated with stroke were increased age, preexisting cerebrovascular disease, ascending aortic atherosclerosis, prolonged cardiopulmonary bypass time, and severe perioperative hypotension.

Tuman et al in 1992[2] investigated the effects of age on the incidence of low cardiac output, myocardial infarction, and neurologic injury in coronary bypass patients. Whereas the incidence of low cardiac output and myocardial infarction was constant as patient age increased, the risk of neurologic damage rose exponentially after age 65. The stroke rate rose from 0.9% for patients younger than 65 years to 8.9% for patients older than 75.

To place the problem of the increasing age of coronary bypass patients into a more contemporary context, at the Massachusetts General Hospital the mean age of patients having coronary artery bypass grafting has risen from 56 years in 1980 to over 68 years in 2001. In addition, in 1980 only 6% of patients were age 70 or older, whereas by 2001 over 45% were age 70 or older and 13% were age 80 or older.

John et al[3] reported that the New York State Cardiac Surgical Database recorded a stroke rate of 1.4% in 19,224 patients having coronary artery bypass grafting in 1995. Multivariable predictors of stroke included aortic calcification, renal failure, prior stroke, smoking, carotid vascular disease, age, peripheral vascular disease, and diabetes. In their review of 10,860 patients having primary myocardial revascularization between 1986 and 1996, Puskas et al[4] noted that stroke occurred in 2.2%. Multivariable predictors of stroke were age, previous transient ischemic attack, and carotid bruits.

Cost of Perioperative Stroke

In the study cited above by Puskas et al,[4] perioperative stroke was associated with significantly more in-hospital morbidity, longer length of stay, and almost twice the hospital cost. Patients in that study who suffered a perioperative stroke had a 23% hospital mortality rate. Roach et al[5] noted a 21% mortality rate for patients suffering a perioperative stroke following coronary artery bypass grafting and a mean hospital stay of 25 days among survivors.

Causes of Perioperative Stroke

Given that the rate of perioperative stroke is a function of patient age, it is useful to consider the possible causes of perioperative neurologic injury (Table 23-1). The most common cause of perioperative stroke is atherosclerotic or thrombotic embolic debris from the heart or major vessels. Less commonly, entrained air may cause neurologic events, although rarely focal deficits. Intracardiac emboli can arise from mural thrombus secondary to myocardial infarction, left atrial thrombus associated with mitral valve disease or atrial fibrillation, or suture lines in the left atrium or left ventricle for venting the left heart or for access to left-sided structures. Catheters in the left side of the heart can also be a source of postoperative emboli.

TABLE 23–1 Potential causes of perioperative neurologic injury during coronary artery bypass grafting

Vascular occlusion, usually embolic
Heart
Aorta
Inominate, carotid, or vertebral arteries
Low flow phenomenon
Insufficient perfusion pressure on cardiopulmonary bypass
Poor collateral circulation
Vascular spasm
Intracranial hemorrhage

The aorta has been increasingly recognized as a source of embolic debris. Cannulation of the ascending aorta for cardiopulmonary bypass, the use of aortic occlusion clamps, and intra-aortic cardioplegia delivery devices increase the risk of dislodging any existing atherosclerotic material from the aortic wall. Wareing et al have demonstrated that aortic atherosclerosis is an important contributor to perioperative neurologic injury.[6] Routine use of intraoperative echocardiography of the ascending aorta to identify the degree of atherosclerosis of the aorta and the subsequent alteration of operative techniques to accommodate to the identified problems led to an improved stroke risk in their patients.

Embolism from diseased carotid arteries is a well-defined cause of perioperative neurologic injury. Evidence exists that the carotid plaque morphology has an important impact on the stroke risk for patients with carotid stenosis. A companion study to the North American Symptomatic Carotid Endarterectomy Trial found that ulcerated carotid plaques were significant incremental risk factors for stroke across all degrees of carotid stenosis.[7]

Neurologic injury can result from inadequate blood flow on cardiopulmonary bypass. The importance of adequate perfusion pressure on bypass has been emphasized by Schwartz et al.[8] They noted that cerebral blood flow is dependent on arterial perfusion pressures, not on cardiopulmonary bypass flow rates. Low cerebral blood flow occurred with perfusion pressures less than 60 mm Hg and was not influenced by the pump flow rate. Obviously, adequate perfusion pressure is even more of an issue in the presence of carotid stenosis. When there is occlusion of carotid or intracerebral arteries, blood flow to portions of the brain is dependent upon collateral circulation, which in turn is dependent on perfusion pressure. Whether carotid or intracerebral vascular spasm can contribute to neurologic injury is open to question.

Finally, the development of intracranial hemorrhage may contribute to neurologic injury following cardiopulmonary bypass, but the fact that this does not occur more frequently is surprising, given that patients are fully anticoagulated for cardiopulmonary bypass. In fact, in our institution, where CT scanning is routine following the clinical suspicion of a perioperative stroke to guide the use of heparin for cerebrovascular accident, the finding of intracerebral bleeding is extremely uncommon.

From a surgical point of view, of all the potential causes of perioperative neurologic injury listed in Table 23-1, carotid stenosis is the one anatomic situation about which the surgeon can routinely take action to remove the pathology. Thus the importance of defining carotid disease as a true potential risk factor for perioperative stroke becomes obvious.

Relationship of Carotid Stenosis to Perioperative Stroke

Early studies related the presence of carotid stenosis to development of perioperative neurologic injuries using auscultatory evidence of carotid disease as the method of diagnosis. In 1988 Reed et al from our institution investigated the relationship between carotid bruits and perioperative stroke,[9] and documented a 3.9-fold increase in the odds ratio for stroke in the presence of a carotid bruit.

Unfortunately, carotid bruits are not reliable indicators of internal carotid stenosis, nor are they discriminatory as to the degree of stenosis. In 1994, Sauve et al, in the North American Symptomatic Carotid Endarterectomy Trial, found poor correlation between auscultatory findings and the degree of carotid stenosis, as defined by carotid angiography.[10] Indeed, as carotid lesions progress to high degrees of stenosis, a carotid bruit may become inaudible.

Much better definition of the degree of carotid stenosis is obtained with noninvasive carotid testing using Doppler ultrasound techniques. The reliability of these methods to quantify the degree of stenosis and provide visual images of the stenosis has made these methods the initial method of choice in evaluating patients suspected of having carotid occlusive disease.

Brener et al studied 4047 cardiac surgical patients and found a 9.2% rate of stroke or transient ischemic attack in patients with asymptomatic carotid stenosis, which was significantly greater than the 1.3% rate in patients with no carotid stenosis.[11]

Faggioli et al published an important study in 1990 on the efficacy of routine carotid noninvasive testing in coronary artery bypass patients with no ischemic neurologic symptoms.[12] The odds ratio for stroke increased 9.9-fold in the presence of a greater than 75% carotid stenosis. For patients over age 60 with a greater than 75% carotid stenosis, the stroke rate was 15%, versus 0.6% for patients of the same age with no carotid disease. Perioperative strokes occurred in 4 (14.3%) of the 28 patients who had a greater than 75% carotid stenosis who did not have concomitant carotid endarterectomy, compared to no strokes in the 19 patients with a greater than 75% carotid stenosis who had a prophylactic carotid endarterectomy with their coronary artery bypass grafting.

In 1992 Berens et al reported their results with routine carotid duplex scanning for all cardiac surgical patients 65 years of age or older.[13] The risk of stroke was 2.5% for carotid lesions that were greater than 50%, 7.6% for carotid stenoses that were greater than 50%, 10.9% for carotid stenoses greater than 80%, and 10.9% for unilateral carotid artery occlusion.

Thus, adequate evidence exists that significant carotid artery stenosis is an important incremental risk factor for the development of perioperative neurologic injury following coronary artery bypass grafting. In addition, the study by Faggioli et al[12] suggests that carotid endarterectomy performed with coronary grafting yields a lower stroke rate.

Mechanism of Perioperative Stroke with Carotid Stenosis

Exactly how carotid stenoses cause perioperative strokes is not well understood, especially since patients are fully anticoagulated while on cardiopulmonary bypass. Perioperative strokes due to carotid artery disease may result from emboli from the carotid plaque itself. Loss of pulsatile perfusion or failure to maintain an adequate perfusion pressure on bypass may lead to diminished flow distal to a significant stenosis, resulting in a watershed stroke. However, Reed et al[9] reported that more than half of the strokes occur following the immediate postoperative period. These delayed strokes in patients with uncorrected carotid stenoses may be related to the prothrombotic milieu that is thought to occur in the early days after cardiopulmonary bypass.

Relationship of Uncorrected Carotid Stenosis to Late Stroke

In 1985 Barnes et al assessed the late risk of untreated asymptomatic carotid stenosis in 65 patients who had cardiovascular operations, of whom 40 had coronary artery bypass grafting.[14] At a mean follow-up of only 22 months, 10% of the coronary bypass patients had died, and 17.5% had suffered a stroke. Late noninvasive carotid testing revealed progression of the carotid artery disease in half of the patients within four years.

CAROTID STENOSIS IN CORONARY ARTERY BYPASS PATIENTS

Incidence of Carotid Stenosis in Coronary Artery Bypass Patients

In 1977 Mehigan et al reported that routine noninvasive testing in 874 patients prior to myocardial revascularization revealed a 6% incidence of significant extracranial cerebrovascular disease.[15] Ivey et al reported in 1984 that routine screening for a history of neurologic events and for cervical bruits in 1035 patients having isolated coronary artery bypass grafting revealed significant carotid stenosis confirmed by ultrasonic duplex scanning in 86 patients (8.3%).[16] In addition in the study noted above, Faggioli et al[12] evaluated 539 neurologically asymptomatic coronary artery bypass patients using noninvasive methods. In their study 8.7% of the patients had a carotid stenosis greater than 75%. The incidence rose from 3.8% for patients younger than 60 years to 11.3% for patients over 60.

Berens et al reported the results of routine carotid duplex ultrasonography in 1087 candidates for cardiac surgery who were 65 years of age or older (91% with coronary artery disease).[13] In their population with a mean age of 72 years, 186 (17.0%) had a greater than 50% carotid stenosis and 65 (5.9%) had a greater than 80% carotid stenosis. Predictors of severe carotid disease were female gender, peripheral vascular disease, history of transient ischemic attacks or stroke, smoking history, and left main coronary artery disease.

D'Agostino et al performed nonivasive carotid testing in 1279 coronary bypass candidates and found that 262 (20.5%) had greater than 50% stenosis in at least one carotid artery and 23 (1.8%) had bilateral stenoses greater than 80%.[17] Significant multivariable predictors of significant carotid disease were age, diabetes, female sex, left main coronary disease, prior stroke, peripheral vascular disease, and smoking.

Diagnosis of Carotid Artery Disease

PHYSICAL EXAMINATION

Auscultation of a bruit over the neck may provide some evidence of a carotid artery stenosis, but it is neither diagnostic nor capable of revealing the degree of carotid stenosis.[10] Indeed, as the degree of stenosis increases and approaches total occlusion, the bruit may fade and become inaudible. Palpation of the carotid artery provides no useful information and theoretically can dislodge thrombus or embolic debris.

NONINVASIVE TESTING

Given that auscultatory examination of carotid bruits is not a reliable way to assess the degree of carotid stenosis, and that direct carotid angiography is both too expensive and invasive to serve as an initial test for all patients suspected to have carotid artery disease, noninvasive methods of assessing carotid stenosis are the procedures of choice for screening patients.

Indirect testing One method of noninvasive indirect testing that has some usefulness in assessing the degree of carotid stenosis is oculoplethysmography, an indirect measurement of the pressure in the ophthalmic artery, which in turn reflects the pressure in the distal internal carotid artery. The test compares pressure in the contralateral normal artery to decreased pressures on the side of the carotid stenosis and can provide an estimate of the severity of the carotid stenosis.

Another indirect testing method is transcranial Doppler, which assesses ophthalmic and intracranial arterial flow and is useful in elucidating the status of collateral flow above a lesion at the origin or in the siphon of the internal carotid artery. This method can detect additional disease in the intracranial extension of the internal carotid system, especially the middle cerebral artery. Evaluation of the vertebral and basilar arteries with this method can also provide information about disease in those arterial systems that may be contributory to neurologic symptoms.

Direct testing Direct testing usually takes the form of either duplex ultrasonography or triplex ultrasound scanning. In duplex ultrasound scanning, a range-gated Doppler probe is directed at the bifurcation of the common carotid artery, the origins of the internal and external carotid arteries, and the more distal portions of those vessels. The Doppler probe samples a small volume of flowing blood in the artery at the point of maximum stenosis, just distal to the point of maximal stenosis where there is the greatest turbulence, and then further distally in the artery where laminar flow is reestablished. A higher flow velocity means a tighter stenosis, and a tighter stenosis creates greater turbulence. This mode of testing provides information about residual lumen diameter and plaque morphology. Plaque ulceration and calcification can also be identified. The value of the study is very dependent on patient cooperation and the skill of the technician. Duplex scanning cannot easily distinguish between complete occlusion and near occlusion with only a minimal residual lumen.

Triplex ultrasound scanning, or color flow Doppler, combines the B-mode imaging of duplex scanning with a multigated pulse Doppler, which allows flow measurements across the entire vascular structure. As an added advantage over duplex scanning, the data can be converted to color-coded flow displays over the B-mode image of the vessel. Although the method can reveal turbulence over a larger area, this technique cannot differentiate near from total occlusion.

Indications for noninvasive testing Current indications for performing noninvasive carotid testing include patients with:

1. An audible bruit in the neck
2. History of a prior stroke
3. History of transient ischemic attacks
4. Patients with severe peripheral vascular disease
5. Elderly patients

All of the above are quite self-explanatory, except the last. Because the incidence of carotid stenosis rises dramatically in patients over age 65, there must be an age at which it becomes cost-effective to screen all patients for carotid disease. This fact is particularly pertinent since the publication of numerous randomized trials verifying the efficacy of carotid endarterectomy as treatment for both symptomatic and asymptomatic severe carotid stenoses (a topic that will be discussed in detail below.) However, that age limit has not yet been clearly determined. Such a determination will have to demonstrate the cost advantage of routine carotid endarterectomy versus allowing uncorrected carotid stenoses to lead to expensive cerebrovascular accidents in some patients.

DIRECT CAROTID ANGIOGRAPHY

Until several years ago in our institution, a noninvasive test suggesting severe carotid stenosis was an indication for direct carotid angiography. For patients with an audible bruit who were actively neurologically symptomatic, direct carotid angiography was utilized without the need for noninvasive testing. Direct carotid angiography yields detailed images of the carotid arteries and their pathology and can identify ulcerative lesions, the degree of stenosis, and often the presence of mural thrombus. The technique also provides information on the distal vessels and collateral circulation. Unfortunately, carotid angiography is not without risks, including aortic dissection or embolization of debris from carotid lesions. Cholesterol embolization due to catheter manipulation in a diseased aorta can cause embolic compromise of other vascular distributions, especially the renal arteries. Finally, the technique is quite expensive.

MAGNETIC RESONANCE ANGIOGRAPHY

Beginning in the early 1990s, magnetic resonance angiography was increasingly used to define the degree and location of carotid lesions. The advantage of magnetic resonance angiography over direct carotid angiography is that it is essentially noninvasive, thereby eliminating the risk of procedure-related strokes. A severe stenosis is usually manifested by signal dropout when the stenosis is greater than 70%. Unfortunately, this technique cannot distinguish total from near total occlusion. In addition there is little true cost savings over direct angiographic techniques.

Definition of Severe Carotid Artery Stenosis

The definition of severe carotid stenosis varies from study to study and has changed as techniques used to investigate carotid artery disease have changed. When direct carotid angiography is used to define the degree of stenosis, severe stenosis was judged to be one that reduced residual diameter to less than 1.5 mm or one that reduced residual lumen diameter by more than 70%. Using magnetic resonance angiography, a severe stenosis is one that causes signal dropout.

EFFICACY OF CAROTID ENDARTERECTOMY AS A TREATMENT FOR CAROTID STENOSIS

Until the 1990s, there was considerable debate as to whether or not carotid endarterectomy improved survival and yielded a lower incidence of neurologic events in patients with documented carotid stenosis. This controversy existed both for patients with symptomatic and, more particularly, asymptomatic carotid lesions. Several studies and randomized trials addressed this issue and reported results that supported the operative approach as the more efficacious.

Carotid Endarterectomy for Symptomatic Carotid Stenosis

In 1986 Hertzer et al studied 211 previously unoperated patients with transient ischemic attacks or strokes and a carotid stenosis greater than 50% on digital subtraction angiography.[18] Nonoperative treatment was continued in 126 patients, while 85 had carotid endarterectomy. Although there was no difference in survival between the two groups at a mean follow-up of 36 months, carotid endarterectomy yielded significantly better freedom from late neurologic events for patients with (1) greater than 70% unilateral stenosis, (2) greater than 50% bilateral stenoses, and (3) a greater than 50% carotid stenosis in association with contralateral internal carotid occlusions.

In 1991 the results of the randomized North American Symptomatic Carotid Endarterectomy Trial of medical treatment or carotid endarterectomy in 659 patients were reported.[19] All patients had either hemispheric, retinal transient ischemic attacks or nondisabling strokes within 120 days of entry into the trial in association with a 70% to 99% stenosis in the symptomatic carotid artery. The actuarial cumulative risk of any ipsilateral stroke at two years was significantly lower at 9% in the 328 surgical patients versus 26% in the 331 medical patients. For major or fatal ipsilateral strokes, the risk was 2.5% for surgical patients versus 13.1% for medical patients ($p < .001$). When all strokes and deaths were included in the analysis, carotid endarterectomy was still found to be better than continued medical treatment.

Also in 1991, the Veterans Affairs Cooperative Study of symptomatic carotid stenosis reported its results of randomization of 189 men with stenoses greater than 50% ipsilateral to the presenting symptoms to medical or surgical treatment.[20] After one year there was a significant reduction in stroke or crescendo transient ischemic attacks in the patients having carotid endarterectomy (7.7%) compared to nonsurgically treated patients (19.4%). The results were even more divergent for patients with a carotid stenosis greater than 70%.

The European Carotid Surgery Trial randomized to medical or surgical treatment 2518 patients with a nondisabling stroke, transient ischemic attack, or retinal infarction in conjunction with stenosis in the ipsilateral carotid artery.[21] For the 778 patients with severe stenoses of 70% to 99%, the cumulative risk of stroke at carotid endarterectomy of 7.5%, plus an additional late stroke rate at three years of 2.8%, was less than the 16.8% rate for medically treated patients. At three years the cumulative risk of operative death, operative stroke, ipsilateral ischemic stroke, and any other stroke was 12.3% for the surgical cohort versus 21.9% for the medical group ($p < .01$). Finally the risk of fatal or disabling ipsilateral stroke at three years was 6.0% for the carotid endarterectomy patients versus 11.0% for the medical control patients ($p < .05$).

Therefore, one retrospective and three randomized trials have clearly established the superiority of carotid endarterectomy over continued medical treatment for patients with symptomatic severe carotid artery stenoses.

Carotid Endarterectomy for Asymptomatic Carotid Stenosis

Hertzer's group also studied operative and nonoperative treatment in 290 previously unoperated patients who had greater than 50% asymptomatic carotid artery stenoses identified by digital subtraction angiography.[22] During follow-up to about three years, prophylactic carotid endarterectomy in 95 patients yielded a significantly reduced incidence of subsequent neurologic events compared to continued medical treatment in 195 patients ($p = .05$).

The results of Veterans Affairs Cooperative Study of randomized medical treatment or carotid endarterectomy in 444 men with asymptomatic carotid artery stenosis, defined as greater than 50% in diameter reduction by angiography, were reported in 1993.[23] At a mean follow-up of four years, the combined incidence of ipsilateral neurologic events was 8.0% for the surgical patients versus 20.6% for the medical patients ($p < .001$). There was no significant difference between groups when all strokes and deaths were analyzed. Total mortality, including operative deaths, was due mostly to coronary artery ischemic events.

In 1995 the results of the Asymptomatic Carotid Atherosclerosis Study, which randomized 1662 patients to either carotid endarterectomy or continued medical treatment, were published.[24] In that trial a stenosis of more than 60% was defined as severe. After a mean follow-up of 2.7 years, the aggregate risk for ipsilateral stroke and any perioperative stroke or death for the surgical group was 5.1%, which was significantly lower than the rate of ipsilateral stroke of 11.0% for the medical group.

In summary, one retrospective and two randomized trials have documented a significant advantage of carotid endarterectomy over continued medical management for patients with severe asymptomatic carotid artery stenoses.

CAROTID STENTING

Following the success of percutaneous transluminal coronary angioplasty, particularly with adjunctive stenting, to treat coronary artery disease, interventionalists have attempted to treat carotid artery stenosis with angioplasty and stenting.[25–27] Early experience with combined coronary and carotid angioplasty has been reported.[28] Unlike coronary angioplasty, which if it leads to coronary artery embolism or occlusion may not significantly impact global left ventricular function, any carotid embolus or occlusion can result in disastrous neurologic complications. The issue of relative efficacy of carotid stenting versus conventional surgical endarterectomy is currently under investigation.[29]

MYOCARDIAL ISCHEMIC EVENTS IN PATIENTS WITH CAROTID ARTERY DISEASE

Although this chapter is primarily directed at the management of patients with known coronary artery disease who also have significant extracranial cerebrovascular disease, some comment on the contribution of ischemic heart disease to the short- and long-term risks of carotid endarterectomy patients is appropriate.

Incidence of Coronary Artery Disease in Carotid Endarterectomy Patients

Utilizing only clinical history and electrocardiographic studies in 614 carotid endarterectomy patients, Mackey et al found that 324 (53%) had overt evidence of coronary artery disease.[30] Assessing coronary disease in 106 carotid endarterectomy patients with thallium exercise testing, Urbinati et al found that 27 (25%) had significant defects on myocardial scanning.[31] In 1985 the Cleveland Clinic reported the results of routine preoperative coronary angiography in 506 carotid endarterectomy patients.[32] In that study only 7% of patients had normal coronary arteries, and 28% had mild to moderate coronary disease. However, 30% had advanced but compensated disease, 28% had severe, correctable disease, and 7% had severe, inoperable coronary disease.

Risk of Myocardial Ischemic Events

SHORT-TERM RISKS

The significant contribution of coronary artery ischemic events to the short-term risks of carotid endarterectomy has been well documented. In 1981 Hertzer et al assessed the myocardial risks in 335 carotid endarterectomy patients.[33] Hospital mortality occurred in 1.8%, of which 60% were due to coronary artery disease. Ennix et al[34] reported the mortality rate following carotid endarterectomy to be 4.9%, and the perioperative myocardial infarction rate to be 8.4%. In the study by Mackey et al cited above, carotid endarterectomy patients with clinically overt coronary artery disease had an operative mortality of 1.5% and a myocardial infarction rate of 4.3% compared with no mortality and an infarction rate of 0.5% for patients without overt coronary disease.[30] The incidence of myocardial infarction following carotid endarterectomy has been summarized to range from 1.5% to 5%.[35]

LONG-TERM RISKS

Mackey's study of carotid endarterectomy patients reported the 5-year and 10-year survival rates of patients with clinically overt coronary artery disease to be 68.6% and 44.9%, respectively, versus 86.4% and 72.3% for patients with no overt coronary disease.[30] When Urbinati et al followed their carotid endarterectomy patients, the 7-year freedom from all cardiac events was 51% for patients with silent myocardial ischemia compared to 98% for patients with normal thallium exercise testing.[31]

In the study cited above by Hertzer et al,[33] the 5-year mortality rate for hospital survivors was 27%, and 37% of those late deaths were due to myocardial infarction. In that same study 209 patients had clinically suspected coronary artery disease. Actuarial survival and reduction in the late mortality rate at 11 years were significantly better for the subgroup of patients with coronary artery disease who had myocardial revascularization. A later study from the same surgical group of 329 carotid endarterectomy patients followed to 10 years confirmed that myocardial infarction caused more late deaths (37%) than did stroke (15%).[36] Again, 10-year survival was significantly better for patients having coronary artery bypass grafting.

TIMING OF CAROTID AND CORONARY SURGERY

If one accepts that: (1) uncorrected carotid stenosis poses an important risk of neurologic events for patients with severe carotid and coronary artery disease who have only isolated coronary artery bypass grafting; (2) carotid endarterectomy is the indicated treatment for severe symptomatic and asymptomatic carotid stenosis; (3) coronary artery disease is a significant contributor to the short- and long-term risk for carotid endarterectomy patients; and (4) coronary artery bypass grafting is an indicated treatment for severe coronary artery disease, then the important question becomes not the indication for but the timing of the two operative procedures.

Staged Carotid and Coronary Operations

One approach is to perform the carotid endarterectomy and coronary artery bypass operations as staged procedures. Situations exist for which one can present a rationale for either operative procedure being the initial operation. By convention, performing the carotid endarterectomy before the coronary artery bypass grafting is referred to as a "staged procedure," while performing the coronary grafting followed by the carotid operation is called a "reversed staged procedure."

Most surgeons who advocate a sequential operative approach to patients with severe combined disease usually do the carotid endarterectomy initially (staged operation) if the patient is hemodynamically stable and not ischemic. Improvements in patient management, particularly better anesthetic techniques or the use of local anesthesia, have made some vascular surgeons comfortable doing carotid endarterectomy on patients who are stable from a cardiac point of view. However, the risk of a perioperative coronary ischemic event remains a real issue.

For patients with unstable cardiac symptoms, particularly those whose carotid stenoses are asymptomatic, some cardiac surgeons have opted to perform an initial myocardial revascularization followed by an interval carotid endarterectomy (reversed staged operation). The principal risk with this approach is the potential for neurologic complications either during or shortly after the myocardial revascularization.

Currently we advocate concomitant carotid and coronary bypass operations for virtually all patients with severe combined disease. However, in patients found to have severe bilateral carotid stenosis, a staged approach may be appropriate to deal with the second carotid lesion, especially if the patient is stable from a cardiac point of view. We occasionally treat the more severe of the two carotid lesions with initial isolated endarterectomy, followed by combined coronary artery bypass grafting and endarterectomy of the other carotid artery within a few days. Utilizing a reversed staged approach, namely, doing one carotid endarterectomy with myocardial revascularization followed several days later by the other carotid endarterectomy, is rarely utilized because of the increased stroke risk with reversed staged procedures (to be discussed below).

Concomitant Carotid and Coronary Operations

In 1972 Bernhard et al published the first report of successful combined carotid endarterectomy and coronary bypass grafting in 15 patients.[37] Since then, numerous groups have added their results to the published literature. The strategy of performing both operative procedures during one anesthetic is based upon the premise that only such an approach in patients with severe combined disease can minimize cardiac events that frequently complicate isolated carotid endarterectomy and neurologic events that complicate isolated coronary bypass grafting.

As reported by Daily et al,[38] one can also make a strong case that doing the two operative procedures together is more cost-effective than a staged or reversed staged approach, which requires two anesthetics and incurs the additional costs associated with extra days in the hospital between operations.

OPERATIVE TECHNIQUES FOR CONCOMITANT CAROTID AND CORONARY OPERATIONS

Standard Approach

The usual operative technique for concomitant carotid endarterectomy and coronary artery bypass grafting has been to perform the carotid endarterectomy during harvesting of coronary bypass conduits prior to cardiopulmonary bypass. This is the approach we routinely use at our institution, where the carotid operation is performed by peripheral vascular surgeons as the cardiac surgical team harvests whatever saphenous vein or other conduits may be needed.

The actual technique of carotid endarterectomy varies among our vascular surgeons. Several surgeons desire electroencephalographic monitoring and place an intravascular shunt if changes are noted on that study. Others routinely employ an intravascular shunt without using electroencephalographic monitoring. The decision to patch the carotid artery is usually based upon the size or tortuosity of the vessel. When vascular patches are used, they are usually saphenous vein.

After the carotid endarterectomy is completed, the neck incision is loosely approximated over a sponge. Final closure of the neck incision, usually over a temporary plastic drain, is performed after cardiopulmonary bypass is completed and heparinization is reversed.

Alternative Approaches

Minami et al reported using some perceived advantages of cardiopulmonary bypass, namely, heparinization, hypothermia, and hemodynamic control, to perform carotid endarterectomy in 116 patients while on bypass for myocardial revascularization.[39] Operative mortality was 1.7%, and total stroke risk was 4.3%. Weiss et al advocate performing the carotid endarterectomy on bypass with systemic hypothermia to 20°C and with the heart protected with retrograde blood cardioplegia.[40] In 23 patients they had no neurologic events and one postoperative death. Several surgical groups have adopted this approach, feeling that hypothermia on cardiopulmonary bypass provides an extra margin of ischemic protection for the brain during the carotid endarterectomy and avoids the need for intravascular shunting. The level of systemic hypothermia utilized has varied among surgical groups using this approach.

Whether or not this approach of performing the carotid and coronary operations on cardiopulmonary bypass saves total operative time is not proven, but it does prolong aortic occlusion and cardiopulmonary bypass times, something most cardiac surgeons would preferably avoid. A deeper level of hypothermia is not favored by most cardiac surgeons, particularly as the trend to using lesser degrees of hypothermia has become more popular.

HIGHLIGHTS OF POSTOPERATIVE MANAGEMENT

In our institution postoperative management of patients following concomitant carotid endarterectomy and coronary artery bypass grafting does not differ importantly from the management of patients having isolated myocardial revascularization. We believe that maintenance of a good coronary perfusion pressure, and by extension good cerebral perfusion pressure, in the early postoperative hours is beneficial. Early clearing of perioperative edema with diuresis seems to be efficacious.

The routine anticoagulation protocol for our myocardial revascularization patients, consisting of aspirin begun within six hours of completion of the operation, unless the patient is continuing to bleed, is adequate for patients who have either primary or saphenous vein patch closure of the carotid arterotomy. In cases in which a prosthetic patch is used, or the patient has considerable residual disease higher in the carotid system that cannot be removed, or there is uncorrected contralateral carotid disease, especially if the plaque is ulcerated, some surgeons prefer early anticoagulation with heparin, followed by long-term warfarin anticoagulation.

If a surgeon decides not to perform a carotid endarterectomy for a severe stenosis either as a staged approach or with a concomitant operation, then the increased incidence of stroke in the early days after isolated myocardial revascularization seen with the reversed staged approach would seem to suggest that heparinization of the patient would be appropriate once the acute bleeding risk of the coronary bypass operation is past.

RESULTS OF STAGED AND CONCOMITANT CAROTID AND CORONARY ARTERY OPERATIONS

Early Results

STAGED CAROTID AND CORONARY OPERATIONS

Several studies report the results of staged operations for concomitant carotid and coronary disease, but patients were randomized to concomitant or reversed staged operations in only one. Hertzer et al published a study containing a randomized subgroup of patients with unstable coronary syndromes and incidental asymptomatic carotid stenosis.[41] Over a five-year period they treated 275 patients with severe combined disease. Their criteria for carotid endarterectomy was either symptomatic and/or severe (greater than 70%) carotid disease. Only 24 (9%) of the patients were judged to have coronary disease stable enough to allow carotid endarterectomy prior to coronary artery bypass grafting. Of those 24 patients, one (4.2%) suffered a perioperative stroke after the preliminary carotid endarterectomy and died of a myocardial infarction while awaiting myocardial revascularization.

Symptomatic or severe bilateral carotid disease in 122 patients was treated with combined carotid and coronary operation with an operative mortality rate of 6.1% and a perioperative stroke rate of 7.1%.

The remaining 129 patients with unstable coronary symptoms and unilateral, asymptomatic, severe carotid stenoses were randomized to either a combined operation or a reversed staged operation. Patients having concomitant carotid and coronary operations had a mortality rate of 4.2% versus a combined rate of 5.3% for the two operations in the staged patients. The incidence of stroke in the concomitant operations was 2.8%, which was significantly lower than the 14% risk of the reversed staged operations (6.9% during the isolated coronary artery bypass grafting and 7.5% during the delayed isolated carotid endarterectomy). This study emphasizes the advantage of concomitant operations over reversed staged procedures.

In 1999 Borger et al reported the results of a meta-analysis of nonrandomized, observational studies published between 1972 and 1998 from centers that documented results with both staged and concomitant operations.[42] They identified a trend toward increased risk of stroke and death with combined operations. The results of this study need to be viewed with caution for several reasons. First, using meta-analysis to compare observational and not randomized studies limits its statistical power. Second, the surgical care strategy in most of these series was to treat unstable patients with combined operations and use staged procedures for stable patients. Third, the main criteria for entry into these studies was operations completed, not intention to treat. Thus one cannot be sure if some patients were eliminated from the study for whom a staged approach was planned, but the second operation was never performed because of a poor result from the first procedure.

CONCOMITANT CAROTID AND CORONARY OPERATIONS

Since the late 1970s some cardiac surgeons in our group have been aggressive in their approach to the patients with combined severe carotid and coronary artery disease, utilizing concomitant operative repair as the standard approach. Staged operations were reserved for the few patients with very stable coronary artery disease. In 1995 we published our early results with the first 200 consecutive patients having combined operations between 1979 and 1993.[43]

The average age of our patients having the combined operations was 67 years, about 6 years older than the mean age for all coronary bypass patients during that time period. Two thirds of the patients presented with unstable angina pectoris, and 42% had a prior myocardial infarction. Although the distribution of single-, double-, and triple-vessel disease was expected at 6%, 28%, and 65%, respectively, 43% of patients had significant left main coronary artery disease. Of the 200 patients, 115 (58%) were neurologically asymptomatic, 32% were having transient ischemic attacks, and 16% had a prior stroke. Unilateral severe carotid stenosis was found in 156 patients (78%), whereas 22% had some disease in the contralateral carotid artery.

Urgent or emergency operations were required in 33% of patients, of whom 4% were on the intra-aortic balloon pump. The average number of grafts per patient was 3.8. Only 50% overall received at least one mammary artery graft, but of the last 100 patients, 81% received a mammary graft.

Hospital mortality was 3.5%, perioperative myocardial infarction 2.5%, and perioperative stroke 4.0%, of which three quarters were permanent. Significant multivariate predictors of hospital death were postoperative stroke, failure to use an internal mammary graft, requirement for intraoperative intra-aortic balloon pumping, and nonelective operation. Peripheral vascular disease and unstable angina predicted postoperative stroke. Significant predictors of prolonged postoperative hospital stay were postoperative stroke, advanced age, and nonelective operation.

Vermeulen et al found the only significant multivariate predictor of hospital death in their study of 230 combined operations to be left main coronary artery disease.[44] Postoperative neurologic events were predicted by the presence of severe left ventricular dysfunction and preoperative neurologic events, either stroke or transient ischemic attacks.

Several series of concomitant carotid endarterectomy and coronary artery bypass grafting published since 1985 are noted in Table 23-2. In addition to our published results,[43] the table also includes our total results with concomitant carotid and coronary operations through 2001 in 500 consecutive patients.

We performed 500 consecutive combined operations for carotid and coronary disease between 1979 and 2001. The mean age of these patients was 69 years. The in-hospital complication rates were: mortality, 3.0%; myocardial infarction, 2.0%; and permanent stroke, 3.6 %. Of the 18 strokes, 9 were ipsilateral to the carotid endarterectomy while 9 were bilateral or contralateral, suggesting that our approach has neutralized unilateral carotid stenosis as a risk factor for perioperative stroke in these patients with complex, coexistent disease.

TABLE 23–2 Series since 1985 of combined carotid and coronary operations with >100 patients

Reference	Year	Patients (no.)	Mean age (y)	Deaths, no. (%)	MI,* no. (%)	Total CVA,** no. (%)	Permanent CVA,** no. (%)
Dunn[46]	1986	130	60	6 (4.6)	–	13 (10.0)	5 (3.8)
Hertzer[41]	1989	170	65	9 (5.3)	–	12 (7.1)	9 (5.3)
Vermeulen[44]	1992	230	63	8 (3.5)	4 (1.8)	13 (5.6)	7 (3.0)
Rizzo[45]	1992	127	65	7 (5.5)	6 (4.7)	8 (6.3)	7 (5.5)
Takach[47]	1997	255	66	10 (3.9)	12 (4.7)	10 (3.9)	10 (3.9)
Darling[48]	1998	420	69	10 (2.4)	1 (0.2)	13 (3.1)	5 (1.2)
Khaitan[49]	2000	121	69	7 (5.8)	–	9 (7.4)	7 (5.8)
Minami[50]	2000	340	65	9 (2.6)	2 (0.6)	16 (4.7)	11 (3.2)
TOTAL		1793	65	66 (3.7)	25 (1.4)	94 (5.2)	61 (3.4)
Akins[43]	1995	200	67	7 (3.5)	5 (2.5)	8 (4.0)	6 (3.0)
Akins, current		500	69	15 (3.0)	10 (2.0)	22 (4.4)	18 (3.6)

*Myocardial infarction.
**Cerebrovascular accident.

Late Results

Follow-up in our series of combined operations was 99% complete and revealed the following 10-year actuarial freedom from late events: death, 59%; myocardial infarction, 81%; percutaneous transluminal coronary angioplasty, 98%; reoperative myocardial revascularization, 94%; total stroke, 96%; ipsilateral stroke, 96%; and carotid endarterectomy, 94%.[43] Ten-year actuarial freedom from combined cardiac and neurologic morbidity and mortality was 57%.

Vermeulen et al found their 10-year actuarial freedom from cardiac events to be 50%, freedom from neurologic events to be 81%, and freedom from all events to be 41%.[44] The only significant multivariate predictors of late cardiac mortality in their study were the presence of severe left ventricular dysfunction and advanced age.

In a study of 127 combined carotid and coronary operations, Rizzo et al reported a 5-year survival rate of 70%, freedom from myocardial infarction of 84%, and freedom from stroke of 88%.[45] Survival was worse for patients with low ejection fractions. Late strokes were least common in patients who were neurologically asymptomatic preoperatively, more common in patients who were transiently symptomatic, and most frequent in patients with prior stroke.

SUMMARY

The risk of perioperative stroke following myocardial revascularization is directly related to the increasing age of coronary artery bypass patients, and this increasing age is accompanied by an increased incidence of carotid artery disease. Several studies have defined severe, uncorrected carotid stenosis as a major risk factor for perioperative stroke. Therefore, in addition to patients with audible carotid bruits or a history of ischemic neurologic events, patients who are 65 years old or older ought to have noninvasive carotid evaluation prior to surgical myocardial revascularization. In addition, excellent randomized trials have established the safety and efficacy of carotid endarterectomy as the most appropriate treatment for both symptomatic and asymptomatic severe carotid stenosis. Another randomized study has demonstrated the advantage of concomitant carotid endarterectomy and coronary artery bypass grafting over reversed staged operations. Thus, we advocate combined carotid and coronary operations for virtually all patients who present for coronary artery bypass grafting and who have significant carotid artery stenosis.

ACKNOWLEDGMENTS

This work was supported in part by a grant from the John F. Welch/GE Fund for Cardiac Surgical Research.

REFERENCES

1. Gardner TJ, Horneffer PJ, Manolio TA, et al: Major stroke after coronary artery bypass surgery: changing magnitude of the problem. *J Vasc Surg* 1986; 3:684.
2. Tuman KJ, McCarthy RJ, Najafi H, Ivankovich AD: Differential effects of advanced age on neurologic and cardiac risks on coronary artery operations. *J Thorac Cardiovasc Surg* 1992; 104:1510.
3. John R, Choudhri AF, Weinberg AD, et al: Multicenter review of preoperative risk factors for stroke after coronary artery bypass grafting. *Ann Thorac Surg* 2000; 69:30.
4. Puskas JD, Winston D, Wright CE, et al: Stroke after coronary artery operation: incidence, correlates, outcome, and cost. *Ann Thorac Surg* 2000; 69:1053.
5. Roach GW, Kanchuger M, Mangano CM, et al: Adverse cerebral outcomes after coronary bypass surgery. *N Engl J Med* 1996; 335:1857.
6. Wareing TH, Davila-Roman VG, Barzilai B, et al: Management of the severely atherosclerotic ascending aorta during cardiac operations. *J Thorac Cardiovasc Surg* 1992; 103:453.
7. Eliasziw M, Streifler JY, Fox AJ, et al: Significance of plaque ulceration in symptomatic patients with high-grade carotid stenosis. *Stroke* 1994; 25:304.

8. Schwartz AE, Sandhu AA, Kaplon RJ, et al: Cerebral blood flow is determined by arterial pressure and not cardiopulmonary bypass flow rate. *Ann Thorac Surg* 1995; 60:165.
9. Reed GL, Singer DE, Picard EH, DeSanctis RW: Stroke following coronary artery bypass surgery. *N Engl J Med* 1988; 319:1246.
10. Sauve JS, Thorpe KE, Sackett DL, et al: Can bruits distinguish high-grade from moderate symptomatic carotid stenosis? *Ann Intern Med* 1994; 120:633.
11. Brener BJ, Brief DK, Alpert J, et al: The risk of stroke in patients with asymptomatic carotid stenosis undergoing cardiac surgery: a follow-up study. *J Vasc Surg* 1987; 5:269.
12. Faggioli GL, Curl GR, Ricotta JJ: The role of carotid screening before coronary artery bypass. *J Vasc Surg* 1990; 12:724.
13. Berens ES, Kouchoukos NT, Murphy SF, Wareing TH: Preoperative carotid artery screening in elderly patients undergoing cardiac surgery. *J Vasc Surg* 1992; 15:313.
14. Barnes RW, Nix ML, Sansonetti D, et al: Late outcome of untreated asymptomatic carotid disease following cardiovascular operations. *J Vasc Surg* 1985; 2:843.
15. Mehigan JT, Buch SW, Pipkin RD, et al: A planned approach to coexistent cerebrovascular disease in coronary artery bypass candidates. *Arch Surg* 1977; 112:1403.
16. Ivey TD, Strandness DE, Williams DB, et al: Management of patients with carotid bruit undergoing cardiopulmonary bypass. *J Thorac Cardiovasc Surg* 1984; 87:183.
17. D'Agostino RS, Svensson LG, Neumann DJ, et al: Screening carotid ultrasonography and risk factors for stroke in coronary artery surgery patients. *Ann Thorac Surg* 1996; 62:1714.
18. Hertzer NR, Flanagan RA, O'Hara PJ, Beven EG: Surgical versus nonoperative treatment of symptomatic carotid stenosis. *Ann Surg* 1986; 204:154.
19. North American Symptomatic Carotid Endarterectomy Trial Collaborators: Beneficial effect of carotid endarterectomy in symptomatic patients with high-grade carotid stenosis. *N Engl J Med* 1991; 325:445.
20. Mayberg MR, Wilson SE, Yatsu F, et al: Carotid endarterectomy and prevention of cerebral ischemia in symptomatic carotid stenosis. *JAMA* 1991; 266:3289.
21. European Carotid Surgery Trialists' Collaborative Group: MRC European Carotid Surgery Trial: interim results for symptomatic patients with severe (70–99%) or with mild (0–29%) carotid stenosis. *Lancet* 1991; 337:1235.
22. Hertzer NR, Flanagan RA, O'Hara PJ, Beven EG: Surgical versus nonoperative treatment of asymptomatic carotid stenosis. *Ann Surg* 1986; 204:163.
23. Hobson RW, Weiss DG, Fields WS, et al: Efficacy of carotid endarterectomy for asymptomatic carotid stenosis. *N Engl J Med* 1993; 328:221.
24. Executive Committee for the Asymptomatic Carotid Atherosclerosis Study: Endarterectomy for asymptomatic carotid artery stenosis. *JAMA* 1995; 273:1421.
25. Namaguchi Y, Puyau FA, Provenza LJ, Richardson DE: Percutaneous transluminal angioplasty of the carotid artery: its application to post surgical stenosis. *Neuroradiology* 1984; 26:527.
26. Roubin GS, Yadav S, Iyer SS, et al: Carotid stent-supported angioplasty: a neurovascular intervention to prevent stroke. *Am J Cardiol* 1996; 78:8.
27. Mathur A, Roubin GS, Piamsomboom C, et al: Predictors of stroke following carotid stenting: univariate and multivariate analysis. *Circulation* 1997; 96:A1710.
28. Shawl FA, Efstratiou A, Hoff S, Dougherty K: Combined percutaneous carotid stenting and coronary angioplasty during acute ischemic neurologic and coronary syndromes. *Am J Cardiol* 1996; 77:1109.
29. Hobson RW 2nd: Update on the Carotid Revascularization Endarterectomy Versus Stent Trial (CREST) protocol. *J Am Coll Surg* 2002; 194(suppl):S9.
30. Mackey WC, O'Donnell TF, Callow AD: Cardiac risk in patients undergoing carotid endarterectomy: impact on perioperative and long-term mortality. *J Vasc Surg* 1990; 11:226.
31. Urbinati S, DiPasquale G, Andreoli A, et al: Frequency and prognostic significance of silent coronary artery disease in patients with cerebral ischemia undergoing carotid endarterectomy. *Am J Cardiol* 1992; 69:1166.
32. Hertzer NR, Young JR, Beven EG, et al: Coronary angiography in 506 patients with extracranial cerebrovascular disease. *Arch Intern Med* 1985; 145:849.
33. Hertzer NR, Lees CD: Fatal myocardial infarction following carotid endarterectomy. *Ann Surg* 1981; 194:212.
34. Ennix CL, Lawrie GM, Morris GC, et al: Improved results of carotid endarterectomy in patients with symptomatic coronary disease: an analysis of 1,546 consecutive carotid operations. *Stroke* 1979; 10:122.
35. Yeager R, Moneta R: Assessing the cardiac risk in vascular surgical patients: current status. *Perspec Vasc Surg* 1989; 2:18.
36. Hertzer NR, Arison R: Cumulative stroke and survival ten years after carotid endarterectomy. *J Vasc Surg* 1985; 2:661.
37. Bernhard VM, Johnson WD, Peterson JJ: Carotid artery stenosis: association with surgery for coronary artery disease. *Arch Surg* 1972; 105:837.
38. Daily PO, Freeman RK, Dembitsky WP, et al: Cost reduction by combined carotid endarterectomy and coronary artery bypass grafting. *J Thorac Cardiovasc Surg* 1996; 111:1185.
39. Minami K, Gawaz M, Ohlmeier H, et al: Management of concomitant occlusive disease of coronary and carotid arteries using cardiopulmonary bypass for both procedures. *J Cardiovasc Surg* 1989; 30:723.
40. Weiss SJ, Sutter FP, Shannon TO, Goldman SM: Combined cardiac operation and carotid endarterectomy during aortic cross-clamping. *Ann Thorac Surg* 1992; 53:813.
41. Hertzer NR, Loop FD, Beven EG, et al: Surgical staging for simultaneous coronary and carotid disease: a study including prospective randomization. *J Vasc Surg* 1989; 9:455.
42. Borger MA, Tremes SE, Weisel RD, et al: Coronary bypass and carotid endarterectomy: does a combined approach increase risk? A meta-analysis. *Ann Thorac Surg* 1999; 68:14.
43. Akins CW, Moncure AC, Daggett WM, et al: Safety and efficacy of concomitant carotid and coronary artery operations. *Ann Thorac Surg* 1995; 60:311.
44. Vermeulen FEE, Hamerlijnck RPHM, Defauw JJHM, Ernst SMPG: Synchronous operation for ischemic cardiac and cerebrovascular disease: early results and long-term follow-up. *Ann Thorac Surg* 1992; 53:381.
45. Rizzo RJ, Whittemore AD, Couper GS, et al: Combined carotid and coronary revascularization: the preferred approach to the severe vasculopath. *Ann Thorac Surg* 1992; 54:1099.
46. Dunn EJ: Concomitant cerebral and myocardial revascularization. *Surg Clin North Am* 1986; 66:385.
47. Takach TJ, Reul GJ, Cooley DA, et al: Is an integrated approach warranted for concomitant carotid and coronary artery disease? *Ann Thorac Surg* 1997; 64:16.
48. Darling RC, Dylewski M, Chang BB, et al: Combined carotid endarterectomy and coronary bypass grafting does not increase the risk of perioperative stroke. *Cardiovasc Surg* 1998; 6:448.
49. Khatian L, Sutter FP, Goldman SM, et al: Simultaneous carotid endarterectomy and coronary revascularization. *Ann Thorac Surg* 2000; 69:421.
50. Minami K, Fukahara K, Boethig D, et al: Long-term results of simultaneous carotid endarterectomy and myocardial revascularization with cardiopulmonary bypass used for both procedures. *J Thorac Cardiovasc Surg* 2000; 119:764.

Chapter 24

Myocardial Revascularization after Acute Myocardial Infarction

Daniel C. Lee/Windsor Ting/Mehmet C. Oz

The ability of surgical interventions to minimize myocardial loss following myocardial infarction has advanced dramatically over the past two decades. Acute myocardial infarctions still afflict approximately 1.1 million individuals each year in the United States.[1] About 250,000 Americans a year die before reaching the hospital.[1] Prompt medical attention, including transport to the hospital, diagnosis, and treatment of the myocardial infarction, is critical to patient survival. Since 1989, the death rate due to acute myocardial infarctions has declined 24%, while the actual number of deaths declined only 7%.[1] Over the last 40 years, especially during the 1980s, new pharmacologic agents, interventional cardiology procedures, and coronary artery bypass surgical techniques have advanced and have led to a decrease in the overall morbidity and mortality associated with acute myocardial infarction.[2,3] Despite this overall improvement, mechanical and electrical complications such as cardiogenic shock, rupture of the ventricular septum or free wall, acute mitral regurgitation, pericarditis, tamponade, and arrhythmias challenge the medical community caring for patients presenting with acute myocardial infarction on a daily basis.[2,3] Of these complications, cardiogenic shock complicating acute myocardial infarctions has the most significant impact on in-hospital mortality and long-term survival. Loss of more than 40% of functioning left ventricular mass is the major cause of cardiogenic shock and is determined by both the degree of preinfarction ventricular dysfunction and the size of the infarcted vessel.[4,5]

Restoration of blood flow to the threatened myocardium offers the best chance of survival following acute coronary occlusion, but the means and timing of revascularization continue to be a highly debated and studied topic. Thrombolytics, percutaneous transluminal coronary angioplasty, and coronary artery bypass surgery have decreased the mortality associated with acute myocardial infarctions. Advances in myocardial preservation and mechanical support lead the surgical armamentarium in the treatment of acute myocardial infarctions.

PATHOGENESIS OF ACUTE OCCLUSION

Myocardial ischemia due to coronary occlusion for as little as 60 seconds causes ischemic zone changes from a state of active systolic shortening to one of passive systolic lengthening.[6] Occlusions for less than 20 minutes usually cause reversible cellular damage and depressed function with subsequent myocardial stunning. Furthermore, reperfusion of the infarct leads to variable amounts of salvageable myocardium. After 40 minutes of ischemia followed by reperfusion, 60% to 70% of the ultimate infarct is salvageable, but this decreases dramatically to 10% after 3 hours of ischemia.[7,8] Animal model evidence has also demonstrated that 6 hours of regional ischemia produces extensive transmural necrosis.[9] The exact timing in humans is even more difficult to analyze because of collateral flow, which is a major determinant of myocardial necrosis in the area at risk in humans.[8] The collateral blood supply is extremely variable, especially in patients with long-standing coronary disease. However, collateral flow is jeopardized with arrhythmias, hypotension, or the rise of left ventricular end-diastolic pressure above tissue capillary pressure.[7] Thus loss of collateral flow to the infarct area may lead to the cellular death of salvageable myocardium. Control of blood pressure and prevention of arrhythmias are vital during this immediate time after infarction.

Many clinical trials have shown the beneficial effects of early reperfusion within 24 hours after acute myocardial infarction.[10] Although benefits of late reperfusion beyond 24 hours, particularly in asymptomatic patients, have yet to be shown in large clinical studies, advocates for aggressive management believe that reperfusion is warranted to preserve the border areas that may be underperfused during the early days after an infarction. While some of these patients may develop objective evidence of ischemia, the clinical assumption that a hypotensive patient with a suddenly dilated and pressure-overloaded ventricle is prone to losing more muscle mass in border zones of the infarct is reasonable. This is true even in patients who have had complete revascularization. Conservative measures, such as nitroglycerin and intra-aortic balloon pumps, have demonstrated their efficacy in this population of patients without clearly salvageable myocardium by improving coronary blood supply and reducing the work demand of the left ventricle. More radical approaches such as insertion of a left ventricular assist device (LVAD) have been advocated as well. At our center, placement of long-term assist devices into this group of patients has sometimes resulted in significantly improved ventricular function at the time of device explantation months later.[11,12]

TABLE 24–1 Factors that influence the evolution and severity of acute myocardial infarction

Anatomic
Site of lesion
Size of myocardium at risk
Collateral circulation
Physiologic
Arrhythmias
Coronary perfusion pressure
Myocardial oxygen consumption
Reperfusion injury
Stunned myocardium
Therapeutic options
Medical management
Revascularization
Thrombolysis
Percutaneous coronary angioplasty
Coronary artery surgery
Controlled reperfusion
Buckberg solution and technique
Mechanical circulatory support

Table 24-1 outlines the effects of anatomical, physiological, and therapeutic variables on the evolution of final infarct size. Anatomically, the location of the coronary obstructive lesion and additional diseased vessels and the presence of collateral flow will determine the extent of early injury, especially for borderline areas. However, ventricular remodeling of the infarct has important consequences influencing ventricular function after myocardial infarction.[13] Thus appropriate and aggressive invasive therapies such as PTCA, IABP, CABG, controlled reperfusion, and LVAD insertion can mitigate myocardial injury and salvage borderline areas even if the interventions occur many hours or days after the initial infarction, particularly in patients with ongoing ischemia.

Reperfusion injury also contributes to myocardial damage as free oxygen radicals are released and destroy endothelial cells and produce interstitial edema. The timing and management of reperfusion effects on myocardial damage may have an impact on both survival and functional recovery of individuals following acute myocardial infarction.[14] Some centers have argued convincingly that controlled reperfusion with specially designed perfusate and a decompressed, energy-conserving ventricle resting on cardiopulmonary bypass is the best means to preserve muscle mass.[15]

CARDIOGENIC SHOCK

Definition

Cardiogenic shock is defined clinically as a systolic blood pressure below 80 mm Hg in the absence of hypovolemia, peripheral vasoconstriction with cold extremities, changes in mental status, and urine output of less than 20 mL/h. Hemodynamic parameters for cardiogenic shock include cardiac index less than 1.8 L/min/m^2, stroke volume index less than 20 mL/m^2, mean pulmonary capillary wedge pressure greater than 18 mm Hg, tachycardia, and a systemic vascular resistance of over 2400 dyn·sec/cm^5. These patients are defined as type IV by the Killip classification, a widely used system to classify myocardial infarctions.[16]

Prevalence

Shock is the most common cause of in-hospital mortality following myocardial infarction.[17] The in-hospital mortality associated with cardiogenic shock has remained unchanged at approximately 80% despite the development of new treatment modalities.[17] Cardiogenic shock occurs in 2.4% to 12.0% of patients with acute myocardial infarction.[18] Since 1975, the incidence of cardiogenic shock complicating acute myocardial infarctions has remained constant at 7.5%, ranging between 5% and 15% (Table 24-2).[17] One reason these figures may have remained constant is the increasing efficiency of emergency medical systems in resuscitating patients in the community and bringing them to the hospital. Previously, these patients would have died before reaching the hospital. Similarly, there has been a decrease in the incidence of out-of-hospital deaths due to coronary disease between 1975 and 1988.[17] The key to success in patients in shock is early intervention and revascularization. In a prospective randomized study, Hochman et al showed that revascularization within 6 hours of diagnosis of cardiogenic shock confers survival benefits, particularly in those patients under 75 years of age.[19,20] Use of mechanical circulatory support also may play a role by resting stunned myocardium to allow its recovery and to prevent the irreversible end-organ injury that may result from prolonged shock.[11,12]

TABLE 24–2 Crude incidence rates and adjusted risk estimates for cardiogenic shock resulting from acute myocardial infarction

Year studied	Patients (no.)	Incidence (%)	Relative risk (95% CI)
1975	780	7.3	1.0*
1978	845	7.1	0.83 (0.54-1.28)
1981	999	7.5	0.96 (0.63-1.48)
1984	714	6.7	0.68 (0.42-1.12)
1986	765	7.6	1.16 (0.70-1.92)
1988	659	9.1	1.65 (0.99-2.77)
Total	4762	7.5	–

*Reference category.

Source: Reproduced with permission from Goldberg RJ, Gore JM, Alpert JS, et al: Cardiogenic shock after acute myocardial infarction. N Engl J Med 1991; 325:1117.

Infarct Size and Shock

Shock is directly related to the extent of the myocardium involved. Myocardial infarctions resulting in loss of at least 40% of the left ventricle have been shown to result in cardiogenic shock.[4,5,21] Autopsy findings also revealed marginal extension of the recent infarct and focal areas of necrosis in patients with cardiogenic shock.[4] Extensive three-vessel disease is usually found in individuals with cardiogenic shock, and extension of the infarct is an important determinant in those individuals.[4,5,21] Limiting the size of the infarct and its extension is the key to therapeutic interventions in patients with myocardial infarction. By following creatinine phosphate kinase (CPK) levels, Gutovitz et al[22] showed that the progression/extension of myocardial damage results in cardiogenic shock. Patients who develop shock have higher peak values.

MEDICAL MANAGEMENT OF MYOCARDIAL INFARCTION

The management of patients with acute myocardial infarctions demands expeditious treatment and decision making. With the ultimate goal of reperfusing the ischemic myocardium, treatment strategies should be directed toward reducing myocardial oxygen demand, maintaining circulatory support, and protecting the threatened myocardium before irreversible damage and expansion of the infarct occur.

Both clinical and basic science research have demonstrated that reperfusion is the main treatment option for acute myocardial infarction. Unfortunately, the majority of patients with myocardial infarction receive only conservative medical management; only 40% of patients having an acute myocardial infarction receive thrombolytic therapy, the most common means of reperfusion.[23]

A major tenet of medical management is the provision of adequate arterial oxygenation, defined as greater than 90% saturation. Supplemental oxygen and mechanical ventilation, including positive end-expiratory pressure and endotracheal intubation, aid in the management of pulmonary edema.

Nitroglycerin dilates epicardial arteries, increases collateral flow, and decreases ventricular preload. Although clearly beneficial in the treatment of myocardial infarction, nitrates may increase ventilation-perfusion mismatch and cause hypotension due to preload reduction.

Adequate analgesia is also beneficial. Morphine sulfate, the most commonly used analgesic, reduces preload and afterload, myocardial oxygen demand, anxiety, and circulating catecholamines. Side effects include hypotension and respiratory depression, each of which is treatable with basic resuscitative efforts.

Antiarrhythmic therapy, including lidocaine, is indicated under certain guidelines, along with atropine and countershock therapy when arrhythmias occur. Since arrhythmias are one of the most common complications after myocardial infarction, electrocardiographic (ECG) monitoring is recommended for the first 48 to 72 hours.

Arterial monitoring and the balloon flotation catheter aid in the management of patients who are hemodynamically unstable, developing congestive heart failure, or developing mechanical complications of a myocardial infarction. Long-term therapy for uncomplicated myocardial infarction includes the use of beta blockers, calcium channel blockers, and angiotensin-converting enzyme inhibitors.

Medical management includes the use of vasopressors and inotropic agents as first-line treatment strategies for cardiogenic shock. Optimizing filling pressure by balancing fluid management and diuretics is essential. Pulmonary capillary wedge pressures should be kept in the 16- to 22-mm Hg range.[2]

The use of dobutamine and dopamine is part of the pharmacologic armamentarium. These agents affect adrenergic receptors in different ways. Dopamine at doses of 5 to 8 μ/kg/min stimulates beta-adrenergic receptors; at higher doses, alpha-adrenergic receptors are activated. At rates of more than 10 μ/kg/min, left ventricular filling pressures rise and increase myocardial oxygen consumption. Dobutamine affects beta-adrenergic receptors and thus decreases afterload while stimulating the myocardium. Although vasopressors are necessary to maintain adequate perfusion pressures, they also increase afterload of the heart and increase myocardial oxygen demand, potentially worsening ischemia and extending the area of infarction.

While medical management of cardiogenic shock complicating acute myocardial infarctions is associated with high mortality, early revascularization will reduce mortality. As will be discussed later, early revascularization with PTCA or CABG has been shown to be the treatment of choice in this cohort.

In contrast to using inotropic agents to improve circulation, beta blockers have been used successfully to reduce death after infarction, probably due to their ability to reduce myocardial oxygen demand and arrhythmias. In hypotensive patients or individuals suffering bradycardia after infarctions involving the right coronary artery, beta blockade is contraindicated. Other mainstay therapies mentioned earlier—heparin, nitrates, and morphine—also comprise the traditional medical management of these critically ill patients.

STATES OF IMPAIRED MYOCARDIUM

Coronary insufficiency can result in three states of impaired myocardium: infarcted, hibernating, and stunned. Each state requires separate clinical interventions and carries different prognostic implications. Infarcted myocardium is irreversible myocardial cell death due to prolonged ischemia. Hibernating myocardium is a state of impaired myocardial and left ventricular function at rest due to reduced coronary blood flow that can be restored to normal if a normal myocardial oxygen supply-demand relationship is reestablished.[24,25] Hibernating myocardium is defined as contractility-depressed myocardial function secondary to severe chronic ischemia that improves clinically immediately following myocardial revascularization. Stunned myocardium is left ventricular dysfunction without cell death that occurs following restoration of blood flow after an ischemic episode. If a patient survives the insult resulting from a temporary period of ischemia followed by reperfusion, the previously ischemic areas of cardiac muscle eventually demonstrate improved contractility (Table 24-3).

Hibernating Myocardium

Hibernation may be acute or chronic. Carlson et al[26] showed that hibernating myocardium was present in up to 75% of patients with unstable angina and 28% with stable angina. The entity also occurs after myocardial infarction. Angina after myocardial infarction commonly occurs at a distance from the area of infarction.[27] In fact, mortality is significantly higher in patients with ischemia at a distance (72%) compared with ischemia adjacent to the infarct zone (33%).[27] It is the hibernating myocardium that may be in jeopardy and salvageable, although its presence is usually incidental to the occurrence of the acute infarction. By distinguishing between hibernating myocardium and irreversibly injured myocardium, a more aggressive approach to restoring or improving blood flow to the area at risk is reasonable. Function often improves immediately after revascularization of appropriately selected regions.

TABLE 24–3 States of myocardial cells after periods of ischemia

Condition	Viability of cells	Cause of injury	Return of function
Infarcted	Nonviable	Prolonged ischemia	No recovery
Stunned viable	Limited ischemia	Delayed with reperfusion	Recovery
Hibernating	Viable	Ongoing ischemia	Prompt, sometimes unpredictable recovery

Stunned Myocardium

In the 1970s it was observed that after brief episodes of severe ischemia, prolonged dysfunction with gradual return of contractile activity occurred. In 1982 Braunwald and Kloner[28] coined the phrase stunned myocardium. Stunning is a fully reversible process despite the severity and duration of the insult if the cells remain viable. However, myocardial dysfunction, biochemical alterations, and ultrastructural abnormalities continue to persist after return of blood flow. Within 60 seconds of coronary occlusion, the ischemic zone changes from a state of active shortening to one of passive shortening.[6] Coronary occlusion lasting less than 20 minutes is the classic model reproducing the stunning phenomenon.[28–30]

The most likely mechanisms of myocardial stunning are calcium overload, generation of oxygen-derived free radicals, excitation-contraction uncoupling due to sarcoplasmic reticulum dysfunction, or a combination thereof. Other mechanisms that may contribute to the stunning phenomenon include insufficient energy production, impaired energy use by myofibrils, impaired sympathetic neural responsiveness, impaired myocardial perfusion, damaged extracellular collagen matrix, and decreased sensitivity of myofilaments to calcium (Table 24-4).[29,31,32]

Stunned myocardium can occur adjacent to necrotic tissue after prolonged coronary occlusion and can be associated with demand-induced ischemia, coronary spasm, and cardioplegia-induced cardiac arrest during cardiopulmonary bypass. Clinically these regions are edematous and even hemorrhagic. They also have a propensity for arrhythmias, which can lead to more extensive ventricular stunning and hypotension with subsequent infarction of these regions.

In summary, infarcted myocardium is nonviable myocardium, while hibernating myocardium is viable myocardium that is chronically dysfunctional due to impaired blood supply. Stunned myocardium is viable myocardium that is acutely dysfunctional after adequate blood supply has been restored.

TABLE 24–4 Mechanisms of contractile dysfunction after myocardial stunning

Mechanism
Generation of oxygen-derived free radicals*
Excitation-contraction uncoupling due to sarcoplasmic reticulum dysfunction
Calcium overload
Insufficient energy production by mitochondria
Impaired energy use by myofibrils
Impairment of sympathetic neural responsiveness
Impairment of myocardial perfusion
Damage of the extracellular collagen matrix
Decreased sensitivity of myofilaments to calcium

*Regarded as the primary mechanism of myocardial stunning.

Source: Modified with permission from Bolli R: Mechanism of myocardial stunning. Circulation 1990; 82:723.

Diagnosis of Viable Myocardium

Mechanisms to identify patients with myocardial stunning and hibernation include ECG findings, radionuclide imaging, positron emission tomography (PET), dobutamine echocardiography, and more recently MRI. Thallium identifies perfusion-related defects of the myocardium and can distinguish between viable and scarred myocardium as well. However, early redistribution of thallium does not distinguish between hibernating and scarred myocardium since many segments with irreversible defects by thallium improve after reperfusion.[33] Redistribution imaging and reinjection imaging improve the predictive value of thallium imaging in distinguishing hibernating myocardium.

PET measures the metabolic activity of myocardial cells. It has high positive and negative predictive values.[34] Many studies have suggested that PET is perhaps the best diagnostic tool to assess myocardial viability.[35]

Dobutamine echocardiography identifies hibernating and stunned myocardium by monitoring changes in segmental wall motion while the heart is stressed inotropically and chronotropically by dobutamine infusion. It has comparable specificity, sensitivity, and, more importantly, positive predictive value.[36]

MRI, a recently emerging technique, also has demonstrated effectiveness in distinguishing hibernating myocardium.[37] To date, it has not been proved to be sensitive and specific enough for routine use.

Treatment of Stunned Myocardium

Several approaches to management of this critically ill group should be taken. Blocking the production of oxygen free radicals will reduce both additional cell death and edema in stunned myocardium. By reducing inflammation, the prothrombotic effects on injured endothelial cells also can be reduced and thus enhance ventricular recovery. Several techniques attack the production or effects of these oxygen free radicals. Allopurinol blocks the xanthine oxidase-hypoxanthine pathway and decreases superoxide anion radicals; however, clinical trials have yielded conflicting results.[38–40]

Iloprost, an analogue of prostacyclin, has demonstrated some effectiveness in reducing stunning in animals. The proposed mechanism is inhibition of neutrophil and platelet function and reduction in the production of oxygen free radicals. In the Thrombolysis and Angioplasty in Myocardial Infarction (TAMI) trial, iloprost did not show improved ventricular function after reperfusion with tissue plasminogen activator (t-PA).[41]

Recombinant superoxide dismutase (SOD), an oxygen free radical scavenger, is a hydrophilic enzyme that does not cross the cell membrane. Additionally, SOD works most effectively if it is in tissue prior to reperfusion injury and oxygen free radical production.[42,43] Perhaps because of these two limitations, the use of SOD has not yet shown clinical effectiveness.[44]

Other pharmacologic agents, including calcium antagonists, nitrates, beta-blocking agents, and angiotensin-converting enzyme inhibitors, also have been studied with some beneficial results.[45–49] Recent clinical studies have shown that patients receiving calcium channel blockers had improved recovery from stunning over nitrate therapy.[50,51] Intracellular adhesion molecule blockers and p-selectin blockers also may prove beneficial in the coming years.

The use of inotropic agents can overcome stunning in both animal experiments and human observation. It is recognized that contractility of reversibly injured myocardium can be enhanced by catecholamines. Thus inotropic agents may have a role in supporting the patient with borderline function until the stunned myocardium can recover.[43]

Hemodynamic stability must be maintained while stunned myocardium is recovering or being treated by one of the above-mentioned means. Short-term mechanical circulatory devices can aid in the support of patients until the myocardium has sufficiently recovered.

Summary

Differentiation between infarcted, hibernating, and stunned myocardium guides therapeutic options in patients with poor ventricular function. If adequate regions of hibernating myocardium are present as documented by PET, thallium scanning, or dobutamine echocardiography, revascularization may allow ventricular recovery. In patients without evidence of hibernating or stunned myocardium, medical management or transplantation is a better option.

Further distinction is required between stunned and hibernating myocardium. Hibernating myocardium requires revascularization to restore blood supply to this area. Stunned myocardium requires only support, which may take the form of pharmacologic manipulations, including addition of epinephrine, dobutamine, and/or amrinone. If conservative measures fail, the intra-aortic balloon pump (IABP) or short-term LVAD support becomes necessary.

RATIONALE FOR AGGRESSIVE MANAGEMENT OF MYOCARDIAL INFARCTION

Randomized trials have shown beneficial effects of early reperfusion within 12 hours and possibly up to 24 hours after acute myocardial infarction.[10] Early reperfusion clearly reduces infarct size in the major areas at risk. Controlled reperfusion may be even superior. The arguments are more difficult to make for patients outside the 24-hour window; however, patients with ongoing ischemia often have ischemic border regions that are prone to arrhythmias and necrosis. In addition, these patients are at risk for prolonged periods of hypotension with resulting end-organ injury and further left ventricular dysfunction. Even if revascularization does not appear critical, ventricular unloading with IABP or LVAD may provide the bridge to recovery needed in patients dying after myocardial infarction. The major limiting factors to aggressive surgical management are major comorbidities, which make continuation of life undesirable or unlikely, and an unclear neurologic status, especially after a period of cardiopulmonary arrest.

REPERFUSION

Although restoration of blood flow to ischemic regions is essential, the accompanying reperfusion injury initially can worsen rather than improve myocardial dysfunction. The area at risk is affected not only by reperfusion but also by the conditions of reperfusion and the composition of the reperfusate.[14] Thus controlling reperfusion itself may aid in reducing myocardial infarct size and ventricular injury.

At the cellular level, myocardial ischemia results in a change in energy production from aerobic to anaerobic metabolism. The consequences of ischemia vary from decreased adenosine triphosphate production and increased intracellular calcium to decreased amino acid precursors such as aspartate and glutamate. These changes can be reversed only by reperfusion.

However, as oxygen is reintroduced into a region, oxygen free radical generation ensues with resulting cellular damage. Cellular swelling and/or contracture leads to a "no-reflow phenomenon" that limits the recovery of some myocytes and possibly adds to irreversible injury of others. The production of oxygen free radicals during ischemia and at the time of reperfusion is the leading mechanism proposed to explain cellular injury. Four basic types of reperfusion injury have been described: lethal cell death, microvascular injury, stunned myocardium, and reperfusion arrhythmias (Table 24-5).

Buckberg et al[14,15,52–68] conducted studies of controlled reperfusion after ischemia and produced a clinical application for controlled reperfusion. The conditions of reperfusion and the composition of the reperfusate allowed more

TABLE 24–5 Potential types of reperfusion injury

Lethal	Cell death secondary to reperfusion
Vascular	Progressive damage causes an expanding zone of "no reflow" and deterioration of coronary flow reserve during the phase of reperfusion
Reperfusion arrhythmias	Arrhythmias, mainly ventricular, that occur shortly after reperfusion
Stunned myocardium	Postischemic ventricular dysfunction

Source: Modified with permission from Kloner RA: Does reperfusion injury exist in humans? J Am Coll Cardiol 1993; 21:537.

TABLE 24–6 Buckberg cardioplegic solution to decrease reperfusion injury

Principle	Method	Final concentration
Provide oxygenation	Blood	20%-30% Hct
Maintain arrest	KCl	8-10 mEq/L
Buffer acidosis	THAM	pH 7.5-7.6
Limit Ca^{2+}	CPD	0.15-0.25 mmol/L Ca^{2+}
Substrate	Aspartate	13 mmol/L
	Glutamate	13 mmol/L
Hyperglycemia	Glucose	>400 mg/dL
Reduce edema	Osmolarity	350-400 mosmol

THAM, tris(hydroxymethyl)aminomethane; CPD, citrate-phosphate-dextrose.

TABLE 24–7 Reperfusion with Buckberg cardioplegic solution in patients with acute myocardial infarction

Classification	Patients (no.)	%
Overall mortality	6/156	3.9
Subgroups		
LAD occlusion	5/95	5.3
Three-vessel disease	0/66	0.0
Age >70 years	1/22	4.5
Preoperative shock	6/66	9.1

This table represents the clinical experience using the Buckberg cardioplegic solution in patients undergoing surgical revascularization for acute myocardial infarction. Time from infarct to surgical revascularization averaged 6 hours in this group of patients.

Source: Modified with permission from Allen BS, Buckberg GD, Fontan FM, et al: Superiority of controlled surgical reperfusion versus percutaneous transluminal coronary angioplasty in acute coronary occlusion. J Thorac Cardiovasc Surg 1993; 105:864.

muscle salvage, less postischemic edema, and greater immediate recovery of systolic shortening than uncontrolled reperfusion.[52] The composition of the reperfusate was designed to provide oxygen, reduce calcium influx, reverse acidosis, mobilize edema, and replenish substrates. To accomplish this, the cardioplegic solution was hyperosmolar and basic and contained blood, a chelating agent, aspartate, and glutamate (Table 24-6).[53] The duration of reperfusion, 20 minutes, as well as the dose, was critical.[60]

The surgical strategy of controlled reperfusion, especially as espoused by Buckberg et al, includes several elements. First, extracorporeal circulation is established as expeditiously as possible with venting of the left ventricle as required. Initially, antegrade cardioplegia is delivered using either a warm Buckberg solution to rebuild ATP stores or cold, high-potassium cardioplegia to achieve rapid diastolic arrest. We routinely add retrograde cardioplegia to ensure global cooling, even in areas of active ischemia. The temperatures of the anterior and inferior walls of the ventricle are measured to ensure adequate cooling. After each distal anastomosis, cold cardioplegia is infused into each graft and the aorta at 200 mL/min over 1 minute. This is followed by retrograde infusion through the coronary sinus for 1 minute. After completion of the final distal anastomosis, warm substrate-enriched blood cardioplegia is given at 150 mL/min for 2 minutes into each anastomosis and the aorta. After removal of the aortic cross-clamp, regional blood cardioplegia is given at 50 mL/min into the graft supplying the region at risk for 18 minutes. The proximal vein grafts are then completed, followed by reestablishment of normal blood flow. To decrease oxygen demand, the heart is allowed to beat in the empty state for 30 minutes. After this time, the patient is weaned off bypass.

Application of the Buckberg solution and technique has been shown to be effective in improving mortality rates and myocardial function after acute coronary occlusion. With ischemic times averaging 6 hours, a prevalence of multivessel disease, and cardiogenic shock, the overall mortality in patients with acute coronary arterial occlusions who underwent surgical revascularization applying this method of reperfusion was 3.9%. Postoperative ejection fractions averaged 50%.[15] Surgical revascularization in this series using controlled reperfusion compared favorably with percutaneous transluminal coronary angioplasty (PTCA) in several large series.[15] The superior results of this method for the treatment of cardiogenic shock, a 9% mortality, have brought this method to the forefront in the treatment of cardiogenic shock (Table 24-7).[15]

Methods of Reperfusion

ROLE OF THROMBOLYTIC THERAPY

Since myocardial salvage depends on reperfusion of occluded coronary arteries, rapid dissolution of an occluding thrombus with thrombolytic therapy is an appealing intervention. Intracoronary streptokinase in patients with acute myocardial infarction demonstrates that thrombolytic therapy is a safe and efficient way to achieve the desired early reperfusion.[69] Following this study, a number of multi-institutional megatrials showed the effectiveness of thrombolytic therapy in treating acute myocardial infarctions.

The trial of the Italian Group for the Study of Streptokinase in Myocardial Infarction (Gruppo Italiano per lo Studio della Streptochinasi nell'Infarto Miocardio, GISSI)[70] and the Second International Study of Infarct Survival (ISIS-2)[71] found a reduced hospital mortality in patients treated with streptokinase. The effectiveness of tissue-type plasminogen activator (t-PA) also has been evaluated in randomized studies. The Thrombolysis in Myocardial Infarction (TIMI) study[72] and the European Cooperative Study Group (ECSG)[73] demonstrated the effectiveness of t-PA for the treatment of acute myocardial infarction.

When streptokinase and t-PA were compared, two studies failed to demonstrate any difference in mortality.[74,75]

A third study, however, the Global Utilization of Streptokinase and Tissue Plasminogen Activator for Occluded Coronary Arteries (GUSTO) trial, supported the use of t-PA by demonstrating a more rapid and complete restoration of coronary flow that resulted in improved ventricular performance and reduced mortality.[76,77] After 90 minutes, 54% of the group receiving t-PA and heparin had normal flow, compared with less than 40% in the other groups. While patency rates were similar after 3 hours, 30-day mortality was lowest in patients whose flow was normal at 90 minutes (4.4%).[76,77] This supports the importance of rapid restoration of flow. Although the actual difference in patient survival between the two groups was small (6% vs. 7% mortality), the number of lives saved each year may justify the added expense of t-PA.[76,77] The mode of delivery of t-PA has been credited for the differences in the outcomes in these trials. Differences in methods of delivery between t-PA and streptokinase and adjuvant therapy with aspirin and heparin, along with cost factors of each agent, have stimulated a continuing debate over these two drugs.[23] Table 24-8 summarizes some of the previously mentioned trials.

While thrombolyis improves survival and ventricular function, the patency of infarct-related arteries is reported to be between 50% and 85%.[70–77] Normal flow should be achieved in 60% of patients by today's standards. Thrombolytic therapy works well but is not without complications, including bleeding and intracranial hemorrhage.[78] Bleeding is usually minor and occurs mostly at the sites of vascular puncture. Intracranial hemorrhage and stroke rates are around 1% and are an "acceptable" risk.

CARDIOGENIC SHOCK

Thrombolytic therapy for patients presenting in cardiogenic shock or heart failure does not appear to improve survival in this population but may decrease the incidence of patients developing heart failure after myocardial infarction.[79] However, a recent randomized SHOCK (Should We Emergently Revascularize Occluded Coronaries for Cardiogenic Shock) trial found clear survival benefits for early revascularization by PTCA or CABG over initial medical stablization by thrombolytic therapy.[18,19]

TABLE 24–8 Trials comparing thrombolytic therapy with conventional therapy

Trial	Death (%)	Total stroke (%)	Cerebral hemorrhage (%)
GISSI-2[74]			
SK	9.2	0.94	0.29
t-PA	9.6	1.33	0.42
ISIS-3[75]			
SK	10.6	1.04	0.24
t-PA	10.3	1.39	0.66
GUSTO[76,77]			
SK + SQH	7.2	7.9	0.5
SK + IVH	7.4	8.2	0.9
t-PA + IVH	6.3	7.2	0.0
SK + t-PA	7.0	7.9	1.3

SK, streptokinase; t-PA, tissue plasminogen activator; SQH, subcutaneous heparin; IVH, intravenous heparin.

SUMMARY

Thrombolytic agents for the treatment of myocardial infarction have demonstrated several important points. Survival is improved by decreasing time to reperfusion. The GUSTO trial showed that patients treated within the first hour had the greatest improvement in survival, with a 1% reduction in mortality for each hour of time saved.[76,77] Thrombolytic therapy is easy to administer in the community by trained personnel. Since the time to reperfusion is a critical element in preserving myocardium, thrombolytic therapy is ideal for most communities. One study evaluated the use of prehospital-administered thrombolytics and found a trend toward improved survival.[80] Further large-scale trials must be initiated before recommendations are made. However, in communities, thrombolytics should be used for treatment of patients with acute myocardial infarction.

Role of PTCA

Since the first reported use of percutaneous transluminal coronary angioplasty (PTCA) by Gruntzig et al[81] in 1979, the efficacy of this procedure in the treatment of coronary artery disease has been well recognized. A number of studies have evaluated the efficacy of primary PTCA in the treatment of acute myocardial infarction. Overall, PTCA hospital mortality rates range from 6% to 9%.[82–87]

Several different strategies employing PTCA for acute myocardial infarction have been developed and examined through clinical trials. Primary, rescue, immediate, delayed, and elective PTCA are options for the treatment of acute myocardial infarction. Primary PTCA uses angioplasty as the method of reperfusion in patients presenting with acute myocardial infarction. Rescue, immediate, delayed, and elective PTCA all are done in conjunction with or following thrombolytic therapy. Rescue PTCA is done following recurrent angina or hemodynamic instability following thrombolytic therapy. Immediate PTCA is performed in conjunction with thrombolytic therapy, and delayed PTCA occurs during the intervening hospitalization. Finally, elective PTCA is done following thrombolytic therapy and medical management when a positive stress test is obtained during the same hospitalization or soon thereafter.

Primary PTCA functions in several roles for the treatment of acute myocardial infarctions. Since there are some absolute and relative contraindications to thrombolytics, PTCA is the best method of reperfusion in patients with acute myocardial infarction, according to studies that evaluated PTCA as first-line therapy. Several studies evaluated the role of PTCA compared with thrombolytic therapy. The Primary Angioplasty in Myocardial Infarction Study Group trial concluded that immediate PTCA without thrombolytics reduced occurrence of reinfarction and death and was associated with a lower rate of intracranial hemorrhage. The trial did not show any differences in left ventricular systolic function.[83] Myocardial salvage is similar for PTCA and thrombolytic therapy[84]; however, primary PTCA may be slightly less costly than thrombolytic therapy.[85]

There are limits to the use of primary PTCA. Logistic and economic constraints apply to invasive modes of therapy. Catheterization laboratories and personnel must be ready at all times. This is not practical in most communities, and transportation to tertiary care centers raises costs considerably.

Immediate PTCA following thrombolytic therapy does not improve clinical outcome and is associated with increased complication rates. The ECSG,[73] the TAMI trial,[86] and the TIMI-IIA trial[87] demonstrated that immediate angioplasty does not improve clinical outcome or left ventricular function compared with delayed angioplasty.[73,86,87] Immediate angioplasty is also associated with a higher risk of bleeding and emergent bypass. The ECSG trial demonstrated a lower incidence of bleeding, hypotension, and ventricular fibrillation as well as lower mortality with delayed PTCA.[73] The TAMI trial, which compared immediate versus delayed PTCA after thrombolysis, showed no difference in global ventricular function at 1 week between the two groups in patients with angiographically patent infarct arteries.[86] Overall, immediate angioplasty does not lead to better ventricular function or clinical outcome compared with elective PTCA. Finally, TIMI-IIA concluded that immediate PTCA after thrombolytic therapy for acute myocardial infarction does not improve survival or ventricular function[87] and is associated with increased bleeding, reinfarction, and emergency coronary artery bypass grafting (CABG) (Table 24-9).

TABLE 24–9 Comparison of percutaneous transluminal coronary angioplasty and thrombolytic therapy

Trial	Death (%)	Reinfarction (%)
TIMI[72]		
T + A	5.2	6.4
T	4.7	5.8
TAMI[86]		
T + A	4.0	11.0
T	1.0	13.0
ECSGS[73]		
T + A	7.0	4.0
T	3.0	7.0
TIMI IIA[87]		
T + A	7.7	5.6
T	5.2	3.1

T. thrombolysis only; T + A, thrombolysis and angioplasty.

Delayed PTCA does not improve clinical outcome either. The Treatment of Post-Thrombolytic Stenoses (TOPS) study group concluded that there is no functional or clinical benefit from routine late PTCA after acute myocardial infarction treated with thrombolytic therapy in patients who did not have ischemia on stress testing before hospital discharge.[88] However, the TIMI-IIB trial indicated that thrombolytic therapy followed by angioplasty in individuals with symptomatic or provokable ischemia is appropriate.[87]

CARDIOGENIC SHOCK

Primary PTCA may play a greater role in patients presenting in cardiogenic shock. The GISSI I and II trials demonstrated no benefit from intravenous thrombolysis, with mortality rates of 70%.[70,74] In patients presenting in or developing cardiogenic shock after acute myocardial infarction, PTCA improved survival to 40% and 60%.[89,90] This improvement was even greater when angioplasty was successful; in-hospital survival rates increased to 70%. In most of these series an IABP was used in conjunction with PTCA. The SHOCK trial showed that revascularization by PTCA or CABG within 6 hours of the onset of cardiogenic shock results in improved 1-year survival (46.7% versus 33.6% for initial medical stablization followed by revascularization) in this high-risk group, particularly for those under the age of 75 years.[19,20]

SUMMARY

Primary PTCA should be performed in patients with acute myocardial infarction and contraindications to thrombolytic therapy. Patients with established or developing cardiogenic shock should be revascularized early by PTCA rather than initial medical stablization by thrombolytic therapy. Specialized centers that have 24-hour catheterization facilities can provide primary PTCA as a first-line therapy. Rescue PTCA after failed thrombolytic therapy for patients with ongoing ischemia or clinical compromise is also recommended. Finally, elective PTCA should be performed on patients who have recurrent or provokable angina prior to hospital discharge.

INTRACORONARY STENTS

Intracoronary stents may be useful for acute coronary arterial dissections and have proven benefits in lowered rates of restenosis, abrupt closure, and emergent CABG following PTCA. However, critics have argued that stent trials often involved selection bias leading to better outcomes.[91] At this time, identification of patients who may or may not require stents and the optimal rate of stent use remains unclear.

Role of Coronary Artery Bypass Grafting (CABG)

The role of surgical revascularization in the treatment acute myocardial infarction has changed considerably over the past

30 years. Improvements in intraoperative management and myocardial preservation techniques have strengthened the surgeon's armamentarium. However, the development and use of thrombolytic therapy and PTCA offer alternatives to surgery.

Early studies reported increased morbidity and mortality for patients undergoing surgical revascularization within 30 days of the infarct.[92] A concern arose over a high risk of extension and hemorrhage into infarction after surgical revascularization of acute myocardial infarction.[93] Medical management was believed the more prudent therapy. The only absolute indications for emergent operative intervention treatment of acute myocardial infarctions during this era were papillary muscle rupture, ventricular septal defect, and left ventricular rupture. For these entities, surgery was the only hopeful option.

During the 1980s, reports appeared recommending surgical revascularization in preference to medical therapy for acute myocardial infarction.[94–100] Mortality rates under 5% were reported. Critics argued that these studies lacked randomization or consecutive entry of patients, that preoperative stratification was absent, and that enzyme levels were not included. Inherent bias that favored surgery in low-risk patients was believed to be the reason for the excellent outcomes.[101]

At the time these reports surfaced, thrombolytic therapy and interventional cardiology were emerging as alternative options for acute infarction. With the availability of thrombolytics and PTCA, large multicenter trials began looking at the efficacy and usefulness of these two techniques. Randomized trials using CABG were not done, and thus this option was never established as an option for acute myocardial infarction.

However, several centers continued to use surgical revascularization to treat acute myocardial infarction. Excellent results were achieved by coordinated community and hospital systems. However, practical, logistic, and economic constraints relegate surgical revascularization to a third option behind thrombolytics and PTCA for the primary treatment of acute myocardial infarction.

There continue to be several scenarios that require emergent or urgent surgical revascularization. Failure of thrombolytics and PTCA with acute occlusion may require surgical intervention. Additionally, CABG for postinfarction angina has became a critical step in the pathway of treating acute myocardial infarction.

TIMING AFTER INFARCTION

If surgical revascularization within 6 hours after the onset of symptoms is feasible, the mortality rate is improved over that of medically treated, nonrevascularized patients.[94–97] While these early studies were not controlled and were criticized for selection bias, they did demonstrate that surgical revascularization may be performed with an acceptable mortality in the presence of acute myocardial infarction with improved myocardial protection, anesthesia, and surgical techniques. However, with the advent of thrombolytic therapy, PTCA, and an aging population, the surgical patient we encounter today bears little resemblance to the patient population represented in these early data.

Recent analyses of the New York State Cardiac Surgery Registry, which included every patient undergoing a cardiac operation in the last decade in the state of New York, had resulted in valuable information regarding the optimal timing of CABG in acute myocardial infarction. In this large and contemporary patient population, there is a significant correlation between hospital mortality and time interval from acute myocardial infarction to time of operation, particularly if CABG was performed within one week of acute myocardial infarction. In addition, patients with transmural and nontransmural acute myocardial infarction have different trends in mortality when the time course is taken into consideration. Mortality for the nontransmural group peaked if the operation was performed within 6 hours of acute myocardial infarction, then decreased precipitously (Table 24-10).[102] On the other hand, mortality for the transmural group remained high during the first 3 days before returning to baseline (Fig. 24-1).[103] Multivariable analyses confirmed that CABG within 6 hours for the nontransmural group and 3 days for the transmural group were independently associated with in-hospital mortality.[102,103] Optimal timing of CABG in patients with acute myocardial infarction is a controversial subject. Early surgical intervention has the advantage of limiting the infarct expansion and ventricular remodeling that may result in possible ventricular aneurysm and rupture.[104] However, there is the theoretical risk of reperfusion injury, which may lead to hemorrhagic infarction resulting in extension of infarct size, poor infarct healing, and scar development.[105] The data from these studies caution against early revascularization, particularly among patients with transmural acute myocardial infarction within 3 days of onset. Some have

TABLE 24–10 Comparison of hospital mortality with respect to time of surgery—transmural vs. nontransmural myocardial infarction

Time between CABG and MI	Mortality	
	Transmural MI (%)	Nontransmural MI (%)
<6 h	14	13
6-23 h	14*	6*
1-7 d	5	4
>7 d	3	3

*$p < .01$ nontransmural vs. transmural.

Source: Data compiled from the New York State Cardiac Surgery Registry, which included every patient undergoing a cardiac operation in the last decade in the state of New York.

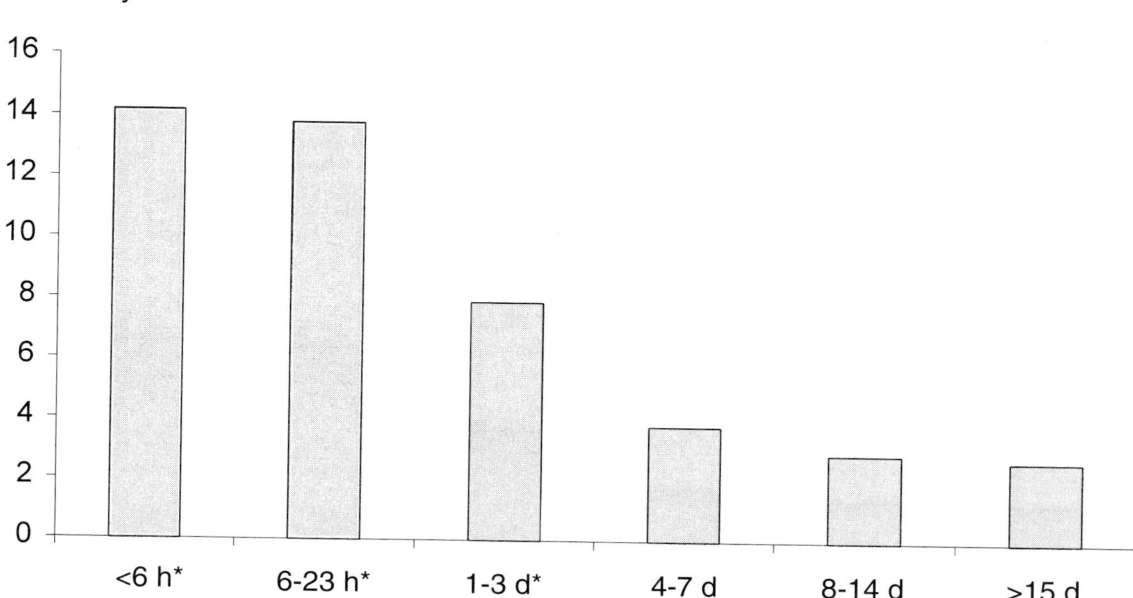

FIGURE 24–1 Hospital mortality versus timing of CABG after transmural MI. Among patients who underwent CABG after transmural MI in New York State, mortality was more than doubled that of the baseline value when surgery was performed within 3 days of transmural MI.

advocated the use of mechanical support to stabilize and allow elective rather than emergent surgery.[106] Utilizing mechanical support "prophylactically" instead of CABG to improve outcome, however, would require placement of such support in many unnecessary cases. If revascularization cannot be delayed, aggressive mechanical support such as a left ventricular assist device (LVAD) must be available since mortality is most likely due to pump failure. Furthermore, mechanical circulatory support has been shown to be efficacious as a bridge to ventricular recovery or transplantation for this patient cohort.[12] While emergent cases such as structure complications and ongoing ischemia clearly cannot be delayed, nonemergent cases, particularly patients with transmural acute myocardial infarction, may benefit from delay of surgery. Early surgery after transmural acute myocardial infarction has a significantly higher risk and surgeons should be prepared to provide aggressive cardiac support including LVADs in this ailing population. Waiting in some may be warranted.

RISK FACTORS

In addition to timing of surgery as discussed above, risk factors include urgency of the operation, increasing patient age, renal insufficiency, number of previous myocardial infarctions, hypertension,[107] reoperation, cardiogenic shock, depressed left ventricular function and the need for cardiopulmonary resuscitation,[108] left main disease, female sex, left ventricular wall motion score,[109] IABP, and transmural infarction.[110] Characteristics associated with better outcome early after myocardial infarction include preservation of left ventricular ejection fraction, male gender, left main disease, younger patients, and subendocardial versus transmural myocardial infarction.

CARDIOGENIC SHOCK

Surgical revascularization in acute myocardial infarction complicated by cardiogenic shock has been shown to improve survival. Cardiogenic shock, as discussed earlier, is accompanied by 80% to 90% mortality rates. DeWood et al[111] were the first to demonstrate improved results with revascularization in patients in cardiogenic shock complicating acute myocardial infarction. Patients who were stabilized with an IABP and underwent emergent surgical revascularization had survival rates of 75%. Early surgical revascularization is associated with survival rates of 40% to 88% in patients in cardiogenic shock due to nonmechanical causes. Guyton et al[112] reported an 88% in-hospital survival and a 3-year survival of 88%, with no late deaths reported. Furthermore, the SHOCK trial demonstrated survival benefit in early revascularization by CABG or PTCA within 6 hours of the diagnosis of cardiogenic shock for those under 75 years of age.[19,20] Thus, for patients in cardiogenic shock, surgical revascularization is a viable option.

ADVANTAGES OF CABG

Reported survival rates are similar for CABG and PTCA in the treatment of acute myocardial infarction. To date there have been no large randomized clinical trials comparing CABG with PTCA and thrombolytics. Due to the lack of prospective, randomized trials, recommendations must be based on retrospective and observational studies. CABG offers several potential advantages. First, surgical revascularization is the most definite form of treatment of the occlusion. CABG offers the longest patency of revascularized stenotic and occluded arteries in elective cases; 90% of internal mammary arteries are patent at 10 years. Second, CABG also offers more complete revascularization, since all the vessels are treated. Third, difficult distal obstructions can be reached. Fourth, there is controlled reperfusion to reverse ischemic injury and reduce reperfusion injury. Fifth, as with other forms of reperfusion, CABG interrupts the progression of ischemia and necrosis and limits infarct size.

DISADVANTAGES OF CABG

Disadvantages of immediate surgical revascularization include the high mortality associated with early CABG. Rapid availability of catheterization and operating room personnel for emergency procedures imposes logistic and economic constraints. Thus CABG is not readily applicable to the vast majority of patients in the community, and to provide this would strain health care resources. Second, it is difficult to analyze published results of CABG for acute myocardial infarction because randomized trials have not been done. Comparisons thus far have used medically treated patients as controls. Patients in the surgical group may be at lower risk; this might explain their progression to operation rather than continuing medical treatment. Crossover of patients from medical to surgical treatment also may have skewed the data.

SUMMARY

Surgical revascularization following acute myocardial infarction can be performed with excellent results when the timing and patient cohort are appropriate. Most patients do not need such measures and would not benefit from this aggressive form of therapy. However, patients with mechanical complications, those in cardiogenic shock, and those with postinfarction angina are likely to benefit from early CABG.

USE OF THE INTRA-AORTIC BALLOON PUMP

The early use of aortic counterpulsation with an intra-aortic balloon pump (IABP) demonstrated the safety but not efficacy of this device for patients in cardiogenic shock following acute myocardial infarction.[113] While survival was not improved, aortic counterpulsation did improve the myocardial oxygen requirements and myocardial energetics were reduced in patients in shock.[113] As revascularization techniques for the repair of occluded coronary arteries of patients in cardiogenic shock have improved, use of aortic counterpulsation has found a role as an adjuvant to treatment protocols.

IABP counterpulsation in combination with early reperfusion is effective in the treatment of acute myocardial infarction complicated by cardiogenic shock.[111,114] While the major improvement in survival is due to early reperfusion, patients who had combined reperfusion and IABP additionally have improved long-term survival. IABP improves circulatory physiology and decreases end-organ damage in the early shock period before the myocardium is reperfused and recovers function.

Aortic counterpulsation decreases the reocclusion rate, recurrent ischemia, and need for emergency PTCA in patients who have coronary artery patency established by emergency cardiac catheterization following acute myocardial infarction.[115] Prophylactic counterpulsation for 48 hours sustains patency in coronary arteries after patency is reestablished following myocardial infarction. No increase in vascular or hemorrhagic complications is observed as compared with controls.[115]

Weaning from the IABP should take place only after there is clear evidence of myocardial and end-organ recovery. In general, inotropic requirements should be reduced first in order to minimize myocardial stress. The one exception is the development of limb ischemia due to the IABP catheter.

ROLE OF CIRCULATORY ASSIST

Circulatory support devices are reserved for patients who are hemodynamically unstable; however, intervention should not be delayed until after irreversible end-organ injury occurs. This group of shock patients has a mortality rate of 80%, and survival data with the use of assist devices reflect the critical condition of patients treated. Mortality rates have changed very little in the last 20 years despite improvements in medical and surgical therapy.

Patients in cardiogenic shock who are candidates for circulatory assist devices may be divided into two groups: individuals who have stunned myocardium and need a bridge to recovery, and those who have irreversible myocardial damage and need a bridge to cardiac transplantation. For example, if a patient with a previously normal ventricle develops a large myocardial infarction, we prefer short-term support, since enough recovery may occur to allow a fruitful existence with the native heart. However, if a patient with preexisting heart failure has another infarction, the need to definitively bridge the patient to transplant with a long-term implantable device is apparent. Difficulty arises in assessing the results of mechanical assistance for patients following acute myocardial infarction and cardiogenic shock because of these different objectives.

Mechanical assist devices augment systemic perfusion and prevent end-organ damage while resting the stunned ventricle.[116] Early studies on implantable LVADs have shown that end-organ function is an early predictor of mortality. Treatment of patients prior to end-organ deterioration is essential for improving the odds for long-term survival. In addition to affecting end-organ function, assist devices also may improve myocardial contractility of postischemic hearts.[116] Recent studies have shown that circulatory support early after myocardial infarction improved survival and offered a feasible bridge to recovery or transplantation.[11,12]

Decisions regarding specific device use depend on the degree of circulatory support needed and many other factors. Selection criteria for device placement include:

1. Potential reversibility of cardiac dysfunction
2. Cause of the cardiac dysfunction
3. Degree of right and left ventricular dysfunction
4. Amount of circulatory support needed
5. Importance of the device for myocardial functional recovery
6. Patient size
7. Anatomic location of collapse or deterioration
8. Whether the patient is a candidate for cardiac transplantation
9. Whether the patient can be anticoagulated
10. Expected duration of support
11. Patient's age and severity of comorbid conditions[117]

At New York Presbyterian Hospital (Columbia Center), several circulatory assist devices are available to aid treatment of each group. Short-term devices that can be placed percutaneously include the IABP and extracorporeal membrane oxygenation. Devices that require sternotomy and are beneficial for short-term use include the ABIOMED and Thoratec pumps. Both these devices primarily treat stunned myocardium, but they are capable of bridging to transplant. These devices are easy to insert, do not require excision of ventricular muscle, and do not compromise ventricular function following device removal. These devices can be removed without the need to reinstitute cardiopulmonary bypass. These devices are effective in patients who require emergency support secondary to cardiogenic shock.

Another device that requires thoracotomy is a direct mechanical ventricular actuation device. This elliptically shaped cup that fits over both ventricles compresses and relaxes the ventricles, simulating directed cardiac actuation. Reports document improved cardiac outputs using this device and survival of several patients over prolonged periods of support.[118] (A complete discussion of temporary and long-term ventricular assist devices is found in Chs. 17 and 62.)

The Heartmate (Thoratec, Pleasanton, CA) and Novacor (Ottawa Heart, Ottawa, Canada) LVADs are long-term implantable assist devices that we use for bridging to transplantation. Initial reports of increased mortality in this high-risk patient population have been refuted by studies reporting higher than usual survival in acute MI patients who received VAD support. At our facility, over 80% of this patient cohort have survived until transplantation, a result 3-fold better than databases of extracorporeal systems.

Weaning of Circulatory Support

Cardiac enzyme levels at the time of infarction, ECG changes, and the preinfarction condition of the ventricle help determine the likelihood of LV recovery. If the ventricle is considered not likely to recover, early use of a long-term device is rational. On the other hand, if recovery is possible, the heart should be rested for 3 to 5 days, loaded with the institution's choice of inotropic support, including a phosphodiesterase inhibitor, and allowed to beat and eject. If a transesophageal echocardiogram demonstrates recovery, the short-term support device should be removed in the operating room and kept available for 1 hour while the patient is observed for signs of decompensation. If the device cannot be removed within a week, the heart is not likely to recover. In this event, either a longer-term device is placed or patient support is discontinued.

We have reported a baseline LV recovery in more than half of patients supported for a prolonged period with implantable devices. Upon removal of the device, most of these patients have redeveloped CHF in our experience[12] although other centers have reported high success rates.[119,120] As our understanding of the underlying causes of LV failure improve, we will be able to design targeted therapies that can be used with temporary device support to facilitate sustainable recovery.

Ethical Considerations

Programs that aggressively pursue surgical approaches to high-risk patients also must aggressively seek termination of care in futile cases. A liaison should be developed with a medical ethics individual or group to provide support for primary caregivers; however, the burden of medical decisions must rest with the attending physician. The family should not be forced to sign declarations withdrawing care unless significant controversy and/or the potential of legal action encumbers the decision. In the case of mechanical circulatory support, each pump of the device can be interpreted as a new intervention and therefore can be terminated if necessary. A precedent for this course of action has been set with mechanical ventilation. If significant neurologic or other end-organ dysfunction has developed and cardiac function has not returned, termination of support is reasonable and appropriate.

The Ethics Committee of the Columbia Presbyterian Center of The New York Presbyterian Hospital has drafted a statement that patients and physicians must review together prior to placement of a ventricular assist device (VAD), or, when circumstances do not permit, immediately thereafter. The statement asserts that VAD restoration of hemodynamic stability in a patient with critical myocardial dysfunction may, for various reasons, not reach the goal of enabling the patient to receive a heart transplant or achieve adequate stability to be discharged home on the device.

The statement reads as follows:

> Every effort will be made to help our patients on ventricular assist devices (VAD) to improve to the point where they meet the criteria to receive a heart transplant, or stabilize enough to be discharged from the hospital on the VAD. However, if despite all our efforts, a patient has no reasonable chance of achieving either of these goals, we will discontinue the VAD, as it will, under these circumstances, no longer be serving the purpose for which it was originally used. When this occurs, the VAD will be discontinued only after the physicians caring for the patient are in agreement that the goals for VAD use cannot be met, and have consulted with the patient, or, when the patient is too ill, with the family or friends of the patient.

We believe such a document is needed at the beginning of the patient's care to make clear to the family the goals of VAD use. Specifically, a VAD should not be used solely to prolong a patient's dying. Once a medical determination has been made by both the attending cardiac surgeon and the attending cardiologist that the patient cannot survive to leave the hospital, continued use of the VAD is inappropriate.

If the patient or his health care proxy or surrogates disagree with the decision to discontinue the VAD, the case is submitted to the ethics committee for arbitration.

SURGICAL MANAGEMENT

New York Presbyterian (Columbia Center) Approach

Patients who are potential transplant candidates and who are dying of cardiogenic shock after myocardial infarction are all candidates for placement of a long-term implantable left ventricular assist device (LVAD). If at all possible, a coronary angiogram is obtained to allow revascularization with or without LVAD insertion. Surgery is delayed if the culprit vessel can be opened with angioplasty and the patient stabilized in the catheterization laboratory. If hemodynamics continue to deteriorate, the patient is taken directly to the operating suite, even if infarction occurred earlier than 6 hours before the planned procedure. Hemodynamic observations that favor early CABG are pulmonary artery pressures of less than 60/30 mm Hg and cardiac output of more than 3 L/min. If the hemodynamics are worse, early implantation of a long-term implantable LVAD may be needed, especially if the mixed venous oxygen saturation is less than 50%. The decision to place a long-term LVAD is influenced by the patient score on a screening scale designed for this purpose (Table 24-11). These scores were selected to identify end-organ dysfunction (lung, liver, kidney) and operative constraints (right-sided heart failure and bleeding). We have nearly a 90% survival if the summed scores are less than 5 points versus 30% survival with summed scores of greater than 5 points.[121] For this reason, if the total score is greater than 5 points, an attempt is made to stabilize the patient prior to beginning long-term LVAD insertion. Patients with lower scores are offered temporary LVAD.

TABLE 24–11 Preoperative risk scale for left ventricular assist device placement*

Criteria	Points
Urine output <30 cc/h	3
Intubated	2
Prothrombin time >16 sec	2
Central venous pressure >16 mm Hg	2
Reoperation	1

*A combined score of >5 is associated with a 70% mortality risk.

If a patient is not a potential transplant candidate, our approach is more conservative, since we do not have a safety net if coronary revascularization fails and a temporary support device is inserted. An angiogram must be obtained; if hemodynamics are not favorable and no acute ischemia is present, we delay surgery until pulmonary arterial pressures fall. If the patient is ischemic, we proceed with CABG as described below. If the patient cannot be separated from bypass without high-dose inotropic support including alpha agonists, if the cardiac index is less than 2 L/min/m^2, and if left-sided filling pressures remain high with mixed venous oxygen saturations of less than 50%, short-term LVAD support with the ABIOMED system is instituted (Fig. 24-2). IABP alone in this patient population often does not prevent death and almost always results in significant renal, hepatic, and pulmonary dysfunction that significantly complicates patient recovery even if adequate cardiac function returns. Most important, stressing the heart with high-dose inotropic agents and high filling pressures when it is weakest during the early reperfusion period after acute infarction may compromise border zone regions. This concern is especially true of patients with older infarctions (more than 6 hours). We err on the side of implanting this short-term device early, since the survival

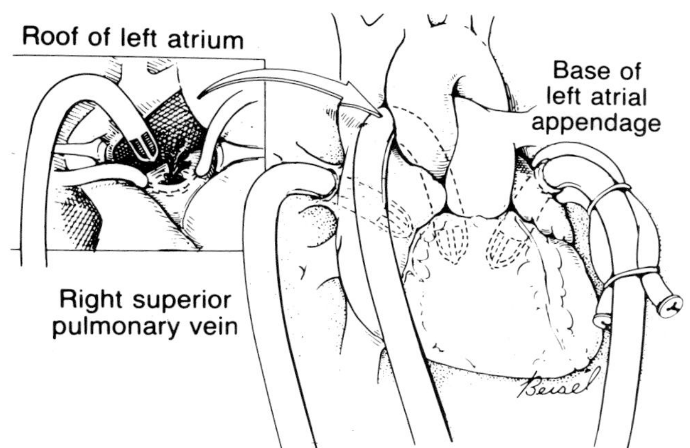

FIGURE 24–2 The inflow cannula for short-term left ventricular assist device support can be placed through the right superior pulmonary vein, the dome of the left atrium, or the left atrial appendage. Lighthouse tip cannulas allow improved venous return.

rate is only 7% if the device is inserted after a cardiac arrest in the recovery room.

Operative Techniques for Acute Myocardial Infarction

ANESTHESIA

Anesthesia is provided by a rapid narcotics-based regimen with perfusion and surgical teams prepared to respond to catastrophic hypotension or cardiac arrest. Transesophageal probes are always placed in these patients if possible. As the patient is prepped, a test dose followed by a loading dose of aprotinin is given.

BLEEDING

Bleeding is a significant complication of emergency CABG and often results in further myocardial depression and pulmonary hypertension. Cytokine release induced by infusion of blood products and thromboxane A2 released by cardiopulmonary bypass stimulate pulmonary hypertension, which can be catastrophic in the setting of right ventricular ischemia. Use of aprotinin decreases bleeding during CABG[122,123] and reduces right-sided heart failure and death after LVAD insertion.[124] There are reported cases of aprotinin use following thrombolytic therapy for acute myocardial infarction.[125] Successful use of aprotinin for reoperative, emergency, or high-risk CABG is common in many institutions.

CHOICE OF CONDUITS

For emergency cases, the choice of conduit should not differ from elective cases in most circumstances. The internal mammary artery is not associated with a higher number of complications compared with saphenous vein grafting in emergent situations and can be used in most circumstances.[126,127] There is one reported case of successful use of polytetrafluoroethylene for coronary revascularization in a patient in shock.[128]

INTRAOPERATIVE CONSIDERATIONS

Decompression of the ventricle during revascularization after acute coronary occlusion decreases muscle damage and improves functional outcome by decreasing wall tension and reducing oxygen consumption (Figs. 24-3 and 24-4).[62] Indeed, ventricular decompression reduces metabolic energy consumption by 60%. Diastolic basal arrest, by avoiding the energy of contraction, is the second most important means of minimizing oxygen consumption and further reduces metabolic energy consumption by 30%. Cooling of the patient and heart has an impact only on the final 10% of basal energy requirements.

Reduction of myocardial energy consumption is best achieved by early institution of cardiopulmonary bypass to maintain a high perfusion pressure. If a coronary salvage catheter has been placed across a tight coronary lesion, the catheter is left in place until just before cross-clamping. Antegrade and retrograde catheters are placed prior to cross-clamping to allow quick instillation of retrograde cardioplegia and protection of the territory supplied by the occluded or compromised vessel. The standard Buckberg protocol is

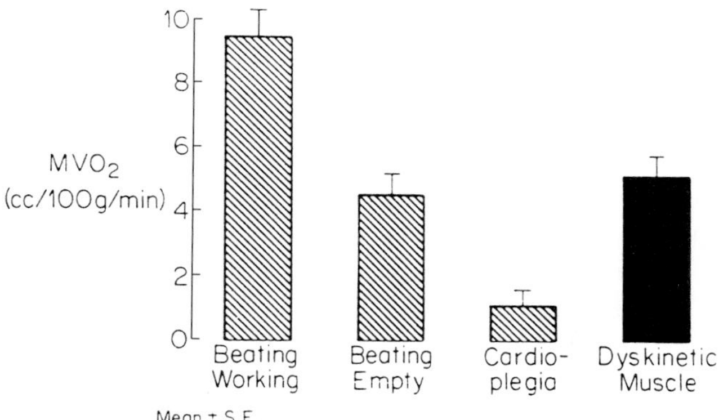

FIGURE 24–3 Myocardial oxygen uptake (measured in cc/100 g/min) in beating and working, beating and empty, and arrested hearts. Values after cardioplegia were determined both during cardiopulmonary bypass (cardioplegia) and during regional cardioplegic reperfusion in the working heart (paradoxing muscle). Note (1) marked fall in Mvo_2 with cardioplegia in the decompressed heart and (2) O_2 requirements of dyskinetic muscle increase 5-fold over cardioplegia alone and equal almost 55% of beating, working needs. *(Reproduced with permission from Allen BS, Rosenkranz ER, Buckberg GD, et al: Studies of controlled reperfusion after ischemia, VII: high oxygen requirements of dyskinetic cardiac muscle. J Thorac Cardiovasc Surg 1986; 92:543.)*

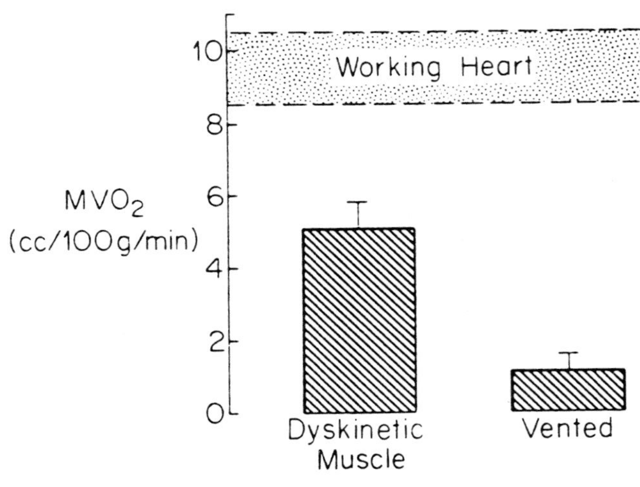

FIGURE 24–4 Regional oxygen uptake during selective cardioplegic reperfusion in dyskinetic and vented cardiac muscle. Stippled areas show requirements in working heart (8.5 to 10.5 cc/100 g/min). Note (1) high O_2 demands of dykinetic muscle and (2) marked reduction in demands when noncontracting muscle is decompressed by venting. *(Reproduced with permission from Allen BS, Rosenkranz ER, Buckberg GD, et al: Studies of controlled reperfusion after ischemia, VII: high oxygen requirements of dyskinetic cardiac muscle. J Thorac Cardiovasc Surg 1986; 92:543.)*

followed, including warm induction to allow regeneration of depleted ATP (adenosine triphosphate) stores.

If the territory at risk is grafted by saphenous vein, this anastamosis is performed first to allow direct instillation of cardioplegia into the territory at risk. The proximal anastomoses should be performed prior to removal of the cross-clamp to allow complete perfusion of the entire heart upon removal of the cross-clamp. The role of off-pump CABG in this setting is appealing, but remains unproven.

While large ventricular aneurysms are treated by resection and patch, debate surrounds smaller aneurysms. Our group does not resect small aneurysms, but some groups are more aggressive. If an aneurysm is resected, the defect is repaired with a patch of bovine pericardium sewn to the fibrotic rim of the endoaneurysm surface. The native left ventricular wall is closed over the patch.

Utilization of the Dor procedure (endoventricular circular patch plasty repair) in the post MI setting is a controversial subject. Recent data have shown surgical remodeling may improve systolic pump function.[129] However, a large clinical trial is needed to definitively answer this question.

POSTOPERATIVE CARE

A higher incidence of complications in shock patients compared with nonshock emergencies has been reported. Guyton et al[112] report a 47% complication rate associated with cardiogenic shock compared with 13% for patients with nonshock emergencies. This increase in complications probably reflects the preoperative condition of the patients rather than the treatment itself. Long-term follow-up in patients following emergency surgical revascularization shows that survival rates are closely correlated with postoperative ejection fraction and left ventricular size.[130,131]

CONCLUSION

The treatment of acute myocardial infarction should be divided into two approaches (Fig. 24-5). Uncomplicated acute myocardial infarction can be treated in most community hospitals. In most areas of the country, these patients are treated effectively with thrombolytic therapy and medical management. For communities and facilities that have catheterization laboratories, primary angioplasty may be more cost-effective and produce similar results. At this time, emergency coronary artery bypass surgery is not the most cost-effective approach; randomized, controlled studies to demonstrate

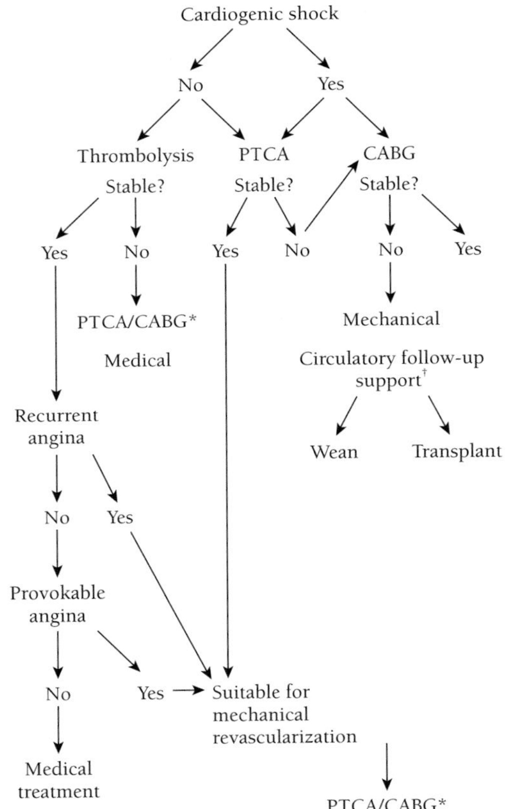

*PTCA = percutaneous transluminal coronary angioplasty; CABG = coronary artery bypass grafting. Choice of therapy is made based on the lesion(s) and comorbid factors.

†Choice of mechanical support is based on many factors (see text, along with other chapters).

FIGURE 24–5 Acute myocardial infarction algorithm.

advantages of emergency CABG have not yet been performed.

The approach to acute myocardial infarctions complicated by cardiogenic shock presents a more difficult problem. Mortality rates are high with medical management. Reperfusion therapy is the only real hope for improved survival in this group of patients. Thrombolytic therapy is associated with poor outcomes. Early PTCA and CABG are the primary options in patients under the age of 75. Mechanical circulatory assistance has an important role for supporting patients until the myocardium recovers. Use of pharmacologic agents and means to control reperfusion are important areas of current research and development. Assist devices and artificial heart programs offer indispensible options and must be considered in this patient population, especially since all therapies offer suboptimal results.

REFERENCES

1. American Heart Association: *Heart Disease and Stroke Statistics—2002 Update.* Dallas, TX, American Heart Association, 2002.
2. Lavie CJ, Gersh BJ: Mechanical and electrical complications of acute myocardial infarction. *Mayo Clin Proc* 1990; 65:709.
3. Goldberg RJ, Gore JM, Alpert JS, et al: Cardiogenic shock after acute myocardial infarction. *N Engl J Med* 1991; 325:1117.
4. Page DL, Caulfield JB, Kastor JA, et al: Myocardial changes associated with cardiogenic shock. *N Engl J Med* 1971; 285:133.
5. Alonso DR, Scheidt S, Post M, Killip T: Pathophysiology of cardiogenic shock: quantification of myocardial necrosis, clinical, pathologic and electrocardiographic correlations. *Circulation* 1973; 48:588.
6. Tennant T, Wiggers CJ: Effect of coronary occlusion on myocardial contraction. *Am J Physiol* 1935; 112:351.
7. Jennings RB, Reimer KA: Factors involved in salvaging ischemic myocardium: effect of reperfusion of arterial blood. *Circulation* 1983; 68(suppl I):I-25.
8. Schaper W: Experimental coronary artery occlusion, III: the determinants of collateral blood flow in acute coronary occlusion. *Basic Res Cardiol* 1978; 73:584.
9. Reimer KA, Jennings RB: The wavefront phenomenon of myocardial ischemic cell death, II: transmural progression of necrosis within the framework of ischemic bed size (myocardium at risk) and collateral flow. *Lab Invest* 1979; 40:633.
10. Sadanandan S, Hochman JS: Early reperfusion, late reperfusion, and the open artery hypothesis: an overview. *Prog Cardiovasc Dis* 2000; 42:397.
11. Mancini DM, Beniaminovitz A, Levin H, et al: Low incidence of myocardial recovery after left ventricular assist device implantation in patients with chronic heart failure. *Circulation* 1998; 98:2383.
12. Chen JM, DeRose JJ, Slater JP, et al: Improved survival rates support left ventricular assist device implantation early after myocardial infarction. *J Am Coll Cardiol* 1999; 33:1903.
13. Eaton LW, Weiss JL, Bulkley BH, et al: Regional cardiac dilation after acute myocardial infarction. *N Engl J Med* 1979; 300:57.
14. Buckberg GD: Studies of controlled reperfusion after ischemia, I: when is cardiac muscle damaged irreversibly? *J Thorac Cardiovasc Surg* 1986; 92:483.
15. Allen BS, Buckberg GD, Fontan FM, et al: Superiority of controlled surgical reperfusion versus percutaneous transluminal coronary angioplasty in acute coronary occlusion. *J Thorac Cardiovasc Surg* 1993; 105:864.
16. Killip T 3rd, Kimball JT: Treatment of myocardial infarction in a coronary care unit: a two-year experience with 250 patients. *Am J Cardiol* 1972; 20:457.
17. Goldberg RJ, Gore JM, Alpert JS, et al: Cardiogenic shock after acute myocardial infarction. *N Engl J Med* 1991; 325:1117.
18. Gacioch GM, Ellis SG, Lee L, et al: Cardiogenic shock complicating acute myocardial infarction: the use of coronary angioplasty and the integration of the new support devices into patient management. *J Am Coll Cardiol* 1992; 19:647.
19. Hochman JS, Sleeper LA, Webb JG, et al: Early revascularization in acute myocardial infarction complicated by cardiogenic shock. SHOCK Investigators. Should We Emergently Revascularize Occluded Coronaries for Cardiogenic Shock. *N Engl J Med* 1999; 341:625.
20. Hochman JS, Sleeper LA, White HD, et al: One-year survival following early revascularization for cardiogenic shock. *JAMA* 2001; 285:190.
21. Wackers FJ, Lie KI, Becker AE, et al: Coronary artery disease in patients dying from cardiogenic shock or congestive heart failure in the setting of acute myocardial infarction. *Br Heart J* 1976; 38:906.
22. Gutovitz AL, Sobel BE, Roberts R: Progressive nature of myocardial injury in selected patients with cardiogenic shock. *Am J Cardiol* 1978; 41:469.
23. Hennekens CH, O'Donnell CJ, Ridker PM, Marder VJ: Current issues concerning thrombolytic therapy for acute myocardial infarction. *J Am Coll Cardiol* 1995; 25(suppl):18S.
24. Rahimtoola SH: The hibernating myocardium. *Am Heart J* 1989; 117:211.
25. Rahimtoola SH: The hibernating myocardium in ischemia and congestive heart failure. *Eur Heart J* 1993; 14 (suppl A):22.
26. Carlson EB, Cowley MJ, Wolfgang TC, Vetrovec GW: Acute changes in global and regional rest ventricular function after successful coronary angioplasty: comparative results in stable and unstable angina. *J Am Coll Cardiol* 1989; 13:1262.
27. Schuster EH, Bulkley BH: Early post-infarction angina: ischemia at a distance and ischemia in the infarct zone. *N Engl J Med* 1981; 305:1101.
28. Braunwald E, Kloner RA: The stunned myocardium: prolonged postischemic ventricular dysfunction. *Circulation* 1982; 66:1146.
29. Bolli R: Mechanism of myocardial stunning. *Circulation* 1990; 82:723.
30. Heyndrickx GR, Millard RW, McRitchie RJ, et al: Regional myocardial function and electrophysiological alterations after brief coronary artery occlusion in conscious dogs. *J Clin Invest* 1975; 56:978.
31. Marban E: Myocardial stunning and hibernation: the physiology behind the colloquialisms. *Circulation* 1991; 83:681.
32. Conti CR: The stunned and hibernating myocardium: a brief review. *Clin Cardiol* 1991; 14:708.
33. Gibson RS, Watson DD, Taylor GJ, et al: Prospective assessment of regional myocardial perfusion before and after coronary revascularization surgery by quantitative thallium-201 scintigraphy. *J Am Coll Cardiol* 1983; 1:804.
34. Dilsizian V, Bonow RO: Current diagnostic techniques of asssessing myocardial viability in patients with stunned and hibernating myocardium. *Circulation* 1993; 87:1.
35. Bergmann SR: Cardiac positron emission tomography. *Semin Nucl Med* 1998, 28:320.
36. Charney R, Schwinger ME, Cohen MV, et al: Dobutamine echocardiography predicts recovery of hibernating myocardium following coronary revascularization. *J Am Coll Cardiol* 1992; 19:176A.

37. Klein C, Nekolla SG, Bengel FM, et al: Assessment of myocardial viability with contrast-enhanced magnetic resonance imaging: comparison with positron emission tomography. *Circulation* 2002; 105:162.
38. Johnson WD, Kayser KL, Brenowitz JB, et al: A randomized controlled trial of allopurinol in coronary bypass surgery. *Am Heart J* 1991; 121:20.
39. Eddy LJ, Stewart JR, Jones HP, et al: Free radical-producing enzyme, xanthine oxidase, is undetectable in human hearts. *Am J Physiol* 1987; 253:H709.
40. Muxfeldt M, Schaper W: The activity of xanthine oxidase in hearts of pigs, guinea pigs, rats, and humans. *Basic Res Cardiol* 1987; 82:486.
41. Topol EJ, Ellis SH, Califf RM, et al: Combined tissue-type plasminogen activator and prostacyclin therapy for acute myocardial infarction. *J Am Coll Cardiol* 1989; 14:877.
42. Scott BD, Kerber RE: Clinical and experimental aspects of myocardial stunning. *Prog Cardiovasc Dis* 1992; 35:61.
43. Bolli R, Jeroudi MO, Patel BS, et al: Marked reduction of free radical generation and contractile function by antioxidant therapy begun at the time of reperfusion. *Circ Res* 1989; 65:607.
44. Werns S, Brinker J, Gruber J, et al: A randomized, double-blind trial of recombinant human superoxide dismutase in patients undergoing PTCA for acute myocardial infarction. *Circulation* 1989; 80 (suppl 2):113.
45. Taylor AL, Golino P, Eckels R, et al: Differential enhancement of postischemic segmental systolic thickening by diltiazem. *J Am Coll Cardiol* 1990; 15:737.
46. Westlin W, Mullane K: Does captopril attenuate reperfusion induced myocardial dysfunction by scavenging free radicals? *Circulation* 1988; 77(suppl I): I-30.
47. Stahl LD, Aversano TR, Becker LC: Selective enhancement of function of stunned myocardium by increased flow. *Circulation* 1986; 74:843.
48. Al-Wathiqui MH, Farber N, Pelc L, et al: Improvement in functional recovery of stunned canine myocardium by long-term pretreatment with oral propranolol. *Am Heart J* 1989; 117:791.
49. Lamping KA, Gross GJ: Improved recovery of myocardial segment function following a short coronary occlusion in dogs by nicorandil, a potential new antianginal agent, and nifedipine. *J Cardiovasc Pharmacol* 1985; 7:158.
50. Sheiban I, Tonni S, Marini A, et al: Clinical and therapeutic implications of chronic left ventricular dysfunction in coronary artery disease. *Am J Cardiol* 1995; 73:23E.
51. Rinaldi CA, Linka AZ, Masaini ND, et al: Randomized, double-blind crossover study to investigate the effects of amlodipine and isosorbide mononitrate on the time course and severity of exercise-induced myocardial stunning. *Circulation* 1998; 98:749.
52. Vinten-Johansen J, Buckberg GD, Okamoto F, et al: Studies of controlled reperfusion after ischemia, V: superiority of surgical versus medical reperfusion after regional ischemia. *J Thorac Cardiovasc Surg* 1986; 92:525.
53. Vinten-Johansen J, Rosenkranz ER, Buckberg GD, et al: Studies of controlled reperfusion after ischemia, VI: metabolic and histochemical benefits of regional blood cardioplegic reperfusion without cardiopulmonary bypass. *J Thorac Cardiovasc Surg* 1986; 92:535.
54. Acar C, Partington MT, Buckberg GD: Studies of controlled reperfusion after ischemia, XX: reperfusate composition: detrimental effects of initial asanguineous cardioplegic washout after acute coronary occlusion. *J Thorac Cardiovasc Surg* 1991; 101:294.
55. Acar C, Partington MT, Buckberg GD: Studies of controlled reperfusion after ischemia, XVIII: reperfusion conditions: attention of the regional ischemia effect by temporary total vented bypass before controlled reperfusion. *J Thorac Cardiovasc Surg* 1990; 100:737.
56. Acar C, Partington MT, Buckberg GD: Studies of controlled reperfusion after ischemia, XVII: reperfusion conditions: controlled reperfusion through an internal mammary artery graft: a new technique emphasizing fixed pressure versus fixed flow. *J Thorac Cardiovasc Surg* 1990; 100:724.
57. Allen BS, Buckberg GD, Schwaiger M, et al: Studies of controlled reperfusion after ischemia, XVI: early recovery of regional wall motion in patients following surgical revascularization after eight hours of acute coronary occlusion. *J Thorac Cardiovasc Surg* 1986; 92:636.
58. Allen BS, Okamoto F, Buckberg GD, et al: Studies of controlled reperfusion after ischemia, XV: immediate functional recovery after six hours of regional ischemia by careful control of conditions of reperfusion and composition of reperfusate. *J Thorac Cardiovasc Surg* 1986; 92:621.
59. Allen BS, Okamoto F, Buckberg GD, et al: Studies of controlled reperfusion after ischemia, XIII: reperfusion conditions: critical importance of total ventricular decompression during regional reperfusion. *J Thorac Cardiovasc Surg* 1986; 92:605.
60. Allen BS, Okamoto F, Buckberg GD, et al: Studies of controlled reperfusion after ischemia, XII: effects of "duration" of reperfusate administration versus reperfusate "dose" on regional, functional, biochemical, and histological recovery. *J Thorac Cardiovasc Surg* 1986; 92:594.
61. Allen BS, Okamoto F, Buckberg GD, et al: Studies of controlled reperfusion after ischemia, IX: reperfusate composition benefits of marked hypocalcemia and diltiazem on regional recovery. *J Thorac Cardiovasc Surg* 1986; 92:564.
62. Allen BS, Rosenkranz ER, Buckberg GD, et al: Studies of controlled reperfusion after ischemia, VII: high oxygen requirements of dyskinetic cardiac muscle. *J Thorac Cardiovasc Surg* 1986; 92:543.
63. Okamoto F, Allen BS, Buckberg GD, et al: Studies of controlled reperfusion after ischemia, XIV: reperfusion conditions: importance of ensuring gentle versus sudden reperfusion during relief of coronary occlusion. *J Thorac Cardiovasc Surg* 1986; 92:613.
64. Okamoto F, Allen BS, Buckberg GD, et al: Studies of controlled reperfusion after ischemia, X: reperfusate composition: supplemental role of intravenous and intracoronary coenzyme Q10 in avoiding reperfusion damage. *J Thorac Cardiovasc Surg* 1986; 92:573.
65. Okamoto F, Allen BS, Buckberg GD, et al: Studies of controlled reperfusion after ischemia, VIII: regional blood cardioplegic reperfusion during total vented bypass without thoracotomy: a new concept. *J Thorac Cardiovasc Surg* 1986; 92:553.
66. Okamoto F, Allen BS, Buckberg GD, et al: Studies of controlled reperfusion after ischemia, XI: reperfusate composition: interaction of marked hyperglycemia and marked hyperosmolarity in allowing immediate contractile recovery after four hours of regional ischemia. *J Thorac Cardiovasc Surg* 1986; 92:583.
67. Rosenkranz ER, Okamoto F, Buckberg GD, et al: Studies of controlled reperfusion after ischemia, II: biochemical studies: failure of tissue adenosine triphosphate levels to predict recovery of contractile function after controlled reperfusion. *J Thorac Cardiovasc Surg* 1986; 92:488.
68. Quillen J, Kofsky ER, Buckberg GD, et al: Studies of controlled reperfusion after ischemia, XXIII: Deleterious effects of simulated thrombolysis preceding simulated coronary artery bypass grafting with controlled blood cardioplegic reperfusion. *J Thorac Cardiovasc Surg* 1991; 101:455.

69. Rentrop P, Blanke H, Karsch KR, et al: Selective intracoronary thrombolysis in acute myocardial infarction and unstable angina pectoris. *Circulation* 1981; 63:307.
70. Gruppo Italiano per lo Studio della Streptokinasi: The effectiveness of intravenous thrombolytic treatment in acute myocardial infarction. *Lancet* 1986; 1:397.
71. ISSI-2 (Second International Study of Infarct Survival): Randomized trial of intravenous streptokinase, oral aspirin, both, or neither among 17187 cases of suspected acute myocardial infarction. *Lancet* 1988; 2:349.
72. The TIMI Study Group: Comparison of invasive and conservative strategies after treatment with intravenous tissue plasminogen activator in acute myocardial infarction. *N Engl J Med* 1989; 320:618.
73. Simoons ML, Betriu A, Col J, et al: Thrombolysis with tissue plasminogen activator in acute myocardial infarction: no additional benefit from immediate percutaneous coronary angioplasty. *Lancet* 1988; 1:197.
74. Gruppo Italiano per lo Studio della Streptokinasi: GISSI-2: a factorial randomized trial of altepase versus streptokinase and heparin versus no heparin among 12,490 patients with acute myocardial infarction. *Lancet* 1990; 336:65.
75. ISIS-3 (Third International Study of Infarct Survival): ISIS-3: a randomized comparison of streptokinase vs tissue plasminogen activator vs anistreplase and of aspirin plus heparin vs aspirin alone among 41,299 cases of suspected acute myocardial infarction. *Lancet* 1993; 339:753.
76. The GUSTO Angiographic Investigators: The effects of tissue plasminogen activator, streptokinase, or both on coronary patency, ventricular function, and survival after acute myocardial infarction. *N Engl J Med* 1993; 329:1615.
77. The GUSTO Investigators: An international randomized trial comparing four thrombolytic strategies for acute myocardial infarction. *N Engl J Med* 1993; 329:673.
78. Rentrop KP: Restoration of antegrade flow in acute myocardial infarction: the first 15 years. *J Am Coll Cardiol* 1995; 25(suppl): 1S.
79. Bates ER, Topol EJ: Limitations of thrombolytic therapy for acute myocardial infarction complicated by congestive heart failure and cardiogenic shock. *J Am Coll Cardiol* 1991; 18:1077.
80. Weaver WD, Cerueira M, Hallstrom AP, et al: Prehospital-initiated versus hospital-initiated thrombolytic therapy: the myocardial infarction, triage, and intervention trial (MITI). *JAMA* 1993; 270:1211.
81. Gruntzig AR, Senning A, Siegenthaler WE: Nonoperative dilation of coronary-artery stenoses. *N Engl J Med* 1979; 301:61.
82. O'Keefe JH Jr, Bailey WL, Rutherford BD, Hartzler GO: Primary angioplasty for acute myocardial infarction in 1000 consecutive patients. *Am J Cardiol* 1993; 72:107G.
83. Grines CL, Browne KF, Marco J, et al: A comparison of immediate angioplasty with thrombolytic therapy in acute myocardial infarction. *N Engl J Med* 1993; 328:673.
84. Gibbons RJ, Holmes DR, Reeder GS, et al: Immediate angioplasty compared with the administration of a thrombolytic agent followed by conservative treatment for myocardial infarction. *N Engl J Med* 1993; 328:685.
85. Goldman L: Cost and quality of life: thrombolysis and primary angioplasty. *J Am Coll Cardiol* 1995; 25(suppl):38S.
86. Topol EJ, Califf RM, George BS, et al: A randomized trial of immediate versus delayed elective angioplasty after intravenous tissue plasminogen activator in acute myocardial infarction. *N Engl J Med* 1987; 317:581.
87. Rogers WJ, Baim DS, Gore JM, et al: Comparison of immediate invasive, delayed invasive, and conservative strategies after tissue-type plasminogen activator: results of the thrombolysis in myocardial infarction (TIMI) phase II-a trial. *Circulation* 1990; 81:1457.
88. Ellis SG, Mooney MR, George BS, et al: Randomized trial of late elective angioplasty versus conservative management for patients with residual stenoses after thrombolytic treatment of myocardial infarction. *Circulation* 1992; 86:1400.
89. Lee L, Bates ER, Pitt B, et al: Percutaneous transluminal coronary angioplasty improves survival in acute myocardial infarction complicated by cardiogenic shock. *Circulation* 1988; 78:1345.
90. Lee L, Erbel R, Brown TM, et al: Multicenter registry of angioplasty therapy of cardiogenic shock: initial and long-term survival. *J Am Coll Cardiol* 1991; 17:599.
91. Cantor WJ, Peterson ED, Popma JJ, et al: Provisional stenting strategies: systemic overview and implications for clinical decision-making. *J Am Coll Cardiol* 2000, 36:1142.
92. Dawson JT, Hall RJ, Hallman GL, Cooley DA: Mortality in patients undergoing coronary artery bypass surgery after myocardial infarction. *Am J Cardiol* 1974; 33:483.
93. Levine FH, Gold HK, Leinbach RC, et al: Safe early revascularization for continuing ischemia after acute myocardial infarction. *Circulation* 1979; 60(suppl I): I-5.
94. Berg R Jr, Selinger SL, Leonard JJ, et al: Immediate coronary artery bypass for acute evolving myocardial infarction. *J Thorac Cardiovasc Surg* 1981; 81:493.
95. DeWood MA, Notske RN, Berg R, et al: Medical and surgical management of early Q wave myocardial infarction, I: effects of surgical reperfusion on survival, recurrent myocardial infarction, sudden death and functional class at 10 or more years of follow-up. *J Am Coll Cardiol* 1989; 14:65.
96. DeWood MA, Spores J, Berg R Jr, et al: Acute myocardial infarction: a decade of experience with surgical reperfusion in 701 patients. *Circulation* 1983; 68(suppl II): II-8.
97. DeWood MA, Spores J, Notske RN, et al: Prevalence of total coronary occlusion during the early hours of transmural myocardial infarction. *N Engl J Med* 1980; 303:897.
98. Phillips SJ, Kongtahworn C, Skinner JR, Zeff RH: Emergency coronary artery reperfusion: a choice therapy for evolving myocardial infarction. *J Thorac Cardiovasc Surg* 1983; 86:679.
99. Phillips SJ, Kongtahworn C, Zeff RH, et al: Emergency coronary artery revascularization: a possible therapy for acute myocardial infarction. *Circulation* 1979; 60:241.
100. Phillips SJ, Zeff RH, Skinner JR, et al: Reperfusion protocol and results in 738 patients with evolving myocardial infarction. *Ann Thorac Surg* 1986; 41:119.
101. Spencer FC: Emergency coronary bypass for acute infarction: an unproved clinical experiment. *Circulation* 1983; 68(suppl II): II-17.
102. Lee DC, Oz MC, Weinberg AD, et al: Optimal timing of revascularization: transmural versus nontransmural acute myocardial infarction. *Ann Thorac Surg* 2001; 71:1198.
103. Lee DC, Oz MC, Weinberg AD, et al: Appropriate timing of surgical intervention after transmural acute myocardial infarction. *J Thorac Cardiovasc Surg (in press)*.
104. Weiss JL, Marino N, Shapiro EP: Myocardial infarct expansion: recognition, significance and pathology. *Am J Cardiol* 1991; 68:35.
105. Roberts CS, Schoen FJ, Kloner RA: Effects of coronary reperfusion on myocardial hemorrhage and infarct healing. *Am J Cardiol* 1983; 52:610.
106. Creswell LL, Rosenbloom M, Cox JL, et al: Intraaortic balloon counterpulsation: patterns of usage and outcome in cardiac surgical patients. *Ann Thorac Surg* 1992; 54:11.
107. Creswell LR, Moulton MJ, Cox JL, Rosenbloom M: Revascularization after acute myocardial infarction. *Ann Thorac Surg* 1995; 60:19.

108. Dresdale AR, Paone G: Surgical treatment of acute myocardial infarction. *Henry Ford Hosp Med J* 1991; 39:245.
109. Kouchoukos NT, Murphy S, Philpott T, et al: Coronary artery bypass grafting for postinfarction angina pectoris. *Circulation* 1989; 79(suppl I):I-68.
110. Stuart RS, Baumgartner WA, Soule L, et al: Predictors of perioperative mortality in patients with unstable postinfarction angina. *Circulation* 1988; 78(suppl I):I-163.
111. DeWood MA, Notske RN, Hensley GR, et al: Intraaortic balloon counterpulsation with and without reperfusion for myocardial infarction shock. *Circulation* 1980; 61:1105.
112. Guyton RA, Arcidi JM, Langford DA, et al: Emergency coronary bypass for cardiogenic shock. *Circulation* 1987; 76(suppl V):V-22.
113. Scheidt S, Wilner G, Mueller H, et al: Intra-aortic balloon counterpulsation in cardiogenic shock. *N Engl J Med* 1973; 288:979.
114. Waksman R, Weiss AT, Gotsman MS, Hasin Y: Intra-aortic balloon counterpulsation improves survival in cardiogenic shock complicating acute myocardial infarction. *Eur Heart J* 1993; 14:71.
115. Ohman EM, George BS, White CJ, et al: Use of aortic counterpulsation to improve sustained coronary artery patency during acute myocardial infarction. *Circulation* 1994; 90:792.
116. Ratcliffe MB, Bavaria JE, Wenger RK, et al: Left ventricular mechanics of ejecting postischemic hearts during left ventricular circulatory assistance. *J Thorac Cardiovasc Surg* 1991; 101:245.
117. Goldenberg IF: Nonpharmacologic management of cardiac arrest and cardiogenic shock. *Chest* 1992; 102:596S.
118. Lowe JE, Anstadt MP, Van Tright P, et al: First successful bridge to cardiac transplantation using direct mechanical ventricular actuation. *Ann Thorac Surg* 1991; 52:1237.
119. Loebe M, Hennig E, Muller J, et al: Long-term mechanical circulatory support as a bridge to transplantation, for recovery from cardiomyopathy, and for permanent replacement. *Eur J Cardiothorac Surg* 1997; 11:S18.
120. Yacoub MH: A novel strategy to maximize the efficacy of left ventricular assist devices as a bridge to recovery. *Eur Heart J* 2001; 22:534.
121. Oz MC, Pepino P, Goldstein DJ, et al: Selection scale predicts patients successfully receiving long-term, implantable left ventricular assist devices. *Circulation* 1994; 90:I-308.
122. Lemmer JH Jr, Stanford W, Bonney SL, et al: Aprotinin for coronary artery bypass operations: efficacy, safety, and influence on early saphenous vein graft patency. *J Thorac Cardiovasc Surg* 1994; 107:543.
123. Murkin JM, Lux J, Shannon NA, et al: Aprotinin significantly decreases bleeding and transfusion requirements in patients recieving aspirin and undergoing cardiac operations. *J Thorac Cardiovasc Surg* 1994; 107:554.
124. Goldstein DJ, Seldomridge JA, Chen JM, et al: Use of aprotinin in LVAD recipients reduces blood loss, blood product requirement, and perioperative mortality. *Ann Thorac Surg* 1995; 59:1063.
125. Efstratiadis T, Munsch C, Crossman D, Taylor K: Aprotinin used in emergency coronary operation after streptokinase treatment. *Ann Thorac Surg* 1991; 52:1320.
126. Caes FL, Van Nooten GJ: Use of internal mammary artery for emergency grafting after failed coronary angioplasty. *Ann Thorac Surg* 1994; 57:1295.
127. Zaplonski A, Rosenblum J, Myler RK, et al: Emergency coronary artery bypass surgery following failed balloon angioplasty: role of the internal mammary artery graft. *J Cardiac Surg* 1995; 10:32.
128. Hartman AR, Vlay SC, Dervan JP, et al: Emergency coronary revasculariztion using polytetrafluoroethylene conduits in a patient in cardiogenic shock. *Clin Cardiol* 1991; 14:75.
129. Di Donato M, Sabatier M, Dor V, et al: Effects of the Dor procedure on left ventricular dimension and shape and geometric correlates of mitral regurgitation one year after surgery. *J Thorac Cardiovasc Surg* 2001; 121:91.
130. Applebaum R, House R, Rademaker A, et al: Coronary artery bypass grafting within thirty days of acute myocardial infarction. *J Thorac Cardiovasc Surg* 1991; 102:745.
131. Hochberg MS, Parsonnet V, Gielchinsky I, et al: Timing of coronary revascularization after acute myocardial infarction. *J Thorac Cardiovasc Surg* 1984; 88:914.

Chapter 25

Coronary Artery Reoperations

Bruce W. Lytle

Coronary reoperations are more complicated than primary operations. Patients undergoing reoperations have distinct, more dangerous pathologies; reoperations are technically more difficult to perform; and the risks are greater.[1–12] Vein graft atherosclerosis, present in most reoperative candidates, is a unique and dangerous lesion. Reoperative candidates commonly have severe and diffuse native vessel distal coronary artery disease, a problem that has had the time to develop only because those patients did not die from their original proximal coronary lesions. Aortic and noncardiac atherosclerosis are also often far advanced in many reoperative candidates. Some technical hazards, including the presence of patent arterial grafts and sternal reentry, are unique to reoperations, and others, such as lack of bypass conduits and difficult coronary exposure, are common.

INCIDENCE OF REOPERATION

After a primary bypass operation the likelihood of a patient undergoing a reoperation is dependent on patient-related variables, primary operation–related variables, the possibility of alternative treatments, physician opinion about the feasibility of reoperation, and time. Review of 4000 patients who had primary bypass surgery at The Cleveland Clinic Foundation during the years 1971 through 1974 documented a cumulative incidence of reoperation of 3% by 5 years, 10% by 10 years, and 25% by 20 postoperative years (Fig. 25-1).[13] Factors associated statistically with an increased likelihood of reoperation have been variables predicting a favorable long-term survival (young age, normal left ventricular function, single- or double-vessel disease), variables designating an imperfect primary operation (no interior thoracic artery graft, incomplete revascularization), and symptom status (Class III or IV symptoms at primary operation). Young age at primary operation and incomplete revascularization are also markers of a severe atherogenic diathesis.

Surgery has changed in directions that will decrease the rate of reoperation. Use of the left internal thoracic artery (LITA) to graft the left anterior descending (LAD) coronary artery decreases the risk of reoperation compared to the strategy of using only vein grafts, and the LITA-LAD graft has become a standard part of operations for coronary revascularization.[14] Furthermore, it now appears that the use of bilateral ITA grafts decreases the likelihood of death and reoperation when compared to the single LITA-LAD strategy (Fig. 25-2).[15] The use of other arterial conduits such as the radial artery and the gastroepiploic artery in the context of total arterial revascularization may further decrease the risk of reoperation, but as yet the long-term data are insufficient to answer that question.

The patient population of reoperative candidates has evolved. Cleveland Clinic Foundation studies have shown that in the early years of bypass surgery (1967–1978) only 28% of patients underwent reoperation solely because of

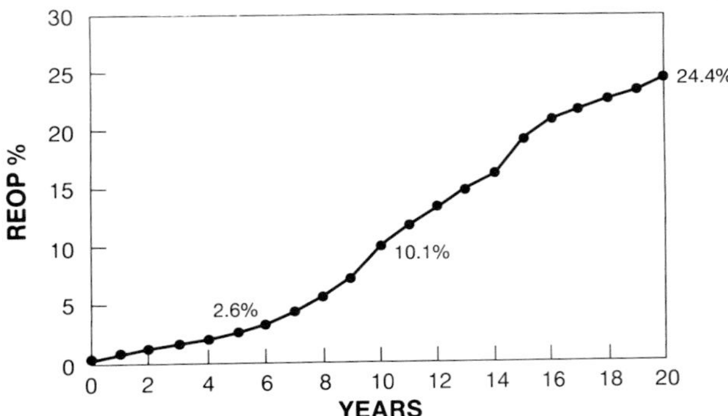

FIGURE 25–1 Study of 4000 patients who underwent bypass surgery from 1971–1974 showed that 25% of patients had undergone a reoperation within a period of 20 years after primary operation. *(Data from Cosgrove DM, Loop FD, Lytle BW, et al: Predictors of reoperation after myocardial revascularization. J Thorac Cardiovasc Surg 1986; 92:811.)*

graft failure, and that graft failure often occurred early after the primary operation (mean postoperative interval of 28 months after primary operation). Reoperation because of the progression of atherosclerosis in nongrafted coronary arteries was common in the 1967-1978 time period (55% of patients).[1,2] Today early graft failure and progression of disease in nongrafted vessels are not common causes of reoperation. In our cohort of reoperative patients examined most recently (1988–1991), almost all had graft failure as at least part of the indication for reoperation (92%), but that graft failure occurred late after the primary operation with a mean interval of 116 months.[3] Thus, patients undergoing reoperation today usually had a successful primary operation at least 10 years previously for the treatment of multivessel coronary artery disease, and the angiographic indications for reoperation are progression of native vessel distal coronary artery disease in combination with late graft failure caused by vein graft atherosclerosis.

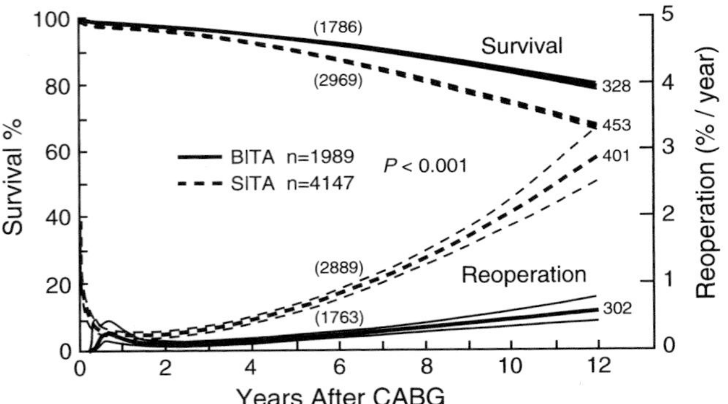

FIGURE 25–2 Comparison of survival and reoperation hazard function curves in the propensity-matched patients undergoing bilateral (BITA, n = 1989) or single ITA (SITA, n = 4147) coronary bypass grafting. *(Reproduced with permission from Lytle BW, Blackstone EH, Loop FD, et al: Two internal thoracic artery grafts are better than one. J Thorac Cardiovasc Surg 1999;117:855.)*

GRAFT FAILURE

An understanding of the pathology and causes of saphenous vein graft failure is important not only for an understanding of the causes of the need for reoperation but also to understand the dangers inherent in either the interventional or conservative treatment of patients with previous bypass surgery.

Saphenous vein to coronary artery grafts exhibit different pathologies at different intervals after operation.[16–19] Within a few months they often have diffuse endothelial disruptions with associated mural thrombus. The mural thrombus is usually not obstructing, and when grafts do become occluded early after operation due to thrombosis it may not be a result of these intimal changes but rather it is related to hemodynamic factors. Most saphenous vein grafts examined more than 2 to 3 months after operation have developed a proliferative intimal fibroplasia. This is a concentric cellular process and it is diffuse, extending the entire length of the graft (Fig. 25-3). It evolves with time to a more fibrous lesion. It is not friable, and although intimal fibroplasia involves most vein grafts, it causes stenoses or occlusions of only a few.

Vein graft atherosclerosis is a distinct pathologic process that is often recognized as early as 3 to 4 years after operation and is characterized by lipid infiltration of areas of intimal fibroplasia (Fig. 25-3). The distribution of vein graft atherosclerosis mimics that of intimal fibroplasia in that it is concentric and diffuse, although as vein graft atherosclerosis progresses, stenotic lesions may become eccentric. In addition, vein graft atherosclerosis is a superficial lesion, it is very friable, and it is often associated with overlying mural thrombus. These characteristics make it different from native vessel coronary atherosclerosis, a process that is segmental and proximal, eccentric, encapsulated, usually not friable, and usually not associated with overlying mural thrombus. Vein graft atherosclerosis is seen in a majority of grafts explanted more than 10 years after surgery whether or not those grafts are stenotic, and atherosclerotic lesions appear to account for almost all late saphenous vein graft (SVG) stenoses. The extreme friability of vein graft atherosclerosis creates a substantial risk of distal coronary artery embolization during percutaneous interventions to treat stenotic lesions and during reoperations for patients with atherosclerotic vein grafts. It is also probable that spontaneous coronary embolization may occur from atherosclerotic grafts. In addition, atherosclerotic stenoses in vein grafts appear to predispose to graft thrombosis. Vein graft atherosclerosis appears to be an "active" event-producing lesion.

The exact incidence of late SVG stenoses and occlusions is difficult to determine even with prospective studies because death and reoperation are nonrandom events that

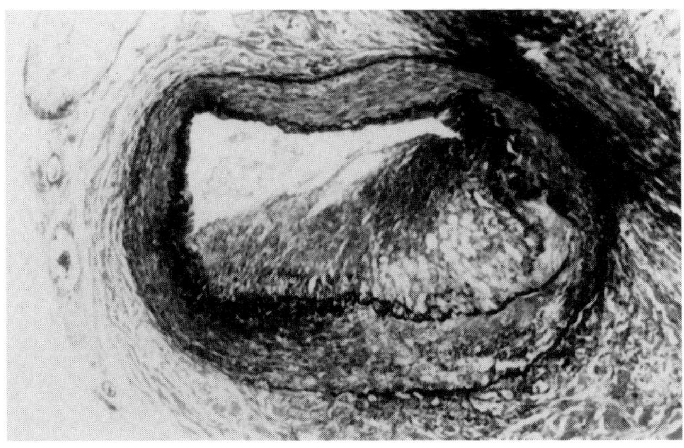

A

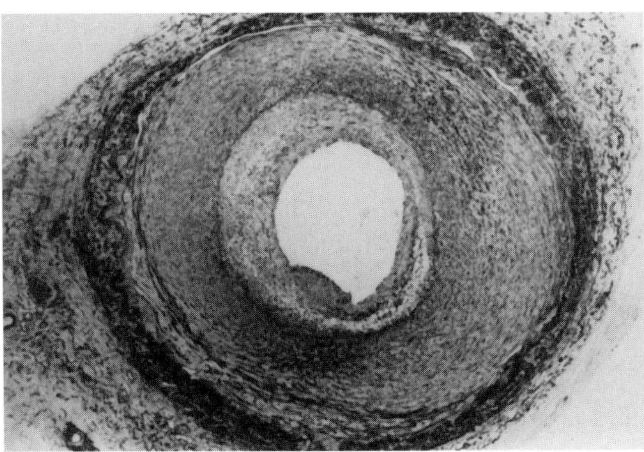

B

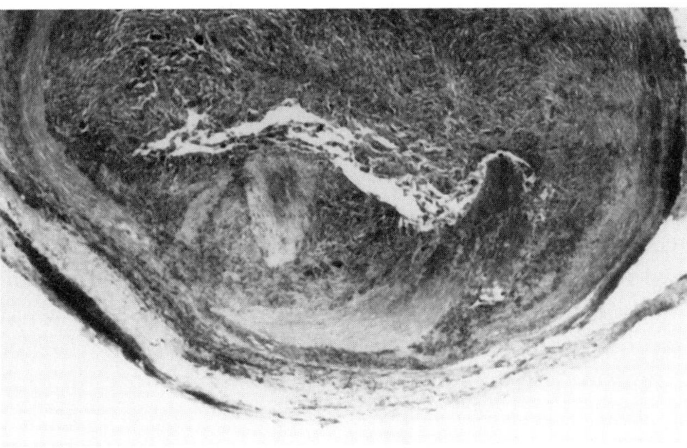

C

FIGURE 25–3 Pathology of (A) native coronary artery atherosclerosis; (B) vein graft intimal fibrosis; and (C) severe vein graft atherosclerosis. *(Reproduced with permission from Lytle BW, Cosgrove DM: Coronary artery bypass surgery, in Wells SA (ed): Current Problems in Surgery. Philadelphia, WB Saunders, 1992; p 733.)*

remove patients from prospective populations available for late coronary angiography. However, it appears that by 10 years after operation approximately 30% of vein grafts are totally occluded, and 30% of patent grafts exhibit some degree of stenosis or intimal irregularities characteristic of vein graft atherosclerosis.[20,21] Although vein graft atherosclerosis is not the only factor related to late SVG occlusion, it is an important one. Native vessel stenoses distal to the insertion site of vein grafts may decrease SVG graft outflow and contribute to graft failure, but late graft occlusion usually occurs in the presence of vein graft atherosclerosis. Furthermore, when stenotic vein grafts are replaced at reoperation, the late patency rate of the new vein grafts is good.[2]

Progress has been made toward decreasing the rate of vein graft failure. The early patency rates of SVGs have been improved by the use of perioperative and long-term platelet inhibitors,[22–24] but even recent data involving patients receiving platelet inhibitors indicate that the 10-year vein graft failure rate is approximately 35%. Some studies have shown that lipid lowering regimens decrease late vein graft disease and the risk of late cardiac events. However, the overall level of improvement has been small.[25,26] So far, the only way known to avoid vein graft atherosclerosis is to avoid using vein grafts.

ITA grafts rarely develop late atherosclerosis and the late attrition rate of patent ITA grafts is extremely low. Left ITA to LAD grafts have a very high late (20 years) patency rate, and for most patients the LAD is a profoundly important coronary artery.[20,27] These factors account for the impact of the LITA-LAD graft not only in decreasing the rate of late death after primary bypass surgery but also in decreasing the rate of reoperation.[14] Multiple ITA grafts provide incremental benefit in decreasing the risk of reoperation.[15] It is also important that ITA grafts do not develop graft atherosclerosis and, therefore, do not create the risk of coronary embolization during reoperation. The presence of patent arterial grafts may create other technical problems during repeat surgery, but embolization is not among them.

INDICATIONS FOR REOPERATION

The randomized trials of bypass surgery versus medical management that were initiated in the 1970s provided a framework of information concerning the indications for bypass surgery, and subsequent observational studies have added substance to that framework. However, no randomized trials of medical versus surgical management pertain to patients with prior surgery. The coronary pathology of patients with previous bypass surgery is different than that for patients with only native vessel stenoses, and we cannot assume that the natural history of, for example, triple-vessel disease based on atherosclerotic vein grafts is equivalent to that of patients with triple-vessel, native-vessel disease.

There are two nonrandomized retrospective studies of patients who had angiograms post–bypass surgery that addressed the issue of late survival.[28,29] One study showed that patients with early (less than 5 years after operation) stenoses in vein grafts and patients with no stenotic vein grafts had approximately the same outcomes, and that these outcomes were relatively good.[28] However, the presence of late (5 years or more after operation) stenoses in vein grafts predicted poor long-term outcomes, particularly if a stenotic vein graft supplied the LAD coronary artery. When late stenoses in LAD vein grafts were combined with other high-risk characteristics, the late survival rate was particularly dismal. For example, patients with a 50% to 99% stenosis in a LAD vein graft combined with abnormal left ventricular function, triple-vessel or left main stenoses had only a 46% 2-year survival without reoperation. Patients with late stenoses in an LAD vein graft had significantly worse long-term outcomes than did patients with the LAD jeopardized by a native lesion (Fig. 25-4). This study showed that the difference in the pathology of early (intimal fibroplasia) and late (vein graft atherosclerosis) vein graft stenoses is associated with a difference in clinical outcome and that late stenoses in vein grafts are dangerous lesions.

A second study compared the outcomes of patients with stenotic vein grafts treated with reoperation (REOP group) versus those treated with medical treatment (MED group).[29] Again, this was a nonrandomized, retrospective study, and the patients in the REOP group were older and more symptomatic, had worse left ventricular function, and had fewer patent grafts than the patients in the MED group did.

The survival of patients with early (less than 5 years) SVG stenoses was not different in the two groups. The operative risk for the REOP group was low (no deaths among the 59 patients) and the long-term survival was good, but late survival was just as good for the patients treated medically (Fig. 25-5). It is important to note that the patients in the REOP group were more symptomatic to start with and at late follow-up they were less symptomatic than the patients in the MED group. Thus, reoperation for patients with early vein graft stenosis was an effective way of relieving symptoms of angina, but it appears that patients without symptoms can be treated medically with safety, at least over the short term.

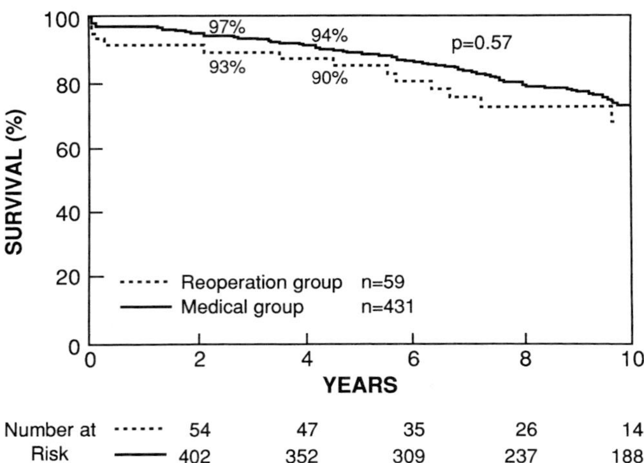

FIGURE 25–5 The survival of patients with early (<5 years after operation) stenoses in vein grafts was favorable with and without reoperation (p = NS). *(Reproduced with permission from Lytle BW, Loop FD, Taylor AC, et al: The effect of coronary reoperation on the survival of patients with stenoses in saphenous vein to coronary bypass grafts. J Thorac Cardiovasc Surg 1993; 105:605.*

However, the overall outcomes were worse for patients with late stenoses in vein grafts, and many subgroups had improved survival rates with reoperation. By multivariate testing (Table 25-1), a stenotic (20% to 99%) LAD vein graft predicted late death, and performing a reoperation increased late survival for those patients. Multivariate testing of smaller subgroups showed that the survival advantage for the REOP group was true even for patients with only Class I or Class II symptoms and that reoperation still improved survival for the remaining patients when patients with stenoses in LAD vein grafts were excluded from the analysis.

Univariate comparisons for the REOP and MED subgroups of patients with stenotic LAD grafts are shown in Figure 25-6, demonstrating the improved survival for the REOP group. When patients with stenotic LAD vein grafts were subgrouped on the basis of severity of the stenotic lesions (Fig. 25-7), the patients with severely (50% to 99%) stenotic vein grafts obviously benefitted from surgery, exhibiting a decreased risk of death even early in the follow-up period. For patients with moderate (20% to 49%) stenoses in LAD vein grafts, the survival of the MED and REOP groups were equivalent for about 2 years but after that point the

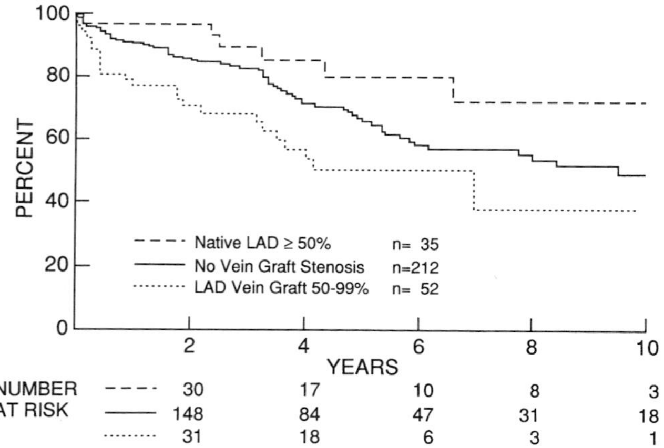

FIGURE 25–4 Patients with late stenoses in vein grafts to the LAD coronary artery had worse survival when compared to either patients with native coronary LAD stenoses or patients with no stenotic vein grafts. *(Reproduced with permission from Lytle BW, Loop FD, Taylor PC, et al: Vein graft disease: the clinical impact of stenoses in saphenous vein bypass grafts to coronary arteries. J Thorac Cardiovasc Surg 1992; 103:831.)*

TABLE 25–1 Patients with late stenoses (≥5 y) in saphenous vein to coronary artery bypass grafts: multivariate model of variables influencing late survival

	p-value	Relative risk
Variables decreasing survival		
LVF moderate/severe	.0001	2.58
Age (at catheterization)	.0001	1.04*
3 VD/LMT	.0011	2.87
LAD-SVG stenosis (20%–99%)	.0019	1.90
Variable increasing survival		
Reoperation	.0007	0.51

LVF = left ventricular function; 3VD/LMT = triple-vessel disease and/or left main stenosis.

* per year of age.

Source: Reproduced with permission from Lytle BW, Loop FD, Taylor PC, et al: The effect of coronary reoperation on the survival of patients with stenoses in saphenous vein to coronary bypass grafts. J Thorac Cardiovasc Surg 1993; 105:605.

survival of the patients in the MED group became rapidly worse, so that by 3 to 4 years of follow-up the survival benefit of reoperation became apparent. Although the patients in the studies noted above did not have consistent functional testing, there is evidence that myocardial perfusion and functional studies can help identify patients likely to benefit from reoperation. Lauer et al studied 873 symptom-free postoperative patients with symptom-limited exercise thallium-201 studies and found that patients with reversible perfusion defects were more likely to die or experience major cardiac events during a 3-year follow-up.[30] Impaired exercise capacity was also strongly predictive of unfavorable outcomes.

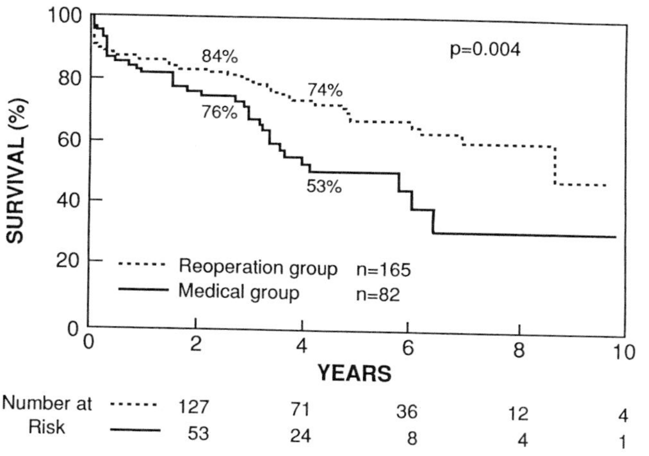

FIGURE 25–6 If patients had late (≥5 years after operation) stenoses in LAD vein grafts, they had a better survival rate ($p = .004$) with immediate reoperation than if they received initial nonoperative treatment. *(Reproduced with permission from Lytle BW, Loop FD, Taylor AC, et al: The effect of coronary reoperation on the survival of patients with stenoses in saphenous vein to coronary bypass grafts. J Thorac Cardiovasc Surg 1993; 105:605.*

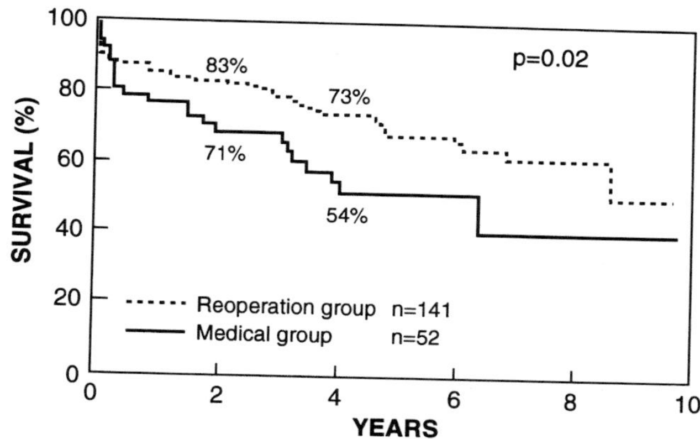

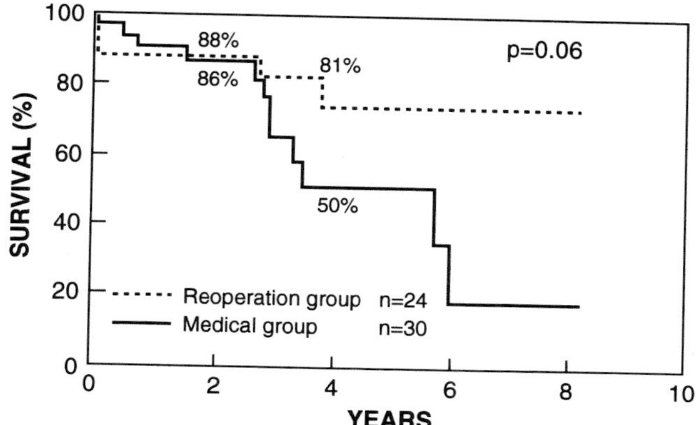

FIGURE 25–7 Patients with late stenoses in LAD vein grafts (*top*) had immediate improvement in their survival rate. Patients with moderate (20% to 49%) stenoses in LAD vein grafts had equivalent survival with or without reoperation for approximately 2 years, but after that point the patients who did not have reoperation did poorly. *(Reproduced with permission from Lytle BW, Loop FD, Taylor PC, et al: The effect of coronary reoperation on the survival of patients with stenoses in saphenous vein to coronary bypass grafts. J Thorac Cardiovasc Surg 1993;105:605.)*

PERCUTANEOUS TREATMENT OF POSTOPERATIVE PATIENTS

Percutaneous treatments (PCT) represent alternative anatomical treatments for postoperative patients and are often useful. The effectiveness of PCT is related to the vascular pathology to be treated and the clinical implications of treatment failure. Today, native coronary artery stenoses can often be treated with a low restenosis rate as long as those vessels are large enough to allow intracoronary stenting. Unfortunately, many postoperative patients have very diffuse native coronary atherosclerosis that makes PCT difficult or ineffective. Also, PCT has not been effective in the treatment of diabetic native coronary artery disease.

The reliability of PCT in the treatment of vein grafts is related to the age and the pathology of the vein grafts. In an early study of percutaneous transluminal coronary angioplasty (PTCA) for stenotic vein grafts, Platko et al found that patients treated with balloon angioplasty who had late stenoses in saphenous vein grafts (more than 36 months after operation) had a 4% risk of death, 12.5% risk of myocardial infarction, and 4% risk of bypass surgery versus no procedure-related complications for 53 patients with vein grafts treated within 36 months after operation.[31] In this study repeat angiography documented restenosis in 42.3% of patients treated for early stenosis versus 82.6% of those treated for late stenosis ($p < .01$). Furthermore, the late event-free survival was substantially worse for the patients with late SVG stenoses.

The rate of technologic change in interventional cardiology has been rapid, and multiple percutaneous technologies have been used to treat stenotic vein grafts. Not all new technologies have produced improved outcomes. Direct coronary atherectomy (DCA) increased the risk of coronary embolization without improving the restenosis rate.[32] It has been hoped that the use of intracoronary stents in stenotic vein grafts might achieve a better result in terms of lumen diameter at the time of intervention that would translate into a lower recurrence rate. A nonrandomized comparison of stenting and PTCA to treat vein grafts in place for 5 years and longer appears to show a decrease in procedure-related complications (PTCA 17% vs. stenting 10%) and a decrease in the 1-year incidence of death, myocardial infarction, and revascularization (45% vs. 23%, $p < .001$).[33] However, the kinetics of treatment failure after PCT for vein grafts are different than for native coronary vessels. Restenosis and new stenotic lesions in vein grafts continue to appear with time, and the shoulder on the adverse outcome curve that appears at 6 months to 1 year after PCT for native vessels does not appear for vein grafts. Thus, there is still some uncertainty about the clinical impact of percutaneous treatments of stenotic vein grafts. Patients with previous bypass surgery are an extremely heterogeneous group; some subgroups are at low risk without any anatomical treatment at all, and some subgroups are at high risk without effective therapy. To date the reported studies of PCT of SVG lesions have not included clinical risk stratifications that would allow comparison of patient survival rates.

SUMMARY OF CURRENT INDICATIONS FOR REOPERATION

There are no randomized prospective studies comparing medical, interventional, and reoperative management for patients with previous bypass surgery. It does appear that the presence of atherosclerotic vein grafts compresses the natural history of coronary artery disease, because progression of atherosclerotic lesions in vein grafts is often rapid. Combining this observation with data from the randomized studies of patients without previous bypass surgery allows some conclusions to be made on the basis of logic.

TABLE 25–2 Reoperation vs. PTCA for patients with stenotic vein grafts

Factors favoring reoperation	Factors favoring PTCA
Late (≥5 years) stenoses	Early (<5 years) stenoses
Multiple stenotic vein grafts	Single stenotic vein graft
Diffusely atherosclerotic vein grafts	Other patent vein grafts
Stenotic LAD vein graft	Focal graft lesions
No patent ITA graft	Patent ITA-LAD graft
Abnormal left ventricular function	Normal left ventricular function

There are data to support some anatomic indications for reoperation including: (1) atherosclerotic (late) stenoses in vein grafts that supply the LAD; (2) multiple stenotic vein grafts that supply large areas of myocardium; and (3) multivessel disease with a proximal LAD lesion and/or abnormal left ventricular function based on either native vessel lesions or stenotic vein grafts, or a combination of the two pathologies. Reoperation is also effective in other anatomical situations in which severe symptoms are the indication for invasive treatment, including patients with a patent ITA to LAD graft combined with other ischemia-producing pathology and multiple early vein graft stenoses. The combination of the anatomical characteristics noted above and reversible ischemia and/or worsening left ventricular function during stress constitutes a particularly strong indication for reoperation.

Despite persistently high restenosis rates following percutaneous interventions, there are still many indications for their use in the treatment of patients with previous bypass surgery. Realistically, the ideal uses of percutaneous treatments are in situations in which failure of the anatomical treatment is not likely to be catastrophic. These situations include symptomatic patients with (1) early vein graft stenoses, (2) native coronary stenoses, or (3) focal late SVG stenoses in vein grafts not supplying the LAD. There are many patients with previous surgery who will fall into a middle ground where it is not clear whether PTCA or reoperation is likely to yield the best outcome, and judgments must be made on the specific advantages and disadvantages of the treatments for those particular patients. Factors making PTCA more attractive than reoperation are listed in Table 25-2.

TECHNICAL ASPECTS OF CORONARY REOPERATIONS

Reoperations are more complicated than primary operations. The specific technical challenges that surgeons must recognize and solve that are unique to or more common during coronary reoperation are:

1. Sternal reentry
2. Stenotic or patent vein or arterial bypass grafts

3. Aortic atherosclerosis
4. Diffuse native vessel coronary artery disease
5. Coronary arteries located amid old grafts and epicardial scarring
6. Lack of bypass conduits

The overall problem of myocardial protection is more difficult during reoperations, with perioperative myocardial infarction still being the most common cause of in-hospital death.[3,6] The metabolic concepts of myocardial protection in use today are valid, but the reasons that myocardial protection sometimes fails during reoperation are related to anatomic causes of myocardial infarction. Those anatomical causes of perioperative myocardial infarction include injury to bypass grafts, atherosclerotic embolization from vein grafts or the aorta to distal coronary arteries, myocardial devascularization secondary to graft removal, hypoperfusion through new grafts, failure to deliver cardioplegic solution, early vein graft thrombosis, incomplete revascularization, diffuse air embolization, and technical error.[3,34–38] To be consistently successful, coronary reoperations must be designed to avoid these causes of myocardial infarction.

Preoperative Assessment

A complete understanding of the patient's native coronary and bypass graft anatomy is essential. Achieving that goal is sometimes not as easy as it sounds, particularly if the patient has had multiple previous coronary operations. If bypass grafts, venous or arterial, are not demonstrated by a preoperative coronary angiogram, it usually means that they are occluded, but it is also possible that the angiogram has simply failed to demonstrate their location. Examination of old angiograms performed prior to previous operations and review of previous operative records often help to understand the patient's coronary anatomy.

It is also important to know that graftable stenotic coronary arteries supply viable myocardium. Myocardial scar and viability can be differentiated by thallium scanning, positron emission tomography, and stress (exercise or dobutamine) echocardiography. The intricacies of establishing myocardial viability are beyond this discussion, but it is an important issue. Before embarking on a reoperation, it makes sense to be reasonably sure that there is a matchup between the patient's graftable arteries and some viable myocardium, such that grafting those arteries will provide some long-term benefits.

It is also wise to have a preoperative plan for bypass conduit selection and to document that potential bypass conduits are available. ITA angiography is often helpful. Venous Doppler studies can be used to assess the presence of greater and lesser saphenous vein segments, and arterial Doppler studies can assess the radial and inferior epigastric arteries and establish the adequacy of flow to the digits during radial artery occlusion.

Median Sternotomy Incision, Conduit Preparation, and Cannulation

Most coronary reoperations are performed through a median sternotomy. Situations associated with increased risk during a repeat median sternotomy include right ventricular or aortic enlargement, a patent vein graft to the right coronary artery, an *in situ* right ITA graft patent to a left coronary artery branch, an *in situ* left ITA graft that curls under the sternum, multiple previous operations, and difficulty reopening the sternum during a previous reoperation. In such situations vessels for arterial (via the femoral or axillary artery) and venous access for cardiopulmonary bypass are dissected out prior to sternal reentry. All bypass grafts except for the internal thoracic arteries may be prepared prior to sternal reentry. The preparation of radial artery and greater and lesser saphenous vein segments can be carried out simultaneously.

When reopening a median sternotomy the incision is made to the level of the sternal wires; the wires are cut anteriorly and bent back but are not removed (Fig. 25-8). An oscillating saw is used to divide the anterior table of the sternum. When the anterior table has been divided, ventilation is stopped and the assistants elevate each side of the sternum with rake retractors while the posterior table of the sternum is divided in a caudal-cranial direction. The sternal wires that have been left in place posterior to the sternum help to protect underlying structures. Once the posterior table of the sternum has been divided with the saw, the wires are removed and sharp dissection with scissors is used to separate each side of the sternum from underlying structures. Once the sternum has been divided it is important that the assistants retract in an upward direction, not laterally. The right ventricle is more often injured by lateral retraction while it is still adherent to the underside of the sternum than it is by a direct saw injury.

In high-risk situations it can be helpful to perform a small anterolateral right thoracotomy (Fig. 25-9) prior to the repeat median sternotomy. Underlying structures, such as the aorta, patent bypass grafts, and the right atrium and ventricle, can be dissected away from the sternum via this approach and thus, with the surgeon's hand placed behind the sternum, reentry is safe. This small additional incision contributes little morbidity.

Another technique for sternal reentry in high-risk situations is to heparinize, cannulate, and initiate cardiopulmonary bypass prior to median sternotomy. The advantages of this strategy are that the heart can be emptied and allowed to fall away from the sternum, and cardiopulmonary bypass has already been initiated for protection if an injury does occur. The disadvantages of this approach are that extensive mediastinal dissection must be carried out in a heparinized patient including the dissection of the right internal thoracic artery if that is to be used. We rarely employ this approach except in situations in which adherence of an aortic aneurysm to the sternum or a patent right ITA to LAD graft creates a specific danger.

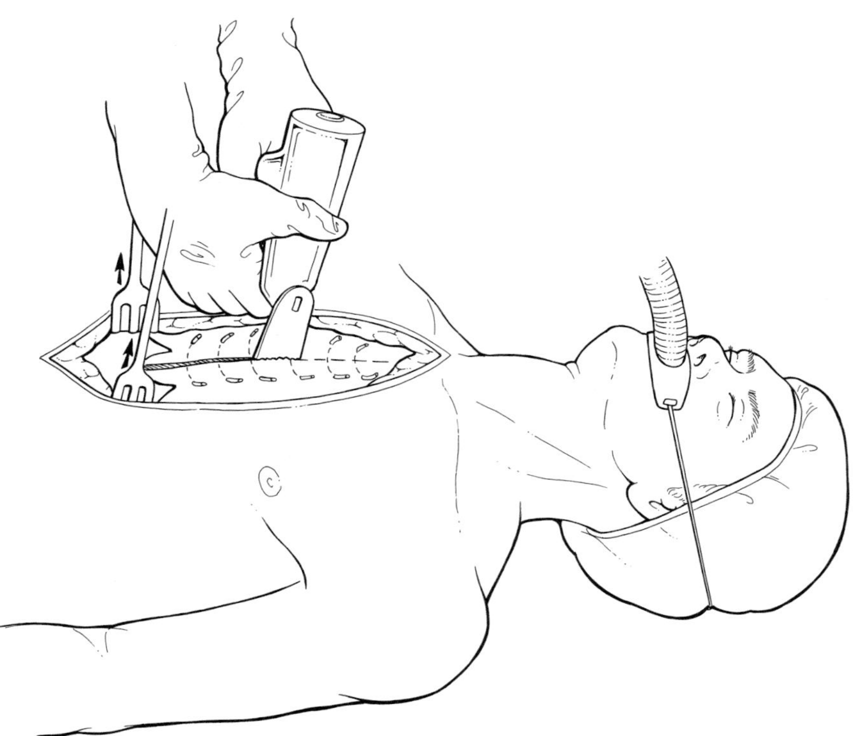

FIGURE 25–8 Leaving the sternal wires in place posteriorly helps protect underlying structures while the posterior table of the sternum is divided with an oscillating saw. The direction of retraction with "rake" retractors should be anterior, not lateral.

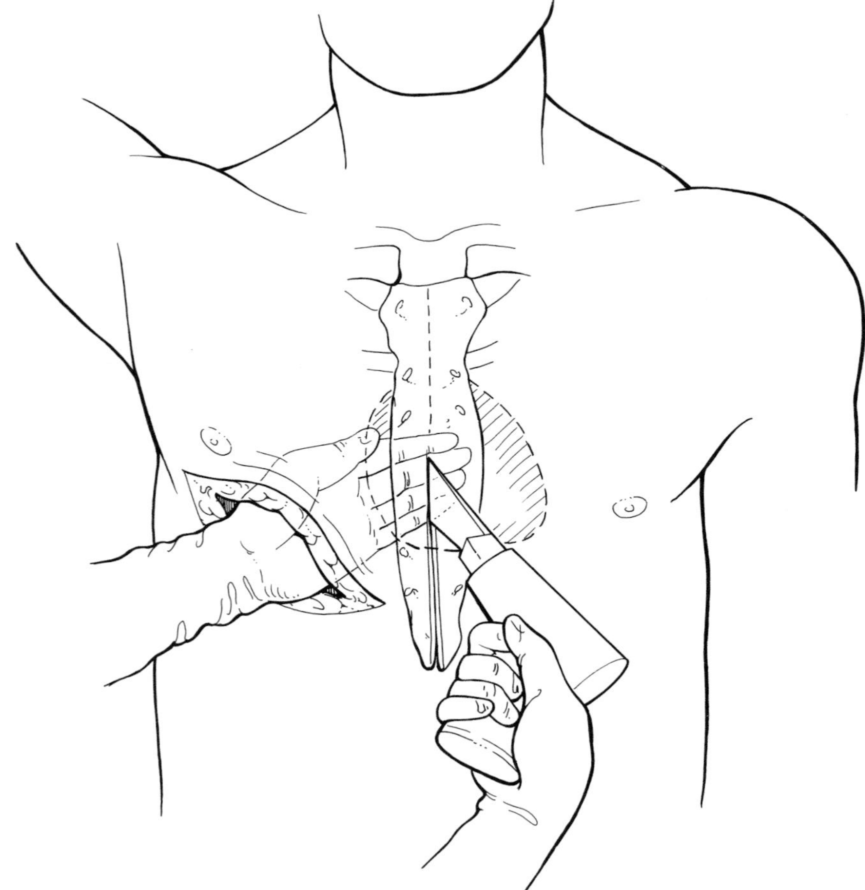

FIGURE 25–9 A small anterior-lateral right thoracotomy allows dissection of substernal structures such as patent grafts and the right ventricle or aorta away from the sternum under direct vision. While the sternum is being divided, the surgeon may place a hand behind the sternum for further safety.

Once the sternum has been divided, the pleural cavities are entered. A general principle of dissection during reoperation is that starting at the level of the diaphragm and proceeding in a cranial direction is usually the safest approach. At the level of the diaphragm there are few critical structures that are injured if the wrong plane is entered. Therefore, at this point in the operation we usually dissect along the level of the diaphragm to the patient's right side until we enter the pleural cavity and then detach the pleural reflection from the chest wall in a cranial direction to the level of the innominate vein. The innominate vein is dissected away from both sides of the sternum with scissors, a maneuver that prevents a "stretch" injury to that vein.

Once the right side of the sternum is separated from the cardiac structures, it is usually possible to prepare a right ITA graft. Because of parietal pleural thickening, it is often more difficult to obtain length on ITA grafts during reoperation than it is during primary procedures, and the right ITA is frequently used as a "free" graft. Once the right ITA dissection is completed to the superior border of the first rib, an incision is made in the parietal pleura to separate the proximal ITA from the area of the phrenic nerve. Thus, if right ITA needs to be converted to a "free" graft during aortic cross-clamping, it makes division at that point easier because the proximal ITA is easily identifiable. Although intrapericardial dissection of the left side of the heart is left until later, freeing the left side of the anterior chest wall from the underlying structures (that may include a patent ITA graft) is undertaken now. This is difficult only if there is a patent ITA graft that is densely adherent to the chest wall. Again, it is best to enter the left pleural cavity at the level of the diaphragm and proceed in a cranial direction.

The most difficult point of dissection is usually at the level of the sternal angle, where a patent ITA graft may approach the midline and be adherent to the sternum or to the aorta. There are no tricks for dissecting out a patent ITA graft except being careful. The danger to a patent left ITA graft during sternal reentry and mediastinal dissection is entirely related to the location of the graft at the time of the primary operation. Ideally the pericardium should be divided at a primary operation and the left ITA graft allowed to run posterior to the lung through the incision in the pericardium and to the

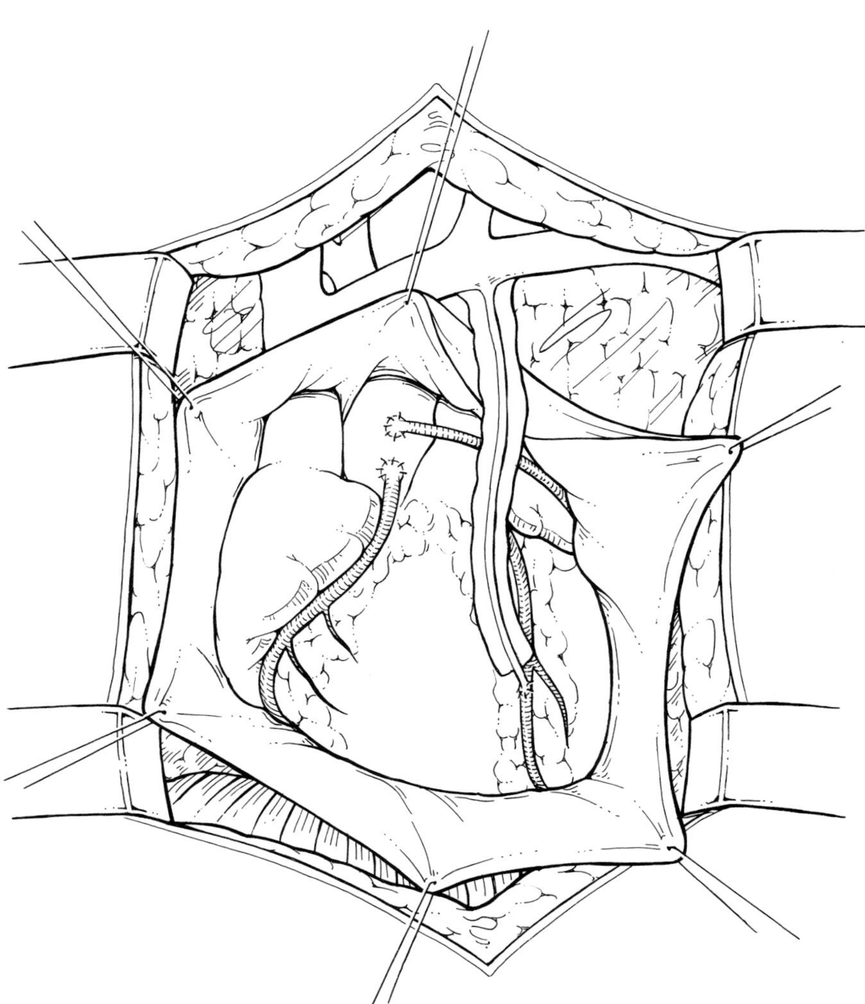

FIGURE 25–10 A patent left ITA to LAD graft should not pose a threat during reoperation. At a primary operation the pericardium should be divided in a posterior direction and the ITA graft should be placed in that incision. The ITA graft will then lie posterior to the lung and will not be pushed toward the midline by the lung or become adherent to the sternum.

LAD or circumflex artery (Fig. 25-10). When that is done, the lung will lie anterior to the left ITA and that graft will not become adherent to the aorta or to the chest wall.

Once the left side of the chest wall is free, the left IMA is prepared (if it has not been used at a previous operation), the sternal spreader is inserted, and the intrapericardial dissection of the aorta and right atrium is accomplished. Again, in most cases it is safest to find the correct dissection plane at the level of the diaphragm and then to continue around the right atrium to the aorta. The one situation in which that strategy may be dangerous is if an atherosclerotic vein graft to the right coronary artery lies over the right atrium. Manipulation of atherosclerotic vein grafts can cause embolization of atherosclerotic debris into coronary arteries, and it is best to employ a "no touch" technique with such grafts. If a vein graft to the right coronary artery lies in an awkward position over the right atrium, it is best to leave the right atrium alone and to use femoral vein and superior vena cava cannulation to establish venous drainage (Fig. 25-11). Once cardiopulmonary bypass has been established, the aorta cross-clamped, and cardioplegia given, the atherosclerotic vein graft can then be disconnected.

The goal of dissection of the ascending aorta is to obtain enough length for cannulation and cross-clamping, and to avoid the most common error, aortic subadventitial dissection. The correct level of dissection on the aorta is usually found either by following the right atrium to the aorta in a caudal to cranial direction, or by identifying the innominate vein and leaving all the tissue beneath the innominate vein on the aorta. At the level of the innominate vein the pericardial reflection on each side of the aorta will be identifiable. Division of the pericardial reflection on the left side in a posterior direction will lead to the plane between the aorta and the pulmonary artery. Once the left side of the aorta is identified, the surgeon may then dissect posteriorly on the medial aspect of the left lung toward the hilum. The segment of tissue between these two dissection planes will usually include a patent left ITA graft, if present, and clamping that tissue will produce occlusion of the ITA graft.

When the aorta has been dissected out, heparin is given and cannulation is undertaken. Cannulation of an atherosclerotic ascending aorta may cause atherosclerotic embolization leading to stroke, myocardial infarction, or multiorgan failure, and so the ascending aorta should be studied with palpation and echocardiography to detect atherosclerosis before cannulation.[39,40] Although the most widely used alternative arterial cannulation site is the femoral artery, arteriopathic patients often have severe femoral artery atherosclerosis. The axillary artery is an alternative arterial cannulation site that we have used with

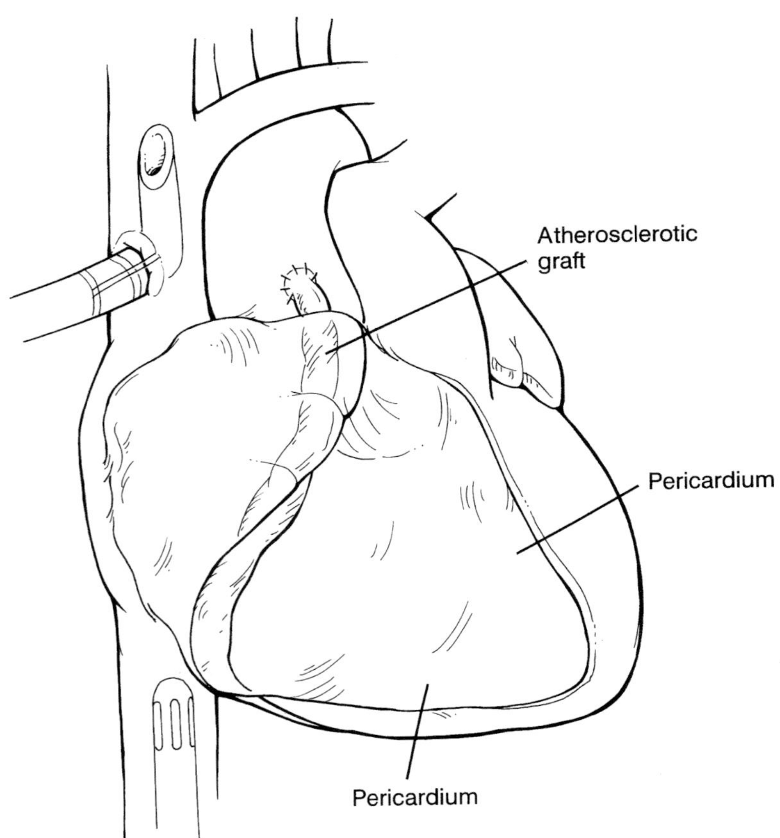

FIGURE 25–11 Manipulation of patent but atherosclerotic vein grafts should be avoided. If an atherosclerotic right coronary vein graft blocks access to the right atrium, femoral vein and direct superior vena cava cannulation are safer than than mobilizing the vein graft in order to achieve right atrial cannulation.

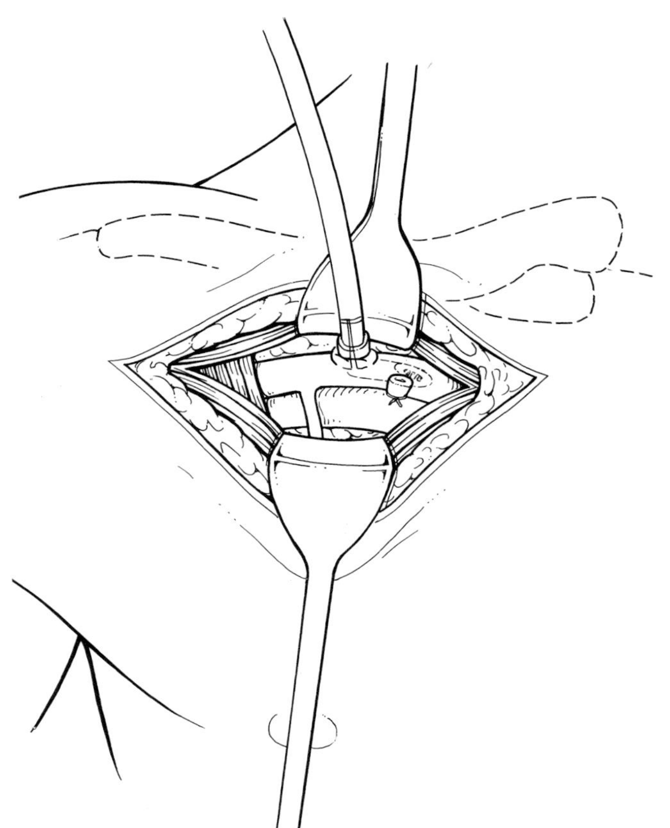

FIGURE 25–12 The axillary artery is an important alternative arterial cannulation site for patients with aortic and femoral artery atherosclerosis. A 21-gauge cannula will fit the axillary artery in most patients.

increasing frequency because atherosclerotic disease is usually not present in that vessel and its cannulation allows antegrade perfusion (Fig. 25-12).[41] If atherosclerotic disease or calcification of the aorta makes any aortic occlusion hazardous, the options are off-pump bypass surgery (see "Other Options" section below) or replacement of the aorta with axillary artery cannulation, hypothermia, and circulatory arrest. Venous cannulation is usually accomplished with a single two-stage right atrial cannula. A transatrial coronary sinus cardioplegia cannula is inserted via a right atrial purse string with the aid of a stylet, and a needle is placed in the ascending aorta for delivery of antegrade cardioplegia and for use as a vent (Fig. 25-13).

Myocardial Protection

The myocardial protection strategy used by the author during most coronary reoperations is a combination of antegrade and retrograde delivery of intermittent cold blood cardioplegia combined with a dose of warm reperfusion cardioplegia (hot shot) given prior to aortic unclamping, principles developed by Buckberg et al.[42,43] Multiple types of cardioplegic solutions have been described and most appear to provide a metabolic environment that effectively protects the myocardium. Because of the potential anatomical challenges to cardioplegic myocardial protection during reoperations, the details of how the cardioplegic solution is delivered are very important. In most primary bypass operations, antegrade cardioplegia works well by itself. During reoperations, however, antegrade cardioplegia may not be effective for areas of myocardium that are supplied by patent *in situ* arterial grafts and may be dangerous because of the risk of embolization of atherosclerotic debris into the coronary arteries from old vein grafts. The delivery of cardioplegia through the coronary sinus and through the cardiac venous system to the myocardium (retrograde cardioplegia) has been a step forward in myocardial protection during reoperations.[44,45] Retrograde cardioplegia delivery avoids atheroembolism from vein grafts, can be helpful in removing atherosclerotic debris and air from the coronary system, and can deliver cardioplegia to areas supplied by *in situ* arterial grafts. The biggest disadvantage of retrograde cardioplegia is that it is not always possible to place a catheter in the coronary sinuses that will deliver cardioplegia consistently. It is important to monitor the adequacy of cardioplegia delivery by measuring the pressure in the coronary sinus, noting the distention of cardiac veins with arterial blood, the cooling of the myocardium, and the return of desaturated blood from open coronary arteries.

Cardiopulmonary bypass is begun, the perfusionist empties the heart and produces mild systemic hypothermia (34°C), and the aorta is cross-clamped. We usually initiate cardioplegia induction with aortic root cardioplegia. To induce and maintain cardioplegic protection, it is helpful to be able to occlude patent arterial grafts. If it has not yet been possible to dissect out a patent arterial graft so it can be clamped, the systemic perfusion temperature is decreased to 25°C until control of the graft is achieved. After antegrade cardioplegia has been given for 2 to 3 minutes, we shift to retrograde induction for another 2 to 3 minutes. Giving any antegrade cardioplegia does risk embolization from atherosclerotic vein grafts, but if these grafts have not yet been manipulated that danger is relatively small. Once the adequacy of retrograde cardioplegia delivery has been established, it is often possible to use that route predominantly for maintenance doses.

Intrapericardial Dissection

When the heart has been completely arrested, intrapericardial dissection of the left ventricle is undertaken, starting at the diaphragm and extending out to the left of the apex of the heart. After the apex is identified, the surgeon divides the pericardium in a cranial direction on the left side of the LAD coronary artery (Fig. 25-14). A patent LITA to LAD graft will be contained within the strip of pericardium that lies over the LAD. Dissection of this pedicle from the anterior aspect of the pulmonary artery will allow an atraumatic

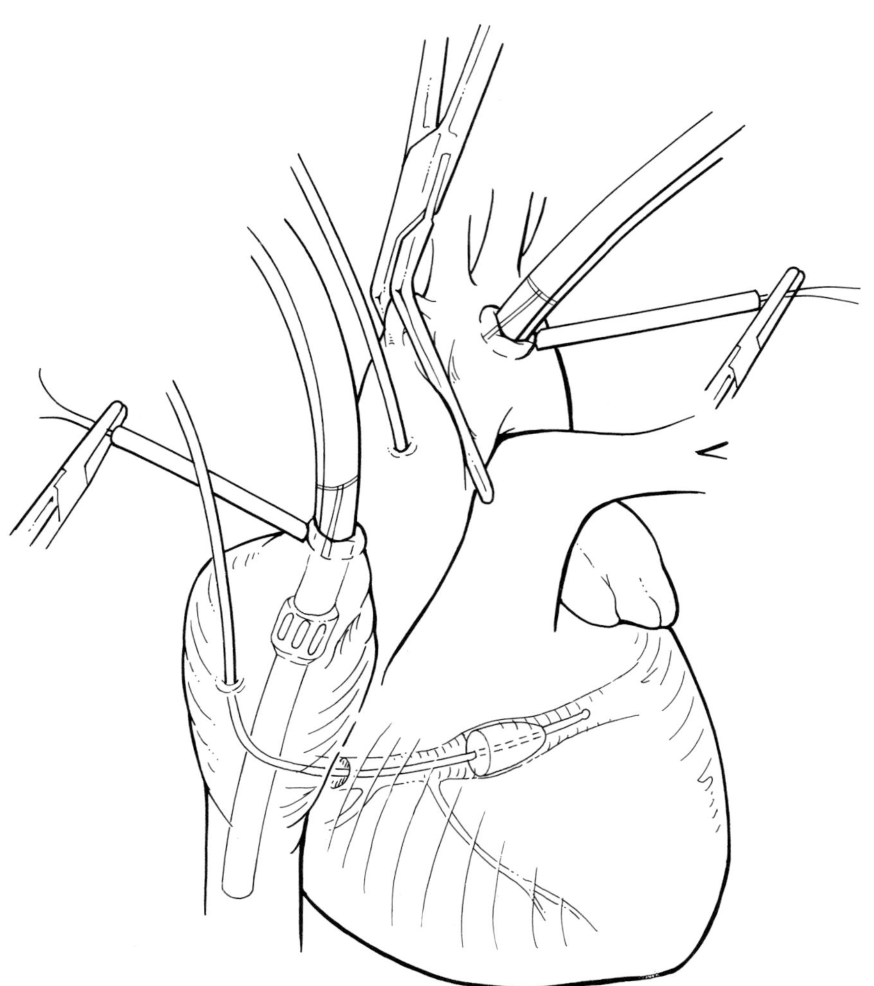

FIGURE 25–13 Standard cannulation for coronary reoperation includes aortic arterial cannulation, an aortic needle for antegrade delivery of cardioplegia and aortic root venting, a single two-stage venous cannula, and a transatrial coronary sinus catheter with a self-inflating balloon for delivery of retrograde cardioplegia. Cannulation is accomplished prior to dissection of the left ventricle.

clamp to be placed across the patent ITA graft and also will allow the passage of new bypass grafts from the aorta underneath the patent ITA graft to left-sided coronary arteries. The advantages of waiting until after aortic clamping and arrest to dissect out the left ventricle are that dissection is more accurate, there is less damage to the epicardium and less bleeding, manipulation of atherosclerotic vein grafts is less likely to cause coronary embolization, and the dissection of patent ITA grafts is safer.

After the heart is completely dissected out, the coronary arteries to be grafted can be identified, the lengths that bypass conduits need to reach those vessels may be assessed, and the final operative plan can be established. The old grafts and epicardial scarring that are present during reoperations make the preoperative prediction of the lengths of conduits needed for bypass grafts quite difficult, particularly the lengths of arterial grafts, and it is wise to have some flexibility in the operative plan. Prior to the construction of the anastomoses, those patent but atherosclerotic vein grafts that are going to be disconnected are identified and are disconnected with a scalpel. The order of anastomosis construction that is used by the author is: first, distal vein graft anastomoses; second, distal free arterial graft anastomoses; third, distal *in situ* arterial graft anastomoses; and, fourth, proximal (aortic) anastomoses.

Stenotic Vein Grafts

When should patent or stenotic vein grafts be replaced and what should they be replaced with? Atherosclerosis in vein grafts is common if those grafts are more than 5 years old, and leaving them in place risks embolization of atherosclerotic debris at the time of reoperation and subsequent development of premature graft stenoses or occlusions after reoperation. On the other hand, replacement of all vein grafts extends the operation and may use up available bypass conduits.

In the past, our general rule has been to replace all vein grafts more than 5 years old at the time of reoperation, even if those grafts are not angiographically diseased. However,

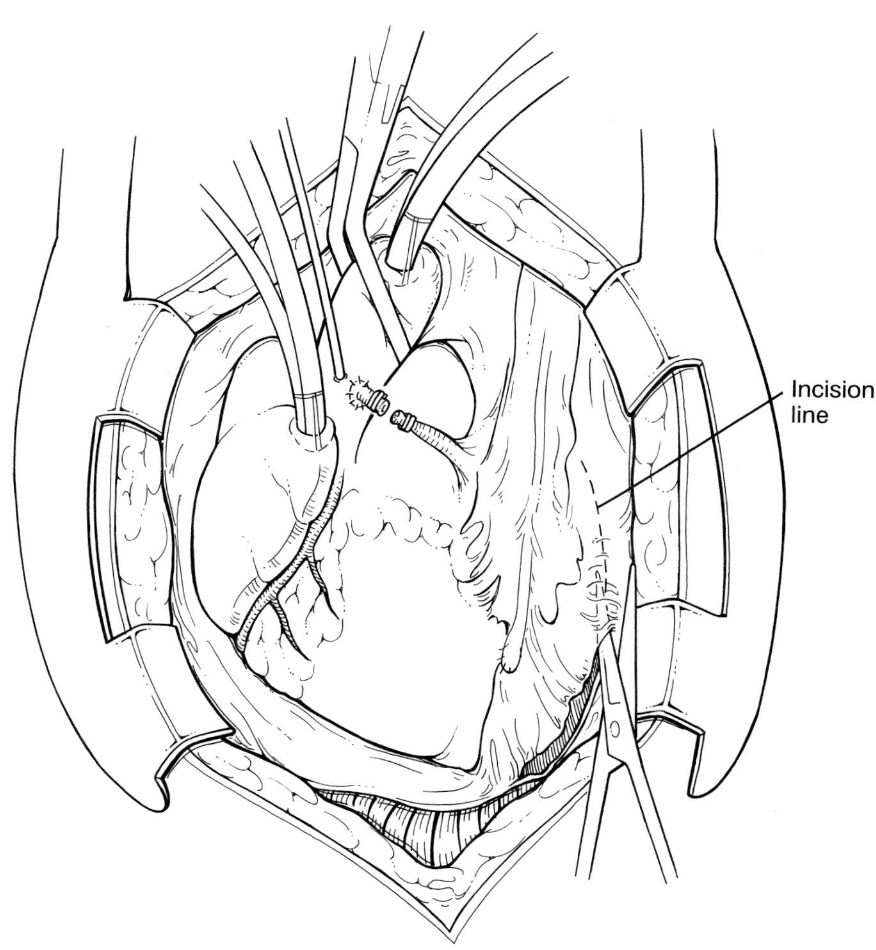

FIGURE 25–14 Division of the pericardium along the diaphragm allows the surgeon to reach a point to the left of the cardiac apex. From that point the pericardium can be divided in a cranial direction to the left of the LAD, leaving a patent ITA graft in the strip of tissue overlying the LAD. Atherosclerotic vein grafts that are going to be replaced may be divided once a dose of antegrade cardioplegia is given.

that strategy assumes that there are conduits available that can replace these old grafts. Today many patients have very limited conduits at reoperation because of the large numbers of vein grafts used at primary surgery or because of multiple previous operations. Thus, graft replacement must be individualized. Inspection of vein grafts at reoperation will occasionally identify a graft that looks angiographically normal and does not appear to have any thickening or atherosclerosis on visual inspection. Often those vein grafts will be left alone.

Replacing old vein grafts with new vein grafts is often best accomplished by creating the new vein to coronary anastomosis at the site of the previous distal anastomosis, leaving only 1 mm or so of the old vein in place (Fig. 25-15). If significant native vessel stenoses have developed distal to the old vein graft, it is often best to place a new graft to the distal vessel in addition to replacing the vein graft. Many reoperative candidates have proximal occlusions of the native coronary system and multiple stenoses throughout the vessel, and if only new distal grafts are constructed, the proximal segments of coronary arteries and their branches that are supplied by atherosclerotic vein grafts may be jeopardized. More than one graft to a major coronary artery may be desirable during reoperation (Fig. 25-16).

Sequential vein grafts are often very helpful during reoperation because they allow more distal anastomoses and fewer proximal anastomoses. Sites for proximal anastomoses are often at a premium in the scarred reoperative aorta.

Arterial to coronary artery bypass grafts have many advantages during reoperations. First, they are often available. Second, the tendency of arterial grafts to remain patent even when used as grafts to diffusely diseased coronary arteries makes them particularly applicable to reoperative candidates. Third, *in situ* arterial grafts don't require a proximal anastomosis. If the left ITA has not been used as a graft at a previous operation, a strong attempt should be made to use it as an *in situ* graft to the LAD coronary artery. During primary operations the right ITA can usually be crossed over as an *in situ* graft to left-sided vessels, but that plan is more difficult during repeat surgery, and so the right ITA is often used as a free graft.

Arterial graft proximal anastomoses are a problem at reoperation, because the scarring and thickening of the reoperative aorta often makes direct anastomoses of arterial grafts

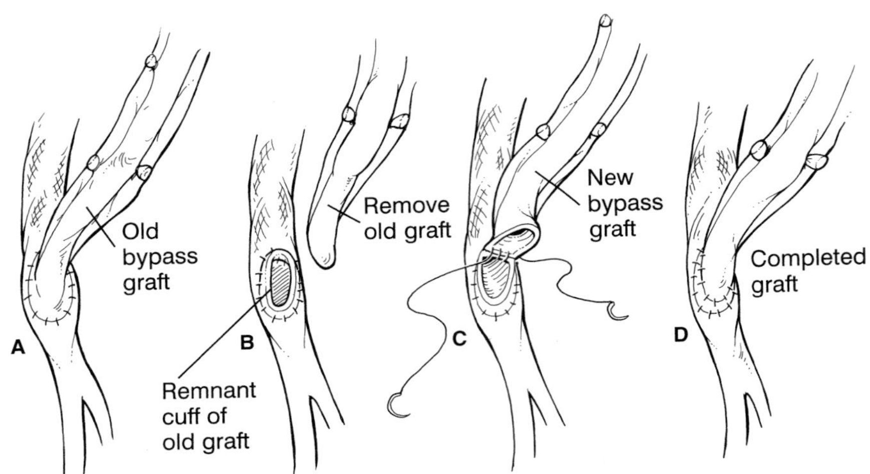

FIGURE 25–15 For patients with extensive native coronary atherosclerosis the distal anastomotic site of an old vein graft is often the best spot for the distal anastomosis of a new graft. Only a small rim of the old graft should be left in place.

to the aorta unsatisfactory. However, when old vein grafts become occluded there is usually a "bubble" of the hood of the old vein graft that is not atherosclerotic and that is often a good spot for construction of a free (aorta to coronary) arterial graft anastomosis (Fig. 25-17). In addition, if new vein grafts are performed, the hood of that new vein graft represents a favorable location for an arterial graft anastomosis. Late angiographic data regarding this strategy are not available, but the relative freedom of the hood of vein grafts from the development of atherosclerosis means these grafts are likely to be successful.

Another effective strategy is to use either an old arterial graft or a newly constructed arterial graft for the proximal anastomosis of a free arterial graft (Fig. 25-18). Composite arterial grafts, usually using a new *in situ* left ITA graft at the proximal anastomotic site for a free right ITA graft,

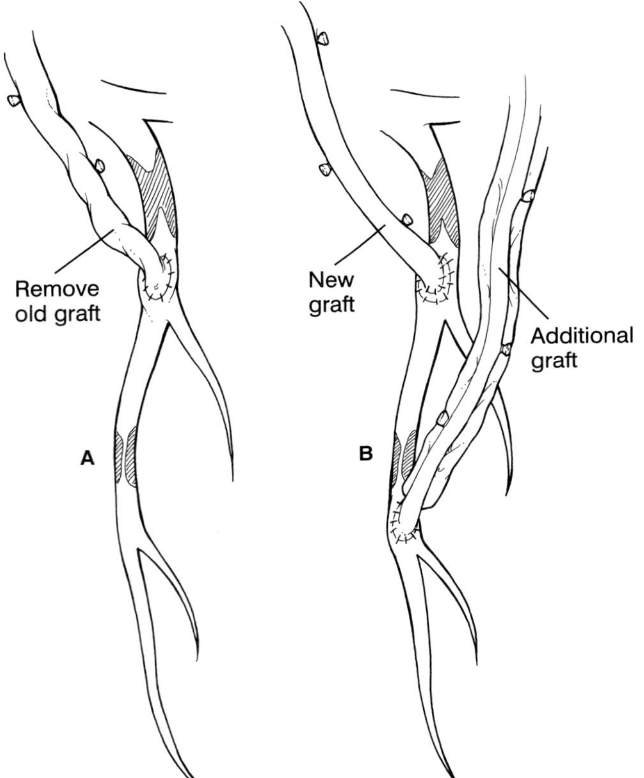

FIGURE 25–16 Extension of native vessel coronary artery disease may indicate the placement of new distal grafts as well as replacement of diseased vein grafts supplying proximal coronary artery segments.

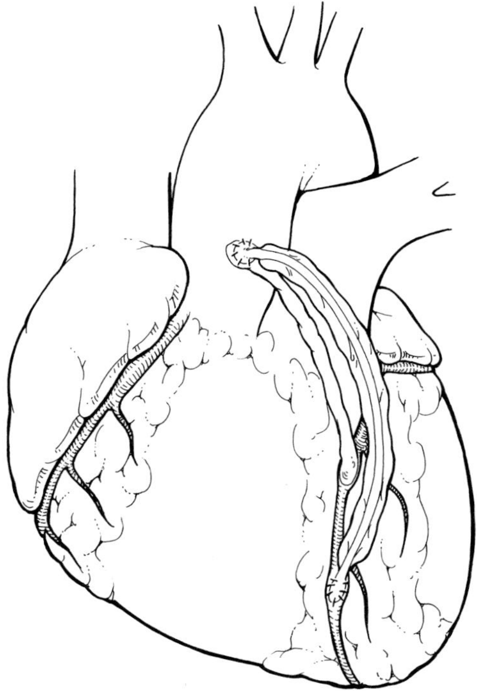

FIGURE 25–17 The hood of new or old vein grafts is often the best spot for the aortic anastomosis of free arterial grafts. Atherosclerosis rarely occurs in that "bubble" of vein.

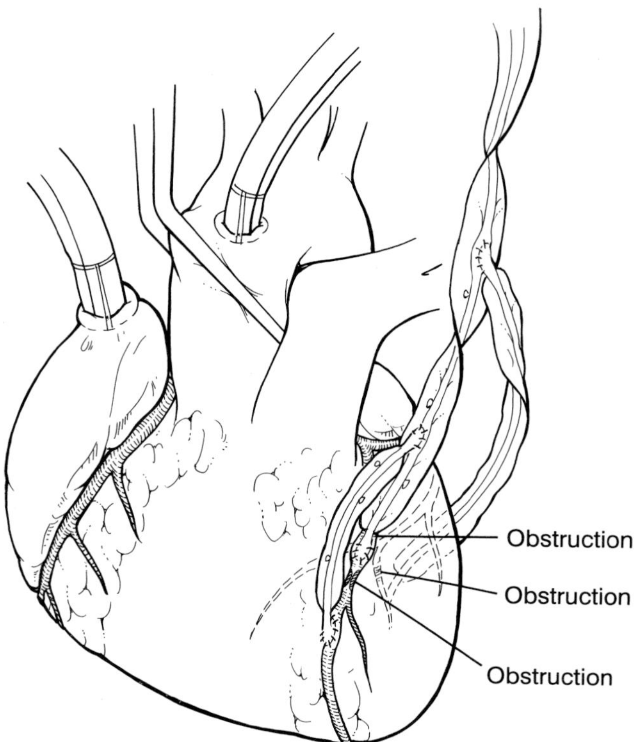

FIGURE 25–18 Composite arterial grafts can be constructed using a new or old left ITA graft as the inflow source. With its proximal anastomosis to the left ITA, a right ITA graft will easily reach the circumflex branches. Furthermore, a shorter segment of inferior epigastric artery or radial artery can be used to reach the distal LAD if intervening native LAD stenoses have limited the effectiveness of an old ITA graft.

have been employed with increasing frequency and early outcomes have been favorable.[46,47] This method is particularly useful during reoperations because it may avoid an aortic anastomosis and less right ITA graft length is needed to reach distal circumflex arteries. Other advantages of using a previously performed patent ITA graft for the proximal anastomosis of a new arterial graft are that the old left ITA graft has often increased in size and the preoperative angiogram has demonstrated its integrity. In situations where the effectiveness of an LITA to LAD graft has been jeopardized by a distal LAD lesion, a short segment of a new arterial graft can be used to bridge that stenosis from the old arterial graft to the distal LAD (Fig. 25-18).

Can an ITA graft be used to replace a vein graft during reoperation? When faced with replacing a stenotic or patent vein graft during reoperation, the surgeon has a number of options, all of which have some potential disadvantages:

1. The surgeon may leave the old vein graft in place and add an arterial graft to the same coronary vessel. The dangers of this approach are that atherosclerotic embolization from the old vein may occur during the reoperation, and competitive flow between the vein graft and the arterial graft may jeopardize the ITA graft after reoperation.
2. The surgeon may remove the old vein graft and replace it with an ITA graft. This decreases the likelihood of atherosclerotic embolization and competitive flow but risks hypoperfusion during reoperation if the arterial graft cannot supply all the flow that previously had been generated by the vein graft.
3. Replace the old vein graft with a new vein graft. The disadvantage of this approach is a long-term one: the coronary vessel is left dependent upon a vein graft.

When we examined these choices in a retrospective study of operations for patients with atherosclerotic vein grafts supplying the LAD coronary artery, we found that the worst outcomes resulted from removing a patent (although stenotic) vein graft and replacing it with only an ITA graft.[37] That strategy was associated with a significant incidence of hypoperfusion and severe hemodynamic difficulties during reoperation that were effectively treated only by adding a vein graft to the same coronary artery. The incidence of myocardial infarction associated with leaving a stenotic vein graft in place was low. Thus, atherosclerotic embolization from an atherosclerotic vein graft is a danger, but it appears that with the use of retrograde cardioplegia it is not commonly a major catastrophe.

Another potential disadvantage of the strategy of adding an ITA graft to a stenotic vein graft is that competition in flow from the stenotic vein graft may lead to failure of the new ITA graft. However, that is unlikely to occur as long as the stenosis in the SVG is severe.[48] Our usual approach, therefore, is to remove atherosclerotic vein grafts when replacing them with a new vein graft but leave stenotic vein grafts in place when grafting the same vessel with an arterial graft (Fig. 25-19).

Alternative arterial grafts are often very useful during reoperation. The radial artery has particular advantages during repeat surgery because it is larger and longer than other free arterial grafts. Those qualities increase the range of coronary arteries that can be grafted. Early studies of radial artery grafts have shown favorable patency rates but few long-term data currently exist. If the high patency rates that have been documented by the early studies are confirmed by the tests of time, the radial artery will be used extensively during reoperations. The inferior epigastric artery is often too short to function as a separate aorta to coronary graft during reoperation but can be extremely useful as a short composite arterial graft, as illustrated in Fig. 25-18.

The right gastroepiploic artery (RGEA) has established a good mid-term graft patency rate record and is often useful during reoperation because it is an *in situ* graft.[49] Furthermore, it can be prepared prior to the median sternotomy. It is most often effective as an *in situ* graft to the posterior descending branch of the right coronary artery or to the distal LAD (Fig. 25-20).

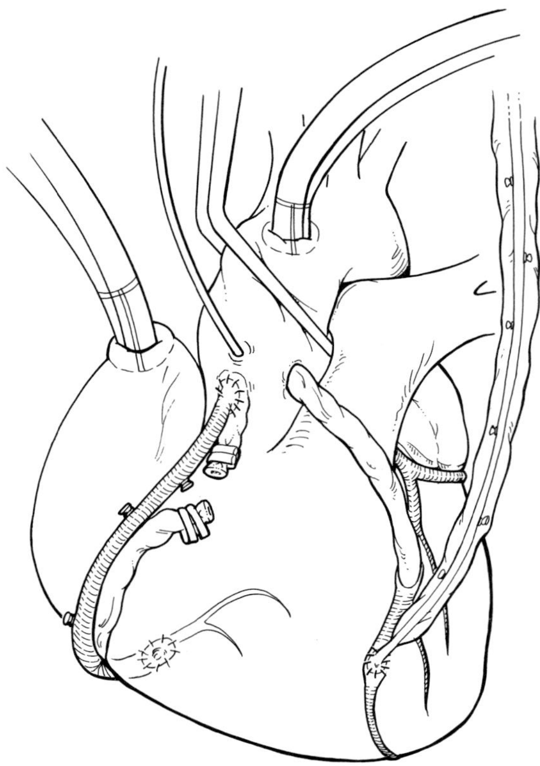

FIGURE 25–19 In this example, an atherosclerotic right coronary artery vein graft is disconnected and is replaced with a new vein graft. However, the stenotic vein graft to the LAD is left in place to avoid hypoperfusion and a new ITA graft is added to the LAD.

The aortic anastomoses of the vein and arterial grafts are performed last during the single period of aortic cross-clamping. Sites for aortic anastomoses are often at a premium due to previous scarring, atherosclerotic disease, or the use of Teflon felt during the primary operation, and often the locations of the previous vein graft proximal anastomoses are the best locations for the new ones. The advantages of constructing aortic anastomoses during a single period of aortic cross-clamping are that it minimizes aortic trauma and allows excellent visualization of the proximal anastomoses. In addition, if patent or stenotic vein grafts have been removed and replaced, reperfusion is not accomplished by aortic declamping until the aortic anastomoses have been completed.

The disadvantage of this approach is that it prolongs the period of aortic cross-clamping. However, our strategies for reoperation are not based on trying to minimize myocardial ischemic time. If cardioplegia can be effectively delivered, its metabolic concepts are valid and myocardial protection is secure. Failure of myocardial protection is usually caused by anatomical events, not by metabolic failure. Once the proximal anastomosis has been constructed, a "hot shot" of substrate-enhanced blood cardioplegia is given and the aortic cross-clamp is removed.

Other Options

Although most reoperations are performed through a median sternotomy with the use of cardiopulmonary bypass, the strategies of small incision surgery and off-pump surgery that have been gaining increasing use for primary coronary operations can also be helpful during reoperations.

Reoperations in situations in which a limited area of myocardium needs revascularization can often be accomplished through a limited incision and without the use of cardiopulmonary bypass (known as the minimally invasive direct coronary artery bypass, or MIDCAB, operation). The distal LAD coronary artery may be exposed with a small anterior thoracotomy and the LAD or diagonal grafted with a left ITA graft. A stabilizing device is usually used for anastomotic construction although the intrapericardial adhesions provide some stability during reoperations. If the left ITA is not available, a segment of saphenous vein can be anastomosed to the subclavian artery and routed in a transthoracic path to the LAD. If the right ITA is to be used as an *in situ* graft to the LAD, a median sternotomy is indicated, but if that is the only graft, off-pump surgery is usually possible.

The lateral wall of the heart can be exposed through a left lateral thoracotomy (Fig. 25-21) and the circumflex and distal right coronary artery branches grafted with this approach. Often the LITA has already been used for a graft, but the descending thoracic aorta may be used as a site for the proximal anastomosis of a vein graft or a radial artery graft using a partial occluding clamp. The disadvantages of this approach are that the right ITA is difficult to use as an *in situ* graft, and if the circumflex vessels are deeply intramyocardial they may be difficult to expose and isolate with the off-pump strategy.

In addition to avoiding potential complications of cardiopulmonary bypass, the "limited area–off-pump" approach also avoids extensive dissection of the heart and possible manipulation of atherosclerotic vein grafts. The disadvantage of this approach is that most patients who are candidates for reoperation need grafts to multiple vessels in multiple myocardial areas.

Use of a median sternotomy and the off-pump strategy to graft multiple myocardial areas is now a standard approach to primary coronary revascularization and also can be used during reoperation. However, because of the need to access all areas, extensive dissection is sometimes necessary for lysis of adhesions to be able to mobilize the heart. If patients have atherosclerotic vein grafts, dissection and manipulation create the dangers of embolization of atherosclerotic debris and myocardial infarction. This problem was encountered during the early years of bypass surgery when the risks of atherosclerotic embolization were less recognized. Another disadvantage of off-pump reoperative strategies is that reoperative candidates often have very distal and diffuse coronary disease, which leave intramyocardial segments as the

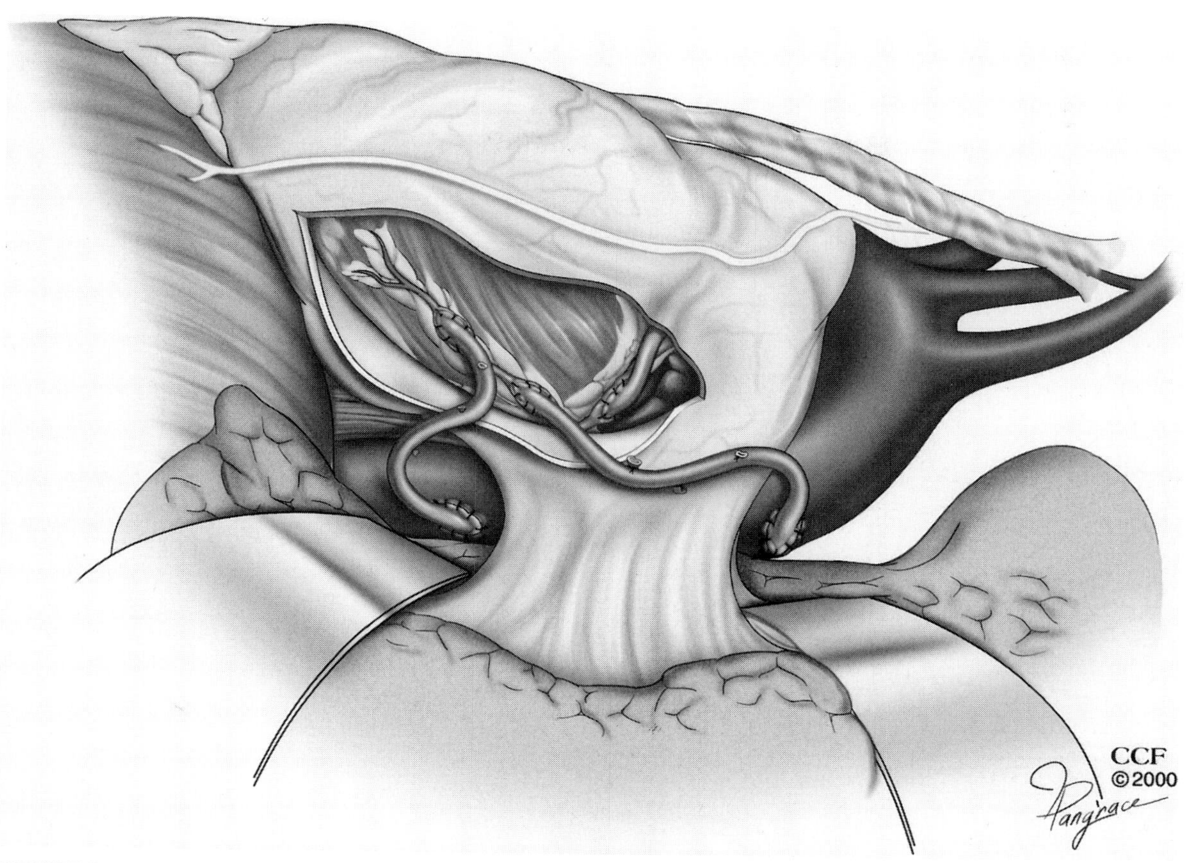

FIGURE 25–20 Circumflex vessels may be grafted through a left thoracotomy incision without cardiopulmonary bypass.

best areas for grafting. These characteristics stress off-pump isolation and immobilization techniques. In addition, the aortic anastomoses of vein or free arterial grafts may be difficult because of aortic atherosclerosis, adhesions, or previous aortic anastomoses that may limit the application of a partial occluding clamp. On the other hand, the use of off-pump techniques may minimize aortic trauma, particularly if *in situ* arterial grafts can be employed to provide inflow to new grafts.

In an individual case, the disadvantages of off-pump surgery may be important or irrelevant. Surgeons who perform reoperative coronary surgery in a wide spectrum of situations will find both on- and off-pump strategies helpful.

THE RESULTS OF CORONARY REOPERATIONS

Coronary reoperations are riskier than primary operations. A study from the Society of Thoracic Surgeons (STS) database reported an in-hospital mortality of 6.95% associated with reoperations for the years 1991-1993, and in a multivariate analysis of all isolated coronary bypass surgery identified "previous operation" as a factor increasing the mortality rate.[12] At the Cleveland Clinic Foundation, the in-hospital mortality rate of a first reoperation ranged between 3% and 4% from 1967 through 1991, and 3.7% for 1663 patients having repeat surgery from 1988 through 1991.[1–3] Progress during the last decade has continued to lower that risk to approximately 2%. Recent mortality rates from other large series range from 6.9% to 11.4%, most being around 7%.[4–9] All of these figures are 2 to 3 times higher than the rates we would expect for the risk of primary bypass surgery.

Coronary reoperations are associated with a higher in-hospital mortality mostly because of an increased risk of perioperative myocardial infarction. In the Cleveland Clinic Foundation series, the cause of perioperative death was cardiovascular in 85% of cases in the most recent cohort of patients undergoing reoperation, a figure that contrasts with recent studies of primary operations in which noncardiac causes of death have been increasingly important.[3,14] Furthermore, in the reoperative series in-hospital mortality was associated with new perioperative myocardial infarction in 67% of cases. Multiple causes of myocardial infarction have been identified, including incomplete revascularization due to distal coronary artery disease, vein graft thrombosis, ITA graft failure, atherosclerotic embolization from vein grafts, injury to bypass grafts, hypoperfusion from arterial grafts,

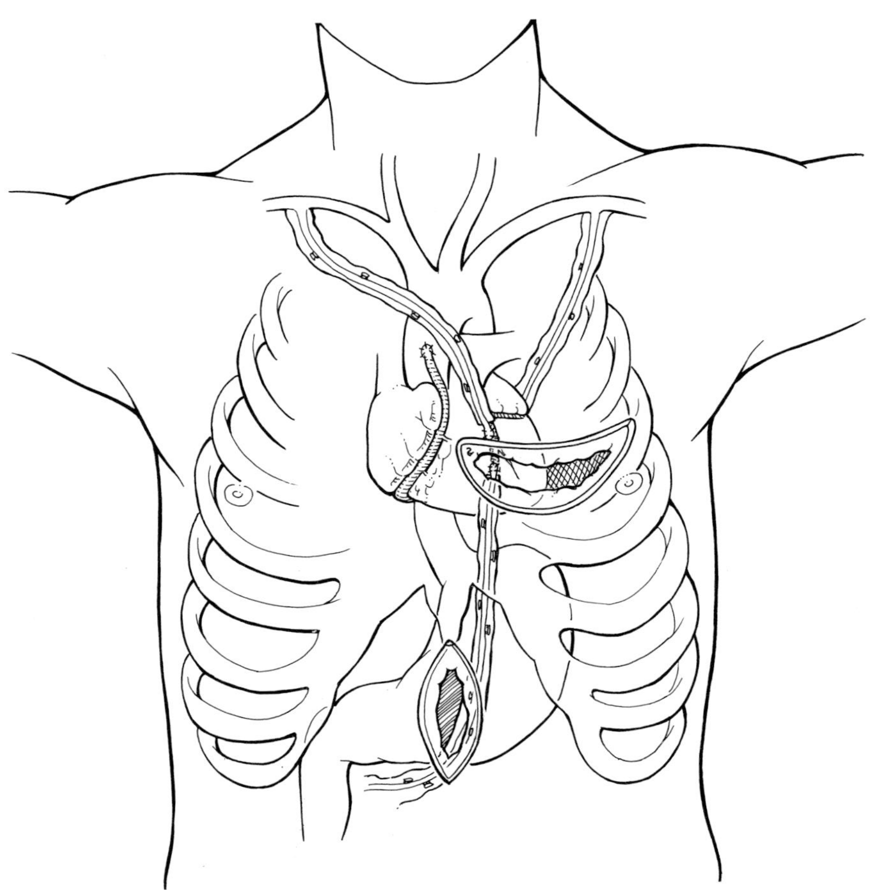

FIGURE 25–21 An in-situ GEA graft may be used for an on- or off-pump anastomosis to the distal LAD coronary artery.

preoperative myocardial infarction, and complications of PTCA.

Multiple studies of patients undergoing reoperation have identified increased age, female gender, and emergency operation as clinical variables that have a high association with in-hospital mortality. Emergency operation is a particularly strong factor. Although there is not a standard definition of "emergency," mortality rates after emergency reoperations that have been reported range from 13% to 40%.[3,5–8] Data from the Society of Thoracic Surgeons for the year 1997 documented a risk of 5.2% for elective reoperations, 7.4% for urgent reoperations, 13.5% for emergency reoperations, and 40.7% for "salvage" reoperations. There is clearly a major increment in risk associated with emergency reoperations, a larger increment than has existed for patients undergoing primary surgery.

Advanced age, by itself, does not substantially increase the risk of reoperation but does so when combined with other variables. In a review of 739 patients aged 70 years or older undergoing reoperation, we noted an overall in-hospital mortality rate of 7.6% and identified emergency operation, female gender, left ventricular dysfunction, creatinine greater than 1.6 μg/dL, and left main coronary artery stenosis as specific factors increasing risk. For patients with none of these characteristics the in-hospital mortality rate was only 1.5%.[50]

Specific anatomical situations, in particular the presence of patent ITA grafts and atherosclerotic vein grafts, can increase the risk of reoperation, but with experience these technical factors have largely been neutralized. We have never documented an increased mortality rate for patients with patent ITA grafts but have noted that the risk of ITA damage has dropped from 8% in our early experience to 3.7% more recently, an improvement almost entirely related to increased surgical experience. With proper positioning of an ITA graft at primary operation, a patent LITA to LAD or circumflex graft should not represent an impediment to reoperation. Situations where a patent *in situ* right ITA graft crosses the midline to supply the LAD or circumflex system are more difficult and require extreme care in reoperating using a median sternotomy incision. Although these situations are uncommon and provide difficult technical challenges, the risks for these patients have not been increased.

Studies from the past noted that the presence of atherosclerotic vein grafts did increase perioperative risk. Perrault et al documented mortality rates of 7%, 17%, and 29% for patients with 1, 2, or 3 stenotic vein grafts, respectively, and in a previous study of patients with atherosclerotic vein grafts we noted that the presence of an atherosclerotic vein graft to the LAD increased in-hospital risk.[34,29] However, in our more recent study we found that atherosclerotic vein grafts did not increase mortality, although there was a nonsignificant trend toward increased risk for patients with multiple stenotic grafts.[3] The favorable results for these patients have been based on a combination of improved technology, the use of retrograde cardioplegia delivery, and increased surgeon experience.

Although arterial grafts may offer advantages at reoperation, their use may prolong an already complex operation and the influence of arterial grafting on perioperative risk has been a concern. However, we have specifically studied this issue and found that the use of single or double ITA grafts at reoperation does not increase perioperative risk and, in fact, not having an ITA graft at either the first or second operation appeared to be a factor associated with increased in-hospital mortality.[3] Graft selection in that study was not randomized, and it is certainly possible that the increased risk for patients receiving only vein grafts was related to patient-related variables rather than surgical strategy. It does appear, however, that the use of arterial grafts does not increase risk. Except for an increased incidence of perioperative myocardial infarction, in-hospital morbidity does not seem to be increased for patients undergoing reoperation. One important observation relates to wound complications. Multiple groups, including ours, have noted an increased risk of wound complications when diabetic patients have received bilateral (simultaneous) ITA grafts. However, there does not appear to be an increased risk of wound complications for diabetic patients who receive staged ITA grafts, one at the first and another at a second operation.

It is important to note that only the variables that can be identified and quantified are included in studies consistently enough to be identified as risk factors. For example, experience and logic dictate that severe atherosclerosis of the ascending aorta is a major risk factor, but that is rarely identified in large studies because patients do not routinely undergo echocardiography to identify the presence of aortic atherosclerosis.

Late Results

Patients who are undergoing reoperation are at a later stage in the progression of their native coronary atherosclerosis compared to the point when they underwent primary surgery, and the anatomical corrections achieved at reoperation are less perfect. Although the definition of "complete revascularization" varies widely, few reoperative candidates undergo an operation in which all diseased segments of all arteries receive bypass grafts. It is not surprising that the long-term results of reoperation have not been as favorable as the long-term results of primary operations.

The likelihood of recurrent angina after any bypass operation is related to time, but angina symptoms are more common after repeat surgery than they are after primary operation. Follow-up of our reoperative patients at a mean interval of 72 months after reoperation showed that 64% of patients were in NYHA Functional Class I, although only 10% of patients had Class III or Class IV symptoms.[2] Weintraub et al also noted at a 4-year follow-up that 41% of reoperative patients had experienced some angina.[6]

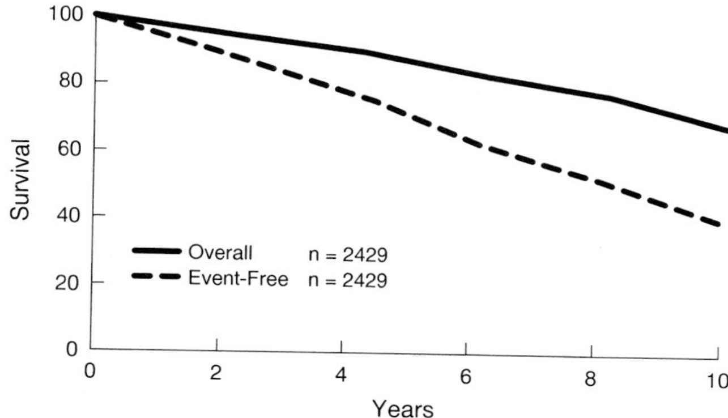

FIGURE 25–22 For 2429 hospital survivors who underwent reoperation between 1967 and 1987, the 10-year survival was 69% and event-free survival was 41%. *(Reprinted with permission from Loop FD, Lytle BW, Cosgrove DM, et al: Reoperation for coronary atherosclerosis: changing practice in 2509 consecutive patients. Ann Surg 1990; 212:378.)*

Late survival rates after reoperation are also inferior to those after primary surgery. Weintraub et al noted a 76% 5-year and 55% 10-year survival rate, and our most recent follow-up study found a 10-year survival of 69% for in-hospital survivors (Fig. 25-22).[2,6] The predictors of late survival have varied among studies, but left ventricular dysfunction, advanced age, and diabetes have been consistently associated with a decreased late survival rate. The variables identified by multivariate testing as decreasing the late survival for 2429 hospital survivors of a first reoperation are

TABLE 25–3 Factors decreasing late survival after reoperation: 1967–1987[2]

Factor	*p*-value	Relative risk
LV dysfunction	.0001	1.9
Age	.0001	1.04
Current cigarette smoking	.0001	1.6
Hypertension	.0002	1.4
Left main ≥50%	.0001	2.0
Triple-vessel disease	.0001	1.6
NYHA III/IV symptoms	.003	1.4
Peripheral vascular disease	.001	1.5
Interval >60 months	.006	1.003
No ITA at first operation	0.03	1.5

LV = left ventricular; MI = myocardial infarction.

Source: Reproduced with permssion from Loop FD, Lytle BW, Cosgrove DM, et al: Reoperation for coronary atherosclerosis: changing practice in 2509 consecutive patients. Ann Surg 1990; 212:378.

listed in Table 25-3. The influence of ITA grafts on late survival has been difficult to determine for reoperations. We found a positive influence of a single ITA graft on late survival, as have others,[51] but the effect was not as dramatic as has been noted after primary operations. Weintraub et al did not document an improved survival associated with ITA grafting.[6]

Multiple Coronary Reoperations

Patients who have had more than one previous coronary operation are like patients undergoing first reoperations, only more so. Many patients undergoing multiple reoperations had their first procedure more than 15 years ago, and severe native vessel disease and lack of bypass conduits are a common combination of problems. Selection criteria vary widely among institutions, but in-hospital mortality rates are increased relative to first reoperations.[10,11] Through 1993, we reoperated on 392 patients who had more than one previous bypass operation, with an in-hospital mortality rate of 8%. Follow-up of the in-hospital survivors found a late survival of 84% at 5 and 66% at 10 postoperative years. So although the in-hospital risks were increased for these patients, the long-term outcome has been relatively favorable. Age was a major determinant of outcome. Recently in-hospital mortality for patients younger than 70 years has decreased to 1% to 2%, but for patients over age 70 it has remained higher than 10%. Furthermore, patients over age 70 who did survive operation in our series had only a 50% 5-year late survival.

CONCLUSION

Coronary reoperations continue to present adult cardiac surgeons with their most difficult challenges in part because of the many technical pitfalls that exist but also because coronary reoperations are so common. The population of patients who have had previous bypass surgery is huge, and patients who develop recurrent ischemic syndromes expect that they will be effectively treated. Although we now understand the long-term implications of using vein grafts, technical and operative time considerations make it unlikely that a wave of total arterial revascularization will engulf primary coronary surgery. Thus, the numbers of reoperations are likely to continue to increase, and improvement over the principles outlined in this chapter will continue to be an important goal.

REFERENCES

1. Lytle BW, Loop FD, Cosgrove DM, et al: Fifteen hundred coronary reoperations: results and determinants of early and late survival. *J Thorac Cardiovasc Surg* 1987; 93:847.
2. Loop FD, Lytle BW, Cosgrove DM, et al: Reoperation for coronary atherosclerosis: changing practice in 2509 consecutive patients. *Ann Surg* 1990; 212:378.
3. Lytle BW, McElroy D, McCarthy PM, et al: The influence of arterial coronary bypass grafts on the mortality of coronary reoperations. *J Thorac Cardiovasc Surg* 1994; 107:675.
4. Salomon NW, Page US, Bigelow JC, et al: Reoperative coronary surgery: comparative analysis of 6591 patients undergoing primary bypass and 508 patients undergoing reoperative coronary artery bypass. *J Thorac Cardiovasc Surg* 1990; 100: 250.
5. Grinda JM, Zegdi R, Couetil JP, et al: Coronary reoperations: indications, techniques and operative results: retrospective study of 240 coronary reoperations. *J Cardiovasc Surg* 2000; 41:703.
6. Weintraub WS, Jones EL, Craver JM, et al: In-hospital and long-term out come after reoperative coronary artery bypass graft surgery. *Circulation* 1995; 92(suppl II); II-50.
7. He GW, Acuff TE, Ryan WH, et al: Determinants of operative mortality in reoperative coronary artery bypass grafting. *J Thorac Cardiovasc Surg* 1995; 110:971.
8. Akins CW, Buckley MJ, Daggett WM, et al: Reoperative coronary grafting: changing patient profiles, operative indications, techniques, and results. *Ann Thorac Surg* 1994; 58:359.
9. Levy JH, Pifarre R, Schaff HV, et al: A multicenter double-blind placebo-controlled trial of aprotinin for reducing blood loss and the requirement for donor-blood transfusion in patients undergoing repeat coronary artery bypass grafting. *Circulation* 1995; 92: 2236.
10. Lytle BW, Cosgrove DM, Taylor PC, et al: Multiple coronary reoperations: early and late results. *Circulation* 1989; 80(supp.II):626.
11. Yau TM, Borger MA, Weisel RD, et al: The changing pattern of reoperative coronary surgery: trends in 1230 consecutive reoperations. *J Thorac Cardiovasc Surg* 2000; 120:156.
12. Edwards FH, Clark RE, Schwartz M: Coronary artery bypass grafting: the Society of Thoracic Surgeons National Database experience. *Ann Thorac Surg* 1994; 57:12.
13. Cosgrove DM, Loop FD, Lytle BW, et al: Predictors of reoperation after myocardial revascularization. *J Thorac Cardiovasc Surg* 1986; 92:811.
14. Loop FD, Lytle BW, Cosgrove DM, et al: Influence of the internal mammary artery graft on 10-year survival and other cardiac events. *N Engl J Med* 1986; 314:1.
15. Lytle BW, Blackstone EH, Loop FD, et al: Two internal thoracic artery grafts are better than one. *J Thorac Cardiovasc Surg* 1999; 117:855.
16. Neitzel GF, Barboriak JJ, Pintar K, et al: Atherosclerosis in aortocoronary bypass grafts: morphologic study and risk factor analysis 6 to 12 years after surgery. *Arteriosclerosis* 1986; 6:594.
17. Ratliff NB, Myles JL: Rapidly progressive atherosclerosis in aortocoronary saphenous vein grafts: possible immuno-mediated disease. *Arch Pathol Lab Med* 1989; 113:772.
18. Solymoss BC, Leung TK, Pelletier LC, et al: Pathologic changes in coronary artery saphenous vein grafts and related etiologic factors. *Cardiovasc Clin* 1991; 21:45.
19. Bourassa MG, Campeau L, Lesperance J: Changes in grafts and in coronary arteries after coronary bypass surgery. *Cardiovasc Clin* 1991; 21:83.
20. Lytle BW, Loop FD, Cosgrove DM, et al: Long-term (5 to 12 years) serial studies of internal mammary artery and saphenous vein coronary bypass grafts. *J Thorac Cardiovasc Surg* 1985; 89:248.
21. Fitzgibbon GM, Leach AJ, Kafka HP, et al: Coronary bypass graft fate: long-term angiographic study. *J Am Coll Cardiol* 1991; 17:1075.
22. Chesebro JH, Fuster V, Elveback LR, et al: Effect of dipyridamole and aspirin on late vein graft patency after coronary bypass operations. *N Engl J Med* 1984; 310:209.

23. Goldman S, Copeland J, Moritz T, et al: Saphenous vein graft patency 1 year after coronary artery bypass surgery and effects of antiplatelet therapy. *Circulation* 1989; 80:1190.
24. Gavaghan TP, Gebski V, Baron DW: Immediate postoperative aspirin improves vein graft patency early and late after coronary artery bypass graft surgery: a placebo-controlled, randomized study. *Circulation* 1991; 83:1526.
25. The Post Coronary Artery-Bypass Graft Trial Investigators: The effect of aggressive lowering of low-density lipoprotein cholesterol levels and low-dose anti-coagulation on obstructive changes in saphenous-vein coronary artery bypass grafts. *N Engl J Med* 1997; 336:153.
26. Flaker GC, Warnica JW, Sacks EM, et al: Provastatin prevents clinical events in revascularized patients with average cholesterol concentrations: cholesterol and recurrent events (CARE) investigators. *J Am Coll Cardiol* 1999;34:106.
27. Dion R, Verhelst R, Rousseau M, et al: Sequential mammary grafting: clinical, functional and angiographic assessment 6 months postoperatively in 231 consecutive patients. *J Thorac Cardiovasc Surg* 1989; 98:80.
28. Lytle BW, Loop FD, Taylor PC, et al: Vein graft disease: the clinical impact of stenoses in saphenous vein bypass grafts to coronary arteries. *J Thorac Cardiovasc Surg* 1992; 103:831.
29. Lytle BW, Loop FD, Taylor PC, et al: The effect of coronary reoperation on the survival of patients with stenoses in saphenous vein to coronary bypass grafts. *J Thorac Cardiovasc Surg* 1993; 105: 605.
30. Lauer MS, Lytle B, Pashkow F, et al: Prediction of death and myocardial infarction by screening exercise-thallium testing after coronary-artery-bypass grafting. *Lancet* 1998; 351: 615.
31. Platko WP, Hollman J, Whitlow PL, Franco I: Percutaneous vs transluminal angioplasty of saphenous vein graft stenosis: long-term follow-up. *J Am Coll Cardiol* 1989; 14:1645.
32. Holmes DR Jr, Topol EJ, Califf RM, et al: A multicenter, randomized trial of coronary angioplasty versus directional atherectomy for patients with saphenous vein bypass graft lesions. *Circulation* 1995; 91:1966.
33. Brener SJ, Ellis SG, Apperson-Hansen C, et al: Comparison of stenting and balloon angioplasty for narrowings in aortocoronary saphenous vein conduits in place for more than five years. *Am J Cardiol* 1997; 79:13.
34. Perrault L, Carrier M, Cartier R, et al: Morbidity and mortality of reoperation for coronary artery bypass grafting: significance of atheromatous vein grafts. *Can J Cardiol* 1991; 7:427.
35. Jones EL, Lattouf OM, Weintraub WS: Catastrophic consequences of internal mammary artery hypoperfusion. *J Thorac Cardiovasc Surg* 1989; 98:902.
36. Jain U, Sullivan HJ, Pifarre R, et al: Graft atheroembolism as the probable cause of failure to wean from cardiopulmonary bypass. *J Cardiothorac Anesth* 1990; 4:476.
37. Navia D, Cosgrove DM, Lytle BW, et al: Is the internal thoracic artery the conduit of choice to replace a stenotic vein graft? *Ann Thorac Surg* 1994; 57:40.
38. Keon WJ, Heggtveit HA, Leduc J: Perioperative myocardial infarction caused by atheroembolization. *J Thorac Cardiovasc Surg* 1982; 84:849.
39. Blauth CI, Cosgrove DM, Webb BW, et al: Atheroembolism from the ascending aorta: an emerging problem in cardiac surgery. *J Thorac Cardiovasc Surg* 1992; 103:1104.
40. Barzilai B, Marshall WG Jr, Saffitz JE, et al: Avoidance of embolic complications by ultrasonic characterization of the ascending aorta. *Circulation* 1989; 80(suppl I):I-275.
41. Sabik JF, Lytle BW, McCarthy PM, et al: Axillary artery: an alternative site of arterial cannulation for patients with extensive aortic and peripheral vascular disease. *J Thorac Cardiovasc Surg* 1995; 109:885.
42. Buckberg GD: Strategies and logic of cardioplegic delivery to prevent, avoid and reverse ischemic and reperfusion damage. *J Thorac Cardiovasc Surg* 1987; 93:127.
43. Partington MT, Acar C, Buckberg GD, et al: Studies of retrograde cardioplegia, II: advantages of antegrade/retrograde cardioplegia to optimize distribution in jeopardized myocardium. *J Thorac Cardiovasc Surg* 1989; 97:613.
44. Menasche P, Kural S, Fauchet M, et al: Retrograde coronary sinus perfusion: a safe alternative for ensuring cardioplegic delivery in aortic valve surgery. *Ann Thorac Surg* 1982; 34:647.
45. Gundry SR, Razzouk AJ, Vigesaa RE, et al: Optimal delivery of cardioplegic solution for "redo" operations. *J Thorac Cardiovasc Surg* 1992; 103:896.
46. Tector AJ, Amundsen S, Schmahl TM, et al: Total revascularization with T grafts. *Ann Thorac Surg* 1994; 57:33.
47. Calafiore AM, DiGiammarco G, Teodori G, Vitolla G: Myocardial revascularization with composite arterial grafts, in Possat GF, Suma H, Alessandria F (eds): Proceedings of the Workshop on Arterial Conduits for Myocardial Revascularization. Rome, Italy, 1995.
48. Turner FE, Lytle BW, Navia D, et al: Coronary reoperations: results of adding an internal mammary artery graft to a stenotic vein graft. *Ann Thorac Surg* 1994; 58:1353.
49. Suma H, Wanibuchi Y, Terada Y, et al: The right gastroepiploic artery graft; clinical and angiographic midterm results in 200 patients. *J Thorac Cardiovasc Surg* 1993; 105:615.
50. Yamamuro M, Lytle BW, Sapp SK, et al: Risk factors and outcomes after coronary reoperation in 739 elderly patients. *Ann Thorac Surg* 2000; 69:464.
51. Dougenis D, Brown AH: Long term results of reoperations for recurrent angina with internal mammary artery versus saphenous vein grafts. *Heart* 1998; 80:9.

Chapter **26**

Surgical Treatment of Complications of Acute Myocardial Infarction: Postinfarction Ventricular Septal Defect and Free Wall Rupture

Arvind K. Agnihotri/Joren C. Madsen/Willard M. Daggett, Jr.

Rupture of the ventricular septum following myocardial infarction is a relatively infrequent condition, which results in variable amounts of left-to-right shunting at the ventricular level and causes heart failure. The clinical presentation ranges from an asymptomatic murmur to cardiogenic shock. The first step in the evolution of surgical techniques to repair an acute postinfarction ventricular septal rupture involved differentiating the surgical treatment of these acquired lesions from the surgical approaches used to repair congenital ventricular septal defects, which are, for the most part, not applicable. Next, understanding the significance of differing anatomic locations of postinfarction ventricular septal defects led to innovations in terms of the location of the cardiotomy and the type of repair necessary to achieve a successful result in any given patient. Then, the gradual appreciation of different clinical courses pursued by patients after postinfarction ventricular septal rupture, both in terms of location of the defect and the degree of right ventricular functional impairment, led to an increased urgency relative to the timing of surgical repair. More recently, improved results have been reported using the technique of endocardial patching with infarct exclusion, which may signify progress in the evolution of the surgical management of postinfarction ventricular septal defects. The incorporation of specific anatomic concepts of surgical repair and a better understanding of the physiologic basis of the disease has led to an integrated approach to the patient that has improved salvage of patients suffering this catastrophic complication of acute myocardial infarction.[1]

An *acute* postinfarction ventricular septal defect is a perforation of the muscular ventricular septum occurring in an area of acutely infarcted myocardium. A ventricular septal rupture may be termed *chronic* when it has been present for more than 4 to 6 weeks. A *postinfarction ventricular rupture* is a perforation of the ventricular free wall occurring in an area of acutely infarcted myocardium.

POSTINFARCTION VENTRICULAR SEPTAL DEFECT

History

In 1845 Latham[2] described a postinfarction ventricular septal rupture at autopsy, but it was not until 1923 that Brunn[3] first made the diagnosis antemortem. Sager[4] in 1934 added the 18th case to the world literature and established specific clinical criteria for diagnosis, stressing the association of postinfarction septal rupture with coronary artery disease.

The treatment of this entity was medical and strictly palliative until 1956, when Cooley et al[5] performed the first successful surgical repair in a patient 9 weeks after the diagnosis of septal rupture. These first patients who underwent similar repairs in the early 1960s usually presented with congestive heart failure, having survived for more than a month after acute septal perforation.[6,7] The success of operation in these patients and the precipitous, acute course of other patients with this complication[8] gave rise to the belief that operative repair should be limited to patients surviving for 1 month or longer.[6,9] This, purportedly, allowed for scarring at the edges of the defect, which was thought to be crucial to the secure and long-lasting closure of the septal rupture.[10,11]

In the late 1960s, more rapid recognition of septal rupture following infarction led to the recommendation that operation be attempted earlier in patients who were hemodynamically deteriorating.[1,3,12] The use of improved prosthetic materials accompanied the successful surgical repair of defects from 1 to 11 days old, as reported by Allen and Woodwark[12] in 1966, Heimbecker et al[13] in 1968, and Iben et al[14] in 1969. Notable among these was a superb early study by Heimbecker et al of infarctectomy and its clinical application to patients with postinfarction ventricular septal defects. The surgical management of these patients was further refined by the inclusion of infarctectomy[13,15,16] and aneurysmectomy[17,18] and the development of techniques to repair perforations in different areas of the septum.[19,20a,20b]

Over the last 15 years, it has become increasingly clear that in the majority of cases postinfarction ventricular septal rupture constitutes a surgical emergency. More recently, improved surgical techniques, newer prosthetic materials, enhanced myocardial protection, and improved perioperative mechanical and pharmacologic support have led to more favorable results in the surgical management of patients with postinfarction septal rupture.[21,22]

Incidence

Postinfarction ventricular septal defects complicate approximately 1% to 2% of cases of acute myocardial infarctions and account for about 5% of early deaths after myocardial infarction.[23,24] The average time from infarction to rupture has been reported to be between 2 and 4 days, but it may be as short as a few hours or as long as 2 weeks.[24–27] These observations correlate well with the pathological findings, which demonstrate that necrotic tissue is most abundant and ingrowth of blood vessels and connective tissue is only beginning 4 to 21 days following a myocardial infarction.[28,29] Postinfarction ventricular septal defects occur in men more often than women (3 to 2), but more women experience rupture than what would be expected from the incidence of coronary artery disease in women.[8] The age of patients with this complication ranges from 44 to 81 years, with a mean of 62.5 years. However, there is some evidence that the average age is increasing.[22,24,30,31] The vast majority of patients who experience ventricular septal rupture do so after their initial infarction.[24,31] The overall incidence of postinfarction ventricular septal rupture may have decreased slightly during the past decade as a result of aggressive pharmacologic treatment of ischemia and thrombolytic and interventional therapy in patients with evolving myocardial infarction, as well as the prompt control of hypertension in these patients.[31]

Angiographic evaluation of patients with postinfarction ventricular rupture indicates that septal rupture is usually associated with complete occlusion rather than severe stenosis of a coronary artery.[32] On average, these patients have slightly less extensive coronary artery disease, as well as less developed septal collaterals than do other patients with coronary artery disease.[33] The lack of collateral flow noted acutely may be secondary to anatomic configuration, edema, or associated arterial disease. Hill et al,[34] in reviewing 19 cases of postinfarction ventricular septal rupture, found single-vessel disease in 64%, double-vessel disease in 7%, and triple-vessel disease in 29%. However, the frequency of single-, double-, and triple-vessel coronary artery disease is more evenly distributed in other series.[27,35]

Postinfarction ventricular septal defects are most commonly located in the anteroapical septum as the result of a full-thickness anterior infarction (in approximately 60% of cases). These anterior septal ruptures are caused by anteroseptal myocardial infarction following occlusion of the left anterior descending artery. In about 20% to 40% of patients, the rupture occurs in the posterior septum following an inferoseptal infarction, which is usually due to occlusion of a dominant right coronary artery or, less frequently, a dominant circumflex artery.[36] Thus, ventricular septal perforations occur most frequently in 65-year-old men with single-vessel coronary disease and poor collateral flow who present 2 to 4 days following their first anterior myocardial infarction.

Pathogenesis

The infarct associated with septal rupture is transmural and generally quite extensive, involving, on average, 26% of the left ventricular wall in hearts with septal rupture, compared with only 15% in other acute infarctions.[24] In an autopsy study, Cummings et al[37] found that in patients with acute anterior or inferior infarctions, the amount of right ventricular infarction was much greater in the hearts with septal ruptures as compared to those without septal defects. Likewise, hearts with posterior septal rupture had more extensive left ventricular necrosis than did hearts with inferior infarctions and no septal defects.

Why certain hearts rupture and others do not is unclear at present. Slippage of myocytes during infarct expansion[38] may allow blood to dissect through the necrotic myocardium and enter either the right ventricle or pericardial space.[39] Hyaline degeneration of cardiomyocytes with subsequent fragmentation and enzymatic digestion may allow fissures to form, predisposing to rupture.[40]

There are two types of rupture: simple, consisting of a direct through-and-through defect usually located anteriorly; and complex, consisting of a serpiginous dissection tract remote from the primary septal defect, which is usually located inferiorly.[41] Multiple defects, which may develop within several days of each other, occur in 5% to 11% of cases and are probably due to infarct extension. Since a successful surgical outcome is related to adequacy of closure of septal defects, multiple defects must be sought preoperatively if possible, and certainly at the time of operative repair.

Of the small number of patients who survive the early period of ventricular septal rupture, 35% to 68% go on to develop ventricular aneurysms[25,34] through the process of ventricular remodeling.[42] This compares with a 12% incidence of aneurysm formation in patients suffering an infarction but no septal rupture,[43] and probably relates to the size and transmural nature of the infarction associated with septal rupture. Postinfarction septal rupture, especially in the posterior septum, may be accompanied by mitral valve regurgitation due to papillary muscle infarction or dysfunction. In approximately one third of cases of septal rupture, there is a degree of mitral insufficiency, usually functional in nature, secondary to left ventricular dysfunction with mitral annular dilation, which usually resolves with repair of the defect.[33]

Pathophysiology

The most important determinant of early outcome following postinfarction ventricular septal rupture is the development of heart failure (left, right, or both). The associated cardiogenic shock leads to end-organ malperfusion, which may be irreversible. The degree to which heart failure develops depends on the size of the ventricular infarction and the magnitude of the left-to-right shunt. Left ventricular dysfunction due to extensive necrosis of the left ventricle is the primary determinant of congestive heart failure and cardiogenic shock in patients with anterior septal rupture, while right ventricular dysfunction secondary to extensive infarction of the right ventricle is the principal determinant of heart failure and cardiogenic shock in patients with posterior septal rupture.[35,44,45] However, the development of congestive heart failure and cardiogenic shock in a patient with postinfarction ventricular septal defects is not explained solely by the degree of damage sustained by the ventricle.[46]

The magnitude of the left-to-right shunt is the other key variable in the development of hemodynamic compromise. With the opening of a ventricular septal defect, the heart is challenged by an increase in pulmonary blood flow, and a decrease in system blood flow as a portion of each stroke volume is diverted to the pulmonary circuit. As a consequence of the sudden increase in hemodynamic load imposed upon a heart already compromised by acute infarction, and possibly by a ventricular aneurysm, mitral valve dysfunction, or a combination of these problems, a severe low cardiac output state results. The normally compliant right ventricle is especially susceptible to failure in this circumstance.[47,48] Patients with posterior ventricular septal rupture and right ventricular dysfunction may display shunt reversal during diastole because the end-diastolic pressure in the right ventricle can be higher than in the left.[39,49] Ultimately, persistence of a low cardiac output state results in peripheral organ failure.

Diagnosis

The typical presentation of a ventricular septal rupture is that of a patient who has suffered an acute myocardial infarction and who, after convalescing for a few days, develops a new systolic murmur, recurrent chest pain, and an abrupt deterioration in hemodynamics. The development of a loud systolic murmur, usually within the first week following an acute myocardial infarction, is the most consistent physical finding of postinfarction ventricular septal rupture (present in over 90% of cases). The murmur is usually harsh, pansystolic, and best heard at the left lower sternal border. The murmur is often associated with a palpable thrill. Depending on the location of the septal defect, the murmur may radiate to the left axilla, thereby mimicking mitral regurgitation.[26] Up to half of these patients experience postinfarction chest pain in association with the appearance of the murmur.[24]

Coincident with the onset of the murmur, there is usually an abrupt decline in the patient's clinical course, with the onset of congestive failure and often cardiogenic shock. The findings of cardiac failure that occur acutely in these patients are primarily the result of right-sided heart failure, with pulmonary edema being less prominent than that occurring in patients with acute mitral regurgitation due to ruptured papillary muscle.[50]

The electrocardiographic findings in patients with acute septal rupture relate to the changes associated with antecedent anterior, inferior, posterior, or septal infarction. The localization of infarction by ECG correlates highly with the location of the associated septal perforation. In our review[31] of 55 patients with postinfarction septal rupture, the location of the defect corresponded to the territory of transmural infarction as determined by ECG in all but three patients. Up to one third of patients develop some degree of atrioventricular conduction block (usually transient) that may precede rupture,[51] but there is no pathognomonic prognostic indicator of impending perforation. The chest radiograph usually shows increased pulmonary vascularity consistent with pulmonary venous hypertension.

It is important to realize that the sudden appearance of a systolic murmur and hemodynamic deterioration following infarction may also result from acute mitral regurgitation due to ruptured papillary muscle. Distinguishing these two lesions clinically is difficult, but a number of points may help. First, the systolic murmur associated with a septal rupture is more prominent at the left sternal border, whereas the murmur resulting from a ruptured papillary muscle is best heard at the apex. Second, the murmur associated with septal perforation is loud and associated with a thrill (in over 50% of patients), whereas the murmur of acute mitral regurgitation is softer and has no associated thrill.[8] Third, septal rupture is often associated with anterior infarctions and conduction abnormalities, whereas papillary muscle rupture is commonly associated with an inferior infarction and no conduction defects.[52] Finally, it should be noted that septal rupture and papillary muscle rupture may coexist following infarction.[20,53,54]

Until recently, the mainstay of differentiating septal rupture from mitral valve dysfunction has been right heart catheterization using the Swan-Ganz catheter.[55] With septal rupture, there is an oxygen saturation step-up between the right atrium and pulmonary artery. Step-up in oxygen saturation greater than 9% between the right atrium and pulmonary artery confirms the presence of a shunt.[56] The pulmonary-to-systemic flow ratios (Qp/Qs), obtained from oxygen saturation samples, range from 1.4:1 to greater than 8:1 and roughly correlate with the size of the defect.[57] In contrast, with acute mitral regurgitation secondary to papillary muscle rupture, there are classic giant V-waves in the pulmonary artery wedge pressure trace. It should be noted, however, that up to one third of patients with septal rupture also have mild mitral regurgitation secondary to left ventricular dysfunction.[58]

Advances in transthoracic and transesophageal echocardiography, especially color flow Doppler mapping, have revolutionized the diagnosis of both the presence and site of septal rupture.[58–61] Echocardiography can detect the defect, localize its site and size, determine right and left ventricular function, assess pulmonary artery and right ventricular pressures, and exclude coexisting mitral regurgitation or free wall rupture. Smyllie et al[60] reported a 100% specificity and 100% sensitivity when color flow Doppler mapping was used to differentiate ventricular septal rupture from acute severe mitral regurgitation following acute myocardial infarction. It also correctly demonstrated the site of septal rupture in 41 of 42 patients. Widespread use of this technology has, for the most part, replaced thermodilution catheter insertion, which in outlying hospitals, where patients are often seen first, may be time consuming and difficult to accomplish. Indeed, the trend toward early surgical referral and prompt operative repair is at least partially explained by the more widespread use of color Doppler echocardiography for diagnosis in peripheral centers.[22]

The necessity of preoperative left heart catheterization with coronary angiography has been a matter of debate. On one hand, left heart catheterization provides important information concerning associated coronary artery disease, left ventricular wall motion, and specifics of valvular dysfunction, which are all important in planning operative correction of postinfarction septal rupture. In most series[62] over 60% of patients with septal rupture have significant involvement of at least one vessel other than the one supplying the infarcted area. Bypassing associated coronary artery disease may increase long-term survival when compared with patients with unbypassed coronary artery disease.[62] However, left heart catheterization has disadvantages—it is time consuming and can contribute to both the mortality and morbidity of these already compromised patients.[22] Thus, some centers do not carry out preoperative left heart catheterization.[63,64] Others use it selectively, avoiding invasive studies in patients with septal rupture caused by anterior wall infarction, which is associated with a much lower incidence of multiple-vessel disease than septal defects resulting from posterior infarctions.[22] The issue of concomitant coronary bypassing is discussed in greater detail below.

Natural History

Reviews by Oyamada and Queen,[65] Sanders et al,[8] and Kirklin et al[66] reveal that nearly 25% of patients with postinfarction septal rupture and no surgical intervention died within the first 24 hours, 50% died within 1 week, 65% within 2 weeks, 80% within 4 weeks; only 7% lived longer than one year. Lemery et al[67] reported that of 25 patients with postinfarction ventricular septal defects treated medically, 19 died within one month. Thus, the risk of death following postinfarction ventricular septal defect (VSD) is highest immediately after infarction and septal rupture, and then gradually declines. Interestingly, there are reports of spontaneous closure of small defects, though this is so rare that it would be unreasonable to manage a patient with the expectation of closure.

Recently, the SHOCK Trial (Should We Emergently Revascularize Occluded Coronaries in Cardiogenic Shock) provided intriguing data on the outcome of medically managed patients with shock and postinfarction VSD.[68] The multi-institutional study tracked 55 patients in cardiogenic shock from postinfarction VSD. Rupture occurred a median of 16 hours after infarction, and the median time to the onset of shock was 7.3 hours. Twenty-four patients were managed medically; the remaining 31 patients comprised a high-risk surgical group. There were only 7 survivors, of whom 6 had surgery to the repair the defect.

Despite the many advances in the nonoperative treatment of congestive heart failure and cardiogenic shock, including the intra-aortic balloon pump and a multitude of new inotropic agents and vasodilators, these do not supplant the need for operative intervention in these critically ill patients.

Management

It has become clear that the early practice of waiting for several weeks after ventricular septal rupture before proceeding with surgery only selects out the small minority of patients in whom the hemodynamic insult is less severe and is better tolerated.[19,35,69] Likewise, it has also become clear that to manage most patients supportively, in hopes of deferring operation, is to deprive the great majority of those with postinfarction ventricular septal rupture of the benefits of definitive surgery before irreversible damage due to peripheral organ ischemia has occurred.[62,70]

While we[21] as well as others[69] have advocated early surgery since the middle of the 1970s, some continue to prefer to defer operation in patients who are easily supported and exhibit no further hemodynamic deterioration.[71,72] Persistence of congestive heart failure or marginal stabilization with rising blood urea nitrogen (BUN) and borderline urine output necessitate aggressive therapy and prompt operation. The routine use of the intra-aortic balloon pump, whenever technically feasible, frequently results in *transient* reversal of the hemodynamic deterioration. This period of stability often makes it possible to complete left heart catheterization before proceeding to operation but should not significantly delay definitive surgical treatment. Patients with septal rupture rarely die of cardiac failure per se, but rather of end-organ failure as a consequence of shock. Shortening the duration of shock by operating early is the only therapeutic solution for this group of patients and can yield dramatic results.[31,73]

Our experience and the experience of others suggest that patients in cardiogenic shock represent a true surgical emergency requiring immediate operative repair. Because deaths in these patients result from multisystem failure secondary to organ hypoperfusion, delay in operative repair for patients in cardiogenic shock represents a "failed therapeutic strategy." Those few patients who are completely stable, with no clinical deterioration, and who require no hemodynamic support, can undergo operative repair when convenient during that hospitalization. The large group of patients who are in an intermediate position between those with shock and those in stable condition should be operated on early (usually within 12 to 24 hours) after appropriate preoperative evaluation. Since the group of patients in stable condition constitutes 5% or less of the total population of patients with postinfarction ventricular septal rupture, the overwhelming majority of patients require prompt surgical treatment.

Rarely, because of a delayed referral, a patient will be seen for surgical therapy who is already in a state of multisystem failure or has developed septic complications. Such a patient is unlikely to survive an emergency operation and thus may benefit from prolonged support with an intra-aortic balloon pump before an attempted operative repair. We have found it necessary to treat a small number of patients (3 of 92) in this fashion. Baillot et al[72] have reported individual successes with such an approach, which we consider the exception rather than the rule.

Preoperative Management

Because the natural course of the disease in unoperated patients is so dismal, the diagnosis of postinfarction ventricular septal rupture can be regarded as its own indication for operation.[70] Preoperative management is directed towards stabilization of the hemodynamic condition so that peripheral organ perfusion can be best maintained while any further diagnostic studies are obtained and while deciding on the optimal time for surgical intervention. Although the early clinical course of patients with postinfarction ventricular septal rupture can be quite variable, 50% to 60% present with severe congestive heart failure and a low cardiac output state requiring intensive therapy.[74]

The goals of preoperative management are to: (1) reduce the systemic vascular resistance, and thus the left-to-right shunt; (2) maintain cardiac output and arterial pressure to ensure peripheral organ perfusion; and (3) maintain or improve coronary artery blood flow. This is best accomplished by the intra-aortic balloon pump (IABP). Counterpulsation reduces left ventricular afterload, thereby increasing cardiac output and decreasing the left-to-right shunt, as reported by Gold et al in 1973.[75] In addition, IABP support is associated with decreased myocardial oxygen consumption, as well as improved myocardial and peripheral organ perfusion. Although counterpulsation produces an overall improvement in the patient's condition, a complete correction of the hemodynamic picture cannot be obtained.[76] Peak improvement occurs within 24 hours and no further benefit has been observed with prolonged balloon pumping.[77] Pharmacologic therapy with inotropic agents and diuretics should be instituted promptly. The addition of vasodilators (i.e., sodium nitroprusside or intravenous nitroglycerine) makes good

TABLE 26–1 Principles of repair of postinfarction ventricular septal defects

1. Expeditious establishment of total cardiopulmonary bypass with moderate hypothermia and meticulous attention to myocardial protection.
2. Transinfarct approach to ventricular septal defect with the site of ventriculotomy determined by the location of the transmural infarction.
3. Thorough trimming of the left ventricular margins of the infarct back to viable muscle to prevent delayed rupture of the closure.
4. Conservative trimming of the right ventricular muscle as required for complete visualization of the margins of the defect.
5. Inspection of the left ventricular papillary muscles and concomitant replacement of the mitral valve only if there is frank papillary muscular rupture.
6. Closure of the septal defect without tension, which in most instances will require the use of prosthetic material.
7. Closure of the infarctectomy without tension with generous use of prosthetic material as indicated, and epicardial placement of the patch to the free wall to avoid strain on the friable endocardial tissue.
8. Buttressing of the suture lines with pledgets or strips of Teflon felt or similar material to prevent sutures from cutting through friable muscle.

Source: Reproduced with permission from Heitmiller R, Jacobs ML, Daggett WM: Surgical management of postinfarction ventricular septal rupture. Ann Thorac Surg 1986; 41:683.

theoretical sense, because it can decrease the left-to-right shunting associated with the mechanical defect, and thus increase cardiac output. However, these effects are often associated with a marked fall in mean arterial blood pressure and reduced coronary perfusion, both poorly tolerated in these critically ill patients. It must be stressed that pharmacologic therapy is intended primarily to support the patient in preparation for operation and should not in any way delay urgent operation in the critically ill patient. We now admit patients with postinfarction septal rupture directly to the surgical intensive care unit rather than to the coronary care or medical intensive care unit.

Other techniques that have been tried in an effort to improve the hemodynamics of patients with interventricular septal rupture include venoarterial extracorporeal membrane oxygenation (ECMO),[78] and inflation of a balloon in the right ventricular outflow tract to decrease the left-to-right shunt.[79] Neither has been proven reliable in clinical application. Use of a catheter-mounted axial flow pump (Hemopump) in stabilizing these patients is controversial because of the risk of acute pump failure due to catheter blockage from pieces of necrotic tissue.[80]

Operative Techniques

The first repair by Cooley et al[5] of an acquired ventricular septal defect was accomplished using an approach through the right ventricle with incision of the right ventricular outflow tract. This approach, which was adapted from surgical techniques for closure of congenital ventricular septal defects, proved to be disadvantageous for many reasons. Exposure of the defect was frequently less than optimal, particularly for defects located in the apical septum. It involved unnecessary injury to normal right ventricular muscle and interruption of collaterals from the right coronary artery. Finally, it failed to eliminate the paradoxical bulging segment of infarcted left ventricular wall. Subsequently, Heimbecker et al[13] introduced, and others adopted,[16,25,81] a left-sided approach (left ventriculotomy) with incision through the area of infarction. Such an approach frequently incorporates infarctectomy and aneurysmectomy, together with repair of septal rupture.

Experience with a variety of techniques for closure of postinfarction ventricular septal rupture has led us to the evolution of eight basic principles (Table 26-1). Adherence to these principles in the closure of septal defects in different locations has led to the evolution of individualized approaches to apical, anterior, and inferoposterior septal defects.

GENERAL TECHNIQUES

Patients are anesthetized using a fentanyl-based regimen. Pancuronium is selected as the muscle relaxant so as to prevent bradycardia. Pulmonary bed vasodilators such as dobutamine are avoided to minimize the left-to-right shunt fraction. Preoperative antibiotics include both cefazolin and vancomycin given the fact that prosthetic material may be left in the patient.

Cardiopulmonary bypass is accomplished with bicaval venous drainage. Systemic cooling to 25°C is employed. Cardiac standstill is achieved with cold, oxygenated, dilute blood cardioplegia[82,83] using antegrade induction followed by retrograde perfusion via the coronary sinus. Although a number of myocardial protection strategies are currently available, we[82] and others[45,84,85] continue to use cold oxygenated, dilute blood cardioplegia to protect the heart during surgical correction of a ventricular septal defect. A total of 1200 to 2000 mL of cardioplegia solution is delivered depending on the size of the heart and the degree of hypertrophy.[86] Although we have not employed warm cardioplegic induction,[87] we do administer warm reperfusion cardioplegia just before removing the aortic cross-clamp.[88] Patients with multivessel coronary disease and critical

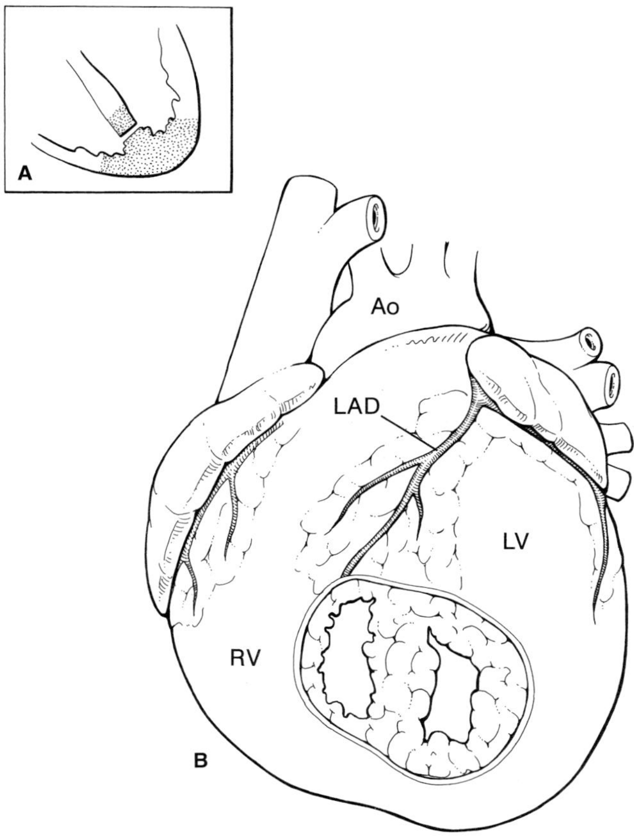

FIGURE 26–1 (A) Apical postinfarction ventricular septal defect. (B) View of the apical septal rupture, which is exposed by amputating apex of left and right ventricles. Stippled region, infarcted myocardium; Ao, aorta; LAD, left anterior descending coronary artery; RV, right ventricle; LV, left ventricle.

coronary stenoses are revascularized before opening the heart in order to optimize myocardial protection. In most of these patients, saphenous vein rather than the left internal mammary artery is utilized.

APICAL SEPTAL RUPTURE

The technique of apical amputation was described by Daggett et al in 1970.[16] An incision is made through the infarcted apex of the left ventricle. Excision of the necrotic myocardium back to healthy muscle results in amputation of the apical portion of the left ventricle, right ventricle, and septum (Fig. 26-1A and B). The remaining apical portions of the left and right ventricle free walls are then approximated to the apical septum. This is accomplished by means of a row of interrupted mattress sutures of 0 Tevdek that are passed sequentially through a buttressing strip of Teflon felt, the left ventricular wall, a second strip of felt, the interventricular septum, a third strip of felt, the right ventricular wall, and a fourth strip of felt (Fig. 26-2A and B). After all sutures have been tied, the closure is reinforced with an additional over-and-over suture, as in ventricular aneurysm repair, to insure hemostasis of the ventriculotomy closure (not shown).

ANTERIOR SEPTAL RUPTURE

The approach to these defects is by a left ventricular transinfarct incision with infarctectomy (Fig. 26-3). Small defects beneath anterior infarcts can be closed by the technique of plication as suggested by Shumaker.[89] This involves approximation of the free anterior edge of the septum to the right ventricular free wall using mattress sutures of 0 Tevdek over strips of felt (Fig. 26-4A). The transinfarct incision is then closed with a second row of mattress sutures buttressed with strips of felt (Fig. 26-4B-D). An over-and-over running suture completes the ventriculotomy closure (not shown).

Most anterior defects require closure with a prosthetic patch (DeBakey Elastic Dacron fabric made by U.S.C.I., Division of C.R. Bard, Inc., Billerica, MA) in order to avoid tension that could lead to disruption of the repair (Fig. 26-5). After debridement of necrotic septum and left ventricular muscle, a series of pledgeted interrupted mattress sutures are placed around the perimeter of the defect (Fig. 26-5A). Along the posterior aspect of the defect, sutures are passed through the septum from right side to left. Along the anterior edge of the defect, sutures are passed from the epicardial surface of the right ventricle to the endocardial surface. All sutures are placed before the patch is inserted, and then passed through the edge of a synthetic patch, which is seated on the left side of the septum (Fig. 26-5B). Each suture is then passed through an additional pledget and all are tied. We use additional pledgets on the left ventricular side overlying the patch (Fig. 26-4B) to cushion each suture as it is tied down to prevent cutting through the friable muscle. The edges of the ventriculotomy are then approximated by a two-layer closure consisting of interrupted mattress sutures passed through buttressing strips of Teflon felt (or glutaraldehyde preserved bovine pericardium) and a final over-and-over running suture (not shown).

POSTERIOR/INFERIOR SEPTAL RUPTURE

Closure of inferoposterior septal defects, which result from transmural infarction in the distribution of the posterior descending artery, has posed the greatest technical challenge.[20a,20b] Early attempts at primary closure of these defects by simple plication techniques similar to those used in the repair of anterior defects were frequently unsuccessful because of the sutures tearing out of soft, friable myocardium that had been closed under tension. This resulted in either reopening of the defect or catastrophic disruption of the infarctectomy closure. It was, in large part, the analysis of such early results that led to the evolution of the operative principles enumerated in Table 26-1.

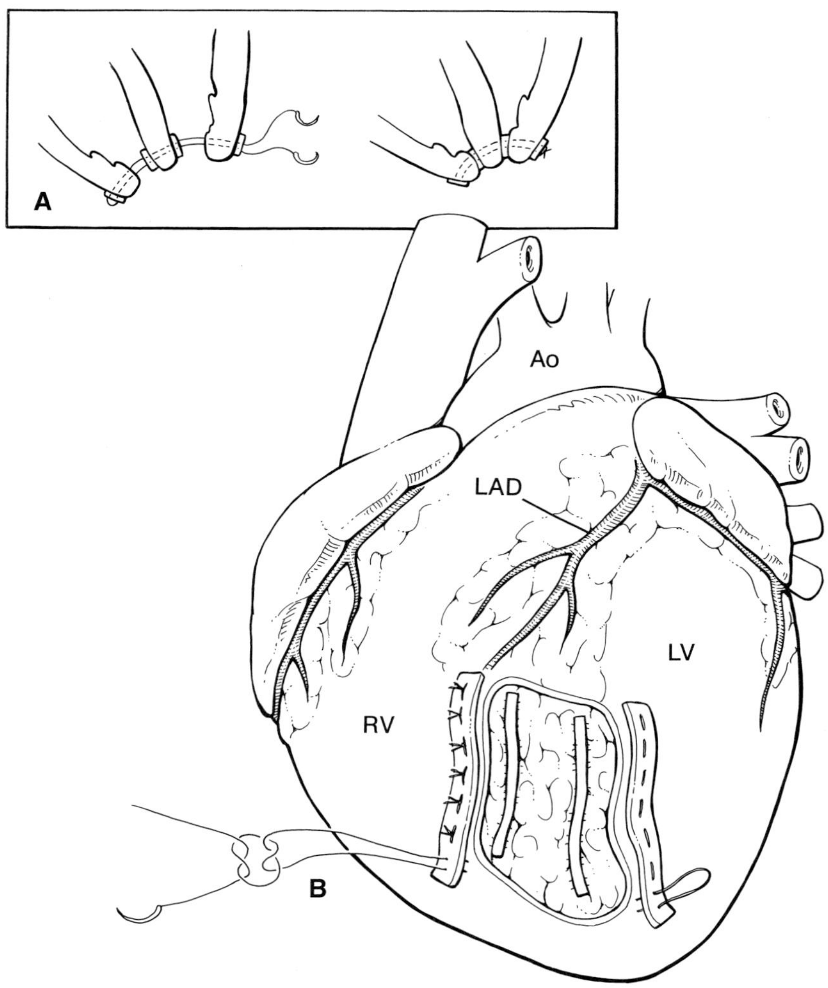

FIGURE 26–2 (A) Necrotic infarct and apical septum have been debrided back to healthy muscle. Repair is made by approximating the left ventricle, apical septum, and right ventricle using interrupted mattress sutures of 0 Tevdek with buttressing strips of Teflon felt. Felt strips are used within the interior of the left and right ventricles as well as on the epicardial surface of each ventricle. (B) All sutures are placed before any are tied. A second running over and over suture (not shown) is used, as in left ventricular aneurysm repair, to ensure a secure hemostatic ventriculotomy closure. Ao, aorta; LAD, left anterior descending coronary artery; RV, right ventricle; LV, left ventricle. *(Adapted with permission from Daggett WM, Burwell LR, Lawson DW, Austen WG: Resection of acute ventricular aneurysm and ruptured interventricular septum after myocardial infarction. N Engl J Med 1970; 283:1507.)*

Use of the following techniques has been associated with an improved operative survival. After the establishment of bypass with bicaval cannulation, the left side of the heart is vented via the right superior pulmonary vein. The heart is retracted out of the pericardial well as for bypass to the posterior descending coronary artery. The margins of the defect may involve the inferior aspects of both ventricles, or of the left ventricle only (Fig. 26-6A). A transinfarct incision is made in the left ventricle, and the left ventricular portion of the infarct is excised (Fig. 26-6B), exposing the septal defect. The left ventricular papillary muscles are inspected. Only if there is frank papillary muscle rupture is mitral valve replacement performed. When it is indicated, we prefer to perform mitral valve replacement through a separate conventional left atrial incision, to avoid trauma to the friable ventricular muscle. After all infarcted left ventricular muscle has been excised, a less aggressive debridement of the right ventricle is accomplished, with the goal of resecting only as much muscle as is necessary to afford complete visualization of the defect(s). Using this technique, delayed rupture of the right ventricle has not been a problem. If the posterior septum has cracked or split from the adjacent ventricular free wall without loss of a great deal of septal tissue, then the septal rim of the posterior defect may be approximated to the edge of the diaphragmatic right ventricular free wall using mattress sutures buttressed with strips of Teflon felt or bovine pericardium (Fig. 26-6C and D).

Larger posterior defects require patch closure (Fig. 26-7). Pledgeted mattress sutures are placed from the right side of the septum and from the epicardial side of the right ventricular free wall (Fig. 26-7B). All sutures are passed through the perimeter of the patch and then through additional pledgets, and are then tied (Fig. 26-7C). Thus, as in closure of large anterior defects, the patch is secured on the left ventricular side of the septum. Direct closure of the remaining infarctectomy is rarely possible because of tension required to pull together the edges of the gaping defect. A prosthetic patch is generally required. Originally, we cut an oval patch from a Cooley low-porosity woven Dacron tube graft (Meadox Medicals, Inc. Oakland, NJ). Currently, we cut this patch from

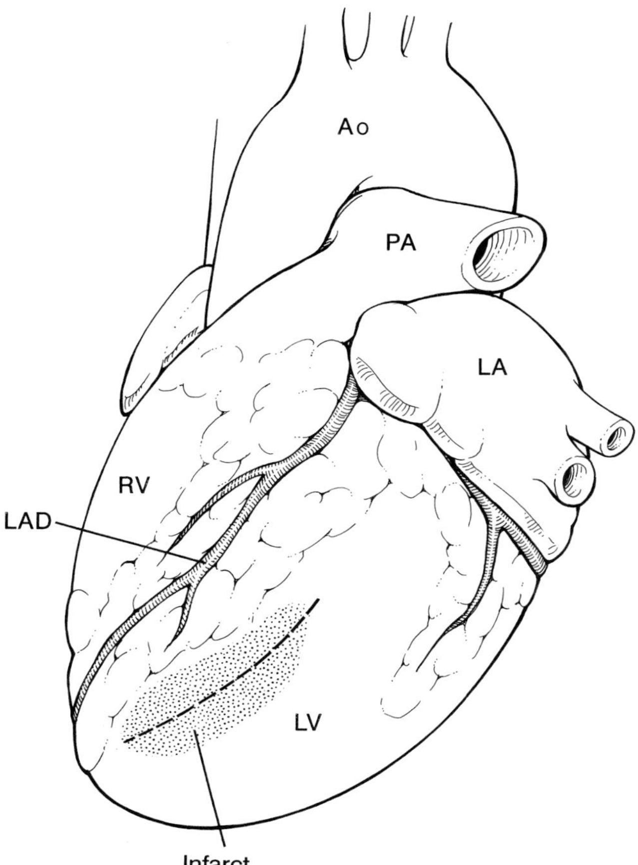

FIGURE 26–3 Transinfarct left ventricular incision to expose an anterior septal rupture. An incision (dashed line) is made parallel to anterior descending branch of left coronary artery (LAD) through center of infarct (stippled area) in anterior left ventricle (LV). Ao, aorta; RV, right ventricle; PA, pulmonary artery.

a Hemashield woven Dacron collagen impregnated graft (Meadox Medicals, Inc.). Pledgeted mattress sutures are passed out through the margin of the infarctectomy (endocardium to epicardium) and then through the patch (Fig. 26-7D), which is seated on the epicardial surface of the heart. After each suture is passed through an additional pledget, all sutures are tied (Fig. 26-7E). The cross-sectional view of the completed repair (Fig. 26-8) illustrates the restoration of relatively normal ventricular geometry, which is accomplished by the use of appropriately sized prosthetic patches.

ENDOCARDIAL PATCH REPAIR WITH INFARCT EXCLUSION

The concept that the preservation of left ventricular geometry plays a crucial role in the preservation of left ventricular function[19,90] has laid the groundwork for a recent evolution in the surgical approach to postinfarction ventricular septal defects—the technique of endocardial patch repair of postinfarction ventricular septal defects described by David,[81,84] Cooley,[91,92] and then by Ross[93] in the early 1990s. This operative technique, which is an application to ventricular septal rupture repair of Dor's technique of ventricular endoaneurysmorrhaphy,[90] involves intracavitary placement of an endocardial patch to exclude infarcted myocardium while maintaining ventricular geometry. Thus, instead of closing the septal defect, it is simply *excluded* from the high-pressure zone of the left ventricle. The recent impressive results obtained using infarct exclusion[45] mandate that a detailed description of the technique be provided here. The following descriptions are taken from the work of David et al (with permission).[39,45,84]

In patients with anterior septal rupture, the interventricular septum is exposed via a left ventriculotomy, which is made through the infarcted anterolateral wall starting at the apex and extending proximally parallel to but 1 to 2 cm away from the anterior descending artery (Fig. 26-9A). Stay sutures are passed through the margins of the ventriculotomy to aid in the exposure of the infarcted septum. The septal defect is located and the margins of the infarcted muscle identified. A glutaraldehyde-fixed bovine pericardial patch is tailored to the shape of the left ventricular infarction as seen from the endocardium but 1 to 2 cm larger. The patch is usually oval and measures approximately 4 × 6 cm in most patients. The pericardial patch is then sutured to healthy endocardium all around the infarct (Fig. 26-9B). Suturing begins in the lowest and most proximal part of the noninfarcted endocardium of the septum with a continuous 3-0 polypropylene suture. Interrupted mattress sutures with felt pledgets may be used to reinforce the repair.[92] The patch is also sutured to the noninfarcted endocardium of the anterolateral ventricular wall. The stitches should be inserted 5 to 7 mm deep in the muscle and 4 to 5 mm apart. The stitches in the patch should be at least 5 to 7 mm from its free margin so as to allow the patch to cover the area between the entrance and exit of the suture in the myocardium.[39] This technique minimizes the risk of tearing muscle as the suture is pulled taut. If the infarct involves the base of the anterior papillary muscle, the suture is brought outside of the heart and buttressed on a strip of bovine pericardium or Teflon felt applied to the epicardial surface of the left ventricle. Once the patch is completely secured to the endocardium of the left ventricle, the left ventricular cavity becomes largely excluded from the infarcted myocardium. The ventriculotomy is closed in two layers over two strips of bovine pericardium or Teflon felt using 2-0 or 3-0 polypropylene sutures as illustrated in Figure 26-9C. No infarctectomy is performed unless the necrotic muscle along the ventriculotomy is sloughing at the time of its closure, and even then it is minimized, since infarcted muscle will not be exposed to left ventricular pressures when the heart begins to work (Fig. 26-9D). Alternatively, sutures can be passed through the ventricular free wall and through a tailored external patch of Teflon or pericardium (Fig. 26-10).[71,88]

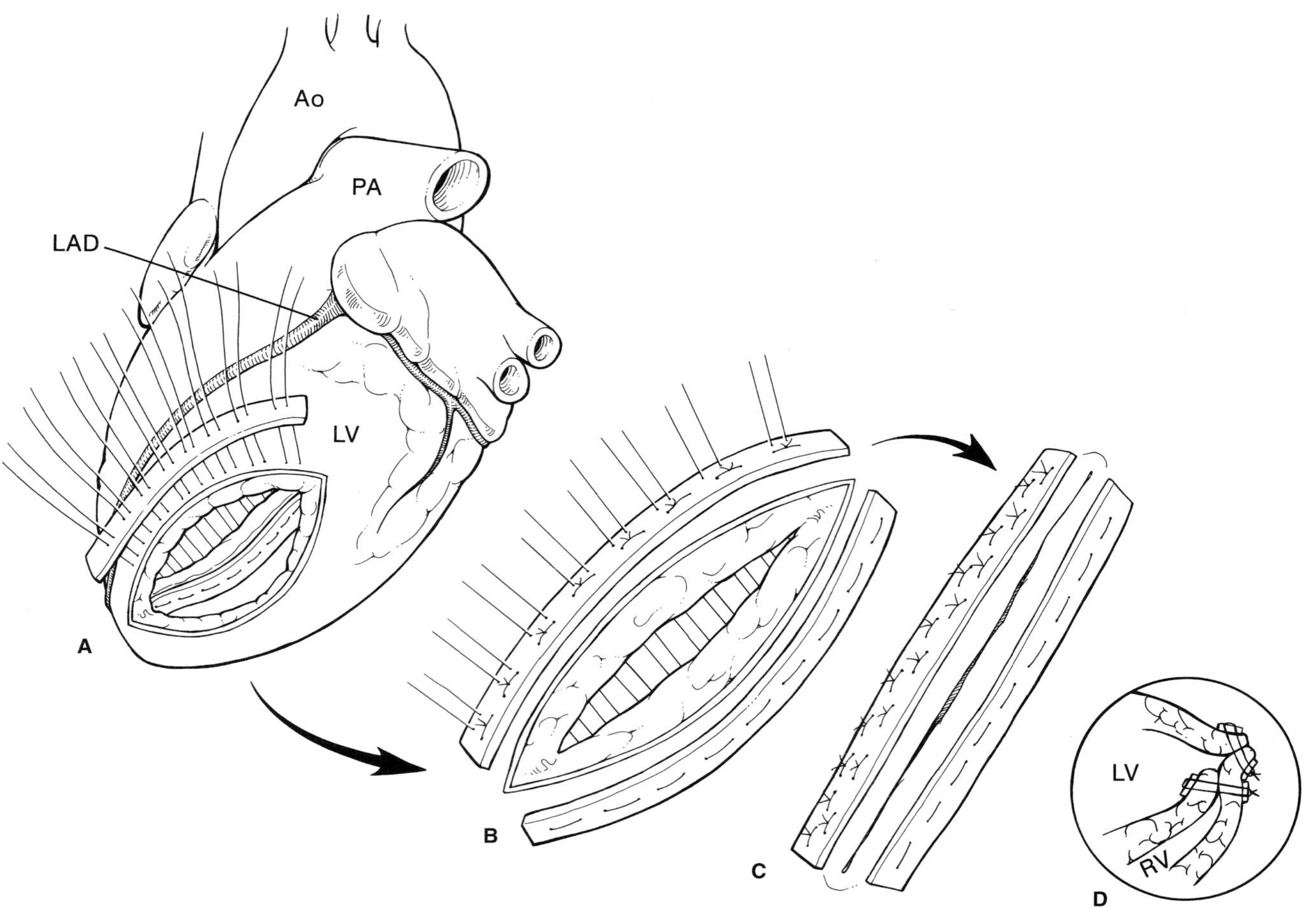

FIGURE 26–4 (A) Repair of an anterior septal rupture by placating the free anterior edge of septum to right ventricular free wall with interrupted 0 Tevdek mattress sutures buttressed with strips of Teflon felt. (B, C, and D) The left ventriculotomy is then closed as a separate suture line, again with interrupted mattress sutures of 0 Tevdek buttressed with felt strips. A second running suture (not shown) is used to ensure a secure left ventriculotomy closure. Ao, aorta; LAD, left anterior descending coronary artery; PA, pulmonary artery; LV, left ventricle. *(Adapted with permission from Guyton SW, Daggett WM: Surgical repair of post-infarction ventricular septal rupture, in Cohn LH (ed): Modern Techniques in Surgery: Cardiac/Thoracic Surgery. Mt. Kisco, NY, Futura, 1983; installment 9, p 61–1.)*

In patients with posterior septal defects, an incision is made in the inferior wall of the left ventricle 1 or 2 mm from the posterior descending artery (Fig. 26-11A). This incision is started at the midportion of the inferior wall and extended proximally toward the mitral annulus and distally toward the apex of the ventricle. Care is taken to avoid damage to the posterolateral papillary muscle. Stay sutures are passed through the fat pad of the apex of the ventricle and margins of the ventriculotomy to facilitate exposure of the ventricular cavity. In most cases, the rupture is found in the proximal half of the posterior septum and the posteromedial papillary muscle is involved by the infarction.[45] A bovine pericardial patch is tailored in a triangular shape of approximately 4 × 7 cm in most patients. The base of the triangular-shaped patch is sutured to the fibrous annulus of the mitral valve with a continuous 3-0 polypropylene suture starting at a point corresponding to the level of the posteromedial papillary muscle and moving medially toward the septum until the noninfarcted endocardium is reached (Fig. 26-11B). At that level, the suture is interrupted and any excess patch material trimmed. The medial margin of the triangular-shaped patch is sewn to healthy septal endocardium with a continuous 3-0 or 4-0 polypropylene suture taking bites the same size as described for anterior defects. In this area of the septum, reinforcing pledgeted sutures may be required.[92] The lateral side of the patch is sutured to the posterior wall of the left ventricle along a line corresponding to the medial margin of the base of the posteromedial papillary muscle. Because the posterior wall of the left ventricle is infarcted, it is usually necessary to use full-thickness bites and anchor the sutures on a strip of pericardium or Teflon felt applied on the epicardial surface of the posterior wall of the left

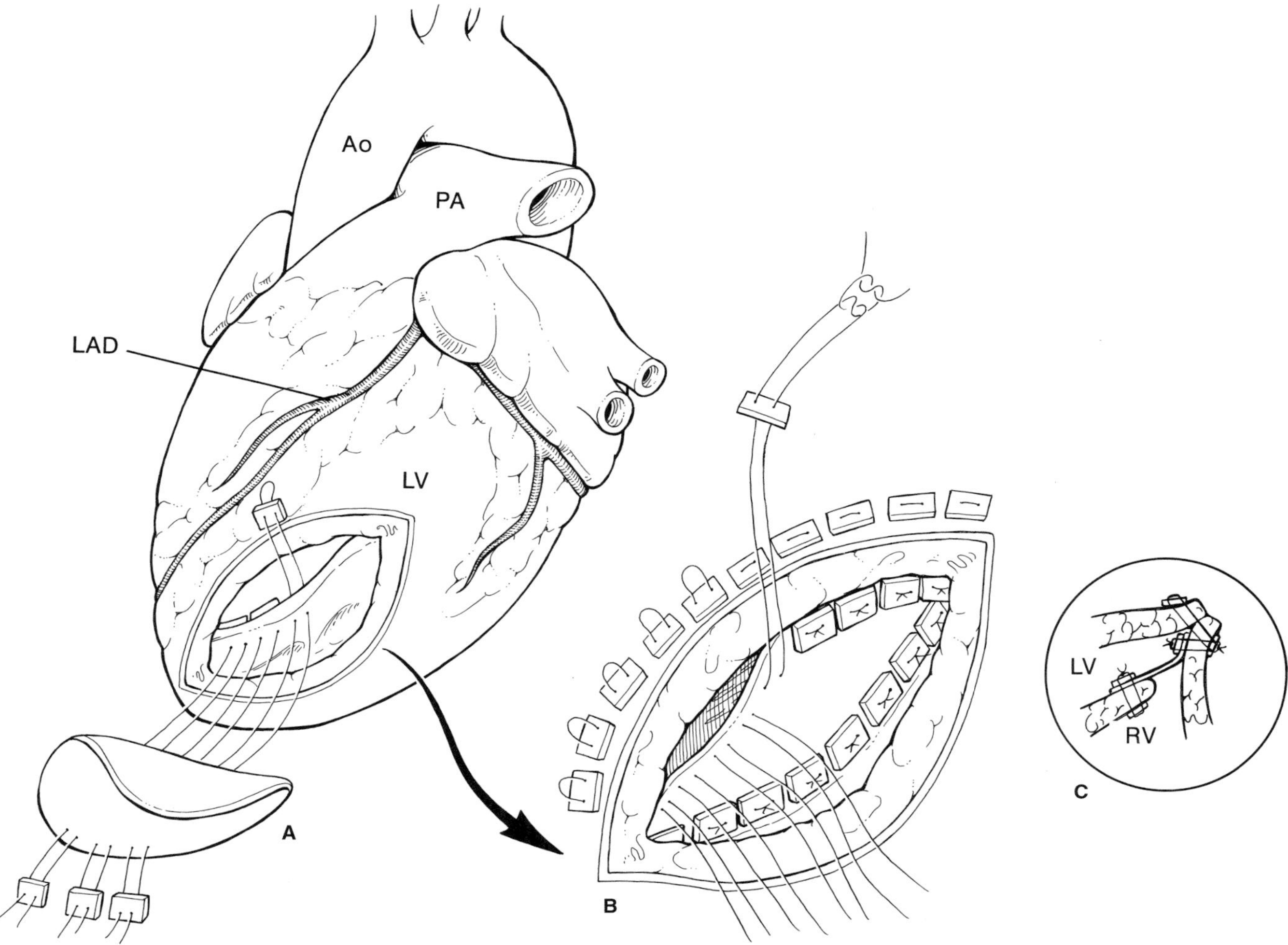

FIGURE 26–5 (A) Larger anterior septal defects require a patch (DeBakey Dacron, United States Catheter and Instrument Corporation, Billerica, MA), which is sewn to the left side of the ventricular septum with interrupted mattress sutures, each of which is buttressed with a pledget of Teflon felt on the right ventricular side of the septum and anteriorly on the epicardial surface of the right ventricular free wall. All sutures are placed before the patch is inserted. (B and C) We use additional pledgets on the left ventricular side overlying the patch to cushion each suture as it is tied down to prevent cutting through the friable muscle. Ao, aorta; LAD, left anterior descending coronary artery; PA, pulmonary artery; LV, left ventricle. *(Adapted with permission from Guyton SW, Daggett WM: Surgical repair of post-infarction ventricular septal rupture, in Cohn LH (ed): Modern Techniques in Surgery: Cardiac/Thoracic Surgery. Mt. Kisco, NY, Futura, 1983; installment 9, p 61–1.)*

ventricle right at the level of the posteromedial papillary muscle insertion, as shown in Figure 26-11B. Once the patch is completely sutured to the mitral valve annulus, the endocardium of the interventricular septum, and the full thickness of the posterior wall (Fig. 26-11C), the ventriculotomy is closed in two layers of full thickness sutures buttressed on strips of pericardium or Teflon felt (Fig. 26-11D). The infarcted right ventricular wall is left undisturbed. If the posteromedial papillary muscle is ruptured, mitral valve replacement is necessary.[84]

There are several theoretical advantages in the technique of infarct exclusion. (1) It does not require resection of myocardium; excessive resection results in depression of ventricular function and insufficient resection predisposes to recurrence of septal rupture. (2) It maintains ventricular geometry, which enhances ventricular function.[42] (3) It avoids tension on friable muscle, which may diminish postoperative bleeding.[45]

OTHER TECHNIQUES

Most other operative techniques that have resulted in successful management of postinfarction of ventricular septal rupture have adhered to the same general principles

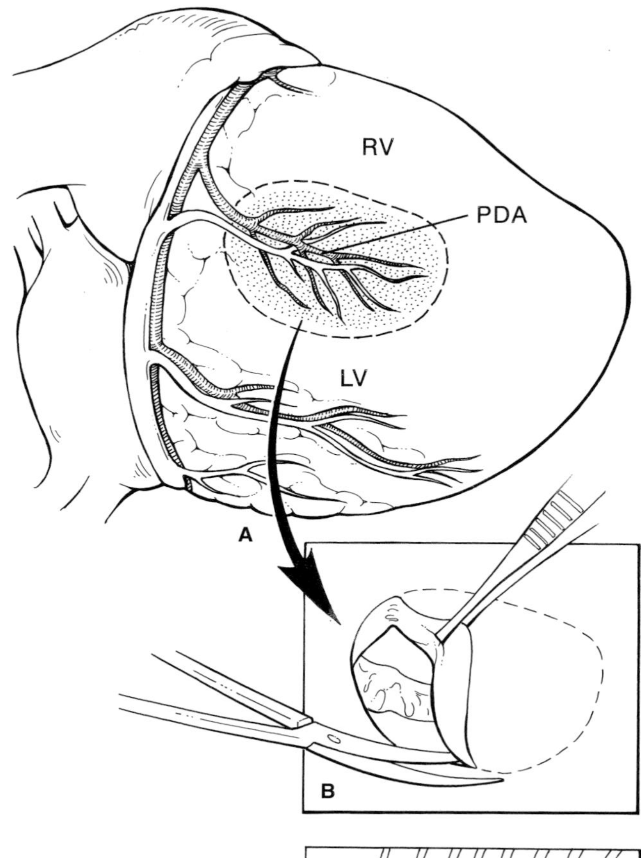

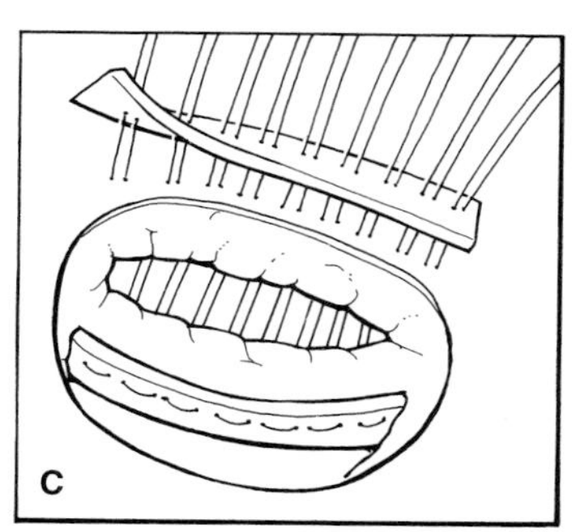

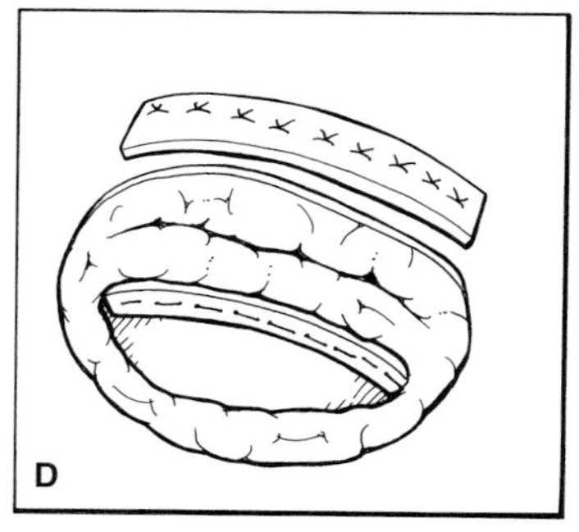

FIGURE 26–6 (A) View of an inferior infarct (stippled area) associated with posterior septal rupture. Apex of the heart is to the right. Exposure at operation is achieved by dislocating the heart up and out of the pericardial sac, and then retracting it cephalad, as in the performance of distal vein bypass and anastomosis to the posterior descending artery. (B) The inferoposterior infarct is excised to expose the posterior septal defect. Complete excision of the left ventricular portion of the infarct is important to prevent delayed rupture of the ventriculotomy repair. The free edge of the right ventricle is progressively shaved back to expose the margins of the defect clearly. (C and D) Repair of the posterior septal rupture by approximating the edge of the posterior septum to the free wall of the diaphragmatic right ventricle with felt-buttressed mattress sutures. The repair is possible when the septum has cracked or split off from the posterior ventricular wall without necrosis of a great deal of septal muscle. The surgeon can perform repair of posterior septal rupture to best advantage by standing at the left side of the supine patient. The left ventriculotomy is then closed as a separate suture line, again with interrupted mattress sutures of 0 Tevdek buttressed with felt strips. A second running suture (not shown) is used to ensure a secure left ventriculotomy closure (not shown). RV, diaphragmatic surface of right ventricle; LV, posterior left ventricle; PDA, posterior descending artery. *(Adapted with permission from Daggett WM: Surgical technique for early repair of posterior ventricular septal rupture. J Thorac Cardiovasc Surg 1982; 84:306.)*

described above. For example, da Silva et al[94] report a technique whereby a nontransfixing running suture has been used to secure a large prosthetic patch to the left side of the ventricular septum, with little or no resection of septum muscle. Tashiro et al[95] described an extended endocardial repair in which a *saccular* patch of glutaraldehyde-fixed equine pericardium was used to exclude an anterior septal rupture. Usui et al[96] reported the successful repair of a posterior septal rupture using two sheets of equine pericardium to sandwich the infarcted myocardium, including the septal

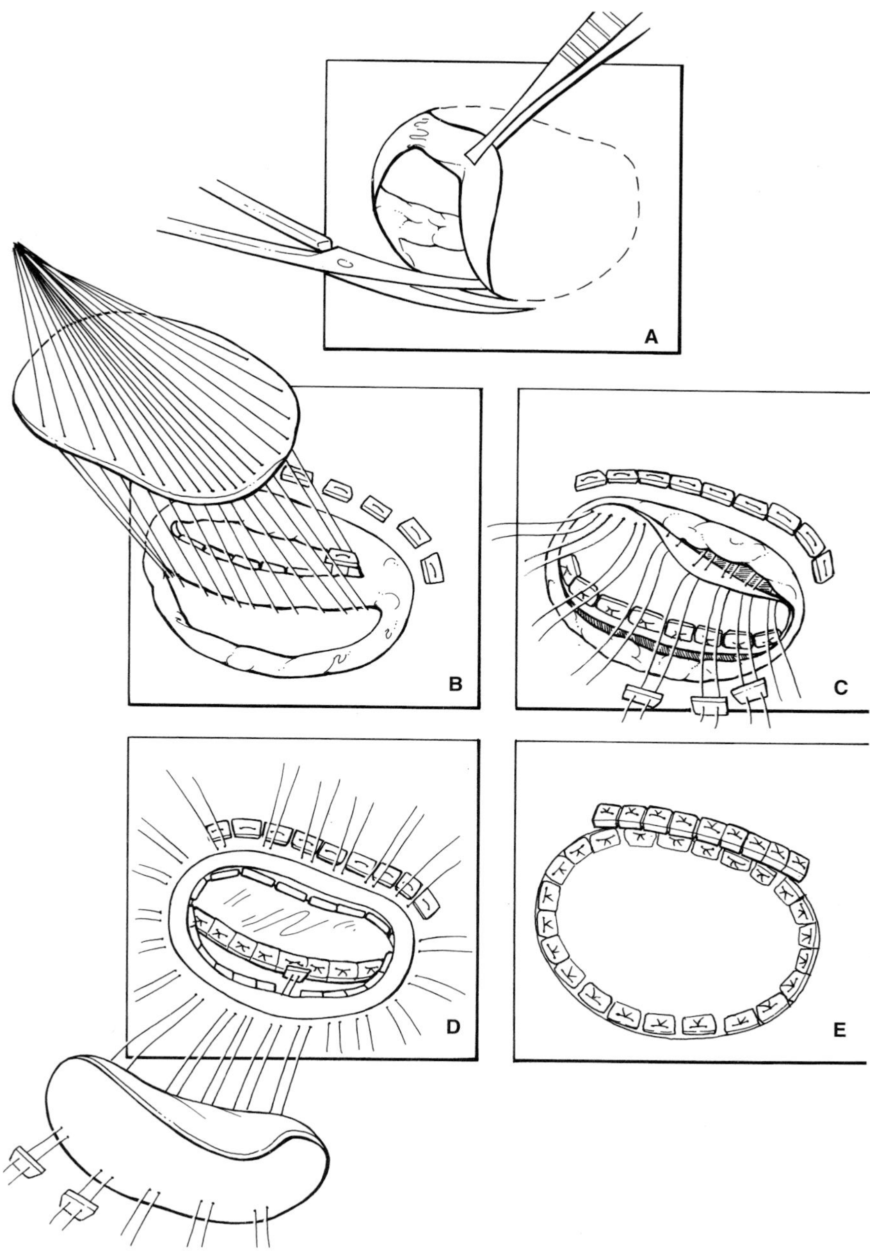

FIGURE 26–7 (A) Repair of posterior septal rupture when necrosis of a substantial portion of the posterior septum requires the use of patches. (B) Interrupted mattress sutures of 2-0 Tevdek are placed circumferentially around the defect. These sutures are buttressed with felt pledgets on the right ventricular side of the septum and on the epicardial surface of the diaphragmatic right ventricle. (C) All sutures are placed and then the patch (DeBakey elastic Dacron fabric) is slid into place on the left ventricular side of the septum. The patch sutures are tied down with an additional felt pledget placed on top of the patch (left ventricular side), as each suture is tied, to cushion the tie and prevent cutting through the friable muscle. These maneuvers are viewed by the authors as essential to the success of early repair of the posterior septal rupture. (D) Remaining to be repaired is the posterior left ventricular free wall defect created by infarctectomy. Mattress sutures of 2-0 Tevdek are placed circumferentially around the margins of the posterior left ventricular free wall defect. Each suture is buttressed with a Teflon felt pledget on the endocardial side of the left ventricle. With all sutures in place, a circular patch, fashioned from a Hemashield woven double velour Dacron collagen impregnated graft (Meadox Medicals Inc., Oakland, NJ), is slid down onto the epicardial surface of the left ventricle. An additional pledget of Teflon felt is placed under each suture (on top of the patch) as it is tied to cushion the tie and prevent cutting through the friable underlying muscle. This onlay technique of patch placement prevents the cracking of friable left ventricular muscle that occurred with the eversion technique of patch insertion. (E) Completed repair. *(Adapted with permission from Daggett WM: Surgical technique for early repair of posterior ventricular septal rupture. J Thorac Cardiovasc Surg 1982; 84:306.)*

defect and ventriculotomy. Others have modified the exclusion technique by use of tissue sealants to aid in the septal closure.[97]

PERCUTANEOUS CLOSURE

Successful transcatheter closure of postinfarction ventricular septal rupture has been reported using several types of catheter-deployed devices. The largest experience is with the CardioSEAL device, a nitinol, double umbrella prosthesis.[98] The device consists of two attached and opposing umbrellas formed by hinged steel arms covered in a Dacron meshwork that, theoretically, promotes endothelization. The arms are manually everted to allow the device to be passed through a narrow percutaneous deployment system. When extruded from the guiding catheter, the arms spring backward, resembling a "clamshell." The device approaches the septum via the systemic veins and through the atrial septum (or alternatively via the arterial system through the aortic valve). As reported by Landzberg and Lock,[98] the experience at Boston Children's Hospital and Brigham and Women's Hospital indicates that, while the device can be routinely deployed in the setting of an acute infarction, the continued necrosis of septal tissue led to decompensation and death in

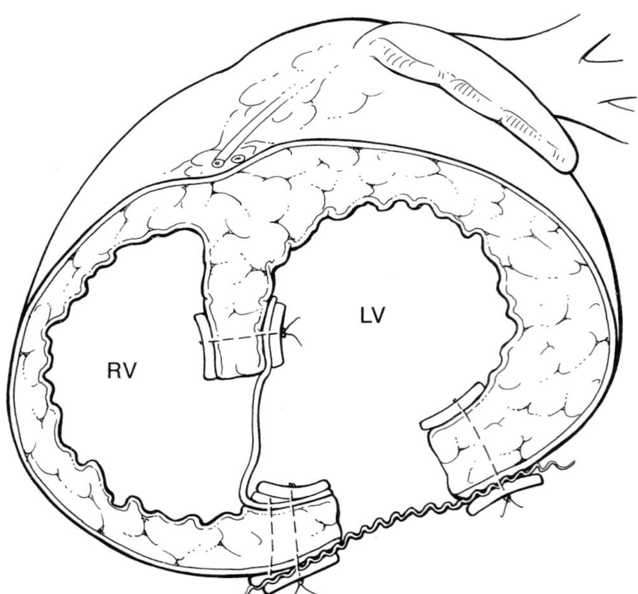

FIGURE 26–8 Cross-sectional view of the completed repair of posterior septal rupture with prosthetic patch placement of the posterior left ventricular free wall defect created by infarctectomy. RV, right ventricular cavity; LV, left ventricular cavity. *(Adapted with permission from Daggett WM: Surgical technique for early repair of posterior septal rupture. J Thorac Cardiovasc Surg 1982; 84:306.)*

4 of 7 patients. In contrast, they reported success in 6 of 6 patients treated for residual or recurrent septal defects discovered after primary operative repair. Other catheter devices have also been attempted, which variable success, including the Amplatzer septal occluder and the Rashkind double umbrella.[99]

The best use of such devices in an overall treatment strategy is unclear. As a primary treatment, data suggest the devices have a high early failure rate, but their potential role in improving the risk of an unstable surgical patient is not yet well characterized. Currently, catheter approaches appear to be most effective in treatment of recurrent or residual defects, and we preferentially employ them for these conditions. Device development is an ongoing process, and the future undoubtedly will see use of new devices, especially in the high-risk patient with multisystem failure.

Of interest, two centers have reported using a standard Swan-Ganz balloon catheter from the groin to abolish the shunt in unstable patients with postinfarction septal rupture.[100,101] Hemodynamic improvement was immediate in both patients, who underwent subsequent surgical repair of the defect.

Role of Ventricular Assist Devices

In patients who present for operation with evidence of potentially reversible multiorgan dysfunction, or in patients who have intractable failure following repair, there may be a role for temporary mechanical heart support. There have been anecdotal cases of unstable patients being successfully managed by mechanical support followed by definitive operation.[102]

The theoretical advantages that make mechanical support attractive as an initial therapy in very sick patients with postinfarction VSD include: (1) the potential to reverse end-organ dysfunction; (2) maturation of the infarct leading to firmer tissue, making the closure less prone to technical failure; and (3) recovery of the stunned and energy-depleted myocardium. In our limited experience, this strategy has shown promise, and we are evaluating its broader application based on careful preoperative risk assessment. However, there are potential hazards with mechanical support that are specific to the patient with postinfarction VSD. High right-to-left shunting across the ventricular septum has been reported to cause hypoxic brain injury in a postinfarction VSD patient placed on a HeartMate LVAD.[103] This anecdotal observation suggests that either partial left heart support or preferably biventricular support should be considered when using mechanical assistance in these patients. In a report using the Hemopump axial flow device, 2 of 2 patients supported experienced lethal pump failure. Examination of the device at autopsy disclosed necrotic material clogging the catheter system.[104]

Simultaneous Myocardial Revascularization

There has been controversy in the literature concerning the advantages and disadvantages of concurrent coronary artery grafting in patients undergoing emergent repair of postinfarction ventricular septal rupture.[25,30,64,73,105] Some have argued that revascularization provides no survival benefit and subjects patients to preoperative left heart catheterization, a time-consuming and potentially dangerous diagnostic procedure.[63,64] Loisance et al[105] base their policy of not revascularizing patients with postinfarction septal ruptures on the fact that none of their 20 long-term survivors (5 of whom were bypassed) had incapacitating angina or recurrent myocardial infarction. Piwnica et al[106] reported a series of 28 survivors of early operative closure of postinfarction ventricular septal rupture, among whom only one had coronary artery grafting. Among the 24 patients for whom follow-up was complete, there were only 2 late deaths of cardiac origin. However, it is not clear from their report what the impact of associated coronary artery disease (revascularized or not) may have been on the course of the other 32 patients who did not survive operation.

Some groups use left heart catheterization and coronary bypassing selectively.[22,30] Davies et al[30] found that of 60 long-term survivors (median 70 months; range 1 to 174 months), only five patients developed exertional angina during follow-up and none required revascularization. Their

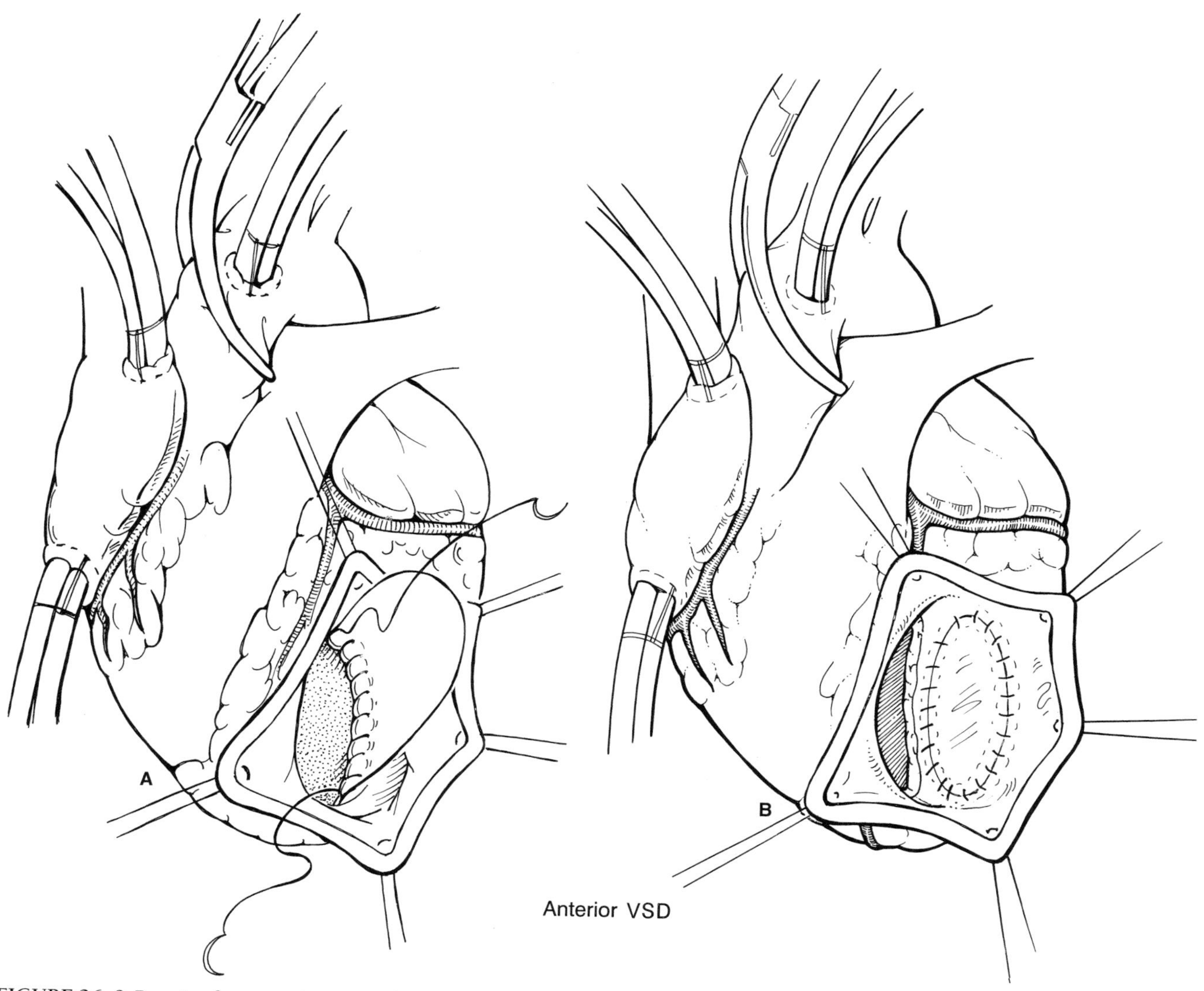

FIGURE 26–9 Repair of an anterior postinfarction ventricular septal rupture using the technique of infarct exclusion. (A) The standard ventriculotomy is made in the infarcted area of left ventricular free wall. An interior patch of Dacron (Meadox Medicals Inc., Oakland, NJ), polytetrafluoroethylene, or glutaraldehyde-fixed pericardium is fashioned to replace and/or cover the diseased areas (septal defect, septal infarction, or free wall infarction). (B) The internal patch is secured to normal endocardium with a continuous monofilament suture, which may be reinforced with pledgeted mattress sutures. There is little, if any, resection of myocardium and no attempt is made to close the septal defect.

current policy is to avoid left heart catheterization on patients in whom an acquired septal defect is suspected to be a consequence of their first anterior infarction, provided that the patient has no history of angina or electrocardiographic evidence of previous infarction in another territory.[30] This approach is also based on the findings that multivessel disease is much less prevalent in those with an apical septal rupture as a result of anterior infarction.[22]

We and others[35,45,74,93,107] have tended to employ coronary revascularization with increasing frequency. Our policy is to place aortocoronary grafts to principal epicardial coronary arteries that have severe proximal stenoses. In order to investigate the early and late effects of coronary artery revascularization, we previously reviewed our experience in patients undergoing repair of postinfarction septal rupture,[73] and concluded that revascularization was of early and long-term benefit. In a more recent review, the effect of bypass was less dramatic, not achieving statistical significance (manuscript in preparation). Nevertheless, there is no information that would suggest any negative impact of bypass grafting, and we continue to perform bypasses routinely when the clinical presentation permits catheterization.

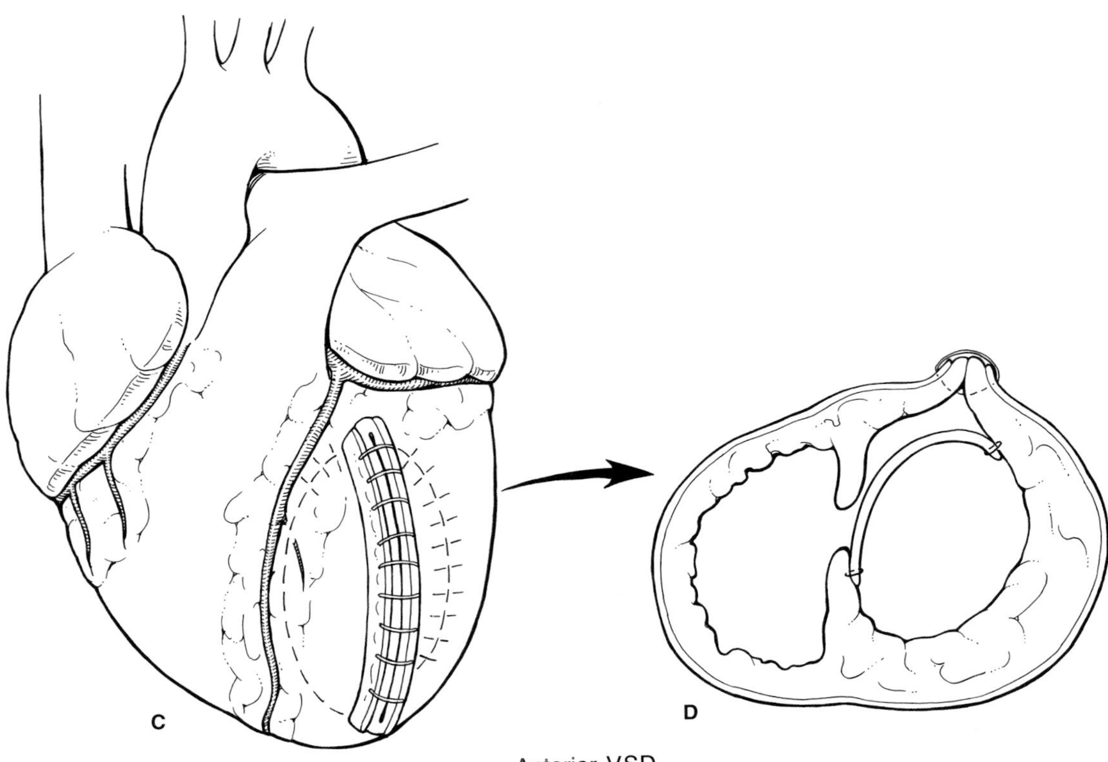

FIGURE 26–9 (Continued) Repair of an anterior postinfarction ventricular septal rupture using the technique of infarct exclusion. (C) The ventriculotomy, which is outside the pressure zone of the left ventricle, may be repaired with a continuous suture. (D) On transverse section, one can see that the endocardial patch is secured at three levels, above and below the septal rupture and beyond the ventriculotomy. *(Adapted with permission from David TE, Dale L, Sun Z: Postinfarction ventricular septal rupture: repair by endocardial patch with infarct exclusion. J Thorac Cardiovasc Surg 1995; 110:1315.)*

Weaning from Cardiopulmonary Bypass

Intraoperative transesophageal echocardiography is essential to assess ventricular function, ventricular dimensions, residual shunt, and mitral regurgitation when weaning from bypass. The two most common problems encountered in separating from bypass following repair of a postinfarction ventricular septal defect are low cardiac output and bleeding. Although the treatment of low cardiac output following cardiac surgery is beyond the scope of this chapter, a few agents and principles are worth mentioning. First, most of these patients will have had an intra-aortic balloon pump (IABP) inserted before surgery. If not, one should be inserted in the operating room, especially if the low output state is secondary to left ventricular dysfunction. Also, IABP may benefit patients with right ventricular failure by improving right coronary artery blood flow due to diastolic augmentation. We have found intravenous milrinone, a phosphodiesterase inhibitor, to be very effective in reversing low output states secondary to left ventricular dysfunction. Milrinone possesses a balance of inotropic and vasodilatory properties that together produce an increase in cardiac output and reduction in right and left filling pressures and systemic vascular resistance. It is less arrhythmogenic than dobutamine, causes less hypotension than amrinone, and is not associated with thrombocytopenia.[108]

Posterior defects are commonly associated with mitral regurgitation and right heart dysfunction secondary to extensive right ventricular infarction.[37] Management of right heart failure is aimed at reducing right ventricular afterload while maintaining systemic pressure.[100] Initial steps to manage right ventricular dysfunction include volume loading, inotropic support, and correction of acidosis, hypoxemia, and hypercarbia. If patients remain unresponsive to these measures, we have successfully treated right ventricular failure with a prostaglandin E_1 infusion (0.5-2.0 μg/min) into the right heart, counterbalanced with a norepinephrine infusion titrated into the left atrium.[109] Inhaled nitric oxide (20-80 ppm), which selectively dilates the pulmonary circuit, has also proven efficacious in the treatment of right heart failure.[110]

In our experience, inability to separate from bypass has been uncommon if the repair has been successful. However,

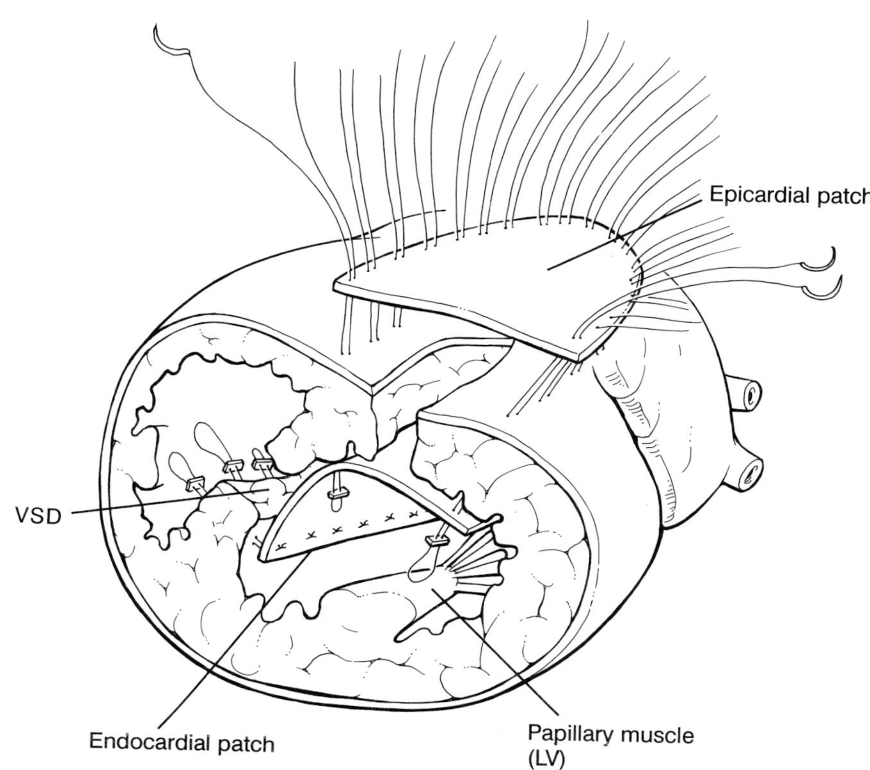

FIGURE 26–10 Repair of an anterior postinfarction ventricular septal rupture using the technique of infarct exclusion with external patching of the ventricular free wall with tailored Teflon or pericardium. *(Adapted with permission from Cooley DA: Repair of postinfarction ventricular septal defect. J Card Surg 1994; 9:427.)*

if a patient cannot be weaned from bypass using conventional therapy and is less than 70 years old with no residual hemodynamically significant lesion, we consider using a ventricular assist device. Indications for a left ventricular assist device are a cardiac index less than 1.8 L/min per m^2, a left atrial pressure above 18 to 25 mm Hg, a right atrial pressure below 15 mm Hg, and an aortic pressure below 90 mm Hg peak systolic. Indications for a right ventricular assist device are a cardiac index less than 1.8 L/min per m^2, an aortic pressure below 90 mm Hg peak systolic, and a left atrial pressure less than 15 mm Hg despite volume loading to a right atrial pressure of 25 mm Hg with a competent tricuspid valve. Important points to remember when instituting ventricular assistance are:

1. Right ventricular failure may not become evident until left ventricular assistance is instituted.
2. Once refractory ventricular failure has been identified, delay in initiating support is associated with increased morbidity and mortality.
3. Closure of a patent foramen ovale is mandatory prior to left ventricular support.
4. Postoperative hemorrhage should be treated aggressively and completely controlled.
5. Residual septal defects may result in right-to-left shunting and severe hypoxia when only left heart support is used.[111]

To prevent postpump coagulopathy, we begin antifibrinolytic therapy with either aprotinin or ε-aminocaproic acid (Amicar) before commencing cardiopulmonary bypass. Half-dose aprotinin is administered by first giving an intravenous test dose of 10,000 KIU over 10 minutes (before administering blockers), and then loading patients with 1 million KIU over 20 minutes prior to bypass. Another 1 million KIU is given in the pump prime, and then 250,000 KIU/hr is administered for the duration of the surgery. Heparin is managed in the usual fashion with activated clotting times (ACT), but kaolin, not Celite, is used as the ACT activator. Since controversy surrounds the issue of increased renal dysfunction and perioperative thrombotic events in patients receiving aprotinin,[112] we prefer to use Amicar in patients who (1) require aortocoronary bypasses, (2) are diabetic, or (3) have known renal dysfunction. Amicar is administered by loading patients with 10 g prior to commencing bypass and then adding another 10 g to the pump prime. During the procedure Amicar is continuously infused at 1 g/h for the duration of surgery. We avoid giving over 30 g of Amicar. Postpump suture line bleeding may be reduced by application of a fibrin sealant to the ventricular septum around the septal defect *prior* to formal repair.[113] Biological glue may be effective in controlling bleeding suture lines following repair.[114] As a last resort, Baldwin and Cooley[115] have suggested insertion of a left ventricular assist device solely as an adjunct to the repair of friable or damaged myocardium to reduce left ventricular distension and thus control bleeding.

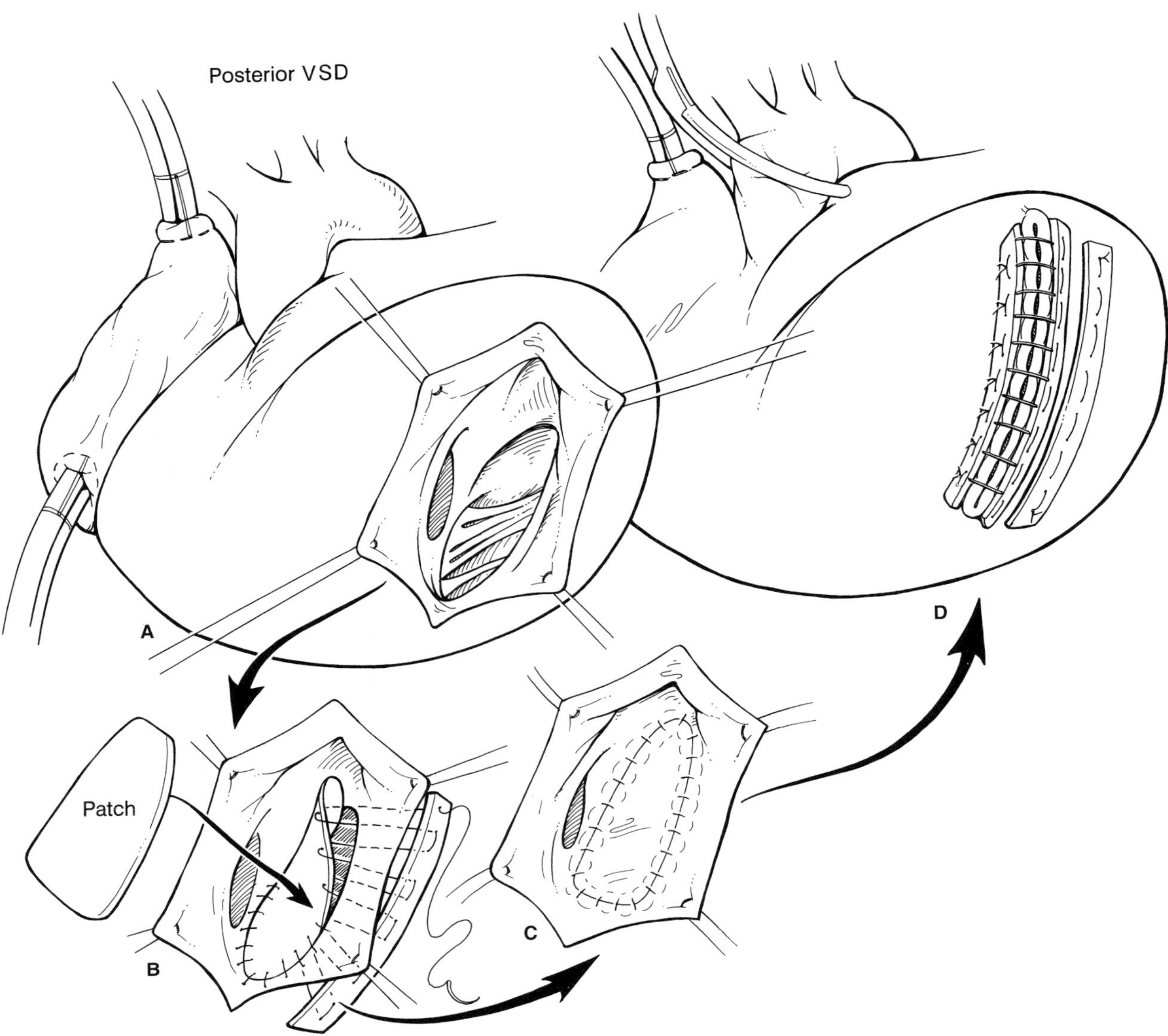

FIGURE 26–11 Endocardial repair of a posterior postinfarction ventricular septal rupture using the technique of infarct exclusion. (A) An incision is made in the inferior wall of the left ventricle 1 or 2 mm from the posterior descending artery starting at the midportion of the inferior wall and extended proximally toward the mitral annulus and distally toward the apex of the ventricle. Care is taken to avoid damage to the posterolateral papillary muscle. (B) A bovine pericardial patch is tailored in a triangular shape. The base of the triangular-shaped patch is sutured to the fibrous annulus of the mitral valve with a continuous 3-0 polypropylene suture starting at a point corresponding to the level of the posteromedial papillary muscle and moving medially toward the septum until the noninfarcted endocardium is reached. (C) The medial margin of the triangular-shaped patch is sewn to healthy septal endocardium with a continuous 3-0 or 4-0 polypropylene suture. The lateral side of the patch is sutured to the posterior wall of the left ventricle along a line corresponding to the medial margin of the base of the posteromedial papillary muscle. At this point, it is usually necessary to use full-thickness bites and anchor the sutures on a strip of pericardium or Teflon felt applied on the epicardial surface of the posterior wall of the left ventricle. (D) Once the patch is completely sutured to the mitral valve annulus, the endocardium of the interventricular septum, and the full thickness of the posterior wall, the ventriculotomy is closed in two layers of full thickness sutures buttressed on strips of pericardium or Teflon felt. The infarcted right ventricular wall is left undisturbed. *(Adapted with permission from David TE, Dale L, Sun Z: Postinfarction ventricular septal rupture: repair by endocardial patch with infarct exclusion. J Thorac Cardiovasc Surg 1995; 110:1315.)*

TABLE 26–2 Summary of recent clinical experience with surgical repair of postinfarction VSD

Institution	City	Year	N	Hospital mortality	5-y survival	Reference
Massachusetts General Hospital	Boston	2002	114	37%	45%	184
Papworth Hospital	Cambridge	2002	25	48%	–	185
University Hospital	Zurich	2000	54	26%	52%*	186
Sakurabashi Watanabe Hospital	Osaka	2000	16	38%	–	187
Glenfield General Hospital	Leicester	2000	117	37% (30 day)	46%	188
Evangelismos General Hospital	Athens	1999	14	50%	–	189
Texas Heart Institute	Houston	1998	126	46%	–	124
The Toronto Hospital	Toronto	1998	52	19%	65%*	190
Southhampton General	Southampton	1998	179	27%	49%	121
Cedars-Sinai	Los Angeles	1998	31	32%	–	191
Mid America Heart Institute	Kansas City	1997	76	41%	41%	192
St. Anthonius Hospital	Nieuwegein	1996	109	28% (30 day)	–	193
Green Lane Hospital	Auckland	1995	35	31% (30 day)	60%*	194
Hospital Cardiologique du Haut-Lévèque	Bordeaux	1991	62	38%	44%	35
CHU Henri Mondor	Créteil	1991	66	45%	44%	195

*Value estimated from published graphical or tabular data.
Note: Series with less than 10 patients were excluded from the table.

Highlights of Postoperative Care

Early postoperative diuresis and positive end-expiratory pressure ventilation are used to decrease the arterial-alveolar gradient induced by the increased extravascular pulmonary water associated with cardiopulmonary bypass. Once the patient has warmed, we commonly use an intravenous infusion of Lasix combined with mannitol (1 g of Lasix in 400 cc of 20% mannitol) at a rate of 1 to 20 cc per hour to keep the urine output greater than 100 cc per hour. If renal function has been compromised preoperatively, continuous venovenous hemofiltration (CVVH) is employed postoperatively.

Intractable postoperative ventricular arrhythmias secondary to reperfusion injury are sometimes difficult to control using standard therapy. We have been impressed with the efficacy of intravenous amiodarone in these situations (10-20 mg/kg over 24 hours).[116]

Operative Mortality and Risk Factors for Death

Table 26-2 summarizes recently reported experience from several centers. Operative mortality, defined as death prior to discharge *or* within 30 days of operation, ranged from 30% to 50%. In the MGH experience of 114 patients, operative mortality was 37% (Fig. 26-12A). The risk for death was found to be very high initially, but dropped rapidly (Fig. 26-12B). We identified independent risk factors for early and late death using multivariate methods (Table 26-3). The most important predictor of operative mortality in our study, and in other reports, was preoperative *hemodynamic instability*. Patients in this group are usually in cardiogenic shock, are emergency cases, are on inotropic support, and usually have intra-aortic balloon pumps. Several variables are highly correlated with hemodynamic instability, and different multivariate models may use one or more of these indicators of severe hemodynamic failure in their final model. As previously discussed, the degree to which the patient's hemodynamics suffer depends both on the magnitude of the shunt and the size of the infarction.[35,45,74,117–119]

Additional risk factors for early and late death include the presence of *left main coronary artery disease, previous myocardial infarction, renal dysfunction,* and *right heart failure* (Fig. 26-13). Other factors have been found to increase the risk of early death. *Posterior location* of the septal rupture has been associated with an increased operative mortality.[35,37,47,49] This has been attributed to a more technically difficult repair,[19,120] to the increased risk of associated mitral regurgitation, and to associated right ventricular dysfunction that is an independent predictor of early mortality following posterior infarction.[48,121] *A short time interval between infarction and operation* selects for sicker patients unable to be managed medically. Patient *age* has also been associated with an increased early mortality.[21,78,119,122] In our analysis, we found that the impact of age was more pronounced in the "high-risk" patient, and should not be used as a reason for denying surgery in an otherwise low-risk elderly candidate (Fig. 26-14).

Interestingly, a retrospective analysis of 109 patients in which the location of the septal defect was divided into four separate sites—proximal, posterior, distal, and anterior—revealed that proximal location of the septal defect (not posterior) was the main predictor for cardiogenic shock, which in turn was the strongest determinant of early mortality (34.3% vs. 16.7% for distal septal defects).[119] Presumably, this relationship results from the fact that proximal septal defects are associated with larger infarctions.

Our review of the MGH experience underscored the large variability of risk to which patients could be segregated using a few clinical variables (Figs. 26-15 and 26-16), most notably indicators of hemodynamic instability (emergency

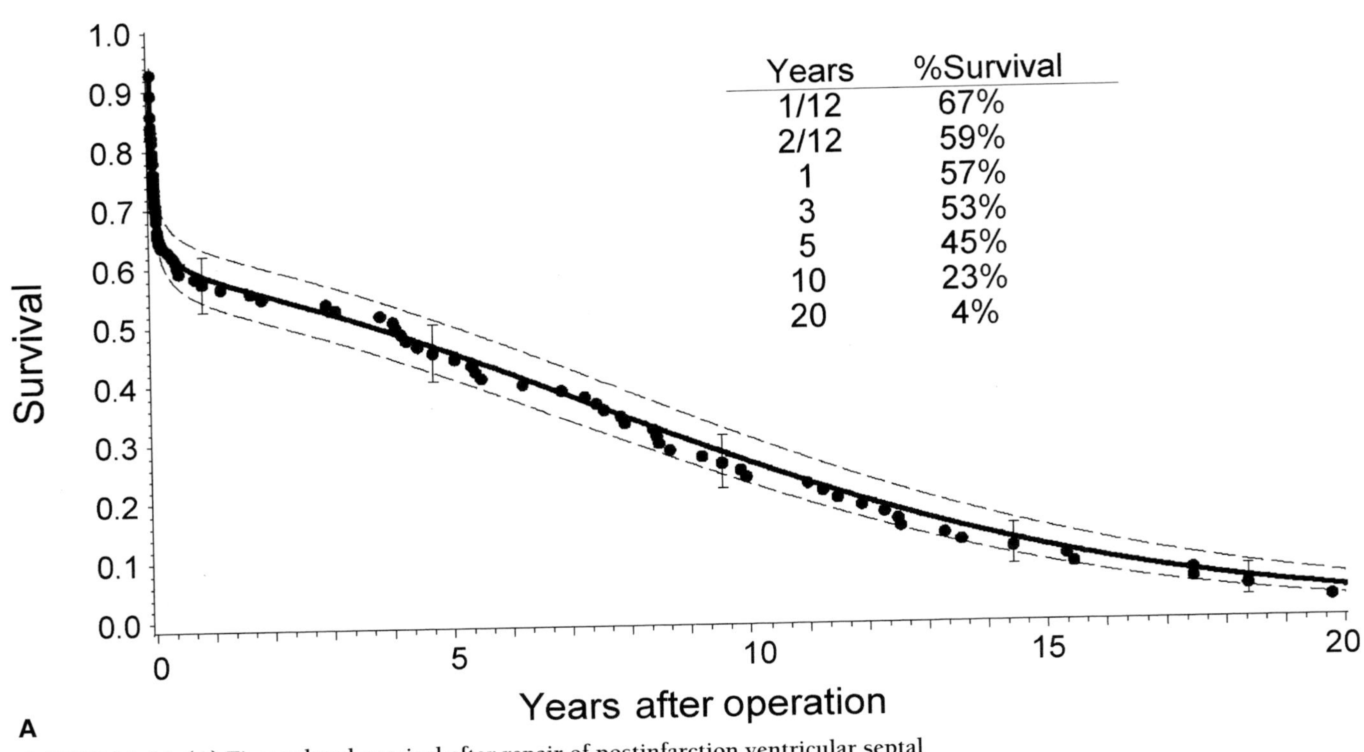

FIGURE 26–12 (A) Time-related survival after repair of postinfarction ventricular septal defect at the Massachusetts General Hospital (MGH, n = 114). Note that the horizontal axis extends to 20 years. Circles represent each death, positioned on the horizontal axis at the interval from operation to death, and actuarially (Kaplan-Meier method) along the vertical axis. The vertical bars represent 70% confidence limits (± 1 SD). The solid line represents the parametrically estimated freedom from death, and the dashed lines enclose the 70% confidence limits of that estimate. The table shows the nonparametric estimates at specified intervals.

surgery and use of inotropics). The result was that a small group of high-risk patients dramatically affected the overall mortality rate. We believe that this phenomenon makes it very difficult to compare mortality between institutions. A slight difference in practice patterns, such as a tendency of a surgeon or referring cardiologist to deny operation, could substantially affect results. Additionally, any difference in transport dynamics to certain centers could lead to loss of unstable patients, which could create another type of selection bias. In our opinion, these issues are by far the most important source of mortality differences in modern series.

One clinical experience stands out as having a particularly low mortality. Using the infarct exclusion technique, David's group in Toronto reported an overall operative mortality of 19%. David et al attribute their low operative mortality, especially for posterior ruptures, to the fact that infarct exclusion results in less ventricular dysfunction than repairs that require infarctectomy.[45]

There is limited information from other centers on results using the exclusion technique. Ross commented that he was enjoying improved results with the method, although instead of using a running suture he used interrupted buttressed mattress sutures, and added an epicardial patch.[123] Cooley and others have also modified the method due to difficulty with the continuous suture line, and noted improved results with a decrease in mortality to 36.4% from a historical level of 46%.[124] Our group has not been able to replicate the excellent Toronto results, with a disappointing 60% mortality in 10 patients who underwent the "exclusion" type repair (higher than the rate achieved historically with traditional techniques).

Regardless of the technique, the most common cause of death following repair of acute postinfarction ventricular septal defect was low cardiac output syndrome (52%). Technical failures, most commonly recurrent or residual VSD but including bleeding, were the second most common (23%). Other causes of death include sepsis (17%), recurrent infarction (9%), cerebrovascular complications (4%), and intractable ventricular arrhythmias.

Long-Term Results

Long-term results have been favorable as regards both mortality risk and functional rehabilitation. Actuarial survival at 5 years for most recent series generally ranges between 40%

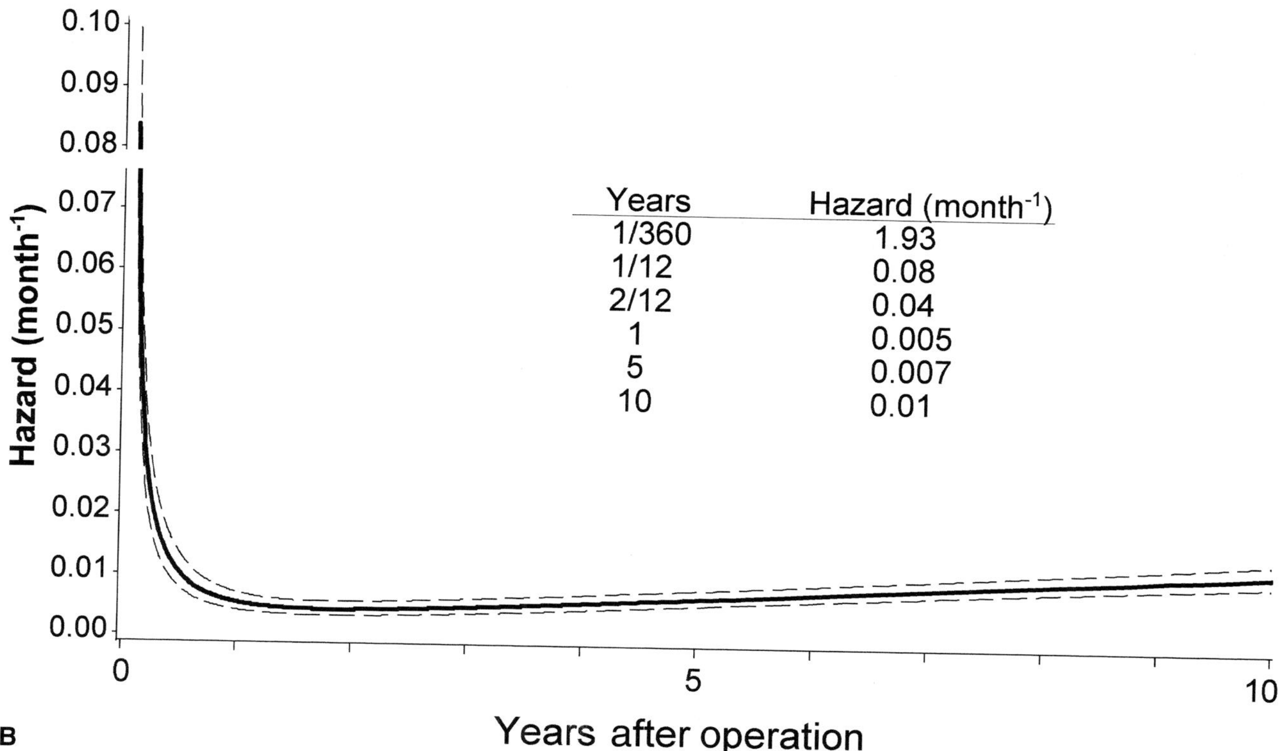

FIGURE 26–12 (continued) (B) Hazard function for death after repair of postinfarction ventricular septal defect (MGH; n = 114). The horizontal axis is expanded for better visualization of early risk. The hazard function has two phases, consisting of an early, rapidly declining phase, which gives way to a slowly rising phase at about 6 months. The estimate is shown with 70% confidence limits.

and 60% (see Table 26-2). Due to the overall high risk of the operation, it is rewarding to note that hospital survivors enjoy excellent longevity, with 1-, 5-, and 10-year survival of 91%, 70%, and 37%. They also are quite functional—among 15 of our patients contacted during the most recent follow-up of long-term survivors, 75% were in NYHA functional class I, and 12.5% were class II.[31]

TABLE 26–3 Incremental risk factors for death following repair of postinfarction VSD*

Risk factor	Hazard phase	
	Early	Late
Demographic		
Age (older)	•	•
Clinical History		
Previous MI		•
Clinical Status		
BUN (higher)	•	
Creatinine (higher)		•
"Emergency"	•	
Right atrial P (higher)	•	•
Catecholamines	•	
Coronary/VSD Anatomy		
Left main Dz		•

*MGH experience; N = 114; 95 events.

Gaudiani et al[74] reported similar long-term results using an early operative approach. In their series, 88% of hospital survivors were alive at 5 years, with 74% of survivors in NYHA functional class I and 21% of survivors in class II. In the series of patients reported by Piwnica et al,[105] there were 20 long-term survivors, of whom 8 were in class I and 12 were in class II. David et al[45] have reported a 66% 6-year survival rate in patients operated on since 1980. Finally, Davies et al[30] reported 5-, 10-, and 14-year survivals of 69%, 50%, and 37%. Eighty-two percent of patients were in NYHA functional class I or II.

Recurrent Ventricular Septal Defects

Recurrent or residual septal defects have been diagnosed by Doppler color flow mapping early or late postoperatively in 10% to 25% of patients.[22] They may be due to reopening of a closed defect, to the presence of an overlooked defect, or to the development of a new septal rupture during the early postoperative period. These recurrent defects should be closed when they cause symptoms or signs of heart failure or when the calculated shunt fraction is large

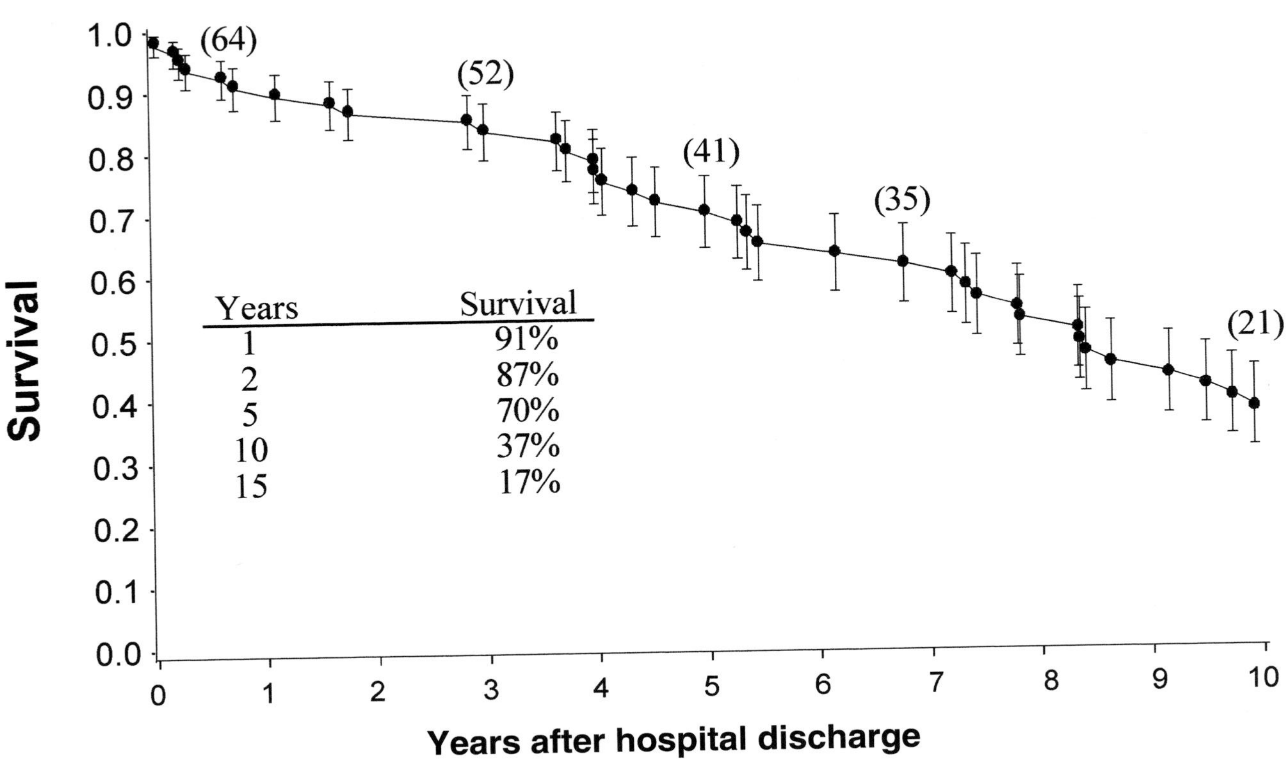

FIGURE 26–13 Survival in patients who were discharged after repair of postinfarction ventricular septal defect (MGH, n = 72). The horizontal axis is expanded and represents the time from hospital discharge to death. The depiction is otherwise similar to Figure 26-12A.

(Qp: Qs > 2.0). When they are small (Qp:Qs < 2.0) and either asymptomatic or controlled with minimal diuretic therapy, a conservative approach is reasonable and late spontaneous closure can occur.[22] Intervention in the catheterization laboratory may be useful in closing symptomatic residual or recurrent defects postoperatively.

Chronic Ventricular Septal Defects

In 1987 Rousou et al reported successful closure of an acquired posterior ventricular septal defect by means of a right transatrial approach.[125] Filgueira et al have used the transatrial approach for *delayed* repair of chronic acquired posterior septal defects.[126] Approaching a postinfarction ventricular septal defect through the tricuspid valve should not be used in acute cases because of the friability of the necrotic septum, poor exposure, and because this technique does not involve infarctectomy, and thus cannot achieve the hemodynamic advantages of elimination of a paradoxically bulging segment of ventricular wall. However, the right heart approach can be used in chronic postinfarction ventricular septal defects when the septum is well scarred and the patch can be safely sutured to it from the right atrium. We emphasize that while the transatrial approach may be used selectively for the closure of chronic defects, it is unlikely to be an appropriate choice for the closure of acute defects, except perhaps in the rare circumstance when an infarct is localized to the septum with no evidence of necrosis of the free wall of the left ventricle.[39]

POSTINFARCTION VENTRICULAR FREE WALL RUPTURE

History

William Harvey first described rupture of the free wall of the heart after acute myocardial infarction in 1647.[127] In 1765, Morgagni reported 11 cases of myocardial rupture found at postmortem.[128] Ironically, Morgagni later died of myocardial rupture.[129] Hatcher and colleagues from Emory University reported the first successful operation for free wall rupture of the right ventricle in 1970.[130] FitzGibbon et al[131] in 1971 and Montegut[132] in 1972 reported the first successful repairs of a left ventricular rupture associated with ischemic heart disease.

Incidence

Autopsy studies reveal that ventricular free wall rupture occurs about 10 times more frequently than postinfarction ventricular septal rupture, occurring in about 11% of patients

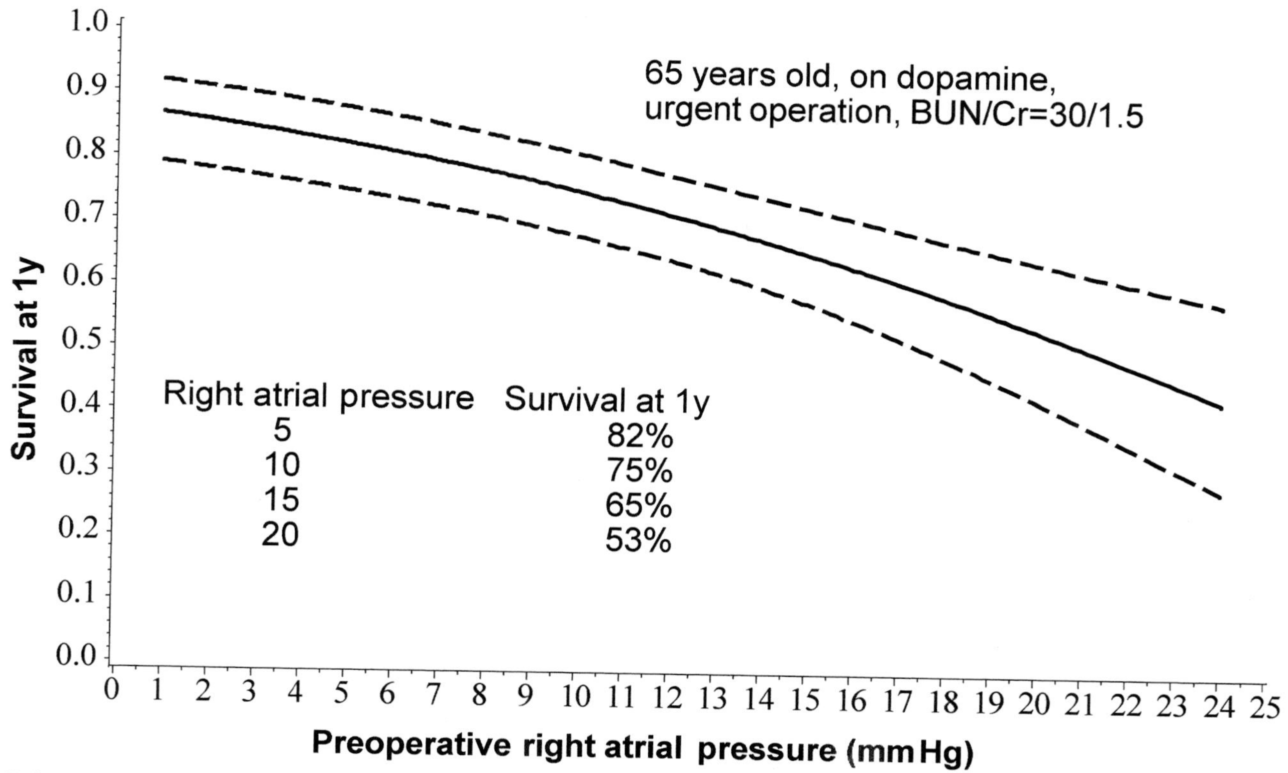

FIGURE 26–14 Survival at 1 year vs. preoperative right atrial pressure (MGH; n = 114). The depiction is a solution of the multivariate equation for a 65-year-old with a BUN of 30, a creatinine of 1.5, not on catecholamines, not an "emergency" case, and without a history of myocardial infarction or left main coronary artery disease.

following acute myocardial infarction.[23,133] The incidence has been found to be as high as 31% in autopsy studies of anterior myocardial infarction.[134] Ventricular rupture and cardiogenic shock are now the leading causes of death following acute myocardial infarction, and together account for over two thirds of early deaths in patients suffering their first acute infarction.[135] Postinfarction ventricular ruptures are more common in elderly women (mean age of 63 years) suffering their first infarction.[136,137] In the prethrombolytic era, 90% of ruptures occurred within 2 weeks after infarction with the peak incidence at 5 days.[138] In contrast, the time to cardiac rupture (not frequency of rupture) seems to be accelerated by thrombolysis and coronary reperfusion, sometimes occurring within hours from the onset of symptoms.[139] Thus, free ventricular ruptures occur most frequently in hypertensive women over the age of 60 who develop symptoms within 5 days of their first transmural myocardial infarction.

Opinions differ as to the most common site of left ventricular rupture. The older literature suggests that the anterior wall is the most frequent site.[140] However, more recent series have observed a preponderance of lateral and posterior wall ruptures.[27,133,138] David[141] has suggested that a lateral wall infarction is more likely to rupture than is an anterior or inferior one, but since anterior infarctions are much more frequent than lateral infarctions, overall the commonest site of rupture is the anterior wall. Like postinfarction ventricular septal rupture, free wall ruptures may be simple or complex.[41] A simple rupture results from a straight through-and-through tear which is perpendicular to the endothelial and epicardial surfaces, whereas a complex rupture results from a more serpiginous tear, often oblique to the endocardial and epicardial surfaces.[141] Batts et al[138] reported 100 consecutive cases of left ventricular free wall rupture and found that half were simple ruptures and the rest were complex.

Pathogenesis and Pathophysiology

Left ventricle free wall rupture can be divided into three clinicopathological categories: acute, subacute, and chronic.[142,143] An *acute* or "blow-out" rupture is characterized by sudden recurrent chest pain, electrical mechanical dissociation, profound shock, and death within a few minutes due to massive hemorrhage into the pericardial cavity. This type of rupture is probably not amenable to current management. A *subacute* rupture is characterized by a smaller tear, which may be temporarily sealed by clot or fibrinous pericardial adhesions. These usually present with the signs and symptoms of cardiac tamponade and, eventually,

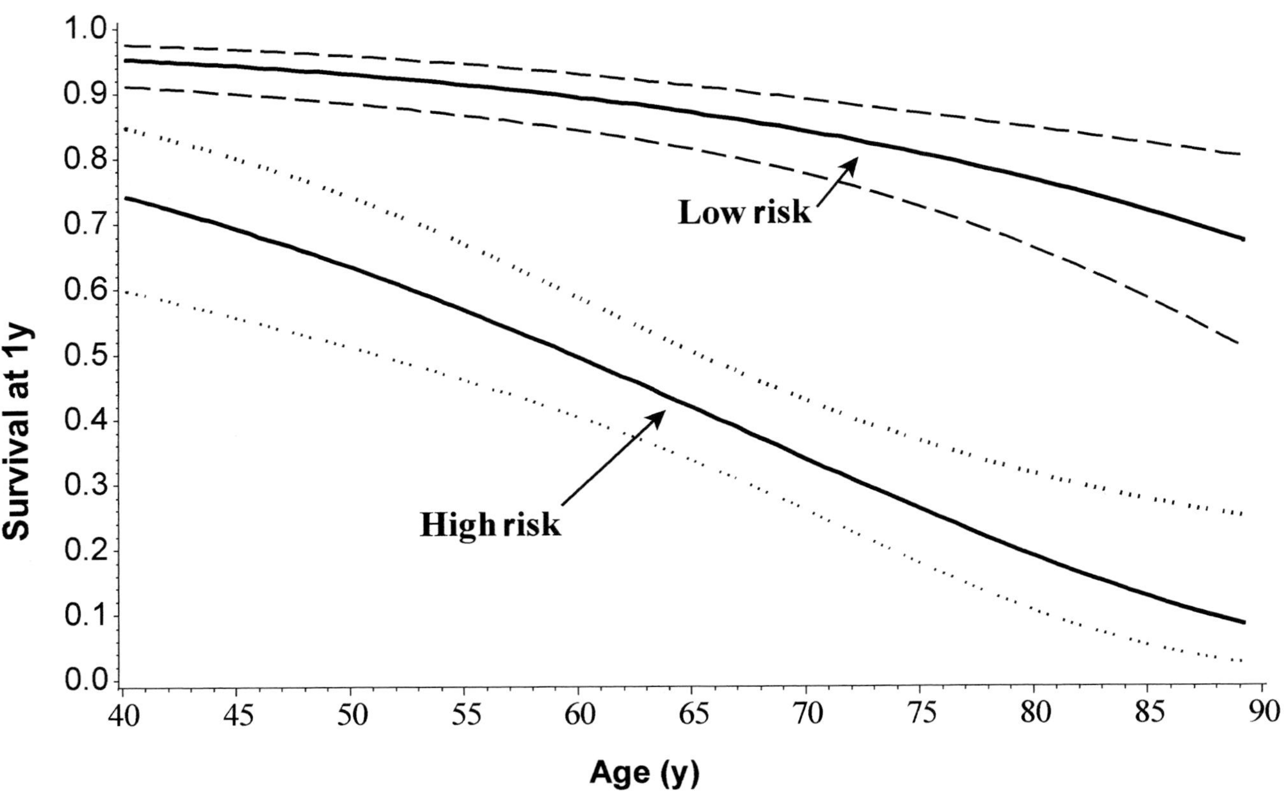

FIGURE 26–15 Nomograms (specific solutions to the multivariate equation) depicting the effect of age on risk in two different hypothetical patients. In both curves the patient was considered to have no left main disease, a BUN of 30, Cr of 1.5, and no history of previous myocardial infarction. The curve for "low-risk" was solved for a patient who was not emergent and not on catecholamines. The curve for "high-risk" was for an emergent patient on inotropes. The vertical axis represents the calculated survival at 1 year.

cardiogenic shock. Subacute rupture may mimic other complications of acute myocardial infarction such as infarct extension and right ventricular failure, and may be compatible with life for several hours or days or even longer.[141] A *chronic* rupture with *false aneurysm* formation occurs when the leakage of blood is slow and when surrounding pressure on the epicardium temporarily controls the hemorrhage. Adhesions form between the epicardium and pericardium, which reinforce and contain the rupture.[29] The most common clinical presentation of patients with false aneurysms of the left ventricle is congestive heart failure.[144] A false aneurysm may also be an echocardiographic finding in an otherwise asymptomatic patient recovering from acute myocardial infarction. Angina, syncope, arrhythmias, and thromboembolic complications occur in a small percentage of patients.[144] There are four major differences between a true and false aneurysm of the left ventricle:

1. The wall of a false aneurysm contains no myocardial cells.
2. False aneurysms are more likely to form posteriorly.
3. False aneurysms usually have a narrow neck.
4. False aneurysms have a great propensity for rupture.[145–147]

Rupture of the free wall of the left ventricle may occur in isolation or with rupture of other ventricular structures such as the interventricular septum, papillary muscles, or right ventricle.[144,147]

The pathogenesis of cardiac rupture remains poorly understood. However, cardiac rupture occurs only with transmural myocardial infarctions and infarction expansion appears to play an important role in its pathogenesis.[38,42,148] Infarct expansion is an acute regional thinning and dilatation of the infarct zone, seen as early as 24 hours following acute transmural myocardial infarction and not related to additional myocardial necrosis.[149] This regional thinning and dilatation of the infarct zone is a consequence of slippage between muscle bundles, resulting in a reduction in the number of myocytes across the infarcted area.[150] Infarct expansion increases the size of the ventricular cavity, with a consequent increase in wall tension (Laplace effect) that subjects the infarct zone to more tension and predisposes to endocardial tearing.[141] Systemic hypertension aggravates

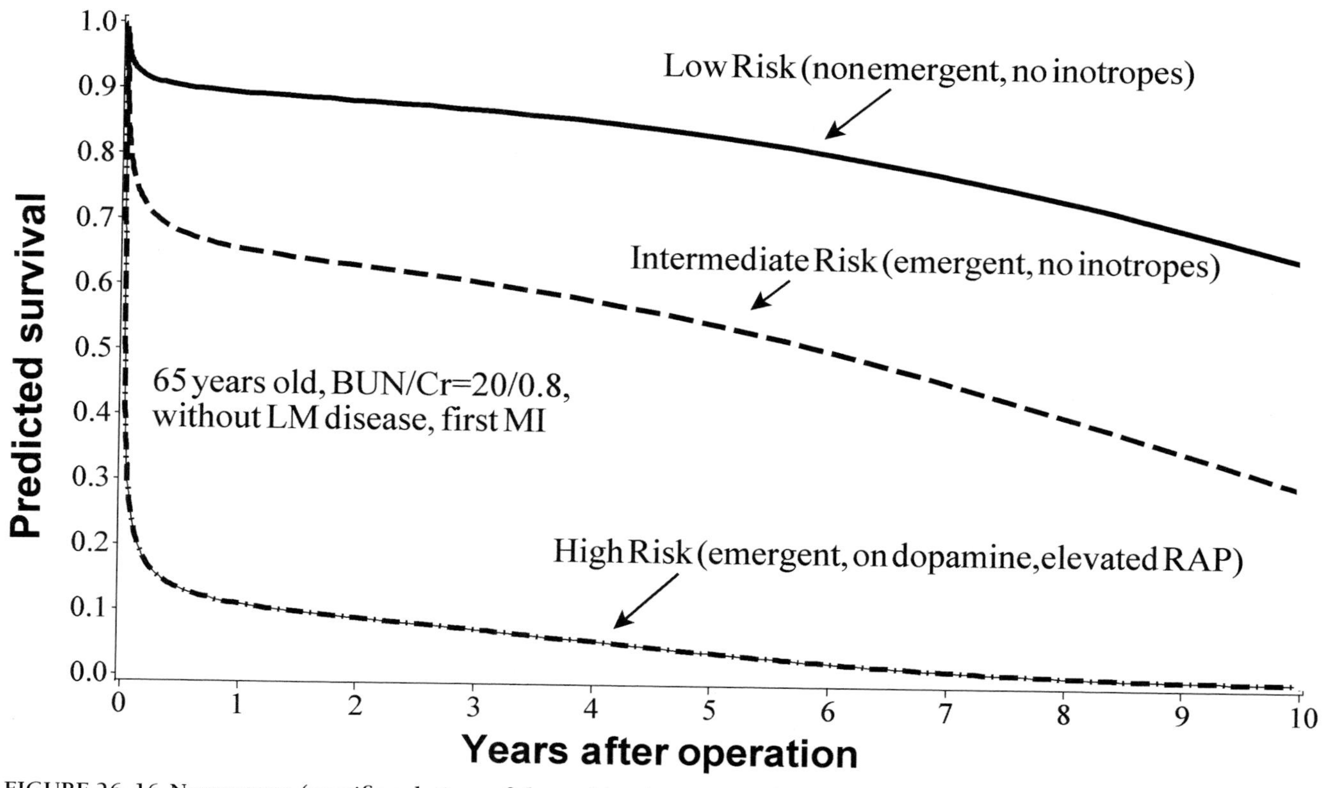

FIGURE 26–16 Nomograms (specific solutions of the multivariate equation) depicting the predicted survival in three hypothetical 65-year-old patients who present with VSD. Each solution is for a patient who has no history of myocardial infarction and without left main coronary artery disease, normal BUN, and Cr of 20 and 0.8, respectively. The "low-risk" patient is nonemergent, not on inotropes, with right atrial pressure of 8. The "intermediate risk" patient is emergent, not on inotropes, with right atrial pressure of 12. The "high-risk patient" is emergent, on inotropes, with right atrial pressure of 20. Confidence limits have been eliminated to improve clarity.

the problem of thinning and dilatation of the infarct wall and increases the probability of rupture.[151] Lack of collateral flow may also promote ventricular rupture.[152]

Since myocardial rupture occurs in regions of complete transmural myocardial necrosis, usually after extensive hemorrhagic transformation of the acute infarct,[148,153,154] and because thrombolytic therapy is associated with the conversion of a bland infarct into a hemorrhagic infarct,[155] there has been an ongoing concern that thrombolysis might increase the likelihood of ventricular rupture.[156] Honan et al[153] performed a meta-analysis of four large clinical trials (1638 patients) in which streptokinase was used to treat acute myocardial infarctions and concluded that the risk of cardiac rupture was directly related to the timing of thrombolytic therapy. Early treatment (within 7 hours from the onset of symptoms) decreased the risk of cardiac rupture, whereas late treatment (after 17 hours) increased the risk of this complication even though, surprisingly, the overall mortality rate was diminished when streptokinase was given late after acute infarction. In a prospective ancillary study of 5711 patients, Late Assessment of Thrombolytic Efficacy (LATE), Becker et al[139] were unable to show an increased risk of cardiac rupture in patients treated with rt-PA 6 to 24 hours after the onset of symptoms. Thus, there is general agreement that early successful thrombolysis decreases the overall risk of cardiac rupture, probably by limiting the extent of necrosis resulting in a nontransmural instead of transmural infarct, but the impact of late thrombolytic therapy on cardiac rupture remains unclear.

Diagnosis

The clinical picture of a subacute ventricular rupture is primarily that of pericardial tamponade with pulsus paradoxus, distended neck veins, and cardiogenic shock. The hemodynamics of tamponade include hypotension, right atrial and pulmonary capillary pressures greater than10 mm Hg, equalization of right atrial and pulmonary capillary pressures (with a difference of less than 5 mm Hg between both pressures), and right atrial pressure waveform exhibiting a deep *x* descent and blunted *y* descent.[157] The identification of clinical or hemodynamic findings of cardiac tamponade should be followed by transthoracic or transesophageal echocardiography to confirm the presence of a pericardial effusion. Although 5% to 37% of patients with acute myocardial infarction but no rupture may develop a pericardial effusion,[158] echocardiographic signs that increase the sensitivity and specificity for cardiac rupture include effusion thickness greater than 10 mm, echo-dense masses in the effusion, ventricular wall defects, and signs of tamponade (e.g., right atrial and right ventricular early diastolic collapse and increased respiratory variation in transvalvular blood flow velocities).[136,159,160] Pericardiocentesis and aspiration of uncoagulated blood has been considered the most reliable criterion of subacute ventricular rupture[161,162]; however, false-positive and false-negative diagnoses have been reported.[136,159] The demonstration of a clear pericardial fluid on pericardiocentesis definitively excludes cardiac rupture.[159] Pericardiocentesis is of therapeutic value in some patients, often providing a short-term circulatory improvement.[163] The certainty of diagnosis of cardiac rupture can be provided promptly using echocardiography.[136]

In an attempt to define symptomatic, electrocardiographic, and hemodynamic markers that may permit the prospective identification of patients prone to rupture of the heart after acute myocardial infarction, Oliva et al[134] retrospectively studied 70 consecutive patients with rupture and 100 comparison patients with acute myocardial infarction but without rupture. They found a number of markers that were associated with a significant increase in the risk of rupture (Table 26-4). The presence of a lateral infarction, especially with associated inferior or posterior infarction, identified a subset of patients at increased risk for rupture. Persistent, progressive, or recurrent ST-segment elevation and, especially, persistent T-wave changes after 48 to 72 hours, or the gradual reversal of initially inverted T waves, are associated with an increased risk of rupture. Finally, the development of pericarditis, repetitive emesis, or restlessness and agitation, particularly two or three of these symptoms, conveyed predictive value.[134] In a similar type of study, Pollak et al[160] identified lateral wall involvement, history of hypertension, and age older than 65 years to be associated with a high risk of subacute left ventricular rupture following acute myocardial infarction.

TABLE 26–4 Sensitivity, specificity, and predictive value of symptoms and electrocardiographic criteria for cardiac rupture

	Sensitivity (%)	Specificity (%)	Predictive value (%)
Pericarditis	86	72	68
Repetitive emesis	64	95	90
Restlessness, agitation	55	95	86
Two or more symptoms	84	97	95
ST-segment deviations	61	72	58
T-wave deviations	94	66	66
ST-T–wave deviations	61	68	64

Source: Reproduced with permission from Oliva PB, Hammill SC, Edwards WD: Cardiac rupture, a clinically predictable complication of acute myocardial infarction: report of 70 cases with clinicopathologic correlations. J Am Coll Cardiol 1993; 22:720.

Diagnosis of a left ventricular false aneurysm can be made preoperatively with a variety of techniques including echocardiography, computed tomography, magnetic resonance imaging, radionucleotide studies, and contrast ventriculography.[146,164,165]

Natural History

Acute rupture of the free wall of the left ventricle is invariably fatal, with death usually occurring within minutes of the onset of recurrent chest pain.[138,141,152] In most of these cases, the sequence of events leading to death is so rapid that there is not enough time for surgical intervention. In contrast, patients with a subacute rupture usually survive hours or days, rarely weeks, following the myocardial tear.[143] Pollak et al[160] found that in 24 cases of postinfarction subacute rupture, survival time (i.e., time from critical event to death) varied between 45 minutes and 6.5 weeks, with a median survival of 8 hours. Núñez et al[166] found that in 29 cases of subacute rupture, 20 (69%) died within minutes of the onset of symptoms and 9 (31%) lived several hours, allowing time for treatment. Subacute ventricular ruptures are generally considered to be less common than acute free wall ruptures. In recent studies, with high autopsy rates, 21% to 42% of all postinfarction free wall ruptures followed a subacute course.[160,167,168]

Because of its rarity, the natural history of false aneurysm of the left ventricle has not been established.[141] It is believed to have a poor prognosis because of its high probability of rupture[145,169,170]; however, there are patients in whom the diagnosis was made many years after myocardial infarction.[144,171,172] The increasingly wide application of echocardiography after acute myocardial infarction gives promise of altering clinical outcome for many patients with the various forms of ventricular wall rupture.

Preoperative Management

Usually, the sequence of events leading to death is so rapid in patients with acute rupture of the free wall of the left ventricle that there is not time enough for surgical intervention.[141] These patients usually die within minutes of the onset of recurrent chest pain.[166] However, a high index of suspicion, combined with a novel technique of percutaneous intrapericardial infusion of fibrin glue immediately following pericardiocentesis,[173,174] may afford at least a chance of survival in this surgically untreatable subgroup of patients.

In contrast, patients with subacute left ventricular rupture can be saved with surgery. Once the diagnosis of rupture of the free wall is established, the patient should be immediately transferred to the operating room. No time should be wasted attempting to perform coronary angiography.[136,141,166,175] Inotropic agents and fluids should be started while preparing for surgery. Pericardiocentesis often improves hemodynamics temporarily,[175] and insertion of an intra-aortic balloon pump may be beneficial, even though the principal problem is cardiac tamponade.[162]

The timing of surgery following the diagnosis of false aneurysm of the left ventricle is dependent upon the age of the myocardial infarction. When a false aneurysm is discovered within the first 2 to 3 months after coronary infarction, surgery is urgently recommended after coronary angiography and ventriculography because of the unpredictability of rupture.[144,172] However, when the diagnosis is made several months or years after myocardial infarction, the urgency of the operation is not determined so much by the risk of rupture, but rather by symptoms and the severity of the coronary artery disease.[141,171]

Operative Techniques

SUBACUTE RUPTURE OF THE FREE WALL

As soon as the diagnosis of rupture of the free wall of the left ventricle is confirmed by echocardiography, the patient should be transferred to the operating room. In patients with tamponade, severe hypotension may result during the induction of anesthesia. Therefore, we usually complete the sterile preparation and draping of the patient before inducing anesthesia. Some even advocate femoral artery cannulation before the induction of anesthesia.[176] A median sternotomy is performed and upon decompressing the pericardium, the blood pressure commonly rises quickly. This should be anticipated and controlled because hypertension can cause ventricular bleeding to start again, or may even increase the size of the ventricular rent.[141] In most cases, however, the ventricular tear is sealed off by clot, and there is no active bleeding.

Traditionally, postinfarction rupture of the free wall of the left heart has been repaired on cardiopulmonary bypass[136,143,157,161,162,166,176,177]; however, some surgeons have suggested that cardiopulmonary bypass is not necessary except perhaps in patients with posterior wall rupture, severe mitral regurgitation, ventricular septal rupture, or graftable coronary artery disease.[141,175] Although the ventricular tear can be repaired without aortic cross-clamping, cardiac standstill and left ventricular decompression make the procedure easier when the rupture is in the posterior wall of the left ventricle.[141]

Four surgical techniques have been used to control ventricular rupture. The first technique involves closing the rent with large horizontal mattress sutures buttressed with two strips of Teflon felt.[130,178] This method is not recommended because the sutures are placed into necrotic, friable myocardium and can easily tear.[136] The second method combines infarct excision and closure of the defect with interrupted, pledgeted sutures[131,136,162,176] or a Dacron patch.[179,180] This method usually requires aortic cross-clamping and is probably best reserved for those patients who have an associated ventricular septal defect.[166] The third technique, described by Núñez et al,[166] involves closing the defect with horizontal mattress sutures buttressed with two strips of Teflon felt, and then covering the closed ventricular tear and surrounding infarcted myocardium with a Teflon patch sutured to healthy epicardium with a continuous polypropylene suture (Fig. 26-17).

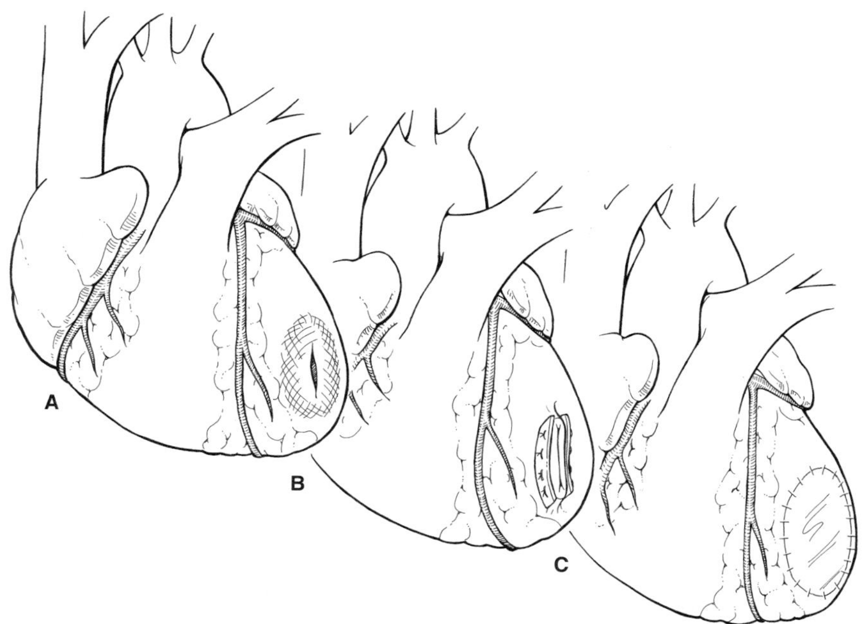

FIGURE 26–17 Technique to repair rupture of the free wall of the left ventricle. (A) Left ventricular free wall rupture. (B) A limited infarctectomy is closed with horizontal mattress sutures buttressed with two strips of felt. (C) Then the whole area is covered with a Teflon patch sutured to healthy epicardium with a continuous propylene suture. Alternatively, the Teflon patch can be glued to the ventricular tear and the infarcted area using a biocompatible glue. *(Adapted from David TE: Surgery for postinfarction rupture of the free wall of the ventricle, in David TE (ed): Mechanical Complications of Myocardial Infarction. Austin, TX, RG Landes Company, 1993; p 142.)*

Good control of active ventricular hemorrhage has been achieved with this method.[136] The fourth method consists of simply gluing a patch of either Teflon[175] or autologous gluteraldehyde-preserved bovine pericardium[136,181,182] to the ventricular tear and infarcted area using a biocompatible glue of either fibrin (Tissucol, Immuno AG, Vienna, Austria), butyl-2-cyanoacrylate monomer (Histoacryl Blue, B. Braun, Melsungen AG, Germany), or gelatin-resorcin-formaldehyde (Pharmacie Centrale, C.H.V. Henry Mondor, Créteil, France). This technique does not necessarily require institution of cardiopulmonary bypass and may be the repair of choice when the ventricle is not actively bleeding.[136,175]

FALSE ANEURYSM OF THE LEFT VENTRICLE

Acute false aneurysms are probably best repaired with an endocardial patch using the same methods as are used in repairing true ventricular aneurysms.[141] Chronic anterior false aneurysms can usually be closed primarily if the neck is fibrotic. However, primary closure of the neck of a posterior false aneurysm may exacerbate mitral regurgitation, and therefore probably should be reconstructed with a patch of Dacron graft or glutaraldehyde-fixed bovine pericardium.[144,147]

Results

SUBACUTE RUPTURE OF THE FREE WALL

The surgical experience with this entity is largely anecdotal. The single largest experience with surgical repair of postinfarction left ventricular free wall rupture was reported by Padró et al.[175] They treated 13 patients using a Teflon patch glued onto the ventricular tear and surrounding infarcted muscle, and utilized cardiopulmonary bypass in only 1 patient who presented with a posterior defect. All of their patients survived and were alive after a mean follow-up of 26 months. Eleven of them were asymptomatic and 2 had exertional angina.[175] Núñez et al[166] operated on 7 patients, 4 of whom survived. Recently the group at McGill University reported hospital discharge in 5 of 6 patients who received unsupported felt secured with cyanoacrylate glue.[183] Coletti et al[136] treated 5 patients and 4 survived. Pifarre et al[162] treated 4 patients successfully, while Pappas et al[180] treated 4 patients of whom 2 survived.

Although operative risk can not be determined from these small numbers, it is likely that without surgery all these patients would have died.[141] It appears that patients who survive surgery tend to do well afterwards.[141]

FALSE ANEURYSM OF THE LEFT VENTRICLE

Komeda and David[144] treated 12 patients with postinfarction left ventricular false aneurysms; 4 of them also had mitral valve replacements, 1 had repair of a fistula between the false aneurysm and the right ventricle, and 9 had coronary artery bypass surgery. There were 3 operative deaths, all in patients who needed mitral valve replacements. Of the 8 patients who underwent isolated repair of false aneurysms, all were alive after a mean follow-up of 62 months. Seven patients were asymptomatic and 1 had angina pectoris.[144] Mackenzie and Lemole[146] reported 14 cases of left ventricular false aneurysm, 12 of which were related to a previous myocardial infarction. There were 3 operative deaths. Long-term follow-up was not reported.

Overall, the literature suggests that patients who have isolated repair of false aneurysms of the left ventricle have low operative mortality.[141]

REFERENCES

1. Daggett WM: Postinfarction ventricular septal defect repair: retrospective thoughts and historical perspectives. *Ann Thorac Surg* 1990; 50:1006.
2. Latham PM: *Lectures on Subjects Connected with Clinical Medicine Comprising Diseases of the Heart*. London, Longman Rees, 1845.
3. Brunn F: Diagnostik der erworbenen ruptur der kammerscheidewand des herzens. *Wien Arch Inn Med* 1923; 6:533.
4. Sager R: Coronary thrombosis: perforation of the infarcted interventricular septum. *Arch Intern Med* 1934; 53:140.
5. Cooley DA, Belmonte BA, Zeis LB, Schnur S: Surgical repair of ruptured interventricular septum following acute myocardial infarction. *Surgery* 1957; 41:930.
6. Effler DB, Tapia FA, McCormack LJ: Rupture of the ventricular myocardium and perforation of the interventricular septum complicating acute myocardial infarction. *Circulation* 1959; 20:128.
7. Payne WS, Hunt JC, Kirklin JW: Surgical repair of ventricular septal defect due to myocardial infarction: report of a case. *JAMA* 1963; 183:603.
8. Sanders RJ, Kern WH, Blount SG: Perforation of the interventricular septum complicating myocardial infarction. *Am Heart J* 1956; 51:736.
9. Lee WY, Cardon L, Slodki SV: Perforation of infarcted interventricular septum. *Arch Intern Med* 1962; 109:135.
10. Dobell ARC, Scott HJ, Cronin RFP, Reid EAS: Surgical closure of interventricular septal perforation complicating myocardial infarction. *J Thorac Cardiovasc Surg* 1962; 43:802.
11. Daicoff AR, Rhodes ML: Surgical repair of ventricular septal rupture and ventricular aneurysms. *JAMA* 1968; 203:457.
12. Allen P, Woodwark G: Surgical management of postinfarction ventricular septal defects. *J Thorac Cardiovasc Surg* 1966; 51:346.
13. Heimbecker RO, Lemire G, Chen C: Surgery for massive myocardial infarction. *Circulation* 1968; 11(suppl 2):37.
14. Iben AB, Pupello DF, Stinson EB, Shumway NE: Surgical treatment of postinfarction ventricular septal defects. *Ann Thorac Surg* 1969; 8:252.
15. Lojos TZ, Greene DG, Bunnell IL, et al: Surgery for acute myocardial infarction. *Ann Thorac Surg* 1969; 8:452.
16. Daggett WM, Burwell LR, Lawson DW, Austen WG: Resection of acute ventricular aneurysm and ruptured interventricular septum after myocardial infarction. *N Engl J Med* 1970; 283:1507.
17. Stinson EB, Becker J, Shumway NE: Successful repair of postinfarction ventricular septal defect and biventricular aneurysm. *J Thorac Cardiovasc Surg* 1969; 58:20.

18. Freeny PC, Schattenberg TT, Danielson GK, et al: Ventricular septal defect and ventricular aneurysm secondary to acute myocardial infarction. *Circulation* 1971; 43:360.
19. Daggett WM, Guyton RA, Mundth ED, et al: Surgery for post-myocardial infarct ventricular septal defects. *Ann Surg* 1977; 186:260.

20a. Daggett WM, Mundth ED, Gold HK, et al: Early repair of ventricular septal defects complicating inferior myocardial infarction. *Circulation* 1974; 50(suppl 3):112.

20b. Daggett WM: Surgical technique for early repair of posterior ventricular septal rupture. *J Thorac Cardiovasc Surg* 1982; 84:306.

21. Daggett WM: Surgical management of ventricular septal defects complicating myocardial infarction. *World J Surg* 1978; 2:753.
22. Skillington PD, Davies RH, Luff AJ, et al: Surgical treatment for infarct-related ventricular septal defects. *J Thorac Cardiovasc Surg* 1990; 99:798.
23. Lundberg S, Sodestrom J: Perforation of the interventricular septum in myocardial infarction: a study based on autopsy material. *Acta Med Scand* 1962; 172:413.
24. Hutchins GM: Rupture of the interventricular septum complicating myocardial infarction: pathological analysis of 10 patients with clinically diagnosed perforation. *Am Heart J* 1979; 97:165.
25. Kitamura S, Mendez A, Kay JH: Ventricular septal defect following myocardial infarction: experience with surgical repair through a left ventriculotomy and review of the literature. *J Thorac Cardiovasc Surg* 1971; 61:186.
26. Selzer A, Gerbode F, Keith WJ: Clinical, hemodynamic and surgical considerations of rupture of the ventricular septum after myocardial infarction. *Am Heart J* 1969; 78:598.
27. Mann JM, Robert WC: Acquired ventricular septal defect during acute myocardial infarction: analysis of 38 unoperated necropsy patients and comparison with 50 unoperated necropsy patients without rupture. *Am J Cardiol* 1988; 62:8.
28. Mallory GK, White PD, Salcedo-Salgar J: The speed of healing of myocardial infarction: a study of the pathologic anatomy in seventy cases. *Am Heart J* 1939; 18:647.
29. Silver MD, Butany J, Chiasson DA: The pathology of myocardial infarction and its mechanical complications, in David TE (ed): *Mechanical Complications of Myocardial Infarction*. Austin, TX, RG Landes, 1993; p 4.
30. Davies RH, Dawkins KD, Skillington PD, et al: Late functional results after surgical closure of acquired ventricular septal defect. *J Thorac Cardiovasc Surg* 1992; 106:592.
31. Daggett WM, Buckley MJ, Akins CW, et al: Improved results of surgical management of postinfarction ventricular septal rupture. *Ann Surg* 1982; 196:269.
32. Skehan JD, Carey C, Norrell MS, et al: Patterns of coronary artery disease in post-infarction ventricular septal rupture. *Br Heart J* 1989; 62:268.
33. Miller S, Dinsmore RE, Grenne RE, Daggett WM: Coronary, ventricular, and pulmonary abnormalities associated with rupture of the interventricular septum complicating myocardial infarction. *Am J Radiol* 1978; 131:571.
34. Hill JD, Lary D, Keith WJ, Gerbode F: Acquired ventricular septal defects: evolution of an operation, surgical technique and results. *J Thorac Cardiovasc Surg* 1975; 70:440.
35. Deville C, Fontan F, Chevalier JM, et al: Surgery of post-infarction ventricular defect: risk factors for hospital death and long-term results. *Eur J Cardiothorac Surg* 1991; 5:167.
36. Swithingbank JM: Perforation of the interventricular septum in myocardial infarction. *Br Heart J* 1959; 21:562.
37. Cummings RG, Reimer KA, Catliff R, et al: Quantitative analysis of right and left ventricular infarction in the presence of postinfarction ventricular septal defect. *Circulation* 1988; 77:33.
38. Weisman HF, Healy B: Myocardial infarct expansion, infarct extension, and reinfarction: pathophysiologic concepts. *Prog Cardiovasc Dis* 1987; 30:73.
39. David TE: Surgery for postinfarction ventricular septal defects, in David TE (ed): *Mechanical Complications of Myocardial Infarction*. Austin, TX, RG Landes, 1993; p 175.
40. Beranek JT: Hyaline degeneration of myocardium is implicated in the pathogenesis of postinfarction heart rupture. *Cor Notes* 1994; 9:3.
41. Edwards BS, Edwards WD, Edwards JE: Ventricular septal rupture complicating acute myocardial infarction: identification of simple and complex types in 53 autopsied hearts. *Am J Cardiol* 1984; 54:1201.
42. Pfeffer MA, Braunwald E: Ventricular remodeling after myocardial infarction: clinical observations and clinical implications. *Circulation* 1990; 81:1161.
43. Abrams D, Edilist A, Luria M, Miller A: Ventricular aneurysms. *Circulation* 1963; 27:164.
44. Fanapazir L, Bray CL, Dark JF: Right ventricular dysfunction and surgical outcome in postinfarction ventricular septal defect. *Eur J Cardiothorac Surg* 1983; 4:155.
45. David TE, Dale L, Sun Z: Postinfarction ventricular septal rupture: repair by endocardial patch with infarct exclusion. *J Thorac Cardiovasc Surg* 1995; 110:1315.
46. Radford MJ, Johnson RA, Daggett WM, et al: Ventricular septal defect following myocardial infarction: factors affecting survival. *Clin Res* 1978; 26:262A.
47. Moore CA, Nygaard TW, Kaiser DL, et al: Postinfarction ventricular septal rupture: the importance of location of infarction and right ventricular function in determining survival. *Circulation* 1986; 74:45.
48. Zehender M, Kasper W, Kauder E: Right ventricular infarction as an independent predictor of prognosis after acute inferior myocardial infarction. *N Engl J Med* 1993; 328:981.
49. Anderson DR, Adams S, Bhat A, Pepper JR: Postinfarction ventricular septal defect: the importance of site of infarction and cardiogenic shock on outcome. *Eur J Cardiothorac Surg* 1989; 3:554.
50. Campion BL, Harrison CE, Guiliani ER, et al: Ventricular septal defect after myocardial infarction. *Ann Intern Med* 1969; 70:251.
51. Vlodaver Z, Edwards JE: Rupture of ventricular septum or papillary muscle complicating myocardial infarction. *Circulation* 1977; 55:815.
52. Honey M, Belcher JR, Hasa M, Gibbons JRP: Case reports: successful early repair of acquired ventricular septal defect after myocardial infarction. *Br Heart J* 1967; 29:453.
53. Rawlins MO, Mendel D, Braimbridge MV: Ventricular septal defect and mitral regurgitation secondary to myocardial infarction. *Br Heart J* 1972; 34:323.
54. Taylor FH, Citron DS, Robicsek F, Sanger PW: Simultaneous repair of ventricular septal defect and left ventricular aneurysm following myocardial infarction. *Ann Thorac Surg* 1965; 1:72.
55. Meister SG, Helfant RH: Rapid differentiation of ruptured interventricular septum from acute mitral insufficiency. *N Engl J Med* 1972; 287:1024.
56. Hillis LD, Firth BG, Winniford MD: Variability of right-sided cardiac oxygen saturations in adults with and without left-to-right intracardiac shunt. *Am J Cardiol* 1986; 58:129.
57. Heiffila J, Karesoja M: Ruptured interventricular septum complicating acute myocardial infarction. *Chest* 1974; 66:675.
58. Buckley MJ, Mundth ED, Daggett WM, et al: Surgical therapy for early complications of myocardial infarction. *Surgery* 1971; 70:814.
59. Harrison MR, MacPhail B, Gurley JC, et al: Usefulness of color Doppler flow imaging to distinguish ventricular septal defect from acute mitral regurgitation complicating acute myocardial infarction. *Am J Cardiol* 1989; 64:697.

60. Smyllie JH, Sutherland GR, Geuskens R, et al: Doppler color flow mapping in the diagnosis of ventricular septal rupture and acute mitral regurgitation after myocardial infarction. *J Am Coll Cardiol* 1990; 15:1455.
61. Fortin DF, Sheikh KH, Kisslo J: The utility of echocardiography in the diagnostic strategy of postinfarction ventricular septal rupture: a comparison of two-dimensional versus Doppler color flow imaging. *Am Heart J* 1991; 121:25.
62. Blanche C, Khan SS, Matloff JM, et al: Results of early repair of ventricular septal defect after an acute myocardial infarction. *J Thorac Cardiovasc Surg* 1992; 104:961.
63. Matsui K, Kay JH, Mendez M, et al: Ventricular septal rupture secondary to myocardial infarction: clinical approach and surgical results. *JAMA* 1981; 245:1537.
64. Kaplan MA, Harris CN, Kay JH, et al: Postinfarctional septal rupture: clinical approach and surgical results. *Chest* 1976; 69:734.
65. Oyamada A, Queen FB: Spontaneous rupture of the interventricular septum following acute myocardial infarction with some clinico-pathologic observations on survival in five cases [unpublished]. 1961.
66. Berger TJ, Blackstone EH, Kirklin JW: Postinfarction ventricular septal defect, in Kirklin JW, Barratt-Boyes BG (eds): *Cardiac Surgery.* New York, Churchill Livingstone, 1993; p 403.
67. Lemery R, Smith HC, Giuliani ER, Gersh BJ: Prognosis in rupture of the ventricular septum after acute myocardial infarction and role of early surgical intervention. *Am J Cardiol* 1992; 70:147.
68. Menon V, Webb J, Hillis D, et al: Outcome and profile of ventricular septal rupture with cardiogentic shock after myocardial infarction: a report from the SHOCK Trial Registry. *J Am Coll Cardiol* 2000; 36:1010.
69. Kay HR: In discussion of Daggett WM: Surgical management of ventricular septal defects complicating myocardial infarction. *World J Surg* 1978; 2:753.
70. Heitmiller R, Jacobs ML, Daggett WM: Surgical management of postinfarction ventricular septal rupture. *Ann Thorac Surg* 1986; 41:683.
71. Estrada-Quintero T, Uretsky BF, Murali S, Hardesty RL: Prolonged intraaortic balloon support for septal rupture after myocardial infarction. *Ann Thorac Surg* 1992; 53:335.
72. Baillot R, Pelletier C, Trivino-Marin J, Castonguay Y: Postinfarction ventricular septal defect: delayed closure with prolonged mechanical circulatory support. *Ann Thorac Surg* 1983; 35:138.
73. Muehrcke DD, Daggett WM, Buckley MJ, et al: Postinfarct ventricular septal defect repair: effect of coronary artery bypass grafting. *Ann Thorac Surg* 1992; 54:876.
74. Gaudiani VA, Miller DC, Oyer PE, et al: Post-infarction ventricular septal defect: an argument for early operation. *Surgery* 1981; 89:48.
75. Gold HK, Leinbach RC, Sanders CA, et al: Intra-aortic balloon pumping for ventricular septal defect or mitral regurgitation complicating acute myocardial infarction. *Circulation* 1973; 47:1191.
76. Montoya A: Ventricular septal rupture secondary to acute myocardial infarction, in Pifarre R (ed): *Cardiac Surgery: Acute Myocardial Infarction and Its Complications.* Philadelphia, Hanley & Belfus, 1992; p 159.
77. Scanlon PJ, Monatoya A, Johnson SA: Urgent surgery for ventricular septal rupture complicating myocardial infarction. *Circulation* 1985; 72(suppl 2):185.
78. Loisance DY, Cachera JP, Poulain H, et al: Ventricular septal defect after acute myocardial infarcion. *J Thorac Cardiovasc Surg* 1980; 80:61.
79. Babb JD, Waldhausen JA, Zelis R: Balloon induced right ventricular outflow obstruction: a new approach to control of acute interventricular shunting after myocardial infarction in canines and swine. *Circ Res* 1977; 40:372.
80. Meyns B, Vanermen H, Vanhaecke J, et al: Hemopump fails as bridge to transplantation in postinfarction ventricular septal defect. *J Heart Lung Transplant* 1994; 13:1133.
81. David H, Hunter JA, Najafi H, et al: Left ventricular approach for the repair of ventricular septal performation and infarctectomy. *J Thorac Cardiovasc Surg* 1972; 63:14.
82. Daggett WM, Randolph JD, Jacobs ML, et al: The superiority of cold oxygenated dilute blood cardioplegia. *Ann Thorac Surg* 1987; 43:397.
83. Hendren WG, O'Keefe DD, Geffin GA, et al: Maximal oxygenation of dilute blood cardioplegia solution. *Ann Thorac Surg* 1994; 58:1558.
84. David TE: Surgical treatment of postinfarction ventricular septal rupture. *Australas J Card Thorac Surg* 1991; 1:7.
85. Weisel RD: Myocardial protection during surgery for mechanical complications of myocardial infarction, in David TE (ed): *Mechanical Complications of Myocardial Infarction.* Austin, TX, RG Landes, 1993; p 120.
86. Torchiana DF, Geffin GA, O'Keefe DD, Daggett WM: Cardioplegia for repair of postinfarction ventricular septal defect, in Engleman RM, Levitsky S, (eds): *A Textbook of Cardioplegia for Difficult Clinical Problems.* Mount Kisco, NY, Futura, 1992; p 115.
87. Rosenkranz ER, Buckberg GD, Mulder DG, Laks H: Warm induction of cardioplegia with glutamate-enriched blood in coronary patients with cardiogenic shock who are dependent on inotropic drugs and intraaortic ballon support: initial experience and operative strategy. *J Thorac Cardiovasc Surg* 1983; 86:507.
88. Teoh KH, Christakis GT, Weisel RD, et al: Accelerated myocardial metabolic recovery with terminal warm blood cardioplegia. *J Thorac Cardiovasc Surg* 1986; 91:888.
89. Shumacker H: Suggestions concerning operative management of postinfarction ventricular septal defects. *J Thorac Cardiovasc Surg* 1972; 64:452.
90. Dor V, Saab M, Coste P, et al: Left ventricular aneurysm: a new surgical approach. *Thorac Cardiovasc Surg* 1989; 37:11.
91. Cooley DA: Repair of the difficult ventriculotomy. *Ann Thorac Surg* 1990; 49:150.
92. Cooley DA: Repair of postinfarction ventricular septal defect. *J Card Surg* 1994; 9:427.
93. Alvarez JM, Brady PW, Ross DE: Technical improvements in the repair of acute postinfarction ventricular septal rupture. *J Card Surg* 1992; 7:198.
94. daSilva JP, Cascudo MM, Baumgratz JF, et al: Postinfarction ventricular septal defect: an efficacious technique for early surgical repair. *J Thorac Cardiovasc Surg* 1989; 97:86.
95. Tashiro T, Todo K, Haruta Y, et al: Extended endocardial repair of postinfarction ventricular septal rupture: new operative technique modification of the komeda-david operation. *J Card Surg* 1994; 9:97.
96. Usui A, Murase M, Maeda M, et al: Sandwich repair with two sheets of equine pericardial patch for acute posterior postinfarction ventricular septal defect. *Eur J Cardiothorac Surg* 1993; 7:47.
97. Fujimoto K, Kawahito K, Yamaguchi A, et al: Percutaneous extracorporeal life support for treatment of fatal mechanical complications associated with acute myocardial infarction. *Artif Organs* 2001; 25:1000.
98. Landzberg MJ, Lock JE: Transcatheter management of ventricular septal rupture after myocardial infarction. *Semin Thorac Cardiovasc Surg* 1998; 10:128.
99. Lock JE, Block PC, McKay RG, et al: Transcatheter closure of ventricular septal defects. *Circulation* 1988; 78:361.
100. Hachida M, Nakano H, Hirai M, Shi CY: Percutaneous transaortic closure of postinfarction ventricular septal rupture. *Ann Thorac Surg* 1991; 51:655.

101. Abhyankar A, Jagtap P: Post-infarction ventricular septal defect: percutaneous transvenous closure using a Swan-Ganz catheter. *Cathet Cardiovasc Interv* 1999; 47:208.
102. Aliabadi D, Roland C, Pett S, et al: Percutaneous cardiopulmonary support for the management of catastrophic mechanical complications of acute myocardial infarction. *Cathet Cardiovasc Diagn* 1996; 37:223.
103. Kshettry V, Salerno C, Bank A: Risk of left ventricular assist device as a bridge to heart transplant following postinfarction ventricular septal rupture. *J Card Surg* 1997; 12:93.
104. Meyns B, Vanermen H, Vanhaecke J, et al: Hemopump fails as bridge to transplantation in postinfarction ventricular septal defect. *J Heart Lung Transplant* 1994:13:1133.
105. Loisance DP, Lordez JM, Deleuze PH, et al: Acute postinfarction septal rupture: long-term results. *Ann Thorac Surg* 1991; 52:474.
106. Piwnica A, Menasche P, Beaufils P, Julliard JM: Long-term results of emergency surgery for postinfarction ventricular septal defect. *Ann Thorac Surg* 1987; 44:274.
107. Weintraub RM, Thurer RL, Wei J: Repair of postinfarction ventricular septal defect in the elderly: early and long term results. *J Thorac Cardiovasc Surg* 1983; 85:191.
108. Marchetti A, Wechsler AS. Pharmacologic intervention for acute low cardiac output [abstract]. *Adv Card Surg* 1996; 7:21.
109. D'Ambra MN, LaRaia PJ, Philbin DM, et al: Prostaglandin E_1: a new therapy for refractory right heart failure and pulmonary hypertension after mitral valve replacement. *J Thorac Cardiovasc Surg* 1985; 89:567.
110. Rich GF, Murphy GD Jr, Roos CM, Johns RA: Inhaled nitric oxide: selective pulmonary vasodilatation in cardiac surgical patients. *Anesthesiology* 1993; 78:1028.
111. Pae WE Jr, Pierce WS, Sapirstein JS: Intra-aortic balloon counterpulsation, ventricular assist pumping, and the artificial heart, in Baue AE, Geha AS, Hammond GL, Laks H, Naunheim KS, (eds): *Glenn's Thoracic and Cardiovascular Surgery*. Stamford, CT, Appleton & Lange, 1996; p 1825.
112. Sundt TM 3rd, Kouchoukos NT, Saffitz JE, et al: Renal dysfunction and intravascular coagulation with aprotinin and hypothermic circulatory arrest. *Ann Thorac Surg* 1993; 55:1418.
113. Seguin JR, Frapier JM, Colson P, Chaptal PA: Fibrin sealant for early repair of acquired ventricular septal defect. *J Thorac Cardiovasc Surg* 1992; 104:748.
114. Fabiani J-N, Jebara VA, Deloche A, et al: Use of surgical glue without replacement in the treatment of type A aortic dissection. *Circulation* 1989; 80:264.
115. Baldwin RT, Cooley DA: Mechanical support for intraventricular decompression in repair of left ventricular disruption. *Ann Thorac Surg* 1992; 54:176.
116. Saksena S, Rothbart ST, Shah Y: Clinical efficacy and electropharmacology of continuous intravenous amiodarone infusion and chronic oral amiodarone in refractory ventricular tachycardia. *Am J Cardiol* 1984; 54:347.
117. Komeda M, Fremes SE, David TE: Surgical repair of the postinfarction ventricular septal defect. *Circulation* 1990; 82(suppl 4):243.
118. Radford MJ, Johnson RA, Daggett WM, et al: Ventricular septal rupture: a review of clinical and physiological features and an analysis of survival. *Circulation* 1981; 64:545.
119. Cox FF, Morshuis WJ, Plokker HWT, et al: Early mortality after surgical repair of post-infarction ventricular septal rupture: importance of rupture location. *Ann Thorac Surg* 1996; 61:1752.
120. Jones MT, Schofield PM, Dark JF: Surgical repair of acquired ventricular septal defect: determinants of early and late outcome. *J Thorac Cardiovasc Surg* 1987; 93:680.
121. Dalrymple-Hay MJR, Monro JL, Livesey SA, Lamb RK: Postinfarction ventricular septal rupture: the Wessex experience. *Semin Thorac Cardiovasc Surg* 1998; 10:111.
122. Hill JD, Stiles QR: Acute ischemic ventricular septal defect. *Circulation* 1989; 79(suppl 1):112.
123. Ross D: Overlay patch technique for ventricular septal defect repair. *Australas J Card Thorac Surg* 1992; 1:11.
124. Cooley DA: Postinfarction ventricular septal rupture. *Semin Thorac Cardiovasc Surg* 1998; 10:100.
125. Rousou JA, Engelman RM, Breyer RH, et al: Transatrial repair of postinfarction posterior ventricular septal defect. *Ann Thorac Surg* 1987; 43:665.
126. Filgueira JL, Battistessa SA, Estable H, et al: Delayed repair of an acquired posterior septal defect through a right atrial approach. *Ann Thorac Surg* 1986; 42:208.
127. Willius FA, Dry TJ: *A History of the Heart and Circulation*. Philadelphia, WB Saunders, 1948.
128. Morgagni JB: *The Seat and Causes of Disease Investigated by Anatomy*. London, A. Millau & T. Cadell, 1769; p 811.
129. Willius FA, Dry TJ: *A History of the Heart and Circulation*. Philadelphia, WB Saunders, 1948.
130. Hatcher CR Jr, Mansour K, Logan WD Jr, et al: Surgical complications of myocardial infarction. *Am Surg* 1970; 36:163.
131. FitzGibbon GM, Hooper GD, Heggtveit HA: Successful surgical treatment of postinfarction external cardiac rupture. *J Thorac Cardiovasc Surg* 1972; 63:622.
132. Montegut FJ Jr: Left ventricular rupture secondary to myocardial infarction. *Ann Thorac Surg* 1972; 14:75.
133. Oliva PB, Hammill SC, Edwards WD: Cardiac rupture, a clinically predictable complication of acute myocardial infarction: report of 70 cases with clinicopathologic correlations. *J Am Coll Cardiol* 1993; 22:720.
134. Hutchins KD, Skurnick J, Lavendar M, et al: Cardiac rupture in acute myocardial infarction: a reassessment. *Am J Forensic Med Pathol* 2002; 23:78–82.
135. Stevenson WG, Linssen GCM, Havenith MG, et al: The spectrum of death after myocardial infarction: a necropsy study. *Am Heart J* 1989; 118:1182.
136. Coletti G, Torracca L, Zogno M, et al: Surgical management of left ventricular free wall rupture after acute myocardial infarction. *Cardiovasc Surg* 1995; 3:181.
137. Herlitz J, Samuelsson SO, Richter A, Hjalmarson Å: Prediction of rupture in acute myocardial infarction. *Clin Cardiol* 1988; 11:63.
138. Batts KP, Ackermann DM, Edwards WD: Post-infarction rupture of the left ventricular free wall: clinicopathologic correlates in 100 consecutive autopsy cases. *Hum Pathol* 1990; 21:530.
139. Becker RC, Charlesworth A, Wilcox RG, et al: Cardiac rupture associated with thrombolytic therapy: impact of time to treatment in the late assessment of thrombolytic efficacy (LATE) study. *J Am Coll Cardiol* 1995; 25:1063.
140. Krumbahaar EB, Crowell C: Spontaneous rupture of the heart: a clinicopathologic study based on 22 unpublished cases and 632 from the literature. *Am J Med Sci* 1925; 170:828.
141. David TE: Surgery for postinfarction rupture of the free wall of the ventricle, in David TE (ed): *Mechanical Complications of Myocardial Infarction*. Austin, TX, RG Landes, 1993; p 142.
142. Bashour T, Kabbani SS, Ellertson DG, et al: Surgical salvage of heart rupture: report of two cases and review of the literature. *Ann Thorac Surg* 1983; 36:209.
143. O'Rourke MF: Subacute heart rupture following myocardial infarction: clinical features of a correctable condition. *Lancet* 1973; 22:124.
144. Komeda M, David TE: Surgical treatment of postinfarction false aneurysm of the left ventricle. *J Thorac Cardiovasc Surg* 1993; 106:1189.
145. Van Tassel RA, Edwards JE: Rupture of heart complicating myocardial infarction: analysis of 40 cases including nine examples of left ventricular false aneurysm. *Chest* 1972; 61:104.

146. Mackenzie JW, Lemole GM: Pseudoaneurysm of the left ventricle. *Tex Heart Inst J* 1994; 21:286.
147. Mascarenhas DAN, Benotti JR, Daggett WM, et al: Postinfarction septal aneurysm with delayed formation of left-to-right shunt. *Am Heart J* 1991; 122:226.
148. Schuster EH, Bulkley BH: Expansion of transmural myocardial infarction: a pathophysiologic factor in cardiac rupture. *Circulation* 1979; 60:1532.
149. Hutchins GM, Bulkley BH: Infarct expansion versus extension: two different complications of acute myocardial infarction. *Am J Cardiol* 1978; 41:1127.
150. Weisman HF, Bush DE, Mannisi JA, et al: Cellular mechanisms of myocardial infarct expansion. *Circulation* 1988; 78:186.
151. Christensen DJ, Ford M, Reading J, Castle CH: Effects of hypertension in myocardial rupture after acute myocardial infarction. *Chest* 1977; 72:618.
152. Pohjola-Sintonen S, Muller JE, Stone PH, et al: Ventricular septal and free wall rupture complicating acute myocardial infarction: experience in the multicenter investigation of limitation of infarct size. *Am Heart J* 1989; 117:809.
153. Honan MB, Harrell FE, Reimer KA, et al: Cardiac rupture, mortality and timing of thrombolytic therapy: a meta-analysis. *J Am Coll Cardiol* 1990; 16:359.
154. Wessler S, Zoll PM, Schlesinger MJ: Expansion of transmural myocardial infarction: a pathophysiological factor in cardiac rupture. *Circulation* 1952; 6:334.
155. Mathey DG, Schofer J, Kuck KH, et al: Transmural hemorrhagic infarction after intracoronary streptokinase: clinical, angiographic,and necropsy findings. *Br Heart J* 1982; 48:546.
156. Westaby S, Parry A, Ormerod O, et al: Thrombolysis and postinfarction ventricular septal rupture. *J Thorac Cardiovasc Surg* 1992; 104:1506.
157. Abel RM, Buckley MJ, Friedlich AL, Austen WG: Survival following free rupture of left ventricular aneurysm: report of a case. *Ann Thorac Surg* 1976; 21:175.
158. Wunderink RG: Incidence of pericardial effusions in acute myocardial infarction. *Chest* 1984; 85:494.
159. López-Sendón J, González A, López De Sá E, et al. Diagnosis of subacute ventricular wall rupture after acute myocardial infarction: sensitivity and specificity of clinical, hemodynamic and echocardiographic criteria. *J Am Coll Cardiol* 1992; 19:1145.
160. Pollack H, Diez W, Spiel R, et al: Early diagnosis of subacute free wall rupture complicating acute myocardial infarction. *Eur Heart J* 1993; 14:640.
161. Kendall RW, DeWood MA: Postinfarction cardiac rupture: surgical success and review of the literature. *Ann Thorac Surg* 1978; 25:311.
162. Pifarré R, Sullivan HJ, Grieco J, et al: Management of left ventricular rupture complicating myocardial infarction. *J Thorac Cardiovasc Surg* 1983; 86:441.
163. Coma-Canella I, López-Sendón J, González A: Hemodynamic effect of dobutamine, dextran and pericardiocentesis in cardiac tamponade following acute myocardial infarction. *Am Heart J* 1987; 114:78.
164. Rueda B, Panidis I, Gonzales R, McDonough M: Left ventricular pseudoaneurysm: detection and postoperative follow-up by color Doppler echocardiography. *Am Heart J* 1990; 120:990.
165. Pollak H, Mayr H, Binder T, et al: Diagnosis of a false left ventricular aneurysm with magnetic resonance imaging. *Am Heart J* 1990; 120:706.
166. Núñez L, de la Llana R, López Sendón J, et al: Diagnosis and treatment of subacute free wall ventricular rupture after infarction. *Ann Thorac Surg* 1982; 35:525.
167. Feneley MP, Chang VP, O'Rourke MF: Myocardial rupture after acute myocardial infarction: ten year review. *Br Heart J* 1983; 49:550.
168. Dellborg M, Held P, Swedberg K, Vedin A: Rupture of the myocardium: occurrence and risk factors. *Br Heart J* 1985; 54:11.
169. Chesler E, Korns ME, Semba T, Edwards JE: False aneurysm of the left ventricle following myocardial infarction. *Am J Cardiol* 1969; 23:76.
170. Epstein JI, Hutchins GM: Subepicardial aneurysms: a rare complication of myocardial infarction. *Am J Cardiol* 1983; 75:639.
171. Harper RW, Sloman G, Westlake G: Successful surgical resection of a chronic false aneurysm of the left ventricle. *Chest* 1975; 67:359.
172. Shabbo FP, Dymond DS, Rees GM, Hill IM: Surgical treatment of false aneurysm of the left ventricle after myocardial infarction. *Thorax* 1983; 38:25.
173. Kyo S, Ogiwara M, Miyamoto N, et al: Percutaneous intrapericardial fibrin-glue infusion therapy for rupture of the left ventricle free wall following acute myocardial infarction [abstract]. *J Am Coll Cardiol* 1996; 27:327A.
174. Kyo S, Ogiwara M, Miyamoto N, et al: Treatment of rupture of left ventricle free wall with fibrin-glue: experimental study and clinical experience [abstract]. *J Am Coll Cardiol* 1994; 1:484A.
175. Padró JM, Mesa J, Silvestre J, et al: Subacute cardiac rupture: repair with a sutureless technique. *Ann Thorac Surg* 1993; 55:20.
176. Eisenmann B, Bareiss P, Pacifico AD, et al: Anatomic, clinical, and therapeutic features of acute cardiac rupture. *J Thorac Cardiovasc Surg* 1978; 76:78.
177. Pugliese P, Tommassini G, Macrì R, et al: Successful repair of postinfarction heart rupture. *J Cardiovasc Surg* 1986; 27:332.
178. Pierli C, Lisi G, Mezzacapo B: Subacute left ventricular free wall rupture: surgical repair prompted by echocardiographic diagnosis. *Chest* 1991; 100:1174.
179. Levett JM, Southgate TJ, Jose AB, et al: Technique for repair of left ventricular free wall rupture. *Ann Thorac Surg* 1988; 46:248.
180. Pappas PJ, Cernaianu AC, Baldino WA, et al: Ventricular free-wall rupture after mycardial infarction: treatment and outcome. *Chest* 1991; 4:892.
181. Zogno M, LaCanna G, Ceconi C, et al: Postinfarction left ventricular free wall rupture: original management and surgical technique. *J Card Surg* 1991; 6:396.
182. Del Rizzo DF, Goldman BS, Hare G: Autologous pericardial patch without infarctectomy for the treatment of acute cardiac rupture. *Can J Cardiol* 1995; 11:702.
183. Lachapelle K, deVarennes B, Ergina PL: Sutureless patch technique for postinfarction left ventricular rupture. *Ann Thorac Surg* 2002; 74:96.
184. Agnihotri AK, Madsen J, Daggett WM: Unpublished data from Massachusetts General Hospital experience.
185. Rhydwen GR, Charman S, Schofeild PM: Influence of thrombolytic therapy on the patterns of ventricular septal rupture after acute myocardial infarction. *Postgrad Med J* 2002; 79:408.
186. Pretre R, Ye Q, Grünefelfder J, et al: Role of myocardial revascularization in postinfarction ventricular septal rupture. *Ann Thorac Surg* 2000; 69:51.
187. Hirata N, Sakai K, Sakkakis, et al: Assesment of perioperative predictive factors influencing survival in patients with postinfarction septal perforation. *J Cardiovasc Surg* 2000; 41:547.
188. Deja MA, Szostek J, Widenka K, et al: Post infarction ventricular septal defect—can we do better? *Eur J Cardiothorac Surg* 2000; 18:194.
189. Athanassiadi K, Apostolakis E, Kalavrouziotis G, et al: Surgical repair of postinfarction ventricular septal defect: 10-year experience. *World J Surg* 1999; 23:64.

190. David TE, Armstrong S: Surgical repair of postinfarction ventricular septal defect by infarct exclusion. *Semin Thorac Cardiovasc Surg* 1998; 10:105.
191. Chaux A, Blanch C, Matloff JM, et al: Postinfarction ventricular septal defect. *Semin Thorac Cardiovasc Surg* 1998; 10:93.
192. Killen DA, Piehler JM, Borkon AM, et al: Early repair of postinfarction ventricular septal rupture. *Ann Thorac Surg* 1997; 63:138.
193. Cox FF, Morshuis WJ, Plokker T, et al: Early mortality after repair of postinfarction ventricular septal rupture: importance of rupture location. *Ann Thorac Surg* 1996; 61:1752.
194. Ellis CJ, Parkinson GF, Jaffe WM, et al: Good long-term outcome following surgical repair of post-infarction ventricular septal defect. *Aust NZ J Med* 1995; 25:330.
195. Loisance DY, Lordex JM, Deluze PH, et al: Acute postinfarction septal rupture: long-term results. *Ann Thorac Surg* 1991; 52:474.

Chapter 27

Therapeutic Angiogenesis, Transmyocardial Laser Revascularization, and Cell Therapy

Marc Ruel/Ralph A. Kelly/Frank W. Sellke

Despite increased awareness and better management of cardiovascular risk factors, coronary artery disease (CAD) may involve the epicardial vasculature of some patients so diffusely that repeated attempts at catheter-based interventions and coronary artery bypass grafting (CABG) can prove unsuccessful at alleviating ischemic symptoms and preventing complications. Although this situation may be encountered in any given subgroup of patients (particularly those who have previously undergone CABG), it is more common in diabetics,[1,2] heart transplant recipients with cardiac allograft vasculopathy,[3,4] and patients of Indian descent or with a family history of early-onset CAD.[5,6] Overall, it is estimated that patients with ungraftable coronary artery disease account for approximately 5% of patients who undergo coronary angiography at large referral centers.[7] The failure to revascularize even a single ischemic myocardial territory due to poor graftability is associated with a decrease in both survival and freedom from angina in these patients, regardless of the presence of a patent left internal thoracic artery bypass to the left anterior descending artery.[8] Consequently, patients with ungraftable coronary disease may potentially benefit from alternative therapies such as therapeutic angiogenesis and transmyocardial laser revascularization, either of which could serve as the sole therapy or as an adjunct towards complete myocardial revascularization.

There are also a large number of patients with poor left ventricular function and congestive symptoms due to one or several myocardial infarctions for whom medical therapy or conventional revascularization procedures have been unsuccessful or are likely to fail in the context of an unfavorable myocardial viability profile. Although many of these patients may be eligible for orthotopic heart transplantation, current waiting times for donor hearts and limitations in organ availability render this option unlikely to occur before the patient has become severely ill and reached status I priority level. Cell-based modalities for heart failure, collectively referred to as cell therapy, may eventually constitute a therapeutic option for these patients by enabling repopulation of their infarcted myocardial territories with functional cardiomyocytes.

Therapeutic angiogenesis, transmyocardial laser revascularization, and cell therapy share a common goal of directly restoring perfusion and function to chronically ischemic myocardial territories without intervening on the epicardial coronary arteries. In spite of these approaches having received considerable scientific attention over the last several years, they have not yet been proven to provide clinical benefit and are consequently reserved for patients who have failed conventional therapies. Nevertheless, as the understanding of the physiologic mechanisms that constitute their scientific foundations improves over time, their more widespread applications could potentially revolutionize the practice of cardiovascular medicine. For these reasons, all members of the multidisciplinary cardiac team may be called to play a role in their development and implementation, and will benefit from an understanding of the mechanistic basis, current status of research, clinical data, and therapeutic potential behind these approaches. This chapter provides a synopsis of these key points as they pertain to each of these three modalities.

THERAPEUTIC ANGIOGENESIS

Vasculogenesis, Arteriogenesis, and Angiogenesis

At least three different processes may result in the growth of new blood vessels: vasculogenesis, arteriogenesis, and true angiogenesis (Table 27-1).[9,10] *Vasculogenesis* occurs early in fetal development, within new avascular tissue, and consists of the differentiation of endothelial cells from angioblasts and endothelial progenitor cells, followed by their proliferation, coalescence, and recruitment of other cell types to complete the process of vascular formation in situ.[11] Although long considered to play little or no role in the response to chronic ischemia in adult tissues, vasculogenesis has been shown to occur in adult mice from the recruitment of circulating bone marrow endothelial progenitor cells after cutaneous wounding and hindlimb ischemia.[12]

Arteriogenesis refers both to the process by which an individual's postnatal vascular network is remodeled later in life by the maturation of preexisting collaterals in response to supply-demand imbalances ("angiogenic remodeling"), and to the de novo formation (by sprouting) of mature blood vessels that contain pericytes and smooth muscle cells, which in fact constitutes the true goal of "therapeutic angiogenesis."

Angiogenesis, in its strictest definitional meaning, refers to the sprouting into surrounding tissues of newly formed capillaries derived from preexisting vessels, which spontaneously occurs at the border zone of myocardial infarction or in granulation tissue during wound healing. However, these newly formed capillaries lack a fully developed medial layer, have abnormal permeability, and do not undergo vasomotor regulation. Thus the term "therapeutic *angiogenesis*" may

TABLE 27–1 Biological processes leading to the formation of new blood vessels

	Vasculogenesis	Arteriogenesis	Angiogenesis
Cell types involved	Endothelial stem cells	Endothelial cells; pericytes; smooth muscle cells; other	Endothelial cells
Primary stimulus	Development	Not known (ischemia? inflammation?)	Inflammation, Ischemia
End result	Fully formed vessels	Arterioles	Capillaries
Occurrence in adult tissues	Minimal (?)	Yes	Yes
Contribution to effective perfusion	Minimal (?)	Major	Likely minimal
Growth factors involved	VEGF, Ang-1, Ang-2	PDGF, Ang-1, Ang-2, FGFs (?)	FGFs, VEGFs

Ang = angiopoietin; FGF = fibroblast growth factor; PDGF = platelet-derived growth factor; VEGF = vascular endothelial growth factor.

Source: Modified with permission from Simons M, Bonow RO, Chronos NA, et al: Clinical trials in angiogenesis: issues, problems, consensus: an expert panel summary. Circulation 2000; 102: E73.

constitute a misnomer, and "therapeutic *arteriogenesis*" better decribes a process that is likely to result in the alleviation of ischemia; nevertheless, the former designation is widely accepted and the distinction will not be carried further in this text.

Mechanisms of Angiogenesis

Vasodilation and increased capillary permeability from the sequestration of intercellular adhesion molecules such as vascular endothelial (VE)-cadherin and platelet endothelial cell adhesion molecule (PECAM)-1 are believed to constitute initial steps in the physiologic angiogenic process (Fig. 27-1).[13] These events are mediated by the combined actions of nitric oxide (NO) and vascular endothelial growth factor (VEGF) on endothelial and smooth muscle cells and result in the extravasation of plasma proteins, although limited by the negative feedback actions of angiopoietin-1 (Ang1), an agonist for the Tie2 receptor of endothelial cells.[14] The detachment of smooth muscle cells and the degradation of the surrounding perivascular matrix constitute a next step that involves the Tie2 antagonist angiopoietin-2 (Ang2) and several metalloproteinases. This allows for the migration of endothelial cells and the liberation of endogenous growth factors such as fibroblast growth factor (FGF)-2 and VEGF from the matrix.[13]

The subsequent proliferation of endothelial cells and their migration to distant sites are induced by several growth factors including VEGFs, FGFs (which recruit endothelial, mesenchymal, and inflammatory cells),[15] Ang1 (chemotactic for endothelial cells and an inducer of sprouting),[16] and platelet-derived growth factors (which recruit pericytes and smooth muscle cells around nascent vessel sprouts).[17] Endothelial cells can then assemble into cords, form a lumen, and reexpress adhesion molecules such as VE-cadherin, three processes believed to make endothelial cells resistant to apoptosis and mediated by VEGF, FGF-2, and Ang1.[18,19] These rudimentary cords can remain dormant or develop, branch, recruit periendothelial cells, and mature as functional vessels in order to meet local demands. The signals and mechanisms responsible for these maturation processes are incompletely understood, but may involve the combined actions of PDGF-BB (smooth muscle chemotaxis),[17] Ang1 and Tie2 (smooth muscle to endothelial cell interactions),[16] and FGF-2 (smooth muscle growth and vessel enlargement).[13] Table 27-2 summarizes the role of select substances involved in the angiogenic process.

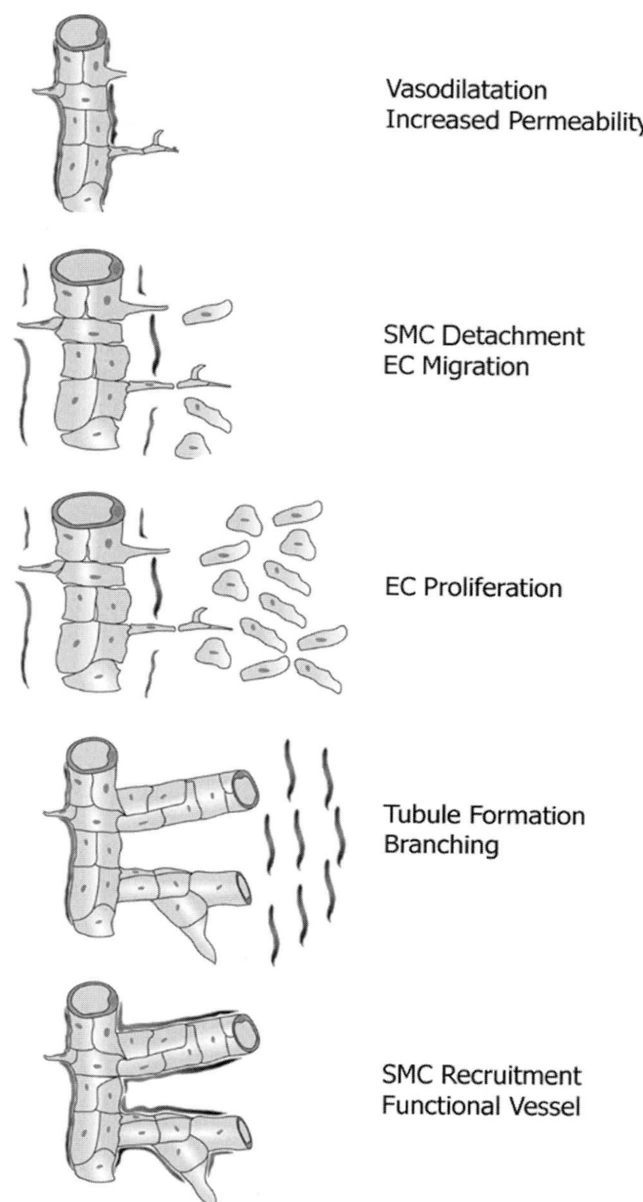

FIGURE 27–1 Mechanisms implicated in the angiogenic process. SMC = smooth muscle cell; EC = endothelial cell.

Spontaneous Angiogenesis in Adult Tissues

While vasculogenesis may not significantly contribute to increasing the vascularity of adult tissues under ischemic or inflammatory conditions, the spontaneous occurrence of both arteriogenesis and angiogenesis has been demonstrated in animals models and humans under a variety of stresses that include wound healing and inflammation,[20] peripheral vascular disease, chronic coronary insufficiency,[21,22] and acute myocardial ischemia.[23–28]

Spontaneous angiogenesis may be enhanced by a number of commonly encountered substances. Nicotine, for instance, is proangiogenic and may worsen atherosclerotic plaques by promoting intimal proliferation.[29,30] Moderate ethanol concentrations and low-dose statins also have proangiogenic properties, and the use of statins has been associated with increased tissue perfusion in a hindlimb ischemia model.[31,32] Adenosine and heparin appear to stimulate angiogenesis in the presence of ischemia. In a trial of

TABLE 27–2 Substances involved in the angiogenic process (partial listing)

	Function
Nitric oxide	Vasodilation; cofactor for VEGFs, FGFs, and other angiogens (?)
Vascular endothelial growth factors	Vasodilation; increased permeability; sequestration of VE-cadherin and PECAM-1; endothelial cell proliferation; formation of cords and lumens
Fibroblast growth factors	Endothelial cell proliferation; formation of cords and lumens (?); recruitment of inflammatory cells, pericytes, and smooth muscle cells; vessel maturation and enlargement (?)
Angiopoietin-1	Prevention of excessive vascular permeability; endothelial cell chemotaxis; formation of cords and lumens; vessel stabilization via smooth muscle to endothelial cell interactions
Angiopoietin-2	Vessel destabilization; detachment of smooth muscle cells; degradation of extracellular matrix (in conjunction with matrix metalloproteinases)
Platelet-derived growth factors	Chemotaxis/recruitment of pericytes and smooth muscle cells; branching of nascent rudimentary vessels
Cyclooxygenase-2	Vasodilation; stimulation of angiogenesis

FGF = fibroblast growth factor; PECAM = platelet endothelial cell adhesion molecule; VE = vascular endothelial; VEGF = vascular endothelial growth factor.

IV adenosine and heparin administered daily for 10 days in patients with chronic stable angina, a 9% reduction in the extent and a 14% improvement in the severity of perfusion defects was noted on exercise thallium imaging in patients who received adenosine and heparin versus those who received placebo.[33]

A number of commonly used medications have been shown to potentially interfere with the angiogenic process. These include captopril,[34] isosorbide dinitrate,[35] furosemide,[36] spironolactone,[37] as well as ASA and other anti-inflammatory drugs whose antiangiogenic effects relate to the inhibition of COX-2, the inducible isoform of cyclooxygenase.[38,39]

Growth Factors and Delivery Strategies

Despite the complexity of the angiogenic process, therapeutic angiogenesis regimens have mainly focused on the administration of a single growth factor, with select isoforms of VEGF-A ($VEGF_{121}$, $VEGF_{165}$) and FGF (FGF-1, FGF-2) having been most extensively studied.[40] Delivery strategies may involve the actual angiogenic protein or the gene encoding for it; while proteins are administered directly, gene-based approaches usually employ naked plasmid DNA or a viral vector that encodes the gene to be incorporated by the host endothelial cells. Several routes of administration have been developed to deliver angiogenic substances to the ischemic myocardium in a single or repeated fashion, and include intravenous, intracoronary, left atrial, surgical perivascular, intrapericardial (via a catheter placed under echo guidance), and catheter-based intramyocardial approaches. Table 27-3 outlines the relative advantages and disadvantages of protein- versus gene-based approaches.

Gene Delivery Vectors

Gene-based approaches require vectors in order to incorporate an angiogenic gene into a target host cell and induce production of the encoded protein. Although naked plasmid DNA can be used for these purposes, its efficiency is limited by the small fraction of plasmid DNA that actually enters the cell nucleus.[41] The use of adenoviruses as vectors is associated with much higher transfection efficiency, and these viruses can be readily produced as replication-deficient mutants for gene transfer applications. However, elevated titers of circulating antibodies to adenoviruses are common in the

TABLE 27–3 Protein vs. gene therapy for therapeutic angiogenesis

	Protein therapy	Gene therapy
Duration of expression	+ (++ if sustained-release)	++
Regulation of expression	+++	+
Dose-response	Defined	Unpredictable
Choice of delivery routes	+++	+++
Inflammatory reaction	+	+++
Potential for multiagent and repeated administration	++	+

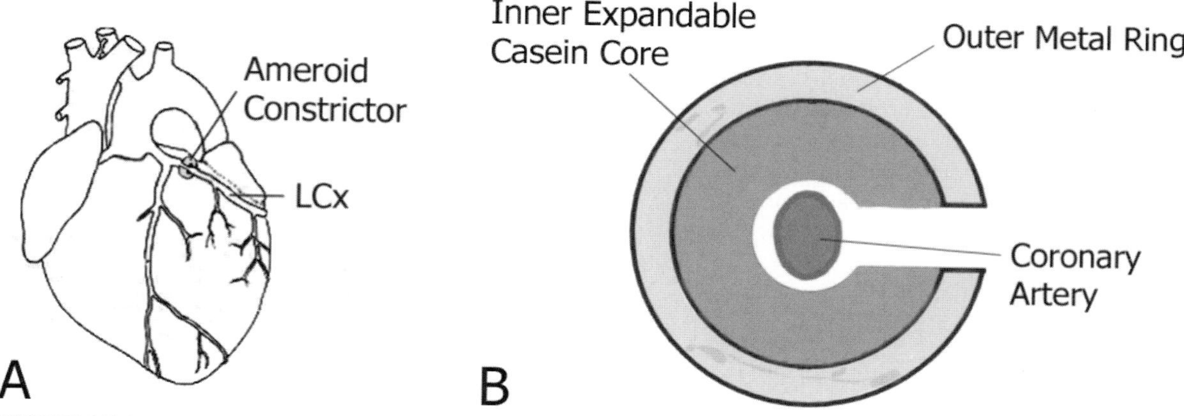

FIGURE 27–2 Ameroid constrictor model of chronic myocardial ischemia. (A) The ameroid is surgically inserted around the proximal left circumplex artery (LCx). (B) Expansion of the inner casein core is limited by the outer metal ring, resulting in progressive occlusion of the vessel.

general population and can elicit an inflammatory response that may compromise the incorporation and expression of the gene.[42] Alternatives have therefore been developed that include adeno-associated viruses, which are unique in their ability to transduce nondividing cells (thereby allowing for a more prolonged transgene expression), and retroviral vectors.[41] Retroviruses differ from plasmid and other viral vectors in that their RNA is reverse transcribed to DNA and integrated into the host cell genome. While this induces long-lasting expression of the incorporated gene, it also raises legitimate safety concerns linked to potentially deleterious overexpression.[10] In an attempt to increase the efficacy and safety profile of gene delivery vectors, several laboratories are now focusing on the development of viral vectors that would allow for up- or downregulation of the gene of interest.

Preclinical Studies

AMEROID CONSTRICTOR MODEL OF CHRONIC MYOCARDIAL ISCHEMIA

A large animal model of chronic myocardial ischemia constitutes one of the requirements for the preclinical evaluation of direct revascularization modalities such as therapeutic angiogenesis. Since laboratory animals do not spontaneously develop CAD, some intervention that leads to coronary insufficiency must be performed. Vessel embolization, surgical ligation, or thrombogenic copper coil implantation results in acute coronary occlusion and myocardial infarction; although a chronic ischemic area exists at the border zone of this infarct, it does not adequately model the ischemic myocardial territory of patients with severe angina.

A collateral-dependent, chronically ischemic myocardial territory with minimal infarction can be created with the surgical implantation and intermittent inflation of an external pneumatic coronary occluder,[43,44] or by inserting an ameroid constrictor around a major coronary artery (usually the proximal left circumflex).[45] The ameroid method results in progressive stenosis and occlusion of the encircled vessel over a period of 2 to 4 weeks (Fig. 27-2A). The constrictor consists of hygroscopic compressed casein made into a cylindrical shape and enclosed within a stainless steel collar; when in contact with fluid, the casein expands in an inward radial direction as a result of the fixed metal ring and occludes the artery (Fig. 27-2B). Ameroid constrictors have been used clinically to produce gradual occlusion of the portal vein in conjunction with hepatic artery ligation for the palliation of unresectable hepatic tumors in children.[46]

Pigs are an ideal model for the study of chronic myocardial ischemia due to their relatively few native collateral vessels (unlike dogs, which have an extensively interconnected coronary network) and their lack of propensity to develop normal perfusion to the collateral-dependent myocardium induced by the placement of an ameroid constrictor. Even so, swine mount an endogenous angiogenic response to chronic myocardial ischemia that results in increased intercoronary collateral flow, and which mandates for the use of ischemic controls in preclinical studies.[47,48] Compared to normal vessels, these collaterals have less medial smooth muscle, impaired endothelial-mediated vasodilatation, and altered endothelium-independent relaxation properties.[48,49]

STUDIES WITH VASCULAR ENDOTHELIAL GROWTH FACTOR

Preclinical experience with VEGF has mainly involved its $VEGF_{165}$ and $VEGF_{121}$ isoforms derived from alternative splicing of the VEGF-A gene. Both protein- and gene-based approaches have been employed, and success has been observed using either modality in limb ischemia models as well as in the setting of myocardial ischemia.[50–57] For instance, 2 μg of VEGF were administered perivascularly over 4 weeks to swine whose lateral myocardial territory had been rendered ischemic by a circumflex ameroid occluder.[52] Treated animals developed higher coronary flow and a 4-fold increase in capillary density of the collateral-dependent myocardium when compared with controls; furthermore, a decrease in the size of the ischemic zone was demonstrated on magnetic resonance imaging.[55]

The use of intracoronary or intrapericardial routes for the administration of VEGF has not consistently led to similar preclinical success. In dog studies, a 28-day course of intracoronary VEGF injections was effective in increasing flow to the collateral-dependent territory above that of controls,[57] but a 7-day course did not produce any effect and actually exacerbated neointimal accumulation following endothelial injury.[58] In another study, the same authors reported that while injection of an adenoviral vector encoding for $VEGF_{165}$ through an indwelling pericardial catheter resulted in sustained pericardial transgene expression, no increase in perfusion of the collateral-dependent territory could be demonstrated.[59]

STUDIES WITH FIBROBLAST GROWTH FACTOR

Like VEGF, several isoforms of fibroblast growth factor exist, of which FGF-1 and FGF-2 have been the most studied. Both FGFs are believed to induce angiogenesis as well as arteriogenesis by stimulating the growth of a variety of cell types, including vascular smooth muscle cells and endothelial cells.[13]

FGF-1 is strongly expressed in ischemic myocardium and may play a key role in the spontaneous formation of collaterals.[60] Its initial use to stimulate angiogenesis in large animals produced disappointing results that were perhaps due to the instability of wild-type FGF-1, which has a biologic half-life of 15 min at 37°C.[61–63] Following recognition that heparin binding and the replacement of a single cysteine residue with a serine increased the half-life of FGF-1 1000-fold,[63] perivascular administration of its S^{117} mutant form was studied in a porcine ameroid model and resulted in improvements of collateral-dependent myocardial blood flow and left ventricular function.[64]

FGF-2 has been extensively studied in canine and porcine models of myocardial ischemia using a variety of delivery strategies. Unger et al gave daily intracoronary bolus injections of 110 μg of FGF-2 in the distal circumflex artery of dogs starting 10 days after placement of an ameroid constrictor and continuing for 28 days.[65] The transmural collateral flow in FGF-2-treated dogs significantly exceeded that of controls by the second week of treatment and was associated with an increase in the density of distribution ($>20\ \mu$m) vessels. These investigators also conducted chronic studies with daily left atrial injections of FGF-2 for up to 13 weeks, in which the maximum effect attributable to the growth factor was temporally related to the presence of myocardial ischemia.[66] In these prolonged studies, chronic FGF-2 therapy was not associated with the occurrence of any structural or vasoproliferative adverse effect for up to 6 months after treatment initiation.[66]

Local perivascular administration of FGF-2 using 10 sustained-release heparin-alginate capsules that each contained 1 or 10 μg of FGF-2 was studied in swine, and was associated with increased perfusion of the collateral-dependent territory and a dose-dependent improvement in left ventricular ejection fraction both at rest and during pacing.[67–69] Furthermore, perivascular FGF-2 administration resulted in normalization of ischemia-induced impairments of endothelial-dependent vasodilatation in the collateral-dependent territory.[70] Single-dose intrapericardial and intracoronary delivery of FGF-2 were also studied and led to comparable perfusion and contractility improvements; however, single-dose intravenous infusion was not effective.[71,72]

The myocardial and tissue distribution of I^{125} labeled FGF-2 after intracoronary and intravenous administration in swine were studied with organ autoradiography.[73] The liver accounted for the majority of I^{125}-labeled FGF-2 activity at 1 hour after injection with either route; total cardiac-specific activity at 1 hour was 0.88% for intracoronary and 0.26% for intravenous administration, and further decreased to 0.05% and 0.04% at 24 hours, respectively (Fig. 27-3A). In another study, the distribution of intravenous injections of FGF-2 was compared with that of perivascular sustained-release delivery.[74] The amount of FGF-2 deposited in arteries adjacent to sustained-release devices was 40 times that deposited in animals who received a single intravenous bolus of FGF-2 (Fig. 27-3B). FGF-2 was also 5- to 30-fold more abundant in the kidney, liver, and spleen after intravenous injection than following perivascular release, supporting perivascular delivery as being far more efficient and specific than intravenous delivery at achieving local deposition of FGF-2.

SAFETY PROFILE

Although overexpression of VEGF in mice has been associated with the formation of angiomas and vascular tumors,[75,76] the occurrence of these adverse events or of proliferative retinopathy has not been reported in any study of growth factor therapy that has involved large animals. Most of these studies were of short-term duration, however, and may not have involved a sufficient number of animals to detect a rare occurrence of these events.

VEGF and FGF-2 are known to be associated with systemic hypotension that occurs in a dose-dependent fashion; in this regard, the doses of FGF-2 leading to hypotension are substantially higher than for VEGF.[77,78] FGF-2 has also been associated with proliferative membranous nephropathy leading to proteinuria in mice, but this has not been observed in preclinical or clinical studies.[79,80]

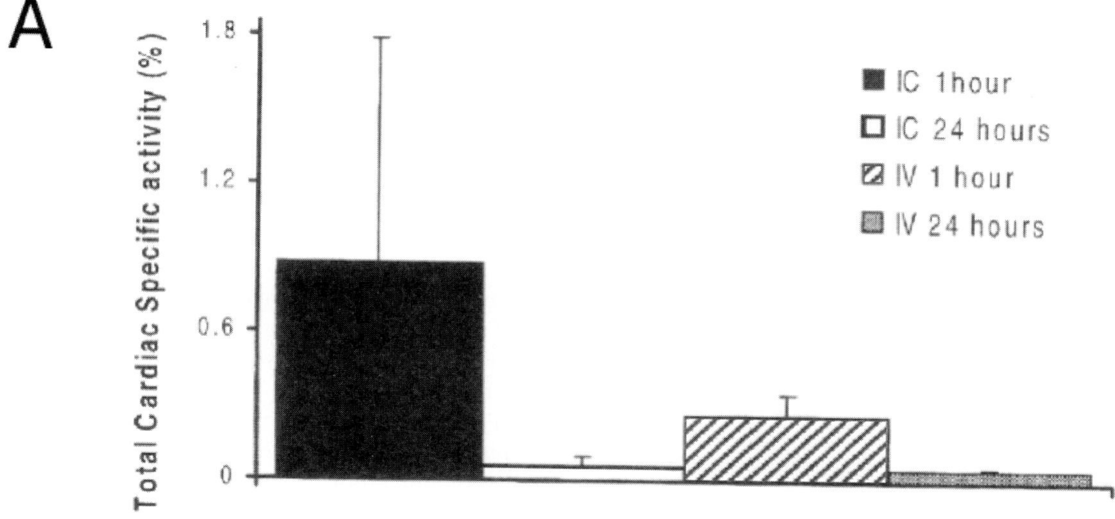

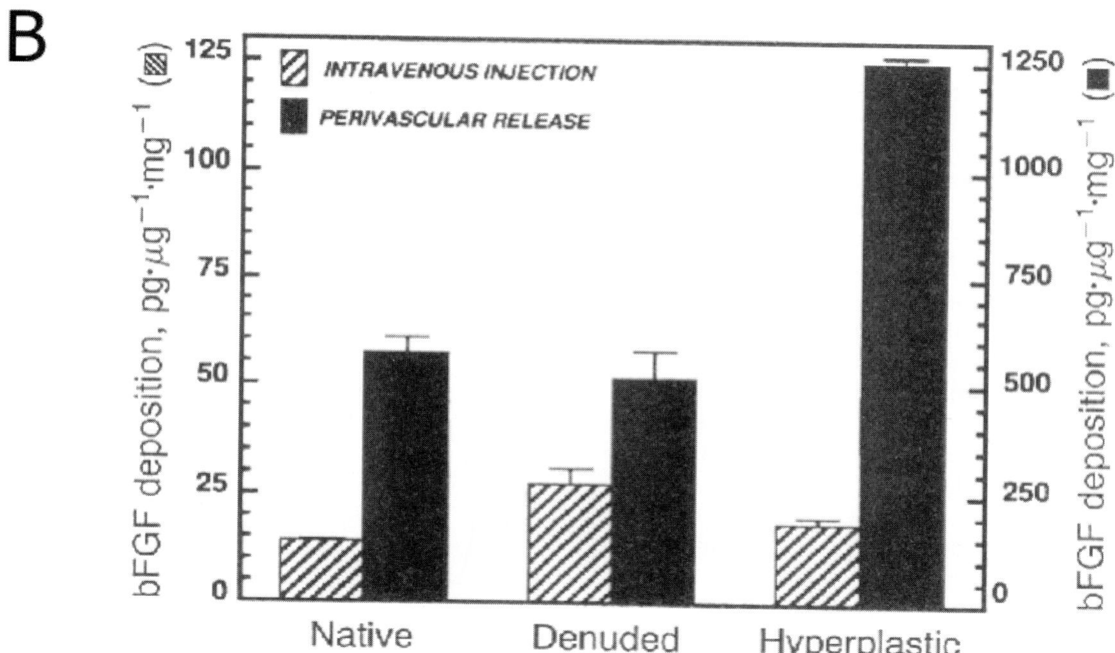

FIGURE 27–3 Tissue deposition after intravenous (IV), intracoronary (IC), and perivascular (using heparin-alginate sustained released capsules) administration of FGF-2. (A) Total cardiac specific activity after IC and IV injection of 25-μg Ci of I^{125}-FGF-2 in swine. Total specific cardiac activity with either method was less than 1% at 1 hour and 0.1% at 24 hours, with the liver accounting for most of the I^{125}-FGF-2 activity. (*Reproduced with permission from Laham RJ, Rezaee M, Post M, et al: Intracoronary and intravenous administration of basic fibroblast growth factor: myocardial and tissue distribution. Drug Metab Dispos 1999; 27:821.*) (B) Tissue deposition after a single intravenous injection versus perivascular administration of FGF-2 in intact carotid arteries ("native"), in arteries whose endothelium was denuded, and in arteries allowed to develop intimal hyperplasia 2 weeks after endothelial denudation. Deposition of FGF-2 was substantially lower with IV injection than with perivascular release for native arteries (factor of 40.0 less), denuded arteries (factor of 18.9 less), and hyperplastic arteries (factor of 67.1 less). bFGF = FGF-2. (*Reproduced with permission from Edelman ER, Nugent MA, Karnovsky MJ: Perivascular and intravenous administration of basic fibroblast growth factor: vascular and solid organ deposition. Proc Natl Acad Sci U S A 1993; 90:1513.*)

TABLE 27–4 Potential indications and contraindications to angiogenic therapy

Potential indications	Contraindications
Chronic stable angina in the presence of ungraftable CAD in a major coronary distribution, with:	Malignancy within past 5 years
Documentation of ischemia in the ungraftable territory	Vascular proliferative lesions: Diabetic retinopathy; Arteriovenous malformations; Hemangiomas
Evidence of ungraftability, such as previous failed attempts at PTCA and CABG	LVEF <30 %
Presence of viable myocardium in the ungraftable territory	Chronically low BP
	Impaired renal function (FGF-2)

Indications and Surgical Technique

INDICATIONS FOR ANGIOGENIC THERAPY

Table 27-4 outlines the current potential indications and contraindications to angiogenic therapy. As of this writing, the clinical effectiveness of this modality has not yet been proven. Therapeutic angiogenesis should therefore be considered experimental and reserved only for patients who have failed or are not amenable to conventional revascularization procedures.

Patients considered for therapeutic angiogenesis should have persistent, severe chronic stable angina imputed to a myocardial territory that can not adequately or safely be revascularized by conventional methods.[81] Dobutamine-stress echocardiography or nuclear imaging to confirm ischemia and viability in the target territory is recommended. Since therapeutic angiogenesis implies a slow course of new vessel development, it should not be employed to attempt emergency revascularization or salvage of threatened proximal coronary occlusion.[10]

Absolute contraindications to the administration of angiogenic growth factors include a history of malignancy within the last 5 years, with the exception of basal or early-stage squamous skin cancers that are considered cured. Therapeutic angiogenesis should not be carried out in patients with proliferative retinopathy, vascular malformations, and chronically low blood pressure. In addition, FGF-2 is contraindicated in patients with decreased creatinine clearance or proteinuria. Severely compromised left ventricular ejection fraction constitutes a relative contraindication to angiogenic therapy, since most delivery techniques involve procedural stress that could precipitate cardiac decompensation.

TECHNIQUE OF SURGICAL PERIVASCULAR IMPLANTATION

The surgical perivascular implantation of angiogenic growth factors can be performed in conjunction with CABG or as sole therapy.[82,83] Both strategies are amenable to the use of minimally invasive approaches in combination with multivessel off-pump CABG, ipsi- or contralateral minimally invasive direct coronary artery bypass (MIDCAB), or as sole therapy (through a subxiphoid or small thoracotomy incision). In the future, the safe implantation of angiogenic growth factors via a closed-chest, videoscopic approach may constitute an ideal method of delivery.

Although a surgical approach can be used for the administration of virtually any type of angiogenic protein or gene vector, most of the experience has involved the perivascular delivery of FGF-2 protein using sustained-release beads implanted at the time of CABG (Fig. 27-4).[81,82,84] Controlled release of the FGF-2 is derived from its avidity for heparin, which is bound to sepharose beads and hardened into a capsule using a calcium chloride–alginate solution, without causing any substantial reduction in the biological activity of the growth factor.[67,74,85] Once implanted, release of FGF-2 from the polymer occurs via first-order kinetics over a 4- to 5-week period, without any inflammatory reaction resulting from polymer placement.

The perivascular implantation of FGF-2 using this delivery system in conjunction with CABG has been carried out through a median sternotomy.[82,84] After the institution of total cardiopulmonary bypass and cardioplegic arrest, distal coronary anastomoses were performed to graftable coronaries and the nongraftability of the target territory was confirmed by direct inspection of the vessel. Multiple linear incisions were made in the epicardial fat surrounding the

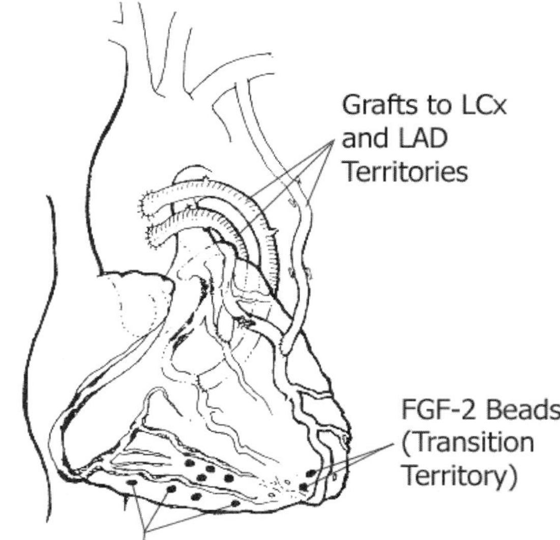

FIGURE 27–4 Implantation of sustained-release FGF-2 beads in the myocardial distribution of an ungraftable right coronary artery, in conjunction with CABG. PDA = posterior descending artery; LVB = left ventricular branches of the right coronary artery. (*Adapted with permission from Sellke FW, Laham RJ, Edelman ER, et al: Therapeutic angiogenesis with basic fibroblast growth factor: technique and early results. Ann Thorac Surg 1998; 65:15.*)

ungraftable vessel and in the transition zone between the target territory and that supplied by a grafted or patent coronary artery in order to enable the development of subepicardial collaterals between ischemic and normally perfused myocardium. Ten heparin-alginate beads, each containing 1 or 10 μg of human recombinant FGF-2, were inserted in the subepicardium and secured in place with a 6-0 polypropylene suture, with up to 3 beads being placed in a single incision. Proximal anastomoses were then constructed, the patient separated from cardiopulmonary bypass, and routine closure performed. As a quality control measure, 2 to 6 heparin-alginate beads from each batch were cultured aerobically and anaerobically to ensure sterility.

Clinical Studies

PROTEIN THERAPY

Perivascular delivery The safety of surgical FGF-1 administration was demonstrated in a series of 20 patients conducted by Schumacher et al, who injected 0.01 mg/kg of FGF-1 directly into the myocardium along a diffusely diseased left anterior descending (LAD) coronary artery to which the left internal thoracic artery (LITA) was also grafted.[86,87] Patients were followed up 12 weeks and 3 years later, when the LITA was selectively injected and the degree of anterior myocardial collateralization quantitatively evaluated by digital subtraction angiography. Although a local increase in collateral blush was observed along the LAD, the investigators did not report nuclear imaging assessments of ischemia or functional parameters such as exercise capacity, CCS angina class, or freedom from angina recurrence.

The safety and efficacy of perivascular FGF-2 administration was evaluated in a phase I, double-blind, randomized controlled trial that involved 24 patients concomitantly undergoing CABG.[84] In this study, patients in whom high-dose FGF-2 sustained-release capsules had been implanted in an ungraftable territory at the time of CABG had complete relief from angina and showed significant improvements in stress nuclear perfusion defect size at 3-month follow-up. These patients were subsequently followed up to a mean of 32 months postoperatively with clinical assessment and nuclear imaging.[81] At this late follow-up, patients treated with either dose of FGF-2 had experienced significantly greater freedom from angina recurrence than controls (Fig. 27-5). Double-blinded late nuclear imaging studies revealed that all but one patient in the control group had either persistence of a reversible perfusion defect or evidence of a new fixed defect in the ungraftable myocardial territory; in contrast, this was observed in only 1 of 9 patients treated with FGF-2

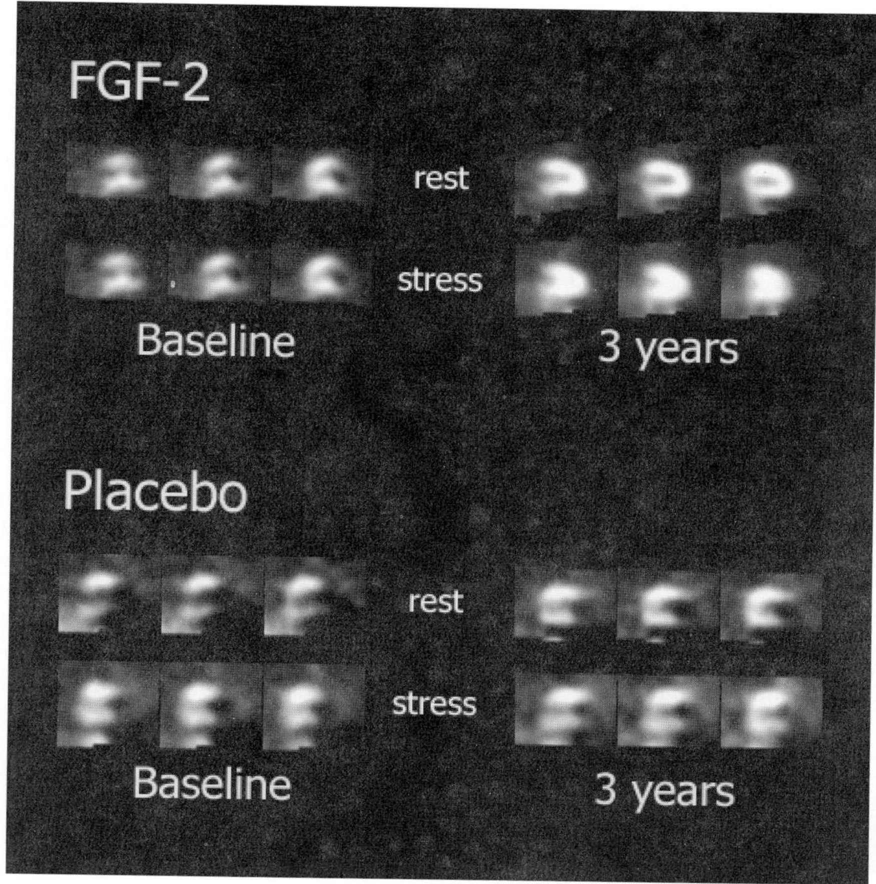

FIGURE 27–5 Baseline and 3 years postoperative SPECT images of patients who received FGF-2 versus placebo beads implanted in an ungraftable inferoapical myocardial territory at the time of CABG.[81] Horizontal long-axis views show complete resolution of the large inferoapical perfusion defect at rest and stress in the patient who received FGF-2, and no detectable change from baseline in the patient who received placebo.

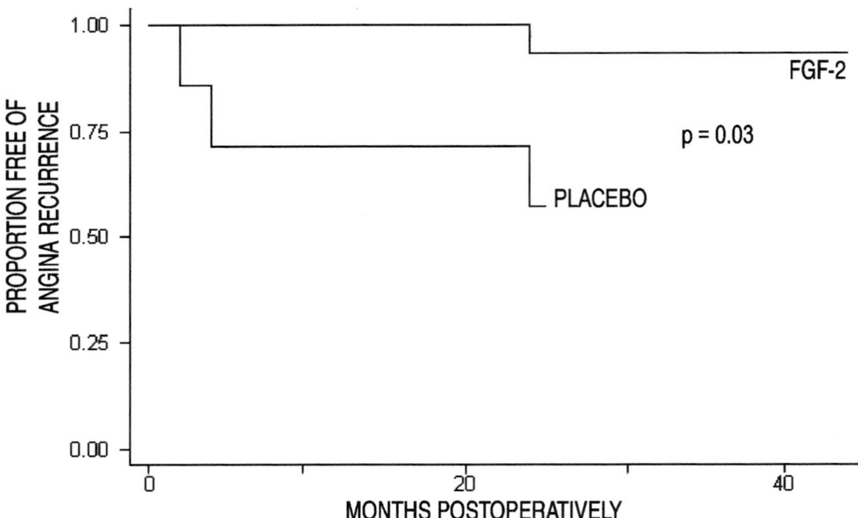

FIGURE 27–6 Freedom from angina in patients who underwent implantation of FGF-2 versus placebo in a major, nongraftable myocardial territory at the time of CABG. (*Reproduced with permission from Ruel M, Laham RJ, Parker JA, et al: Long-term effects of surgical angiogenic therapy with FGF-2 protein. J Thorac Cardiovasc Surg 2002; 124:28.*)

(Fig. 27-6). The remaining FGF-treated patients had disappearance of their ungraftable territory reversible perfusion defect and stability or decrease in the size of their fixed defect. FGF-treated patients also showed better late global left ventricular perfusion scores during pharmacologic stress.[81] Although this study only involved a small number of patients and may have been confounded by concomitant CABG, it nevertheless suggested that perivascular FGF-2 therapy may be associated with persistent freedom from angina recurrence and sustained improvements in left ventricular perfusion.

Intravascular delivery Laham et al conducted a phase I, open-label dose-escalation trial that evaluated the efficacy and safety of a single-bolus intracoronary administration of FGF-2 in 52 patients. Their results suggested that this therapy may improve symptoms and myocardial perfusion.[88] These investigators proceeded with a multicenter, randomized, double-blind, placebo-controlled trial of a single intracoronary infusion of FGF-2 at 0, 0.3, 3, or 30 μg/kg in 337 patients (FGF-2 Initiating Revascularization Support [FIRST]trial).[89] Efficacy was evaluated at 90 and 180 days by exercise tolerance test, nuclear perfusion imaging, and angina questionnaire. Exercise tolerance was increased at 90 days in all groups but was not significantly different between placebo and FGF-treated groups. FGF-2 reduced angina symptoms, and these differences were more pronounced in highly symptomatic patients with baseline CCS angina class scores of III or IV. However, this benefit did not persist at 180 days because of continued improvement in the placebo group, and the trial was considered negative with respect to all main end points. Adverse events were similar across all groups, except for hypotension, which occurred more frequently in the 30-μg/kg FGF-2 group.

Intravenous and intracoronary administration of VEGF was studied in a randomized, double-blind, phase II trial (VEGF in Ischemia for Vascular Angiogenesis [VIVA]trial), which was also completely negative with respect to symptom improvement, exercise time, and nuclear imaging end points.[90] It is possible that the effects of FGF-2 and VEGF in the FIRST and VIVA trials may have been compromised by the choice of intravascular delivery routes, which not only are nonspecific in their tissue distribution, but also carry the potential to worsen atherosclerosis.[30]

GENE THERAPY

Perivascular delivery Rosengart et al have examined the effects of direct administration of an adenoviral vector encoding for $VEGF_{121}$, either as an adjunct to conventional CABG (in 15 patients) or as sole therapy (in 6 patients).[83] There was no control group and the principal end points of this phase I trial were related to safety. In this regard, no systemic or cardiac-related adverse events related to vector administration were observed. All patients reported improvements in angina class, and postoperative nuclear imaging suggested increased contractility during stress conditions in the area of vector administration, but did not reveal an increase in myocardial perfusion.

Losordo et al initiated a small phase 1 trial to determine the safety and bioactivity of direct myocardial gene transfer (using naked plasmid DNA) of $VEGF_{165}$ as the sole therapy in 5 patients with inoperable CAD and symptomatic myocardial ischemia.[91] The vector was administered by four 2.0-mL needle injections into the anterolateral left ventricular free wall through a small left anterolateral thoracotomy. The injections were not associated with any side effect other than isolated premature ventricular complexes at the time of needle penetration. All patients had a significant reduction in angina as measured by nitroglycerin use, improved collateral scores on angiography, and reduced size of the ischemic defect on dobutamine nuclear imaging. These data were reproduced in another open-label, uncontrolled study in which 20 patients received either 125 or 250 μg of naked plasmid $VEGF_{121}$ injected directly into the myocardium via a minimally invasive thoracotomy.[92] Plasma VEGF concentrations increased at 14 days to a level 2-fold over pretreatment values and returned to baseline by 3 months. As in the previous study, patients reported decreased angina and reduced nitroglycerine use, and improvement was seen on radionuclide perfusion imaging.[92]

Catheter-based delivery A pilot study of catheter-based myocardial gene transfer involved 6 patients with chronic myocardial ischemia who were randomized to receive 200 μg of VEGF-2 or placebo.[93] A steerable, deflectable 8F catheter incorporating a 27-gauge needle was advanced percutaneously and guided into the left ventricular myocardium by left ventricular electromechanical mapping. Despite the small number of patients, end points of angina frequency, nitroglycerin consumption, and stress myocardial perfusion on nuclear imaging showed a trend in favor of the group of subjects transfected with VEGF-2 versus controls. These trends were confirmed by the same group of investigators in a subsequent phase 1/2 trial involving 19 patients.[93a]

Efficacy Issues

CHOICE OF DELIVERY ROUTES

From the evidence currently available, perivascular administration of angiogenic proteins may arguably constitute the route of choice for angiogenic therapy, since it presents a more specific tissue distribution profile than intravascular techniques, does not result in rapid washout, is not limited by the endothelial barrier, and does not carry the potential of exacerbating intimal plaques. Protein administration also offers safety advantages over gene-based approaches, and may be delivered perivascularly using a sustained-delivery system without provoking an inflammatory response.[10,82,84] Although a surgical approach is required, it allows for the precise placement of beads within the ischemic territory as well as at the transition between normally perfused and collateral-dependent myocardium, thereby promoting the formation of subepicardial collaterals that may provide arterial inflow to the ischemic zone. Overall, these properties may account for the greater efficacy of perivascular over intravascular approaches in preclinical and clinical studies,[81,84] which in our opinion makes it the currently preferred route for angiogenic therapy (in patients with end-stage CAD who have no alternative treatment option).

No tangible evidence currently exists that clearly supports the clinical efficacy of myocardial gene transfer modalities. Furthermore, these approaches have fallen into public and scientific disfavor following the highly publicized deaths of an 18-year-old patient and other subjects enrolled in gene transfer angiogenesis studies.[94] At the present time, gene-based approaches should only be used in an experimental and closely regulated setting until further safety and efficacy data are available.

ROLE OF NO IN ANGIOGENESIS

There is an interaction between the local availability of NO and the regulation of blood vessel growth mediated by the actions of VEGF and to a lesser extent FGF-2.[95–98] Diminished NO availability has been implicated in the inhibition of spontaneous and exogenous angiogenic responses in hypercholesterolemic rodents,[99,100] and recently in preclinical, large-animal models of hypercholesterolemia-induced endothelial dysfunction (Ruel M, Sellke FW: submitted data). Given these data and the fact that therapeutic angiogenesis is not nearly as effective in patients with inoperable CAD as it has been in laboratory animals, the failure of effect observed in clinical trials may relate to a deficiency in the stimulated release of NO, whose production as well as that of other endothelium-derived substances is altered in advanced CAD. The current clinical indications for angiogenic therapy may therefore paradoxically target a subgroup of patients for whom the modality therapy is least likely to work, and it is plausible that the clinical efficacy of therapeutic angiogenesis may depend on the concomitant modulation of the coronary microvascular endothelium in patients with end-stage CAD. Research aimed at elucidating these questions is ongoing and may help clarify the missing link between successful animal models and disappointing clinical trials of angiogenic therapy.

MULTIAGENT THERAPY AND MASTER-SWITCH GENES

Although the physiological events that result in angiogenesis are incompletely understood and likely of formidable complexity, therapeutic approaches so far have mostly concentrated on the administration of a single growth factor. While this strategy was made necessary by safety considerations and limited knowledge of potential interactions between growth factors, it is debatable whether it will ever result in clinically reproducible de novo formation of functionally competent vessels.[40] Alternatively, the safety and efficacy of therapeutic approaches could be increased by stimulating *endogenous* angiogenesis in response to ischemia or by using combinations of exogenous growth factors. For instance, the experimental stimulation of endogenous angiogenesis without administration of exogenous growth factors was recently achieved by modulating the proangiogenic properties of the gastric submucosa in order to accomplish myocardial revascularization in a swine model of chronic ischemia (Fig. 27-7).[101]

A developing alternative is the use of angiogenesis master-switch genes, which are capable of inducing whole cascades of angiogenesis-related genes.[40] These master-switch genes are physiologically induced by ischemia and mediate

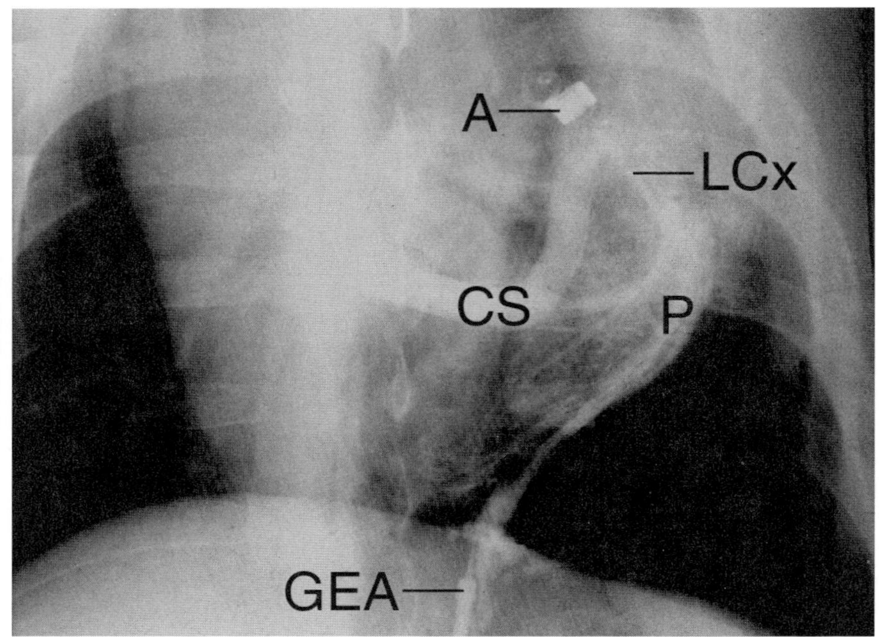

FIGURE 27–7 Gastroepiploic (GEA) arteriogram of a swine with chronic myocardial ischemia 7 weeks after apposition of a pedicled gastric submucosal patch. Patch contour (P), circumflex artery reconstitution (LCx) and occlusion at the ameroid constrictor (A) level, and drainage of contrast via the coronary sinus (CS) are seen.[101] The rationale for this model was to evaluate whether endogenous angiogenesis could be stimulated without the need for growth factors. (*Reproduced with permission from Ruel M, Sellke FW, Bianchi C, et al: Endogenous myocardial angiogenesis and revascularization using a gastric submucosal patch. Ann Thorac Surg (in press).*)

the endogenous angiogenic responses of animals and humans.[28,102] One example is hypoxia-induced factor (HIF)-1α, a gene expressed in tissues subjected to ischemia, which initiates the cascade of VEGF-dependent angiogenesis.[40] PR39 and relaxin are two other master-switch genes that have the propensity to induce both VEGF and FGF systems.[40,103–105] However, the therapeutic use of exogenous master-switch genes may potentially lead to excessive, uncontrolled angiogenesis by upregulating hundreds of proangiogenic genes. Their use should therefore be restricted until they are better understood and their tissue distribution reliably confined to a predetermined myocardial territory.

TRANSMYOCARDIAL LASER REVASCULARIZATION

History

The notion of achieving myocardial revascularization by directly creating channels into the myocardium dates back more than half a century. Arthur Vineberg had long suggested that some application of this concept could result in the alleviation of angina[106] when Sen et al, after studying the reptilian heart, reported in 1965 on the experimental use of "transmyocardial acupuncture" for myocardial revascularization.[107,108] Hershey and White demonstrated that multiple myocardial punctures with an 18-gauge needle could allow for chronic survival in dogs after total excision of the LAD, as well as following ameroid occlusion of all 3 coronary arteries.[109–112] Nevertheless, the interpretation of these experimental data was already controversial and the concept termed "a physiologic impossibility" as early as 1969.[113]

The limited success of these procedures was overshadowed by the invention and widespread popularity of CABG until interest in them was revived in 1981 by Mirhoseini,[114] who used a 450-W carbon dioxide laser to revascularize the hypokinetic anterior wall of a patient with a nongraftable LAD in conjunction with the construction of bypass grafts to other territories.[115,116] Still, interest in transmyocardial laser revascularization (TMR) did not rise until 1995, largely catalyzed by the work of Frazier and Cooley.[117] These authors reported promising preliminary results on 21 patients in whom TMR had been used as sole therapy, which suggested that this modality may improve anginal status, endocardial perfusion as measured by photon emission tomography (PET), and regional contractile function during stress. Following subsequent phase I studies, the FDA approved TMR as a therapy for angina in the presence of ungraftable coronary disease in 1998.[118]

Types of Lasers

Although historically involving mechanical needle punctures,[107,108] TMR has since used lasers to create a series of 1-mm channels placed approximately 1 cm apart in the myocardial territory to be lased. Three main types of lasers exist: carbon dioxide (CO_2), holmium:yttrium-aluminum garnet (YAG) and xenon-chloride (excimer).[119–122] The key characteristics of these lasers are outlined in Table 27-5. Regardless of the type of laser, the end result is generally the creation of a channel approximately 1 mm in diameter, surrounded by a 1- to 2-mm rim of necrosis and a 1- to 3-mm

TABLE 27–5 Main types of lasers used for TMR

	CO_2	Holmium:YAG	Xe:CI (Excimer)
Spectrum	Infrared	Infrared	Ultraviolet
Energy level	High	Low	Low
No. pulses/channel	Usually 1	6-8	6-8
Mechanics	Continuous thermal	Pulsed thermal	Continuous cold
Thermal injury	++	+++	+
Fiberoptic	No	Yes	Yes
R-wave sync	Yes	No	No

zone of myofibrillary degeneration in the periphery of this rim.[123] The CO_2 laser has the advantage of producing high-energy pulses that create a transmural channel with a single pulse, low peak power, and high photonic absorption that may, in comparison to other laser types, minimize structural tissue trauma. The pulse can be synchronized with the R wave of the ECG and delivered during end diastole to transect the heart within 10 to 60 milliseconds, thereby minimizing the interference with ventricular conduction. The holmium:YAG and excimer lasers are low-energy, require multiple firing for the creation of a single channel, and cannot be synchronized with the ECG; however, they have the capacity of being coupled to a fiberoptic catheter for transluminal endocardial delivery.[124] To avoid uncontrolled pericardial hemorrhage, channels created by a percutaneous approach are not transmural; it has been hypothesized that this may lead to less stimulation of subepicardial collateralization and arteriogenesis between normally perfused and collateral-dependent myocardial territories after TMR.

Mechanisms of TMR

PATENT CHANNELS

Since the initial experimental evaluation of this modality, a major matter of debate has been whether the channels created with TMR remained patent or not. Cooley reported in 1994 a patient who died of an extracardiac cause 3 months after undergoing TMR, and in whom histologic analysis revealed multiple patent channels running perpendicular to and interconnecting with the native vasculature.[125] Although reactive fibrous scar tissue had caused narrowing of the original laser tract, the channels had endothelialized and contained red blood cells, suggesting that they were functional. Amid support from other investigators[126,127] and the documentation of patent channels 2 hours after TMR,[123] this mechanism was called into question by autopsy results obtained 4 1/2 weeks after TMR, which did not show patency.[128] Canine studies with CO_2 and holmium:YAG lasers also showed that, regardless of the laser source, channels were occluded by thrombus within 6 to 24 hours, after which organization and neovascularization of the channel region occurred.[129,130] In swine studies by another group, all channels became occluded by scar within 6 weeks.[131] Furthermore, in an excised canine heart model, channels created with a CO_2 laser did not provide acute myocardial perfusion or preserve myocardial viability in the presence of acute ischemia secondary to LAD ligation.[129,130]

Subsequent histologic studies of patients who died after TMR validated these experimental findings and showed that laser-induced channels were filled with abundant granulocytes and thrombocytes, fibrinous network, clots, and detritus as early as 3 days after operation.[132] This was also documented in a report of three patients who had died 1 to 11 days following laser revascularization and in whom the internal lining surface of laser channels was not endothelialized, was composed of vacuolated and condensed myocardial debris, and was surrounded by zones of necrotic cardiomyocytes, without any obvious connections between laser channels and the ventricular cavity.[133] It is now widely recognized that the postulated long-term patency of TMR channels is a myth; in this regard, it is possible that early reports may have confused thebesian veins with the so-called ventriculo-myocardial connections that would have resulted from TMR.[134]

ANGIOGENESIS

TMR could stimulate angiogenesis by a specific mechanism or by a wound-healing response to injury.[135] In a study of TMR in swine, Hughes et al found a highly disorganized pattern of neovascularization consistent with angiogenesis located predominantly at the periphery of the channels.[136] Immunohistochemistry confirmed the presence of endothelial cells within these neovessels, and a higher vascular density was demonstrated in lased ischemic myocardium than in nonlased ischemic myocardium. Horvath et al found a 2-fold increase in VEGF mRNA expression in the ischemic territory of swine treated with TMR using a CO_2 laser versus control animals subjected to ameroid constriction of the left circumflex alone.[137] There was a 3-fold increase in the number of new blood vessels in the ischemic zone of the TMR group compared with the control group. TMR also resulted in a higher number of von Willebrand factor–positive microvessels with increased expression of matrix metalloproteinases and platelet-derived endothelial cell growth factor in dogs at 2 weeks,[138] and TMR led to a significantly greater vascular density and increased expression of FGF-2 and transforming growth factor-beta in rats.[139]

Whether this angiogenic response is specific to TMR, enhanced by the use of one specific type of laser versus another, or equivalently brought on by the mechanical (versus laser) creation of channels remains controversial. It has been found that both mechanical and laser transmyocardial revascularization lead to an increase in the expression of VEGF and FGF-2.[140,141] This was, however, contradicted by Horvath et al, who showed that only laser TMR resulted in a significant increase in new blood vessels in the ischemic zone at 6 weeks, in addition to causing less fibrosis and better preserving the contractility of the collateral-dependent zone than mechanical TMR using a hot needle, a normothermic needle, or an ultrasonic needle.[142]

DENERVATION

The denervation of cardiac sympathetic afferent fibers is another mechanism that has been proposed to explain the relief of anginal symptoms imputed to TMR. TMR with a holmium:YAG laser has been shown in dogs to result in a decreased response to the epicardial application of bradykinin and a 66% decrease in the protein expression of tyrosine hydroxylase in lased regions, consistent with a destruction of cardiac nerve fibers.[143,144] However, these findings were refuted by subsequent studies that suggested that TMR does not acutely change sympathetic or parasympathetic efferent neuronal activation in the affected ventricle either after electrical or chemical, combined with isoproterenol, stimulation.[145] Furthermore, TMR had no acute effect on reflexes mediated by left ventricular receptors with sympathetic afferent fibers after epicardial and intracoronary administration in anesthetized dogs.[146]

The chronic neural response was studied by Aurora et al, who showed that TMR made the intrinsic cardiac nervous system less responsive to chemical stimulation with nicotine, although it did not alter responses to electrical stimulation.[147] A human correlate of this finding was suggested by the report of decreased myocardial PET hydroxyephedrine uptake (a marker of sympathetic innervation) in patients treated with TMR in excess of perfusion defects.[148] Critics of the denervation theory maintain that the myocardial area treated by TMR represents less than 1% of the left ventricular mass and that denervation is unlikely to account for the alleviation of ischemia.

FIBROSIS

TMR produces fibrosis in the lased segments,[135,149] and it has been hypothesized that the resultant diastolic tethering of the left ventricle may improve wall stress characteristics, prevent further ischemia and dilatation of the ischemic segment, and promote favorable remodeling.[150] No experimental model has been used to test this hypothesis, however.

Preclinical Studies

STUDIES WITH CO_2 LASER

The use of a CO_2 laser has been championed in preclinical and clinical studies by Horvath et al. These investigators have shown in a porcine ameroid model of chronic ischemia that TMR improved myocardial perfusion and wall motion at rest.[151] These findings were supported by Hughes et al, who used a hibernating myocardium model and reported significantly improved regional stress function in the lased segments (using both CO_2 and holmium:YAG lasers) at 6 months postoperatively, consistent with a reduction in ischemia. Global left ventricular wall motion at peak stress improved as well.[152] TMR was reported to prevent necrosis and scarring and to improve myocardial function in a sheep model of acute myocardial infarction,[153] but these findings were not reproduced in other studies.[154–156] Horvath also developed a closed thoracoscopic technique for TMR that proved feasible in swine.[157]

STUDIES WITH HOLMIUM:YAG AND EXCIMER LASERS

Like the CO_2 laser, the preclinical feasibility and efficacy of these two types of lasers were demonstrated in several studies.[152,158–161] However, one report involving the holmium:YAG laser failed to show that TMR increased perfusion assessed by thermal imaging and postmortem MRI, both acutely after occlusion of the first diagonal branch in sheep, as well as 28 days later.[162] Rosengart et al reported that TMR with an excimer laser resulted in increased channel derivatives and neovascularization compared with nonlased channels while preserving normal ventricular function, and that there was a dose-response relationship with the number of channels created.[158] The feasibility of percutaneous TMR using a holmium:YAG laser in dogs was reported in 1997.[163]

COMPARISON OF LASERS

A comparison of the three main types of lasers in swine showed that the CO_2 laser synchronized with the R wave was significantly less arrhythmogenic than the Ho:YAG and excimer lasers.[164] In addition, the interaction of the CO_2 laser with porcine cardiac tissue appeared significantly less traumatic than that of the Ho:YAG and excimer lasers. Ho:YAG channels were highly irregular and were surrounded by a relatively wide ring of coagulation necrosis, which was also observed after use of the excimer laser. In contrast, the CO_2 channels were straight, well demarcated, and the zone of structural and thermal damage was smaller than with the other two types of laser. These lasers were also compared in another study, which found that only TMR performed with CO_2 and holmium:YAG lasers resulted in a significant improvement in myocardial blood flow to the lased left circumflex regions, with no increase observed in sham- or excimer-lased animals.[165] Furthermore, there was significant improvement in regional stress function on dobutamine stress echocardiography of the lased segments 6 months postoperatively in animals undergoing holmium:YAG and CO_2 laser TMR, but no change in wall motion in sham- or excimer-lased animals.

COMBINATION OF TMR AND THERAPEUTIC ANGIOGENESIS

Experience in preclinical models of TMR combined with angiogenic therapy has been mixed, with some investigators reporting an increased inflammatory response from the addition of VEGF therapy to TMR in lieu of the enhanced angiogenic response that was anticipated.[166] Yamamoto et al combined TMR and intramyocardial FGF-2 treatment (directly into the channels) in chronically ischemic dogs and found that this combination resulted in an increase in the density of large vessels (>50 μm), in keeping with the postulated arteriogenic effects of FGF-2 in ischemic tissues, but no augmentation of myocardial blood flow.[167] The combination of gene transfer vectors with TMR also produced mixed results, with one group showing that TMR enhanced the transfection efficiency of an expression plasmid encoding for VEGF at 6 weeks,[168] but another reporting impaired transgene expression of an adenoviral vector gene and increased myocardial inflammation from combination of the two therapies.[169]

Indications and Surgical Technique

INDICATIONS FOR TMR

The potential indications and contraindications to TMR are outlined in Table 27-6. As in the case of therapeutic angiogenesis, data confirming the effectiveness of TMR in double-blind, randomized controlled trials have not been produced. Although the procedure has been approved by the FDA since 1998, TMR is best considered semiexperimental and reserved for patients who have failed or are not amenable to conventional revascularization procedures.

Patients eligible for TMR should have persistent, severe chronic stable angina imputed to a myocardial territory that cannot be adequately or safely revascularized by conventional methods. Most patients have previously had CABG.[170] The procedure should not be employed to attempt emergency revascularization or salvage of threatened proximal coronary occlusion. TMR has been used for the relief of unstable angina when attempts at weaning intravenous antianginal medications have failed; intermediate results for this indication have showed a two-class improvement in angina severity in 82% of patients and a mortality of 13% to 22.4% at 1 year, but were associated with an increased in perioperative mortality compared to when the procedure is used for chronic stable angina.[171,172]

TMR has been proposed as a therapeutic adjunct for the heart transplant patient population, either as a bridge to transplant for patients with a low ejection fraction and ungraftable coronary disease,[173,174] or for the treatment of allograft vasculopathy.[175–178] Hetzer's group, in a report of 30 patients with ischemia and reduced left ventricular ejection fraction (<30%) who were treated with TMR as a sole therapy, showed that myocardial perfusion and ejection fraction did not significantly improve.[179] Survival was only 50% at 1 year, and the authors did not recommend the use of TMR for this indication. Similarly, the use of TMR for the treatment of cardiac allograft arteriosclerosis appeared feasible in initial case series,[175–178] but did not lead to any benefit 24 months after treatment.[180]

It is unknown whether redo TMR should be considered for select patients; one case performed 4 years following initially successful TMR resulted in angina class and functional improvements.[181]

TABLE 27–6 Potential indications and contraindications to TMR

Potential indications	Contraindications
Chronic stable angina in the presence of ungraftable CAD in a major coronary distribution, with:	LVEF <30 %
Evidence of ungraftability from previous failed attempts at PTCA and CABG	Emergency revascularization
Documentation of ischemia in the ungraftable territory	Bridge to transplant
	Allograft vasculopathy

TECHNIQUE OF SURGICAL TMR

Surgical TMR may be performed via a small anterolateral thoracotomy,[182] in conjunction with CABG through a sternotomy, or using a videoscopic approach. Attentive anesthetic management is crucial in order to minimize intraoperative cardiac ischemia. In this regard, particular attention should be given to the constant optimization of coronary perfusion pressure and ventricular afterload, oxygenation (in anticipation of one-lung ventilation), and potassium and magnesium levels (to prevent ventricular irritability). The monitoring of mixed venous oxygen saturation with a Swan-Ganz catheter and the assessment of regional contractility and mitral valve function with transesophageal echocardiography (TEE) are recommended; TEE is also mandated to confirm endocardial penetration by the laser beam. If intraoperative ischemia arises despite these measures and leads to hemodynamic instability, an intra-aortic balloon pump (IABP) is inserted. Postoperative pain should be managed attentively, and the use of a thoracic epidural catheter is advisable unless contraindicated by coagulopathy or heparin use.

The patient is positioned in a 45-degree right lateral decubitus position with the left arm suspended at a right angle to retract the latissimus dorsi laterally. External defibrillator

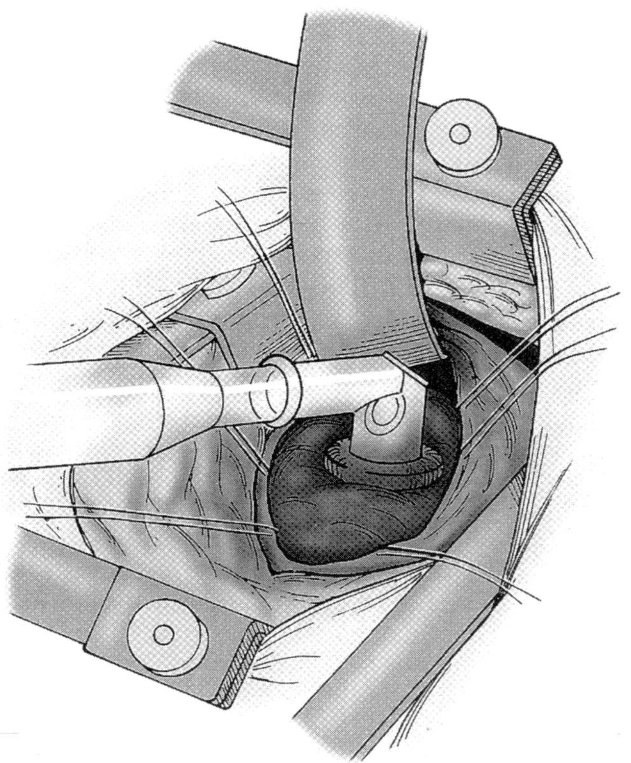

FIGURE 27–8 Exposure of the left ventricle for TMR using a CO_2 laser is obtained by progressively opening the thoracotomy incision with two small rib spreaders placed at right angle to each other and by suspending the pericardium. (*Reproduced with permission from March RJ: Laser revascularization of ischemic myocardium, in Naunheim KS (ed): Minimal Access Cardiothoracic Surgery. Philadelphia, WB Saunders, 2000.*)

pads are placed over the right chest and left shoulder. The left groin is prepared and available for the establishment of femoro-femoral cardiopulmonary bypass or the placement of an IABP. A cell-saver suction and a carbon canister smoke evacuator are installed, and the operating room personnel are provided with protective eyewear.

A 6- to 10-cm anterolateral thoracotomy is performed in the fifth intercostal space at a level over the point of maximum impulse, which brings the inferior border of the incision to the level of the diaphragm and left ventricular apex. The ribs are progressively opened with two small rib spreaders placed at right angles to each other (Fig. 27-8). Since many of these patients have previously undergone CABG, care is taken to avoid lung or internal thoracic artery pedicle injury that could result from the shearing of adhesions, as well as to avoid the manipulation of diseased saphenous vein grafts. The left lung is selectively decompressed or reduced tidal volume ventilation is used, and the pericardium is exposed and incised vertically anterior to the left phrenic nerve. The pericardium is freed and retracted laterally, and the diaphragm retracted caudally, thereby allowing for exposure of the entire free wall of the left ventricle (Fig. 27-9). Complete dissection of all epicardial adhesions is essential to prevent dimpling of the left ventricle wall, which can bring mitral valve chordae closer to the endocardial surface and make them susceptible to injury during activation of the laser (Fig. 27-10).

The laser handpiece is put against the myocardial area to be lased with care taken to avoid epicardial vessels, the anticipated location of papillary muscles (Fig. 27-11), and the indentation of the left ventricular wall. One channel is created per every cm^2 of myocardial surface to be treated. With the CO_2 laser, each 30-J pulse is gated on the R wave of the ECG (when the ventricle is distended with blood and electrically quiescent), and creates a transmural scar without causing arrhythmias. Transmural penetration is confirmed with TEE; a

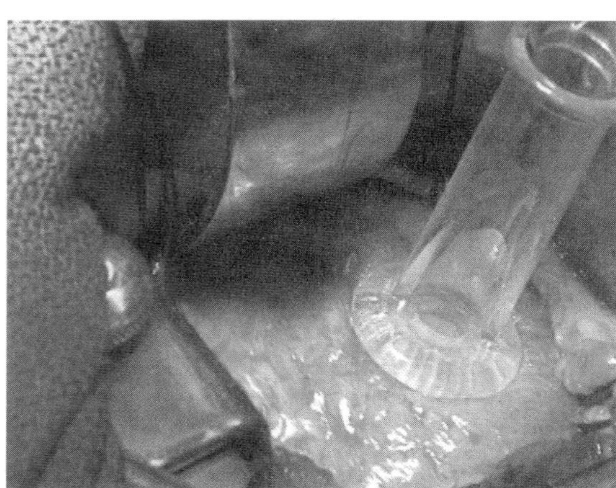

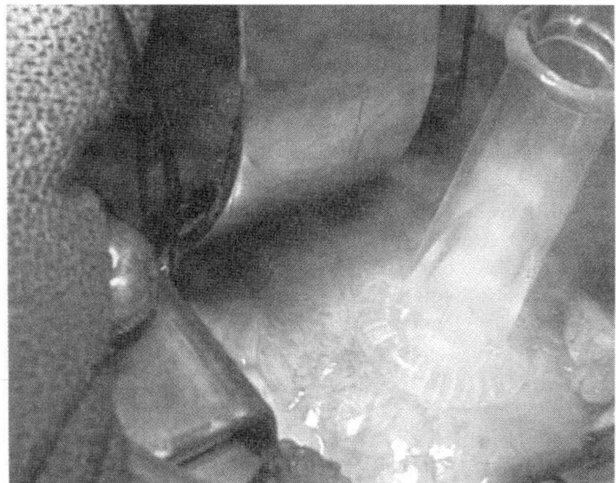

FIGURE 27–9 Surgical exposure and performance of TMR using a holmium:YAG laser. (*Reproduced with permission from March RJ: Laser revascularization of ischemic myocardium, in Naunheim KS (ed): Minimal Access Cardiothoracic Surgery. Philadelphia, WB Saunders, 2000.*)

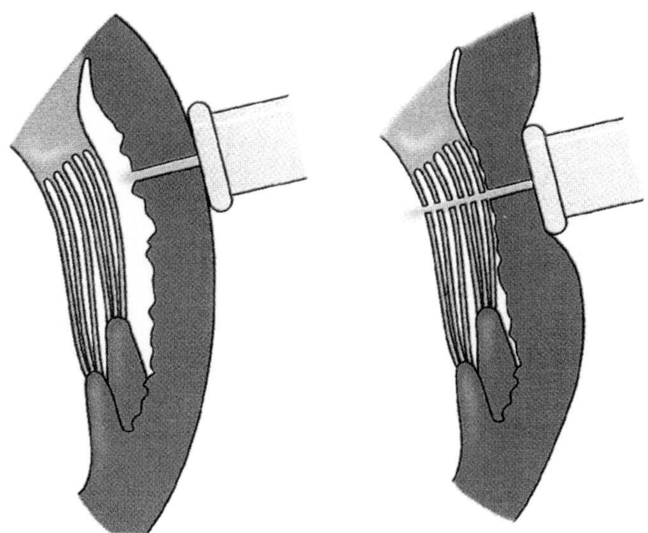

FIGURE 27–10 Complete dissection of all epicardial adhesions is essential to prevent dimpling of the left ventricle wall during TMR, which can bring mitral valve chordae close to the endocardial surface and make them susceptible to injury during activation of the laser. (*Reproduced with permission from March RJ: Laser revascularization of ischemic myocardium, in Naunheim KS (ed): Minimal Access Cardiothoracic Surgery. Philadelphia, WB Saunders, 2000.*)

higher energy level may be used depending on the amount of epicardial fat and wall thickness (which is thicker towards the apex), or a lower energy employed if the procedure is performed on CPB in order to minimize bleeding. With the holmium:YAG, 3 to 8 pulses are usually needed to result in a transmural penetration at a rate of 5 pulses per second. Arrhythmias are minimized if these channels are created slowly. Once approximately 5 channels are made in an area, direct pressure with a sponge is used to control the bleeding and the laser procedure restarted once hemostasis is achieved. If necessary, a 6-0 polypropylene horizontal mattress suture may be used to close the epicardium. A typical TMR procedure involves the placement of 30 to 50 channels. The pericardial cavity is then irrigated with warm saline, and each channel is checked for bleeding. The pericardium is loosely reapproximated, and a single chest tube is left in the pleural space in communication with the pericardial space.

Surgical TMR has also been performed though a sternotomy in conjunction with CABG[183–185] and thoracoscopically with minimal morbidity.[186–189] Percutaneous direct myocardial revascularization involves the insertion of a 9F deflectable guiding catheter in the common right femoral artery under local anesthesia. An optical fiber connected to a holmium:YAG laser is passed over a guide wire into the left ventricle and electromechanical mapping is used to create non-transmural channels in the desired area, each channel being approximately 1 mm in diameter and 2 to 5 mm in depth.[190]

PERIOPERATIVE MANAGEMENT AND RESULTS

TMR is associated with a considerable risk (up to 47%) of perioperative cardiac morbidity, which consists mostly of myocardial infarction, low cardiac output syndrome, and ventricular arrhythmias (Table 27-7).[170,191] Pericardial tamponade, delayed chordal rupture from laser injury, and micro air emboli from the creation of channels on the beating left ventricle have also been reported.[192] TMR is associated with universal rises in CPK-MB and a 50% incidence of ischemic

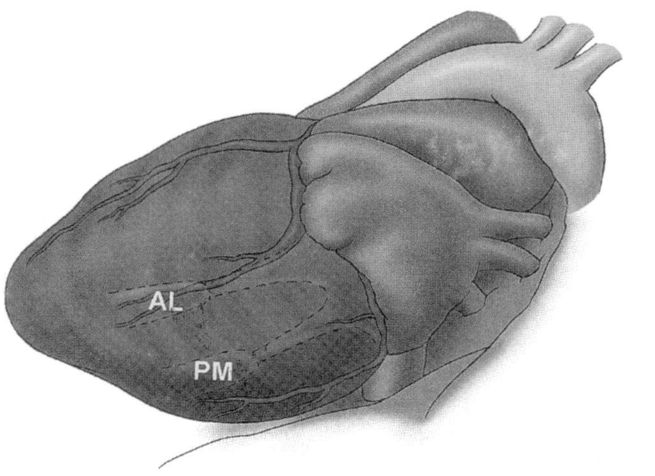

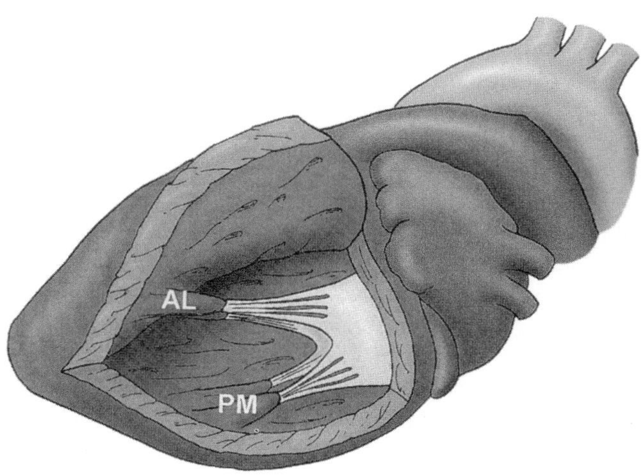

FIGURE 27–11 Anticipated location of the anterolateral (AL) and posteromedial (PM) papillary muscles, which should be excluded from the area of myocardium to be lased during TMR. (*Reproduced with permission from March RJ: Laser revascularization of ischemic myocardium, in Naunheim KS (ed): Minimal Access Cardiothoracic Surgery. Philadelphia, WB Saunders, 2000.*)

TABLE 27–7 Perioperative complications of TMR

Myocardial infarction
Low cardiac output syndrome
Ventricular arrhythmias
Pericardial tamponade
Papillary muscle or chordal injury
Cerebrovascular event (micro–air emboli)
Atrial fibrillation

electrocardiographic changes in the first 48 hours.[193] A TEE should be performed and compared to the last operative view whenever the suspicion of a mechanical cardiac complication is raised. Low cardiac output and ischemia are indications for the insertion of an IABP. If chordal rupture has occurred, IABP insertion and aggressive afterload reduction are carried out, and the necessity of surgical repair is reevaluated under these conditions; the prognosis with this complication is poor regardless of the approach elected. The use of TMR for unstable angina and the presence of poor LVEF (<40%) have been identified as independent predictors of perioperative morbidity[170,191]; conversely, good blood flow to at least one myocardial territory, female gender, and prior CABG have been associated with a decreased risk of mortality after TMR.[194,195]

Clinical Studies

CO_2 LASER

Case series The feasibility and safety of TMR with a CO_2 laser have been evaluated in a number of case series published over the last 7 years.[196–198] Overall, these have shown that TMR is associated with a perioperative mortality of approximately 9% to 15%[197,199–201] (reduced to 3% to 5% in subsequent randomized trials),[202–204] significant decreases in angina class at 3, 6, and 12 months compared to pretreatment,[197,199–201] improvements in exercise tolerance,[200,201] a decrease in the number of perfusion defects in the lased areas of the left ventricle,[197–199] and a significant decrease in the number of admissions for angina in the year following the procedure when compared with the year before treatment.[197,205] However, a conflicting report noted that technetium perfusion scans in 94 TMR patients were significantly worse than those of matched controls both at rest and during stress at 3-, 6-, and 12-month follow-up.[206] This was also supported by Landolfo et al, who reported that despite improvements in mean anginal class at 3, 6, and 12 months, no improvement in perfusion imaging parameters could be demonstrated at any time point after TMR.[205] Furthermore, TMR has been associated in other series with no improvement[200] or an actual decrease in left ventricular ejection fraction.[207]

The long-term effects of TMR were evaluated by Horvath et al in a series of 78 patients treated with a CO_2 laser and followed up to a mean of 5 years.[208] Benefits similar to those observed at 1-year follow-up were noted, including a persistent improvement in angina class and Seattle Angina Questionnaire scores. Eighty-one percent of patients were of CCS class II or better, and 17% of the patients had no angina 5 years after TMR. Late nuclear imaging studies were not conducted.

Clinical trials Randomized controlled trials of TMR using a CO_2 laser have been less numerous than case series, and were all open-label. A multicenter randomized controlled trial that involved 91 patients who underwent transmyocardial revascularization and 101 patients who received continued medical treatment showed impressive results: angina had improved by at least two CCS classes at 12 months in 72% of the patients assigned to TMR versus 13% of the patients who received medical treatment, and was associated with a significantly improved quality of life in the TMR group.[202] In the first year of follow-up, only 2% of patients who underwent TMR were hospitalized because of unstable angina, compared with 69% of patients assigned to medical treatment. Myocardial perfusion improved by 20% in the TMR group and worsened by 27% in the medical treatment group. These differences were all statistically significant.

Almost simultaneously, a randomized controlled trial that involved a total of 188 patients showed that TMR was associated with only modest improvements in angina class in TMR-treated patients at 12 months, and with no significant difference in treadmill exercise time.[203] Another open-label randomized controlled trial demonstrated that TMR was associated with a decrease in angina symptoms, and decreased time to chest pain during exercise, but no difference in total exercise time or $M\text{V}O_2$ during exercise.[204] These investigators subsequently reported a small but significant reduction in left ventricular ejection fraction and an increase in left-ventricular end-diastolic volume in the TMR group on nuclear imaging at 12-month follow-up, without any myocardial perfusion benefit attributable to this modality.[207]

HOLMIUM:YAG LASER

Case series The feasibility of TMR using a holmium:YAG laser either as sole therapy or in conjunction with CABG has been reported compared to that of TMR with a CO_2 laser. Perioperative mortality ranged from zero to 12%,[170,209–212] improvements in angina class[170,172,209–211] and exercise tolerance were noted,[210,211] but lack of improvement[210,212] or worsening[170] in perfusion of the lased areas and in left ventricular ejection fraction was also documented.[210,212] Furthermore, Mohr et al did not find any sustained benefits in angina relief 36 months after the performance of TMR with a holmium:YAG laser as sole therapy.[212]

Percutaneous direct myocardial revascularization has been evaluated in a number of case series and was associated with a periprocedural mortality ranging from zero to 2.9%[213,214] and improved time to onset of angina during exercise with improved exercise duration,[190,213,214] but again with some conflicting nuclear imaging results that showed either no improvement at 1 and 6 months[213,214] or improvement at stress only.[215] However, decreased size of the ischemic zone on cardiac MRI was reported by another group,[216] whose authors also documented the feasibility of combining percutaneous direct myocardial revascularization with coronary angioplasty and stenting.[217,218]

Clinical trials Open-label, randomized controlled trials of surgical TMR using a holmium:YAG laser have shown benefit in reducing angina and improving exercise tolerance.[219,220] A large, nonblinded trial that involved 275 patients demonstrated that surgical TMR with a holmium:YAG laser was also associated with a significantly higher survival without major cardiac events, and freedom from rehospitalization at one year.[220] These surprising results were not supported by any myocardial perfusion differences between TMR and control patients, however. These investigators subsequently evaluated surgical TMR in combination with CABG versus CABG alone (i.e., where an ungraftable myocardial territory was not addressed) and found that the TMR-CABG combination was associated with a trend towards greater survival and freedom from major adverse cardiac events at 1 year, but no difference in angina relief and treadmill improvement.[221]

The Angina Treatments—Lasers and Normal Therapies in Comparison (ATLANTIC) trial recruited 182 patients who were randomized either to surgical TMR or best medical therapy.[222] All patients had an ejection fraction of over 30%, no severe congestive symptoms, and at least one myocardial territory supplied by a normal or mildly diseased graft or coronary artery. Angina class and exercise tolerance were significantly improved in the TMR versus the medical treatment group at all study time points, but on nuclear imaging the changes in the percentage of myocardium with fixed and reversible defects from baseline to the 3-month, 6-month, and 12-month visits did not differ significantly between the two treatment groups. In the TMR group, a small but significant decrease in ejection fraction was noted from baseline to 3 months, and the rate of heart failure or new onset left ventricular dysfunction was higher in the TMR group. As a sequel to the ATLANTIC study, the Potential Class Improvement from Intramyocardial Channels (PACIFIC) trial was conducted to evaluate the efficacy of percutaneous TMR in a total of 221 patients randomized to undergo this modality or receive medical treatment.[223] The percutaneous procedure was associated with low morbidity, increased exercise tolerance time, lower angina scores, and improved quality of life.

The only double-blind, randomized controlled trial of any type of direct myocardial revascularization modality is the Direct Myocardial Revascularization in Regeneration of Endomyocardial Channels Trial (DIRECT), whose final results were presented at the 2001 meeting of the American College of Cardiology.[224] This multicenter trial conducted by Leon et al examined whether percutaneous myocardial revascularization using a holmium:YAG laser improved exercise duration or angina frequency when compared to medical management. It also evaluated the incidence of major adverse cardiac events; nuclear perfusion imaging was conducted at 6 months. The trial involved 298 predominantly male patients with a mean age of 63 years and preserved LV function who had coronary disease and severe symptoms despite best medical therapy, were no longer candidates for either PTCA or CABG, and had reproducible positive exercise tests associated with reversible ischemia. Patients were randomized into three arms: placebo (sham procedure), low-dose PDMR (10–15 channels/zone), or high-dose PDMR (20–25 channels/zone). No crossovers were permitted for the full year of follow-up. The trial was essentially negative with respect to all end points, with no differences in angina class and exercise duration among the three groups at baseline, 6 months, or 12 months, although there were statistically significant improvements in each group in terms of 6-month and 12-month to baseline differences for these two end points. The magnitude of ischemia on nuclear perfusion imaging at 6 months also showed no consistent differences that would suggest a therapeutic effect related to percutaneous direct myocardial revascularization. Although it is possible that the results of the DIRECT trial may not be entirely generalizable to surgical TMR, especially if involving a CO_2 laser, they are highly suggestive that a strong placebo effect may have plagued most if not all case series and open-label clinical trials in this field, whose results should therefore be viewed with caution and skepticism until efficacy is reevaluated in a blinded and randomized fashion.

CELL THERAPY

At the beginning of the 21st century, while large gains have been made in treating or preventing the most common underlying causes of many forms of heart failure, particularly ischemic vascular disease, the treatment of established heart failure of any cause remains unsatisfactory. Drug treatment with vasodilators and "neurohormonal" antagonists resulted in important but largely marginal gains in mortality and the functional status of many patients with heart failure. In contrast, drugs that markedly improved symptoms and functional status were associated with *increased* mortality.[225] The development of mechanical devices to assist or replace heart function has also had an impact, and indeed has saved lives in patients with end-stage disease.[226–228] However, much additional development will be necessary to lower patient morbidity and achieve economies of scale before widespread adoption of these devices is possible. Finally, while gene therapy approaches to either the prevention of heart failure (e.g., by inducing angiogenesis in ischemic but viable muscle) or the improvement of heart function directly (e.g., by inhibiting myocyte apoptosis or manipulation of adrenergic signaling) remain promising, none has yet proven safe and effective in humans.[229]

An alternative approach is to examine the possibility of replacing damaged myocardial cells with either newly formed cardiac myocytes (e.g., either by inducing cardiac myocytes to divide or by de novo generation of myocytes from a stem cell population), or by adding other cell types to damaged heart tissue that may prevent further ventricular dilation and deleterious "remodeling." In this section, we review the current literature on "cell therapy" approaches to the treatment of heart failure, some of which have now entered clinical trials. While a detailed description of earlier literature on this topic is beyond the scope of this chapter, the reader is referred to a comprehensive review of the data up to 2000 by P.D. Kessler and B.J. Byrne.[230]

Skeletal Myoblast Implants for Heart Failure

Cardiac myocytes in adult hearts *may* have a limited ability to undergo DNA synthesis and cytokinesis.[231,232] Moreover, recent data document that a reservoir of pluripotent stem cells, whether derived from the bone marrow or resident in tissues of adult humans, may be able to repopulate damaged cardiac muscle (vide infra). Regardless, none of these mechanisms is normally sufficient to replace the function of more than a small number of damaged myocytes. In contrast, fetal or neonatal myocytes, which retain a substantial proliferative capacity, can "replace" damaged cardiac tissue, by integrating into areas of myocyte necrosis and forming gap junctions with adjacent viable cells.[233–236] For obvious reasons, use of fetal or neonatal human tissue for this purpose is impractical, while transplanting fetal cells from other species remains problematic due to issues of tissue rejection and the possibility of infectious agents crossing a species barrier.

The cell type that has been most extensively examined to date for "repair" of injured cardiac muscle is immature skeletal muscle cells known as skeletal myoblasts, a lineage-restricted form of stem cell that serves as a reservoir of cells for injured striated muscle or muscle placed under increased mechanical stress. Chiu et al were among the first to systematically examine the effects of skeletal myoblast transplantation, documenting in both canine and rat models that transplanted skeletal myoblasts survived in scar tissue created by cryoinjury.[237,238] Field et al documented the engraftment of an immortalized skeletal myocyte cell line (C2C12 cells) into cardiac muscle, including the formation of intercalated discs.[233,234,239–242] Murry et al also demonstrated that myoblasts derived from fetal skeletal muscle would integrate into cardiac muscle damaged by cryoinjury. The transplanted myoblasts altered their typical fast-twitch muscle phenotype to include some slow-twitch, β-myosin heavy chain (β-MHC)–containing fibers as well.

Since slow-twitch fibers are much less resistant to fatigue, this held the promise that autologous skeletal myoblasts from juvenile or adult humans might also exhibit the ability to "adapt" to the microenvironment within the human heart. However, although undifferentiated skeletal myoblasts in vitro express connexin 43, which facilitates formation of electromechanical ("gap") junctions with cardiac myocytes in tissue culture, connexin 43 was rapidly downregulated when myoblasts were implanted in vivo, making it unlikely that skeletal myoblasts would spontaneously integrate with cardiac myocytes in situ in the heart.[235,242,243] Indeed, when injected into normal cardiac muscle in a syngeneic rat model, skeletal myoblasts initially engrafted and adopted a slow-twitch phenotype, but clearly did not adopt a characteristic cardiac myocyte phenotype. Furthermore, again, when injected into normal cardiac muscle, the skeletal muscle grafts never expressed intercalated disc proteins such as N-cadherin and connexin 43, and typically atrophied over time.[244,245]

Taylor et al have reported the most detailed hemodynamic assessments of the consequences of implantation of autologous skeletal myoblasts into the injured heart.[246–249] Autologous skeletal myoblast grafts were examined in rabbit hearts scarred by cryoinjury, a model that replicates with some fidelity the hemodynamics observed in infarcted human hearts. Successful engraftment of skeletal myoblasts into infarcted muscle resulted in improved ventricular compliance with limited diastolic "creep" or progressive remodeling and dilatation of infarcted ventricular muscle, and appeared to be superior to a nonmyocyte cell type (i.e., fibroblasts).[250] These authors also performed a comprehensive analysis of myocardial function in the in situ rabbit heart. In addition to the improvement in diastolic strain and stiffness, Taylor et al noted a modest improvement in systolic function in some animals, although this remains a controversial finding.[249,251]

Apstein et al[252] also examined the effects of transplantation of skeletal myoblasts from syngeneic donor animals into adult rat hearts following a myocardial infarction in an ischemia-reperfusion model. Thus, this model differs from that of Taylor by using a more clinically relevant mode of injury, and by using myoblasts of fetal origin, which may have had a higher replicative potential, and also may integrate more readily into adult myocardium. Using echocardiographic analysis of the rat heart in situ, and ex vivo Langendorff retrograde (blood) perfused heart function analysis, the data indicated both less global ventricular dilatation and improved ex vivo systolic pressure generation in hearts that had received myoblast implants (Figs. 27-12 and 27-13). Interestingly, exercise tolerance (i.e., running time on a treadmill in animals conditioned to perform the test) was also enhanced in animals that had been treated with myoblast injections. Although the use of fetal skeletal myoblasts might have confounded the analysis of these data, this laboratory has repeated these studies using skeletal myoblasts from adult syngeneic donor animals, with similar results (Apstein C, Liao R, et al: manuscript in preparation).

Another group that has contributed extensively to this literature is the laboratory of Weisel et al, beginning with a

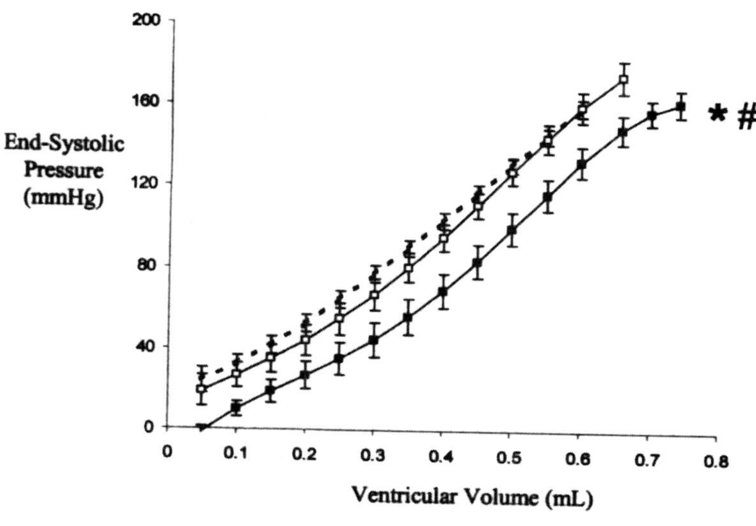

FIGURE 27–12 Systolic pressure–volume relationship at 6 weeks following cell transplantation. Data are shown for three groups of animals in the study by Jain et al, which compared the ex vivo systolic pressure volume relationship among hearts from control, noninfarcted hearts (dashed line), control infarcted hearts (dark boxes), and infarcted hearts that received injections of fetal skeletal myoblasts (light boxes).[252] *, $p < .05$ vs. control at any given systolic volume; #, $p < .05$ vs MI+cells at any given systolic volume. *(Reproduced with permission from Jain M, DerSimonian H, Brenner DA, et al: Cell therapy attenuates deleterious ventricular remodeling and improves cardiac performance after myocardial infarction. Circulation 2001; 103:1920.)*

report in 1996 on the hemodynamic effects of fetal rat cardiac myocytes implanted into cryoinjured muscle and scar tissue of adult rats.[253] Additional studies from this laboratory have compared the effects on cardiac function and angiogenesis of a variety of cell types, including fetal rat enteric smooth muscle cells, fetal and adult skeletal myoblasts, and skin fibroblasts, among other cell types.[254,255] As expected, not all cell types contributed equally to the maintenance of systolic and diastolic function, and animals that received injections of enteric smooth muscle cells or skin fibroblasts showed no significant improvement over controls.[255] Importantly for the design of clinical trials of cell therapies, in a study in an adult rat heart cryoinjury model using syngeneic fetal cardiac myocytes, in which cells were given either immediately,

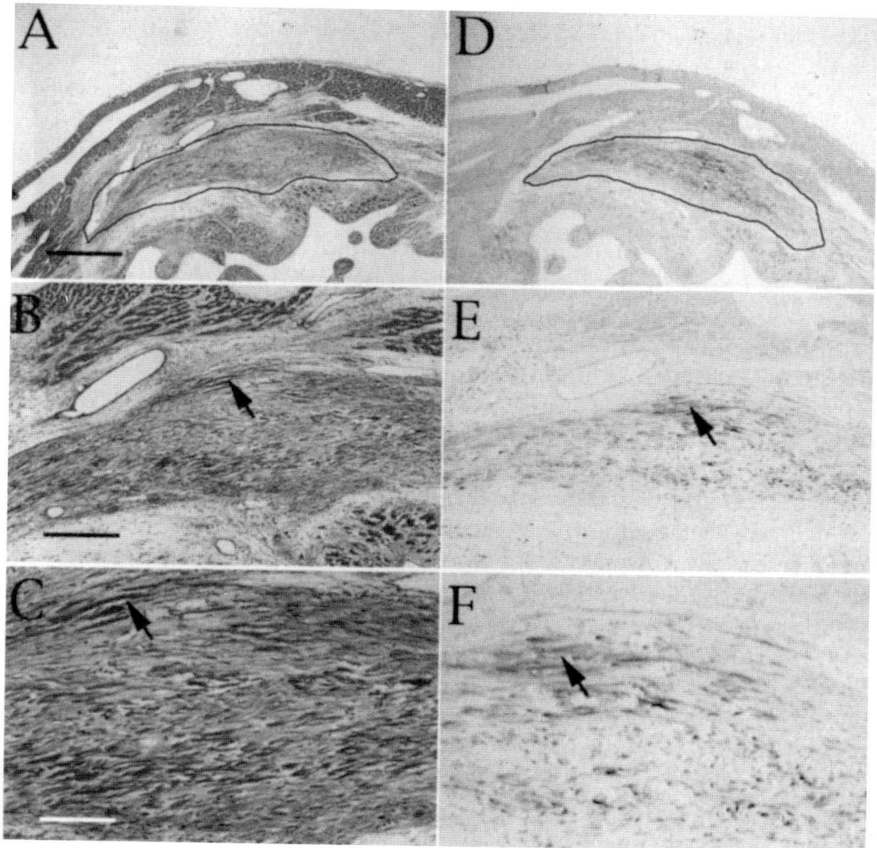

FIGURE 27–13 Skeletal myoblast survival following transplantation. Immunohistochemical analysis of skeletal myoblast survival in the infarcted hearts of rats 9 days following cell injections. Panels A-C show trichrome staining at progressively increasing magnification in which fibrotic tissue stains blue, and viable muscle stains red (bars represent 1 mm, 200 μm, and 100 μm, respectively). Panels D-F show staining for myogenin, a skeletal muscle–specific transcription factor.

or at 2 weeks or 4 weeks following injury, Li et al determined that neonatal myocytes transplanted immediately (i.e., at the time of injury) could not be detected at 8 weeks, nor did these "0" time point transplanted hearts perform better that control animals that had received injections of culture medium alone. Animals transplanted at 2 weeks after cryoinjury exhibited the greatest functional improvement.[256] The presumed reason for the absence of benefit of myocytes transplanted immediately following injury was the presence of a robust inflammatory response in the recently infarcted muscle, a process that takes a week or more to completely resolve in rodents (this observation contrasts with results obtained with immediate injection of some stem cell populations, as discussed below).

Finally, although it is often assumed that skeletal myoblasts in these preparations are the "active" cell type responsible for the diastolic and possibly systolic functional improvements observed in hearts that had received transplants, this remains a hypothesis. In all the experiments described above that used skeletal "myoblast" preparations, other cell types (mostly fibroblasts) account for the large minority or even a majority of the cells injected, depending on the preparation. Apstein et al have directly compared relatively pure populations of fibroblasts with skeletal myoblasts, both prepared from adult rat tissues, in their rat infarct/reperfusion model of cardiac injury. When examined at 8 weeks following the infarct, as determined by both echocardiography and Langedorff retrograde (blood) perfusion hemodynamics, both cell types yielded nearly identical improvements in cardiac function, when compared to infarcted control hearts that received culture medium alone (Apstein C, Wentworth BM, Liao R: manuscript in preparation).

Perhaps the most extensive experience to date with skeletal myoblast transfer for the treatment of heart failure has been accrued by the laboratory of Menasche et al. In a series of reports, they have documented that syngeneic skeletal myoblasts from neonatal rats were equivalent to fetal cardiac myocytes in their ability to delay maladaptive ventricular remodeling.[257,258] Although neither group of cells is directly relevant to the currently proposed clinical trials in humans, these results did address whether fetal cardiac myocytes (which retain a significant proliferative capacity compared to adult cardiac myocytes, and can integrate with surviving myocytes in the injured myocardium) were clearly superior to skeletal myoblasts. The answer is: apparently not, at least based on these data.

In one of the first rodent experiments to use autologous skeletal myoblasts (analogous to currently ongoing trials in humans), Menasche et al also documented an improvement in cardiac function in animals that received myoblast injections compared to animals that received injections of cell culture medium alone.[258] In these experiments, on average 3.5×10^6 cells were injected, a "dose" that when adjusted for heart size approximates that being used in their clinical trials. Note however that, once again, only approximately 50% of the cells were desmin positive (a characteristic of muscle, as opposed to fibroblasts), again raising the issue of the relative contribution of skeletal myoblasts versus other cell types in these primary cultures.

While encouraging, these data begged the question of whether the appropriate comparisons were being done in animal studies in which skeletal myoblast implantation was compared to untreated control animals. Since virtually all heart failure patients now receive at a minimum an angiotensin-converting enzyme (ACE) inhibitor, Menasche et al next asked whether skeletal myoblast therapy added anything in addition to current medical therapy for heart failure.[259] The rat infarct model was a relevant animal model in which to test this hypothesis, since proof-of-concept animal studies validating the survival benefit of ACE inhibitors (ACEI) in heart failure had first been done in the rat by Pfeffer et al (reviewed in Bristow et al[225]). Menasche et al[259] studied 4 groups of animals ($n = 99$ animals): MI controls, MI with ACEI, MI with myoblast injections, and MI with myoblast injections and ACEI. Although mortality was not a primary end point at 8 weeks of follow-up, there was a clear separation of groups based on 2D echocardiography. Control animals that received injections of culture medium alone exhibited a continuing decline in ejection fraction (to an average of 19%) compared to either ACE inhibitor–treated or myoblast-treated animals (ejection fractions of 32% vs. 37%, respectively). The animals that received both ACEI and myoblast injections had an average ejection fraction of 44%, clearly indicating a biological and—if transferable to humans—clinically meaningful improvement (Fig. 27-14).[259]

To validate whether the observations made in rodents were applicable to larger animals, Menasche et al have also examined the effect of autologous skeletal myoblasts in an ovine circumflex artery embolization infarct model. Cells were injected through a lateral thoracotomy 2 weeks following the infarct, with injections both within and surrounding the infarct zone. Although the number of animals was relatively small, and the primary end point for most animals was just 4 months, there was a statistically significant improvement in ejection fraction and end-diastolic volume in the animals that received myoblasts, when compared to control sheep.[260]

In separate studies in rodents, two groups have independently shown that transplantation of skeletal myoblasts also can improve cardiac function in animals with cardiomyopathies not of ischemic origin. Scorsin et al[261] demonstrated that direct intramyocardial injection of fetal murine cardiomyocytes improved LV function compared to medium-injected control mice, as measured by echocardiography, in animals with heart failure induced by doxorubicin, an anthracycline antibiotic widely used in cancer chemotherapy.[261] Data similar to these were subsequently published by Weisel et al.[262] Neonatal ventricular myocytes were injected directly into the hearts of hamsters

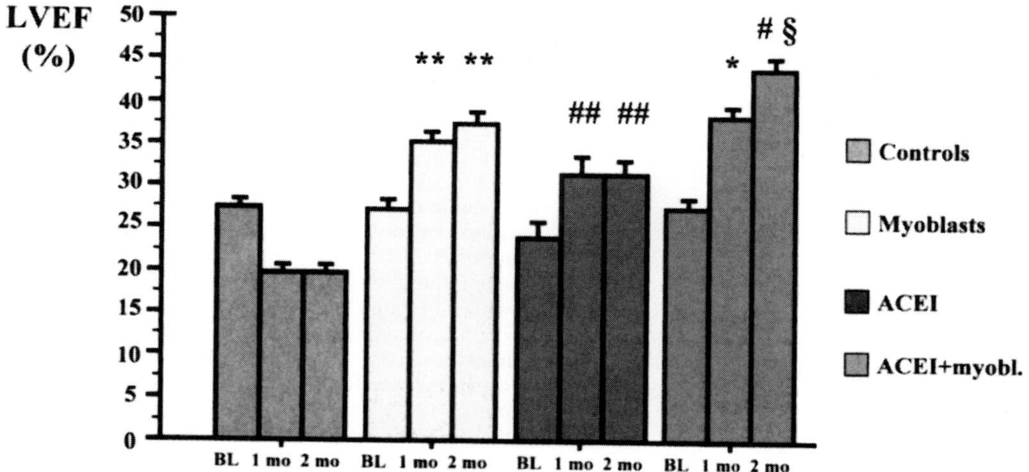

FIGURE 27–14 Heart failure, ACE inhibitors, and skeletal myoblast injections. The data shown are the left ventricular ejection fractions (LVEF) for four groups of animals at three time points: baseline (BL), 1, and 2 months: (1) control infarcted animals; (2) infarcted animals treated with myoblast injections alone; (3) infarcted animals treated with ACE inhibitors alone; and (4) infarcted animals treated with both skeletal myoblast injections and ACE inhibitors. *, $p = .0048$ vs. ACEI; #, $p < .0001$ vs. ACE inhibitors; §, $p = .0084$ vs. skeletal myoblasts; ** $p < .000$ vs. control rats; ##, $p < .0001$ vs. control rats. (*Reproduced with permission from Masferrer JL, Koki A, Seibert K: COX-2 inhibitors: a new class of antiangiogenic agents. Ann NY Acad Sci 1999; 889:84.*)

with a cardiomyopathy due to an abnormal delta-sarcoglycan gene. Although both sets of experiments were performed on animals with distinctly different global cardiomyopathies, ventricular function, as measured in situ by fractional shortening on echo[261] or on ex vivo Langendorff isolated perfused heart functional analysis,[262] was improved in both experimental models following injections of neonatal cardiac myocytes when compared to controls, at least during the time course of these experiments (1 month for both sets of experiments). Once again, however, it is not clear that cardiac myocytes are essential for modifying the progressive decline in cardiac function in the cardiomyopathy model, since Weisel et al noted that smooth muscle cells harvested from the vas deferens of cardiomyopathic hamsters and implanted into the hearts of recipient animals of the same hamster strain maintained smaller ventricular dimensions and better contractile function than controls.[262]

Similar data have been obtained by Suzuki et al[263] in a rat model of doxorubicin toxicity, in which syngeneic neonatal rat skeletal myoblasts were injected in a heterotopic cardiac transplant model, in which the transplanted heart was obtained from rats treated for 2 weeks with high doses of the anthracycline. Once again, function of the transplanted heart was improved compared to controls, as measured by end-of-life Langendorff perfusion studies. One important difference in the experimental protocol employed by Suzuki et al was that the transplanted cells (approximately 10^6 cells) were injected into the coronary arteries using a Langendorff retrograde perfusion technique. Presumably a proportion of the injected cells were trapped in the microcirculation of the heart, and subsequently migrated into the surrounding muscle, a technique that this group had previously demonstrated resulted in successful cell transplantation.[264]

Enhancing the Survival of Transplanted Cells

Suzuki et al have also investigated several methods that might enhance survival of cells transplanted into ischemic muscle. Reasoning that exposing cells ex vivo to increased temperature (i.e., to a "heat shock" stimulus, induced by incubation at 42°C for 60 minutes) might enhance graft viability, they demonstrated greater survival of heat-shocked L6 rat myoblasts after 28 days, as judged by staining for β galactosidase (used to track the injected cells), compared to untreated myoblasts.[265] Carrying this line of experimentation to its logical next step, this group then demonstrated that ex vivo transfection of intact rat hearts with a protein known to play an important role in the heat shock response, HSP70, encoded within a viral/liposome complex, resulted in an improvement in myocardial function following ischemic stress compared to control hearts.[266] This group has also employed skeletal myoblasts that had been transfected with a gene encoding a protein that could have enhanced the function or survival of implanted myoblasts. Rat skeletal myoblasts transfected with connexin 43, a gap junction protein, enhanced myotube development in vitro (i.e., the cells adopted a differentiated phenotype more readily).[267]

With regard to survival of transplanted cells, particularly in animal models of coronary ischemia, one primary determinant will be the blood supply to cells transplanted into

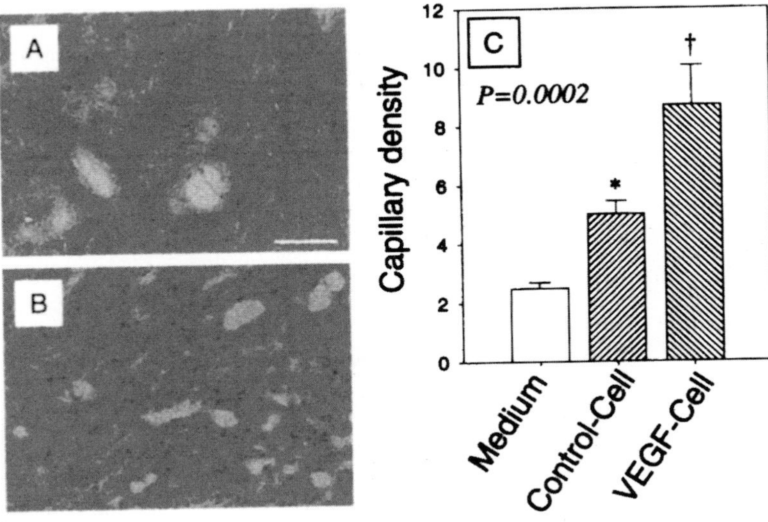

FIGURE 27–15 Ex vivo transfection of skeletal myoblasts with a VEGF-A isoform. Suzuki et al tested the hyopothesis that ex vivo transfection of primary cultures of skeletal myoblasts isolated from juvenile rats with an angiogenic gene—in this case, the VEGF-A_{165} isoform—would induce a greater angiogenic response than myoblast therapy alone, and thereby improve myocardial contractile function. Panels A and B illustrate sections from hearts treated with (A) myoblasts alone or (B) myoblasts treated ex vivo with VEGF-A_{165}. Scale bar = 50 μm. (C) Capillary density is illustrated for animals treated with injections of culture medium alone (i.e., no cells), skeletal myoblasts alone (Control–Cell), and skeletal myoblasts transfected with VEGF-A_{165} (VEGF–Cell).*, $p < .05$ vs. medium alone control; +, $p < .05$ vs. both medium alone and myoblast alone groups. (*Reproduced with permission from Suzuki K, Murtuza B, Smolenski RT, et al: Cell transplantation for the treatment of myocardial infarction using vascular endothelial growth factor-expressing skeletal myoblasts. Circulation 2001; 104:1207.*)

an ischemic environment. Weisel et al have shown that implantation of (allogeneic) aortic endothelial cells in cryoinjured rat hearts resulted in increased regional blood flow as measured by microsphere analysis,[138] suggesting that cell transplantation alone induces at least a moderate angiogenic response. Suzuki et al have transfected skeletal myoblasts with a vascular endothelial growth factor (VEGF) type-A isoform (VEGF-A_{165}) ex vivo, which were then injected into the peri-infarct border zone of rats hour following LAD occlusion.[268] This VEGF-A isoform retains the heparin binding motif (unlike VEGF-A_{121}) and has been demonstrated to induce angiogenesis in a number of animal models (clinical trials with this reagent are currently ongoing [269]). Infarcted animals treated with myoblasts that had been transfected ex vivo with VEGF-A_{165} had a reduced mortality rate at 28 days, and a significant reduction in infarct size, possibly due in part to an increased angiogenic response, as judged by counting capillary density (a relatively insensitive technique for detecting angiogenesis) (Fig. 27-15).[268] Similar data were reported by Li et al following ex vivo transfection of cardiac myoyctes and fibroblasts with plasmids encoding VEGF-A_{165}.[270]

One caveat to this approach has been raised by the work of Blau et al. They examined the effects of high levels of VEGF-A expression observed in mice whose hearts had been implanted with primary cultures of murine skeletal myoblasts that had been transfected ex vivo with the murine VEGF-A gene driven by a retroviral promoter.[271,272] Animals that received the VEGF-A gene-transfected myoblasts all exhibited highly vascularized intramural tumors. It is presumed that the continuous high levels of all VEGF-A isoforms within the hearts of these mice, possibly the consequence of using a retroviral promoter, were the reason for the observed increase in angioma formation. There have been no reports of similar tumors in humans treated with recombinant proteins, or either plasmid or viral vectors encoding a VEGF-A isoform, although most of the studies reported to date are relatively small Phase I and Phase II clinical trials. Despite this caveat, the current safety profile of this technology is encouraging. Moreover, it is reasonable to assume that with the development of tissue-specific and regulatable promoter technologies, it will be possible in the future to calibrate the amount of transgene expression—and therefore target protein levels—within a given cell type and tissue. This should enhance the safety of adjunctive gene therapy, whether given in vivo or ex vivo, when applied to cell transplantation protocols.

Finally, an alternative approach to the induction of angiogenesis by cell therapy is to inject relatively undifferentiated autologous bone marrow cells into the myocardium. Chiu et al documented increased neovascularization in infarcted rat hearts following injection of a population of "mesenchymal" bone marrow–derived cells from syngeneic rat donors.[238] Fuchs et al also demonstrated that endomyocardial injections of autologous bone marrow resulted in enhanced myocardial perfusion in a porcine ameroid constrictor model, as judged by microsphere analysis.[273] The presumptive mechanisms include the likelihood that a number of injected cells secrete cytokines such as GM-CSF that are known to facilitate angiogenesis, as well as the presence of a population of "endothelial progenitor cells" or "EPCs" present in relatively undifferentiated bone marrow preparations, which may undergo amplification and differentiation in the ischemic intracellular milieu of the healing, postinfarct scar tissue, and contribute to angiogenesis and arteriogenesis.[274,275]

Inducing Proliferation of Adult Cardiac Myocytes

Although recent data, noted above, support the hypothesis that cardiac myocytes may possess a limited capacity for cell division (cytokinesis), the inability of the large majority of myocytes within the heart—and the limited recruitment of pluripotent stem cells from within the heart itself or other tissue sources—to contribute to repair of the injured myocardium is an important cause of morbidity and mortality. A number of approaches have been attempted to induce "terminally differentiated" cardiomyocytes to divide, but most myocytes typically undergo programmed cell death (apoptosis) when "forced" into the cell cycle. One approach to addressing this problem that has provided important insights into the signaling pathways that regulate cardiomyocyte division has been developed by Field.[276,277] This laboratory has reported on the actions of several "tumor suppressor" cell cycle regulatory genes,[278] and had identified a 193-kDa protein, in addition to other known tumor suppressor proteins within cardiac myocytes (such as p53 and p107), which participated in the induction of apoptosis following exposure to agents such as simian virus 40 (SV40) large T antigen, or the adenoviral E1A oncoprotein. In a screening assay to determine which portions of the p193 protein were important for the bioactivity of this tumor suppressor protein, Field et al generated a truncated mutant termed 1152stp that, instead of inducing apoptosis, enhanced myocyte proliferation, particularly in combination with a known prosurvival mutant of p53 (termed CB7). Cotransfection of both mutant proteins into embryonic stem (ES) cell-derived cultures of beating cardiomyocytes prevented apoptosis in cells exposed to a potent growth stimulus, such as adenoviral E1A. Thus, despite the recent demonstration that stem cells derived from bone marrow—and possibly a reservoir of cells within the myocardium itself, reviewed below—may contribute to cardiac repair following injury, the controlled induction of DNA synthesis, karyokinesis, and cytokinesis of adult cardiac myocytes in situ in the adult heart remains a promising if daunting therapeutic challenge.

Stem Cell Approaches to Cardiac Repair and Regeneration

The ability of the human heart to repair damaged muscle after injury is limited after the first year or two of life. This had been attributed to an irreversible exit from the cell cycle in "terminally differentiated" cardiac myocytes, although the underlying mechanism(s) limiting further myocyte replication remained unclear. However, recent evidence from a number of sources has cast doubt on this long-held tenet of cardiac cell biology. As will be discussed briefly below, cardiac "regeneration" following injury may be possible using several approaches.

Since myocardial ischemia and infarction due to advanced coronary atherosclerosis are among the commonest causes of death and disability in adult humans, the ability to induce new blood vessel formation—angiogenesis—particularly when accompanied by progressive vascular remodeling that contributes to the growth of larger arterioles and conduit vessels, a process termed arteriogenesis,[279–281] would be an important advance on current therapeutic alternatives. "Angiogenesis" induced by cytokines such as isoforms of the VEGF-A gene or members of the fibroblast growth factor (FGF) family, whether given as gene therapy or as recombinant proteins, or transcription factors such as hypoxia-inducible factor-1 (HIF-1), all have potential to induce new blood vessel growth, and clinical trials employing each of these approaches are now underway.[269,274] There is now good evidence that further remodeling of new blood vessels into large-caliber vessels is dependent upon recruitment of inflammatory cells[279–281] and a discrete lineage-restricted bone marrow stem cell population termed "angioblasts,"[282] or "endothelial progenitor cells" (EPCs) by Asahara et al.[275,283] There also is increasing evidence that recruitment of EPCs by cytokines, or ex vivo expansion of EPCs, followed by direct injection into ischemic tissue or by systemic administration, accelerates new blood vessel formation and minimizes cardiac damage.[282,283]

Following large amounts of tissue damage due to ischemia or infarction, even restoration of adequate blood flow will not restore normal cardiac function and is often insufficient to prevent subsequent ventricular remodeling. However, as noted above, the received wisdom that the heart—like the brain—is a "terminally differentiated" tissue, incapable of substantive repair with restoration of function, must be reevaluated based on recent data (for both organs). It is well known, of course, that cardiac myocytes in juvenile and adult mammals, including humans, can undergo a limited degree of DNA synthesis and even karyokinesis (nuclear division), but the capacity for cytokinesis—actual cell division—was believed to be quite limited or nil. This assumption has been challenged by a wealth of recent evidence, reviewed below.

Perhaps the most striking example from the recent literature is in a specific strain of mouse known as the "MRL"strain. This strain has been well known for years to have a remarkable ability to heal wounds, a capacity that has been likened to that of amphibians. To determine whether MRL mice also have the capacity to regenerate injured cardiac muscle, Haber-Katz et al[284] induced full-thickness right ventricular infarctions using a cryoprobe, and compared the response in this mouse strain to a control mouse strain (C57Bl/6). Remarkably, within 60 to 90 days following the injury, the MRL mice had essentially completely regrown replacement, vascularized muscle with restoration of normal right ventricular function, while control animals went on to develop a thinned, scarred, and dysfunctional right ventricular remnant. Note that myocardial infarcts in the mouse, whether due to cryoinjury or ischemia, undergo a repair process and induce progressive ventricular remodeling elsewhere in the ventricle that is similar to that observed in humans, although the time course is "telescoped" into days to weeks, as opposed to months or years in patients. This strain is now being intensively examined for clues to its remarkable ability for repairing damaged tissues.

The data reviewed above in the MRL strain do not mean that human hearts do not exhibit any capacity for cardiac myoycte replacment following injury. Anversa et al have demonstrated that, following a myocardial infarction, cardiac myocytes in adult human hearts (harvested at autopsy) express the nuclear antigen Ki-67, a marker limited to cells undergoing replication. Moreover, myocytes caught in the act of cell division, with clearly identifiable mitotic spindles and division into daughter cells, could also be identified. Ki-67–positive cells were most readily identifiable in the peri-infarct region (i.e., the "border zone"), but could be identified, at lower frequencies, in areas of the heart remote from the infarct. In contrast, hearts harvested from subjects who had died from noncardiac causes exhibited little or no Ki-67.

While these observations suggested that myocytes in situ within the heart were being induced to replicate, albeit at a rate inadequate to replace the damaged tissue, there was another, not mutually exclusive, possibility—that myocytes were being formed by a reservoir of pluripotent stem cells recruited from within the heart itself and/or other tissues, such as bone marrow. In male heart transplant recipients, for example, who had received a heart from a female donor and who later came to autopsy, the transplanted hearts were found to contain a number of cell types, including fully differentiated cardiac myocytes, that contained a "Y" chromosome, indicating that that particular cell must have been of host origin.[285] While it is possible that at least some of the Y-chromosome–positive cardiac cells had migrated from the atrial remnant of the recipient—a hypothesis for which Anversa et al provide intriguing evidence—some proportion of the cells had likely been recruited from other tissues, with the bone marrow the most obvious candidate.

In support of this hypothesis, recent data in experimental animals and humans document that bone marrow–derived cells in recipient animals can populate organ grafts. Krause et al[286] demonstrated that female mice, following doses of radiation sufficient to ablate the bone marrow and subsequently infused with bone marrow constituents from syngeneic male donors, had cells that exhibited Y-chromosome positivity in virtually all tissue beds, when examined several months later. Similar data have been generated by Goodell et al,[287] who performed a myocardial infarction in female mice that had previously been lethally irradiated and subsequently reconstituted with bone marrow, once again from male donor mice. Although the percentage of male donor–derived myocytes in the hearts of the female bone marrow recipient mice was low (about 0.02%), they were easily detectable. That this process clearly occurs in humans has been demonstrated by Grimm et al,[288] who examined male recipients of kidney allografts from a female donor, who also documented the presence of Y-chromosome–positive cells in all cellular constituents of the kidney, including blood vessels, mesangial cells, endothelial cells, and tubular epithelium.

This phenomenon of bone marrow–derived pluripotent progenitor cells continuously repopulating tissues may have important implications for other disease processes of relevance to cardiac and vascular surgeons, such as transplant arteriopathy. Long-term survival of, for example, cardiac allografts is limited by the development of an arteriopathy that involves neointimal thickening and gradual occlusion of coronary arteries and arterioles. The source of the neointimal cells has been presumed to be inflammatory cells of host origin as well as vascular smooth muscle cells derived from the media of vessels within the allograft itself. However, Mitchell et al,[289] in a murine model of aortic transplant arteriopathy, in which aortas from a standard strain of laboratory mice were transplanted into HLA mismatched mice that also constitutively express the marker gene β-galactosidase ("βGal"), demonstrated that virtually all the smooth muscle cells populating the neointima of the aortic allograft were of recipient origin; i.e., they were all βGal-positive, indicating that the neointimal cells must have been of host origin—presumably from bone marrow—and not due to increased replication of smooth muscle cells of donor origin within the graft (Fig. 27-16).[289]

What then is the potential of pluripotent stem cells, whether of marrow origin or recruited from peripheral tissues, for inducing repair of damaged cardiac tissue? Once again, recent data provide reason for optimism. Anversa et al,[290] in a murine myocardial infarction model, examined whether a specific subset of bone marrow derived cells that were negative for common hematopoietic lineage markers (i.e., "lin^-"), but positive for stem cell factor (i.e., "$c\text{-}kit^+$"), when injected within hours of a myocardial infarction in mice, would induce the formation of new cardiac muscle replete with regenerated cardiac myocytes, blood vessels, and stromal cells (Figs. 27-17 and 27-18). A similar bone marrow–derived cell population that also contained "lin^-" cells, but was, however, negative for c-kit (i.e., "$c\text{-}kit^-$"), did not result in substantive cardiac repair. The injected cells were tracked over time using bone marrow cells from syngeneic donor mice that were sex mismatched (i.e., male donors into female recipients) and that constitutively expressed enhanced green fluorescent protein (EGFP), providing an additional marker with which to track the injected cells. Interestingly, injections of lin^-, $c\text{-}kit^+$ cells were ineffective if given after the reparative inflammatory response had begun in the infarcted tissue, typically after 12 hours or longer following the infarction.[290]

An extensive discussion of the cell biology of mammalian stem cell populations is beyond the scope of this chapter. However, the advances in our understanding of the phenotypic plasticity of many "committed" stem cell lineages are also requiring the construction of new paradigms.[291,292]

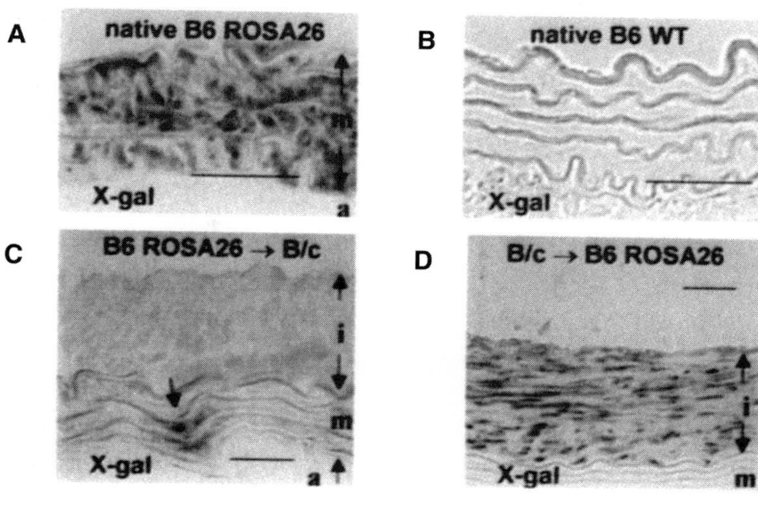

FIGURE 27–16 Recipient (presumably bone marrow origin) of intimal hyperplasia in aortic allografts. To determine whether cells contributing to the intimal hyperplasia characteristic of solid organ transplants were of graft or host origin, Mitchell et al transplanted portions of the thoracic aortic from one strain of mice, BALB/c ("B/c"), into another MHC mismatched strain, C57Bl/6, and vice versa. The C57Bl/6 mice were also ROSA 26 β-galactosidase transgenic animals ("B6 ROSA26"); the cells from those animals can be tracked because they stain blue with the appropriate reagents (X-gal). Sections of the native aortas of B6 ROSA26 mice and B/c mice are shown in (A) and (B), respectively. Note the absence of any neointimal proliferation in either panel. Panels (C) and (D) show a B6 ROSA 26 aorta transplanted into a B/c recipient, and a B/c aorta transplanted into a B6 ROSA 26 recipient. Note that in both cases the robust neointimal proliferation present in panels (C) and (D) exhibited the phenotype of the recipient animal; i.e., the cells comprising the neointimal proliferation did not originate from cells migrating into the neointima from the media of the graft, but were of host origin—presumably recruited from the bone marrow of the recipient animal. (*Reproduced with permission from Shimizu K, Sugiyama S, Aikawa M, et al: Host bone-marrow cells are a source of donor intimal smooth-muscle-like cells in murine aortic transplant arteriopathy. Nat Med 2001; 7:738.*)

The phenotypic "barriers" that are assumed to exist among, for example, the mesenchymal, hematopoietic, and neurologic lineages have also yielded to new data, as highlighted by Moore's evocative 1999 editorial entitled "Turning brain into blood."[293] In addition to bone marrow, Verfaille et al have recently shown that pluripotent stem cells also reside in bone marrow and in other tissues in adult humans, cells that exhibit a remarkable ability to assume any of the three principal germline lineages,[291] which she has termed "multipotential adult progenitor cells" or "MAPCs."

Whether MAPCs are indeed a unique reservoir of pluripotent stem cells in the adult animal, or represent just a more thorough understanding of the phenotypic plasticity of the conventional stem cell lineages, will require additional experimentation. For example, Condorelli et al[294] have demonstrated that even apparently differentiated cells of one "traditional" lineage—endothelial cells, of hematopoietic lineage origin—can be induced to form a cell type of mesenchymal lineage—cardiac myocytes—under specific culture conditions in vitro or when injected into injured, ischemic myocardium. Importantly, MAPCs isolated from both juvenile and adult human bone marrow could be propogated through at least 80 population doublings in vitro, without any sign of senescence, indicating that this reservoir of stem cells in the adult animal could provide a renewable resource for facilitating tissue repair.[292]

Indeed, our understanding of stem cell biology is now expanding so rapidly that it is unclear whether a cell phenotype such as that described for MAPCs is importantly different than bone marrow– or other tissue-derived adult stem cells that can undergo differentiation into a number of phenotypes, such as "mesenchymal" stem cells, a stem cell phenotype that had been reported earlier.[295] Toma et al[296] have documented that human bone marrow–derived mesenchymal stem cells will engraft in infarcted hearts of immunocompromised (CB17 SCID/beige) adult mice when injected directly into ventricular muscle. A portion of the injected human cells became immunohistochemically indistinguishable from the resident murine cardiac myocytes, expressing a number of (human) cardiac myocyte-specific markers.[296]

Alternatively, Ogawa et al have demonstrated that "mesenchymal" stem cells, isolated from murine bone marrow, can undergo differentiation into a cardiac myocyte-like phenotype after exposure to a demethylating agent, 5-azacytidine.[297,298] Although these cells expressed a number of characteristics of cardiac myoyctes, including the expected complement of adrenergic and muscarinic receptors, among other markers, the safety of this approach, which uses a demethylating agent to induce expression of cardiac-specific genes, may limit its application in studies in humans.

Although the data reviewed above suggest that it may be possible to repair damaged myocardium, as noted by Anversa et al in the infarcted mouse heart, the timing of therapeutic interventions may be critical to the repair process. Since

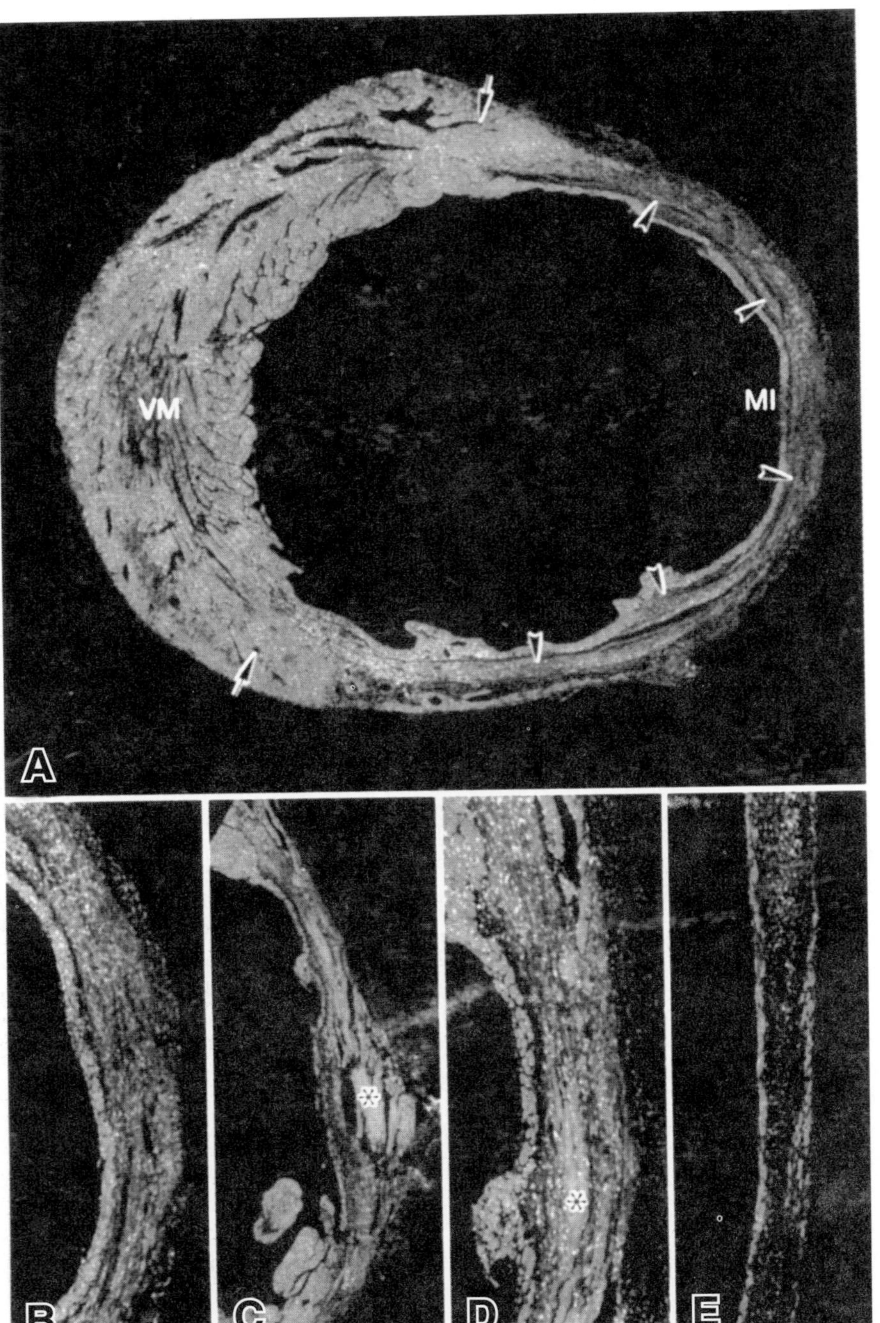

FIGURE 27–17 Bone marrow-derived cells reconstitute infarcted cardiac muscle. (A) In a murine model of myocardial infarction, Orlic et al injected a specific subset of bone marrow–derived cells (lin$^-$, c-kit$^+$) into the newly infarcted muscle shortly after the infarct was created directly. Compared to control animals that received a different subset of bone marrow–derived cells (lin$^-$, c-kit$^-$) whose infarcts exhibited only normal healing (E), animals that received injections of lin$^-$, c-kit$^+$ cells exhibited evidence of reconstitution of the infarct area with newly formed cardiac myocytes, vasculature, and stromal cells (A-D). The asterisk denotes necrotic myocytes. Arrowheads note the placement of lin$^-$, c-kit$^+$ cells. VM = viable muscle; MI = myocardial infarction. Magnification is × 12 (A), × 25 (C), × 50 (B, D, and E); red, cardiac myosin; green: propidium iodide labeling of nuclei. (*Reproduced with permission from Orlic D, Kajstura J, Chimenti S, et al: Bone marrow cells regenerate infarcted myocardium. Nature 2001; 410:701.*)

collection and ex vivo expansion of autologous stem cell populations would of necessity take time, certainly days and perhaps weeks, this approach may have practical limitations for limiting, for example, the extent of tissue necrosis following a myocardial infarction accompanied by pharmacologic, percutaneous, or surgical revascularization. Interestingly, cells of the "mesenchymal" lineage appear to induce a remarkable degree of immunologic tolerance; i.e., they appear not to elicit rejection as allografts or even as xenografts.[299,300] While the mechanism(s) by which selected subsets of adult stem cells induce tolerance remains unknown, if this were true, it would permit the development of "off-the-shelf" stem cell products, thereby eliminating the 2- to 4-week period required to harvest, culture, and expand lineage-restricted autologous stem cells (such as skeletal myoblasts). Regardless, these new data suggest that repair of diseased or damaged tissues by cellular therapeutics holds substantial promise for the future.

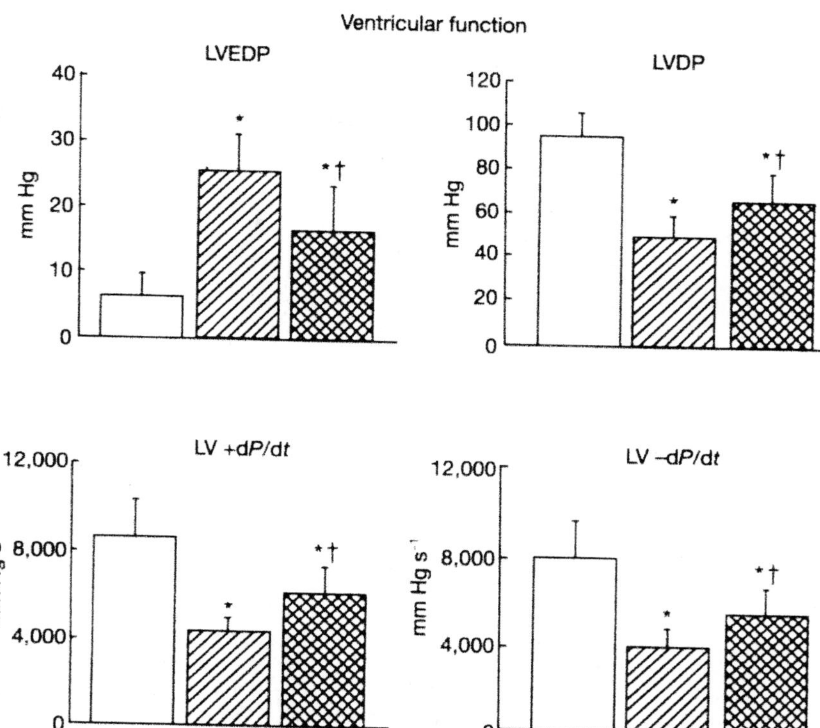

FIGURE 27–18 Ventricular function was analyzed in sham-operated mice (SO; n = 11), control mice that had a myocardial infarction but received control injections of (lin^-, c-kit^-) cells (MI; n = 6), and in mice that had had a myocardial infarction and received injections of (lin^-, c-kit^+) bone marrow–derived cells (MI+BM; n = 9), Hemodynamic testing was performed prior to sacrifice on anaesthetized animals with a Millar microtip pressure transducer in the ventricular cavity (*, $p < .05$ vs. SO; +, $p < .05$ vs. MI; mean ± SD). (*Reproduced with permission from Orlic D, Kajstura J, Chimenti S, et al: Bone marrow cells regenerate infarcted myocardium. Nature 2001; 410:701.*)

REFERENCES

1. Natali A, Vichi S, Landi P, et al: Coronary atherosclerosis in Type II diabetes: angiographic findings and clinical outcome. *Diabetologia* 2000; 43:632.
2. Kip KE, Faxon DP, Detre KM, et al: Coronary angioplasty in diabetic patients. The National Heart, Lung, and Blood Institute Percutaneous Transluminal Coronary Angioplasty Registry. *Circulation* 1996; 94:1818.
3. Musci M, Loebe M, Wellnhofer E, et al: Coronary angioplasty, bypass surgery, and retransplantation in cardiac transplant patients with graft coronary disease. *Thorac Cardiovasc Surg* 1998; 46:268.
4. Musci M, Pasic M, Meyer R, et al: Coronary artery bypass grafting after orthotopic heart transplantation. *Eur J Cardiothorac Surg* 1999; 16:163.
5. Shaukat N, Lear J, Lowy A, et al: First myocardial infarction in patients of Indian subcontinent and European origin: comparison of risk factors, management, and long term outcome. *BMJ* 1997; 314:639.
6. Varghese PJ, Arumugam SB, Cherian KM, et al: Atheromatous plaque reflects serum total cholesterol levels: a comparative morphologic study of endarterectomy coronary atherosclerotic plaques removed from patients from the southern part of India and Caucasians from Ottawa, Canada. *Clin Cardiol* 1998; 21:335.
7. Mukherjee D, Bhatt DL, Roe MT, et al: Direct myocardial revascularization and angiogenesis–how many patients might be eligible? *Am J Cardiol* 1999; 84:598.
8. Scott R, Blackstone EH, McCarthy PM, et al: Isolated bypass grafting of the left internal thoracic artery to the left anterior descending coronary artery: late consequences of incomplete revascularization. *J Thorac Cardiovasc Surg* 2000; 120:173.
9. Risau W: Mechanisms of angiogenesis. *Nature* 1997; 386:671.
10. Simons M, Bonow RO, Chronos NA, et al: Clinical trials in coronary angiogenesis: issues, problems, consensus: an expert panel summary. *Circulation* 2000; 102:E73.
11. Yancopoulos GD, Davis S, Gale NW, et al: Vascular-specific growth factors and blood vessel formation. *Nature* 2000; 407:242.
12. Asahara T, Masuda H, Takahashi T, et al: Bone marrow origin of endothelial progenitor cells responsible for postnatal vasculogenesis in physiological and pathological neovascularization. *Circ Res* 1999; 85:221.
13. Conway EM, Collen D, Carmeliet P: Molecular mechanisms of blood vessel growth. *Cardiovasc Res* 2001; 49:507.
14. Thurston G, Suri C, Smith K, et al: Leakage-resistant blood vessels in mice transgenically overexpressing angiopoietin-1. *Science* 1999; 286:2511.
15. Carmeliet P: Fibroblast growth factor-1 stimulates branching and survival of myocardial arteries: a goal for therapeutic angiogenesis? *Circ Res* 2000; 87:176.
16. Suri C, Jones PF, Patan S, et al: Requisite role of angiopoietin-1, a ligand for the TIE2 receptor, during embryonic angiogenesis. *Cell* 1996; 87:1171.
17. Lindahl P, Bostrom H, Karlsson L, et al: Role of platelet-derived growth factors in angiogenesis and alveogenesis. *Curr Top Pathol* 1999; 93:27.
18. Carmeliet P, Collen D: Molecular basis of angiogenesis: role of VEGF and VE-cadherin. *Ann N Y Acad Sci* 2000; 902:249.
19. Goto F, Goto K, Weindel K, Folkman J: Synergistic effects of vascular endothelial growth factor and basic fibroblast growth factor on the proliferation and cord formation of bovine capillary endothelial cells within collagen gels. *Lab Invest* 1993; 69:508.
20. Folkman J, Shing Y: Angiogenesis. *J Biol Chem* 1992; 267:10931.
21. Gibson CM, Ryan K, Sparano A, et al: Angiographic methods to assess human coronary angiogenesis. *Am Heart J* 1999; 137:169.
22. Nishigami K, Ando M, Hayasaki K: Effects of antecedent anginal episodes and coronary artery stenosis on left ventricular function during coronary occlusion. *Am Heart J* 1995; 130:244.

23. Banai S, Shweiki D, Pinson A, et al: Upregulation of vascular endothelial growth factor expression induced by myocardial ischaemia: implications for coronary angiogenesis. *Cardiovasc Res* 1994; 28:1176.
24. Tofukuji M, Metais C, Li J, et al: Myocardial VEGF expression after cardiopulmonary bypass and cardioplegia. *Circulation* 1998; 98:II242.
25. Kranz A, Rau C, Kochs M, Waltenberger J: Elevation of vascular endothelial growth factor-A serum levels following acute myocardial infarction: evidence for its origin and functional significance. *J Mol Cell Cardiol* 2000; 32:65.
26. Hojo Y, Ikeda U, Zhu Y, et al: Expression of vascular endothelial growth factor in patients with acute myocardial infarction. *J Am Coll Cardiol* 2000; 35:968.
27. Xu X, Li J, Simons M, et al: Expression of vascular endothelial growth factor and its receptors is increased, but microvascular relaxation is impaired in patients after acute myocardial ischemia. *J Thorac Cardiovasc Surg* 2001; 121:735.
28. Lee SH, Wolf PL, Escudero R, et al: Early expression of angiogenesis factors in acute myocardial ischemia and infarction. *N Engl J Med* 2000; 342:626.
29. Heeschen C, Jang JJ, Weis M, et al: Nicotine stimulates angiogenesis and promotes tumor growth and atherosclerosis. *Nat Med* 2001; 7:833.
30. O'Brien ER, Garvin MR, Dev R, et al: Angiogenesis in human coronary atherosclerotic plaques. *Am J Pathol* 1994; 145:883.
31. Gu JW, Elam J, Sartin A, et al: Moderate levels of ethanol induce expression of vascular endothelial growth factor and stimulate angiogenesis. *Am J Physiol Regul Integr Comp Physiol* 2001; 281:R365.
32. Kureishi Y, Luo Z, Shiojima I, et al: The HMG-CoA reductase inhibitor simvastatin activates the protein kinase Akt and promotes angiogenesis in normocholesterolemic animals. *Nat Med* 2000; 6:1004.
33. Barron HV, Sciammarella MG, Lenihan K, et al: Effects of the repeated administration of adenosine and heparin on myocardial perfusion in patients with chronic stable angina pectoris. *Am J Cardiol* 2000; 85:1.
34. Volpert OV, Ward WF, Lingen MW, et al: Captopril inhibits angiogenesis and slows the growth of experimental tumors in rats. *J Clin Invest* 1996; 98:671.
35. Pipili-Synetos E, Papageorgiou A, Sakkoula E, et al: Inhibition of angiogenesis, tumour growth and metastasis by the NO-releasing vasodilators, isosorbide mononitrate and dinitrate. *Br J Pharmacol* 1995; 116:1829.
36. Panet R, Markus M, Atlan H: Bumetanide and furosemide inhibited vascular endothelial cell proliferation. *J Cell Physiol* 1994; 158:121.
37. Klauber N, Browne F, Anand-Apte B, D'Amato RJ: New activity of spironolactone: inhibition of angiogenesis in vitro and in vivo. *Circulation* 1996; 94:2566.
38. Masferrer J: Approach to angiogenesis inhibition based on cyclooxygenase-2. *Cancer J* 2001; 7(suppl 3):S144.
39. Masferrer JL, Koki A, Seibert K: COX-2 inhibitors: a new class of antiangiogenic agents. *Ann N Y Acad Sci* 1999; 889:84.
40. Simons M: Therapeutic coronary angiogenesis: a fronte praecipitium a tergo lupi? *Am J Physiol Heart Circ Physiol* 2001; 280:H1923.
41. Laham RJ, Simons M, Sellke F: Gene transfer for angiogenesis in coronary artery disease. *Annu Rev Med* 2001; 52:485.
42. Gilgenkrantz H, Duboc D, Juillard V, et al: Transient expression of genes transferred in vivo into heart using first-generation adenoviral vectors: role of the immune response. *Hum Gene Ther* 1995; 6:1265.
43. Fujita M, McKown DP, McKown MD, Franklin D: Changes in coronary flow following repeated brief coronary occlusion in the conscious dog. *Heart Vessels* 1986; 2:87.
44. Cohen MV, Yang XM, Liu Y, et al: A new animal model of controlled coronary artery occlusion in conscious rabbits. *Cardiovasc Res* 1994; 28:61.
45. Sellke FW, Li J, Stamler A, et al: Angiogenesis induced by acidic fibroblast growth factor as an alternative method of revascularization for chronic myocardial ischemia. *Surgery* 1996; 120:182.
46. Ikeda K, Hayashida Y, Suita S, Shimoda H: Gradual occlusion of the portal branch with hepatic artery ligation for unresectable hepatic tumour in children. *Z Kinderchir* 1981; 32:121.
47. Sharma HS, Wunsch M, Brand T, et al: Molecular biology of the coronary vascular and myocardial responses to ischemia. *J Cardiovasc Pharmacol* 1992; 20(suppl 1):S23.
48. White FC, Carroll SM, Magnet A, Bloor CM: Coronary collateral development in swine after coronary artery occlusion. *Circ Res* 1992; 71:1490.
49. Sellke FW, Kagaya Y, Johnson RG, et al: Endothelial modulation of porcine coronary microcirculation perfused via immature collaterals. *Am J Physiol* 1992; 262:H1669.
50. Takeshita S, Zheng LP, Brogi E, et al: Therapeutic angiogenesis: a single intraarterial bolus of vascular endothelial growth factor augments revascularization in a rabbit ischemic hind limb model. *J Clin Invest* 1994; 93:662.
51. Takeshita S, Weir L, Chen D, et al: Therapeutic angiogenesis following arterial gene transfer of vascular endothelial growth factor in a rabbit model of hindlimb ischemia. *Biochem Biophys Res Commun* 1996; 227:628.
52. Harada K, Friedman M, Lopez JJ, et al: Vascular endothelial growth factor administration in chronic myocardial ischemia. *Am J Physiol* 1996; 270:H1791.
53. Lee LY, Patel SR, Hackett NR, et al: Focal angiogen therapy using intramyocardial delivery of an adenovirus vector coding for vascular endothelial growth factor 121. *Ann Thorac Surg* 2000; 69:14.
54. Lopez JJ, Laham RJ, Stamler A, et al: VEGF administration in chronic myocardial ischemia in pigs. *Cardiovasc Res* 1988; 40:272.
55. Pearlman JD, Hibberd MG, Chuang ML, et al: Magnetic resonance mapping demonstrates benefits of VEGF-induced myocardial angiogenesis. *Nat Med* 1995; 1:1085.
56. Sato K, Wu T, Laham RJ, Johnson RB, et al: Efficacy of intracoronary or intravenous VEGF165 in a pig model of chronic myocardial ischemia. *J Am Coll Cardiol* 2001; 37:616.
57. Banai S, Jaklitsch MT, Shou M, et al: Angiogenic-induced enhancement of collateral blood flow to ischemic myocardium by vascular endothelial growth factor in dogs. *Circulation* 1994; 89:2183.
58. Lazarous DF, Shou M, Scheinowitz M, et al: Comparative effects of basic fibroblast growth factor and vascular endothelial growth factor on coronary collateral development and the arterial response to injury. *Circulation* 1996; 94:1074.
59. Lazarous DF, Shou M, Stiber JA, et al: Adenoviral-mediated gene transfer induces sustained pericardial VEGF expression in dogs: effect on myocardial angiogenesis. *Cardiovasc Res* 1999; 44:294.
60. Schaper W, Ito WD: Molecular mechanisms of coronary collateral vessel growth. *Circ Res* 1996; 79:911.
61. Unger EF, Banai S, Shou M, et al: A model to assess interventions to improve collateral blood flow: continuous administration of agents into the left coronary artery in dogs. *Cardiovasc Res* 1993; 27:785.
62. Unger EF, Shou M, Sheffield CD, et al: Extracardiac to coronary anastomoses support regional left ventricular function in dogs. *Am J Physiol* 1993; 264:H1567.
63. Ortega S, Schaeffer MT, Soderman D, et al: Conversion of cysteine to serine residues alters the activity, stability, and heparin

dependence of acidic fibroblast growth factor. *J Biol Chem* 1991; 266:5842.

64. Lopez JJ, Edelman ER, Stamler A, et al: Angiogenic potential of perivascularly delivered aFGF in a porcine model of chronic myocardial ischemia. *Am J Physiol* 1998; 274:H930.
65. Unger EF, Banai S, Shou M, et al: Basic fibroblast growth factor enhances myocardial collateral flow in a canine model. *Am J Physiol* 1994; 266:H1588.
66. Lazarous DF, Scheinowitz M, Shou M, et al.: Effects of chronic systemic administration of basic fibroblast growth factor on collateral development in the canine heart. *Circulation* 1995; 91:145.
67. Edelman ER, Mathiowitz E, Langer R, Klagsbrun M: Controlled and modulated release of basic fibroblast growth factor. *Biomaterials* 1991; 12:619.
68. Harada K, Grossman W, Friedman M, et al: Basic fibroblast growth factor improves myocardial function in chronically ischemic porcine hearts. *J Clin Invest* 1994; 94:623.
69. Lopez JJ, Edelman ER, Stamler A, et al: Basic fibroblast growth factor in a porcine model of chronic myocardial ischemia: a comparison of angiographic, echocardiographic and coronary flow parameters. *J Pharmacol Exp Ther* 1997; 282:385.
70. Sellke FW, Wang SY, Friedman M, et al: Basic FGF enhances endothelium-dependent relaxation of the collateral-perfused coronary microcirculation. *Am J Physiol* 1994; 267:H1303.
71. Laham RJ, Rezaee M, Post M, et al: Intrapericardial delivery of fibroblast growth factor-2 induces neovascularization in a porcine model of chronic myocardial ischemia. *J Pharmacol Exp Ther* 2000; 292:795.
72. Sato K, Laham RJ, Pearlman JD, et al: Efficacy of intracoronary versus intravenous FGF-2 in a pig model of chronic myocardial ischemia [in process citation]. *Ann Thorac Surg* 2000; 70:2113.
73. Laham RJ, Rezaee M, Post M, et al: Intracoronary and intravenous administration of basic fibroblast growth factor: myocardial and tissue distribution. *Drug Metab Dispos* 1999; 27:821.
74. Edelman ER, Nugent MA, Karnovsky MJ: Perivascular and intravenous administration of basic fibroblast growth factor: vascular and solid organ deposition. *Proc Natl Acad Sci U S A* 1993; 90:1513.
75. Lee RJ, Springer ML, Blanco-Bose WE, et al: VEGF gene delivery to myocardium: deleterious effects of unregulated expression. *Circulation* 2000; 102:898.
76. Carmeliet P: VEGF gene therapy: stimulating angiogenesis or angioma-genesis? *Nat Med* 2000; 6:1102.
77. Lopez JJ, Laham RJ, Carrozza JP, et al: Hemodynamic effects of intracoronary VEGF delivery: evidence of tachyphylaxis and NO dependence of response. *Am J Physiol* 1997; 273:H1317.
78. Cuevas P, Garcia-Calvo M, Carceller F, et al: Correction of hypertension by normalization of endothelial levels of fibroblast growth factor and nitric oxide synthase in spontaneously hypertensive rats. *Proc Natl Acad Sci U S A* 1996; 93:11996.
79. Floege J, Kriz W, Schulze M, et al: Basic fibroblast growth factor augments podocyte injury and induces glomerulosclerosis in rats with experimental membranous nephropathy. *J Clin Invest* 1995; 96:2809.
80. Sasaki T, Jyo Y, Tanda N, et al: Changes in glomerular epithelial cells induced by FGF2 and FGF2 neutralizing antibody in puromycin aminonucleoside nephropathy. *Kidney Int* 1997; 51:301.
81. Ruel M, Laham RJ, Parker JA, et al: Long-term effects of surgical angiogenic therapy with FGF-2 protein. *J Thorac Cardiovasc Surg* 2002; 124:28.
82. Sellke FW, Laham RJ, Edelman ER, et al: Therapeutic angiogenesis with basic fibroblast growth factor: technique and early results. *Ann Thorac Surg* 1998; 65:1540.
83. Rosengart TK, Lee LY, Patel SR, et al: Angiogenesis gene therapy: phase I assessment of direct intramyocardial administration of an adenovirus vector expressing VEGF121 cDNA to individuals with clinically significant severe coronary artery disease. *Circulation* 1999; 100:468.
84. Laham RJ, Sellke FW, Edelman ER, et al: Local perivascular delivery of basic fibroblast growth factor in patients undergoing coronary bypass surgery: results of a phase I randomized, double-blind, placebo-controlled trial. *Circulation* 1999; 100:1865.
85. Lopez JJ, Edelman ER, Stamler A, et al: Local perivascular administration of basic fibroblast growth factor: drug delivery and toxicological evaluation. *Drug Metab Dispos* 1996; 24:922. [Published erratum appears in *Drug Metab Dispos* 1996; 24:1166.]
86. Schumacher B, Pecher P, von Specht BU, Stegmann T: Induction of neoangiogenesis in ischemic myocardium by human growth factors: first clinical results of a new treatment of coronary heart disease. *Circulation* 1998; 97:645.
87. Pecher P, Schumacher BA: Angiogenesis in ischemic human myocardium: clinical results after 3 years. *Ann Thorac Surg* 2000; 69:1414.
88. Laham RJ, Chronos NA, Pike M, et al: Intracoronary basic fibroblast growth factor (FGF-2) in patients with severe ischemic heart disease: results of a phase I open-label dose escalation study. *J Am Coll Cardiol* 2000; 36:2132.
89. Simons M, Annex BH, Laham RJ, et al: Pharmacological treatment of coronary artery disease with recombinant fibroblast growth factor-2: double-blind, randomized, controlled clinical trial. *Circulation* 2002; 105:788.
90. Henry TD, Abraham JA: Review of preclinical and clinical results with vascular endothelial growth factors for therapeutic angiogenesis. *Curr Interv Cardiol Rep* 2000; 2:228.
91. Losordo DW, Vale PR, Symes JF, et al: Gene therapy for myocardial angiogenesis: initial clinical results with direct myocardial injection of phVEGF165 as sole therapy for myocardial ischemia. *Circulation* 1998; 98:2800.
92. Symes JF, Losordo DW, Vale PR, et al: Gene therapy with vascular endothelial growth factor for inoperable coronary artery disease. *Ann Thorac Surg* 1999; 68:830.
93. Vale PR, Losordo DW, Milliken CE, et al: Randomized, single-blind, placebo-controlled pilot study of catheter-based myocardial gene transfer for therapeutic angiogenesis using left ventricular electromechanical mapping in patients with chronic myocardial ischemia. *Circulation* 2001; 103:2138.

93a. Losordo DW, Vale PR, Hendel RC, et al: Phase 1/2 placebo-controlled, double-blind, dose-escalating trial of myocardial vascular endothelial growth factor 2 gene transfer by catheter delivery in patients with chronic myocardial ischemia. *Circulation* 2002; 105: 2012.

94. Shalala D: Protecting research subjects–what must be done. *N Engl J Med* 2000; 343:808.
95. Arnal JF, Yamin J, Dockery S, Harrison DG: Regulation of endothelial nitric oxide synthase mRNA, protein, and activity during cell growth. *Am J Physiol* 1994; 267:C1381.
96. Sellke FW, Wang SY, Stamler A, et al: Enhanced microvascular relaxations to VEGF and bFGF in chronically ischemic porcine myocardium. *Am J Physiol* 1996; 271:H713.
97. Granger HJ, Ziche M, Hawker JR Jr, et al: Molecular and cellular basis of myocardial angiogenesis. *Cell Mol Biol Res* 1994; 40:81.
98. Murohara T, Witzenbichler B, Spyridopoulos I, et al: Role of endothelial nitric oxide synthase in endothelial cell migration. *Arterioscler Thromb Vasc Biol* 1999; 19:1156.
99. Duan J, Murohara T, Ikeda H, et al: Hypercholesterolemia inhibits angiogenesis in response to hindlimb ischemia: nitric oxide-dependent mechanism. *Circulation* 2000; 102:III370.
100. Jang JJ, Ho HK, Kwan HH, et al: Angiogenesis is impaired by hypercholesterolemia: role of asymmetric dimethylarginine. *Circulation* 2000; 102:1414.

101. Ruel M, Sellke FW, Bianchi C, et al: Endogenous myocardial angiogenesis and revascularization using a gastric submucosal patch. *Ann Thorac Surg (in press)*.
102. Lee YM, Jeong CH, Koo SY, et al: Determination of hypoxic region by hypoxia marker in developing mouse embryos in vivo: a possible signal for vessel development. *Dev Dyn* 2001; 220:175.
103. Li J, Post M, Volk R, et al: PR39, a peptide regulator of angiogenesis. *Nat Med* 2000; 6:49. [Published erratum appears in *Nat Med* 2000; 6:356.]
104. Unemori EN, Lewis M, Constant J, et al: Relaxin induces vascular endothelial growth factor expression and angiogenesis selectively at wound sites. *Wound Repair Regen* 2000; 8:361.
105. Gavino ES, Furst DE: Recombinant relaxin: a review of pharmacology and potential therapeutic use. *BioDrugs* 2001; 15:609.
106. Vineberg AM: Development of an anastomosis between the coronary vessels and a transplanted internal mammary artery. *Can Med Assoc J* 1946; 55:117.
107. Sen PK, Udwadia TE, Kinare SG, Parulkar GB: Transmyocardial acupuncture: a new approach to myocardial revascularization. *J Thorac Cardiovasc Surg* 1965; 50:181.
108. Sen PK, Daulatram J, Kinare SG, et al: Further studies in multiple transmyocardial acupuncture as a method of myocardial revascularization. *Surgery* 1968; 64:861.
109. Hershey JE, White M: Transmyocardial puncture revascularization: a possible emergency adujct to arterial implant surgery. *Geriatrics* 1969; 24:101.
110. Hershey JE: Multiple transmyocardial puncture revascularization. *Ann Thorac Surg* 1999; 68:1890.
111. Hershey JE: Transmyocardial revascularization: could mechanical puncture be more effective than puncture by laser? *Tex Heart Inst J* 2000; 27:80.
112. White M, Hershey JE: Multiple transmyocardial puncture revascularization in refractory ventricular fibrillation due to myocardial ischemia. *Ann Thorac Surg* 1968; 6:557.
113. Pifarre R, Jasuja ML, Lynch RD, Neville WE: Myocardial revascularization by transmyocardial acupuncture: a physiologic impossibility. *J Thorac Cardiovasc Surg* 1969; 58:424.
114. Mirhoseini M, Cayton MM: Revascularization of the heart by laser. *J Microsurg* 1981; 2:253.
115. Mirhoseini M, Fisher JC, Cayton M: Myocardial revascularization by laser: a clinical report. *Lasers Surg Med* 1983; 3:241.
116. Mirhoseini M, Cayton MM: Transmyocardial laser revascularization: historical background and future directions. *J Clin Laser Med Surg* 1997; 15:245.
117. Frazier OH, Cooley DA, Kadipasaoglu KA, et al: Myocardial revascularization with laser. Preliminary findings. *Circulation* 1995; 92:II58.
118. Josefson D: FDA approves heart laser treatment. *BMJ* 1998; 316:1409.
119. Yano OJ, Bielefeld MR, Jeevanandam V, et al: Prevention of acute regional ischemia with endocardial laser channels. *Ann Thorac Surg* 1993; 56:46.
120. Whittaker P, Kloner RA, Przyklenk K: Laser-mediated transmural myocardial channels do not salvage acutely ischemic myocardium. *J Am Coll Cardiol* 1993; 22:302.
121. Lee LY, O'Hara MF, Finnin EB, et al: Transmyocardial laser revascularization with excimer laser: clinical results at 1 year. *Ann Thorac Surg* 2000; 70:498.
122. Martin JS, Sayeed-Shah U, Byrne JG, et al: Excimer versus carbon dioxide transmyocardial laser revascularization: effects on regional left ventricular function and perfusion. *Ann Thorac Surg* 2000; 69:1811.
123. Lutter G, Schwarzkopf J, Lutz C, et al: Histologic findings of transmyocardial laser channels after two hours. *Ann Thorac Surg* 1998; 65:1437.
124. Kadipasaoglu KA, Frazier OH: Transmyocardial laser revascularization: effect of laser parameters on tissue ablation and cardiac perfusion. *Semin Thorac Cardiovasc Surg* 1999; 11:4.
125. Cooley DA, Frazier OH, Kadipasaoglu KA, et al: Transmyocardial laser revascularization: anatomic evidence of long-term channel patency. *Tex Heart Inst J* 1994; 21:220.
126. Beranek JT: Long-lasting patent channels created by transmyocardial laser revascularization. *Lasers Surg Med* 1999; 25:375.
127. Beranek JT: In situ DNA nick-end labeling positive reaction around laser channels. *Thorac Cardiovasc Surg* 2001; 49:318.
128. Burkhoff D, Fisher PE, Apfelbaum M, et al: Histologic appearance of transmyocardial laser channels after 4 1/2 weeks. *Ann Thorac Surg* 1996; 61:1532.
129. Fisher PE, Khomoto T, DeRosa CM, et al: Histologic analysis of transmyocardial channels: comparison of CO2 and holmium:YAG lasers. *Ann Thorac Surg* 1997; 64:466.
130. Kohmoto T, Fisher PE, Gu A, et al: Physiology, histology, and 2–week morphology of acute transmyocardial channels made with a CO2 laser. *Ann Thorac Surg* 1997; 63:1275.
131. Genyk IA, Frenz M, Ott B, et al: Acute and chronic effects of transmyocardial laser revascularization in the nonischemic pig myocardium by using three laser systems. *Lasers Surg Med* 2000; 27:438.
132. Gassler N, Wintzer HO, Stubbe HM, et al: Transmyocardial laser revascularization: histological features in human nonresponder myocardium. *Circulation* 1997; 95:371.
133. Cherian SM, Bobryshev YV, Liang H, et al: Ultrastructural and immunohistochemical analysis of early myocardial changes following transmyocardial laser revascularization. *J Card Surg* 2000; 15:341.
134. Ansari A: Anatomy and clinical significance of ventricular Thebesian veins. *Clin Anat* 2001; 14:102.
135. Malekan R, Reynolds C, Narula N, et al: Angiogenesis in transmyocardial laser revascularization: a nonspecific response to injury. *Circulation* 1998; 98:I162.
136. Hughes GC, Lowe JE, Kypson AP, et al: Neovascularization after transmyocardial laser revascularization in a model of chronic ischemia. *Ann Thorac Surg* 1998; 66:2029.
137. Horvath KA, Chiu E, Maun DC, et al: Up-regulation of vascular endothelial growth factor mRNA and angiogenesis after transmyocardial laser revascularization. *Ann Thorac Surg* 1999; 68:825.
138. Kim EJ, Li RK, Weisel RD, et al: Angiogenesis by endothelial cell transplantation. *J Thorac Cardiovasc Surg* 2001; 122:963.
139. Pelletier MP, Giaid A, Sivaraman S, et al: Angiogenesis and growth factor expression in a model of transmyocardial revascularization. *Ann Thorac Surg* 1998; 66:12.
140. Chu V, Kuang J, McGinn A, et al: Angiogenic response induced by mechanical transmyocardial revascularization. *J Thorac Cardiovasc Surg* 1999; 118:849.
141. Chu VF, Giaid A, Kuang JQ, et al: Thoracic Surgery Directors Association Award. Angiogenesis in transmyocardial revascularization: comparison of laser versus mechanical punctures. *Ann Thorac Surg* 1999; 68:301.
142. Horvath KA, Belkind N, Wu I, et al: Functional comparison of transmyocardial revascularization by mechanical and laser means. *Ann Thorac Surg* 2001; 72:1997.
143. Kwong KF, Kanellopoulos GK, Nickols JC, et al: Transmyocardial laser treatment denervates canine myocardium. *J Thorac Cardiovasc Surg* 1997; 114:883.
144. Kwong KF, Schuessler RB, Kanellopoulos GK, et al: Nontransmural laser treatment incompletely denervates canine myocardium. *Circulation* 1998; 98:II67.
145. Hirsch GM, Thompson GW, Arora RC, et al: Transmyocardial laser revascularization does not denervate the canine heart. *Ann Thorac Surg* 1999; 68:460.

146. Minisi AJ, Topaz O, Quinn MS, Mohanty LB: Cardiac nociceptive reflexes after transmyocardial laser revascularization: implications for the neural hypothesis of angina relief. *J Thorac Cardiovasc Surg* 2001; 122:712.
147. Arora RC, Hirsch GM, Hirsch K, Armour JA: Transmyocardial laser revascularization remodels the intrinsic cardiac nervous system in a chronic setting. *Circulation* 2001; 104:I115.
148. Al-Sheikh T, Allen KB, Straka SP, et al: Cardiac sympathetic denervation after transmyocardial laser revascularization. *Circulation* 1999; 100:135.
149. Gassler N, Rastar F, Hentz MW: Angiogenesis and expression of tenascin after transmural laser revascularization. *Histol Histopathol* 1999; 14:81.
150. Laham RJ, Simons M: Laser myocardial revascularization: fact or fiction? *Card Vasc Regener* 2000; 1:70.
151. Horvath KA, Greene R, Belkind N, et al: Left ventricular functional improvement after transmyocardial laser revascularization. *Ann Thorac Surg* 1998; 66:721.
152. Hughes GC, Kypson AP, St Louis JD, et al: Improved perfusion and contractile reserve after transmyocardial laser revascularization in a model of hibernating myocardium. *Ann Thorac Surg* 1999; 67:1714.
153. Horvath KA, Smith WJ, Laurence RG, et al: Recovery and viability of an acute myocardial infarct after transmyocardial laser revascularization. *J Am Coll Cardiol* 1995; 25:258.
154. Landreneau R, Nawarawong W, Laughlin H, et al: Direct CO2 laser "revascularization" of the myocardium. *Lasers Surg Med* 1991; 11:35.
155. Hattan N, Ban K, Tanaka E, et al: Transmyocardial revascularization aggravates myocardial ischemia around the channels in the immediate phase. *Am J Physiol Heart Circ Physiol* 2000; 279:H1392.
156. Malekan R, Kelley ST, Suzuki Y, et al: Transmyocardial laser revascularization fails to prevent left ventricular functional deterioration and aneurysm formation after acute myocardial infarction in sheep. *J Thorac Cardiovasc Surg* 1998; 116:752.
157. deGuzman BJ, Lautz DB, Chen FY, et al: Thoracoscopic transmyocardial laser revascularization. *Ann Thorac Surg* 1997; 64:171.
158. Mack CA, Magovern CJ, Hahn RT, et al: Channel patency and neovascularization after transmyocardial revascularization using an excimer laser: results and comparisons to nonlased channels. *Circulation* 1997; 96:II65.
159. Hamawy AH, Lee LY, Samy SA, et al: Transmyocardial laser revascularization dose response: enhanced perfusion in a porcine ischemia model as a function of channel density. *Ann Thorac Surg* 2001; 72:817.
160. Mueller XM, Bettex D, Tevaearai HT, von Segesser LK: Acute effects of transmyocardial laser revascularization on left-ventricular function: a haemodynamic and echocardiographic study. *Thorac Cardiovasc Surg* 1998; 46:126.
161. Hughes GC, Shah AS, Yin B, et al: Early postoperative changes in regional systolic and diastolic left ventricular function after transmyocardial laser revascularization: a comparison of holmium:YAG and CO2 lasers. *J Am Coll Cardiol* 2000; 35:1022.
162. Eckstein FS, Scheule AM, Vogel U, et al: Transmyocardial laser revascularization in the acute ischaemic heart: no improvement of acute myocardial perfusion or prevention of myocardial infarction. *Eur J Cardiothorac Surg* 199; 15:702.
163. Kim CB, Kesten R, Javier M, et al: Percutaneous method of laser transmyocardial revascularization. *Cathet Cardiovasc Diagn* 1997; 40:223.
164. Kadipasaoglu KA, Sartori M, Masai T, et al: Intraoperative arrhythmias and tissue damage during transmyocardial laser revascularization. *Ann Thorac Surg* 1999; 67:423.
165. Hughes GC, Kypson AP, Annex BH, et al: Induction of angiogenesis after TMR: a comparison of holmium:YAG, CO2, and excimer lasers. *Ann Thorac Surg* 2000; 70:504.
166. Fleischer KJ, Goldschmidt-Clermont PJ, et al: One-month histologic response of transmyocardial laser channels with molecular intervention. *Ann Thorac Surg* 1996; 62:1051.
167. Yamamoto N, Kohmoto T, Roethy W, et al: Histologic evidence that basic fibroblast growth factor enhances the angiogenic effects of transmyocardial laser revascularization. *Basic Res Cardiol* 2000; 95:55.
168. Sayeed-Shah U, Mann MJ, Martin J, et al: Complete reversal of ischemic wall motion abnormalities by combined use of gene therapy with transmyocardial laser revascularization. *J Thorac Cardiovasc Surg* 1998; 116:763.
169. Hughes GC, Annex BH, Yin B, et al: Transmyocardial laser revascularization limits in vivo adenoviral-mediated gene transfer in porcine myocardium. *Cardiovasc Res* 1999; 44:81.
170. Nagele H, Stubbe HM, Nienaber C, Rodiger W: Results of transmyocardial laser revascularization in non-revascularizable coronary artery disease after 3 years follow-up [see comments]. *Eur Heart J* 1998; 19:1525.
171. Hattler BG, Griffith BP, Zenati MA, et al: Transmyocardial laser revascularization in the patient with unmanageable unstable angina. *Ann Thorac Surg* 1999; 68:1203.
172. Dowling RD, Petracek MR, Selinger SL, Allen KB: Transmyocardial revascularization in patients with refractory, unstable angina. *Circulation* 1998; 98:II73.
173. Kalangos A, Schweizer A, Licker M, et al: Partial left ventriculectomy combined with transmyocardial laser revascularization. *Ann Thorac Surg* 1999; 68:1397.
174. Lutter G, Saurbier B, Nitzsche E, et al: Transmyocardial laser revascularization (TMLR) in patients with unstable angina and low ejection fraction. *Eur J Cardiothorac Surg* 1998; 13:21.
175. Frazier OH, Kadipasaoglu KA, Radovancevic B, et al: Transmyocardial laser revascularization in allograft coronary artery disease. *Ann Thorac Surg* 1998; 65:1138.
176. Malik FS, Mehra MR, Ventura HO, et al: Management of cardiac allograft vasculopathy by transmyocardial laser revascularization. *Am J Cardiol* 1997; 80:224.
177. March RJ, Guynn T: Cardiac allograft vasculopathy: the potential role for transmyocardial laser revascularization. *J Heart Lung Transplant* 1995; 14:S242.
178. McFadden PM, Robbins RJ, Ochsner JL, et al: Transmyocardial revascularization for cardiac transplantation allograft vasculopathy. *J Thorac Cardiovasc Surg* 1998; 115:1385.
179. Grauhan O, Krabatsch T, Lieback E, Hetzer R: Transmyocardial laser revascularization in ischemic cardiomyopathy. *J Heart Lung Transplant* 2001; 20:687.
180. Mehra MR, Uber PA, Prasad AK, et al: Long-term outcome of cardiac allograft vasculopathy treated by transmyocardial laser revascularization: early rewards, late losses. *J Heart Lung Transplant* 2000; 19:801.
181. Lee R, Fischer KC, Moon MR: Reoperative transmyocardial laser revascularization for late recurrent angina. *Ann Thorac Surg* 2002; 73:650.
182. March RJ: Laser revascularization of ischemic myocardium, in Naunheim KS (ed): *Minimal Access Cardiothoracic Surgery*. Philadelphia, WB Saunders, 2000; p 598.
183. Saatvedt K, Dragsund M, Nordstrand K: Transmyocardial laser revascularization and coronary artery bypass grafting without cardiopulmonary bypass. *Ann Thorac Surg* 1996; 62:323.
184. Trehan N, Mishra M, Bapna R, et al: Transmyocardial laser revascularisation combined with coronary artery bypass grafting without cardiopulmonary bypass. *Eur J Cardiothorac Surg* 1997; 12:276.

185. Trehan N, Mishra Y, Mehta Y, Jangid DR: Transmyocardial laser as an adjunct to minimally invasive CABG for complete myocardial revascularization. *Ann Thorac Surg* 1998; 66:1113.
186. Horvath KA: Thoracoscopic transmyocardial laser revascularization. *Ann Thorac Surg* 1998; 65:1439.
187. Milano A, Pietrabissa A, Bortolotti U: Transmyocardial laser revascularization using a thoracoscopic approach. *Am J Cardiol* 1997; 80:538.
188. Milano A, Pietrabissa A, Bortolotti U: Thoracoscopic transmyocardial revascularization. *Ann Thorac Surg* 1998; 65:1510.
189. Milano A, Pratali S, De Carlo M, et al: Transmyocardial holmium laser revascularization: feasibility of a thoracoscopic approach. *Eur J Cardiothorac Surg* 1998; 14(suppl 1):S105.
190. Bortone AS, D'Agostino D, Schena S, et al: Instrumental validation of percutaneous transmyocardial revascularization: follow-up data at one year. *Ann Thorac Surg* 2000; 70:1115.
191. Hughes GC, Landolfo KP, Lowe JE, et al: Perioperative morbidity and mortality after transmyocardial laser revascularization: incidence and risk factors for adverse events. *J Am Coll Cardiol* 1999; 33:1021.
192. von Knobelsdorff G, Brauer P, Tonner PH, et al: Transmyocardial laser revascularization induces cerebral microembolization. *Anesthesiology* 1997; 87:58.
193. Hughes GC, Landolfo KP, Lowe JE, et al: Diagnosis, incidence, and clinical significance of early postoperative ischemia after transmyocardial laser revascularization. *Am Heart J* 1999; 137:1163.
194. Burkhoff D, Wesley MN, Resar JR, Lansing AM: Factors correlating with risk of mortality after transmyocardial revascularization. *J Am Coll Cardiol* 1999; 34:55.
195. Kraatz EG, Misfeld M, Jungbluth B, Sievers HH: Survival after transmyocardial laser revascularization in relation to nonlasered perfused myocardial zones. *Ann Thorac Surg* 2001; 71:532.
196. Cooley DA, Frazier OH, Kadipasaoglu KA, et al: Transmyocardial laser revascularization: clinical experience with twelve-month follow-up. *J Thorac Cardiovasc Surg* 1996; 111:791.
197. Horvath KA, Cohn LH, Cooley DA, et al: Transmyocardial laser revascularization: results of a multicenter trial with transmyocardial laser revascularization used as sole therapy for end-stage coronary artery disease. *J Thorac Cardiovasc Surg* 1997; 113:645.
198. Donovan CL, Landolfo KP, Lowe JE, et al: Improvement in inducible ischemia during dobutamine stress echocardiography after transmyocardial laser revascularization in patients with refractory angina pectoris. *J Am Coll Cardiol* 1997; 30:607.
199. Horvath KA, Mannting F, Cummings N, et al: Transmyocardial laser revascularization: operative techniques and clinical results at two years. *J Thorac Cardiovasc Surg* 1996; 111:1047.
200. Agarwal R, Ajit M, Kurian VM, et al: Transmyocardial laser revascularization: early results and 1–year follow-up. *Ann Thorac Surg* 1999; 67:432.
201. Burns SM, Sharples LD, Tait S, et al: The transmyocardial laser revascularization international registry report. *Eur Heart J* 1999; 20:31.
202. Frazier OH, March RJ, Horvath KA: Transmyocardial revascularization with a carbon dioxide laser in patients with end-stage coronary artery disease. *N Engl J Med* 1999; 341:1021.
203. Schofield PM, Sharples LD, Caine N, et al: Transmyocardial laser revascularisation in patients with refractory angina: a randomised controlled trial. *Lancet* 1999; 353:519.
204. Aaberge L, Nordstrand K, Dragsund M, et al: Transmyocardial revascularization with CO2 laser in patients with refractory angina pectoris: clinical results from the Norwegian randomized trial. *J Am Coll Cardiol* 2000; 35:1170.
205. Landolfo CK, Landolfo KP, Hughes GC, et al: Intermediate-term clinical outcome following transmyocardial laser revascularization in patients with refractory angina pectoris. *Circulation* 1999; 100:II128.
206. Burns SM, Brown S, White CA, et al: Quantitative analysis of myocardial perfusion changes with transmyocardial laser revascularization. *Am J Cardiol* 2001; 87:861.
207. Aaberge L, Rootwelt K, Smith HJ, et al: Effects of transmyocardial revascularization on myocardial perfusion and systolic function assessed by nuclear and magnetic resonance imaging methods. *Scand Cardiovasc J* 2001; 35:8.
208. Horvath KA, Aranki SF, Cohn LH, et al: Sustained angina relief 5 years after transmyocardial laser revascularization with a CO(2) laser. *Circulation* 2001; 104:I81.
209. Allen KB, Dowling RD, Heimansohn DA, et al: Transmyocardial revascularization utilizing a holmium:YAG laser. *Eur J Cardiothorac Surg* 1998; 4(suppl 1):S100.
210. Diegeler A, Schneider J, Lauer B, et al: Transmyocardial laser revascularization using the Holium-YAG laser for treatment of end stage coronary artery disease. *Eur J Cardiothorac Surg* 1998; 13:392.
211. Jones JW, Richman BW, Crigger NA, Baldwin JC: Technique of transmyocardial revascularization: avoiding complications in high-risk patients. *J Cardiovasc Surg* (Torino) 2001; 42:353.
212. Schneider J, Diegeler A, Krakor R, et al: Transmyocardial laser revascularization with the holmium:YAG laser: loss of symptomatic improvement after 2 years. *Eur J Cardiothorac Surg* 2001; 19:164.
213. Kornowski R, Baim DS, Moses JW, et al: Short- and intermediate-term clinical outcomes from direct myocardial laser revascularization guided by biosense left ventricular electromechanical mapping. *Circulation* 2000; 102:1120.
214. Lauer B, Junghans U, Stahl F, et al: Catheter-based percutaneous myocardial laser revascularization in patients with end-stage coronary artery disease. *J Am Coll Cardiol* 1999; 34:1663.
215. Kluge R, Lauer B, Stahl F, et al: Changes in myocardial perfusion after catheter-based percutaneous laser revascularisation. *Eur J Nucl Med* 2000; 27:1292.
216. Laham RJ, Simons M, Pearlman JD, et al: Magnetic resonance imaging demonstrates improved regional systolic wall motion and thickening and myocardial perfusion of myocardial territories treated by laser myocardial revascularization. *J Am Coll Cardiol* 2002; 39:1.
217. Laham RJ, Baim DS: Combined percutaneous biosense-guided laser myocardial revascularization and coronary intervention. *Cathet Cardiovasc Interv* 2001; 53:235.
218. Dixon SR, Schreiber TL, Rabah M, et al: Immediate effect of percutaneous myocardial laser revascularization on hemodynamics and left ventricular systolic function in severe angina pectoris. *Am J Cardiol* 2001; 87:516.
219. Jones JW, Schmidt SE, Richman BW, et al: YAG laser transmyocardial revascularization relieves angina and improves functional status. *Ann Thorac Surg* 1999; 67:1596.
220. Allen KB, Dowling RD, Fudge TL, et al: Comparison of transmyocardial revascularization with medical therapy in patients with refractory angina. *N Engl J Med* 1999; 341:1029.
221. Allen KB, Dowling RD, DelRossi AJ, et al: Transmyocardial laser revascularization combined with coronary artery bypass grafting: a multicenter, blinded, prospective, randomized, controlled trial. *J Thorac Cardiovasc Surg* 2000; 119:540.
222. Burkhoff D, Schmidt S, Schulman SP, et al: Transmyocardial laser revascularisation compared with continued medical therapy for treatment of refractory angina pectoris: a prospective randomised trial. ATLANTIC Investigators. Angina Treatments—Lasers and Normal Therapies in Comparison. *Lancet* 1999; 354:885.
223. Oesterle SN, Sanborn TA, Ali N, et al: Percutaneous transmyocardial laser revascularisation for severe angina: the PACIFIC

randomised trial. Potential Class Improvement from Intramyocardial Channels. *Lancet* 2000; 356:1705.

224. Leon MB, Baim DS, Moses JW, et al: A randomized blinded clinical trial comparing percutaneous laser revascularization vs. placebo in patients with refractory coronary ischemia (DIRECT trial). Presentation at the 50th meeting of the American College of Cardiology, Orlando, FL, March 2001.
225. Bristow MR, Port JD, Kelly RA: Drugs used in the treatment of heart failure, in Braunwald E (ed): *Heart Disease: A Textbook of Cardiovascular Medicine*. Philadelphia, W.B. Saunders, 2001; p 562.
226. Rose EA: Randomized evaluation of mechanical assistance for the treatment of congestive heart failure (REMATCH). *Circulation* 2002; 105:E38.
227. Rose EA, Moskowitz AJ, Packer M, et al: The REMATCH trial: rationale, design, and end points. Randomized Evaluation of Mechanical Assistance for the Treatment of Congestive Heart Failure. *Ann Thorac Surg* 1999; 67:723.
228. Louis AA, Manousos IR, Coletta AP, et al: Clinical trials update: The Heart Protection Study, IONA, CARISA, ENRICHD, ACUTE, ALIVE, MADIT II and REMATCH. Impact Of Nicorandil on Angina. Combination Assessment of Ranolazine In Stable Angina. ENhancing Recovery In Coronary Heart Disease patients. Assessment of Cardioversion Using Transoesophageal Echocardiography. AzimiLide post-Infarct surVival Evaluation. Randomised Evaluation of Mechanical Assistance for Treatment of Chronic Heart failure. *Eur J Heart Fail* 2002; 4:111.
229. Rockman HA, Koch WJ, Lefkowitz RJ: Seven-transmembrane-spanning receptors and heart function. *Nature* 2002; 415:206.
230. Kessler PD, Byrne BJ: Myoblast cell grafting into heart muscle: cellular biology and potential applications. *Annu Rev Physiol* 1999; 61:219.
231. Anversa P, Nadal-Ginard B: Myocyte renewal and ventricular remodelling. *Nature* 2002; 415:240.
232. Beltrami AP, Urbanek K, Kajstura J, et al: Evidence that human cardiac myocytes divide after myocardial infarction. *N Engl J Med* 2001; 344:1750.
233. Soonpaa MH, Koh GY, Klug MG, Field LJ: Formation of nascent intercalated disks between grafted fetal cardiomyocytes and host myocardium. *Science* 1994; 264:98.
234. Koh GY, Soonpaa MH, Klug MG, et al: Stable fetal cardiomyocyte grafts in the hearts of dystrophic mice and dogs. *J Clin Invest* 1995; 96:2034.
235. Reinecke H, Zhang M, Bartosek T, Murry CE: Survival, integration, and differentiation of cardiomyocyte grafts: a study in normal and injured rat hearts. *Circulation* 1999; 100:193.
236. Scorsin M, Hagege AA, Marotte F, Mirochnik N, Copin H, Barnoux M, Sabri A, Samuel JL, Rappaport L, Menasche P: Does transplantation of cardiomyocytes improve function of infarcted myocardium? *Circulation* 96:II, 1997.
237. Chiu RC, Zibaitis A, Kao RL: Cellular cardiomyoplasty: myocardial regeneration with satellite cell implantation. *Ann Thorac Surg* 1995; 60:12.
238. Wang JS, Shum-Tim D, Chedrawy E, Chiu RC: The coronary delivery of marrow stromal cells for myocardial regeneration: pathophysiologic and therapeutic implications. *J Thorac Cardiovasc Surg* 122:699, 2001.
239. Koh GY, Klug MG, Soonpaa MH, Field LJ: Differentiation and long-term survival of C2C12 myoblast grafts in heart. *J Clin Invest* 1993; 92:1548.
240. Murry CE, Kay MA, Bartosek T, et al: Muscle differentiation during repair of myocardial necrosis in rats via gene transfer with MyoD. *J Clin Invest* 1996; 98:2209.
241. Murry CE, Wiseman RW, Schwartz SM, Hauschka SD: Skeletal myoblast transplantation for repair of myocardial necrosis. *J Clin Invest* 1996; 98:2512.
242. Reinecke H, MacDonald GH, Hauschka SD, Murry CE: Electromechanical coupling between skeletal and cardiac muscle. Implications for infarct repair. *J Cell Biol* 2000; 149:731.
243. Reinecke H, Murry CE: Transmural replacement of myocardium after skeletal myoblast grafting into the heart: too much of a good thing? *Cardiovasc Pathol* 2000; 9:337.
244. Zhang M, Methot D, Poppa V, et al: Cardiomyocyte grafting for cardiac repair: graft cell death and anti-death strategies. *J Mol Cell Cardiol* 2001; 33:907.
245. Reinecke H, Poppa V, Murry CE: Skeletal muscle stem cells do not transdifferentiate into cardiomyocytes after cardiac grafting. *J Mol Cell Cardiol* 2002; 34:241.
246. Taylor DA, Atkins BZ, Hungspreugs P, et al: Regenerating functional myocardium: improved performance after skeletal myoblast transplantation. *Nat Med* 1998; 4:929.
247. Atkins BZ, Lewis CW, Kraus WE, et al: Intracardiac transplantation of skeletal myoblasts yields two populations of striated cells in situ. *Ann Thorac Surg* 1999; 67:124.
248. Atkins BZ, Hueman MT, Meuchel J, et al: Cellular cardiomyoplasty improves diastolic properties of injured heart. *J Surg Res* 1999; 85:234.
249. Atkins BZ, Hueman MT, Meuchel JM, Cottman MJ, Hutcheson KA, Taylor DA: Myogenic cell transplantation improves in vivo regional performance in infarcted rabbit myocardium. *J Heart Lung Transplant* 1999; 18:1173.
250. Hutcheson KA, Atkins BZ, Hueman MT, et al: Comparison of benefits on myocardial performance of cellular cardiomyoplasty with skeletal myoblasts and fibroblasts. *Cell Transplant* 200; 9:359.
251. Scarborough JE, Colgrove SL, Lowe M, et al: Autologous skeletal myoblast transplantation prevents ventricular dilatation in a porcine model of myocardial infarction. *J Heart Lung Transplant* 2002; 21:163.
252. Jain M, DerSimonian H, Brenner DA, et al: Cell therapy attenuates deleterious ventricular remodeling and improves cardiac performance after myocardial infarction. *Circulation* 2001; 103:1920.
253. Li RK, Mickle DA, Weisel RD, et al: In vivo survival and function of transplanted rat cardiomyocytes. *Circ Res* 1996; 78:283.
254. Li RK, Jia ZQ, Weisel RD, et al: Cardiomyocyte transplantation improves heart function. *Ann Thorac Surg* 1996; 62:654.
255. Sakai T, Li RK, Weisel RD, et al: Fetal cell transplantation: a comparison of three cell types. *J Thorac Cardiovasc Surg* 1999; 118:715.
256. Li RK, Mickle DA, Weisel RD, et al: Optimal time for cardiomyocyte transplantation to maximize myocardial function after left ventricular injury. *Ann Thorac Surg* 2001; 72:1957.
257. Scorsin M, Hagege A, Vilquin JT, et al: Comparison of the effects of fetal cardiomyocyte and skeletal myoblast transplantation on postinfarction left ventricular function. *J Thorac Cardiovasc Surg* 2000; 119:1169.
258. Pouzet B, Vilquin JT, Hagege AA, et al: Factors affecting functional outcome after autologous skeletal myoblast transplantation. *Ann Thorac Surg* 2001; 71:844.
259. Pouzet B, Ghostine S, Vilquin JT, et al: Is skeletal myoblast transplantation clinically relevant in the era of angiotensin-converting enzyme inhibitors? *Circulation* 2001; 104:I223.
260. Ghostine S, Carrion C, Souza LCG, et al: Long-term efficacy of myoblast transplantation on regional structure and function after myocardial infarction. *Circulation* 2002; 106:1131.
261. Scorsin M, Hagege AA, Dolizy I, et al: Can cellular transplantation improve function in doxorubicin-induced heart failure? *Circulation* 1998; 98:II151.
262. Yoo KJ, Li RK, Weisel RD, et al: Heart cell transplantation improves heart function in dilated cardiomyopathic hamsters. *Circulation* 2000; 102:III204.

263. Suzuki K, Murtuza B, Suzuki N, et al: Intracoronary infusion of skeletal myoblasts improves cardiac function in doxorubicin-induced heart failure. *Circulation* 2001; 104:I213.
264. Suzuki K, Brand NJ, Smolenski RT, et al: Development of a novel method for cell transplantation through the coronary artery. *Circulation* 2000; 102:III359.
265. Suzuki K, Smolenski RT, Jayakumar J, et al: Heat shock treatment enhances graft cell survival in skeletal myoblast transplantation to the heart. *Circulation* 2000; 102:III216.
266. Jayakumar J, Suzuki K, Khan M, et al: Gene therapy for myocardial protection: transfection of donor hearts with heat shock protein 70 gene protects cardiac function against ischemia-reperfusion injury. *Circulation* 2000; 102:III302.
267. Suzuki K, Brand NJ, Allen S, et al: Overexpression of connexin 43 in skeletal myoblasts: relevance to cell transplantation to the heart. *J Thorac Cardiovasc Surg* 2001; 122:759.
268. Suzuki K, Murtuza B, Smolenski RT, et al: Cell transplantation for the treatment of acute myocardial infarction using vascular endothelial growth factor-expressing skeletal myoblasts. *Circulation* 2001; 104:I207.
269. Vincent KA, Feron O, Kelly RA: Harnessing the tissue response to hypoxia: HIF-1alpha and therapeutic angiogenesis. *Trends Cardiovasc Sci* 2002; 12:362.
270. Yau TM, Fung K, Weisel RD, et al: Enhanced myocardial angiogenesis by gene transfer with transplanted cells. *Circulation* 2001; 104:I218.
271. Lee RJ, Springer ML, Blanco-Bose WE, et al: VEGF gene delivery to myocardium: deleterious effects of unregulated expression. *Circulation* 2000; 102:898.
272. Banfi A, Springer ML, Blau HM: Myoblast-mediated gene transfer for therapeutic angiogenesis. *Methods Enzymol* 2002; 346:145.
273. Fuchs S, Baffour R, Zhou YF, et al: Transendocardial delivery of autologous bone marrow enhances collateral perfusion and regional function in pigs with chronic experimental myocardial ischemia. *J Am Coll Cardiol* 2001; 37:1726.
274. Freedman SB, Isner JM: Therapeutic angiogenesis for coronary artery disease. *Ann Intern Med* 2002; 136:54.
275. Luttun A, Carmeliet G, Carmeliet P: Vascular progenitors: from biology to treatment. *Trends Cardiovasc Med* 2002; 12:88.
276. Pasumarthi KB, Nakajima H, Nakajima HO, et al: Enhanced cardiomyocyte DNA synthesis during myocardial hypertrophy in mice expressing a modified TSC2 transgene. *Circ Res* 2000; 86:1069.
277. Pasumarthi KB, Tsai SC, Field LJ: Coexpression of mutant p53 and p193 renders embryonic stem cell-derived cardiomyocytes responsive to the growth-promoting activities of adenoviral E1A. *Circ Res* 2001; 88:1004.
278. Tsai SC, Pasumarthi KB, Pajak L, et al: Simian virus 40 large T antigen binds a novel Bcl-2 homology domain 3–containing proapoptosis protein in the cytoplasm. *J Biol Chem* 2000; 275:3239.
279. Buschmann IR, Hoefer IE, van Royen N, et al: GM-CSF: a strong arteriogenic factor acting by amplification of monocyte function. *Atherosclerosis* 2001; 159:343.
280. Deindl E, Buschmann I, Hoefer IE, et al: Role of ischemia and of hypoxia-inducible genes in arteriogenesis after femoral artery occlusion in the rabbit. *Circ Res* 2001; 89:779.
281. Lindner V, Maciag T: The putative convergent and divergent natures of angiogenesis and arteriogenesis. *Circ Res* 2001; 89:747.
282. Kocher AA, Schuster MD, Szabolcs MJ, et al: Neovascularization of ischemic myocardium by human bone-marrow-derived angioblasts prevents cardiomyocyte apoptosis, reduces remodeling and improves cardiac function. *Nat Med* 2001; 7:430.
283. Kawamoto A, Gwon HC, Iwaguro H, et al: Therapeutic potential of ex vivo expanded endothelial progenitor cells for myocardial ischemia. *Circulation* 2001; 103:634.
284. Leferovich JM, Bedelbaeva K, Samulewicz S, et al: Heart regeneration in adult MRL mice. *Proc Natl Acad Sci U S A* 2001; 98:9830.
285. Quaini F, Urbanek K, Beltrami AP, et al: Chimerism of the transplanted heart. *N Engl J Med* 2002; 346:5.
286. Krause DS, Theise ND, Collector MI, et al: Multi-organ, multi-lineage engraftment by a single bone marrow-derived stem cell. *Cell* 2001; 105:369.
287. Jackson KA, Majka SM, Wang H, et al: Regeneration of ischemic cardiac muscle and vascular endothelium by adult stem cells. *J Clin Invest* 2001; 107:1395.
288. Grimm PC, Nickerson P, Jeffery J, et al: Neointimal and tubulointerstitial infiltration by recipient mesenchymal cells in chronic renal-allograft rejection. *N Engl J Med* 2001; 345:93.
289. Shimizu K, Sugiyama S, Aikawa M, et al: Host bone-marrow cells are a source of donor intimal smooth-muscle-like cells in murine aortic transplant arteriopathy. *Nat Med* 2001; 7:738.
290. Orlic D, Kajstura J, Chimenti S, et al: Bone marrow cells regenerate infarcted myocardium. *Nature* 2001; 410:701.
291. Reyes M, Dudek A, Jahagirdar B, et al: Origin of endothelial progenitors in human postnatal bone marrow. *J Clin Invest* 2002; 109:337.
292. Moore MA: Putting the neo into neoangiogenesis. *J Clin Invest* 2002; 109:313.
293. Moore MA: "Turning brain into blood"—clinical applications of stem-cell research in neurobiology and hematology. *N Engl J Med* 1999; 341:605.
294. Condorelli G, Borello U, De Angelis L, et al: Cardiomyocytes induce endothelial cells to trans-differentiate into cardiac muscle: implications for myocardium regeneration. *Proc Natl Acad Sci U S A* 2001; 98:10733.
295. Pittenger MF, Mackay AM, Beck SC, et al: Multilineage potential of adult human mesenchymal stem cells. *Science* 1999; 284:143.
296. Toma C, Pittenger MF, Cahill KS, et al: Human mesenchymal stem cells differentiate to a cardiomyocyte phenotype in the adult murine heart. *Circulation* 2002; 105:93.
297. Makino S, Fukuda K, Miyoshi S, et al: Cardiomyocytes can be generated from marrow stromal cells in vitro. *J Clin Invest* 1999; 103:697.
298. Hakuno D, Fukuda K, Makino S, et al: Bone marrow-derived regenerated cardiomyocytes (CMG cells) express functional adrenergic and muscarinic receptors. *Circulation* 2002; 105:380.
299. Lazarus HM, Koc ON: Culture-expanded human marrow-derived MSCs in clinical hematopoietic stem cell transplantation. *Graft Rev* 2000; 3:329.
300. McIntosh K, Bartholomew A: Stromal cell modulation of the immune system: a potential role for mesenchymal stem cells. *Graft Rev* 2000; 3:324.

Chapter 28

Ischemic Mitral Regurgitation

Robert C. Gorman/Joseph H. Gorman III/L. Henry Edmunds, Jr.

Ischemic mitral regurgitation (IMR) is an ominous disease that is associated with poor long-term survival irrespective of treatment. Its progressive and often insidious nature and the frequent association with coronary artery disease (CAD) and mitral regurgitation (MR) of nonischemic origin have generated confusion and a poor understanding of the disease mechanism and natural history.

Ischemic mitral regurgitation is mitral insufficiency *caused by* myocardial infarction.[1–7] Myocardial infarction always precedes ischemic MR. The leaflets and subvalvular apparatus are by definition normal. The disease must be distinguished from MR *associated with* coronary artery disease in which no cause and effect relationship exists. The prevalence of coronary arterial disease[8] makes the association of myocardial infarction and nonischemic mitral insufficiency very common. The term ischemic mitral regurgitation excludes degenerative, myxomatous, and connective tissue valvular disease, spontaneous ruptured chordae tendineae, and other causes of acute or chronic mitral regurgitation due to infection, inflammation, trauma, congenital abnormalities (including mitral valve prolapse), annular calcification, or tumors. Mitral regurgitation associated with dilated cardiomyopathy and profound left ventricular (LV) dysfunction is a related phenomenon but should be considered etiologically distinct from IMR.

Intermittent MR that is completely attributable to transient ischemia is an infrequent[6] associated condition that is a manifestation of coronary insufficiency similar to angina and should be treated as such.

The wide and often confusing clinical spectrum of IMR is due to the fact that the disease is a manifestation of postinfarction ventricular remodeling. The size, location, and transmurality of the myocardial infarction (MI) sets in motion left ventricular remodeling that determines the severity, time course, and clinical manifestation of IMR. The presentation may be either acute (with and without papillary muscle rupture and immediately life-threatening) or develop insidiously over time in association with congestive heart failure (CHF).

Ischemic mitral regurgitation is a disease of the myocardium (both infarcted and normally perfused) that disturbs mitral valvular function; MR to due other etiologies is a valvular disease that affects the myocardium. The cellular, molecular, and genetic effects on the myocardium of these two different causes of MR are probably unrelated. Lessons learned from experience with MR of nonischemic origin are not likely applicable to IMR. Recent clinical and laboratory studies are beginning to improve our understanding and approach to this vexing clinical problem.

PREVALENCE

All except the most recently reported series[6,7] of IMR are "contaminated" with large numbers of patients with CAD and *associated* structural mitral valve disease. Inclusion of such patients produces a heterogeneous population that is difficult to analyze.[9–14] With this caveat, we present the available data. Suffice to say, the problem is large and likely to grow as survival after acute myocardial infarction continues to improve.

Between 17% and 55% of patients develop a mitral systolic murmur or echocardiographic evidence of IMR early after acute myocardial infarction (AMI).[2,15–18] Of patients who have cardiac catheterization within 6 hours of the onset of symptoms of AMI, 18% have IMR.[5] In 3.4% of these patients, the degree of mitral insufficiency is severe.[5] Many of the murmurs early after acute myocardial infarction are transient and disappear by the time of discharge.[2,16]

In one study, 19% of 11,748 patients who had elective cardiac catheterization for symptomatic coronary artery disease had ventriculographic evidence of mitral regurgitation.[19] In most of these patients the degree of mitral insufficiency was mild, but in 7.2% of all patients the degree of regurgitation was 2+ or greater, and in 3.4% MR was severe with evidence of heart failure.[19] In another study of consecutive cardiac catheterizations, 10.9% of 1739 patients with CAD had MR.[20]

Collectively, these data indicate that IMR is frequent early after AMI, but in many patients is mild or disappears completely. The relatively high incidence of IMR (10.9% to 19%) in catheterized patients with symptomatic coronary artery disease suggests that chronic IMR persists in many patients after acute infarction and may subsequently develop in others.[16] Approximately 12.6 million Americans have angina or a history of myocardial infarction, and untold millions more have asymptomatic coronary atherosclerosis.[8] Using these figures,[8,19,20] the incidence of IMR in the United States is estimated to be 1.2 to 2.1 million patients, with approximately 425,000 patients having moderate or severe IMR with heart failure.[8,19]

PATHOLOGY

Ischemic mitral regurgitation may present suddenly in association with AMI or chronically with CHF as a late manifestation of postinfarction ventricular remodeling. In all cases (by definition) the valve leaflets and subvalvular apparatus are structurally normal. Whether, when, and to what degree IMR develops is dependent on the size, transmurality, and location of the MI. Attempts to correlate IMR with the severity and distribution of coronary stenoses have added little to understanding of the disease.[19,20] Studies evaluating the distribution of wall motion abnormalities associated with IMR have been much more enlightening. Clinical studies published in the 1970s and 1980s were the first to suggest an association of IMR with posteroinferior myocardial infarctions. By auscultatory criteria IMR was found to be more common and severe after posterior infarction.[4,10,20,21] These studies also demonstrated that posterior infarctions were more likely to involve the papillary muscle and be transmural. Recent laboratory and clinical reports have confirmed and strengthened the association between IMR and transmural posteroinferior myocardial infarction.[6,22,23]

In sheep, which have unvarying, left dominant coronary arterial anatomy,[23] ligation of the two most distal circumflex marginal arteries infarcts 21% of the left ventricular (LV) mass, includes the posterior papillary muscle, and produces progressively more severe MR as the left ventricle dilates over the subsequent 8 weeks.[23] Ligation of these vessels and the posterior descending coronary artery infarcts 32% of the LV mass and produces immediate MR.[24] Comparably sized infarctions in any other ventricular location, including those involving the anterior papillary muscle, do not produce significant MR.[25] These well-controlled animal experiments confirm the importance of infarct location on the development of IMR. They also suggest that infarct size is relevant to the acuity of presentation.

A report by Gillinov et al involving nearly 500 patients treated over 13 years at the Cleveland Clinic confirmed the clinical importance of infarct location and size on the development of IMR.[6] In this study, 73% of patients had posterior wall motion abnormalities and 63% had inferior wall motion abnormalities. Virtually all were found by echocardiography to have evidence of posterior and/or inferior myocardial infarctions. While infarctions in other locations occurred, they were less common and probably represent the diffuse nature of coronary atherosclerosis that is present in most patients with IMR.[6]

Ruptured papillary muscle causes acute, often life-threatening IMR after AMI. The posterior papillary muscle is involved three to six times more commonly than is the anterior muscle.[26–30] Either the entire trunk of the muscle or one of the heads to which chordae attach may rupture; in most series partial rupture is more common[27,28,30]; in a few the reverse is true.[26,31] The extent of the infarct averages approximately 20%[21,25] but varies widely. Complete rupture occurs most commonly within the first week after acute infarction.[25,30] Partial rupture may be delayed up to 3 months.[27,30]

AMI may also produce sudden, severe mitral insufficiency without rupture of a papillary muscle. These patients are usually described euphemistically as having "papillary muscle dysfunction,"[16,26,27,30] and, indeed, the papillary muscle does not contract, but this expression tends to minimize a dangerous clinical situation. The associated (again, usually posterior) left ventricular wall at the base of the affected papillary muscle is invariably involved with a large infarction[28,30] that is often hemorrhagic and friable.[28]

In chronic IMR, sizes and ages of infarcts vary widely, but as Gillinov has documented the wall motion abnormalities are overwhelmingly located in the posteroinferior aspect of the LV, and usually involve the posterior papillary muscle.[6] Wall motion scores in these patients vary widely,[22,32] but the more severe degrees of MR are associated with larger areas of myocardial asynergy.[22] Kono et al noted that the LV is more spherical in patients with chronic IMR and heart failure than in patients with previous infarctions that do not produce MR.[33] Surgeons usually describe a dilated mitral annulus at reparative operations for chronic IMR,[34,35] but detailed measurements and information regarding prior infarctions, the electrocardiogram, and ventricular dimensions during the cardiac cycle are not reported. Izumi et al observed significant annular dilatation (>3 cm) in 11 of 43 patients with chronic IMR and noted a high correlation with increased LV volume and centralization of the regurgitant jet.[22] Severe LV enlargement may occur without any dilatation of the mitral annulus.[16,36] Unlike dilated cardiomyopathies[37] or degenerative or connective tissue MR,[38] the mitral annulus may or may not be dilated in chronic IMR.[16] The annulus tends to dilate in proportion to LV volume[22] and in these patients the left atrium is often enlarged.

PATHOGENESIS

Normal Valve Function

The mitral valve has six anatomic components: leaflets, chordae tendineae, annulus, papillary muscles, left ventricle (LV), and left atrium. The mitral annulus is saddle-shaped (actually a hyperbolic parabloid with two-directional curvature) with cephalad promontories near the mid portions of the anterior and posterior leaflets and caudad depressions at the commissures (Fig. 28-1).[39] This unique shape is present in all mammalian mitral valves and has been shown, using finite element analysis, to reduce leaflet, annular, and chordal stress.[40] Function of the normal mitral valve is wonderfully complex and involves precisely timed interactions among the six components. These interactions are most easily described by relating the changes in each of the six components during a cardiac cycle. For this description the cardiac cycle is divided into four periods: systole, diastole, isovolemic relaxation (IVR), and isovolemic contraction (IVC), as defined below.

End systole (ES) is defined as the maximum negative left ventricular *dP/dt*[41] and *end diastole* (ED) is defined as the peak of the QRS complex. *End isovolemic contraction* (EIVC) is defined as the first time point at which the aortic root *dP/dt* is greater than zero. *End isovolemic relaxation* (EIVR) is defined as the time at which the LVP is 10% of LVP_{max} and the left ventricular $dP/dt < 0$.[41]

During isovolemic contraction (IVC), *left atrial* filling begins immediately after the mitral valve closes and before the aortic valve opens.[42] Flow through the mitral valve briefly reverses as the leaflets coapt and bulge toward the atrium.[43] During systole the left atrium rapidly fills[42] and reaches maximum near ES. The position of the *annulus* ascends (away from the apex) slightly during atrial contraction,[44–46] which occurs during late diastole, does not change during IVC, and descends progressively 1 to 1.5 cm toward the apex throughout systole.[42,46,47] The annulus asymmetrically[44] contracts[47] during atrial and ventricular systole and in humans reaches a minimal area (mean reduction of 27%)

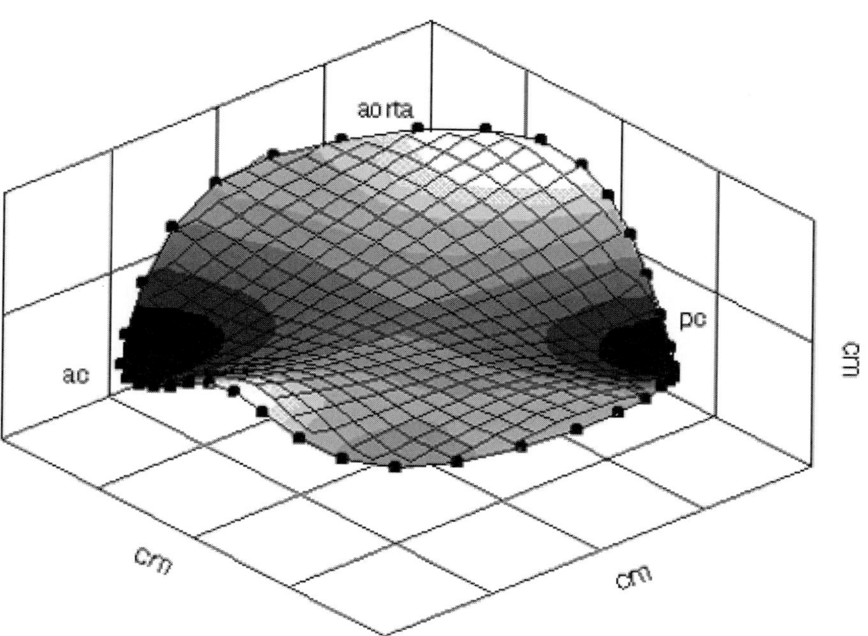

FIGURE 28–1 Image of a human mitral annulus obtained using three-dimensional transesophageal echocardiography (TEE). The image is reconstructed from two-dimensional images sampled every 10 degrees using a rotational omni-probe gated for heart rate and respiration. The annulus is viewed from posterior annulus (near) to aorta (far). The pronounced saddle shape of the human mitral annulus is well demonstrated.

in mid systole.[48] Immediately after atrial contraction, the mitral *leaflets* approach each other and close within 20 to 60 milliseconds after pressure crossover when LV pressure exceeds LA pressure.[42] Since the total area of leaflet tissue is approximately twice the total area of the annulus,[36,49] the apposition point of the two leaflets at the time of pressure crossover is very near the plane of the annulus.[50,51] At closure approximately 30% of the anterior cusp and 50% of the longer posterior cusp are in apposition.[50] *Chordae tendineae* attached to the free edges and body of the leaflets[50] restrict the upward movement of the slightly compliant leaflets and produce a tight seal along the line of apposition.[50] Chordal tension peaks in early systole and begins to fall slowly in late systole and rapidly during IVR.[52] *Papillary muscles* begin to shorten during late IVC and throughout systole in synchrony with shortening of the adjacent ventricular wall.[53] The actual distance papillary muscles shorten is small and ranges between 2 and 4 mm.[37,54] During systole, the directions and timing of *left ventricular* contraction are not necessarily uniform throughout systole because of the complex anatomic arrangement of muscle bundles[55,56] and the timing produced by the impulse conduction pattern.[57] LV shortening is greater in both equatorial axes than in the long axis.[57] LV wall thickness increases during IVC and decreases rapidly during IVR.[58] Peak wall thickness occurs near ES, but timing of the exact peak varies slightly between ventricular wall segments. During systole the ventricle progressively twists counterclockwise (as viewed from the apex) along its longitudinal axis to reach a maximum at ES.[59]

During IVR the *left atrium* begins to empty when left atrial pressure crosses over and exceeds LV pressure.[42,43] The atrium empties rapidly in early diastole and further diminishes with atrial contraction in late diastole just before IVC.[60] The LV may actually generate negative pressure in early diastole if left atrial pressures are low.[61] During IVR, the *mitral annulus* to LV apex distance lengthens as the mitral annulus ascends in early diastole, descends slightly, and ascends again with atrial contraction.[42,45] The area of the mitral orifice increases slightly during IVR and continues to increase during diastole until it reaches a maximum just before the left atrium contracts.[44,48] In humans, the annular area index reaches a maximum of 3.9 ± 0.7 cm^2/m^2.[48] As the annular area increases, its shape changes asymmetrically; most of the area increase is due to lengthening in the posterior and lateral parts of the annulus (away from the fibrous trigone).[44] During IVR the *mitral leaflets* separate approximately 30 milliseconds before left atrial pressure exceeds LV pressure.[42] Peak blood flow through the valve occurs early in diastole, but the mitral leaflets reach their maximal open position *before* peak flow occurs and begin closing while flow is still accelerating.[62]

The *papillary muscles* may shorten very slightly during early IVR,[41,53,54,63] but do not begin to lengthen until the beginning of diastole. Papillary muscles reach maximum length shortly after ED during IVC. *Chordal tension* decreases rapidly during IVR and remains near zero until late diastole, when a small increase occurs.[52,62] The *left ventricle* relaxes and dilates after ES and reverses the complex deformations of LV shape produced by systole. During early diastole, and the period of rapid filling, the ventricle dilates primarily along both equatorial axes and much less along the longitudinal, base-to-apex axis.[57] Only a little shape change occurs in mid diastole and after atrial contraction. Ventricular wall thickness decreases[58] primarily during IVR. Lastly, the ventricle rapidly untwists (rotating clockwise) during early diastole and more gradually during mid and late diastole.[59]

Mechanism of Ischemic Mitral Regurgitation

The pathogenesis of both acute IMR in the absence of papillary muscle rupture and chronic IMR is complex. Experimental analysis of clinically relevant ovine models using tantalum marker imaging, sonomicrometry array localization, and three-dimensional echocardiography[64–69] as well as detailed clinical echocardiographic studies has more clearly elucidated the mechanism of the complex geometric and temporal perturbations that cause a structurally normal mitral valve to leak, often massively, early or late after a myocardial infarction.

ACUTE ISCHEMIC MITRAL REGURGITATION

Numerous studies have conclusively demonstrated that loss of papillary muscle shortening alone as result of acute ischemia does not cause MR.[49,70–74] The term "papillary muscle dysfunction" is, therefore, erroneous and should be avoided. With ischemia or infarction, the posterior papillary muscle elongates 2 to 4 mm in the sheep and dog[53,54]; the tip moves 1.5 to 3 mm closer to the annulus.[54,75] These are very small changes, and echocardiographic studies in dog, sheep, and man uniformly fail to show mitral valve prolapse with acute IMR in the absence of papillary muscle rupture.[3,33,51,76] In the sheep model of acute IMR, the uninfarcted anterior papillary muscle contracts earlier and more vigorously than before infarction. This moves the tip 4 to 5 mm further away from the annular plane at mid systole than before infarction.[64] This discoordination of normal synchronous papillary muscle contraction has a complex effect on leaflet coaptation that has been meticulously characterized by Miller et al[67,68] using tantalum marker technology. It is sufficient to say that the interaction of these rather small changes in papillary muscle contraction dynamics and location cause subtle distortions of valvular leaflet coaptation that are not simply leaflet prolapse and tethering. Annular dilatation is at best mild (10% to 15%) and located primarily along the posterior annulus in the ovine model of acute IMR.[64–66,77] This degree of dilatation is within the physiologic range achieved by varying loading conditions in sheep.[78] Leaflet area in sheep exceeds the maximum annular area by 50% to 100%.[77] These data suggest that acute IMR results from a complex interaction of very small geometric and temporal changes that for the most part are not demonstrable by standard imaging techniques and are not discernible in a flaccid heart at the time of surgery.

CHRONIC ISCHEMIC MITRAL REGURGITATION

In chronic IMR mitral valve prolapse has been described[79] in occasional patients, but the vast majority have incomplete mitral valve closure due to papillary muscle and chordal restriction of leaflet motion.[33,71,76,79–82] Pathologic studies consistently show fibrosis and atrophy of infarcted papillary muscles,[3,16,36,70] and none demonstrate papillary muscle or chordal elongation. Nevertheless, surgeons describe elongated chordae in some patients with myocardial infarction and MR.[6,34,35] Elongated chordae and mitral valve prolapse without MR probably antedate the infarction in these patients.[83,84] In a patient with preexisting mitral valve prolapse, ventricular infarction may cause the previously competent valve to leak. This hypothesis explains sporadic observations of mitral valve prolapse in patients with chronic IMR, but needs preinfarction echocardiograms for confirmation.

Ovine experiments using sonomicrometry array localization to study postinfarction MR that evolves during the first 8 weeks after infarction have added insight relevant to the pathogenesis of chronic IMR. In this model, a combination of asymmetric annular dilatation and leaflet tethering by *both* papillary muscles occurs to produce chronic IMR. The annular area dilates by at least 60% at all time points during systolic ejection, but the dilatation involves all of the muscular annulus. The posterior or mural portion of the annulus directly adjacent to the infarct moves away from the relatively fixed anterior commissure (at the anterior fibrous trigone) and stretches the anterior portion of the mural annulus and the posterior portion of the aortic-based annulus, which are remote from the infarct. This finding illustrates how a moderately sized (21% of the LV mass) localized infarct remodels and distorts remote, uninfarcted myocardium including the mitral valve annulus (Fig. 28-2A).[85]

Interestingly, the posterior papillary muscle tip to posterior commissure relationship does not change significantly. Both these points are displaced *together,* away from the relatively fixed anterior commissure as a result of the remodeling process (Fig. 28-2B). This indicates that the posterior papillary muscle tethering is more pronounced at its most anterior connection with both leaflets near the center of the coaptation line and not at the commissure. The anterior papillary muscle tip is displaced significantly from both commissures but further from the posterior commissure. This indicates the tethering effect of the anterior papillary muscle is greatest along both leaflets from the anterior commissure to the middle of the coaptation line. Together, these findings suggest that in this model the postinfarction ventricular remodeling process tethers the anterior portion of both leaflets.

The concept of leaflet tethering as a contributing factor in the pathogenesis of chronic IMR is not new.[86–88] Two recent echocardiographic reports, one studying the same sheep model presented here and one human study, demonstrated findings very consistent with the experimental results cited above. Otsuji et al applied a very effective three-dimensional echocardiographic technique to quantify leaflet tethering in the same ovine model.[86] These authors also reported mid-systolic distortions between both papillary muscle tips and the anterior commissure, but did not observe changes between papillary muscle tips and the posterior commissure or annular dilatation. Yiu used quantitative two-dimensional echocardiography to corroborate these findings clinically by comparing normal controls with a cohort of patients with varying degrees of chronic IMR.[88] They found that ventricular distortions, which most closely correlated with the degree of MR, occurred between the posterior papillary muscle tip and anterior commissure ($R = 0.55$) and posterior displacement of the anterior papillary muscle tip ($R = 0.65$).

To summarize, the geometric changes that lead to acute IMR are multiple but extremely subtle (<5 mm) and are not reliably imaged by currently available clinical modalities. Chronic IMR involves larger changes (1-2 cm) that cause moderate annular dilatation and complex leaflet tethering along the anterior and mid leaflet coaptation line.

NATURAL HISTORY

After acute myocardial infarction (AMI), approximately 15% of mitral murmurs disappear by hospital discharge and another 15% are gone within several months.[16] In patients with AMI who do not have an early mitral murmur, approximately 12% develop an MR murmur later.[16] Thus roughly 15% of patients have some degree of MR months after AMI.[19]

The presence of MR after AMI as determined by color flow Doppler velocity mapping or cardiac catheterization increases the likelihood of pulmonary edema, cardiogenic shock, and death.[2,5,89] However, when adjusted for age, ejection fraction, heart failure, and other variables that affect mortality, the presence of MR is not an incremental risk factor for early death.[5] Nevertheless, even mild or moderate MR after AMI doubles the 30-day and 3-year mortality to approximately 15% and 20%, respectively,[5] as compared to patients without MR.[90]

Without surgery, median survival following rupture of a papillary muscle trunk is three to four days.[26,27] Some patients with partial rupture or rupture of one head survive several weeks or a few months.[27,91] Overall, acute moderate or severe (3+ or 4+) IMR has a 30-day mortality of 24% and a 1-year mortality of 52%.[5] The onset of cardiogenic shock reduces survival to a few days.

Chronic IMR of 2+ severity discovered at cardiac catheterization for symptomatic coronary artery disease has

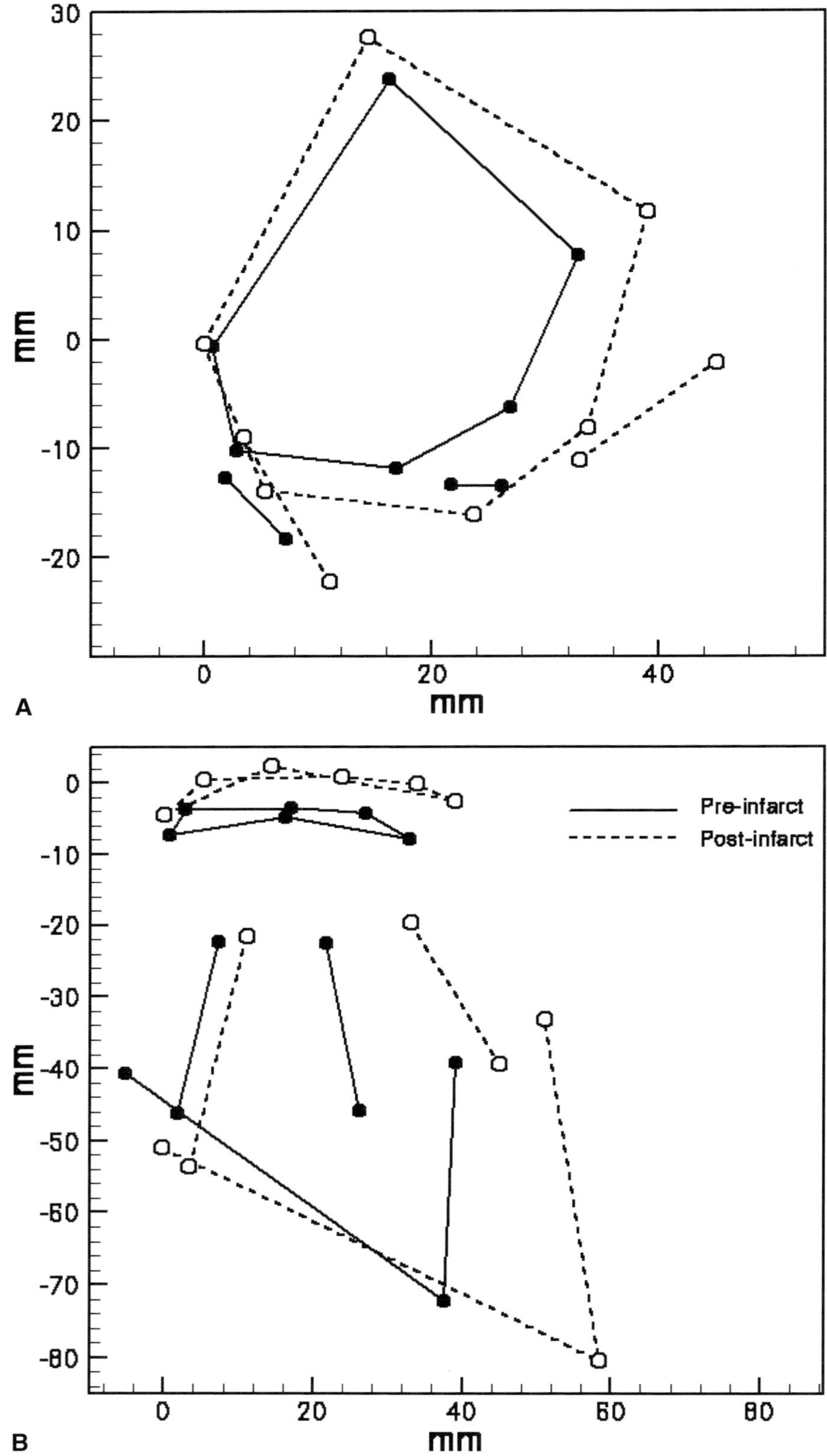

FIGURE 28–2 (A) Two-dimensional axial view of the mitral valve annulus and papillary muscle transducers before (solid line) and 8 weeks after infarction. Note the stretching of both the posterior part of the aortic portion of the annulus (Ao to PC) and the anterior part of the mural portion of the annulus (Ao to P1 to P2). Also, note how the portion of the annulus between P2 and PC along with the posterior papillary muscle tip (PPT) pulls away from the relatively fixed anterior commissure. (B) Two-dimensional saggital view of the sheep mitral annulus and its relationship to the LV and papillary muscles before and 8 weeks after infarction. Note how the PPT and the posterior annulus are retracted away form the anterior commissure. The heart shown in this figure is the same one shown in Figure 28-1.

a 1-year mortality of approximately 17%; 1+ severity increases mortality to approximately 10% from about 6% if MR is not present.[19] The one-year mortality for 3+ and 4+ IMR is approximately 40%,[19] which is only slightly less than severe MR after acute infarction.[5]

DIAGNOSIS AND MANAGEMENT

As noted above, acute IMR and chronic IMR are clinically related entities that are pathophysiologically and etiologically distinct. Their presentation, diagnosis, treatment, and outcome are discussed separately below to emphasize this distinction.

Acute Postinfarction Mitral Regurgitation

In most patients, the presence of MR does not affect management of AMI. Postinfarction angina with mild or moderate MR without symptoms or signs of heart failure is managed similarly to postinfarction angina without MR. A minority of patients develop severe (3+ or 4+) MR with symptoms of heart failure, low cardiac output, or both.

Severe MR following AMI may be due to rupture of a papillary muscle trunk or tip or to displacement of a papillary muscle and distortion of subvalvular structures. Rupture of the trunk of a papillary muscle (Fig. 28-3) invariably causes immediate, severe MR with pulmonary edema and cardiogenic shock and requires prompt intervention for survival. Rupture of a papillary muscle tip usually produces severe MR, but can, rarely, be consistent with longer survival.[27,91] Acute, severe postinfarction MR without rupture is more common than papillary muscle rupture and may be associated with both large and small infarctions. Although the specific pathology varies, acute, severe postinfarction MR is a distinct, highly lethal clinical entity that invariably requires surgery for survival.

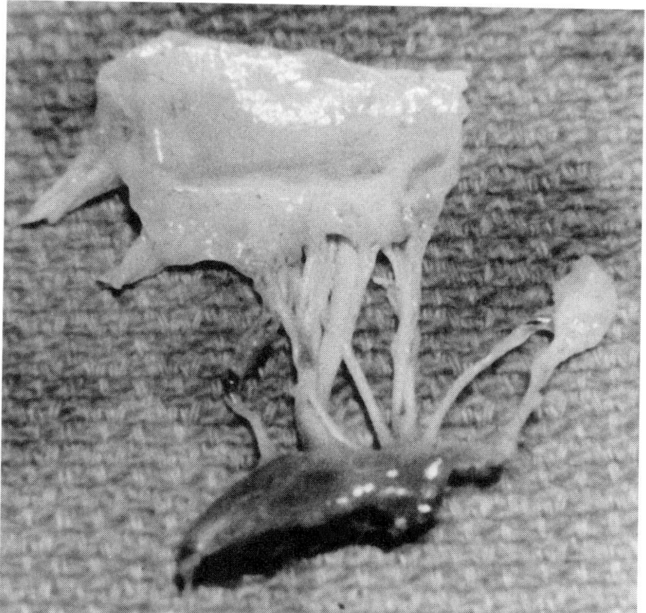

FIGURE 28–3 Surgical specimen from a patient who ruptured the trunk of the posterior papillary muscle three days after acute postero-inferior myocardial infarction.

Acute, severe IMR occurs in 0.1% of patients with symptomatic coronary arterial disease[19] and complicates 0.4% to 0.9% of all patients with AMI.[92] However, in contemporary practice the incidence actually may be higher as more patients with AMI survive. Wei observed papillary muscle rupture in 5% of all fatal myocardial infarctions at Johns Hopkins Hospital.[26] Approximately two-thirds of acute, severe IMR involve the posterior papillary muscle[16,26,30,93] even though anterior myocardial infarctions are more common. An average of 20% of the LV mass is infarcted, but in autopsy series the size of the infarct varies widely.[26]

PATHOPHYSIOLOGY

Acute, severe mitral regurgitation produces acute LV volume overload and immediately increases LV end-diastolic volume and preload and decreases end-systolic volume.[94] Volume of regurgitant flow depends upon the size of the incompetent valve opening during systole and the pressure difference between the LV and left atrium. This pressure difference is influenced by LV afterload, forward flow past the aortic valve, and myocardial contractile force. Acute MR enhances early diastolic filling of the ventricle and decreases end-systolic wall stress (afterload) and end-systolic elastance.[95] Myocardial oxygen consumption does not change because of reduced wall stress in late systole.[94] Stroke volume increases and initially cardiac output may be maintained by a tremendous increase in stroke volume. However, if the regurgitant fraction of the increased stroke volume is very large, the amount of forward flow past the aortic valve (i.e., cardiac output) decreases. With MR, ejection fraction increases in animals without LV infarction; in patients with infarction, ejection fraction varies widely.[31] Left atrial, pulmonary capillary wedge, and LV end-diastolic pressures increase abruptly with acute MR; end-diastolic wall stress also increases markedly, and end-diastolic wall thickness and stiffness decrease slightly.[96] In patients with small atria, a prominent "v" wave appears.[28,97] Pulmonary vascular resistance increases rapidly and may cause right heart failure.[94]

CLINICAL PRESENTATION

Acute, severe IMR usually presents abruptly with an acute onset of chest pain and/or shortness of breath. The age range of patients reflects the age range of myocardial infarction; the mean age is around 60. The syndrome is slightly more common in men than women. Recent series report that 17% to 20% of ischemic mitral regurgitation cases coming to surgery are for acute IMR.[6,7] Only a few patients have historical or electrocardiographic evidence of prior myocardial infarction and less than half have angina.[26,28,30] The disease presents as an acute myocardial infarction and occasionally may be silent.[28,30] Papillary muscle rupture may occur as early as the first day after infarction and nearly always within 7 days (mean approximately 4 days).[26,28,30]

Typically, patients are short of breath and many rapidly develop pulmonary edema complicated by systemic hypotension. Most patients have a loud apical, holosystolic murmur that radiates to the left axilla[97]; in some the murmur occurs in mid or late systole, and in others it may be absent[90] or difficult to hear because of pulmonary rales.[28] The most compelling findings are those of low cardiac output and congestive heart failure in the setting of AMI. Many patients develop cardiogenic shock characterized by systemic hypotension, oliguria, acidosis, and poor peripheral pulses and perfusion.[93] A few have cardiac arrest.[31]

DIAGNOSTIC STUDIES

Nearly all electrocardiograms are abnormal,[26,28,30] but only slightly more than half are diagnostic of AMI. Some of the nondiagnostic changes include right or left bundle branch block and nonspecific ST- and T-wave changes in the anteroseptal, lateral, or inferior leads.[26–28,30] Most patients are in sinus rhythm.[28,94] In autopsy series, the incidence of subendocardial infarctions is approximately equal to the incidence of transmural infarctions.[26,30] Frequently patients with ruptured papillary muscle have electrocardiographic evidence of an inferior infarction. When the ECG is diagnostic, inferior wall infarctions are much more common than anterior and lateral wall infarctions. Conduction abnormalities are relatively uncommon and are more often found in patients with postinfarction ventricular septal defects.[98]

Chest x-rays nearly always show signs of pulmonary congestion, interstitial pulmonary edema, and pulmonary venous engorgement.[28] The heart may or may not be enlarged[26] and usually is not massively enlarged.

The differential diagnosis includes postinfarction ventricular septal defect, massive AMI without significant MR, and ruptured chordae tendineae without AMI. Right heart catheterization usually shows elevated pulmonary arterial pressures with prominent "v" waves reaching 40 mm Hg or higher.[28,31] Mean pulmonary artery wedge pressures are greater than 20 mm Hg unless cardiac output is very low. Mixed venous oxygen saturations are often well below 50% and reflect low cardiac output with indices that range from 1.0 to 2.9 $L/m^2/min$.[31] In the presence of a loud systolic murmur, absence of an oxygen step-up in the pulmonary artery is strong evidence against the diagnosis of postinfarction ventricular septal defect. Electrocardiographic evidence of AMI distinguishes acute IMR from acute chordal rupture, but in some instances the two diseases cannot be distinguished until after operation or death.[28]

Transthoracic echocardiography (TTE) assesses the degree of MR, confirms wall motion abnormalities, and often demonstrates flail mitral leaflets. Transesophageal (TEE) echocardiography is the diagnostic imaging tool of choice. This modality definitively documents the degree of MR, associated wall motion abnormalities, and the status of the posterior papillary muscle.[99,100] Typically the left atrium is not enlarged, but the left ventricle shows signs of volume overload and segmental wall motion abnormalities. Color flow Doppler velocity mapping documents the presence of MR after myocardial infarction[90] and semiquantitates its severity.[101] Ejection fractions vary widely, but do not reflect the extent of the LV infarction.

Despite hemodynamic instability, most patients have a diagnostic cardiac catheterization primarily for definition of coronary arterial anatomy; however, the wisdom of prescribing cardiac catheterization for patients in cardiogenic shock is highly questionable in that revascularization of obstructed, remote coronary vessels is not likely to improve a patient's chances for immediate survival.[93] Approximately half of catheterized patients have single-vessel disease, most often of the right coronary artery.[28,31] Most of the remainder have three-vessel disease.[26–28,30] Ventriculography shows increased LV volume at both end diastole and end systole, severe MR, segmental wall motion abnormalities,[102] and a wide range of ejection fractions, which are generally over 40% and frequently over 60%.[27,31] LV end-diastolic pressures are elevated with prominent left atrial "v" waves and moderate pulmonary hypertension. Occasional patients have mild or moderate tricuspid regurgitation. Cardiac output is usually low.

MEDICAL MANAGEMENT

The urgency and aggressiveness of initial management depends upon the presence or absence of cardiogenic shock and/or congestive heart failure. Because of the severity of MR, definitive therapy means surgery or rarely interventional cardiac catheterization. Beyond the need for diagnosis and brief attempts to stabilize the circulation, there is nothing to gain by deferring definitive therapy. In an intensive care unit, patients are monitored by continuous electrocardiogram, measurement of peripheral oxygen saturation, an arterial catheter with continuous display of arterial blood pressure, and a Swan-Ganz catheter to monitor central venous pressure, pulmonary arterial pressure, cardiac output (intermittently or ongoing), and mixed venous oxygen saturations. An additional intravenous access may be needed. If surgery is possible or probable, a blood sample should be sent for type and cross-match and routine blood work for hematology, electrolytes, glucose, renal function, and coagulation studies. Blood gases for arterial oxygen saturation, Pa_{CO_2}, and pH are also obtained. Nasal prongs or mask provides supplemental oxygen. The decision to intubate and ventilate the patient is made on the basis of clinical assessment of respiratory distress, findings of pulmonary edema, low Pa_{O_2}, or elevated Pa_{CO_2}.

The adequacy or inadequacy of the circulation must be assessed early before arrhythmias or cardiac arrest intervenes. The criteria for cardiogenic shock vary slightly between specialists, but systemic hypotension (peak pressure <80 mm Hg; mean pressure <55 mm Hg), mixed venous oxygen saturation less than 50%, thermodilution cardiac index less than 2.0 L/m^2/min, metabolic acidosis, oliguria, and poor peripheral perfusion (pallor, cool extremities, faint peripheral pulses) are findings that collectively or in various combinations indicate that the circulation is not adequate. Even if the criteria for cardiogenic shock are not present, patients must be promptly worked up and carefully monitored to avoid either progressive or abrupt deterioration of the circulation. Necessary diagnostic studies are best performed as promptly as possible.

Circulatory performance must be optimized and carefully monitored. Drugs that least impair myocardial contractility or cause hypotension should be used to control arrhythmias. Electrical cardioversion is often the first choice for tachyarrhthmias when cardiac output is low. Temporary pacing via skin electrodes or an intravenous catheter may be the best treatment of bradyarrhythmias and atrial flutter. Appropriate inotropic therapy should be used to optimize cardiac output. If organ perfusion is still unacceptable, an intra-aortic balloon pump may be needed to maintain coronary perfusion pressure, unload the LV, and to increase cardiac output. For patients who are not hypotensive, pharmacologic reduction of afterload using intravenous nitroglycerin[103] or nitroprusside improves cardiac output. Management of fluid volume is critical and best guided by ongoing measurements of central venous and pulmonary capillary wedge or diastolic pressures. Additional volume must be given cautiously in critically ill patients to avoid volume overload and acute decompensation of the ventricle. In less ill patients, additional crystalloid or colloid may improve cardiac output and restore urine flow.

DEFINITIVE THERAPY

Prompt surgery is the best chance for survival for most patients with acute, severe postinfarction MR. A few, highly selected patients without papillary muscle rupture early in their presentation have been treated by emergency percutaneous transluminal coronary angioplasty (PTCA) and/or thrombolytic therapy in an attempt to reduce the size of the infarct and thereby reduce MR.[5,79,104,105]

PTCA or thrombolysis carried out within 4 hours of the onset of AMI may on occasion produce spectacular reversal of both the infarction and MR.[79,104,105] However, less rapid PTCA may not succeed in preempting the infarct and aborting MR.[105] PTCA and thrombolysis in catheterized patients are potentially worth trying if patients reach medical attention soon after the onset of symptoms, are sufficiently stable, and can be followed by echocardiography. However, in many patients PTCA and thrombolysis do not provide a favorable outcome.[5] In one study, 17% of patients with acute IMR and successful thrombolysis died in hospital; in those with successful PTCA, 50% died shortly afterward, and 77% were dead in one year.[5] Of the survivors, the majority continue to have 3+ or 4+ MR.[5]

For patients who have acute postinfarction angina with 1+ or 2+ MR, urgent myocardial revascularization is indicated to relieve angina and to prevent extension of the infarction. It is important to prevent progression of MR and the development of congestive heart failure or cardiogenic shock. This is usually accomplished by thrombolysis, PTCA, or an intracoronary arterial stent. If these measures are unsuccessful, operation is rarely completed in time to reverse the infarction, but early operation may reduce the size of the ultimate infarct.[106–108] The presence of mild to moderate IMR does not increase operative mortality,[109–111] but the presence of congestive heart failure is a risk factor.[112] In these patients, the mitral valve is generally not addressed unless intraoperative transesophageal echocardiography indicates 3+ or 4+ MR.

Indications for emergency surgery for acute, severe postinfarction MR vary among institutions[5,28,29,31,93,113,114] and probably explain wide discrepancies in reports of hospital mortality.[32,113] In this group of patients, medical therapy does not produce survivors[27,28] and patients denied operation are not reported.[28] Aged patients are less likely to survive operation,[32,79] and there are only anecdotal reports of successful operation in octogenarians (Gorman JH III, personal communication). Other risk factors for hospital death are severe congestive heart failure, the number and severity of comorbid diseases such as renal or pulmonary problems, presence of an intra-aortic balloon pump, reduced ejection fraction, and greater number of diseased coronary arteries.[33] Contemporary concerns regarding costs and longevity beyond immediate hospital survival also influence indications for operation and reported mortality.

Operation for acute (within 30 days) severe, postinfarction MR consists of mitral valve repair or replacement with or without myocardial revascularization. Nearly all surgeons recommend revascularization of all significantly obstructed coronary vessels away from the site of the infarction,[113] and improved methods of cardioplegia and the open-artery hypothesis support this recommendation even in patients with preoperative cardiogenic shock who have had cardiac catheterization. The wisdom of blind revascularization of remote coronary vessels in patients who have not had preoperative cardiac catheterization and revascularization of the infarct artery more than 4 to 6 hours after onset of pain is less clear.[93] On a statistical basis, only half of patients with acute IMR have multivessel coronary artery disease.[26,28,31] Revascularization of completed infarctions favorably influences subsequent ventricular remodeling.[107–109]

OPERATION

Operation for acute, severe postinfarction MR is often urgent or an emergency; a high percentage of patients have an intra-aortic balloon pump inserted before induction of anesthesia.[31,93] Monitors include the electrocardiogram, arterial blood pressure, a Swan-Ganz catheter with mixed venous oxygen electrode, nasopharyngeal and rectal (or bladder) temperature, and a catheter for urine output. The heart is exposed through a midline sternotomy and needed saphenous vein is harvested simultaneously. Mammary arteries are less often used for revascularization because of the extra time needed and typically precarious condition of the patient. Both cavae are cannulated separately and the pericardial attachments around the superior and inferior cavae and the right pulmonary veins are dissected back. Most patients with acute IMR have small left atria. During cardiopulmonary bypass moderate systemic hypothermia is employed; the aorta is cross-clamped; and the heart is protected by cardioplegia (e.g., retrograde and antegrade cold blood with myocardial temperature monitoring). After opening the left atrium for decompression of the heart, planned coronary bypass grafts are constructed prior to exposing the mitral valve.

The left atrium is usually opened after dissecting the lateral interatrial septum. The incision extends behind the inferior vena cava. Valvular exposure can in some cases be difficult; better exposure may be obtained by opening the right atrium just anterior to the interatrial septum and then cutting the septum transversely toward (but not to) the anterior commissure of the tricuspid valve. Improved exposure may also be obtained by extending the atrial incision superiorly behind the superior caval–right atrial junction. The mobilized cava may be retracted strongly anteriorly or, if cannulated directly, it may be divided at the right atrial junction.

Replacement of the diseased valve is the most reliable option in these often critically ill patients regardless of the pathology of the acute IMR.[7] It is important to preserve the chordal attachments to the annulus (Fig. 28-4). The prosthetic valve (usually mechanical) is sutured to the annulus with running or interrupted sutures. The choice of a mechanical or bioprosthetic valve is optional since durability and anticoagulation issues are relatively minor concerns in these patients. The atrial incisions are closed with running sutures and any proximal anastomses are completed before weaning the patient off cardiopulmonary bypass.

During weaning, transesophageal echocardiography is helpful for assessing LV function and loading. Inotropic drugs and systemic and coronary arterial vasodilators are used initially, but if the LV cannot easily maintain an adequate cardiac output, mechanical circulatory assistance is instituted immediately. If the intra-aortic balloon pump is not adequate, left atrial to aorta or femoral artery perfusion or another temporary left ventricular assist device is used promptly and before the weakened heart is subjected to

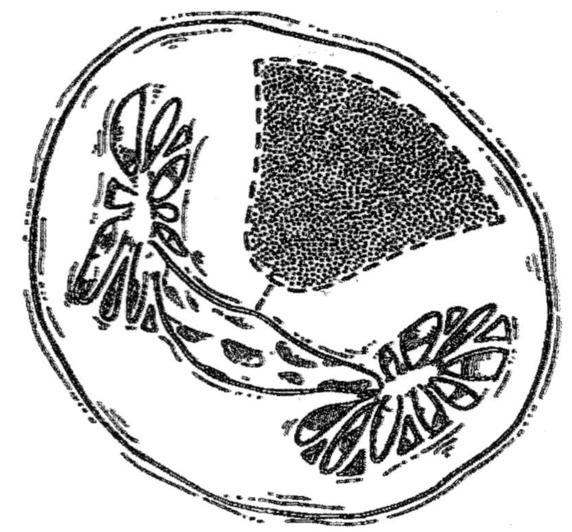

A

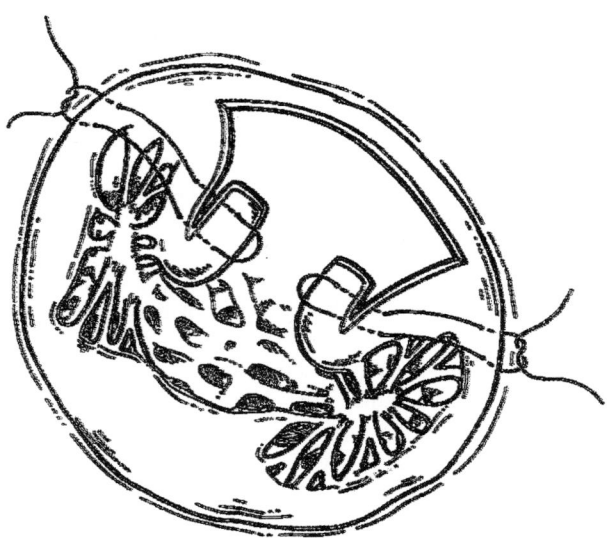

B

FIGURE 28–4 Okita's method for retaining chordal attachment to the mitral annulus during replacement of the mitral valve. (A) Diagram showing the mitral valve from the left atrium. The center of the anterior leaflet is excised (shaded area) and the leaflet is divided retaining the chordae from each papillary muscle attached to the residual anterior leaflet tissue. The posterior leaflet may be divided at its midpoint if necessary. (B) Remnants of the anterior leaflets are sutured to the annulus using a single stitch as shown. This tissue is later included in sutures used in sewing the valve to the annulus. *(Modified slightly with permission from Okita Y, Miki S, Kusuhara K, et al. Analysis of left ventricular motion after mitral valve replacement with a technique of preservation of all chordae tendineae. J Thorac Cardiovasc Surg 1992; 104:786.)*

injury from transitory volume or pressure overload or coronary ischemia.

RESULTS

Published results of mitral valve replacement, which is recommended by many surgeons for acute, severe IMR, are poor.[28,29,31,32,93,113,115] Hospital mortality ranges from 31% to 69% and probably reflects the selection process more than quality of care. Variables that increase early mortality include patient age, cardiogenic shock, comorbid conditions, the amount of infarcted myocardium, and delay in operation.[27,28,31,32] More recent experience may be better[6,7,116] because of prompt diagnosis, early surgery, complete revascularization, and application of chordal preservation techniques that better preserve LV function.[117–121] Several techniques are available for preserving chordae (Fig. 28-4).[117,122,123] David reports a hospital mortality of 22% in 18 patients using chordal preservation techniques.[116]

Many surgeons do not recommend mitral valve repair for acute IMR,[7,29,93,114,116] but others do.[6,33,122,124] Repair of the valve in acute IMR poses difficult problems. As demonstrated above, the anatomical derangements may be very subtle. A reasonable repair option is, therefore, undersized ring annuloplasty. In cases of papillary muscle rupture, successful reimplantation in conjunction with ring annuloplasty has been reported, but these patients are uncommon and usually much less ill.[6] Intraoperative transesophageal echocardiography and color flow Doppler velocity mapping are essential adjuncts to operation to assess quality of the repair.[99,100] Long-term (5-year) survival in patients who survive the perioperative period is poor and even in modern reports hovers around 50%.[6,7]

Chronic Ischemic Mitral Regurgitation

Between 10.9% and 19.0% of patients with symptomatic coronary arterial disease who have cardiac catheterization[19,20] and 3.5% to 7.0% of patients who have myocardial revascularization have IMR.[125–128] The majority of patients with IMR have chronic IMR, and most of these patients have 1+ or 2+ MR without heart failure.[19,20,125–127]

In patients with chronic IMR, three major variables interrelate to produce the clinical spectrum of patients with varying combinations of symptomatic ischemia and heart failure. As with acute IMR, the three variables are: (1) the presence and severity of ischemia, (2) the severity of MR, and (3) the magnitude of LV dysfunction. Patients with obstructive coronary artery disease may have no symptoms or have stable, progressive, unstable, or postinfarction angina or its equivalent. Because of disabling symptoms, threat to LV mass or statistically shortened survival ischemia is a compelling problem that must be addressed therapeutically. The approach and methods do not materially differ from similar patients who do not have IMR. The severity of MR is the second variable. At present, 1+ or 2+ MR in patients without symptoms of heart failure does not compel invasive therapy for MR. More severe MR and/or symptoms of heart failure require evaluation for possible operation irrespective of the therapy needed for ischemia. The degree of LV dysfunction is the last variable and the most difficult to assess in the presence of MR. Symptoms of heart failure may be due to LV dysfunction, MR, or both.

PATHOPHYSIOLOGY

It is important to realize the clinical and laboratory data regarding mitral regurgitation without prior myocardial infarction are not confidently extrapolated to patients with chronic IMR. It is possible (and recently laboratory studies suggest likely)[129] that the myocardial insult of progressive MR is dwarfed by the dramatic changes inflicted on normally perfused myocardium as a result of postinfarction ventricular remodeling.[130]

In patients with chronic IMR, LV volume and wall stress increase at end diastole[20,89,96,131] and LV mass increases progressively without an increase in end-diastolic wall thickness.[131] Infarction contributes to LV dilatation by increasing diastolic wall stress and by stimulating myocyte hypertrophy and myocyte slippage in uninfarcted, remote areas.[132] In patients with IMR who maintain a near normal ejection fraction, peak systolic wall stress increases[132] and the velocity of shortening decreases,[133] but end-systolic volume and stress remain near normal.[131] Cardiac output is reduced but maintained at asymptomatic or minimally symptomatic levels by an increase in preload (increased end-diastolic wall stress).[131] However, in patients with reduced ejection fractions, both end-diastolic and end-systolic volumes and stresses increase and cardiac output and stroke volume fall; the increase in afterload cannot be overcome by increased myocardial contractility produced by the increased preload.[131] Left atrial, LV end-diastolic, and pulmonary wedge pressures increase to two or three times normal values independent of ejection fraction[131]; often the atrial "v" wave disappears[97] as does atrial contraction. The left atrium enlarges.[97] In patients with chronic IMR, the LV enlarges asymmetrically,[16,20] particularly in the infarct and borderzone myocardium around the infarct.[134] Over time both the severity of MR[20] and loss of myocardial contractile strength worsen.[16,20,130,133] The degree to which the MR exacerbates loss of contractile function induced by ventricular remodeling is an area of intense laboratory and clinical investigation.

CLINICAL PRESENTATION

Most published series of chronic "ischemic mitral regurgitation" are of limited value because of "contamination" by inclusion of patients with nonischemic MR. Gillinov et al reported on 482 consecutive patients operated on for ischemic mitral regurgitation at the Cleveland Clinic over a 13-year period.[6] The report is unique and highly informative because the authors excluded patients with nonischemic MR. All patients had normal leaflet and subvalvular structure and all had a previous myocardial infarction. A clear distinction was also made between patients having operation within 2 weeks of their infarction. In this study 78% of patients were over 60 years old and 54% were male. NYHA class II, II, or IV heart failure symptoms were present in 32%, 30%, and 36%, respectfully. Chronic IMR was present in 80% and 12% had an intra-aortic balloon pump placed prior to surgery. There was a history of an inferior MI in 73% and superior MI in 63%, and essentially all patients had posterior, inferior, or both types of infarction. The procedure was a reoperation in 23% and an emergency in 8%. Triple- or double-vessel coronary artery disease was present in 89%. Atrial fibrillation occurred in one third of the patients. Myocardial revascularization was performed at the time of valve surgery in 95%. These demographic data are remarkably similar to another excellent report published by Grossi et al from New York University.[7]

DIAGNOSTIC STUDIES

The primary purpose of diagnostic studies is to determine the severity of coronary arterial disease and its anatomy, the severity and mechanism of MR, and the degree of LV dysfunction. In chronic IMR, the ventricular geometry and function reflect remodeling due to both the MR and infarction; therefore, these patients may require diagnostic studies and perhaps operative procedures that are different from patients with CAD *associated* with MR. It is also important to define comorbidity of other organ systems by appropriate diagnostic studies dictated by the patient's history, physical examination, and screening laboratory findings.

In patients with IMR, the ECG usually shows evidence of a prior myocardial infarction.[126,127,135,136] The incidence of arrhythmias varies but atrial fibrillation as noted earlier is quite common. In patients without failure and mild MR, heart size by chest x-ray is normal or slightly enlarged; the left atrium is seldom enlarged. In those with moderate or severe MR and/or severe LV dysfunction, the heart is enlarged and usually the left atrium is also enlarged.[97]

Transthoracic echocardiography and TEE are useful in determining the etiology of MR. Two-dimensional echocardiography reliably detects ruptured chordae, annular calcification, and myxomatous degeneration, which are not features of chronic IMR, and differentiates rheumatic valve disease, endocarditis, and congenital deformities. Echocardiography also effectively assesses regional wall motion abnormalities and global LV function. The degree of MR is also well-quantified by color flow Doppler measurements.

Cardiac catheterization defines the coronary arterial pathology. Ventriculograms add little to the data provided by TTE or TEE and should be avoided especially in patients with impaired renal function. Measurements of chamber pressures and estimates of cardiac output contribute to the overall evaluation of LV function. Pulmonary hypertension, when present, is typically moderate and correlates with the degree of LV dysfunction and/or severity of MR.

INDICATIONS FOR SURGERY

Patients with symptomatic coronary artery disease that is not amenable to interventional cardiology are candidates for operation. The criteria for revascularization do not differ from patients without IMR; however, the presence of MR and/or severe LV dysfunction increases the risk of operation.[126,125,135] A decision not to expose the mitral valve is generally made preoperatively if the severity of MR is 1+ or 2+, and is confirmed in the operating room by transesophageal echocardiography and color flow Doppler velocity mapping before and after cardiopulmonary bypass and after manipulating afterload and preload.

The presence of severe IMR (3+ or 4+) and significant LV dysfunction has been a conventional indication for operative therapy on the mitral valve in addition to any bypass grafts needed to ameliorate symptoms of coronary ischemia. Valve repair or replacement in these patients simplifies weaning from cardiopulmonary bypass and early postoperative management. Whether or not restoring valve competency in these patients reduces heart failure symptoms or improves longevity has not been resolved by available clinical and laboratory data.

OPERATION

Operation is usually elective except in patients with uncontrolled symptoms of coronary ischemia who may require emergency or urgent operation to prevent infarction. Preoperative preparation and intraoperative monitors do not differ from other cardiac operations with the exception of transesophageal echocardiography and color flow Doppler velocity mapping. After induction of anesthesia, the degree of MR, anatomy of the valve, and dimensions and segmental wall motion of the LV are carefully assessed to determine whether or not the mitral valve needs to be addressed. Since anesthesia generally reduces systemic vascular resistance and afterload, assessment of the valve after administration of phenylephrine may unmask more severe MR. If the amount of MR is 2+, transfusion after aortic cannulation to increase preload to 1.5 to 2.0 times resting pulmonary capillary wedge pressure may unmask more severe MR and prompt a decision to expose and repair the valve.[137] If there is a significant discrepancy between the intraoperative degree of MR and that diagnosed by preoperative TEE, it is probably best to treat according to the preoperative value since this likely what the patient experiences under normal loading conditions. In patients with marginal LV function, a Swan-Ganz catheter with an oxygen electrode and a femoral arterial catheter for possible intra-aortic balloon insertion are recommended.

The heart is exposed via midline sternotomy; other incisions may be used to expose the mitral valve, but these compromise the ability to revascularize the heart. For patients who have only revascularization, cannulation, administration of cardioplegia, depth of systemic hypothermia, choice of conduit, and conduct of operation do not differ from revascularization operations without IMR. However, if there is any possibility that the mitral valve will be exposed, separate cannulation of both cavae through the right atrium may save time later.

For patients who require mitral valve repair or replacement, two venous cannulas are preferred and one of the specialized retractors for facilitating exposure of the mitral valve is used after the sternotomy and mammary arterial dissection. Pericardial attachments to both cavae and the right pulmonary veins are dissected away to mobilize the heart. After starting cardiopulmonary bypass, the left atrium is opened for decompression of the ventricle; the aorta is clamped and cardioplegia is given. Both antegrade and retrograde cold blood cardioplegia are recommended with myocardial temperature monitoring to minimize myocardial stunning and post–bypass LV dysfunction. Distal coronary arterial anastomoses are done first to reduce manipulation of the heart with possible rupture of the ventricle at the atrioventricular groove after mitral valve repair or replacement.

The left atrium is usually enlarged and accommodates a generous incision behind the interatrial septum. The atrial septum and right atrium are retracted to expose the valve. An initial inspection reveals the amount of annular dilatation and may indicate segments of the mural annulus that appear disproportionately elongated. Traction sutures in the annulus at each commissure elevate the valve and facilitate exposure of the leaflets, chordae, and papillary muscles. Careful inspection searching for ruptured, elongated, or sclerosed chordae; fibrotic, atrophied papillary muscle; and redundant or defective leaflet tissue is made. Most often the entire valve appears normal; sometimes the posterior papillary muscle seems slightly more yellowish brown than the rest of the ventricle and the posterior part of the mural annulus seems slightly elongated.

The decision to repair or replace the valve is often difficult. Replacement is recommended in older patients with severe LV dysfunction, who do not easily tolerate prolonged cardiopulmonary bypass with cardioplegic arrest. A short operation ending with a competent valve offers the greatest chance of success. In other patients, repair is preferred if a competent valve is produced. Since repair of IMR does not address the primary pathology causing MR, a decision to repair carries the caveat of immediate replacement if unsuccessful

Gillinov's report demonstrated that mitral valve repair is effective (at least in the short term) in 97% of patients undergoing elective surgery for 3+ to 4+ chronic IMR. Ring annuloplasty was employed in 98% of these repairs and was the sole surgical maneuver on the valve in over 80%. There was a distinct inclination in this study to undersize the valvuloplasty ring; 79% of the rings were 30 mm or less. Iatrogenic mitral stenosis was not seen even in the patients who received 26-mm annuloplasty devices.[6]

Chordal sparing techniques[117–119,122,123,138] are used if the valve is replaced. These methods have significantly reduced postoperative ventricular dysfunction observed after valve excision in the past and produce no more LV dysfunction than reparative operations.[123] Aged patients in sinus rhythm and patients with a life expectancy of less than 5 or 6 years who otherwise do not need anticoagulation are candidates for bioprosthetic valves; mechanical valves are recommended for others. The valve is inserted after excising[118,123] or transposing[122] anterior leaflet tissue using running over and over sutures. Pledgeted interrupted mattress sutures are used only in patients with extremely friable atrial and annular tissue. The mural leaflet is plicated into the valve insertion suture line to prevent interference with the valve mechanism.

Prior to removing the aortic clamp, all air is evacuated from the ventricle and the mitral valve is kept incompetent using a transvalvular catheter with ventricular and atrial holes. Absence of air and assessment of ventricular wall motion is made by transesophageal echocardiography. Anticipated pharmacologic support is started and satisfactory LV contractility is established before loading the heart. After weaning, cardiopulmonary bypass is restarted if the LV begins to dilate and wall motion deteriorates; every effort is made to prevent any distention of the ventricle that might reduce myocardial contractile force.[138] Decisions for using intra-aortic balloon pumping or even temporary left ventricular assistance are better made early than after multiple attempts to wean from cardiopulmonary bypass have failed.

RESULTS

Myocardial revascularization alone in patients with chronic IMR has a higher hospital mortality than in patients without IMR.[128] Mild (1+) IMR increases operative mortality to 3.4% to 4.5%[126–128,139] and moderate (2+) IMR raises operative mortality to 6% to 11%.[126–128,140] Five-year survival is influenced by the severity of LV dysfunction at the time of operation, age, and comorbid disease.[33]

Two-year survival for revascularization alone in patients with 1+ and 2+ MR is 88% and 78%, respectively.[141] Five-year survival rates for patients with mild MR range between 70% and 80%.[19,126,135,142] For moderate IMR, five-year survival ranges between 60% and 70%.[143,144] There are little data regarding the functional class and quality of life in revascularized patients with mild to moderate MR and no data regarding rates of progressive worsening of MR.

Historically, repair and revascularization of chronic IMR has an operative mortality that ranges from 3.0% to

29.4%[37,38,114,142,145,146] and a rate of reoperation up to 14.7%.[122,145,147] These values are confirmed in the most recent reports.[6,7] The long-term durability of repairs for chronic (and acute) IMR is difficult to assess since death is a strong competing end point and repair failure is usually defined as a need for reoperation. The incidence and severity of recurrent MR that does not require reoperation are almost never reported. Mitral valve replacement and revascularization have a hospital mortality between 3% and 33%[35,114,116,126–128,132,148–151] and average around 20%. Most of this reported experience with valve replacement occurred before chordal sparing became standard practice.[126,127,148–151] In addition, many series combined patients who had myocardial revascularization and mitral valve replacement for any type of mitral disease.[147–149,151–153] However, Grossi's recent report using modern techniques and a rigorous definition of IMR confirmed these statistics.[7] In general, operation for IMR has a higher mortality than for other causes of mitral valve malfunction.[129,138,143] The choice of valve prosthesis does not appear to influence results. Risk factors for hospital death include age, congestive heart failure, severity of LV dysfunction, preoperative intra-aortic balloon pump, ejection fraction, number of diseased coronary arteries, and comorbid conditions.[32,101,137]

Most reports indicate the 5-year survival after revascularization and mitral valve repair or replacement is between 30% and 40%.[19,34,126,127,135] Gillinov's report again confirms these statistics. In his series 5-year survival in the propensity-matched best risk group was 58% for valve repair and 36% for replacement. This group had significantly fewer NYHA class IV patients and less severe MR preoperatively. In the propensity-matched poorer risk groups (more severe CHF, MR, and emergency surgery) and for the group as a whole (Fig. 28-5) there was no difference between repair and replacement and 5-year survival was uniformly less than 50%.[6] These sobering 5-year survival data are depressingly similar to those for medically treated heart failure patients. As Miller has aptly stated, "successful revascularization and correction of IMR does relatively little in terms of ameliorating the ravages of previous LV infarction. . . ."[154]

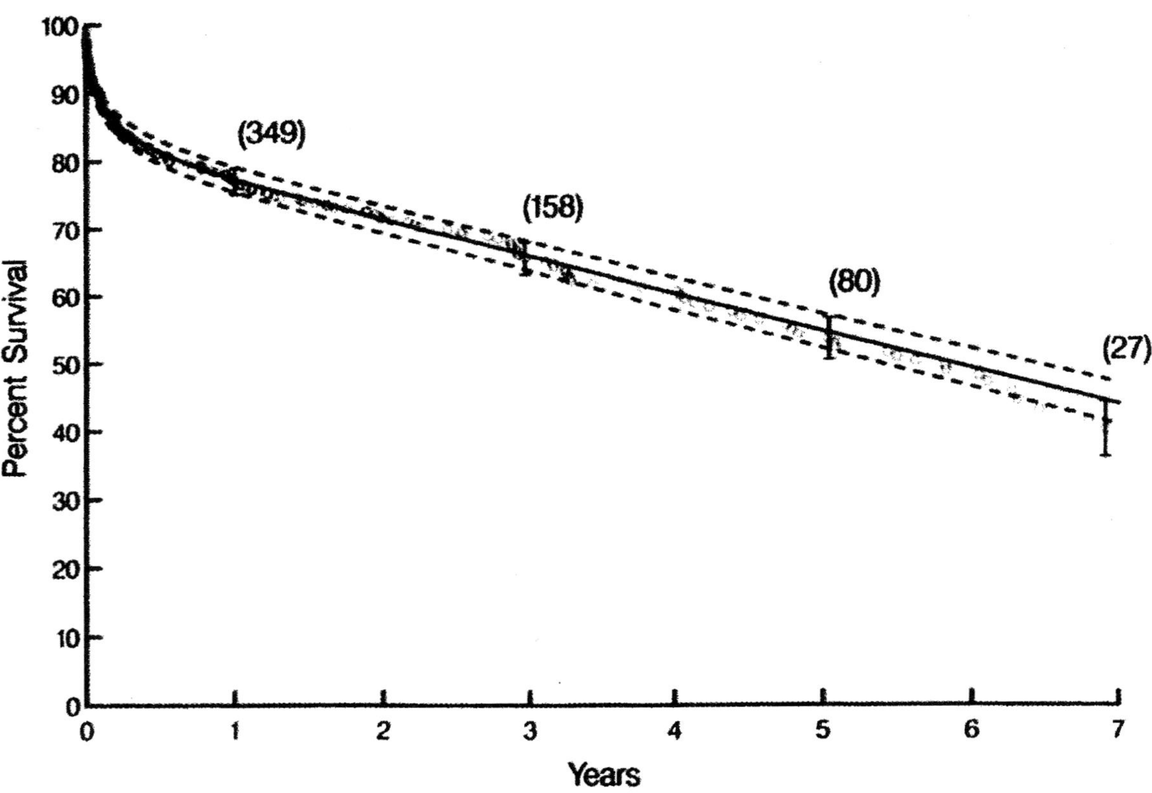

FIGURE 28–5 Survival after mitral valve surgery for all patients with ischemic mitral regurgitation. Each symbol represents a death according to Kaplan-Meier estimator. Vertical bars enclose asymmetric 68% confidence limits. Solid lines represent parametric survival estimates; these are enclosed between dashed 68% confidence limits. Numbers in parentheses are numbers of patients traced beyond that point. *(Reproduced with permission from Gillinov AM, Wierup PN, Blackstone EH, et al: Is repair preferable to replacement for ischemic mitral regurgitation? J Thorac Cardiovasc Surg 2001; 122:1125.)*

A LOOK TO THE FUTURE

In spite of best efforts the 5-year survival for medical and/or surgical therapies for infarction-induced heart failure has hovered stubbornly around 50% (worse than for most types of cancer). This reflects a lack of understanding of the basic pathophysiology of postinfarction left ventricular remodeling. Why are some regional acute myocardial infarctions tolerated without severe loss of function initially, but progress to severe ventricular dysfunction during postinfarction remodeling in the absence of further infarctions? Recent clinical,[155] theoretical,[156] and experimental[130,157] studies have shed new light on this problem. These studies suggest that a transmural myocardial infarction that expands soon after infarction initiates a myopathic process in normal perfused myocardium that cannot be explained solely on the basis of mechanical disadvantage due to geometric shape change. Whether this process is reversible remains to be seen, but unimpressive results with LV volume reduction[158] and LV aneurysm[159] operations strongly suggest that it is not.

Recent work supports the concept that regional increases in wall stress of normally perfused myocardium adjacent to the infarction initiates production of oxygen free radicals, apoptosis, and alterations in collagen metabolism.[130,160–163] Although much more work is needed to prove this hypothesis, the concept introduces the possibility of early surgical and/or medical interventions before LV remodeling occurs, rather than afterwards. Reperfusion of completed infarctions, although too late to save myocytes, attenuates LV dilatation,[109] improves survival, and alters collagen metabolism of the extracellular matrix.[163] Restraining infarct expansion preserves LV resting function and stabilizes LV geometry in a sheep model of anteroapical infarction,[164] alters collagen metabolism,[162] and reduces the severity of chronic remodeling MR.[165] Preliminary work suggests that preventing infarct expansion using a partial LV wrap significantly reduces subsequent development of both MR and ventricular dilatation. These approaches, which address the hypothesis of stress-induced apoptosis, better address the pathogenesis of chronic ischemic MR and may eventually improve results in this large group of difficult patients.

REFERENCES

1. Selzer A, Katayama E: Mitral regurgitation; clinical patterns, pathophysiology and natural history. *Medicine* 1972; 51:337.
2. Maisel AS, Gilpin EA, Klein L, et al: The murmur of papillary muscle dysfunction in acute myocardial infarction; clinical features and prognostic implications. *Am Heart J* 1986; 112:705.
3. Sharma SK, Seckler J, Israel DH, et al: Clinical, angiographic and anatomic findings in acute severe ischemic mitral regurgitation. *Am J Cardiol* 1992; 70:277.
4. Becker AE: Anatomy of the coronary arteries with respect to chronic ischemic mitral regurgitation, in Vetter HO, Hetzer R, Schmutzler H (eds): *Ischemic Mitral Incompetence.* New York, Springer-Verlag, 1991; p 17.
5. Tcheng JE, Jackman JD Jr, Nelson CL, et al: Outcome of patients sustaining acute ischemic mitral regurgitation during myocardial infarction. *Ann Int Med* 1992; 117:18.
6. Gillinov AM, Wierup PN, Blackstone EH, et al: Is repair preferable to replacement for ischemic mitral regurgitation? *J Thorac Cardiovasc Surg* 2001; 122:1125.
7. Grossi EA, Goldberg JD, LaPietra A, et al: Ischemic mitral valve reconstruction and replacement: comparison of long-term survival and complications. *J Thorac Cardiovasc Surg* 2001; 122:1107.
8. *Heart and Stroke Facts: 1995 Statistical Supplement.* Dallas, TX, American Heart Association, 1996.
9. Lytle BW, Cosgrove DM, Gill CC, et al: Mitral valve replacement combined with myocardial revascularization: early and late results for 300 patients, 1970–1983. *Circulation* 1985; 71:1179.
10. Akins CW, Hilgenberg AD, Buckley MJ, et al: Mitral valve reconstruction versus replacement for degenerative or ischemic mitral regurgitation. *Ann Thorac Surg* 1994; 58:668.
11. Czer LSC, Gray RJ, DeRobertis MA, et al: Mitral valve replacement: impact of coronary artery disease and determinants of prognosis after revascularization. *Circulation* 1984; 70(suppl I): I-198.
12. Angell WW, Oury JH: A comparison of replacement and reconstruction in patients with mitral regurgitation. *J Thorac Cardiovasc Surg* 1987; 93:665.
13. Karp RB: Mitral valve replacement and coronary artery bypass grafting. *Ann Thorac Surg* 1982; 34:480.
14. Enriquez-Sarano M, Schaff HV, Orszulak TA: Valve repair improves the outcome of surgery for mitral regurgitation. *Circulation* 1995; 91:1022.
15. Gahl I, Sutton R, Pearson M, et al: Mitral regurgitation in coronary disease. *Br Heart J* 1977; 39:13.
16. Heikkila J: Mitral incompetence as a complication of acute myocardial infarction. *Acta Medica Scand Suppl* 1967; 475:1.
17. Loperfido R, Biasucci LM, Pennestri F, et al: Pulsed Doppler echocardiographic analysis of mitral regurgitation after myocardial infarction. *Am J Cardiol* 1986; 58:692.
18. Barzilai B, Gessler C, Perez JE, et al: Significance of Doppler-detected mitral regurgitation in acute myocardial infarction. *Am J Cardiol* 1988; 61:220.
19. Hickey M StJ, Smith LR, Muhlbaier LH, et al: Current prognosis of ischemic mitral regurgitation. *Circulation* 1988; 78:I-51.
20. Frantz E, Weininger F, Oswald H, Fleck E: Predictors for mitral regurgitation in coronary artery disease, in Vetter HO, Hetzer R, Schmutzler H (eds): *Ischemic Mitral Incompetence.* New York, Springer-Verlag, 1991; p 57.
21. Davies MJ: The pathology of the mitral valve, in Ionescu MI, Cohn LH (eds): *Mitral Valve Disease.* London, Butterworths, 1985; p 27.
22. Izumi S, Miyatake K, Beppu S, et al: Mechanism of mitral regurgitation in patients with myocardial infarction: a study using real time two-dimensional Doppler flow imaging and echocardiography. *Circulation* 1987; 76:777.
23. Llaneras MR, Nance ML, Streicher JT, et al: Pathogenesis of ischemic mitral insufficiency. *J Thorac Cardiovasc Surg* 1993; 105:439.
24. Gorman RC, Mc Caughan JS, Ratcliffe MB, et al: Pathogenesis of acute ischemic mitral regurgitation in three dimensions. *J Thorac Cardiovasc Surg* 1995; 109:684.
25. Gorman JH 3rd, Gorman RC, Plappert T, et al: Infarct size and location determine development of mitral regurgitation in the sheep model. *J Thorac Cardiovasc Surg* 1998; 115:615.
26. Wei JY, Hutchins GM, Bulkley BH: Papillary muscle rupture and fatal acute myocardial infarction. *Ann Intern Med* 1979; 90:149.
27. Nishimura RA, Schaff HV, Shub C, et al: Papillary muscle rupture complicating acute myocardial infarction: analysis of 17 patients. *Am J Cardiol* 1983; 51:373.

28. Loisance DY, Deleuze PH, Hillion ML, Cachera JP: Are there indications for reconstructive surgery in severe mitral regurgitation after acute myocardial infarction? *Eur J Cardiothorac Surg* 1990; 4:394.
29. Clements SD, Story WE, Hurst JW, et al: Ruptured papillary muscle, a complication of myocardial infarction: clinical presentation, diagnosis, and treatment. *Clin Cardiol* 1985; 8:93.
30. Barbour DJ, Roberts WC: Rupture of a left ventricular papillary muscle during acute myocardial infarction; analysis of 22 necropsy patients. *J Am Coll Cardiol* 1886; 8:558.
31. Tepe NA, Edmunds LH Jr: Operation for acute postinfarction mitral insufficiency and cardiogenic shock. *J Thorac Cardiovasc Surg* 1985; 89:525.
32. Rankin JS, Hickey MSJ, Smith LR, et al: Ischemic mitral regurgitation. *Circulation* 1989; 79 (suppl I):I-116.
33. Kono T, Sabbah HN, Stein PD, et al: Left ventricular shape as a determinant of functional mitral regurgitation in patients with severe heart failure secondary to either coronary artery disease or idiopathic dilated cardiomyopathy. *Am J Cardiol* 1991; 68:355.
34. Hendren WG, Memec JJ, Lytle BW, et al: Mitral valve repair for ischemic mitral insufficiency. *Ann Thorac Surg* 1991; 52:1246.
35. Rankin JS, Fenely MP, Hickey MS, et al: A clinical comparison of mitral valve repair versus valve replacement in ischemic mitral regurgitation. *J Thorac Cardiovasc Surg* 1988; 95:165.
36. Roberts WC, Cohen LS: Left ventricular papillary muscles. *Circulation* 1972; 46:138.
37. Boltwood CM, Tei C, Wong M, Shah PM: Quantitative echocardiography of the mitral complex in dilated cardiomyopathy: the mechanism of functional mitral regurgitation. *Circulation* 1983; 68:498.
38. Bulkley BH, Roberts WC: Dilatation of the mitral annulus. *Am J Med* 1975; 59:457.
39. Levine RA, Handschumacher MD, Sanfilippo AJ, et al: Three-dimensional echocardiographic reconstruction of the mitral valve, with implications for the diagnosis of mitral valve prolapse. *Circulation* 1989; 80:589.
40. Salgo IS, Gorman JH 3rd, Gorman RC, et al: The effect of annular shape on leaflet curvature in reducing mitral leaflet stress. *Circulation* 2002; 106:711.
41. Rayhill SC, Daughters GT, Castro LJ, et al: Dynamics of normal and ischemic canine papillary muscles. *Circ Res* 1994; 74:1179.
42. Tsakiris AG, Gordon DA, Padiyar R, Frechette D: Relation of mitral valve opening and closure to left atrial and ventricular pressures in the intact dog. *Am J Physiol Heart Circ Physiol* 1978; 234:H146.
43. Nolan SP, Dixon SH Jr, Fisher RD, Morrow AG: The influence of atrial contraction and mitral valve mechanics on ventricular filling. *Am Heart J* 1969; 77:784.
44. Tsakiris AG, von Bernuth G, Rastelli GC, et al: Size and motion of the mitral valve annulus in anesthetized intact dogs. *J Appl Physiol* 1971; 30:611.
45. Hinds JE, Hawthorne EW, Mullins CB, Mitchell JH: Instantaneous changes in the left ventricular lengths occurring in dogs during the cardiac cycle. *Fed Proc* 1969; 28:1351.
46. Keren G, Sonnenblick EH, LeJemtel TH: Mitral annulus motion. *Circulation* 1988; 78:621.
47. Tsakiris AG, Sturm RE, Wood EH: Experimental studies on the mechanisms of closure of cardiac valves with use of Roentgen videodensitometry. *Am J Cardiol* 1973; 32:136.
48. Ormiston JA, Shah Pravin M, Tei C, Wong M: Size and motion of the mitral valve annulus in man. *Circulation* 1982; 65:713.
49. Perloff JK, Roberts WC: The mitral apparatus. *Circulation* 1972; 46:227.
50. Frater RWM: Functional anatomy of the mitral valve, in Ionescu MI, Cohn LH (eds): *Mitral Valve Disease*. London, Butterworths, 1985; p 127.
51. Kono T, Sabbah HN, Rosman H, et al: Mechanism of functional mitral regurgitation during acute myocardial ischemia. *J Am Coll Cardiol* 1992; 19:1101.
52. Salisbury PF, Cross CE, Rieben PA: Chorda tendinea tension. *Am J Physiol* 1963; 205:385.
53. Hirakawa S, Sasayama S, Tomoike H, et al: In situ measurement of papillary muscle dynamics in the dog left ventricle. *Am J Physiol Heart Circ Physiol* 1977; 2:H384.
54. Gorman RC, McCaughan JS, Ratcliffe MB, et al: A three-dimensional analysis of papillary muscle spatial relationships in acute postinfarction mitral insufficiency. *Surg Forum* 1994; 45:330.
55. Davies MJ: *Cardiovascular Pathology*. New York, Harvey Miller Publishers, Oxford University Press, 1986.
56. Gould SE, Ioannides G: Ischemic heart disease, in Gould SE (ed): *Pathology of the Heart and Blood Vessels*. Springfield, IL, Charles C Thomas, 1968.
57. Walley KR, Grover M, Raff GL, et al: Left ventricular dynamic geometry in the intact and open chest dog. *Circ Res* 1982; 50:573.
58. Pandian NG, Kerber RE: Two-dimensional echocardiography in experimental coronary stenosis. *Circulation* 1982 ;66:597.
59. Moon MR, Ingels NB Jr, Daughters GHT 2nd, et al: Alterations in left ventricular twist mechanics with inotropic stimulation and volume loading in human subjects. *Circulation* 1994; 89:142.
60. Tsakiris AG, Gordon DA, Padiyar R, et al: The role of displacement of the mitral annulus in left atrial filling and emptying in the intact dog. *Can J Physiol Pharmacol* 1978; 56:447.
61. Ingels NB Jr, Daughters GT 2nd, Nikolic SD, et al: Left atrial pressure-clamp servomechanism demonstrates LV suction in canine hearts with normal mitral valves. *Am J Physiol Heart Circ Physiol* 1994; 267:H354.
62. Yellin EL, Peskin C, Yoran C, et al: Mechanisms of mitral valve motion during diastole. *Am J Physiol Heart Circ Physiol* 1981; 241:H389.
63. Marzilli M, Sabbah HN, Lee T, Stein PD: Role of the papillary muscle in opening and closure of the mitral valve. *Am J Physiol Heart Circ Physiol* 1980; 238: H348.
64. Gorman JH 3rd, Gorman RC, Jackson BM, et al: Papillary muscle discoordination rather than increased annular area facilitates mitral regurgitation after acute posterior infarction. *Circulation* 1997; 96 (suppl II): 124.
65. Gorman JH 3rd, Gorman RC, Jackson BM, et al: Three-dimensional annular changes in acute ischemic mitral regurgitation. *Surg Forum* 1996; 47:288.
66. Gorman RC, McCaughan J, Ratcliffe MB, et al: Pathogenesis of acute ischemic mitral regurgitation in three dimensions. *J Thorac Cardiovasc Surg* 1995; 109:684.
67. Glasson JR, Komeda M, Daughters GT, et al: Early systolic mitral leaflet "loitering" during acute ischemic mitral regurgitation. *J Thorac Cardiovasc Surg* 1998; 116:193.
68. Komeda M, Glasson JR, Bolger AF, et al: Geometric determinants of ischemic mitral regurgitation. *Circulation* 1997; 96(suppl): II-128.
69. Otsuji Y, Handschumacher MD, Liel-Cohen N, et al: Mechanism of ischemic mitral regurgitation with segmental left ventricular dysfunction: three-dimensional echocardiographic studies in models of acute and chronic progressive regurgitation. *J Am Coll Cardiol* 2001; 37:641.
70. Llaneras MR, Nance ML, Streicher JT, et al: A large animal model of ischemic mitral regurgitation. *Ann Thorac Surg* 1994; 57:432.

71. Godley RW, Wann LS, Rogers EW, et al: Incomplete mitral leaflet closure in patients with papillary muscle dysfunction. *Circulation* 1981; 63:565.
72. Mittal AK, Langston M Jr, Cohn KE, et al: Combined papillary muscle and left ventricular wall dysfunction as a cause of mitral regurgitation. *Circulation* 1971; 44:174.
73. Tsakiris AG, Rastelli GC, Amorim DD, et al: Effect of experimental papillary muscle damage on mitral valve closure in intact anesthetized dogs. *Mayo Clin Proc* 1970; 45:275.
74. Kaul S, Spotnitz WD, Glasheen WP, Touchstone DA: Mechanism of ischemic mitral regurgitation. *Circulation* 1991; 84:2167.
75. Tei C, Sakamaki T, Shah PM, et al: Mitral valve prolapse in short-term experimental coronary occlusion: a possible mechanism of ischemic mitral regurgitation. *Circulation* 1983; 68:183.
76. Kinney EL, Frangi MJ: Value of two-dimensional echocardiographic detection of incomplete mitral leaflet closure. *Am Heart J* 1985; 109:87.
77. Gorman JH 3rd, Gorman RC, Jackson BM, et al: Distortions of the mitral valve in acute ischemic mitral regurgitation. *Ann Thorac Surg* 1997; 64:1026.
78. Gorman JH 3rd, Gorman RC, Jackson BM, et al: The effect of inotropic state on the size of the mitral annulus. *J Am Coll Cardiol* 2001; 37:1087.
79. LeFeuvre C, Metzger JP, Lachurie ML, et al: Treatment of severe mitral regurgitation caused by ischemic papillary muscle dysfunction: indications for coronary angioplasty. *Am Heart J* 1992; 123:860.
80. Grigioni F, Enriquez-Sarano M, Zehr KJ, et al: Ischemic mitral regurgitation: long-term outcome and prognostic implications with quantitative Doppler assessment. *Circulation* 2001; 103:1759.
81. Yiu SF, Enriquez-Sarano M, Tribouilloy C, et al: Determinants of the degree of functional mitral regurgitation in patients with systolic left ventricular dysfunction: a quantitative clinical study. *Circulation* 2000; 102:1400.
82. Calafiore AM, Gallina S, Di Mauro M, et al: Mitral valve procedure in dilated cardiomyopathy: repair or replacement? *Ann Thorac Surg* 2001; 71:1146.
83. Savage DD, Garrison RJ, Devereux RB, et al: Mitral valve prolapse in the general population, I: epidemiologic features: the Framingham Study. *Am Heart J* 1983; 106:571.
84. Braunwald E: Valvular heart disease, in Braunwald E (ed): *Heart Disease,* 4th ed. Philadelphia, WB Saunders, 1992; p 1007.
85. Jackson BM, Gorman JH 3rd, Moainie SL, et al: Extension of borderzone myocardium in postinfarction dilated cardiomyopathy. *J Am Coll Cardiol (in press).*
86. Otsuji Y, Handschumacher MD, Schwammenthal E, et al: Insights from three-dimensional echocardiography into the mechanism of functional mitral regurgitation: direct in vivo demonstration of altered leaflet tethering geometry. *Circulation* 1997; 96:1999.
87. He S, Fontaine AA, Schwammenthal E, et al: Integrated mechanism for functional mitral regurgitation: leaflet restriction versus coapting force: in vitro studies. *Circulation,* 1997; 96:1826.
88. Yiu SF, Enriquez-Sarano M, Tribouilloy C, et al: Determinants of the degree of functional mitral regurgitation in patients with systolic left ventricular dysfunction: a quantitative clinical study. *Circulation* 2000; 102:1400.
89. Barzilai B, Gessler C, Perez JE, et al: Significance of Doppler-detected mitral regurgitation in acute myocardial infarction. *Am J Cardiol* 1988; 61:220.
90. Lamas GA, Mitchell GF, Flaker GC, et al: Clinical significance of mitral regurgitation after acute myocardial infarction. Survival and Ventricular Enlargement Investigators. *Circulation* 1997; 96:827.
91. Austen WG, Sokol DM, De Sanctis RW, Sanders CA: Surgical treatment of papillary-muscle rupture complicating myocardial infarction. *N Engl J Med* 1968; 278:1137.
92. Cederqvist L, Soderstrom J: Papillary muscle rupture in myocardial infarction: a study based on autopsy material. *Acta Med Scand* 1964; 176:287.
93. Piwnica A, Menasche PH, Kucharski C, et al: Surgery for acute ischemic mitral incompetence, in Vetter HO, Hetzer H, Schmutzler H (eds): *Ischemic Mitral Incompetence.* New York, Springer-Verlag, 1991; p 193.
94. Braunwald E: Mitral regurgitation. *N Engl J Med* 1969; 281:425.
95. Katayama K, Tajimi T, Guth BD, et al: Early diastolic filling dynamics during experimental mitral regurgitation in the conscious dog. *Circulation* 1988; 78:390.
96. Zile MR, Monita M, Nakano K, et al: Effects of left ventricular overload produced by mitral regurgitation on diastolic function. *Am J Physiol Heart Circ Physiol* 1991; 261:H1471.
97. DeBusk RF, Harrison EC: The clinical spectrum of papillary muscle disease. *N Engl J Med* 1969; 281:1458.
98. Sanders RJ, Neubergen KT, Ravin A: Rupture of papillary muscle: occurrence of rupture of the posterior papillary muscle as a complication of posterior myocardial infarction. *Chest* 1957; 31:316.
99. Stewart WJ, Currie PJ, Salcedo EE, et al: Intraoperative Doppler color flow mapping for decision-making in valve repair for mitral regurgitation. *Circulation* 1990; 81:556.
100. Maurer G, Siegel RJ, Czer LSC: The use of color mapping for intraoperative assessment of valve repair. *Circulation* 1991; 81: I-250.
101. Bargiggia GS, Tronconi L, Sahn DJ, et al: A new method for quantitation of mitral regurgitation based on color flow Doppler imaging of flow convergence proximal to regurgitant orifice. *Circulation* 1991; 84:1481.
102. Swanson JS, Starr A: Surgical results with severe ischemic mitral regurgitation, in Vetter HO, Hetzer H, Schmutzler H (eds): *Ischemic Mitral Incompetence.* New York, Springer-Verlag, 1991; p 187.
103. Keren G, Bier A, Strom JA, et al: Dynamics of mitral regurgitation during nitroglycerin therapy: a Doppler echocardiographic study. *Am Heart J* 1986; 112:517.
104. Heuser RR, Maddoux GL, Goss JE, et al: Coronary angioplasty for acute mitral regurgitation due to myocardial infarction. *Ann Intern Med* 1987; 107:852.
105. Shawl FA, Forman MB, Punja S, Goldbaum TS: Emergent coronary angioplasty in the treatment of acute ischemic mitral regurgitation: long-term results in five cases. *J Am Coll Cardiol* 1989; 986:986.
106. Bates, ER, Califf RM, Stack RS, et al: The Thrombolysis and Angioplasty in Myocardial Infarction (TAMI-1) Trial; influence of infarct location on arterial patency, left ventricular function and mortality. *J Am Coll Cardiol* 1989; 13:12.
107. Pfeffer MA, Braunwald E: Ventricular remodeling after myocardial infarction. *Circulation* 1990; 81:1161.
108. Marino P, Zanolla L, Zardini P, on behalf of GISSI: Effect of streptokinase on left ventricular modeling and function after myocardial infarction: the GISSI (Gruppo Italiano per lo studio della Streptochinaisi nell; Infarto Miocardico) Trial. *J Am Coll Cardiol* 1989; 14:1149.
109. Hochman JS, Choo H: Limitation of myocardial infarct expansion by reperfusion independent of myocardial salvage. *Circulation* 1987; 75:299.
110. Kaiser GC, Schaff HV, Killip T: Myocardial revascularization for unstable angina pectoris. *Circulation* 1989; 79(suppl I): I-60.

111. Kouchoukos NT, Murphy S, Philpott T, et al: Coronary artery bypass grafting for postinfarction angina pectoris. *Circulation* 1989; 79(suppl I): I-68.
112. Kennedy JW, Ivey TD, Misbach G, et al: Coronary artery bypass graft surgery early after acute myocardial infarction. *Circulation* 1989; 79(suppl I): I-73.
113. Replogle RL, Campbell CD: Surgery for mitral regurgitation associated with ischemic heart disease. *Circulation* 1989; 79(suppl I):I-122.
114. Siniawski H, Weng Y, Hetzer R: Decision-making aspects in the surgical treatment of ischemic mitral incompetence, in Vetter HO, Hetzer H, Schmutzler H (eds): *Ischemic Mitral Incompetence*. New York, Springer-Verlag, 1991; p 137.
115. Kay GL, Zubiate P, Prejean CA Jr, et al: Probability of repair for pure mitral regurgitation. *J Thorac Cardiovasc Surg* 1994; 108:871.
116. David TE: Techniques and results of mitral valve repair for ischemic mitral regurgitation. *J Cardiac Surg* 1994; 9:274.
117. Lillehei CW, Levy MJ, Bonnabeau RC Jr: Mitral valve replacement with preservation of papillary muscles and chordae tendineae. *J Thorac Cardiovasc Surg* 1964; 47:532.
118. David TE, Uden DE, Strauss HD: The importance of the mitral apparatus in left ventricular function after correction of mitral regurgitation. *Circulation* 1983; 68(suppl II):II-76.
119. Sarris GE, Fann JI, Niczyporuk MA, et al: Global and regional left ventricular systolic performance in the in situ ejecting canine heart. *Circulation* 1989; 80(suppl I):I-24.
120. Yun KL, Niczyporuk MA, Sarris GE, et al: Importance of mitral subvalvular apparatus in terms of cardiac energetics and systolic mechanics in the ejecting canine heart. *J Clin Invest* 1991; 87:247.
121. Yun KL, Rayhill SC, Niczyporuk MA, et al: Mitral valve replacement in dilated canine hearts with chronic mitral regurgitation. *Circulation* 1991; 84(suppl III):III-112.
122. Oury JH, Cleveland, JC, Duran CG, Angell WW: Ischemic mitral valve disease: classification and systemic approach to management. *J Cardiac Surg* 1994; 9:262.
123. Okita Y, Miki S, Kusuhara K, et al: Analysis of left ventricular motion after mitral valve replacement with a technique of preservation of all chordae tendineae. *J Thorac Cardiovasc Surg* 1992; 104:786.
124. Kay GL, Kay JH, Zubiate P, et al: Mitral valve repair for mitral regurgitation secondary to coronary artery disease. *Circulation* 1986; 74(suppl I):I-88.
125. Balu V, Hershowitz S, Zaki Masud AR, et al: Mitral regurgitation in coronary artery disease. *Chest* 1982; 81:550.
126. Pinson CW, Cobanoglu A, Metzdorff MT, et al: Late surgical results for ischemic mitral regurgitation. *J Thorac Cardiovasc Surg* 1984; 88:663.
127. Connolly MW, Gelbfish JS, Jacobowitz IJ, et al: Surgical results for mitral regurgitation from coronary artery disease. *J Thorac Cardiovasc Surg* 1986; 91:379.
128. Karp RB, Mills N, Edmunds LH Jr: Coronary artery bypass grafting in the presence of valvular disease. *Circulation* 1989; 79:(suppl I): I-182.
129. Guy TS, Moainie SL, Jackson BM, et al: Prophylactic mitral annuloplasty prevents mitral regurgitation but not heart failure after posterolateral myocardial infarction. *Surg Forum* 2001; 52:102.
130. Jackson BM, Gorman JH 3rd, Moainie S, et al: Extension of borderzone myocardium in postinfarction dilated cardiomyopathy. *J Am Coll Cardiol* 2002; 40:1160.
131. Corin WJ, Monrad ES, Murakami T, et al: The relationship of afterload to ejection performance in chronic mitral regurgitation. *Circulation* 1987; 76:59.
132. Olivetti G, Capasso JM, Sonnenblick EH, Anversa P: Side-to-side slippage of myocytes participates in ventricular wall remodeling acutely after myocardial infarction in rats. *Circ Res* 1990; 67:23.
133. Eckberg, DL, Gault JH, Bouchard RL, et al: Mechanics of left ventricular contraction in chronic severe mitral regurgitation. *Circulation* 1973; 47:1252.
134. Fehrenbacher G, Schmidt DH, Bommer WJ: Evaluation of transient mitral regurgitation in coronary artery disease. *Am J Cardiol* 1991; 68:868.
135. Arcidi JM Jr, Hebler RF, Craver JM, et al: Treatment of moderate mitral regurgitation in coronary disease by coronary bypass alone. *J Thorac Cardiovasc Surg* 1988; 95:951.
136. Czer LSC, Maurer G, Trento A, et al: Comparative efficacy of ring and suture annuloplasty for ischemic mitral regurgitation. *Circulation* 1992; 86(suppl II):II-46.
137. Rankin JS, Hickey MSJ, Smith LR, et al: Current concepts in the pathogenesis and treatment of ischemic mitral regurgitation, in Vetter HO, Hetzer H, Schmutzler H (eds): *Ischemic Mitral Incompetence*. New York, Springer-Verlag, 1991; p 157.
138. Cooley DA, Ingram MT: Intravalvular implantation of mitral valve prostheses. *Tex Heart Inst J* 1987; 14:188.
139. Waibel AW, Hausdorf G, Vetter HO, et al: Results of surgical therapy in ischemic mitral regurgitation, in Vetter HO, Hetzer H, Schmutzler H (eds): *Ischemic Mitral Incompetence*. New York, Springer-Verlag, 1991; p 149.
140. Downing SW, Savage EB, Streicher JS, et al: The stretched ventricle; myocardial creep and contractile dysfunction after acute nonischemic ventricular distention. *J Thorac Cardiovasc Surg* 1992; 104:996.
141. Adler DS, Goldman L, O'Neil A, et al: Long-term survival of more than 2,000 patients after coronary artery bypass grafting. *Am J Cardiol* 1986; 58:195.
142. Dion R: Ischemic mitral regurgitation: when and how should it be corrected? *J Heart Valve Dis* 1993; 2:536.
143. Tamaki N, Kawamoto M, Tadamura E, et al: Prediction of reversible ischemia after revascularization. *Circulation* 1995; 91:1697.
144. Schelbert HR: Different roads to the assessment of myocardial viability. *Circulation* 1995; 91:1894.
145. Cohn LH: Surgical treatment of ischemic mitral regurgitation by repair and replacement, in Vetter HO, Hetzer H, Schmutzler H (eds): *Ischemic Mitral Incompetence*. New York, Springer-Verlag, 1991; p 179.
146. David TE, Ho WC: The effect of preservation of chordae tendineae on mitral valve replacement for postinfarction mitral regurgitation. *Circulation* 1986; 74(suppl I):I-116.
147. Angell WW, Oury JH: A comparison of replacement and reconstruction in patients with mitral regurgitation. *J Thorac Cardiovasc Surg* 1987; 93:665.
148. Lytle BW, Cosgrove DM, Gill CC, et al: Mitral valve replacement combined with myocardial revascularization: early and late results for 300 patients, 1970–1983. *Circulation* 1985; 71:1179.
149. Czer LSC, Gray RJ, DeRobertis MA, et al: Mitral valve replacement: impact of coronary artery disease and determinants of prognosis after revascularization. *Circulation* 1984; 70(suppl I):I-198.
150. Magovern JA, Pennock JL, Campbell DB, et al: Risks of mitral valve replacement and mitral valve replacement with coronary artery bypass. *Ann Thorac Surg* 1985; 39:346.
151. Karp RB: Mitral valve replacement and coronary artery bypass grafting. *Ann Thorac Surg* 1982; 34:480.
152. Akins CW, Hilgenberg AD, Buckley MJ, et al: Mitral valve reconstruction versus replacement for degenerative or ischemic mitral regurgitation. *Ann Thorac Surg* 1994; 58:668.
153. Enriquez-Sarano M, Schaff HV, Orszulak TA: Valve repair improves the outcome of surgery for mitral regurgitation. *Circulation* 1995; 91:1022.
154. Miller DC: Ischemic mitral regurgitation redux—to repair or to replace? *J Thorac Cardiovasc Surg* 2001; 122:1059.

155. Narula J, Dawson MS, Singh BK, et al: Noninvasive characterization of stunned, hibernating, remodeled and nonviable myocardium in ischemic cardiomyopathy. *J Am Coll Cardiol* 2000; 36:1913.
156. Guccione JM, Moonly SM, Moustakidis P, et al: Mechanism underlying mechanical dysfunction in the border zone of left ventricular aneurysm: a finite element model study. *Ann Thorac Surg* 2001; 71:654.
157. Moainie SL, Gorman JH 3rd, Guy TS, et al: An ovine model of postinfarction dilated cardiomyopathy. *Ann Thorac Surg* 2002; 74:753.
158. Athanasuleas CL, Stanley AW Jr, Buckberg GD, et al: Surgical anterior ventricular endocardial restoration (SAVER) in the dilated remodeled ventricle after anterior myocardial infarction. *J Am Coll Cardiol* 2001; 37:1199.
159. Couper GS, Bunton RW, Birjiniuk V, et al: Relative risks of left ventricular aneurysmectomy in patients with akinetic scars versus true dyskinetic aneurysms. *Circulation* 1990; 82(suppl 5): IV248-56.
160. Narula J, Arbustini E, Chandrashekhar Y, Schwaiger M: Apoptosis and systolic dysfunction in congestive heart failure: the story of apoptosis interruptus and zombie myocytes. *Cardiol Clin* 2001; 19:113.
161. Saraste A, Pulkki K, Kallajoki M, et al: Apoptosis in human acute myocardial infarction. *Circulation* 1997; 95:320.
162. Bowen F, Jones SC, Narula N, et al: Restraining acute infarct expansion decreases collagenase activity in borderzone myocardium. *Ann Thorac Surg* 2001; 72:1950.
163. Bowen FW, Hattori T, Narula N, et al: Reappearance of myocytes in ovine infarcts produced by six hours of complete ischemia followed by reperfusion. *Ann Thorac Surg* 2001; 71:1845.
164. Kelley ST, Malekan R, Gorman JH 3rd, et al: Restraining infarct expansion preserves left ventricular geometry and function after acute anteroapical infarction. *Circulation* 1999; 99:135.
165. Moainie SL, Guy TS, Gorman JH 3rd, et al: Infarct restraint attenuates remodeling and reduces chronic ischemic mitral regurgitation following postero-lateral infarction. *Ann Thorac Surg* 2002; 74:444.

Chapter 29

Left Ventricular Aneurysm

Donald D. Glower/James E. Lowe

DEFINITION

Left ventricular aneurysm has been strictly defined as a distinct area of abnormal left ventricular diastolic contour with systolic dyskinesia or paradoxical bulging (Fig. 29-1).[1] Yet, a growing number of authors favor defining left ventricular aneurysm more loosely as any large area of left ventricular akinesia or dyskinesia that reduces left ventricular ejection fraction.[2–4] This broader definition has been justified by data suggesting that the pathophysiology and treatment may be the same for ventricular akinesia and for ventricular dyskinesia.[3,5] Intraoperatively, a left ventricular aneurysm may also be defined as an area that collapses upon left ventricular decompression.[2,5,6] True left ventricular aneurysms involve bulging of the full thickness of the left ventricular wall, while a false aneurysm of the left ventricle is, in fact, a rupture of the left ventricular wall contained by surrounding pericardium.

HISTORY

Left ventricular aneurysms have long been described at autopsy, but left ventricular aneurysm was not recognized to be a consequence of coronary artery disease until 1881.[7] The angiographic diagnosis of left ventricular aneurysm was first made in 1951.[7] A congenital left ventricular aneurysm was first treated surgically by Weitland in 1912 using an aneurysm ligation. In 1944, Beck[8] described fasciae latae plication to treat left ventricular aneurysms. Likoff and Bailey[9] successfully resected a left ventricular aneurysm through a thoracotomy in 1955 using a special clamp without cardiopulmonary bypass. The modern treatment era began in 1958 when Cooley et al[10] successfully performed a linear repair of a left ventricular aneurysm using cardiopulmonary bypass. More geometric ventricular reconstruction techniques were subsequently devised by Stoney et al,[11] Daggett et al,[12] Dor et al,[13] Jatene,[14] and Cooley et al.[15,16]

INCIDENCE

The incidence of left ventricular aneurysm in patients suffering myocardial infarction has varied between 10% and 35% depending on the definition and the methods used. Of patients undergoing cardiac catheterization in the Coronary Artery Surgery Study (CASS), 7.6% had angiographic

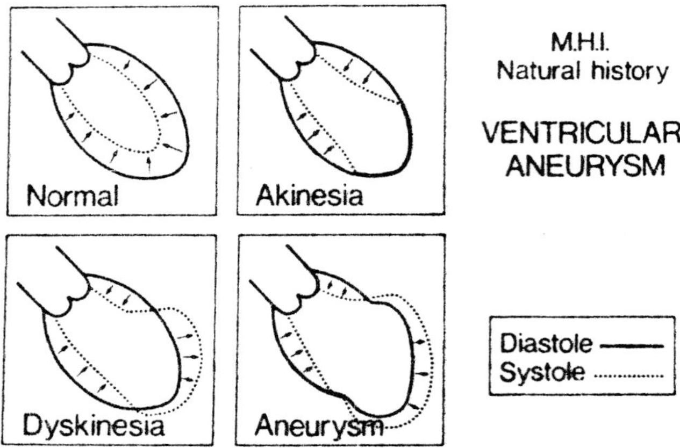

FIGURE 29–1 Diagrammatic distinction between aneurysm and other states of the left ventricle. (*Reproduced with permission from Grondin P, Kretz JG, Bical O, et al: Natural history of saccular aneurysm of the left ventricle. J Thorac Cardiovasc Surg 1979; 77:57.*)

evidence of left ventricular aneurysms.[17] The absolute incidence of left ventricular aneurysms may be declining due to the increased use of thrombolytics and revascularization after myocardial infarction.[18,19]

ETIOLOGY

Over 95% of true left ventricular aneurysms reported in the English literature result from coronary artery disease and myocardial infarction. True left ventricular aneurysms also may result from trauma,[20] Chagas' disease,[21] or sarcoidosis.[22] A very small number of congenital left ventricular aneurysms also have been reported and have been termed *diverticula* of the left ventricle.[23]

False aneurysms of the left ventricle result most commonly from contained rupture of the ventricle 5 to 10 days after myocardial infarction and often occur after circumflex coronary arterial occlusion. False aneurysm of the left ventricle also may result from submitral rupture of the ventricular wall, a dramatic event that generally occurs after mitral valve replacement with resection of the mitral valve apparatus.[24] Left ventricular pseudoaneurysm may also result from septic pericarditis[25] or any prior operation on the left ventricle, aortic annulus, or mitral annulus.

PATHOPHYSIOLOGY

The development of a true left ventricular aneurysm involves two principal phases: early expansion and late remodeling.

Early Expansion Phase

The early expansion phase begins with the onset of myocardial infarction. Ventriculography can demonstrate left ventricular aneurysm formation within 48 hours of infarction in 50% of patients who develop ventricular aneurysms. The remaining patients have evidence of aneurysm formation by 2 weeks after infarction.[26]

True aneurysm of the left ventricle generally follows transmural myocardial infarction due to acute occlusion of the left anterior descending or dominant right coronary artery. Lack of angiographic collaterals is strongly associated with aneurysm formation in patients with acute myocardial infarction and left anterior descending artery occlusion,[27] and absence of reformed collateral circulation is probably a prerequisite for formation of a dyskinetic left ventricular aneurysm (Table 29-1). At least 88% of dyskinetic ventricular aneurysms result from anterior infarction, while the remainder follow inferior infarction.[7] Posterior infarctions that produce a distinct dyskinetic left ventricular aneurysm are relatively unusual.

In experimental transmural infarction without collateral circulation, myocyte death begins 19 minutes after coronary occlusion. Infarctions that result in dyskinetic aneurysm formation are almost always transmural and may show gross thinning of the infarct zone within hours of infarction. Within a few days, the endocardial surface of the developing aneurysm becomes smooth with loss of trabeculae and deposition of fibrin and thrombus on the endocardial surface in at least 50% of patients. While most myocytes within the infarct are necrotic, viable myocytes often remain within the infarct zone. In a minority of patients, extravascular hemorrhage occurs in the infarcted tissue and may further depress systolic and diastolic function of involved myocardium. Inflammatory cells migrate into the infarct zone by 2 to 3 days after infarction and contribute to lysis of necrotic myocytes by 5 to 10 days after infarction. Electron microscopy demonstrates disruption of the native collagen network several days after infarction. Collagen disruption and myocyte necrosis produce a nadir of myocardial tensile strength between 5 and 10 days after infarction, when rupture of the myocardial wall is most common. Left ventricular rupture is relatively rare after the ventricular aneurysmal wall becomes replaced with fibrous tissue.

Loss of systolic contraction in the large infarcted zone and preserved contraction of surrounding myocardium cause systolic bulging and thinning of the infarct. By Laplace's

TABLE 29–1 Factors contributing to left ventricular aneurysm formation

Preserved contractility of surrounding myocardium
Transmural infarction
Lack of collateral circulation
Lack of reperfusion
Elevated wall stress
Hypertension
Ventricular dilation
Wall thinning

law ($T = Pr/2h$), at a constant ventricular pressure (P), increased radius of curvature (r) and decreased wall thickness (h) in the infarcted zone both contribute to increased muscle fiber tension (T) and further stretch the infarcted ventricular wall.

Relative to normal myocardium, ischemically injured or infarcted myocardium displays greater *plasticity* or *creep*, defined as deformation or stretch over time under a constant load.[28] Thus increased systolic and diastolic wall stress in the infarcted zone tends to produce progressive stretch of the infarcted myocardium (termed *infarct expansion*)[29] until healing reduces its plasticity.

Transmural infarction without significant hibernating myocardium within the infarct region is necessary for subsequent development of a true left ventricular aneurysm. Angiographic ventricular aneurysms with evidence of hibernating myocardium (lack of Q waves or presence of uptake on technetium scan) may resolve over several weeks and thus do not represent true left ventricular aneurysms by strict criteria.[30]

Due to increased diastolic stretch or preload and elevated catecholamines, remaining noninfarcted myocardium may demonstrate increased fiber shortening and, ultimately, myocardial hypertrophy in the presence of a left ventricular aneurysm.[31] This increased shortening and increased wall stress increase oxygen demand for noninfarcted myocardium and for the left ventricle as a whole.

In addition to increased regional wall stresses, left ventricular aneurysm can increase ventricular oxygen demand and decrease net forward cardiac output by producing a ventricular volume load because a portion of the stroke volume goes into the aneurysm instead of out through the aortic valve. Net mechanical efficiency of the left ventricle (external stroke work minus myocardial oxygen consumption) is decreased by reducing external stroke work (volume times pressure) and increasing myocardial oxygen consumption.

Left ventricular aneurysms can produce both systolic and diastolic ventricular dysfunction. Diastolic dysfunction results from increased stiffness of the distended and fibrotic aneurysmal wall, which impairs diastolic filling and increases left ventricular end-diastolic pressure.

Late Remodeling Phase

The remodeling phase of ventricular aneurysm formation begins 2 to 4 weeks after infarction, when highly vascularized granulation tissue appears. This granulation tissue is subsequently replaced by fibrous tissue 6 to 8 weeks after infarction. As myocytes are lost, ventricular wall thickness decreases as the myocardium becomes largely replaced by fibrous tissue. In larger infarcts, the thin scar is often lined with mural thrombus.[32]

After acute myocardial infarction, animal studies show that ventricular load reduction with 8 weeks of nitrate therapy may reduce expected infarct thinning, decrease infarct stretch, and lessen hypertrophy of noninfarcted myocardium.[33] Interestingly, nitrate therapy for only 2 weeks after infarction does not prevent aneurysm formation. This observation emphasizes the importance of late remodeling from 2 to 8 weeks after infarction. Angiotensin-converting enzyme (ACE) inhibitors also reduce infarct expansion and subsequent development of ventricular aneurysm. Because animal studies show that ACE inhibitors nonspecifically suppress ventricular hypertrophy, it is not clear whether suppression of the compensatory hypertrophy of surrounding myocardium is ultimately beneficial or harmful.

Lack of coronary reperfusion is probably prerequisite for development of left ventricular aneurysm. In humans, reperfusion of the infarct vessel, whether spontaneously,[30] by thrombolysis,[34] or by angioplasty,[35] has been associated with a lower incidence of aneurysm formation. It is speculated that coronary reperfusion as late as 2 weeks after infarction prevents aneurysm formation by improving blood flow and fibroblast migration into the infarcted myocardium. The role of delayed infarct healing in aneurysm development is supported by observations that steroids after myocardial infarction may increase the likelihood of aneurysm formation.[36]

Arrhythmias such as ventricular tachycardia may occur at any time during the development of ventricular aneurysm, and all these patients have the substrate for reentrant conduction pathways within the heterogeneous ventricular myocardium. These pathways tend to involve border zones surrounding the ventricular aneurysm (see Ch. 54).

NATURAL HISTORY

The excellent prognosis of asymptomatic patients with dyskinetic ventricular aneurysms who were treated medically was demonstrated in a series of 40 patients followed for a mean of 5 years.[37] Of 18 initially asymptomatic patients, 6 developed class II symptoms while 12 remained asymptomatic. Ten-year survival was 90% for these patients but was only 46% at 10 years in patients who presented with symptoms (Fig. 29-2).

Although earlier autopsy series reported relatively poor survival in patients with medically managed left ventricular dyskinetic aneurysms (12% at 5 years), most recent studies report 5-year survival from 47% to 70%.[17,37–39] Causes of death include arrhythmia in 44%, heart failure in 33%, recurrent myocardial infarction in 11%, and noncardiac causes in 22%.[37] The natural history of patients with akinetic rather than dyskinetic left ventricular aneurysms is less well documented.

Factors that influence survival with medically managed left ventricular dyskinetic aneurysm include age, heart failure score, extent of coronary disease, duration of angina, prior infarction, mitral regurgitation, ventricular arrhythmias, aneurysm size, function of residual ventricle, and left

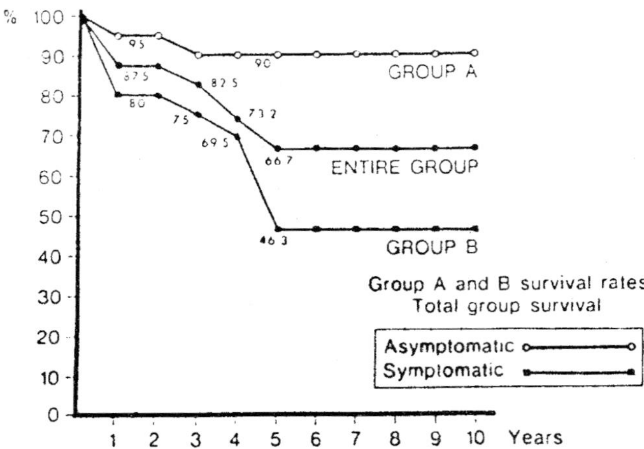

FIGURE 29–2 Survival in medically treated patients with left ventricular aneurysm based on presence (group B) or absence (group A) of symptoms. (*Reproduced with permission from Grondin P, Kretz JG, Bical O, et al: Natural history of saccular aneurysm of the left ventricle. J Thorac Cardiovasc Surg 1979; 77:57.*)

ventricular end-diastolic pressure.[37,40] Early development of aneurysm within 48 hours after infarction also diminishes survival.[26]

In general, the risk of thromboembolism is low for patients with aneurysms (0.35% per patient-year),[38] and long-term anticoagulation is not usually recommended. However, in the 50% of patients with mural thrombus visible by echocardiography after myocardial infarction, 19% develop thromboembolism over a mean follow-up period of 24 months.[41] In these patients, anticoagulation and close echocardiographic follow-up may be indicated. Atrial fibrillation and large aneurysmal size are additional risk factors for thromboembolism.

The natural history of left ventricular pseudoaneurysm is not well documented. Frank rupture of chronic left ventricular pseudoaneurysms is less common than one might expect.[42] Rupture of left ventricular pseudoaneurysms may be most likely in the acute phase or in large-sized pseudoaneurymsms.[43] Left ventricular pseudoaneurysms tend to behave similarly to true aneurysms in that they may present a volume load to the left ventricle or may be a source of embolization or endocarditis. Left ventricular pseudoaneurysms after prior cardiac surgery have also been reported to compress adjacent structures such as the pulmonary artery or esophagus.

CLINICAL PRESENTATION

Angina is the most frequent symptom in most series of patients operated upon for left ventricular aneurysm. Given that three-vessel coronary disease is present in 60% or more of these patients, the frequency of angina is not surprising.[44]

Dyspnea is the second most common symptom of ventricular aneurysm and often develops when 20% or more of the ventricular wall is infarcted. Dyspnea may occur from a combination of decreased systolic function and diastolic dysfunction.

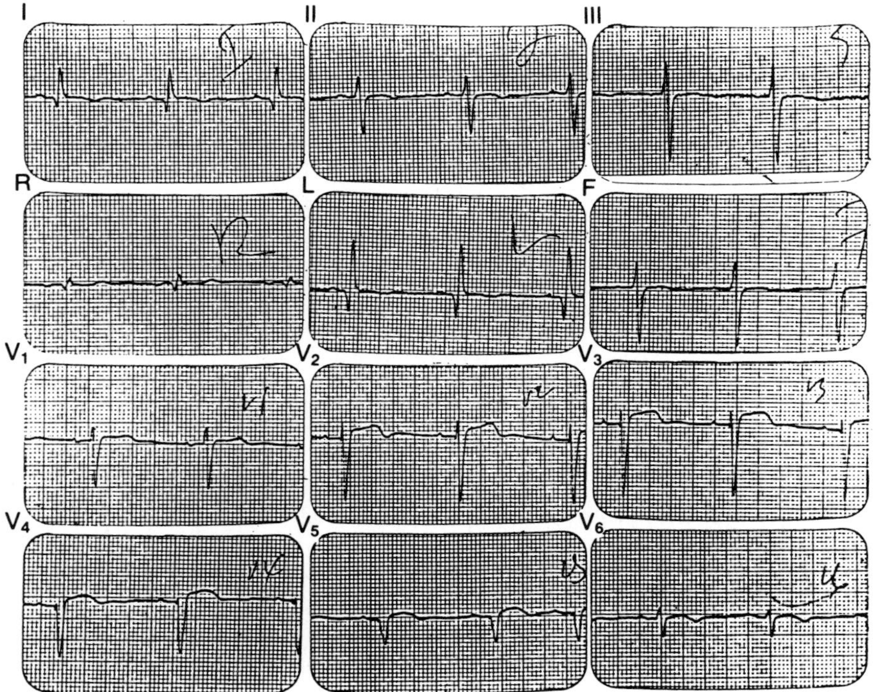

FIGURE 29–3 Electrocardiogram showing persistent ST-segment elevation with pathologic Q waves in a 60-year-old woman with left ventricular aneurysm. (*Reproduced with permission from Ba'albaki HA, Clements SD Jr: Left ventricular aneurysm: a review. Clin Cardiol 1989; 12:5.*)

Either atrial or ventricular arrhythmias may produce palpitations, syncope, or sudden death, or aggravate angina and dyspnea in up to one third of patients.[44] Thromboembolism is unusual but may produce symptoms of stroke, myocardial infarction, or limb or visceral ischemia.

DIAGNOSIS

The electrocardiogram frequently demonstrates Q waves in the anterior leads along with persistent anterior ST-segment elevation (Fig. 29-3). The chest radiograph may show left ventricular enlargement and cardiomegaly (Fig. 29-4), but the chest radiograph is not usually specific for left ventricular aneurysm.

Left ventriculography is the gold standard for diagnosis of left ventricular aneurysm. The diagnosis is made by demonstrating a large, discrete area of dyskinesia (or akinesia), generally in the anteroseptal-apical walls. Occasionally, left ventriculography also may demonstrate mural thrombus. Quantitative definition of left ventricular aneurysms has been accomplished using a centerline analysis of left ventricular wall motion on left ventriculography in the 30-degree right anterior oblique view.[4] Hypocontractile segments contracting more than 2 standard deviations out of normal range are defined as aneurysmal (Fig. 29-5).[45] Outward motion is termed dyskinetic, and remaining aneurysmal segments are termed akinetic. The fraction of total left ventricular circumference that is aneurysmal can thus be computed as the value %A.[4]

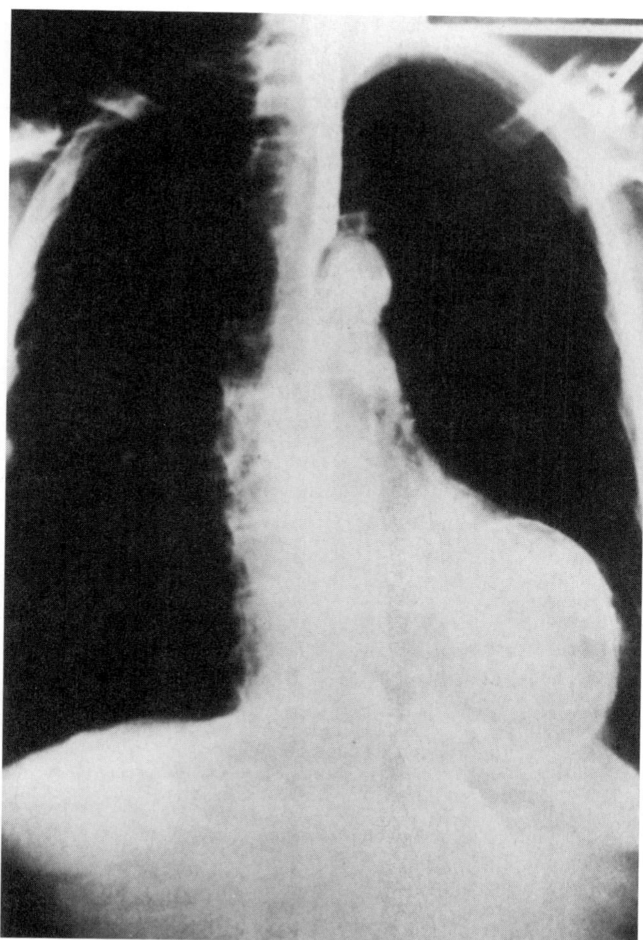

FIGURE 29–4 Posteroanterior chest radiograph in a patient with a calcified left ventricular aneurysm. (*Reproduced with permission from Ba'albaki HA, Clements SD Jr: Left ventricular aneurysm: a review. Clin Cardiol 1989; 12:5.*)

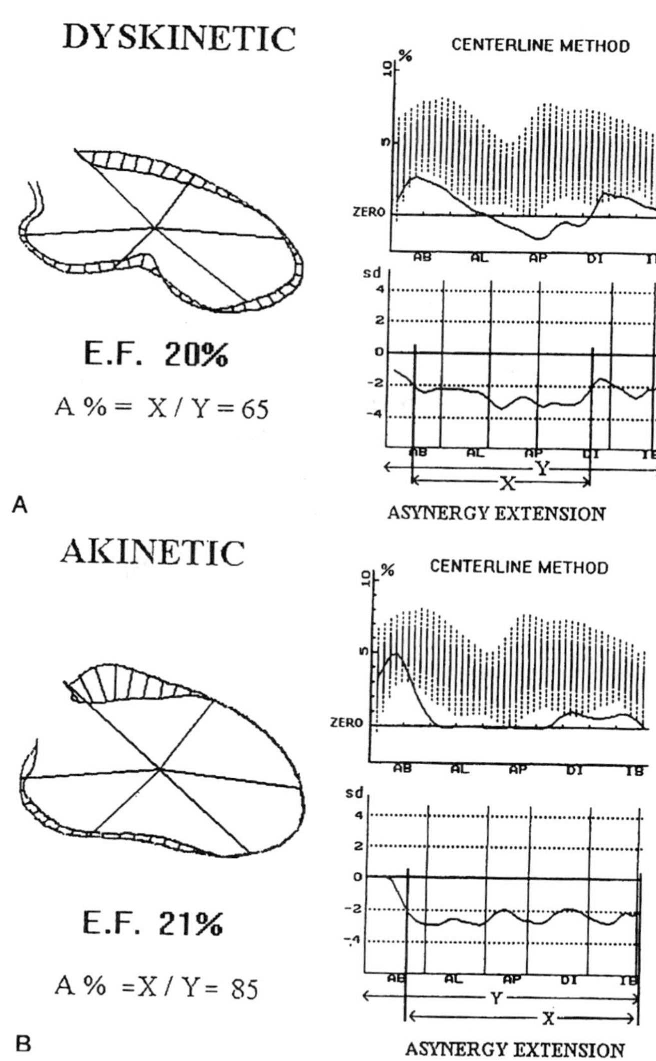

FIGURE 29–5 Examples of preoperative centerline analysis in dyskinetic (A) and akinetic (B) LV aneurysms. Vertical lines indicate the extent of asynergy. E.F., ejection fraction; AB anterobasal; AL anterolateral; AP apical; DI diaphragmatic; IB inferobasal. (*Reproduced with permission from Dor V, Sabatier M, DiDonato M: Efficacy of endoventricular patch plasty in large postinfarction akinetic scar and severe left ventricular dysfunction: comparison with a series of large dyskinetic scars. J Thorac Cardiovasc Surg 1998; 116:50.*)

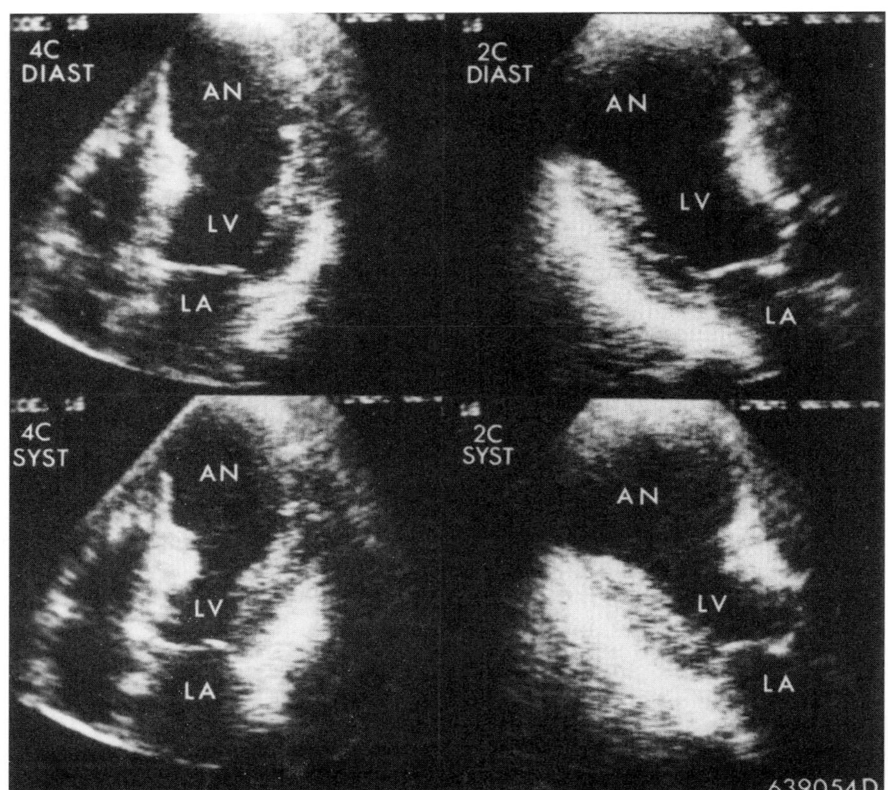

FIGURE 29–6 Four-chamber (4C) and two-chamber (2C) two-dimensional echocardiograms demonstrating a left ventricular aneurysm (AN) during systole (SYST) and diastole (DIAST) (LV, left ventricle; LA, left atrium). (*Reproduced with permission from Feigenbaum H: Echocardiography. Philadelphia, Lea & Febiger, 1986; p 484.*)

Two-dimensional echocardiography is also a sensitive and specific means of diagnosing left ventricular aneurysm (Fig. 29-6). Mural thrombus and mitral valve regurgitation are detected most readily by echocardiography. Echocardiography is also useful for distinguishing false aneurysm from true aneurysm by demonstrating a defect in the true ventricular wall. Tomographic three-dimensional echocardiography and magnetic resonance imaging are the most reliable means of assessing left ventricular volume in the presence of left ventricular aneurysm.[46] Gated radionuclide angiography reliably detects left ventricular aneurysms, and thallium scanning or positron emission tomography (PET) can be helpful early after infarction to differentiate true aneurysm from hibernating myocardium with reversible dysfunction. Magnetic resonance imaging (MRI) accurately depicts left ventricular aneurysms and is a reliable means for detecting mural thrombus.[47]

INDICATIONS FOR OPERATION

Because of the relatively good prognosis for asymptomatic left ventricular aneurysm,[37] no indications for repairing chronic, asymptomatic aneurysms are established. Yet, in low-risk patients during operation for associated coronary disease, investigators report repairing large, minimally symptomatic aneurysms.[7,48]

On the other hand, operation is indicated for symptoms of angina, congestive heart failure, or selected ventricular arrhythmias (see Ch. 54) (Table 29-2). For these symptomatic patients, operation offers better outcome than medical therapy. To be worthy of operation, a dyskinetic or akinetic left ventricular aneurysm should significantly enlarge left ventricular end-systolic volume index (over 80 mL/m^2) and end-diastolic volume (over 120 mL/m^2). These volume criteria are, however, poorly defined and limited by technical difficulty measuring left ventricular volume in aneurysmal left ventricles. Because results are not affected by whether aneurysms are akinetic versus dyskinetic, Dor et al feel that dyskinesia is not a prerequisite for aneurysm repair.[3,4]

Operation is also indicated in viable patients with contained cardiac rupture, with or without development of a

TABLE 29–2 Relative indications for ventricular aneurysm operation

Documented expansion/large size
Angina
Congestive heart failure
Arrhythmia
Rupture
Pseudoaneurysm
Congenital aneurysm
Embolism

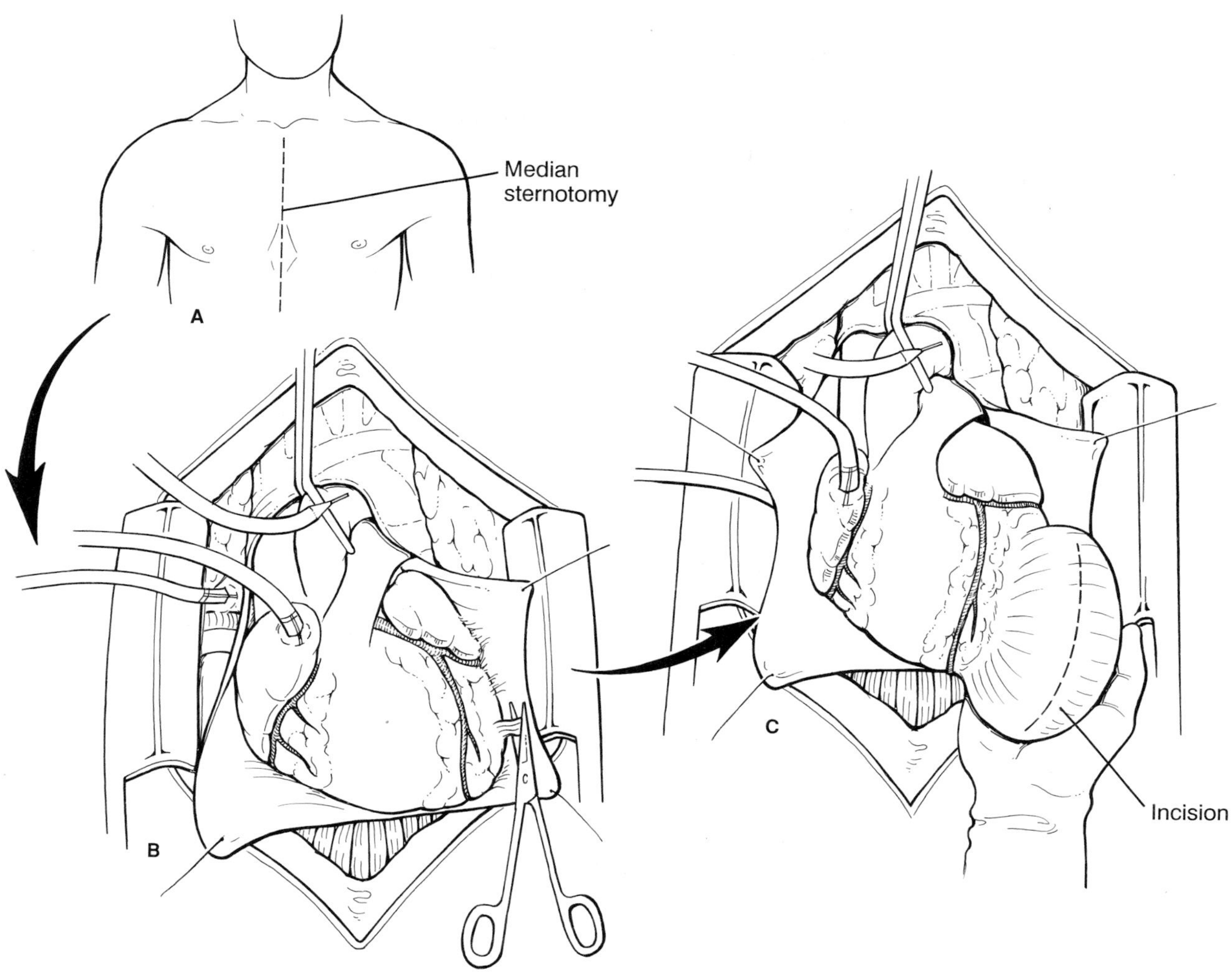

FIGURE 29–7 Technique of exposure for left ventricular aneurysm repair through a median sternotomy. The ascending aorta and right atrium are cannulated. A left ventricular vent is placed through the right superior pulmonary vein. Pericardial adhesions are divided, and the aneurysm is opened.

false aneurysm. Because left ventricular pseudoaneurysms may have a tendency to rupture when acute or of larger size (either with or without symptoms), operation is indicated.[42,43,49] Similarly, congenital aneurysms have a presumed risk of rupture and should undergo repair independently of symptoms. Rarely, embolism is an indication for operation in medically treated patients at high risk for repeated thromboembolism. The role of operation in asymptomatic patients with very large aneurysms or documented expansion of aneurysms is uncertain.

Relative contraindications to operation for left ventricular aneurysm include excessive anesthetic risk, impaired function of residual myocardium outside the aneurysm, resting cardiac index less than 2.0 L/min/m^2, significant mitral regurgitation, evidence of nontransmural infarction (hibernating myocardium), and lack of a discrete, thin-walled aneurysm with distinct margins. Global ejection fraction may be less useful than ejection fraction of the basal, contractile portion of the heart in determining operability.[50]

Angioplasty has an uncertain role in the treatment of left ventricular aneurysms but may be indicated in patients with suitable coronary anatomy, one- or two-vessel disease, a contraindication for operation, or asymptomatic status with inducible ischemia.

PREPARATION FOR OPERATION

All patients being considered for operation should undergo right- and left-sided heart catheterization with coronary arteriography and left ventriculography. Patients with 2+ or greater mitral regurgitation at cardiac catheterization should have echocardiography to assess the mitral valve and to look for intrinsic mitral valve disease not amenable to annuloplasty.

Preoperative electrophysiologic study is clearly indicated in any patient with preoperative ventricular tachycardia or ventricular fibrillation. The decision to perform an electrophysiologic study in patients without preoperative ventricular arrhythmias is controversial, because the incidence of postoperative ventricular arrhythmias is low and not changed by endocardial resection at the time of operation.[7] Electrophysiologic study is frequently not helpful in patients with polymorphic ventricular tachycardia occurring within 6 weeks of myocardial infarction.[7]

OPERATIVE TECHNIQUES

General

Operation for left ventricular aneurysm requires cardiopulmonary bypass and a balanced anesthetic technique, as generally used for coronary bypass grafting. After induction of anesthesia and endotracheal intubation, an electrocardiogram monitor, a Foley catheter, a radial arterial line, and a Swan-Ganz catheter are placed. A median sternotomy is performed, and the patient is given heparin. Saphenous vein or arterial conduits are prepared.

Cardiopulmonary bypass is begun after cannulating the ascending aorta. A single, two-stage cannula is generally adequate to cannulate the right atrium, but dual venous cannulation should be considered if the right ventricle is to be opened. Epicardial mapping is performed if necessary. The left ventricle is inspected to identify an appropriate area of thinned ventricular wall. A linear vertical ventriculotomy, generally on the anterior wall 3 to 4 cm from the left anterior descending coronary artery, is made (Fig. 29-7). The left ventricle is opened (Fig. 29-8), all mural thrombus is carefully removed, and endocardial mapping is performed if necessary. A left ventricular vent is now placed through the right superior pulmonary vein–left atrial junction after mural thrombus is removed. Coronary arteries to be grafted are identified. Endocardial scar, if present, is resected, and afterwards,

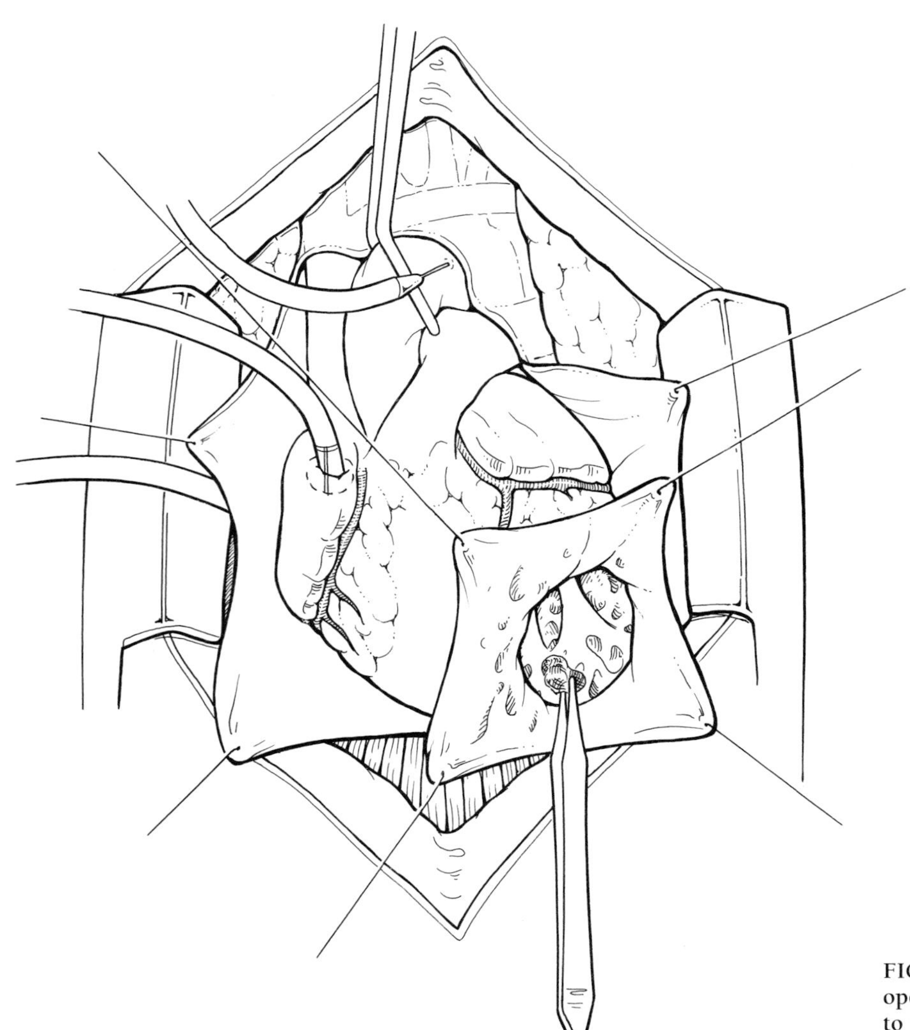

FIGURE 29–8 With the aneurysm wall opened, thrombus is removed, without injury to the papillary muscles.

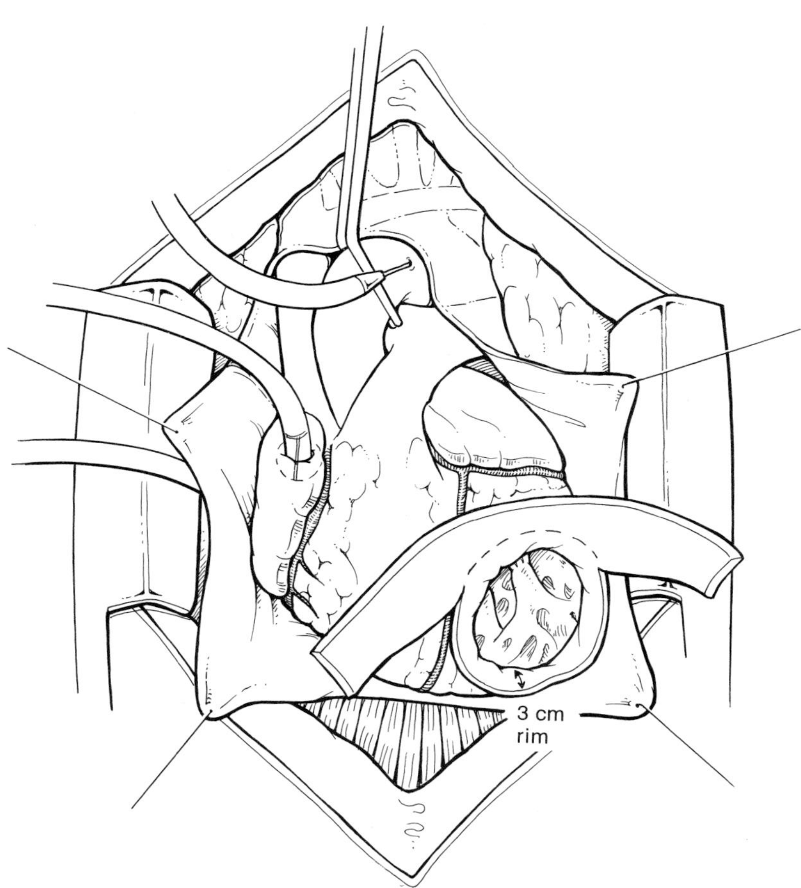

FIGURE 29–9 Linear repair. The fibrous aneurysm wall is excised, leaving a 3-cm rim of fibrous aneurysm wall attached to healthy muscle.

endocardial mapping is repeated. Body temperature is maintained at 37°C until intraoperative mapping is completed; thereafter, temperature is decreased to 28°C to 32°C.

The ascending aorta is clamped, and the heart is arrested with cold antegrade cardioplegic solution. Alternatively, the aorta is not clamped and the entire procedure is done during hypothermic fibrillation. The left ventricular aneurysm is repaired using one of the techniques described below. The distal coronary anastomoses are performed, followed by aortic declamping.[51] Air is removed by venting the ascending aorta and left ventricle while filling the heart and ventilating the lungs with the patient in the Trendelenburg position. The patient is rewarmed, and proximal coronary anastomoses are performed. Once normothermia is achieved, an electrophysiologic study may be repeated if indicated. Temporary pacing wires are placed on the right atrium and right ventricle, cardiopulmonary bypass is discontinued, and heparin is reversed. The heart is decannulated, and the median sternotomy is closed.

Weaning from cardiopulmonary bypass frequently requires some degree of inotropic support. Typically, 5 μg/kg/min of dopamine, nitroglycerin to prevent coronary spasm, and nitroprusside for afterload reduction are used. An intra-aortic balloon pump may be needed in patients with borderline ventricular function. Transesophageal echocardiography is useful for assessing left ventricular function and to detect residual intracardiac air.

Additional inotropic support may not increase cardiac output significantly because of abnormal ventricular compliance and may produce arrhythmias and poorly tolerated tachycardia. Because the left ventricle is poorly distensible, stroke volume is relatively fixed, and a resting heart rate between 90 and 115 beats per minute is not unusual to maintain a cardiac index of approximately 2.0 L/min/m^2.

Growing experience suggests that the ultimate size of the left ventricular cavity at the end of the procedure is critical to patient outcome. Using preoperative and postoperative three-dimensional techniques to image the left ventricle, Cherniavsky et al proposed that the aneurysm resection or patch should produce a postoperative left ventricular end-diastolic volume of about 150 mL.[52]

Plication

Plication without opening the aneurysm is reserved for only the smallest aneurysms that do not contain mural thrombus. A two-layer suture line of 0 monofilament is placed across the aneurysm using a strip of Teflon felt on either side. The suture line is oriented to reconstruct a relatively normal left ventricular contour and does not exclude all aneurysmal tissue.

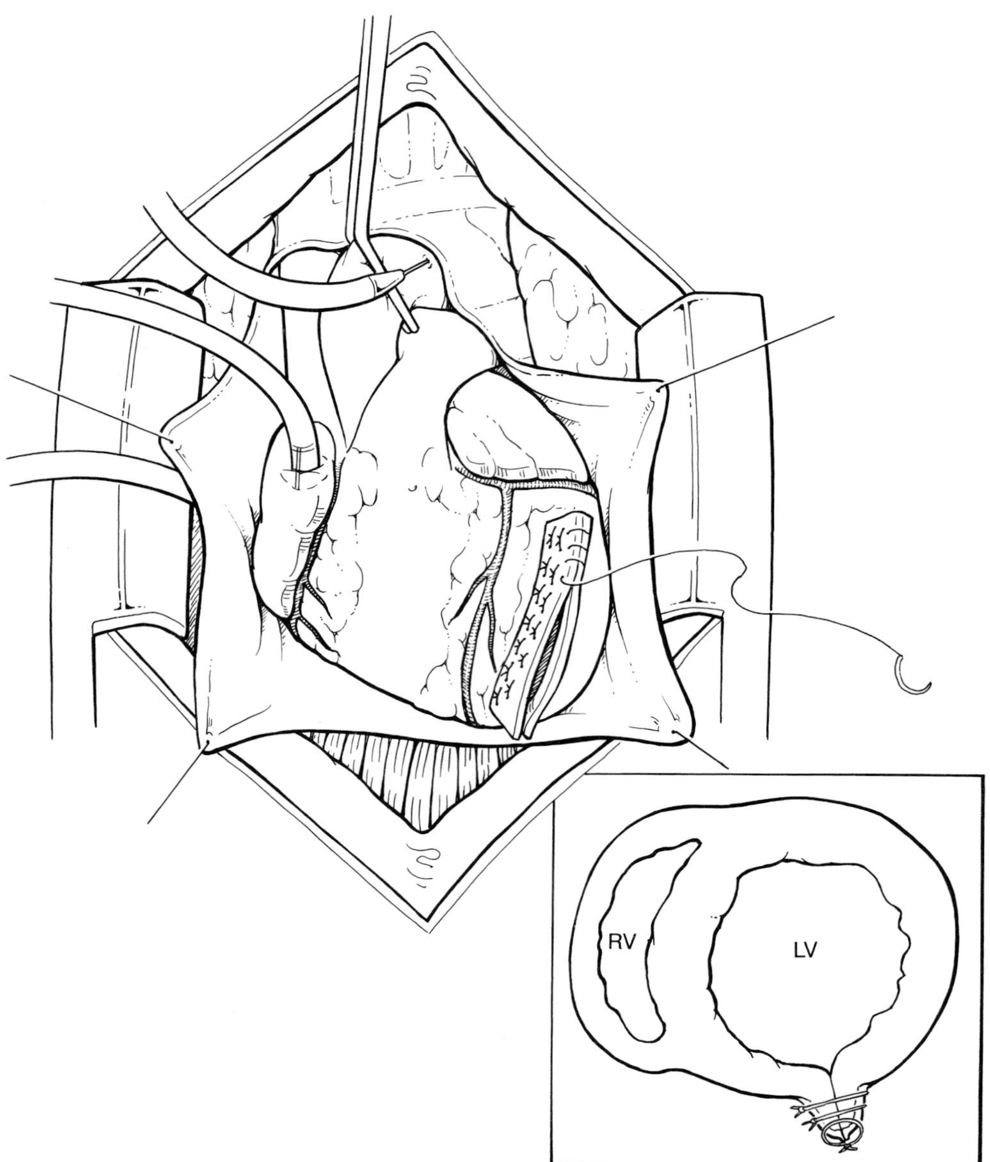

FIGURE 29–10 Linear repair. The aneurysm walls are closed in a vertical line between two layers of Teflon felt. Two layers of 0 monofilament interrupted horizontal mattress sutures are reinforced with two layers of running 2-0 monofilament sutures.

Linear Closure

After removing all mural thrombus, the aneurysmal wall is trimmed, leaving a 3-cm rim of scar to allow reconstruction of the normal left ventricular contour (Fig. 29-9). Care is taken not to resect too much aneurysmal wall and overly reduce ventricular cavity size. A monofilament 2-0 suture may be used to reduce the neck of the aneurysm to the proper size before closure of the ventricular wall.[14] Anterior aneurysm defects are closed vertically between two external 1.5-cm strips of Teflon felt, two layers of 0 monofilament horizontal mattress sutures, and finally, two layers of running 2-0 monofilament vertical sutures with large-diameter needles (Fig. 29-10).

Circular Patch

Inferior or posterior aneurysms generally require circular patch closure, which also can be applied to anterior aneurysms. After opening the aneurysm (Fig. 29-11) and after debridement of thrombus and aneurysm wall (Fig. 29-12), a Dacron (Hemashield) patch is cut to be 2 cm greater in diameter than the ventricular opening. Interrupted,

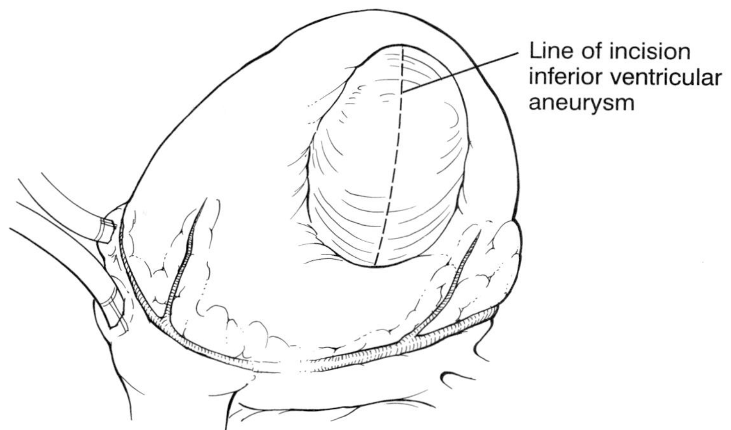

FIGURE 29–11 Circular patch repair. The aneurysm wall is incised. An inferior aneurysm is shown.

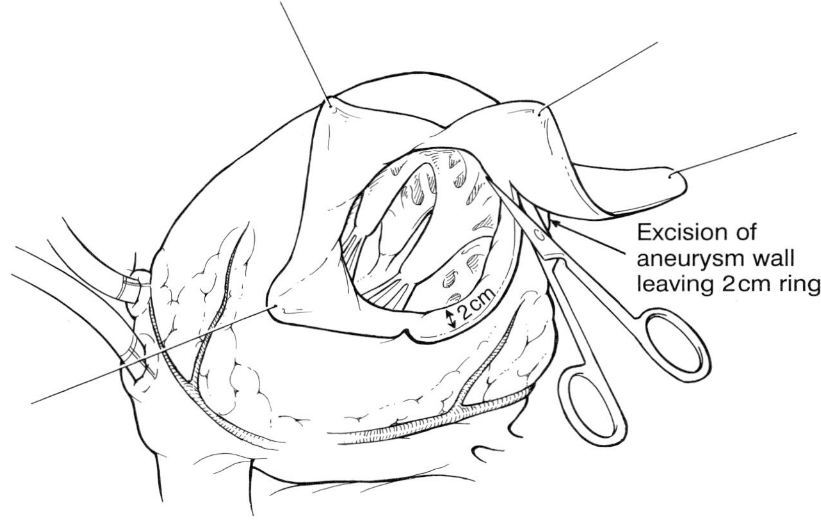

FIGURE 29–12 Circular patch repair. The aneurysmal wall is excised, leaving a 2-cm rim of fibrous aneurysmal wall attached to healthy muscle.

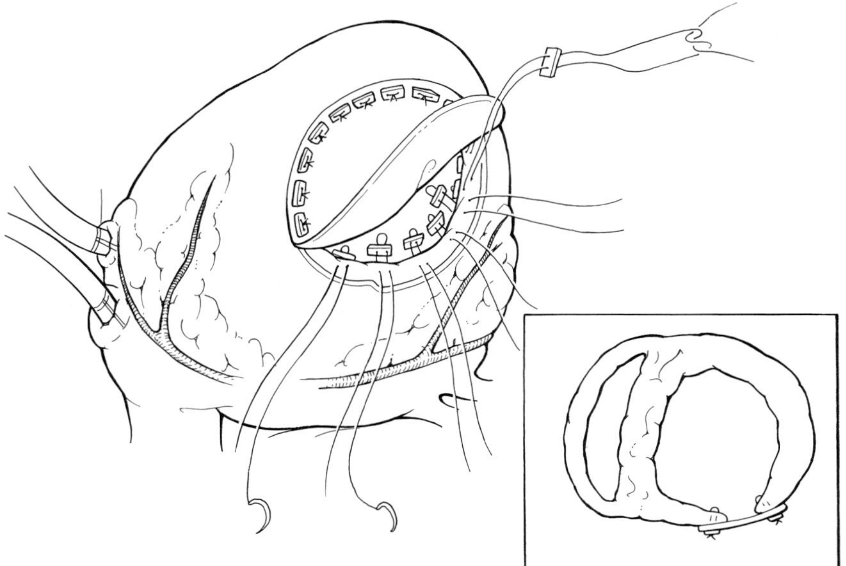

FIGURE 29–13 Circular patch repair. The aneurysmal defect is closed with a Dacron patch using interrupted 2-0 monofilament horizontal mattress sutures with reinforcing pledgets.

pledgeted 0 monofilament horizontal mattress sutures are placed through the ventriculotomy rim and then through the patch, leaving the pledgets outside the ventricular cavity (Fig. 29-13). Sutures are tied, and additional interrupted sutures or a second layer of running 2-0 monofilament is placed for hemostasis.

Endoventricular Patch

The endoventricular patch technique is suitable for anterior aneurysms but is less suited for inferior or posterior aneurysms, for which the standard (circular) patch technique is used. After debridement of thrombus, a running 2-0 polypropylene suture may be placed at the aneurysm rim to optimize left ventricular size.[3,14,45,50] If the remaining ventricular defect is small (<3 cm), then the ventricular wall may be closed linearly.[14] More commonly, a patch (bovine pericardium, Dacron cloth, or polytetrafluoroethylene) is cut to size sufficient to restore normal ventricular size and geometry when secured to the aneurysmal rim (Fig. 29-14). The patch is sutured to normal muscle at the aneurysmal circumference using a running 3-0 polypropylene suture that is secured with single sutures at three or four places around the patch circumference. The patch may extend onto the interventricular septum,[3,45,50] or the aneurysmal septum may be plicated.[14] Interrupted 3-0 sutures are placed as needed to ensure good fit. Care is taken not to distort the papillary muscles. The aneurysmal rim is trimmed to allow primary closure of the native aneurysmal wall over the patch using two layers of running 2-0 monofilament suture without pledgets (Fig. 29-15).

As compared with linear and circular patch techniques, the endoventricular patch technique has technical advantages. An endoventricular patch preserves the left anterior descending artery for possible grafting and leaves no external prosthetic material to produce heavy pericardial adhesions.

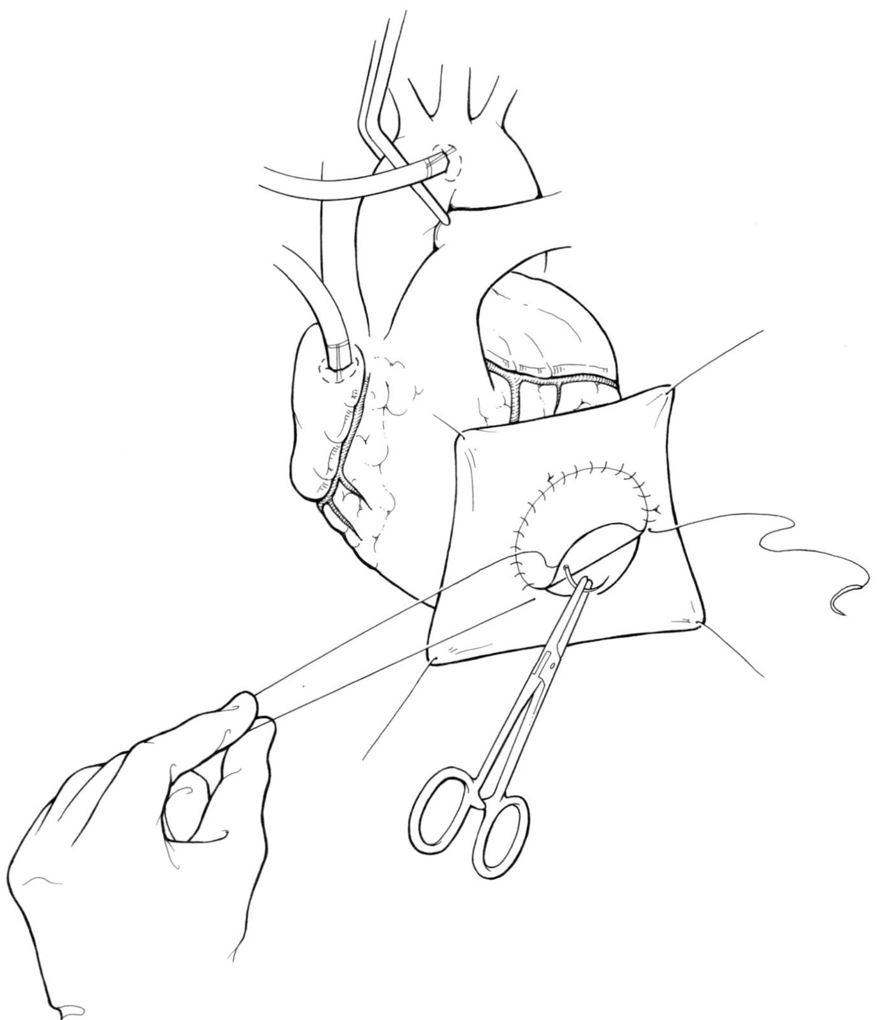

FIGURE 29–14 Endocardial patch. Without excising the aneurysm wall, the ventricular defect is closed with a Teflon felt patch using 3-0 polyproplyene suture secured at three or four points along the suture line. Additional 3-0 pledgeted horizontal mattress sutures may be used to achieve hemostasis.

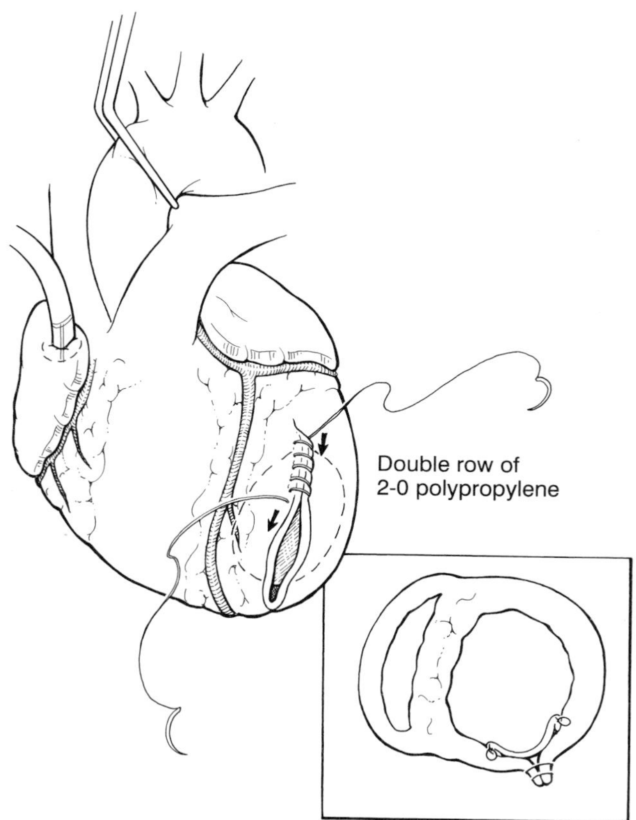

FIGURE 29–15 **Endocardial patch. The aneurysm wall is closed over a Teflon patch after resecting excess aneurysm tissue. A double row of running vertical 2-0 polyproplyene suture is used.**

The technique facilitates patching the interventricular septum, and is suitable for acute infarctions when tissues are friable.[7,16,53]

Other Ventricular Remodeling Techniques

In addition to the techniques listed above, in which left ventricular infarct tissue is excised and/or replaced with patch material, an alternative is to alter the biological properties of the infarct scar. Remaining infarct scar (whether aneurysmal or not) can then be seeded with myoblasts or stem cells, which offer the potential to restore cardiac muscle mass and contraction. This technique has been termed cellular cardiomyoplasty and has been done only on a limited basis in humans.[54] In animals, cellular cardiomyoplasty has successfully improved global left ventricular performance and geometry using either myoblasts, stem cells that differentiate into myocytes, or even fibrocytes.[55–57] Only myoblasts or stem cells that differentiate into myocytes have improved regional ventricular contractility. Cellular cardiomyoplasty could be done by direct injection of cells at the time of coronary revascularization, or even by transcoronary or intramyocardial injection in the cardiac catheterization laboratory.

TABLE 29–3 In-hospital complications of ventricular aneurysm repair

Low cardiac output	22%-39%
Ventricular arrhythmias	9%-19%
Respiratory failure	4%-11%
Bleeding	4%-7%
Dialysis-dependent renal failure	4%
Stroke	3%-4%

Mitral Regurgitation

The severity of mitral regurgitation should be evaluated by intraoperative transesophageal echocardiography before cardiopulmonary bypass. The mitral valve is also inspected from below after opening the aneurysm and beginning repair of the aneurysm. Transventricular mitral valve repair may be done by placing pledgeted polypropylene sutures at both mitral commissures to reduce the circumference of the annulus.[58] This technique produces satisfactory short-term results, but long-term results are not known. Usually the mitral valve is repaired via left atriotomy after completion of the distal coronary anastomoses and before releasing the aortic cross-clamp. If mitral regurgitation results from annular dilatation and systolic restriction of leaflet motion (Carpentier type IIIB), Carpentier mitral annuloplasty is done.[59]

Ventricular False Aneurysm

Ventricular false aneurysms are repaired with the same techniques used for true ventricular aneurysms according to the

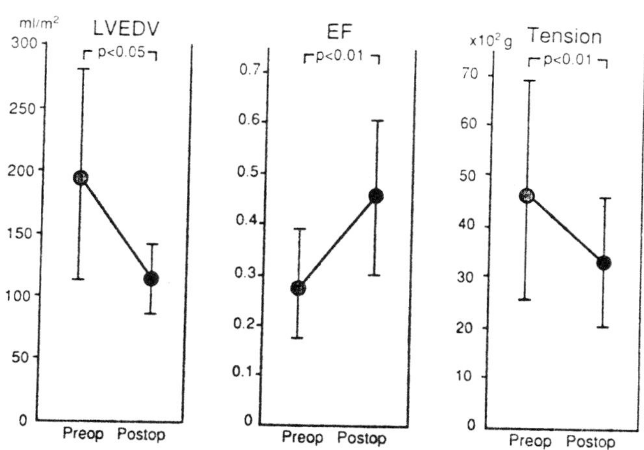

FIGURE 29–16 **Effects of linear aneurysmectomy on left ventricular end-diastolic volume (LVEDV), ejection fraction (EF), and wall tension.** (*Reproduced with permission from Kawachi K, Kitamura S, Kawata T, et al: Hemodynamic assessment during exercise after left ventricular aneurysmectomy. J Thorac Cardiovasc Surg 1994; 107:178.*)

location and size of the aneurysm. The circular patch technique is particularly useful in that inferior false aneurysms are common and typically have narrow necks. Usually the wall of the false aneurysm is inadequate to use to close the defect.

Ventricular Rupture

Any of the techniques described above may be used to manage a contained ventricular rupture. Because infarcted tissue is particularly friable 5 to 10 days after rupture, closure may be difficult. The endoventricular technique is particularly well suited for this uncommon operation because the patch can be sewn to the margins of healthy endocardium, which may be at some distance from the site of rupture. Patient survival also has been reported by gluing a biological patch to the ventricular epicardium over the site of the rupture.

EARLY RESULTS

Hospital Mortality

In a compilation of 3439 operations for left ventricular aneurysm performed between 1972 and 1987, hospital mortality was 9.9% and ranged from 2% to 19%.[18] More recent reports indicate that hospital mortality has fallen to 3% to 7% in the last decade using either patch[7,16,60,61] or linear closures.[19,48,61] The most common cause of hospital mortality was left ventricular failure, which occurred in 64% of deaths.[48]

Risk factors for hospital mortality include increased age,[18,48,61] incomplete revascularization,[48] increased heart failure class,[18,61–63] female gender,[18] emergent operation,[18] ejection fraction less than 20% to 30%,[61,62] concurrent mitral valve replacement,[7,18] preoperative cardiac index <2.1 L/min/m^2,[4] mean pulmonary artery pressure >33 mm Hg,[4] serum creatinine >1.8 mg/dL,[4] and failure to use the internal mammary artery.[63]

In-Hospital Complications

The most common in-hospital complications are shown in Table 29-3 and include low cardiac output, ventricular arrhythmias, and respiratory failure.[18,19,60,61,64] Low cardiac output may be more common in patients undergoing intraoperative mapping due to perioperative cardiac injury.[65]

Left Ventricular Function

The preponderance of data from the last two decades has shown that left ventricular function improves in most patients undergoing operation for left ventricular aneurysm. Operation improves ejection fraction whether linear

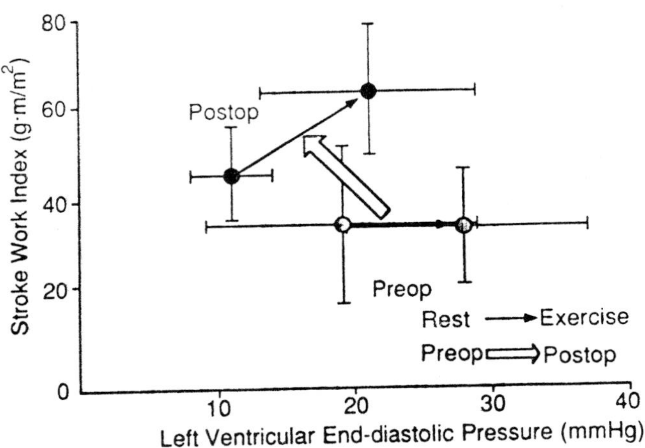

FIGURE 29–17 Relationship between stroke work index and left ventricular end-diastolic pressure. Data are shown at rest and during exercise before (preop) and after (postop) linear aneurysmectomy. Stroke work index increased only with exercise postoperatively. (*Reproduced with permission from Kawachi K, Kitamura S, Kawata T, et al: Hemodynamic assessment during exercise after left ventricular aneurysmectomy. J Thorac Cardiovasc Surg 1994; 107:178.*)

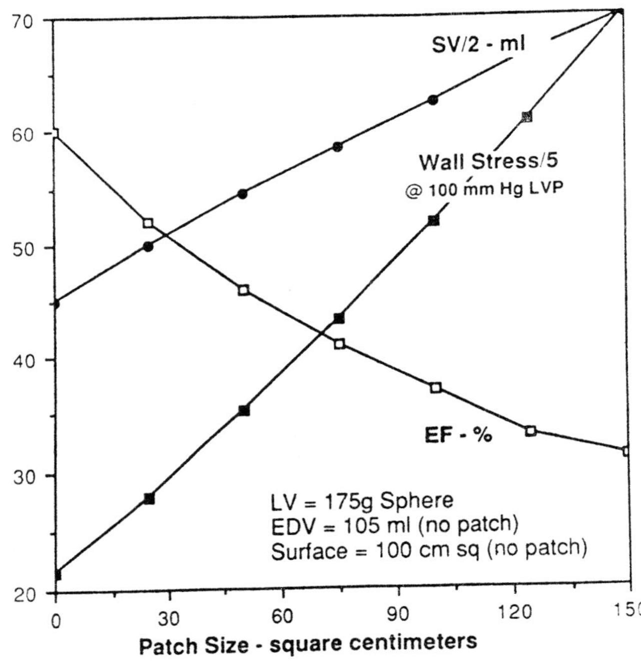

FIGURE 29–18 Computer prediction of the effects of patch size on stroke volume (SV), ejection fraction (EF), and wall stress (afterload) at a chamber pressure of 100 mm Hg. Predictions are based on data from an animal model of simulated aneurysm repair, neglecting the effects of afterload on stroke volume. Because increasing afterload in reality decreases muscle shortening, patch reconstruction can increase stroke volume only if contractile reserve is sufficient to overcome the afterload from increased ventricular size. (*Reproduced with permission from Nicolosi AC, Weng ZC, Detwiler PW, et al: Simulated left ventricular aneurysm and aneurysm repair in swine. J Thorac Cardiovasc Surg 1990; 100:745.*)

repair[5,8,66–68] or patch repair[13,16,69–71] is used (Fig. 29-16). Both techniques decrease end-diastolic and end-systolic volumes[67,70] and improve exercise response[16,68] (Fig. 29-17). Aneurysmal repair in general also improves diastolic filling, left ventricular diastolic compliance, left ventricular contractility, and effective arterial elastance (Ea).[31,71,72]

Controversy remains strong regarding whether patch techniques provide results superior to those achieved with linear closures. Stoney et al[11,73] noted lower left ventricular end-diastolic pressure when more geometric reconstructions were performed. Hutchins and Brawley[74] first noted at autopsy that some patients had severe reduction and distortion of ventricular volume after linear repair. The authors proposed that a more geometric repair might avert these problems. Although no prospective studies compare results from the two procedures, several very experienced groups attribute improved symptoms, less low cardiac output, and greater improvement in ejection fraction to a switch to patch techniques.[7,16,75–78] In other retrospective comparisons, no differences were seen in postoperative symptoms, ejection fraction, echocardiographic ventricular dimensions, or late survival between linear and patch repairs.[67,79,80] In an animal model of simulated aneurysm repair, Nicolosi et al[81] found no difference in left ventricular systolic or diastolic function between linear and patch techniques. Two groups reported that a switch to patch techniques was associated with increased operative mortality, perhaps due to excessive volume reduction.[82,83]

The durability of functional benefit from aneurysm repair remains poorly documented. In animals and humans, there is a tendency for the initial improvement in ejection fraction, ventricular volume, and filling pressures to diminish over the next 6 weeks to 6 months.[84,85]

Although technical differences exist between patch and linear repairs, good functional results are possible with either technique. Suboptimal outcomes result from either technique when left ventricular cavitary volume is overly reduced with resultant decreased stroke volume and impaired diastolic filling.[74,77,85] Excessively small patches reduce stroke volume and impair diastolic filling, but excessively large patches reduce ejection fraction and increase wall stress (Fig. 29-18).

LATE RESULTS

Survival

Survival after operation for left ventricular aneurysm is variable, largely due to differences between patient populations. Five-year survival in recent series varies between 58% and 80%,[5,62] 10-year overall survival is 34%,[62] and 10-year cardiac survival is 57%[48] (Fig. 29-19). Cardiac causes are responsible for 57% of late deaths,[65] and most cardiac deaths result from new myocardial infarctions. In aneurysm patients

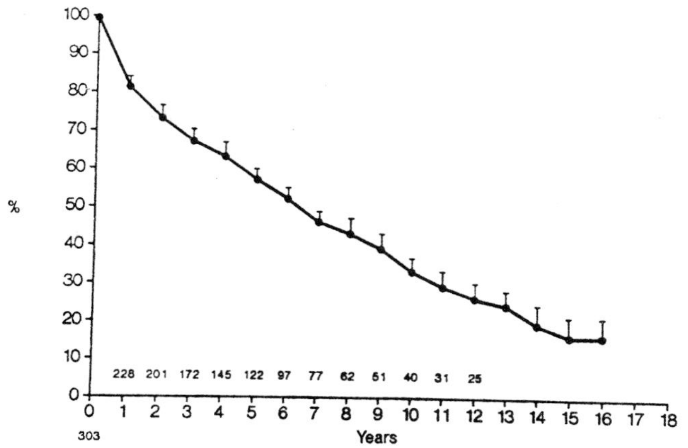

FIGURE 29–19 Survival in 303 patients undergoing left ventricular aneurysmectomy. (*Reproduced with permission from Couper GS, Bunton RW, Birjiniuk V, et al: Relative risks of left ventricular aneurysmectomy in patients with akinetic scars versus true dyskinetic aneurysms. Circulation 1990; 82(suppl IV):248.*)

randomized to medical or surgical therapy in the CASS study (most of the patients had minimal symptoms), survival was not different between medical or surgical therapy, except for patients with three-vessel disease.[40] These patients had better survival with surgery (Fig. 29-20).

Preoperative risk factors for late death include age, heart failure score, ejection fraction less than 35%, cardiomegaly on chest radiograph, left ventricular end-diastolic pressure greater than 20 mm Hg, and mitral regurgitation[40,48,65,79] (Fig. 29-21).

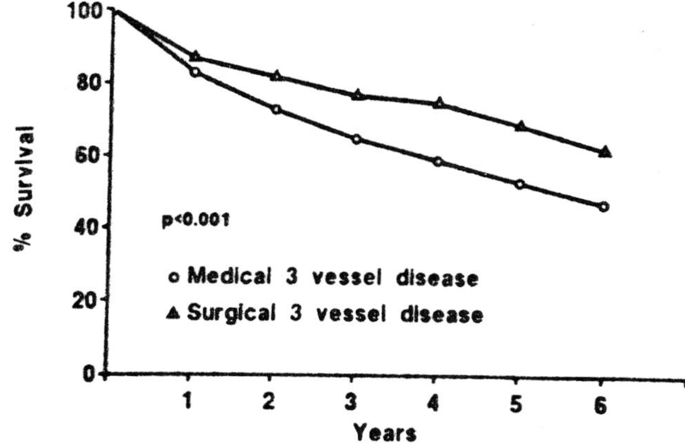

FIGURE 29–20 Survival in patients with left ventricular aneurysm and three-vessel coronary disease treated with medical or surgical therapy. (*Reproduced with permission from Faxon DP, Myers WO, McCabe CH: The influence of surgery on the natural history of angiographically documented left ventricular aneurysm: the Coronary Artery Surgery Study. Circulation 1986; 74:110.*)

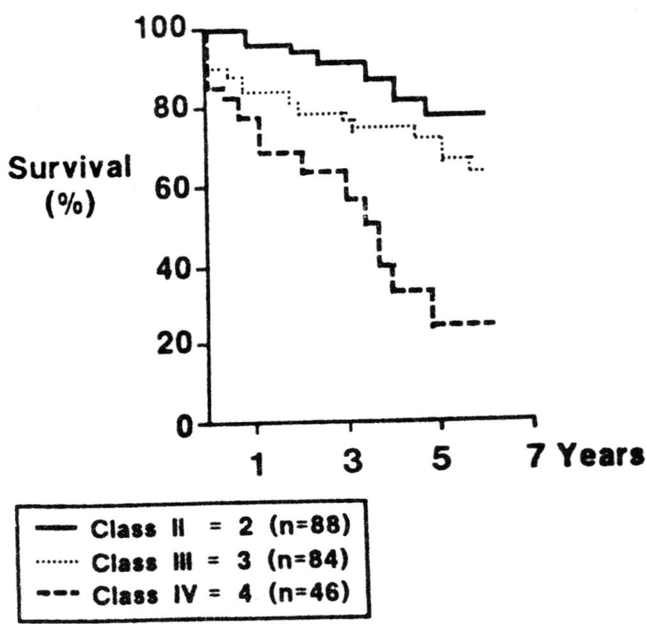

FIGURE 29–21 Effects of preoperative NYHA functional class on survival after ventricular aneurysm repair and myocardial revascularization. (*Reproduced with permission from Vauthy JN, Berry DW, Snyder DW, et al: Left ventricular aneurysm repair with myocardial revascularization: an analysis of 246 consecutive patients over 15 years. Ann Thorac Surg 1988; 46:29.*)

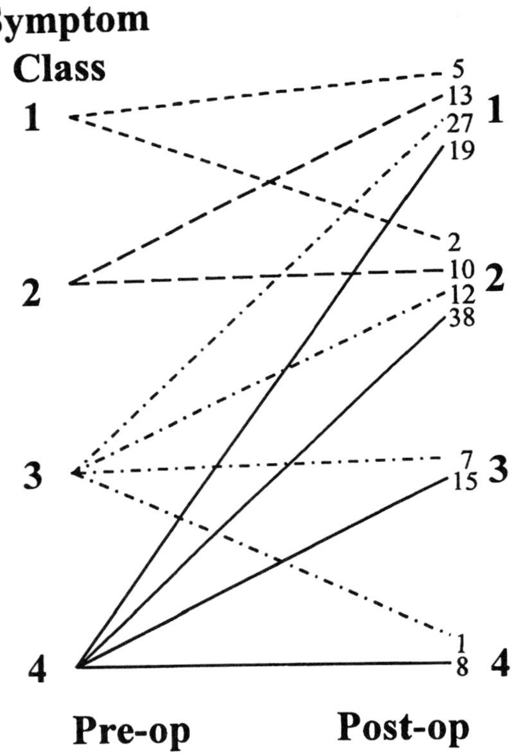

FIGURE 29–22 Preoperative (Pre-op) and postoperative (Post-op) symptoms of congestive heart failure (NYHA class) in patients undergoing left ventricular aneurysmectomy. (*Reproduced with permission from Mickleborough LL, Carson S, Ivanov J: Repair of dyskinetic or akinetic left ventricular aneurysm: results obtained with a modified linear closure. J Thorac Cardiovasc Surg 2001; 121:675.*)

Symptomatic Improvement

Studies consistently demonstrate improvement in symptoms after operation relative to preoperative symptoms[5,66] (Fig. 29-22). In the study of Elefteriades et al,[66] who used a linear repair, mean angina class improved from 3.5 to 1.2 and mean CHF class improved from 3.0 to 1.7. In the randomized CASS study, the subset of patients with left ventricular aneurysm achieved a better heart failure class with surgical therapy than with medicine, and rehospitalization for heart failure was less common for the surgical therapy group than for the medicine group.[40]

REFERENCES

1. Rutherford JD, Braunwald E, Cohn PE: Chronic ischemic heart disease, in Braunwald E (ed): *Heart Disease: A Textbook of Cardiovascular Medicine*. Philadelphia, WB Saunders, 1988; p 1364.
2. Buckberg GD: Defining the relationship between akinesia and dyskinesia and the cause of left ventricular failure after anterior infarction and reversal of remodeling to restoration. *J Thorac Cardiovasc Surg* 1998; 116:47.
3. Dor V, Sabatier M, DiDonato M: Efficacy of endoventricular patch plasty in large postinfarction akinetic scar and severe left ventricular dysfunction: comparison with a series of large dyskinetic scars. *J Thorac Cardiovasc Surg* 1998; 116:50.
4. Di Donato M, Sabatier M, Dor V, et al: Akinetic versus dyskinetic postinfarction scar: relation to surgical outcome in patients undergoing endoventricular circular patch plasty repair. *J Am Coll Cardiol* 1997; 29:1569.
5. Mickleborough LL, Carson S, Ivanov J: Repair of dyskinetic or akinetic left ventricular aneurysm: results obtained with a modified linear closure. *J Thorac Cardiovasc Surg* 2001; 121:675.
6. Cox JL: Left ventricular aneurysms: pathophysiologic observations and standard resection. *Sem Thorac Cardiovasc Surg* 1997; 9:113.
7. Mills NL, Everson CT, Hockmuth DR: Technical advances in the treatment of left ventricular aneurysm. *Ann Thorac Surg* 1993; 55:792.
8. Beck CS: Operation for aneurysm of the heart. *Ann Surg* 1944; 120:34.
9. Likoff W, Bailey CP: Ventriculoplasty: excision of myocardial aneurysm. *JAMA* 1955; 158:915.
10. Cooley DA, Collins HA, Morris GC, et al: Ventricular aneurysm after myocardial infarction: surgical excision with use of temporary cardiopulmonary bypass. *JAMA* 1958; 167:557.
11. Stoney WS, Alford WC Jr, Burrus GR, et al: Repair of anteroseptal ventricular aneurysm. *Ann Thorac Surg* 1973; 15:394.
12. Daggett WM, Guyton RA, Mundth ED: Surgery for post-myocardial infarct ventricular septal defect. *Ann Surg* 1977; 86:260.
13. Dor V, Saab M, Coste P, et al: Left ventricular aneurysm: a new surgical approach. *Thorac Cardiovasc Surg* 1989; 37:11.
14. Jatene AD: Left ventricular aneurysmectomy: resection of reconstruction. *J Thorac Cardiovasc Surg* 1985; 89:321.

15. Cooley DA: Ventricular endoaneurysmorrhaphy: a simplified repair for extensive postinfarction aneurysm. *J Cardiac Surg* 1989; 4:200.
16. Cooley DA, Frazier OH, Duncan JM, et al: Intracavitary repair of ventricular aneurysm and regional dyskinesia. *Ann Surg* 1992; 215:417.
17. Faxon DP, Ryan TJ, David KB: Prognostic significance of angiographically documented left ventricular aneurysm from the Coronary Artery Surgery Study (CASS). *Am J Cardiol* 1982; 50:157.
18. Cosgrove DM, Lytle BW, Taylor PC, et al: Ventricular aneurysm resection: trends in surgical risk. *Circulation* 1989; 79(suppl I):97.
19. Coltharp WH, Hoff SJ, Stoney WS, et al: Ventricular aneurysmectomy: a 25-year experience. *Ann Surg* 1994; 219:707.
20. Grieco JG, Montoya A, Sullivan HJ, et al: Ventricular aneurysm due to blunt chest injury. *Ann Thorac Surg* 1989; 47:322.
21. de Oliveira JA: Heart aneurysm in Chagas' disease. *Rev Inst Med Trop Sao Paulo* 1998; 40:301.
22. Silverman KJ, Hutchins GM, Bulkley BH: Cardiac sarcoid: a clinicopathological study of 84 unselected patients with systemic sarcoidosis. *Circulation* 1978; 58:1204.
23. Davila JC, Enriquez F, Bergoglio S, et al: Congenital aneurysm of the left ventricle. *Ann Thorac Surg* 1965; 1:697.
24. Antunes MJ: Submitral left ventricular aneurysms. *J Thorac Cardiovasc Surg* 1987; 94:241.
25. de Boer HD, Elzenga NJ, de Boer WJ, et al: Pseudoaneurysm of the left ventricle after isolated pericarditis and Staphylococcus aureus septicemia. *Eur J Cardiothorac Surg* 1999; 15:97.
26. Meizlish JL, Berger MJ, Plaukey M, et al: Functional left ventricular aneurysm formation after acute anterior transmural myocardial infarction: incidence, natural history, and prognostic implications. *N Engl J Med* 1984; 311:1001.
27. Forman MB, Collins HW, Kopelman HA, et al: Determinants of left ventricular aneurysm formation after anterior myocardial infarction: a clinical and angiographic study. *J Am Coll Cardiol* 1986; 8:1256.
28. Glower DD, Schaper J, Kabas JS, et al: Relation between reversal of diastolic creep and recovery of systolic function after ischemic myocardial injury in conscious dogs. *Circ Res* 1987; 60:850.
29. Eaton LW, Weiss JL, Bulkley BH, et al: Regional cardiac dilation after acute myocardial infarction: recognition by two-dimensional echocardiography. *N Engl J Med* 1979; 300:57.
30. Iwasaki K, Kita T, Taniguichi G, Kusachi S: Improvement of left ventricular aneurysm after myocardial infarction: report of three cases. *Clin Cardiol* 1991; 14:355.
31. Sakaguchi G, Young RL, Komeda M, et al: Left ventricular aneurysm repair in rats: structural, functional, and molecular consequences. *J Thorac Cardiovasc Surg* 2001; 121:750.
32. Markowitz LJ, Savage EB, Ratcliffe MB, et al: Large animal model of left ventricular aneurysm. *Ann Thorac Surg* 1989; 48:838.
33. Jugdutt BI, Khan MI: Effect of prolonged nitrate therapy on left ventricular modeling after canine acute myocardial infarction. *Circulation* 1994; 89:2297.
34. Kayden DS, Wackers FJ, Zaret BL: Left ventricular aneurysm formation after thrombolytic therapy for anterior infarction. TIMI phase I and open label 1985–1986. *Circulation* 1987; 76(suppl IV):97.
35. Chen JS, Hwang CL, Lee DY, et al: Regression of left ventricular aneurysm after delayed percutaneous transluminal coronary angioplasty (PTCA) in patients with acute myocardial infarction. *Int J Cardiol* 1995; 48:39.
36. Bulkley BH, Roberts WC: Steroid therapy during acute myocardial infarction: a cause of delayed healing and of ventricular aneurysm. *Am J Med* 1974; 58:244.
37. Grondin P, Kretz JG, Bical O, et al: Natural history of saccular aneurysm of the left ventricle. *J Thorac Cardiovasc Surg* 1979; 77:57.
38. Lapeyre AC III, Steele PM, Kazimer FJ, et al: Systemic embolism in chronic left ventricular aneurysm: incidence and the role of anticoagulation. *Am J Cardiol* 1985; 6:534.
39. Benediktsson R, Eyjolfsson O, Thorgeirsson G: Natural history of chronic left ventricular aneurysm: a population based cohort study. *J Clin Epidemiol* 1991; 44:1131.
40. Faxon DP, Myers WO, McCabe CH: The influence of surgery on the natural history of angiographically documented left ventricular aneurysm: the Coronary Artery Surgery Study. *Circulation* 1986; 74:110.
41. Keren A, Goldberg S, Gottlieb S, et al: Natural history of left ventricular thrombi: their appearance and resolution in the posthospitalization period of acute myocardial infarction. *J Am Coll Cardiol* 1990; 15:790.
42. Yeo TC, Malouf JF, Reeder GS, et al: Clinical characteristics and outcome in postinfarction pseudoaneurysm. *Am J Cardiol* 1999; 84:592.
43. Pretre R, Linka A, Jenni R, et al: Surgical treatment of acquired left ventricular pseudoaneurysms. *Ann Thorac Surg* 2000; 70:553.
44. Ba'albaki HA, Clements SD Jr: Left ventricular aneurysm: a review. *Clin Cardiol* 1989; 12:5.
45. Dor V: Reconstructive left ventricular surgery for post-ischemic akinetic dilatation. *Semin Thorac Cardiovasc Surg* 1997; 9:139.
46. Buck T, Hunold P, Wentz KU, et al: Tomographic three-dimensional echocardiographic determination of chamber size and systolic function in patients with left ventricular aneurysm: comparison to magnetic resonance imaging, cineventriculography, and two-dimensional echocardiography. *Circulation* 1997; 96:4286.
47. Frances CD, Shlipak MG, Grady D: Left ventricular pseudoaneurysm: diagnosis by cine magnetic resonance imaging. *Cardiology* 1999; 92:217.
48. Baciewicz PA, Weintraub WS, Jones EL, et al: Late follow-up after repair of left ventricular aneurysm and (usually) associated coronary bypass grafting. *Am J Cardiol* 1991; 68:193.
49. Vlodaver Z, Coe JE, Edwards JE: True and false left ventricular aneurysm: propensity for the latter to rupture. *Circulation* 1975; 51:567.
50. Dor V, Saab M, Coste P, et al: Endoventricular patch plasties with septal exclusion for repair of ischemic left ventricle: technique, results and indications from a series of 781 cases. *Jpn J Thorac Cardiovasc Surg* 1998; 46:389.
51. Akins CW: Resection of left ventricular aneurysm during hypothermic fibrillatory arrest without aortic occlusion. *J Thorac Cardiovasc Surg* 1986; 91:610.
52. Cherniavsky AM, Karaskov AM, Marchenko AV, et al: Preoperative modeling of an optimal left ventricle volume for surgical treatment of ventricular aneurysms. *Eur J Cardiothorac Surg* 2001; 20:777.
53. Cox JL: Surgical management of left ventricular aneurysms: a clarification of the similarities and differences between the Jatene and Dor techniques. *Semin Thorac Cardiovasc Surg* 1997; 9:131.
54. Menasche P, Hagege A, Scorsin M, et al: Autologous skeletal myoblast transplantation for cardiac insufficiency: first clinical case. *Arch Mal Coeur Vaiss* 2001; 94:180.
55. Wang JS, Shum-Tim D, Chedrawy E, et al: The coronary delivery of marrow stromal cells for myocardial regeneration: pathophysiologic and therapeutic implications. *J Thorac Cardiovasc Surg* 2001; 122:699.
56. Yokomuro H, Li RK, Mickle DA, et al: Transplantation of cryopreserved cardiomyocytes. *J Thorac Cardiovasc Surg* 2001; 121:98.
57. Taylor DA, Atkins BZ, Hungspreugs P, et al: Regenerating functional myocardium: improved performance after skeletal myoblast transplantation. *Nat Med* 1998; 4:929.
58. Rankin JS, Hickey MSJ, Smith LR, et al: Current management of mitral valve incompetence associated with coronary artery disease. *J Cardiac Surg* 1989; 4:25.

59. Wellens F, Degreick Y, Deferm H, et al: Surgical treatment of left ventricular aneurysm and ischemic mitral incompetence. *Acta Chir Belg* 1991; 91:44.
60. Dor V: Left ventricular aneurysms: the endoventricular circular patch plasty. *Semin Thorac Cardiovasc Surg* 1997; 9:123.
61. Komeda M, David TE, Malik A, et al: Operative risks and long-term results of operation for left ventricular aneurysm. *Ann Thorac Surg* 1992; 53:22.
62. Couper GS, Bunton RW, Birjiniuk V, et al: Relative risks of left ventricular aneurysmectomy in patients with akinetic scars versus true dyskinetic aneurysms. *Circulation* 1990; 82(suppl IV): 248.
63. Stahle E, Bergstrom R, Nystrom SO, et al: Surgical treatment of left ventricular aneurysm assessment of risk factors for early and late mortality. *Eur J Cardiothorac Surg* 1994; 8:67.
64. Silveira WL, Leite AF, Soares EC, et al: Short-term follow-up of patients after aneurysmectomy of the left ventricle. *Arq Bras Cardiol* 2000; 75:401.
65. Vauthy JN, Berry DW, Snyder DW, et al: Left ventricular aneurysm repair with myocardial revascularization: an analysis of 246 consecutive patients over 15 years. *Ann Thorac Surg* 1988; 46:29.
66. Elefteriades JA, Solomon LW, Salazar AM, et al: Linear left ventricular aneurysmectomy: modern imaging studies reveal improved morphology and function. *Ann Thorac Surg* 1993; 56:242.
67. Kesler KA, Fiore AC, Naunheim KS, et al: Anterior wall left ventricular aneurysm repair: a comparison of linear versus circular closure. *J Thorac Cardiovasc Surg* 1992; 103:841.
68. Kawachi K, Kitamura S, Kawata T, et al: Hemodynamic assessment during exercise after left ventricular aneurysmectomy. *J Thorac Cardiovasc Surg* 1994; 107:178.
69. David TE: Surgical treatment of mechanical complications of myocardial infarction, in Spence PA, Chitwood RA (eds): *Cardiac Surgery: State of the Art Reviews,* vol 5. Philadelphia, Hanley and Belfus, 1991; p 423.
70. DiDonato M, Barletta G, Maioli M, et al: Early hemodynamical results of left ventricular reconstructive surgery for anterior wall left ventricular aneurysm. *Am J Cardiol* 1992; 69:886.
71. Kawata T, Kitamura S, Kawachi K, et al: Systolic and diastolic function after patch reconstruction of left ventricular aneurysms. *Ann Thorac Surg* 1995; 59:403.
72. Fantini F, Barletta G, Toso A, et al: Effects of reconstructive surgery for left ventricular anterior aneurysm on ventriculoarterial coupling. *Heart* 1999; 81:171.
73. Walker WE, Stoney WS, Alford WC, et al: Results of surgical management of acute left ventricular aneurysm. *Circulation* 1978; 62(suppl II):75.
74. Hutchins GM, Brawley RK: The influence of cardiac geometry on the results of ventricular aneurysm repair. *Am J Pathol* 1980; 99: 221.
75. Vural KM, Sener E, Ozatik MA, et al: Left ventricular aneurysm repair: an assessment of surgical treatment modalities. *Eur J Cardiothorac Surg* 1998; 13:49.
76. Turkay C, Mete A, Yilmaz M, et al: Comparative methods of repairing left ventricular aneurysms. *Texas Heart Inst J* 1997; 24:343.
77. Sinatra R, Macrina F, Braccio M, et al: Left ventricular aneurysmectomy: comparison between two techniques: early and late results. *Eur J Cardiothorac Surg* 1997; 12:291.
78. Shapira OM, Davidoff R, Hilkert RJ, et al: Repair of left ventricular aneurysm: long-term results of linear repair versus endoaneurysmorrhaphy. *Ann Thorac Surg* 1997; 63:701.
79. Pasini S, Gagliardotto P, Punta G, et al: Early and late results after surgical therapy of postinfarction left ventricular aneurysm. *J Cardiovasc Surg* 1998; 39:209.
80. Doss M, Martens S, Sayour S, et al: Long term follow up of left ventricular function after repair of left ventricular aneurysm: a comparison of linear closure versus patch plasty. *Eur J Cardiothorac Surg* 2001; 20:783.
81. Nicolosi AC, Weng ZC, Detwiler PW, et al: Simulated left ventricular aneurysm and aneurysm repair in swine. *J Thorac Cardiovasc Surg* 1990; 100:745.
82. Vicol C, Rupp G, Fischer S, et al: Linear repair versus ventricular reconstruction for treatment of left ventricular aneurysm: a 10-year experience. *J Cardiovasc Surg* 1998; 39:461.
83. Salati M, Paje A, DiBiasi P, et al: Severe diastolic dysfunction after endoventriculoplasty. *J Thorac Cardiovasc Surg* 1995; 109:694.
84. Ratcliffe MB, Wallace AW, Salahieh A, et al: Ventricular volume, chamber stiffness, and function after anteroapical aneurysm plication in the sheep. *J Thorac Cardiovasc Surg* 2000; 119:115.
85. Di Mattia DG, Di Biasi P, Salati M, et al: Surgical treatment of left ventricular post-infarction aneurysm with endoventriculoplasty: late clinical and functional results. *Eur J Cardiothorac Surg* 1999; 15:413.

Part IVa

Valvular Heart Disease: Aortic Valve Disease

Chapter 30

Pathophysiology of Aortic Valve Disease

Tomislav Mihaljevic/Subroto Paul/Lawrence H. Cohn/Andrew Wechsler

Although the aortic valve is simple in structure, its proper function is one of the critical elements determining efficient cardiac function. This chapter explores the aortic valve from many viewpoints, and provides an understanding of its intrinsic mechanical and physiologic properties. Alteration of these properties leads to a pathophysiologic process and aortic valve disease.

EMBRYOLOGIC DEVELOPMENT

Embryologic development of the aortic valve is closely associated with the development of the left ventricular outflow tract. During the early stages, the main arterial segment (truncus arteriosus) of the primary heart tube is connected to the primitive right ventricle. With subsequent cardiac loop formation, the truncus arterious together with distal segments of the ventricular outlet component is divided by endocardiac cushion tissue into subaortic and pulmonary outflow tracts. The truncus arteriousus eventually develops into the pulmonary arteries and aorta. As seen in Figure 30-1, a septum develops within the truncus arteriosus and subsequently fuses with the underlying ventricular septum. At the point of fusion between these two septal components, separation of the ventricular chamber is accomplished by the development of the aortic valve.

The right and left cusps of the aortic valve develop from the aortic side of the truncal septum. Opposing this septum, the embryonic posterior aortic valve develops from the truncoconal lining. As development continues, the aortic valve leaflets grow to become nearly uniform in size and dimensions.

ANATOMY

The aortic valve separates the terminal portion of the left ventricular outflow tract from the aorta. Since the subaortic outflow tract has both muscular and fibrous components, all

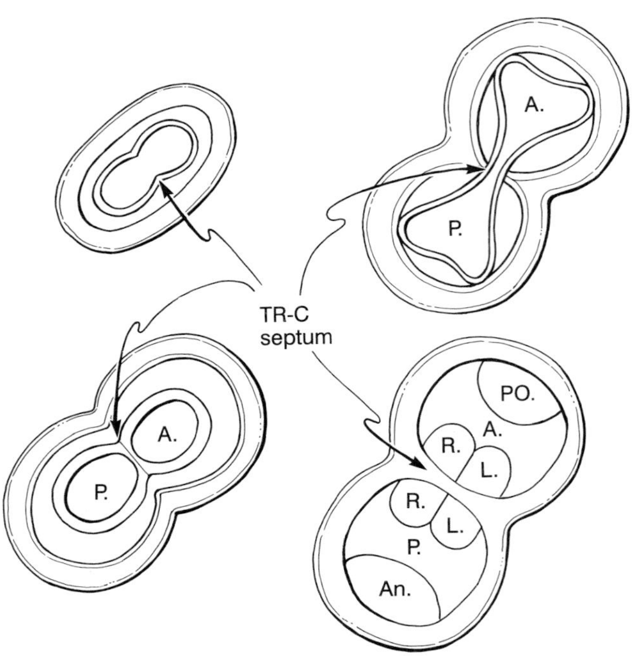

FIGURE 30–1 Development of the aorta and pulmonary artery is shown, with subsequent development of the aortic valve leaflets. (Top left) The truncoconal (TR-C) septum is beginning to divide the truncococonal segment. (Top right) This septum continues until division of the aorta and pulmonary artery is completed (shown at bottom left). (Bottom right) The right and left aortic valve leaflets are derived from the truncoconal septum, whereas the posterior leaflet is derived from the endocardial tissue opposite the truncoconal segment.

three aortic valve cusps also have in part fibrous and in part muscular attachments. The aortic valve lies anterosuperior and slightly to the right of the mitral atrioventricular orifice. It is composed of three semilunar cusps (leaflets) and the aortic valve annulus. The cusps themselves are attached within the expanded aortic sinuses. The sinus of Valsalva is defined as the space between the edge of the leaflets and the aorta. Because two of these sinuses give rise to coronary arteries, they have been conventionally named as the right coronary, left coronary, and noncoronary sinuses. Because of the oblique position of the aortic root, the sinuses themselves are rarely in strictly right and left position. The ostia of the coronary arteries usually open from the upper part of the sinus of origin, the ostium of the left coronary artery often being a little lower than the ostium of the right.

Areas where attachments of two adjacent cusps to the aorta meet comprise commissures. The commissure between the noncoronary and left coronary leaflets is positioned along the area of aortic–mitral valve continuity. Beneath this commissure is the so-called fibrous aortomitral curtain. To the right of this commissure, the noncoronary leaflet is attached to the posterior diverticulum of the left ventricular outflow tract. This is the part where the aortic valve is directly related to the right atrial wall. The commissure between the noncoronary and right coronary cusp is positioned directly above the penetrating atrioventricular bundle and membranous septum. The commissure between the right and the left coronary cusp is positioned opposite a facing commissure of the pulmonary valve. The adjacent parts of these two aortic cusps are directly related to the right ventricular infundibulum. The lateral part of the left coronary sinus is the only part of the aortic valve that is not related to another cardiac chamber, but is in direct relationship with the free pericardial space.

The aortic valve may be described as having a passive valve mechanism that is quite different from the mitral valve. Because of its passive mechanism, the structure of the aortic valve must open and close with minimal pressure differences between the ventricle and aorta. During closing, this same mechanism must prevent backflow by perfectly aligning the cusps, which must have enough structural integrity to withstand systemic pressures.

There is no true aortic valve annulus, in contrast to the mitral valve. The commonly designated "annulus of the aortic valve" is actually an aortic ring and is the last impediment to the flow prior to blood reaching the aorta.

The junction between the ventricular chamber and the aorta is designated as the ventricular arterial junction. This must be viewed as either an anatomic or physiologic junction. The physiologic junction is marked by attachments of the semilunar valves that define the separation between ventricular outflow chamber and the proximal aorta. However, there is a discrepancy between this physiologic junction and the anatomic junction, in part due to muscular tissue of the ventricle and in part due to fibrous tissue of the septum and mitral valve. As can be seen in Figure 30-2, the commissures are above the anatomic junction, but the bases of the semilunar attachments of the aortic leaflets are at the true anatomic junction.[1] The fibrous skeleton of the heart forms the posterior wall of the outflow tract where the leaflets are in fibrous continuity with those of the mitral valve (Fig. 30-2).[1]

A valve leaflet is composed of collagen, elastin, and glycosaminoglycans. These are the main components for the three principal layers of the leaflet: the fibrosa or arteriosa, the spongiosa, and the ventricularis (Figs. 30-3 and 30-4). As can be seen in Figure 30-3, the arterial and ventricular sides of the aortic leaflet are associated with the corresponding aortic and ventricular wall. There is no demarcation between the outer layers of the leaflet and the corresponding wall.[2] The outer layers of the leaflet form a continuum with the aortic endothelium or ventricular endothelium.

The ventricular side of each aortic valve cusp contains elastin-rich fibers aligned in a radial direction, perpendicular to the leaflet free margin. Elastin is mechanically coupled to collagen. The purpose of elastin in the aortic valve leaflet is to maintain a specific collagen fiber configuration and return the fibers to their initial state, once the external

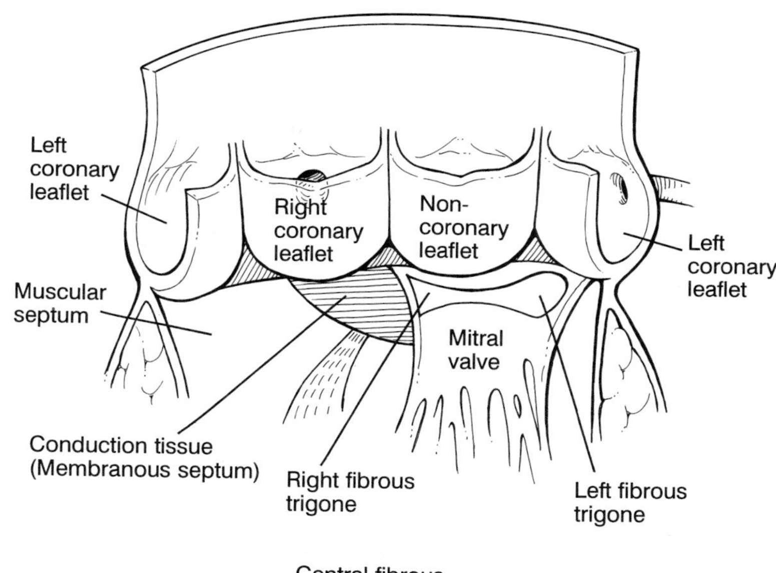

FIGURE 30–2 A schematic diagram of the relationship of the aortic valve leaflets to the structures underlying the commissures. The noncoronary leaflet straddles the central fibrous body overlying the anterior leaflet of the mitral valve. The conduction tissue traverses the membranous septum between the right coronary and noncoronary leaflets.

forces of blood flow subside.[3] In addition, there is a collagen component lying parallel to the free margin in a circumferential direction. The aortic side contains a collagen-rich layer referred to as the corrugated fibrosa. These fibers are in a circumferential direction and, in a relaxed state, assume a waveform pattern. The middle layer, referred to as the spongiosa, consists of mainly loose connective tissue or mucopolysaccharides. These principal layers of the aortic leaflet provide the necessary biomechanical properties for proper valve function.

On the arteriosa (fibrosa) side of the valve leaflet, endothelial cells are present. Endothelial cells normally align in the direction of stress. In an artery, endothelial cells are aligned in the direction of blood flow because flow stress is the major stress. However, endothelial cells on the aortic valve leaflet are arranged in a circumferential pattern; i.e., they are arranged perpendicular to the blood flow. Therefore, shear stress of blood flow across the aortic valve is not the major stress. The major stress across the aortic valve is in the circumferential direction and is perpendicular to blood flow.[4]

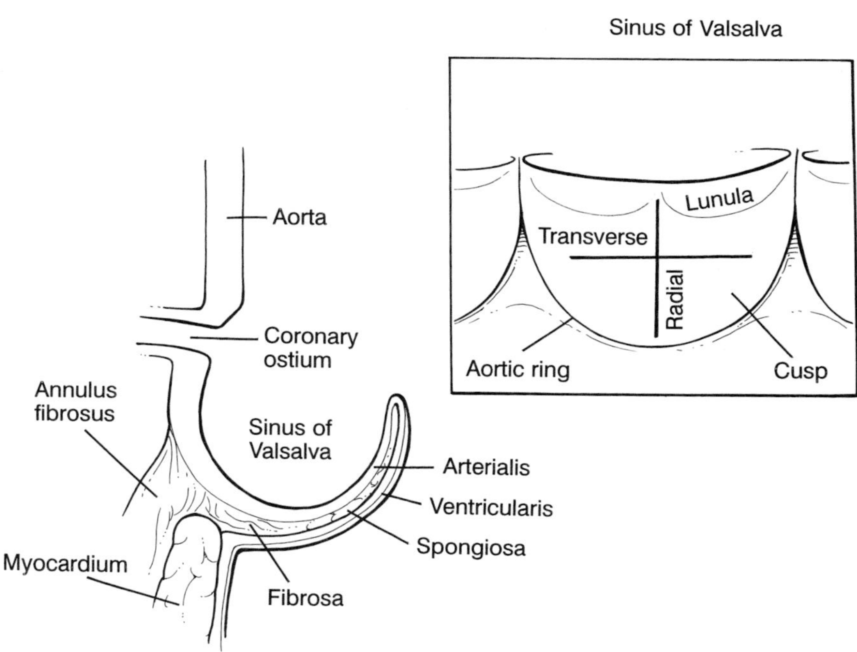

FIGURE 30–3 Schematic representation of a cross section through the aortic valve leaflet, showing the continuity of endocardial and endothelial components with the aortic valve. Inset illustrates the radial and transverse (circumferential) axes of the valve leaflet and the line of attachment to the aortic wall.

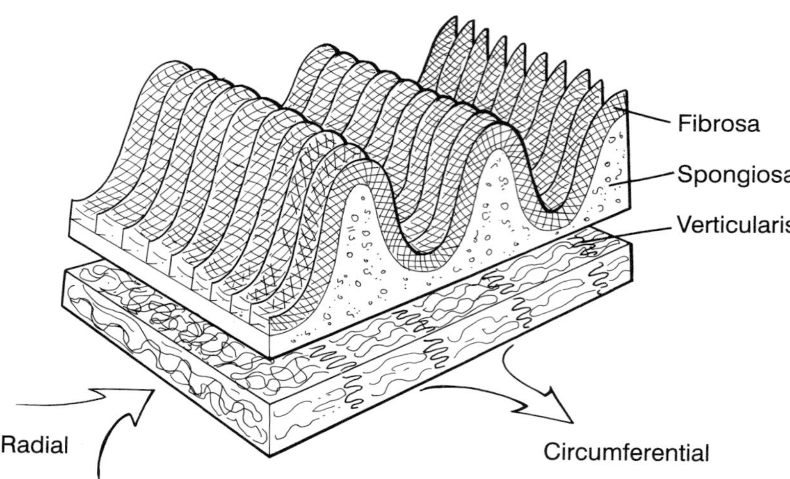

FIGURE 30–4 Schematic representation of the different layers of the aortic valve leaflet, showing that the fibrosa layer is corrugated, enhancing the ability to stretch in a radial direction. (*Reproduced with permission from Broom ND: Connective tissue function and malfunction: a biomechanical perspective. Pathology 1988; 20:93.*)

BIOMECHANICAL PROPERTIES

The mechanical properties of the aortic valve must allow the valve to open with minimal transvalvular pressure differences and to close completely with minimal flow reversal. Although these functional requirements are simple, the mechanical properties also must provide durability. The pressure drop across the aortic valve generates large stress within the leaflets. These stresses are too great for the leaflets and must be distributed to the fibrous skeleton of the surrounding structures by the valve anatomy.[2]

The valve leaflets demonstrate anisotropic properties because equal leaflet strain distribution would not allow the valve to close properly during diastole. Differences in strain properties allow the cusps to stretch during closure to completely coapt along the free margins. Strain distribution is in two directions: circumferential and radial. The radial vector is perpendicular to blood flow, and the circumferential vector is in the direction of blood flow. Circumferential stiffness is increased relative to radial stiffness. These anisotropic properties allow the valve to stretch in a radial direction, whereas downward movement is relatively restricted. This facilitates leaflet coaptation, and sealing during diastole. As seen in Figure 30-4, the fibrosa layer of the valve leaflet is corrugated. This property allows the fibrosa layer to stretch in a radial direction and allows each leaflet to billow toward the other leaflets. Although this layer is the principal load-bearing layer, these properties do not prevent it from stretching. The ventricularis layer determines the stiffness in the circumferential direction.[2] These properties are demonstrated in Figure 30-5, where different layers of the valve leaflet are severed and strain properties measured.

Because the principal stresses are oriented in a radial direction, endothelial cells on the fibrosa layer of the leaflets are oriented in a radial direction. Most of the stress on the leaflets occurs at the interface between the two coapting edges of the cusp. These stresses are reduced by several factors. By mutual coaptive support, each leaflet reduces the stresses of the other. These stresses are then distributed along the leaflet edges to corners of the commissures.

Further stress reduction is also accomplished by the interaction of the sinus of Valsalva with the leaflet assembly. The sinus of Valsalva changes its radius of curvature from systole to diastole, decreasing approximately 16%.[5] This change in radius of curvature allows distribution of stresses within the sinus in accordance with the Laplace formula. By coaptation of the valve leaflets in diastole, there is an inward bending of each sinus at the commissural attachments and outward bowing of the aortic wall within the sinus between commissures. This decreases the radius of curvature of the aortic wall of the sinus and verifies that each sinus of Valsalva shares the stresses during diastole.

These mechanisms of stress reduction are important for valve durability. If stresses are unabated due to abnormalities, such as improper coaptation of the valve leaflets or congential anatomic abnormalities, the normal mechanism of stress reduction cannot operate. Stress reduction is important because endothelial damage on valve leaflets is directly proportional to the amount of stress. With turnover of endothelial cells and fibroblastic activity, repair of the valve incorporates calcium, which further reduces the mechanical efficiency of the valve. Inability to manage stresses efficiently explains why abnormal leaflets produce progressive deterioration of valve function.

Mechanics of Movement

The opening and closing of the aortic valve constitute a passive mechanism responding to the pressure fluctuations of the cardiac cycle and pressure differences between the ventricular chamber and the aorta. Although pressure changes during the cardiac cycle may create some structural changes of the valve mechanism to facilitate opening or closing, the principal component is the pressure difference between the

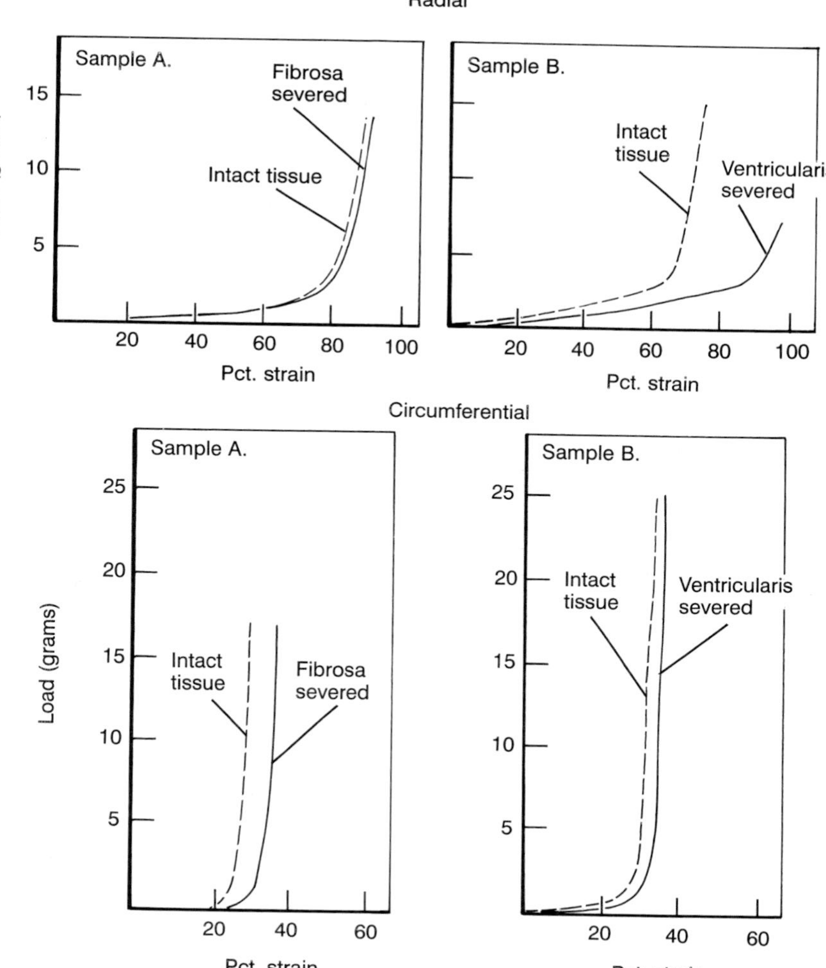

FIGURE 30–5 Illustrated data from Broom and Christie[109] showing the effect of severing specific layers of the aortic valve leaflet in radial and circumferential directions. In the top panels (sample A), when the fibrosa is severed in a radial direction, the stress-strain relationship is unchanged, indicating that in a radial direction the ventricularis layer is the strain-limiting component. This is verified in sample B. When the ventricularis is severed, the strain of the leaflet increases per given load. This is in contrast to a circumferential incision (bottom panels), in which there is relatively little change when either the fibrosa or ventricularis is severed.

ventricle and aorta. Under normal circumstances, the valve leaflets offer little impediment to flow because the specific gravity of the leaflets is equal to that of blood.[6] Proper function depends on rapid closure in response to minimal forces moving the valve leaflets.

OPENING

During diastole, the pressure difference between the aorta and the ventricle creates stress on the valve leaflets. This stress toward the central portion of the aortic opening constricts the base of the aortic root. In addition, the elastic properties of the aortic root contribute to this decrease in diameter. During late diastole, as the blood fills the ventricle, a 12% expansion of the aortic root occurs approximately 20 to 40 milliseconds prior to aortic valve opening.[7,8] Dilatation of the root alone helps in opening the leaflet to about 20%. Actually, the leaflets begin to open even before any positive pressure is applied, due primarily to the effect of aortic root dilatation.[9] As pressure rises in the ventricular outflow tract, tension across the leaflets lessens. As pressure continues to rise, the pressure difference across the valve leaflets is minimal, and no tension is present within the leaflet.[7] At this point, without constriction of the aortic root at the leaflet attachments due to redistributed stress during diastole, the aortic root expands to allow the valve to open rapidly at the beginning of ejection. Ejection takes place with a brisk upward movement of straightened leaflets, and the angle at their bases becomes more acute. These mechanisms permit the valve to open quickly and to offer minimal resistance to ejection.[10]

CLOSING

Closure of the aortic valve is one of the more elegant mechanisms of the valve apparatus.[11] A principal theory involved in closure is the vortex theory. The vortex theory recognizes the importance of the sinus of Valsalva in providing a reservoir of blood for small developing vortices. These small vortices allow full expansion of the opened valve leaflets. However, by maintaining the space between the edge of the leaflet and the aortic wall, reversal of flow at the end of systole provides rapid closure. As ejection occurs, deceleration of blood at the stream edge creates small eddy currents of vortices. These small vortices along the aortic wall gradually move toward the base of the ventricular arterial junction to the edge of the leaflet and top of the sinus of Valsalva. As flow declines at end systole, the pressure difference across the opened aortic valve leaflet decreases. At the end of ejection and prior to valve closure, the vortices within the sinus of Valsalva balloon the valve leaflets toward the center of the aorta. The angle at the base of the leaflet becomes more obtuse and rounded, in contrast to the sharp angle at maximal valve opening. This point of flexure begins to move up the valve leaflet and eventually terminates at the free margin of the valve cusp.[10] Therefore, the mechanism of valve closure begins during ejection with the development of vortices within the sinus of Valsalva that prime the leaflets for valve closure. When pressure between the ventricular outflow tract and aorta equalizes, a small reversal of flow occurs due to the deceleration of ejected blood. This small flow reversal causes the leaflets to close rapidly.

Apposition of the valve leaflets occurs briskly. The second heart sound occurs after complete closure of the aortic valve.[12] The valve leaflets act as an elastic membrane, with stretch and recoil producing the sound; the sound is not produced by physical apposition of the valve leaflets. The second heart sound depends on the elasticity of the valve leaflet and diastolic blood pressure to cause reverberation of the leaflet.

Rheology

Blood flow across the aortic valve is pulsatile and differs from classic laminar flow such as flow through pipe at a constant rate. Analysis of flow characteristics is difficult because structural components above and below the aortic valve differ from patient to patient. In addition, the dynamics of the valve mechanism and rate of ejection force vary considerably. However, while recognizing these limitations, certain characteristics of normal aortic flow rheology can be described.

As ventricular contraction occurs, blood pressure within the chamber increases. As the pressurized blood moves through the ventricular outflow tract, velocity increases until the blood is ejected at the aortic valve. The ventricular outflow tract acts as a funnel to increase blood flow velocity. As blood passes through the relatively fixed aortic valve ring to the slightly larger aorta, a laminar flow profile develops.

The ejected blood produces a skewed peak systolic velocity profile that varies in its location along the aortic wall and during the course of ejection. This velocity profile becomes more blunt at the end of the ejection. Because the effective valve orifice is normally smaller than the aorta, the ejection flow pattern interacts with the blood column along the aortic wall that has relatively low velocity. This interaction between blood moving at varying velocities causes turbulence.[13] Therefore, it is normal to have some turbulence; however, the degree of turbulence is directly proportional to both the velocity of ejected blood and the interface between ejected blood and the relatively stagnant blood in the aorta.

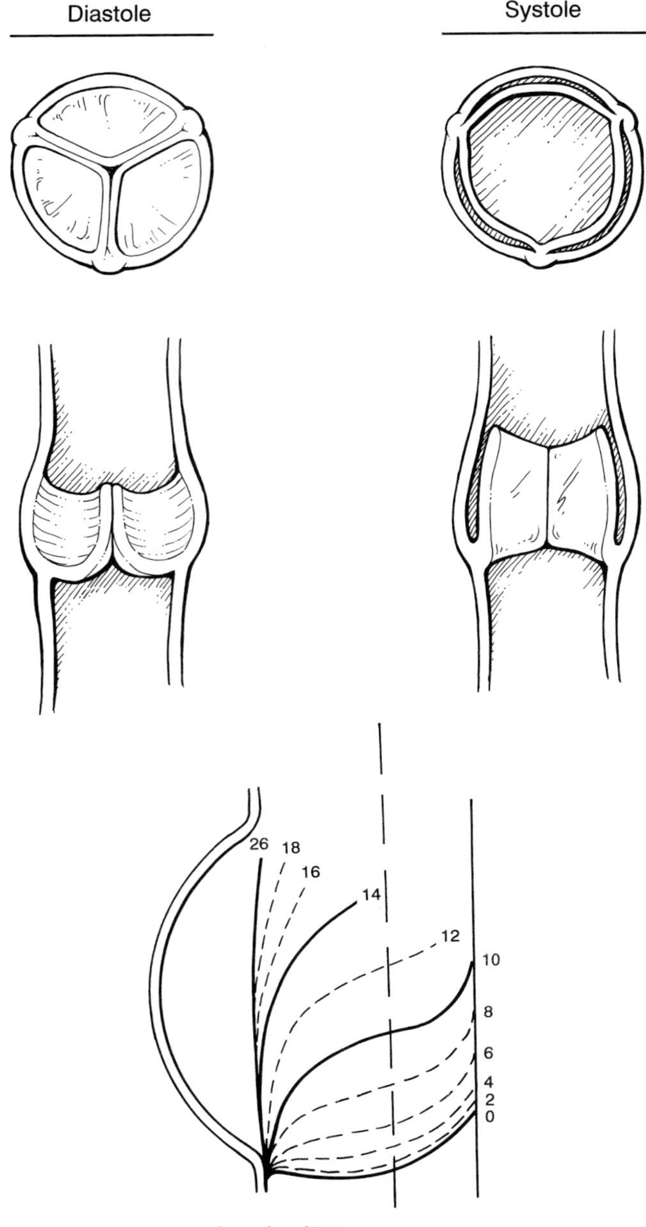

FIGURE 30–6 Positions of the aortic valve leaflets at end diastole and end systole and of a single leaflet in profile during ejection as the leaflet moves from the closed position (0) to full opening (26). Note how the fully opened leaflet tends to produce a uniform diameter above the ventricular-arterial junction to reduce turbulence that otherwise would be increased by the sinuses of Valsalva.

Figure 30-6 demonstrates that as blood is ejected through the valve orifice, the position of the leaflets helps to reduce turbulence by masking the dilatation of the sinuses to produce an aortic root of nearly uniform diameter. Under these normal circumstances, the effective valve orifice is minimally smaller than the aorta. Once the flow profile reaches the aortic wall, the interaction between stagnant blood and high-velocity blood no longer occurs, and turbulence is diminished.

When high-velocity blood interacts with low-velocity blood, energy transfer occurs and contributes to turbulence. This energy density can be up to 14 times greater in highly turbulent blood as compared with normal blood turbulence. This energy density is obviously transferred to the surrounding structures, particularly the endothelium of the aorta, but this high turbulence may initiate damage to intimal surfaces to produce intimal thickening and platelet deposition with subsequent thrombosis.[14]

Throughout systole and early diastole, a bidirectional velocity profile is present. Retrograde velocities present around the wall of the aorta subsequently contribute to closure of the aortic valve leaflets. Bidirectional velocity is present under normal circumstances. However, if it is severe, it may contribute to early systolic closure of the aortic valve.

Abnormalities in blood rheology are present in patients with heart valve disease; plasma fibrinogen, plasma viscosity, and red cell aggregation are all elevated. These abnormalities might be related to the increased incidence of thromboembolism in patients with valvular disease.[15]

AORTIC STENOSIS

Prevalence and Etiology

Valvular aortic stenosis (AS) without accompanying mitral valve disease is more common in men than in women, and is rarely rheumatic in etiology. Instead, the isolated aortic stenosis is most commonly degenerative or congenital in origin. The prevalence of aortic valve abnormality as detected by echocardiography increases with age, with aortic sclerosis seen in 26% of adults older than 65 years and stenosis present in 4% percent of adults over 84 years of age.[16–18]

ACQUIRED AORTIC STENOSIS

Age-related degenerative aortic stenosis is now the most common cause of isolated aortic valve disease in the adult population, and the most frequent reason for aortic valve replacement. Aortic sclerosis and aortic stenosis most likely represent different stages of the same disease process. The characteristic pathologic findings are discrete, focal lesions on the aortic side of the leaflet, which can extend deep into the aortic annulus. Typically, there is displacement of the subendothelial elastica by protein and lipid infiltration in conjunction with cellular infiltration with macrophages and T lymphocytes. Gradual increase in size and calcification of subendothelial lesions leads to increased valve stiffness and increasing valvular obstruction.[19–21] Both diabetes and hypercholesterolemia are risk factors for development of degenerative calcific aortic stenosis. Aortic sclerosis as well as calcific aortic stenosis are associated with traditional risk factors for development of atherosclerosis: hypertension, cigarette smoking, and hypercholesterolemia.[22]

Acquired aortic stenosis is associated with some other less frequent conditions, including end-stage renal failure, Paget disease of the bone, and rheumatic fever.[23–25] Ochronosis is a rare cause of isolated aortic stenosis, which can also cause a rare greenish discoloration of aortic valve.[26]

CONGENITAL AORTIC STENOSIS

Calcified bicuspid aortic valve represents the most common form of congenital aortic stenosis, which presents in adulthood. The abnormal structure of the aortic valve induces turbulent flow, which traumatizes leaflets and leads to fibrosis and calcification.[27] Calcifications progress to produce clinically evident stenosis by the fifth or sixth decade of life. The calcification of the valve is usually most severe at the site of commissural fusion, and often extends deep into aortic valve annulus. Tricuspid aortic valve with unequal size cusps with some degree of commissural fusion represents a rare form of congenital aortic stenosis with presentation in adulthood.

RHEUMATIC AORTIC STENOSIS

Rheumatic aortic stenosis represents the least common form of aortic stenosis in the adult population. Aortic stenosis is the consequence of pathologic processes, which cause the fusion of the aortic valve cusps and subsequent narrowing of the valve orifice. Rheumatic aortic valve stenosis is rarely an isolated disease, and usually occurs in conjunction with mitral valve stenosis.[22]

Overall distribution of causes of aortic stenosis varies significantly among different age groups. Among patients younger than 70 years, congenitally calcified bicuspid valves were responsible for half of surgical cases. In contrast, in patients over 70 years of age, degenerative calcific stenosis is by far the most prevalent cause of stenosis, accounting for 48% of all surgical cases.[22]

Hemodynamics

Aortic stenosis, regardless of etiology, results in obstruction to left ventricular outflow. The stenotic process is usually gradual in onset and progression, allowing enough time for the adaptation of the left ventricle. Chronic pressure overload of the left ventricle with resulting increase in the ventricular pressure during systole causes hypertrophy of the left ventricular myocardium. This compensatory response maintains cardiac output and end-diastolic volume of the left ventricle for a prolonged time despite a systolic pressure gradient between the left ventricle and aorta. Pressures in the ventricular chamber and outflow tract are not equal during systole. Since the outflow tract is tapered, flow velocity is increased as compared with that in the left ventricle.[28] Because of this increase in flow velocity, measured pressure is less than pressure measured in lower portions of the ventricle.[29] Thus the location of the ventricular pressure measurement is critical in determining the pressure difference across the valve. The most accurate measurement for determining aortic valve area using the Gorlin formula is that taken just below the valve.

An appreciation of the velocity profile in aortic stenosis is needed not only to understand the consequences of the high-velocity ejection, but also because noninvasive measures of velocity are used to assess the degree of stenosis. The velocity of blood ejected through the aortic valve is determined by several factors. The first factor is the contractile force of the left ventricle. With normal ventricular function, aortic stenosis is associated with a highly asymmetric flow profile. Because this flow profile is asymmetric, different velocities occur within the ejection stream, depending on location. A low ejection fraction demonstrates a lower velocity profile and more symmetry. In this situation, the flow velocity profile at any point is similar despite the same degree of stenosis as a normally ejecting heart

Pressure differences occur within domains of blood, within the valve orifice, and above the valve. These pressure differences are important because blood with high velocity and relatively low pressure interacts with fluid with lower velocity and higher pressure and may produce turbulence. The critical Reynolds number that depends on flow velocity determines whether turbulence will occur.[30] As blood velocity increases, from an increase in either ejection force or more severe stenosis, the critical Reynolds number is reached and turbulence occurs. As mentioned previously, a high degree of turbulence causes deterioration of the valvular intimal lining and induces changes within the aortic wall.

As the effective valve orifice decreases with increasing aortic stenosis, flow separation occurs at the junction between the ejection stream and nonejected blood present in the aorta. This flow separation may cause stagnation and sometimes flow reversal. Retrograde flow in the ascending aorta occurs during both systole and diastole and is enhanced by both the degree of aortic stenosis and the ejection velocity. Retrograde flow also occurs along the wall of the aorta and in regions of vortex formation. These deviations from normal flow characteristics can cause dramatic changes within aortic endothelium and in aortic size.

Prolonged aortic stenosis may produce poststenotic dilatation. Two factors determine the diameter of a vessel: the distending pressure acting perpendicular to the vessel wall, and the intrinsic elastic properties of the wall itself. Pressure fluctuations caused by aortic stenosis produce a wide range of fluid movements that vibrate the vessel wall at various frequencies.[31,32] With deterioration of elastic properties, the aortic wall tends dilate more at any given distending pressure. Poststenotic dilatation is usually seen distal to the aortic valve and most likely where the ejection stream interacts with the aorta directly to modulate elastin.

Ventricular Adaptations

As previously mentioned, aortic stenosis causes a chronic pressure overload of the left ventricle. Myocardial hypertrophy, defined as increased cardiac mass and cardiomyocyte volume associated with characteristic changes in gene and protein expression, represents the response of the left ventricle to the hemodynamic stress (Fig. 30-7). Ventricular adaptive remodeling can be analyzed from the viewpoint of classic hemodynamic measurements, as well as from the perspective of cellular and molecular responses.

The initial phase of ventricular response to aortic stenosis is marked by enhanced myocardial force-generating capacity and favorable geometry in the hypertrophied heart, which compensates for increased pressure load, and thus permits preservation of normal cardiac output. Because mature cardiac myocytes do not undergo cell division, hypertrophy occurs by an increase in myocyte volume through increased synthesis of sarcomeres. These changes occur almost immediately after increasing pressure load and have both short- and long-term adaptive roles. These adaptive mechanisms recapitulate a fetal pattern of gene expression and alter both cellular contractile elements such as myosin and the biochemistry that affects the relaxation capabilities of the left ventricle. The stimulus for reexpression of a fetal gene type appears to be development of increased left ventricular stress. The exact mechanisms by which increased stress induces genetic reexpression are under active investigation. Stressed myocytes are thought to upregulate protein kinase A and C. These kinases activate transcription factors that stimulate promoter genes to produce hypertrophy and normalize stress.[33–35] A change in transcriptional activation probably upregulates cardiac genes to increase protein synthesis and the total concentration of cardiac RNA.[36–39] These changes correspond with increase in protein synthesis and oncogene activation.

Severe, long-standing aortic stenosis causes progressively more isometric contraction of the left ventricle. Subsequent elevation of the left ventricular end-diastolic pressures, which is characteristic of severe AS, is a marker of diminished compliance of hypertrophied left ventricle. Diastolic dysfunction is an important feature of severe aortic stenosis, which is a dominant cause of heart failure in 15% to 40% of patients. The passive elastic properties of the left ventricle during diastole do not depend on preload or afterload but are directly proportional to the degree of hypertrophy present.[40] In patients with severe AS, enhanced contraction of the left atrium plays an important role in filling of the poorly compliant left ventricle. Loss of normal atrial contraction, such as occurs in atrial fibrillation, can lead to acute clinical deterioration in patients with severe aortic stenosis.

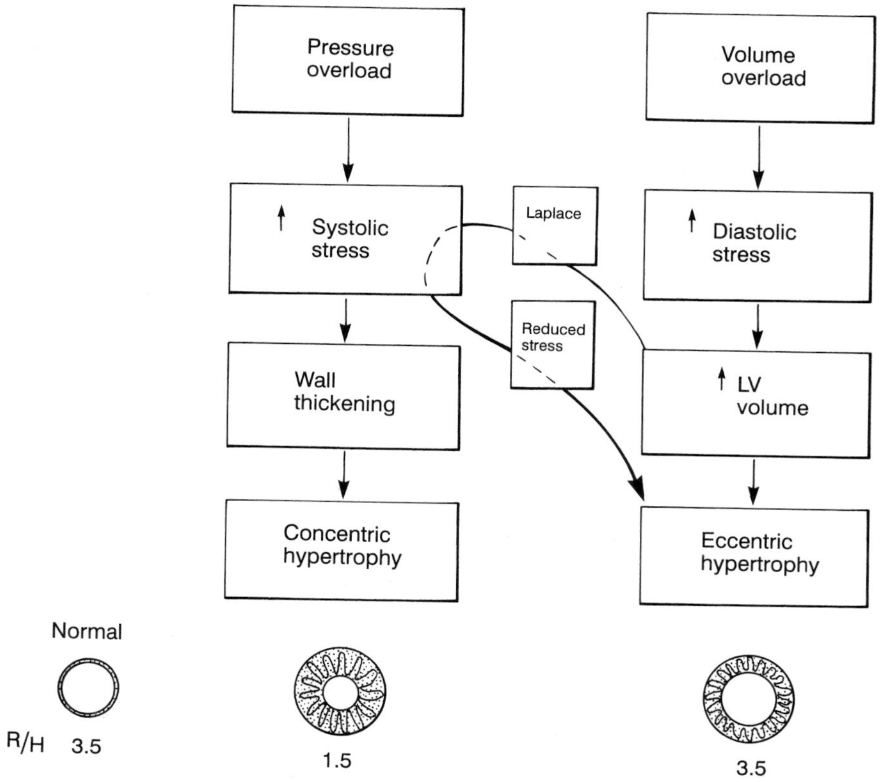

FIGURE 30–7 Schematic representation of the pathophysiology of pressure and volume overload. With pressure overload, an increase in systolic wall stress provides the stimulus to increase wall thickness and normalizes peak systolic stress. This progresses to concentric hypertrophy, where the ratio of the radius to wall thickness is markedly less than normal. This development is in sharp contrast to volume overload, wherein the increase in diastolic stress provides a stimulus for elongation of myofibrils to increase left ventricular volume. Because of the increase in left ventricular volume, by Laplace's law, systolic stress increases to induce wall thickening, which reduces stress and produces eccentric hypertrophy. Eccentric hypertrophy increases left ventricular volume and wall thickness; however, the ratio of ventricular radius to wall thickness (R/H) remains normal. *(Modified with permission from Grossman W, McLaurin LP, Stefadouros MA: Left ventricular stiffness associated with chronic pressue and volume overloads in man. Circ Res 1974; 35:793.)*

Cardiac tissue in this phase is highly active metabolically, and mechanical stretch promotes cardiac fibroblast proliferation and enhances collagen production.

Later in the course of untreated severe aortic stenosis, compensated hypertrophy inexorably and inevitably fails, leading to dilated cardiomyopathy and decompensation. The cardiac output and stroke volume decline, with simultaneous increase in the mean left atrial and pulmonary artery wedge pressure. As a consequence, pulmonary hypertension develops, leading to right ventricular failure. Loss of cardiomyocytes contributes to decompensation of hypertrophied ventricle. Recent studies have increasingly suggested an important role for cardiomyocyte apoptosis in progression of aortic stenosis to heart failure. Hypetrophy-induced molecular triggers for cardiomyocyte suicide were recently identified in an animal model.[41] In addition to the triggering of apoptotic mechanism, the transition from the compensatory hypertrophy to the failure is mediated by downregulation of peptide growth factors like neuregulins.[42]

Further understanding of molecular mechanisms of myocardial failure of hypertrophied myocardium may allow new therapeutic approaches as an important adjunct to standard surgical therapy.

Coronary Blood Flow

Severe left ventricular hypertrophy causes significant associated changes in coronary blood flow. Abnormalities in coronary blood flow are responsible for the occurrence of angina, which occurs in approximately 35% to 50% of patients with aortic stenosis.[43]

Increased oxygen demand due to increased muscle mass causes the coronary arteries to increase in diameter in hearts with left ventricular hypertrophy secondary to aortic stenosis. Data demonstrate that the circumflex and left anterior descending (LAD) coronary arteries are both increased in diameter. This increase is greater in circumflex territory as compared with the LAD artery. This observation may explain the propensity for sudden death and increased episodes of ventricular ectopy in patients with aortic stenosis.[44] The cross-sectional area of the coronary arteries is increased in proportion to the left ventricular mass in asymptomatic patients with left ventricular hypertrophy, but this proportional increase is not present in patients with left ventricular hypertrophy and angina.[45] The cause for the increase in coronary artery diameter is not totally known, but vessel growth factors are supposedly responsible. The larger coronary cross-sectional diameters decrease after aortic valve replacement.[46,47] Patients with angina have a higher peak systolic pressure that may reflect possible reverse flow or markedly decreased systolic coronary blood flow.[48] Patients with angina also have a higher diastolic peak coronary artery flow velocity that may be reflective of a relative functional stenosis of the coronary arteries.

A decrease in the driving pressure of coronary blood flow also may be responsible for angina. The pressure in the sinus of Valsalva, particularly during systole, may be depressed due to rheologic factors (Bernoulli theorem). This contributes to

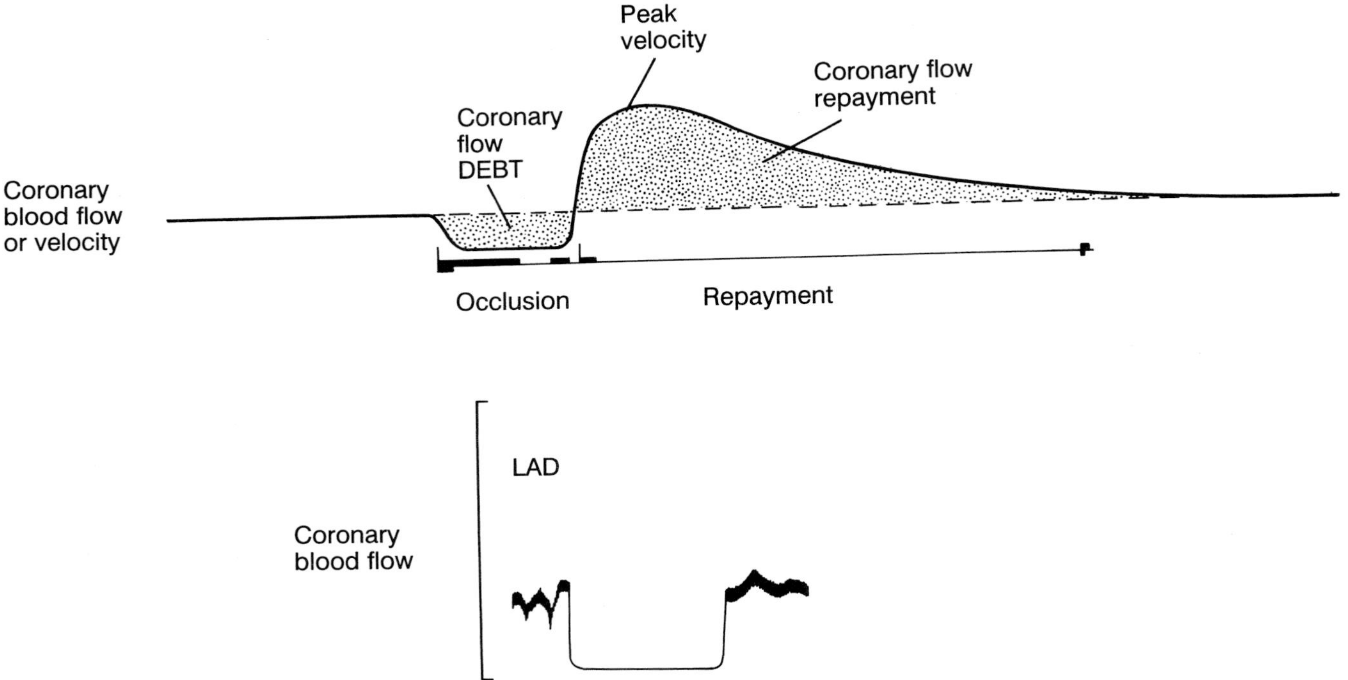

FIGURE 30–8 (Top) Coronary flow dynamics during temporary coronary occlusion in a normal heart. (Bottom) Coronary blood flow is interrupted in the left anterior descending coronary artery in a patient with aortic stenosis. In the normal heart, during 10 seconds of occlusion the myocardium incurs a coronary flow deficit that is more than repaid during a hyperemic response after flow resumes. In a patient with aortic stenosis, either an attenuated or no hyperemic response occurs after 10 seconds of occlusion, indicating little or no coronary artery flow reserve.

a decrease in the driving pressure of blood flow, particularly during systole and early diastole, when intraventricular pressures are elevated. Coronary blood flow is further reduced by abnormal relaxation during diastole and this may contribute to early diastolic dysfunction.[45]

The coronary vascular bed does not keep pace with the increase in myocardial mass. The density of capillaries is reduced in hypertrophied hearts, and this may explain the development of angina with exercise. The distribution of capillaries is usually not altered unless left ventricular muscle grows 75% or more. The greatest coronary blood flow occurs in midwall layers, with lesser but approximately equal flow to the endocardium and epicardium.

One of the major physiologic consequences of hypertrophy is decreased coronary reserve. As shown in Figure 30-8, the normal hyperemic response after a ten-second coronary artery occlusion is severely blunted in a coronary artery distributing blood flow to hypertrophied myocardium.[49] The peak velocity of coronary blood flow following coronary artery occlusion is decreased by more than 50%.[50] These changes in flow reserve are reversed after surgery.

Left ventricular hypertrophy impairs subendocardial blood flow. There is a decrease in the endocardial-epicardial flow ratio from 1.2 to 0.9. This accounts for an increase in the oxygen extraction that is highest in endocardium.[51,52] The change in the endocardial-epicardial flow ratio is due to hypertrophy and is not due to an increase in left ventricular pressure.[52] Thus endocardium is more vulnerable to ischemia because most of its blood supply occurs during diastole.[53]

Signs and Symptoms

Patients with aortic stenosis are asymptomatic for a prolonged period of time despite the obstruction and an increased pressure load to left ventricle. However, progressive and long-standing obstruction with compensatory left ventricular hypertrophy can lead to one or more main symptoms associated with aortic stenosis:

1. Syncope
2. Angina
3. Dsypnea and congestive heart failure

Exertional dizziness or syncope appears to be due to an inappropriate ventricular baroreceptor response leading to peripheral vasodilatation and consequent hypotension and decreased cerebral perfusion. It can also result from arrhythmia, particularly ventricular tachycardia or nonsustained ventricular fibrillation.

Angina with effort occurs in about two thirds of patients with severe aortic stenosis. Approximately one half of these patients have underlying coronary artery disease. Angina in patients who do not have coronary artery disease is due to myocardial oxygen supply-demand imbalance. This imbalance can be the product of various factors: increased ventricular oxygen demand as a result of increased left ventricular mass; compression of intramyocardial portions of coronary arteries during prolonged systole; or reduced diastolic coronary perfusion time during tachycardia.

Heart failure is usually manifested initially as decreased exercise tolerance, which with time progresses to frank dyspnea. Decreased exercise tolerance can be viewed as a sign of diastolic dysfunction of the ventricle leading to an increase in end-diastolic pressure with exercise. Systolic left ventricular dysfunction occurs late in the course of the disease and is manifested by shortness of breath, debilitation, and other signs and symptoms of low cardiac output state.

Other less common symptoms include gastrointestinal bleeding due to angiodysplasia (most commonly of the right colon). Infective endocarditis can occur in younger patients with aortic stenosis; it is less common in elderly patients with severely calcified valves. On rare occasions, a stenotic valve can be a source of calcium emboli to any organ.

Diagnostic Evaluation

PHYSICAL EXAMINATION

Physical examination is very helpful in the assessment of the severity of aortic stenosis. An important clinical finding, which reflects the severity of stenosis, is the quality of the arterial pulse. The arterial pulse is weak and rises slowly ("parvus and tardus"), which reflects the obstruction of blood flow into the peripheral circulation.

Stenosis of aortic leaflets is associated with reduced mobility and delayed valve closure. The S_1 is usually normal. The S_2 is soft and single since aortic closure (A_2) is delayed and tends to occur simultaneously with P_2. Vigorous left atrial contraction can be heard as the fourth heart sound (S_4). Systolic ejection murmur is best heard at the base of the heart and is harsh in quality, but does not correlate with severity of stenosis.

ELECTROCARDIOGRAPHY

The principal electrocardiographic findings in aortic stenosis are related to the presence of left ventricular hypertrophy and are therefore nonspecific. The voltage is usually significantly increased, with common findings of associated ST-segment changes suggestive of subendocardial ischemia. It is important to emphasize that the absence of signs of left ventricular hypertrophy on electrocardiogram does not exclude the diagnosis of aortic stenosis.

CHEST X-RAY

The chest radiograph has a normal appearance in the vast majority of patients with aortic stenosis, with some common although nonspecific findings. Left ventricular hypertrophy is suggested by the rounding of the left ventricular free wall. Severe calcification of the aortic valve can frequently be seen in adult patients with severe or critical aortic stenosis. The absence of calcification on an overpenetrated chest x-ray essentially eliminates the diagnosis of severe aortic stenosis.

ECHOCARDIOGRAPHY

Echocardiography is the most commonly used noninvasive diagnostic method for assessing the significance of aortic stenosis. Two-dimensional echocardiography may determine abnormal valvular motion and morphology but cannot assess the severity of aortic stenosis. Doppler echocardiography became the first noninvasive test of choice for the assessment of the severity of aortic stenosis. This method identifies increased velocity of flow across stenotic valves from which the severity of stenosis may be calculated.

The recommendations for the diagnostic use of echocardiography in symptomatic and asymptomatic patients were established by an ACC/AHA Task force in 1998.[54] In echocardiographic evaluation of aortic stenosis the purpose of examination is to: (1) define the severity and etiology of the primary valvular lesion; (2) define hemodynamics; (3) define coexisting abnormalities; (4) detect secondary lesions; (5) evaluate cardiac chamber size and function; and (6) reevaluate the patient after intervention. There are several typical and important echocardiographic findings in patients with aortic stenosis: the aortic leaflets are thickened and calcified with reduced movement; the reduced valve orifice can often be visualized; in the case of bicuspid aortic valve, the cusps are asymmetric; and the left ventricle shows significant myocardial hypertrophy with usually preserved systolic function.

Transthoracic Doppler echocardiography allows precise estimation of the transvalvular pressure gradient using a simplified Bernoulli equation:

$$\Delta P = 4 \times (VAV)^2$$

where ΔP = peak pressure gradient between the left ventricle and the aorta (mm Hg), and VAV = maximum stenotic jet velocity.

The main Doppler gradient correlates highly with the catheter-derived values. Eccentric stenotic jets may cause the underestimation of the true gradient. On the other hand, the overestimation of the gradient may result from: (1) mistaken identification of the jet; (2) inappropriate jet selection (jet of the extrasystolic beat); or (3) failure to consider subvalvular velocities (e.g., subaortic stenosis in patients with hypertrophic obstructive cardiomyopathy).

Doppler-derived velocities can be directly applied to an estimation of aortic valve area by the continuity principle. The orifice area of the stenotic valve can be calculated by this simple formula:

$$AVA = (AOT \times VOT)/VAV$$

where AVA = area of the stenotic valve, AOT = area of the left ventricular outflow tract, VOT = velocity in the outflow tract, and VAV = maximum velocity across the aortic valve.

The accuracy of this method for the estimation of the aortic valve area has been well established. The continuity equation may be expected to be less susceptible to flow variations, since the empiric constant of the Gorlin formula is avoided. However, the overestimation of the severity of stenosis in patients with severe left ventricular dysfunction and low output states remains an important clinical problem.

CARDIAC CATHETERIZATION

The accuracy and noninvasive nature of echocardiography has reduced the importance of hemodynamic measurements obtained at the time of cardiac catheterization and left ventricular angiography. Current indications include assessment of coronary circulation and confirmation or clarification of the clinical or echocardiographic diagnosis. Coronary angiography is indicated in patients undergoing aortic valve replacement who are suspected to have coronary artery disease. Combined right and left heart catheterization may be needed if there is a discrepancy between clinical and echocardiographic data, or in cases of severe biventricular failure, concomitant other valvular disease, or suspected pulmonary hypertension.

The classic method of evaluating the severity of aortic stenosis is a calculation of aortic valve area (AVA) based on Gorlin equation:

$$AVA = (SV/SEP)/(44.3(\sqrt{\Delta}P))$$

where SV = stroke volume (mL per beat), SEP = systolic ejection period, and ΔP = mean systolic pressure gradient between the left ventricle and aorta (mm Hg). The average area of the adult aortic valve is 3.0 cm^2.

Cardiac catheterization can be used to obtain several important pieces of information including: (1) number of leaflets; (2) presence of calcification; (3) presence of associated disease (coronary artery disease and poststenotic dilatation); and (4) accurate measurements of aortic valve gradients and presence and severity of aortic regurgitation.

Severe AS and low cardiac output often result in a low transvalvular pressure gradient, which makes it difficult to distinguish from low cardiac output and mild aortic stenosis. The standard Gorlin formula is known to underestimate the valve area in low flow states. In patients with low gradient stenosis and what appears to be moderate to severe aortic stenosis, it may be useful to determine the transvalvular pressure gradient and calculate the valve area during the baseline state, as well as under pharmacologically induced stress (dobutamine challenge). Alternatively, stress echocardiography can be performed.

GRADING THE DEGREE OF AORTIC STENOSIS

The normal area of the adult aortic valve measures on average 3.0 to 4.0 cm^2. Reduction of the normal area usually does not produce symptoms until it reaches one fourth of its normal dimension. Currently accepted criteria for the gradation of aortic stenosis are:

1. Mild aortic stenosis: area >1.5 cm^2
2. Moderate aortic stenosis: area 1 to 1.5 cm^2
3. Severe aortic stenosis: area <1.0 cm^2

Therapeutic decisions regarding the need for aortic valve replacement are based largely on the presence or absence of symptoms. Some patients with severe aortic stenosis may remain asymptomatic for a long period of time, while some with only moderate aortic stenosis may develop symptoms relatively early in the course of the disease. Therapeutic decisions are largely based on the absence or presence of the symptoms, rather than on the size of the aortic valve area. Natural progression of the disease usually causes the decrease in the aortic valve area by an average of 0.12 cm^2 per year. In patients with severe stenosis and preserved left ventricular function, the mean transvalvular gradient is usually higher than 50 mm Hg. The systolic pressure gradient usually increases by 15 mm Hg per year, provided that left ventricular function remains preserved. However, the variation in the rate of the progression of the disease is great, and many patients show little or no progression over a number of years.

Eventually the patient develops symptoms of syncope, heart failure, or angina. After the onset of symptoms, the average survival without aortic valve replacement is usually less than 2 to 3 years. Patients who present with heart failure have the worst prognosis, with average survival of less than 2 years. Those who present with angina and syncope have a somewhat better prognosis, with an average survival of 3 and 4 years, respectively.

Sudden death is the known, tragic outcome in some patients with aortic stenosis. Sudden death is rarely the presenting symptom of the aortic stenosis. Most patients had had some symptoms in the past. The risk of sudden death of patients with severe aortic stenosis is likely less than 1% per year.

Indications for Surgery

Aortic valve replacement is the only effective treatment for severe aortic stenosis in the adult population. Percutaneous balloon aortic valvotomy has a role in the treatment of children with aortic stenosis and in the temporization of some symptomatic adults who are poor surgical candidates.

Aortic valve replacement is usually recommended for patients who have any symptoms due to aortic stenosis in the absence of major comorbidities. Patients undergoing aortic valve replacement have an improvement in symptoms and increased survival after valve replacement surgery. Patients with moderately depressed ventricular function do as well as those with normal function. Depressed ventricular function may be due to afterload mismatch or an intrinsic depression of contractility. Both the safety and prognosis of aortic valve replacement relate to distinguishing between these two causes of reduced ventricular function. Patients with true afterload mismatch do well after aortic valve replacement despite very low ejection fractions. Depressed contractility from myocardial disease does not respond as well to aortic valve replacement. Nevertheless, patients with low ejection fractions and low wall stress often do well, with improved hemodynamics and functional status.[54,55]

Aortic valve replacement in patients without symptoms is controversial. Many authors recommend surgery only for symptomatic patients, since ventricular changes are reversible. However, others argue that there is a subset of patients with asymptomatic aortic stenosis who may be at high risk of sudden death or irreversible depression of ventricular function who may benefit from aortic valve replacement prior to the onset of symptoms. There are no clear criteria that define this subset of patients. However, many argue that an aortic valve area of 0.60 cm^2 or less, evidence of an abnormal hypotensive response to exercise or left ventricular dysfunction, ventricular tachycardia, or excessive left ventricular hypertrophy ($>$15 mm) are indications for operation. Further studies are needed to better define guidelines for this subgroup of patients.[54]

Given the high prevalence of coronary artery disease in the adult population with aortic stenosis, aortic valve replacement is also recommended in asymptomatic patients with moderate aortic stenosis (valve area 1 to 1.5 cm^2) who are undergoing concomitant coronary artery bypass surgery or other valve (typically mitral valve) or aortic root surgery.[54] Controversy currently exists are to whether asymptomatic patients with mild aortic stenosis should also undergo aortic valve replacement at the time of coronary artery bypass grafting.[56]

AORTIC REGURGITATION

Aortic regurgitation results from the improper or inadequate coaptation of the aortic valve leaflets during diastole. Inadequate closure of the valve leaflets allows previously ejected blood to flow retrograde into the left ventricle. Effective stroke volume is reduced from regurgitant blood flow. Unlike aortic stenosis, both volume and pressure overload of the left ventricular chamber occurs. Volume overload occurs secondary to regurgitant flow, while the pressure overload is due to the increased wall stress of the increased volume of blood according to the law of Laplace. Acute overload leads to immediate decompensation and signs of left-sided failure as left ventricular end-diastolic volume is exceeded. Chronic volume and pressure overload allows for compensatory changes in left ventricular volume, leading to eccentric hypertrophy of the chamber.

Prevalence and Etiology

Aortic regurgitation has numerous causes, which can be grouped according to the structural components of the valve affected. The valve leaflets may be distorted, thereby preventing proper valve coaptation. Calcific aortic disease, idiopathic degenerative disease, active or chronic aortic valve endocarditis, rheumatic disease, a biscuspid aortic valve, and myxomatous proliferation of aortic valve tissue all prevent the valve cusps from closing properly.[27,57–59] More recently, anorectic medications, such as fenfluramine and phentermine, have been found to cause aortic valve distortion from accelerated degeneration of valve leaflets leading to regurgitation similar to that seen in carcinoid syndrome.[60,61] Aortic annular dilatation will prevent the aortic cusps from closing properly as well leading to valve insufficiency. Aortic dissection; trauma; chronic systemic hypertension; aortitis from syphilis, viral syndromes, or other systemic arteritides (giant cell, Takayasu's); connective tissue disorders such as Marfan syndrome, Reiter's disease, and Ehlers-Danlos syndrome; osteogenesis imperfecta; and rheumatoid arthritis syndromes all lead to annular dilatation that causes valvular insufficiency.[57,62–67] Pure aortic regurgitation is rare and commonly seen only in aortic dissection or in pathophysiologic processes causing annular dilatation. Most commonly, aortic valvular insufficiency is seen in combination with aortic stenosis as often seen in aortic disease, rheumatic valvular disease, or myxomatous degenerative disease.

Hemodyamics

Despite the etiology, aortic regurgitation leads to similar hemodynamic consequences. With acute regurgitation, the left ventricular chamber cannot dilate rapidly and hence is unable to accommodate the large regurgitant flows. This inability to adapt is worse for the concentrically thickened hypertrophic myocardium typically seen in those with chronic hypertension. Disease states that typically present in this acute fashion include endocarditis, trauma, and aortic dissection. Even with small regurgitant volumes, left ventricular diastolic pressures increase dramatically. The mitral valve may close earlier in late diastole to reduce the amount of left atrial blood entering the ventricle, thereby preventing backflow into the left atrium and pulmonary veins. The normally widened pulse pressure of chronic aortic regurgitation is attenuated or nonexistent in the acute regurgitation due to the rapid rise in diastolic pressure.[68] Effective cardiac output is less than that of the chronic state as compensatory dilatation has not occurred and hence left ventricular end-diastolic volume remains larger than normal but small in comparison to effective stroke volume. Compensatory changes in heart rate occur, higher than those of chronic regurgitation, to augment cardiac output. Overall, the hemodyamic effects of acute aortic insufficiency produce a low effective cardiac output with an elevated diastolic ventricular pressure and heart rate, which are maintained in a precarious balance leading to the onset of early congestive heart failure with any perturbation in diastolic filling or heart rate.

Chronic aortic insufficiency allows the left ventricular chamber to develop eccentric ventricular hypertrophy to accommodate to the increased volume and pressure caused by the regurgitant flow. Consequently, large end-diastolic volumes are present. Despite these large volumes, left ventricular compliance is normal so that end-diastolic pressure is not elevated in well-compensated chronic aortic regurgitation. Left ventricular end-diastolic pressure does not approach aortic diastolic pressure, as can occur in acute insufficiency, leading to the widened pulse pressure that is an associated physical sign of this disease. Aortic regurgitation also impairs early diastolic function as eccentric hypertrophy leads to impaired left ventricular relaxation during later stages of the disease process.[69] Unlike acute aortic insufficiency, premature closure of the mitral valve does not occur. However, flutter of the anterior leaflet of the mitral valve may occur due to a Bernoulli effect.

Aortic regurgitation leads to changes in diastolic perfusion pressure, and coronary blood flow may be reduced, leading to chest pain in patients. Myocardial oxygen demands are high in hearts with aortic insufficiency due to large end-diastolic volumes and pressures, which lead to increased ventricular wall tension, according to the law of Laplace. With only a moderate reduction in aortic diastolic perfusion pressure, myocardial blood flow is usually adequate to meet the metabolic demands of the myocardium. However, with a severe reduction in diastolic pressure, a decrease in diastolic coronary perfusion occurs that is only partially compensated by increased coronary arterial flow during systole. With decreased diastolic pressure, coronary perfusion is now unable to meet the oxygen demands of the overloaded ventricular myocardium. In experimental models, diastolic aortic pressures of 40 mm Hg or less dramatically reduce coronary artery blood flow and increase myocardial ischemia as measured by lactate production.[44] Severe regurgitant flow may even lead to a reversal of diastolic coronary arterial flow. This is seen more often in degenerative and bicuspid valve disease as the morphology of the valve shapes allows for more regurgitant flow than for valves made incompetent by rheumatic disease.[70] Left ventricular hypertrophy not only increases myocardial oxygen demand but also reduces coronary artery vascular reserve in proportion to the degree of hypertrophy, most likely by compression of capillary blood flow.[71] Superimposed coronary artery disease only exacerbates the effect of decreased diastolic coronary perfusion pressure and myocardial hypertrophy.

As seen from the hemodynamic effects of aortic insufficiency, effective forward cardiac output is enhanced by any physiological changes that decrease afterload or increase heart rate, which in and of itself increases cardiac output and decreases diastolic filling time and hence regurgitant flow time. The peripheral vasodilatation and increased heart rate that accompany exercise increase effective cardiac output in this manner.[72] This is the physiologic basis for vasodilator therapy for the treatment of acute and chronic aortic insufficiency. It also becomes clear why bradycardia and negative inotropic and chronotropic agents are to be carefully used or avoided in aortic regurgitation as increased filling times leads to increased regurgitative flow and pulmonary congestion.

Ventricular Adaptations

Aortic regurgitant flow causes increased end-diastolic volume and pressure leading to wall stress, according to Laplace's law as mentioned earlier. Chronically, these changes lead to eccentric myocardial hypertrophy through myocytes adding myofibrils in series that extend the full length of each myocyte. The exact molecular and biochemical mechanisms underlying mechanical stress-induced myocardial hypertrophy are unknown. Recent advances in molecular biology have shown that mechanical stress activates numerous protein kinases, such as calcium-dependent protein kinase and calcineurin, a calcium-dependent phosphatase that is the target of cyclosporine.[31,73] The activation of these kinases results in the induction of various vasoactive peptides, including angiotensin II, neuregulin, and other growth factors leading to increased myofibril production and decreased degradation at a cellular level and consequent hypertrophy.[42] Clearly, differences exist at the molecular and cellular level in the differing pathways resulting in eccentric versus concentric hypertrophy. Myocyte hypertrophy in response to pressure overload, as in aortic stenosis, leads to an increase in the rate of myofibrillar protein synthesis and occurs rapidly within three days. However, in chronic aortic regurgitation, the increase in myofibrillar protein content in 1 month is not due to increased rate of synthesis but decreased rate of degradation.[74] These divergent pathways are only now beginning to be elucidated. It is hoped that with better understanding of these molecular responses, new therapeutic agents can be found to target these pathways and modulate the course of the disease.

Although the exact molecular and cellular responses to increased wall stress are unclear, the myocardial response is not. Myofibril addition in series in each myocyte leads to increases in the left ventricular internal diameter and the length to width ratio of each myocyte changes to accommodate increasing left ventricular volume.[75] Initially, ventricular wall thickness remains unchanged. As systolic stress within the ventricular gradually increases, the ventricle hypertrophies with subsequent reduction of wall stress.[75,76] The adaptive process of progressive left ventricular dilatation and increasing wall thickness creates an enormous ventricular chamber. This large chamber is capable of generating total (not effective) cardiac outputs as high as 20 L/min in well-compensated chronic aortic regurgitation with normal or near-normal ejection fractions.

With continued dilatation from untreated aortic regurgitation, fibrosis develops within the myocardium, possibly as a result of subclinical ischemia, myofibrillar degeneration, or myocyte apoptosis triggered by increasing ventricular dilatation and mediated through death proteins, such as the mitochondrial death protein Nix.[41] With continued fibrosis, left ventricular compliance diminishes, as well as the likelihood of postoperative return of cardiac function. Severe myocardial fibrosis also correlates with metabolic deficiencies that include the mitochondrial enzymes ATP and succinyl dehydrogenase. These enzyme deficiencies and increased myocardial fibrosis portend poor prognosis but are not predictive.[77]

As aortic insufficiency progresses, the preload reserve of the left ventricle is eventually reached. Thereafter, any further increase in afterload creates afterload mismatch. In general, patients with aortic insufficiency have slightly depressed ventricular function when compared to normal subjects if ventricular function is evaluated in terms of end-systolic pressure-volume relationships (ESPVR). A depressed ejection fraction with a near-normal ESPVR indicates afterload mismatch.[78] Hence, ejection fraction may not be a good indicator of ventricular function.[79] However, a depressed ejection fraction with a depressed ESPVR indicates intrinsic myocardial disease, especially in patients with large end-systolic and end-diastolic volumes. At this stage, prolonged aortic insufficiency has lead to further increases in wall stress without compensatory hypertrophy, leading to eventual myofibrillar slippage. Subsequent molecular events lead to fibrosis and irreversible changes in ventricular function.

It is at this point in the natural history of aortic insufficiency when valve replacement will not improve cardiac function. Identifying these patients is somewhat difficult at the clinical level. Ejection fraction alone is a poor indicator of postoperative functional recovery because it depends on preload and afterload. Irreversible changes decrease both the ejection fraction and the ability to develop peak systolic stress in relation to chamber size. Attempts to identify these patients include studies illustrating that patients with left ventricular end-systolic volumes exceeding 60 mL/m^2 remain in functional class IV postoperatively. Other studies have suggested that when the ratio of chamber volume to wall thickness exceeds 3.8, postoperative recovery may be compromised.[80] This ratio is indicative of progressive dilatation with myofibrillar slippage. Some echocardiographic studies have found that an end-systolic left ventricular dimension of greater than 55 mm and a fractional shortening of less than 25% are associated with decreased ventricular recovery postoperatively and increased mortality.[81] This is based on the belief that left ventricular end-systolic volume is an indicator of left ventricular function. Other studies have refuted this finding, but current guidelines recommend aortic valve replacement in asymptomatic patients when left ventricular end-systolic volume is greater than 55 mm.[54]

Signs and Symptoms

Physical exam findings of aortic regurgitation vary with the chronicity of the disease process. The widened pulse pressure seen in chronic aortic regurgitation results from the augmentation of total cardiac output that leads to the distention of the peripheral arterial system followed by a quick collapse from regurgitant flow. This leads to many classic physical findings such as a "waterhammer" pulse (Corrigan's pulse), head bobbing with each heartbeat (DeMusset's sign), and capillary pulsations at the lips and fingers (Quincke's pulses). Other findings are associated with congestive heart failure if present (rales, S_3, etc).[82] Many of the classic signs and symptoms of chronic aortic insufficiency are absent in the acute manifestation of this valvular disorder. In acute insufficiency, as discussed earlier, pulse pressure is not widened and hence the signs associated with this pathologic physiology are absent. Instead, the signs of acute congestive heart failure predominate.

Patients with compensated aortic regurgitation remain asymptomatic for prolonged periods of time. However, with ventricular decompensation occurring with large regurgitant volumes, patients may experience palpitations, an awareness of each heartbeat especially at the ventricular apex, or atypical chest pain syndromes.[82] Chest pain is rare in aortic insufficiency, unlike aortic stenosis. The eccentric hypertrophic myocardium of compensated aortic insufficiency is by no means as thick as that of aortic stenosis, leading to lower degrees of increased oxygen requirement, and the coronary circulation is maximally dilated. However, turbulent flow patterns and diminished diastolic perfusion pressure may at some point lead to insufficient coronary and myocardial perfusion. Most symptoms of aortic insufficiency occur from underlying heart failure and pulmonary congestion as the ventricular chamber decompensates.

Diagnostic Evaluation

Often, the signs and symptoms of aortic insufficiency are all that is needed to make the diagnosis. However, if additional testing is required for diagnosis or quantification of the severity of disease, other diagnostic tests can be employed including electrocardiograms (ECG), echocardiography, magnetic resonance imaging (MRI), and cardiac catheterization, which are discussed below.

ELECTROCARDIOGRAPHY

Chronic aortic regurgitation results in left axis deviation. Q waves in leads I, V_1, and V_3 to V_6 are indicative of diastolic volume overload.[83] Left ventricular conduction defects are usually associated with left ventricular dysfunction. The QRS amplitude is linearly correlated with left ventricular mass. The finding of a strain pattern in relation to a reduction in the QRS amplitude is indicative of severe depression of ejection fraction and contractility.[84] Overall, the ECG is not an accurate predictor of the severity of aortic regurgitation.

ECHOCARDIOGRAPHY

Echocardiography is the most useful diagnostic modality in the both the initial diagnosis and continued monitoring of patients with aortic regurgitation. Transthoracic echocardiography (TTE) is the most commonly used imaging tool. Transesophageal echocardiography (TEE) is invasive and used only when patient body habitus does not allow for adequate assessment of the valvular function or when evaluation of aortic valve and ascending aorta is needed in a patient with suspected aortic dissection. TTE is indispensable in the diagnosis of the presence and degree of aortic insufficiency, its etiology, valve morphology, and presence of vegetations and calcification, the quantification of pulmonary hypertension, and determination of ventricular function. But most importantly, it allows for the noninvasive monitoring of valvular disease and left ventricular function in asymptomatic patients. This is critically important in determining the timing of surgery in asymptomatic patients prior to the onset of permanent ventricular decompensation.

The etiology of aortic insufficiency is defined by failure of leaflets to coapt versus stiffness of fibrotic or calcified leaflets. The quality of the regurgitant murmur is evaluated by color-flow techniques. Measurements of end-systolic and end-diastolic volumes, as well as measurements of wall thickness, can be obtained. These measurements are useful for determining irreversible changes in left ventricular function.[84–87] Premature closure of the mitral valve, as seen in acute aortic regurgitation, can be recognized. Fluttering of the anterior mitral leaflet from regurgitant flow may also occur during diastole and can be appreciated. This is a sensitive indicator of both acute and chronic aortic regurgitation. Although fluttering of the open mitral valve is classically seen during diastole, fluttering also may occur with the mitral valve closed. Fluttering of the posterior mitral valve leaflet is also described.[88]

MAGNETIC RESONANCE IMAGING

With current improvements in MRI technology, MRI cineangiography is able to provide some the same information provided by TTE and TEE. MRI in some aspects provides superior resolution of the valves and better quantification of regurgitant flow and left ventricular function. However, MRI is costly and expertise is not available in most centers. Future improvements in technology may reduce costs and increase its availability, thereby making it a standard imaging modality along with or replacing echocardiography.[89–91]

CARDIAC CATHETERIZATION

Cardiac catheterization is important to estimate the severity of aortic insufficiency if echocardiographic studies are equivocal or there is concomitant coronary artery disease. The amount of regurgitant flow can be determined by calculating the angiographic stroke volume minus a measured fixed stroke volume. The difference between these two measured volumes divided by the angiographic stroke volume determines the regurgitant fraction. In general, a regurgitant fraction less than 20% is 1+ aortic insufficiency. An increase in regurgitant fraction to 60% corresponds to 4+ insufficiency.[92] Left ventricular end-diastolic pressure is measured directly, and ejection fraction is estimated roughly. Radionucleotide imaging with ventriculography can be substituted for angiography if there is a contradiction to cardiac catherization or serial follow-up of patients is required.[54] This imaging modality, like echocardiography, allows for the noninvasive monitoring of aortic insufficiency and ventricular function, although it does not visualize the valvular apparatus directly.

Indications for Operation

Acute aortic regurgitation is treated by early valve replacement. With inadequate time for the left ventricle to compensate by myocardial hypertrophy, progressive congestive heart failure, tachycardia, and diminished cardiac output ensue rapidly.

Compensated chronic aortic regurgitation is well tolerated by most patients.[93,94] Aortic valve replacement is currently not recommended for patients who are asymptomatic, even with severe chronic aortic regurgitation. These patients, however, must have normal ventricular function and good exercise tolerance. In asymptomatic patients, aortic valve replacement is indicated for deteriorating ventricular function.[54,95] An ejection fraction of less than 55% with a diastolic diameter approaching 75 mm or an end-systolic diameter approaching 55 mm is an indication for operation.[54,81,96–99]

Predictive indicators of impending symptoms in asymptomatic patients are not available. One potential indicator is measurement of left ventricular wall stress at rest and after exercise. Some studies have shown that patients with increased wall stress during exercise develop decompensated left ventricular failure within 5 years.[100] Aortic valve replacement is indicated if patients develop symptoms of congestive heart failure or decreased exercise tolerance. However, decreased ejection fraction during exercise is not a good measure to indicate need for valve replacement in asymptomatic patients with normal systolic function at rest. The lack of correlation between exercise ejection fraction and need for operation lies in the fact that exercise ejection fraction depends on multiple factors and no studies have shown conclusive proof showing that exercise ejection fraction is either linked with mortality preoperatively or is of prognostic value postoperatively.

Ideally, aortic valve replacement should be performed before irreversible myocardial damage from myocyte apoptosis with resulting fibrosis occurs. Although patients with impaired ventricular function are at an increased perioperative risk, survival is prolonged when compared to patients undergoing medical management. Nonoperative management of patients with severe aortic regurgitation and abnormal left ventricular function is associated with a 50% mortality in 1 year.[101] Risk factors for postoperative mortality include a radius-to-wall thickness ratio of 3.8 or greater.[80,102] However, despite aortic valve replacement, impaired left ventricular dysfunction may continue in some. These patients are difficult to identify preoperatively and their hearts as expected show increased interstitial fibrosis.

In those patients in whom ventricular remodeling occurs after aortic valve replacement, the regression of left ventricular dimension and cross-sectional area can take as long as three years. The best predictor for persistent, postoperative left ventricular enlargement is preoperative enlargement of the end-diastolic dimension, but this measurement is not always predictive of outcome. Duration of symptoms of left ventricular dysfunction preoperatively is also an indicator for poor reversibility of ventricular function postoperatively.[103]

Early postoperative studies of left ventricular size and function reveal that end-diastolic volumes decrease significantly with valve replacement. With the decrease in preload, subsequent ejection fraction decreases; however, if the operation is correctly timed, ejection fraction eventually recovers to near-normal values in selected patients.[55,104] Further recovery includes regression of myocardial hypertrophy, reduction in left ventricular size, normalization of the mass/volume ratio, and increased diastolic coronary flow.[105,106] If improvement is going to occur after aortic valve replacement, it occurs within the first 6 months as the ventricular end-diastolic dimension decreases. A decrease in the peak systolic wall stress and increase in ejection fraction also occur within the first six months.[2,107–109]

REFERENCES

1. Anderson RH, Devine WA, Ho SY, et al: The myth of the aortic annulus: the anatomy of the subaortic outflow tract. *Ann Thorac Surg* 1991; 52:640.
2. Broom ND: The Third George Swanson Christie memorial lecture. Connective tissue function and malfunction: a biomechanical perspective. *Pathology* 1988; 20:93.
3. Vesely I: The role of elastin in aortic valve mechanics. *J Biomech* 1998; 31:115.
4. Deck JD: Endothelial cell orientation on aortic valve leaflets. *Cardiovasc Res* 1986; 20:760.
5. Thubrikar MJ, Nolan SP, Aouad J, Deck JD: Stress sharing between the sinus and leaflets of canine aortic valve. *Ann Thorac Surg* 1986; 42:434.
6. Zimmerman J: The functional and surgical anatomy of the aortic valve. *Isr J Med Sci* 1969; 5:862.
7. Deck JD, Thubrikar MJ, Schneider PJ, Nolan SP: Structure, stress, and tissue repair in aortic valve leaflets. *Cardiovasc Res* 1988; 22:7.
8. Thubrikar M, Harry R, Nolan SP: Normal aortic valve function in dogs. *Am J Cardiol* 1977; 40:563.
9. Gnyaneshwar R, Kumar RK, Komarakshi RB: Dynamic analysis of the aortic valve using a finite element model. *Ann Thorac Surg* 2002; 73:1122.
10. Mercer JL: The movements of the dog's aortic valve studied by high speed cineangiography. *Br J Radiol* 1973; 46:344.
11. Jones CJ, Sugawara M: "Wavefronts" in the aorta—implications for the mechanisms of left ventricular ejection and aortic valve closure. *Cardiovasc Res* 1993; 27:1902.
12. Sabbah HN, Stein PD: Investigation of the theory and mechanism of the origin of the second heart sound. *Circ Res* 1976; 39:874.
13. Segadal L, Matre K: Blood velocity distribution in the human ascending aorta. *Circulation* 1987; 76:90.
14. Von Bernuth G, Tsakiris AG, Wood EH: Effects of variations in the strength of left ventricular contraction on aortic valve closure in the dog. *Circ Res* 1971; 28:705.
15. Koppensteiner R, Moritz A, Moidl R, et al: Blood rheology in patients with native heart valve disease and after valve replacement. *Am J Cardiol* 1998; 81:250.
16. Otto CM: Aortic stenosis; clinical evaluation and optimal timing of surgery. *Cardiol Clin* 1998; 16:354.
17. Otto CM: *Valvular Heart Disease*. Philadelphia, W.B. Saunders, 1999; p 135.
18. Epperlein S, Mohr-Kahaly S, Erbel R, et al: Aorta and aortic valve morphologies predisposing to aortic dissection: an in vivo assessment with transoesophageal echocardiography. *Eur Heart J* 1994; 15:1520.
19. Otto CM, Kuusisto J, Reichenbach DD, et al: Characterization of the early lesion of "degenerative" valvular aortic stenosis: histological and immunohistochemical studies. *Circulation* 1994; 90:844.
20. Olsson M, Dalsgaard CJ, Haegerstrand A, et al: Accumulation of T lymphocytes and expression of interleukin-2 receptors in nonrheumatic stenotic aortic valves. *J Am Coll Cardiol* 1994; 23:1162.
21. Robicsek F, Thubrikar MJ, Fokin AA: Cause of degenerative disease of the trileaflet aortic valve: review of subject and presentation of a new theory. *Ann Thorac Surg* 2002; 73:1346.
22. Passik CS, Ackermann DM, Pluth JR, Edwards WD: Temporal changes in the causes of aortic stenosis: a surgical pathologic study of 646 cases. *Mayo Clin Proc* 1987; 62:119.

23. Mohler ER 3rd, Adam LP, McClelland P, Detection of osteopontin in calcified human aortic valves. *Arterioscler Thromb Vasc Biol* 1997; 17:547.
24. Hultgren HN: Osteitis deformans (Paget's disease) and calcific disease of the heart valves. *Am J Cardiol* 1998; 81:1461.
25. Maher ER, Young G, Smyth-Walsh B, et al: Aortic and mitral valve calcification in patients with end-stage renal disease. *Lancet* 1987; 2:875.
26. Hangaishi M, Taguchi J, Ikari Y, et al: Aortic valve stenosis in alkaptonuria: images in cardiovascular medicine. *Circulation* 1998; 98:1148.
27. Roberts WC, Morrow AG, McIntosh CL, et al: Congenitally bicuspid aortic valve causing severe, pure aortic regurgitation without superimposed infective endocarditis: analysis of 13 patients requiring aortic valve replacement. *Am J Cardiol* 1981; 47:206.
28. Clark C: The propagation of turbulence produced by a stenosis. *J Biomech* 1980; 13:591.
29. Pasipoularides A, Murgo JP, Bird JJ, Craig WE: Fluid dynamics of aortic stenosis: mechanisms for the presence of subvalvular pressure gradients. *Am J Physiol* 1984; 246:H542.
30. Clark C: Turbulent wall pressure measurements in a model of aortic stenosis. *J Biomech* 1977; 10:461.
31. Zhou YQ, Faerestrand S, Matre K: Velocity distributions in the left ventricular outflow tract in patients with valvular aortic stenosis: effect on the measurement of aortic valve area by using the continuity equation. *Eur Heart J* 1995; 16:383.
32. Boughner DR, Roach MR: Effect of low frequency vibration on the arterial wall. *Circ Res* 1971; 29:136.
33. Komuro I, Yazaki Y: Control of cardiac gene expression by mechanical stress. *Annu Rev Physiol* 1993; 55:55.
34. Komuro I, Katoh Y, Kaida T, et al: Mechanical loading stimulates cell hypertrophy and specific gene expression in cultured rat cardiac myocytes: possible role of protein kinase C activation. *J Biol Chem* 1991; 266:1265.
35. Komuro I, Kaida T, Shibazaki Y, et al: Stretching cardiac myocytes stimulates protooncogene expression. *J Biol Chem* 1990; 265:3595.
36. Schunkert H, Jahn L, Izumo S, et al: Localization and regulation of c-fos and c-jun protooncogene induction by systolic wall stress in normal and hypertrophied rat hearts. *Proc Natl Acad Sci U S A* 1991; 88:11480.
37. Chien KR, Knowlton KU, Zhu H, Chien S: Regulation of cardiac gene expression during myocardial growth and hypertrophy: molecular studies of an adaptive physiologic response. *FASEB J* 1991; 5:3037.
38. Hannan RD, Stennard FA, West AK: Expression of c-fos and related genes in the rat heart in response to norepinephrine. *J Mol Cell Cardiol* 1993; 25:1137.
39. Mansier P, Chevalier B, Mayoux E, et al: Membrane proteins of the myocytes in cardiac overload. *Br J Clin Pharmacol* 1990; 30(suppl 1):43S.
40. Fifer MA, Borow KM, Colan SD, Lorell BH: Early diastolic left ventricular function in children and adults with aortic stenosis. *J Am Coll Cardiol* 1985; 5:1147.
41. Yussman MG, Toyokawa T, Odley A, et al: Mitochondrial death protein Nix is induced in cardiac hypertrophy and triggers apoptotic cardiomyopathy. *Nat Med* 2002; 8:725.
42. Rohrbach S, Yan X, Weinberg EO, et al: Neuregulin in cardiac hypertrophy in rats with aortic stenosis: differential expression of erbB2 and erbB4 receptors. *Circulation* 1999; 100:407.
43. Alyono D, Anderson RW, Parrish DG, et al: Alterations of myocardial blood flow associated with experimental canine left ventricular hypertrophy secondary to valvular aortic stenosis. *Circ Res* 1986; 58:47.
44. Griggs DM Jr, Chen CC, Tchokoev VV: Subendocardial anaerobic metabolism in experimental aortic stenosis. *Am J Physiol* 1973; 224:607.
45. Brazier JR, Buckberg GD: Effects of tachycardia on the adequacy of subendocardial oxygen delivery in experimental aortic stenosis. *Am Heart J* 1975; 90:222.
46. Isaaz K, Bruntz JF, Paris D, et al: Abnormal coronary flow velocity pattern in patients with left ventricular hypertrophy, angina pectoris, and normal coronary arteries: a transesophageal Doppler echocardiographic study. *Am Heart J* 1994; 128:500.
47. Villari B, Hess OM, Meier C, et al: Regression of coronary artery dimensions after successful aortic valve replacement. *Circulation* 1992; 85:972.
48. Kimball BP, LiPreti V, Bui S, Wigle ED: Comparison of proximal left anterior descending and circumflex coronary artery dimensions in aortic valve stenosis and hypertrophic cardiomyopathy. *Am J Cardiol* 1990; 65:767.
49. Reichek N, Devereux RB: Left ventricular hypertrophy: relationship of anatomic, echocardiographic and electrocardiographic findings. *Circulation* 1981; 63:1391.
50. Johnson LL, Sciacca RR, Ellis K, et al: Reduced left ventricular myocardial blood flow per unit mass in aortic stenosis. *Circulation* 1978; 57:582.
51. Grover GJ, Scholz PM, Mackenzie JW, Weiss HR: Effect of aortic stenosis on oxygen balance in partially ischemic myocardium. *Ann Thorac Surg* 1987; 43:270.
52. Hongo M, Goto T, Watanabe N, et al: Relation of phasic coronary flow velocity profile to clinical and hemodynamic characteristics of patients with aortic valve disease. *Circulation* 1993; 88:953.
53. Carroll RJ, Falsetti HL: Retrograde coronary artery flow in aortic valve disease. *Circulation* 1976; 54:494.
54. Bonow RO, Carabello B, de Leon AC Jr, et al: Guidelines for the management of patients with valvular heart disease: executive summary. A report of the American College of Cardiology/American Heart Association Task Force on Practice Guidelines (Committee on Management of Patients with Valvular Heart Disease). *Circulation* 1998; 98:1949.
55. Boucher CA, Bingham JB, Osbakken MD, et al: Early changes in left ventricular size and function after correction of left ventricular volume overload. *Am J Cardiol* 1981; 47:991.
56. Filsoufi F, Aklog L, Adams DH, Byrne JG: Management of mild to moderate aortic stenosis at the time of coronary artery bypass grafting. *J Heart Valve Dis* 2002; 11(suppl 1):S45.
57. Waller B: Rheumatic and nonrheumatic conditions producing valvular heart disease, in Frankl W, Brest AN (eds): *Cardiovascular Clinics: Valvular Heart Disease: Comprehensive Evaluation and Management*. Philadelphia, FA Davis, 1986, p 30.
58. Tonnemacher D, Reid C, Kawanishi D, et al Frequency of myxomatous degeneration of the aortic valve as a cause of isolated aortic regurgitation severe enough to warrant aortic valve replacement. *Am J Cardiol* 1987; 60:1194.
59. Stein PD, Sabbah HN: Turbulent blood flow in the ascending aorta of humans with normal and diseased aortic valves. *Circ Res* 1976; 39:58.
60. Mast ST, Jollis JG, Ryan T, et al: The progression of fenfluramine-associated valvular heart disease assessed by echocardiography. *Ann Intern Med* 2001; 134:261.
61. Khan MA, Herzog CA, St Peter JV, et al: The prevalence of cardiac valvular insufficiency assessed by transthoracic echocardiography in obese patients treated with appetite-suppressant drugs. *N Engl J Med* 1998; 339:713.
62. Carter JB, Sethi S, Lee GB, Edwards JE: Prolapse of semilunar cusps as causes of aortic insufficiency. *Circulation* 1971; 43:922.
63. Roberts WC: Aortic dissection: anatomy, consequences, and causes. *Am Heart J* 1981; 101:195.

64. Roldan CA, Chavez J, Wiest PW, et al: Aortic root disease and valve disease associated with ankylosing spondylitis. *J Am Coll Cardiol* 1998; 32:1397.
65. Roldan CA: Valvular disease associated with systemic illness. *Cardiol Clin* 1998; 16:531.
66. Heppner RL, Babitt HI, Bianchine JW, Warbasse JR: Aortic regurgitation and aneurysm of sinus of Valsalva associated with osteogenesis imperfecta. *Am J Cardiol* 1973; 31:654.
67. Emanuel R, Ng RA, Marcomichelakis J, et al: Formes frustes of Marfan's syndrome presenting with severe aortic regurgitation: clinicogenetic study of 18 families. *Br Heart J* 1977; 39:190.
68. Reimold SC, Maier SE, Fleischmann KE, et al: Dynamic nature of the aortic regurgitant orifice area during diastole in patients with chronic aortic regurgitation. *Circulation* 1994; 89:2085.
69. Rousseau MF, Pouleur H, Charlier AA, Brasseur LA: Assessment of left ventricular relaxation in patients with valvular regurgitation. *Am J Cardiol* 1982; 50:1028.
70. Grayburn PA, Eichhorn EJ, Eberhart RC, et al: Aortic valve morphology influences regurgitant volume in aortic regurgitation: in vitro evaluation. *Cardiovasc Res* 1991; 25:73.
71. Pichard AD, Smith H, Holt J, et al: Coronary vascular reserve in left ventricular hypertrophy secondary to chronic aortic regurgitation. *Am J Cardiol* 1983; 51:315.
72. Slordahl SA, Piene H: Haemodynamic effects of arterial compliance, total peripheral resistance, and glyceryl trinitrate on regurgitant volume in aortic regurgitation. *Cardiovasc Res* 1991; 25:869.
73. Sussman MA, Lim HW, Gude N, et al: Prevention of cardiac hypertrophy in mice by calcineurin inhibition. *Science* 1998; 281:1690.
74. Magid NM, Wallerson DC, Borer JS: Myofibrillar protein turnover in cardiac hypertrophy due to aortic regurgitation. *Cardiology* 1993; 82:20.
75. Feiring AJ, Rumberger JA: Ultrafast computed tomography analysis of regional radius-to-wall thickness ratios in normal and volume-overloaded human left ventricle. *Circulation* 1992; 85:1423.
76. Magid NM, Wallerson DC, Borer JS, et al: Left ventricular diastolic and systolic performance during chronic experimental aortic regurgitation. *Am J Physiol* 1992; 263:H226.
77. Donaldson RM, Florio R, Rickards AF, et al: Irreversible morphological changes contributing to depressed cardiac function after surgery for chronic aortic regurgitation. *Br Heart J* 1982; 48:589.
78. Branzi A, Lolli C, Piovaccari G, et al: Echocardiographic evaluation of the response to afterload stress test in young asymptomatic patients with chronic severe aortic regurgitation: sensitivity of the left ventricular end-systolic pressure-volume relationship. *Circulation* 1984; 70:561.
79. Wisenbaugh T, Spann JF, Carabello BA: Differences in myocardial performance and load between patients with similar amounts of chronic aortic versus chronic mitral regurgitation. *J Am Coll Cardiol* 1984; 3:916.
80. Gaasch WH, Carroll JD, Levine HJ, Criscitiello MG: Chronic aortic regurgitation: prognostic value of left ventricular end-systolic dimension and end-diastolic radius/thickness ratio. *J Am Coll Cardiol* 1983; 1:775.
81. Henry WL, Bonow RO, Borer JS, et al: Observations on the optimum time for operative intervention for aortic regurgitation, I: evaluation of the results of aortic valve replacement in symptomatic patients. *Circulation* 1980; 61:471.
82. DeGowin RL, DeGowin EL, Brown DD, Christensen J: *DeGowin & DeGowin's Diagnostic Examination*. New York, McGraw-Hill, 1994; pp xix, 1033.
83. Schamroth L, Schamroth CL, Sareli P, Hummel D: Electrocardiographic differentiation of the causes of left ventricular diastolic overload. *Chest* 1986; 89:95.
84. Scognamiglio R, Fasoli G, Bruni A, Dalla-Volta S: Observations on the capability of the electrocardiogram to detect left ventricular function in chronic severe aortic regurgitation. *Eur Heart J* 1988; 9:54.
85. Aurigemma G, Whitfield S, Sweeney A, et al: Color Doppler mapping of aortic regurgitation in aortic stenosis: comparison with angiography. *Cardiology* 1992; 81:251.
86. Bouchard A, Yock P, Schiller NB, et al: Value of color Doppler estimation of regurgitant volume in patients with chronic aortic insufficiency. *Am Heart J* 1989; 117:1099.
87. Enriquez-Sarano M, Bailey KR, Seward JB, et al: Quantitative Doppler assessment of valvular regurgitation. *Circulation* 1993; 87:841.
88. Chia BL: Mitral valve fluttering in aortic insufficiency. *J Clin Ultrasound* 1981; 9:198.
89. Wyttenbach R, Bremerich J, Saeed M, Higgins CB: Integrated MR imaging approach to valvular heart disease. *Cardiol Clin* 1998; 16:277.
90. Wisenbaugh T, Essop R, Middlemost S, et al: Excessive vasoconstriction in rheumatic mitral stenosis with modestly reduced ejection fraction. *J Am Coll Cardiol* 1992; 20:1339.
91. Schwitter J: Valvular heart disease: assessment of valve morphology and quantification using MR. *Herz* 2000; 25:342.
92. Holm S, Eriksson P, Karp K, et al: Quantitative assessment of aortic regurgitation by combined two-dimensional, continuous-wave and colour flow Doppler measurements. *J Intern Med* 1992; 231:115.
93. Goldschlager N, Pfeifer J, Cohn K, et al: The natural history of aortic regurgitation. A clinical and hemodynamic study. *Am J Med* 1973; 54:577.
94. Bonow RO, Rosing DR, McIntosh CL, et al: The natural history of asymptomatic patients with aortic regurgitation and normal left ventricular function. *Circulation* 1983; 68:509.
95. Bonow RO, Epstein SE: Is preoperative left ventricular function predictive of survival and functional results after aortic valve replacement for chronic aortic regurgitation? *J Am Coll Cardiol* 1987; 10:713.
96. Pugliese P, Negri A, Muneretto C, et al: Aortic insufficiency: a multivariate analysis of incremental risk factors for operative mortality and functional results. *J Cardiovasc Surg* (Torino) 1990; 31:213.
97. Grossman W: Aortic and mitral regurgitation: how to evaluate the condition and when to consider surgical intervention. *JAMA* 1984; 252:2447.
98. Carabello BA: The changing unnatural history of valvular regurgitation. *Ann Thorac Surg* 1992; 53:191.
99. Bonow RO, Lakatos E, Maron BJ, Epstein SE: Serial long-term assessment of the natural history of asymptomatic patients with chronic aortic regurgitation and normal left ventricular systolic function. *Circulation* 1991; 84:1625.
100. Percy RF, Miller AB, Conetta DA: Usefulness of left ventricular wall stress at rest and after exercise for outcome prediction in asymptomatic aortic regurgitation. *Am Heart J* 1993; 125:151.
101. Aronow WS: Usefulness of M-mode, 2-dimensional, and Doppler echocardiography in the diagnosis, prognosis, and management of valvular aortic stenosis, aortic regurgitation, and mitral annular calcium in older patients. *J Am Geriatr Soc* 1995; 43:295.
102. Borow KM: Surgical outcome in chronic aortic regurgitation: a physiologic framework for assessing preoperative predictors. *J Am Coll Cardiol* 1987; 10:1165.
103. Bonow RO, Rosing DR, Maron BJ, et al: Reversal of left ventricular dysfunction after aortic valve replacement for chronic aortic regurgitation: influence of duration of preoperative left ventricular dysfunction. *Circulation* 1984; 70:570.

104. Borer JS, Rosing DR, Kent KM, et al: Left ventricular function at rest and during exercise after aortic valve replacement in patients with aortic regurgitation. *Am J Cardiol* 1979; 44:1297.
105. Schuler G, Peterson KL, Johnson AD, et al: Serial noninvasive assessment of left ventricular hypertrophy and function after surgical correction of aortic regurgitation. *Am J Cardiol* 1979; 44:585.
106. Fujiwara T, Nogami A, Masaki H, et al: Coronary flow characteristics of left coronary artery in aortic regurgitation before and after aortic valve replacement. *Ann Thorac Surg* 1988; 46:79.
107. Bonow RO, Dodd JT, Maron BJ, et al: Long-term serial changes in left ventricular function and reversal of ventricular dilatation after valve replacement for chronic aortic regurgitation. *Circulation* 1988; 78:1108.
108. Bonow RO, Picone AL, McIntosh CL, et al: Survival and functional results after valve replacement for aortic regurgitation from 1976 to 1983: impact of preoperative left ventricular function. *Circulation* 1985; 72:1244.
109. Broom N, Christie, GW: The structure/function relationship of fresh and glutaraldehyde-fixed aortic valve leaflets, in Cohn L, Gallucci V (eds): *Cardiac Bioprostheses: Proceedings of the 2nd International Symposium*. New York, Yorke Medical, 1982; p 477.

Chapter 31

Aortic Valve Repair and Aortic Valve-Sparing Operations

Tirone E. David

FUNCTIONAL ANATOMY OF THE AORTIC VALVE

The aortic valve is a complex structure that is best described as a functional and anatomic unit called the aortic root. The aortic root has four components: aortic annulus, aortic cusps, aortic sinuses (sinuses of Valsalva), and sinotubular junction.

The aortic annulus unites the aortic cusps and aortic sinuses to the left ventricle. The aortic annulus is attached to ventricular myocardium (interventricular septum) in approximately 45% of its circumference and to fibrous structures (mitral valve and membranous septum) in the remaining 55% (Fig. 31-1). The aortic annulus has a scalloped shape. Histologic examination of the aortic annulus reveals that it is a fibrous structure with strands attaching itself to the muscular interventricular septum and has a fibrous continuity with the anterior leaflet of the mitral valve and membranous septum. The fibrous tissue that separates the aortic root from the mitral valve is called intervalvular fibrous body. An important structure immediately below the membranous septum is the bundle of His. The atrioventricular node lies in the floor of the right atrium between the annulus of the septal leaflet of the tricuspid valve and the coronary sinus. This node gives origin to the bundle of His, which travels through the right fibrous trigone along the posterior edge of the membranous septum to the muscular interventricular septum. At this point the bundle of His divides into left and right bundle branches that extend subendocardially along both sides of the interventricular septum.

The aortic cusps are attached to the aortic annulus in a scalloped fashion (see Fig. 31-1). The aortic cusps have a semilunar shape whereby the length of the base is approximately 1.5 times longer than the length of the free margin, as illustrated in Figure 31-2. There are three aortic cusps and three aortic sinuses: left, right, and noncoronary. The aortic sinuses are also referred to as sinuses of Valsalva. The left coronary artery arises from the left aortic sinus and the right coronary artery arises from the right aortic sinus. The left coronary artery orifice is closer to the aortic annulus than is the right coronary artery orifice. The highest point where two cusps meet is called the commissure, and it is located immediately below the sinotubular junction. The scalloped shape of the aortic annulus creates three triangular spaces

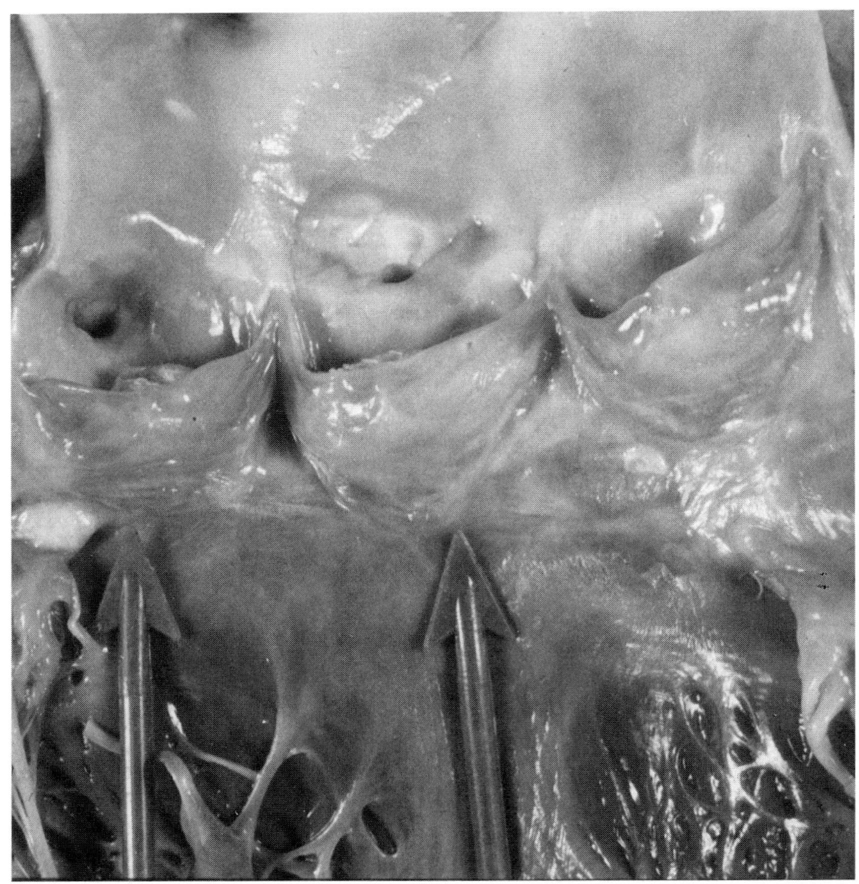

FIGURE 31–1 A photograph of a human open left ventricular outflow tract and aortic root. *(Reproduced from David TE: Aortic valve repair for management of aortic insufficiency. Adv Card Surg 1999; 11:129, with permission from Mosby Inc.)*

underneath the commissures. The two triangles beneath the commissures of the noncoronary cusp are fibrous structures, whereas the triangular space beneath the commissure between the right and left aortic cusps is muscular. These three triangles are seen in Figure 31-1. The sinotubular junction is the end of the aortic root. It is an important component of the aortic root because the commissures of the aortic cusps are immediately below it.

The geometry of the aortic root and its anatomic components varies among individuals, but the geometry of these components is somewhat interrelated.[1–4] For instance, the larger the aortic cusps, the larger are the diameters of the aortic annulus and sinotubular junction.[4] The aortic cusps are semilunar (crescent shaped), their bases are attached to the annulus, the free margins extend from commissure to commissure, and the cusps coapt centrally during diastole. The size of the aortic cusps varies among individuals and within the same person, but as a rule the noncoronary cusp is slightly larger than the right and left. The left is usually the smallest of the three. Because of the crescent shape of the aortic cusps and the fact that their free margins extend from commissure to commissure, the diameter of the aortic orifice must be smaller than the length of the free margins. Indeed, anatomic studies of fresh human aortic roots demonstrated

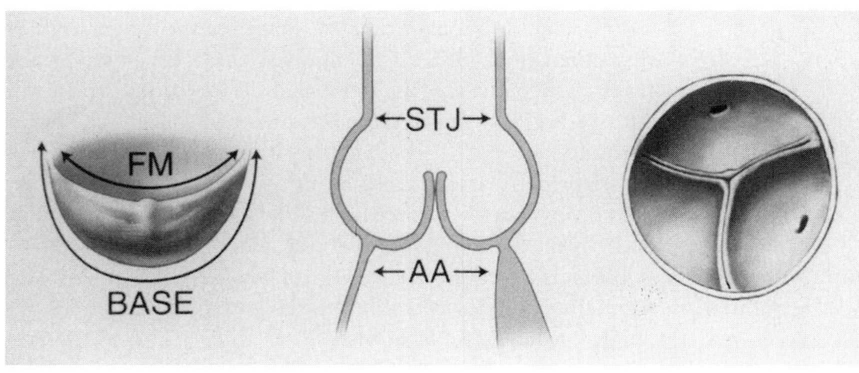

FIGURE 31–2 Geometric relationships of various components of the aortic root. The base of the aortic cusp is 1.5 times longer than its free margin. The diameter of the aortic annulus is 10% to 15% larger than the diameter of the sinotubular junction, but it tends to become equal with aging. Three semilunar cusps seal the aortic orifice. *(Reproduced from David TE: Aortic valve repair for management of aortic insufficiency. Adv Card Surg 1999; 11:129, with permission from Mosby Inc.)*

that the average length of the free margins of the aortic cusps was one-third longer than the diameter of the aortic orifice.[1]

The diameter of the aortic annulus is 15% to 20% larger than the diameter of the sinotubular junction in normal aortic roots of young persons, but these diameters tend to become equal in older ones. All components of the aortic root are very elastic and compliant in young patients but this compliance decreases with age as elastic fibers are replaced by fibrous tissue.

The aortic annulus, the aortic cusps, and the sinotubular junction play an important role in maintaining valve competence. On the other had, the aortic sinuses play no role in valve competence,[5] but they are believed to be important in minimizing mechanical stress on the aortic cusps during the cardiac cycle.[2]

AORTIC VALVE PATHOLOGY IN ADULTS

Anatomically normal aortic cusps may become calcified late in life and cause aortic stenosis. This type of lesion is called dystrophic calcification, senile calcification, or degenerative calcification. The range of histopathologic lesions includes calcification, chondroid and osseous metaplasia, neorevascularization, inflammation, and lipid deposition.[6] The pathogenesis of this lesion is not well understood. Aging is certainly the most important epidemiologic factor.[6–9] Degenerative calcification is an active inflammatory process with similarities and dissimilarities to atherosclerosis.[7–9] Aging and high levels of lipoprotein *a* were found to be correlated with aortic valve sclerosis.[7] Degenerative calcification of the aortic valve is the most common cause of aortic stenosis in elderly patients in North America.[10,11]

Bicuspid aortic valve is common and occurs in 1% to 2% of the population.[12] It usually functions satisfactorily and does not cause hemodynamic problems until late in life when it becomes calcified and stenotic. Calcified bicuspid aortic valve is the second most common cause of aortic stenosis in elderly patients.[10] Bicuspid aortic valve can also cause aortic insufficiency, particularly in young patients in whom mild to moderate dilation of the aortic root is often present.[13] Most patients with bicuspid aortic valve have three aortic sinuses. The two cusps are of different sizes and the larger one often contains a raphe instead of a commissure. The raphe extends from the mid portion of the cusp to the aortic annulus, and its insertion in the aortic root is at a lower level than the other two commissures. Bicuspid aortic valves with two aortic sinuses and no raphe are uncommon. The right coronary artery is nondominant in most patients with a bicuspid aortic valve.

Unicusp aortic valve is another congenital anomaly of the aortic valve. It often contains only one commissure and causes aortic stenosis. Bicuspid and unicusp aortic valves are frequently associated with premature degenerative changes of the media of the aortic root and ascending aorta. They increase the risk of aneurysms and type A aortic dissection.[14]

Quadricusp aortic valve is a rare anomaly that may cause aortic insufficiency. Three of the four cusps are usually of similar size and the other is hypoplastic.

Subaortic membranous ventricular septal defect with aortic insufficiency is uncommon in adults. The interventricular septal defect causes distortion of the aortic annulus, and the right aortic cusp is often elongated and may prolapse and cause aortic insufficiency.

Dilation of the aortic root is the most common cause of aortic insufficiency in North America.[10–11] Older patients with ascending aortic aneurysm may develop aortic insufficiency because of dilation of the sinotubular junction. The aortic sinuses and aortic annulus may remain relatively normal in these patients. Aortic aneurysm in young patients usually begins with dilation of the aortic sinuses, which progresses into the sinotubular junction and ultimately the aortic annulus. Annuloaortic ectasia is a term used to describe dilation of the aortic annulus. Aortic root aneurysm is common in patients with Marfan syndrome.

Aortic dissections involving the ascending aorta can cause aortic insufficiency because of preexisting aortic root aneurysm or by detachment of one or more commissures with consequent prolapse of the cusps.[15]

Rheumatic aortic valve disease is still prevalent in developing countries. The rheumatic process causes fibrosis, thickening, and contraction of the aortic cusps, often with commissural fusion. In advanced cases, the valve becomes calcified. It is possible that some postinflammatory aortic valve lesions are not rheumatic in origin.[16]

Numerous connective tissue disorders (ankylosing spondylitis, osteogenesis imperfecta, rheumatoid arthritis, Reiter's syndrome, lupus, etc.) can cause aortic insufficiency. The anorexigenic drugs phentermine and fenfluramine can also cause aortic insufficiency.[16]

NATURAL HISTORY OF AORTIC VALVE DISEASE

Aortic Stenosis

Several studies showed that asymptomatic patients with aortic stenosis have a good prognosis.[17,18] Sudden death in asymptomatic patients is uncommon.[18] However, when symptoms develop, the prognosis becomes poor and the average survival is 2 to 3 years for patients with symptoms of angina or syncope, and 1 to 2 years for those who develop congestive heart failure.[19]

Aortic Insufficiency

The prognosis of symptomatic patients is poor with death occurring within 4 years after development of angina and within 2 years after the onset of congestive heart failure.[20] Since aortic insufficiency may cause ventricular damage, asymptomatic patients should be operated on when ventricular function begins to deteriorate.

INDICATIONS FOR AORTIC VALVE SURGERY

Aortic Stenosis

Patients with symptoms should be considered for surgery. Asymptomatic patients with an aortic valve area of less than 0.8 cm^2 or a mean systolic gradient greater than 50 mm Hg with left ventricular hypertrophy should also be considered for surgery if it can be performed with low operative risk. An echocardiographic flow velocity across the aortic valve greater than 4 m/s is also indication for surgery.[21]

Aortic Insufficiency

Symptomatic patients should be operated on. Asymptomatic patients should also be operated on when left ventricular function begins to deteriorate.[22]

Aortic Root Aneurysm

Patients with aortic root aneurysm with or without Marfan syndrome should undergo surgery when the aortic root diameter reaches 55 mm.[23] If an aortic valve-sparing operation is likely to be feasible, the operation is justifiable when the aneurysm reaches 50 mm in diameter.[24] Patients with Marfan syndrome and a family history of aortic dissection should also have surgery when the diameter of the aortic root reaches 50 mm even if a valve-sparing procedure is not feasible.[25]

Ascending Aortic Aneurysm

Patients with ascending aortic aneurysm should undergo surgery when the transverse diameter reaches 60 mm.[26] If moderate or severe aortic insufficiency is present and the valve is deemed repairable, surgery should be performed before the diameter reaches 60 mm to avoid further damage to the aortic cusps.

SELECTION OF PATIENTS FOR AORTIC VALVE SURGERY

Only a small proportion of adult patients with aortic valve disease are candidates for aortic valve repair. Stenotic aortic valves, particularly senile calcific valves, are not suitable for aortic valve repair. However, mechanical decalcification of a mildly or moderately stenotic aortic valve is sometimes possible in patients in whom the primary indication for operation is myocardial revascularization. The calcific deposits should be limited to small segments of the aortic cusps and most areas should be free of calcification. Decalcification of these valves should be done mechanically and care must be exercised to avoid damage to the cusps. The calcium on the annulus should also be removed to make it more pliable. Long-term therapy with cholesterol-lowering agents may prevent recurrence of the aortic stenosis. Ultrasonic decalcification of aortic valve often causes scarring with retraction of the cusps and aortic insufficiency within a few months after surgery and it has been largely abandoned.[27]

Incompetent aortic valves due to dilation of one or more components of the aortic root or due to aortic cusp prolapse are amenable to aortic valve-conserving procedures. Since surgery in asymptomatic patients with aortic insufficiency is justifiable if the aortic valve can be repaired, it is important to identify these patients preoperatively. Transesophageal echocardiography is the best tool to study the aortic root and determine the mechanism of aortic insufficiency.[28] The echocardiographer has to carefully interrogate each component of the aortic valve in multiple views to evaluate the number, quality, and morphology of the aortic cusps as well as to measure the diameters of the aortic annulus, aortic sinuses, sinotubular junction, and ascending aorta. In addition, the height of the cusps and the level of their coaptation should be measured. The most important information needed is related to the thickness, mobility, and general appearance of the aortic cusps.

Aortic insufficiency due to prolapse of one cusp, regardless of whether the valve has three or two cusps, is amenable to valve repair if the cusps are thin, pliable, and without calcification. Rugged and thickened free margins usually preclude a good repair. Cusp prolapse can also be caused by acute type A aortic dissection. Echocardiography not only diagnoses the dissection, but it also can aid the surgeon in planning the type of procedure in the aortic root.[15]

Dilation of the sinotubular junction in patients with ascending aortic aneurysm may cause aortic insufficiency by pulling the cusps apart, as shown in Figure 31-3. The aortic annulus is usually normal in these patients. Aortic valve repair is certainly feasible if transesophageal echocardiography shows the aortic cusps to be thin, mobile, and without calcification.

Aneurysm of the aortic root is the most common indication for aortic valve-sparing operations. These patients may or may not have aortic insufficiency and, when insufficiency is present, the cusps may already be overstretched or contain stress fenestrations in their commissural areas and their free margins may be elongated. Patients with aortic root aneurysm and mild or no aortic insufficiency are better candidates for aortic valve-sparing than patients with more severe aortic insufficiency.

TECHNIQUES OF AORTIC VALVE REPAIR

Cusp Perforation

Occasionally a cusp perforation is the sole reason for aortic insufficiency. The perforation may be iatrogenic, a sequelae of healed endocarditis, or the result of resection of a papillary fibroelastoma. A simple patch of fresh or glutaraldehyde-fixed autologous pericardium has been adequate to correct the problem.

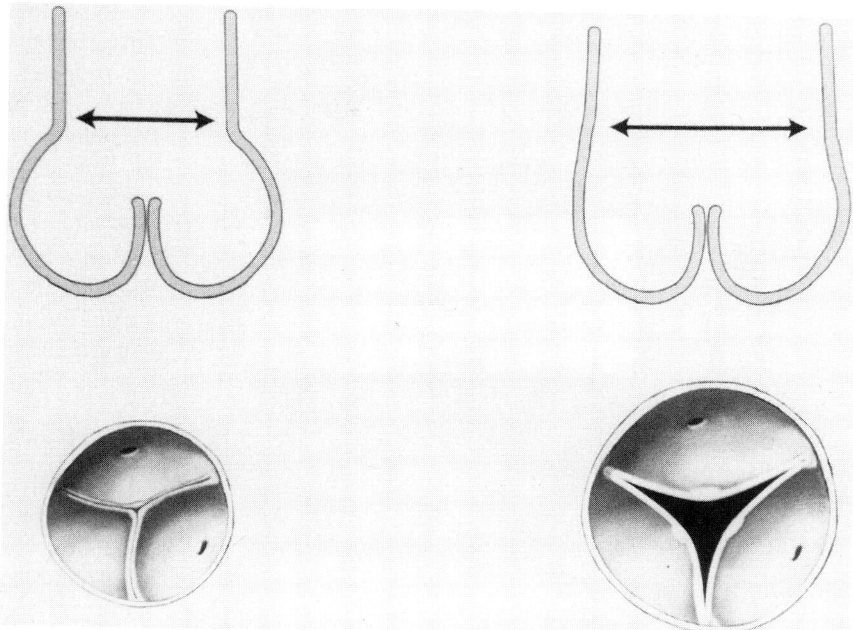

FIGURE 31–3 Dilation of the sinotubular junction pulls the aortic cusps apart and causes aortic insufficiency. *(Reproduced from David TE: Aortic valve repair for management of aortic insufficiency. Adv Card Surg 1999; 11:129, with permission from Mosby Inc.)*

Cusp Extension

Cusp extension has been used to repair rheumatic aortic insufficiency. Glutaraldehyde-fixed bovine or autologous pericardium has been used for this purpose.[29]

Cusp Prolapse

Isolated prolapse of a single cusp in adult patients with a tricuspid aortic valve is rare. Repair is accomplished by plication of the elongated free margin of the cusp (Fig. 31-4). The prolapsed cusp is usually thicker than normal and simple interrupted sutures with a 5-0 polypropylene are adequate. If the cusp is very thin, it may be safer to use mattressed sutures on pledgets of autologous pericardium. If the subcommissural triangles of the prolapsing cusps appear widened, they can be reduced with plicating sutures, leaving the knots on the outside of the left ventricular outflow tract. If the free margin is thinned and overstretched, it can be reinforced and shortened with a double layer of a 6-0 expanded polytetrafluoroethylene suture (Fig. 31-5).

Bicuspid Aortic Valve

The most commonly performed aortic valve repair in adults is for congenitally bicuspid aortic valve with prolapse of one of the cusps. Although the anatomic arrangement of bicuspid

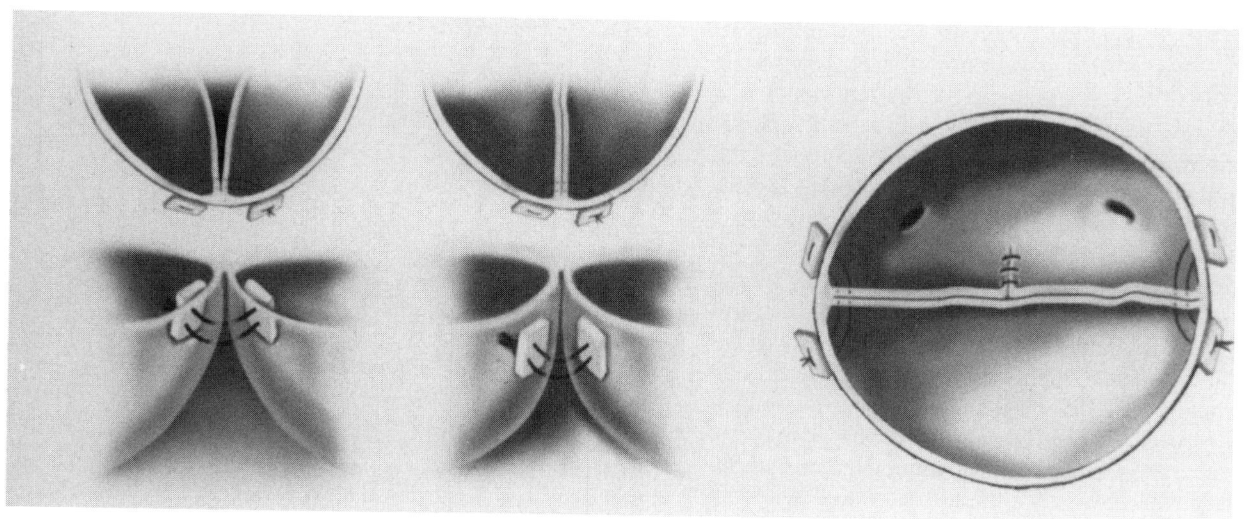

FIGURE 31–4 Repair of cusp prolapse.

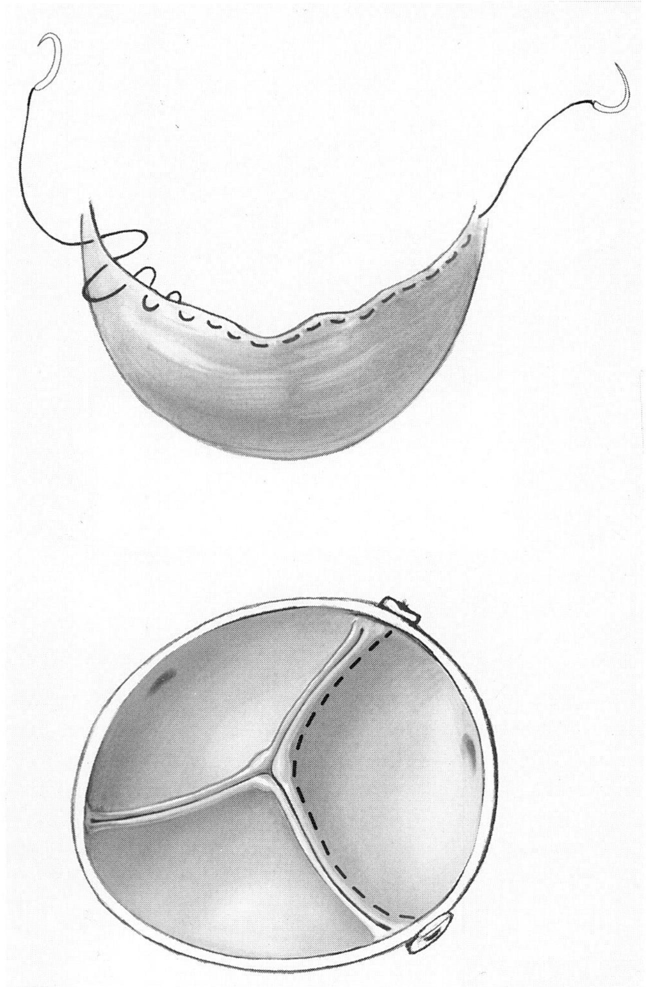

FIGURE 31–5 Reinforcement of the free margin of the aortic cusp with a single or double layer of a fine suture of expanded polytetrafluoroethylene.

aortic valves varies, most patients have an anterior cusp attached to the interventicular septum and a posterior cusp attached to the fibrous components of the left ventricular outflow tract. The anterior cusp often contains a raphe at approximately where the commissure between the right and left cusps would be. This cusp is usually the one that is elongated and prolapsed. As long as the posterior cusp is normal, repair is feasible and relatively simple. The raphe is excised and the free margin of the anterior cusp is shortened with plicating sutures (see Fig. 31-4). The lengths of the free margins of both cusps should be the similar and should coapt at the same level. This is determined by passing a suture through the arterial wall immediately above each of the two commissures, and then pulling them upward and gently apart.

Since most of these patients have some degree of annuloaortic ectasia, the two subcommissural triangles should also be plicated if possible to reduce the diameter of the aortic annulus and increase coaptation of the aortic cusps. This can be done with horizontal mattress sutures of 4-0 polypropylene with Teflon felt pledgets on the outside of the aortic root (see Fig. 31-4). The suture is initially passed from the outside to the inside of the aortic root 2 or 3 mm below the commissure and 1 mm above the aortic annulus into the aortic sinus, and then through the annulus of both cusps and outside of the aorta. The same suture is brought back 4 or 5 mm below that level on both sides of the annulus and the ends are tied together on the outside of the aorta. If the aortic root diameter exceeds 45 mm, the sinuses should be excised and an aortic valve-sparing operation performed.

AORTIC VALVE-SPARING OPERATIONS

"Aortic valve-sparing operations" encompass various procedures used to preserve the aortic valve in patients with ascending aortic aneurysm and aortic insufficiency or aortic root aneurysm with or without aortic insufficiency.[30–33] The complexity of these operations varies with the pathologic process. Sometimes all that is needed is a simple reduction in the diameter of the sinotubular junction, which is often the case in older patients with ascending aortic aneurysm and normal aortic sinuses and aortic annulus. Other times more extensive procedures, which may include an aortic

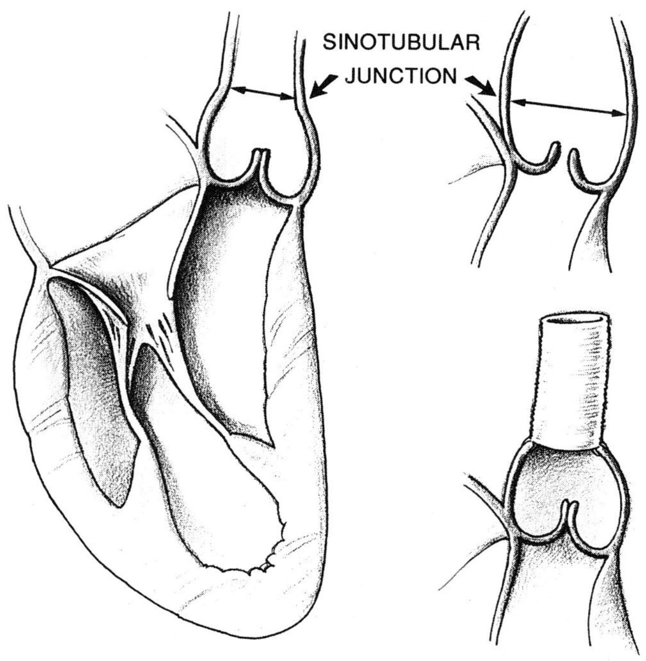

FIGURE 31–6 Simple adjustment of the diameter of the sinotubular junction by a graft of appropriate diameter corrects aortic insufficiency in patients with ascending aortic aneurysm if the aortic cusps are normal. *(Reproduced from David TE, Feindel CM, Bos J: Repair of the aortic valve in patients with aortic insufficiency and aortic root aneurysm. J Thorac Cardiovasc Surg 1995; 109:345, with permission from Mosby Inc.)*

annuloplasty, replacement of the aortic sinuses, reimplantation of the coronary arteries, adjustment of the sinotubular junction, and correction of aortic cusp prolapse, are needed in young patients with aortic root aneurysm.

Ascending Aortic Aneurysm with Aortic Insufficiency

Dilation of the sinotubular junction displaces the commissures of the aortic valve outward and prevents the cusps from coapting during diastole (see Fig. 31-3). Most of these patients have normal or mildly stretched aortic cusps. If the aortic sinuses and annulus are not dilated, simple adjustment of the sinotubular junction restores aortic valve competence. This is accomplished by transecting the ascending aorta 5 mm above the commissures and pulling the three commissures upward and close to each other until the aortic cusps coapt. The three commissures form a triangle. The diameter of the circle that includes this triangle is the diameter of the graft that should be used to remodel the sinotubular junction. Because the aortic cusps frequently have different sizes, this triangle is not always equilateral and the commissures must be spaced according to the length of the free margin of each cusp. The diameter of the graft and the space between commissures are facilitated by sizing the diameter of the circle that contains all three commissures with a transparent valve sizer, such as the one for the Toronto SPV bioprosthesis (St Jude Medical, St Paul, MN). That particular sizer has three equidistant marks, and one can determine the space between the commissures by comparing to the distance between the marks. The tubular Dacron graft is sutured right at the level of the sinotubular junction with a continuous 4-0 polypropylene (Fig. 31-6). If after adjusting the sinotubular junction, one aortic cusp appears to prolapse, shortening of its free margin should be performed as described above. Valve competence can be checked at this time by injecting cardioplegia solution into the graft under pressure and observing the left ventricle for distension.

Grafts smaller than 24 mm in diameter should be avoided in these patients because they may increase left ventricular afterload, particularly if long segments are used, such as with concomitant transverse arch replacement using the elephant trunk technique. If the estimated diameter of the sinotubular junction is less than 24 mm, a larger graft should be used, and the end that is anastomosed to the sinotubular junction reduced to the necessary diameter.

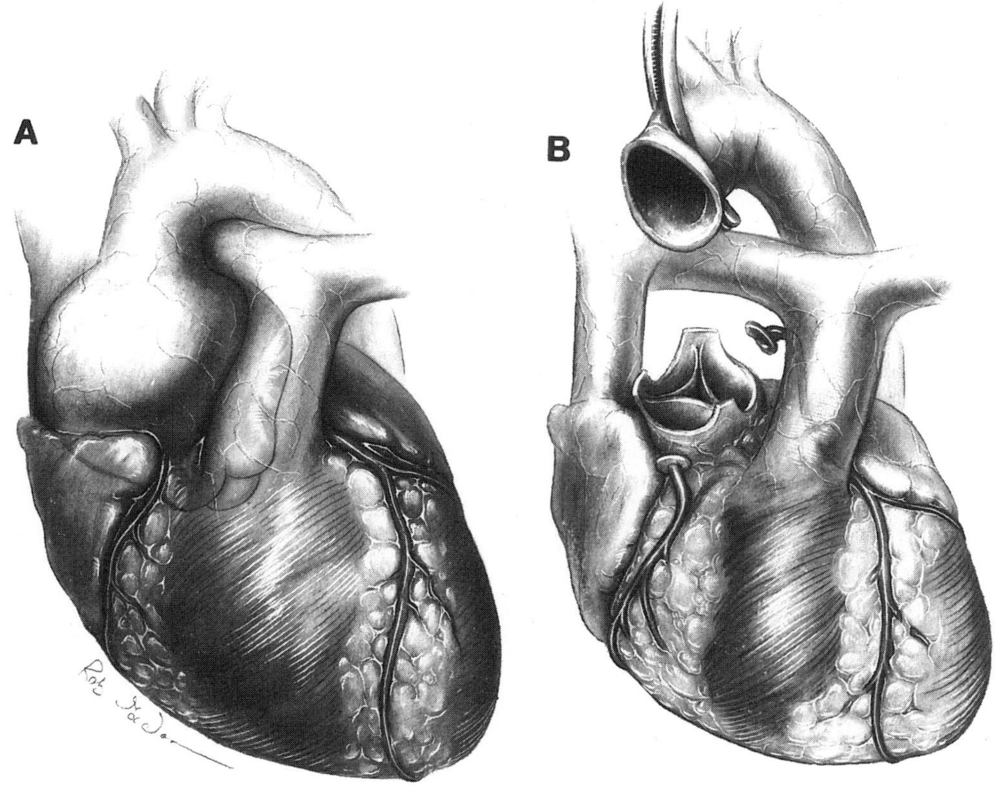

FIGURE 31–7 (A) Remodeling of the aortic root for aortic root aneurysm. (B) The aortic sinuses are excised. *(Reproduced from David TE: Remodeling of the aortic root with preservation of the native aortic valve. Op Tech Cardiac Thorac Surg 1996; 1:44, with permission from WB Saunders.)*

Aortic Root Aneurysm

Patients with aortic root aneurysm can have the aortic cusps preserved during surgery as long as they are reasonably normal. A common problem with these cusps is that stress fenestration may appear near the commissural areas. As long as the tissues are of good quality, it is possible to reinforce the free margins of the cusps and preserve the native valve (see Fig. 31-5). Although it is not always simple to determine intraoperatively if an aortic cusp is elongated or not, a fair estimation is obtained by pulling all three commissures vertically and approximating them to each other until the cusps coapt. The coaptation level should be well above the level of the aortic annulus, and if one cusp is elongated it can be identified. It is important to maintain the normal scalloped shape of the aortic annulus while the commissures are pulled upward.

Assessing dilation of the aortic annulus is even more difficult than assessing cusp prolapse. The aortic orifice is sealed by three aortic cusps, and the larger the cusps, the larger the aortic annulus. The geometric relationship between these two components of the aortic root is variable, but the diameter of the annulus must be smaller than the average lengths of the free margins of the aortic cusps and the radius of the annulus must be smaller than the height of the cusps. Using these two parameters, it is possible to estimate whether the annulus is dilated or not.

There are two general types of aortic valve-sparing operations for patients with aortic root aneurysms: remodeling of the aortic root and reimplantation of the aortic valve.[31]

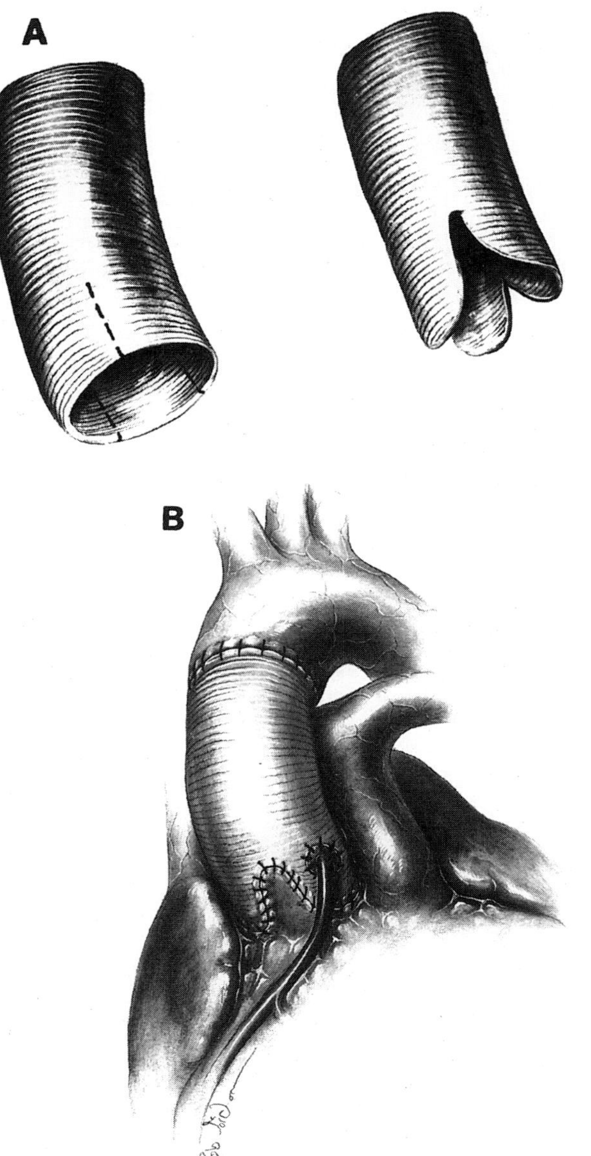

FIGURE 31–8 **(A) A tubular Dacron graft is tailored to create three neo-aortic sinuses. (B) The complete repair.** *(Reproduced from David TE: Remodeling of the aortic root with preservation of the native aortic valve. Op Tech Cardiac Thorac Surg 1996; 1:44, with permission from WB Saunders.)*

REMODELING OF THE AORTIC ROOT

After the aorta is cross-clamped, the ascending aorta is transected and the aortic root is dissected circumferentially down to the level of the aortic annulus. All three aortic sinuses are excised, leaving approximately 4 to 6 mm of arterial wall attached all around the aortic annulus, as shown in Figure 31-7. If it the aortic annulus is not dilated, the three commissures are gently pulled vertically and approximated until the cusps coapt. The three commissures form a triangle and the diameter of the circle that contains that triangle is the diameter of the graft to be used for remodeling. Here again the sizers of the Toronto SPV are very useful to determine the diameter of the graft and also the distance between commissures, because they may not be equidistant. The spaces in between the commissures are marked in one of the ends of the graft, and the graft is tailored to create three neoaortic sinuses (Fig. 31-8A). The heights of these neosinuses should be approximately equal to the diameter of the graft. The three commissures are suspended in the graft (Fig. 31-9A), which is then sutured to the aortic annulus and remnants of the aortic wall with a continuous 4-0 polypropylene suture (Fig. 31-9B). After suturing the Dacron graft to the aortic annulus, the coronary arteries are reimplanted into their respective neoaortic sinuses. The three aortic cusps are then examined and their central coaptation evaluated. If one or more cusps appear to prolapse, the free margin should be shortened as described above. The coronary arteries are reimplanted into their sinuses. Aortic valve competence can be assessed by injecting cardioplegia under pressure into the graft and observing the left ventricle for distension. The graft is then anastomosed to the distal ascending aorta or transverse aortic arch graft depending on the extent of the aneurysm (Fig. 31-8B).

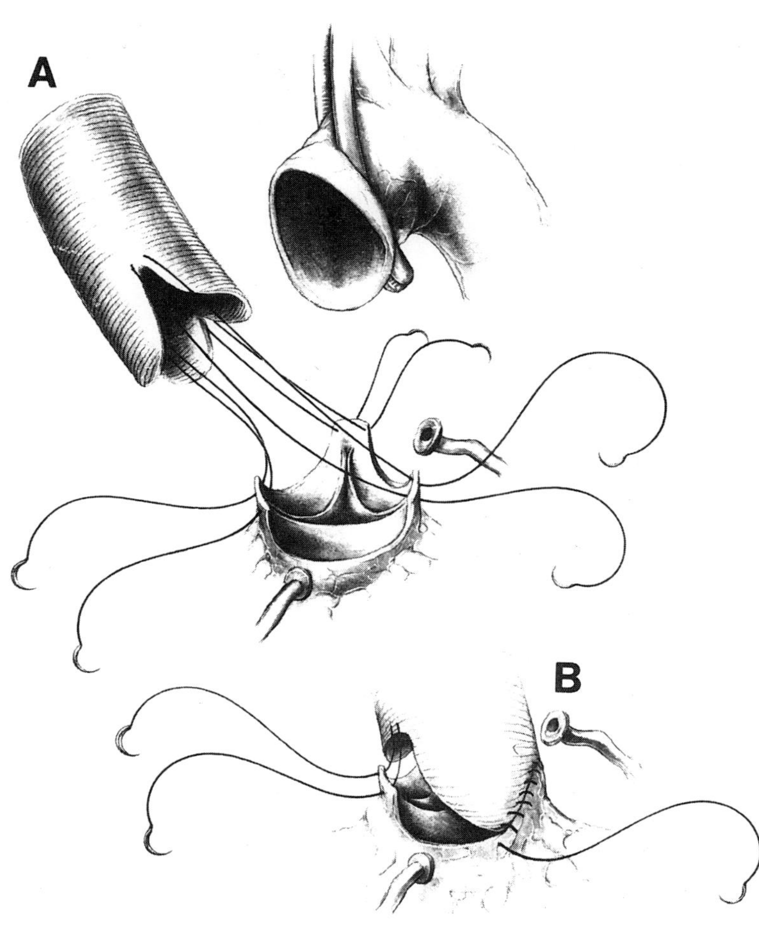

FIGURE 31–9 (A) The three commissures are secured to the tailored end of the Dacron graft, and (B) the neo-aortic sinuses are sutured to the aortic annulus and remnants of the aortic sinuses. *(Reproduced from David TE: Remodeling of the aortic root with preservation of the native aortic valve. Op Tech Cardiac Thorac Surg 1996; 1:44, with permission from WB Saunders.)*

If the patient has Marfan syndrome or annuloaortic ectasia, an aortic annuloplasty is necessary before the remodeling procedure is performed. A band of Dacron fabric is sutured on the outside of the ventricular outflow tract (Fig. 31-10). Multiple interrupted horizontal mattress sutures are placed through a single horizontal plane on the fibrous components of the left ventricular outflow tract and through the Dacron band. Most of the dilation of the aortic annulus occurs beneath the commissures of the noncoronary cusps. The aortic annulus should be reduced to a diameter approximately 20% less than the average lengths of the free margins of the aortic cusps and to a radius equal to approximately two thirds of the average heights of the aortic cusps. Clinical experience has demonstrated that these estimates of the diameter of the aortic annulus appear to correct the problem of annular dilation. Figure 31-11 illustrates the completed procedure.

REIMPLANTATION OF THE AORTIC VALVE

This procedure can be performed in all patients with aortic root aneurysm, but it is particularly valuable in patients with annuloaortic ectasia and in those with acute type A aortic dissection. The three aortic sinuses are excised as described for the remodeling procedure. Multiple horizontal mattress sutures of 3-0 or 4-0 polyester are passed from the inside to the outside of the left ventricular outflow tract, immediately below the nadir of the aortic annulus, through a single horizontal plane along the fibrous portion of the outflow tract and along its scalloped shape in the interventricular septum (Fig. 31-12). If the fibrous portion is thin, sutures with small Teflon felt pledgets should be used. Next, the three commissures are pulled vertically and approximated to each other until the cusps coapt, in order to estimate the diameter of the sinotubular junction. A tubular graft with a diameter 3 or 4 mm larger than the estimated diameter of the sinotubular junction is selected, and three equidistant marks are placed in one of its ends to correspond approximately to each commissure. If one cusp is larger than the others, the distance between the three marks should reflect that. A small triangular wedge is trimmed off in the mark that corresponds to the commissure between the left and right cusps (Fig. 31-12). The polyester sutures passed through the left ventricular outflow tract are then passed through the graft from the inside to the outside, making an effort to space them correctly. One should remember that most of the dilation of the aortic annulus occurs beneath the commissures of the noncoronary

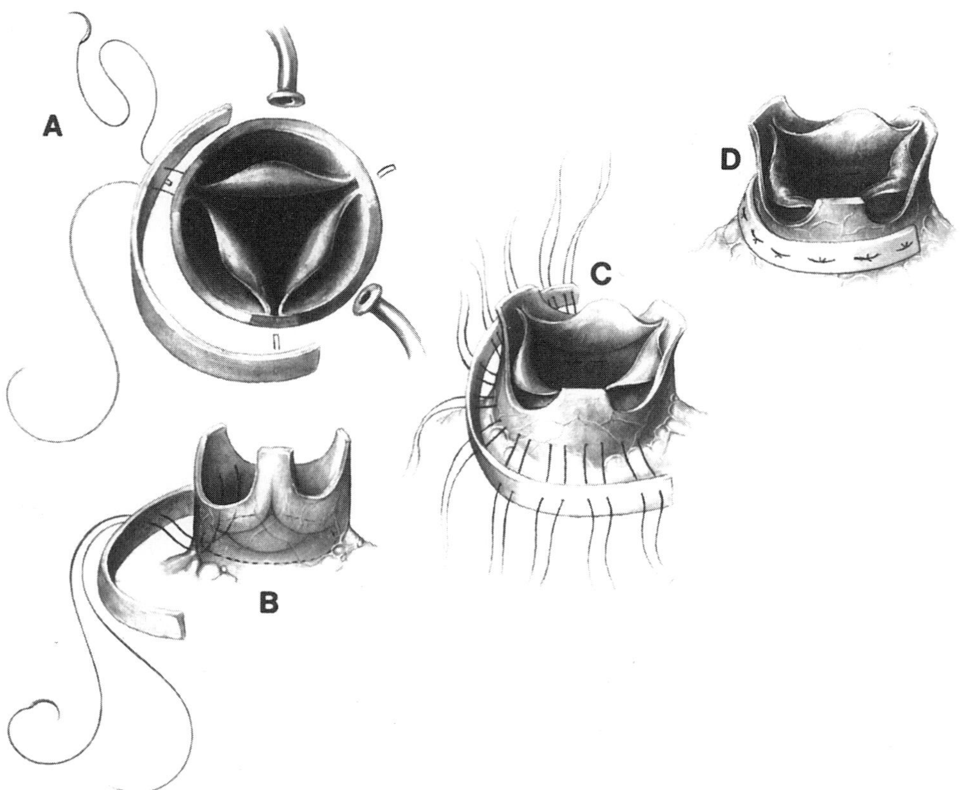

FIGURE 31–10 Aortic annuloplasty: a strip of Dacron fabric is secured to the fibrous components of the left ventricular outflow tract, immediately below the aortic annulus (A, B, C, and D). *(Reproduced from David TE: Remodeling of the aortic root with preservation of the native aortic valve. Op Tech Cardiac Thorac Surg 1996; 1:44, with permission from WB Saunders.)*

cusp, and if any annular reduction is needed, those are the areas in which to do it. The sutures are tied on the outside of the graft. Care must be exercised not to purse-string this suture line. The graft is then cut in a length of approximately 6 to 7 cm and pulled upward gently, and the three commissures are pulled vertically and secured to the graft with transfixing 4-0 polypropylene sutures, but they are not tied. The appropriate position of the commissures is determined by observing the aortic cusps and the level of the free margins and where they coapt. If all three commissures are on a correct level, the remnants of the aortic wall are sutured to the graft using a full-thickness, transfixing continuous suture. The coronary arteries are reimplanted into their respective neosinuses (Fig. 31-13). The spaces between commissures immediately above their highest point is plicated to create neosinuses. For every 3 mm that are plicated, the diameter of the sinotubular junction is reduced by 1 mm. The coaptation level of the aortic cusps is checked again and valve competence can be assessed by injecting cardioplegia under pressure into the graft and observing the left ventricle for distension. The graft is then sutured to the distal ascending aorta or to the graft used to replace the transverse aortic arch.

RESULTS OF AORTIC VALVE SURGERY

Bicuspid Aortic Valve Repair

The largest published series on aortic valve repair for aortic insufficiency due to prolapse of bicuspid valve is from the Cleveland Clinic.[34,35] Investigators from that institution reported on 94 patients with a mean age of 38 years. The freedom from reoperation was 84% at 7 years.[35] The only factor predictive of reoperation was residual aortic insufficiency after the repair. There was no operative mortality in that series. Our experience with repair of bicuspid aortic valve is limited to 45 patients over the past decade. Six of them also required reconstruction of the aortic root. There were no operative or late deaths. During a mean follow-up of 3.7 years, one patient required aortic root replacement after cusp repair with remodeling of the aortic root.

Ascending Aortic Aneurysm with Aortic Insufficiency

We recently reported our experience with aortic valve-sparing operations in patients with ascending aortic

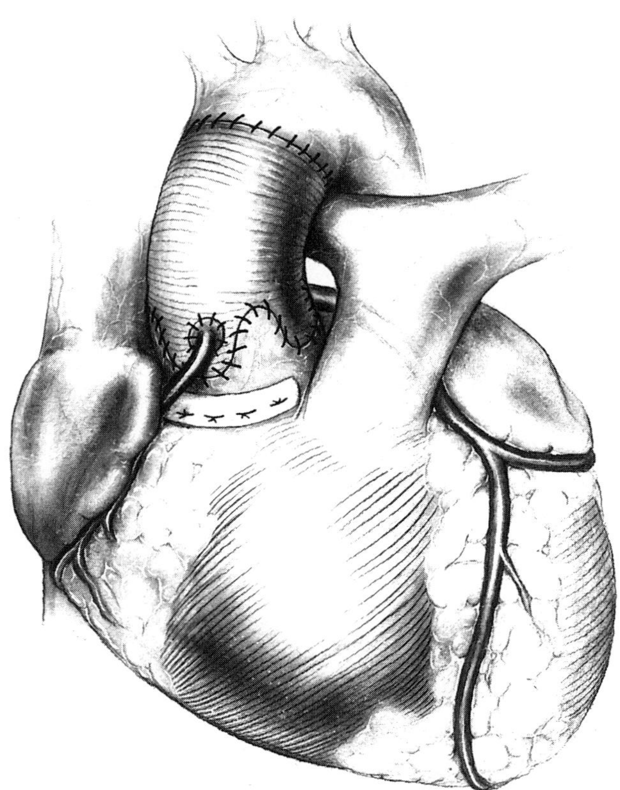

FIGURE 31–11 Remodeling of the aortic root with aortic annuloplasty. *(Reproduced from David TE: Remodeling of the aortic root with preservation of the native aortic valve. Op Tech Cardiac Thorac Surg 1996; 1:44, with permission from WB Saunders.)*

aneurysm and aortic insufficiency.[32] Replacement of the ascending aorta with adjustment of the sinotubular junction was performed in 68 patients.[32] The mean age of 38 men and 30 women was 68 years. Thirteen patients had type A aortic dissection, 17 had coronary artery disease, 43 had transverse arch aneurysm, and 22 had mega-aorta syndrome. Six patients had bicuspid aortic valve. The aortic insufficiency was graded as moderate (3+) in 31 patients and severe (4+) in 37. There was one operative death. The survival at 5 years was 68% and the freedom from aortic valve replacement 97%. The freedom from moderate or severe aortic insufficiency at 5 years was 98%.

Aortic Root Aneurysm

We recently reported the results of aortic valve-sparing operations in 120 patients operated on from 1988 to 2000.[33] Eleven patients had previous cardiac surgery: replacement of the ascending aorta in 10, and the Ross procedure in 1. Twenty-two patients had aortic dissection, 48 had Marfan syndrome, 17 had coronary artery disease, and 8 had severe mitral regurgitation. The mean diameter of the aortic root was 53 ± 8 mm and the aortic insufficiency was moderate or severe in 41% of the patients. Remodeling of the aortic root was used in 56 patients and reimplantation of the aortic valve in 64 patients. There were 2 operative deaths due to perioperative myocardial infarction. There was 1 operative failure early on in our experience, which required valve replacement. During a mean follow-up of 3 years, there were 5 late deaths (aortic dissection in 2 cases, sudden death in 1, and noncardiovascular causes in 2). The survival at 10 years was 88% ± 4%. The type of valve sparing had no effect on survival. The freedom from aortic valve replacement was 99% at 10 years. Late echocardiographic studies in 112 survivors showed no aortic insufficiency in 19, trace in 47, mild in 39, and moderate in 7. The freedom from moderate aortic insufficiency at 10 years was 83% ± 8%.

Yacoub et al,[36] who used the remodeling procedure without an aortic annuloplasty in 158 patients, reported a freedom from aortic valve replacement of 89% at 10 years, and moderate aortic insufficiency in one third of the patients. It is conceivable that the development of aortic insufficiency and ultimately valve failure leading to reoperation in that series is due to the lack of annuloplasty in patients with annuloaortic ectasia. Actually, we presently use only the reimplantation technique in patients with Marfan syndrome or its forme fruste with dilated aortic annulus, including those with bicuspid aortic valve and aortic insufficiency, because we believe that the aortic annulus may dilate after remodeling of the aortic root.

Pethig et al reported their experience with 75 consecutive patients who had the reimplantation technique and were followed for at least one year.[37] They found a correlation between the level of coaptation of the aortic cusps and the late development of aortic insufficiency, which was likely to occur if the coaptation level was below the level of the tubular graft. Our impression is that the level of coaptation after any type of valve-sparing procedure is a function of two factors: length of the free margins of the aortic cusps and size of the graft used for reconstruction. If the aortic cusps are elongated and/or if the graft is too small in diameter, the cusps will coapt at a low level within the reconstructed aortic root. Graeter et al found similar clinical and echocardiographic results after aortic root remodeling and reimplantation of the aortic valve at 5 years in patients with aortic root aneurysm.[38]

Finite element analysis of the aortic root by Grande-Allen et al suggested that placement of the aortic valve inside a cylindrical structure, such as used in the technique of reimplantation of the aortic valve, is associated with increased stress on the aortic cusps.[2] In addition, since nature created the aortic root with sinuses of Valsalva, it may be prudent to create neoaortic sinuses during the reconstruction of the aortic root with preservation of the aortic cusps. Neoaortic sinuses are easily created during the remodeling procedure by tailoring the tubular Dacron graft in such a way that the perimeter of the scalloped end of the graft is longer than the perimeter of the aortic annulus. Neoaortic sinuses can also be created during reimplantation of the aortic valve by using

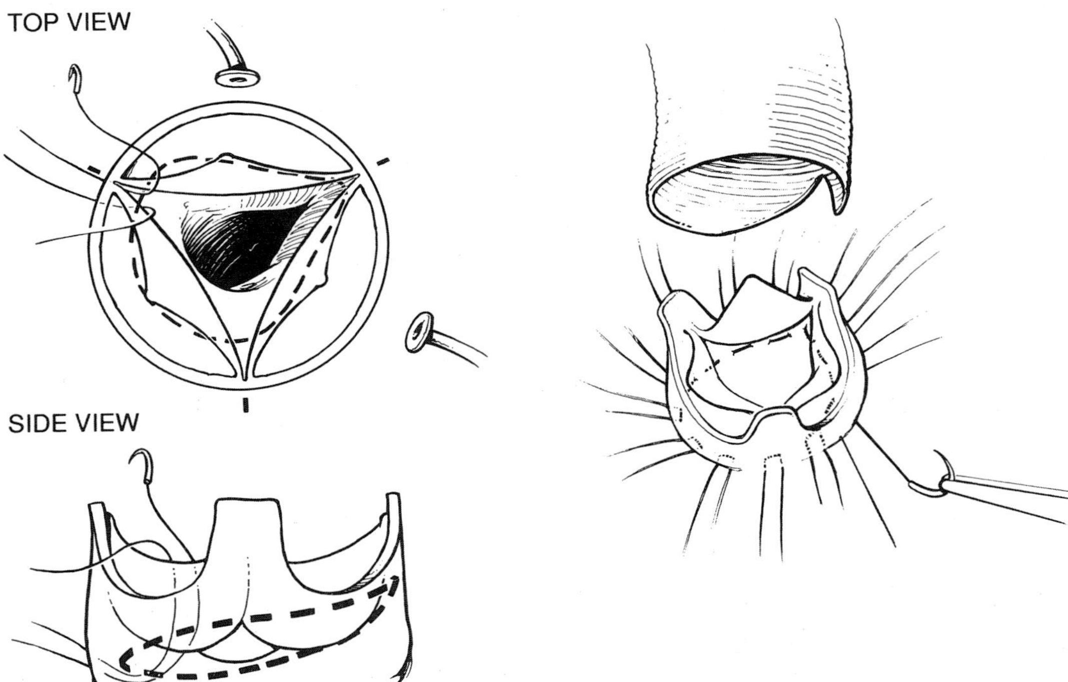

FIGURE 31–12 Reimplantation of the aortic valve. Multiple horizontal mattress sutures are placed in the left ventricular outflow tract, immediately below the aortic annulus and in a single horizontal plane along the fribrous components and following the scalloped shape of the annulus along the muscular attachments.

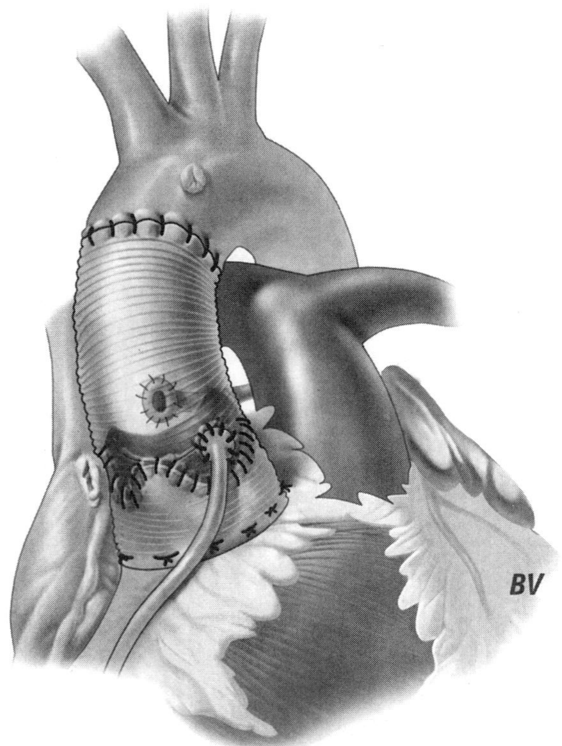

FIGURE 31–13 Reimplantation of the aortic valve. The three commissures are resuspended inside the graft and the remnants of the aortic sinuses are secured to the Dacron graft. The coronary arteries are reimplanted.

a graft larger than needed, and then reducing it at the level of the aortic annulus and at the sinotubular junction as described earlier in the section on reimplantation of the aortic valve. De Paulis et al have developed a Dacron graft with neosinuses that is now commercially available (Gelweave Valsalva; Sulzer Vascutek, Renfrewshire, Scotland). Their initial experience with that prosthesis is satisfactory.[39]

REFERENCES

1. Kunzelman KS, Grande J, David TE, et al: Aortic root and valve relationships: impact on surgical repair. *J Thorac Cardiovasc Surg* 1994; 107:162.
2. Grande-Allen KJ, Cochran RP, Reinhall PG, et al: Recreation of sinuses is important for sparing the aortic valve: a finite element study. *J Thorac Cardiovasc Surg* 2000; 119:753.
3. Swanson M, Clark RW: Dimensions and geometric relationships of the human aortic valve as a function of pressure circulation. *Circ Res* 1974; 34:871.
4. Silver MA, Roberts WC: Detailed anatomy of the normally functioning aortic valve in hearts of normal and increased weight. *Am J Cardiol* 1985; 55:454.
5. Furukawa K, Ohteki H, Cao ZL, et al: Does dilatation of the sinotubular junction cause aortic insufficiency? *Ann Thorac Surg* 1999; 68:949.
6. Warren BA, Hong JL: Calcification of the aortic valve: its progression and grading. *Pathology* 1997; 29:360.
7. Gotoh T, Kuroda T, Yamasawa M, et al: Correlation between lipoprotein (a) and aortic valve sclerosis assessed by echocardiography: the JMS Cardiac Echo and Cohort Study. *Am J Cardiol* 1995; 76:928.

8. Otto CM, Kuusisto J, Reichenbach DD, et al: Characterization of the early lesion of "degenerative" valvular aortic stenosis: histological and immuno-histochemical studies. *Circulation* 1994; 90:844.
9. Olsson M, Dalsgaard CJ, Haegerstrand A, et al: Accumulation of T lymphocytes and expression of interleukin-2 receptors in non-rheumatic stenotic aortic valves. *J Am Coll Cardiol* 1994; 23:1162.
10. David TE: Surgery of the aortic valve. *Curr Probl Surg* 1999; 36:421.
11. Dare AJ, Veinot PJ, Edwards WD, et al: New observations on the etiology of aortic valve disease: a surgical pathologic study of 236 cases from1990. *Hum Pathol* 1993; 24:1330.
12. Roberts WC: The congenitally bicuspid aortic valve: a study of 85 autopsy cases. *Am J Cardiol* 1970; 26:72.
13. Nistri S, Sorbo MD, Marin M, et al: Aortic root dilatation in young men with normally functioning bicuspid aortic valves. *Heart* 1999; 82:19.
14. Edwards WD, Leaf DS, Edwards JE: Dissecting aortic aneurysm associated with congenital bicuspid aortic valve. *Circulation* 1978; 57:1022.
15. Mousowitz HO, Levine RA, Hilgenberg AD, et al: Transeptal echocardiographic description of the mechanisms of aortic regurgitation in acute type A aortic dissection: implications for aortic repair. *J Am Coll Cardiol* 2000; 36:884.
16. Volmar KE, Hutchins GM: Aortic and mitral fenfluramine-phentermine valvulopathy in 64 patients treated with anorectic agents. *Arch Pathol Lab Med* 2001; 125:1555.
17. Davies SW, Gershlick AH, Balcon R: The progression of valvular aortic stenosis: a long-term retrospective study. *Eur Heart J* 1991; 12:10.
18. Pellika PA, Nishimura RA, Bailey KR, et al: The natural history of adults with asymptomatic hemodynamically significant aortic stenosis. *J Am Coll Cardiol* 1990; 15:1018.
19. Frank S, Johnson A, Ross J Jr: Natural history of valvular aortic stenosis. *Br Heart J* 1997; 35:41.
20. Goldschlager N, Pfeifer J, Cohn K, et al: The natural history of aortic regurgitation: a clinical and hemodynamic study. *Am J Med* 1973; 54:577.
21. Otto CM, Burwash IG, Legget ME, et al: Prospective study of asymptomatic valvular aortic stenosis: clinical, echocardiographic, and exercise predictors of outcome. *Circulation* 1997; 95: 2262.
22. Bonow RO, Lakatos E, Maron BJ, et al: Serial long-term assessment of the natural history of asymptomatic patients with chronic aortic regurgitation and normal left ventricular systolic function. *Circulation* 1991; 84:1625.
23. Gott VL, Greene PS, Alejo DE, et al: Replacement of the aortic root in patients with Marfan's syndrome. *N Engl J Med* 1999; 340:1307.
24. Tambeur L, David TE, Unger M, et al: Results of surgery for aortic root aneurysm in patients with Marfan syndrome. *Eur J Cardiothorac Surg* 2000; 17;415.
25. Pyeritz RE: Predictors of dissection of the ascending aorta in Marfan syndrome [abstract]. *Circulation* 1991; 84(2 suppl):351.
26. Coady MA, Rizzo JA, Hammond GL, et al: What is the appropriate size criterion for resection of thoracic aortic aneurysms? *J Thorac Cardiovasc Surg* 1997; 113:476.
27. McBride LR, Nauheim KD, Fiore AC, et al: Aortic valve decalcification. *J Thorac Cardiovasc Surg* 1990; 100:36.
28. David TE: Aortic valve repair for management of aortic insufficiency. *Adv Card Surg* 1999; 11:129.
29. Duran CM, Gometza B, Shahid M, Al-Halees Z: Treated bovine and autologous pericardium for aortic valve reconstruction. *Ann Thorac Surg* 1998; 66(6 suppl):S166.
30. David TE, Feindel CM: An aortic valve-sparing operation for patients with aortic incompetence and aneurysm of the ascending aorta. *J Thorac Cardiovasc Surg* 1992; 103:617.
31. David TE, Feindel CM, Bos J: Repair of the aortic valve in patients with aortic insufficiency and aortic root aneurysm. *J Thorac Cardiovasc Surg* 1995; 109:345.
32. David TE, Armstrong S, Ivanov J, et al: Results of aortic valve-sparing operations. *J Thorac Cardiovasc Surg* 2001; 122:39.
33. David TE: Aortic valve sparing operations for aortic root aneurysm. *Sem Thorac Cardiovasc Surg* 2001; 13:291.
34. Cosgrove DM, Rosenkranz ER, Hendren WG, et al: Valvuloplasty for aortic insufficiency. *J Thorac Cardiovasc Surg* 1991; 102:571.
35. Casselman FP, Gillinov AM, Akhrass R, et al: Intermediate-term durability of bicuspid aortic valve repair for prolapsing leaflet. *Eur J Cardiothorac Surg* 1999; 15:302.
36. Yacoub MH, Gehle P, Chandrasekaran V, et al: Late results of a valve-preserving operation in patients with aneurysms of the ascending aorta and root. *J Thorac Cardiovasc Surg* 1998; 115:1080.
37. Pethig K, Milz A, Hagl C, et al: Aortic valve reimplantation in ascending aortic aneurysm: risk factors for early valve failure. *Ann Thorac Surg* 2002; 73:29.
38. Graeter T, Aicher D, Langer F, et al: Mid-term results of aortic valve preserving: remodeling versus reimplantation. *Thorac Cardiovasc Surg* 2002; 50:21.
39. De Paulis R, De Matteis GM, Nardi P, et al: One-year appraisal of a new aortic root conduit with sinuses of Valsalva. *J Thorac Cardiovasc Surg* 2002; 123:33.

Chapter 32

Stented Mechanical/Bioprosthetic Aortic Valve Replacement

Nimesh D. Desai/George T. Christakis

This chapter provides an overview of aortic valve replacement with mechanical and stented bioprostheses. Detailed anatomy and pathophysiology of aortic valve disease are presented in previous chapters. The indications for aortic valve surgery are reviewed with an emphasis on evidence-based guidelines. The techniques of aortic valve implantation are illustrated for mechanical and stented bioprostheses, and postoperative medical management is reviewed. Currently approved mechanical and stented aortic prostheses are described. Clinical and physiologic outcomes of aortic valve surgery are reviewed to create a rational basis for prosthesis selection. Techniques of allograft and stentless bioprosthesis implantation, advanced surgery of the aortic root, and aortic valve repair are presented in subsequent chapters.

NATURAL HISTORY AND INDICATIONS FOR OPERATION

Aortic Stenosis

Aortic stenosis may be caused by degenerative calcification, congenital malformations, or rheumatic fever. It may also be found in association with systemic diseases such as Paget's disease of bone and end-stage renal disease. Congenital malformations include unicommisural and, more commonly, bicuspid valves. Detailed descriptions of these pathologies are presented earlier in this volume. Regardless of the initial pathology, there is a progressive reduction of effective orifice area caused by cusp calcification and/or commissural fusion.[1,2] The normal human aortic valve has an area between 3.0 and 4.0 cm^2. Mild, moderate, and severe aortic stenosis are defined as aortic valve areas greater than 1.5 cm^2, 1.0 to 1.5 cm^2, and less than 1.0 cm^2, respectively.[3] In the presence of normal cardiac output, transvalvular gradient is greater than 50 mm Hg when the aortic valve area is less than 1.0 cm^2.[4] There is a rapid increase in transvalvular gradient when the aortic valve area is less than 0.8 cm^2.[5] Exposure to elevated intracavitary pressures causes increased wall stress leading to parallel replication of sarcomeres and concentric hypertrophy.[6,7] Concentric hypertrophy compensates for the obstruction to flow created by the reduced orifice area of the aortic valve and maintains normal cardiac output. With progressive hypertrophy, the compliance of the ventricle decreases and end-diastolic pressure rises.[8,9] In this situation, the contribution of atrial contraction to preload becomes more significant and loss of sinus rhythm may lead to rapid progression of symptoms.[7]

SYMPTOMATIC PATIENTS

Hemodynamically significant aortic stenosis is initially counteracted by left ventricular hypertrophy. Progression of outflow obstruction and ventricular hypertrophy lead to the cardinal symptoms of aortic stenosis: angina, syncope, and congestive heart failure. The average aortic valve area is 0.6 cm^2 at the onset of symptoms.[7] Classic natural history studies have shown that the average life expectancy in patients with hemodynamically significant aortic stenosis is 4 years if anginal symptoms are present, 3 years if they have experienced syncope, and 2 years with the onset of congestive heart failure.[10] Symptomatic patients should therefore undergo aortic valve replacement (AVR)in a timely fashion.[11] Excessive waiting periods for AVR in symptomatic patients are associated with increased mortality. The rate of sudden death is greater than 10% per year in symptomatic patients. Once a patient is symptomatic, average survival is less than 3 years.[12–15]

ASYMPTOMATIC PATIENTS

Managing asymptomatic patients with hemodynamically significant aortic stenosis can be a challenging problem as there is often a prolonged latent period before symptoms emerge. During the latent period, there is a progression of concentric left ventricular hypertrophy as the ventricle adapts to elevated chamber pressures. Studies by Otto et al have shown that 7% of asymptomatic patients experience death or aortic valve surgery within 1 year after diagnosis.[16] After 5 years, the incidence of death or aortic valve surgery increases to 38%. The average decrease in aortic valve area is 0.12 cm^2 per year, while the average increase in transvalvular pressure is often 10 to 15 mm Hg per year.[17] Sudden death is quite uncommon and occurs in asymptomatic patients at a rate of approximately 0.4% per year.[18] The vast majority of patients who experience sudden death will become symptomatic in the months prior to death.[19] There is considerable variation in disease progression and many patients do not experience any change in gradient for several years. Rosenhek et al identified that, among asymptomatic patients, patients with an increase in peak jet velocity greater than 0.45 m/s per year on serial echocardiography were substantially more likely to need operation than patients with lesser changes in jet velocity.[20]

LOW-GRADIENT SEVERE AORTIC STENOSIS

The significance of aortic stenosis is often unclear in patients with very poor ventricular function (ejection fraction less than 20%) who have severely stenotic valves but small (<30 mm Hg) transvalvular gradients. The compromised left ventricular function in these patients may be caused by afterload mismatch created by the stenotic valve, or by an intrinsic cardiomyopathy, particularly in the setting of chronic ischemia from diffuse coronary disease. In these patients, measurement of transvalvular gradient and valve area at rest and with positive inotropy (i.e., dobutamine infusion) may distinguish whether cardiomyopathy or true valvular stenosis is the most responsible lesion. Patients with a preponderance of cardiomyopathy often do not experience significant benefit from valve replacement.[21] Hwang et al, using a multivariate analysis to determine factors that predict poor functional outcome after aortic valve replacement for aortic stenosis, identified that poor preoperative left ventricular function was the most significant predictor, followed by preoperative myocardial infarction, preoperative low transvalvular gradient, and incomplete coronary revascularization.[22]

INDICATIONS FOR OPERATION

In 1998, a joint task force of the American College of Cardiology (ACC) and the American Heart Association (AHA) developed evidence-based consensus guidelines for management of valvular heart disease.[23] Their recommendations for aortic valve replacement in the setting of aortic stenosis are summarized in Table 32-1. A class I recommendation indicates there is good evidence and general agreement that the treatment is useful and effective; class IIA indicates there may be some disagreement but the weight of evidence

TABLE 32–1 ACC/AHA guidelines for aortic valve replacement in patients with aortic stenosis

Indication	Class
1. Symptomatic patients with severe AS	I
2. Patients with severe AS undergoing coronary bypass surgery	I
3. Patients with severe AS undergoing surgery on the aorta or other heart valves	I
4. Patients with moderate AS undergoing coronary artery bypass or other aortic or valvular surgery	IIa
5. Asymptomatic patients with severe AS and:	
LV dysfunction	IIa
Abnormal response to exercise (hypotension)	IIa
Ventricular tachycardia	IIb
LVH >15 mm	IIb
Valve area <0.6 cm^2	IIb
6. Prevention of sudden death in an asymptomatic patient with none of the findings in 5.	III

Source: Adapted with permission from Bonow RO, Carbello B, De Leon AC Jr, et al: ACC/AHA guidelines for the management of patients with valvular disease. J Am Coll Cardiol 1998; 32:1486.

supports the usefulness/efficacy of the treatment in that setting; class IIB indicates that the usefulness/efficacy of the treatment is less well established; and a class III recommendation indicates that the treatment is either not useful or may be potentially harmful.

Aortic valve replacement is indicated in all symptomatic patients or patients with severe asymptomatic aortic stenosis who require concomitant coronary bypass, aortic surgery, or other valve replacement. It is our practice to perform aortic valve replacement on patients with moderate aortic stenosis requiring concomitant cardiac surgery. We do not routinely perform aortic valve replacement in patients with mild aortic stenosis undergoing concomitant cardiac surgery. Aortic valve replacement should be performed in otherwise asymptomatic patients with severe aortic stenosis and severe left ventricular dysfunction, exercise-induced symptoms, significant hypertrophy, or ventricular arrhythmia. Asymptomatic patients with very high transvalvular gradients (>60 mm Hg) or highly stenotic valves (valve area less than 0.6 cm^2) are at higher risk for progression to symptoms and should have valve replacement prior to significant ventricular decompensation or sudden death.

Aortic Regurgitation

ACUTE AORTIC REGURGITATION

Acute aortic regurgitation occurs in the setting of acute aortic dissection, infective endocarditis, trauma, active connective tissue disease, aortic cusp prolapse associated with ventricular septal defects, aortitis (syphilitic or giant cell), Marfan syndrome, Ehlers-Danlos syndrome, or iatrogenically after aortic balloon valvotomy.[7] It may be caused by acute dilatation of the aortic annulus preventing adequate cusp coaptation or by disruption of the valve cusps themselves. The heart cannot readily tolerate acute aortic regurgitation as the left ventricle is unable to cope with the sudden increase in end-diastolic volume caused by the regurgitant volume load. The normal ventricular chamber cannot acutely dilate sufficiently to prevent the Frank-Starling mechanism from being overwhelmed.[24] Hence, a dramatic reduction in forward stroke volume occurs. If there is poor left ventricular compliance from hypertrophy prior to the onset of acute aortic regurgitation, hemodynamic decompensation is significantly more dramatic.

To compensate for the acute decline in forward stroke volume, tachycardia ensues. Volume overload causes the left ventricular diastolic pressure to acutely rise above left atrial pressure resulting in early closure of the mitral valve.[25] While early mitral valve closure protects the pulmonary venous circulation from high end-diastolic pressures, rapid progression of pulmonary edema and cardiogenic shock are often unavoidable.

Death is the common end point of all etiologies of acute aortic regurgitation. Progressive cardiogenic shock and malignant ventricular arrhythmias are common causes of death. Urgent surgical treatment is warranted for all causes of hemodynamically significant acute aortic regurgitation.

CHRONIC AORTIC REGURGITATION

Chronic aortic regurgitation is caused by either slow enlargement of the aortic root or dysfunction of the valve cusps. Common etiologies include congenital abnormalities, calcific cusp degeneration, rheumatic fever, endocarditis, degenerative aortic dilatation as seen in the elderly, Marfan syndrome, Ehlers-Danlos syndrome, myxomatous proliferation, osteogenesis imperfecta, ankylosing spondylitis, Behcet syndrome, Reiter syndrome, psoriatic arthritis, severe systemic hypertension, and idiopathic aortic root dilatation.[7] The anorectic drugs fenfluramine and dexfenfluramine have been implicated in left- and right-sided valvular disease, including aortic regurgitation.[26,27] Bicuspid aortic valve is the most common congenital abnormality, but unicommissural, quadricuspid, and fenestrated valves may also occur.[28]

Chronic aortic regurgitation causes a chronic volume overload of the left ventricle. This leads to progressive chamber enlargement without increasing end-diastolic pressure during the asymptomatic phase of the disease.[29] Progressive chamber enlargement is accompanied by eccentric hypertrophy, with sarcomere replication and elongation of myocytes.[30] The combination of chamber dilatation and hypertrophy leads to a massive increase in left ventricular mass. Initially, the ratio of wall thickness to chamber diameter, ejection fraction, and fractional shortening are all maintained.[31] However, this degenerates into a repetitive cycle of enlarging chamber radius with continually increasing wall stress. This wall stress is compensated by ventricular hypertrophy. Interstitial fibrosis limits the ability of the ventricle to further dilate and this cycle becomes overwhelmed, leading to elevated end-diastolic pressure, left ventricular systolic dysfunction, and congestive heart failure.[32] Vasodilator therapy may delay progression of ventricular dysfunction by decreasing afterload and decreasing regurgitant flow. This therapy is not recommended in patients with severe aortic regurgitation and left ventricular dysfunction as it does not improve survival.[33] Vasodilator therapy is currently indicated in patients with severe left ventricular dysfunction who are not operative candidates, asymptomatic patients with hypertension, asymptomatic patients with severe aortic regurgitation, ventricular dilatation, and preserved systolic function, and for short-term hemodynamic tailoring prior to operation.[33]

SYMPTOMATIC CHRONIC AORTIC REGURGITATION

The time course from diagnosis of aortic regurgitation to the development of symptoms is highly variable. Since symptoms, such as angina and dyspnea, develop only after significant ventricular decompensation, surgery is advocated prior to the symptomatic phase of the disease. Symptomatic patients experience greater than 10% mortality per year without surgical management.[34,35]

ASYMPTOMATIC CHRONIC AORTIC REGURGITATION

Natural history studies of asymptomatic aortic regurgitation show that symptoms, left ventricular dysfunction, or both develop in less than 6% of patients per year.[36] Progression to asymptomatic left ventricular dysfunction occurs in less than 4% of patients per year.[37] Sudden death occurs in less than 0.2% per year.[38] Age, left ventricular end-systolic dimension, rate of change in end-systolic dimension, and rest ejection fraction are all independent predictors of progression to symptoms, left ventricular dysfunction, or death in asymptomatic patients.[39] Asymptomatic patients with left ventricular systolic dysfunction experience onset of symptoms at a rate exceeding 25% per year.[40]

TABLE 32–2 AHA/ACC recommendations for aortic valve replacement in chronic severe aortic regurgitation

Indication	Class
1. Patients with NYHA functional class III or IV symptoms and preserved LV systolic function, defined as normal ejection fraction at rest (ejection fraction >50%)	I
2. Patients with NYHA functional class II symptoms and preserved LV systolic function (ejection fraction >50% at rest) but with progressive LV dilatation or declining ejection fraction at rest on serial studies or declining effort tolerance on exercise testing	I
3. Patients with Canadian Cardiovascular Society functional class II or greater angina with or without CAD	I
4. Asymptomatic or symptomatic patients with mild to moderate LV dysfunction at rest (ejection fraction 25% to 50%)	I
5. Patients undergoing coronary artery bypass surgery or surgery on the aorta or other heart valves	I
6. Patients with NYHA functional class II symptoms and preserved LV systolic function (ejection fraction>50% at rest) with stable LV size and systolic function on serial studies and stable exercise tolerance	IIa
7. Asymptomatic patients with normal LV systolic function (ejection fraction >50%) but with severe LV dilatation (end-diastolic dimension >75 mm or end-systolic dimension >55 mm)*	IIa
8. Patients with severe LV dysfunction (ejection fraction <25%)	IIb
9. Asymptomatic patients with normal systolic function at rest (ejection fraction >50%) and progressive LV dilatation when the degree of dilatation is moderately severe (end-diastolic dimension 70-75 mm, end-systolic dimension 50-55 mm)	IIb
10. Asymptomatic patients with normal systolic function at rest (ejection fraction >50%) but with decline in ejection fraction during:	
Exercise radionuclide angiography	IIb
Stress echocardiography	III
11. Asymptomatic patients with normal systolic function at rest (ejection fraction >50%) and LV dilatation when degree of dilatation is not severe (end-diastolic dimension <70 mm, end-systolic dimension <50 mm)	III

*Consider lower threshold values for patients of small stature of either gender. Clinical judgment is required.

Source: Adapted with permission from Bonow RO, Carbello B, De Leon AC Jr, et al: ACC/AHA guidelines for the management of patients with valvular disease. J Am Coll Cardiol 1998; 32:1486.

INDICATIONS FOR OPERATION

A summary of the ACC/AHA Task Force guidelines for aortic valve replacement for aortic regurgitation is presented in Table 32-2.[41] Symptomatic patients (NYHA class II or higher) with mild to moderate left ventricular systolic dysfunction (ejection fraction >20% to 30% or end-systolic dimension <55 mm) should have aortic valve replacement. Mild to moderately symptomatic patients with significant ventricular dysfunction often experience significant benefit from surgery. Patients with more severe symptoms or left ventricular dysfunction have decreased survival due to irreversible changes to the ventricle including hypertrophy and interstitial fibrosis.[42] Aortic valve replacement in patients with NYHA class IV symptoms and severe left ventricular dysfunction is associated with increased perioperative mortality and poor prognosis.[42,43] The decision to operate on such patients is dependent on individual variables as the outcomes are poor with surgery or medical therapy.

All patients with moderate to severe symptoms (NYHA class III or IV) and preserved left ventricular function should undergo aortic valve replacement. Patients with mild symptoms should have valve replacement if there is evidence of declining left ventricular systolic function (ejection fraction approaching 50%) or increasing chamber size (end-systolic diameter approaching 55 mm, end-diastolic dimension approaching 70 mm) on serial assessment.

Asymptomatic patients with systolic dysfunction (ejection fraction <50%) or severe left ventricular enlargement (end-systolic diameter >55 mm, end-diastolic dimension >70 mm) should have aortic valve replacement. Patients with serial deterioration of ventricular function or chamber size should have valve replacement prior to the onset of irreversible ventricular depression. Hwang et al identified poor preoperative left ventricular function and left ventricular systolic pressure as determinants of poor postoperative functional outcome in patients undergoing aortic valve replacement for aortic regurgitation.[44]

CORONARY ANGIOGRAPHY AND AORTIC VALVE REPLACEMENT

Many patients requiring aortic valve replacement have coexistent coronary artery disease. At our institution, more than one third of aortic valve replacement procedures are combined with coronary bypass surgery. This proportion may increase as the surgical population continues to age. Risk assessment for ischemic heart disease is complicated in patients with aortic valve disease since angina may be related to true ischemia from hemodynamically significant coronary lesions or other causes such as left ventricular wall stress with subendocardial ischemia or chamber enlargement in the setting of reduced coronary flow reserve. Since traditional coronary risk stratification is unreliable in aortic valve patients, it is our practice to routinely perform diagnostic coronary angiography on all patients over the age of 35. ACC/AHA Task Force guidelines for preoperative angiography are presented in Table 32-3.[45]

TABLE 32–3 ACC/AHA task force guidelines on coronary angiography in patients with valvular heart disease

Indication	Class
1. Before valve surgery (including infective endocarditis) or mitral balloon commissurotomy in patients with: Chest pain Other objective evidence of ischemia Decreased LV systolic function History of CAD Coronary risk factors (including advanced age)	I
2. Patients with apparently mild to moderate valvular heart disease but with: Progressive (class II or greater) angina Objective evidence of ischemia Decreased LV systolic function Overt congestive heart failure	I
3. Patients undergoing catheterization to confirm the severity of valve lesions before valve surgery without preexisting evidence of CAD, multiple coronary risk factors, or advanced age	IIb
4. Young patients undergoing nonemergent valve surgery when no further hemodynamic assessment by catheterization is deemed necessary and no coronary risk factors, no history of CAD, and no evidence of ischemia are present	III
5. Asymptomatic patients with valvular heart disease when valve surgery or balloon commissurotomy is not being considered	III
6. Patients having emergency valve surgery for acute valve regurgitation, aortic root disease, or infective endocarditis when there are no coronary risk factors, angina, objective evidence of ischemia, evidence of coronary embolization, LV systolic dysfunction, or age <35 years	

Source: Adapted with permission from Bonow RO, Carbello B, De Leon AC Jr, et al: ACC/AHA guidelines for the management of patients with valvular disease. J Am Coll Cardiol 1998; 32:1486.

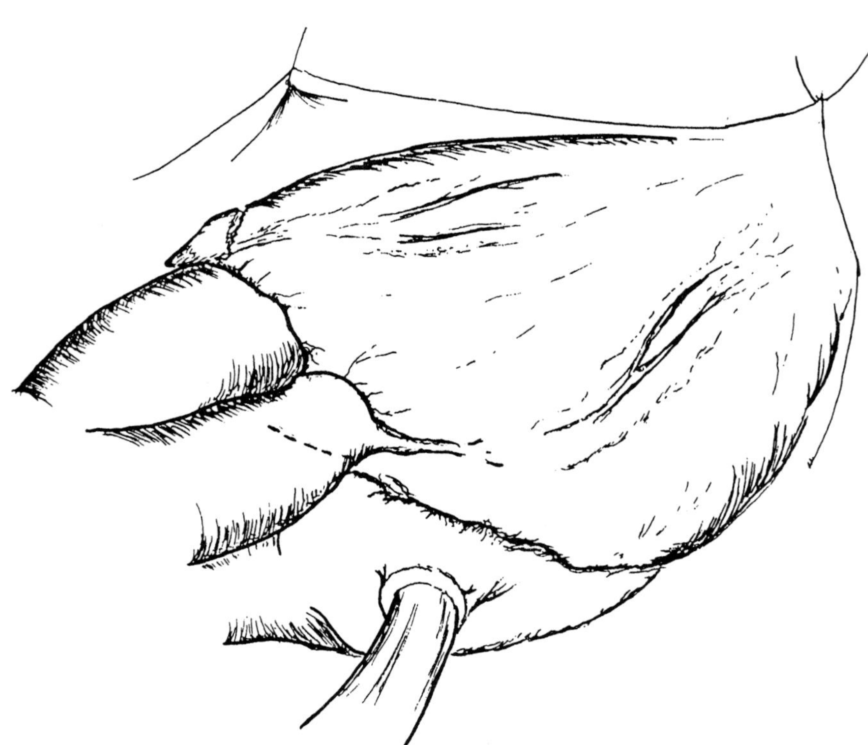

FIGURE 32–1 Exposure and aortotomy incision. A two-stage venous cannula is in place in the right atrial appendage. The aortotomy (dashed line) is started approximately 5 mm above the origin of the right coronary artery. (*Courtesy of Dr. C. Hayman.*)

TECHNIQUE OF OPERATION

Myocardial Protection and Cardiopulmonary Bypass

Isolated aortic valve replacement is performed using a single two-stage venous cannula inserted into the right atrium for venous return and a standard arterial cannula into the ascending aorta for systemic perfusion of oxygenated blood. A venting cannula is placed in the right superior pulmonary vein to ensure a bloodless field. After the cross-clamp is applied, myocardial protection is initially delivered as a single dose of high-potassium blood through the ascending aorta.[46–48] This will achieve prompt diastolic arrest unless there is significant aortic regurgitation. Our group does not routinely use retrograde cardioplegia for all aortic valve cases, but this strategy is helpful in patients with significant aortic regurgitation or severe concomitant coronary disease.[49] Myocardial protection is maintained by continuous infusion of tepid oxygenated blood delivered via direct cannulation of both coronary ostia after the aorta has been opened.[50] If retrograde perfusion is employed, this is also used in a continuous manner. Right ventricular myocardial protection via retrograde perfusion is often inadequate and can lead to significant right ventricular dysfunction after cardiopulmonary bypass is discontinued.[51–54]

Aortotomy, Valve Excision, and Debridement

The aorta and pulmonary artery are dissected to expose the anterior aortic root to the left coronary artery prior to initiating cardioplegia. After arrest has been achieved, the aorta is opened with a transverse incision approximately 5 mm above the origin of the right coronary artery that may be extended posteriorly to the noncoronary sinus of Valsalva (Fig. 32-1). Morphology of the valve is then inspected (Fig. 32-2). Excision of the valve cusps starts at the commisure between the right and noncoronary cusps (Fig. 32-3). Mayo scissors are usually used at this stage. A moistened radioopaque sponge is placed into the outflow area to catch

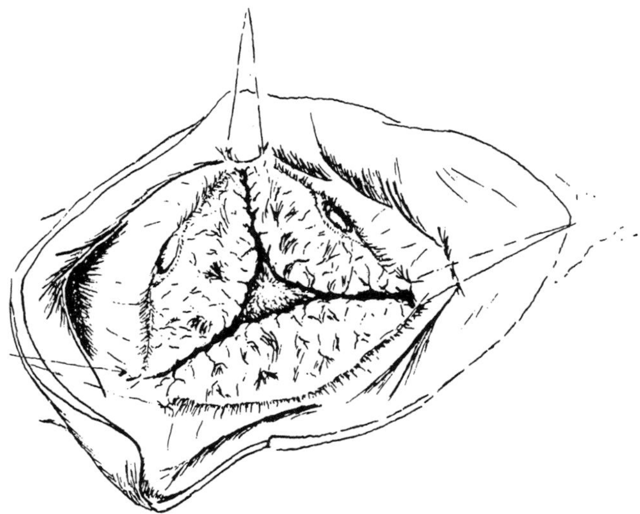

FIGURE 32–2 The exposed aortic valve. (*Courtesy of Dr. C. Hayman.*)

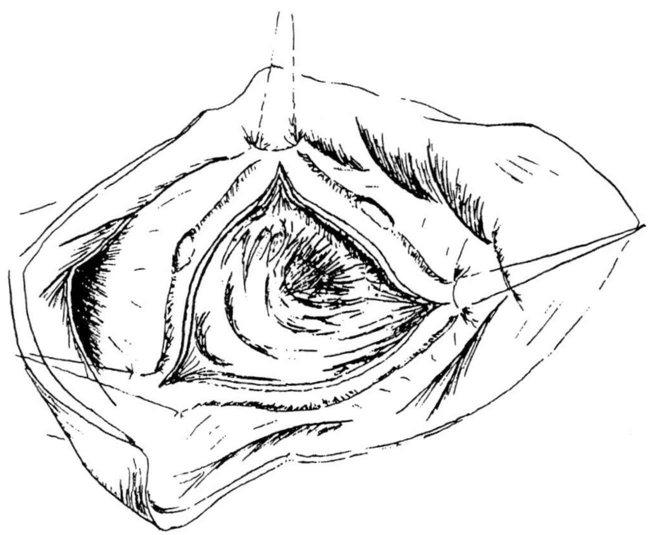

FIGURE 32–3 The aortic valve after debridement. (*Courtesy of Dr. C. Hayman.*)

debris. Thorough decalcification to soft tissue improves seating of the prosthesis, and decreases the incidence of paravalvular leak and dehiscense. Care must be taken to prevent aortic perforation while all calcific deposits are debrided off the aortic wall, particularly at the commissure between the left and noncoronary cusps. Careful use of a scalpel or rongieurs may also be required. It is important to note that the bundle of His (conduction system) is located below the junction of the right and noncoronary cusp at the membranous septum. The anterior leaflet of the mitral valve is in direct continuity with the left aortic valve cusp. If it is damaged during decalcification, an autologous pericardial patch is used to repair the defect.

Valve Implantation

After the native valve has been excised, the annulus is sized with a valve sizer appropriate to the selected mechanical or bioprosthetic device. The valve is secured to the annulus

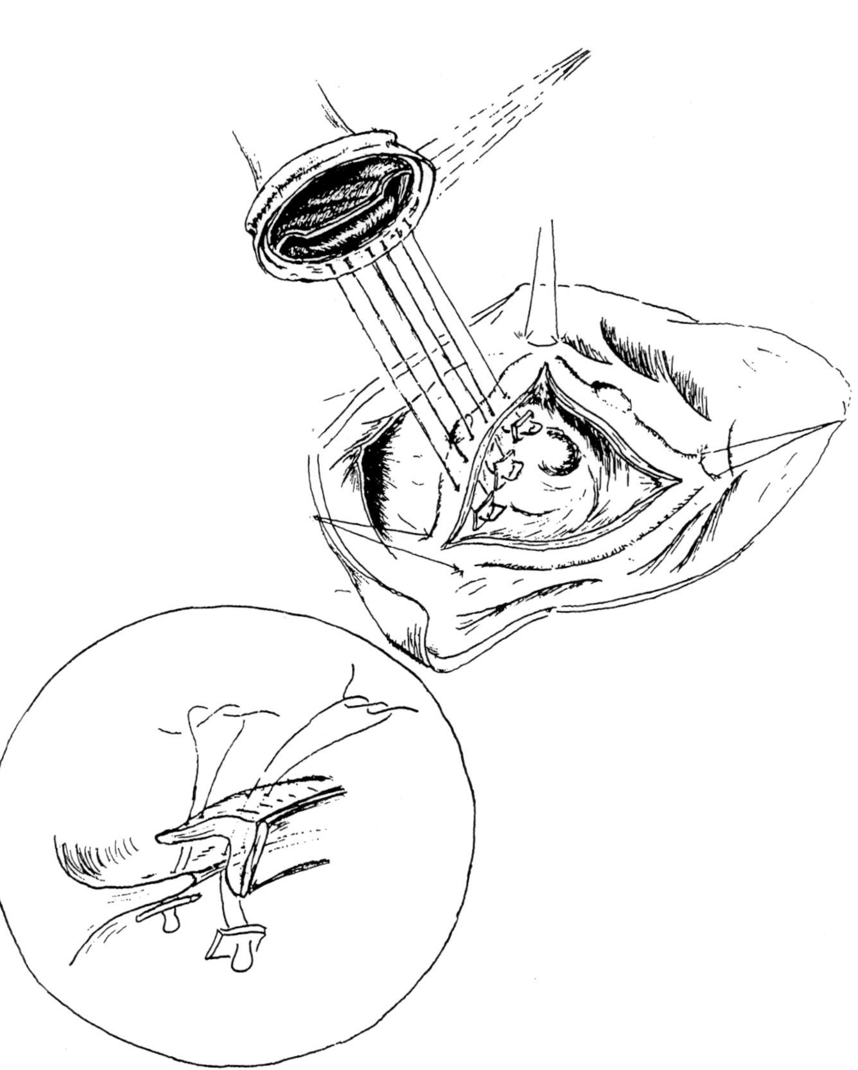

FIGURE 32–4 Placement of sutures with pledgets below the annulus. (*Courtesy of Dr. C. Hayman.*)

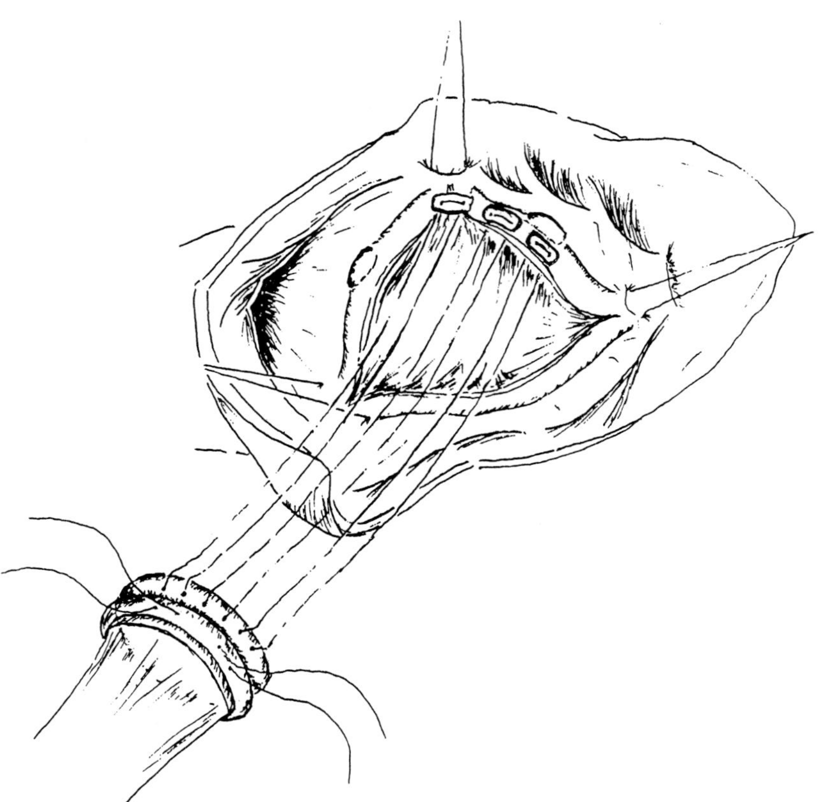

FIGURE 32–5 Placement of sutures with pledgets above the annulus. (*Courtesy of Dr. C. Hayman.*)

using 12 to 16 double-needled interrupted 2-0 synthetic braided pledgeted sutures. The pledgets can be left on the inflow/ventricular side or the outflow/aortic side of the aortic annulus (Figs. 32-4 and 32-5). Placing the pledgets on the inflow side of the annulus allows the placement of a larger prosthesis and this technique is routinely used at our institution. The aorta is closed with a double row of synthetic polypropelene sutures.

De-airing

During AVR, air may be entrained into the left atrium and ventricle and the aorta. This must be removed to prevent potential catastrophic air embolization. Immediately prior to tying the suture of the aortotomy, the heart is allowed to fill, the vent in the superior pulmonary vein is stopped, the lungs are inflated, and the cross-clamp is briefly partially opened. The subsequent influx of blood should expel most air from these cavities out of the partially open aortotomy. Closure of the aortotomy is then completed and the cross-clamp is fully removed. The cardioplegia cannula in the ascending aorta and the LV vent are then placed on suction to remove any residual air as the heart begins electrical activity. A small needle (21 gauge) is used to aspirate the apex of the left ventricle and the dome of the left atrium.

Technical Considerations with Concomitant Coronary Artery Bypass Grafting

Operative technique is modified to optimize myocardial protection when there is concomitant coronary disease. Distal anastomoses are performed prior to aortic valve replacement so that cardioplegia may be administered through these grafts during the operation. We routinely use the left internal thoracic artery for revascularization of the left anterior descending artery as this may improve long-term survival.[55] This anastomosis is performed after the aortotomy is closed to ensure that the coronary circulation is not exposed to systemic circulation during cardioplegic arrest and to prevent trauma to the anastomosis during manipulation of the heart. All surgeons at our institution use a single cross-clamp technique for performing proximal anastomoses.

Aortic Root Enlargement Procedures

Detailed descriptions of aortic root enlargement procedures are presented in a later chapter. Either an anterior or posterior annular enlargement procedure may be performed in a patient with small aortic root to allow for implantation of a larger valve. The posterior approach is the most commonly used aortic root enlargement procedure in adults and can increase the annular diameter by 2 to 4 mm. With the posterior approach, first described by Nicks et al in 1970, the aortotomy is extended downward through the noncoronary cusp, through the aortic annulus, and into the anterior mitral leaflet.[56] Manouguian, in 1979, described a procedure extending the aortotomy incision in a downward direction through the commissure between the left and noncoronary cusps into the interleaflet triangle and anterior leaflet of the mitral valve.[57,58] The anterior approach is generally used in the pediatric population. Described by Konno et al in 1975, this technique, which is also known as aortoventriculoplasty, is used when greater than 4 mm of annular enlargement is required.[59] Instead of a transverse incision, a longitudinal incision is made in the anterior aorta and extended to the right coronary sinus of Valsalva and then through the anterior wall of the right ventricle to open the right ventricular outflow tract. The ventricular septum is incised allowing significant expansion of the aortic annulus and left ventricular outflow tract.

Reoperative Aortic Valve Surgery

Repeat sternotomy after aortic valve replacement may be performed for valve-related complications, progressive ascending aortic disease, or coronary disease. Valve-related causes include structural valve deterioration, prosthetic endocarditis, prosthesis thrombosis, or paravalular leak. Chest reentry is the most hazardous portion of any repeat cardiac procedure. It is our practice to obtain an adequate lateral chest roentgenogram to determine the proximetry of cardiac structures to the posterior sternum. If the right ventricle or an ascending aortic graft is close to the sternum, a computed tomography scan is performed to accurately determine the risk of injury upon entry. Cardiopulmonary bypass is instituted through the femoral vessels when there is concern about chest reentry. An oscillating saw is used to open the sternum and the dissection is kept as limited as possible. Extreme caution must be employed during dissection when there are patent bypass grafts.

The prosthesis is excised with sharp dissection. Care must be taken to remove all sutures and pledgets from the annulus. Annular injuries caused while excising the prosthesis are repaired with pledgeted interrupted sutures.

In the setting of endocarditis, aggressive debridement of infected tissue must be performed with appropriate annular reconstruction with pericardium when root abscesses are present.[60,61] All foreign graft material, including Dacron aortic grafts, must be excised in the presence of active endocarditis.[62]

In the presence of a Dacron prosthesis in the ascending aorta, chest reentry is extremely hazardous since exsanguination will occur if the graft is accidentally opened during dissection. To limit the systemic consequences of exsanguination at normothermia, the patient should be placed on femoral-femoral cardiopulmonary bypasss and cooled to 20°C prior to chest reentry.[63] If the Dacron graft is accidentally opened, local control of the bleeding is established and cardiopulmonary bypass is stopped. Under circulatory arrest, atrial venous cannulation is instituted and the graft is controlled distal to the tear. Cardiopulmonary bypass may then be restarted.

In all repeat aortic procedures, rigorous myocardial protection must be applied because these procedures often have very long ischemic times. Antegrade cold blood cardioplegia is usually employed in a continuous fashion throughout the case by selective cannulation of the coronary ostia.

Aortic Balloon Valvotomy

Aortic balloon valvotomy may be performed percutaneously via a femoral artery puncture in the interventional angiography suite to treat aortic stenosis.[64] Inflation of the balloon within the valve orifice can stretch the annular tissue and fracture calcified areas or open fused commissures. There is no role for valvotomy in the patient with significant aortic regurgitation as this will become significantly worse after the procedure.[65–67] Balloon valvotomy is rarely successful if significant calcification is present and carries a prohibitive risk of stroke from calcific emboli.[67,68] The long-term outcomes of this procedure in adult patients are dismal, with restenosis usually occurring within 1 year.[67,69,70] Patients with severe symptomatic aortic stenosis who are too hemodynamically unstable to tolerate operation or have comorbid illnesses, such as advanced malignancy, which contraindicate operation, may benefit from palliative balloon valvotomy.[71–74]

POSTOPERATIVE MANAGEMENT

Special consideration must be given to the underlying pathologic changes to the ventricle during the immediate postoperative period. The severely hypertrophied, noncompliant left ventricle found in aortic stenosis is highly dependent on sufficient preload for adequate filling. Filling pressures should be carefully titrated between 15 mm Hg and 18 mm Hg with intravenous volume infusion. Maintenance of sinus rhythm is also essential as up to one third of cardiac output is derived from atrial contraction in a noncompliant ventricle. Up to 10% of patients will experience low cardiac output syndrome in the immediate postoperative period.[75] If pacing is required postoperatively, synchronous atrioventricular pacing is beneficial in preventing low cardiac output syndrome. In cases of severe hypertrophy, subvalvular left ventricular outflow obstruction with systolic anterior wall motion of the mitral valve may occur. Intravenous beta-adrenergic blockade may relieve this obstruction by decreasing inotropy. In extreme cases, surgical myectomy may be required.[62]

Profound peripheral vasodilation, often seen in patients with aortic insufficiency, is treated with vasoconstrictors including alpha-adrenergic agonists or vasopressin. Adequate filling of the dilated left ventricle may also require volume infusion.

Complete heart block occurs in 3% to 5% of AVR patients. This complication may be due to suture placement or injury from aggressive debridement near the conduction system. Transient complete heart block caused by perioperative edema usually resolves in 4 to 6 days, after which insertion of a permanent pacemaker is recommended. Optimal antithrombotic therapy will be addressed later in this chapter.

AORTIC VALVE REPLACEMENT DEVICES

Mechanical Prostheses

Currently available mechanical prostheses include caged-ball, single tilting disc, and bileaflet prostheses.

CAGED-BALL PROSTHESIS

The Starr-Edwards caged-ball prosthesis was developed in the early 1960s and was the first commercially available heart valve. Although it initially underwent minor modifications, it has not been changed since 1965 and is still actively implanted throughout the world. It is associated with a very low incidence of mechanical failure but may have a higher risk of thromboembolism than other currently available mechanical prostheses.[33]

TILTING MONOLEAFLET PROSTHESES

Tilting monoleaflet prostheses were initially developed in the late 1960s and current models include the Medtronic Hall (Medtronic, Minneapolis, MN), Omnicarbon (MedicalCV, Inc., Inver Grove Heights, MN), and Allcarbon Monodisc (Sorin Biomedica, Saluggia, Italy) prostheses. These valves incorporate a single pyrolite carbon-coated tungsten-impregnated leaflet into a titanium or solid pyrolite housing. The leaflet of the Medtronic Hall valve slides along an open-ended central guide strut. The leaflet of Omnicarbon valve rotates about pivots located in the housing, while the leaflet of the Allcarbon Monodisc valve is contained by struts from the valve housing. The opening angle of these monoleaflet valves is between 75° and 80°.

BILEAFLET PROSTHESES

Bileaflet prostheses currently available in North America include the St. Jude Medical Standard, Masters, Regent, and Hemodynamic Plus valves (St. Jude Medical Inc., Minneapolis, Minnesota); Carbomedics and Top-Hat Supra-annular valves (Sulzer Carbomedics, Inc., Austin, Texas); ATS valve (ATS Medical Inc., Minneapolis, Minnesota); Bicarbon valve (Sorin Biomedica, Saluggia, Italy); Edwards MIRA valve (Edwards Lifesciences, Irvine CA.); and the On-X valve (Medical Carbon Research Institute, Austin, Texas). Modern bileaflet prostheses are typically comprised of two pyrolite-carbon coated leaflets made of radiopaque tungsten-impregnated graphite substrate inside a solid pyrolite carbon or pyrolite carbon-coated titanium housing. The leaflets rotate around pivots located within the housing. Retrograde washing decreases thrombogenicity by decreasing stasis of blood around the valve and pivot mechanisms.

Recent design changes include the ability to rotate the valve within the housing for optimum alignment of the leaflets. Most bileaflet valves have opening angles between 75° and 85°. Modifications to the sewing cuffs of current prostheses include narrower sewing cuffs to increase valve internal diameter and allow supra-annular placement. Several valves including the Edwards MIRA and Bicarbon valves incorporate curved leaflets to potentially improve laminar flow and allow for faster closure.

Stented Bioprostheses

Stented biologic prostheses may be constructed of porcine aortic valves or bovine pericardium. Over the past 40 years, advances in tissue fixation methodology and chemical treatments to prevent calcification have yielded improvements in the longevity of bioprostheses. All heterograft valves are preserved with glutaraldehyde, which cross-links collagen fibers and reduces the antigenicity of the tissue. Glutaraldehyde also reduces the rate of in vivo enzymatic degradation and causes the loss of cell viability, thereby preventing normal turnover and remodeling of extracellular matrix tissues.[76,77] Calcification occurs when nonviable glutaraldehyde-fixed cells cannot maintain low intracellular calcium.[78] Calcium-phosphate crystals form at the phospholipid-rich membranes and their remnants, and collagen also calcifies.[79]

Glutaraldehyde fixation in porcine valves can be performed at high pressure (60-80 mm Hg), low pressure (0.1-2 mm Hg), or zero pressure (0 mm Hg). Pericardial prostheses are fixed in pressure-free conditions. Porcine prostheses fixed at zero pressure retain the collagen architecture of the relaxed aortic valve cusp.[80] Higher fixation pressures cause tissue flattening and compression with loss of transverse cuspal ridges and collagen crimp.[81–83]

Multiple chemical treatments have been proposed to decrease the calcification process that invariably leads to material failure and valvular dysfunction. These include sodium dodecyl sulfate, polysorbate-80, Triton X-100 and N-lauryl sarcosine, amino-oleic acid, aminopropanehydroxydiphosphonate, toluidine blue, controlled-release diphosphonates, ferric chloride, aluminum chloride, and phosphocitrate.[84–98]

FIRST-GENERATION PROSTHESES

First-generation bioprostheses were preserved with high-pressure fixation and were placed in the annular position. They include the Medtronic Hancock Standard and Modified Orifice (Medtronic, Minneapolis, MN) and Carpentier-Edwards Standard porcine prostheses (Edwards Lifesciences, Irvine, CA).

SECOND-GENERATION PROSTHESES

Second-generation prostheses are treated with low- or zero-pressure fixation. Several second-generation prostheses may also be placed in the supra-annular position, which allows placement of a slightly larger prosthesis. Porcine second-generation prostheses include the Medtronic Hancock II (Medtronic, Minneapolis, MN) and Carpentier-Edwards Supra-annular (SAV) (Edwards Lifesciences, Irvine, CA) valves. Second-generation pericardial prostheses include the Carpentier-Edwards Perimount (Edwards Lifesciences, Irvine, CA) and Mitroflow Synergy (Sulzer Carbomedics, Austin, TX) valves.

THIRD-GENERATION PROSTHESES

Newer generation prostheses incorporate zero- or low-pressure fixation with antimineralization processes that are designed to reduce material fatigue and calcification. They include the Medtronic Mosiac porcine (Medtronic, Minneapolis, MN), Medtronic Intact porcine (Medtronic, Minneapolis, MN), St. Jude Medical X-Cell porcine (St. Jude Medical, Minneapolis, MN), Sulzer Synergy ST porcine (Sulzer Carbomedics, Austin, TX), and Pericarbon MORE (Sorin Biomedica Saluggia, Italy) pericardial valves.

OUTCOMES OF AORTIC VALVE REPLACEMENT

Operative Mortality

Operative mortality is defined as all-cause mortality within 30 days of operation or during the same hospital admission.[99] Contemporary series describe a low or very low operative mortality for isolated aortic valve replacement. The mortality from aortic valve replacement varies between 1% and 6%, depending on the patient population and era of study.[100–111] A recent publication from the Society of Thoracic Surgeons database reviewing the results of 86,580 valve procedures found an overall mortality of 4.3% for isolated aortic valve replacement and 8.0% for aortic valve replacement with coronary bypass surgery.[110] Aortic valve replacement with ascending aortic aneurysm repair had an operative mortality of 9.7%.[110] The results of this study are summarized in Table 32-4. It is important to note that information in this database is voluntarily submitted and includes academic, nonacademic, low-volume, and high-volume centers.

Advanced patient age, poor preoperative left ventricular function, NYHA class IV symptoms, concomitant coronary artery disease, severe preoperative renal dysfunction, active endocarditis, female sex, emergent or salvage operation, and previous aortic valve replacement have been associated with increased operative mortality in several series.[75,102,110–117] In the absence of major comorbidities and preserved left ventricular function, isolated aortic valve replacement can be performed with an expected mortality of less than 1%.[62] Kouchoukos et al have shown that operative mortality is not further increased if simple resection of an ascending aortic aneurysm is performed at an experienced center.[118] Concomitant coronary bypass surgery is associated with approximately double the operative mortality of isolated aortic valve replacement.[109,110,119–121] Table 32-5 presents the

TABLE 32–4 Operative mortality rates for aortic valve procedures from the Society of Thoracic Surgeons' database

Operative category	No.	Operative mortality (%)
AVR (isolated)	26,317	4.3
Multiple valve replacement	3,840	9.6
AVR + CAB	22,713	8.0
Multiple valve replacement + CAB	1,424	18.8
AVR + any valve repair	938	7.4
Aortic valve repair	597	5.9
AVR + aortic aneurysm repair	1,723	9.7
AVR + other*	356	8.4

AVR = aortic valve replacement; CAB = coronary artery bypass; MVR = mitral valve replacement.

*Other includes left ventricular aneurysm, ventricular septal defect, atrial septal defect, congenital, cardiac trauma, cardiac transplant, permanent pacemaker, automatic implanted cardioverter defibrillator, aortic aneurysm, or carotid endarterectomy. Isolated aortic valve replacement and aortic aneurysm are not included in aortic valve replacement + other.

Source: Adapted with permission from Jameison WR, Edwards FH, Schwartz M, et al: Risk stratification for cardiac valve replacement. National Cardiac Surgery Database. Ann Thorac Surg 1999; 67:943.

TABLE 32–5 Independent risk factors for operative mortality (odds ratios) for isolated aortic valve replacement and aortic valve replacement plus coronary artery bypass from the Society of Thoracic Surgeons' database

Aortic valve replacement			Aortic valve replacement plus coronary artery bypass		
Risk factor	Odds ratio	CI	Risk factor	Odds ratio	CI
Salvage status	7.12	4.69–10.68	Salvage status	7.00	4.74–10.33
DDRF	4.32	2.83–6.43	DDRF	4.60	3.10–6.70
ES	3.46	2.62–4.52	Reoperation	2.40	2.11–2.73
Mult reop	2.27	1.57–3.21	NDRF	2.11	1.77–2.51
NDRF	2.20	1.76–2.73	ES	1.89	1.50–2.36
Resuscitation	1.77	1.05–2.91	Preop IABP	1.82	1.43–2.30
First reoperation	1.70	1.44–1.99	Female gender	1.61	1.45–1.80
CS	1.67	1.14–2.40	CS	1.57	1.14–2.13
NYHA IV	1.56	1.35–1.81	NYHA IV	1.36	1.21–1.52
Inotropic agent used	1.47	1.10–1.95	TVD	1.31	1.18–1.45
CVA	1.44	1.14–1.80	CVA	1.24	1.03–1.48
MI	1.36	1.12–1.65	Diabetes	1.23	1.10–1.38
Female gender	1.25	1.10–1.42	Obesity	1.23	1.04–1.44
US	1.25	1.05–1.48	COPD	1.21	1.06–1.37
Diabetes	1.23	1.04–1.44	LMD	1.20	1.04–1.38
CHF	1.22	1.07–1.40	PVD	1.17	1.00–1.36
Arr	1.16	1.01–1.31	Diuretics	1.16	1.05–1.29
Age	1.03	1.03–1.04	MI	1.16	1.03–1.29
EF	0.99	0.99–1.00	Arr	1.14	1.01–1.29
			Age	1.04	1.03–1.05
			EF	1.00	0.99–1.00

Arr = arrhythmia; CHF = congestive heart failure; CI = 95% confidence interval; COPD = chronic obstructive pulmonary disease; CS = cardiogenic shock; CVA = cerebrovascular accident; CVD = cerebrovascular disease; DDRF = dialysis-dependent renal failure; EF = ejection fraction; ES = emergency status; HI = hemodynamic instability; LMD = left main disease; MI = myocardial infarction; Mult reop = multiple reoperation; NDRF = non-dialysis-dependent renal failure; NYHA IV = New York Heart Association class IV; PH = pulmonary hypertension; Preop IABP = preoperative intraaortic balloon pump; PVD = peripheral vascular disease; TVD = triple-vessel disease; US = urgent status.

Source: Adapted with permission from Jameison WR, Edwards FH, Schwartz M, et al: Risk stratification for cardiac valve replacement. National Cardiac Surgery Database. Ann Thorac Surg 1999; 67:943.

preoperative risk factors of operative mortality derived from the Society of Thoracic Surgeons database. Most early deaths are attributable to postoperative low cardiac output syndrome, neurologic injury, or infection.

Long-Term Survival

Longitudinal analysis shows there is no difference in survival over 10 years of follow-up between patients receiving mechanical and bioprosthetic valves when they are implanted in similar age cohorts.[122] However, after 15 years of follow-up, structural valve deterioration in bioprosthetic valves leads to a survival benefit for patients with mechanical valves. In a prospective trial by Hammermeister et al, 11-year mortality was 62% and 57% for bioprosthetic and mechanical valves, respectively.[123] At 15 years, mortality in the bioprosthetic group rose to 79% while mortality in the mechanical valve group rose to 66%.[124] There were substantially more bleeding events in patients with mechanical valves. In is important to note that the effect of bioprosthetic structural deterioration on mortality in this series was influenced by the actual prosthesis used in the study (Medtronic Hancock porcine). This is a first-generation prosthesis and may be more prone to structural failure than new devices.[125,126]

In most published series, the expected survival after aortic valve replacement is approximately 80% to 85% at 5 years, 65% to 75% at 10 years, and 45% to 55% at 15 years. [125,127–129] The outcomes of AVR are highly dependent on the functional status and comorbidities of each individual patient.[129,130] Cohen et al studied the impact of age, concomitant coronary artery disease, left ventricular dysfunction, and poor functional status on survival after bioprosthetic aortic valve replacement. Their results, presented in Table 32-6, show an additive risk for each of these comorbid factors.[131] Other studies have shown that concomitant renal disease, female gender, concomitant cardiac or vascular procedure, and atrial fibrillation are also risk factors for late mortality.[102,120,130,132,133]

TABLE 32–6 Survival probability calculated from the accelerated time failure model with the log-logistic distribution for combinations of risk factors

CAD	Age >65	NYHA class IV	Left ventricular grade III or IV	Predicted 5-y survival (%)	Predicted 10-y survival (%)
				89.1 (73, 100)	83.9 (73, 95)
X				83.4 (70, 97)	76.2 (67, 85)
	X			84.5 (71, 98)	77.7 (69, 86)
		X		83.6 (70, 97)	76.6 (68, 85)
			X	82.3 (69, 96)	74.8 (66, 84)
X	X			77.1 (66, 88)	68.2 (61, 75)
X		X		75.9 (65, 87)	66.8 (60, 74)
X			X	74.1 (63, 85)	64.6 (58, 72)
	X	X		77.4 (66, 88)	68.6 (62, 76)
	X		X	75.7 (65, 86)	66.5 (59, 74)
		X	X	74.5 (64, 85)	65.1 (58, 72)
X	X	X		67.8 (59, 77)	57.4 (52, 63)
X	X		X	65.7 (57, 75)	55.0 (49, 61)
	X	X	X	66.2 (57, 75)	55.5 (50, 61)
X	X	X	X	54.6 (47, 62)	43.5 (39, 48)

Each of these 4 risk factors was entered into the model as a dichotomous variable (i.e. NYHA IV versus NYHA I, II, or III; left ventricular grades 3 or 4 versus left ventricular grades 1 or 2). The (X) indicates the risk factor is present. These 4 risk factors are not present for the first row of estimates. The upper and lower 95% CI for the predicted survival probabilities are given in parentheses.

Source: Reproduced with permission from Cohen G, David TE, Ivanov J, et al: The impact of age, coronary artery disease, and cardiac comorbidity on late survival after bioprosthetic aortic valve replacement. J Thorac Cardiovasc Surg 1999; 117:273.

Valve-Related Mortality

Long-term survival data distinguishes between valve-related mortality, nonvalve-related cardiac mortality, and mortality from other causes. A revised consensus document from the Society of Thoracic Surgeons (STS) and the American Association of Thoracic Surgeons (AATS) was published in 1996 outlining a standardized method to report valve-related complications in prosthetic and repaired heart valves.[134] This panel defined valve-related mortality as all deaths caused by structural valve deterioration, nonstructural valve dysfunction, valve thrombosis, embolism, bleeding event, operated valvular endocarditis, or death related to reoperation of an operated valve. Sudden, unexplained, unexpected deaths of patients with an operated valve are included as valve-related mortality. Deaths caused by progressive heart failure in patients with satisfactorily functioning cardiac valves are not included. In the Hammermeister series, valve-related deaths accounted for 37% of all deaths in patients with a mechanical valve and 41% of all deaths in patients with a bioprosthesis at 15 years.[124] Nonvalvular cardiac deaths accounted for 17% and 21% of deaths at 15 years in patients with mechanical valves and bioprostheses, respectively.[124]

Nonfatal Valve Events

The joint STS/AATS panel defined specific guidelines for reporting outcomes on structural and nonstructural valve deterioration, valve thrombosis, embolic events, bleeding events, and prosthetic endocarditis.[135] These definitions are summarized below.

1. *Structural valve deterioration:* Any change in function of an operated valve resulting from an intrinsic abnormality of the valve that causes stenosis or regurgitation, such as wear, leaflet tears, or suture line disruption of components.
2. *Nonstructural dysfunction:* Any abnormality of an operated valve resulting in stenosis or regurgitation that is caused by factors not intrinsic to the valve itself, such as pannus overgrowth, inappropriate sizing, or paravalvular leak.
3. *Valve thrombosis:* Any thrombus attached to or near an operated valve that interferes with valve function in the absence of infection.
4. *Embolism:* Any embolic event that occurs after the immediate postoperative period when perioperative anesthesia has been completely reversed. Emboli may be peripheral (noncerebral) or cerebral. Myocardial infarction is excluded unless the event occurs after the perioperative period and coronary artery embolus is unequivocally documented.

Cerebral embolic events are subclassified into:

a. *Transient ischemic attacks*: Fully reversible neurologic events lasting less than 24 hours.

TABLE 32–7 Structural deterioration of stented bioprosthetic valves in the aortic position: long-term follow-up over 12-15 years

Reference	Prosthesis	Patients (no.)	Mean age (y)	Mean follow-up (mo.)	Time of SVD estimate (y)	Actuarial freedom from SVD	Actuarial freedom from reoperation
David, 1998[125]	Hancock II Porcine	723	65 ± 12	68 ± 40	12	94 ± 2	89 ± 5
Dellgren, 2002[127]	CE Pericardial	254	71 ± 9	60 ± 31	12	86 ± 9	83 ± 9
Poirier, 1998[138]	CE Pericardial	598	65*	57.7	12	93 ± 2	91 ± 2
Corbineau, 2002[291]	Medtronic Intact	188	72 ± 8	86.4 ± 50.4	13	91 ± 3.3	
Jamieson, 1998[156]	CE SAV Porcine	1657	65.5 ± 11.9	70.8 ± 58.8	12	83.4 ± 2.1	
Burdon, 1992[292]	Hancock I and MO	857	59 ± 11	87.6	15	63 ± 3	57 ± 3

b. *Reversible ischemic neurological deficit*: Fully reversible neurologic events lasting more than 24 hours and less than 3 weeks.
c. *Stroke*: Permanent neurologic deficit lasting longer than three weeks or causing death.

5. *Bleeding event*: Any episode of major internal or external bleeding that causes death, hospitalization, or permanent injury, or requires transfusion regardless of the patient's anticoagulation status. This does not include embolic stroke followed by hemorrhagic transformation and intracranial bleed.
6. *Operated valvular endocarditis*: Any infection involving an operated valve. Any structural/nonstructural valvular dysfunction, thrombosis, or embolic event associated with operated valvular endocarditis is included only in this category.

Time-related analysis of nonfatal complications is often expressed by the Kaplan-Meier actuarial method or by the recently described cumulative incidence method proposed by Grunkemeier.[136] Cumulative incidence (or actual) reporting provides more meaningful information as it censors the impact of mortality on nonfatal outcomes. This is most relevant in higher risk groups such as elderly patients, in which many patients will die from other causes prior to the occurrence of nonfatal valve-related events. Kaplan-Meier actuarial methods tend to exaggerate nonfatal events by continuing to assume that patients who have died are still at risk for these nonfatal events.

Structural Valve Deterioration

MECHANICAL PROSTHESES

Currently available mechanical prosthesis are extremely resistant to material fatigue or structural valve deterioration (SVD). Long-term follow-up in the Starr-Edwards caged-ball prosthesis, the Medtronic Hall tilting disc prosthesis, and the St. Jude bileaflet mechanical prosthesis show that these valves are exceedingly resilient to structural failure. Some discontinued mechanical prostheses, such as the Bjork-Shiley convexo-concave valve, had high rates of structural failure due to fracture of the outlet strut.[137]

STENTED BIOPROSTHESES

There are several large series describing long-term follow-up of first- and second-generation bioprostheses. Most of these series are not comparable to each other as they took place in different patient populations or in different eras. Structural valve deterioration is the most common nonfatal valve-related complication in bioprosthetic aortic valves. Table 32-7 summarizes the long-term SVD outcomes of commonly used first- and second-generation stented bioprostheses. Long-term follow-up of currently available second-generation stented bioprostheses, including the Medtronic Hancock II porcine and Carpentier-Edwards pericardial valves, show that these prostheses have a freedom from structural valve deterioration greater than 90% at 12-year follow-up.[125,127,138]

There is an important predisposition for premature bioprosthetic SVD in younger patients, particularly those under the age of 40 years.[139,140] Table 32-8 summarizes the effect of patient age on structural valve deterioration. SVD may be less common in elderly patients due to decreased hemodynamic stress placed on the valve. Also, the freedom from SVD

TABLE 32–8 Bioprosthetic valve failure 10 years after valve replacement according to the patient's age at the time of implantation

Patient's age (y)	Percentage with valve failure after 10 y
<40	42
40-49	30
50-59	21
60-69	15
>70	10

Source: Adapted with permission from Vongpatanasin W, Hillis LD, Lange RA et al: Medical progress: prosthetic heart valves. N Engl J Med 1996; 335:407, based on data from Grunkemeier GL, Jamieson WR, Miller DC, Starr A: Actuarial versus actual risk of porcine structural valve deterioration. J Thorac Cardiovasc Surg 1994; 108:709.

may be underestimated in the literature since most series report SVD by the actuarial method instead of the actual or cumulative incidence method.[136] Actuarial statistical analysis overestimates SVD in older patients since it assumes that patients who have died of other causes will continue to be at risk for SVD.[141]

Freedom from Reoperation

Freedom from reoperation for currently available mechanical valves is greater than 95% at 10 years and greater than 90% at 15 years.[124,142–147] Bioprostheses have a significantly higher rate of reoperation due to structural valve dysfunction. In large series, freedom from reoperation is greater than 95% at 5 years, greater than 90% at 10 years, but less than 70% at 15 years.[138,148–166] The long-term freedom from reoperation for several commonly available valves is presented in Table 32-7.

Optimal Antithrombotic Therapy

MECHANICAL VALVES

All mechanical valves require formal anticoagulation with warfarin for the lifetime of the patient as these valves are inherently thrombogenic. The overall linearized risk of thromboembolism in patients on warfarin therapy is 1% to 2% per year in most published series.[124,167–184] A meta-analysis of over 13,000 patients showed that the incidence of major embolism in mechanical valves without antithrombotic therapy was 4 per 100 patient-years.[185] With antiplatelet therapy this risk was 2.2 per 100 patient-years, and with warfarin therapy it was reduced to 1 per 100 patient-years. The incidence of thromboembolism was slightly higher in patients with caged-ball prostheses than other mechanical prostheses.[186]

The embolic risk is highest in the first few months, before the exposed cloth sewing ring and valve components have fully endothelialized.[187] Antithrombotic therapy is initiated on the second postoperative day with oral warfarin. In the presence of complicating factors such as gastrointestinal or mediastinal bleeding or perioperative neurologic injury, anticoagulation may be held initially. If the target level of anticoagulation is not achieved by the fourth postoperative day, intravenous heparin is instituted to achieve a partial thromboplastin time (PTT) between 60 and 90 seconds. If the patient is at high risk for thromboembolism, heparin is started concurrently with warfarin on the second postoperative day. High-risk patients include those with atrial fibrillation, intracardiac thrombus, left atrial enlargement, severe left ventricular dysfunction, and history of systemic emboli or hypercoagulable state.[33]

The target level of anticoagulation for each individual patient is dependent on the thrombotic risk profile and the type of valve employed. It is our practice to establish an international normalized ratio (INR) of 3.0 (acceptable range 2.5 to 3.5) for high-risk patients with mechanical valves and additionally institute low-dose aspirin therapy (80-100 mg once daily). For lower risk patients, the target INR is 2.5 (acceptable range 2.0 to 3.0) and low-dose aspirin is started on an individual basis.

Several articles suggest that caged-ball valves in the aortic position require a higher level of anticoagulation than tilting monoleaflet or bileaflet prostheses.[33,179] These valves should be anticoagulated to an INR of 3.5 to 4.5. Although older tilting monoleaftlet prostheses were associated with an increased rate of thromboembolism, currently available prostheses, such as the Medtronic Hall valve, do not appear to have increased thomboembolism risk versus bileaflet prostheses and should have the same target INR.[182,188,189]

Aspirin, an antiplatelet agent, is routinely used at a low dose to minimize the risk of thromboembolic events. Randomized trials have shown that low-dose aspirin significantly reduces fatal cardiovascular and embolic events for all patients with mechanical valves, particularly in patients with concomitant coronary or vascular disease.[190–193] There are increased bleeding events when higher doses of aspirin are used in patients formally anticoagulated with warfarin.[194,195] The linearized risk of a bleeding event is 0.1% to 3.5% per year depending on how these events are defined, the range of anticoagulation used, and how often coagulation parameters are measured.[194,196–198]

BIOPROSTHETIC VALVES

Bioprosthetic valves are less thrombogenic than mechanical prostheses and do not require long-term anticoagulation with warfarin unless the patient is at high risk for thromboembolism or has had a thromboembolic event with their prosthesis.[199] Stented bioprostheses have a linearized risk for thromboembolism between 0.5% and 1% per year.[100,138,149,200–203] This risk appears to be lower in patients with stentless heterograft, allograft, or autograft valves.[204–209] Anticoagulant management of bioprostheses during the first three months after implantation remains variable between institutions. There is an increased hazard function for thromboembolism before the exposed surfaces of stented bioprosthesis endothelialize.[187] The current American College of Cardiology/American Heart Association guidelines recommend anticoagulation with warfarin to an INR between 2.0 and 3.0 for the first 3 months for bioprosthetic valves.[33] This is discontinued at the end of the third month unless the patient is at high risk for thromboembolism. Low-dose aspirin is continued as monotherapy in low-risk patients and in conjunction with warfarin in high-risk patients for the lifetime of the patient. Combined aspirin and warfarin have a survival benefit over warfarin alone in high-risk patients with bioprosthetic heart valves.[33] Aspirin significantly decreases the risk of thromboembolism in low-risk patients with bioprostheses versus no antiplatelet therapy.[199,210–212] If a patient has identified high-risk factors for thrombosis preoperatively, a mechanical prosthesis should be implanted unless the risk factor is amenable to correction, because formal anticoagulation with warfarin will still be necessary. With aspirin, patients with bioprosthetic valves have approximately the same risk of thromboembolism as patients with mechanical valves on full anticoagulation, with fewer bleeding complications.[33]

Prosthesis Thrombosis

Prosthesis thrombosis is a rare but potentially devastating outcome after aortic valve replacement. The incidence of prosthesis thrombosis is less than 0.2% per year and it occurs more often in mechanical prostheses.[213–215] Thrombolytic therapy may be used in some patients but it is often ineffective. Thrombolysis is recommended in patients with left-sided thrombosis who are experiencing significant heart failure (NYHA class III or higher) and are considered too high risk for surgery.[33,216] Cerebral or peripheral thromboembolism occurs in 12% of patients after thrombolytic therapy.[33] Surgical treatment includes replacement of the valve or open thrombectomy, and mortality from either procedure is similar at approximately 10% to 15%.[217] Recurrent thrombosis after declotting occurs in up to 40% of patients, and we recommend valve replacement in virtually all patients who are managed operatively.[218]

Prosthetic Valve Endocarditis

Prosthetic valve endocarditis (PVE) is separated into two time frames: early (less than 60 days postimplantation) and late (greater than 60 days postimplantation). Early PVE is usually a sequela of perioperative bacterial seeding of the valve either during implantation or postoperatively from wound or intravascular catheter infections.[62] *Staphylococcus aureus, Staphylococcus epidermidis,* gram-negative bacteria, and fungal infections are common in this period.[33,219–223] Although most cases of late PVE are caused by septicemia from noncardiac sources, a small proportion of late PVE in the first year is attributable to less virulent organisms introduced in the perioperative period, particularly *Staphylococcus epidermidis*.[224] Organisms responsible for late PVE include *Streptococcus* and *Staphylococcus* species and other organisms commonly found in native valve infectious endocarditis.[33] All unexplained fevers should be meticulously investigated for PVE with serial blood cultures and transesophageal and/or transthoracic echocardiography. Transesophageal echocardiography provides more detailed anatomic information such as the presence of vegetations, abscesses, and fistulas, but often does not provide adequate views of the anterior portion of the valve.[225] Transthoracic views may be helpful in these cases. Mechanical valves are particularly difficult to visualize by echocardiography due to shadowing created by valve components.

The annual risk of PVE in the aortic position is 0.6% to 0.9% per patient-year.[10,138,180,188,201,202,226–234] The 5-year freedom from PVE reported in many major series is greater than 97%.[100,127,235,236] Mechanical valves have a slightly higher early hazard for PVE than stented bioprostheses.[237] However, there is no difference in risk between patients with mechanical and stented bioprostheses after the early phase. Stentless porcine heterografts and human allografts are less likely to develop PVE since they have less prosthetic material that may serve as a nidus of infection.[238–245] These valves may be particularly helpful in valve re-replacement for PVE.

Outcome for patients with PVE is very poor. Invasive paravalvular infection occurs in up to 40% of cases of PVE.[246] Early PVE is associated with 30% to 80% mortality while late PVE is associated with 20% to 40% mortality.[62,247]

Surgery is indicated for PVE in the following circumstances:

1. All cases of early (<60 days postimplantation) prosthetic endocarditis.
2. Concomitant heart failure and valvular dysfunction.
3. Paravalvular leak or partial dehiscence, even in a stable patient, requires operative management, particularly if more than 40% of the valve annular circumference is involved.
4. The presence of a new conduction defect, abscess, aneurysm, or fistula mandates operative management. All fungal infections and those caused by the most virulent strains of *Staphylococcus aureus, Serratia marcescens,* and *Pseudomonas aeruginosa* also require operation as these organisms are highly invasive and antibiotic therapy is generally ineffective.
5. Any case of persistent bacteremia despite a maximum of 5 days of appropriate antibiotic therapy and no other source of infection.
6. Vegetations larger than10 mm are not well penetrated by antibiotics and usually need operative management.
7. Multiple systemic emboli.

Paravalvular Leak and Hemolysis

Paravalvular leak is uncommon outside of the setting of infective endocarditis. Technical errors may result in inappropriately large gaps between sutures, leaving a small portion of the prosthesis unattached to the annulus. If paravalvular leak is sufficient to cause significant hemolysis, surgical correction may be performed with a few interrupted pledgeted sutures. Hemolysis is uncommon with the currently available mechanical or stented bioprosthetic valves if they are functioning well. Pannus overgrowth and prosthetic structural degeneration interfering with normal valve opening and closure may cause hemolysis severe enough to warrant reoperation. Milder cases of hemolysis may be managed conservatively by dietary supplementation with iron and folic acid and routine measurement of hemoglobin, serum haptoglobin, and lactate dehydrogenase (LDH).

TABLE 32–9 The effective orifice area and mean systolic gradient of commonly available bioprostheses

	19 mm		21 mm		23 mm		25 mm		27 mm	
Prosthesis[ref no]	EOA (cm^2)	MSG (mm Hg)	EOA (cm^2)	MSG (mm Hg)	EOA (cm^2)	MSG (mm Hg)	EOA (cm^2)	MSG (mm Hg)	EOA (cm^2)	MSG (mm Hg)
Hancock Standard[293–295]	1.0	25	1.0-1.3	18-30	1.3-1.5	7-24	-	13-17		
Hancock Modified Orifice[295,296]	0.9	12-19	1.4	10-17	1.4	11-16	1.7	10-12		
Hancock II[162]			1.2		1.3		1.5		1.6	
Medtronic Intact[297,298]			1.5	17	1.6	19	17	1.9	15	
Medtronic Mosaic[299–301]	1.2	16	1.3	14-15	1.5	12-13	1.8	11-12	2.0	9-10
CE Standard[302–304]	0.85	26	1.3-1.4	18-21	1.3-1.6	15-30	1.2-2.1	13-21		
CE Supraannular[305–307]		17	1.2	11	1.4	12	2.1	16		9
CE Pericardial [308–310]	0.95	18-19	1.1	13-14	1.5	11-14	1.4	10-11	1.6	10
Mitroflow Pericardial[311]	1.3		1.4		1.7					
Toronto SPV[258,312,313]				8	1.6-1.8	3-7	1.4-1.9	3.5-7	1.7-2.3	3-5
Medtronic Freestyle[108,313–315]	1.0-1.4	18-22	1.3-1.4	7-13	1.4-1.5	7-14	1.7-2.0	5-9	2.0-2.3	5-7
Edwards Prima Valve[316]	1.6	9	1.6	9	1.9	6	2.1	6	2.4	5

EOA = effective orifice area; MSG = mean systolic gradient; CE = Carpentier-Edwards

HEMODYNAMIC PERFORMANCE AND VENTRICULAR REMODELLING

Pressure and/or volume overloading caused by aortic valve disease leads to increased intracavitary left ventricular pressures and compensatory left ventricular hypertrophy. Severe aortic regurgitation causes volume overload with an increase in left ventricular end-diastolic volume and eccentric hypertrophy, but may not change the ratio of ventricular wall thickness to cavity radius. In severe aortic stenosis, concentric ventricular hypertrophy occurs without increasing end-diastolic dimension until late in the disease process, thus increasing the ventricular wall thickness to cavity radius ratio.

Both pathologies result in an increase in left ventricular mass. Studies from the hypertension literature indicate that increased left ventricular mass has a strong negative prognostic effect. Several reports, including the Framingham Heart Study, indicate that increased left ventricular mass was a predictor of all cardiac events including sudden cardiac death.[248–250] The overall goal of aortic valve replacement is to alleviate the pressure and volume overload on the left ventricle allowing myocardial remodeling and regression of left ventricular mass.

The clinical impact of left ventricular mass regression is not as well understood, despite its widespread acceptance as a measure of outcome after aortic valve surgery. Smaller studies have shown that in hypertensive patients undergoing medical treatment, patients with a reduction of left ventricular mass had fewer cardiac events than those whose left ventricular mass did not change or increased.[251] The prognostic implications of left ventricular mass regression after aortic valve surgery have not been rigorously studied, but logic would suggest that poor left ventricular mass regression is associated with poor clinical outcome. There are no studies showing that there is incremental clinical benefit with greater degrees of ventricular mass regression.

Left ventricular mass regresses significantly over the first 18 months and returns to within normal limits in many patients after aortic valve replacement for isolated aortic stenosis.[252–257] Ventricular mass regression may continue for up to 5 years after valve replacement.[258] However, some patients do not experience adequate ventricular mass regression and may experience poorer prognosis. Several authors have identified a situation, referred to as patient-prosthesis mismatch, in which the poor hemodynamic performance of a prosthesis results in poor regression of left ventricular hypertrophy and poor patient outcome.

Patient-Prosthesis Mismatch

The term patient-prosthesis mismatch has been applied to several different clinical situations. It has been used to describe absolute small valve size (i.e., less than 21 mm), small valve size in a patient with a large body surface area, excessive transvalvular gradient immediately postimplantation,

TABLE 32–10 Patient-prosthesis mismatch: patient characteristics by postoperative gradient

Characteristic	Normal gradient	Abnormal gradient	*p* Value
Preoperative			
Age (y)	65.2 ± 11.5	62.0 ± 12.5	
Age >70y	36.0%	33.7%	
Female	30.3%	50.0%	0.001
Body surface area (m^2)	1.88 ± 0.22	1.83 ± 0.23	
Urgent surgery	18.6%	21.7%	
NYHA class III or IV	68.7%	72.8%	
Congestive heart failure	17.1%	21.7%	
Diabetes	13.3%	14.1%	
Hypertension	44.9%	50.0%	
COPD	7.1%	4.4%	
Peripheral vascular disease	10.9%	14.1%	
LV grade (3 or 4)	12.7%	12.0%	
Coronary artery disease	41.4%	31.5%	
Stenosis	69.0%	75.0%	
Regurgitation	26.2%	20.2%	
Prosthetic valve	1.7%	2.3%	
Operative			
Pump time (min)	145.1 ± 46.8	146.3 ± 48.2	
Cross-clamp time (min)	117.1 ± 38.6	114.7 ± 39.2	
Valve size (mm)	24.4 ± 2.5	23.0 ± 2.3	0.0001
Internal diameter (mm)	21.3 ± 2.5	19.6 ± 2.8	0.0001
Mechanical	36.0%	38.9%	
Toronto SP valve	23.4%	23.3%	
Tissue valve (stented)	40.2%	37.8%	
Bentall or ascending aorta	8.9%	1.8%	0.01
Annulus enlargement	4.9%	6.5%	
Postoperative			
Early mortality	0.6%	2.2%	
ICU stay (d)	2.8 ± 5.1	2.8 ± 2.1	
Hospital stay (d)	11.5 ± 16.3	10.2 ± 7.3	
Cerebrovascular accident	4.6%	5.4%	
Low output syndrome	17.3%	23.9%	
Mean aortic gradients (mm Hg)	11.9 ± 4.2	29.7 ± 13.7	
Follow-up			
Mean follow-up time (y)	39.1 ± 31.5	47.2 ± 39.4	

COPD = chronic obstructive pulmonary disease; ICU = intensive care unit; LV = left ventricle; NYHA = New York Heart Association.

Source: Hanayama N, Christakis GT, Mallidi HR, et al: Patient prosthesis mismatch is rare after aortic valve replacement: valve size may be irrelevant. Ann Thorac Surg 2002; 73:1822.

increased transvalvular gradient with exercise, indexed effective orifice area (IEOA), and various combinations of these variables (Table 32-9).

IEOA is calculated by dividing the echocardiographically determined effective orifice area (EOA) by the body surface area (BSA). Effective orifice area is calculated by a reconfiguration of the continuity equation:

$$EOA = (CSA_{LVOT} \times TVI_{LVOT})/TVI_{AO}$$

where EOA is effective orifice area in cm^2, CSA_{LVOT} is the cross-sectional area of the left ventricular outflow tract (LVOT) in cm^2 determined by two-dimensional measurement of the LVOT diameter, TVI_{LVOT} is the velocity time integral of forward blood flow in cm derived from pulse-wave Doppler in the LVOT, and TVI_{AO} is the velocity time integral of forward blood flow in cm derived from software integration of transvalvular continuous wave Doppler.[259] Although the aortic annular dimensions can be used instead of LVOT, several studies have shown that LVOT is a more accurate measure for estimating effective orifice area in bioprosthetic heart valves.[260,261]

Rahimtoola defined patient-prosthesis mismatch as a condition that occurs when the valve area of a prosthetic valve is less than the area of that patient's normal valve.[262] In this situation, the prosthesis may be too small for the patient's cardiac output requirements, as estimated by their body surface area. The prosthesis creates a residual stenosis that results in an elevated transvalvular gradient.

To some extent, all mechanical and stented biological prostheses are inherently stenotic.[62] The presence of rigid sewing rings and, in the case of stented bioprostheses, struts to hold the valve commissures causes obstruction to outflow and will therefore cause a residual gradient despite normal prosthesis function. The problem is exacerbated by annular fibrosis, annular calcification, and left ventricular hypertrophy, as seen in aortic stenosis, which cause contraction of the native annulus leading to the implantation of a smaller prosthesis. Larger patients are also more likely to have lower IEOA based on their larger body surface areas. The significance of patient-prosthesis mismatch is controversial as there is little evidence that lower IEOA causes diminished clinical results in many patients.

Several authors suggest that patient-prosthesis mismatch occurs at an indexed effective orifice area of less than 0.85 cm^2/m^2.[263,264] This definition is based on the assumption that transvalvular gradients begin to rise substantially at IEOA below this value and these elevated gradients cause increased left ventricular work that prevents adequate regression of left ventricular hypertrophy.[265]

Using this criteria, Pibarot and Dumesnil prospectively studied 72 patients over 7 years and found no difference in survival between patients with patient-prosthesis mismatch and those without.[266] Mean gradients were higher in the patient-prosthesis mismatch group (22 ± 8 mm Hg vs. 15 ± 7 mm Hg). The clinical relevance of a 7 mm Hg difference in gradient in otherwise asymptomatic patients is unclear and certainly would not warrant any treatment. Also, the difference in gradient is within the measurement error for this echocardiographically derived variable. In this study, lower IEOA was an independent predictor of poorer NYHA class early after aortic valve replacement, but this relationship was not present at 7-year follow up. No objective testing of function was performed on these patients.

Rao et al studied patient-prosthesis mismatch in patients undergoing aortic valve replacement.[267] A total of 2145 patients were reviewed including 227 patients with patient-prosthesis mismatch and 1927 without. Overall survival was the same in both groups, but valve-related mortality was higher in the patient-prosthesis mismatch group at 10 years. This retrospective study was not randomized, and valve-related mortality included mechanisms of death that are totally unrelated to patient-prosthesis mismatch (embolic stroke, valve failure, endocarditis, bleeding, reoperation). Furthermore, this study had no echocardiographic data.

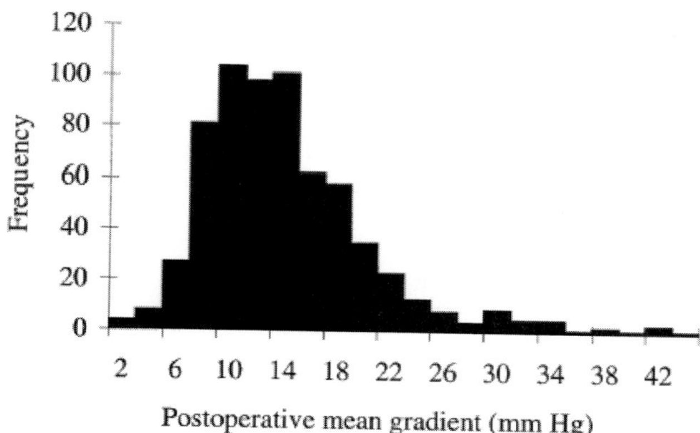

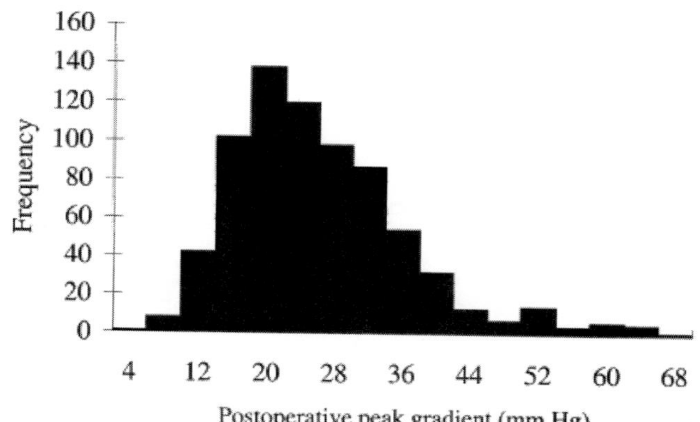

FIGURE 32–6 Distribution of postoperative peak gradients and mean gradients. (*Reproduced with permission from Hanayama N, Christakis GT, Mallidi HR, et al: Patient prosthesis mismatch is rare after aortic valve replacement: valve size may be irrelevant. Ann Thorac Surg 2002; 73:1822.*)

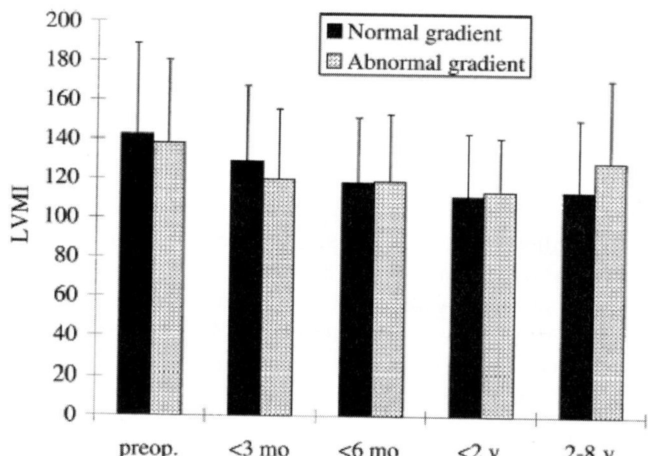

FIGURE 32–7 Left ventricular mass index in the normal gradient group and the abnormal gradient group. There was no significant difference between the two groups. LVMI = left ventricular mass index; preop. = preoperative. (*Reproduced with permission from Hanayama N, Christakis GT, Mallidi HR, et al: Patient prosthesis mismatch is rare after aortic valve replacement: valve size may be irrelevant. Ann Thorac Surg 2002; 73:1822.*)

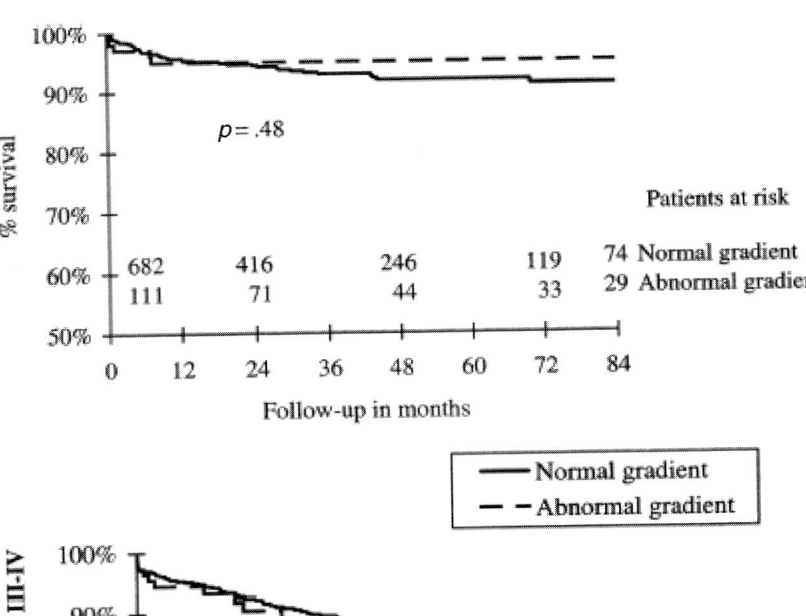

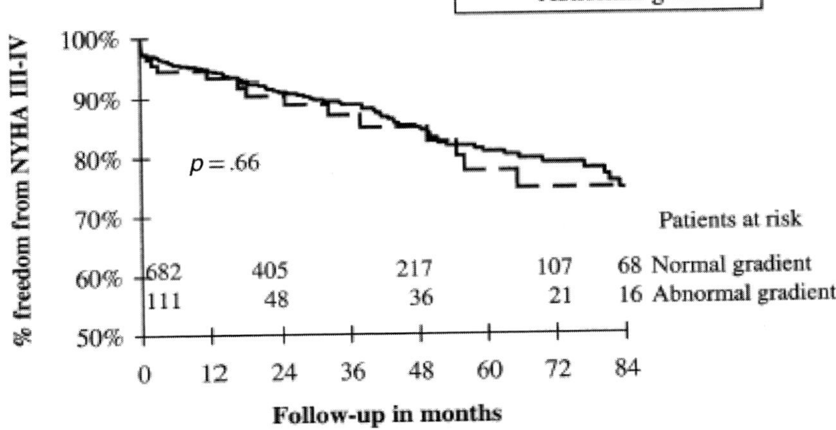

FIGURE 32–8 Actuarial survival and freedom from New York Heart Association (NYHA) class III or IV in the normal gradient group and the abnormal gradient group. Seven-year survival was 91.2% ± 1.5% (normal gradient) and 95.0% ± 2.2% (abnormal gradient). Seven-year freedom from NYHA class III or IV was 74.5% ± 3.1% and 74.6% ± 6.2%, respectively. There were no significant differences in the two groups. (*Reproduced with permission from Hanayama N, Christakis GT, Mallidi HR, et al: Patient prosthesis mismatch is rare after aortic valve replacement: valve size may be irrelevant. Ann Thorac Surg 2002; 73:1822.*)

Effective orifice area was obtained from in vitro data supplied by the manufacturers according to the valve size implanted. Patient-prosthesis mismatch was simply assumed on the basis of calculated numbers unrelated to individual patients.

Several well-designed multivariate studies have not shown that patient-prosthesis mismatch influences survival. Medalion et al studied 892 aortic valve replacements and demonstrated that although 25% of patients received valves with an indexed internal orifice area less than two standard deviations below predicted normal aortic valve size, there were no differences in 15-year survival between patients with or without patient-prosthesis mismatch.[268]

We have recently reported our institutional experience with patient-prosthesis mismatch in 1129 patients who were prospectively studied over a 10-year period.[269] We defined patient-prosthesis mismatch as an IEOA less than the 90th percentile in our patient population. The cutoff value for IEOA to define patient-prosthesis mismatch was 0.6 cm^2/m^2, which would be considered very severe by most groups. Preoperative patient characteristics comparing those with normal and abnormal gradients are presented in Table 32-10. The only preoperative predictor of abnormal gradient was small valve size. Postoperative mean and peak gradients are outlined in Figure 32-6. Figures 32-7 and 32-8 illustrate that there were no differences in left ventricular mass index or survival at midterm follow-up between patients with normal and abnormal gradients. Thus, although valve size is a predictor of abnormal postoperative gradient, no clinical significance can be correlated to this finding. The distribution of indexed effective orifice areas in these patients is presented in Figure 32-9. Figures 32-10 and 32-11 show that there were no differences in left ventricular mass index or survival at midterm follow-up between patients with or without patient-prosthesis mismatch defined as IEOA less than 0.6 cm^2/m^2.

Many authors have expressed concern about a high incidence of patient-prosthesis mismatch in the small aortic root. He et al assessed 30-year survival after aortic valve replacement in the small aortic root and concluded that body surface area in this high-risk group influenced survival only in patients with concomitant coronary artery bypass grafting.[270] Sawant et al demonstrated that in patients with small aortic roots, body surface area and valve size were not determinants of long-term survival.[271]

Studies by De Paulis et al have shown that there was no difference in left ventricular mass regression between patients

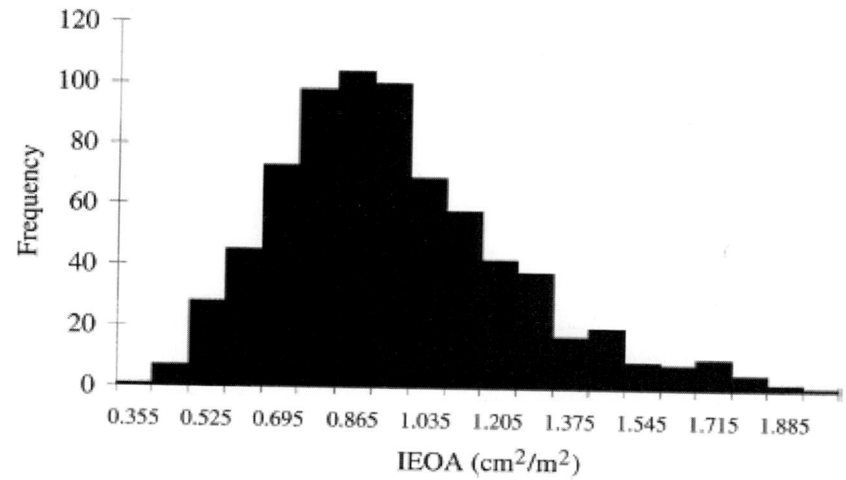

FIGURE 32–9 **Distribution of postoperative indexed effective orifice area (IEOA).** *(Reproduced with permission from Hanayama N, Christakis GT, Mallidi HR, et al: Patient prosthesis mismatch is rare after aortic valve replacement: valve size may be irrelevant. Ann Thorac Surg 2002; 73:1822.)*

receiving 19-mm and 21-mm mechanical valves and those with 23-mm or 25-mm valves.[272] Hence, there is little clinical benefit derived from implantation of a one-size larger prosthesis, particularly if the potential operative morbidity is increased to do this. There is no evidence in the literature suggesting that small differences in the degree of left ventricular mass regression have any clinical significance in patients after aortic valve replacement or hypertension.

Foster et al showed that in patients with 17-mm and 19-mm prostheses who had resting transvalvular gradients greater than 30 mm Hg, 93% were in NYHA class I at late follow-up.[273] Kratz et al also reported that small valve size was not predictive of congestive heart failure or late death.[274] Khan et al studied 19-mm to 23-mm Carpentier-Edwards pericardial valves and found that significant left ventricular

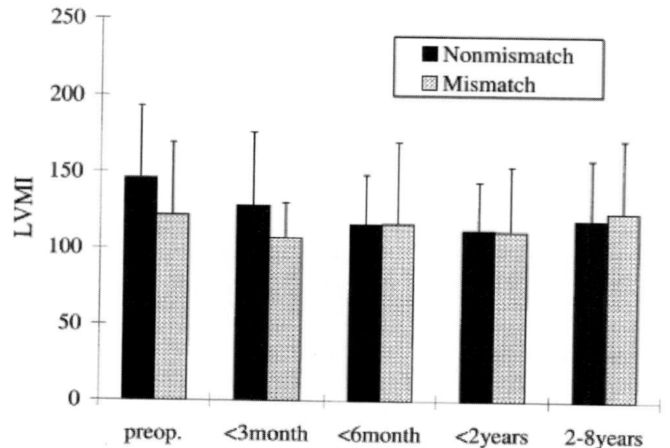

FIGURE 32–10 **Left ventricular mass index (LVMI) in the mismatch and the nonmismatch group. There were no significant differences in the two groups. preop. = preoperative.** *(Reproduced with permission from Hanayama N, Christakis GT, Mallidi HR, et al: Patient prosthesis mismatch is rare after aortic valve replacement: valve size may be irrelevant. Ann Thorac Surg 2002; 73:1822.)*

mass regression occurred with each valve size, including 19-mm valves.[275]

Complex operations of the aortic root including root enlargement procedures and stentless porcine prostheses have been proposed to enable the implantation of valves with a larger IEOA. The rationale for choosing a more complex operation, which carries an increased perioperative risk, is predicated on the assumption that the patient will experience improved long-term outcome. However, there is no clear evidence to suggest that a patient receiving a prosthesis with an IEOA as low as 0.6 cm^2/m^2 will experience any decrease in life expectancy based on prosthesis size.[269]

Aortic root enlargement procedures may carry excessive mortality, particularly when performed by less experienced surgeons. In a large series, David et al performed aortic root enlargement procedures in almost 20% of aortic valve replacements without any increase in mortality.[276] The prognostic benefit of root enlargement procedures in decreasing left ventricular mass or preventing cardiac events has not been established.[277]

Walther et al performed a small randomized trial comparing the ability of stented porcine and stentless porcine valves to cause regression of left ventricular hypertrophy.[278] They showed that despite equivalent annular dimensions in the stented and stentless groups, larger valves (by labeled size) were implanted in the stentless group. The patients receiving stentless valves had a greater degree of left ventricular mass regression than those receiving stented valves. No clinical follow-up was provided.

Rao et al compared hemodynamic data among 19-mm to 23-mm Carpentier-Edwards pericardial valves and Toronto SPV stentless valves of equivalent internal diameter and found no hemodynamic differences in peak or mean gradient.[49] At the same institution, Cohen et al randomized patients to receive Carpentier-Edwards pericardial valves and Toronto SPV stentless valves and compared clinical outcomes.[279] There were no differences in the size of the aortic root between the two groups. Postoperative

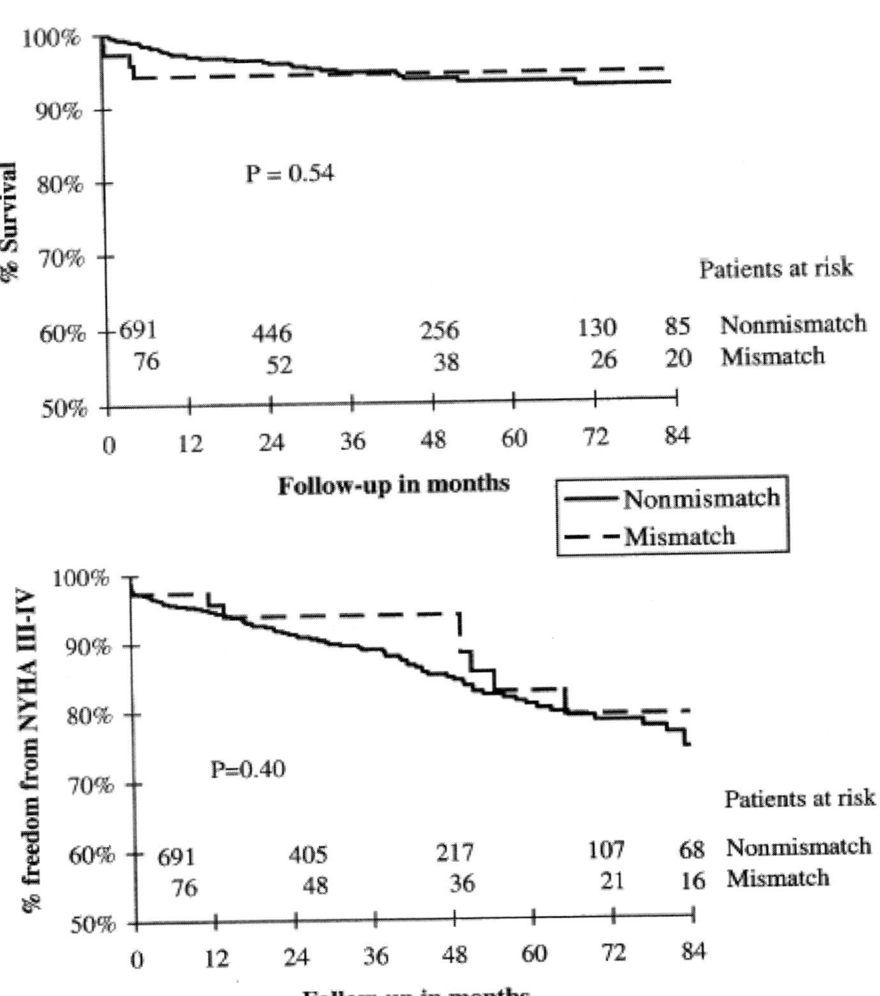

FIGURE 32–11 Actuarial survival and freedom from New York Heart Association (NYHA) class III or IV in the nonmismatch group and the mismatch group. Seven-year survival was 94.7% ± 3.0% (nonmismatch group) and 95.1% ± 1.3% (mismatch group). Seven-year freedom from New York Heart Association class III or IV was 79.3% ± 6.6% and 74.5% ± 2.5%, respectively. There were no significant differences in the two groups. (*Reproduced with permission from Hanayama N, Christakis GT, Mallidi HR, et al: Patient prosthesis mismatch is rare after aortic valve replacement: valve size may be irrelevant. Ann Thorac Surg 2002; 73:1822.*)

echocardiography showed that there was no difference in indexed effective orifice area or left ventricular mass regression between groups (Fig. 32-12). They also found no difference in functional outcome between valves at 1-year follow-up (Fig. 32-13). These findings challenge the notion that stentless porcine valves provide increased IEOA, or either hemodynamic or clinically significant benefits. Some reports have shown that transvalvular gradients in patients with lower IEOA often increase substantially with exercise.[280,281] Although the majority of patients undergoing aortic valve replacement are elderly and unlikely to experience function limitations from this situation, in younger, highly active patients either root enlargement or stentless prostheses may provide better functional outcome.

PROSTHESIS SELECTION

An ideal aortic prosthesis would be simple to implant, widely available, possess long-term durability, would have no intrinsic thrombogenicity, would not have a predilection for endocarditis, and would have no residual transvalvular pressure gradient. Such a valve does not currently exist. Currently available options include mechanical valves, stented biologic heterograft valves, stentless biologic heterograft valves, allograft valves, and pulmonary autograft valves. Among these options, pulmonary autograft valves and allograft valves are the most physiologic prostheses. They are less prone to thrombosis or endocarditis and have excellent hemodynamic characteristics.[206,240,282–288] The longevity of such valves is dependent on patient factors, the preparation of the valve, and the technical skill of the operating surgeon. Despite their potential benefits, these prostheses are not readily available and can be very technically demanding to implant compared to standard mechanical or stented bioprostheses. They are most beneficial in children and younger adults. Allograft valves may also improve the results of aortic valve replacement in active endocarditis.[239] A further discussion of these valves is presented in subsequent chapters. As their use has remained confined to a few centers that perform

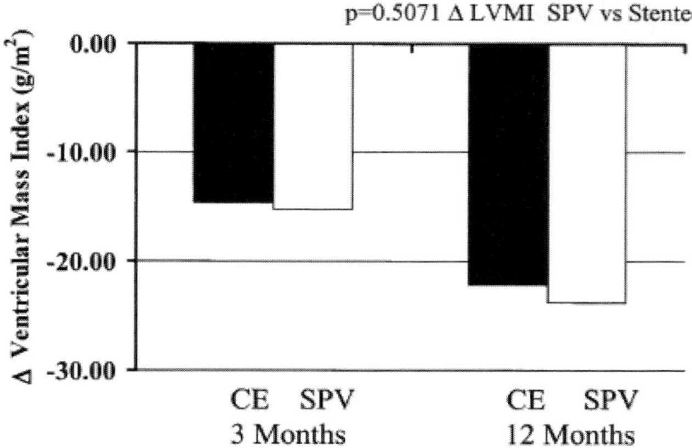

FIGURE 32–12 Indexed ventricular mass regression in both groups over time. CE = Carpentier-Edwards stented valve; LVMI = left ventricular mass index; SPV = Toronto stentless porcine valve. (*Reproduced with permission from Cohen G, Christakis GT, Joyner CD, et al: Are stentless valves hemodynamically superior to stented valves? A prospective randomized trial. Ann Thorac Surg 2002; 73:767.*)

such operations regularly, the remainder of this discussion will focus on issues regarding selection of mechanical or bioprosthetic valves.

Mechanical versus Stented Biologic Valves

When selecting between mechanical and biologic heart valves, the surgeon and patient must balance the risks and benefits of each choice. Mechanical valves are much less likely to undergo structural deterioration than bioprosthetic valves, and reoperation for structural valve deterioration is more common in patients with bioprosthetic valves.

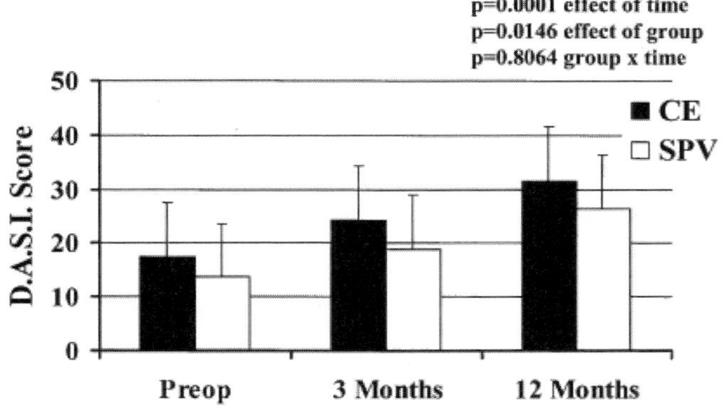

FIGURE 32–13 Change in Duke Activity Status Index (D.A.S.I.) scores in both groups over time. CE = Carpentier-Edwards stented valve; SPV = Toronto stentless porcine valve; Preop = preoperative. (*Reproduced with permission from Cohen G, Christakis GT, Joyner CD, et al: Are stentless valves hemodynamically superior to stented valves? A prospective randomized trial. Ann Thorac Surg 2002; 73:767.*)

Mechanical valves are more thrombogenic than bioprosthetic valves and require formal anticoagulation with oral warfarin. Anticoagulated patients have a significantly increased risk of bleeding complications. Patients with mechanical valves and adequate anticoagulation do not have significantly greater risk of thromboembolic events than bioprosthetic valves. There is no difference in actuarial freedom from bacterial endocarditis between mechanical and bioprosthetic valves.

Patients with an absolute requirement for long-term anticoagulation such as atrial fibrillation, previous thromboembolic events, hypercoagulable state, severe left ventricular dysfunction, another mechanical heart valve in place, or intracardiac thrombus, should receive a mechanical valve regardless of age. Patients with end-stage renal failure and hypercalcemia have a significantly elevated risk for early bioprosthetic structural valve deterioration and should also receive a mechanical prosthesis unless they are not expected to outlive their bioprosthesis.

Currently available second-generation bioprostheses, such as the Medtronic Hancock II porcine and Carpentier-Edwards pericardial valves, have greater than 90% freedom from structural valve dysfunction and greater than 90% freedom from reoperation at 12-year follow-up.[138,158,165] The rate of structural deterioration is lower in patients older than 65 to 70 years. Hence, patients over 70 years old at the time of surgery should receive a biologic valve. Patients between 65 and 70 years of age who have comorbidities such as coronary artery disease are less likely to outlive their prosthesis and should receive a biologic valve. Patients between 65 and 70 years old who are otherwise quite healthy and have isolated aortic valve disease without significant ventricular dysfunction are at higher risk to outlive a bioprosthesis and should receive a mechanical valve. Patients under the age of 65 years should have a mechanical prosthesis to minimize the risk of structural failure requiring repeat aortic valve replacement in an octogenarian. Also, patients in whom anticoagulation is contraindicated, such as women of childbearing age wishing to become pregnant, or those who refuse anticoagulation, should receive a bioprosthesis.

A detailed discussion of these risks and benefits of prosthesis selection should occur with all patients and their families prior to surgery.

Stented versus Stentless Biologic Valves

Stentless porcine valves have gained popularity in cardiac surgery due to pioneering work by David at the Toronto General Hospital in 1988.[289] Since they do not have obstructive stents and strut posts, stentless valves provide residual gradients and effective orifice areas that are similar to freehand allografts. Since stentless valves are more difficult to implant and require a longer cross-clamp time, the risks of operation must be matched to a specific benefit the patient may receive with a stentless valve. As discussed earlier in this chapter, there is conflicting evidence that the use of stentless valves results in improved left ventricular mass regression over stented bioprostheses. Several studies have shown adequate left ventricular mass regression in patients receiving small stented bioprostheses. There is also no evidence that incremental improvements in left ventricular mass provide additional clinical benefit. Thus, the routine use of stentless bioprostheses cannot be recommended for most patients with small aortic roots with the currently available data. At this time, stentless porcine valves are most useful in a relatively younger patient with a small aortic root who is active and likely to be limited by the elevated residual gradient a stented bioprosthesis will create. Long-term durability data are not available to fairly compare current generation stented and stentless bioprostheses. There are reports of decreased thromboembolic events in stentless valves.[290] The final role of stentless aortic valves will be decided based on their long-term freedom from structural valve deterioration and clinical outcomes.

REFERENCES

1. Selzer A, Lombard JT: Clinical findings in adult aortic stenosis—then and now. *Eur Heart J* 1988; 9(suppl E):53.
2. Selzer A: Changing aspects of the natural history of valvular aortic stenosis. *N Engl J Med* 1987; 317:91.
3. Bonow RO, Carabello B, de Leon AC, et al: ACC/AHA guidelines for the management of patients with valvular heart disease: executive summary. A report of the American College of Cardiology/American Heart Association Task Force on Practice Guidelines (Committee on Management of Patients With Valvular Heart Disease). *J Heart Valve Dis* 1998; 7:672.
4. Rahimtoola SH. Valvular heart disease: a perspective. *J Am Coll Cardiol* 1983; 1:199.
5. Bonow RO, Carabello B, de Leon AC, et al: ACC/AHA guidelines for the management of patients with valvular heart disease: executive summary. A report of the American College of Cardiology/American Heart Association Task Force on Practice Guidelines (Committee on Management of Patients With Valvular Heart Disease). *J Heart Valve Dis* 1998; 7:672.
6. Hess OM, Villari B, Krayenbuehl HP: Diastolic dysfunction in aortic stenosis. *Circulation* 1993; 87(5 suppl):IV73.
7. Braunwald E: Valvular heart disease, in Braunwald E (ed): *Heart Disease: A Textbook of Cardiovascular Medicine*, 6th ed. Philadelphia, WB Saunders, 2001; p 1643.
8. Hess OM, Ritter M, Schneider J, et al: Diastolic stiffness and myocardial structure in aortic valve disease before and after valve replacement. *Circulation* 1984; 69:855.
9. Villari B, Vassalli G, Monrad ES, et al: Normalization of diastolic dysfunction in aortic stenosis late after valve replacement. *Circulation* 1995; 91:2353.
10. Horstkotte D, Loogen F: The natural history of aortic valve stenosis. *Eur Heart J* 1988; 9(suppl E):57.
11. Lund O, Nielsen TT, Emmertsen K, et al: Mortality and worsening of prognostic profile during waiting time for valve replacement in aortic stenosis. *Thorac Cardiovasc Surg* 1996; 44:289.
12. Schwarz F, Baumann P, Manthey J, et al: The effect of aortic valve replacement on survival. *Circulation* 1982; 66:1105.
13. Horstkotte D, Loogen F: The natural history of aortic valve stenosis. *Eur Heart J* 1988; 9(suppl E):57.
14. Iivanainen AM, Lindroos M, Tilvis R, et al: Natural history of aortic valve stenosis of varying severity in the elderly. *Am J Cardiol* 1996; 78:97.
15. Pellikka PA, Nishimura RA, Bailey KR, Tajik AJ: The natural history of adults with asymptomatic, hemodynamically significant aortic stenosis. *J Am Coll Cardiol* 1990; 15:1012.
16. Otto CM, Burwash IG, Legget ME, et al: Prospective study of asymptomatic valvular aortic stenosis: clinical, echocardiographic, and exercise predictors of outcome. *Circulation* 1997; 95:2262.
17. Otto CM, Burwash IG, Legget ME, et al: Prospective study of asymptomatic valvular aortic stenosis: clinical, echocardiographic, and exercise predictors of outcome. *Circulation* 1997; 95:2262.
18. ACC/AHA guidelines for the management of patients with valvular heart disease. A report of the American College of Cardiology/American Heart Association. Task Force on Practice Guidelines (Committee on Management of Patients with Valvular Heart Disease). *J Am Coll Cardiol* 1998; 32:1486.
19. Rosenhek R, Binder T, Porenta G, et al: Predictors of outcome in severe, asymptomatic aortic stenosis. *N Engl J Med* 2000; 343:611.
20. Rosenhek R, Binder T, Porenta G, et al: Predictors of outcome in severe, asymptomatic aortic stenosis. *N Engl J Med* 2000; 343:611.
21. deFilippi CR, Willett DL, Brickner ME, et al: Usefulness of dobutamine echocardiography in distinguishing severe from nonsevere valvular aortic stenosis in patients with depressed left ventricular function and low transvalvular gradients. *Am J Cardiol* 1995; 75:191.
22. Hwang MH, Hammermeister KE, Oprian C, et al: Preoperative identification of patients likely to have left ventricular dysfunction after aortic valve replacement. Participants in the Veterans Administration Cooperative Study on Valvular Heart Disease. *Circulation* 1989; 80(3 pt 1):I65.
23. ACC/AHA guidelines for the management of patients with valvular heart disease. A report of the American College of Cardiology/American Heart Association. Task Force on Practice Guidelines (Committee on Management of Patients with Valvular Heart Disease). *J Am Coll Cardiol* 1998; 32:1486.
24. Braunwald E: Aortic valve replacement: an update at the turn of the millennium. *Eur Heart J* 2000; 21:1032.
25. Downes TR, Nomeir AM, Hackshaw BT, et al: Diastolic mitral regurgitation in acute but not chronic aortic regurgitation: implications regarding the mechanism of mitral closure. *Am Heart J* 1989; 117:1106.
26. Loke YK, Derry S, Pritchard-Copley A: Appetite suppressants and valvular heart disease—a systematic review. *BMC Clin Pharmacol* 2002; 2:6.
27. Connolly HM, Crary JL, McGoon MD, et al: Valvular heart disease associated with fenfluramine-phentermine. *N Engl J Med* 1997; 337:581.
28. Braunwald E: Valvular heart disease, in Braunwald E (ed): *Heart Disease: A Textbook of Cardiovascular Medicine*, 6th ed. Philadelphia, WB Saunders, 2001; p 1643.
29. Borow KM, Marcus RH: Aortic regurgitation: the need for an integrated physiologic approach. *J Am Coll Cardiol* 1991; 17:898.
30. Grossman W, Jones D, McLaurin LP: Wall stress and patterns of hypertrophy in the human left ventricle. *J Clin Invest* 1975; 56:56.
31. Grossman W, Jones D, McLaurin LP: Wall stress and patterns of hypertrophy in the human left ventricle. *J Clin Invest* 1975; 56:56.
32. Starling MR, Kirsh MM, Montgomery DG, Gross MD: Mechanisms for left ventricular systolic dysfunction in aortic

regurgitation: importance for predicting the functional response to aortic valve replacement. *J Am Coll Cardiol* 1991; 17:887.
33. ACC/AHA guidelines for the management of patients with valvular heart disease. A report of the American College of Cardiology/American Heart Association. Task Force on Practice Guidelines (Committee on Management of Patients with Valvular Heart Disease). *J Am Coll Cardiol* 1998; 32:1486.
34. Rapaport E: Should valvular replacement be reserved for symptomatic valvular heart disease? *Cardiovasc Clin* 1977; 8:269.
35. Rapaport E: Natural history of aortic and mitral valve disease. *Am J Cardiol* 1975; 35:221.
36. Bonow RO: Asymptomatic aortic regurgitation: indications for operation. *J Card Surg* 1994; 9(2 suppl):170.
37. Bonow RO, Rosing DR, McIntosh CL, et al: The natural history of asymptomatic patients with aortic regurgitation and normal left ventricular function. *Circulation* 1983; 68:509.
38. Bonow RO, Rosing DR, McIntosh CL, et al: The natural history of asymptomatic patients with aortic regurgitation and normal left ventricular function. *Circulation* 1983; 68:509.
39. Bonow RO, Lakatos E, Maron BJ, Epstein SE: Serial long-term assessment of the natural history of asymptomatic patients with chronic aortic regurgitation and normal left ventricular systolic function. *Circulation* 1991; 84:1625.
40. Tornos MP, Olona M, Permanyer-Miralda G, et al: Clinical outcome of severe asymptomatic chronic aortic regurgitation: a long-term prospective follow-up study. *Am Heart J* 1995; 130:333.
41. ACC/AHA guidelines for the management of patients with valvular heart disease. A report of the American College of Cardiology/American Heart Association. Task Force on Practice Guidelines (Committee on Management of Patients with Valvular Heart Disease). *J Am Coll Cardiol* 1998; 32:1486.
42. Bonow RO, Nikas D, Elefteriades JA: Valve replacement for regurgitant lesions of the aortic or mitral valve in advanced left ventricular dysfunction. *Cardiol Clin* 1995; 13:73.
43. Cohn PF, Gorlin R, Cohn LH, Collins JJ Jr: Left ventricular ejection fraction as a prognostic guide in surgical treatment of coronary and valvular heart disease. *Am J Cardiol* 1974; 34:136.
44. Hwang MH, Burchfiel CM, Sethi GK, et al: Comparison of the causes of late death following aortic and mitral valve replacement. VA Co-operative Study on Valvular Heart Disease. *J Heart Valve Dis* 1994; 3:17.
45. ACC/AHA guidelines for the management of patients with valvular heart disease. A report of the American College of Cardiology/American Heart Association. Task Force on Practice Guidelines (Committee on Management of Patients with Valvular Heart Disease). *J Am Coll Cardiol* 1998; 32:1486.
46. Weisel RD, Fremes SE, Baird RJ, et al: Improved myocardial protection with blood and crystalloid cardioplegia. *J Vasc Surg* 1984; 1:656.
47. Fremes SE, Weisel RD, Mickle DA, et al: Myocardial metabolism and ventricular function following cold potassium cardioplegia. *J Thorac Cardiovasc Surg* 1985; 89:531.
48. Myers ML, Fremes SE: Myocardial protection for cardiac surgery. *EXS* 1996; 76:345.
49. Rao V, Christakis GT, Sever J, et al: A novel comparison of stentless versus stented valves in the small aortic root. *J Thorac Cardiovasc Surg* 1999; 117:431.
50. Lichtenstein SV, Fremes SE, Abel JG, et al: Technical aspects of warm heart surgery. *J Card Surg* 1991; 6:278.
51. Allen BS, Winkelmann JW, Hanafy H, et al: Retrograde cardioplegia does not adequately perfuse the right ventricle. *J Thorac Cardiovasc Surg* 1995; 109:1116.
52. Lee J, Gates RN, Laks H, et al: A comparison of distribution between simultaneously or sequentially delivered antegrade/retrograde blood cardioplegia. *J Card Surg* 1996; 11:111.
53. Borger MA, Wei KS, Weisel RD, et al: Myocardial perfusion during warm antegrade and retrograde cardioplegia: a contrast echo study. *Ann Thorac Surg* 1999; 68:955.
54. Mullen JC, Fremes SE, Weisel RD, et al: Right ventricular function: a comparison between blood and crystalloid cardioplegia. *Ann Thorac Surg* 1987; 43:17.
55. Gall S Jr, Lowe JE, Wolfe WG, et al: Efficacy of the internal mammary artery in combined aortic valve replacement-coronary artery bypass grafting. *Ann Thorac Surg* 2000; 69:524.
56. Nicks R, Cartmill T, Bernstein L: Hypoplasia of the aortic root: the problem of aortic valve replacement. *Thorax* 1970; 25:339.
57. Mayumi H, Toshima Y, Kawachi Y, et al: Simplified Manouguian's aortic annular enlargement for aortic valve replacement. *Ann Thorac Surg* 1995; 60:701.
58. Manouguian S, Seybold-Epting W. Patch enlargement of the aortic valve ring by extending the aortic incision into the anterior mitral leaflet: new operative technique. *J Thorac Cardiovasc Surg* 1979; 78:402.
59. Konno S, Imai Y, Iida Y, et al: A new method for prosthetic valve replacement in congenital aortic stenosis associated with hypoplasia of the aortic valve ring. *J Thorac Cardiovasc Surg* 1975; 70:909.
60. David TE: Surgical management of aortic root abscess. *J Card Surg* 1997; 12(2 suppl):262.
61. David TE, Bos J, Christakis GT, et al: Heart valve operations in patients with active infective endocarditis. *Ann Thorac Surg* 1990; 49:701.
62. David TE: Surgery of the aortic valve. *Curr Probl Surg* 1999; 36:426.
63. David TE: Reoperations on the aortic valve combined with replacement of the ascending aorta. *J Card Surg* 2002; 17:46.
64. Safian RD, Berman AD, Diver DJ, et al: Balloon aortic valvuloplasty in 170 consecutive patients. *N Engl J Med* 1988; 319:125.
65. Lababidi Z, Wu JR, Walls JT: Percutaneous balloon aortic valvuloplasty: results in 23 patients. *Am J Cardiol* 1984; 53:194.
66. Kuntz RE, Tosteson AN, Berman AD, et al: Predictors of event-free survival after balloon aortic valvuloplasty. *N Engl J Med* 1991; 325:17.
67. Percutaneous balloon aortic valvuloplasty: acute and 30-day follow-up results in 674 patients from the NHLBI Balloon Valvuloplasty Registry. *Circulation* 1991; 84:2383.
68. Safian RD, Mandell VS, Thurer RE, et al: Postmortem and intraoperative balloon valvuloplasty of calcific aortic stenosis in elderly patients: mechanisms of successful dilation. *J Am Coll Cardiol* 1987; 9:655.
69. Bernard Y, Etievent J, Mourand JL, et al: Long-term results of percutaneous aortic valvuloplasty compared with aortic valve replacement in patients more than 75 years old. *J Am Coll Cardiol* 1992; 20:796.
70. Diethrich EB: The treatment of aortic stenosis: is valvuloplasty ever an alternative to surgery? *J Interv Cardiol* 1993; 6:7.
71. Sathe S, Wong J, Warren R, Hunt D: Immediate and long-term results of percutaneous balloon aortic valvuloplasty: a report of 33 procedures. *Aust N Z J Med* 1992; 22:647.
72. Smedira NG, Ports TA, Merrick SH, Rankin JS: Balloon aortic valvuloplasty as a bridge to aortic valve replacement in critically ill patients. *Ann Thorac Surg* 1993; 55:914.
73. Cormier B, Vahanian A: Indications and outcome of valvuloplasty. *Curr Opin Cardiol* 1992; 7:222.
74. Hayes SN, Holmes DR Jr, Nishimura RA, Reeder GS: Palliative percutaneous aortic balloon valvuloplasty before noncardiac operations and invasive diagnostic procedures. *Mayo Clin Proc* 1989; 64:753.
75. Rao V, Christakis GT, Weisel RD, et al: Changing pattern of valve surgery. *Circulation* 1996; 94(9 suppl):II113.

76. Hilbert SL, Ferrans VJ: Porcine aortic valve bioprostheses: morphologic and functional considerations. *J Long Term Eff Med Implants* 1992; 2:99.
77. Schoen FJ, Levy RJ: Tissue heart valves: current challenges and future research perspectives. Founder's Award, 25th Annual Meeting of the Society for Biomaterials, perspectives (Providence, RI, April 28-May 2, 1999). *J Biomed Mater Res* 1999; 47:439.
78. Schoen FJ, Levy RJ: Tissue heart valves: current challenges and future research perspectives. Founder's Award, 25th Annual Meeting of the Society for Biomaterials, perspectives (Providence, RI, April 28-May 2, 1999). *J Biomed Mater Res* 1999; 47:439.
79. Schoen FJ, Levy RJ, Nelson AC, et al: Onset and progression of experimental bioprosthetic heart valve calcification. *Lab Invest* 1985; 52:523.
80. Flomenbaum MA, Schoen FJ: Effects of fixation back pressure and antimineralization treatment on the morphology of porcine aortic bioprosthetic valves. *J Thorac Cardiovasc Surg* 1993; 105:154.
81. Flomenbaum MA, Schoen FJ: Effects of fixation back pressure and antimineralization treatment on the morphology of porcine aortic bioprosthetic valves. *J Thorac Cardiovasc Surg* 1993; 105:154.
82. Hilbert SL, Sword LC, Batchelder KF, et al: Simultaneous assessment of bioprosthetic heart valve biomechanical properties and collagen crimp length. *J Biomed Mater Res* 1996; 314:503.
83. Hilbert SL, Barrick MK, Ferrans VJ: Porcine aortic valve bioprostheses: a morphologic comparison of the effects of fixation pressure. *J Biomed Mater Res* 1990; 24:773.
84. Chen W, Schoen FJ, Myers DJ, Levy RJ: Synergistic inhibition of calcification of porcine aortic root with preincubation in FeCl3 and alpha-amino oleic acid in a rat subdermal model. *J Biomed Mater Res* 1997; 38:43.
85. Chen W, Kim JD, Schoen FJ, Levy RJ: Effect of 2-amino oleic acid exposure conditions on the inhibition of calcification of glutaraldehyde cross-linked porcine aortic valves. *J Biomed Mater Res* 1994; 28:1485.
86. Chen W, Schoen FJ, Levy RJ: Mechanism of efficacy of 2-amino oleic acid for inhibition of calcification of glutaraldehyde-pretreated porcine bioprosthetic heart valves. *Circulation* 1994; 90:323.
87. Golomb G, Dixon M, Smith MS, et al: Controlled-release drug delivery of diphosphonates to inhibit bioprosthetic heart valve calcification: release rate modulation with silicone matrices via drug solubility and membrane coating. *J Pharm Sci* 1987; 76:271.
88. Gott JP, Girardot MN, Girardot JM, et al: Refinement of the alpha aminooleic acid bioprosthetic valve anticalcification technique. *Ann Thorac Surg* 1997; 64:50.
89. Hirsch D, Drader J, Thomas TJ, et al: Inhibition of calcification of glutaraldehyde pretreated porcine aortic valve cusps with sodium dodecyl sulfate: preincubation and controlled release studies. *J Biomed Mater Res* 1993; 27:1477.
90. Hirsch D, Drader J, Pathak YV, et al: Synergistic inhibition of the calcification of glutaraldehyde pretreated bovine pericardium in a rat subdermal model by FeCl3 and ethanehydroxydiphosphonate: preincubation and polymeric controlled release studies. *Biomaterials* 1993; 14:705.
91. Hirsch D, Schoen FJ, Levy RJ: Effects of metallic ions and diphosphonates on inhibition of pericardial bioprosthetic tissue calcification and associated alkaline phosphatase activity. *Biomaterials* 1993; 14:371.
92. Levy RJ, Schoen FJ, Lund SA, Smith MS: Prevention of leaflet calcification of bioprosthetic heart valves with diphosphonate injection therapy: experimental studies of optimal dosages and therapeutic durations. *J Thorac Cardiovasc Surg* 1987; 94:551.
93. Vyavahare N, Ogle M, Schoen FJ, Levy RJ: Elastin calcification and its prevention with aluminum chloride pretreatment. *Am J Pathol* 1999; 155:973.
94. Webb CL, Schoen FJ, Flowers WE, et al: Inhibition of mineralization of glutaraldehyde-pretreated bovine pericardium by AlCl3: mechanisms and comparisons with FeCl3, LaCl3, and Ga(NO3)3 in rat subdermal model studies. *Am J Pathol* 1991; 138:971.
95. Webb CL, Phelps LL, Schoen FJ, Levy RJ: Aminodiphosphonate or Al preincubation inhibits calcification of aortic homografts in the rat subdermal model. *ASAIO Trans* 1988; 34:851.
96. Webb CL, Benedict JJ, Schoen FJ, et al: Inhibition of bioprosthetic heart valve calcification with covalently bound aminopropanehydroxydiphosphonate. *ASAIO Trans* 1987; 33:592.
97. Jones M, Eidbo EE, Hilbert SL, et al: Anticalcification treatments of bioprosthetic heart valves: in vivo studies in sheep. *J Card Surg* 1989; 4:69.
98. Jones M, Eidbo EE, Hilbert SL, et al: The effects of anticalcification treatments on bioprosthetic heart valves implanted in sheep. *ASAIO Trans* 1988; 34:1027.
99. Edmunds LH Jr, Clark RE, Cohn LH, et al: Guidelines for reporting morbidity and mortality after cardiac valvular operations. Ad Hoc Liaison Committee for Standardizing Definitions of Prosthetic Heart Valve Morbidity of The American Association for Thoracic Surgery and The Society of Thoracic Surgeons. *J Thorac Cardiovasc Surg* 1996; 112:708.
100. David TE, Armstrong S, Sun Z: The Hancock II bioprosthesis at 12 years. *Ann Thorac Surg* 1998; 66(6 suppl):S95.
101. Bloodwell RD, Okies JE, Hallman GL, Cooley DA. Aortic valve replacement: long-term results. *J Thorac Cardiovasc Surg* 1969; 58:457.
102. Gonzalez-Lavin L, Gonzalez-Lavin J, McGrath LB, et al: Factors determining in-hospital or late survival after aortic valve replacement. *Chest* 1989; 95:38.
103. Hammermeister KE, Henderson WG, Burchfiel CM, et al: Comparison of outcome after valve replacement with a bioprosthesis versus a mechanical prosthesis: initial 5 year results of a randomized trial. *J Am Coll Cardiol* 1987; 10:719.
104. Christakis GT, Weisel RD, David TE, et al: Predictors of operative survival after valve replacement. *Circulation* 1988; 78(3 pt 2):I25.
105. Bessone LN, Pupello DF, Blank RH, et al: Valve replacement in patients over 70 years. *Ann Thorac Surg* 1977; 24:417.
106. Elayda MA, Hall RJ, Reul RM, et al: Aortic valve replacement in patients 80 years and older: operative risks and long-term results. *Circulation* 1993; 88(5 pt 2):II11.
107. Meurs AA, Grundemann AM, Bezemer PD, et al: Early and 8 year results of aortic valve replacement: a clinical study of 232 patients. *Eur Heart J* 1985; 6:870.
108. Doty JR, Flores JH, Millar RC, Doty DB: Aortic valve replacement with Medtronic freestyle bioprosthesis: operative technique and results. *J Card Surg* 1998; 13:208.
109. Craver JM, Weintraub WS, Jones EL, et al: Predictors of mortality, complications, and length of stay in aortic valve replacement for aortic stenosis. *Circulation* 1988; 78(3 pt 2):I85.
110. Edwards FH, Peterson ED, Coombs LP, et al: Prediction of operative mortality after valve replacement surgery. *J Am Coll Cardiol* 2001; 37:885.
111. Scott WC, Miller DC, Haverich A, et al: Determinants of operative mortality for patients undergoing aortic valve replacement: discriminant analysis of 1,479 operations. *J Thorac Cardiovasc Surg* 1985; 89:400.
112. Wideman FE, Blackstone EH, Kirklin JW, et al: Hospital mortality of re-replacement of the aortic valve: incremental risk factors. *J Thorac Cardiovasc Surg* 1981; 82:692.
113. Bloomstein LZ, Gielchinsky I, Bernstein AD, et al: Aortic valve replacement in geriatric patients: determinants of in-hospital mortality. *Ann Thorac Surg* 2001; 71:597.
114. Cohn LH, Allred EN, DiSesa VJ, et al: Early and late risk of aortic valve replacement: a 12 year concomitant comparison of

the porcine bioprosthetic and tilting disc prosthetic aortic valves. *J Thorac Cardiovasc Surg* 1984; 88(5 pt 1):695.

115. Khan S, Chaux A, Matloff J, et al: The St. Jude Medical valve: experience with 1,000 cases. *J Thorac Cardiovasc Surg* 1994; 108:1010.
116. He GW, Acuff TE, Ryan WH, et al: Aortic valve replacement: determinants of operative mortality. *Ann Thorac Surg* 1994; 57:1140.
117. Lytle BW, Cosgrove DM, Loop FD, et al: Replacement of aortic valve combined with myocardial revascularization: determinants of early and late risk for 500 patients, 1967–1981. *Circulation* 1983; 68:1149.
118. Kouchoukos NT, Marshall WG Jr, Wedige-Stecher TA: Eleven-year experience with composite graft replacement of the ascending aorta and aortic valve. *J Thorac Cardiovasc Surg* 1986; 92:691.
119. Stahle E, Bergstrom R, Nystrom SO, Hansson HE: Early results of aortic valve replacement with or without concomitant coronary artery bypass grafting. *Scand J Thorac Cardiovasc Surg* 1991; 25:29.
120. Aranki SF, Rizzo RJ, Couper GS, et al: Aortic valve replacement in the elderly: effect of gender and coronary artery disease on operative mortality. *Circulation* 1993; 88(5 pt 2):II17.
121. Loop FD, Phillips DF, Roy M, et al: Aortic valve replacement combined with myocardial revascularization: late clinical results and survival of surgically-treated aortic valve patients with and without coronary artery disease. *Circulation* 1977; 55:169.
122. Hammermeister KE, Sethi GK, Henderson WG, et al: A comparison of outcomes in men 11 years after heart-valve replacement with a mechanical valve or bioprosthesis. Veterans Affairs Cooperative Study on Valvular Heart Disease. *N Engl J Med* 1993; 328:1289.
123. Hammermeister KE, Sethi GK, Henderson WG, et al: A comparison of outcomes in men 11 years after heart-valve replacement with a mechanical valve or bioprosthesis. Veterans Affairs Cooperative Study on Valvular Heart Disease. *N Engl J Med* 1993; 328:1289.
124. Hammermeister K, Sethi GK, Henderson WG, et al: Outcomes 15 years after valve replacement with a mechanical versus a bioprosthetic valve: final report of the Veterans Affairs randomized trial. *J Am Coll Cardiol* 2000; 36:1152.
125. David TE, Ivanov J, Armstrong S, et al: Late results of heart valve replacement with the Hancock II bioprosthesis. *J Thorac Cardiovasc Surg* 2001; 121:268.
126. Bortolotti U, Milano A, Mossuto E, et al: Porcine valve durability: a comparison between Hancock standard and Hancock II bioprostheses. *Ann Thorac Surg* 1995; 60 (2 suppl):S216.
127. Dellgren G, David TE, Raanani E, et al: Late hemodynamic and clinical outcomes of aortic valve replacement with the Carpentier-Edwards Perimount pericardial bioprosthesis. *J Thorac Cardiovasc Surg* 2002; 124:146.
128. Stahle E, Kvidal P, Nystrom SO, Bergstrom R: Long-term relative survival after primary heart valve replacement. *Eur J Cardiothorac Surg* 1997; 11:81.
129. Thulin LI, Sjogren JL: Aortic valve replacement with and without concomitant coronary artery bypass surgery in the elderly: risk factors related to long-term survival. *Croat Med J* 2000; 41:406.
130. Abdelnoor M, Hauge SN, Hall KV: Prognostic variables in late follow-up of aortic valve replacement using the proportional hazard model: a study on patients using the Medtronic-Hall cardiac prosthesis. *Life Support Syst* 1986; 4:103.
131. Cohen G, David TE, Ivanov J, et al: The impact of age, coronary artery disease, and cardiac comorbidity on late survival after bioprosthetic aortic valve replacement. *J Thorac Cardiovasc Surg* 1999; 117:273.
132. Verheul HA, van den Brink RB, Bouma BJ, et al: Analysis of risk factors for excess mortality after aortic valve replacement. *J Am Coll Cardiol* 1995; 26:1280.
133. Lytle BW, Cosgrove DM, Taylor PC, et al: Primary isolated aortic valve replacement: early and late results. *J Thorac Cardiovasc Surg* 1989; 97:675.
134. Edmunds LH Jr, Clark RE, Cohn LH, et al: Guidelines for reporting morbidity and mortality after cardiac valvular operations. *Eur J Cardiothorac Surg* 1996; 10:812.
135. Edmunds LH Jr, Clark RE, Cohn LH, et al: Guidelines for reporting morbidity and mortality after cardiac valvular operations. Ad Hoc Liaison Committee for Standardizing Definitions of Prosthetic Heart Valve Morbidity of The American Association for Thoracic Surgery and The Society of Thoracic Surgeons. *J Thorac Cardiovasc Surg* 1996; 112:708.
136. Grunkemeier GL, Wu Y: Actual versus actuarial event-free percentages. *Ann Thorac Surg* 2001; 72:677.
137. Ericsson A, Lindblom D, Semb G, et al: Strut fracture with Bjork-Shiley 70 degrees convexo-concave valve: an international multi-institutional follow-up study. *Eur J Cardiothorac Surg* 1992; 6:339.
138. Poirer NC, Pelletier LC, Pellerin M, Carrier M: 15-year experience with the Carpentier-Edwards pericardial bioprosthesis. *Ann Thorac Surg* 1998; 66(6 Suppl):S57.
139. Grunkemeier GL, Jamieson WR, Miller DC, Starr A: Actuarial versus actual risk of porcine structural valve deterioration. *J Thorac Cardiovasc Surg* 1994; 108:709.
140. Vongpatanasin W, Hillis LD, Lange RA: Prosthetic heart valves. *N Engl J Med* 1996; 335:407.
141. Mahoney CB, Miller DC, Khan SS, Hill JD, Cohn LH: Twenty-year, three-institution evaluation of the Hancock Modified Orifice aortic valve durability: comparison of actual and actuarial estimates. *Circulation* 1998; 98(19 suppl):II88.
142. Masters RG, Pipe AL, Walley VM, Keon WJ: Comparative results with the St. Jude Medical and Medtronic Hall mechanical valves. *J Thorac Cardiovasc Surg* 1995; 110:663.
143. Hurle A, Abad C, Feijoo J, et al: Long-term clinical performance of Sorin tilting-disc mechanical prostheses in the mitral and aortic position. *J Cardiovasc Surg* (Torino) 1997; 38:507.
144. Milano A, Guglielmi C, De Carlo M, et al: Valve-related complications in elderly patients with biological and mechanical aortic valves. *Ann Thorac Surg* 1998; 66(6 suppl):S82.
145. Jamieson WR, Fradet GJ, Miyagishima RT, et al: CarboMedics mechanical prosthesis: performance at eight years. *J Heart Valve Dis* 2000; 9:678.
146. Khan SS, Trento A, DeRobertis M, et al: Twenty-year comparison of tissue and mechanical valve replacement. *J Thorac Cardiovasc Surg* 2001; 122:257.
147. Tatoulis J, Chaiyaroj S, Smith JA: Aortic valve replacement in patients 50 years old or younger with the St. Jude Medical valve: 14-year experience. *J Heart Valve Dis* 1996; 5:491.
148. Gallo I, Ruiz B, Duran CM: Clinical experience with the Carpentier-Edwards porcine bioprosthesis: short-term results (from 2 to 4.5 years). *Thorac Cardiovasc Surg* 1983; 31:277.
149. Jamieson WR, Munro AI, Miyagishima RT, et al: The Carpentier-Edwards supraannular porcine bioprosthesis: a new generation tissue valve with excellent intermediate clinical performance. *J Thorac Cardiovasc Surg* 1988; 96:652.
150. Akins CW, Carroll DL, Buckley MJ, et al: Late results with Carpentier-Edwards porcine bioprosthesis. *Circulation* 1990; 82 (5 suppl):IV65.
151. Perier P, Mihaileanu S, Fabiani JN, et al: Long-term evaluation of the Carpentier-Edwards pericardial valve in the aortic position. *J Card Surg* 1991; 6(4 suppl):589.
152. Jamieson WR, Miyagishima RT, Munro AI, et al: The Carpentier-Edwards supra-annular porcine bioprosthesis: clinical performance to 8 years of a new generation porcine bioprosthesis. *J Card Surg* 1991; 6(4 suppl):562.

153. Jamieson WR, Hayden RI, Miyagishima RT, et al: The Carpentier-Edwards standard porcine bioprosthesis: clinical performance to 15 years. *J Card Surg* 1991; 6(4 suppl):550.
154. Glower DD, White WD, Hatton AC, et al: Determinants of reoperation after 960 valve replacements with Carpentier-Edwards prostheses. *J Thorac Cardiovasc Surg* 1994; 107:381.
155. Pellerin M, Mihaileanu S, Couetil JP, et al: Carpentier-Edwards pericardial bioprosthesis in aortic position: long-term follow-up 1980 to 1994. *Ann Thorac Surg* 1995; 60(2 suppl):S292.
156. Jamieson WR, Ling H, Burr LH, et al: Carpentier-Edwards supraannular porcine bioprosthesis evaluation over 15 years. *Ann Thorac Surg* 1998; 66(6 suppl):S49.
157. Corbineau H, De La TB, Verhoye JP, et al: Carpentier-Edwards supraannular porcine bioprosthesis in aortic position: 16-year experience. *Ann Thorac Surg* 2001; 71(5 suppl):S228.
158. Dellgren G, David TE, Raanani E, et al: Late hemodynamic and clinical outcomes of aortic valve replacement with the Carpentier-Edwards Perimount pericardial bioprosthesis. *J Thorac Cardiovasc Surg* 2002; 124:146.
159. Gallo I, Ruiz B, Duran CM: Five- to eight-year follow-up of patients with the Hancock cardiac bioprosthesis. *J Thorac Cardiovasc Surg* 1983; 86:897.
160. Milano AD, Bortolotti U, Mazzucco A, et al: Performance of the Hancock porcine bioprosthesis following aortic valve replacement: considerations based on a 15-year experience. *Ann Thorac Surg* 1988; 46:216.
161. Cohn LH, DiSesa VJ, Collins JJ Jr: The Hancock modified-orifice porcine bioprosthetic valve: 1976–1988. *Ann Thorac Surg* 1989; 48(3 suppl):S81.
162. David TE, Armstrong S, Sun Z: Clinical and hemodynamic assessment of the Hancock II bioprosthesis. *Ann Thorac Surg* 1992; 54:661.
163. David TE, Armstrong S, Sun Z: The Hancock II bioprosthesis at ten years. *Ann Thorac Surg* 1995; 60(2 suppl):S229.
164. David TE, Armstrong S, Sun Z: The Hancock II bioprosthesis at 12 years. *Ann Thorac Surg* 1998; 66(6 suppl):S95.
165. David TE, Ivanov J, Armstrong S, et al: Late results of heart valve replacement with the Hancock II bioprosthesis. *J Thorac Cardiovasc Surg* 2001; 121:268.
166. Thulin LI, Thilen UJ, Kymle KA: Mitroflow pericardial bioprosthesis in the aortic position: low incidence of structural valve deterioration in elderly patients during an 11-year follow-up. *Scand Cardiovasc J* 2000; 34:192.
167. Cannegieter SC, Rosendaal FR, Briet E: Thromboembolic and bleeding complications in patients with mechanical heart valve prostheses. *Circulation* 1994; 89:635.
168. Edmunds LH Jr: Thrombotic and bleeding complications of prosthetic heart valves. *Ann Thorac Surg* 1987; 44:430.
169. Edmunds LH Jr: Thromboembolic complications of current cardiac valvular prostheses. *Ann Thorac Surg* 1982; 34:96.
170. Ibrahim M, O'kane H, Cleland J, et al: The St. Jude Medical prosthesis: a thirteen-year experience. *J Thorac Cardiovasc Surg* 1994; 108:221.
171. Abdelnoor M, Hall KV, Nitter-Hauge S, et al: Morbidity in valvular heart replacement: risk factors of systemic emboli and thrombotic obstruction. *Int J Artif Organs* 1988; 11:303.
172. Ahram J, Blatt JM, Borman JB: Comparative study of Bjork-Shiley and Starr-Edwards prostheses for aortic valve replacement. *Isr J Med Sci* 1983; 19:45.
173. Andersen PV, Alstrup P: Long-term survival and complications in patients with mechanical aortic valves without anticoagulation: a follow-up study from 1 to 15 years. *Eur J Cardiothorac Surg* 1992; 6:62.
174. Antunes MJ: Valve replacement in the elderly: is the mechanical valve a good alternative? *J Thorac Cardiovasc Surg* 1989; 98:485.
175. Aosaki M, Koyanagi H, Terada K, et al: Present status of thromboembolic complications in patients with prosthetic heart valves. *Jpn Circ J* 1986; 50:884.
176. Bernal JM, Rabasa JM, Gutierrez-Garcia F, et al: The CarboMedics valve: experience with 1,049 implants. *Ann Thorac Surg* 1998; 65:137.
177. Dewall R, Pelletier LC, Panebianco A, et al: Factors influencing thromboembolic complications in Omniscience cardiac valve patients. *Eur Heart J* 1984; 5 (suppl D):53.
178. Douglas PS, Hirshfeld JW Jr, Edie RN, et al: Clinical comparison of St. Jude and porcine aortic valve prostheses. *Circulation* 1985; 72(3 pt 2):II135.
179. Fuster V, Pumphrey CW, McGoon MD, et al: Systemic thromboembolism in mitral and aortic Starr-Edwards prostheses: a 10–19 year follow-up. *Circulation* 1982; 66(2 pt 2):I157.
180. Kazui T, Komatsu S, Inoue N: Clinical evaluation of the Omniscience aortic disc valve prosthesis. *Scand J Thorac Cardiovasc Surg* 1987; 21:173.
181. Milano A, Bortolotti U, Mazzucco A, et al: Heart valve replacement with the Sorin tilting-disc prosthesis: a 10-year experience. *J Thorac Cardiovasc Surg* 1992; 103:267.
182. Semb BK, Hall KV, Nitter-Hauge S, Abdelnoor M: A 5-year follow-up of the Medtronic-Hall valve: survival and thromboembolism. *Thorac Cardiovasc Surg* 1983; 31 (spec 2):61.
183. Sinci V, Halit V, Kalaycioglu S, et al: Eight year experience with the CarboMedics bileaflet valvular prosthesis. *Ann Thorac Cardiovasc Surg* 1999; 5:382.
184. Thevenet A: Lillehei-Kaster prosthesis in the aortic position with and without anticoagulants. *J Cardiovasc Surg* (Torino) 1980; 21:669.
185. Cannegieter SC, Rosendaal FR, Briet E: Thromboembolic and bleeding complications in patients with mechanical heart valve prostheses. *Circulation* 1994; 89:635.
186. Cannegieter SC, Rosendaal FR, Briet E: Thromboembolic and bleeding complications in patients with mechanical heart valve prostheses. *Circulation* 1994; 89:635.
187. Heras M, Chesebro JH, Fuster V, et al: High risk of thromboemboli early after bioprosthetic cardiac valve replacement. *J Am Coll Cardiol* 1995; 25:1111.
188. Antunes MJ: Clinical performance of St. Jude and Medtronic-Hall prostheses: a randomized comparative study. *Ann Thorac Surg* 1990; 50:743.
189. Nitter-Hauge S, Semb B, Abdelnoor M, Hall KV: A 5 year experience with the Medtronic-Hall disc valve prosthesis. *Circulation* 1983; 68(3 pt 2):II169.
190. Hayashi J, Nakazawa S, Oguma F, et al: Combined warfarin and antiplatelet therapy after St. Jude Medical valve replacement for mitral valve disease. *J Am Coll Cardiol* 1994; 23:672.
191. Albertal J, Sutton M, Pereyra D, et al: Experience with moderate intensity anticoagulation and aspirin after mechanical valve replacement: a retrospective, non-randomized study. *J Heart Valve Dis* 1993; 2:302.
192. Chesebro JH, Adams PC, Fuster V: Antithrombotic therapy in patients with valvular heart disease and prosthetic heart valves. *J Am Coll Cardiol* 1986; 8(6 suppl B):41B.
193. Turpie AG, Gent M, Laupacis A, et al: A comparison of aspirin with placebo in patients treated with warfarin after heart-valve replacement. *N Engl J Med* 1993; 329:524.
194. Cannegieter SC, Torn M, Rosendaal FR: Oral anticoagulant treatment in patients with mechanical heart valves: how to reduce the risk of thromboembolic and bleeding complications. *J Intern Med* 1999; 245:369.
195. Brott WH, Zajtchuk R, Bowen TE, et al: Dipyridamole-aspirin as thromboembolic prophylaxis in patients with aortic valve prosthesis: prospective study with the Model 2320 Starr-Edwards prosthesis. *J Thorac Cardiovasc Surg* 1981; 81:632.

196. Acar J, Iung B, Boissel JP, Samama MM, et al: AREVA: multicenter randomized comparison of low-dose versus standard-dose anticoagulation in patients with mechanical prosthetic heart valves. *Circulation* 1996; 94:2107.
197. Casselman FP, Bots ML, Van Lommel W, et al: Repeated thromboembolic and bleeding events after mechanical aortic valve replacement. *Ann Thorac Surg* 2001; 71:1172.
198. Horstkotte D, Schulte H, Bircks W, Strauer B: Unexpected findings concerning thromboembolic complications and anticoagulation after complete 10 year follow up of patients with St. Jude Medical prostheses. *J Heart Valve Dis* 1993; 2:291.
199. David TE, Ho WI, Christakis GT: Thromboembolism in patients with aortic porcine bioprostheses. *Ann Thorac Surg* 1985; 40:229.
200. Bortolotti U, Milano A, Mazzaro E, et al: Hancock II porcine bioprosthesis: excellent durability at intermediate-term follow-up. *J Am Coll Cardiol* 1994; 24:676.
201. Aupart M, Neville P, Dreyfus X, et al: The Carpentier-Edwards pericardial aortic valve: intermediate results in 420 patients. *Eur J Cardiothorac Surg* 1994; 8:277.
202. Glower DD, Landolfo KP, Cheruvu S, et al: Determinants of 15-year outcome with 1,119 standard Carpentier-Edwards porcine valves. *Ann Thorac Surg* 1998; 66(6 suppl):S44.
203. Neville PH, Aupart MR, Diemont FF, et al: Carpentier-Edwards pericardial bioprosthesis in aortic or mitral position: a 12-year experience. *Ann Thorac Surg* 1998; 66(6 suppl):S143.
204. Dellgren G, Feindel CM, Bos J, et al: Aortic valve replacement with the Toronto SPV: long-term clinical and hemodynamic results. *Eur J Cardiothorac Surg* 2002; 21:698.
205. Doty DB, Michielon G, Wang ND, et al: Replacement of the aortic valve with cryopreserved aortic allograft. *Ann Thorac Surg* 1993; 56:228.
206. O'Brien MF, Stafford EG, Gardner MA, et al: Allograft aortic valve replacement: long-term follow-up. *Ann Thorac Surg* 1995; 60 (2 suppl):S65.
207. Bodnar E, Wain WH, Martelli V, Ross DN: Long term performance of 580 homograft and autograft valves used for aortic valve replacement. *Thorac Cardiovasc Surg* 1979; 27:31.
208. Gonzalez-Lavin L, Geens M, Ross D: Aortic valve replacement with a pulmonary valve autograft: indications and surgical technique. *Surgery* 1970; 68:450.
209. Gross C, Harringer W, Beran H, et al: Aortic valve replacement: is the stentless xenograft an alternative to the homograft? Midterm results. *Ann Thorac Surg* 1999; 68:919.
210. Blair KL, Hatton AC, White WD, et al: Comparison of anticoagulation regimens after Carpentier-Edwards aortic or mitral valve replacement. *Circulation* 1994; 90(5 pt 2):II214.
211. Goldsmith I, Lip GY, Mukundan S, Rosin MD: Experience with low-dose aspirin as thromboprophylaxis for the Tissuemed porcine aortic bioprosthesis: a survey of five years' experience. *J Heart Valve Dis* 1998; 7:574.
212. Nunez L, Gil AM, Larrea JL, et al: Prevention of thromboembolism using aspirin after mitral valve replacement with porcine bioprosthesis. *Ann Thorac Surg* 1984; 37:84.
213. Martinell J, Fraile J, Artiz V, et al: Reoperations for left-sided low-profile mechanical prosthetic obstructions. *Ann Thorac Surg* 1987; 43:172.
214. Gharagozloo F, Mullany CJ, Orszulak TA: Early thrombotic stenosis of aortic bioprosthetic valves: report of two cases. *Mayo Clin Proc* 1993; 68:703.
215. Lengyel M, Vandor L: The role of thrombolysis in the management of left-sided prosthetic valve thrombosis: a study of 85 cases diagnosed by transesophageal echocardiography. *J Heart Valve Dis* 2001; 10:636.
216. Lengyel M, Fuster V, Keltai M, et al: Guidelines for management of left-sided prosthetic valve thrombosis: a role for thrombolytic therapy. Consensus Conference on Prosthetic Valve Thrombosis. *J Am Coll Cardiol* 1997; 30:1521.
217. Lengyel M, Fuster V, Keltai M, et al: Guidelines for management of left-sided prosthetic valve thrombosis: a role for thrombolytic therapy. Consensus Conference on Prosthetic Valve Thrombosis. *J Am Coll Cardiol* 1997; 30:1521.
218. Martinell J, Jimenez A, Rabago G, et al: Mechanical cardiac valve thrombosis. Is thrombectomy justified? *Circulation* 1991; 84 (5 suppl):III70.
219. Bower SP, Tucker PE: Fungal meningitis and intracerebral hemorrhage complicating prosthetic valve endocarditis. *Pathology* 1993; 25:87.
220. Calderwood SB, Swinski LA, Waternaux CM, et al: Risk factors for the development of prosthetic valve endocarditis. *Circulation* 1985; 72:31.
221. George T, Burch K, Magilligan DJ Jr: Rifampin in the management of early prosthetic staphylococcus epidermidis endocarditis. *Ann Thorac Surg* 1980; 29:74.
222. Otaki M: Prosthetic valve endocarditis: surgical procedures and clinical outcome. *Cardiovasc Surg* 1994; 2:212.
223. Sobrino J, Marco F, Miro JM, et al: Prosthetic valve endocarditis caused by Corynebacterium pilosum. *Infection* 1991; 19:247.
224. Vongpatanasin W, Hillis LD, Lange RA: Prosthetic heart valves. *N Engl J Med* 1996; 335:407.
225. Zabalgoitia M, Garcia M: Pitfalls in the echo-Doppler diagnosis of prosthetic valve disorders. *Echocardiography* 1993; 10:203.
226. al Khaja N, Belboul A, Larsson S, Roberts D: Eleven years' experience with Carpentier-Edwards biological valves in relation to survival and complications. *Eur J Cardiothorac Surg* 1989; 3:305.
227. Bernal JM, Rabasa JM, Cagigas JC, et al: Valve-related complications with the Hancock I porcine bioprosthesis: a twelve- to fourteen-year follow-up study. *J Thorac Cardiovasc Surg* 1991; 101:871.
228. Jamieson WR, Burr LH, Munro AI, et al: Cardiac valve replacement in the elderly: clinical performance of biological prostheses. *Ann Thorac Surg* 1989; 48:173.
229. Klepetko W, Moritz A, Khunl-Brady G, et al: Implantation of the Duromedics bileaflet cardiac valve prosthesis in 400 patients. *Ann Thorac Surg* 1987; 44:303.
230. Levy MJ, Vidne B: Late results of aortic valve replacement by prosthesis. *Isr J Med Sci* 1973; 9:998.
231. Mazzucotelli JP, Bertrand PC, Loisance DY: Durability of the Mitroflow pericardial valve at ten years. *Ann Thorac Surg* 1995; 60(2 suppl):S303.
232. Myken PS, Caidahl K, Larsson S, Berggren HE: 10-year experience with the Biocor porcine bioprosthesis in the aortic position. *J Heart Valve Dis* 1994; 3:648.
233. Otto TJ, Cleland WP, Bentall HH: Results of aortic valve replacement with Starr-Edwards prosthesis. *J Cardiovasc Surg* (Torino) 1969; 10:339.
234. Zussa C, Ottino G, di Summa M, et al: Porcine cardiac bioprostheses: evaluation of long-term results in 990 patients. *Ann Thorac Surg* 1985; 39:243.
235. Blackstone EH, Kirklin JW: Death and other time-related events after valve replacement. *Circulation* 1985; 72:753.
236. Ivert TS, Dismukes WE, Cobbs CG, et al: Prosthetic valve endocarditis. *Circulation* 1984; 69:223.
237. Ivert TS, Dismukes WE, Cobbs CG, et al: Prosthetic valve endocarditis. *Circulation* 1984; 69:223.
238. O'Brien MF, Stafford EG, Gardner MA, et al: A comparison of aortic valve replacement with viable cryopreserved and fresh allograft valves, with a note on chromosomal studies. *J Thorac Cardiovasc Surg* 1987; 94:812.
239. Lupinetti FM, Lemmer JH Jr: Comparison of allografts and prosthetic valves when used for emergency aortic valve replacement for active infective endocarditis. *Am J Cardiol* 1991; 68:637.

240. Haydock D, Barratt-Boyes B, Macedo T, et al: Aortic valve replacement for active infectious endocarditis in 108 patients: a comparison of freehand allograft valves with mechanical prostheses and bioprostheses. *J Thorac Cardiovasc Surg* 1992; 103:130.
241. Ladowski JS, Deschner WP: Allograft replacement of the aortic valve for active endocarditis. *J Cardiovasc Surg* (Torino) 1996; 37(6 suppl 1):61.
242. Dearani JA, Orszulak TA, Schaff HV, et al: Results of allograft aortic valve replacement for complex endocarditis. *J Thorac Cardiovasc Surg* 1997; 113:285.
243. Santini F, Musazzi A, Bertolini P, et al: Stentless porcine bioprostheses in the treatment of aortic valve infective endocarditis. *J Card Surg* 1995; 10:205.
244. Santini F, Bertolini P, Vecchi B, et al: Results of Biocor stentless valve replacement for infective endocarditis of the native aortic valve. *Am J Cardiol* 1998; 82:1136.
245. Strelich K, Deeb GM, Bach DS: Echocardiographic correlates of Freestyle stentless tissue aortic valve endocarditis. *Semin Thorac Cardiovasc Surg* 2001; 13(4 suppl 1):113.
246. Vongpatanasin W, Hillis LD, Lange RA: Prosthetic heart valves. *N Engl J Med* 1996; 335:407.
247. Vongpatanasin W, Hillis LD, Lange RA: Prosthetic heart valves. *N Engl J Med* 1996; 335:407.
248. Levy D, Garrison RJ, Savage DD, et al: Prognostic implications of echocardiographically determined left ventricular mass in the Framingham Heart Study. *N Engl J Med* 1990; 322:1561.
249. Haider AW, Larson MG, Benjamin EJ, Levy D: Increased left ventricular mass and hypertrophy are associated with increased risk for sudden death. *J Am Coll Cardiol* 1998; 32:1454.
250. Casale PN, Devereux RB, Milner M, et al: Value of echocardiographic measurement of left ventricular mass in predicting cardiovascular morbid events in hypertensive men. *Ann Intern Med* 1986; 105:173.
251. Verdecchia P, Schillaci G, Borgioni C, et al: Prognostic significance of serial changes in left ventricular mass in essential hypertension. *Circulation* 1998; 97:48.
252. Kurnik PB, Innerfield M, Wachspress JD, et al: Left ventricular mass regression after aortic valve replacement measured by ultrafast computed tomography. *Am Heart J* 1990; 120:919.
253. Christakis GT, Joyner CD, Morgan CD, et al: Left ventricular mass regression early after aortic valve replacement. *Ann Thorac Surg* 1996; 62:1084.
254. Lee JW, Choi KJ, Lee SG, et al. Left ventricular muscle mass regression after aortic valve replacement. *J Korean Med Sci* 1999; 14:511.
255. Kuhl HP, Franke A, Puschmann D, et al: Regression of left ventricular mass one year after aortic valve replacement for pure severe aortic stenosis. *Am J Cardiol* 2002; 89:408.
256. Kennedy JW, Doces J, Stewart DK: Left ventricular function before and following aortic valve replacement. *Circulation* 1977; 56:944.
257. Pantely G, Morton M, Rahimtoola SH: Effects of successful, uncomplicated valve replacement on ventricular hypertrophy, volume, and performance in aortic stenosis and in aortic incompetence. *J Thorac Cardiovasc Surg* 1978; 75:383.
258. Dellgren G, David TE, Raanani E, et al: The Toronto SPV: hemodynamic data at 1 and 5 years' postimplantation. *Semin Thorac Cardiovasc Surg* 1999; 11(4 suppl 1):107.
259. Hanayama N, Christakis GT, Mallidi HR, et al: Patient prosthesis mismatch is rare after aortic valve replacement: valve size may be irrelevant. *Ann Thorac Surg* 2002; 73:1822.
260. Henneke KH, Pongratz G, Bachmann K: Limitations of Doppler echocardiography in the assessment of prosthetic valve hemodynamics. *J Heart Valve Dis* 1995; 4:18.
261. Henneke KH, Pongratz G, Pohlmann M, Bachmann K: Doppler echocardiographic determination of geometric orifice areas in mechanical aortic valve prostheses. *Cardiology* 1995; 86:508.
262. Rahimtoola SH: The problem of valve prosthesis-patient mismatch. *Circulation* 1978; 58:20.
263. Pibarot P, Dumesnil JG, Lemieux M, et al: Impact of prosthesis-patient mismatch on hemodynamic and symptomatic status, morbidity and mortality after aortic valve replacement with a bioprosthetic heart valve. *J Heart Valve Dis* 1998; 7:211.
264. Yun KL, Jamieson WR, Khonsari S, et al: Prosthesis-patient mismatch: hemodynamic comparison of stented and stentless aortic valves. *Semin Thorac Cardiovasc Surg* 1999; 11(4 suppl 1):98.
265. Pibarot P, Dumesnil JG: Hemodynamic and clinical impact of prosthesis-patient mismatch in the aortic valve position and its prevention. *J Am Coll Cardiol* 2000; 36:1131.
266. Pibarot P, Honos GN, Durand LG, Dumesnil JG: The effect of prosthesis-patient mismatch on aortic bioprosthetic valve hemodynamic performance and patient clinical status. *Can J Cardiol* 1996; 12:379.
267. Rao V, Jamieson WR, Ivanov J, et al: Prosthesis-patient mismatch affects survival after aortic valve replacement. *Circulation* 2000; 102(19 suppl 3):III5.
268. Medalion B, Blackstone EH, Lytle BW, et al: Aortic valve replacement: is valve size important? *J Thorac Cardiovasc Surg* 2000; 119:963.
269. Hanayama N, Christakis GT, Mallidi HR, et al: Patient prosthesis mismatch is rare after aortic valve replacement: valve size may be irrelevant. *Ann Thorac Surg* 2002; 73:1822.
270. He GW, Grunkemeier GL, Gately HL, et al: Up to thirty-year survival after aortic valve replacement in the small aortic root. *Ann Thorac Surg* 1995; 59:1056.
271. Sawant D, Singh AK, Feng WC, et al: St. Jude Medical cardiac valves in small aortic roots: follow-up to sixteen years. *J Thorac Cardiovasc Surg* 1997; 113:499.
272. De Paulis R, Sommariva L, Colagrande L, et al: Regression of left ventricular hypertrophy after aortic valve replacement for aortic stenosis with different valve substitutes. *J Thorac Cardiovasc Surg* 1998; 116:590.
273. Foster AH, Tracy CM, Greenberg GJ, et al: Valve replacement in narrow aortic roots: serial hemodynamics and long-term clinical outcome. *Ann Thorac Surg* 1986; 42:506.
274. Kratz JM, Sade RM, Crawford FA Jr, et al: The risk of small St. Jude aortic valve prostheses. *Ann Thorac Surg* 1994; 57:1114.
275. Khan SS, Siegel RJ, DeRobertis MA, et al: Regression of hypertrophy after Carpentier-Edwards pericardial aortic valve replacement. *Ann Thorac Surg* 2000; 69:531.
276. Cohen G, David TE, Ivanov J, et al: The impact of age, coronary artery disease, and cardiac comorbidity on late survival after bioprosthetic aortic valve replacement. *J Thorac Cardiovasc Surg* 1999; 117:273.
277. Sommers KE, David TE: Aortic valve replacement with patch enlargement of the aortic annulus. *Ann Thorac Surg* 1997; 63:1608.
278. Walther T, Falk V, Langebartels G, et al: Prospectively randomized evaluation of stentless versus conventional biological aortic valves: impact on early regression of left ventricular hypertrophy. *Circulation* 1999; 100(19 suppl):II6.
279. Cohen G, Christakis GT, Joyner CD, et al: Are stentless valves hemodynamically superior to stented valves? A prospective randomized trial. *Ann Thorac Surg* 2002; 73:767.
280. Pibarot P, Dumesnil JG, Jobin J, et al: Hemodynamic and physical performance during maximal exercise in patients with an aortic bioprosthetic valve: comparison of stentless versus stented bioprostheses. *J Am Coll Cardiol* 1999; 34:1609.
281. Pibarot P, Dumesnil JG: Effect of exercise on bioprosthetic valve hemodynamics. *Am J Cardiol* 1999; 83:1593.
282. Angell WW, Oury JH, Duran CG, Infantes-Alcon C: Twenty-year comparison of the human allograft and porcine xenograft. *Ann Thorac Surg* 1989; 48(3 suppl):S89.

283. Angell WW, Oury JH, Lamberti JJ, Koziol J: Durability of the viable aortic allograft. *J Thorac Cardiovasc Surg* 1989; 98:48.
284. Lund O, Chandrasekaran V, Grocott-Mason R, et al: Primary aortic valve replacement with allografts over twenty-five years: valve-related and procedure-related determinants of outcome. *J Thorac Cardiovasc Surg* 1999; 117:77.
285. Mair R, Harringer W, Wimmer-Greinecker G, et al: Aortic valve replacement with cryopreserved pulmonary allografts: five years' follow-up. *Ann Thorac Surg* 1995; 60(2 suppl):S185.
286. Mair R, Harringer W, Gross C, et al: Early results of cryopreserved pulmonary allografts as aortic valve substitute. *Eur J Cardiothorac Surg* 1992; 6:485.
287. McGiffin DC, O'Brien MF, Stafford EG, et al: Long-term results of the viable cryopreserved allograft aortic valve: continuing evidence for superior valve durability. *J Card Surg* 1988; 3(3 suppl):289.
288. Miller DC, Shumway NE: "Fresh" aortic allografts: long-term results with free-hand aortic valve replacement. *J Card Surg* 1987; 2(1 suppl):185.
289. David TE, Ropchan GC, Butany JW: Aortic valve replacement with stentless porcine bioprostheses. *J Card Surg* 1988; 3:501.
290. Dellgren G, Feindel CM, Bos J, et al: Aortic valve replacement with the Toronto SPV: long-term clinical and hemodynamic results. *Eur J Cardiothorac Surg* 2002; 21:698.
291. Corbineau H, Verhoye JP, Tauran A, et al: Medtronic intact porcine bioprosthesis in the aortic position: 13-year results. *J Heart Valve Dis* 2002; 11:537.
292. Burdon TA, Miller DC, Oyer PE, et al: Durability of porcine valves at fifteen years in a representative North American patient population. *J Thorac Cardiovasc Surg* 1992; 103:238.
293. Johnson A, Thompson S, Vieweg WV, et al: Evaluation of the in vivo function of the Hancock porcine xenograft in the aortic position. *J Thorac Cardiovasc Surg* 1978; 75:599.
294. Jones EL, Craver JM, Morris DC, et al: Hemodynamic and clinical evaluation of the Hancock xenograft bioprosthesis of aortic valve replacement (with emphasis on management of the small aortic root). *J Thorac Cardiovasc Surg* 1978; 75:300.
295. Rossiter SJ, Miller DC, Stinson EB, et al: Hemodynamic and clinical comparison of the Hancock modified orifice and standard orifice bioprostheses in the aortic position. *J Thorac Cardiovasc Surg* 1980; 80:54.
296. Zusman DR, Levine FH, Carter JE, Buckley MJ: Hemodynamic and clinical evaluation of the Hancock modified-orifice aortic bioprosthesis. *Circulation* 1981; 64 (2 pt 2):II189.
297. Lemieux MD, Jamieson WR, Landymore RW, et al: Medtronic Intact porcine bioprosthesis: clinical performance to seven years. *Ann Thorac Surg* 1995; 60(2 suppl):S258.
298. Kadir I, Izzat MB, Wilde P, et al: Dynamic evaluation of the 21-mm Medtronic Intact aortic bioprosthesis by dobutamine echocardiography. *Ann Thorac Surg* 1997; 63:1128.
299. Jasinski MJ, Kadziola Z, Keal R, Sosnowski AW: "Mosaic" medtronic bioprosthetic valve replacement clinical results and hemodynamical performance. *J Cardiovasc Surg* (Torino) 2000; 41:181.
300. Corbineau H, Lelong B, Langanay T, et al: Echocardiographic assessment and preliminary clinical results after aortic valve replacement with the Medtronic Mosaic bioprosthesis. *J Heart Valve Dis* 2001; 10:171.
301. Nardi C, Scioti G, Milano AD, et al: Hemodynamic assessment of the Medtronic Mosaic bioprosthesis in the aortic position. *J Heart Valve Dis* 2001; 10:100.
302. Pelletier C, Chaitman BR, Baillot R, et al: Clinical and hemodynamic results with the Carpentier-Edwards porcine bioprosthesis. *Ann Thorac Surg* 1982; 34:612.
303. Bove EL, Marvasti MA, Potts JL, et al: Rest and exercise hemodynamics following aortic valve replacement: a comparison between 19 and 21 mm Ionescu-Shiley pericardial and Carpentier-Edwards porcine valves. *J Thorac Cardiovasc Surg* 1985; 90:750.
304. Chaitman BR, Bonan R, Lepage G, et al: Hemodynamic evaluation of the Carpentier-Edwards porcine xenograft. *Circulation* 1979; 60:1170.
305. Kallis P, Sneddon JF, Simpson IA, et al: Clinical and hemodynamic evaluation of the 19-mm Carpentier-Edwards supraannular aortic valve. *Ann Thorac Surg* 1992; 54:1182.
306. Plume SK, Sanders JH: The Carpentier-Edwards stented supra-annular pericardial aortic valve prosthesis: clinical durability and hemodynamic performance. *Curr Opin Cardiol* 2002; 17:183.
307. Williams RJ, Muir DF, Pathi V, et al: Randomized controlled trial of stented and stentless aortic bioprotheses: hemodynamic performance at 3 years. *Semin Thorac Cardiovasc Surg* 1999; 11(4 suppl 1):93.
308. Cosgrove DM, Lytle BW, Williams GW: Hemodynamic performance of the Carpentier-Edwards pericardial valve in the aortic position in vivo. *Circulation* 1985; 72(3 pt 2):II146.
309. Pelletier LC, Leclerc Y, Bonan R, et al: Aortic valve replacement with the Carpentier-Edwards pericardial bioprosthesis: clinical and hemodynamic results. *J Card Surg* 1988; 3(3 suppl):405.
310. Marquez S, Hon RT, Yoganathan AP: Comparative hydrodynamic evaluation of bioprosthetic heart valves. *J Heart Valve Dis* 2001; 10:802.
311. Jennings LM, El Gatit A, Nagy ZL, et al: Hydrodynamic function of the second-generation mitroflow pericardial bioprosthesis. *Ann Thorac Surg* 2002; 74:63.
312. Danton MH, Sarsam MA, Byrne JG, et al: Clinical and hemodynamic performance of the Toronto SPV bioprosthesis. *J Heart Valve Dis* 2000; 9:644.
313. Del Rizzo DF, Abdoh A: Clinical and hemodynamic comparison of the Medtronic Freestyle and Toronto SPV stentless valves. *J Card Surg* 1998; 13:398.
314. Cartier PC, Dumesnil JG, Metras J, et al: Clinical and hemodynamic performance of the Freestyle aortic root bioprosthesis. *Ann Thorac Surg* 1999; 67:345.
315. Legare JF, Wood JW, Koilpillai C, et al: St. Jude SPV versus Medtronic Freestyle: a single institution comparison of two stentless aortic valves. *J Card Surg* 1998; 13:392.
316. Jin XY, Ratnatunga C, Pillai R: Performance of Edwards prima stentless aortic valve over eight years. *Semin Thorac Cardiovasc Surg* 2001; 13(4 suppl 1):163.

Chapter 33

Surgical Treatment of Aortic Valve Endocarditis

Tirone E. David

DEFINITION

Infective endocarditis is a disease in which a microorganism colonizes a focus in the heart, producing fever, heart murmur, splenomegaly, embolic manifestations, and bacteremia or fungemia. Early diagnosis of this condition is extremely important because it almost invariably leads to devastating complications and death if not treated properly.

EPIDEMIOLOGY

Predisposing factors for infective endocarditis are cardiac abnormalities that disrupt the endocardium by means of a jet injury as well as the presence of blood-borne microorganism that colonize these abnormal surfaces. Congenitally bicuspid aortic valve is the most common predisposing lesion for endocarditis of the aortic valve.[1] Other congenital abnormalities of the aortic valve, degenerative calcific aortic stenosis, aortic insufficiency secondary to connective tissue disorders, and rheumatic aortic valve disease, are also predisposing lesions for infection. Depending on the virulence of the offending microorganism, normal aortic valves can also be affected. Patients with prosthetic heart valves have a constant risk of developing infective endocarditis.

It is difficult to determine the incidence and prevalence of native aortic valve endocarditis in the general population because this disease is continuously changing.[2] The annual incidence of infective endocarditis is estimated to range from 1.7 to 6.2 episodes per 100,000 patient-years in North America.[3–4]

Patients with prosthetic aortic valves are reported to have an incidence of infective endocarditis of 0.2 to 1.4 episodes per 100 patient-years, which varies with the type of aortic valves.[5–11] Approximately 1.4% of patients undergoing aortic valve replacement develop prosthetic valve endocarditis during the first postoperative year.[12]

Dental extractions have been demonstrated to produce bacteremia, however, even simple mastication, teeth brushing or cleaning, and oral irrigation can produce transient bacteremia. Endoscopic procedures may also produce bacteremia. Intravenous drug users are particularly susceptible to infective endocarditis, which often occurs in structurally normal heart valves. Infective endocarditis in hemodialysis patients is relatively infrequent but it is associated with high mortality.[13]

PATHOGENESIS AND PATHOLOGY

In 1928, Grant et al[14] theorized that platelet-fibrin thrombi on the heart valve served as a nidus for bacteria adherence. In 1963, Angrist and Oka[15] introduced the term "nonbacterial thrombotic endocarditis" to describe sterile vegetations on a heart valve and provided experimental animal evidence supporting the role of these vegetations in the pathogenesis of endocarditis. Experimental inoculation in animals with preexisting "nonbacterial thrombotic endocarditis" produced by mechanical abrasion of the endothelial covering of heart valves causes a prompt leukocytic infiltration of the thrombi.[16] As the microorganism multiplies, more leukocytes and thrombotic material accumulate in the area and a verrucous vegetation begins to form.

Depending on the virulence of the microorganism and the resistance of the host, the aortic valve can be destroyed and the infection may spread into the annulus and surrounding structures with abscess formation. The abscess may rupture into the pericardial cavity or into a cardiac cavity.

Infective endocarditis of the aortic valve not only causes destruction of the aortic cusps, paravalvular abscess, and cardiac fistulas, but also can cause coronary and systemic embolization of vegetations.[17] Cerebral infarction, either ischemic due to arterial occlusion or hemorrhagic due to rupture of the mycotic aneurysm, is common in these patients.[18,19] Mycotic aneurysms, infarcts, and abscesses of other organs such as spleen, liver, kidneys, and limbs are also common.[17] Aortic valve endocarditis with a large vegetation that prolapses into the left ventricle and comes in contact to the anterior leaflet of the mitral valve can cause secondary involvement of this valve.[20,21]

Infection of a mechanical heart valve is usually located in its sewing ring.[22,23] Infection of a porcine or pericardial valve may involve the cusps, the sewing ring, or both.[24,25] Infection in aortic valve homografts and pulmonary autografts resembles that of native aortic valve: it begins in the aortic cusps and destroys them, causing aortic insufficiency, but it may also extend into surrounding structures.[26] Endocarditis after aortic root replacement with mechanical valves frequently causes dehiscence of the valve from the aortic annulus with consequent false aneurysm.[27]

MICROBIOLOGY

Staphylococcus aureus and *Streptococcus viridans* are the most common microorganisms responsible for native aortic valve endocarditis.[28–32] *Staphylococcus aureus* is extremely virulent and able to cause infection in patients with normal aortic valves. *Streptococcus viridans* is not as virulent and causes infection that often follows a protracted course. *Staphylococcus epidermidis* and various other streptococci can also cause endocarditis.

Endocarditis due to gram-negative bacteria is uncommon, but it is often resistant to antibiotic therapy and may cause serious complications. *Haemophillus, Actinobacillus, Cardiobacterium, Eikenella,* and *Kingella* (HACEK group) are gram-negative bacilli grouped together for their characteristic fastidiousness requiring prolonged incubation period before growth. Endocarditis by the HACEK group is also uncommon. Fungal endocarditis is rare but extremely serious. *Candida albicans* and *Aspergillus fumigatus* are the usual agents.

The microbiology of prosthetic aortic valve endocarditis is different from that of the native valve.[23,28–33] Prosthetic valve endocarditis has been arbitrarily classified as *early* when it occurs within the first two months after surgery and *late* when it occurs after two months.[34] However, it is possible that many cases of prosthetic valve endocarditis that occur during the first year after surgery are acquired at the time of implantation of the artificial heart valve. This may be particularly true when the infection is caused by the HACEK group of bacteria. Early prosthetic valve endocarditis is caused by contamination of the valve at the time of implantation of by perioperative bacteremia.[12,33] *Staphylococcus epidermidis, Staphylococcus aureus,* and *Enterococcus faecalis* are among the more common microorganisms responsible for early prosthetic valve endocarditis.[12,28–33] The sources of late prosthetic valve endocarditis are more difficult to determine. Bacteremia is probably the principal cause of late endocarditis. Although streptococci and staphylococci are commonly encountered in these patients, a myriad of microorganisms can cause late prosthetic valve endocarditis.[23,28,33]

In a small proportion of cases of aortic valve endocarditis, no microorganism can be cultured from either the blood or surgical specimens.[28–33] This is called "culture-negative endocarditis," but it is important to rule out fastidious microorganisms and every effort should be made to identify them.

CLINICAL PRESENTATION AND DIAGNOSIS

It is helpful to classify infective endocarditis as acute and subacute because there are major differences between these two clinical presentations. Subacute endocarditis is often caused by less virulent microorganism such as *S. viridans*. When this organism affects a diseased aortic valve, the clinical course is protracted and antibiotics alone cure most cases. On the other hand, acute endocarditis is frequently caused by a virulent microorganism such as *S. aureus* and may affect a normal aortic valve. The clinical course is acute, and antibiotics alone seldom cure the infection.

The onset of subacute endocarditis in most cases is subtle, with low-grade fever and malaise. Patients think they have the "flu" and are often treated with oral antibiotics for a week to 10 days with improvement of symptoms. However, in most cases the symptoms recur a few days after stopping antibiotics. In the majority of cases no predisposing factor is identified. An aortic valve murmur is present in nearly all patients because they have preexisting aortic valve disease. Splenomegaly is common. Clubbing of the fingers and toes may develop in long-standing cases. Skin and mucous membrane signs occur late in this form of endocarditis. Petechiae appear on any part of the body. Small areas of hemorrhage may be seen in the ocular fundi. Hemorrhages in the nail beds usually have a linear distribution near the distal end, hence the name splinter hemorrhages. Osler's nodes are acute, tender, barely palpable nodular lesions in the pulp of the fingers and toes. Bacteria have been cultured from these lesions. Embolization of large vegetation fragments may cause dramatic clinical events such as acute myocardial infarction, stroke, or splenic or hepatic infarcts. Any other organ also may be involved. Destruction of the aortic cusps causes aortic insufficiency and heart failure. The blood picture is not distinctive in subacute endocarditis. Anemia without reticulocytosis develops in patients untreated for more than a few weeks. The leukocyte count is moderately elevated. Blood cultures frequently identify the offending microorganism.

The clinical course of acute endocarditis is often fulminating. A preexisting source of bacteremia may be identified. This form of endocarditis can present all symptoms and signs described under subacute endocarditis, but they are more acute and patients are often sicker with overwhelming signs of sepsis. Early metastatic infections are common. Two physical signs are seen only in acute endocarditis: the Janeway lesion (a painless red-blue hemorrhagic lesion of a few millimeters in diameter found in the palms of the hands and in the soles of the feet) and the Roth spot (an oval pale area near the optic disc surrounded by hemorrhage). Acute endocarditis is common in patients with no preexisting aortic valve disease. Early cardiac decompensation due to aortic insufficiency is common. Paravalvular abscess is also common, and, depending on the location of the abscess, the electrocardiogram may show an increased PR interval or heart block. The blood picture is one of acute sepsis. Blood culture often isolates the infecting agent.

Prosthetic valve endocarditis may present as acute or subacute endocarditis.

Doppler echocardiography is extremely useful in the diagnosis and management of infective endocarditis.[35–38] Transesophageal echocardiography is usually better than transthoracic echocardiography, and multiplane is better than monoplane for the diagnosis of endocarditis. Echocardiography can detect vegetations as small as 1 or 2 mm in size, but it is more reliable in native than in prosthetic valve endocarditis. It is more useful for tissue than for mechanical valves because of the acoustic shadowing of ball, disc, or leaflet motion of mechanical heart valves. Echocardiography is also extremely sensitive for detecting paravalvular abscess and cardiac fistulas.[38,39]

Clinical investigators from Duke University proposed certain criteria for confirming or rejecting the diagnosis of infective endocarditis.[40] These criteria have been confirmed by other investigators and are now widely used.[41,42] Table 33-1 summarizes the Duke University criteria for the diagnosis of infective endocarditis.

TABLE 33–1 Duke University criteria for diagnosis of infective endocarditis

DEFINITE DIAGNOSIS

A. Pathologic criteria
   1. Identification of a microorganism in the blood, vegetation, or embolus
   2. Pathologic lesions: vegetations or cardiac abscess confirmed by histology

B. Clinical criteria: 2 major or 1 major + 3 minor or 5 minor

   Major criteria
   1. Positive blood culture: typical microorganism for infective endocarditis
   2. Persistent positive blood culture from blood drawn more than 12 hours apart or all of 3 or the majority of 4 blood cultures drawn at least 1 hour apart
   3. Evidence of endocardial involvement: vegetation, abscess, or new partial dehiscence of prosthetic heart valve
   4. New valvular regurgitation

   Minor criteria
   1. Predisposing condition
   2. Fever ≥38°C
   3. Vascular phenomena: major arterial emboli, septic emboli, mycotic aneurysm, intracranial hemorrhage, conjunctival hemorrhage, Janeway lesions
   4. Immunological phenomena: glumeronephritis, Osler's nodes, Roth spots, rheumatoid factor
   5. Microbiologic phenomena: positive blood culture but not meeting major criterion or serologic evidence of active infection with organism consistent with infective endocarditis
   6. Echocardiogram consistent with endocarditis but not meeting major criterion

POSSIBLE DIAGNOSIS

Finding consistent with infective endocarditis that falls short of "definite"

REJECTED DIAGNOSIS: One or more of the following:
1. Firm alternate diagnosis for manifestations of endocarditis
2. Resolution of manifestations of endocarditis with antibiotics for 4 days or less
3. No pathologic evidence of infective endocarditis at surgery or autopsy after antibiotics for 4 days or less

Heart catheterization and coronary angiography increase the risk of embolization in patients with aortic valve vegetations and should be avoided.

TREATMENT

An appropriate antibiotic is the most important aspect of the management of patients with infective endocarditis.[17,28,29] Antibiotic therapy should be started soon after obtaining several blood cultures. The initial choice of antibiotics is based on clinical circumstances and the suspected source of infection. Patients who had recent dental work should receive antibiotics to counteract bacteria from the oral cavity; those who had recent urinary or colonic procedures should be treated with antibiotics that are effective against gram-negative bacteria. Intravenous drug users are usually infected with *S. aureus* or *S. epidermidis*, and antibiotics should be chosen accordingly. Once the microorganism is identified by blood cultures and its sensitivity to specific antibiotics is known, antibiotic therapy is adjusted accordingly. A combination of two or three antibiotics that potentiate each other is often needed in the treatment of endocarditis caused by virulent microorganisms. Intravenous antibiotic therapy is continued for 6 weeks.

It is difficult to eradicate infection caused by virulent microorganisms with antibiotics alone because they often destroy the native aortic valve very rapidly and cause aortic insufficiency and congestive heart failure. These infections are usually due to *S. aureus*, *Pseudomonas aeruginosa*, *Serratia marcescens*, or fungi.

Surveillance blood cultures are performed in 48 hours to monitor the efficacy of antibiotic therapy. The patient must be watched closely for signs of congestive heart failure, coronary and systemic embolization, and persistent infection. Daily electrocardiograms and frequent echocardiograms are performed during the first two weeks of treatment. At any evidence of increasing aortic insufficiency, enlarging vegetations, recurrent embolism, paravalvular abscess, or persistent infection, surgery should be immediately performed. It is important to operate on patients before they develop intractable heart failure, cardiogenic or septic shock, or extensive aortic root abscesses. Patients with vegetations larger than 10 mm present a clinical problem because they are more likely to develop serious complications and early surgery is justifiable.[35–37]

Anticoagulation is not effective in preventing embolization of vegetations in native and biological valves and is associated with an increased risk of neurologic complications.[43]

Early surgical treatment should be considered in patients with signs of congestive heart failure, acute valve dysfunction, paravalvular abscess or cardiac fistulas, recurrent systemic embolization when aortic valve vegetations are present, and persistent sepsis despite adequate antibiotic therapy for more than 4 to 5 days. Prosthetic valve endocarditis is best treated by early surgery, particularly in patients with mechanical valves.[23,29,30] Acute endocarditis of the aortic valve due to *S. aureus* is also best treated with early surgery because of the destructive power of the bacteria.[27,28]

Patients with neurologic deficits should have computed tomography scan or magnetic resonance imaging to determine if the cerebrovascular accident is ischemic or hemorrhagic. Ischemic damages are far more common than hemorrhagic, but both are associated with increased mortality and morbidity.[44–46] Mycotic aneurysms should be treated before valve surgery. Aortic valve replacement should be postponed for 2 weeks after an ischemic stroke and 4 weeks after a hemorrhagic stroke if possible.[46]

SURGICAL TREATMENT

Patients who need surgery are often very sick and may be in congestive heart failure. For this reason and because they often require complex and long operative procedures, myocardial protection is of utmost importance. Another important aspect of surgery for endocarditis is avoidance of contamination of the surgical field, instruments, drapes, and gloves with vegetations and pus. Instruments used to extirpate contaminated areas in the heart should be discarded before reconstruction of the ventricle and aortic root begins. In addition, local drapes, suction equipment, and surgical gloves should all be changed.

When the infection is limited to the cusps of the native aortic valve or a bioprosthetic valve, complete removal of the valve and implantation of a biological or mechanical valve usually resolve the problem. There is no evidence that bioprostheses are better than mechanical valves in patients with active infective endocarditis,[32] but aortic valve homograft is believed to be ideal for patients with endocarditis.[47] Some surgeons favor the pulmonary autograft, particularly in young patients.[48]

If the aortic annulus is involved in the infective process, resection of the necrotic or inflamed area is needed before a prosthetic valve can be implanted. The defect created by the resection should be patched before a prosthetic valve is implanted. We prefer to use fresh autologous pericardium to patch small defects (1 or 2 cm wide) in the aortic root and left ventricular outflow tract, and glutaraldehyde-fixed bovine pericardium for larger defects.[49,50] Some surgeons also use Dacron fabric to reconstruct the aortic root.[48–52] Here again, aortic valve homograft is believed to be ideal for reconstruction of the aortic root and left ventricular outflow tract.[53–55] The mitral valve of the aortic valve homograft can be used to patch defects in the left ventricular outflow tract by correctly orienting the homograft. The pulmonary autograft has also been used in cases of extensive destruction of the aortic root.[56] However, an aortic valve homograft or a pulmonary autograft is by no means a substitute for radical resection of all infected tissues, because persistent infection can occur with these biological grafts.[57,58]

Surgery for aortic root abscess and/or cardiac fistulas is challenging. The most important aspect in the surgical treatment of these patients is radical resection of all infected tissues.[23,29,50] We believe that the type of valve implanted is less important than complete extirpation of all infected and edematous tissues.[50] These patients frequently require replacement of the entire aortic root and reconstruction of the surrounding structures that are also involved by the abscess. These operations must be individualized because the pathology of aortic root abscess is variable. Extensive resection and reconstruction may be needed.[49,50] Thus, patching of the interventricular septum, dome of the left atrium, intervalvular fibrous body, right atrium, and pulmonary artery may be necessary, as well as repair of the left and/or right coronary arteries. The aortic root is often replaced with a valved conduit.

Figure 33-1 illustrates a procedure in which the dome of the left atrium and noncoronary sinus was patched before implanting a mechanical aortic valve.

Figure 33-2 illustrates an operation in which the entire aortic annulus and dome of the left atrium were reconstructed before a new valved conduit was implanted. An aortic valve homograft is ideal in this circumstance because the patch in the aortic annulus may not be necessary.

Aortic root abscess extending into the intervalvular fibrous body or into a prosthetic aortic and mitral valve is particularly difficult to treat.[59] In these cases, the resection and reconstruction can be performed through the aortic root and dome of the atrium.[59,60] After removing the native or prosthetic aortic valve, the aortotomy is extended into the intervalvular fibrous body and dome of the left atrium as illustrated in Figure 33-3. The abscess is best excised en bloc even if it is necessary to resect an excessive amount of tissue. If the abscess is limited to the intervalvular fibrous body, it may be possible to save the mitral valve. The proximal third of the anterior leaflet of the mitral valve can be safely resected and reconstructed. However, when in doubt, it is safer to remove the entire anterior leaflet than to leave infected tissue behind. If the native or prosthetic mitral valve is removed (Fig. 33-4), the base of the left ventricle becomes widely open without separation between its inflow and outflow tracts. It is necessary to create a new intervalvular fibrous body, and this can be accomplished by suturing two triangular shaped patches of bovine pericardium to the fibrous trigones (Fig. 33-5). A mitral valve prosthesis is secured to the posterior mitral annulus and to the double patch superiorly. The incision in the dome of the left atrium is closed with the outer patch and the aortic root reconstructed with the inner patch (Fig. 33-6). An aortic valve prosthesis is secured to the patch and normal aortic annulus (Fig. 33-7). When an aortic valve homograft is used for this type of reconstruction, the anterior leaflet of the mitral valve of the homograft can be used as patch material for the new fibrous body between the aortic and mitral valves. Actually, aortic and valve homografts in a single bloc of tissue have been used to treat this condition.[61]

Postoperative complications are common after surgery for active infective endocarditis. Septic patients may have severe coagulopathy and may bleed excessively after cardiopulmonary bypass. Antifibrinolytic agents, particularly aprotonin, should be used. Transfusion of platelets, cryoprecipitate, and fresh frozen plasma is often necessary to obtain hemostasis. Radical resection of aortic root abscess may cause heart block, for which a permanent pacemaker will be needed postoperatively. Depending on the patient's clinical condition before surgery, multiorgan failure may develop postoperatively. Neurologic deterioration may occur in patients with preexisting cerebral emboli. Pulmonary, splenic, hepatic, and other metastatic abscesses seldom require surgical treatment. Large metastatic abscesses, may have to be drained, and in the case of the spleen, splenectomy should be performed because of the risk of rupture.[62]

Clinical Results

The prognosis of aortic valve endocarditis depends largely on when the disease is diagnosed and how promptly it is treated.[27] Patients with prosthetic aortic valve endocarditis have a more serious prognosis than patients with native aortic valve endocarditis.[28,29] The results of surgery for infective endocarditis have improved significantly during the past three decades.[17] The operative mortality for patients with infection limited to the cusps of the aortic valve is as low as for aortic valve replacement without endocarditis[28,29]; it is higher in patients with prosthetic valve endocarditis[23,24,29–32] and in those with aortic root abscess.[50–53] In recent series of surgically treated patients the operative mortality for native valve endocarditis was under 10% and for prosthetic valve endocarditis was 20% to 30%.[23,29–32]

A review of our experience with surgery for active infective endocarditis in 122 patients found a 10-year survival of 61% ± 6%. Patients operated on for active infective endocarditis have a higher risk of developing endocarditis again than do patients with prosthetic valves who never had endocarditis.[29,30] In our experience, 8 of 122 patients developed recurrent infection after a mean interval of 47 months; freedom from recurrent endocarditis at 10 years was 79% ± 9%.[29] In most of these patients, a different microorganism caused the second episode of endocarditis.

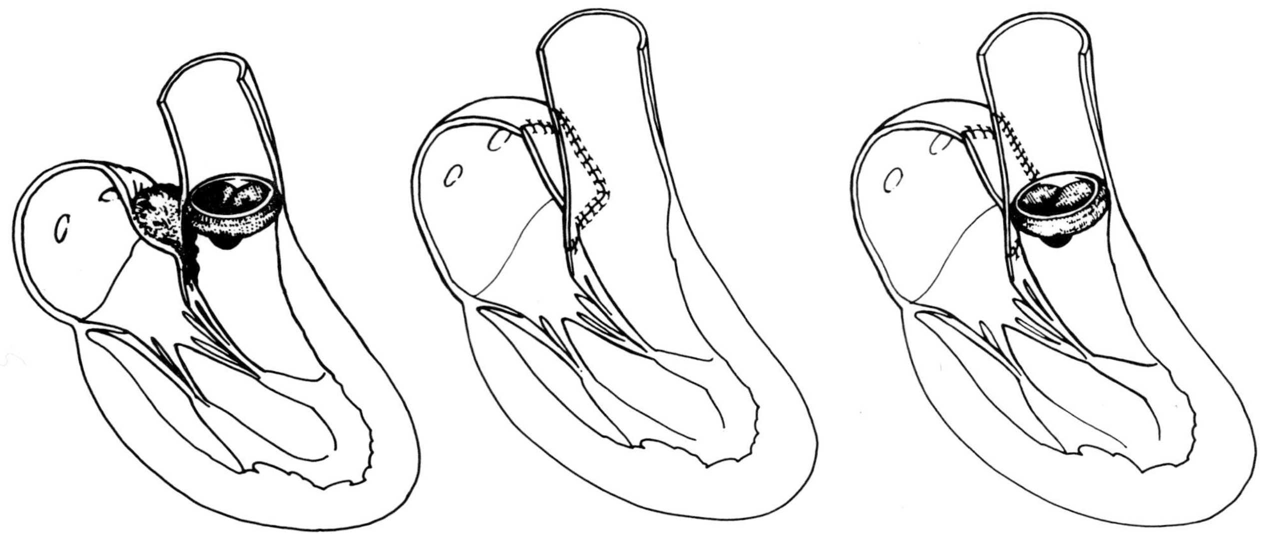

FIGURE 33–1 Repair of a localized aortic root abscess. One patch is used to reconstruct the dome of the left atrium and one for the aortic root. *(Reproduced from David TE: Aortic valve surgery. Curr Probl Surg 1999; 336:421, with permission from Mosby.)*

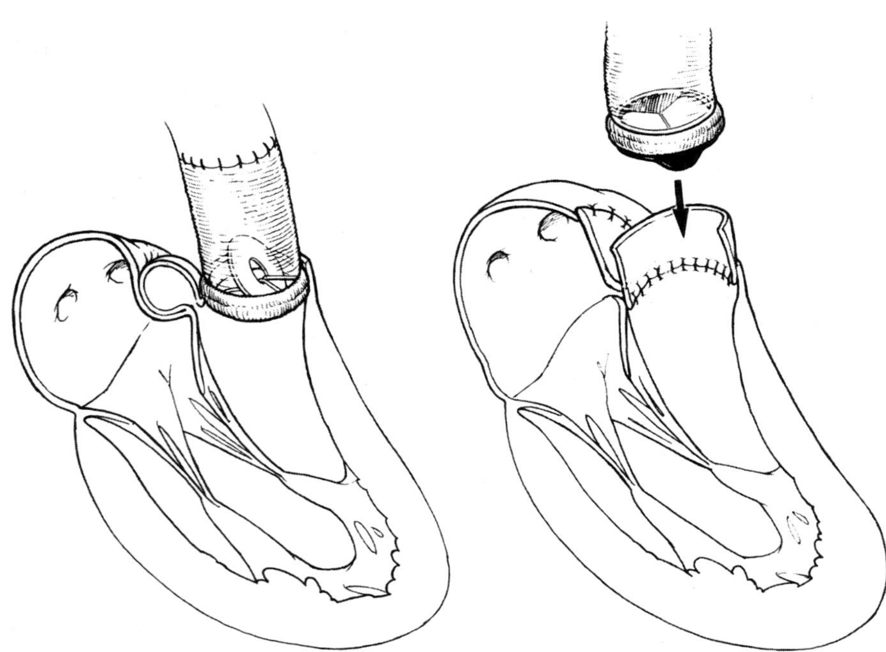

FIGURE 33–2 Repair of aortic annular abscess after aortic root replacement. One patch is used to reconstruct the dome of the left atrium and one to reconstruct the left ventricular outflow tract before a new valved conduit is implanted. *(Reproduced from David TE: Aortic valve surgery. Curr Probl Surg 1999;336:421, with permission from Mosby.)*

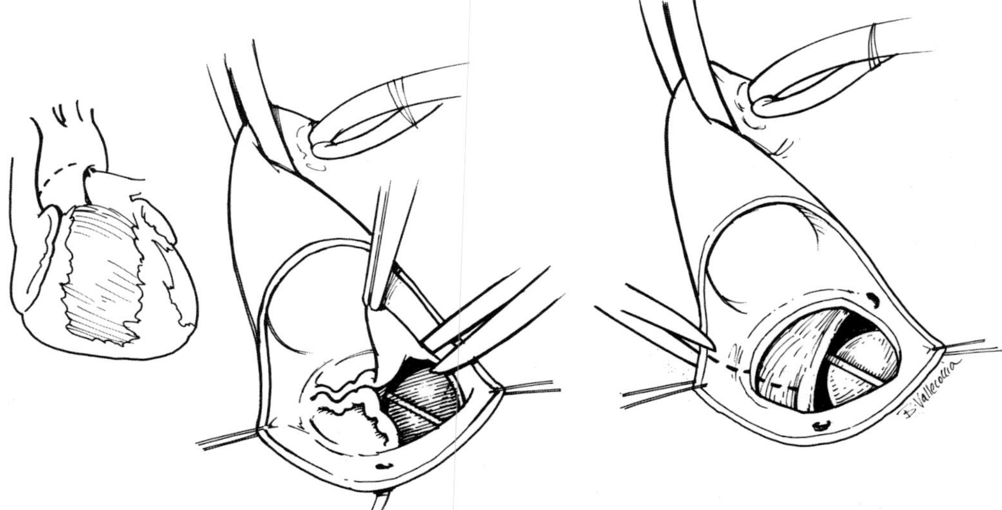

FIGURE 33–3 Double valve endocarditis with reconstruction of the intervalvular fibrous body. The aortic and mitral valves are excised through the aortic root and dome of the left atrium. *(Reproduced from David TE, Kuo J, Armstrong S: Aortic and mitral valve replacement with reconstruction of the intervalvular fibrous body. J Thorac Cardiovasc Surg 1997;114:766, with permission from Mosby.)*

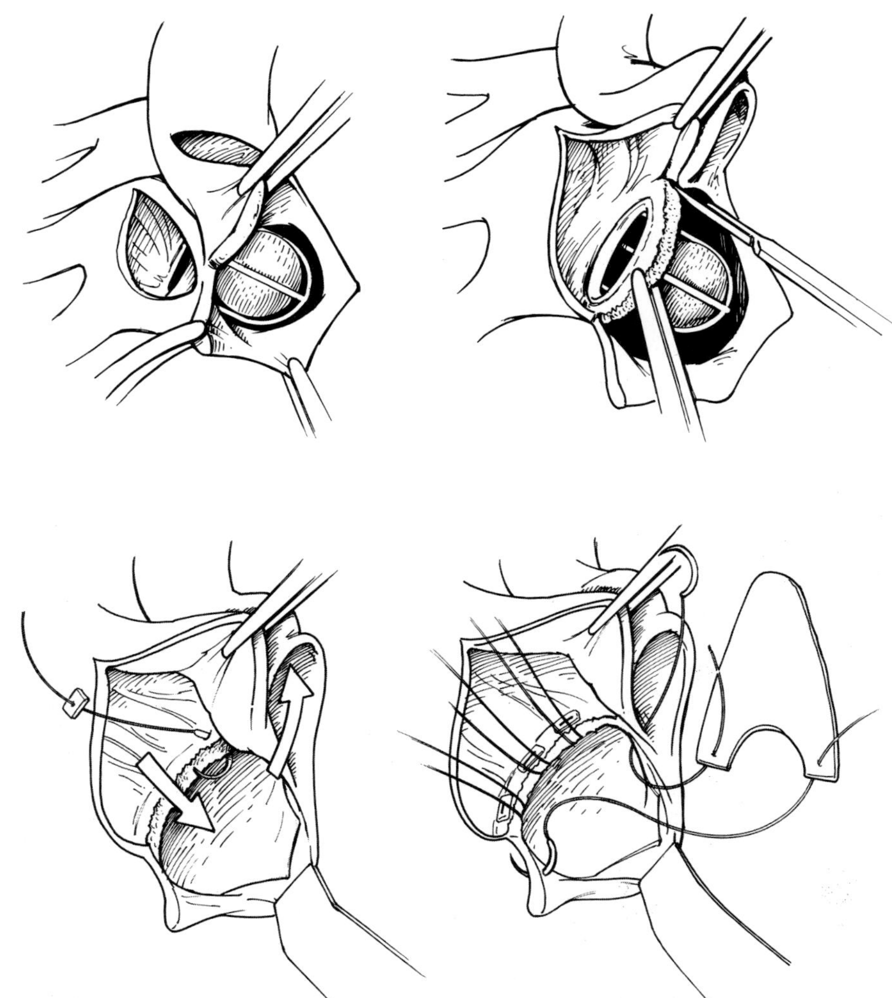

FIGURE 33–4 Both valves are excised along with any infected surrounding tissues. *(Reproduced from David TE, Kuo J, Armstrong S: Aortic and mitral valve replacement with reconstruction of the intervalvular fibrous body. J Thorac Cardiovasc Surg 1997;114:766, with permission from Mosby.)*

FIGURE 33–5 The left ventricular inflow and outflow tracts become a single orifice that is divided into mitral and aortic orifices with two triangular shape patches sutured to the lateral and medial fibrous trigones or endocardium of the left ventricle depending on the extensiveness of the resection. *(Reproduced from David TE, Kuo J, Armstrong S: Aortic and mitral valve replacement with reconstruction of the intervalvular fibrous body. J Thorac Cardiovasc Surg 1997;114:766, with permission from Mosby.)*

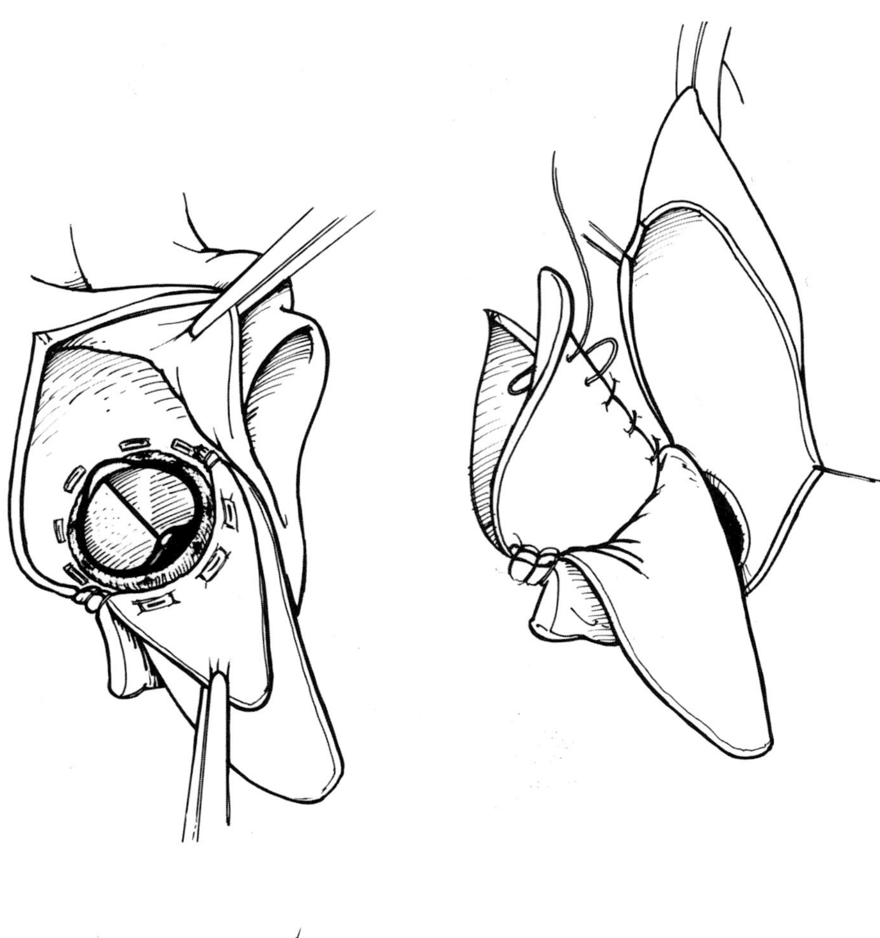

FIGURE 33–6 A prosthetic mitral valve is secured in the mitral annulus posteriorly and patches superiorly. The outer patch is used to close the dome of the left atrium. *(Reproduced from David TE, Kuo J, Armstrong S: Aortic and mitral valve replacement with reconstruction of the intervalvular fibrous body. J Thorac Cardiovasc Surg 1997;114:766, with permission from Mosby.)*

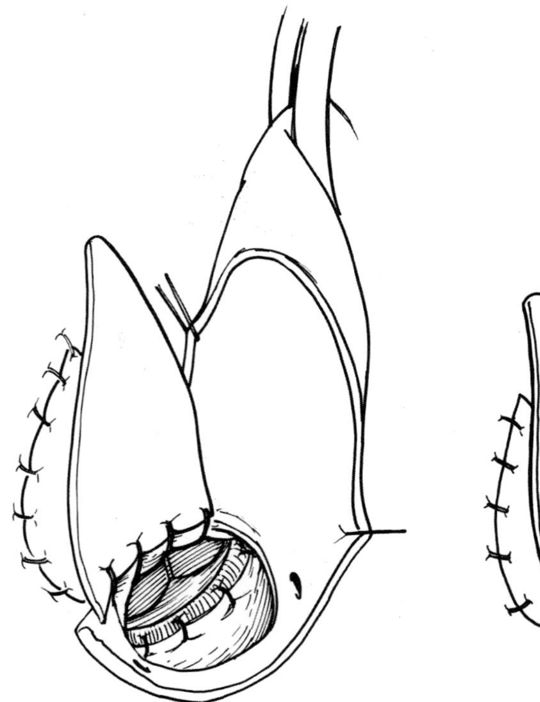

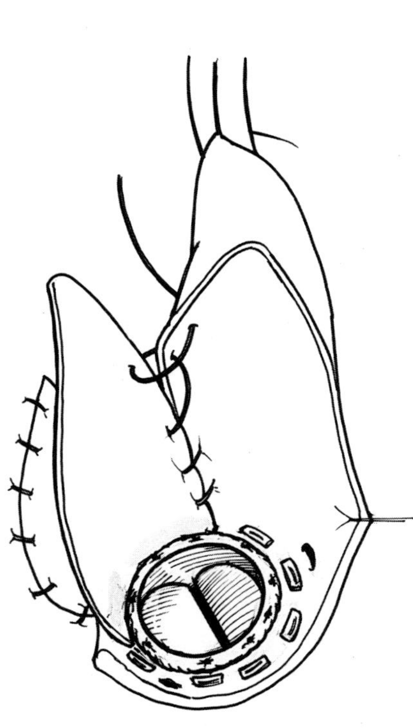

FIGURE 33–7 A prosthetic aortic valve is secured to the aortic annulus and medial patch, which is in turn used to close the aortotomy. *(Reproduced from David TE, Kuo J, Armstrong S: Aortic and mitral valve replacement with reconstruction of the intervalvular fibrous body. J Thorac Cardiovasc Surg 1997;114:766, with permission from Mosby.)*

REFERENCES

1. Lamas CC, Eykyn SJ: Bicuspid aortic valve—a silent danger: analysis of 50 cases of infective endocarditis. *Clin Infect Dis* 2000; 30:336.
2. Dyson C, Barnes RA, Harrison GA: Infective endocarditis: an epidemiological review of 128 episodes. *J Infect* 2000; 40:99.
3. King JW, Nguyen VQ, Conrad SA: Results of a prospective statewide reporting system for infective endocarditis. *Am J Med Sci* 1988; 295:517.
4. Berlin JA, Abrutyn E, Strom BL, et al: Incidence of infective endocarditis in the Delaware Valley, 1988–1990. *Am J Cardiol* 1995; 76:933.
5. Chamber JC, Sommerville J, Stone S, et al: Pulmonary autograft procedure for aortic valve disease: long-term results of a pioneer series. *Circulation* 1997; 96:2206.
6. Yacoub M, Rasmi NRN, Sundt TM, et al: Fourteen-year experience with homovital homograft for aortic valve replacement. *J Thorac Cardiovasc Surg* 1995; 110:186.
7. David TE, Ivanov J, Armstrong S, et al: Late results of heart valve replacement with the Hancock II bioprosthesis. *J Thorac Cardiovasc Surg* 2001; 121:268.
8. Jamieson WRE, Janusz MT, Burr LH, et al: Carpentier-Edwards supra-annular porcine bioprosthesis: second generation prosthesis in aortic valve replacement. *Ann Thorac Surg* 2001; 71:S224.
9. Poirier NC, Pelletier LC, Pellerin M, et al: 15-year experience with the Carpentier-Edwards pericardial bioprosthesis. *Ann Thorac Surg* 1998; 66:S57.
10. Khan S, Chaux A, Matloff J, et al: The St. Jude Medical valve: experience with 1,000 cases. *J Thorac Cardiovasc Surg* 1994; 109:1010.
11. Hammermeister KE, Sethi GK, Henderson WG, et al: Outcomes 15 years after valve replacement with a mechanical versus a bioprosthetic valve: final report of the Veterans Affairs randomized trial. *J Am Coll Cardiol* 2000; 36:1152.
12. Gordon SM, Serkey JM, Longworth DL, et al: Early onset prosthetic valve endocarditis: the Cleveland Clinic experience 1992–1997. *Ann Thorac Surg* 2000; 69:1388.
13. McCarthy JT, Steckelberg JM: Infective endocarditis in patients receiving long-term hemodialysis. *Mayo Clin Proc* 2000; 75:1008.
14. Grant RT, Wood JR Jr, Jones TS: Heart valve irregularities in relation to subacute bacterial endocarditis. *Heart* 1928; 14:247.
15. Angrist AA, Oka M: Pathogenesis of bacterial endocarditis. *JAMA* 1963; 181:249.
16. Durack DT, Beeson PB, Petersdorf RG: Experimental bacterial endocarditis, III: production and progress of the disease in rabbits. *Br J Exp Pathol* 1973; 54:142.
17. Mylonakis E, Calderwood SB: Infective endocarditis in adults. *N Eng J Med* 2001; 345:1318.
18. Salgado AV, Furlan AJ, Keys TF, et al: Neurologic complications of endocarditis: a 12-year experience. *Neurology* 1989; 39:173.
19. Kanter MC, Hart RG: Neurologic complications of infective endocarditis. *Neurology* 1991; 41:1015.
20. Piper C, Hetzer R, Korfer R, et al: The importance of secondary mitral valve involvement in primary aortic valve endocarditis: the mitral kissing vegetation. *Heart* 2002; 23:79.
21. Gillinov AM, Diaz R, Blackstone EH, et al: Double valve endocarditis. *Ann Thorac Surg* 2001; 71:1874.
22. Arnett EN, Roberts WC: Prosthetic valve endocarditis: clinicopathologic analysis of 22 necropsy patients with active infective endocarditis involving natural left-sided cardiac valves. *Am J Cardiol* 1976; 38:282.
23. David TE: The surgical treatment of patients with prosthetic valve endocarditis. *Semin Thorac Cardiovasc Surg* 1995; 7:47.
24. Sett SS, Hudon MPJ, Jamieson WRE, et al: Prosthetic valve endocarditis: experience with porcine bioprostheses. *J Thorac Cardiovasc Surg* 1993; 105:428.
25. Fernicola DJ, Roberts WC: Frequence of ring abscess and cuspal infection in active infective endocarditis involving bioprosthetic valves. *Am J Cardiol* 1993; 72:314.
26. Clarkson PM, Barratt-Boyes BG: Bacterial endocarditis following homograft replacement of the aortic valve. *Circulation* 1970; 42:987.
27. Ralph-Edwards A, David TE, Bos J: Infective endocarditis in patients who had replacement of the aortic root. *Ann Thorac Surg* 1994; 35:429.
28. Watanakunakorn C, Burket T: Infective endocarditis at a large community teaching hospital, 1980–1990: a review of 210 episodes. *Medicine* 1993; 72:90.
29. D'Udekem Y, David TE, Feindel CM, et al: Long-term results of surgery for active infective endocarditis. *Eur J Cardiothorac Surg* 1997; 11:46.
30. Larbalestier RJ, Kinchla NM, Aranki SF, et al: Acute bacterial endocarditis: optimizing surgical results. *Circulation* 1992; 86(suppl II):68.
31. Alexiou C, Langley SM, Stafford H, et al: Surgery for active culture-positive endocarditis: determinants of early and late outcome. *Ann Thorac Surg* 2000; 69:1448.
32. Moon MR, Miller DC, Moore KA, et al: Treatment of endocarditis with valve replacement: the question of tissue versus mechanical prosthesis. *Ann Thorac Surg* 2001; 71:1164.
33. Fang G, Keys TF, Gentry LO, et al: Prosthetic valve endocarditis resulting from nosocomial bacteremia: a prospective, multicenter study. *Ann Intern Med* 1993; 119:560.
34. Calderwood SB, Swinsk LA, Waternaux CM, et al: Risk factors for development of prosthetic valve endocarditis. *Circulation* 1985; 72:31.
35. Buda AJ, Zotx RJ, Lemire MS, Back DS: Prognostic significance of vegetations detected by two-dimensional echocardiography in infective endocarditis. *Am Heart J* 1986; 112:1291.
36. Lowry RW, Zoghbi WA, Baker WB, et al: Clinical impact of transesophageal echocardiography in the diagnosis and management of infective endocarditis. *Am J Cardiol* 1994; 73:1089.
37. DiSalvo G, Habib G, Pergola V, et al: Echocardiography predicts embolic events in infective endocarditis. *J Am Coll Cardiol* 2001; 15:1069.
38. Daniel WG, Mugge A, Martin RP, et al: Improvement in the diagnosis of abscesses associated with endocarditis by transesophageal echocardiography. *N Engl J Med* 1991; 324:795.
39. Anguera I, Quaglio G, Miro JM, et al: Aortocardiac fistulas complicating infective endocarditis. *Am J Cardiol* 2001; 87:652.
40. Durack DT, Lukes AS, Bright DK: New criteria for diagnosis of infective endocarditis: utilization of specific echocardiographic findings. *Am J Cardiol* 1994; 96:200.
41. Sekeres MA, Abrutyn Em Berlin JA, et al: An assessment of the usefulness of the Duke criteria for diagnosing active infective endocarditis. *Clin Infect Dis* 1997; 24:1185.
42. Habib G, Derumeaux G, Avierinos JF, et al: Value and limitations of the Duke criteria for the diagnosis of infective endocarditis. *J Am Coll Cardiol* 1999; 33:2023.
43. Davenport J, Hart RG: Prosthetic valve endocarditis 1976–1987: antibiotics, anticoagulation, and stroke. *Stroke* 1990; 21:993.
44. Ting W, Silverman N, Levistky S: Valve replacement in patients with endocarditis and cerebral septic emboli. *Ann Thorac Surg* 1991; 51:18.
45. Matsushita K, Kuriyama Y, Sawada T, et al: Hemorrhagic and ischemic cerebrovascular complications of active infective endocarditis of native valve. *Eur Neurol* 1993; 33:267.
46. Gillinov AM, Shah RV, Curtis WE et al: Valve replacement in patients with endocarditis and acute neurologic deficit. *Ann Thorac Surg* 1996; 61:1125.
47. Haydock D, Barratt-Boyes B, Macedo T, et al: Aortic valve replacement for active infective endocarditis in 108 patients: a comparison

of free-hand allograft valves with mechanical prostheses and bioprostheses. *J Thorac Cardiovasc Surg* 1992; 103:130.

48. Oswalt JD, Dewan SJ, Mueller MC, et al: Highlights of a ten-year experience with the Ross procedure. *Ann Thorac Surg* 2001; 71:S332.
49. David TE, Komeda M, Brofman PR: Surgical treatment of aortic root abscess. *Circulation* 1989; 80(suppl 1):269.
50. D'Udekem Y, David TE, Feindel CM, et al: Long-term results of operation for paravalvular abscess. *Ann Thorac Surg* 1996; 62:48.
51. Jault F, Gandjbakhch I, Chastre JC, et al: Prosthetic valve endocarditis with ring abscesses: surgical management and long-term results. *J Thorac Cardiovasc Surg* 1993; 105:1106.
52. Fiore AC, Ivey TD, McKeown PP, et al: Patch closure of aortic annulus mycotic aneurysm. *Ann Thorac Surg* 1986; 42:372.
53. Glazier JJ, Verwilghen J, Donaldson RM, et al: Treatment of complicated prosthetic aortic valve endocarditis with annular abscess formation by homograft root replacement. *J Am Coll Cardiol* 1991; 17:1177.
54. Dossche KM, Defauw JJ, Ernst SM, et al: Allograft aortic root replacement in prosthetic aortic valve endocarditis: a review of 32 patients. *Ann Thorac Surg* 1997; 63:1644.
55. Knosalla C, Weng Y, Yankah AC, et al: Surgical treatment of active infective aortic valve endocarditis with associated periannular abscess—11 year results. *Eur Heart J* 2000; 21:421.
56. Pettersson G, Tingleff J, Joyce FS: Treatment of aortic valve endocarditis with the Ross procedure. *Eur J Cardiothorac Surg* 1998; 13:678.
57. Ritter M, von Segesser L, Lenni R: Persistent root abscess after emergency repair with an aortic homograft. *Br Heart J* 1994; 72:495.
58. Joyce FS, McCarthy PM, Stewart WJ, et al: Left ventricle to right atrial fistula after aortic homograft replacement for endocarditis. *Eur J Cardiothorac Surg* 1994; 8:100.
59. David TE, Kuo J, Armstrong S: Aortic and mitral valve replacement with reconstruction of the intervalvular fibrous body. *J Thorac Cardiovasc Surg* 1997; 114:766.
60. David TE, Feindel CM, Armstrong S, et al: Reconstruction of the mitral annulus: a ten-year experience. *J Thorac Cardiovasc Surg* 1995; 110:1323.
61. Obadia JF, Raisky O, Sebbag L, et al: Monobloc aorto-mitral homogaft as a treatment of complex cases of endocarditis. *J Thorac Cardiovasc Surg* 2001; 121:584.
62. Ting W, Silverman NA, Levitsky S: Splenic septic emboli in endocarditis. *Circulation* 1990; 82(suppl V):105.

Chapter 34

Stentless Aortic Valve Replacement: Homograft/Autograft

Craig R. Hampton/Albert J. Chong/Edward D. Verrier

The number of heart valve procedures performed annually in the United States surpassed 80,000 in 1998 and continues to increase. Despite this increasing experience, the search for an ideal valve replacement for a diseased aortic valve continues. Currently, there are essentially five choices for replacement of the aortic valve: a mechanical valve prosthesis (e.g., the St. Jude bileaflet); a stented bioprosthetic valve (i.e., a xenograft); a stentless bioprosthetic valve (e.g., the Toronto stentless porcine valve); an aortic homograft; and a pulmonary autograft (i.e., the Ross procedure). Since there is no single ideal valve choice, the selection of a suitable valve for aortic valve replacement must be individualized through consideration of the relative advantages and disadvantages of these five options. To this end, we believe there are six valve-related issues to be considered when selecting a valve replacement option: durability; risk of thromboembolism and need for anticoagulation; technical ease of insertion; infectibility; availability; and valve-related noise. Consideration of these issues in the context of an individual patient will allow prudent selection of a suitable valve, with all choices having their relative advantages and disadvantages.

HISTORICAL PERSPECTIVE

Gordon Murray was the first to utilize an aortic homograft for treatment of aortic valvular disease.[1] After successful attempts in the animal laboratory, Murray placed valve-bearing aortic homograft segments in the descending aorta for treatment of severe aortic insufficiency (AI) with good results up to 4 years postoperatively.[2] Subsequently, the hemodynamic benefits of heterotopic placement of aortic homograft in the descending aorta for AI were confirmed by Beall et al, also in the animal laboratory.[3] Kerwin et al of Toronto extended the clinical experience of heterotopic homograft to 9 patients, with good results in 6 patients up to 6 years postoperatively.[4] At nearly the same time, Bigelow of Toronto reported placing an aortic homograft in the orthotopic position, but the patient died of a coronary thrombosis within a day.[5] Successful orthotopic placement of an aortic homograft was soon performed independently and nearly simultaneously[6] by Ross of Guy's Hospital in London[7] and Barratt-Boyes of Green Lane Hospital in Auckland,[8] followed a few months later by Paneth and O'Brien of the Brompton Hospital. In 1964, Barratt-Boyes reported his early experience with aortic homografts in 44 patients, with good/fair results in all but 3 patients.[8]

Since these initial efforts to utilize homografts in the aortic position, the procurement and preservation of these biologic valves have changed significantly. Initially, aortic valves were implanted shortly after collection.[9] This technique fell out of favor and was rapidly supplanted by techniques to sterilize and preserve the valve for later use—a fundamental strategy of contemporary tissue banking. Valves were collected cleanly and then were sterilized with beta-propiolactone[8,10] or 0.02% chlorhexidine,[11] followed by ethylene oxide[11] or radiation exposure.[12] After chemical sterilization, valves were placed in Hanks' balanced salt solution at 4°C for up to 4 weeks, followed by freeze-drying.[8,13] Recognizing that the incidence of valve rupture was high in chemically treated valves, Barratt-Boyes introduced antibiotic sterilization of homografts in 1968.[14] Cryopreservation of allografts was introduced in 1975 by O'Brien in an attempt to increase the cell viability of preserved allografts.[15] Cryopreservation continues to be the most commonly used method for aortic allografts.

Recognizing that homografts may incite alloreactivity, it was suggested that autologous biologic valves would diminish this risk while maintaining the superior hemodynamic profile. Use of the pulmonic valve to replace another valve was first reported in 1961 when Lower et al of Stanford transposed the pulmonic valve to the mitral position in dogs.[16] Shortly thereafter, Pillsbury and Shumway, also of Stanford, experimentally transposed the autologous pulmonic valve to replace a diseased aortic valve.[17] Ross extended this work to humans, reporting in 1967 a series of 14 patients in whom he replaced a diseased aortic valve with autologous pulmonic valve.[18] Since that time, this procedure has come to bear his name—the Ross procedure—and is also described as a pulmonary autograft. Widespread early fervor about this procedure was quickly tempered when surgeons appreciated its technical demands as well as considering it to be a "double valve" replacement. In the last decade, however, there has been renewed interest in the Ross procedure due to its proven durability and its hemodynamic superiority over alternative valve replacement options. Currently, over 240 surgeons worldwide have performed the Ross procedure, as reported in the Ross Procedure International Registry, which was established in the early 1990s to catalog these procedures and follow the outcomes.

ALLOGRAFTS

Procurement and Preservation

In the United States, the majority of allograft valves are obtained from beating-heart organ donors whose hearts are not suitable for transplantation. Allografts obtained from cadavers less than 24 hours old comprise the second primary source of valves. The processing of cadaveric tissue is increasingly performed by regional tissue centers that specialize in the procurement and preservation of human tissues for ultimate allotransplantation. The increasing prevalence of cardiac allotransplantation has allowed the use of fresh "homovital" allografts,[19] which may have enhanced preservation of cellular viability. Ideally, fresh valves would be implanted within 24 hours, but even at centers with significant experience, the interval between harvesting and implantation is up to 60 days, with an average interval of 3.9 days.[19] Cryopreservation is the most common technique used, which optimizes cellular viability[15] and prolongs shelf life, which is an obvious advantage given the shortage of organ donors.

The heart is procured under sterile (multiorgan donor) or clean (cadaveric donor) conditions and gently rinsed with cold isotonic salt solution (e.g., Ringers lactate) to remove the blood and its elements from the cardiac chambers. The heart is then placed in a bag containing ice-slush solution to be kept cold until further processing. Warm ischemia time does not exceed 12 hours, unless the donor is in an environment with temperature of 8°C or lower within six hours of death, which can extend the "warm" ischemia time to 24 hours. Donor blood is obtained for culture and serologic testing of common infectious agents (e.g., viral hepatitis B and C, HIV, HTLV, and *Treponema pallidum*).

The following details concerning tissue center processing are based on procedural protocols of the Northwest Tissue Center, Seattle, Washington,[20] and are similar to other institutions.[21] Once at the tissue center, an aortic block is dissected in a controlled environment (Class 100 clean room environment). Donor tissue and the transport solution are cultured for aerobic and anaerobic organisms, fungus, and acid-fast bacilli (AFB). Proximally the dissection includes the aortic ring and the anterior leaflet of the mitral valve with a variable amount of ventricular muscle, and extends distally to the left subclavian artery, including the branches of the thoracic aorta. The coronary ostia are ligated, allowing a subsequent interposition "free-root" allograft if needed. The base of the graft contains a variable amount of ventricular muscle that may be trimmed at the time of graft implantation. The valve is inspected for leaflet fenestrations, atheroma, or damage, which may make it unsuitable for implantation. Of these, leaflet atheroma absolutely contraindicates use of the allograft, while fenestrations or other damage are relative contraindications, and depend on their severity and magnitude. Obturators are then used to size both the valve and the aorta (Fig. 34-1).

After harvesting, the allograft block undergoes a series of rinses and is then placed in a nutrient medium (e.g., RPMI-1640) with low levels of antibiotics (polymyxin B sulfate 250,000 units, cefoxitin sodium 60 mg, vancomycin HCl 12.5 mg, lincomycin HCl 30 mg)[22] for sterilization. Although this regimen (CLPVA) originally included amphotericin B, it is often omitted to optimize cellular viability.[23] The allograft can then either be used as a fresh homovital allograft, or prepared for cryopreservation. Throughout this process, cultures are serially obtained to rule out contamination that may preclude use of the graft.

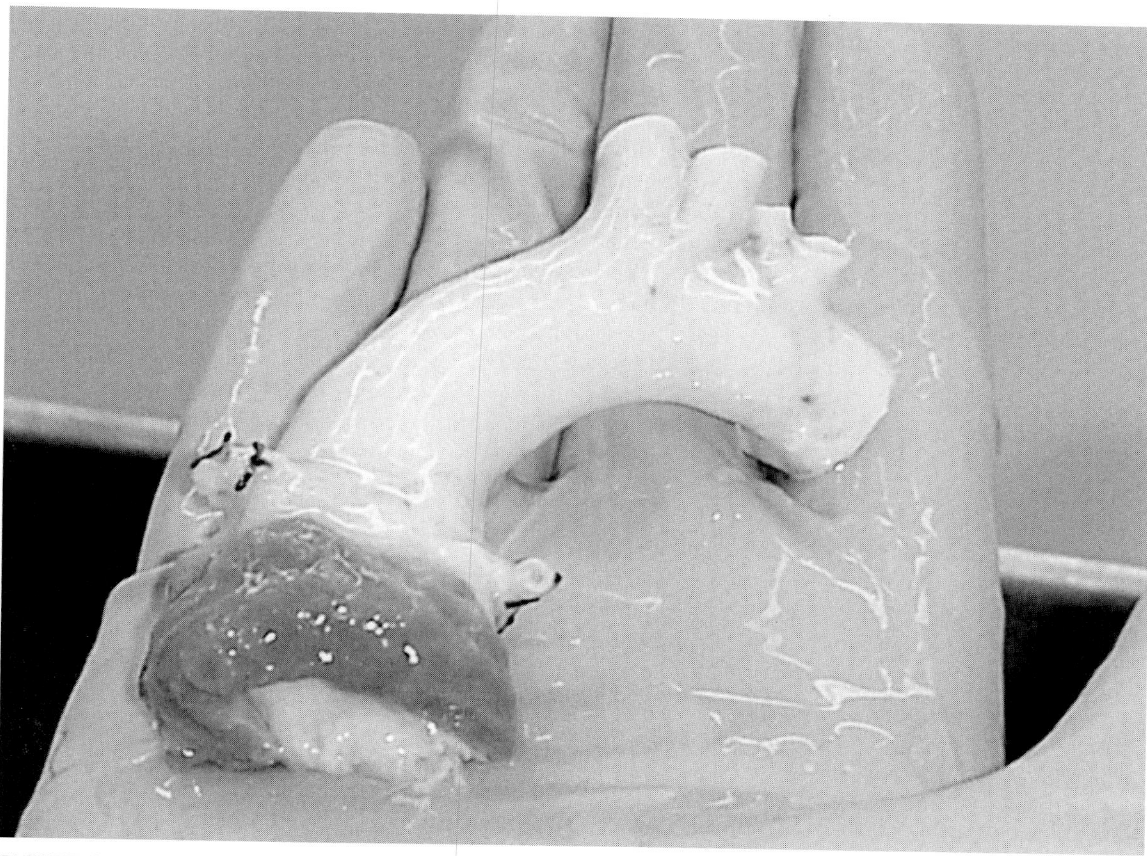

FIGURE 34–1 Aortic valve allograft after harvesting from the donor. The block includes a variable amount of ventricular muscle and the anterior leaflet of the mitral valve. Additional trimming for replacement is performed at the time of implantation. (*Reproduced with permission from The Northwest Tissue Center, Puget Sound Blood Center.*)

The *sine qua non* of cryopreservation is controlled rate freezing, as introduced by O'Brien et al in 1975.[15] Prior to packaging, the air in the packaging room, the gloves of the technologist, and three designated locations in the sterile packaging field are sampled for viable particles. The allograft is transferred from the antibiotics to a sterile storage pouch containing culture medium (e.g., RPMI-1640), 10% fetal calf serum, and 7.5% DMSO (a cryoprotectant). These substrates are designed to provide nutritive support to the allograft and minimize crystal formation and tissue damage during the freezing process. A final sample is taken of the packaging solution for aerobic and anaerobic organisms. Within two hours of exposure to DMSO, the allograft is frozen at −1°C per minute down to −40°C and then placed in vapor-phase liquid nitrogen storage (about −195°C) until it is used. After tissue cultures and serology results are available (about 4 to 6 weeks) and negative, the valve may be used for implantation; if there are any positive culture or serology results, the valve is discarded.

After release of the allograft from the tissue center, it is shipped in a container validated to maintain temperatures below −100°C for ten days. Two temperature-sensitive indicators, which turn red if temperatures rise above −100°C, are included with each shipment to ensure maintenance of shipping temperatures. Upon arrival to the institution where it will be used, the storage pouch is removed from the liquid nitrogen and placed in warm saline (37°C to 42°C). The allograft size and number are confirmed. After removal from the storage pouch, the allograft then undergoes a series of gentle rinses and thawing, in solutions that have increasingly dilute DMSO, followed by a final rinse in pure nutrient media prior to use. The allograft is then ready for final trimming and implantation.

Cellular and Immunologic Aspects of Allografts

Normal valves are ultrastructurally comprised of cellular components, including endothelium, fibroblasts, and smooth muscle cells (SMCs), and an amorphous and fibrillar extracellular matrix (ECM) derived primarily from fibroblasts and SMCs.[24] In nonpathologic states, there is a steady state between destruction of these elements and remodeling, which underlies an overall structure and function. In accordance with the paradigm that structural integrity, and thus function, depends on cellular viability of an allograft, preservation techniques have attempted to optimize the preservation of viable cellular elements to improve function and durability.

As mentioned, earlier methods of chemical sterilization and irradiation had a prohibitive incidence of cusp rupture[14] and histologic analysis of these allograft valves reveals nonviable cellular elements.[25] Antibiotic sterilization of allografts and storage in a balanced salt solution or nutrient medium at 4°C does not maintain cellular viability beyond a few days.[26,27] The durability of these valves is improved from chemically sterilized valves with a freedom from reoperation for valve degeneration at 10 years of 89%.[15] Gentle procurement and cryopreservation of allografts has been shown to maintain donor fibroblast viability up to 9.5 years after implantation in one patient, and viable fibroblasts have been consistently demonstrated in a small number of other patients.[15] More recently, persistence of viable, functional donor fibroblasts in allografts harvested up to 70 months has been reported.[28] Also, using in situ hybridization technology, the viable fibroblasts in the explanted allografts were demonstrated to be of both recipient and donor origin. Other investigators have demonstrated no cellular viability of allograft valves after antibiotic treatment[26] or after explantation.[29] Of note, however, is the fact that the methods of valvular preservation in the latter investigation[29] were not reported, and these valves were explanted primarily for deterioration, contributing to significant selection bias. In the end, the extent to which viable cellular elements persist in allografts after cryopreservation is not clear. Given the occasional findings of viable cells, particularly fibroblasts, up to 9 years after implantation,[15] it is likely that some viable cells persist in allografts, at least some of the time. Moreover, when viable cells are present, they are likely of both donor and recipient origin.[15,28] The discrepant findings with respect to the persistence of viable cells in the allograft may relate to warm ischemia times or differences in procurement and preservation techniques. More importantly, when present, the extent to which these viable fibroblasts remain functional and contribute to the structural integrity of the allograft components is not known.

While modifications of valve preservation techniques have attempted to maintain cellular viability of the allograft[15] to improve long-term structural integrity and function,[30] the presence of viable donor cells may be detrimental by inciting an allograft rejection reaction.[31] Multiple studies have demonstrated the generation of donor-specific alloantibodies directed against human leukocyte antigens (HLA) class I (A and B antigens) and II (DR antigens) in allograft valve recipients.[32,33] The development of panel-reactive antibodies (PRA) seems to increase with time,[33] approximating 82% at 6 years after graft implantation,[34] occurs in both adults and children, and is irrespective of the method of cryopreservation.[35] Despite consistent evidence of antibody formation directed against the HLA antigens of the allograft, the clinical significance is not clear.

Dignan et al reported a significant association between HLA class II antigen mismatch and postoperative fever and homograft dysfunction in recipients of cryopreserved allografts.[36] In recipients of homovital allografts, Smith et al reported no significant association between HLA class I or II antigens with long-term (6 years) valve function,[34] although there was an increased prevalence of valve degeneration in those patients with HLA antibodies. In HLA antibody-negative patients, the actuarial freedom from valve degeneration at 1, 5, and 10 years was 100%. In patients with PRA less than 50%, freedom from valve degeneration at 1, 5, and 10 years was 100%, 97%, and 92%; in those patients who were highly sensitized, it was 98%, 94%, and 88%.[34] Taken together, these data suggest that antibody-mediated alloreactivity may play a causal role in allograft valve dysfunction over time, but larger studies are certainly needed with adequate power to detect small (i.e., 5% at 10 years) differences between allograft recipients who are HLA matched and mismatched. In the meantime, until such data are available, it has been suggested that prospective matching of HLA antigens may be warranted.[34] Recognizing that investigation of allografts in humans is limited to preimplanation analysis (i.e., during procurement or preservation) or valves that require explantation due to valve failure, heart transplantation of the recipient, or recipient death, investigators have developed alternative models for this inquiry.

Accordingly, to better understand the immunologic aspects of allograft valve dysfunction, numerous investigators have used animal models of allograft implantation. Multiple studies of allograft implantation across MHC barriers in rats demonstrate significant cellular infiltration into thickened valve leaflets over the first 28 days, which is temporally followed by valve degeneration and failure.[37–40] The cellular infiltration may be phasic, characterized by early monocyte infiltration,[37] and followed by progressive monocyte/macrophage and T-lymphocyte infiltration, which is maximal by 7 days after implantation.[37,40] There is a coincidental decline in allograft donor cell viability over this time that is paralleled by declining valve structure and function.[37] Importantly, in T-cell–deficient rats, these cellular events do not occur and allograft function is preserved, providing additional support for immune-mediated valvular destruction.[38] Moreover, immune modulation with cyclosporine and anti-adhesion molecule (anti-$\alpha 4/\beta 2$ integrin) therapy attenuates leaflet cellular infiltration and prevents allograft structural failure.[41] Taken together, these data strongly support a donor-specific, cell-mediated (primarily T lymphocytes) immune reaction directed against the donor alloantigens that is followed by structural valve failure—a cellular cascade typical of solid organ rejection.

In summary, despite intensive investigation over the past three decades, the relative contribution of the immune response, preservation techniques, and warm ischemia time to ultimate valve degeneration (i.e., sclerosis, calcification, etc.) is not clear. More importantly, after consideration of the structural benefits and the immune-reaction risks, the net advantage of maintaining cellular (particularly fibroblasts) viability in the allograft is not well defined.[31] Future investigations should endeavor to further clarify the relative contributions of these factors to allograft valve antigenicity, immunogenicity, and durability. Further, the impact of immune modulation on long-term allograft function warrants further study.

Indications

Aortic valve replacement with an allograft has a number of advantages including excellent hemodynamic profile with low transvalvular gradients, low risk of thromboembolism without the need for systemic anticoagulation, possibly enhanced regression of LV mass,[42] and low risk of prosthetic valve infection. Allograft durability is limited, however, with a freedom from reoperation at 20 years of 38% to 50% and a freedom from structural valve failure at 20 years of 18% to 32%.[43,44] The incidence of structural failure is proportional to recipient and donor age; that is, increased structural failure over time in older recipients that receive allografts from older donors. As a result, we believe allografts should be considered in: (1) treatment of active endocarditis of either a native or prosthetic valve; (2) patients 30 to 60 years old, with at least 10-year life expectancy, who cannot be anticoagulated, for whatever reason; (3) patients with small aortic annuli; and (4) patients requiring composite replacement of the aortic valve and aortic root. Further, we believe allografts should be avoided in: (1) patients who have a heavily calcified, noncompliant aortic root and (2) patients younger than 20 years old, because of the likelihood of valve degeneration over time.

Preoperative Evaluation

Preoperative preparation for placement of an aortic allograft is similar to other aortic valve operations. Invariably, a transthoracic echocardiogram (TTE) will be available. TTE is invaluable diagnostic tool for evaluation of valvular morphology and function, etiology of valvular dysfunction, and ventricular function. Further, preoperative TTE may also accurately predict aortic annulus diameter, and thus, the size of the homograft required. However, the accuracy of TTE in predicting aortic annulus size is not entirely clear.

Greaves et al demonstrated that two independent observers, interpreting identical echocardiograms, predicted annulus diameter within 2 mm 57% or 70% of the time, and up to 12% of the measurements were discordant from actual valve diameter by more than 4 mm.[45] Moreover, there was significant interobserver variability. Others, however, have demonstrated accurate prediction of actual valve size, or within 2 mm, 80% to 100% of the time.[46,47]

More recently, the predictive value of transesophageal echocardiography (TEE) has been assessed. In 20 patients

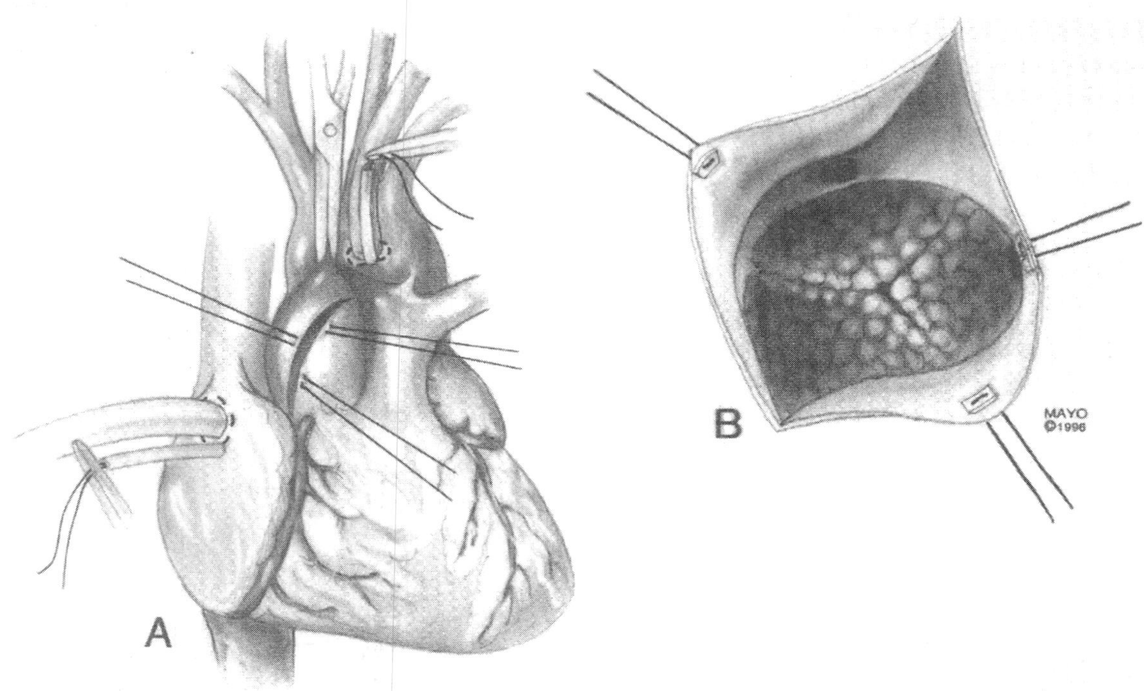

FIGURE 34–2 Standard cardiopulmonary bypass is performed. A "lazy-S" or oblique aortotomy is performed beginning above the right coronary cusp with the transverse portion just cephalad to the noncoronary cusp. This incision provides excellent exposure for all techniques when replacing the aortic valve and root. (*Reproduced with permission from Schaff HV, Cable DG: Aortic valve replacement with homograft, in Kaiser LR, Kron IL, Spray TL (eds): Mastery of Cardiothoracic Surgery. Philadelphia, Lippincott-Raven, 1998.*)

evaluated before cardiopulmonary bypass (CPB), Abraham et al demonstrated that both biplane and multiplane TEE predicted surgical obturator measurement, within 1 mm, 100% of the time and was superior to TTE.[48] Oh et al have recently demonstrated similar results with intraoperative TEE, accurately predicting size of the homograft in all patients.[49] Taken together, these data suggest that TEE is superior to TTE in predicting homograft size, and may be an excellent tool to optimize the efficiency of homograft placement by reducing ischemic and cross-clamp times. However, given the limited data, correlation with direct surgical measurement is still warranted, since accurate sizing of homografts is absolutely critical for good long-term function.

Operative Technique

GENERAL PREPARATION

A full median sternotomy is used with standard techniques of cardiopulmonary bypass (CPB). Aortic cannulation is obtained as far distally as possible, near the innominate artery, and a two-stage cannula is placed into the right atrial appendage. A ventricular vent is placed into the right superior pulmonary vein. Both antegrade and retrograde cardioplegia are delivered. The aortotomy incision is a reverse "lazy-S" that begins 4 to 5 cm above the coronary ostia (Fig. 34-2). The transverse aspect of the "lazy-S" lies just above the right coronary ostia and continues downwards along the right lateral aorta to the center of the noncoronary sinus. After retraction of the aorta, facilitated with silk stay sutures, the valve is excised. The aortic root and annulus are then closely examined for geometric morphology and symmetry, indicating feasibility of a good result with a homograft. Next, the aortic ring is sized with standardized obturators or Hagar dilators, taking care not to stretch the annulus or the leaflets. Since this represents an external diameter of the recipient, and allografts are sized based on internal diameters, an allograft 2 to 4 mm smaller than the recipient measurement is obtained. The appropriately sized allograft can then be thawed. If the allograft was selected based on accurate TTE or TEE measurements, it should already have been thawed. The allograft is then trimmed.

Because the allograft block contains a variable amount of ventricular muscle, mitral leaflet, and the arch, the goal of trimming is to remove excess tissue and shape the allograft appropriately for placement. To this end, the mitral leaflet is shaved and trimmed, and the ventricular septum is debulked. A straight lower margin, which will contain the lower suture line, is created 2 to 3 mm below the nadir of each aortic cusp. If the freehand scalloped techniques (i.e., scalloped or intact noncoronary sinus) are to be used, the sinuses are removed from the ascending aorta, leaving three pillars of aorta supporting each commissure of the cusps. For the intact noncoronary sinus technique, the noncoronary sinus is spared (Fig. 34-3).

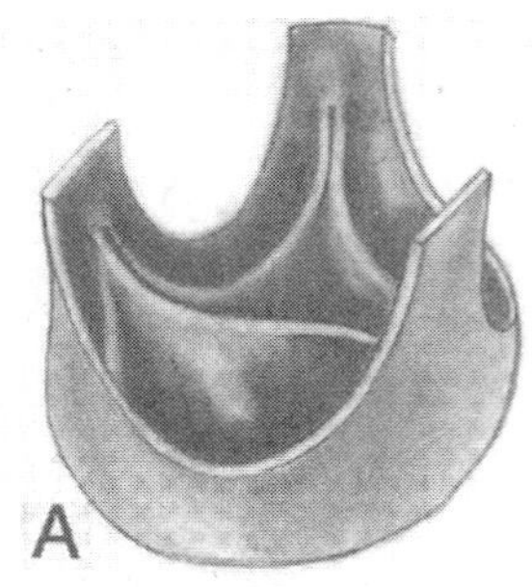

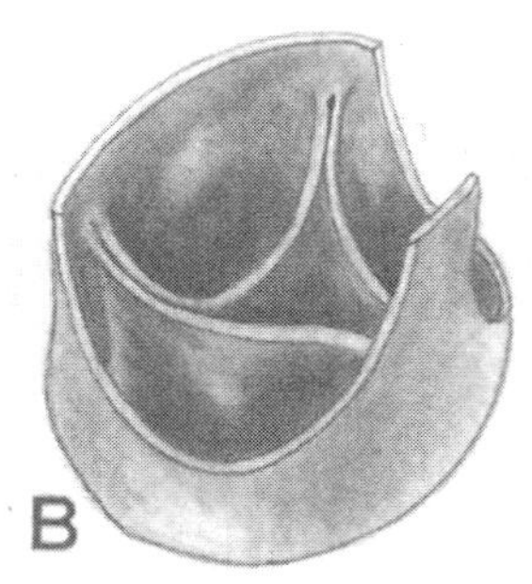

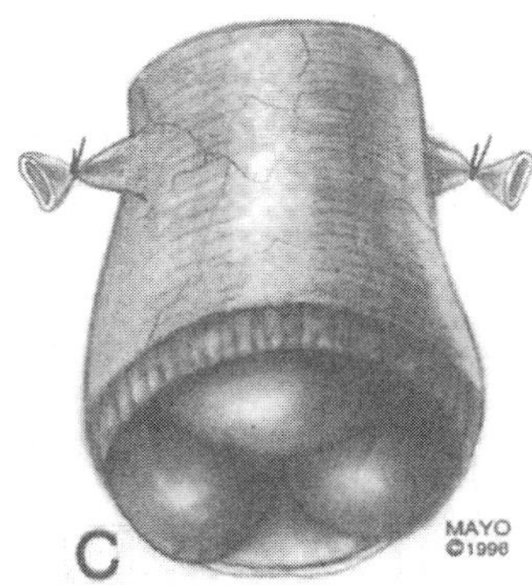

FIGURE 34–3 Preparation of an aortic homograft from the aortic block. The ventricular muscle and mitral leaflet are removed. (A) The "free-hand" subcoronary insertion technique involves removal of sinus aorta within 5 mm of the cusp attachments down to within 3 mm of the cusp bases, thus removing all three sinuses. (B) The intact noncoronary sinus technique involves preservation of the noncoronary sinus. (C) For aortic root replacement, the entire aortic wall can be retained, and then be implanted as an "inclusion cylinder" or "mini-root" insertion. (*Reproduced with permission from Schaff HV, Cable DG: Aortic valve replacement with homograft, in Kaiser LR, Kron IL, Spray TL (eds): Mastery of Cardiothoracic Surgery. Philadelphia, Lippincott-Raven, 1998.*)

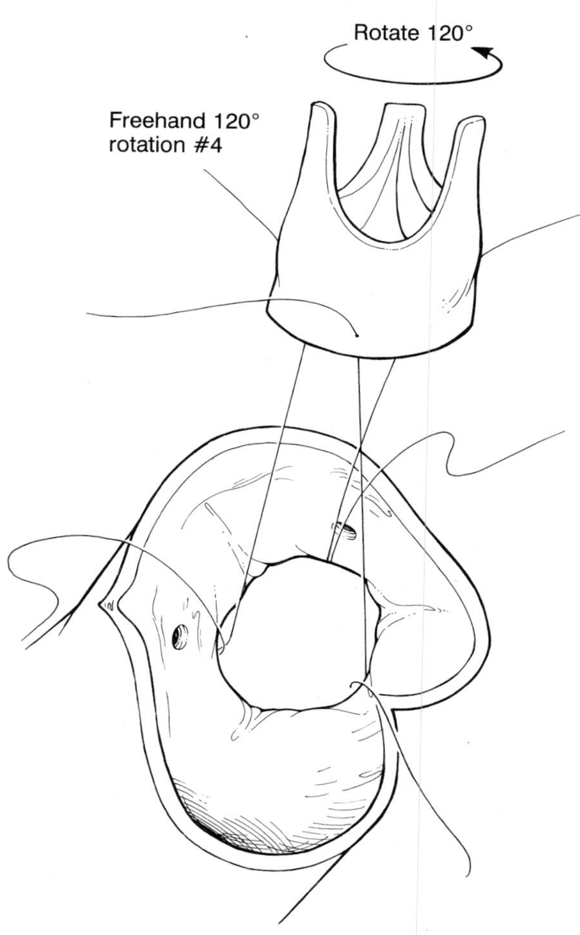

FIGURE 34–4 For the scalloped 120° rotation "freehand" technique, the allograft is rotated 120° counterclockwise so that the donor right sinus lies below the recipient left coronary sinus. Three orientation stay sutures are placed below the nadir of each cusp. (*Reproduced with permission from Albertucci M, Karp RB: Aortic valvular allografts and pulmonary autografts, in Edmunds LH (ed): Cardiac Surgery in the Adult. New York, McGraw-Hill, 1997.*)

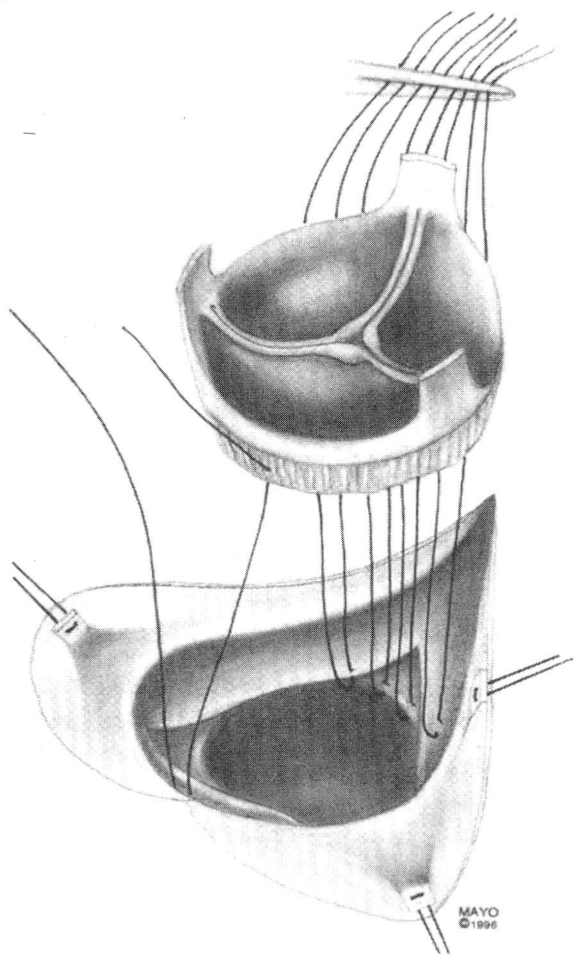

FIGURE 34–5 The inferior suture line with simple interrupted sutures. (*Reproduced with permission from Schaff HV, Cable DG: Aortic valve replacement with homograft, in Kaiser LR, Kron IL, Spray TL (eds): Mastery of Cardiothoracic Surgery. Philadelphia, Lippincott-Raven, 1998.*)

TECHNIQUES OF ALLOGRAFT PLACEMENT

There are multiple techniques for placing the allograft in the aortic position, and the strategies have continued to evolve over time. Ross[7] and Barrat-Boyes[50] originally described the 120° rotation scalloped freehand technique. Numerous groups later modified this technique, whereby the right and left coronary sinuses were scalloped, but the noncoronary sinus was left intact—the intact noncoronary sinus technique. Later, this technique was further altered to preserve all the sinuses on the donor and insert the allograft as a cylinder within the recipient aortic root, with reimplantation of the coronary ostia as needed. More recently, the allograft has been implanted as a mini-root interposition graft when the severely diseased aortic root must be excised. Thus, there are essentially four techniques for placing an aortic allograft: (1) 120° rotation scalloped implant; (2) intact noncoronary sinus scalloped technique; (3) aortic root inclusion cylinder technique, with reimplantation of the coronary ostia as needed; and (4) aortic "mini-root" replacement with interposition allograft.

Scalloped 120° rotation freehand technique For the scalloped 120° freehand rotation technique, the sinus aorta is trimmed within 5 mm of the cusp attachments down to within 3 mm of the cusp bases, effectively removing all three sinuses.[50] The valve is then rotated 120° in the counterclockwise direction, so that the donor right sinus lies below the recipient left coronory sinus (Fig. 34-4). This critical maneuver brings the weaker muscular portion of the allograft posteriorly adjacent to the fibrous trigone and anterior leaflet of the mitral valve.[50,51] Two suture lines are required for this technique. The lower suture line can either be a continuous, running suture or simple interrupted sutures can be used,

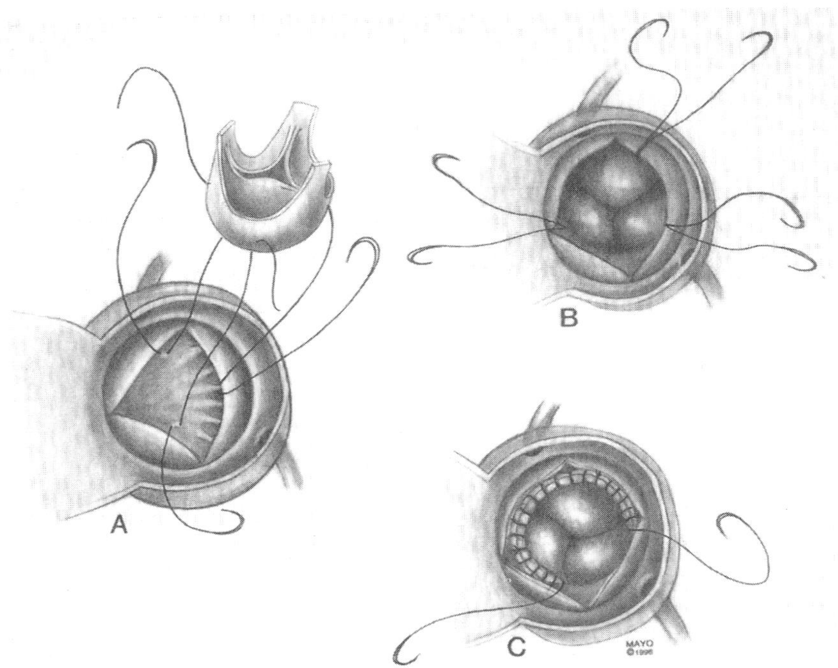

FIGURE 34–6 The inferior suture line with continuous suture. (A) The double-arm orientation stay sutures facilitate placement. (B) The allograft is inverted into the ventricle and the stay sutures are tied. (C) The stay sutures are then "run" in a clockwise manner to complete the lower suture line. *(Reproduced with permission from Schaff HV, Cable DG: Aortic valve replacement with homograft, in Kaiser LR, Kron IL, Spray TL (eds): Mastery of Cardiothoracic Surgery. Philadelphia, Lippincott-Raven, 1998.)*

usually of 4-0 or 5-0 polypropylene (Figs. 34-5, 34-6, and 34-7). For the running suture, the homograft can be turned inside out to facilitate the lower suture line. In the area of the membranous septum, sutures are placed more superficially to avoid the conduction system.

As Dearani,[51] McGiffin,[52] and others[53,54] have emphasized, proper alignment of the commissures in the aortic root is absolutely critical for proper coaptation of the aortic valve leaflets to ensure good long-term graft function. Accordingly, if the commissures are malaligned or kinked, the leaflets will

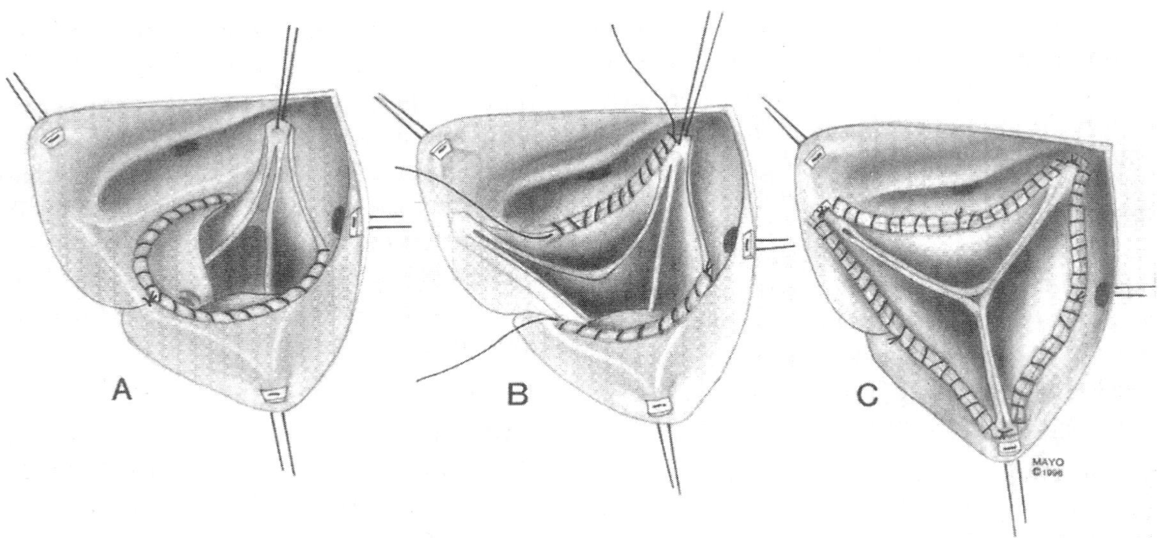

FIGURE 34–7 The downstream continuous suture line. (A) The allograft is everted after completion of the inferior suture line, by applying traction to the commissural posts. (B) A continuous suture completes the implantation. (C) Completed suture line. *(Reproduced with permission from Schaff HV, Cable DG: Aortic valve replacement with homograft, in Kaiser LR, Kron IL, Spray TL (eds): Mastery of Cardiothoracic Surgery. Philadelphia, Lippincott-Raven, 1998.)*

not coapt properly and a regurgitant valve ensues. Moreover, if there is only slight malalignment initially with a competent valve, the free cusp edges may be subjected to increased stresses over time, leading to premature structural deterioration and aortic regurgitation.[51] Similarly, size discrepancy between the donor allograft and the recipient sinotubular junction is likely to result in aortic insufficiency.[55] For these reasons, the scalloped 120° freehand rotation technique is considered more demanding than the other allograft placement techniques and may have poorer long-term results than the other methods of allograft placement.[44,51–54] Recognizing these technical and physiologic aspects of the scalloped subcoronary implant, it is a good technique for patients with small, symmetric aortic roots and sinotubular junctions, while it is a poor choice for those with dilated, asymmetric, or severely diseased roots or sinotubular junctions.

Freehand intact noncoronary sinus technique Scalloping of the coronary sinuses while preserving the noncoronary sinus is a technical extension of the scalloped 120° subcoronary implant technique (Fig. 34-8). This modification increases stability of the homograft and maintains symmetry more easily. Further, the risk for noncoronary cusp prolapse is attenuated in patients with a dilated or abnormal sinotubular junction.[56] Accordingly, it is a reasonable choice for patients with mildly dilated or asymmetric aortic roots and those with AI. For the intact noncoronary sinus technique, the allograft is prepared as above, except the noncoronary sinus is preserved. The allograft is then inserted into the aortic root, maintaining anatomic alignment without any rotation, and is sutured as described above. Additionally, mattress sutures are placed through the native aorta and the noncoronary sinus of the allograft to obliterate the space between the noncoronary sinus and the native aorta.

Aortic root replacement In patients who have dilated or geometrically distorted aortic roots, root replacement techniques are a good alternative. In many ways, these techniques

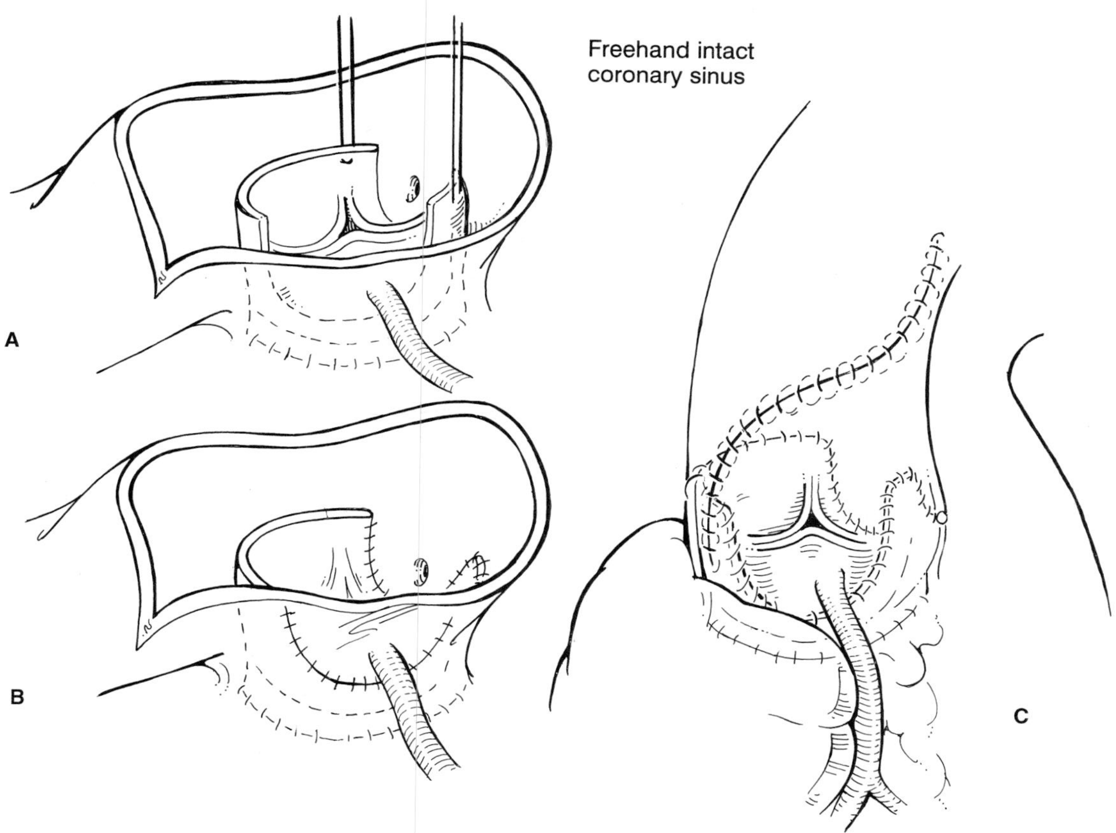

FIGURE 34–8 The intact noncoronary sinus technique. (A) This technique is nearly identical to the scalloped freehand technique, except the anatomic alignment of the donor allograft is maintained. (B) The noncoronary sinus is sutured to the corresponding aortic wall after partial closure of the aortotomy. This ensures minimal tension on this suture line. (C) The space behind the noncoronary sinus is obliterated with a U-stitch and the aortotomy is closed. (*Reproduced with permission from Albertucci M, Karp RB: Aortic valvular allografts and pulmonary autografts, in Edmunds LH (ed): Cardiac Surgery in the Adult. New York, McGraw-Hill, 1997.*)

are technically easier to perform than the freehand techniques described above. Further, a 2- to 3-mm disparity in donor-recipient root size is tolerated reasonably well, which increases the effective donor pool, and reduces the probability of not having an allograft available. Despite earlier concerns about increased perioperative morbidity with root replacement techniques, recent reports from experienced surgeons do not support this to be true.[51,57] Root replacement techniques have become the most commonly used techniques for placement of a homograft in the aortic position.

Aortic root replacement with inclusion cylinder technique Ross et al modified the aforementioned techniques to place the allograft as a sleeve or cylinder within the aortic root. The technique of implantation is very similar to that outlined above. For the inclusion cylinder technique, the sinuses are retained, and the cusp-sinus relationships are preserved (Fig. 34-9). Depending on the length of the cylinder, the recipient coronary ostia may need reimplantation into a buttonhole in the side of the allograft or directly into the donor coronary ostia. Conversely, if the distal aspect of the allograft is caudal to, or near the recipient coronary ostia, then minimal scalloping of the allograft wall will suffice to ensure coronary flow. The two suture lines are created with simple interrupted 4-0 polypropylene suture.

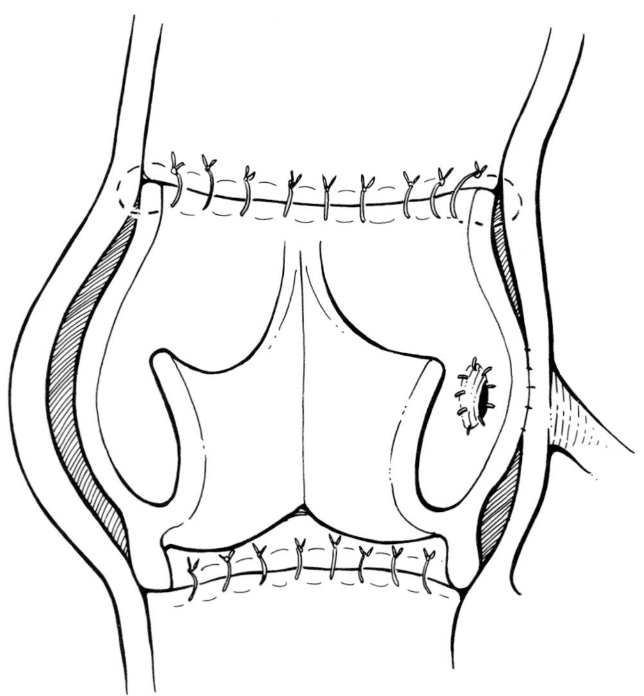

FIGURE 34–9 The inclusion cylinder technique for aortic root replacement. The cylinder retains the aortic allograft anatomic relationship. Depending on the length of the cylinder, the recipient coronary ostia may require reimplantation. *(Reproduced with permission from Albertucci M, Karp RB: Aortic valvular allografts and pulmonary autografts, in Edmunds LH (ed): Cardiac Surgery in the Adult. New York, McGraw-Hill, 1997.)*

Aortic root replacement with freestanding (interposition) root replacement The aforementioned techniques have been further modified to allow complete, or freestanding, replacement of the aortic root. To this end, the aortic root is completely excised and the homograft is interposed as a cylinder between the left ventricular outflow tract (LVOT) and the ascending aorta. Again, the two suture lines are created with simple interrupted 4-0 polypropylene suture, although some use a continuous suture for the distal anastomosis. The coronary arteries are then removed from the native aorta as buttons, and reimplanted into the side of the allograft using 5-0 polypropylene suture. In all the aforementioned techniques, the aortotomy is closed with a running 4-0 polypropylene suture.

Postreplacement Assessment

Intraoperative TEE with Doppler color flow measurement is the most valuable postreplacement assessment tool. Recognizing that the primary determinants of regurgitation are the valvular orifice area, the transvalvular pressure gradient, and the duration of diastole,[58] it is important to assess the aortic valve hemodynamics after the patient is weaned from cardiopulmonary bypass. The accuracy of the TEE assessment can be further enhanced with volume loading and administration of phenylephrine to effect vasoconstriction. Moreover, the transvalvular gradient, orifice area, subvalvular structures, and presence of regurgitation may all be accurately determined with TEE. With appropriate loading conditions, moderate to severe AI warrants reinstitution of CPB with inspection and revision of the allograft as needed. Mild AI is usually tolerated well and does not warrant reexploration.

Postoperative Management

Postoperative management following allograft placement is similar to that for other aortic valve replacements, and is dictated by the antecedent physiology that resulted from the aortic stenosis or regurgitation that required surgery. Aortic stenosis produces a hypertrophied, noncompliant ventricle that requires adequate preload and maintenance of sinus rhythm for adequate cardiac output. In contrast, aortic regurgitation results in a dilated left ventricle that may be coincidentally hypertrophied. Again, ensuring adequate preload and aggressively treating arrhythmias are imperative. Since patients with aortic regurgitation are chronically vasodilated to maintain systemic perfusion, vasoconstricting agents may be required after the patient is normothermic in the intensive care unit.

In both of these groups, systolic hypertension should be treated aggressively to protect the aortic suture line. Other than atrial arrhythmias, these patients are also susceptible to heart block, since the conduction system lies just near the right coronary cusp. When this occurs, epicardial pacing is employed as needed, and when persistent beyond a few days, a permanent pacer may be placed.

Long-term anticoagulation is not required and once-daily aspirin is sufficient.

Perioperative Complications

In patients without endocarditis at the time of allograft placement, operative mortality is 1% to 5%.[43,44,57] Notably, numerous experienced and talented groups have reported that the root replacement technique does not impact early mortality.[44,57] In contrast, patients with endocarditis at the time of allograft valve placement have a much higher early mortality, from 8% to 16%.[19,44,59–61] In these patients, early mortality was higher in patients with cardiogenic shock[61] or prosthetic valve endocarditis (18.8%), as compared to native valve endocarditis (10%).[59]

Early postoperative AI occurs infrequently and most often results from technical factors, like inaccurate sizing of the allograft, or valve distortion during placement, particularly with the scalloped subcoronary implant technique. This complication should be appreciated intraoperatively with loading maneuvers and intraoperative TEE, as previously mentioned.

Hemorrhage, heart block, stroke, myocardial infarction, and infectious complications occur with similar frequency to other aortic valve replacements, and are not unique to homografts.

Results

As mentioned, 30-day mortality following homograft placement is less than 5% in patients without endocarditis (Table 34-1). Crude survival at 10 and 20 years is reported to be 67% and 35%, respectively,[44] while in other studies actuarial survival at 10, 20 and 25 years is 81%,[43] 58%,[43] and 19%.[57]

The durability of allografts is limited. Structural valve failure (primary valve failure or deterioration) of allografts increases with time, and approximates 19% to 38% at 10 years and 69% to 82% at 20 years.[43,44] Structural deterioration over time may increase as recipient age decreases at time of allograft placement,[57] while Lund et al have found that recipient age older than 65 years and increasing donor age may increase structural failure.[44]

Hemodynamic characteristics of allografts are excellent at short- and-medium term follow-up, both at rest and during exercise.[62,63] However, progressive allograft dysfunction develops over time, coinciding with increasing structural failure. Freedom from repeat aortic valve replacement (AVR), for any reason, parallels structural valve failure and is 86.5% and 38.8% at 10 and 20 years, respectively.[43]

Infectibility of allografts is low, with freedom from endocarditis at 10 years of 93% to 98%[43,44] and at 20 years of 89% to 95%.[43,44,57] Similarly, freedom from thromboembolism at 15 and 20 years in patients undergoing AVR with coronary artery bypass grafting is 92% and 83%, respectively.[57] O'Brien et al found that neither preservation methods nor implantation techniques affected overall 20-year rates of thromboembolism, endocarditis, or structural valve deterioration.[57]

In patients with active endocarditis requiring aortic valve replacement, results are much poorer. Operative mortality is nearly twice that of patients without endocarditis, from 8% to 17%,[59–61] and higher in patients with prosthetic valve endocarditis.[60] Late survival ranges from 58% at 5 years[59] to 91% at 10 years,[61] and is significantly lower in patients with prosthetic valve endocarditis.[60] Importantly, the risk of recurrent endocarditis is less than 4% up to 4 years postoperatively.[51,60,61] As a result of these outcomes, the homograft is the preferred valve for aortic replacement in patients with active endocarditis.

Conclusions

Replacement of a diseased aortic valve with an allograft is not a perfect solution. However, there are many advantages,

TABLE 34–1 Long-term follow-up of homograft valves: summary of large experiences

Reference	Patients (no.)	Follow-up (y) Max	Follow-up (y) Mean	Overall survival 10 y	15 y	20 y	Freedom from: Structural valve failure 10 y	15 y	20y	Reoperation AVR 10 y	15 y	20 y	Thromboembolism 10 y	15 y	20 y
Lund et al[44]	618	27.1	10.1	67%	48%	35%	62%	34%	18%	81%	55%	35%	89%	85%	80%
Langley et al[43]	200		15.6	81%	68%	58%	81%	62%	32%	87%	70%	39%	Overall, 99% freedom		
O'Brien et al[57]	1022	29	7.3	77%	60%	42%				Overall, 87%			94%	92%	83%

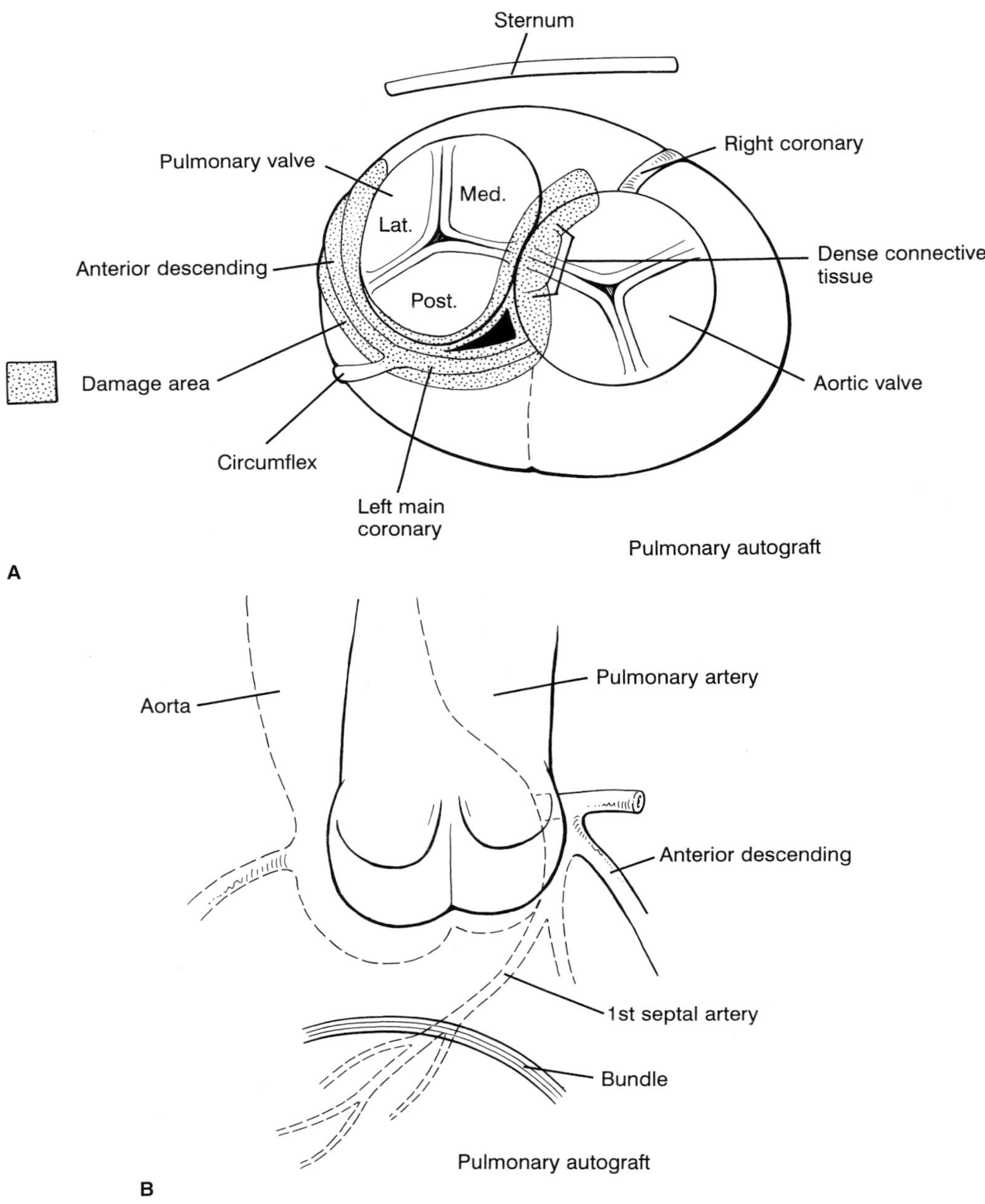

FIGURE 34–10 (A) The anatomic relationship of the pulmonary and aortic valves. The free space separating the pulmonary artery from the main coronary artery is bounded by the left sinus of Valsalva, the left main coronary artery, and the posterior sinus of the pulmonary root. (B) The position of the first septal artery and the conduction system (bundle). (*Reproduced with permission from Albertucci M, Karp RB: Aortic valvular allografts and pulmonary autografts, in Edmunds LH (ed): Cardiac Surgery in the Adult. New York, McGraw-Hill, 1997.*)

including low operative mortality rate, excellent early and mid-term hemodynamics across the allograft, and low infectibility. The primary shortcoming of aortic allografts is progressive deterioration of valve structure and function over time, which limits its use in younger patients with long life expectancy. This structural deterioration is likely a result of a donor-specific immune-mediated rejection reaction, which may be a potential target for targeted immunosuppressive agents to increase valve durability. Increased investigation in this area is needed. Lack of availability is also a limiting factor in the selection of allograft valves, in contrast to the alternatives. For patients with active endocarditis of either the native or prosthetic aortic valve, allograft replacement is the procedure of choice.

PULMONARY AUTOGRAFT

Theoretical Considerations

Replacement of a diseased aortic valve with a pulmonary autograft has a number of advantages including: (1) freedom from thromboembolism without the need for anticoagulation; (2) improved hemodynamics through the valve orifice without obstruction or turbulence; (3) growth of the autograft with time, particularly beneficial for young patients who will continue to grow after receiving the aortic autograft[64]; (4) and the assumption that replacement of the aortic valve with living autologous tissue is preferential to prosthetic or xenogeneic materials.

A theoretical concern of this repair is the ability of the pulmonic valve, usually subjected to relatively low pressures from the right ventricle, to withstand the increased stresses of the systemic circulation beyond the high-pressure left ventricle when placed in the aortic position (Fig. 34-10).

Patient Selection

In addition to individual surgeon experience, a number of patient factors influence consideration of the Ross procedure for replacement of a diseased aortic valve. Table 34-2 summarizes the important patient factors to bear in mind when considering the Ross procedure. The only absolute contraindications are significant pulmonary valve disease, congenitally abnormal pulmonary valves (e.g., bicuspid or quadricuspid), Marfan syndrome, unusual coronary artery anatomy, and probably severe coexisting autoimmune disease, particularly if it is the cause of the aortic valve disease. Of note, bacterial endocarditis is not a contraindication for the Ross procedure, though, when present, it usually dictates that the root replacement technique is used. Additional minor considerations often come into play including patient age, associated medical conditions, physiologic reserve, suitability for anticoagulation, and underlying ventricular function, because the time on cardiopulmonary bypass (CPB) is potentially long.

After 1988, there was a steady increase in the number of Ross procedures performed until the peak frequency in 1996, then a steady and small decline until 2000 (Fig. 34-11). The recent decline in the number of Ross procedures performed temporally coincides with the increased appreciation of abnormal flow dynamics across the components of

TABLE 34–2 Patient factors influencing Ross operation selection

Favorable	Unfavorable
Young	Age < 1 or > 70 years
Anticoagulation contraindicated	No contraindications to anticoagulation
Good LV function	Severe LV dysfunction
Aortic stenosis	Aortic insufficiency
Small-normal aorta and aortic annulus	Larger than normal or dilated aorta or annulus
No pulmonic valve pathology	Pulmonic valve pathology
>20 years life expectancy	Limited life expectancy
No other valvular disease	Other valvular disease present (e.g., mitral)
No systemic autoimmune disease present	Autoimmune disease

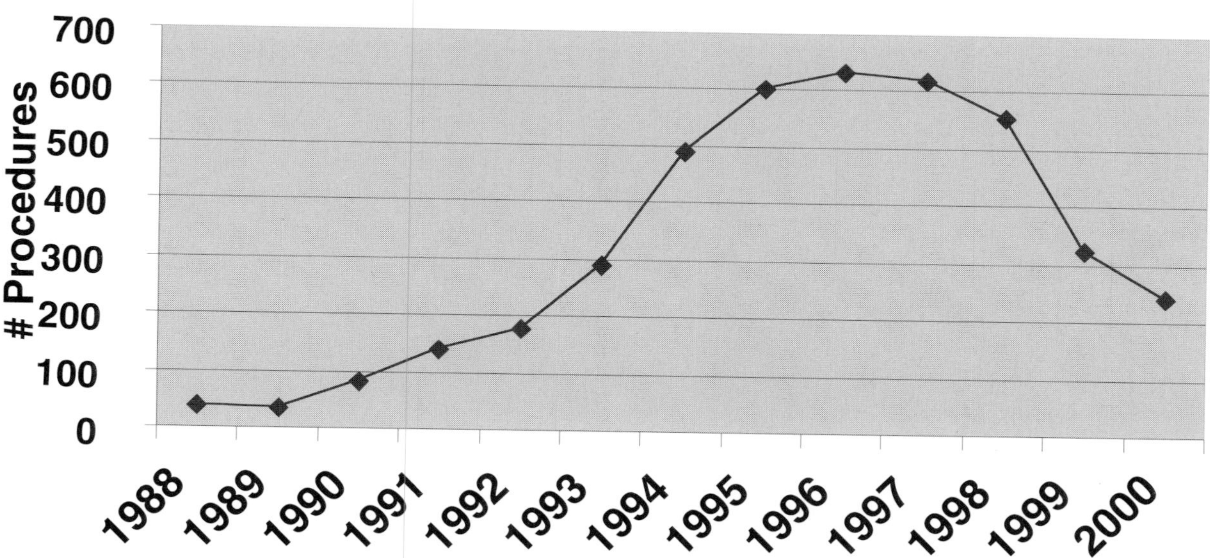

FIGURE 34–11 Ross procedures performed according to Ross Registry 1988–1999. (*Adapted from the Ross Procedure International Registry; http://www.rossregistry.com.*)

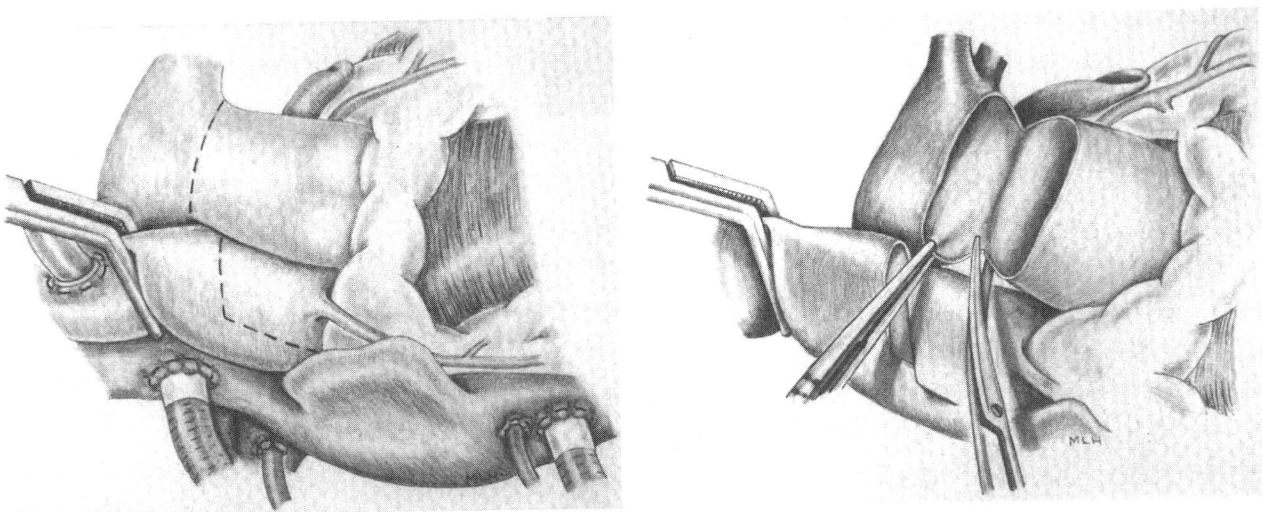

FIGURE 34–12 The distal pulmonary artery is incised at the origin of the right pulmonary artery. A transverse arteriotomy is made to allow careful inspection of the pulmonary artery. Shown from the surgeons' perspective, as though standing on the patients' right side. (*Reproduced with permission from Elkins RC, Aortic valve: Ross procedure, in Kaiser LR, Kron IL, Spray TL (eds): Mastery of Cardiothoracic Surgery. Philadelphia, Lippincott-Raven, 1998.*)

the Ross repair, particularly the right ventricle to pulmonary artery (RV-PA) conduit.

Techniques

Since the initial description by Ross of the scalloped subcoronary implant, a number of modifications have been described, including the inclusion cylinder technique and the root replacement technique. These techniques are performed identically to those outlined above for aortic homografts. According to the Ross Procedure International Registry, the root replacement technique is the most commonly performed variation owing to its superior versatility and possible decreased incidence of early and late graft failure.[65]

The conduct of the operation is similar to placement of aortic homograft. Full CPB is utilized with arterial cannulation of the distal aorta. Again, the ventricular vent is placed through the right superior pulmonary vein. Cardioplegia is delivered antegrade and retrograde, via the coronary sinus catheter. A reverse "lazy-S" aortotomy is performed similarly to placing an allograft. After retraction of the aorta, facilitated with stay sutures, the aortic valve and root are inspected and the suitability of the pulmonary autograft for repair is confirmed. The aortic valve is then excised, along

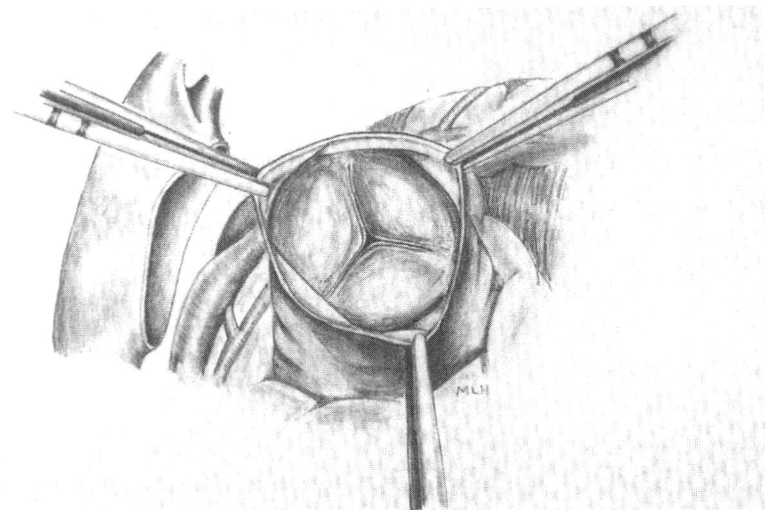

FIGURE 34–13 The normal trileaflet pulmonic valve with three equal sinuses and no fenestrations or other abnormalities. (*Reproduced with permission from Schaff HV, Cable DG: Aortic valve replacement with homograft, in Kaiser LR, Kron IL, Spray TL (eds): Mastery of Cardiothoracic Surgery. Philadelphia, Lippincott-Raven, 1998.*)

with the coronary ostia as buttons. When the root replacement technique is used, the aortic root is excised as previously described for the allograft. Attention is then turned to the pulmonary artery (PA) and pulmonic valve.

After institution of CPB, the PA is mobilized to its bifurcation. The PA is then sharply divided transversely just proximal to the origin of the right and left pulmonary arteries (Fig. 34-12). This allows visual inspection of the pulmonic valve endoluminally, which is normally tricuspid, without fenestrations or atheroma (Fig. 34-13). The discovery of a bicuspid or quadricuspid valve, or the presence of large fenestrations or atheroma precludes use of the valve as an autograft. The mobilization of the pulmonary artery then begins distally, near the transverse arteriotomy, and continues proximally towards the valve. The dissection is initiated posteriorly, staying very close to the pulmonary artery, and taking care not to buttonhole the wall (Fig. 34-14). The left main coronary artery and its bifurcation into the left anterior descending (LAD) artery, with its septal perforators, and the circumflex arteries should be identified and avoided. When these are not easily appreciated, a probe may be placed into the left coronary os, through the aortotomy, to facilitate identification of the left main coronary artery and its branches. The dissection continues proximally until septal musculature is reached, taking care to avoid injury to the conal branch of the right coronary artery. A point 3 to 4 mm below the pulmonic annulus is identified, often facilitated by passing a probe through the pulmonic valve, and the right ventricular outflow tract (RVOT) is divided (Fig. 34-15). Where the RVOT meets the septum, the dissection must be kept superficial (i.e., on the right ventricular side) to avoid injury to the septal perforators of the LAD. The adventitia of the autograft is preserved. After complete division, the autograft is then accurately sized at its base, as well as the RVOT, and an appropriately sized allograft is obtained.

ROOT REPLACEMENT TECHNIQUE

The steps in this technique are illustrated in Figure 34-16. The autograft is oriented so that the posterior pulmonary sinus becomes the noncoronary sinus. The proximal suture line is performed first. In adults, this is performed with a running 4-0 or 5-0 polypropylene, while an absorbable monofilament suture (e.g., Maxon, Davis + Geck, Manati, PR) is used in children and adolescents, recognizing future growth of the autograft with the patient.[64] The left coronary artery is then implanted at the midpoint of the left coronary sinus, as previously described. Again, 5-0 polypropylene is used in adults and 6-0 Maxon is used in children. The distal suture line is then performed, after the autograft is trimmed 4 to 5 mm beyond the sinotubular junction of the autograft. A running 4-0 or 5-0 polypropylene suture is used in adults, while Maxon is used in children. The importance of similarly sized aortic and pulmonary valves has recently been suggested.[66] If a size or geometric mismatch between valves occurs, the diameter of the aortic annulus and/or sinotubular junction may be surgically reduced, with a reduction aortoplasty, as described and performed by Elkins.[67] Also, if the ascending aorta is aneurysmal, it may be replaced with an interposition Dacron graft bridging between the distal autograft

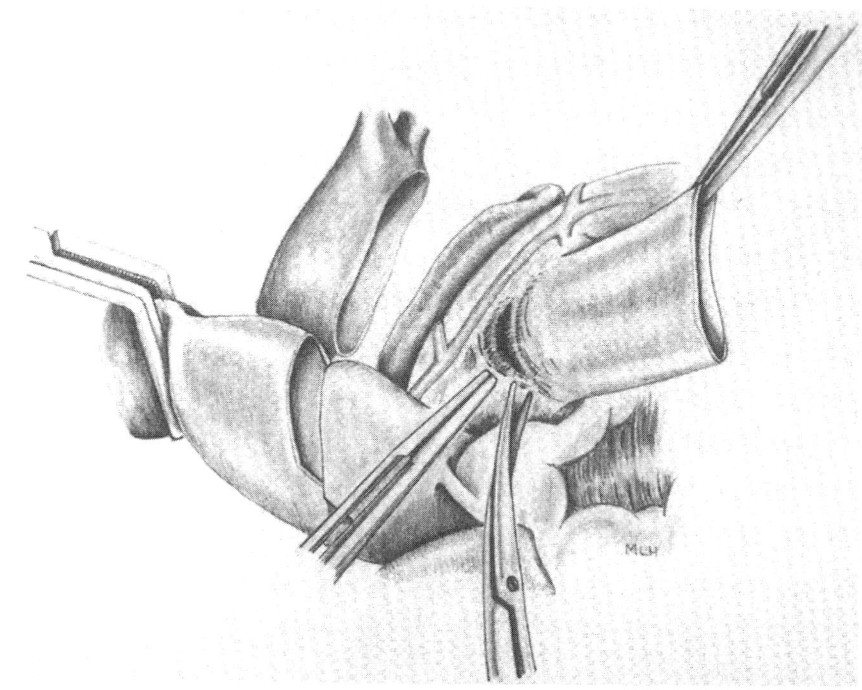

FIGURE 34–14 Dissection of the pulmonary autograft is initiated on the posterior aspect of the proximal pulmonary artery. Dissection is continued in this plane, adjacent to the pulmonary artery, until the septal myocardium is encountered. The left main coronary artery and left anterior descending artery are protected. ***(Reproduced with permission from Schaff HV, Cable DG: Aortic valve replacement with homograft, in Kaiser LR, Kron IL, Spray TL (eds): Mastery of Cardiothoracic Surgery. Philadelphia, Lippincott-Raven, 1998.)***

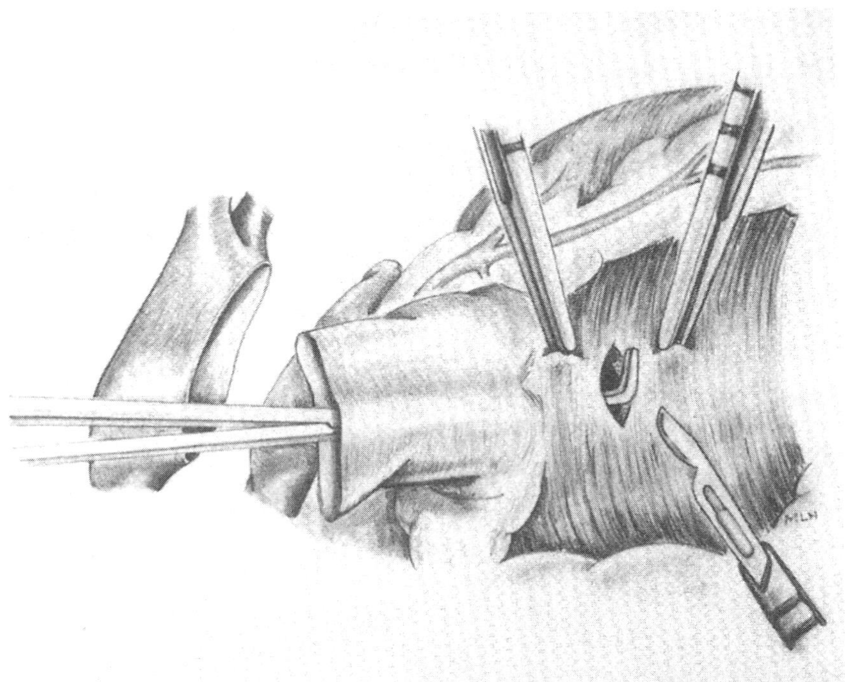

FIGURE 34–15 Identification of the anterior right ventriculotomy is facilitated by placement of a right-angled clamp through the pulmonary valve and indenting the myocardium 3 mm to 4 mm below the pulmonary valve annulus. (*Reproduced with permission from Schaff HV, Cable DG: Aortic valve replacement with homograft, in Kaiser LR, Kron IL, Spray TL (eds): Mastery of Cardiothoracic Surgery. Philadelphia, Lippincott-Raven, 1998.*)

and the ascending aorta just proximal to the innominate artery. This is followed by reimplantation of the right coronary artery, similar to that described for the left coronary artery. After the suture lines are inspected, the cross-clamp is removed and the operation is completed during rewarming.

A pulmonary homograft, oversized by 4 to 6 mm, is then obtained. The homograft is trimmed, and the proximal anastomosis is performed to the RVOT with running 4-0 polypropylene. Again, the left coronary artery and its branches lie close to the posterior aspect of the anastomosis, and sutures must be precisely placed in the endocardium to avoid kinking or injuring these structures. The distal suture line is then completed with a running 4-0 or 5-0 polypropylene suture. De-airing and weaning from CPB are performed in a standard fashion.

INCLUSION CYLINDER TECHNIQUE

The inclusion cylinder technique is nearly identical to that previously described for the allograft (Figs. 34-17 and 34-18).

Results

Ross initially reported his results in 1991, setting the standard for outcomes after the Ross procedure.[68] He reported follow-up in 339 patients up to 24 years with an 80% survival and an 85% freedom from reoperation. More recently, a longer follow-up report from this initial series included 131 patients (long-term survivors) with a mean follow-up of 20 years (range 9-26 years).[69] In this report, freedom from reoperation was 76% and 62% at 10 and 20 years, respectively. Freedom from autograft replacement was 88% and 75% at 10 and 20 years, respectively. The main indication prompting autograft replacement was severe regurgitation, which occurred in 28 of 30 patients. At 25 years, the pulmonary homograft was free of replacement in 69% of patients. Indeed, these outcome results have set the benchmark for aortic valve repairs using autologous pulmonic valve. It is worth noting that most of the patients in Ross's series were repaired by the scalloped subcoronary implant technique, whereas the root replacement technique is the most commonly performed technique today.

Current data from the Ross Registry resemble Ross's initial results with an 68% survival, 84% freedom from right ventricular outflow tract (RVOT) repair/replacement, and an 82% freedom from autograft explant over 25 years.

Operative Risk

With increasing experience and improved perioperative care, operative risk has declined since Ross first described this procedure. According to the International Ross Registry, overall perioperative mortality (i.e., <30 days) is now 4.1% (129 deaths in 3922 patients). Although 4.1% perioperative mortality is acceptable for some cardiac operations, many believe it is unacceptably high for the younger patients that are most often subjected to the Ross procedure. This controversial point highlights the need for individualized therapy with respect to valve replacement through consideration of all the risks and benefits associated with the available options. We do not believe that the risks of the

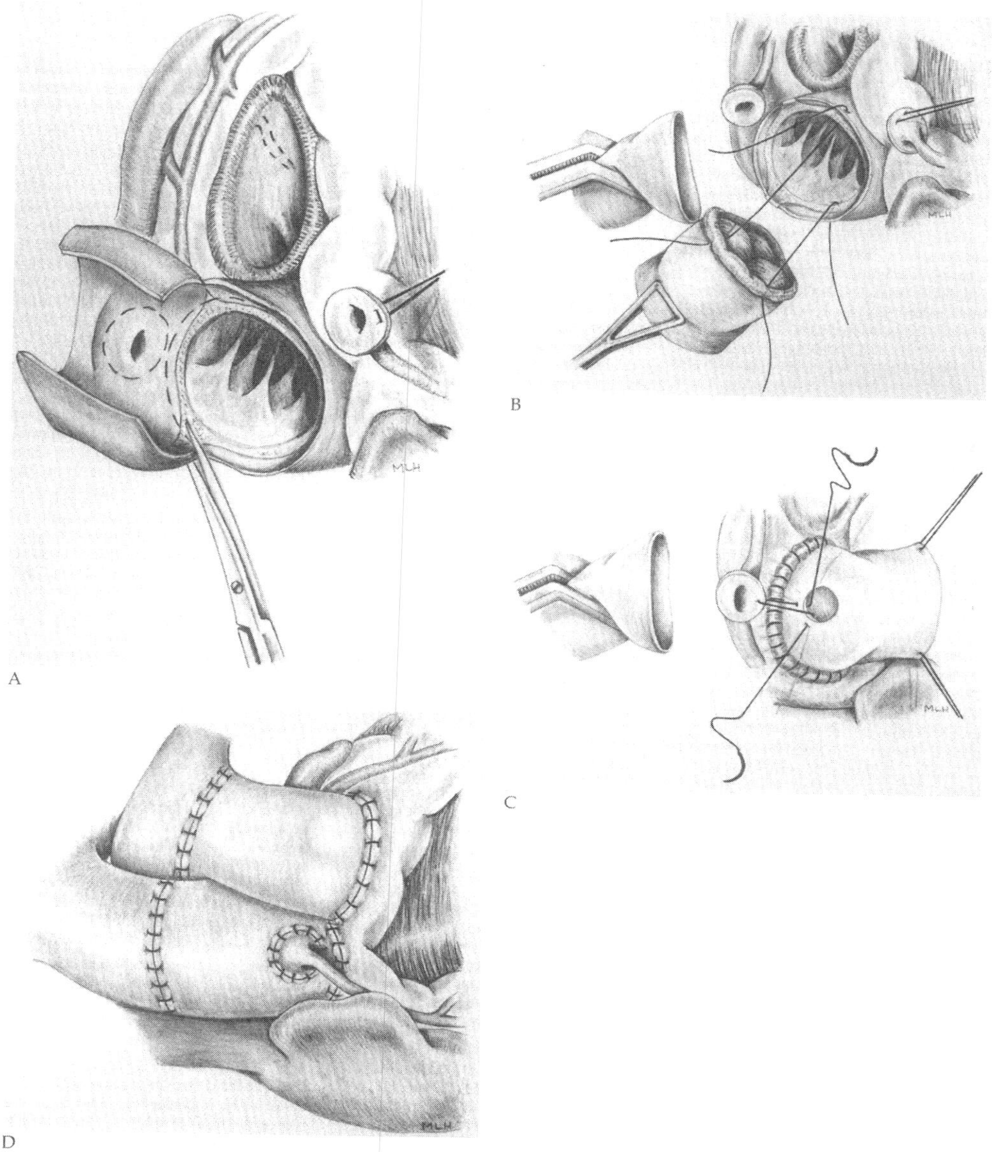

FIGURE 34–16 Root replacement technique. (A) Generous cuffs of aorta are left attached to the right and left coronary ostia. Minimal mobilization of these arteries is performed. The remaining proximal aorta is excised, transecting the aorta below the aortic annulus in the interleaflet triangle. (B) The pulmonary autograft is in an anatomic position with the posterior sinus of the autograft becoming the new left coronary sinus (stay sutures omitted from drawing). The remaining sutures for orientation are placed to position the new right coronary sinus and to trifurcate the aortic annulus. (C) Completion of the pulmonary autograft root implantation with selection of the site of implantation of the right coronary artery with the autograft distended. (D) The pulmonary homograft reconstruction of the right ventricle outflow tract is done with two continuous suture lines. *(Reproduced with permission from Schaff HV, Cable DG: Aortic valve replacement with homograft, in Kaiser LR, Kron IL, Spray TL (eds): Mastery of Cardiothoracic Surgery. Philadelphia, Lippincott-Raven, 1998.)*

Ross procedure are prohibitive in appropriately selected patients. Further, as more experience is gained with this procedure, a volume-outcome relationship may be apparent, supporting regional specialization and referrals to "centers of excellence."

Pulmonary Autograft Dysfunction

Early autograft dysfunction occurs infrequently. Elkins reported early autograft dysfunction (<6 months) in 3 of 195 patients (1.5%).[64]

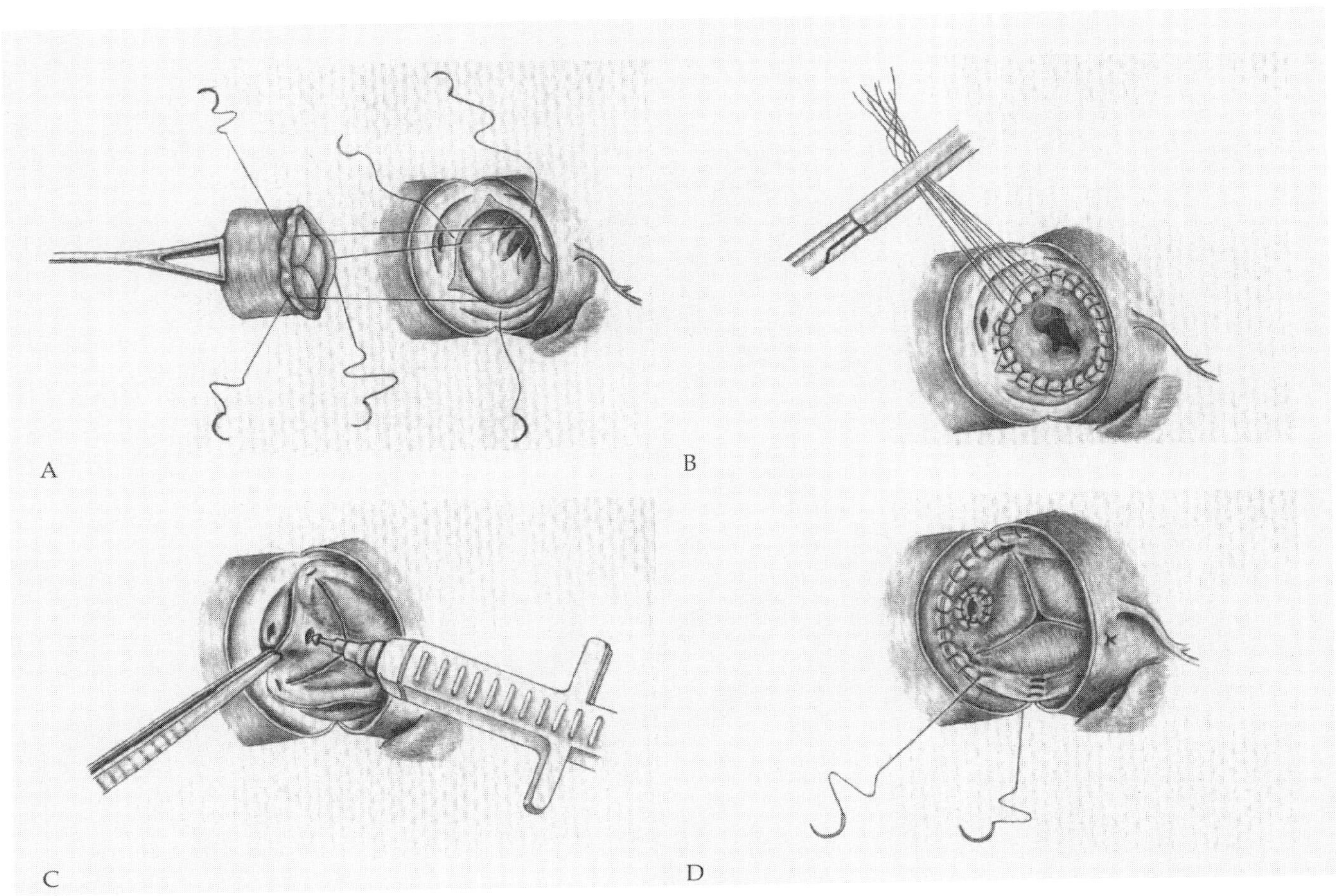

FIGURE 34–17 Inclusion cylinder technique. (A) Placement of three polypropylene sutures to orient the pulmonary autograft. The posterior sinus of the pulmonary autograft becomes the new left coronary sinus. (B) The autograft is inverted into the left ventricle and the proximal sutures are tied and divided. (C) The pulmonary autograft is reinverted. Horizontal mattress sutures are placed to secure the height and position of the autograft (but not tied until the right and left coronary arteries are implanted). An aortic punch (4 mm or 5 mm) is used to create an opening in the autograft to allow attachment of the coronary artery ostia. (D) Completion of coronary artery anastomosis. Commissural stay sutures are tied and divided, and the distal suture line is initiated at the commissure between the left and right coronary artery. This is continued to the aortotomy extension into the noncoronary sinus. This portion of the aortotomy is closed with a running suture line with the suture including a full-thickness "bite" of the noncoronary sinus of the pulmonary autograft. (*Reproduced with permission from Schaff HV, Cable DG: Aortic valve replacement with homograft, in Kaiser LR, Kron IL, Spray TL (eds): Mastery of Cardiothoracic Surgery. Philadelphia, Lippincott-Raven, 1998.*)

Late autograft dysfunction is an increasingly recognized phenomenon following the Ross procedure, although few studies have followed patients longitudinally with routine evaluations. A recent report of midterm follow-up (mean 2.47 years) in 132 consecutive patients who underwent routine echocardiographic evaluations of the pulmonary autograft revealed mild aortic insufficiency (graded 1 out of 4) in 39.2% to 53.6% of patients, depending on follow-up interval.[70] Three percent of patients had moderate insufficiency early after surgery, increasing to 14.3% at 5 years. The mean transvalvular gradient across the aortic valve was minimal (3 mm Hg) early and remained stable during follow-up.

In Elkins' series of 289 patients, 6% (16) of the patients required autograft reoperation.[65] In the patients who received root replacement implants, 97% had no change in autograft function during follow-up, while only 1% had severe insufficiency (3+). In contrast, of those who received scalloped subcoronary or inclusion cylinder implants, 86% had no change in autograft function, while 8% had progressed to severe insufficiency (3+).

David et al have provided additional insight into late autograft dysfunction following the Ross procedure, by assessing dilatation of the pulmonary autograft.[71] From 1990 to 1997, 118 patients with a mean age of 34 years (range 17-57)

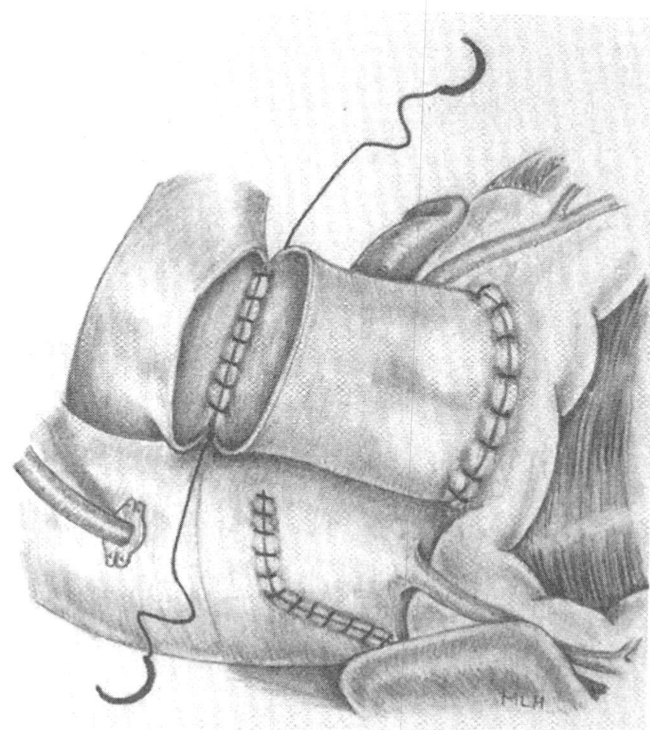

FIGURE 34–18 Completion of the closure of the aortotomy for the inclusion cylinder technique. The aortic cross-clamp is removed. The pulmonary homograft reconstruction of the outflow tract is accomplished with two continuous sutures of polypropylene. The proximal suture line is completed first. *(Reproduced with permission from Schaff HV, Cable DG: Aortic valve replacement with homograft, in Kaiser LR, Kron IL, Spray TL (eds): Mastery of Cardiothoracic Surgery. Philadelphia, Lippincott-Raven, 1998.)*

underwent the Ross procedure. Of note, if there was a 2-mm or greater size mismatch between the aortic and pulmonic sinotubular junction or annuli, they were surgically reduced prior to implantation. The root replacement technique was most commonly used (71/118, 60%), followed by the root inclusion technique (45/118, 38%); the subcoronary implant was the least common technique (2/118, 1.7%). Follow-up was 12 to 96 months (mean 44 months) including annual echocardiography. Over the observation period the diameter of the sinuses of Valsalva significantly increased from 31.4 mm to 33.7 mm. Further, with respect to operative techniques, aortic root replacement was significantly positively correlated with increased risk of dilatation. No interpretable changes were seen in the aortic annulus over time. However, the diameter of the sinotubular junction increased in patients who had aortic root replacement and decreased in those subjected to root inclusion technique. During the observation period, only 5.9% (7/118) of patients developed moderate AI. However, all the patients with AI had dilatation of the aortic annulus and/or the sinotubular junction.

Taken together, these data indicate that the autologous pulmonic valve in the aortic position is quite durable and able to withstand the increased stresses at this position. Further, although valve effective orifice area (EOA) does not seem to change, up to 50% of patients may develop mild AI, which seems to increase with time, likely resulting from dilatation of the pulmonary autograft sinotubular junction and/or sinuses of Valsalva. Although it is suggested that this may be affected by surgical technique, it is unclear whether the use of the root replacement technique or root inclusion technique impacts the development of late pulmonary autograft dysfunction. Additional investigation is needed to elucidate risk factors for this complication and surgical interventions that may attenuate the frequency of this complication (e.g., reduction aortoplasty or Dacron banding of aortic annulus and sinotubular junction).

Homograft Dysfunction

Although the cryopreserved homograft has many advantages for an RV-PA conduit, it has become increasingly clear that it is susceptible to stenosis, degeneration, and calcification. Since current cryopreservation techniques result in varying degrees of donor cell viability, these effects may be immunologically mediated, although this remains controversial.[72] Again, the precise incidence of this phenomenon is likely underappreciated due to lack of routine echocardiographic screening.

Midterm echocardiographic follow-up results of 132 patients (mean follow-up 2.47 years) after the Ross procedure demonstrated early minimal transvalvular gradients (+3± 4 mm Hg) with significant worsening (+6± 8 mm Hg) over time.[70] Further, there was decreasing valve EOA (−0.74± 0.82 cm^2), mostly within the first 6 months. This resulted in 19.3% of patients having an EOA index of less than 0.85 cm^2/m^2 at 1-year follow-up. Put another way, after 2 years the pulmonary valve EOAs were, on average, 31% less than they were immediately following surgery. Through multivariate analysis, only small homograft size and hypertension were found to be significant negative predictors of EOA at 1-year follow-up.

Raanani et al followed 109 consecutive patients after the Ross procedure to identify the incidence and risk factors for homograft stenosis.[73] Echocardiographic follow-up (mean 39 ± 20 months) was available in 105 (97%) patients. The primary abnormality identified was homograft stenosis. In support, they identified a peak systolic transvalvular gradient of more than 20 mm Hg in 28.5% (30/105) of patients and more than 40 mm Hg peak gradient in 3.8% (4/105) of patients. This obstruction occurred at all levels of the homograft, as opposed to just at anastomotic sites, and was associated with homograft thickening. Moderate or severe homograft insufficiency was identified in 9.5% (10/105) of patients. Through multivariate analysis, the only independent significant predictors of homograft stenosis that approached statistical significance were cryopreservation duration of less than 20 months, donor age younger than 30 years, and small homograft size.

Taken together, these data indicate that pulmonary homograft stenosis may develop in up to 30% of patients following the Ross operation. More importantly, the clinical significance of these data is not clear. For example, in the context of congenital pulmonary stenosis, it appears that peak transvalvular gradients of less than 50 mm Hg are usually well tolerated.[74] However, it would be erroneous to extrapolate these data to the demographic of the Ross procedure, as many of these patients are into adulthood when they undergo this procedure. Further, similar to the pulmonic autograft in the aortic position, the incidence and severity of pulmonic insufficiency appears to increase with time. Clearly, these data suggest that future endeavors to improve the Ross procedure should be directed to elucidating the mechanisms underlying the pulmonary homograft stenosis and towards therapy to minimize these untoward effects.

Summary

The search for the ideal valve to replace the diseased aortic valve is ongoing and available techniques are imperfect. Nonetheless, the Ross operation, in which the pulmonic valve is transposed to the aortic position and the RVOT is replaced with cryopreserved homograft (most commonly), has proven to be a durable solution for complex congenital abnormalities and disease isolated to the aortic valve, particularly in children and young adults.

Observations of the long-term durability of the pulmonic autograft in the aortic position affirm its ability to withstand the increased physical stresses at this location and maintain near normal hemodynamics over time, making it an excellent choice for replacement of a diseased aortic valve. The incidence of AI is low and increases with time, likely resulting from dilatation of the pulmonary autograft sinotubular junction and/or the sinuses of Valsalva. Further studies are needed to discern the risk factors for this occurrence, but utilizing the root replacement technique compared to the root inclusion technique may affect it.

The homograft in the pulmonic position is more susceptible to complications, namely stenosis, which occurs primarily within the first year. Up to 30% of patients may have a hemodynamically significant stenosis at this location that is likely to be immunologically mediated, though the clinical significance of these findings remains unclear. Small homograft size is consistently a risk factor for stenosis, thereby supporting the current practice of oversizing the homograft by 2 to 3 mm. Future attempts to improve outcome after the Ross procedure should be directed towards reducing homograft stenosis.

The Ross procedure remains an excellent option for replacement of the diseased aortic valve, particularly in children and young adults. As longer follow-up continues to accumulate, the risks and benefits of this procedure relative to other treatment options for replacement of a diseased aortic valve will be better characterized.

REFERENCES

1. Murray G, Roschlau W, Lougheed W: Homologous aortic-valve-segment transplants as surgical treatment for aortic and mitral insufficiency. *Angiology* 1956; 7:466.
2. Murray G: Aortic valve transplants. *Angiology* 1960; 11:99.
3. Beall ACJ, Morris GJ, Cooley D, DeBakey M: Homotransplantation of the aortic valve. *J Thorac Cardiovasc Surg* 1961; 42:497.
4. Kerwin AJ, Lenkei SC, Wilson DR: Aortic-valve homograft in the treatment of aortic insufficiency. *N Engl J Med* 1962; 266:852.
5. Bigelow WG, Kuypers PG, Heimbecker RO, Gunton RW: Clinical assessment of the efficiency and durability of direct vision annuloplasty. *Ann Surg* 1961; 154:320.
6. Shumacker HBJ: *The Evolution of Cardiac Surgery*. Bloomington, IN, Indiana University Press, 1992.
7. Ross DN: Homograft replacement of the aortic valve. *Lancet* 1962; 2:487.
8. Barratt-Boyes BG: Homograft aortic valve replacement in aortic incompetence and stenosis. *Thorax* 1964; 19:131.
9. Kirklin JW, Barratt-Boyes BG (eds): *Cardiac Surgery*, 2d ed. New York, Churchill Livingstone, 1993.
10. LoGrippo GA, Rupe CE: Procedure for sterilization of arterial homografts with beta-propiolactone. *Lab Invest* 1955; 4:217.
11. Davies H, Lessof MH, Roberts CI, Ross DN: Homograft replacement of the aortic valve. *Lancet* 1965 (1 May); 926.
12. Pacifico AD, Karp RB, Kirklin JW: Homografts for replacement of the aortic valve. *Circulation* 1972; 45/46:I-36.
13. Sands MP, Nelson RJ, Mohri H, Merendino KA: The procurement and preparation of aortic valve homografts. *Surgery* 1967; 62:839.
14. Barratt-Boyes BG: Long-term follow-up of aortic valvar grafts. *Br Heart J* 1971; 33:60.
15. O'Brien MF, Stafford EG, Gardner MA, et al: A comparison of aortic valve replacement with viable cryopreserved and fresh allograft valves, with a note on chromosomal studies. *J Thorac Cardiovasc Surg* 1987; 94:812.
16. Lower RR Sr, Shumway NE: Total excision of the mitral valve and replacement with the autologous pulmonic valve. *J Thorac Cardiovasc Surg* 1961; 42:696.
17. Pillsbury RC, Shumway NE: Replacement of the aortic valve with the autologous pulmonic valve. *Surg Forum* 1966; 17:176.
18. Ross DN: Replacement of aortic and mitral valves with a pulmonary autograft. *Lancet* 1967; 2:956.
19. Yacoub MH, Rasmi NRH, Sundt TM, et al: Fourteen-year experience with homovital homografts for aortic valve replacement. *J Thorac Cardiovasc Surg* 1995; 110:186.
20. Personal communication to the authors from DM Johnson. Procuring, processing, packaging, cryopreserving, storing, and distributing cardiovascular tissue: a summary of the Northwest Tissue Center Procedures. March 27, 2002.
21. Edmunds LH Jr (ed): *Cardiac Surgery in the Adult*. New York, McGraw-Hill, 1997.
22. Strickett MG, Barratt-Boyes BG, MacCulloch D: Disinfection of human heart valve allografts with antibiotics in low concentration. *Pathology* 1983; 15:457.
23. Gall KL, Smith SE, Willmette CA, O'Brien MF: Allograft heart valve viability and valve-processing variables. *Ann Thorac Surg* 1998; 65:1032.

24. Mitchell RN, Jonas RA, Schoen FJ: Structure-function correlations in cryopreserved allograft cardiac valves. *Ann Thorac Surg* 1995; 60:S108.
25. Smith JC: The pathology of human aortic valve homografts. *Thorax* 1967; 22:114.
26. Armiger LC: Viability studies of human valves prepared for use as allografts. *Ann Thorac Surg* 1995; 60:S118.
27. O'Brien MF, Stafford G, Gardner M, et al: The viable cryopreserved allograft aortic valve. *J Card Surg* 1987; 2:153.
28. Koolbergen DR, Hazekamp MG, Kurvers M, et al: Tissue chimerism in human cryopreserved homograft valve explants demonstrated by in situ hybridization. *Ann Thorac Surg* 1998; 66:S225.
29. Mitchell RN, Jonas RA, Schoen FJ: Pathology of explanted cryopreserved allograft heart valves: comparison with aortic valves from orthotopic heart transplants. *J Thorac Cardiovasc Surg* 1998; 115:118.
30. O'Brien MF, Johnston N, Stafford G, et al: A study of the cells in the explanted viable cryopreserved allograft valve. *J Card Surg* 1988; 3:279.
31. Armiger LC: Postimplantation leaflet cellularity of valve allografts: are donor cells beneficial or detrimental? *Ann Thorac Surg* 1998; 66:S233.
32. Hoekstra F, Witvliet M, Knoop C, et al: Donor-specific anti-human leukocyte antigen class I antibodies after implantation of cardiac valve allografts. *J Heart Lung Transplant* 1997; 16:570.
33. Shaddy RE, Hunter DD, Osborn KA, et al: Prospective analysis of HLA immunogenicity of cryopreserved valved allografts used in pediatric heart surgery. *Circulation* 1996; 94:1063.
34. Smith JD, Hornick PI, Rasmi N, et al: Effect of HLA mismatching and antibody status on "homovital" aortic valve homograft performance. *Ann Thorac Surg* 1998; 66:S212.
35. Smith JD, Ogino H, Hunt D, et al: Humoral immune response to human aortic valve homografts. *Ann Thorac Surg* 1995; 60:S127.
36. Dignan R, O'Brien M, Hogan P, et al: Influence of HLA matching and associated factors on aortic valve homograft function. *J Heart Valve Dis* 2000; 9:504.
37. Green MK, Walsh MD, Dare A, et al: Histologic and immunohistochemical responses after aortic valve allografts in the rat. *Ann Thorac Surg* 1998; 66:S216.
38. Legare JF, Lee TD, Creaser K, Ross DB: T lymphocytes mediate leaflet destruction and allograft aortic valve failure in rats. *Ann Thorac Surg* 2000; 70:1238.
39. Legare JF, Lee TD, Ross DB: Cryopreservation of rat aortic valves results in increased structural failure. *Circulation* 2000; 102:III75.
40. Oei FB, Stegmann AP, Vaessen LM, et al: Immunological aspects of fresh and cryopreserved aortic valve transplantation in rats. *Ann Thorac Surg* 2001; 71:S379.
41. Legare JF, Ross DB, Issekutz TB, et al: Prevention of allograft heart valve failure in a rat model. *J Thorac Cardiovasc Surg* 2001; 122:310.
42. Maselli D, Pizio R, Bruno LP, et al: Left ventricular mass reduction after aortic valve replacement: homografts, stentless and stented valves. *Ann Thorac Surg* 1999; 67:966.
43. Langley SM, McGuirk SP, Chaudhry MA, et al: Twenty-year follow-up of aortic valve replacement with antibiotic sterilized homografts in 200 patients. *Semin Thorac Cardiovasc Surg* 1999; 11:28.
44. Lund O, Chandrasekaran V, Grocott-Mason R, et al: Primary aortic valve replacement with allografts over twenty-five years: valve-related and procedure related determinants of outcome. *J Thorac Cardiovasc Surg* 1999; 117:77.
45. Greaves SC, Reimold SC, Lee RT, et al: Preoperative prediction of prosthetic aortic valve annulus diameter by two-dimensional echocardiography. *J Heart Valve Dis* 1995; 4:14.
46. Moscucci M, Weinert L, Karp RB, Neumann A: Prediction of aortic annulus diameter by two-dimensional echocardiography: application in the preoperative selection and preparation of homograft aortic valves. *Circulation* 1991; 84:III76.
47. Weinert L, Karp R, Vignon P, et al: Feasibility of aortic diameter measurement by multiplane transesophageal echocardiography for preoperative selection and preparation of homograft aortic valves. *J Thorac Cardiovasc Surg* 1996; 112:954.
48. Abraham TP, Kon ND, Nomeir AM, et al: Accuracy of transesophageal echocardiography in preoperative determination of aortic anulus size during valve replacement. *J Am Soc Echocardiogr* 1997; 10:149.
49. Oh CC, Click RL, Orszulak TA, et al: Role of intraoperative transesophageal echocardiography in determining aortic annulus diameter in homograft insertion. *J Am Soc Echocardiogr* 1998; 11:638.
50. Barratt-Boyes BG: A method for preparing and inserting a homograft aortic valve. *Br J Surg* 1965; 52:847.
51. Dearani JA, Orszulak TA, Daly RC, et al: Comparison of techniques for implantation of aortic valve allografts. *Ann Thorac Surg* 1996; 62:1069.
52. McGiffin DC, O'Brien MF: A technique for aortic root replacement by an aortic allograft. *Ann Thorac Surg* 1989; 47:625.
53. Daicoff GR, Botero LM, Quintessenza JA: Allograft replacement of the aortic valve versus the miniroot and valve. *Ann Thorac Surg* 1993; 55:855.
54. Rubay JE, Raphael D, Sluysmans T, et al: Aortic valve replacement with allograft/autograft: subcoronary versus intraluminal cylinder or root. *Ann Thorac Surg* 1995; 60:S78.
55. Yankah AC, Klose H, Musci M, et al: Geometric mismatch between homograft (allograft) and native aortic root: a 14 year clinical experience. *Eur J Cardiothorac Surg* 2001; 20:835.
56. Doty DB: Aortic valve replacement with homograft and autograft. *Semin Thorac Cardiovasc Surg* 1996; 8:249.
57. O'Brien MF, Harrocks S, Stafford EG, et al: The homograft aortic valve: a 29-year, 99.3% follow up of 1,022 valve replacements. *J Heart Valve Dis* 2001; 10:334.
58. Gaasch WH, Sundaram M, Meyer TE: Managing asymptomatic patients with chronic aortic regurgitation. *Chest* 1997; 111:1702.
59. Dearani JA, Orszulak TA, Schaff HV, et al: Results of allograft aortic valve replacement for complex endocarditis. *J Thorac Cardiovasc Surg* 1997; 113:285.
60. Niwaya K, Knott-Craig CJ, Santangelo K, et al: Advantage of autograft and homograft valve replacement for complex aortic valve endocarditis. *Ann Thorac Surg* 1999; 67:1603.
61. Yankah AC, Klose H, Petzina R, et al: Surgical management of acute aortic root endocarditis with viable homograft: 13-year experience. *Eur J Cardiothorac Surg* 2002; 21:260.
62. Eriksson MJ, Kallner G, Rosfors S, et al: Hemodynamic performance of cryopreserved aortic homograft valves during midterm follow-up. *J Am Coll Cardiol* 1998; 32:1002.
63. Hasegawa J, Kitamura S, Taniguchi S, et al: Comparative rest and exercise hemodynamics of allograft and prosthetic valves in the aortic position. *Ann Thorac Surg* 1997; 64:1753.
64. Elkins RC, Lane M, McCue C: Pulmonary autograft reoperation: incidence and management. *Ann Thorac Surg* 1996; 62:450.
65. Franco KL, Verrier ED: *Advanced Therapy in Cardiac Surgery*. Hamilton, Ont., BC Decker, 1999; p 183.
66. David TE, Omran A, Webb G, et al: Geometric mismatch of the aortic and pulmonary roots causes aortic insufficiency after the Ross procedure. *J Thorac Cardiovasc Surg* 1996; 112:1231.
67. Elkins RC, Lane MM, McCue C, Chandrasekaran K: Ross operation and aneurysm or dilation of the ascending aorta. *Semin Thorac Cardiovasc Surg* 1999; 11:50.
68. Ross D, Jackson M, Davies J: Pulmonary autograft aortic valve replacement: long-term results. *J Card Surg* 1991; 6:529.

69. Chambers JC, Somerville J, Stone S, Ross DN: Pulmonary autograft procedure for aortic valve disease: long-term results of the pioneer series. *Circulation* 1997; 96:2206.
70. Briand M, Pibarot P, Dumesnil JG, Cartier P: Midterm echocardiographic follow-up after Ross operation. *Circulation* 2000; 102:III10.
71. David TE, Omran A, Ivanov J, et al: Dilation of the pulmonary autograft after the Ross procedure. *J Thorac Cardiovasc Surg* 2000; 119:210.
72. Lang SJ, Giordano MS, Cardon-Cardo C, et al: Biochemical and cellular characterization of cardiac valve tissue after cryopreservation or antibiotic preservation. *J Thorac Cardiovasc Surg* 1994;108: 63.
73. Raanani E, Yau TM, David TE, et al: Risk factors for late pulmonary homograft stenosis after the Ross procedure. *Ann Thorac Surg* 2000; 70:1953.
74. Bonow RO, Carabello B, de Leon AC Jr, et al: Guidelines for the management of patients with valvular heart disease: executive summary. A report of the American College of Cardiology/American Heart Association Task Force on Practice Guidelines (Committee on Management of Patients with Valvular Heart Disease). *Circulation* 1998; 98:1949.

Chapter 35

Stentless Aortic Valve Replacement: Bioprostheses

Donald B. Doty/John R. Doty

After nearly 40 years of experience with bioprosthetic heart valves, it would seem reasonable that a single design of bioprosthesis, ideal for all circumstances in which it is necessary to replace the aortic valve, should have emerged. Unfortunately, this is not the case. The surgeon must choose from an ever-increasing number of replacement devices. There seems to be no end to the new devices that are being designed, tested, and added to the market availability after short-term clinical trials. By the time medium-term or in some cases long-term performance data are known, an equal number of valves have been discarded in favor of new and unproven devices.

The porcine aortic valve, directly implanted into the aortic root, was originally proposed for aortic valve replacement by Binet et al in 1965.[1] O'Brien subsequently developed a heterograft valve bank for continued use of both bovine and porcine nonstented valves.[2] Direct heterograft valve implantation was abandoned because of unsatisfactory results, likely due to inadequate tissue preservation, in favor of heterograft valves that were mounted on a stent frame. Stented bioprostheses manufactured to provide a standard device that is easily implanted and provide reproducible results in the aortic position were associated with good short- and medium-term results. Unfortunately, stented heterograft tissue failure with calcification and cusp rupture became apparent with longer follow-up, particularly in younger patients. Hemodynamic performance of stent-mounted porcine valves was less than ideal when the aortic root was small.

David et al revived the concept of direct insertion of a nonstented porcine heterograft into the aortic root in 1990.[3] This valve, originally manufactured on a limited trial basis by Hancock Laboratory, was subsequently produced for clinical use by St. Jude Medical as the Toronto SPV (stentless porcine valve). Other devices were developed soon thereafter.

The search for the ideal prosthesis for aortic valve replacement continues, and recent advances in tissue valve technology have engineered the development of a new generation of stentless bioprosthetic valves. Traditionally, bioprosthetic valves are mounted on a semirigid stent, which maintains the valve geometry and assists the surgeon in implanting the valve. The new stentless xenograft valves do not have these prosthetic stents, allowing for larger valves to be implanted with presumably better hemodynamic performance than if a stented bioprosthesis is used.

STENTLESS AORTIC BIOPROSTHESES

A partial listing of commercially available stentless aortic bioprostheses follows. Some are available in the United States and others are available only in international markets. Three basic techniques are used for implantation depending on the construction of the stentless bioprostheses: (1) subcoronary valve replacement; (2) root inclusion; and (3) root replacement.

St. Jude Medical Toronto SPV

This device (from St. Jude Medical, St. Paul, MN) is derived from the porcine aortic root. The porcine tissue is fixed in glutaraldehyde with the aortic valve in the closed position by applying low pressure to the fixative solution. No anticalcification agent is added. The aorta is removed from all three sinuses of Valsalva and the exterior is covered completely with fine polyester fabric. The device is used for aortic valve replacement only as a subcoronary implant in the essentially normal aortic root without dilation of the sinotubular junction. Modifications of the device are planned to offer a full aortic root and to add BioLinx anticalcification treatment to the bioprosthesis.[4] The anticalcification agents include treatment of the aortic wall with aluminum chloride ($AlCl_3$) and curing the aortic leaflets with ethanol.

Medtronic Freestyle Aortic Root Bioprosthesis

This valve (from Medtronic, Minneapolis, MN) is a stentless valve derived from a porcine aortic root preserved in glutaraldehyde and has a ring of polyester at the inflow and covering the septal myocardium, which provides strength and ease of implantation. The Freestyle device is presented as an intact porcine aortic root with ligated coronary arteries. The aortic root is preserved in a buffered 0.2% glutaraldehyde solution to which an antimineralization agent, alpha amino oleic acid, has been added. Zero net pressure is applied to the valve leaflets while the aortic root contour is maintained in a slightly dilated position by applying a pressure of 40 mm Hg to the intra-aortic solution. This process is designed to retard calcium deposition[5,6] and retain the natural collagen crimp and flexibility[7] in the valve leaflets. The device may be implanted as a subcoronary valve replacement, as an inclusion root, or as an aortic root replacement.

Edwards Lifesciences Prima Plus

This prosthesis (from Edwards Lifesciences, Irvine, CA) consists of an extended porcine aortic root fixed in glutaraldehyde at low pressure. The "Plus" designation indicates treatment with the proprietary XenoLogiX FET-80, a combination of agents including ethanol and Tween-80 (surfactant) to retard calcification.[8] A minimum of polyester fabric is used to enhance pliability. There are markings on the outside of the aortic root to guide trimming of the aorta. It can be implanted subcoronary, as an inclusion root, or as an aortic root replacement.

CryoLife-O'Brien

This stentless porcine aortic valve (from CryoLife, Inc., Kennesaw, GA) is a manufactured composite of the noncoronary sinus and leaflet from three porcine aortic roots. It is fixed in glutaraldehyde at low pressure without calcium retardant. The bioprosthesis has no polyester cloth support and the only synthetic material is the suture that holds the leaflets together. It is designed to be implanted below the coronary arteries in a supra-annular position in the sinuses of Valsalva by a single suture line. Experience is limited to a few centers and the technical aspects of implantation appear to be somewhat more difficult than the other stentless bioprostheses in spite of only a single suture line being employed.

AorTech Freesewn Porcine Elan

This porcine aortic valve (from AorTech, Bellshill, Scotland, UK) is fixed at low pressure in glutaraldehyde and is designed for subcoronary implantation as a valve replacement. The aorta from all three sinuses of Valsalva is removed and a cuff of pericardium is attached to the inflow tract. A valve holding device is supplied.

Shelhigh No-React Stentless Bioprosthesis

This prosthesis (from Shelhigh Inc., Millburn NJ) is a porcine aortic valve or aortic root fixed in glutaraldehyde at low pressure. The tissue is "skeletonized" and covered with fixed pericardium for support. No-React[9,10] is a proprietary surfactant/heparin binding chemical process. The device is implanted in the subcoronary position.

Biocor PSB/SJM

This heterograft (from Biocor Industria e Pesquisa Ltda, Belo Horizonte, MG, Brazil) was originally developed in Brazil and is a composite valve constructed from three individual porcine leaflets fixed at zero pressure in glutaraldehyde. Now marketed by St. Jude Medical, the prosthesis is treated with the proprietary No-React[9,10] surfactant treatment to reduce calcification. The leaflets are secured to a strip of bovine pericardium to create a slightly conical conduit. Subcoronary implantation is employed.

Sorin Pericarbon Stentless Bioprosthesis

This is a stentless all-bovine pericardial valve (from Sorin Biomedica, Saluggia, Italy). A glutaraldehyde-fixed sheet of bovine pericardium is formed into a valve that is supported by a second sheet of bovine pericardium attached using pyrolite carbon-coated suture. This device is implanted as an aortic valve replacement in the subcoronary position, tailoring the patient noncoronary sinus to reduce the diameter of the sinotubular junction for a discrepancy of less than 10% compared with the annular diameter.[11]

OPERATIVE TECHNIQUE

Subcoronary Valve Replacement

In this technique the bioprosthesis is used only as a valve supported by the sinus aorta of the patient.[11–18] A transverse aortotomy is made 5 to 10 mm above the sinus rim. Alternatively, the ascending aorta is transected for exposure of the aortic root and coronary arteries. The diseased aortic valve is excised and calcium depositions are thoroughly debrided from the aortic root. The diameter of the aortic root is measured at the ventriculoaortic junction (valve annulus) using obturators provided by the manufacturer. The diameter at the sinotubular junction is measured when the Toronto SPV valve is considered for implantation. Major dilation of the sinotubular junction contraindicates use of this bioprosthesis but not the use of the Freestyle device. An equal or slightly larger diameter size of the bioprosthesis is selected for implantation. Associated procedures are performed while the bioprosthesis is rinsed in saline solution to remove glutaraldehyde.

The Toronto SPV, CryoLife-O'Brien, Shelhigh, AorTec, Biocor, and Sorin devices are pretrimmed and ready for implantation. The Freestyle and Prima Plus valve must be tailored by removing the sinus aorta from the right and left coronary sinuses of the bioprosthesis. The noncoronary sinus is usually left intact so that the position and spatial relationships of the commissures on either side of the noncoronary sinus are fixed, making implantation more reproducible. The bioprosthesis is implanted in anatomic position without rotation unless the right coronary artery is positioned so low that the prosthesis will not fit under it. The prosthesis could be rotated 120 degrees in that situation to place the right coronary sinus of the graft into the noncoronary sinus of the patient.

The cloth sewing rim at the inflow margin of the graft is attached to the patient aortic root using continuous or interrupted suture technique. The suture line is kept in a level plane through the lowest points of the dense fibrous tissue of the hinge of the native valve (annulus). The suture line is below the annulus in the interleaflet triangle except in the region of the membranous septum, where the suture line must follow the annulus directly in order to protect the conduction system from injury. During suture placement, the bioprosthesis is held away from the native root because it is too stiff to work with conveniently when lowered into the aortic root. The exception is the Sorin Pericarbon Stentless Bioprosthesis, which is flexible enough to be inverted into the left ventricular outflow tract during proximal suture line placement.[11]

When all of the stitches are placed, the graft is attached to the aortic root by lowering it into place and adjusting suture loop tension on continuous suture or tying down interrupted stitches. The sinus aorta of the graft is attached to the sinus aorta of the patient below the coronary arteries. When the Toronto SPV or the other fully trimmed devices are used, the sinus aorta must also be contoured into the noncoronary sinus of Valsalva. Continuous stitches of polypropylene suture are placed in radial fashion below the coronary artery ostium. The stitches are often quite close to the ostium because the cloth covering on the graft raises the graft. This position of the graft cannot be forced to a lower position without risking graft buckling. The suture line is carried to the top of both adjacent commissures. When the noncoronary sinus remains intact, the position of two of the commissures is fixed so that proper location of the commissure between the right and left coronary sinuses ensures a competent valve. The preservation characteristics of the bioprostheses aid in proper implantation, because even the trimmed graft aorta holds its shape well. This also holds for grafts in which all three sinuses have been removed. The patient aorta may be conformed and approximated to the aorta of the graft in reproducible fashion. The noncoronary sinus of the patient may be closed over the graft as there is sufficient space to accommodate the graft without distortion. The graft is trimmed above the sinotubular junction (sinus rim) and approximated to the inside of the closed aorta of the patient or to the cut edge of the divided aorta. If the aorta has been divided, it is reanastomosed in end-to-end fashion. Valve function is checked by intraoperative echocardiography in all cases.

Root Inclusion

Root inclusion technique refers to placement of the Freestyle or Prima Plus bioprosthesis as a tube inside the native aorta.[19] This technique is performed least frequently and may be more difficult than the other techniques. It is done in an attempt to reduce the possibility of distortion of the graft. The only modification to the graft is openings made in the sinus aorta to accommodate anastomosis of the patient coronary arteries to the graft. This technique is useful for a patient with a dilated aortic root and ascending aorta that is not aneurysmal.

A transverse incision of about two thirds of the aortic circumference is made in the ascending aorta about 4 cm above the annulus. The aorta may also be divided completely to obtain better exposure of the aortic root. The aortic valve is excised and the annulus debrided of all calcareous deposits. The size of the annulus is measured as described above. An appropriate size bioprosthesis is chosen and rinsed. The aorta in the right and left sinus of the graft is completely excised from just below the sinotubular junction to the cloth covering below. Continuous stitches of monofilament suture are used to attach the inflow sewing ring of the graft to the left ventricular outflow tract at a level plane at the level of the annulus. The three commissures of the bioprosthesis are then aligned within the aortic root by placing separate mattress sutures from the graft to an appropriate position above the commissures of the patient through the aortic wall. The sinus aorta of the graft is attached to the sinus aorta of the patient by continuous suture working from within the graft. The position of the sutures is governed by the appropriate anatomic fit of the graft to the aortic root. The distal end of the graft is shortened to approximate the aortic incision. The graft is incorporated into the aorta by continuous suture taking up excess patient aorta to the graft. The aortotomy is closed or the aorta reanastomosed. Valve function is checked by intraoperative echocardiography.

Root Replacement

Root replacement means that the entire native aortic root and valve are excised and replaced with the Freestyle or Prima Plus bioprosthesis.[20] Full-root replacement technique is employed for the treatment of aortic root pathology that precludes the use of other techniques that require relatively normal patient aorta to support the graft. It is also employed because there is the least chance for aortic valve distortion of any of the implant techniques. Full-root replacement technique is possible only with the Freestyle and the Prima Plus devices.

The aorta is divided above the sinotubular junction. Both coronary ostia are mobilized on generous buttons of aortic wall. The remaining sinus aorta is removed. The aortic valve is excised and the annulus debrided. The size of the annulus is measured and an appropriate size valve is chosen. A larger prosthesis may be employed because the device will stand by itself and is not enclosed within the aorta. The inflow sewing ring of the graft is attached to the aortic annulus with multiple interrupted stitches of 3-0 braided polyester suture or a continuous stitch of 3-0 polypropylene suture. It is important to line up the position of the left coronary artery of the graft with the left coronary artery of the patient during construction of the proximal suture line. The left coronary ostia of the graft is opened and an anastomosis of the left coronary artery made to the graft using continuous stitches of 5-0 polypropylene suture. Location of the proper position for the right coronary anastomosis is aided by filling the right ventricle. The right coronary artery ostium of the graft is opened if it is properly positioned, or another opening is made in the right coronary sinus. The right coronary artery is anastomosed to the graft. An end-to-end anastomosis of the distal end of the graft is constructed to the ascending aorta. It is usually necessary to make some size adjustment of the patient aorta or the graft to achieve a good fitting anastomosis. In some cases, the graft is extended with a polyester graft for replacement of the ascending aorta. Intraoperative echocardiography is performed to assess aortic valve function and segmental left ventricular wall motion. Abnormal left ventricular wall motion or ventricular arrhythmia suggests coronary artery blood flow compromise, which should be treated by reconstruction of coronary artery-to-graft anastomoses or by coronary artery bypass grafts.

CLINICAL RESULTS

Several authors have now reported large series with mid-term follow-up on the Medtronic Freestyle and the Toronto SPV valves.[12,21–34] There is less experience with the other valves.[35–43] Mid-term (5-year) studies have shown excellent performance for all devices. Early mortality is low and comparable to mechanical or stented bioprostheses. Freedom from valve-related mortality is low with the stentless xenografts, although there has not been sufficient long-term follow-up to identify late hazards or associated risk factors. The Toronto SPV bioprosthesis and the Medtronic Freestyle aortic root bioprosthesis have been implanted in a large number of patients, mostly over the age of 61 years. Follow-up extends to 10 years for the Toronto SPV valve[12] and over 7 years in some patients with the Freeestyle valve.[21,22] Investigators have compared these two stentless bioprostheses in single-institution trials and have found very little difference in hemodynamic or clinical results. Del Rizzo and Abdoh[44] found no differences in clinical outcome or hemodynamic performance between these two valves and both devices offer excellent results with normalization of left ventricular function. Legare et al[45] reported that the hemodynamic performance of both valves was excellent and equivalent, but there was slightly more aortic valve regurgitation with the Toronto SPV valve. Bach et al[46] recently presented data suggesting increased aortic valve regurgitation at 8 years after operation using the Toronto SPV valve, which may be attributed to dilation of the unsupported sinotubular junction. At mid-term follow-up, however, there seems to be little difference in clinical results for the two valves.

There was an acceptable risk of operation in the Freestyle experience (5.7% overall), considering that most of the patients were elderly.[21] The aortic valve lesion for which aortic valve replacement was required was pure stenosis in 43% or mixed stenosis and insufficiency in 45% (total stenotic lesions = 88%). There was a remarkable improvement in functional capacity after operation with 95% of patients in functional class I or II; 73% had been in class III or IV prior to operation.

The most popular method of implantation has been subcoronary valve replacement.[21] Although this method requires knowledge of the spatial relationships of the aortic root, it does not alter the natural tissues of the aortic root substantially. In that sense, it is somewhat less of an operation than aortic root replacement techniques, but in another sense, it may be more difficult to perform reproducibly. The data from the Freestyle series[22] show that there is remarkably high probability (95% to 100%) that the bioprosthetic valve will be competent or have no more than mild regurgitation regardless of the technique chosen for implantation. Risk of hemorrhage may be less and it may be more easily controlled with subcoronary valve replacement or root inclusion technique than with full-root replacement technique because the bioprosthesis is completely enclosed within the natural aorta so that the only source of major bleeding is the readily accessible aortotomy. Risk of operation was lowest using subcoronary valve implant techniques (5.0% vs. 9.3% for full root), even though the patients were older with two thirds being over the age of 70 years.[21] Subcoronary technique also required less myocardial ischemia time by about 20 minutes compared to the aortic root techniques.[21] Less xenograft aorta is inserted when the subcoronary valve replacement is used and may account for a somewhat less frequency of thromboembolism. Xenograft aorta will ultimately calcify even though anticalcification agents are added to the fixative because retardation of calcification in the aorta is less effective than in the leaflet tissue. The possible exception may be the use of BioLinx technology,[4] because $AlCl_3$ appears to be more effective than other agents in inhibiting aortic calcification. This may also be in favor of using a subcoronary valve implantation technique so that more of the patient's own flexible aorta is preserved. On the other hand, the most perfect early and late implants in terms of valve competence were achieved by full-root replacement technique.

Aortic root pathology encountered at operation surely affected choice of operation.[22] Aortic root pathology often dictates replacement of the aortic root or ascending aorta, favoring full-root replacement compared to the other techniques in which the bioprosthesis is enclosed within the aortic root. Aortic root replacement operations, however, require more time to perform by about 20 to 30 minutes. This was especially important when aortic valve replacement was accompanied by aortocoronary bypass. Taken in sum, a longer procedure, more complex aortic root pathology, and more exposed suture lines in complete aortic root replacement procedures may extract a higher early death rate after operation than when other methods are employed. By 7 years, however, actuarial analysis[22] indicates little difference in survival when subcoronary implant technique is compared to full-root technique (62.0% vs. 67.7% freedom from death).

Hemodynamic Performance

The remarkable functional improvement may be related to excellent hemodynamic performance of the stentless bioprosthesis. These xenografts have very favorable hemodynamic performance, even in the smallest sizes, and are therefore ideally suited for the patient with a small aortic root.[47,48] By eliminating the stent, a larger valve can be implanted in the patient's aortic root. Mean systolic gradients are low, generally less than 10 mm Hg. Mean gradients across the various sizes of the Medtronic Freestyle valve[22] have shown about 15 mm Hg for 19-mm bioprostheses, with the larger valves having lower mean transvalvular gradients. These gradients approach those of homograft valves, which are only slightly higher than the normal aortic valve. Low transvalvular gradients were sustained during mid-term follow-up. Over the first several months after implantation of a stentless heterograft, effective valve orifice area actually increases and there is measurable regression in left ventricular hypertrophy as the left ventricle undergoes remodeling with improved function.[49–53] In general, a 10% to 20% reduction in left ventricular mass occurs over the first 6 to 12 months and stabilizes at that point. In a prospective, randomized study Walther et al[54] found a greater regression of left ventricular hypertrophy in patients receiving stentless bioprostheses compared to other types of valve prostheses. Maselli et al[55] and Jin et al[56] both reported a more rapid and complete resolution of left ventricular hypertrophy and greater improvement in left ventricular function when either aortic homograft or a stentless porcine bioprosthesis was used for aortic valve replacement as compared to stented bioprostheses or mechanical valves. A previously reported reduction in transvalvular gradient observed in the first year after operation stabilized and remained constant up to the 4-year mark.[21] Effective valve area has been consistently good even in small size valves allowing implantation of 19-mm or 21-mm prostheses without enlargement of the aortic root with expectation that hemodynamic performance will be good.[16] Low transvalvular gradient and large effective orifice area even in 19-mm and 21-mm valves reduce the possibility of patient-to-prosthesis size mismatch and are associated with rapid resolution of left ventricular hypertrophy.

Echocardiographic Functional Assessment

The absence of a sewing ring and stents on the new stentless bioprosthesis results in an echocardiographic image that is very similar to the native aortic valve. There are, however, some important characteristics of a stentless bioprosthesis that should be evaluated with intraoperative transesophageal echocardiography during the initial implantation and subsequently with either transesophageal or transthoracic echocardiography during follow-up.

Evaluation of global left ventricular function either in the preoperative setting or by transesophageal echocardiography in the operating room prior to the initiation of cardiopulmonary bypass is important to determine overall and segmental left ventricular function. Reduced left ventricular function prior to the ischemic period required for aortic valve replacement may affect the choice of operation, favoring more simplified approaches. Intraoperative imaging should also assess the status of the left ventricular outflow tract including subvalvular obstruction, associated valvular heart disease, and the condition of the aortic root and ascending aorta.

The stentless bioprosthesis should be assessed after implantation and separation from cardiopulmonary bypass, but before administration of protamine, to examine for the presence and degree of valve regurgitation as well as to establish a baseline for the specific anatomic characteristics of that valve. The stentless bioprosthesis should be carefully evaluated with intraoperative echocardiography for the presence of paravalvular leak. Bach[57] has extensively described the variants in paravalvular anatomy with these valves, noting that there is creation of a potential space between the native aortic wall and the porcine aortic wall. The size, extent, and echo characteristics of this potential space vary depending on the specific bioprosthesis and how much of the porcine root is actually inside the native aortic root. Valves that are implanted using the subcoronary technique have the smallest amount of tissue overlap, while root inclusion techniques produce the greatest amount. This tissue overlap results in a "double lumen" appearance that gradually resolves over time, with near-complete resolution at 6 months as demonstrated by Bauer et al.[58] Accumulation of fluid and hematoma in the space between the graft and the aorta results in an echo-lucent area. These collections should be carefully interrogated with color flow Doppler to assess the presence of diastolic flow, which indicates a paravalvular leak. It is difficult to determine the precise origin of such leaks, but paravalvular leaks always originate at the distal suture line, above the prosthetic valve. The stentless bioprostheses, with the exception of the Cryolife-O'Brien valve, all require both a proximal and distal suture line. A paravalvular leak can be demonstrated either by the presence of diastolic flow between the porcine wall and the native aortic wall or at the level of the annulus. Both findings are indicative of valve dehiscence at the distal suture line and are an indication for resumption of cardiopulmonary bypass and revision of the distal suture line. If there is no evidence of paravalvular leak and valve function is otherwise normal, paravalvular edema and/or hematoma do not require intervention.

Stentless bioprostheses can be inserted with a high degree of diastolic competence. In one study, the bioprosthesis was competent or only mildly incompetent in 96% to 100% of the patients, with the highest levels of competence achieved when the device was implanted by the full-root replacement technique.[22] Moderate valve regurgitation was present in only 8% of patients at the 6-year mark and there were no patients with severe valve regurgitation. The Sorin Pericarbon device showed somewhat higher incidence of aortic valve regurgitation[11] with 69% having no regurgitation, 23% mild, and 8% moderate regurgitation.

COMPLICATIONS

Reoperation for Valve Explant

Eight valves were explanted in the Freestyle series[22] for technical problems resulting in valvular incompetence or unsatisfactory hemodynamic performance. This is a very low incidence of valve explantation, indicating that surgeons can master the techniques of insertion and become confident that this bioprosthesis will have good hemodynamic performance and will not leak. An additional 6 valves were explanted for infective endocarditis. None were removed for structural deterioration of the bioprosthesis. Total valve explant rate was 0.5% per patient-year, leaving 92% to 99% of patients free of valve explant at the 7-year mark.

Thromboembolism

Thromboembolic rate for the Freestyle bioprosthesis was low,[22] in spite of the fact that patients were not given warfarin unless there was persistent atrial fibrillation or flutter. Early thromboembolism was noted in only 1.9% of patients having subcoronary valve implantation when very rigid criteria were applied. Late thromboembolism occurred at a rate of 1.6 events per patient-year, with permanent neurologic events at an even lower rate of 0.6 per patient-year. Actuarial analysis of thromboembolism rate showed 78% to 87% of patients free of this complication at 7 years after valve implantation.

Endocarditis

Endocarditis was an infrequent event in the Freestyle experience.[22] The freedom from endocarditis was greater than 94.5% at 7 years. This indicates that the Freestyle bioprosthesis is quite resistant to infection, and that infection on this bioprosthesis can be treated and cured. Endocarditis, however, accounted for nearly one half of the valves that were explanted (6 of 14).

Structural Deterioration

Structural deterioration during the 5-year follow-up has been rare,[21] with no valves explanted for this cause. These data imply that if the Freestyle bioprosthesis can be implanted with technical accuracy and without bacterial contamination, it can be expected to function very well up to the 7-year mark. It is too early to know if the durability of the Freestyle bioprosthesis will compare favorably with other bioprostheses. The hope and expectation are that the zero-net pressure fixation of the porcine aortic valve leaflets and the addition of alpha amino oleic acid to the tissues, technology unique to this bioprosthesis, will favorably affect durability, but many more years of detailed follow-up are needed before this can be known.

SURVIVAL

There is increasing evidence of the hemodynamic benefits of the stentless bioprostheses. Retrospective data suggest improved survival compared to standard aortic valve replacement with either mechanical or stented bioprostheses.[54,59,60] This could be related to improved hemodynamics and/or resolution of left ventricular hypertrophy. Del Rizzo et al[60] reported on over 1100 patients undergoing stentless aortic valve replacement, and documented that baseline left ventricular mass index and patient-prosthetic mismatch have significant effects on the regression of left ventricular hypertrophy. For a given body mass index, there is a predicted normal size for the aortic annulus. Patient-prosthesis mismatch is defined as a postoperative indexed valve effective orifice area of less than or equal to 0.85 cm^2/m^2, as described by Pibarot et al.[61] Inserting a prosthesis that is smaller than the predicted normal size produces patient-prosthesis mismatch, which can result in higher transvalvular gradients and left ventricular outflow obstruction, preventing regression of left ventricular hypertrophy. Del Rizzo et al[60] showed a survival advantage for stentless valves over stented valves, with approximately a 5-fold greater probability of death at 5 years in patients younger than 60 years of age who received stented valves.

CHOOSING A BIOPROSTHESIS

The comparative information concerning performance specifications of the various valves is confusing. The body of literature on valve performance and outcome statistics is enormous. It is nearly impossible for an individual surgeon to know enough of these data to make informed choices. A few constants are of some value in interpreting performance characteristics of the various cardiac valve replacement devices. The manufacturer's label size (mm) expresses only an approximate size (diameter) of the prosthesis. For a stent-mounted bioprosthesis the label size correlates with the outside diameter of the stent, not the real outer diameter including the sewing ring. Stentless valves are measured by the actual diameter at the outside of the bioprosthesis, and that is the label size. The label size is always larger than the primary orifice or inside diameter of the device. The primary orifice is often referred to as the internal orifice area or the measured geometric orifice in square centimeters. The primary orifice is difficult, if not impossible, to measure in any bioprosthetic valve. The internal orifice area is always larger than the in vitro orifice area, which is measured by testing the valve in the laboratory in a pulse duplicator. The in vitro orifice area is always larger than the area measured in vivo by Doppler ultrasound after the valve is implanted. The orifice area measured either in vitro or in vivo is also called the effective orifice area (EOA), expressed in square centimeters, and may be "indexed" to body size by dividing by the body surface area (indexed EOA = EOA/BSA). It is noted, however, that body surface area is calculated from both height and weight, so obesity may distort this figure.

Pibarot and Dumesnil[61] showed that when valve size and body size are used to calculate an indexed effective valve area, there is a strong relationship between small (19-mm or 21-mm) mechanical or stented bioprosthetic valve size and pressure gradient over the valve during rest and exercise. Del Rizzo et al[60] showed that indexed effective orifice area smaller than 0.8 cm^2/m^2 had a major effect on the extent of left ventricular mass regression after aortic valve replacement with stentless bioprostheses. Dumesnil and Yoganathan have shown that the indexed effective orifice area (cm^2/m^2) predicts the performance of prosthetic valves during exercise.[62] Indexed effective orifice area larger than 0.85 will keep the pressure gradient from rising during exercise on the steep part of performance curves. Indexed effective orifice areas smaller than 0.85 are considered to represent patient-prosthesis mismatch because of the rapid rise in mean pressure gradient observed during exercise.

Stented bioprostheses tend to be on the ascending portion of performance curves more frequently than stentless bioprostheses, homografts, or autografts. The choice of the size of bioprosthesis that can be inserted in the aortic root is actually determined by the size of the aortic root. Inserting an oversized bioprosthesis is of no advantage because stentless bioprostheses may be distorted and therefore obstructive. A stented bioprosthesis that is too large will erode the aortic root tissues, creating immediate problems in adjacent structures or later problems should change of the valve be required. Stented bioprostheses in current use have contoured sewing rings designed to facilitate implantation in a supra-annular position, thereby allowing insertion of a larger device owing to the increased space above the valve annulus provided by the sinus of Valsalva. Stentless bioprostheses must be inserted in an intra-annular position. This may allow devices of similar internal orifice to be implanted and may account for some studies that show equivalent hemodynamic performance of these devices.

Stented xenografts are easy to implant in standard aortic valve replacement procedures and give reproducible results. As noted earlier, however, it is difficult to use a stented heterograft in the small aortic root and it is subject to structural deterioration over time. Homografts are difficult to implant and are in short supply, being dependent on the donor pool. The homograft, however, offers superior hemodynamics and is ideally suited for reconstruction of the small aortic root or for extensive root destruction from prior operation or due to endocarditis. Stentless xenografts, although more difficult to implant than a traditional stented valve, are easier to secure than a homograft due to the stiffness imparted by the fixation technique and also from the cloth covering which is found on some of the valves. As with any valve prosthesis, meticulous technique is required, but the stentless xenografts are more flexible than the stented variety and can therefore be implanted into a smaller aortic root without sacrificing effective valve orifice area.[13]

Several authors have compared hemodynamics and outcomes between stented and stentless xenografts.[63–65] Although these studies were retrospective in nature and were not randomized clinical trials, stentless valves have lower rest and exercise gradients than stented valves. In addition, patients receiving stentless valves had lower hospital mortality, fewer reoperations, and lower valve-related mortality than patients receiving stented valves. Long-term survival benefits from stentless valves compared to stented valves have not been reported in a prospective, randomized fashion. There has been one prospective randomized study published to date comparing stentless bioprostheses with stented valves for aortic valve replacement. Cohen et al[66] randomized 99 total patients to receive either a stented pericardial valve or a stentless Toronto SPV valve. No difference was shown between the two valves for survival, regression of left ventricular mass, or decrease in transvalvular gradient over the 12-month study period.

Others[67–70] have compared similar outcomes between stentless xenografts and homografts. Survival, freedom from valve-related complications, and left ventricular remodeling were similar between the two types of valves, although the stentless xenografts had slightly higher gradients. Two of the studies showed a trend toward a higher incidence of aortic valve insufficiency in the Toronto SPV valves. One study[71] compared the Toronto SPV, the Biocor PSB, and the Cryolife-O'Brien valves, reporting that the first two were essentially equivalent, while the Cryolife-O'Brien valve had a higher incidence of reoperation and valve deterioration.

CONCLUSION

In summary, stentless xenografts are being more widely used for replacement and reconstruction of aortic valve and root pathology. Some of the stentless bioprostheses can be tailored by the surgeon to repair part or all of the aortic root, and all of the stentless valves are suitable for patients with a small aortic root. Although the implantation technique is more difficult than standard aortic valve replacement with a stented xenograft, it is not as demanding as homograft implantation. Stentless xenografts in patients have resulted in improved functional class and exercise performance presumably due to excellent hemodynamic performance, and reoperation for valve-related causes is unusual. There is high freedom from valve-related complications such as thromboembolism and endocarditis. Stentless bioprostheses do not require anticoagulation. Mechanical stress to the leaflets is theoretically less due to the absence of the stent, although long-term data are not yet available to support this contention. Newer anticalcification treatments developed for the stentless xenografts may reduce or prevent valve and/or aortic calcification over time. Survival, functional classification, and freedom from valve deterioration are excellent at midterm follow-up (5-10 years) for all types of stentless bioprostheses. Long-term follow-up will ultimately determine the role of these valves. At present, however, stentless bioprostheses should be carefully considered whenever aortic valve replacement is required and may be the device of choice in patients older than 70 years having a 19- to 21-mm aortic annulus.

REFERENCES

1. Binet JP, Duran CG, Carpentier A, et al: Heterologous aortic valve transplantation. *Lancet* 1965; 2:1275.
2. O'Brien MF: Heterograft aortic valves for human use. *J Thorac Cardiovasc Surg* 1967; 53:392.
3. David TE, Pollick C, Bos J: Aortic valve replacement with stentless porcine aortic bioprosthesis. *J Thorac Cardiovasc Surg* 1990; 99:113.
4. Walther T, Falk V, Autschbach R, et al: Comparison of different anticalcification treatments for stentless bioprostheses. *Ann Thorac Surg* 1998; 66:S249.
5. Girardot MN, Torrianni MW, Girardot JM: Effect of AOA on glutaraldehyde-fixed bioprosthetic heart valve cusps and walls: binding and calcification studies. *Int J Artif Organs* 1994; 17:76.
6. Chen W, Schoen FJ, Levy RJ: Mechanism of efficacy of 2-amino oleic acid for inhibition of calcification of glutaraldehyde pretreated porcine bioprosthestic heart valves. *Circulation* 1994; 90:323.
7. Mayne ASD, Christie GW, Smaille BH, et al: An assessment of the mechanical properties of leaflets from four second generation porcine bioprostheses using biaxial testing techniques. *J Thorac Cardiovasc Surg* 1989; 98:170.
8. Carpentier A, Nashef A, Carpentier S, et al: Techniques for prevention of calcification of valvular bioprostheses. *Circulation* 1984; 70(suppl I):165.
9. Herijgers P, Ozaki S, Verbeken E, et al: The No-React anticalcification treatment: a comparison of Biocor No-React II and Toronto SPV stentless bioprostheses implanted in sheep. *Semin Thorac Cardiovasc Surg* 1999; 11:171.
10. Abolhoda A, Yu S, Oyarzun JR, et al: No-React detoxification process: a superior anticalcification method for bioprostheses. *Ann Thorac Surg* 1996; 62:1724.
11. Westaby S, Jin XY, Vaccari G, Katsumota T: The Sorin stentless pericardial valve: implant techniques and hemodynamic profile. *Semin Thorac Cardiovasc Surg* 1999; 11:62.
12. David TE, Feindel CM, Scully HE, et al: Aortic valve replacement with stentless porcine aortic valves: a ten-year study. *J Heart Valve Dis* 1998; 7:250.
13. Doty JR, Flores JH, Millar RC, Doty DB: Aortic valve replacement with Medtronic Freestyle bioprosthesis: operative technique and results. *J Card Surg* 1998; 13:208.
14. Krause AH Jr: Technique for complete subcoronary implantation of the Medtronic Freestyle porcine bioprosthesis. *Ann Thorac Surg* 1997; 64:1495.
15. Pepper JR: The stentless porcine valve. *J Card Surg* 1998; 13:352.
16. Sintek CF, Fletcher AD, Khonsari S: Small aortic root in the elderly: use of stentless bioprosthesis. *J Heart Valve Dis* 1996; 5(suppl III):S308.
17. Westaby S, Amarasena N, Ormerod O, et al: Aortic valve replacement with the Freestyle stentless xenograft. *Ann Thorac Surg* 1995; 60:S422.
18. Flynn M, Iaccovoni A, Pathi V, et al: The aortic Elan stentless aortic valve: excellent hemodynamics and ease of implantation. Semin Thorac Cardiovasc Surg 2001; 13(4 suppl):48.

19. Huysmans H: Implanting the Freestyle bioprosthesis: root-inclusion technique: the Freestyle aortic root bioprosthesis implant technique monograph. Minneapolis, MN, Medtronic, Inc., 1997.
20. Kon ND, Westaby S, Amarasena N, et al: Comparison of implantation techniques using Freestyle stentless porcine aortic valve. *Ann Thorac Surg* 1995; 59:857.
21. Doty DB, Cafferty A, Cartier P, et al: Aortic valve replacement with Medtronic Freestyle bioprosthesis: 5-year results. *Semin Thorac Cardiovasc Surg* 1999; 2(suppl 1):35.
22. Doty DB, Cafferty A, Cartier P, et al: Aortic valve replacement with Medtronic Freestyle bioprosthesis: seven year results. Presentation at Medtronic Freestyle Valve Symposium, Salt Lake City, UT, May 18, 2001.
23. Doty DB, Cafferty A, Kon ND, et al: Medtronic Freestyle aortic root bioprosthesis: implant techniques. *J Card Surg* 1998; 13:369.
24. Dagenais F, Cartier P, Dumesnil JG, et al: A single center experience with the Freestyle bioprosthesis: midterm results at the Quebec Heart Institute. *Semin Thorac Cardiovasc Surg* 2001; 13(4 suppl):156.
25. Kappetein AP, Braun J, Baur LHB, et al: Outcome and follow-up of aortic valve replacement with the Freestyle stentless bioprosthesis. *Ann Thorac Surg* 2001; 71:691.
26. Cartier PC, Dumesnil JG, Metras J, et al: Clinical and hemodynamic performance of the Freestyle aortic root bioprosthesis. *Ann Thorac Surg* 1999; 67:345.
27. Kon ND, Cordell AR, Adair SM, et al: Aortic root replacement with the Freestyle stentless porcine aortic root bioprosthesis. *Ann Thorac Surg* 1999; 67:1609.
28. Westaby S, Jin XY, Katsumata T, et al: Valve replacement with a stentless bioprosthesis: versatility of the porcine aortic root. *J Thorac Cardiovasc Surg* 1998; 116:477.
29. Goldman BS, David TE, Wood JR, et al: Clinical outcomes after aortic valve replacement with the Toronto stentless porcine valve. *Ann Thorac Surg* 2001; 71:S302.
30. Sintek CF, Pfeffer TA, Kochamba GS, et al: Freestyle valve experience: technical considerations and mid-term results. *J Card Surg* 1998; 13:360.
31. Goldman B, Christakis G, David T, et al: Will stentless valves be durable? The Toronto Valve (TSPV) at 5 to 6 years. *Semin Thorac Cardiovasc Surg* 1999; 11:42.
32. Shargall Y, Goldman B, Christakis G, David T: Analysis of explants and causes of mortality during long-term follow-up of the Toronto stentless porcine valve. *Semin Thorac Cardiovasc Surg* 2001; 13(4 suppl):106.
33. Williams RJ, McLean AD, Pathi VL, et al: Six-year follow-up of the Toronto stentless porcine valve. *Semin Thorac Cardiovasc Surg* 2001; 13(4 suppl):168.
34. David TE, Feindel CM, Bos J, et al: Aortic valve replacement with a stentless porcine aortic valve. *J Thorac Cardiovasc Surg* 1994; 108:1030.
35. Gelsomino S, Frassani R, DaCol P, et al: The Cryolife-O'Brien stentless porcine aortic bioprosthesis: 5-year follow-up. *Ann Thorac Surg* 2001; 71:86.
36. Hvass U, Palatianos GM, Frassani R, et al: Multicenter study of stentless valve replacement in the small aortic root. *J Thorac Cardiovasc Surg* 1999; 117:267.
37. O'Brien MF, Gardner MAH, Garlick RB, et al: The Cryolife-O'Brien stentless aortic porcine xenograft valve. *J Card Surg* 1998; 13:376.
38. Jin XY, Ratnatunga C, Pillai R: Performance of Edwards prima stentless aortic valve over eight years. *Semin Thorac Cardiovasc Surg* 2001; 13(4 suppl):163.
39. Bortolotti U, Scioti G, Milano A, et al: The Edwards Prima stentless valve: hemodynamic performance at one year. *Ann Thorac Surg* 1999; 68:2147.
40. Jin XY, Dhital K, Bhattacharya K, et al: Fifth-year hemodynamic performance of the Prima stentless aortic valve. *Ann Thorac Surg* 1998; 66:805.
41. Dossche K, Vanermen H: Experience with the Edwards Prima stentless aortic bioprosthesis: a 2-year review. *J Heart Valve Dis* 1995; 4:S85.
42. Vrandecic M, Fantini FA, Filho BG, et al: Long-term results with the Biocor-SJM stentless porcine aortic bioprosthesis. *J Heart Valve Dis* 2002; 11:47.
43. Bertolini P, Luciani GB, Vecchi B, et al: Aortic valve replacement with the Biocor PSB stentless xenograft. *Ann Thorac Surg* 1998; 66:425.
44. Del Rizzo DF, Abdoh A: Clinical and hemodynamic comparison of the Medtronic Freestyle and Toronto SPV stentless valves. *J Card Surg* 1998; 13:398.
45. Legare JF, Wood JW, Koilpillai C, et al: St. Jude SPV versus Medtronic Freestyle: a single institution comparison of two stentless aortic valves. *J Card Surg* 1998; 13:392.
46. Bach DS, Goldman B, Verrier E, et al: Eight-year hemodynamic follow-up after aortic valve replacement with the Toronto SPV stentless aortic valve. *Semin Thorac Cardiovasc Surg* 2001; 13(suppl 1):173.
47. Barratt-Boyes BG, Christie GW: What is the best bioprosthetic operation for the small aortic root? Allograft, autograft, porcine or pericardial? Stented or unstented? *J Card Surg* 1994; 9:158.
48. Sintek CF, Fletcher AD, Khonsari S: Stentless porcine aortic root: valve of choice for the elderly patient with small aortic root. *J Thorac Cardiovasc Surg* 1995; 109:871.
49. Westaby S, Amarasena N, Long V, et al: Time-related hemodynamic changes after aortic replacement with the Freestyle stentless xenograft. *Ann Thorac Surg* 1995; 60:1633.
50. Del Rizzo DF, Goldman BS, Christakis GT, et al: Hemodynamic benefits of the Toronto stentless valve. *J Thorac Cardiovasc Surg* 1996; 112:1431.
51. Fries R, Wendler O, Schieffer H, et al: Comparative rest and exercise hemodynamics of 23-mm stentless versus 23-mm stented aortic bioprostheses. *Ann Thorac Surg* 2000; 69:817.
52. Nagy ZL, Fisher J, Walker PG, et al: The effect of sizing on the hydrodynamic parameters of the Medtronic Freestyle valve in vitro. *Ann Thorac Surg* 2000; 69:1408.
53. De Paulis R, Sommariva L, Colagrande L, et al: Regression of left ventricular hypertrophy after aortic valve replacement for aortic stenosis with different valve substitutes. *J Thorac Cardiovasc Surg* 1998; 116:590.
54. Walther T, Falk V, Langebartels G, et al: Regression of left ventricular hypertrophy after stentless versus conventional aortic valve replacement. *Semin Thorac Cardiovasc Surg* 1999; 11:18.
55. Maselli D, Pizio R, Bruno LP, et al: Left ventricular mass reduction after aortic valve replacement: homografts, stentless and stented valves. *Ann Thorac Surg* 1999; 67:966.
56. Jin XY, Zhang ZM, Gibson DG, et al: Effects of valve substitute on changes in left ventricular function and hypertrophy after aortic valve replacement. *Ann Thorac Surg* 1996; 62:683.
57. Bach DS: Echocardiographic assessment of stentless aortic bioprosthetic valves. *J Am Soc Echocardiogr* 2000; 13:941.
58. Bauer LHB, Jin XY, Houdas Y, et al: Echocardiographic parameters of the Freestyle stentless bioprosthesis in aortic position: the European experience. *J Am Soc Echocardiogr* 1999; 12:729.
59. Westaby S, Horton M, Jin XY, et al: Survival advantage of stentless aortic bioprostheses. *Ann Thorac Surg* 2000; 70:785.
60. Del Rizzo DF, Abdoh A, Cartier P, et al: Factors affecting left ventricular mass regression after aortic valve replacement with stentless valves. *Semin Thorac Cardiovasc Surg* 1999; 8:114.
61. Pibarot P, Dumesnil JG, Lemieux M, et al: Impact of prosthesis-patient mismatch on hemodynamic and symptomatic status,

morbidity and mortality after aortic valve replacement with a bioprosthetic heart valve. *J Heart Valve Dis* 1998; 7:211.

62. Dumesnil JG, Yoganathan AP: Valve prosthesis hemodynamics and the problem of high transprosthetic pressure gradients. *Eur J Cardiothorac Surg* 1992; 6(suppl I):S34.
63. David TE, Psuchmann R, Ivanov J, et al: Aortic valve replacement with stentless and stented porcine valves: a case-match study. *J Thorac Cardiovasc Surg* 1998; 116:236.
64. Rao V, Christakis GT, Sever J, et al: A novel comparison of stentless versus stented valves in the small aortic root. *J Thorac Cardiovasc Surg* 1999; 117:431.
65. Vrandecic M, Fantini FA, Filho BG, et al: Retrospective clinical analysis of stented vs. stentless porcine aortic bioprostheses. *Eur J Cardiothorac Surg* 2000; 18:46.
66. Cohen G, Christakis GT, Joyner CD, et al: Are stentless valves superior to stented valves? A prospective randomized trial. *Ann Thorac Surg* 2002; 73:676.
67. Gross C, Harringer W, Beran H, et al: Aortic valve replacement: is the stentless xenograft an alternative to the homograft? Midterm results. *Ann Thorac Surg* 1999; 68:919.
68. Kon ND, Cordell AR, Adair SM, et al: Comparison of results using "Freestyle" stentless porcine aortic root bioprosthesis with cryopreserved aortic allograft. *Semin Thorac Cardiovasc Surg* 1999; 11:69.
69. Rajappan K, Melina G, Bellenger NG, et al: Evaluation of left ventricular function and mass after Medtronic Freestyle versus homograft aortic root replacement using cardiovascular magnetic resonance. *J Heart Valve Dis* 2002; 11:60.
70. Riley RD, Hammon JW Jr, Adair SM, et al: Stentless aortic valve replacement with Freestyle or Toronto SPV: an early comparison. *Ann Thoracic Surg* 2000; 70:48.
71. Luciani GB, Bertolini P, Vecchi B, et al: Midterm results after aortic valve replacement with freehand stentless xenografts: a comparison of three prostheses. *J Thorac Cardiovasc Surg* 1998; 115:1287.

Part ***IVb***

Valvular Heart Disease: Mitral Valve Disease

Chapter 36

Pathophysiology of Mitral Valve Disease

James I. Fann/Neil B. Ingels, Jr./D. Craig Miller

THE NORMAL MITRAL VALVE

Anatomy

The mitral annulus is a pliable junctional zone of fibrous and muscular tissue joining the left atrium and ventricle that anchors the hinge portion of the anterior and posterior mitral leaflets.[1–11] The annulus has two major collagenous structures: (1) the right fibrous trigone, which is part of the central fibrous body and is located at the intersection of the atrioventricular membranous septum, the mitral and tricuspid valves, and the aortic root; and (2) the left fibrous trigone at the junction of the mitral valve and left coronary cusp of the aortic valve (Fig. 36-1). The anterior mitral leaflet spans the distance between the commissures (including the trigones) and is in direct fibrous continuity with most of the left and noncoronary aortic valve cusps. Fine tendon-like collagen bundles, the fila of Henle, extend out circumferentially from each fibrous trigone a variable distance towards the corresponding side of the mitral orifice. The posterior one half to two thirds of the annulus, which subtends the posterior leaflet, is primarily muscular with little or no fibrous tissue.[10] This muscle is arranged mainly perpendicularly to the annulus, but a less prominent group of muscle fibers is arranged parallel to the annulus.

The mitral valve has two major leaflets, the much larger anterior (or aortic) leaflet and the smaller posterior (or mural) leaflet; the latter usually contains three (or sometimes more) scallops separated by fetal clefts or "subcommissures," which are developed to variable degrees in different individuals.[12] The central portions of the leaflets on the atrial surface are termed the *rough zone*, with the remainder of the free edge leaflet surface being the *bare, membranous, smooth,* or *clear zone*. The ratio of the height of the rough zone to the height of the clear zone is 0.6 for the anterior leaflet and 1.4 for the posterior leaflet, as the clear zone on the posterior scallops is only about 2 mm high.[12] The two leaflets are separated at the annulus by the posteromedial and anterolateral commissures, which are usually distinctly developed.

The histologic structure of the leaflets includes three layers: (1) the fibrosa, the solid collagenous core that is continuous with the chordae tendineae; (2) the spongiosa, which covers the atrial aspect and forms the leaflet leading edge (it consists of few collagen fibers but has abundant proteoglycans, elastin, and mixed connective tissue cells);

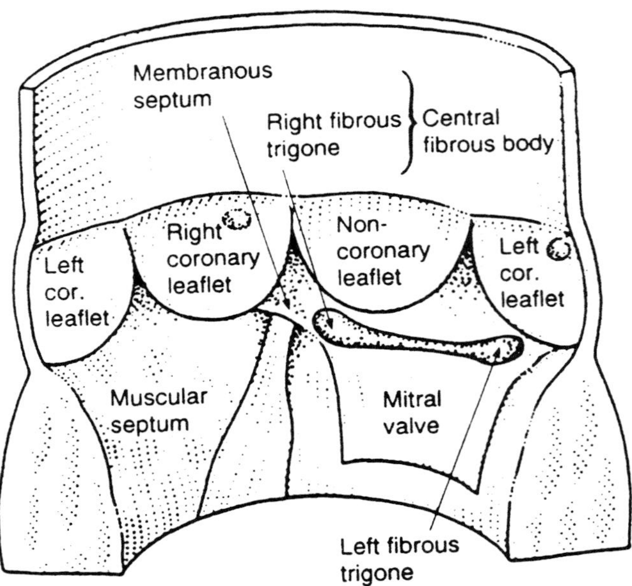

FIGURE 36–1 Diagram from a pathological perspective with division of the septum illustrating the fibrous continuity between the mitral and aortic valves. *(Reproduced with permission from Anderson RH, Wilcox BR: The anatomy of the mitral valve, in Wells FC, Shapiro LM (eds): Mitral Valve Disease. Oxford, England, Butterworth-Heinemann, 1996; p 4.)*

and (3) a thin fibroelastic covering of most of the leaflets.[10] On the atrial aspect of both leaflets, this surface (the *atrialis*) is rich in elastin. The ventricular side of the fibroelastic cover (the *ventricularis*) is much thicker; it is confined mostly to the anterior leaflet and is densely packed with elastin. The fibroelastic layers become thickened with advanced age due to elaboration of more elastin and collagen formation; similar accelerated changes also accompany the progression of myxomatous (or degenerative or "floppy") mitral valvular disease. In addition to these complex connective tissue structures, the mitral leaflets contain myocardium, smooth muscle, contractile interstitial cells, and blood vessels, as well as both adrenergic and cholinergic afferent and efferent nerves.[13–19] Leaflet contractile tissue is neurally controlled and may play a role in mitral valve function.[6,16–25] The atrial surface of the anterior leaflet exhibits a depolarizing spike shortly before the onset of the QRS complex, and the resulting contraction of leaflet muscle, along with contraction of smooth muscle and interstitial cells, possibly aids leaflet coaptation before the onset of systole, as well as stiffens the leaflet in response to rising left ventricular (LV) pressure.[16–19,24,26–29] Mitral leaflet stretch of 10% or more also leads to an action potential that initiates leaflet muscle contraction.[28]

Annular Size, Shape, and Dynamics

The average mitral annulus cross-sectional area ranges from 5.0 to 11.4 cm^2 in normal human hearts (average is 7.6 cm^2).[30] The annular perimeter of the posterior leaflet is longer than that subtending the anterior leaflet by a 2:1 ratio; i.e., the posterior annulus circumscribes about two thirds of the mitral annulus.[12] Annular area varies during the cardiac cycle and is influenced directly by both left atrial and LV size and pressure.[4,31] The magnitude of change in mitral annular area is in the 20% to 40% range.[4,8,9,31–38] Annular size increases beginning in late systole and continues through isovolumic relaxation and into diastole; maximal annular area occurs in late diastole around the time of the P wave on the electrocardiogram.[4,8,33,35,36,39] Importantly, one half to two thirds of the total decrease in annular area may occur during atrial contraction (thereby actually being *presystolic*); this component of annular area change is smaller when the PR interval is short, and is completely abolished when atrial fibrillation is present or ventricular pacing is employed. Annular area decreases further (if LV end-diastolic volume is not abnormally elevated) to a minimum in early to mid systole.[4,7,8,31,33]

The human mitral annulus is roughly elliptical (or D- or kidney-shaped), with greater eccentricity (i.e., being less circular) in systole than in diastole.[3,4,8,30,31,35,37,40] In its most elliptical configuration, the ratio of minor to major diameters is approximately 0.75. In three-dimensional space, the annulus is somewhat saddle-shaped (or, more precisely, a hyperbolic paraboloid), with the highest point (i.e., farthest from the LV apex) located anteriorly; this point is termed the "fibrosa" or the "saddle horn" in the echocardiography literature, is located in the middle of the anterior annulus, and is readily identified in echocardiographic images due to the common surface it shares with the aortic valve. The low points are located posteromedially and anterolaterally near the commissures, and another less prominent high point is located directly posterior.[4,41,42] During the cardiac cycle, annular regions adjacent to the posterior leaflet (where the leaflet attaches directly to the atrial and ventricular endocardium) move toward (during systole) and away from (during diastole) the relatively immobile anterior annulus.[4,37] Certain annular segments located near the left fibrous trigone (or area of aortic-mitral continuity), however, may actually lengthen slightly during LV ejection, at least in canine and ovine hearts.[43]

The mitral annulus moves upward into the left atrium in diastole and toward the LV apex during systole; the duration, average rate, and magnitude of annular displacement correlate with (and perhaps influence) the rate of left atrial filling and emptying.[4,8,33,36,44,45] The annulus moves little during late diastole (2 to 4 mm toward the left atrium during atrial systole). This movement does not occur in the presence of atrial fibrillation and thus may be an atriogenic contractile property. The annulus moves a greater distance (3 to 16 mm toward the LV apex) during isovolumic contraction and ventricular ejection. This systolic motion, which subsequently aids left atrial filling, occurs in the presence or absence of atrial fibrillation and is related to the extent of ventricular emptying; thus it is likely driven by LV contraction.[4,8,35,36,44–50] Subsequently, the annulus moves very little during isovolumic relaxation but then exhibits rapid recoil back toward the left atrium in early diastole. This recoiling increases the net velocity of mitral inflow by as much as 20%.[9,36]

Dynamic Leaflet Motion

The posterior mitral leaflet is attached to thinner chordae tendineae than the anterior leaflet, and its motion is restrained by chordae during both systole and diastole.[12,44] Regions of both leaflets are concave toward the left ventricle during systole,[51–53] but leaflet shape is complex and some regional anterior leaflet curvature may actually be convex to the left ventricle during systole.[39,41,42] Leaflet opening does not start with the free margin but rather in the center of the leaflet; leaflet curvature initially flattens and then becomes reversed (making the leaflet convex toward the left ventricle) while the edges are still approximated.[39,52,53] The leading edge then moves into the left ventricle (like a traveling wave), and the leaflet straightens. The leaflet edges in the middle of the valve appear to separate before those portions closer to the commissures, and posterior leaflet opening occurs approximately 8 to 40 milliseconds later.[53–55] Once reaching maximum opening, the edges exhibit a slow to-and-fro movement (like a flag flapping in a breeze) until another less forceful opening impulse occurs, associated with the *a* wave. During late diastole, the leaflets move gradually away from the LV wall.

Valve closure starts with the leaflet bulging toward the atrium at its attachment point to the annulus. The closure rate of the anterior leaflet is almost twice that of the posterior leaflet, thereby ensuring arrival of both cusps at their closed positions simultaneously (since the anterior leaflet is opened more widely than the posterior leaflet at the onset of ventricular systole).[55] The anterior leaflet actually arrives at the plane of the annulus in a bulged shape (concave to the ventricle), but as the closing movement proceeds and the leaflet ascends toward the atrium, this curvature appears to run through the whole leaflet, from the annulus toward the edge, in a rolling manner. The leaflet edge is the last part of the leaflet to approach the annular plane. Leaflet curvature is more pronounced with the onset of systolic ejection.[52,53]

Mitral valve closure is completed 10 to 40 milliseconds after the initial systolic rise of LV pressure, but, surprisingly, leaflet opening motion may actually precede the diastolic pressure crossover point by up to 60 milliseconds.[53,56,57] While the onset of mitral valve closure at the end of diastole appears to be initiated by atrial contraction, competent leaflet closure requires an increase in ventricular pressure above that in the atrium (irrespective of whether or not a normal atrial electrical and mechanical sequence is present) and a proper valve annular size to permit apposition of the valve leaflets at the onset of and during ventricular ejection.[16,31,55]

Chordae Tendineae and Papillary Muscles

Epicardial fibers in the left ventricle descend from the base of the heart and proceed inward at the apex to form the two papillary muscles, which are characterized by vertically oriented myocardial fibers.[11,58] The anterolateral papillary muscle usually has one major head and is a more prominent structure; the posteromedial papillary muscle can have two or more subheads and is flatter.[12] A loop from the papillary muscles to the mitral annulus is completed by the chordae tendineae continuing into the mitral leaflets, which are then attached to the annular ring. The distance from the tip of the human papillary muscle to its corresponding mitral annulus averages 23.5 mm from the tip of the anterolateral papillary muscle to the left trigone, and 23.2 mm to the point between the anterior and middle scallops of the posterior leaflet.[59] The distance from the tip of the posteromedial papillary muscle to the right trigone is 23.5 mm and to the annular point between the middle and posteromedial scallops of the posterior leaflet is 23.5 mm. The posteromedial papillary muscle is usually supplied by the right coronary artery (or a dominant left circumflex artery in 10% of cases); the anterolateral papillary muscle is supplied by both the left anterior descending and circumflex coronary arteries.[11,60,61]

The posteromedial and anterolateral papillary muscles give rise to chordae tendineae going to both leaflets (Fig. 36-2).[12] The chordae are classically and functionally divided into three groups.[11,62] First-order chordae originate near the papillary muscle tips, divide progressively, and insert on the leading edge of the leaflets; these primary chordae prevent valve edge prolapse during systole. The second-order chordae (including two or more larger and less branched "strut" chordae) originate from the same location and tend to be thicker and fewer in number[12,62]; they insert on the ventricular surface of the leaflets at the junction of the rough and clear zones, which is demarcated by a ridge corresponding to the line of leaflet coaptation. The second-order chordae (including the strut chordae) serve to anchor the valve and are more prominent on the anterior leaflet; second-order chordae may also arborize from large chordae that go to the leaflet free edge (first-order chordae). The third-order chordae, also called tertiary or basal chordae, originate directly from the trabeculae carnae of the ventricular wall, attach to the posterior leaflet near the annulus, and can be identified by their fan-shaped patterns.[62] Additionally, distinct commissural chordae and cleft chordae exist in the commissures. Chordae contain nerve fibers, and some chordae, considered to be immature forms, may contain muscle tissue.[17] In total, about 25 major chordal trunks (range 15 to 32) arise from the papillary muscles in humans, equally divided between those going to the anterior and posterior leaflets[62]; on the other end, over 100 smaller individual chordae attach to the leaflets.

During diastole, the papillary muscles form an inflow tract; during systole, they create an outflow tract, which

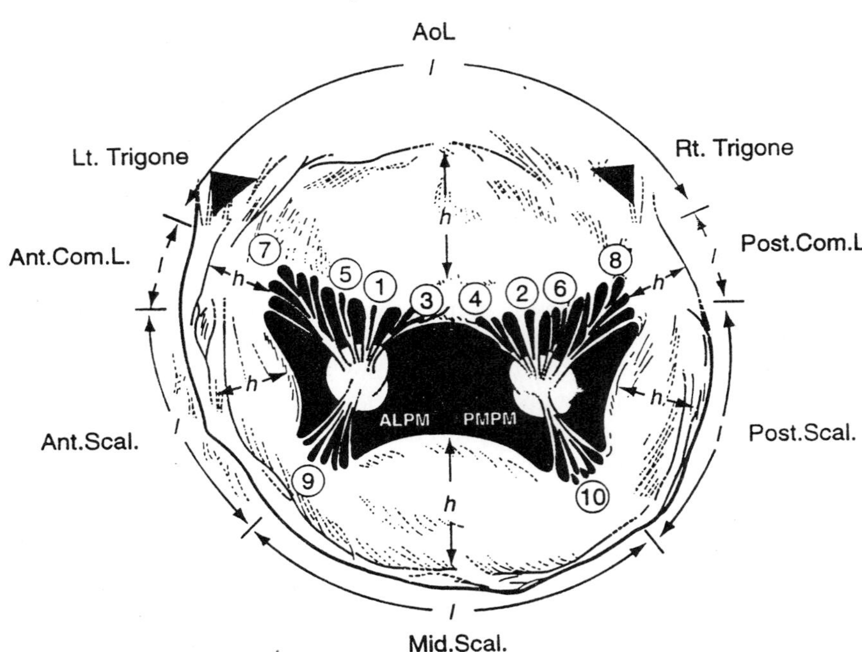

FIGURE 36–2 Mitral valve and subvalvular apparatus. Anterolateral papillary muscle (ALPM); posteromedial papillary muscle (PMPM); aortic leaflet (AoL); anterior commissural leaflet (Ant.Com.L.); posterior commissural leaflet (Post.Com.L.); anterior scallop (Ant.Scal.); middle scallop (Mid.Scal.); height of leaflet (*h*); length of attachment of leaflet (l) l posterior scallop (Post.Scal.); right fibrous trigone (Rt.Trigone); left fibrous trigone (Lt.Trigone); anterior main chorda (1); posterior main chorda (2); anterior paramedial chorda (3); posterior paramedial chorda (4); anterior paracommissural chorda (5); posterior paracommissural chorda (6); anterior commissural chorda (7); posterior commissural chorda (8); anterior cleft chorda (9); and posterior cleft chorda (10). (*Reproduced with permission from Sakai T, Okita Y, Ueda Y, et al: Distance between mitral annulus and papillary muscles: anatomic study in normal human hearts. J Thorac Cardiovasc Surg 1999; 118: 636.*)

later becomes obliterated due to systolic thickening of the papillary muscles and augments LV ejection by volume displacement.[58] The contribution of the papillary muscles to LV chamber volume is 5% to 8% during diastole, but 15% to 30% during systole.[58,63] The anterior and posterior papillary muscles contract simultaneously; they are innervated by sympathetic and parasympathetic (vagal) nerves.[64,65]

Previous analyses of papillary muscle function during the cardiac cycle yielded widely discordant results.[64,66–70] Although the papillary muscles shorten at some point during systole (by upwards of one fourth of their maximum length),[66,69,71–74] some suggest that this contraction may be isometric or substantially less than that of the LV free wall fibers.[68,74] In addition, there is no consensus as to the exact

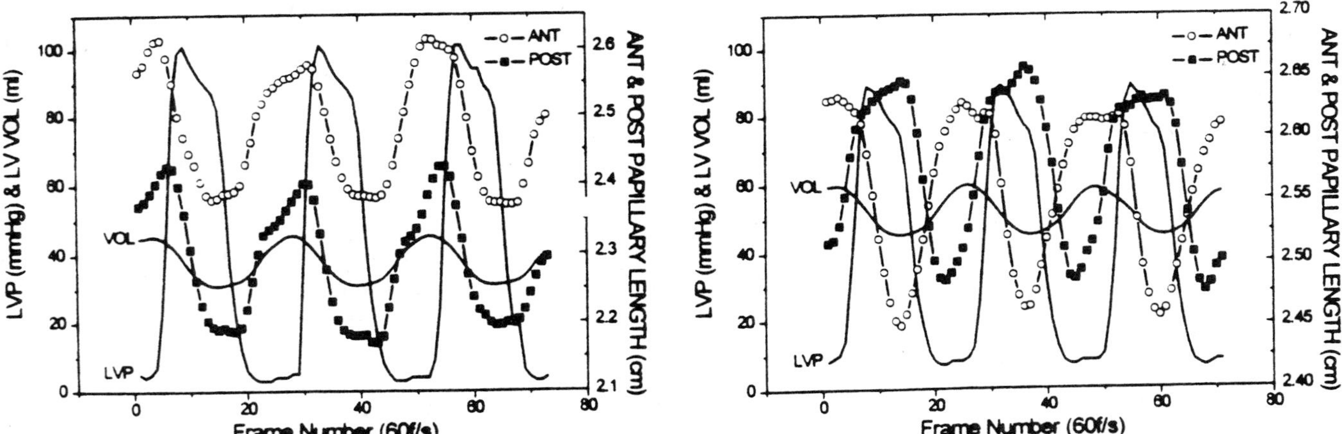

FIGURE 36–3 Graphs showing typical dynamics of the left ventricle and papillary muscles from a control run (left panel) and 2 minutes after left circumflex coronary artery occlusion (right panel). In the left panel, papillary muscle lengths are temporally related closely to changes in LV volume (LV VOL). In the right panel, the dynamics of the ischemic posterior papillary muscle are markedly different and more closely track changes in LV pressure (LVP). ANT, anterior papillary muscle; POST, posterior papillary muscle. (*Reproduced with permission from Rayhill SC, Daughters GT, Castro LJ, et al: Dynamics of normal and ischemic canine papillary muscles. Circ Res 1994; 74:1179.*)

timing of papillary muscle contraction and elongation during the cardiac cycle.[64–67,69,70,72,73] Some suggest that papillary muscles contract before the LV free wall so that the mitral valve leaflets are supported during early LV ejection[70]; others, however, report that papillary muscles lengthen during isovolumic contraction and shorten during ejection as well as during isovolumic relaxation.[65,67,69] From the standpoint of electromechanics, although papillary muscle excitation occurs simultaneously with the rest of the endocardial surface of the ventricle, the papillary muscles may contract just after the onset of LV contraction.[64,72] Maximal shortening and elongation of the papillary muscle may follow thickening and thinning of an adjacent LV free wall segment.[72,73] Papillary muscle shortening throughout isovolumic relaxation may play a role in opening the mitral valve, and elongation in late diastole may be necessary to permit proper valve closure.[72]

In the experimental setting, it has been shown that both papillary muscles closely mimic general LV dynamics; i.e., the papillary muscles shorten during ejection, lengthen during diastole, and change length minimally during the isovolumic periods (Fig. 36-3).[66] These findings suggest that earlier studies purporting papillary muscle lengthening during isovolumic contraction and shortening during isovolumic relaxation may have been confounded by some form of myocardial injury or surgical trauma.[66]

MITRAL STENOSIS

Etiology

Mitral stenosis is generally the result of rheumatic heart disease.[75–81] Nonrheumatic causes of mitral stenosis or LV inflow obstruction include severe mitral annular and/or leaflet calcification, congenital mitral valve deformities, malignant carcinoid syndrome, neoplasm, left atrial thrombus, endocarditic vegetations, certain inherited metabolic diseases, and causes related to a previous commissurotomy or implanted prosthetic valve (Fig. 36-4).[79–83] A definite history of rheumatic fever can be obtained in only about 50% to 60% of patients; women are affected more often than men by a 2:1 to 3:1 ratio. Nearly always acquired before age 20, rheumatic valvular disease becomes clinically evident one to three decades later.

Approximately 20 million cases of rheumatic fever occur in third world countries annually, with a correspondingly high incidence of advanced mitral stenosis later in life.[84] In the United States, Western Europe, and other developed countries, the frequency of mitral stenosis has decreased markedly. The etiologic agent for acute rheumatic fever is group A beta-hemolytic streptococcus, but the specific immunologic and inflammatory mechanisms leading to the valvulitis are unknown.[84] Streptococcal antigens cross-react with human tissues and may stimulate or modify immunologic responses. Differences in the cellular and extracellular

Normal mitral valve

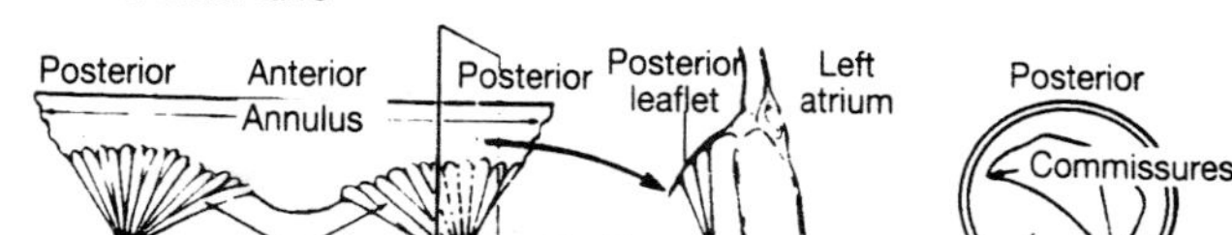

Rheumatic

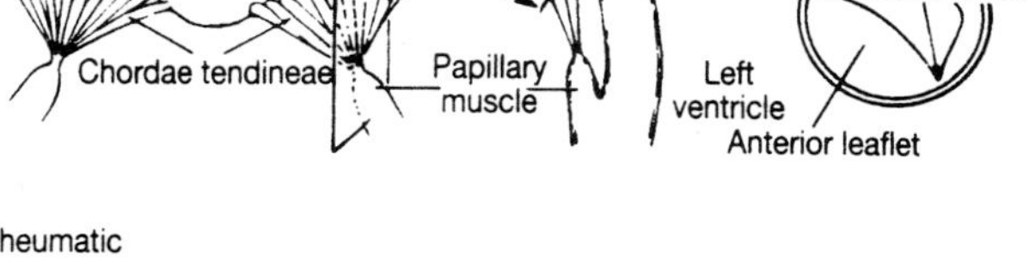

Active infective endocarditis (massive obstructing vegetation)

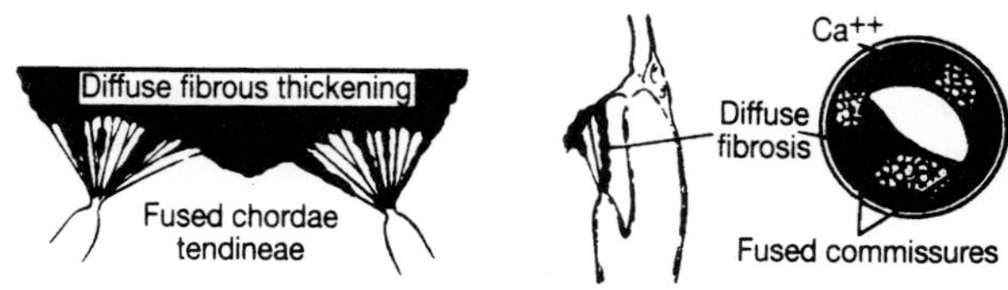

Massive annular calcium

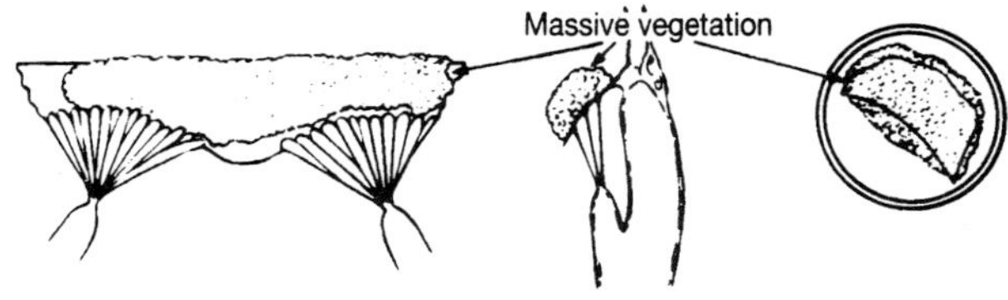

Congenital "parachute" (single papillary muscle)

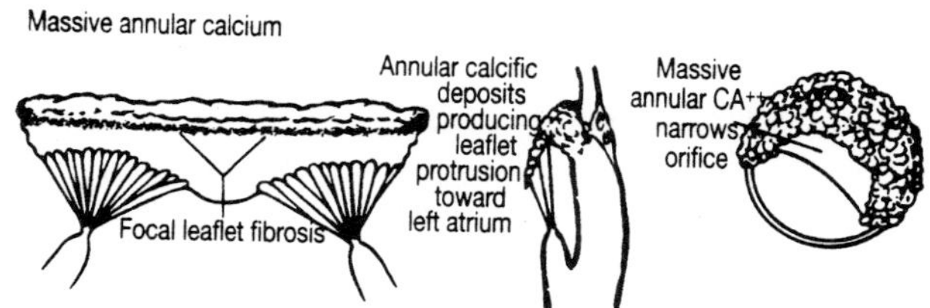

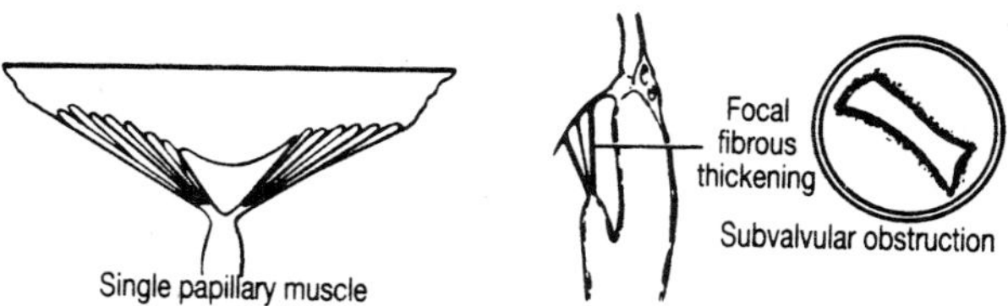

FIGURE 36–4 Diagrams demonstrating causes of mitral stenosis, including rheumatic heart disease, active infective endocarditis, massive mitral annular calcification, and congenital single papillary muscle syndrome. (*Modified from Waller BF, Howard J, Fess S: Pathology of mitral valve stenosis and pure mitral regurgitation, part I. Clin Cardiol 17:330, 1994. Copyrighted and reprinted with the permission of Clinical Cardiology Publishing Company, Inc., and/or the Foundation for Advances in Medicine and Science, Inc., Mahwah, NJ 07430-0832, USA.*)

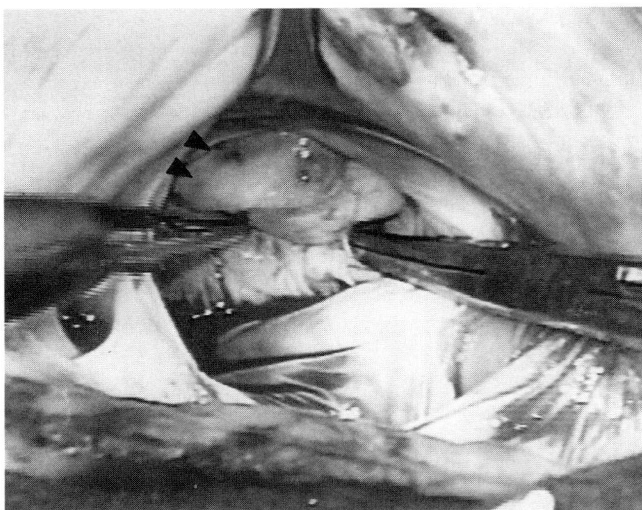

FIGURE 36–5 Intraoperative photograph of mitral stenosis as a result of rheumatic heart disease. The mitral leaflets are markedly restricted. The arrowheads point to the anterior leaflet near the anterolateral commissure.

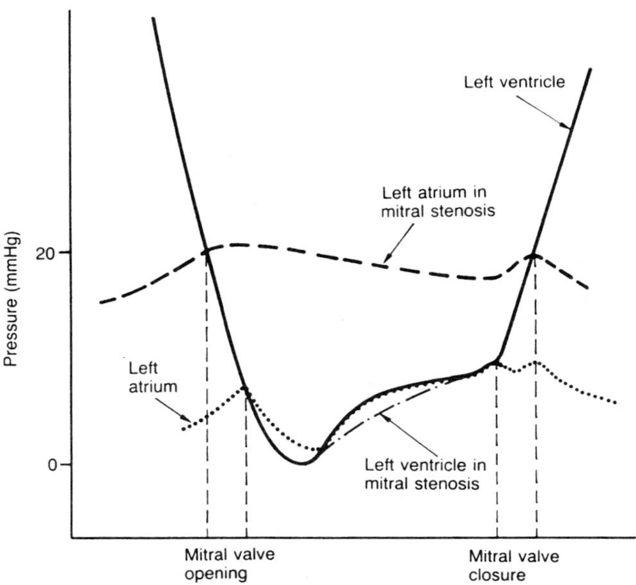

FIGURE 36–6 Left ventricular and left atrial pressures in mitral stenosis. The higher left atrial pressure results in earlier opening and later closure of the mitral valve. The left ventricular diastolic pressure in mitral stenosis rises slowly because of the absence of a rapid filling wave. (*Reproduced with permission from Schofield PM: Invasive investigation of the mitral valve, in Wells FC, Shapiro LM (eds): Mitral Valve Disease. Oxford, England, Butterworth-Heinemann, 1996; p 84.*)

proteins in the many strains of group A streptococcus may be important in the development of rheumatic heart disease. Components implicated in the organism's virulence include the hyaluronic acid capsule and the serotype of the antigenic capsular M protein, which resists phagocytosis and opsonization.[84] Along with the individual's immunologic responsiveness, other genetic factors are likely to be involved in the susceptibility to disease development or progression.

In addition to affecting the cardiac valves, rheumatic heart disease is a pancarditis affecting to various degrees the endocardium, myocardium, and pericardium (Fig. 36-5).[75,77,78] In rheumatic valvulitis, mitral valve involvement is the most common (isolated mitral stenosis is found in 40% of cases), followed by combined aortic and mitral valve disease, and, least frequently, isolated aortic valve disease. Pathoanatomic changes characteristic of mitral valvulitis include commissural fusion, leaflet fibrosis with stiffening and retraction, and chordal fusion and shortening.[77] Leaflet stiffening and fibrosis can be exacerbated over time by increased flow turbulence. Valvular regurgitation can develop due to chordal fusion and shortening. The chordae tendineae may become so retracted that the leaflets appear to insert directly into the papillary muscles. The degree of calcification varies; it is more common and of greater severity in men, older patients, and those with a higher transvalvular gradient.[78] In some cases, rheumatic myocarditis results in cardiac dilation and progressive heart failure.

Mitral annular calcification may progress to mitral sclerosis and eventually stenosis in elderly patients.[76,83] The anterior leaflet can becomes thick and immobile; LV inflow obstruction also results from calcification of the posterior mitral valve leaflet. Calcific protrusions into the ventricle and extension of the calcium into the leaflets further narrow the valve orifice resulting in mitral stenosis.[83] In these cases, the left ventricle is typically small, hypertrophied, and noncompliant.

Hemodynamics

In patients with mitral stenosis, an early, mid-, and late diastolic transvalvular gradient is present between the left atrium and ventricle, and as the degree of mitral stenosis worsens, a progressively higher gradient, especially late in diastole, occurs (Fig. 36-6).[79,85–87] The average left atrial pressure in patients with severe mitral stenosis may be in the range of 15 to 20 mm Hg at rest, with a mean transvalvular gradient of 10 to 15 mm Hg.[85,87] With exercise, the left atrial pressure and gradient rise substantially. LV end-diastolic pressure is usually normal.

Another physiological measurement in patients with mitral stenosis is the (derived) cross-sectional valve area, which is calculated from the mean transvalvular pressure gradient and cardiac output. The transvalvular pressure gradient is a function of the square of the transvalvular flow rate; for instance, doubling the flow quadruples the gradient. At a given flow rate, a smaller valve area corresponds to a higher pressure gradient. Mitral transvalvular flow depends on cardiac output and heart rate. An increase in heart rate decreases the duration of transvalvular LV filling during diastole, thereby reducing forward cardiac output; the transvalvular mean gradient increases and, consequently, so does left atrial pressure.[86,88] A high transvalvular gradient may be associated with a normal cardiac output; conversely, if cardiac output is low, only a modest transvalvular gradient may be present.

Because of effective atrial contraction, the mean left atrial pressure in patients with mitral stenosis and normal sinus rhythm is lower compared to that of patients in atrial fibrillation.[89,90] Sinus rhythm further augments flow through the stenotic valve, thereby helping to maintain adequate forward cardiac output. The development of atrial fibrillation decreases cardiac output by 20% or more; atrial fibrillation with a rapid ventricular response can lead to acute dyspnea and pulmonary edema.[75,89,90]

Ventricular Adaptation

In patients with isolated mitral stenosis and restricted LV inflow, LV chamber size (end-diastolic volume) is normal or decreased, and the end-diastolic pressure is typically low.[79,91,92] The peak filling rate is reduced, as is stroke volume. Cardiac output is thus diminished as a result of inflow obstruction rather than LV pump failure.[93] LV mass is normal or slightly subnormal in the majority of these patients.[91] During exercise, the ejection fraction may increase slightly; however, LV filling is compromised by the shorter diastolic periods at higher heart rates, resulting in a smaller end-diastolic volume (or LV preload). Therefore, stroke volume and a blunted increase (or even decrease) in cardiac output can occur.[92]

Approximately 25% to 50% of patients with severe mitral stenosis have LV systolic dysfunction as a consequence of associated diseases (e.g., mitral regurgitation, aortic valve disease, ischemic heart disease, rheumatic myocarditis or pancarditis, and myocardial fibrosis).[78,87,92] In these patients, LV end-systolic and end-diastolic volumes may be larger than normal. Also, because right ventricular afterload increases as pulmonary hypertension develops in these patients, right ventricular systolic performance deteriorates.[79,94] Clinically, however, increased right ventricular afterload as a result of mitral stenosis is usually associated with normal right ventricular contractility.[79]

Atrial Adaptation

In patients with mitral stenosis who are in normal sinus rhythm, the left atrial pressure tracing is characterized by an elevated mean left atrial pressure with a prominent *a* wave, which is followed by a gradual pressure decline.[75,90] The *a* wave pressure largely reflects the kinetic energy dissipated in overcoming the resistance across the valve. Because of the stenotic valve, coordinated left atrial contraction is important in maintaining transvalvular flow.[90] The high left atrial pressure gradually leads to left atrial hypertrophy and dilation, atrial fibrillation, and atrial mural thrombi formation.[78,92,95] The degree of left atrial enlargement and fibrosis does not correlate with the severity of the valvular stenosis, partly because of the marked variation in duration of the stenotic lesion and atrial involvement by the underlying rheumatic inflammatory process.[92] Disorganization of atrial muscle fibers is associated with abnormal conduction velocities and inhomogeneous refractory periods. Premature atrial activation due to increased automaticity or reentry eventually may lead to atrial fibrillation, which is present in over one half of patients with either pure mitral stenosis or mixed mitral stenosis and regurgitation.[95,96] Major determinants of atrial fibrillation in patients with rheumatic heart disease include older age and larger left atrial diameter.[95]

Pulmonary Changes

In patients with mild to moderate mitral stenosis, pulmonary vascular resistance is not increased, and pulmonary arterial pressure may remain normal at rest, rising only with exertion or increased heart rate.[85] In severe chronic mitral stenosis with elevated pulmonary vascular resistance, pulmonary arterial pressure is elevated at rest and can approach systemic pressure with exercise. A pulmonary arterial systolic pressure greater than 60 mm Hg significantly elevates impedance to right ventricular emptying and produces high right ventricular end-diastolic and right atrial pressures.

Left atrial hypertension produces pulmonary vasoconstriction, which exacerbates the elevated pulmonary vascular resistance.[78,94] As the mean left atrial pressure exceeds 30 mm Hg above oncotic pressure, transudation of fluid into the pulmonary interstitium occurs, leading to reduced lung compliance. Pulmonary hypertension develops as a result of passive transmission of high left atrial pressure, pulmonary venous hypertension, pulmonary arteriolar constriction, and, eventually, pulmonary vascular obliterative changes. Early changes in the pulmonary vascular bed may be considered protective in that the elevated pulmonary vascular resistance protects the pulmonary capillary bed from excessively high pressures; however, the pulmonary hypertension progressively worsens, leading to right-sided heart failure, tricuspid insufficiency, and occasionally pulmonic valve insufficiency.[79,94] Severe mitral stenosis ultimately causes irreversible pulmonary vascular changes; cardiac output is low at rest and remains subnormal during exercise.[85]

Clinical Evaluation

Because of the gradual development of mitral stenosis, patients may remain asymptomatic for many years.[75,85,96] Characteristic symptoms of mitral stenosis eventually develop and are associated primarily with pulmonary venous congestion or low cardiac output, e.g., dyspnea on exertion, orthopnea, or paroxysmal nocturnal dyspnea and fatigue.

Dyspnea is often precipitated by events that elevate left atrial pressure, such as physical or emotional stress or atrial fibrillation. In patients with mild mitral stenosis, symptoms usually occur only with extreme exertion. With progressive stenosis (valve area between 1 and 2 cm^2), patients become symptomatic with less effort. When mitral valve area decreases to about 1 cm^2, symptoms become more pronounced. As pulmonary hypertension and right-sided heart failure subsequently develop, signs of tricuspid regurgitation, hepatomegaly, edema, and ascites can be found.

As a result of high left atrial pressure and increased pulmonary blood volume in the early phases of the disease, hemoptysis may develop secondary to rupture of dilated bronchial veins (or submucosal varices).[75,94] Over time, pulmonary vascular resistance increases and the likelihood of hemoptysis decreases. Hemoptysis also may result from pulmonary infarction, which is a late complication of chronic heart failure. Acute pulmonary edema with pink frothy sputum can occur due to rupture of alveolar capillaries.

Systemic thromboembolism, occurring in approximately 20% of cases, may be the first symptom of mitral stenosis; recurrent embolization occurs in 25% of patients.[75,97,98] The incidence of thromboembolic events is higher in patients with mitral stenosis or mixed mitral stenosis–regurgitation than in those with pure mitral regurgitation. At least 40% of all clinically important embolic events involve the cerebral circulation, approximately 15% involve the visceral vessels, and 15% affect the lower extremities.[75,99] Embolization to coronary arteries may lead to angina, arrhythmias, or myocardial infarction; renal embolization can result in hypertension.[75] Factors that increase the risk of thromboembolic events include low cardiac output, left atrial dilation, atrial fibrillation, left atrial thrombus, absence of tricuspid or aortic regurgitation, and the presence of echocardiographic "smoke," an indicator of stagnant flow. Patients with these risk factors should be anticoagulated.[75,97–99] If an episode of systemic embolization occurs in patients in sinus rhythm, infective endocarditis, which is more common in mild than in severe mitral stenosis, should be considered.

Patients with chronic mitral stenosis are often thin and frail (cardiac cachexia), indicative of long-standing low cardiac output, congestive heart failure, and inanition.[75] The peripheral arterial pulse is generally normal, except in patients with a decreased LV stroke volume, in which case the pulse amplitude is diminished. Heart size is usually normal, with a normal apical impulse on chest palpation. An apical diastolic thrill may be present. In patients with pulmonary hypertension, a right ventricular lift can be felt in the left parasternal region. Auscultatory findings include a presystolic murmur, an increased first sound, an opening snap, and an apical diastolic rumble.[75,100–102] The presystolic murmur, which occurs due to closing of the anterior mitral leaflet, is a consistent finding and begins earlier in those in sinus rhythm compared with patients in atrial fibrillation.[102] The first heart sound (S_1) is accentuated in mitral stenosis when the leaflets are pliable, but diminished in later phases of the disease when the leaflets are thickened or calcified. As pulmonary artery pressure becomes elevated, S_2 becomes prominent.[103] With progressive pulmonary hypertension, the normal splitting of S_2 narrows because of reduced pulmonary vascular compliance. Other signs of pulmonary hypertension include a murmur of tricuspid and/or pulmonic regurgitation and an S_4 originating from the right ventricle. Best heard at the apex, the early diastolic mitral opening snap is due to sudden tensing of the pliable leaflets during valve opening and is absent when the leaflets are rigid or immobile.[75,100,101] In mild mitral stenosis, the diastolic murmur is soft and of short duration; a long or holo-diastolic murmur indicates severe mitral stenosis. The intensity of the murmur does not necessarily correlate with the severity of the stenosis; indeed, no diastolic murmur may be detectable in patients with severe stenosis, calcified leaflets, or low cardiac output.[102]

On chest radiography, left atrial enlargement is the earliest change found in patients with mitral stenosis; it is suggested by posterior bulging of the left atrium seen on the lateral view, a double contour of the right heart border seen on the posteroanterior film, and elevation of the left mainstem bronchus.[76,85,104] The overall cardiac size is often normal. Prominence of the pulmonary arteries coupled with left atrial enlargement may obliterate the normal concavity between the aorta and left ventricle to produce a straight left heart border. In the lung fields, pulmonary congestion may be recognized as distension of the pulmonary arteries and veins in the upper lung fields and pleural effusions. If mitral stenosis is severe, engorged pulmonary lymphatics are seen as distinct horizontal linear opacities in the lower lung fields (Kerley B lines).

The electrocardiogram is not accurate in assessing the severity of mitral stenosis and in many cases may be completely normal. In patients with severe mitral stenosis and in normal sinus rhythm, left atrial enlargement is the earliest change (a wide notched P wave in lead II and a biphasic P wave in lead V_1).[85,105] Atrial arrhythmias are more common in patients with advanced degrees of mitral stenosis. In those with pulmonary hypertension, right ventricular hypertrophy may develop and is associated with right-axis deviation, a tall R wave in V_1, and secondary ST-T wave changes; however, the electrocardiogram is not a sensitive indicator of right ventricular hypertrophy or the degree of pulmonary hypertension.[105] Because multivalvular disease may be present in patients with rheumatic heart disease, signs of left and right ventricular hypertrophy can be identified on the electrocardiogram in cases of combined mitral and aortic stenosis. Right atrial enlargement and right ventricular dilation and hypertrophy, however, also can mask the changes indicative of LV hypertrophy on the electrocardiographic tracing in patients with multivalvular disease.[105]

Echocardiography has become the primary noninvasive technique for assessing mitral valve pathology and pathophysiology.[76,106–109] Cross-sectional valve area and left

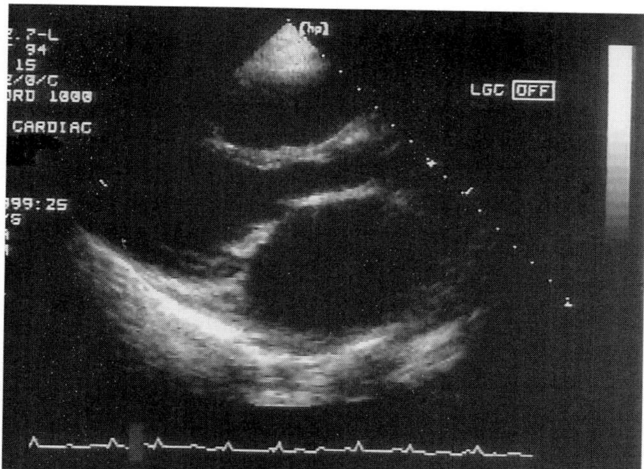

FIGURE 36–7 Echocardiogram (long axis) of a patient with severe mitral stenosis due to rheumatic heart disease. A thickened, stenotic valve separates an enlarged left atrium (right) and the left ventricle (left) and outflow tract (above).

atrial and ventricular dimensions can be quantified using two-dimensional echocardiography. Best appreciated in the parasternal long-axis view, the features of rheumatic mitral stenosis include reduced diastolic excursion of the leaflets and thickening or calcification of the valvular and subvalvular apparatus (Figs. 36-7 and 36-8). M-mode findings include thickening, reduced motion, and parallel movement of the anterior and posterior leaflets during diastole. The mitral valve area can be planimetered directly in the short-axis view, but this measurement has limited clinical value. Doppler echocardiography accurately determines peak and mean transvalvular mitral pressure gradients that correlate closely with cardiac catheterization measurements.[75,107] To estimate mitral valve area, the pressure half-time (time required for the initial diastolic gradient to decline by 50%) is employed; the more prolonged the half-time, the more severe is the reduction in orifice area.[107] Using the pressure half-time determination, mitral valve area is equal to 220 (an empirical value) divided by the pressure half-time. Deriving mitral valve area using the pressure half-time method has generally fallen out of popularity. In patients with combined aortic regurgitation and mitral stenosis, the pressure half-time method may be unreliable because the regurgitant jet may interfere with the valve area calculation.[107]

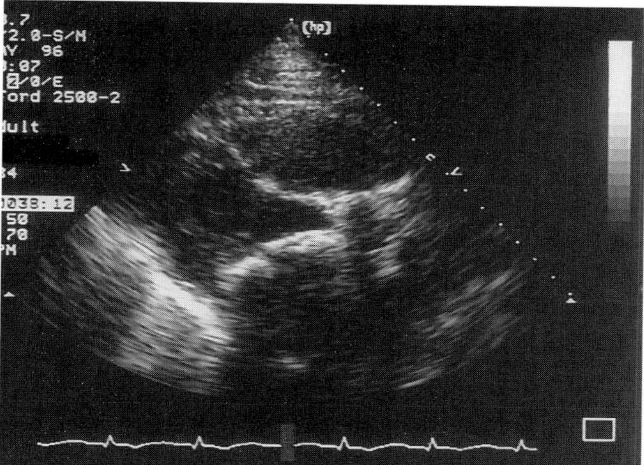

FIGURE 36–8 Echocardiogram (long axis) of a patient with severe mitral stenosis due to mitral annular calcification.

Today, the mean mitral gradient at rest and with bicycle or supine exercise measured using Doppler echocardiography is more clinically useful than estimating mitral valve area; the simultaneous increase in right ventricular systolic pressure (estimated from continuous wave or pulse wave Doppler envelopes of the tricuspid regurgitation signal) during exercise is also very revealing. Transesophageal echocardiography (TEE) can provide even more information in the evaluation of mitral stenosis; it is better than the transthoracic approach for visualizing details of valvular pathology, such as valve mobility and thickness, subvalvular apparatus involvement, and extent of leaflet or commissural calcification.[107,109] In addition, TEE is more reliable in detecting left atrial thrombi. Three-dimensional echocardiography facilitates spatial recognition of intracardiac structures, thereby enhancing conventional echocardiographic findings.[110] The accuracy of three-dimensional images has been validated both in vitro and in vivo. This modality may provide additional information regarding fusion of the mitral commissures in patients with mitral stenosis. Measurements of LV volume using three-dimensional echocardiography correlate with those obtained using both contrast ventriculography and magnetic resonance imaging (MRI).

Cardiac catheterization is not necessary to establish the diagnosis of mitral stenosis; however, it can provide valuable data regarding associated coronary artery disease.[76,104] Left ventriculography permits assessment of the mitral valve and LV contractility and calculation of ejection fraction, but today its role has been replaced by echocardiography. Left-sided heart catheterization allows determination of LV end-diastolic pressure; right-sided heart catheterization is performed to measure cardiac index and the degree of pulmonary hypertension. Therefore, the only real need for cardiac catheterization in these patients currently is to study coronary arteries or, rarely, to evaluate the reversibility of severe pulmonary hypertension using pharmacological interventions.

Postoperative Outcome

Whereas indexes of LV systolic function are used to determine the natural history and surgical prognosis of patients with other valvular lesions, there are few data linking LV function to outcome in those with mitral stenosis. Not surprisingly, the best indicator is related to the degree of clinical impairment. Surgical intervention (open mitral commissurotomy or mitral valve replacement) substantially improves the functional capacity and long-term survival of patients with mitral stenosis; 67% to 90% of patients are alive at 10 years.[105,111–113] However, patients who received an open commissurotomy have a higher rate of reoperation at 10 years compared to those who underwent mitral valve replacement (42% versus 4%).[113]

Generally, a valve area of 1 cm^2 is considered critical mitral stenosis and is associated with significant symptoms and morbidity. In physically active or larger patients, somewhat larger valve areas ($\leq$1.2 cm^2) may produce symptoms.[79] The LV cavity may become foreshortened and more globular; these morphologic changes, however, rarely dictate operative timing and do not influence surgical outcome. Despite a higher operative risk in those with severe pulmonary hypertension and right-sided heart failure, these patients usually improve postoperatively with a reduction in pulmonary vascular pressures.[79,114]

Summary

Mitral stenosis is generally due to rheumatic heart disease. In rheumatic valvulitis, the mitral valve is most commonly involved, followed by combined aortic and mitral valve disease. With worsening mitral stenosis, a progressively higher transvalvular pressure gradient occurs. Mitral transvalvular flow depends on cardiac output and heart rate; an increase in heart rate decreases the duration of transvalvular filling during diastole and reduces forward cardiac output. In mild to moderate mitral stenosis, pulmonary vascular resistance may not be elevated, and pulmonary arterial pressure may be normal at rest and rise only with exertion or increased heart rate. In severe mitral stenosis with elevated pulmonary vascular resistance, pulmonary arterial pressure is usually high at rest. Characteristic symptoms of mitral stenosis are primarily associated with pulmonary venous congestion or low cardiac output. Echocardiography remains the best noninvasive technique for assessing mitral valve pathology and pathophysiology. Surgical intervention can substantially improve the functional capacity and long-term survival of patients with mitral stenosis.

MITRAL REGURGITATION

Etiology

The functional competence of the mitral valve relies on proper, coordinated interaction of the mitral annulus and leaflets, chordae tendineae, papillary muscles, left atrium, and left ventricle.[11,60,115,116] Normal LV geometry and alignment of papillary muscles and chordae tendineae permit leaflet coaptation and prevent leaflet prolapse during ventricular systole. Dysfunction of any one or more components of this valvular-ventricular complex can lead to mitral regurgitation. Regurgitation can also occur in diastole. Diastolic regurgitation results from delayed ventricular contraction, but this phenomenon appears to have few clinical implications.[117]

The most common etiology of systolic mitral regurgitation in patients undergoing surgical evaluation is myxomatous degeneration, also termed "flail leaflet," floppy mitral valve, or mitral valve prolapse (29% to 70% of cases); other causes include ischemic heart disease with ischemic mitral regurgitation (IMR), dilated cardiomyopathy (in which the term "functional mitral regurgitation" [FMR] is used), rheumatic valve disease, mitral annular calcification, infective endocarditis, idiopathic chordal rupture (usually associated with fibroelastic deficiency), congenital anomalies, endocardial fibrosis, and collagen-vascular disorders (Fig. 36-9).[76,80,81,104,116,118–122] IMR is a specific subset of FMR, but both are usually associated with morphologically normal mitral leaflets.

Four different types of structural changes of the mitral valve apparatus may produce regurgitation: leaflet retraction from fibrosis and calcification, annular dilation, chordal abnormalities (including rupture, elongation, shortening, or apical tethering or "tenting" as seen in FMR and IMR), and possibly papillary muscle dysfunction.[11,60,115,116] Carpentier et al classified mitral regurgitation into three pathoanatomic types based on leaflet and chordal motion: normal leaflet motion (type I), leaflet prolapse or excessive motion (type II), and restricted leaflet motion (type III).[123,124] Type III is further subdivided into "a" and "b" based on leaflet restriction during diastole (type IIIa) or during systole (type IIIb, as typically seen in patients with IMR) (Fig. 36-10). Mitral regurgitation with normal leaflet motion is caused by annular dilation, which is often secondary to LV dilation; as a rule, insufficient leaflet coaptation area or incomplete mitral leaflet coaptation is present. Examples include patients with dilated cardiomyopathy and some with ischemic heart disease complicated by IMR. Normal leaflet motion is also associated with leaflet perforation secondary to endocarditis. Leaflet prolapse typically results from a floppy mitral valve with chordal elongation and/or rupture, but can be seen in patients with coronary artery disease who have papillary muscle rupture or, rarely, papillary muscle elongation. Mitral regurgitation due to restricted leaflet motion is associated with rheumatic valve disease (type IIIa and type IIIb), ischemic heart disease (IMR with type IIIb restricted systolic leaflet motion with or without annular dilation), and dilated cardiomyopathy (type IIIb plus annular dilation).[124–126]

MYXOMATOUS DEGENERATION

Myxomatous degeneration (floppy mitral valve or mitral valve prolapse) is the most common cause of mitral regurgitation in the United States.[11,118,119,127] The cause of mitral valve prolapse is most likely congenital with defective

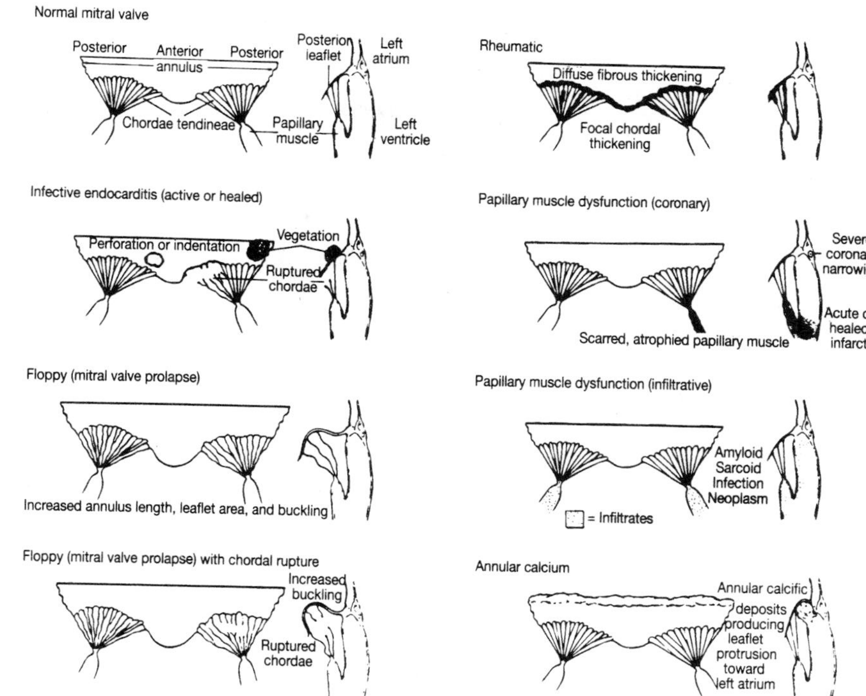

FIGURE 36–9 Diagram demonstrating causes of pure mitral regurgitation, including infective endocarditis, floppy mitral valve, floppy mitral valve with ruptured chordae, rheumatic heart disease, papillary muscle dysfunction, hypertrophic cardiomyopathy, dilated cardiomyopathy, endocardial disorders, and annular calcification. (*Modified from Waller BF, Howard J, Fess S: Pathology of mitral valve stenosis and pure mitral regurgitation, part II. Clin Cardiol 17:395, 1994. Copyrighted and reprinted with the permission of Clinical Cardiology Publishing Company, Inc., and/or the Foundation for Advances in Medicine and Science, Inc., Mahwah, NJ 07430-0832, USA.*)

fibroelastic connective tissue in the leaflets, chordae, and annulus (Fig. 36-11).[78,128–130] Some degree of mitral valve prolapse is seen echocardiographically in 5% to 6% of the normal female population[128,129,131]; it can be familial and is associated with hypertension. Although mitral valve prolapse appears to be more widespread in women, severe mitral regurgitation due to mitral valve prolapse is more common in men. Heart failure, usually manifest as declining stamina and fatigue, may be the presenting complaint in 25% to 40% of symptomatic patients with mitral valve prolapse. The risk of endocarditis is increased only if valvular regurgitation is present and accompanied by a murmur. The syndrome of mitral valve prolapse includes palpitations, chest pain, syncope or dyspnea, and a mid-systolic click (with or without a late systolic murmur of mitral regurgitation).[128,129] These latter findings are typically seen in patients with Barlow's syndrome, where extensive hooding and billowing of both leaflets are the rule.

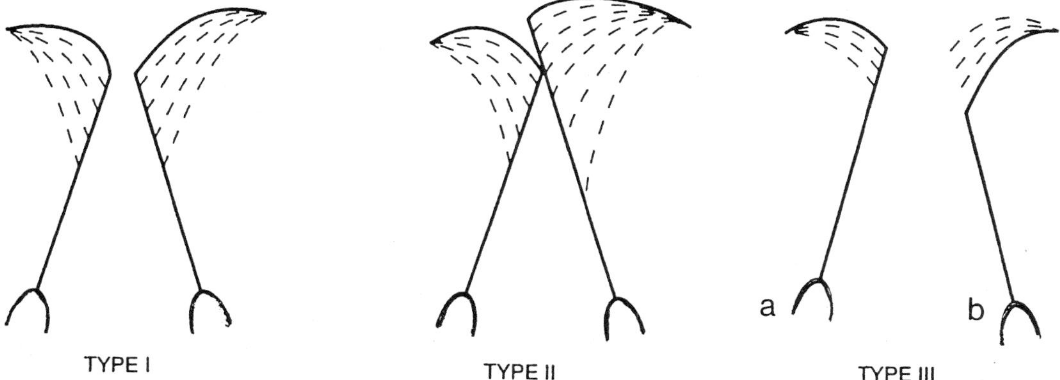

FIGURE 36–10 Carpentier's functional classification of the types of leaflet and chordal motion associated with mitral regurgitation. In type I, the leaflet motion is normal. Type II mitral regurgitation is due to leaflet prolapse or excessive motion. Type III (restricted leaflet motion) is subdivided into restriction during diastole ("a") or systole ("b"). Type IIIb is typically seen in patients with ischemic mitral regurgitation. The course of the leaflets during the cardiac cycle is represented by the dotted lines. (*Modified with permission from Carpentier A: Cardiac valve surgery: the "French correction." J Thorac Cardiovasc Surg 86: 323, 1983.*)

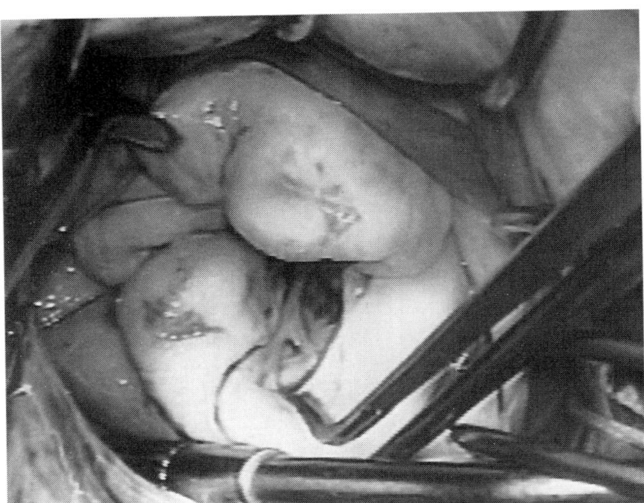

FIGURE 36–11 Intraoperative photograph of mitral regurgitation due to floppy mitral valve.

Pathologically, the atrial aspect of the prolapsed mitral leaflet is often focally thickened.[78,128,130] The changes on the ventricular surface of the leaflet consist of connective tissue thickening or pads forming primarily on the interchordal segments, with proliferation of fibrous tissue extending into adjacent chordae and occasionally onto the ventricular endocardium.[78] Myxomatous degeneration commonly also involves the annulus, resulting in annular thickening and dilation. The leaflets become thickened and opaque, occasionally with yellow plaque formation. Histologically, elastic fiber and collagen fragmentation and disorganization are present; acid mucopolysaccharide material accumulates in the leaflets.

Only 5% to 10% of patients with mitral valve prolapse progress to severe mitral regurgitation, and the majority remain asymptomatic.[76,128,129] Mechanisms accounting for severe mitral regurgitation in persons with mitral valve prolapse include annular dilation and rupture or elongation of the first-order chordae (58%), annular dilation without chordal rupture (19%), and chordal rupture without annular dilation (19%).[130] Chordal rupture is probably related to defective collagen, underlying papillary muscle fibrosis or dysfunction, or bacterial endocarditis.[11,60,78,80,81,119,121,132–134] Elongation without rupture of other first-order as well as many second-order chordae frequently accompanies chordal rupture. Chordal rupture is typically the culprit when mitral regurgitation develops acutely in patients without any previous symptoms of heart disease and in those with known mitral valve prolapse.[76,80,121] Chordal rupture was evident in 14% to 23% of surgically excised purely regurgitant valve specimens; in 73% to 93% of these cases, the underlying pathology was degenerative or floppy mitral valve syndrome.[80,81,121] Posterior chordal rupture was the most frequent finding, followed by anterior chordal rupture and then combined anterior and posterior chordal rupture.[80,81,119,121]

FUNCTIONAL AND ISCHEMIC MITRAL REGURGITATION

Functional mitral regurgitation (FMR), or regurgitation in the setting of structurally normal valve leaflets, is due to incomplete mitral leaflet coaptation in patients with LV dysfunction and dilation (e.g., dilated cardiomyopathy and ischemic heart disease).[135–138] Often clinically silent, FMR or IMR portends a poor prognosis. Similar degrees of LV systolic dysfunction and dilation may also be associated with long-standing severe mitral regurgitation simply due to the chronic volume overload of the ventricle.

In patients with acute myocardial infarction, IMR occurs in about 15% of cases of anterior wall involvement but is present in up to 40% of patients with an inferior infarct.[80,81] The severity of mitral regurgitation is generally related to the size of the area of LV akinesia or dyskinesia. Experimentally, the papillary-annular distances remain relatively constant in the normal heart throughout the cardiac cycle.[136] In acute ischemia, however, the papillary-annular distances differ from the nonischemic state, suggesting a repositioning of the papillary muscle tips relative to the mitral annulus. These papillary tip displacements can tether or "tent" the leaflets apically during systole, e.g., Carpentier "type IIIb" restricted systolic leaflet motion.[123,136] Furthermore, during acute ischemia, alterations in mitral apparatus geometry are seen not only in late or end systole, but in early systole as well.[139] Systolic mitral annular dilation and shape change and altered posterior papillary muscle position and motion may be the primary mechanisms for incomplete mitral leaflet coaptation causing acute IMR during acute inferior or posterolateral ischemia.

Chronic ischemic heart disease results in LV dilation, regional LV systolic wall motion abnormalities, and occasionally papillary muscle fibrosis and shortening, which can lead to papillary muscle malalignment and mitral regurgitation. Mechanisms implicated in chronic IMR include simple annular dilation from LV enlargement, which causes incomplete mitral leaflet coaptation and is associated with normal leaflet motion (Carpentier type I); local LV remodeling with papillary muscle displacement producing apical tethering or tenting of the leaflets (Carpentier type IIIb restricted leaflet motion); or both mechanisms.[123,135] Experimentally, IMR increases over time as the left ventricle dilates and changes shape due to ischemia and previous infarction.[137,138] Geometric changes associated with LV remodeling include an increased distance over which the mitral leaflets are tethered from the papillary muscles (usually the posterior papillary muscle) to the middle of the anterior annulus (or "fibrosa," an easily identified echocardiographic landmark), as well as an increased mitral annular diameter.[137,138] The leaflets cannot coapt normally during systole due to apical leaflet tenting (Fig. 36-12).

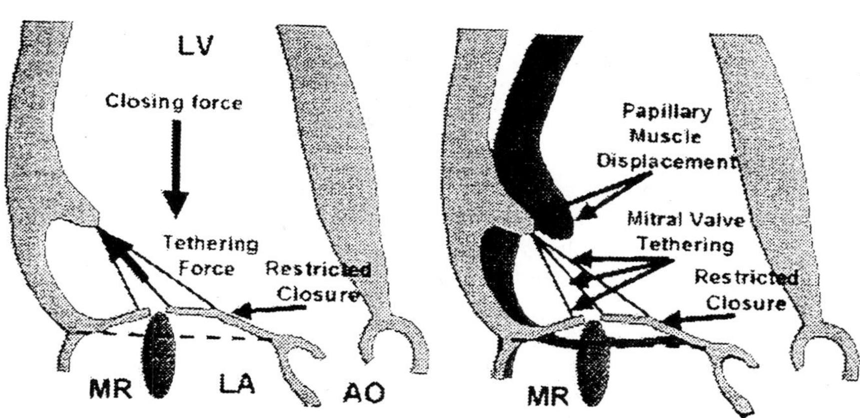

FIGURE 36–12 Drawing of balance of forces in mitral apparatus in the left panel. In the right panel, potential effect of papillary muscle displacement to restrain leaflet closure, causing mitral regurgitation. *(Reproduced with permission from Liel-Cohen N, Guerrero JL, Otsuji Y, et al: Design of a new surgical approach for ventricular remodeling to relieve ischemic mitral regurgitation. Circulation 2000; 101: 2756.)*

Papillary muscle dysfunction in patients with coronary artery disease may possibly also contribute to IMR.[11,60,61,80,81,140] The papillary muscles are particularly susceptible to ischemia; the posteromedial papillary muscle (generally supplied by the posterior descending artery) is more vulnerable to the effects of acute ischemia than is the anterolateral papillary muscle (which is customarily supplied by branches of the left anterior descending and the circumflex arteries).[11,60,61,141] The posteromedial papillary muscle is perfused by one major coronary artery in 63% of cases and by two vessels in the remainder; on the other hand, the anterior papillary muscle has two-vessel perfusion in 71% of normal individuals.[61]

Myocardial infarction leading to papillary muscle dysfunction occurs more frequently when the blood supply to the papillary muscle is provided by one vessel, as is more frequently the case with the posteromedial papillary muscle after an inferior myocardial infarction. Also, coronary artery disease involving both the right and circumflex coronary arteries (as opposed to single-vessel disease) can cause posteromedial papillary muscle dysfunction.[141] Although papillary muscle necrosis frequently complicates myocardial infarction, frank rupture of a papillary muscle is rare. Total papillary muscle rupture is usually fatal due to the resulting severe mitral regurgitation and LV pump failure; survival is possible with rupture of one or two of the subheads of a papillary muscle, which is associated with a lesser degree of mitral regurgitation. Papillary muscle rupture usually occurs 2 to 7 days after myocardial infarction; without urgent surgery, approximately 50% to 75% of such patients may die within 24 hours.[142,143]

RHEUMATIC DISEASE

Although the incidence is decreasing in the United States, rheumatic fever remains a common cause of mitral regurgitation around the world.[11,80,81,116,120–122] It is unknown why rheumatic fever leads to valvular stenosis in some patients and pure regurgitation in others. The pathoanatomic changes of the purely regurgitant rheumatic valve differ from those in a stenotic valve. Regurgitant rheumatic valves have diffuse fibrous thickening of leaflets with minimal calcific deposits and relatively nonfused commissures; chordae tendineae are usually not extremely thickened nor fused.[80,81] There also may be shortening of the chordae tendineae, infiltration of the papillary muscle, and asymmetric annular dilation that develops primarily in the posteromedial portions.

MITRAL ANNULAR CALCIFICATION

Mitral annular calcification is a degenerative disease that is essentially limited to the elderly.[11,76,83] Most patients are older than 60 years of age, and women are affected more often than men. The pathogenesis of mitral annular calcification is not known, but it appears to be a stress-induced phenomenon; annular calcification is associated with systemic hypertension, hypertrophic cardiomyopathy, and aortic stenosis. Other predisposing conditions include chronic renal failure and diabetes mellitus. Aortic valve calcification is an associated finding in 50% of patients with severe mitral annular calcification.

The gross appearance of mitral annular calcification may vary from small, localized calcified spicules to rigid bars up to 2 cm in thickness.[76,83] Initially, calcification begins at the mid portion of the posterior annulus; as the process progresses, the leaflets become upwardly deformed, stretching the chordae tendineae, and a rigid curved bar surrounding the entire posterior annulus or even a complete ring of calcium may encircle the entire mitral orifice. Invasion of the calcific spurs into the myocardium and impingement on the conduction system can result in atrioventricular and/or intraventricular conduction defects. Annular calcification causes mitral regurgitation by displacing the mitral leaflets, immobilizing the peripheral portion of the mitral leaflets (thereby preventing their normal systolic coaptation), or impairing the presystolic sphincteric action of the annulus.[76,83] As the degree of mitral regurgitation gets worse over time, LV volume overload can lead to heart failure. Systemic embolization can occur if annular calcific debris is extensive and friable.

Hemodynamics

The pathophysiology of acute mitral regurgitation markedly differs from that of chronic mitral regurgitation. Acute regurgitation may result from spontaneous chordal rupture, myocardial ischemia, infective endocarditis, or chest trauma.[11,60,133,142,143] The clinical impact of acute mitral incompetence is largely modulated by the compliance of the left atrium. In a normal left atrium with a relatively low compliance, acute mitral regurgitation results in high left atrial pressure, which can rapidly lead to pulmonary edema. Such is not the situation in patients with chronic mitral regurgitation, in whom compensatory changes over time increase left atrial and pulmonary venous compliance so that the symptoms of pulmonary congestion can be negligible for several years.

In mitral regurgitation, the impedance to LV emptying is decreased because the mitral orifice is in parallel with the LV outflow tract.[11,87,144] The volume of mitral regurgitation depends on the square root of the systolic pressure gradient between the left ventricle and the atrium, the time duration of regurgitation, and the effective regurgitant orifice (termed "ERO").[11,145,146] Regurgitation into the left atrium increases left atrial pressure and reduces forward systemic flow. Left atrial pressure rises significantly during ventricular systole, followed by an abrupt decline in early diastole. At end-diastole, left atrial pressure may remain elevated with a transient 5- to 10-mm Hg transvalvular gradient, representing a flow gradient associated with the increased diastolic flow rate.

If the mitral annulus is not rigid, various diagnostic and therapeutic interventions can alter the size of the ERO. Altered loading conditions (elevated preload and afterload) and decreased contractility result in progressive LV dilation and a larger ERO.[147] When LV size is reduced by medical management (e.g., digoxin, diuretics, and most importantly vasodilators), the ERO and regurgitant volume are reduced.[148,149] Importantly, stress echocardiography using an inotropic drug like dobutamine usually decreases the ERO and degree of mitral regurgitation in patients with FMR and IMR because the LV chamber is smaller and the viable LV walls are thickening and contracting better.

Ventricular Adaptation

The loading conditions in mitral regurgitation are favorable to LV ejection because LV preload is increased whereas LV afterload is normal or decreased. In terms of cardiac energetics, reduced LV impedance in patients with mitral regurgitation allows a greater proportion of contractile energy to be expended in myocardial fiber shortening than in tension development.[11,144] Because this increased shortening is less of a determinant of myocardial oxygen consumption than other components, such as tension (or pressure) development and heart rate, mitral regurgitation causes only small increases in myocardial oxygen consumption.[144] Simultaneous reductions in developed tension due to lower LV systolic wall stress (or afterload) associated with mitral regurgitation allow the ventricle to adapt to the substantial regurgitant volume by increasing LV end-diastolic volume to maintain adequate forward output. Along with lower afterload, this substantial increase in preload (LV end-diastolic volume or, more precisely, LV end-diastolic wall stress) allows the heart to compensate for the chronic mitral regurgitation for long periods of time before severe symptoms occur.[11,150,151] A fundamental response of the ventricle to augmented preload is to increase stroke volume and stroke work, although effective forward stroke volume may be normal or actually subnormal. High LV preload eventually leads to LV dilation and shape changes of the ventricle, i.e., more spherical remodeling, due to replication of sarcomeres in series as a consequence of chronic elevation of LV end-diastolic wall stress.[150,151] This is in contrast to LV hypertrophy secondary to chronic pressure overload (elevated systolic wall stress), which leads to sarcomere replication in parallel.

In chronic mitral regurgitation, LV mass also increases; however (and unlike the situation in patients with LV pressure overload), the degree of hypertrophy correlates with the amount of chamber dilation so that the ratio of LV mass to end-diastolic volume remains in the normal range.[152–154] The contractile dysfunction that ultimately evolves is accompanied by increased myocyte length as well as reduced myofibril content.[151,152] The basic changes thus are a combination of myofibrillar loss and the absence of significant hypertrophy in response to the progressive decrease in ventricular pump function; experimental work indicates that the defect is intrinsic to the myocyte per se.[155] Conversely, in acute mitral regurgitation, the ratio of LV mass to end-diastolic volume is reduced because chamber dilation can occur rapidly and the LV wall becomes acutely thinned; this increase in LV end-diastolic volume is associated with sarcomere lengthening along the length-tension curve.[151]

After the initial compensatory phase, LV systolic contractility becomes progressively more impaired with chronic mitral regurgitation.[153–156] Because of the low impedance during systole, however, clinical indexes of myocardial systolic function, such as ejection fraction and fractional circumferential fiber shortening (%FSc), can still be normal even if severely depressed LV systolic contractility is present.[155,157,158] An ejection fraction of less than 40% to 50% or %FSc under 28% indicates an advanced degree of myocardial dysfunction in the presence of severe mitral regurgitation. The commonly used ejection-phase indexes of LV performance, e.g., ejection fraction, %FSc, cardiac output, stroke volume, stroke work, etc., are all affected by changes in LV preload and afterload that accompany all forms of valvular heart disease. End-systolic dimension or LV end-systolic volume (LVESV) is less dependent on preload than is ejection fraction and can be used as a better measure of left ventricular systolic contractile function.[159]

To avoid the pitfalls imposed by abnormal LV loading conditions, load-independent indexes of LV contractility (e.g., end-systolic elastance derived from the end-systolic pressure-volume relationship [ESPVR]) are preferable to measure LV systolic functional mechanics in the face of mitral regurgitation.[153,154,159–161] In hypertrophied and dilated hearts, as seen in chronic mitral regurgitation, however, the utility of end-systolic elastance may be limited due to the geometric changes and hypertrophy that occur; using the end-systolic stress-volume relationship in these circumstances yields more precise estimates. One other problem inherent in the use of end-systolic elastance or stress-volume data is that end systole and end ejection are dissociated in patients with mitral regurgitation; *end ejection* is defined as minimum LV volume, and *end systole* is defined as the instant when LV elastance reaches its maximal value. Because of this dissociation of end systole from minimal ventricular volume, end ejection pressure-volume relations do not correlate with maximal elastance values derived using isochronal methods.[160]

Using load-independent indexes of LV contractility in an experimental mitral regurgitation preparation, Yun et al demonstrated that the normalized end-systolic pressure-volume relationships decreased by 36% and end-systolic stress-volume relationships declined by 21% after 3 months of mitral regurgitation (Fig. 36-13).[153] There was a 26% reduction in LV preload-recruitable stroke work (the relation of stroke work to LV end-diastolic volume) and a 14% drop in preload-recruitable pressure-volume area (the relation of stroke work to LV pressure-volume area). The efficiency of energy transfer from pressure-volume area to external pressure-volume work at matched LV end-diastolic volume decreased by 25%. Furthermore, there was deterioration in ventriculoarterial coupling over time; i.e., a mismatch developed between the ventricle and the total (forward and regurgitant) vascular load. Although the overall (systemic plus left atrial) effective arterial elastance decreased, there was a proportionally greater reduction in LV end-systolic elastance. Thus LV systolic mechanics were impaired, global LV energetics and efficiency deteriorated, and a mismatch in coupling between the left ventricle and arterial bed emerged.[153] Further analysis demonstrated that progression from acute to chronic mitral regurgitation at 3 months was associated with a decrease in maximum torsional deformation from 6.3 degrees to 4.7 degrees and a decrease in early diastolic recoil from +3.8 degrees to –1.5 degrees (Fig. 36-14).[162]

Because torsion is a mechanism by which the left ventricle equalizes transmural gradients of fiber strain and oxygen demand, a decrease in torsion in chronic mitral regurgitation may play a role in the progressive decline of ventricular performance. Loss of torsion would be associated with a larger

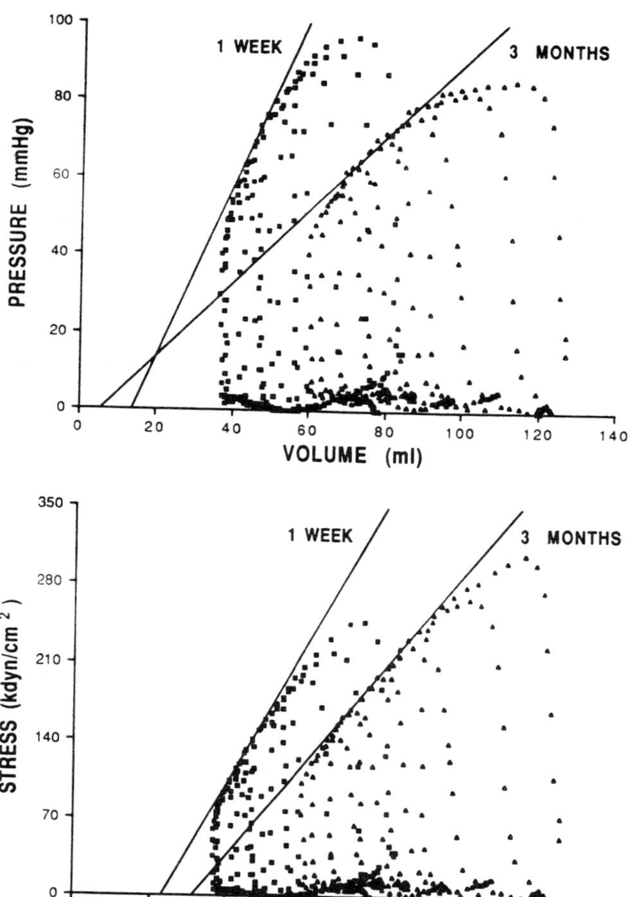

FIGURE 36–13 Pressure-volume (top panel) and stress-volume (bottom panel) loops obtained during caval occlusion at 1 week (squares) and 3 months (triangles) after surgically creating mitral regurgitation in dogs along with the corresponding end-systolic pressure-volume (ESPV) relationship (top) and end-systolic stress-volume (ESSV) relationship (bottom). In each animal, there was a rightward and downward shift of the ESPV and ESSV relationships along with a decline in their slopes at 3 months. *(Reproduced with permission from Yun KL, Rayhill SC, Niczyporuk MA, et al: Left ventricular mechanics and energetics in the dilated canine heart: acute versus chronic mitral regurgitation. J Thorac Cardiovasc Surg 1992; 104:26.)*

transmural gradient of fiber strain and imbalance of oxygen supply and demand. Decreased torsion may contribute to a deleterious feedback loop of ventricular mechanics.[162] The left ventricle responds to decreased forward cardiac output due to mitral regurgitation with dilation. Ventricular dilation tends to equalize the lengths of the endocardial and epicardial radii and decreases torsion. The associated increase in transmural gradients of fiber strain and oxygen supply-demand imbalance results in a further decrease in forward cardiac output, leading to more dilation, thus continuing the cycle.

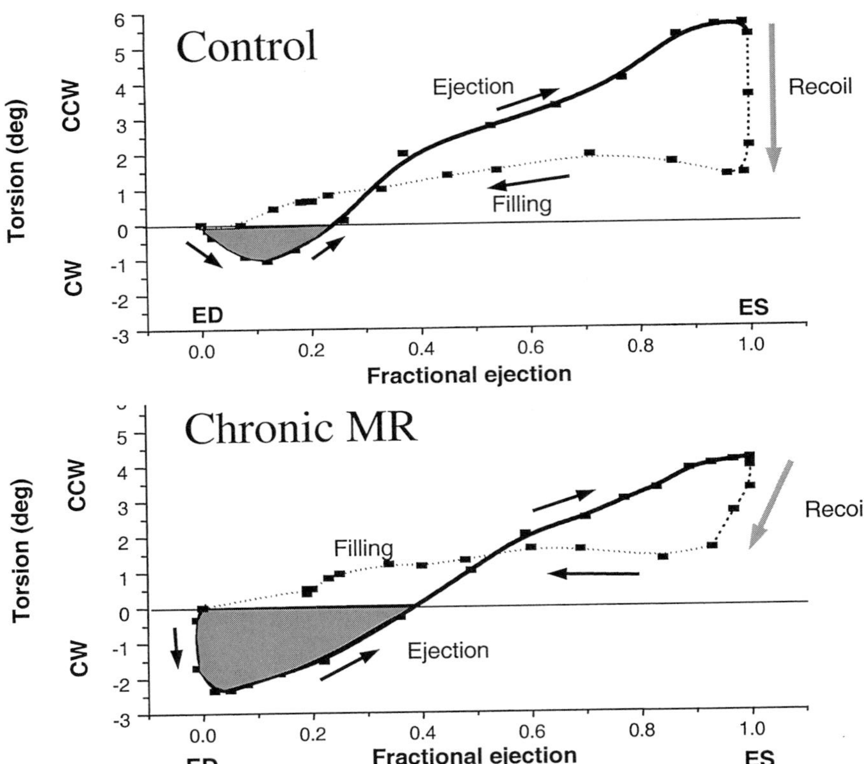

FIGURE 36–14 Torsional deformation versus fractional ejection with acute (top) and chronic (bottom) mitral regurgitation in a representative animal. With acute mitral regurgitation, systole (solid line) is characterized by a slight clockwise rotation followed be counterclockwise torsion that peaks at end ejection. Early diastole (dashed line) shows steeper torsional recoil than mid-to-late diastole (dotted line). With chronic mitral regurgitation, the initial clockwise torsion is larger, the maximum positive torsion is decreased, and less recoil occurs during early diastole. (*Reproduced with permission from Tibayan FA, Yun KL, Lai DTM, et al: Torsional dynamics in the evolution from acute to chronic mitral regurgitation. J Heart Valve Dis 2002; 11:39.*)

Clinically, LVESV accurately reflects changes in LV systolic function; it is independent of preload and varies directly and linearly with afterload (Fig. 36-15).[159,163–166] The larger the LVESV becomes, the worse the LV systolic function or contractility. Correcting LVESV for afterload (i.e., end-systolic wall stress [ESS]) and body size (LV end-systolic volume index [LVESVI]) provides an excellent index of LV systolic function that is less influenced by loading conditions and variation in patient size. [163,164] Preoperative LVESV or LVESVI has been shown to be a better predictor of postoperative outcome in terms of postoperative LV systolic performance and cardiac death than is ejection fraction, LV end-diastolic volume, or LV end-diastolic pressure.[166]

LV diastolic function is also affected by chronic mitral regurgitation.[167–171] Diastolic inflow into the ventricle must increase as total stroke volume increases during the evolution of mitral regurgitation. To compensate, the left ventricle dilates. Early on, mitral regurgitation enhances LV diastolic function by increasing the early diastolic filling rate and decreasing LV chamber stiffness. Flow across the mitral valve during early diastole is chiefly determined by the left atrial-ventricular pressure gradient, even though other factors, such as diastolic restoring forces and isovolumic relaxation, also influence early LV filling.[167] In mid and late diastole, the lower LV chamber stiffness found in patients with acute mitral regurgitation (evidenced by a shift of the LV diastolic pressure-dimension or pressure-volume relationship to the right) allows the LV mean and end-diastolic pressures (and stresses) to remain in the normal range. On the other hand, in patients with chronic mitral regurgitation and preserved ejection fraction, a decrease in LV chamber stiffness (similar to that expected during acute mitral regurgitation) is observed; in those with impaired systolic function, chamber stiffness is usually normal.[169] During the period of passive filling, maximal rates of circumferential fiber lengthening and strain are increased only in the group with preserved ejection fraction.[169] The absence of augmented filling rate in patients with depressed LV systolic function probably reflects underlying myocyte abnormalities. In general, chronic mitral regurgitation causes a decrease in LV systolic contractile function but an increase in early diastolic function (as evidenced by an increase in early diastolic filling rate and a decrease in chamber stiffness).[170,172] The reduced chamber stiffness may be the result of altered ventricular geometry (the more spherical or less eccentric shape)[169]; however, this shape change can exacerbate the degree of mitral regurgitation by altering annular shape and producing papillary muscle malalignment.[115,173] Although the LV chamber becomes less stiff due to the change in geometry, the LV myocardium may actually be stiffer due to myocyte hypertrophy and interstitial fibrosis.[169,170] Experiments using muscle strips from epicardial biopsy specimens in patients with mitral regurgitation revealed that the myosin-actin interaction may be prolonged and that there may be decreased energy supply on

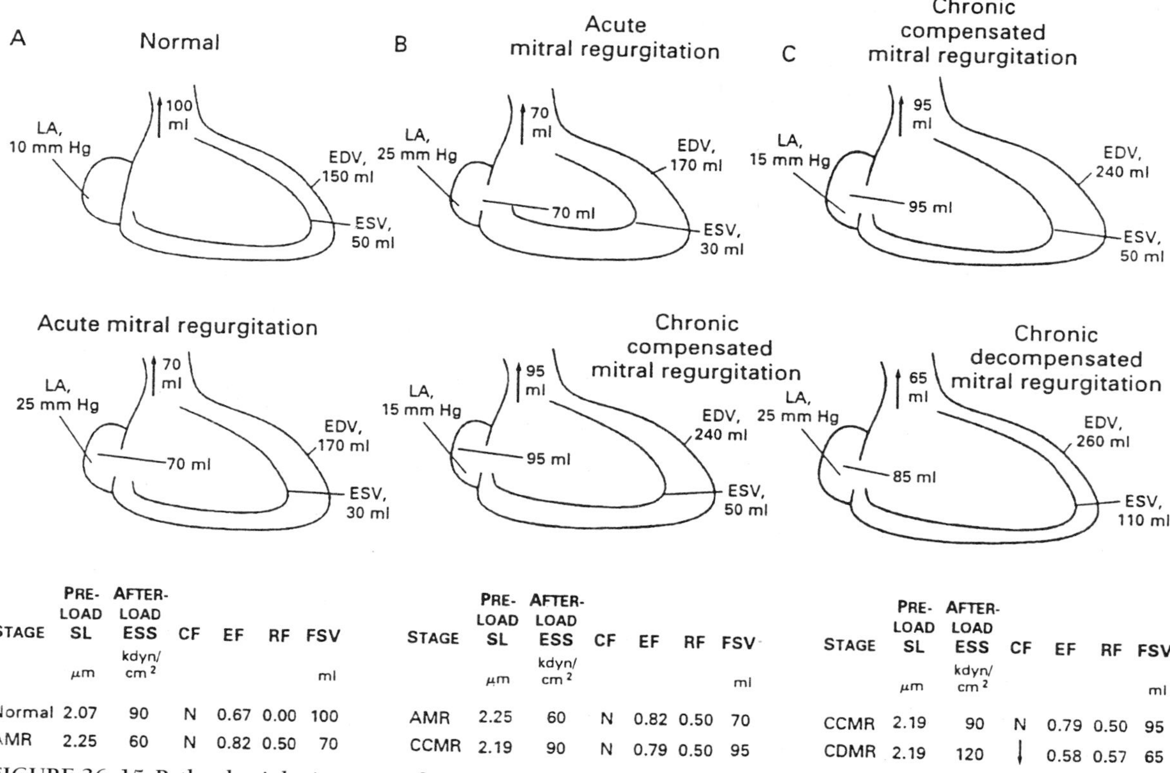

STAGE	PRELOAD SL (μm)	AFTERLOAD ESS (kdyn/cm²)	CF	EF	RF	FSV (ml)
Normal	2.07	90	N	0.67	0.00	100
AMR	2.25	60	N	0.82	0.50	70

STAGE	PRELOAD SL (μm)	AFTERLOAD ESS (kdyn/cm²)	CF	EF	RF	FSV (ml)
AMR	2.25	60	N	0.82	0.50	70
CCMR	2.19	90	N	0.79	0.50	95

STAGE	PRELOAD SL (μm)	AFTERLOAD ESS (kdyn/cm²)	CF	EF	RF	FSV (ml)
CCMR	2.19	90	N	0.79	0.50	95
CDMR	2.19	120	↓	0.58	0.57	65

FIGURE 36–15 Pathophysiologic stages of mitral regurgitation. Panel A shows the transition from normal physiology to acute mitral regurgitation (AMR). The volume overload of acute regurgitation increases preload sarcomere length (SL) so that end-diastolic volume (EDV) increases from 150 to 170 mL. Ejection of blood into the left atrium (LA) reduces afterload [or end-systolic stress (ESS)], and therefore end-systolic volume (ESV) is reduced from 50 to 30 mL. Ejection fraction (EF) increases acutely, but because 50% of the stroke volume is regurgitated into the left atrium (regurgitant fraction of 0.50), forward stroke volume (FSV) is reduced from 100 to 70 mL. Increased left atrial volume raises left atrial pressure from normal to 25 mm Hg. Panel B shows the transition from acute mitral regurgitation to chronic compensated mitral regurgitation (CCMR). Development of eccentric hypertrophy has increased end-diastolic volume from 170 to 240 mL. The larger ventricle has an increased afterload because the radius applied in the Laplace equation for stress is larger. In turn, end-systolic volume is returned to normal. The presence of eccentric hypertrophy, however, allows for increase in total stroke volume and forward stroke volume. Left atrial enlargement allows the left atrial volume overload to be accommodated at a lower filling pressure (15 mm Hg). The LV ejection fraction is supernormal. Panel C shows the transition to chronic decompensated mitral regurgitation (CDMR). The now weakened ventricle can no longer contract well, and LV end-systolic volume increases from 50 to 110 mL. Forward stroke volume is reduced, and cardiac dilation leads to an increased mitral regurgitant fraction. These favorable loading conditions, however, still permit the ejection fraction to remain normal (0.58). CF: contractile function; N: normal; downward arrow: depressed. (*Modified with permission from* Carabello BA: Mitral regurgitation, pt.1: basic pathophysiological principles. *Mod Concepts Cardiovasc Dis* 1998; 57:53.)

the cellular level, resulting in increased myocardial stiffness and reduced ejection fraction.[174] Regarding the impact of mitral regurgitation on right ventricular contractility, reduction in right ventricular systolic function is associated with a worse prognosis, emphasizing the adverse impact of pulmonary hypertension in this disease.[175] Patients with right ventricular ejection fraction of less than 30% are especially at risk for a suboptimal outcome.

Atrial Adaptation

Regurgitant flow into the left atrium leads to progressive atrial enlargement, the degree of which does not correspond directly with the severity of mitral regurgitation.[91,144] Also, the left atrial *v* wave in mitral regurgitation does not correlate with left atrial volume. Compared to patients with mitral stenosis, left atrial size can be larger in patients with long-standing mitral regurgitation; conversely, thrombus formation and systemic thromboembolization occur less frequently because of the absence of atrial stasis.[91,94] Also, atrial fibrillation occurs less often in those with mitral regurgitation and does not affect the clinical course as dramatically as in individuals with mitral stenosis.[94]

Left atrial compliance is an important component of the patient's overall hemodynamic status with mitral regurgitation.[11,133,144,176,177] With sudden development of mitral regurgitation due to chordal rupture, papillary muscle infarction, or leaflet perforation, left atrial compliance is normal or reduced. The left atrium is not enlarged, but the mean left atrial pressure (and the *v* wave) is elevated. Gradually, the left atrial myocardium becomes hypertrophied; proliferative changes develop in the pulmonary vasculature, and pulmonary vascular resistance rises. As the mitral regurgitation becomes chronic and more severe, left atrial compliance increases and left atrial enlargement occurs. In patients with severe, long-standing mitral regurgitation, the left atrium is markedly enlarged, atrial compliance is increased, the atrial wall is fibrotic, but left atrial pressure is normal or only slightly above normal.[176] In this situation, pulmonary artery pressure and pulmonary vascular resistance usually still remain in the normal range or are only modestly elevated. Atrial fibrillation and a low cardiac output, however, can be present.

Pulmonary Changes

Because chronic mitral regurgitation is associated with left atrial enlargement and mild elevation in left atrial pressure, pronounced increases in pulmonary vascular resistance usually do not develop. In patients with acute mitral regurgitation with normal or reduced left atrial compliance, a sudden increase in left atrial pressure initially may modulate an elevation in pulmonary vascular resistance and acute right-sided heart failure.[11,133] Acute pulmonary edema occurs less frequently in patients with chronic mitral regurgitation than in those with mitral stenosis because a sudden increase in left atrial pressure is uncommon. Pulmonary vascular resistance is increased more often in patients with mitral stenosis than in those with mitral regurgitation due to the chronically high left atrial pressure. From the standpoint of pulmonary parenchymal function and respiratory mechanics in patients with chronic mitral regurgitation, there is a decline in vital capacity, total lung capacity, forced expiratory volume, and maximal expiratory flow at 50% vital capacity.[178] These patients also may have a positive response to methacholine challenge; this bronchial hyperresponsiveness may result from increased vagal tone due to chronic pulmonary congestion.

Clinical Evaluation

Patients with mild to moderate mitral regurgitation may remain asymptomatic for many years as the left ventricle adapts to the increased workload. Gradually, symptoms reflective of decreased cardiac output with physical activity and/or pulmonary congestion develop, such as weakness, fatigue, palpitations, and dyspnea on exertion. If right-sided heart failure appears, hepatomegaly, peripheral edema, and ascites occur and can be associated with rapid clinical deterioration.[96,98] With acute mitral regurgitation, pulmonary congestion and pulmonary edema are prominent. Clinically, acute papillary muscle rupture may mimic the presentation of a patient with a postinfarction ventricular septal defect.[179]

On physical examination, the cardiac impulse in patients with mitral regurgitation is hyperdynamic and displaced to the left; the forcefulness of the apical impulse is indicative of the degree of LV enlargement. In patients with chronic mitral regurgitation, S_1 is usually diminished. S_2 may be single, closely split, normally split, or even widely split as a consequence of the reduced resistance to LV ejection; a common finding is a widely split S_2 that results from shortening of LV systole and early closure of the aortic valve.[180] An S_3 may be appreciated due to the increased transmitral diastolic flow rate during the rapid filling phase. The apical systolic murmur is blowing, moderately harsh, and radiates to the axilla and the inferior angle of the scapula, left sternal border, occasionally to the neck, and to the vertebral column.[180] With rupture of posterior leaflet first-order chordae, the mitral regurgitation jet is directed anteriorly and impinges on the atrial septum near the base of the aorta, which can produce a murmur prominent in the aortic area radiating to the neck.[180,181] In ruptured anterior leaflet first-order chordae, the leakage is aimed toward the posterior left atrial wall, and the murmur may be transmitted posteriorly. Although there is little correlation between the intensity of the systolic murmur and the hemodynamic severity of the mitral regurgitation, a holosystolic murmur is characteristic of more regurgitant flow.[180,182] Because of the relatively noncompliant left atrium in acute mitral regurgitation, the murmur is often early and mid-systolic.[11] In patients with the Barlow syndrome (severe bileaflet mitral billowing and/or prolapse) and mitral regurgitation, a characteristic mid-systolic click is heard followed by a late systolic murmur.

On chest radiography, cardiomegaly indicative of LV and left atrial enlargement is commonly found in patients with long-standing moderate to severe mitral regurgitation.[180,183] Acute mitral regurgitation often is not associated with an enlarged heart shadow and may produce only mild left atrial enlargement, despite an elevated left atrial pressure. Chest x-ray findings of congestive changes in the lung fields are less prominent in patients with mitral regurgitation compared with those with mitral stenosis, but interstitial edema is frequently seen in individuals with acute mitral regurgitation or those with progressive LV failure secondary to chronic mitral regurgitation.

Changes on the electrocardiogram are generally not reliable and depend on the etiology, severity, and duration of the mitral regurgitation.[105,180] Atrial fibrillation is a common

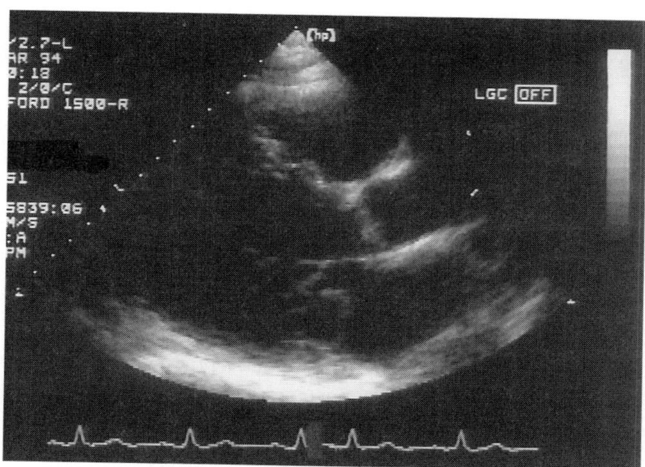

FIGURE 36–16 Echocardiogram (long axis) of a patient with mitral regurgitation due to floppy mitral valve. The leaflets billow back into the left atrium during systole.

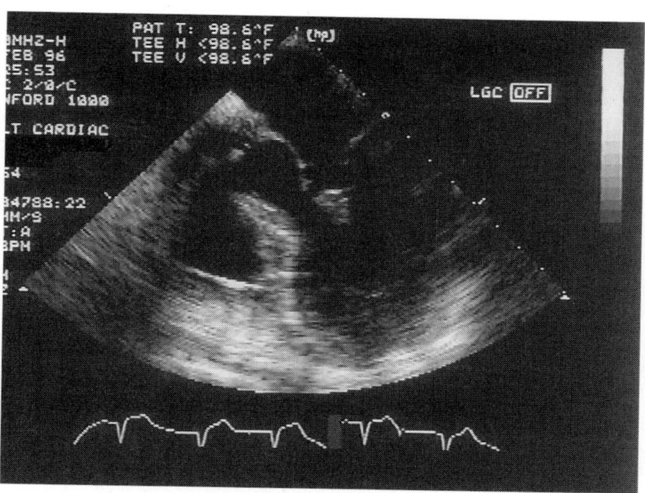

FIGURE 36–17 Echocardiogram (two-chamber view) of a patient with mitral regurgitation due to ruptured papillary muscle.

finding late in the natural history of the disease. In cases of chronic mitral regurgitation, LV volume overload leads to left atrial and ventricular dilation and, eventually, some degree of LV hypertrophy. Evidence of LV enlargement or hypertrophy occurs in one half of patients; 15% have right ventricular hypertrophy due to increased pulmonary vascular resistance, and 5% have combined left and right ventricular hypertrophy.[105] Complex ventricular arrhythmias may be noted on ambulatory electrocardiogram recordings, especially in patients with LV systolic dysfunction. In acute mitral regurgitation, left atrial and/or LV dilation may not be evident, and the electrocardiogram may be normal or show only nonspecific findings, including sinus tachycardia or ST-T wave alterations.[105] Findings of myocardial ischemia or infarction, more commonly noted in the inferior leads, may be present when acute mitral regurgitation is related to ischemic heart disease; in these cases, first-degree AV block is a common coexisting finding.

In the majority of individuals with mitral valve prolapse, particularly those who are asymptomatic, the resting electrocardiogram is normal.[105,131,184] In symptomatic patients, a variety of ST-T wave changes, including T-wave inversion and sometimes ST-segment depression, particularly in the inferior leads, can be found.[128,131] QTc prolongation also may be seen. Arrhythmias may be observed on ambulatory electrocardiograms, including premature atrial contractions, supraventricular tachycardia, AV block, bradyarrhythmias, and premature ventricular contractions.[131] Complex atrial arrhythmias may be present in upwards of 14% of patients, and complex ventricular arrhythmias are present in 30% of patients.[124] Age correlates with the incidence of complex atrial arrhythmias; female gender and anterior mitral valve thickening are predictors of complex ventricular arrhythmias.[124]

Transthoracic echocardiography is used to follow accurately the progression of left atrial and LV dilation in patients with chronic mitral regurgitation.[11,106,108,185,186] Echocardiography confirms enlargement of the chamber, and color flow Doppler examination of the mitral valve establishes the pattern, direction, and magnitude of regurgitant flow. Two-dimensional echocardiography identifies abnormalities of leaflet and chordal morphology and function, including myxomatous degeneration with or without leaflet prolapse, restricted leaflet motion and lack of adequate coaptation from rheumatic valvulitis (fused leaflets), ischemic heart disease, and leaflet destruction by endocarditis (Fig. 36-16).[11,107,126,187] Chordal rupture causing a flail leaflet is characterized by excessive motion of the leaflet tip beyond the normal coaptation point and mitral annular level into the left atrium. Papillary muscle rupture following myocardial infarction and annular dilation also can be visualized by echocardiography (Fig. 36-17).[107] Pulsed wave or continuous wave Doppler echocardiography tends to overestimate the severity of mitral regurgitation in patients with depressed LV ejection fraction and low cardiac output; it is extremely sensitive and specific in diagnosing mild or severe mitral regurgitation, but not as accurate in assessing moderate degrees of regurgitation.[11] The most commonly used method to assess the degree of regurgitation is echocardiographic Doppler color-flow mapping, which permits visualization of the origin, extent, direction, duration, and velocity of disturbed flow (regurgitant jet) within the left atrium.[107,185,186] In patients with LV dysfunction and FMR, apical leaflet tenting, leaflet tenting area, tenting height, and estimated ERO can be quantitatively measured.[145,146] Tenting is characterized by restriction of normal leaflet displacement towards the annulus during systole, with resultant mitral regurgitation (Fig. 36-18). The degree of systolic leaflet tenting is determined by apical and posterior papillary muscle displacement. Further, the degree of mitral regurgitation can be quantitatively measured by calculating mitral and

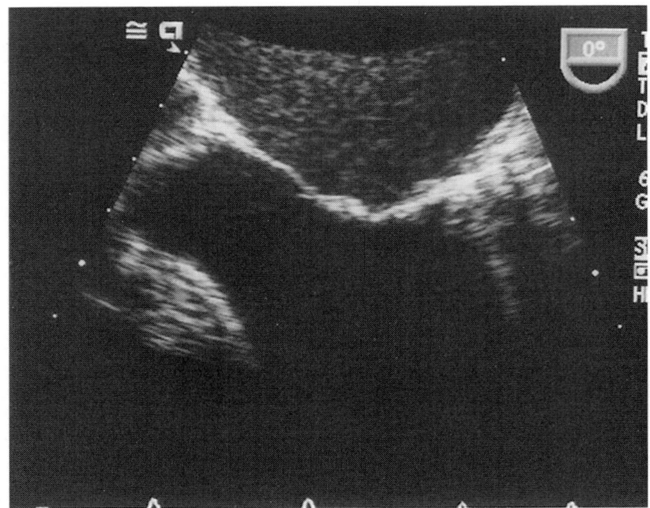

FIGURE 36–18 Echocardiogram of a patient with ischemic mitral regurgitation and apical systolic leaflet tenting.

aortic stroke volumes; regurgitant volume is the difference between these two stroke volumes. The ERO area is the ratio of regurgitant volume to regurgitant time-velocity integral. Additionally, examination of the proximal isovelocity surface area analyzes the proximal flow convergence below the valve leaflets as the blood accelerates towards the leaking site, and ERO is calculated as the ratio of regurgitant flow to regurgitant velocity.[145]

Transesophageal echocardiography (TEE) is superior to transthoracic echocardiography in defining the details of the valvular pathoanatomy and the severity of mitral regurgitation.[11,108,185,187,188] It can detect mitral vegetations, a flail leaflet segment, ruptured chordae, leaflet perforations, calcification, and other inflammatory changes. TEE is particularly useful in patients with annular or leaflet calcification and those with a previously implanted aortic valve prosthesis that can interfere with assessment of mitral regurgitation due to acoustic shadowing. Although intraoperative TEE is essential in the assessment of mitral regurgitation and the adequacy of mitral valve repair, a major limitation is that the vascular unloading effects of general anesthesia frequently downgrade the severity of the mitral regurgitation.[189,190] A thorough preoperative assessment of the degree of regurgitation is thus imperative in deciding whether to proceed with mitral valve surgery at the time of coronary artery bypass grafting. For patients in whom the degree of mitral regurgitation has been downgraded by the effects of anesthesia or after valve repair, intraoperative provocative testing using TEE and vasoconstrictor drugs with or without volume infusion can assist surgical decision making. Testing consists of attempts to reproduce the normal or active ambulatory hemodynamic condition with preload and afterload challenges.[189,190] The preload challenge is performed after aortic cannulation for cardiopulmonary bypass by rapidly infusing volume from the pump until the pulmonary capillary wedge pressure reaches 15 to 18 mm Hg. If severe mitral regurgitation is produced, LV afterload is simultaneously increased by an intravenous bolus of phenylephrine until the arterial systolic pressure climbs to the 130 to 150 mm Hg range. In patients undergoing coronary artery bypass grafting, if both tests are negative, or if regurgitation is induced but associated with new regional LV systolic wall motion abnormalities or electrocardiographic changes (i.e., the regurgitation is due to acute ischemia of viable myocardium), the valve may not require visual inspection as coronary revascularization is usually all that is necessary. If these tests confirm the presence of moderate to severe mitral regurgitation, the valve is inspected and usually repaired using a small ring annuloplasty at the time of coronary revascularization.

Three-dimensional echocardiography continues to evolve and shows some promise in the assessment of congenital and acquired heart disease.[110] This technique facilitates spatial recognition of intracardiac structures and has been validated experimentally. In patients with mitral regurgitation, three-dimensional echocardiography has been shown to be fairly accurate in elucidating the dynamic mechanisms of the mitral regurgitation leaks, but only offers qualitative information.

Cardiac catheterization and left ventriculography have been important in the assessment of mitral regurgitation in the past,[11,103,150,183,191] but echocardiography has basically replaced the need for left-heart catheterization in the vast majority of patients. It usually is indicated only to determine coronary artery anatomy in older patients. The severity of mitral regurgitation can be estimated during left ventriculography by the degree of opacification of the left atrium and pulmonary veins (Table 36-1),[191] but this is far inferior to echocardiographic imaging methods. Other techniques, such as calculating mitral regurgitant fraction, have many limitations (regurgitant volume is determined as the

TABLE 36–1 Angiographic grading system for mitral regurgitation

Grade	Definition
0+	No evidence of mitral regurgitation.
1+	Mild—Contrast clears with each heartbeat and never opacifies atrium.
2+	Moderate—Contrast does not clear with one beat and generally opacifies the entire left atrium faintly after several beats.
3+	Moderately severe—Contrast opacifies the left atrium completely and achieves equal opacification with the left ventricle.
4+	Severe—Contrast opacifies the entire left atrium within one beat, the opacification becomes more dense with each beat, and contrast refluxes into the pulmonary veins during ventricular systole.

difference between total LV angiographic stroke volume and the effective forward stroke volume measured by the Fick principle). By measuring rest and (supine bicycle) exercise pulmonary artery pressures and cardiac outputs, left- and right-sided heart catheterization can occasionally be useful to identify patients with primary myocardial disease who present with LV dilation and relatively mild degrees of mitral regurgitation (who therefore may not have a high likelihood of benefiting from mitral valve surgery).

Magnetic resonance imaging (MRI) is a noninvasive modality that can be employed to assess the cardiovascular system, including cardiac structure and function.[192–194] MRI and newer advanced techniques, such as moving slice velocity mapping, control volume method, or real-time color flow MRI, have been used to evaluate and quantify the degree of mitral regurgitation. The presence of valvular regurgitation can be determined, LV volumes and mitral regurgitant fraction can be estimated, and information can be obtained concerning mitral and coronary anatomy. MRI quantitative measurements, such as LV end-diastolic and end-systolic volumes and regurgitant fraction, correlate well with those determined at cardiac catheterization; however, further clinical experience with this diagnostic modality is necessary.

Postoperative Changes in Left Ventricular Function

Mitral regurgitation due to flail leaflet is frequently asymptomatic yet is associated with a risk of progressive LV dysfunction and a suboptimal natural history if not treated surgically. Treated medically, mitral regurgitation due to flail leaflet is associated with high annual mortality (6.3%) and morbidity rates.[195,196] In these patients, the strategy of early surgery after diagnosis is associated with improved long-term rates of survival and morbidity after diagnosis.

Successful mitral valve repair or replacement is generally associated with clinical improvement, augmented forward stroke volume with lower total stroke volume, smaller LV end-diastolic volume, and regression of LV hypertrophy.[197,198] Surgical correction of chronic mitral regurgitation can preserve LV contractility, particularly in patients with a normal preoperative ejection fraction who have minimal ventricular dilation. On the other hand, in patients with impaired preoperative LV contractile function, improvement in LV function may not necessarily occur after operation.[199] An LVESVI exceeding 30 mL/m^2 is associated with decreased postoperative LV function, which is proportional to the degree of elevated preoperative LVESVI.[166,199] Patients with chronic mitral regurgitation should be referred for mitral valve surgery when LVESVI is no higher than 40 to 50 mL/m^2; when LVESVI exceeds 60 mL/m^2, a poor outcome is likely.[166] LVESVI corrected for LV wall stress, a single-point ratio of end-systolic wall stress to end-systolic volume index, or ESS/LVESVI, is a good predictor of LV systolic function and an accurate predictor of surgical outcome in patients with mitral regurgitation.[163,164] Specifically, an ESS/LVESVI less than 2.6 portends a poor medium-term prognosis; conversely, a normal or high ESS/LVESVI ratio is associated with a favorable outcome, suggesting that LV contractile function had been relatively normal preoperatively.[164] Other predictors of increased operative risk include older age, higher NYHA functional class, associated coronary artery disease, increased LV end-diastolic pressure, elevated LV end-diastolic volume index, elevated LV end-systolic dimension, reduced LV ESS index, depressed resting ejection fraction, decreased fractional shortening, reduced cardiac index, elevated capillary wedge or right ventricular end-diastolic pressure, concomitant operative procedures, and previous cardiac surgery.[140,166,197,199–210]

Regarding long-term outcome, identified risk factors portending postoperative cardiac deterioration include larger LV end-diastolic dimension, increased LV end-systolic dimension, increased LVESV, diminished fractional shortening, reduced LV ESS index, large left atrial size, decreased LV wall thickness/cavity dimension at end systole, and associated coronary artery disease.[166,202,207–209,211,212] Although coronary artery disease portends a higher incidence of late death, simultaneous coronary revascularization improves this prognosis.[202]

Mitral valve repair for patients with myxomatous mitral regurgitation is feasible in the large majority of patients and offers excellent early and late functional results.[119,213–215] Because fewer complications and a lower operative mortality rate are associated with valve repair compared with valve replacement, operation should be considered earlier in the natural history of the disease if the pathological anatomy is judged favorable for valve repair.[116,118,124,195,196,202,213,216–218] When preoperative LVESVI indicates the presence of advanced LV systolic dysfunction, every effort should be made to repair the valve, or at least preserve all chordae tendineae (to both the anterior and posterior leaflets) at time of valve replacement.[116,219]

IMR is associated with higher operative risk (9% to 30%) than nonischemic forms of chronic mitral regurgitation.[140,197,198,200,201,220,221] This higher mortality rate reflects concomitant adverse consequences of previous myocardial infarction and ischemia on LV function. Valve repair should be considered in these patients when feasible because it can potentially reduce complications and improve long-term survival.[140,200,220,222] In the Brigham and Women's Hospital experience, patients with IMR and annular dilation or restricted leaflet motion (not chordal or papillary muscle rupture) who underwent valve repair, however, had a worse long-term outcome than those who underwent valve replacement.[221] Therefore, the pathophysiology of the IMR was a strong determinant (more so than the type of valve procedure) of long-term survival. The NYU group showed higher complication-free survival rates of 64% at 5 years for patients undergoing mitral valve repair compared to 47% at 5 years for those undergoing valve replacement.[222] The analysis of the early mortality rates of patients undergoing mitral

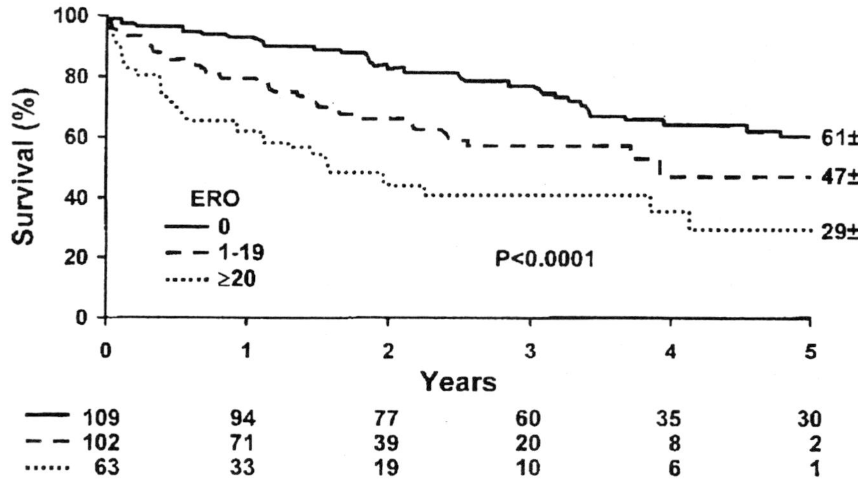

FIGURE 36–19 Survival after diagnosis according to degree of mitral regurgitation as graded by effective regurgitant orifice (ERO) being 20 mm^2 or higher, or less than 20 mm^2. Numbers at bottom indicate patients at risk for each interval. *(Reproduced with permission from Grigioni F, Enriquez-Sarano M, Zehr KJ, et al: Ischemic mitral regurgitation: long term outcome and prognostic implications with quantitative Doppler assessment. Circulation 2001; 103:1759.)*

valve repair and those undergoing valve replacement for IMR was confounded by the variables of functional class and presence of angina. Excluding these two variables, further analysis showed that the early mortality rate was lower for patients undergoing valve repair compared to that of patients undergoing valve replacement.[222] In the Cleveland Clinic experience, in the "better-risk" group of patients with IMR, there was a survival advantage of the mitral valve repair group (58% at 5 years) compared to those who underwent valve replacement (36% at 5 years); however, in the most complex, high-risk cases, late survival rates after valve repair and valve replacement were similarly poor.[223]

In a recent Mayo Clinic report, the group of medically managed patients who developed IMR in the chronic phase after myocardial infarction had a considerably higher mortality rate (62% at 5 years) compared to those who sustained myocardial infarctions and did not develop IMR (39% at 5 years).[146] Medium-term survival for patients with IMR and LV dysfunction was inversely related to the ERO and regurgitant volume. At 5 years, the survival rate was 47% for patients with ERO less than 20 mm^2 and 29% for those with ERO 20 mm^2 or higher (Fig. 36-19). Survival rates at 5 years were 35% when the regurgitant volume was 30 mL or higher compared to 44% for regurgitant volume less than 30 mL.[146] The risk ratio of cardiac death for patients with IMR was 1.56 for patients with ERO less than 20 mm^2 and 2.38 for those with ERO higher than 20 mm^2.[146] Comparatively, in patients with organic mitral regurgitation, ERO higher than 40 mm^2 has been considered severe, presumably the result of different LV and left atrial function and compliance compared to those with IMR.[224]

Experimentally, normalization of LV contractile function is associated with increased myocyte length, augmented myocyte cross-sectional area, and significantly increased contractile protein content.[152] The changes in LV diastolic properties (including early diastolic filling rate, myocardial relaxation, chamber stiffness, myocardial stiffness, and end-diastolic pressure) are reversible after mitral valve replacement surgery.[170] Furthermore, valve replacement normalizes LV volume and the volume-to-mass (or dimension-to-thickness) ratio, but mild LV hypertrophy persists.[170] If surgical correction of mitral regurgitation is carried out before the volume-overload myopathy reaches an irreversible stage, LV diastolic filling characteristics and systolic contractile function return toward normal values.

Even after mitral valve surgery, some patients continue to be limited by heart failure symptoms and have a less than optimal long-term postoperative course. The incidence of congestive heart failure in patients who survived surgery (combined series of valve repair and valve replacement) for pure mitral regurgitation was 23%, 33%, and 37% at 5, 10, and 14 years in the Mayo Clinic experience.[225] Valve repair (vs. replacement) was not an independent predictor of a decreased incidence of congestive heart failure; however, using a combined end point of congestive heart failure and death, valve repair compared to replacement in patients with organic mitral regurgitation appeared to confer a survival advantage. Patient survival after the first episode of congestive heart failure was dismal, being only 44% at 5 years. Causes of congestive heart failure include LV dysfunction in two thirds of the patients and valvular dysfunction in the other third. Predictors of postoperative heart failure were preoperative ejection fraction, coronary artery disease, and functional class.[225] Importantly, preoperative functional class III/IV symptoms are associated with markedly decreased postoperative medium- and long-term survival independent of all baseline characteristics.[226] Because mitral regurgitation in these patients was associated with late manifestation of advanced LV dysfunction, it historically was thought that mitral valve surgery could not help those with pronounced LV dilation and severe global systolic dysfunction. On the other hand, Bolling et al reported favorable medium-term results after mitral valve repair using an undersized flexible annuloplasty ring with resultant decreased LV volume and

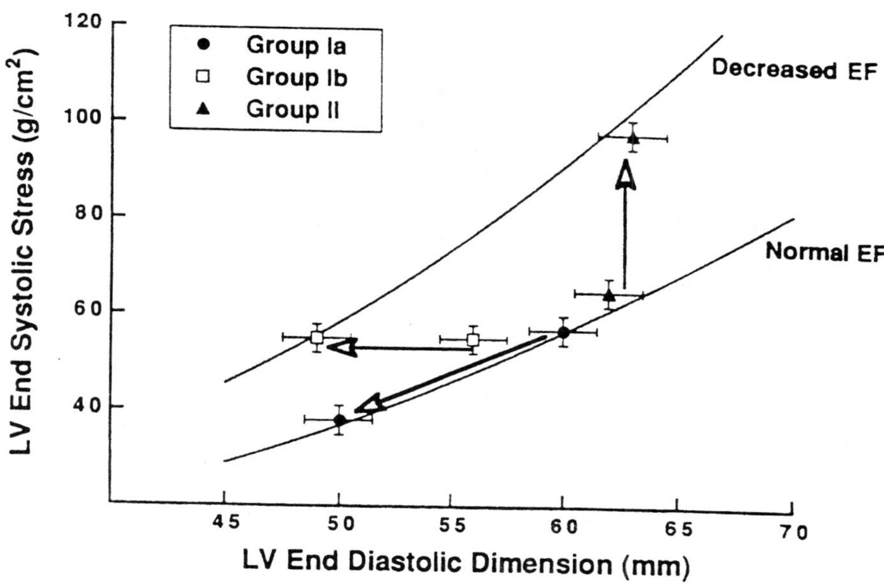

FIGURE 36–20 Illustration using the preload reserve-afterload mismatch concept of John Ross, Jr., of the potential responses of the left ventricle after surgical correction of chronic mitral regurgitation by mitral valve replacement (MVR) with or without chordal preservation. Left ventricular end-systolic stress (LV afterload) is plotted on the vertical axis and LV end-diastolic dimension (LV preload) is on the horizontal axis. The curves relate ejection fraction (EF) to both LV preload and afterload: the lower curve represents a ventricle with a normal EF and the upper curve indicates one with a decreased EF. The average preoperative and postoperative values of end-diastolic dimension, end-systolic stress, and EF are plotted for two different patient groups who underwent MVR: group I (end-diastolic dimension declined after MVR, a salutary response) and group II (no postoperative reduction in end-diastolic dimension, an undesired response). Group I consisted of two subgroups: group Ia (MVR with chordal preservation) and Ib (MVR with chordal division). The optimal postoperative response—a decrease in chamber size, lower afterload, and preserved EF—occurred only in group Ia (closed circles), where some or all of the chordae to one or both mitral leaflets were preserved. Group Ib (MVR with chordal division) also had smaller ventricles postoperatively (open squares), but experienced no decline in LV afterload; therefore, the LV systolic pump performance deteriorated (moving to the lower EF curve postoperatively). Finally, LV chamber size did not change and LV end-systolic stress actually increased postoperatively in group II (MVR with chordal division), indicative of impaired LV ejection performance (lower EF). The salutary response in group Ia was due in part to chordal preservation during MVR; additionally, it is possible that these patients could have been referred earlier in the natural history of their disease. The less favorable response seen in group Ib could potentially have been prevented if the chordae had been preserved during MVR, or if the valve could have been repaired. Finally, the most deleterious post-MVR response observed in group II was due to chordal severing during MVR, very late surgical referral (after irreversible myocardial dysfunction had occurred), or both. Data are shown as mean ± 1 standard error. (*Clinical data were extracted from Rozich JD, Carabello BA, Usher BW, et al: Mitral valve replacement with and without chordal preservation in chronic mitral regurgitation. Circulation 1992; 86:1718. Reproduced with permission from Goldfine H, Aurigemma GP, Zile MR, et al: Left ventricular length-force-shortening relations before and after surgical correction of chronic mitral regurgitation. J Am Coll Cardiol 1998; 31:180.*)

sphericity and increased ejection fraction and cardiac output in a challenging patient population who had dilated or ischemic cardiomyopathy and congestive heart failure.[227]

The decline in ejection fraction after mitral valve replacement for chronic mitral regurgitation is believed to be a result of postoperative increase in afterload, which historically was thought to be secondary to closure of the low resistance "pop-off" into the left atrium. A spherical mathematical model of the left ventricle has been used to define the relations between LV end-diastolic dimension, systolic wall stress, and ejection fraction (Fig. 36-20).[228] In patients undergoing mitral valve replacement, concordant echocardiographic data and mathematical model results indicate that postoperative changes in systolic stress are directly related to changes in chamber size and that LV afterload may actually decrease if chordal preservation mitral

TABLE 36–2 Neurohormone levels before and after surgery

	Before	After	Controls (n = 24)
Norepinephrine (pg/L)	520 (400-650)*	430 (380-610)*	130 (100-260)
PRA (ng/mL/h)	3.1 (2.0-4.5)*	1.2 (0.9-2.2)*#	0.88 (0.56-1.22)
Aldosterone (pg/mL)	160 (118-180)*	93 (58-133)*#	78 (49-107)
ANP (pmol/L)	75 (47-128)*	62 (48-79)*#	14 (8-21)
Endothelin-1 (pmol/L)	2.1 (1.9-2.4)*	1.8 (1.6-2.2)	1.7 (1.2-2.1)

Data are median value (95% confidence interval).

ANP: atrial natriuretic peptide; PRA: plasma renal activity.

* $p < .05$ vs. control.

# $p < .05$ after vs. before.

Source: Reproduced with permission from Le Tourneau T, de Groote P, Millaire A, et al.: Effect of mitral valve surgery on exercise capacity, ventricular ejection fraction and neurohumoral activation in patients with severe mitral regurgitation. J Am Coll Cardiol 2000; 36:2263.

valve replacement techniques are used. In terms of exercise performance after mitral valve surgery for nonischemic mitral regurgitation, it has been shown that although the patients are symptomatically improved, cardiopulmonary exercise testing at 7 months actually was not better.[229] Furthermore, abnormal neurohumoral activation (norepinephrine, plasma renin activity, aldosterone, atrial natriuretic peptide, and endothelin-1) persisted at 7 months postoperatively (Table 36-2). Plasma renin activity, aldosterone, and ANP decreased somewhat after surgery but were still elevated compared to control. Neurohumoral activation may contribute to the impairment of exercise performance in patients with heart failure by limiting exercise-induced vasodilation or by contributing to maldistribution of peripheral blood flow.[229] The persistence of abnormal neurohumoral activation probably reflects incomplete recovery of LV contractility 7 months after surgery; whether or not this pathological state with exercise will thereafter return to normal is unknown.

Mitral Subvalvular Apparatus

Since the concept was originally proposed by Lillehei et al in 1964, the mitral subvalvular apparatus is recognized as an important functional component of LV systolic and diastolic performance.[153,154,230–248] The subvalvular apparatus, including normal chordal and papillary muscle function, is necessary to maintain optimal postoperative LV geometry and optimize postoperative LV systolic pump function. After conventional mitral valve replacement with total chordal excision, a significant decline in LV performance occurs with depression of regional and global elastance, dysynergy of contraction, and dyskinesia at the papillary muscle insertion sites; conversely, after valve replacement with (total or partial) chordal preservation, LV contractile function is preserved.[172,236–240,242,248] Differences in LV systolic function between patients undergoing mitral valve repair and those having valve replacement without chordal preservation are attributed to disruption of the subvalvular apparatus. In a porcine experiment, severing either the anterior or the posterior leaflet chordae was detrimental to global LV systolic function (reduced maximal elastance), but function returned to normal after chordal reattachment.[239] The contributions of the chordae subtending the anterior mitral leaflet are slightly greater than (but additive to) the contributions of the posterior leaflet chordae.[238]

In a canine experimental model of chronic mitral regurgitation, Yun et al demonstrated that mitral valve replacement with chordal preservation optimizes postoperative LV energetics and ventriculo-vascular coupling in addition to enhancing systolic performance.[154] After chordal interruption, global LV end-systolic elastance and the end-systolic stress-volume relationship fell by 46% and 33%, respectively. In terms of myocardial energetics, the slopes of the LV stroke work–end-diastolic volume and pressure-volume area–end-diastolic volume relations declined significantly by 20% and 11% (indicating reduced external stroke work and mechanical energy generated at any given level of preload) after valve replacement with chordal excision. Chordal severing in dilated canine hearts (secondary to chronic mitral regurgitation) after valve replacement resulted in impaired LV systolic mechanics and decreased LV energetics and efficiency due to an exacerbated mismatch in ventriculo-vascular coupling between the left ventricle and the systemic arterial bed.[154]

Mitral valve replacement with chordal division results in a decline in segmental LV systolic function, not only in the areas subtending papillary muscle insertion but also in remote LV regions.[232] Clinically, valve replacement with chordal transection is associated with reduced rest and exercise ejection fraction due in part to an increase in ESS.[247] Mitral valve repair improves rest and exercise ejection indexes, primarily due to a marked reduction in ESS and maintenance of a more ellipsoidal chamber geometry. Additionally, mitral valve replacement with complete chordal transection caused no postoperative change in LV end-diastolic volume, an increase in LVESV, an increase in ESS (89 to 111 g/m^2), and a decrease in ejection fraction (from 60% to 36%).[246] Conversely, patients in whom the chordae tendineae were preserved during valve replacement had a smaller LV end-diastolic volume and LVESV, decreased ESS (from 95 to 66 g/m^2), and unchanged ejection fraction (63% and 61%). These findings suggest that reduced chamber size, reduced systolic afterload, and preservation of ventricular contractile function act in concert to maintain ejection performance after chordal-sparing valve replacement procedures. Conversely, increased LV chamber size, increased systolic afterload, and probable reduction in chamber contractile function combine to reduce ejection performance after mitral valve replacement with chordal transection.[246]

The loss of ventricular function after mitral valve replacement with chordal division may be due to heterogeneity of regional LV wall stress, and not to local depression of regional contractile function.[249] After valve replacement with chordal transection in an experimental canine preparation, outward displacement of the ventricular wall and transverse shearing deformation were observed in the LV region of papillary muscle insertion during isovolumic contraction.[249] Circumferential and radial strains during ejection were maintained at the basal LV site and enhanced on the apical LV site. Chordal transection induced an unloading effect on the myocardium at the papillary muscle insertion site; the resulting heterogeneity of regional systolic function was felt to be the mechanism for reduced global LV function and slowed ventricular relaxation. Anterior chordal transection with mitral valve replacement impaired not only regional LV function, but also regional right ventricular function.[250] Using radionuclide angiography before and after mitral valve repair, LV ejection fraction did not change and right ventricular ejection fraction improved. In contrast, LV ejection fraction decreased after valve replacement with anterior chordal transection, and right ventricular ejection fraction was unchanged. In the region of the anterior papillary muscle insertion, local LV contractile function was impaired after valve replacement; additionally, the right ventricular apicoseptal region was impaired.[250]

Summary

The functional competence of the mitral valve relies on the interaction of the mitral annulus and leaflets, the subvalvular apparatus, the left atrium, and the left ventricle. The etiology of pure mitral regurgitation is variable, including myxomatous degeneration or floppy mitral valve, FMR or IMR, and rheumatic valve disease. Reduced LV impedance in patients with mitral regurgitation allows a greater proportion of contractile energy to be expended in myocardial fiber shortening rather than in tension development. Because increased shortening is a smaller determinant of myocardial oxygen consumption than the other components, mitral regurgitation causes only small increases in myocardial oxygen consumption. The augmented preload in chronic mitral regurgitation eventually leads to LV dilation. After the initial compensatory phase, LV systolic contractility becomes progressively more depressed as chronic mitral regurgitation evolves. Preoperative LVESV or LVESVI is a good predictor of postoperative outcome in terms of LV systolic performance. Operation for symptomatic patients should be performed before severe, irreversible LV systolic dysfunction develops, especially if the pathological anatomy appears to favor valve repair.

The mitral subvalvular apparatus is recognized as an important component of LV ejection performance; an intact mitral subvalvular apparatus, including chordae to both leaflets, is necessary to maintain optimal postoperative LV geometry and optimize LV systolic pump function. After mitral valve replacement with chordal transection, which hopefully is not performed commonly today, a decline in LV systolic performance occurs with depression of regional and global LV myocardial elastance, dysynergy of contraction, and dyskinesia at the papillary muscle insertion sites. A large cascade of experimental and clinical findings suggests that reduced LV chamber size, reduced LV systolic afterload, and preservation of ventricular contractile function act in concert to maintain ejection performance if chordal-sparing valve replacement techniques are carried out.

REFERENCES

1. Zimmerman J, Bailey CP: The surgical significance of the fibrous skeleton of the heart. *J Thorac Cardiovasc Surg* 1962; 44:701.
2. Davila JC, Plamer ET: The mitral valve: anatomy and pathology for the surgeon. *Arch Surg* 1962; 84:174.
3. Silverman ME, Hurst JW: The mitral complex: interaction of the anatomy, physiology, and pathology of the mitral annulus, mitral valve leaflets, chordae tendineae, and papillary muscles. *Am Heart J* 1968; 76:399.
4. Tsakiris AG, Von Bernuth G, Rastelli GC, et al: Size and motion of the mitral valve annulus in anesthetized intact dogs. *J Appl Physiol* 1971; 30:611.
5. Perloff JK, Roberts WC: The mitral apparatus: functional anatomy of mitral regurgitation. *Circulation* 1972; 46:227.
6. Fenoglio J Jr, Tuan DP, Wit AL, et al: Canine mitral complex: ultrastructure and electromechanical properties. *Circ Res* 1972; 31:417.
7. Walmsley R: Anatomy of human mitral valve in adult cadaver and comparative anatomy of the valve. *Br Heart J* 1978; 40:351.
8. Ormiston JA, Shah PM, Tei C, et al: Size and motion of the mitral valve annulus in man: I. A two-dimensional echocardiographic method and findings in normal subjects. *Circulation* 1981; 64:113.
9. Toumanidis ST, Sideris DA, Papamichael CM, et al: The role of mitral annulus motion in left ventricular function. *Acta Cardiol* 1992; 47:331.
10. Anderson RH, Wilcox BR: The anatomy of the mitral valve, in Wells FC, Shapiro LM (eds): *Mitral Valve Disease.* Oxford, England, Butterworth-Heinemann, 1996; p 4.
11. Fenster MS, Feldman MD: Mitral regurgitation: an overview. *Curr Probl Cardiol* 1995; 20:193.
12. Ranganathan N, Lam JH, Wigle ED, et al: Morphology of the human mitral valve, II: the valve leaflets. *Circulation* 1970; 41:459.
13. Williams TH: Mitral and tricuspid valve innervation. *Br Heart J* 1964; 26:105.
14. Cooper T, Napolitano L, Fitzgerald M, et al: Structural basis for cardiac valvular function. *Arch Surg* 1966; 93:767.

15. Wit AL, Fenoglio J Jr, Hordof AJ, Reemtsma K: Ultrastructure and transmembrane potentials of cardiac muscle in the human anterior mitral valve leaflet. *Circulation* 1979; 59:1284.
16. Curtis MB, Priola DV: Mechanical properties of the canine mitral valve: effects of autonomic stimulation. *Am J Physiol* 1992; 262 (1 pt 2):H56.
17. Marron K, Yacoub MH, Polak JM, et al: Innervation of human atrioventricular and arterial valves. *Circulation* 1996; 94:368.
18. Ahmed A, Johansson O, Folan-Curran J: Distribution of PGP 9.5, TH, NPY, SP and CGRP immunoreactive nerves in the rat and guinea pig atrioventricular valves and chordae tendinae. *J Anat* 1997; 191:547.
19. Filip DA, Radu A, Simionescu M: Interstitial cells of the heart valves possess characteristics similar to smooth muscle cells. *Circ Res* 1986; 59:310.
20. Erlanger J: A note on the contractility of the musculature of the auriculo-ventricular valves. *Am J Physiol* 1916; 40:150.
21. Dean AL Jr: The movements of the mitral cusps in relation to the cardiac cycle. *Am J Physiol* 1916; 40:206.
22. Sarnoff SJ, Gilmore JP, Mitchell JH: Influence of atrial contraction and relaxation on closure of mitral valve. *Circ Res* 1962; 11:26.
23. Sonnenblick EH, Napolitano LM, Daggett WM, Cooper T: An intrinsic neuromuscular basis for mitral valve motion in the dog. *Circ Res* 1967; 21:9.
24. Cooper T, Sonnenblick EH, Priola DV, et al: An intrinsic neuromuscular basis for mitral valve motion, in Brewer LA (ed): *Prosthetic Heart Valves*. Springfield, IL, Charles C Thomas, 1969; Ch. 2.
25. Anderson RH: The disposition and innervation of atrioventricular ring specialized tissue in rats and rabbits. *J Anat* 1972; 113:197.
26. Priola DV, Fulton RL, Napolitano LM, Cooper T: Electrical activity of the canine mitral valve in situ. *Am J Physiol* 1969; 216:238.
27. Priola DV, Fellows C, Moorehouse J, Sanchez R: Mechanical activity of canine mitral valve in situ. *Am J Physiol* 1970; 219:1647.
28. Wit AL, Fenoglio J Jr, Wagner BM, Bassett AL: Electrophysiological properties of cardiac muscle in the anterior mitral valve leaflet and the adjacent atrium in the dog: possible implications for the genesis of atrial dysrhythmias. *Circ Res* 1973; 32:731.
29. Rozanski GJ: Electrophysiological properties of automatic fibers in rabbit atrioventricular valves. *Am J Physiol* 1987; 253:H720.
30. Police C, Piton M, Filly K, et al: Mitral and aortic valve orifice area in normal subjects and in patients with congestive cardiomyopathy: determination by two-dimensional echocardiography. *Am J Cardiol* 1982; 49:1191.
31. Tsakiris AG, Strum RE, Wood EH: Experimental studies on the mechanisms of closure of cardiac valves with use of roentgen videodensitometry. *Am J Cardiol* 1973; 32:136.
32. Hamilton WF, Rompf JH: Movements of the base of the ventricle and the relative constancy of the cardiac volume. *Am J Physiol* 1932; 102:559.
33. Davis PKB, Kinmonth JB: The movements of the annulus of the mitral valve. *J Cardiovasc Surg* 1963; 4:427.
34. Padula RT, Cowan G Jr, Camishion RC: Photographic analysis of the active and passive components of cardiac valvular action. *J Thorac Cardiovasc Surg* 1968; 56:790.
35. Ormiston JA, Shah PM, Tei C, Wong M: Size and motion of the mitral valve annulus in man, II: abnormalities in mitral valve prolapse. *Circulation* 1982; 65:713.
36. Keren G, Sonnenblick EH, LeJemtel TH: Mitral annulus motion: relation to pulmonary venous and transmitral flows in normal subjects and in patients with dilated cardiomyopathy. *Circulation* 1988; 78:621.
37. van Rijk-Zwikker GL, Mast F, Schipperheyn JJ, et al: Comparison of rigid and flexible rings for annuloplasty of the porcine mitral valve. *Circulation* 1990; 82(suppl V):V-58.
38. Oe M, Asou T, Kawachi Y, et al: Effects of preserving mitral apparatus on ventricular systolic function in mitral valve operations in dogs. *J Thorac Cardiovasc Surg* 1993; 106:1138.
39. Karlsson MO, Glasson JR, Bolger AF, et al: Mitral valve opening in the ovine heart. *Am J Physiol* 1998; 274: H552.
40. Roberts WC, Perloff JK: Mitral valvular disease: a clinicopathologic survey of the conditions causing the mitral valve to function abnormally. *Ann Intern Med* 1972; 77:939.
41. Levine RA, Triulzi MO, Harrigan P, Weyman AE: The relationship of mitral annular shape to the diagnosis of mitral valve prolapse. *Circulation* 1987; 75:756.
42. Levine RA, Handschumacher MD, Sanfilippo AJ, et al: Three-dimensional echocardiographic reconstruction of the mitral valve, with implications for the diagnosis of mitral valve prolapse. *Circulation* 1989; 80:589.
43. Glasson JR, Komeda M, Daughters GT, et al: Three-dimensional regional dynamics of the normal mitral annulus during left ventricular ejection. *J Thorac Cardiovasc Surg* 1996; 111:574.
44. Rushmer R, Finlayson B, Nash A: Movements of the mitral valve. *Circ Res* 1956; 4:337.
45. Tsakiris AG, Gordon DA, Padiyar R, et al: The role of displacement of the mitral annulus in left atrial filling and emptying in the intact dog. *Can J Physiol Pharmacol* 1978; 56:447.
46. Rushmer RF: Initial phase of ventricular systole: asynchronous contraction. *Am J Physiol* 1956; 184:188.
47. Zaky A, Nasser WK, Feigenbaum H: A study of mitral valve action recorded by reflected ultrasound and its application in the diagnosis of mitral stenosis. *Circulation* 1968; 37:789.
48. Hinds JE, Hawthorne EW, Mullins CB, Mitchell JH: Instantaneous changes in the left ventricular lengths occurring in dogs during the cardiac cycle. *FASEB J* 1969; 28:1351.
49. Popp RL, Harrison DC: Ultrasonic cardiac echography for determining stroke volume and valvular regurgitation. *Circulation* 1970; 41:493.
50. Tsakiris AG, Padiyar R, Gordon DA, et al: Left atrial size and geometry in the intact dog. *Am J Physiol* 1977; 232:H167.
51. Chiechi MA, Lees M, Thompson R: Functional anatomy of the normal mitral valve. *J Thorac Cardiovasc Surg* 1956; 32:378.
52. Sovak M, Lynch PR, Stewart GH: Movement of the mitral valve and its correlation with the first heart sound: selective valvular visualization and high-speed cineradiography in intact dogs. *Invest Radiol* 1973; 8:150.
53. Pohost GM, Dinsmore RE, Rubenstein JJ, et al: The echocardiogram of the anterior leaflet of the mitral valve: correlation with hemodynamic and cineroentgenographic studies in dogs. *Circulation* 1975; 51:88.
54. Edler I, Gustafson A, Karlefors T, et al: Mitral and aortic valve movements recorded by an ultra-sonic echo method: an experimental study in ultrasound cardiology. *Acta Med Scand* 1961; 370(suppl):68.
55. Tsakiris AG, Gordon DA, Mathieu Y, et al: Motion of both mitral valve leaflets: a cineroentgenographic study in intact dogs. *J Appl Physiol* 1975; 39:359.
56. Laniado S, Yellin EL, Miller H, et al: Temporal relation of the first heart sound to closure of the mitral valve. *Circulation* 1973; 47:1006.
57. Tsakiris AG, Gordon DA, Padiyar R, et al: Relation of mitral valve opening and closure to left atrial and ventricular pressures in the intact dog. *Am J Physiol* 1978; 234:H146.
58. Armour JA, Randall WC: Structural basis for cardiac function. *Am J Physiol* 1970; 218:1517.
59. Sakai T, Okita Y, Ueda Y, et al: Distance between mitral annulus and papillary muscles: anatomic study in normal human hearts. *J Thorac Cardiovasc Surg* 1999; 118:636.
60. Luther RR, Meyers SN: Acute mitral insufficiency secondary to ruptured chordae tendineae. *Arch Intern Med* 1974; 134:568.

61. Voci P, Bilotta F, Caretta Q, et al: Papillary muscle perfusion pattern: a hypothesis for ischemic papillary muscle dysfunction. *Circulation* 1995; 91:1714.
62. Lam JHC, Ranganathan N, Wigle ED, et al: Morphology of the human mitral valve, I: chordae tendineae: a new classification. *Circulation* 1970; 41:449.
63. Ross J Jr, Sonnenblick EH, Covell JW, et al: The architecture of the heart in systole and diastole. *Circ Res* 1967; 21:409.
64. Armour JA, Randall WC: Electrical and mechanical activity of papillary muscle. *Am J Physiol* 1978; 218:1710.
65. Cronin R, Armour JA, Randall WC: Function of the in-situ papillary muscle in the canine left ventricle. *Circ Res* 1969; 25:67.
66. Rayhill SC, Daughters GT, Castro LJ, et al: Dynamics of normal and ischemic canine papillary muscles. *Circ Res* 1994; 74:1179.
67. Fisher VJ, Stuckey JH, Lee RJ, et al: Length changes of papillary muscles of the canine left ventricle during the cardiac cycle [abstract]. *Fed Proc* 1965; 24:278.
68. Karas S, Elkins RC: Mechanism of function of the mitral valve leaflets, chordae tendineae and left ventricular papillary muscles in dogs. *Circ Res* 1970; 26:689.
69. Semafuko WEB, Bowie WC: Papillary muscle dynamics: in situ function and responses of the papillary muscle. *Am J Physiol* 1975; 228:1800.
70. Burch GE, DePasquale NP: Time course of tension in papillary muscle of the heart. *JAMA* 1965; 192:701.
71. Grimm AF, Lendrum BL, Lin HL: Papillary muscle shortening in the intact dog. *Circ Res* 1975; 36:49.
72. Marzilli M, Sabbah HN, Lee T, et al: Role of the papillary muscle in opening and closure of the mitral valve. *Am J Physiol* 1980; 238:H348.
73. Marzilli M, Sabbah HN, Goldstein S, et al: Assessment of papillary muscle function in the intact heart. *Circulation* 1985; 71:1017.
74. Hirakawa S, Sasayama S, Tomoike H, et al: In situ measurement of papillary muscle dynamics in the dog left ventricle. *Am J Physiol* 1977; 233:H384.
75. Wood P: An appreciation of mitral stenosis. *Br Med J* 1954; 1:1051.
76. Marzo KP, Herling IM: Valvular disease in the elderly. *Cardiovasc Clin* 1993; 23:175.
77. Spencer FC: A plea for early, open mitral commissurotomy. *Am Heart J* 1978; 95:668.
78. Roberts WC: Morphologic aspects of cardiac valve dysfunction. *Am Heart J* 1992; 123:1610.
79. Carabello BA: Timing of surgery in mitral and aortic stenosis. *Cardiol Clin* 1991; 9:229.
80. Waller BF, Howard J, Fess S: Pathology of mitral valve stenosis and pure mitral regurgitation, part I. *Clin Cardiol* 1994; 17:330.
81. Waller BF, Howard J, Fess S: Pathology of mitral valve stenosis and pure mitral regurgitation, part II. *Clin Cardiol* 1994; 17:395.
82. Khalil KG, Shapiro I, Kilman JW: Congenital mitral stenosis. *J Thorac Cardiovasc Surg* 1975; 70:40.
83. Korn D, DeSanctis RW, Sell S: Massive calcification of the mitral annulus. *N Engl J Med* 1962; 267:900.
84. Burge DJ, DeHoratious RJ: Acute rheumatic fever. *Cardiovasc Clin* 1993; 23:3.
85. Hygenholtz PG, Ryan TJ, Stein SW, et al: The spectrum of pure mitral stenosis. *Am J Cardiol* 1962; 10:773.
86. Arani DT, Carleton RA: The deleterious role of tachycardia in mitral stenosis. *Circulation* 1967; 36:511.
87. Schofield PM: Invasive investigation of the mitral valve, in Wells FC, Shapiro LM (eds): *Mitral Valve Disease.* Oxford, England, Butterworth-Heineman, 1996; p 84.
88. Braunwald E, Turi ZG: Pathophysiology of mitral valve disease, in Wells FC, Shapiro LM (eds): *Mitral Valve Disease.* Oxford, England, Butterworth-Heineman, 1996; p 28.
89. Thompson ME, Shaver JA, Leon DF: Effect of tachycardia on atrial transport in mitral stenosis. *Am Heart J* 1977; 94:297.
90. Stott DK, Marpole DGF, Bristow JD, et al: The role of left atrial transport in aortic and mitral stenosis. *Circulation* 1970; 41:1031.
91. Kennedy JW, Yarnall SR, Murray JA, et al: Quantitative angiocardiography: relationships of left atrial and ventricular pressure and volume in mitral valve disease. *Circulation* 1970; 41:817.
92. Choi BW, Bacharach SL, Barcour DJ, et al: Left ventricular systolic dysfunction: diastolic filling characteristics and exercise cardiac reserve in mitral stenosis. *Am J Cardiol* 1995; 75:526.
93. Bolen JL, Lopes MG, Harrison DC, et al: Analysis of left ventricular function in response to afterload changes in patients with mitral stenosis. *Circulation* 1975; 52:894.
94. Schwartz R, Myerson RM, Lawrence LT, et al: Mitral stenosis, massive pulmonary hemorrhage, and emergency valve replacement. *N Engl J Med* 1966; 275:755.
95. Diker E, Aydogdu S, Ozdemir M, et al: Prevalence and predictors of atrial fibrillation in rheumatic valvular heart disease. *Am J Cardiol* 1996; 77:96.
96. Gray RJ, Helfant RH: Timing of surgery in valvular heart disease. *Cardiovasc Clin* 1993; 23:209.
97. Neilson GH, Galea EG, Hossack KF: Thromboembolic complications of mitral valve disease. *Aust NZ J Med* 1978; 8:372.
98. Chiang CW, Lo SK, Kuo CT, et al: Noninvasive predictors of systemic embolism in mitral stenosis. *Chest* 1994; 106:396.
99. Daley R, Mattingly TW, Holt CL, et al: Systemic arterial embolism in rheumatic heart disease. *Am Heart J* 1951; 42:566.
100. McCall BW, Price JL: Movement of mitral valve cusps in relation to first heart sound and opening snap in patients with mitral stenosis. *Br Heart J* 1967; 29:417.
101. Kalmanson D, Veyrat C, Bernier A, et al: Opening snap and isovolumic relaxation period in relation to mitral valve flow in patients with mitral stenosis. *Br Heart J* 1976; 38:135.
102. Toutouzas P, Koidakis A, Velimezis A, et al: Mechanism of diastolic rumble and presystolic murmur in mitral stenosis. *Br Heart J* 1974; 36:1096.
103. Perloff JK: Auscultatory and phonocardiographic manifestations of pulmonary hypertension. *Prog Cardiovasc Dis* 1967; 9:303.
104. Amplatz K: The roentgenographic diagnosis of mitral and aortic valvular disease. *Am Heart J* 1962; 64:556.
105. Goldstein MA, Michelson EL, Dreifus LS: The electrocardiogram in valvular heart disease. *Cardiovasc Clin* 1993; 23:55.
106. Wann LS, Weyman AE, Feigenbaum H, et al: Determination of mitral valve area by cross-sectional echocardiography. *Ann Intern Med* 1978; 88:337.
107. Kotler MN, Jacobs LE, Podolsky LA, et al: Echo-Doppler in valvular heart disease. *Cardiovasc Clin* 1993; 23:77.
108. Karalis DG, Ross JJ, Brown BM, et al: Transesophageal echocardiography in valvular heart disease. *Cardiovasc Clin* 1993; 23:105.
109. Stoddard MF, Prince CR, Ammash NM, et al: Two-dimensional transesophageal echocardiographic of mitral valve area in adults with mitral stenosis. *Am Heart J* 1994; 127:1348.
110. Lange A, Palka P, Burstow DJ, et al: Three-dimensional echocardiography: historical development and current applications. *J Am Soc Echocardiogr* 2001; 14:403.
111. Cohn LH, Allred EN, Cohn LA, et al: Long-term results of open mitral valve reconstruction for mitral stenosis. *Am J Cardiol* 1985; 55:731.
112. Detter C, Fischlein T, Feldmeier C, et al: Mitral commissurotomy, a technique outdated? Long-term follow-up over a period of 35 years. *Ann Thorac Surg* 1999; 68:2112.
113. Glower DD, Landolfo KP, Davis RD, et al: Comparison of open mitral commissurotomy with mitral valve replacement with or without chordal preservation in patients with mitral stenosis. *Circulation* 1998; 98:II-120.

114. Zener JC, Hancock EW, Shumway NE, et al: Regression of extreme pulmonary hypertension after mitral valve surgery. *Am J Cardiol* 1972; 30:820.
115. Perloff JK, Roberts WC: The mitral apparatus: functional anatomy of mitral regurgitation. *Circulation* 1972; 46:227.
116. Galloway AC, Colvin SB, Baumann FG, et al: Current concepts of mitral valve reconstruction for mitral insufficiency. *Circulation* 1988; 78:1087.
117. Covalesky VA, Ross J, Chandrasekaran, et al: Detection of diastolic atrioventricular valvular regurgitation by M-mode color Doppler echocardiography. *Am J Cardiol* 1989; 64:809.
118. Chavez AM, Cosgrove DM, Lytle BW, et al: Applicability of mitral valvuloplasty techniques in a North American population. *Am J Cardiol* 1988; 62:253.
119. Cosgrove DM: Surgery for degenerative valve disease. *Semin Thorac Cardiovasc Surg* 1989; 1:183.
120. Hanson TP, Edwards BS, Edwards JE: Pathology of surgically excised mitral valves: one hundred consecutive cases. *Arch Pathol Lab Med* 1985; 109:823.
121. Olson LJ, Subramanian R, Ackermann DM, et al: Surgical pathology of the mitral valve: a study of 812 cases spanning 21 years. *Mayo Clin Proc* 1987; 62:22.
122. Waller BF, Morrow AG, Maron BJ, et al: Etiology of clinically isolated, severe, chronic, pure, mitral regurgitation: analysis of 97 patients over 30 years of age having mitral valve replacement. *Am Heart J* 1982; 104:188.
123. Carpentier A: Cardiac valve surgery: the French correction. *J Thorac Cardiovasc Surg* 1983; 86:323.
124. Carpentier A, Chauvaud S, Fabiani J, et al: Reconstructive surgery of mitral valve incompetence: ten year appraisal. *J Thorac Cardiovasc Surg* 1980; 79:338.
125. Wells FC: Conservation and surgical repair of the mitral valve, in Wells FC, Shapiro LM (eds): *Mitral Valve Disease.* Oxford, England, Butterworth-Heineman, 1996; p 114.
126. Stewart WJ, Sun JP, Mayer E, et al: Mitral regurgitation with normal leaflets results from apical displacement of coaptation, not annular dilation [abstract]. *Circulation* 1994; 90(suppl I):I-311.
127. Olsen LJ, Subramanian R, Ackerman DM, et al: Surgical pathology of the mitral valve: a study of 712 cases spanning 21 years. *Mayo Clin Proc* 1987; 62:22.
128. Barlow JB, Pocock WA: Mitral valve prolapse, the specific billowing mitral leaflet syndrome, or an insignificant non-ejection systolic click. *Am Heart J* 1979; 97:277.
129. Abrams J: Mitral valve prolapse: a plea for unanimity. *Am Heart J* 1976; 92:413.
130. Roberts WC, McIntosh CL, Wallace RB: Mechanisms of severe mitral regurgitation in mitral valve prolapse determined from analysis of operatively excised valves. *Am Heart J* 1987; 113:1316.
131. Procacci PM, Savran SV, Schreiter SL, et al: Prevalence of clinical mitral-valve prolapse in 1169 young women. *N Engl J Med* 1976; 294:1086.
132. Marchand P, Barlow JB, DuPlessis LA, et al: Mitral regurgitation with rupture of normal chordae tendineae. *Br Heart J* 1966; 28:746.
133. Roberts WC, Braunwald E, Morrow AG: Acute severe mitral regurgitation secondary to ruptured chordae tendineae. *Circulation* 1966; 33:58.
134. Gallagher PJ, Caves PK, Stinson EB: Pathological changes in spontaneous rupture of chordae tendineae. *Ann Chir Gynaecol* 1977; 66:135.
135. Miller DC: Ischemic mitral regurgitation redux—to repair or to replace? *J Thorac Cardiovasc Surg* 2001; 122:1059.
136. Dagum P, Timek TA, Green GR, et al: Coordinate-free analysis of mitral valve dynamics in normal and ischemic hearts. *Circulation* 2000; 102:III-62.
137. Otsuji Y, Handschumacher MD, Liel-Cohen N, et al: Mechanism of ischemic mitral regurgitation with segmental left ventricular dysfunction: three-dimensional echocardiographic studies in models of acute and chronic progressive regurgitation. *J Am Coll Cardiol* 2001; 37:641.
138. Liel-Cohen N, Guerrero JL, Otsuji Y, et al: Design of a new surgical approach for ventricular remodeling to relieve ischemic mitral regurgitation. *Circulation* 2000; 101:2756.
139. Glasson J, Komeda M, Daughters GT, et al: Early systolic mitral leaflet "loitering" during acute ischemic mitral regurgitation. *J Thorac Cardiovasc Surg* 1998; 116:193.
140. Hickey MS, Smith LR, Muhlbaier LH, et al: Current prognosis of ischemic mitral regurgitation. *Circulation* 1988; 78(suppl I): I-51.
141. Sharma SK, Seckler J, Israel DH, et al: Clinical, angiographic and anatomic findings in acute severe ischemic mitral regurgitation. *Am J Cardiol* 1992; 70:277.
142. Kishon Y, Oh JK, Schaff HV, et al: Mitral valve operation in postinfarction rupture of a papillary muscle: immediate results and long-term follow-up in 22 patients. *Mayo Clin Proc* 1992; 67:1023.
143. LeFeuvre C, Metzger JP, Lachurie ML, et al: Treatment of severe mitral regurgitation caused by ischemic papillary muscle dysfunction: indications for coronary angioplasty. *Am Heart J* 1992; 123:860.
144. Braunwald E: Mitral regurgitation: physiologic, clinical and surgical considerations. *N Engl J Med* 1969; 281:425.
145. Yiu SF, Enriquez-Sarano M, Tribouilloy C, et al: Determinants of the degree of functional mitral regurgitation in patients with systolic left ventricular dysfunction. *Circulation* 2000; 102:1400.
146. Grigioni F, Enriquez-Sarano M, Zehr KJ, et al: Ischemic mitral regurgitation: Long term outcome and prognostic implications with quantitative Doppler assessment. *Circulation* 2001; 103:1759.
147. Yoran C, Yellin EL, Becker RM, et al: Dynamic aspects of acute mitral regurgitation: effects of ventricular volume, pressure and contractility on the effective regurgitant orifice area. *Circulation* 1979; 60:170.
148. Keren G, Laniado S, Sonnenblick EH, et al: Dynamics of functional mitral regurgitation during dobutamine therapy in patients with severe congestive heart failure: a Doppler echocardiographic study. *Am Heart J* 1989; 118:748.
149. Keren G, Katz S, Strom J, et al: Dynamic mitral regurgitation: an important determinant of the hemodynamic response to load alterations and inotropic therapy in severe heart failure. *Circulation* 1989; 80:306.
150. Grossman W: Profiles in valvular heart disease, in Baim DS, Grossman W (eds): *Cardiac Catheterization, Angiography and Intervention,* 5th ed. Baltimore, Williams & Wilkins, 1996; p 735.
151. Ross J Jr: Adaptations of the left ventricle to chronic volume overload. *Circ Res* 1974; 34/35(suppl II):II-64.
152. Spinale FG, Ishihra K, Zile M, et al: Structural basis for changes in left ventricular function and geometry because of chronic mitral regurgitation and after correction of volume overload. *J Thorac Cardiovasc Surg* 1993; 106:1147.
153. Yun KL, Rayhill SC, Niczyporuk MA, et al: Left ventricular mechanics and energetics in the dilated canine heart: acute versus chronic mitral regurgitation. *J Thorac Cardiovasc Surg* 1992; 104:26.
154. Yun KL, Rayhill SC, Niczyporuk MA, et al: Mitral valve replacement in dilated canine hearts with chronic mitral regurgitation. *Circulation* 1991; 84(suppl III):III-112.
155. Urabe Y, Mann DL, Kent RL, et al: Cellular and ventricular contractile dysfunction in experimental canine mitral regurgitation. *Circ Res* 1992; 70:131.
156. Carabello BA, Nakano K, Corin W, et al: Left ventricular function in experimental volume overload hypertrophy. *Am J Physiol* 1989; 256:H974.

157. Starling MR, Kirsh MM, Montgomery DG, et al: Impaired left ventricular contractile function in patients with long-term mitral regurgitation and normal ejection fraction. *J Am Coll Cardiol* 1993; 22:239.
158. Nakano K, Swindle MM, Spinale F, et al: Depressed contractile function due to canine mitral regurgitation improves after correction of the volume overload. *J Clin Invest* 1991; 87:2077.
159. Carabello BA, Crawford FA Jr: Valvular heart disease. *N Eng J Med* 1997; 337:32.
160. Brickner ME, Starling MR: Dissociation of end systole from end-ejection in patients with long-term mitral regurgitation. *Circulation* 1990; 81:1277.
161. Sagawa K: The end-systolic pressure-volume relation of the ventricle: definition, modifications and clinical use. *Circulation* 1981; 63:1223.
162. Tibayan FA, Yun KL, Lai DTM, et al: Torsion dynamics in the evolution from acute to chronic mitral regurgitation. *J Heart Valve Dis* 2002; 11:39.
163. Carabello BA, Nolan SP, McGuire LB: Assessment of preoperative left ventricular function in patients with mitral regurgitation: value of the end-systolic wall stress–end-systolic volume ratio. *Circulation* 1981; 64:1212.
164. Carabello BA, Williams H, Gash AK, et al: Hemodynamic predictors of outcome in patients undergoing valve replacement. *Circulation* 1986; 74:1309.
165. Grossman W, Braunwald E, Mann T, et al: Contractile state of the left ventricle in man as evaluated from end-systolic pressure-volume relations. *Circulation* 1977; 56:845.
166. Borow KM, Green LH, Mann T, et al: End-systolic volume as a predictor of postoperative left ventricular performance in volume overload from valvular regurgitation. *Am J Med* 1980; 68:655.
167. Yellin EL, Nikolic S, Frater RWM: Left ventricular filling dynamics and diastolic function. *Prog Cardiovasc Dis* 1990; 32:333.
168. Zile MR, Tomita M, Nakano K, et al: Effects of left ventricular volume overload produced by mitral regurgitation on diastolic function. *Am J Physiol* 1991; 261:H471.
169. Corin WJ, Murakami T, Monrad ES, et al: Left ventricular passive diastolic properties in chronic mitral regurgitation. *Circulation* 1991; 83:797.
170. Zile MR, Tomita M, Ishihara K, et al: Changes in diastolic function during development and correction of chronic left ventricular volume overload produced by mitral regurgitation. *Circulation* 1993; 87:1378.
171. Tsutsui H, Urabe Y, Mamu D, et al: Effects of chronic mitral regurgitation on diastolic function in isolated cardiocytes. *Circ Res* 1993; 72:1110.
172. Corin WJ, Sutsch G, Murakami T, et al: Left ventricular function in chronic mitral regurgitation: preoperative and postoperative comparison. *J Am Coll Cardiol* 1995; 25:113.
173. Sabbah HN, Kono T, Rosman H, et al: Left ventricular shape: a factor in the etiology of functional mitral regurgitation in heart failure. *Am Heart J* 1992; 123:961.
174. Komeda M, Glasson JR, Bolger AF, et al: Papillary muscle-left ventricular wall "complex". *J Thorac Cardiovasc Surg* 1997; 113:292.
175. Borer JS, Hochreiter C, Rosen S: Right ventricular function in severe non-ischemic mitral insufficiency. *Eur Heart J* 1991; 12:22.
176. Braunwald E, Awe WC: The syndrome of severe mitral regurgitation with normal left atrial pressure. *Circulation* 1963; 27:29.
177. Sasayama S, Takahashi M, Osakada G, et al: Dynamic geometry of the left atrium and left ventricle in acute mitral regurgitation. *Circulation* 1979; 60:177.
178. Rolla G, Bucca C, Caria E, et al: Bronchial responsiveness in patients with mitral valve disease. *Eur Respir J* 1990; 3:127.
179. Harrison MR, MacPhail B, Gurley JC, et al: Usefulness of color Doppler flow imaging to distinguish ventricular septal defect from acute mitral regurgitation complicating acute myocardial infarction. *Am J Cardiol* 1989; 64:697.
180. Perloff JK, Harvey WP: Auscultatory and phonocardiographic manifestations of pure mitral regurgitation. *Prog Cardiovasc Dis* 1962; 5:172.
181. Antman EM, Angoff GH, Sloss LJ: Demonstration of the mechanism by which mitral regurgitation mimics aortic stenosis. *Am J Cardiol* 1978; 42:1044.
182. Aravanis C: Silent mitral insufficiency. *Am Heart J* 1965; 70:620.
183. Ross RS, Criley JM: Contrast radiography in mitral regurgitation. *Prog Cardiovasc Dis* 1962; 5:195.
184. Zuppiroli A, Mori F, Favilli S, et al: Arrhythmias in mitral valve prolapse: relation to anterior mitral leaflet thickening, clinical variables, and color Doppler echocardiographic parameters. *Am Heart J* 1994; 128:919.
185. Smith MD, Cassidy JM, Gurley JC, et al: Echo Doppler evaluation of patients with acute mitral regurgitation: superiority of transesophageal echocardiography with color flow imaging. *Am Heart J* 1995; 129:967.
186. Smith MD: Evaluation of valvular regurgitation by Doppler echocardiography. *Cardiol Clin* 1991; 9:193.
187. Stewart WJ, Currie PJ, Salcedo EE, et al: Evaluation of mitral leaflet motion by echocardiography and jet direction by Doppler color flow mapping to determine the mechanism of mitral regurgitation. *J Am Coll Cardiol* 1992; 20:1353.
188. Pieper EPG, Hellemans IM, Hamer HPM, et al: Additional value of biplane transesophageal echocardiography in assessing the genesis of mitral regurgitation and the feasibility of valve repair. *Am J Cardiol* 1995; 75:489.
189. Grewal KS, Malkowsi MJ, Piracha AR, et al: Effect of general anesthesia on the severity of mitral regurgitation by transesophageal echocardiography. *Am J Cardiol* 2000; 85:199.
190. Byrne JG, Aklog L, Adams DH: Assessment and management of functional or ischemic mitral regurgitation. *Lancet* 2000; 355:1743.
191. Grossman W, Baim DS: *Cardiac Catheterization Angiography and Intervention*, 4th ed. Philadelphia, Lea & Febiger, 1991; p 563.
192. Hundley WG, Li HF, Willard JE, et al: Magnetic resonance imaging assessment of the severity of mitral regurgitation. *Circulation* 1995; 92:1151.
193. Kozerke S, Schwitter J, Pedersen EM, et al: Aortic and mitral regurgitation: quantification using moving slice velocity mapping. *J Magn Reson Imaging* 2001; 14:106.
194. Nayak KS, Pauly JM, Kerr AB, et al: Real-time color flow MRI. *J Magn Reson Med* 2000; 43: 251.
195. Ling LH, Enriquez-Sarano M, Seward JB, et al: Clinical outcome of mitral regurgitation due to flail leaflet. *N Eng J Med* 1996; 335:1417.
196. Ling LH, Enriquez-Sarano M, Seward JB, et al: Early surgery in patients with mitral regurgitation due to flail leaflets. *Circulation* 1997; 96:1819.
197. van Herwerden LA, Tjan D, Tjissen JG, et al: Determinants of survival after surgery for mitral valve regurgitation in patients with and without coronary artery disease. *Eur J Cardiothorac Surg* 1990; 4:329.
198. Lytle BW: Impact of coronary artery disease on valvular heart surgery. *Cardiol Clin* 1991; 9:301.
199. Starling MR: Effects of valve surgery on left ventricular contractile function in patients with long-term mitral regurgitation. *Circulation* 1995; 92:811.
200. Rankin JS, Hickey MS, Smith LR, et al: Ischemic mitral regurgitation. *Circulation* 1989; 79(suppl I):I-116.
201. Replogle RL, Campbell CD: Surgery for mitral regurgitation associated with ischemic heart disease. *Circulation* 1989; 79(suppl I): I-122.

202. Salomon NW, Stinson EB, Griepp RB, et al: Patient-related risk factors as predictors of results following isolated mitral valve replacement. *Ann Thorac Surg* 1977; 24:520.
203. Wisenbaugh T, Skudicky D, Sarelli P: Prediction of outcome after valve replacement for rheumatic mitral regurgitation in the era of chordal preservation. *Circulation* 1994; 89:191.
204. Acar J, Michel PL, Luxereau P, et al: Indications for surgery in mitral regurgitation. *Eur Heart J* 1991; 12(suppl B):52.
205. Nair CK, Biddle WP, Kaneshige A, et al: Ten-year experience with mitral valve replacement in the elderly. *Am Heart J* 1992; 124:154.
206. Crawford MH, Souchek J, Oprian CA, et al: Determinants of survival and left ventricular performance after mitral valve replacement. *Circulation* 1990; 81:1173.
207. Michel PL, Iung B, Blanchard B, et al: Long-term results of mitral valve repair for non-ischemic mitral regurgitation. *Eur Heart J* 1991; 12(suppl B):39.
208. Zile MR, Gaasch WH, Carroll JD, et al: Chronic mitral regurgitation: predictive value of preoperative echocardiographic indexes of left ventricular function and wall stress. *J Am Coll Cardiol* 1984; 3:235.
209. Levine HJ: Is valve surgery indicated in patients with severe mitral regurgitation even if they are asymptomatic? *Cardiovasc Clin* 1990; 21:161.
210. Davis EA, Gardner TJ, Gillinov AM, et al: Valvular disease in the elderly: influence on surgical results. *Ann Thorac Surg* 1993; 55:333.
211. Vanderberg BF, Dellsperger KD, Chandran KB, et al: Detection, localization and quantitation of bioprosthetic mitral valve regurgitation: an in vitro two-dimensional color-Doppler flow mapping study. *Circulation* 1988; 78:528.
212. Reed D, Abbott R, Smucker M, et al: Prediction of outcome after mitral valve replacement in patients with symptomatic chronic mitral regurgitation: the importance of left atrial size. *Circulation* 1991; 84:23.
213. Cohn LH, Couper GS, Aranki SF, et al: Long-term results of mitral valve reconstruction for regurgitation of the myxomatous mitral valve. *J Thorac Cardiovasc Surg* 1994; 107:143.
214. Deloche A, Jebara V, Relland J, et al: Valve repair with Carpentier techniques: the second decade. *J Thorac Cardiovasc Surg* 1990; 99:990.
215. David TE, Armstrong S, Sun Z, et al: Late results of mitral valve repair for mitral regurgitation due to degenerative disease. *Ann Thorac Surg* 1993; 56:7.
216. Akins CW, Hilgenberg AD, Buckley MJ, et al: Mitral valve reconstruction versus replacement for degenerative or ischemic mitral regurgitation. *Ann Thorac Surg* 1994; 58:668.
217. Xu M, McHaffie DJ, Hilless AD: Mitral valve repair: a clinical and echocardiographic study. *Br Heart J* 1994; 71:51.
218. Skoularigis J, Sinovich V, Joubert G, et al: Evaluation of the long-term results of mitral valve repair in 254 young patients with rheumatic mitral regurgitation. *Circulation* 1994; 90(suppl II): II-167.
219. Zile MR: Chronic aortic and mitral regurgitation: choosing the optimal time for surgical correction. *Cardiol Clin* 1991; 9:239.
220. Hendren WG, Nemec JJ, Lytle BW, et al: Mitral valve repair for ischemic mitral insufficiency. *Ann Thorac Surg* 1991; 52: 1246.
221. Cohn LH, Rizzo RJ, Adams DH, et al: The effect of pathophysiology on the surgical treatment of ischemic mitral regurgitation: operative and late risks of repair versus replacement. *Eur J Cardiothorac Surg* 1995; 9:568.
222. Grossi EA, Goldberg JD, LaPietra A, et al: Ischemic mitral valve reconstruction and replacement: comparison of long-term survival and complications. *J Thorac Cardiovasc Surg* 2001; 122:1107.
223. Gillinov AM, Wieryp PN, Blackstone EH, et al: Is repair preferable to replacement for ischemic mitral regurgitation? *J Thorac Cardiovasc Surg* 2001; 122:1125.
224. Dujardin KS, Enriquez-Sarano M, Bailey KR, et al: Grading of mitral regurgitation by quantitative Doppler echocardiography; calibration by left ventricular angiography in routine clinical practice. *Circulation* 1997; 96:3409.
225. Enriquez-Sarano M, Schaff HV, Orszulak TA, et al: Congestive heart failure after surgical correction of mitral regurgitation. *Circulation* 1995; 92:2496.
226. Tribouilloy CM, Enriquez-Sarano M, Schaff HV, et al: Impact of preoperative symptoms on survival after surgical correction of organic mitral regurgitation. *Circulation* 1999; 99:400.
227. Bolling SF, Pagani FD, Deeb GM, et al: Intermediate-term outcome of mitral reconstruction in cardiomyopathy. *J Thorac Cardiovasc Surg* 1998; 115:383.
228. Goldfine H, Aurigemma GP, Zile MR, et al: Left ventricular length-force-shortening relations before and after surgical correction of chronic mitral regurgitation. *J Am Coll Cardiol* 1998; 31:180.
229. LeTourneau T, deGroote P, Millaire A, et al: Effect of mitral valve surgery on exercise capacity, ventricular ejection fraction and neurohumoral activation in patients with severe mitral regurgitation. *J Am Coll Cardiol* 2000; 36:2263.
230. Lillehei CW, Levy MJ, Bonnabeau RC: Mitral valve replacement with preservation of papillary muscles and chordae tendineae. *J Thorac Cardiovasc Surg* 1964; 47:532.
231. Moon MR, DeAnda A, Daughters GT, et al: Experimental evaluation of different chordal preservation methods during mitral valve replacement. *Ann Thorac Surg* 1994; 58:931.
232. Yun KL, Fann JI, Rayhill SC, et al: Importance of the mitral subvalvular apparatus for left ventricular segmental systolic mechanics. *Circulation* 1990; 82(suppl IV):IV-89.
233. Yun KL, Niczyporuk MA, Sarris GE, et al: Importance of mitral subvalvular apparatus in terms of cardiac energetics and systolic mechanics in the ejecting canine heart. *J Clin Invest* 1991; 87:247.
234. Horskotte D, Schulte HD, Bircks W, et al: The effect of chordal preservation on late outcome after mitral valve replacement: a randomized study. *J Heart Valve Dis* 1993; 2:150.
235. DeAnda A, Komeda M, Nikolic SD, et al: Left ventricular function, twist, and recoil after mitral valve replacement. *Circulation* 1995; 92(suppl II):II-458.
236. Komeda M, David TE, Rao V, et al: Late hemodynamic effects of the preserved papillary muscles during mitral valve replacement. *Circulation* 1994; 90(suppl II):II-190.
237. Hansen DE, Cahill PD, DeCampli WM, et al: Valvular-ventricular interaction: importance of the mitral apparatus in canine left ventricular systolic performance. *Circulation* 1986; 73:1310.
238. Hansen DE, Cahill PD, Derby GC, et al: Relative contributions of the anterior and posterior mitral chordae tendineae to canine global left ventricular systolic function. *J Thorac Cardiovasc Surg* 1987; 93:45.
239. Sarris GE, Cahill PD, Hansen DE, et al: Restoration of left ventricular systolic performance after reattachment of the mitral chordae tendinae. *J Thorac Cardiovasc Surg* 1988; 95:969.
240. David TE, Uden DE, Straus HD: The importance of the mitral apparatus in left ventricular function after correction of mitral regurgitation. *Circulation* 1983; 68(suppl II):II-76.
241. David TE, Burns RJ, Bacchus CM, et al: Mitral valve replacement for mitral regurgitation with and without preservation of chordae tendinae. *J Thorac Cardiovasc Surg* 1984; 88:718.
242. Hansen DE, Sarris GE, Niczyporuk MA, et al: Physiologic role of the mitral apparatus in left ventricular regional mechanics, contraction synergy, and global systolic performance. *J Thorac Cardiovasc Surg* 1989; 97:521.

243. Spence PA, Peniston CM, David TE, et al: Toward a better understanding of the etiology of left ventricular dysfunction after mitral valve replacement: an experimental study with possible clinical implications. *J Thorac Cardiovasc Surg* 1986; 41:363.
244. David TE, Komeda M, Pollick C, et al: Mitral valve annuloplasty: the effect of the type on left ventricular function. *Ann Thorac Surg* 1989; 47:524.
245. Okita Y, Miki S, Kusuhara K, et al: Analysis of left ventricular motion after mitral valve replacement with a technique of preservation of all chordae tendinae. *J Thorac Cardiovasc Surg* 1992; 104:786.
246. Rozich JD, Carabello BA, Usher BW, et al: Mitral valve replacement with and without chordal preservation in chronic mitral regurgitation. *Circulation* 1992; 86:1718.
247. Tischler MD, Cooper KA, Rowen M, et al: Mitral valve replacement versus mitral valve repair: a Doppler and quantitative stress echocardiographic study. *Circulation* 1994; 89:132.
248. Pitarys CJ, Forman ZMB, Panayiotou H, et al: Long-term effects of excision of the mitral apparatus on global and regional ventricular function in humans. *J Am Coll Cardiol* 1990; 15:557.
249. Takayama Y, Holmes JW, LeGrice I, et al: Enhanced regional deformation at the anterior papillary muscle insertion site after chordal transection. *Circulation* 1996; 93:585.
250. Le Tourneau T, Grandmougin D, Foucher C, et al: Anterior chordal transection impairs not only regional left ventricular function but also regional right ventricular function in mitral regurgitation. *Circulation* 2001; 104:I-41.

Chapter 37

Mitral Valve Repair

A. Marc Gillinov/Delos M. Cosgrove III

Mitral valve repair is the procedure of choice to treat mitral valve dysfunction of all etiologies.[1–5] Advantages of mitral valve repair over mitral valve replacement include improved long-term survival, better preservation of left ventricular function, and greater freedom from endocarditis, thromboembolism, and anticoagulant-related hemorrhage.[1–8] With the introduction of standardized surgical techniques by Carpentier, Duran, and others,[7–11] mitral valve repair has become reproducible and widely disseminated. Repairable lesions in adult patients are caused by degenerative, rheumatic, ischemic, and endocarditic processes. Congenital mitral lesions in the adult are uncommon and will not be discussed.

SURGICAL ANATOMY OF THE MITRAL VALVE

The mitral apparatus includes the leaflets, annulus, chordae tendineae, papillary muscles, and left ventricle.

Leaflets

The mitral valve has two leaflets, the anterior (aortic) and posterior (mural) leaflets. The leaflets are attached directly to the mitral annulus and to the papillary muscles by primary and secondary chordae. The anterior mitral leaflet is in direct continuity with the fibrous skeleton of the heart. This leaflet is contiguous with the left and noncoronary cusps of the aortic valve and the area beneath the intervening aortic commissure, termed the fibrous subaortic curtain. Although the anterior leaflet occupies only 35% to 45% of the annular circumference, its leaflet area is almost identical to that of the posterior leaflet.[12]

The posterior leaflet is rectangular. The free margin of the posterior leaflet has two variable indentations or clefts that divide the posterior leaflet into three scallops: the largest or middle scallop, the posteromedial scallop, and the anterolateral scallop. Fan-shaped chordae insert into and define the clefts between the individual posterior scallops. Motion of the posterior leaflet is more restricted than that of the anterior leaflet; however, both mitral leaflets contribute importantly to effective valve closure.

The surface of the mitral leaflet is divided into three zones corresponding to areas of chordal insertion and leaflet coaptation. The rough zone is the leading edge of the anterior and posterior mitral leaflets. This zone is the contact surface of the mitral leaflets during systole. The clear zone is peripheral to the rough zone and represents most of the body of the leaflet; this portion of the mitral valve billows into the atrium during ventricular contraction. The basal zone, between the clear zone and the annulus, receives the insertion of the basal chordae tendineae (tertiary chordae), which originate directly from the trabeculae of the left ventricle. The basal zone is found only on the posterior leaflet.

Annulus

The mitral annulus is the site of leaflet attachment to muscular fibers of the atrium and ventricle. The annulus is flexible and decreases in diameter during each systolic contraction by approximately 26%.[13] The orifice of the mitral valve also changes shape, from elliptical during ventricular systole to circular during late diastole. This flexibility increases leaflet coaptation during systole and maximizes orifice area during diastole. Changes in size and shape of the annulus result from relaxation and contraction of the basoconstrictor muscles (bulbospiral and sinospiral bundles).[14] In the horizontal plane the annulus is saddle-shaped. Anteriorly, the annulus is attached to the fibrous skeleton of the heart.[15] This limits its flexibility and its capacity to dilate with mitral regurgitation (MR). The posterior annulus is more flexible and is not attached to rigid surrounding structures. This accounts for the clinical observation that dilation of the annulus occurs posteriorly with MR.[16]

Knowledge of the anatomy of the mitral annulus and surrounding structures is critical to avoiding inadvertent injury during mitral valve repair. The circumflex coronary artery courses laterally around the mitral annulus in the posterior atrioventricular groove (Fig. 37-1). The coronary sinus runs more medially in the same groove. The artery to the atrioventricular node, usually a branch of the right coronary artery, runs a course parallel and close to the annulus of the anterior leaflet near the posteromedial commissure. The aortic valve is situated between the anterior and posterior fibrous trigones. The bundle of His is located near the posterior trigone.

Chordae Tendineae

The chordae tendineae are chords of fibrous connective tissue that attach the mitral leaflets to either the papillary muscles or the left ventricular free wall. They often

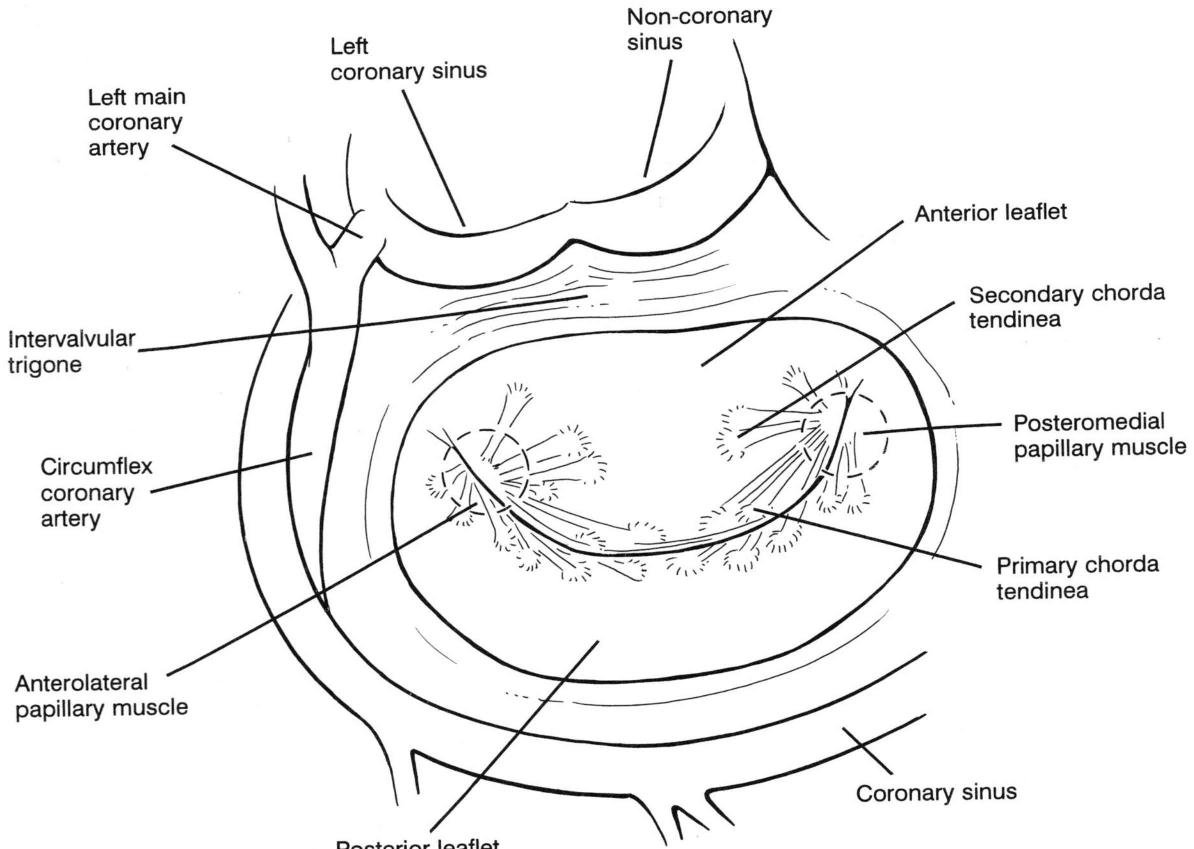

FIGURE 37–1 Surgical anatomy of the mitral valve. Note proximity of the aortic valve and circumflex coronary artery.

subdivide and interconnect before they attach to the leaflets. The chordae are divided into primary chordae, secondary chordae, and tertiary chordae. Primary chordae attach directly to the fibrous band running along the free edge of the leaflets. These chordae ensure that the contact surfaces (rough zone) of the leaflets coapt without leaflet prolapse or flail. Secondary chordae attach to the ventricular surface of the leaflets at the junction between the rough and clear zones. These chordae contribute to ventricular function. Secondary chordae enable the ventricle to contract in an efficient cone-shaped fashion; when secondary chordae are excised, the left ventricle assumes a globular shape.[17,18] Tertiary chordae are unique to the posterior leaflet. They arise as strands directly from the left ventricular wall or from small trabeculae to insert into the ventricular surface of the leaflet near the annulus.

Papillary Muscles

The anterolateral and posteromedial papillary muscles each supply chordae tendineae to both leaflets. The two groups of papillary muscles subtend the anterolateral and posteromedial commissures and arise from the junction of the apical and middle thirds of the ventricular wall. The anterolateral papillary muscle receives a dual blood supply from the anterior descending coronary artery and either a diagonal branch or a marginal branch of the left circumflex artery.[19–21] The posteromedial papillary muscle receives its blood supply from either the left circumflex artery or a distal branch of the right coronary artery. Because of the single blood supply to the posteromedial papillary muscle, infarction of the posteromedial papillary muscle is much more common.

Left Ventricle

The posterior left ventricular wall and papillary muscles play an important role in leaflet coaptation and valve competence. Papillary muscles are aligned parallel to the ventricular wall and attach via chordae to the free edges of the valve leaflets. These muscles project from the trabeculae and may be single, bifid, or a row of muscles arising from the ventricular wall. During isovolumetric contraction the mitral leaflets are pulled downward and together by this interaction. Ventricular dilatation may affect the alignment and tension on the papillary muscles and valve competence.

DIAGNOSIS AND ASSESSMENT OF MITRAL VALVE DISEASE

Clinical Findings

Patients with mitral valve dysfunction may be asymptomatic or present with manifestations of heart failure. Those with endocarditis generally have additional signs and symptoms caused by infection and embolization. Auscultation reveals murmurs typical of mitral regurgitation and/or mitral stenosis.

Echocardiography

Echocardiography is the standard diagnostic test for the evaluation of patients with suspected valvular heart disease. This technology provides a noninvasive method to evaluate the extent and cause of mitral valve dysfunction.[22] In most cases, a preoperative transthoracic echocardiogram is sufficient to assess the mechanisms and degree of dysfunction and the feasibility of repair; if further morphologic information is necessary, a transesophageal echocardiogram is obtained.

Several qualitative, semiqualitative, and quantitative approaches are available to determine the severity of regurgitation and stenosis.[23,24] Color flow Doppler mapping provides a rapid, semiqualitative evaluation of the size of the regurgitant jet.[25] The maximal area of the regurgitant jet is expressed as a percentage of the area of the left atrium. The duration of the jet is also important. Pan-systolic jets involve a greater volume of regurgitant flow than jets of equal size but brief duration. Pulmonary venous flow is another index of the severity of mitral regurgitation.[26] In severe MR, flow in the pulmonary veins reverses. There is no single method to quantitate the magnitude of MR; however, several techniques exist that, when taken together, provide an overall echocardiographic assessment of MR severity.

In addition to determining the *degree* of MR, echocardiography demonstrates the *mechanism* of dysfunction. The direction of the regurgitant jet is particularly helpful. In degenerative disease, the direction of the jet is usually opposite to the leaflet that prolapses. Thus, posterior leaflet prolapse causes an anteriorly directed jet, and anterior leaflet prolapse causes a posteriorly directed jet. Jet direction accurately predicts the mechanism of regurgitation in 80% of patients. Some patients have bileaflet prolapse; in these cases, there may be two or more jets within the atrium or a broad, central jet. Restricted leaflet motion characteristic of functional ischemic mitral regurgitation tends to cause a central jet.[6] Eccentric jets occur occasionally when the jet originates from a commissure or from a leaflet perforation caused by endocarditis.

Echocardiography is also used to assess the severity and mechanisms of mitral valve dysfunction in patients with mitral stenosis. The severity of mitral stenosis is determined by measuring the mitral valve orifice area in the short-axis view during diastole.[27] In mitral stenosis, valve leaflets are thickened or calcified and produce dense echo images. Leaflet excursion during diastole is reduced and opening of the valve is restricted. Doming of the anterior leaflet in diastole, i.e., the body of the leaflet moving more than the edge, is a pathognomonic feature of mitral stenosis. Using echocardiography, the feasibility of mitral valve repair is determined and information is obtained about chamber size, function, and other valvular abnormalities.

Cardiac Catheterization

Preoperative coronary angiography is recommended in all patients over 40 years of age and any patient with a history or clinical presentation suggesting the presence of coronary artery disease. While left ventriculography may demonstrate MR, much more information is gleaned from echocardiography. Mitral annular calcification visible on fluoroscopy indicates that mitral valve surgery will be complex.

MITRAL VALVE OPERATION

Anesthesia and Monitoring

Patients undergoing mitral valve surgery are monitored with an arterial pressure line and transesophageal echocardiography; a pulmonary artery catheter is employed if there is ventricular dysfunction or an extensive operation is anticipated. Low-dose, short-acting narcotic anesthesia is supplemented by inhalation agents intraoperatively and short-acting intravenous sedation postoperatively to facilitate early extubation after surgery.

Mitral Valve Exposure

Excellent, consistent exposure of the mitral valve is essential for successful mitral valve repair. The traditional approach to the mitral valve includes median sternotomy, and that approach will be described here. Patients presenting for isolated, primary heart valve surgery are frequently candidates for minimally invasive approaches, and these will be discussed later.

After median sternotomy, the pericardium is opened slightly to the right of center and the right-sided pericardium tacked to the drapes under tension. Cardiopulmonary bypass is established with bicaval cannulation, and the heart is arrested with antegrade and retrograde blood cardioplegia. Thereafter, intermittent blood cardioplegia is delivered retrograde. The superior and inferior vena cavae are mobilized widely. A tourniquet is placed around the inferior vena cava with traction directed toward the patient's feet; this further elevates the right side of the heart.

To reduce the possibility of embolization of left atrial thrombus, the left atrium is not manipulated until after the aortic cross-clamp is applied. The field is flooded with CO_2 at 6 L per minute; the CO_2 displaces air, reducing the volume of intracardiac air.[28] The left atrium is incised parallel to the interatrial groove. The incision is extended behind the superior vena cava and a considerable distance below the inferior vena cava. A specifically designed self-retaining retractor with three blades is used to facilitate exposure.[29] The operating table is rotated away from the surgeon.

Exposure of the papillary muscles and the anterolateral commissure may require additional maneuvers.[30] Exposure of the posteromedial papillary muscle is facilitated by sponges placed between the diaphragm and the diaphragmatic surface of the left ventricle. Gentle pressure with a sponge stick on the right ventricular outflow tract exposes the anterolateral commissure for annuloplasty suture placement.

Alternative Methods to Expose the Mitral Valve

Other approaches, often including alternative cardiac incisions, may be used to expose the mitral valve in particular circumstances. A right anterolateral thoracotomy is useful in patients with a previous sternotomy and patent coronary artery bypass grafts in the midline. Using this incision, cardiopulmonary bypass is established by peripheral cannulation, and the mitral valve is approached via the left atrium during a period of ventricular fibrillation. This approach may be quite challenging, as the mitral valve is at a distance from the skin incision.

In patients with a small left atrium and/or in a reoperative setting, an extended transseptal approach provides excellent exposure of the mitral valve. When this incision is used in a reoperation, left-sided cardiac adhesions need not be dissected. After opening the right atrium, the interatrial septum is incised and this incision is taken onto the dome of the left atrium. The incision on the dome of the left atrium should be kept at least 1 cm from the aorta to facilitate closure. Although the extended transseptal incision divides the artery to the sinus node and increases the incidence of postoperative junctional rhythm, the need for permanent pacemakers is not increased over a standard left atriotomy.[31]

Valve Analysis

Preoperative and intraoperative echo define the mechanism of mitral valve dysfunction before the valve is visualized. However, before beginning the repair, the surgeon performs a systematic examination of the valve. Although the mitral pathology is usually obvious, it is important to perform a complete assessment before committing to a repair strategy. The annulus is systematically evaluated for dilatation and/or deformity. Leaflets and leaflet motion are examined next. Nerve hooks are used to assess leaflet pliability and to assess leaflet prolapse or restriction. The motion of each leaflet is classified as normal (type I), prolapsed (type II), or restricted (type III).[32] Lesions that produce MR with normal leaflet motion include annular dilatation and leaflet perforation. Lesions that produce regurgitation with prolapse include chordal rupture, chordal elongation, papillary muscle rupture, and papillary muscle elongation. Lesions that produce regurgitation with restricted leaflet motion include ventricular dilatation and dysfunction and rheumatic involvement of the subvalvular apparatus. After assessing the leaflets, the chordae are examined to evaluate length, thickening, fusion, or rupture. Finally, the papillary muscles are assessed, looking for elongation or rupture secondary to infarction.

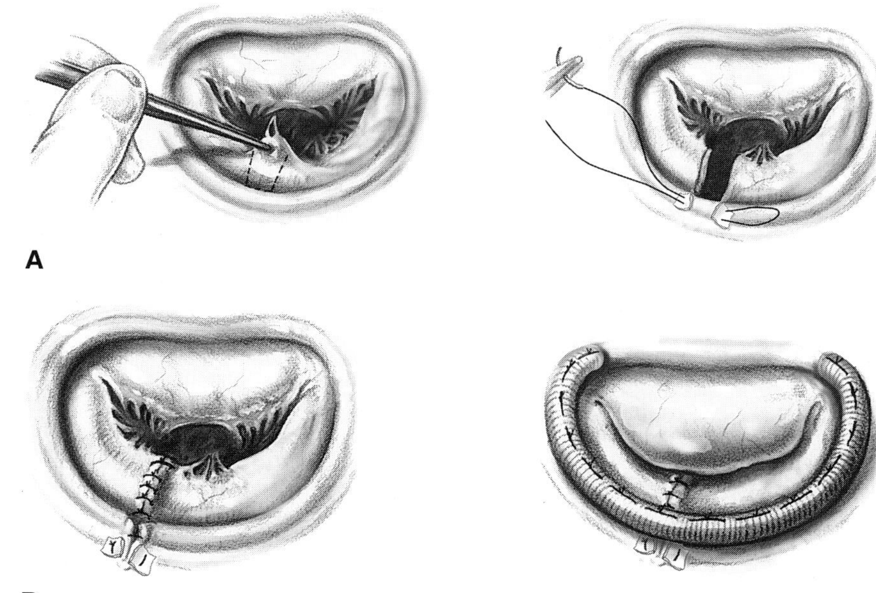

FIGURE 37–2 Posterior leaflet quadrangular resection. (Top) After leaflet resection, the annulus is plicated with one or two pledgeted sutures. (Bottom) The leaflet edges are approximated, and an annuloplasty completes the repair.

ETIOLOGY OF MITRAL VALVE DYSFUNCTION AND VALVE REPAIR

Degenerative Mitral Valve Disease

Also termed myxomatous mitral valve disease and floppy mitral valve disease, degenerative mitral valve disease is the most common indication for mitral valve surgery in North America and Europe.[7,8,33–36] Mitral valve prolapse occurs in 4% to 5% of the general population.[37] Approximately 5% of patients with prolapse ultimately develop MR that requires surgery.[37–41]

Ninety percent of degenerative mitral valves are amenable to repair.[36] However, pathology in degenerative valve disease varies considerably and influences the complexity of repair. The classic features of degenerative mitral valve disease include leaflet prolapse and annular dilatation.[7–9] Chordae may be elongated and thinned, ruptured, or thickened. The posterior leaflet and its chordae are affected more commonly than is the anterior leaflet. Posterior chordal rupture is the most common finding, occurring in 50% of patients.[7] Such patients most commonly have prolapse or flail of the middle scallop of the posterior leaflet.

SURGICAL INDICATIONS

Symptomatic patients with degenerative mitral valve disease and 3+ or 4+ mitral regurgitation should be referred for surgery. Asymptomatic patients with 3+ or 4+ mitral regurgitation and a decrease in left ventricular function as demonstrated by resting or stress echocardiography, left ventricular dilatation, or new onset atrial fibrillation should also be referred for surgery.[42–47]

REPAIR TECHNIQUES

Quadrangular resection Posterior leaflet prolapse is treated by quadrangular resection (Fig. 37-2). The portion of the posterior leaflet with elongated or ruptured chordae is identified. Stay sutures are placed around normal chordae on either side of the diseased chordae to demarcate the area of resection. The segment of posterior leaflet with diseased chordae is then resected using a knife and scissors. The resulting gap in the annulus is closed with 1 or 2 pledgeted sutures; this annular plication is a critical step in the repair, and these sutures must be placed in firm annular tissue. After tying the annular plication sutures, the leaflet edges should not be under tension. The leaflet edges are reapproximated using running 5-0 braided suture. An annuloplasty completes the repair. Occasionally, two posterior leaflet quadrangular resections are performed in the same patient.

Quadrangular resection may also be performed to treat ruptured chordae at a commissure. However, commissural prolapse is most easily managed by simple closure of the commissure.

Sliding leaflet repair The sliding leaflet repair, a variant of posterior leaflet quadrangular resection, was devised by Carpentier to prevent left ventricular outflow tract obstruction caused by systolic anterior motion (SAM) of the anterior leaflet of the mitral valve.[48] SAM occurs only in patients having quadrangular resection for degenerative disease, and, before development of the sliding leaflet repair, SAM complicated repair in 5% to 10% of cases.[49–51] SAM develops in patients with excess leaflet tissue; in such cases, after the repair, the line of leaflet coaptation is displaced anteriorly by redundant posterior leaflet tissue, and the long anterior leaflet obstructs the left ventricular outflow tract.[52,53] SAM may occur with a rigid annuloplasty ring, a flexible annuloplasty ring, or no annuloplasty ring.[50,54–56] In patients at risk, SAM is potentiated by hypovolemia, vasodilatation, and administration of inotropes. In mild cases of SAM occurring after repair, volume loading, inotrope cessation, and administration of afterload-increasing agents suffice to reduce or eliminate the hemodynamic consequences of SAM.[54] In such mild cases, SAM will usually regress with time.[54]

The best strategy in patients at risk for SAM is prevention by sliding leaflet repair.[57] The sliding leaflet repair is used as an adjunct to quadrangular resection in patients with excess leaflet tissue and a posterior leaflet with a height of more than 1.5 cm (Fig. 37-3). The primary purpose of the sliding leaflet repair is to reduce the height of the posterior leaflet, thereby moving the point of systolic leaflet coaptation posteriorly. After quadrangular resection, the posterior leaflet is detached from the annulus for a distance of 1.5 to 2 cm on either side of the resection. Annuloplasty sutures are easily placed once the leaflet is detached. Then the leaflet is reapproximated to the annulus using running 4-0 polypropylene suture. Deep bites are taken in the posterior leaflet, thereby reducing its height. The leaflet edges at the site of resection are reapproximated with running 5-0 multifilament suture, and an annuloplasty completes the repair. This procedure has virtually eliminated the risk of SAM in patients with degenerative disease.[57,58]

Anterior leaflet prolapse A variety of techniques have been used to treat anterior leaflet prolapse. The most popular include chordal transfer, chordal replacement, and chordal shortening. Anterior leaflet resection is rarely indicated.

Chordal transfer is our favored technique for treating anterior leaflet prolapse. Normal primary chordae from the posterior leaflet or secondary chordae from the anterior leaflet are transposed to the unsupported region of the anterior leaflet. The advantage to this procedure is that precise measurement of the transfered chordae is unnecessary; provided that they are not diseased, the transferred chordae are always the right length.

For posterior chordal transfer, a segment of the posterior leaflet and its normal chordae are detached from the posterior annulus (Fig. 37-4). The detached segment is then sewn to the unsupported portion of the anterior leaflet using interrupted 4-0 braided suture. The defect in the posterior leaflet is repaired as for standard quadrangular resection. When anterior leaflet secondary chordae are transposed to the free edge of the anterior leaflet, they are simply detached and sutured into place (Fig. 37-5).

Chordal replacement is another option for correction of anterior leaflet prolapse. David and others have extensive favorable experience with this technique.[59,60] PTFE suture (4-0 or 5-0) is the preferred material for chordal replacement. The neochordae are affixed to the fibrous portion of the papillary muscle and then passed through the leaflet one or more times and tied. The primary challenges with this technique are judging the length of the chordae and tying the PTFE. Several authors have reported ingenious solutions to these problems.[59,60]

Chordal shortening was one of the original techniques described by Carpentier for management of anterior leaflet prolapse.[36] The pathologic, elongated chord is shortened by tucking it into a papillary muscle trench or affixing a portion of the chord to the side of the papillary muscle. Alternatively, the chord may be shortened at its insertion into the mitral leaflet.[61] Durablility of these techniques is jeopardized by late rupture of previously shortened chordae.[7,62,63] At The Cleveland Clinic Foundation, we prefer chordal transfer for correction of anterior leaflet prolapse.

Annuloplasty Annular enlargement is present in patients with degenerative disease. Usually, annular dilatation occurs only along the posterior annulus because the anterior annulus is attached to the fibrous skeleton of the heart. Annuloplasty is a component of the repair in all patients with degenerative disease. Annuloplasty is performed to correct annular dilatation, increase leaflet coaptation, reinforce suture lines, and prevent further annular dilatation. A variety of annuloplasty rings are available; all provide excellent results in patients with degenerative disease.[7,8,64] Rings may be flexible or rigid, complete or incomplete.[64–67]

When placing annular sutures, relatively deep bites through the annulus are required. Posteriorly, the needle should be directed toward the ventricular cavity in order to avoid injury to the circumflex coronary artery (see Fig. 37-1). It is important to place sutures in the fibrous trigones, which are located near the commissures and may be visible as indentations in the endocardium. If a circumferential annuloplasty is used, care must be taken not to injure the aortic valve anteriorly.

Calcified annulus In patients with degenerative disease, the posterior mitral annulus may be calcified. Annular decalcification is necessary to facilitate annuloplasty placement. When calcium is not extensive, simple debridement suffices. In the setting of dense posterior annular calcification, the calcium may be removed piecemeal or en bloc.[68–70] In order to facilitate debridement, the posterior leaflet is detached from the annulus as in a sliding leaflet repair. After debridement, if there is a concern about posterior ventricular rupture, a pericardial patch is used to cover the weakened area. The patch is affixed to ventricular and left atrial muscle. The leaflets are then attached to the patch at the annular level.

Alfieri edge-to-edge repair Alfieri et al described the edge-to-edge repair.[71,72] When employed to correct anterior leaflet prolapse, a suture affixes the free edge of a segment of normal posterior leaflet to the free edge of a prolapsing portion of the anterior leaflet. The normal posterior leaflet with its chordae serves to anchor the anterior leaflet, restricting its motion. This technique is particularly useful when anterior leaflet prolapse is the primary pathology and posterior annular calcification renders chordal transfer problematic.

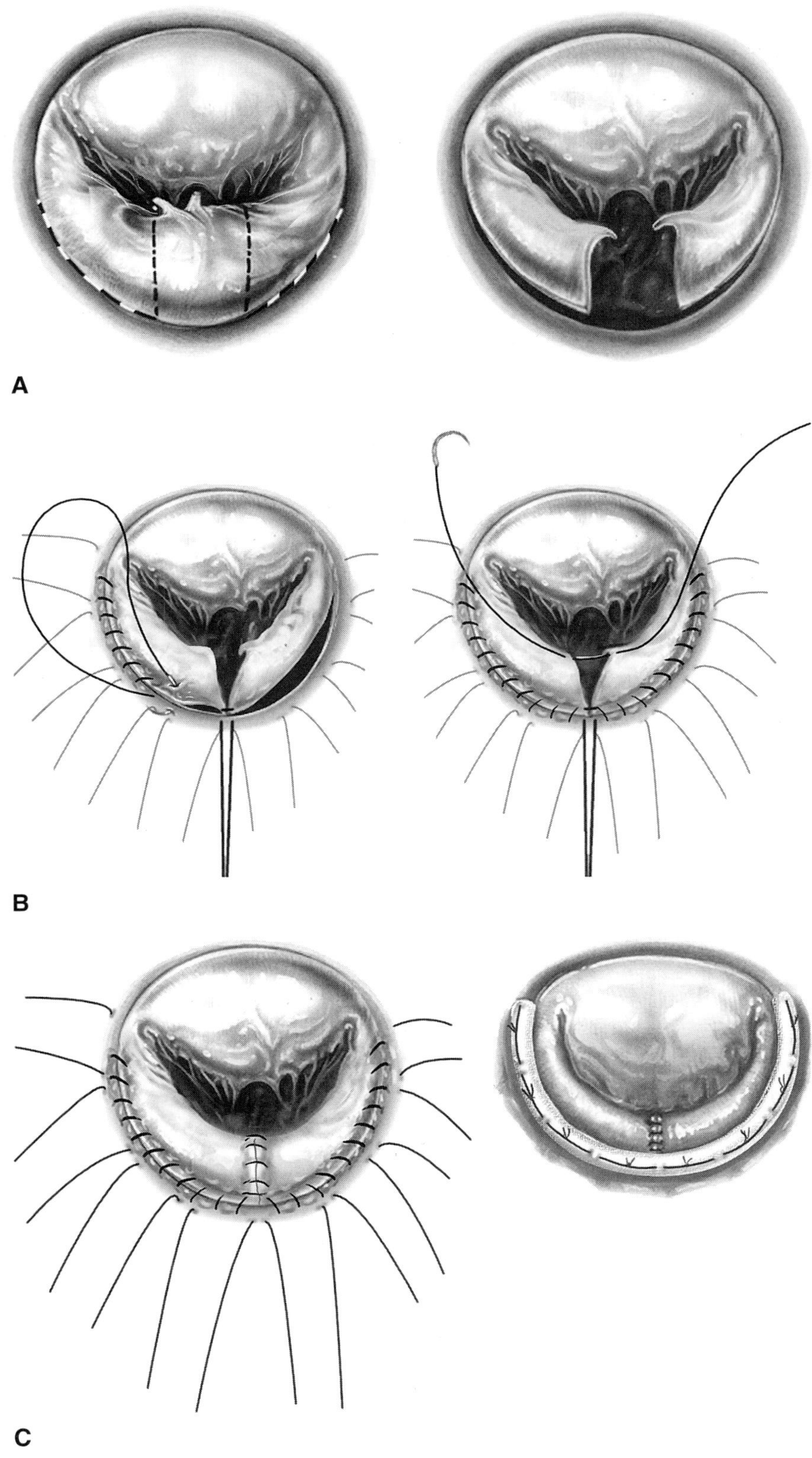

FIGURE 37–3 Sliding leaflet repair to prevent SAM. (Top) After leaflet resection, the posterior leaflet is detached from the annulus for a distance of 1 to 2 cm toward each commissure. (Middle) Annuloplasty sutures are placed, and the leaflet is reattached to the annulus. (Bottom) The leaflet edges are reapproximated, and annuloplasty completes the repair.

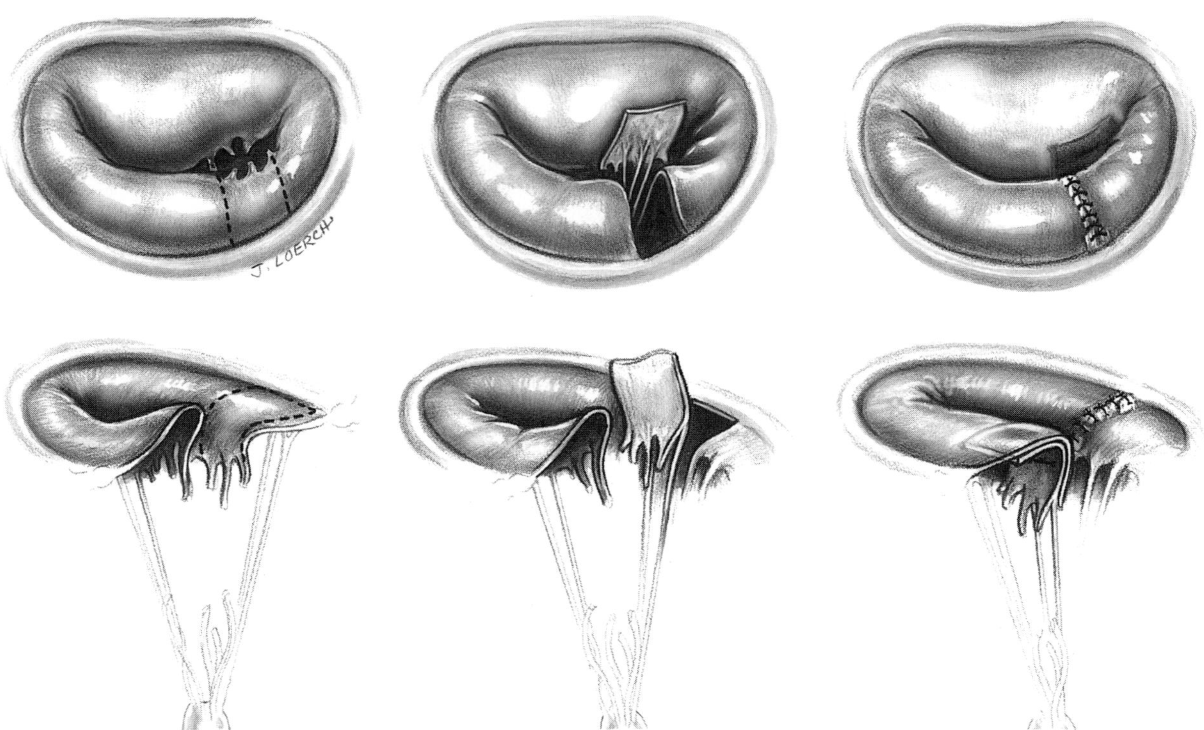

FIGURE 37–4 Chordal transfer from posterior to anterior leaflet. In order to support a portion of anterior leaflet with ruptured chordae, a segment of the posterior leaflet with its attached chordae is transferred to the anterior leaflet.

RESULTS

Using these techniques, 90% of degenerative mitral valves can be repaired. For isolated mitral valve repair, hospital mortality is less than 1%, and repair results in survival curves similar to those of the general population.[7,8] Degenerative disease is associated with the most durable mitral valve repairs. Overall, 10-year freedom from reoperation is 93%; posterior leaflet repair with quadrangular resection and annuloplasty and echocardiographic assessment results in 98% 10-year and 97% 20-year freedoms from reoperation.[7,8,33,36]

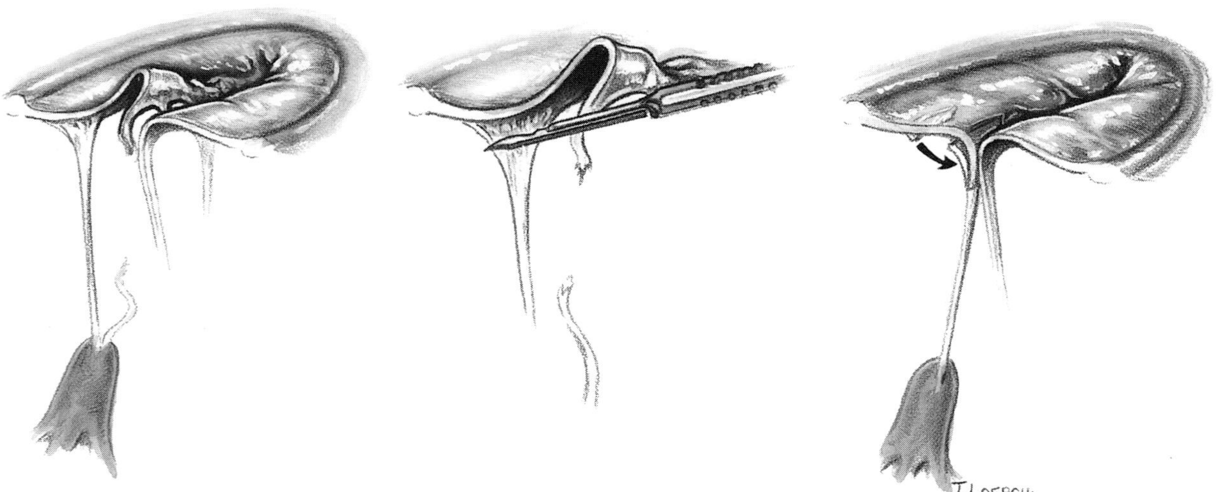

FIGURE 37–5 Chordal transfer from anterior leaflet. A normal secondary chord is transferred from the body to the free edge of the anterior leaflet to correct prolapse caused by anterior chordal rupture.

Risk of repair failure is increased by anterior leaflet prolapse, chordal shortening, and failure to use an annuloplasty or intraoperative echocardiography.[7,8,73] After repair, patients should not leave the operating room with more than 1+ MR.[74,75]

Rheumatic Mitral Valve Disease

The prevalence of rheumatic mitral valve disease has been decreasing in surgical practice in North America and Europe. This is attributable to the reduced incidence of the disease and the advent of percutaneous balloon mitral valvuloplasty to treat mitral stenosis.[76,77]

Pathologic features of rheumatic mitral valve disease produce varying degrees of regurgitation, stenosis, or mixed lesions.[78] Acute rheumatic valvitis produces leaflet prolapse and MR; these features are uncommon in North America.[79] Most patients presenting for evaluation have some component of restricted leaflet motion, producing mitral stenosis or a mixed lesion.[80] Restricted leaflet motion is caused by thickening of the subvalvular apparatus, thickening of the leaflets, and commissural fusion; there may also be calcification of any component of the valve.

SURGICAL INDICATIONS

Symptomatic mitral stenosis or regurgitation is an indication for intervention. New onset atrial fibrillation is also an indication for intervention. Patients with mitral stenosis and low echocardiographic scores should have percutaneous balloon valvotomy.[81,82] Patients with higher echo scores (>8) should be offered surgery. In such patients, if the anterior leaflet and chordae are pliable, repair is considered.[80,83] In contrast, if the valve is severely distorted, the leaflets heavily calcified, or the papillary muscles fused to the leaflet edges, the valve should be replaced.

Pure rheumatic mitral regurgitation is uncommon. Durability of repair for this entity is limited.[84] In such patients, repair may be offered as a palliative option, particularly if there are compelling reasons to provide a period of time during which the patient will not require anticoagulation (e.g., childbearing).

Patients with mixed rheumatic stenosis and regurgitation present a particular technical challenge and are least amenable to repair.[85] If valve distortion is not severe and the anterior leaflet and chordae are pliable, repair may be considered.

REPAIR TECHNIQUES

In North America, most patients who present for surgical treatment of rheumatic mitral valve disease have severely deformed valves that are best suited to replacement.[80] However, in patients with primary mitral stenosis and limited calcification and subvalvular thickening, open mitral commissurotomy is a good option. The commissurotomy should extend to 2 mm from the annulus; more extensive commissurotomy may cause MR. If there is MR after commissurotomy, an annuloplasty is added. Debridement of calcium and fibrous peel from the leaflets is an adjunctive measure employed in some patients.

Rheumatic MR from leaflet prolapse is repaired using techniques such as chordal transfer and creation of artificial chordae.[79] An annuloplasty is incorporated in these repairs.

Patients with combined mitral stenosis and regurgitation are usually best served by replacement. When repair is attempted, a combination of techniques described above is necessary.

RESULTS

Mitral valve repair may confer a survival advantage when compared to mitral valve replacement in patients with rheumatic disease.[80,86] Overall, 10-year freedom from reoperation in patients with repaired rheumatic valves is 72%.[80] However, the feasibility and durability of repair are influenced strongly by the valve pathology. In appropriately selected patients with pure mitral stenosis, open mitral commissurotomy provides excellent results, with 78% to 91% 10-year freedom from reoperation.[87,88] However, durability is particularly limited in young patients with acute rheumatic carditis and prolapse; nearly half of these patients develop severe recurrent MR within 5 years.[84] In patients with mixed lesions, valve morphology usually limits the ability to achieve a satisfactory repair; when repair is attempted in such patients, durability is limited, with half of patients requiring reoperation within 14 years.[83,85]

Ischemic Mitral Regurgitation

Ischemic mitral regurgitation is MR that is caused by coronary artery disease.[6] As such, ischemic MR must be distinguished from organic mitral valve disease with coexisting coronary artery disease. In patients with ischemic MR, the valve leaflets and chordae appear normal.[89,90] The MR is a direct consequence of left ventricular dysfunction. Ischemic MR may be transient, a result of reversible ischemia that causes ventricular dysfunction. In this setting, relief of ischemia generally causes MR to decrease or disappear, and a mitral valve procedure is unnecessary. More commonly, ischemic MR is a consequence of previous myocardial infarction.

Ischemic MR caused by previous myocardial infarction is subdivided into three mechanisms: (1) ruptured papillary muscle, (2) infarcted papillary muscle without rupture, and (3) functional regurgitation (Table 37-1). Ruptured papillary muscle is most frequently caused by infarction in the circumflex or right coronary artery distribution. Patients with elongated and infarcted but unruptured papillary

TABLE 37–1 Mechanisms of ischemic mitral regurgitation

Mechanism
Reversible ischemia
Transient left ventricular dilatation/dysfunction
Myocardial infarction
Ruptured papillary muscle
Infarcted but unruptured papillary muscle
Functional
Left ventricular dilatation/dysfunction
Annular dilatation
Left ventricular dilatation/dysfunction and annular dilatation

muscles have leaflet prolapse. Patients with isolated functional MR have normal papillary muscles, chordae, and leaflets; however, the leaflets fail to coapt. Failure of coaptation is caused by annular dilatation, leaflet tethering, or both (Fig. 37-6). Myocardial infarction produces ventricular dilatation and dysfunction, and the resulting geometric changes prevent leaflet coaptation. These changes in annular and ventricular geometry are usually caused by myocardial infarction in the circumflex or right coronary artery distributions.[6,91,92] Using echocardiography, the majority of patients with ischemic MR can be placed into one of these groups.

SURGICAL INDICATIONS

Patients with acute ischemic MR and active myocardial ischemia are most commonly treated by a combination of medical therapy and percutaneous coronary intervention. However, in instances of important left main coronary artery disease or severe three-vessel coronary artery disease, they may require urgent surgical revascularization. When surgery is required in these patients, a mitral valve procedure is deferred until examination of the postbypass echocardiogram; if MR of 2+ or higher persists, a mitral procedure is then performed.

Papillary muscle rupture causes cardiogenic shock. After diagnosis by echocardiography and coronary angiography, an intra-aortic balloon pump is placed and emergency surgery is performed. When patients with papillary muscle infarction and elongation without rupture develop 3+ or 4+ MR and congestive symptoms, surgery is indicated.

Surgical indications for patients with functional ischemic MR are controversial. The degree of MR should be established by *preoperative* echocardiogram, as intraoperative echocardiogram tends to result in downgrading of MR due to changes in loading conditions.[6,92] These patients present for combined coronary artery bypass grafting and mitral valve surgery or isolated mitral valve surgery. In patients undergoing coronary artery bypass grafting, 3+ or 4+ MR should be addressed. In patients with 2+ MR, we favor mitral valve repair at the time of coronary artery bypass grafting. Currently, however, data are lacking to support an advantage to this approach.

Selected patients with ischemic cardiomyopathy and functional MR should be offered mitral valve repair.[93–96] These patients should be offered surgery only if they have 3+ or 4+ MR. Such patients should have a preoperative viability study to assess the need for coronary artery bypass grafting.

REPAIR TECHNIQUES

Papillary muscle rupture should usually be managed by mitral valve replacement with a bioprosthesis.[6,97] Although occasional patients may be treated by reimplantation of a ruptured papillary muscle head into adjacent viable myocardium, such a strategy subjects a critically ill patient to the possibility of catastrophic early or late repair failure caused by recurrent rupture.

Papillary muscle infarction with elongation is managed using the techniques described for patients with degenerative mitral valve disease and prolapse. If a portion of the posterior leaflet is affected, quadrangular resection is indicated.

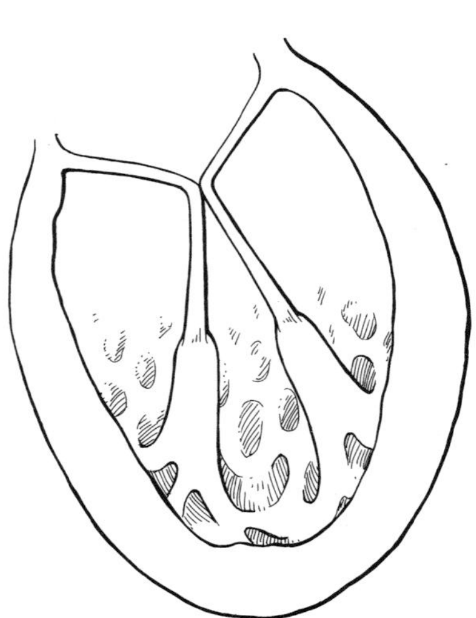

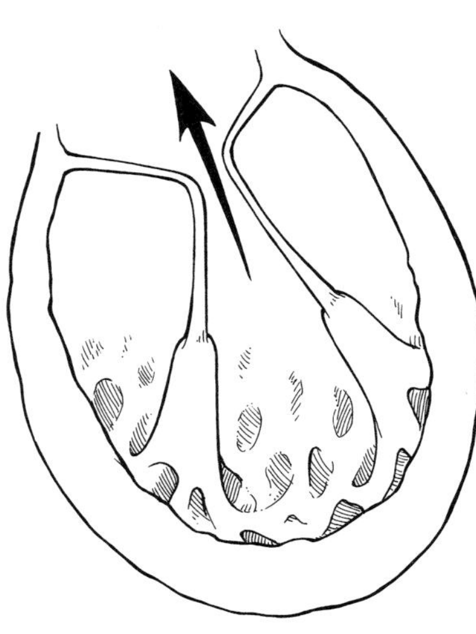

FIGURE 37–6 Functional ischemic mitral regurgitation occurs when ventricular dilatation and dysfunction cause leaflet tethering, preventing normal leaflet coaptation.

If there is anterior leaflet prolapse, chordal transfer or chordal replacement suffices. Occasionally, papillary muscle shortening is employed.[98]

Functional ischemic MR is generally managed with annuloplasty alone. The annuloplasty should be undersized in order to increase maximally leaflet coaptation.[6,93] The precise type of annuloplasty (flexible vs. rigid, complete vs. incomplete) is controversial.[6,93] We favor an undersized, flexible, posterior annuloplasty. If, on static testing in the arrested heart, it appears likely that a leak will remain after annuloplasty, an Alfieri stitch may be added. This is generally placed in the middle of the valve, or, occasionally, toward the posteromedial commissure.[96] If leaflet tethering is extensive and annuloplasty fails, mitral valve replacement with a bioprosthesis and preservation of the subvalvular apparatus is indicated.[99]

RESULTS

Surgical treatment of ischemic MR is associated with poor long-term survival. Hospital mortality after valve repair in patients with ischemic MR is 3% to 6%.[6] However, 5-year survival is only 58%.[6] The mechanism of MR influences survival.[6,89,91] Patients with ruptured papillary muscle have the best long-term survival, likely related to better preservation of left ventricular function.[6] Patients with functional ischemic MR have more LV damage and correspondingly reduced longevity. The majority of patients with ischemic MR benefit from mitral valve repair versus replacement. Replacement should be reserved for patients in whom repair fails or is not feasible. In addition, the most critically ill patients should receive bioprostheses; in such patients, there is no survival benefit to repair.

Because long-term survival is limited, the durability of mitral valve repair in patients with ischemic MR is difficult to establish. Bolling and others report excellent freedom from recurrent MR in patients with ischemic cardiomyopathy.[93,96] This success is attributed to a combination of small annuloplasty ring size and favorable ventricular remodeling. There is no large study documenting long-term echocardiographic follow-up in patients having mitral valve repair for ischemic MR.

Endocarditis

Native valve endocarditis is generally caused by streptococcal or staphylococcal species.[100–103] Pathologic findings include chordal rupture (70%), vegetation (62%), leaflet perforation (53%), and abscess (7%).[100]

SURGICAL INDICATIONS

Surgical indications are well established.[104–107] They include heart failure unresponsive to medical therapy, multiple embolic events, uncontrolled sepsis, and extension of infection into surrounding structures. In addition, early operation is indicated for fungal and staphylococcal infections. Potential advantages of mitral valve repair in the setting of infection include preservation of the native, living valve apparatus, which is resistant to infection, and corresponding avoidance of prosthetic material.[100–103]

REPAIR TECHNIQUES

Radical debridement is the cornerstone of operative treatment of endocarditis.[103] All infected material must be removed. If there are ruptured chordae to the posterior leaflet, quadrangular resection is performed. Anterior chordal rupture is repaired with standard techniques. Anterior leaflet perforations are repaired with autologous pericardial patches; it is not necessary to fix or tan the pericardium. Abscess cavities are debrided and excluded with a pericardial patch.[108] We favor posterior pericardial annuloplasty in both active and chronic endocarditis.[100]

RESULTS

Eighty percent of infected mitral valves are amenable to repair.[100] Hospital mortality is 0% to 7%.[100–103] Recurrent endocarditis is rare after mitral valve repair.[100–103] When compared to replacement, repair of the infected mitral valve results in greater freedom from recurrent infection and higher early and late survival.[100]

MINIMALLY INVASIVE MITRAL VALVE SURGERY

A variety of less invasive approaches have been developed to perform isolated mitral valve surgery or combined mitral and aortic valve surgery. Chest wall incisions include right parasternal,[109] right thoracotomy,[110–112] partial lower sternotomy,[113] and partial upper sterntomy.[31,114] Adjunctive techniques employed for mitral valve surgery include Port-Access instrumentation,[115,116] video assistance,[110,111] and robotic assistance.[117–119] Excellent results have been reported with each of these approaches.

We favor partial upper sternotomy access for isolated valve surgery. This approach affords the surgeon a familiar orientation. Central cannulation is possible in all cases, and exposure of the mitral valve is excellent. Through a 6-cm skin incision, a partial upper sternotomy extends from the sternal notch to the left 4th intercostal space (Fig. 37-7). Cardiopulmonary bypass is accomplished via bicaval and aortic cannulation. Vacuum-assisted venous drainage allows the use of smaller, less obstructive cannulae, reduces the priming volume of the cardiopulmonary bypass circuit, prevents air locks, and keeps the field dry. After opening the right atrium, a cannula is placed in the coronary sinus for delivery of retrograde cardioplegia. The mitral valve is approached through a transseptal incision that is extended onto the dome of the left atrium. This exposure of the mitral valve facilitates both simple and complex repair procedures.

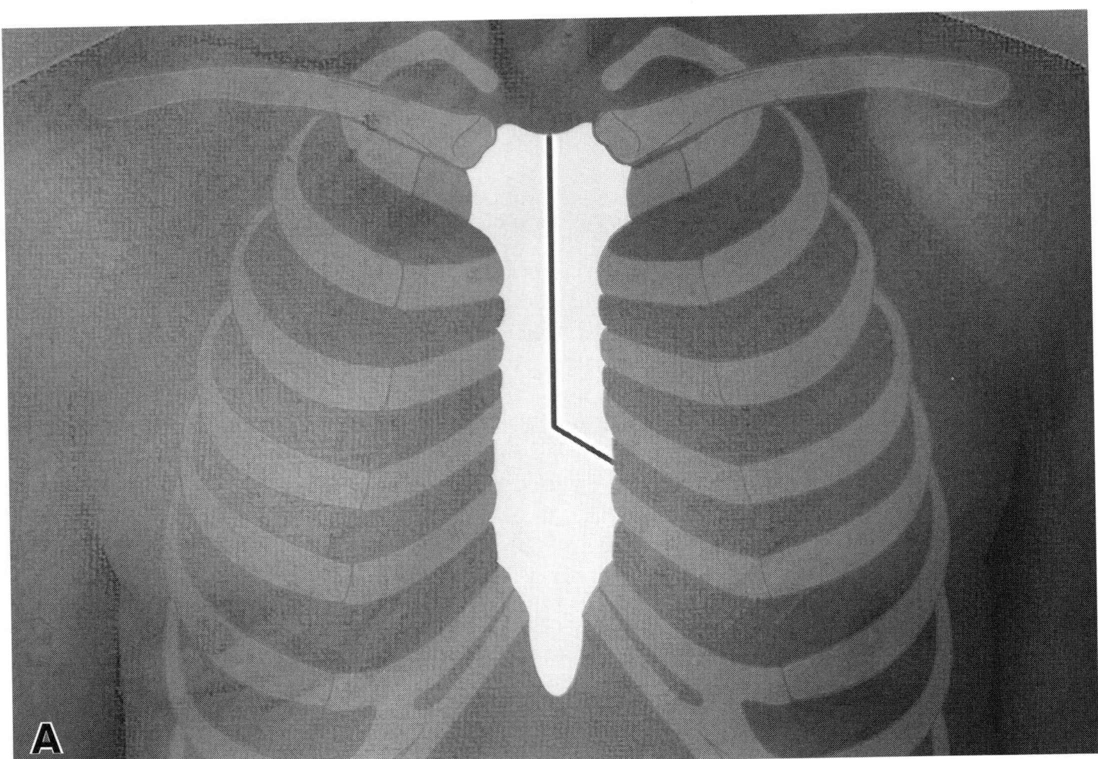

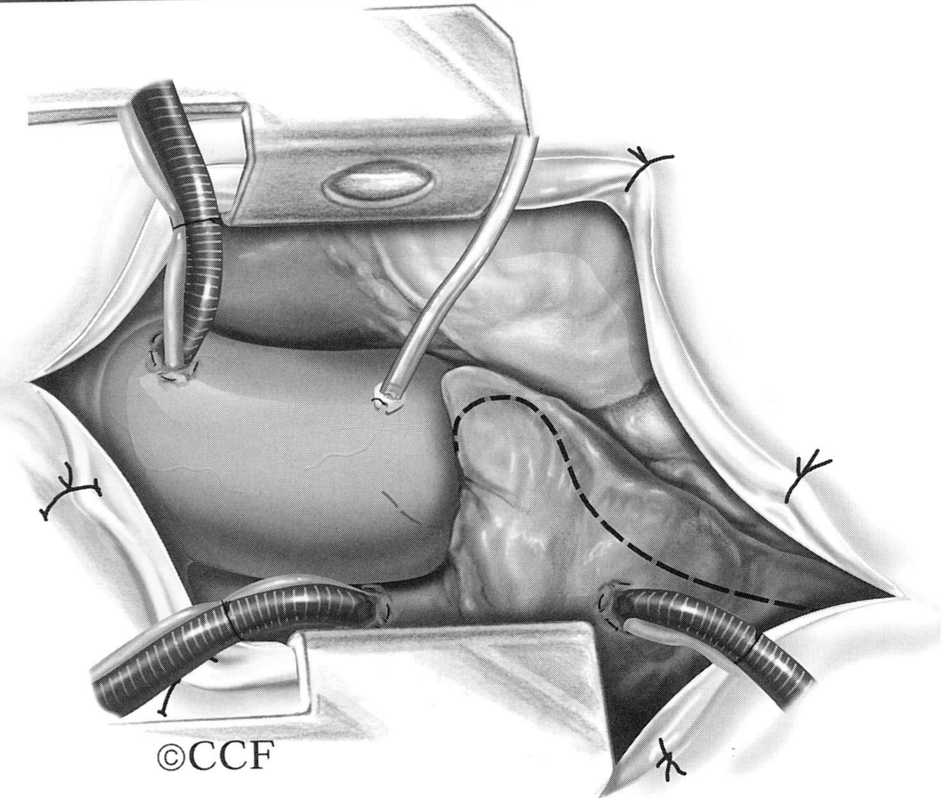

FIGURE 37–7 Minimally invasive mitral valve repair. Partial upper sternotomy provides access. The mitral valve is approached via an extended transseptal incision.

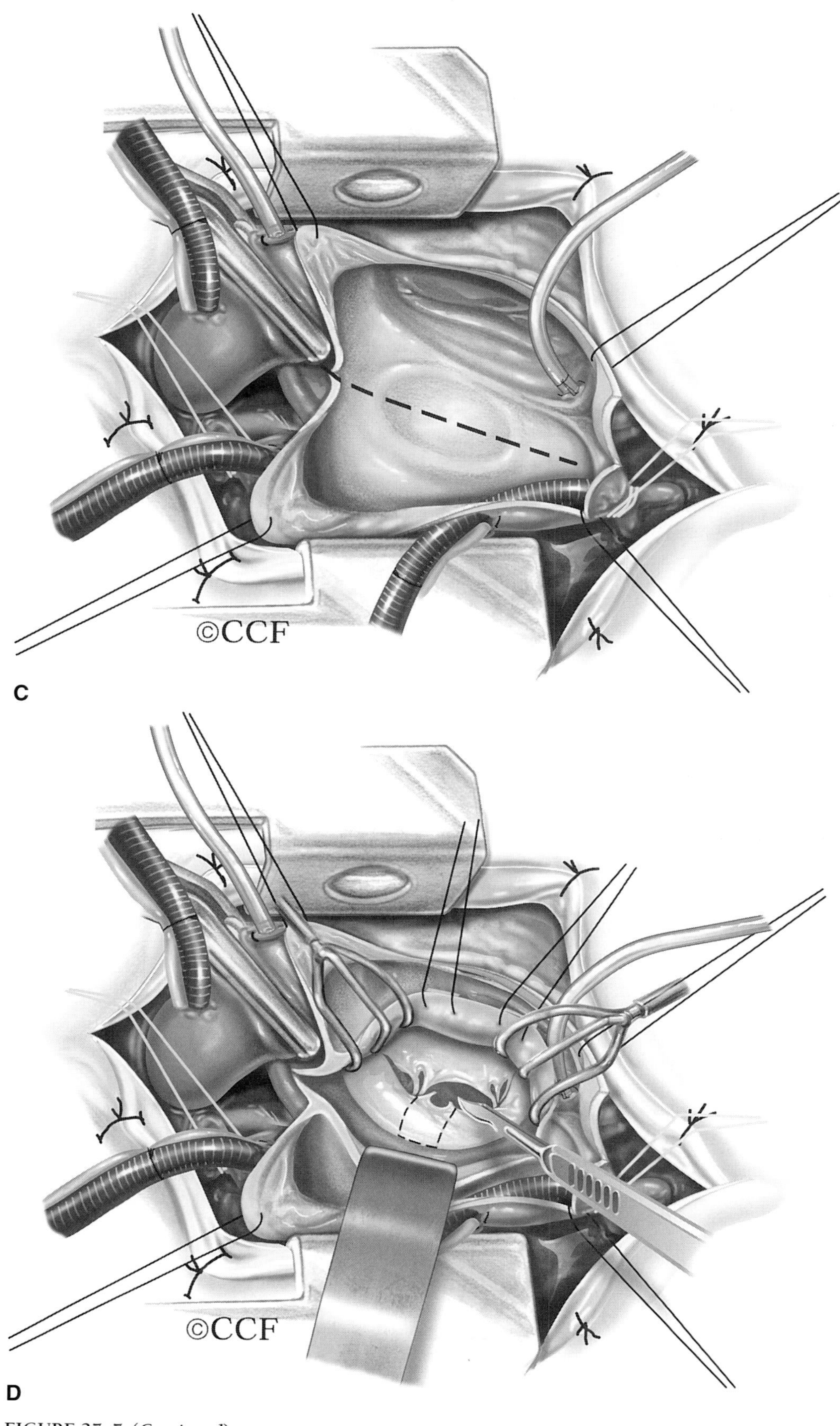

FIGURE 37–7 (*Continued*)

This approach has been used in more than 1400 mitral valve procedures at the Cleveland Clinic Foundation; 90% of these patients had mitral valve repair. Conversion to full sternotomy was necessary in 1% of cases. Hospital mortality was 0.3%. This is now our approach of choice in patients with isolated heart valve disease.

MITRAL VALVE REPAIR AND ATRIAL FIBRILLATION

Thirty to fifty percent of patients presenting for mitral valve surgery have atrial fibrillation.[120] In such patients, an important goal of the procedure is ablation of atrial fibrillation in addition to mitral valve repair. When atrial fibrillation has been present for less than 1 year, mitral valve repair alone is likely to cure the atrial fibrillation.[120–123] In contrast, when atrial fibrillation has been present for more than 1 year, 80% of patients will remain in atrial fibrillation, requiring coumadin after mitral valve repair.[121] Therefore, surgical ablation of atrial fibrillation is indicated in patients having mitral valve surgery who have a history of more than 1 year of paroxysmal, persistent, or permanent atrial fibrillation.

A variety of surgical procedures are available for ablation of atrial fibrillation, ranging from the Cox-Maze III procedure to pulmonary vein isolation using alternative energy sources.[120,124–130] Alternative energy sources currently available to create lines of conduction block include microwave, radiofrequency, cryothermy, and laser. Use of alternative energy sources decreases the operative time and reduces the risk of bleeding. These are generally used to create left atrial lesion sets that include pulmonary vein isolation and connecting lesions to the left atrial appendage and to the mitral annulus.[120,130] This is based upon current concepts regarding the pulmonary veins and left atrium in the genesis of atrial fibrillation.[131,132] Right atrial lesions are frequently omitted, as atrial fibrillation rarely arises from the right atrium.

The Cox-Maze III procedure cures atrial fibrillation in 80% to 100% of patients having concomitant mitral valve surgery.[124,125] Increased left atrial size and rheumatic disease may limit success. Early data suggest that use of alternative energy sources to create left atrial lesion sets ablates atrial fibrillation in 70% to 80% of patients.[120] Given these data, patients with preoperative atrial fibrillation of more than 1 year's duration should have surgical ablation of atrial fibrillation in addition to mitral valve repair. In such patients, this strategy is the only means to avoid lifelong anticoagulation and its attendant risks.

REFERENCES

1. Sand ME, Naftel DC, Blackstone EH, et al: A comparison of repair and replacement for mitral valve incompetence. *J Thorac Cardiovasc Surg* 1987; 94:208.
2. Perier P, Deloche A, Chauvaud S, et al: Comparative evaluation of mitral valve repair and replacement with Starr, Bjork, and porcine valve prostheses. *Circulation* 1984; 70(suppl I):I-187.
3. Lawrie GM: Mitral valve repair vs replacement: current recommendations and long-term results. *Cardiol Clin* 1998; 16:437.
4. Goldsmith IRA, Lip GYH, Patel RL: A prospective study of changes in the quality of life of patients following mitral valve repair and replacement. *Eur J Cardiothoracic Surg* 2001; 20:949.
5. Ren JF, Aksut S, Lighty GW, et al: Mitral valve repair is superior to valve replacement for the early preservation of cardiac function: relation of ventricular geometry to function. *Am Heart J* 1996; 131:974.
6. Gillinov AM, Wierup PN, Blackstone EH, et al: Is repair preferable to replacement for ischemic mitral regurgitation? *J Thorac Cardiovasc Surg* 2001; 122:1125.
7. Gillinov AM, Cosgrove DM, Blackstone EH, et al: Durability of mitral valve repair for degenerative disease. *J Thorac Cardiovasc Surg* 1998; 116:734.
8. Braunberger E, Deloche A, Berrebi A, et al: Very long-term results (more than 20 years) of valve repair with Carpentier's techniques in nonrheumatic mitral valve insufficiency. *Circulation* 2001; 104 (Suppl I): I-B.
9. Carpentier A, Deloche A, Dauptain J, et al: A new reconstructive operation for correction of mitral and tricuspid insufficiency. *J Thorac Cardiovasc Surg* 1971; 61:1.
10. Duran CM, Gometza B, DeVol EB: Valve repair in rheumatic mitral disease. *Circulation* 1991; 84(suppl):III-125.
11. David TE, Armstrong S, Sun Z, Daniel L: Late results of mitral valve repair for mitral regurgitation due to degenerative disease. *Ann Thorac Surg* 1993; 56:7.
12. Du Plessis LA, Marchano P: The anatomy of the mitral valve and its associated structures. *Thorax* 1964; 19:221.
13. Ormiston JA, Shah PM, Tei C, et al: Size and motion of the mitral annulus in man: a two-dimensional echocardiographic method and findings in normal subjects. *Circulation* 1981; 64:113.
14. Sonnenblick EA, Napolitano LN, Dagett WR: An intrinsic neuromuscular basis for mitral valve motion in the dog. *Circulation* 1969; 21:9.
15. Levine RA, Triulz MO, Harringan P, et al: The relationship of mitral annular shape to the diagnosis of mitral valve prolapse. *Circulation* 1987; 75:756.
16. Carpentier A, Deloche A, Dauptain J, et al: A new reconstructive operation for correction of mitral and tricuspid insufficiency. *J Thorac Cardiovasc Surg* 1971; 61:1.
17. David TE, Ho WC: The effects of preservation of chordae tendineae on mitral valve replacement for postinfarction mitral regurgitation. *Circulation* 1986; 74(suppl 1):116.
18. Rozich JD, Carabello BA, Uscher BW, et al: Mitral valve replacement with and without chordal preservation in patients with chronic mitral regurgitation: mechanics for differences in postoperative ejection performance. *Circulation* 1992; 86:1718.
19. Estes EH, Dalton FM, Entman ML, et al: The anatomy and blood supply of the papillary muscles of the left ventricle. *Am Heart J* 1966; 71:356.
20. James TN: Anatomy of the coronary arteries in health and disease. *Circulation* 1955; 32:1020.
21. Fulton WFM: *The Coronary Arteries: Arteriography, Microanatomy and Pathogenesis of Obliterative Coronary Artery Disease.* Springfield, IL, Charles C Thomas, 1955.
22. Stewart WS, Chavez AM, Currie PJ, et al: Echo determination of mitral pathology and feasibility of repair for mitral regurgitation. *Circulation* 1987; 76:III-434.
23. Ascah KJ, Steward WJ, Jiang L, et al: A Doppler two-dimensional echocardiographic method for quantitation of mitral regurgitation. *Circulation* 1985; 72:377.

24. Bargiggia GS, Tronconi L, Sahn DJ, et al: A new method for quantification of mitral regurgitation based on color flow Doppler imaging of flow convergence proximal to regurgitation orifice. *Circulation* 1991; 84:1481.
25. Helmcke F, Nanda MC, Hsiung MC, et al: Color Doppler assessment of mitral regurgitation with orthogonal planes. *Circulation* 1987; 75:175.
26. Sarano EM, Seward JB, Bailey KR, et al: Effective regurgitant orifice area: a noninvasive Doppler development of an old hemodynamic concept. *J Am Coll Cardiol* 1994; 23:443.
27. Martin RP, Rakowski H, Kleinman JH, et al: Reliability and reproducibility of two-dimensional echocardiographic measurement of the stenotic valve orifice area. *Am J Card* 1979; 43:560.
28. Cosgrove DM, Gillinov AM: Partial sternotomy for mitral valve operations. *Op Techniques Card and Thorac Surg* 1998; 3:62.
29. Cosgrove DM: A self-retaining retractor for mitral valve operations. *J Thorac Cardiovasc Surg* 1986; 92:305.
30. Gillinov AM, Cosgrove DM: Mitral valve repair. *Op Techniques Card and Thorac Surg* 1998; 3:95.
31. Gillinov AM, Cosgrove DM: Minimally invasive mitral valve surgery: mini-sternotomy with extended transseptal approach. *Semin Thorac Cardiovasc Surg* 1999; 11:206.
32. Carpentier A: Cardiac valve surgery: the French correction. *J Thorac Cardiovasc Surg* 1983; 86:323.
33. Gillinov AM, Cosgrove DM: Mitral valve repair for degenerative disease. *J Heart Valve Dis* 2002; 11(suppl 1): S15.
34. Cohn LH, Couper GS, Aranki SF, et al: The long-term results of mitral valve reconstruction for the "floppy" valve. *J Card Surg* 1994; 4(suppl):278.
35. Cohn LH, DiSesa VJ, Couper GS, et al: Mitral valve repair for myxomatous degeneration and prolapse of the mitral valve. *J Thorac Cardiovasc Surg* 1989; 98:987.
36. Deloche A, Jebara VA, Relland JYM, et al: Valve repair with Carpentier techniques: the second decade. *J Thorac Cardiovasc Surg* 1990; 99:990.
37. Braunwald E: *Heart Disease,* 3rd ed. Philadelphia, WB Saunders, 1988; p 1045.
38. Nishimura RA, McGoon DC, Shub C, et al: Echocardiographically documented mitral-valve prolapse: long-term follow up of 237 patients. *N Engl J Med* 1985; 313:1306.
39. Mills P, Rose J, Hollingsworth J, et al: Long-term prognosis of mitral-valve prolapse. *N Engl J Med* 1977; 297:13.
40. Allen H, Harris A, Leatham A: Significance and prognosis of an isolated late systolic murmur: a 9-to-22 year followup. *Br Heart J* 1974; 36:525.
41. Appelblatt NH, Willis PW III, Lenhart JA, et al: Ten to 40-year follow up of patients with systolic click with or without apical late systolic murmur. *Am J Cardiol* 1979; 35:119.
42. Ling LH, Enriquez-Sarano M, Seward JB: Early surgery in patients with mitral regurgitation due to flial leaflets: a long-term outcome study. *Circulation* 1997; 96:1819.
43. Smoles IA, Pagani FD, Deeb GM, et al: Prophylactic mitral reconstruction for mitral regurgitation. *J Thorac Cardiovasc Surg* 2001; 72:1210.
44. Ling LH, Enriquez-Sarano M, Seward JB, et al: Clinical outcome of mitral regurgitation due to flail leaflet. *N Engl J Med* 1996; 335:1417.
45. Ross J Jr: The timing of surgery for severe mitral regurgitation [editorial]. *N Engl J Med* 1996; 335:1456.
46. Uva MS, Dreyfus G, Rescigno G, et al: Surgical treatment of asymptomatic and mildly symptomatic mitral regurgitation. *J Thorac Cardiovasc Surg* 1996; 112:1240.
47. Dalrymple-Hay, MJR, Bryant M, Jones RA, et al: Degenerative mitral regurgitation: when should we operate? *Ann Thorac Surg* 1998; 66:1579.
48. Carpentier A: The sliding leaflet technique. *Le Club Mitrale Newsletter,* August 1988: I-5.
49. Kreindel MS, Schiavone WA, Lever HM, Cosgrove DM: Systolic anterior motion of the mitral valve after Carpentier ring valvuloplasty for mitral valve prolapse. *Am J Cardiol* 1986; 57:408.
50. Kronzon I, Cohen ML, Winer HE, Colvin SB: Left ventricular outflow tract obstruction: a complication of mitral valvuloplasty. *J Am Coll Cardiol* 1984; 4:825.
51. Stewart WJ, Currie PJ, Lytle BW, et al: Intraoperative Doppler color flow mapping for decision making in valve repair for mitral regurgitation: techniques and results in 100 patients. *Circulation* 1990; 81:556.
52. Lee KS, Stewart WJ, Lever HM, et al: Mechanism of outflow obstruction following failed valve repair: anterior displacement of leaflet coaptation. *Circulation* 1993; 88:(suppl II):II24.
53. Mihaileanu S, Marino JP, Chauvaud S, et al: Left ventricular outflow obstruction after mitral repair (Carpentier's technique): proposed mechanism of disease. *Circulation* 1988; 78:(suppl I):78.
54. Grossi EA, Galloway AC, Parish MA, et al: Experience with twenty-eight cases of systolic motion after mitral valve construction by Carpentier technique. *J Thorac Cardiovasc Surg* 1992; 103:466.
55. Lopez JA, Schnee M, Gaos CM, Wilansky S: Left ventricular outflow tract obstruction and hemolytic anemia after mitral valve repair with a Duran ring. *Ann Thorac Surg* 1994; 58:876.
56. Kupferschmid JP, Carr T, Connelly GP, Shemin RJ: Systolic anterior motion of the mitral valve after valve repair without an annular ring. *Ann Thorac Surg* 1994; 57:484.
57. Gillinov AM, Cosgrove DM III: Modified sliding leaflet technique for repair of the mitral valve. *Ann Thorac Surg* 1999; 68:2356.
58. Perier P, Clausnizer B, Mistarz K: Carpentier sliding leaflet technique for repair of the mitral valve: early results. *Ann Thorac Surg* 1994; 57:383.
59. Zussa C: Artificial chordae. *J Heart Valve Dis* 1995; 4(suppl II): S249.
60. David TE, Omran A, Armstrong S, et al: Long-term results of mitral valve repair for myxomatous disease with and without chordal replacement with expanded polytetrafluoroethylene sutures. *J Thorac Cardiovasc Surg* 1998; 115:1279.
61. Gregori F Jr, da Silva SS, Goulart MP, et al: Grafting of chordae tendineae: a new technique for repair of mitral insufficiency caused by ruptured chordae of the anterior leaflet [letter]. *J Thorac Cardiovas Surg* 1994; 107:635.
62. Smedira NG, Selman R, Cosgrove DM, et al: Repair of anterior leaflet prolapse: chordal transfer is superior to chordal shortening. *J Thorac Cardiovasc Surg* 1996; 112:287.
63. El Khoury G, Noirhomme P, Verhelst R, et al: Surgical repair of the prolapsing anterior leaflet in degenerative mitral valve disease. *J Heart Valve Di* 2000; 9:75.
64. Raffoul R, Uva MS, Rescigno G, et al: Clinical evalutation of the physio annuloplasty ring. *Clin Invest* 1998; 113:1296.
65. Gorton ME, Piehler JM, Killen DA, et al: Mitral valve repair using a flexible and adjustable annuloplasty ring. *Ann Thorac Surg* 1993; 55:860.
66. Cosgrove DM III, Arcidi JM, Rodriquez L, et al: Initial experience with the Cosgrove-Edwards annuloplasty system. *Ann Thorac Surg* 1995; 60:499.
67. Gillinov AM, Cosgrove DM, Takahiro S, et al: Cosgrove-Edwards annuloplasty system: midterm results. *Ann Thorac Surg* 2000; 69:717.
68. Bichell DP, Adams DH, Aranaki SF, et al: Repair of mitral regurgitation for myxomatous degeneration in the patient with a severely calcified posterior annulus. *J Card Surg* 1995; 10:281.
69. El Asmar B, Acker N, Couetil JP, et al: Mitral valve repair in the extensively calcified mitral annulus. *Ann Thorac Surg* 1991; 52:66.

70. Carpentier AF, Pellerin M, Fuzellier JF, et al: Extensive calcification of the mitral valve annulus: pathology and surgical management. *J Thorac Cardiovasc Surg* 1996; 111:718.
71. Fucci C, Sandrelli L, Pardini A, et al: Improved results with mitral valve repair using new surgical techniques. *Eur J Cardiothorac Surg* 1995; 9:621.
72. Alfieri O, Maisano F, De Bonis M, et al: The double-orifice technique in mitral valve repair: a simple solution for complex problems. *J Thorac Cardiovasc Surg* 2001; 122: 674.
73. Gillinov AM, Cosgrove DM, Lytle BW, et al: Reoperation for failure of mitral valve repair. *J Thorac Cardiovasc Surg* 1997; 113:467.
74. Saiki Y, Kasegawa H, Kawase M, et al: Intraoperative TEE during mitral valve repair: does it predict early and late postoperative mitral valve dysfunction? *Ann Thorac Surg* 1998; 66:1277.
75. Fix J, Isada L, Cosgrove DM, et al: Do patients with less than "echo perfect" results from mitral valve repair by intraoperative echocardiography have a different outcome? *Circulation* 1993; 88(part 2):II39.
76. Gordis L: The virtual disappearance of rheumatic fever in the United States: lessons in the rise and fall of disease. T. Duckett Jones Memorial Lecture. *Circulation* 1985; 72:1155.
77. Edwards JE: Pathology of mitral incompetence, in Silver MD (ed): *Cardiovascular Pathology*, Vol 1. New York, Churchill Livingstone, 1983; p 575.
78. Duran CMG, Gometza B, Saad E: Valve repair in rheumatic mitral disease: an unsolved problem. *J Card Surg* 1994; 9(suppl):282.
79. Kalangos A, Beghetti M, Vala D, et al: Anterior mitral leaflet prolapse as a primary cause of pure rheumatic mitral insufficiency. *Ann Thorac Surg* 2000; 69:755.
80. Yau TM, El-Ghoneimi YAF, Armstrong S, et al: Mitral valve repair and replacement for rheumatic disease. *J Thorac Cardiovasc Surg* 2000; 119:53.
81. Palacios IF, Block PC, Wilkins GT, et al: Follow-up of patients undergoing percutaneous mitral balloon valvuloplasty: analysis of factors determining restenosis. *Circulation* 1989; 79:573.
82. Wilkins GT, Weyman E, Abascal VM, et al: Percutaneous mitral valvuloplasty: an analysis of echocardiographic variables related to outcome and the mechanism of dilatation. *Br Heart J* 1988; 60:299.
83. David TE: The appropriateness of mitral valve repair for rheumatic mitral valve disease [editorial]. *J Heart Valve Dis* 1997; 6:373.
84. Gometza B, Al-Halees Z, Shahid M, et al: Surgery for rheumatic mitral regurgitation in patients below twenty years of age: an analysis of failures. *J Heart Valve Dis* 1996; 5: 294.
85. Nakano S, Kawashima Y, Hirose H, et al: Reconsiderations of indications for open mitral commissurotomy based on pathologic features of the stenosed mitral valve. *J Thorac Cardiovasc Surg* 1987; 94:336.
86. Grossi EA, Galloway AC, Miller JS, et al: Valve repair versus replacement for mitral insufficiency: when is a mechanical valve still indicated? *J Thorac Cardiovasc Surg* 1998; 115:389.
87. Hickey MSJ, Blackstone EH, Kirklin JW, et al: Outcome probabilities and life history after surgical mitral commissurotomy: implications for balloon commissurotomy. *J Am Coll Card* 1991; 17:29.
88. Herrera JM, Vega JL, Bernal JM, et al: Open mitral commissurotomy: fourteen-to-eighteen-year follow-up clinical study. *Ann Thorac Surg* 1993; 55:641.
89. Edmunds LH Jr: Ischemic mitral regurgitation, in Edmunds LH Jr (ed): *Cardiac Surgery in the Adult*. New York, McGraw-Hill, 1997; p 657.
90. Miller DC: Ischemic mitral regurgitation redux—to repair or to replace? *J Thorac Cardiovasc Surg* 2001; 122:1059.
91. Cohn LH, Rizzo RJ, Adams DH, et al: The effect of pathophysiology on the surgical treatment of ischemic mitral regurgitation: operative and late risks of repair versus replacement. *Eur J Cardiothorac Surg* 1995; 9:568.
92. Dion R: Ischemic mitral regurgitation: when and how it should be corrected? *J Heart Valve Dis* 1993; 2:536.
93. Bolling SF, Pagani FD, Deeb GM, et al: Intermediate-term outcome of mitral reconstruction in cardiomyopathy. *J Thorac Cardiovasc Surg* 1998; 115:381.
94. Chen FY, Adams DH, Aranki SF, et al: Mitral valve repair in cardiomyopathy. *Circulation* 1998; 98:II-124.
95. Bitran D, Merin O, Klutstein MW, et al: Mitral valve repair in severe ischemic cardiomyopathy. *J Card Surg* 2001; 16:79.
96. Bishay ES, McCarthy PM, Cosgrove DM, et al: Mitral valve surgery in patients with severe left ventricular dysfunction. *Eur J Cardiothorac Surg* 2000; 17:213.
97. David TE: Techniques and results of mitral valve repair for ischemic mitral regurgitaion. *J Card Surg* 1994; 9(suppl):274.
98. Fasol R, Wild T, Pfannmuller B, et al: Papillary muscle shortening for mitral valve reconstruction in patients with ischaemic mitral insufficiency. *Eur Heart J* 1998; 19:1730.
99. David TE, Ho WC: The effect of preservation of chordae tendineae on mitral valve replacement for postinfarction mitral regurgitation. *Circulation* 1986; 74(suppl I):I-116.
100. Muehrcke DD, Cosgrove DM III, Lytle BW, et al: Is there an advantage to repairing infected mitral valves? *Ann Thorac Surg* 1997; 63:1718.
101. Hendren WG, Morris AS, Rosencranz ER, et al: Mitral valve repair for bacterial endocarditis. *J Thorac Cardiovasc Surg* 1992; 103:124.
102. Dreyfus G, Serraf A, Jebara VA, et al: Valve repair in acute endocarditis. *Ann Thorac Surg* 1990; 49:706.
103. David TE, Bos J, Christakis GT, et al: Heart valve operations in patients with active infective endocarditis. *Ann Thorac Surg* 1990; 49:701.
104. Middlemost S, Wisenbaugh T, Meyerowitz C, et al: A case for early surgery in native left-sided endocarditis complicated by heart failure: results in 203 patients. *J Am Coll Card* 1991; 18:663.
105. Suryapranata H, Roelandt J, Haalebos M, et al: Early cardiac valve replacement in ineffective endocarditis: a 10-year experience. *Eur Heart J* 1987; 8:464.
106. Raychaudhury T, Faichney A, Cameron EWJ, et al: Surgical management of native valve endocarditis. *Thorax* 1983; 38:168.
107. Bogers AJJC, Van Vreeswijk H, Verbaan CJ, et al: Early surgery for active infective endocarditis improves early and late results. *Thorac Cardiovasc Surg* 1991; 39:284.
108. d'Udekem Y, David TE, Feindel CM, et al: Long-term results of operation for paravalvular abscess. *Ann Thorac Surg* 1996; 62:48.
109. Cosgrove DM III, Sabik JF, Navia JL: Minimally invasive valve operations. *Ann Thorac Surg* 1998; 65:1535.
110. Chitwood WR Jr, Wixon CL, Elbeery JR, et al: Video-assisted minimally invasive mitral valve surgery. *J Thorac Cardiovasc Surg* 1997; 114:773.
111. Chitwood WR Jr, Elbeery JR, Chapman WHH, et al: Video-assisted minimally invasive mitral valve surgery: The 'micro-mitral' operation. *J Thorac Cardiovasc Surg* 1997; 113:413.
112. Loulmet DF, Carpentier A, Cho PW, et al: Less invasive techniques for mitral valve surgery. *J Thorac Cardiovasc Surg* 1998; 115:772.
113. Gillinov AM, Banbury MK, Cosgrove DM, et al: Is minimally invasive heart valve surgery a paradigm for the future? *Curr Cardiol Rep* 1999; 1:318.
114. Gundry SR, Shattuck OH, Razzouk AJ, et al: Facile minimally invasive cardiac surgery via ministernotomy. *Ann Thorac Surg* 1998; 65:1100.
115. Fann JI, Pompili MF, Burdon TA, et al: Minimally invasive mitral valve surgery. *Semin Thorac Cardiovasc Surg* 1997; 9:320.
116. Mohr FW, Falk V, Diegeler A, et al: Minimally invasive port-access mitral valve surgery. *J Thorac Cardiovasc Surg* 1998; 115:567.

117. Falk V, Walther T, Autschbach R, et al: Robot-assisted minimally invasive solo mitral valve operation. *J Thorac Cardiovasc Surg* 1998; 115:470.
118. Mehmanesh H, Henze R, Lange R: Totally endoscopic mitral valve repair. *J Thorac Cardiovasc Surg* 2002; 123:96.
119. Felger JE, Chitwood WR Jr, Nifong LW, et al: Evolution of mitral valve surgery: toward a totally endoscopic approach. *Ann Thorac Surg* 2001; 72:1203.
120. Cox JL: Intraoperative options for treating atrial fibrillation associated with mitral valve disease. *J Thorac Cardiovasc Surg* 2001; 122:212.
121. Obadia JF, El Farra M, Bastien OH, et al: Outcome of atrial fibrillation after mitral valve repair. *J Thorac Cardiovasc Surg* 1997; 114:179.
122. Chua YL, Schaff HV, Orszulak TA, Morris JJ: Outcome of mitral valve repair in patients with preoperative atrial fibrillation: should the Maze procedure be combined with mitral valvuloplasty? *J Thorac Cardiovasc Surg* 1994; 107:408.
123. Vogt PR, Brunner-LaRocca HP, Rist M, et al: Preoperative predictors of recurrent atrial fibrillation late after successful mitral valve reconstruction. *Eur J Cardiothorac Surg* 1998; 13:619.
124. Cox JL, Ad N, Palazzo T, et al: Current status of the Maze procedure for the treatment of atrial fibrillation. *Semin Thorac Cardiovasc Surg* 2000; 12:15.
125. McCarthy PM, Gillinov AM, Castle L, et al: The Cox-Maze procedure: the Cleveland Clinic experience. *Semin Thorac Cardiovasc Surg* 2000; 12:25.
126. Kosakai Y, Kawaguchi AT, Isobe F, et al: Cox-Maze procedure for chronic atrial fibrillation associated with mitral valve disease. *J Thorac Cardiovasc Surg* 1994; 108:1049.
127. Kobayashi J, Kosakai Y, Nakano K, et al: Improved success rate of the Maze procedure in mitral valve disease by new criteria for patients' selection. *Eur J Cardiothorac Surg* 1998; 13:247.
128. Takami Y, Yasuura K, Takagi Y, et al: Partial Maze procedure is effective treatment for chronic atrial fibrillation associated with valve disease. *J Card Surg* 1999; 14:103.
129. Tuinenburg AE, Van Gelder IC, Tieleman RG, et al: Mini-Maze suffices as adjunct to mitral valve surgery in patients with preoperative atrial fibrillation. *J Cardiovasc Electrophysiol* 2000; 11:960.
130. Sueda T, Nagata H, Orihashi K, et al: Efficacy of a simple left atrial procedure for chronic atrial fibrillation in mitral valve operations. *Ann Thorac Surg* 1997; 63:1070.
131. Haissaguerre M, Jais P, Shah DC, et al: Spontaneous initiation of atrial fibrillation by ectopic beats originating in the pulmonary veins. *N Engl J Med* 1998; 339:659.
132. Harada A, Sasaki K, Fukushima T, et al: Atrial activiation during chronic atrial fibrillation in patients with isolated mitral valve disease. *Ann Thorac Surg* 1996; 61:104.

Chapter 38

Mechanical/Bioprosthetic Mitral Valve Replacement

Tomas Gudbjartsson/Sary Aranki/Lawrence H. Cohn

HISTORICAL BACKGROUND

Mitral valve surgery in the twentieth century began with Elliot Cutler's first operation at the Peter Bent Brigham Hospital in 1923.[1] This was a mitral valvulotomy he had worked on for two years in the laboratory together with Samuel Levine, a Boston cardiologist. Two years later Dr. Suttar, an English surgeon, performed a mitral valvulotomy using his fingers to open up the commissures.[2,3] The patient made an uneventful recovery, but Dr. Suttar did not perform any more mitral valvulotomies. It took two more decades until Dwight Harken and Charles Bailey independently continued the development of digital valvulotomy for rheumatic mitral stenosis.[4,5] The results were dramatic and the operation gained popularity. This launched the modern area of cardiac surgery. But recurrence of the stenosis was still a major problem, even after the development of the cardiopulmonary bypass in the early 1950s, which enabled more complete open valvulotomy.

The next major step in the development of mitral valve surgery was the development of reliable, quality-controlled prosthetic heart valve devices in the late 1950s and early 1960s. For the first time devices were available that could effectively replace a diseased, nonreparable mitral valve with relative ease of implantation and assurance that the hemodynamic abnormalities from either mitral stenosis or regurgitation were corrected and maintained indefinitely.

The first successful prosthetic mitral valve replacement was a device implanted by Nina Braunwald at the National Institute of Health in 1959.[6] This was a homemade device with artificial chordae made of polyurethane. Two years later the first reliable device for replacement of the mitral valve was produced on a commercial basis. This was the Starr-Edwards ball-and-cage mitral valve that resulted from the collaboration of Albert Starr, a cardiac surgeon in Portland,

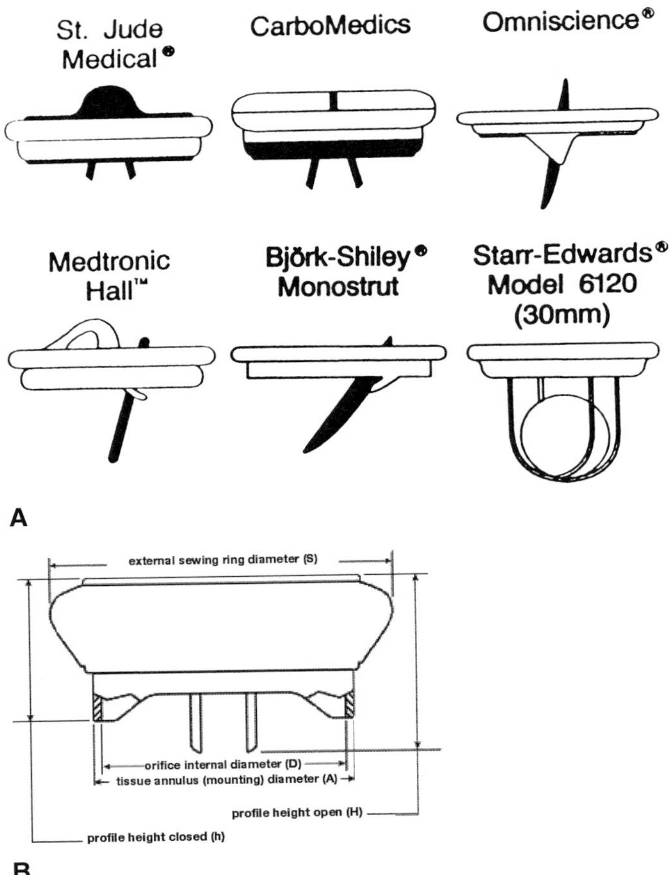

FIGURE 38–1 (A) Profiles of mechanical mitral valve prostheses. (B) Profile of the ON-X mitral valve.

and Lowell Edwards, a mechanical engineer in Southern California.[7] This prosthesis was a great success and became the "gold standard" for many years, until the late 1960s, when second- and third-generation prosthetic valves began to appear. Although reliable hemodynamically, it was soon found that the Starr-Edwards valve had significant thromboembolic potential, particularly in the small ventricle, and aggressive anticoagulation was required to control thromboembolic events.[8,9] The Silastic ball in the original prosthesis also had to be corrected because of inadequate durability.

During the next decade a vide variety of different ball-and-disk valves were developed, and their profile was considerably reduced by alterations in both the height of the valve and the type of occluder (Fig. 38-1). After a number of experimental valves were evaluated (without Food and Drug Administration supervision), one valve emerged as the leading prototype for the 1970s: the Björk-Shiley tilting-disk valve, which was developed by Viking Björk in Stockholm and Earl Shiley in California.[10] This valve had better hemodynamics (larger cross-sectional area and less hemolysis) than the Starr-Edwards valve and consequently had a lower thromboembolic potential.[11–13] However, problems with thrombosis occurred when the anticoagulation was altered. When an engineering change was made to correct this problem in a later model (a concave-convex disk), a fracture in the strut ensued and the Björk-Shiley prosthesis was taken off the market.[14]

A third-generation prosthetic valve was developed in the late 1970s that became the valve of the 1980s: the bileaflet St. Jude Medical valve, which had improved hemodynamics compared to older valves with less stagnation of blood, more complete opening of the leaflets, and reduced incidence of thromboembolism.[15–25] Several other disk prostheses are currently available (see Fig. 38-1), all with flow characteristics similar to the St. Jude valve but still with a small but definite risk of hemorrhage related to anticoagulant therapy and thromboembolism.

As the first, second, and third generations of prosthetic valves were developed, biologic or tissue replacement devices were developed concomitantly. The biologic valves showed a much lower frequency of thromboembolism and long-term anticoagulation seemed to be unnecessary.

In the 1960s, investigators began to use formalin fixation to sterilize and fixate fresh heterograft tissue.[26,27] But when it became apparent that this fixation was unrealiable because of collagen breakdown in valve cusps resulting in fibrosis and calcifications, glutaraldehyde fixation of porcine tissue began.[28] This fixative stabilized collagen bonding in the valve cusps and led to increased durability. The glutaraldehyde-fixed porcine aortic valve, principally developed by Hancock in the United States (1970) and Carpentier in Paris (1976), was the first commercially available bioprosthetic valve.[29,30] These valves revolutionized mitral valve surgery by providing a biologic alternative that allowed long-term use without the need for lifelong warfarin anticoagulation. Both the Hancock and the Carpentier-Edwards valves became enormously popular in the 1970s and studies showed excellent 5-year durability (95%). But in the early 1980s structural valve dysfunction (SVD) became more apparent, with 15% to 20% of the prostheses failing within 10 years. The rate of deterioration seemed to accelerate in younger patients, with the valve gradually wearing down as a result of different biologically mediated dysfunctional processes.[31–40]

The first- and second-generation biologic valves were constructed from porcine aortic valves. Because of limited durability these valves have mostly been replaced by the third generation of biological valves, which still include porcine valves in addition to biomechanically engineered bovine pericardial valves. For this third generation of valves new technology has been incorporated aimed at improving valve longevity and hemodynamic function This has resulted in better mid-term results.[41–48] These techniques include low-pressure or no-pressure fixation, antimineralization processes of the tissues, and low-profile, semiflexible stents that better define the biomechanical properties of the leaflets.

This chapter discusses the surgical indications, operative techniques, and early and late follow-up after implantation of mechanical and bioprosthetic mitral valve devices. The valves that are discussed are those that are currently (2002) approved by the U.S. Food and Drug Administration (FDA). Figure 38-2 shows the current FDA-approved prosthetic mitral valve devices, including the Starr-Edwards ball-and-cage valve, the Omnicarbon tilting-disk valve, the Medtronic Hall tilting-disk valve, the St. Jude Medical bileaflet valve, the Carbomedics bileaflet valve, the ATS bileaflet valve, and the On-X bileaflet valve. The FDA-approved bioprosthetic valve devices are shown in Figure 38-3, and include the Hancock II porcine valve, the Carpentier-Edwards porcine valve, the Carpentier-Edwards pericardial valve, and the Mosaic porcine valve.

INDICATIONS FOR MITRAL VALVE REPLACEMENT

The indications for mitral valve replacement are variable and undergoing evolution. Because of increasing use of reparative techniques, particularly for mitral regurgitation, replacement or repair of a mitral valve often depends on the experience of the operating surgeon. Current indications for valve replacement pertain to those types of valve problems that are unlikely to be repaired by most surgeons or which have been shown to have poor long-term success after reconstruction. Indications are discussed according to (1) pathophysiologic states for needing operation, and (2) type of valve required (i.e., mechanical or bioprosthetic).

Mitral Stenosis

Mitral stenosis is almost exclusively caused by rheumatic fever, even though a definite clinical history only can be obtained in about 50% of patients. The incidence of mitral stenosis has decreased substantially in the United States in the last several decades because of effective prophylaxis of rheumatic fever. In some African and Asian countries, especially India, mitral stenosis is still very common. Two thirds of patients with rheumatic mitral stenosis are female.

The pathologic changes in rheumatic valvulitis are mainly fusion of the valve leaflets at the commissures; shortening and fusion of the cordae tendinae; and thickening of the leaflets due to fibrosis with subsequent stiffening, contraction, and calcification. Approximately 25% of patients have pure mitral stenosis, but an additional 40% have combined mitral stenosis and mitral regurgitation.[49]

Stenosis usually develops one or two decades after the acute illness of rheumatic fever with no or slow onset of symptoms until the stenosis becomes more severe. Limitation of exercise tolerance is usually the first symptom followed by dyspnea that can progress to pulmonary edema. New onset atrial fibrillation and risk for thromboembolism, hemoptysis, and pulmonary hypertension are other common symptoms in patients with mitral stenosis.

The diagnostic workup of the symptomatic patient with mitral stenosis should include a complete cardiac catheterization, including coronary angiography in any patient over the age of 40. Under age 40, echocardiographic findings of the mitral valve suffice in most symptomatic patients for the definition of mitral valve pathology unless there is a history of chest pain or coronary artery disease. Cardiac catheterization establishes the extent of mitral valve stenosis by determining valve gradients and valve area. Pulmonary artery pressure, which may be extremely high in long-standing cases of mitral stenosis, is also documented. In general, operation is prescribed when the mean valve area is 1.0 cm^2 or less[50,51] (normal mitral valve area: 4-6 cm^2); however, with a "mixed" lesion of mitral stenosis and mitral regurgitation, the valve area in symptomatic patients occasionally may be as large as 1.5 cm^2. Asymptomatic patients are generally not considered for surgery,[50] but some authors recommend operation in asymptomatic patients with significant hemodynamic mitral stensosis (see Ch. 36).[52] The degree of pulmonary artery pressure elevation secondary to mitral stenosis continues to be an area of concern for the mitral valve surgeon. Is there any level of pulmonary hypertension

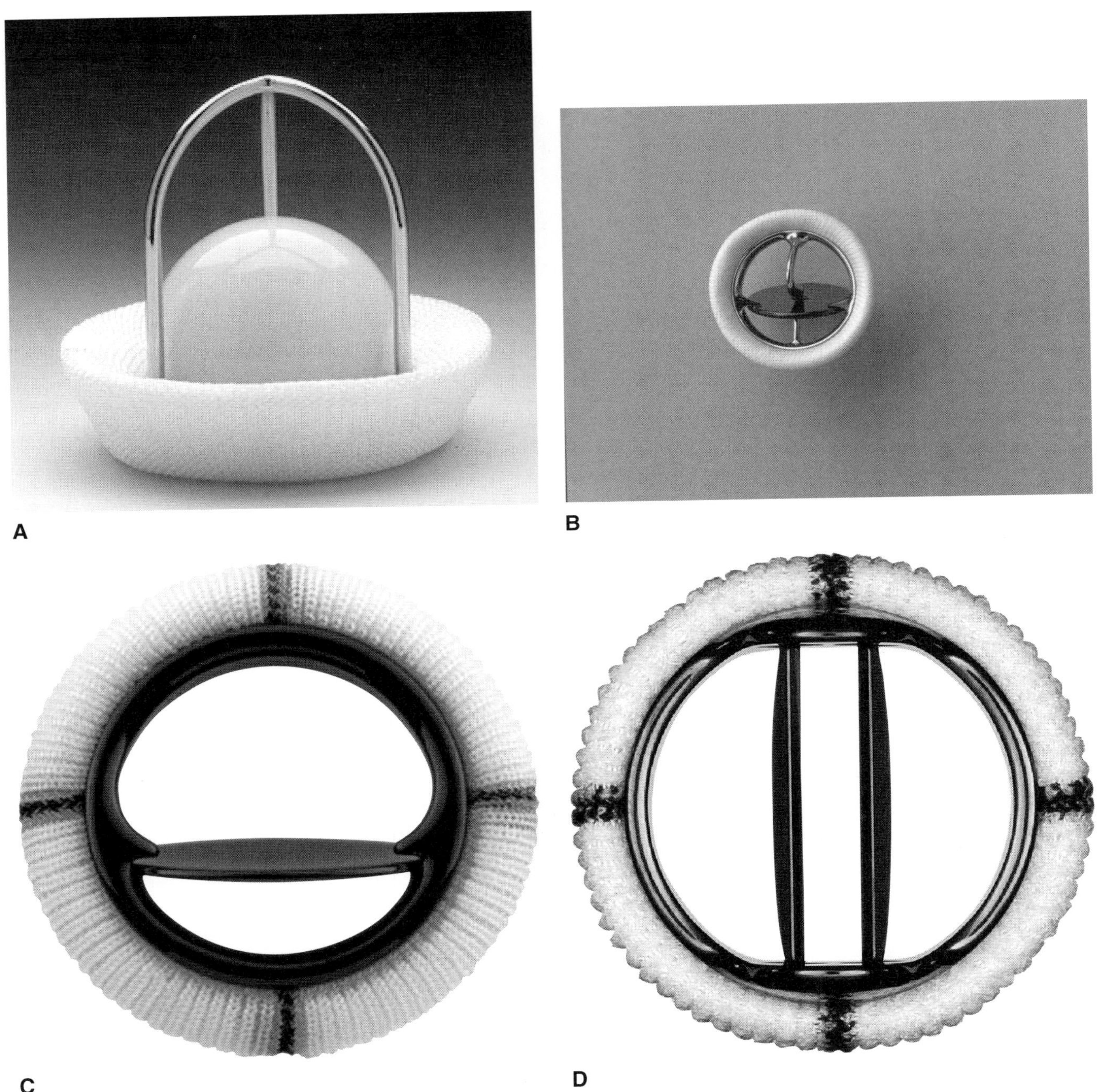

FIGURE 38–2 FDA-approved mechanical mitral valves. (A) Starr-Edwards ball-and-cage. (B) Medtronic-Hall tilting-disk. (C) Omnicarbon tilting-disk. (D) St. Jude Medical bifleaflet.

that is too high for mitral valve replacement in the current surgical era of improved intraoperative and postoperative care? There is still no definitive answer to this question, but most surgeons operate on patients with severe pulmonary hypertension (suprasystemic) with the knowledge that intensive postoperative respiratory and diuretic therapy are necessary to maintain relatively dry lungs and to reduce the risk of severe right ventricular failure. It has been known for over 25 years that after mitral valve replacement for mitral stenosis, pulmonary artery pressure decreases within hours in most patients and decreases more gradually over weeks and months in others.[53–58]

The success with closed commissurectomies after World War II and the development of the Starr-Edwards valve in the early 1960s led to an enormous increase in operations for rheumatic mitral valve disease; that pattern became a

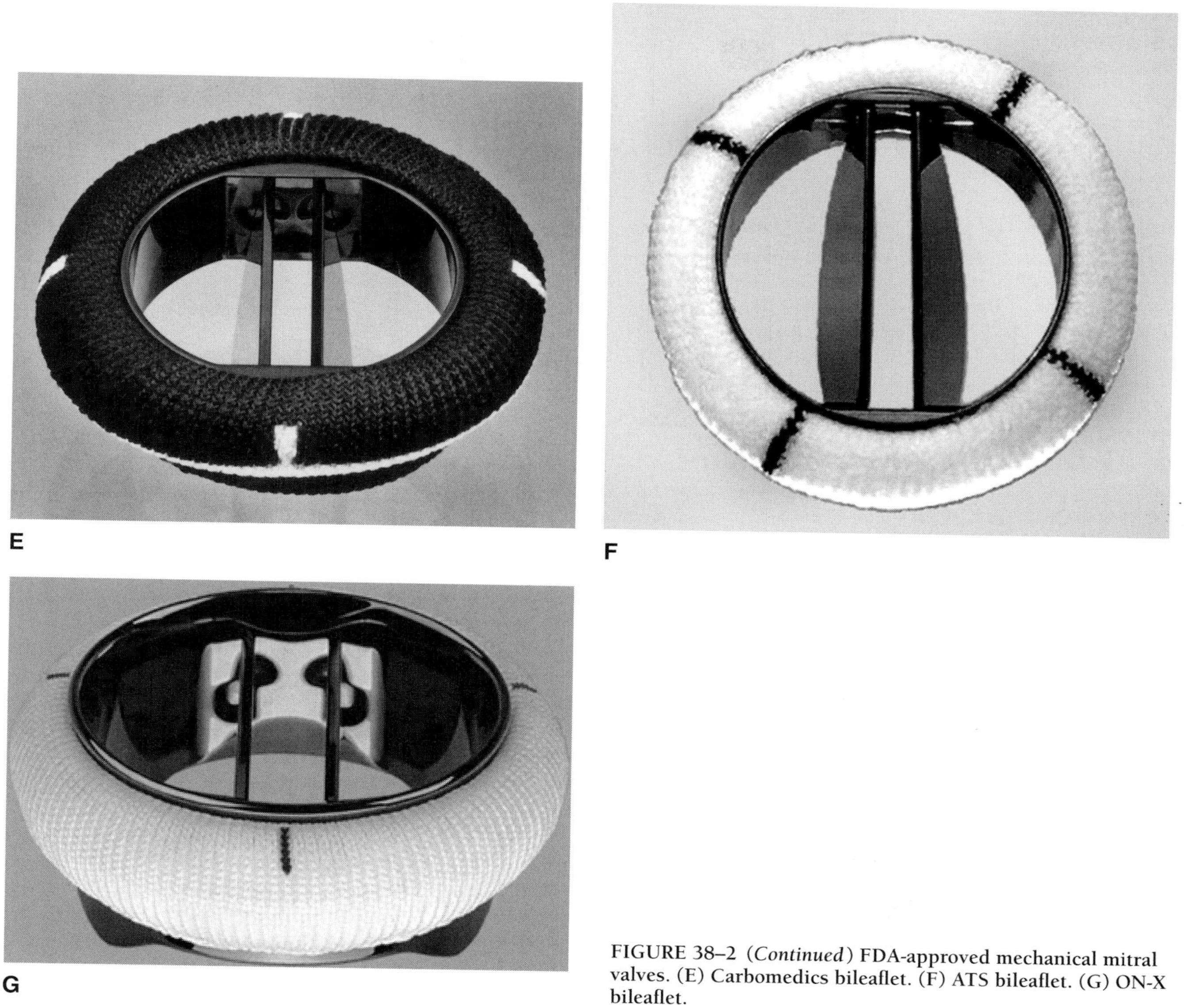

E

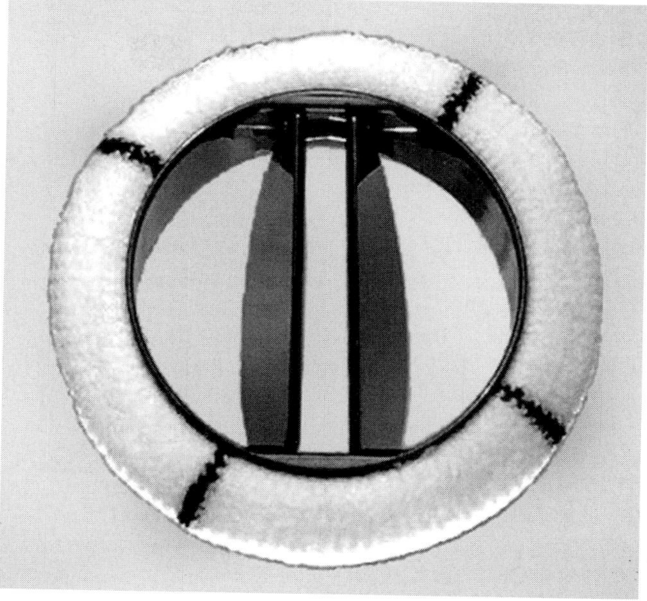

F

G

FIGURE 38–2 (*Continued*) FDA-approved mechanical mitral valves. (E) Carbomedics bileaflet. (F) ATS bileaflet. (G) ON-X bileaflet.

decrease as rheumatic disease declined. In recent years, a small resurgence in rheumatic valve disease has been observed in emigrés from Southeast Asia and Latin America. In the 1990s, balloon dilation of fibrotic, stenotic mitral valves became increasingly utilized.[50,59,60] At the present time, percutaneous mitral balloon valve dilation is used in most cases of symptomatic noncalcified, fibrotic mitral stenosis. But even though this technique has been shown to be equivalent in the short run to closed mitral commissurectomy, especially in young patients, it is only indicated in a minority of patients, i.e., those with optimal valvular characteristiscs.[50,61,62] Open mitral commissurotomy and valvuloplasty for such patients can be a successful operation,[63] but other studies have shown better long-term results with mitral valve replacement using a mechanical valve.[64] Many patients with chronic mitral stenosis now require valve replacement because the valve has developed significant dystrophic changes, including marked thickening and shortening of all chordae, obliteration of the subvalvular space, agglutination of the papillary muscles, and calcification in both annular and leaflet tissue. Aggressive decalcification and heroic reconstructive techniques for these extremely advanced pathologic valves generally have produced poor long-term results; nevertheless, some surgeons still advocate aggressive repairs in this subset of patients.[65]

Mitral Regurgitation

The etiology of mitral regurgitation is very diverse and the decision to recommend operation for patients with mitral regurgitation is more complex than for patients with

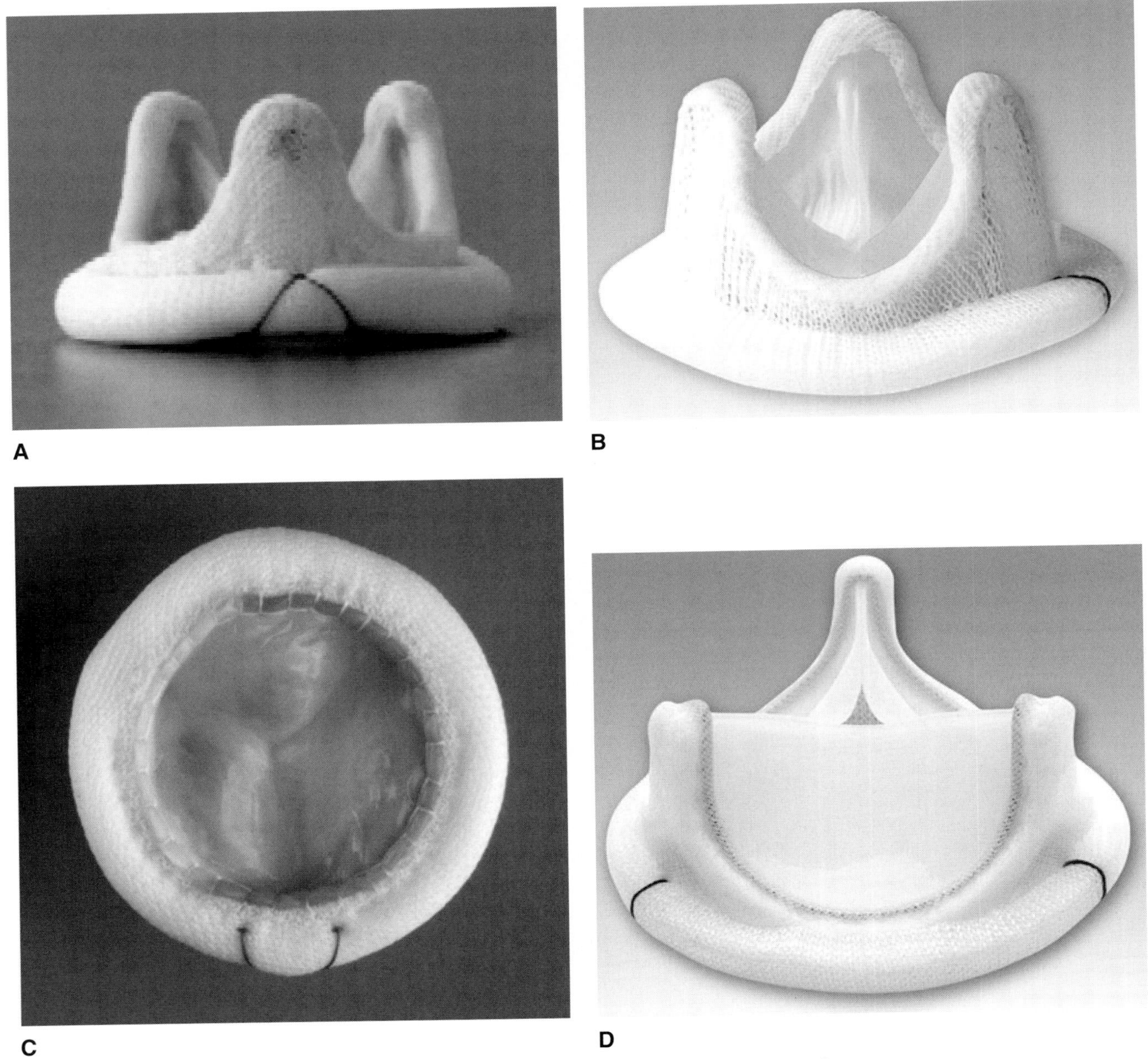

FIGURE 38–3 FDA-approved bioprosthetic mitral valves. (A) Hancock II porcine heterograft. (B) Carpentier-Edwards standard porcine heterograft. (C) Mosaic porcine heterograft. (D) Carpentier-Edwards pericardial bovine heterograft.

mitral stenosis, except in cases of acute ischemic mitral regurgitation and endocarditis, where indications are more straightforward. The pathologic subsets that produce mitral regurgitation are related to a number of metabolic, functional, and anatomic abnormalities.[66] These can be categorized into degenerative (mitral prolapse, ruptured/elongated chordae), rheumatic, infectious, and ischemic diseases of the mitral valve. Most of these entities are now amenable to mitral valve repair and reconstruction with and without the use of annuloplasty rings, as mentioned elsewhere in this book (see Ch. 37).

For any of the preceding major pathologic subsets, indications for surgery in patients with mitral regurgitation vary from the asymptomatic patient with an enlarging but well-functioning left ventricle and atrium to severely depressed left ventricular function. Any symptomatic patient with significant mitral regurgitation (3+ to 4+) should be operated on, and operation should be considered in any relatively symptom-free individual if there is objective evidence of left ventricular deterioration and documented and significant increases in left ventricular end-systolic and end-diastolic volumes.[67–72]

Regurgitation through the valve is usually measured with Doppler echocardiography, but MRI is another noninvasive technology for measuring the regurgitant flow and can provide measurements of ventricular end-diastolic/systolic volumes and ventricular mass.[73] Left ventricular angiography can be helpful but is otherwise indicated for evaluating the coronary arteries preoperatively in patients older than 40 years.

It is important to stress that ejection fraction is a poor indicator of left ventricular function in patients with mitral regurgitation. Ejection fraction can be preserved in patients with irreversible left ventricular failure because of regurgitant flow through the valve.[74,75] Depressed cardiac output (<40%) therefore usually indicates severe left ventricular dysfunction, and results of surgery are not as favorable in these patients as they are in patients with normal ventricles.[76] Compared to ejection fraction, measurements of end-systolic volume and diameter are more reliable noninvasive parameters to evaluate the status of the left ventricle and determine the optimal time for operation (see Ch. 36).[77,78]

Once the valve is exposed, indications for mitral valve replacement in patients with mitral regurgitation depend on the extent of the pathology in each patient and the reparative experience of the operating surgeon. Thus, in regurgitation from degenerative prolapsing myxomatous valves that have a high probability of reconstruction, mitral valve repair is indicated if the prolapse is generalized and local findings that decrease the probability of a successful repair are absent.[63,79–82] Similarly, if rheumatic mitral regurgitation, calcific deposits throughout the leaflet substance, and shortened chordae and papillary muscles are encountered, mitral valve replacement is the most prudent operation because the probability of successful repair is low.[83] In ischemic mitral regurgitation, pathology that precludes satisfactory repair includes restrictive valve motion from shortened, scarred papillary muscles, an acutely infarcted papillary muscle, and rupture of chordae associated with extensive calcification of valve leaflets.[84–86] In endocarditis, mitral valve replacement may be required because of destruction of the valve leaflets and subvalvular mechanisms and annular abscess formation. Although repair of the valve and avoidance of prosthetic material are very desirable in septic situations, the extent of the destruction may preclude repair. Therefore, mitral valve replacement is required after careful debridement of the infectious tissue and reconstruction of the valve annulus.[87,88]

CHOICE OF VALVE TYPE

Indications for Mechanical Valve Replacement

Worldwide prosthetic (mechanical) mitral valve replacement is more common today than bioprosthetic mitral valve replacement, about 60% versus 40%, but in the United States the ratio is inverse. Currently available prosthetic valves in the United States, in descending order of popularity, are the bileaflet, the tilting-disk, and the ball-and-cage valve. For the young patient, the patient in chronic atrial fibrillation who requires long-term anticoagulation, or any patient who wants to minimize the chance of reoperation, a prosthetic valve should be chosen if valve replacement is required. The St. Jude Medical bileaflet valve is the most widely used prosthetic mitral valve at present because it has good hemodynamic characteristics and is easy to insert. Indications to choose one prosthetic or another vary primarily by surgeon preference and occasionally depending on the state of the annulus and whether or not there have been multiple previous operations. For example, infrequently the mitral annulus provides poor anchorage with subsequent perivalvular leak with the bileaflet or tilting-disk valve, which requires an everting suture technique. In this instance, the central-flow Starr-Edwards ball-and-cage valve with a bulky sewing ring may be chosen to reduce the probability of subsequent perivalvular leak. A low-profile mechanical valve is on the other hand preferable in a patient with a small left ventricular cavity to prevent obstruction of left ventricular outflow and impingement of the myocardium.

Indications for Bioprosthetic Valve Replacement

Patients in any age group in sinus rhythm who wish to avoid anticoagulation may prefer a bioprosthetic valve. This is especially true for patients in whom anticoagulation is contraindicated, for instance in patients with a history of gastrointestinal bleeding or those who have a high-risk occupation or lifestyle.[89] A bioprosthetic valve is preferred in patients over age 70 and in sinus rhythm, since these valves deteriorate more slowly in older patients. In addition, as observed by Grunkemeier et al, some 60-year-olds may not outlive their prosthetic valves because of comorbid disease.[90,91] Specifically, patients who require combined mitral valve replacement and coronary bypass grafting for ischemic mitral regurgitation and coronary artery disease have significantly reduced long-term survival as compared with patients who do not have concomitant coronary artery disease.[92–102] These individuals may avoid anticoagulation with little risk of reoperation.

As 20-year results have become available for various bioprostheses, it is clear that structural valve degeneration (SVD) is the most prominent drawback of these valves.[31,33,103–107] The durability of porcine valves is less with mitral bioprostheses than with aortic bioprostheses. The more rapid deterioration of mitral bioprostheses may be due to higher ventricular systolic pressures against the mitral cusps as compared with the diastolic pressures resisted by aortic bioprosthetic leaflets. Durability of bioprosthetic valves is directly proportional to age;[108] deterioration occurs within months or a few years in children and young adults and only gradually over years in septuagenarians and octogenarians.[33,40,42,43,92,93,103,109] Essentially all valves implanted into patients less than 60 years of age have to be replaced ultimately and valve failure is prohibitively rapid in children and in adults under 35 to 40 years of age; therefore, bioprosthesis are not advisable in these age groups.[110,111] Nevertheless, there are still indications for mitral porcine bioprosthetic valves in young patients. In a woman who desires to become pregnant, a bioprosthesis may be used to avoid warfarin anticoagulation and fetal damage during pregnancy.[112–115] In patients with chronic renal failure and hypercalcemia related to hyperparathyroidism, bioprostheses have extremely limited durability and should therefore be avoided.

For the last decade there are several reports, mainly from European centers, utilizing unstented cryopreserved homografts[116–121] and stentless heterografts[122–124] for mitral valve replacements, particularly in patients with endocarditis. The prosthetic valve is transplanted, donor papillary muscles are reattached to recipient papillary muscles, and the annulus is sutured circumferentially. Only a few patients are included in these studies with a short follow-up, and long-term results are therefore not available. But recent reports suggest that these operations may be a feasible alternative to stented valve replacement in patients with endocarditis. Pulmonary autografts have also been used for replacing the mitral valve (Ross II procedure) but only in a few patients with very short follow-up.[125,126]

HEMODYNAMICS OF MITRAL VALVE DEVICES

Mechanical Protheses

The designs of mechanical and bioprosthetic heart valves have evolved over the last four decades in an effort to develop the ideal replacement for the pathologic mitral valve. Biochemical and engineering advances have produced hemodynamic improvements and reduced morbidity from valve-related complications. The ideal valve, however, is not available, and the positive and negative characteristics of current valves must be considered when choosing the most appropriate valve for an individual patient. The optimal heart valve exerts minimal resistance to forward blood flow and allows only trivial regurgitant backflow as the occluder closes. The design must cause minimal turbulence and stasis in vivo during physiologic flow conditions. The valve must be durable enough to last a lifetime and must be constructed of biomaterials that are nonantigenic, nontoxic, nonimmunogenic, nondegradable, and noncarcinogenic. The valve also must have a low incidence of thromboembolism.

The opening resistance to blood flow is determined by the orifice diameter; the size, shape, and weight of the occluder; the opening angle; and the orientation of leaflet or disk occluders with respect to the plane of the mitral annular orifice for any given annular size. Least resistance to transvalvular blood flow during diastole for valves in the mitral position is provided by a large ratio of orifice to total annular area. A wide opening angle also improves the effective orifice area and results in decreased diastolic pressure gradients. With an increasing orifice diameter, however, more energy is lost across the valve as more backflow passes through the valve at end diastole and early systole. Table 38-1 shows hemodynamic assessments of each of the FDA-approved mitral valve prostheses for the most commonly used mitral valve sizes.[16,24,25,46,47,127–154] The results of in vivo assessments at rest by invasive (catheterization) or noninvasive (Doppler echocardiography) techniques are tabulated.

Blood turbulence flowing across mitral valve devices results from impedance to forward or reverse flow. This impedance can be minimized by occluder design and orientation, central flow through the orifice, and limited struts or pivots extending into flow areas (Fig. 38-4). Hemolysis is the product of red blood cell destruction that is caused by cavitation and shearing stresses of turbulence, high-velocity flow, regurgitation, and mechanical damage during valve closure.[155] Areas of perivalvular blood stagnation and turbulence increase platelet aggregation, activation of the coagulation proteins, and thrombus formation.

Dynamic regurgitation is a feature of all prosthetic valves and is the sum of the closing volume during occluder closure and the leakage volume that passes through the valve while it is closed. The closing volume is a function of the effective orifice area and the time needed for closure. Closure time is influenced by the difference between the opening and closing angles of the occluder and valve ring. Leakage volume is inherent to the design of the valve and depends on the amount of time the valve remains in the closed position.[156] A small amount of regurgitant volume can be beneficial by minimizing stasis and reducing platelet aggregation; this decreases the incidence of valve thrombosis and valve-related thromboembolism.[137]

The Starr-Edwards Model 6120 is the only ball-and-cage mitral valve prosthesis currently approved for use in the United States by the FDA. It was introduced with its current design in 1965 after undergoing several engineering modifications and has been in use longer than any other type of mechanical valve (see Fig. 38-2A). The occluder is a barium-impregnated Silastic ball in a Stellite alloy cage that projects into the left ventricle. This valve has a large Teflon/polypropylene sewing ring that produces a relatively small effective orifice and larger diastolic pressure gradients as compared with other prosthetic valves of similar annular sizes. Leakage volumes are not inherent in the ball-and-cage design, and in contrast to other mechanical valves, the presence of regurgitation may indicate a pathologic process. The central ball occluder causes lateralization of forward flow and results in turbulence and cavitation that increase the risk of hemolysis and thromboembolic complications (see Fig. 38-4A). The incidence of thromboembolism has been shown to be higher with the Starr-Edwards valve compared to the bileaflet valves.[9,157] Because the cage projects into the

TABLE 38–1 Hemodynamics of mitral valve prostheses

Valve	Reference (year)	EOA (cm^2)					Mean diastolic gradient (mm Hg)				
		25 mm	27 mm	29 mm	31 mm	33 mm	25 mm	27 mm	29 mm	31 mm	33 mm
Starr-Edwards	Pyle[128] (1978)		1.4	1.4	1.9			8.0	10.0	5.0	
	Sala[132] (1982)							7.9	6.7	5.0	
	Horskotte[137] (1987)			1.8				6.3			
Omniscience/ Omnicarbon	Mikhail[139] (1989)							6.1		5.4	
	Messner-Pellenc[145] (1993)		1.9	2.2	2.0	2.0	4.3	3.6	3.5	2.0	
	Fehske[148] (1994)						6	6	5	6	4
Medtronic Hall	Hall[135] (1985)							3.0	2.7	2.0	
	Fiore[24] (1998)						4.0	4.3	3.1	2.9	2.7
St. Jude	Chaux[16] (1981)			2.1	2.8	3.1			1.9	1.8	1.6
	Horskotte[137] (1987)			3.1					2.3		
	Fiore[24] (1998)						3.0	3.3	3.8	1.5	2.5
	Hasegawa[153] (2000)	2.6	2.5	2.4							
Carbomedics	Johnston[141] (1992)			3.3					3.8		
	Chambers[143] (1993)		2.1	2.1	1.8			3.9	3.3	3.3	
	Carbomedics[142] (1993)		2.9	3.0	3.0			3.9	4.6	4.6	
ATS	Westaby[151] (1996)		3	2	2	2					
	Shiono[149] (1996)						5	6	4.5		
	Hasegawa[153] (2000)	2.3	2.6	2.7							
	Emery[154] (2001)						7.8	5	6	4	3
Hancock standard	Johnson[127] (1975)		1.0	2.5	1.8			12.0	5.0	5.0	
	Ubago[133] (1982)		1.3	1.0	1.0			7.0	7.6	7.4	
	Khuri[138] (1988)		1.5	2.0	1.8			7.0	7.0	7.0	
Carpentier-Edwards porcine	Chaitman[129] (1979)		1.7	2.2	2.8			7.0	6.7	5.0	
	Levine[130] (1981)			3.0	3.2				2.0	2.6	
	Pelletier[131] (1982)		1.7	2.4	2.5			6.5	7.4	5.3	
Carpentier-Edwards pericardial	Aupart[146] (1997)	2.6	2.7	2.6	3.1		4.1	3.0	3.0	3.0	???
Mosaic	Thomson[47] (2001)			1.7 (all sizes)							
	Fradet[46] (2001)	1.6	1.7	1.8	1.7	1.9	5.7	4.6	4.4	3.7	3.4
Normal				4.6					0		
Severe stenosis				>1.0					>12		
Desired postoperative				>1.5					>10		

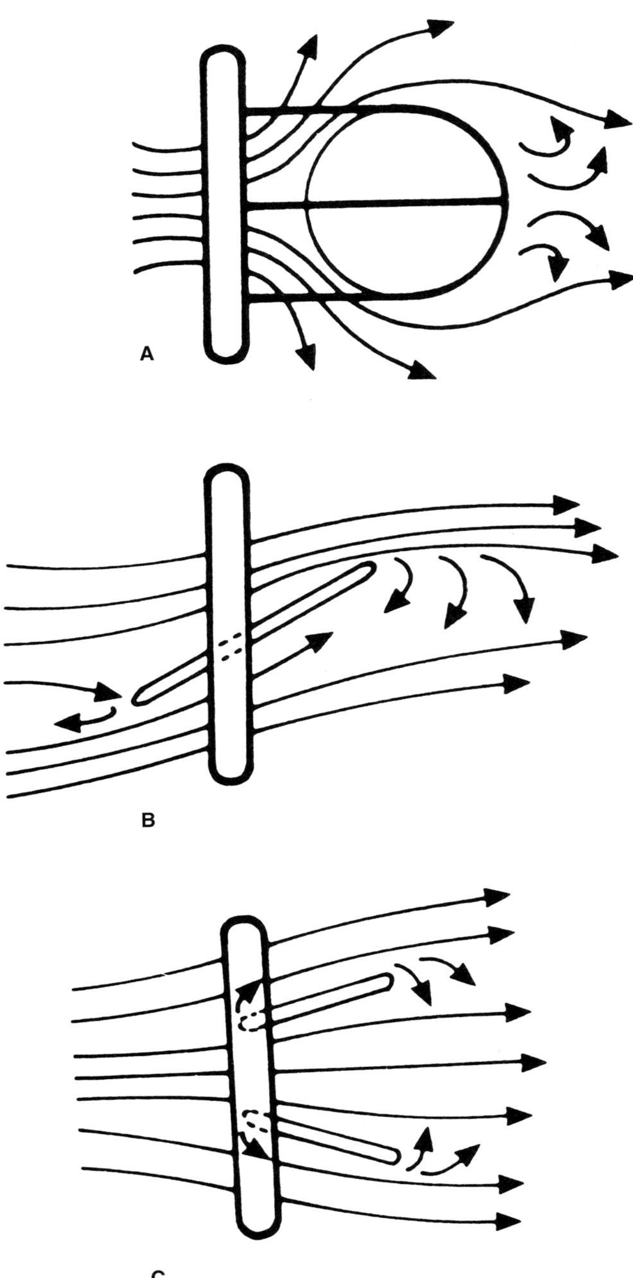

FIGURE 38–4 Flow characteristics of different mechanical valve designs. (a) Ball-and-cage. (B) Tilting-disk. (C) Bileaflet.

left ventricle, it is unwise to implant this valve in small left ventricles, where the cage may contact the ventricular wall or cause ventricular outflow obstruction.[144]

Tilting-disk mitral valve prostheses have better hemodynamic characteristics as compared with ball-and-cage valves (see Fig.38-4B). The Medtronic Hall central pivoting-disk valve was introduced in 1977 and is based on engineering design modifications of the earlier Hall-Kaster valve (see Fig. 38-2B).[158] The axis of the tilting disk was moved more centrally to allow greater blood flow through the minor orifice and to reduce stagnation in areas of low flow. The opening angle was originally increased to 78 degrees to decrease resistance to forward flow and later narrowed to 70 degrees when in vitro studies revealed an unacceptable regurgitant volume. The opening angle of 70 degrees produced regurgitation volumes of less than 5% of left ventricular stroke volume without significantly compromising forward flow. The disk occluder was allowed to slide out of the housing at the end of the closing cycle to provide a gap through which blood could flow to minimize stasis at the contact surfaces.[158] The large opening angle and slim disk occluder along with a thinner sewing ring provide improved hemodynamics with comparably larger effective orifice areas and lower mean diastolic pressure gradients for each valve size. During implantation, the larger orifice should be oriented posteriorly when using the larger valve sizes to minimize the potential for disk impingement. Smaller valves (27 mm or less) should be oriented with the larger orifice anteriorly to optimize in vivo hemodynamics.[136,159]

The Omniscience tilting-disk valve is a second-generation device derived from improvements to the design of the Lillehei-Kaster pivoting-disk valve.[160] This low-profile device has a pyrolytic disk eccentrically located in a one-piece titanium housing attached to a seamless Teflon sewing ring. Introduced in 1978, the Omniscience prosthesis includes several engineering modifications from prior devices in an effort to improve its hemodynamic function. The orifice-to-annular area ratio was increased to minimize resistance to forward flow. The opening angle of 80 degrees is relatively large to allow flow reserve in patients with high cardiac outputs and during exercise. Resulting increases in regurgitant volumes are minimized by the disk design. Turbulence is reduced by the curvature of the disk, and areas of stasis and shear stress are reduced by the eccentric location of the pivot axis, in an effort to decrease the risk of thrombosis, thromboembolism, and hemolysis. Retaining prongs are not utilized, and the lower profile reduces the risk of impingement.[139] A potential hemodynamic disadvantage that has been the subject of debate is the possibility of incomplete disk opening in vivo. Clinical studies report postoperative mean opening angles of between 44.8 degrees[136] and 75.9 degrees.[161] Implicated factors causing this variation include valve sizing, orientation during implantation, and anticoagulation status.[161,162] A subsequent generation of the Omniscience valve is the all-carbon Omnicarbon monoleaflet valve that was released in 2001 in the United States but has been in clinical use in Europe since 1984 (see Fig. 38-2C). The housing material is made of pyrolytic carbon instead of titanium. As a result of this change, the incidence of thromboembolism, valvular thrombosis, and reoperations was significantly decreased compared with that of the Omniscience valve protheses.[163] For all of the tilting-disk valves meticulous surgical technique is important because retained leaflets or chordae can cause subvalvular interference and leakage.

The unique design of the bileaflet St. Jude Medical valve was introduced in 1977 and it is currently the prosthesis used most commonly worldwide (see Fig. 38-2D). Two separate pyrolytic carbon semi-disks in a pyrolytic carbon housing are attached to a Dacron sewing ring. The housing has two pivot guards that project into the left atrium. The bileaflet design produces three different flow areas through the valve orifice that provide overall a more uniform, central, and laminar flow than in the caged-ball and monleaflet tilting-disk design. The improved flow results in less turbulence and decreased transmitral diastolic pressure gradients[156,164] (see Fig. 38-4C) at any annulus diameter size and cardiac output compared to caged-ball or single-leaflet tilting valves.[165] The favorable hemodynamics in smaller sizes makes it especially useful in children.[166] The central opening angle is 85 degrees, with a closing angle of 30 to 35 degrees, which, along with a thin sewing ring, provides a large effective orifice area for each valve size at the expense of greater regurgitant volumes, especially at low heart rates. Asynchronous closure of the valve leaflets in vivo also contributes to the regurgitant volume.[167] The design of this prosthesis provides excellent hemodynamic function even in small sizes, in any rotational plane.[168] The antianatomic plane, however, with the central slit between the leaflets oriented perpendicular to the opening axis of the native valve leaflets, decreases the potential risk of leaflet impingement by the posterior left ventricular wall.[169]

The Carbomedics bileaflet valve was approved by the FDA in 1986 (see Fig. 38-2E). This low-profile device is constructed of pyrolytic carbon and has no pivot guards, struts, or orifice projections to decrease blood flow impedance and turbulence through the valve.[156] It has a rotatable sewing cuff design and is available with a more generous and flexible sewing cuff (the OptiForm variant) that confirms more easily to different patient anatomies. The leaflet opening angle is 78 degrees, which, with the bileaflet design, provides a relatively large effective orifice area and transvalvular diastolic pressure differences only slightly greater than the St. Jude Medical bileaflet valve. Rapid synchronous leaflet closure reduces closing regurgitant volumes to less than that of the Björk-Shiley pivoting-disk prosthesis, which has an opening angle of 60 degrees. Leakage volume, however, is greater with Carbomedics valves because of backflow through gaps around pivots. Because of its narrow closing angle and large leakage volume, the Carbomedics valve does not reduce the relatively large regurgitant volume associated with the bileaflet design. Although this valve has good hemodynamic function overall, in the mitral position, the 25-mm Carbomedics valve has a relatively high diastolic pressure gradient and large regurgitant energy loss across the valve, especially at high flows. Hemodynamic studies suggest that the Carbomedics valve should be avoided in patients with a small mitral valve orifice.[156]

The ATS (Advancing The Standard) mechanical prosthesis has been in clinical use in the United States since 2000. Similar to the Carbomedics valve, the ATS valve is a low-profile bileaflet prosthesis with a pyrolytic housing and pyrolytic carbon leaflets containing graphite substrate (see Fig. 38-2F). The pivot areas are located entirely within the orifice ring and the valve leaflets hinge on convex pivot guides on the carbon orifice ring. This design minimizes the overall height of the valve and provides wider orifice area, and the absence of cavities in the valve ring theoretically reduces stasis or eddy currents that may develop. Valve noise, a bothersome problem for some patients, is also reduced by this design.[170] The opening angle is up to 85 degrees and the sewing cuff is constructed of double velour polyester fabric that is mounted to a titanium stiffening ring, which enables the surgeon to rotate the valve orifice during and after implantation.

The prosthesis most recently approved by the FDA (2002) is the On-X valve. It has a bileaflet design similar to the St. Jude Medical, Carbomedics, and ATS prostheses with comparable hemodynamic performance, i.e., a relatively large orifice diameter and a wide opening angle (90 degrees) (see Fig. 38-2F). Instead of silicon-alloyed pyrolytic carbon, as used in the other mechanical prosthesis, the On-X valve is made of pure pyrolytic carbon. This material is stronger and tougher than silicon alloyed carbon[171] and allows incorporation of hydrodynamically efficient features to the valve orifice, such as increased orifice length and a flared inlet that reduces transvalvular gradient.[152] Early clinical results are promising[172] and the valve produces very little hemolysis with postoperative levels of serum lactate dehydrogenase in the normal range.[173]

Bioprostheses

PORCINE VALVES

The porcine bioprosthetic mitral valves are designed to mimic the flow characteristics of the in situ aortic valve. The Hancock I mitral valve bioprosthesis was introduced in 1970. It has three glutaraldehyde-preserved porcine aortic valve leaflets on a polypropylene stent attached to a Dacron-covered silicone sewing ring. The design allows for central laminar flow through the valve, which tends to decrease diastolic pressure gradients and minimize turbulence.[164] The stent, however, impedes forward flow and results in relatively large diastolic pressure gradients across the bioprosthesis. The stent and the large sewing ring contribute to effective orifice areas that are smaller than those of size-matched mechanical valves (see Table 38-1).

The Hancock II porcine bioprosthesis is the more modern version of the Hancock I prosthesis (see Fig. 38-3A). The stent is made of Delrin with a scalloped sewing ring and reduced stent profile. The leaflets are fixated in glutaraldehyde at low pressure and subsequently for a prolonged period at high pressure. To retard calcification, the leaflets are treated with sodium dodecyl sulfate.

The Carpentier-Edwards porcine valve utilizes a flexible stent to decrease the stress of leaflet flexion while maintaining its overall configuration (see Fig. 38-3B).[144] The effective orifice-to-total-annulus area ratio for the Carpentier-Edwards valve is relatively small, but exercise studies show that the effective orifice area increases significantly with increased blood flow across the valve; diastolic gradients also increase, although to a lesser degree.[131,138,174] Porcine bioprostheses in the mitral position should be avoided in patients with small left ventricles because of the possibility of ventricular rupture or left ventricular outflow obstruction caused by the large struts.[174]

The Mosaic porcine bioprosthesis is a third-generation bioprosthesis utilizing the Hancock II stent (see Fig. 38-3C). It was introduced in the United States in 2000 and has a Delrin stent, scalloped sewing ring, and reduced stent profile. The valve tissue is pressure-free fixed with glutaraldehyde and the prosthesis is treated with alpha oleic acid (AOA) to retard calcification.

PERICARDIAL VALVES

Previous studies indicated poor durability of pericardial valves, namely, the Ionescu-Shiley valve, caused by leaflet tearing. This led to significant changes in design, including mounting of the pericardium completely within the stent, causing less leaflet abrasion and increased durability. The Carpentier-Edwards pericardial valve uses bovine pericardium as material to fabricate a trileaflet valve that is cut, fitted, and sewn onto a flexible Elgiloy wire frame for stress reduction (see Fig. 38-3D). The tissue is preserved with glutaralderhyde with no applied pressure and the leaflets are treated with the calcium mitigation agent XenoLogiX. Compared to the Carpentier-Edwards porcine bioprosthesis, the stent profile is reduced. Long-term durability for the Carpentier-Edwards pericardial valve is strong and compared to third-generation porcine valves, valve-related complications are similar (see discussion later in this chapter).

Hemodynamically, pericardial valves provide the best solution to flow problems. The design maximizes use of the flow area, which results in minimal flow resistance.[175] Figure 38-5A shows how the cone shape of the open valve and circular valve orifice minimize flow disturbance compared to more irregular cone shape for the porcine valves that allow for central unimpeded flow (Fig. 38-5B).

Structural valve deterioration is seen after long-term follow-up of patients with both porcine and pericardial bioprostheses and results in mitral stenosis or regurgitation or both. Hemodynamic studies early after operation and at 5 years reveal higher average diastolic pressure gradients and smaller effective orifice areas when compared in the same patients at the follow-up study. In some patients these changes are sufficiently severe to require reoperation as soon as 4 to 5 years postoperatively, and by 10 years the rate of primary tissue failure averages 30%. It then accelerates, and by 15 years postoperatively the actuarial freedom from bioprosthetic primary tissue failure has ranged from 35% to 71% (see Table 38-2). Most of these patients show hemodynamic evidence of valvular deterioration prior to any clinical signs or symptoms.[131] Bioprosthetic valves have the advantage of low thrombogenicity, which must be weighed against poor long-term durability and subsequent hemodynamic deterioration and the risk of reoperation.

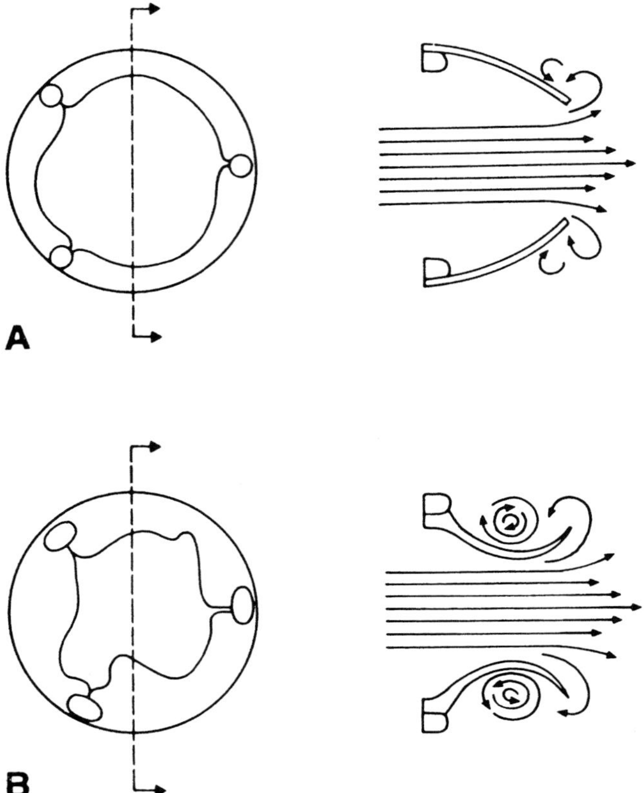

FIGURE 38–5 Flow patterns for bioprosthetic valves. (A) Pericardial bioprosthesis. (B) Porcine bioprosthesis.

OPERATIVE TECHNIQUES

Preoperative Management and Anesthetic Preparation

Congestive heart failure secondary to mitral stenosis can usually be treated with aggressive diuretic therapy and sodium restriction preoperatively. If the patient is in rapid atrial fibrillation, digoxin, beta blockers, and calcium channel antagonists can be used to slow down the ventricular rate. Patients with acute mitral regurgitation are often in cardiogenic shock, and they can be stabilized preoperatively with inotropes and arterial vasodilators to reduce systemic afterload. Intra-aortic balloon counterpulsation can also be used for this purpose. Symptoms of congestive heart failure

TABLE 38–2 **Freedom from structural valve detorioration after mitral valve replacement with bioprotheses**

Valve	Reference (year)	5 y	10 y	15 y	20 y
Hancock Standard	Cohn[242] (1989)	98%	75%	45%	
	Burdon[103] (1992)	98%	80%	44%	
	Bortolotti[274] (1995)	94%	73%	35%	
	Khan[106] (1998)				65%
Hancock II	David[45] (2001)	100%	86%	66%	
Carpentier-Edwards porcine	Perier[287] (1989)	89%	65%		
	Sarris[251] (1993)	97%	60%		
	Jamieson[38] (1995)	98%	72%	49%	
	Van Doorn[104] (1995)	97%	71%		
	Corbineau[107] (2001)	98%	83%	48%	
Carpentier-Edwards pericardial	Pelletier[41] (1995)	100%	79% (8 y)		
	Takahara[48] (1995)		84% (9 y)		
	Aupart[146] (1997)	100%	76%		
	Marchand[43] (1998)	98%	85% (11 y)		
	Neville[44] (1998)	100%	78% (12 y)		
	Poirer[42] (1998)	100%	81%		
Mosaic	Jasinski[147] (2000)	100% (2 y)			
	Fradet[46] (2001)	100% (4 y)			
	Thomson[47] (2001)	100% (4 y)			

in patients with chronic mitral regurgitation are treated with diuretics and oral vasodilators. The vasodilators lower the peripheral vascular resistance, and forward cardiac output is increased by reducing the regurgitant volume into the left atrium.

Preferred anesthesia for mitral valve replacement typically involves a combination of narcotic and inhalational agents.[176] Ultimately, anesthetic management is dictated by the wide range of functional disabilities and hemodynamic abnormalities of patients who present for mitral valve replacement. For example, a cachectic patient with functional class IV mitral stenosis and severe pulmonary hypertension may require postoperative positive-pressure mechanical ventilation for 1 or 2 days to remove excess pulmonary fluid by diuresis, facilitate bronchial toileting, and provide optimal conditions for adequate gas exchange. Alternatively, young patients who require mitral valve surgery and present with less preoperative comorbidity may benefit from a short-acting, balanced anesthetic that can facilitate extubation within 6 hours following surgery.[177]

Monitoring should include arterial and venous lines, a urinary catheter, and a pulmonary artery catheter placed before bypass to measure pulmonary pressures and cardiac output. Following valve replacement, occasionally a left atrial catheter directly inserted through the left atrial incision can be helpful to allow measurement of pulmonary vascular resistance, but we do not use it routinely. Preoperative intravenous prophylactic antibiotics are administered to all patients and are continued for 2 postoperative days until lines are removed. Temporary ventricular pacing wires are placed, and in many instances temporary atrial pacing wires are placed for possible pacing or diagnosis of various atrial arrhythmias.

Management of Cardiopulmonary Bypass for Mitral Valve Replacement

Cardiopulmonary bypass is instituted by placing two right-angle cannulas into the superior and inferior venae cavae. We place a small (22F) plastic or metal cannula directly into the superior vena cava, above the sinoatrial node. The inferior caval cannula is placed at the entrance of the inferior vena cava, low in the right atrium. These insertion sites keep the caval catheters out of the operative field and yet maintain excellent bicaval drainage. An arterial cannula is placed in the distal ascending aorta. Bypass flows are approximately 1.5 L/min per m^2, and moderate hypothermia (30°C) is used with vacuum-assisted suction. Myocardial protection includes antegrade and retrograde blood cardioplegia and profound myocardial hypothermia.[178–181] Retrograde cardioplegia is useful for all valve surgery to protect the ischemic left ventricle and to help remove ascending aorta bubbles. Antegrade cardioplegia, used as an initial loading dose, is augmented by intermittent retrograde cardioplegia every 20 minutes. This provides safer delivery of cardioplegia, because when the atrium is retracted during valve replacement, the aortic valve is distorted, and antegrade cardioplegia tends to fill the ventricle.

Exposure of the Mitral Valve

Evolution of meticulous and complicated methods of mitral valve repair and reconstruction has required optimal

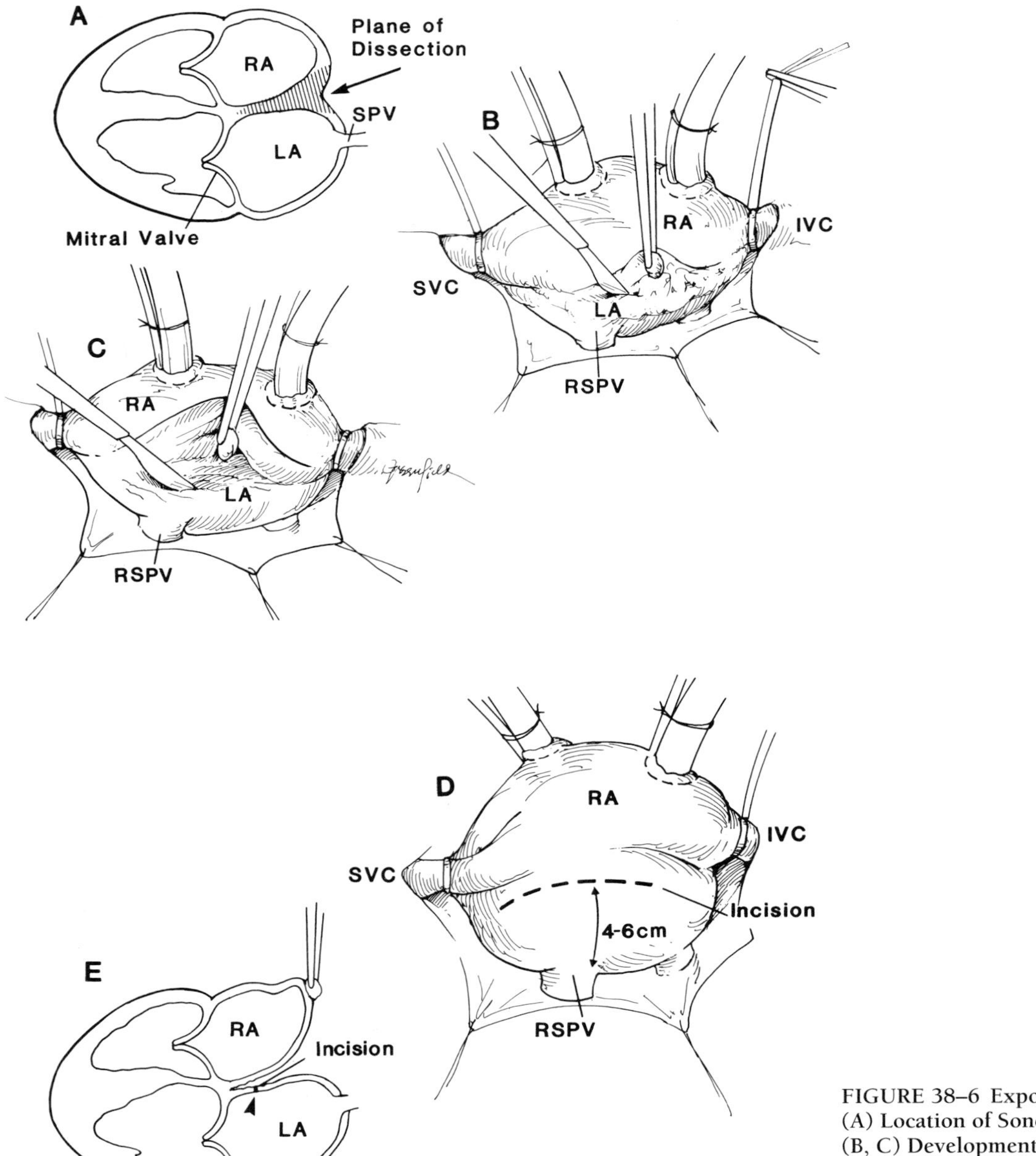

FIGURE 38–6 Exposure of the mitral valve. (A) Location of Sondergaard's plane. (B, C) Development of the interatrial plane. (D) Location of the left atrial incision. (E) Cross-sectional view.

exposure of the mitral valve. In primary operations, median sternotomy, development of Sondergaard's plane, and incision of the left atrium close to the atrial septum provide excellent exposure.[182,183] (Fig. 38-6). This incision is a ubiquitous one, and we have rarely seen indications for use of other incisions, such as the superior approach through the dome of the left atrium,[184–186] the so-called biatrial incision popularized by Guiraudon et al,[187] division of the superior vena cava,[188,189] and the less common but occasionally useful trans-right atrial septal incision.[186,190] The trans-right atrial incision has in some studies been related to higher incidence of junctional and nonsinus rhythm postoperatively,[191] although this has not been confirmed by other studies.[192]

Minimally Invasive Mitral Valve Replacement

Following advances in videoscopic and other minimally invasive techniques in many areas of surgery in the 1990s, similar techniques are now being increasingly used in cardiac surgery, especially in mitral valve surgery.

In 1996 we began minimally invasive valve surgery for patients who have isolated valvular pathology without concomitant coronary artery disease. Our experience at Brigham and Women's Hospital now totals over 400 patients, including mitral valve repairs and aortic and mitral valve replacements.

The minimally invasive approach for mitral valve surgery is usually accomplished with a 5- to 7-cm midline skin incision (Fig. 38-7A). The superior margin of the incision is 2 cm distal to the angle of Louis, and the incision then extends caudally to a point that is 2 cm proximal to the sterno-xyphoid junction. Partial lower sternotomy is performed with an oscillitating saw from the xyphoid process, up to the manubrium with angled incision made into the right 2nd intercostal space. The pericardium is incised vertically and pericardial stay sutures are placed at the right side of the pericardial edge (Fig. 38-7B). Suspension of the right side of the pericardial cradle to the sternal edges allows better exposure of the base of the heart. This approach allows excellent exposure of the left and right atrium and proximal ascending aorta. A slightly different approach is to access the right atrium through a right parasternal incision, excising the 3rd and 4th costal cartilage. This approach, which was used in some of the early cases of minimally invasive mitral surgery, was associated with significant incidence of lung herniation, and has been abandoned.

Cardiopulmonary bypass can be established in several different ways, depending upon the exposure of the ascending aorta and superior vena cava. The exposure depends on the habitus of the patient, as well as upon the relative sizes of the right atrium and ascending aorta. If easily accessible, the ascending aorta can be cannulated directly using a Seldinger technique with a flexible aortic cannula. Both femoral and internal jugular vein are cannulated percutaneously (see Fig. 38-7A). Percutaneous venous cannulation allows better visualization of the operative field, since none of the cannulas exit the sternotomy incision. We routinely use vacuum-assisted venous drainage, which allows the use of smaller diameter cannulas (21F femoral venous cannula, and 14F right internal jugular cannula). Tips of the cannulas are positioned in the distal parts of the superior and inferior vena cavae, respectively. The positioning of the cannulas is done under transesophageal echocardiographic guidance. After fibrillating the heart, the aortic cross-clamp is applied and antegrade blood cardioplegia is administered through the aortic root. Systemic temperature is lowered to 28°C. The valve is approached through the left atrium as described above, or more often the right atrium with a transseptal incision (see Fig. 38-7B). After the valve has been replaced with a standard technique, the atrium and septum (if opened) are closed with running 4-0 Prolene. Intracardiac air is always monitored by transesophageal echocardiography and alternate filling used to evacuate the air by manipulating the volume of the heart on bypass.

Safety and efficacy of minimally invasive mitral valve surgery have been confirmed in several reports.[192–195] Trauma seems to be less with the minimally invasive incisions, which is beneficial in regard to infections (including mediastinitis) and bleeding from the incision and the operative field, leading to lesser usage of homologous blood.[193] There is also improved cosmesis with these incisions and postoperative pain seems to be considerably less than in patients with the median sternotomy. This can result in less requirement for pain medication, faster return to normal activity with less dependence on after-hospital stay, and after-hospital care without compromising results.

Femoral arterial and venous cannulation are tolerated well in the vast majority of patients, and are associated with minimal morbidity. One of the important technical aspects of cannulation is the use of a limited (2-3 cm) oblique suprainguinal incision just above femoral vessels. This incision, in contrast to the standard vertical incision, has been associated with minimal discomfort and low wound infection rate, since it does not transverse the inguinal skin crease, and is not exposed to stretching during hip flexion and ambulation. One of the rare potential risks of femoral arterial cannulation is the development of retrograde aortic dissection, or retrograde plaque embolization in patients with severe atherosclerotic disease of the descending aorta. We perform routine assessment of descending aorta with transesophageal echocardiography prior to cannulation. Deairing the heart is more complex because the apex of the heart is not accessible, the heart is only partially visible through the 5- to 7-cm incision, and the left atrial appendage cannot be invaginated. Flooding the operative field with continuous CO_2 can be beneficial in reducing intracardial air, and by manipulating the volume of the heart on bypass and alternating the position of the patient, air can be effectively evacuated. This is done under the guidance of transesophageal echocardiography, which is used in most patients undergoing minimally invasive mitral surgery. If transesophageal echocardiography is contraindicated, for instance because of esophageal diverticulum, the assessment of the mitral apparatus as well as de-aring of the heart chambers can be performed with direct epicardial echocardiography. If concomitant coronary artery bypass graft is needed, a full sternotomy is necessary.

Intracardiac Technique

Operation entails secure fixation of a valve prosthesis to the annulus by reliable suture techniques without damage to adjacent structures or myocardium and without tissue interference with valve function. Implantation should prevent injury to anatomic structures surrounding the mitral valve annulus. Figure 38-8 shows the proximity of important cardiac structures near the mitral valve annulus. These include the circumflex coronary artery within the atrioventricular (AV) groove, the left atrial appendage, the aortic valve in continuity with the anterior mitral curtain, and the AV node.

An accumulation of laboratory and clinical evidence indicates that preservation of papillary muscle–chordal attachments to the annulus is important for maintenance of left

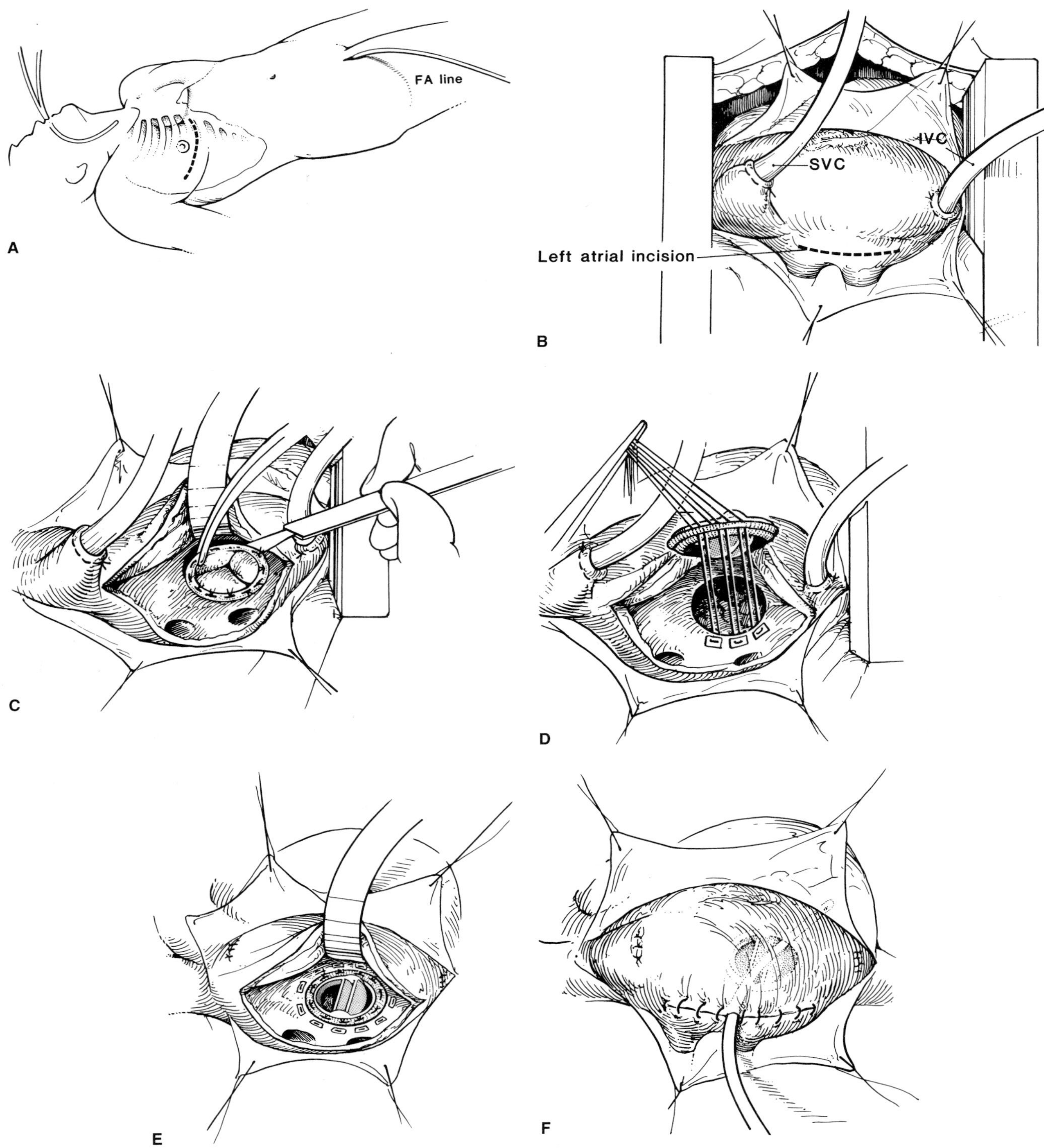

FIGURE 38–7 (A) Minimally invasive right thoracotomy and groin cannulation. (B) A right atrial incision is used to gain access to the mitral valve through the septum. (C) When the right atrium is incised, an incision is made in the atrial septum through the fossa ovalis. Retraction sutures, on both the right atrium and the atrial septum, of 2-0 silk, are then used to elevate the septum and to keep the left atrium open. The mitral valve will then be exposed (inset).

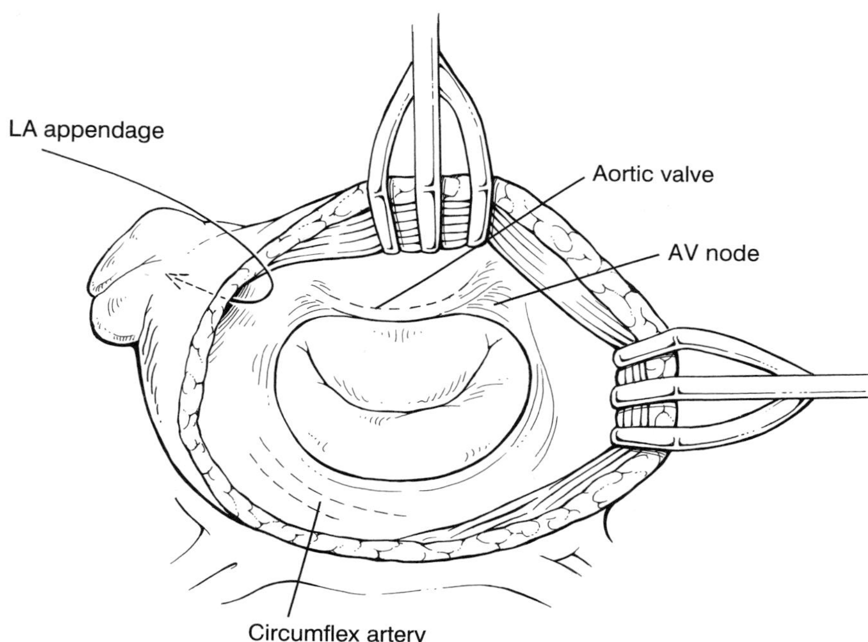

FIGURE 38–8 Location of important structures surrounding the mitral annulus. (*Courtesy of David Bichell, M.D.*)

ventricular function. In patients with mitral stenosis with agglutinated, fibrotic chordae and papillary muscles, preservation of these structures probably has little effect on left ventricular dysfunction but does protect the AV groove from rupture by preserving the posterior leaflet. However, preservation of the posterior mitral leaflet may preclude an adequately sized prosthesis. If fibrotic, agglutinated chordae and the posterior leaflet are excised, placement of artificial Gore-Tex chordae to reattach the papillary muscles to the annulus may improve early and late preservation of cardiac output.[196,197] In patients with mitral regurgitation, however, it is important to preserve as much of the papillary muscle and annular interaction as possible. This can be achieved by a variety of techniques, as shown in Figure 38-9. The anterior leaflet may be partially excised and brought to the posterior leaflet[198] (Fig. 38-9) or can be partially excised and "furled" to the anterior annulus by a running Prolene suture (Fig. 38-9B).[199–201]

Experimental and clinical evidence suggest that preservation of the conical shape of the ventricle is important to maintain normal cardiac output,[202–208] and that assumption of a globular shape from cutting papillary muscles is deleterious to left ventricular function. Furthermore, preservation of the posterior leaflet and chordae has dramatically reduced the incidence of perforation of the left ventricle and atrioventricular separation during mitral valve replacement.[64,209–212]

Suturing techniques vary according to the type of valve that is implanted. The bioprosthetic valve is preferentially inserted with the sutures placed from ventricle to atrium (noneverting or subannular). This has been shown to be the strongest type of suturing technique to the mitral annulus and is used with this valve and the central-flow Starr-Edwards ball-and-cage valve (Fig. 38-10A).[213]

To ensure adequate function of bileaflet or tilting-disk valves, everting sutures (atrium to ventricle to sewing ring) should be used (Fig. 38-10B). This technique pushes the prosthetic valve out into the center of the orifice and minimizes any tissue interference of the prosthetic valve leaflets. This is particularly important if annular-chordal attachments are preserved. Teflon pledgeted sutures, particularly with the thin sewing rings of the currently available bileaflet and tilting-disk valves, should be used. If a bioprosthetic valve is inserted, a dental mirror is used to ensure that no annular suture is wrapped around a stent strut. A running Prolene suture for implantation of mitral valves has been advocated by some surgeons.[214–216] This technique makes a very clean suture line with minimal knots but runs the risk of valve dehiscence if an infection occurs.[217]

Prior to closure, the left atrial appendage is ligated by suture or stapled to prevent clot formation in patients with chronic atrial fibrillation, enlarged left atrium, or left atrial thrombus.[218,219] The atrium is closed by a running Prolene suture, making sure that endocardial surfaces are approximated. If needed, a left atrial catheter can be inserted through the suture line.

Associated Operations/Procedures

Coronary bypass is the most common procedure performed with mitral valve replacement and should be performed first. This reduces lifting of the heart after the rigid mitral valve prosthesis is in place, which can cause rupture of the

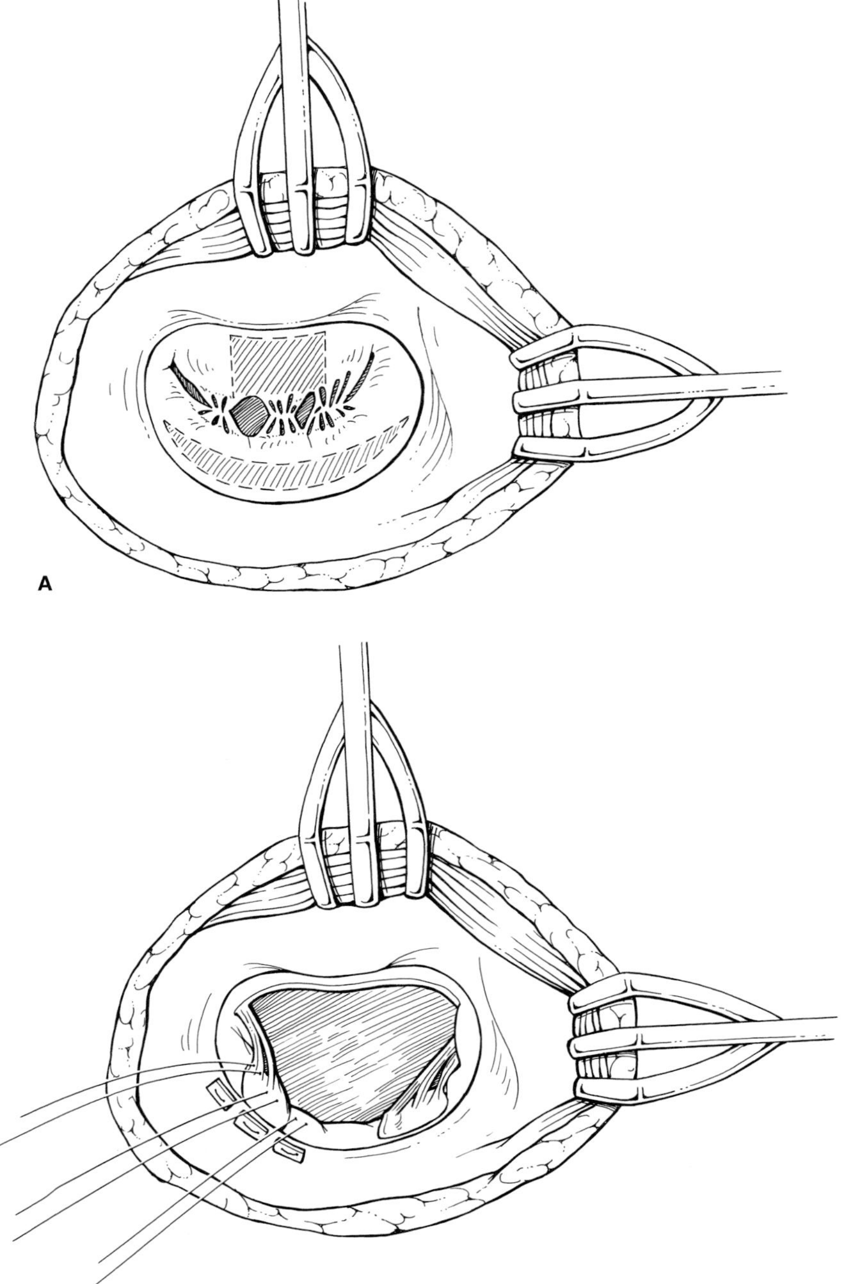

FIGURE 38–9 Techniques to maintain annular–papillary muscle continuity. (A) An ellipse is removed from the posterior leaflet, and a flap is cut form the central portion of the anterior leaflet. The anterior flap is flipped to the posterior annulus and tacked to the caudad edge of the posterior leaflet and the posterior annulus. Sutures anchoring the prosthesis include the annulus and anterior and posterior leaflet remnants to which chordae are attached. (B) The anterior leaflet is partially excised, and remnants are "furled" to the annulus by sutures used to insert the prosthesis.

myocardium or the atrioventricular groove. This also allows cardioplegia to be delivered through the bypass grafts.

Tricuspid valve repair or replacements are usually performed after replacing the mitral valve. In these cases the mitral valve is often approached through the right atrium and a transseptal incision. After the mitral valve prosthesis is in place, the septum is closed and the aortic crossclamp removed before proceeding with the tricuspid valve procedure.[220]

When both the aortic and mitral valves are replaced at the same operation, most surgeons begin with excising the aortic valve before proceeding with the mitral valve procedure. When excising the anterior mitral valve leaflet care must be taken not to injure the aortic annulus and the intra-annular region. The aortic valve is then sewn in after the mitral valve is in place.

Weaning Off Cardiopulmonary Bypass

We use transesophageal echocardiography for every valve operation and particularly for mitral valves, where excellent images can be obtained. If transesophageal echocardiography

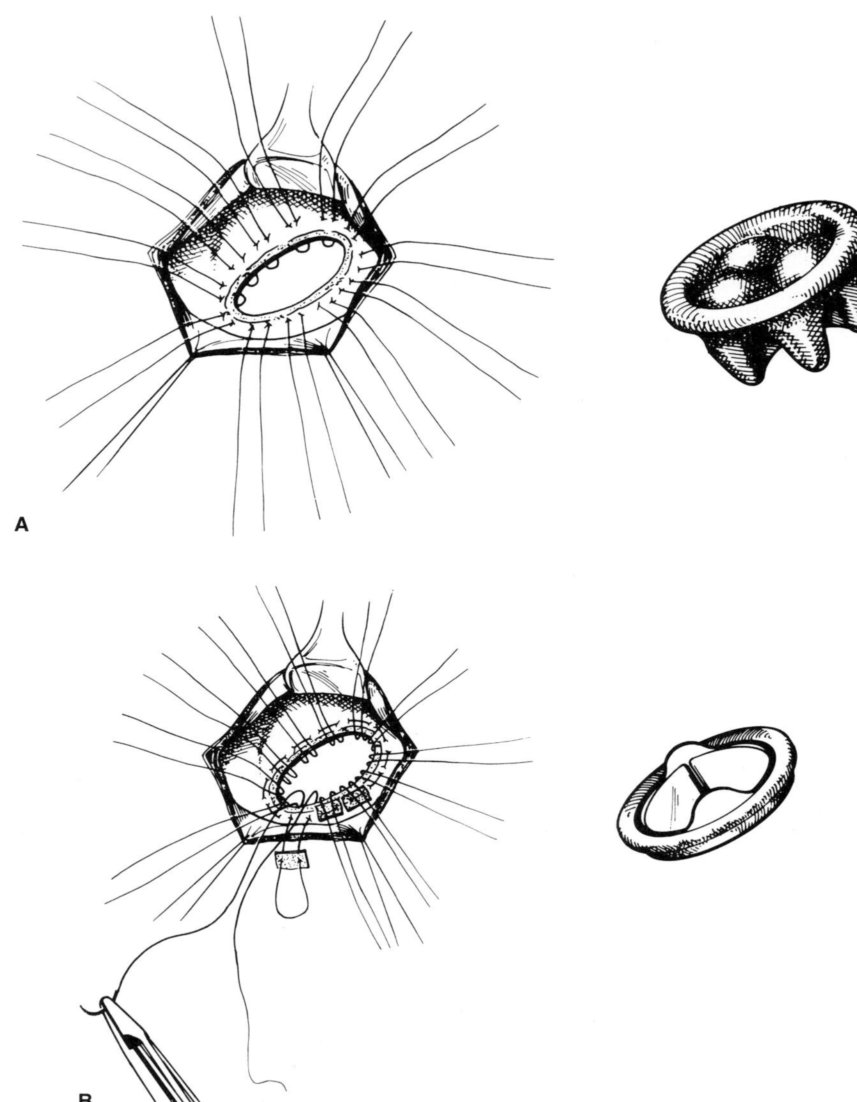

FIGURE 38–10 Suturing techniques for prosthetic mitral valve implantation. Noneverting (subannular) sutures placed from ventricle to atrium for bioprosthetic or Starr-Edwards valves. Everting (supra-annular) sutures placed from atrium to ventricle for bileaflet or tilting-disk valves.

is contraindicated (e.g., because of esophageal disease), direct epicardial echocardiography can be used. The echocardiograms provide information about valve and left ventricular function, possible retained material in the left atrium including thrombus, and removal of intracardiac air.[221–223]

A careful de-airing at the end of the operation is essential. The heart is vented through the left atrium and the ascending aorta and sometimes the left ventricle. Before the aortic cross-clamp is removed, the patient's head is lowered and the lungs inflated carefully to dislodge any air bubbles in the pulmonary vein. The operation table is then tilted from side to side, the left atrial appendage inverted, and the cardiac chambers aspirated if necessary. Once de-airing maneuvers are completed, and after the patient is completely rewarmed, venous return is partially occluded, and the heart is gradually volume loaded. Pulmonary artery pressures are monitored carefully. Pharmacologic agents, such as amrinone or dobutamine, particularly for right ventricular overload, are often used.

POSTOPERATIVE CARE

Postoperative care is directed toward the resumption of normal cardiac output, respiratory function, temperature control, electrolyte management, adequate renal flow, and prophylaxis against bleeding. Patients with low cardiac output are managed with a variety of pharmacologic agents after providing adequate volume loading. Left atrial and especially pulmonary arterial catheters are particularly helpful in determining optimal balancing of volume loading and myocardial function in the first hours following operation.[224]

Reduction of pulmonary interstitial fluid is aggressively pursued by diuresis in the intensive care unit in patients with severe pulmonary hypertension. Most patients with severe pulmonary hypertension can be extubated within 48 hours following surgery. Nutritional, respiratory, and general metabolic support are provided. Many patients with severe, long-standing mitral disease are cachectic and, despite preoperative nutritional support, are severely catabolic at the time of operation. These patients generally require longer periods of ventilatory support due to lack of respiratory muscle strength. They need aggressive nutritional support with nasogastric hyperalimentation to increase respiratory muscle strength. In patients with severe pulmonary hypertension and cardiac cachexia who require prolonged intubation, tracheostomy may be necessary to reduce ventilatory dead space and facilitate faster weaning and better pulmonary toilet. Tracheostomy is usually performed by the end of the first postoperative week.

Postoperative atrial arrhythmias are so common that their absence is unusual. Arrhythmias vary from rapid supraventricular tachycardias, usually atrial fibrillation, to junctional rhythm and heart block. These arrhythmias are treated by pharmacologic agents, pacemakers, or both. If rapid atrial fibrillation cannot be controlled pharmacologically and is destabilizing hemodynamically, emergency cardioversion is done to improve cardiac output. Pharmacologic management of supraventricular tachycardia is usually required but may precipitate the need for a prophylactic transvenous pacemaker if severe slowing of the heart rate occurs.

Anticoagulation is prescribed for all patients undergoing mitral valve replacement with either a mechanical or a bioprosthetic valve. In the first 6 weeks following operation, the incidence of atrial and other arrhythmias is high; thus these fluctuating rhythms mandate anticoagulation even if the basic rhythm is sinus. In addition to rhythm concerns, the left atrial incisions and the possibility of stasis in the left atrial appendage justify full anticoagulation with warfarin for all patients. Some surgeons advocate immediate intravenous heparin until therapeutic warfarin doses can be reached.[225,226] Low molecular weight heparin (LMWH) can also be used.[227] In our patients who are at high risk for thromboembolism, e.g., those with a large left atrium or an intra-atrial thrombus, we use dextran (500 mL every 24 hours) until the patient is anticoagulated with warfarin. We believe that this is safer than heparin in the early postoperative period and avoids blood accumulation in the pericardium.

The therapeutic International Normalized Ratio (INR) after mitral valve replacement is 2.5 to 3.5 depending on the type of valve, cardiac rhythm, and presence or absence of the aforementioned intraoperative risk factors for thromboembolism.[51,218,219,225,227] Anticoagulation levels are in the low range for patients in sinus rhythm who received tissue valves. Patients who have mechanical valves need lifelong anticoagulation. Patients who have bioprosthetic valves are evaluated at 6 to 12 weeks for cardiac rhythm abnormalities. If they are in predominantly sinus rhythm, warfarin is stopped, and one aspirin tablet is given daily indefinitely. If the patient has continuous atrial fibrillation or fluctuating rhythms, anticoagulation with warfarin is continued. This is also true for patients with history of previous embolism or in whom thrombus is found in the left atrium at operation.

Warfarin is usually started on the second postoperative day. Addition of aspirin, 80 to 150 mg daily, together with warfarin may reduce the risk of thromboembolism.[228] and should be given to all patients with prosthetic valves.[166]

RESULTS

Early Results

The hospital mortality for mitral valve replacement with and without coronary bypass grafting has decreased significantly since inception of mitral valve surgery. The current risk (2002) of elective primary mitral valve replacement with and without coronary bypass grafting is 5% to 9% in most studies (range 3.3% to 13.1%).[24,25,42,43,47,104–106,146,204,229–233] Operative (30-day) mortality is related to myocardial failure, multisystem organ failure, bleeding, respiratory failure in the chronically ill, debilitated individual, diabetes, infection, stroke, and, very rarely, technical problems.[102,234] Mortality is correlated with preoperative functional class, age, and preexisting coronary artery disease.[233,235]

Published results on mitral valve surgery have improved in recent years,[236] probably because of preservation of papillary muscles, preventing midventricular rupture,[209–212] and preservation of the normal geometry of the left ventricle, which aids in the maintenance of early postoperative cardiac output.[199,202,204–206,208] Mitral valve replacement and coronary artery bypass surgery 15 to 20 years ago had an associated mortality of about 10% to 20%.[17,94,237] This mortality risk also has decreased as myocardial protection has improved with the use of blood cardioplegia and retrograde methods of administration.[178–180] Some studies have indicated that the risk of combined mitral valve replacement–coronary artery bypass grafting is now no greater than that of mitral valve repair with an annuloplasty ring or mitral valve replacement without coronary artery bypass grafting.[204,238] Other studies have shown significantly increased morbidity and mortality with the addition of coronary artery bypass graft.[101] Figures from the database of the Society of Thoracic Surgeons indicate that both reoperation and emergency operation increase operative mortality (Fig. 38-11).[239]

Late Results

FUNCTIONAL IMPROVEMENT

In over 90% of patients following mitral valve replacement, functional class improves to at least class II. A small group of

TABLE 38–3 Actuarial survival following mitral valve replacement

			Actuarial survival			
Valve	**Reference (year)**	**5 y**	**10 y**	**15 y**	**20 y**	**30 y**
Starr-Edwards	Teply[240] (1981)	78%	56%			
	Sala[132] (1982)	78%	72%			
	Miller[9] (1983)	71%	47%			
	Godje[259] (1997)	85%	75%	56%	37%	23%
Omniscience/Omnicarbon	Damle[241] (1987)	91% (4 y)				
	Peter[250] (1993)	77% (4 y)				
	Otaki[264] (1993)	82% (6 y)				
	Misawa[263] (1993)	94% (3 y)				
	Thevenet[265] (1995)		88% (9 y)			
	Iguro[266] (1999)	88%				
	Torregrosa[267] (1999)		81%			
Medtronic Hall	Vallejo[244] (1990)	79%				
	Masters[253] (1995)	70%	67%			
	Fiore[24] (1998)	70%	58%			
	Butchart[233] (2001)		58%	36%		
St. Jude	DiSesa[243] (1989)	65% (4 y)				
	Kratz[249] (1993)	80%	63%			
	Aoyagi[231] (1994)	88%	81%			
	Masters[253] (1995)	75%				
	Fiore[24] (1998)	65%	53%			
	Camilleri[262] (2001)	89% (4 y)				
	Remadi[???] (2001)	88%	76%	61%		
Carbomedics	Bortolotti[245] (1991)	90%				
	Rabelo[246] (1991)	75% (4 y)				
	De Luca[248] (1993)	93% (3 y)				
	Copeland[255] (1994)	86% (2 y)				
	Copeland[254] (1995)	81%				
	Nistal[232] (1996)	83%				
	Yamauchi[258] (1996)	92%				
	Santini[230] (2002)	86%				
Hancock standard	Cohn[242] (1989)	82%	60%			
	Burdon[103] (1992)	74%	55%			
	Sarris[251] (1993)	79%	58%			
	Khan[106] (1998)		50%	29%	14%	
Hancock II	David[45] (2001)	69%	52%	30%		
Carpentier-Edwards standard	Akins[40] (1990)	53%	45%			
	Louagie[247] (1992)	61%	46%			
	Bernal[33] (1995)	89%	80%			
	Pelletier[41] (1995)	83%	62% (8 y)			
	van Doorn[104] (1995)	75%	53%			
	Murakami[257] (1996)		75%			
	Marchand[43] (1998)		53% (11 y)			
Carpentier-Edwards pericardial	Takahara[48] (1995)		59% (9 y)			
	Aupart[146] (1997)	78%	71%			
	Marchand[43] (1998)		53 (11 y)			
	Neville[44] (1998)		54% (12 y)			
	Porier[42] (1998)	84%	58%			
Mosaic	Jasinski[147] (2000)	100% (3 y)				
	Fradet[46] (2001)	83 (4 y)				
	Thomson[47] (2001)	79% (4 y)				

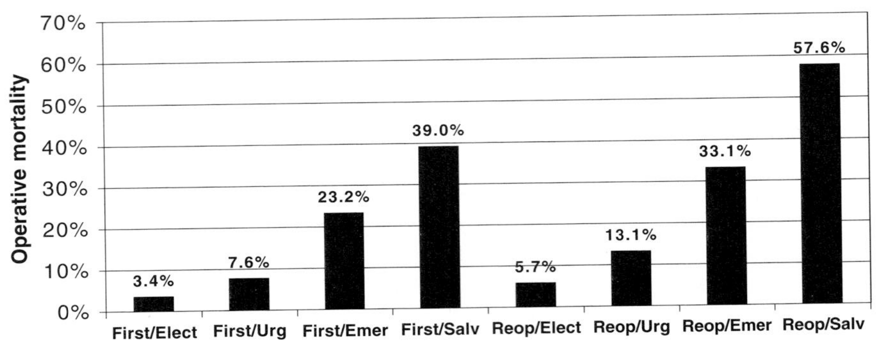

FIGURE 38–11 Operative mortality for elective, urgent, emergency, and salvage procedures for primary operations and reoperations for mitral vavlular replacements. (Data used with permission from Society of Thoracic Surgeons.)

patients remain in class III or IV depending on left ventricular function prior to surgery or other coexisting morbidity.

SURVIVAL

The causes of late death in patients following mitral valve replacement are primarily chronic myocardial dysfunction, thromboemboli and stroke, endocarditis, anticoagulant-related hemorrhage, and coronary artery disease. The extent of left ventricular dysfunction and patient age, particularly if myocardial and coronary diseases are combined, also correlates with late mortality. The probability of survival after mitral valve replacement at 10 years is usually around 50% to 60% (range 42% to 81%, Table 38-3).[9,24,25,33,40–48,103–106,132,146,147,152,154,172,230–233,240–267] Long-term patient survival seems to be similar for patients with biologic and mechanical mitral valves.[268–271] Unlike patients with severe aortic regurgitation or aortic stenosis, arrhythmias seldom cause sudden death in patients following mitral valve replacement; however, a few die from thromboembolic stroke due to chronic atrial fibrillation.[253] The fact that more than 50% of patients following mitral valve replacement are in chronic atrial fibrillation increases the propensity for thromboembolic stroke despite anticoagulation and for mechanical valve thrombosis if the anticoagulation protocol is altered. In addition, patients with older types of prosthetic valves who receive higher-intensity anticoagulation may develop severe anticoagulant hemorrhage.[9,272]

In patients with bioprosthetic valves, one of the important determinants of mortality is reoperation secondary to structural valve degeneration (Table 38-4).[33,40,269,273–276] Reoperative mitral valve replacement mortality has decreased

TABLE 38–4 Freedom from reoperation

Valve	Reference (year)	Actuarial freedom from reoperation		
		5 y	10 y	15 y
Hancock	Cohn[242] (1989)	96%	79%	41%
	Perier[287] (1989)	88%	59%	
	Bernal[304] (1991)	92%	69%	25%
	Sarris[251] (1993)	93%	69%	
	Khan[106] (1998)			44%
Hancock II	David[45] (2001)	98%	85%	69%
Carpentier-Edwards standard	Perier[287] (1989)	91%	64%	
	Jamieson[37] (1991)	94%	64%	39%
	Sarris[251] (1993)	91%	57% (8 y)	
	Van Doorn[104] (1995)	95%	69%	
	Glower[260] (1998)	94%	65%	30%
Carpentier-Edwards pericardial	Pelletier[41] (1995)	98%	67% (8 y)	
	Murakami[257] (1996)	100%	77%	
	Aupart[146] (1997)		90%	
	Marchand[43] (1998)		83% (11 y)	
	Neville[44] (1998)		76% (12 y)	
	Poirer[42] (1998)	99%	76%	
Mosaic	Fradet[46] (2001)	97% (4 y)		
	Jasinski[147] (2001)	100% (3 y)		

TABLE 38–5 Incidence of thromboembolism and anticoagulant-related hemorrhage

Valve	Reference (year)	Incidence of thromboembolism (%/pt-y)	Incidence of anticoagulant-related bleeding (%/pt-y)
Starr-Edwards	Miller[9] (1983)	5.7	3.7
	Akins[283] (1987)	3.9	2.4
	Agathos[157] (1993)	6.6	2.2
	Godje[259] (1997)	1.3	0.6
Omniscience/Omnicarbon	Cortina[282] (1986)		2.7
	Damle[241] (1987)	2.5	
	Akalin[161] (1992)	1.0	2.7
	Peter[251] (1993)	1.7	0.9
	Otaki[264] (1993)	0.7	0.0
	Misawa[263] (1993)	1.8	0.0
	Ohta[291] (1995)	1.1	0.8
	Thevenet[265] (1995)	0.9	1.1
	Iguro[266] (1999)	1.0	0.6
	Torregrosa[267] (1999)	0.6	0.8
Medtronic Hall	Antunes[285] (1988)	4.2	1.5
	Beaudet[286] (1988)	2.1	3.2
	Akins[288] (1991)	1.8	3.2
	Butchart[233] (2001)	4.0	1.4
St. Jude	Czer[20] (1990)	1.9	2.1
	Kratz[249] (1993)	2.9	2.2
	Jegaden[225] (1994)	1.5	0.9
	Aoyagi[231] (1994)	1.1	0.3
	Nistal[232] (1996)	3.7	2.8
	Camilleri[262] (2001)	1.9	1.5
	Khan[290] (2001)	3.0	1.9
	Ramadi[???] (2001)	0.7	0.9
Carbomedics	De Luca[248] (1993)	0.8	0.0
	Copeland[255] (1994)	4.3	2.4
	Copeland[254] (1995)	0.6	1.5
	Nistal[232] (1996)	0.9	2.8
	Yamauchi[258] (1996)	1.6	1.5
	Jamieson[289?303?] (2000)	4.6	2.7
ATS	Shiono[149] (1996)		0.0
	Westaby[151] (1996)	0.0	
	Emery[154] (2001)	3.3	4.9
ON-X	Laczkovics[172] (2001)	1.8	0.0
Hancock standard	Cohn[242] (1989)	2.4	0.4
	Perier[287] (1989)	1.1	1.0
	Bortolotti[274] (1995)	1.4	0.7
Carpentier-Edwards Porcine	Perier[287] (1989)	0.8	1.0
	Akins[40] (1990)	1.4	1.2
	Jamieson[284] (1987)	2.4	0.7
	van Doorn[104] (1995)	1.9	
	Glower[260] (1998)	1.7	0.7
Carpentier-Edwards Pericardial	Pelletier[41] (1995)	1.5	0.3
	Murakami[96] (1996)	0.6	0.0
	Aupart[146] (1997)	0.7	1.2
	Marchand[43] (1998)	1.2	1.0
	Neville[44] (1998)	0.6	1.1
	Poirer[42] (1998)	1.7	0.3
Mosaic	Fradet[46] (2001)	1.4	1.1
	Thomson[47] (2001)	0.2	0.9

significantly in the last 10 years to under 10%, even in patients who have required multiple mitral valve reoperations.[178,180,277,278] At the Brigham and Women's Hospital, operative mortality was less than 6% for reoperative mitral valve operations from 1990 to 1995.[178] Improved myocardial protection, earlier selection of patients for reoperation, and better perfusion techniques including frequent femorofemoral bypass to protect the right ventricle during incision and dissection of the heart are factors contributing to decreased mortality.[178,204,275,276,279,280]

LATE MORBIDITY

The major morbidity in patients following mitral valve replacement is structural valve deterioration of a bioprosthetic valve and thromboembolism and anticoagulant hemorrhage with a mechanical prosthesis. Both valve types develop perivalvular leak and infection.

THROMBOEMBOLISM

Thromboembolism is perhaps the most common complication of both biologic and mechanical mitral prostheses but is more frequent in patients with mechanical valves. Chronic atrial fibrillation and local atrial factors, already discussed, increase the risk of thromboembolism in patients with mitral prostheses.[20,31,40,249,273] A number of recent studies have summarized the thromboembolic potential of various valves.[9,20,25,40–44,46,47,104,105,146,149,151,154,157,161,172,225,230–234,241,246,248–250,252,254,255,257–267,274,281–291] (Table 38-5), and it appears that the better the valve hemodynamics, the lower is the probability of thromboemboli. The incidence of thromboemboli in currently available bileaflet valves and tilting-disk valves is similar to that of bioprosthetic valves—about 1.5% to 2.0% per patient-year. Thromboembolism in patients with mitral valve replacement is lower in those with a small left atrium, sinus rhythm, and normal cardiac output. It is much higher in patients with large left atria, chronic atrial fibrillation, and the presence of intra-atrial clot.[218,219,292] Thrombosis of a mechanical valve, once a feared complication of tilting-disk valves,[293–295] is now relatively rare unless anticoagulation is stopped for any period of time. Valve thrombosis can be treated with thrombolytic agents if the patient is not in cardiogenic shock but requires surgery if the circulation is inadequate.[296–300]

ANTICOAGULANT HEMORRHAGE

Bleeding related to anticoagulation is most commonly seen in the gastrointestinal, urogenital, and central nervous system and is usually proportionate to the INR. The incidence of anticoagulant-related hemorrhage has decreased markedly with hemodynamic improvements in mitral valve prostheses. New valves do not require the intensity of anticoagulation of older prostheses. For example, the distinctive Starr-Edwards ball-and-cage valve requires an INR of 3.5 to 4.5.[272] Patients with streamlined bileaflet or tilting-disk valves require an INR of between 2.5 and 3.5; thus the incidence of anticoagulant hemorrhage is significantly reduced in the newer, hemodynamically improved prostheses.[243,301] Table 38-5 lists the incidence of anticoagulant hemorrhage with various bioprostheses and mechanical valves.

STRUCTURAL VALVE DEGENERATION

Structural valve degeneration (SVD) is the most important complication of the bioprosthetic valve. The probability of structural failure with currently available porcine valves (Hancock or Carpentier-Edwards) begins to increase 8 years after operation and reaches over 60% at 15 years.[45,98,106,107,302] This finite durability is a major impediment to long-term success of these biologic prostheses, even though the failure rate in the patient 70 years of age or older is significantly less than in younger age groups.[41–45,95–98,105,107,146,260,303] Structural valve degeneration presents as either mitral regurgitation from leaflet tear or as calcific mitral stenosis due to calcification of valve leaflets or as both. The appearance of a new murmur with new congestive symptoms should prompt a noninvasive investigation of the prosthesis and elective re-replacement if dysfunction is documented. Structural valve degeneration leading to reoperation is the cause for at least two thirds of the reoperations in patients with bioprostheses.[40,276,278] The probabilities of structural valve degeneration at 5, 10, and 15 years of the four most commonly used biologic prostheses are shown in Table 38-6.[38,40–48,103–107,146,147,242,251,257,274,287,296–300,304,305] With current quality controls, the incidence of structural valve degeneration is virtually zero for bileaflet, tilting-disk, and ball-and-cage valves.

PERIVALVULAR LEAK

Perivalvular leak is an uncommon complication that is usually dependent on technical factors. Patient-related factors such as endocarditis or calcifications involving the annulus are also important. Perivalvular leak usually causes refractory hemolytic anemia in contrast to the more mild chronic hemolysis that is seen after implantation of some of the mechanical valves, especially the tilting-disk valves.[306]

Because of improved surgical techniques and the use of Teflon pledgets, the incidence of perivalvular leak has fallen, and is about 0% to 1.5% per patient-year for both mechanical and biologic valves.[20,216,246,267,284,285,307] Perivalvular leak is slightly more common with the bileaflet valve than with the porcine valve because of the need for the everting suture technique and less bulky sewing ring.[308,309] Surgery should be offered to all symptomatic patients and even patients with mild symptoms that require blood transfusions.[310]

TABLE 38–6 Freedom from SVD by age

Valve	Reference (year)	Age	Freedom from SVD		
			5 y	10 y	15 y
Hancock	Cohn[242] (1989)	≤40		68%	
		41–69		84%	
		≥70		84%	
Hancock II	David[45] (2001)	<65			76%
		≥65			89%
Carpentier-Edwards standard					
	Akins[40] (1990)	≤40		71%	
		41–50		82%	
		51–60		65%	
		61–70		79%	
		≥70		98%	
	Jamieson[38] (1995)	≤35	79%	51%	
		36–40	99%	68%	48%
		51–64	98%	72%	42%
		65–69	98%	74%	64%
		≥70	100%	90%	90%
	Corbineau[107] (2001)	≤35			0% (14 y)
		36–50			22% (14 y)
		51–60			34% (14 y)
		61–65			50% (14 y)
		66–70			93% (14 y)
		≥70			96% (14 y)
Carpentier-Edwards pericardial	Aupart[146] (1997)	<60	47%		
		≥60	100%		
	Marchand[43] (1998)	≤60		78% (11 y)	
		61–70		89% (11 y)	
		>70		100% (11 y)	
	Pelletier[41] (1995)	≤59	100%	64% (8 y)	
		60–69	100%	91% (8 y)	
		≥70	100%	100% (8 y)	
	Neville[44] (1998)	<60		70%	
		≥60		100%	
	Poirer[42] (1998)	<60	100%	78%	
		60–69	100%	78%	
		≥70	100%	100%	

ENDOCARDITIS

Endocarditis is a feared complication after valve replacement, and prosthetic mitral valve endocarditis often presents difficult management problems related to timing of operation, type of operation, ability to securely fix the prosthesis, and operative and late survival. Mitral valve endocarditis is considerably less common than aortic prosthetic valve endocarditis,[311,312] but when it does appear, it may present as septicemia, malignant burrowing infections, abscess formation, and septic emboli. With better antibiotic prophylaxis at the time of mitral surgery and improved prophylaxis for all patients having dental or other surgical procedures, the incidence of endocarditis is relatively low.

The incidence of prosthetic endocarditis is usually higher during the initial 6 months after surgery and thereafter declines to a lower but persistent risk.[49] The probability of freedom from this morbid event is shown in Table 38-7 for both mechanical and bioprosthetic valves.[9,24,25,40–47,104,105,135,146,147,154,157,172,230–233,239,241,242,247–251,253–255,257–260,262–265,267,274,283,285,288,290,291,303,304,313–315] Biologic and mechanical valves seem to have a similar incidence of endocarditis, except for the initial months after valve implantation when mechanical prostheses carry a greater risk of infection.[49,316]

The diagnosis and treatment of mitral perivalvular endocarditis are related to the infecting organism. The diagnosis is made by symptoms or the appearance of a new murmur, a septic embolus, or a large vegetation on echocardiogram. Blood cultures usually are positive, although a small

TABLE 38–7 Prosthetic valve endocarditis

Valve	Reference (year)	PVE rate (%/pt-y)	Freedom from PVE at 5 y	
Starr-Edwards	Miller[9] (1983)	0.5	97%	
	Akins[283] (1987)	0.4	95%	
	Agathos[157] (1993)	0.6		
	Godje[259] (1997)		99% (10 y)	
Omniscience/Omnicarbon	Carrier[313] (1987)	0.8	98%	
	Damle[241] (1987)	0.8	98%	
	Peter[250] (1993)	0.0	100%	
	Otaki[264] (1993)	1.5		
	Misawa[263] (1993)	0.0	100% (3 y)	
	Ohta[291] (1995)	0.5		
	Thenevet[265] (1995)	0.2		
	Torregrosa[267] (1999)	0.2	99% (10 y)	
Medtronic Hall	Keenan[315] (1990)	0.5	98%	
	Akins[288] (1991)	0.1	100%	
	Masters[253] (1995)		96%	
	Fiore[24] (1998)		94% (10 y)	
	Butchart[233] (2001)	0.4	94% (10 y)	
St. Jude	Antunes[285] (1988)	0.5	97%	
	Kratz[249] (1993)	0.4		
	Aoyagi[231] (1994)	0.1	100%	
	Masters[253] (1995)		97%	
	Fiore[24] (1998)		100% (10 y)	
	Camilleri[262] (2001)	0.8		
	Khan[290] (2001)	0.3		
Carbomedics	De Luca[248] (1993)	0.0	100%	
	Copeland[255] (1994)	0.0	100%	
	Copeland[254] (1995)	0.3	96%	
	Nistal[232] (1996)	0.0	100%	
	Yamauchi[258] (1996)	0.0	100%	
	Jamieson[289] (2000)	0.4		
	Santini[230] (2002)		100%	
ATS	Emery[154] (2001)	0.81		
ON-X	Laczkovics[172] (2001)	0.5		
Hancock standard	Cohn[242] (1989)		93%	
	Bernal[304] (1991)	0.3		
	Sarris[251] (1993)		93%	
	Bortolotti[274] (1995)	0.3		
Hancock II	David[45] (2001)		91% (15 y)	
Carpentier-Edwards porcine	Pelletier[314] (1989)	0.4		
	Akins[40] (1990)	1.0		
	Louagie[247] (1992)	0.0	100%	
	Sarris[251] (1993)		91%	
	van Doorn[104] (1995)		97%	92% (10 y)
	Glower[260] (1998)	0.3	97%	96% (10 y)
Carpentier-Edwards pericardial	Pelletier[41] (1995)	0.3%	93% (10 y)	
	Murakami[257] (1996)	0.86	94% (10 y)	
	Aupart[146] (1997)	0.4%	97% (10 y)	
	Marchand[43] (1998)	0.1%		
	Neville[44] (1998)	0.6%	94% (12 y)	
	Poirer[42] (1998)	0.3%	95% (10 y)	
Mosaic	Jasinski[147] (2000)		100% (3 y)	
	Fradet[46] (2001)	0.8	97%	
	Thomson[47] (2001)	0.8		

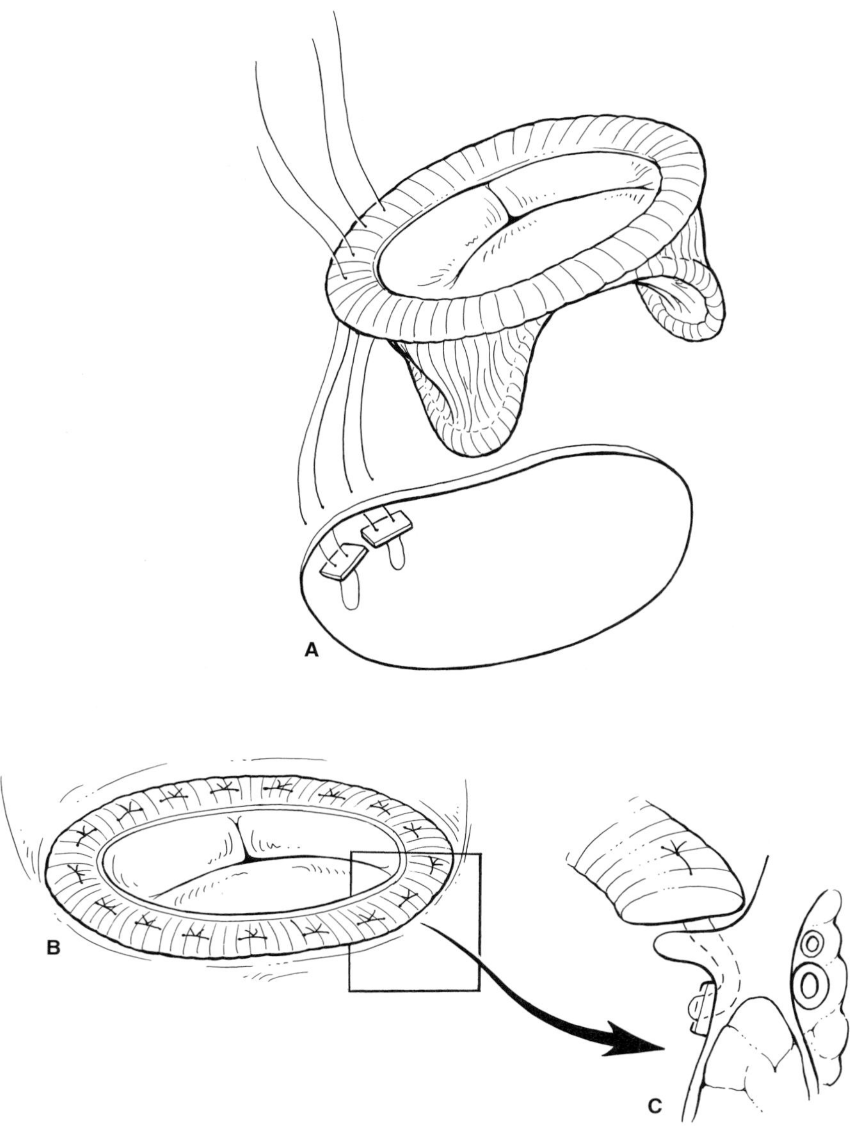

FIGURE 38–12 Preferred technique for inserting a mitral bioprosthesis in a patient with bacterial endocarditis. Pledgets are made from pericardium to minimize foreign material.

percentage of patients have culture-negative endocarditis. Echocardiograms may show a rocking motion of the prosthesis and the presence of vegetations. The most frequent organisms are still *Streptococcus* and *Staphylococcus;* the latter is usually hospital acquired.[317] Antibiotic therapy depends on the sensitivity of the organisms, but immediate high-dose intravenous therapy must begin as soon as possible. Experience indicates that a number of patients with bioprosthetic valvular endocarditis can be "cured" of low-potency organisms such as *Streptococcus*. However, it is unlikely that antibiotics alone can sterilize more virulent mitral valve infections, particularly *Staphylococcus*. These infections usually require urgent and sometimes emergent surgery because of invasion of the cardiac exoskeleton.

The surgical indications for mitral valve prosthetic endocarditis are persistent sepsis, congestive failure, perivalvular leak, large vegetations, or systemic infected emboli.[87,318,319]

Operative technique is similar to other mitral procedures with respect to anesthesia, monitoring, cardioplegia, left atrial incision, and exposure of the valve. Usually biologic valves are used for patients older than 65 years of age or younger patients with short life expectancy.[311] Mechanical valves can be used in younger patients. Excision of the valve and debridement of the annulus and abscesses must be meticulous and extensive. All necrotic and infected tissue must be removed. After local application of an antibacterial solution such as Betadine and local antibiotic irrigation, the annulus and areas of tissue loss are reconstructed using autologous pericardium. Pericardium must be used to reconstruct the mitral valve annulus, and all sutures must be placed through the pericardial-lined annulus to obtain secure anchorage of the new prosthesis. Autologous pericardial pledgets can be made and used instead of conventional cloth pledgets to avoid synthetic material as much as

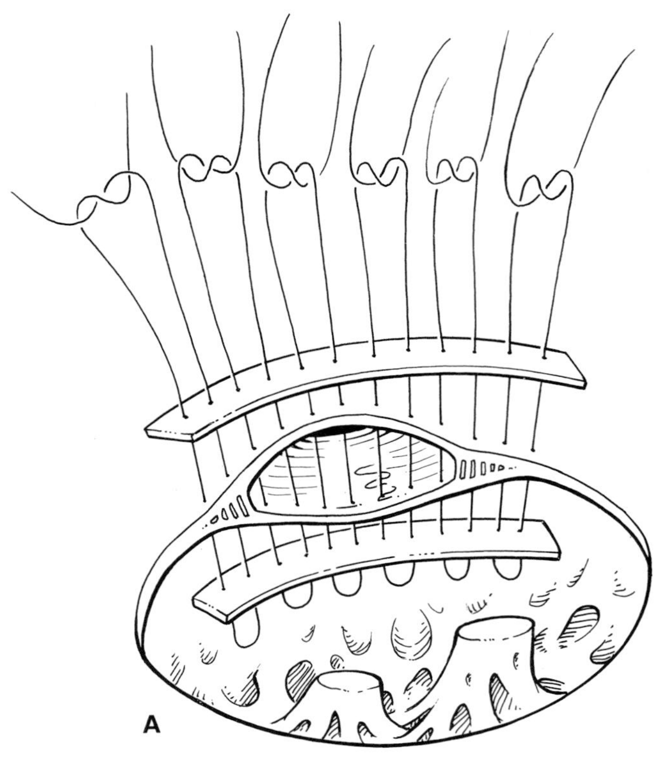

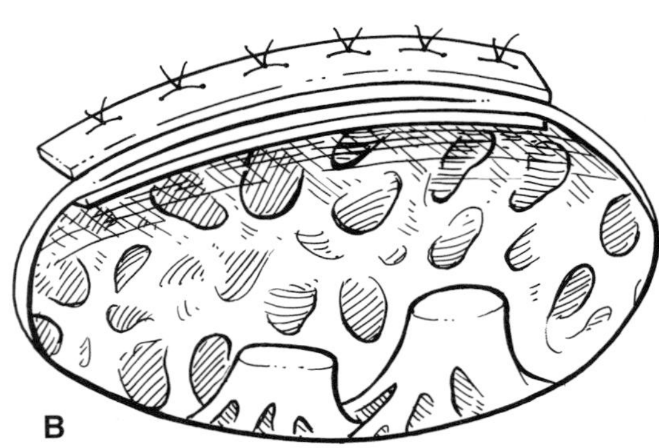

FIGURE 38–13 Repair of a mitral annular abscess using strips of pericardium. (A) Reconstruction of the annulus after debridement of the annulus. (B) The reconstructed annulus before insertion of the prosthesis.

possible. Examples of operative techniques for closure and repair of local abscesses and infectious destruction of the mitral valve annulus are shown in Figures 38-12 and 38-13.[320]

Postoperative care should include at least 6 weeks of appropriate intravenous antibiotics. Hospital mortality is related primarily to ongoing sepsis, multisystem organ failure, or failure to eradicate the local infection and subsequent recurrent perivalvular leak.[321,322] Recurrence of infection depends on the type of organism and the surgeon's ability to completely remove all areas of infection.[318] Recurrence of infection is the single most important long-term complication.

CONCLUSIONS

Mitral valve replacement by mechanical or bioprosthetic valves revolutionized the care of patients with severe mitral valve disease. Reconstructive operations of the mitral valve have now assumed an equally important role for mitral regurgitation. A number of advanced lesions of the mitral valve still require mitral valve replacement with reliable devices. The bileaflet, tilting-disk, and ball-and-cage prosthetic valves are extremely reliable in terms of durability but require long-term anticoagulation and have a high risk of thromboembolism or thrombosis without anticoagulation. Bioprosthetic porcine valves, conversely, in patients in sinus rhythm do not need long-term anticoagulation and are used mainly in elderly patients who are not likely to outlive the valve and in women who plan to become pregnant and do not wish to accept the risks of warfarin or heparin. The long-term durability of these valves is limited, and the probability of valve failure at 15 years is at least 40%. Improvements in mechanical valve design and biologic valve preservation of collagen structure and resistance to calcification are ongoing and are the hopes for the future. In addition, there is renewed interest in homograft mitral valves, which may offer better long-term durability, as has been observed with cryopreserved homograft aortic valves. Improved valve design and development of better biomaterials will eventually improve clinical results; however, current FDA restrictions on the development and evaluation of new prosthetic valves have an important impact on this process.

REFERENCES

1. Cutler E, Levine S: Cardiotomy and valvulotomy for mitral stenosis: experimental observations and clinical notes concerning an operated case with recovery. *Boston Med Surg* 1923; 188:1023.
2. Suttar H: Surgical treatment of mitral stenosis. *BMJ* 1925; 2:603.
3. Harken DE, Ellis LE, Ware PF, Norman LR: The surgical treatment of mitral stenosis, I: valvuloplasty. *N Engl J Med* 1948; 239:801.
4. Harken DE, Ellis LE, Ware PF, Norman LR: The surgical treatment of mitral stenosis, I: valvuloplasty. *N Engl J Med* 1948; 239:801.
5. Bailey C: The surgical treatment of mitral stenosis (mitral comissurotomy). *Dis Chest* 1949; 15:377.
6. Braunwald N, Cooper T, Morrow A: Complete replacement of the mitral valve. *J Thorac Surg* 1960; 40:1.
7. Starr A, Edwards M: Mitral replacement: clinical experience with a ball valve prosthesis. *Ann Thorac Surg* 1961; 154:726.
8. Cobanoglu A, Grunkemeier GL, Aru GM, et al: Mitral replacement: clinical experience with a ball-valve prosthesis: twenty-five years later. *Ann Surg* 1985; 202:376.

9. Miller DC, Oyer PE, Stinson EB, et al: Ten to fifteen year reassessment of the performance characteristics of the Starr-Edwards Model 6120 mitral valve prosthesis. *J Thorac Cardiovasc Surg* 1983; 85:1.
10. Bjork VO, Lindblom D The Monostrut Bjork-Shiley heart valve. *J Am Coll Cardiol* 1985; 6:1142.
11. Nakano S, Kawashima Y, Matsuda H, et al: A five-year appraisal and hemodynamic evaluation of the Bjork-Shiley Monostrut valve. *J Thorac Cardiovasc Surg* 1991; 101:881.
12. Jacobs M, Buckley M, WG Austen, et al: Mechanical valves: ten year follow-up of Starr-Edwards and Bjork-Shiley protheses. *Circulation* 1995; 72(suppl III):III-1.
13. Thulin LI, Bain WH, Huysmans HH, et al: Heart valve replacement with the Bjork-Shiley Monostrut valve: early results of a multicenter clinical investigation. *Ann Thorac Surg* 1988; 45: 164.
14. Ostermeyer J, Horstkotte D, Bennett J, et al: The Bjork-Shiley 70 degree convexo-concave prosthesis strut fracture problem (present state of information). *Thorac Cardiovasc Surg* 1987; 35:71.
15. Gabbay S, McQueen DM, Yellin EL, et al: In vitro hydrodynamic comparison of mitral valve prostheses at high flow rates. *J Thorac Cardiovasc Surg* 1978; 76:771.
16. Chaux A, Gray RJ, Matloff JM, et al: An appreciation of the new St. Jude valvular prosthesis. *J Thorac Cardiovasc Surg* 1981; 81:202.
17. Arom KV, Nicoloff DM, Kersten TE, et al: Six years of experience with the St. Jude Medical valvular prosthesis. *Circulation* 1985; 72:II153.
18. Duncan JM, Cooley DA, Reul GJ, et al: Durability and low thrombogenicity of the St. Jude Medical valve at 5-year follow-up. *Ann Thorac Surg* 1986; 42:500.
19. Edmunds LH Jr: Thrombotic and bleeding complications of prosthetic heart valves. *Ann Thorac Surg* 1987; 44:430.
20. Czer LS, Chaux A, Matloff JM, et al: Ten-year experience with the St. Jude Medical valve for primary valve replacement. *J Thorac Cardiovasc Surg* 1990; 100:44.
21. Fiore AC, Naunheim KS, D'Orazio S, et al: Mitral valve replacement: randomized trial of St. Jude and Medtronic-Hall prostheses. *Ann Thorac Surg* 1992; 54:68.
22. Hayashi J, Oguma F, Tsuchida S, et al: Review of ten years' use of the St. Jude Medical prosthetic valve replacement and postoperative management at Nigata University Hospital. *Acta Med Biol* 1993; 41:81.
23. O'Kane BC, Gladstone D, et al: The St. Jude prosthesis: a thirteen year experience. *J Thorac Cardiovasc Surg* 1994; 108:221.
24. Fiore AC, Barner HB, Swartz MT, et al: Mitral valve replacement: randomized trial of St. Jude and Medtronic Hall prostheses. *Ann Thorac Surg* 1998; 66:707.
25. Remadi JP, Baron O, Roussel C, et al: Isolated mitral valve replacement with St. Jude medical prosthesis: long-term results: a follow-up of 19 years. *Circulation* 2001; 103:1542.
26. Carpentier A: From valvular xenograft to valvular bioprosthesis: 1965–1970. *Ann Thorac Surg* 1989; 48:S73.
27. Binet JP: Pioneering in heterografts. *Ann Thorac Surg* 1989; 48:S71.
28. Carpentier A, Lemaigre G, Robert L, et al: Biological factors affecting long-term results of valvular heterografts. *J Thorac Cardiovasc Surg* 1969; 58:467.
29. Kaiser GA HW, Lukban SB, Litwak RS: Clinical use of a new design stented xenograft heart valve prosthesis. *Surg Forum* 1969; 20:137.
30. Carpentier A: *Principles of Tissue Valve Transplantation*. London, Butterworths, 1971.
31. Cohn LH: Atrioventricular valve replacement with a Hancock porcine xenograft. *Ann Thorac Surg* 1991; 51:683.
32. Pupello P, Bessone L, Blank R, et al: The porcine bioprosthesis: patient age as a factor in predicting failure in Bodnar E, Yacoub M (eds): Biological and Bioprosthetic Valves. New York, Yorke Medical Books, 1986; p 130.
33. Bernal JM, Rabasa JM, Lopez R, et al: Durability of the Carpentier-Edwards porcine bioprosthesis: role of age and valve position. *Ann Thorac Surg* 1995; 60:S248.
34. Geha AS, Laks H, Stansel HC Jr, et al: Late failure of porcine valve heterografts in children. *J Thorac Cardiovasc Surg* 1979; 78:351.
35. Thandroyen FT, Whitton IN, Pirie D, et al: Severe calcification of glutaraldehyde-preserved porcine xenografts in children. *Am J Cardiol* 1980; 45:690.
36. Jamieson WR, Rosado LJ, Munro AI, et al: Carpentier-Edwards standard porcine bioprosthesis: primary tissue failure (structural valve deterioration) by age groups. *Ann Thorac Surg* 1988; 46: 155.
37. Jamieson WR, Tyers GF, Janusz MT, et al: Age as a determinant for selection of porcine bioprostheses for cardiac valve replacement: experience with Carpentier-Edwards standard bioprosthesis. *Can J Cardiol* 1991; 7:181.
38. Jamieson WR, Burr LH, Miyagishima RT, et al: Structural deterioration in Carpentier-Edwards standard and supraannular porcine bioprostheses. *Ann Thorac Surg* 1995; 60:S241.
39. Glower DD, White WD, Hatton AC, et al: Determinants of reoperation after 960 valve replacements with Carpentier-Edwards prostheses. *J Thorac Cardiovasc Surg* 1994; 107:381.
40. Akins CW, Carroll DL, Buckley MJ, et al: Late results with Carpentier-Edwards porcine bioprosthesis. *Circulation* 1990; 82:IV65.
41. Pelletier LC, Carrier M, Leclerc Y, Dyrda I: The Carpentier-Edwards pericardial bioprosthesis: clinical experience with 600 patients. *Ann Thorac Surg* 1995; 60:S297.
42. Poirer NC, Pelletier LC, Pellerin M, Carrier M: 15-year experience with the Carpentier-Edwards pericardial bioprosthesis. *Ann Thorac Surg* 1998; 66:S57.
43. Marchand M, Aupart M, Norton R, et al: Twelve-year experience with Carpentier-Edwards PERIMOUNT pericardial valve in the mitral position: a multicenter study. *J Heart Valve Dis* 1998; 7: 292.
44. Neville PH, Aupart MR, Diemont FF, et al: Carpentier-Edwards pericardial bioprosthesis in aortic or mitral position: a 12-year experience. *Ann Thorac Surg* 1998; 66:S143.
45. David TE, Ivanov J, Armstrong S, et al: Late results of heart valve replacement with the Hancock II bioprosthesis. *J Thorac Cardiovasc Surg* 2001; 121:268.
46. Fradet GJ, Bleese N, Burgess J, Cartier PC: Mosaic valve international clinical trial: early performance results. *Ann Thorac Surg* 2001; 71:S273.
47. Thomson DJ, Jamieson WR, Dumesnil JG, et al: Medtronic Mosaic porcine bioprosthesis: midterm investigational trial results. *Ann Thorac Surg* 2001; 71:S269.
48. Takahara Y, Sudou Y, Murayama H, Nakamura T: [Long-term evaluation of the Carpentier-Edwards pericardial bioprosthesis]. *Nippon Kyobu Geka Gakkai Zassh* 1995; 43:1097.
49. Braunwald E: Valvular heart disease, in Braunwald E (ed): *Heart Disease, A Textbook of Cardiovascular Medicine,* 6th ed. Philadelphia, WB Saunders, 2001.
50. Braunwald E: Valvular heart disease, in Braunwald E (ed): *Heart Disease, A Textbook of Cardiovascular Medicine,* 6th ed. Philadelphia, WB Saunders, 2001.
51. Bonow RO, Carabello B, de Leon AC Jr, et al: Guidelines for the management of patients with valvular heart disease: executive summary. A report of the American College of Cardiology/American Heart Association Task Force on Practice Guidelines (Committee on Management of Patients with Valvular Heart Disease). *Circulation* 1998; 98:1949.
52. Spencer FC: A plea for early, open mitral commissurotomy. *Am Heart J* 1978; 95:668.

53. Dalen JE, Matloff JM, Evans GL, et al: Early reduction of pulmonary vascular resistance after mitral-valve replacement. *N Engl J Med* 1967; 277:387.
54. Kaul TK, Bain WH, Jones JV, et al: Mitral valve replacement in the presence of severe pulmonary hypertension. *Thorax* 1976; 31:332.
55. Braunwald E, Braunwald N, Ross JJ, Morrow A: Effects of mitral valve replacement on the pulmonary vascular dynamics of patients with pulmonary hypertension. *N Engl J Med* 1965; 273: 509.
56. Pasaoglu I, Demircin M, Dogan R, et al: Mitral valve surgery in the presence of pulmonary hypertension. *Jpn Heart J* 1992; 33:179.
57. Aris A, Camara ML: As originally published in 1988: Long-term results of mitral valve surgery in patients with severe pulmonary hypertension. Updated in 1996. *Ann Thorac Surg* 1996; 61:1583.
58. Vincens JJ, Temizer D, Post JR, et al: Long-term outcome of cardiac surgery in patients with mitral stenosis and severe pulmonary hypertension. *Circulation* 1995; 92:II137.
59. Reyes VP, Raju BS, Wynne J, et al: Percutaneous balloon valvuloplasty compared with open surgical commissurotomy for mitral stenosis. *N Engl J Med* 1994; 331:961.
60. Palacios IF, Tuzcu ME, Weyman AE, et al: Clinical follow-up of patients undergoing percutaneous mitral balloon valvotomy. *Circulation* 1995; 91:671.
61. National Heart, Lung, Blood Institute Ballon Valvuloplasty Registry: Complications and mortality of percutaneous balloon commissurotomy. *Circulation* 1992; 85:2014.
62. Tuzcu EM, Block PC, Palacios IF: Comparison of early versus late experience with percutaneous mitral balloon valvuloplasty. *J Am Coll Cardiol* 1991; 17:1121.
63. Cohn LH, Allred EN, Cohn LA, et al: Long-term results of open mitral valve reconstruction for mitral stenosis. *Am J Cardiol* 1985; 55:731.
64. Glower DD, Landolfo KP, Davis RD, et al: Comparison of open mitral commissurotomy with mitral valve replacement with or without chordal preservation in patients with mitral stenosis. *Circulation* 1998; 98:II120.
65. el Asmar B, Acker M, Couetil JP, et al: Mitral valve repair in the extensively calcified mitral valve annulus. *Ann Thorac Surg* 1991; 52:66.
66. Braunwald E: Valvular heart disease, in Braunwald E (ed): *Heart Disease, A Textbook of Cardiovascular Medicine,* 6th ed. Philadelphia, WB Saunders, 2001.
67. Carabello BA: Preservation of left ventricular function in patients with mitral regurgitation: a realistic goal for the nineties. *J Am Coll Cardiol* 1990; 15:564.
68. Mudge GH Jr: Asymptomatic mitral regurgitation: when to operate? *J Card Surg* 1994; 9:248.
69. Stewart WJ: Choosing the "golden moment" for mitral valve repair. *J Am Coll Cardiol* 1994; 24:1544.
70. Ling LH, Enriquez-Sarano M, Seward JB, et al: Clinical outcome of mitral regurgitation due to flail leaflet. *N Engl J Med* 1996; 335:1417.
71. Tavel ME, Carabello BA: Chronic mitral regurgitation: when and how to operate. *Chest* 1998; 113:1399.
72. Tribouilloy CM, Enriquez-Sarano M, Schaff HV, et al: Impact of preoperative symptoms on survival after surgical correction of organic mitral regurgitation: rationale for optimizing surgical indications. *Circulation* 1999; 99:400.
73. Kizilbash AM, Hundley WG, Willett DL, et al: Comparison of quantitative Doppler with magnetic resonance imaging for assessment of the severity of mitral regurgitation. *Am J Cardiol* 1998; 81:792.
74. Enriquez-Sarano M, Tajik AJ, Schaff HV, et al: Echocardiographic prediction of survival after surgical correction of organic mitral regurgitation. *Circulation* 1994; 90:830.
75. Timmis SB, Kirsh MM, Montgomery DG, Starling MR: Evaluation of left ventricular ejection fraction as a measure of pump performance in patients with chronic mitral regurgitation. *Cathet Cardiovasc Interv* 2000; 49:290.
76. Kontos GJ Jr, Schaff HV, Gersh BJ, Bove AA: Left ventricular function in subacute and chronic mitral regurgitation: effect on function early postoperatively. *J Thorac Cardiovasc Surg* 1989; 98: 163.
77. Borrow KM, Green LH, Mann T, et al: End-systolic volume as a predictor of postoperative left ventricular performance in volume overload from valvular regurgitation. *Am J Med* 1980; 68:655.
78. Wisenbaugh T, Skudicky D, Sareli P: Prediction of outcome after valve replacement for rheumatic mitral regurgitation in the era of chordal preservation. *Circulation* 1994; 89:191.
79. David TE, Armstrong S, Sun Z, Daniel L: Late results of mitral valve repair for mitral regurgitation due to degenerative disease. *Ann Thorac Surg* 1993; 56:7.
80. Cohn LH, Couper GS, Aranki SF, et al: The long-term results of mitral valve reconstruction for the "floppy" valve. *J Card Surg* 1994; 9:278.
81. Cosgrove DM, Chavez AM, Lytle BW, et al: Results of mitral valve reconstruction. *Circulation* 1986; 74:I82.
82. Braunberger E, Deloche A, Berrebi A, et al: Very long-term results (more than 20 years) of valve repair with Carpentier's techniques in nonrheumatic mitral valve insufficiency. *Circulation* 2001; 104:I8.
83. Asmar BE, Perrier P, Couetil J, Carpentier A: Failures in reconstructive mitral valve surgery. *J Med Liban* 1991; 39:7.
84. Cohn LH, Rizzo RJ, Adams DH, et al: The effect of pathophysiology on the surgical treatment of ischemic mitral regurgitation: operative and late risks of repair versus replacement. *Eur J Cardiothorac Surg* 1995; 9:568.
85. David T: Techniques and results of mitral valve repair for ischemic mitral regurgitation. *J Card Surg* 1994; 9(suppl II):II.
86. Byrne JG, Aranki SF, Cohn LH: Repair versus replacement of mitral valve for treating severe ischemic mitral regurgitation. *Coron Artery Dis* 2000; 11:31.
87. Aranki SF, Adams DH, Rizzo RJ, et al: Determinants of early mortality and late survival in mitral valve endocarditis. *Circulation* 1995; 92:II143.
88. Alexiou C, Langley SM, Stafford H, et al: Surgical treatment of infective mitral valve endocarditis: predictors of early and late outcome. *J Heart Valve Dis* 2000; 9:327.
89. Braunwald E: Valvular heart disease, in Braunwald E (ed): *Heart Disease, A Textbook of Cardiovascular Medicine,* 6th ed. Philadelphia, WB Saunders, 2001.
90. Grunkemeier GL, Jamieson WR, Miller DC, Starr A: Actuarial versus actual risk of porcine structural valve deterioration. *J Thorac Cardiovasc Surg* 1994; 108:709.
91. Peterseim DS, Cen YY, Cheruvu S, et al: Long-term outcome after biologic versus mechanical aortic valve replacement in 841 patients. *J Thorac Cardiovasc Surg* 1999; 117:890.
92. Schoen FJ, Collins JJ Jr, Cohn LH: Long-term failure rate and morphologic correlations in porcine bioprosthetic heart valves. *Am J Cardiol* 1983; 51:957.
93. Jones EL, Weintraub WS, Craver JM, et al: Ten-year experience with the porcine bioprosthetic valve: interrelationship of valve survival and patient survival in 1,050 valve replacements. *Ann Thorac Surg* 1990; 49:370.
94. DiSesa VJ, Cohn LH, Collins JJ Jr, et al: Determinants of operative survival following combined mitral valve replacement and coronary revascularization. *Ann Thorac Surg* 1982; 34:482.
95. Jamieson WR, Burr LH, Munro AI, et al: Cardiac valve replacement in the elderly: clinical performance of biological prostheses. *Ann Thorac Surg* 1989; 48:173.

96. Holper K, Wottke M, Lewe T, et al: Bioprosthetic and mechanical valves in the elderly: benefits and risks. *Ann Thorac Surg* 1995; 60:S443.
97. Helft G, Tabone X, Georges JL, et al: Bioprosthetic valve replacement in the elderly. *Eur Heart J* 1995; 16:529.
98. David TE, Armstrong S, Sun Z: The Hancock II bioprosthesis at ten years. *Ann Thorac Surg* 1995; 60:S229.
99. Angell WW, Pupello DF, Bessone LN, et al: Influence of coronary artery disease on structural deterioration of porcine bioprostheses. *Ann Thorac Surg* 1995; 60:S276.
100. Jones EL, Weintraub WS, Craver JM, et al: Interaction of age and coronary disease after valve replacement: implications for valve selection. *Ann Thorac Surg* 1994; 58:378.
101. Thourani VH, Weintraub WS, Craver JM, et al: Influence of concomitant CABG and urgent/emergent status on mitral valve replacement surgery. *Ann Thorac Surg* 2000; 70:778.
102. Edwards FH, Peterson ED, Coombs LP, et al: Prediction of operative mortality after valve replacement surgery. *J Am Coll Cardiol* 2001; 37:885.
103. Burdon TA, Miller DC, Oyer PE, et al: Durability of porcine valves at fifteen years in a representative North American patient population. *J Thorac Cardiovasc Surg* 1992; 103:238.
104. van Doorn CA, Stoodley KD, Saunders NR, et al: Mitral valve replacement with the Carpentier-Edwards standard bioprosthesis: performance into the second decade. *Eur J Cardiothorac Surg* 1995; 9:253.
105. Jamieson WR, Burr LH, Munro AI, Miyagishima RT: Carpentier-Edwards standard porcine bioprosthesis: a 21-year experience. *Ann Thorac Surg* 1998; 66:S40.
106. Khan SS, Chaux A, Blanche C, et al: A 20-year experience with the Hancock porcine xenograft in the elderly. *Ann Thorac Surg* 1998; 66:S35.
107. Corbineau H, Du Haut Cilly FB, Langanay T, et al: Structural durability in Carpentier Edwards Standard bioprosthesis in the mitral position: a 20-year experience. *J Heart Valve Dis* 2001; 10:443.
108. Cohn LH, Collins JJ Jr, Rizzo RJ, et al: Twenty-year follow-up of the Hancock modified orifice porcine aortic valve. *Ann Thorac Surg* 1998; 66:S30.
109. Pupello DF, Bessone LN, Hiro SP, et al: Bioprosthetic valve longevity in the elderly: an 18-year longitudinal study. *Ann Thorac Surg* 1995; 60:S270.
110. Jamieson WR, Tyers GF, Janusz MT, et al: Age as a determinant for selection of porcine bioprostheses for cardiac valve replacement: experience with Carpentier-Edwards standard bioprosthesis. *Can J Cardiol* 1991; 7:181.
111. Braunwald E: Valvular heart disease, in Braunwald E (ed): *Heart Disease, A Textbook of Cardiovascular Medicine,* 6th ed. Philadelphia, WB Saunders, 2001.
112. Jamieson WR, Miller DC, Akins CW, et al: Pregnancy and bioprostheses: influence on structural valve deterioration. *Ann Thorac Surg* 1995; 60:S282.
113. Salazar E, Zajarias A, Gutierrez N, Iturbe I: The problem of cardiac valve prostheses, anticoagulants, and pregnancy. *Circulation* 1984; 70:I169.
114. Sareli P, England MJ, Berk MR, et al: Maternal and fetal sequelae of anticoagulation during pregnancy in patients with mechanical heart valve prostheses. *Am J Cardiol* 1989; 63:1462.
115. Badduke BR, Jamieson WR, Miyagishima RT, et al: Pregnancy and childbearing in a population with biologic valvular prostheses. *J Thorac Cardiovasc Surg* 1991; 102:179.
116. Acar C, Farge A, Ramsheyi A, et al: Mitral valve replacement using a cryopreserved mitral homograft. *Ann Thorac Surg* 1994; 57:746.
117. Deac RF, Simionescu D, Deac D: New evolution in mitral physiology and surgery: mitral stentless pericardial valve. *Ann Thorac Surg* 1995; 60:S433.
118. Gulbins H, Kreuzer E, Uhlig A, Reichart B: Mitral valve surgery utilizing homografts: early results. *J Heart Valve Dis* 2000; 9:222.
119. Plunkett MD, Bond LM, Geiss DM: Allograft mitral valve replacement. *Semin Thorac Cardiovasc Surg Pediatr Card Surg Annu* 1999; 2:95.
120. Kumar AS, Choudhary SK, Mathur A, et al: Homograft mitral valve replacement: five years' results. *J Thorac Cardiovasc Surg* 2000; 120:450.
121. Doty DB, Doty JR, Flores JH, Millar RC: Cardiac valve replacement with mitral homograft. *Semin Thorac Cardiovasc Surg* 2001; 13:35.
122. Vrandecic MO, Fantini FA, Gontijo BF, et al: Surgical technique of implanting the stentless porcine mitral valve. *Ann Thorac Surg* 1995; 60:S439.
123. Walther T, Walther C, Falk V, et al: Early clinical results after stentless mitral valve implantation and comparison with conventional valve repair or replacement. *Circulation* 1999; 100:II178.
124. Hofmann B, Cichon R, Knaut M, et al: Early experience with a quadrileaflet stentless mitral valve. *Ann Thorac Surg* 2001; 71:S323.
125. Kumar AS, Aggarwal S, Choudhary SK: Mitral valve replacement with the pulmonary autograft: the Ross II procedure. *J Thorac Cardiovasc Surg* 2001; 122:378.
126. Mestres CA, Pomar JL: Mitral valve replacement with a pulmonary autograft: initial experience. *J Heart Valve Dis* 2000; 9:169.
127. Johnson AD, Daily PO, Peterson KL, et al: Functional evaluation of the porcine heterograft in the mitral position. *Circulation* 1975; 52:I40.
128. Pyle RB, Mayer JE Jr, Lindsay WG, et al: Hemodynamic evaluation of Lillehei-Kaiser and Starr-Edwards prosthesis. *Ann Thorac Surg* 1978; 26:336.
129. Chaitman BR, Bonan R, Lepage G, et al: Hemodynamic evaluation of the Carpentier-Edwards porcine xenograft. *Circulation* 1979; 60:1170.
130. Levine FH, Carter JE, Buckley MJ, et al: Hemodynamic evaluation of Hancock and Carpentier-Edwards bioprostheses. *Circulation* 1981; 64:II192.
131. Pelletier C, Chaitman B, Bonan R, Dyrda I: Hemodynamic evaluation of the Carpentier-Edwards standard and improved annulus bioprostheses, in Cohn LH, Gallucci V (eds): *Cardiac Bioprostheses; Proceedings of the Second International Symposium.* New York, Yorke Medical Books, 1982; p 96.
132. Sala A, Schoevaerdts JC, Jaumin P, et al: Review of 387 isolated mitral valve replacements by the Model 6120 Starr-Edwards prosthesis. *J Thorac Cardiovasc Surg* 1982; 84:744.
133. Ubago J, Figueroa A, Colman T, et al: Hemodynamic evaluation of the Hancock bioprosthesis in the mitral position, in Cohn LH, Gallucci V (eds): *Cardiac Bioprostheses; Proceedings of the Second International Symposium.* New York, Yorke Medical Books, 1982; p 87.
134. *Medtronic Hall Prosthetic Heart Valve: 8 Year Experience.* New York, Medtronic, 1985.
135. Hall KV, Nitter-Hauge S, Abdelnoor M: Seven and one-half years' experience with the Medtronic-Hall valve. *J Am Coll Cardiol* 1985; 6:1417.
136. Cordoba M, Almeida P, Martinez P, et al: Invasive assessment of mitral valve prostheses, in Rabago G, Cooley DA (eds): *Heart Valve Replacement and Future Trends in Cardiac Surgery.* New York, Futura, 1987.
137. Horskotte D, Curtis J, Bircks W, Loogen F: Noninvasive evaluation of prosthetic heart valves, in Rabago G, Cooley DA (eds): *Heart Valve Replacement and Future Trends in Cardiac Surgery.* New York, Futura, 1987.
138. Khuri SF, Folland ED, Sethi GK, et al: Six month postoperative hemodynamics of the Hancock heterograft and the Bjork-Shiley

prosthesis: results of a Veterans Administration cooperative prospective randomized trial. *J Am Coll Cardiol* 1988; 12:8.

139. Mikhail AA, Ellis R, Johnson S: Eighteen-year evolution from the Lillehei-Kaster valve to the Omni design. *Ann Thorac Surg* 1989; 48:S61.
140. Tatineni S, Barner HB, Pearson AC, et al: Rest and exercise evaluation of St. Jude Medical and Medtronic Hall prostheses: influence of primary lesion, valvular type, valvular size, and left ventricular function. *Circulation* 1989; 80:116.
141. Johnston RT, Weerasena NA, Butterfield M, et al: Carbomedics and St. Jude Medical bileaflet valves: an in vitro and in vivo comparison. *Eur J Cardiothorac Surg* 1992; 6:267.
142. Carbomedics Inc: Carbomedics prosthetic heart valve FDA-PMA summary of safety and effectiveness, thromboembolism and valve thrombosis complications. Application approved by FDA, September 29, 1993.
143. Chambers J, Cross J, Deverall P, Sowton E: Echocardiographic description of the CarboMedics bileaflet prosthetic heart valve. *J Am Coll Cardiol* 1993; 21:398.
144. Kirklin J, Barratt-Boyes B: Mitral valve disease with or without tricuspid valve disease, in Kirklin JW, Barratt-Boyes BG (eds): *Cardiac Surgery*, 2d ed. New York, Churchill Livingstone, 1993; p 463.
145. Messner-Pellenc P, Wittenberg O, Leclercq F, et al: Doppler echocardiographic evaluation of the Omnicarbon cardiac valve prostheses. *J Cardiovasc Surg* (Torino). 1993; 34:195.
146. Aupart MR, Neville PH, Hammami S, et al: Carpentier-Edwards pericardial valves in the mitral position: ten-year follow-up. *J Thorac Cardiovasc Surg* 1997; 113:492.
147. Jasinski MJ, Kadziola Z, Keal R, Sosnowski AW: "Mosaic" Medtronic bioprosthetic valve replacement clinical results and hemodynamical performance. *J Cardiovasc Surg* (Torino) 2000; 41:181.
148. Fehske W, Kessel D, Kirchhoff PG, et al: Echocardiographic profile of the normally functioning Omnicarbon valve. *J Heart Valve Dis* 1994; 3:263.
149. Shiono M, Sezai Y, Sezai A, et al: Multi-institutional experience of the ATS open pivot bileaflet valve in Japan. *Ann Thorac Cardiovasc Surg* 1996; 1:21.
150. Van Nooten G, Caes F, Francois K, et al: Clinical experience with the first 100 ATS heart valve implants. *Cardiovasc Surg* 1996; 4:288.
151. Westaby S, Van Nooten G, Sharif H, et al: Valve replacement with the ATS open pivot bileaflet prosthesis. *Eur J Cardiothorac Surg* 1996; 10:660.
152. Chambers J, Ely JL: Early postoperative echocardiographic hemodynamic performance of the On-X prosthetic heart valve: a multicenter study. *J Heart Valve Dis* 1998; 7:569.
153. Hasegawa M: Clinical evaluation of ATS prosthetic valve by Doppler echocardiography: comparison with St. Jude Medical (SJM) valve. *Ann Thorac Cardiovasc Surg* 2000; 6:247.
154. Emery RW, Petersen RJ, Kersten TE, et al: The initial United States experience with the ATS mechanical cardiac valve prosthesis. *Heart Surg Forum* 2001; 4:346.
155. Horskotte D, Loogen F, Birckson B: Is the late outcome of heart valve replacement influenced by the hemodynamics of the heart valve substitute? in Horskotte D, Loogen F (eds): *Update in Heart Valve Replacement: Proceedings of the 2nd European Symposium on the St. Jude Heart Valve*. New York, Springer-Verlag, 1986; p 55.
156. Butterfield M, Fisher J, Davies GA, Spyt TJ: Comparative study of the hydrodynamic function of the CarboMedics valve. *Ann Thorac Surg* 1991; 52:815.
157. Agathos EA, Starr A: Mitral valve replacement. *Curr Probl Surg* 1993; 30:481.
158. Hall KV: The Medtronic-Hall valve: a design in 1977 to improve the results of valve replacement. *Eur J Cardiothorac Surg* 1992; (6 suppl 1):S64.
159. Butchart E: Early clinical and hemodynamic results with Hall-Kaster valve, in *Medtronic International Valve Symposium*. Lisbon, Portugal, Congress Books, 1981.
160. Grunkemeier GL, Starr A, Rahimtoola SH: Prosthetic heart valve performance: long-term follow-up. *Curr Probl Cardiol* 1992; 17:329.
161. Akalin H, Corapcioglu ET, Ozyurda U, et al: Clinical evaluation of the Omniscience cardiac valve prosthesis: follow-up of up to 6 years. *J Thorac Cardiovasc Surg* 1992; 103:259.
162. DeWall R, Pelletier LC, Panebianco A, et al: Five-year clinical experience with the Omniscience cardiac valve. *Ann Thorac Surg* 1984; 38:275.
163. Watanabe N, Abe T, Yamada O, et al: Comparative analysis of Omniscience and Omnicarbon protsthesis after aortic valve replacement. *Jpn J Artif Organs* 1989; 18:773.
164. Emery RW, Nicoloff DM: St. Jude Medical cardiac valve prosthesis: in vitro studies. *J Thorac Cardiovasc Surg* 1979; 78:269.
165. Nair CK, Mohiuddin SM, Hilleman DE, et al: Ten-year results with the St. Jude Medical prosthesis. *Am J Cardiol* 1990; 65:217.
166. Braunwald E: Valvular heart disease, in Braunwald E (ed): *Heart Disease, A Textbook of Cardiovascular Medicine,* 6th ed. Philadelphia, WB Saunders, 2001.
167. Champsaur G, Gressier M, Niret J, et al: When are hemodynamics important for the selection of a prosthetic heart valve? in Horskotte D, Loogen F (eds): *Update in Heart Valve Replacement: Proceedings of the 2nd European Symposium on the St. Jude Heart Valve.* New York, Springer-Verlag, 1986; p 71.
168. D'Alessandro L, Narducci C, Pucci A, et al: The use of mechanical valves in the treatment of valvular heart disease in Horskotte D, Loogen F (eds): *Update in Heart Valve Replacement: Proceedings of the 2nd European Symposium on the St. Jude Heart Valve.* New York, Springer-Verlag, 1986.
169. Laub GW, Muralidharan S, Pollock SB, et al: The experimental relationship between leaflet clearance and orientation of the St. Jude Medical valve in the mitral position. *J Thorac Cardiovasc Surg* 1992; 103:638.
170. Sezai A, Shiono M, Orime Y, et al: Evaluation of valve sound and its effects on ATS prosthetic valves in patients' quality of life. *Ann Thorac Surg* 2000; 69:507.
171. Ely JL, Emken MR, Accuntius JA, et al: Pure pyrolytic carbon: preparation and properties of a new material, On-X carbon for mechanical heart valve prostheses. *J Heart Valve Dis* 1998; 7:626.
172. Laczkovics A, Heidt M, Oelert H, et al: Early clinical experience with the On-X prosthetic heart valve. *J Heart Valve Dis* 2001; 10:94.
173. Birnbaum D, Laczkovics A, Heidt M, et al: Examination of hemolytic potential with the On-X(R) prosthetic heart valve. *J Heart Valve Dis* 2000; 9:142.
174. Gallucci V, Valfre C, Mazzucco A, et al: Heart valve replacement with the Hancock bioprosthesis: a 5- to 11-year follow-up. Cohn LH, Gallucci V (eds): *Cardiac Bioprostheses: Proceedings of the Second International Symposium.* New York, Yorke Medical Books, 1982.
175. Black MM, Cochrame TT, Lawford PV: Design and flow characteristics, in Bodner E, Frater R (eds): *Replacement Cardiac Valves.* New York, McGraw-Hill, 1992; p 1.
176. Jacson JM, Thomas SJ: Valvular heart disease, in Kaplan J, Reich D, Konstadt S (ed): *Cardiac Anaesthesia.* Philadelphia, WB Saunders, 1999; p 727.
177. D'Attellis N, Nicolas-Robin A, Delayance S, et al: Early extubation after mitral valve surgery: a target-controlled infusion of propofol and low-dose sufentanil. *J Cardiothorac Vasc Anesth* 1997; 11:467.

178. Cohn LH, Aranki SF, Rizzo RJ, et al: Decrease in operative risk of reoperative valve surgery. *Ann Thorac Surg* 1993; 56:15.
179. Buckberg GD: Antegrade/retrograde blood cardioplegia to ensure cardioplegic distribution: operative techniques and objectives. *J Card Surg* 1989; 4:216.
180. Singh AK: Warm retrograde cardioplegia: protection of the right ventricle in mitral valve operations. *J Thorac Cardiovasc Surg* 1993; 106:370.
181. Buckberg GD: Development of blood cardioplegia and retrograde techniques: the experimenter/observer complex. *J Card Surg* 1998; 13:163.
182. Sondergaard T, Gotzsche M, Ottosen P, Schultz J: Surgical closure of interatrial septal defects by circumclusion. *Acta Chir Scand* 1955; 109:188.
183. Larbalestier RI, Chard RB, Cohn LH: Optimal approach to the mitral valve: dissection of the interatrial groove. *Ann Thorac Surg* 1992; 54:1186.
184. Hirt SW, Frimpong-Boateng K, Borst HG: The superior approach to the mitral valve—is it worthwhile? *Eur J Cardiothorac Surg* 1988; 2:372.
185. Saksena DS, Tucker BI, Lindesmith GG, et al: The superior approach to the mitral valve: a review of clinical experience. *Ann Thorac Surg* 1971; 12:146.
186. Utley JR, Leyland SA, Nguyenduy T: Comparison of outcomes with three atrial incisions for mitral valve operations: right lateral, superior septal, and transseptal. *J Thorac Cardiovasc Surg* 1995; 109:582.
187. Guiraudon GM, Ofiesh JG, Kaushik R: Extended vertical transatrial septal approach to the mitral valve. *Ann Thorac Surg* 1991; 52:1058.
188. Selle JG: Temporary division of the superior vena cava for exceptional mitral valve exposure. *J Thorac Cardiovasc Surg* 1984; 88:302.
189. Barner HB: Combined superior and right lateral left atriotomy with division of the superior vena cava for exposure of the mitral valve. *Ann Thorac Surg* 1985; 40:365.
190. Kon ND, Tucker WY, Mills SA, et al: Mitral valve operation via an extended transseptal approach. *Ann Thorac Surg* 1993; 55:1413.
191. Kumar N, Saad E, Prabhakar G, et al: Extended transseptal versus conventional left atriotomy: early postoperative study. *Ann Thorac Surg* 1995; 60:426.
192. Cosgrove DM 3rd, Sabik JF, Navia JL: Minimally invasive valve operations. *Ann Thorac Surg* 1998; 65:1535.
193. Cohn LH, Adams DH, Couper GS, et al: Minimally invasive cardiac valve surgery improves patient satisfaction while reducing costs of cardiac valve replacement and repair. *Ann Surg* 1997; 226:421.
194. Tam RK, Ho C, Almeida AA: Minimally invasive mitral valve surgery. *J Thorac Cardiovasc Surg* 1998; 115:246.
195. Greelish JG, Cohn LH, Leacche M, et al: Early and late results of minimally invasive mitral valve surgery suggests earlier operations for mitral valve disease. *J Thorac Cardiovasc Surg (in press)*.
196. Cohn LH, Couper GS, Aranki SF, et al: The long-term results of mitral valve reconstruction for the "floppy" valve. *J Card Surg* 1994; 9:278.
197. David TE, Bos J, Rakowski H: Mitral valve repair by replacement of chordae tendineae with polytetrafluoroethylene sutures. *J Thorac Cardiovasc Surg* 1991; 101:495.
198. Douglas JJ: *Mitral Valve Replacement*. Philadelphia, WB Saunders, 1995.
199. David TE: Mitral valve replacement with preservation of chordae tendinae: rationale and technical considerations. *Ann Thorac Surg* 1986; 41:680.
200. David TE, Armstrong S, Sun Z: Left ventricular function after mitral valve surgery. *J Heart Valve Dis* 1995; 4(suppl 2):S175.
201. Reardon MJ, David TE: Mitral valve replacement with preservation of the subvalvular apparatus. *Curr Opin Cardiol* 1999; 14:104.
202. Lillehei C, Levy M, Bonnabeau R: Mitral valve replacement with preservation of papillary muscles and chordae tendinae. *J Thorac Cardiovasc Surg* 1964; 47:532.
203. Cohn LH, Kowalker W, Bhatia S, et al: Comparative morbidity of mitral valve repair versus replacement for mitral regurgitation with and without coronary artery disease. *Ann Thorac Surg* 1988; 45:284.
204. Cohn LH, Couper GS, Kinchla NM, Collins JJ Jr: Decreased operative risk of surgical treatment of mitral regurgitation with or without coronary artery disease. *J Am Coll Cardiol* 1990; 16:1575.
205. Miki S, Ueda Y, Tahata T, Okita Y: Mitral valve replacement with preservation of chordae tendineae and papillary muscles. Updated in 1995. *Ann Thorac Surg* 1995; 60:225.
206. Horskotte D, Schulte HD, Bircks W, Strauer BE: The effect of chordal preservation on late outcome after mitral valve replacement: a randomized study. *J Heart Valve Dis* 1993; 2:150.
207. Okita Y, Miki S, Ueda Y, et al: Left ventricular function after mitral valve replacement with or without chordal preservation. *J Heart Valve Dis* 1995; 4(suppl 2):S181.
208. Okita Y, Miki S, Ueda Y, et al: Mid-term results of mitral valve replacement combined with chordae tendineae replacement in patients with mitral stenosis. *J Heart Valve Dis* 1997; 6:37.
209. Asano K, Yagyu K: [Mitral valve replacement with preservation of the posterior leaflet, chordae tendineae and papillary muscles (modified MVP)]. *Nippon Geka Gakkai Zasshi* 1985; 86:233.
210. Cobbs BW Jr, Hatcher CR Jr, Craver JM, et al: Transverse midventricular disruption after mitral valve replacement. *Am Heart J* 1980; 99:33.
211. Spencer FC, Galloway AC, Colvin SB: A clinical evaluation of the hypothesis that rupture of the left ventricle following mitral valve replacement can be prevented by preservation of the chordae of the mural leaflet. *Ann Surg* 1985; 202:673.
212. Karlson KJ, Ashraf MM, Berger RL: Rupture of left ventricle following mitral valve replacement. *Ann Thorac Surg* 1988; 46:590.
213. Chambers EP Jr, Heath BJ: Comparison of supraannular and subannular pledgeted sutures in mitral valve replacement. *Ann Thorac Surg* 1991; 51:60.
214. Cooley DA: Simplified techniques of valve replacement. *J Card Surg* 1992; 7:357.
215. Antunes MJ: Technique of implantation of the Medtronic-Hall valve and other modern tilting-disc prostheses. *J Card Surg* 1990; 5:86.
216. Ibrahim M, O'Kane H, Cleland J, et al: The St. Jude Medical prosthesis: a thirteen-year experience. *J Thorac Cardiovasc Surg* 1994; 108:221.
217. Dhasmana JP, Blackstone EH, Kirklin JW, Kouchoukos NT: Factors associated with periprosthetic leakage following primary mitral valve replacement: with special consideration of the suture technique. *Ann Thorac Surg* 1983; 35:170.
218. Spencer F: *Acquired Disease of the Mitral Valve,* 4th ed. Philadelphia, WB Saunders, 1983.
219. DiSesa VJ, Tam S, Cohn LH: Ligation of the left atrial appendage using an automatic surgical stapler. *Ann Thorac Surg* 1988; 46:652.
220. Cohn LH: Tricuspid regurgitation secondary to mitral valve disease: when and how to repair. *J Card Surg* 1994; 9:237.
221. Bach DS, Deeb GM, Bolling SF: Accuracy of intraoperative transesophageal echocardiography for estimating the severity of functional mitral regurgitation. *Am J Cardiol* 1995; 76:508.
222. Jaggers J, Chetham PM, Kinnard TL, Fullerton DA: Intraoperative prosthetic valve dysfunction: detection by transesophageal echocardiography. *Ann Thorac Surg* 1995; 59:755.

223. Orsinelli DA, Pasierski TJ, Pearson AC: Spontaneously appearing microbubbles associated with prosthetic cardiac valves detected by transesophageal echocardiography. *Am Heart J* 1994; 128:990.
224. Meister S, Wolf N: Postoperative management of patients with implanted valvular prostheses, in Morse D, Steiner RM, Fernandez J (eds): *Guide to Prosthetic Cardiac Valves*. New York, Springer-Verlag, 1985; p 179.
225. Jegaden O, Eker A, Delahaye F, et al: Thromboembolic risk and late survival after mitral valve replacement with the St. Jude Medical valve. *Ann Thorac Surg* 1994; 58:1721.
226. Heras M, Chesebro JH, Fuster V, et al: High risk of thromboemboli early after bioprosthetic cardiac valve replacement. *J Am Coll Cardiol* 1995; 25:1111.
227. Ezekowitz MD: Anticoagulation management of valve replacement patients. *J Heart Valve Dis* 2002; 11(suppl 1):S56.
228. Laffort P, Roudaut R, Roques X, et al: Early and long-term (one-year) effects of the association of aspirin and oral anticoagulant on thrombi and morbidity after replacement of the mitral valve with the St. Jude medical prosthesis: a clinical and transesophageal echocardiographic study. *J Am Coll Cardiol* 2000; 35:739.
229. Peterffy A, Nagy Z, Vaszily M, et al: Valve surgery combined with myocardial revascularisation: report of 62 cases. *Scand J Thorac Cardiovasc Surg* 1989; 23:25.
230. Santini F, Casali G, Viscardi F, et al: The Carbomedics prosthetic heart valve: experience with 1,084 implants. *J Heart Valve Dis* 2002; 11:121.
231. Aoyagi S, Oryoji A, Nishi Y, et al: Long-term results of valve replacement with the St. Jude Medical valve. *J Thorac Cardiovasc Surg* 1994; 108:1021.
232. Nistal JF, Hurle A, Revuelta JM, Gandarillas M: Clinical experience with the CarboMedics valve: early results with a new bileaflet mechanical prosthesis. *J Thorac Cardiovasc Surg* 1996; 112:59.
233. Butchart EG, Li HH, Payne N, et al: Twenty years' experience with the Medtronic Hall valve. *J Thorac Cardiovasc Surg* 2001; 121:1090.
234. Cohn LH, Allred EN, Cohn LA, et al: Early and late risk of mitral valve replacement: a 12 year concomitant comparison of the porcine bioprosthetic and prosthetic disc mitral valves. *J Thorac Cardiovasc Surg* 1985; 90:872.
235. Remadi JP, Bizouarn P, Baron O, et al: Mitral valve replacement with the St. Jude Medical prosthesis: a 15-year follow-up. *Ann Thorac Surg* 1998; 66:762.
236. Birkmeyer NJ, Marrin CA, Morton JR, et al: Decreasing mortality for aortic and mitral valve surgery in Northern New England. Northern New England Cardiovascular Disease Study Group. *Ann Thorac Surg* 2000; 70:432.
237. Brais MP, Bedard JP, Goldstein W, et al: Mitral valve replacement with Hancock porcine bioprostheses: up to 7-year follow-up. *Can J Surg* 1985; 28:119.
238. Oury JH, Cleveland JC, Duran CG, Angell WW: Ischemic mitral valve disease: classification and systemic approach to management. *J Card Surg* 1994; 9:262.
239. Society of Thoracic Surgeons: *Data Analysis of the Society of Thoracic Surgeons National Cardiac Surgery Database: The Fifth Year–January 1996*. Minneapolis, Summit Medical Systems, 1996.
240. Teply JF, Grunkemeier GL, Sutherland HD, et al: The ultimate prognosis after valve replacement: an assessment at twenty years. *Ann Thorac Surg* 1981; 32:111.
241. Damle A, Coles J, Teijeira J, et al: A six-year study of the Omniscience valve in four Canadian centers. *Ann Thorac Surg* 1987; 43:513.
242. Cohn LH, Collins JJ Jr, DiSesa VJ, et al: Fifteen-year experience with 1678 Hancock porcine bioprosthetic heart valve replacements. *Ann Surg* 1989; 210:435.
243. DiSesa VJ, Collins JJ Jr, Cohn LH: Hematological complications with the St. Jude valve and reduced-dose Coumadin. *Ann Thorac Surg* 1989; 48:280.
244. Vallejo JL, Gonzalez-Santos JM, Albertos J, et al: Eight years' experience with the Medtronic-Hall valve prosthesis. *Ann Thorac Surg* 1990; 50:429.
245. Bortolotti U, Milano A, Testolin L, et al: The CarboMedics bileaflet prosthesis: initial experience at the University of Padova. *Clin Rep* 1991; 4.
246. Rabelo R, Brasil J, Castro A, et al: CarboMedics bileaflet prosthesis: initial experience at the University of Padova. *Clin Rep* 1991; 4.
247. Louagie Y, Noirhomme P, Aranguis E, et al: Use of the Carpentier-Edwards porcine bioprosthesis: assessment of a patient selection policy. *J Thorac Cardiovasc Surg* 1992; 104:1013.
248. de Luca L, Vitale N, Giannolo B, et al: Mid-term follow-up after heart valve replacement with CarboMedics bileaflet prostheses. *J Thorac Cardiovasc Surg* 1993; 106:1158.
249. Kratz JM, Crawford FA Jr, Sade RM, et al: St. Jude prosthesis for aortic and mitral valve replacement: a ten-year experience. *Ann Thorac Surg* 1993; 56:462.
250. Peter M, Weiss P, Jenzer HR, et al: The Omnicarbon tilting-disc heart valve prosthesis: a clinical and Doppler echocardiographic follow-up. *J Thorac Cardiovasc Surg* 1993; 106:599.
251. Sarris GE, Robbins RC, Miller DC, et al: Randomized, prospective assessment of bioprosthetic valve durability: Hancock versus Carpentier-Edwards valves. *Circulation*. 1993; 88:II55.
252. Khan S, Chaux A, Matloff J, et al: The St. Jude Medical valve: experience with 1,000 cases. *J Thorac Cardiovasc Surg* 1994; 108:1010.
253. Masters RG, Pipe AL, Walley VM, Keon WJ: Comparative results with the St. Jude Medical and Medtronic Hall mechanical valves. *J Thorac Cardiovasc Surg* 1995; 110:663.
254. Copeland JG 3rd: An international experience with the CarboMedics prosthetic heart valve. *J Heart Valve Dis* 1995; 4:56.
255. Copeland JG 3rd, Sethi GK: Four-year experience with the CarboMedics valve: the North American experience. North American team of clinical investigators for the CarboMedics prosthetic heart valve. *Ann Thorac Surg* 1994; 58:630.
256. Hayashi J, Nakazawa S, Eguchi S, et al: Long-term outcome of patients who received Starr-Edwards valves between 1965 and 1977. *Cardiovasc Surg* 1996; 4:281.
257. Murakami T, Eishi K, Nakano S, et al: Aortic and mitral valve replacement with the Carpentier-Edwards pericardial bioprosthesis: 10-year results. *J Heart Valve Dis* 1996; 5:45.
258. Yamauchi M, Eishi K, Nakano K, et al: Valve replacement with the CarboMedics bileaflet mechanical prosthesis: clinical results at midterm. *J Cardiovasc Surg* (Torino). 1996; 37:285.
259. Godje OL, Fischlein T, Adelhard K, et al: Thirty-year results of Starr-Edwards prostheses in the aortic and mitral position. *Ann Thorac Surg* 1997; 63:613.
260. Glower DD, Landolfo KP, Cheruvu S, et al: Determinants of 15-year outcome with 1,119 standard Carpentier-Edwards porcine valves. *Ann Thorac Surg* 1998; 66:S44.
261. Kuntze CE, Ebels T, Eijgelaar A, et al: Rates of thromboembolism with three different mechanical heart valve prostheses: randomised study. *Lancet* 1989; 1:514.
262. Camilleri LF, Bailly P, Legault BJ, et al: Mitral and mitro-aortic valve replacement with Sorin Bicarbon valves compared with St. Jude Medical valves. *Cardiovasc Surg* 2001; 9:272.
263. Misawa Y, Hasegawa T, Kato M: Clinical experience with the Omnicarbon prosthetic heart valve. *J Thorac Cardiovasc Surg* 1993; 105:168.
264. Otaki M, Kitamura N: Six years' experience with the Omnicarbon valve prosthesis. *Cardiovasc Surg* 1993; 1:594.

265. Thevenet A, Albat B: Long term follow up of 292 patients after valve replacement with the Omnicarbon prosthetic valve. *J Heart Valve Dis* 1995; 4:634.
266. Iguro Y, Moriyama Y, Yamaoka A, et al: Clinical experience of 473 patients with the omnicarbon prosthetic heart valve. *J Heart Valve Dis* 1999; 8:674.
267. Torregrosa S, Gomez-Plana J, Valera FJ, et al: Long-term clinical experience with the Omnicarbon prosthetic valve. *Ann Thorac Surg* 1999; 68:881.
268. Hammermeister K, Sethi GK, Henderson WG, et al: Outcomes 15 years after valve replacement with a mechanical versus a bioprosthetic valve: final report of the Veterans Affairs randomized trial. *J Am Coll Cardiol* 2000; 36:1152.
269. Cen YY, Glower DD, Landolfo K, et al: Comparison of survival after mitral valve replacement with biologic and mechanical valves in 1139 patients. *J Thorac Cardiovasc Surg* 2001; 122:569.
270. Grossi EA, Galloway AC, Miller JS, et al: Valve repair versus replacement for mitral insufficiency: when is a mechanical valve still indicated? *J Thorac Cardiovasc Surg* 1998; 115:389.
271. Sidhu P, O'Kane H, Ali N, et al: Mechanical or bioprosthetic valves in the elderly: a 20-year comparison. *Ann Thorac Surg* 2001; 71:S257.
272. Starr A: The Starr-Edwards valve. *J Am Coll Cardiol* 1985; 6:899.
273. Myken PS, Caidahl K, Larsson P, et al: Mechanical versus biological valve prosthesis: a ten-year comparison regarding function and quality of life. *Ann Thorac Surg* 1995; 60:S447.
274. Bortolotti U, Milano A, Mossuto E, et al: Porcine valve durability: a comparison between Hancock standard and Hancock II bioprostheses. *Ann Thorac Surg* 1995; 60:S216.
275. Wideman FE, Blackstone EH, Kirklin JW, et al: Hospital mortality of re-replacement of the aortic valve: incremental risk factors. *J Thorac Cardiovasc Surg* 1981; 82:692.
276. Perier P, Swanson J, Takriti A, et al: Decreasing operative risk in isolated valve re-replacement, in Bodnar E, Yacoub M (eds): *Biological and Bioprosthetic Valves: Proceedings of the Third International Symposium*. New York, Yorke Medical Books, 1986.
277. Kazui T, Kimura N, Morikawa M, et al: [Reoperation of primary tissue failure of bioprosthesis in the mitral position]. *Nippon Kyobu Geka Gakkai Zasshi* 1991; 39:862.
278. Tyers GF, Jamieson WR, Munro AI, et al: Reoperation in biological and mechanical valve populations: fate of the reoperative patient. *Ann Thorac Surg* 1995; 60:S464.
279. Cohn LH, Peigh PS, Sell J, DiSesa VJ: Right thoracotomy, femorofemoral bypass, and deep hypothermia for re-replacement of the mitral valve. *Ann Thorac Surg* 1989; 48:69.
280. McGiffin DC, O'Brien MF, Galbraith AJ, et al: An analysis of risk factors for death and mode-specific death after aortic valve replacement with allograft, xenograft, and mechanical valves. *J Thorac Cardiovasc Surg* 1993; 106:895.
281. Gallucci V, Bortolotti U, Milano A, et al: Isolated mitral valve replacement with the Hancock bioprosthesis: a 13-year appraisal. *Ann Thorac Surg* 1984; 38:571.
282. Cortina JM, Martinell J, Artiz V, et al: Comparative clinical results with Omniscience (STM1), Medtronic-Hall, and Bjork-Shiley convexo-concave (70 degrees) prostheses in mitral valve replacement. *J Thorac Cardiovasc Surg* 1986; 91:174.
283. Akins C, Buckley M, Daggett W, et al: Ten-year follow-up of the Starr-Edwards prosthesis, in Rabago G, Cooley DA (eds): *Heart Valve Replacement and Future Trends in Cardiac Surgery*. New York, Futura, 1987.
284. Jamieson W, Burr L, Allen P, et al: Quality of life afforded by porcine bioprostheses illustrated by the new-generation Carpentier-Edwards porcine bioprosthesis, in Rabago G, Cooley DA (eds): *Heart Valve Replacement and Future Trends in Cardiac Surgery*. New York, Futura, 1987.
285. Antunes MJ, Wessels A, Sadowski RG, et al: Medtronic Hall valve replacement in a third-world population group: a review of the performance of 1000 prostheses. *J Thorac Cardiovasc Surg* 1988; 95:980.
286. Beaudet RL, Nakhle G, Beaulieu CR, et al: Medtronic-Hall prosthesis: valve related deaths and complications. *Can J Cardiol* 1988; 4:376.
287. Perier P, Deloche A, Chauvaud S, et al: A 10-year comparison of mitral valve replacement with Carpentier-Edwards and Hancock porcine bioprostheses. *Ann Thorac Surg* 1989; 48:54.
288. Akins CW: Mechanical cardiac valvular prostheses. *Ann Thorac Surg* 1991; 52:161.
289. Jamieson WR, Fradet GJ, Miyagishima RT, et al: CarboMedics mechanical prosthesis: performance at eight years. *J Heart Valve Dis* 2000; 9:678.
290. Khan SS, Trento A, DeRobertis M, et al: Twenty-year comparison of tissue and mechanical valve replacement. *J Thorac Cardiovasc Surg* 2001; 122:257.
291. Ohta S, Ohuchi M, Katsumoto K, et al: [Comparison of long-term clinical results of the three models of the Bjork-Shiley valve prosthesis and the Omnicarbon valve prosthesis]. *Nippon Kyobu Geka Gakkai Zasshi* 1995; 43:1569.
292. Cohn LH, Sanders JH, Collins JJ Jr: Actuarial comparison of Hancock porcine and prosthetic disc valves for isolated mitral valve replacement. *Circulation*. 1976; 54:III60.
293. Levantino M, Tartarini G, Barzaghi C, et al: Survival despite almost complete occlusion by chronic thrombosis of a Bjork-Shiley mitral prosthesis. *J Heart Valve Dis* 1995; 4:103.
294. Copans H, Lakier JB, Kinsley RH, et al: Thrombosed Bjork-Shiley mitral prostheses. *Circulation* 1980; 61:169.
295. Edmunds L: Thrombotic complications with the Omniscience valve. *J Thorac Cardiovasc Surg* 1989; 98:300.
296. Martinell J, Jimenez A, Rabago G, et al: Mechanical cardiac valve thrombosis: is thrombectomy justified? *Circulation* 1991; 84:III70.
297. Roudaut R, Labbe T, Lorient-Roudaut MF, et al: Mechanical cardiac valve thrombosis: is fibrinolysis justified? *Circulation* 1992; 86:II8.
298. McKay C: Prosthetic heart valve thrombosis: "what can be done with regard to treatment?" *Circulation* 1993; 87:294.
299. Silber H, Khan SS, Matloff JM, et al. The St. Jude valve: thrombolysis as the first line of therapy for cardiac valve thrombosis. *Circulation* 1993; 87:30.
300. Manteiga R, Carlos Souto J, Altes A, et al: Short-course thrombolysis as the first line of therapy for cardiac valve thrombosis. *J Thorac Cardiovasc Surg* 1998; 115:780.
301. Horstkotte D, Schulte HD, Bircks W, Strauer BE: Lower intensity anticoagulation therapy results in lower complication rates with the St. Jude Medical prosthesis. *J Thorac Cardiovasc Surg* 1994; 107:1136.
302. Jamieson WR, Miyagishima RT, Munro AI, et al: The Carpentier-Edwards supra-annular porcine bioprosthesis: clinical performance to 8 years of a new generation porcine bioprosthesis. *J Card Surg* 1991; 6:562.
303. Jamieson WR, Miyagishima RT, Burr LH, et al: Carpentier-Edwards porcine bioprostheses: clinical performance assessed by actual analysis. *J Heart Valve Dis* 2000; 9:530.
304. Bernal JM, Rabasa JM, Cagigas JC, et al: Valve-related complications with the Hancock I porcine bioprosthesis: a twelve- to fourteen-year follow-up study. *J Thorac Cardiovasc Surg* 1991; 101:871.
305. Jamieson WR, Hayden RI, Miyagishima RT, et al: The Carpentier-Edwards standard porcine bioprosthesis: clinical performance to 15 years. *J Card Surg* 1991; 6:550.

306. Ahmad R, Manohitharajah SM, Deverall PB, Watson DA: Chronic hemolysis following mitral valve replacement: a comparative study of the Bjork-Shiley, composite-seat Starr-Edwards, and frame-mounted aortic homograft valves. *J Thorac Cardiovasc Surg* 1976; 71:212.
307. Beaudet R, Nakhle G, Beaulieu R, et al: The Medtronic-Hall valve: evaluation of its complications and their effect on quality of life, in Rabago G, Cooley DA (eds): *Heart Valve Replacement: Current Status and Future Trends.* New York, Futura, 1987.
308. Gallucci V, Mazzucco A, Bortolotti U, et al: The standard Hancock porcine bioprosthesis: overall experience at the University of Padova. *J Card Surg* 1988; 3:337.
309. Burckhardt D, Striebel D, Vogt S, et al: Heart valve replacement with St. Jude Medical valve prosthesis: long-term experience in 743 patients in Switzerland. *Circulation* 1988; 78:I18.
310. Genoni M, Franzen D, Vogt P, et al: Paravalvular leakage after mitral valve replacement: improved long-term survival with aggressive surgery? *Eur J Cardiothorac Surg* 2000; 17:14.
311. Baumgartner WA, Miller DC, Reitz BA, et al: Surgical treatment of prosthetic valve endocarditis. *Ann Thorac Surg* 1983; 35:87.
312. Dismukes WE, Karchmer AW, Buckley MJ, et al: Prosthetic valve endocarditis: analysis of 38 cases. *Circulation* 1973; 48:365.
313. Carrier M, Martineau JP, Bonan R, Pelletier LC: Clinical and hemodynamic assessment of the Omniscience prosthetic heart valve. *J Thorac Cardiovasc Surg* 1987; 93:300.
314. Pelletier LC, Carrier M, Leclerc Y, et al: Porcine versus pericardial bioprostheses: a comparison of late results in 1,593 patients. *Ann Thorac Surg* 1989; 47:352.
315. Keenan RJ, Armitage JM, Trento A, et al: Clinical experience with the Medtronic-Hall valve prosthesis. *Ann Thorac Surg* 1990; 50:748.
316. Calderwood SB, Swinski LA, Waternaux CM, et al: Risk factors for the development of prosthetic valve endocarditis. *Circulation* 1985; 72:31.
317. Bayliss R, Clarke C, Oakley CM, et al: The microbiology and pathogenesis of infective endocarditis. *Br Heart J* 1983; 50:513.
318. Miller DC: Determinants of outcome in surgically treated patients with native valve endocarditis (NVE). *J Card Surg* 1989; 4:331.
319. Verheul HA, van den Brink RB, van Vreeland T, et al: Effects of changes in management of active infective endocarditis on outcome in a 25-year period. *Am J Cardiol* 1993; 72:682.
320. Cachera JP, Loisance D, Mourtada A, et al: Surgical techniques for treatment of bacterial endocarditis of the mitral valve. *J Card Surg* 1987; 2:265.
321. Jault F, Gandjbakhch I, Rama A, et al: Active native valve endocarditis: determinants of operative death and late mortality. *Ann Thorac Surg* 1997; 63:1737.
322. Edwards MB, Ratnatunga CP, Dore CJ, Taylor KM: Thirty-day mortality and long-term survival following surgery for prosthetic endocarditis: a study from the UK heart valve registry. *Eur J Cardiothorac Surg* 1998; 14:156.

Chapter 39

Surgical Treatment of Mitral Valve Endocarditis

Farzan Filsoufi/David H. Adams

Infective endocarditis is a well-established cause of valvular heart disease and carries a high risk of morbidity and mortality. During the last 50 years, the introduction and wide use of antimicrobial therapy have significantly changed the course of this disease. The majority of patients can be successfully treated medically with total eradication of the disease process. In certain clinical presentations, however, surgical intervention remains an indispensable adjunct to the management of acute and subacute endocarditis.

Despite the use of preventative measures such as antibiotic prophylaxis in patients with valvular heart disease undergoing invasive procedures, the overall incidence of infective endocarditis continues to rise. Infective endocarditis affects primarily the left-sided valves with a higher incidence of aortic versus mitral valve involvement. When the mitral valve is involved, the existence of predisposing conditions such as rheumatic heart disease or degenerative mitral disease is a common finding. Infective endocarditis can also occur in patients with a mitral prosthetic valve. Epidemiologic studies estimate the actuarial cumulative incidence of prosthetic valve endocarditis from 1.4% to 3.1% at 1 year and 3.2% to 5.7% at 5 years.[1–3] The risk is greatest during the first 6 months following surgery and declines over time to a lower rate of around 0.2% to 0.35% per year.

Valvular endocarditis is most often due to infection by either streptococcal or staphylococcal bacteria. The principal organisms involved in native valve endocarditis are *Streptococcus viridans*, *Streptococcus bovis*, and *Staphylococcus aureus*.[4,5] However, during the last decade, *Staphylococcus epidermidis* has assumed an increasing role in native mitral valve endocarditis in patients with underlying degenerative mitral valve disease. The microbiology of infective endocarditis is relatively predictable in some patients with additional risk factors. *Staphylococcus aureus* is the most common cause of infection in patients who abuse intravenous drugs as well as in patients with insulin-dependent diabetes mellitus. Early prosthetic valve endocarditis, defined as endocarditis during the first 2 months following surgery, is frequently due to coagulase-negative staphylococci, primarily *Staphylococcus epidermidis*.[4,5] The microbiology profile of late prosthetic endocarditis is similar to that of native valve endocarditis with the addition of gram-negative bacilli, particularly the HACEK group (*Haemophilus*, *Actinobacillus*, *Cardiobacterium*, *Eikenella*, and *Kingella*), and fungi (*Candida* species).[4–7]

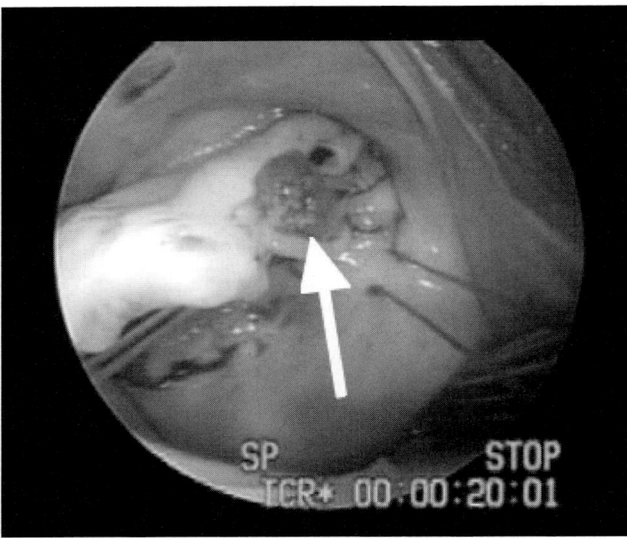

FIGURE 39–1 Vegetation on the atrial side of the A3 segment of the anterior leaflet (posterior paracommissural area).

PATHOLOGY

The pathology of mitral valve endocarditis varies with the route of infection.

Isolated Native Mitral Endocarditis

In isolated mitral valve endocarditis, the infectious process begins on and remains localized to the mitral valve. Mitral valve endocarditis can cause several types of lesions including vegetations, chordal rupture, leaflet abscess/perforation, and mitral annulus abscess.

Vegetations are made up bacteria, altered polynuclear cells, and fibrin deposits, and are indicators of the acute nature of the infectious process. They are often localized on the atrial side of mitral leaflets, particularly the anterior leaflet (Fig. 39-1). They may be mobile or adherent with a sessile or pedicled base of insertion. Vegetations can vary in size and rate of growth. Highly virulent organisms such as HACEK, MRSA (methicillin-resistant *Staphylococcus aureus*), and fungal infections cause particularly large vegetations and are at high risk for embolization. Occasionally, these large vegetations can cause mitral valve obstruction with congestive heart failure. Vegetations may remain on the mitral valve and become organized and calcified despite the eradication of the infectious process.

If the infectious process starts at the free margin of the leaflets, or directly at the level of subvalvular apparatus, chordal rupture with leaflet prolapse can occur. These lesions are usually located at the middle scallop of anterior or posterior leaflets as well as the posterior commissural area.

The valvular abscess consists of a mass of necrotic tissue and active inflammation located underneath the endocardial surface of the valve. It most often involves the anterior leaflet of the mitral valve. Occasionally, leaflet abscess causes a true aneurysm of the body of the anterior leaflet (Fig. 39-2). Locally, leaflet perforation can be the final stage in the evolution of an abscess, although extension into the annulus and/or intervalvular fibrous body may also occur.

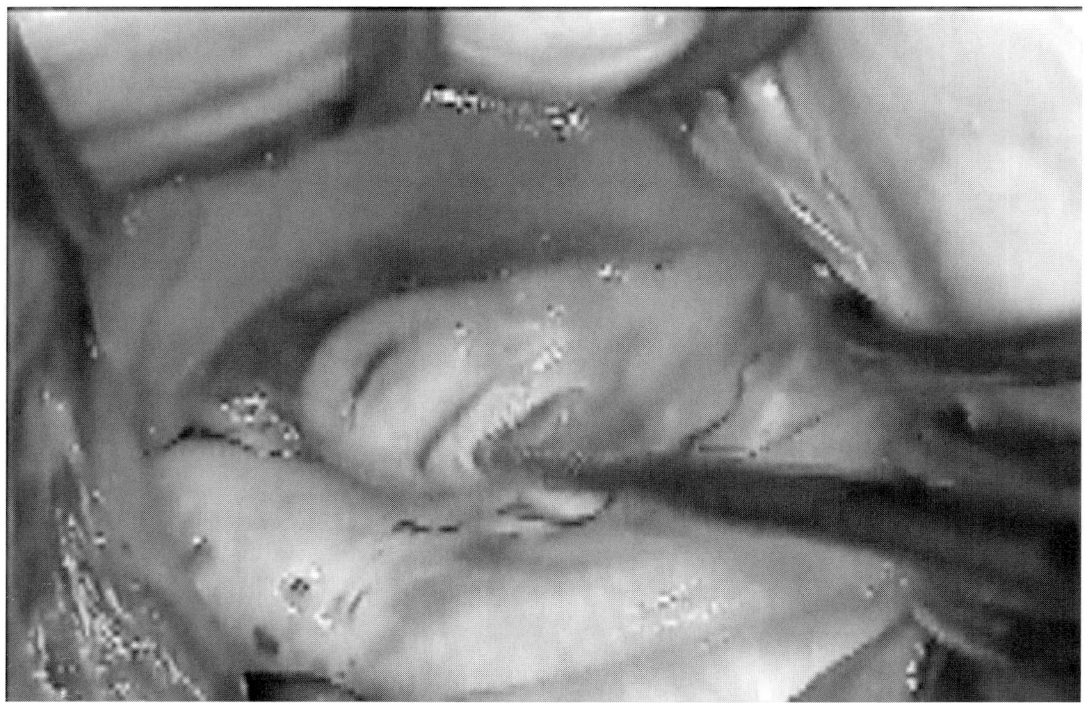

FIGURE 39–2 Aneurysm of the body of the anterior leaflet, complicated by leaflet perforation.

Two different patterns explain the formation of mitral annular abscess. The most common is extension of infection from the body of the leaflet toward the annulus. The second mechanism is primary infection of calcified annular lesions. In the absence of appropriate surgical treatment, an annular abscess can cause false aneurysm of the left ventricle or the atrioventricular groove.

Secondary Native Mitral Endocarditis

Because of the close anatomic relationship between the aortic and mitral valves, aortic valve endocarditis can lead to concomitant mitral valve endocarditis. The localization of the infectious process to the mitral valve can be explained by two different mechanisms. In the first, an aortic annular abscess can extend to the intervalvular fibrous body and then to the mitral annulus. Subsequent infection can spread to the anterior leaflet of the mitral valve, which may result in its partial/complete detachment from the annulus.

In the second mechanism, the diastolic jet of aortic regurgitation due to the primary aortic endocarditis can produce a secondary lesion on the ventricular surface of the anterior mitral leaflet. This lesion can be a vegetation, leaflet abscess, and/or leaflet perforation. This so-called "kissing lesion" is observed in 10% to 15% of patients with endocarditis.[8,9]

Prosthetic Mitral Valve Endocarditis

Prosthetic valve endocarditis often produces three types of lesions: vegetation, valve dehiscence with paravalvular leak, and paravalvular abscess.[4,6,10,11] Early bioprosthetic endocarditis usually involves the sewing ring and leads to an annular abscess and paravalvular leak. Conversely, late bioprosthetic endocarditis often starts at the level of the leaflets, potentially leading to valve obstruction or regurgitation secondary to a large vegetation or leaflet perforation, respectively. In these late cases, the risk remains for extension of infection to the sewing ring with subsequent annular abscess and valve dehiscence. Mechanical mitral prosthetic endocarditis usually involves the sewing ring with complications similar to those mentioned above.

INDICATIONS FOR SURGERY

Surgical intervention plays an important role in the overall management of native mitral valve endocarditis. Several clinical presentations are currently considered absolute indications for surgical intervention. They are:

1. Significant mitral regurgitation, with or without symptoms of congestive heart failure
2. Uncontrolled sepsis despite proper antibiotic therapy
3. Presence of an antibiotic-resistant organism
4. Endocarditis caused by fungus, *Staphylococcus aureus*, or gram-negative bacteria
5. Evidence of mitral annular abscess, extension of infection to intervalvular fibrous body, or formation of intracardiac fistulas
6. Onset of a new conduction disturbance
7. Large vegetations (>1 cm), particularly those that are mobile and located on the anterior leaflet, and thus at high risk for embolic complications
8. Multiple emboli after appropriate antibiotic therapy

In these situations, surgical therapy has dramatically improved both morbidity and mortality over medical treatment alone.

Indications for surgical intervention in patients with prosthetic valve endocarditis include those stated above as well as unstable prosthesis with paravalvular leak. It should be emphasized that surgical intervention is rarely avoided in the setting of prosthetic endocarditis because the infection of foreign material cannot be treated effectively with antibiotics alone.

TIMING OF SURGERY

When there is an indication for surgery, the procedure should be performed soon after the diagnosis is made regardless of the duration of antimicrobial therapy. Even in the setting of severe valvular regurgitation with minimal clinical symptoms, early surgical intervention is justified. Surgery should be delayed, however, in patients who present with recent neurologic injury.[12,13] There is a significant correlation between the interval of neurologic event and surgery and the exacerbation of cerebral complications.[13] Patients who have suffered a recent ischemic or hemorrhagic cerebral injury should not be operated upon for at least 2 or 4 weeks, respectively. Daily neurologic examination, CT scans, and MRI at regular intervals should be performed to determine the appropriate timing of surgery.

PREOPERATIVE INVESTIGATION

Echocardiography (transthoracic or transesophageal), the principal preoperative examination, must be performed in every patient. Echocardiography provides evidence of new valvular regurgitation and/or detects valvular lesions such as vegetations, leaflet or annular abscess, and new partial dehiscence of prosthetic valve (Figs. 39-3 and 39-4).[5,14–16] In the presence of sepsis, these findings are strongly suggestive of infective endocarditis.

In patients with mitral insufficiency, Carpentier's functional classification can be used to describe the mechanism of regurgitation (Fig. 39-5).[17] This functional classification determines valvular dysfunction based on an assessment of the amplitude of anterior and posterior leaflet motion during systole and can be applied to patients with mitral regurgitation secondary to endocarditis. The precise location

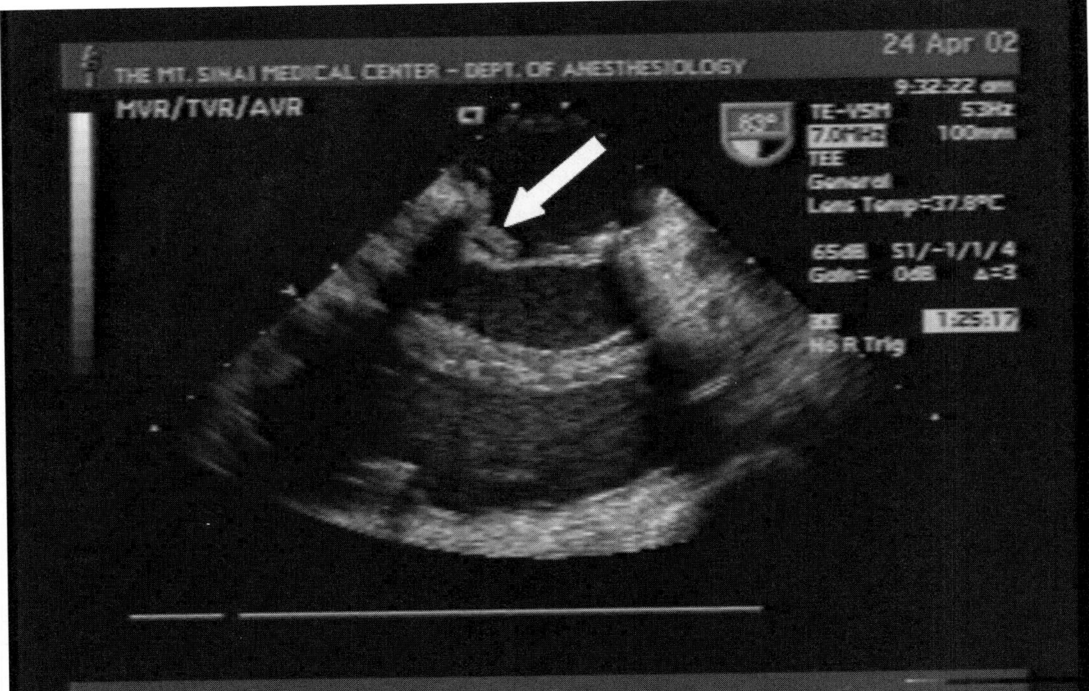

FIGURE 39–3 Vegetation on the atrial surface of the anterior leaflet seen on transesophageal imaging.

of valve dysfunction is then established using segmental valve analysis. The mitral valve is composed of two commissures (anterior and posterior) and two leaflets. The presence of two indentations at the free margin of the posterior leaflet divides the leaflets into three segments. P1 and A1 are the anterior paracommissural segments of the posterior and anterior leaflet, respectively. P2 and A2 are middle scallops and P3/A3 are posterior paracommissural segments. During echocardiography, the transgastric view best visualizes these different components of the mitral valve.

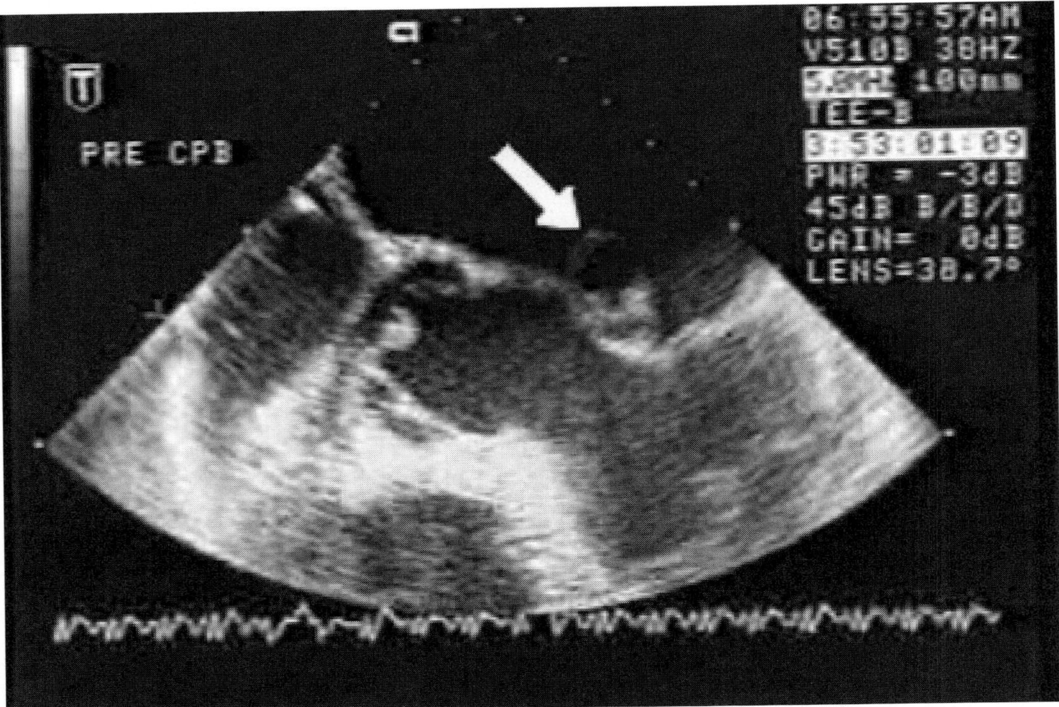

FIGURE 39–4 Four-chamber mid-esophageal view showing a true aneurysm of the body of the anterior leaflet.

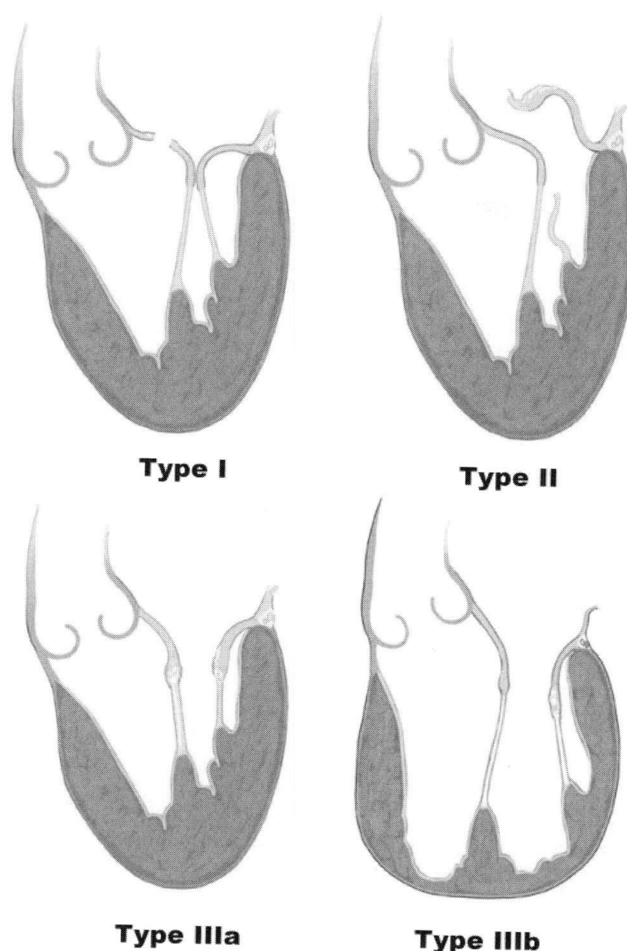

FIGURE 39–5 Carpentier's functional classification of mitral regurgitation. Type I: normal leaflet motion. Type II: increased leaflet motion (leaflet prolapse). Type III: restricted leaflet motion; IIIa, restriction in diastole and systole; IIIb, restriction in systole. Types I and II valvular dysfunctions are due to leaflet perforation and chordal rupture, respectively, in the setting of mitral endocarditis.

In native mitral endocarditis, lesions are usually extensive. Patients often present with a combination of lesions, which may include perforation of the anterior leaflet (type I valvular dysfunction) in association with posterior leaflet prolapse secondary to ruptured chordae (type II dysfunction). Typically, one or more vegetations may also be present. In patients with preexisting valve pathology (e.g., degenerative or ischemic mitral disease), annular dilatation is a common finding and constitutes a secondary lesion, which is not related directly to the infectious process. Rarely, type IIIa dysfunction is seen in patients with chronic healed mitral endocarditis due to calcified vegetations located on leaflets or subvalvular apparatus. Mitral valve endocarditis does not cause type IIIb valvular dysfunction.

Transthoracic echocardiography (TTE) has an excellent specificity for vegetation. However, TTE cannot exclude several aspects of endocarditis, including prosthetic valve infection, annular abscess, and intracardiac fistula. Patients at risk of perivalvular extension or prosthetic valve endocarditis should undergo transesophageal echocardiography (TEE). TEE has a significantly higher sensitivity (76% to 100%) and specificity (94%) than TTE for perivalvular infection.[5] TEE also improves visualization of prosthetic valves, with 86% to 94% sensitivity and 88% to 100% specificity for vegetations. Echocardiography is also used to diagnose the potential concurrent infective endocarditis on aortic and tricuspid valves.

The preoperative examination also consists of a complete sepsis workup (i.e. serial blood cultures, urinalysis, dental exam, etc.) in order to confirm the diagnosis and identify potential sources of infection. Other studies may be necessary to rule out potential complications of endocarditis, such as renal dysfunction, peripheral septic emboli including cerebral embolism, thrombocytopenia, and coagulopathy.

OPERATIVE TECHNIQUE

Principles

Surgery of both native and prosthetic mitral valve endocarditis may be challenging and requires experience with mitral reconstructive and reoperative procedures, respectively. However, regardless of the type of surgery, a systematic approach using the following principles should be applied to optimize surgical results:

1. Intraoperative transesophageal echocardiography should be performed in every patient. It can be used initially to determine the mechanism of mitral regurgitation and at the completion of the procedure to evaluate the quality of repair or assess prosthetic valve function.
2. Cardiac manipulation before aortic cross-clamping should be minimized to prevent peripheral embolization of vegetations. This is particularly important in patients with large, mobile, and friable vegetations.
3. Following valve exposure, an accurate valve analysis should be performed to confirm the echocardiographic data and to assess the extent of lesions (perivalvular abscess, intervalvular fibrous body/ventricular involvement, and presence of intracardiac fistula).
4. Radical resection of all infected and necrotic tissues is performed with a 1- to 2-mm margin of normal tissue. An infected prosthetic valve should be removed completely. Multiple specimens including vegetation and valvular debris should be sent for further microbiologic analysis. Local application of an antiseptic solution may be used.
5. Surgical instruments including suction tips should be changed after debridement of infected tissue.
6. The aortic valve may need to be inspected to rule out the extension of infection to the aortic root and the presence of any secondary lesions on the cusps.

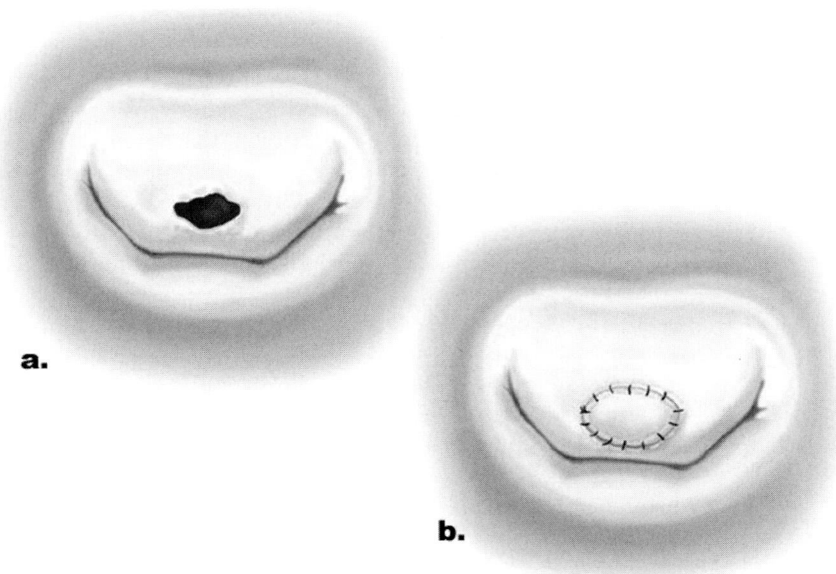

FIGURE 39–6 Leaflet perforation (anterior leaflet) treated by autologous pericardial patch.

Native Mitral Valve Endocarditis

A full sternotomy is performed. Cardiopulmonary bypass is established after the cannulation of the distal ascending aorta and superior/inferior vena cava with moderate systemic hypothermia. Myocardial protection is achieved with warm and cold blood cardioplegia delivered in an antegrade fashion (caution must be used when placing a retrograde cannula not to dislodge mitral vegetations). The mitral valve is exposed via a left atriotomy through the interatrial groove.

All macroscopically involved tissues are widely excised without any concern about the possibility of repair. Once the debridement is performed, reconstructive surgery using Carpentier's technique should be considered.[18] The feasibility of mitral repair depends on the availability of healthy tissue following debridement. In the event of entire leaflet involvement or extensive destruction of the subvalvular apparatus, prosthetic valve replacement is performed using standard techniques. Because multiple studies have failed to identify differences in the recurrence of infection between mechanical and bioprosthetic valves, standard criteria should be applied for valve selection.[7,19,20] There have also been reports of mitral homograft replacement in the setting of acute endocarditis, but at this time clinical experience remains limited.[21]

Mitral valve repair can be performed safely in multiple anatomic presentations provided sufficient tissue remains to allow valvular reconstruction without excessive tension on the suture lines.[18,22–25]

LEAFLET PERFORATION OR DETACHMENT

This lesion affects primarily the anterior leaflet. A common clinical presentation is a simultaneous aortic and mitral endocarditis. After adequate debridement, the leaflet defect is repaired with a patch of autologous pericardium. A piece of pericardium is preserved in 0.625% glutaraldehyde for 10 minutes and then rinsed in a saline bath for a total of 15 minutes. The patch is fixed to the remaining leaflet with polypropylene suture (Fig. 39-6). The smooth surface of the pericardium is turned toward the atrium to decrease the potential risk of thromboembolic complication. Occasionally, a large surface area of the anterior leaflet is destroyed in the setting of aortic and mitral valve endocarditis. If a homograft is used to reconstruct the aortic root, the homograft's attached mitroaortic curtain can be used to reconstruct the body of the native anterior leaflet. Mitral detachment from the fibrous skeleton can also occur in the setting of aortic and mitral endocarditis due to the extensions of aortic annular lesions. This typically occurs in a localized fashion around the anterior commissure of the mitral valve. Resuspension of the mitral apparatus to the fibrous skeleton can be accomplished in most circumstances with interrupted sutures (Fig. 39-7).

POSTERIOR LEAFLET PROLAPSE

The middle scallop of the posterior segment (P2 segment) is often involved in the infectious process with one or several ruptured chordae. A quadrangular resection of P2 segment is performed. Plication or compression sutures are placed along the posterior annulus of the mitral valve. A sliding plasty of P1 and P3 segments is performed and the gap between the two scallops is closed with polypropylene suture (Fig. 39-8).

ANTERIOR LEAFLET PROLAPSE

Limited infection of the free margin of the anterior leaflet is best treated with a triangular resection followed by closure

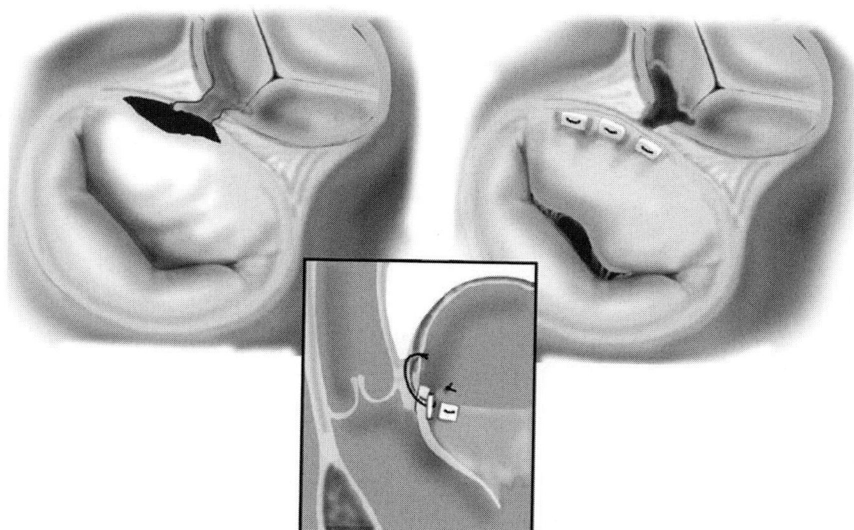

FIGURE 39–7 Mitral detachment from the fibrous skeleton treated by resuspension using interrupted sutures.

with interrupted polypropylene suture. In the event of chordal rupture, chordal transfer of the secondary chordae of anterior leaflet to the free margin or chordal transposition from the posterior leaflet may be required to provide adequate support.

COMMISSURAL PROLAPSE

When the commissure is involved, the prolapsed area is resected and reconstructed using leaflet sliding plasty (Fig. 39-9).

ANNULOPLASTY

In the setting of mitral valve endocarditis, prosthetic ring annuloplasty following reconstruction remains controversial. In patients with acute endocarditis without annular dilatation or deformation, the use of a prosthetic ring can be avoided. However, in patients with chronic mitral regurgitation and dilated annulus, prosthetic ring annuloplasty should be utilized to restore proper coaptation and assure long-term durability of the repair. Alternatively, in the setting of acute endocarditis, a pericardial strip fixed in glutaraldehyde can be used to fashion a posterior annuloplasty.

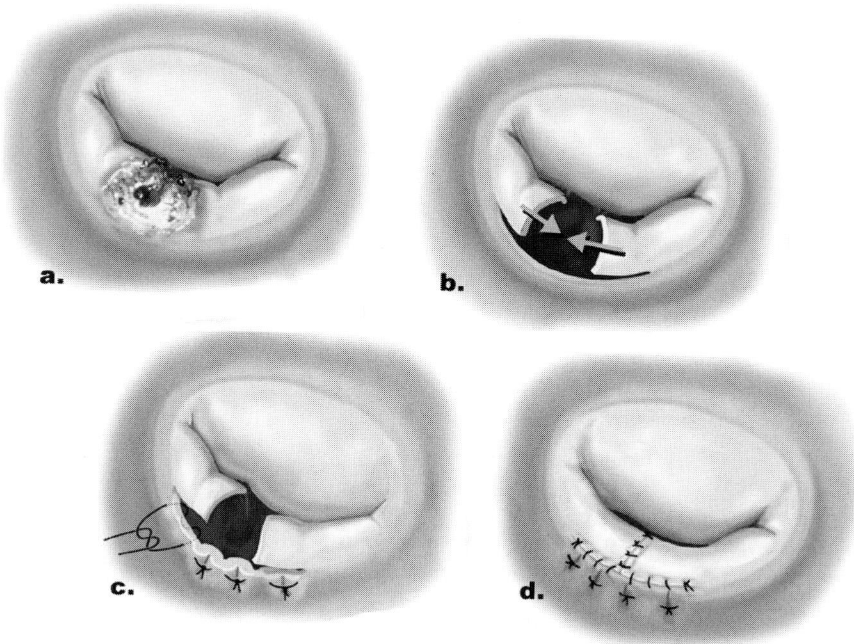

FIGURE 39–8 (A) Posterior leaflet endocarditis with P2 segment prolapse. (B) P2 segment is resected. (C) Compression sutures are placed along the posterior annulus. (D) Sliding plasty of segments P1 and P3 is performed.

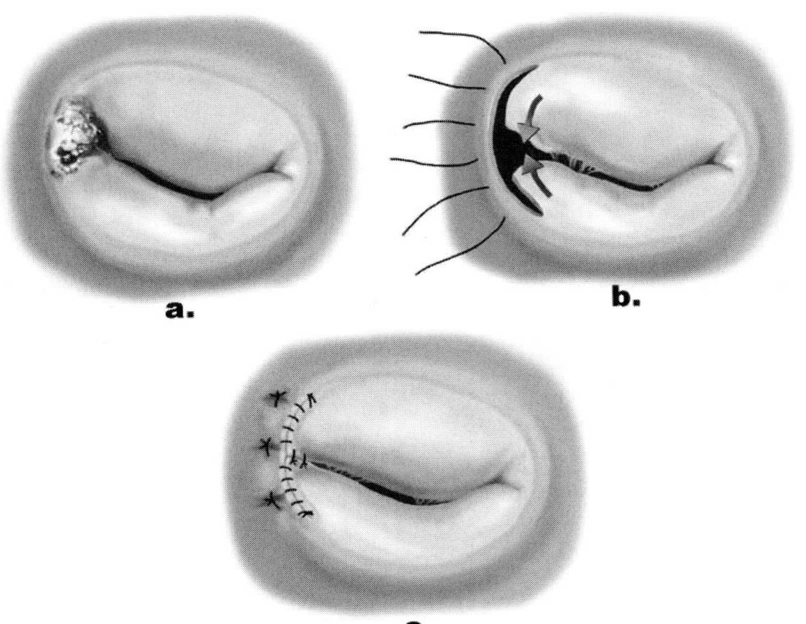

FIGURE 39–9 (A) Anterior commissure endocarditis with prolapse. (B) Infected area is resected and compression sutures are placed. (C) Sliding commissuroplasty in the paracommissural area is performed.

Prosthetic Mitral Valve Endocarditis

Reoperative mitral valve surgery can be performed through a redo sternotomy or right anterolateral thoracotomy. In patients with previous isolated mitral valve surgery, either redo sternotomy or right anterolateral thoracotomy (provided that the aortic valve is not affected by the infectious process) can be performed safely with low operative risk. Redo sternotomy is the approach of choice if concomitant procedures such as coronary artery bypass grafting and/or aortic valve surgery are required. Right anterolateral thoracotomy is the preferred approach if the patient presents with multiple previous sternotomies, history of bypass grafting with patent grafts, or possibility of severe mediastinal adhesions (recent sternotomy, mediastinitis, and mediastinal radiation).[26,27] The latter approach is relatively contraindicated in the setting of previous right-sided chest surgery, severe chronic obstructive pulmonary disease, or moderate to severe aortic insufficiency.

REDO STERNOTOMY

Femoral vessels are exposed in selective cases (e.g., suspicion of severe mediastinal adhesions or prior bypass surgery with patent grafts). If the femoral artery is not suitable because of atheroslerotic disease, the axillary artery may be used for an arterial cannulation site. After redo sternotomy, mediastinal dissection is limited to the ascending aorta and the right lateral aspect of the heart. Further dissection of the left side of the heart to drop the left ventricular apex may improve mitral valve exposure in some patients.

RIGHT ANTEROLATERAL THORACOTOMY

An anterolateral thoracotomy is performed through the 4th intercostal space. The interatrial groove and the right superior pulmonary vein are dissected. Direct cannulation of the ascending aorta and percutaneous femoral vein and direct superior vena cava cannulation are performed. If the ascending aorta is not suitable for cannulation (inaccessible, inadequate exposure, calcification), the femoral or axillary arteries are alternative sites for arterial cannulation. Peripheral cannulation is done using the Seldinger technique with a small, high-flow cannula specifically designed for percutaneous insertion. Cardiopulmonary bypass is instituted with vacuum-assisted drainage and the temperature is lowered. Once the heart fibrillates, the left atrium is opened. Brief periods of low-flow bypass may be necessary to ensure adequate exposure of the mitral valve in the presence of mild aortic regurgitation, particularly when operating near the anterior commissure.

MITRAL VALVE EXPOSURE

In both redo sternotomy and right anterolateral thoracotomy approaches, the mitral valve can be exposed transseptally[28] or via a left atriotomy through the interatrial groove. The left atrium approach is the preferred technique. A complete dissection of the interatrial groove, which enables a left atriotomy closer to the valve, and posterior extension of the atriotomy are two maneuvers that significantly improve the valve exposure. The transseptal approach is useful in the setting of a small left atrium, prior aortic valve replacement, or when concomitant tricuspid valve surgery is also required.

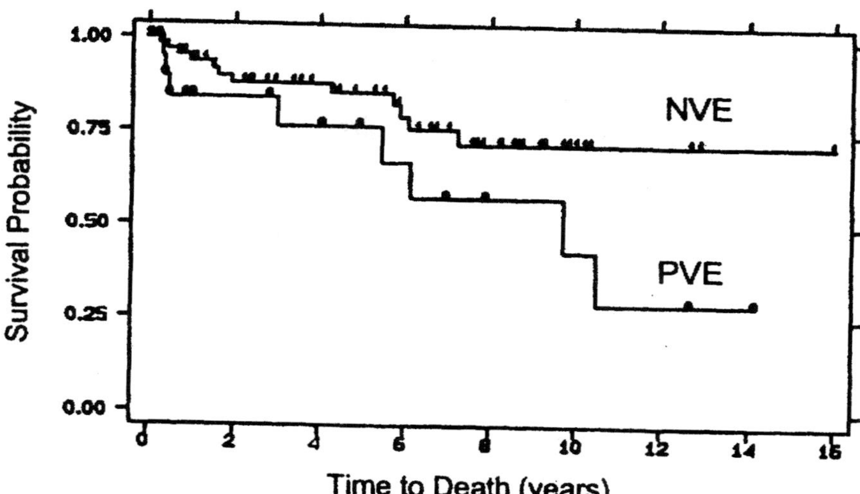

FIGURE 39–10 Kaplan-Meier survival curves for discharged native valve endocarditis (NVE) and prosthetic valve endocarditis (PVE) patients. (*Reproduced with permission from Aranki SF, Adams DH, Rizzo RJ, et al: Determinants of early mortality and late survival in mitral valve endocarditis. Circulation 1995; 92(suppl II): II-143.*)

RECONSTRUCTION OF THE MITRAL ANNULUS

Following mitral valve exposure, the infected prostheses should be excised. Because prosthetic valve endocarditis typically causes partial or total destruction of the mitral annulus, one may need to reconstruct the annulus before performing a reoperative mitral valve replacement. There are numerous techniques for annular reconstruction.

Mitral annular reconstruction using autologous or glutaraldehyde-fixed bovine pericardium (David technique)[29,30] In patients with posterior annular destruction, a semicircular-shaped pericardial patch is used to reconstruct the annulus. While ensuring the patch is large enough to completely cover the defect, one side of the patch is sutured to the endocardium of the left ventricle and the other side is used to secure the prosthetic valve.

In patients with complete destruction of the annulus, a circumferential patch is tailored for annular reconstruction.

Mitral annular reconstruction using figure-of-eight atrial and ventricular sutures (Carpentier technique)[31] With this technique, after careful debridement, the AV junction is reconstructed by a series of figure-of-eight 2-0 braided sutures placed into the atrial and ventricular edges. These sutures are the brought out on the atrial side. The ventricular bites of theses sutures should only involve one third of the thickness of the myocardial wall and be as wide as possible, taking advantage of any fibrous tissue present on the surface of the myocardium. Exerting traction on these sutures reduces the size of the annulus and closes the AV groove without injury to the circumflex vessels. The closure of the AV groove is facilitated by downward displacement of the atrial edge toward the ventricular edge with forceps. By means of this technique the circumflex vessels and surrounding fat are displaced outward and the AV junction is restored as a firm fibrous structure available for valve replacement.

If the infectious process involves the ventricular myocardium, the atrial edge is dissected free to mobilize an atrial

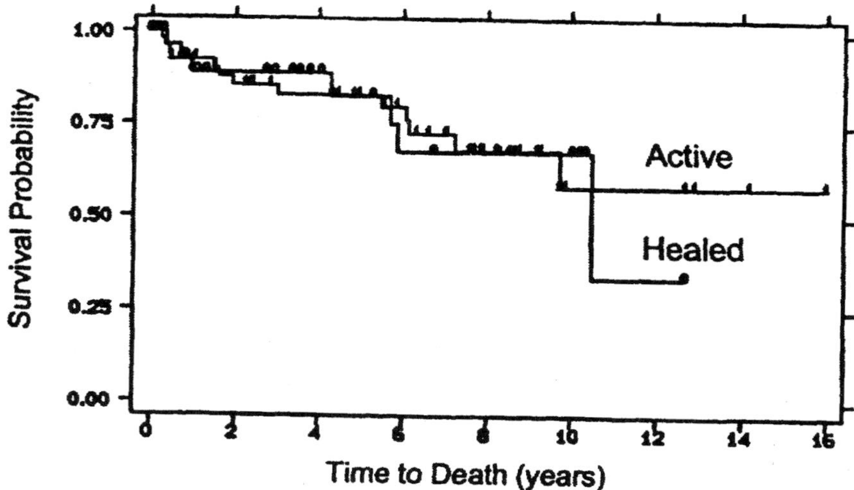

FIGURE 39–11 Kaplan-Meier survival curves for discharged active and healed endocarditis patients. (*Reproduced with permission from Aranki SF, Adams DH, Rizzo RJ, et al: Determinants of early mortality and late survival in mitral valve endocarditis. Circulation 1995; 92(suppl II):II-143.*)

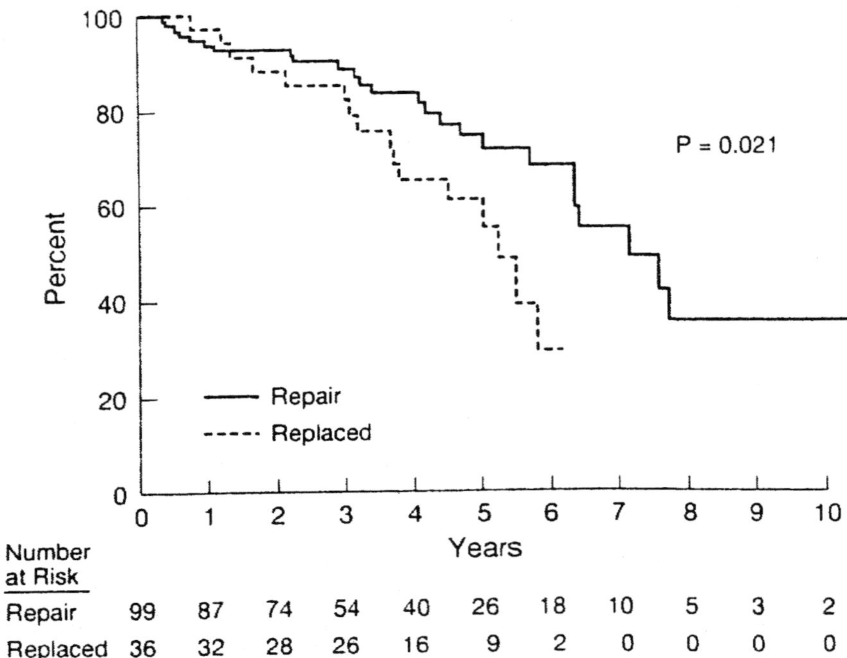

FIGURE 39–12 Event-free survival for all patients with endocarditis undergoing mitral valve repair or replacement. (*Reproduced with permission from Muehrcke DD, Cosgrove DM III, Lytle BW, et al: Is there an advantage to repairing infected mitral valves? Ann Thorac Surg 1997;63:1718.*)

flap (sliding atrium technique), which is used to cover the destroyed area. The fat and connective tissue surrounding the circumflex vessels are left attached to the ventricular side. Figure-of-eight sutures as described earlier are used to reconstruct the annulus and cover the ventricular area.

After mitral annular reconstruction, mitral valve replacement is performed using a standard technique.

RESULTS

Hospital mortality rates ranging to approximately 50% have been previously reported in patients with mitral valve endocarditis, although recent series described improved results with mortality rates typically ranging between 0% and 20%.[4,6,7,10,18,22–25,32,33] Several variables, including improvements in antimicrobial therapy, patient selection, myocardial protection, and surgical techniques, have all likely contributed to decreasing the operative mortality rate. Prosthetic valve endocarditis remains associated with a much higher operative mortality rate than native valve endocarditis (Fig. 39-10).[4,6,7,33] Interestingly, the activity of mitral endocarditis (i.e., active vs. healed) does not appear to have an effect on short- or long-term survival, and therefore the activity of endocarditis is not of primary concern in the decision-making process regarding timing of surgery (Fig. 39-11).[4] In patients with native mitral valve endocarditis, valve repair is preferable to valve replacement whenever feasible, because repair is associated with a lower hospital mortality and improved long-term survival (Fig. 39-12).[24] Series from Broussais Hospital and the Cleveland Clinic have reported repair rates of 80% and 45%, respectively, demonstrating the feasibility of an aggressive approach to valve repair in patients with mitral valve endocarditis.[18,24] Several recent series have documented outstanding results with valve repair in the setting of mitral endocarditis, with mortality rates ranging between 0% and 9%.[18,22–25] In terms of infection-free survival, mitral valve repair is associated with a less than 1% per year reinfection rate, and appears to be preferable to mitral valve replacement.[24] Preserving native mitral valve tissue by means of repair and avoiding a valve prosthesis in the setting of active infection most likely accounts for this observation.

REFERENCES

1. Rutledge R, Kim J, Applebaum RE: Actuarial analysis of the risk of prosthetic valve endocarditis in 1,598 patients with mechanical and bioprosthetic valves. *Arch Surg* 1985; 120:469.
2. Arvay A, Lengyel M: Incidence and risk factors of prosthetic valve endocarditis. *Eur J Cardiothoracic Surg* 1988; 2:340.
3. Horskotte D, Piper C, Niehues R, et al: Late prosthetic valve endocarditis. *Eur Heart J* 1995; 16(suppl B):39.
4. Aranki SF, Adams DH, Rizzo RJ, et al: Determinants of early mortality and late survival in mitral valve endocarditis. *Circulation* 1995;92(suppl II):II-143.
5. Bayer AS, Bolger AF, Taubert KA, et al: Diagnosis and management of infective endocarditis and its complications. *Circulation* 1998; 98:2936.
6. David TE: The surgical treatment of patients with prosthetic valve endocarditis. *Semin Thorac Cardiovasc Surg* 1995; 7:47.
7. Moon MR, Miller DC, Moore KA, et al: Treatment of endocarditis with valve replacement: the question of tissue versus mechanical prosthesis. *Ann Thorac Surg* 2001; 71:1164.
8. Oakley C: The mitral kissing vegetation. *Eur Heart J* 2002; 23:11.

9. Gillinov AM, Diaz R, Blackstone EH, et al: Double valve endocarditis. *Ann Thorac Surg* 2001; 71:1874.
10. David TE, Bos J, Christakis GT, et al: Heart valve operations in patients with active infective endocarditis. *Ann Thorac Surg* 1990; 49:701.
11. David TE, Kuo J, Armstrong S: Aortic and mitral valve replacement with reconstruction of the intervalvular fibrous body. *J Thorac Cardiovasc Surg* 1997; 114:766.
12. Cabell CH, Pond KK, Peterson GE, et al: The risk of stroke and death in patients with aortic and mitral valve endocarditis. *Am Heart J* 2001; 142:75.
13. Eishi K, Kawazoe K, Kuriyama Y, et al: Surgical management of infective endocarditis associated with cerebral complications: a multi-center retrospective study in Japan. *J Thorac Cardiovasc Surg* 1995; 110:1745.
14. Durack DT, Lukes AS, Bright DK, et al: New criteria for diagnosis of infective endocarditis: utilization of specific echocardiographic findings. *Am J Med* 1994; 96:200.
15. DiSalvo G, Habib G, Pergola V, et al: Echocardiography predicts embolic events in infective endocarditis. *J Am Coll Cardiol* 2001; 37:1069.
16. Senni M, Merlo M, Sangiorgi G, et al: Mitral valve repair and transesophageal echocardiographic findings in a high-risk subgroup of patients with active, acute infective endocarditis. *J Heart Valve Dis* 2001; 10:72.
17. Carpentier A: Cardiac valve surgery—the "French correction." *J Thorac Cardiovasc Surg* 1983; 86:323.
18. Dreyfus G, Serraf A, Jebara VA, et al: Valve repair in acute endocarditis. *Ann Thorac Surg* 1990; 49:706.
19. Grover FL, Cohen DJ, Oprian C, et al: Determinants of the occurrence of and survival from prosthetic valve endocarditis: experience of the Veterans Affairs Cooperative Study on Valvular Heart Disease. *J Thorac Cardiovasc Surg* 1994; 108:207.
20. Shumway NE, Reitz BA: Treatment of endocarditis with valve replacement: the question of tissue versus mechanical prosthesis. *Ann Thorac Surg* 2001; 71:1164.
21. Acar C, Tolan M, Berrebi A, et al: Homograft replacement of the mitral valve: graft selection, technique of implantation, and results in forty-three patients. *J Thorac Cardiovasc Surg* 1996; 111:367.
22. Hendren WG, Morris AS, Rosenkranz ER, et al: Mitral valve repair for bacterial endocarditis. *J Thorac Cardiovasc Surg* 1992; 103:124.
23. Pagani FD, Monaghan HL, Deeb GM, et al: Mitral valve reconstruction for active and healed endocarditis. *Circulation* 1996; 94(suppl):II133.
24. Muehrcke DD, Cosgrove DM III, Lytle BW, et al: Is there an advantage to repairing infected mitral valves? *Ann Thorac Surg* 1997; 63:1718.
25. Sternik L, Zehr KJ, Orszulak TA, et al: The advantage of repair of mitral valve in acute endocarditis. *J Heart Valve Dis* 2002; 11:91.
26. Byrne JG, Karavas AN, Adams DH, et al: The preferred approach for mitral valve surgery after CABG: right thoracotomy, hypothermia and avoidance of LIMA-LAD graft. *J Heart Valve Dis* 2001; 10:584.
27. Adams DH, Filsoufi F, Byrne JG, et al: Mitral valve repair in redo cardiac surgery. *J Card Surg* 2002; 17:40.
28. Guiraudon G, Ofiesh JG: Extended vertical transatrial septal approach to the mitral valve. *Ann Thorac Surg* 1991; 52:1058.
29. David TE, Feindel CM: Reconstruction of the mitral annulus. *Circulation* 1987; 76(suppl III):III-102.
30. David TE, Feindel CM, Armstrong S, et al: Reconstruction of the mitral annulus: a ten year experience. *J Thorac Cardiovasc Surg* 1995; 110:1323.
31. Carpentier AF, Pellerin M, Fuzellier JF, et al: Extensive calcification of the mitral valve annulus: pathology and surgical management. *J Thorac Cardiovasc Surg* 1996; 111:718.
32. d'Udekem Y, David TE, Feindel CM, et al: Long-term results of operation for paravalvular abscess. *Ann Thorac Surg* 1996; 62:48.
33. Delay D, Pellerin M, Carrier M, et al: Immediate and long-term results of valve replacement for native and prosthetic valve endocarditis. *Ann Thorac Surg* 2000; 70:1219.

Part **IVc**

Valvular Heart Disease: Other Valve Lesions

Chapter 40

Tricuspid Valve Disease

Richard J. Shemin

The tricuspid valve is composed of three leaflets (anterior, posterior, and septal) attached to a fibrous annulus. The leaflets usually attach via chordae tendineae to three papillary muscles that are an integral part of the right ventricular wall. Surrounding structures of surgical importance are the coronary sinus, atrioventricular node, and right coronary artery (Fig. 40-1).

The tricuspid valve may malfunction due to structural malformation or secondary to other cardiac pathology. Congenital abnormalities such as atrial septal defect (ASD), ventricular septal defect (VSD), and Ebstein's disease lead to malfunction and tricuspid regurgitation. Cases of isolated tricuspid disease associated with systemic lupus erythematosus, cor pulmonale, inferior myocardial infarction, scleroderma, or methysergide intake are noteworthy but rarely encountered in surgical practice.[1–12]

ETIOLOGY

The most common presentation of tricuspid regurgitation is secondary to cardiac valvular pathology (mostly mitral valve disease) on the left side of the heart. As pulmonary hypertension develops leading to right ventricular dilatation, the tricuspid valve annulus will dilate. The circumference of the annulus lengthens primarily along the attachments of the anterior and posterior leaflets. The septal leaflet is fixed between the fiberous trigones, preventing lengthening. As the annular and ventricular dilation progresses, the chordal papillary muscle complex becomes functionally shortened. This combination prevents leaflet apposition, resulting in valvular incompetence.[13–18]

Eisenmenger's syndrome and primary pulmonary hypertension lead to the same pathophysiology of progressive right ventricular dilation, tricuspid annular enlargement, and valvular incompetence. A right ventricular infarction produces either disruption of the papillary muscle or a severe regional wall motion abnormality preventing normal leaflet apposition by a tethering effect on the leaflets, leading to regurgitation. Marfan syndrome and other variations of myxomatous disease affecting the mitral and tricuspid valve can lead to prolapsing leaflets, elongation of chordae, or chordal rupture producing valvular incompetence. Blunt or penetrating chest trauma may structurally disrupt the structural components of the tricuspid valve. Dilated cardiomyopathy in the late stages of biventricular failure and pulmonary hypertension produces tricuspid regurgitation.[19–22] Infectious endocarditis can destroy leaflet tissue, mostly in drug addicts with staphylococcal infection.[23–26]

The carcinoid syndrome leads to either focal or diffuse deposits of fibrous tissue on the endocardium of valve cusps, cardiac chambers, intima of the great vessels, and coronary sinus. The white fiberous carcinoid plaques, if present on the ventricular side of the tricuspid valve cusps, adhere the

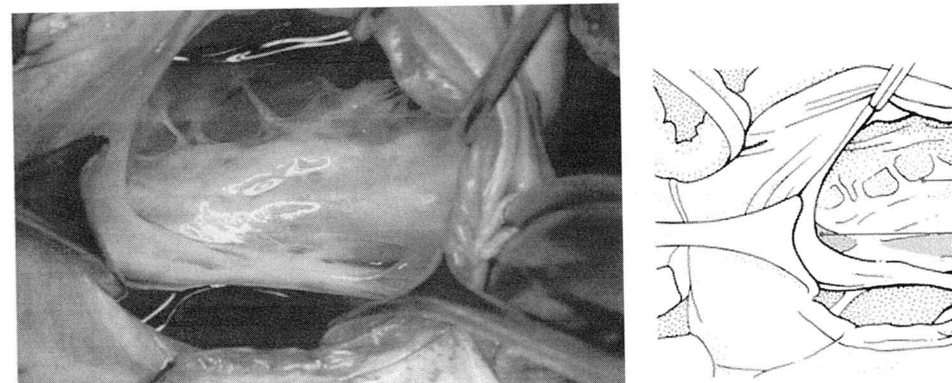

FIGURE 40–1 View of the tricuspid valve and labeled structures of surgical importance.

leaflet tissue to the right ventricular wall, preventing leaflet coaptation.[27–29] Rheumatic disease of the tricuspid valve is always associated with mitral valve involvement, and the deformity of the tricuspid tissue results in a tricuspid valve stenosis as well as regurgitation.[30]

CLINICAL PRESENTATION AND PATHOPHYSIOLOGY

Tricuspid Regurgitation

Patients with tricuspid regurgitation have the presenting symptoms of fatigue and weakness related to a reduction in cardiac output. Right heart failure leads to ascites, congestive hepatosplenomegaly, pulsatile liver, pleural effusions, and peripheral edema. In the late stages these patients are wasted with cachexia, cyanosis, and jaundice. Atrial fibrillation is common. Impressive jugular venous distention with an *s* wave or fused *c* and *v* waves, followed by a prominent *y* descent, is present. During inspiration this finding is accentuated because of the physiologic increase in venous return. The cardiac oscillatory exam is notable for an S_3 that increases with inspiration and decreases with a Valsalva maneuver, increased P_2 if pulmonary hypertension has developed, and a parasternal pansystolic murmur increasing with inspiration.

The chest x-ray demonstrates cardiomegaly, increased right atrial and ventricular size, a prominent azygous vein, possible pleural effusion, and upward diaphragmatic displacement due to ascites. Echocardiography best assesses the degree of regurgitation, structural abnormalities of the valve, pulmonary artery pressures, and right ventricular function both preoperatively and intraoperatively. A shift in the atrial septum to the left and paradoxical septal motion are consistent with right ventricular diastolic overload. Pulsed Doppler and color flow help identify systolic right ventricular to right atrial flow with inferior vena cava and hepatic vein flow reversal. Contrast echocardiography can be useful with a rapid saline bolus injection producing microcavities that are visible on echo, demonstrating to-and-fro motion across the valve orifice and reversal into the inferior vena cava and hepatic veins. Possible ASD or patent foramen ovale should be sought. Endocarditic lesions and vegetations are clearly visible by echo; the valve may be destroyed and septic pulmonary emboli are a common feature. The tricuspid valve in carcinoid syndrome is thickened with retracted leaflets fixed in a semiopen position throughout the cardiac cycle.[31–42]

Cardiac catheterization will document increased right atrial and right ventricular end-diastolic pressure.[43] The right atrial pressure tracing has an absent X descent, prominent V wave, and "ventricularization" of the right atrial tracing, and the degree of pulmonary artery hypertension is documented. Pulmonary artery pressures of over 60 mm Hg are usually due to left-sided lesions leading to secondary tricuspid regurgitation. A right ventriculogram has been used but is unnecessary with current echocardiographic evaluation.

Tricuspid Stenosis

Tricuspid stenosis is most commonly rheumatic. It is extremely rare to have isolated tricuspid stenosis, as some degree of tricuspid regurgitation will be present.[44–47] Mitral valve disease coexists with occasional involvement of the aortic valve. The third world and especially the Indian subcontinent still have a significant prevalence of rheumatic tricuspid valvular disease. The anatomic features are similar to mitral stenosis with fusion and shortening of the chordae and leaflet thickening. Fusion along the free edges and calcific deposits on the valve are found late in the disease. The preponderance of cases are in young women.

The diastolic gradient between the right atrium and right ventricle is significantly elevated even at 2 to 5 mm Hg mean pressure. As the right atrial pressure increases, venous congestion leads to distention of the jugular veins, ascites, pleural effusion, and peripheral edema. The right atrial wall thickens and the atrial chamber dilates.

If the patient remains in normal sinus rhythm, the right atrial tracing and jugular venous pulse have prominent *a* waves that accentuate with inspiration. The cardiac murmur is mid-diastolic, increases with inspiration, is heard maximally along the left sternoid border, and may have an opening snap.

Clinical features are consistent with reduced cardiac output producing the symptoms of fatigue and malaise. Significant liver engorgement produces right upper quadrant tenderness with a palpable liver with a presystolic pulse. Ascites produces increased abdominal girth. Significant peripheral edema or anasarca can develop. Severe tricuspid stenosis may mask or reduce the pulmonary congestion of mitral stenosis due to reduced blood flow to the left side of the heart. The low output state of the patient is prominent.

The chest x-ray demonstrates cardiomegaly with an increase in the right atria and pulmonary artery size. The EKG will demonstrate increased P-wave amplitude if the patient is in normal sinus rhythm. Echocardiography reveals the diagnostic features of diastolic doming of the thickened tricuspid valve leaflets, reduced leaflet mobility, and a reduced orifice of flow. The Doppler flow pattern across the tricuspid valve has a prolonged slope of antegrade flow.

The patient's ability to tolerate stenotic lesions of the tricuspid valve is dictated to a large degree by the natural history of the mitral or aortic valve disease. In patients with predominant tricuspid regurgitation, the negative consequences of right ventricular volume overload develop slowly. Acute tricuspid regurgitation due to traumatic rupture or complete excision of the tricuspid valve as the treatment for infective endocarditis can be well tolerated for years if the pulmonary artery pressure is not elevated. Functional tricuspid incompetence is progressive. Surgical treatment of left-sided valvular lesions is not always adequate to resolve or prevent progressive tricuspid regurgitation. This is particularly true when pulmonary hypertension persists.

SURGICAL DECISIONS

The cardiologist and the cardiac surgeon face the decision of when to intervene and when to surgically repair or replace the tricuspid valve. The choice of the reparative technique to use for a durable result must be evaluated as well as evaluation of which type of valve, mechanical or bioprosthesis, to employ to maximize durability and minimize complications (i.e., thrombosis and thromboembolism). The surgical literature can be misleading due to case selection bias and the various time frames of retrospective reviews. This is particularly true during the era that cage-ball and single-disc mechanical valves were in use.

SURGICAL EXPOSURE

Tricuspid valve annuloplasty performed with either mitral and/or aortic valve operations is accomplished either through a full or partial lower sternotomy approach or less invasive right minithoracotomy exposure. Bicaval venous cannulation with caval snares is essential to isolate the right atrium. The cannula can be conventionally placed via the right atrium or less invasively via the femoral vein and a superior vena cava cannula inserted via the internal jugular vein.

The left-sided valve repair or replacement is performed under blood cardioplegic arrest with antegrade and/or retrograde administration, moderate systemic hypothermia, and topical cold saline surface cooling. The mitral valve can be exposed through a left atrial incision posterior to the intra-atrial septum or through a transseptal incision (Fig. 40-2). After unclamping the aorta and completing de-airing maneuvers, attention can be turned to the tricuspid valve during rewarming and return of a cardiac rhythm. During the tricuspid valve suturing, misplacement of a suture adversely affecting the cardiac conduction system can be immediately assessed and corrected. In a reoperative setting, approaching the tricuspid valve through a right minithoracotomy has the advantage of avoiding adhesions and possible injury to the right ventricle during repeat sternotomy. If the operation will include the mitral valve, exposure can be simplified by using a right atrial incision and transseptal approach. If atrial fibrillation is present, a Maze procedure using the Cox-Maze III technique or radiofrequency ablation can be added to the technical maneuvers.

ANNULOPLASTY TECHNIQUES

Techniques to deal with a dilated tricuspid valve annulus with normal leaflets and chordal structures include plication of the posterior leaflet's annulus (bicuspidization), partial purse-string reduction of the anterior and posterior leaflet annulus (DeVega technique), and rigid or flexible rings or bands placed to reduce the annular size and achieve leaflet coaptation. The preoperative and intraoperative echocardiograms are valuable assessment tools to help the surgeon understand the structure and function of the valve.[34–42]

The degree of pulmonary hypertension, right ventricular dilatation, and systolic function coupled with the size of the right atrium must be factored into the surgical decision making. The classical technique of inserting a finger via a purse-string suture into the right atrium to palpate the tricuspid valve and withdrawing the finger tip 2 to 3 cm from the valve orifice trying to access the force of the regurgitant jet is of less importance in the current era of cardiac surgery than previously. After repair, the intraoperative transesophogeal echocardiogram allows the surgeon to leave the operating room with confidence that the repair is functioning satisfactorily.[48–63]

Minimal right atrial enlargement and +1 to +2 regurgitation will usually resolve after surgery on left-sided valve lesions, especially if the pulmonary hypertension resolves. Otherwise, tricuspid annuloplasty should be performed to help improve the early postoperative course and prevent residual or progressive tricuspid regurgitation. Special note should be taken in assessing the foramen ovale for patency.

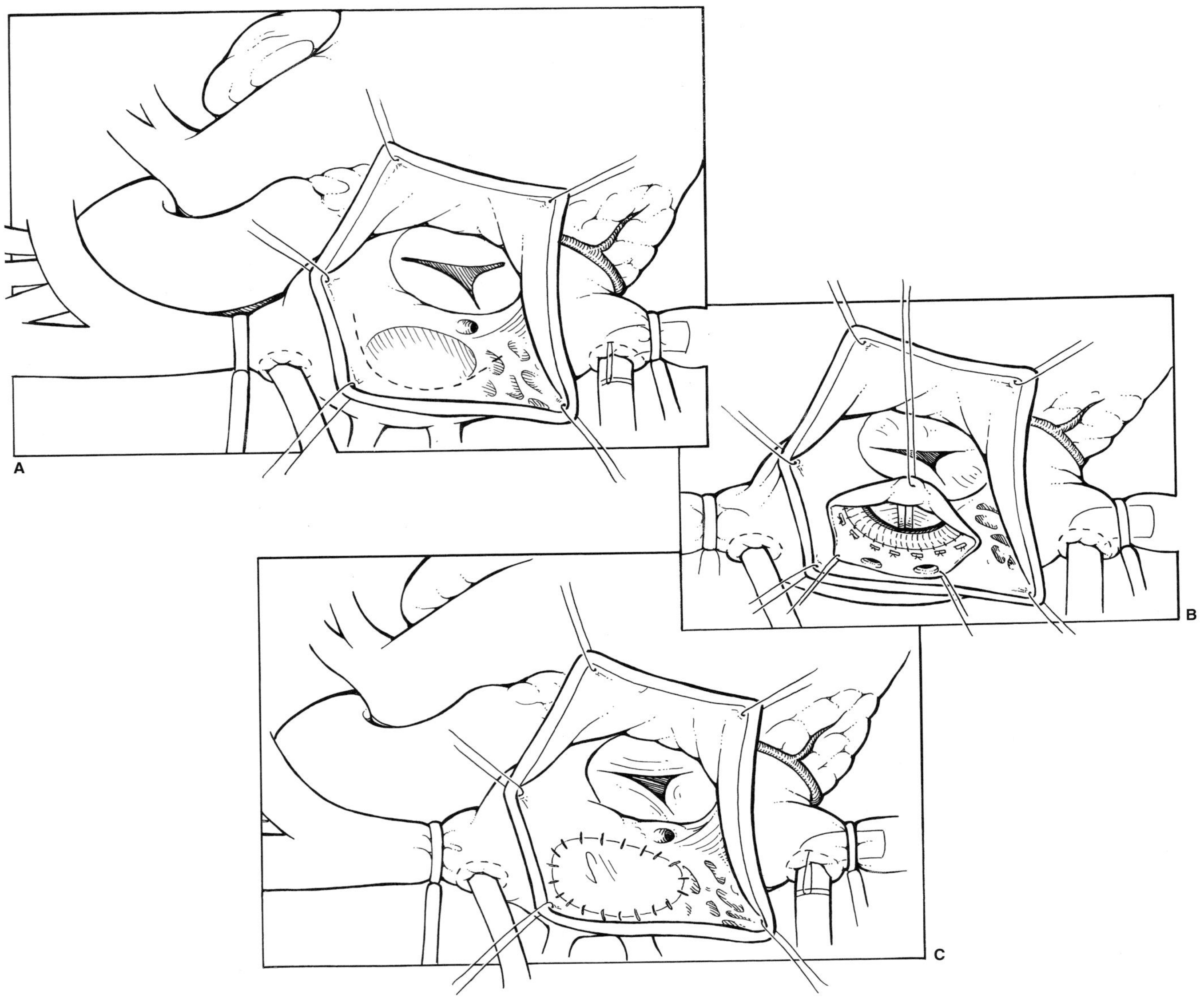

FIGURE 40–2 (A) The superior and inferior vena cava are cannulated, an oblique atriotomy incision is made, and stay sutures are placed on the right atrial wall to aid exposure. For transatrial exposure of the mitral valve, an incision is placed in the fossa ovale and extended superiorly through the interatrial septum. The superior aspect of the septal incision is extended if necessary into the dome of the left atrium behind the aorta. (B) Stay sutures in the interatrial septum are used for retraction. Use of retractors is avoided to prevent injury to the atrioventricular node. The mitral prosthesis is implanted in an antianatomic orientation. (C) The interatrial septum is closed primarily or using a pericardial patch with a continuous 4-0 Prolene suture.

These lesions should always be sutured closed, reducing the possibility of arterial desaturation from right to left shunting or paradoxical embolization.

Bicuspidization

After the caval snares are tightened, the right atrium is opened via an oblique incision. Exposure and assessment of all aspects of the tricuspid valve structure should be performed prior to choosing the technique of annuloplasty. Suture plication to deal with mild dilation of the annulus is accomplished by placing pledgeted mattress sutures from the center of the posterior leaflet to the commissure between the septal and posterior leaflets. A second suture is often necessary to further reduce the annulus, ensuring proper leaflet coaptation while providing an adequate orifice for flow. An annuloplasty ring can be inserted to further support the annular reduction (Fig. 40-3).

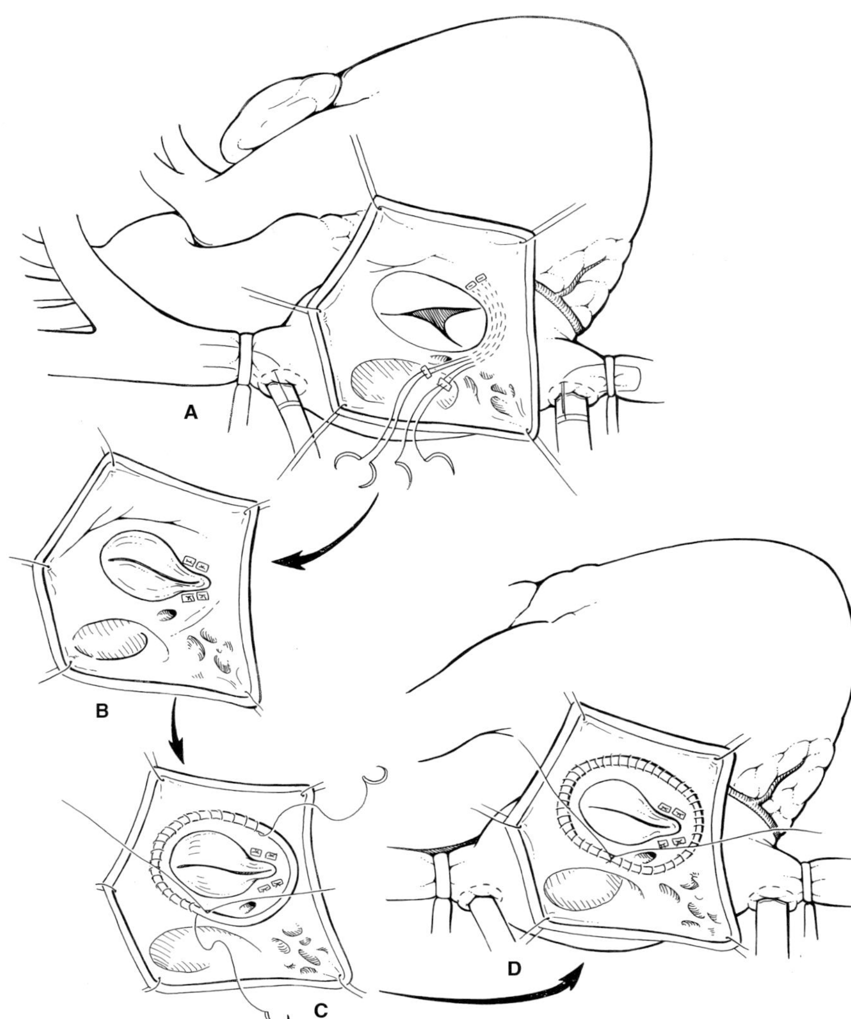

FIGURE 40–3 (A) Tricuspid valve bicuspidization is accomplished by plicating the annulus along the posterior leaflet. Two concentric, pledgeted 2-0 Ethibond sutures are utilized. (B) The sutures are tied, obliterating the posterior leaflet, effectively creating a bicuspid atrioventricular valve. Saline is injected into the right ventricle to test the competency of the repair. (C) As an option to support the bicuspidization repair, a flexible ring may be placed. Prior to ring implantation, measuring the intertrigonal distance chooses the annular size. As an option the ring can be inserted using a continuous 4-0 Prolene suture. Care is taken to avoid the atrioventricular node. As another option, the ring can be implanted above the coronary sinus.

DeVega Technique

The DeVega technique can also be employed for mild to moderate annular dilation.[52] The technique employs a 2-0 Prolene or Dacron polyester suture placed at the junction of the annulus and right ventricular free wall, running from the anterior septal commissure to the posterior septal commissure. The second limb of the suture is placed through a pledget and run parallel and close to the first suture line in the same clockwise direction, placing it through a second pledget at the posterioseptal commissure. The suture is tightened, producing a purse-string effect and reducing the length of the anterior and posterior annulus to provide adequate leaflet coaptation and orifice of flow (Fig. 40-4).

The judgment regarding the degree of annular reduction has varied from the guideline of being able to insert 2-1/2 to 3 fingerbreadths snugly through the valve orifice to using the ring annuloplasty sizers designed for the tricuspid valve. An annuloplasty sizer, chosen by measuring of the intertrigonal distance, can be used as a template while tying the purse-string suture to achieve the proper degree of reduction. The DeVega and suture plication techniques should be reserved for mild annular reductions and situations in which the structural integrity of the annulus is not absolutely necessary for long-term success (i.e., functional tricuspid regurgitation expected to resolve over time). In these situations the annuloplasty provides a competent tricuspid valve during the early postoperative course while the heart remodels after surgical treatment of the left-sided valvular lesions.[63–65]

Rings and Bands

Significant degrees of annular reduction requiring durability are best accomplished with rigid rings (Carpentier-Edwards), flexible rings (i.e., Duran), or flexible bands (i.e., Cosgrove annuloplasty system). The length of the base of the septal leaflet (intertrigonal distance) determines the size

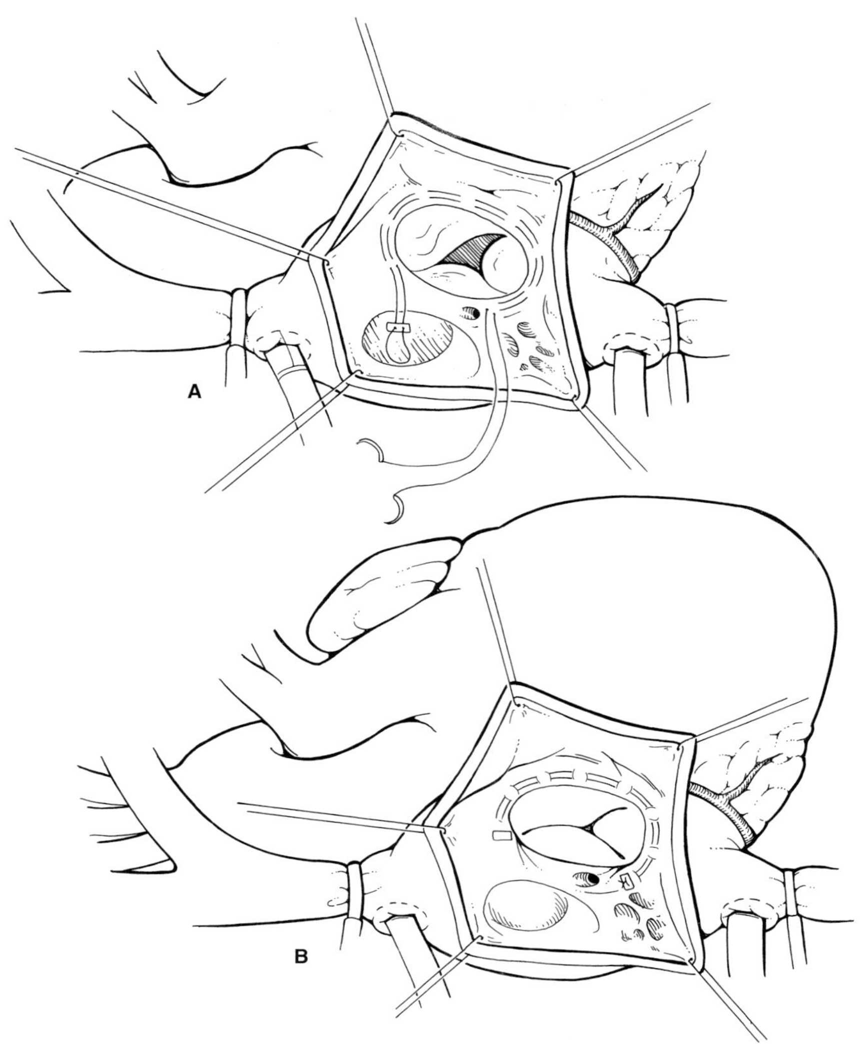

FIGURE 40–4 (A) A modified DeVega annuloplasty technique is shown. A single pledgeted 2-0 Prolene suture is placed. Care is taken to avoid the area of the atrioventricular node. (B) The suture is tied, completing the annuloplasty. Injecting saline into the right ventricle using a bulb syringe tests valve competency.

of the ring or band. These devices avoid suture placement in the region of the AV node (apex of the triangle of Koch) to avoid postoperative conduction problems. The mattress sutures are placed circumferentially, with wider bites on the annulus and smaller corresponding bites through the fabric of the ring or band, producing the annular plication mostly along the length of the posterior leaflet. The result allows the tricuspid valve orifice to be primarily occluded by the leaflet tissue of the anterior and septal leaflets. Overly aggressive annular reduction can lead to ring dehiscence due to excessive tension on the tenuous tricuspid valve tissue (Fig. 40-5).[66–75]

INTRAOPERATIVE ASSESSMENT OF THE REPAIR

Assessment of tricuspid valve competence after the annuloplasty requires filling the right ventricle with saline and observing the leaflet coaptation. This assessment is best performed with the heart beating and the pulmonary artery clamped to allow right ventricular volume to generate enough intracavitary pressure to close the tricuspid valve tightly. If the result appears inadequate, replacement should be performed. Final assessment is by TEE examination after completely weaning from cardiopulmonary bypass with appropriate volume and afterload adjustment.

TRICUSPID VALVE REPLACEMENT

The technique for secure fixation of a tricuspid valve is with pledgeted mattress sutures, using an everting suture technique for mechanical valves and either a supra-annular or an intra-annular everting technique for a bioprosthesis. The tricuspid valve leaflets are left in place, preserving the subvalvular structures and helping to avoid injury to the conduction system (Fig. 40-6)

Tricuspid valve replacement with a homograft is more complicated. The homograft tissue is a mitral valve.[76–79] Sizing is performed by measuring the intratrigonal distances. Fixation of the papillary muscles is either intracavity (right

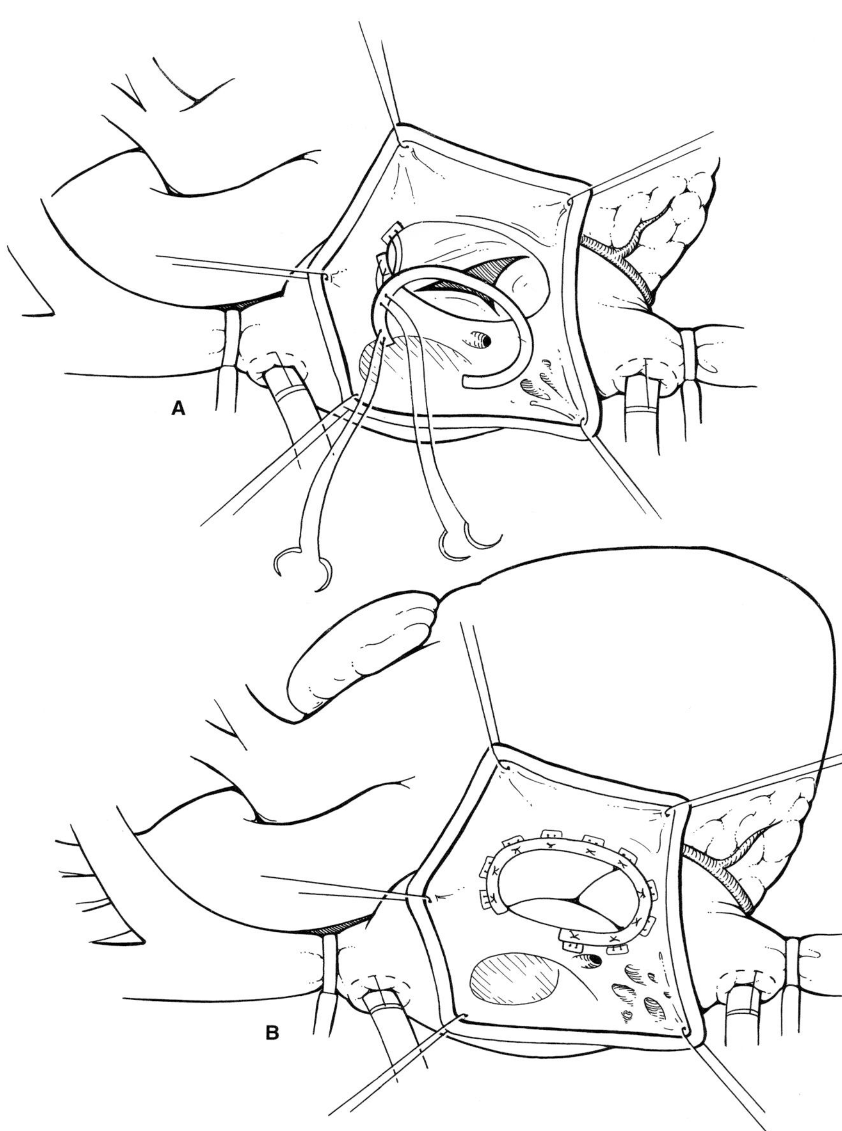

FIGURE 40–5 (A) The Carpentier-Edwards ring annuloplasty is shown. A sizer measuring the intertrigonal distance was utilized to determine the ring size. Multiple interrupted, pledgeted 2-0 Ethibond sutures are placed at the atrioannular junction. All sutures are inserted prior to seating the ring. (B) The valve is seated, and the sutures are tied.

ventricle) or through the wall of the right ventricle. This requires judgment and experience to gauge proper chordal length. The annulus is run with a monofilament suture line. An annuloplasty ring is inserted to prevent dilatation and ensure adequate leaflet coaptation. Special care is necessary in suture placement to avoid conduction disturbances. Suture placement and tying with the heart beating provide immediate detection of rhythm disturbances. Similar to mitral valve replacement, leaflet and chordal preservation should be performed or Gore-Tex suture used as an artificial chorda to maintain annular papillary muscle continuity.

Carpentier techniques for mitral valve repair can be applied to the tricuspid valve. Traumatic disruptions, occasionally endocarditis with healed lesions and perforations, or the rare myxomatous valve can be repaired. Pericardial patching of perforations, partial leaflet resections of the anterior (limited) or posterior (extensive) leaflets, and ring annuloplasty are standard techniques to produce competent valves and avoid replacement.[80–82]

ENDOCARDITIS

Tricuspid valve excision is possible if pulmonary pressures are not elevated and the degree of infection is extensive.[83–91] Blood flows passively through the right heart to the lungs. After eradication of the infection, a second-stage procedure with valve replacement can be performed months to years later when all infection is eradicated. In patients with tricuspid valve endocarditis due to drug addiction, the second-stage valve insertion should be performed preferably after controlling the drug dependence or hopefully curing the accompanying addiction. Late survival and reinfection are directly correlated with continued drug use. Less severe cases

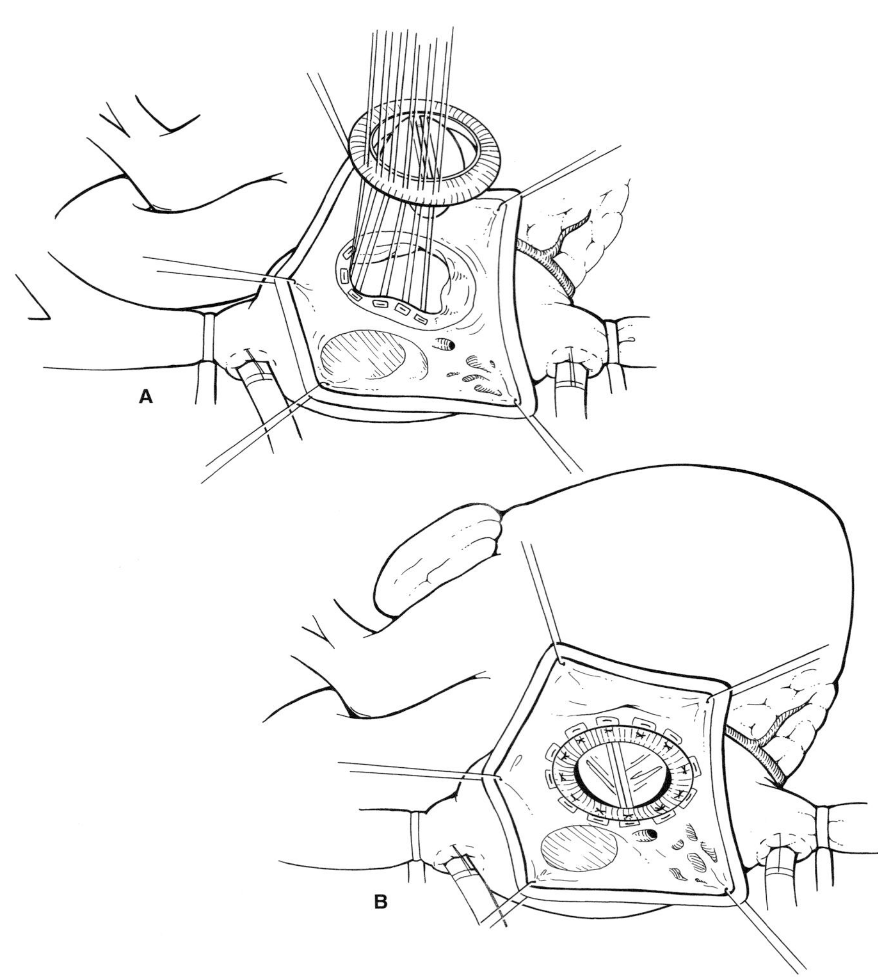

FIGURE 40–6 (A) Tricuspid valve replacement is performed with a St. Jude Medical valve. The native leaflets are left in situ, and the pledgeted 2-0 Ethibond sutures are passed through the annulus and the edges of the leaflets. (B) The valve is seated, and the sutures are tied. The subvalvular apparatus is visualized to ensure that there is no impingement of the prosthetic valve leaflets. The valve can be rotated if necessary to prevent leaflet contact with tissue.

can have one-stage procedures with prosthetic replacement, or localized leaflet excision and repair.[92,93] Homograft tissue is often versatile for partial or total tricuspid valve repair or replacement.

PROSTHETIC VALVE CHOICE

The choice of prosthesis follows an algorithm similar to that used for valve replacement in other cardiac valve positions. The patient's age, anticoagulation considerations, whether the patient is a young woman during her childbearing years, and social issues must be considered. The previously reported poor results with mechanical valves in the tricuspid position were due to valve thrombosis. Most of these reports were during the era of cage-ball and tilting-disc prosthesis.[94] More recent reports with the St. Jude bileaflet valve have provided encouraging data, allowing the surgeon to recommend a mechanical valve with confidence to younger patients who do not have a contraindication to anticoagulation.[95–101] This strategy will avoid the not uncommon situation in the past in which patients received a bioprothesis on the right side and a mechanical prosthesis on the left. Bioprostheses, both porcine and of pericardial tissue, have functioned well in the tricuspid position.[102–105] The data demonstrate a longer duration of freedom from structural valve dysfunction or re-replacement for a bioprosthetic valve in the tricuspid compared to the mitral valve position.[106]

Table 40-1 summarizes multiple reports from the literature. The reports either compare bioprosthetic and mechanical valves in the tricuspid position or follow-up of bioprosthetic valves alone. The bioprostheses, either porcine or pericardial valves, have excellent freedom from degeneration and re-replacement for structural valve degeneration. In 1984, Cohen et al reported on 6 simultaneously implanted and then explanted valves from the mitral and tricuspid position. Degenerative changes were less extensive for the bioprosthetic valve in the tricuspid position than in the mitral position. However, thrombus formation and pannus formation (interpreted as organized thrombotic material) were observed more frequently in the tricuspid position.[106]

Nakano's review of the Carpentier-Edwards pericardial xenograft reported a freedom from structural degeneration

TABLE 40–1 Reports of bioprosthetic and mechanical valves in the tricuspid position

			Operative mortality						Actuarial freedom from								
						Death			Structural degeneration			Nonstructural degeneration			Tricuspid reoperation		
Reference	Series dates	Patients (no.)	Bioprosthesis (B)	Mechanical (M)	Overall (A)	B	M	A	B	M	A	B	M	A	B	M	A
Nakano[98]	1979–92	39		8%			55% @14y		100%			72%				100% @14y	
Nakano[103]	1978–95	98	15%			77% @5y; 69% @10y and 18y			98% @5y 96% @18y			99% @5y 82% @10y 77% @18y*			97% @5y; 76% @10y; 63% @18y		
Ratnatanga[101]	1966–97	425	19%	16%	17%	71% @1y; 62% @5y; 48% @10y	74% 58% 34%	72% 60% 43%							99% @1y; 98% @10y;	98% 97%	
Glower[102]	1972–93	129			27% (14% 1st operation)	56% @5y; 48% @10y; 31% @14y									96% @5y; 93% @10y; 49% @14y		

(*Continued*)

TABLE 40–1 (*Continued*)

Reference	Series dates	Patients (no.)	Operative mortality: Bioprosthesis (B)	Mechanical (M)	Overall (A)	Actuarial freedom from: Death B	Death M	Death A	Structural degeneration B	Structural degeneration M	Structural degeneration A	Nonstructural degeneration B	Nonstructural degeneration M	Nonstructural degeneration A	Tricuspid reoperation B	Tricuspid reoperation M	Tricuspid reoperation A
Ohata[105]	1984–98	88	7%			88% @5y; 81% @10y; 69% @14y			100% @14y			†			88% @14y		
Van Nooton[93]	1967–87	146			16%			74% @5y; 23% @10y									
Singh[96]	1981–84	14		8%			50% @10y										
Munro[99]	1975–92	94	15%	14%	14%				97% @5, 7y, and 10y	100%					97%	87%	
Kaplan[94]	1980–2000	122			25%	55% @20y	68% @20y	65% @20y	90% @20y	97%‡ @20y							
Scully[95]	1975–93	60			27%		50% @15y										

*Thick fibrous pannus in 35% of survivors; freedom from nonstructural valve dysfunction at 18 y = 24%.

†Thick pannus noted in reoperative case.

‡Freedom from deterioration, endocarditis, leakage, and thromboembolism 93% @20 y.

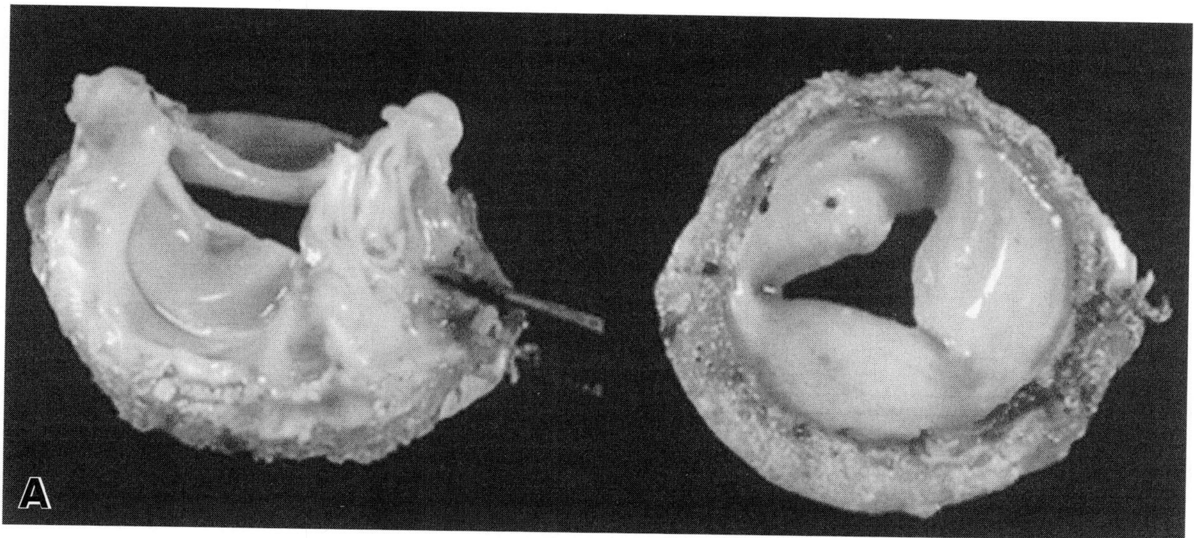

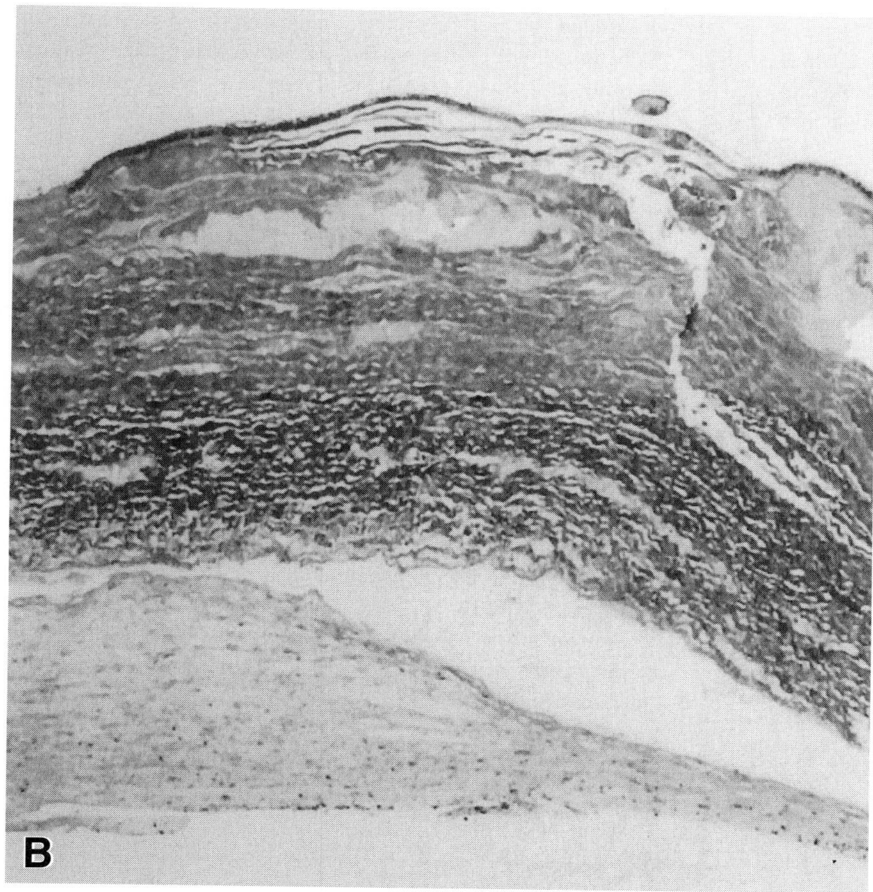

FIGURE 40–7 (A) Fibrous pannus observed 8 years after implantation of a Carpentier-Edwards pericardial valve. (B) Photomicrograph of a pericardial leaflet. The bottom of the leaflet has pannus, a dense fibrous tissue on the ventricular side. (*Reprinted with permission from the Society of Thoracic Surgeons. Nakano K, Ishibashi-Ueda H, Kobayashi J, et al: Tricuspid valve replacement with bioprostheses: long-term results and causes of valve dysfunction. Ann Thor Surg 2001; 71:105.*)

of 100% at 9 years but nonstructural dysfunction was 72.8%. The cause of nonstructural dysfunction was pannus formation on the ventricular side of the cusps. This finding is often subclinical. Echocardiographic follow-up revealed a 35% incidence of this anatomic finding in patients with at least 5 years of follow-up.[104] Guerra reported similar changes in simultaneously explanted porcine valves. The tricuspid position had less structural tissue degeneration and calcification than the mitral. The report described the presence of pannus formation on the ventricular side of the cusps in tricuspid porcine valves. The pannus interfered with cuspal pliability and function.[107]

Nakano's 2001 report of bioprosthetic tricuspid valves reported an 18-year freedom from reoperation of 63%.[103] The freedom from structural deterioration was 96%, and nonstructural dysfunction was 77%. Reoperation replacing previously placed bioprosthetic valves occurred in 12 of 58 survivors. In 6 of the 12 patients, the primary indication for reoperation was tricuspid dysfunction, and 7 of the 12 had pannus formation on the ventricular side of the cusps (Fig. 40-7). This rate of degeneration and the subclinically high incidence of pannus formation, often eventually leading to reoperation, are major concerns. Tricuspid bioprosthetic valves require echocardiographic follow-up. Possible anticoagulation of bioprosthetic valves in the tricuspid position can reduce the incidence of pannus formation. The reported data in the literature categorize this pannus formation as nonstructural degeneration; therefore, clinical surgeons should be aware of future reports following this potentially serious clinical problem.

In the tricuspid position it is always possible to place large bioprosthetic or mechanical valves. Prostheses with more than a 27-mm internal diameter do not have clinically significant gradients. Therefore hemodynamic performance is rarely an issue for tricuspid valve replacement. The data demonstrate excellent results with modern bileaflet mechanical valves. Series comparing bioprosthetic and mechanical valves have been consistent in demonstrating equality during the period of follow-up. The development of thrombus on a bileaflet valve can be successfully treated with thrombolysis.

Some patients with mitral valve disease undergoing surgery with tricuspid regurgitation do not require surgical treatment of the tricuspid valve. Guidelines to identify these patients are poorly developed. Experience has shown that careful observation of the patient preoperatively is quite valuable. Absence of tricuspid valve regurgitation during periods of good medical control, absence of tricuspid regurgitation by transesophageal echo (TEE) at the time of operation, minimal elevation of pulmonary vascular resistance, and absence of right atrial enlargement are helpful findings permitting the surgeon to confidently replace the mitral valve without performing an annuloplasty or replacement of the tricuspid valve. If left unrepaired, reassessment of the tricuspid valve by TEE after weaning from cardiopulmonary bypass (CPB) is essential.

Temporary right ventricular dysfunction due to right coronary air embolism often requires a brief return to CPB, repeat of air maneuvers, elevation of the blood pressure, TEE evaluation for residual intra-cavity air, and search for the characteristic echogenic brightness in the myocardial distribution of the right coronary artery confirming the suspicion of air embolism. Treatment should include 10 to 15 minutes of cardiopulmonary bypass (CPB) support and reweaning from CPB, with inotropic support for right ventricular dysfunction and reassessment of the tricuspid regurgitation and cardiac function. If tricuspid regurgitation persists and elevated right atrial pressures greater than the left atrial pressures are encountered with an underfilled well-contracting left ventricle, tricuspid repair should be performed. A patent foramen ovalae with interatrial shunting needs to be identified and surgically closed. Hemodynamically, when right atrial pressure is greater than left atrial pressure, the foramen may open, leading to systemic desaturation from a right to left shunt.

RESULTS

Clinical experience has demonstrated that up to 20% of patients undergoing mitral valve replacement receive a tricuspid annuloplasty but less than 2% require replacement. The surgeon's clinical judgment and experience guide the approach to tricuspid valve surgery and ultimately lead to variability in reported clinical data. The accuracy of the judgments can be guided by assessment of the risk factors for persistent or progressive tricuspid valve regurgitation. They are related to unresolved or recurrent mitral valve pathology, the degree of preoperative tricuspid regurgitation or the misjudgment of its severity, failure of the pulmonary hypertension and pulmonary vascular resistance to resolve, resulting in persistent impairment in right ventricular function (often with right ventricular dilatation), and failure to recognize organic tricuspid valve disease.

Patients undergoing a tricuspid valve annuloplasty during a mitral valve replacement have more advanced disease than those having mitral valve replacement alone. This is evidenced by the elevation in operative mortality (approximately 12% vs. 3%) and the progressive increased hazard of late death (5-year survival of 80% vs. 70%) in spite of good valve function. However, these patients achieved good functional results (class 1-2). It is unknown what the survival and functional result would have been if tricuspid repair had not been performed in these patients, but one presumes it would have been worse.

The durability of simple annuloplasty techniques such as bicuspidization and the DeVega has been good when employed only for mild to moderate degrees of functional tricuspid regurgitation with successful resolution of pulmonary hypertension after the mitral valve operation. Extensive experience with the tricuspid annuloplasty using the Duran, Carpentier-Edwards, or Cosgrove rings or bands resulted in an 85% freedom from moderate to severe tricuspid regurgitation at 6 years. The subsequent requirement for tricuspid reoperation is very low. Inadequate resolution of the mitral disease and persistent pulmonary hypertension with right ventricular dilation and dysfunction are the major predictors of poor late results.

Patients requiring tricuspid and mitral replacement have operative mortalities from 5% to 10% by current standards. Actuarial survival rates are 55% at 10 years. Advanced right ventricular failure or arrhythmia causes late death. Patients who need valve replacement for endocarditis comprise a unique subgroup with the additional risk for death due to sepsis, reinfection, and the complications related to drug addiction.

Complete heart block can occur immediately postoperatively due to damage to the conduction system during mitral and tricuspid valve surgery. This complication can be minimized intraoperatively by performing the tricuspid valve procedure on the perfused beating heart as described earlier. Late heart block remains a persistent risk with a 25% actuarial incidence at 10 years for patients with mitral and tricuspid prostheses.[108] Late development of heart block rarely occurs after mitral valve replacement and tricuspid annuloplasty. The presence of two rigid prosthetic sewing rings can produce ongoing trauma and lead to atrioventricular node dysfunction over time.

The surgical treatment of tricuspid valve disease presents the surgeon with challenges requiring clinical and intraoperative judgment. Following the guidelines presented in this chapter for when to repair or replace the tricuspid valve should lead to optional clinical outcome. The data support the safe use of mechanical bileaflet prostheses. A lingering concern is the pannus formation on the ventricular side of bioprosthetic cusps. This observation should be followed closely as future clinical series are reported.

REFERENCES

1. Starr A, Herr R, Wood J: Tricuspid replacement for acquired valve disease. *Surg Gynecol Obstet* 1966; 122:1295
2. Bigelow JC, Herr RH, Wood JA, et al: Multiple valve replacement: review of five years' experience. *Circulation* 1968; 38:656.
3. Braunwald NS, Ross J, Morrow AG: Conservation management of tricuspid regurgitation in patients undergoing mitral valve replacement. *Circulation* 1967; 35-36(suppl):1–63.
4. Kay GL, Morita S, Mendez M, et al: Tricuspid regurgitation associated with mitral valve disease: repair and replacement. *Ann Thorac Surg* 1989; 48–593.
5. Chan P, Igilby JD, Segal B: Tricuspid valve endocarditis. *Am Heart J* 1988; 117:1140.
6. Van Son JAM, Danielson GK, Schaff HV, et al: Traumatic tricuspid valve insufficiency. *J Thorac Cardiovasc Surg* 1994; 108:893.
7. Collins P, Daly JJ: Tricuspid incompetence complicating acute myocardial infarction. *Postgrad Med J* 1977; 53:51.
8. DiSesa VJ, Mills RM, Collins JJ: Surgical management of carcinoid heart disease. *Chest* 1985; 88:789.
9. Asmar BE, Acker M, Couetil JP, et al: Tricuspid valve myxoma: a rare indication for tricuspid valve repair. *Ann Thorac Surg* 1991; 52:1315.
10. Sackner MA, Heinz ER, Steinberg AJ: The heart in scleroderma. *Am J Cardiol* 1966; 1:542.
11. Solley GO, Maldonado JE, Gleich GJ, et al: Endomyocardiopathy with eosinophilia. *Mayo Clin Proc* 1976; 51:697.
12. Mason JW, Billingham ME, Friedman JP: Methysergide induced heart disease: a case of multivalvular and myocardial fibrosis. *Circulation* 1977; 56:889.
13. Cohen ST, Sell JE, McIntosh CL, et al: Tricuspid regurgitation in patients with acquired, chronic, pure mitral regurgitation, I: prevalence, diagnosis, and comparison of preoperative clinical and hemodynamic features in patients with and without tricuspid regurgitation. *J Thorac Cardiovasc Surg* 1987; 94:481
14. Cohen SR, Sell JE, McIntosh CL, et al: Tricuspid regurgitation in patients with acquired, chronic, pure mitral regurgitation, II: nonoperative management, tricuspid valve annuloplasty, and tricuspid valve replacement. *J Thorac Cardiovasc Surg* 1987; 94:488.
15. Silver M.D., Lam JHC, Ranganathan, et al: Morphology of the human tricuspid valve. *Circulation* 1971; 53:333.
16. Tsakiris AG, Mair DD, Seki S, et al: Motion of the tricuspid valve annulus in anesthetized intact dogs. *Circulation* 1975; 36:43.
17. Tei C, Pilgrim JP, Shah PM, et al: The tricuspid valve annulus; study of size and motion in normal subjects and in patients with tricuspid regurgitation. *Circulation* 1982; 66:665.
18. Ubago JL, Figueroa A, Ochotcco A, et al: Analysis of the amount of tricuspid valve annular dilation required to produce functional tricuspid regurgitation. *Am J Cardiol* 1983; 52:155.
19. Come PC, Riley MF: Tricuspid annular dilatation and failure of tricuspid leaflet coaptation in tricuspid regurgitation. *Am J Cardiol* 1985; 55:599.
20. Waller BF, Moriarty AT, Able JN, et al: Etiology of pure tricuspid regurgitation based on annular circumference and leaflet area: analysis of 45 necropsy patients with clinical and morphologic evidence of pure tricuspid regurgitation. *J Am Coll Cardiol* 1986; 7:1063.
21. Miller MJ, McKay RG, Ferguson JJ, et al: Right atrial pressure-volume relationships in tricuspid regurgitation. *Circulation* 1986; 73:799.
22. Morrison DA, Ovit T, Hammermeister KE, et al: Functional tricuspid regurgitation and right ventricular dysfunction in pulmonary hypertension. *Am J Cardiol* 1988; 62:108.
23. Atbulu A, Holmes RJ, Asfaw I: Surgical treatment of intractable right-sided infective endocarditis in drug addicts: 25 years experience. *J Heart Valve Dis* 1993; 2:129.
24. Carrel T, Schaffner A, Vogt P, et al: Endocarditis in intravenous drug addicts and HIV infected patients: possibilities and limitation of surgical treatment. *J Heart Valve Dis* 1993; 2:140.
25. Bayer AS, Blomquist IK, Bello E, et al: Tricuspid valve endocarditis due to *Staphylococcus aureus*. *Chest* 1988; 93:247.
26. Tanaka M, Abe T, Hosokawa ST, et al: Tricuspid valve *Candida* endocarditis cured by valve-sparing debridement. *Ann Thorac Surg* 1989; 48:857.
27. Robiolio PA, Rigolin VH, Harrison JK, et al: Predictors of outcome of tricuspid valve replacement in carcinoid heart disease. *Am J Cardiol* 1995, 75:485.
28. Ohri SK, Schofield JB, Hodgson H, et al: Carcinoid heart disease: early failure of an allograft valve replacement. *Ann Thorac Surg* 1994; 58:1161.
29. Lundin I, Norheim I, Landelius J, et al: Carcinoid heart disease: relationship of circulating vasoactive substances to ultrasound-detectable cardiac abnormalities. *Circulation* 1988; 77:264.
30. Fujii S, Funaki K, Denzunn N: Isolated rheumatic tricuspid regurgitation and stenosis. *Clin Cardiol* 1966; 9:353.
31. Cha SD, Desai BS, Gooch AS, et al: Diagnosis of severe tricuspid regurgitation. *Chest* 1982; 82:726.
32. Brown AK, Anderson V: The value of contrast cross-sectional echocardiography in the diagnosis of tricuspid regurgitation. *Eur Heart J* 1984; 5:62.
33. Wilkins GT, Gillam LD, Kutzer GI, et al: Validation of continuous-wave Doppler echocardiography measurements of mitral and tricuspid prosthetic valve gradients: a simultaneous Doppler-catheter study. *Circulation* 1986; 74:786.
34. Child JS: Improved guides to tricuspid valve repair: two-dimensional echocardiographic analysis of tricuspid annulus function and color flow imaging of severity of tricuspid regurgitation. *J Am Coll Cardiol* 1989; 14:1275.

35. Chopra HK, Nanda NC, Fan P, et al: Can two-dimensional echocardiography and Doppler color flow mapping identify the need for tricuspid valve repair? *J Am Coll Cardiol* 1989; 14:1266.
36. Fisher EA, Goldman ME: Simple, rapid method for quantification of tricuspid regurgitation by two-dimensional echocardiography. *Am J Cardiol* 1989; 3:1375.
37. Wong M, Matsumura M, Kutsuzawa S, et al: The value of Doppler echocardiography in the treatment of tricuspid regurgitation in patients with mitral valve replacement. *J Thorac Cardiovasc Surg* 1990; 99:1003.
38. Goldman ME, Guarino I, Foster V, et al: The necessity for tricuspid valve repair can be determined intraoperatively by two-dimensional echocardiography. *J Thorac Cardiovasc Surg* 1987; 94:542.
39. Czer LSC, Maurer G, Bolger A, et al: Tricuspid valve repair, operative and follow-up evaluation by Doppler color flow mapping. *J Thorac Cardiovasc Surg* 1989; 98:101.
40. DeSimone R, Lange R, Saggau W, et al: Intraoperative transesophageal echocardiography for the evaluation of mutual, aortic and tricuspid valve repair. *Eur J Cardiothorac Surg* 1992; 6:665.
41. Maurer G, Siegel RJ, Czer LSC: The use of color flow mapping for intraoperative assessment of valve repair. *Circulation* 1991; 84(suppl I):I-250.
42. DeSimone R, Lange R, Lanzeem A, et al: Adjustable tricuspid valve annuloplasty assisted by intraoperative transesophageal color Doppler echocardiography. *Am J Cardiol* 1993; 71:926.
43. McGrath LB, Chen C, Bailey B, et al: Determination of the need for tricuspid valve replacement: value of preoperative right ventricular angiocardiography. *J Invas Cardiol* 1991; 3:21.
44. Gibson R, Wood P: The diagnosis of tricuspid stenosis. *Br Heart J* 1955; 17:552.
45. Keefe JF, Wolk MJ, Levine HJ: Isolated tricuspid valvular stenosis. *Am J Cardiol* 1970; 25:252.
46. Shore D, Rigby MI, Lincoln C: Severe tricuspid stenosis presenting as tricuspid atresia: echocardiography diagnosis and surgical management. *Br Heart J* 1982; 48:404.
47. Roberts WC, Sullivan MF; Combined mitral valve stenosis and tricuspid valve stenosis: morphologic observations after mitral and tricuspid valve replacements or mitral replacement and tricuspid valve commissurotomy. *Am J Cardiol* 1986; 58:850.
48. McGrath LB, Gonzalez-Lavin L, Bailey BM, et al: Tricuspid valve operations in 530 patients. *J Thorac Cardiovasc Surg* 1990; 99:124.
49. Kay JH, Mendez AM, Zubiate P: A further look at tricuspid annuloplasty. *Ann Thorac Surg* 1976; 22:498.
50. Simon R, Oelert H, Borst HG, et al: Influence of mitral valve surgery on tricuspid incompetence concomitant with mitral valve disease. *Circulation* 1980; 62(suppl I):I-152.
51. King RM, Schaff HV, Danielson GK, et al: Surgery for tricuspid regurgitation late after mitral valve replacement. *Circulation* 1984;70(suppl):I-193.
52. Cohn L: Tricuspid regurgitation secondary to mitral valve disease: when and how to repair. *J Card Surg* 1994; (suppl):237.
53. Breyer RH, McClenathan JH, Michaelis LL, et al: Tricuspid regurgitation: a comparison of nonoperative management, tricuspid annuloplasty and tricuspid valve replacement. *J Thorac Cardiovasc Surg* 1976; 72:867.
54. Duran CMG, Pomar JL, Colman T, et al: Is tricuspid valve repair necessary? *J Thorac Cardiovasc Surg* 1980; 80:849.
55. Carpentier A, Deloche A, Hanania G, et al: Surgical management of acquired tricuspid valve disease. *J Thorac Cardiovasc Surg* 1974; 67:53.
56. Boyd AD, Engelman RM, Isom OW, et al: Tricuspid annuloplasty: five and one-half years' experience with 78 patients. *J Thorac Cardiovasc Surg* 1974; 68:344
57. Kay JH, Mendez AM, Zubiate P: A further look at tricuspid annuloplasty. *Ann Thorac Surg* 1976; 22:498.
58. Haerten K, Seipel L, Loogen F, et al: Hemodynamic studies after DeVega's tricuspid annuloplasty. *Circulation* 1978; 58(suppl): I-28.
59. Yousof AM, Shafei MZ, Endrys G, et al: Tricuspid stenosis and regurgitation in rheumatic heart disease: a prospective cardiac catheterization study in 525 patients. *Am Heart J* 1985; 110:60.
60. Kratz JM, Crawford FA, Stroud MR, et al: Trends and results in tricuspid valve surgery. *Chest* 1985; 88:837.
61. Sullivan MF, Roberts WC: Mitral valve stenosis and pure tricuspid valve regurgitation: comparison of necropsy patients having simultaneous mitral and tricuspid valve replacements with necropsy patients having simultaneous mitral valve replacement and tricuspid valve annuloplasty. *Am J Cardiol* 1986; 58:768.
62. Abe T, Tukamoto M, Yanagiya M, et al: DeVega's annuloplasty for acquired tricuspid disease: early and late results in 110 patients. *Ann Thorac Surg* 1989; 48:670.
63. Duran CM, Kumar N, Prabhakar G, et al: Vanishing DeVega annuloplasty for functional tricuspid regurgitation. *J Thorac Cardiovasc Surg* 1993; 106:609.
64. Chidambaram M, Abdulali SA, Baliga BG, et al: Long-term results of DeVega tricuspid annuloplasty. *Ann Thorac Surg* 1987; 43:185.
65. Carpentier A, Deloche A, Dauptain J, et al: A new reconstructive operation for correction of mitral and tricuspid insufficiency. *J Thorac Cardiovasc Surg* 1971; 61:1.
66. Grondin P, Meere C, Limet R, et al: Carpentier's annulus and DeVega's annuloplasty. *J Thorac Cardiovasc Surg* 1975; 70:852.
67. Brugger JJ, Egloff L, Rothlin M, et al: Tricuspid annuloplasty: results and complications. *Thorac Cardiovasc Surg* 1982; 30:284.
68. Autunes MJ, Girdwood RW: Tricuspid annuloplasty: a modified technique. *Ann Thorac Surg* 1983; 35:676.
69. Henze A, Peterffy A, Orinius I: The adjustable half-moon: an alternative device for tricuspid annuloplasty. *Scand J Thorac Cardiovasc Surg* 1984; 18:29.
70. Nakano S, Kawashima Y, Huose H, et al: An effective adjunct to tricuspid annuloplasty. *Ann Thorac Surg* 1984; 18:68.
71. Rivera R, Duran E, Ajuria M, et al: Carpentier's flexible ring versus DeVega's annuloplasty. *J Thorac Cardiovasc Surg* 1985; 89:196.
72. Bex JP, Lecompte LY: Tricuspid valve repair using a flexible linear reducer. *J Card Surg* 1986; I:151.
73. Rabago G, Fraile J, Martinell J, et al: Technique and results of tricuspid annuloplasty. *J Card Surg* 1986; I:247.
74. Gatti G, Maffei G, Lusa A, et al: Tricuspid valve repair with Cosgrove-Edwards annuloplasty system: early clinical and echocardiographic results. *Ann Thorac Surg* 2001; 72:764.
75. Kurlansky P, Rose EA, Malm JR: Adjustable annuloplasty for tricuspid insufficiency. *Ann Thorac Surg* 1987; 44:404.
76. Pomar JI, Mestres C: Tricuspid valve replacement using a mitral homograft surgical technique and initial results. *J Heart Valve Dis* 1993; 2:125.
77. Pomar JI, Mestres CA, Pate JC, et al: Management of persistent tricuspid endocarditis with transplantation of cryopreserved mitral homografts. *J Thorac Cardiovasc Surg* 1994; 107:1460.
78. Hvass U, Baron F, Fourchy D, et al: Mitral homografts for total tricuspid valve replacement: comparison of two techniques. *J Thorac Cardiovasc Surg* 2001; 3:592.
79. Katz NM, Pallas RS: Traumatic rupture of the tricuspid valve: repair by chordal replacements and annuloplasty. *J Thorac Cardiovasc Surg* 1986; 91:310.
80. Sutlic Z, Schmid C, Borst HG: Repair of flail anterior leaflets of tricuspid and mitral valves by cusp remodeling. *Ann Thorac Cardiovasc Surg* 1990; 50:927.
81. Doty JR, Cameron DE, Elmaci T, et al: Penetrating trauma to the tricuspid valve and ventricular septum: delayed repair. *Ann Thorac Surg* 1999; 67:252.

82. Arbulu A, Asfaw I: Tricuspid valvulectomy without prosthetic replacement. *J Thorac Cardiovasc Surg* 1981; 82:684.
83. Arbulu A, Thoms NW, Wilson RI: Valvulectomy without prosthetic replacement: a lifesaving operation for tricuspid *Pseudomonas* endocarditis. *J Cardiovasc Surg* 1972; 74:103.
84. Lai D, Chard RB: Commissuroplasty: a method of valve repair for mitral and tricuspid endocarditis. *Ann Thorac Surg* 1999; 68:1727.
85. Walther T, Falk V, Schneider J, et al: Stentless tricuspid valve replacement. *Ann Thorac Surg* 1999; 68:1858.
86. Arneborn P, Bjork VO, Rodriquez I, et al: Two-stage replacement of tricuspid valve in active endocarditis. *Br Heart J* 1977; 39:1276.
87. Wright JS, Glennie JS: Excision of tricuspid valve with later replacement in endocarditis of drug addition. *Thorax* 1978; 33:518.
88. Sethia B, Williams BI: Tricuspid valve excision without replacement in a case of endocarditis secondary to drug abuse. *Br Heart J* 1978; 40:579.
89. Arbulu A, Holmes RJ, Asfaw I: Tricuspid valvulectomy without replacement: twenty years' experience. *J Thorac Cardiovasc Surg* 1991; 102:917.
90. Yee ES, Khonsari S: Right-sided infective endocarditis: valvuloplasty, valvectomy or replacement. *J Cardiovasc Surg* 1989; 30:744.
91. Evora PRBK, Brasil JCF, Elias MLC, at al: Surgical excision of the vegetation as treatment of tricuspid valve endocarditis. *Cardiology* 1988; 74:287.
92. Turley K: Surgery of right-sided endocarditis: valve preservation versus replacement. *J Card Surg* 1989; 4:317.
93. Van Nooten G, Caes F, Tacymans Y, et al: Tricuspid valve replacement: postoperative and long-term results. *J Thorac Cardiovasc Surg* 1995; 110:672.
94. Kaplan M, Kut MS, Demirtas MM, et al: Prosthetic replacement of tricuspid valve: bioprosthetic or mechanical. *Ann Thorac Surg* 2002; 73:467.
95. Scully HE, Armstrong CS: Tricuspid valve replacement: fifteen years of experience with mechanical prostheses and bioprostheses. *J Thorac Cardiovasc Surg* 1995; 109:1035.
96. Singh AK, Feng WC, Sanofsky SJ: Long-term results of St. Jude Medical valve in the tricuspid position. *Ann Thorac Surg* 1992; 54:538.
97. Kaplan M, Kut MS, Demirtas MM, et al: Prosthetic replacement of tricuspid valve: bioprosthetic or mechanical. *Ann Thorac Surg* 2002; 73:467.
98. Nakano K, Koyanagi H, Hashimoto A, et al: Tricuspid valve replacement with the bileaflet St. Jude Medical valve prosthesis. *J Thorac Cardiovasc Surg* 1994; 108:888.
99. Munro AI, Jamieson WRE, Tyers FO, et al: Tricuspid valve replacement: porcine bioprostheses and mechanical prostheses. *Ann Thorac Surg* 1995; 59:S470.
100. Ohata T, Kigawa I, Tohda E, et al: Comparison of durability of bioprostheses in tricuspid and mitral positions. *Ann Thorac Surg* 2001; 71:S240.
101. Ratnatunga C, Edwards M-B, Dore C, et al: Tricuspid valve replacement: UK heart valve registry mid-term results comparing mechanical and biological prostheses. *Ann Thorac Surg* 1998; 66:1940.
102. Glower DD, White WD, Smith LR, et al: In-hospital and long-term outcome after porcine tricuspid valve replacement. *J Thorac Cardiovasc Surg* 1995; 109:877.
103. Nakano K, Ishibashi-Ueda H, Kobayashi J, et al: Tricuspid valve replacement with bioprostheses: long-term results and causes of valve dysfunction. *Ann Thorac Surg* 2001; 71:105.
104. Nakano K, Eishi K, Kosakai Y, et al: Ten-year experience with the Carpentier-Edwards pericardial xenograft in the tricuspid position. *J Thorac Cardiovasc Surg* 1996; 111:605.
105. Ohata T, Kigawa I, Yamashita Y, et al: Surgical strategy for severe tricuspid valve regurgitation complicated by advanced mitral valve disease: long-term outcome of tricuspid valve supra-annular implantation in eighty-eight cases. *J Thorac Cardiovasc Surg* 2000; 120:280.
106. Cohen SR, Silver MA, McIntosh CL, Roberts WC: Comparison of late (62 to 104 months) degenerative changes in simultaneously implanted and explanted porcine (Hancock) bioprosthesis in the tricuspid and mitral positions in six patients. *Am J Cardiol* 1984; 53:1599.
107. Guerra F, Bortolotti U, Thiene G, et al: Long-term performance of the Hancock porcine bioprosthesis in the tricuspid position: a review of 45 patients with 14 visit follow-up. *J Thorac Cardiovasc Surg* 1990; 99:838.
108. Kirklin JW, Barratt-Boyes BG (eds): *Cardiac Surgery*, Vol. 1, 2d ed. New York, Churchill Livingstone, 1992; p 598.

Chapter 41

Multiple Valve Disease

Hartzell V. Schaff/Dale H. Marsh

Pathologic changes in the cardiac valves requiring surgical correction of more than one valve can result from rheumatic heart disease, degenerative valve diseases, infective endocarditis, and a number of miscellaneous causes. Further, valve dysfunction may be primary, i.e., a direct result of a disease process, or secondary, caused by cardiac enlargement and/or pulmonary hypertension. Surgical management is influenced both by the underlying cause of valve dysfunction and, when valves are secondarily involved, the anticipated response to replacement or repair of the primary valve lesion. In addition, the consequences of various combinations of diseased valves on left and right ventricular geometry and function frequently are different from the remodeling as a result of single valve disease. This chapter addresses pathophysiologic considerations in multivalvular heart disease, surgical techniques, and management of commonly encountered etiologies.

Repair of multiple lesions was necessary even in the early development of operative management of valvular heart disease (Table 41-1). The first triple valve replacement during a single operation was reported in 1960, and simultaneous replacement of all four valves was reported in 1992.[1,2]

Experience from clinical practice indicates that multiple valve disease requiring surgical correction occurs in a few common combinations. As seen in Table 41-2, multiple procedures account for approximately 15% of all operations on cardiac valves; 80% of these operations involve the aortic and mitral positions. Replacement of the mitral and tricuspid valves (with or without aortic replacement) accounts for 20% of operations. Only rarely is the combination of aortic and tricuspid disease encountered.

TABLE 41–1 History of multiple valve operations

Event	Year	Institution
Staged mitral then tricuspid commissurotomy	1952	Doctor's Hospital Philadelphia, PA[165]
Simultaneous mitral and tricuspid commissurotomy	1953	Cleveland, OH[166]
Simultaneous mitral commissurotomy and aortic valvuloplasty using cardiopulmonary bypass	1956	University of Minnesota Minneapolis, MN[167]
Simultaneous mitral and aortic valve replacement	1961	St. Francis General Hospital Pittsburgh, PA[129]
Simultaneous triple valve replacement	1963	University of Oregon Portland, OR
Simultaneous quadruple valve replacement	1992	Mayo Clinic Rochester, MN[126]

Source: Modified with permission from Acker M, Hargrove WC, Stephenson LW: Multiple valve replacement. Cardiol Clin 1985; 3:425.

PATHOPHYSIOLOGY OF MULTIPLE VALVE DISEASE

Valvular regurgitation may result from the pathologic process affecting the valve directly or may be secondary to alterations in ventricular morphology caused by other valve lesions; this secondary or functional regurgitation affects the atrioventricular valves. In some patients, secondary valvular regurgitation may be expected to improve with repair or replacement of the primarily diseased valve. In other patients, the secondary disease process may have advanced to the stage that valve function will not improve following correction of the primary lesion, and thus simultaneous surgical correction should be considered.

Primary Aortic Valve Disease with Secondary Mitral Regurgitation

Isolated aortic valve lesions can cause secondary regurgitation of the mitral valve and, rarely, of the tricuspid valve.

TABLE 41–2 Prevalence of multiple cardiac valve replacement according to institution

	University of Alabama	Mayo Clinic	Texas Heart Institute	University of Oregon	Percentage of all valve surgery (11,026 cases)	Percentage of multiple valve surgery (1662 cases)
Years involved	1967–1976	1963–1972	1962–1974	1960–1980		
Total number of all valve operations	2555	2166	4170	2135		
All multiple valve procedures	383 (15%)	437 (20%)	541 (13%)	301 (14%)	15 (1662)	100
M-A	298 (11.6%)	320 (14.7%)	459 (11%)	253 (11.8%)	12 (1330)	80
M-A-T	40 (1.6%)	55 (2.5%)	55 (2.5%)	48 (2.2%)	2 (198)	12
M-T	41 (1.6%)	58 (2.5%)	26 (0.6%)	—	1.5 (125)	8
A-T	4 (0.1%)	4 (0.2%)	1 (0.02%)	—	0.1 (9)	5

M = mitral valve; A = aortic valve; T = tricuspid valve.

Source: Modified with permission from Acker M, Hargrove WC, Stephenson LW: Multiple valve replacement. Cardiol Clin 1985; 3:425.

Severe aortic valve stenosis with or without left ventricular dilatation is frequently associated with some degree of mitral valve regurgitation. In one series, 67% of patients with severe aortic valve stenosis had associated mitral valve leakage.[3]

When the mitral valve is structurally normal, its regurgitation would be expected to improve with relief of left ventricular outflow obstruction[4]; mild mitral valve regurgitation would be expected to resolve almost completely following aortic valve replacement. Improvement in mitral valve regurgitation results both from decreased intraventricular pressure and ventricular remodeling.[5] If mitral valve regurgitation is severe, some degree of persistent regurgitation is expected following aortic valve replacement, and mitral valve annuloplasty may be required. In contrast, with aortic valve stenosis and mitral valve regurgitation associated with a structurally abnormal mitral valve, repair or replacement of the mitral valve usually is necessary.

Thus, determination of the morphology and pathophysiologic severity of each valve lesion is critically important in planning surgical management, and preoperative and intraoperative echocardiographic studies are necessary in all patients suspected of having multiple valve disease. Often, transthoracic echocardiography can define the etiology of mitral and tricuspid valvular regurgitation. When valve regurgitation is entirely secondary, the mitral valve leaflets will appear thin and freely mobile, without prolapsing segments. Mitral (and tricuspid) valve regurgitation secondary to rheumatic disease is readily identified when leaflets are thickened and chordae are shortened; fibrosis of these structures restricts leaflet mobility. Leaflet prolapse with or without ruptured chordae tendineae may also cause atrioventricular valve regurgitation.

Transesophageal echocardiography images the heart from a retrocardiac position, which avoids interference from interposed ribs, lungs, and subcutaneous tissue. A high-frequency (5-MHz) transducer is employed, which yields better resolution than that of images obtained with routine transthoracic imaging utilizing 2.25- to 3.5-MHz transducers.[6] Thus, transesophageal echocardiography provides the best image of the mitral and tricuspid valves and may be obtained preoperatively. Intraoperative transesophageal Doppler echocardiography should be employed in all patients having valve replacement or repair, and the technique is especially important for assessment of response of mitral regurgitation to relief of left ventricular outflow obstruction.[7] In some cases, preoperative left ventriculography may help to quantify left atrioventricular valve leakage. Right ventricular angiocardiography also can be useful in determining the degree of tricuspid valve dysfunction, but it is rarely employed in current practice.[8]

Tricuspid Valve Regurgitation Secondary to Other Valvular Disease

Secondary tricuspid valve regurgitation commonly is associated with rheumatic mitral valve stenosis, and the exact cause is unknown.[9,10] Some authors believe that secondary tricuspid valve regurgitation is a result of pulmonary artery hypertension and right ventricular dilatation.[11] As with the mitral valve, tricuspid valve annular dilatation is asymmetrical. Most enlargement occurs in the annulus subtended by the free wall of the right ventricle, and there is little dilatation of the annulus adjacent to the septal leaflet of the tricuspid valve.[12,13]

Although pulmonary artery hypertension with secondary enlargement of the right ventricle and tricuspid valve annulus may be an important contributing factor in secondary tricuspid regurgitation, it is not the sole mechanism. For example, congenital heart lesions such as tetralogy of Fallot produce systemic pressure in the right ventricle, yet severe tricuspid valve regurgitation rarely is seen in these patients. Similarly, important tricuspid valve regurgitation is uncommon in children with ventricular septal defects who have enlargement of the right ventricle associated with variable degrees of pulmonary hypertension.

Furthermore, clinical experience suggests that other mechanisms must play a role in development of secondary tricuspid valve regurgitation. Patients who have had mitral valve replacement for rheumatic mitral valve stenosis may develop regurgitation of their native tricuspid valve years after initial operation, and many patients have only modest elevation of pulmonary artery pressure.[14,15]

It is useful to classify secondary mitral and tricuspid valve regurgitation as mild, moderate, and severe.[13] Usually, patients with mild tricuspid valve regurgitation do not have clinical signs and symptoms of right heart failure. Also, mild tricuspid regurgitation demonstrated by preoperative echocardiography may appear even less severe in the operating room under general anesthesia. In most instances, mild secondary tricuspid regurgitation does not require intervention.

Patients with echocardiographic evidence of significant regurgitation who do not have symptoms or have their symptoms controlled by medical treatment can be classified as having moderate tricuspid regurgitation. These patients usually are managed with a deVega suture annuloplasty or a partial ring annuloplasty.[16] Patients with severe secondary tricuspid regurgitation and clinical evidence of right heart failure (pulsatile liver, distended neck veins, and peripheral edema with or without ascites) are managed by concomitant ring annuloplasty or tricuspid valve replacement.

The degree of pulmonary hypertension may influence surgical management of secondary tricuspid valve regurgitation. Kaul et al grouped 86 patients with functional tricuspid regurgitation in association with rheumatic mitral valve disease according to the degree of pulmonary hypertension. One group had severe pulmonary hypertension (mean pulmonary pressure 78 mm Hg), and a second group had moderate pulmonary hypertension (mean pulmonary artery pressure 41 mm Hg). Patients with moderate pulmonary hypertension preoperatively had more advanced right heart failure and right ventricular dilatation, and many of these patients continued to have tricuspid valve regurgitation following mitral valve surgery without tricuspid valve surgery. The patients with severe pulmonary hypertension all showed regression of tricuspid regurgitation, and 28% had complete resolution following mitral valve surgery without operation on the tricuspid valve.[12]

Excluding hospital mortality, about 40% of patients undergoing tricuspid valve surgery have premature death.[8]

It is also important to understand that mild-to-moderate (2+) regurgitation is a risk factor for late failure of tricuspid valve repair, and severe (4+) regurgitation preoperatively is a predictor of early residual regurgitation.[17]

VALVE SELECTION FOR MULTIPLE VALVE REPLACEMENT

When multiple valve replacement is confined to the left ventricle, replacement valves should be chosen from the same class with respect to the need for anticoagulation and projected longevity. There are no theoretical or practical advantages to use of a tissue valve and a mechanical valve for mitral and aortic valve replacement, and studies show no reduction in the risk of thromboembolism, valve-related morbidity, or late death.[18,19] In addition, a lower reoperation rate is reported for patients with two mechanical valves in the left ventricle compared to patients with one mechanical and one tissue valve.[18]

For tricuspid valve replacement, alone or in conjunction with other valve procedures, use of a bioprosthesis may have advantages as regards minimizing risk of valve thrombosis.[20,21] Furthermore, there are few hemodynamic considerations in selecting a tricuspid prosthesis; the greater hemodynamic efficiency of mechanical valves compared to bioprostheses rarely is an issue in atrioventricular valve replacement, especially the tricuspid valve, in which the annulus diameter in adults is often 33 mm or more. In vitro studies demonstrate only minimal hemodynamic improvement with atrioventricular valves larger than 25 mm.[22]

SURGICAL METHODS

Aortic and Mitral Valve Replacement

CANNULATION

Arterial inflow is established by cannulation of the distal ascending aorta near the pericardial reflection just to the left of the origin of the innominate artery (Fig. 41-1A). Venous cannulation is simplified by using a two-stage cannula in the right atrium for venous return. Individual cannulation of the superior and inferior venae cavae is reserved for operations that require right atrial or ventricular incisions (Fig. 41-2A).

Cardiopulmonary bypass is commenced at 2.4 L/min/m^2, and systemic hypothermia is induced according to requirements of the operation. The authors prefer maintaining systemic temperature near normal (35°C to 37°C) for most operations including multiple valve procedures. Provisions for intraoperative autotransfusion are used routinely, and antifibrinolytic drugs such as aprotinin or epsilon-aminocaproic acid (Amicar) may be useful, especially in reoperations where pericardial adhesions may worsen bleeding.[23]

CARDIOPLEGIA

If the aortic valve is competent, myocardial protection during aortic cross-clamping is achieved by initial infusion of cold (4°C to 8°C) blood cardioplegia through a tack vent placed in the aorta proximal to the clamp. The volume of cardioplegia needed to achieve diastolic arrest and uniform hypothermia depends upon the heart size and the presence of aortic valve regurgitation. Generally, the initial volume of cardioplegia required for hearts with multiple valve disease is higher than that required for coronary revascularization because of myocardial hypertrophy. For patients without cardiac enlargement, we infuse approximately 10 mL per kg body weight, whereas 15 mL per kg body weight is used for patients with significant degrees of myocardial hypertrophy. Repeat infusions of 400 mL of cardioplegia are given directly into the coronary ostia at 20-minute intervals during aortic occlusion. We use custom-designed, soft-tipped coronary perfusion catheters to minimize the potential for trauma to the coronary ostia during intubation and infusion.[24]

If aortic valve regurgitation is moderate or severe, cardioplegia is infused directly into the coronary ostia. Initial aortotomy is facilitated by emptying the heart, using suction on an aortic tack vent, and temporarily reducing cardiopulmonary bypass flow rate to maximize venous return. Some surgeons prefer retrograde infusion of cardioplegia,[25] and if this method is used, even larger volumes are necessary because of non-nutritive flow through the coronary venous system and variation in coronary venous anatomy.[26,27]

PROCEDURE

After cardioplegia, the aortic valve is inspected through an oblique aortotomy extended into the noncoronary aortic sinus (Fig. 41-1B). Aortic valve regurgitation caused by cuspal perforation or prolapse of a congenitally bicuspid valve can often be repaired,[28] but the decision for or against aortic valve repair should take into consideration whether or not a mitral valve prosthesis will be needed. For example, even though aortic valve repair might seem technically possible, prosthetic replacement may be the best option for a patient who requires mitral valve replacement and will be maintained on warfarin for long-term anticoagulation.

Severe calcification of the valve, whether it is bicuspid or tricuspid, necessitates replacement,[29] and the cusps therefore are excised and annular calcium debrided carefully.

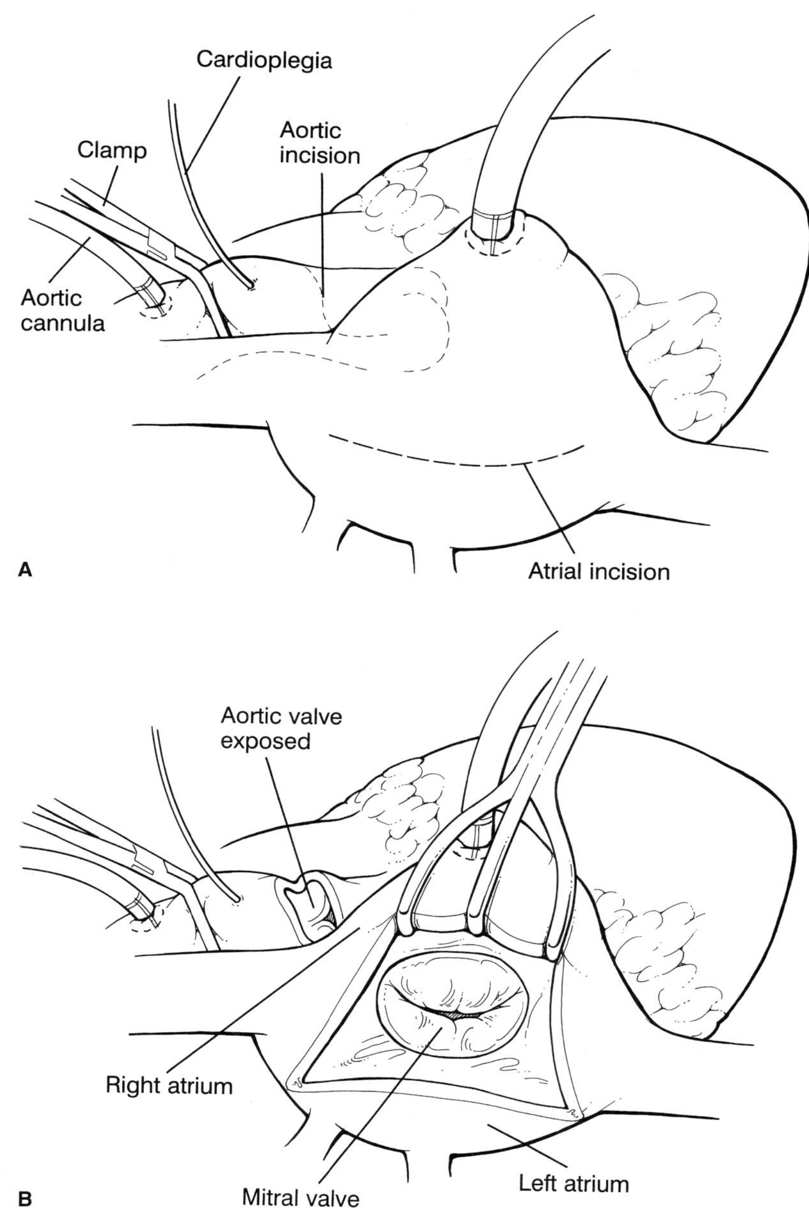

FIGURE 41–1 Aortic and mitral valve replacements showing the sequence of cannulation (A) and exposure of valves (B).

The aortic annulus is then calibrated; experience has shown that subsequent replacement of the mitral valve usually reduces the aortic annular diameter by shortening the circumference that is in continuity with the attachment of the anterior mitral valve leaflet. Therefore, we routinely identify (but do not break the sterile packaging of) two aortic prostheses: one corresponds to the calibrated dimension, and the other is the next size smaller. Final selection of the aortic prosthesis is made after mitral valve replacement or repair.

Although first exposed, the aortic valve usually is replaced after mitral valve repair or insertion of the mitral valve prosthesis. Sutures placed in the portion of the aortic valve annulus that is continuous with the anterior leaflet of the mitral valve pull the anterior leaflet superiorly toward the left ventricular outflow area and thus hinder exposure of this area as viewed through the left atriotomy.

If the aortic annulus is small, it can be enlarged with a patch of pericardium.[30] This technique increases annular diameter by 2 to 4 mm or more, and only rarely are more radical techniques necessary.[31–33] Another maneuver to accommodate as large a prosthesis as possible is to place the necessary sutures for the mitral valve repair or replacement but not secure the mitral prosthesis until the aortic valve is implanted. This eliminates downsizing of the aortic prosthesis but does not compromise insertion of sutures in the superior portion of the mitral valve annulus.

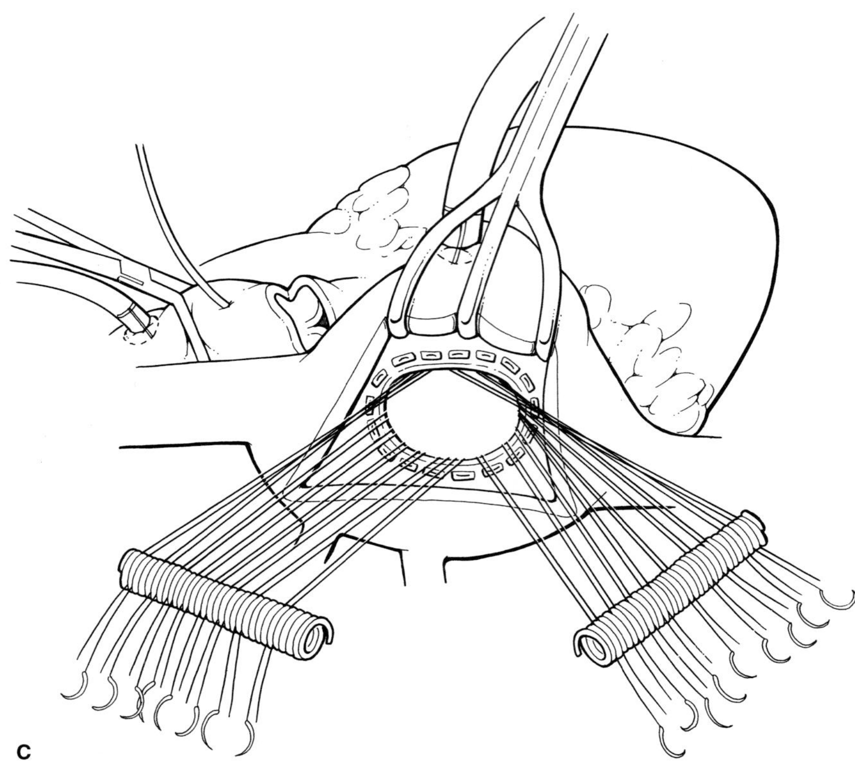

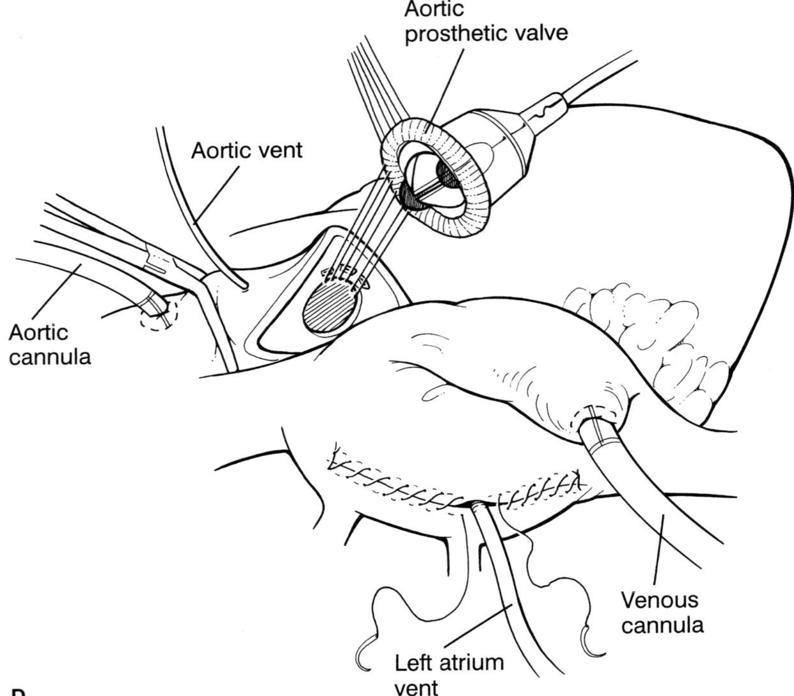

FIGURE 41–1 (*Continued*) Aortic and mitral valve replacements showing the sequence of replacement of the mitral (C) and aortic valves (D).

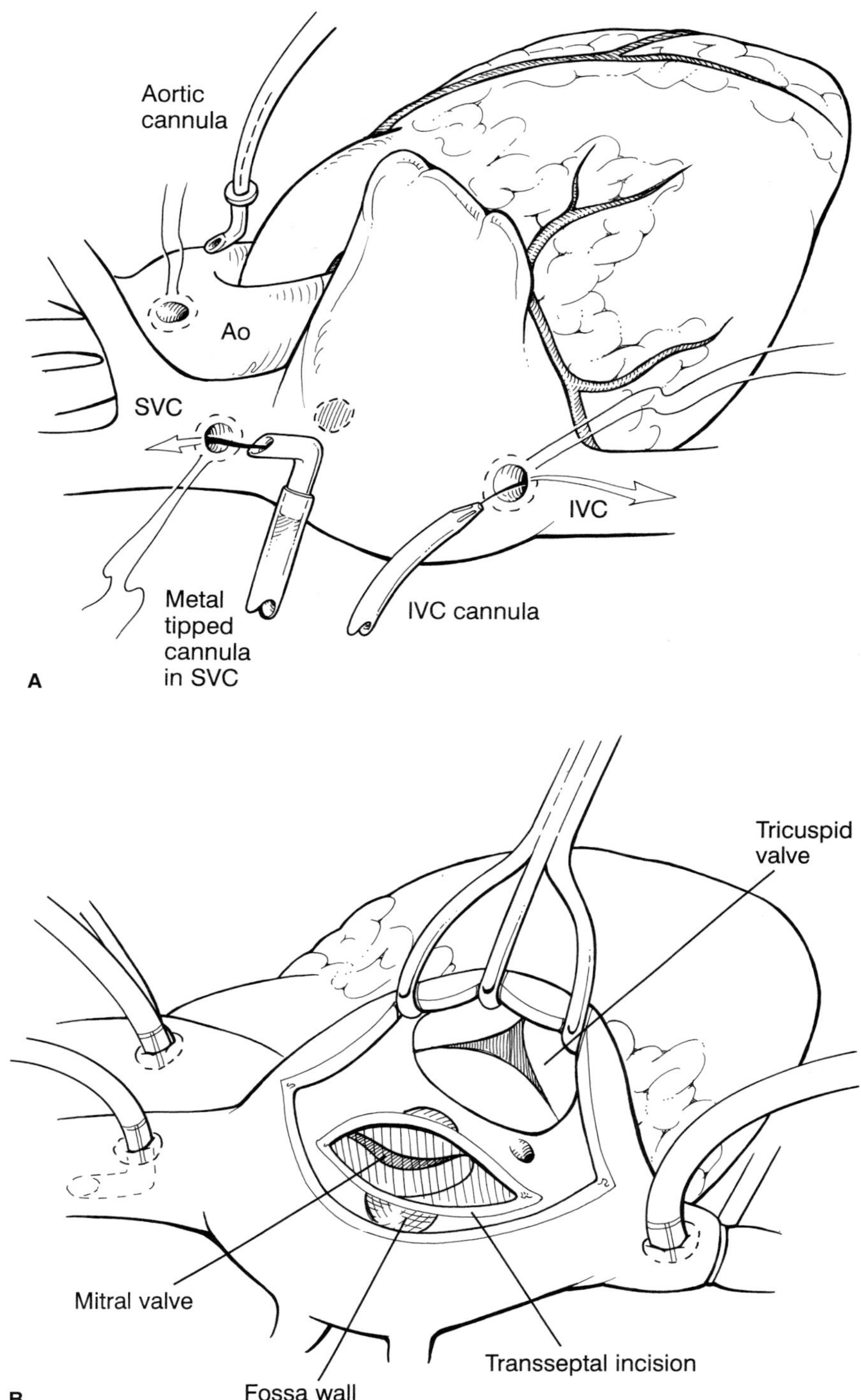

FIGURE 41–2 Combined mitral valve and tricuspid operation. The panels illustrate cannulation (A) and transseptal incision (B).

After removal of the aortic valve, the right atrial cannula is repositioned, and the mitral valve is exposed through an incision posterior to the interatrial groove (see Fig. 41-1B). The presence or absence of thrombi in the left atrium is noted, and the mitral valve is inspected. When there is rheumatic disease of the aortic valve, the mitral valve almost always will be involved to some extent. If aortic valve replacement is necessary, the surgeon should have a low threshold for replacing a diseased mitral valve because scarring and fibrosis of the rheumatic process is progressive, and mitral valve repair (commissurotomy for stenosis or leaflet repair and annuloplasty for regurgitation) is less durable than repair for

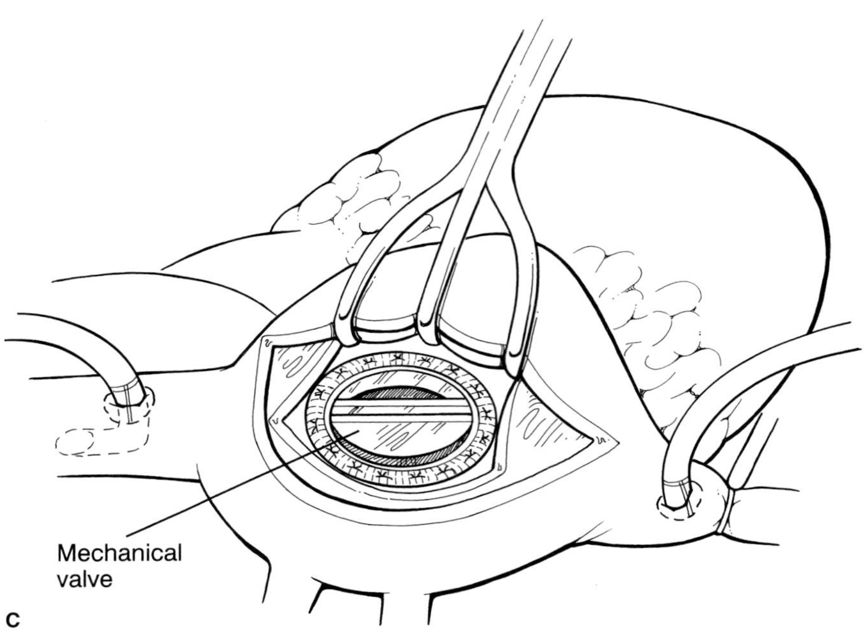

FIGURE 41–2 (*Continued*) Combined mitral valve and tricuspid operation: mitral replacement (C). (Superior vena cava snare not shown.)

degenerative disease.[34–36] In contrast, when aortic valve replacement is necessary because of calcification of a bicuspid valve or because of senescent calcification, repair of mitral valve regurgitation owing to degenerative causes can be expected to give predictably good long-term results. Repair of the mitral valve is described in Chapter 37.

In preparation for replacement, the anterior leaflet of the mitral valve is excised, and, when possible, a portion of the posterior leaflet with its chordal attachments is preserved to maintain left ventricular papillary muscle–annular continuity.[37–39] Some surgeons make special effort to preserve the anterior leaflet and its chordal attachments, believing this has a further beneficial effect on ventricular performance.[40] The mitral prosthesis is implanted using interrupted mattress sutures of 2-0 braided polyester reinforced with felt pledgets, which can be situated on the atrial or ventricular side of the valve annulus (Fig. 41-1C). The leaflets of mechanical valves should be tested for free mobility following valve seating.

When atrial fibrillation is present preoperatively, we obliterate the left atrial appendage by oversewing its orifice from within the left atrium or by ligating it externally. The left atriotomy is closed from each end with running polypropylene sutures. Vent tubing is inserted through the partially closed left atriotomy and left in place while the aortic valve is being replaced (Fig. 41-1D).

After appropriate exposure, the aortic prosthesis is sewn in place with interrupted 2-0 polyester mattress sutures backed with felt pledgets, and the aortotomy is closed, usually with two layers of 4-0 polypropylene. Any remaining air is evacuated from the heart with the usual maneuvers, and a tack vent in the ascending aorta is placed on suction as the aortic clamp is removed. The vent is removed from the left atrium and closure of the left atriotomy is secured.

In patients with annuloaortic ectasia, the mitral valve sometimes can be visualized and replaced through the enlarged aortic annulus.[41]

Aortic Valve Replacement and Mitral Valve Repair

Intraoperative transesophageal echocardiography is useful in assessing the degree of mitral regurgitation and, importantly, in identifying the cause of valve leakage. When mitral valve regurgitation is only moderate and leaflet morphology normal, we expect mitral valve function to improve following relief of severe aortic stenosis. In all other instances, the valve should be inspected directly to determine need for repair or replacement.

Sternotomy, cannulation, and assessment of the aortic valve proceed as previously described. When there is no indication of tricuspid valve disease and no other right atrial procedures are planned, venous return is obtained through a single two-staged cannula (Fig. 41-3A). Specific techniques of mitral valve repair depend on operative findings.[42] Localized prolapse of a portion of the posterior leaflet with or without ruptured chordae usually is managed by triangular excision of that segment and repair with continuous 4-0 polypropylene suture. Ruptured chordae to the anterior leaflet are replaced with 4-0 or 5-0 PTFE sutures inserted into papillary muscle and through the free edge of the prolapsing leaflet.[43]

Almost all leaflet repairs are supplemented with a posterior annuloplasty. Interrupted 2-0 braided polyester mattress sutures are placed along the posterior circumference

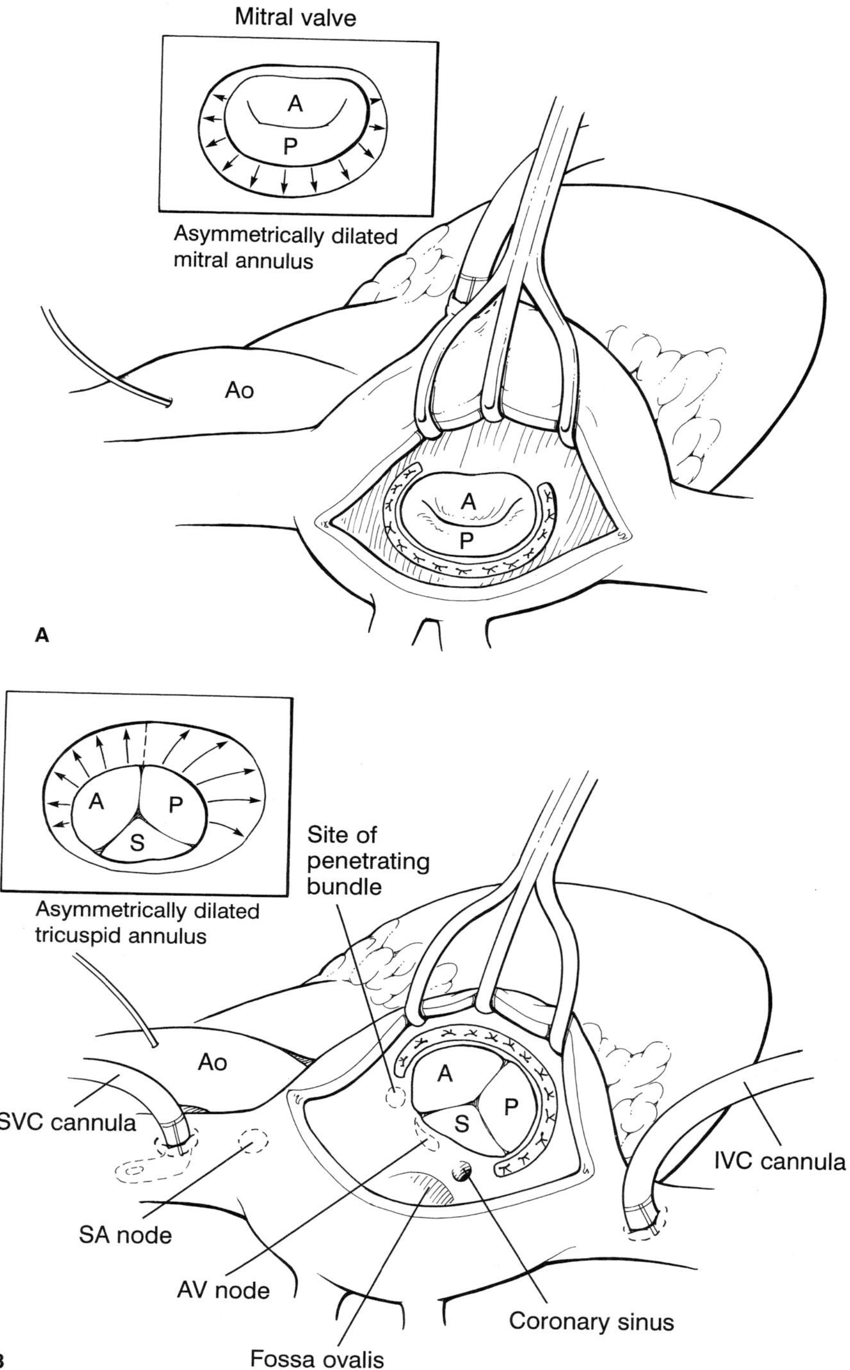

FIGURE 41–3 Mitral valve repair (A) and tricuspid valve repair (B) using a partial ring annuloplasty. (Superior and inferior vena cava snares not shown.)

of the annulus ending at the right and left fibrous trigones (Fig. 41-3A). Sutures then are spaced evenly through a flexible 6.0- to 6.5-cm long partial ring; this standard length can be obtained by using a 32-mm Cosgrove-Edwards ring or two thirds of a 27-mm Duran ring.[44] Following annuloplasty, competence of the mitral valve is tested by filling the ventricle with saline or blood; the atrium then is closed, and the aortic valve prosthesis is sewn into place.

Mitral Valve Replacement and Tricuspid Valve Replacement or Repair

In most instances, tricuspid valve regurgitation is caused by annular dilatation.[45] The severity of tricuspid valve leakage can be determined by transesophageal echocardiography prior to bypass and by digital exploration of the right atrium just prior to venous cannulation. Under general anesthesia, changes in blood volume and cardiac output can cause significant changes in the amount of regurgitation, and most often the severity of tricuspid valve leakage is lessened in the immediate prebypass period.

The patient's clinical condition must be correlated with echocardiographic findings and intraoperative assessment of the tricuspid valve. Patients with enlarged, pulsatile liver, peripheral edema, and jugular venous distention are likely to require tricuspid valvuloplasty following mitral valve replacement or repair. Those patients without the stigmata of right heart failure usually have less severe valve leakage, and tricuspid valve function may improve without direct repair or replacement after left-sided valvular lesions are corrected.

The decision for repair or replacement of functional tricuspid valve regurgitation at the time of mitral valve replacement is important because risk of subsequent reoperation is high. In our earlier experience, operative mortality was 25% in patients who required later reoperation for tricuspid valve regurgitation. Further, tricuspid regurgitation progresses in 10% to 15% of patients after replacement of rheumatic mitral valves.[46] Therefore, we maintain a liberal policy for annuloplasty or prosthetic replacement at initial operation.[47]

PROCEDURE

For operations on the tricuspid valve, insertion of a Swan-Ganz catheter is optional; if it is used, the catheter is withdrawn from the right heart chambers during inspection and assessment of the tricuspid valve. We prefer direct cannulation of the inferior and superior venae cavae.[48] After commencement of cardiopulmonary bypass and cardioplegia, the cavae are snared around the venous cannulae, and the interatrial septum and tricuspid valve are exposed through a right atriotomy (Fig. 41-2A). A decision for repair or replacement of the tricuspid valve is made and the necessary prosthesis identified.

Usually we expose the mitral valve through an incision in the interatrial septum, which crosses the fossa ovalis and can be extended superiorly (Fig. 41-2B). Care should be taken during retraction to avoid tearing the septum inferiorly toward the coronary sinus and triangle of Koch. Alternatively, the mitral valve can be exposed through a standard left atriotomy posterior to the interatrial groove.

After repair or replacement of the mitral valve (Fig. 41-2C), the septal or left atrial incision is closed, and the tricuspid valve is repaired or replaced. For tricuspid valve repair, we use either the deVega method or ring annuloplasty.[11,16,49,50] Both techniques are based on the observation that the anterior and posterior valve portions of the tricuspid valve annulus are more prone to dilation than the septal leaflet portion of the annulus as previously described. When ring annuloplasty is indicated, we prefer a flexible device such as the Cosgrove-Edwards prosthesis[51] or a partial Duran ring (Fig. 41-3B). The use of a partial ring avoids placement of sutures in the annulus near the penetrating bundle of His and reduces risk of injury to conduction tissue.

Tricuspid Valve Replacement and Pulmonary Valve Replacement for Carcinoid Heart Disease

If there is no involvement of the mitral and aortic valves,[52] tricuspid and pulmonary valve replacement can usually be performed without the need for aortic occlusion and cardioplegic arrest. It is important to exclude the presence of a patent foramen ovale to eliminate risk of air entering the left atrium, and if a defect in the atrial septum is identified, it is closed using a brief period of aortic occlusion. In the past, our strategy for patients with carcinoid heart disease was to replace the tricuspid valve and excise the diseased pulmonary valve. Subsequent experience suggests that right ventricular function is better preserved with a functioning pulmonary valve, so we now favor pulmonary valve replacement rather than valvectomy.[53] Tricuspid valve replacement always is indicated, and it is usually necessary only to remove the anterior leaflet. Carcinoid disease produces fibrosis and retraction of the leaflets, so that anchoring sutures (interrupted mattress of 2-0 braided polyester backed with felt pledgets) can be inserted into the remaining septal and posterior leaflets. We prefer to position the pledgets on the ventricular side of the valve annulus. If exposure is difficult, a brief period of aortic clamping and cardioplegic arrest is utilized during placement of sutures in the posterior and septal leaflets; the aortic cross-clamp is removed, and the heart is allowed to beat rhythmically. The remaining sutures are placed, and all sutures are secured with observation of the electrocardiogram. If atrioventricular block develops, the sutures in the area of the penetrating bundle of His are removed and reinserted in a more superficial location.

Pulmonary valve replacement is performed through a longitudinal incision across the valve annulus on to the outflow portion of the right ventricle. We prefer to insert the prosthetic valve using continuous 3-0 polypropylene suture, anchoring the sewing ring to the native valve annulus for approximately two thirds of the valve annulus and then anteriorly to a pericardial patch that is used routinely to augment the valve annulus and to facilitate closure of the pulmonary artery and right ventricle.

Triple Valve Replacement

Operative preparation is similar to that previously described. Usually left-sided valvular lesions are corrected prior to tricuspid valve procedures. Again, if there is aortic valve regurgitation, the aortotomy is performed first, and cardioplegia is administered; simultaneously, we snare the cavae and open the right atrium. After excision of the aortic valve and calibration of the annulus, the interatrial septum is incised,

TABLE 41–3 Reports of operations for multiple valve disease, showing the high incidence of rheumatic heart disease

Study	Patients (no.)	Patients with rheumatic heart disease, % (no.)
Combined mitral and aortic replacement[157]	86	100 (86)
Combined mitral and aortic replacement[133]	92	100 (92)
Combined mitral and aortic replacement with tricuspid repair[48]	109	98 (107)
Triple valve replacement[159]	48	100 (48)
Combined mitral and aortic replacement[95]	54	85 (46)
Multiple valve procedures[138]	50	86 (43)
Triple valve replacement[20]	91	100 (91)
Combined mitral and aortic replacement[137]	65	80 (52)
Mitral replacement and tricuspid surgery[14]	32	81 (26)
Combined mitral and aortic replacement[168]	166	64 (106)
Mitral and aortic procedures[66]	124	100 (124)
Multiple valve procedures[169]	102	100 (102)
Combined mitral and aortic replacement[170]	33	82 (27)
Mitral and aortic regurgitation[85]	39	67 (26)
Mitral and aortic stenosis[78]	32	100 (32)
Mitral and aortic stenosis[76]	141	100 (141)

and the mitral valve is repaired or replaced. Next, the aortic valve is implanted, and after closure of the aortotomy and septotomy, the tricuspid valvuloplasty or prosthetic replacement can be performed without aortic cross-clamping.[54]

RHEUMATIC HEART DISEASE AFFECTING MULTIPLE VALVES

As shown in Table 41-3, rheumatic valvulitis is a common cause of multiple valve disease. Autopsy studies show that almost all patients with rheumatic heart disease have some involvement of the mitral valve, although it is not always evident clinically.[55] The percentages of multiple valve involvement in two autopsy studies of patients with rheumatic heart disease are shown in Table 41-4. Forty-seven percent of those studied had involvement of more than one valve. Mitral and aortic valve disease was the most common combination and was present in 34% of patients; the second most common combination was mitral, aortic, and tricuspid valve disease (9%).

Long-term follow-up of children with rheumatic heart disease suggests that approximately 50% of patients have multivalvular involvement.[56,57] In a study of patients undergoing mitral valvotomy for rheumatic mitral stenosis (Table 41-5), 13% had clinical evidence of other rheumatic valve stenosis or regurgitation. Most of these patients had associated rheumatic aortic disease.[58]

Rheumatic heart disease can cause valve stenosis, regurgitation, or a combination of lesions. The percentages of 290 patients with specific valvular lesions from four studies of multiple valve disease are shown in Table 41-6. Mixed lesions producing stenosis and regurgitation were encountered most commonly in both aortic and mitral valves.

TABLE 41–4 Results of autopsy series (1910–1937) showing multiple valve involvement in 996 patients with rheumatic heart disease

Valve lesion at autopsy	Clawson[171]	Cooke and White[172]	Percentage of 996 patients studied
All combinations	321	147	47
M-A	221	100	32
M-A-T	52	35	9
M-T	31	7	4
M-A-T-P	14	5	2
A-T	2	0	0.2
A-M-P	1	0	0.1

M = mitral valve; A = aortic valve; T = tricuspid valve; P = pulmonary valve.

Source: Modified with permission from Acker M, Hargrove WC, Stephenson LW: Multiple valve replacement. Cardiol Clin 1985; 3:425.

TABLE 41–5 Patients with rheumatic mitral stenosis undergoing valvotomy with clinical evidence of multiple valve disease

Valve lesion at surgery	No.	Percentage of 1000 patients with rheumatic mitral stenosis
All combinations	127	12.7
M-A	121	12.1
M-T	6	0.6

M = mitral valve; A = aortic valve; T = tricuspid valve.
Does not include patients with tricuspid regurgitation.

Source: Modified with permission from Ellis LB, Harken DE, Black H: A clinical study of 1000 consecutive cases of mitral stenosis two to nine years after mitral valvuloplasty. Circulation 1959; 19:803.

TABLE 41–6 Hemodynamic classification in patients undergoing multiple valve surgery for rheumatic valvular disease

	Combined mitral and aortic surgery[66]	Triple valve replacement[159]	Combined mitral and aortic replacement[170]	Triple valve replacement[20]	Totals
Number in study	124	48	27	91	290
MS	53% (66)	19% (9)	30% (8)	22% (20)	35.5% (103/290)
MR	47% (58)	10% (5)	52% (14)	12% (11)	30.3% (88/290)
MS/MR	—	71% (34)	19% (5)	66% (169)	34.1% (99/290)
AS	53% (66)	10% (5)	44% (12)	10% (9)	31.7% (92/290)
AR	47% (58)	35% (17)	41% (11)	33% (30)	40% (116/290)
AS/AR	—	54% (26)	15% (4)	57% (52)	28.3% (82/290)

MS = mitral stenosis; MR = mitral regurgitation; AS = aortic stenosis; AR = aortic regurgitation.

Rheumatic Mitral Stenosis with Rheumatic Aortic Regurgitation

Approximately 10% of patients with rheumatic mitral valve stenosis also have rheumatic aortic regurgitation.[59] Clinical and laboratory characteristics of patients with mitral stenosis and aortic regurgitation are summarized in Table 41-7.

DIAGNOSIS, SIGNS, AND SYMPTOMS

Physical findings An early blowing diastolic murmur is present along the left sternal border in about 75% of patients with rheumatic mitral stenosis.[60,61] This murmur can mimic a Graham Steell murmur of pulmonary valve regurgitation; however, this diastolic murmur usually originates from the aortic valve and represents mild aortic regurgitation.[62] In patients with aortic regurgitation, a late diastolic murmur can either be the murmur of mitral stenosis or the Austin Flint murmur caused by a regurgitant jet directed toward the anterior mitral leaflet.[63] Exercise or amyl nitrite inhalation intensifies the murmur of organic mitral stenosis while diminishing the murmur of aortic regurgitation and the Austin Flint murmur.[61] Doppler echocardiography differentiates mild aortic regurgitation and pulmonic regurgitation.[64] Occasionally the murmur and peripheral signs of aortic regurgitation are absent because of mitral stenosis.[60,65]

Electrocardiography Electrocardiographic and roentgenographic evidence of eccentric left ventricular hypertrophy in patients with mitral stenosis is an important clue to associated aortic valve regurgitation. Also, atrial fibrillation early in the course of aortic regurgitation is a clue to associated mitral stenosis.[61,66]

TABLE 41–7 Characteristics of patients with combined mitral stenosis and aortic regurgitation

Mitral stenosis and aortic regurgitation	Terzaki[66]
Number of patients	26
Symptom of dyspnea	100% (26)
Electrocardiographic evidence of LVH	62% (16)
Roentgenographic evidence of LVH	54% (14)
Symptom of angina	23% (6)
Aortic diastolic pressure >70 mmHg	46% (12)
Elevated LVEDP	38% (10)

LVH = left ventricular hypertrophy; LVEDP = left ventricular end-diastolic pressure.

Echocardiography Left ventricular hypertrophy and volume overload detected by echocardiography suggest severe aortic valve regurgitation because these findings are not normally associated with mitral stenosis.[61] Diastolic fluttering of the anterior leaflet of the mitral valve and the ventricular septum is an additional finding suggesting aortic valve regurgitation in patients with mitral stenosis.[61,67] In the presence of aortic valve regurgitation, the Doppler determination of mitral valve area is overestimated when pressure half-time measurements are used.[68]

Catheterization data With current echocardiographic methods, cardiac catheterization to determine severity of valvular heart disease is rarely indicated; however, hemodynamic profiles of such patients have been studied thoroughly. Characteristically, the left ventricular diastolic pressure is elevated in about 35% of patients with mitral stenosis and aortic regurgitation. This can cause the transmitral gradient at rest to be small even when significant stenosis of the mitral valve is present.[41,69] In patients with isolated aortic valve regurgitation, the left ventricular diastolic pressure is elevated more frequently than in patients with concomitant mitral stenosis and aortic regurgitation.[45] Aortography may underestimate the severity of aortic regurgitation in patients with associated mitral stenosis because low cardiac output and low stroke volume produce a concomitant reduction in regurgitant volume.[38]

PATHOPHYSIOLOGY

In patients with mitral valve stenosis and aortic valve regurgitation, decreased cardiac output minimizes the classic signs of aortic regurgitation (waterhammer pulse, head bobbing, or visibly pulsating capillaries). Also, concomitant mitral stenosis reduces left ventricular volume overload that is a characteristic of isolated aortic regurgitation.[69] The underfilling of the left ventricle characteristic of mitral stenosis is offset by overfilling secondary to aortic valve regurgitation.

TABLE 41–8 **Clinical characteristics of patients with combined mitral and aortic stenosis**

Mitral stenosis and aortic stenosis	Uricchio[76]	Katznelson[74]	Terzaki[66]	Honey[78]	Totals
Number of patients	141	22	40	35	198
Dyspnea	94% (132)	100% (22)	—	97% (34)	95% (188/198)
Fatigue	87% (122)	—	—	—	87% (122/141)
Edema	60% (85)	—	73% (29)	—	63% (114/181)
Palpitations	—	64% (14)	58% (23)	—	60% (37/62)
Orthopnea	—	55% (12)	—	63% (22)	60% (34/57)
Atrial fibrillation	47% (66)	68% (15)	65% (26)	—	53% (107/203)
PND	36% (51)	55% (12)	—	40% (14)	39% (77/198)
Hemoptysis	32% (45)	32% (7)	—	60% (21)	37% (73/198)
Angina	23% (32)	23% (5)	68% (27)	17% (6)	29% (70/238)
Vertigo, dizziness, or syncope	25% (35)	32% (7)	25% (10)	23% (8)	25% (60/238)
Emboli	20% (27)	27% (6)	—	17% (6)	20% (39/198)

PND = paroxysmal nocturnal dyspnea.
Number of patients in parentheses.

Pulmonary artery hypertension characteristic of mitral stenosis usually is present.

OPERATIVE DECISION MAKING

Patients with rheumatic mitral stenosis and rheumatic aortic regurgitation of more than a mild degree usually require replacement of both valves. Aortic valve repair is possible using techniques such as cuspal extension with glutaraldehyde-treated bovine or autologous pericardium.[70] Although early results with cuspal extension have been good, inexorable progression of valve fibrosis will necessitate later prosthetic replacement for many patients.[71]

Preoperative transthoracic and intraoperative transesophageal echocardiography aids in assessing function of the aortic valve in patients requiring surgery for mitral stenosis. At operation, the degree of ventricular fullness and amount of aortic root distention with infusion of cardioplegia are clues to important aortic valve regurgitation. As stated previously, if mitral valve replacement is necessary, strong consideration should be given to replacement of the aortic valve when there is moderate or worse leakage owing to rheumatic valvulitis.

Great care should be exercised to avoid ventricular distention if ventricular fibrillation occurs prior to aortic clamping. If ventricular fibrillation develops, distention of the heart can be prevented by inserting a left ventricular vent and by manually compressing the heart. Also, even mild or moderate degrees of aortic regurgitation can complicate cardioplegia delivery through the proximal aorta.

Rheumatic Mitral Stenosis with Rheumatic Aortic Stenosis

DIAGNOSIS, SIGNS, AND SYMPTOMS

Physical findings When rheumatic valve disease produces the combination of mitral valve stenosis and aortic stenosis, the signs and symptoms of both lesions can be present; however, those of mitral stenosis (dyspnea) tend to predominate, and the signs and symptoms of aortic stenosis (syncope, angina) occur less frequently. Table 41-8 outlines the clinical characteristics of patients in four studies of combined mitral and aortic stenosis. Dyspnea, the most frequently observed symptom, was present in 95% of patients, and angina and syncope were observed in 29% and 25% of patients, respectively. Mitral valve stenosis may even mask the signs and symptoms of aortic stenosis, making the clinical recognition of aortic stenosis difficult in patients with combined disease.[72]

In addition, auscultatory findings may be confusing if the elevated end-diastolic pressure caused by aortic stenosis minimizes the opening snap of mitral stenosis.[72–74] Clinical signs of aortic stenosis, delayed carotid upstroke, systolic thrill, and ejection murmur, may be less prominent in patients with coexisting mitral valve stenosis compared to those with isolated aortic valve stenosis.[73] Some clinical features raising suspicion of multiple valve involvement in patients with mitral stenosis or aortic stenosis are shown in Table 41-9 and Table 41-10.

Radiographic findings in patients with combined rheumatic mitral and aortic valve stenosis are summarized in Table 41-11. Left atrial enlargement is observed in 85% of patients, and dilatation of the proximal ascending aorta, common in patients with congenitally bicuspid valves, is relatively infrequent (22%). Calcification of the mitral or aortic valves is identified in approximately 35% of patients.

Electrocardiography Atrial fibrillation is not common in patients with isolated aortic valve stenosis but is observed in

TABLE 41–9 **Features raising suspicion of mitral stenosis in a patient with known aortic stenosis**[74]

ECG	Atrial fibrillation, P-mitrale
Chest roentgenogram	Left atrial enlargement, right ventricular enlargement, or calcification of mitral valve

TABLE 41–10 Features raising suspicion of aortic stenosis in a patient with known mitral valve disease[61]

Symptoms	Angina or syncope
Physical findings	Delayed carotid upstroke Prolonged ejection murmur
ECG	Left ventricular hypertrophy in presence of mitral stenosis
Chest roentgenogram	Aortic valve calcification Poststenotic aortic root dilation

52% of patients with combined disease (Table 41-12). Approximately one third of patients will exhibit electrocardiographic evidence of left ventricular hypertrophy, and right ventricular hypertrophy occurs in 18% of patients. Atrial enlargement manifested by P-mitrale is observed in 32% of patients.

Echocardiography Echocardiography provides definitive information on valve structure, function, and hemodynamics. In patients with combined mitral and aortic stenosis, estimation or measurement of valve area may be more reliable than the pressure gradient because cardiac output may be low, and atrial fibrillation produces variable stroke volume from one cardiac cycle to the next. Severity of mitral valve stenosis is determined by directly measuring the mitral valve orifice on the short-axis view of two-dimensional echocardiography. This method is reliable and reproducible, and there is excellent correlation between mitral valve area measured from a two-dimensional echocardiogram and the area measured directly from a pathologic specimen.[75]

PATHOPHYSIOLOGY

In contrast to isolated mitral stenosis in which ventricular function frequently is preserved, the combination of mitral and aortic stenosis is associated with ventricular hypertrophy and diastolic dysfunction. The pressure load from the aortic stenosis causes a concentric hypertrophy with a small, noncompliant ventricular cavity.[66] Mitral stenosis compromises the ventricle's ability to maintain cardiac output (in contrast to isolated aortic stenosis in which cardiac output is maintained).[74,76] The decrease in cardiac output minimizes the signs and symptoms of aortic stenosis and may make the diagnosis of aortic stenosis difficult.[77] Other hemodynamic parameters are similar to isolated mitral stenosis, e.g., elevation of left atrial and pulmonary arterial pressures.[76,78]

OPERATIVE DECISION MAKING

Although mitral valve stenosis sometimes can be treated effectively with valvuloplasty, commissurotomy for rheumatic aortic stenosis is rarely indicated. Thus, for patients with both aortic and mitral valve stenoses caused by rheumatic heart disease, we favor prosthetic replacement with mechanical prostheses if patients can manage long-term anticoagulation. If aortic valve stenosis is only mild in severity and the decision is made not to replace the aortic valve at the time of mitral valve replacement, then the patient should be followed carefully because over 50% will develop moderate to severe disease by 15 years postoperatively.[79]

The combination of aortic stenosis and mitral stenosis may present unique problems for the surgeon. First, concentric hypertrophy of the left ventricle may displace the mitral valve orifice anteriorly, producing poor exposure through a standard atriotomy; several maneuvers and alternative incisions are described for patients in whom mitral valve exposure is difficult.[77,80–84] Also, the small left ventricular cavity may impinge upon struts of caged-ball or stent-mounted bioprostheses. There is the potential for left ventricular outflow obstruction from high-profile prostheses in the mitral position in patients with aortic and mitral valve stenoses and small left ventricular cavity size.

Rheumatic Mitral Regurgitation with Rheumatic Aortic Regurgitation

DIAGNOSIS, SIGNS, AND SYMPTOMS

Physical findings When mitral regurgitation and aortic regurgitation are both present, the cardinal signs of either lesion may be masked by the other,[66] and when the clinical features of aortic regurgitation predominate, it may be difficult to determine whether coexisting mitral regurgitation requires surgical treatment.[66] The clinical characteristics of

TABLE 41–11 Frequency of radiographic findings in patients with combined aortic and mitral stenosis

	Honey[78]	Katznelson[74]	Terzaki[66]	Zitnik[72]	Total
Number of patients	35	22	40	10	107
Left atrial enlargement^{2+}	—	64% (14)	100% (40)	70% (7)	85% (61/72)
LVH^{2+}	9% (3)	59% (13)	76% (31)	60% (6)	50% (53/107)
Mitral valve calcification	—	36% (8)	38% (15)	50% (5)	39% (28/72)
Aortic valve calcification	6% (2)	55% (12)	43% (17)	30% (3)	32% (34/107)
Aortic dilation	11% (4)	32% (7)	—	40% (4)	22% (15/67)

Number of patients in parentheses.

TABLE 41–12 Frequency of electrocardiographic findings in patients with combined aortic and mitral stenosis

	Honey[78]	Katznelson[74]	Uricchio[76]	Terzaki[66]	Zitnik[72]	Total
Number of patients	35	22	144	40	10	251
Atrial fibrillation	21	15	66	26	3	52% (131/251)
LVH	13	12	26	34	3	35% (88/251)
P-mitrale or left atrial hypertrophy	—	6	—	10	7	32% (23/72)
RVH	11	1	21	9	4	18% (46/251)

LVH = left ventricular hypertrophy; RVH = right ventricular hypertrophy.

patients with combined mitral and aortic regurgitation are summarized in Table 41-13. Dyspnea and congestive heart failure are most common, whereas angina, syncope, and evidence of emboli occur less frequently.

Mitral valve regurgitation produces a characteristic systolic blowing murmur and may also be associated with a diastolic flow murmur. Aortic valve regurgitation produces a characteristic diastolic murmur and may also cause a systolic flow murmur. The combination of two simultaneous murmurs during both diastole and systole may confuse clinical diagnosis. Most patients have a long, pansystolic murmur heard best at the apex, often with a diastolic rumble and decreased intensity of aortic closure. In general, when aortic regurgitation is the dominant lesion, the early diastolic rumble is prominent; when mitral regurgitation prevails, the aortic diastolic murmur is less intense.[85–87] However, the severity of the two lesions does not always correlate with the relative intensity of murmurs.[66] Additionally, a prominent S3 gallop can be heard, whereas an S4 is unusual.[88]

Combined aortic and mitral regurgitation also results in significant left ventricular enlargement,[86] which is evident on both electrocardiogram[66,85] and chest x-ray.[66,85,87,88] Characteristic electrocardiographic findings are summarized in Table 41-14. On chest x-ray, nearly all patients have cardiomegaly and left atrial enlargement.[66,85] Calcification of the mitral or aortic valve is relatively uncommon.[66]

Echocardiography Mitral valve motion and diastolic orifice configuration may be altered in aortic regurgitation with a decrease in the opening amplitude of the anterior leaflet, and an abnormal mitral orifice configuration with diastolic leaflet oscillation.[88] The mitral valve orifice image is deformed because restriction in anterior leaflet excursion is most pronounced in the center of the leaflet, where peak vertical separation normally occurs. This restriction causes the anterior leaflet to appear flattened rather than convex anteriorly, and in severe cases it may actually be concave toward the left ventricular outflow tract.[88]

TABLE 41–13 Clinical characteristics of patients with combined mitral and aortic regurgitation due to rheumatic valvular disease

Mitral and aortic regurgitation	Shine[85]	Terzaki[66]	Totals
Number of patients	39	32	71
Dyspnea	—	100% (32)	100% (32/32)
CHF	90% (35)	38% (12)	66% (47/71)
Angina	28% (11)	25% (8)	27% (19/71)
Syncope	8% (3)	19% (6)	13% (9/71)
Emboli	5% (2)	—	5% (2/39)

CHF = congestive heart failure.
Number of patients in parentheses.

Catheterization data Most patients have elevated right atrial and pulmonary arterial capillary wedge pressure. There is usually a prominent *v* wave in pulmonary capillary wedge tracing. Approximately 75% of patients have an elevated left ventricular end-diastolic pressure.[59,66]

PATHOPHYSIOLOGY

The combination of mitral and aortic valve regurgitation produces severe volume overload of the left ventricle. The reduction of impedance to ejection allows the ventricle to empty further, reducing ventricular wall tension with a resultant increase in the velocity of shortening.[89] Chronic volume overload increases stroke volume and distention of the left ventricle so that a larger stroke volume can be achieved with less myocardial fiber shortening compared to normal hearts.[66] Patients who respond to increased volume load by left ventricular dilation appear to tolerate surgical correction better than patients with left ventricular hypertrophy owing to an increased pressure load.[66]

TABLE 41–14 Frequency of electrocardiographic findings in patients with combined aortic and mitral regurgitation

Electrocardiographic finding	Shine[85]	Terzaki[66]	Total
Number of patients	39	32	71
LVH	79% (31)	81% (26)	80% (57/71)
Left atrial enlargement	—	69% (22)	69% (22/32)
Atrial fibrillation	59% (23)	68% (22)	63% (45/71)
LBBB	5% (2)	—	5% (2/39)

LVH = left ventricular hypertrophy; LBBB = left bundle branch block.
Number of patients in parentheses.

TABLE 41–15 Incidence of echocardiographic evidence of aortic valve prolapse in patients with mitral valve prolapse

	Ogawa[98]	Rippe[97]	Mardelli[173]	Total
Number of patients with MVP	50	400	75	525
Aortic valve prolapse	24% (12)	3% (11)	20% (15)	7% (38/525)
Aortic regurgitation	16% (8)	1% (4)	—	3% (12/450)
Aortic and mitral valve replacement	2% (1)	—	—	2% (1/50)

MVP = mitral valve prolapse.
Number of patients in parentheses.

Patients with aortic valve regurgitation have augmented stroke volume to maintain an adequate cardiac output, but when mitral regurgitation coexists, part of the augmented stroke regurgitates into the left atrium and pulmonary veins. For this reason, when aortic regurgitation is severe, concomitant mitral regurgitation greatly reduces systemic cardiac output and can produce severe pulmonary congestion.[90]

OPERATIVE DECISION MAKING

As stated previously, aortic valves involved with rheumatic disease usually require replacement. When the mitral valve also has rheumatic involvement, we replace the mitral valve at the time of aortic valve operation. After the aortic valve is excised, the mitral valve is visually inspected if it is suspected of being diseased or if the degree of regurgitation is severe.

MYXOMATOUS AND PROLAPSING VALVE DISEASE AFFECTING MULTIPLE VALVES

Myxomatous degeneration is the most common etiology of mitral regurgitation requiring surgical correction in North America, and myxomatous aortic valve disease with annular dilatation is, perhaps, the most common cause of aortic regurgitation.[91–93] Most cases of either isolated mitral or isolated aortic valve prolapse are not associated with known connective tissue disorders. Mitral and aortic valvular prolapse coexist frequently with connective tissue disorders such as Marfan syndrome, Ehlers-Danlos syndrome, osteogenesis imperfecta, and others.[90]

Aortic valve regurgitation in patients with Marfan syndrome is caused by progressive enlargement of the sinus portion of the aorta and the aortic valve annulus, i.e., annuloaortic ectasia.[94,95] The principal causes of mitral regurgitation in patients with Marfan syndrome are mitral annular dilation, floppy or prolapsing leaflets, and mitral annular calcification.[95] The pathological lesion in Marfan syndrome is cystic medial necrosis, which is characterized by degeneration of elastic fibers and infrequent cysts.[95] Alterations in the synthesis and cellular secretion of fibrillin are responsible for the phenotypic characteristics of many patients with Marfan syndrome.[96] Some patients have myxomatous cardiovascular lesions and annuloaortic ectasia without the other clinical characteristics of Marfan syndrome.

Two-dimensional echocardiographic studies show that the frequency of aortic valve prolapse in patients with mitral valve prolapse varies between 3% and 24% (Table 41-15).[97,98] In one necropsy study, the frequency of mitral regurgitation in Marfan patients with aortic aneurysms (most with aortic regurgitation) was 54% (7 of 13).[95] About 17% of patients who undergo surgery for myxomatous aortic valve require surgical correction of mitral regurgitation (Table 41-16). Although multiple valve involvement with myxomatous degeneration usually manifests itself as mitral regurgitation in combination with aortic regurgitation, in some cases all four valves may be involved.[99] It is not clear whether the underlying pathology of isolated mitral valve prolapse is the same as the cardiovascular lesions that occur in the Marfan syndrome and other multiple floppy valve syndromes.[100,101]

Diagnosis, Signs, and Symptoms

Signs and symptoms of aortic and mitral valve regurgitation are reviewed in the section on rheumatic valvular disease. In addition to complete evaluation of the aortic and mitral valves and proximal aorta, patients with Marfan syndrome should have assessment of the descending aorta for aneurysm or chronic dissection.

TABLE 41–16 Frequency of mitral valve procedures in patients undergoing aortic valve repair or replacement for myxomatous degeneration, prolapse, or root dilation

	David[174]	Gott[175]	Shigenobu[91]	Agozzino[94]	Bellitti[93]	Total
All aortic surgery	18	270	13	69	25	395
Number requiring concomitant mitral surgery	3 (17%)	36 (13%)	5 (38%)	16 (23%)	3 (12%)	63 (16%)

Operative Decision Making

If annuloaortic ectasia is not present, patients with mitral and aortic valve regurgitation caused by myxomatous degeneration are candidates for repair of both valves. The aortic valve is inspected initially, and the decision for repair or prosthetic replacement is made depending on cuspal morphology. If tissue is sturdy and there is little prolapse or prolapse is limited to one cusp, repair can be undertaken with commissural narrowing and cusp resuspension. Often, aortic valve regurgitation is central, and simply narrowing the annulus by commissural plication restores valvular competence. Outcome of repair of both mitral and aortic valves has been good as regards patient survival and freedom from valve-related complications, but reoperation is necessary in 35% of patients 10 years after the initial procedure; patients with most severe aortic valve regurgitation have increased risk of late reoperation.[102] If tissue is attenuated or if multiple cusps have severe prolapse, the valve is replaced.

In most instances, patients with Marfan syndrome and aortic regurgitation require composite replacement of the aortic valve and ascending aorta.[103] Occasionally, moderate aortic regurgitation can be repaired at the time of aortic replacement by suspending the aortic valve inside a tube graft or remodeling the sinus portion of the aorta.[104] Even if the aortic valve is replaced with a composite graft and mechanical valve, the surgeon should favor repair of associated mitral regurgitation. Gillinov et al report that valvuloplasty is possible in approximately 80% of patients with mitral regurgitation and Marfan syndrome, and that 5 years postoperatively, 88% of patients are free of significant mitral valve insufficiency.[105]

Myxomatous Mitral Regurgitation with Tricuspid Regurgitation

Myxomatous degeneration may also involve the tricuspid valve, and presentation of mitral and tricuspid valve regurgitation owing to degenerative disease is not uncommon. In one study, 54% of patients with mitral valve prolapse also had tricuspid prolapse; however, most of these patients did not have significant regurgitation.[90] As with tricuspid regurgitation associated with rheumatic mitral disease, preoperative and intraoperative echocardiography is important in evaluating tricuspid disease in patients with myxomatous mitral regurgitation. In contrast to rheumatic disease, myxomatous mitral and tricuspid regurgitation almost always lends itself to valve repair.

SENILE CALCIFIC AORTIC VALVE DISEASE WITH MULTIPLE VALVE INVOLVEMENT

Unlike aortic stenosis caused by rheumatic disease in which associated mitral valve disease is common, senile calcific aortic stenosis usually presents as an isolated lesion. Although the combination of mitral valve disease and senile calcific aortic stenosis is uncommon, senile aortic calcification is a frequent cause of aortic valve stenosis.[92] The incidence of senile calcific aortic disease has steadily increased in the last 20 years. Therefore, although mitral valve disease associated with calcific aortic stenosis is less common than that seen with rheumatic disease of the aortic valve, as the incidence of calcific aortic stenosis increases, so does the likelihood of encountering patients with disease of both valves.

Patterns of Multiple Valve Involvement with Calcific Aortic Stenosis

CALCIFIC AORTIC STENOSIS WITH INFECTIVE ENDOCARDITIS OF THE MITRAL VALVE

Stenotic aortic valves are frequently sites of infective endocarditis. As discussed in the section on endocarditis, the mitral valve may become involved with infective endocarditis by common abscess, by verrucous extension, or from a jet lesion, and infection may cause mitral valve aneurysm, perforation, and chordae disruption.[106] Management of these patients usually requires aortic valve replacement and assessment of the mitral valve at the time of operation. Vegetations of the mitral valve can sometimes be removed and perforations patched if the remaining tissue is sturdy and appears healthy.

CALCIFIC AORTIC STENOSIS WITH FUNCTIONAL MITRAL VALVE DISEASE

Senile calcification of the aortic valve may lead to mixed stenosis and regurgitation,[92] and the volume load from regurgitation may lead to left ventricular dilatation and secondary mitral regurgitation of an otherwise normal mitral valve.[92] Mitral regurgitation secondary to aortic valvular disease is discussed in the section on pathophysiology of multiple valve disease.

CALCIFIC AORTIC STENOSIS WITH CALCIFICATION OF THE MITRAL VALVE

Degenerative calcification is an age-related process usually affecting the aortic and mitral valves. In a study of patients over 75 years of age, one third had degenerative aortic or mitral calcification.[90] About 25% to 50% of patients with calcific aortic stenosis have calcification of the mitral valve annulus. Generally, patients with associated mitral annular calcification are older, have more severe aortic stenosis, and are more often female when compared with patients with aortic stenosis without mitral annular calcification.[98] Mills reported 17 patients undergoing mitral valve replacement for valvular disease related to severe annular calcification. Four of these patients also had concomitant aortic valve replacement.[107] Patients with mitral annular calcification have increased incidence of conduction defects[108] and aortic outflow murmurs, and annular calcification may exist in combination with rheumatic or myxomatous disease.[109]

Diagnosis, Signs, and Symptoms

PHYSICAL FINDINGS

Auscultatory findings in aortic stenosis and mitral regurgitation consist of two systolic murmurs that can be distinguished by location of maximum intensity and radiation. Characteristically, aortic stenosis produces a crescendo-decrescendo murmur at the base, and mitral regurgitation produces a holosystolic murmur at the apex. Occasionally, a prolonged ejection murmur of aortic stenosis may simulate a holosystolic murmur at the apex, and the murmur of severe mitral regurgitation may radiate toward the base and may take on a crescendo-decrescendo pattern simulating an ejection murmur.[61,64]

ELECTROCARDIOGRAPHY

Atrial fibrillation is uncommon in isolated aortic stenosis, and its presence is a clue to associated mitral valve disease.[61] Both aortic stenosis and mitral regurgitation produce left ventricular hypertrophy and left atrial enlargement.

ECHOCARDIOGRAPHY

Echocardiography is necessary to delineate mitral valve morphology and presence of flail segments, and to assess the severity of aortic valve stenosis. Transesophageal echocardiography, either preoperatively or intraoperatively, may be required to fully evaluate the mitral valve.

INFECTIVE ENDOCARDITIS AFFECTING MULTIPLE VALVES

As with infection of a single valve, multiple valve infective endocarditis may occur in previously diseased valves, normal valves, and prosthetic valves. Infective endocarditis requiring multiple valvular procedures occurs in about 10% to 25% of all patients having operation and usually involves the mitral and aortic valves (Table 41-17 and Table 41-18).[12,109–115] Conduction defects on electrocardiogram may be a clue to abscess involvement of both the aortic and mitral annulus.[116]

About 1% to 5% of patients who require surgery for multiple valve endocarditis have biventricular involvement, and most instances of tricuspid valve infections are owing to intravenous drug use.[113,117] Patients with multiple valve infective endocarditis more frequently have congestive heart failure as an indication for surgery and are more likely to have intracardiac abscess when compared to single valve infective endocarditis.[113]

TABLE 41–17 Locations and combinations of valvular infective endocarditis

	NVE	PVE	Total
Number of patients	131	47	178
Aortic	51% (68)	68% (32)	56% (100)
Mitral	27% (36)	23% (11)	26% (47)
Multiple	24% (31)	9% (4)	20% (35)
Aortic and mitral	18% (24)	9% (4)	16% (28)
Tricuspid	3% (4)	0% (0)	2% (4)
Mitral and tricuspid	1% (2)	0% (0)	1% (2)
Aortic, mitral, and tricuspid	1% (1)	0% (0)	0.6% (1)

NVE = native valve endocarditis; PVE = prosthetic valve endocarditis. Number of patients in parentheses.

Source: Modified with permission from Karp RB: Role of surgery in infective endocarditis [review]. Cardiovasc Clin 1987; 17:141.

Aortic Regurgitant Jet Lesion of the Mitral Valve

Perforation of the anterior leaflet of the mitral valve may occur from the regurgitant jet of aortic valve endocarditis, and the diagnosis can be made from transesophageal echocardiography.[118] Often, the perforation in the mitral valve can be debrided and repaired with a patch of pericardium or prosthetic material.

Prosthetic Valve Endocarditis

Risk of prosthetic valve endocarditis is greatest approximately 4 to 6 weeks postoperatively and decreases to a stable rate by about one year after operation.[119,120] *Staphylococcus epidermidis* and *Staphylococcus aureus* account for 20% to 30% of cases, respectively.[121] Transesophageal echocardiography can identify vegetations caused by infection as well as prosthetic valve dysfunction and associated abscess cavities.[121] In general, management of patients with endocarditis affecting multiple valves is similar to management of patients with infection of one valve. There are, however, some special considerations. When aortic valve endocarditis is complicated by abscess formation, infections may extend into the mitral annulus and necessitate concomitant mitral

TABLE 41–18 Incidence of multiple valve replacement for native valve infective endocarditis from 1961–1974 at the Mayo Clinic

	No. of patients	Percent
Valve replacement for IE	138	
Aortic	99	71% (99/138)
Mitral	16	12% (16/138)
Multiple	23	17% (23/138)

IE = infective endocarditis.

Source: Modified with permission from Wilson WR, Danielson GK, Giuliani ER, et al: Cardiac valve replacement in congestive heart failure due to infective endocarditis. Mayo Clin Proc 1979; 54:223.

valve replacement; this occurs in approximately 12% of patients with aortic root abscess[122] and is especially prevalent when there is involvement of the aorticomitral junction or subannular interventricular septum.[113,122]

Tricuspid Valve with Left-Sided Valve Replacement

When the tricuspid valve is excised at the time of left-sided valve replacement, there remains a question of whether the tricuspid valve needs to be replaced. Simple excision of the tricuspid valve seems appropriate only in the absence of pulmonary hypertension and left-sided failure. A prosthetic left-sided valve is intrinsically stenotic, and many patients with tricuspid valve endocarditis can have pulmonary hypertension secondary to septic pulmonary emboli. Silverman found that patients who had tricuspid excision alone with left-sided valve replacement required perioperative inotropic support, and management of their postoperative congestive heart failure was more difficult than that of the patients who had tricuspid replacement.[113]

Results

Early mortality following surgery for multiple valve endocarditis is in the range of 20% to 30%, and Table 41-19 compares NYHA-class matched groups that had multiple valve procedures for infective endocarditis and for other reasons.

CARCINOID HEART DISEASE AFFECTING MULTIPLE VALVES

Valvular heart disease develops in about 50% of patients with carcinoid tumors; patients with primary carcinoid tumor in the small intestine are more likely to have carcinoid heart disease than those with carcinoid tumors in other locations.[2] In most cases, the tricuspid and pulmonary valves are involved. We have offered valvular surgery to patients with severe symptoms of right heart failure caused by carcinoid heart disease whose systemic carcinoid symptoms are controlled by octreotide and/or hepatic dearterialization.[123]

TABLE 41–19 Comparison of early outcome between patients having multiple valve surgery for infective endocarditis and patients having multiple valve surgery for other reasons[8,102]

	Class II	Class III	Class IV
Multiple valve procedures for infective endocarditis	20% (15)	33% (3)	20% (5)
Multiple valve procedures for other causes	16% (25)	12% (25)	36% (25)

Operative mortality is expressed as percentage, and numbers of patients are in parentheses.

Signs and Symptoms/Diagnosis

Jugular venous distention with *v* waves (from tricuspid regurgitation) and *a* waves (from tricuspid stenosis) can be evident. Right ventricular enlargement can produce a pericardial lift. Most patients have murmurs from the tricuspid and pulmonary valves.[123] Patients often demonstrate ascites and liver enlargement as a result of either right-sided heart failure or hepatic metastases, or both. Therefore, these findings are not necessarily indicative of severe tricuspid valve regurgitation.

The electrocardiogram of patients with carcinoid heart disease often shows low voltage (85%), right bundle branch block (42%), and evidence of right atrial enlargement (35%).[2,123] The chest x-ray characteristically shows cardiomegaly (69%), pleural effusions (58%), and pleural thickening (35%).[123]

Echocardiography

Echocardiographic findings of carcinoid heart disease include thickening and reduced motion of the tricuspid valve leaflets; the pulmonic valve cusps may be thickened and retracted. Fusion of the pulmonary valve commissures results in a stiff fibrotic ring that may cause a stricture in the entire pulmonary orifice. Pulmonary regurgitation and stenosis may both be present.[124]

Invasive Studies

Cardiac catheterization is not necessary unless ischemic symptoms or a history of myocardial infarction suggest coronary artery disease.

Pathophysiology

Carcinoid heart disease results from deposition of plaques on the endocardium of the valves and atria; this usually occurs on the right side of the heart. However, plaques can develop on the mitral and aortic valves when there is carcinoid tumor in the lungs, or in the presence of intracardiac shunting that bypasses the lungs. Valves are damaged by exposure to circulating substances released from carcinoid tumors such as serotonin and bradykinin. Both of these components are inactivated by the lungs and the liver; the relationship between tumor location and the location of cardiac lesions is summarized in Table 41-20.[125] The plaques usually deposit on the downstream side of the cardiac valves causing adherence of the leaflet to the underlying structures, producing functional regurgitation. Carcinoid plaque deposition also may constrict the valve annulus and produce stenosis.[2]

The dominant functional lesion of carcinoid heart disease is tricuspid valve regurgitation; the valve is fixed in a semi-open position, so that some degree of stenosis is present. Fibrosis and plaque deposition also affect the pulmonary

TABLE 41–20 A comparison of venous drainage, presence of liver metastases, and carcinoid plaque location in relation to location of primary carcinoid tumor[125]

Tumor location	Venous drainage	Liver metastases	Plaque location
Gut	Portal	Yes	Right-sided
Ovary	Systemic	No	Right-sided
Bronchial	Pulmonary	No	Left-sided

valve, causing mixed stenosis and regurgitation, which increases the degree of tricuspid regurgitation.[2]

Operative Decision Making

TIMING OF OPERATION

The primary indications for surgery are increasing symptoms of congestive failure with objective evidence of valvular disease.[126] Again it should be noted that some of the signs of right heart failure, such as peripheral edema, ascites, and hepatomegaly, can be caused by the primary disease. Another indication for operation may be progressive right ventricular enlargement in the absence of symptoms. In a small series of carcinoid patients, right ventricular size and function did not correlate with operative or late mortality.[123] Currently we employ exercise testing to provide an objective assessment of the functional status and a guideline to the timing of cardiac surgery. If the primary cause for debilitation is right heart failure, it is reasonable to offer valve replacement even though the prognosis may be guarded.[126]

TRICUSPID VALVE OPERATION

The tricuspid valve always requires replacement, and in our earlier experience we used mechanical prostheses because of the possibility of carcinoid plaque formation on a bioprosthesis. However, review of our patients and those reported previously shows little difference in patient survival with mechanical or tissue valves. Bioprostheses are selected for patients who have liver dysfunction that would complicate anticoagulation with Coumadin and for patients who will undergo subsequent hepatic resection or hepatic artery embolization.

PULMONARY VALVE OPTIONS

As stated previously, we now advise valve replacement rather than excision when the pulmonary valve is involved.

Management of the carcinoid syndrome during and early after operation is critically important, and this has been simplified greatly by treatment with long-acting octreotide; this is supplemented intraoperatively with intravenous administration of short-acting octreotide when there is evidence of flushing and vasodilation.[127] Preoperative steroids and antihistamines can also be used to prevent adverse effects from tumor-released mediators.[127,128] We usually give octreotide, 500 μg intravenously, prior to induction of anesthesia with additional intravenous doses as needed at the onset and termination of cardiopulmonary bypass. Postoperatively, octreotide is continued and the dose is adjusted according to the severity of the flushing and vasodilation. Aprotinin, a kallikrein inhibitor, may mitigate the effects of substances released by carcinoid tumors during anesthesia and reduce intraoperative and postoperative bleeding.[127]

RARE CAUSES OF MULTIPLE VALVE DISEASE

Table 41-21 lists some rare causes of multiple heart valve disease that require surgical correction.

RESULTS OF MULTIPLE VALVE SURGERY

Long- and Short-Term Mortality

Survival following multiple valve surgery has improved along with refinements in myocardial protection; for example, mortality for multiple valve operations performed using normothermic ischemic arrest was approximately 40%[129]; the use of cardioplegic arrest reduced operative risk by three-quarters.[66,129,130] In recent reports, operative mortality (30-day mortality or hospital mortality) ranges from about 6% to 17% (Table 41-22, part A). The 5-year actuarial survival is 60% to 88% (Table 41-22, part B), and the 10-year actuarial survival is 43% to 81% (Table 41-22, part C). Risk factors identified for morbidity and mortality following multiple valve surgery include advanced NYHA

TABLE 41–21 Rare causes of multiple valve disease requiring surgery

Disease	Valves replaced or repaired
Methysergide/ergotamine toxicity[90]	Aortic and mitral
Radiation injury[125,176]	Mitral and tricuspid
Q-fever endocarditis[177]	Aortic and mitral
Ectodermal anhydrotic dysplasia[178]	Aortic and mitral
Maroteaux-Lamy syndrome (mucopoly-saccharidosis type VI)[179]	Aortic and mitral
Werner's syndrome (adult progeria)[180]	Aortic and mitral
Blunt trauma[181]	Mitral and tricuspid
Lymphoma[182]	Aortic and mitral
Relapsing polychondritis[183]	Aortic and mitral
Systemic lupus erythematosus[184]	Mitral and tricuspid
Secondary hyperparathyroidism[185]	Aortic and mitral
Urticarial vasculitis syndrome (HUVS) with Jaccoud's hands deformity[186]	Aortic and mitral

TABLE 41–22 Summary of morbidity and mortality following multiple valve surgery

	DVR	MVR	AVR	*P* value	Valve type	Reference
A. Operative mortality (percent)	5.6				Various*	Teoh[136]
	5.9	4.3	2	—	SJM	Horstkotte[152]
	6.3	5.2	3.1	—	SJM	Smith[146]
	6.5				SJM	Armenti[133]
	7.2	4.7	3.9	—	SJM	Aoyagi[21]
	8.2	4.3	2.4	—	SJM	Ibrahim[187]
	10				Hancock II	David[188]
	10.5				C-E	Jamieson[189]
	10.8	11.3	7.8	—	Sorin Disc	Milano[190]
	10.8				Various*	Galloway[134]
	11.5	13.0	4.9	$p < .001$	SJM	Khan[132]
	11.6	7.5	5.1	—	C-E	Bernal[153]
	15.3				Various	Donahoo[137]
	17.5				Various*	Mattila[138]
B. 5-year actuarial survival (percent)	88	88	91	N.S.	SJM	Aoyagi[21]
	86	86	94	MVR or DVR < AVR $p < .05$	SJM	Smith[146]
	86				SJM	Khan[132]
	78				Various*	Galloway[134]
	75				C-E	Bernal[153]
	73				Hancock II	David[188]
	70				C-E	Jamieson[189]
	62				MIPB	Lemieux[191]
	61	65	75	DVR < MVR or AVR $p < .01$	SJM	Khan[132]
	60				SJM	Armenti[133]
	****	****	****	DVR < AVR or MVR $p < .006$	B-S	Alvarez[140]
C. 10-year actuarial survival (percent)	81	80	81	N.S.	SJM	Aoyagi[21]
	72	78	85	—	SJM	Horstkotte[152]
	60	59	71	N.S.	SJM	Ibrahim[184]
	55	63	65	—	B-S	Orszulak[192]
	43	42	43	N.S.	SJM	Khan[132]
D. Thromboembolism (percent per patient-year)	0.3	0.3	0.6	—	SJM	Smith[146]
	0.79	1.6	1.3	—	SJM	Nakano[193]
	1.3	1.1	1.0	N.S.	SJM	Aoyagi[21]
	2.1				Various*	Mattila[138]
	2.1	1.2	1.3	N.S.	Sorin Disc	Milano[190]
	3.2	2.4	2.5	N.S.	SJM	Khan[132]
	4.5				Various*	Mullany[48]
	4.6				SJM	Armenti[133]
	4.6	4.3	2.1	—	B-S	Orszulak[192]
	5.0	4.4	2.4	—	SJM	Ibrahim[187]
	6.6	5.1	3.7	—	SJM	Horstkotte[152]
E. 10-year freedom from thromboembolism (percent)	89	92	91	—	C-E pericardial	Pelletier[194]
	89	89	94	N.S.	SJM	Aoyagi[21]
	89	83		—	C-E	van Doorn[145]
	86	88	80	—	Hancock II	David[188]
	77	83	76	N.S.	SJM	Khan[132]
	77	79	87	—	B-S	Orszulak[192]
	§	§	§	N.S.	B-S	Alvarez[140]
F. Anticoagulation-related hemorrhage (percent per patient-year)	0.1	0.2	0.1	—	SJM	Nakano[193]
	0.5	0.3	0.4	—	SJM	Aoyagi[21]
	0.9	0.9	0.9	N.S.	Sorin Disc	Milano[190]
	1.2				SJM	Armenti[132]
	1.2	0.7	0.2	—	SJM†	Horstkotte[152]
	2.3	1.2	2.0	N.S.	SJM	Khan[132]
	4.5	2.1	1.2	—	SJM‡	Horstkotte[152]
	§	§	§	DVR > AVR or MVR $p < .05$	B-S	Alvarez[140]

TABLE 41–22 (*Continued*)

	DVR	MVR	AVR	*P* value	Valve type	Reference
G. Endocarditis (percent per patient-year)	0.2	0.06	0.21	—	St. Jude	Nakano[193]
	0.3	0.03	0.4	—	St. Jude	Aoyagi[21]
	2.1				Various*	Mattila[138]
	2.5				SJM	Armenti[133]
	§	§	§	DVR > AVR or MVR $p < .05$	B-S	Alvarez[140]
H. 8-,10-, and 15-year freedom from structural deterioration for bioprostheses (percent)	77	79	87	—	C-E pericardial	Pelletier[194]
	59.6	70.8		—	C-E	van Doorn[195]
	44	33	62	$p < .03$	C-E	Bernal[153]
	38	58	80	DVR < MVR < AVR $p < .05$	MP	Pomar[149]

DVR = double valve replacement; AVR = isolated aortic valve replacement; MVR = isolated mitral valve replacement; N.S. = not statistically significant; SJM = St. Jude Medical; C-E = Carpentier-Edwards; B-S = Björk-Shiley; MP = Mitroflow pericardial; MIPB = Medtronic intact porcine bioprosthesis.

* = Includes some patients with concomitant tricuspid procedures.

† = INR 1.75 = 2.75.

‡ = INR 4 = 6.

§ = Results reported graphically.

Comparisons to isolated aortic and mitral valve procedures from the same series are included when available. If statistical analysis between the results of multiple and single valve procedures was reported, the *p* values are included. If a series was limited to a single valve type, it is listed.

class,[131–133] advanced age,[131–135] current or prior myocardial revascularization,[134] ejection fraction 11% to 35%,[131] presence of coronary artery disease,[131,132] aortic stenosis,[136] elevated pulmonary artery pressure,[134] tricuspid regurgitation,[136] and diabetes mellitus.[134]

Clearly, operative mortality is influenced by patient selection,[133] and comparisons between studies are of limited value.[133] Causes of death following multiple valve surgery are low cardiac output,[21,133,136–139] myocardial infarction,[138] technical failure,[139] multiple organ failure,[21] ventricular rupture,[95,134,137] and mechanical obstruction of prosthetic leaflet.[95,138]

Comparisons of late survival between patients having multiple valve versus single valve replacement are inconsistent. Some studies show poorer survival[132] after multiple valve replacement, and others report no significant difference in survival.[21,130,132,139–144] The discrepancy in these results may be because the majority of deaths in many reports are secondary to progression of coronary artery disease and noncardiac causes rather than valve-related deaths.[130,132] The presence of coronary artery disease and concomitant coronary artery surgery increases mortality following multiple valve surgery.[134,145,146]

Some causes of early death following multiple valve surgery are perhaps less common today owing to changes in practice. In a necropsy study from 1963 to 1985 of patients who died early following double valve replacement, prosthetic valve dysfunction secondary to mechanical interference was evident in almost 50%, and ventricular rupture had occurred in 15% of cases.[95] Most of these patients received Starr-Edwards caged-ball prosthetic valves. Mechanical failure of low-profile tilting-disc prostheses that are in current use is rare, and early valve-related death with this type of prosthesis is very unusual.[21,132,133,147] The current practice of preserving the posterior leaflet and chordal attachments of the mitral valve during prosthetic replacement may decrease the chance of ventricular disruption.[148]

Thromboembolism

Thromboembolic rates following multiple valve replacement are shown in Table 41-22, part D, and range from 1% to 7% per patient-year for double valve replacement. Ten years postoperatively, freedom from thromboembolic events ranges from 77% to 89% (Table 41-22, part E). Although the data presented in Table 41-22, part D, along with other sources,[149] do not indicate significant differences between single and multiple valve replacement, some reports suggest that both mechanical[150] and bioprosthetic[151] valves have an increased risk of thromboembolism in the mitral position. This risk is present early (90 days after operation) in patients undergoing multiple valve replacement that includes a bioprosthetic mitral valve.[151]

Anticoagulation-Related Hemorrhage

Rates of anticoagulant-related hemorrhage following multiple valve replacement, as with single valve surgery, are dependent on target INR.[152] Risks of hemorrhage are reported to be 0.1% to 4.5% per patient-year following multiple valve surgery (Table 41-22, part F). Alvarez reported a significantly higher rate of anticoagulant-related hemorrhage following multiple valve replacement compared to single valve replacement.[140]

Prosthetic Valve Infective Endocarditis

Rates of infective endocarditis following multiple valve surgery range from 0.2% to 2.5% per patient-year as shown in Table 41-22, part G. In comparison to isolated valve surgery, Alvarez reports prosthesis infection is more frequent following double valve replacement when compared to either isolated aortic ($p < .05$) or mitral replacement ($p < .001$).[140]

Valve Performance

Rates of bioprosthetic structural deterioration relate to valve position; tissue valves appear to fail earlier in the mitral position than in the aortic position. When multiple valve replacements include the mitral valve, the rates of deterioration are similar[153] or even worse than[149] isolated mitral valve replacement (Table 41-22, part H).

COMPARISON OF BIOPROSTHETIC VALVES TO MECHANICAL VALVES

Comparisons of outcomes of patients with two or more mechanical prostheses to patients with two or more bioprostheses show similar rates of thromboembolism,[18,154] but freedom from operation favors those with multiple mechanical valves.[18,154] As might be expected, anticoagulation-related hemorrhage is less in patients with two bioprosthetic valves,[154,155] but there is no clear advantage of one prosthesis over the other as regards early and late mortality.[18,154,155]

Results of Tricuspid Valve Procedures with Other Valve Procedures

RESULTS OF MITRAL AND TRICUSPID SURGERY

Reported operative mortality following mitral valve replacement and tricuspid valve repair or replacement is approximately 12% to 15%,[156] and 65% to 75% of patients are alive 5 years postoperatively.[134,156] Outlook for patients with lesser degrees of tricuspid regurgitation at the time of mitral valve replacement is good; 5-year actuarial survival for patients with tricuspid regurgitation who do not have tricuspid repair or replacement is 80% to 84%, and 10-year survival is 62% to 77%.[157]

TRIPLE VALVE REPLACEMENT

The operative mortality following triple valve replacement is higher than that for double valve replacement and ranges from 5% to 25%.[20,134] As with double valve replacement, advanced age and higher NYHA class are associated with a risk factor for early mortality.[20,158] Causes of perioperative death are similar to those following double valve replacement and include low cardiac output, multiorgan failure, hemorrhage, and dysrhythmia.[20]

Five-year actuarial survival after triple valve replacement is 53% to 78%, and 10- and 15-year survival are 40% and 25%, respectively (Table 41-23). Considering only perioperative survivors of triple valve replacement, late survival is comparable to that of patients undergoing isolated valve replacement.[20,159] Reports of thromboembolic rates following triple valve replacement range from 5% to 12% per patient-year (Table 41-23).

DOUBLE VALVE REPLACEMENT AND TRICUSPID ANNULOPLASTY

Operative mortality for patients undergoing double valve replacement with tricuspid valve repair is about 25%,[48] and the 10- and 15-year survival rates are 35% and 27%, generally comparable to those of patients having triple valve replacement.[48] Rates of thromboembolism in this group are reported to be 5% per patient-year.[48]

Other Results

The operative mortality for double re-replacement is about 10% to 20%.[132,160] Incidence of postoperative ventricular arrhythmias is higher in patients having combined valve surgery compared to single valve surgery.[161] Hemolysis may be more common with multiple valve disease or following multiple valve replacement.[162,163]

The incidence of perivalvular leak following multiple valve surgery is about 4% per patient-year and may be more frequent following multiple valve surgery compared to single valve surgery.[138,140]

When multiple valve surgery is combined with myocardial revascularization, the morbidity and mortality are 12% to 24%.[145,164] Early death in this group of patients is associated with prolonged perfusion time, the need for postoperative inotropic support, and high blood loss.[164]

SUMMARY

The challenges of multiple valve replacement and repair include not only the technical maneuvers of operation but also the identification of associated valve lesions and correct judgment in surgical management. Echocardiography is the essential tool in preoperative diagnosis, and surgeons should become as familiar and facile with interpretation of ultrasound assessment of cardiac valves as with analysis of coronary angiograms. Finally, the various etiologies of multiple valve disease occur in certain combinations, and understanding the pathophysiology and pathologic anatomy is necessary to select the best procedure and to optimize early and late operative results.

TABLE 41–23 Results of triple valve surgery by author

	Col[196]	Gersh[20]	Galloway[134]	Brown[154]	Mullany[48]	Kara[158]
Years studied	1970–1984	1962–1984	1976–1985		1965–1984	1972–1983
Number of patients	37	91	61	40	109	107
Type of procedure	Triple valve replacement	Triple valve replacement	Triple valve procedure	Triple valve replacement	Double valve replacement with tricuspid repair	Triple valve procedure
Valve type		Various (mostly S-E)	Various	Various	Various (60% S-E)	S-E, Björk, or St. Jude
Operative mortality	5%	24%	23%		21%	20%
Actuarial 5-year survival	75%	55%	62%	78%	70%	53%
Thromboembolism rate		12.3% pt-y		32% at 5 years combined with hemorrhage	4.5% pt-y	
Prosthetic infective endocarditis rate		6%			3%	
Hemorrhage rate		22%			17%	
Significant risk factors		Age, NYHA Class IV			Age, NYHA Class IV	Higher NYHA class, emergent operation, tricuspid replacement

S-E = Starr-Edwards; NYHA = New York Heart Association functional class.

REFERENCES

1. Starr A, Edwards LM, McCord CW, et al: Multiple valve replacement. *Circulation* 1964; 29(suppl):30.
2. Knott-Craig CJ, Schaff HV, Mullany CJ, et al: Carcinoid disease of the heart. Surgical management of ten patients. *J Thorac Cardiovasc Surg* 1992; 104:475.
3. Schulman DS, Remetz MS, Elefteriades J, et al: Mild mitral insufficiency is a marker of impaired left ventricular performance in aortic stenosis. *J Am Coll Cardiol* 1989; 13:796.
4. Christenson JT, Jordan B, Bloch A, et al: Should a regurgitant mitral valve be replaced simultaneously with a stenotic aortic valve? *Tex Heart Inst J* 2000; 27:350.
5. Harris KM, Malenka DJ, Haney MF, et al: Improvement in mitral regurgitation after aortic valve replacement. *Am J Cardiol* 1997; 80:741.
6. Freeman WK, Seward JB, Khandheria BK, et al: *Transesophageal Echocardiography*. Boston, Little, Brown, 1994.
7. Nowrangi SK, Connolly HM, Freeman WK, et al: Impact of intraoperative transesophageal echocardiography among patients undergoing aortic valve replacement for aortic stenosis. *J Am Soc Echocardiogr* 2001; 14:863.
8. McGrath L, Gonzalez-Lavin L, Bailey B, et al: Tricuspid valve operations in 530 patients: twenty-five-year assessment of early and late phase events. *J Thorac Cardiovasc Surg* 1990; 99:124.
9. Farid L, Dayem MK, Guindy R, et al: The importance of tricuspid valve structure and function in the surgical treatment of rheumatic mitral and aortic disease. *Eur Heart J* 1992; 13:366.
10. Pellegrini A, Colombo T, Donatelli F, et al: Evaluation and treatment of secondary tricuspid insufficiency. *Eur J Cardiothorac Surg* 1992; 6:288.
11. Carpentier A, Deloche A, Hannia G, et al: Surgical management of acquired tricuspid valve disease. *J Thorac Cardiovasc Surg* 1974; 67:53.
12. Wilson WR, Danielson GK, Giuliani ER, et al: Cardiac valve replacement in congestive heart failure due to infective endocarditis. *Mayo Clin Proc* 1979; 54:223.
13. Cohn LH: Tricuspid regurgitation secondary to mitral valve disease: when and how to repair. *J Card Surg* 1994; 9 (suppl):237.
14. King RM, Schaff HV, Danielson GK, et al: Surgery for tricuspid regurgitation, late after mitral valve replacement. *Circulation* 1984; (suppl I):193.
15. Izumi C, Iga K, Konishi T: Progression of isolated tricuspid regurgitation late after mitral valve surgery for rheumatic mitral valve disease. *J Heart Valve Dis* 2002; 11:353.
16. DeVega NG: La anuloplastia selectiva reguable y permanente. *Rev Esp Cardiol* 1972; 25:6.
17. Kuwaki K, Morishita K, Tsukamoto M, et al: Tricuspid valve surgery for functional tricuspid valve regurgitation associated with left-sided valvular disease. *Eur J Cardiothorac Surg* 2001; 20:577.
18. Bortolotti U, Milano A, Testolin L, et al: Influence of type of prosthesis on late results after combined mitral-aortic valve replacement. *Ann Thorac Surg* 1991; 52:84.
19. Brown PJ, Roberts CS, McIntosh CL, et al: Relation between choice of prostheses and late outcome in double-valve replacement. *Ann Thorac Surg* 1993; 55:631.
20. Gersh BJ, Schaff HV, Vatterott PJ, et al: Results of triple valve replacement in 91 patients: perioperative mortality and long-term follow-up. *Circulation* 1985; 72:130.
21. Kawano H, Oda T, Fukunaga S, et al: Tricuspid valve replacement with the St. Jude Medical valve: 19 years of experience. *Eur J Cardiothorac Surg* 2000; 18:565.
22. Struber M, Campbell A, Richard G, et al: Hydrodynamic performance of Carbomedics valves in double valve replacement. *J Heart Valve Dis* 1994; 3:667.
23. Levi M, Cromheecke ME, de Jonge E, et al: Pharmacological strategies to decrease excessive blood loss in cardiac surgery: a meta-analysis of clinically relevant endpoints. *Lancet* 1999; 354:1940.
24. Tyner JJ, Hunter JA, Najafi H: Postperfusion coronary stenosis. *Ann Thorac Surg* 1987; 44:418.
25. Talwalkar NG, Lawrie GM, Earle N: Can retrograde cardioplegia alone provide adequate protection for cardiac valve surgery? *Chest* 1999; 115:1359.
26. Villanueva FS, Spotnitz WD, Glasheen WP, et al: New insights into the physiology of retrograde cardioplegia delivery. *Am J Physiol* 1995; 268 (4 pt 2):H1555.
27. Ruengsakulrach P, Buxton BF: Anatomic and hemodynamic considerations influencing the efficiency of retrograde cardioplegia. *Ann Thorac Surg* 2001; 71:1389.
28. Fraser CD Jr, Wang N, Mee RB, et al: Repair of insufficient bicuspid aortic valves. *Ann Thorac Surg* 1994; 58:386.
29. Cosgrove DM, Ratliff NB, Schaff HV, Eards WD: Aortic valve decalcification: history repeated with a new result. *Ann Thorac Surg* 1994; 49:689.
30. Piehler JM, Danielson GK, Pluth JR, et al: Enlargement of the aortic root or annulus with autogenous pericardial patch during aortic valve replacement: long-term follow-up. *J Thorac Cardiovasc Surg* 1983; 86:350.
31. Ross DB, Trusler GA, Coles JG, et al: Successful reconstruction of aorto-left atrial fistula following aortic valve replacement and root enlargement by the Manouguian procedure. *J Card Surg* 1994; 9:392.
32. de Vivie ER, Borowski A, Mehlhorn U: Reduction of the left-ventricular outflow-tract obstruction by aortoventriculoplasty—long-term results of 96 patients. *Thorac Cardiovasc Surg* 1993; 41:216.
33. Manouguian S: [A new method for patch enlargement of hypoplastic aortic annulus. An experimental study (author's translation)]. *Thoraxchirurgie Vaskulare Chirurgie* 1976; 24(5):418.
34. Skoularigis J, Sinovich V, Joubert G, Sareli P: Evaluation of the long-term results of mitral valve repair in 254 young patients with rheumatic mitral regurgitation. *Circulation* 1994; 90(5 pt 2): II-167.
35. Enriquez-Sarano M, Tajik AJ, Schaff HV, et al: Echocardiographic prediction of survival after surgical correction of organic mitral regurgitation. *Circulation* 1994; 90:830.
36. Enriquez-Sarano M, Schaff HV, Orszulak TA, et al: Valve repair improves the outcome of surgery for mitral regurgitation: a multivariate analysis. *Circulation* 1995; 91:1022.
37. Liao K, Wu JJ, Frater RW: Comparative evaluation of left ventricular performance after mitral valve repair or valve replacement with or without chordal preservation. *J Heart Valve Dis* 1993; 2:159.
38. David TE: Papillary muscle-annular continuity: is it important? *J Card Surg* 1994; 9 (2 suppl):252.
39. Suzuki N, Takanashi Y, Tokuhiro K, et al: Mitral valve replacement with and without chordal preservation in patients with chronic mitral regurgitation: mechanisms for differences. *Circulation* 1992; 86:1718.
40. Wasir H, Choudhary SK, Airan B, et al: Mitral valve replacement with chordal preservation in a rheumatic population. *J Heart Valve Dis* 2001; 10:84.
41. Crawford ES, Coselli JS: Marfan's syndrome: combined composite valve graft replacement of the aortic root and transaortic mitral valve replacement. *Ann Thorac Surg* 1988; 45:296.
42. Seccombe JF, Schaff HV: Mitral valve repair: current techniques and indications, in Franco L, Verrier ED (eds): *Advanced Therapy in Cardiac Surgery*. Hanover, PA, The Sheridan Press, 1999; p 220.
43. Phillips MR, Daly RC, Schaff HV, et al: Repair of anterior leaflet mitral valve prolapse: chordal replacement versus chordal shortening. *Ann Thorac Surg* 2000; 69:25.

44. Odell JA, Schaff HV, Orszulak TA: Early results of a simplified method of mitral valve annuloplasty. *Circulation* 1995; 92 (suppl II):150.
45. Acar C, Perier P, Fontaliran F, et al: Anatomical study of the tricuspid valve and its variations. *Surg Radiol Anat* 1990; 12:229.
46. Izumi C, Iga K, Konishi T: Progression of isolated tricuspid regurgitation late after mitral valve surgery for rheumatic mitral valve disease. *J Heart Valve Dis* 2002; 11:353.
47. King RM, Schaff HV, Danielson GK, et al: Surgical treatment of tricuspid insufficiency late after mitral valve replacement. *Circulation* 1983; 68:III.
48. Mullany CJ, Gersh BJ, Orszulak TA, et al: Repair of tricuspid valve insufficiency in patients undergoing double (aortic and mitral) valve replacement: perioperative mortality and long-term (1 to 20 years) follow-up in 109 patients. *J Thorac Cardiovasc Surg* 1987; 94:740.
49. Duran CG, Ubago JL: Clinical and hemodynamic performance of a totally flexible prosthetic ring for atrio-ventricular valve reconstruction. *Ann Thorac Surg* 1976; 22:458.
50. Kay JH, Maselli-Capagna G, Tsuji HK: Surgical treatment of tricuspid insufficiency. *Ann Surg* 1965; 162:53.
51. McCarthy JF, Cosgrove DM: Tricuspid valve repair with the Cosgrove-Edwards annuloplasty system. *Ann Thorac Surg* 1997; 64:267.
52. Connolly HM, Schaff HV, Mullany CJ, et al: Surgical management of left-sided carcinoid heart disease. *Circulation* 2001; 104(12 suppl S):136.
53. Connolly HM, Schaff HV, Larson RA, et al: Carcinoid heart disease: impact of pulmonary valve replacement on right ventricular function and remodeling. *Circulation*. 2001; 104:II-685.
54. Kirklin J, Barratt-Boyes B: Combined aortic and mitral valve disease with and without tricuspid valve disease, in Kirklin JW, Barratt-Boyes B (eds): *Cardiac Surgery*. New York, Wiley, 1993; p 431.
55. Roberts WC, Virmani R: Aschoff bodies at necropsy in valvular heart disease. *Circulation* 1978; 57:803.
56. Bland EF, Jones TD: Rheumatic fever and rheumatic heart disease: a twenty year report on 1000 patients followed since childhood. *Circulation* 1951; 4:836.
57. Wilson MG, Lubschez R: Longevity in rheumatic fever. *JAMA* 1948; 121:1.
58. Ellis LB, Harken DE, Black H: A clinical study of 1000 consecutive cases of mitral stenosis two to nine years after mitral valvuloplasty. *Circulation* 1959; 19:803.
59. Kern MJ, Aguirre F, Donohue T, et al: Interpretation of cardiac pathophysiology from pressure waveform analysis: multivalvular regurgitant lesions. *Cathet Cardiovasc Diag* 1993; 28(2):167.
60. Segal B, Harvey WP, Hufnagel CA: Clinical study of 100 cases of severe aortic insufficiency. *Am J Med* 1956; 21:200.
61. Paraskos JA: Combined valvular disease, in Dalen JE, Alpert JS (eds): *Valvular Heart Disease,* vol 2. Boston, Little, Brown, 1987; p 439.
62. Brest AN, Udhoji V, Likoff W: A re-evaluation of the Grahm Steell murmur. *N Engl J Med* 1962; 263:1229.
63. Rahko PS: Doppler and echocardiographic characteristics of patients having an Austin Flint murmur. *Circulation* 1991; 83:1940.
64. Hall R: Other valvular disorders, in Julian D, Camm J, Fox K, et al (eds): *Diseases of the Heart*. London, Bailliere Tindall, 1989; p 838.
65. Cohn LH, Mason DT, Ross J Jr, et al: Pre-operative assessment of aortic regurgitation in patients with mitral valve disease. *Am J Cardiol* 1967; 19:177.
66. Terzaki AK, Cokkinos DV, Leachman RD, et al: Combined mitral and aortic valve disease. *Am J Cardiol* 1970; 25:588.
67. Braunwald E: *Heart Disease: A Textbook of Cardiovascular Medicine*. Philadelphia, WB Saunders, 1988.
68. Mego DM, Johns JP, Rubal BJ: Pharmacodynamic Doppler determination of mitral valve area in patients with significant aortic regurgitation. *J Am Soc Echocardiogr* 1993; 6(2):142.
69. Gash AK, Carabello BA, Kent RL, et al: Left ventricular performance in patients with coexistent mitral stenosis and aortic insufficiency. *J Am Coll Cardiol* 1984; 67:148.
70. Grinda JM, Latremouille C, Berrebi AJ, et al: Aortic cusp extension valvuloplasty for rheumatic aortic valve disease: midterm results. *Ann Thorac Surg* 2002; 74:438.
71. Prabhakar G, Kumar N, Gometza B, et al: Triple-valve operation in the young rheumatic patient. *Ann Thorac Surg* 1993; 55:1492.
72. Zitnik RS, Piemme TE, Messer RJ, et al: The masking of aortic stenosis by mitral stenosis. *Am Heart J* 1965; 69:22.
73. Schattenberg TT, Titus JL, Parkin TW: Clinical findings in acquired aortic valve stenosis. *Am Heart J* 1967; 73:322.
74. Katznelson G, Jreissaty RM, Levinson GE, et al: Combined aortic and mitral stenosis: a clinical and physiological study. *Am J Med* 1960; 29:242.
75. Brandenburg RO, Giuliani ER, Nishimura RA, et al: Acquired valvular heart disease: mitral stenosis, in Giuliani ER, Fuster V, Gersh BJ, et al (eds): *Cardiology: Fundamentals and Practice*. St. Louis, Mosby Yearbook, 1991; p 1543.
76. Uricchio JF, Sinha KP, Bentivoglio L, et al: A study of combined mitral and aortic stenosis. *Ann Intern Med* 1959; 51:668.
77. Kumar N, Saad E, Prabhakar G, et al: Extended transseptal versus conventional left atriotomy: early postoperative study. *Ann Thorac Surg* 1995; 60:426.
78. Honey M: Clinical and haemodynamic observations on combined mitral and aortic stenoses. *Br Heart J* 1961; 23:545.
79. Choudhary SK, Talwar S, Juneja R, et al: Fate of mild aortic valve disease after mitral valve intervention. *J Thorac Cardiovasc Surg* 2001; 122:583.
80. Larbalestier RI, Chard RB, Cohn LH: Optimal approach to the mitral valve: dissection of the interatrial groove. *Ann Thorac Surg* 1992; 54:1186.
81. Barner HB: Combined superior and right lateral left atriotomy with division of the superior vena cava for exposure of the mitral valve. *Ann Thorac Surg* 1992; 54:594.
82. Smith CR: Septal-superior exposure of the mitral valve: the transplant approach. *J Thorac Cardiovasc Surg* 1992; 103:623.
83. Couetil JP, Ramsheyi A, Tolan MJ, et al: Biatrial inferior transseptal approach to the mitral valve. *Ann Thorac Surg* 1995; 60:1432.
84. Brawley RK: Improved exposure of the mitral valve in patients with a small left atrium. *Ann Thorac Surg* 1980; 29:179.
85. Shine KI, DeSanctis RW, Sanders CA, et al: Combined aortic and mitral incompetence: clinical features and surgical. *Am Heart J* 1968; 76:728.
86. Hess O, Scherrer U, Nicod P: Combined valvular disease, in Willerson J, Cohn J (eds): *Cardiovascular Medicine*. New York, Churchill Livingstone, 1995; p 225.
87. Rackley C, Edwards J, Karp R: *Multivalvular Disease*. New York, McGraw-Hill, 1994.
88. Weyman AE: *Principles and Practice of Echocardiography*. Philadelphia, Waverly, 1994.
89. Urschel CW, Covell JW, Sonnenblick EH, et al: Myocardial mechanics in aortic and mitral valvular regurgitation: the concept of instantaneous impedance as a determinant of the performance of the intact heart. *J Clin Invest* 1968; 47:867.
90. Boucher C: Multivalvular heart disease, in Eagle K, Haber E, DeSanctis R, et al (eds): *The Practice of Cardiology,* 2nd ed. Boston, Little, Brown, 1989; p 765.
91. Shigenobu M, Senoo Y, Teramoto S: Results of surgery for aortic regurgitation due to aortic valve prolapse. *Acta Medica Okayama* 1988; 42:343.

92. Dare AJ, Veinot JP, Edwards WD, et al: New observations on the etiology of aortic valve disease: a surgical pathologic study of 236 cases from 1990. *Hum Pathol* 1993; 24:1330.
93. Bellitti R, Caruso A, Festa M, et al: Prolapse of the floppy aortic valve as a cause of aortic regurgitation: a clinico-morphologic study. *Int J Cardiol* 1985; 9:399.
94. Agozzino L, de Vivo F, Falco A, et al: Non-inflammatory aortic root disease and floppy aortic valve as cause of isolated regurgitation: a clinico-morphologic study. *Int J Cardiol* 1994; 45:129.
95. Roberts WC, Sullivan MF: Clinical and necropsy observations early after simultaneous replacement of the mitral and aortic valves. *Am J Cardiol* 1986; 58:1067.
96. Milewicz DM, Pyeritz RE, Crawford ES, et al: Marfan syndrome: defective synthesis, secretion, and extracellular matrix formation of fibrillin by cultured dermal fibroblasts. *J Clin Invest* 1992; 89:79.
97. Rippe LM, Angoff G, Sloss LJ: Multiple floppy valves: an echocardiographic syndrome. *Am J Med* 1979; 66:817.
98. Ogawa S, Hayashi J, Sasaki H, et al: Evaluation of combined valvular prolapse syndrome by two-dimensional echocardiography. *Circulation* 1982; 65:174.
99. Suzuki K, Murakami Y, Mori K, et al: Multiple floppy valves with all cardiac valves prolapsing: clinical course and treatment. *Pediatr Cardiol* 1991; 12:110.
100. Lakier JB, Copans H, Rosman HS, et al: Idiopathic degeneration of the aortic valve: A common cause of isolated aortic regurgitation. *J Am Coll Cardiol* 1985; 5(2 pt 1):347.
101. Tomaru T, Uchida Y, Mohri N, et al: Postinflammatory mitral and aortic valve prolapse: a clinical and pathological study. *Circulation* 1987; 76:68.
102. Gillinov AM, Blackstone EH, White J, et al: Durability of combined aortic and mitral valve repair. *Ann Thorac Surg* 2001; 72:20.
103. Gott VL, Cameron DE, Alejo DE, et al: Aortic root replacement in 271 Marfan patients: a 24-year experience. *Ann Thorac Surg* 2002; 73:438.
104. David TE: Aortic valve-sparing operations for aortic root aneurysm. *Semin Thorac Cardiovasc Surg* 2001; 13:291.
105. Gillinov AM, Hulyalkar A, Cameron DE, et al: Mitral valve operation in patients with the Marfan syndrome. *J Thorac Cardiovasc Surg* 1994; 107:724.
106. Fernicola DJ, Roberts WC: Pure mitral regurgitation associated with a malfunctioning congenitally bicuspid aortic valve necessitating combined mitral and aortic valve replacement. *Am J Cardiol* 1994; 74:619.
107. Mills NL, McIntosh CL, Mills LJ: Techniques for management of the calcified mitral annulus. *J Card Surg* 1986; 1:347.
108. Nair CK, Aronow WS, Sketch MH, et al: Clinical and echocardiography characteristics of patients with mitral annular calcification: comparison with age- and sex-matched control subjects. *Am J Cardiol* 1983; 51:992.
109. Utley JR, Mills J, Hutchinson JC, et al: Valve replacement for bacterial and fungal endocarditis: a comparative study. *Circulation* 1973; 3:42.
110. Buchbinder NA, Roberts WC: Left-sided valvular active infective endocarditis: a study of forty-five necropsy patients. *Am J Med* 1972; 53:20.
111. Mathew J, Addai T, Anand A, et al: Clinical features, site of involvement, bacteriologic findings, and outcome of infective endocarditis in intravenous drug users. *Arch Int Med* 1995; 155:1641.
112. Karp RB: Role of surgery in infective endocarditis [review]. *Cardiovasc Clin* 1987; 17:141.
113. Silverman NA, Levitsky S, Mammana R: Acute endocarditis in drug addicts: surgical treatment for multiple valve infection. *J Am Coll Cardiol* 1984; 4:680.
114. Yoshida K, Yoshikawa J, Akasaka T, et al: Infective endocarditis—analysis of 116 surgically and 26 medically treated patients. *Jpn Circ J* 1991; 55:794.
115. Abe T, Tsukamoto M, Komatsu S: Surgical treatment of active infective endocarditis—early and late results of active native and prosthetic valve endocarditis. *Jpn Circ J* 1993; 57:1080.
116. Steckelberg JM, Giuliani ER, Wilson WR: Infective endocarditis, in Giuliani ER, Fuster V, Gersh BJ, et al (eds): *Cardiology: Fundamentals and Practice*. St. Louis, Mosby Year Book, 1991; p 1739.
117. Richardson JV, Karp RB, Kirklin JW, et al: Treatment of infective endocarditis: a 10-year comparative analysis. *Circulation* 1978; 58:589.
118. Nomeir AM, Downes TR, Cordell AR: Perforation of the anterior mitral leaflet caused by aortic valve endocarditis: diagnosis by two-dimensional, transesophageal echocardiography and color flow Doppler. *J Am Soc Echocardiogr* 1992; 5:195.
119. Aoyagi S, Oryoji A, Nishi Y, et al: Long-term results of valve replacement with the St. Jude Medical valve. *J Thorac Cardiovasc Surg* 1994; 108:1021.
120. Kratz J, Crawford F, Sade R, et al: St. Jude prosthesis for aortic and mitral replacement: a ten-year experience. *Ann Thorac Surg* 1993; 56:462.
121. Chastre J, Trouillet JL: Early infective endocarditis on prosthetic valves [review]. *Eur Heart J* 1995; 16 (suppl B):32.
122. Watanabe G, Haverich A, Speier R, et al: Surgical treatment of active infective endocarditis with paravalvular involvement. *J Thorac Cardiovasc Surg* 1994; 107:171.
123. Connolly HM, Nishimura RA, Smith HC, et al: Outcome of cardiac surgery for carcinoid heart disease. *J Am Coll Cardiol* 1995; 25:410.
124. Pellikka PA, Tajik AJ, Khandheria BK, et al: Carcinoid heart disease: clinical and echocardiographic spectrum in 74 patients. *Circulation* 1993; 87:1188.
125. Schoen FJ, Berger BM, Guerina NG: Cardiac effects of noncardiac neoplasms [review]. *Cardiol Clin* 1984; 2:657.
126. Connolly HM: Carcinoid heart disease: medical and surgical considerations. *Cancer Control* 2001; 8:454.
127. Propst JW, Siegel LC, Stover EP: Anesthetic considerations for valve replacement surgery in a patient with carcinoid syndrome. *J Cardiothorac Vasc Anesth* 1994; 8:209.
128. Neustein SM, Cohen E, Reich D, et al: Transoesophageal echocardiography and the intraoperative diagnosis of left atrial invasion by carcinoid tumour. *Can J Anaesth* 1993; 40:664.
129. Cartwright RS, Giacobine JW, Ratan RS, et al: Combined aortic and mitral valve replacement. *J Thorac Cardiovasc Surg* 1963; 45:35.
130. Stephenson LW, Edie RN, Harken AH, et al: Combined aortic and mitral valve replacement: changes in practice and prognosis. *Circulation* 1984; 69:640.
131. LaSalle CW, Csicsko JF, Mirro MJ: Double cardiac valve replacement: a community hospital experience. *Ind Med* 1993; 86:422.
132. Khan S, Chaux A, Matloff J, et al: The St. Jude medical valve: experience with 1,000 cases. *J Thorac Cardiovasc Surg* 1994; 108:1010.
133. Armenti F, Stephenson LW, Edmunds LH Jr: Simultaneous implantation of St. Jude Medical aortic and mitral prostheses. *J Thorac Cardiovasc Surg* 1987; 94:733.
134. Galloway A, Grossi E, Bauman F, et al: Multiple valve operation for advanced valvular heart disease: results and risk factors in 513 patients. *J Am Coll Cardiol* 1992; 19:725.
135. Fiore AC, Swartz MT, Sharp TG, et al: Double-valve replacement with Medtronic-Hall or St. Jude valve. *Ann Thorac Surg* 1995; 59:1113.
136. Teoh KH, Christakis GT, Weisel RD, et al: The determinants of mortality and morbidity after multiple-valve operations. *Ann Thorac Surg* 1987; 43:353.
137. Donahoo JS, Lechman MJ, MacVaugh H 3rd: Combined aortic and mitral valve replacement: a 6-year experience. *Cardiol Clin* 1985; 3:417.
138. Mattila S, Harjula A, Kupari M, et al: Combined multiple-valve procedures: factors influencing the early and late results. *Scand J Thorac Cardiovasc Surg* 1985; 19:33.

139. He G, Acuff T, Ryan W, et al: Aortic valve replacement: determinants of operative mortality. *Ann Thorac Surg* 1994; 57:1140.
140. Alvarez L, Escudero C, Figuera D, et al: The Bjork-Shiley valve prosthesis: analysis of long-term evolution. *J Thorac Cardiovasc Surg* 1992; 104:1249.
141. Jegaden O, Eker A, Delahaye F, et al: Thromboembolic risk and late survival after mitral valve replacement with the St. Jude medical valve. *Ann Thorac Surg* 1994; 58:1721.
142. Copeland J 3rd: An international experience with the Carbo-Medics prosthetic heart valve. *J Heart Valve Dis* 1995; 4:56.
143. Bernal JM, Rabasa JM, Cagigas JC, et al: Valve-related complications with the Hancock I porcine bioprosthesis: a twelve- to fourteen-year follow-up study. *J Thorac Cardiovasc Surg* 1991; 101:871.
144. Loisance DY, Mazzucotelli JP, Bertrand PC, et al: Mitroflow pericardial valve: long-term durability [see comments]. *Ann Thorac Surg* 1993; 56:131.
145. Akins CW, Buckley MJ, Daggett WM, et al: Myocardial revascularization with combined aortic and mitral valve replacements. *J Thorac Cardiovasc Surg* 1985; 90:272.
146. Smith JA, Westlake GW, Mullerworth MH, et al: Excellent long-term results of cardiac valve replacement with the St. Jude Medical valve prosthesis. *Circulation* 1993; 88(5 pt 2):II49.
147. Sante P, Renzulli A, Festa M, et al: Acute postoperative block of mechanical prostheses: incidence and treatment. *Cardiovasc Surg* 1994; 2:403.
148. Craver JM, Jones EL, Guyton RA, et al: Avoidance of transverse midventricular disruption following mitral valve replacement. *Ann Thorac Surg* 1985; 40:163.
149. Pomar JL, Jamieson WR, Pelletier LC, et al: Mitroflow pericardial bioprosthesis: clinical performance to ten years. *Ann Thorac Surg* 1995; 60 (2 suppl):S305.
150. Cannegieter SC, Rosendaal FR, Briet E: Thromboembolic and bleeding complications in patients with mechanical heart valve prostheses [review]. *Circulation* 1994; 89:635.
151. Heras M, Chesebro JH, Fuster V, et al: High risk of thromboembolism early after bioprosthetic cardiac valve replacement. *J Am Coll Cardiol* 1995; 25:1111.
152. Horstkotte D, Schulte HD, Bircks W, et al: Lower intensity anticoagulation therapy results in lower complication rates with the St. Jude medical prosthesis. *J Thorac Cardiovasc Surg* 1994; 107:1136.
153. Bernal JM, Rabasa JM, Lopez R, et al: Durability of the Carpentier-Edwards porcine bioprosthesis: role of age and valve position. *Ann Thorac Surg* 1995; 60 (2 suppl):S248.
154. Brown PJ, Roberts CS, McIntosh CL, et al: Late results after triple-valve replacement with various substitute valves. *Ann Thorac Surg* 1993; 55:502.
155. Munro AI, Jamieson WR, Burr LH, et al: Comparison of porcine bioprostheses and mechanical prostheses in multiple valve replacement operations. *Ann Thorac Surg* 1995; 60(2 suppl):S459.
156. Pellegrini A, Colombo T, Donatelli F, et al: Evaluation and treatment of secondary tricuspid insufficiency. *Eur J Cardiothorac Surg* 1992; 6:288.
157. Kaul TK, Ramsdale DR, Mercer JL: Functional tricuspid regurgitation following replacement of the mitral valve. *Int J Cardiol* 1991; 33:305.
158. Kara M, Langlet MF, Blin D, et al: Triple valve procedures: an analysis of early and late results. *Thorac Cardiovasc Surg* 1986; 34:17.
159. Macmanus Q, Grunkemeier G, Starr A: Late results of triple valve replacement: a 14-year review. *Ann Thorac Surg* 1978; 25:402.
160. Cohn L, Aranki S, Rizzo R, et al: Decrease in operative risk of reoperative valve surgery. *Ann Thorac Surg* 1993; 56:15.
161. Konishi Y, Matsuda K, Nishiwaki N, et al: Ventricular arrhythmias late after aortic and/or mitral valve replacement. *Jpn Circ J* 1985; 49:576.
162. Konstantopoulos K, Kasparian T, Sideris J, et al: Mechanical hemolysis associated with a bioprosthetic mitral valve combined with a calcified aortic valve stenosis. *Acta Haematol* 1994; 91:164.
163. Skoularigis J, Essop M, Skudicky D, et al: Valvular heart disease: frequency and severity of intravascular hemolysis after left-sided cardiac valve replacement with Medtronic Hall and St. Jude medical prostheses, and influence of prosthetic type, position, size and number. *Am J Cardiol* 1993; 71:587.
164. Page RD, Jeffrey RR, Fabri BM, et al: Combined multiple valve procedures and myocardial revascularisation. *Thorac Cardiovasc Surg* 1990; 38:308.
165. Trace HD, Bailey CP, Wendkos MH: Tricuspid valve commissurotomy with one year followup. *Am Heart J* 1954; 47:613.
166. Brofman BL: Right auriculoventricular pressure gradient with special reference to tricuspid stenosis. *J Lab Clin Med* 1953; 42:789.
167. Lillehei CW, Gott VL, DeWall RA, et al: The surgical treatment of stenotic and regurgitant lesions of the mitral and aortic valves by direct utilization of a pump oxygenator. *J Thorac Surg* 1958; 35:154.
168. Aberg B: Surgical treatment of combined aortic and mitral valvular disease. *Scand J Thorac Cardiovasc Surg* 1980; 25(suppl):1.
169. West PN, Ferguson TB, Clark RE, et al: Multiple valve replacement: changing status. *Ann Thorac Surg* 1978; 26:32.
170. Lemole GM, Cuasay R: Improved technique of double valve replacement. *J Thorac Cardiovasc Surg* 1976; 71:759.
171. Clawson BJ: Rheumatic heart disease: an analysis of 796 cases. *Am Heart J* 1940; 20:454.
172. Cooke WT, White PD: Tricuspid stenosis with particular reference to diagnosis and prognosis. *Br Heart J* 1941; 3:141.
173. Mardelli TJ, Morganroth J, Naito M, et al: Cross-sectional echocardiographic identification of aortic valve prolapse [abstract]. *Circulation* 1979; 60 (suppl II):II-204.
174. David TE: Aortic valve repair in patients with Marfan syndrome and ascending aorta aneurysms due to degenerative disease. *J Card Surg* 1994; 9 (2 suppl):182.
175. Gott VL, Gillinov AM, Pyeritz RE, et al: Aortic root replacement: risk factor analysis of a seventeen-year experience with 270 patients. *J Thorac Cardiovasc Surg* 1995; 109:536.
176. Raviprasad GS, Salem BI, Gowda S, et al: Radiation-induced mitral and tricuspid regurgitation with severe ostial coronary artery disease: a case report with successful surgical treatment [review]. *Cathet Cardiovasc Diag* 1995; 35:146.
177. Blanche C, Freimark D, Valenza M, et al: Heart transplantation for Q fever endocarditis. *Ann Thorac Surg* 1994; 58:1768.
178. Rozycka CB, Hryniewiecki T, Solik TA, et al: Mitral and aortic valve replacement in a patient with ectodermal anhydrotic dysplasia: a case report. *J Heart Valve Dis* 1994; 3:224.
179. Tan C, Schaff H, Miller F, et al: Clinical investigation: valvular heart disease in four patients with maroteaux-lamy syndrome. *Circulation* 1992; 85:188.
180. Carrel T, Pasic M, Tkebuchava T, et al: Aortic homograft and mitral valve repair in a patient with Werner's syndrome. *Ann Thorac Surg* 1994; 57:1319.
181. Pellegrini RV, Copeland CE, DiMarco RF, et al: Blunt rupture of both atrioventricular valves. *Ann Thorac Surg* 1986; 42:471.
182. Gabarre J, Gessain A, Raphael M, et al: Adult T-cell leukemia/lymphoma revealed by a surgically cured cardiac valve lymphomatous involvement in an Iranian woman: clinical, immunopathological and viromolecular studies. *Leukemia* 1993; 7:1904.
183. Lang LL, Hvass U, Paillole C, et al: Cardiac valve replacement in relapsing polychondritis: a review [review]. *J Heart Valve Dis* 1995; 4:227.
184. Ames DE, Asherson RA, Coltart JD, et al: Systemic lupus erythematosus complicated by tricuspid stenosis and regurgitation:

successful treatment by valve transplantation. *Ann Rheum Dis* 1992; 51:120.

185. Fujise K, Amerling R, Sherman W: Rapid progression of mitral and aortic stenosis in a patient with secondary hyperparathyroidism. *Br Heart J* 1993; 70:282.
186. Palazzo E, Bourgeois P, Meyer O, et al: Hypocomplementemic urticarial vasculitis syndrome, Jaccoud's syndrome, valvulopathy: a new syndromic combination. *J Rheumatol* 1993; 20:1236.
187. Ibrahim M, O'Kane H, Cleland J, et al: The St. Jude Medical prosthesis: a thirteen-year experience. *J Thorac Cardiovasc Surg* 1994; 108:221.
188. David TE, Armstrong S, Sun Z: The Hancock II bioprosthesis at ten years. *Ann Thorac Surg* 1995; 60 (2 suppl):S229.
189. Jamieson WR, Burr LH, Tyers GF, et al: Carpentier-Edwards supraannular porcine bioprosthesis: clinical performance to twelve years. *Ann Thorac Surg* 1995; 60:S235.
190. Milano A, Bortolotti U, Mazzucco A, et al: Heart valve replacement with the Sorin tilting-disc prosthesis: a 10-year experience. *J Thorac Cardiovasc Surg* 1992; 103:267.
191. Lemieux MD, Jamieson WR, Landymore RW, et al: Medtronic intact porcine bioprosthesis: clinical performance to seven years. *Ann Thorac Surg* 1995; 60 (2 suppl):S258.
192. Orszulak TA, Schaff HV, DeSmet JM, et al: Late results of valve replacement with the Bjork-Shiley valve (1973 to 1982) [see comments]. *J Thorac Cardiovasc Surg* 1993; 105:302.
193. Nakano K, Koyanagi H, Hashimoto A, et al: Twelve years' experience with the St. Jude medical valve prosthesis. *Ann Thorac Surg* 1994; 57:697.
194. Pelletier LC, Carrier M, Leclerc Y, et al: The Carpentier-Edwards pericardial bioprosthesis: clinical experience with 600 patients. *Ann Thorac Surg* 1995; 60 (2 suppl):S297.
195. van Doorn C, Stoodley K, Saunders N, et al: Mitral valve replacement with the Carpentier-Edwards standard bioprosthesis: performance into the second decade. *Eur J Cardiothoracic Surg* 1995; 9:253.
196. Coll MJ, Jegaden O, Janody P, et al: Results of triple valve replacement: perioperative mortality and long term results. *J Cardiovasc Surg* 1987; 28:369.

Chapter 42

Reoperative Valve Surgery

John G. Byrne/Bradley J. Phillips/Lawrence H. Cohn

The number of patients undergoing reoperation for valvular heart disease is increasing and will continue to increase as the general population ages.[1] These reoperations most commonly involve progression of native valve disease after nonvalve surgery and structural deterioration of a bioprosthesis. In fact, structural failure of a biological valve should be considered as part of their natural evolution and fully appreciated by both the surgeon and patient prior to implantation.[2] Reoperations are technically more difficult than primary operations because of adhesions around the heart and the common association of pulmonary hypertension with valve dysfunction. Also, replacement operations are often performed in functionally compromised patients who tolerate complications poorly or have little reserve. In the past, reoperative valve surgery has been associated with a considerably higher operative mortality than primary valve surgery, particularly in patients who have had multiple prior replacements.[3] However, in the modern era there has been some improvement in both morbidity and mortality.[4,5]

Reductions in operative risk and postoperative morbidity after reoperative valve surgery have been made in the past few years by advances in myocardial protection, as well as the proper use of deep hypothermic cardiac arrest.[6] Utilization of peripheral cannulation techniques to institute cardiopulmonary bypass has become a relatively standard practice.[7–9] Early institution of partial cardiopulmonary bypass is thought to prevent injury to the hypertensive right ventricle or patent coronary artery bypass grafts during reoperative sternotomy. This technique decreases myocardial distension, thereby reducing oxygen consumption.[3]

Successful replacement of the diseased cardiac valve usually results in gratifying symptomatic and hemodynamic improvement. Maintenance of this improved state, however, depends on acceptable prosthetic valve function. Improvements in valve design have lessened, but not eliminated, the incidence of primary bioprosthetic valve failure.[10–12] Thus, the risk of re-replacement for bioprosthetic failure remains a factor to be considered in the selection of valve type.[13]

MECHANICAL VS. BIOLOGICAL VALVES

Mechanical valvular prostheses have the distinct advantage of longevity but carry a risk of anticoagulant-related bleeding as well as thromboembolic events (TE), which are dependent on valve design, structural materials, and host-related interactions.[14] While endocarditis, dehiscence, perivalvular leak, and pannus formation are common to both biological and mechanical valves, acute prosthetic thrombosis is mostly a complication of mechanical valves.[15,16] Mechanical prostheses are usually selected in younger recipients because of their proven durability over time, yet thrombogenecity remains a persistent risk that requires lifelong anticoagulation. In a 12-year comparison of Björk-Shiley versus porcine valves, Bloomfield et al documented severe bleeding complications of 18.6% versus 7.1%, respectively.[17] These rates, however, must be balanced with the known risk of tissue valve failure and expected risks of further intervention.

In evaluating reoperations for bioprosthetic failure, Husebye et al reviewed their 20-year experience.[13] Operative mortality for the first reoperation (n = 530 patients) was 5.9% for the aortic position and 19.6% for the mitral position. Overall operative mortality was 14% (n = 69 patients) and 7% (n = 14 patients) for the second and third reoperations, respectively. In the aortic position, operative mortality was 2.4% for NYHA I patients, 1.6% for NYHA II, 6.3% for NYHA III, and 20.8% for NYHA IV. The mortality for elective mitral valve reoperation was 1.4%; urgent procedures, 8%; and emergency procedures, 37.5%. Based on this, the authors recommended that reoperation should be undertaken when valve dysfunction is first noted.[13]

Jones et al also reviewed their experience with first heart valve reoperations involving 671 patients between 1969 and 1998.[4] Their overall operative mortality for first-time heart valve reoperation was 8.6%, which is similar to the results published by Lytle[18] (10.9%), Cohn[3] (10.1%), Akins[19] (7.3%), Pansini[2] (9.6%), and Tyers[20] (11.0%). In their series, mortality increased from 3.0% for reoperation on a failed repair or reoperation at a new valve site to 10.6% for prosthetic valve dysfunction or periprosthetic leak; mortality increased to 29.4% for associated endocarditis or valve thrombosis. Concomitant coronary artery bypass grafting was associated with a mortality of 15.4% compared to 8.2% when it was not required. Among 336 patients requiring re-replacement of prosthetic valves, mortality was 26.1% for re-replacement of a mechanical valve compared with 8.6% for re-replacement of a tissue valve. The authors found through multivariate analysis that significant predictors of mortality were year of reoperation, age, indication, concomitant coronary artery bypass grafting, and the replacement of a mechanical valve rather than a tissue valve.[4]

Structural degeneration of a bioprosthesis is the leading cause and the most frequent indication for reoperation in patients with tissue valves.[21,22] The most appropriate valve substitute for the individual patient is still a source of much controversy. This choice should be adapted to each individual patient depending on age, life expectancy, valve size, and cardiac as well as noncardiac comorbidities.[23] Some studies comparing the long-term outcome between biological and mechanical aortic valve prostheses have yielded similar results in regards to overall valve-related complications.[22,24–27] However, most recent large studies have documented that anticoagulant-related bleeding with mechanical valves must be balanced against life expectation and the risk of biological valve re-replacement.[28–31] Bioprosthetic valves are known to undergo a time-dependent process of structural deterioration that results in dysfunction and requires re-replacement in 12 to 15 years.[24] Furthermore, encouraged by the availability of stentless valves and homografts, more surgeons are placing an aortic bioprosthesis in progressively younger age groups.[23,32–35] In addition, many patients do not accept the risks of an anticoagulant-related hemorrhage, which are 0.5% per patient-year for a major event and 2% to 4% per patient-year for a minor event.[14]

REOPERATIVE AORTIC VALVE SURGERY

Historical Points

Historically, aortic valve surgery usually involved the placement of a mechanical valve. In the past, there were only a few generally accepted indications to use a bioprosthesis for primary, isolated aortic valve replacement: (1) the presence of well-established contraindications to continuous anticoagulation; (2) the inability to adequately monitor prothrombin levels; and (3) patients whose survival was limited and more dependent on issues unrelated to their valve dysfunction.[22,23] However, in recent years the use of biological valves in the aortic position has become more common.[29,30]

Reoperations are technically demanding and many patients present in a poor functional state that increases the reoperative mortality rate of a failing aortic bioprosthesis, in some series up to 19%.[17,36,37] However, elective re-replacement of malfunctioning aortic bioprostheses can be performed with results similar to the primary operation.[23,38] The presence of concomitant coronary artery disease and pulmonary hypertension have been shown to be independent risk factors.[23] These patients need careful surveillance once the probability of bioprosthetic dysfunction begins increasing 6 to 10 years after implantation.[12] In regards to valve surveillance and timing of reoperation, the following variables are clinically relevant to managing patients with an aortic bioprosthesis: a history of endocarditis prior to the first operation; perioperative infectious complications; coronary artery disease acquired after the first operation; an increase in pulmonary artery pressure; and a decrease in left ventricular function during the interval.[23] Proper timing of the reoperation is important, because duration of clinical signs with a dysfunctional aortic bioprosthesis may be misleading. The need for an emergency reoperation of a biological valve, itself, is the most important factor in contributing to poor patient outcome yielding a consistently high early mortality rate of 25% to 44%.[39]

Approaches and Techniques

THE STANDARD: RESTERNOTOMY

The evolution of cardiac surgery through the last few decades has led to the popularization of various surgical approaches. Thoracotomy was once used extensively to gain access to mediastinal structures. Then, median sternotomy became the standard approach. However, in reoperative cases, repeating the sternotomy carries definite risks. Prior to proceeding with a resternotomy, the relationship between anterior mediastinal structures and the posterior aspect of the sternum, as visualized on chest radiograph or computed tomography (CT), must be assessed carefully.[40] Preparations for emergency femorofemoral cardiopulmonary bypass should be completed prior to beginning the resternotomy.

Sternal wires from the previous operation should be carefully undone, but left in place as a safeguard during sternal division. An oscillating (not reciprocating) bone saw can be used to divide the anterior sternal table. Most authors recommend dividing the posterior table using a combination of scissors and lateral retraction.[40–42] Following this, other mediastinal structures should be carefully dissected using rake retraction. The pericardial dissection plane can be developed by starting at the cardiophrenic angle and then slowly advanced cephalad and laterally on the surface of the right heart. Cephalad dissection should start with innominate vein identification and then carried down the superior vena cava, noting location of the right phrenic nerve. Repairing small ventricular or atrial lacerations should not be attempted before releasing the tension of the surrounding adhesions. Repair of great vessel injuries is best done under CPB.[40] Active hemorrhage during a second sternotomy is usually due to adherence of the heart or great vessels to the posterior sternum. Whether this could be prevented by interposition of pericardium or other mediastinal tissue at time of the first operation is debatable.[42] The incidence of resternotomy hemorrhage is between 2% and 6% per patient reoperation.[43–45]

In a report of 552 patients who had undergone reoperative prosthetic valve surgery, 23 (4%) had complications related directly to sternal opening.[13] Of these, 5 patients had entry into the right atrium, 7 patients had lacerated right ventricles, 9 patients had injuries to the aorta, and there were 2 patients in whom a previously placed coronary graft was divided. Nineteen of the 23 complications occurred during a first-time reoperation. Overall, there were 2 operative deaths related to resternotomy. The first death involved division of a previously placed coronary graft during reentry. The second death was due to laceration of the aorta with subsequent exsanguination.[13]

Macanus et al reviewed their experience with 100 patients undergoing repeat median sternotomy.[44] Eighty-one patients had one repeat sternotomy while the others had undergone multiple sternotomies. All had a previous valve procedure in the past and were reoperated upon for progressive rheumatic valvular disease or for complications related to the prosthesis. Complications included operative hemorrhage in 8 patients, postoperative hemorrhage in 2, seroma in 4, and dehiscence, wound infection, and hematoma in 1 patient each. There was one operative death directly related to resternotomy hemorrhage.[44]

When major hemorrhage does occur upon sternal entry, attempts at resternotomy should be abandoned. The patient should be immediately heparinized while obtaining femoral arterial and venous cannulation. Blood lost from the resternotomy should be aspirated with cardiotomy suction and returned to the pump-oxygenator. Once bypass has been established, core cooling can commence, flow rates are reduced, and the sternal division completed, followed by direct repair of the underlying injury.[42] Accepting the risk of this scenario, we routinely expose peripheral cannulation sites prior to beginning a resternotomy.

MINIMALLY INVASIVE REOPERATIVE AORTIC VALVE REPLACEMENT

"Minimally invasive" valve procedures have gradually become more accepted as new technologies and instrumentation develop.[46] Reoperative procedures pose an area in which minimally invasive procedures may be of direct benefit.[47,48] Our surgical approach for reoperative AVR is shown in Figure 42-1.[46] In all patients, peripheral cannulation sites

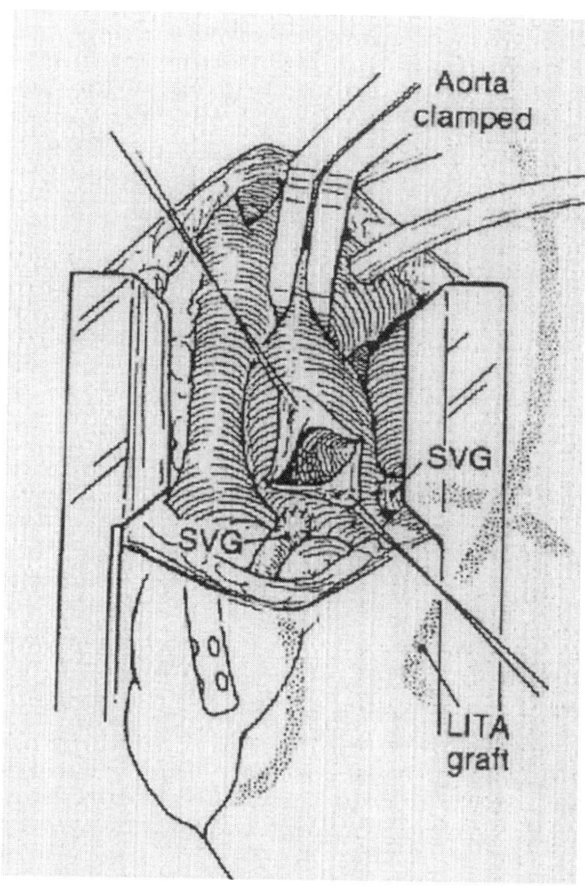

FIGURE 42–1 Partial upper resternotomy for reoperative AVR. The previous sternotomy incision is exposed to the 3rd or 4th intercostal space, depending on the position of the aortic valve as documented by transesophageal echocardiography. After dissection of the ascending aorta, paying particular attention to the position of CAB grafts and their proximal anastomoses, cannulation is carried out. In this illustration, the ascending aorta and innominate vein are cannulated. Frequently, however, other cannulation sites are required due to space limitations in the chest. The ascending aorta is cross-clamped and the aortic valve re-replacement is conducted in the standard fashion. *(Reproduced with permission from Byrne J, Karavas A, Adams D, et al: Partial upper re-sternotomy for aortic valve replacement or re-replacement after previous cardiac surgery. Eur J Cardiothorac Surg 2000; 18:282.)*

are exposed and dissected prior to beginning the partial upper resternotomy. An external defibrillator is placed on the patient prior to draping for subsequent defibrillation, as necessary. A transesophageal echo (TEE) probe is used in every patient. An "inverted T"[49] partial upper resternotomy is carried out to the 3rd or 4th intercostal space depending on the estimated position of the aortic valve as documented by TEE. The oscillating saw is used to divide the anterior sternal table while the straight Mayo scissors, under direct visualization, divide the posterior sternal table. The chest wall incision is then extended laterally into the intercostal spaces on both sides. In the setting of a patent LIMA-LAD graft, or other anterior CAB grafts, patients are placed on cardiopulmonary bypass (CPB) prior to partial resternotomy. Mediastinal dissection is limited to the ascending aorta for clamping and aortotomy. The right atrium (RA) is dissected only if it is cannulated. Although intrathoracic cannulation is preferred, we frequently use peripheral cannulation to avoid clutter in the chest. Retrograde cardioplegia, if necessary, is delivered via a transjugular coronary sinus catheter. Vacuum assistance for venous drainage is used in the majority of cases. On CPB, all patients are systemically cooled to 20°C to 25°C. Patients with patent LIMA-LAD grafts are routinely cooled to 20°C. If collateral flow from the patent LIMA-LAD graft flows out of the left main ostium on CPB and obscures the operative field, pump flows are turned down temporarily to allow visualization. Venting is accomplished by placing a pediatric vent through the aortic annulus.

The aortic valve surgery is then performed based on patient indications. While closing the aortotomy, intracardiac air is removed by insufflating the lungs and decreasing flows on CPB. Patients are also tilted from side to side to help with de-airing, and the ascending aortic vent is left open until separation from CPB. Temporary epicardial pacing wires are placed on the anterior surface of the right ventricle before the aortic cross-clamp is removed. Two 32F right-angled submammary chest tubes are then placed through the right pleural space, one angled medially into the mediastinum and one angled posterior into the pleural space. Decannulation and closure is then performed in the standard manner.

Reoperative procedures are challenging due to diffuse mediastinal and pericardial adhesions. A large incision that increases the operative field has also been associated with a higher risk of injury to cardiac structures, CAB grafts, and greater bleeding with subsequent transfusion requirements.[50–53] A smaller incision, on the other hand, will reduce the area of pericardiolysis, thus limiting these effects. The remaining intact lower sternum will preserve integrity of the caudal chest wall, thereby enhancing sternal stability and promoting an earlier extubation.[46,54]

With our increasing experience in minimally invasive reoperative AVR, we have refined our technique as an alternative to conventional full resternotomy.[46] In doing so, we have ascertained certain technical details of the partial upper resternotomy approach (Table 42-1). By following these guidelines, we have yet to convert any patient to a full resternotomy. Lateral chest x-ray and/or TEE is helpful in locating the level of the aortic valve and determining the proximity of the aorta to the posterior aspect of the sternum.[49] If necessary, additional information can be obtained with CT scanning or magnetic resonance imaging (MRI). Also, extension of the sternal incision laterally on both sides through the intercostal spaces helps to later reapproximate the sternum. We have tried to limit mediastinal and pericardial dissection primarily to the aorta, believing that this is the principal reason for decreased bleeding and transfusion requirements postoperatively.[46,48,55,56] The right ventricle, which is often attached to the sternum, does not need to be dissected. Also, injuries to patent but atherosclerotic vein grafts can be reduced with this "no-touch technique."[57]

Arterial and venous cannulation sites can vary considerably, reflecting the individual choice of the operating surgeon

TABLE 42–1 Thirteen technical details for successful aortic valve replacement after previous cardiac surgery by use of partial upper resternotomy

1. Routine exposure of peripheral cannulation sites prior to partial upper resternotomy
2. Placement of Zoll (Zoll, Inc, Burlington, MA) defibrillator pads prior to prepping
3. Use of intraoperative transesophageal echocardiography for air removal and inspection of valve
4. In patients with patent left internal mammary artery to left anterior descending coronary artery (LIMA-LAD) graft, peripheral cannulation and cardiopulmonary bypass (CPB) established prior to partial upper resternotomy
5. Mediastinal dissection limited to ascending aorta for clamping and aortotomy, and right atrium (RA) only if RA is cannulated
6. Use of peripheral cannulation to avoid clutter in the chest
7. Use of vacuum assistance on CPB
8. Use of retrograde cardioplegia (CP) delivered by transjugular retrograde CP catheter in addition to antegrade CP
9. Use of aprotinin unless absolute contraindication
10. Cooling to at least 25°C in all patients primarily for myocardial protection; if a patent LIMA-LAD graft is present, cooling to 20°C without isolation and clamping LIMA graft
11. If visualization is poor due to LIMA-LAD collaterals flowing from coronary ostia, temporary low flows on CPB to improve visualization
12. Venting with a pediatric vent placed through the aortic annulus
13. Placement of temporary pacing wires on the right ventricular free wall before aortic clamp removal

Source: Reproduced with permission from Byrne J, Karavas A, Adams D, et al: Partial upper re-sternotomy for aortic valve replacement or re-replacement after previous cardiac surgery. Eur J Cardiothorac Surg 2000; 18:282.

and the sufficiency of intrathoracic space. Possible cannulation sites, other than standard ones, include the axillary artery, innominate vein, and percutaneous femoral vein.[58,59] The use of innominate vein or percutaneous femoral vein cannulation and the use of the retrograde cardioplegia coronary sinus catheter have been extremely helpful in minimizing the dissection of the right atrium. At present, we consider this approach to be our standard for isolated, elective reoperative aortic valve surgery.[46]

REPLACEMENT OF HOMOGRAFTS AND ALLOGRAFTS

Aortic valve replacement with a homograft or autograft has been used increasingly because of their excellent freedom from thromboembolism, resistance to infection, and superior hemodynamic performance.[32] Although in younger patients durability is superior to that of stented xenografts,[35,60] many patients will subsequently require aortic valve re-replacement for structural degeneration of the homograft or autograft valve.[61]

The requirement for a second aortic valve operation for patients with previous homograft or autograft is expected to increase, as popularity and availability of these valves increase. Recently, Hasnet et al documented the results of 144 patients who underwent a second aortic homograft replacement, with a hospital mortality rate of 3.5%.[61] However, since this is a relatively rare operation at most centers, we believe that a simplified approach may be optimal. Our approach to this rare problem has been to perform aortic valve re-replacement using a mechanical valve or stented xenograft, while reserving a second homograft for specific indications such as endocarditis, associated root pathology, or a very young patient with contraindications to a mechanical valve.

It is expected that approximately one third of patients less than 40 years of age will require aortic valve re-replacement within 12 years after homograft. This is primarily due to structural valve degeneration. Thus, the issue of homograft or autograft durability is particularly pertinent for this subgroup of younger patients who are expected to live beyond 15 years from time of operation.[60]

Hospital mortality of homograft re-replacement varies widely across many centers, and ranges between 2.5% and 50%.[34,62,63] Variations in sample size, valve selection, surgical techniques, and patient factors, as well as the experience of the surgeons, may account for these wide differences. Currently, there is no consensus as to the optimal surgical method of primary homograft AVR. The technique of primary homograft operation may have relevance at reoperation because calcification or aneurysmal dilation of the homograft may pose surgical challenges at reoperation. Sundt and others[34,62,63] have documented the feasibility of aortic valve re-replacement after full root replacement with a homograft. In our own series of 18 patients, full root, mini-root, and subcoronary techniques were all amenable to valve re-replacement.[32]

REOPERATIVE MITRAL AND TRICUSPID VALVE SURGERY

Historical Points

Fundamental to a flawless surgical procedure is excellent and consistent exposure of the mitral valve.[64] Historically, the mitral valve has been exposed through a variety of surgical approaches, including median sternotomy, right thoracotomy, left thoracotomy, and transverse sternotomy.[65] The median sternotomy and right thoracotomy will be discussed in detail below; however, a brief description of the other approaches is warranted.

The left thoracotomy has been used in recent years to gain access to the mitral valve. This incision is made through the fourth intercostal space and the left pleural cavity is entered in the standard fashion.[65] However, this approach provides limited access to the other cardiac chambers as well as poor visibility of the mitral valve apparatus, which is anatomically directed towards the right. This left-sided approach is typically reserved for cases in which reoperative sternotomy or right thoracotomy is considered unacceptable. A bilateral anterior thoracotomy (i.e., transverse sternotomy) carried out through the fourth intercostal space has also been described.[66] Rarely used today, this incision transects the sternum transversely requiring ligation of both internal mammary arteries. Regardless of the actual approach, once CPB has been established and the heart exposed, there are several incisions that can be employed to view the underlying mitral valve. The standard left atriotomy begins with blunt dissection of the interatrial groove, allowing the right atrium to be retracted medially and anteriorly. The right superior pulmonary vein at its junction with the left atrium is then exposed and the left atrium is opened at the midpoint between the right superior pulmonary vein insertion and the interatrial groove. This incision is extended longitudinally both superiorly and inferiorly to give enough exposure of the mitral valve. Care must be taken to avoid inadvertent injury to the posterior wall of the left atrium and, when closing, one must avoid including the posterior wall of the right pulmonary vein.

The right atrial transseptal approach has become more popular in recent years especially in reoperative valve surgery. After opening the RA, the interatrial septum is incised starting at the fossa ovalis and directed vertically upward for a few centimeters (Fig. 42-2). This technique is especially helpful in reoperative surgery, since it minimizes the amount of dissection required. Superior, biatrial atriotomy, left ventriculotomy, and aortotomy have all been well described[11,53,64,65,67,68] as approaches to the mitral valve; each one has varying advantages and disadvantages.

Approaches and Techniques

RESTERNOTOMY

Resternotomy is still the most common approach in reoperative mitral valve surgery. In many cases, this incision provides full and adequate exposure. This is especially true when concomitant procedures are necessary. However, reoperative median sternotomy has known risks, including injury to or embolism from prior grafts, sternal dehiscence, excessive hemorrhage, and inadvertent cardiac injury.[69] Patients with valvular heart disease may be especially prone to these complications because atrial dilatation can result in significant cardiomegaly, atrial thinning, and adherence of the heart to the posterior sternum. As we have previously discussed, patients undergoing prosthetic valve reoperation have a 4% incidence of complications directly related to sternal reentry, which can cause intraoperative death.[13,18] Resternotomy has also been noted to be particularly hazardous in the presence of patent internal mammary grafts. Injury to a patent LIMA graft has an associated mortality rate approaching 50%.[42,69] Furthermore, manipulation of patent but diseased saphenous vein grafts can result in embolization into the native coronary circulation with resulting morbidity and mortality.[70,71] In the setting of reoperative surgery, the initial resternotomy is likely to be the most dangerous part of the operation.[72] In this situation, we have tried to employ techniques that avoid resternotomy.

RIGHT THORACOTOMY

The right anterolateral thoracotomy approach was one of the first surgical approaches to the mitral valve, and it has become a safe alternative to resternotomy for mitral valve replacement (Fig. 42-3).[6,42,73,75] This approach provides excellent exposure of the valves (mitral and tricuspid) with minimal need for dissection within the pericardium. In our recent experience with this approach,[72,76,77] all patients had double-lumen endotracheal tubes placed and operations were performed in the right lateral thoracotomy position. We routinely prepared and draped the right groin to allow femoral cannulation, if necessary. Preoperative and intraoperative Doppler transesophageal echocardiography was performed in all patients, as well as standard intraoperative cardiac monitoring and thermodilution Swan-Ganz catheterization. A right thoracotomy was made and the chest entered through the bed of the fifth rib. Adhesions of the right lung to the chest wall or pericardium were divided by electrocautery. The pericardium was entered anterior to the phrenic nerve. Arterial cannulation was performed via the ascending aorta with the use of a flexible aortic cannula. Bicaval venous

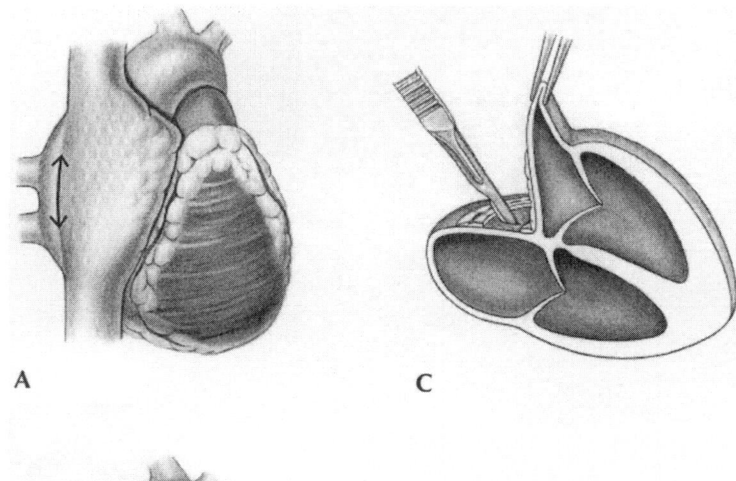

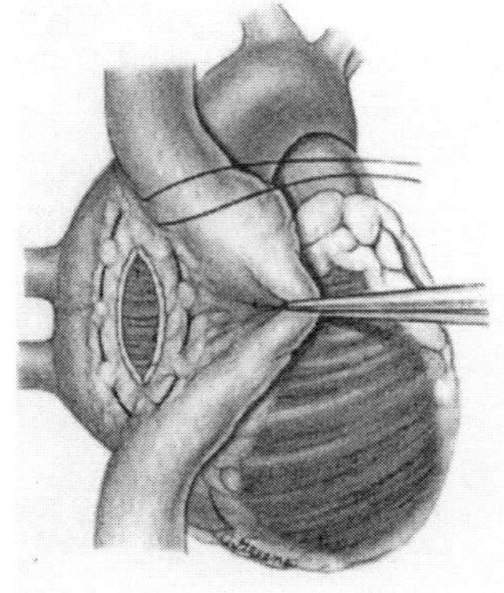

FIGURE 42–2 Sondergaard's groove approach. (A) The left atrium enlarges to the right, increasing visualization from the right thoracotomy approach. (B) The interatrial groove (Sondergaard's groove) is dissected approximately 1 cm deep, down to the left atrial wall. The purse-string suture is placed in the nondissected area. This prevents tearing of the dissected left atrial wall when the suture is tied down. (C) Sagittal view shows location of the mitral valve in relation to the atriotomy. *(Reproduced with permission from Hanh D, Pezzella T: Closed mitral commissurotomy utilizing right thoracotomy approach. Asian Cardiovasc Thorac Ann 2000; 8:192.)*

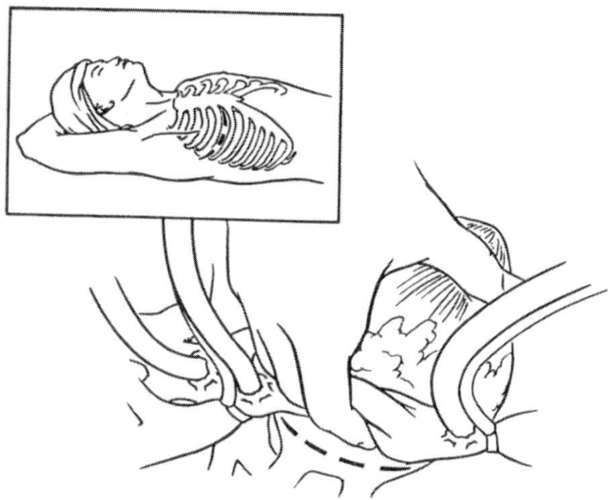

FIGURE 42–3 Right anterolateral thoracotomy. Right anterolateral thoracotomy through the 4th intercostal space and standard left atriotomy. *(Reproduced with permission from Balasundaram SG, Duran C: Surgical approaches to the mitral valve. J Card Surg 1990; 5:163.)*

cannulation was carried out with a 28F (DLP) cannula in the superior vena cava and a 32F (USCI) flexible cannula in the inferior vena cava. Patients were then cooled to 25°C. Fibrillatory arrest occurred spontaneously in the majority of patients. Aortic cross-clamping was usually not required. The mitral valve was then approached through the left atrium by dissection of the intra-atrial groove or through the atrial septum (Fig. 42-4). As the valve procedure was completed, we began rewarming (Fig. 42-5).

The left ventricular vent was positioned across the valve while an air needle, on suction in the ascending aorta, was used to remove any ejected air. The patient was then placed in the Trendelenburg position and de-airing accomplished under two-dimensional transesophageal echocardiography guidance. When core temperatures reached 36°C, the patient was weaned from cardiopulmonary bypass. Temporary atrial and ventricular pacing wires were placed and exteriorized through the chest wall. Closure was then routine. At the conclusion of the procedure, patients were returned to the supine position and reintubated with a single-lumen endotracheal tube for postoperative ventilation.

The use of a small right anterior thoracotomy, femorofemoral bypass, and deep hypothermia has increased since our initial report in 1989.[78] Reduced blood use, and decreased risk of LIMA or cardiac structural injury during sternal reentry, makes it a desirable approach for almost all complicated mitral reoperations. Deep hypothermia (approximately 20°C) and low-flow femorofemoral bypass perfusion, without the necessity of aortic cross-clamping, provides adequate myocardial protection.[79] Cardiopulmonary bypass times, blood loss, blood product usage, and LIMA injury rates have been lower in reoperative patients undergoing right thoracotomy than in those with resternotomy.[69,73,79,80]

Certain issues must be considered before the right thoracotomy approach can be utilized. Patients who require simultaneous coronary artery bypass grafting will generally require a median sternotomy, although isolated right-sided grafting may be performed. Simultaneous replacement of the aortic valve is difficult from a thoracotomy approach and

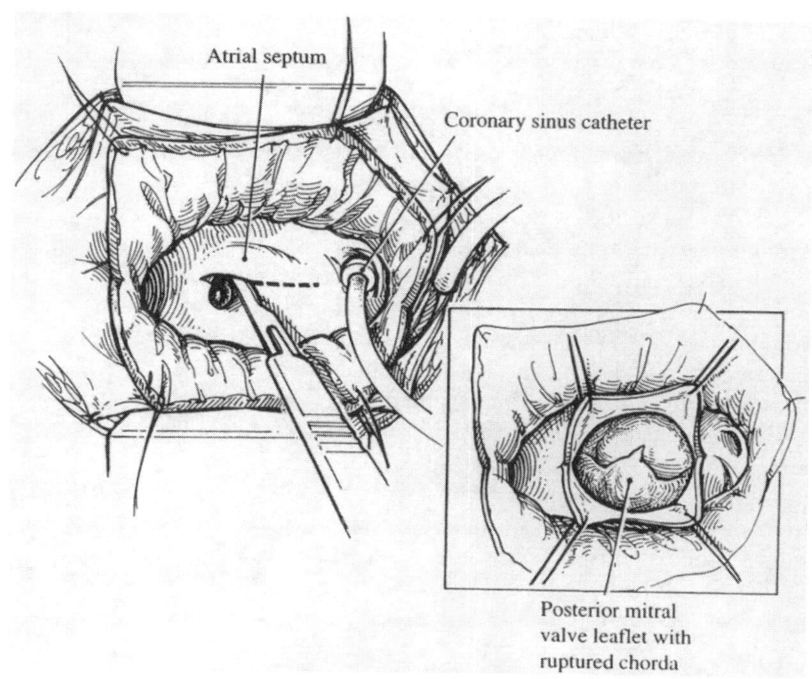

FIGURE 42–4 Atrial incision through the fossa ovalis. When the right atrium is incised, an incision is made in the atrial septum through the fossa ovalis. Retraction sutures, on both the right atrium and the atrial septum, of 2-0 silk, are then used to elevate the septum and to keep the left atrium open. The mitral valve will then be exposed (inset). *(Reproduced with permission from Byrne JG, Mitchell ME, Adams DH, et al: Minimally invasive direct access mitral valve surgery. Semin Thorac Cardiovasc Surg 1999; 11:212.)*

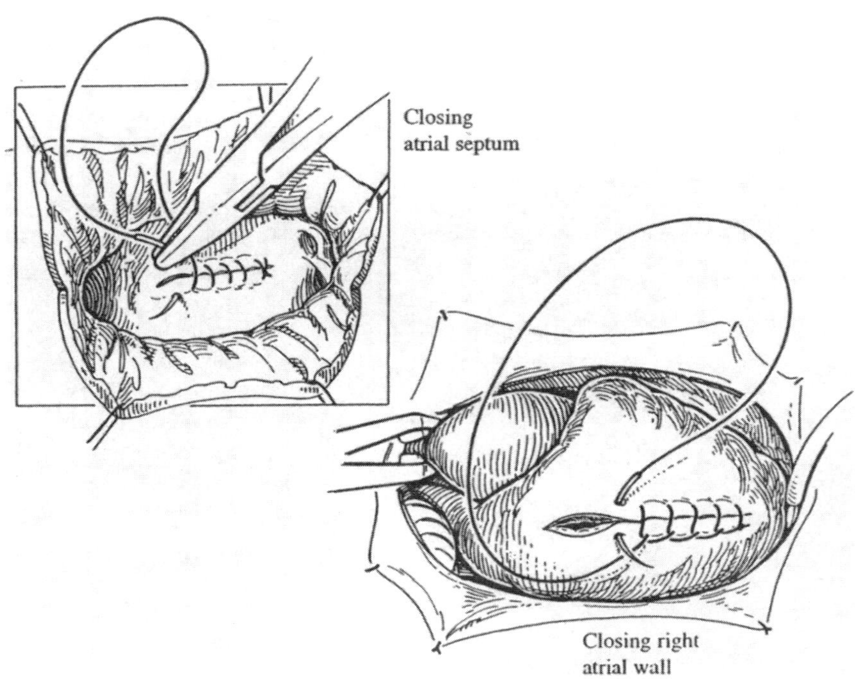

FIGURE 42–5 Closure. In the transeptal approach, the atrial septum is approximated with running 4-0 Prolene sutures and is left open until the aortic cross-clamp is removed and the air is evacuated. The left ventricle should be filled with fluid before removal of the cross-clamp to help dislodgment of intraventricular air. Once the cross-clamp has been removed, air is evacuated vigorously from the left atrium through the septum or the left atrium itself, and the sutures are tied. The right atrium is then closed with running 4-0 Prolene sutures in two layers. Transesophageal echocardiogram has been very important in helping to monitor the clearing of air from the intracardiac structures. We consider it mandatory in the minimally invasive technique in which access to the entire cardiac structure is limited. *(Reproduced with permission from Byrne JG, Mitchell ME, Adams DH, et al: Minimally invasive direct access mitral valve surgery. Semin Thorac Cardiovasc Surg 1999; 11:212.)*

should generally be performed through a resternotomy. Significant aortic insufficiency can make effective perfusion on CPB difficult because, after opening the left atrium, blood will be returned to the pump oxygenator via cardiotomy suction. Unless the ascending aorta is clamped, effective end-organ perfusion will not be achieved. Also, in the setting of aortic insufficiency (AI), exposure of the mitral valve may be difficult and require core cooling to allow low flow rates. Left ventricular distension and injury can also occur with fibrillatory arrest. Patients with greater than minimal aortic insufficiency should either be excluded from a right thoracotomy approach or expected to require aortic cross-clamping either with traditional clamping or balloon occlusion. Significant right pleural disease, especially scarring in the right hemithorax, has previously been a relative contraindication to a right thoracotomy, although our series includes two patients with a previous right thoracotomy who did not represent an overwhelming challenge.[69]

Vleissus reported on 22 patients who underwent a minimally invasive right thoracotomy approach to the atrioventricular valves.[81] The procedures performed included mitral valve repair (n = 12), mitral valve replacement (n = 5), prosthetic mitral valve re-replacement (n = 4), repair of perivalvular leak (n = 3), tricuspid valve repair (n = 5), and closure of an atrial septal defect (n = 7). Mean bypass time was 109 minutes with a mean fibrillatory time of 62 minutes. Operative mortality in this group was 0% and none of the patients experienced a wound complication. At follow-up, all patients thought their recovery from this approach was more rapid and less painful than their original sternotomy.[81]

Holman et al reported their experience in 84 patients undergoing reoperative mitral valve surgery via right thoracotomy.[82] Myocardial management included ventricular fibrillation in 10 patients, beating heart in 58 patients, and hypothermic blood cardioplegia in 16 patients. The mean duration of cardiopulmonary bypass was 63 ± 56 minutes. There were no perioperative strokes and the operative risk for patients who received cardioplegic arrest was significantly greater than in the other two groups ($p = .007$). The authors concluded that procedures on the beating or fibrillating heart were feasible in most patients and are at least as safe as surgery using cardioplegic arrest.[82]

CONCLUSION

The most common indication for valve re-replacement is structural valve degeneration of porcine bioprostheses.[3] After 8 to 10 years of follow-up, biological valves begin to structurally deteriorate, especially in young patients and in the mitral position. Accelerated follow-up intervals should be the rule in these patients to avoid missing early degeneration. When patients have been allowed to fall into NYHA class IV, reoperative mortality has been directly affected.

REFERENCES

1. Fremes SE, Goldman BS, Ivanov J, et al: Valvular surgery in the elderly. *Circulation* 1989; 80(3 Pt 1):177.
2. Pansini S, Ottino G, Forsennati PG, et al: Reoperations on heart valve prostheses: an analysis of operative risks and late results. *Ann Thorac Surg* 1990; 50:590.

3. Cohn LH, Aranki SF, Rizzo RJ, et al: Decrease in operative risk of reoperative valve surgery. *Ann Thorac Surg* 1993; 56:15.
4. Jones JM, O'Kane H, Gladstone DJ, et al: Repeat heart valve surgery: risk factors for operative mortality. *J Thorac Cardiovasc Surg* 2001; 122:913.
5. Weerasinghe A, Edwards MB, Taylor KM: First redo heart valve replacement: a 10-year analysis. *Circulation* 1999; 99:655.
6. Cohn LH, Peigh PS, Sell J, DiSesa VJ: Right thoracotomy, femorofemoral bypass, and deep hypothermia for re-replacement of the mitral valve. *Ann Thorac Surg* 1989; 48:69.
7. Jones RE, Fitzgerald D, Cohn LH: Reoperative cardiac surgery using a new femoral venous right atrial cannula. *J Card Surg* 1990; 5:170.
8. Aranki SF, Adams DH, Rizzo RJ, et al: Femoral veno-arterial extracorporeal life support with minimal or no heparin. *Ann Thorac Surg* 1993; 56:149.
9. Bichell DP, Balaguer JM, Aranki SF, et al: Axilloaxillary cardiopulmonary bypass: a practical alternative to femorofemoral bypass [see comments]. *Ann Thorac Surg* 1997; 64:702.
10. Cohn LH, Koster JK Jr, VandeVanter S, Collins JJ Jr: The in-hospital risk of rereplacement of dysfunctional mitral and aortic valves. *Circulation* 1982; 66(2 pt 2):1153.
11. Antunes MJ: Reoperations on cardiac valves. *J Heart Valve Dis* 1992; 1:15.
12. Turina J, Hess OM, Turina M, Krayenbuehl HP. Cardiac bioprostheses in the 1990s. *Circulation* 1993; 88:775.
13. Husebye DG, Pluth JR, Piehler JM, et al: Reoperation on prosthetic heart valves: an analysis of risk factors in 552 patients. *J Thorac Cardiovasc Surg* 1983; 86:543.
14. Edmunds LH Jr: Thrombotic and bleeding complications of prosthetic heart valves. *Ann Thorac Surg* 1987; 44:430.
15. Rizzoli G, Guglielmi C, Toscano G, et al: Reoperations for acute prosthetic thrombosis and pannus: an assessment of rates, relationship and risk. *Eur J Cardiothorac Surg* 1999; 16:74.
16. Deviri E, Sareli P, Wisenbaugh T, Cronje SL: Obstruction of mechanical heart valve prostheses: clinical aspects and surgical management. *J Am Coll Cardiol* 1991; 17:646.
17. Bloomfield P, Wheatley DJ, Prescott RJ, Miller HC: Twelve-year comparison of a Bjork-Shiley mechanical heart valve with porcine bioprostheses. *N Engl J Med* 1991; 324:573.
18. Lytle BW, Cosgrove DM, Taylor PC, et al: Reoperations for valve surgery: perioperative mortality and determinants of risk for 1,000 patients, 1958–1984. *Ann Thorac Surg* 1986; 42:632.
19. Akins CW, Buckley MJ, Daggett WM, et al: Risk of reoperative valve replacement for failed mitral and aortic bioprostheses. *Ann Thorac Surg* 1998; 65:1545.
20. Tyers GF, Jamieson WR, Munro AI, et al: Reoperation in biological and mechanical valve populations: fate of the reoperative patient. *Ann Thorac Surg* 1995; 60(2 suppl):S464.
21. Borkon AM, Soule LM, Baughman KL, et al: Aortic valve selection in the elderly patient. *Ann Thorac Surg* 1988; 46:270.
22. Cohn LH, Couper GS, Aranki SF, et al: The long-term follow-up of the Hancock Modified Orifice porcine bioprosthetic valve. *J Card Surg* 1991; 6(4 suppl):557.
23. Vogt PR, Brunner-LaRocca H, Sidler P, et al: Reoperative surgery for degenerated aortic bioprostheses: predictors for emergency surgery and reoperative mortality. *Eur J Cardiothorac Surg* 2000; 17:134.
24. Starr A, Grunkemeier GL: The expected lifetime of porcine valves. *Ann Thorac Surg* 1989; 48:317.
25. Myken PS, Caidahl K, Larsson P, et al: Mechanical versus biological valve prosthesis: a ten-year comparison regarding function and quality of life. *Ann Thorac Surg* 1995; 60(2 suppl):S447.
26. Myken P, Larsson P, Larsson S, et al: Similar quality of life after heart valve replacement with mechanical or bioprosthetic valves. *J Heart Valve Dis* 1995; 4:339.
27. Milano A, Guglielmi C, De Carlo M, et al: Valve-related complications in elderly patients with biological and mechanical aortic valves. *Ann Thorac Surg* 1998; 66(6 suppl):S82.
28. Barwinsky J, Cohen M, Bhattacharya S, et al: Bjork-Shiley cardiac valves long term results: Winnipeg experience. *Can J Cardiol* 1988; 4:366.
29. Birkmeyer NJ, Birkmeyer JD, Tosteson AN, et al: Prosthetic valve type for patients undergoing aortic valve replacement: a decision analysis. *Ann Thorac Surg* 2000; 70:1946.
30. Birkmeyer NJ, Marrin CA, Morton JR, et al: Decreasing mortality for aortic and mitral valve surgery in Northern New England. Northern New England Cardiovascular Disease Study Group. *Ann Thorac Surg* 2000; 70:432.
31. Peterseim DS, Cen YY, Cheruvu S, et al: Long-term outcome after biologic versus mechanical aortic valve replacement in 841 patients. *J Thorac Cardiovasc Surg* 1999; 117:890.
32. Byrne JG, Karavas AN, Aklog L, et al: Aortic valve reoperation after homograft or autograft replacement. *J Heart Valve Dis* 2001; 10:451.
33. Kouchoukos NT: Aortic allografts and pulmonary autografts for replacement of the aortic valve and aortic root. *Ann Thorac Surg* 1999; 67:1846.
34. Albertucci M, Wong K, Petrou M, et al: The use of unstented homograft valves for aortic valve reoperations: review of a twenty-three-year experience. *J Thorac Cardiovasc Surg* 1994; 107:152.
35. O'Brien MF, McGiffin DC, Stafford EG, et al: Allograft aortic valve replacement: long-term comparative clinical analysis of the viable cryopreserved and antibiotic 4 degrees C stored valves. *J Card Surg* 1991; 6(4 suppl):534.
36. Cohn LH, Collins JJ, Jr., DiSesa VJ, et al: Fifteen-year experience with 1678 Hancock porcine bioprosthetic heart valve replacements. *Ann Surg* 1989; 210:435.
37. Jamieson WR, Munro AI, Miyagishima RT, et al: Carpentier-Edwards standard porcine bioprosthesis: clinical performance to seventeen years. *Ann Thorac Surg* 1995; 60:999.
38. Antunes MJ, Magalhaes MP: Isolated replacement of a prosthesis or a bioprosthesis in the mitral valve position. *Am J Cardiol* 1987; 59:346.
39. Bortolotti U, Guerra F, Magni A, et al: Emergency reoperation for primary tissue failure of porcine bioprostheses. *Am J Cardiol* 1987; 60:920.
40. Ban T, Soga Y: [Re-sternotomy]. *Nippon Geka Gakkai Zasshi* 1998; 99:63.
41. Elami A, Laks H, Merin G: Technique for reoperative median sternotomy in the presence of a patent left internal mammary artery graft. *J Card Surg* 1994; 9:123.
42. Dobell AR, Jain AK: Catastrophic hemorrhage during redo sternotomy. *Ann Thorac Surg* 1984; 37:273.
43. English TA, Milstein BB: Repeat open intracardiac operation: analysis of fifty operations. *J Thorac Cardiovasc Surg* 1978; 76:56.
44. Macmanus Q, Okies JE, Phillips SJ, Starr A: Surgical considerations in patients undergoing repeat median sternotomy. *J Thorac Cardiovasc Surg* 1975; 69:138.
45. Wideman FE, Blackstone EH, Kirklin JW, et al: Hospital mortality of re-replacement of the aortic valve: incremental risk factors. *J Thorac Cardiovasc Surg* 1981; 82:692.
46. Byrne J, Karavas A, Adams D, et al: Partial upper re-sternotomy for aortic valve replacement or re-replacement after previous cardiac surgery. *Eur J Cardiothorac Surg* 2000; 18:282.
47. Tam RK, Garlick RB, Almeida AA: Minimally invasive redo aortic valve replacement. *J Thorac Cardiovasc Surg* 1997; 114:682.
48. Byrne JG, Aranki SF, Couper GS, et al: Reoperative aortic valve replacement: partial upper hemisternotomy versus conventional full sternotomy. *J Thorac Cardiovasc Surg* 1999; 118:991.

49. Gundry SR, Shattuck OH, Razzouk AJ, et al: Facile minimally invasive cardiac surgery via ministernotomy. *Ann Thorac Surg* 1998; 65:1100.
50. Cosgrove DM 3rd, Sabik JF, Navia JL: Minimally invasive valve operations. *Ann Thorac Surg* 1998; 65:1535.
51. Cosgrove DM 3rd, Sabik JF: Minimally invasive approach for aortic valve operations. *Ann Thorac Surg* 1996; 62:596.
52. Hearn CJ, Kraenzler EJ, Wallace LK, et al: Minimally invasive aortic valve surgery: anesthetic considerations. *Anesth Analg* 1996; 83:1342.
53. Aklog L, Adams DH, Couper GS, et al: Techniques and results of direct-access minimally invasive mitral valve surgery: a paradigm for the future. *J Thorac Cardiovasc Surg* 1998; 116:705.
54. Machler HE, Bergmann P, Anelli-Monti M, et al: Minimally invasive versus conventional aortic valve operations: a prospective study in 120 patients. *Ann Thorac Surg* 1999; 67:1001.
55. Luciani GB, Casali G, Santini F, Mazzucco A: Aortic root replacement in adolescents and young adults: composite graft versus homograft or autograft. *Ann Thorac Surg* 1998; 66(6 suppl): S189.
56. Byrne JG, Karavas AN, Cohn LH, Adams DH: Minimal access aortic root, valve, and complex ascending aortic surgery. *Curr Cardiol Rep* 2000; 2:549.
57. Byrne JG, Aranki SF, Cohn LH: Aortic valve operations under deep hypothermic circulatory arrest for the porcelain aorta: "no-touch technique" [see comments]. *Ann Thorac Surg* 1998; 65:1313.
58. Bichell DP, Balaguer JM, Aranki SF, et al: Axilloaxillary cardiopulmonary bypass: a practical alternative to femorofemoral bypass. *Ann Thorac Surg* 1997; 64:702.
59. Zlotnick AY, Gilfeather MS, Adams DH, et al: Innominate vein cannulation for venous drainage in minimally invasive aortic valve replacement. *Ann Thorac Surg* 1999; 67:864.
60. McGiffin DC, Galbraith AJ, O'Brien MF, et al: An analysis of valve re-replacement after aortic valve replacement with biologic devices. *J Thorac Cardiovasc Surg* 1997; 113:311.
61. Hasnat K, Birks EJ, Liddicoat J, et al: Patient outcome and valve performance following a second aortic valve homograft replacement. *Circulation* 1999; 100(19 suppl):II42.
62. Sundt TM 3rd, Rasmi N, Wong K, et al: Reoperative aortic valve operation after homograft root replacement: surgical options and results. *Ann Thorac Surg* 1995; 60(2 suppl):S95.
63. Yacoub M, Rasmi NR, Sundt TM, et al: Fourteen-year experience with homovital homografts for aortic valve replacement. *J Thorac Cardiovasc Surg* 1995; 110:186.
64. McCarthy JF, Cosgrove DM 3rd: Optimizing mitral valve exposure with conventional left atriotomy [see comments]. *Ann Thorac Surg* 1998; 65:1161.
65. Balasundaram SG, Duran C: Surgical approaches to the mitral valve. *J Card Surg* 1990; 5:163.
66. Brawley RK: Improved exposure of the mitral valve in patients with a small left atrium. *Ann Thorac Surg* 1980; 29:179.
67. Praeger PI, Pooley RW, Moggio RA, et al: Simplified method for reoperation on the mitral valve. *Ann Thorac Surg* 1989; 48:835.
68. Bonchek LI. Mitral valve reoperation [letter]. *Ann Thorac Surg* 1991; 51:160.
69. Steimle CN, Bolling SF: Outcome of reoperative valve surgery via right thoracotomy. *Circulation* 1996; 94(9 suppl):II126.
70. Grondin CM, Pomar JL, Hebert Y, et al: Reoperation in patients with patent atherosclerotic coronary vein grafts: a different approach to a different disease. *J Thorac Cardiovasc Surg* 1984; 87:379.
71. Keon WJ, Heggtveit HA, Leduc J: Perioperative myocardial infarction caused by atheroembolism. *J Thorac Cardiovasc Surg* 1982; 84:849.
72. Byrne JG, Aranki SF, Adams DH, et al: Mitral valve surgery after previous CABG with functioning IMA grafts. *Ann Thorac Surg* 1999; 68:2243.
73. Tribble CG, Killinger WA Jr, Harman PK, et al: Anterolateral thoracotomy as an alternative to repeat median sternotomy for replacement of the mitral valve. *Ann Thorac Surg* 1987; 43:380.
74. Londe S, Sugg WL: The challenge of reoperation in cardiac surgery. *Ann Thorac Surg* 1974; 17:157.
75. Berreklouw E, Alfieri O: Revival of right thoracotomy to approach atrio-ventricular valves in reoperations. *Thorac Cardiovasc Surg* 1984; 32:331.
76. Byrne JG, Hsin MK, Adams DH, et al: Minimally invasive direct access heart valve surgery. *J Card Surg* 2000; 15:21.
77. Byrne JG, Mitchell ME, Adams DH, et al: Minimally invasive direct access mitral valve surgery. *Semin Thorac Cardiovasc Surg* 1999; 11:212.
78. Cohn LH: As originally published in 1989: Right thoracotomy, femorofemoral bypass, and deep hypothermia for re-replacement of the mitral valve. Updated in 1997. *Ann Thorac Surg* 1997; 64:578.
79. Byrne JG, Karavas AN, Adams DH, et al: The preferred approach for mitral valve surgery after CABG: right thoracotomy, hypothermia and avoidance of LIMA-LAD graft. *J Heart Valve Dis* 2001; 10:584.
80. Braxton JH, Higgins RS, Schwann TA, et al: Reoperative mitral valve surgery via right thoracotomy: decreased blood loss and improved hemodynamics [see comments]. *J Heart Valve Dis* 1996; 5:169.
81. Vleissis AA, Bolling SF: Mini-reoperative mitral valve surgery. *J Card Surg* 1998; 13:468.
82. Holman WL, Goldberg SP, Early LJ, et al: Right thoracotomy for mitral reoperation: analysis of technique and outcome. *Ann Thorac Surg* 2000; 70:1970.
83. Hanh D, Pezzella T: Closed mitral commissurotomy utilizing right thoracotomy approach. *Asian Cardiovasc Thorac Ann* 2000; 8:192.

Chapter 43

Valvular and Ischemic Heart Disease

Martin LeBoutillier III/Verdi J. DiSesa

In recent years, there has been a great deal of progress in coronary artery surgery, nonsurgical treatment of coronary artery disease, and the surgical treatment of valvular heart disease. As thoroughly described in previous chapters, beating heart surgery has become commonplace. Interventional therapies for coronary artery obstruction have extended to multivessel disease and continue to change the number and the nature of patients referred for bypass surgery. The options for treatment of valvular disease have continued to expand with advances in techniques for repair of aortic and mitral valves as well as increases in the choices of valve type for replacement. Other areas of rapidly growing interest are surgical treatment of atrial arrhythmias and the surgical approach to the failing ventricle in dilated ischemic cardiomyopathy. Some of these topics will be discussed in subsequent chapters. All are issues that the surgeon must consider when planning strategy for the treatment of the patient with combined valvular and coronary artery disease. More patients are now presenting with increasingly complex pathology. It is less often that the surgeon sees a patient with simple aortic stenosis and proximal coronary artery disease. Rather, that patient now may have been managed with more aggressive medical therapy or even catheter interventions and is referred at an older age and is sicker, with more diffuse disease, arrhythmias, and worsening ventricular function. As a result those patients who present for surgery have a higher risk profile than was previously the case, and require a more flexible and thoughtful approach.

The interaction between the pathophysiologies of valvular heart disease and coronary artery disease is complex. Valvular heart disease alters ventricular function. Coronary artery disease may have an additional impact because of its potential to affect ventricular morphology and physiology. In addition to decreases in contractile strength, regional myocardial infarction may lead to distortion of ventricular shape with resulting effects not only on ventricular function but also on mitral valve performance. In patients with valvular heart disease, coronary obstructions may be symptomatic or asymptomatic, but the decision to intervene surgically is often made regardless of the presence of symptoms and in order to have a positive effect on the pathophysiology of both diseases.

Under most circumstances, surgeons attempt to treat both valvular and coronary artery diseases simultaneously. At the least, this makes for a longer and more complicated operation with longer myocardial ischemia times. Because of this, combined coronary artery and valve operations usually have a higher risk for early and late mortality than operations for valvular heart disease alone (Fig. 43-1). The increased complexity increases the need for careful preoperative assessment of myocardial function and an understanding of the impact of changing afterload and preload associated with valve surgery on ventricular function. In adult patients with combined valvular and ischemic heart disease, therefore, the assessment of intrinsic left ventricular function assumes paramount importance. Clinical signs and symptoms of left ventricular failure should be sought. In addition to history, physical examination, and routine lab tests, preoperative echocardiography is mandatory. Transesophageal echocardiography allows for accurate planning

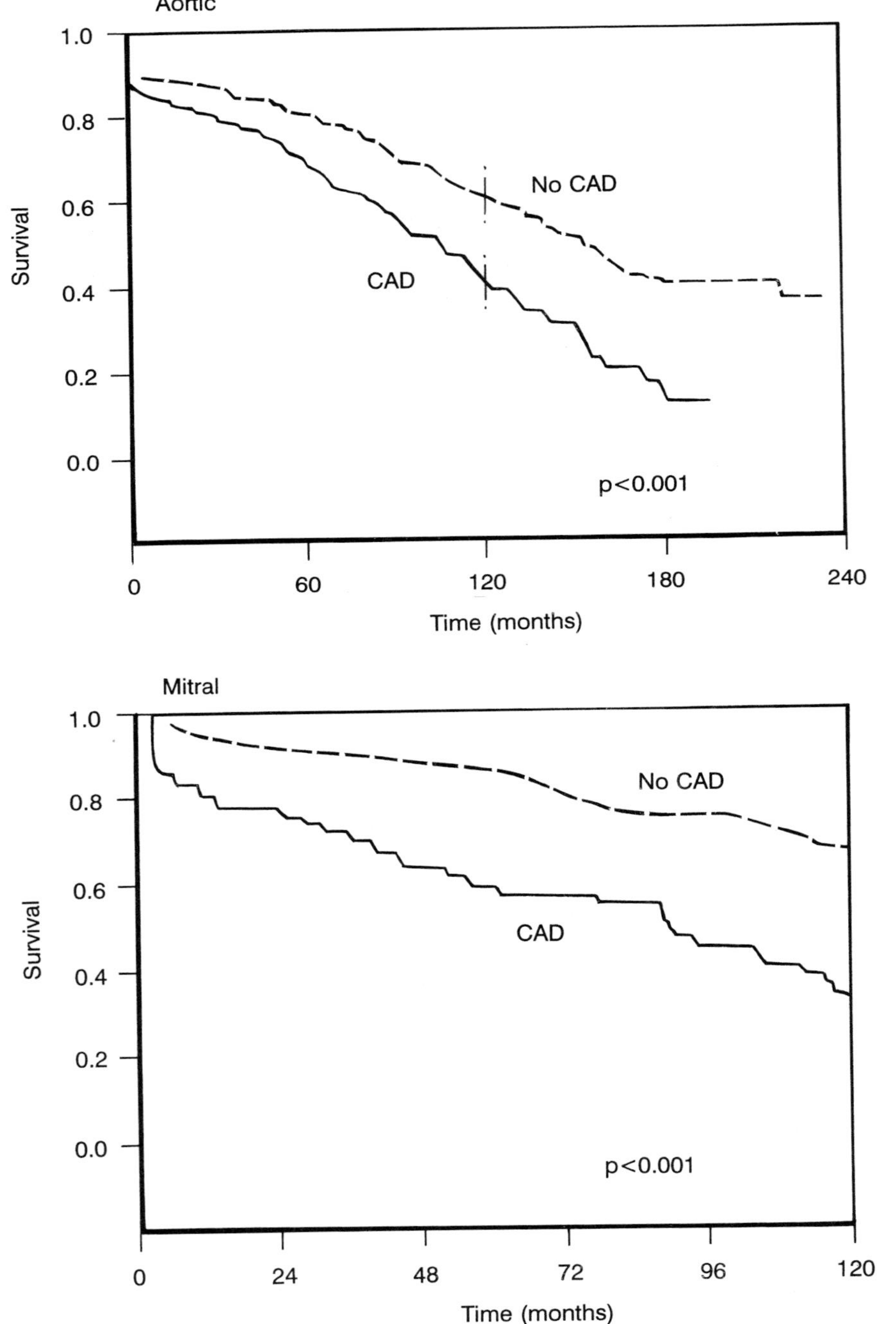

FIGURE 43–1 Survival after aortic or mitral valve replacement in patients with and without coronary artery disease. In both cases, long-term survival is significantly worse in patients with coronary disease. (*Adapted with permission from Jones EL, Weintraub WS, Craver JM, et al: Interaction of age and coronary disease after valve replacement: implications for valve selection. Ann Thorac Surg 1994; 58:378.*)

when operative repair is considered. It is also important to distinguish heart failure due to valvular disease from reversible or irreversible myocardial dysfunction due to coronary ischemia. Dobutamine stress echocardiography may be useful in eliciting ventricular size and shape changes that occur under stress and any resultant exacerbation of underlying valve pathology. At cardiac catheterization, left ventricular end-diastolic pressure and pulmonary pressures give additional information about left and right ventricular function and supplement noninvasive evaluation of valve function and coronary anatomy. In centers where it is available, positron-emission tomography (PET) helps detect areas of viable myocardium with reversible ischemia and ischemic dysfunction as distinguished from irreversibly scarred muscle. These assessments are important prior to embarking on combined valve and coronary artery surgery, for they are crucial in estimating operative risk and planning the operative approach.

The assessment of valve pathology is covered in detail in previous chapters on isolated valvular heart disease. As has been noted earlier, coronary angiography is not necessarily required in all patients with valvular pathology who are about to undergo valve surgery. However, given the prevalence of coronary artery disease in aging Western populations, a high index of suspicion leads to the generalized use of coronary angiography in all patients over 40 years of age, and in select younger patients as well.

With present technology and techniques, myocardial revascularization can be added to any valve operation. For the most part, all that is needed is a rational approach, more time, and good myocardial protection. Because of the wide pathophysiologic spectrum of valvular and coronary artery diseases, several frequently encountered valve and coronary artery combinations are considered in this chapter, including (1) aortic stenosis with coronary artery disease (CAD), (2) aortic regurgitation plus CAD, (3) mitral regurgitation plus CAD, (4) mitral stenosis plus CAD, (5) aortic stenosis and mitral regurgitation plus CAD, and (6) aortic regurgitation and mitral regurgitation plus CAD. Of course, patients may have combined lesions of stenosis and insufficiency, but to avoid unproductive complexity, and because one lesion usually dominates, the somewhat arbitrary categorization noted above will be maintained during the ensuing discussion. For each entity, the clinical presentation, the pathophysiology of the disease state and its correction, the operative and management approach, and short- and long-term results are discussed.

AORTIC STENOSIS AND CORONARY ARTERY DISEASE

Aortic stenosis is one of the more frequently encountered valvular lesions in adult populations. Since degenerative calcific aortic stenosis is most common in patients in their 60s, 70s, and 80s,[1,2] and since congenitally bicuspid valves that become stenotic are more frequent in men who are susceptible to coronary artery disease at an earlier age,[3] it is not surprising that the combination of aortic stenosis and coronary artery disease is encountered frequently. This disease combination is usually gratifying to treat because the response to surgical relief of aortic stenosis and coronary artery obstructions is significant, immediate, and relatively durable.

Clinical Presentation

Patients with aortic stenosis are asymptomatic initially but eventually present with angina pectoris, congestive heart failure, syncope, or some combination of these. When significant coronary artery obstructions are present in addition to valvular obstruction, angina pectoris is almost always present. However, angina pectoris can occur in the absence of significant coronary artery obstructions. It is relatively easy to identify symptoms of myocardial ischemia or congestive heart failure in these patients. Neurologic symptoms may be more difficult to elicit, and careful questioning regarding transient symptomatology is required. Symptoms suggestive of carotid artery obstruction should be sought. Specific studies of the carotid arteries may be necessary, especially since the murmur of aortic stenosis may radiate into the carotids and obscure the detection of bruits.

Prominent findings on physical examination include the typical crescendo/decrescendo systolic murmur heard in the aortic area. Signs of congestive heart failure with rales and edema may be present. The electrocardiogram may show left ventricular strain. If the patient suffered recent or old myocardial infarction, electrocardiographic abnormalities typical of infarction also may be present. The echocardiogram typically shows calcified and immobile aortic valve leaflets producing a constricted aortic orifice with the resultant hypertrophied left ventricle. All patients with angina pectoris and all patients with aortic valve disease who are over 40 years of age should have coronary angiography to define coronary anatomy. Right- and left-sided heart catheterization should be performed simultaneously so that complete evaluation of myocardial performance, including measurement of left ventricular end-diastolic pressure and the pulmonary artery pressures, can be obtained. Transaortic valvar gradient also can be determined at catheterization.

The preoperative evaluation of patients with aortic stenosis, coronary artery disease, and poor ventricular function is complicated. Patients with poor ventricular function often generate relatively low transaortic valve gradients. This renders the calculation of valve area and the assessment of critical aortic stenosis less accurate. The morphology of the valve with immobile leaflets and heavy calcification as seen on echocardiography is often an important confirmatory sign that critical aortic stenosis is present. Even in the presence of a small gradient, if echocardiographic signs of significant valve stenosis are present, and if left ventricular intracavitary pressure exceeds 120 mm Hg in systole, mortality rates are acceptable, and response to valve replacement surgery is usually good. A poorly contractile, thinned-out ventricle with low transvalvular gradient and low intracavitary systolic pressure usually suggests that operation is of high risk and may be of limited or no benefit. A poorly contractile ventricle with normal or increased wall thickness may recover contractile force if a substantial amount of reversibly ischemic myocardium is present and if the degree of aortic stenosis is significant. In addition to ventricular function, other important determinants of the risks and advisability of surgery include patient age, presence of previous cardiac operations, and overall organ functions, especially renal function.

Pathophysiology

Aortic stenosis produces high ventricular afterload, which ultimately is the source of all the symptoms and signs of aortic stenosis. Most patients with aortic stenosis have hypertrophied and thick-walled left ventricles. Contractile function is initially good, and ejection fraction may be maintained. In later stages of the disease, the ventricle begins to fail with enlargement and global diminution of contractile function. At any stage of the disease, the presence of critical coronary artery obstruction can cause regional wall motion abnormalities. Significant three-vessel coronary artery disease of long-standing duration may itself lead to global ventricular dysfunction.

In patients with critical aortic stenosis and good ventricular function, the increased left ventricular afterload is immediately reduced by valve replacement. Since most patients with aortic stenosis have hypertrophied and thick-walled ventricles, intraoperative subendocardial ischemia is more difficult to avoid during aortic cross-clamping. Although revascularization should not decrease left ventricular contractility and may increase it, some myocardial stunning with a temporary decrease in global and regional left ventricular contractility inevitably results from the surgical procedure.[4–7] This, of course, assumes more important pathophysiologic significance in patients with poor ventricular function preoperatively.

Postoperatively, patients may have dramatic improvement in symptoms. Relief of left ventricular outflow obstruction immediately leads to enhanced cardiac output and perfusion of vital organs. In addition, left ventricular function improves both immediately and over time after relief of outflow obstruction and as remodeling ensues. Correction of myocardial ischemia can lead to recruitment of formerly hibernating myocardium[7] with further enhancement of ventricular function.[3]

Operative Management

Monitoring for surgery of the aortic valve and coronary arteries includes catheters and measurements that have become standard for most cardiac surgical operations. These include arterial lines (usually in the radial artery for blood pressure and blood gases), and a pulmonary artery catheter for measurement of pulmonary artery pressures, cardiac output by thermodilution, with optical sensors for continuous estimation of mixed venous oxygen saturation. While the pulmonary artery catheter has a balloon at its tip, occlusion wedge pressure is rarely measured in the perioperative period because of the danger of pulmonary artery rupture. Particularly useful information is provided by continuous measurement of mixed venous oxygen saturation.

The perfusion setup is standard and similar to that for isolated coronary artery bypass (Fig. 43-2). A single aortic cannula is ordinarily placed in the distal ascending aorta. A single two-stage venous cannula is placed via the right atrial appendage with its tip positioned in the inferior vena cava. After establishment of cardiopulmonary bypass, the patient is usually cooled to 32°C to 34°C, during which time a left ventricular vent is positioned via the right superior pulmonary vein. With the heart well emptied, the aortic cross-clamp is applied during a temporary reduction in pump flow. Thereafter, the heart is arrested with cold (4°C) potassium blood cardioplegia and topical irrigation is applied with iced saline solution. After the aorta is opened, the endocardium is intermittently irrigated with iced saline solution to enhance myocardial cooling.

A combination of antegrade and retrograde cardioplegia is optimal. The initial dose of cardioplegia usually is given both ways, half antegrade and half retrograde. Approximately 15 mL/kg is given as the initial dose. Subsequent doses of cardioplegia are given retrograde throughout the operation. This is particularly convenient because retrograde cardioplegia can be given even after the aortic root is opened without significantly disrupting the flow of the operation. Cardioplegia may also be given antegrade via radial and vein grafts after they are attached. This is especially important if a graft has been placed in the right coronary system, as retrograde cardioplegia may not fully protect the right ventricle.

The left internal mammary artery is almost always used to graft the left anterior descending artery when it has a significant obstruction. In general, reversed greater saphenous veins and radial arteries are used for other bypass grafts. The reasoning behind the choice of valve prosthesis is nearly identical to that in the treatment of isolated valvular heart disease. Any type of prosthesis may be used. However, several issues must be considered. The indications for all types of tissue valves are stronger as these patients' life expectancies are often shorter. However, these sicker patients may not well tolerate the longer clamp times necessary for the more complex implantation of nonstented tissue valves.

The multiple steps in the combined operation follow a logical sequence. After establishment of cardiopulmonary bypass and insertion of the left ventricular vent, the aorta is clamped and the heart arrested with antegrade and retrograde cold blood cardioplegia and topical hypothermia with iced saline. The first step in the operation is performance of the distal radial artery and saphenous vein bypass grafts.

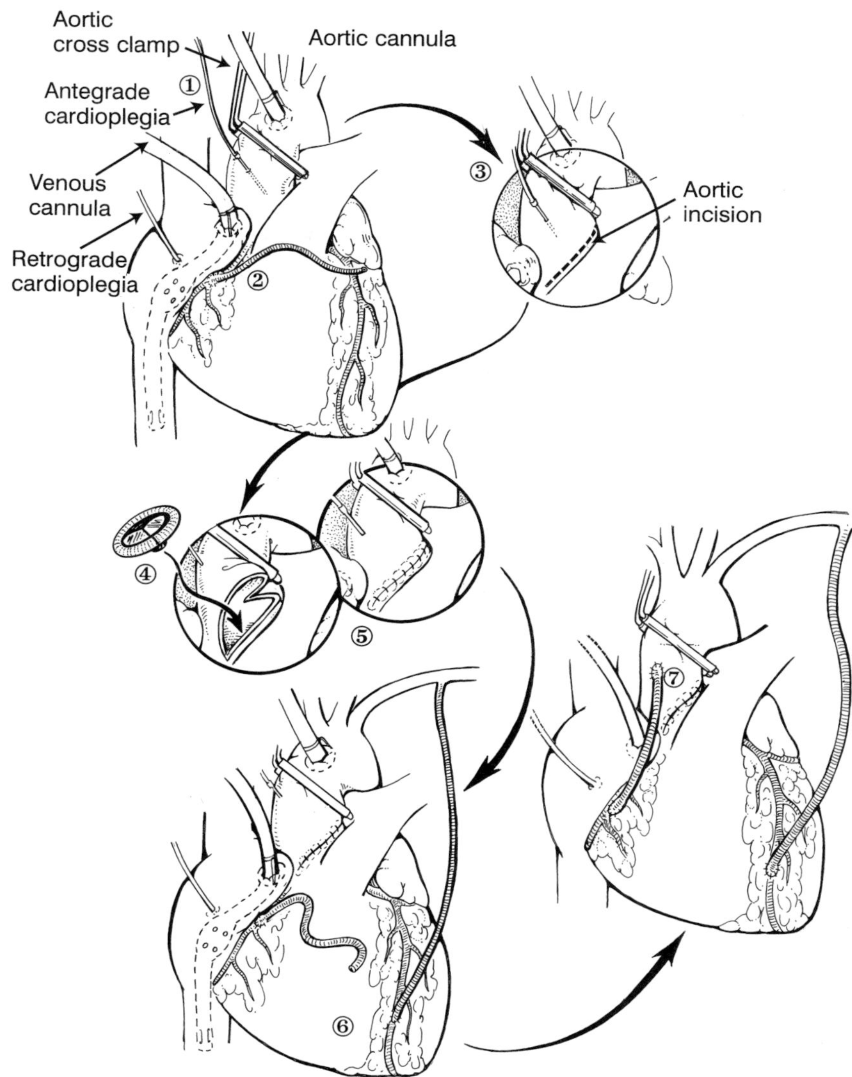

FIGURE 43–2 Operative sequence for aortic valve replacement and coronary artery bypass grafting: (1) aorta is cross-clamped and cardioplegia administered antegrade and retrograde, (2) distal graft anastomoses are performed, (3) the aortotomy is made with an oblique incision into the noncoronary sinus of Valsalva, (4) aortic valve replacement is carried out using the prosthesis of choice, (5) the aortotomy is closed, (6) the distal mammary artery anastomosis is performed, and (7) the proximal graft anastomoses are done. In this case, the proximal anastomoses are done with the aortic cross-clamp in place.

When these are complete, the ventricles may be wrapped in a cooling pad after which the aorta is opened, and aortic valve replacement is carried out using the prosthesis of choice. The aorta is closed completely at this point. The distal anastomosis of the internal mammary artery graft is then made. Following completion of this, air is evacuated from the heart and the aortic cross-clamp is released. A partially occluding clamp is applied to the aorta, and proximal anastamoses are performed, when necessary. Alternatively, the proximal anastomoses can be performed with the aortic cross-clamp still in place. While this prolongs the ischemia time, it avoids application of a second clamp to the aorta with the potential for disruption of atheromatous debris or injury to the aortic suture line. This consideration is particularly important in patients undergoing reoperations, since the presence of previous bypass grafts can make application of a partially occluding clamp on the aorta difficult. Coordinated sinus rhythm is established after temporary atrial and ventricular pacing wires are positioned. After de-airing is confirmed by TEE, the left ventricular vent is removed. Of note, atrial-ventricular sequential activation is particularly important to optimize hemodynamic performance in patients with aortic stenosis because as much as 30% of the cardiac output may be derived from atrial kick as a result of the hypertrophied and noncompliant ventricle that is typical of the patient with aortic stenosis.

Weaning from cardiopulmonary bypass is performed gradually with stepwise diminution of pump flow and increased left ventricular filling. Simultaneous monitoring of the appearance of the heart, pulmonary artery and systemic blood pressures, and mixed venous oxygen saturation is done during weaning. In patients with hypertrophied ventricles, it may be important to keep the left ventricle filled to prevent excessive left ventricular outflow tract obstruction in systole and to provide adequate preload in the noncompliant heart.

In patients with particularly severe ventricular dysfunction who do not wean from bypass, the intra-aortic balloon pump may be used. Two to three attempts to wean from cardiopulmonary bypass using inotropic drugs should be made over a period of 20 to 30 minutes. If weaning from cardiopulmonary bypass is not successful at this point, an intra-aortic balloon pump should be inserted. In some patients, a ventricular assist device is required. Persistent attempts to wean from bypass without mechanical support may be counterproductive because complications from prolonged cardiopulmonary bypass may ensue beyond 30 minutes of elapsed time. As the hypertrophied heart recovers following the ischemic insult, inotropic and mechanical support often can be weaned rapidly. In patients with more impaired ventricular function, weaning, of necessity, occurs more gradually and may take days.

Results

Early hospital mortality after aortic valve replacement and coronary bypass grafting ranges from approximately 2% to 10%.[3,8] Higher mortality is observed in patients with more severe symptoms of heart failure and impaired ventricular function preoperatively. Most frequent causes of operative death are low-output cardiac failure, myocardial infarction, and arrhythmia. Incremental risk factors for hospital death include patient age, functional class, and several measures of ventricular function. In a number of studies, late survival has ranged from 60% to 80% at 5 years and from 50% to 75% at 8 years postoperatively (Fig. 43-3).[9–14] By multivariate analysis, variables leading to reduced late survival include older age, cardiac enlargement, and more severe preoperative clinical symptoms. The use of a mechanical prosthesis at valve replacement has been associated with lower long-term survival and lower long-term event-free survival (Fig. 43-4). As discussed earlier, choice of valve type is a complex issue in combined valve–coronary artery surgery. This is a decision that cannot be made without consultation with the patient. A frank discussion of the advantages and drawbacks of each approach continues to be an important component of the preoperative evaluation and planning for this type of surgery.

AORTIC REGURGITATION AND CORONARY ARTERY DISEASE

Significant aortic regurgitation occurs less often in older populations, and is also less often encountered with coronary artery disease. Most series of patients undergoing aortic valve replacement and coronary artery bypass surgery include a relatively small number (10% to 25%) of patients with aortic insufficiency[3,8–11] While the operative management of patients with aortic regurgitation and coronary artery bypass surgery is similar to that previously described, aortic insufficiency produces different pathophysiology that has implications for perioperative management, and the presence of an incompetent aortic valve introduces subtle nuances to the intraoperative management of these patients.

Clinical Presentation

Patients with aortic regurgitation and coronary artery disease usually present in one of three ways. The aortic regurgitation may be asymptomatic and detected incidentally during evaluation for symptomatic coronary disease. Second, the patient may be asymptomatic, yet a routine physical examination reveals a murmur of aortic insufficiency that leads to cardiac evaluation and detection of coronary disease. Finally, patients may present relatively late in the course of

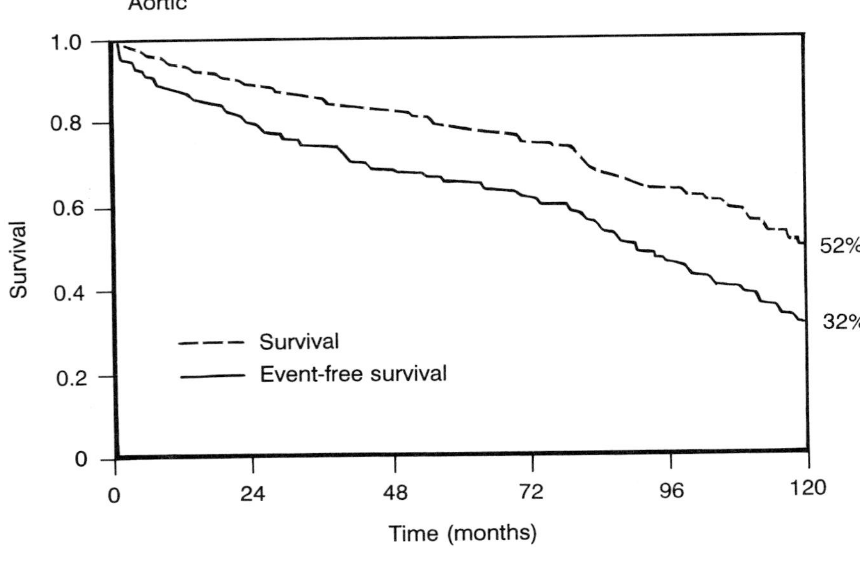

FIGURE 43–3 Long-term survival and event-free survival after aortic valve replacement and coronary artery bypass grafting in 471 patients. (*Adapted with permission from Lytle BW, Cosgrove DM, Gill CC, et al: Aortic valve replacement combined with myocardial revascularization. J Thorac Cardiovasc Surg 1988; 95:402.*)

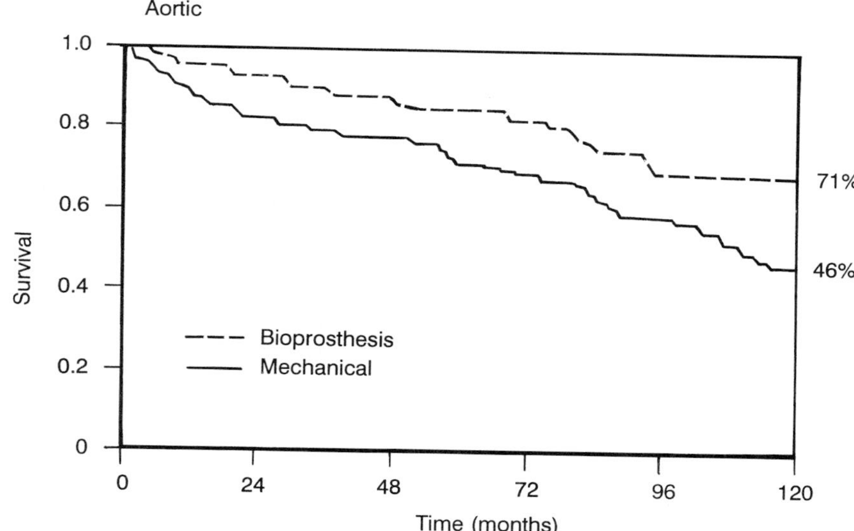

FIGURE 43–4 Long-term survival advantage for patients undergoing aortic valve replacement and coronary artery bypass grafting using a bioprosthesis ($n = 218$) versus a mechanical valve ($n = 253$). (*Adapted with permission from Lytle BW, Cosgrove DM, Gill CC, et al: Aortic valve replacement combined with myocardial revascularization. J Thorac Cardiovasc Surg 1988; 95:402.*)

valvular heart disease with congestive heart failure due to decompensation of the volume-overloaded left ventricle or ischemic damage or both. Patients therefore may present with no symptoms and essentially normal physiology, a classic ischemic syndrome, or congestive heart failure. The physical signs also will depend on the nature of the presentation. In general, all patients with aortic insufficiency have an audible early diastolic blowing murmur. In late stages of the disease, signs of congestive heart failure, including rales and peripheral edema, may be present.

The preoperative evaluation of a patient with aortic insufficiency and coronary artery disease is not different from that previously described for patients with aortic stenosis and ischemic heart disease. Echocardiography is particularly useful in detecting aortic regurgitation because the murmur is sometimes subtle and difficult to detect. In addition, echocardiography gives important information regarding both ventricular contractile function and ventricular size. Since many patients with aortic regurgitation are asymptomatic, careful evaluation for changes in ventricular size or function is important because the presence of these changes may constitute an indication to proceed with surgical intervention in the absence of symptoms.

Pathophysiology

Aortic regurgitation increases left ventricular preload and causes left ventricular dilatation. Dilatation does not occur acutely, and patients with acute aortic insufficiency are often severely symptomatic due to a sudden increase in left ventricular end-diastolic pressure and decrease in net forward cardiac output. Left ventricular dysfunction due to coronary artery disease also can produce left ventricular dilatation. Valve replacement relieves some of the preload but does not immediately result in improved left ventricular contractility. Revascularization may produce improved contractility by recruitment of hibernating myocardium.[4,7] This operation does not increase left ventricular afterload.

The indications for surgery in aortic regurgitation continue to be somewhat controversial, and are reviewed in depth in the section on aortic valve disease. The evaluation of valvular pathology proceeds along similar lines as described above, with emphasis on echocardiographic results. However, this evaluation is somewhat more difficult when coronary artery disease is also present, because there might be an impact on ventricular function that revascularization may or may not improve. Nevertheless, except in advanced stages of diffuse three-vessel coronary artery disease, myocardial abnormalities due to coronary artery obstructions are usually regional and can be distinguished from global dysfunction due to volume overload from the insufficient valve. Making this distinction is of paramount importance in the preoperative assessment and risk stratification of these patients. Again, decisions about timing of aortic valve surgery in the presence of coronary artery disease are different than in cases of isolated valvular disease, with emphasis on fixing the valve earlier in the course of the disease.

Operative Management

The operation is conducted in a fashion similar to that described for aortic stenosis and coronary artery disease. However, in the presence of aortic insufficiency, antegrade cardioplegia in the aortic root cannot be given because the cardioplegia solution leaks into the left ventricle. In general, retrograde cardioplegia is used under these circumstances with doses of antegrade cardioplegia given into the coronary ostia with hand-held catheters after the aorta has been opened.

Considerations in weaning from cardiopulmonary bypass are somewhat different from those described for aortic stenosis. Patients with aortic regurgitation are more likely to have dilated ventricles that tolerate increases in afterload poorly. Successful perioperative management of these patients, therefore, requires careful attention to adjustments in preload and afterload. In patients with volume-overloaded ventricles due to aortic insufficiency, vasodilators may be an important component of postoperative management. Drugs such as milrinone and dobutamine have a role because they provide both inotropic support and ventricular unloading. The mechanical ventricular unloading device—the intra-aortic balloon pump—also may be used. It is rare that mechanical circulatory assistance with a ventricular assist device is required. Its use should be reserved for younger patients without comorbid conditions in whom prompt improvement in ventricular function is anticipated.

Results

Early results after operation for aortic regurgitation and coronary artery disease include an expected hospital mortality rate of less than 10%.[3,8] Incremental risk factors for hospital death are similar to those described previously, with advanced age and poor ventricular function having the greatest impact. Late survival after this operation is similar to that for aortic stenosis and coronary artery disease (see Fig. 43-3).[9–14] Despite the impression that patients with aortic insufficiency and coronary artery disease do not do as well as those with aortic stenosis, aortic insufficiency has not been an independent risk factor for early or late mortality.[3] Interestingly, recovery of ventricular ejection fraction does have a favorable impact on late mortality. When ventricular dilatation and diminution in ventricular systolic function occur in the setting of aortic regurgitation, these often are irreversible changes. While some improvement of function can occur with elimination of the volume overload and with revascularization in patients with combined valvular and coronary artery diseases, there may be less recovery of ejection fraction in patients with aortic insufficiency compared with aortic stenosis. Failure of recovery of ventricular function in this setting may have an impact on long-term survival but not one so great as to render aortic insufficiency an independent risk factor for late death.

MITRAL REGURGITATION AND CORONARY ARTERY DISEASE

Successful management of patients with mitral regurgitation and coronary artery disease remains one of the greater challenges in adult cardiac surgery. This group of patients tends to be sicker, and their surgical care is accomplished at higher risk.[1,15–18] This is almost certainly because of the complex interaction between the left ventricle and the mitral valve. Normal valve function depends on normal function of the entire mitral apparatus, which includes the ventricular wall and the papillary muscles. Similarly, normal ventricular function depends on competence of the mitral valve. Therefore, there is unique potential for coronary artery disease and mitral valve disease to interact, making the patient sicker, the pathophysiology more complicated, and the surgical management more difficult.

In patients with preserved ventricular function, the pathophysiology and management strategies are not significantly different from those for treatment of isolated mitral regurgitation or coronary artery disease. Of course, the operation is more complex and longer, and therefore, as has been described previously, a carefully conceived operative plan with special attention to myocardial preservation is important. However, the more interesting problems are in those patients with mitral insufficiency and coronary artery disease who do not have normal hearts, and in fact, most patients with this disease combination do not have normal ventricular function.

Clinical Presentation

The spectrum of clinical presentation ranges from patients who are asymptomatic to those who are moribund in cardiogenic shock. The patient may have no signs or symptoms of heart disease, or may have predominant symptoms of failure, ischemia, or both. Finally, patients may present with acute syndromes often related to myocardial infarction and the sudden development of mitral insufficiency. These patients are extremely ill when they present in congestive heart failure and cardiogenic shock. Management of these patients is the most difficult.

Findings on physical examination obviously relate to the nature of the presentation, and can range from signs of mild mitral insufficiency to severe congestive failure or cardiogenic shock. An electrocardiogram may show evidence of ischemic heart disease. All patients should undergo echocardiography. The echocardiogram is particularly useful because it gives information both about the valve and about ventricular geometry and function. Transesophageal echocardiography is especially useful in the evaluation of mitral function. Assessments of mitral valve leaflet structure and function, chordal anatomy, and functioning of the papillary muscles and adjacent ventricular wall via TEE are invaluable. All these data are important in planning the operative approach to the mitral valve and assessing the risk of surgery. Cardiac catheterization is performed in these patients for the same reasons outlined for patients with aortic valve disease. Any patient with angina pectoris or a positive stress test and any patient with mitral insufficiency over the age of 40 should have coronary angiography before surgery. As noted previously, cardiac catheterization also provides information about hemodynamics that is important in planning the operation.

Pathophysiology

Mitral regurgitation increases left ventricular preload and decreases afterload at the expense of cardiac output. Ischemic damage causes ventricular dilatation with decreased contractility and an increase in left ventricular filling pressures. These lesions combined cause synergistic decompensation and can produce pulmonary hypertension and secondary tricuspid regurgitation. Cardiac output may be very low, especially in patients with acute mitral insufficiency. Mitral insufficiency may occur in association with coronary artery disease, but often the coronary artery disease is the cause of mitral insufficiency. The pathophysiology of primary mitral insufficiency can be due to involvement of the valve leaflets, the annulus, the subvalvular apparatus, or some combination of all of the above. A detailed understanding of the pathophysiology of primary mitral insufficiency is important for planning the operative approach.

When coronary artery disease is the cause of mitral insufficiency by its effect on regional and global ventricular function, the pathophysiology is more complicated. Global ventricular dysfunction from coronary artery disease can produce ventricular dilatation with mitral annular dilatation and subsequent mitral insufficiency. The jet of mitral regurgitation is usually central and often can be managed with annuloplasty. Alternatively, regional wall motion abnormalities involving the papillary muscle and the adjacent ventricular wall can produce dynamic changes that produce insufficiency of the mitral valve. These abnormalities are now becoming better understood and are discussed more completely in Chapter 36.

Correction of mitral insufficiency either by valve repair or valve replacement produces an instantaneous increase in left ventricular afterload. The ventricle no longer has the low-impedance left atrial chamber in which to eject blood and must overcome systemic afterload in systole. Even when myocardial ischemia is reversible, recruitment of hibernating myocardium may take time. These factors in combination with the sudden increase in left ventricular afterload are responsible for the difficulty and increased risk of managing this entity. Secondary right ventricular failure may be present or ensue because pulmonary hypertension does not decrease immediately after mitral valve repair or replacement, and coronary artery disease also may affect right ventricular function.

Symptomatic mitral insufficiency and symptomatic coronary artery disease are the usual indicators for combined surgery. As noted, patients with acute illnesses may be *in extremis*. Ventricular dysfunction is not per se a contraindication to surgery, especially if it is due to reversible ischemia. Patients with global irreversible cardiomyopathy and mitral insufficiency should not be operated on because the ventricle tolerates the increase in afterload poorly and results are unsatisfactory. Estimation of the viability of the myocardium and demonstration of reversible ischemia using thallium or PET scanning therefore are important.

Finally, with the left atrial enlargement that is common in these patients, they often present with chronic or recent onset atrial fibrillation. This further acts to reduce cardiac output and may also benefit from being addressed at the time of surgery by ablation therapy.

Operative Management

One important preoperative decision in patients with mitral regurgitation and coronary artery disease is whether there is, in fact, any need for valve surgery. Since mitral regurgitation in the presence of coronary artery disease may be functional and due to reversible myocardial ischemia, revascularization alone may improve mitral regurgitation. It is important, therefore, to distinguish organic from functional mitral insufficiency. Intraoperative transesophageal echocardiography is an essential tool for assessment of mitral valve function in this setting.[19] Patients with no preoperative congestive heart failure, absent or only transient murmurs of mitral insufficiency, normal pulmonary pressures in the operating room, and trace to mild mitral insufficiency by transesophageal echocardiography after induction of anesthesia probably do not need mitral valve surgery at all.[20] Many of these patients will appear to have more mitral regurgitation and higher pulmonary pressures at catheterization or when they are ischemic than when they are under anesthesia. Clearly, however, those with moderate to severe insufficiency will need to have the valve regurgitation addressed.[21] Some patients with ventricular enlargement and annular dilation secondary to coronary artery disease and/or mitral insufficiency may be managed with annuloplasty alone. Patients with organic mitral valve disease such as leaflet prolapse, chordal rupture, or chordal elongation need primary repair. Restricted leaflet motion is frequently a complication of ischemic changes in ventricular shape. Standard leaflet resection techniques for posterior flail segments are indicated. In sicker patients, and those with restricted leaflet motion or more complex lesions (severe myxomatous degeneration), an edge-to-edge leaflet approximation (the "Alfieri stitch") may be appropriate.[22] This is especially true in patients with extensive calcification of the posterior annulus or severely restricted posterior leaflet motion.[23] As noted elsewhere, results of mitral repair and coronary artery bypass surgery are superior to those of mitral valve replacement, which should be avoided except in the setting of acute, severe mitral insufficiency due to papillary muscle rupture.[24]

Anesthetic considerations are similar to those described previously, although it must be recognized that these patients are, in general, sicker than patients with aortic valve

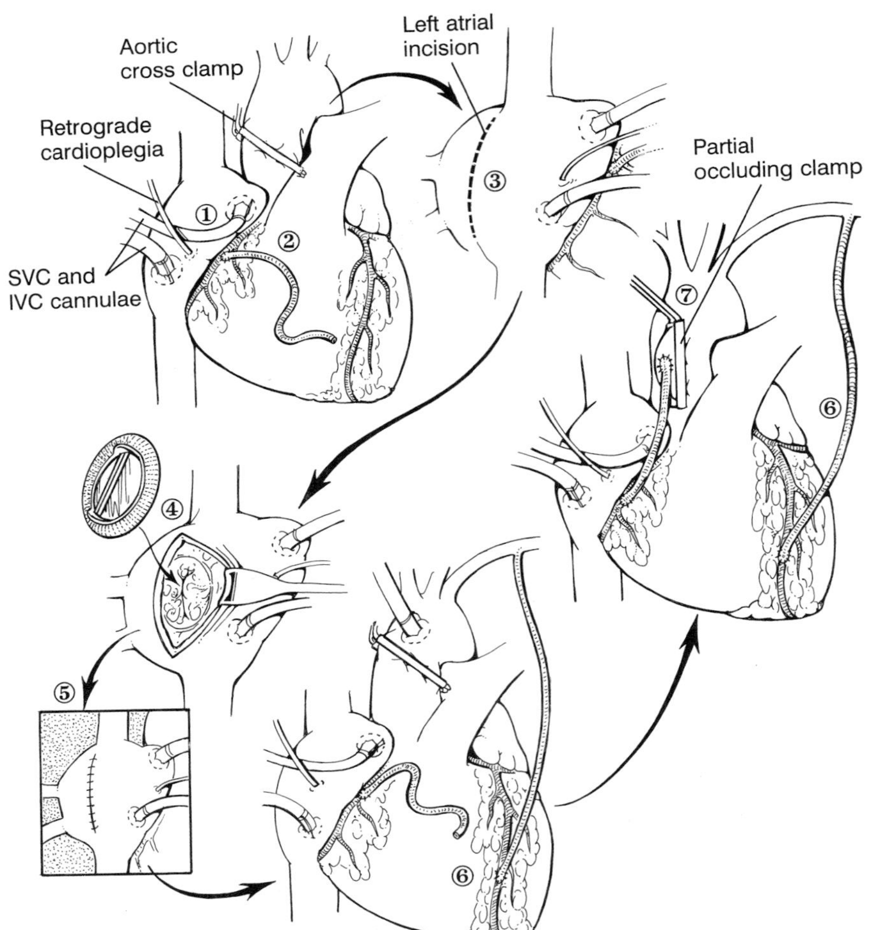

FIGURE 43–5 Operative sequence for mitral valve replacement and coronary artery bypass grafting: (1) cannulation and cross-clamping of the aorta with antegrade and retrograde cardioplegia, (2) distal vein graft anastomoses are performed, (3) left atriotomy is performed after dissection in the interatrial groove, (4) mitral valve repair or replacement with the prosthesis of choice, (5) closure of left atriotomy, (6) distal anastomosis using the mammary artery is performed, and (7) proximal graft anastomosis is done. In this case, the cross-clamp has been removed and a partially occluding aortic clamp used.

disease and in some cases are among the sickest patients treated. Monitoring includes a radial artery line and a pulmonary artery catheter. As suggested earlier, transesophageal echocardiography is particularly important in this group of patients. Setup for cardiopulmonary bypass is similar to that described. However, both venae cavae are cannulated for venous return (Fig. 43-5). This is usually accomplished by introducing the cannulas through purse strings in the superior vena cava and low in the right atrium. After clamping the aorta, cardioplegia is administered antegrade and then retrograde. Subsequent doses of cardioplegia are given retrograde. As with aortic disease, special attention must be paid to protecting the right ventricle during periods of prolonged retrograde cardioplegia.

The most common incision is in the wall of the left atrium anterior to the right pulmonary veins. Preparative dissection of the interatrial groove usually facilitates exposure using this incision. Another choice for exposure of the mitral valve is the trans-septal approach. This allows for direct visual insertion of the retrograde cardioplegia catheter through a purse string, and affords an excellent view of the mitral valve, especially if the left atrium is not enlarged, without excessive stretching of the right atrium or the cavae. If necessary, the incision can be carried up into the dome of the left atrium for even greater exposure. Other incisions are discussed in the section on mitral valve disease. Choice of coronary artery grafts is similar to that for aortic disease.

The first choice in surgery for mitral insufficiency is valve repair. When valve repair is impossible, valve replacement follows the same guidelines set forth in Chapter 38. However, in patients with this disease combination and an abbreviated life expectancy, a stronger rationale for use of a tissue prosthesis may exist.[25] Regardless of the type of prosthesis, an effort should be made to retain continuity between the papillary muscles and the mitral annulus. The attachments to the posterior leaflet usually can be retained in their entirety without interfering with prosthesis function. The anterior leaflet must be resected either in whole or in part to avoid left ventricular outflow tract obstruction or interference with mechanical valve function. However, major chordal attachments may still be preserved and incorporated into the annular suture line. Regardless, standard practice is to retain continuity between the mitral annulus and the subvalvular apparatus whenever the mitral valve is replaced. Short- and long-term ventricular functions appear to be better when this is done. Obviously, in this clinical setting where ventricular function has a significant impact on short- and long-term results, all steps should be taken to ensure optimal myocardial performance postoperatively.

Patients with papillary muscle rupture due to infarction are usually extremely sick. Valve replacement is almost always required. Some surgeons have reported success with reimplantation of the papillary muscle. This strategy is risky in these sick patients because the operation must be both expeditious and effective. Multiple attempts to achieve mitral valve competence are tolerated poorly. A reimplanted, infarcted papillary muscle does not necessarily restore mitral valve competence and also may be subject to late breakdown.

As in combined aortic valve and coronary artery surgery, distal graft anastomoses are performed first (see Fig. 43-5). At this point, after the atrium has been opened, it may be prudent to undertake an arrhythmia ablation procedure in selected patients. Radiofrequency or cryoablation probes can be used to create a lesion set within the left and right atria, as described elsewhere in this text (Chapter 53). The left atrial appendage may be oversewn as necessary. Valve repair or replacement is then carried out, followed by performance of the mammary artery anastomosis. Proximal graft anastomoses can be done either after release of the cross-clamp and application of a partially occluding clamp or with the cross-clamp in place. Weaning from cardiopulmonary bypass is similar to that in patients with aortic insufficiency and coronary artery disease. Again, in this group of patients, afterload reduction using drugs or the intra-aortic balloon pump may be required. Inotropic drugs with afterload-reducing capabilities such as dobutamine and milrinone may be particularly indicated. The surgeon should have a low threshold for adding a drug such as milrinone to epinephrine because this combination has some theoretical advantages as a result of positive inotropic and unloading effects, as well as a reduction in pulmonary artery pressures. Alternatively, dobutamine, which has both central inotropic and peripheral afterload-reducing effects, may be a first-choice drug. Since some of these patients are particularly sick, little time should be wasted in futile attempts to wean from cardiopulmonary bypass on medications and without the intra-aortic balloon. There should be a low threshold for insertion of the intra-aortic balloon in patients whose hemodynamics may be quite tenuous for hours to days after surgery, especially when the operation is an emergency.

Another consideration for a select subset of patients with this disease is the incorporation of ventricular remodeling into the operation. A large body of work is now emerging indicating that patients with anterior infarctions and dilated cardiomyopathy, mitral insufficiency, and coronary artery disease will benefit from exclusion of the infarcted area and remodeling of the left ventricle with return to elliptical shape.[26] This can be performed safely, along with mitral repair and coronary revascularization, in carefully selected patients. The result can be a dramatic increase in ejection fraction with greatly improved postoperative function.

Strict attention must be paid to right ventricular function in this group of patients, although right ventricular failure is more common in the setting of mitral stenosis. Right ventricular failure must be anticipated and correctly diagnosed and managed. The presence of a falling systemic blood pressure and cardiac output with falling pulmonary artery pressure and/or pulmonary capillary wedge pressure should prompt a search for right ventricular failure, which is manifested by a rising central venous pressure. Failure to recognize this and inappropriate administration of fluid can lead to irreversible right ventricular failure.

Results

Hospital mortality for this group of patients is higher than for most other forms of acquired heart disease. Early mortality rates range from 3% in good-risk patients to 60% in the sickest patients.[12–14,15–18,27] The higher mortality is seen in patients with acute ischemic mitral valve disease and severe ventricular dysfunction who require emergency operation. Incremental risk factors for early death include age, functional class, ventricular function, pulmonary pressures, and cardiogenic shock. Late survival in this entity is 55% to 85% at 5 years and 30% to 45% at 10 years (Fig. 43-6).[12–14,15–18,28] In general, patients who survive surgery have good relief of symptoms. Significant risk factors for late death include preoperative functional class, left ventricular function, and an ischemic as opposed to a degenerative etiology for mitral insufficiency (Fig. 43-7).

MITRAL STENOSIS AND CORONARY ARTERY DISEASE

Patients with mitral stenosis and coronary artery disease usually have good left ventricular function and often are a relatively easy group of patients to take care of because the mitral stenosis protects the left ventricle from hemodynamic loads. Coronary artery disease may cause left ventricular dysfunction, but this is unusual. A more usual concern is right ventricular dysfunction postoperatively, since in patients with mitral stenosis, pulmonary hypertension, with its potential to produce right ventricular failure and tricuspid insufficiency, is often encountered.

Clinical Presentation

As implied earlier, mitral stenosis is usually the dominant lesion in patients with mitral stenosis and coronary artery disease. Therefore, symptoms usually are due to the valvular lesion. Patients may have congestive heart failure with shortness of breath and orthopnea and fatigue. Atrial fibrillation is

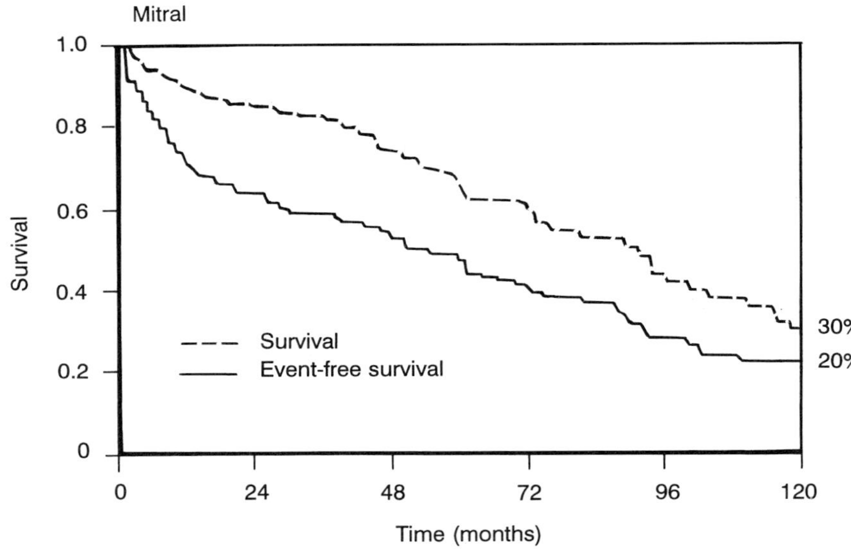

FIGURE 43–6 Survival and event-free survival after mitral valve replacement combined with coronary artery bypass grafting in 278 patients. (*Adapted with permission from Lytle BW, Cosgrove DM, Gill CC, et al: Mitral valve replacement combined with myocardial revascularization: early and late results for 300 patients, 1970 to 1983. Circulation 1985; 71:1179.*)

a common presenting symptom with mitral stenosis. Patients with mitral stenosis and coronary artery disease infrequently have angina as a presenting symptom. The electrocardiogram may show evidence of right ventricular strain and hypertrophy. Transesophageal echocardiography confirms the diagnosis of mitral stenosis and usually shows a small left ventricle with preserved contractile function. The right ventricle may be enlarged and hypertrophied. Cardiac catheterization further confirms the diagnosis by showing a gradient across the mitral valve. Other important information gleaned from invasive catheterization includes a measurement of the pulmonary artery pressures and central venous pressure. The degree of pulmonary hypertension is a marker of the severity and duration of mitral stenosis and alerts the surgeon to the potential for right ventricular failure postoperatively. An elevated central venous pressure is a potential sign that right ventricular decompensation has already occurred. Coronary angiography should be done in all patients with angina pectoris and, as noted before, in any patient over age 40 in whom mitral valve surgery is anticipated.

Pathophysiology

Unlike the other entities described, mitral stenosis and coronary artery disease do not have significantly synergistic pathologic effects on the heart. Coronary artery disease

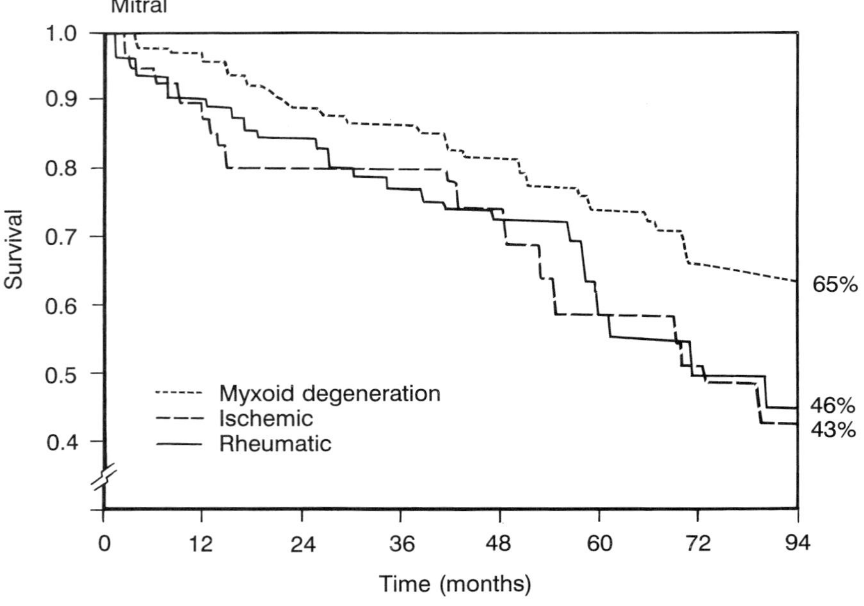

FIGURE 43–7 Survival after mitral valve replacement and coronary artery bypass grafting based on the etiology of mitral valve disease. A survival advantage for patients with myxoid degeneration of the mitral valve is demonstrated. (*Adapted with permission from Lytle BW, Cosgrove DM, Gill CC, et al: Mitral valve replacement combined with myocardial revascularization: early and late results for 300 patients, 1970 to 1983. Circulation 1985; 71:1179.*)

usually has more profound effects on the left ventricle, which remains protected in patients with mitral stenosis until late in the disease. The right ventricle is the chamber most vulnerable to the effects of long-standing mitral stenosis, as noted. However, even with right ventricular hypertension, the potential impact of coronary artery disease on right ventricular function in adults is relatively insignificant. In the rare patient with diffuse coronary artery disease and ischemic cardiomyopathy, the risk of surgery is enhanced because of global ventricular dysfunction. The indications for surgery, not surprisingly, are determined usually by the severity of the mitral stenosis. Patients with significant heart failure and low cardiac output from mitral stenosis whose calculated valve area is less than 1 cm^2 should have a mitral valve operation and associated bypass grafting if significant coronary artery disease is present. A rare patient may have significant coronary artery disease and mild mitral stenosis detected incidentally. These patients may be managed with coronary artery bypass surgery and mitral commissurotomy if this is technically feasible.

Operative Management

Monitoring, perfusion setup, and operative sequence are identical to those described for treatment of mitral regurgitation and coronary artery disease. Transesophageal echocardiography is useful to assess both the feasibility of mitral commissurotomy (or more extensive mitral repair) and the results of valvuloplasty. In most patients with mitral stenosis, valve replacement is required because irreversible damage to the leaflets and subvalvar apparatus is usually extensive. A mechanical prosthesis is used most often because the majority of patients have chronic atrial fibrillation from left atrial enlargement, and long-term anticoagulation is indicated. However, an ablation procedure (as discussed above) within the left and right atria may be indicated, which also may have an impact on prosthetic choice.

Transesophageal echocardiography is often important in monitoring both right and left ventricular function postoperatively. The early differentiation between left and right ventricular failure is facilitated by the use of this modality during weaning from cardiopulmonary bypass. If inotropic drugs are required, their selection should be based in part on the consideration that pulmonary hypertension and right ventricular failure might be an important component of the clinical syndrome postoperatively. Drugs such as isoproterenol, dobutamine, and especially milrinone (the latter often in combination with norepinephrine) may be indicated for their combined beneficial effects on right ventricular contractility and pulmonary vascular resistance. Judicious use of inotropic drugs and careful administration of fluid should result in optimal cardiac output. The intra-aortic balloon is almost never useful in these patients because right ventricular problems predominate, and the intra-aortic balloon has little direct effect on right ventricular function. Temporary support with a right ventricular assist device may be employed because mitral valve replacement can lead to dramatic decreases in pulmonary artery pressures and subsequent recovery of right ventricular function.

Results

Early mortality after combined surgery for mitral stenosis and coronary artery disease is approximately 8%.[12–14,15–18,27] This is not significantly different from results of surgery in better-risk patients with mitral regurgitation and coronary artery disease. Long-term probability of survival is approximately 50% at 7 years and in one series was not significantly different from that for patients with ischemic mitral insufficiency.[12–14,16–18,28] Interestingly, long-term survival of patients with myxoid degeneration of the mitral valve and coronary artery disease (65%) was significantly better than survival of the patients with rheumatic or ischemic mitral valve disease and coronary artery disease in at least one series (see Fig. 43-7).[16] As implied, rheumatic valve pathology is a risk factor for late death, as is poor preoperative left ventricular function and the presence of ventricular arrhythmias. Interestingly, the use of a bioprosthesis without anticoagulants confers both a survival advantage and an event-free survival advantage in these patients (Fig. 43-8). These data lend support to the hypothesis that biologic valves may be appropriate for mitral replacement in older patients and in those with coronary artery disease, whose expected life span may be shorter than the expected durability of the replacement device.[25]

AORTIC STENOSIS, MITRAL REGURGITATION, AND CORONARY ARTERY DISEASE

Patients with aortic stenosis, mitral regurgitation, and coronary artery disease often present with aortic stenosis as the predominant lesion. It is important to note that functional mitral regurgitation may improve after relief of aortic stenosis with concomitant reduction in left ventricular systolic pressure. If the mitral valve is not intrinsically diseased, it may not require operation.

Clinical Presentation

Patients with these diseases often present identically to patients with aortic stenosis and coronary artery disease but may do so earlier because of the combined valvular lesions. Angina, congestive heart failure, and syncope may be presenting symptoms alone or together. It is relatively uncommon for symptoms due to mitral insufficiency to be predominant. Echocardiography is an extremely important tool in this disease combination. Careful evaluation of the mitral valve, often using transesophageal echocardiography, is

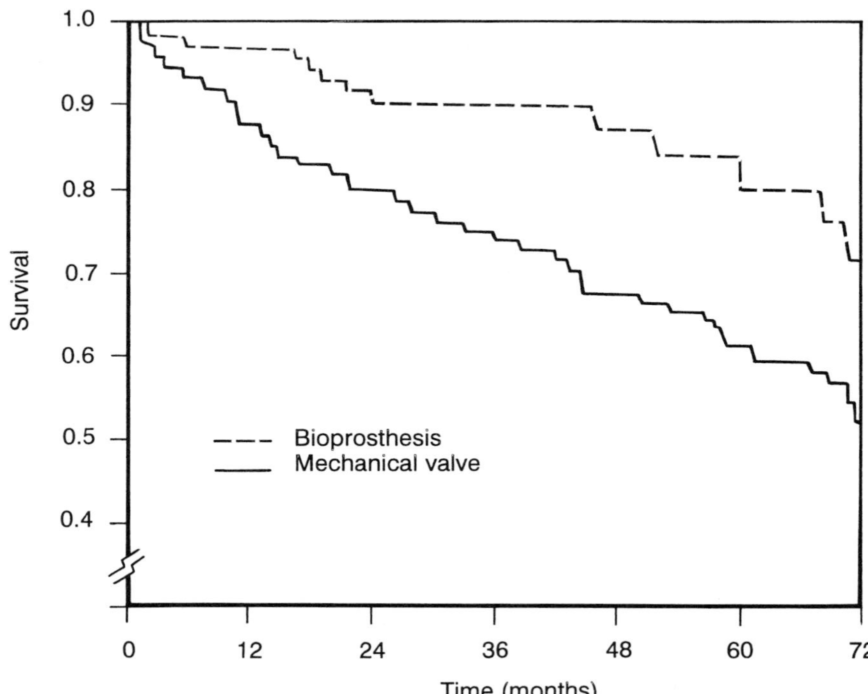

FIGURE 43–8 Comparative survival after mitral valve replacement and coronary artery bypass grafting for patients having mitral valve replacement with a bioprosthesis (n = 82) or mechanical valve (n = 100). (*Adapted with permission from Lytle BW, Cosgrove DM, Gill CC, et al: Mitral valve replacement combined with myocardial revascularization: early and late results for 300 patients, 1970 to 1983. Circulation 1985; 71:1179.*)

necessary to determine the degree of intrinsic mitral valve disease, since improvement in mitral insufficiency is expected after aortic valve replacement and relief of left ventricular obstruction. It is critical to determine whether or not anatomic abnormalities of the mitral valve are present that might not reverse with aortic surgery alone. Of course, cardiac catheterization is required, as it is for the other disease entities described.

Pathophysiology

Aortic stenosis increases left ventricular afterload and the potential amount of mitral regurgitation. The left ventricle may be better preserved in this setting than in patients with isolated mitral insufficiency and coronary artery disease. Also as noted, the mitral valve may not be structurally diseased. Because of earlier presentation, pulmonary hypertension and subsequent right ventricular failure and tricuspid valve incompetence are usually not prominent features. Because relief of outflow obstruction helps left ventricular function immediately, these patients often do quite well.

The indications for surgery are usually the same as for aortic stenosis and coronary artery disease. Critical aortic stenosis, when documented, requires valve replacement; if significant coronary artery disease is present, coronary artery bypass grafts are also done. Mitral valve repair is almost always necessary and possible when mitral insufficiency is moderate to severe and/or anatomic abnormalities of the valve are detected. If absolutely necessary, valve replacement may be performed. End-stage ventricular dysfunction with ventricular dilatation and myocardial thinning is the only cardiac contraindication to surgery.

Operative Management

Anesthesia and perfusion setup are identical to those described for mitral valve and coronary artery surgery. In this entity, intraoperative transesophageal echocardiographic monitoring plays an important role because the intraoperative assessment of mitral valve function before and after bypass is critical. The choice of valves for aortic replacement is the same as described previously. In almost all situations, however, bioprosthetic valves should be considered, especially if the mitral valve is to be repaired.

Under almost all circumstances in which anatomic abnormalities of the mitral valve are detected or in which mitral insufficiency is severe, mitral valve repair should be considered. Annuloplasty may be all that is required if the mitral insufficiency is due to annular dilatation and there is a symmetric central jet of regurgitation. More complex disease may require more extensive repair or even replacement of the mitral valve. When the decision is made not to operate on the mitral valve, transesophageal echocardiography is done to assess residual mitral valve dysfunction following aortic valve replacement and coronary artery bypass surgery. If moderate or severe mitral regurgitation remains, the valve is repaired or replaced. This is technically more difficult after the aortic valve has been replaced, since the prosthesis in the aortic position hinders exposure of the mitral valve.

Therefore, every effort must be made to assess mitral valvular morphology and function before starting cardiopulmonary bypass.

As in the other entities described, distal graft anastomoses are performed first (Fig. 43-9). After these grafts are completed, the aorta is opened, and the aortic valve is resected. Replacement of the aortic valve, however, is deferred until after the mitral valve operation. However, it is important to resect the aortic valve before replacing the mitral valve to improve exposure of the latter. In addition, sutures used for mitral valve repair or replacement may become disrupted during resection or debridement of the aortic valve and annulus. After resection of the aortic valve, the atrium is opened, and the mitral operation is performed. The atrium is closed with a vent across the mitral valve. The aortic valve is then replaced, and the aorta is closed. The internal mammary artery graft is done last. Proximal graft anastomoses can be done with the aortic cross-clamp in place or after removal of the cross-clamp and placement of a partially occluding clamp, as described previously.

As noted, this group of patients may have preserved ventricular function, and weaning from cardiopulmonary bypass may be relatively easy. Inotropic drugs and the intra-aortic balloon can be used as indicated.

Results

Early hospital mortality is 12% to 16%.[29,30] Not surprisingly, predictors of early death include severe mitral regurgitation, lower ejection fraction with more severe symptoms of heart failure, and the presence of triple-vessel coronary artery disease. Late survival is approximately 60% at 72 months (Fig. 43-10). Multivariate predictors of late mortality include advanced symptoms of heart failure and increased severity of mitral insufficiency.

AORTIC AND MITRAL REGURGITATION AND CORONARY ARTERY DISEASE

Not many patients have regurgitation of both the aortic and mitral valves and coronary artery disease. These patients usually have rheumatic heart disease and present early in the course of the disease. Aortic regurgitation may be the primary valve pathology in a patient with significant coronary artery disease. Patients may have mitral disease secondary to left ventricular dilatation from ischemia as well as from aortic regurgitation. Organic mitral valve disease may not be present. Assessment of left ventricular contractility may be difficult because of the alterations in preload and afterload produced by this combination of lesions. In addition, the presence of reversible ischemia may obscure accurate assessment of ventricular function. Therefore, assessment of myocardial viability is important.

Clinical Presentation

Most patients with this combination of cardiac lesions present with congestive heart failure. It is unusual to see a patient with angina as the primary symptom who also has significant insufficiency of both the aortic and mitral valves. Typical murmurs of aortic and mitral insufficiency are present, and the patient may have other signs of chronic congestive heart failure, including rales and peripheral edema. If myocardial infarction is a significant component of the pathophysiology and presentation of the disease, evidence of it on electrocardiogram and echocardiogram may be seen. On echocardiography, patients may have regional wall motion abnormalities if infarction has occurred, as well as global ventricular dilatation and dysfunction from the combined valvular lesions. Cardiac catheterization defines the coronary anatomy, and helps define the severity of the valvular insufficiency and ventricular dysfunction. Accurate assessment of true left ventricular function is difficult in this entity. Mitral insufficiency may abnormally inflate visual measurements of ejection fraction because the ventricle can eject into the low-pressure pulmonary venous circuit. The misleading ejection fraction combined with the multiple volume overloads of leaking aortic and mitral valves and the potential contribution of dysfunctional myocardium from ischemia make it very difficult to get an accurate perception of preoperative left ventricular function. Thallium or PET scans may be useful to assess which areas of dysfunctional myocardium may be viable and potentially recruitable after revascularization.

Pathophysiology

Symptoms and signs of left ventricular failure develop as the left ventricle dilates. In patients with rheumatic disease with both valves intrinsically damaged, ischemic disease may be minimal. In the more common setting of patients with aortic regurgitation and severe ischemia, mitral regurgitation is likely to be secondary to both of these processes, and valve repair should be possible. Correction of aortic regurgitation reduces preload, whereas correction of mitral insufficiency increases afterload. The dilated myopathic ventricle may not have sufficient reserves to maintain adequate output under these circumstances. Higher postoperative preload may need to be maintained while afterload is reduced. Any additional contractility as a result of revascularization, given a smaller left ventricle, should further improve output. Hence, forward flow should improve if ventricular contractility is maintained or increased. However, because of the multiple, uncontrollable variables that inhibit preoperative assessment of ventricular function, prediction of expected improvement from this operation is difficult.

This consideration is extremely important. Patients with severe and irreversible ischemic myocardial disease and poor ventricular function will not do well with operative

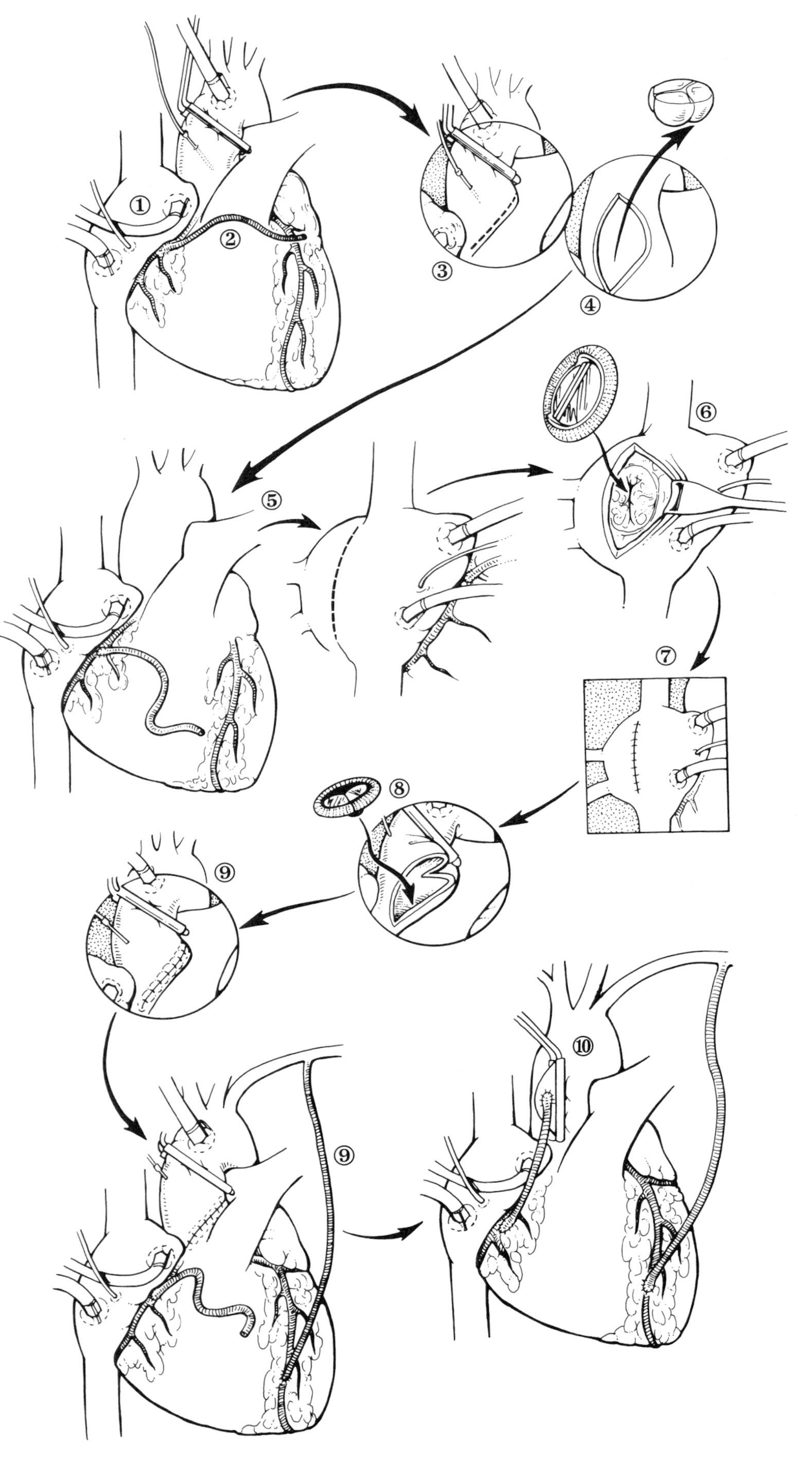
①
②
③
④
⑤
⑥
⑦
⑧
⑨
⑨
⑩

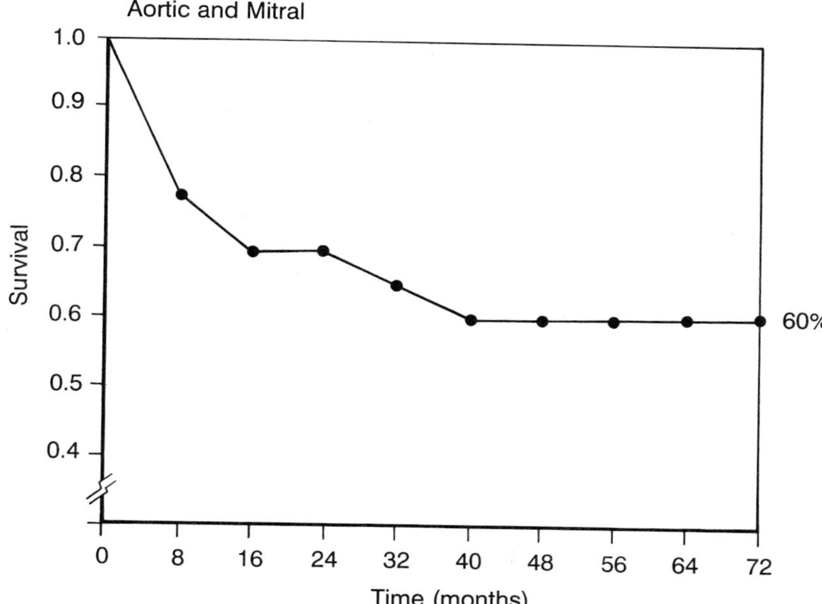

FIGURE 43–10 Long-term survival after combined aortic and mitral valve replacement and coronary artery bypass grafting. (*Adapted with permission from Akins CW, Buckley MJ, Daggett WM, et al: Myocardial revascularization with combined aortic and mitral valve replacements. J Thorac Cardiovasc Surg 1985; 90:272.*)

treatment of this entity. Therefore, preoperative assessments of myocardial viability and reversible ischemia are important. It is also important to assess whether organic mitral valve disease is present. The best results in these patients are in those in whom no mitral operation, or at most annuloplasty, is required.

Operative Management

Details of the operative technique are similar to those described previously. Because of the presence of aortic insufficiency, retrograde cardioplegia must be used in conjunction with handheld antegrade ostial cannulae as necessary. Transesophageal echocardiography is required in the operating room for the assessment of mitral valve function. Residual 1+ to 2+ mitral regurgitation may be acceptable in certain patients because relief of aortic regurgitation can be expected to reduce ventricular size, which may lead to improvement of mitral regurgitation with time. Similarly, myocardial revascularization also may lead to ultimate improvement in ventricular and mitral valve function.

In weaning from cardiopulmonary bypass, afterload reduction is extremely important because of the large preoperative volume overload of the heart. Drugs that reduce ventricular afterload, including vasodilators and inotropic drugs such as milrinone, may be particularly appropriate. The intra-aortic balloon pump may be needed.

Results

Early hospital mortality in this group of patients may be high, and if myocardial failure is severe, overall mortality rates exceed the range already noted for double-valve and coronary artery surgery.[29,30] Important determinants of risk in these patients are the familiar ones. In several series, predictors of hospital death and late events included severe mitral regurgitation, lower ejection fraction, more severe symptoms of congestive heart failure, and severe triple-vessel coronary artery disease.

SUMMARY

This chapter has reviewed the management of patients with valvular and ischemic heart disease. The discussion has focused on management of disease of the aortic and mitral valves, since these are the valves most frequently affected in adults who present with these combined diseases.

Rather than concentrate on the details of the technical aspects of valve implantation or coronary artery grafting,

FIGURE 43–9 Operative sequence for aortic valve replacement, mitral valve replacement, and coronary artery bypass grafting: (1) cannulation with cross-clamping of the aorta and administration of antegrade and retrograde cardioplegia, (2) distal graft anastomoses are performed, (3) aortotomy with standard oblique incision, (4) aortic valve is resected but not replaced, (5) standard left atriotomy after dissection in the interatrial groove, (6) mitral valve repair or replacement with the prosthesis of choice, (7) closure of left atriotomy, (8) aortic valve replacement with prosthesis of choice, (9) closure of aortotomy and performance of distal anastomosis with the internal mammary artery, and (10) proximal graft anastomoses performed. In this illustration, a partially occluding clamp has been applied to the aorta.

the discussion has focused on the particular problems for surgical management that the combined pathophysiology of valvular and ischemic heart disease produces. As has been noted often during the discussion, there is usually an interaction between valve function, myocardial perfusion, and ventricular performance. Dysfunction of the aortic and mitral valves has secondary effects on ventricular function, and the addition of coronary artery disease can make this interaction more complex. Therefore, the pathophysiology of these disease states can be complicated. In order to manage these entities successfully, this pathophysiology must be understood so that accurate estimates of risk and reasonable expectations for results can be achieved.

In almost every case, ventricular function and severity of mitral incompetence are important short- and long-term risk factors. Also, functional mitral insufficiency in the absence of anatomic abnormalities of the mitral valve may resolve after aortic and/or coronary artery surgery, and therefore an operation on the mitral valve may not be required. Finally, data from several sources suggest that patients with both coronary artery and valvular heart disease should be considered for a tissue prosthesis because of reduced life expectancy.

In addition, the complex interaction between ventricular function, valvular function, and coronary ischemia requires that the operation be well planned with attention paid to expeditious surgery with short myocardial ischemia times and good myocardial preservation. Much of the discussion in this chapter, therefore, has focused on the operative plan and the development of a rational approach to intraoperative and postoperative management of these patients.

REFERENCES

1. Davis EA, Gardner TJ, Gillinov AM, et al: Valvular disease in the elderly: influence on surgical results. *Ann Thorac Surg* 1993; 55:333.
2. Freeman WK, Schaff HV, O'Brien PC, et al: Cardiac surgery in the octogenarian: perioperative outcome and clinical follow-up. *J Am Coll Cardiol* 1991; 18:29.
3. Morris JJ, Schaff HV, Mullany CJ, et al: Determinants of survival and recovery of left ventricular function after aortic valve replacement. *Ann Thorac Surg* 1993; 56:22.
4. Ren JF, Panidis IP, Kotler MN, et al: Effect of coronary bypass surgery and valve replacement on left ventricular function: assessment by intraoperative two-dimensional echocardiography. *Am Heart J* 1985; 103:281.
5. Braunwald E, Kloner RA: The stunned myocardium: prolonged postischemic ventricular dysfunction. *Circulation* 1982; 66:1146.
6. Braunwald E: The stunned myocardium: newer insights into mechanisms and clinical applications. *J Thorac Cardiovasc Surg* 1990; 100:310.
7. Marban E: Myocardial stunning and hibernation: the physiology behind the colloquialisms. *Circulation* 1991; 83:681.
8. Shahle E, Bergstrom R, Nystrom SO, Hansson HE: Early results of aortic valve replacement with or without concomitant coronary artery bypass grafting. *Scand J Thorac Cardiovasc Surg* 1991; 25:29.
9. Lytle BW, Cosgrove DM, Gill CC, et al: Aortic valve replacement combined with myocardial revascularization. *J Thorac Cardiovasc Surg* 1988; 95:402.
10. Kay PH, Nunley D, Grunkemeier GL, et al: Ten-year survival following aortic valve bypass as a risk factor: a multivariate analysis of coronary replacement. *J Cardiovasc Surg* 1986; 27:494.
11. Mullany CJ, Elveback LR, Frye FL, et al: Coronary artery disease and its management: influence on survival in patients undergoing aortic valve replacement. *J Am Coll Cardiol* 1987; 10:66.
12. Kirklin JK, Nartel DC, Blackstone EH, et al: Risk factors for mortality after primary combined valvular and coronary artery surgery. *Circulation* 1989; 79(suppl I):I-180.
13. Karp RB, Mills N, Edmunds LH Jr: Coronary artery bypass grafting in the presence of valvular disease. *Circulation* 1989; 79(suppl I): I-182.
14. Tsai TP, Matloff JM, Chaux A, et al: Combined valve and coronary artery bypass procedures in septuagenarians and octogenarians: results in 120 patients. *Ann Thorac Surg* 1986; 42:681.
15. Andrade IG, Cartier R, Panisi P, et al: Factors influencing early and late survival in patients with combined mitral valve replacement and myocardial revascularization and in those with isolated replacement. *Ann Thorac Surg* 1987; 44:607.
16. Lytle BW, Cosgrove DM, Gill CC, et al: Mitral valve replacement combined with myocardial revascularization: early and late results for 300 patients, 1970 to 1983. *Circulation* 1985; 71:1179.
17. Ashraf SS, Shaukat N, Odom N, et al: Early and late results following combined coronary bypass surgery and mitral valve replacement. *Eur J Cardiothorac Surg* 1994; 8:57.
18. Szecsi J, Herrijgers P, Sergeant P, et al: Mitral valve surgery combined with coronary bypass grafting: multivariate analysis of factors predicting early and late results. *J Heart Valve Dis* 1994; 3:236.
19. Sheikh KH, Bengtson JR, Rankin JS, et al: Intraoperative transesophageal Doppler color flow imaging used to guide patient selection and operative treatment of ischemic mitral regurgitation. *Circulation* 1991; 84:594.
20. Dion R: Ischemic mitral regurgitation: when and how should it be corrected? *J Heart Valve Dis* 1993; 2:536.
21. Aklog L, Filsoufi F, Flores KQ, et al: Does coronary artery bypass grafting alone correct moderate ischemic mitral regurgitation? *Circulation* 2001; 75:I-68.
22. Maisano F, Schreuder JJ, Oppizzi M, et al: The double-orifice technique as a standardized approach to treat mitral regurgitation due to severe myxomatous disease: surgical technique. *Eur J Cardiothorac Surg* 2000; 17:201.
23. Alfieri O, Maisano F, DeBonis M, et al: The double-orifice technique in mitral valve repair: a simple solution for complex problems. *J Thorac Cardiovasc Surg* 2001; 122:674.
24. Cohn LH, Kowalker W, Bhatia S, et al: Comparative morbidity of mitral valve repair versus replacement for mitral regurgitation with and without coronary artery disease. *Ann Thorac Surg* 1988; 45:284.
25. Jones EL, Weintraub WS, Craver JM, et al: Interaction of age and coronary disease after valve replacement: implications for valve selection. *Ann Thorac Surg* 1994; 58:378.
26. Cox JL, Buckberg GD: Ventricular shape and function in health and disease. *Semin Thorac Cardiovasc Surg* 2001; 13:298.
27. Cohn LH, Couper GS, Kinchla NM, Collins JJ Jr: Decreased operative risk of surgical treatment of mitral regurgitation with or without coronary artery disease. *J Am Coll Cardiol* 1990; 16:1575.
28. Kay PH, Nunley DL, Grunkemeier GL, et al: Late results of combined mitral valve replacement and coronary bypass surgery. *J Am Coll Cardiol* 1985; 5:29.
29. Akins CW, Buckley MJ, Daggett WM, et al: Myocardial revascularization with combined aortic and mitral valve replacements. *J Thorac Cardiovasc Surg* 1985; 90:272.
30. Johnson WD, Kayser KL, Pedraza PM, Brenowitz JB: Combined valve replacement and coronary bypass surgery: results in 127 operations stratified by surgical risk factors. *Chest* 1986; 90:338.

Chapter 44

Minimally Invasive and Robotic Valve Surgery

W. Randolph Chitwood, Jr./L. Wiley Nifong

Surgeons and their patients have become energized by the benefits and possibilities of minimally invasive heart valve surgery (MIHVS). Until 1995, cardiac surgery lagged far behind other specialties in the development of minimal access methods. Then, Cohn and Cosgrove, along with several European colleagues, first modified cardiopulmonary bypass techniques and reduced incision sizes to enable safe, effective minimally invasive valve surgery.[1–3] Concurrently, Port-Access methods, using endoaortic balloon occluders, were developed and rapidly became popular.[4,5] Despite early enthusiasm for MIHVS, most surgeons were skeptical and many were very critical of cardiac surgery done through small incisions, owing to possibilities of unsafe operations and/or inferior results.[6–9] Despite this circumspect reticence, significant advances occurred in a short time and encouraging clinical series began to emerge. Concurrent advances in cardiopulmonary perfusion, intracardiac visualization, instrumentation, and robotic telemanipulation hastened a technologic shift toward efficient, safe MIHVS. Today, both replacing and repairing cardiac valves through small incisions have become standard practice for many surgeons, and patients are becoming more aware of the increasing availability.

EVOLUTION OF MINIMALLY INVASIVE VALVE SURGERY

To perform the *ideal cardiac valve operation* (Table 44-1) surgeons need to operate in restricted spaces through tiny incisions, which requires assisted vision and advanced instrumentation. Although this goal has not been achieved widely, MIHVS has continued to evolve toward video-assisted or video-directed operations. Moreover, new robotic methods now offer near endoscopic possibilities for mitral valve surgeons. Both video-assisted and direct-vision limited-access valve surgery are now within the reach of most cardiac surgeons.

Minimally invasive cardiac surgery has not enjoyed a standard nomenclature. The terms *minimally invasive* or *limited-access* cardiac surgery have referred to the size of the incision, the avoidance of a sternotomy, use of a partial sternotomy, or abstention from cardiopulmonary bypass. However, the development of MIHVS may be considered analogous to an Everest ascent, embarking from a conventional or "base camp" operation and advancing progressively toward less invasiveness through experience and acclimatization. A nomenclature that parallels this "mountaineering" analogy is shown in Table 44-2. In this scheme, levels of technical complexity are mastered starting with small incision, direct vision approaches (level 1), then moving toward more complex video-assisted procedures (level 2 or 3), and finally

TABLE 44–1 **Ideal cardiac valve operation**

Tiny incisions; endoscopic ports
Central antegrade perfusion
Tactile feedback
Eye-brain–"like" visualization
Facile, secure valve attachment
Intracardiac access
Dexterous valve and subvalvular topographic access
No instrument conflicts
Minimal:
Cardiopulmonary perfusion
Use of blood products
Ventilation and ICU care
Hospital time
Same or better quality
Valve repairs in 60%-80%
Few reoperations (1%-2%)
Low mortality (1%-2%)
Computerized surgical pathway memory
Instrument navigation systems

to robotic valve operations (level 4). With the constant evolution of new technology and surgical expertise, many established surgeons already have attained serial "comfort zones" along this MIHVS trek.

Level 1: Direct-Vision

Early MIHVS was based solely on modifications of previous incisions, and nearly all operations were done under direct vision. In 1996 the first truly minimally invasive aortic valve operations were reported.[1–3,10–12] At that time surgeons found that minimal-access incisions also provided adequate exposure of the mitral valve.[10,11,13,14] Using either ministernal or parasternal incisions, Cosgrove, Cohn, Gundry, and Arom each showed encouraging results with low surgical mortality (1%-3%) and morbidity for valve surgery.[1,2,10,15] In Cosgrove's first 50 minimally invasive aortic operations, perfusion and cardioplegia times approximated conventional operations, and his operative mortality was only 2%. Over half the patients were discharged by the fifth postoperative day.[2] In early 1997, Cohn presented 41 minimally invasive aortic operations and first defined the economic benefits of these operations.[1]

The Stanford group performed the first minimally invasive mitral valve replacements, using intra-aortic balloon occlusion (Port-Access) and cardioplegia in early 1996.[14–17] Subsequently, surgeons at the University of Leipzig reported 24 mitral valve repairs done through a minithoracotomy using Port-Access techniques.[5] This group later reported a high incidence of retrograde aortic dissections and neurologic complications, which seemed to be related to new catheter technology and limited surgeon experience.[18] By early 1997, Colvin and Galloway had performed 27 direct-vision, Port-Access mitral repairs or replacements with a single death. They experienced no aortic dissections, and 63% of patients had mitral valve repairs with no reoperations for leakage.[19] By December of 1998, Cosgrove had done 250 minimally invasive mitral valve operations using either a ministernotomy or parasternal incision with no mortality.[3] The successes of these early MIHVS procedures became the springboard to the current direct-vision techniques described herein.

TABLE 44–2 **Minimally invasive cardiac surgery**

Level 1
Direct-vision
Mini (10-12 cm) incisions
Level 2
Video-assisted
Micro (4-6 cm) incisions
Level 3
Video-directed and robot-assisted
Micro or port (1-cm) incisions
Level 4
Robotic telemanipulation
Port (1-cm) incisions

Level 2: Video-Assisted

Avant-garde endoscopic surgical techniques in the 1980s became routine general, urologic, orthopedic, and gynecologic operations in the 1990s. This was related primarily to successes with extirpative endoscopic operations. In contrast, fine anastomotic and complex reparative procedures are the centerpieces of cardiac surgery. Because of difficulty in acquiring the fine video dexterity needed for these operations, cardiac surgeons have been the last to explore the benefits of operative video assistance.

As mentioned, most Port-Access, sternal modification, and parasternal mitral valve operations have been done using direct vision. In early 1996, Carpentier performed the first video-assisted *mitral valve repair* through a minithoracotomy using hypothermic ventricular fibrillation.[20] Shortly thereafter, we completed the first video-assisted mitral valve surgery through a minithoracotomy, using a new percutaneous transthoracic aortic clamp and retrograde cardioplegia.[21,22] This clamping and visualization technique was simple and cost-effective, and has remained the mainstay of isolated mitral valve operations at our center.

In 1997 Mohr reported 51 minimally invasive mitral operations, done using Port-Access cardioplegia techniques, a 4-cm incision, and for the first time three-dimensional videoscopy.[23] In this series three-dimensional (3-D) assistance aided mitral replacements; however, these surgeons found that less complex reconstructions were significantly more difficult than sternotomy-based operations. At about the same time Loulmet and Carpentier deployed an intracardiac "mini-camera" for lighting and subvalvular visualization; however, they concluded that two-dimensional visualization was inadequate for detailed repairs.[24] Concurrently, our group reported 31 successful mitral operations done using two-dimensional video assistance.[25] Complex repairs were possible and these included quadrangular resections, sliding valvuloplasties, chordal transfers, and synthetic chordal replacements. Our initial results were encouraging.

Level 3: Video-Directed and Robot-Assisted

In 1997 Mohr first used the Aesop 3000 voice-activated camera robot in minimally invasive videoscopic mitral valve surgery.[23] Six months later we began using the Aesop 3000 to perform both video-assisted and video-directed minimally invasive mitral valve repairs.[26] We have continued to use this device during most isolated mitral valve surgery. This instrument provides the surgeon with camera-site voice activation, precluding the translation errors that are inherent with verbal transmission to an assistant. Camera motion has been shown to be much smoother and more predictable, and requires less lens cleaning than during manual direction. Currently, if necessary, we are able to do over 90% of a mitral repair under video direction with the Aesop 3000. Mohr termed this method "solo mitral surgery" and reported 8 patients undergoing successful mitral repairs using this robotic technique.[23] Since these early procedures, over 1500 videoscopic and robot-assisted mitral valve repairs have been done worldwide with excellent results.

Level 4: Telemanipulation and Robotic

In June of 1998 Carpentier and Mohr did the first true robotic mitral valve operations using the da Vinci surgical system.[27,28] In May of 2000 the East Carolina University group performed the first da Vinci mitral repair in the United States.[29] This system provides both tele- and micromanipulation of tissues in small spaces. The surgeon operates from a console through micro wrist instruments that are mounted on robotic arms inserted through the chest wall. These devices emulate human X-Y-Z axis wrist activity throughout seven full degrees of manipulative excursion. These motions occur through two joints that each affect pitch, yaw, and rotation. Additionally, arm insertion and rotation, as well as variable grip strength, give additive freedom to the operating "wrist." Mohr and Chitwood have the largest experiences in this area and independently have determined this device effective for performing complex mitral valve repairs.[28,30] Using the Zeus system, Grossi et al performed a partial mitral valve repair but had limited ergonomic freedom.[31] Lange et al in Munich were the first to perform a totally endoscopic mitral valve repair using only 1-cm ports and da Vinci.[32]

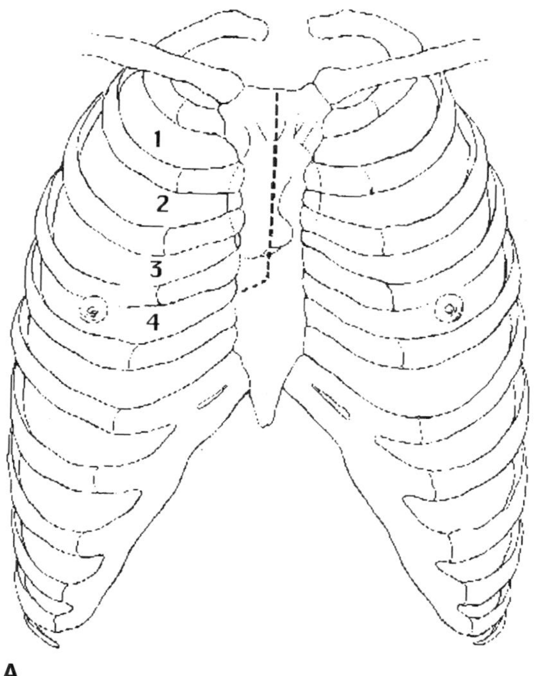

A

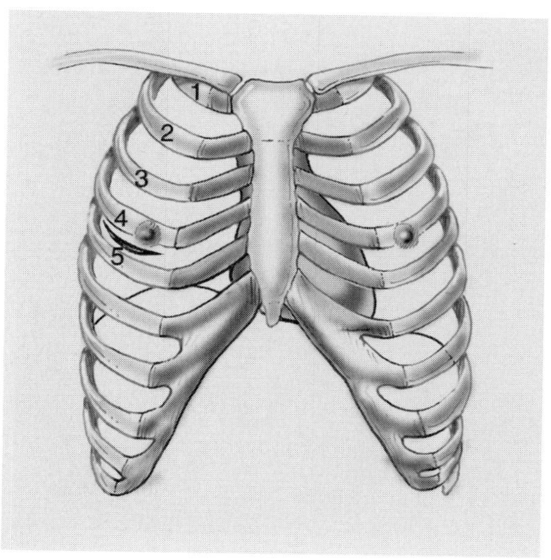

B

FIGURE 44–1 **(A) Hemisternotomy for minimally invasive mitral and aortic valve surgery. (B) Minithoracotomy for minimally invasive mitral valve surgery.**

INCISIONS FOR MINIMALLY INVASIVE VALVE SURGERY

The type and size of the musculoskeletal incision remain central to MIHVS discussions. A myriad of modified small sternal, parasternal, and thoracotomy incisions have been used for cardiac valve access. To date, most minimal-access cardiac surgery has been done under direct vision (level 1), requiring larger incisions than needed for videoscopic operations (levels 2-4).

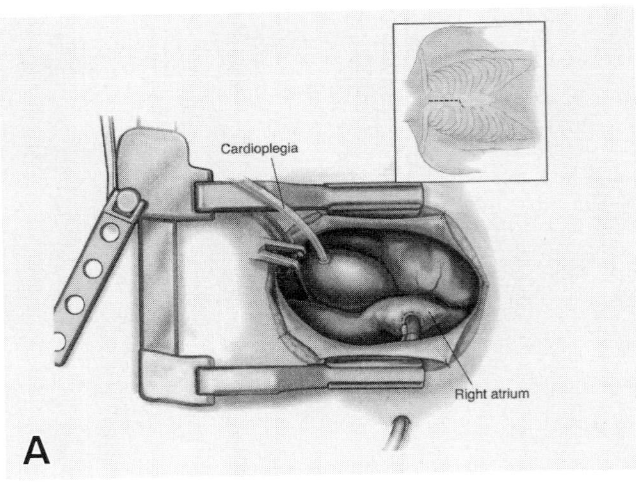

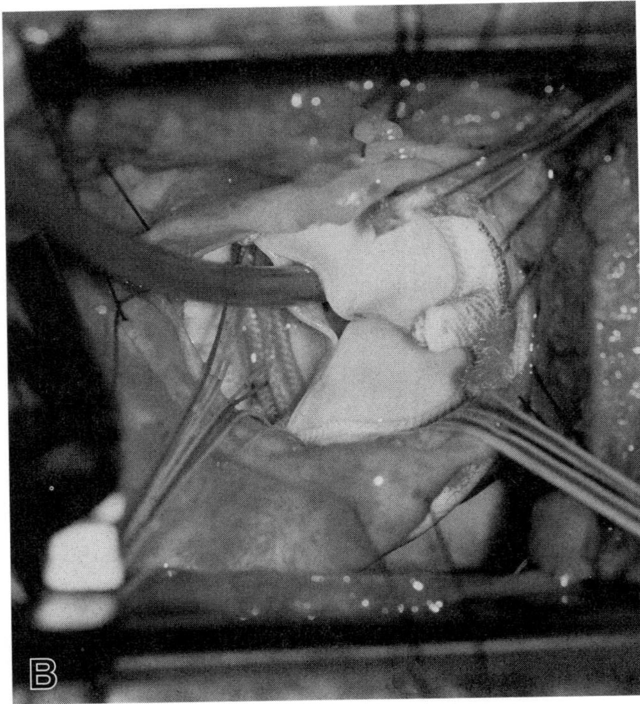

FIGURE 44–2 (A) Hemisternotomy and surgical exposure for direct-vision access during aortic valve surgery. Note that pericardial retraction sutures pull the aorta toward the operative field. (*Courtesy of Dr. L.H. Cohn.*) (B) Minimally invasive prosthetic aortic valve replacement via a hemisternotomy. A suction catheter is placed into the ventricle for venting. We prefer antegrade cardioplegia via frequent ostial administrations.

Aortic Valve

Initially, Cohn and Cosgrove reported both excellent valve exposure and clinical results using parasternal or transsternal incisions.[1–3,33] However, these incisions largely have been abandoned because of cosmetic dissatisfaction, pain, and sternal nonunion. Currently, most minimal-access aortic and mitral valve operations are performed either through a ministernotomy or minithoracotomy (Fig. 44-1).

Our group uses an upper hemisternotomy for most aortic valve operations. Following an 8- to 10-cm skin incision, the longitudinal midsternal cut is made from the notch into the 3rd to 5th interspace (ICS), deviating to the right, often without transecting the sternum. Care is taken not to injure the internal thoracic vessels. For direct aortic and right atrial venous cannulation, the sternal incision must be carried at least to the 4th ICS. When the sternal incision ends at the 3rd ICS, femoral vein cannulation is usually required because of limited atrial access. Gundry and Sardari suggested that optimal sites of either sternal division or ICS deviation are best determined echocardiographically.[15,34] However, we have found that crossing into the right 4th or 5th ICS always provides excellent right atrial exposure. After pericardial edges are approximated tightly to the skin edges, a small Finochietto retractor is used to spread the sternal halves laterally. This maneuver "pulls" both the aorta and valve annulus toward the surgical field (Fig. 44-2). Generally, we cannulate the aorta near the innominate artery using a flexible guidewire-directed cannula. Early placement of commissure retraction sutures facilitates aortic valve exposure. Doty and Karagoz prefer a lower hemisternotomy to reach both aortic and mitral valves.[35,36] Bennetti first reported aortic valve access through a right 2nd ICS minithoracotomy and the New York University group uses this approach routinely.[37,38]

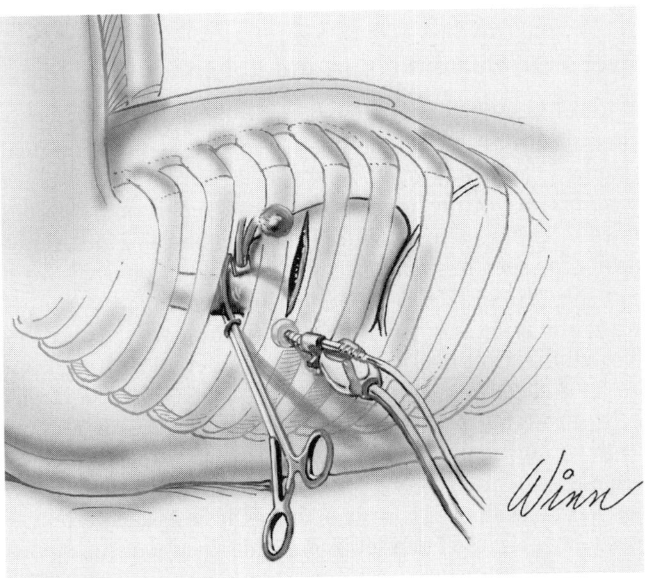

FIGURE 44–3 Right minithoracotomy and video access. The right minithoracotomy allows aortic access for the transthoracic clamp shown here as well as the video camera. With this arrangement minimal rib spreading is needed to perform mitral surgery.

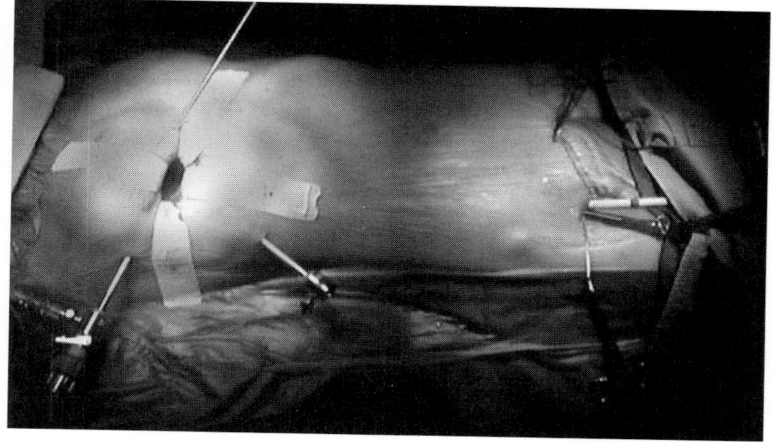

FIGURE 44–4 Small "nonretracted" minithoracotomy for video-directed mitral surgery. Using videoscopic techniques, a small nonretracted minithoracotomy provides excellent access for long instrument manipulation. Here, a soft tissue retractor mobilizes skin edges away from the incision. (*Courtesy of Dr. H Vanermen.*)

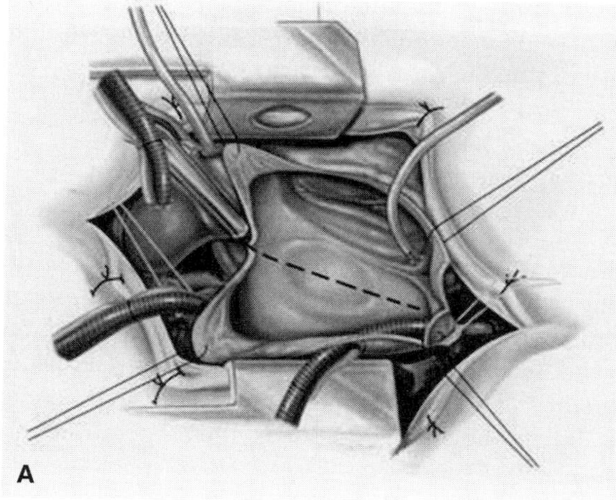

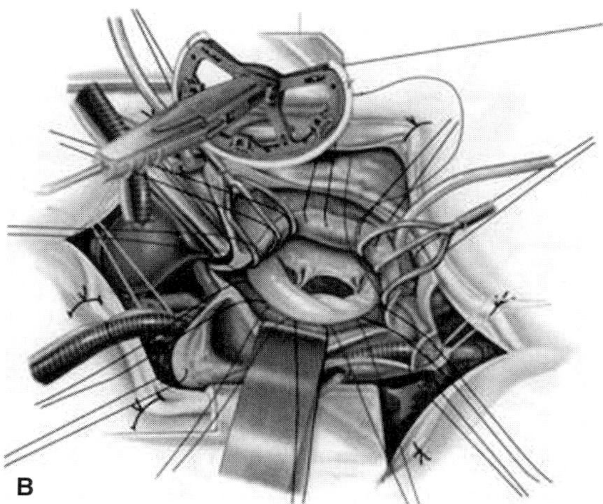

FIGURE 44–5 (A) Hemisternotomy with an extended atrial incision. Popularized by Dr. Cosgrove, the incision begins along the ventral right atrium and extends over the dome of the left atrium and through the left atrial wall and interatrial septum. (B) Mitral valve exposure is excellent through this hemisternotomy with an extended atrial incision, and complex repairs are similar in difficulty to full sternotomy operations. (*Courtesy of Dr. D.M. Cosgrove.*)

Mitral Valve and Tricuspid Valve

Although many surgeons prefer the hemisternotomy approach, a right minithoracotomy yields excellent direct-vision and videoscopic mitral valve access (Figs. 44-1B and 44-3). To access the left atrium for direct vision, while maintaining a limited-access minithoracotomy, a 6- to 8-cm incision should be placed in the submammary fold along the anterior axillary line. The pectoralis and intercostal muscle fibers are divided, and the thorax is entered through the 4th ICS with minimal rib distraction and no rib cutting. The New York University group has been quite successful in combining this incision, Port-Access methods, and direct vision for both mitral and tricuspid repairs/replacements.[39] A smaller 4- to 5-cm incision with minimal rib retraction can be used in video-assisted cases and is large enough for prosthesis passage (Fig. 44-4). Vanermen and Mohr perform video-assisted mitral operations routinely through 4-cm, nonretracted thoracic incisions with excellent results.[40–42] Minimal rib spreading, prevention of intercostal nerve injury, and intraoperative local anesthetics are the keys to minimizing postoperative discomfort. Tricuspid operations can be performed through this incision as long as bicaval cannulation with isolation is used.

The author considers the term "minimally invasive" to include the size of the actual cardiac incision. Most superior and trans-septal mitral valve approaches require a larger cardiac incision. For aortic, mitral, and tricuspid valve operations, Cosgrove uses a 4th ICS ministernotomy with direct aortic arch and right atrial cannulation.[3,12,43] To access the mitral valve, he extends the atriotomy from the right atrium across the left atrial roof, continuing caudally to divide the interatrial septum (Fig. 44-5). This incision provides excellent exposure for aortic, mitral, and tricuspid valve replacements as well as repairs. Although the septal artery is divided, the incidence of atrial arrhythmias seems to parallel traditional interatrial groove atriotomies. For mitral and aortic surgery Gundry uses a similar hemisternotomy and a

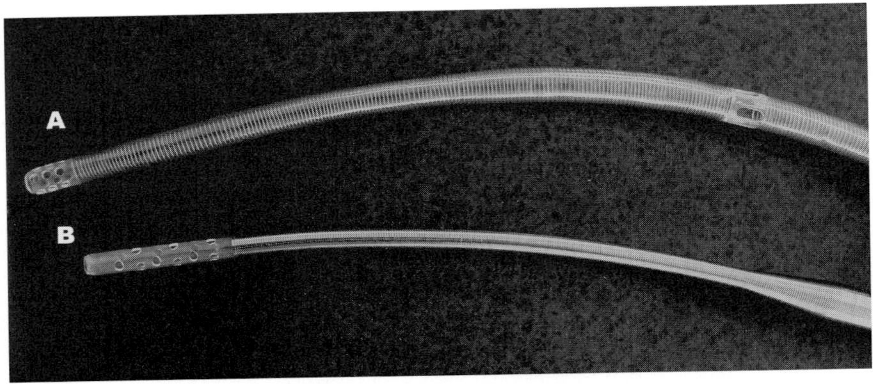

FIGURE 44–6 (A) Percutaneous Carpentier dual-stage venous drainage cannula (Medtronic Inc., Minneapolis, MN). This cannula is inserted from the femoral approach using the Seldinger guidewire method. (B) Thin-walled 19F arterial perfusion cannula (Bio-Medicus; Medtronic Minneapolis, MN). A smaller 17F version is used for percutaneous internal jugular vein cannulation.

single right atrial cannula. He gains exposure similar to that described by opening the atrial roof, between the superior vena cava and aorta, without entering the right atrium.[15] Cohn now prefers sternal modification incisions for both aortic and mitral surgery and uses a trans-septal approach for mitral exposure.[44] Loulmet and Carpentier reported using a midsternal, C-shaped, partial sternotomy for exposing mitral valves through the interatrial septum.[24] All of these incisions provide generous direct-vision exposure, if combined with optimal pericardial retraction.

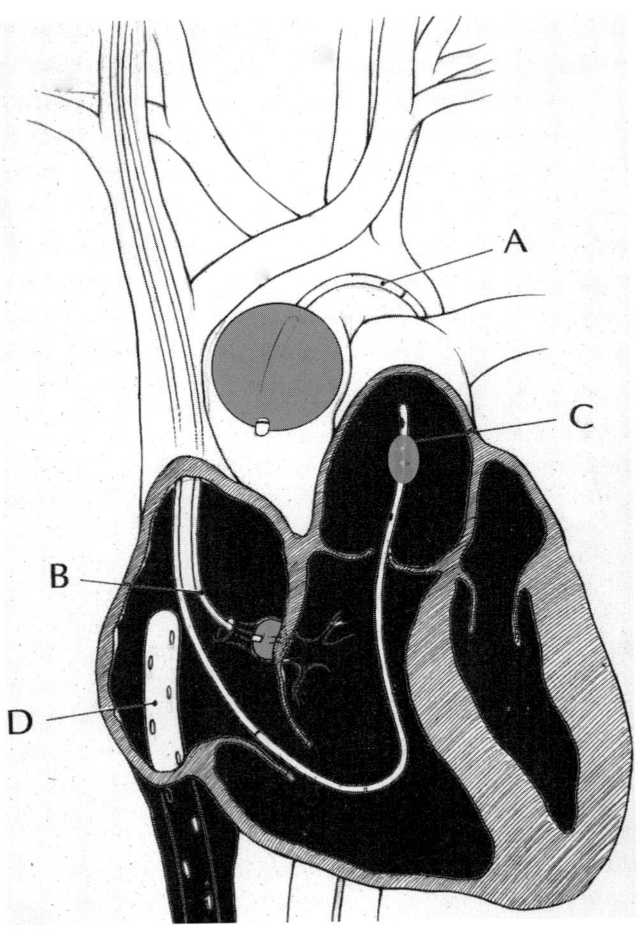

FIGURE 44–7 Port-Access system with transfemoral artery endoaortic balloon occluder, femoral venous drainage catheter, percutaneous internal jugular retrograde coronary sinus cardioplegia catheter, and pulmonary artery vent (Cardiovations, Ethicon Inc., Norwalk, CT).

PERFUSION TECHNOLOGY

By combining modified traditional perfusion methods and new technology, surgeons have been able to speed the development of MIHVS. Thin-walled arterial and venous cannulas, transthoracic aortic cannulas, endoaortic balloon occluders, modified aortic clamping devices, percutaneous coronary sinus cardioplegia catheters, and assisted venous drainage all have aided in evolution of these operations.

Arterial Access

As ministernotomy incisions lend themselves to facile antegrade aortic cannulation, most surgeons prefer central arterial cannulation. For minimally invasive aortic surgery, we cannulate the transverse aortic arch, just distal to the innominate artery through the upper incision and use either a 17F or 19F nonkinking Bio-Medicus cannula (Fig. 44-6). Port-Access surgical systems initially required retrograde femoral arterial perfusion, femoral-atrial venous drainage, and intraluminal aortic balloon occlusion (Fig. 44-7).[45] However, current specialized direct aortic cannulas can provide combined antegrade perfusion, balloon aortic occlusion, and antegrade cardioplegia.[46]

For minimally invasive mitral surgery, we prefer retrograde femoral perfusion, employing small wire-wound Bio-Medicus arterial cannulas (17F or 19 F) inserted over a guidewire (Figs. 44-6 and 44-8). In our patients excellent flow rates with acceptable perfusion pressures have been attained with no retrograde aortic dissections. Mitral patients with peripheral atherosclerosis or small iliac vessels may require direct aortic cannulation, either placed through the incision or via a transthoracic approach. Recently, a long 21F femoral cannula has been developed for remote access

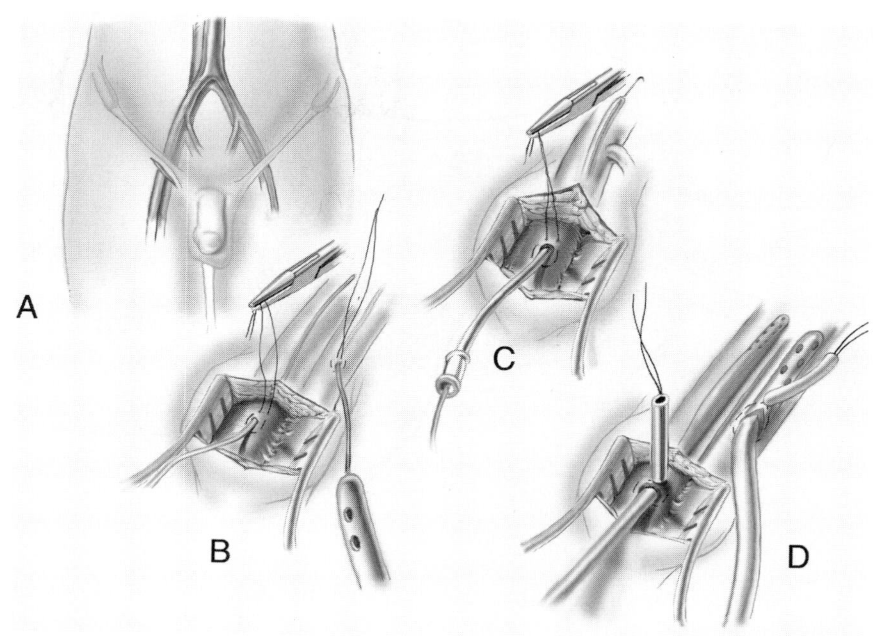

FIGURE 44–8 Femoral artery cannulation for minimally invasive mitral valve surgery. Both the (17F-19 F) perfusion cannula and (23 F) venous cannula are inserted over a guidewire using the Seldinger technique after progressive coaxial dilations. Nonpenetrating oval purse-string sutures are placed in both the artery and vein for hemostasis. Echocardiographic guidance is essential for safe passage of the venous cannula to the right atrium.

antegrade perfusion through fenestrations located in the proximal catheter (Fig. 44-9).[47]

Venous Drainage

Venous access can be established in a variety of ways. At the Brigham and Women's Hospital, for aortic and mitral surgery, the right atrium is cannulated directly through the incision or separate skin incisions may be used for the isolated caval cannulation, when needed (Fig. 44-10). Cosgrove introduces a small (23F) cannula directly into the right atrium through the ministernotomy. Koernitz and Gundry insert an oval-flat or "pancake" cannula into the right atrium to minimize incision space loss.[12,15]

For a first aortic valve operation, we use a 23F direct right atrial cannula and apply suction venous return. In aortic valve reoperations, we pass a 23F percutaneous femoral venous cannula to the right atrium, using the Seldinger technique and echocardiographic guidance. For minimally invasive mitral valve surgery we always establish bicaval venous drainage using a percutaneous 17F internal jugular cannula and a femoral vein to right atrial catheter (Fig. 44-11).[48,49] For safety it is important to use the Seldinger guidewire method with echocardiographic guidance to assure optimal venous catheter tracking and atrial position. Using internal jugular and femoral venous catheters, combined either with caval tapes or balloon occluders, minimally invasive tricuspid surgery can be performed alone or in combination with mitral operations using a 5-cm minithoracotomy. Carpentier designed a specialized percutaneous femoral venous cannula with dual-stage drainage ports (see Fig. 44-6).[24] This catheter can be combined with caval snares to perform atrial septal and tricuspid surgery, as well. After heparin reversal both jugular and femoral percutaneous venous cannulas can be removed with local pressure applied for hemostasis.

Assisted venous drainage has been a major advance as this technique enhances the efficiency of smaller cannulas. We prefer to use the Bio-Medicus centrifugal vortex pump to create variable negative pressures for venous drainage. Also, by combining wall suction (less than −40 cm H_2O pressure) and a hard-shell cardiotomy reservoir, a safe, simple, and economical assisted venous drainage system can be developed.[43] Using these altered cannulation methods and a

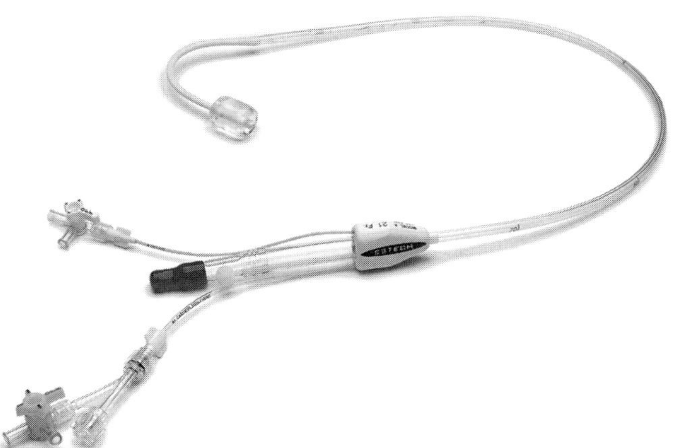

FIGURE 44–9 The Remote Access Balloon Perfusion Cannula (ESTECH Corp., Danville, CA) is inserted retrograde via the femoral artery and is unique in that antegrade arterial perfusion is established. In the same catheter a proximal balloon aortic occluder that delivers antegrade cardioplegia establishes protected cardiac arrest. Holes in the proximal catheter are the sole source of antegrade aortic perfusion, minimizing risks of retrograde aortic dissection during cardiopulmonary bypass.

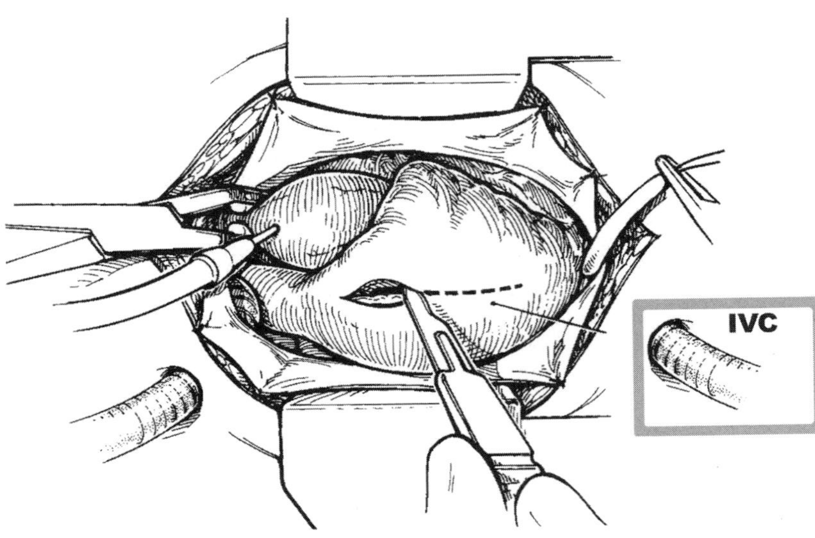

FIGURE 44–10 For direct-vision minimally invasive mitral or aortic valve surgery, traditional cannulation methods may be modified. Here, smaller venous drainage cannulas are inserted through auxiliary incisions. Standard caval occlusion and venous drainage are usually effective. However, additive active venous suction allows usage of smaller cannulas. (*Courtesy of Dr. L.H. Cohn.*)

vortex pump, venous drainage has been excellent for aortic, mitral, and tricuspid surgery.

Myocardial Preservation

Myocardial preservation techniques used with MIHVS are similar to sternotomy-based operations. For both aortic and mitral valve patients, we cool systemically to 28°C, as the ambient cardiac temperature generally is warmer than during conventional valve operations. With either a ministernotomy or minithoracotomy, a retrograde coronary sinus cardioplegia catheter can be inserted *directly* into the right atrium and position confirmed echocardiographically. Also, Port-Access technology provides a percutaneous retrograde cardioplegia catheter, which is introduced using echo via the internal jugular vein preoperatively (see Fig. 44-7). Although retrograde cardioplegia seems preferable, to assure uniform cardiac cooling and even distribution of cardioplegia solutions, we have found antegrade cardioplegia preferable and efficient. Exposure limitations make direct retrograde coronary sinus catheter insertion more difficult and with less control should sinus complications arise. We prefer cold antegrade blood cardioplegia for both minimally invasive aortic and mitral surgery. During aortic valve surgery, supplemental ostial cardioplegia can be delivered intermittently using a soft catheter. In mitral patients we

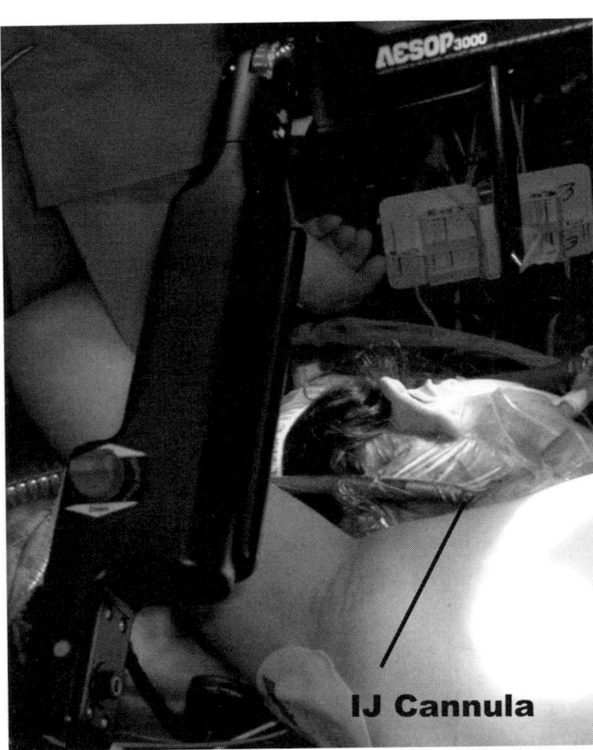

FIGURE 44–11 A right internal jugular venous catheter (17F) is combined with femoral-atrial active venous drainage for full bicaval access. This is important during atrial retraction in a near closed chest where the cavae can be kinked with distraction. The Aesop 3000 robotic camera arm is seen in the foreground.

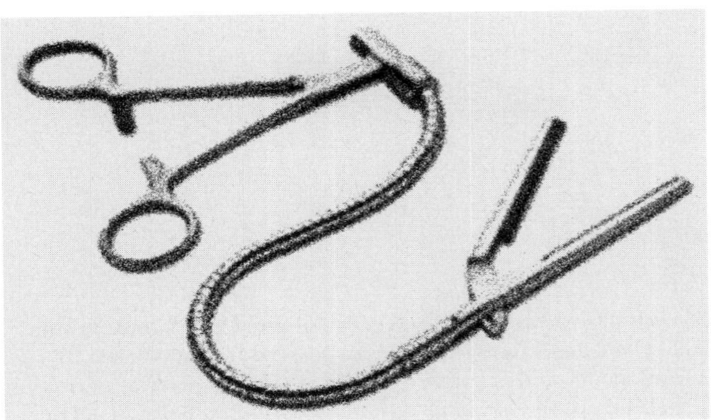

FIGURE 44–12 Flexible arm Cosgrove Aortic Clamp (Allegiance Healthcare Corp., McGaw Park, IL). This mobile arm clamp allows complete aortic occlusion through limited-access incisions, such as the ministernotomy. We have also used it for transthoracic aortic occlusion in mitral surgery.

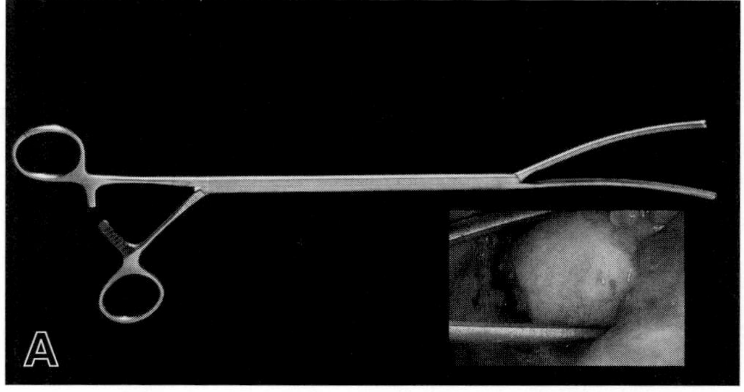

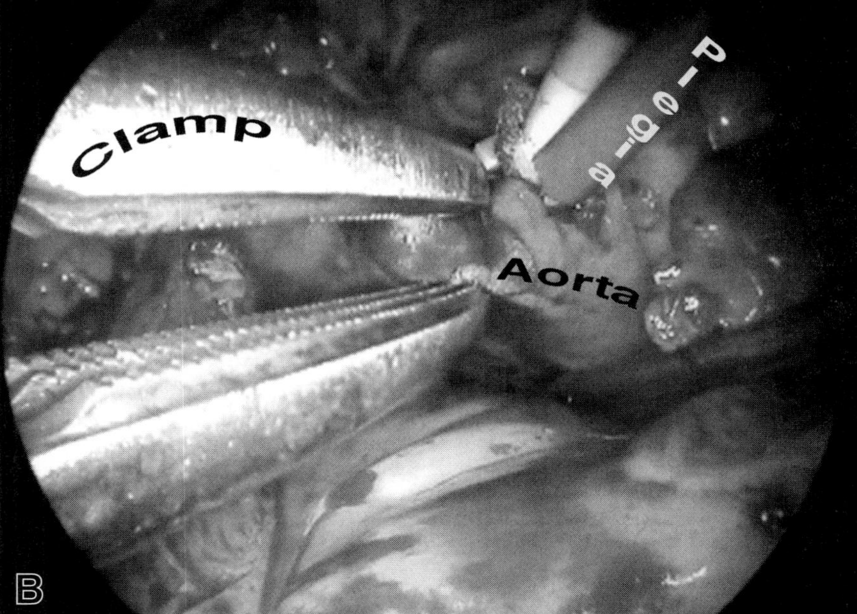

FIGURE 44–13 (A) The Chitwood transthoracic aortic cross-clamp (Scanlan International Inc., Minneapolis, MN). The shaft, which is 4 mm in diameter, is passed through the 3rd intercostal space. (Inset) The posterior or fixed prong of the clamp is passed through the transverse sinus, under direct or video visualization to avoid injury to the right pulmonary artery, left atrial appendage, or left main coronary artery. The mobile prong is passed ventral to the aorta as far as the main pulmonary artery. (B) A videoscopic view of the deployed transthoracic aortic clamp (Clamp). The aorta is fully compressed and an antegrade cardioplegia needle is shown (Plegia), in position just distal to the right coronary artery origin.

insert an antegrade cardioplegia/aortic vent catheter into the aortic root directly through the incision. For aortic valve operations, we rarely vent either the left ventricle or pulmonary artery. However, we keep the operative field clear using a small catheter, placed across the valve annulus into the left ventricle. Should additional venting be required, the ministernotomy provides excellent exposure to the superior pulmonary vein. To keep the surgical field clear during mitral surgery, we place a flexible sucker directly into the left atrium.

Aortic Occlusion

For MIVHS most surgeons use a standard cross-clamp, placed through the incision (see Figs. 44-2 and 44-5). Specialized flexible-handle aortic clamps have been developed to increase exposure through the hemisternotomy and minimize inadvertent dislodgement (Fig. 44-12). For minithoracotomy mitral operations, we use a percutaneous, transthoracic aortic cross-clamp. The clamp is inserted through a 4-mm incision placed in the right lateral 3rd intercostal space. The posterior immobile "tine" of the clamp is positioned through the transverse sinus dorsal to the aorta (Figs. 44-3 and 44-13).[48] During placement, attention is necessary to prevent injury to the left atrial appendage and right pulmonary artery behind the aorta. This clamp has provided very secure occlusion without any aortic injuries.

Intra-aortic balloon occluders generally are introduced retrograde through the femoral artery. The occlusive balloon should be positioned, under echocardiographic control, just above the tubulosinus ridge in the ascending aorta (Fig. 44-14).[5,45] Balloon pressures often approximate 300 torr during complete occlusion, and the catheter tip position must be monitored continuously. Antegrade cardioplegia is given via the catheter central lumen. Balloon dislodgement can cause innominate artery occlusion, resulting in neurologic injury, or prolapse into the left ventricle with inferior myocardial preservation. Thus continuous echocardiographic monitoring is essential to detect balloon migration.

Cardiac Air Removal

Meticulous cardiac air removal is particularly important in minimally invasive valve operations. Difficulty exists in

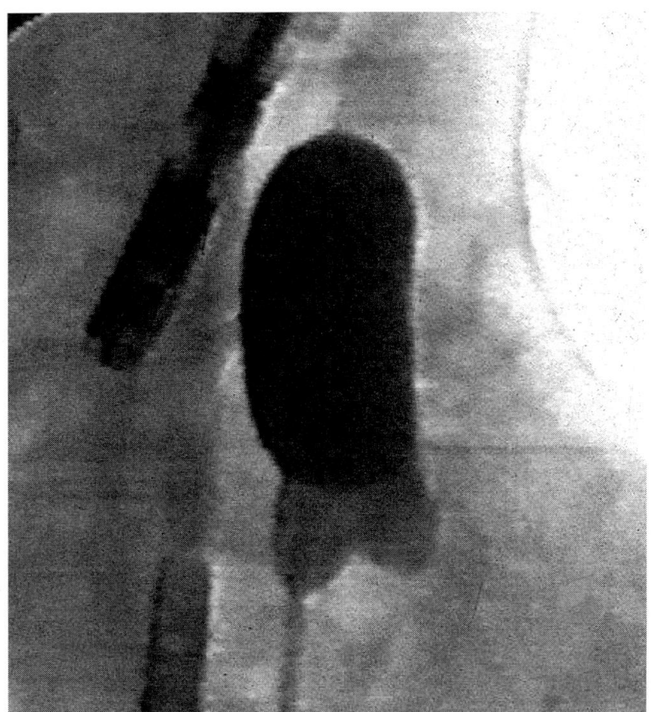

FIGURE 44–14 Radiograph of an expanded Port-Access balloon occluder in the ascending aorta. Optimal positioning, with the proximal balloon at the aortic tubulosinus ridge and the distal segment below the innominate artery, is confirmed either by angiography or more commonly by transesophageal echocardiography. An echo probe is also seen in this illustration, as is the venous drainage catheter.

manipulating and de-airing the cardiac apex, as it cannot be elevated. Also, with a right anterolateral minithoracotomy, air tends to be retained along the more dorsal ventricular septum and in the right pulmonary veins. Continuous carbon dioxide (CO_2)insufflation has been particularly helpful in minimizing cardiac air and should be begun before cardiac chambers are opened. CO_2 is much more soluble in blood than is air and displaces it very efficiently. We infuse CO_2 continuously (4-5 L/min) into the thorax, and prior to cross-clamp release ventilate both lungs vigorously to draw the gas deep into all pulmonary veins. After atriotomy closure and following cross-clamp release, suction is applied to the aortic root vent, and we then compress the right coronary artery origin during early ejection. As the heart beats, nonatherosclerotic aortas are reclamped gently to expel residual air into the vent suction. Constant transesophageal echocardiographic monitoring is essential to assure adequate air removal before weaning from cardiopulmonary bypass.

ROBOTIC TECHNOLOGY

The Aesop 3000 robotic camera manipulator (Computer Motion, Inc., Santa Barbara, CA) has remained a pillar of control during our minimally invasive video-assisted mitral surgery. Figure 44-15 shows how this device is arranged during these operations. Even though video assistance with robotic vision control has proved valuable, surgeons still must operate with long instruments in a two-dimensional operative field. The da Vinci Surgical System (Intuitive Surgical, Inc., Mountain View, CA) is comprised of three components: a surgeon console, an instrument cart, and a visioning platform (Fig. 44-16).[49] The operative console is removed physically from the patient and allows the surgeon to sit comfortably, resting the arms ergonomically with his/her head positioned in a three-dimensional (3-D) vision array. The surgeon's finger and wrist movements are registered, through sensors, in computer memory banks, and then these actions are transferred efficiently to an instrument cart, which operates the synchronous end-effector instruments (Fig. 44-17). Through 1-cm ports, instruments are positioned near cardiac operative sites in the thorax, and the camera is passed via a 4-cm working port used for suture and prosthesis passage (Fig. 44-18). Every analog finger movement, along with inherent human tremor at 8 to 10 Hz/sec, is converted to binary digital data, which are smoothed and filtered to increase microinstrument precision. Wrist-like instrument articulation emulates precisely the surgeon's actions at the tissue level, and dexterity becomes enhanced through combined tremor suppression and motion scaling. This allows both increased precision and dexterity, with the surgeon becoming truly ambidextrous. A clutching mechanism enables readjustment of hand positions to maintain an optimal ergonomic attitude with respect to the visual field. This clutch acts very much like a computer mouse, which can be reoriented by lifting and repositioning it to reestablish unrestrained freedom of computer activation.

The 3-D digital visioning system enables natural depth perception with high-power magnification (10X). Both 0° and 30° endoscopes can be manipulated electronically to look either "up" or "down" within the heart. Access to and visualization of the internal thoracic artery, coronary arteries, and mitral apparatus have been shown to be excellent. The operator becomes ensconced in the 3-D operative topography and can perform extremely precise surgical manipulations, devoid of traditional distractions. Figure 44-19 shows the surgeon's operative field during a da Vinci mitral repair. Perfusion technology is the same as described above for video-assisted operations and a larger minithoracotomy.

CURRENT STATUS

Minimally Invasive Aortic Valve Surgery

Most cardiac surgeons already have the innate abilities needed to perform direct-vision MIHVS. Valve exposure, repair methods, prosthesis insertion, and perfusion technology differ little from traditional aortic operations. The

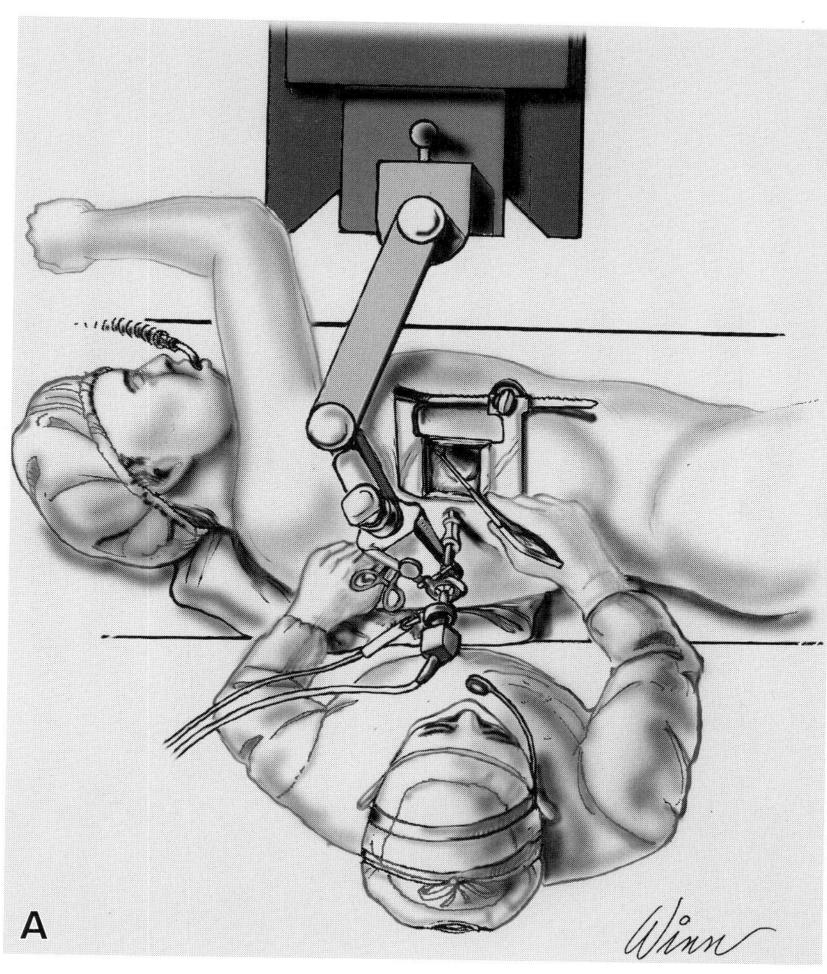

FIGURE 44–15 (A) During minimally invasive video-assisted mitral surgery, the camera is voice activated and positioned by the surgeon using the Aesop 3000 robot. Operative maneuvers are made through the 5-cm incision using long instruments and secondary vision.

hemisternotomy approach, initially described by Cosgrove, Cohn, Gundry, Koernitz, Machler, von Sagesser, and others, has been the most common incision used by minimally invasive aortic valve surgeons.[1,2,12,15,50,51] In a randomized study, comparing the conventional sternotomy (N = 60 patients) to an upper hemisternotomy (N = 60 patients), Machler found the latter to provide reduced trauma, less ventilation requirements, less blood loss, and better cosmesis.[50] Comparatively, Aris found no differences in results; however, he used two different hemisternotomy approaches, therefore seemingly confounding his conclusions.[52] Christiansen concluded the only benefit remaining 1 year following minimally invasive aortic surgery in 25 patients to be cosmesis.[53]

Currently, at the Cleveland Clinic 90% of aortic valve patients undergo a minimally invasive operation.[54] By early 2002 Dr. Cosgrove's team had performed a total of 607 MIS aortic operations, of which 76% either had homograft, mechanical, or xenograft tissue replacements and 24% were repairs. A number of these were combined with ascending aortic root operations. Only 1.7% required conversion to a full sternotomy, and the most common reason was for adjunctive coronary revascularization. Interestingly, only 2 patients were converted for poor exposure and none for bleeding. Cardiac arrest and perfusion times averaged 60 and 70 minutes, respectively, and these data were similar to his conventional aortic valve operations. Their overall mortality for minimally invasive aortic valve operations was 0.8%. Complications included bleeding (4.9%), respiratory insufficiency (1.5%), stroke (2.5%), and wound problems (0.7%). Of these patients 11% required transfusions, and the average hospitalization was 6.2 days with 30% being discharged before the fourth postoperative day. Mortality and length of stay data have been superior to risk-adjusted cohorts from the STS National Adult Cardiac Surgery Database for conventional aortic valve operations, which were 4% and 7 days, respectively. Since minimally invasive aortic surgery was first introduced in 1996 at the Cleveland Clinic, perfusion times have fallen there more than cross-clamp intervals, indicating learning curves to be related more to optimizing perfusion technology and aortic valve exposure than the actual repair/replacement. For aortic valve surgery the upper hemisternotomy has supplanted both parasternal and transsternal incisions at most institutions.

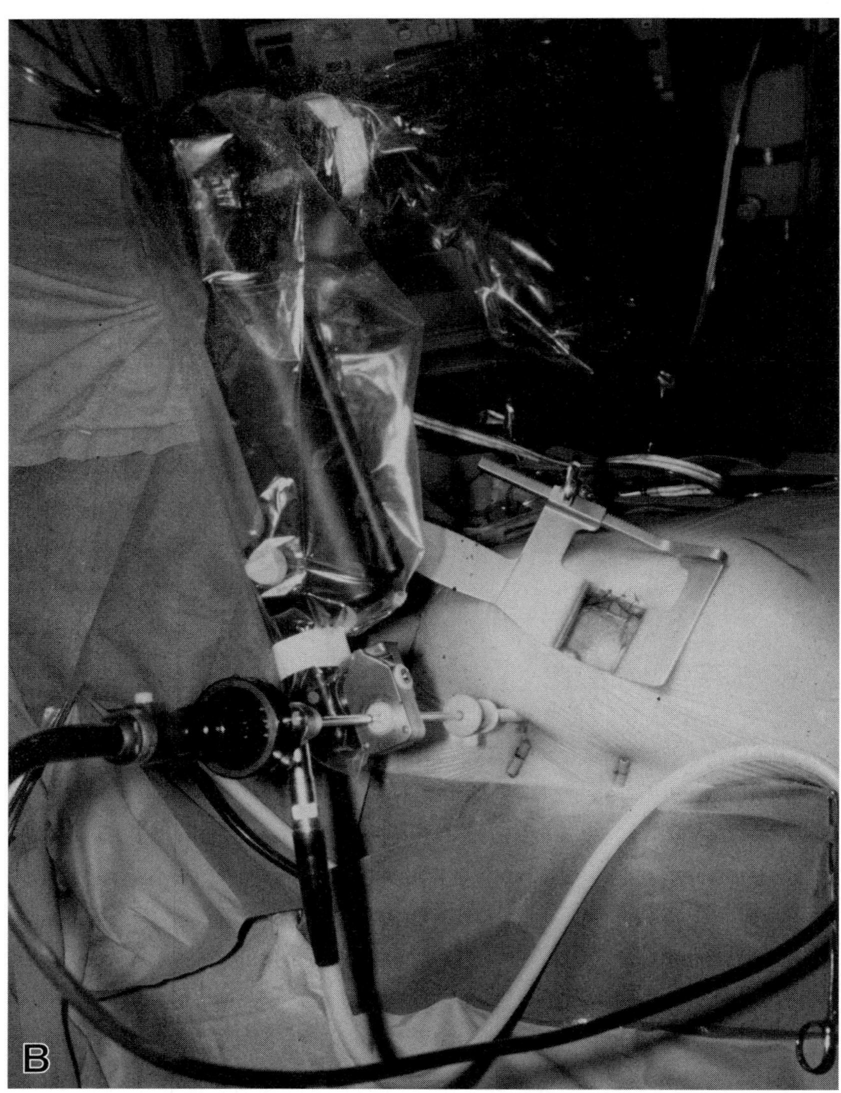

FIGURE 44–15 (*Continued*) (B) Here the Aesop 3000 is attached to a 5-mm 0° two-dimensional telescope. For mitral valve surgery the pericardial edges are retracted using transthoracic sutures.

Independently, Cohn began performing minimally invasive aortic valve surgery at the Brigham and Women's Hospital in June of 1996.[1,14,33] First he preferred the parasternal approach, but for the last five years he has used the upper hemisternotomy.[14,44,55] His series of 425 aortic valve operations has yielded equally impressive results to those described above. Nearly all patients underwent valve replacements with pericardial prostheses dominating the series and bileaflet pyrolytic carbon prostheses used next in frequency. The operative mortality was 2.4% and complications included bleeding (3.1%), stroke (1.6%), heart block (5.2%), and wound problems (2.6%). In this series 50% of patients were transfused, and the average length of hospitalization was 7 days. Of these patients 11% were minimally invasive aortic valve *reoperations*, which were facilitated by avoiding patent internal thoracic arterial graft clamping.[55,56] The mean age was 10 years older in reoperative patients, and complications and operative mortality (6.4%) were higher than for first operations.

Other surgeons with smaller series have reported results similar to those of Cosgrove and Cohn. Using a lower hemisternal incision (8-cm), Bonnachi found significant cosmetic benefits, compared with conventional sternotomies (24-cm incision), and noted reduced transfusions, ventilator time, pain management, and hospital stay. In both cohorts he reported similar perfusion and cross-clamp times as well.[57] In contradistinction, Ferdinand found no difference between conventional and MIHVS with three different types of stentless aortic valve replacements.[58] Using modified Port-Access methods, the New York University group performed 153 aortic valve replacements with a conventional cross-clamp placed through a right second ICS incision.[38] In this series both a 6.5% perioperative mortality and a 2.6% stroke rate were reported. They had good surgical access but

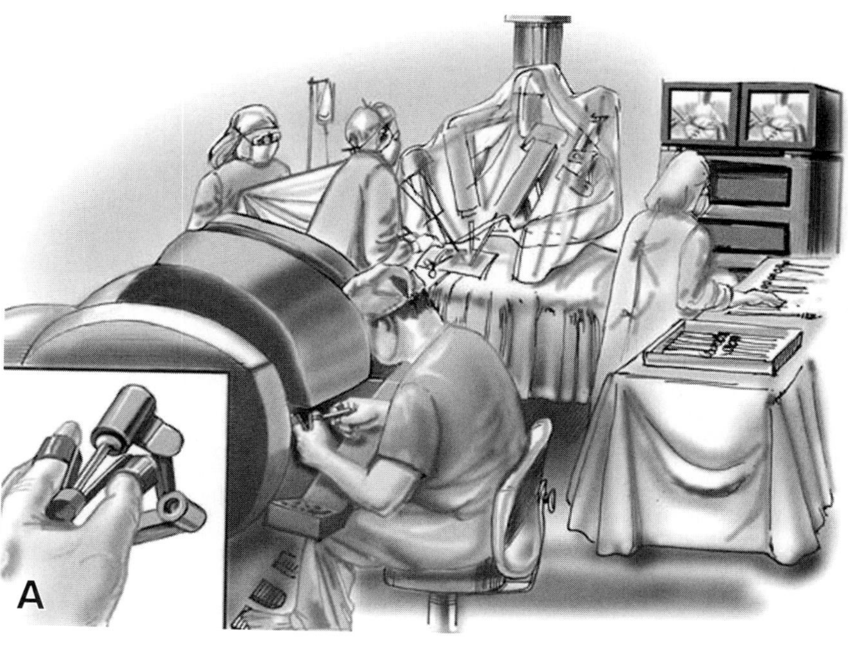

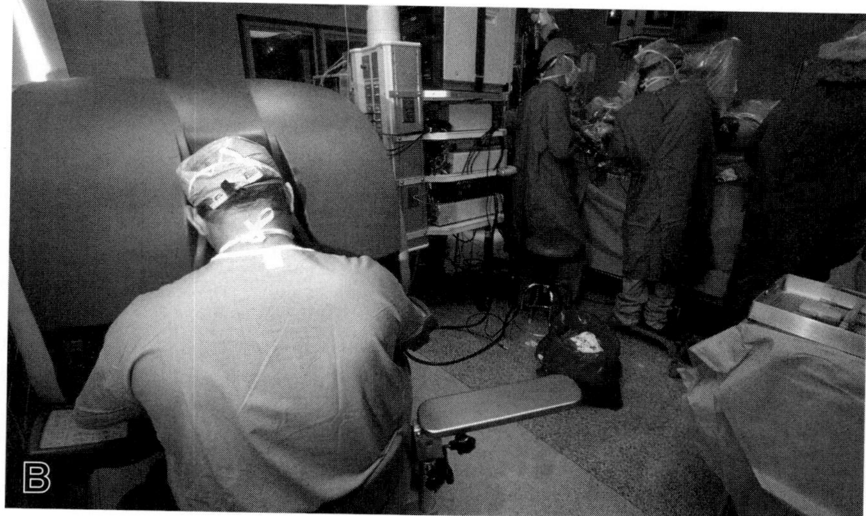

FIGURE 44–16 (A) da Vinci Robotic telemanipulation system. The operative console is in the foreground while the instrument cart is at the table. Both the operating surgeon and patient side assistant are shown. (B) da Vinci Robotic mitral valve repair. The surgeon is positioned approximately 10 feet from the patient. The instrument cart is placed on the left side of the tilted patient with arms entering the right thorax.

found mild or greater aortic insufficiency by echocardiography in 24% of their postoperative patients. In a parallel editorial, Chitwood concluded that the second intercostal minithoracotomy might have limited their exposure, resulting in more residual leaks than expected.[59]

For aortic valve surgery our group has preferred a small incision and either an upper sternotomy with deviation to the right or near complete sternal division with simple spreading of each upper half, "springing" the lower part without division. From these series we can conclude that the upper hemisternotomy provides excellent exposure for simple aortic valve operations and most surgeons can master this technique easily without compromising results. More complex operations involving the aortic root and/or Ross autograft method can be done by this route but should be reserved for surgeons who are very experienced with minimally invasive techniques.

Minimally Invasive Mitral Valve Surgery

Again, Cosgrove and Gundry have been consistent proponents of using the ministernotomy for mitral surgery. They have considered the ministernotomy technique more reproducible for surgeons with variable experiences and abilities. Both complex replacements and repairs have been done through this incision and to date few operative failures have resulted from this exposure. Between 1996 and early 2002, Cosgrove and his Cleveland Clinic group had done 1427

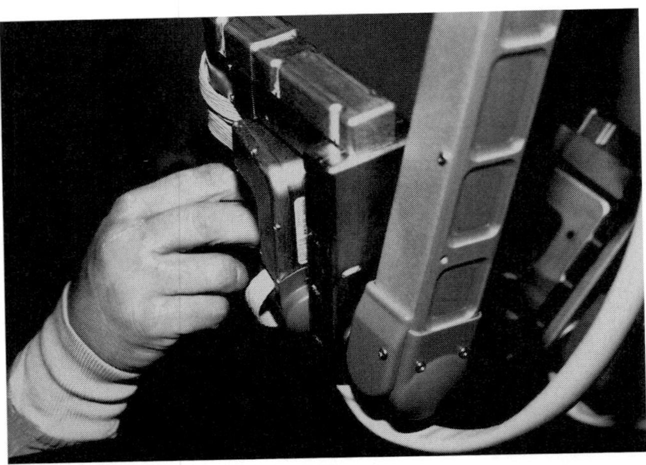

FIGURE 44–17 The operating surgeon manipulates instrument tips in the patient's thorax via ergonomic "handpieces" that transfer filtered digitized data into smoothed movements.

minimally invasive mitral operations, using direct vision, upper hemisternotomy, and modified perfusion methods. As noted earlier, the extended atriotomy, used by Cosgrove, apparently has not eventuated in additional atrial arrhythmias. Of these patients, 82% had degenerative and 9% had rheumatic disease. Of all mitral valves, 90% were insufficient and nearly all were repaired, with 98% having a band annuloplasty and 85% undergoing leaflet resections. Perfusion and aortic occlusion times averaged 80 and 60 minutes, respectively. These times are shorter than those of many experienced surgeons using a full sternal approach. As seen earlier in their aortic operations, perfusion times have fallen more significantly than arrest times since 1996. This mitral valve series presents an impressive mortality (0.3%) and complication rate (bleeding [3.1%], strokes [1.8 %], respiratory insufficiency [0.8%]). Conversions to a full sternotomy have fallen at the Cleveland Clinic from 5 % in 1997 to 0.5% in 2002 (1.5% overall), and most of these have been related to poor exposure, not bleeding. Only 7% of patients were transfused, and the mean hospitalization was 6.5 days, with 20% being discharged in less than 4 days.

After initially using a right parasternal incision with bicaval cannulation and left atrial entry via the interatrial septum, Cohn et al now prefer modified hemisternal approaches for mitral valve surgery. Of the 411 mitral patients operated between 1996 and early 2002, 201 had hemisternotomies and 201 had parasternal incisions, with 8 having a minithoracotomy. Myxomatous (81%), rheumatic (10%), and endocarditic (4%) were the most common etiologies. In 88% repairs were done, and in the remaining 12%, replacements were done using mechanical valves (84%). Their operative mortality was an impressive 0.2% with no deaths in the repair group. Bleeding occurred in 2% and 38% were transfused with an average of one packed cell unit per patient. Strokes occurred in 2.2% of patients, with myocardial infarctions in 1.0%. Patients were hospitalized for a mean of 6 days and 8.3% required additional rehabilitation prior to discharge.

Grossi et al at New York University compared 100 minimally invasive mitral operations, done through a 6- to 8-cm minithoracotomy using direct-vision and Port-Access methods, to a cohort of 100 conventional mitral operations.[39] They reported a perioperative mortality of 1.0%. In these patients 80% had a posterior leaflet procedure and 30% had an anterior leaflet reconstruction. This ratio did not differ from that of their full sternotomy patients, nor did the status of repairs 1 year following surgery. Their results suggest minimally invasive mitral operations can be done safely using Port-Access methods with similar results as conventional

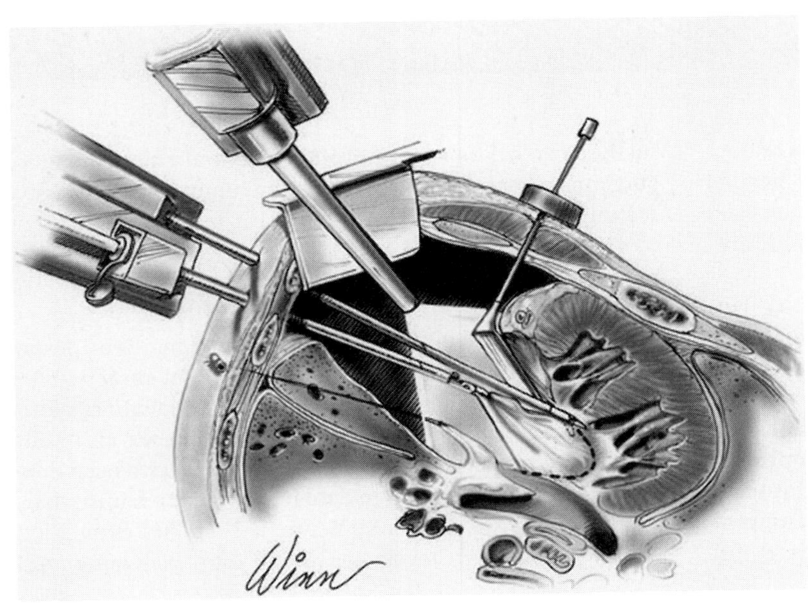

FIGURE 44–18 This thoracic cross section during a da Vinci mitral operation shows how both instrument arms and the visual field converge at the operative plane to effect an unobstructed topographic view with full access to valvular and subvalvular structures.

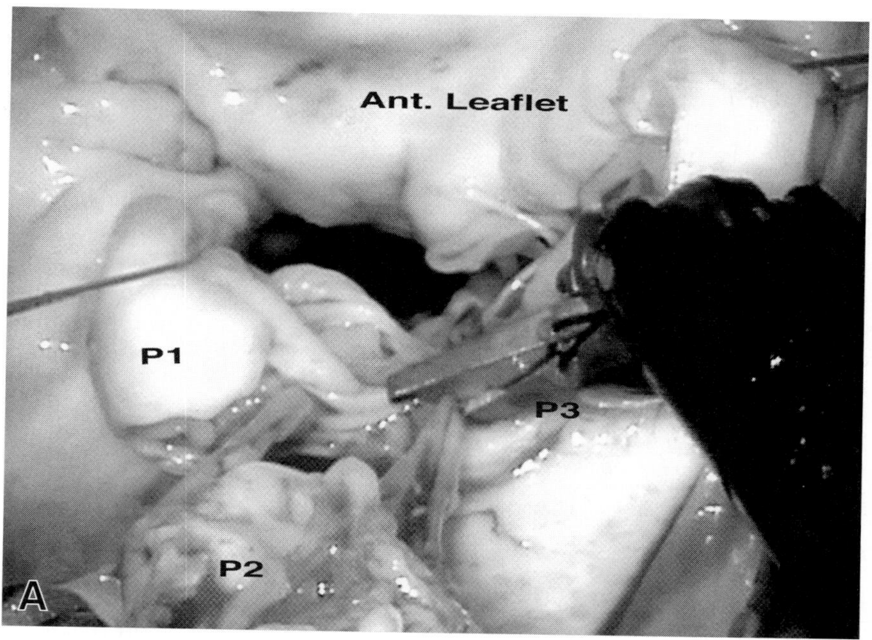

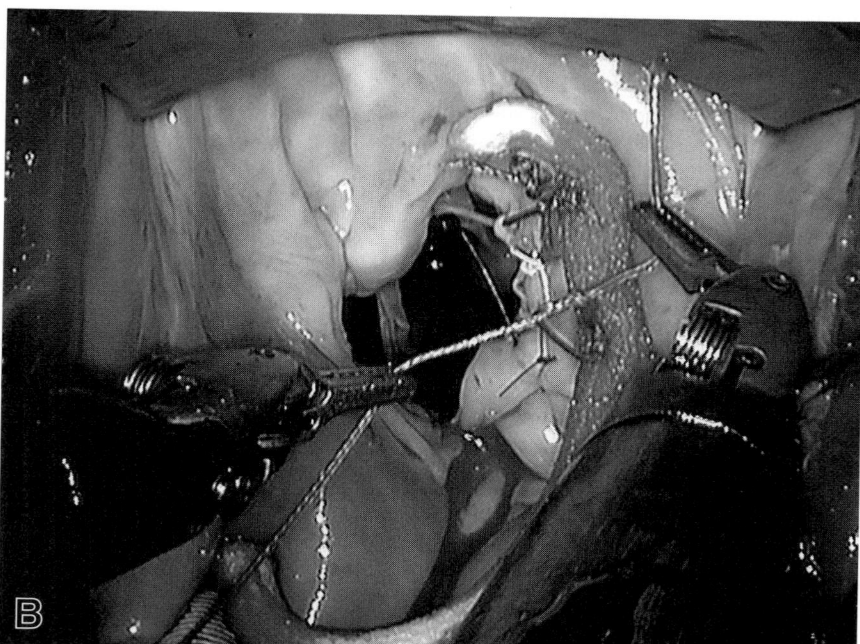

FIGURE 44–19 (A) da Vinci mitral valve repair. The P_2 segment of the posterior leaflet is being resected by robotic microscissors. The annulus is reduced and both P_1 and P_3 approximated. (B) Instrument arms of the da Vinci are tying sutures to secure an annuloplasty band along the posterior annulus.

operations and with no added mortality or morbidity. At the same time they had fewer transfusions, shorter lengths of stay, and less septic complications, despite longer cardiopulmonary bypass times. In a multi-institutional analysis of 491 Port-Access mitral repairs from 104 centers, Glower reported that 86% of all valves were repaired with aortic cross-clamp times of 90 minutes and perfusion times of 137 minutes.[60,61] The overall mortality for repairs was 1.6% and was 5.5% for replacements. Age was the only independent predictor of strokes (2.7%) in these patients. Neurologic complications associated with early use of this technique have diminished with the advent of better devices and more experience. The overall length of stay for this large group of mitral patients was 7 days.

In early 2001 the East Carolina University (ECU) group reported their 128 successful video-assisted mitral valve operations.[26] At first patients with anterior leaflet pathology and annular calcification were avoided. However, now we consider these patients within the realm of video-assisted surgery. Table 44-3 details our current criteria for patient selection. In our series repairs have included quadrangular resections, annuloplasties, and complex chordal operations.

TABLE 44–3 Current patient selection: videoscopic or video-assisted mitral valve surgery

Unsuitable candidates
Highly calcified mitral annulus
Severe pulmonary hypertension, especially with a small right coronary
Significant untreated coronary disease
Severe peripheral atherosclerosis
Prior right chest surgery
Suitable candidates
Patients with primary mitral valve disease
Reoperative mitral valve patients
Bileaflet and/or anterior leaflet disease
Combined tricuspid and mitral operations
Mild annular calcification
Obese or large patients
Elderly patients

The majority of the patients had myxomatous disease, and 61% of the total group underwent a repair. Figure 44-20 shows a videoscopic bileaflet repair utilizing two (P_1 and P_2) sliding plasties as well as a P_2 segment transfer to A_2 for Type 2 anterior leaflet prolapse. When the early series is combined with the subsequent 100 video-assisted mitral operations, repairs have been done in 81% of patients at ECU. The operative and 30-day mortalities for our entire series have been 0.4% and 1.7%, respectively. After implementing the Aesop 3000 robot to voice-direct the endoscopic camera, cross-clamp and perfusion times fell secondary to improved visualization and reduced lens cleaning. However, in the latter half of the early series cross-clamp (90 minutes) and perfusion (143 minutes) times still remained longer than conventional operations. Currently, cardiac arrest and perfusion times have fallen to 70 and 100 minutes, respectively. Interestingly, we have seen no difference in bleeding and transfusion requirements between our conventional and MIHVS patients. However, the hospital lengths of stays have averaged 4.9 days compared to 8 days for conventional operations. Of these 228 patients, there have been two conversions to a sternotomy, two strokes, and no aortic dissections. We have had one vena caval injury during cannulation. Included in this series are 28 patients having had either prior coronary or mitral surgery. These patients underwent video-assisted *reoperations* with a 3.5% mortality and markedly less blood loss than conventional reoperations.

Mohr et al reported on 154 video-assisted mitral valve operations using Aesop 3000 robotic camera control.[23,28,62] In these patients the aortic cross-clamp and perfusion times were similar to his conventional operations, and the operative mortality was 1.2%. He considered three-dimensional visualization to be the key to excellent results during videoscopic valve reconstructions. In a study comparing the Port-Access technique to transthoracic clamping, Wimmer-Greinecker obtained similar repair results but with faster operations, less technical difficulties, and lower cost using the clamping method.[63] In early 2002 Vanermen reported success in 187 patients undergoing totally endoscopic repairs using the Port-Access method and no rib spreading. He used a holder-mounted, two-dimensional endoscopic camera and performed complex repairs with excellent results at follow-up 19 months later.[41] The hospital mortality was 0.5%, and there were two conversions to a sternotomy for bleeding. Freedom from reoperation was 95% at four years. Over 90% of patients had minimal postoperative pain. Although this and other series have not been randomized, there are strong

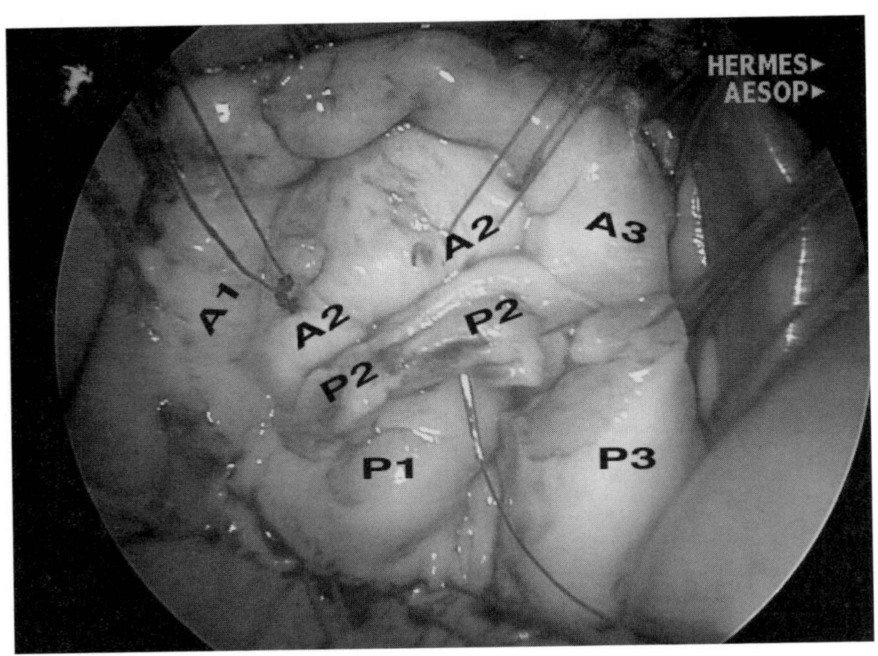

FIGURE 44–20 Videoscopic (Aesop 3000) complex mitral valve repair. Here, both the anterior and posterior leaflets are redundant with severe type 2 prolapse. The posterior part of P_2 was resected, leaving the anterior quarter of the leaflet with chords attached along the coapting edge. This segment of P_2 is then transferred along the coapting edge of A_2. Securing mattress sutures are being placed. Finally, a height-reducing sliding plasty is done for both P_1 and P_3 before central approximation. A band annuloplasty is done last. We have found this method very effective for treating severe anterior prolapse minimally invasively.

suggestions that mitral valve surgery has entered a new era and that video techniques can facilitate these operations.

Robotic Mitral Valve Surgery

At our institution, as part of an FDA trial, mitral repairs have been performed in 50 patients using the robotic da Vinci Surgical System.[29,30] Quadrangular leaflet resections, leaflet sliding plasties, chordal transfers, PTFE chord replacements, and annuloplasty band insertions have been done with facility. Difficult commissural and trigone sutures dissolved into simple efforts using da Vinci. Robotic repair and total operating times decreased from 1.9 and 5.1 hours, respectively, for the first 25 patients to 1.5 and 4.4 hours, respectively, in the last 25 patients. Excepting times required to place annuloplasty bands, all time intervals decreased significantly with experience. In the last cohort, cross-clamp and perfusion times were 1.8 and 2.7 hours, respectively. This time course paralleled improvements experienced with our videoscopic series reported above. We have had no major complications and the mean length of stay has been 3.8 days. Two valves were replaced either because of hemolysis (19 days) or a new grade 3 leak (2 months). Mohr has successfully completed 22 mitral repairs in Leipzig with da Vinci.[28] Lange in Munich has performed a totally endoscopic mitral repair using only 1-cm port incisions.[32] A multicenter da Vinci trial, enlisting approximately 120 patients, is nearing completion and to date demonstrates efficacy and safety in performing these operations by multiple surgeons at various centers. To date aortic and tricuspid valves have not held widespread interest for robotic surgeons.

CONCLUSIONS

The above information suggests that minimally invasive valve surgery is well on the way to reality. Although operative philosophies, patient populations, and surgeon abilities differ between centers, the compendium of recent results remains very encouraging. The advent of true three-dimensional vision with tactile instrument feedback will be the major bridge to truly "tele-micro-access" operations. Also, to perform these operations optimally, "extracorporeal" surgeons and engineers will need to improve methods by which instruments are directed by computers. Recent successes with direct-vision, videoscopic, and robotic minimally invasive surgery all have reaffirmed that this evolution can be extremely fast, albeit through various pathways. In fact catheter-based technology is even moving toward treating aortic valve disease, and mitral annuloplasties have been done experimentally through the coronary sinus.[64]

Patient requirements, technology developments, and surgeon capabilities all must become aligned to drive these needed changes. In addition we must work closer with our cardiology colleagues in these developments. This is an evolutionary process, and even the greatest skeptics must concede that progress has been made. However, curmudgeons and surgical scientists alike must continue to interject their concerns. Caution cannot be overemphasized. Traditional valve operations enjoy long-term success with ever-decreasing morbidity and mortality, and remain our measure for comparison. Surgeons and cardiologists must remember that less invasive approaches to treating valve disease cannot capitulate to poorer operative quality or unsatisfactory valve and/or patient longevity.

REFERENCES

1. Cohn LH, Adams DH, Couper GS, Bichell DP: Minimally invasive aortic valve replacement. *Semin Thorac Cardiovasc Surg* 1997; 9:331.
2. Cosgrove DM, Sabik JF: Minimally invasive approach for aortic valve operations. *Ann Thorac Surg* 1996; 62:596.
3. Cosgrove DM, Sabik JF, Navia J: Minimally invasive valve surgery. *Ann Thorac Surg* 1998; 65:1535.
4. Pompili MF, Stevens JH, Burdon TA, et al: Port-access mitral valve replacement in dogs. *J Thorac Cardiovasc Surg* 1996; 112:1268.
5. Falk V, Walther T, Diegeler R, et al: Echocardiographic monitoring of minimally invasive mitral valve surgery using an endoaortic clamp. *J Heart Valve Dis* 1996; 5:630.
6. Baldwin JC: Minimally invasive port-access mitral valve surgery [editorial; comment]. *J Thorac Cardiovasc Surg* 1998; 115:563.
7. Baldwin JC: Defining "minimally invasive" in valvular heart disease. *Curr Opin Cardiol* 2001; 16:125.
8. Ullyot DJ: Look ma, no hands! [editorial]. *Ann Thorac Surg* 1996; 61:10.
9. Cooley DA: Antagonist's view of minimally invasive heart valve surgery. *J Card Surg* 2000; 15:3.
10. Arom KV, Emery RW: Minimally invasive mitral operations. *Ann Thorac Surg* 1996; 62:1542.
11. Arom KV, Emery RW, Kshettry VR, Janey PA: Comparison between port access and less invasive valve surgery. *Ann Thorac Surg* 1999; 68:1525.
12. Konertz W, Waldenberger F, Schmutzler M, et al: Minimal access valve surgery through superior partial sternotomy: a preliminary study. *J Heart Valve Dis* 1996; 6:638.
13. Navia JL, Cosgrove DM: Minimally invasive mitral valve operations. *Ann Thorac Surg* 1996; 62:1542.
14. Cohn LH, Adams DH, Couper GS, et al: Minimally invasive cardiac valve surgery improves patient satisfaction while reducing costs of cardiac valve replacement and repair. *Ann Surg* 1997: 226:421.
15. Gundry SR, Shattuck OH, Razzouk AJ, et al: Facile minimally invasive cardiac surgery via mini-sternotomy. *Ann Thorac Surg* 1998; 65:1100.
16. Fann JI, Pompili MF, Stevens JH, et al: Port-access cardiac operations with cardioplegic arrest. *Ann Thorac Surg* 1997; 63(6 suppl):35.
17. Fann JI, Pompili MF, Burdon TA, et al: Minimally invasive mitral valve surgery. *Semin Thorac Cardiovasc Surg* 1997; 9:320.
18. Mohr FW, Falk V, Diegeler A, et al: Minimally invasive port-access mitral valve surgery. *J Thorac Cardiovasc Surg* 1998: 115:567.
19. Spencer FC, Galloway AC, Grossi EA, et al: Recent developments and evolving techniques of mitral valve reconstruction. *Ann Thorac Surg* 1998; 65:307.
20. Carpentier A, Loulmet D, Le Bret E, et al: Chirugie à coeur ouvert par vidéo-chirurgie et mini-thoracotomie—primier cas (valvuloplastie mitrale) opéré avec succès [First open heart operation (mitral valvuloplasty) under videosurgery through a minithoracotomy]. *Comptes Rendus De L'Academie des Sciences: Sciences de la vie* 1996; 319:219.

21. Chitwood WR, Elbeery JR, Moran JM: Minimally invasive mitral valve repair: using a mini-thoracotomy and trans-thoracic aortic occlusion. *Ann Thorac Surg* 1997; 63:1477.
22. Chitwood WR, Elbeery JR, Chapman WHH, et al: Video-assisted minimally invasive mitral valve surgery: the "micro-mitral" operation. *J Thorac Cardiovasc Surg* 1997;113:413.
23. Falk V, Walther T, Autschbach R, et al: Robot-assisted minimally invasive solo mitral valve operation. *J Thorac Cardiovasc Surg* 1998; 115:470.
24. Loulmet DF, Carpentier A, Cho PW, et al: Less invasive methods for mitral valve surgery. *J Thorac Cardiovasc Surg* 1998; 115:772.
25. Chitwood WR Jr, Wixon CL, Elbeery JR, et al: Video-assisted minimally invasive mitral valve surgery. *J Thorac Cardiovasc Surg* 1997; 114:773.
26. Felger JE, Chitwood WR, Nifong LW, Holbert D: Evolution of mitral valve surgery: toward a totally endoscopic approach. *Ann Thorac Surg* 2001; 72:1203.
27. Carpentier A, Loulmet D, Aupecle B, et al: Computer assisted open-heart surgery: first case operated on with success. *Comtes Rendus de L'Académe des Sciences III* 1998; 321:437.
28. Mohr FW, Falk V, Diegler A, Walther T, et al: Computer-enhanced "robotic" cardiac surgery: experience in 148 patients. *J Thorac Cardiovasc Surg* 2001; 121:842.
29. Chitwood WR, Nifong LW, Elbeery JE, et al: Robotic mitral valve repair: trapezoidal resection and prosthetic annuloplasty with the da Vinci surgical system. *J Thorac Cardiovasc Surg* 2000; 120:1171.
30. Nifong LW, Chitwood WR, Chu VF, et al: Robotic mitral valve repair: experience with the da Vinci system. *Ann Thorac Surg (in press).*
31. Grossi E, Lapietra A, Applebaum RM, et al: Case report of robotic instrument-enhanced mitral valve surgery. *J Thorac Cardiovasc Surg* 2000; 120:1169.
32. Mehmanesh H, Henze R, Lange R: Totally endoscopic mitral valve repair. *J Thorac Cardiovasc Surg* 2002; 123:96.
33. Cohn LH: Parasternal approach for minimally invasive aortic valve surgery, in Cox JL, Sundt TM (eds): *Operative Techniques in Cardiac and Thoracic Surgery: A Comparative Atlas.* Philadelphia, WB Saunders, 1998; p 1.
34. Sardari FF, Schlunt ML, Applegate RL 2nd, Gundry SR: The use of transesophageal echocardiography to guide sternal division for cardiac operations via mini-sternotomy. *J Card Surg* 1997; 12:67.
35. Doty DB, Flores JH, Doty JR: Cardiac valve operations using a partial sternotomy (lower half) technique. *J Card Surg* 2000; 15:35.
36. Karagoz HY, Bayazit K, Battaloglu B, et al: Minimally invasive mitral valve surgery: the subxiphoid approach. *Ann Thorac Surg* 1999; 67:1328.
37. Benetti FJ, Mariani MA, Rizzardi JL, Benetti I: Minimally invasive aortic valve replacement. *J Thorac Cardiovasc Surg* 1997; 113:806.
38. Kort S, Applebaum RM, Grossi EA, et al: Minimally invasive aortic valve replacement: echocardiographic and clinical results. *Am Heart J* 2001; 142:476.
39. Grossi E, LaPietra A, Ribakove GH, et al: Minimally invasive sternotomy approaches for mitral reconstruction: comparison of intermediate term results. *J Thorac Cardiovasc Surg* 2001; 121:708.
40. Schoeyers P, Wellens F, De Geest R, et al: Minimally invasive video-assisted mitral valve surgery: our lessons after a 4 year experience. *Ann Thorac Surg* 2001; 72:S1050.
41. Casselman FP, van Slyche S, Dom H, et al: Totally endoscopic mitral valve repair: feasible, reproducible, and durable. *J Thorac Cardiovasc Surg (in press).*
42. Mohr FW, Onnasch JF, Falk V, et al: The evolution of minimally invasive valve surgery—2 year experience. *Eur J Cardiothorac Surg* 1999; 15:233.
43. Cosgrove DM, Gillinov AM: Partial sternotomy for mitral valve operations, in Cox JL, Sundt TM (eds): *Operative Techniques in Cardiac and Thoracic Surgery: A Comparative Atlas.* Philadelphia, WB Saunders, 1998; p 62.
44. Cohn LH: Minimally invasive valve surgery. *J Card Surg* 2001; 16:260.
45. Grossi EA, Ribakove G, Schwartz DS, et al: Port-access approach for minimally invasive mitral valve surgery, in Cox JL, Sundt TM (eds): *Operative Techniques in Cardiac and Thoracic Surgery: A Comparative Atlas.* Philadelphia, WB Saunders, 1998; p 32.
46. Glower DD, Komtebedde J, Clements C, et al: Direct aortic cannulation for port-access mitral or coronary artery bypass grafting. *Ann Thorac Surg* 1999; 68:1878.
47. Van Nooten G, Van Belleghem Y, Van Overbeke H, et al: Redo mitral surgery using the ESTECH endoclamp. *Heart Surg Forum* 2001; 4:31.
48. Chitwood WR: Minimally invasive video-assisted mitral valve surgery using the Chitwood clamp, in Cox JL, Sundt TM (eds): *Operative Techniques in Cardiac and Thoracic Surgery: A Comparative Atlas.* Philadelphia, WB Saunders, 1998; p 1.
49. Chitwood WR, Nifong LW: Robotic assistance in cardiac surgery, in Talamini MA (ed): *Problems in General Surgery.* Philadelphia, Lippincott Williams & Wilkins, 2001; 18:9.
50. Machler HE, Bergmann P, Anelli-Monti M, et al: Minimally invasive versus conventional aortic valve operations: a prospective study in 120 patients. *Ann Thorac Surg* 1999; 67:1001.
51. Von Sagesser LK, Westaby S, Pomar J, et al: Less invasive aortic valve surgery: rationale and technique. *Eur J Cardiothorac Surg* 1999; 15:781.
52. Aris A, Camara ML,Casan P, Litvan H: Pulmonary function following aortic valve replacement: a comparison between ministernotomy and median sternotomy. *J Heart Valve Dis* 1999; 8:605.
53. Christiansen S, Stypmann J, Tjan TD, et al: Minimally-invasive versus conventional aortic valve replacement—perioperative course and mid-term results. *Eur J Cardiothorac Surg* 1999; 16:647.
54. Gillinov AM, Banbury MK, Cosgrove DM: Hemi-sternotomy approach for aortic and mitral valve surgery. *J Card Surg* 2000; 15:15.
55. Bryne JG, Karavas AN, Filsoufi F, et al: Aortic valve surgery after previous coronary artery bypass grafting with functioning internal mammary artery grafts. *Ann Thorac Surg* 2002; 73:779.
56. Bryne JG, Karavas AN, Adams DH, et al: Partial upper re-sternotomy for aortic valve replacement or re-replacement after previous cardiac surgery. *Eur J Cardiothorac Surg* 2000; 18:282.
57. Bonacchi M, Prifti E, Giumti G, et al: Does mini-sternotomy improve postoperative outcome in aortic valve operation? A prospective randomized study. *Ann Thorac Surg* 2002; 73:460.
58. Ferdinand FD, Sutter FP, Goldman SM: Clinical use of stentless aortic valves with standard and minimally invasive surgical techniques. *Semin Thorac Cardiovasc Surg* 2001; 13:283.
59. Chitwood WR: Minimally invasive aortic valve surgery: what is "port access"? *Am Heart J* 2001; 142:391.
60. Glower DD, Siegel LC, Galloway AC, et al: Predictors of operative time in multicenter Port-access valve registry: institutional differences in learning. *Heart Surg Forum* 2001; 4:40.
61. Glower DD, Siegel LC, Frischmerer KL, et al: Predictors of outcome in a multicenter Port-access valve registry. *Ann Thorac Surg* 2000; 70:1054.
62. Autschbach R, Onnasch JF, Falk V, et al: The Leipzig experience with robotic valve surgery. *J Card Surg* 2000; 15:82.
63. Aybek T, Dogan S, Wimmer-Greineker G, et al: The micro-mitral operation: comparing the Port-access technique and the transthoracic clamp technique. *J Card Surg* 2000; 15:76.
64. Lutter G, Kuklinski D, Berg G, et al: Percutaneous aortic valve replacement: an experimental study, I: studies on implantation. *J Thorac Cardiovasc Surg* 2002; 123:768.

Part V

Disease of the Great Vessels

Chapter 45

Aortic Dissection

G. Randall Green/Irving L. Kron

Thoracic aorta dissection occurs as blood flow is redirected from the aorta (true lumen) through an intimal tear into the media of the aortic wall (false lumen). A dissection plane that separates the intima from the overlying adventitia along a variable length of the aorta is created within the media. The acute form of aortic dissection is often rapidly lethal, while those surviving the initial event go on to develop a chronic dissection with more protean manifestations. The purpose of this chapter is to review the etiology and pathogenesis of aortic dissection, examine current diagnostic algorithms, and provide detailed descriptions of contemporary surgical techniques for treatment. Additional information regarding follow-up and the subsequent management of these patients is presented to provide a comprehensive understanding of a clinical entity that has challenged physicians and surgeons for centuries.

HISTORY

Sennertus is credited with the first description of the dissection process, but the earliest detailed descriptions of the clinical entity appeared in the 17th and 18th centuries, during which time Maunoir named the process aortic "dissection."[1,2] Laennec defined the propensity of the chronically dissected aorta to become aneurysmal.[3] Aortic dissection was exclusively a postmortem diagnosis until the first part of the 20th century, but in 1935 Gurin attempted surgical intervention with the first aortic fenestration procedure to treat malperfusion syndrome.[4] In 1949 Abbott and Paulin advanced surgical treatment by theoretically preventing aortic rupture by wrapping the aorta with cellophane.[5] Other attempts at surgical treatment over the years met with limited clinical success while certain concepts regarding surgical management are still in use today. With the advent of cardiopulmonary bypass, DeBakey and Cooley forever altered the natural history of aortic dissection by successfully performing primary surgical repair using techniques not remarkably different from contemporary procedures.[6,7] Investigators such as Wheat made substantial contributions by defining physiologically based medical management

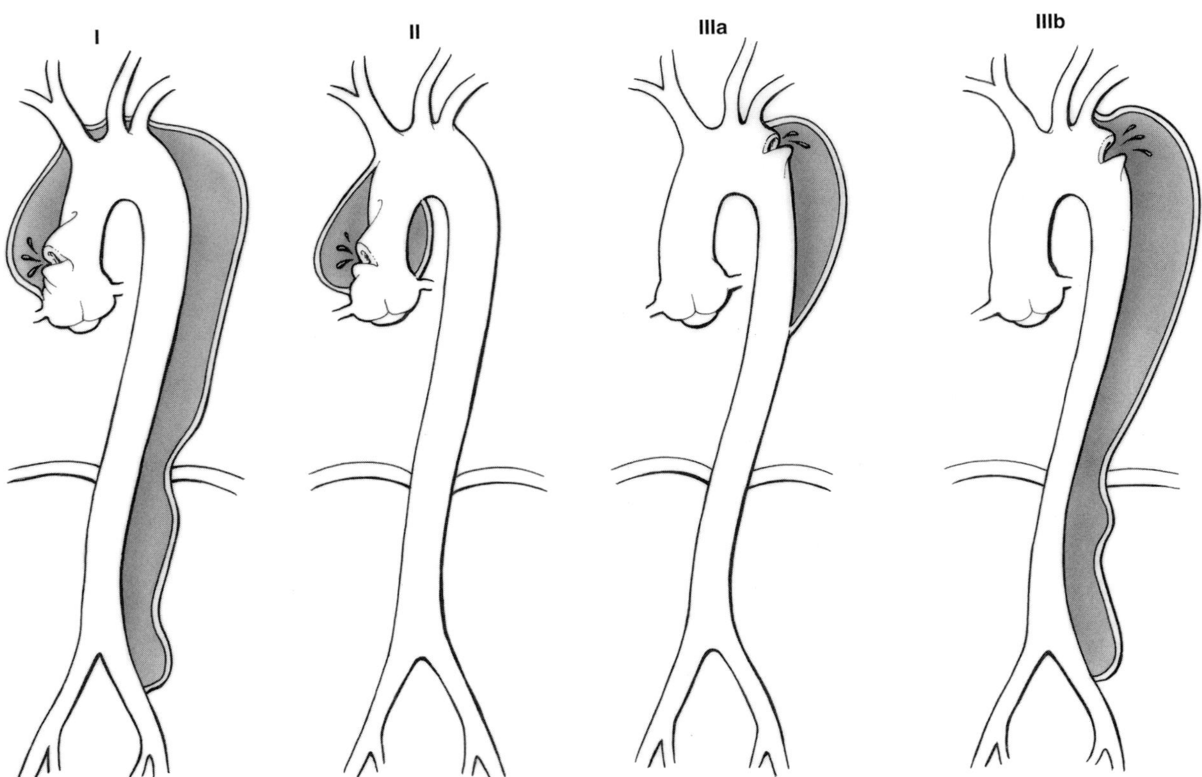

FIGURE 45–1 Classification of aortic dissection. DeBakey type I and Stanford type A include dissections that involve the proximal aorta, arch, and descending thoracic aorta. DeBakey type II only involves the ascending aorta; this dissection is included in Stanford type A. DeBakey type III and Stanford type B include dissections that originate in the descending thoracic and thoracoabdominal aorta regardless of any retrograde involvement of the arch. These are subdivided into a and b depending on abdominal aortic involvement. (*Reproduced with permission from Stone C, Borst H: Dissecting aortic aneurysm, in Edmunds LJ Jr (ed): Cardiac Surgery in the Adult. New York, McGraw-Hill, 1997; p 1125.*)

algorithms to complement surgical correction.[8] There is still considerable controversy regarding surgical versus medical treatment of certain forms of acute thoracic aortic dissection.

CLASSIFICATION

The classification systems used for aortic dissection are based on the location and extent of dissection. The particular type is then subclassified based on the timing of dissection. Acute dissection has traditionally been used to describe presentation within the first 2 weeks, while the term chronic is reserved for those patients presenting at greater than 2 months following the initial event. The more recently added subacute designation is sometimes used to describe the period between 2 weeks and 2 months.

Two classification systems are most frequently used in clinical practice: the DeBakey and the Stanford systems (Fig. 45-1). The DeBakey system differentiates patients based upon the location and extent of aortic dissection.[9] The advantage of this system is that four different groups of patients with different forms of aortic dissection emerge and provide the greatest opportunity for subsequent comparative research. In contrast, the Stanford system proposed by Daily et al is a functional classification system.[10] All dissections that involve the ascending aorta are grouped together as type A, regardless of where the primary tear occurs. Proponents of the simpler Stanford system contend that the clinical behavior of patients with aortic dissection is essentially determined by involvement of the ascending aorta. Critics, however, suggest that individual patients in the type A classification may be quite different from one another depending upon the distal extent of dissection. Drawing clinical conclusions from such a potentially heterogeneous patient population has inherent limitations. The Stanford system will be used throughout this chapter.

INCIDENCE

Aortic dissection is the most frequently diagnosed lethal condition of the aorta and occurs nearly three times as frequently

TABLE 45–1 Clinical characteristics of patients presenting with acute type A and B thoracic aortic dissections

	Type A	Type B
Frequency	60–75%	25–40%
Sex (M:F)	1.7–2.6:1	2.3–3:1
Age (y)	50–56	60–70
Hypertension	++	+++
Connective tissue disorder	++	+
Pain		
Retrosternal	+++	+, −
Interscapular	+, −	+++
Syncope	++	+, −
Cerebrovascular accident	+	−
Congestive heart failure	+	−
Aortic valve regurgitation	++	+, −
Myocardial infarction	+	−
Pericardial effusion	+++	−
Pleural effusion	+, −	+++
Abdominal pain	+, −	+, −
Peripheral pulse deficit	Upper and lower extremities	Lower extremities

TABLE 45–2 Risk factors for type A and B thoracic aortic dissection

Risk factor
Hypertension
Connective tissue disorders
Ehlers-Danlos syndrome
Marfan disease
Turner's syndrome
Cystic medial disease of aorta
Aortitis
Iatrogenic
Atherosclerosis
Thoracic aortic aneurysm
Bicuspid aortic valve
Trauma
Pharmacologic
Coarctation of aorta
Hypervolemia (pregnancy)
Congenital aortic stenosis
Polycystic kidney disease
Pheochromocytoma
Sheehan's syndrome
Cushing's syndrome

as does rupture of abdominal aortic aneurysm in the United States.[11] There is an estimated worldwide prevalence of 0.5 to 2.95 per 100,000 per year; the prevalence ranges from 0.2 to 0.8 per 100,000 per year in the United States, resulting in roughly 2000 new cases per year. These figures are, however, only an estimate. In one autopsy series, the antemortem diagnosis was made in only 15% of patients, revealing that many immediately fatal events go undiagnosed.[12] Clinically, type A dissections occur with an overall greater frequency (Table 45-1).

ETIOLOGY AND PATHOGENESIS

There are several hypotheses regarding the etiology of the intimal disruption (primary tear) that permits aortic blood flow to create a cleavage plane within the media of the aortic wall. This was originally viewed as a consequence of a biochemical abnormality within the media upon which normal mechanical forces in the aorta acted to create an intimal tear. The link between the abnormal media, termed cystic medial necrosis or degeneration, and the primary tear has not been scientifically established. In fact, medial degeneration is found in only a minority of patients with acute aortic dissection and most are children.[13] This theory has lost support over the years.

Alternatively, there are data supporting a relationship between aortic dissections and intramural hematoma. Advocates of this theory suggest that bleeding from vasa vasorum into the media creates a mass, which results in localized areas of increased stress in the intima during diastole. These areas then permit intimal disruption. In fact, between 10% and 20% of patients thought to have acute aortic dissection are found to have intramural hematoma suggesting that it may be a precursor to dissection.[14] Penetrating atherosclerotic ulcers have been implicated as the source of intimal disruption in certain cases, yet support for the concept has waned over the years. The pattern of atherosclerotic involvement of the thoracic aorta resulting in penetrating ulcer and the frequency of dissection throughout the aorta do not support this theory.

While no single disorder is responsible for aortic dissection, several risk factors have been identified that can damage the aortic wall and lead to dissection (Table 45-2). These include direct mechanical forces on the aortic wall (i.e., hypertension, hypervolemia, derangements of aortic flow) and forces that affect the composition of the aortic wall (i.e., connective tissue disorders or direct chemical destruction). Hypertension is the mechanical force most often associated with dissection and is found in greater than 75% of cases. Although the role of increased strain on the aortic wall is intuitive, the mechanism by which hypertension actually leads to dissection is unclear. Similarly, hypervolemia, high cardiac output, and an abnormal hormonal milieu certainly contribute to the increased incidence of dissection in pregnancy, but the mechanism is unclear. Atherosclerosis is not a risk factor for aortic dissection except in preexisting aneurysms or in the case of atherosclerotic ulceration, which may lead to dissection in the descending thoracic aorta. Iatrogenic trauma to the aortic intima may result in dissection. Catheterization procedures, aortic root and femoral artery cannulation for cardiopulmonary bypass, aortic

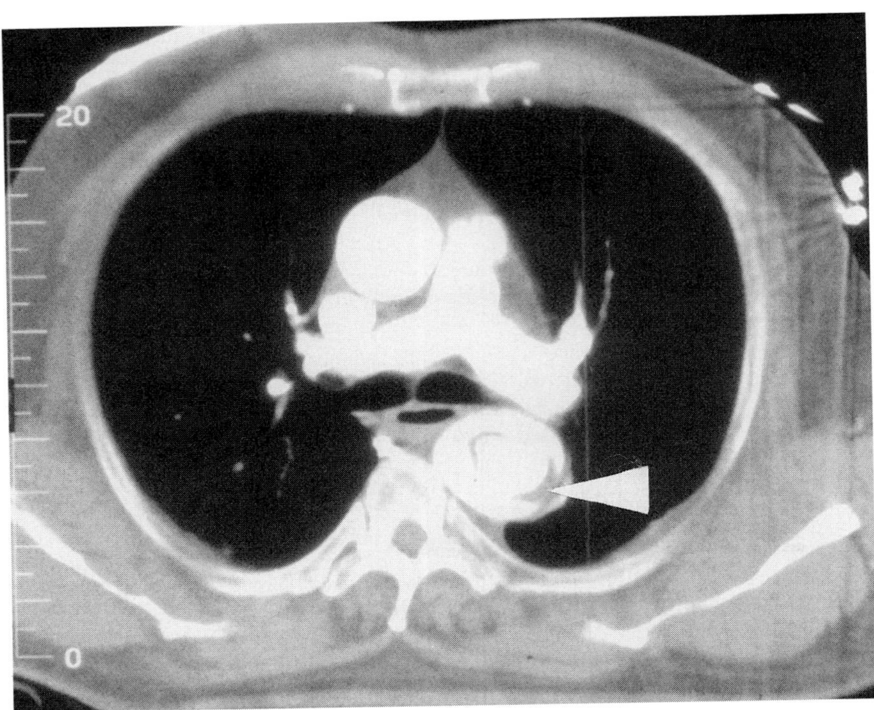

FIGURE 45–2 Axial image of CT arteriogram showing a nearly circumferential dissection flap (arrowhead) as a result of acute traumatic aortic transection. (*Reproduced with permission from Stone C, Borst H: Dissecting aortic aneurysm, in Edmunds LJ Jr (ed): Cardiac Surgery in the Adult. New York, McGraw-Hill, 1997; p 1125.*)

cross-clamping, surgical procedures performed on the aorta (aortic valve replacement and aorto-coronary bypass grafting), and placement of intra-aortic balloon pumps have all been reported to result in dissection. Aortic transection as a result of trauma rarely results in excessive dissection and deserves differentiation from the process of aortic dissection. This process is usually limited to the aortic isthmus and in addition to the risk of rupture may present as a circular prolapse of the intima and media producing aortic obstruction referred to as "pseudo-coarctation" (Fig. 45-2).

Once a cleavage plane exists in the media, the aortic wall floating within the lumen is termed the dissection flap and is composed of the aortic intima and partial thickness media. The primary tear is usually greater than 50% of the circumference of the aorta, but the full circumference is rarely involved. The primary tear in type A dissection is usually located on the right anterior aspect of the ascending aorta and follows a somewhat predictable course, spiraling around the arch and into the descending thoracic and abdominal aorta on the left and posteriorly. The dissection may propagate in a retrograde fashion for a variable distance as well to involve the coronary ostia; this occurs in roughly 11% of all dissections.[15] Myocardial ischemia and rupture into the pericardium are the cause of death in as many as 80% of deaths from acute dissection. Often the distal false lumen communicates with the true lumen through one or more fenestrations within the dissection flap. The false lumen may also end blindly in as many as 4% to 12% of patients, in which case blood in the false lumen frequently becomes thrombotic. The false lumen may also penetrate the adventitia causing rupture and death. Regardless of whether the true and false lumen communicate, perfusion of aortic side branches may be compromised by the dissection causing end-organ ischemia (Fig. 45-3). If these acute complications are avoided, the weakened outer aortic wall, composed of partial media and the adventitia, may dilate over time resulting in aneurysm formation. This long-term complication is the reason for operation in the majority of chronic dissections regardless of type.

The adventitia provides most of the tensile strength of the aortic wall with little contribution from the media. The media is composed of concentrically arranged smooth muscle interposed with connective tissue proteins such as collagen, elastin, and fibrillin within the ground substance. Abnormal constituents of the media, as in certain connective tissue disorders such as Marfan disease and Ehlers-Danlos syndrome, are associated with aortic dissection. Marfan syndrome is an autosomal dominant inherited disorder in which a point mutation in the fibrillin-1 gene (FBN1) located on the long arm of chromosome 15 results in an abnormal media. The incidence of Marfan syndrome is approximately 1 per 5000 live births. There are, however, many incomplete forms of the disease and as many as 25% may be sporadic in which no known fibrillin abnormalities are observed. Type IV Ehlers-Danlos syndrome is a connective tissue disorder of the proα1(III) chain of Type III collagen with an incidence of 1 in 5000. The structurally abnormal media is susceptible to dissection. There are also familial aggregations of dissection without discernable biochemical or genetic abnormalities.

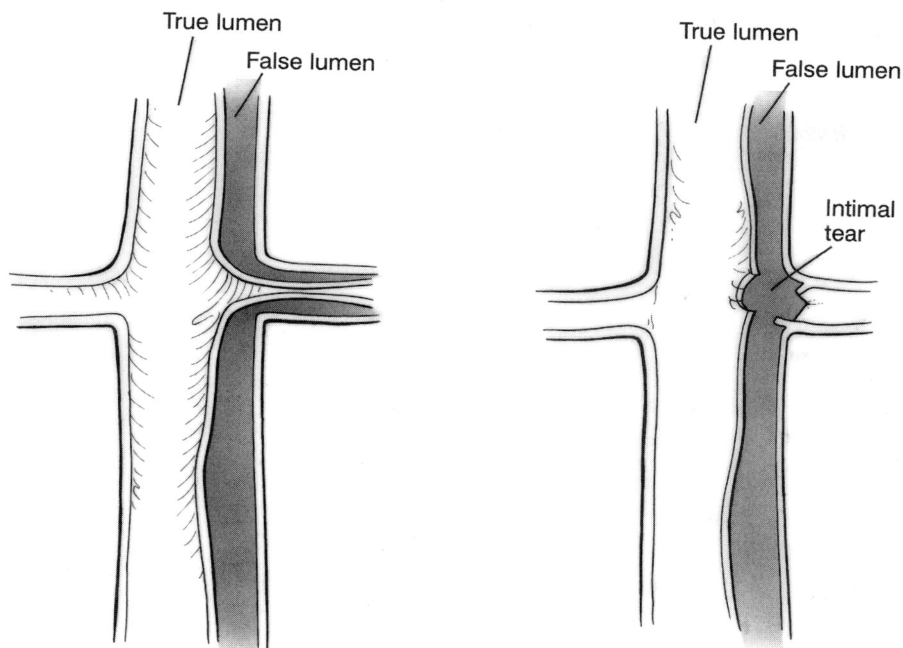

FIGURE 45–3 Diagram of aortic dissection. (A) An intact dissection membrane compresses the true lumen and causes malperfusion of a branch artery. (B) Rupture of the dissection membrane that may or may not restore blood flow to the branch.

ACUTE AORTIC DISSECTION

Clinical Presentation

SIGNS AND SYMPTOMS

As many as 40% of patients suffering acute aortic dissection die immediately. Those surviving the initial event may be stabilized with medical management, and it is these patients in whom subsequent therapeutic intervention of aortic dissection has altered the natural history of the disease. The clinical outcome is eventually determined by dissection type and timing of presentation, patient-related factors, and the quality and experience of the individuals and institution providing care.

The initial evaluation of a stable patient suspected of having aortic dissection includes a detailed history and physical examination focusing on those elements likely to rule in the diagnosis. The diagnosis of aortic dissection requires a high level of suspicion. As many as 30% of patients ultimately diagnosed with acute dissection are first thought to have another diagnosis. Aortic dissection should always be considered in the setting of severe, unrelenting chest pain, which is present in most patients. Patients usually have no previous episodes of similar pain and are often quite anxious. Pain is generally located in the mid-sternum for ascending aortic dissection and in the interscapular region for descending thoracic aortic dissection (see Table 45-1). It is not unusual for the location of maximum pain to change as the dissection extends in an antegrade or retrograde direction and such "migratory pain" should arouse clinical suspicion. The character of the pain is often described as "ripping" or "tearing" and is constant with greatest intensity at the onset.

Painless dissection has been described and usually occurs in the setting of an existing aneurysm where the pain of a new dissection may not be differentiated from chronic aneurysm pain. Patients may also have signs or symptoms related to malperfusion of the brain, limbs, or visceral organs. These findings may dominate the presentation following an initial episode of pain.

Elements of the past medical history such as primary hypertension, presence of aneurysmal disease of the aorta, or familial connective tissue disorders are useful as risk factors to help establish the diagnosis. Illicit drug use is an increasingly important predisposing factor to ascertain during the initial evaluation. The differential diagnosis of chest pain as a result of aortic dissection includes diagnoses such as myocardial ischemia, aortic aneurysm, acute aortic regurgitation, pericarditis, musculoskeletal pain, and pulmonary embolus. It is essential to consider aortic dissection in each case as specific therapy (e.g., thrombolytic therapy for acute myocardial infarction) may impact the survivability of acute dissection.

Patients suffering acute dissection appear ill. Tachycardia is usually accompanied by hypertension in the setting of baseline essential hypertension and increased catecholamine levels from pain and anxiety. Hypotension and tachycardia may result from aortic rupture, pericardial tamponade, acute aortic valve regurgitation, or even acute myocardial ischemia with involvement of the coronary ostia. An abnormal peripheral vascular examination is present in less than 20% to 40% of patients with acute aortic dissection but when present may indicate the type of dissection. Absence of pulses in the upper extremity suggests ascending aortic involvement, whereas pulse deficits in the lower extremities speak to involvement

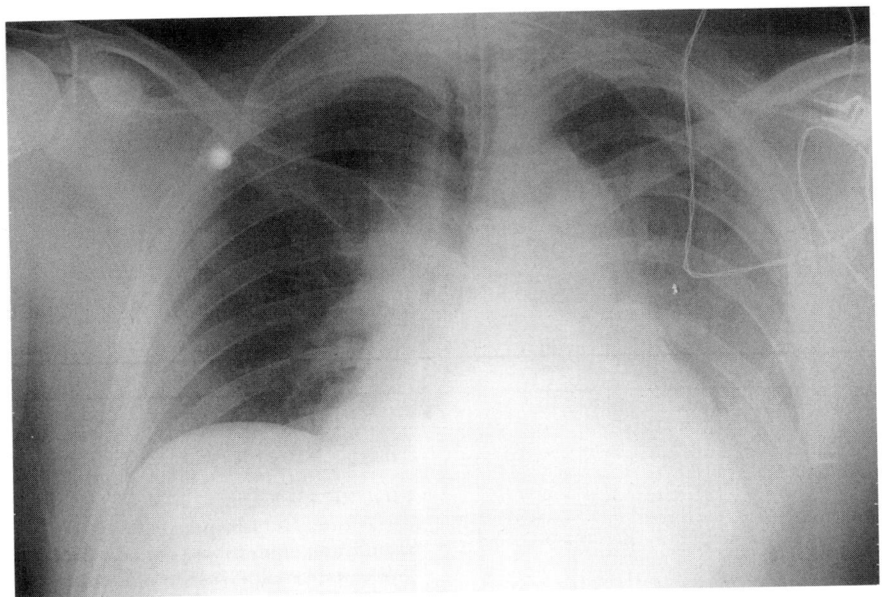

FIGURE 45–4 Plain chest x-ray exhibiting many features of acute type A dissection such as a widened mediastinum, rightward tracheal displacement, irregular aortic contour with loss of the aortic knob, an indistinct aortopulmonary window, and a left pleural effusion.

of the distal aorta. These findings are subject to change as the dissection progresses or reentry into the true lumen occurs. Auscultation of the heart may reveal a diastolic murmur consistent with acute aortic regurgitation or an S3 indicating left heart volume overload. Physical exam findings such as jugular venous distension and a pulsus paradoxus are signs of pericardial tamponade that should be identified in any unstable patient to initiate the correct diagnostic and treatment algorithms. Unilateral loss of breath sounds, usually the left, may indicate hemothorax as a result of aortic leak or rupture with hemothorax. Alternatively, a pleural effusion may exist secondary to pleural inflammation related to the dissection. This finding requires additional evaluation prior to treatment.

A complete central and peripheral neurologic exam is critical in that abnormalities are present in up to 40% of acute type A dissections. Involvement of the brachiocephalic vessels with loss of brain perfusion may result in transient syncope or stroke. Syncope may also result from rupture into the pericardium and is an ominous sign. Stroke rarely improves with restoration of blood flow and may even cause hemorrhage and brain death, yet surgery is indicated in such patients. Fortunately, stroke is a presenting feature in fewer than 5% of patients with acute type A dissection. Loss of perfusion to intercostal or lumbar arteries may result in spinal cord ischemia and paraplegia. Peripheral nerve ischemia as a result of malperfusion may yield findings similar to spinal cord malperfusion and should be discerned as these patients often improve with restoration of blood flow. Acute aortic dissection may also cause superior vena cava syndrome, vocal cord paralysis, hematemesis, Horners syndrome, hemoptysis, and airway compression as a result of local compression and mass effect.

DIAGNOSTIC STUDIES

Routine diagnostic studies including blood tests, chest x-ray, and ECG should be obtained but are often not sufficient to establish the diagnosis of acute aortic dissection. Electrocardiogram often reveals no ischemic changes. Obvious ischemic changes are present in up to 20% of acute type A dissections, while only nonspecific repolarization abnormalities are present in nearly one third of patients with coronary ostial involvement. The ECG may also reveal left ventricular hypertrophy in those patients with long-standing hypertension. The chest x-ray is abnormal in 60% to 90% of patients with acute dissection (Fig. 45-4). Although most patients have at least one, if not several abnormal findings, a normal chest x-ray does not rule out the diagnosis. Blood should be drawn and sent for complete blood count, serum electrolytes, creatine kinase with myocardial isoenzymes, and troponin, and a blood type and screen are obtained. These tests obtained at the time of initial observation are usually unremarkable. There is frequently a mild to moderate leukocytosis. Anemia may result from sequestration of blood or hemolysis. Liver function tests, serum creatinine, myoglobin, and lactic acid may all be abnormal in the setting of certain malperfusion syndromes depending on duration.

DIAGNOSTIC IMAGING

Diagnostic imaging is essential to classify acute aortic dissection, regardless of the clinical certainty with which the diagnosis is made or the acuity of the patient. The diagnosis should be made rapidly and with minimal distress for the patient. Two imaging modalities currently meet these criteria and are used to diagnose acute aortic dissection:

TABLE 45–3 Sensitivity and specificity of various imaging modalities useful for the diagnosis of thoracic aortic dissection

Imaging study	Sensitivity	Specificity
Aortography	80%–90%	88%–95%
Computerized tomography (CT)	90%–100%	90%–100%
Intravascular ultrasound (IVUS)	94%–100%	97%–100%
Echocardiogram		
Transthoracic	60%–80%	80%–96%
Transesophageal	90%–99%	85%–98%
Magnetic resonance imaging (MRI)	98%–100%	98%–100%

computerized tomography and echocardiography. Magnetic resonance imaging and aortography, with or without intravascular ultrasound, are used to diagnose acute aortic dissection but are second-line modalities for various reasons. The benefits, disadvantages, and diagnostic accuracy of each are useful when choosing the most appropriate study for a particular clinical situation (Table 45-3). Each test provides unique information, which may include the site of intimal disruption, reentry points, whether there is flow or thrombus in the false lumen, status of the aortic valve, presence and nature of myocardial ischemia, and brachiocephalic and aortic branch vessel involvement. Specific data may be necessary for operative planning and subsequent management to define the imaging study most appropriate for a particular patient.

Helical computerized tomography scanning (CT) is widely available and now the most frequently utilized test to diagnose acute aortic dissection. It requires intravenous contrast medium that may limit its use in certain clinical situations but generates images familiar to most practitioners and has a high sensitivity and specificity. This technique can be performed quickly fulfilling the requirements for use in the early management of acute dissection. Additional structures such as the pleural and pericardial spaces are imaged. When performed and formatted as an arteriogram, aortic branch vessels may also be evaluated; involvement of the brachiocephalic vessels is identified with nearly 96% accuracy. The diagnosis of dissection requires two or more channels separated by a dissection flap (Fig. 45-5). Transaxial two-dimensional images can be reconstructed to display three-dimensional images of the aorta that not only aid in diagnosis but also are useful for operative planning.

Transesophageal echocardiography (TEE) is currently the second most frequently utilized study for making the diagnosis of acute aortic dissection. It is widely available, requires no intravenous contrast or radiation, and generates dynamic images of the aorta from which the diagnosis can be made (Fig. 45-6). It requires operator expertise both to acquire the necessary images and to conduct of the examination safely. Although the safest setting in which to perform TEE is the operating room under general anesthesia, it can be performed in a monitored setting using topical anesthesia and light sedation. Patient comfort is paramount in this situation as rupture has been reported during difficult studies and a complete examination of the entire aorta is necessary to exclude the diagnosis of acute dissection. Absolute contraindications to TEE include esophageal abnormalities

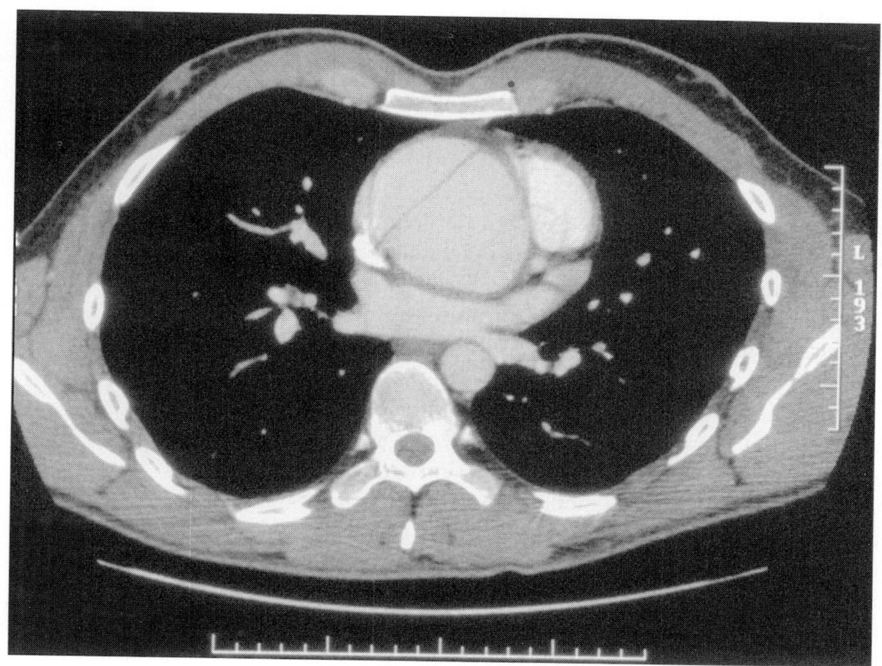

FIGURE 45–5 Axial image of CT arteriogram of acute type A dissection showing a dissection flap in the mid-ascending aorta.

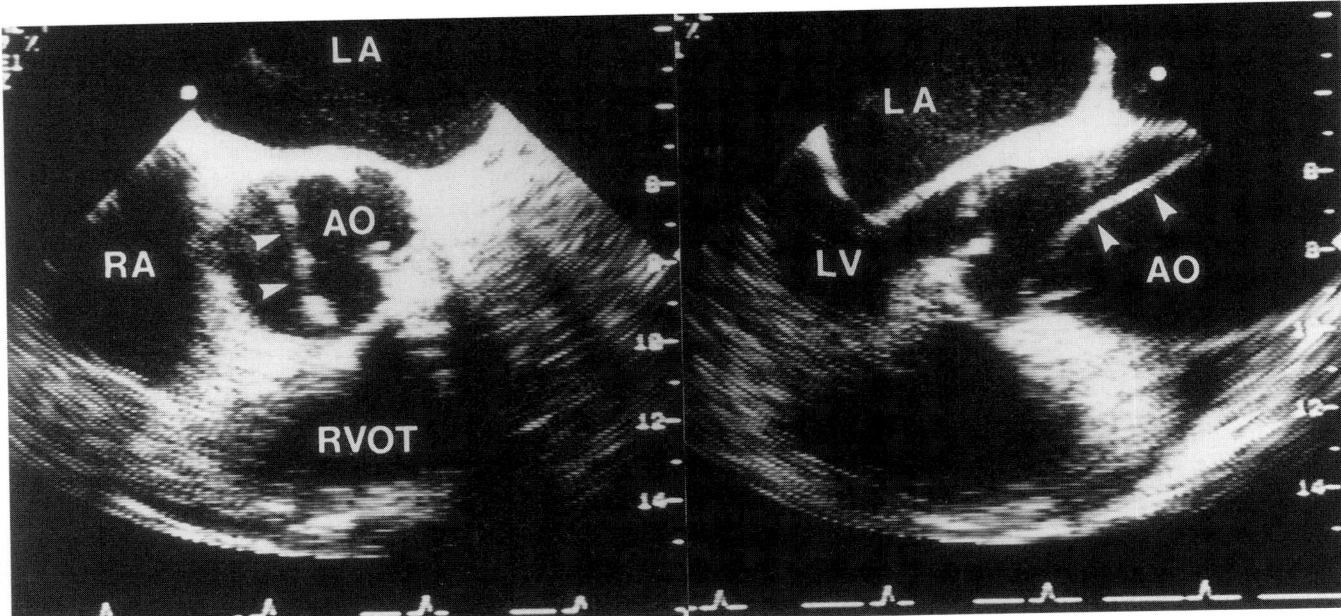

FIGURE 45–6 Transesophageal echocardiogram showing the dissection membrane (arrows) in the short (left panel) and long (right panel) views of a type A dissection.

such as varices, stricture, or tumor. A full stomach or recent meal are relative contraindications, but recognition of these conditions permits safe examination with few complications in the vast majority of patients. Criteria for making the diagnosis of acute aortic dissection include visualization of an echogenic surface separating two distinct lumens, repeatedly, in more than one view, and which can be differentiated from normal surrounding cardiac structures. The true lumen is identified by expansion during systole and collapse in diastole. Communication of the false lumen is found by identifying distal tears in the flap and flow in the false lumen with the addition of color Doppler; similarly, the absence of flow indicates false lumen thrombosis. TEE additionally may provide high-quality images of the aortic valve and pericardial space. The coronary ostia are directly evaluated and regional left ventricular function may be assessed to identify myocardial ischemia indirectly. Color flow Doppler reliably quantifies aortic regurgitation and may be used to assess for additional valvular abnormalities. The pericardium and pleural space are also visualized and therefore effusions may be identified.

Transthoracic echocardiography provides images of the ascending aorta and sections of the aortic arch that may yield the diagnosis but with much less sensitivity than transesophageal imaging. As such, transthoracic imaging may prove useful but is generally insufficient to reliably establish the diagnosis. Transthoracic evaluation is additionally limited by patient-related factors including body habitus, emphysema, and mechanical ventilation. A negative transthoracic study should be complemented by a transesophageal study, which provides greater detail of the entire aorta.

Aortography was the first study used to diagnose acute dissection in 1939 and until recently was considered the gold standard for diagnosis. It is an invasive test requiring nephrotoxic contrast media in which the aorta is visualized

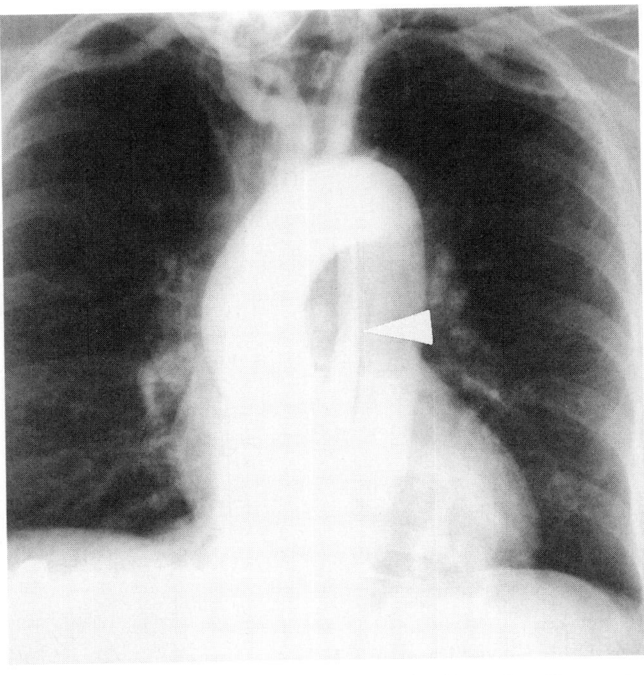

FIGURE 45–7 Aortogram of acute type B dissection illustrating differential contrast enhancement of the true and false lumens in the descending thoracic aorta. The intimal flap (arrowhead) can be seen separating the two lumens.

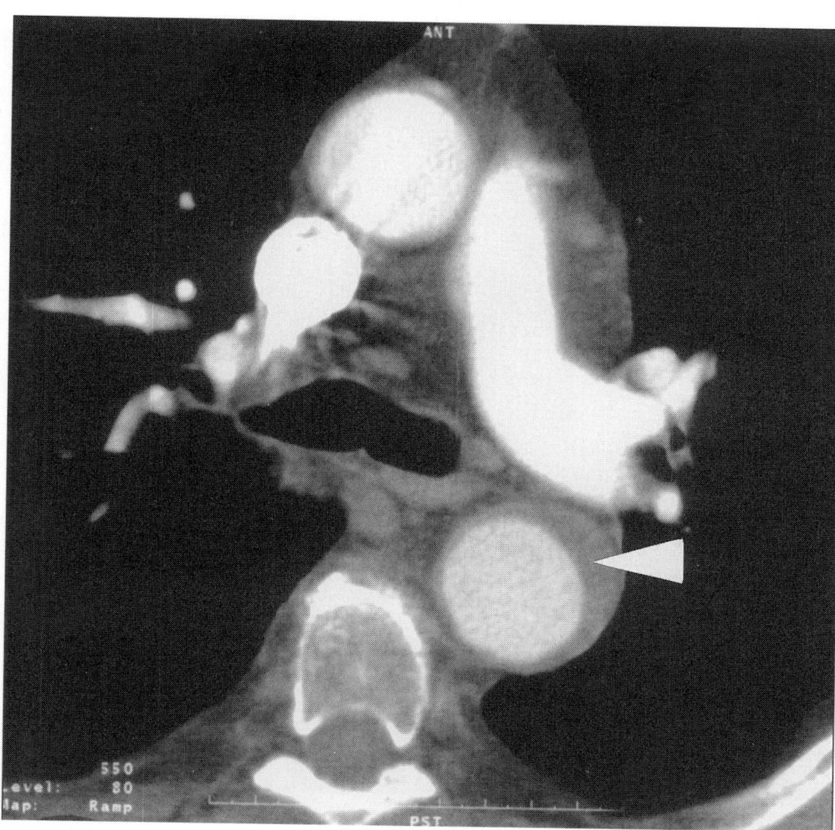

FIGURE 45–8 Axial image from CT arteriogram showing an intramural hematoma of the descending thoracic aorta (arrowhead).

in multiple two-dimensional projections. The diagnosis of dissection depends upon visualization of the intimal flap, two distinct lumens, or compression of the true lumen by flow through an adjacent false lumen (Fig. 45-7). Indirect signs of dissection include the presence of branch vessel abnormalities and abnormal intimal contour on injection of the false lumen. The status of the aortic valve may be evaluated and coronary angiography in the setting of type A dissections is possible only with this diagnostic test. Coronary angiography is, however, not recommended given that the coronary ostia are involved in 10% to 20% of acute type A dissections and are easily evaluated at the time of surgery. Coronary atherosclerosis is present in 25% of all patients with acute aortic dissection, but even in those patients repair of the dissection should take precedence. Aortography is sometimes useful in acute type B dissections with evidence of mesenteric ischemia or oliguria and in type A dissection with signs of malperfusion because catheter-based intervention may be possible. Aortography may yield false-negative results with thrombosis of one lumen or when contrast equally opacifies each lumen, impairing distinction of a separate true and false lumen. The diagnosis of intramural hematoma may also be difficult given the absence of intimal disruption, while penetrating atherosclerotic ulcer is usually easily visualized. Visualization of the dissection variants is best with either CT scanning or MRI (Figs. 45-8 and 45-9). One major limitation to the use of aortography in the acute setting is the need for skilled personnel. The time required to assemble this team varies with each institution, rendering aortography less useful when compared to other immediately available diagnostic tests. Aortography also requires arterial access, which can be painful and precipitate rupture or dissection extension.

Intravascular ultrasound is a catheter-based imaging tool that provides dynamic imaging of the aortic wall and an intimal flap in patients with aortic dissection. It is particularly useful in delineating the proximal and distal extent of dissection and for identifying the true and false lumens in questionable cases during aortography. High-resolution images of the normal three-layered aortic wall are differentiated to identify the abnormally thin wall adjacent to the false lumen. Because the aortic wall itself is imaged, intramural hematoma and penetrating atherosclerotic ulcers may also be identified. Currently, as an isolated imaging study, it is time consuming and requires skilled personnel, as with aortography, and generally is not useful as an initial study in the acute setting. It may be most useful in combination with aortography when the initial imaging studies are negative yet there remains a high clinical suspicion of dissection.

Magnetic resonance imaging (MRI) and the newer contrast-enhanced magnetic resonance angiography generate superior images reliably demonstrating aortic dissection (Fig. 45-10). In fact, some consider this the "gold-standard"

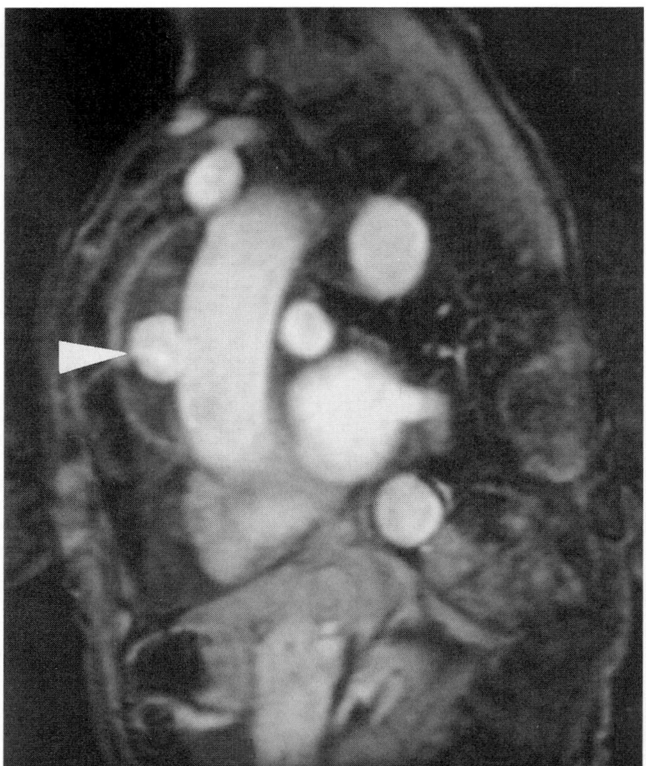

FIGURE 45–9 Sagittal contrast-enhanced MRI of penetrating atherosclerotic ulcer of the ascending aorta (arrowhead).

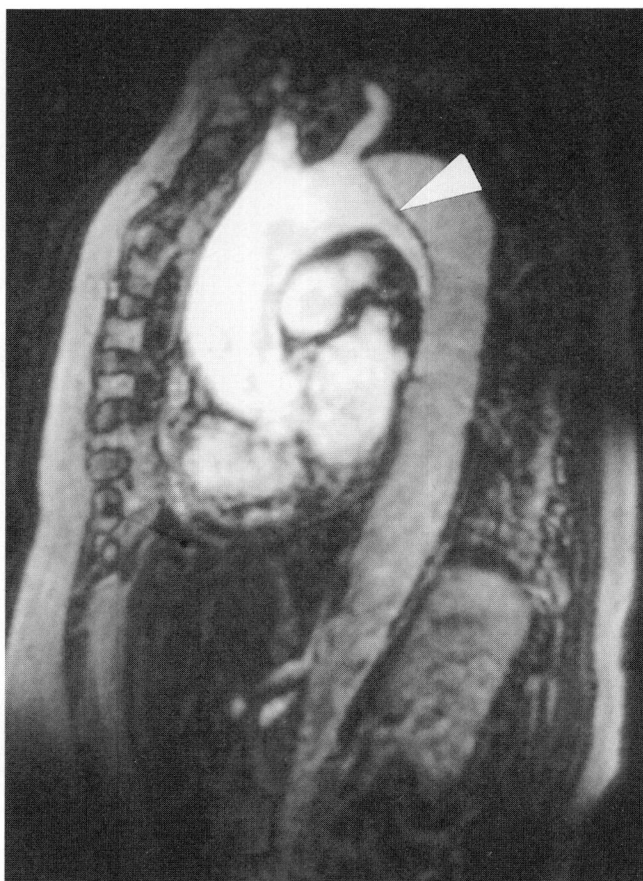

FIGURE 45–10 Sagittal contrast-enhanced magnetic resonance image of chronic type B dissection. The dissection flap (arrowhead) is clearly identified and the false lumen appears to extend the entire length of the thoracic and abdominal aorta (darker posterior lumen).

imaging study given the published diagnostic accuracy. Dissection is identified as an intralumenal membrane separating two or more channels (Fig. 45-11). MRI provides detailed images of the entire aorta, the pericardium, and pleural spaces similar to those obtained with CT. Cine imaging may also be used to evaluate left ventricular function, the status of the aortic valve, and flow in aortic branch vessels as well as flow in the false lumen. It is, however, not widely available and the presence of ferromagnetic metal contraindicates its use. Another disadvantage of MRI is that artifact is identified in up to 64% of studies, which underscores the need for expert radiologic interpretation of the images. These factors account for its infrequent use in the acute setting.

DIAGNOSTIC STRATEGY

The evaluation of suspected acute aortic dissection begins with a determination of the clinical likelihood that the diagnosis is correct and an evaluation of the hemodynamic stability of the patient. The unstable patient should undergo ECG to rule out acute coronary syndrome and be transferred immediately to the operating room. Medical management may be initiated as soon as the diagnosis is suspected. It is our practice to intubate and mechanically ventilate such patients while essential monitoring lines are placed. A transesophageal echocardiogram is then performed. If TEE fails to reveal acute aortic dissection, a hemodynamically unstable patient will then have a protected airway and invasive monitoring lines for subsequent evaluation of alternative diagnoses and continued resuscitation. If, however, acute dissection is suspected despite a negative TEE, CT arteriogram or aortography (potentially with intravascular ultrasound) is the next study of choice.

Clinically and hemodynamically stable patients permit a more detailed history and physical examination with imaging decisions tailored to specific aspects of the presentation. At the University of Virginia, such patients are first evaluated with a CT arteriogram. A CT scanner is located in the emergency room and these data may be obtained in less than 15 minutes. If that study is negative yet the diagnosis still entertained, transesophageal echocardiography is performed. In a recent review, an average of 1.8 imaging studies was used to correctly diagnose acute aortic dissection.[12] Although TTE is a relatively insensitive study (especially in the descending thoracic aorta), patients with suspected acute type A dissection may first undergo that study. If

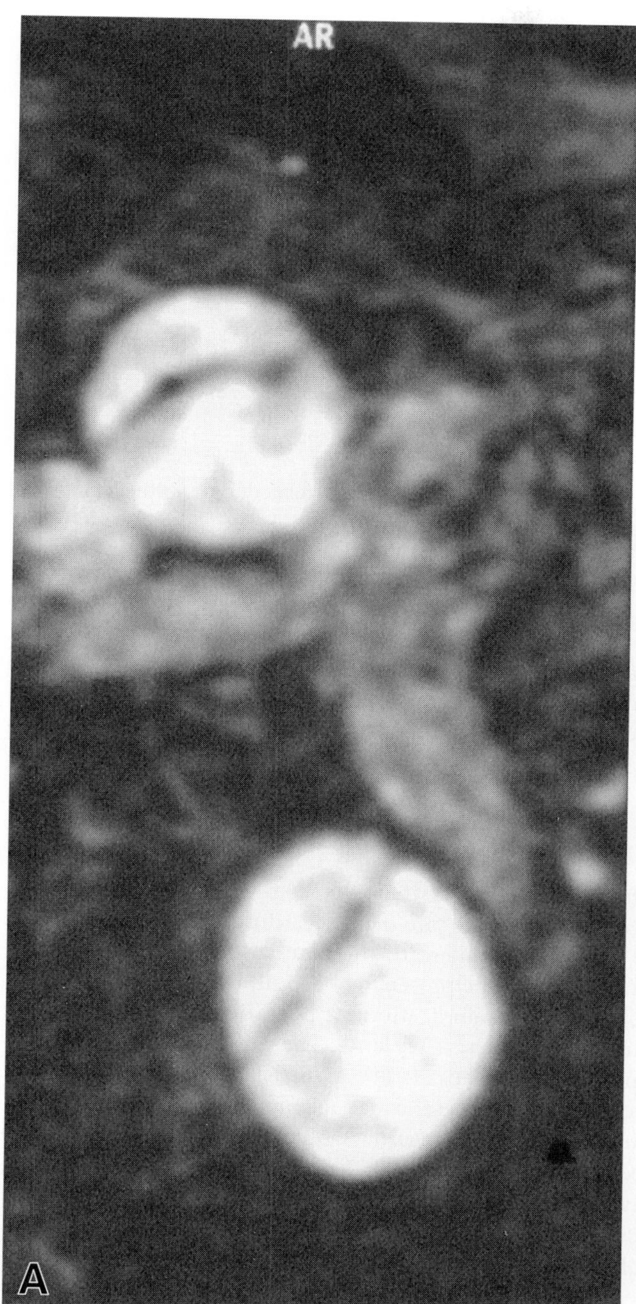

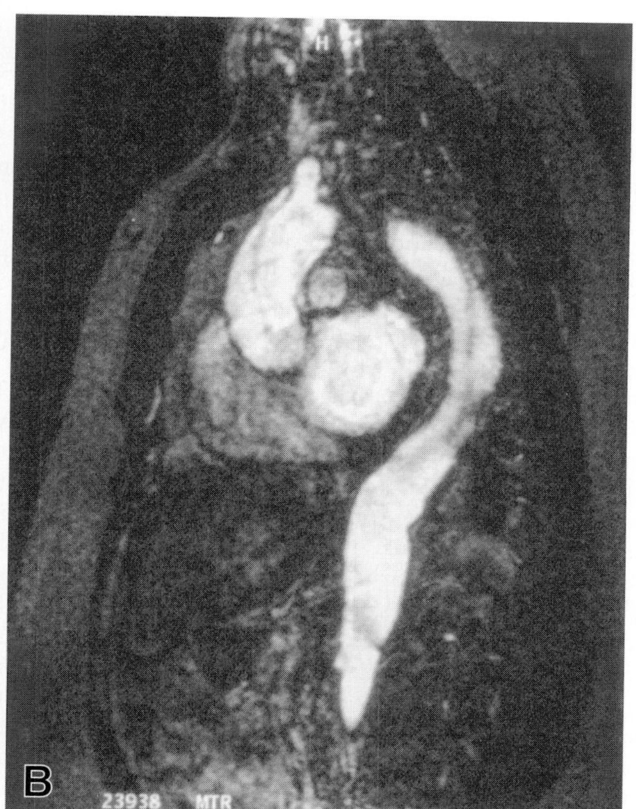

FIGURE 45–11 Axial (A) and sagittal (B) contrast-enhanced magnetic resonance images of a chronic type A dissection.

positive, subsequent confirmation using TEE may be performed in the operating room to expedite surgical management; if negative, either CT scanning or TEE performed in the ICU is appropriate.

Natural History

Fifty percent of patients suffering acute type A aortic dissection are dead within 48 hours.[16] A conventional wisdom has evolved that acute type A dissection carries a "1% per hour" mortality. Newer data, however, reveal a different prognosis such that medical management may be considered in certain high-risk groups. In one such study, type A dissection was managed medically in 28% of patients for various reasons with a 58% in-hospital mortality.[17] Regardless, this relatively high mortality demonstrates that patients surviving acute type A dissection must be quickly and aggressively diagnosed and managed.

The natural history of acute type B dissection is difficult to determine primarily because early autopsy series failed to analyze these patients as a distinct group. As a result, most of the studies estimate a 50% mortality for untreated acute type B dissection. More contemporary data from Elefteriades et al, however, reveal a 9% initial hospital mortality for acute type B dissection with 66% of the remaining patients having no specific aortic complications requiring surgery.[18] These data are obviously influenced by modern medical treatment but speak to a more benign clinical course when compared to type A dissection.

Initial Medical Management

Recognizing the natural history of patients with aortic dissection dictates that management occurs as part of the initial diagnostic evaluation. The initial patient encounter therefore focuses as much on making the diagnosis as in identifying factors that require immediate treatment. The site of this initial evaluation and resuscitation is determined primarily by the hemodynamic stability of the patient. The unstable patient belongs in the operating room, whereas a more detailed diagnostic approach from which management follows on an urgent basis can be undertaken in stable patients. Therefore, the hypotensive patient who may be hypovolemic as a result of blood loss into the thorax or pericardium undergoes the aforementioned evaluation and resuscitation on transfer to the operating room. It is preferable to avoid procedures such as transesophageal echocardiography or central line placement on an awake patient outside the operating room because hypertension resulting from patient discomfort may precipitate aortic rupture or propagation of dissection.

In the stable patient, blood pressure is measured in both arms and immediately treated to achieve a target systolic blood pressure between 90 and 110 mm Hg. Blood pressure control in hypertensive patients with pain should first be treated with narcotic analgesics. In general, the goals of hypertension management in acute aortic dissection are 2-fold.[8] First, aortic wall stress is lowered by decreasing the systolic blood pressure, which reduces the possibility of rupture. Second, shear stress on the aorta is decreased by minimizing the rate of rise of aortic pressure to decrease the likelihood of dissection propagation, so-called anti-impulse therapy. The drugs most commonly used for these purposes are sodium nitroprusside and esmolol. Sodium nitroprusside is a direct arterial vasodilator with a short onset and duration of action, which make it ideal to rapidly achieve the target systolic blood pressure. The rate of rise of aortic pressure, however, is increased when sodium nitroprusside is used alone. Esmolol is added to decrease the inotropic state of the myocardium and to decrease the heart rate. This drug is a beta-1 selective blocking agent with a short half-life that can easily be titrated to achieve the target blood pressure. Loading doses for esmolol and sodium nitroprusside should be avoided to prevent hypotension. Alternative beta-1 blocking drugs such as propranolol or metoprolol, and the combined alpha and beta blocker labetolol are appropriate in the subacute phase. Alternatively, calcium channel blockers may be necessary to reduce systolic blood pressure in those patients with a contraindication to beta-blocker use. There are, however, no compelling data supporting their efficacy in acute dissection.

TABLE 45–4 Operative indications for acute and chronic type A and B thoracic aortic dissections

Dissection type	Operative indication
Acute	
Type A	Presence
Type B	Rupture Malperfusion Progressive dissection Failure of medical management
Chronic	
Type A	Symptoms related to dissection (congestive failure, angina, aortic regurgitation, stroke, pain) Malperfusion Aneurysm
Type B	Symptoms related to dissection Malperfusion Aneurysm

Operative Indications

The goals of surgery in acute type A dissection are to prevent aortic rupture into the pericardium or pleural space and to avoid involvement of the coronary ostia or aortic valve (Table 45-4). The presence of ascending aortic involvement is, therefore, an indication for operative management in all but the highest-risk patients. The difficulty arises in determining which patients are high risk and which additional factors should affect the management algorithm. Patient age, for example, is not regarded as an absolute contraindication to surgery. This fact should perhaps be considered, however, given the few reported survivors of operative treatment for acute type A dissection greater than 80 years of age. Neurologic status at the time of presentation can also affect the decision to operate. While most agree that obtunded or comatose patients are unlikely to improve with surgical repair, complications such as stroke or paraplegia at the time of presentation are not contraindications to surgical correction. The status of the dissection should not be a factor; thrombosis of either lumen occurs but these patients remain at risk for lethal complications and surgery is indicated. Similarly, patients with subacute type A dissection who present or are referred longer than 2 weeks following the event require operation. Scholl et al demonstrated that these patients have avoided the early complications of dissection and may safely undergo elective operation rather than emergency repair.[19]

The goals of surgical management of complicated acute type B dissection are the prevention of free rupture and perfusion of end organs in the absence of symptoms. The most frequent causes of death in acute type B dissection are aortic rupture and visceral malperfusion. These, however, occur much less frequently with medical management than do complications of acute type A dissection treated nonoperatively. Between 70% and 80% of patients with acute type B dissection survive the acute and subacute phases with medical management alone. Such success with medical management has traditionally relegated surgical treatment for acute type B dissections to the complications of medical management or progression of disease (see Table 45-4). The indications for repair include contained or free aortic rupture, acute aortic expansion, malperfusion syndrome, pain or progression of dissection despite maximal medical management, and failure of medical management to control hypertension. Although medical management of acute type B dissection is the rule in most centers, some centers advocate immediate surgical intervention in selected patients with uncomplicated acute type B dissection. Factors which may favor early operation in acute type B dissection are the presence of Marfan syndrome, a large false aneurysm, arch involvement, and presumed medical compliance issues.[20] As in acute type A dissection, acute paralysis does not contraindicate surgery because patients can have remarkable improvement following revascularization.

There is some debate regarding the treatment of patients diagnosed with intramural hematoma and penetrating atherosclerotic ulcer. Recent data regarding the natural history of these dissection variants have made the issue less confusing. Intramural hematoma may lead to acute rupture in up to 35% of patients, whereas regression or no change in the hematoma is seen in the majority of medically managed patients surviving the initial period. Similarly, patients with penetrating atherosclerotic ulcer were found to have a 42% rate of acute rupture.[21] As a result of these relatively high acute rupture rates, the Yale group currently recommends early operative intervention for intramural hematoma and penetrating ulcer involving the ascending aorta. In the descending aorta, medical management with anti-impulse therapy and a low threshold for operative intervention result in the lowest mortality. These patients require continuous observation and repeat diagnostic imaging after 3 to 5 days in the hospital to monitor the lesion.

Operative Technique

ANESTHESIA AND MONITORING

Anesthesia used during the repair of aortic dissections is often narcotic-based with inhalational agents for maintenance. Single-lumen endotracheal tubes are used for procedures performed through a median sternotomy while double-lumen endotracheal tubes are useful but not mandatory for procedures performed through a left thoracotomy. Monitoring lines often include central venous access with a pulmonary artery catheter and one or more arterial pressure monitoring lines specific to the operation performed. One or two radial arterial lines and at least one femoral line are required to ensure adequate perfusion of the upper and lower body. All patients require a transesophageal echocardiography probe for various reasons. Core body temperature is monitored in the bladder using a Foley catheter and in the esophagus using a nasopharangeal probe. A wide skin preparation to include the axillary and femoral arteries is essential to provide all possible cannulation options.

HEMOSTASIS

Surgical procedures for aortic dissection can be associated with significant blood loss. Strict blood conservation is an important aspect of the operation and at least one cell-saver device should be available. Packed red blood cells, platelets, and fresh frozen plasma should be in the operating room at the start of the operation. Coagulopathy as a result of the preoperative status of the patient, cardiopulmonary bypass, and deep hypothermic circulatory arrest contribute to excessive blood loss. Improvements in vascular graft material have all but eliminated this as a reason for intra- and postoperative blood loss. Antifibrinolytic drugs such as epsilon-aminocaproic acid and aprotinin are useful hemostatic adjuncts. Aprotinin is particularly useful when used in either the full or one-half Hammersmith regimen and is most effective when administered prior to the operation. In cases where deep hypothermic circulatory arrest is used, aprotinin is administered in our practice only after the period of circulatory arrest. Patients will often require transfusion of fresh frozen plasma, platelets, and possibly cryoprecipitate. Fibrin glues and hemostatic materials such as Surgicel and Gelfoam are useful as systemic coagulopathy is corrected.

CARDIOPULMONARY BYPASS

There are various options for arterial and venous cannulation sites based upon the type of dissection. Arterial cannulation of the uninvolved distal aortic arch is preferable in acute type A dissection. Cannulation of the true lumen of the dissected ascending aorta is possible and can be accomplished quite easily using the Seldinger technique over a long wire introduced and guided by transesophageal echocardiography. Alternative sites include the right subclavian and the innominate artery for antegrade perfusion, or either femoral artery with retrograde aortic perfusion. In any case of retrograde aortic perfusion, it is essential to monitor proximal perfusion with a functioning radial arterial catheter.

There is debate over which femoral artery to cannulate in the setting of lower extremity malperfusion with a pulse deficit. Dissection of the abdominal aorta often leaves the left femoral artery originating from the false lumen and therefore cannulation of the right femoral artery will most often perfuse the true lumen. Perfusion of the false lumen can cause retrograde dissection and malperfusion of aortic branch vessels arising from the true lumen. In that event, cardiopulmonary bypass should be stopped for aortic cannulation through an alternative site to achieve whole body perfusion. If the chest has been opened, direct cannulation of the ascending aorta is often successful when guided by transesophageal echocardiography. An alternative cannulation technique is through the left ventricular apex and aortic valve. The cannula is then held in position with an ascending aortic tourniquet. Fortunately, there are usually multiple reentry tears throughout the dissection flap which permit perfusion of both lumen regardless of the lumen cannulated.

Venous cannulation is most often through the right atrium using a two-stage venous cannula, while bicaval cannulation is reserved for certain cases in which retrograde cerebral perfusion is preferred during circulatory arrest. A left ventricular vent is necessary in the setting of aortic valve incompetence and is easily placed through the right superior pulmonary vein or rarely through the left ventricular apex wall. Cardioplegia is administered retrograde through a coronary sinus catheter with additional protection via direct cannulation of the undissected coronary ostia.

The formerly popular "clamp and sew" technique used for repair of acute type B dissection has largely been replaced by the use of partial left heart bypass. Arterial cannulation sites for this technique include the distal thoracic aorta for limited dissections of the proximal descending thoracic aorta or the femoral artery for those extending into the abdomen. Venous drainage of oxygenated blood is through the left inferior pulmonary vein or the left atrium via the appendage when accessible. This technique does not require an oxygenator or pump suction and therefore the dose of heparin (100 U/kg) is less than with full cardiopulmonary bypass.

CEREBRAL PROTECTION

Surgical repair of aortic dissection involving the arch requires disruption of adequate blood flow to the brain during a period of circulatory arrest. Cerebral protection during that period is paramount and may be achieved through either deep hypothermia with cessation of electrical activity or some form of continued cerebral perfusion. Deep hypothermia during circulatory arrest was the first method used to perform operations on the aortic arch and remains an effective method for shorter procedures. Generally, periods of circulatory arrest up to 14 minutes are acceptable at 25°C, and periods up to 31 minutes appear to result in only transient neurologic sequelae at 15°C in a small number of patients.[22] Specifically, the risk of transient neurologic dysfunction on cognitive testing following a period of circulatory arrest is roughly 10% at less than 30 minutes, but increases to 15% at 40 minutes, 30% at 50 minutes, and 60% at 60 minutes.[23]

It is critical to correctly estimate brain temperature for expected outcome. Nasopharyngeal and tympanic temperatures are measured to estimate brain temperature but are imperfect. For that reason, some groups use electroencephalographic silence to determine the appropriate point at which to discontinue cooling and perfusion. Slow systemic cooling on cardiopulmonary bypass (20-25 minutes) while maintaining a maximal temperature gradient between perfusate and patient of less than 10°C is ideal. The head is then packed in ice to maintain a low brain temperature. While cooler temperatures increase the safe interval of circulatory arrest, cooling to lower than 15°C may result in a form of nonischemic brain injury and is therefore not recommended. Methylprednisolone and thiopental administration during cooling are adjunctive measures thought by some to decrease cerebral metabolic requirements during the period of circulatory arrest, but we currently do not use either. Reinstitution of cardiopulmonary bypass with systemic rewarming following repair proceeds without exceeding a 10°C temperature gradient to at least 37°C as core body temperature often falls briefly after cessation of active warming and separation from cardiopulmonary bypass. Furosemide and mannitol are administered to initiate diuresis and to promote free radical scavenging following circulatory arrest.

Continued cerebral perfusion during the period of circulatory arrest is an alternative technique for cerebral protection. Cerebral blood flow may be delivered in either a retrograde or antegrade fashion. The technique for retrograde cerebral perfusion depends upon the venous cannulation strategy. If bicaval cannulation is required, reversing flow through the superior vena caval cannula with a proximally placed tourniquet is simple and effective. Dual-stage venous cannulation requires placement of a retrograde coronary sinus catheter into the superior vena cava through a purse-string suture. Retrograde cerebral perfusion has the added benefit of flushing atherosclerotic material and air from the brachiocephalic vessels. A flow rate necessary to produce a superior vena caval pressure of 15 to 25 mm Hg is considered optimal. Selective antegrade cerebral perfusion has recently gained popularity. Once the aortic arch is open, the innominate artery and the left common carotid artery are encircled with vessel occluders and each lumen cannulated with a retrograde coronary sinus cannula. With the left subclavian artery occluded, flow rates are slowly increased to achieve perfusion pressures of 50 to 70 mm Hg at the desired circulatory arrest temperature. These cannulae are then removed just prior to completing the anastomosis of the brachiocephalic vessels to the vascular graft, at which time cardiopulmonary bypass may be reinstituted.

TECHNIQUES FOR TYPE A DISSECTION

The exposure for procedures performed on the ascending aorta and the proximal arch is through a median sternotomy.

This can be modified with supraclavicular, cervical, or trapdoor incisions to gain exposure to brachiocephalic vessels or the descending thoracic aorta. When dissecting the distal arch, it is important to identify and protect both the left vagus nerve with its recurrent branch and the left phrenic nerve. Replacement of the ascending aorta in type A dissections is best performed by an open distal anastomosis technique if the arch is involved (30%) or if arch involvement is unknown. The open distal anastomotic technique requires clamping the mid ascending aorta and cardiac arrest via administration of antegrade and/or retrograde cardioplegic solution. The dissected ascending aorta proximal to the clamp is then opened. Evaluation and surgical correction of the aortic valve is ideally performed at this time while systemic cooling continues. If dissection does not involve the aortic root, the aorta is transected 5 to 10 mm distal to the sinotubular ridge. If dissection involves the sinotubular ridge, the proximal aorta is reconstructed by reuniting the dissected aortic layers between one or two strips of Teflon felt using either 3.0 or 4.0 Prolene suture. Safi et al use a technique of interrupted pledgeted horizontal mattress sutures as compared to the felt sandwich technique. In their experience, this provides superior stabilization and decreases the potential for subsequent aortic stenosis. There has also been a great deal of enthusiasm for reuniting the dissected layers using gelatin-resorcinol-formalin (GRF) glue or the newer BioGlue (Cryolife International Inc., Kennesaw, GA). There are, however, concerns regarding each of the commercially available types of glue in that redissection and toxicity from constituents of the glue (formalin) have been reported.

Once the temperature reaches 18°C to 20°C, perfusion is discontinued during a brief period of circulatory arrest. The aortic clamp is released and the intima of the aortic arch is inspected and repaired accordingly (Fig. 45-12). If the intima is intact, the distal anastomosis is performed and the graft is cannulated, de-aired, and clamped for resumption of cardiopulmonary bypass with systemic warming. If the intima of the arch is violated, then a hemiarch reconstruction is performed (Fig. 45-13). We have only rarely found it necessary to perform a complete arch resection for an acute dissection. If a complex aortic root procedure is required, it is often useful to repair the aortic root with one vascular graft and use a separate graft to create the distal aortic anastomosis. The two grafts are then measured, cut, and anastomosed to provide the correct length and orientation for aortic replacement.

If the ascending aorta cannot be cross-clamped, the patient is cooled to 20°C with subsequent circulatory arrest. The distal aortic reconstruction is performed first in this circumstance, at which time the graft is cannulated and proximally clamped with resumption of cardiopulmonary bypass and systemic rewarming. Cannulation of the graft for antegrade systemic perfusion and rewarming is associated with improved neurologic outcome compared to retrograde perfusion and should be performed whenever possible. Newly available vascular grafts include 7- to 8-mm Dacron side-arm grafts for easy cannulation to facilitate this technique. Because a cross-clamp is not applied, the left ventricle must be decompressed once fibrillation starts during systemic cooling (approximately 20°C) to prevent distension and irreversible myocardial injury. Proximal ascending aortic repair is completed during the period of rewarming.

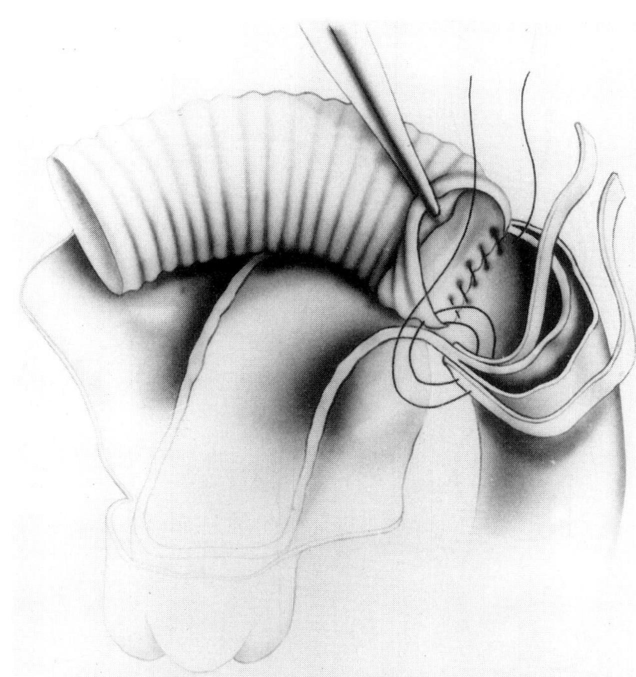

FIGURE 45–12 The false lumen of the distal aorta is closed and the aortic wall is reconstructed with inside and outside felt strips. *(Reproduced with permission from Stone C, Borst H: Dissecting aortic aneurysm, in Edmunds LJ Jr (ed): Cardiac Surgery in the Adult. New York, McGraw-Hill, 1997; p 1125.)*

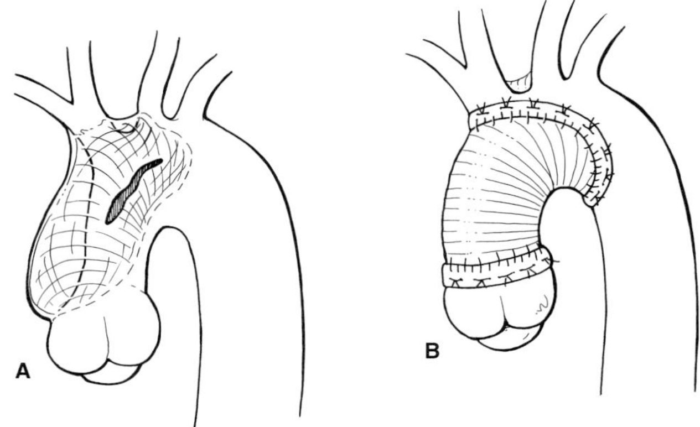

FIGURE 45–13 (A) The type A dissection extends into the proximal aortic arch. (B) The distal dissected aortic wall is reconstructed with inside and outside felt strips to replace part of the arch and ascending aorta. *(Reproduced with permission from Stone C, Borst H: Dissecting aortic aneurysm, in Edmunds LJ Jr (ed): Cardiac Surgery in the Adult. New York, McGraw-Hill, 1997; p 1125.)*

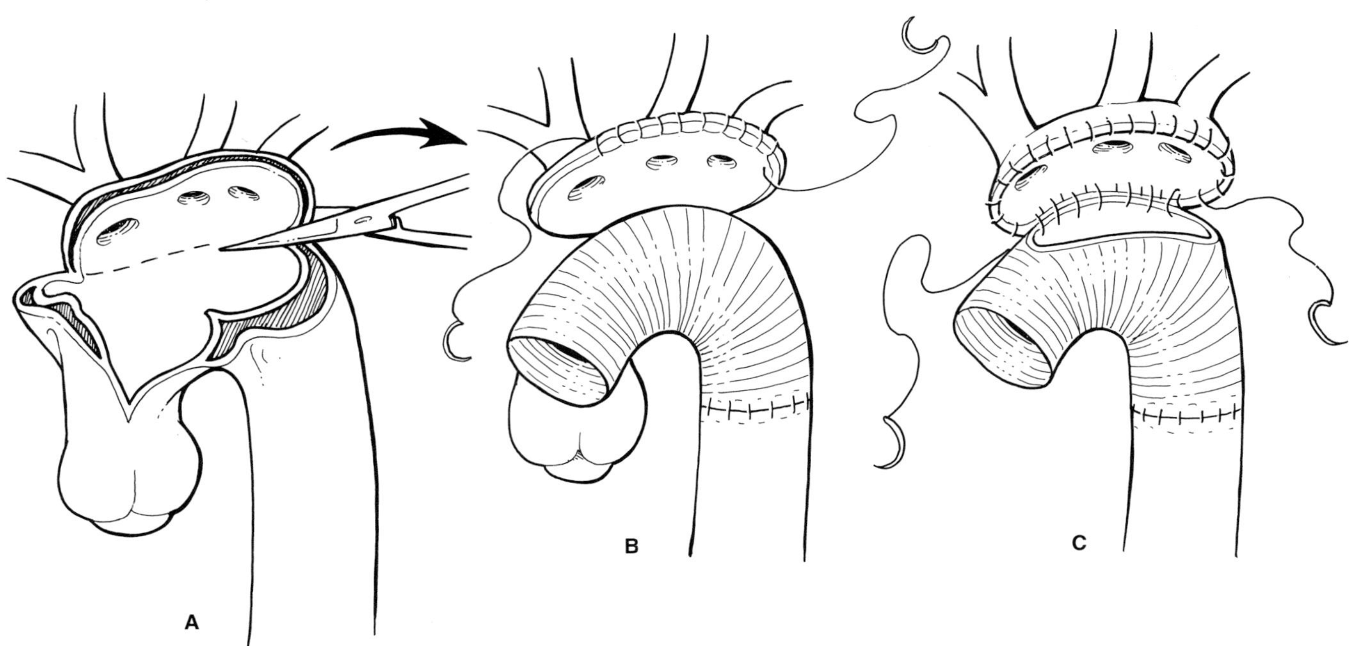

FIGURE 45–14 Brachiocephalic vessels can be reattached to an arch graft as a unit if the inner cylinder of origin of each vessel remains intact. (A) The arch vessels are excised as a unit from the superior surface of the dissected aortic arch. (B) The separated layers of the brachiocephalic patch are reunited using inner and outer felt strips and continuous suture. (C) A corresponding hole is cut into the aortic graft and the brachiocephalic unit is sutured into place. (*Reproduced with permission from Stone C, Borst H: Dissecting aortic aneurysm, in Edmunds LJ Jr (ed): Cardiac Surgery in the Adult. New York, McGraw-Hill, 1997; p 1125.*)

An alternative to the open distal technique is possible when dissection is limited to the ascending aorta or the proximal arch away from the origin of the brachiocephalic vessels. Antegrade arterial perfusion is achieved through distal arch or right subclavian artery cannulation; retrograde perfusion via cannulation of a femoral artery has traditionally provided acceptable results. An aortic cross-clamp is applied tangentially just proximal to the innominate artery. The ascending aorta is resected to include the inferior aspect of the arch. The layers of the dissected aorta proximal to the clamp are then reunited if necessary and the ascending aorta replaced with an appropriately sized, beveled vascular graft. The proximal reconstruction and anastomosis may then be performed and the entire procedure performed without requiring deep hypothermia and circulatory arrest.

Isolated dissection of the aortic arch is rare. Classified as a type A dissection, it requires resection of the arch at the site of intimal disruption and aortic replacement. Surgical management of the brachiocephalic vessels is determined by the integrity of the adjacent intima. If intact, the brachiocephalic vessels are reimplanted as a Carrel patch into a vascular graft after repair (Fig. 45-14). If the dissection involves individual vessels, each may require repair and reimplantation individually into the graft used for arch replacement (Fig. 45-15).

Aortic root dissection often fails to violate the intima of the coronary ostia. Repair of the ascending aorta at the sinotubular junction is therefore sufficient to reunite the aortic root layers and provide uninterrupted coronary blood flow. Minimal disruption of the coronary ostial intima should be repaired primarily with 5-0 or 6-0 Prolene suture. If, however, the ostium is circumferentially dissected and an aortic root replacement is necessary, an aortic button should be excised and the layers reunited with running 5-0 Prolene suture, glue, or both. Coronary buttons are then reimplanted into the vascular graft or to a separate 8-mm vascular graft as part of a Cabrol repair (Fig. 45-16). Aortocoronary bypass grafting is performed only when the coronary ostium is not reconstructable and as a last resort.

Acute type A dissection is complicated by aortic valve insufficiency in up to 75% of patients. Fortunately, preservation of the native valve is successful nearly 85% of the time. The mechanism of aortic insufficiency in most cases is the loss of commissural support of the valve leaflets. This is repaired using pledgeted 4-0 Prolene sutures to reposition each of the commissures at the sinotubular ridge (Fig. 45-17). The dissected aortic root layers are then reunited using 3-0 Prolene suture and either one or two strips of Teflon felt. Bioglue is placed between the layers prior to suture repair of the sinotubular ridge to buttress the repair and reform the sinuses of Valsalva. Aortic valve preservation must always be performed using intraoperative transesophageal echocardiography to assess the valve postoperatively. No more than mild

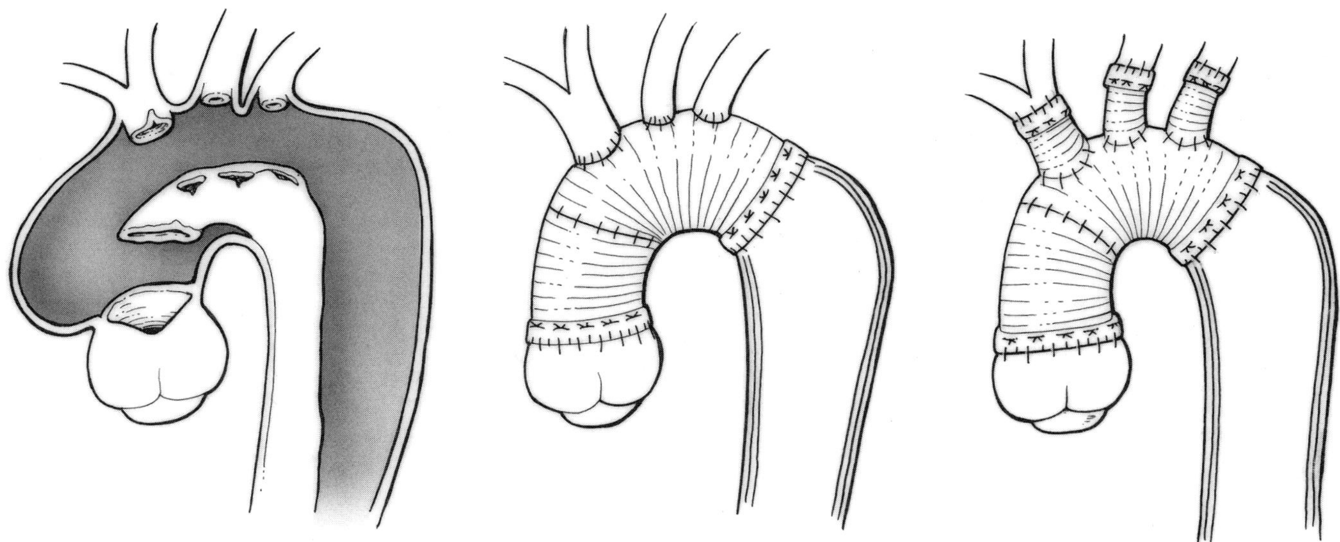

FIGURE 45–15 **The brachiocephalic vessels are separated from the true lumen by the dissected false lumen (left panel). If individual brachiocephalic vessels also are damaged beyond repair, short, interposition grafts are added to reconnect each artery to the aortic graft (right panel).** *(Reproduced with permission from Stone C, Borst H: Dissecting aortic aneurysm, in Edmunds LJ Jr (ed): Cardiac Surgery in the Adult. New York, McGraw-Hill, 1997; p 1125.)*

aortic insufficiency should be present. In addition to commissural resuspension, techniques exist to spare the aortic valve and replace the aortic root in acute type A dissection, but the experience is early and the number of patients few. This topic is covered in greater detail in the section on surgical techniques for chronic type A dissection.

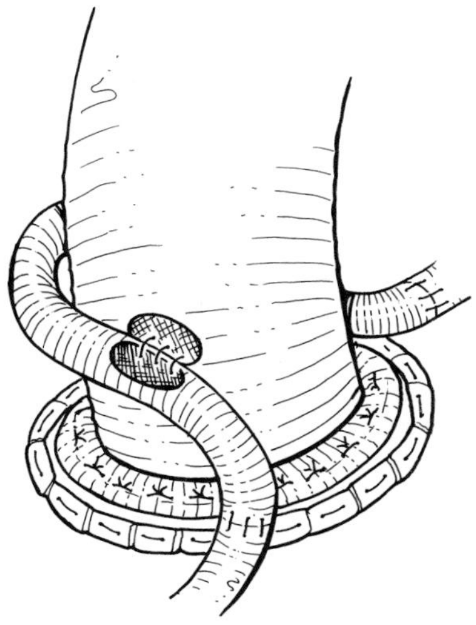

FIGURE 45–16 **Illustration showing attachment of the coronary ostia to the graft using the Cabrol technique. The ends of a 60-mm Dacron graft are sewn end-to-end to each coronary ostium. A side-to-side anastomosis is made between the intercoronary tube graft and the aortic graft.** *(Reproduced with permission from Stone C, Borst H: Dissecting aortic aneurysm, in Edmunds LJ Jr (ed): Cardiac Surgery in the Adult. New York, McGraw-Hill, 1997; p 1125.)*

If the aortic valve cannot be spared, replacement of the ascending aorta and valve should be performed using a composite valve graft or homograft. The composite valve graft is implanted using horizontal mattress 2-0 Tycron sutures to encircle the annulus and to seat the valved conduit (Fig. 45-18). The previously excised and reconstituted coronary buttons are reimplanted into the vascular graft with running 5-0 Prolene suture (Fig. 45-19). The left coronary button is implanted first, at which time the graft is clamped and placed under pressure to define the proper orientation and position of the right coronary button. The aortic homograft is similarly implanted using horizontal mattress 2.0 Tycron sutures, except that a generous margin of aortic root below the coronary buttons is retained for a second hemostatic suture line of running 4-0 Prolene. This is an ideal solution for individuals who have a contraindication to anticoagulation or for young females. The Ross procedure (pulmonary autograft) is not applicable in those patients with connective tissue disorders and not recommended in acute dissection.

Endovascular stent grafting is currently under investigation as a definitive form of management in acute type B dissection and in conjunction with surgery for acute type A dissection. Long-term data and prospective comparisons to surgery will be necessary before percutaneous management can be recommended as an alternative to surgery.

TECHNIQUES FOR TYPE B DISSECTION

The right lateral decubitus position is optimal for surgical treatment of acute type B dissections requiring operation. The pelvis is canted posteriorly to allow access to both sets of

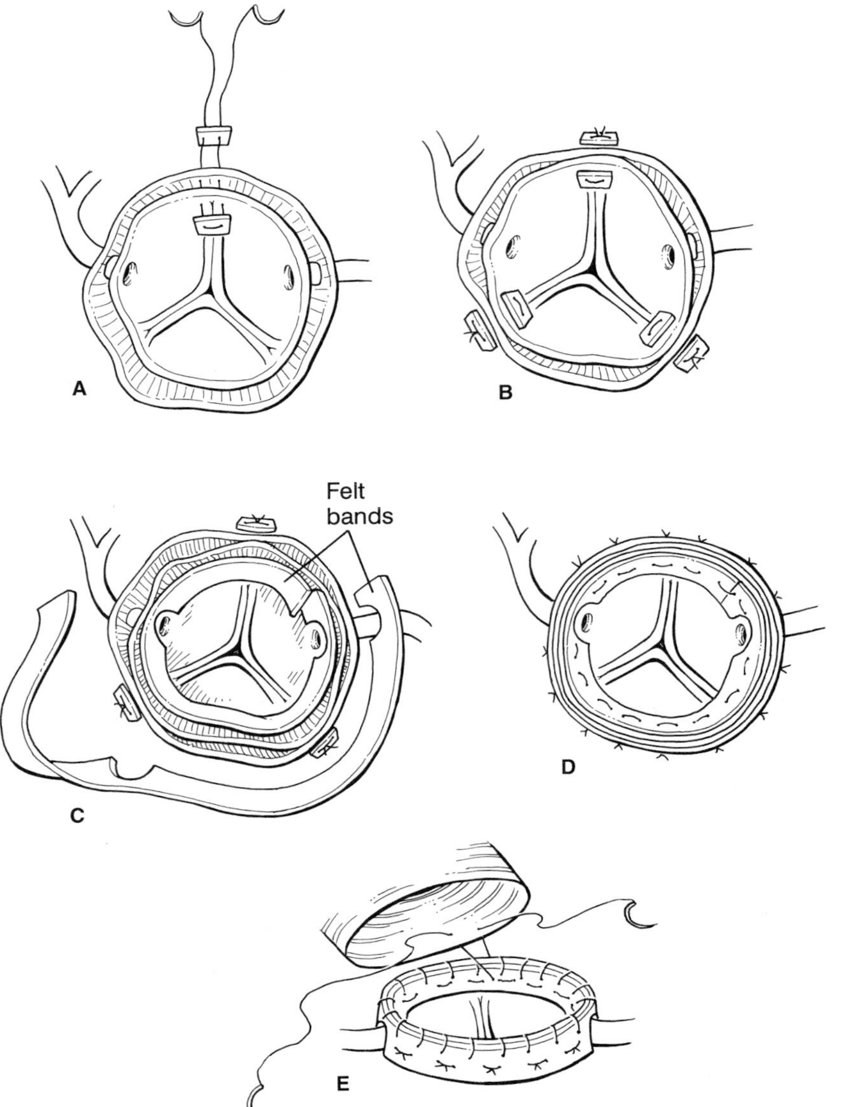

FIGURE 45–17 Resuspension and preservation of the native aortic valve in a type A dissection. The dissected layers are approximated at each commissure with double pledgeted mattress sutures. Completed resuspension of the aortic valve commissures. Thin felt strips (8-10 mm wide) are placed inside and outside around the circumference of the aorta. The coronary ostia are not compromised. The aortic walls are sandwiched between the felt strips with horizontal mattress sutures. A vascular graft is sutured to the reconstructed proximal aorta. (*Reproduced with permission from Stone C, Borst H: Dissecting aortic aneurysm, in Edmunds LJ Jr (ed): Cardiac Surgery in the Adult. New York, McGraw-Hill, 1997; p 1125.*)

femoral vessels. A posterolateral thoracotomy in the 4th intercostal space provides sufficient access to the aorta; notching the 5th and 6th ribs posteriorly permits visualization of the entire thoracic aorta distally. A thoracoabdominal incision may be required to access the abdominal aorta in the case of visceral malperfusion. This may be performed either through the abdomen or the retroperitoneum. The left hemidiaphragm must be carefully divided in a radial fashion while marking adjacent sites on each side of the division with metal clips. This provides all necessary exposure and facilitates subsequent diaphragm approximation at the end of the case.

The ideal operation for acute type B dissection is replacement of as little of the descending thoracic aorta as is necessary. The extent of replacement rarely exceeds the proximal third and includes the primary tear in most cases. Such a strategy optimizes preservation of intercostal arteries perfusing the spinal cord to combat an incidence of paraplegia that may be as high as 19% following surgery for acute type B dissections.[24] This point is controversial, however, and some groups advocate replacement of the entire thoracic aorta. Any less extensive aortic replacement leaves dissected aorta with the potential for late aneurysmal dilatation when there is perfusion of the false lumen. The ideal strategy to minimize spinal cord malperfusion yet resect all involved aorta has not been devised.

Once the thoracic aorta has been exposed, the operation continues with division of the mediastinum between the left subclavian and the left common carotid arteries. The left subclavian artery is encircled with an umbilical tape

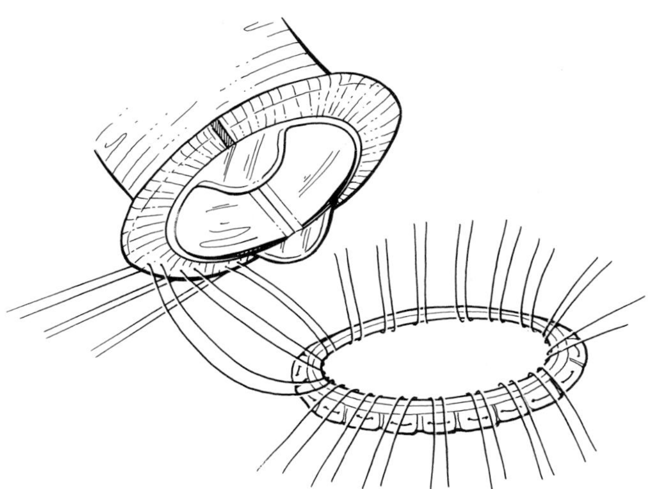

FIGURE 45–18 Everting 2-0 pledgeted mattress sutures are placed shoulder-to-shoulder around the aortic annulus to anchor a composite graft containing a St. Jude prosthesis. (*Reproduced with permission from Stone C, Borst H: Dissecting aortic aneurysm, in Edmunds LJ Jr (ed): Cardiac Surgery in the Adult. New York, McGraw-Hill, 1997; p 1125.*)

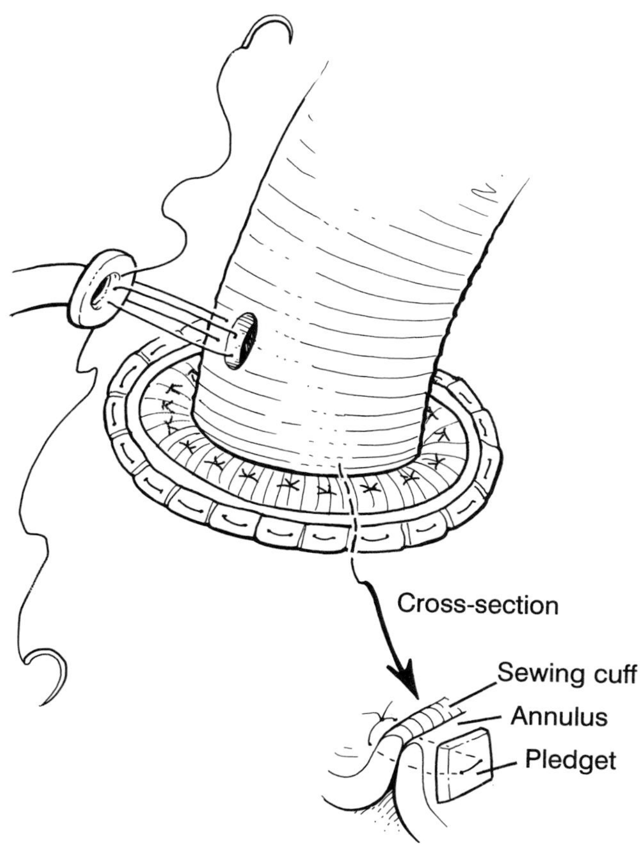

FIGURE 45–19 The coronary ostia are attached to the graft by the button technique using a continuous 5-0 Prolene suture. (*Reproduced with permission from Stone C, Borst H: Dissecting aortic aneurysm, in Edmunds LJ Jr (ed): Cardiac Surgery in the Adult. New York, McGraw-Hill, 1997; p 1125.*)

and Rommell tourniquet. It is essential that the left vagus and recurrent laryngeal nerves are identified and preserved during the course of the dissection. Ultimately, the entire distal arch must be free enough to place an aortic clamp between the left common carotid and left subclavian arteries. Next, the proximal descending thoracic aorta is circumferentially mobilized, dividing intercostal arteries in the segment to be excised. The left inferior pulmonary vein is then dissected and a 4-0 Prolene purse-string suture placed posteriorly to cannulate for partial left heart bypass. Following the administration of 100 U/kg of intravenous heparin, 14F cannulae are inserted into the left inferior pulmonary vein and either a normal appearing area of descending thoracic aorta or percutaneously into either femoral artery. Bypass is then initiated with flow rates between 1 and 2 L/min. The left subclavian artery is controlled and vascular clamps are placed on the aorta proximally and distally on the mid-thoracic aorta. Right radial artery pressure is measured to maintain proximal aortic systolic pressure between 100 and 140 mm Hg and mean femoral artery pressure greater than 60 mm Hg.[25] The aorta is then opened longitudinally and bleeding from intercostal arteries is controlled by suture ligation. Transection of the aorta distal to the origin of the left subclavian artery provides a site for the proximal anastomosis. This is performed using 3-0 Prolene suture and may require external reinforcement with Teflon felt strips.

The graft inclusion technique is another technique in which the posterior aspect of the proximal aorta is not fully transected. The proximal anastomosis is then made to the intact posterior aspect of the aorta. We do not recommend this technique since one cannot be certain of anastomosing all layers of the aorta. The size of the vascular graft is based on the diameter of the distal aorta and beveled to match the aorta proximally. This anastomosis may include the origin of the left subclavian to treat dissection in this vessel. A separate 6- to 8-mm Dacron graft can be used if there is intimal disruption involving the proximal segment of the left subclavian artery. Once the proximal anastomosis is complete, the proximal clamp is released and repositioned on the vascular graft to inspect the anastomosis. Attention is then turned to repairing the distal aorta with Teflon felt or glue. The distal anastomosis is completed, the clamps are released, and partial left heart bypass is terminated. Decannulation is routine except that percutaneously placed femoral artery cannulae 14F or smaller may be removed without direct repair. When cannulae larger than 15F are required, open surgical repair of the femoral arteriotomy is indicated.

Acute type B dissection extending into the abdominal aorta may be approached using total cardiopulmonary bypass and deep hypothermic circulatory arrest to prevent potential cerebral, spinal cord, and intra-abdominal organ ischemia.[26] After creation of a thoracoabdominal incision, the thoracic and abdominal aorta are exposed from the left subclavian artery to the aortic bifurcation. The femoral artery and vein are cannulated for cardiopulmonary bypass with systemic cooling. With the head packed in ice, cardiopulmonary bypass is then interrupted and the aorta opened proximally. The arch is repaired if necessary with Teflon felt or glue and the proximal anastomosis created. The graft is then clamped distal to the anastomosis and cannulated for proximal perfusion with resumption of cardiopulmonary bypass. Intercostal arteries to the upper third of the thoracic aorta are divided; larger vessels below T9 are reimplanted into the back of the graft with 4-0 Prolene suture. As vessels are reimplanted, the proximal clamp is moved distally to maximize spinal cord perfusion. Abdominal aortic branch vessels are divided from the wall of the aorta with a 5-mm cuff for reimplantation. Usually the right renal, superior mesenteric, and celiac arteries and adjacent intercostal and lumbar arteries are removed as a patch and reimplanted into the graft. The left renal artery often originates from a dissected segment of the aorta and is reimplanted individually after repair. The inferior mesenteric artery is often ligated as are bleeding lumbar vessels below L3. Intimal disruption of any abdominal aortic branch vessel requires repair with 5-0 Prolene suture prior to reimplantation. Once all side branches have been secured, the distal anastomosis to the aortic bifurcation is performed reuniting the aortic layers distally with Teflon felt or glue if necessary.

Rupture of the thoracic aorta prior to or during repair is a catastrophic event often leading to operative death. Successful management requires immediate cannulation of the femoral artery and vein for cardiopulmonary bypass and eventual deep hypothermic circulatory arrest, but only if the ruptured area can be locally controlled. Assisted venous drainage through the femoral vein is often adequate but direct cannulation of the right ventricle through the pulmonary artery may also be performed. A left atrial vent is placed through the left inferior pulmonary vein once the heart begins to fibrillate; the left ventricle may vented as well directly through the apex. Once the nasopharyngeal temperature reaches 15°C, the vent is occluded and cardiopulmonary bypass is stopped. The head is placed down and the aorta opened for repair under circulatory arrest. The distal aorta should be clamped to minimize blood loss. Once the proximal anastomosis is performed, the proximal clamp is moved onto the graft and the graft cannulated to resume cardiopulmonary bypass.

Spinal cord ischemia resulting in paraplegia or paraparesis is a recognized complication of acute dissection repair that may be partially preventable and even reversible. The incidence of spinal cord ischemia is between 19% and 36% following repair of acute type B dissection.[24,25] Whereas various strategies exist to prevent spinal cord ischemia during repair of chronic dissection, very few are feasible in the acute setting. Pharmacologic agents such as steroids, free radical scavengers, vasodilators, and adenosine are promising adjuncts to prevent spinal cord ischemia but presently have little to no proven clinical utility. We presently use left atrial to femoral artery bypass and reimplant key intercostals arteries and selectively use cerebrospinal fluid drainage as outlined by Safi et al.[27]

TABLE 45–5 Frequency and location of malperfusion in acute type A and B thoracic aortic dissection

Vascular system	Frequency
Renal	23%–75%
Extremities (upper and lower)	25%–60%
Mesenteric	10%–20%
Coronary	5%–11%
Cerebral	3%–13%
Spinal	2%–9%

MALPERFUSION SYNDROME

Malperfusion of aortic branch vessels may occur from the coronary ostia to the aortic bifurcation and may dominate the presentation of certain patients. Although autopsy series yield a greater percentage of patients with evidence of malperfusion, clinical series reveal that dissection is not infrequently complicated by malperfusion of at least one organ system (Table 45-5).[15,28] Compression of the true lumen by the false lumen is the mechanism by which aortic branch vessel occlusion occurs in the majority of cases. Branch vessels may also be completely sheared off the true lumen and perfused to various degrees by the false lumen. Malperfusion is most often treated with primary surgical repair of the dissection, but catheter-based or open fenestration is reappearing as a potentially more effective treatment.

Percutaneous fenestration and stenting are relatively new adjuncts to the surgical management of malperfusion syndromes. Renewed interest in these procedures grew from the recognition that hospital mortality of patients presenting with malperfusion was as high as 60%.[29] Surgical fenestration to treat malperfusion, however, reduced the mortality to under 20%.[30,31] Indications for percutaneous fenestration and endovascular stent placement were developed to treat malperfusion syndrome with the goal of improving outcome even further. Direct stenting of obstructed branch vessels and percutaneous fenestration with or without placement of a stent in the true lumen are the procedures most commonly performed. In certain situations, stents may be placed across an existing distal reentry tear to maintain patency and perfusion of the true lumen and the branch vessels. Balloon fenestration may be required to create such a communication between the lumen or to prevent thrombosis of the false lumen from which branch vessels may originate. Early results indicate that this procedure is both safe and effective, with restoration of flow in up to 90% of patients and an average 30-day mortality of 10% to 25%.[32,33] Given that the majority of postoperative mortality in patients with acute dissection and malperfusion is related to the duration of concomitant malperfusion, one strategy is percutaneous reperfusion followed by surgical repair.[34] Percutaneous treatment of malperfusion may also be performed following surgical repair of dissection but with less success in most reports.

The techniques used for surgical treatment of malperfusion depend upon location of the affected branch vessel but are generally quite similar. Malperfusion of the brachiocephalic vessels as a result of acute type A dissection is treated by repairing the dissection proximally if the intima is intact. If the intima is violated or if dissection extends into any brachiocephalic vessel, the artery should be resected from the arch, the layers reunited, and the vessel reimplanted into the arch, perhaps with an interposition vascular graft if necessary. Extra-anatomic bypass to the carotid arteries is an option in unreconstructable cases.

Malperfusion of the intra-abdominal viscera may be apparent at presentation but may also complicate surgical repair of acute type A or B dissections. Again, proximal repair of the dissection is standard treatment, but if this fails or if malperfusion persists despite repair, an additional procedure is necessary. Either open surgical or percutaneous fenestration of the dissection flap is necessary. Percutaneous fenestration is performed by pulling an inflated balloon or a fenestration knife through the dissection flap to create a communication between the two lumens. Surgical fenestration procedure is performed through a midline laparotomy or left flank incision to provide exposure of the infrarenal aorta (Fig. 45-20). Occasionally, fenestration of intra-abdominal aortic branch vessels may be required if the intima is violated beyond the ostia. If the dissection flap cannot be completely excised, the distal vessel layers must be reunited. Consideration should be given to patch angioplasty to prevent narrowing when closing smaller vessels. In the event that perfusion is not reestablished, extra-anatomic bypass may be required.

Obstruction of the terminal aorta or malperfusion of the lower extremities following operative repair is best treated with percutaneous fenestration. Surgical fenestration remains an option if percutaneous techniques fail to reestablish blood flow. In the event that surgical fenestration fails, the best solution is femoral-femoral bypass grafting in the setting of unilateral malperfusion or axillo-femoral and femoral-femoral bypass grafting if bilateral lower extremity malperfusion exists.

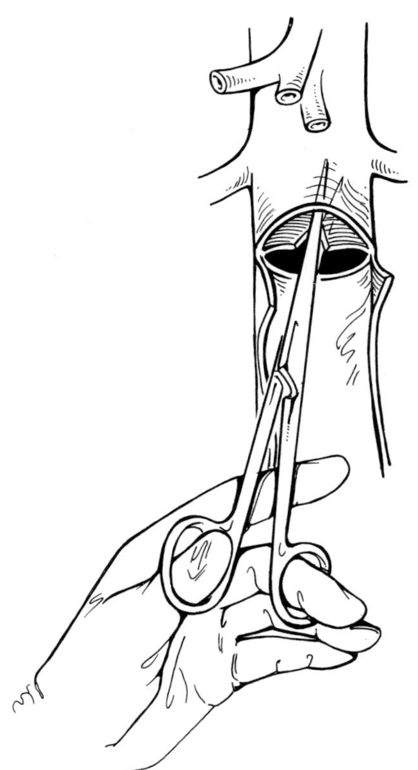

FIGURE 45–20 Fenestration of the abdominal aorta for visceral malperfusion. A transverse incision is made into the aorta, preferably into nondissected aorta. The proximal dissection membrane is incised and then excised to decompress the false lumen as far proximally as possible. The dissected layers are reconstructed with Teflon felt or glue and the aortotomy is closed directly. *(Reproduced with permission from Stone C, Borst H: Dissecting aortic aneurysm, in Edmunds LJ Jr (ed): Cardiac Surgery in the Adult. New York, McGraw-Hill, 1997; p 1125.)*

Postoperative Management

Invasive hemodynamic monitoring is used to ensure adequate end-organ perfusion with a target systolic blood pressure between 90 and 110 mm Hg. Early postoperative blood pressure control begins with adequate analgesia and sedation using narcotics and sedative/hypnotic agents. The patient should, however, be allowed to emerge from general anesthesia briefly for a gross neurologic examination. The patient is then sedated for a period to ensure continued hemodynamic stability and to facilitate hemostasis. Coagulopathy is aggressively treated with blood products and antifibrinolytic agents as necessary and by warming the patient. Hematocrit, platelet count, coagulation studies, and serum electrolytes are obtained and corrected as necessary. An ECG and chest radiograph are used to assess for abnormalities and to serve as baseline studies. A full physical exam including complete peripheral vascular exam is performed upon arrival. Despite adequate repair of the dissection, perfusion of the false lumen may persist and therefore malperfusion syndrome remains possible. If an abdominal malperfusion syndrome is suspected postoperatively, this should be aggressively evaluated with ultrasound and subsequent angiography if positive. A strong clinical suspicion is enough to warrant this evaluation given the consequences of failed recognition. In the morning, if the patient has been hemodynamically stable without excessive bleeding and the results of a neurologic exam are normal, the patient may be weaned from the ventilator and extubated. Management is routine from that point forward.

Long-term Management

Surviving the operation for acute dissection represents the beginning of a lifelong requirement for meticulous medical management and continued close observation. It has been estimated that replacement of the ascending aorta for type A dissection obliterates flow in the distal false lumen in fewer than 10% of patients. As a result, the natural history of repaired dissection may involve dilatation and potential rupture of the chronically dissected distal aorta. This was the reason for late death in nearly 30% of DeBakey's original series in 1982 and is currently the leading cause of late death following surgical repair.[35] Often a multidrug antihypertensive regimen including beta-blocking agents is required to maintain systolic blood pressure below 120 mm Hg. There are some data indicating that blood pressure control within a narrow range may alter the natural history of chronic dissection by diminishing the rate of aneurysmal dilatation. The long-term durability of the aortic valve following supracoronary reconstruction is quite good with freedom from aortic valve replacement of 80% to 90% at 10 years. Progressive aortic insufficiency of the native valve is, however, possible and should be followed with transthoracic echocardiography in some patients.

Follow-up diagnostic imaging is required to monitor aortic diameter in patients with chronic dissection. Spiral CT arteriogram and MRI are the imaging studies of choice. MRI and ultrasound are useful in patients with renal insufficiency and in those requiring only imaging of the abdominal aorta. Echocardiography is useful for imaging the ascending aorta and provides additional information regarding the aortic valve. It is important to recognize the resolution limitations of each imaging modality and inherent imprecision of comparing different imaging modalities to evaluate changes. In general, measurements should be made at the same anatomical level with respect to reproducible anatomical structures (i.e., the sinotubular ridge, proximal to the innominate or left subclavian arteries or at the diaphragmatic hiatus). It is important to recognize that the false lumen should be included in measurements of aortic diameter whether it is perfused or not. Three-dimensional reconstruction of spiral CT and MRI scans minimizes the error introduced by aortic eccentricity when comparing imaging studies and has simplified following this patient population. The current recommendations are to obtain a baseline study prior to hospital discharge and at 6-month intervals during the first year. If the aortic diameter remains unchanged at 1 year, studies are obtained yearly. Aortic enlargement of more than 0.5 cm within a 6-month period and greater eccentricity on comparison of 3-D reconstruction images are high-risk changes for which the interval is decreased to 3 months if surgery is not indicated.

Results

The operative mortality for repair of acute aortic dissection has fallen since DeBakey's original 40% mortality was reported in 1965. Improved ICU and floor care of these patients, earlier recognition of dissection through improved imaging modalities, development of hemostatic vascular graft material, more effective hemostatic agents, and improvements in the safety of cardiopulmonary bypass are likely responsible. In the last two decades, most centers consistently report an operative mortality for acute type A dissection of around 20%. The high early mortality in acute dissection parallels the number of patients who present profoundly hypotensive and in shock. The mode of death is stroke, myocardial ischemia/heart failure, or malperfusion in most cases. The operative mortality of patients suffering acute type B dissection (28%–65%) is higher than for type A dissection because the indications for surgery have traditionally been failure of medical management or complications of dissection as previously discussed.[18] The most recent data from a mulitcenter international registry, however, reveal that such a disparity in operative mortality between acute type A and B dissections may be disappearing. The mortality in that study was 27% for acute type A and 29% for acute type B dissection ($p = \text{NS}$).[36] Early death following acute dissection occurs as a result of aortic rupture or as a consequence of malperfusion.[7]

The published results for long-term survival following acute type A dissection surgically treated over the last decade is roughly 55% to 75% at 5 years and between 32% and 65% at 10 years.[37,38] Operative repair of acute type B dissection yields 5-year survival of 48% with a 10-year survival of 29%.[38]

CHRONIC AORTIC DISSECTION

Clinical Presentation

SIGNS AND SYMPTOMS

Chronic aortic dissection is usually asymptomatic. It may be incidentally discovered following an asymptomatic acute dissection; this most often occurs in patients with a preexisting aortic aneurysm. Some patients eventually require surgical treatment for chronic dissection and most do so as a result of aneurysmal dilatation of a chronically dissected aortic segment. Presenting complaints often include intermittent, dull chest pain or even severe skeletal pain from erosion into the bony thorax with large or rapidly expanding aneurysms. Aortic insufficiency may develop with chronic type A dissection

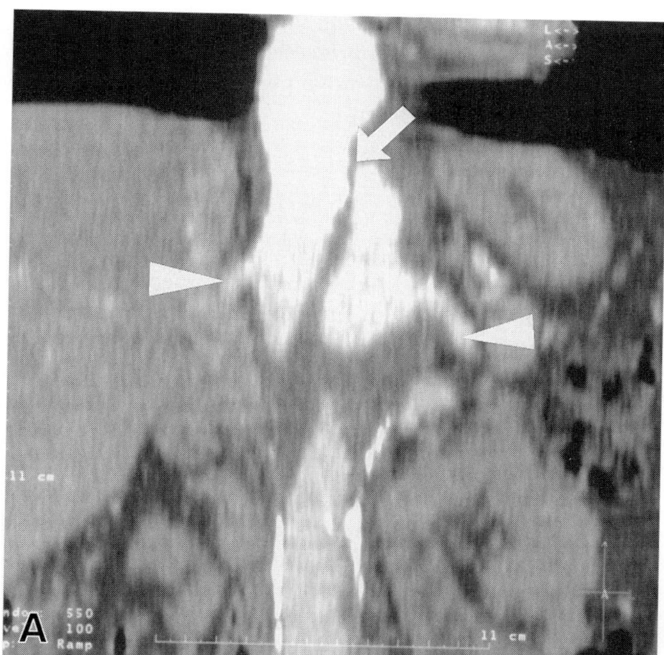

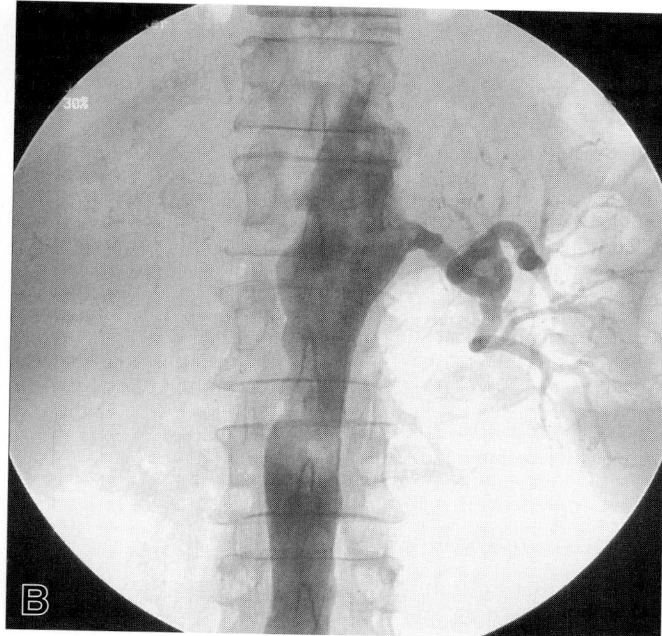

FIGURE 45–21 Coronal view of contrast enhanced MRI (A) demonstrating chronic type B dissection with renal arteries (arrowheads) separated by dissection flap (arrow). Aortogram (B) of the same patient revealing that each renal artery is perfused exclusively by either the true or false lumen. Such tests are often complementary and may influence surgical strategy.

and present with typical features of congestive failure including fatigue, dyspnea, and mild, dull chest pain. Infrequently, chronic dissection may result in paralysis/paraplegia from loss of vital intercostal arteries or even distal embolization of thrombus or atheroma from the false lumen. Malperfusion syndrome is an uncommon presentation for patients with chronic dissection given the likelihood that the true and false lumens communicate.

DIAGNOSTIC IMAGING

Diagnostic imaging of chronic aortic dissection is usually performed for surveillance but may also be necessary in patients with symptoms attributable to dissection and for operative planning. As previously discussed, routine follow-up for acute dissection occurs on a scheduled basis and is usually done with either CT or MRI. We prefer CT scanning for patients with normal renal function and no contrast allergy because CT is usually the original imaging study obtained during the acute dissection. The improved accuracy that comes with comparing similar studies combined with the availability, cost, and patient satisfaction make CT favorable for this purpose. MRI is utilized mostly as a follow-up study for patients with renal insufficiency but is the study of choice to provide precise anatomical detail for operative planning. Transthoracic echocardiography is useful to follow chronic type A dissection when there is aortic insufficiency. It can provide cross-sectional images of the ascending aorta but generating images useful for comparison to previous studies is highly dependent on the skill of the operator. For that reason, we use echocardiography to follow patients with aortic insufficiency but also obtain a CT scan to assess ascending aortic diameter. Aortography is used primarily for operative planning. Patients older than 50 years and those with risk factors for coronary artery disease routinely undergo coronary arteriography prior to operation and images of the aorta are obtained at that time. Aortography is especially useful to determine the origin of aortic branch vessels for operative planning when noninvasive imaging is inadequate (Fig. 45-21).

Natural History

Chronic type A dissection develops in patients who fail to undergo immediate surgical treatment of the acute dissection. In contrast, chronic type B dissection may occur in patients successfully treated medically for the acute process and in those with repaired type A dissection who have a retained dissected descending thoracic aorta. The natural history of acute dissection rarely involves spontaneous healing. This phenomenon is observed in 4% to 31% of medically treated patients. Many patients with distal communication of the false lumen go on to develop aneurysmal dilatation of the aorta. The natural history of this process has been examined and reveals that there is an annual rate of expansion of 2 to 3 mm per year in communicating dissections and the rate is 1 mm per year in those not communicating. Despite appropriate medical management and close follow-up, 20% to 40% of patients with chronic dissection require operation for aneurysmal dilatation at 10 years. This number is probably even higher in those patients with connective tissue disorder. In one study of 50 patients over a period of 40 months, 18% had fatal rupture and another 20% underwent surgical repair because of symptoms or aneurysm enlargement, emphasizing the need for diligent follow-up care. Risk factors for rupture of chronic type B dissection in that study included older age, COPD, hypertension, and marginally pain. Chronic beta-blocker treatment reduces the rate of aortic dilatation as well as the incidence of dissection-related hospital admissions and procedures.[39]

Operative Indications

The operative indications for chronic type A and B dissection are shown in Table 45-4. Chronic type A dissection is rarely symptomatic yet a minority will present with chest pain as a result of aneurysm expansion or heart failure related to aortic regurgitation. Chronic type B dissection may also present with back pain or infrequently with a malperfusion syndrome. While each of these findings is an indication for intervention, the most common indication for surgical management is aneurysmal dilatation. The Yale group recently reviewed the size criteria indicating operative intervention for thoracic aortic aneurysms.[40] These criteria dictate replacement should be performed for ascending aortic size greater than 5.5 cm, or 5 cm if a connective tissue disorder is present. Similarly, the two most frequent indications for operative repair of chronic type B dissection are aneurysmal dilatation and malperfusion. In the descending thoracic aorta, replacement is indicated at 6.5 cm, or 6 cm if there is a family history or physical stigmata of a connective tissue disorder. Eccentricity of the aorta was also predictive of rupture as was rapid expansion (more than 1 cm per year) and continued smoking. Such factors should therefore be considered when deciding to operate based on aneurysm size alone.

Operative Technique

GENERAL CONSIDERATIONS

The purpose of operation in chronic aortic dissection is to replace all segments of dissected aorta at risk for rupture and to prevent the possibility of subsequent malperfusion syndrome. The conduct of the operation including surgical approach, monitoring lines required, anesthetic technique, and cardiopulmonary bypass is similar to that described for acute dissection. Aprotinin or epsilon aminocaproic acid is routinely administered even in cases using deep hypothermic circulatory arrest. Greater emphasis is placed on methods of cerebral and spinal cord protection and various technical differences exist for aortic valve preservation and to avoid postoperative malperfusion.

CEREBRAL AND SPINAL CORD PROTECTION

The incidence of paraplegia following repair of thoracoabdominal aneurysms resulting from aortic dissection is reportedly as high as 10%. Both mechanical and pharmacologic interventions have been advocated over the last decade to reduce this risk. It appears that partial left heart bypass alone as previously described is sufficient for patients with aneurysmal dilatation of the thoracic aorta above the level of T9 and results in a paraplegia rate between 5% and 8%.[41] Aneurysms involving the distal aortic arch require full cardiopulmonary bypass and deep hypothermic circulatory arrest for spinal cord protection. In such cases and in the case of the more extensive thoracoabdominal aneurysms, additional measures have variably reduced paraplegia rates lower than observed with cord hypothermia alone. Drainage of cerebrospinal fluid as described by Safi et al is routinely used in our practice for aneurysms extending lower than T9. Reimplanting intercostal and lumbar arteries between T9 and L1 is also important.[42] The aortic cross-clamp is moved progressively distal to perfuse branches as they are implanted. Preoperative identification of the anterior spinal artery origin has been suggested but the combination of distal perfusion, cerebrospinal fluid drainage, and reimplanting large intercostal and lumbar arteries has provided adequate success at our institution. Additional techniques used for spinal cord protection include measurement of sensory and motor evoked potentials, regional epidural cooling, and the use of a variety of pharmacologic agents for cellular protection.

TECHNIQUES FOR TYPE A DISSECTION

Chronic type A dissection, with or without aneurysmal enlargement, is treated using similar operative techniques described for acute dissection. The particular operation performed depends upon the specific pathology involving the aortic root, status of the aortic valve, distal extent of dissection, and brachiocephalic vessel involvement. The pathology of each of these components can be very different in a chronic dissection as compared to the acute process. These differences underlie the need for surgical techniques appropriate to each unique abnormality. In general, the ascending aorta is replaced using a vascular graft to include the entire diseased segment as in acute dissection, but surgical treatment of the aortic valve and creation of the distal anastomosis differ.

Whereas the aortic valve can be repaired in most cases of acute type A dissection by simple commissural resuspension, the rate of aortic valve replacement is much higher in patients with chronic dissection. Preservation of the aortic valve is complicated by morphologic changes in the valvular apparatus such as leaflet elongation and annuloaortic ectasia, which render the valve irreparable in as many as 50%. More severe grades of preoperative aortic regurgitation portend a lower probability of valve preservation. In cases where the aortic valve cannot be preserved with simple commissural reattachment, three options exist to treat aortic insufficiency: composite valve-graft replacement, aortic valve replacement with separate ascending aortic replacement, and finally valve-sparing aortic root repair. The technical aspects of composite valve-graft repair were covered under acute type A dissection. Separate aortic valve and ascending aortic replacement are appropriate when there is an operative indication to repair the ascending aorta in the setting of a normal aortic root and structural aortic valve disease. Note that this operation is not appropriate for patients with connective tissue disease. In this situation aortic root replacement is required.

There are several methods for aortic valve preservation when aortic root replacement is indicated. One such technique is performed by reimplanting the valve commissures into an appropriately sized vascular graft, which is secured to the left ventricular outflow tract using multiple horizontal mattress sutures.[43] A more elegant yet time-consuming technique requires resection of the sinuses of Valsalva leaving a 5-mm rim of aorta circumferentially around the leaflets. Scallops are then created in the vascular graft to resuspend the commissures and remodel the aortic root. David et al advocate Teflon felt reinforcement of the aortic annulus to prevent late annular dilatation and recurrent aortic insufficiency for the remodeling technique. The mid-term outcome of such operations revealed a freedom from reoperation of 97% to 99% at 5 years and a 5-year survival for the aortic dissection subgroup of 84%.[44] Cochran et al devised a similar technique to recreate the sinuses of Valsalva which may be more important than previously recognized and contribute to improved long-term valve durability.[45] Such data in patients with chronic dissection are lacking. These techniques appear appropriate for patients with Marfan disease and in those with congenitally bicuspid aortic valves.

Treatment of the distal aorta in chronic type A dissection is somewhat controversial. Some advocate obliteration of flow in the false lumen with distal aortic repair, whereas others purposely maintain flow into both the true and false lumen using distal resection of the intimal flap. Those who reunite the chronically dissected aortic layers to perfuse only the true lumen maintain that false lumen perfusion continues through distal reentry tears in over 50%. There is a theoretical concern that important side branches arise exclusively from the false lumen and perfusion may be interrupted with this technique. Our practice at the University of Virginia is to resect the distal chronic dissection flap to obviate such concerns. The distal anastomosis is therefore made to the outer wall of the aorta, which has a great deal of structural integrity. Malperfusion of the brachiocephalic vessels as a result of chronic type A dissection is treated with resection of the dissection flap from the arch. Infrequently, the chronic dissection flap extends into more distal branch vessels and may present as transient ischemic attacks or stroke. In such cases it is often necessary to resect the dissection flap into the branch vessel or reunite the layers distally prior to reimplantation.

Infrequently, chronic type A dissection results in extensive aneurysmal dilatation of the aorta extending from the ascending aorta through the arch and into the descending thoracic aorta. Surgical treatment of such extensive disease has traditionally been performed as a staged procedure in which the ascending aorta and arch are replaced first through a sternotomy. The second stage of the so-called elephant trunk procedure is performed 6 weeks later through a left thoracotomy for replacement of the descending aorta using a second vascular graft. Originally described by Borst et al, this technique has been used extensively with good results.[46] In some cases, the aorta distal to the left subclavian artery may be so large as to preclude the use of a two-stage repair. Kouchoukos et al recently described a single-stage repair performed through a bilateral anterior thoracotomy in which the arch is repaired first during a brief period of circulatory arrest. Right subclavian and femoral artery cannulation for cardiopulmonary bypass provide proximal and distal perfusion during the subsequent ascending and descending aortic replacement. The hospital mortality was 6.2% and there were no adverse neurologic outcomes in this small series.[47]

TECHNIQUES FOR TYPE B DISSECTION

The techniques used for replacement of the descending thoracic aorta are identical to those described for treatment of acute type B dissection. The extent of resection, however, for chronic type B dissection is usually greater with the goal to remove all dissected aorta at risk for rupture or symptoms. Usually these operations can be performed through the left chest, but more extensive aneurysms or cases of visceral malperfusion require a thoracoabdominal incision or a staged repair similar to the elephant trunk. The proximal anastomosis is ideally made to undissected normal aorta but infrequently the distal arch is involved, which requires alteration in surgical strategy. Most of the technical controversy regarding repair of chronic type B dissection centers on methods of spinal cord protection during these operations.

As mentioned, we prefer the combination of partial left heart bypass and cerebrospinal fluid drainage. Sites for cannulation are the left inferior pulmonary vein and the left femoral artery or descending thoracic aorta. Depending upon location and extent of aneurysm, the distal arch is mobilized first. The area between the left common carotid and left subclavian artery is circumferentially dissected, and the left subclavian artery is independently controlled. Partial left heart bypass is then initiated. Ideally clamps are placed

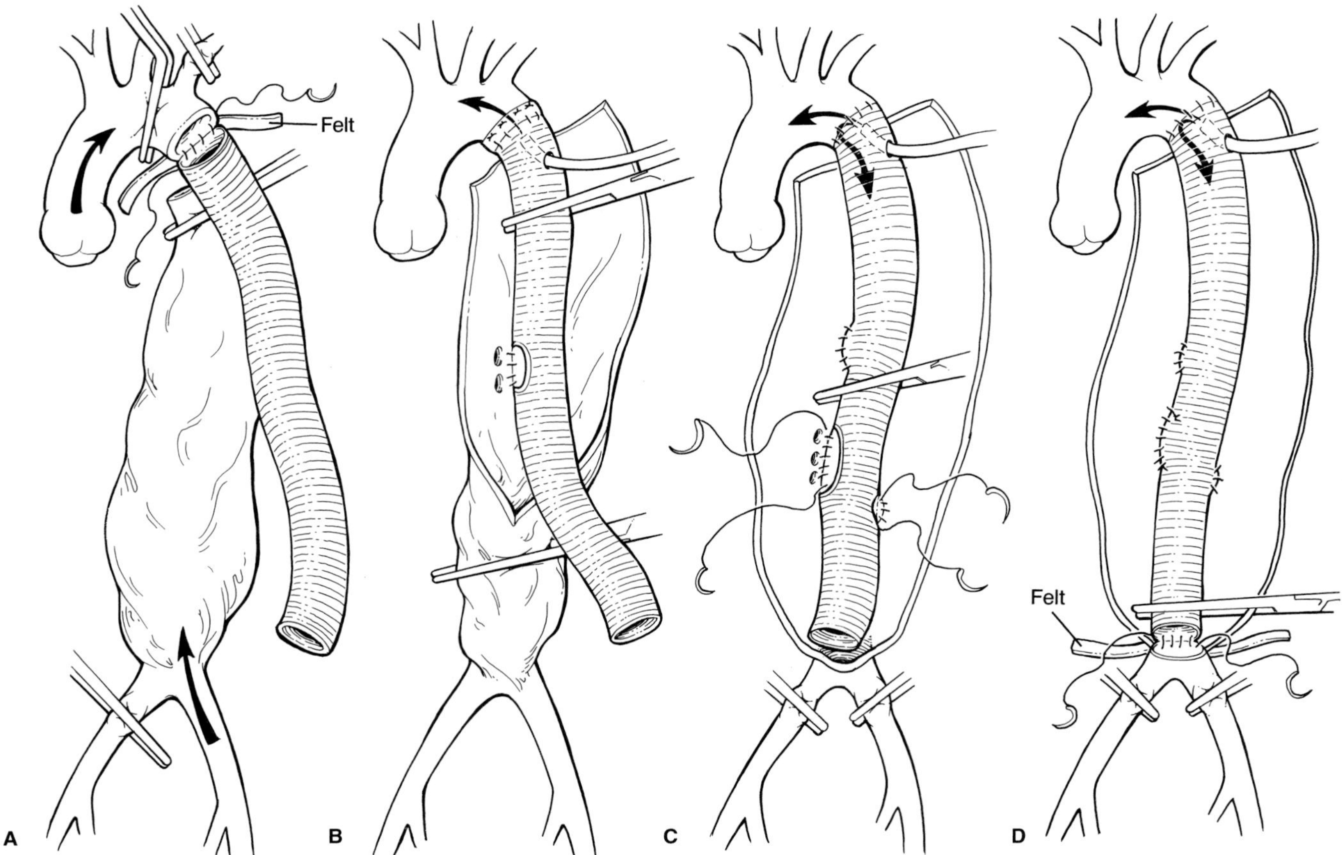

FIGURE 45–22 Replacement of the thoracoabdominal aorta. (A) A left femoral cannula perfuses the lower body and viscera while the heart continues to eject. The arch is transected near or at the left subclavian and any dissection involving the proximal cuff is repaired. The graft is sewn end-to-end to the proximal aorta. (B) The clamp is moved down and a second arterial cannula is inserted into the proximal graft to perfuse the upper body and heart. The anterior wall of the dissection is incised longitudinally and bleeding intercostals of the upper six pairs are oversewn. A group of lower intercostal arteries above the celiac axis is sutured to the graft. (C) The clamp is moved down and the distal aortic clamp is moved to the left common iliac artery. A patch of aorta containing the celiac, superior mesenteric, and right renal artery is sewn to an opening in the graft. The left renal artery is sutured separately to the graft. (D) The proximal clamp is moved below the visceral anastomoses and the distal aortic anastomosis is made to the aortic bifurcation. *(Reproduced with permission from Stone C, Borst H: Dissecting aortic aneurysm, in Edmunds LJ Jr (ed): Cardiac Surgery in the Adult. New York, McGraw-Hill, 1997; p 1125.)*

between the left subclavian and left common carotid arteries and on the aorta distal to the involved segment. If the entire descending thoracic aorta is diseased, the clamp is placed on the mid-thoracic aorta to perform the proximal anastomosis first. The aorta is opened and small intercostal arteries are oversewn. The proximal anastomosis is made to normal aorta whenever possible with running 3-0 Prolene; 4-0 Prolene is used if the tissue is fragile. The clamp is moved distally onto the graft to inspect the proximal anastomosis and achieve hemostasis. Several centimeters of the dissection flap is then resected from the lumen of the distal aorta and the distal anastomosis created to the adventitia of the chronic dissection. In more extensive thoracoabdominal disease, the clamp is progressively moved distal as intercostals arteries below T7 to L2 and visceral vessels are reimplanted (Fig. 45-22). Bypass is terminated and the operation completed.

Full cardiopulmonary bypass with deep hypothermic circulatory arrest may be necessary in cases where the proximal anastomosis cannot be safely or adequately performed with a clamp in the usual position. Kouchoukas et al have a large experience in this area and cite a 6.2% 30-day mortality, 1.9% stroke rate, and no paraplegia in the subgroup of patients with aortic dissection.[48] These data strongly support this simple and elegant technique as one of the most efficacious for spinal cord and visceral organ protection in these complicated procedures.

Results

The operative mortality for chronic type A dissection is between 4% and 17% and on average is very similar to that reported for chronic type B repair at 11% to 15%.[37,49] The actuarial survival following operation for chronic type A and B dissections is not different at 5 years (59%–75%) or at 10 years (45%).[38] The stroke rate following repair of chronic type A is 4%. Early neurologic complications occurred in 9%.[49] Regular follow-up of the aortic valve is necessary when the native valve is preserved at the initial operation. This is best performed using transthoracic echocardiography on a yearly basis. Early reports indicated that nearly 20% of patients require reoperation secondary to progressive aortic regurgitation. The most recent data from David et al, however, reveal a 90% ± 4% 5-year freedom from severe or moderate aortic insufficiency in patients with aortic root aneurysm and 98% ± 2% in patients with ascending aortic aneurysm following valve-sparing operation.[50]

CONCLUSION

Considerable improvement in the treatment of patients with acute and chronic aortic dissection has occurred over the last 50 years. Continued progress is inevitable and technologies such as endovascular repair may eventually achieve results comparable to surgery. Complex forms of dissection that include aortic root and valvular pathology, however, will require surgical treatment for the foreseeable future. These patients will undoubtedly benefit from the novel basic and clinical research taking place in the areas of spinal cord and cerebral protection, strategies for cardiopulmonary bypass, improved vascular graft technology, and procedures for preservation of the aortic valve. Such progress may even permit advancement in our greatest remaining clinical challenge, those patients who are hemodynamically unstable following aortic dissection.

REFERENCES

1. Sennertus D: Cap. *42 Op Omn Lib* 1650; 5:306.
2. Maunoir JP: *Memoires Physiologiques et Practiques sur l'Aneurysme at la Ligature des Arteres*. Geneva, JJ Paschoud, 1802.
3. Laennec R: *Traite de l'Ausculattion Mediate*, 2d ed. 1826; T.2:693.
4. Gurin D: Dissecting aneurysms of the aorta: diagnosis and operative relief of acute arterial obstruction due to this cause. *N Y State J Med* 1935; 35:1200.
5. Abbott OA: Clinical experiences with application of polythene cellophane upon aneurysms of thoracic vessels. *J Thorac Surg* 1949; 18:435.
6. DeBakey ME, Cooley DA, Creech O: Surgical considerations of dissecting aneurysm of the aorta. *Ann Surg* 1955; 142:586.
7. Creech O, DeBakey ME, Cooley DA: Surgical treatment of dissecting aneurysm of the aorta. *Texas State J Med* 1956; 52:287.
8. Wheat MW, Palmer RF, Bartley TD, et al: Treatment of dissecting aneurysms of the aorta without surgery. *J Thorac Cardiovasc Surg* 1965; 50:364.
9. DeBakey ME, Beall AC Jr, Cooley DA, et al: Dissecting aneurysms of the aorta. *Surg Clin North Am* 1966; 46:1045.
10. Daily PO, Trueblood HW, Stinson EB, et al: Management of acute aortic dissections. *Ann Thorac Surg* 1970; 10:237.
11. Coady MA, Rizzo JA, Goldstein LJ, et al: Natural history, pathogenesis, and etiology of thoracic aortic aneurysms and dissections. *Cardiol Clin* 1999; 17:615.
12. Erbel R, Alfonso F, Boileau C, et al: Diagnosis and management of aortic dissection: Recommendations of the Task Force on Aortic Dissection, European Society of Cardiology. *Eur Heart J* 2001; 22:1642.
13. Larson EW, Edwards WD: Risk factors for aortic dissection: a necropsy study of 161 cases. *Am J Cardiol* 1984; 53:849.
14. Coady MA, Rizzo JA, Elefteriades JA: Pathologic variants of thoracic aorta dissection: penetrating atherosclerotic ulcers and intramural hematomas. *Cardiol Clin* 1999; 17:637.
15. Neri E, Toscono T, Papilia U, et al: Proximal aortic dissection with coronary malperfusion: presentation, management, and outcome. *J Thorac Cardiovasc Surg* 2001; 121:552.
16. Anagnostopoulos CE, Prabhakar MJ, Kittle CF: Aortic dissections and dissecting aneurysms. *Am J Cardiol* 1972; 30:263.
17. Hagan PG, Nienaber CA, Isselbacher EM, et al: The international registry of acute aortic dissection (IRAD): new insights into an old disease. *JAMA* 2000; 283:897.
18. Elefteriades JA, Lovoulos CJ, Coady MA: Management of descending aortic dissection. *Ann Thorac Surg* 1999; 67:2002.
19. Scholl FG, Coady MA, Davies RR, et al: Interval or permanent nonoperative management of type A aortic dissection. *Arch Surg* 1999; 134:402.
20. Miller DC: The continuing dilemma concerning medical versus surgical management of patients with acute type B dissections. *Semin Thorac Cardiovasc Surg* 1993; 5:33.
21. Coady MA, Rizzo JA, Hammond GL, et al: Penetrating ulcer of the thoracic aorta: what is it? how do we recognize it? how do we manage it? *J Vasc Surg* 1998; 27:1006.
22. McCullough JN, Zhang N, Reich D, et al: Cerebral metabolic suppression during circulatory arrest in humans. *Ann Thorac Surg* 1999; 67:1895.
23. Ergin MA, Griepp EB, Lansman SL, et al: Hypothermic circulatory arrest and other methods of cerebral protection during operations on the thoracic aorta. *J Card Surg* 1994; 9:525.
24. Coselli JS, LeMarie SA, de Figueiredo LP, et al: Paraplegia after thoracoabdominal aneurysm repair: is dissection a risk factor? *Ann Thorac Surg* 1997; 63:28.
25. Cunningham JN Jr, Laschinger JC, Spencer FC, et al: Monitoring of somatosensory evoked potentials during surgical procedures on the thoracoabdominal aorta, IV: Clinical observations and results. *J Thorac Cardiovasc Surg* 1987; 94:275.
26. Crawford ES, Svensson LG, Hess KR, et al: A prospective randomized study of cerebrospinal fluid drainage to prevent paraplegia after high-risk surgery on the thoracoabdominal aorta. *J Vasc Surg* 1991; 13:36.
27. Safi HJ, Hess KR, Randel M, et al: Cerebrospinal fluid drainage and distal aortic perfusion: reducing neurologic complications in repair of thoracoabdominal aortic aneurysms types I and II. *J Vasc Surg* 1996; 23:223.
28. Cambria RP, Brewster DC, Gertler J, et al: Vascular complications associated with spontaneous aortic dissection. *J Vasc Surg* 1988; 7:199.
29. Fann JI, Sarris GE, Mitchell RS, et al: Treatment of patients with aortic dissection presenting with peripheral vascular complications. *Ann Surg* 1990; 212:705.
30. Lauterbach SR, Cambria RP, Brewster DC, et al: Contemporary management of aortic branch compromise resulting from acute aortic dissection. *J Vasc Surg* 2001; 33:1185.

31. Elefteriades JA, Hartleroad J, Gusberg RJ, et al: Long-term experience with descending aortic dissection: the complication-specific approach. *Ann Thorac Surg* 1992; 53:11.
32. Slonim SM, Miller DC, Mitchell RS, et al: Percutaneous balloon fenestration and stenting for life-threatening ischemic complications in patients with acute aortic dissection. *J Thorac Cardiovasc Surg* 1999; 117:1118.
33. Williams DM, Lee DY, Hamilton BH, et al: The dissected aorta: percutaneous treatment of ischaemic complications: principles and results. *J Vasc Interv Radiol* 1997; 8:605.
34. Deeb GM, Williams DM, Bolling SF, et al: Surgical delay for acute type A dissection with malperfusion. *Ann Thorac Surg* 1997; 64:1669.
35. DeBakey ME, McCollum CH, Crawford ES, et al: Dissection and dissecting aneurysms of the aorta: twenty-year follow-up of five hundred and twenty-seven patients treated surgically. *Surgery* 1982; 92:1118.
36. Eagle KA, Burkmann D, Isselbacher E, et al: Predictive of mortality in patients with type A acute aortic dissections: results from the International Registry of Acute Aortic Dissection (IRAD). *J Am Coll Cardiol* 2000; 35:223.
37. Sabik JF, Lytle BW, Blackstone EH, et al: Long-term effectiveness of operations for ascending aortic dissections. *J Thorac Cardiovasc Surg* 2000; 119:946.
38. Fann JI, Smith JA, Miller DC, et al: Surgical management of aortic dissection during a 30-year period. *Circulation* 1995; 92:II113.
39. Genoni M, Paul M, Jenni R, et al: Chronic β-blocker therapy improves outcome and reduces treatment costs in chronic type B dissection. *Eur J Cardiothoracic Surg* 2001; 19:606.
40. Coady MA, Rizzo JA, Hammond GL, et al: What is the appropriate size criterion for resection of thoracic aortic aneurysms? *J Thorac Cardiovasc Surg* 1997; 113:476.
41. Coselli JS, LeMarie SA: Left heart bypass reduces paraplegia rates following thoracoabdominal aortic aneurysm repair. *Ann Thorac Surg* 1999; 67:1931.
42. Safi HJ, Miller CC 3rd, Carr C, et al: Importance of intercostal artery reattachment during thoracoabdominal aortic aneurysm repair. *J Vasc Surg* 1998; 27:58.
43. David TE, Feindel CM: An aortic valve sparing operation for patients with aortic incompetence and aneurysm of the ascending aorta. *J Thorac Cardiovasc Surg* 1992; 103:617.
44. David TE, Armstrong S, Ivanov J, et al: Results of aortic valve-sparing operations. *J Thorac Cardiovasc Surg* 2001; 122:39.
45. Cochran RP, Kunzelman KS, Eddy AC, et al: Modified conduit preparation creates a pseudosinus in an aortic valve-sparing procedure for aneurysm of the ascending aorta. *J Thorac Cardiovasc Surg* 1995; 109:1049.
46. Borst HG, Walterbusch G, Schaps D. Extensive aortic replacement using "elephant trunk" prosthesis. *Thorac Cardiovasc Surg* 1983; 31:37.
47. Kouchoukos NT, Masetti P, Rokkas CK, et al: Single-stage reoperative repair of chronic type A aortic dissection by means of the arch-first technique. *J Thorac Cardiovasc Surg* 2001; 122: 578.
48. Kouchoukos NT, Masetti P, Rokkas CK, et al: Safety and efficacy of hypothermic cardiopulmonary bypass and circulatory arrest for operations on the descending thoracic and thoracoabdominal aorta. *Ann Thorac Surg* 2001; 72:699.
49. Safi HJ, Miller CC III, Reardon MJ, et al: Operation for acute and chronic dissection: recent outcome with regard to neurologic deficit and early death. *Ann Thorac Surg* 1998; 66:402.
50. David TE, Armstrong S, Ivanov J, et al: Results of aortic valve-sparing operations. *J Thorac Cardiovasc Surg* 2001; 122:39.

Chapter 46

Ascending Aortic Aneurysms

Curtis A. Anderson/Robert J. Rizzo/Lawrence H. Cohn

HISTORY

Early Descriptions and Surgical Interventions

Galen is credited as the first to describe arterial aneurysms. This was based on his observation of false aneurysms in gladiators injured during battle in the 2nd century A.D.[1] Antyllus, during the same time period, made the distinction between traumatic aneurysms and those of a degenerative etiology. Antyllus was also the first to attempt surgical treatment of aneurysms with proximal and distal ligation,[2] but his techniques were not broadly applied at the time. Ambroise Paré in the late 1700s proposed that syphilis played a causative role in some aortic aneurysms, but this was not generally accepted until many years later when Dohle described the histology of syphilitic aortitis.[1]

The earliest surgical treatment of aneurysms consisted of interruption of arterial flow via either ligation or the stimulation of thrombosis. These procedures met with variable success depending upon the position of the aneurysm and the extent of collateral circulation.[2] Arterial ligation was popularized in the 1800s by John Hunter, who demonstrated safe and reproducible means of ligating certain peripheral arteries.[3] Innovative measures used to cause thrombosis of aneurysms included the insertion of long segments of wire[4] with the application of an electric current,[5] and wrapping of aneurysms with cellophane or other irritating materials.[6,7]

In 1888, Rudolph Matas introduced a very different approach. In an operation he referred to as obliterative endoaneurysmorraphy,[8,9] stitches placed from within the aneurysm sac obliterated the arterial openings. This provided more secure closure of large aneurysms that would have been difficult to ligate externally. Recognizing the importance of maintaining arterial continuity for certain aneurysms, he subsequently devised techniques of restorative or reconstructive endoaneurysmorraphy[10] in which diseased segments of the aneurysm wall were resected and the remaining vessel wall was reconstructed to reestablish flow. The number of aneurysms to which these techniques could be applied, however, was very limited. The broad application of surgical treatment for major arterial aneurysms would have to await the development of satisfactory conduits and the techniques to insert them.

Evolution of Modern Surgical Techniques

Replacement of the ascending aorta, which had to await the development and refinement of cardiopulmonary bypass technology, was first performed by Cooley and DeBakey using an aortic allograft in 1956.[11] Mueller et al combined allograft insertion with aortic valve repair in 1960 in a patient with Marfan syndrome.[12] As the need for conduits grew, attention was shifted to the development of a suitable artificial conduit. The first fabric to be utilized was Vinyon N cloth by Blakemore and Voorhees.[13] Dacron was subsequently introduced by DeBakey,[2] who discovered it in a Houston department store, and it soon became the artificial conduit of choice for aortic replacement.

Replacement of the supracoronary ascending aorta with a synthetic graft and separate mechanical aortic valve replacement was performed by Starr et al in 1963.[14] Wheat et al[15] in 1964 resected the ascending aorta and entire aortic root except for small tongues of aortic tissue surrounding the coronary arteries. They then performed a mechanical valve insertion and fashioned the proximal tube graft to accommodate the coronary arteries, which were left in situ. The first use of a composite valve-graft conduit to replace the aortic root and ascending aorta was by Bentall and De Bono in 1968.[16] The coronaries were left intact in the aortic wall and the surrounding aortic tissue was sewn to orifices that were created in the tube graft. The remaining aorta was wrapped tightly around the tube graft, creating an inclusion cylinder arrangement. In 1981 Cabrol used an 8- to 10-mm Dacron graft to facilitate the restoration of coronary blood flow following aortic root replacement.[17] Variations of these pioneering procedures using modern low-profile mechanical valves and hemostatic collagen- or gelatin-impregnated woven Dacron grafts are commonly performed today.

INCIDENCE AND RISK FACTORS

Aortic aneurysms are the 13th leading cause of mortality in the United States.[18] The incidence of thoracic aortic aneurysms is estimated to be 5.9 cases per 100,000 person-years,[19] and replacement of the ascending aorta accounts for the majority of thoracic aortic procedures.[20] The mean age at the time of diagnosis ranges from 59 to 69 years.[21] Men are typically diagnosed at a younger age and there is a 2:1 to 4:1 male predominance.[21]

Traditional risk factors have included smoking, hypertension, atherosclerosis, and well-defined genetic disorders such as Marfan syndrome and Ehlers-Danlos syndrome.[19,22–25] Subtler forms of inherited metabolic disorders are being elucidated,[26] and perhaps play a role in more instances than was previously suspected. Syphilis, at one time the predominant etiology of ascending aortic aneurysms, has become very uncommon with the development of effective antibiotics. Bicuspid and unicuspid aortic valves are associated with ascending aortic aneurysms and dissections beyond that which can be attributed to simple hemodynamic disturbance, suggesting an underlying abnormality of the aortic wall.[27]

ETIOLOGY AND PATHOPHYSIOLOGY

General

Most of the elasticity and tensile strength of the aorta is derived from its medial layer, which consists of approximately 45 to 55 lamellar units of elastin, collagen, smooth muscle cells, and ground substance. In the ascending aorta, the elastin content is high, consistent with its compliant nature, and diminishes as one proceeds distally into the descending thoracic and abdominal aorta. The media also becomes thinner distally, and in the abdominal aorta the total number of lamellae is reduced by approximately one half.[28]

The aortic wall is a biologically active environment. Smooth muscle cells synthesize and degrade elastin, collagen, and proteoglycans.[29] In the media of a typical ascending aortic aneurysm there is fragmentation of elastic fibers, and loss of smooth muscle cells[30] or alteration in smooth muscle cell function.[29] The resulting pathologic entity is referred to as cystic medial degeneration or cystic medial necrosis. In advanced forms there is a dramatic loss of elastic fibers and smooth muscle cells with the accumulation of a basophilic amorphous material giving the media a true cystic appearance.[30] Subtler degrees of elastic fiber fragmentation are normal, and the diameter of the ascending aorta typically increases with age.[31] Smoking has been associated with increased concentrations of elastolytic enzymes within the aortic wall, possibly hastening this process.[31,32] The role of atherosclerosis is controversial.

During systole, the ascending aorta expands, converting a portion of the kinetic energy of left ventricular contraction into potential energy in the aortic wall. During diastole the aorta recoils, converting this potential energy once again into the kinetic energy of forward flow.[33] This coupling of the left ventricle and aorta ensures efficient forward flow during both phases of the cardiac cycle. With weakening of the aortic wall and loss of elasticity, dilation ensues. Dilation results in increased wall tension relative to intra-aortic pressure according to the law of Laplace. This amplifies the injurious forces on the aortic wall produced by hypertension and results in progressive dilation. These pathologic changes in the aortic wall can result in inefficient ventricular-aortic coupling, aortic valve incompetence, and the potential for rupture or dissection.

Idiopathic Cystic Medial Degeneration

Elastic fiber fragmentation is a normal process of aging,[31] but is accelerated in some individuals for poorly understood reasons. This results in premature weakening of the aortic wall, aneurysmal dilation, and the potential for rupture or dissection. Many cases that are now considered idiopathic may in the future be described as subtle disorders of metabolism that accelerate aortic wall degeneration in response to common risk factors.

Genetic Disorders

MARFAN SYNDROME

Marfan syndrome is an autosomal dominant connective tissue disorder, with potentially life-threatening cardiovascular manifestations.[34] The estimated frequency is 1 per 10,000 births.[35] This disorder has been traced to the fibrillin gene of chromosome 15,[36–40] with more than 70 different defects identified thus far.[41] It is believed that one third of cases are secondary to spontaneous mutations.[42] Fibrillin is one of the major structural components of the elastic fiber.[43] The resulting abnormal elastic fibers are prone to disruption and result in histologic findings consistent with cystic medial degeneration at an early age.[30] Seventy-five to eighty-five percent of patients with Marfan syndrome have dilation of the aortic sinuses and annulus in addition to the ascending aorta. This morphology, referred to as annuloaortic ectasia, is the classic presentation of Marfan syndrome, but can occur in the absence of a known connective tissue disorder. Because of the frequent aortic root involvement, aortic insufficiency is common.[44] One third of patients with Marfan syndrome also have mitral regurgitation.[44]

EHLERS-DANLOS SYNDROME

Ehlers-Danlos syndrome is an inherited disorder of connective tissue with multiple subtypes. Type IV Ehlers-Danlos may be associated with life-threatening cardiovascular manifestations.[45] Spontaneous arterial rupture is the most common cause of death and usually involves the mesenteric vessels.[45] Less commonly, patients develop abdominal or thoracic aortic aneurysms or dissections.[46,47] Surgical treatment is challenging because of the friable nature of the vascular tissue.

FAMILIAL ANEURYSMS

Certain families, without phenotypic expression of Marfan syndrome, exhibit strong histories of ascending aortic aneurysm formation and dissection transmitted in an autosomal dominant fashion. In a recent study of 15 such families, 9 demonstrated evidence of linkage to the 5q locus, although the specific gene and product have not been identified.[26] None of the 15 families demonstrated linkage to the fibrillin gene. Further investigation will likely reveal other examples of more subtle inherited or spontaneously occurring disorders of metabolism that result in accelerated deterioration of the aortic wall.

Atherosclerosis

Atherosclerosis is less commonly seen in ascending aortic aneurysms than in descending thoracic or abdominal aortic aneurysms. It has long been theorized that the development of invasive atheromas results in destruction of elastic fibers and smooth muscle cells in the media, resulting in weakening and dilation.[19] This process was proposed as the primary etiology of descending thoracic and abdominal aortic aneurysms, and the second most common cause of ascending aortic aneurysms.[19,48] These theories are now challenged by the concept that atherosclerosis is a concomitant process that infiltrates a diseased media with altered barriers.[49] This would explain the divergent course of the atherosclerotic abdominal aorta towards obstructive versus aneurysmal disease.

Aneurysms Associated with Aortic Dissection

Patients who survive acute dissection of the ascending aorta often have or will develop an associated aneurysm. The rate of expansion is higher than other types of ascending aortic aneurysms as the barrier to dilation and rupture is only the outer one third of the media and the adventitia.[19,50] Aortic dissection is discussed in Chapter 45.

Aneurysms Associated with Aortic Valve Disease

Bicuspid and unicuspid aortic valves are associated with ascending aortic aneurysm formation. Although initially thought to be secondary to poststenotic dilation, a primary structural abnormality of the aortic wall appears contributory. Aortic enlargement occurs at an accelerated pace in congenitally stenosed valves compared to trileaflet valves with equivalent degrees of stenosis.[27,51] Aortic dissection occurs in patients with bicuspid aortic valves at a rate 10-fold the normal population, a trend that is not found in other forms of aortic stenosis.[22] This strongly implies an inherent weakness in the aortic wall.

Infection

BACTERIAL (MYCOTIC) ANEURYSMS

True primary bacterial infection of the ascending aortic wall resulting in aneurysm formation is rare. This is believed to occur either after an episode of bacterial endocarditis or from an aortic jet lesion causing endothelial trauma.[52] The most common organisms include, in order of decreasing frequency, *Staphylococcus aureus, Staphylococcus epidermidis, Salmonella,* and *Streptococcus*.[53] Infection of laminar clot within a previously formed aneurysm may also occur after transient bacteremia.[53]

SYPHILITIC ANEURYSMS

Syphilitic aortitis, caused by the spirochete *Treponema pallidum,* was once the most common cause of ascending aortic aneurysms. It has now become a rarity in developed countries because of effective antibiotic therapy. In this disease an obliterative endarteritis of the vasa-vasorum results in ischemic injury to the aortic media with subsequent destruction of elastic and muscular elements.[30] The media is replaced by a thickened fibrous tissue, which begins to dilate. This process most commonly involves the ascending aorta and arch,[54] but may involve the root as well. If the regions of the coronary ostia are involved, significant coronary obstruction may occur.[1] Antibiotic therapy does not reverse the vascular pathology.

Arteritis

Takayasu's arteritis most commonly involves the aortic arch and its major branches, but may involve any or all segments of the aorta. Takayasu's usually produces obstructive lesions, but may have a dilative component in 15% of cases.[55] Giant cell arteritis (temporal arteritis) may lead to weakening of the aortic wall and eventual aneurysm formation or dissection.[56,57] In one population-based study temporal arteritis was associated with a greater than 17-fold increase in the risk of developing a thoracic aneurysm.[58]

Trauma

Chronic traumatic aneurysms of the ascending aorta are rare. Although the ascending aorta is the site of rupture in 20% of blunt aortic injuries, survival beyond the initial injury is unusual, with the patient usually succumbing to acute cardiac tamponade.[59] This subject is covered in Chapter 51.

Pseudoaneurysms

The wall of a pseudoaneurysm is composed primarily of adventitia, thrombus, and surrounding structures.[30] Postoperative pseudoaneurysms may occur at an aortic suture line or at the site of aortic cannulation. Causes include technical error, acute dissection, native tissue degeneration, or deterioration of the graft or suture material.[60,61] The use of modern monofilament suture and low-porosity collagen- or gelatin-impregnated Dacron grafts,[62] as well as the abandonment of the inclusion cylinder technique,[63,64] have lessened the incidence of this complication. Less commonly, pseudoaneurysms of the ascending aorta occur after trauma or infection.

NATURAL HISTORY

General

The appropriate application of surgical treatment depends upon an understanding of the relative risks of surgery versus the natural history of the disease. The natural history of untreated aneurysms of the thoracic aorta often concludes with patient death because of rupture or dissection.

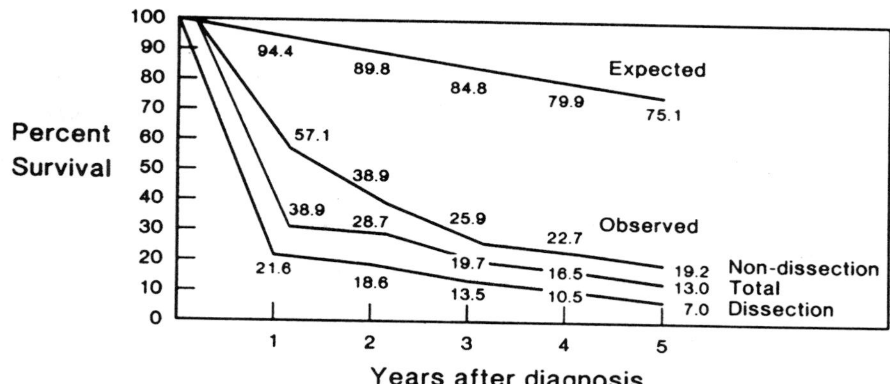

FIGURE 46–1 Actuarial survival estimates of 72 patients followed nonoperatively with thoracic aneurysms and dissections. (*Reproduced with permission from Bickerstaff LK, Pairolero PC, Hollier LH, et al: Thoracic aortic aneurysms: a population-based study. Surgery 1982; 92:1103.*)

Figure 46-1 shows the estimated actuarial survival curve for 72 patients who were diagnosed with thoracic aneurysms from 1951 to 1980 and were followed nonoperatively. Seventy-four percent of the patients experienced rupture, and 94% of these patients died.[19] The potential for complications of rupture or dissection is primarily dependent upon size and the underlying etiology of the aneurysm.

Size

Based on the law of Laplace, wall tension increases as the diameter of an aneurysm increases. It is therefore intuitive that larger aneurysms have a greater risk of rupture. This was first established for abdominal aortic aneurysms by Szilagyi et al in 1966.[65] Subsequent natural history studies have confirmed this finding and have found also that larger aneurysms have a higher rate of expansion.[66,67] Coady et al[68] have written extensively on the natural history of thoracic aortic aneurysms. The incidence of acute dissection or rupture according to size in their cohort of patients is shown in Figure 46-2. Logistic regression analysis revealed a 4.3-fold increased risk of rupture or dissection in an aneurysm 6.0 to 6.9 cm in diameter compared to an aneurysm 4.0 to 4.9 cm in diameter. Growth rates varied from 0.08 cm per year for aneurysms less than 4.0 cm to 0.16 cm per year for aneurysms greater than 8.0 cm in diameter. Mean growth rates as great as 0.42 cm per year have been reported in other series.[69,70] Dapunt et al [50] also noted an increased rate of growth in smokers and patients with a history of hypertension.

The Influence of Etiology on Natural History

MARFAN SYNDROME

Although size criteria are perhaps most important, the underlying etiology must be considered. Patients with Marfan syndrome have accelerated aneurysm growth and tend to rupture or dissect at smaller sizes.[71] This is particularly true for those with a family history of early complications.[71] The average age of death for untreated patients with Marfan syndrome is 32 years[72] with complications of the aortic root being responsible for 60% to 80% of these deaths.[44,72]

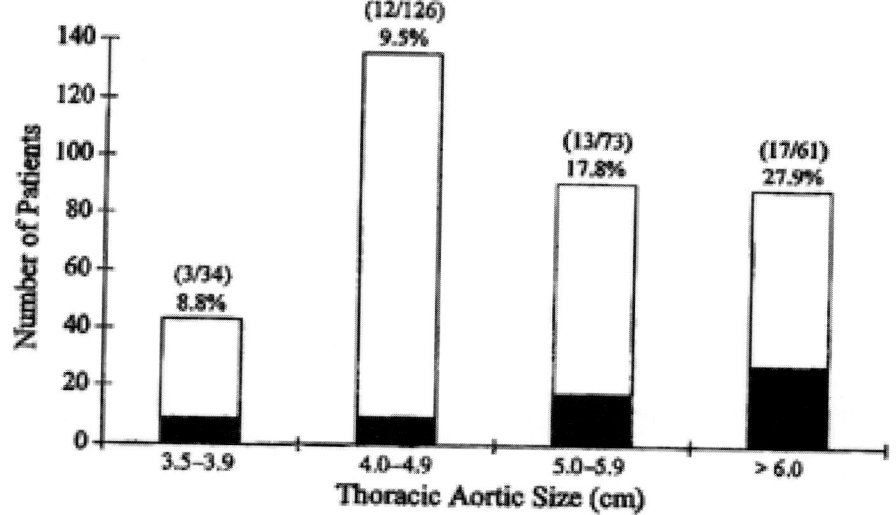

FIGURE 46–2 The incidence of acute dissection or rupture of thoracic aneurysms according to size. The height of the column corresponds to the total number of patients and the black area to the proportion of patients who suffered complications of dissection or rupture. (*Reproduced with permission from Coady MA, Rizzo JA, Elefteriades JA: Developing surgical intervention criteria for thoracic aortic aneurysms. Cardiol Clin 1999; 17:827.*)

FAMILIAL ANEURYSMS

The inheritance of aneurysmal disease without an associated phenotypic syndrome such as Marfan syndrome was first noted for abdominal aortic aneurysms.[73,74] In 1997 familial aggregation of thoracic aneurysms was noted by Biddinger et al.[75] Coady et al[76] estimated that 19% of their study population fit criteria for familial aneurysms by pedigree analysis. The primary mode of inheritance was autosomal dominant, but X-linked and recessive patterns were also evident in some cases. This subgroup had an annual growth rate almost double the growth rate for the entire population.

AORTIC DISSECTION

In chronic dissections, the barrier to rupture is the outer third of the media and the adventitia. Dissections are therefore associated with an accelerated rate of expansion and rupture. Comparisons between dissecting and nondissecting thoracic aneurysms of similar size have revealed as much as a 6-fold greater growth rate for dissections.[21]

SYPHILITIC ANEURYSMS

The average time from the diagnosis of advanced syphilis to cardiovascular symptoms is 10 to 20 years.[1] The average survival from the onset of cardiac symptoms is only six to eight months.[1] Saccular aneurysms, which are common in this disease, may have a more rapid rate of expansion and greater risk of rupture.[77] Dissection is less likely because of the scarring that occurs within the media.[30] Modern studies of growth rates and size at the time of rupture are not feasible because of the rarity of this condition

CLINICAL PRESENTATION

Signs and Symptoms

Many ascending aortic aneurysms are asymptomatic when diagnosed, being incidentally noted on chest x-ray or other imaging study.[24] Echocardiographic evaluation of aortic insufficiency is also a frequent mode of diagnosis. Between 25% and 75% of patients, however, present with chest pain that results in the diagnosis of an aneurysm.[24,78,79] Pain from the ascending aorta is usually localized to the anterior chest. The pain may be acute in onset signifying impending rupture, or a chronic gnawing pain from compression of the overlying sternum. Occasionally signs of superior vena caval or airway compression are present.[79] Less commonly, aneurysms of the ascending aorta or aortic root can rupture into the right atrium or the superior vena cava, presenting with high output cardiac failure or into the lungs with ensuing hemoptysis. Hoarseness resulting from stretch injury of the left recurrent laryngeal nerve suggests involvement of the distal aortic arch or proximal descending thoracic aorta. In contrast, dissection of the ascending aorta presents with severe "tearing" pain in 75% of patients.[23,24]

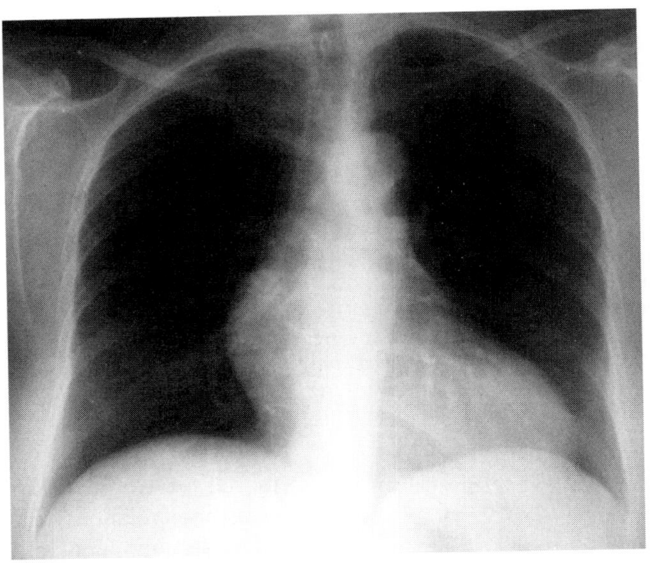

A

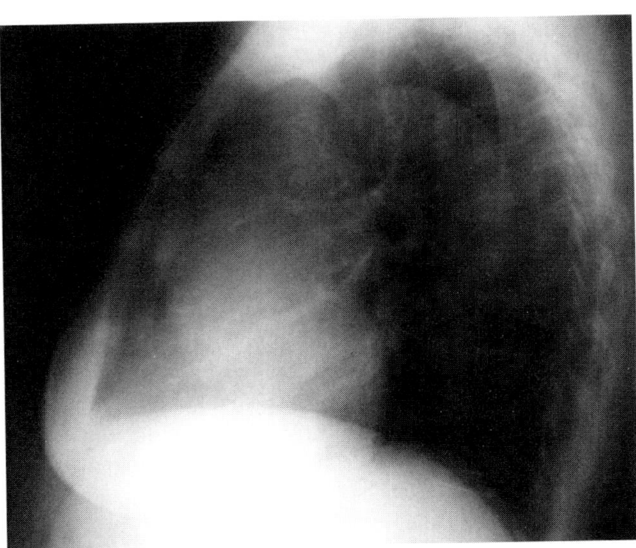

B

FIGURE 46–3 PA and lateral chest radiograph of a patient with an ascending aortic aneurysm. The PA view (A) shows convexity of the right mediastinum, and the lateral view (B) shows loss of the normal retrosternal air space. (*Reproduced with permission from Downing SW, Kouchokos NT: Ascending aortic aneurysm, in Edmunds LH Jr (ed): Cardiac Surgery in the Adult. New York, McGraw-Hill, 1997; p 1163.*)

Physical Examination

In the case of rupture, the patient will present in extremis. In a patient without rupture, the examination is often unremarkable. If the sinotubular ridge or aortic root is dilated, a widened pulse pressure or diastolic murmur signifying aortic insufficiency may be noted. If dilation is isolated to the ascending aorta, however, the aneurysm can reach large dimensions without producing physical findings. A thorough vascular exam should be carried out to look for any concomitant peripheral vascular disease, carotid disease, or sequelae of distal embolization. Abdominal aortic aneurysms are present in 10% to 20% of patients with atherosclerotic involvement of an ascending aortic aneurysm,[23,80] and this should also be sought on physical examination. In rare cases, aneurysms may cause compression necrosis of the overlying sternum and ribs. Syphilitic aneurysms have been noted to erode through the chest wall and rupture externally.[1]

DIAGNOSTIC STUDIES

Electrocardiogram

With significant aortic insufficiency, left ventricular hypertrophy or strain is evident. Patients with generalized atherosclerosis may show evidence of concomitant coronary artery disease, or previous myocardial injury.

Chest Radiography

Many asymptomatic ascending aortic aneurysms are first detected on chest x-ray. The enlarged ascending aorta produces a convex contour of the right superior mediastinum (Fig. 46-3A). In the lateral view, there is loss of the retrosternal air space (Fig. 46-3B). Aneurysms confined to the aortic root can be obscured by the cardiac silhouette and may not be evident on chest radiograph.[81]

Echocardiography

Ascending aortic aneurysms are the most common cause of isolated aortic insufficiency,[82] and therefore aneurysms are frequently detected during evaluation of a regurgitant aortic valve. Transesophageal echocardiography (TEE) can accurately detect and differentiate between ascending aortic aneurysms, dissections, and intramural hematoma.[83] Imaging of the distal ascending aorta is obscured by air in the tracheobronchial tree with up to 40% of its distal extent not well visualized.[84] Transthoracic echocardiography is far less reliable.[78]

Aortography

Aortography provides precise delineation of the aortic lumen, and certain diseases have very characteristic arteriographic patterns. Annuloaortic ectasia has a "pear-shaped" morphology (Fig. 46-4) with prominent dilation of the aortic sinuses and less severe dilation of the ascending aorta tapering to normal caliber at the origin of the innominate artery. Pseudoaneurysms appear as saccular outpouchings with an irregular contour.[85] Syphilitic aneurysms involving the aortic root are often associated with coronary ostial stenosis.[30]

One of the beneficial aspects of aortography is accurate demonstration of the relationship of the aneurysm to the arch vessels. Aortography also detects aortic regurgitation and cephalad displacement of the coronary ostia. In patients over the age of 40 or with a pertinent history, the opportunity is afforded to check for coronary disease and left ventricular dysfunction. Disadvantages include contrast and radiation exposure, puncture site complications, underestimation of

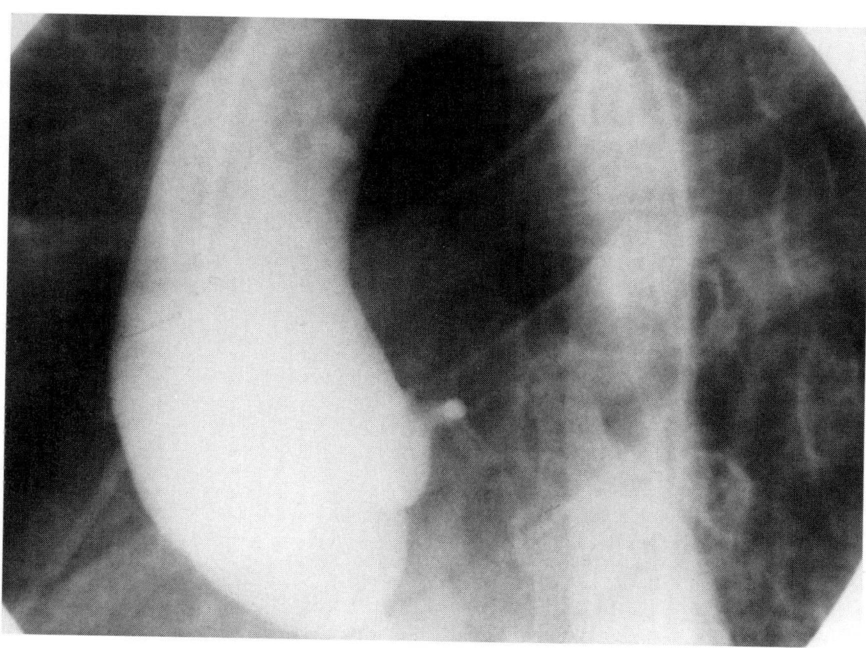

FIGURE 46–4 Aortic angiogram of patient with classic annuloaortic ectasia. The aortic root is dilated and the ascending aorta tapers to a normal caliber at the origin of the innominate artery giving the classic "pear-shaped" morphology. *(Reproduced with permission from Downing SW, Kouchokos NT: Ascending aortic aneurysm, in Edmunds LH Jr (ed): Cardiac Surgery in the Adult. New York, McGraw-Hill, 1997; p 1163.)*

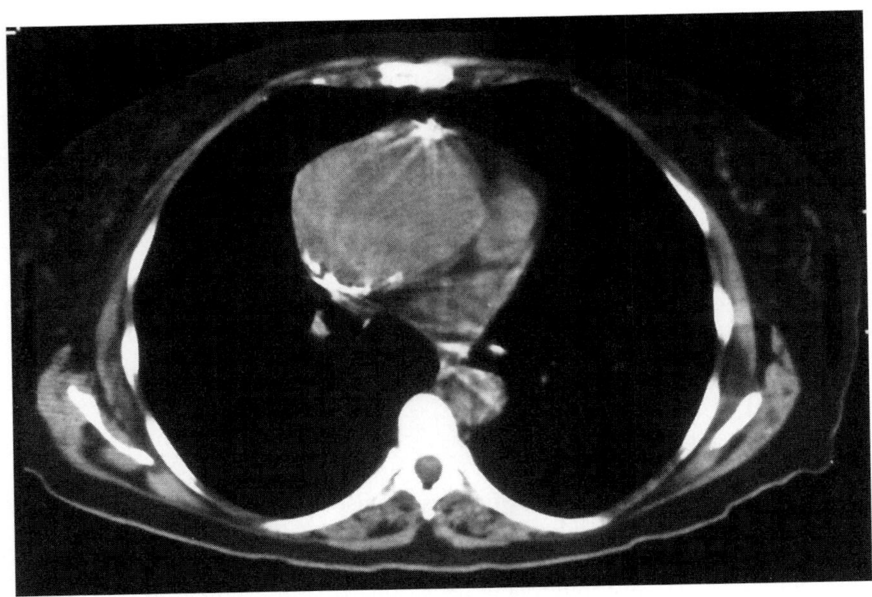

FIGURE 46–5 Computed tomographic scan of an 8-cm ascending aortic aneurysm. *(Reproduced with permission from Downing SW, Kouchokos NT: Ascending aortic aneurysm, in Edmunds LH Jr (ed): Cardiac Surgery in the Adult. New York, McGraw-Hill, 1997; p 1163.)*

aneurysm size in the presence of laminar clot, and the likelihood of missing dissections.

Computed Tomography

Contrast-enhanced computed tomography (CT) provides rapid and precise evaluation of the ascending aorta (Fig. 46-5). CT scanning detects areas of calcification, and accurately identifies dissections and mural thrombus. When laminar clot is present, CT scanning provides a more accurate assessment of aneurysm size than aortography. However, because structures are visualized in an axial view only, the diameter of a tortuous aorta can be grossly overestimated. Three-dimensional reconstruction of CT scans may prove useful in determining the proximal and distal extent of aortic disease relative to the arch vessels, which can aid the surgeon in operative planning.[78]

Magnetic Resonance Imaging

The benefits of magnetic resonance imaging (MRI) over CT scanning include visualization in the sagittal and coronal planes (Fig. 46-6), and the avoidance of contrast and radiation exposure. Cardiac imaging with MRI is evolving, and may provide evaluation of cardiac perfusion, myocardial function, and coronary and valve anatomy with a single modality in the future.[86–88] Currently, however, MRI is expensive, less readily available, and more time consuming than CT scanning.

INDICATIONS FOR OPERATION

Symptoms

Emergent operation is indicated in the setting of acute ascending aortic dissection or rupture. Ascending aortic aneurysms rupture into the pericardial space and result in death from acute cardiac tamponade. Aortic dissections may rupture or may compromise coronary or cerebral circulation. Operative mortality is significant in this setting, but death is certain in the case of rupture and probable in the case of acute dissection if not surgically addressed.

Symptomatic aortic insufficiency or stenosis may be the primary indication for operation. When replacing or repairing a diseased valve a decision must be made regarding the moderately dilated aorta. Michel et al [89] reported that 25% of patients undergoing surgery for aortic insufficiency who had ascending aortic diameters greater than 4 cm required subsequent operation for aortic replacement. Prenger et al [90] reported a 27% incidence of aortic dissection following aortic valve replacement in patients with aortic diameters greater than 5 cm. Based on these findings it is recommended that aortic diameters of 4 to 5 cm be dealt with at the time of aortic valve surgery. Further incentive for earlier surgery is the improved possibility of native valve preservation.

Size/Growth Rate

Because the diameter of an aneurysm strongly correlates with the risk of rupture or dissection, size has long been used as the criteria for elective surgical intervention. Although size criteria for the abdominal aorta have been well established and generally agreed upon, less of a consensus has emerged for the thoracic aorta. Variable growth rates and propensities for rupture in different regions of the thoracic aorta and with different underlying pathologies are perhaps to blame. The average size of rupture of the thoracic aorta reported in the literature is highly variable.[50,91,92] Coady et al[68] report rupture or dissection at a median size of 5.9 cm in the ascending aorta (Fig. 46-7 and 7.2 cm in the descending aorta. Because intervention at these diameters would

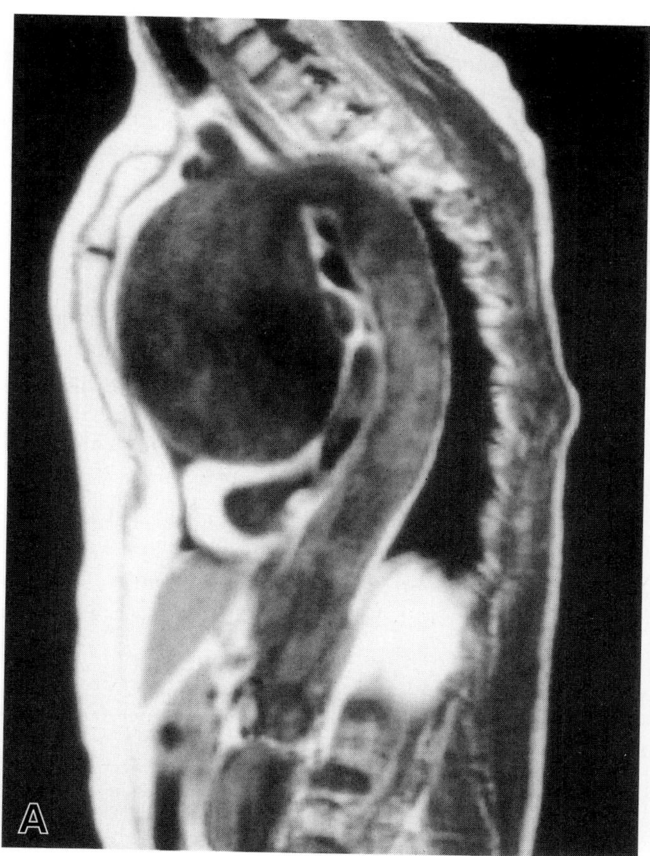

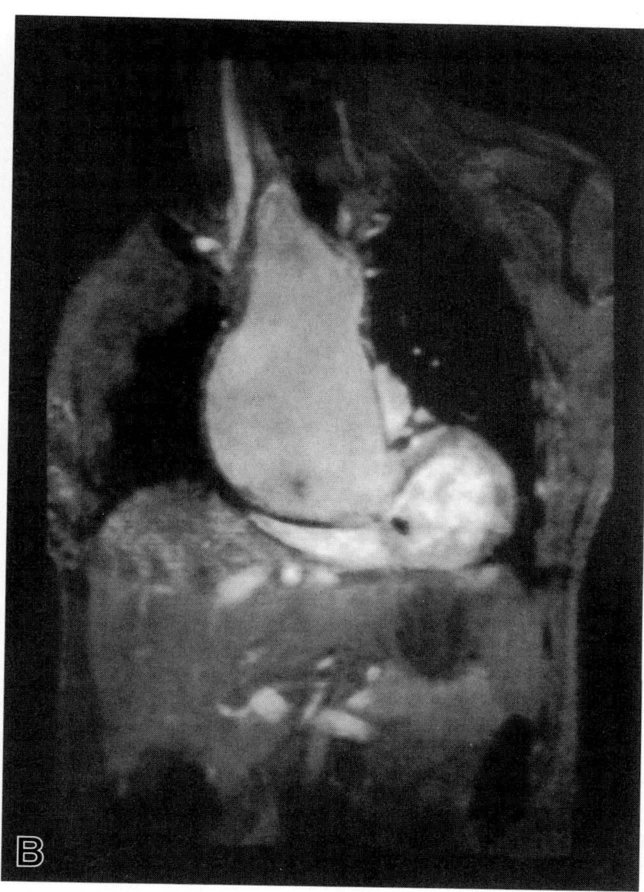

FIGURE 46–6 Magnetic resonance image of ascending aortic aneurysms demonstrating saggital (A) and coronal (B) views. The origin of the innominate and its relationship to the distal portion of the aneurysm can be appreciated on the saggital view. (*Images provided courtesy of Kent E. Yucel, M.D.*)

have by definition resulted in rupture or dissection in 50% of patients, preemptive surgical therapy at 5.5 cm and 6.5 cm, respectively, for ascending and descending aneurysms seems appropriate.

As opposed to absolute size criteria, some surgeons prefer the use of ratios of measured to expected size. The expected size is based on the body surface area and age of the patient. The ratio indicating intervention is adjusted based on

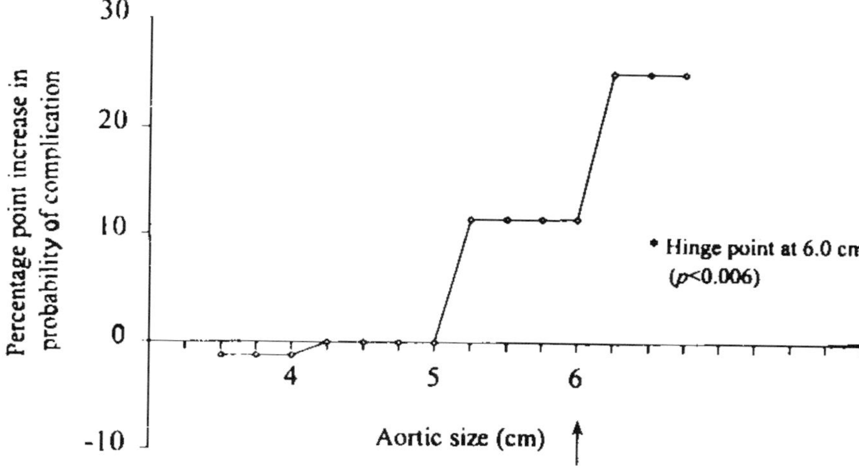

FIGURE 46–7 Logistic regression analysis of initial aneurysm size for risk of rupture or dissection. The probability of rupture or dissection is 25% higher in patients who present with aneurysms 6.0 cm or larger versus a comparison group with aneurysms 4.0 to 4.9 cm in diameter. Six centimeters appears to be a "hinge point" beyond which the risk of complications greatly increases. (*Reproduced with permission from Coady MA, Rizzo JA, Hammond GL, Kopf GS, Elefteriades JA: Surgical intervention criteria for thoracic aortic aneurysms: a study of growth rates and complications. Ann Thorac Surg 1999; 67:1922.*)

the underlying etiology. Ergin et al[93] advocate a ratio of 1.5 for the average patient with an asymptomatic incidentally discovered ascending aortic aneurysm. This leads to intervention at a size of only 4.8 to 5.0 cm in an adult less than 40 years of age with a body surface area of 2 m^2. Because the ascending aorta normally increases in size with age, the diameter for intervention would be higher in a patient more than 40 years old.

The rate of expansion is also an important consideration. Reported mean growth rates of thoracic aneurysms vary from 0.10 to 0.42 cm per year.[50,69,70,94–96] The rate of expansion is usually greater in the descending aorta and in conditions with a weakened aortic wall, such as Marfan syndrome or chronic dissection.[68] Growth at a rate of greater than 1.0 cm per year is certainly an accepted indication for surgical intervention,[50] but more often the rate of dilation is used by the surgeon as supplementary information that helps to guide the timing of surgery rather than serve as an absolute indication.

The Influence of Etiology

Patients with Marfan syndrome or with familial aneurysms, particularly when there is a history of early dissection or rupture, should undergo earlier intervention. Gott et al [97,98] recommend intervention in patients with Marfan syndrome at an ascending aortic diameter of 5.0 to 6.0 cm. Coady et al[99] recommend intervention at 5.0 cm. Ergin et al[93] recommend a measured to expected size ratio of 1.3. Patients with chronic dissection should be considered to have similar intervention criteria as those with Marfan syndrome. Patients with bicuspid and unicuspid aortic valves are probably at intermediate risk, and Ergin et al[93] recommend intervention at a ratio of 1.4 in these patients. Pseudoaneurysms are at a high risk of rupture and should be treated when discovered.

PREOPERATIVE PREPARATION

A careful preoperative evaluation of the patient is important to minimize the risks of surgery. Nearly one third of patients undergoing surgery for thoracic aortic disease have chronic obstructive pulmonary disease.[80] Patients with suspect pulmonary function should have spirometery and room air arterial blood gases. Smoking cessation, antibiotic treatment of chronic bronchitis, and chest physiotherapy may prove beneficial in elective situations. Normal renal function should be ensured with the appropriate blood work, and abnormal results should prompt further investigation. Because unaddressed severe carotid disease is a risk factor for stroke during ascending aortic operations,[100] patients over the age of 65 should have duplex imaging of their carotids. Younger patients with peripheral vascular disease, extensive coronary artery disease, carotid bruits, or history suspicious for cerebral ischemia should be investigated as well.[101] Abdominal aortic aneurysms occur in 10% to 20% of patients with ascending aortic aneurysms.[23,80] Patients with "atherosclerotic aneurysms" that extend into the aortic arch have a greater than 50% probability of having distal thoracic or abdominal aortic aneurysms.[80] CT or MRI of the abdominal aorta is indicated if disease is suspected.

CHOICE OF PROCEDURE

The specific procedure that is performed depends on the distal extent of aortic involvement, condition of the aortic root and the aortic valve, underlying pathology, life expectancy of the patient, desired anticoagulation status, and surgeon preference. Specific procedures and their indications are listed in Table 46-1.

Ascending Aortic Aneurysms

Ascending aortic aneurysms with normal sinuses and aortic annulus require only replacement of the ascending aorta

TABLE 46–1 Specific procedures and indications

Procedure	Potential indications
Simple tube graft*	Ascending aortic aneurysm with normal aortic root May correct central AI resulting from dilation of the ST junction
Composite valve-graft conduit	Involvement of ascending aorta and the root with aortic valve that cannot be spared
Separate ascending aorta-aortic valve replacement*	Ascending aortic aneurysm with normal root and aortic valve that requires replacement
Aortic allograft	Endocarditis with root destruction or infection of previous composite graft Root replacement for younger patients with active lifestyle or patients with contraindications to warfarin
Pulmonary autograft**	Root replacement for young patients who will benefit from growth potential of autograft Root replacement for younger patients with active lifestyle or patients with contraindications to warfarin
Aortic valve-sparing procedure Reimplantation Root remodeling	Diseased ascending aorta and root with grossly normal aortic valves
External wrapping of the ascending aorta	Debilitated patients with limited survival who may not tolerate more extensive procedures

AI = aortic insufficiency; ST = sinotubular junction.
*Sparing the aortic root is contraindicated in Marfan syndrome.
**The use of a pulmonary autograft is contraindicated in Marfan syndrome.

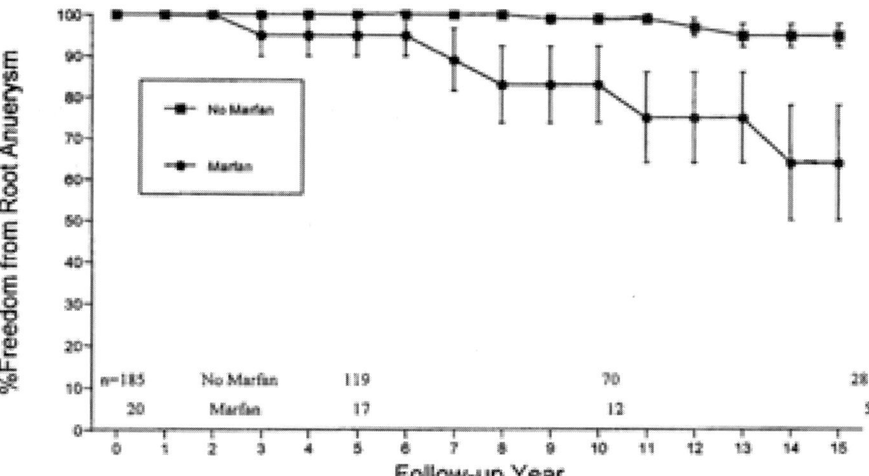

FIGURE 46–8 Actuarial estimate of freedom from late aortic root aneurysm for patients with and without Marfan syndrome who have undergone ascending aortic operations ($p < .0001$). (*Reproduced with permission from Yun KL, Miller DC: Ascending aortic aneurysm and aortic valve disease: what is the most optimal surgical technique? Semin Thorac Cardiovasc Surg 1997; 9:233.*)

from the sinotubular ridge to the origin of the innominate artery with a Dacron tube graft. If the aortic valve is diseased, this can be replaced separately. The sinuses in patients with Marfan syndrome should not be preserved because of the frequent need for reoperation (Fig. 46-8).[102,103]

Annuloaortic Ectasia

COMPOSITE VALVE-GRAFT CONDUIT

Patients who have significant dilation of the aortic root in addition to an aneurysm of the ascending aorta or patients with Marfan syndrome should undergo replacement of the ascending aorta and root. This is usually done with a composite graft consisting of a mechanical valve inserted into a collagen- or gelatin-impregnated Dacron graft that comes preassembled. The coronary arteries are reimplanted as buttons.

AORTIC ALLOGRAFT

The ascending aorta and root can be replaced with an aortic allograft with coronary reimplantation.[104] Accepted indications include patients with endocarditis, women anticipating pregnancy, young adults with active lifestyles, or patients with any other contraindications to anticoagulation.[105]

PULMONARY AUTOGRAFTS (ROSS PROCEDURE)

A pulmonary autograft can be used to replace the aortic root and proximal ascending aorta. More distal replacement of the ascending aorta requires addition of a Dacron graft. The Ross procedure is most commonly performed for congenital surgery because of the proposed growth potential of the autograft. The use of the Ross procedure in adults with aneurysmal disease is more controversial. Potential indications include young adults with active lifestyles and life expectancies exceeding 15 to 20 years, women anticipating pregnancy, or patients with any contraindication to warfarin therapy.[105] The Ross procedure is contraindicated in patients with Marfan syndrome or inherited weakness of the aortic wall that may affect durability of the autograft.[105,106]

VALVE-SPARING PROCEDURES

If the aortic valve leaflets are grossly normal and aortic insufficiency is secondary to dilation of the sinotubular ridge or aortic root, then the native valve can often be spared.[107,108] Yacoub has been able to apply valve-sparing techniques in almost 80% of patients operated on for ascending aortic aneurysms.[109] A variety of procedures are used to preserve the aortic valve. Reduction of the diameter of the sinotubular ridge via ascending aorta replacement[110] may be all that is required to correct central insufficiency. If the aortic root is involved, it may be completely replaced by inserting the scalloped native valve into a Dacron graft,[111] or dilated sinuses may be individually remodeled with tongues of the proximal Dacron graft.[112] If significant annular dilation is present, an aortic annuloplasty can be performed with the external application of a strip of graft material.[113] The application of valve-sparing procedures to patients with Marfan syndrome is controversial as the durability of the leaflets is in question.[114] These procedures are discussed in detail in Chapter 31.

ALTERNATIVE PROCEDURES

In older patients who are high risk, or who have limited life expectancy, external wrapping of the aorta or separate valve and ascending aorta replacement may be appropriate without addressing the aortic root.[93,103,115]

Management of Associated Conditions

CORONARY ARTERY DISEASE

Twenty-five percent of patients undergoing surgery for ascending aortic aneurysms will have concomitant coronary artery disease.[80] These patients should have appropriate bypass grafting performed at the time of ascending aneurysm surgery.

MITRAL VALVE DISEASE

Mitral valve disease is frequently encountered in patients with aortic aneurysms. This is particularly true for patients with Marfan syndrome, where the incidence approaches 30%.[44] Patients who have evidence of moderate to severe mitral regurgitation should undergo mitral valve repair or replacement at the time of aortic replacement.[61,116] Gilinov et al [117] reported results of mitral valve repair in patients with Marfan syndrome, many of whom also had simultaneous replacement of the aortic root. They observed an 88% actuarial rate of freedom from significant mitral regurgitation at 5 years.

OPERATIVE TECHNIQUE

General

MONITORING AND ANESTHESIA

Venous access consists of two large-bore peripheral lines and a central line. We monitor filling pressures and cardiac output with a pulmonary artery catheter. A radial artery line provides blood pressure monitoring and determination of activated clotting times. Systemic temperature is monitored with nasopharyngeal and bladder probes. Transesophageal echocardiographic assessment of myocardial and valvular function is routine. Anesthesia is maintained with isoflurane and intravenous fentanyl.

INCISION

A median sternotomy is the preferred incision. Extension into the left 4th or 5th interspace facilitates exposure of the distal aortic arch or descending aorta when required.

PERFUSION

Cannulation is performed following heparinization (350 U/kg) and confirmation of an activated clotting time greater than 450 seconds. If the distal ascending aorta is not involved, this region or the proximal arch is cannulated. The aortic cannulation site must allow enough room proximally for the cross-clamp and a sufficient cuff of aortic tissue to sew to, while still allowing all diseased aorta to be resected. Epiaortic ultrasound assists in finding safe areas for clamping and cannulation. If the arch is involved and circulatory arrest will be required, the femoral artery or the aneurysm itself is cannulated. Before retrograde perfusion of the femoral artery is considered, however, TEE assessment of the descending aorta is performed. Venous cannulation is performed with a 21F or 24F two-stage cannula in the right atrial appendage. The superior and inferior vena cavae are cannulated separately if circulatory arrest or mitral valve intervention will be required. This allows for retrograde cerebral perfusion and a transeptal approach to the mitral valve.

The cardiopulmonary bypass circuit is primed with lactated Ringer's and 25 g of mannitol. No glucose is added to the prime to prevent exacerbation of neurological injury.[118] The cannulas are attached, and low-flow cardiopulmonary bypass is initiated. A left ventricular vent is inserted via the right superior pulmonary vein and a balloon-tipped catheter is inserted into the coronary sinus for retrograde cardioplegia delivery. Cardiopulmonary bypass flow is increased to 2.2 to 2.5 L/min/m^2 and moderate systemic hypothermia (28°C) and hemodilution (hematocrit 15%-25%) are established.

MYOCARDIAL PROTECTION

Cold blood hyperkalemic cardioplegia (4°C) is given antegrade into the aortic root at a rate of 300 mL/min for 2 minutes and then retrograde at a rate of 200 mL/min for an additional 2 minutes. A cooling jacket may be used to facilitate this process. If the aortic valve is grossly incompetent, and prompt arrest is not achieved with retrograde cardioplegia, the aorta is opened and the coronary ostia are cannulated directly. During the procedure, retrograde cardioplegia is administered every 20 minutes.

CHOICE OF GRAFT

Woven double velour Dacron grafts impregnated with collagen or gelatin are relatively impervious to blood and have excellent handling characteristics. If root replacement is required, prefabricated composite grafts with mechanical valves are available. Bioprosthetic valves can be inserted into a Dacron graft if desired. The indications for pulmonary autograft or aortic allograft use have been previously discussed.

Specific Operative Techniques

REPLACEMENT OF THE ASCENDING AORTA

After cardiopulmonary bypass is established the aorta is clamped just proximal to the innominate artery, and the heart is arrested with cold blood cardioplegia. The aorta is transected below the clamp leaving a sufficient cuff for subsequent anastomosis (Fig. 46-9A). The proximal aorta is then transected just above the commissures. An appropriately sized Dacron graft is selected and sewn to the distal aorta with a continuous 3-0 or 4-0 polypropylene, incorporating a strip of felt (Fig. 46-9B). If required, the aortic valve is replaced at this time (Figs. 46-9C and 46-9D). The proximal

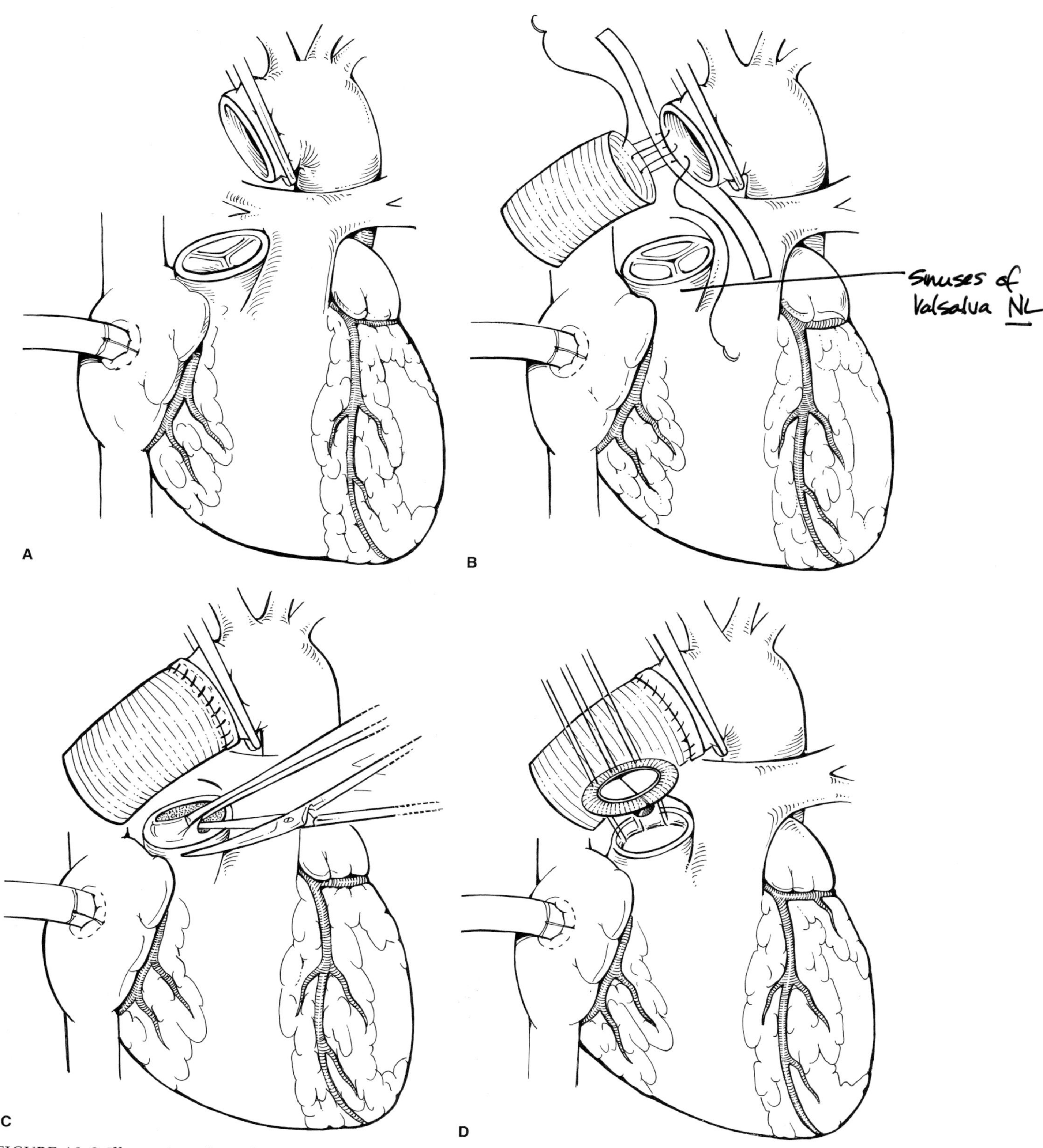

FIGURE 46–9 Illustration of simple aortic tube graft placement with separate replacement of the aortic valve. (A) The aorta is clamped proximal to the innominate artery (aortic perfusion cannula not shown) and the diseased aorta is resected down to just above the aortic valve commissures. (B) A Dacron graft is sewn to the distal aorta with a 3-0 or 4-0 polypropylene suture reinforced with a strip of Teflon felt. (C) If aortic valve replacement is indicated, the diseased valve is excised. (D) The valve is replaced with the valve of the surgeon's choice.

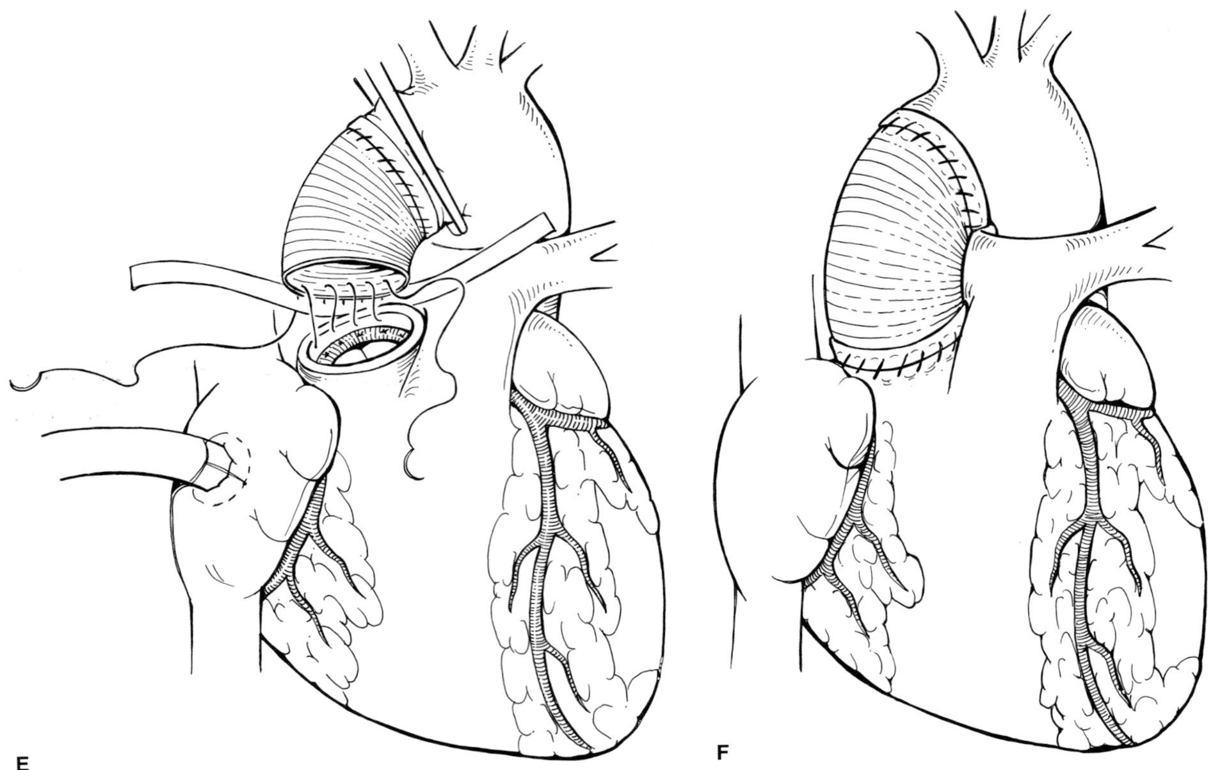

FIGURE 46–9 (*Continued*) (E, F) The graft is sewn to the proximal aorta with 3-0 or 4-0 polypropylene reinforcing the aortic tissue with a strip of Teflon felt. (*Reproduced with permission from Downing SW, Kouchokos NT: Ascending aortic aneurysm, in Edmunds LH Jr (ed): Cardiac Surgery in the Adult. New York, McGraw-Hill, 1997; p 1163.*)

anastomosis is performed in the same fashion after the graft is cut to the appropriate length (Figs. 46-9E and 46-9F). The graft is de-aired and the patient is weaned from cardiopulmonary bypass. After decannulation and protamine administration, suture line hemostasis is ensured.

REPLACEMENT OF THE ASCENDING AORTA AND AORTIC ROOT WITH A COMPOSITE VALVE-GRAFT CONDUIT

After establishing cardiopulmonary bypass, the aorta is clamped just proximal to the innominate artery and the heart is arrested with cold blood cardioplegia. The aorta is transected beneath the clamp ensuring an adequate cuff of aortic tissue. Proximally the aortic root is excised leaving only buttons of aortic tissue surrounding each of the coronary arteries (Fig. 46-10A). The coronaries are mobilized for 1 to 2 cm to prevent tension during reimplantation. A composite graft is selected based on the size of the aortic annulus. The sewing ring of the composite graft is sutured to the annulus with 2-0 pledgeted polyester mattress sutures placed immediately adjacent to each other (Fig 46-10B). The adjacent placement of sutures and the selection of a conduit that snugly fits within the annulus help to ensure hemostasis. Openings for coronary reimplantation are made in the appropriate position in the Dacron graft with an ophthalmic cautery (Fig. 46-10C). First the left and then the right coronary arteries are attached using 4-0 or 5-0 polypropylene suture in continuous fashion incorporating a thin strip of felt (Fig. 46-10D). The distal anastomosis is then performed with a continuous 3-0 or 4-0 polypropylene suture also incorporating a strip of felt. The graft is vented with a needle and the left atrium and ventricle are de-aired. After the patient is decannulated and protamine has been administered, suture line hemostasis is scrutinized.

REPLACEMENT OF THE ASCENDING AORTA AND AORTIC ROOT WITH AN ALLOGRAFT OR AUTOGRAFT

The muscular tissue at the base of the conduit is sutured to the aortic annulus with a continuous or interrupted 4-0 polypropylene or braided synthetic suture. The suture line is reinforced with a strip of Dacron or pericardium. Coronary ostia are created and coronary buttons are inserted with a continuous 4-0 or 5-0 polypropylene suture. Extension with a Dacron tube graft may be required to successfully replace the entire diseased aorta.

OPEN TECHNIQUE FOR DISTAL ANASTOMOSIS

The distal aortic anastomosis may need to be sewn under circulatory arrest as an “open technique” if clamping of the distal ascending aorta is not safe, or if partial or complete

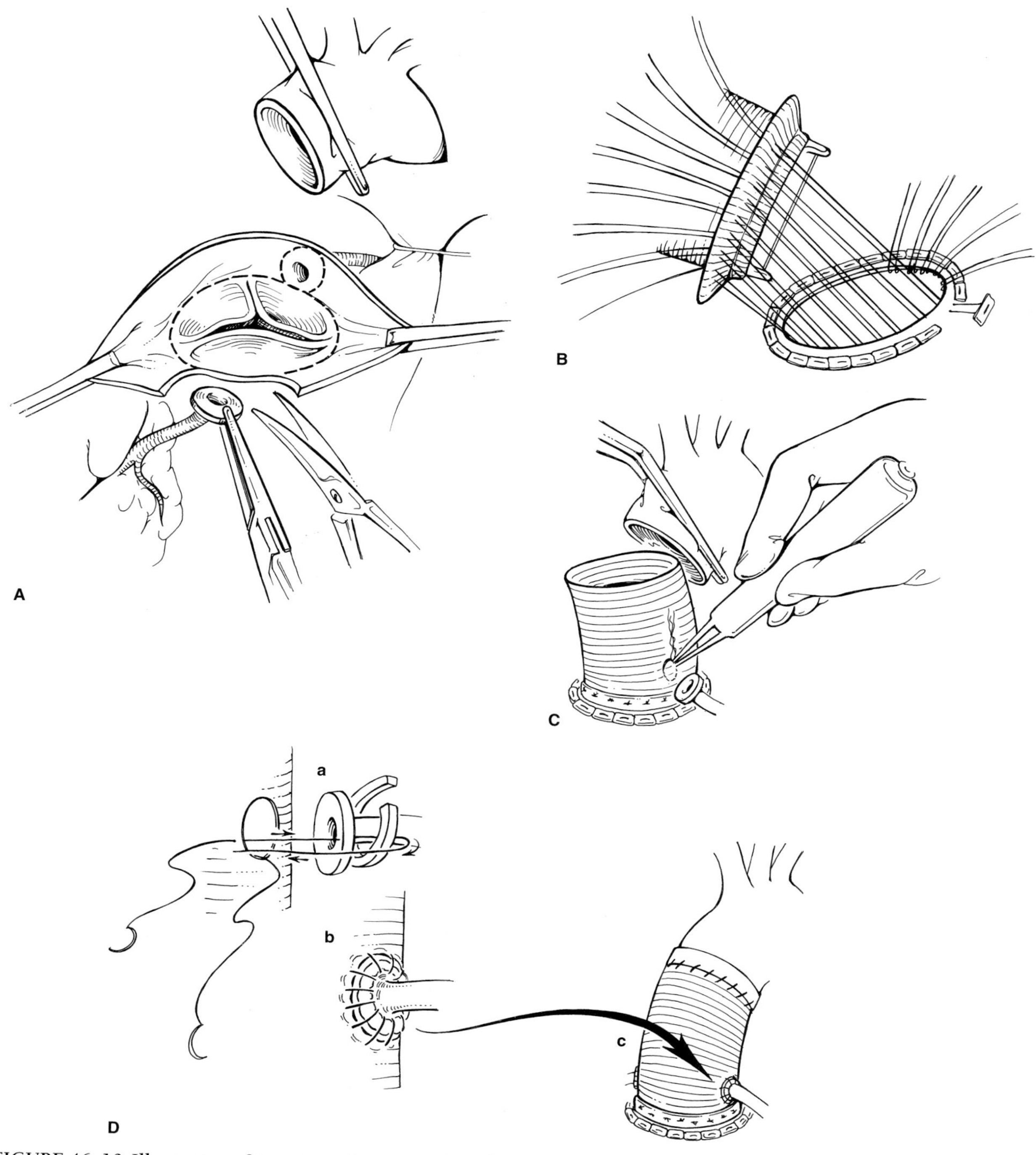

FIGURE 46–10 Illustration of insertion of a composite valve-graft conduit with coronary artery reimplantation. (A) A full-thickness button of aortic wall adjacent to each coronary ostium is fashioned. The aortic valve and sinuses are then excised. (B) Pledgeted 2-0 braided polyester sutures are placed in the supra-annular position and immediately adjacent to one another to ensure a watertight closure. The sutures are placed in the upper half of the sewing ring helping to seat the valve deep within the aortic annulus. Note that no knots or suture material are exposed to the bloodstream. (C) Ophthalmic cautery is used to create an orifice in the graft in the appropriate position for left coronary reimplantation. (D) The left coronary anastomosis is performed first with a continuous 4-0 or 5-0 polypropylene suture incorporating a thin strip of felt. The right coronary anastomosis is then performed in a similar fashion. (*Reproduced with permission from Downing SW, Kouchokos NT: Ascending aortic aneurysm, in Edmunds LH Jr (ed): Cardiac Surgery in the Adult. New York, McGraw-Hill, 1997; p 1163.*)

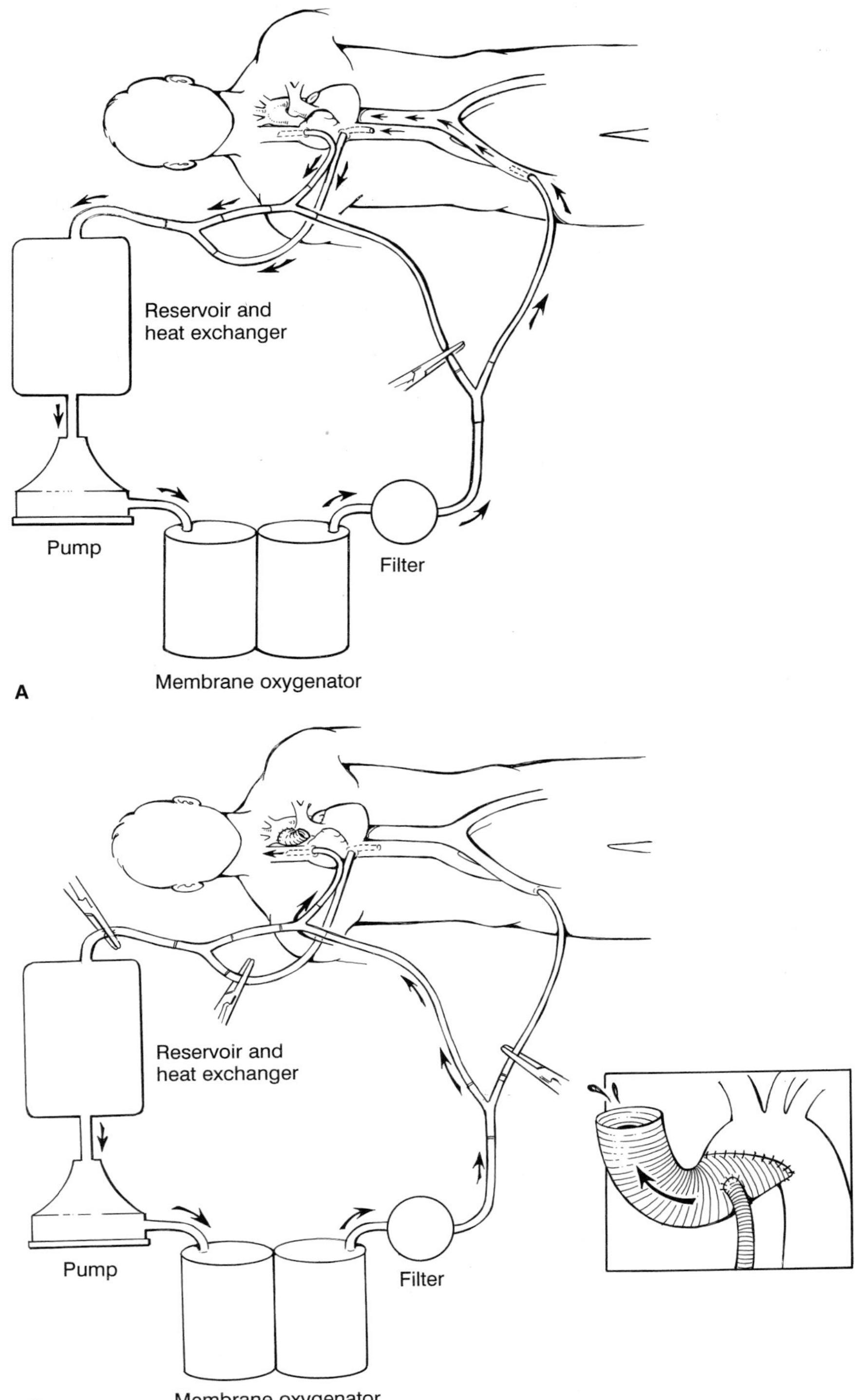

FIGURE 46–11 Schematic representation of the cardiopulmonary bypass circuit used for circulatory arrest when a portion or all of the aortic arch is to be replaced, or when it is unsafe to clamp the ascending aorta. (A) Cardiopulmonary bypass is established using two vena cava cannulas and a femoral artery cannula. A shunt connecting the venous and arterial lines is clamped. (B) The arterial and inferior vena caval lines are clamped and the shunt is opened allowing retrograde cerebral perfusion of cold oxygenated blood through the superior vena cava cannula. Air and atherosclerotic debris are evacuated from the brachiocephalic arteries (inset). A separate 8-mm Dacron graft is sewn to the side of the Dacron graft to allow antegrade reperfusion of the brain once the distal anastomosis is done.

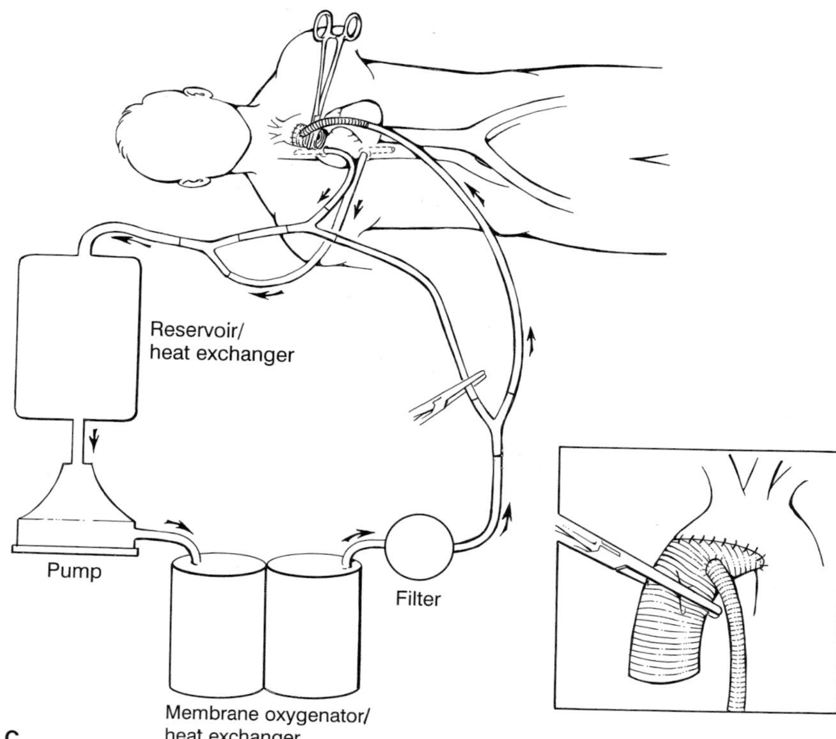

FIGURE 46–11 *(Continued)* (C) **Cardiopulmonary bypass is reestablished in an antegrade fashion. The femoral arterial cannula is removed and the shunt is occluded.** *(Reproduced with permission from Downing SW, Kouchokos NT: Ascending aortic aneurysm, in Edmunds LH Jr (ed): Cardiac Surgery in the Adult. New York, McGraw-Hill, 1997; p 1163.)*

arch replacement is indicated. Clamping may be dangerous because of atherosclerotic disease or clot, or may not be possible because of the distal extent of the aneurysm. Cardiopulmonary bypass is initiated with femoral artery cannulation or direct cannulation of the ascending aneurysm depending on the indication for circulatory arrest. The typical cardiopulmonary bypass setup for a case requiring circulatory arrest is shown in Figure 46-11A. Central nervous system protection is enhanced by maintaining the blood glucose below 200 mg/dL, as well as by the administration of methylprednisolone (7mg/kg) and thiopental (7-15 mg/kg). Mannitol (0.3-0.4 g/kg) and furosemide (100 mg) are given for renal preservation. Once nasopharyngeal temperature reaches 15°C and the electroencephalogram has been isoelectric for 5 minutes, the patient is placed in Trendelenburg position and the circulation arrested. Approximately 25% of the patient's volume is drained into the venous reservoir. The superior vena cava is clamped to raise central venous pressure prior to opening the aorta to prevent air embolism.

The aorta is divided distally in a region dictated by the distal extent of disease. If the aneurysm ends at the takeoff of the innominate artery, the aorta can be transected here and the graft sewn, leaving the arch intact. If the aneurysm extends to the proximal undersurface of the arch, the distal end of the graft is beveled to conform to the resected surface of the arch (Fig. 46-11B). If the arch in the region of the origin of the brachiocephalic vessels is involved, then the aorta is divided distal to the origin of the left subclavian artery. The distal anastomosis is performed with a running 3-0 polypropylene suture enforced with a felt strip. An elliptical portion of the graft is then excised which corresponds to a single island of aortic tissue that has been fashioned around the origin of the brachiocephalic vessels. This anastomosis is performed with felt-enforced running 3-0 polypropylene sutures as well. During this anastomosis, slow retrograde perfusion of the superior vena cava is performed to remove any air or particulate debris (Fig. 46-11B). Antegrade perfusion is then initiated via direct cannulation of the graft or insertion of a cannula into a previously placed 8-mm side graft (Fig. 46-11C). Femoral perfusion is not resumed in order to prevent cerebral embolization of distal aortic debris that may have occurred during previous manipulations.

The patient is rewarmed, and any additional procedures that are required such as coronary revascularization or mitral valve interventions are performed now that cerebral circulation has been restored. The proximal graft is sewn to the ascending aorta just above the sinotubular ridge or the aortic annulus in the case of composite graft placement. Thorough de-airing is performed and the patient is weaned from cardiopulmonary bypass. After protamine, suture lines are inspected closely.

CABROL TECHNIQUE FOR REESTABLISHING CORONARY FLOW

Avoidance of tension at the site of coronary reimplantation after aortic root replacement is essential to prevent postoperative bleeding and pseudoaneurysm formation. In the Cabrol technique, a single 8- to 10-mm Dacron graft is anastomosed

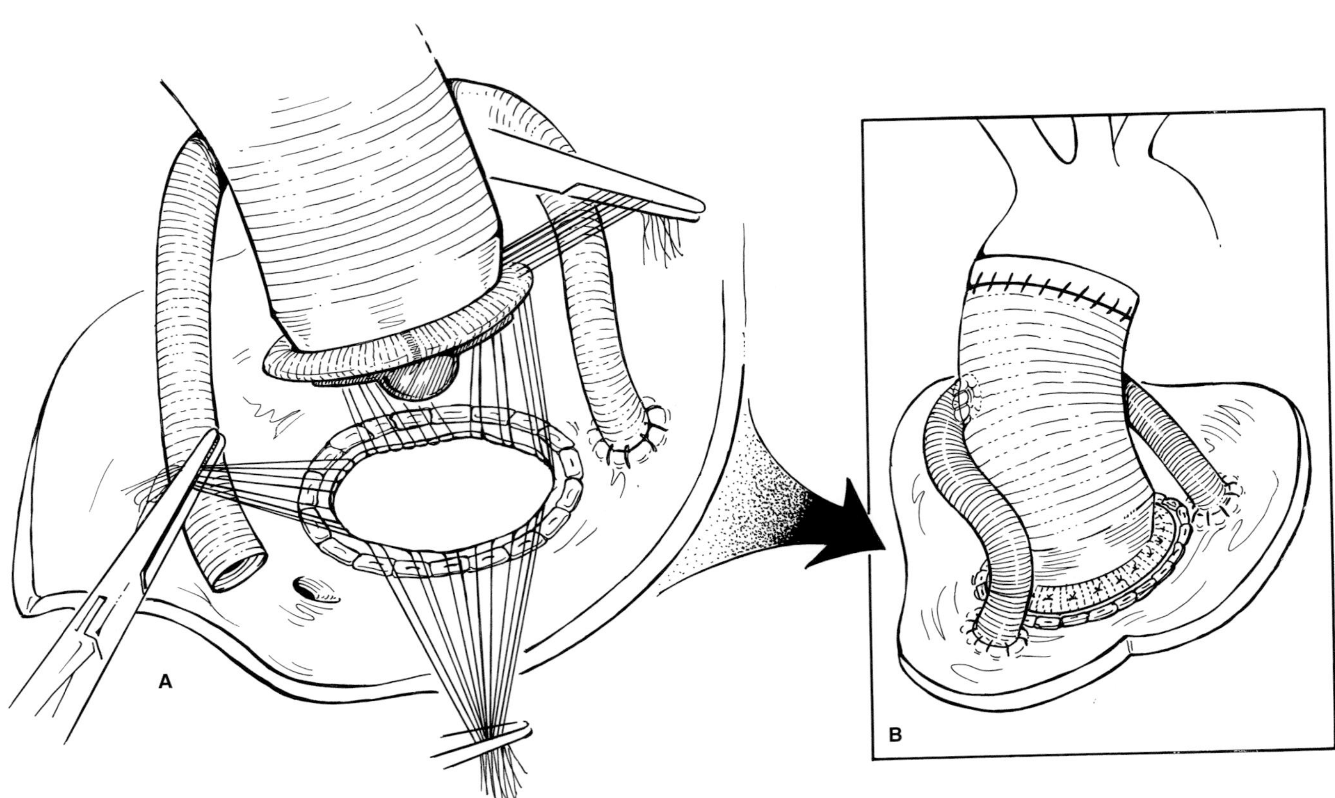

FIGURE 46–12 Classic Cabrol technique for coronary reimplantation. (A) An 8- to 10-mm Dacron tube graft is anastomosed end-to-end to the aortic tissue surrounding the left and right coronary ostia. (B) An opening is made in the mid portion of the coronary graft and in an appropriate position in the aortic graft and an anastomosis is formed. The modified Cabrol technique involves the formation of individual coronary buttons allowing the small caliber Dacron graft to be sewn to the full thickness of the aortic tissue surrounding the coronary ostia. (*Reproduced with permission from Downing SW, Kouchokos NT: Ascending aortic aneurysm, in Edmunds LH Jr (ed): Cardiac Surgery in the Adult. New York, McGraw-Hill, 1997; p 1163.*)

end-to-end to the coronary arteries and then the mid segment of the coronary graft is anastomosed side-to-side to the aortic graft (Fig. 46-12). This technique is often required when the coronary ostia are low or when there is scarring from a previous operation preventing adequate mobilization. Tension on the left coronary anastomosis is more common, and a small Dacron interposition graft may be required on this side in isolation in certain cases.

REOPERATION ON THE ASCENDING AORTA AND AORTIC ROOT

Reoperative surgery on the ascending aorta and aortic root can be particularly challenging, but is becoming more frequent. Because of improved outcomes,[61,64,100,119,120] the criteria for treatment of ascending aortic disease have been liberalized to include more elderly patients and more patients who have had previous cardiac surgery.[121,122] Increasing use of allografts, pulmonary autografts, and valve-preserving techniques may also result in an increased need for subsequent reintervention as these patients age. Indications for reoperation include aortic insufficiency, development of aneurysms or dissections in remaining segments of the thoracic aorta, false aneurysms, prosthetic valve malfunction or infection, or degeneration of biologic prostheses.[121]

To maximize safety, preemptive femoral exposure or cannulation is required. In the case of large pseudoaneurysms or grafts tethered to the posterior sternal wall, significant blood loss may be unavoidable upon entry. In such situations it is necessary to go on "pump-sucker bypass" until structures are dissected out and bleeding is controlled. Fifty percent of patients undergoing reoperation have significant aortic insufficiency, making myocardial preservation more challenging. In such cases, the perfusate temperature must not be reduced until exposure is sufficient to allow either clamping of the aorta or venting in order to prevent fibrillation and distension of the left ventricle. Reimplantation of coronary buttons in the case of root replacement is often not possible without use of a modified Cabrol technique or an interposition graft.

Management of Complications

BLEEDING

Woven Dacron grafts impregnated with collagen or gelatin are relatively impervious to blood and have reduced blood loss following replacement of the ascending aorta. Anastomotic bleeding is lessened with the use of Teflon pledgets at the aortic and coronary anastomoses. When composite valve-graft insertion is indicated, choosing a valve size that snugly fits the annulus and placing mattress stitches immediately adjacent to each other are helpful. Tension must be avoided at the sites of coronary reimplantation, as this is a frequent site of bleeding. The modified Cabrol method or an interposition graft should be used when any tension is present. The inclusion technique of graft insertion is associated with an increased incidence of bleeding and pseudoaneurysm formation and has largely been abandoned.[61,123,124] All coronary and aortic anastomoses should be sewn to the full thickness of the aorta, and wrapping of the graft with residual aorta is not indicated. After the administration of protamine, all anastomoses must be evaluated closely.

Suspected coagulopathy should be documented by laboratory tests and treated accordingly. In cases of refractory coagulopathy, the anastomosis can be wrapped tightly with a small segment of Dacron to reduce tension on the suture line and reduce needle hole bleeding. Homologous blood donation can be avoided in a significant number of patients with the use of blood conservation techniques such as cell savers, autologous blood donation, platelet pheresis, the reinfusion of chest tube drainage, and the use of antifibrinolytics.[64]

STROKE

Neurologic injury following proximal aortic surgery remains a significant cause of morbidity and mortality. Embolization of atherosclerotic debris or thrombus from the ascending aorta and arch produces focal neurologic deficits. Diffuse injury can be attributed to microemboli of air or cellular debris, insufficient or uneven cooling, and a prolonged circulatory arrest period. After circulatory arrest periods exceeding 40 minutes the incidence of stroke greatly increases.[125] Profound hypothermia may itself be injurious to the central nervous system without associated circulatory arrest.[125]

Stroke due to embolization is diminished when the aorta is evaluated via epiaortic ultrasound or other imaging modality to detect atherosclerotic plaques and thrombus. This allows appropriate adjustments to be made in clamping and cannulation strategies.[126] The utility of retrograde cerebral perfusion as an adjunct to hypothermic circulatory arrest is controversial, but some groups report an increase in the safe period of circulatory arrest.[127–129] Laboratory evidence suggests that the primary benefits of retrograde cerebral perfusion are flushing of embolic material and perhaps more homogeneous cooling, rather than effective nutrient delivery, which is far superior with antegrade circulation.[130] Resumption of antegrade circulation through the graft once the distal aortic anastomosis is complete, rather than retrograde via the femoral vessels, after a period of circulatory arrest avoids embolization of distal aortic debris. Patients with severe carotid artery occlusive disease are at increased risk of stroke during ascending aortic procedures,[100] and patients older than 65, those with peripheral vascular disease, or those with pertinent histories should be evaluated.

PULMONARY DYSFUNCTION

Cardiopulmonary bypass is known to cause alterations in pulmonary function as evidenced by changes in alveolar-arterial oxygen gradients, pulmonary vascular resistance, pulmonary compliance, and intrapulmonary shunting. Usually these changes are subclinical, but a full-blown adult respiratory distress-like syndrome is reported in 0.5% to 1.7% of patients following cardiopulmonary bypass.[131] The specific cause is the subject of much investigation and debate, but it is generally accepted that exposure of blood elements to the foreign surface of the cardiopulmonary circuit results in the activation of inflammatory cells and the complement cascade resulting in pulmonary injury.[131] The duration of cardiopulmonary bypass, urgency of the procedure, and general condition of the patient may roughly correlate with the occurrence and severity of pulmonary dysfunction, but it can be unpredictable.[132]

Treatment is supportive, with early diagnosis and treatment of any subsequent pulmonary infections. Preventative measures may include preoperative optimization of pulmonary function, minimization of pump time, judicious use of blood products, heparin-coated bypass circuits,[133,134] and leukocyte depletion.[135,136]

POSTOPERATIVE CORONARY INSUFFICIENCY

Coronary insufficiency is uncommon in the postoperative period, but may occur following root replacement and coronary reimplantation. Ischemia may be due to kinking of a Dacron or saphenous vein interposition graft. Coronaries implanted under tension, or aortic suture lines, may bleed resulting in compression from an expanding hematoma. Suspicion of coronary insufficiency must be promptly evaluated with angiography and/or reoperation.

RESULTS OF OPERATION

Perioperative Morbidity

The primary causes of significant morbidity in the early postoperative period are neurologic injury and bleeding. Stroke has been reported in 1.8% to 5.9% of patients in various series.[64,80,120,137–139] Antegrade reperfusion following completion of the distal aortic anastomosis[64] and the use of retrograde cerebral perfusion[127,128] may lower the risk of stroke in patients requiring circulatory arrest. Postoperative bleeding requiring reoperation ranges from 2.4% to 11.1%.[61,64,120,137–140] The use of the exclusion technique of graft insertion and blood impervious grafts has resulted in lower bleeding rates in more recent series. Ten to eighteen percent of patients require prolonged mechanical ventilation,[64,139] and 18% to 25% require prolonged (more than 6 hours) inotropic support.[61,139] Postoperative myocardial infarction, reported in up to 2.5%, may be related to technical problems with coronary reimplantation.[64,120,137]

Perioperative Mortality

Contemporary surgical series on ascending aortic disease using modern grafting techniques and methods of cerebral and myocardial protection report hospital mortality rates of 1.7% to 17.1%.[41,64,93,119,120,140–142] Comparison of outcomes is difficult, however, because of heterogeneity of patients. Some series do not include dissection,[120] and the proportion of emergent operations, reoperations, and arch replacements is highly variable. The most common cause of early death is clearly cardiac failure. Other frequent causes of early death include stroke, bleeding, and pulmonary insufficiency.[61,80,119,137–139]

Risk Factors for Hospital Mortality

Emergent operation after the onset of acute dissection or rupture is the clearest risk factor for early death.[80,93,137] Risk of death following elective intervention is increased by increasing NYHA classification,[119,137,143] increasing age,[80,93,138,139,143] prolonged cardiopulmonary bypass time,[61,137,138] dissection,[119] previous cardiac surgery,[80,139] and need for concomitant coronary revascularization.[137,139] Major risk factors are shown in Table 46-2.

Late Mortality

Reported actuarial survival, like early mortality, is variable and dependent upon the patient cohort. Survival rates are 81% to 95% at 1 year,[80,137] 73% to 92% at 5 years,[80,93,119,137] 60% to 73% at 8 to 10 years,[93,119,139] and 48% to 67% at 12 to 14 years.[61,119] Predictors of late mortality include elevated NYHA,[61,139] requirement for arch reconstruction,[139] Marfan syndrome,[61] and extent of distal disease.[80,137] The most common cause of late death is cardiac, but distal aortic disease accounted for 32% of late deaths in one series.[80]

Reoperation

Reoperations may be required because of pseudoaneurysm formation, valve thrombosis or endocarditis, progression of

TABLE 46–2 Independent predictors of early mortality

Risk factor	*p*-value (range)
Emergent operation	000-.0017
NYHA	.0001-.015
Age	.01-.045
CPB time	<.001-.018
Dissection	<.001-.04
Concomitant CABG	.001-.0014
Previous cardiac operation	<.001-.0068
Arch replacement	<.001
Reoperation for bleed	.0009-.032

NYHA = New York Heart Association classification; CPB = cardiopulmonary bypass; CABG = coronary artery bypass grafting. Only risk factors found to be predictive on multivariate analysis are reported. Some of the reported risk factors were not significant in some series. Data are from the following references: 41, 61, 80, 119, 137, 138, 139, 141, 142, 143.

disease in the native valve or remaining aortic segments, or because of degeneration of a bioprosthesis. Reported mortality for reoperative ascending aortic surgery varies between 6% and 22%, but has been reported as low as 3% for elective reoperations[122] and as high as 100% for emergent reoperations.[144] Predictors of poor outcome have included emergent reoperation, requirement for arch replacement, preoperative functional class III/IV, and duration of cardiopulmonary bypass.[121,122] Freedom from reoperation is 86% to 90% at 9 to 10 years.[119,139] Predictors of late reoperation have included Marfan syndrome (Fig. 46-13), the inclusion cylinder technique (Fig. 46-14),[61,145] and chronic dissection. Surveillance of patients who have undergone previous aortic surgery to minimize the need for urgent reoperations and appropriate resection of all diseased aortic tissue at the time of original operation will improve outcomes. In one series it was estimated that nearly 60% percent of redo aortic cases were required because of inadequate repair during previous operations.[121]

Thromboembolism

Major thromboembolic events following replacement of the aortic root with a composite graft are currently uncommon. Unlike simple aortic valve replacement, suture material and pledgets are excluded from the bloodstream. Freedom from thromboembolism was 82% to 83% at 10 to 12 years in two older series.[61,138] The incidence in more recent series is considerably lower.[64] Gott et al [119] reported an incidence of only 0.42 thromboembolic events per 100 patient years.

Prosthetic Valve Endocarditis

Prosthetic valve endocarditis is not reported in some series, but was the most common late complication occurring after root replacement reported by Gott et al.[119] The actuarial

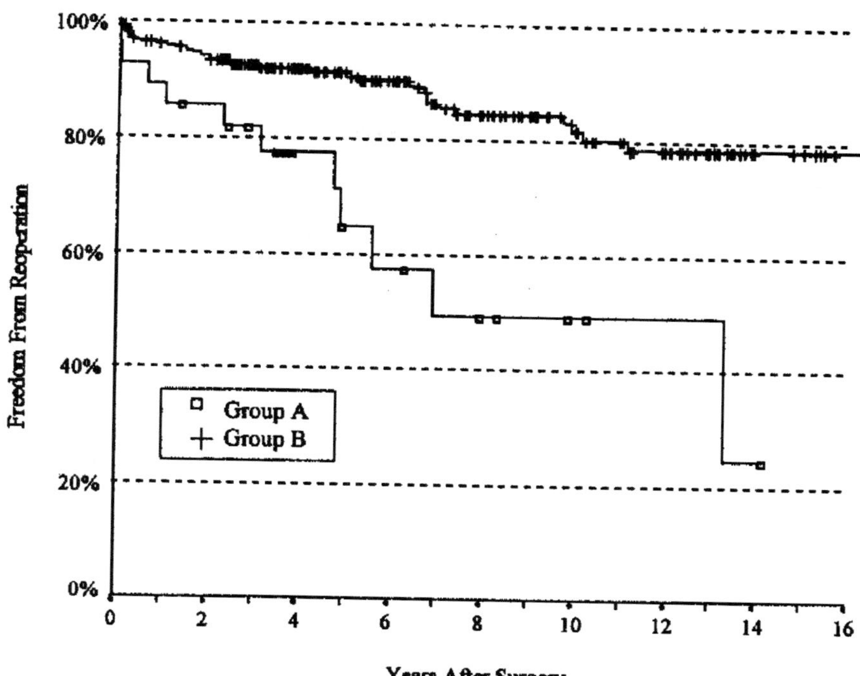

FIGURE 46–13 Freedom from reoperation (Kaplan-Meier) of patients with Marfan syndrome (group A) versus those without fibrillinopathic etiologies (group B). (*Reproduced with permission from Detter C, Mair H, Klein H, et al: Long-term prognosis of surgically-treated aortic aneurysms and dissections in patients with and without Marfan syndrome. Eur J Cardiothorac Surg 1998; 13:416.*)

freedom from endocarditis in 270 patients was 88% at 14 years.

Results of Operation in Patients with Marfan Syndrome

Gott et al [97] reviewed the experience of 10 surgical centers with regards to root replacement in 675 patients with Marfan syndrome from 1968 to 1996. The 30-day mortality was 3.3%, but was only 1.5% for elective repair. Emergency surgery resulted in a 30-day mortality of nearly 12%. The survival rate was 93% at 1 year, 84% at 5 years, 75% at 10 years, and 59% at 20 years. Complications related to the residual thoracic aorta and arrhythmias were the leading causes of death. The most frequent late complication was thromboembolism. Advanced NYHA at the time of original operation was the only predictor of late death. This very complete multicenter review demonstrates that root replacement in Marfan syndrome can be performed with a low mortality and good long-term survival. Kaplan-Meier survival analysis is shown in Figure 46-15.

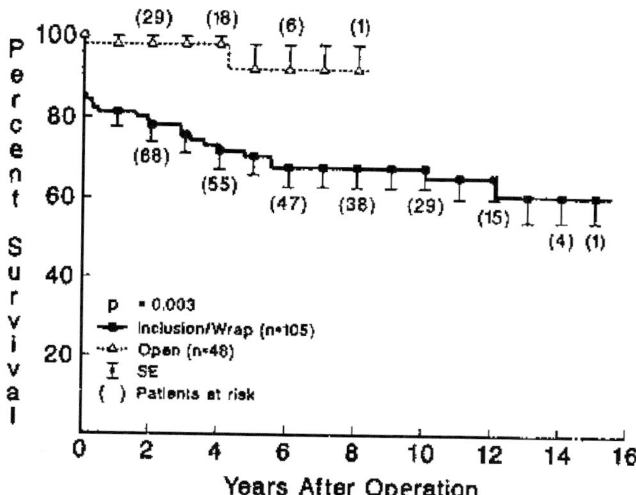

FIGURE 46–14 Actuarial freedom from reoperation on the ascending aorta or aortic valve. Patients are divided into those who had inclusion versus exclusion grafting techniques. (*Reproduced with permission from Kouchoukos NT, Wareing TH, Murphy SF, Perrillo JB: Sixteen-year experience with aortic root replacement: results of 172 operations. Ann Surg 1991; 214:308.*)

LONG-TERM SURVEILLANCE AFTER ASCENDING AORTIC OPERATIONS

All patients who have undergone thoracic aortic surgery must have long-term follow-up. Residual aortic tissue is often not normal and patients are prone to subsequent development of dissections or aneurysms. Pseudoaneurysms are frequently asymptomatic in the early stages and may initially present as periprosthetic hematomas. A significant proportion of patients will require reoperation, and emergent operation is associated with a very high mortality. Periodic CT or MRI is ideal for assessing progression of disease in the residual aorta and for discovering the development of complications. Patients at increased risk of reoperation, such as those with Marfan syndrome, familial aneurysms, or dissections, require more vigilant follow-up.

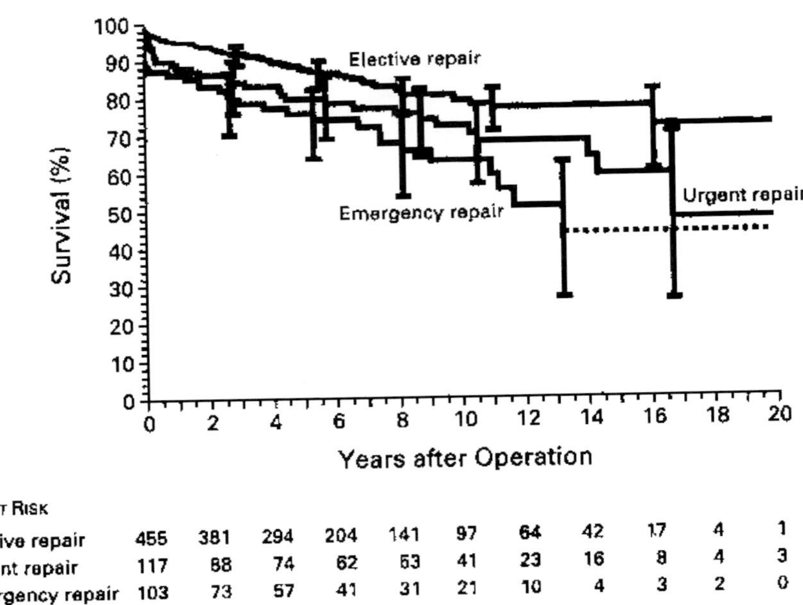

FIGURE 46–15 Kaplan-Meier survival analysis for 675 patients with Marfan syndrome from ten different surgical centers according to the urgency of the procedure. (*Reproduced with permission from Gott VL, Greene PS, Alejo DE, et al: Replacement of the aortic root in patients with Marfan's syndrome. N Engl J Med 1999; 340:1307.*)

THE INFECTED AORTIC GRAFT

Incidence

Graft infections are reported in 0.9% to 1.9% of patients following surgery of the thoracic aorta[146,147] and are associated with a mortality rate ranging from 25% to 75%.[147,148] Most graft infections become evident in the first month after operation,[148,149] but may occur years after graft insertion.[150]

Risk Factors

The risk of infection with any graft is increased with breaks in sterile technique and postoperative infectious complications. In one series 55% of patients had previous significant infectious complications including wound infection, line sepsis, pneumonia, empyema, or septicemia.[150] The ascending aortic graft may be particularly vulnerable because of proximity to the wound and poor natural tissue coverage. The major infectious agents are *Staphylococcus aureus, Staphylococcus epidermidis,* and less commonly *Pseudomonas.*[148–150] Infections may also be polymicrobial, fungal, or indeterminate.

Diagnosis

The majority of patients present with clinical signs of infection such as fever, chills, and elevated white blood cell count.[149–151] CT or MRI may demonstrate fluid collections or air in the periprosthetic space, but these are nonspecific findings, particularly in the early postoperative period. Confirmation of infection may require CT-guided aspiration of suspicious fluid collections. Associated pseudoaneurysms are detected by aortography or transesophageal echocardiography. Nuclear imaging techniques are endorsed by some,[152] but can be nonspecific for infection versus normal postoperative inflammation.[150]

Treatment

The traditional treatment of infected ascending aortic grafts, originally described by Hargrove and Edmunds in 1984,[147] includes removal of the infected prosthetic material, aggressive tissue debridement, local irrigation, systemic antibiotic therapy, replacement of the infected conduit, and utilization of autologous tissue to surround the new conduit and obliterate deadspace. Most surgeons prefer replacement of the infected graft with a cryopreserved homograft, as it may be more resistant to subsequent infection.[153–155] The ideal autogenous tissue filler is the greater omentum because of its physical properties and its proposed ability to help combat infection.[156] In some cases small pseudoaneurysms have been resected and the graft locally repaired,[150] although this is controversial. Mortality rates remain substantial despite these aggressive measures.[150]

REFERENCES

1. Kampmeier RH: Saccular aneurysms of the thoracic aorta: a clinical study of 635 cases. *Ann Int Med* 1938; 12:624.
2. Westaby S, Cecil B. Surgery of the thoracic aorta, in Westaby S (ed): *Landmarks in Cardiac Surgery.* Oxford, Isis Medical Media, 1997; p 223.
3. Cooper A: *Lectures on the Principles and Practice of Surgery,* 2d ed. London, FC Westley, 1830; p 110.
4. Moore C: On a new method of procuring the consolidation of fibrin in certain incurable aneurysms. *Med Chir Trans* (London) 1864; 47:129.
5. Matas R: Surgery of the vascular system, in Matas R (ed): *Surgery, Its Principles and Practice,* vol. 5. Philadelphia, WB Saunders, 1914.

6. Harrison P, Chandy J: A subclavian aneurysm cured by cellophane fibrosis. *Ann Surg* 1943; 118:478.
7. Poppe J, De Oliviera H: Treatment of syphilitic aneurysms by cellophane wrapping. *J Thorac Surg* 1946; 15:186.
8. Matas R: Traumatic aneurysm of the left brachial artery. *Med News* 1888; 53:462.
9. Matas R: An operation for the radical cure of aneurism based upon arteriorrhaphy. *Ann Surg* 1903; 37:161.
10. Matas R: Endo-aneurismorrhaphy. *Surg Gynecol Obstet* 1920; 30:456.
11. Cooley DA, DeBakey ME: Resection of the entire ascending aorta in fusiform aneurysm using cardiac bypass. *JAMA* 1956; 162: 1158.
12. Mueller WH, Dammann FJ, Warren WD: Surgical correction of cardiovascular deformities in Marfan's syndrome. *Ann Surg* 1960; 152:506.
13. Blakemore AH, Voorhees AB: Aneurysm of the aorta: review of 356 cases. *Angiology* 1954; 5:209.
14. Starr A, Edwards ML, McCord CW: Aortic replacement. *Circulation* 1963; 27:779.
15. Wheat MWJ, Wilson JR, Bartley TD: Successful replacement of the entire ascending aorta and aortic valve. *JAMA* 1964; 188:717.
16. Bentall H, De Bono A: A technique for complete replacement of the ascending aorta. *Thorax* 1968; 23:338.
17. Cabrol C, Pavie A, Gandjbakhch I, et al: Complete replacement of the ascending aorta with reimplantation of the coronary arteries: new surgical approach. *J Thorac Cardiovasc Surg* 1981; 81:309.
18. Majumder PP, St Jean PL, Ferrell RE, et al: On the inheritance of abdominal aortic aneurysm. *Am J Hum Genet* 1991; 48:164.
19. Bickerstaff LK, Pairolero PC, Hollier LH, et al: Thoracic aortic aneurysms: a population-based study. *Surgery* 1982; 92:1103.
20. Gillum RF: Epidemiology of aortic aneurysm in the United States. *J Clin Epidemiol* 1995; 48:1289.
21. Coady MA, Rizzo JA, Goldstein LJ, Elefteriades JA: Natural history, pathogenesis, and etiology of thoracic aortic aneurysms and dissections. *Cardiol Clin* 1999; 17:615.
22. Larson EW, Edwards WD: Risk factors for aortic dissection: a necropsy study of 161 cases. *Am J Cardiol* 1984; 53:849.
23. Pressler V, McNamara JJ: Thoracic aortic aneurysm: natural history and treatment. *J Thorac Cardiovasc Surg* 1980; 79:489.
24. Pressler V, McNamara JJ: Aneurysm of the thoracic aorta: review of 260 cases. *J Thorac Cardiovasc Surg* 1985; 89:50.
25. Milewicz DM, Michael K, Fisher N, et al: Fibrillin-1 (FBN1) mutations in patients with thoracic aortic aneurysms. *Circulation* 1996; 94:2708.
26. Guo D, Hasham S, Kuang SQ, et al: Familial thoracic aortic aneurysms and dissections: genetic heterogeneity with a major locus mapping to 5q13-14. *Circulation* 2001; 103:2461.
27. Keane MG, Wiegers SE, Plappert T, et al: Bicuspid aortic valves are associated with aortic dilatation out of proportion to coexistent valvular lesions. *Circulation* 2000; 102:III35-9.
28. Wolinsky H: A lamellar unit of aortic medial structure and function in mammals. *Circ Res* 1967; 20:99.
29. Lesauskaite V, Tanganelli P, Sassi C, et al: Smooth muscle cells of the media in the dilatative pathology of ascending thoracic aorta: morphology, immunoreactivity for osteopontin, matrix metalloproteinases, and their inhibitors. *Hum Pathol* 2001; 32:1003.
30. Schoen F: Blood vessels, in Cotran R, Kanor V, Collins C (eds): *Robbins Pathologic Basis of Disease*. Philadelphia, WB Saunders, 1999.
31. Pearce WH, Slaughter MS, LeMaire S, et al: Aortic diameter as a function of age, gender, and body surface area. *Surgery* 1993; 114:691.
32. Cannon DJ, Read RC: Blood elastolytic activity in patients with aortic aneurysm. *Ann Thorac Surg* 1982; 34:10.
33. O'Rouke MF, Avolio AP, Nichols WW: Left-ventricular-systemic arterial coupling in humans and strategies to improve coupling in desease states, in Yin FCP (ed): *Ventricular/Vascular Coupling: Clinical, Physiological and Engineering Aspects*. New York, Springer-Verlag, 1987.
34. Pyeritz RE, McKusick VA: The Marfan syndrome: diagnosis and management. *N Engl J Med* 1979; 300:772.
35. Pyeritz RE: The Marfan syndrome, in Royce PM, Steinman B (eds): *Connective Tissue and its Heritable Disorders*. New York, Wiley-Liss, 1993; p 437.
36. Kainulainen K, Pulkkinen L, Savolainen A, et al: Location on chromosome 15 of the gene defect causing Marfan syndrome. *N Engl J Med* 1990; 323:935.
37. Tsipouras P, Del Mastro R, Sarfarazi M, et al: Genetic linkage of the Marfan syndrome, ectopia lentis, and congenital contractural arachnodactyly to the fibrillin genes on chromosomes 15 and 5. The International Marfan Syndrome Collaborative Study. *N Engl J Med* 1992; 326:905.
38. Dietz HC, Cutting GR, Pyeritz RE, et al: Marfan syndrome caused by a recurrent de novo missense mutation in the fibrillin gene. *Nature* 1991; 352:337.
39. Dietz HC, Pyeritz RE, Hall BD, et al: The Marfan syndrome locus: confirmation of assignment to chromosome 15 and identification of tightly linked markers at 15q15-q21.3. *Genomics* 1991; 9:355.
40. Lee B, Godfrey M, Vitale E, et al: Linkage of Marfan syndrome and a phenotypically related disorder to two different fibrillin genes. *Nature* 1991; 352:330.
41. Detter C, Mair H, Klein HG, et al: Long-term prognosis of surgically-treated aortic aneurysms and dissections in patients with and without Marfan syndrome. *Eur J Cardiothorac Surg* 1998; 13:416.
42. Sakai LY, Keene DR, Engvall E: Fibrillin, a new 350-kD glycoprotein, is a component of extracellular microfibrils. *J Cell Biol* 1986; 103:2499.
43. Milewicz DM: Inheritable disorders of connective tissue, in Willerson JT, Cohn JN, (eds): *Cardiovascular Medicine*. New York, Churchill Livingstone, 1995; p 1638.
44. Marsalese DL, Moodie DS, Vacante M, et al: Marfan's syndrome: natural history and long-term follow-up of cardiovascular involvement. *J Am Coll Cardiol* 1989; 14:422.
45. Pope FM, Narcisi P, Nicholls AC, et al: Clinical presentations of Ehlers Danlos syndrome type IV. *Arch Dis Child* 1988; 63:1016.
46. Cikrit DF, Miles JH, Silver D: Spontaneous arterial perforation: the Ehlers-Danlos specter. *J Vasc Surg* 1987; 5:248.
47. Raman J, Saldanha RF, Esmore DS, et al: The Bentall procedure: a surgical option in Ehlers-Danlos syndrome. *J Cardiovasc Surg* (Torino) 1988; 29:647.
48. Galloway AC, Colvin SB, LaMendola CL, et al: Ten-year operative experience with 165 aneurysms of the ascending aorta and aortic arch. *Circulation* 1989; 80:I249.
49. Svensson LG, Crawford ES: Degenerative aortic aneurysms, in Svensson LG, Crawford ES (eds): *Cardiovascular and Vascular Disease of the Aorta*. Philadelphia, WB Saunders, 1997.
50. Dapunt OE, Galla JD, Sadeghi AM, et al: The natural history of thoracic aortic aneurysms. *J Thorac Cardiovasc Surg* 1994; 107:1323.
51. Pachulski RT, Weinberg AL, Chan KL: Aortic aneurysm in patients with functionally normal or minimally stenotic bicuspid aortic valve. *Am J Cardiol* 1991; 67:781.
52. Feigl D, Feigl A, Edwards JE: Mycotic aneurysms of the aortic root: a pathologic study of 20 cases. *Chest* 1986; 90:553.
53. Chan FY, Crawford ES, Coselli JS, et al: In situ prosthetic graft replacement for mycotic aneurysm of the aorta. *Ann Thorac Surg* 1989; 47:193.
54. Heggtveit HA: Syphilitic aortitis: a clinicopathologic autopsy study of 100 cases, 1950 to 1960. *Circulation* 1964; 29:346.

55. Isselbacher EM, Eagel KA, Desanctis RW: Diseases of the aorta, in Braunwald E (ed): *Heart Disease: A Textbook of Cardiovascular Medicine*, vol. 2. Philadelphia, WB Saunders, 1997; p 1546.
56. Austen WB, Blennerhasset JB: Giant cell aortitis causing an aneurysm of the ascending aorta and aortic regurgitation. *N Engl J Med* 1964; 272:80.
57. Salisbury RS, Hazleman BL: Successful treatment of dissecting aortic aneurysm due to giant cell arteritis. *Ann Rheum Dis* 1981; 40:507.
58. Evans JM, O'Fallon WM, Hunder GG: Increased incidence of aortic aneurysm and dissection in giant cell (temporal) arteritis: a population-based study. *Ann Intern Med* 1995; 122:502.
59. Turney SZ: Blunt trauma of the thoracic aorta and its branches. *Semin Thorac Cardiovasc Surg* 1992; 4:209.
60. Sato O, Tada Y, Miyata T, Shindo S: False aneurysms after aortic operations. *J Cardiovasc Surg* (Torino) 1992; 33:604.
61. Kouchoukos NT, Wareing TH, Murphy SF, Perrillo JB: Sixteen-year experience with aortic root replacement: results of 172 operations. *Ann Surg* 1991; 214:308.
62. Merrill WH, Achuff SC, White RI Jr, et al: Late false aneurysm following replacement of ascending aorta: the problem of the teflon graft in combination with a silk suture anastomosis. *Ann Thorac Surg* 1985; 39:271.
63. Pokela R, Juvonen T, Satta J, Karkola P: Composite graft replacement for treatment of ascending aortic aneurysms using original Bentall-DeBono procedure or its open button modification. *Eur J Cardiothorac Surg* 1998; 13:484.
64. Stowe CL, Baertlein MA, Wierman MD, et al: Surgical management of ascending and aortic arch disease: refined techniques with improved results. *Ann Thorac Surg* 1998; 66:388.
65. Szulagyi DE, Smith RF, DeRusso FJ, et al: Contribution of abdominal aortic aneurysmectomy to prolongation of life. *Ann Surg* 1966; 4:678.
66. Kalman PG, Taylor BV: Natural history of abdominal aortic aneurysms: do size, sex, age, and family matter? in Calligaro KD, Dougherty MJ, Hollier LH (eds): *Diagnosis and Treatment of Aortic and Peripheral Arterial Aneurysms*. Philadelphia, WB Saunders, 1999.
67. Guirguis EM, Barber GG: The natural history of abdominal aortic aneurysms. *Am J Surg* 1991; 162:481.
68. Coady MA, Rizzo JA, Elefteriades JA: Developing surgical intervention criteria for thoracic aortic aneurysms. *Cardiol Clin* 1999; 17:827.
69. Hirose Y, Hamada S, Takamiya M: Predicting the growth of aortic aneurysms: a comparison of linear vs exponential models. *Angiology* 1995; 46:413.
70. Shores J, Berger KR, Murphy EA, Pyeritz RE: Progression of aortic dilatation and the benefit of long-term beta-adrenergic blockade in Marfan's syndrome. *N Engl J Med* 1994; 330:1335.
71. Child AH: Marfan syndrome—current medical and genetic knowledge: how to treat and when. *J Card Surg* 1997; 12:131.
72. Murdoch JL, Walker BA, Halpern BL, et al: Life expectancy and causes of death in the Marfan syndrome. *N Engl J Med* 1972; 286:804.
73. Clifton MA: Familial abdominal aortic aneurysms. *Br J Surg* 1977; 64:765.
74. Tilson MD, Seashore MR: Fifty families with abdominal aortic aneurysms in two or more first-order relatives. *Am J Surg* 1984; 147:551.
75. Biddinger A, Rocklin M, Coselli J, Milewicz DM: Familial thoracic aortic dilatations and dissections: a case control study. *J Vasc Surg* 1997; 25:506.
76. Coady MA, Davies RR, Roberts M, et al: Familial patterns of thoracic aortic aneurysms. *Arch Surg* 1999; 134:361.
77. Faggioli GL, Stella A, Gargiulo M, et al: Morphology of small aneurysms: definition and impact on risk of rupture. *Am J Surg* 1994; 168:131.
78. von Kodolitsch Y, Simic O, Nienaber CA: Aneurysms of the ascending aorta: diagnostic features and prognosis in patients with Marfan's syndrome versus hypertension. *Clin Cardiol* 1998; 21:817.
79. Joyce JW, Fairburn JF, Kincaid OW, Juergens JL: Aneurysms of the thoracic aorta. A clinical study with a special reference to prognosis. *Circulation* 1964; 29:176.
80. Crawford ES, Svensson LG, Coselli JS, Safi HJ, Hess KR: Surgical treatment of aneurysm and/or dissection of the ascending aorta, transverse aortic arch, and ascending aorta and transverse aortic arch: factors influencing survival in 717 patients. *J Thorac Cardiovasc Surg* 1989; 98:659.
81. Guthaner DF: The plain chest film in assessing aneurysms and dissecting hematomas of the thoracic aorta, in Taveras JN, Ferrucci JT (eds): *Radiology: Diagnosis-Imaging-Intervention*. Philadelphia, JB Lippincott, 1994; Ch. 33.
82. Olson LJ, Subramanian R, Edwards WD: Surgical pathology of pure aortic insufficiency: a study of 225 cases. *Mayo Clin Proc* 1984; 59:835.
83. Schappert T, Sadony V, Schoen F, et al: Diagnosis and therapeutic consequences of intramural aortic hematoma. *J Card Surg* 1994; 9:508.
84. Konstadt SN, Reich DL, Quintana C, Levy M: The ascending aorta: how much does transesophageal echocardiography see? *Anesth Analg* 1994; 78:240.
85. Guthaner DF: Angiography in assessing aneurysms and dissecting hematomas of the thoracic aorta, in Taveras JN, Ferrucci JT (eds): *Radiology: Diagnosis-Imaging-Intervention*. Philadelphia, JB Lippincott, 1994; Ch. 36.
86. Setser RM, Sayre K, Flacke S, et al: Assessment of ventricular contractility during cardiac magnetic resonance imaging examinations using normalized maximal ventricular power. *Ann Biomed Eng* 2001; 29:974.
87. Waller C, Hiller KH, Voll S, et al: Myocardial perfusion imaging using a non-contrast agent MR imaging technique. *Int J Card Imaging* 2001; 17:123.
88. Bunce NH, Lorenz CH, Pennell DJ: MR coronary angiography: 2001 update. *Rays* 2001; 26:61.
89. Michel PL, Acar J, Chomette G, Iung B: Degenerative aortic regurgitation. *Eur Heart J* 1991; 12:875.
90. Prenger K, Pieters F, Cheriex E: Aortic dissection after aortic valve replacement: incidence and consequences for strategy. *J Card Surg* 1994; 9:495.
91. McNamara JJ, Pressler VM: Natural history of arteriosclerotic thoracic aortic aneurysms. *Ann Thorac Surg* 1978; 26:468.
92. Crawford ES, Hess KR, Cohen ES, et al: Ruptured aneurysm of the descending thoracic and thoracoabdominal aorta: analysis according to size and treatment. *Ann Surg* 1991; 213:417.
93. Ergin MA, Spielvogel D, Apaydin A, et al: Surgical treatment of the dilated ascending aorta: when and how? *Ann Thorac Surg* 1999; 67:1834.
94. Coady MA, Rizzo JA, Hammond GL, et al: What is the appropriate size criterion for resection of thoracic aortic aneurysms? *J Thorac Cardiovasc Surg* 1997; 113:476.
95. Hirose Y, Hamada S, Takamiya M, et al: Aortic aneurysms: growth rates measured with CT. *Radiology* 1992; 185:249.
96. Masuda Y, Takanashi K, Takasu J, et al: Expansion rate of thoracic aortic aneurysms and influencing factors. *Chest* 1992; 102:461.
97. Gott VL, Greene PS, Alejo DE, et al: Replacement of the aortic root in patients with Marfan's syndrome. *N Engl J Med* 1999; 340:1307.
98. Baumgartner WA, Cameron DE, Redmond JM, et al: Operative management of Marfan syndrome: the Johns Hopkins experience. *Ann Thorac Surg* 1999; 67:1859.

99. Coady MA, Rizzo JA, Hammond GL, et al: Surgical intervention criteria for thoracic aortic aneurysms: a study of growth rates and complications. *Ann Thorac Surg* 1999; 67:1922.
100. Kouchoukos NT: Adjuncts to reduce the incidence of embolic brain injury during operations on the aortic arch. *Ann Thorac Surg* 1994; 57:243.
101. Berens ES, Kouchoukos NT, Murphy SF, et al: Preoperative carotid artery screening in elderly patients undergoing cardiac surgery. *J Vasc Surg* 1992; 15:313.
102. Lawrie GM, Earle N, DeBakey ME: Long-term fate of the aortic root and aortic valve after ascending aneurysm surgery. *Ann Surg* 1993; 217:711.
103. Yun KL, Miller DC, Fann JI, et al: Composite valve graft versus separate aortic valve and ascending aortic replacement: is there still a role for the separate procedure? *Circulation* 1997; 96:II-368.
104. Gulbins H, Kreuzer E, Uhlig A, Reichart B: Homografts in patients with combined disease of the aortic valve and the ascending aorta: an alternative to the classical Bentall procedure. *J Heart Valve Dis* 2001; 10:650.
105. Kouchoukos NT: Aortic allografts and pulmonary autografts for replacement of the aortic valve and aortic root. *Ann Thorac Surg* 1999; 67:1846.
106. Elkins RC, Lane MM, McCue C: Ross procedure for ascending aortic replacement. *Ann Thorac Surg* 1999; 67:1843.
107. David TE, Feindel CM, Bos J: Repair of the aortic valve in patients with aortic insufficiency and aortic root aneurysm. *J Thorac Cardiovasc Surg* 1995; 109:345.
108. David TE: Aortic valve-sparing operations in patients with ascending aortic aneurysms. *Curr Opin Cardiol* 1997; 12:391.
109. Yacoub MH, Gehle P, Chandrasekaran V, et al: Late results of a valve-preserving operation in patients with aneurysms of the ascending aorta and root. *J Thorac Cardiovasc Surg* 1998; 115:1080.
110. David TE: Aortic root aneurysms: remodeling or composite replacement? *Ann Thorac Surg* 1997; 64:1564.
111. David TE, Feindel CM: An aortic valve-sparing operation for patients with aortic incompetence and aneurysm of the ascending aorta. *J Thorac Cardiovasc Surg* 1992; 103:617.
112. Cochran RP, Kunzelman KS, Eddy AC, et al: Modified conduit preparation creates a pseudosinus in an aortic valve-sparing procedure for aneurysm of the ascending aorta. *J Thorac Cardiovasc Surg* 1995; 109:1049.
113. David TE: Remodeling of aortic root and preservation of the native aortic valve. *Op Tech Cardiac Thorac Surg* 1996; 1:44.
114. Fleischer KJ, Nousari HC, Anhalt GJ, et al: Immunohistochemical abnormalities of fibrillin in cardiovascular tissues in Marfan's syndrome. *Ann Thorac Surg* 1997; 63:1012.
115. Carrel T, von Segesser L, Jenni R, et al: Dealing with dilated ascending aorta during aortic valve replacement: advantages of conservative surgical approach. *Eur J Cardiothorac Surg* 1991; 5:137.
116. Gott VL, Pyeritz RE, Cameron DE, et al: Composite graft repair of Marfan aneurysm of the ascending aorta: results in 100 patients. *Ann Thorac Surg* 1991; 52:38.
117. Gillinov AM, Hulyalkar A, Cameron DE, et al: Mitral valve operation in patients with the Marfan syndrome. *J Thorac Cardiovasc Surg* 1994; 107:724.
118. Steward DJ, Da Silva CA, Flegel T: Elevated blood glucose levels may increase the danger of neurological deficit following profoundly hypothermic cardiac arrest. *Anesthesiology* 1988; 68:653.
119. Gott VL, Gillinov AM, Pyeritz RE, et al: Aortic root replacement: risk factor analysis of a seventeen-year experience with 270 patients. *J Thorac Cardiovasc Surg* 1995; 109:536.
120. Cohn LH, Rizzo RJ, Adams DH, et al: Reduced mortality and morbidity for ascending aortic aneurysm resection regardless of cause. *Ann Thorac Surg* 1996; 62:463.
121. Dougenis D, Daily BB, Kouchoukos NT: Reoperations on the aortic root and ascending aorta. *Ann Thorac Surg* 1997; 64:986.
122. Luciani GB, Casali G, Faggian G, Mazzucco A: Predicting outcome after reoperative procedures on the aortic root and ascending aorta. *Eur J Cardiothorac Surg* 2000; 17:602.
123. Crawford ES, Crawford JL, Safi HJ, Coselli JS: Redo operations for recurrent aneurysmal disease of the ascending aorta and transverse aortic arch. *Ann Thorac Surg* 1985; 40:439.
124. Kouchoukos NT, Marshall WG Jr, Wedige-Stecher TA: Eleven-year experience with composite graft replacement of the ascending aorta and aortic valve. *J Thorac Cardiovasc Surg* 1986; 92:691.
125. Svensson LG: Brain protection. *J Card Surg* 1997; 12:326.
126. Wareing TH, Davila-Roman VG, Daily BB, et al: Strategy for the reduction of stroke incidence in cardiac surgical patients. *Ann Thorac Surg* 1993; 55:1400.
127. Coselli JS, LeMaire SA: Experience with retrograde cerebral perfusion during proximal aortic surgery in 290 patients. *J Card Surg* 1997; 12:322.
128. Usui A, Abe T, Murase M: Early clinical results of retrograde cerebral perfusion for aortic arch operations in Japan. *Ann Thorac Surg* 1996; 62:94.
129. Safi HJ, Letsou GV, Iliopoulos DC, et al: Impact of retrograde cerebral perfusion on ascending aortic and arch aneurysm repair. *Ann Thorac Surg* 1997; 63:1601.
130. Griepp RB, Ergin MA, McCullough JN, et al: Use of hypothermic circulatory arrest for cerebral protection during aortic surgery. *J Card Surg* 1997; 12:312.
131. Asimakopoulos G, Smith PL, Ratnatunga CP, Taylor KM: Lung injury and acute respiratory distress syndrome after cardiopulmonary bypass. *Ann Thorac Surg* 1999; 68:1107.
132. Asimakopoulos G, Taylor KM, Smith PL, Ratnatunga CP: Prevalence of acute respiratory distress syndrome after cardiac surgery. *J Thorac Cardiovasc Surg* 1999; 117:620.
133. Redmond JM, Gillinov AM, Stuart RS, et al: Heparin-coated bypass circuits reduce pulmonary injury. *Ann Thorac Surg* 1993; 56:474.
134. Gott JP, Cooper WA, Schmidt FE Jr, et al: Modifying risk for extracorporeal circulation: trial of four antiinflammatory strategies. *Ann Thorac Surg* 1998; 66:747.
135. Hachida M, Hanayama N, Okamura T, et al: The role of leukocyte depletion in reducing injury to myocardium and lung during cardiopulmonary bypass. *ASAIO J* 1995; 41:M291.
136. Gu YJ, de Vries AJ, Boonstra PW, van Oeveren W: Leukocyte depletion results in improved lung function and reduced inflammatory response after cardiac surgery. *J Thorac Cardiovasc Surg* 1996; 112:494.
137. Lewis CT, Cooley DA, Murphy MC, et al: Surgical repair of aortic root aneurysms in 280 patients. *Ann Thorac Surg* 1992; 53:38.
138. Raudkivi PJ, Williams JD, Monro JL, Ross JK: Surgical treatment of the ascending aorta: fourteen years' experience with 83 patients. *J Thorac Cardiovasc Surg* 1989; 98:675.
139. Jault F, Nataf P, Rama A, et al: Chronic disease of the ascending aorta: surgical treatment and long-term results. *J Thorac Cardiovasc Surg* 1994; 108:747.
140. Bhan A, Choudhary SK, Saikia M, et al: Surgical experience with dissecting and nondissecting aneurysms of the ascending aorta. *Indian Heart J* 2001; 53:319.
141. Budillon AM, Nicolini F, Beghi C, et al: Surgical repair of thoracic aortic aneurysms: results and complications. *Acta Biomed Ateneo Parmense* 2001; 72:33.
142. Okita Y, Ando M, Minatoya K, et al: Early and long-term results of surgery for aneurysms of the thoracic aorta in septuagenarians and octogenarians. *Eur J Cardiothorac Surg* 1999; 16:317.
143. Mingke D, Dresler C, Stone CD, Borst HG: Composite graft replacement of the aortic root in 335 patients with aneurysm or dissection. *Thorac Cardiovasc Surg* 1998; 46:12.

144. Vallely MP, Hughes CF, Bannon PG, et al: Composite graft replacement of the aortic root after previous cardiac surgery: a 20-year experience. *Ann Thorac Surg* 2000; 70:851.
145. Taniguchi K, Nakano S, Matsuda H, et al: Long-term survival and complications after composite graft replacement for ascending aortic aneurysm associated with aortic regurgitation. *Circulation* 1991; 84:III31.
146. Svensson LG, Crawford ES, Hess KR, et al: Experience with 1509 patients undergoing thoracoabdominal aortic operations. *J Vasc Surg* 1993; 17:357.
147. Hargrove WC 3rd, Edmunds LH Jr: Management of infected thoracic aortic prosthetic grafts. *Ann Thorac Surg* 1984; 37:72.
148. Coselli JS, Crawford ES, Williams TW Jr, et al: Treatment of postoperative infection of ascending aorta and transverse aortic arch, including use of viable omentum and muscle flaps. *Ann Thorac Surg* 1990; 50:868.
149. Nakajima N, Masuda M, Ichinose M, Ando M: A new method for the treatment of graft infection in the thoracic aorta: in situ preservation. *Ann Thorac Surg* 1999; 67:1994.
150. Coselli JS, Koksoy C, LeMaire SA: Management of thoracic aortic graft infections. *Ann Thorac Surg* 1999; 67:1990.
151. Vogt PR, Turina MI: Management of infected aortic grafts: development of less invasive surgery using cryopreserved homografts. *Ann Thorac Surg* 1999; 67:1986.
152. McKeown PP, Miller DC, Jamieson SW, et al: Diagnosis of arterial prosthetic graft infection by indium-111 oxine white blood cell scans. *Circulation* 1982; 66:I130.
153. Vogt PR, von Segesser LK, Goffin Y, et al: Cryopreserved arterial homografts for in situ reconstruction of mycotic aneurysms and prosthetic graft infection. *Eur J Cardiothorac Surg* 1995; 9:502.
154. Vogt PR, von Segesser LK, Goffin Y, et al: Eradication of aortic infections with the use of cryopreserved arterial homografts. *Ann Thorac Surg* 1996; 62:640.
155. Riberi A, Caus T, Mesana T, et al: Aortic valve or root replacement with cryopreserved homograft for active infectious endocarditis. *Cardiovasc Surg* 1997; 5:579.
156. Mathisen DJ, Grillo HC, Vlahakes GJ, Daggett WM: The omentum in the management of complicated cardiothoracic problems. *J Thorac Cardiovasc Surg* 1988; 95:677.

Chapter 47

Aneurysms of the Aortic Arch

David Spielvogel/Manu N. Mathur/Randall B. Griepp

The unique considerations in approaching aortic arch surgery concern cerebral protection. The question of how best to protect the brain while providing surgical access to the cerebral vessels is still a subject of controversy and of research. The issues of concern in brain protection involve both minimizing global ischemia during the mandatory arrest of the circulation during aortic arch surgery and preventing embolization of air and atheromatous debris from the often very diseased arch during the repair. Thus, cerebral protection methods are a major focus of discussion in this chapter, which describes in considerable detail the history and rationale for the use of hypothermic circulatory arrest, selective antegrade perfusion, and retrograde cerebral perfusion for prevention of global ischemia. It also discusses use of axillary artery cannulation and of a branched graft technique to minimize possible embolic damage.

Preoperative evaluation, anesthesia and monitoring, and other, more general surgical considerations are not overlooked. Operative technique is addressed chiefly in the last section, in which several specific surgical procedures, appropriate for particular different pathologies, are described in detail.

PREOPERATIVE EVALUATION

A thorough medical history and routine laboratory studies are of extreme importance in evaluating possible symptoms due to the aneurysm and revealing other medical problems in these usually elderly patients. A family history of a ruptured aneurysm is not uncommon, and aids in the decision to recommend surgery. The discovery of other medical conditions may influence the operative approach, allow anticipation and possibly prevention of intraoperative or postoperative complications to which the patient is especially vulnerable, or may contraindicate operation altogether.

Evaluation of an aortic arch aneurysm itself requires a computed tomographic (CT) scan with contrast of the entire aorta. With new multidetector CT scans, the entire aorta can be imaged in tens of seconds with reduced contrast and 3-D reconstructions. However, with advances in MRI, equally detailed images can be obtained, and MRI is becoming the preferred modality for imaging in the view of some surgeons.[1] Disadvantages of MRI are the duration of the examination and the cost, but there are definite indications for MRI in patients with renal dysfunction, since the contrast agents for MRI are not nephrotoxic. Angiograms are not required routinely to visualize the lesion, but if coronary angiography is indicated, an aortogram can be done with very little additional risk.

Cardiac Status and Management of Coronary Artery Disease

All patients being evaluated for aneurysm surgery require a preoperative echocardiogram. This is to assess left ventricular function and to rule out significant valvular heart disease. In patients with aneurysms of the ascending aorta in whom a Bentall procedure may be required, coronary arteriography is carried out to delineate the anatomy of the proximal coronary arteries. All patients over the age of 40 require routine coronary arteriography. Patients younger than 40 who have significant risk factors for coronary disease such as abnormal electrocardiogram, history of angina or smoking, or strong family history should also undergo coronary angiography.

If, on the basis of preoperative evaluation, insignificant coronary artery disease is found, then aneurysm surgery is performed as planned, with care taken to avoid undue cardiac stress. If significant coronary artery disease is present, coronary artery surgery or angioplasty is considered. If the lesions are amenable to angioplasty, this procedure is done two weeks before aneurysm surgery to prevent possible coronary thrombotic sequelae, since thrombotic complications have been observed when surgery involving administration of heparin and protamine is carried out sooner after angioplasty.[2] If the aneurysm can be resected by a median sternotomy, or if the coronary arteries that require bypass are easily accessible through a left thoracotomy, coronary artery bypass grafting can be done at the time of aneurysm repair. If the aneurysm is very extensive, or if access to the relevant coronary arteries will be difficult through an incision that is optimal for aneurysm resection, coronary artery bypass surgery is undertaken in a separate procedure several weeks prior to aneurysm repair.

If severe pulmonary dysfunction is suspected on the basis of pulmonary function tests, or because of a history of severely limited exercise tolerance, pulmonary consultation is requested. Active pulmonary infection is treated prior to surgery. All patients are urged to stop smoking for at least a month before operation. Pulmonary dysfunction increases operative risk and prolongs recovery, but chronic lung disease is not necessarily a contraindication to operation unless oxygen dependence or significant carbon dioxide retention are present.

Cerebral Vessels and Prevention of Stroke

A history of transient ischemic attacks or of strokes, or the presence of carotid bruits on examination, prompts a noninvasive workup of extracranial cerebral vessels. Since emboli are likely to arise from the diseased aorta in the presence of an arch aneurysm, a history of a focal cerebral insult is not a contraindication to surgery. In patients with such a history, a CT scan of the brain is carried out preoperatively; this enables detection of silent fresh cerebral infarcts, which necessitate postponement of surgery in most instances. The preoperative CT scan is also invaluable for identification of old and new lesions, and may be helpful in prognosis if focal neurologic symptoms occur postoperatively. Rather than attempt to identify those patients most at risk for intraoperative and postoperative cerebral embolization because of extensive friable atherosclerotic debris in the ascending aorta and arch, we assume that all patients with arch aneurysms have a very high risk of embolization and take all possible steps to minimize their occurrence. Reasonably accurate preoperative identification of those patients at highest risk is possible using transesophageal echocardiography, and even better visualization of the ascending aorta and arch is possible using epiaortic ultrasound intraoperatively.[3–5]

Cannulation Sites

For arterial cannulation in the management of arch aneurysms, we use the right axillary artery almost exclusively. The axillary artery is usually soft and rarely involved in the generalized atherosclerotic process. Its use avoids retrograde perfusion through a diseased abdominal and descending thoracic aorta and the turbulent flow patterns in the arch associated with ascending aortic cannulation, which we—as well as others—believe reduces the risk of atheroembolism.[6,7] Another advantage of axillary artery cannulation is its usefulness for selective antegrade cerebral perfusion during arch reconstruction.

Many surgeons still use the femoral vessels for cannulation. However, these are often calcified and atherosclerotic, and associated with the inherent risk of local dissection, retrograde dissection, and cerebral embolization. Cannulation can also be carried out in the ascending aorta using intraoperative epiaortic ultrasound to select a site free of atheroma in a segment of aorta adjacent to or even included in the anticipated resection; the perfusion cannula can subsequently be moved to the graft during the procedure. Despite the accuracy of epiaortic ultrasound, we are still concerned about using the aorta as a cannulation site and prefer to use the right axillary artery.

ANESTHESIA AND MONITORING

In general, anesthesia for repair of aortic arch aneurysms is not different from that for conventional open heart surgery, which relies primarily on the use of high doses of narcotics. Routine hemodynamic monitoring includes a Swan-Ganz catheter, a jugular venous bulb catheter, and left radial and femoral arterial catheters. Transesophageal echocardiography is used to monitor left ventricular function and distention, to confirm adequate flow in the arch and arch vessels, and to guard against malperfusion. Although we do not rely on EEG surveillance, it is still used by some surgeons to determine maximum cerebral metabolic suppression in conjunction with hypothermic circulatory arrest, and to assess adequacy of cerebral protection.

We no longer administer barbiturates because, at the doses recommended to enhance cerebral protection, they significantly depress myocardial function, and also because there are conflicting laboratory data with regard to their effectiveness in the presence of hypothermia.[8] We give 2 g of methylprednisolone at the beginning of the case and before the start of perfusion in all cases where use of HCA is anticipated. If HCA exceeds 30 minutes, we continue to administer steroids for 48 hours postoperatively (125 mg every 6 hours for 24 hours, then 125 mg every 12 hours for 24 hours).

In patients in whom a thoracotomy is utilized, use of a double-lumen tube that permits selective ventilation of the right lung is helpful if substantial dissection and mobilization of the descending thoracic aorta are necessary before institution of cardiopulmonary bypass.

Although some controversy exists about whether pH during cooling should be maintained according to alpha stat or pH stat principles, we continue to utilize values uncorrected for temperature, the alpha stat approach. We rely on a long duration of cooling, a low esophageal temperature, a high jugular venous oxygen saturation, and topical hypothermia to ensure adequate cerebral protection during HCA.

Perfusion

The routine perfusion protocol for intracardiac operations is also utilized for repair of arch aneurysms; a membrane oxygenator is used in all cases. In the past, for all arch aneurysm cases, we placed a shunt between the arterial and venous perfusion lines. By moving clamps appropriately, this setup allowed us to institute whole body retrograde perfusion. Although we no longer use retrograde cerebral perfusion routinely, some surgeons still advocate its use, and it may have a role in de-airing and flushing out atheroembolic debris. For aortic arch reconstruction, a "Y" connector in the arterial line enables a second antegrade perfusion catheter to be used if needed. With right axillary artery cannulation, the site of arterial perfusion is constant and allows retrograde flushing of the brachiocephalic vessels. Distal arch descending aneurysms require transfer of the perfusion cannula from the femoral artery to the proximal graft following DHCA.

OPERATIVE TECHNIQUES

Incision

In 80% to 90% of aortic arch cases, an extended median sternotomy is used. This incision gives access to the ascending aorta, the arch, and the proximal descending thoracic aorta as far as 5 cm beyond the origin of the left subclavian artery. The conventional median sternotomy is extended along the border of the sternocleidomastoid muscle on the left side of the neck. The strap muscles of the left side of the neck are incised, and the left innominate vein is temporarily ligated and divided.

If the anticipated surgical procedure involves both intracardiac pathology and/or extensive resection of the ascending aorta and the arch as well as resection of aorta beyond the proximal descending thoracic aorta, some surgeons advocate a thoracosternotomy incision.[9] This incision is a bilateral anterior thoracotomy in the 3rd or 4th intercostal space joined by dividing the sternum. It gives excellent exposure to the entire ascending aorta, arch, and most of the descending aorta.[9] However, it may have a deleterious effect on pulmonary function, and puts both phrenic nerves at risk. We have preferred to carry out the repair in this situation in two stages using the elephant trunk approach,[10] and to reserve the thoracosternotomy incision for reoperations. In patients with a lesion primarily in the descending aorta that extends no farther proximally than the distal arch, a left lateral thoracotomy in the 4th or 5th intercostal space is the incision of choice; this can be extended inferiorly across the costochondral site if necessary.

Cooling and Rewarming

We cool using a perfusate at 10°C, and monitor both bladder and esophageal temperatures. After HCA, we utilize a period of hypothermic reperfusion, since our laboratory data have shown this may be beneficial.[11] During rewarming, we never raise blood temperature above 37°C, and we avoid creating a gradient exceeding 10°C between blood and esophagus. Warming is discontinued when the patient reaches an esophageal temperature higher than 35°C, and a bladder temperature of 30°C to 32°C. We prefer the patient to rewarm gradually in the ICU following closure.

Graft and Suture Materials

We use collagen-impregnated grafts. We excise the aneurysmal portion of the aorta completely and a carry out a full-thickness anastomosis to the remaining normal aorta. We use Teflon felt on the outside of the aortic wall for reinforcement, and place the graft within the cuff of aorta. Although some surgeons feel that reinforcing anastomoses with Teflon felt is not necessary, pseudoaneurysms are extremely rare with this technique. Most anastomoses are carried out using 3-0 Prolene, but 2-0 Prolene is used for suturing one large graft to another because the lifetime integrity of a graft-to-graft anastomosis depends upon the sutures.

Myocardial Protection

We use antegrade blood for cardioplegia if the coronary ostia are readily accessible. Otherwise, 60 mEq of potassium is infused into the pump over 1 to 2 minutes just prior to circulatory arrest; this effectively converts ventricular fibrillation to asystole. For the remainder of the procedure, we rely upon total body hypothermia—supplemented with antegrade blood cardioplegia and topical cooling—for myocardial protection. Other surgeons use more elaborate cardioplegia protocols with good results.

Prevention of Paraplegia

Although the possible development of paraplegia is not a major concern with most operations involving the aortic arch, it is a consideration with procedures involving the descending thoracic and thoracoabdominal aorta. In these patients, some protection of the spinal cord is afforded by the use of total body hypothermia, but additional safeguards are warranted. During operations for resection of the distal arch plus a significant portion of the descending aorta, we routinely monitor somatosensory evoked potentials (SSEPs). Motor evoked potentials (MEPs) have recently been introduced and may provide superior monitoring of anterior cord integrity.[12,13] Intercostal vessels are sacrificed gradually prior to institution of cardiopulmonary bypass: each vessel is clamped initially, and the vessel is sacrificed only if no change in SSEPs is seen for more than 10 minutes after its temporary occlusion.[14,15] Postoperatively, SSEP monitoring is continued until the patient awakens. Thereafter, function of the lower extremities is assessed clinically on an hourly basis, for a total of 72 hours of postoperative monitoring. If a change in SSEPs or deterioration in motor function of the lower extremities is seen, blood pressure is increased, and intrathecal pressure is decreased by withdrawal of cerebral spinal fluid via an intrathecal catheter. These maneuvers to increase spinal cord perfusion pressure have proven successful in reversing the manifestations of late onset paraparesis in the majority of our patients,[15] and also have been effective in the hands of others.[16–18]

Control of Hemorrhage

Most current aortic surgery is carried out using antifibrinolytic agents to inhibit bleeding. We routinely use epsilon-aminocaproic acid, but others have reported that tranexamic acid is as effective. The use of aprotinin remains controversial. Some surgeons have observed an untoward incidence of renal dysfunction and intravascular thrombosis when using this protease inhibitor in conjunction with HCA,[19,20] but others feel that the drug is safe if adequate doses of heparin are used concurrently.[14–16] The demonstration of benefit associated with use of aprotinin with HCA has not been consistent.[21] Severe allergic reactions to aprotinin have been reported.[22] In simple cases involving only a short interval of hypothermia, such as ascending aortic and hemiarch replacement, blood and clotting factors are usually not required. If an interval of HCA longer than 30 minutes or duration of perfusion exceeding 3 hours is anticipated, 2 to 4 units of fresh frozen plasma and 5 to 10 units of platelets are brought to the operating room at the end of perfusion. These are infused if any question arises concerning the adequacy of hemostasis after protamine is given.

Use of Glue

European surgeons have enthusiastically used gelatin resorcinol formaldehyde (GRF) and other biological glues predominantly in strengthening aortic tissue after aortic dissection. Excellent results have been reported with the use of these glues in acute type A dissection.[23] Recently, however, there has been concern that the formaldehyde component of the GRF glue may be toxic to the aortic media and cause tissue necrosis, leading to late redissection.[24,25] We have not found any of these agents to be necessary. The availability of Bioglue warrants further evaluation of the usefulness of glue in elective aortic arch repair. Our current use reduces bleeding from long suture lines and graft-to-graft anastomoses.

Treatment of Infected Grafts and Mycotic Aneurysms

In patients in whom a previously inserted graft has become infected, or if a mycotic aneurysm is suspected, our initial strategy is to treat the patient for several days with specific intravenous antibiotics when the organism is known, and with broad-spectrum antibiotics otherwise. At the time of surgery, the entire infected aneurysm or graft is removed and replaced with a new graft. Often the organism causing the infection can be cultured from the resected specimen. Intravenous antibiotics are continued for at least 6 weeks, and, if a suitable agent can be found, oral antibiotic therapy is instituted for an additional 3 to 6 months. In cases of a frankly purulent operating field, the omentum may be brought into the wound and tacked over the implanted prosthetic graft. Others report the successful use of cryopreserved homografts in this setting.[26,27]

CEREBRAL PROTECTION TECHNIQUES

Hypothermic Circulatory Arrest

HISTORICAL AND THEORETICAL CONSIDERATIONS

Hypothermic circulatory arrest (HCA) was first introduced in the early days of open heart surgery as an alternative to extracorporal circulation. In the 1960s, isolated case reports described the use of HCA in repair of aortic arch aneurysms.[28,29] The merit of HCA as a technique for correction of complex congenital heart lesions in infants was advocated by Barrat-Boyes et al.[30] This prompted renewed interest in its use in adults with aneurysms of the aortic arch. The first series of such cases was reported by Griepp et al.[31]

Since that time, the efficacy of HCA in protecting the brain in adults with aortic aneurysms has been widely accepted. Increasing utilization of HCA also revealed some of its limitations, however, and raised concerns about its safety, especially when longer durations are required. A combination of hypothermia and circulatory arrest with selective antegrade cerebral perfusion may allow one to take optimal advantage of the benefits of both cerebral protection strategies.

The basis for the initial enthusiasm for the use of hypothermia to protect the brain during circulatory arrest was a series of investigations in adult dogs that documented profound inhibition of cerebral metabolism with lowering of brain temperature.[32] Using a ratio of normothermic metabolic rate and hypothermic metabolic rate at various temperatures, Michenfelder and Milde postulated that complete arrest of the cerebral circulation for as long as 30 minutes at 18°C would not result in any permanent neurologic injury, and in subsequent experiments they provided evidence indicating that periods of HCA as long as 60 minutes should be safe.[33]

Subsequent laboratory investigations in puppies[34] and piglets,[35] however, showed that suppression of cerebral metabolic function by hypothermia is less complete than predicted by the formula proposed by Michenfelder. In puppies, cerebral metabolic rate is reduced only to 40% of control levels at 18°C, and HCA for 60 minutes at 18°C results in detectable early behavioral dysfunction following surgery and in quantitative electroencephalographic (EEG) changes.[34,36] More prolonged HCA at 20°C in young piglets produces unequivocal behavioral sequelae as well as histologic evidence of cerebral damage.[37] HCA for even short intervals is followed by severe cerebral vasoconstriction that may last for hours. During this period, normal levels of cerebral metabolism are maintained by means of increased oxygen extraction, and the animals are vulnerable to hypoxic insults.[36,38–40] A period of cold reperfusion has been shown to reduce intracranial pressure (ICP) during the recovery phase following HCA.[11] In this and other experimental studies, high ICP correlates with delayed neurologic recovery and subsequent cerebral histopathologic abnormalities. Oxygen saturation data also imply that cerebral blood flow several hours postoperatively is better following cold reperfusion, suggesting improved recovery from HCA.

In a review of 200 adults who underwent HCA during operations on the thoracic aorta, our group found that 19% of the patients had temporary neurologic dysfunction (TND) postoperatively, with varying degrees of obtundation, confusion, agitation, or transient parkinsonism. Occurrence of these symptoms correlated significantly with age and duration of HCA; the interval of HCA averaged 47 minutes in patients with symptoms of TND, and was 33 minutes in those without symptoms. Duration of HCA did not correlate with mortality or with permanent neurologic injury; permanent neurologic injury was usually focal, and was significantly more frequent in older patients and in those with obvious atheromatous debris in the arch or descending aorta at the time of operation.

More sensitive neuropsychologic testing after deep hypothermic circulatory arrest showed that HCA duration of more than 25 minutes and advanced age were significant predictors of poor performance in exams of memory and fine motor function.[41] Impairment of memory function may be related to injury of the hippocampus, which is particularly sensitive to ischemic injury because of its high metabolic rate.[42] Patients with impaired neurocognitive function several weeks postoperatively were significantly more likely to have manifested TND immediately postoperatively. Therefore, TND is a reflection of subtle brain injury, possibly as a result of inadequate cerebral protection. Based on these findings, a duration of circulatory arrest exceeding 25 minutes must be considered a risk factor for long-term albeit subtle deficits in cognitive function.

Past projections of the theoretical safe duration of circulatory arrest based on rates of oxygen consumption at various brain temperatures are now considered to have been misleading. McCullough et al[43] recalculated Q_{10} for the adult human brain based on direct measurements of $CMRO_2$ during HCA. Q_{10} describes the temperature-dependent decrease in cerebral metabolism. The Q_{10} for $CMRO_2$ is defined as the ratio of two $CMRO_2$ measurements differing by 10°C. These data predict that the safe period of arrest at 15°C is about 30 minutes, and that at 10°C it is 40 minutes. Beyond this limit, cerebral cellular anoxia occurs. These observations support the use of truly profound hypothermia before a period of circulatory arrest to achieve maximum cerebral metabolic suppression, particularly if arrest time will exceed 30 minutes. Intracranial temperatures should be protected from rising during HCA by packing the head in ice.[37,38,44,45]

USE OF CORTICOSTEROIDS

High-dose methylprednisolone given at 2 and 8 hours before CPB reduces the change in cerebrovascular resistance and improves cerebral blood flow, cerebral arteriovenous oxygen difference, and oxygen metabolism following deep hypothermic circulatory arrest, and may serve as a neuroprotective agent.[46] Additionally, in 4-week-old piglets, pretreatment with corticosteroids 4 hours prior to CPB—compared to steroids in the CPB prime—reduced total body edema and cerebral vascular leakage, with improved immunohistochemical indices of neuroprotection.[47] The beneficial effect of corticosteroid pretreatment requires alterations in de novo protein synthesis at the level of the mRNA,[48] and inhibition of adhesion molecule expression in the endothelial cells, which impacts on the trafficking of leukocytes into the injured areas.[49] Other benefits of methylprednisolone given 8 hours prior to CPB and HCA were improved pulmonary compliance and alveolar-arterial gradient, and decreased pulmonary vascular resistance.[50] Consistently, benefits are more apparent when steroids are given several hours prior to the institution of CPB; this has influenced our current practice.

CLINICAL IMPLEMENTATION

In patients with aortic arch aneurysms, we no longer utilize EEG or auditory or sensory evoked potentials to guide the efficacy of cerebral cooling. Based on laboratory studies, we prefer to cool with the perfusate at 10°C to an esophageal temperature of 11°C to 14°C for a minimum of 30 minutes. The head is packed in ice to prevent rewarming during the period of circulatory arrest. Animal studies continue to support this practice.[37,38,44,45] We use jugular venous saturations to indicate adequate cerebral cooling and maximal metabolic suppression, since continuing oxygen extraction is an accurate reflection of significant ongoing cerebral metabolic activity. An association between low preoperative cerebral venous saturation and poor recovery of cerebral function following circulatory arrest was noted in some of our experimental animals[34] and also has been observed clinically by others.[51]

Careful rewarming following HCA, maintaining a gradient of no more than 10°C, reduces the likelihood that oxygen demand will exceed oxygen supply during the interval of inappropriate cerebral vasoconstriction following HCA.[36,38–40,52] Avoidance of high perfusate temperatures is essential.[53] Careful hemostasis and maintenance of normal hemodynamics during the post-bypass period are also important, since the vulnerable period of cerebral recovery during which increased oxygen extraction is relied upon to support adequate cerebral metabolism may extend up to 8 hours postoperatively.

Based on careful laboratory studies and clinical review, optimal cerebral protection and minimizing embolization may best be achieved by liberal use of axillary cannulation; avoiding manipulation of atherosclerotic vessels before HCA; using the above-mentioned safeguards during institution of HCA and rewarming; restricting HCA to less than 25 minutes; and, when more complex arch repairs are required, using hypothermic antegrade selective cerebral perfusion (SCP).[54,55] Use of SCP has been demonstrated to reduce temporary neurologic dysfunction associated with prolonged periods of HCA.[56]

Selective Cerebral Perfusion

HISTORICAL AND THEORETICAL CONSIDERATIONS

The earliest attempts to repair aneurysms of the aortic arch were carried out by DeBakey et al[57] using normothermic cerebral perfusion involving several pumps and cannulation of both subclavian and both carotid arteries. The problems associated with controlling pressure and flow in these separate vascular beds to ensure relatively uniform perfusion as well as the poor outcome of the patient led to early abandonment of this technique. Interest waned, but the technique was revisited by several surgeons in the late 1980s, spurred by the realization that HCA may not be safe for the long durations required for repair of more complex and extensive aneurysms. It was recognized that combining selective cerebral perfusion with hypothermia allowed use of much lower flow rates, and that hypothermic SCP afforded better cerebral protection from global ischemia than HCA alone or HCA and RCP.[58–60]

The resurgence of interest in selective hypothermic cerebral perfusion was pioneered by several surgeons. Bachet's group fashioned the term "cold cerebroplegia" to describe perfusion of the innominate and left carotid arteries with blood between 6°C and 12°C (flow 250-350 cc/min) in 54 patients with arch aneurysms. Mortality was 3%, and only one episode of severe neurologic injury occurred, with a 4% incidence of transient focal lesions.[61] Matsuda et al[62] operated on 34 patients with aortic arch aneurysms using SCP at 16°C to 20°C, with a mortality of 9%, a 3% incidence of stroke, and a TND incidence of 5%. His technique required cannulation of the brachiocephalic and left carotid arteries with a two-pump system, and bilateral temporal artery and continuous internal jugular venous saturation monitoring. The authors pointed out that hypothermic cardiopulmonary bypass may not carry a higher risk of coagulopathy. Kazui et al[63,64] have since championed this technique, first describing its use in 1986. Between 1990 and 1999, 220 patients underwent total arch replacement with SCP and open distal anastomosis, with an in-hospital mortality of 12.7% and permanent neurologic dysfunction of 3.3%. Multivariable analysis showed in-hospital mortality was determined by renal failure, long CPB time, and shock, and permanent neurologic deficit was associated with old CVA and long CPB duration. Kazui et al, perfusing two arteries with flows of 10 mL/kg/min at 22°C—considered 50% of physiologic levels based on experimental studies—found that selective cerebral perfusion time had no significant impact on outcome.[65]

The presence of clot or atheroma in the aorta is a determinant of stroke during operation for aneurysm of the aortic arch. Atherosclerotic lesions often develop at the origin of the brachiocephalic vessels. Complete resection and branch grafting should reduce the rate of neurologic injury. In Dr. Kazui's latest 50 patients with atherosclerotic aortic arch aneurysms,[66] the mortality was 2%, permanent neurologic injury 4%, and TND occurred in 4% (adverse outcome 5%), with a history of cerebrovascular disease a risk factor for permanent neurologic dysfunction. The technique and sequence of reconstruction are as follows: systemic cooling of the patient to 22°C is followed by circulatory arrest and selective cerebral perfusion at 22°C via two cannulas, one in the innominate and one in the left common carotid artery. The left subclavian artery is clamped, distal anastomosis to the descending aorta is performed, and lower body perfusion is achieved via the fourth side arm of the 4-branch graft. Left subclavian anastomosis is followed by perfusion, measurement, and construction of the proximal anastomosis, and then the innominate artery and left common carotid artery anastomoses, with full perfusion restored. Permanent neurologic injury is again an independent risk factor for in-hospital mortality. This technique allows one to perform the transection of the brachiocephalic vessels distal to their origins and free of atherosclerotic disease to avoid dislodgement and embolization of debris. Newly designed cannulas allow superior visibility and simultaneous pressure monitoring (personal communication).

Jacobs et al[67] performed 50 arch replacements with selective antegrade cerebral perfusion and moderate hypothermia to 28°C to 30°C. EEG monitoring guided reconstruction techniques, pump flows, and perfusion pressures. Overall adverse outcome was 6%, TND rate 4%, and pulmonary complications occurred in 25%. Antegrade cerebral perfusion time ranged from 75 to 235 minutes, with a mean of 165 minutes. No correlation between long SCP duration and neurologic injury was noted.

Finally, in patients with extensive aneurysmal disease involving the ascending aorta, arch, and varying amounts of the descending thoracic aorta, a single-stage reconstruction can be performed with the "arch first" technique as described by Rokkas and Kouchoukos.[68] This technique employs an interval of HCA followed by selective cerebral perfusion of the upper body while the aortic reconstruction is completed. The use of brachiocephalic artery perfusion allows unhurried completion of aortic arch repairs.

CLINICAL IMPLEMENTATION

In the current era of aortic arch reconstruction, cerebral injury is most often related to the risk of embolization.[69–71] With liberal use of direct axillary artery cannulation,[72] HCA, and grafting to individual brachiocephalic vessels[73] followed by selective cerebral perfusion, lengthy periods of circulatory arrest are no longer necessary. Diseased origins of the brachiocephalic vessels in the arch are avoided, and the arch repair can proceed in an unhurried fashion.

After cooling, and during a brief period of HCA, the individual brachiocephalic arteries are dissected free and anastomosed to a pre-prepared trifurcated graft beginning either with the left subclavian or the innominate artery. Occasionally, when the left subclavian artery is displaced lateral and cephalad, a preoperative left subclavian to left carotid bypass is performed. The trifurcated graft is clamped, and perfusion selectively restored to the upper body. Typically, flows between 600 and 1000 cc/min are required to maintain a mean pressure of 50 mm Hg while allowing the perfusate temperature to drift upward. At the end of the arch reconstruction, the branch graft is sewn to the ascending aortic graft without interrupting flow.

Retrograde Cerebral Perfusion

The limitations of HCA, the success of retrograde cardioplegia, and isolated encouraging reports of the possible efficacy of retrograde cerebral perfusion (RCP) in mitigating the effects of massive air embolism[74] contributed to widespread interest in and enthusiasm for RCP in the early 1990s.[75] The mechanisms whereby RCP may accomplish neuroprotection include: (1) flushing embolic material from the cerebral circulation,[76] (2) providing cerebral flow sufficient to support cerebral metabolism,[77] and (3) maintaining cerebral hypothermia.[78] There is, however, evidence that RCP may worsen neurologic outcome by inducing cerebral edema.

Initial laboratory results and clinical reports regarding RCP were encouraging. However, upon closer examination, many of the studies that reported improved outcomes with RCP used historical controls and short durations of RCP that are well within the limits defined as safe for HCA alone. There were also some disturbing studies, using various techniques in several different animal species, reporting that no flow to the brain during RCP could be demonstrated.[79,80] In other experimental studies, the most effective conditions for retrograde flow were under circumstances—including clamping of the inferior vena cava and use of high perfusion pressures—that resulted in disturbingly high rates of fluid sequestration, significant cerebral edema, and mild cerebral histopathology; these sequelae were seen even after relatively short intervals of RCP.[81] Studies in our laboratory in which cerebral blood flow was quantitated not only by collecting aortic arch return, but also by counting the number of microspheres trapped in the brain, have demonstrated conclusively that too little capillary flow occurs during RCP (even with occlusion of the inferior vena cava) to confer any meaningful metabolic benefit even during deep hypothermia.[82]

The relationship between the use of RCP and mortality rates is unclear. In some studies, RCP duration was not found to be a predictor of death,[83–85] whereas in others it was.[86,87] Clinical outcome studies comparing RCP and HCA have also yielded mixed results, with some having mortality rates comparable to those with use of other cerebral protection methods,[87–89] and others reporting reduced mortality rates with RCP.[90–92] In three studies that included SCP patients, RCP patients had similar mortality rates.[93–95]

The literature examining the relationship between RCP and neurologic morbidity is also mixed. In some series, RCP duration was not found to be a predictor of neurologic morbidity,[84,85] whereas in others it was.[87,96] RCP has been found to be associated with neurologic morbidity rates that are either similar to those associated with HCA,[89,96] or lower.[88,90–92,97] When patients with SCP were included, RCP patients had similar outcomes in three studies[93–95] and worse outcome in one.[97]

In our own earlier[98] and more recent[99] clinical studies, we have been unable to demonstrate any benefit of RCP in our patients. Experimental data from our laboratory suggest that RCP, especially at high pressures, although successful in removing some emboli, may aggravate cerebral injury.[100] In our recent clinical study,[99] we were unable to demonstrate a decrease in the incidence of stroke with RCP. This may be explained by a greater prevalence of patients with clot or atheroma in the RCP group, but it nevertheless is also possible that RCP may not be effective in preventing stroke. Mortality was higher in the RCP group, and temporary neurologic dysfunction was higher with RCP than with SCP. Furthermore, RCP resulted in no reduction of transient neurologic dysfunction compared with HCA alone,[99] reinforcing the notion that RCP probably has no nutritive value for brain tissue. The induction of cerebral edema documented in our animal studies of RCP[100] cannot easily be demonstrated in the clinical situation, but may be another reason for our repeated observation of delayed neurologic recovery postoperatively in patients treated with RCP. Recently, we studied neuropsychologic dysfunction after retrograde cerebral perfusion; we found that RCP was of no benefit, and probably had a negative impact on cognitive outcome.[101]

We believe that the major benefit of RCP is in providing continued cerebral cooling by veno-arterial and veno-venous anastomoses during arrest of antegrade circulation, which helps to protect the brain especially in those patients in whom systemic cooling is not as thorough and prolonged as it should be. We continue to believe that a major benefit of RCP in the studies of others—usually with a historical control group and with a duration of RCP short enough that good results would be anticipated with use of HCA alone—can be explained largely by the enhanced cooling brought about by continuous bathing of the brain with cold blood during RCP. The effective cooling achieved during RCP may make a difference, especially if the initial cooling interval is short and the head is not packed in ice. Several experimental studies reinforce this view.[78] We no longer routinely use RCP. We believe that an upward drift in temperature during HCA can more safely be prevented by thorough initial cooling and packing the head in ice.

CLINICAL IMPLEMENTATION

Although we do not routinely use RCP for cerebral protection, we do occasionally use a short period of retrograde perfusion in patients who have a high risk of embolization because of clot or atheroma in the aorta, recognized either preoperatively or intraoperatively; this includes only about 10% of our patients. Some clinicians apply RCP very briefly at the end of a period of HCA solely for the purpose of flushing out potentially embolic debris.

Retrograde perfusion is always employed in conjunction with profound systemic hypothermia. To initiate retrograde perfusion, blood is infused into either one or both venae cavae at a flow rate to maintain the SVC pressure between 15 and 20 mm Hg. Given the rich network of collaterals between the SVC and IVC, it probably makes no difference whether inflow is into the SVC, into the IVC, or into both venae cavae. Cardiac distension is avoided by choking both venae cavae. When whole-body retrograde perfusion is carried out in this fashion, the initial flow rate is usually 800 to 1000 mL/min, but once the venous capacitance vessels have been filled, a flow of 100 to 500 mL/min is usually sufficient to maintain SVC pressure at 15 to 20 mm Hg.

REPRESENTATIVE PROCEDURES

Aortic arch reconstruction requires different approaches, techniques, and operative strategies depending upon the arch pathology and the involvement of the aorta proximal and distal to the arch. Thus, we describe five different situations and our approach to reconstruction of the arch in each of these.

Case #1: Bentall Procedure and Hemiarch Replacement

The patient has Marfan syndrome and an aortic root aneurysm associated with severe aortic regurgitation and a dilated ascending aorta and proximal arch (Fig. 47-1A).

A median sternotomy is performed. Cardiopulmonary bypass is initiated via the right axillary artery and a two-stage right atrial cannula. Cooling is begun, and when the heart fibrillates, a ventricular vent is placed via the right superior pulmonary veins. The ascending aorta is cross-clamped and opened. Cardioplegia is infused into both coronary ostia, and this is supplemented with topical cooling. Perfusate temperature is maintained at 10°C until the esophageal temperature reaches 20°C, and is maintained at that level while the Bentall procedure is being performed. After aortic valve removal, a composite prosthesis is sutured to the aortic annulus utilizing interrupted pledgeted sutures. Coronary buttons 1 cm in diameter are fashioned. The remainder of the aorta proximal to the clamp is excised. The coronary buttons are mobilized for 1 cm. Corresponding openings are made on the graft

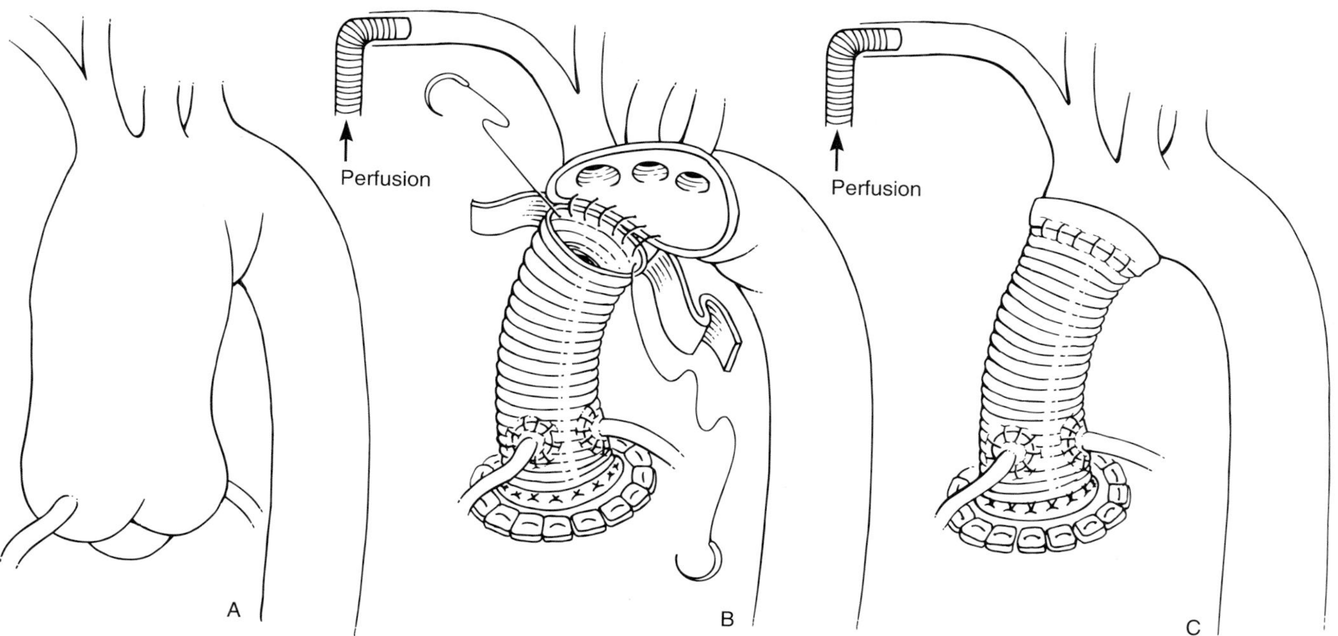

FIGURE 47–1 (A) Ascending aortic aneurysm extending into the underside of the aortic arch. (B) Bentall reconstruction of the aortic root with open resection of the hemiarch. Perfusion via the right axillary artery. (C) Completed repair and full systemic perfusion.

and the coronary buttons are anastomosed to the graft with 4-0 Prolene. Teflon felt buttressing is used to reinforce the buttons from behind. As the coronary button anastomoses are being carried out, jugular venous samples are drawn every 5 minutes and the perfusate temperature is lowered to 10°C.

When the jugular oxygen saturation is above 95% and the esophageal temperature is between 11°C and 14°C, the head is placed downward after being packed in ice, perfusion is discontinued, and the cross-clamp is removed. The distal ascending aorta and proximal arch are mobilized and excised, leaving a beveled aortic cuff extending from the base of the innominate artery on the right to 1 cm proximal to the ligamentum arteriosum and the right recurrent laryngeal nerve on the left. The composite Dacron graft is beveled and anastomosed to the aorta with a continuous 3-0 Prolene suture (Fig. 47-1B). Care is taken to place a 1-cm cuff of Teflon felt outside the aorta and to invaginate the graft within the aorta. The last few loops of the suture line are left loose; the head is placed in steep Trendelenburg position, and perfusion through the axillary artery cannula is restarted at a rate of 500 mL/min to flush all air from the aorta. The heart is also de-aired at this stage. Once all the air is evacuated, the suture line is tied and cold perfusion is commenced for several minutes, followed by rewarming (Fig. 47-1C). A gradient of 10°C or less between the perfusate temperature and esophageal temperature is maintained at all times. Circulatory arrest time is usually about 20 minutes. Approximately 40 minutes of warming is necessary to raise the esophageal temperature to 35°C to 36°C and the bladder temperature to 30°C; at this time, the patient is weaned from cardiopulmonary bypass.

Case #2: Total Arch Replacement for Nonatherosclerotic Pathology

The patient is a young male with an acute type A aortic dissection referred for emergency surgery. The operation we describe has been, in the past, our standard operation for total arch replacement.[102,103] We now use this technique in rare cases in which the arch is free of atherosclerotic debris, and where an unexpected finding such as an arch tear in aortic dissection requires total arch replacement.

Intraoperative transesophageal echo confirms a type A dissection involving the ascending aorta, arch, and descending aorta (Fig. 47-2A). However, the location of the intimal tear is not clearly visualized. Flow is present in both true and false lumens, and there is minimal aortic regurgitation and no pericardial blood or tamponade.

The right axillary artery is prepared for cannulation. A median sternotomy is performed. Cannulation is carried out via the right axillary artery and the right atrium. Cardiopulmonary bypass with cooling is commenced (Fig. 47-2B). When the heart fibrillates, a left ventricular vent is placed via the right superior pulmonary vein. The aorta is cross-clamped and the proximal aorta is opened. Cardioplegia is infused into both coronary ostia and this is supplemented with topical cooling. Careful inspection of the ascending aorta

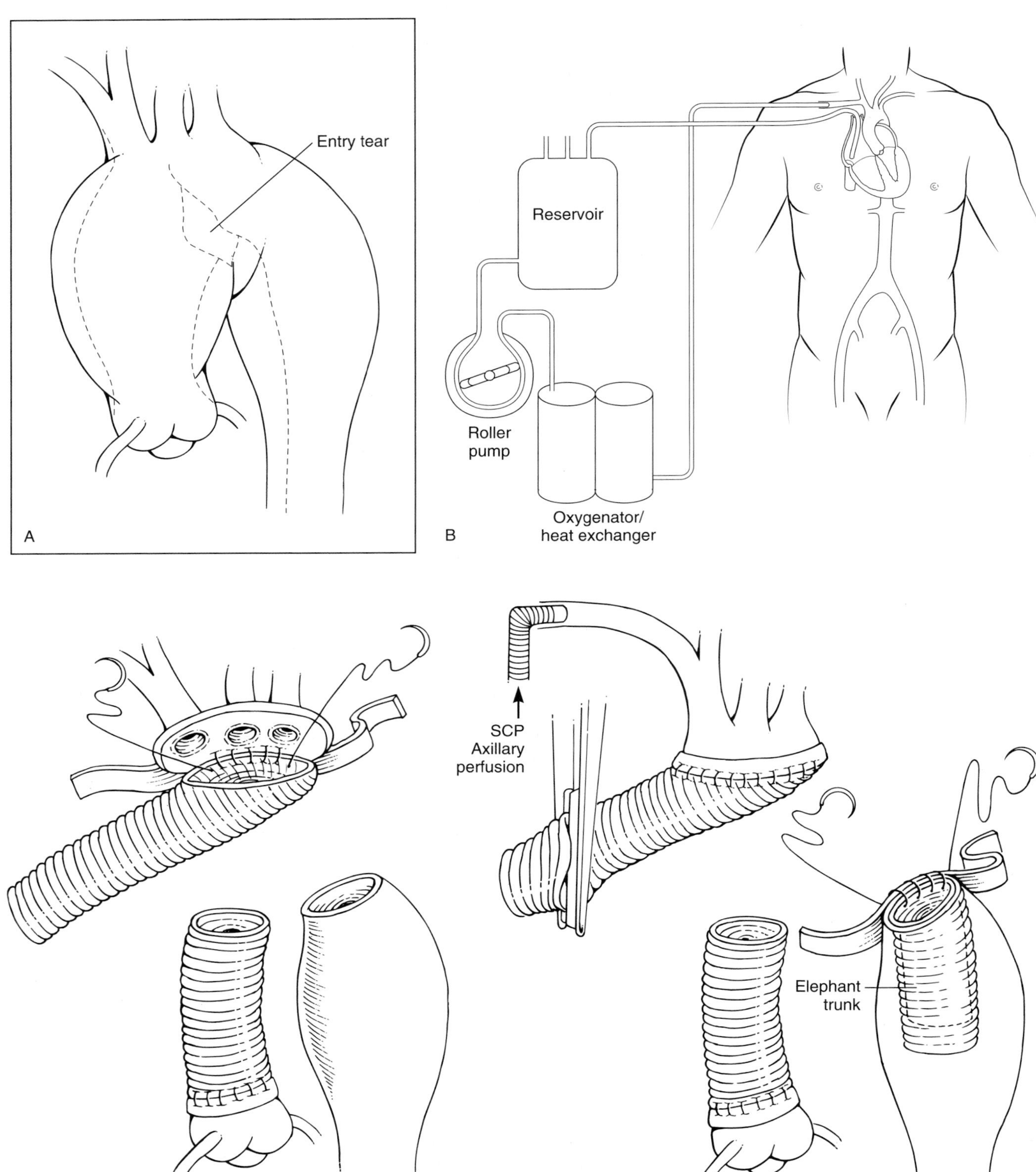

FIGURE 47–2 (A) Acute type A aortic dissection with the entry point located in the aortic arch. (B) Cardiopulmonary bypass via the right axillary artery. (C) Separate graft anastomosis to the brachiocephalic vessels. (D) Selective cerebral perfusion and elephant trunk construction.

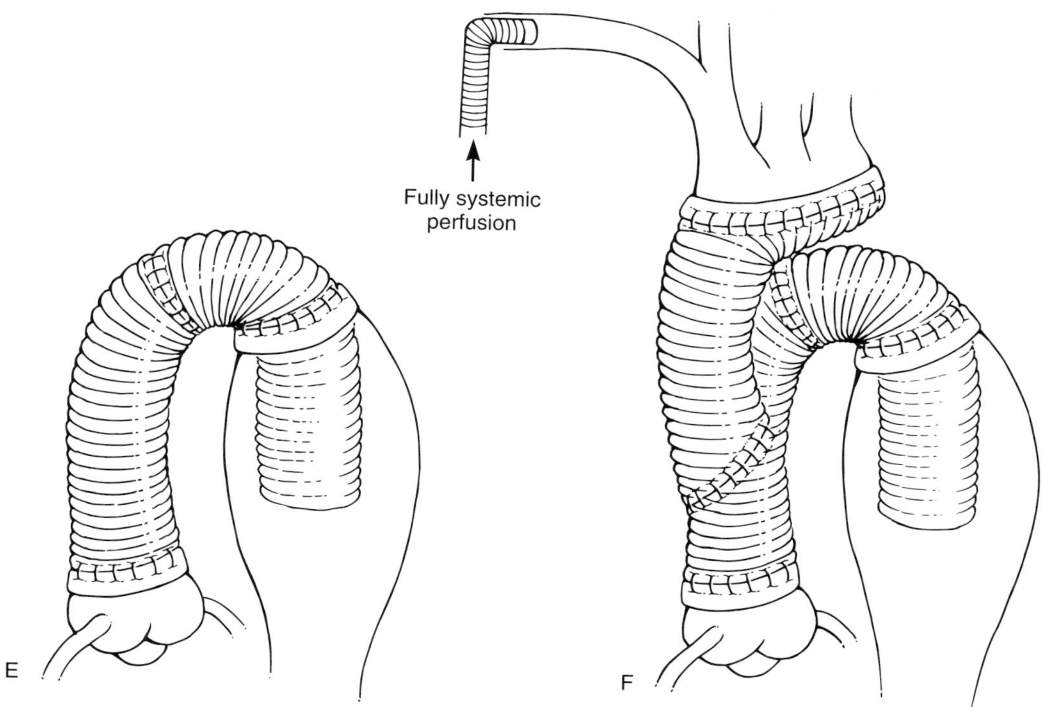

FIGURE 47–2 (*Continued*) (E) Arch reconstruction with graft-to-graft anastomosis. (F) Completed repair.

reveals no intimal tear. Perfusate temperature is maintained at 10°C until the esophageal temperature reaches 20°C, and this temperature is maintained while the proximal aortic reconstruction is performed.

The minimal aortic regurgitation is dealt with by resuspending each commissure with pledgeted horizontal mattress sutures. The root is reconstructed by using a 4-0 Prolene weave to suture a Teflon strip on the outside and a pericardial strip on the inside of the dissected aortic layer. A Hemashield graft is anastomosed with 3-0 Prolene to invaginate the graft within the aortic sandwich. During aortic reconstruction, cooling is continued, and when the esophageal temperature reaches 11°C to 14°C, and the jugular venous oxygen saturation is above 95%, the head is placed downward after being packed in ice, perfusion is discontinued, and the cross-clamp is removed. The aorta is opened into the arch to search for the intimal tear, which is found in the arch opposite the arch vessels. The arch is mobilized and excised, leaving an island of aortic tissue containing the three head vessels. A 16-mm Hemashield graft is then beveled and sutured to the island of aortic tissue with Teflon reinforcement on the outside, once again invaginating the graft within the aorta, so that the dissected layers are sandwiched between the Teflon on the outside and the graft on the inside (Fig. 47-2C). The period of circulatory arrest is usually less than 30 minutes. Antegrade perfusion is then slowly restarted via the right axillary artery, and after careful de-airing, the beveled graft is clamped so that antegrade cerebral perfusion can be instituted at flows between 600 and 1000 mL/min to maintain a proximal perfusion pressure of 50 to 60 mm Hg (Fig. 47-2D).

Attention is now directed to the descending aorta just distal to the left subclavian artery. The aorta is incised circumferentially, Teflon felt is placed outside the aorta, and, to facilitate the distal anastomosis, a small elephant trunk is constructed by invaginating the main arch portion of the graft. On completion of the suture line, the graft is everted, trimmed, and anastomosed to the ascending aortic graft with 2-0 Prolene (Fig. 47-2E). The 16-mm arch graft is then beveled, and a longitudinal opening is made in the ascending aortic portion of the graft. The two grafts are anastomosed to each other with 2-0 Prolene (Fig. 47-2F).

The heart is de-aired, the clamp on the beveled graft is removed, and perfusion to the heart and lower body is resumed. After rewarming, the patient is weaned from cardiopulmonary bypass in the standard fashion.

Case #3: Total Aortic Arch Replacement for Atherosclerotic and Calcified Aneurysms

Our technique for total arch replacement in elderly patients or in patients with atherosclerotic calcified aneurysms has evolved to our current "no-touch" technique (Fig. 47-3A). A trifurcated graft is anastomosed to the arch vessels during hypothermic circulatory arrest in order to reduce the risk of embolization; cerebral ischemia is minimized by permitting antegrade cerebral perfusion as arch reconstruction is completed.[104,105]

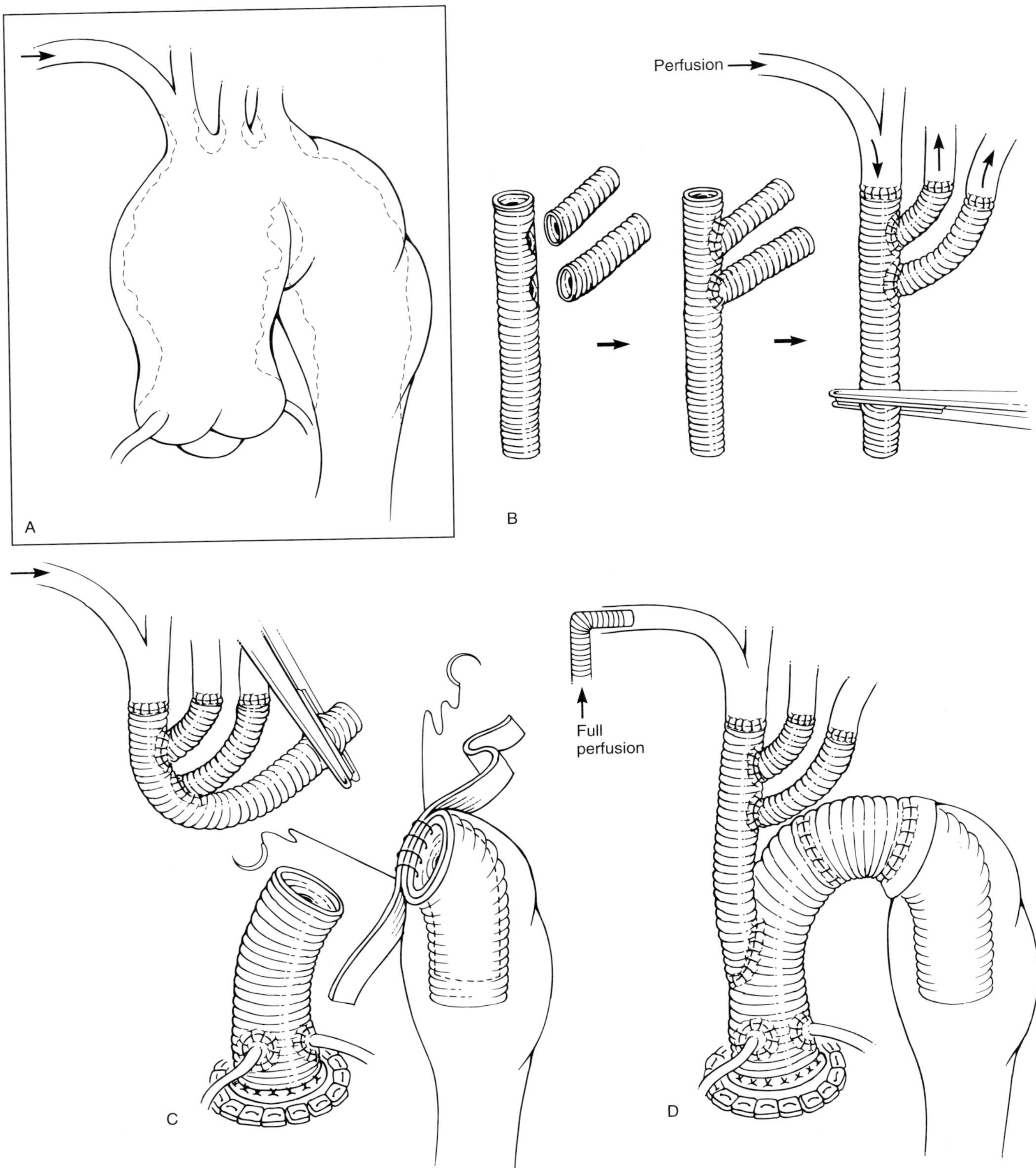

FIGURE 47–3 (A) Atherosclerotic ascending and arch aneurysm. (B) Fabrication of the trifurcated graft. (C) Selective cerebral perfusion and construction of the elephant trunk. (D) Completed repair.

A median sternotomy is performed with extension of the incision superiorly along the medial border of the left sternocleidomastoid muscle. The recurrent laryngeal nerve is preserved as the aortic arch and its branches are exposed. A no-touch technique of dissection is utilized: the patient is dissected away from the aneurysm.

Cardiopulmonary bypass is initiated using the right axillary artery and the right atrium, with a perfusate temperature of 10°C. Examination of the aortic arch with transesophageal echo confirms retrograde flow in the arch, and monitors for dissection or malperfusion. Cardioplegia is given after cross-clamp application, and is supplemented with topical hypothermia. If the ascending aorta is calcified or severely atherosclerotic, no attempt at cross-clamping is made. The patient is cooled, and the heart vented. Just prior to circulatory arrest, 60 mEq of KCl are added to the pump prime to produce diastolic cardiac arrest.

Even in patients with severe atherosclerotic disease of the aortic arch, the arch vessels just beyond their origins are usually spared. This location is ideal for subsequent anastomoses. After carefully sizing the innominate, left carotid, and left subclavian arteries, a trifurcated graft is constructed as illustrated (Fig. 47-3B). Completion of this phase usually coincides with adequate core cooling. The head is packed in ice to prevent rewarming during the ischemic period. When the esophageal temperature reaches 11°C to 14°C, and jugular bulb oxygen saturation is above 95%, maximum cerebral metabolic suppression is achieved. The patient is placed in Trendelenburg position to prevent air trapping during the period of circulatory arrest.

At the beginning of circulatory arrest, the innominate artery is transected just distal to its origin or at the level where atherosclerosis is minimal. The large limb of the trifurcated graft is trimmed and anastomosis is carried out with 4-0 polypropylene suture. The common carotid and the left subclavian artery anastomoses are constructed in a similar fashion. Each anastomosis takes 6 to 10 minutes, depending upon the exposure. Reversing the order of the anastomoses may provide better access to the left subclavian artery in some patients. The trifurcation graft is carefully de-aired, and the proximal portion is clamped, restoring perfusion to the head and upper extremities. Perfusion pressures are maintained at 50 to 60 mm Hg, requiring flows between 600 and 1000 mL/min. Blood temperature is allowed to drift upward. The aortic arch is reconstructed in a variety of ways depending upon the pathology (Fig. 47-3C).

For ascending and arch disease with aortic valve involvement, a Bentall or Yacoub procedure precedes arch reconstruction. If the aortic valve is spared, arch repair begins at the proximal descending thoracic aorta with a suitable cuff of aortic tissue preserving the recurrent laryngeal nerve. If aneurysmal disease involves distal aortic segments, an elephant trunk[106] may be constructed in either the distal or the more proximal aortic arch, or in the distal ascending aorta where the aortic caliber permits. This maneuver, as described by Kuki,[107] avoids potential nerve injury. The anastomosis is constructed with running 3-0 Prolene, reinforced with a strip of Teflon felt, taking great care to place the Dacron graft within the native aorta and the felt on the outside. The inverted graft is then stretched and measured to the appropriate length and sutured to the sinotubular junction or to the graft previously used for aortic root reconstruction. Graft-to-graft anastomoses are constructed with 2-0 Prolene. At this point, the Dacron graft is distended with cardioplegic solution to facilitate choosing the ideal site for anastomosing the trifurcated graft to the ascending portion of the aortic reconstruction interposition graft (Fig. 47-3D). An elliptical opening is made and the trifurcation graft is beveled and trimmed. Cerebral and upper extremity perfusion are not interrupted. On completion of this anastomosis, the patient is placed in Trendelenburg position, the ascending aortic graft is vented, the heart is defibrillated, and rewarming is begun. Cardiopulmonary bypass is discontinued once the patient's esophageal temperature is greater then 35°C.

Case #4: Thoracosternotomy for Arch Reconstruction

For patients with prior ascending aortic replacement presenting with arch and proximal descending aortic pathology (Fig. 47-4A), or patients with arch and proximal descending aortic disease alone, an alternative approach can facilitate a one-stage repair.[108] A bilateral thoracotomy can be used. Both internal mammary arteries are ligated. Exposure of the transverse aortic arch and proximal descending thoracic aorta is outstanding. For brachiocephalic artery reconstruction, either a large Carrell patch to a separate graft or a trifurcated graft to the individual vessels can be used, depending upon the degree of atherosclerotic disease and/or scarring from previous surgery (Figs. 47-4B and C). The patients tolerate the incision well, and exposure of the phrenic and recurrent laryngeal nerves allows easy preservation. The only drawback involves sternal union, and therefore secure stabilization of the sternal tables at the end of the procedure is imperative. Arterial perfusion is the same, through the right axillary artery. Venting of the left ventricle during systemic cooling and cardiac fibrillation can be carried out either via the right superior pulmonary vein or via a small separate thoracotomy overlying the left ventricular apex.

Case #5: Descending Thoracic Aortic Aneurysm Involving the Distal Arch

Descending thoracic aortic aneurysms often involve the distal aortic arch, or are associated with a distal arch that is calcified and severely atherosclerotic, making cross-clamping dangerous (Fig. 47-5A). In these situations we use the following technique.

Operation is carried out through a left thoracotomy in the 4th or 5th intercostal space with the incision extended inferiorly across the costochondral plate to improve exposure. The internal mammary artery is usually preserved. The

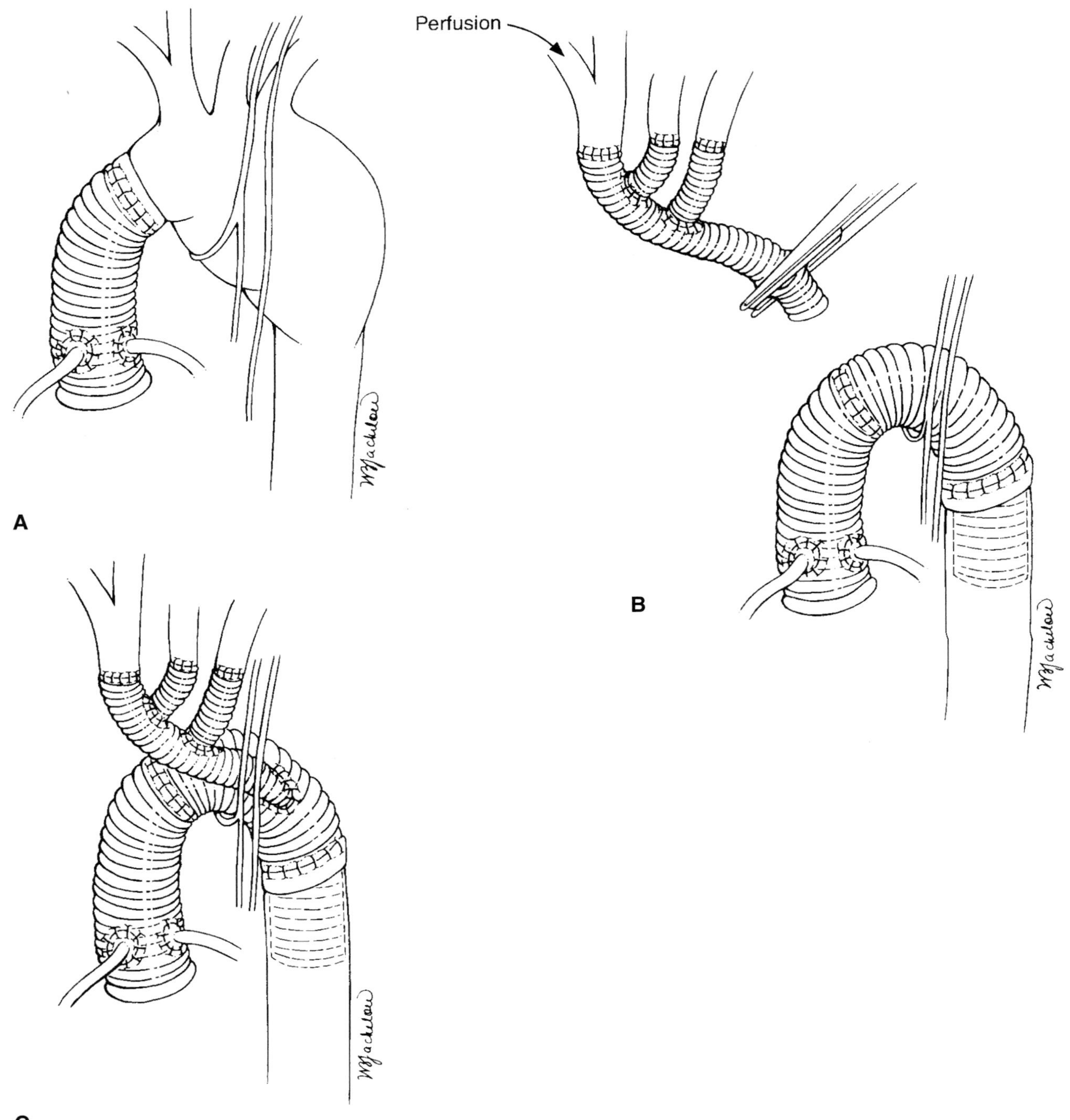

FIGURE 47–4 (A) Recurrent arch proximal descending aneurysm. (B) Selective cerebral perfusion and arch reconstruction. (C) Completed repair.

left femoral artery and vein are dissected out in preparation for cannulation. The descending aorta is gradually mobilized. Intercostal arteries are serially clamped and then sacrificed when no changes in the SSEPs and MEPs develop. Care is taken not to manipulate the distal arch adjacent to the left subclavian artery. Cannulation for cardiopulmonary bypass is carried out with a long perfusion catheter inserted via the femoral vein, and positioned in the right atrium with the aid of a guide wire and transesophageal echo monitoring. Occasionally the main pulmonary artery is used for venous inflow. The left common femoral artery is cannulated. Perfusion is begun gradually to avoid a rapid shift in the perfusion

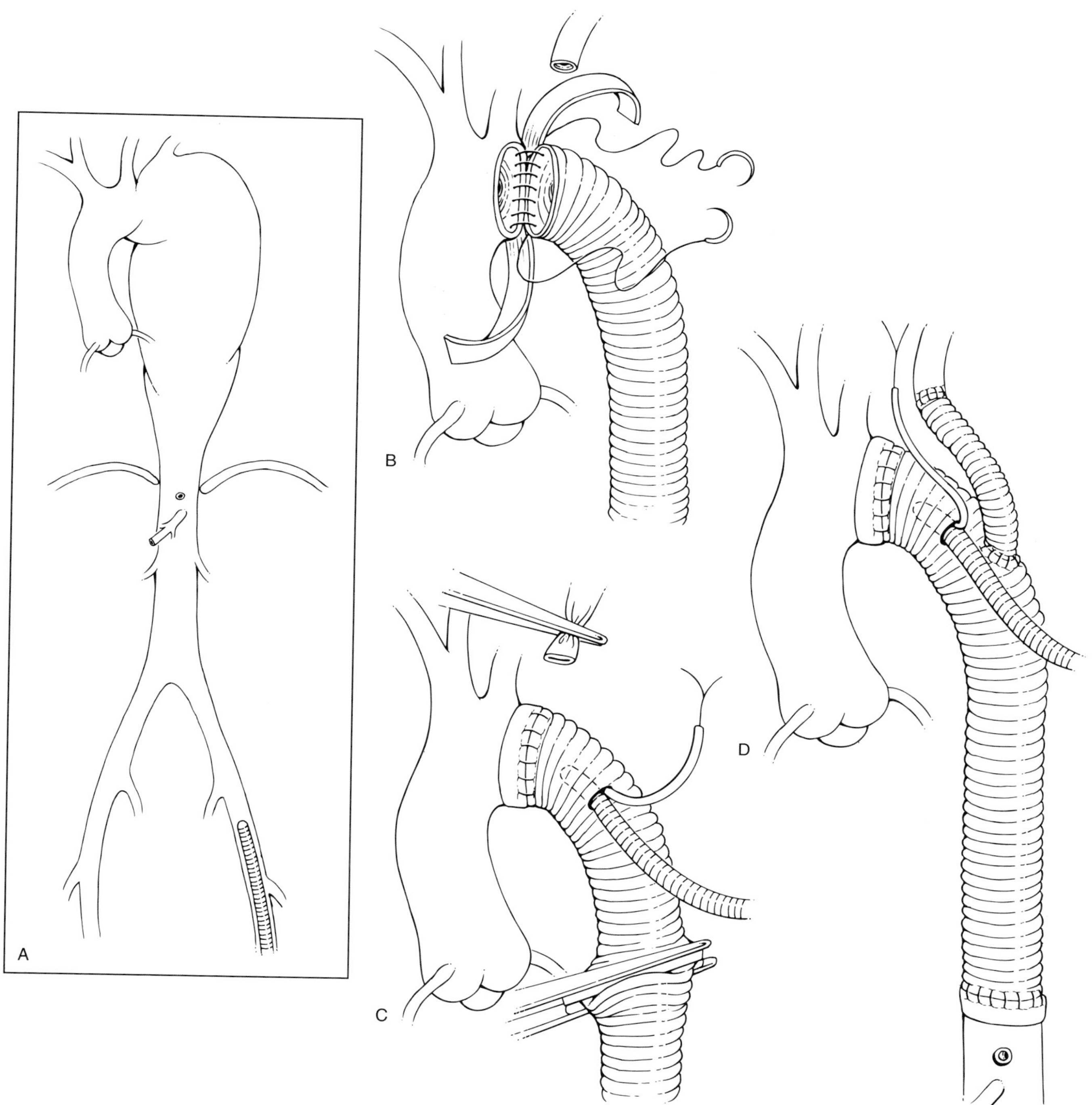

FIGURE 47–5 (A) Distal arch descending thoracic aortic aneurysm with femoral artery perfusion. (B) HCA and anastomosis to the distal arch. (C) Selective cerebral perfusion. (D) Reattachment of the left subclavian artery and completed repair.

patterns in the aorta that might dislodge atheromatous debris. Once perfusion is established, care is exercised to avoid manipulating the descending thoracic aorta, inasmuch as dislodged debris would be carried retrograde toward the arch vessels and the coronary arteries. During cooling and once ventricular fibrillation has occurred, left ventricular distention is closely monitored with transesophageal echo and pulmonary artery pressures. If there is any sign of left ventricular dilatation, a vent is introduced into the left ventricular apex or via the left atrium. After about 30 to 40 minutes of cooling, the esophageal temperature has usually decreased to 11°C to 14°C, and the jugular venous saturation exceeds 95%. Femoral artery perfusion is discontinued.

The left ventricular vent is clamped, and the descending thoracic aorta is opened. A cuff of the underside of the aortic arch, extending inferiorly to the distal ascending aorta and superiorly to the margin of the left carotid artery, is fashioned. An attempt is made to preserve the recurrent laryngeal nerve. A graft is anastomosed to the native aorta with a running suture of 3-0 Prolene (Fig. 47-5B). Teflon felt is used, and the graft is invaginated within the aorta. The graft vessels are carefully aspirated. A perfusion cannula is then placed in the graft, and the arch vessels are de-aired, after which antegrade perfusion is begun through the brachiocephalic and coronary arteries. The subclavian artery is clamped (Fig. 47-5C).

Attention is now turned to the distal descending aorta. Perfusion via the femoral artery catheter is used briefly to wash any loose debris in the descending aorta out into the field. A distal cuff is fashioned, and the graft is anastomosed to it with a running 3-0 Prolene suture. Teflon felt is utilized. The clamp on the graft is removed, and the flow to the entire body is provided through the perfusion catheter placed in the graft. Rewarming, defibrillation, and weaning from cardiopulmonary bypass are carried out in standard fashion. During rewarming, a separate 8-mm graft is sewn to the left subclavian artery, trimmed to the appropriate length, and anastomosed to the descending graft with a side-biting clamp (Fig. 47-5D).

SSEP monitoring is continued throughout the first postoperative night, and arterial pressures are maintained in the high normal range. An intrathecal catheter is placed preoperatively and is used to drain CSF in order to keep CSF pressure below 10 mm Hg for the first 24 to 48 hours.

RESULTS

Over the past 15 years, we have operated on 1131 patients with aneurysms involving the aortic arch. The majority of the lesions have begun in the ascending aorta and have involved either an open distal anastomosis (34%) or replacement of the ascending aorta and the underside of the arch (37%). In 15%, the entire aortic arch required replacement, and in 14% the aortic arch and the descending thoracic aorta were involved. Overall mortality was 9.9%, with a mortality of 8.3% in operations primarily involving the ascending aorta and 14.6% for operations involving the entire arch or the arch and the descending aorta.

The average age of our patients was 64.1 years; 67% were males.Twenty-six percent were operated on as emergencies and another 16% urgently because of acute dissection or impending rupture. In the majority of cases, HCA alone was used for cerebral protection. Recently, 21.6% had selective antegrade cerebral perfusion in addition to HCA, primarily patients with total arch or arch/descending repairs.

The major morbidity following surgery was neurologic; 21.7% of patients suffered strokes, with 6.5% left with permanent focal neurologic impairment. The highest morbidity and mortality were seen in the group of patients with arch and descending thoracic aortic disease, particularly in the subset older than 70 years of age with atherosclerotic disease; temporary neurologic impairment occurred in 31% of this group, and focal lesions in 12.5%.

Renal failure requiring dialysis occurred in 7% overall, and the rate was 9.3% in patients with arch and descending thoracic aneurysms. The incidence of severe respiratory insufficiency requiring tracheostomy differed with the type of incision: 14% in the sternotomy group, 34% in the left thoracotomy patients, and 35% in the bilateral thoracotomy cohort.

Careful retrospective review of 144 patients undergoing total aortic arch replacement since 1988 showed 50 patients using HCA alone between 1988 and 1994, 68 patients using HCA/SCP, and 26 patients using SCP with a trifurcated graft reconstruction and perfusion via the axillary artery since 2000 (SCP/trifurcated graft). The groups were well matched with regard to age (62 vs. 65 vs. 66 years) and urgency (emergent, 18% vs. 15% vs. 12%; urgent, 24% vs. 22% vs. 20%). There were no significant temperature differences between groups. Adverse outcome—hospital death or permanent stroke—occurred in 18%: 24% with HCA versus 16% with HCA/SCP versus 8% with SCP/trifurcated graft ($p = .034$). Transient neurologic dysfunction was significantly lower with SCP/trifurcated graft (9%) than with HCA (28%) versus HCA/SCP (19%) ($p = .031$). Mean duration of HCA fell from 53 minutes (HCA) to 45 minutes (HCA/SCP) to 31 minutes (SCP/trifurcated graft) ($p = .04$). Mean duration of SCP was 57 ± 29 minutes in the HCA/SCP group versus 57 ± 19 minutes with SCP/trifurcated graft (p = NS). The contemporary experience suggests that HCA/SCP is superior to HCA alone for preventing cerebral injury during aortic arch reconstruction and that SCP/trifurcated graft with axillary artery cannulation may be the optimal technique for reducing adverse outcome.

Recently reported series of total aortic arch replacement compare favorably with our results. Safi et al[109] reported a 30-day mortality of 5.1% in 117 patients undergoing stage I elephant trunk reconstruction, with an adverse outcome of 6.8%. Interestingly, 43 (37%) of patients did not return for second-stage repair, and 30.2% died from distal aneurysm rupture in short-term follow-up. Schepens et al[110] reviewed 100 consecutive stage I elephant trunk reconstructions from 1984 to 2001, with an 8% mortality, 12% adverse outcome, and 2% TND. The majority of patients received isolated unilateral or bilateral antegrade cerebral perfusion for cerebral protection.

Ueda et al[111] described 207 consecutive patients with aortic arch repairs from 1988 to 2000, 50% with atherosclerotic aneurysm, and a 12% mortality. The author reemphasized the poor long-term outcome of patients with postoperative neurologic injury. Recently, the use of the anterolateral

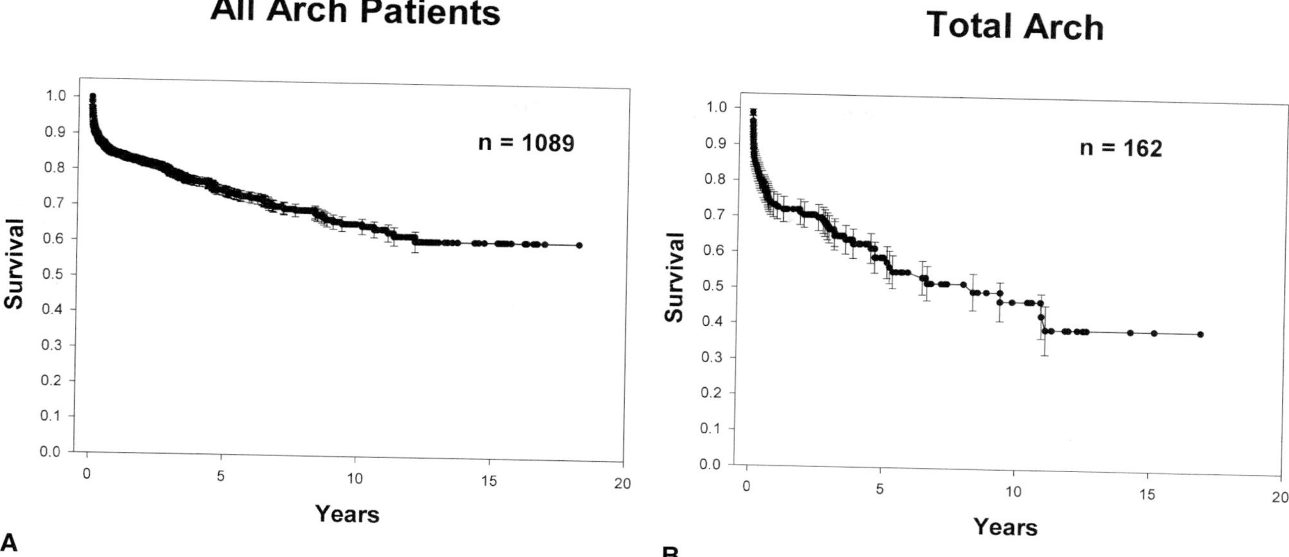

FIGURE 47–6 (A) Life table analysis of long-term survival following aortic arch surgery. (B) Life table analysis of long-term survival following total aortic arch replacement.

approach to complicated arch repair avoided cerebral dysfunction[112]; this is a technique we have employed with contained ruptures and redo arch replacements. Hilgenberg[113] reported adverse outcome in 6% of 67 patients, with 16% experiencing TND with acute dissection, which was the only independent risk factor for neurologic dysfunction. Hirotani et al,[114] using a pharmacologic mixture to improve cerebral protection with HCA, performed a total arch replacement in 43 patients with a mortality of 10.7% and an adverse outcome of 14.7%. The duration of circulatory arrest did not correlate with mortality or postoperative stroke, again illustrating the embolic nature of focal neurologic injury.

Coselli et al,[115] in a series of 227 patients with aortic arch surgery, experienced a 6% early and a 9% late mortality, with a 3% incidence of stroke. The reduction in neurologic injury was attributed to a greater than 50% use of retrograde cerebral perfusion during HCA. Finally, Kazui et al,[66] in his contemporary collection of 50 patients and use of a refined technique of total arch replacement in atherosclerotic aneurysms, achieved outstanding results: 2% mortality, 6% rate of adverse outcome, and 4% incidence of TND. Duration of cardiopulmonary bypass was the only univariate risk factor for TND, and a history of CVA was correlated with permanent neurologic dysfunction.

LONG-TERM FOLLOW-UP

Aortic arch aneurysms may represent a localized manifestation of an often multilevel disease process of the aorta. Therefore, long-term follow-up of the unresected aorta in postoperative patients is mandatory. All patients with aortic aneurysms are entered into our database and follow-up program. Patients with small aneurysms require ongoing radiographic imaging at either 6- or 12-month intervals, depending on the location, rate of progression, and etiology. Baseline CT scan, MRI, or angiograms obtained in the postoperative period document the integrity of the repair and provide a baseline for later comparison. In those patients with no portion of the unresected aorta dilated to a diameter exceeding 4 cm, the first reevaluation is scheduled in 1 year. Patients with significant residual dissection or aneurysmal dilatation are followed more closely at 6-month intervals. Medical therapy includes control of hypertension, beta-blocker therapy in patients with aortic dissection and Marfan syndrome, and encouragement of cessation of cigarette smoking.

Our long-term results are shown in Fig. 47-6A. Life table analysis shows that 84% of patients are alive at 1 year, 74% survive 5 years, and 65% and 61% are still alive after 10 and 15 years, respectively. When examining patients undergoing total arch replacement—reflecting more extensive aneurysmal disease—survival at 1 year is 73%; it is 59% at 5 years, and 47% and 39% at 10 and 15 years, respectively (Fig. 47-6B). Of the 1089 patients surviving aortic arch surgery, 96 patients (8.8%) required additional aortic surgery during follow-up. Fifty-four of 162 patients (33%) required additional aortic surgery following total arch replacement.

Long-term results reported in the literature confirm the importance of continued surveillance of patients following total arch replacement. Crawford et al[116] found that 70% of patients with operations involving the aortic arch had significant disease elsewhere in the aorta. Coselli et al documented that 15% of 227 patients with aortic arch repairs required additional surgery within a mean interval of 17 months.[115] Heinemann et al[117] reoperated on 24% of 82 patients with type A dissection over a 10-year period. Detter et al,[118] examining the long-term prognosis of aortic aneurysm in patients with and without Marfan syndrome, found a reoperation rate of 10.7% and 66.7% respectively, reinforcing the necessity of continued radiographic follow-up, particularly in patients with Marfan syndrome, residual dissection, and aortic arch aneurysms. Late death occurred in 25% of Marfan patients and 14% of non-Marfan patients, with 18% caused by redissection and recurrent aneurysm in the Marfan group. Elective replacement of other aortic segments can be carried out with an acceptable morbidity and mortality, in contrast with the low salvage rate in patients presenting with contained ruptures and untreated comorbid disease.

REFERENCES

1. Roberts DA: Magnetic resonance imaging of thoracic aortic aneurysms and dissection. *Semin Roentgenol* 2001; 36:295.
2. Griepp RB: The aortic arch: panel discussion II. *J Card Surg* 1994; 9:614.
3. Royse C, Royse A, Blake D, Grigg L: Screening the thoracic aorta for atheroma: a comparison of manual palpation, transesophageal and epiaortic ultrasonography. *Ann Thorac Cardiovasc Surg* 1998; 4:347.
4. Bonatti J: Ascending aortic atherosclerosis—a complex and challenging problem for the cardiac surgeon. *Heart Surg Forum* 1999; 2:125.
5. Wilson MJ, Boyd SY, Lisagor PG, et al: Ascending aortic atheroma assessed intraoperatively by epiaortic and transesophageal echocardiography. *Ann Thorac Surg* 2000; 70:25.
6. Sabik JF, Lytle BW, McCarthy PM, Cosgrove DM: Axillary artery: an alternative site of arterial cannulation for patients with extensive aortic and peripheral vascular disease. *J Thorac Cardiovasc Surg* 1995; 109:885.
7. Gillinov AM, Sabik JF, Lytle BW, Cosgrove DM: Axillary artery cannulation. *J Thorac Cardiovasc Surg* 1999; 118:1153.
8. Griepp EB, Griepp RB: Cerebral consequences of hypothermic circulatory arrest in adults. *J Cardiac Surg* 1992; 7:134.
9. Kouchoukos NT, Masetti P, Rokka CK, Murphy SF: Single-stage reoperative repair of chronic type A aortic dissection by means of the arch-first technique. *J Thorac Cardiovasc Surg* 2001; 122:578.
10. Borst HB, Walterbusch G, Scheps D: Extensive aortic replacement using "elephant trunk" prosthesis. *Thorac Cardiovasc Surg* 1983; 31:37.
11. Ehrlich MP, McCullough, Wolfe D, et al: Cerebral effects of cold perfusion after hypothermic circulatory arrest. *J Thorac Cardiovasc Surg* 2001; 121:923.
12. Jacobs MJ, deMol BA, Elenbaas T, et al: Spinal cord blood supply in patients with thoracoabdominal aortic aneurysms. *J Vasc Surg* 2002; 35:30.
13. deHaan P, Kalkmann CJ: Spinal cord monitoring: somatosensory and motor-evoked potentials. *Anesthesiol Clin North Am* 2001; 19:1.
14. Galla JD, Ergin MA, Sadeghi AM, et al: A new technique using somatosensory evoked potential guidance during descending and thoracoabdominal aortic repairs. *J Card Surg* 1994; 9:662.
15. Griepp RB, Ergin MA, Galla JD, Lansman S, et al: Looking for the artery of Adamkiewicz: a quest to minimize paraplegia after operations for aneurysm of the descending thoracic and thoracoabdominal aorta. *J Thorac Cardiovasc Surg* 1996; 112:1202.
16. Safi HJ, Miller CC 3rd, Azizzadeh A, Iliopoulos DC: Observations on delayed neurologic deficit after thoracoabdominal aortic aneurysm repair. *J Vasc Surg* 1997; 26:616.
17. Hill AB, Kalman PG, Johnston KW, Vasi HA: Reversal of delayed onset paraplegia after thoracic aortic surgery with cerebrospinal fluid drainage. *J Vasc Surg* 1994; 20:315.
18. Azizzadeh A, Huynh TTT, Miller CC 3rd, Safi HJ: Reversal of twice-delayed neurologic deficits with cerebrospinal fluid drainage after thoracoabdominal aneurysm repair: a case report and plea for a national database collection. *J Vasc Surg* 2000; 31:592.
19. Sundt TM, Kouchoukos NT, Saffitz JE, et al: Renal dysfunction and intravascular coagulation with aprotinin and hypothermic circulatory arrest. *Ann Thorac Surg* 1993; 55:1418.
20. Alvarez JM, Goldstein J, Mezzatesta J, et al: Fatal intraoperative pulmonary thrombosis after graft replacement of an aneurysm of the arch and descending aorta in association with deep hypothermic circulatory arrest and aprotinin therapy. *J Thorac Cardiovasc Surg* 1998; 115:723.
21. Smith CR, Spanier TB: Aprotinin in deep hypothermic circulatory arrest. *Ann Thorac Surg* 1999; 68:278.
22. Cohen DM, Norberto J, Cartabuke R, Ryu G: Severe anaphylactic reaction after primary exposure to aprotinin. *Ann Thorac Surg*. 1999; 67:837.
23. Westaby S, Saito S, Katsumata T: Acute type A dissection: conservative methods provide consistently low mortality. *Ann Thorac Surg* 2002; 73:707.
24. Kazui T, Washiyama N. Bashar AH, Terada H, et al: Role of biologic glue repair of proximal aortic dissection in the development of early and mid-term redissection of the aortic root. *Ann Thorac Surg* 2001; 72:509.
25. Kirsch M, Ginat M, Lecert L, et al: Aortic wall alterations after use of gelatin-resorcinol-formalin glue. *Ann Thorac Surg* 2002; 73:642.
26. Vogt PR, Brunner-La Rocco HP, Lachat M, et al: Technical details with the use of cryopreserved arterial allografts for aortic infection: influence on early and mid-term mortality. *J Vasc Surg* 2002; 35:80.
27. Ehrlich M, Grabenwoger M, Cartes-Zymelzu F, et al: Operations of the thoracic aorta and hypothermic circulatory arrest: is aprotinin safe? *J Thorac Cardiovasc Surg* 1998; 115:220.
28. Borst GH, Schaudig A, Rudolph W: Arteriovenous fistula of the aortic arch repair during deep hypothermia and circulatory arrest. *J Thorac Cardiovasc Surg* 1964; 3:443.
29. Lillehei CW, Todd DB, Levy MJ, et al: Partial cardiopulmonary bypass, hypothermia and total circulatory arrest: a lifesaving technique for ruptured mycotic aneurysms, ruptured left ventricle, and other complicated aortic pathology. *J Thorac Cardiovasc Surg* 1969; 58:530.
30. Barrat-Boyes BG, Simpson M, Neutze JM: Intracardiac surgery in neonates and infants using deep hypothermia with surface cooling and limited cardiopulmonary bypass. *Circulation* 1971; 43(suppl):1.
31. Griepp RB, Stinson EB, Hollingsworth JF, et al: Prosthetic replacement of the aortic arch. *J Thorac Cardiovasc Surg* 1975; 70:1051.
32. Michenfelder JD, Theye RA: Hypothermia: effect on canine brain and whole body metabolism. *Anesthesiology* 1968; 29:1107.
33. Michenfelder JD, Milde JH: The relationship among canine brain temperature, metabolism and function during hypothermia. *Anesthesiology* 1991; 75:130
34. Mault JR, Ohtake S, Klingensmith MF, et al: Cerebral metabolism and circulatory arrest: effects of duration and strategies for protection. *Ann Thorac Surg* 1993; 55:57.
35. Mezrow CK, Mildulla P, Sadeghi AM, et al: Evaluation of cerebral metabolism and quantitative electroencephalography after circulatory arrest and low-flow cardiopulmonary bypass at different temperatures. *J Thorac Cardiovasc Surg* 1994; 107:1006.
36. Mezrow CK, Midulla PS, Sadeghi AM, et al: Quantitative electroencephalography: a method to assess cerebral injury after

hypothermic circulatory arrest. *J Thorac Cardiovasc Surg* 1995; 109:925.
37. Mildulla PS, Gandsas A, Sadeghi AM, et al: Comparison of retrograde to antegrade cerebral perfusion and hypothermic circulatory arrest in a chronic porcine model. *J Card Surg* 1994; 9:560.
38. Mezrow CK, Gandsas A, Sadeghi AM, et al: Metabolic correlates of neurologic and behavioral injury after prolonged hypothermic circulatory arrest. *J Thorac Cardiovasc Surg* 1995; 109:959.
39. Mezrow CK, Midulla P, Sadeghi A, et al: A vulnerable interval for cerebral injury: comparison of hypothermic circulatory arrest and low flow cardiopulmonary bypass. *Cardiol Young* 1993; 3:287.
40. Mezrow CK, Sadeghi AM, Gandsas A, et al: Cerebral blood flow and metabolism in hypothermic circulatory arrest. *Ann Thorac Surg* 1992; 54:609.
41. Reich DL, Oysal S, Sliwinski M, et al: Neuropsychologic outcome after deep hypothermic circulatory arrest in adults. *J Thorac Cardiovasc Surg* 1998; 117:156.
42. Ergin MA, Uysal S, Reich DL, et al: Temporary neurological dysfunction after deep hypothermic circulatory arrest: a clinical marker of long-term functional deficit. *Ann Thorac Surg* 1999; 67:1887.
43. McCullough JH, Zhang N, Reich DL, et al: Cerebral metabolic suppression during hypothermic circulatory arrest in humans. *Ann Thorac Surg* 1999; 67:1895.
44. Bellinger DC, Wernovsky G, Rapaport LA, et al: cognitive development following repair as neonates of transposition of the great arteries using deep hypothermic circulatory arrest. *Pediatrics* 1991; 87:701.
45. Kawata H, Fackler JC, Aoki M, et al: Recovery of cerebral blood flow and energy state in piglets after hypothermic circulatory arrest versus recovery after low flow bypass. *J Thorac Cardiovasc Surg* 1993; 106:671.
46. Langley SM, Chai PJ, Jaggers JJ, et al: Preoperative high dose methylprednisolone attenuates the cerebral response to DHCA. *Eur J Cardiothorac Surg* 2000; 17:279.
47. Shum-Tim D, Tchervenkov CI, Jamal AM, et al: Systemic steroid pretreatment improves cerebral protection after circulatory arrest. *Ann Thorac Surg* 2001; 72:1465.
48. Temesvari P, Joo F, Koltai M, et al: Cerebroprotective effect of dexamethasone by increasing the tolerance to hypoxia and preventing brain edema in newborn piglets with experimental pneumothorax. *Neurosci Lett* 1984; 49:87.
49. Cronstein BN, Kimmel SC, Levin RI, et al: A mechanism for the anti-inflammatory effects of corticosteroids: the glucocorticoid receptor regulates leukocyte adhesion to endothelial cells and expression of endothelial-leukocyte adhesion molecule 1 and intercellular adhesion molecule. *Proc Natl Acad Sci U S A* 1992; 89:9991.
50. Lodge AJ, Chai PJ, Daggett CW, et al: Methylprednisolone reduces the inflammatory response to cardiopulmonary bypass in neonatal piglets: timing of dose is important. *J Thorac Cardiovasc Surg* 1999; 117:515.
51. Hoka S, Tatebayashi E, Okamoto H, et al: Reduction of jugular venous oxygen saturation coincidental with electroencephalographic abnormality. *Anesth Analg* 1993; 79:387.
52. Jonassen AE, Quaegebeur JM, Young WL, et al: Cerebral blood flow velocity in pediatric patients is reduced after cardiopulmonary bypass with profound hypothermia. *J Thorac Cardiovasc Surg* 1995; 110:934.
53. Shum-Tim D, Hagashima M, Shinoka T, et al: Postischemic hyperthermic exacerbates neurologic injury after deep hypothermic circulatory arrest. *J Thorac Cardiovasc Surg* 1998; 116:780.
54. Griepp RB: Cerebral protection during aortic arch surgery [editorial]. *J Thorac Cardiovasc Surg* 2001; 121:425.
55. Griepp RB: Discussion: Session 3—Aortic Arch I: Aortic Surgery Symposium VI. *Ann Thorac Surg* 1999; 67:1891.
56. Hagl C, Ergin MA, Galla JD, et al: Neurologic outcome after ascending aorta-aortic arch operations: effect of brain protection technique in high-risk patients. *J Thorac Cardiovasc Surg* 2001; 121:1107.
57. DeBakey ME, Crawford ES, Cooley DA, et al: Successful resection of fusiform aneurysm of the aortic arch with replacement homograft. *Surg Gynecol Obstet* 1957; 105:657.
58. Frist, WH, Baldwin, JC, Starnes, VA, et al: A reconsideration of cerebral perfusion in aortic arch replacement. *Ann Thorac Surg* 1986; 42:273.
59. Filgueiras CL, Winsborrow B, Ye J, et al: A ^{31}P magnetic resonance study of antegrade and retrograde cerebral perfusion during aortic arch surgery in pigs. *J Thorac Cardiovasc Surg* 1995; 110:55.
60. Swain JA, McDonald TJ, Griffith PK, et al: Low-flow hypothermic cardiopulmonary bypass protects the brain. *J Thorac Cardiovasc Surg* 1991, 102.
61. Bachet J, Guilmet D, Goudot B, et al: Cold cerebroplegia: a new technique of cerebral protection during operations on the transverse aortic arch. *J Thorac Cardiovasc Surg* 1991; 102:85.
62. Matsuda H, Nakano S, Shirakura R, et al: Surgery for aortic arch aneurysm with selective cerebral perfusion and hypothermic cardiopulmonary bypass. *Circulation* 1989; 80:243.
63. Kazui T, Inoue N, Komatsu S: Surgical treatment of aneurysms of the transverse aortic arch. *J Cardiovasc Surg* 1989; 30:402.
64. Kazui T, Washiyama N, Muhammad BAH, et al: Total arch replacement using aortic arch branched grafts with the aid of antegrade selective cerebral perfusion. *Ann Thorac Surg* 2000; 70:3.
65. Kazui T, Inoue N, Yamada O, et al: Selective cerebral perfusion during operation for aneurysms of the aortic arch: a reassessment. *Ann Thorac Surg* 1992; 53:109.
66. Kazui T, Washiyama N, Muhammad BAH, et al: Improved results of atherosclerotic arch aneurysm operations with a refined technique. *J Thorac Cardiovasc Surg* 2001; 121:491.
67. Jacobs MJ, deMol BA, Veldman DJ: Aortic arch and proximal supraaortic arterial repair under continuous antegrade cerebral perfusion and moderate hypothermia. *Cardiovasc Surg* 2001; 9:396.
68. Rokkas CK, Kouchoukos NT: Single-stage extensive replacement of the thoracic aortic: the arch-first technique. *J Thorac Cardiovasc Surg* 1999; 117:99.
69. Okita Y, Minatoya K, Tagusari O, et al: Prospective comparative study of brain protection in total aortic arch replacement: deep hypothermic circulatory arrest with retrograde cerebral perfusion or selective antegrade cerebral perfusion. *Ann Thorac Surg* 2001; 72:72.
70. Westaby S, Katsumata T: Proximal aortic perfusion for complex arch and descending aortic disease. *J Thorac Cardiovasc Surg* 1998; 115:162.
71. Ueda T, Shimizu H, Ito T, et al: Cerebral complications associated with selective perfusion of the arch vessels. *Ann Thorac Surg* 2000; 70:1472.
72. Gerdes A, Joubert-Hűbner E, Esders K, et al: Hydrodynamics of aortic arch vessels during perfusion through the right subclavian artery. *Ann Thorac Surg* 2000; 69:1425.
73. Kuki S, Taniguchi K, Masai T, et al: A novel modification of elephant trunk technique using a single four-branched arch graft for extensive thoracic aortic aneurysm. *Eur J Cardiothorac Surg* 2000; 18:246.
74. Mills NL, Ochsner JL: Massive air embolism during cardiopulmonary bypass: causes, preventions, and management. *J Thorac Cardiovasc Surg* 1980; 80:708.
75. Udea Y, Miki S, Kusuhara K, et al: Surgical treatment of aneurysm on dissection involving the ascending aorta and aortic arch, utilizing circulatory arrest and retrograde cerebral perfusion. *J Cardiovasc Surg* (Torino) 1990; 31:553.
76. Juvonen T, Weisz D, Wolfe D, et al: Can retrograde perfusion mitigate cerebral injury after particulate embolization: a study in a chronic porcine model. *J Thorac Cardiovasc Surg* 1998; 115:1142.

77. Usui A, Motta T, Miroura M, et al: Retrograde cerebral perfusion through a superior vena caval cannula protects the brain. *Ann Thorac Surg* 1992; 53:47.
78. Anttila V, Pokela M, Kiriluoma K, et al: Is maintained cranial hypothermia the only factor leading to improved outcome after retrograde cerebral perfusion: an experimental study with a chronic porcine model. *J Thorac Cardiovasc Surg* 2000; 119:1021.
79. Boeckxstans CJ, Flameng WJ: Retrograde cerebral perfusion does not protect the brain in non-human primates. *Ann Thorac Surg* 1995; 60:319.
80. Ye J, Yang L, Del Rigio MR, et al: Retrograde cerebral perfusion provides limited distribution of blood to the brain: a study in pigs. *J Thorac Cardiovasc Surg* 1997; 114:660.
81. Juvonen T, Weisz DJ, Wolfe D, et al: Can retrograde perfusion mitigate cerebral injury following particulate embolization: a study ini a chronic porcine model. *Ann Thorac Surg* 1998; 66:38.
82. Ehrlich MP, Hagl C, McCullough JN, et al: Retrograde cerebral perfusion provides negligible flow through brain capillaries in the pig. *J Thorac Cardiovasc Surg* 2001; 122:331.
83. Sasaguri S, Yamamoto S, Hosoda Y: What is the safe time limit for retrograde cerebral perfusion with hypothermic circulatory arrest in aortic surgery? *J Cardiovasc Surg* 1996; 77:441.
84. Deeb GM, Williams DM, Quint LE, et al: Risk analysis for aortic surgery using hypothermic circulatory arrest with retrograde cerebral perfusion. *Ann Thorac Surg* 1999; 67:1883.
85. Okita Y, Takamoto S, Ando M, et al: Mortality and cerebral outcome in patients who underwent aortic arch operations using deep hypothermic circulatory arrest with retrograde cerebral perfusion: no relation of early death, stroke and delirium to the duration of circulatory arrest. *J Thorac Cardiovasc Surg* 1998; 115:129.
86. Wong CH, Bonser RS: Does retrograde cerebral perfusion affect risk factors for stroke and mortality after hypothermic circulatory arrest? *Ann Thorac Surg* 1999; 67:1900.
87. Ueda Y, Okita Y, Aomi S, et al: Retrograde cerebral perfusion for aortic arch surgery: analysis of risk factors. *Ann Thorac Surg* 1999; 67:1879.
88. Grabenwoger M, Ehrlich M, Cartes-Zumelzu F, et al: Surgical treatment of aortic arch aneurysms in profound hypothermia and circulatory arrest. *Ann Thorac Surg* 1997; 64:1967.
89. Shapira OM, Aldea GS, Cutter SM, et al: Improved clinical outcomes after operation of the proximal aorta: a 10-year experience. *Ann Thorac Surg* 1999; 67:1030.
90. Bavaria JE, Woo J, Hall A, et al: Circulatory management with retrograde cerebral perfusion for acute type A aortic dissection. *Circulation* 1996; 94(suppl II):II173.
91. Coselli JS: Retrograde cerebral perfusion is an effective means of neural support during deep hypothermic circulatory arrest. *Ann Thorac Surg* 1997; 64:908.
92. Ehrlich M, Fang C, Grabenwoger M, et al: Perioperative risk factors for mortality in patients with acute type A aortic dissection. *Circulation* 1998; 98(19 suppl):II294.
93. Okita Y, Takamoto S, Ando M, et al: Predictive factors for postoperative cerebral complications in patients with thoracic aortic aneurysm. *Eur J Cardiothorac Surg* 1996; 10:826.
94. Okita Y, Ando M, Minatoya K, et al: Predictive factors for mortality and cerebral complications in arteriosclerotic aneurysm of the aortic arch. *Ann Thorac Surg* 1999; 67:72.
95. Usui A, Yasuura K, Watanabe T, et al: Comparative clinical study between retrograde cerebral perfusion and selective cerebral perfusion in surgery for acute type A aortic dissection. *Eur J Cardiothorac Surg* 1999; 15:571.
96. Wong CH, Rooney SJ, Bosner RS: S-100beta release in hypothermic circulatory arrest and coronary artery surgery. *Ann Thorac Surg* 1999; 67:1911.
97. Safi HJ, Letsou GV, Iliopoulos DC, et al: Impact of retrograde cerebral perfusion on ascending aortic and arch aneurysm repair. *Ann Thorac Surg* 1997; 63:1601.
98. Griepp RB, Ergin MA, McCullough JN, et al: Use of hypothermic circulatory arrest for cerebral protection during aortic surgery. *J Card Surg* 1997; 12:312.
99. Jag C, Ergin MA, Galla JD, et al: Neurologic outcome after ascending aorta-aortic arch operations: effect of brain protection technique in high risk patients. *J Thorac Cardiovasc Surg* 2001; 121:1107.
100. Juvonen T, Weisz DJ, Wolfe D, et al: Can retrograde perfusion mitigate cerebral injury following particulate embolization: a study in a chronic porcine model. *Ann Thorac Surg* 1998; 66:38.
101. Reich DL, Uysal S, Ergin MA, et al: Retrograde cerebral perfusion during thoracic aortic surgery and late neuropsychological dysfunction. *Eur J Cardiothorac Surg* 2001; 19:594.
102. Griepp B, Ergin MA: Aneurysms of the aortic arch, in Edmunds LH Jr (ed): *Cardiac Surgery in the Adult*. New York, McGraw-Hill, 1997; p 1209.
103. Ergin MA, Griepp EB, Lansman SL, et al: Hypothermic circulatory arrest and other methods of cerebral protection during operations of the thoracic aorta. *J Card Surg* 1994; 9:525.
104. Spielvogel D, Strauch JT, Minanov O, et al: Aortic arch replacement using a trifurcated graft and selective cerebral antegrade perfusion. *Ann Thorac Surg* 2002;74:S1810.
105. Mathur MN, Spielvogel D, Lansman SL, et al: Aortic arch reconstruction using a trifurcated graft. *Ann Thorac Surg (in press)*.
106. Borst HG, Walterbusch G, Schaps D. Extensive aortic replacement using "elephant trunk" prosthesis. *Thorac Cardiovasc Surg* 1983; 31:37.
107. Kuki S, Taniguchi K, Masai T, Endo S: A novel modification of "elephant trunk" technique using a single four-branched arch graft for extensive thoracic aortic aneurysm. *Eur J Cardiothoracic Surg* 2000; 18:246.
108. Kouchoukos NT, Masetti, Rokkas CK, Murphy SF: Single-stage reoperative repair of chronic Type A aortic dissection by means of the arch-first technique. *J Thorac Cardiovasc Surg* 2001; 122:578.
109. Safi HJ, Miller CC 3rd, Estrera Al, et al: Staged repair of extensive aortic aneurysms: morbidity and mortality in the elephant trunk technique. *Circulation* 2001; 104:2938.
110. Schepens MA, Dossche KM, Morshuis, WJ, et al: The elephant trunk technique: operative results in 100 consecutive patients. *Eur J Cardiothorac Surg* 2002; 21:276.
111. Ueda Y: Retrograde cerebral perfusion with hypothermic circulatory arrest in aortic arch surgery: operative and long-term results. *Nagoya J Med Sci* 2001; 64:93.
112. Ogino H, Ueda Y, Sugita T, et al: Aortic arch repairs through three different approaches. *Eur J Cardiothorac Surg* 2001; 19:25.
113. Hilgenberg, AD, Logan DL: Results of aortic arch repair with hypothermic circulatory arrest and retrograde cerebral perfusion. *J Card Surg* 2001; 16:246.
114. Hirotani T, Kameda T, Kumamoto T, et al: Aortic arch repair using hypothermic circulatory arrest technique associated with pharmacological brain protection. *Eur J Cardiothorac Surg* 2000; 18:545.
115. Coselli JS, Bueket S, Djukanovic B: Aortic arch surgery: current treatment and results. *Ann Thorac Surg* 1995; 59:19.
116. Crawford ES, Coselli JS, Svennson LG, et al: Diffuse aneurysmal disease (chronic aortic dissection, Marfan, and mega aorta syndromes) and multiple aneurysms. *Ann Surg* 1990; 211:525.
117. Heinemann M, Laas J, Karck M, et al: Thoracic aortic aneurysms after acute type a aortic dissection: necessity for follow-up. *Ann Thorac Surg* 1990; 49:580.
118. Detter C, Mair H, Klein HG, et al: Long term prognosis of surgically-treated aortic aneurysms and dissections in patients with and without Marfan syndrome. *Eur J Cardiothorac Surg* 1998; 13:416.

Chapter 48

Descending and Thoracoabdominal Aneurysm

Joseph S. Coselli/Paulo L. Moreno

The aorta is a simple conduit. When weakened by disease, its wall may dilate, producing an aneurysm. Descending thoracic aortic aneurysms are aneurysms that involve the thoracic aorta from the left subclavian artery to the diaphragm. Aneurysms that simultaneously involve the descending thoracic aorta and varying portions of the abdominal aorta in continuity are referred to as thoracoabdominal aortic aneurysms (TAAA). The extent of such aortic pathology and the formidable operative procedures required for treatment are why this entity continues to represent a significant clinical challenge to the cardiovascular surgeon. Since the first successful TAAA repair by Etheredge et al in 1955, the care of these patients has undergone significant improvements.[1] As our population ages and the availability of diagnostic modalities increases, recognition of thoracic aortic aneurysms and presentation of patients in need of operative intervention are increasing in frequency.

ETIOLOGY AND PATHOGENESIS

In order of frequency, the majority of thoracoabdominal aneurysms are caused by degenerative processes (myxomatous or myxoid degeneration, senile aorta), dissection, Marfan syndrome (cystic medial necrosis), Ehlers-Danlos syndrome, infection (mycotic), aortitis (Takayasu's disease), and trauma (Table 48-1).[2–4] Traditionally, many thoracic aortic aneurysms were termed atherosclerotic aneurysms. Although atherosclerosis and aortic aneurysms share common risk factors and frequently occur concomitantly, thoracic aortic aneurysms primarily are the result of age-related changes in elastin and collagen that lead to a loss of integrity and strength. Subsequent enlargement and aneurysm formation provide fertile ground for superimposed intimal atherosclerosis and further degeneration of the aortic wall.

Although the pathologic processes may differ microscopically and etiologically, the fundamental process of dilatation, continued expansion with local pressure-related symptoms, and eventual rupture is the same for all. Most etiologic conditions produce diffuse, fusiform aneurysmal dilatation. One exception to this is infection (mycotic aneurysm), which frequently produces a saccular aneurysm at localized areas of

TABLE 48–1 Etiology of thoracoabdominal aortic aneurysms in 1773 patients

Medial degeneration	1300 (73.3%)
Dissection	473 (26.7%)
Marfan syndrome	126 (7.1%)
Ehlers-Danlos syndrome	2 (0.1%)
Mycotic	11 (0.6%)
Takayasu's disease	8 (0.5%)

the aortic wall destroyed by the mycotic process. Characteristically, for unknown reasons, such mycotic aneurysms tend to occur along the lesser curvature of the transverse aortic arch or in the upper abdominal aorta immediately posterior to the origin of the visceral vessels. In such cases, only a portion of aortic circumference is affected and consequently localized weakening causes a diverticular or saccular outpouching. Saccular aneurysms of the thoracic aorta, taken as a whole, are more frequently secondary to atherosclerosis, although both mycotic and degenerative saccular aneurysms may be superimposed on or combined with fusiform, more generalized aneurysmal disease of the thoracoabdominal aorta.

Marfan syndrome is a genetic disorder characterized by identifiable connective tissue defects that lead to aneurysm. The aortic wall is weakened by fragmentation of elastic fibers and deposition of extensive amounts of mucopolysaccharides.[5] Many patients with Marfan syndrome have an abnormal mutation of the fibrillin gene located on the long arm of the 15th chromosome.[6] Abnormal fibrillin in the extracellular matrix decreases connective tissue strength in the aortic wall and produces abnormal elastic properties that predispose the aorta to dilatation from wall tension resulting from left ventricular ejection impulses (DP/DT). Laplace's law causes cycles of progressive dilatation as increasing luminal diameters produce greater wall tension. The usual histologic changes of the aging aorta include cystic medial necrosis, elastin fragmentation, fibrosis with increased collagen, and medial necrosis.[7]

An adequate preoperative assessment of the diameter of the aorta remains the single most important factor in the decision to repair a thoracic aortic aneurysm. The Ad Hoc Committee on Reporting Standards of the Society for Vascular Surgery and the North American Chapter of the International Society for Cardiovascular Surgery states that the definition of an aneurysm is a permanent localized dilatation of an artery having at least 50% increase in diameter compared to the expected normal diameter of the artery in question.[8] This definition can be applied to the thoracic aorta, but it is first necessary to know the normal diameter.

The average diameter of the mid-descending thoracic aorta is 28 mm for men and 26 mm for women; at the level of the celiac axis, 23 mm for men and 20 mm for women; and at the infrarenal aorta, 19.5 mm for men and 15.5 mm for women.[9] Normal aortic diameters, however, vary according to age, gender, and body surface area. Aortic enlargement with advancing age is reported in a number of studies.[10] Even when corrected for age and body surface area, aortic size is statistically smaller in women than in men. On average, the aorta is 2 to 3 mm greater in diameter for men than for women. Body surface area is a better predictor of aortic size than height or weight and best correlates with aortic diameter in patients less than 50 years of age.[11]

NATURAL HISTORY

The expected natural history of TAAA is less well defined in the literature than that for aneurysmal disease involving the infrarenal abdominal aorta, but whatever the cause its course is one of progressive enlargement and eventual rupture. Crawford reported 94 patients who were diagnosed with TAAA but did not undergo operative resection and replacement because of patient choice, age, associated comorbidity, or insufficient dilatation to warrant replacement, or because treatment was staged with the more proximal or distal operation performed first, and the thoracoabdominal aneurysm deferred to a second stage.[12] The 2-year survival rate for this group of patients was only 24%, and half of the deaths were owing to rupture of the aneurysm.

Cambria reported 57 patients with nondissecting TAAA preselected for nonoperative management.[13] The overall survival rate was 39%, and the repair-free survival rate was only 17% at 5 years. They found an expansion rate of 0.2 cm per year. Dapunt, however, reported the rate of enlargement of thoracic and thoracoabdominal aortic aneurysms in 67 patients followed by computed tomography scanning, and demonstrated an enlargement rate of 0.43 cm per year.[14] A significantly higher rate of aneurysm expansion was found in smokers and in patients with larger aortic diameters (more than 5 cm) at diagnosis. No correlation was noted between rate of enlargement and age, sex, or the presence of dissection.

In a series of 53 patients with thoracic aneurysms followed for at least 6 months after diagnosis, Masuda found, by univariate analysis, that three variables—initial size of the aneurysm, diastolic blood pressure, and presence of renal failure—were statistically correlated to expansion rate of thoracic aortic aneurysms.[15] In a population-based study, Bickerstaff reported the outcome of thoracic aortic aneurysms in 72 patients.[16] Rupture occurred in 53 patients (74%) and 50 died. The median interval between diagnosis and rupture in 16 patients with known aneurysms was 2 years. Ninety-five percent of aortic dissections ruptured and 51% of nondissecting aneurysms ruptured. The actuarial 5-year survival for all 72 patients was 13%; for patients with aortic dissection it was 7%, and for those without dissection, 19.2%.

Pressler and McNamara compiled data from 176 patients with the diagnosis of thoracic aortic aneurysm.[17] In their study, 90 patients (51%) had arteriosclerotic fusiform aneurysms and 86 (49%) had dissecting aneurysms. Eighty-nine percent of the arteriosclerotic aneurysms and 41% of the dissecting aneurysms were located in the descending thoracic aorta. Seventy-eight percent of patients with dissecting aneurysms had symptoms of pain in the back or chest, whereas only 42% of patients with atherosclerotic aneurysms had back or chest pain. Rupture caused 37 of 48 deaths (77%) in 59 patients with dissecting aneurysms, and 25 of 57 deaths (44%) in 76 patients with atherosclerotic aneurysms. Concomitant cardiovascular disease was the second leading cause of death in patients with atherosclerotic aneurysms not treated surgically (19 deaths out of 86 patients; 22%), but only one of 59 patients with dissecting aneurysms not treated surgically died of heart disease.

Aortic size at the time of diagnosis is related to the development of complications including rupture. Pressler and McNamara reported that 8 of 9 ruptured descending thoracic aortic aneurysms were larger than 10 cm.[17] In the report by Dapunt on descending thoracic and thoracoabdominal aortic aneurysms, mean aortic diameter at the time of rupture was 6.1 cm.[14] Crawford found a mean size of 8 cm at the time of rupture in a series of 117 patients with descending thoracic and thoracoabdominal aortic aneurysms. Since rupture was observed in some 10% of aneurysms smaller than 6 cm in diameter, the authors recommended elective operation when a 5-cm diameter threshold was exceeded.[18] Factors associated with increased morbidity and mortality from rupture and related complications include aneurysm size, presence of dissection, previous rate of expansion, and hypertension (Table 48-2).

In an effort to better assess the risk of rupture in individual patients, Juvonen et al developed a predictive model based on five risk factors: (1) increasing age, (2) diameter of the descending thoracic aorta, (3) diameter of the abdominal aorta, (4) chronic obstructive pulmonary disease, and (5) the presence of symptoms.[19] The Mount Sinai group performed a multivariable analysis that included data from computer-generated three-dimensional computed tomographic reconstructions of the thoracoabdominal aorta. The resulting formula determines the probability of rupture within 1 year based on patient age, the presence of pain and chronic obstructive pulmonary disease, and the maximum true diameters of the descending thoracic and abdominal aortic segments.

Increasing age and preoperative renal insufficiency have remained major risk factors for early mortality throughout the history of TAAA repair. Both were among the predictive variables determined by Svensson et al's multivariable analysis of Crawford's complete experience with TAAA surgery in 1509 patients treated between 1960 and 1991.[20] The recent report by Acher et al confirms that, along with acute presentation, age and elevated creatinine levels remain important predictors of early death.[21]

TABLE 48–2 Preoperative characteristics of thoracoabdominal aortic aneurysms in 1773 patients

Hypertension	1344 (75.8%)
Symptomatic aneurysms	1143 (64.5%)
Chronic obstructive pulmonary disease	655 (36.9%)
Coronary artery disease	629 (35.5%)
Concurrent aneurysm	310 (17.5%)
Prior aneurysm repair	739 (41.7%)
Prior thoracic aneurysm repair	445 (25.1%)
Renal arterial occlusive disease	478 (27.0%)
Renal insufficiency	237 (13.4%)
Cerebrovascular disease	196 (11.1%)
Ruptured aneurysm	109 (6.1%)
Diabetes	99 (5.6%)
Preoperative paraplegia	18 (1.0%)
Peptic ulcer disease	110 (6.2%)

CLINICAL PRESENTATION

Degenerative TAAA is asymptomatic at the time of diagnosis in roughly 43% of patients, but symptomatic in approximately 48%.[4] TAAAs remain asymptomatic for prolonged periods of time; however, most ultimately produce a variety of symptoms prior to rupture and inevitable death. The most frequent symptom is back pain localized between the scapulae. When the aneurysm is largest in the region of the aortic hiatus, mid back and epigastric pain may occur. This symptom is caused by pressure on adjacent structures, aneurysm expansion, intramural hematoma, or contained rupture.

Compression of the trachea or bronchus can produce stridor, wheezing, or cough. Pneumonitis distal to an area of bronchial obstruction develops if secretions cannot be cleared. Hemoptysis occurs when an aneurysm erodes directly into the pulmonary parenchyma or bronchus. Compression of the esophagus may produce dysphasia, whereas erosion into the esophagus causes hematemesis.[22] Similarly, erosion into the duodenum causes either partial obstruction or intermittent/massive gastrointestinal bleeding. Compression of the liver or porta hepatis is uncommon, but when this occurs, jaundice results. Hoarseness is owing to traction on the vagus nerve as the distal aortic arch expands, to produce recurrent laryngeal nerve paralysis. Thoracic or lumbar vertebral body erosion causes back pain, spinal instability, and neurologic deficits from spinal cord compression. Mycotic aneurysms have a peculiar propensity to destroy vertebral bodies. Additionally, neurologic symptoms, including paraplegia and/or paraparesis, may occur with thrombosis of intercostal and spinal arteries. This is most frequently seen with acute aortic dissection, which may occur primarily, or become superimposed on medial degenerative fusiform aneurysmal disease. Erosive fistula formation into the inferior vena cava or iliac vein will present with an abdominal bruit, widened pulse pressure, edema, and heart failure. Thoracic aortic aneurysms, similar to aneurysms in other locations, may produce distal emboli of clot or atheromatous debris that gradually obliterates and thromboses visceral, renal, or lower extremity branches. Secondary infection of atheromatous debris and clot within an aneurysm may produce generalized sepsis. Nine percent of patients with TAAA present with frank rupture at the time of diagnosis.[4]

DIAGNOSTIC EVALUATION

Patients with aortic aneurysms usually require multiple tests to evaluate the aorta. The best method for optimal imaging of the thoracic and thoracoabdominal aorta is somewhat institution-specific, based on the availability of imaging equipment and expertise.[23] Although physical examination may detect large infrarenal abdominal aortic aneurysms, thoracic involvement of a palpable aortic aneurysm is rarely suspected during physical examination unless the abdominal component is so extensive that the cephalic projection cannot be palpated because of the costal margins. Plain chest x-rays may demonstrate widening of the descending thoracic aortic shadow, which may be highlighted by a rim of calcification outlining the dilated aneurysmal aortic wall. Aneurysmal calcium may also be seen in the upper abdomen on a standard x-ray made in the anterior, posterior, or lateral projections (Fig. 48-1). Enough calcification may be present in the aortic wall to make the diagnosis of aneurysms in 65% to 75% of cases. A negative plane chest roentgenogram does not exclude the diagnosis of aortic aneurysm.

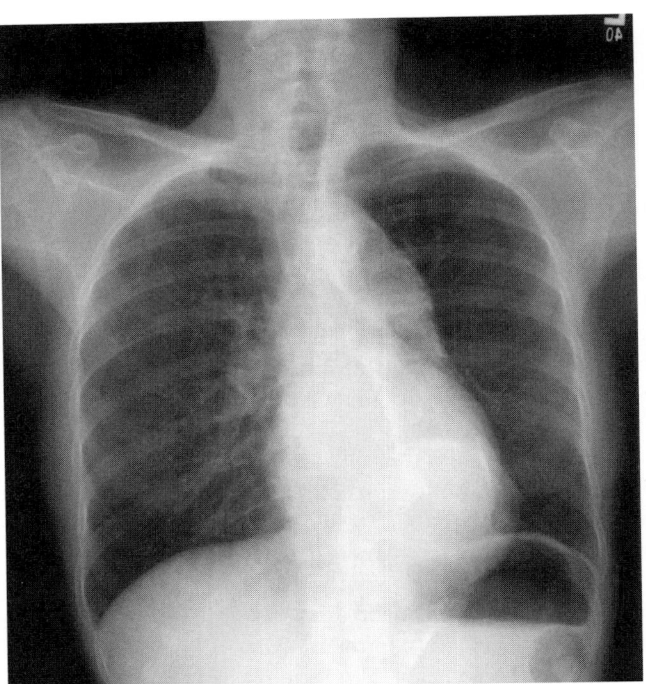

A

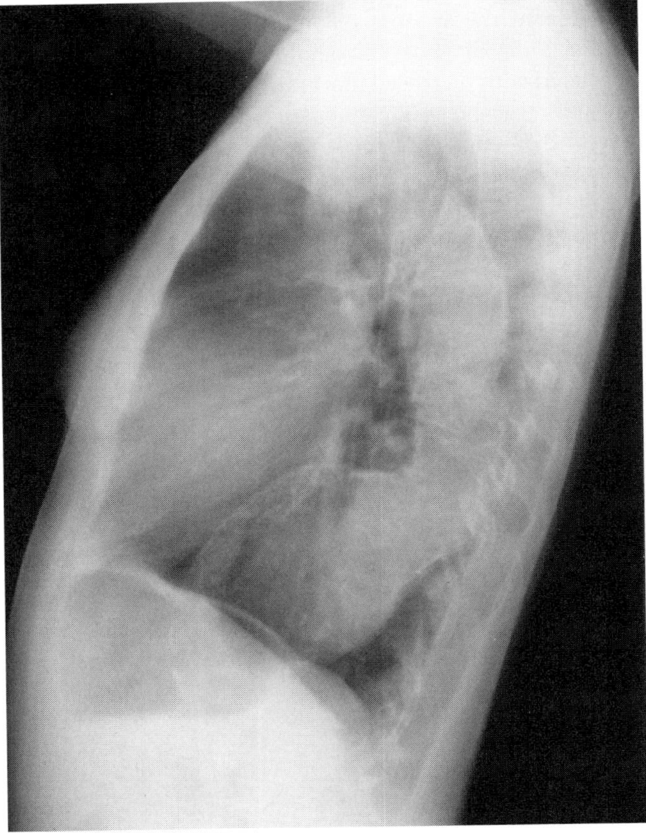

B

FIGURE 48–1 Simple chest roentgenogram, EPA (A) and lateral (B), demonstrating calcified rim in the aortic wall of a thoracoabdominal aortic aneurysm.

Ultrasonography

Ultrasonography, although useful in evaluating infrarenal abdominal aortic aneurysms, is not useful for imaging the thoracic or suprarenal aorta primarily because of overlying lung tissue.[24] The advantages of ultrasonography are wide availability, low cost, portability, noninvasiveness, lack of ionizing radiation, and rapid examination. When the definitive neck of an infrarenal abdominal aortic aneurysm cannot be demonstrated at the level of the renal arteries, thoracoabdominal aortic involvement should be suspected.

Transesophageal Echocardiography

Transesophageal echocardiography provides access to the proximal aorta, and complements transabdominal ultrasonography.[25,26] The technique requires considerable technical skill both in obtaining adequate images and in interpretation. The technique is excellent for determining the presence of dissection but has limitations in evaluating the region of the transverse aortic arch and upper abdominal aorta.

Computed Tomography

Computed tomography scanning is widely available and provides access to the entire thoracic and abdominal aorta. In

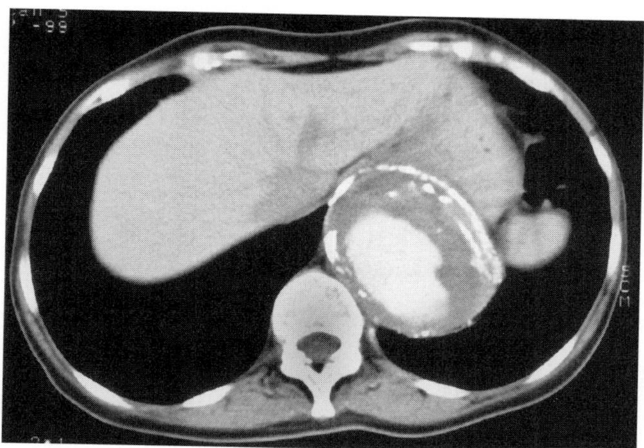

FIGURE 48–2 Computed tomography (CT) scan demonstrating large calcified thoracoabdominal aortic aneurysm with intraluminal laminated thrombus.

addition to diagnosis, information regarding location and extent is provided.[27] Major branch vessels including the celiac, superior mesenteric, renal, and iliac arteries, left subclavian, and virtually all adjacent organs are imaged. Although not widely available, computer programs can construct sagittal, coronal, and oblique images as well as three-dimensional reconstructions.[28,29] Computed tomography scanning, which is contrast-enhanced, provides information regarding the aortic lumen, mural thrombus, presence of aortic dissection, intramural hematoma, mediastinal or retroperitoneal hematoma, aortic rupture, and periaortic fibrosis associated with inflammatory aneurysms (Fig. 48-2).[30] Although angiography remains the "gold standard" for evaluating aortic occlusive disease, improvements in computed tomography (CT) and magnetic resonance imaging (MRI) are leading to strategies that provide excellent images without the morbidity or cost of angiography.[31] Because of improvements in noninvasive imaging modalities and a stroke risk of 0.6% to 1.2% with angiography, the role of diagnostic angiography for aortic arch vessels is becoming limited.[32–34]

A clinically valuable advance in recent times has occurred in the area of spiral CT images. Sophisticated spiral CT hardware and CT protocols are important for good results, but the image quality is equally dependent on software. Traditionally, only limited hard copies of selected views are provided to surgeons; this may exclude a great deal of the information that is available from the volume of data acquired by spiral CT. To make the best use of CT angiography (CTA) and multiplanar reconstructions or multiplanar reformats (MPRs), a CT workstation is used to scroll through multiple axial or sagittal cross-sections in a "cine" mode. This approach to viewing can be very helpful in clarifying the patient's anatomy, following a structure from one slice to the next in rapid succession. For these reconstruction methods, if the spiral CT data are stored digitally in a computer hard drive, they may be viewed from many different perspectives without exposing the patients to any additional radiation or contrast.[35]

Magnetic Resonance Angiography

An important advantage of magnetic resonance angiography (MRA) over computed tomography angiography (CTA) is that it uses nontoxic gadolinium instead of nephrotoxic contrast. Additionally, the patient avoids exposure to ionizing radiation. MRI employs radiofrequency energy and a strong magnetic field to produce images. MRA provides the same volume of information as does CTA with regards to image processing, but further provides information on relative quantity of blood flow and an appearance similar to conventional angiography. Additionally, the technique can provide a three-dimensional anatomical analysis. MRA imaging of the aorta can elucidate information on wall composition, wall thickness, and intraluminal thrombus, whereas conventional aortography only depicts the lumen. A current limitation of MRA is the susceptibility to artifacts created by ferromagnetic materials. Although expensive, the technology is widely available and has the capability of accessing the entire aorta. MRA images can more clearly distinguish arteries and veins from viscera and other surrounding tissue.[36]

Aortography

Classical aortography remains the mainstay for preoperative evaluation of patients with thoracoabdominal aortic aneurysms.[24] It has the ability to define the extent of aneurysm, branch vessel involvement, and branch vessel stenotic lesions. Risks of aortography include renal toxicity from the large volumes of contrast material required to adequately fill large aneurysms. There is the additional risk of embolization from laminated thrombus secondary to manipulation of intraluminal catheters. Anterior, posterior, oblique, and lateral views are obtained simultaneously to obtain satisfactory information regarding branch vessels. Patients with suspected renal and/or visceral ischemia, aorto-iliac occlusive disease, horseshoe kidney, or peripheral aneurysms should be considered for aortography prior to TAAA repair.

Aortography is performed in a well-hydrated patient who is also receiving intravenous fluids. Routinely, 1000 mL of 5% dextrose and Ringer's lactate solution with 25 g of mannitol are given intravenously immediately prior to the procedure and are continued at 100 mL per hour following study. If at all possible, operation is delayed for 24 hours or longer to determine the effects of angiography on renal function and to permit diuresis of the contrast agent. If renal insufficiency occurs or is worsened, the surgical procedure is postponed until renal function returns to normal or is satisfactorily stabilized.

PREOPERATIVE ASSESSMENT AND PREPARATION

An adequate preoperative assessment of physiologic reserve is critical in evaluating patient's operative risk. Preoperatively all patients undergo a thorough evaluation with emphasis placed on cardiac, pulmonary, and renal function.[37]

Heart

A history of coronary artery occlusive disease is present in 30% of patients with thoracoabdominal aortic aneurysms. Additionally, cardiac disease is responsible for 49% of early deaths and 34% of late deaths.[3,4] Transthoracic echocardiography is a satisfactory noninvasive screening method that evaluates both valvular and biventricular function. Dipyridamole-thallium myocardial scanning identifies regions of myocardium that are reversibly ischemic and is more practical than exercise testing in this generally elderly population that commonly is limited by concurrent lower extremity peripheral vascular disease. We routinely employ preoperative screening of all patients for coronary artery disease with cine arteriography; however, in patients with a significant history of angina or an ejection fraction of 30% or less, cardiac catheterization and coronary arteriography are performed with aortography. Patients who have asymptomatic TAAA and severe coronary artery occlusive disease (left main, triple vessel, and proximal left anterior descending) undergo myocardial revascularization prior to aneurysm replacement. In appropriate patients, percutaneous transluminal angioplasty is carried out prior to operation.

Kidney

Renal function is assessed preoperatively by serum electrolytes, blood urea nitrogen (BUN), and creatinine measurements. Renal size may be determined from a CT scan, by ultrasound, or from the nephrogram obtained during aortography. Renal artery patency is confirmed by arteriography.[38] Patients are not rejected as surgical candidates based on renal function. Patients with preoperative renal failure and an established hemodialysis program do not have significantly greater morbidity than patients with normal renal function. Patients with severely impaired renal function, but who are not on chronic hemodialysis, frequently require transient temporary hemodialysis early after operation. Additionally, patients with poor renal function secondary to severe proximal renal occlusive disease are revascularized at operation by either renal arterial endarterectomy or bypass grafting with the expectation that renal function will stabilize or improve.

Lung

All patients undergo pulmonary function screening with arterial blood gases and spirometry.[39–41] Patients with an FEV_1 greater than 1.0 and a P_{CO_2} less than 45 are surgical candidates. In suitable patients, borderline pulmonary function frequently is improved by stopping smoking, progressively treating bronchitis, losing weight, and following a general exercise program for a period of 1 to 3 months before operation. However, operation is not withheld in patients with symptomatic aortic aneurysms and poor pulmonary function. In such patients, preservation of the left recurrent laryngeal nerve, phrenic nerve, and diaphragmatic function is particularly important.

OPERATIVE TREATMENT

Anesthetic Management

Successful conduct of operation requires close coordination between surgeon and anesthesiologist. Advances in anesthetic techniques, monitoring, and perfusion technology have contributed to improved results in the treatment of TAAA. As a result of advanced age and concomitant prevalence of associated coronary artery occlusive disease, anesthesia is induced with narcotic agents (fentanyl) to minimize the risk of myocardial depression. A large-bore central venous line (a three-lumen 12-gauge catheter) and a Swan-Ganz pulmonary artery catheter are placed for access and monitoring. A right radial and, frequently, bilateral radial intra-arterial catheters are placed for monitoring and blood withdrawal. Muscle relaxation is achieved and maintained with pancuronium bromide. Either a double-lumen endobronchial tube is placed for selective ventilation of the right lung and deflation of the left lung, or alternatively a single-lumen endotracheal tube with an intrabronchial blocker is utilized. Deflation of the left lung reduces retraction trauma to the lung, improves exposure, and alleviates the risk of cardiac compression. The patient is turned to a right lateral decubitus position with the shoulders placed at 60° to 80° and the hips flexed to 30° to 40° from horizontal. The position is stabilized using a beanbag. Arterial blood gases, electrolytes, and serum glucose are monitored frequently (30-60 minutes). Intraoperatively the electrocardiogram, arterial and venous blood pressures, and temperature are monitored continuously. In patients with a significant history of cardiac disease and/or known impaired cardiac function, a transesophageal echocardiography probe is inserted following induction of anesthesia.

Shortly after the induction of anesthesia, 25 to 50 g of mannitol are given intravenously to promote a vigorous diuresis. Intravenous crystalloid solutions are begun prior to operation. The first liter consists of lactated Ringer's solution with 5% dextrose, and the remainder, Ringer's solution without dextrose in sufficient volumes to maintain the central venous pressure between 7 and 10 mm H_2O and the pulmonary capillary wedge pressure at normal or preanesthetic levels. Proximal blood pressure, cardiac hemodynamics, and peripheral vascular resistance are maintained at optimal levels by administration of sodium nitroprusside and/or nitroglycerin, and replacement of fluid and blood losses. Nitroprusside is specifically discontinued several minutes before the release of the distal aortic cross-clamp. Sodium bicarbonate solution is administered routinely at a rate of 2 to 3 mEq/kg/h by continuous infusion during aortic cross-clamping to prevent acidosis.

Throughout the procedure, hemoglobin and coagulation parameters are monitored carefully and are adjusted primarily by replacing appropriate blood components. In general, we administer fresh frozen plasma continuously throughout the operation, and at least one pheresis unit of platelets at the time of aortic declamping. This minimizes problems related to coagulopathy produced by dilution of coagulation proteins. A cell-saving device is used throughout the procedure to salvage all shed blood from the operative field. If necessary, during a period of substantial blood loss, the device allows direct reinfusion of unwashed blood from the reservoir. The authors' preference is to use citrate rather than heparin in the autotranfusion device, and so intermittent monitoring of the serum calcium level is important. Mechanized rapid transfusion devices using large-bore central venous catheters for access are particularly valuable in restoring blood volume immediately prior to declamping.

Heparin is administered intravenously (1 mg/kg) before placing the aortic cross-clamp or initiating left heart bypass. Potential benefits of heparinization include preservation of the microcirculation and prevention of embolization; the authors have not encountered increased bleeding or other morbidity related to the heparin. Following this low heparin dose, the activated clotting time generally ranges from 220 to 270 seconds. By avoiding the initiation of the clotting cascade, the use of heparin may have a favorable influence on reducing the incidence of diminished intravascular coagulation.

Classification of Thoracoabdominal Aneurysms

Thoracoabdominal aneurysms can involve the entire thoracoabdominal aorta from the origin of the left subclavian artery to the aortic bifurcation or can involve only one or more segments. The Crawford classification has advanced the surgical treatment of TAAA because it has permitted a standardized reporting of aneurysm extent, allowing for an appropriate stratification of risks, specific treatment modalities based on the extent of the aneurysm, and a type-specific determination of neurologic deficit as well as morbidity and mortality associated with thoracoabdominal aneurysm repair (Fig. 48-3). Extent I thoracoabdominal aortic aneurysms involve most of the descending thoracic aorta from the left subclavian artery down to vessels in the abdomen. Usually the renal arteries are not involved in extent I aneurysms. Extent II aneurysms begin at the left subclavian artery and reach the infrarenal abdominal aorta even as far as the inguinal area. Extent III aneurysms involve the distal half or less of the descending thoracic aorta and substantial segments of the abdominal aorta. Extent IV aneurysms are those that involve the upper abdominal aorta and all or none of the infrarenal aorta.

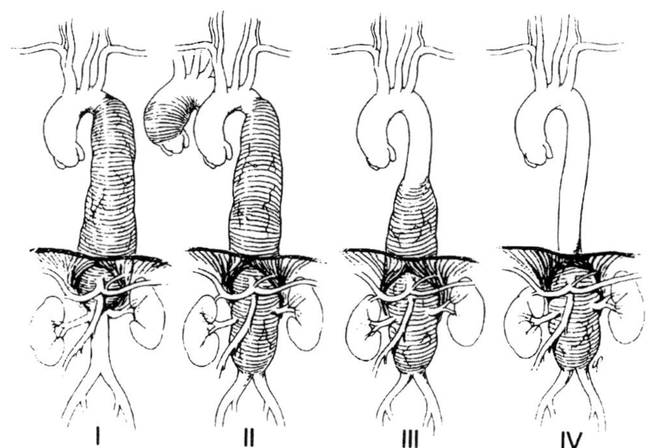

FIGURE 48–3 Crawford classification of thoracoabdominal aneurysms.

Incisions

A fundamental principle is the importance of adequate exposure. The thoracoabdominal incision varies in length and level, depending on the anticipated extent of aortic replacement (Fig. 48-4A). When the aneurysm extends into the superior aspect of the thorax (Crawford extents I and II), the upper portion of the thoracoabdominal incision is through the 6th intercostal space or the bed of the resected 6th rib. In recent years, we have routinely removed a rib. When the interspace is used, the upper rib may be divided at the neck for additional proximal exposure. With lower aneurysms (Crawford extents III and IV), an incision through the 7th, 8th, or 9th interspace is employed according to the desired level of exposure. A straight transverse incision through the 10th or 11th interspace is used in patients with aneurysms between the diaphragm and aortic bifurcation (Crawford extent IV). In all others, a gentle curve to reduce the risk of tissue necrosis at the apex of the lower portion of the musculoskeletal tissue flap is made as the incision crosses the costal margin. In patients with proximal aneurysms, the posterior portion of the incision is located between the scapula and the spinal processes. The distal extent of the incision is carried down to the level of the umbilicus.

Exposure

After entering the chest, the left lung is deflated. Fixed metal retractors attached to the operating table provide consistent static exposure. The diaphragm is divided in a circular fashion to protect the phrenic nerve and to preserve as much diaphragm as possible. Only a 1- to 1.5-cm rim of diaphragmatic tissue is left laterally for closure at the completion of operation.

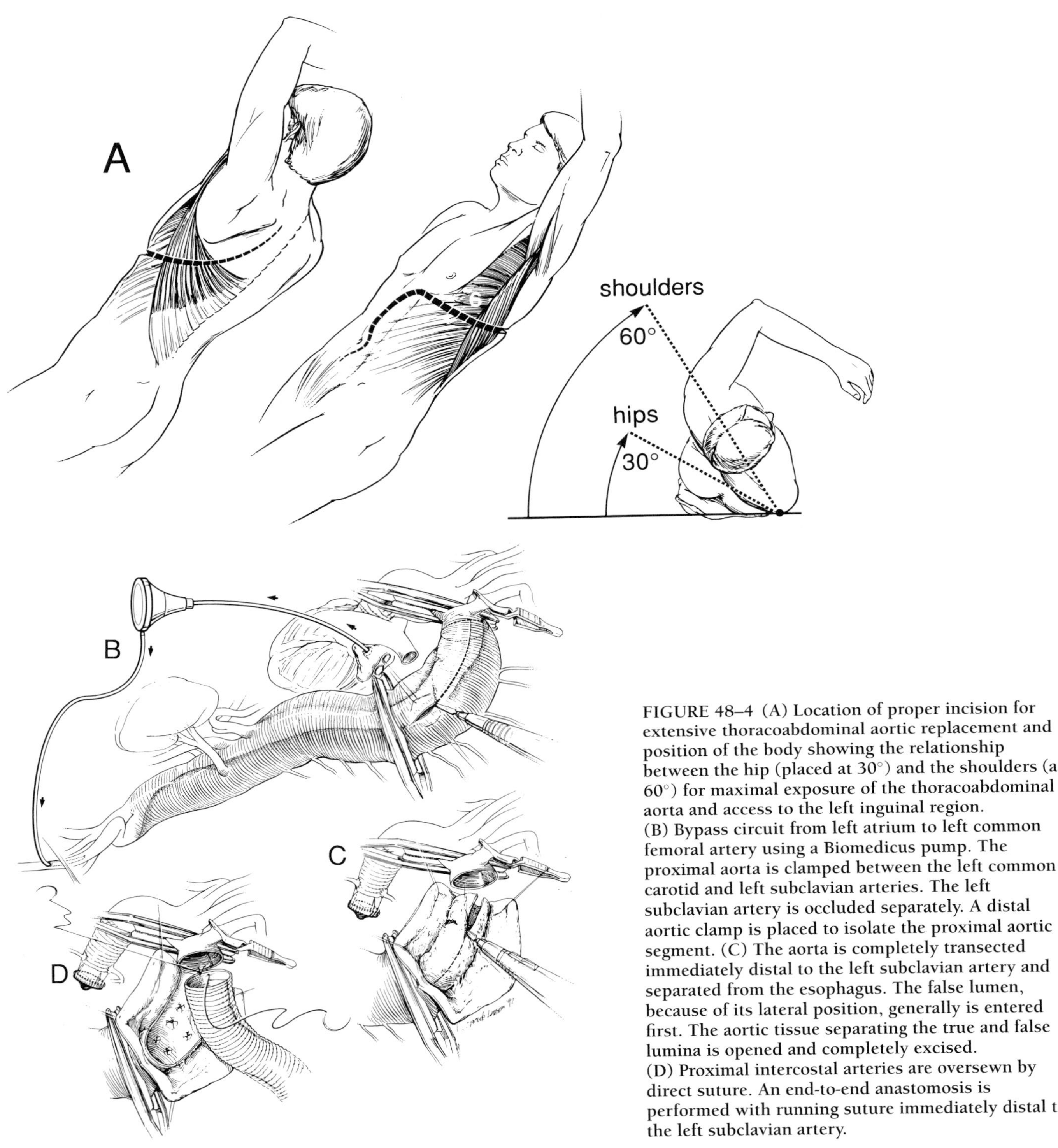

FIGURE 48–4 (A) Location of proper incision for extensive thoracoabdominal aortic replacement and position of the body showing the relationship between the hip (placed at 30°) and the shoulders (at 60°) for maximal exposure of the thoracoabdominal aorta and access to the left inguinal region.
(B) Bypass circuit from left atrium to left common femoral artery using a Biomedicus pump. The proximal aorta is clamped between the left common carotid and left subclavian arteries. The left subclavian artery is occluded separately. A distal aortic clamp is placed to isolate the proximal aortic segment. (C) The aorta is completely transected immediately distal to the left subclavian artery and separated from the esophagus. The false lumen, because of its lateral position, generally is entered first. The aortic tissue separating the true and false lumina is opened and completely excised.
(D) Proximal intercostal arteries are oversewn by direct suture. An end-to-end anastomosis is performed with running suture immediately distal to the left subclavian artery.

The abdominal aortic segment is exposed using a transperitoneal approach; the retroperitoneum is entered lateral to the left colon.[42] A dissection plane is developed in the retroperitoneum anterior to the psoas muscle and posterior to the left kidney. This is extended directly to the left posterolateral aspect of the abdominal aorta. The left colon, spleen, left kidney, and tail of the pancreas are retracted anteriorly and to the right. An open abdominal approach permits direct inspection of the bowel, abdominal viscera, and visceral blood supply following completion of the aortic

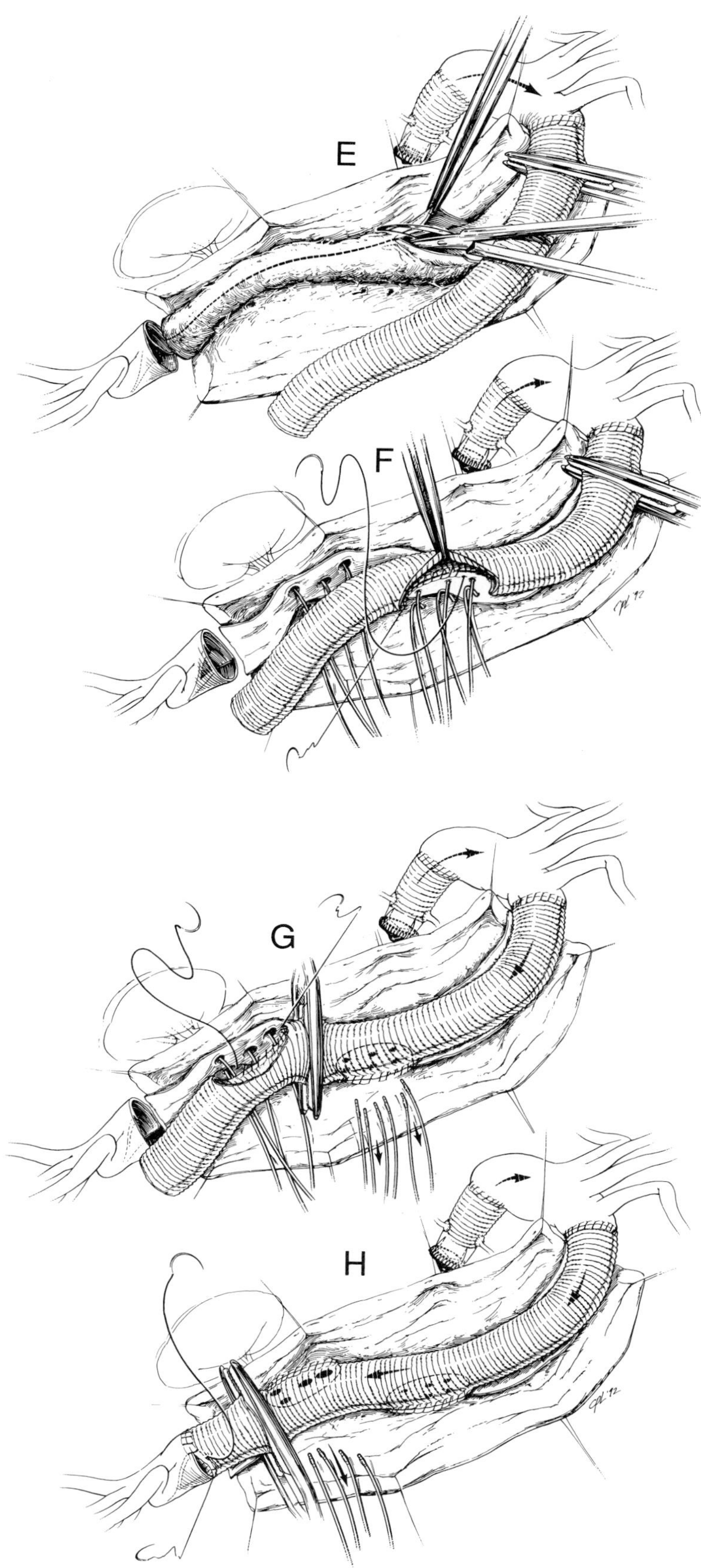

FIGURE 48–4 (*Continued*) (E) The occluding clamp is removed from the distal aortic arch and placed on the graft beyond the left subclavian artery. The left subclavian artery clamp also is removed. Cardiofemoral bypass is discontinued following completion of the proximal anastomosis. The aneurysm is opened for its full length to the aortic bifurcation, and the remaining wall between the true and the false lumina throughout is completely excised. (F) Back bleeding from intercostal, visceral, and renal arteries is controlled with balloon catheters. Patent intercostal arteries in the region from T8 to T12 are reattached to an opening in the aortic graft. (G) The cross-clamp is sequentially moved further down on the aortic graft, to restore flow to reattached intercostal arteries. A separate opening in the graft is made for reattachment of the celiac axis and superior mesenteric and renal arteries. (H) Following reattachment of the visceral and renal arteries, the cross-clamp is again moved down the graft to progressively restore flow. To complete the replacement, an end-to-end distal anastomosis is performed proximal to the aortic bifurcation.

reconstruction. An entirely retroperitoneal approach is used in patients with a so-called hostile abdomen, defined by multiple prior abdominal operations, or a history of extensive adhesions and/or peritonitis.

The crus of the diaphragm is divided and the left renal, superior mesenteric, and celiac arteries are identified but not circumferentially dissected or encircled with tapes. Commonly, a large lumbar branch of the left renal vein courses posteriorly around the aorta. This may be ligated and divided as needed. If a retroaortic left renal vein is encountered, the vessel is divided between vascular clamps if the aortic repair extends below the vein. Direct reanastomosis or interposition grafting of this retroaortic renal vein is necessary if the left kidney appears congested with distended testicular, ovarian, and adrenal collaterals.

Repair

Patients with extensive thoracoabdominal aortic aneurysms (Crawford extents I and II), and particularly those with dissection, are at greatest risk for development of postoperative paraplegia and paraparesis. In such patients, distal aortic perfusion during the proximal aortic portion of the repair is achieved by using temporary bypass from the left atrium to either the femoral artery (most commonly the left) or distal descending thoracic aorta with a closed-circuit in-line centrifugal pump (Biomedicus, Medtronic, Inc., Eden-Prairie, MN) (Fig. 48-4B). If the pericardium was previously entered for coronary artery bypass grafting or valve replacement (Fig. 48-4C), cannulation of the superior or inferior pulmonary vein is equally effective. Cannulation of the distal descending thoracic aorta (usually at the level of the diaphragm) was initially used solely as an alternative to femoral artery cannulation in patients with femoral or iliac artery occlusive disease. Because of the lack of complications using this technique and the elimination of femoral artery exposure and repair, distal aortic cannulation has become the preferred approach. Careful examination of CT or MRI scans assists selection of an appropriate site for direct aortic cannulation and avoidance of intraluminal thrombus with potential for distal embolization. Bypass flows are adjusted to maintain distal arterial pressures of 70 mm Hg, while maintaining normal proximal arterial and venous filling pressures. Flows between 1500 and 2500 mL/min are generally required. Left heart bypass (LHB) flows are targeted toward two thirds of the baseline cardiac output, which is routinely measured shortly after induction. LHB facilitates rapid adjustments in proximal arterial pressure and cardiac preload, thereby reducing the need for pharmacologic intervention. The patient's temperature is allowed to drift down to a rectal temperature of 32°C to 33°C.

When the aneurysm encroaches on the left subclavian artery, the distal aortic arch is mobilized gently by dividing the remnant of the ductus arteriosus. The vagus and recurrent laryngeal nerves are identified. The vagus nerve may be divided below the recurrent nerve to provide additional mobility, consequently protecting it from injury. Preservation of the recurrent laryngeal nerve is particularly important in patients with chronic obstructive pulmonary disease and reduced pulmonary function. Vocal cord paralysis should be suspected in patients with postoperative hoarseness and confirmed by direct examination. Effective treatment can be provided by direct cord medialization (type 1 thyroplasty), or, in higher-risk patients, by polytetrafluoroethylene injection.[43] Careful circumferential dissection of the distal transverse aortic arch separates it from the pulmonary artery and esophagus. If cross-clamping proximal to the left subclavian artery is anticipated, the left subclavian artery is separately and circumferentially mobilized. In patients with a prior left internal mammary arterial bypass graft, either a left common carotid to subclavian bypass or a left subclavian to carotid transfer is necessary to avoid cardiac ischemia when the cross-clamp is applied proximal to the left subclavian artery.

The distal clamp is placed between T4 and T7. Distal aortic perfusion provides circulation to the viscera, kidneys, lower extremities, and lower intercostal and lumbar arteries. The aorta is transected 1 cm distal to the proximal clamp and separated from the esophagus to permit full-thickness sutures through the aortic wall without injuring the esophagus (Fig. 48-4C). A gelatin-impregnated woven Dacron graft (Sulzer Vascutek, Scotland) is selected; 22-mm to 24-mm grafts are used in most patients. The anastomosis and all remaining anastomoses are usually made with a running 3-0 polypropylene suture (Fig. 48-4D). Teflon felt strips are generally not used. In patients with particularly fragile aortic tissues such as those found in Marfan syndrome, 4-0 polypropylene sutures are used. As the aorta is replaced from proximal to distal, the distal aortic clamp is moved sequentially to lower positions along the aorta to maintain distal perfusion and restore proximal blood flow (Fig. 48-4E-H). Sequential distal clamping is often not feasible due to a variety of factors related to the severity of the aortic disease, including aneurysm size and tortuosity, mural calcification, and intraluminal thrombus.

Commonly, atrio-distal bypass is discontinued following completion of the proximal anastomosis. The entire aneurysm then is opened longitudinally, passing posterior to the left renal artery and continuing to the distal extent of the aneurysm. A distal clamp is not used, allowing for an "open" anastomosis. With a chronic dissection, the partition between the true and false lumens is completely removed. Aorto-visceral bypass then is restarted using a Y line off the arterial perfusion line and separate balloon perfusion catheters placed within the origin of the celiac, superior mesenteric, and renal arteries. This provides oxygenated blood to the abdominal viscera and kidneys (Fig. 48-5). With this technique, the total renal and visceral ischemic time can be reduced to just a few minutes during even the most

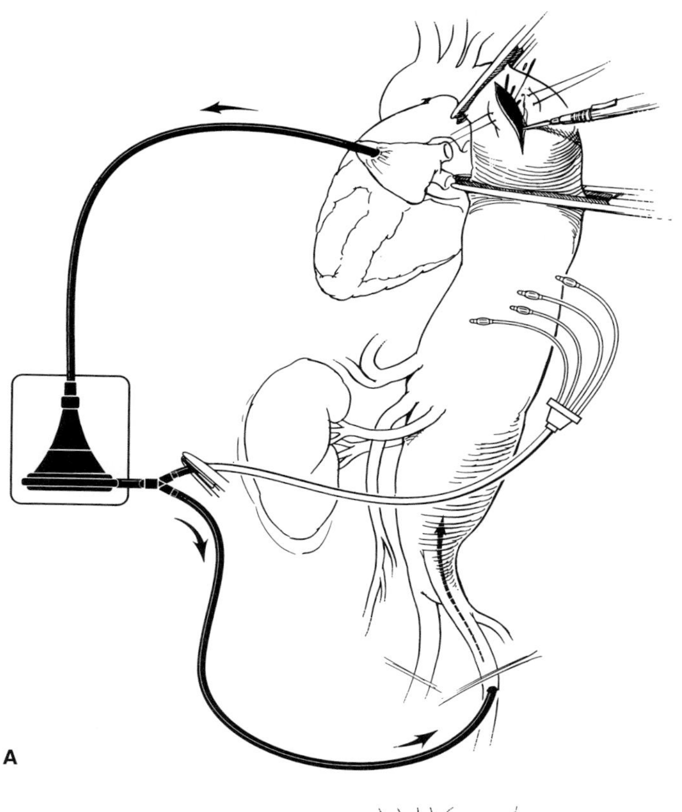

FIGURE 48–5 (A) Technique for extensive thoracoabdominal aortic aneurysm repair utilizing proximal aortic isolation with distal aortic perfusion employing left atrial to left common femoral artery bypass with a centrifugal pump. (B) Following completion of the proximal anastomosis, visceral and renal arteries are perfused using 9 F Pruitt catheters with oxygenated blood from the bypass circuit during intercostal arterial reattachment. (C) Prior to completion of distal reconstruction, visceral and renal perfusion are continued during reattachment of the aortic graft. Sequential clamping provides intercostal perfusion.

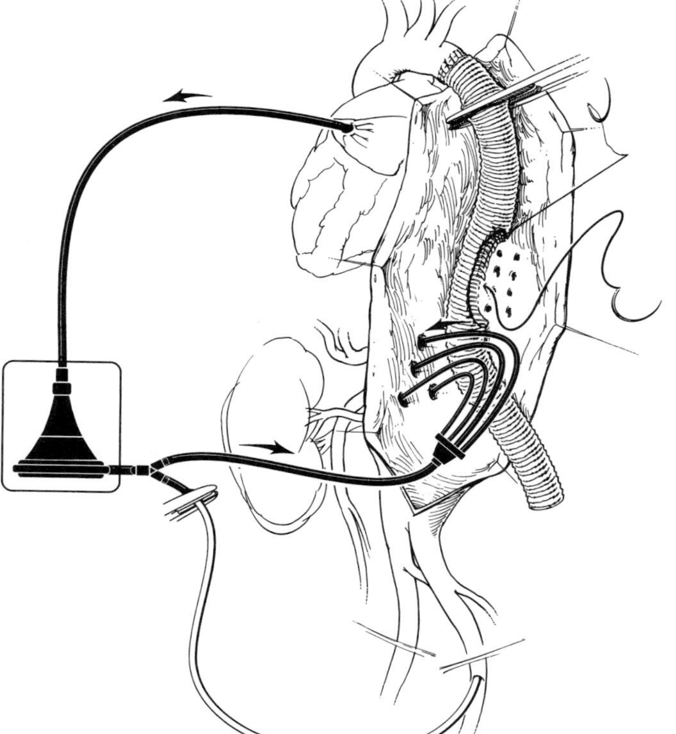

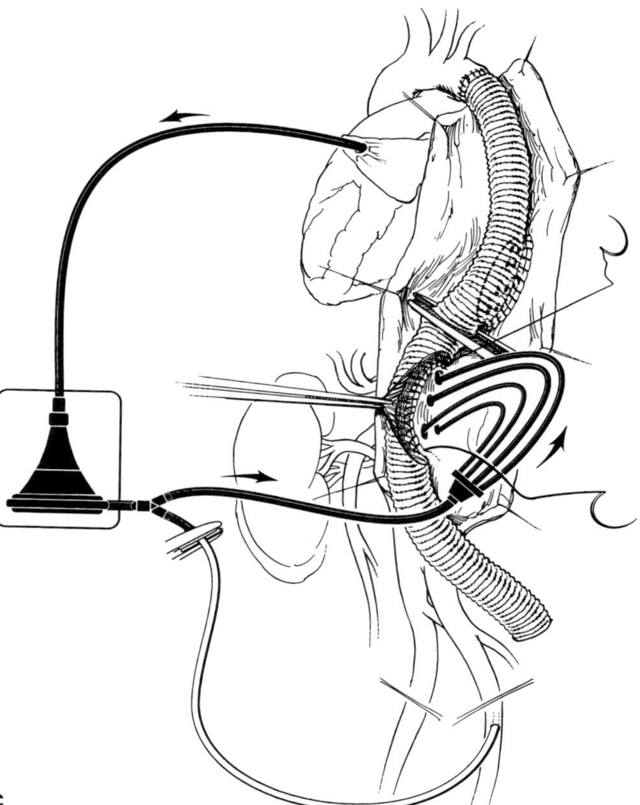

complex aortic reconstructions. The potential benefits of reducing hepatic and bowel ischemia include decreased risks for postoperative coagulopathy and bacterial translocation, respectively.

All patent intercostal arteries from T7 to L2 are reattached to one or more openings made in the graft (Fig. 48-5B). Large intercostal arteries with little or no back bleeding are considered particularly important. After this is done, the proximal clamp is moved down the graft to restore flow to the intercostal arteries (Fig. 48-5C). When none are patent, endarterectomy of the aortic wall with removal of calcified intimal disease should be considered. Subsequently, visceral and renal artery ostia are reattached to one or more openings in the graft. The left renal artery requires a separate opening in the graft in 30% to 40% of the cases. Visceral or renal artery stenosis is encountered in at least 25% of cases and requires either endarterectomy (if anatomically suitable) or interposition bypass grafting.[2,3] In extent I repairs, the reattachment of the visceral arteries is often incorporated into a beveled distal anastomosis, but in extent II and III repairs the visceral and renal artery origins are reattached to one or more oval openings in the graft. After completing the aortic repair, an inline heat exchanger in the bypass circuit may be used to rewarm patients and reduce the risk for arrhythmias or coagulopathy, but in the authors' experience, this has generally not been necessary. Alternatively, warm water may be used to irrigate the operative field, thereby reversing the decrease in temperature and initiating rewarming of the patient.

In patients with lower aortic aneurysms (i.e., Crawford extents III and IV) atrio distal aortic bypass may be modified to provide only atrio visceral and/or renal bypass (Fig. 48-6). This technique avoids distal aortic or femoral cannulation, but reduces cardiac preload, protects the renal parenchyma, reduces post-clamp acidosis, and may reduce the risk of postoperative bacterial translocation by reducing bowel ischemia.

An alternative technique for distal arterial perfusion is employed in selected patients, i.e., primarily those with Crawford extents I, II, or III, and in whom cross-clamping at the diaphragm is technically feasible but is not appropriate at the mid- and upper mid-descending thoracic aorta. Atriofemoral bypass is used but the distal aortic anastomosis is made first to allow for sequential graft clamping as visceral arteries and subsequently intercostal arteries are attached to the graft from below upward (Fig. 48-7A-C).

A staged operative procedure is preferred in patients presenting with extensive aneurysmal disease involving the ascending aorta, arch, and descending thoracic or thoracoabdominal aorta. When the distal thoracic aorta is not disproportionately large compared to the proximal aorta and when the distal thoracic aorta is asymptomatic, proximal aortic repair is carried out as an initial procedure. An important benefit of initial proximal aortic repair is that it allows treatment of valvular and coronary artery occlusive disease at the first operation. In these patients with so-called mega-aorta, the elephant-trunk technique described by Borst is employed (Fig. 48-8).[44] In this technique the ascending and transverse aortic arch are replaced first, leaving a segment of graft within the proximal descending thoracic aorta to be used at the second procedure (Fig. 48-8A). The technique permits access to the distal graft at the second operation without the need to dissect in and around the distal transverse aortic arch. This reduces or eliminates risk of injury to the left recurrent laryngeal nerve, esophagus, and pulmonary artery.

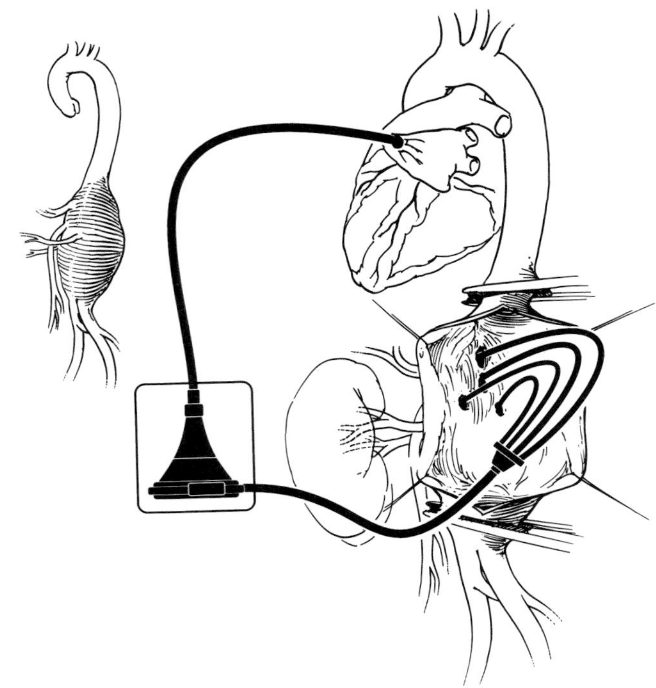

FIGURE 48–6 Crawford extent IV thoracoabdominal aortic aneurysm with visceral and renal oxygenated blood perfusion from left atrium during the ischemic period of aortic reconstruction.

Conversely, in patients with mega-aorta and rupturing, symptomatic (e.g., back pain), or disproportionately large TAAA, this segment is treated during the initial operation and repair of the ascending aorta and transverse aortic arch is performed as a second procedure. During this "reversed" elephant-trunk repair, a portion of the proximal end of the aortic graft is inverted down into the lumen during the first operation and is later used to facilitate second-stage repair of the ascending and transverse aortic arch.[45]

Closure

Following completion of aortic repair, protamine sulfate is administered to reverse heparin. It is imperative that adequate hemostasis is achieved and secured at all suture lines. The renal, visceral, and peripheral circulation are assessed.

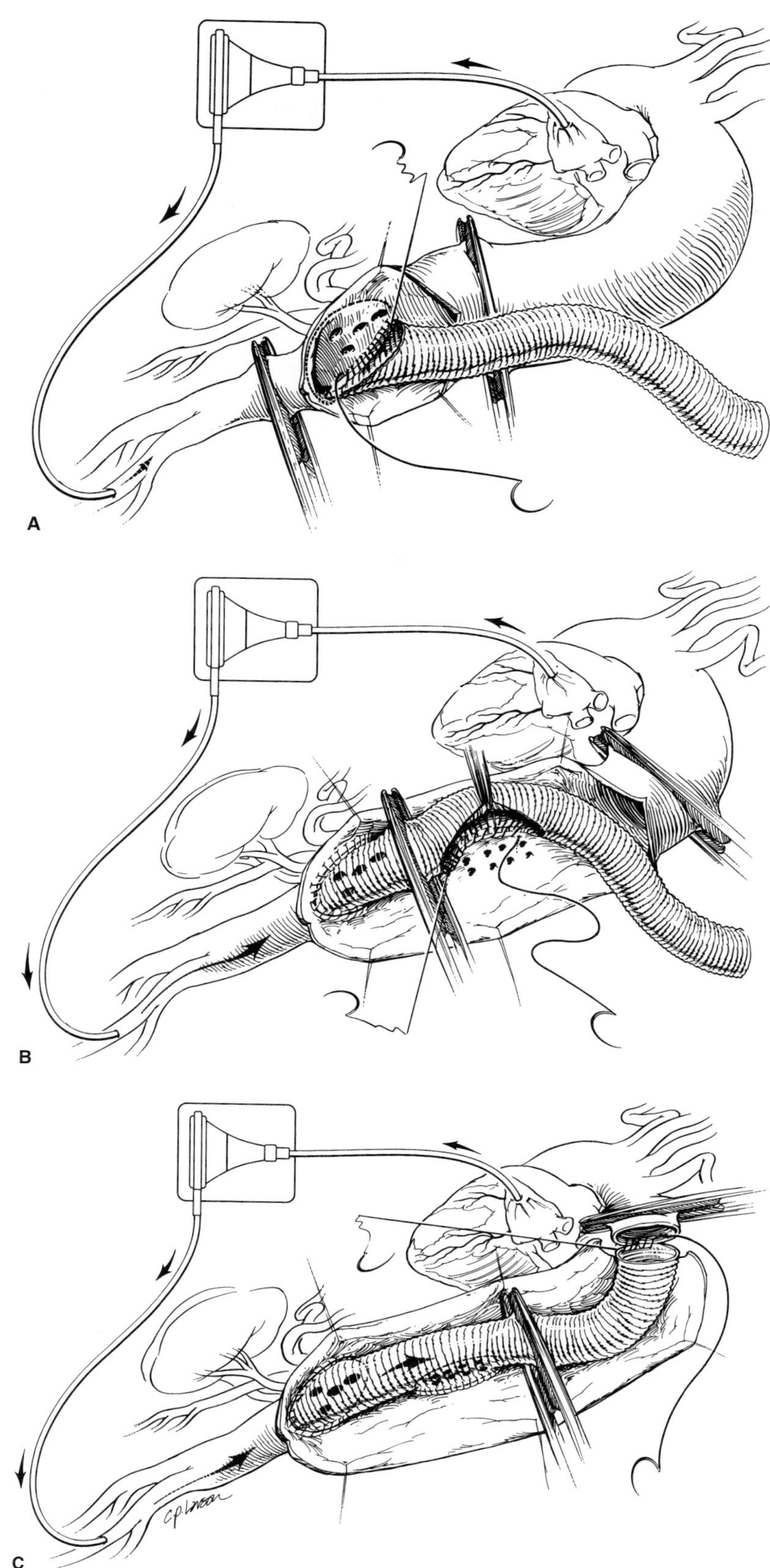

FIGURE 48–7 (A) Crawford extent I thoracoabdominal aortic aneurysm using atrio-femoral bypass, with beveled distal anastomosis, includes visceral and renal arterial reattachment that is carried out first. (B) Sequential clamping of graft provides renal and visceral perfusion during reattachment of a patch of intercostal arteries. (C) Sequential placement of the clamp allows distal perfusion of reattached intercostal arteries during the proximal aortic anastomosis.

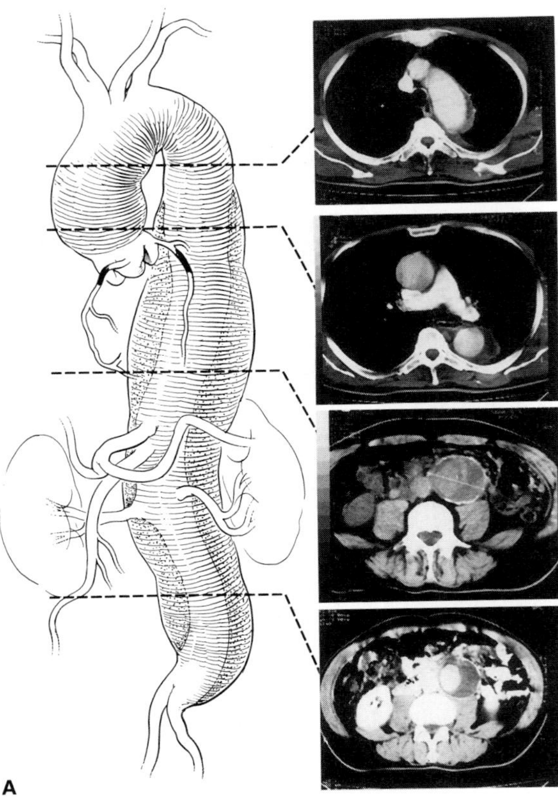

FIGURE 48–8 (A) Computed tomography scan and drawing of a patient with mega aorta–fusiform aneurysmal disease involving the ascending, arch, and all of the thoracoabdominal aorta. (B) First stage of repair including resection and replacement of the ascending aorta and transverse aortic arch using the elephant-trunk technique and coronary artery bypass grafting with vein grafts for coronary artery occlusive disease. (C) Drawing and aortogram following completion of repair including ascending, transverse aortic arch, all of thoracoabdominal aorta, and reattachment of intercostal, visceral, and renal vessels.

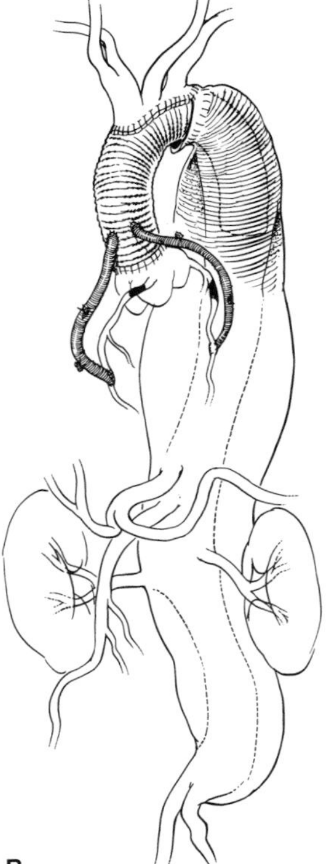

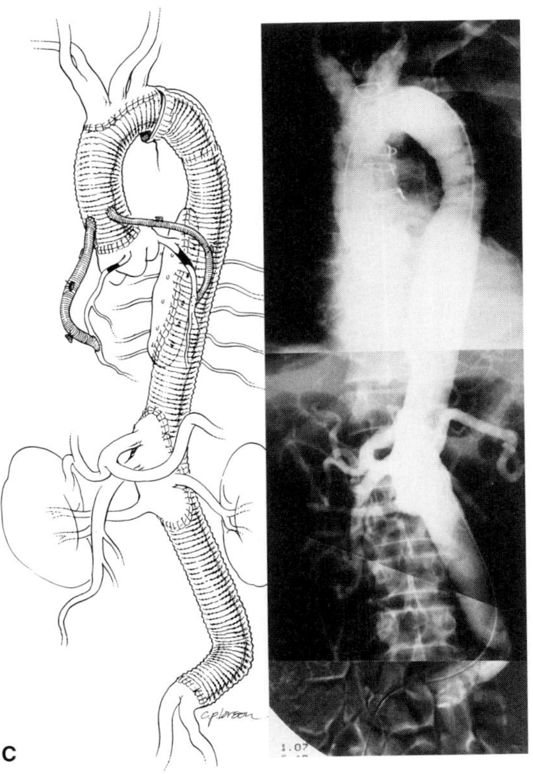

The aneurysmal wall is then loosely wrapped around the aortic graft. Two posteriorly located thoracic drainage tubes and a closed-suction retroperitoneal drain are placed prior to closure. The diaphragm is closed with running nonabsorbable suture; disruption postoperatively is exceedingly rare. To stimulate and maintain renal function, a low-dose dopamine drip of 2 to 3 mg/kg/min is initiated and continued for 24 to 48 hours. Patients are generally weaned from the respirator overnight and extubated the following morning. All drains are removed and antibiotics discontinued at 36 to 48 hours postoperatively. Ambulation is started on the second postoperative day.

The author routinely uses CSF (cerebrospinal fluid) drainage in patients with Crawford extent I or II. In patients in whom this is considered necessary, an 18-gauge intrathecal catheter is placed through the second or third lumbar space. The catheter permits aspiration of cerebrospinal fluid and pressure monitoring throughout the operation, and is continued for 2 to 3 days postoperatively. CSF is allowed to passively drain from the catheter. CSF is aspirated as needed during the period of aortic occlusion to keep the CSF pressure at or below 10 mm Hg using a closed collection system.

Endovascular Repair of Thoracic Aortic Aneurysms

Parodi et al reported the first clinical use of stent grafts for repair of abdominal aortic aneurysm in 1991.[46] Dake et al reported the first endovascular thoracic aortic repair in 1994.[47] Subsequent reports have supported this new less invasive therapy for traumatic, mycotic, and ruptured aneurysms of descending thoracic aorta.[48–50] Theoretically, endovascular repair of thoracic aortic aneurysm with stent grafts is a feasible alternative to standard surgical procedures in the treatment of selected patients with compromised cardiac, pulmonary, or renal status, persons who have undergone previous complex thoracic aortic procedures, and the very elderly. Conceptually, there is the potential to offer potentially reduced operative risk, hospital stay, and procedural cost.

Appropriate anatomy for endovascular repair includes the following: (1) a normal arterial segment proximal to the aneurysm and distal to the left common carotid artery of at least 2 cm in length and less than 38 mm in diameter; (2) a normal arterial segment distal to the aneurysm and proximal to the celiac axis of at least 2 cm in length and less than 38 mm in diameter; and (3) iliac arteries greater than 8 mm in diameter.[51]

The mortality and morbidity of endovascular repair of the thoracic aortic aneurysm are very difficult to determine. Most of the reported series are small and selection of patients may play a major role in determining outcome. The largest series is from the Stanford group, which included 103 patients. They reported a 30-day mortality rate of 9%, paraplegia/paraparesis (3%), myocardial infarction (2%), respiratory insufficiency (12%), and a high incidence of stroke (7%).[52] Balm et al, in a selected group of 144 patients with descending aortic aneurysms treated with endovascular stents, identified an early incidence of endoleak of 23% as documented by angiography or CT scanning.[53] The initial experience with these devices suggest that transluminally placed endovascular stent grafts are an attractive alternative for conventional surgery. However, there are not enough data available to determine the long-term effectiveness of this treatment; that will be established by well-controlled, large-scale studies that compare the open operative repair to this new technique.

PARAPLEGIA AND SPINAL CORD PROTECTION STRATEGIES

Incidence

Irreversible paraplegia is one of the most devastating complications after TAAA repair. The incidence of paraplegia or paraparesis, as reported in the literature, following thoracoabdominal aortic aneurysms varies substantially and ranges from 4% to 32%.[4] Svensson et al's landmark report of Crawford's experience documented on overall 16% incidence of paraplegia or paraparesis; complete paralysis occurred in more than half of patients with deficits.[3] In the author's report of 1108 patients who underwent elective repair, the combined incidence of paraplegia/paraparesis was 3.6% (40 of 1099 patients, excluding 7 patients with preoperative paraplegia and 2 patients who died during operation).[54] Generally, in large series the incidence of paraplegia and paraparesis is equally divided.[2,3] Up to 30% of patients who develop postoperative neurologic deficits initially awake with lower extremity function but develop deficits subsequently, i.e., "delayed paraplegia."[3] Operative factors that contribute to spinal cord injury include the duration and degree of ischemia, reperfusion injury, and loss of critical intercostals and lumbar arteries due to ligation, embolization, or thrombosis.[55] The risk of spinal cord injury averages, based on the Crawford classification, 13% for extent I, 28% to 31% for extent II, 7% for extent III, and 4% for extent IV.[4] Although in the past aortic dissection was identified as a risk factor, in more recent experience, dissection is no longer a risk factor for the development of postoperative paraplegia or paraparesis.[56] This is primarily a consequence of aggressive reattachment of intercostal arteries in patients with aortic dissection. This effort to reattach intercostal arteries has also likely reduced the risk of delayed paraplegia.

Vascular Anatomy of the Spinal Cord

The anatomy of the blood supply to the spinal cord is relevant to prevention of spinal cord ischemia and its sequelae. The major arterial circulation to the spinal cord is the anterior longitudinal spinal artery and the paired posterior longitudinal spinal arteries.[57] These vessels originate from intracranial vertebral arteries, or branches thereof, and course along the spinal cord for its entire length. The segmental spinal arteries supplying the thoracic and lumbar regions of the cord originate from the posterior branches of the intercostal and lumbar arteries, respectively. The anatomy is highly variable from one individual to another. The segmental spinal arteries give rise to the large anterior and smaller posterior radicular arteries. Each then directly supplies the anterior and posterior longitudinal spinal arteries. Not all anterior and posterior radicular arteries, however, reach the cord. It is this fact and the fact that the anterior spinal artery frequently is attenuated, or entirely discontinuous, that makes the spinal cord highly vulnerable to ischemia. The artery of Adamkiewicz is the largest of the radicular medullary arteries.[58] It has a variable origin, arising between T5 and T8 in 12% to 15% of the cases, between T9 and T12 in 60%, at L1 in 14%, at L2 in 10%, at L3 in 1.4%, and between L4 and L5 in 0.2%. The arteria radicularis magna anterior is a decisive factor influencing spinal cord damage during aortic occlusion.[59] When the vessel reaches the anterior spinal artery, generally it bifurcates into a smaller ascending branch and a larger descending branch. Intimal atherosclerosis, particularly in medial degenerative fusiform aneurysms, obliterates many intercostal and lumbar arteries, and complicates matters anatomically.

Pathophysiology of Aortic Cross-Clamping

An understanding of the pathophysiological mechanisms involved in aortic cross-clamping and unclamping is imperative in selecting effective measures to prevent and treat the consequences. Most clinical studies indicate that cardiac output decreases with thoracic aortic cross-clamping, whereas most animal studies show no significant change. The normal heart can withstand large increases in afterload without significant ventricular distention or dysfunction. Although impaired myocardial contractility and reduced coronary reserve are rare in animal experiments, such disorders are frequent in the elderly population undergoing aortic reconstruction.[60] Clamping the aorta increases impedance to aortic flow, increases systemic vascular resistance and afterload, and redistributes blood volume because venous vasculature distal to the aortic clamp collapses and constricts. This effectively increases preload. The increases in afterload and preload demand an increase in myocardial contractility, which causes an autoregulatory increase in coronary blood flow. Impaired subendocardial perfusion caused by high intramyocardial pressure, with resultant acute deterioration in left ventricular function and/or myocardial ischemia, may be the cause of wall motion abnormalities and changes in ejection fraction. If coronary blood cannot increase, cardiac decompensation follows.

Pathophysiology of Spinal Cord Ischemia

Injurious effects to the spinal cord, kidneys, lungs, and abdominal viscera are caused primarily by ischemia and reperfusion of organs distal to the aortic clamp and to a release of mediators from ischemic and reperfused organs. The most challenging and troublesome complication following TAAA replacement remains spinal cord injury and the development of paraplegia or paraparesis.

Spinal cord ischemic injury is the result of permanent or temporary interruption of spinal cord blood supply during aortic cross-clamping and permanent disruption of delicate and variable arteries to the spinal cord. Several pathogenetic mechanisms are related to neuronal cell death after transient spinal cord ischemia: excitotoxicity, intracellular calcium overload, nitric oxide, eicosanoids, apoptosis, inflammation, and reactive oxygen species. These mechanisms should be regarded as pathways that act in both parallel and sequential manners.[61] The duration of cross-clamping influences the magnitude of spinal cord ischemia and reperfusion. Studies suggest that cross-clamping for a period of less than 30 minutes is frequently safe.[62–66] Thoracic aortic occlusion results in increased intracerebral blood flow, which contributes to the increased CSF pressure and decreased spinal cord perfusion pressure.[67] By reducing CSF pressure, therefore, CSF drainage theoretically improves spinal cord perfusion during periods of thoracic aortic clamping.

An alternative explanation proposed by Piano and Gewertz postulates that increased CSF pressure during aortic clamping is related to volume changes in the venous capacitance beds located in the dural space.[68] Based on this model, the benefit of CSF drainage may be related to enhanced patency of these intramural veins. Other authors have suggested that the protective effect of CSF drainage may be attributable to the removal of negative neurotrophic factors that accumulate in the CSF during the ischemic period. Brock et al, for example, observed a strong positive relationship between elevations of CSF excitatory amino acid levels (i.e., glutamate, aspartate, and glycine) during aortic cross-clamping and reperfusion, and subsequent development of clinical signs of spinal cord injury.[69] Our recent prospective randomized trial focused solely on the impact of CSF drainage in preventing neurologic deficits after TAAA repair. The control and treatment groups were extremely well matched and a consistent surgical strategy was used throughout the study. The trial clearly showed that CSF drainage prevents paraplegia after the repair of extent I and II TAAA.[70]

Sodium nitroprusside during thoracic aortic cross-clamping reduces spinal cord perfusion pressure and increases the incidence of neurologic deficits.[71] The decrease in cord perfusion pressure is owing to a decrease in the distal aortic pressure beyond the clamp and an increase in CSF pressure. The increase in CSF pressure occurs from cerebrovasodilatation.[72] Drugs to reduce proximal aortic pressure ideally should possess minimal cerebrovasodilating properties.

Protection Strategies

The neuroprotective effect of hypothermia is presumed to be secondary to decreased tissue metabolism and a generalized reduction in energy-requiring processes in the cell. However, the mechanisms may be more complex and involve membrane stabilization and reduced release of excitatory neurotransmitters.[73] The author uses mild passive hypothermia (31°C-33°C) in all cases. Frank et al report a technique using partial bypass and moderate hypothermia for organ protection during the clamp-induced ischemic period.[74] The advantages of moderate over deep hypothermia include a stable intrinsic cardiac rhythm that eliminates the need for full cardiopulmonary bypass. They report a series of 18 patients undergoing thoracic and thoracoabdominal aortic aneurysm resection and replacement with moderate (30°C) hypothermia and partial bypass (aorto-femoral or atrio-femoral). No patient developed paraplegia or significant renal failure. There were two deaths (11%). The advantages of moderate over deep hypothermia include a stable intrinsic cardiac rhythm that eliminates the need for full cardiopulmonary bypass. Most authors specifically avoid the technique of profound hypothermia and circulatory arrest for TAAA repair, principally because of the threat of coagulopathy, pulmonary dysfunction, and massive fluid shift.

Crawford et al reported the clinical use of cardiopulmonary bypass using hypothermic circulatory arrest in 25 patients treated for thoracic aortic aneurysms through a posterolateral approach.[75] There were 21 early survivors and cerebral protection was entirely satisfactory. The technique was not entirely effective in eliminating paraplegia; 2 (11%) of 18 patients at risk for ischemic spinal cord injury developed neurologic deficits. This may be explained by satisfactory cord protection during the period of ischemia, but spinal cord injury from sacrifice of critical intercostal arteries.

Kouchoukos et al have recently reported on the use of hypothermic cardiopulmonary bypass with circulatory arrest as an adjunct for operations on the distal aortic arch, descending thoracic aorta, and thoracoabdominal aorta.[76] They evaluated 161 patients. Their 30-day mortality rate was 6.2%, and 90-day mortality rate was 11.8%. Paraplegia occurred in 4 and paraparesis in 1 of 156 operative survivors. Renal dialysis was required in 4 (2.5%). They identified hypothermic cardiopulmonary bypass as providing safe and substantial protection against paralysis and renal, cardiac, and visceral organ system failure.

There are two variations of regional spinal cord hypothermia reported in the literature: direct installation of cold perfusate into the epidural or intrathecal space, and intravascular cold perfusion into isolated thoracic aortic segments with the intention that the cold perfusate will be delivered through the intercostals vessels to the spinal cord. Epidural cooling for regional spinal cord hypothermia in the dog model is effective in preventing paraplegia following aortic cross-clamping.[77–79] Davidson et al reported a clinical trial of epidural cooling in eight patients undergoing thoracoabdominal aortic replacement for aneurysm.[80] The technique satisfactorily achieved regional spinal cord hypothermia and adequate protection. Cold perfusion into isolated aortic segments has been used in animal models, with demonstration that cord temperature can be rapidly and effectively diminished.[81]

Intuitively, sacrifice of intercostal or lumbar arteries that are critical to the direct blood supply of the spinal cord is a significant factor in the development of postoperative paraplegia. Maintenance of flow through such arteries during all or part of the anatomical repair potentially keeps the period of spinal cord ischemia within the generally safe 30 minutes.[82,83] This concept is supported by a meta-analysis of the literature reported by von Oppell in a review of 1742 patients treated for traumatic aortic rupture over a 25-year period.[63] Simple aortic cross-clamping produces an incidence of paraplegia of 19.2%, whereas shunting reduces the incidence of paraplegia to 11.1%. Active augmentation of distal aortic perfusion, i.e., left atrial to femoral artery bypass or femoro-femoral bypass, has the lowest incidence of new postoperative paraplegia at 2.3% ($p < .00001$). The cumulative risk of paraplegia increases substantially if the duration of aortic cross-clamping exceeds 30 minutes, but only when distal perfusion is not augmented ($p < .00001$). In using left heart bypass for distal perfusion during replacement of descending thoracic and thoracoabdominal aortic aneurysms, Borst et al found that the technique effectively unloads the proximal circulation during aortic occlusion and maintains adequate perfusion of distal vital organs to reduce early mortality and renal failure.[44] Further, the risk of spinal cord damage decreased with combined distal perfusion and aggressive reattachment of distal intercostal arteries. Clearly, the devastating complication of paraplegia and other organ failure secondary to ischemia is worthy of further research; however, a combination of measures including distal aortic perfusion, aggressive reattachment of intercostal arteries, hypothermia, avoidance of hyperglycemia, and CSF drainage has substantially reduced this devastating complication.

Motor evoked potential (MEP) monitoring has the potential to specifically reflect motor function and motor track blood supply during the period of aortic cross-clamping. MEP uses stimulation of the motor cortex or motor neurons and usually records from a peripheral muscle. In 1997, Haan et al described the technique of transcranial stimulation of the motor cortex with recording of lower extremity myogenic potentials to detect intraoperative spinal cord ischemia.[84] Transcranial stimulation has not yet been approved by the Food and Drug Administration. The method requires special anesthetic techniques, since complete neuromuscular blockade is incompatible with myogenic MEP monitoring. In addition, this technique is generally used in conjunction with left atrium to femoral artery bypass. Recently, Jacobs et al published an excellent series of 184 patients undergoing TAAA repair in which they used a protocol that included left heart bypass, cerebrospinal fluid drainage, and the monitoring of MEPs. They found that MEP was a sensitive technique for the assessment of spinal cord ischemia and the identification of the segmental arteries that critically contributed to spinal cord perfusion. They were able to reduce their incidence of neurologic deficit to less than 3%.[85]

TABLE 48–3 Operative mortality: causes of operative death* in 1773 patients with thoracoabdominal aortic aneurysms

Multiple organ failure	80 (61.4%)
Cardiac complications	24 (18.2%)
Pulmonary complications	13 (9.9%)
Stroke	12 (9.2%)
Hemorrhage	2 (1.5%)

*131 in-hospital and/or 30-day deaths.

RESULTS OF TREATMENT

Mortality following surgical treatment of TAAA averages 13% for elective procedures and 47% for emergent operations.[3,4,56] Intraoperative mortality is 4% to 5%, 30-day mortality 10% to 12%, and in-hospital mortality 12% to 15%.[3,4,56] The etiology of early mortality is primarily multiple organ failure, pulmonary complications, renal failure, myocardial infarction, hemorrhage, and rupture of other aneurysms (Table 48-3). The incidence of postoperative renal dysfunction, defined as a significant increase in postoperative creatinine, averages 20% in reported series and ranges from 4% to 37%.[4,56] Seven to nine percent of patients required postoperative new onset hemodialysis. Prolonged ischemic times, extent of aorta replaced, and preoperative renal dysfunction with elevated creatinine are the primary variables associated with an increased risk of postoperative renal failure.

During the period between January 11, 1986, and December 31, 2001, the author operated on a consecutive series of 1773 patients for treatment of aneurysm of the thoracoabdominal aorta (Table 48-4). There were 1034 male patients (58.3%) and 739 female patients (41.7%). Mean age was 65.5 years (median 68 years) with a range of 18 to 88 years. Thirteen hundred patients (73.3%) were treated for medial degenerative fusiform aneurysms or others of nondissection etiology. Acute dissection was present in 66 patients (3.7%), and chronic dissection occurred in 407 patients (23.0%). There were 126 patients (7.1%) with Marfan syndrome, and 109 patients (6.1%) presented with rupture.

The extent of aortic replacement based on the Crawford classification included 580 with extent I (32.7%), 573 patients with extent II (32.3%), 291 patients with extent III (16.4%), and 329 patients with extent IV (18.6%). The 30-day overall survival was 94.3% and in-hospital survival was 92.9%. There were six (0.3%) intraoperative deaths. The overall incidence of paraplegia or paraparesis was 4.5% (79 patients). CSF drainage was not used in 173 (9.8%) patients. The incidence of paraplegia and paraparesis was evenly divided. Postoperative renal failure requiring hemodialysis occurred in 105 patients (5.9%); in 26 (24.8%), failure was temporary; and 29 patients (1.6%) suffered perioperative stroke. Six hundred eighty-six patients (38.7%) were operated on with the use of left heart bypass, i.e., atriofemoral bypass or femoro-femoral bypass. In 573 patients with extent II aneurysms, the incidence of neurologic deficit was 7.8% (44 patients).

In patients with chronic aortic dissection, paraplegia and paraparesis developed in 3.4% versus 4.6% for patients with chronic fusiform medial degenerative disease. Consequently, the presence of chronic dissection is no longer a variable associated with the development of postoperative neurologic deficits. However, in patients with acute dissection the incidence of spinal cord ischemic sequela remains high (5 of 66; 7.6%). Reattachment of intercostal arteries was accomplished in 61.0% of the entire group of patients, but, as a result of anatomical availability, was achieved as part of the repair in 79.9% of patients with extent I and II aneurysms.

Preoperative, operative, and postoperative variables for this series were analyzed for development of postoperative neurologic deficits and early (30-day) mortality. Multivariate analysis revealed that age, rupture, symptomatic aneurysm, preoperative renal insufficiency, and total clamp time were variables predictive of early mortality, whereas rupture, diabetes, and extent II were variables predictive of paraplegia or paraparesis. In this series of 1773 patients, left heart bypass and aggressive reattachment of lower intercostal and upper lumbar arteries substantially reduced postoperative paraplegia and paraparesis.

The incidence of postoperative renal dysfunction remains a challenge. We recently reported on a group of patients undergoing Crawford extent II TAAA repair with left heart bypass randomized to renal artery perfusion of 4°C lactated Ringer's solution for renal cooling or normothermic blood perfusion from the left heart bypass circuit. Multivariate analysis confirmed that the use of cold crystalloid

TABLE 48–4 Results of thoracoabdominal aortic aneurysm repair in 1200 consecutive patients

Extent	No. of patients	30-day mortality	Paraplegia or paraparesis*	Renal failure†
I	580 (32.7%)	32 (5.5%)	21 (3.7%)	13 (2.3%)
II	573 (32.3%)	43 (7.5%)	44 (7.8%)	50 (8.9%)
III	291 (16.4%)	14 (4.8%)	8 (2.8%)	20 (7.0%)
IV	329 (18.6%)	12 (3.6%)	6 (2.1%)	22 (6.8%)
Total	1773 (100%)	101 (5.7%)	79 (4.5%)	105 (6.0%)

*Excludes 6 patients who died during operation and 18 patients with preoperative paraplegia.
†Excludes 6 patients who died during operation and 27 patients on hemodialysis preoperatively.

perfusion was independently protective against acute renal dysfunction.[86]

Ischemic spinal cord injury following repair remains a devastating complication. One hundred and forty-five patients undergoing extent I or II thoracoabdominal repair with a consistent strategy of moderate heparinization, permissive mild hypothermia, left heart bypass, and reattachment of intercostals arteries were randomized to cerebrospinal fluid (CSF) drainage versus no CSF drainage. In that evaluation, 9 patients (13%) in the control group developed either paraplegia or paraparesis while only 2 patients (2.6%) in the CSF drainage group developed deficits.[87]

A guiding principle for all patient management decisions involves determining whether the risk of the disease's natural history outweighs the risk of its treatment. In the case of TAAA repair, this must be based on each individual's risk of rupture without operation versus their risk of death or paraplegia with operation. A risk factor analysis of mortality and paraplegia after TAAA repair identified predictors of operative mortality to include preoperative renal insufficiency, increasing age, symptomatic aneurysm, and extent II aneurysm, while extent II aneurysm and diabetes were predictors of paraplegia. For patients who are acceptable candidates, contemporary surgical management provides favorable results.[88]

Crawford et al reported a 60% 5-year survival following TAAA replacement. Survival was reduced to 25% in patients with rupture, 40% with renal dysfunction, and 49% with coronary artery disease. The most common causes of late mortality were cardiac, pulmonary, and renal failure, sepsis, and aneurysm rupture of unoperated segments. In addition to the severe impact on lifestyle, the devastating complication of postoperative paraplegia or paraparesis decreased late survival to 44% versus 62% at 5 years.

The evaluation and treatment of patients with TAAA remain a significant challenge and require a great deal of investigative and clinical work to bring about the multifactorial approach necessary to solve the remaining complex problems.

REFERENCES

1. Etheredge et al: Successful resection of a large aneurysm of upper abdominal aorta and replacement with homograft. *Surgery* 1955; 38:1171.
2. Crawford ES, Crawford JL, Safi HJ, et al: Thoracoabdominal aortic aneurysms: preoperative and intraoperative factors determining immediate and long-term results of operations in 605 patients. *J Vasc Surg* 1986; 3:389.
3. Svensson LG, Crawford ES, Hess KR, et al: Experience with 1509 patients undergoing thoracoabdominal aortic operations. *J Vasc Surg* 1993; 17:357.
4. Panneton JM, Hollier LH: Basic data underlying clinical decision making. *Ann Vasc Surg* 1995; 9:503.
5. Sakai LY, Keene DR, Gianville RW, Bachinger HP: Purification and partial characterization of fibrillin, a cysteine-rich structural component of connective tissue microfibrils. *J Biol Chem* 1991; 266:14763.
6. Milewicz DM, Pyeritz RE, Crawford ES, Byers PH: Marfan syndrome: defective synthesis, secretion, and extracellular matrix formation of fibrillin by cultured dermal fibroblasts. *J Clin Invest* 1992; 89:79.
7. Schlatmann TJM, Becker AE: Histologic changes in the normal aging aorta: implications for dissecting aortic aneurysm. *Am J Cardiol* 1977; 39:13.
8. Johnson KW, Rutherford RB, Tilson MD, et al: Suggested standards for reporting on arterial aneurysms. *J Vasc Surg* 1991; 13:452.
9. Pearce WH, Slaughter MS, LeMaire SA, et al: Aortic diameter as a function of age, gender, and body surface area. *Surgery* 1993; 114:691.
10. Cronenwett JL, Garrett HE: Arteriographic measurement of the abdominal aorta, iliac, and femoral arteries in women with atherosclerotic occlusive disease. *Radiology* 1983; 148:389.
11. Liddington MI, Heather BP: The relationship between aortic diameter and body habitus. *Eur J Vasc Surg* 1992; 6:89.
12. Crawford ES, DeNatale RW: Thoracoabdominal aortic aneurysm: observations regarding the natural course of the disease. *J Vasc Surg* 1986; 3:578.
13. Cambria RA, Gloviczki P, Stanson AW, et al: Outcome and expansion rate of 57 thoracoabdominal aortic aneurysms managed nonoperatively. *Am J Surg* 1995; 170:213.
14. Dapunt OE, Galla JD, Sadeghi AM, et al: The natural history of thoracic aortic aneurysms. *J Thorac Cardiovasc Surg* 1994; 107:1323.
15. Masuda Y, Takanashi K, Takasu J, et al: Expansion rate of thoracic aortic aneurysms and influencing factors. *Chest* 1992; 102:461.
16. Bickerstaff LK, Pairolero PC, Hollier LH, et al: Thoracic aortic aneurysms: a population-based study. *Surgery* 1982; 92:1103.
17. Pressler V, McNamara JJ: Thoracic aortic aneurysm: natural history and treatment. *J Thorac Cardiovasc Surg* 1980; 79:489.
18. Crawford ES, Hess KR, Cohen ES, et al: Ruptured aneurysms of the descending thoracic and thoracoabdominal aorta: analysis according to size and treatment. *Ann Surg* 1991; 213:417.
19. Juvonen T, Ergin MA, Galla JD, et al: Prospective study of the natural history of thoracic aortic aneurysms. *Ann Thorac Surg* 1997; 63:1533.
20. Svensson LG, Crawford ES, Hess KR, et al: Experience with 1509 patients undergoing thoracoabdominal aortic operations. *J Vasc Surg* 1988; 46:260.
21. Acher CW, Wynn MM, Hoch JR, Kranner PW: Cardiac function is a risk factor for paralysis in thoracoabdominal aortic replacement. *J Vasc Surg* 1998; 27:821.
22. Coselli JS, Crawford ES: Primary aortoesophageal fistula from aortic aneurysm: successful surgical treatment using omental pedicle graft. *J Vasc Surg* 1990; 12:269.
23. Fillinger MF: Imaging of the thoracic and thoracoabdominal aorta. *Semin Vasc Surg* 2000; 13:247.
24. Goldstone J: Vascular imaging techniques, in Rutherford RB (ed): *Vascular Surgery,* 3d ed. Philadelphia, WB Saunders, 1989; p 119.
25. Wiet SP, Pearce WH, McCarthy WJ, et al: Utility of transesophageal echocardiography in the diagnosis of disease of the thoracic aorta. *J Vasc Surg* 1994; 20:613.
26. Blanchard DG, Kimura BJ, Dittrich HC, DeMaria AN: Transesophagealechocardiography of the aorta. *JAMA* 1994; 272:546.
27. Gomes MN, Choyke PL: Preoperative evaluation of abdominal aortic aneurysms: ultrasound or computed tomography? *J Cardiovasc Surg* 1987; 28:159.
28. Greatorex RA, Dixon AK, Flower CDR, Pulvertaft RW: Limitations of computed tomography in leaking abdominal aortic systems. *BMJ* 1988; 297:284.
29. Clayton MJ, Walsh JW, Brewer WH: Contained rupture of abdominal aortic aneurysms: sonographic and CT diagnosis. *AJR Am J Roentgenol* 1982; 138:154.

30. Weinbaum FI, Dubner S, Turner JW, et al: The accuracy of computed tomography in the diagnosis of retroperitoneal blood in the presence of abdominal aortic aneurysm. *J Vasc Surg* 1987; 6:11.
31. Patel MR, Kuntz KM, Klufas RA, et al: Preoperative assessment of the carotid bifurcation: can magnetic resonance angiography and duplex ultrasonography replace contrast arteriography? *Stroke* 1995; 26:1753.
32. Brott T, Toole JF: Medical compared with surgical treatment of asymptomatic carotid artery stenosis. *Ann Intern Med* 1995; 123:720.
33. Department of Health and Human Services, National Institute of Health: Carotid endarterectomy for patients with asymptomatic internal carotid artery stenosis. *J Neurol Sci* 1995; 129:76.
34. Hertzer NR, O'Hara PJ, Mascha EJ, et al: Early outcome assessment for 2228 consecutive carotid endarterectomy procedures: the Cleveland Clinic experience from 1989 to 1995. *J Vasc Surg* 1997; 26:1.
35. Fillinger MF: Imaging of the thoracic and thoracoabdominal aorta. *Semin Vasc Surg* 2000; 13:247.
36. Danias PG, Eldeman RR, Manning WJ: Magnetic resonance angiography of the great vessels and the coronary arteries, in Pohost GM, O'Rourke RA, Berman DS, Shah PM (eds): *Imaging in Cardiovascular Disease*. Philadelphia, Lippincott Williams & Wilkins, 2000; p 449.
37. Coselli JS: Suprarenal aortic reconstruction: perioperative management, patient selection, patient workup, operative management, and postoperative management. *Sem Vasc Surg* 1992; 5:146.
38. Svensson LG, Crawford ES, Hess KR, et al: Thoracoabdominal aortic aneurysms associated with celiac, superior mesenteric, and renal artery occlusive disease: methods and analysis of results in 271 patients. *J Vasc Surg* 1992; 16:378.
39. Chan FY, Crawford ES, Coselli JS, et al: In-situ prosthetic graft replacement for mycotic aneurysm of the aorta. *Ann Thorac Surg* 1989; 47:193.
40. Coselli JS, Crawford ES: Composite valve graft replacement of aortic root using separate Dacron tube for coronary artery reattachment. *Ann Thorac Surg* 1989; 47:558.
41. Coselli JS, Crawford ES: Thoracic aortic aneurysms, in Haimovici H (ed): *Vascular Surgery,* 3d ed. East Norwalk, CT, Appleton & Lange, 1989; p 591.
42. Coselli JS: Suprarenal aortic reconstruction: endovascular repair. *Semin Vasc Surg* 1992; 5:180.
43. Rosingh HJ, Dikkers FG: Thyroplasty to improve the voice in patients with a unilateral vocal cord paralysis. *Clin Otolaryngol* 1995; 20:124.
44. Borst HG, Frank G, Schaps D: Treatment of extensive aortic aneurysms by a new multiple-stage approach. *J Thorac Cardiovasc Surg* 1988; 95:11.
45. Coselli JS, Oberwalder PJ: Successful repair of mega aorta using reversed elephant trunk procedure. *J Vasc Surg* 1998; 27:183.
46. Parodi JC, Palmaz JC, Barone HD: Transfemoral intraluminal graft implantation for abdominal aortic aneurysms. *Ann Vasc Surg* 1991; 5:491.
47. Dake MD, Miller DC, Semba CP, et al: Transluminal placement of endovascular stent-grafts for the treatment of descending thoracic aortic aneurysms. *N Engl J Med* 1994; 331:1729.
48. Rousseau H, Soula P, Perreault P, et al: Delayed treatment of traumatic rupture of the thoracic aorta with endoluminal covered stent. *Circulation* 1999; 99:498.
49. Semba CP, Sakai T, Slonim SM, et al: Mycotic aneurysm of the thoracic aorta: repair with the use of endovascular stent-grafts. *J Vasc Interv Radiol* 1998; 9:33.
50. Semba CP, Kato N, Kee ST, et al: Acute rupture of the descending thoracic aorta: repair with use of endovascular stent-grafts. *J Vasc Interv Radiol* 1997; 8:337.
51. Rachel ES, Bergamini TM, Kinney EV, et al: Endovascular repair of thoracic aortic aneurysms: a paradigm shift in standard of care. *Vasc Endovasc Surg* 2002; 36:105.
52. Umana JP, Miller DC: Endovascular treatment of aortic dissections and thoracic aortic aneurysms. *Semin Vasc Surg* 2000; 13:290.
53. Balm R, Reekers JA, Jacobs M: Classification of endovascular procedures for thoracic aortic aneurysms, in Branchereau A, Jacobs M (eds): *Surgical and Endovascular Treatment of Aortic Aneurysms*. Armonk, NY, Futura, 2000; p 19.
54. LeMaire SA, Miller CC 3rd, Conklin LD, et al: A new predictive model for adverse outcomes after elective thoracoabdominal aortic aneurysm repair. *Ann Thorac Surg* 2001; 71:1233.
55. Cambria RP, Davison JK: Spinal cord ischemia complications after thoracoabdominal aortic surgery, in Gewertz BL, Schwartz LB (eds): *Surgery of the Aorta and Its Branches*. Philadelphia, WB Saunders, 2000; p 212.
56. Coselli JS: Thoracoabdominal aortic aneurysms: experience with 372 patients. *J Card Surg* 1994; 9:638.
57. Brockstein B, Johns L, Gewertz BL: Blood supply to the spinal cord: anatomic and physiologic correlations. *Ann Vasc Surg* 1994; 8:394.
58. Adamkiewicz A: Die blutgefasse des menschlichen ruckenmarkes, II: Die Gefasse der Rockenmarksoberflache, Sitsungs d.k. *Akad J Wissench Math-Naturw CI,* 1882; p 101.
59. Wadouh F: The arteria radicularis magna anterior as a decisive factor influencing spinal cord damage during aortic occlusion. *J Thorac Cardiovasc Surg* 1984; 88:1.
60. Norris EJ, Frank SM: Anesthesia for vascular surgery, in Miller RD (ed): *Anesthesia*, 5th ed. Philadelphia, Churchill Livingstone, 1999; p 1849.
61. de Haan P: Pharmacologic adjuncts to protect the spinal cord during transient ischemia. *Semin Vasc Surg* 2000; 13:264.
62. Gelman S: The pathophysiology of aortic cross-clamping and unclamping. *Anesthesiology* 1995; 82:1026.
63. von Oppell UO, Dunne TT, De Groot MK, Zilla P: Traumatic aortic rupture: twenty-year metaanalysis of mortality and risk of paraplegia. *Ann Thorac Surg* 1994; 58:585.
64. Kouchoukos NT: Spinal cord ischemic injury: is it preventable? *Semin Thorac Cardiovasc Surg* 1991; 3:323.
65. Hollier LH: Protecting the brain and spinal cord. *J Vasc Surg* 1987; 5:524.
66. Katz NM, Blackstone EH, Kirklin JW, Karp RB: Incremental risk factors for spinal cord injury following operation for acute traumatic aortic transection. *J Thorac Cardiovasc Surg* 1981; 81:669.
67. Saether OD, Juul R, Aadahl P, et al: Cerebral haemodynamics during thoracic- and thoracoabdominal aortic aneurysm repair. *Eur J Vasc Endovasc Surg* 1996; 12:81.
68. Piano G, Gewertz BL: Mechanism of increased cerebrospinal fluid pressure with thoracic aortic occlusion. *J Vasc Surg* 1990; 11:695.
69. Brock MV, Redmond JM, Ishiwa S, et al: Clinical markers in CSF for determining neurologic deficits after thoracoabdominal aortic aneurysm repair. *Ann Thorac Surg* 1997; 64:999.
70. Coselli JS, LeMaire SA, Schmitling ZC, Koksoy C: Cerebrospinal fluid drainage in thoracoabdominal aortic surgery. *Semin Vasc Surg* 2000; 13:308.
71. Martini CP, Grubbs PE, Toporoff B, et al: Effect of sodium nitroprusside on spinal cord perfusion and paraplegia during aortic cross-clamping. *Ann Thorac Surg* 1989; 47:379.
72. Gelman S, Reves JG, Fowler K, et al: Regional blood flow during cross clamping of the thoracic aorta and infusion of sodium nitroprusside. *J Thorac Cardiovasc Surg* 1983; 85:287.
73. Rokkas CK, Sundaresan S, Shuman TA, et al: Profound systemic hypothermia protects the spinal cord in a primate model of spinal cord ischemia. *J Thorac Cardiovasc Surg* 1993; 106:1024.
74. Frank SM, Parker SD, Rock P, et al: Moderate hypothermia, with partial bypass and segmental sequential repair for thoracoabdominal aortic aneurysm. *J Vasc Surg* 1994; 19:687.

75. Crawford ES, Coselli JS, Safi HJ: Partial cardiopulmonary bypass, hypothermic circulatory arrest, and posterolateral exposure for thoracic aortic aneurysm operation. *J Thorac Cardiovasc Surg* 1987; 94:824.
76. Kouchoukos NT, Masetti P, Rokkas CK, et al: Safety and efficacy of hypothermic cardiopulmonary bypass and circulatory arrest for operations on the descending thoracic and thoracoabdominal aorta. *Ann Thorac Surg* 2001; 72:699.
77. Berguer R, Porto J, Fedoronko B, et al: Selective deep hypothermia of the spinal cord prevents paraplegia after aortic cross-clamping in the dog model. *J Vasc Surg* 1992; 15:62.
78. Marsala M, Vanicky I, Galik J, et al: Panmyelic epidural cooling protects against ischemic spinal cord damage. *J Surg Res* 1993; 55:21.
79. Wisselink W, Becker MO, Nguyen JH, et al: Protecting the ischemic spinal cord during aortic clamping; the influence of selective hypothermia and spinal cord perfusion pressure. *J Vasc Surg* 1994; 19:788.
80. Davison JK, Cambria RP, Vierra DJ, et al: Epidural cooling for regional spinal cord hypothermia during thoracoabdominal aneurysm repair. *J Vasc Surg* 1994; 20:304.
81. Ueno T, Furukawa K, Katayama Y, et al: Spinal cord protection: development of a paraplegia-preventive solution. *Ann Thorac Surg* 1994; 58:116.
82. Borst HG, Jurmann M, Bühner B, Laas J: Risk of replacement of descending aorta with a standardized left heart bypass technique. *J Thorac Cardiovasc Surg* 1994; 107:126.
83. Schepens MAAM, Defaus JJAM, Hamerlijnk RPHM, Vermeulen FEE: Use of left heart bypass in the surgical repair of thoracoabdominal aortic aneurysms. *Ann Vasc Surg* 1995; 9:327.
84. de Haan P, Kalkman CJ, DeMol BA, et al: Efficacy of transcranial motor-evoked myogenic potentials to detect spinal cord ischemia during operations for thoracoabdominal aneurysms. *J Thorac Cardiovasc Surg* 1997; 113:87.
85. Jacobs MJ, DeMol BA, Elenbaas T, et al: Spinal cord blood supply in patients with thoracoabdominal aortic aneurysms. *J Vasc Surg* 2002; 35:30.
86. Koksoy C, LeMaire SA, Curling PE, et al: Renal perfusion during thoracoabdominal aortic operations: cold crystalloid is superior to normothermic blood. *Ann Thorac Surg* 2002; 73:730.
87. Coselli JS, LeMaire SA, Koksoy C, et al: Cerebrospinal fluid drainage reduces paraplegia after thoracoabdominal aortic aneurysm repair: results of a randomized clinical trial. *J Vasc Surg* 2002; 35:631.
88. Coselli JS, LeMaire SA, Miller CC 3rd, et al: Mortality and paraplegia after thoracoabdominal aortic aneurysm repair: a risk factor analysis. *Ann Thorac Surg* 2000; 69:409.

Chapter 49

Endovascular Stent Management of Thoracic Aneurysms and Dissections

Susan D. Moffatt/R. Scott Mitchell

The treatment of thoracic aortic pathology is complicated by the morbidity associated with surgical repair, and the fraility of a difficult and elderly population. The modern surgical treatment of disorders of the aorta began in the 1950s when successful treatment of aneurysms using segmental resection and graft replacement was reported by Swan, Lam, DeBakey, and Etheredge.[1–3] In 1956, DeBakey and Cooley reported the first successful resection of an ascending aortic aneurysm using cardiopulmonary bypass.[4] With enhanced diagnostic capability, improved surgical techniques and equipment, and better perioperative care, surgical results have continued to improve. Furthermore, improved understanding of the pathophysiology and natural history of thoracic aortic disease, and analysis of outcomes, has facilitated our treatment decisions in terms of the timing of appropriate intervention.

The patient population afflicted with thoracic aortic disease often harbors multiple comorbidites, including advanced age, renal insufficiency, diabetes, congestive heart disease, hypertension, and chronic obstructive lung disease. Operative intervention in this population frequently results in a significant incidence of death and long-term disability.[5–7] In an effort to reduce the incidence of negative outcomes, minimally invasive techniques in the form of endovascular stenting have been introduced over the past decade.[8–10] The technology, originally described by Parodi, and initially designed for use in abdominal aortic aneurysms, has been adapted for use in the thoracic aorta.[11] Although these techniques were initially envisioned for use in high-risk patients, their decreased morbidity and unique applications make them suitable even for younger patients with complex abnormalities. Fortunately, attracted by the early clinical successes, industry has stepped forward with significant engineering advances over the initial "homemade" mechanical devices.[12] This ongoing effort will likely permit us to expand the applicability of endovascular treatment to the various forms of thoracic aortic pathology including aneurysms and dissections as well as giant penetrating ulcers and intramural hematomas.[13] The worldwide experience is growing and with this a better understanding of the indications and limitations of this innovative therapy will be elucidated.

DEFINITION/PATHOGENESIS/PREVALENCE

Descending Thoracic Aortic Aneurysm

An aortic aneurysm can be defined as an abnormal dilation of the aorta, which undergoes progressive expansion and can be fusiform or saccular in nature.[14] In a Swedish study, performed between 1958 and 1985, with a population autopsy rate of 83%, the incidence of thoracic aortic aneurysm (TAA) was reported as 489 per 100,000 men and 437 per 100,000 women with a median age of 77.7 years for men and 85.3 years for women at autopsy. Approximately 5% of the lesions were thoracoabdominal aneurysms, without any difference between the sexes.[15]

Rupture rates have correlated with size, and a recent population-based study indicates some change in the natural history.[14] In a previous report by Pressler and McNamera, the incidence was noted as 4 per 100,000 population.[16] More recently, from the Olmstead County registry, the actual incidence was noted to have increased 3-fold, although the natural history was somewhat less perilous.[17] Among aneurysms less than 6 cm at discovery, the rupture rate at 3 years was 16%, which increased to 31% at a size of 7 cm.[18,19] Overall the incidence of rupture of thoracic aneurysms has been reported as 0.9 per 100,000 for men and 1.0 per 100,000 for women, whereas the incidence of dissection is 3.2 per 100,000 for both sexes, with fatal dissection occurring earlier in life than rupture.[20]

Approximately 50% of all thoracic aortic aneurysms are located in the descending aorta; these aneurysms more commonly arise at the level of the left subclavian artery and are often associated with atherosclerosis.[16] Histologic examination of aneurysms reveals fragmentation and degeneration of elastic fibers in the arterial media.[14] The mechanisms for this degeneration are unknown. Others have suggested that loss of structural integrity of the adventitia, not the media, is required for aneurysm formation. These pathologic changes must be differentiated from the normal aging process, in which elastic fibers fragment, smooth muscle cells diminish, collagen becomes more prominent, and ground substance increases, thus rendering the aorta less distensible and gradually more weakened.[14]

Heredity is thought to be involved in aortic aneurysm formation; the Yale group has demonstrated a 19% genetic predisposition to the development of familial TAA.[14,20] Other risk factors for aneurysm growth include hypertension, COPD, presence of a chronic dissection, and infection of the aortic wall. Arteriosclerosis has been reported as a risk factor for aneurysms and dissections; however, many have challenged this and the general consensus is that arteriosclerosis may well be a concomitant process and not a direct cause of aneurysm formation and growth.[14,20] Enlarging thoracic aneurysms can present with hoarseness due to stretching of the left recurrent laryngeal nerve, stridor from tracheal compression, dysphagia from esophogeal impingement, dyspnea from compression of the lung, and plethora or edema from compression of the superior vena cava. Patients with aneurysms of the ascending aorta may present with the signs of aortic regurgitation. Thoracic aorta aneurysms can also often be asymptomatic, detected only during work-up for another complaint. Symptomatic states, organ compression, concomitant aortic insufficiency, and acute ascending aortic dissection are widely accepted general indications for surgical intervention regardless of aortic size.[18,19,20]

Penetrating Atherosclerotic Ulcer

Penetrating atherosclerotic ulcer (PAU) and intramural hematoma (IMH) are distinct pathologic entities that are now being diagnosed with increasing frequency.[21–28] PAU was originally described in 1934 by Shennan, who described a pathologic entity in which ulceration penetrates the internal elastic lamina into the media and is associated with a variable amount of hematoma within the aortic wall.[21] It may very well be associated with aortic dissection and aneurysm formation, although it is distinct from those conditions. The ulcers are most often found in the distal descending thoracic aorta but can occur throughout the thoracic and abdominal aorta and have a characteristic appearance on computed tomography (CT) and magnetic resonance imaging (MRI).[23,24]

Intramural Hematoma

Intramural hematoma (IMH) was originally described in 1920 as a dissection without an intimal tear.[24,25] The cause of IMH may be a spontaneous rupture of aortic vasa vasorum that may initiate aortic wall disintegration, eventually leading to dissection with or without an intimal tear. The term "aortic dissection without intimal flap" has frequently been applied to cases that would be classified as IMH by definition.[24] Others have proposed intimal fracture of an atherosclerotic plaque as the primary event that then allows propagation of blood into the aortic media.[25] Moreover, discrete penetrating atheromatous ulcers or "giant penetrating ulcers" have been proposed as a prerequisite for intramural hematoma; both aortic dissection and PAU can be accompanied by aortic wall hematoma.[22,25] Regional thickening of the aortic wall greater than 7 mm in a circular or crescent shape in the absence of an intimal flap and without enhancement after contrast injection in CT and MRI is considered diagnostic of IMH.[23]

Aortic Dissection

Aortic dissection was first described by Nicholls in 1728 and in 1826 Laennec applied the name *Aneurysme Dissequant,* incorrectly associating aortic dissection with aneurysms and not as a distinct entity.[29] Dissection of the aorta is the more appropriate term since entry of blood into the outer two thirds of the aortic media often precedes dilation of the vessel, and dilation of the vessel may never occur. In an acute aortic dissection, the layers of the aortic wall are torn apart, creating a false lumen that runs parallel to the true lumen. The high-pressure entry site into the aortic media allows propagation of the dissection along the entire length of the aorta. Consequently, an acute aortic dissection is the most lethal of events affecting the aorta and many more people die of rupture of dissections than of aneurysms.[30] The prevalence ranges from 0.2% to 0.8% of the population and usually affects males more often than females with ratios similar to that for aortic aneurysms.[30]

Hypertension is the single most important risk factor for thoracic aortic dissection. Aortic dissection is also a known pathology of patients with Ehlers-Danlos syndrome or Marfan syndrome. Other factors known to predispose to dissection include bicuspid aortic valve, aortic coarctation, pregnancy, and surgical manipulation of the thoracic aorta.[31] Intimal tears typically occur at either the right lateral wall of the ascending aorta (type A) or just distal to the ligamentum arteriosum (type B), representing the points of presumed greatest hemodynamic stress.[29]

DIAGNOSIS

Diagnostic modalities for thoracic aortic pathology include chest radiographs, catheter-based angiography, computed tomography (CT), magnetic resonance imaging (MRI), transesophageal echocardiography (TEE), and intravascular ultrasound (IVUS). Although each has relative strengths and weaknesses, stent graft therapies mandate some unique considerations.[32]

Catheter-based angiography, in addition to being invasive and requiring nephrotoxic contrast material, effectively images only the flow lumen, and confers little information regarding the aortic wall, and no information about the mediastinum or pleural and pericardial spaces. Additionally, it requires transport to an angiography suite, and specialty personnel who may not be continuously on site. Exposure to contrast media may be minimized by use of CO_2 and gadolinium.

Computed tomography (CT), although it requires radiation exposure and nephrotoxic contrast material, is usually continuously available and conveniently located. It provides detailed information about the size, location, and extent of the aortic disease, as well as involvement of the mediastinal structures and pericardial and pleural spaces. With the addition of intravenous contrast, the aorta and branch vessels can be readily imaged, and aortic true and false lumens readily distinguished.

Magnetic resonance imaging (MRI) offers many of the advantages of CT but without the necessity for ionizing radiation or nephrotoxic contrast media. However, MRI suites are frequently distant from emergency departments, frequently require more lengthy exam times, are restrictive in terms of accompanying metallic equipment, and may not be continuously available nights and weekends.

Transesophageal echocardiography (TEE), especially with multiplanar capability, offers excellent visualization of the ascending and descending thoracic aorta, cardiac structures, pericardium, and pleural spaces. Tracheal shadowing may limit visualization of the proximal and distal aortic arch, but color duplex imaging allows precise imaging of aortic wall pathology and flow between the true lumen and other areas of interest, such as across the dissection septum, or into an intramural hematoma from a penetrating ulcer.

Intravascular ultrasound, although requiring an arterial puncture and catheter laboratory imaging, provides an unparalleled view of the aortic and branch vessel intima. It can also distinguish true from false lumen, and allows definitive identification of an intimal disruption secondary to blunt aortic trauma.

NATURAL HISTORY AND SURGICAL OUTCOMES OF THORACIC AORTIC DISEASE

Descending Thoracic Aneurysm

Aneurysms of the thoracic aorta, although increasing in prevalence, are incompletely understood. The natural history is often related to the specific location and the primary cause of the disease.[33–38] In patients with Marfan syndrome, dilation of the aortic root is the most penetrant of disease pathologies, and the risk of aortic dissection is directly related to the size of the aortic root.[33,34]

Although the size-rupture correlation is not so well established for thoracic aneurysms as for abdominal aortic aneurysms, recent data have better defined this relationship.[18–20] Clouse et al, from the Olmstead County database, have presented data revealing an increased incidence of thoracic aortic aneurysms, with a 5-year risk for rupture of approximately 30%.[17] Juvonen et al from Mt. Sinai in New York have identified clinical variables that affect the risk for rupture, the most important being increasing age, presence of COPD, maximal thoracic and abdominal aneurysm diameter, and the presence of pain. Utilizing a multivariable equation, the risk of rupture at one year can thus be calculated for any patient.[37]

$$\begin{aligned} \text{Ln}\lambda = &- 21.055 + 0.0093\,(\text{age}) \text{ and } 0.841\,(\text{pain}) \\ &+ 1.282\,(\text{COPD}) + 0.643\,(\text{descending diameter}) \\ &+ 0.405\,(\text{abdominal diameter}) \end{aligned}$$

$$\text{Probability of rupture within 1 year} = e^{-\lambda(365)}$$

Diameters are entered in centimeters, and pain and COPD are 0 if absent and 1 if present.

The Yale Aortic Diseases Group has documented rupture and dissection of ascending or arch aneurysms at a median size of 6 cm and descending or thoracoabdominal aneurysm ruptured or dissected at a median size of 7.2 cm.[18] Overall long-term survival of patients with thoracic aneurysms at 1 and 5 years was 85% and 64%, respectively; patients with descending thoracic aneurysms had lower long-term survivals (82% at 1 year, 39% at 5 years) than did patients with ascending aneurysms (87% at 1 year, 77% at 5 years). Furthermore, the Yale group has recently published a report consisting of 1383 years of patient follow-up before surgical intervention, which permits statistically valid calculation of yearly rates of rupture or other complications.[19] They found that the mean rate of rupture or dissection is 2% per year for small aneurysms, 3% for aneurysms 5.0 to 5.9 cm, and 6.9% for aneurysms of 6.0 cm in diameter or greater. The risk of rupture, dissection, or death from all causes is 6.5% at aneurysm size 5.0 to 5.9 cm and jumps to 14.1% per year for aneurysms of 6.0 cm or greater. Even more striking, when using proportional hazards regression, the odds ratio for rupture is more than 25 times higher in patients with aneurysms of 6.0 cm or greater than in those with aneurysms in the range of 4.0 to 4.9 cm.

Clouse et al reported a population-based cohort study to ascertain if the previously reported poor prognosis for individuals with thoracic aortic aneurysms had changed with better medical therapies and improved surgical techniques.[17] They examined patients with the diagnosis of degenerative thoracic aortic aneurysms among the residents of Olmsted County, Minnesota, between 1980 and 1994 and compared them with a previously reported cohort of similar patients between 1951 and 1980. The cumulative risk of rupture was 20% after 5 years, with 79% of ruptures occurring in women. The interval between initial diagnosis and rupture was 4.3 years, with rupture being the leading cause of death. Of the variables examined in univariate analyses, eventual development of dissection within the aneurysm, female sex, symptoms at diagnosis, and age at diagnosis were related significantly to aneurysm rupture, whereas smoking, chronic obstructive lung disease, hyperlipidemia, family history, and saccular configuration were not. Importantly, the overall 5-year survival improved to 56% between 1980 and 1994 compared with only 19% between 1951 and 1980. In reviewing the outcomes of those patients with thoracic aneurysm who do not undergo surgery, it has been found that 50% to 60% succumb to rupture.[39] By way of comparison, of all those who undergo elective surgery, 70% are alive at 2 years, and 59% are alive at 5 years, which further emphasizes that the natural course of thoracic aortic disease can be favorably altered by appropriate surgical intervention.[40]

Extensive experience has revealed that in patients undergoing thoracoabdominal repairs for aneurysm disease, the survival rate can reach 92% at 30 days and 60% at 5 years.[40–42] The overall incidence of paraplegia and paraparesis ranges from 3% to 16% and the significant predictors were total aortic clamp time, extent of aorta repaired, aortic rupture, patient age, proximal aortic aneurysm, and history of renal dysfunction.[43–45] Despite the advances in surgery, the incidence and attendant morbidity and mortality of postoperative acute renal failure (ARF) have not declined substantially in patients undergoing thoracic aorta surgery. For patients with extensive aortic disease, the risk of hemodialysis is 5% for those with normal preoperative renal function and 17% for those patients with preoperative renal dysfunction.[46]

Traumatic rupture and resultant pseudoaneurysm of the aorta remains a surgical challenge because it is a diagnosis that is not easily made and is frequently associated with other serious injuries, and its repair is associated with high morbidity and mortality.[47] More contemporary theories propose that traumatic aortic rupture is a complex multivariate process secondary to a combination of stresses.[48] The mortality of this injury is in relation to the seriousness of the lesion, associated visceral injury, and the great urgency of the operation. The morbidity is in relation to the difficulty of spinal cord protection, which leads to paraplegia in young patients.[47,48]

Penetrating Atherosclerotic Ulcer

The clinical presentation of penetrating atherosclerotic ulcer (PAU) is similar to that of classic aortic dissection,[21] but very little is known of the natural history of PAU since most patients in the literature have undergone surgical therapy or have had only short-term follow-up. Recently, more follow-up has become available as this disease entity has become better understood.[22] The risk of aortic rupture is higher among patients with PAU (40%) than with patients with type A (7.0%) or type B (3.6%) aortic dissection.[25] However, the progression of PAU is slow and is associated with a low incidence of acute rupture or other life-threatening events. Among patients with PAU who are not treated surgically, the natural history would appear to be that the majority will have enlargement with the formation of saccular or fusiform pseudoaneurysms and intramural thrombus.[22] Age and general health of the patient, the location of the PAU, and the rate of growth should therefore all be considered when deciding whether or when resection is appropriate.[22,26]

Intramural Hematoma

Aggressive control of blood pressure in an ICU setting has been the initial management of intramural hematoma (IMH).[24] The overall mortality of IMH has been shown to be high in the first month after acute onset of symptoms and particularly for IMH of the ascending aorta. Furthermore, the development of mediastinal hemorrhage and pericardial and pleural effusion has been found to be more frequent in patients with aortic IMH than in patients with aortic dissections.[23] The highest mortality rate has been reported among patients in whom the hematoma originated in the ascending aorta and aortic arch. Also, patients with severe artherosclerosis of the ascending aorta and arch have a high prevalence of atheromatous emboli in the cerebral circulation.[25] Experience has therefore suggested that a more aggressive approach with early surgery is warranted in patients who have ascending aortic involvement or in those who have a coexisting aneurysm with IMH.[23,24,27]

Aortic Dissection

For patients with Stanford type A dissections, surgical intervention is performed immediately after diagnosis to avert the high risk of death due to various complications such as cardiac tamponade, aortic regurgitation, and myocardial infarction.[49–51] Untreated, type A dissections are associated with a mortality rate of 1% to 2% per hour during the first 24 to 48 hours. The Stanford experience revealed that the operative mortality for acute type A dissections was 7%; for chronic type A dissections, the operative mortality was 11%. Overall, the 5-year actuarial survival rate for discharged patients was 78% for type A dissections.[52–54]

In contrast, the preferred treatment for most patients with Stanford type B (descending aorta) is less well defined.[53–55] Although anti-impulse therapy, with beta blockade as the primary therapy, has been the most accepted therapy, it is still associated with a 10% to 15% hospital mortality rate, with significant morbidity in the long-term management from aneurysmal dilation of the false lumen.[55] Surgical treatment has been reserved for specific complications, namely, intractable pain, impending rupture, malperfusion syndromes, and early expansion to a diameter greater than 5 cm.[29,54,56] Other conditions that should prompt consideration of early operation include Marfan syndrome, presence of sizable localized false aneurysm in the proximal descending thoracic aorta, arch involvement, and expectations of poor medical compliance.[52,55] For this cohort of complicated patients, however, surgical procedures have been associated with mortality rates as high as 60% to 70%, primarily because of the unpredictable effect a central aortic operation may have on more peripheral perfusion. The actuarial survival for all patients with type B dissection was found to be 65% at 1 year and 50% at 5 years. More specifically, survival was 73% at 1 year and 58% at 5 years for medically treated patients, and 47% at 1 year and 28% at 5 years for surgically treated patients.[53] However, these are not comparable cohorts, as surgical patients are self-selected with their complications.[14,31,53]

ENDOVASCULAR DEVELOPMENT AND THERAPY

The major objective of surgical treatment of thoracic aortic aneurysms is to prevent aortic rupture and avoid complications from compression of adjacent organs. However, surgical procedures on the thoracic aorta are fraught with significant complications, which relate at least in part to the relative inaccessibility of the thoracic aorta. Clearly, less invasive strategies are desirable to avoid these morbid procedures. Endovascular repair is an attractive possibility, as an intravascular access route is readily available.[8–10] Parodi introduced the concept of balloon-expandable stents attached to the ends of a vascular graft for the repair of abdominal aortic aneurysms.[11] There were several attractive features of this concept. The device could be introduced from a peripheral site and advanced under radiographic guidance, eliminating the necessity for an invasive laparotomy or thoracotomy. Aortic cross-clamping, with its physiologic pertubations, could be avoided. Pulmonary trauma and respiratory complications could be minimized, and hospital stay and recovery could be shortened.[57] The initial approach at Stanford Medical Center was a combined effort between the division of interventional radiology and the department of cardiovascular surgery, with the expertise of each complementing the other. Work had already commenced years earlier with the use of uncovered stents for the repair of aortic dissections in an animal model. A stent graft was manufactured using self-expanding Gianturco Z stents (Cook Co., Bloomington, IN), which were fastened together and then covered with a woven Dacron graft (Meadox-Boston Scientific, Natick, MA). An IRB approval was initially obtained for a high-risk study for nonsurgical candidates (Fig. 49-1).[58]

Contrast-enhanced CT with three-dimensional reconstruction was the primary diagnostic tool. Aneurysm size and extent could be evaluated, as well as the distance from critical side branches. Stent grafts were oversized approximately 10% to 15% from the CT cross-sectional diameter in an effort to obtain sufficient radial force to achieve an endoseal and prevent stent graft migration. A minimum of 2 cm

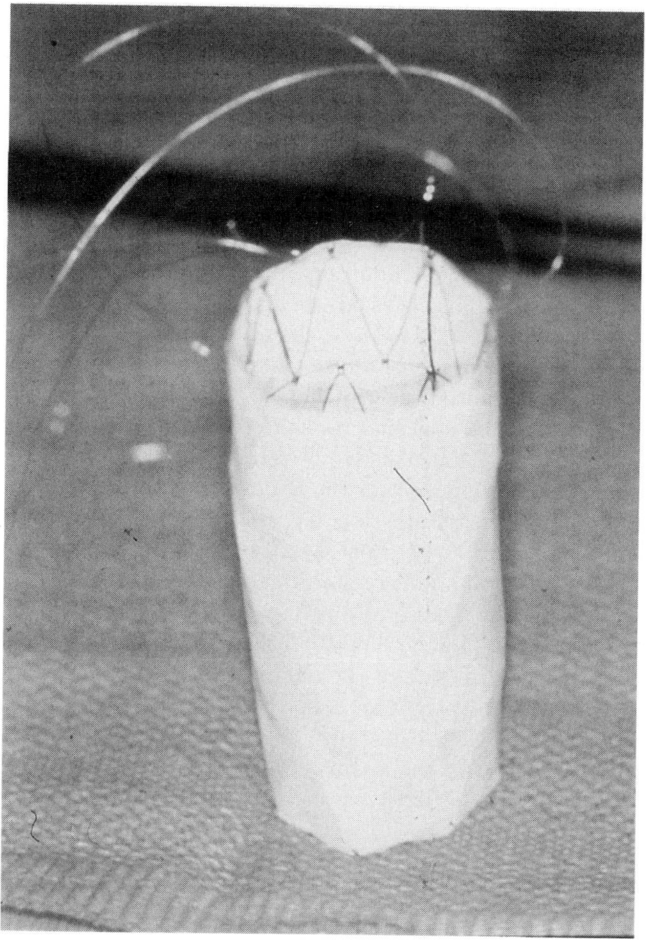

FIGURE 49–1 First-generation stent graft assembled from articulated "Z" stents, and covered with a woven Dacron tube graft.

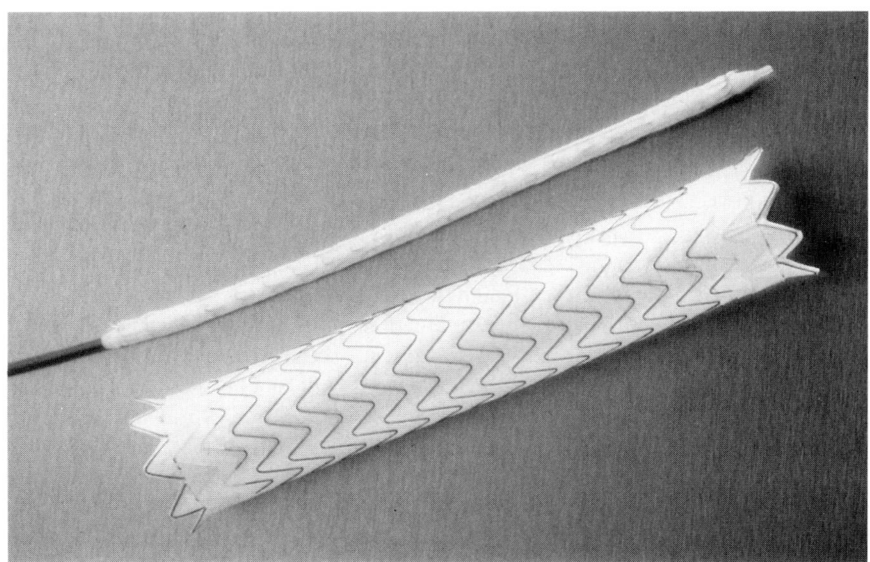

FIGURE 49–2 Second-generation commercially manufactured thoracic stent graft. The thoracic Excluder by W.L. Gore contains a thin-wall PTFE graft covered by a nitinol exoskeleton.

of normal aorta was required for adequate fixation. Digital subtraction angiography was used when necessary to further clarify findings on the CT. Intraoperatively, TEE was an invaluable tool for identifying the true and false lumen, and for verifying guide wire and stent graft placement. Digital fluoroscopy and TEE were used for graft positioning and deployment, and contrast angiography and TEE were used at the conclusion of the operative procedure to assure the absence of type I endoleaks. All patients received a computed tomographic angiogram (CTA) prior to discharge.[58–61]

Some new terminology must be introduced in relation to this technology.[12] Endoleaks, the failure to exclude the aneurysm sac from the blood stream, are classified as types I to IV. Type I endoleaks occur at the proximal or distal attachment sites, and signify a failure to achieve a hemostatic seal at these implantation sites.[9,57–61] Type II endoleaks denote a communication between a branch vessel and the excluded aneurysm sac. These usually occur from a back-bleeding inferior mesenteric artery in the abdomen, or intercostal arteries in the chest. Both an entry and exit vessel are usually necessary for prolonged patency. Type III endoleaks originate from the mid graft sections, and are usually caused by disruption of graft-to-graft overlaps, or by leakage through the graft itself. Finally, Type IV endoleaks are characterized by an increase in size of the aneurysm sac in the absence of an identifiable patent branch vessel, variously ascribed to "endotension." Regardless of type, any endoleak associated with expansion of the aneurysm sac implies a procedural failure.

Descending Thoracic Aortic Aneurysm

The anatomical features of descending thoracic aneurysm make them an almost ideal substrate for this technology. Since they frequently arise distal to the left subclavian artery, and proximal to the celiac axis, adequate landing zones (at least 2 cm in length) are frequently available, usually within relatively straight segments, and with no critical side branches. Femoral and iliac arteries greater than 8 mm in diameter were necessary to allow introduction of a 28F (OD) delivery sheath in Stanford patients. Devices were limited to a maximal diameter of 40 mm; aortas larger than 37 mm in diameter were themselves likely to be aneurysmal, and unlikely to serve as a stable attachment zone. Other anatomical constraints that precluded secure fixation included acute angulation at the distal arch, and severe sigmoid-like tortuosity coursing through the diaphragmatic crura, reflecting the relative inflexibility of these crude first-generation devices.[58–61] Commercially produced second-generation stent grafts (Fig. 49-2) are more flexible, and have a lower profile than these earlier devices.

Within these constraints, stent graft repairs were highly successful (Figs. 49-3 and 49-4). Initially, the greatest limitation was the rather primitive design of the stent graft itself. Since it was composed of articulating "Z" stents 2.5 cm in length, severe angulations could not be accommodated. Acute angulations would frequently result in poor stent graft apposition to the aortic wall within the landing zone, with the expected type I endoleak. Angioplasty balloon inflation was occasionally effective in straightening the stent graft and eliminating these endoleaks.

In our first 103 patients, 60% of whom were absolute nonoperative candidates, operative mortality was approximately 10%.[61] Only one of these deaths was related to the stent graft procedure itself, and most resulted from exacerbation of existent comorbidities. However, embolic strokes occurred in 7 patients, likely secondary to atheroemboli dislodged during guidewire or sheath manipulation within the aortic arch. Subsequent design modifications have eliminated the necessity for passing the introducer sheath into the aortic arch,

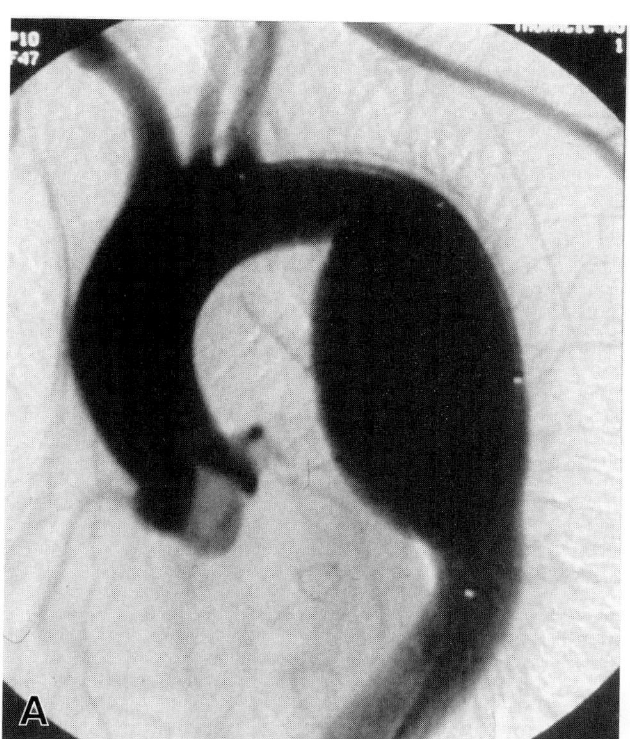

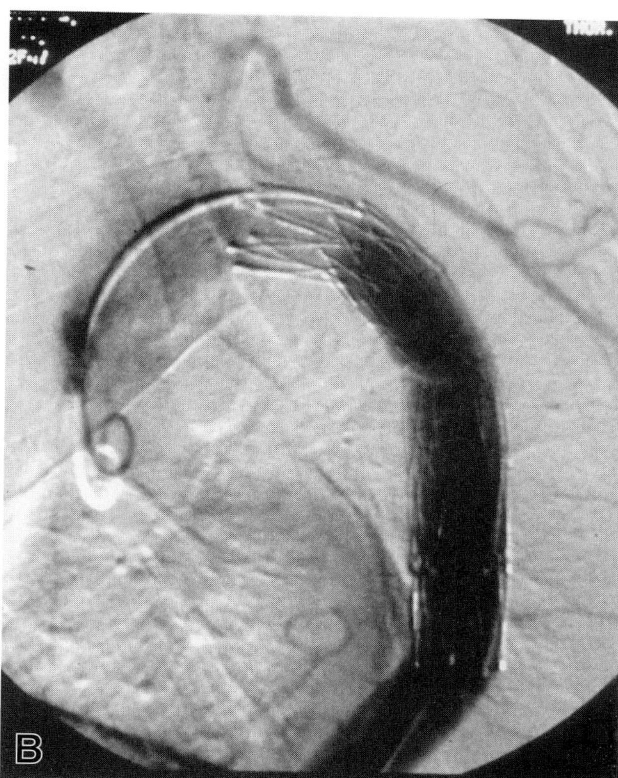

FIGURE 49–3 (A) Thoracic angiogram of a thoracic aortic aneurysm suitable for stent graft repair. (B) Thoracic angiogram illustrating successful exclusion of the aneurysm sac with a thoracic stent graft.

and have significantly reduced this complication. Spinal cord injury was another unknown risk, since critical intercostal arteries in the T-8 to T-12 would be frequently covered, with no possibility for maintaining their perfusion. Fortunately, the actual occurrence of paraplegia/paraparesis was relatively low, appearing in only 3 patients; interestingly, this complication occurred only in patients with concomitant or previous aortic abdominal aneurysm repair. Other authors have reported an incidence up to 2%, including the rather perplexing delayed onset of paraplegia, 12 hours to 28 days following the procedure.[62,63] Although many of these have been reversible with the institution of CSF drainage, naloxone infusion, or steroid administration, their occurrence has remained unpredictable.

Patients with multilevel aortic disease can present a formidable challenge for the cardiothoracic surgeon.[38,64] The morbidity rate of surgical repair can be substantial in these patients, and it is frequently compounded by the requisite second operation. In patients with an abdominal aortic aneurysm, 5% also have a descending thoracic aneurysm; in patients with a descending thoracic aneurysm, 13% to 29% also have abdominal involvement.[35,38] Sequential repair requires an interval period for recovery during which time the second aneurysm can rupture. Crawford found that 30% of early postoperative deaths after isolated repair of a descending thoracic aneurysm were caused by rupture of an untreated infrarenal aneurysm. In asymptomatic patients, Crawford recommended repair of the thoracic aorta initially.[33] While awaiting the second operation, the abdominal aneurysm is easier to observe, and if symptoms or rupture occur, patients could potentially survive for periods sufficient to attempt emergency repair. In contrast, thoracic aneurysms are more likely to rupture without warning and are rapidly fatal within minutes. In the Stanford study, simultaneous repair was successfully undertaken in 17 patients.[61] Utilizing a retroperitoneal approach to the abdominal aorta, an endovascular repair of a thoracic aortic aneurysm could be accomplished through an 8-mm side limb attached to the abdominal graft. A thoracotomy was therefore avoided, and complete aneurysm exclusion was achieved in 94% of patients. One patient died, resulting in a hospital mortality rate of 6%. This may prove to be a valuable addition to the surgical armamentarium for patients with both abdominal and thoracic aortic aneurysms.

Penetrating Atherosclerotic Ulcer

Penetrating ulcers present perhaps one of the most appealing clinical indications for this stent graft technology.[65] Presenting in an elderly population with extensive comorbidities,

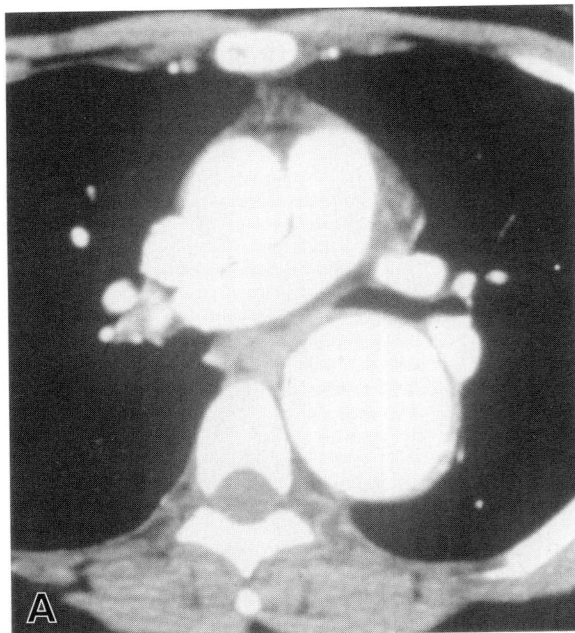

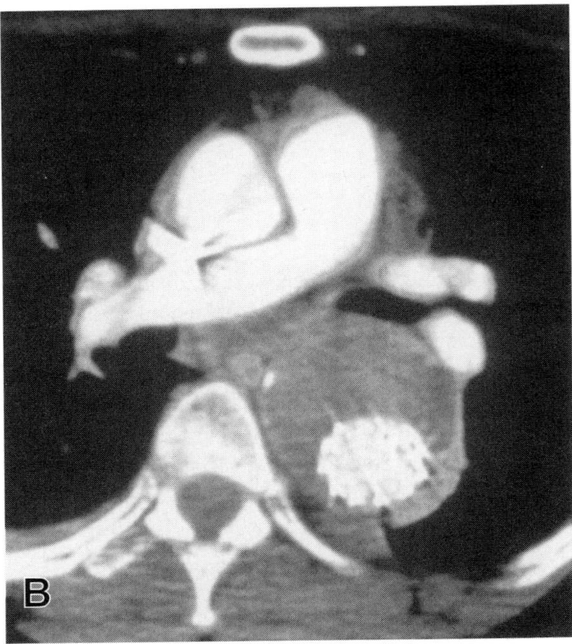

FIGURE 49–4 (A) Computed tomography demonstrating a large descending thoracic aortic aneurysm at the level of the pulmonary artery. (B) CT scan demonstrating complete exclusion of the aneurysm sac after successful repair with a thoracic stent graft as in Figure 49-3B. Complete absence of aneurysm sac enhancement with contrast assures freedom from an endoleak.

these diffusely diseased aortas present significant challenges for conventional repair. Poor tissue integrity combined with a high likelihood for intraoperative thromboembolism is a prime setting for severe complications.[21,22] Additionally, because of the diffuse nature of this process, representing

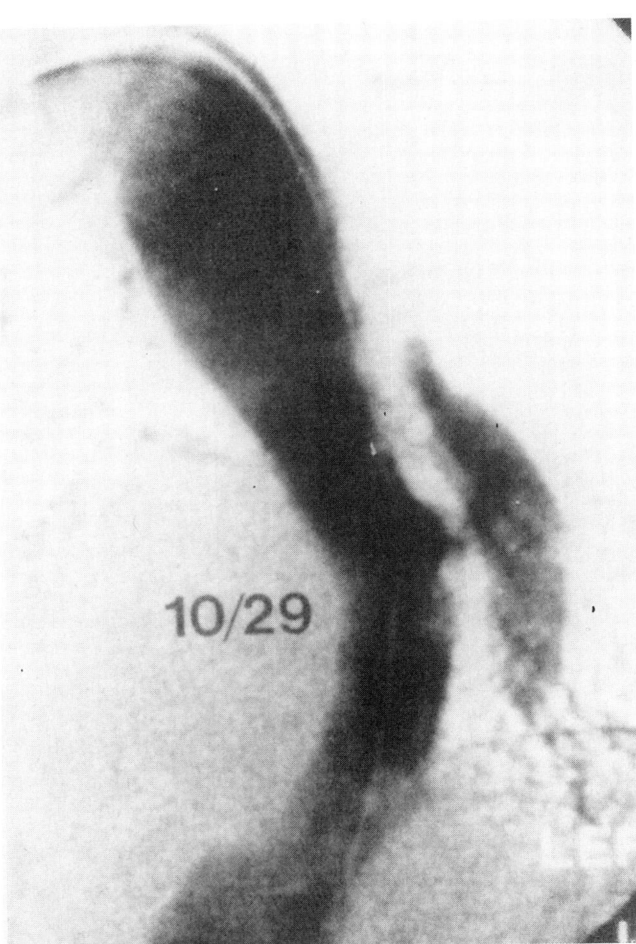

FIGURE 49–5 Thoracic aortogram of a giant penetrating ulcer, with subadventitial contrast collection. Rapid evolution into a saccular aneurysm can be expected, and prevented by coverage of the GPU with a stent graft.

end-stage atherosclerotic disease, it is difficult to limit the extent of resection and consequently the likelihood of complications (Fig. 49-5). Simple stent graft coverage of the penetrating ulcer can limit the progression of IMH and allow healing to occur. Unfortunately, even with successful stent graft implantation, retrograde aortic dissections and new ulcer formation have been noted in a significant percentage of patients, amplifying the diffuse and severe nature of this disease.[65]

Intramural Hematoma

Radiographically, intramural hematomas may be indistinguishable from an acute dissection with a thrombosed false lumen, and in fact may represent one end of a spectrum of disease, with IMH and intact intima at one extreme, and full-blown aortic dissection at the other. Although pure IMH of the thoracic aorta is not amenable to stent graft repair, any secondary intimal defect could be covered, perhaps limiting progression of the disease. IMH of the ascending aorta is problematic, as progression to a classical type A dissection occurs in a significant percentage of patients.[21,25]

Aortic Dissection

Aortic dissections may present the greatest challenge, but also the greatest utility, for thoracic stent grafts.[66–78] For Stanford type A dissections, with involvement of the ascending aorta, open surgical repair is indicated. As more aggressive repairs of acute type A dissections are undertaken in an effort to minimize late aneurysmal complications, as advocated by Kazui et al, stent grafts may play a role.[78] In younger patients, or those afflicted with Marfan disease, aneurysmal complications are more likely to develop late in the time course of a chronic dissection. Aneurysmal changes of the transverse arch are particularly problematic. In an effort to minimize these late complications, Kazui has advocated ascending and arch replacement for these younger, good-risk patients, with very acceptable mortality. Subsequent aneurysmal degenerative changes would be limited to the descending and abdominal aorta, more easily manageable if the arch is already repaired. Some authors have taken this argument one step further, and advocated insertion of a stent graft into the true lumen of the proximal descending thoracic aorta both to minimize late aneurysm formation as well as to promote false lumen thrombosis, potentially avoiding a double lumen aorta.[79] Although such an approach may seem unusually aggressive, if a particular population at risk could be defined, stent graft placement could prevent the late development of aneurysmal complications in a high-risk group.

For Stanford type B dissections, however, this stent graft technology offers many new advantages. Currently, medical management utilizing anti-impulse therapy is the most widely applied therapy for uncomplicated type B dissections. Surgical repair has been reserved for patients presenting with complications, including intractable pain, rapid expansion to a diameter greater than 4.5 to 5 cm, malperfusion syndromes, and leak or impending rupture.[29–31,54] Unfortunately, in this setting, surgical mortality may exceed 60% to 70%.[30] With medical management, which itself carries a 10% hospital mortality, it is estimated that approximately 70% of these patients will have a persistently patent false lumen, and 20% of these will become aneurysmal.[30,55]

The application of this stent graft technology could profoundly affect the natural history of aortic dissections (Fig. 49-6). Coverage of the primary intimal tear redirects flow into the true lumen, which will not only provide protection from rupture, but will also eliminate malperfusion resulting from dynamic obstruction ("true lumen collapse") in nearly all patients.[74] False lumen filling, with the attendant risk for rupture of its aneurysmal dilation, is eliminated, and false lumen thrombosis results in a single-barrel aorta.[80] If the procedure is performed in the catheterization laboratory, subsequent catheter-based investigation can reveal continued malperfusion secondary to uncorrected static obstruction, which can then be expeditiously addressed with uncovered orifice stents into the true lumen.[74] This is clearly a more reliable procedure for restoring visceral perfusion than a central aortic operation, and a less morbid procedure than a direct operation on the visceral arteries themselves. Moreover, the stent graft need not be overly long, rarely extending distal to T-6, thus minimizing the risk for paraplegia. In a previously reported series, 12 of 15 complicated type B dissections were successfully repaired with this approach, with an operative mortality of only 20%, and restoration of a single-lumen aorta in 70% to 80% of patients.[74]

Other interventional therapies are also available to correct malperfusion abnormalities. Localized obstruction to flow at the branch vessel orifice, usually secondary to intussusception of the torn intima, termed static obstruction, may be stented open with an uncovered stent.[81–83] If the only communication to the branch vessel is from the aortic false lumen, which is poorly perfused, a fenestration of the dissection flap can be performed with a catheter-based needle (Rorsch-Uchida, Cook, Bloomington, IN), crossed with a guidewire, and balloon dilated to increase flow into the false lumen. This technique is especially applicable at the distal aorta, with psuedo-occlusion of an iliac artery.

However, one must not discount the possibility for iatrogenic injury during instrumentation for stent graft placement. In the acute phase, the outer layer of the false lumen is a thin and friable adventitia, and its perforation, perhaps even with just a guidewire, would be catastrophic. Similarly, the dissection septum is also quite fragile, and may provide an insufficient distal anchor for a stent graft. There are some examples (Dake; personal communication) of septal perforations at the distal stent graft fixation site, suggesting the susceptibility of the acute dissection septum to repetitive erosive trauma. Even proximal secure placement within a nondissected aorta may pose difficulties, as there have been reports of false aneurysm formation in the transverse arch after placement of an endograft with its proximal portion uncovered. The primary intimal tear may also be quite extensive, and extend proximally to the left subclavian artery orifice. Effective exclusion of false lumen perfusion in these instances may be difficult to achieve, requiring implanting the stent graft just distal to the left carotid artery, and covering the left subclavian orifice. Although it has been suggested that the left subclavian artery may be sacrificed with impunity, the Stanford approach has been to create a left carotid to subclavian transposition or bypass, and then ligate the left subclavian proximal to the vertebral artery takeoff so as to eliminate the possibility of retrograde filling of the aneurysm sac from the left subclavian stump.[57,74,76,77] Another attractive possibility would be that of a branched stent graft for the left subclavian, or even all the arch vessels as advocated by Inoue of Japan.[84]

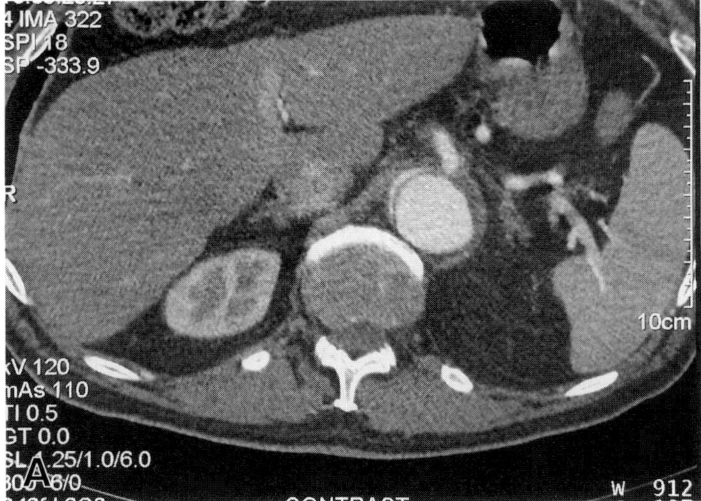

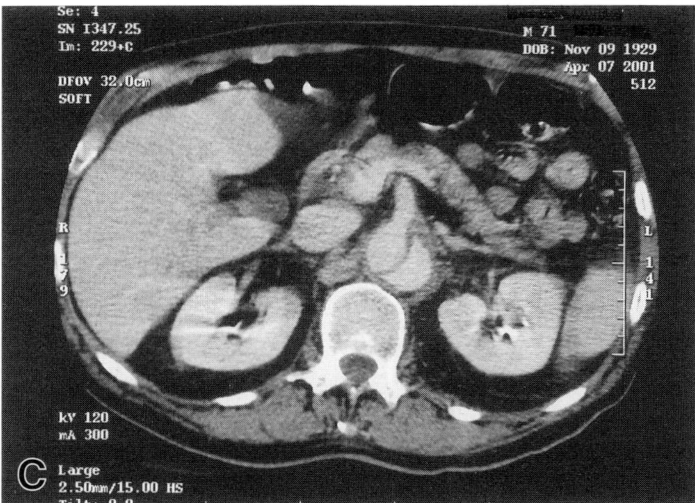

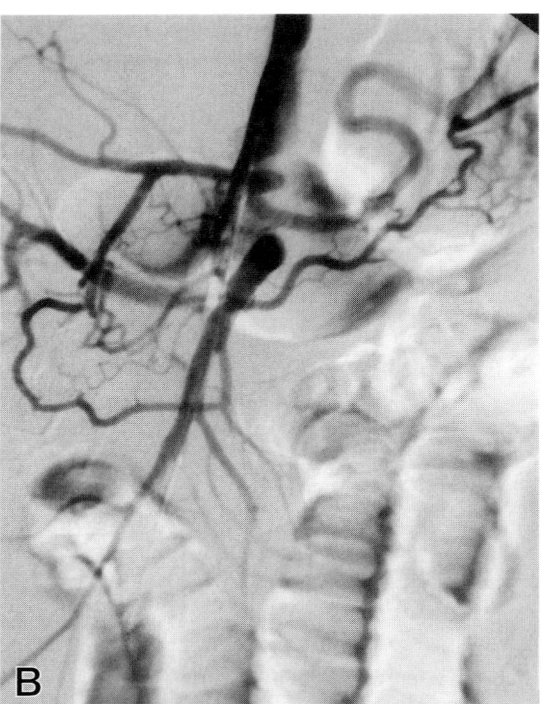

FIGURE 49–6 (A) Intravenous contrast enhanced CT scan of the upper abdomen demonstrating an aortic dissection with severe compression of the true lumen and compromise of perfusion of the celiac axis. (B) Abdominal aortogram in anteroposterior projection showing effacement of the true lumen with no true lumen perfusion below the level of the superior mesenteric artery. (C) CT scan of the abdomen after stent graft implantation into the true lumen in the proximal descending thoracic aorta. Coverage of the primary intimal tear has redirected flow into the true lumen, resulting in expansion of the true lumen and improved perfusion of the superior mesenteric artery.

Many unanswered questions remain. For chronic dissections, and for thickening and fibrosis of the septum, the origin of critical branch vessels from both true and false lumens, as well as the presence of multiple true lumen to false lumen communications, would seemingly markedly limit the utility of this stent graft technology. The presence of critical side branches, especially low intercostal arteries arising from the false lumen, or the presence of critical visceral arteries has tempered enthusiasm for endograft insertion into the true lumen because of the risk for ischemic injury. However, should the motivation for stent graft repair become compelling, stent grafting into the true lumen could be performed, and then false lumen flow could be assured or augmented by angioplasty and stenting of septal perforations. There have been some short-term successes in managing aneurysmal expansion of the false lumen. The proximal portion of the descending thoracic aorta seems inordinately disposed toward false lumen dilation, and stent grafts can frequently be placed to cover the primary entry tear in that aortic segment. Although septal fenestrations usually persist at the level of the diaphragm, as well as more distally around the visceral vessel orifices, thrombosis of a proximal aneurysmal dilation of the false lumen has been achieved in a small number of cases. Whether this thrombosis will remain stable over the long term is unknown.

Ten years of experience with endovascular AAA repair has yielded important information regarding the relationship between stent graft design and stent graft performance.[85–88] For example, tapered, flexible, over-the-wire delivery systems (less than 20F in diameter) rarely fail to traverse tortuous iliac arteries. Hooks at the proximal stent graft appear to provide the most secure means of proximal attachment; column strength is of little value. Although modular stent grafts are more versatile than unibody stent grafts, graft-to-graft attachments and overlaps produce unusual stresses and are similarly prone to late failure. Severe stresses are exerted on thoracic grafts at areas of angulation, predisposing to fatigue fractures. Any movement between the stent body and

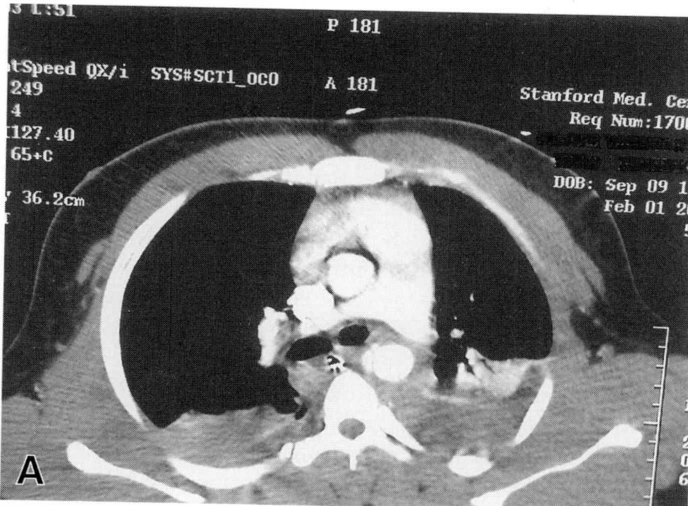

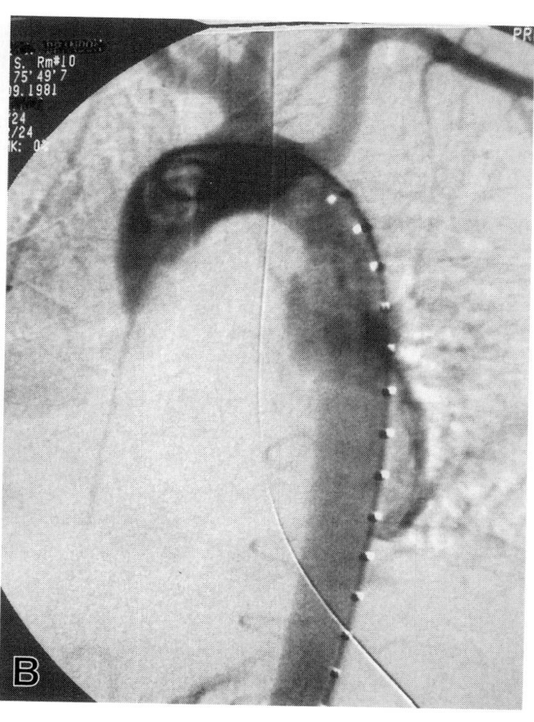

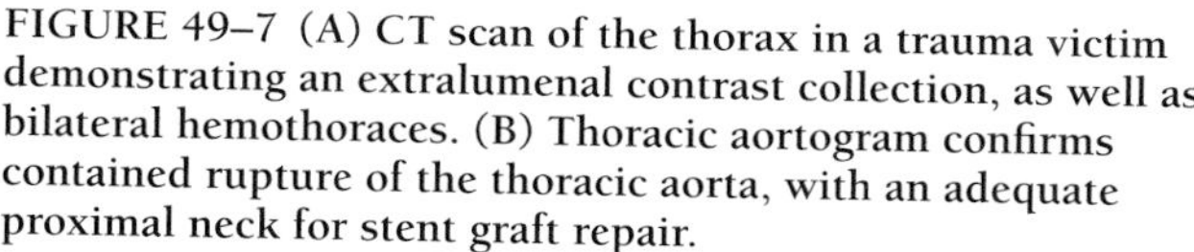

FIGURE 49–7 (A) CT scan of the thorax in a trauma victim demonstrating an extralumenal contrast collection, as well as bilateral hemothoraces. (B) Thoracic aortogram confirms contained rupture of the thoracic aorta, with an adequate proximal neck for stent graft repair.

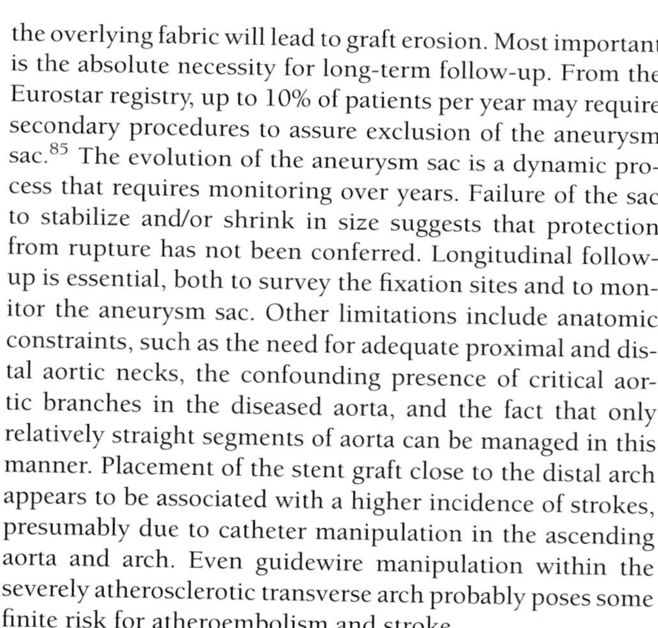

the overlying fabric will lead to graft erosion. Most important is the absolute necessity for long-term follow-up. From the Eurostar registry, up to 10% of patients per year may require secondary procedures to assure exclusion of the aneurysm sac.[85] The evolution of the aneurysm sac is a dynamic process that requires monitoring over years. Failure of the sac to stabilize and/or shrink in size suggests that protection from rupture has not been conferred. Longitudinal follow-up is essential, both to survey the fixation sites and to monitor the aneurysm sac. Other limitations include anatomic constraints, such as the need for adequate proximal and distal aortic necks, the confounding presence of critical aortic branches in the diseased aorta, and the fact that only relatively straight segments of aorta can be managed in this manner. Placement of the stent graft close to the distal arch appears to be associated with a higher incidence of strokes, presumably due to catheter manipulation in the ascending aorta and arch. Even guidewire manipulation within the severely atherosclerotic transverse arch probably poses some finite risk for atheroembolism and stroke.

There are currently no commercially available devices in the United States. Devices under evaluation include the Medtronic Talent, a new iteration of the Gore Excluder, and likely other thoracic stent grafts from the major abdominal stent graft manufacturers. Many of these will likely appear in Europe. In Japan, where this technology has been widely embraced, the vast majority of stent grafts are individually constructed at various centers. The improvements in second- and third-generation devices will likely supplant these devices as they become available. Already, these include lower profile, greater flexibility, increased conformability, and greater ease of insertion and deployment. Whether the perceived advantages of reduced operative time, blood loss, hospital stay, and overall complications and mortality will be confirmed awaits further study. Interestingly, the phase II FDA study of the Gore Excluder included a surgical control arm. Although this was not a randomized surgical cohort, it is the first study to compare results in similar patient populations.

Several authors have reported results of elective stent grafting for Type B aortic dissections using the Talent graft, the Excluder graft, and homemade graft (Fig. 49-6).[63,65,69] Complete coverage of the primary tear was achieved in most instances, and thrombosis of the false lumen was achieved in 70% to 80% of cases. Few complications were noted with the exception of the "postimplantation syndrome," which usually resolved within 4 to 7 days. However, although it is clearly possible to treat type B dissections, more problematic is which patients should be treated. Only further experience, with clear understanding of potential complications and demonstration of long-term durability, will clarify this dilemma.

There is another subset of dissections for which this stent graft technology may have particular utility. For approximately 5% of patients with type A dissections, the primary tear is distal to the left subclavian, with retrograde propagation into the ascending aorta.[78,79] These patients can be quite challenging, as conventional ascending aortic repair leaves the primary intimal tear untouched. Alternatively, proximal descending replacement does not address the dissected ascending aorta. Stent graft coverage of the primary intimal tear has allowed healing of both the ascending and descending aorta.[78,79]

Von Segesser et al have proposed new strategies for the treatment of dissection of the descending thoracic aorta extending back into the ascending aorta such that the dissection should be treated in accordance with the site of the predominant lesion (Fig. 49-7).[89] Replacement of the arch with a variable portion of ascending aorta via median sternotomy is recommended in patients with an enlarged aortic diameter, pericardial effusion, and/or aortic insufficiency. Predominantly distal dissections with a dilated descending thoracic aorta, distal complications, or both are best approached via lateral thoracotomy. Predominantly distal dissection with an almost intact, relatively small ascending aorta, a small aortic arch, and an already thrombosed false ascending aortic lumen is treated in the same manner as type B aortic dissection, in which stent graft repair is an alternative to conventional surgery. Kato et al recently described their experience in 10 type A aortic dissections in which the entry tears were located in the descending thoracic aorta in all cases.[79] Z-stents were placed in the true lumen of the proximal descending thoracic aorta in 9 of 10 patients and in the mid descending thoracic aorta in the remaining patient. Complete closure of the entry tear was achieved at the end of the procedure in all patients and complete thrombosis of the false lumen of the ascending aorta was observed after stent grafting in all patients. No procedure-related complications were observed and, after a mean follow-up of 20 months, no aortic rupture or aneurysm formation was noted. They therefore concluded that stent graft repair of aortic dissection with an entry tear in the descending thoracic aorta is a safe and effective method and may be an alternative to surgical graft replacement in highly selected patients.[79]

These studies have set the stage for randomized trials of stent graft insertion in the treatment of aortic dissection. Both complicated and uncomplicated patients should be randomized, and long-term outcomes assessed. Only then will we know the true utility of this technology.

CONCLUSIONS AND RECOMMENDATIONS

Although impressive results and amazing developments have been achieved in the years since the initial publication of Parodi et al, endograft technology is still in its infancy.[11] Dake's study as well as Nienaber's have been considered milestones in endovascular therapy; they are, however, also starting points.[58–61,63] Device failure and migration and questions about long-term results with respect to endoluminal exclusion and endoleaks constitute the most significant unresolved issues in the field of endograft technology. Refinements in design and improved materials are a certainty in the near future, promising to optimize performance and minimize risks of failure. Further investigations would benefit from longer follow-up and certainly from enrollment of additional patients; an emphasis must be placed on the critical importance of appropriate case selection and the absolute need for lifelong surveillance after endovascular thoracic aorta repair.

It should be emphasized that these patients with thoracic aortic disease represent multidisciplinary efforts involving both surgeons and radiologists. Stent graft placement requires state of the art imaging technology as well as precise manipulation of catheters and positioning of the stent. Aortic dissection remains a surgical disease; even in the context of catheter-based treatment, the management of aortic dissection and its complications requires seasoned judgment and, in some cases, surgical intervention on an urgent basis. Accordingly, surgical specialists must remain involved in the treatment of aortic dissection, irrespective of the type of treatment.

REFERENCES

1. Swan H, Maaske C, Johnson M, Grover R: Arterial homografts, II: resection of thoracic aortic aneurysm using a stored human arterial transplant. *Arch Surg* 1950; 61:732.
2. Lam CR, Aram HH: Resection of a descending thoracic aorta for aneurysm: a report of the use of a homograft in a case and an experimental study. *Ann Surg* 1951; 134:743.
3. DeBakey ME, Cooley DA: Successful resection of aneurysm of thoracic aorta and replacement by graft. *JAMA* 1953; 152:673.
4. Cooley DA, DeBakey ME: Resection of entire ascending aorta in fusiform aneurysm using cardiac bypass. *JAMA* 1956; 162:1158.
5. Gillum RF: Epidemiology of aortic aneurysm in the United States. *J Clin Epidemiol* 1995; 48:1289.
6. Hagan PG, Nienaber CA, Isselbacher EM, et al: The International Registry of Acute Aortic Dissection: new insights into an old disease. *JAMA* 2000; 283:897.
7. Bickerstaff LK, Pairolero PC, Hollier LH, et al: Thoracic aortic aneurysms: a population-based study. *Surgery* 1992; 92:1103.
8. Lawrence DD, Charnsangavej C, Wright KC, Gianturco C: Percutaneous endovascular graft: experimental evaluation. *Radiology* 1987; 163:357.
9. Palmaz JC, Sibbit RR, Tio FO, et al: Expandable intraluminal vascular graft: a feasibility study. *Surgery* 1986; 99:199.
10. Ruiz CE, Zhang HP, Douglas JT, et al: A novel method for treatment of abdominal aortic aneurysms using percutaneous implantation of a newly designed endovascular device. *Circulation* 1995; 91:2470.
11. Parodi JC, Palmaz JC, Barone HD: Transfemoral intraluminal graft implantation for abdominal aortic aneurysms. *Ann Vasc Surg* 1991; 5:491.
12. Chuter TAM: Stent-graft design: the good, the bad and the ugly. *Cardiovasc Surg* 2002; 10:7.
13. Fann JI, Miller DC: Endovascular treatment of descending thoracic aortic aneurysms and dissection. *Surg Clin North Am* 1999; 79:551.
14. Coady MA, Rizzo JA, Goldstein LJ, Elefteriades JA: Natural history, pathogenesis, and etiology of thoracic aortic aneurysms and dissections. *Cardiol Clin North Am* 1999; 17:615.
15. Svensjo S, Bengtsson H, Bergquist D, et al: Thoracic and thoracoabdoimnal aortic aneurysm and dissection: an investigation based on autopsy. *Br J Surg* 1996; 83:68.
16. Pressler V, McNamara JJ: Thoracic aortic aneurysm. *J Thorac Cardiovasc Surg* 1980; 79:489.

17. Clouse WD, Hallett JW, Schaff HV, et al: Improved prognosis of thoracic aortic aneurysms: a population-based study. *JAMA* 1998; 280:1926.
18. Coady MA, Rizzo JA, Elefteriades JA: Developing surgical intervention criteria for thoracic aortic aneurysms. *Cardiol Clin North Am* 1999; 17:827.
19. Davies RR, Goldstein LJ, Coady MA, et al: Yearly rupture or dissection rates for thoracic aortic aneurysms: simple prediction based on size. *Ann Thorac Surg* 2002; 73:17.
20. Coady MA, Rizzo JA, Hammond GL, et al: What is the appropriate size criterion for resection of thoracic aortic aneurysms? *J Thorac Cardiovasc Surg* 1997; 113: 476.
21. Harris JA, Bis KG, Glover JL, et al: Penetrating atherosclerotic ulcers of the aorta. *J Vasc Surg* 1994; 19:90.
22. Coady MA, Rizzo JA, Hammond GL, et al: Penetrating ulcer of the thoracic aorta: What is it? How do we recognize it? How do we manage it? *J Vasc Surg* 1998; 27:1006.
23. Muluk SC, Kaufman JA, Torchiana DF, et al: Diagnosis and treatment of thoracic aortic intramural hematoma. *J Vasc Surg* 1996; 24:1022.
24. Lui RC, Menkis AH, McKenzie FN: Aortic dissection without intimal rupture: diagnosis and management. *Ann Thorac Surg* 1992; 53:886.
25. Coady MA, Rizzo JA, Elefteriades JA: Pathologic variants of thoracic aortic dissections. penetrating atherosclerotic ulcers and intramural hematomas. *Cardiol Clin North Am* 1999; 17:637.
26. Troxler M, Mavor AID, Homer-Vanniasinkam S: Penetrating atherosclerotic ulcers of the aorta. *Br J Surg* 2001; 88:1169.
27. Nienaber CA, von Kodolitsch Y, Petersen B, et al: Intramural hemorrhage of the thoracic aorta: diagnostic and therapeutic implications. *Circulation* 1995; 92:1465.
28. Song JK, Kim HS, Kang DH, et al: Different clinical features of aortic intramural hematoma versus dissection involving the ascending aorta. *J Am Coll Cardiol* 2001; 37:1604.
29. Elefteriades JA, Hartleroad J, Gusberg RJ, et al: Long-term experience with descending aortic dissection: the complication-specific approach. *Ann Thorac Surg* 1992; 53:11.
30. Glower DD, Fann JI, Speier RH, et al: Comparison of medical and surgical therapy for uncomplicated descending aortic dissection. *Circulation* 1990; 82:39.
31. Elefteriades JA, Lovoulos CJ, Coady MA, et al: Management of descending aortic dissection. *Ann Thorac Surg* 1999; 67:2002.
32. Nguyen BT: Computed tomography diagnosis of thoracic aortic aneurysms. *Semin Roentgenol* 2001; 36:309.
33. Crawford ES, DeNatale RW: Thoracoabdominal aortic aneurysm: observations regarding the natural course of the disease. *J Vasc Surg* 1986; 3:578.
34. Griepp RB, Ergin MA, Lansman SL, et al: The natural history of thoracic aortic aneurysms. *Semin Thorac Cardiovasc Surg* 1991; 3:258.
35. Crawford ES, Crawford JS: *Diseases of the Aorta*. Baltimore, Williams & Wilkins, 1984; p 61.
36. Dapunt OE, Galla JD, Sadeghi AM, et al: The natural history of thoracic aortic aneurysms. *J Thorac Cardiovasc Surg* 1994; 107;1323.
37. Jovoenen T, Ergin MA, Galla JD, et al: Prospective study of the natural history of thoracic aortic aneurysms. *Ann Thorac Surg* 1999; 63:551.
38. Crawford ES: Aortic aneurysm: a multifocal disease. *Arch Surg* 1982; 117:1393.
39. Perko MJ, Norgaard M, Herzog TM, et al: Unoperated aortic aneurysm: a survey of 170 patients. *Ann Thorac Surg* 1995; 59:1204.
40. Svensson LG, Crawford ES, Hees KR, et al: Experience with 1509 patients undergoing thoracoabdominal aortic operations. *J Vasc Surg* 1993; 17:357.
41. Crawford ES, Crawford JL, Safi HJ, et al: Thoracoabdominal aortic aneurysm: preoperative and intraoperative factors determining immediate and long-term results of operations in 605 patients. *J Vasc Surg* 1986; 3:389.
42. Svensson LG, Crawford ES, Hess KR, et al: Variables predictive of outcome in 832 patients undergoing repairs of the descending thoracic aorta. *Chest* 1993; 104:1248.
43. Gharagozloo F, Neville RF, Cox JL: Spinal cord protection during surgical procedures on the descending thoracic and thoracoabdominal aorta: a critical overview. *Semin Thorac Cardiovasc Surg* 1998; 10:73.
44. Griepp RB, Ergin MA, Galla JD, et al: Minimizing spinal cord injury during repair of descending thoracic and thoracoabdominal aneurysms: the Mount Sinai approach. *Semin Thorac Cardiovasc Surg* 1998; 10:25.
45. Rokkas CK, Kouchoukos NT: Profound hypothermia for spinal cord protection in operations on the descending thoracic and thoracoabdominal aorta. *Semin Thorac Cardiovasc Surg* 1998; 10:57.
46. Miller DC, Myers BD: Pathophysiology and prevention of acute renal failure associated with thoracoabdominal or abdominal aortic surgery. *J Vasc Surg* 1987; 5:518.
47. Tatou E, Steinmetz E, Jazayeri S, et al: Surgical outcome of traumatic rupture of the thoracic aorta. *Ann Thorac Surg* 2000; 69:70.
48. Richens D, Field M, Neale M, Oakley C: The mechanism of injury in blunt traumatic rupture of the aorta. *Eur J Cardiothorac Surg* 2002; 21:288.
49. Eagle KA, DeSanctis RW: Aortic dissection. *Curr Probl Cardiol* 1989; 14:225.
50. Lansman SL, McCullough JN, Nguyen KH, et al: Subtypes of acute aortic dissection. *Ann Thorac Surg* 1999; 67:1975.
51. Cambria RP, Brewster DC, Gertler J, et al: Vascular complications associated with spontaneous aortic dissection. *J Vasc Surg* 1988; 7:199.
52. Miller DC, Mitchell RS, Oyer PE, et al: Independent determinants of operative mortality for patients with aortic dissections. *Circulation* 1987; 70(suppl I):153.
53. Doroghazi RM, Slater EE, DeSanctis RW, et al: Long-term survival of patients with treated aortic dissections. *J Am Coll Cardiol* 1984; 3:1026.
54. Fann JI, Sarris GE, Mitchell RS, et al: Treatment of patients with aortic dissection presenting with peripheral vascular complications. *Ann Surg* 1990; 212:705.
55. Schor JS, Yerlioglu E, Galla JD, et al: Selective management of acute type b aortic dissection: long-term follow-up. *Ann Thorac Surg* 1996; 61:1339.
56. Lauterback SR, Cambria RP, Brewster DC, et al: Contemporary management of aortic branch compromise resulting from acute aortic dissection. *J Vasc Surg* 2001; 33:1185.
57. Mitchell RS: Endovascular solution for diseases of the thoracic aorta. *Cardiol Clin North Am* 1999; 17:815.
58. Dake MD, Miller DC, Semba CP, et al: Transluminal placement of endovascular stent-grafts for the treatment of descending thoracic aortic aneurysms. *N Engl J Med* 1994; 331:1729.
59. Mitchell RS, Dake MD, Semba CP, et al: Endovascular stent-graft repair of thoracic aortic aneurysms. *J Thorac Cardiovasc Surg* 1996; 111:1054.
60. Dake MD, Miller DC, Mitchell RS, et al: The "first generation" of endovascular stent-grafts for patients with aneurysms of the descending thoracic aorta. *J Thorac Cardiovasc Surg* 1998; 116:689.
61. Mitchell RS, Miller CD, Dake MD, et al: Thoracic aortic aneurysm repair with an endovascular stent graft: the "first generation." *Ann Thorac Surg* 1999; 67:1971.
62. Heijmen RH, Deblier IG, Moll FL, et al: Endovascular stent-grafting for descending thoracic aortic aneurysms. *Eur J Cardiothorac Surg* 2002; 21:5.
63. Nienaber CA, Fattori R, Lund G, et al: Nonsurgical reconstruction of thoracic aortic dissection by stent-graft placement. *N Engl J Med* 1999; 340:1539.

64. Moon MR, Mitchell RS, Dake MD, et al: Simultaneous abdominal aortic replacement and stent-graft placement for multilevel aortic disease. *J Vasc Surg* 1997; 25:332.
65. Sailer J, Peloschek P, Rand T, et al: Endovascular treatment of aortic type b dissection and penetrating ulcer using commercially available stent-grafts. *AJR Am J Roentgenol* 2001; 177:1365.
66. Yoshida H, Yasuda K, Tanabe T: New approach to aortic dissection: development of an insertable aortic prosthesis. *Ann Thorac Surg* 1994; 58:806.
67. Razavi MK, Nishimura E, Slonim S, et al: Percutaneous creation of acute type B aortic dissection: an experimental model for endoluminal therapy. *J Vasc Interv Radiol* 1996; 9:626.
68. Williams DM, Lee DY, Hamilton DH, et al: The dissected aorta: percutaneous treatment of ischemic complications—principles and results. *J Vasc Interv Radiol* 1997; 8:605.
69. Kato N, Hirano T, Shimono T, et al: Treatment of chronic aortic dissection by transluminal endovascular stent-graft placement: preliminary results. *J Vasc Interv Radiol* 2001; 12:835.
70. Dake MD, Kato N, Slonim SM, et al: Endovascular stent-graft placement to obliterate the entry tear: a new treatment for acute aortic dissection. *Circulation* 1998; 98:67.
71. Marty-Anc G, Serres-Cousine O, Laborde JC, et al: Use of endovascular stents for acute aortic dissection: an experimental study. *Ann Vasc Surg* 1994; 8:434.
72. Won JY, Lee DY, Shim WH, et al: Elective endovascular treatment of descending thoracic aortic aneurysms and chronic dissections with stent-grafts. *J Vasc Interv Radiol* 2001; 12:575.
73. Tokui T, Shimono T, Kato N, et al: Less invasive therapy using endovascular stent graft repair and video-assisted thoracoscopic surgery for ruptured acute aortic dissection. *Jpn J Thorac Cardiovasc Surg* 2000; 48:603.
74. Dake MD, Kato NK, Mitchell RS, et al: Endovascular stent-graft placement for the treatment of acute aortic dissection. *N Engl J Med* 1999; 340:1546.
75. Vlahakes GJ: Catheter-based treatment of aortic dissection. *N Engl J Med* 1999; 340:1584.
76. Umana JP, Mitchell RS: Endovascular treatment of aortic dissections and thoracic aortic aneurysms. *Semin Vasc Surg* 2000; 13:290.
77. Fann JI, Miller DC: Endovascular treatment of descending thoracic aortic aneurysms and dissection. *Surg Clin North Am* 1999; 79:551.
78. Kazui T, Tamiya Y, Tanaka T, Komatsu S: Extended aortic replacement for acute type a dissection with the tear in the descending aorta. *J Thorac Cardiovasc Surg* 1996; 112:973.
79. Kato N, Shimono T, Hirano T, et al: Transluminal placement of endovascular stent-grafts for the treatment of type A aortic dissection with an entry tear in the descending thoracic aorta. *J Vasc Surg* 2001; 34:1023.
80. Ergin MA, Phillips RA, Galla JD, et al: Significance of distal false lumen after type A dissection repair. *Ann Thorac Surg* 1994; 57:820.
81. Slonim SM, Miller DC, Mitchell RS, et al: Percutaneous balloon fenestration and stenting for life-threatening ischemic complications in patients with acute aortic dissection. *J Thorac Cardiovasc Surg* 1999; 117:1118.
82. Slonim SM, Nyman U, Semba CP, et al: Aortic dissection: percutaneous management of ischemic complications with endovascular stents and balloon fenestration. *J Vasc Surg* 1996; 23:241.
83. Chavan A, Hausmann D, Dresler C, et al: Intravascular ultrasound-guided percutaneous fenestration of the intimal flap in the dissected aorta. *Circulation* 1997; 96:2124.
84. Inoue K, Sato M, Iwase T, et al: Clinical endovascular placement of branched graft for type B aortic dissection. *J Thorac Cardiovasc Surg* 1996; 112:1111.
85. Blum U, Voshage G, Lammer J, Beyersdorf F, et al: Endoluminal stent-grafts for infrarenal abdominal aortic aneurysms. *N Engl J Med* 1997; 336:13.
86. Zarins CK, White RA, Moll FL, et al: The AneuRx stent graft: four-year results and worldwide experience 2000. *J Vasc Surg* 2001; 33:S135.
87. Parodi JC, Ferreria LM: Ten-year experience with endovascular therapy in aortic aneurysms. *J Am Coll Surg* 2002; 194:S58.
88. Ohki T, Veith FJ, Shaw P, et al: Increasing incidence of midterm and long-term complications after endovascular graft repair of abdominal aortic aneurysms: a note of caution based on a 9-year experience. *Ann Surg* 2001; 234:323.
89. von Segesser LK, Killer I, Ziswiler M, et al: Dissection of the descending thoracic aorta extending into the ascending aorta. *J Thorac Cardiovasc Surg* 1994; 108:755.

Chapter 50

Pulmonary Thromboendarterectomy

Michael M. Madani/Stuart W. Jamieson

Pulmonary thromboendarterectomy (PTE) is the definitive treatment for chronic pulmonary hypertension as the result of thromboembolic disease. Although pulmonary embolism (PE) is one of the more common cardiovascular diseases affecting Americans, pulmonary thromboendarterectomy remains an uncommon procedure, primarily because this form of chronic pulmonary hypertension remains an underdiagnosed condition. These patients may present with a variety of debilitating cardiopulmonary symptoms. However, once diagnosed, there is no curative role for medical management, and surgery remains the only option.

The exact incidence of pulmonary embolism remains unknown, but there are some valid estimates. Acute pulmonary embolism is the third most common cause of death (after heart disease and cancer). Approximately 75% of autopsy-proven PEs are not detected clinically.[1] Dalen[2] calculated that pulmonary embolism results in 630,000 symptomatic episodes in the United States yearly, making it about half as common as acute myocardial infarction, and three times as common as cerebral vascular accidents. This is, however, a low estimate, since in 70% to 80% of the patients in whom the primary cause of death was PE, the diagnosis was unsuspected.[3,4] The disease is particularly common in hospitalized elderly patients. Of hospitalized patients who develop PE, 12% to 21% will die in the hospital, and another 24% to 39% die within 12 months.[5–7] Thus approximately 36% to 60% of the patients who survive the initial episode live beyond 12 months, and may present later in life with a wide variety of symptoms.

More than 90% of clinically detected pulmonary emboli are associated with lower extremity deep vein thrombosis (DVT), but in two thirds of patients with DVT and PE, the DVT is asymptomatic.[8,9] Greenfield estimates that approximately 2.5 million Americans develop DVT each year.[10]

For the most part DVT and acute pulmonary embolisms are managed medically. Cardiac surgeons rarely become involved in hospitalized patients who suffer a massive embolus that causes life-threatening acute right heart failure with low cardiac output. However, the mainstay of treatment for patients with chronic pulmonary thromboembolic disease is the surgical removal of the disease by means of pulmonary thromboendarterectomy. Medical management is only palliative, and surgery by means of transplantation is an inappropriate use of resources with less than satisfactory results.

The prognosis for patients with pulmonary hypertension is poor, and it is worse for those who do not have intracardiac shunts. Thus, patients with primary pulmonary hypertension and those with pulmonary hypertension due to pulmonary emboli fall into a higher risk category than those with Eisenmenger's syndrome, and encounter a higher mortality rate. In fact, once the mean pulmonary pressure in patients with thromboembolic disease reaches 50 mm Hg or higher, the 3-year mortality approaches 90%.[11]

Surgical options are dependent on both the primary disease process and the reversibility of the pulmonary hypertension. With the exception of thromboembolic pulmonary hypertension, lung transplantation is the only effective therapy for patients with pulmonary hypertension when the disease reaches end stage. Pulmonary transplantation is also still used in some centers as the treatment of choice for those with thromboembolic disease. However, a true assessment of the effectiveness of any therapy should take into account the total mortality once the patient has been accepted and put on the waiting list. Thus, the mortality for transplantation (and especially double-lung or heart-lung transplantation) as a therapeutic strategy is much higher than is generally appreciated because of the significant loss of patients awaiting donors. Considering, in addition, the long-term use of antirejection medications with their associated side effects, the higher operative morbidity and mortality, the long waiting time, and inferior prognosis even after transplantation, transplantation is clearly an inferior option to pulmonary thromboendarterectomy. We consider it to be inappropriate therapy for this disease.

DEEP VENOUS THROMBOSIS

Deep venous thrombosis (DVT) primarily affects the veins of the lower extremity or pelvis and rarely affects the venous system elsewhere. The process may involve superficial as well as deep veins, but superficial venous thrombosis does not generally propagate beyond the sapheno-femoral junction and therefore rarely causes PE.[9,12] Venous thrombosis of the upper extremity is almost always associated with trauma, indwelling catheters, or other pathological states and is an uncommon cause of PE, but can be fatal. Pulmonary emboli that do not originate from the deep venous system of the legs and pelvis are thought to come from a diseased right atrium or ventricle or from retroperitoneal and hepatic systems.[12,13]

DVT is most common in hospitalized patients but may occur in ambulatory patients outside the hospital. In recent years improved understanding of the pathogenesis of the disease and better diagnostic tests have identified patients at risk, improved prophylaxis, and increased the percentages of patients who are diagnosed and treated.

Pathology

In careful autopsy studies microscopic thrombi may be found in the pockets of venous valve cusps, in vein saccules, and at vein junctions of pelvic, thigh, and calf veins.[12,14] Calf vein thrombi are most common, and multiple and bilateral thrombi at independent sites within the lower body venous system can occur simultaneously.[12] The initial thrombus grows by accretion of platelets, fibrin, and enmeshed red cells and may detach at any time. Six primary sites of origin of DVT are described: external iliac, common femoral, termination of either the superficial or deep femoral, popliteal, posterior tibial, and intramuscular calf veins.[12] Most calf vein thrombi either do not embolize or produce small often asymptomatic emboli of little clinical significance. However, somewhere between 20% and 30% of calf vein thrombi propagate proximally into upper thigh veins.[9,15] The majority of PEs originate in thigh and pelvic veins.

Thrombi are composed of fibrin, platelets, and usually large numbers of red cells that may form lakes within the clot. In clots that do not embolize, the fibrinolytic system usually dissolves the thrombus. Incomplete dissolution results in the formation of granulation tissue at sites where the thrombus attaches to the vein wall. The organizing thrombus becomes incorporated into the vein wall, but usually destroys the adjacent valve as proliferating vascular channels and fibroblasts invade the site.[14,15]

Pathogenesis

In 1856 Rudolf Virchow made the association between DVT and PE and suggested that the causes of DVT were related to venous stasis, vein wall injury, and hypercoagulopathy. This triad of etiologic factors remains relevant today and is supported by an ever-growing body of evidence.

Injections of contrast material in foot veins require up to 1 hour to clear from venous valves in the soleus muscle of immobilized patients.[16] Venous stasis is also produced by mechanical obstruction of proximal veins, by low cardiac output, by venous dilatation, and by increased blood viscosity.[17] Some pelvic tumors, bulky inguinal adenopathy, the gravid uterus, previous caval or iliac venous disease, and elevated central venous pressures from cardiac causes also enhance venous stasis. Tourniquets, anesthetic agents, pregnancy, high-dose estrogens, and increasing age produce venous dilatation; polycythemia, hyperfibrinogenemia, and some abnormal protein diseases increase the viscosity of blood.[17] It is not clear whether or not superficial varicosities increase the likelihood of DVT in deep veins. However, immobilization is by far the most important cause of venous stasis in hospitalized patients.

The role of vein wall injury is less clear since DVT often begins in the absence of mechanical trauma. Recent work shows that subtle vein wall injuries may occur during operation in veins remote from the operative field.[18,19] In animals,

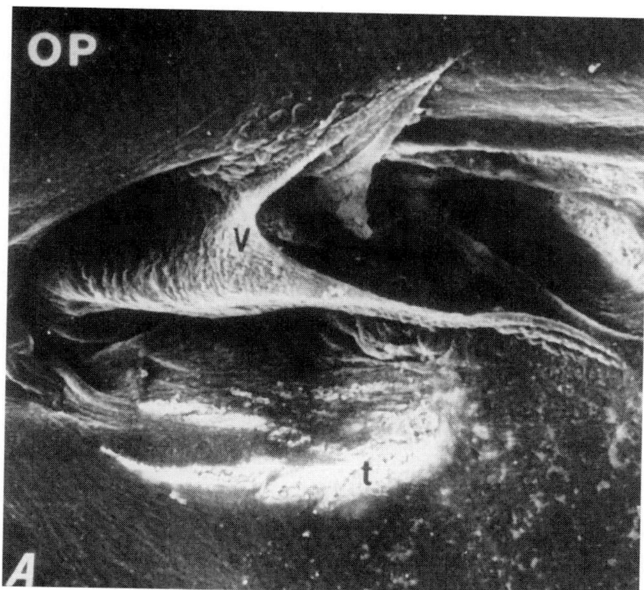

FIGURE 50–1 Scanning electron photomicrograph of a canine jugular vein after total hip replacement with significant operative venous dilatation. An endothelial cell tear (t) is visible near a valve cusp (V). *(Reproduced with permission from Comerota AJ, Stewart GJ, White JV: Combined dihydroergotamine and heparin prophylaxis of postoperative deep vein thrombosis: proposed mechanism of action. Am J Surg 1985; 150:39.)*

endothelial cell tears have been found at junctions of small veins with larger veins at remote sites during sites during hip replacement (Fig. 50-1). The mechanism is thought to be venous dilatation mediated by the production of circulating vasoactive substances, including histamines, bradykinin, activated complement, and the leukotrienes during operation.[20] Exposure of subendothelial tissue factor provides a powerful procoagulant stimulus by activating factor VII and the extrinsic coagulation pathway.[21] The cytokines, interleukin-1 (IL-1), and tumor necrosis factor (TNF) produced by macrophages and other cells in various pathologic conditions stimulate procoagulant activity of endothelial cells. In ways that are still not clear, these processes may combine with venous stasis, microscopic endothelial tears, and blood procoagulant activity to localize the formation of the initial thrombus to venous saccules and valve pockets of the deep leg veins.

Simultaneous maintenance of the fluidity of blood and the integrity of the vascular system requires a balance between blood pro- and anticoagulants. Some patients with DVT have deficiencies in natural anticoagulants. Three uncommon familial deficiencies associated with venous thrombosis are in antithrombin, protein C, and protein S. Antithrombin is a natural plasma protease that inhibits thrombin after it is formed and to a lesser extent before it is formed. Antithrombin is also the cofactor that is accelerated 1000-fold by heparin. Protein C is a potent inhibitor of factor V and platelet-bound factor VII and requires protein S as a cofactor for anticoagulant activity. Both protein C and S are vitamin-K-dependent zymogens that are activated by thrombin and accelerated by thrombomodulin produced by endothelial cells.

A much more common coagulation deficiency, resulting from a mutation of factor V (factor V Leiden) that prevents its degradation by protein C, has been described and is present in approximately 6% to 7% of study populations of Swedes and North American males.[22–24] Both the homozygous and heterozygous mutants are strongly associated with venous thrombosis and pulmonary embolism but are not associated with stroke, myocardial infarction, and other manifestations of arterial thrombosis.[24,25]

Presence of the lupus anticoagulant, which is an acquired IgG or IgM antibody against prothrombinase, increases the likelihood of venous thrombosis by poorly understood mechanisms.[25] The disease may be associated with lupus-like syndromes, immunosuppression, or intake of specific drugs, such as procainamide.

In addition to the three classical risk factors described above, decreased fibrinolytic activity in blood may also contribute to the development of DVT. Fibrinolytic activity is less in leg veins than in arm veins, particularly in older patients.[26] Decreased fibrinolytic activity may be due to decreased production of tissue plasminogen activator (t-PA) or increased concentrations of plasminogen activator inhibitor-1.[27]

Risk Factors for DVT

The presence of major risk factors increases the likelihood of venous thromboembolism in proportion to the number of risk factors present. In patients with clinically suspected DVT, 50% of patients with three risk factors will have a proven diagnosis of DVT; however, without any risk factors DVT is proven in only 11%.[28] The rationale for aggressive prophylactic therapy against the disease is based on the strong association between major risk factors and venous thromboembolism.

Table 50-1 presents a list of major risk factors for the development of DVT or PE. Previous thromboembolism, older age, immobilization for more than one week, orthopedic

TABLE 50–1 Major risk factors for venous thromboembolism

Previous venous thromboembolism
Major hip or knee surgery
Recent major surgery
Congestive heart failure
Pelvis, hip, or leg fracture
High-dose estrogen therapy
Age over 40 years
Bed rest 7 days or longer
Cancer
Paralysis of lower extremity
Multiple trauma

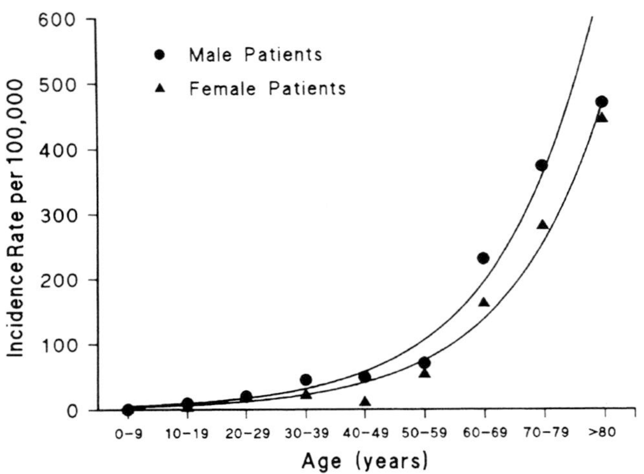

FIGURE 50–2 Annual incidence of venous thromboembolism in the United States stratified for age. Males have a significantly higher incidence rate of venous thromboembolism than females. Both curves fit an exponential function. (*Reproduced with permission from Anderson FA Jr, Wheeler HB, Goldberg RJ, et al: A population based perspective of the hospital incidence and case fatality rates of deep vein thrombosis and pulmonary embolism: the Worcester DVT study. Arch Intern Med 1991; 151:933.*)

surgery of the hip or knee, recent surgery, multiple trauma, and cancer are strong risk factors. In patients with a history of venous thromboembolism the risk of developing a new episode during hospitalization is nearly eight times that of someone without a history.[9,29] Up to 10% of patients with a first episode of DVT or PE and up to 20% of those with a recurrent event develop a new episode of venous thromboembolism within 6 months.[30]

The incidence of DVT and PE increases exponentially with age (Fig. 50-2). Patients in the seventh and eighth decades of life are 200 times more likely to develop venous thromboembolism than patients below age 40. Males are at greater risk than females. Immobility from any cause and prolonged bed rest are major risk factors. Although usually other risk factors are present, the incidence of autopsy-proven venous thrombosis rises from 15% to 80% in patients at bed rest for more than 1 week.[30,31] Surgery, especially orthopedic, abdominal, and multiple trauma, is associated with a significant incidence of DVT and pulmonary embolism. Without prophylaxis the risk of DVT and PE after major abdominal surgery is approximately 25% and 2%, respectively.[8,31] The risk of venous embolism is also increased following urologic surgery and operations for gynecologic cancer.[9] After multiple trauma the risk of DVT and PE is over 50% in patients with pelvic, thigh, or leg injuries.

The incidence of venous thromboembolism increases 3-fold in patients who have operations for cancer.[9] The incidence is highest in patients with advanced or metastatic disease and may be related to the production of procoagulant material or suppression of fibrinolytic activity by some tumors.[9] Patients with congestive heart failure are at higher risk of venous thromboembolism because of venous stasis and higher venous pressures and, if PE occurs, are more likely to die because of reduced cardiac reserve. Acute myocardial infarction may be an independent risk factor for PE, but this is not clear because other risk factors usually are present.[9]

Although the risk of PE is low, women who have just given birth are at higher risk of PE than during pregnancy, and PE remains a major cause of maternal mortality.[17] High-dose estrogen given to treat some malignancies is associated with an increased risk of venous thromboembolism. It is not clear whether oral estrogen contraceptives increase the risk of thromboembolism. Low-dose estrogens, obesity, and varicose veins are probably not independent risk factors for DVT or PE but may be additive.[9]

Of particular interest to cardiac surgeons and cardiologists is the recent observation that clinically silent DVT develops during hospitalization in nearly 50% of patients after myocardial revascularization.[32] Nearly all of the thrombi occur in calf veins and are distributed equally between the saphenous vein donor leg and the opposite extremity. Patients are asymptomatic for DVT and there are no physical clues, but all thrombi in this small series were proven by duplex scanning.[32]

A follow-up study[33] found that the incidence of PE in hospital after coronary arterial bypass operations was 3.2%. Risk factors included prolonged postoperative recovery, previous venous thromboembolism, obesity, and hyperlipidemia. Hospital mortality in patients with PE was 18.7%. Interestingly, valvular surgery was not associated with the development of PE. In a retrospective study of 5694 patients who had open heart surgery, Gillinov et al found the risk of PE proven by V/Q scan (20 patients), angiography (4 patients), or autopsy (8 patients) was 0.56% within 60 days. However, the mortality was 34% in patients with PE.[34]

Diagnosis

Approximately two thirds of patients with DVT do not have clinical symptoms,[9] and thus the diagnosis depends on a high degree of clinical suspicion and a variety of objective diagnostic tests. Venography remains the most reliable test for detecting thrombus in calf veins, but competes with noninvasive tests for detecting DVT in thigh and pelvic veins. Venography, however, is invasive and is not suitable for serial studies, and the contrast material may be thrombogenic if allowed to remain within the deep venous system.[10]

The most popular noninvasive test, which can be done at the bedside, is a combination of ultrasound and color flow Doppler mapping, widely referred to as *duplex scanning*. The method does not detect fresh thrombi directly but infers the presence of clot by flow patterns and the inability to compress the vessel in specific locations.[10] In the hands of skilled examiners, duplex scanning is highly accurate for the detection of thrombus in popliteal, deep femoral, and superficial femoral veins and has a sensitivity between 89% and 100% against venography in symptomatic patients. Diagnostic accuracy is much less in asymptomatic patients for thrombi in these locations and specificity is nearly 100% in both symptomatic and asymptomatic patients.[10,35] Duplex scanning has a sensitivity of 70% for pelvic veins and a specificity of nearly 100% compared to magnetic resonance imaging (MRI).[35] The test is less accurate in the calf and also in patients suspected of recurrent DVT. MRI is a noninvasive method that can image the entire venous system, including upper extremity veins and mediastinum.[36] The method detects flow within the venous system and reliably separates flowing blood from stagnant blood or thrombus.

Impedance plethysmography assesses volume changes in the leg after occlusion of the vein with calf electrodes and a thigh cuff. It is clinically useful in symptomatic patients but has relatively low sensitivity and specificity in asymptomatic patients and those with calf thrombosis.[35] Injection of iodine 125–labeled fibrinogen with subsequent leg scanning is a sensitive test for detecting calf vein thrombus but does not detect iliofemoral vein thrombosis. The combination of these two tests improves sensitivity and specificity, but in most hospitals duplex scanning, venography, and MRI have superseded both tests.

Prophylaxis

The prevalence of DVT, its strong association with PE, and the identification of risk factors in the pathogenesis of the disease provide the basis and rationale for prophylactic measures that are recommended in patients with two or more major risk factors, such as age over 40 years and major surgery.[9] Innocuous measures such as compression stockings probably should be prescribed more often and be used in most nonambulating patients in the hospital. Intermittent pneumatic compression is more expensive and more cumbersome but is effective. Both methods reduce the incidence of DVT after general surgery to approximately 40% of control patients.[9] Low-dose subcutaneous heparin or low molecular weight heparin given once per day reduces the incidence of DVT to approximately 35% and 18% of controls, respectively.[9,31,37] The reduction in PE with subcutaneous standard heparin or low molecular weight heparin is similar.[31,37]

Calf vein DVT that does not propagate has a low risk of PE, and controversy exists as to whether or not these patients should be anticoagulated.[13] Of patients who have DVT without PE diagnosed in the hospital, the probability of clinically diagnosed PE within the next 12 months is 1.7%.[5] If PE occurs, the probability of recurrent PE is 8.0%.[5] Six months of warfarin anticoagulation are recommended for patients who have DVT with or without PE as prophylaxis against recurrent disease.[38]

PULMONARY EMBOLISM

Pathology and Pathogenesis

Partial or complete occlusion of calf or thigh veins reduces the velocity of flow in the more proximal femoral and iliac veins, and enhances the propagation of thrombus toward the direction of the flow. The thrombus is attached to the vein wall at the site of origin, usually does not develop other sites of attachment immediately,[26] and may grow to fill most of the lumen of the vein and extend into the vena cava. The only firm attachment is at the site of origin, usually a venous saccule or venous valve pocket. The degree of organization within the thrombus varies, but recent clots are more likely to migrate than older thrombi that are more firmly attached to the vessel wall.

Detached venous thrombi are carried in the bloodstream through the right heart into the pulmonary circulation. Large thrombi may float as a single embolus or fragment into smaller clots along the way. In autopsy series the percentage of emboli that obstruct two or more lobar arteries (major) ranges between 25% and 67% of all emboli,[39] but this percentage varies with the thoroughness of the examination. The percentage of major emboli is similar and ranges from 30% to 64% in clinical trials based on angiographic data.[40] The majority of pulmonary emboli lodge in the lower lobes,[12] and are slightly more common in the right lung than in the left. Emboli become coated with a layer of platelets and fibrin soon after reaching the lungs.[12]

Simple mechanical obstruction of one or more pulmonary arteries does not entirely explain the often-devastating hemodynamic consequences of major or massive emboli. Humoral factors, specifically serotonin, adenosine diphosphate (ADP), platelet-derived growth factor (PDGF), thromboxane from platelets coating the thrombus, platelet-activating factor (PAF), and leukotrienes from neutrophils are also involved.[41] In animal and early clinical studies serotonin inhibitors, cyproheptadine, and ketanserin partially block constriction of both pulmonary arteries and bronchi associated with pulmonary embolism.[42] Anoxia and tissue ischemia downstream to emboli inhibit endothelium-derived relaxing factor (EDRF) production and enhance release of superoxide anions by activated neutrophils. The combination of these effects contributes to enhanced pulmonary vasoconstriction.[41]

Natural History

The mortality of untreated PE is 18% to 33%, but can be reduced to about 8% if diagnosed and treated.[7,43,44] Seventy-five to ninety percent of patients who die of pulmonary emboli do so within the first few hours of the primary event.[45] It is possible that those who die later do so of recurrent PE. In patients who have sufficient cardiopulmonary reserve and right ventricular strength to survive the initial few hours, autolysis of emboli occurs over the next few days and weeks.[46] On average, approximately 20% of the clot disappears by 7 days, and complete resolution may occur by 14 days.[44,46,47] For many patients, up to 30 days are needed to dissolve small emboli and up to 60 days for massive clots.[48] As the natural fibrinolytic system dissolves the embolic mass, the available cross-sectional area of the pulmonary arterial tree progressively increases, and pulmonary vascular resistance and right ventricular afterload decrease. In the vast majority of patients, pulmonary emboli continue to resolve and thus an immediate interventional therapy, particularly surgical embolectomy, is not necessary for survival except in a minority of patients.

The clot will not lyse in an unknown but small percentage of patients with acute pulmonary embolism, and chronic thromboembolic obstruction of the pulmonary vasculature develops. The reasons for failure of emboli to dissolve are unknown. Patients often are asymptomatic until symptoms of dyspnea, exercise intolerance, or right heart failure develop. Asymptomatic patients may have partial or complete chronic thrombotic occlusion of one or more segmental or lobar arteries. Symptomatic patients usually have over 40% of their pulmonary vasculature obstructed by organized and fresh thrombi.

ACUTE PULMONARY EMBOLISM

Clinical Presentation

Acute pulmonary embolism usually presents suddenly. Symptoms and signs vary with the extent of blockage, the magnitude of the humoral response, and the pre-embolus reserve of the cardiac and pulmonary systems of the patient.[49] Symptoms and signs vary widely, but the clinical diagnosis is often missed or falsely made. Most pulmonary emboli occur without sufficient clinical findings to suggest the diagnosis, and in autopsy series of proven emboli only 16% to 38% of patients were diagnosed during life.[39]

The acute disease is conveniently stratified into minor, major (submassive), or massive embolism on the basis of hemodynamic stability, arterial blood gases, and lung scan or angiographic assessment of the percentage of blocked pulmonary arteries.[40,49,50] Most pulmonary emboli are minor. These patients present with sudden, unexplained anxiety, tachypnea or dyspnea, pleuritic chest pain, cough, and occasionally streak hemoptysis.[39,45,50] Examination may reveal tachycardia, rales, low-grade fever, and sometimes a pleural rub. Heart sounds and systemic blood pressure are often normal; sometimes the pulmonary second sound is increased. Interestingly, less than one third of the patients will have evidence of clinical DVT.[39] Room air arterial blood gases indicate a PaO_2 between 65 and 80 torr and a normal $PaCO_2$ around 35 torr.[50] Pulmonary angiograms show less than 30% occlusion of the pulmonary arterial vasculature.

Major pulmonary embolism is associated with dyspnea, tachypnea, dull chest pain, and some degree of hemodynamic instability manifested by tachycardia, mild to moderate hypotension, and elevation of the central venous pressure.[50] Some patients may present with syncope rather than dyspnea or chest pain. In contrast to massive pulmonary embolism, patients with major embolism (at least two lobar pulmonary arteries obstructed) are hemodynamically stable and have adequate cardiac output.[40] Room air blood gases reveal moderate hypoxia ($PaO_2 < 65$, > 50 torr) and mild hypocarbia ($PaCO_2 < 30$ torr).[50] Echocardiograms may show right ventricular dilatation. Pulmonary angiograms indicate that 30% to 50% of the pulmonary vasculature is blocked; however, in patients with preexisting cardiopulmonary disorders, lesser degrees of vascular obstruction may produce similarly alarming symptoms.

Massive pulmonary embolism is truly life-threatening and is defined as a PE that causes hemodynamic instability.[40] It is sometimes associated with occlusion of more than 50% of the pulmonary vasculature, but may occur with much smaller occlusions, particularly in patients with preexisting cardiac or pulmonary disease. The diagnosis is clinical, not anatomical. Patients develop acute dyspnea, tachypnea, tachycardia, and diaphoresis, and sometimes may lose consciousness. Both hypotension and low cardiac output (<1.8 L/m^2/min) are present. Cardiac arrest may occur. Neck veins are distended, central venous pressure is elevated, and a right ventricular impulse may be present. Room air blood gases show severe hypoxia ($PaO_2 < 50$ torr), hypocarbia ($PaCO_2 < 30$ torr), and sometimes acidosis.[50] Urine output falls; peripheral pulses and perfusion are poor.

Diagnosis

The clinical diagnosis of acute major or massive pulmonary embolism is unreliable and is wrong in 70% to 80% of patients who have angiography subsequently.[49,51] Even in postoperative patients and those with additional major risk factors for DVT, differentiation of major or massive pulmonary embolism from acute myocardial infarction, aortic dissection, septic shock, and other catastrophic states is difficult and uncertain. A plain chest x-ray, an electrocardiogram (ECG), and insertion of a bedside Swan-Ganz catheter may add confirmatory information, but might not necessarily prove the diagnosis.

The chest film may be normal but usually shows some combination of parenchymal infiltrate, atelectasis, and pleural effusion. A zone of hypovascularity or a wedged-shaped pleural-based density raises the possibility of PE. In patients with massive PE and hemodynamic compromise the chest x-ray may actually appear normal. Usually, the ECG shows nonspecific T-wave or RS-T segment changes with PE. A minority of patients with massive embolism (26%) may show evidence of cor pulmonale, right axis deviation, or right bundle branch block.[39] An echocardiogram showing right heart dilatation raises the possibility of major or massive PE. A Swan-Ganz catheter generally shows pulmonary arterial desaturation ($PaO_2 < 25$ torr) but usually does not show pulmonary hypertension over 40 mm Hg because of low cardiac output and cor pulmonale (the unprepared right ventricle cannot generate pulmonary hypertension).

Ventilation-perfusion (V/Q) scans will provide confirmatory evidence, but these studies may be unreliable, since pneumonia, atelectasis, previous pulmonary emboli, and other conditions may cause a mismatch in ventilation and perfusion and mimic positive results. In general, negative V/Q scans essentially exclude the diagnosis of clinically significant PE. V/Q scans usually are interpreted as high, intermediate, or low probability of PE to emphasize the lack of specificity but high sensitivity of the test (Fig. 50-3). Pulmonary angiograms provide the most definitive diagnosis, but collapse of the circulation may not allow time for this procedure, and pulmonary angiograms should not be performed if the patient's circulation cannot be stabilized by pharmacologic or mechanical means. In stable patients, angiograms are associated with a mortality of 0.2%, but similar to a V/Q scan, a normal angiogram will rule out a clinically significant PE.[52,53]

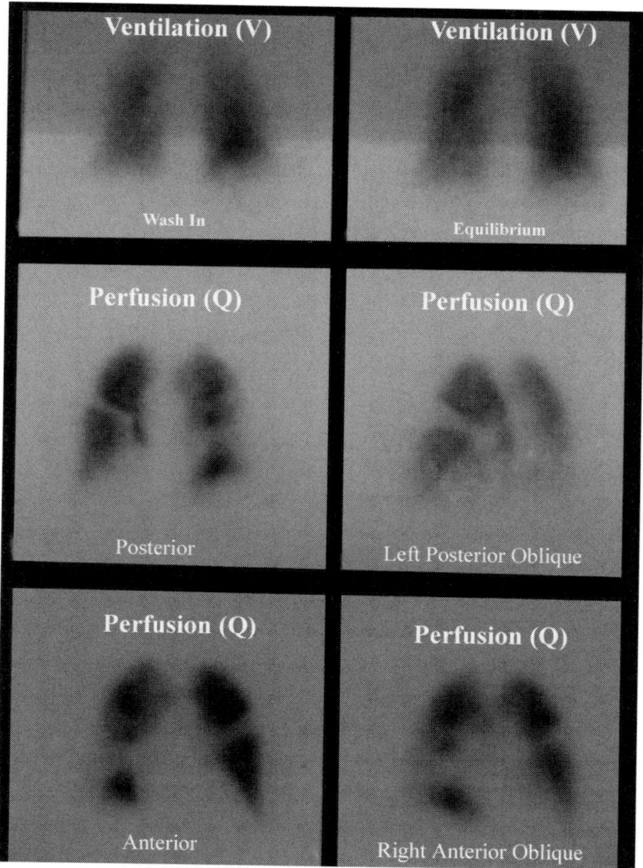

FIGURE 50–3 Anterior and posterior views from a radionuclide perfusion scan in a patient with chronic thromboembolic disease. Note the large punched-out defects.

Magnetic resonance imaging (MRI) is a better noninvasive method for the diagnosis of pulmonary emboli and provides specific information regarding flow within the pulmonary vasculature.[54] Unfortunately, the method is expensive, time consuming, and not widely available. It is thus generally not suitable for hemodynamically unstable patients. Transthoracic (TTE) or transesophageal (TEE) echocardiography with color flow Doppler mapping can provide reliable information about the presence or absence of major thrombi obstructing the main pulmonary artery. More than 80% of patients with clinically significant PE have abnormalities of right ventricular volume or contractility, or acute tricuspid regurgitation by TTE (Fig. 50-4).[55] In some patients abnormal flow patterns can be discerned in major pulmonary arteries during TEE.

Management of Major Pulmonary Embolism

For purposes of this chapter major or submassive pulmonary embolism is defined as an acute episode that causes hypoxia and mild hypotension (systolic arterial pressure >90 mm Hg) but does not cause cardiac arrest or sustained low cardiac output and cardiogenic shock. By definition there is sufficient time in these patients to definitely establish the diagnosis and to attempt pharmacologic therapy and possibly removal of embolic material by catheter suction.

The first priority after sudden collapse of any patient is to establish adequate ventilation and circulation. The first may require intubation and mechanical ventilation. Pharmacologic agents, including cardiovascular pressors and vasoactive agents, are then used to help stabilize the patient's hemodynamics. Once the circulation has been stabilized, both arterial and central venous catheters are placed for access and for continuous pressure monitoring. Usually a Swan-Ganz catheter is also placed to monitor cardiac output and pulmonary arterial oxygen saturation. The ECG is monitored, a Foley catheter is placed for recording urine output, and blood gases are obtained.

If the patient's circulation can be stabilized, intravenous heparin is started with an initial bolus dose of 70 U/kg followed by 18 to 20 U/kg/h if there are no contraindications to heparin. Heparin will prevent propagation and formation of new thromboemboli, but does not dissolve the existing clot. In most instances the patient's own fibrinolytic system lyses fresh thrombi over a period of days or weeks.[46] Heparin is monitored by measurement of activated partial thromboplastin times, which are maintained between 51 and 68 seconds (twice control), every 6 to 8 hours. Platelet counts should be obtained at the beginning of heparin therapy and every 2 to 3 days to detect the presence or appearance of heparin-induced thrombocytopenia. Prothrombin times also are obtained at baseline to prepare for long-term anticoagulation with warfarin later.

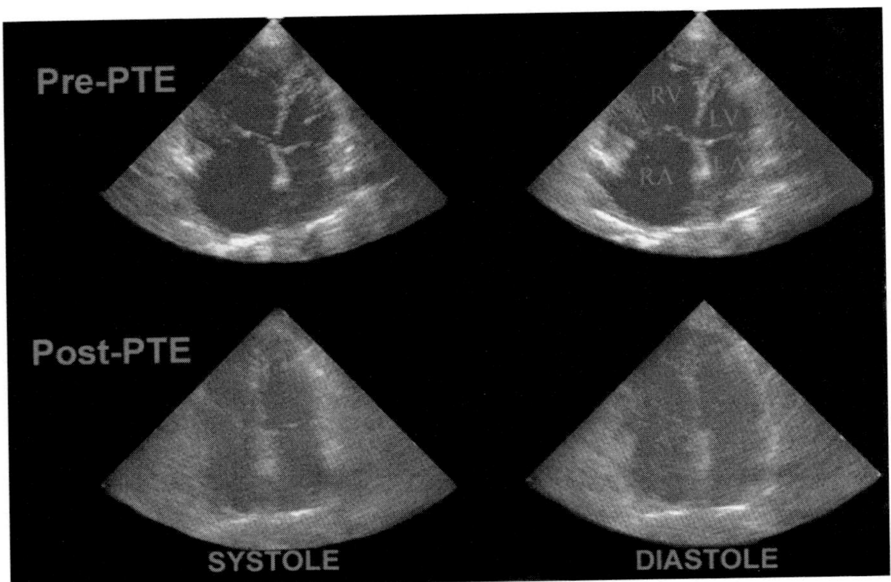

FIGURE 50–4 Appearance of echocardiography before (top) and after (bottom) thromboendarterectomy. Note the shift of the intraventricular septum towards the left in the systole before the operation, together with the relatively small left atrial and left ventricular chambers. After the operation, the septum ahs normalized, and the right-sided chambers are no longer massively enlarged.

The addition of streptokinase, urokinase, or recombinant tissue plasminogen activator (rt-PA) increases the rate of lysis of fresh thrombi and is recommended in patients with a stable circulation and no contraindications. Thrombolytic therapy increases the rate of lysis of fresh pulmonary clots over that of heparin alone during treatment,[56] but there is little difference in the amount of residual thrombus between the two treatments at 5 days or thereafter.[57–60] There is also no statistical difference in mortality or in the incidence of recurrent PE, but more recent experience shows a trend toward better results with thrombolytic therapy because of a more rapid reduction in right ventricular afterload and dysfunction.[56] Furthermore, there are no data that indicate that thrombolysis reduces the subsequent development of chronic pulmonary thromboembolism and pulmonary hypertension. Compared to heparin therapy alone, thrombolytic agents carry a higher risk of bleeding complications. Despite precautions, bleeding complications occur in approximately 20% of patients.[61,62] Contraindications to the use of these agents include patients with fresh surgical wounds, recent stroke, peptic ulcer, or bleeding disorders. Thrombolytics are also contraindicated in severely anemic patients and patients with potential sources of catastrophic intracranial, retroperitoneal, or gastrointestinal bleeding.[56]

Mechanical removal of pulmonary thrombi is possible by a catheter device inserted under local anesthesia into the femoral (preferred) or jugular vein.[63,64] The catheter, which has a small, terminal cup, is steered into the pulmonary artery using fluoroscopy for guidance. Syringe suction is applied to the cup as a thrombus is engaged, and the whole assembly is removed through the venotomy. The procedure may be repeated. Successful extraction of clot with meaningful reduction in pulmonary arterial pressure varies between 61% and 84%.[64]

Management of Massive Pulmonary Embolism

If the circulation cannot be stabilized at survival levels within several minutes or if cardiac arrest occurs after a massive PE, time becomes of paramount importance. Most deaths from acute pulmonary embolism occur before effective treatment is instituted, often as a result of failure of diagnosis. Eleven percent of patients with fatal PE die within the first hour, 43% to 80% within two hours, and 85% within 6 hours.[65] To a great extent, circumstances and the timely availability of necessary equipment and personnel determine therapeutic options. Mitigating factors such as advanced age, irreversible underlying health problems, and the likelihood of brain damage also enter decision making. A decision to treat medically in an effort to stabilize the circulation at a survival level may preempt life-saving surgery, but also may make surgery unnecessary. For many reasons retrospective studies are of limited relevance for this decision. Sometimes surgical treatment is not available immediately; at other times deteriorating patients are referred to surgery too late after failing medical therapy. The relative infrequency of treatment opportunities in massive pulmonary embolism, mitigating factors, and the lack of clear criteria for prescribing medical or surgical therapy leave the management of massive PE unsettled.

Better understanding of the condition and newer technology offer a reasonable, if untried, algorithm for dealing with "probable massive pulmonary embolism with life-threatening hemodynamic instability" in hospitalized patients. In otherwise healthy patients in whom surgery poses little risk of morbidity, emergency thromboembolectomy with preoperative confirmation of the diagnosis in the operating room by transesophageal echocardiography offers the best chance of survival, even though an occasional patient may undergo an unnecessary operation. When surgery is not immediately available, or in patients who may not be surgical candidates or in whom an alternate diagnosis seems more likely, emergency extracorporeal life support (ECLS) using peripheral cannulation is an attractive alternative.[66,67] In prepared institutions ECLS can be instituted rapidly outside the operating room. ECLS compensates for acute cor pulmonale and hypoxia and sustains the circulation until the clot partially lyses, pulmonary vascular resistance falls, and pulmonary blood flow now becomes adequate.

Emergency Pulmonary Thromboembolectomy

Emergency pulmonary thromboembolectomy is indicated for suitable patients with life-threatening circulatory insufficiency, but should not be done without a definitive diagnosis. A clinical diagnosis of PE is often wrong.[47,58,66] If a patient has been taken directly to the operating room without a definitive diagnosis, transesophageal echocardiography and color Doppler mapping can confirm or refute the diagnosis in the operating room.[60,68] Transesophageal echocardiography permits good assessment of right ventricular volume, contractility, and tricuspid regurgitation, which are strongly associated with massive pulmonary embolism and acute cor pulmonale.[58] Echocardiographic detection of a large clot trapped within the right atrium or ventricle is another indication for emergency pulmonary thromboembolectomy.[50,58]

A midline sternotomy incision is used. The ascending aorta and both cavae are cannulated after full heparinization, and cardiopulmonary bypass is initiated. The heart may be electrically fibrillated or arrested with cold cardioplegic solution. Significant hypothermia may not be necessary since only a short period of complete bypass is needed. The main pulmonary artery is then opened 1 to 2 cm downstream to the valve, and the incision is extended into the proximal left pulmonary artery. Forceps and suction catheters remove the clot from the left pulmonary artery and behind the aorta to the right pulmonary artery. The right pulmonary artery can also be exposed and opened between the aorta and superior vena cava to allow better exposure in the distal segments, if necessary. If a sterile pediatric bronchoscope is available, the surgeon can use this instrument to locate and remove thrombi in tertiary and quaternary pulmonary vessels. Alternatively, pleural spaces are entered, and each lung is gently compressed to dislodge small clots into larger vessels and suctioned out. The pulmonary arteriotomy is then closed with a fine running suture (e.g., 6-0 polypropylene). After restarting the heart, the patient is weaned from bypass, decannulated, and closed. Greenfield recommends placement of an inferior vena caval filter before closing the chest.[10,69] European surgeons generally clip the intrapericardial vena cava at the end of pulmonary thromboembolectomy to prevent migration of large clots into the pulmonary circulation.[65] This clip increases venous pressure and stagnant flow in the lower half of the body and causes considerable morbidity in over 60% of patients.[65,70]

Although recurrent PE is always a threat, the likelihood of it occurring during the immediate postoperative period is statistically small. We feel that the diagnosis of proximal DVT, knowledge of risk factors, and efficacy of anticoagulant therapy permit brief deferral of the decision to place a filter. Anticoagulation for 6 months is recommended for most patients with PE, but an inferior vena caval filter is recommended for patients with contraindications to anticoagulation or with recurrent PE, or those who will require pulmonary thromboendarterectomy. The cone-shaped Greenfield filter is most widely used, is associated with a lifetime recurrent embolism rate of 5%, and has 97% patency rate.[71]

Extracorporeal Life Support

The wider availability of long-term extracorporeal perfusion (termed extracorporeal life support, or ELS) using peripheral vessel cannulation to stabilize the circulation offers a compromise position since most massive pulmonary emboli will dissolve in time. ELS can be implemented outside the operating room, but extensive preparations must be made before ELS is available for emergency therapy. An emergency team must be assembled and trained, and needed equipment and supplies must be collected. ELS can be implemented within 15 to 30 minutes by an equipped team of trained personnel.[72]

The femoral vein and artery are rapidly cannulated under sterile conditions using local anesthesia. If the circulation is reasonably stable, both vessels can be cannulated over guidewires inserted via #16 angiographic needle punctures. A small skin incision is made to accommodate the cannulae and, after giving a bolus of heparin (1 mg/kg), first dilators and then cannulae are inserted. Alternatively, surgical cut-down and then cannulation using guidewires under direct vision can expose both femoral vessels. If pulses are absent or weak, a cut-down is usually faster; however, since patients need heparin and possibly fibrinolytic drugs, a minimal wound is preferred. The tip of the venous catheter is advanced into the right atrium to obtain flow rates of 2.5 to 4 L/min using an emergency pump-oxygenator circuit primed with crystalloid.[73] The perfusion circuit consists of a small venous reservoir with intravenous access tubes, a centrifugal pump, and a membrane oxygenator. An arterial filter is not needed, and an electromagnetic flowmeter is usually placed on the arterial line. During ELS, heparin is infused to maintain activated clotting times between 150 and 180 seconds. Activated clotting times are measured every 30 minutes initially and every hour thereafter.

Although the groin wound is minimal, some bleeding occurs. Usually the amount of bleeding is small, but it is often persistent. Theoretically, the addition of thrombolytic drugs accelerates clot lysis and may decrease the duration of ELS; however, these drugs are likely to increase bleeding complications and are not needed once the circulation is stabilized.

An alternative is to give low-dose fibrinolytic therapy directly into the thrombus via a pulmonary arterial catheter. ELS should not be needed beyond a few hours or 1 to 2 days since clot lysis proceeds rapidly. Once pulmonary vascular resistance is adequately reduced, femoral cannulation sites should be closed surgically because of the need for heparin and long-term anticoagulation. ELS should be discontinued in the operating room because vessels should be sutured closed because of the need for heparin and long-term anticoagulation.

Postoperative Care

Postoperative care is not different from care for other patients who require open cardiac surgery. Cardiac output is maintained by pharmacologic means and is usually adequate if the patient can be weaned from cardiopulmonary bypass and has not suffered irreversible myocardial damage. Reperfusion pulmonary edema is not a problem, but renal failure and ischemic brain damage from preoperative periods of inadequate circulation may become apparent. Antibiotics are required, particularly if sterile conditions were compromised in the resuscitation effort.

Results

Mortality rates for emergency pulmonary thromboembolectomy vary widely between 40% and 92%.[66,70,74–77] Results are best if cardiopulmonary bypass is used to support the circulation during pulmonary arteriotomy.[75] The eventual outcome depends largely upon the preoperative condition and circulatory status of the patient. If cardiac arrest occurs and external massage cannot be stopped without ELS, mortality ranges between 45% and 75%, and without cardiac arrest mortality ranges between 8% and 36%.[74,70,77] ELS instituted during cardiac resuscitation is associated with survival rates between 43% and 56%.[74,66] Primary causes of death include brain damage, cardiac failure, bleeding complications, and sepsis. Recurrent embolism is uncommon,[70,78] but approximately 80% of survivors maintain normal pulmonary arterial pressures and exercise tolerance. In these patients postoperative angiograms are normal or show less than 10% obstructed vessels. A minority of patients have 40% to 50% of pulmonary vessels obstructed and have significantly reduced exercise tolerance and pulmonary function.[78]

CHRONIC THROMBOEMBOLIC PULMONARY HYPERTENSION

Incidence

The incidence of pulmonary hypertension caused by chronic pulmonary embolism is even more difficult to determine than that of acute pulmonary embolism. There are more than 500,000 survivors per year of acute symptomatic episodes of acute pulmonary embolization.[79,80] The incidence of chronic thrombotic occlusion in the population depends on what percentage of patients fail to resolve acute embolic material. One estimate is that chronic thromboembolic disease develops in only 0.5% of patients with a clinically recognized acute pulmonary embolism.[79] If these figures are correct and only patients with symptomatic acute pulmonary emboli are counted, approximately 2500 individuals would progress to chronic thromboembolic pulmonary hypertension in the United States each year. However, because many (if not most) patients diagnosed with chronic thromboembolic disease have no antecedent history of acute embolism, the true incidence of this disorder is probably much higher.

Regardless of the exact incidence or the circumstances, it is clear that acute embolism and its chronic relation, fixed chronic thromboembolic occlusive disease, are both much more common than generally appreciated and are seriously underdiagnosed. Houk et al[81] in 1963 reviewed the literature of 240 reported cases of chronic thromboembolic obstruction of major pulmonary arteries and found that only 6 cases had been diagnosed correctly before death. Calculations extrapolated from mortality rates and the random incidence of major thrombotic occlusion found at autopsy would support a postulate that more than 100,000 people in the United States currently have pulmonary hypertension that could be relieved by operation.

Pathology and Pathogenesis

Although most individuals with chronic pulmonary thromboembolic disease are unaware of a past thromboembolic event and give no history of deep venous thrombosis, the origin of most cases of unresolved pulmonary emboli is from acute embolic episodes. Why some patients have unresolved emboli is not certain, but a variety of factors must play a role, alone or in combination.

The volume of acute embolic material may simply overwhelm the lytic mechanisms. The total occlusion of a major arterial branch may prevent lytic material from reaching, and therefore dissolving, the embolus completely. Repetitive emboli may not be able to be resolved. The emboli may be made of substances that cannot be resolved by normal mechanisms (already well-organized fibrous thrombus, fat, or tumor). The lytic mechanisms themselves may be abnormal, or some patients may actually have a propensity for thrombus or a hypercoaguable state. After the clot becomes wedged in the pulmonary artery, one of two processes occurs[82]: (1) the organization of the clot proceeds to canalization, producing multiple small endothelialized channels separated by fibrous septa (i.e., bands and webs), or (2) complete fibrous organization of the fibrin clot without canalization may result, leading to a solid mass of dense fibrous connective tissue totally obstructing the arterial lumen.

In addition, there are other special circumstances. Chronic in-dwelling central venous catheters and pacemaker leads are sometimes associated with pulmonary emboli. More rare causes include tumor emboli; tumor fragments from stomach, breast, and kidney malignancies have also been demonstrated to cause chronic pulmonary arterial occlusion. Right atrial myxomas may also fragment and embolize.

Factors other than the simple hemodynamic consequences of redirected blood flow are probably also involved in this process. For example, after a pneumonectomy, 100% of the right ventricular output flows to one lung, yet little increase in pulmonary pressure occurs, even with follow-up to 11 years.[83] In patients with thromboembolic disease, however, we frequently detect pulmonary hypertension even when less than 50% of the vascular bed is occluded by thrombus. It thus appears that sympathetic neural connections, hormonal changes, or both might initiate pulmonary hypertension in the initially unaffected pulmonary vascular bed. This process can occur with the initial occlusion being in either the same or the contralateral lung.

Regardless of the cause, the evolution of pulmonary hypertension as a result of changes in the previously unobstructed bed is serious because this process may lead to an inoperable situation. Consequently, with our accumulating experience in patients with thrombotic pulmonary hypertension, we have increasingly been inclined towards early operation so as to avoid these changes.

Clinical Presentation

Chronic thromboembolic pulmonary hypertension is an uncommon, frequently under-recognized, but treatable cause of pulmonary hypertension. There are no signs or symptoms specific for chronic thromboembolism. The most common symptom associated with thromboembolic pulmonary hypertension, as with all other causes of pulmonary hypertension, is exertional dyspnea. This dyspnea is out of proportion to any abnormalities found on clinical examination. Like complaints of easy fatigability, dyspnea that initially occurs only with exertion is often attributed to anxiety or being "out of shape." Syncope or presyncope (light-headedness during exertion) is another common symptom in pulmonary hypertension. Generally, it occurs in patients with more advanced disease and higher pulmonary arterial pressures.

Nonspecific chest pains occur in approximately 50% of patients with more severe pulmonary hypertension. Hemoptysis can occur in all forms of pulmonary hypertension and probably results from abnormally dilated vessels distended by increased intravascular pressures. Peripheral edema, early satiety, and epigastric or right upper quadrant fullness or discomfort may develop as the right heart fails (cor pulmonale). Some patients with chronic pulmonary thromboembolic disease present after a small acute pulmonary embolus that may produce acute symptoms of right heart failure. Sometimes hemoptysis occurs. A careful history brings out symptoms of dyspnea on minimal exertion, easy fatigability, diminishing activities, and episodes or angina-like pain or light-headedness. Further examination reveals the signs of pulmonary hypertension.

The physical signs of pulmonary hypertension are the same no matter what the underlying pathophysiology. Initially the jugular venous pulse is characterized by a large A wave. As the right heart fails, the V wave becomes predominant. The right ventricle is usually palpable near the lower left sternal border, and pulmonary valve closure may be audible in the second intercostal space. Occasional patients with advanced disease are hypoxic and slightly cyanotic. Clubbing is an uncommon finding.

The second heart sound is often narrowly split and varies normally with respiration; P2 is accentuated. A sharp systolic ejection click may be heard over the pulmonary artery. As the right heart fails, a right atrial gallop usually is present, and tricuspid insufficiency develops. Because of the large pressure gradient across the tricuspid valve in pulmonary hypertension, the murmur is high-pitched and may not exhibit respiratory variation. These findings are quite different from those usually observed in tricuspid valvular disease. A murmur of pulmonic regurgitation may also be detected.

Pulmonary function tests reveal minimal changes in lung volume and ventilation; patients generally have normal or slightly restricted pulmonary mechanics. Diffusing capacity (DLCO) is often reduced and may be the only abnormality on pulmonary function testing. Pulmonary arterial pressures are elevated and suprasystemic pulmonary pressures are not uncommon. Resting cardiac outputs are lower than the normal range, and pulmonary arterial oxygen saturations are reduced. Most patients are hypoxic; room air arterial oxygen tension ranges between 50 and 83 torr, the average being 65 torr.[84] CO_2 tension is slightly reduced and is compensated by reduced bicarbonate. Dead space ventilation is increased. Ventilation-perfusion studies show moderate mismatch with some heterogeneity among various respirator units within the lung and correlate poorly with the degree of pulmonary obstruction.[85]

Diagnosis

To ensure diagnosis in patients with chronic pulmonary thromboembolism, a standardized evaluation is recommended for all patients who present with unexplained pulmonary hypertension. This workup includes a chest radiograph, which may show either apparent vessel cutoffs of the lobar or segmental pulmonary arteries or regions or oligemia suggesting vascular occlusion. Central pulmonary arteries are enlarged, and the right ventricle may also be enlarged without enlargement of the left atrium or ventricle (Fig. 50-5). However, one should keep in mind that despite these classic findings, a large number of patients might

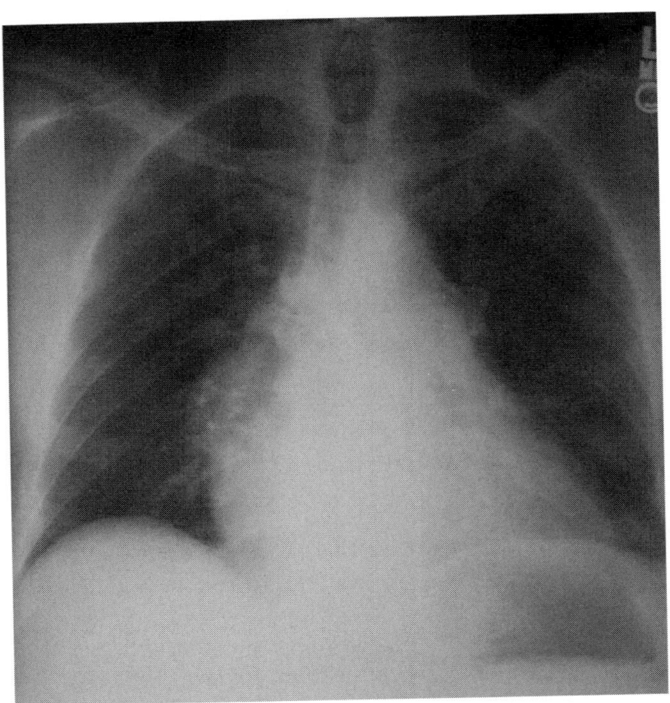

FIGURE 50–5 Chest radiograph of a patient with chronic thromboembolic pulmonary disease and evidence of pulmonary hypertension. Note the enlarged right atrium and right ventricle, disparity of size between the left and right pulmonary arteries, and the hypoperfusion in several areas of the lung fields.

present with a relatively normal chest radiograph, even in the setting of high degrees of pulmonary hypertension. The electrocardiogram demonstrates findings of right ventricular hypertrophy (right axis deviation, dominant R wave in V1). Pulmonary function tests are necessary to exclude obstructive or restrictive intrinsic pulmonary parenchymal disease as the cause of the hypertension.

The ventilation-perfusion lung scan is the essential test for establishing the diagnosis of unresolved pulmonary thromboembolism. An entirely normal lung scan excludes the diagnosis of both acute or chronic unresolved thromboembolism. The usual lung scan pattern in most patients with pulmonary hypertension either is relatively normal or shows a diffuse nonuniform perfusion.[86,87] When subsegmental or larger perfusion defects are noted on the scan, even when matched with ventilatory defects, pulmonary angiography is appropriate to confirm or rule out thromboembolic disease.

Organized thromboembolic lesions do not have the appearance of the intravascular filling defects seen with acute pulmonary emboli, and experience is essential for the proper interpretation of pulmonary angiograms in patients with unresolved, chronic embolic disease. Organized thrombi appear as unusual filling defects, webs, or bands, or completely thrombosed vessels that may resemble congenital absence of the vessel[87] (Fig. 50-6). Organized material along a vascular wall of a recanalized vessel produces a scalloped or serrated lumenal edge. Because of both vessel-wall thickening and dilatation of proximal vessels, the contrast-filled lumen may appear relatively normal in diameter. Distal vessels demonstrate the rapid tapering and pruning characteristic of pulmonary hypertension (Fig. 50-6).

Although some risk remains, the benefit of establishing the presence of a treatable cause of the hypertension far outweighs the small risk; pulmonary angiography should be performed whenever there is a possibility that chronic thromboembolism is the etiology of pulmonary hypertension. Historically, angiography in those with pulmonary

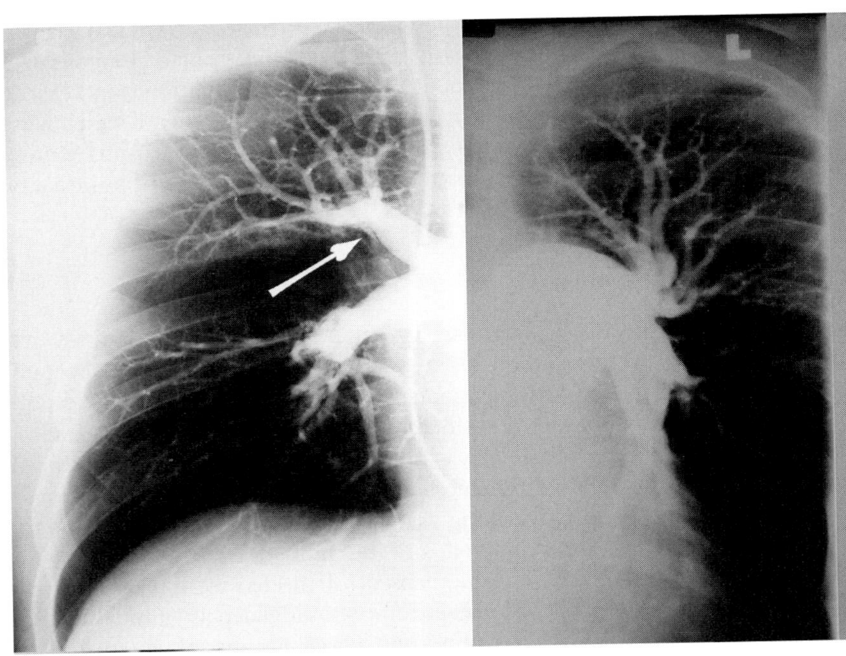

FIGURE 50–6 Right and left pulmonary angiograms demonstrate enlarged pulmonary arteries, poststenotic dilatation of vessels, lack of filling to the periphery in many areas, and abrupt cut-offs of branches. The arrow points to intraluminal filling defects representative of a web or band.

hypertension has been thought to carry disproportionate risk. We have found that not to be the case, and at our institution pulmonary angiographies are performed daily in these patients with minimal associated risks. Several thousand angiograms in pulmonary hypertensive patients have now been performed at our institution without mortality.

In addition to pulmonary angiography, patients over age 35 undergo coronary arteriography and other cardiac investigation as necessary. If significant disease is found, additional cardiac surgery is performed at the time of pulmonary thromboendarterectomy.

In approximately 20% of cases, the differential diagnosis between primary pulmonary hypertension and distal and small-vessel pulmonary thromboembolic disease remains unclear and hard to establish. In these patients, pulmonary angioscopy is often helpful. The pulmonary angioscope is a fiberoptic telescope that is placed through a central line into the pulmonary artery. The tip contains a balloon that is then filled with saline and pushed against the vessel wall. A bloodless field can thus be obtained to view the pulmonary artery wall. The classic appearance of chronic pulmonary thromboembolic disease by angioscopy consists of intimal thickening, with intimal irregularity and scarring, and webs across small vessels. These webs are thought to be the residue of resolved occluding thrombi of small vessels, but are important diagnostic findings. The presence of embolic disease, occlusion of vessels, or the presence of thrombotic material is diagnostic.

Medical Treatment

Chronic anticoagulation represents the mainstay of the medical regimen. Anticoagulation is primarily used to prevent future embolic episodes, but it also serves to limit the development of thrombus in regions of low flow within the pulmonary vasculature. Inferior vena caval filters are used routinely to prevent recurrent embolization. If caval filtration and anticoagulation fail to prevent recurrent emboli, immediate thrombolysis may be beneficial, but lytic agents are incapable of altering the chronic component of the disease.

Right ventricular failure is treated with diuretics and vasodilators, and although some improvement may result, the effect is generally transient[87] because the failure is due to a mechanical obstruction and will not resolve until the obstruction is removed. Similarly, the prognosis is unaffected by medical therapy,[88,89] which should be regarded as only supportive. Because of the bronchial circulation, pulmonary embolization seldom results in tissue necrosis. Surgical endarterectomy therefore will allow distal pulmonary tissue to be used once more in gas exchange.

Natural History

The natural history of chronic thromboembolic pulmonary hypertension is dismal, and nearly all patients die of progressive right heart failure.[90] Because of the insidious onset, the diagnosis is usually made relatively late in the progression of the disease when dyspnea and/or early symptoms of right heart failure develop and pulmonary hypertension is severe (>40 mm Hg mean). In Riedel's series of 13 patients, 9 died a mean of 28 months after the diagnosis of right heart failure.[90] Seven of the 13 had recurrent episodes of fresh emboli demonstrated by new perfusion defects or by autopsy. The severity of pulmonary hypertension at the time of diagnosis inversely correlates with duration of survival.[90]

Pulmonary Thromboendarterectomy

Although there were previous attempts, Allison[91] did the first successful pulmonary "thromboendarterectomy" through a sternotomy using surface hypothermia, but only fresh clots were removed. The operation was 12 days after a thigh injury that led to PE, and there was no endarterectomy. Since then, there have been many occasional surgical reports of the surgical treatment of chronic pulmonary thromboembolism,[92,93] but most of the surgical experience in pulmonary endarterectomy has been reported from the UCSD Medical Center. Braunwald commenced the UCSD experience with this operation in 1970, which now totals more than 1500 cases. The operation described below, using deep hypothermia and circulatory arrest, is now the standard procedure.

INDICATIONS

When the diagnosis of thromboembolic pulmonary hypertension has been firmly established, the decision for operation is made based on the severity of symptoms and the general condition of the patient. Early in the pulmonary endarterectomy experience, Moser et al[93] pointed out that there were three major reasons for considering thromboendarterectomy: hemodynamic, alveolo-respiratory, and prophylactic. The hemodynamic goal is to prevent or ameliorate right ventricular compromise caused by pulmonary hypertension. The respiratory objective is to improve respiratory function by the removal of a large ventilated but unperfused physiologic dead space. The prophylactic goal is to prevent progressive right ventricular dysfunction or retrograde extension of the obstruction, which might result in further cardiorespiratory deterioration or death.[93] Our subsequent experience has added another prophylactic goal: the prevention of secondary arteriopathic changes in the remaining patent vessels.

Most patients who undergo operation are within New York Heart Association (NYHA) class III or class IV. The ages of the patients in our series have ranged from 15 to 85 years. A typical patient will have a severely elevated pulmonary vascular resistance (PVR) level at rest, the absence of significant comorbid disease unrelated to right heart failure, and the appearances of chronic thrombi on angiogram that appear to be in balance with the measured PVR level. Exceptions to this general rule, of course, occur.

Although most patients have a PVR level in the range of 800 dynes/sec/cm-5 and pulmonary artery pressures less than systemic, the hypertrophy of the right ventricle that occurs over time makes pulmonary hypertension to suprasystemic levels possible. Therefore, many patients (perhaps 20% in our practice) have a level of PVR in excess of 1000 dynes/sec/cm-5 and suprasystemic pulmonary artery pressures. There is no upper limit of PVR level, pulmonary artery pressure, or degree of right ventricular dysfunction that excludes patients from operation.

We have become increasingly aware of the changes that can occur in the remaining patent (unaffected by clot) pulmonary vascular bed subjected to the higher pressures and flow that result from obstruction in other areas. Therefore, with the increasing experience and safety of the operation, we are tending to offer surgery to symptomatic patients whenever the angiogram demonstrates thromboembolic disease. A rare patient might have a PVR level that is normal at rest, although elevated with minimal exercise. This is usually a young patient with total unilateral pulmonary artery occlusion and unacceptable exertional dyspnea because of an elevation in dead space ventilation. Operation in this circumstance is performed to reperfuse lung tissue, to reestablish a more normal ventilation/perfusion relationship (thereby reducing minute ventilatory requirements during rest and exercise), and to preserve the integrity of the contralateral circulation.

If not previously implanted, an inferior vena caval filter is routinely placed several days in advance of the operation.

OPERATION

Principles There are several guiding principles for the operation. It must be bilateral because, for pulmonary hypertension to be a major factor, both pulmonary arteries must be substantially involved. The only reasonable approach to both pulmonary arteries is through a median sternotomy incision. Historically, there were many reports of unilateral operation, and occasionally this is still performed, in inexperienced centers, through a thoracotomy. However, the unilateral approach ignores the disease on the contralateral side, subjects the patient to hemodynamic jeopardy during the clamping of the pulmonary artery, and does not allow good visibility because of the continued presence of bronchial blood flow. In addition, collateral channels develop in chronic thrombotic hypertension not only through the bronchial arteries but also from diaphragmatic, intercostal, and pleural vessels. The dissection of the lung in the pleural space via a thoracotomy incision can therefore be extremely bloody. The median sternotomy incision, apart from providing bilateral access, avoids entry into the pleural cavities and allows the ready institution of cardiopulmonary bypass.

Cardiopulmonary bypass is essential to ensure cardiovascular stability when the operation is performed and to cool the patient to allow circulatory arrest. Very good visibility is required, in a bloodless field, to define an adequate endarterectomy plane and to then follow the pulmonary endarterectomy specimen deep into the subsegmental vessels. Because of the copious bronchial blood flow usually present in these cases, periods of circulatory arrest are necessary to ensure perfect visibility. Again, there have been sporadic reports of the performance of this operation without circulatory arrest. However, it should be emphasized that although endarterectomy is possible without circulatory arrest, a complete endarterectomy is not. We always initiate the procedure without circulatory arrest, and a variable amount of dissection (but never complete dissection) is possible before the circulation is stopped. The circulatory arrest periods are limited to 20 minutes, with restoration of flow between each arrest. With experience, the endarterectomy usually can be performed with a single period of circulatory arrest on each side.

A true endarterectomy in the plane of the media must be accomplished. It is essential to appreciate that the removal of visible thrombus is largely incidental to this operation. Indeed, in most patients, no free thrombus is present; on initial direct examination, the pulmonary vascular bed may appear normal. The early literature on this procedure indicates that thrombectomy was often performed without endarterectomy, and in these cases the pulmonary artery pressures did not improve, often with the resultant death of the patient.

Preparation and anesthetic considerations Much of the preoperative preparation is to the same as that for any open heart procedure. Routine monitoring for anesthetic induction includes a surface electrocardiogram, cutaneous oximetry, and radial and pulmonary artery pressures. After anesthetic induction a femoral artery catheter, in addition to a radial arterial line, is also placed. This provides more accurate measurements during rewarming and on discontinuation of cardiopulmonary bypass because of the peripheral vasoconstriction that occurs after hypothermic circulatory arrest. It is generally removed in the ICU when the two readings correlate.

Electroencephalographic recording is performed to ensure the absence of cerebral activity before circulatory arrest is induced. The patient's head is enveloped in a cooling jacket, and cerebral cooling is begun after the initiation of bypass. Temperature measurements are made of the esophagus, tympanic membrane, urinary catheter, rectum, and blood (through the Swan-Ganz catheter). If the patient's condition is stable after the induction of anesthesia, up to 500 mL of autologous whole blood is withdrawn for later use, and the volume deficit is replaced with crystalloid solution.

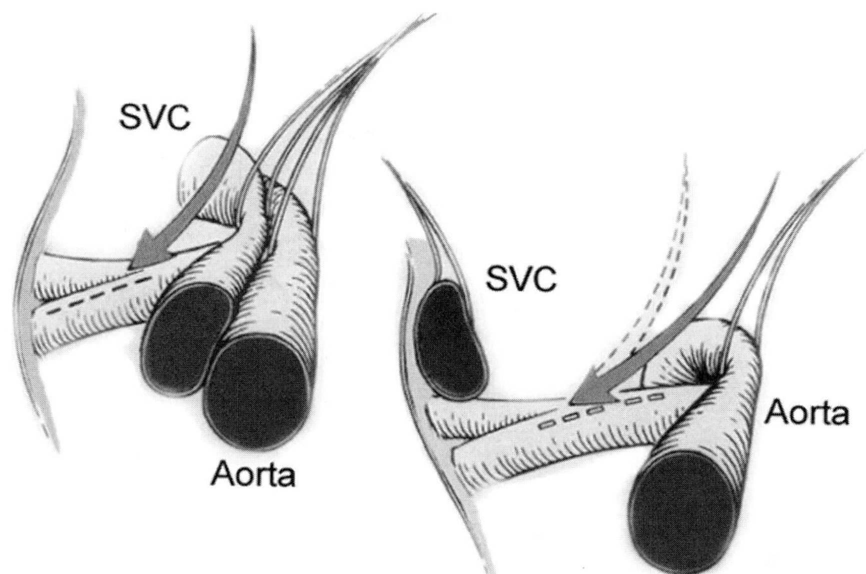

FIGURE 50–7 Recommended surgical approach on the right side. This approach, medial to the superior vena cava (SVC), between the superior vena cava and aorta, provides a direct view into the right pulmonary artery. Note that an approach on the lateral side of the superior vena cava will only provide a restricted view, and should be avoided.

Surgical technique After a median sternotomy incision is made, the pericardium is incised longitudinally and attached to the wound edges. Typically the right heart is enlarged, with a tense right atrium and a variable degree of tricuspid regurgitation. There is usually severe right ventricular hypertrophy, and with critical degrees of obstruction, the patient's condition may become unstable with the manipulation of the heart.

Anticoagulation is achieved with the use of beef-lung heparin sodium (400 U/kg IV) administered to prolong the activated clotting time beyond 400 seconds. Full cardiopulmonary bypass is instituted with high ascending aortic cannulation and two caval cannulae. These cannulae must be inserted into the superior and inferior vena cavae sufficiently to enable subsequent opening of the right atrium. The heart is emptied on bypass, and a temporary pulmonary artery vent is placed in the midline of the main pulmonary artery 1 cm distal to the pulmonary valve. This will mark the beginning of the left pulmonary arteriotomy.

When cardiopulmonary bypass is initiated, surface cooling with both the head jacket and the cooling blanket is begun. The blood is cooled with the pump-oxygenator. During cooling a 10°C gradient between arterial blood and bladder or rectal temperature is maintained.[94] Cooling generally takes 45 minutes to an hour. When ventricular fibrillation occurs, an additional vent is placed in the left atrium through the right superior pulmonary vein. This prevents atrial and ventricular distension from the large amount of bronchial arterial blood flow that is common with these patients.

It is most convenient for the primary surgeon to stand initially on the patient's left side. During the cooling period, some preliminary dissection can be performed, with full mobilization of the right pulmonary artery from the ascending aorta. The superior vena cava is also fully mobilized. The approach to the right pulmonary artery is made medial, not lateral, to the superior vena cava. All dissection of the pulmonary arteries takes place intrapericardially, and neither pleural cavity should be entered. An incision is then made in the right pulmonary artery from beneath the ascending aorta out under the superior vena cava and entering the lower lobe branch of the pulmonary artery just after the take-off of the middle lobe artery (Fig. 50-7). It is important that the incision stays in the center of the vessel and continues into the lower, rather than the middle lobe artery.

Any loose thrombus, if present, is now removed. This is necessary to obtain good visualization. It is most important to recognize, however, that first, an embolectomy without subsequent endarterectomy is quite ineffective, and second, that in most patients with chronic thromboembolic hypertension, direct examination of the pulmonary vascular bed at operation generally shows no obvious embolic material. Therefore, to the inexperienced or cursory glance, the pulmonary vascular bed may well appear normal even in patients with severe chronic embolic pulmonary hypertension.

If the bronchial circulation is not excessive, the endarterectomy plane can be found during this early dissection. However, although a small amount of dissection can be performed before the initiation of circulatory arrest, it is unwise to proceed unless perfect visibility is obtained because the development of a correct plane is essential.

There are four broad types of pulmonary occlusive disease related to thrombus that can be appreciated, and we use the following classification[95–97]: type I disease (approximately

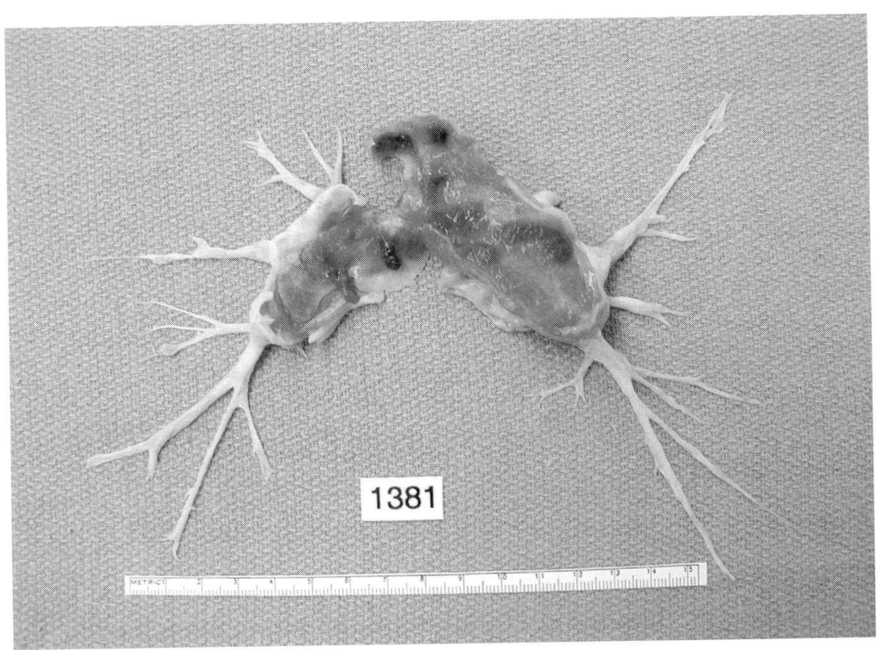

FIGURE 50–8 Surgical specimen removed from a patient showing evidence of some fresh and some old thrombus in the main pulmonary artery. Note that simple removal of the gross disease initially encountered upon pulmonary arteriotomy will not be therapeutic, and any meaningful outcome involves a full endarterectomy into all the distal segments.

20% of cases of thromboembolic pulmonary hypertension; Fig. 50-8) refers to the situation in which major vessel clot is present and readily visible on the opening of the pulmonary arteries. As mentioned earlier, all central thrombotic material has to be completely removed before the endarterectomy. In type II disease (approximately 70% of cases; Fig. 50-9), no major vessel thrombus can be appreciated. In these cases only thickened intima can be seen, occasionally with webs, and the endarterectomy plane is raised in the main, lobar, or segmental vessels. Type III disease (approximately 10% of cases; Fig. 50-10) presents the most challenging surgical situation. The disease is very distal and confined to the segmental and subsegmental branches. No occlusion of vessels can be seen initially. The endarterectomy plane must be carefully and painstakingly raised in each segmental and subsegmental branch. Type III disease is most often associated with presumed repetitive thrombi from indwelling catheters (such as pacemaker wires) or ventriculoatrial shunts. Type IV

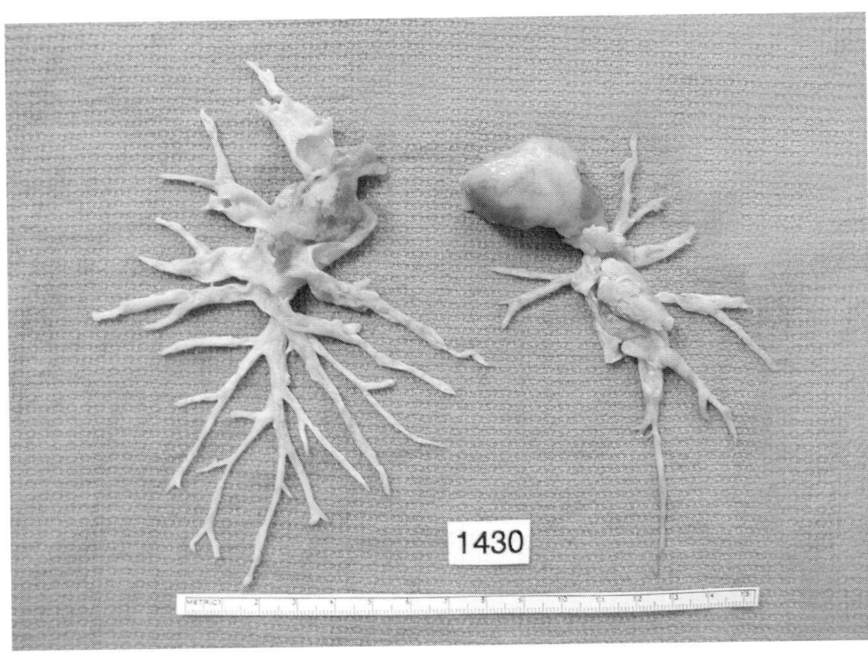

FIGURE 50–9 Specimen removed in a patient with combination of type I and type II disease. The left pulmonary specimen is more representative of type I disease with the central fresh and chronic vessel thrombus, while the right specimen is representative of type II.

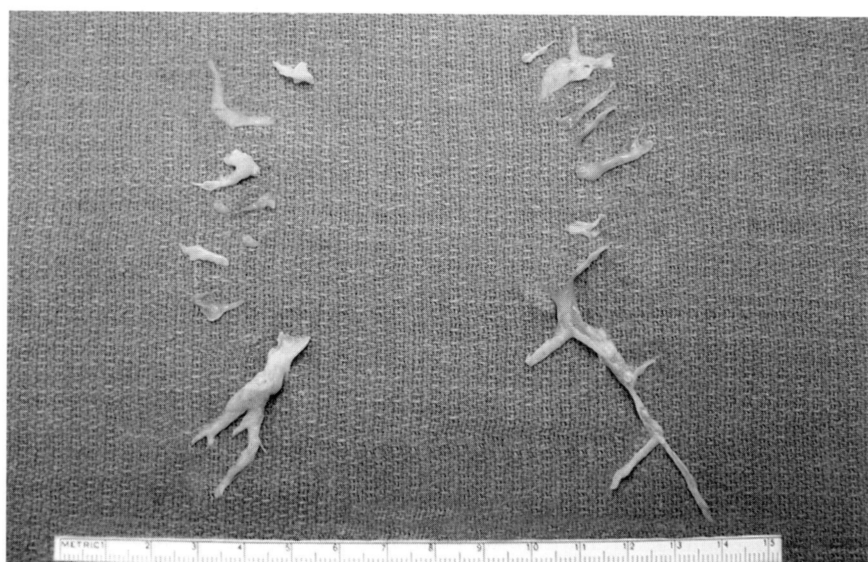

FIGURE 50–10 Specimen removed from a patient with type III disease. Note that the disease is distal, and the plane was raised at each segmental level.

disease (Fig. 50-11) does not represent primary thromboembolic pulmonary hypertension and is inoperable. In this entity there is intrinsic small-vessel disease, although secondary thrombus may occur as a result of stasis. Small-vessel disease may be unrelated to thromboembolic events ("primary" pulmonary hypertension) or occur in relation to thromboembolic hypertension as a result of a high-flow or high-pressure state in previously unaffected vessels similar to the generation of Eisenmenger's syndrome. We believe that there may also be sympathetic "cross-talk" from an affected contralateral side or stenotic areas in the same lung.

When the patient's temperature reaches 20°C, the aorta is cross-clamped and a single dose of cold cardioplegic solution (1 L) is administered. Additional myocardial protection is obtained by the use of a cooling jacket. The entire procedure is now performed with a single aortic cross-clamp period with no further administration of cardioplegic solution.

A modified cerebellar retractor is placed between the aorta and superior vena cava. When blood obscures direct vision of the pulmonary vascular bed, thiopental is administered (500 mg to 1 g) until the electroencephalogram becomes isoelectric. Circulatory arrest is then initiated, and the

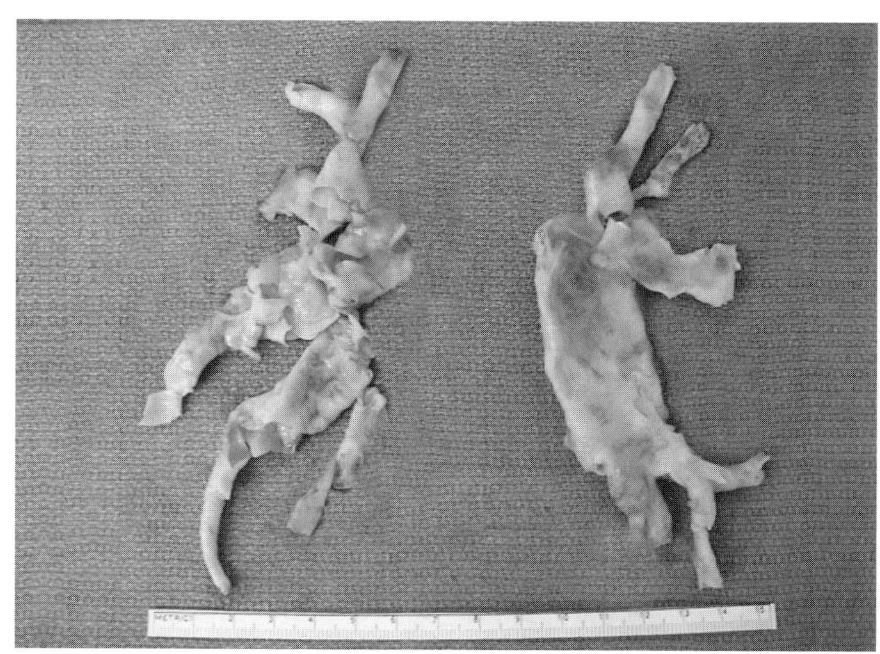

FIGURE 50–11 Note the absence of distal "tails" in this specimen removed from a patient with surgical classification type IV. All "tails" are replaced by "trousers." No clinical benefit was obtained from this procedure and the patient's postoperative hemodynamics were not improved, despite what appears to be an impressive endarterectomy specimen. The patient had primary pulmonary hypertension.

patient undergoes exsanguination. All monitoring lines to the patient are turned off to prevent the aspiration of air. Snares are tightened around the cannulae in the superior and inferior vena cavae. It is rare that more than one 20-minute period is needed for each side. Although retrograde cerebral perfusion has been advocated for total circulatory arrest in other procedures, it is not helpful in this operation because it does not allow a completely bloodless field, and with the short arrest times that can be achieved with experience, it is not necessary.

Any residual loose, thrombotic debris encountered is removed. Then, a microtome knife is used to develop the endarterectomy plane posteriorly, because any inadvertent egress in this site could be repaired readily, or simply left alone. Dissection in the correct plane is critical because if the plane is too deep the pulmonary artery may perforate, with fatal results, and if the dissection plane is not deep enough, inadequate amounts of the chronically thromboembolic material will be removed.

When the proper plane is entered, the layer will strip easily, and the material left with the outer layers of the pulmonary artery will appear somewhat yellow. The ideal layer is marked with a pearly white plane, which strips easily. There should be no residual yellow plaque. If the dissection is too deep, a reddish or pinkish color indicates the adventitia has been reached. A more superficial plane should be sought immediately.

Once the plane is correctly developed, a full-thickness layer is left in the region of the incision to ease subsequent repair. The endarterectomy is then performed with an eversion technique. Because the vessel is everted and subsegmental branches are being worked on, a perforation here will become completely inaccessible and invisible later. This is why the absolute visualization in a completely bloodless field provided by circulatory arrest is essential. It is important that each subsegmental branch is followed and freed individually until it ends in a "tail," beyond which there is no further obstruction. Residual material should never be cut free; the entire specimen should "tail off" and come free spontaneously.

Once the right-sided endarterectomy is completed, circulation is restarted, and the arteriotomy is repaired with a continuous 6-0 polypropylene suture. The hemostatic nature of this closure is aided by the nature of the initial dissection, with the full thickness of the pulmonary artery being preserved immediately adjacent to the incision.

After the completion of the repair of the right arteriotomy, the surgeon moves to the patient's right side. The pulmonary vent catheter is withdrawn, and an arteriotomy is made from the site of the pulmonary vent hole laterally to the pericardial reflection, avoiding entry into the left pleural space. Additional lateral dissection does not enhance intraluminal visibility, may endanger the left phrenic nerve, and makes subsequent repair of the left pulmonary artery more difficult (Fig. 50-12).

The left-sided dissection is virtually analogous in all respects to that accomplished on the right. The duration of circulatory arrest intervals during the performance of the left-sided dissection is subject to the same restriction as the right.

After the completion of the endarterectomy, cardiopulmonary bypass is reinstituted and warming is commenced.

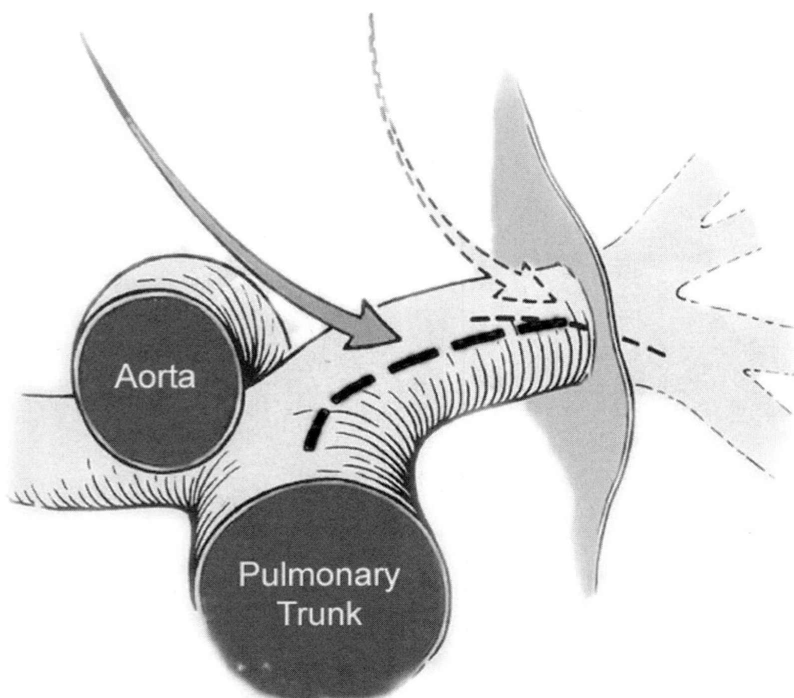

FIGURE 50–12 Surgical approach on the left side. The incision in the left pulmonary artery begins in the midpoint of the main pulmonary trunk, at the insertion site of the pulmonary artery vent. This incision provides better visibility than a more distal approach (dotted line and arrow). Care must be taken to avoid injury to the phrenic nerve.

Methylprednisolone (500 mg IV) and mannitol (12.5 g IV) are administered, and during warming a 10°C temperature gradient is maintained between the perfusate and body temperature. If the systemic vascular resistance level is high, nitroprusside is administered to promote vasodilatation and warming. The rewarming period generally takes approximately 90 minutes but varies according to the body mass of the patient.

When the left pulmonary arteriotomy has been repaired, the pulmonary artery vent is replaced at the top of the incision. The heart is retracted upwards and to the left, and a posterior pericardial window is made, between the aorta and the left phrenic nerve. The right atrium is then opened and examined. Any intra-atrial communication is closed. Although tricuspid valve regurgitation is invariable in these patients and is often severe, tricuspid valve repair is not performed. Right ventricular remodeling occurs within a few days, with the return of tricuspid competence. If other cardiac procedures are required, such as coronary artery or mitral or aortic valve surgery, these are conveniently performed during the systemic rewarming period. Myocardial cooling is discontinued once all cardiac procedures have been concluded. The left atrial vent is removed, and the vent site is repaired. All air is removed from the heart, and the aortic cross-clamp is removed.

When the patient has rewarmed, cardiopulmonary bypass is discontinued. Dopamine hydrochloride is routinely administered at renal doses, and other inotropic agents and vasodilators are titrated as necessary to sustain acceptable hemodynamics. The cardiac output is generally high, with a low systemic vascular resistance. Temporary atrial and ventricular epicardial pacing wires are placed.

POSTOPERATIVE CARE

Meticulous postoperative management is essential to the success of this operation. All patients are mechanically ventilated for at least 24 hours, and all patients are subjected to a maintained diuresis with the goal of reaching the patient's preoperative weight within 24 hours. Although much of the postoperative care is the same as that for other open heart surgery patients, there are some important differences.

The electrocardiogram, systemic and pulmonary arterial and central venous pressures, temperature, urine output, arterial oxygen saturation, chest tube drainage, and fluid balance are monitored. A pulse oximeter is used to continuously monitor peripheral oxygen saturation. Management of cardiac arrhythmias and output and treatment of wound bleeding are identical to other open heart operations. In addition, a higher minute ventilation is often required early after the operation to compensate for the temporary metabolic acidosis that develops after the long period of circulatory arrest, hypothermia, and cardiopulmonary bypass. Tidal volumes higher than those normally recommended after cardiac surgery are therefore generally used to obtain optimal gas exchange. The maximum inspiratory pressure is maintained below 30 cm H_2O if possible.

Although we used to believe that prolonged sedation and ventilation were beneficial and led to less pulmonary edema, subsequent experience has shown this not to be so. Extubation should be performed on the first postoperative day, if possible.

Diuresis Patients have considerable positive fluid balance after operation. After hypothermic circulatory arrest, patients initiate an early spontaneous aggressive diuresis for unknown reasons, but this may, in part, be related to the increased cardiac output related to a now lower PVR level. This should be augmented with diuretics, however, with the aim of returning the patient to the preoperative fluid balance within 24 hours of operation. Because of the increased cardiac output, some degree of systemic hypotension is readily tolerated. Fluid administration is minimized, and the patient's hematocrit level should be maintained above 30% to increase oxygen carrying capacity and mitigate against the pulmonary reperfusion phenomenon.

Arrhythmias The development of atrial arrhythmias, at approximately 10%, is no more common than that encountered in patients who undergo other types of nonvalvular heart surgery. The small, inferior atrial incision, away from the conduction system of the atrium or its blood supply, may be helpful in the reduction of the incidence of these arrhythmias.

Transfusion Despite the requirement for the maintenance of an adequate hematocrit level, transfusion is required in only a few patients if careful blood conservation techniques are used during operation.

Anticoagulation A Greenfield filter is usually inserted before operation, to minimize recurrent pulmonary embolism after pulmonary endarterectomy. However, if this is not possible, it can also be inserted at the time of operation. If the device is to be placed at operation, radiopaque markers should be placed over the spine that correspond to the location of the renal veins to allow correct positioning. Postoperative venous thrombosis prophylaxis with intermittent pneumatic compression devices is used, and the use of subcutaneous heparin is begun on the evening of surgery. Anticoagulation with warfarin is begun as soon as the pacing wires and mediastinal drainage tubes are removed, with a target international normalized ratio of 2.5 to 3.

COMPLICATIONS

Patients are subject to all complications associated with open heart and major lung surgery (arrhythmias, atelectasis, wound infection, pneumonia, mediastinal bleeding, etc.) but also may develop complications specific to this operation.

These include persistent pulmonary hypertension, reperfusion pulmonary response, and neurologic disorders related to deep hypothermia.

Persistent pulmonary hypertension The decrease in PVR level usually results in an immediate and sustained restoration of pulmonary artery pressures to normal levels, with a marked increase in cardiac output. In a few patients, an immediately normal pulmonary vascular tone is not achieved, but an additional substantial reduction may occur over the next few days because of the subsequent relaxation of small vessels and the resolution of intraoperative factors such as pulmonary edema. In such patients, it is usual to see a large pulmonary artery pulse pressure, the low diastolic pressure indicating good runoff, yet persistent pulmonary arterial inflexibility still resulting in a high systolic pressure.

There are a few patients in whom the pulmonary artery pressures do not resolve substantially. We do operate on some patients with severe pulmonary hypertension but equivocal embolic disease. Despite the considerable risk of attempted endarterectomy in these patients, since transplantation is the only other avenue of therapy, there may be a point when it is unlikely that a patient will survive until a donor is found. In our most recent 500 patients, more than one third of perioperative deaths were directly attributable to the problem of inadequate relief of pulmonary artery hypertension. This was a diagnostic rather than an operative technical problem. Attempts at pharmacologic manipulation of high residual PVR levels with sodium nitroprusside, epoprostenol sodium, or inhaled nitric oxide are generally not effective. Because the residual hypertensive defect is fixed, it is not appropriate to use mechanical circulatory support or extracorporeal membrane oxygenation in these patients if they deteriorate subsequently.

The "reperfusion response" A specific complication that occurs in most patients to some degree is localized pulmonary edema, or the "reperfusion response." Reperfusion injury is defined as a radiologic opacity seen in the lungs within 72 hours of pulmonary endarterectomy. This unfortunately loose definition may therefore encompass many causes, such as fluid overload and infection.

True reperfusion injury that directly adversely impacts the clinical course of the patient now occurs in approximately 10% of patients. In its most dramatic form, it occurs soon after operation (within a few hours) and is associated with profound desaturation. Edema-like fluid, sometimes with a bloody tinge, is suctioned from the endotracheal tube. Frank blood from the endotracheal tube, however, signifies a mechanical violation of the blood airway barrier that has occurred at operation and stems from a technical error. This complication should be managed, if possible, by identification of the affected area by bronchoscopy and balloon occlusion of the affected lobe until coagulation can be normalized.

One common cause of the reperfusion pulmonary edema is persistent high pulmonary artery pressures after operation when a thorough endarterectomy has been performed in certain areas, but there remains a large part of the pulmonary vascular bed affected by type IV change. However, the reperfusion phenomenon is often encountered in patients after a seemingly technically perfect operation with complete resolution of high pulmonary artery pressures. In these cases the response may be one of reactive hyperemia, after the revascularization of segments of the pulmonary arterial bed that have long experienced no flow. Other contributing factors may include perioperative pulmonary ischemia and conditions associated with high permeability lung injury in the area of the now denuded endothelium. Fortunately, the incidence of this complication is very much less common now in our series, probably as a result of the more complete and expeditious removal of the endarterectomy specimen that has come with the large experience over the last few years.

Management of the "reperfusion response" Early measures should be taken to minimize the development of pulmonary edema with diuresis, maintenance of the hematocrit levels, and the early use of peak end-expiratory pressure. Once the capillary leak has been established, treatment is supportive because reperfusion pulmonary edema will eventually resolve if satisfactory hemodynamics and oxygenation can be maintained. Careful management of ventilation and fluid balance is required. The hematocrit is kept high (32%-36%), and the patient undergoes aggressive diuresis, even if this requires ultrafiltration. The patient's ventilatory status may be dramatically position sensitive. The FiO_2 level is kept as low as is compatible with an oxygen saturation of 90%. A careful titration of positive end-expiratory pressure is carried out, with a progressive transition from volume-limited to pressure-limited inverse ratio ventilation and the acceptance of moderate hypercapnia. The use of steroids is discouraged because they are generally ineffective and may lead to infection. Infrequently, inhaled nitric oxide at 20 to 40 parts per million can improve the gas exchange. On occasion we have used extracorporeal perfusion support (extracorporeal membrane oxygenator or extracorporeal carbon dioxide removal) until ventilation can be resumed satisfactorily, usually after 7 to 10 days.

Delirium Early in the pulmonary endarterectomy experience (before 1990), there was a substantial incidence of postoperative delirium. A study of 28 patients who underwent pulmonary endarterectomy showed that 77% experienced the development of this complication.[98] Delirium appeared to be related to an accumulated duration of circulatory arrest time of more than 55 minutes; the incidence fell to 11% with significantly shorter periods of arrest time.[99] With the more expeditious operation that has come with our increased experience, postoperative confusion is now encountered no more commonly than with ordinary open heart surgery.

Pericardial effusion Probably because of the lymphatic tissue that is encountered during the dissection of the hilum and the mobilization of the superior vena cava, possibly combined with the diminution of cardiac size that occurs immediately after the operation, we have encountered significant pericardial effusions in several patients. It is now our practice to create a posterior pericardial window at the end of the operation. This has essentially eliminated the problem, and it is much easier to treat the pleural effusion on the left side in the occasional patient who may develop this complication.

RESULTS

More than 1500 pulmonary thromboembolism operations have been performed at UCSD Medical Center since 1970. Most of these cases (over 1300) have been completed since 1990, when the surgical procedure was modified as described earlier in this chapter. The mean patient age in the last 1300 patients was 52 years, with a range of 14 to 85 years. There was a very slight male predominance. In nearly one third of these cases, at least 1 additional cardiac procedure was performed at the time of operation. Most commonly, the adjunct procedure was closure of a persistent foramen ovale or atrial septal defect (26%) or coronary artery bypass grafting (8%).

Hemodynamic results A reduction in pulmonary pressures and resistance to normal levels and a corresponding improvement in pulmonary blood flow and cardiac output are generally immediate and sustained.[99,100] In general, these changes can be assumed to be permanent. Whereas before the operation, more than 95% of the patients were in NYHA functional class III or IV, at 1 year after the operation, 95% of patients remained in NYHA functional class I or II.[100,101] In addition, echocardiographic studies have demonstrated that, with the elimination of chronic pressure overload, right ventricular geometry rapidly reverts toward normal. Right atrial and right ventricular enlargement regresses. Tricuspid valve function returns to normal within a few days as a result of restoration of tricuspid annular geometry after the remodeling of the right ventricle, and tricuspid repair is not therefore part of the operation.

Operative morbidity Severe reperfusion injury was the single most frequent complication in the UCSD series, occurring in 10% of patients. Some of these patients did not survive, and other patients required prolonged mechanical ventilatory support. A few patients were salvaged only by the use of extracorporeal support and blood carbon dioxide removal. Neurologic complications from circulatory arrest appear to have been eliminated, probably as a result of the shorter circulatory arrest periods now experienced, and perioperative confusion and stroke are now no more frequent than with conventional open heart surgery. Early postoperative hemorrhage required reexploration in 2.5% of patients, and only 50% of patients required intra- or postoperative blood transfusion. Despite the prolonged operation, wound infections are relatively infrequent. Only 1.8% experienced the development of sternal wound complications, including sterile dehiscence or mediastinitis.

Deaths In our experience, the overall mortality rate (30 days or in-hospital if the hospital course is prolonged) was 9% for the entire patient group, which encompasses a time span of 30 years. The mortality rate was 9.4% in 1989 and has been 5% to 7% for the more than 1300 patients who have undergone the operation since 1990. In the most recent three years (1999–2001), 378 patients underwent operation, with 17 deaths (4.5%). We generally quote an operative risk of approximately 5%, but some patients predictably fall within a much higher risk. With our increasing experience and many referrals, we continue to accept some patients who, in retrospect, were unsuitable candidates for the procedure (type IV disease). We also accept patients in whom we know that the entire degree of pulmonary hypertension cannot be explained by the occlusive disease detected by angiography but feel that they will be benefited by operation, albeit at higher risk. Residual causes of death are operation on patients in whom thromboembolic disease was not the cause of the pulmonary hypertension (50%) and the rare case of reperfusion pulmonary edema that progresses to a respiratory distress syndrome of long standing, which is not reversible (25%).

LATE FOLLOW-UP

A survey of the surviving patients who underwent pulmonary endarterectomy surgery at UCSD between 1970 and 1995 formally evaluated the long-term outcome.[101] Questionnaires were mailed to 420 patients who were more than 1 year after operation. Responses were obtained from 308 patients. Survival, functional status, quality of life, and the subsequent use of medical help were assessed. Survival after pulmonary thromboendarterectomy was 75% at 6 years or more. Ninety-three percent of the patients were found to be in NYHA class I or II, compared to about 95% of the patients being in NYHA class II or IV preoperatively. Of the working population, 62% of patients who were unemployed before operation returned to work. Patients who had undergone pulmonary endarterectomy scored several quality of life components just slightly lower than normal individuals, but significantly higher than the patients before endarterectomy. Only 10% of patients used oxygen, and in response to the question, "How do you feel about the quality of your life since your surgery?" 77% replied much improved, and 20% replied improved. These data appear to confirm that pulmonary endarterectomy offers substantial improvement in survival, function, and quality of life, with minimal later health care requirements.[101]

CONCLUSION

It is increasingly apparent that pulmonary hypertension caused by chronic pulmonary embolism is a condition that is underrecognized and carries a poor prognosis. Medical therapy is ineffective in prolonging life and only transiently improves the symptoms. The only therapeutic alternative to pulmonary thromboendarterectomy is lung transplantation. The advantages of thromboendarterectomy include a lower operative mortality and excellent long-term results without the risks associated with chronic immunosuppression and chronic allograft rejection. The mortality for thromboendarterectomy at our institution is now in the range of 4.5%, with sustained benefit. These results are clearly superior to those for transplantation both in the short and long term.

Although PTE is technically demanding for the surgeon and requires careful dissection of the pulmonary artery planes and the use of circulatory arrest, excellent short- and long-term results can be achieved. The successive improvements in operative technique developed over the last 4 decades now allow pulmonary endarterectomy to be offered to patients with an acceptable mortality rate and excellent anticipation of clinical improvement. With this growing experience, it has also become clear that unilateral operation is obsolete and that circulatory arrest is essential.

The primary problem remains that this is an underrecognized condition. Increased awareness of both the prevalence of this condition and the possibility of a surgical cure should avail more patients of the opportunity for relief from this debilitating and ultimately fatal disease.

REFERENCES

1. Landefeld CS, Chren MM, Myers A, et al: Diagnostic yield of the autopsy in a university hospital and a community hospital. *N Engl J Med* 1988; 318:1249.
2. Dalen JE, Alpert JS: Natural history of pulmonary embolism. *Prog Cardiovasc Dis* 1975; 17:259.
3. Goldhaber SZ, Hennekens CH, Evens DA, et al: Factors associated with correct antemortem diagnosis of major pulmonary embolism. *Am J Med* 1982; 73:822.
4. Rubinstein L, Murray D, Hoffstein V: Fatal pulmonary emboli in hospitalized patients: an autopsy study. *Arch Intern Med* 1988; 148:1425.
5. Kniffin WD Jr, Baron JA, Barrett J, et al: The epidemiology of diagnosed pulmonary embolism and deep venous thrombosis in the elderly. *Arch Intern Med* 1994; 154:861.
6. Martin M: PHLECO: a multicenter study of the fate of 1647 hospital patients treated conservatively without fibrinolysis and surgery. *Clin Invest* 1993; 71:471.
7. Carson JL, Kelley MA, Duff A, et al: The clinical course of pulmonary embolism. *N Engl J Med* 1992; 326:1240.
8. Clagett GP, Anderson FA Jr, Levine MN, et al: Prevention of venous thromboembolism. *Chest* 1992; 102:391S.
9. Anderson FA Jr, Wheeler HB: Venous thromboembolism; risk factors and prophylaxis, in Tapson VF, Fulkkerson WJ, Saltzman HA (eds): *Clinics in Chest Medicine: Venous Thromboembolism,* vol 16. Philadelphia, WB Saunders, 1995; p 235.
10. Greenfield L: Venous thrombosis and pulmonary thromboembolism, in Schwartz SI (ed): *Principles of Surgery,* 6th ed. New York, McGraw-Hill, 1994; p 989.
11. Trendelenberg F: Uber die operative behandlung der embolie derlungarterie. *Arch Klin Chir* 1908; 86:686.
12. Godleski JJ: Pathology of deep vein thrombosis and pulmonary embolism, in Goldhaber SZ (ed): *Pulmonary Embolism and Deep Venous Thrombosis*. Philadelphia, WB Saunders, 1985; p 11.
13. Moser KM: Venous thromboembolism. *Am Rev Resp Dis* 1990; 141:235.
14. Sevitt S: The structure and growth of valve pocket thrombi in femoral veins. *J Clin Pathol* 1974; 27:517.
15. Philbrick JT, Becker DM: Calf deep vein thrombosis: a wolf in sheep's clothing? *Arch Intern Med* 1988; 148:2131.
16. Kakkar VV, Flan C, Howe CT, Clark MB: Natural history of postoperative deep vein thrombosis. *Lancet* 1969; 2:230.
17. Salzmen EW, Hirsch J: The epidemiology, pathogenesis, and natural history of venous thrombosis, in Colman RW, Hirsch J, Marder VJ, Salzman EW: *Hemostasis and Thrombosis: Basic Principles and Clinical Practice,* 3d ed. Philadelphia, Lippincott, 1994; p 1275.
18. Stewart GJ, Lackman JW, Alburger PD, et al: Intraoperative venous dilation and subsequent development of deep vein thrombosis in patients undergoing total hip or knee replacement. *Ultrasound Med Biol* 1990; 16:133.
19. Comerota AJ, Stewart GJ, Alburger PD, et al: Operative venodilation, a previously unsuspected factor in the cause of postoperative deep vein thrombosis. *Surgery* 1989; 106:301.
20. Comerota AJ, Stewart GJ: Operative venous dilation and its relationship to postoperative deep vein thrombosis, in Goldhaber SZ (ed): *Prevention of Venous Thromboembolism*. New York, Marcel Dekker, 1993; p 25.
21. Weiss HJ, Turitto VT, Baumgartner HR, et al: Evidence for the presence of tissue factor activity on subendothelium. *Blood* 1989; 73;968.
22. Bertina RM, Koeleman BPC, Koster T, et al: Mutation in blood coagulation factor V associated with resistance to activated protein C. *Nature* 1994; 369:64.
23. Svensson PJ, Dahlback B: Resistance to activated protein C as a basis for venous thrombosis. *N Engl J Med* 1994; 330:517.
24. Ridker PM, Hennekens CH, Lindpaintner K, et al: Mutation in the gene coding for coagulation factor V and the risk of myocardial infarction, stroke, and venous thrombosis in apparently healthy men. *N Engl J Med* 1995; 332:912.
25. Feinstein DI: Immune coagulation disorders, in Colman RW, Hirsh J, Marder VJ, Salzman EW: *Hemostasis and Thrombosis: Basic Principles and Clinical Practice,* 3d ed. Philadelphia, Lippincott, 1994; p 881.
26. Robertson BR, Pandolfi M, Nilsson IM: "Fibrinolytic capacity" in healthy volunteers at different ages as studied by standardized venous occlusion of arms and legs. *Acta Med Scand* 1972; 191:199.
27. Prins MH, Hirsh J: A critical review of the evidence supporting a relationship between impaired fibrinolysis and venous thromboembolism. *Arch Intern Med* 1991; 151:1721.
28. Wheeler HB, Anderson FA Jr, Cardullo PA, et al: Suspected deep vein thrombosis: management by impedance plethysmography. *Arch Surg* 1982; 117:1206.
29. Samama MM, Simonneau G, Wainstein JP, et al: SISIUS Study: epidemiology of risk factors of deep vein thrombosis (DVT) of the lower limbs in community practice [abstract]. *Thromb Haemost* 1993; 69:763.
30. Hull R, Hirsh J, Jay R: Different intensities of anticoagulation in the long term treatment of proximal vein thrombosis. *N Engl J Med* 1982; 307:1676.
31. Collins R, Scrimgeor A, Yusuf S, et al: Reduction in fatal pulmonary embolism and venous thrombosis by perioperative

administration of subcutaneous heparin: overview of results and randomized trials in general, orthopedic, and urologic surgery. *N Engl J Med* 1988; 318:1162.
32. Reis SE, Polak JF, Hirsch DR, et al: Frequency of deep vein thrombosis in asymptomatic patients with coronary artery bypass grafts. *Am Heart J* 1991; 122:478.
33. Josa M, Siouffi SY, Silverman AB, et al: Pulmonary embolism after cardiac surgery. *J Am Coll Cardiol* 1993; 21:990.
34. Gillinov AM, Davis EA, Alberg AJ, et al: Pulmonary embolism in the cardiac surgical patient. *Ann Thorac Surg* 1992; 53:988.
35. Burk B, Sostman D, Carroll BA, Witty LA: The diagnostic approach to deep vein thrombosis, in Tapson VF, Fulkkerson WJ, Saltzman HA (eds): *Clinics in Chest Medicine: Venous Thromboembolism,* vol 16. Philadelphia, WB Saunders, 1995; p 253.
36. Evans AJ, Sostman HC, Knelson M, et al: Detection of deep vein thrombosis: a prospective comparison of MR imaging with contrast venography. *Am J Roentgenol* 1993; 161:131.
37. Hirsh J, Levine MN: Low molecular weight heparin. *Blood* 1992; 72:1.
38. Shulman S, Rhedin A-S, Lindmarker P, et al: A comparison of six weeks with six months of oral anticoagulant therapy after a first episode of venous thromboembolism. *N Engl J Med* 1995; 332:1661.
39. Goldhaber SZ: Strategies for diagnosis, in Goldhaber SZ (ed):*Pulmonary Embolism and Deep Vein Thrombosis*. Philadelphia, WB Saunders, 1985; p 79.
40. Hoaglang PM: Massive pulmonary embolism, in Goldhaber SZ (ed); *Pulmonary Embolism and Deep Vein Thrombosis*. Philadelphia, WB Saunders, 1985; p 179.
41. Malik AB, Johnson A: Role of humoral mediators in the pulmonary vascular response to pulmonary embolism, in Weir EK, Reeves JT: *Pulmonary Vascular Physiology and Pathophysiology*. New York, Marcel Dekker, 1989; p 445.
42. Huval WV, Mathieson MA, Stemp LI, et al: Therapeutic benefits of 5-hydroxytryptamine inhibition following pulmonary embolism. *Ann Surg* 1983; 197:223.
43. Barritt DW, Jordan SC: Anticoagulant drugs in treatment of pulmonary embolism: controlled trial. *Lancet* 1960; 1:1309.
44. The urokinase pulmonary embolism trial: a national cooperative study. *Circulation* 1973; 47 (2 suppl): II1.
45. Bell WR, Simon TR. Current status of pulmonary thromboembolic disease: pathophysiology, diagnosis, prevention, and treatment. *Am Heart J* 1982; 103:239.
46. Dalen JE, Banas JS Jr, Brooks HL, et al: Resolution rate of pulmonary embolism in man. *N Engl J Med* 1969; 280:1194.
47. Tow De, Wagner HN: Recovery of pulmonary arterial blood flow in patients with pulmonary embolism. *N Engl J Med* 1967; 276:1053.
48. Dalen JE, Alpert JS: Natural history of pulmonary embolism. *Prog Cardiovasc Dis* 1975; 17:259.
49. Palevsky HI: The problems of the clinical and laboratory diagnosis of pulmonary embolism. *Semin Nucl Med* 1991; 21:276.
50. Greenfield LJ, Proctor MC, Williams DM, Wakefield TW: Longterm experience with transvenous catheter pulmonary embolectomy. *J Vasc Surg* 1993; 18:450.
51. Goodall RJR, Greenfield LJ: Clinical correlations in the diagnosis of pulmonary embolism. *Ann Surg* 1980; 191:219.
52. McCracken S, Bettmen S: Current status of ionic and nonionic intravascular contrast media. *Postgrad Radiol* 1983; 3:345.
53. Novelline RA, Baltarowich OH, Athanasoulis CA, et al: The clinical course of patients with suspect pulmonary embolism and a negative pulmonary arteriogram. *Radiology* 1978; 126:561.
54. Schiebler M, Holland G, Hatabu H, et al: Suspected pulmonary embolism: prospective evaluation with pulmonary MR angiography. *Radiology* 1993; 189:125.
55. Come PC: Echocardiographic evaluation of pulmonary embolism and its response to therapeutic interventions. *Chest* 1992; 101:1515.
56. Goldhaber SZ: Thrombolytic therapy in venous thromboembolism. Clinical trials and current indications, in Tapson VF, Fulkerson WJ, Saltzman HA (eds): *Clinics in Chest Medicine, Venous Thromboembolism,* vol 16. Philadelphia, WB Saunders, 1995; p 307.
57. Marder VJ, Sherry S: Thrombolytic therapy: current status. *N Engl J Med* 1988; 318:1585.
58. Goldhaber SZ, Haire WD, Feldstein ML, et al: Alteplase versus heparin in acute PE; randomized trial assessing right ventricular function and pulmonary perfusion. *Lancet* 1993; 341:507.
59. Tibbutt DA, Davies JA, Anderson JA, et al: Comparison by controlled clinical trial of streptokinase and heparin in treatment of life-threatening PE. *BMJ* 1974: 1:343.
60. Ly B, Arnesen H, Eie H, Hol R: A controlled clinical trial of streptokinase and heparin in the treatment of major PE. *Acta Med Scand* 1978; 203:465.
61. Levine MN: Thrombolytic therapy for venous embolism: complications and contraindications, in Tapson VF, Fulkerson WJ, Saltzman HA (eds): *Clinics in Chest Medicine, Venous Thromboembolism,* vol 16. Philadelphia, WB Saunders, 1995; p 321.
62. Levine M, Hirsh J, Weitz J, et al: A randomized trial of a single bolus dosage regimen of recombinant tissue plasminogen activator in patients with acute PE. *Chest* 1990; 98:1473.
63. Gray JJ, Miller GAH, Paneth M: Pulmonary embolectomy: its place in the management of pulmonary embolism. *Lancet* 1988; 25:1441.
64. Timist J-F, Reynaud P, Meyers G, Sors H: Pulmonary embolectomy by catheter device in massive pulmonary embolism. *Chest* 1991; 100:655.
65. Tapson VF, Witty LA: Massive pulmonary embolism, in Tapson VF, Fulkerson WJ, Saltzman HA (eds): *Clinics in Chest Medicine, Venous Thromboembolism,* vol 16. Philadelphia, WB Saunders, 1995; p 329.
66. Mattox KL, Feldtman RW, Beall AC, De Bakey ME: Pulmonary embolectomy for acute massive pulmonary embolism. *Ann Surg* 1982; 195:726.
67. Boulafendis D, Bastounis E, Panayiotopoulos YP, Papalambros EL: Pulmonary embolectomy: answered and unanswered questions. *Int J Angiol* 1991; 10:187.
68. Kasper W, Meinterz MD, Henkel B, et al: Echocardiographic findings in patients with proved pulmonary embolism. *Am Heart J* 1986; 112:1284.
69. Stewart JR, Greenfield LS: Transvenous vena cava filtration and pulmonary embolectomy. *Surg Clin North Am* 1982; 62:411.
70. Schmid C, Zietlow S, Wagner TOF, et al: Fulminant pulmonary embolism: symptoms, diagnostics, operative technique and results. *Ann Thorac Surg* 1991; 52:1102.
71. Greenfield LJ, Zocco J, Wilk JD, et al: Clinical experience with the Kim-Ray Greenfield vena cava filter. *Ann Surg* 1977; 185:692.
72. Anderson HL III, Delius RE, Sinard JM, et al: Early experience with adult extracorporeal membrane oxygenation in the modern era. *Ann Thorac Surg* 1992; 53:553.
73. Wenger R, Bavaria JB, Ratcliff MB, Edmunds LH Jr: Flow dynamics of peripheral venous catheters during extracorporeal membrane oxygenator (ECMO) with a centrifuge pump. *J Thorac Cardiovasc Surg* 1988; 96:478.
74. Gray HH, Morgan JM, Miller GAH: Pulmonary embolectomy for acute massive pulmonary embolism; an analysis of 71 cases. *Br Heart J* 1988; 60:196.
75. Del Campo C: Pulmonary embolectomy: a review. *Can J Surg* 1985; 28:111.

76. Gulba DC, Schmid C, Borst H-G, et al: Medical compared with surgical treatment for massive pulmonary embolism. *Lancet* 1994; 343:576.
77. Clark DB: Pulmonary embolectomy has a well-defined and valuable place. *Br J Hosp Med* 1989; 41:468.
78. Soyer R, Brunet M, Redonnet JY, et al: Follow-up of surgically treated patients with massive pulmonary embolism, with reference to 12 operated patients. *Thorac Cardiovasc Surg* 1982; 30:103.
79. Benotti JR, Ockene IS, Alpert JS, Dalen JE: The clinical profile of unresolved pulmonary embolism. *Chest* 1983; 84:669.
80. Moser KM, Auger WF, Fedullo PF: Chronic major-vessel thromboembolic pulmonary hypertension. *Circulation* 1990; 81:1735.
81. Houk VN, Hufnnagel CA, McClenathan JE, Moser KM: Chronic thrombosis obstruction of major pulmonary arteries: report of a case successfully treated by thromboendarterectomy and review of the literature. *Am J Med* 1963; 35:269.
82. Dibble JH: Organization and canalization in arterial thrombosis. *J Pathol Bacteriol* 1958; 75:1.
83. Cournad A, Rilev RL, Himmelstein A, Austrian R: Pulmonary circulation in the alveolar ventilation perfusion relationship after pneumonectomy. *J Thorac Surg* 1950; 19:80.
84. Kapitan KS, Buchbinder M, Wagner PD, Moser KM: Mechanisms of hypoxemia in chronic pulmonary hypertension. *Am Rev Respir Dis* 1989; 139:1149.
85. Moser KM, Daily PO, Peterson K, et al: Thromboendarterectomy for chronic, major vessel thromboembolic pulmonary hypertension: immediate and longterm results in 42 patients. *Ann Intern Med* 1987; 107:560.
86. Moser KM: Pulmonary vascular obstruction due to embolism and thrombosis, in Moser KM (ed): *Pulmonary Vascular Disease*. New York, Marcel Dekker, 1979; p 341.
87. Jamieson SW, Kapalanski DP: Pulmonary endarterectomy. *Curr Probl Surg* 2000; 37:165.
88. Dantzker DR, Bower JS: Partial reversibility of chronic pulmonary hypertension caused by pulmonary thromboembolic disease. *Annu Rev Respir Dis* 1981; 124:129.
89. Dash H, Ballentine N, Zelis R: Vasodilators ineffective in secondary pulmonary hypertension. *N Engl J Med* 1980; 303:1062.
90. Reidel M, Stanek V, Widimsky J, Prerovsky I: Long term follow up of patients with pulmonary embolism: late prognosis and evolution of hemodynamic and respiratory data. *Chest* 1982; 81:151.
91. Allison PR, Dunnill MS, Marshall R: Pulmonary embolism. *Thorax* 1960; 15:273.
92. Simonneau G, Azarian R, Bernot F, et al: Surgical management of unresolved pulmonary embolism: a personal series of 72 patients [abstract]. *Chest* 1995; 107:52S.
93. Moser KM, Houk VN, Jones RC, Hufnagel CC: Chronic, massive thrombotic obstruction of the pulmonary arteries: analysis of four operated cases. *Circulation* 1965; 32:377.
94. Winkler MH, Rohrer CH, Ratty SC, et al: Perfusion techniques of profound hypothermia and circulatory arrest for pulmonary thromboendarterectomy. *J Extracorporeal Technol* 1990; 22:57.
95. Jamieson SW: Pulmonary thromboendarterectomy, in Franco KL, Putnam JB (eds): *Advanced Therapy in Thoracic Surgery*. Hamilton, Ontario, BC Decker; 1998; p 310.
96. Levinson RM, Shure D, Moser KM: Reperfusion pulmonary edema after pulmonary artery thromboendarterectomy. *Am Rev Respir Dis* 1986; 134:1241.
97. Wragg RE, Dimsdale JE, Moser KM, Daily PO, et al: Operative predictors of delirium after pulmonary thromboendarterectomy: a model for postcardiotomy syndrome? *J Thorac Cardiovasc Surg* 1988; 96:524.
98. Jamieson SW, Auger WR, Fedullo PF, et al: Experience and results of 150 pulmonary thromboendarterectomy operations over a 29 month period. *J Thorac Cardiovascular Surg* 1993: 106:116.
99. Moser KM, Auger WR, Fedullo PF, Jamieson SW: Chronic thromboembolic pulmonary hypertension: clinical picture and surgical treatment. *Eur Respir J* 1992; 5:334.
100. Fedullo PF, Auger WR, Channick RN, et al: Surgical management of pulmonary embolism, in Morpurgo M (ed): *Pulmonary Embolism*. New York, Marcel Dekker, 1994; p 223.
101. Archibald CJ, Auger WR, Fedullo PF, et al: Long-term outcome after pulmonary thromboendarterectomy. *Am J Respir Crit Care Med* 1999; 160:523.

Chapter 51

Trauma to Great Vessels

Thomas G. Gleason/Joseph E. Bavaria

Eighty-five percent of traumatic injuries to the great vessels in civilian practices are caused by penetrating trauma.[1,2] Fifty-seven percent of penetrating chest injuries are caused by gunshot wounds and 25% by stab wounds.[1,2] These injuries have no distinct pattern of anatomic occurrence but should be approached in a manner consistent with Advanced Trauma Life Support (ATLS) guidelines. Among the remaining 15% of great vessel traumatic injuries, the majority are blunt traumatic aortic ruptures. These injuries should be approached in a uniform manner. One percent of patients presenting with signs of blunt chest trauma will have an aortic injury.[3–5] Vesalius was the first to report on a traumatic injury to the aorta manifesting as a posttraumatic aortic aneurysm in 1557.[6,7] Aortic rupture was a very uncommon injury until travel by motor vehicles increased in the latter half of the 20th century.

The standard reference reporting on traumatic aortic rupture dates to 1958, when Parmley et al reviewed 296 cases from the Armed Forces Institute of Pathology.[6] This injury remains the second leading cause of death from vehicular trauma, representing 15% of motor vehicle–caused deaths.[8–10] Death occurs immediately in 75% to 90% of cases.[6,8–10] Approximately 8% of patients survive more than 4 hours.[6] Those who survive aortic transection typically have two or fewer associated serious injuries, while those who die have four or more serious injuries.[6,10] For example, according to Parmley's original report, 42% of patients with aortic rupture had an associated cardiac injury.[6] The short duration of postaccident survival and the high incidence of fatal associated injuries preclude recovery in most of these patients. Recovery of the select few who survive the first few hours after aortic rupture depends on how they are managed both peri- and intraoperatively.

TRAUMATIC AORTIC DISRUPTION

Incidence

The true incidence of blunt aortic rupture is not known, but based on autopsy series aortic rupture occurs in 12% to 23% of deaths from blunt trauma.[6,11–14] These injuries are primarily caused by motor vehicle accidents or falls. Motor vehicle drivers, passengers, or pedestrians hit by vehicles represent 73% to 92% of all cases.[6,10,11,13,14] Falls causing aortic rupture are typically from greater than 3 m.[6,15–17] Alcohol or other substance abuse is involved in over 40% of motor vehicle accidents.[11,13] Ejection from a vehicle doubles the risk of aortic rupture, and seat belt restraint reduces mortality risk by a factor of four.[11] More recently, aortic rupture of both the ascending and descending aorta has been

TABLE 51–1 **Associated injuries in hospitalized patients with traumatic aortic disruption**

	Associated (surgical) injuries					
	Schmidt[27] (n = 80)	Hilgenberg[26] (n = 51)	Duke[15] (n = 108)	Kirsh[27] (n = 43)	Sturm[28] (n = 37)	AAST[10] (n = 274)
Central nervous system	25%	39%	34%	50%	27%	51%
Thorax						
Diaphragm	13%	2%	12%	9.3%	7%	
Lung	38%	41%	43%	58%	19%	38%
Heart	10%	10%	18%	19%	—	4%
Rib/clavicle fractures	40%	39%	55%	65%	35%	46%
Abdominal						
Spleen	20%	10%	17%	—	14%	14%
Liver	10%	12%	15%	—	22%	22%
Kidney	9%	12%	11%	—	5%	
Bowel	10%	—	15%	—	3%	7%
Other abdominal	11%	—	9%	—	8%	14%
Skeletal						
Extremity	81%	71%	59%	—	—	66%
Spine	5%	10%	20%	—	—	12%
Pelvis	24%	25%	26%	—	22%	31%
Maxillofacial	5%	10%	20%	—	—	13%

attributed to the deployment of an air bag; in some cases the cars were moving at a speed of less than 10 mph.[18–21] Accidental or suicidal falls, crush injuries, airplane accidents, and rare cave-ins are other causes of aortic rupture.[6,10,12,15,16,22] The majority (70%-80%) of victims are male with an average age of 39 (range, 3-88).[10] Recent series demonstrate that 80% of cases are caused by motor vehicle accidents (72% head-on, 24% side impact, and 4% rear impact).[9,10,23] Of the patients with traumatic aortic rupture who make it to the hospital alive, 75% are hemodynamically stable.[10] Compared to autopsy series, these patients have fewer severe associated injuries.[6,9,10,12] Forty percent to 92% of patients are transferred from the original hospital to a level I trauma center.[10,23,24]

Table 51-1 lists the frequency of associated injuries from data accrued from the 1970s to late 1990s in several different series.[10,15,25–28] Data from the American Association for the Surgery of Trauma (AAST) trial were gathered prospectively from 50 trauma centers throughout the United States and Canada.[10] Fifty-one percent of patients have an associated closed head injury. Forty-six percent have multiple rib fractures, and 38% have pulmonary contusions. Compared to older autopsy series, which demonstrated that the majority of patients have associated cardiac contusion, recent data suggest the incidence is only 4%.[10] Orthopedic injuries remain common, occurring in association with aortic rupture in 20% to 35% of cases. Mean Injury Severity Score (ISS) in the AAST trial was 42.1, which is significantly higher than that seen in older retrospective reports, implying that significantly more patients with these types of serious injuries make it to the hospital and are saved in the modern era.[10]

Pathology

ACUTE AORTIC DISRUPTION

In autopsy series aortic disruptions occur in all aortic segments including, rarely, the abdominal aorta. According to autopsy series, 36% to 54% occur at the aortic isthmus, 8% to 27% involve the ascending aorta, 8% to 18% occur in the arch, and 11% to 21% involve the distal descending aorta (Fig. 51-1).[6,12,29,30] However, surgical series demonstrate that 84% to 100% of ruptures occur at the isthmus, and only 3% to 10% occur in the ascending, arch, or distal descending aorta.[9,10,23,26,27,31–33] Among patients who survive, it seems evident that the periadventitial tissue around the isthmus provides some protection against free rupture, allowing for short-term survival and transfer to a hospital.

The aorta is typically transected in a transverse fashion involving all three layers of the aortic wall with the edges often separated by several centimeters (Fig. 51-2).[6,12] Noncircumferential and partial aortic wall disruptions do occur and can vary from only a few millimeters to several centimeters.[6,12,34,35] Spiral lacerations or longitudinal extensions are uncommon. Intramural hematomas and focal dissections occur with partial thickness disruptions but not transections.[6] Partial tears tend to occur posteriorly, involving the intima and media. Aortic wall structure at and around the transection does not differ from uninvolved aorta, and atherosclerotic disease is generally not present.[6,11,12] The aortic adventitia provides the majority of its tensile strength, but there is no evidence to suggest that the adventitia at the aortic isthmus is any weaker than any other area of the aorta.[36,37]

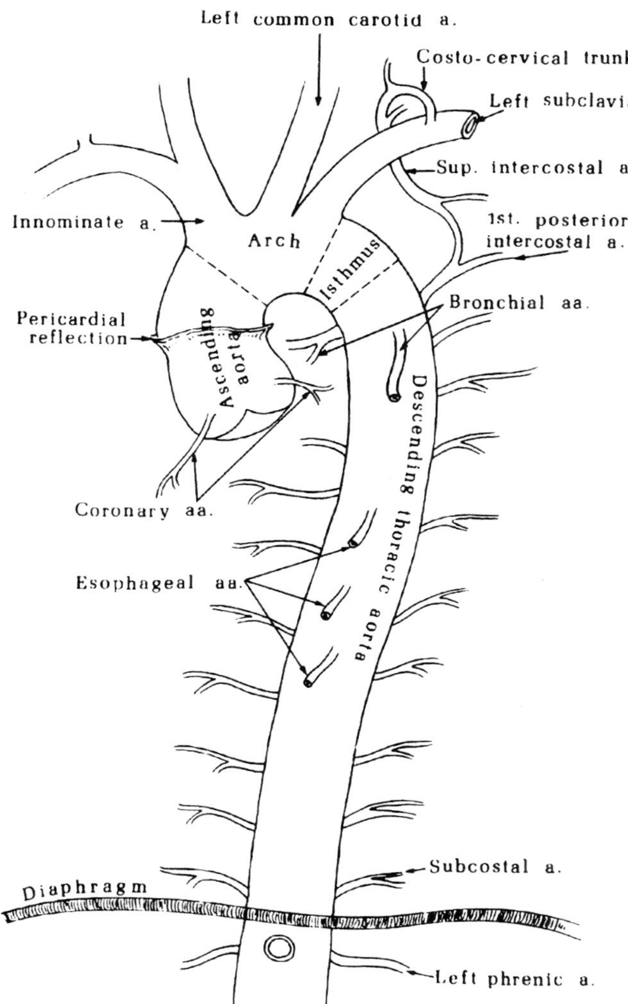

FIGURE 51–1 Anatomic diagram of the thoracic aorta and major branches.

Blunt trauma can also produce trauma to the other great vessels. Disruption at the base of the innominate is the most common, the base of the left subclavian artery less common, and the base of the left carotid the least often disrupted.[38] Central venous injuries are less commonly injured with blunt trauma.[1]

CHRONIC TRAUMATIC AORTIC ANEURYSM

Approximately 2% to 5% of patients with aortic disruptions survive without operation, or even detection, to form chronic false aneurysms.[39] Little is known of the natural history of these chronic pseudoaneurysms. It is likely that an initial false aneurysm with blood flow partially thromboses and organizes to form a fibrous wall. This wall may calcify.[39–41] It can evolve into a saccular or fusiform aneurysm and late expansion or even rupture may occur. Ninety percent involve the aortic isthmus, presumably reflective of some inherent protection afforded to this area by mediastinal periadventitial tissues at the isthmus.[42–44] The patients who develop chronic pseudoaneurysms have fewer associated injuries at the time of the traumatic event.[42–44] In fact, 35% have no other injuries, and 50% have only one.[40]

Pathogenesis

Despite extensive investigation, analysis, and debate, no consensus or unified understanding of the pathogenesis of aortic transection has emerged. Popular opinion has employed the "whiplash" theory, postulating that a combination of traction, torsion, shear, bending, and bursting forces secondary to differential deceleration of tissues within the mediastinum causes an appropriate stress to rupture the aorta at specific sites, the isthmus being the most common.[11,36,37,45–52] The ligamentum arteriosum, the left mainstem bronchus, and

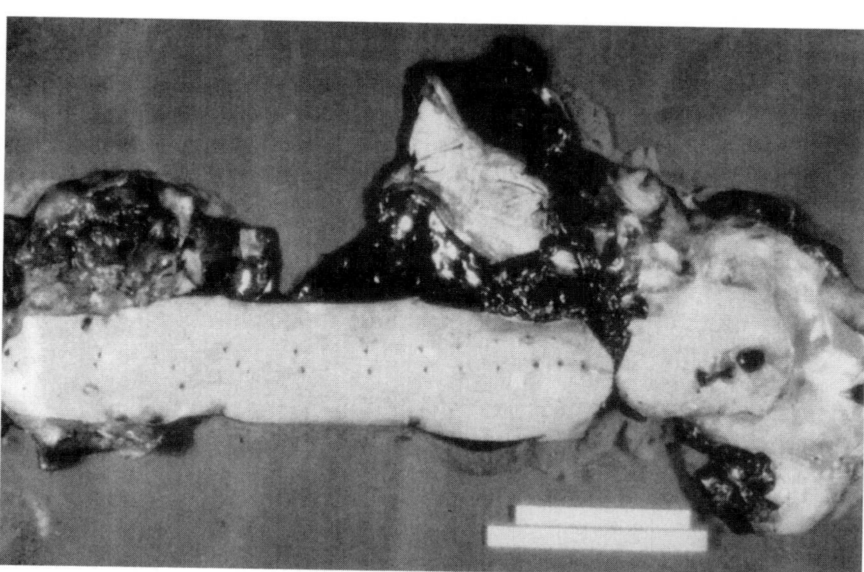

FIGURE 51–2 Photograph of a traumatic aortic disruption at the isthmus. *(Reproduced with permission from Strassman G: Traumatic rupture of the aorta. Am Heart J 1947; 33:508.)*

the paired intercostal arteries limit the mobility of the aorta at the isthmus and just distal to it. Experiments have suggested that the aorta can be displaced in a longitudinal (cranial or caudal) direction sufficient to cause traction tears at the isthmus.[47,49] It has also been recognized that deceleration forces can reach several hundred times the force of gravity, which can produce injury without any direct impact on the chest.[45,46] Alternatively, a "shoveling mechanism" has been postulated to explain cranially directed traction stresses in drivers and front seat passengers in motor vehicle accidents.[53]

Contrarily, Crass et al argue that the forces of differential deceleration, torsion, or hydrostatics have inadequate magnitude in vehicular accidents to result in aortic tearing given the inherent properties of the aorta.[54–56] Several studies have demonstrated that the gravitational forces of vehicular trauma do not approach the tensile strength of the aorta. Oppenheim and Zehnder showed that a normal aorta can withstand pressure of 2000 mm Hg before bursting.[57,58] Crass proposed a new mechanism based on thoracic compression that he coined "the osseous pinch," which was tested in the laboratory. The hypothesis is that anterior thoracic osseous structures (manubrium, first rib, clavicular heads) rotate posteriorly and inferiorly about the axes of the posterior rib attachments. When the force is large enough, these anterior bony structures impact the vertebral column and the portion of the aorta overlying the spine (the isthmus and proximal descending aorta) is pinched between the bones. This causes a direct shearing of the aorta. Crass' group demonstrated in a canine model that a blunt force as small as 20,000 N transected the intima and media of the aorta.[54] In comparison, a 38-mph collision produces a force of 198,000 N in a normal-sized adult.[54]

Other forces may be important in ascending aortic injuries. The anterior location of the ascending aorta and the weight and ease of displacement of the heart downward and to the left facilitate traction stress on and above the aortic root.[49] Hyperextension of the spine and consequent shearing forces may play a role in the distal descending aorta.[54]

It is likely that the majority of victims of motor vehicle accidents experience some combination of differential deceleration forces and thoracic compression forces causing aortic disruption. It is clear that many different mechanisms of trauma (i.e., front impact, side impact, falls, crushing injury, and blasts) have caused aortic disruption. Each of these situations affords different circumstances and different forces. Consequently, it will be difficult to prove the various hypotheses of mechanism in humans.

Natural History

ACUTE AORTIC DISRUPTION

The natural history of aortic transection in a given patient is dependent on many factors, not the least of which is how quickly a diagnosis is made. Our understanding of survival rates is based on data drawn from autopsy series and operative series; autopsy studies tend to underestimate the rate of long-term survival while operative studies tend to overestimate it. Parmley observed that 86% of patients die at the scene, and 11% survive longer than 6 hours.[6] The only survivors in the Parmley series were, in fact, operated on. Mortality rates in most recent surgical series range from 11% to 40%, although the attributable mortality rates are not known.[9,10,16,23] Several groups have reported small series of patients who were treated conservatively with beta blockade and vasodilators in patients deemed unsuitable candidates for surgery or in cases of apparent minimal aortic injury.[3,59–61] Those unsuitable for surgery were too old and morbid or had associated injuries that were too severe for them to tolerate operative repair of the aortic rupture initially and thus underwent delayed repair. When surgery has been delayed with blood pressure control for stabilization of other injuries, the interim mortality rate prior to definitive repair is not clearly known but is probably low. Delays of up to 4 months prior to repair have been reported,[61–68] although in a recent series of patients who were definitively treated nonoperatively for reasons of comorbidity, the mortality rate was 47%.[3] None of the deaths, however, was due to aortic rupture. Another series of 5 patients treated nonoperatively because of associated injuries had an average follow-up of 51 months with no mortality.[64] We conclude that aortic transection can and probably should be treated nonoperatively or with operative delay in certain patients with severe associated injuries or significant comorbidities.

CHRONIC TRAUMATIC AORTIC ANEURYSM

Numerous anecdotal reports confirm long-term survival in self-selected patients who were not diagnosed at the time of injury.[41,44,69–74] A review of the literature by Finkelmeier et al demonstrated that among survivors like these, over 70% survive greater than 5 years from the time of the injury.[40] The inherent survival bias of this group of patients is evident, but it does confirm that some patients can survive long term without surgery. In Finkelmeier's review, the 60 patients who did not have operations for chronic traumatic aortic aneurysms had 5-year, 10-year, and 20-year survival rates of 71%, 66%, and 62%, respectively. Ninety-four percent of chronic traumatic aortic aneurysms were located at the aortic isthmus. Rarely, the arch and ascending aorta were involved.[40]

Clinical Presentation

The presentation of aortic rupture is protean. Aortic rupture itself manifests in the form of specific signs or symptoms in less than 50% of cases.[14,75–78] Patients may develop dyspnea, back pain, or differential hypertension in the lower as compared to the upper extremities.[56,75,76,78–82] Aortic injuries are more commonly identified in the backdrop of a multiple-trauma patient, and the diagnosis is made only if it is suspected. Consequently, aortic injury can easily be missed if patients are not appropriately screened. Identifying the character and mechanism of trauma is the critical first step in making the diagnosis of aortic disruption. If speeds or distances fallen suggest severe impact or high deceleration forces, the possibility of aortic rupture exists, and it should be ruled out. In cases of motor vehicle trauma, falls, blasts, crush injuries, or other acceleration or deceleration forces, aortic rupture should be considered.[3,8,16,60,83–86]

The initial management of a multiple-trauma patient is no different with or without suspected aortic disruption. The patient's airway, breathing, and circulation are addressed first. Primary and secondary surveys are completed. Appropriate venous access is obtained concomitant with initial laboratory and radiographic studies. Priority of injury is based largely on the acute lethal potential of an injury. Exsanguinating hemorrhage in any of the body compartments, perforated viscus, or central neurologic injury take the usual priority. Most patients with aortic disruption also have one or more fractures. These should be stabilized but not definitively treated prior to excluding the diagnosis of aortic rupture or treating an aortic rupture. There are often clues evident in the initial evaluation of a trauma patient that suggest aortic disruption (Table 51-2). In the majority of trauma cases, a supine chest radiograph is obtained as part of the initial evaluation.

TABLE 51–2 Clues that suggest aortic disruption

History
Motor vehicle crash >50 km/h
Motor vehicle crash into fixed barrier
No seat belt
Ejection from vehicle
Broken steering wheel
Motorcycle or airplane crash
Pedestrian hit by motor vehicle
Falls greater than 3 m
Crush or cave-in injuries
Loss of consciousness
Physical signs
Hemodynamic shock (systolic blood pressure < 90 mm Hg)
Fracture of sternum, 1st rib, clavicle, scapula, or multiple ribs
Steering wheel imprint on chest
Cardiac murmurs
Hoarseness
Dyspnea
Back pain
Hemothorax
Unequal extremity blood pressures
Paraplegia or paraparesis

TABLE 51–3 Chest x-ray findings associated with blunt aortic disruption

Widened mediastinum (>8.0 cm)
Mediastinum-to-chest width ratio (M:C) >0.25
Tracheal shift to the patient's right
Blurred aortic contour
Irregularity of loss of the aortic knob
Left apical cap
Depression of the left main bronchus
Opacification of the aortopulmonary window
Right deviation of the nasogastric tube
Wide paraspinal lines
First rib fracture
Any other rib fracture
Clavicle fracture
Pulmonary contusion
Thoracic spine fracture

Source: Adapted from Cook AD, Klein JS, Rogers FB, et al: Chest radiographs of limited utility in the diagnosis of blunt traumatic aortic laceration. J Trauma 2001; 50:843.

Diagnostic Studies

CHEST RADIOGRAPH

A standard supine anteroposterior (AP) chest x-ray does not have the diagnostic sensitivity to rule out aortic injury.[3,5,16,87] Chest x-ray findings are interpreted as normal at the time of initial evaluation of 9% to 40% of patients with aortic rupture in major trauma centers.[3,5,16,77,87–94] At least fifteen distinct signs on a standard AP chest x-ray are associated with blunt aortic injury or rupture (Table 51-3).[87] Unfortunately, none of these signs are sufficiently sensitive, specific, or predictive of aortic rupture. In a series of 188 consecutively evaluated multiple-trauma patients, 10 blunt aortic injuries were identified, and the sensitivities of these plain radiographic findings ranged from 0% to 90%.[87] The specificities ranged from 6% to 93%.[87]

In lieu of attaining an upright chest x-ray, which is typically precluded in a multiple-trauma patient, reverse Trendelenburg 45-degree AP chest x-rays have been suggested to be more accurate than supine films at evaluating the mediastinum.[95] However, this technique is not used routinely in most trauma centers, especially when computed tomography is available.

COMPUTED TOMOGRAPHY

Volumetric helical or spiral computed tomography (CT) has become the standard screening tool to rule out aortic rupture.[5] The technology was introduced in the early 1990s, and since that time it has become the screening modality used in most institutions.[3–5,16,17,59,66,89,93,94,96–106] Its advantages over other sophisticated imaging techniques (e.g., transesophageal echocardiography, magnetic resonance imaging, or aortography) include its wide availability,

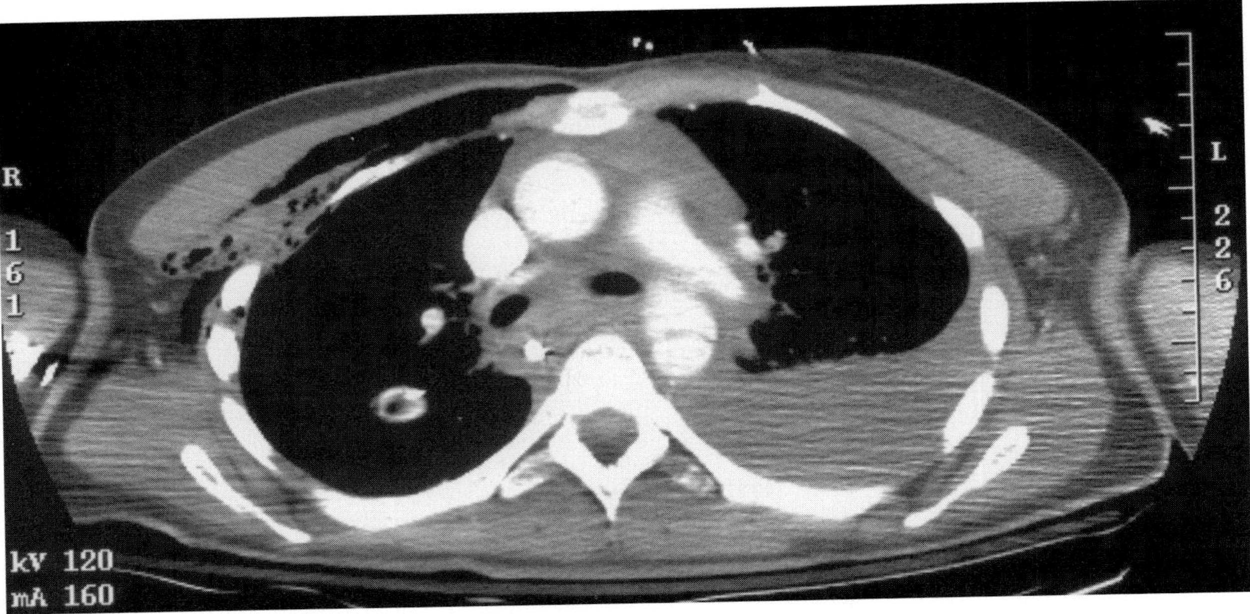

FIGURE 51–3 Helical CT of the chest in a 30-year-old male after a high-speed motor vehicle accident. Aortic transection at the isthmus is clearly seen.

its speed, its sensitivity, its reasonable cost, and its ease of interpretation.

Nonionic contrast media are typically used, and 50 to 60 images with slice thicknesses of 5 to 7 mm can be acquired in less than 1.5 minutes.[5] Normal aorta is depicted with homogeneous enhancement. Several findings are indicative of aortic disruption, including wall thickening, extravasation of contrast, filling defects, para-aortic hematoma, intimal flaps, mural thrombi, pseudoaneurysm, and pseudocoarctation.[5]

Approximately 1% of blunt trauma patients have a thoracic aortic injury identified by helical CT.[3,97] In most prospective series the sensitivity and negative predictive value of helical CT in detecting traumatic aortic rupture are 100%.[3,16,93,107] Aortography has been the standard against which all diagnostic methods have been compared, with sensitivities and specificities approaching 100% in older series.[108] However, in more recent series that have utilized modern imaging techniques of either helical CT or transesophageal echocardiography (TEE), aortography has had sensitivities of only 78% to 92%.[3,109] False-positive CT studies do occur. The specificity, accuracy, and positive predictive value of helical CT range from 50% to 89%.[3,16,93,107] One uncommon finding that mimics aortic injury is a ductus diverticulum remnant.[5] Unlike an aortic injury, a ductus diverticulum will have no intimal irregularity or mediastinal hematoma. When there is a luminal or mural aortic irregularity without evidence of a periaortic hematoma or when there is periaortic hematoma without obvious aortic luminal or mural irregularity, additional aortic imaging either by TEE or aortography should be considered prior to intervention. Minimal aortic injuries (defined as small, less than 1 cm, intimal flaps) are being identified at an increasing rate because of the improved resolution of CT imaging and its widespread use.[3,5,59] These minimal injuries pose another management dilemma. Many of these minor aortic injuries can and probably should be managed medically with antihypertensive medications and wall stress–reducing agents (e.g., beta blockers).[59]

The degree to which thoracic surgeons rely on chest CT to plan repair of thoracic aortic injuries is variable. Our routine practice at the University of Pennsylvania is to obtain a helical chest CT as the initial screen for aortic injury in the hemodynamically stable patient. Studies that unequivocally demonstrate no aortic injury are cleared with CT alone. Studies that show aortic transection with obvious intimal disruption and periaortic hematoma (Fig. 51-3) go to the operating room for definitive repair once other life-threatening injuries have been identified and appropriately addressed. Studies that demonstrate no clear aortic rupture with intimal disruption but show a periaortic, mediastinal hematoma prompt subsequent aortogram. When a patient is hemodynamically unstable due to hemorrhagic shock, the evaluation of thoracic aortic injury is done in the operating room using TEE as described below. The timing of obtaining the chest CT depends on the stability of the patient, associated injuries, and resuscitation issues, but typically will occur at the same time that head and abdominopelvic CTs are obtained.

TRANSESOPHAGEAL ECHOCARDIOGRAPHY

The development of multiplanar transesophageal echocardiography (TEE) has revolutionized cardiothoracic surgery such that its use is now necessary to plan and facilitate

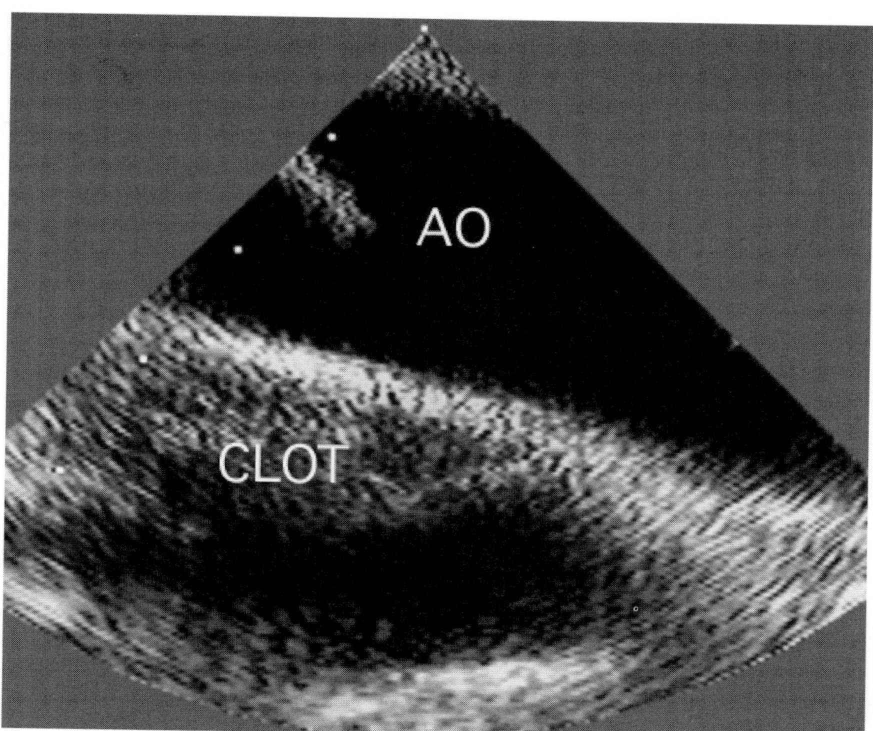

FIGURE 51–4 Transesophageal echocardiographic longitudinal cross-sectional image of the aortic isthmus depicting intimal disruption and para-aortic thrombus. (*Courtesy of B. Milas, University of Pennsylvania.*)

optimal intraoperative management in many cardiothoracic surgical procedures. Its use in cases of aortic transection is no exception. TEE reliably images the entire thoracic aorta except the distal ascending aorta and aortic arch, which are obscured by tracheal and bronchial air artifact. Contrarily, transthoracic echocardiography (TTE) cannot accurately evaluate the distal descending aorta. The accuracy of TEE for diagnosing aortic injury is dependent on the operator. Some report its sensitivity and specificity to be approaching 100%,[107,109,110] while others demonstrate a sensitivity and specificity as low as 63% and 84%, respectively.[111] A recent prospective comparison of the use of helical CT to TEE in evaluating blunt aortic injury in 110 consecutive patients demonstrated a sensitivity, specificity, negative predictive value, and positive predictive value of 93%, 100%, 99%, and 100%, respectively, for TEE compared to 73%, 100%, 95%, and 100% for helical CT.[107]

A major advantage of TEE is its portability. The hemodynamically unstable patient who is taken to the operating room immediately can undergo exploratory laparotomy or other procedures while simultaneously being evaluated by TEE. The major disadvantage of TEE is that it requires an experienced operator. The risk of TEE is low.[107,109] It is contraindicated in cases of concomitant cervical spine, oropharyngeal, esophageal, or severe maxillofacial injury or in patients with esophageal or pharyngeal lesions that would impede passage of the probe.

Multiplanar TEE probes permit acquisition of cross-sectional images at different angles along a single rotational axis (Figs. 51-4 to 51-6). The typical 5- or 7-MHz transducer permits adequate resolution of structures as small as 1 to 2 mm. Time-resolved imaging allows evaluation of the movement of anatomic structures and enhances the ability to determine the physiologic consequences of structural abnormalities. Doppler echocardiography is used to evaluate abnormal blood flow patterns that can aid in identifying intimal flaps (Fig. 51-5).

The most common feature of aortic injury identified by TEE is a mural flap (Figs. 51-4 and 51-6). Thickening of the vessel wall can represent a contained rupture or a mural thrombus (Fig. 51-4). Color Doppler flow mapping can demonstrate alterations in flow patterns including turbulence at the site of injury (Fig. 51-5). Chronic atheromatous changes can produce false positive signs of intimal disruption. When aortic disruption is suspected on TEE, there usually is a surrounding mediastinal hematoma, and its absence should prompt skepticism that transection is the diagnosis.

AORTOGRAPHY

Aortography is the imaging modality by which all other techniques have been compared for evaluation of aortic injury (Fig. 51-7). Temporally, its technique and role in evaluating aortic injuries or other vascular injuries were established long before any of the other sophisticated imaging methodologies. In experienced hands its sensitivity and specificity both approach 100%.[108] Its major disadvantages are that its use requires a highly skilled interventional radiology team, and it is time consuming, rendering the

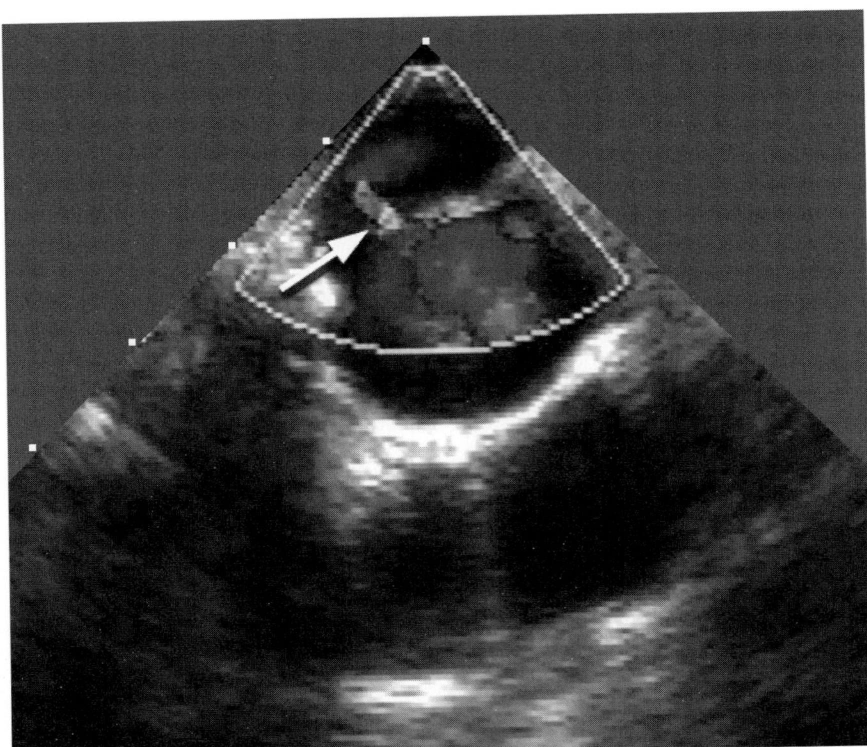

FIGURE 51–5 Transesophageal echocardiographic cross-sectional image in the short axis with color-flow Doppler depicting transection of the aortic isthmus. The transection appears as two distinct lumens, the "double-barrel" sign, and there is flow between the separated aorta. *(Courtesy of B. Milas, University of Pennsylvania.)*

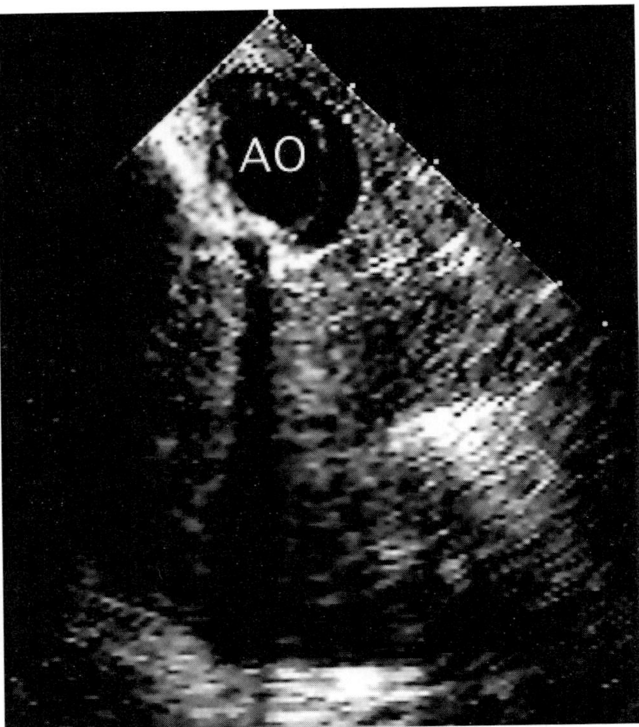

FIGURE 51–6 Transesophageal echocardiographic cross-sectional image in short axis depicting aortic transection with the distal aortic lumen (AO) appearing within the proximal aortic lumen. This is diagnostic of aortic transection. *(Courtesy of B. Milas, University of Pennsylvania.)*

patient inaccessible during the time of the study. Rates of exsanguination and death of up to 10% in the angiography suite have been reported.[82,112,113] Complication rates attributed directly to aortography are low. Contrast reactions, renal insufficiency secondary to contrast material, and groin hematomas or pseudoaneurysms do occur. In the pre–helical CT era, 85% to 95% of aortograms were negative, calling into question the cost- and time-effectiveness of the technique.[17,76,82,105,108,113] False-positive studies are usually attributed to atheromata or ductal diverticula.

The technique of intra-arterial digital subtraction angiography (IADSA) is used by most groups, including our own, and allows for faster generation of images and shorter times in the angiography suite (Fig. 51-7). Intravenous digital subtraction angiography (IVDSA) has been used in the past by some as an even more rapid means of evaluating the aorta in the angiography suite.[113] This technique employs IV contrast instillation with time-delayed images of the arch and descending aorta. The time of study can be reduced by up to 4-fold when compared to conventional biplanar angiography. Unfortunately, the diagnostic quality of IVDSA is less than 70%,[113] and consequently with the near uniform availability of helical CT, the technique has become obsolete.

MAGNETIC RESONANCE ANGIOGRAPHY

Magnetic resonance angiography (MRA) provides excellent images of vascular structures, particularly the thoracic aorta,

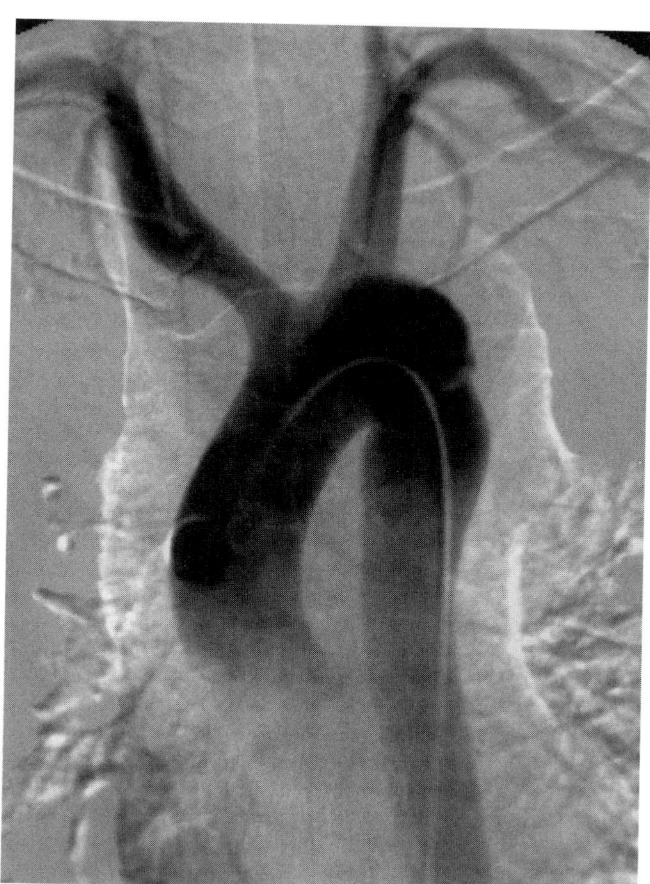

FIGURE 51–7 Intra-arterial digital subtraction angiogram of an acute traumatic aortic disruption at the isthmus. The linear tear is typical.

and its utility in the diagnosis and follow-up of complex aortic disease including aortic dissections and aneurysms is firmly established.[114–117] However, its use in the acute trauma patient has not been justified. The time required to attain images and the confining nature of the scanners preclude its use in this patient population. If MR data acquisition time decreases and patient accessibility within a scanner increases in the future, there may become a role for MRA in acute trauma settings. Alternatively, it is reasonable to follow a patient with traumatic aortic rupture long term using MRA, particularly those patients with minimal aortic injury treated nonoperatively. In the rare patient who presents with aortic aneurysm or pseudoaneurysm remote from the time of aortic injury, MRA is certainly a useful technique.

Management

INITIAL EVALUATION

Ninety-five percent of patients with aortic disruption have associated injuries, and consequently it is imperative that a comprehensive trauma evaluation occur prior to definitive imaging to rule in aortic injury.[9,10,60] The leading cause of death in patients with aortic injury who make it to the hospital is exsanguinating aortic rupture, which occurs in 20% of patients.[10] Among patients who present with an aortic injury and are hemodynamically stable, 4% die in the hospital of aortic rupture prior to surgical repair.[10] These data emphasize that a careful, planned, and expeditious team approach toward these patients is mandatory in order to save as many of these patients as possible. Standard ATLS guidelines for trauma evaluation should be followed. These include performing primary and secondary physical examinations with control of the airway, respiration, and hemodynamics, and obtaining a chest x-ray, baseline chemistry, blood gas, and hematologic studies. The first priorities in these and all trauma patients are to control ventilation and stabilize hemodynamics. This may require intubation, insertion of thoracostomy tubes, resuscitation from cardiac arrest, identification and stabilization of head injuries, laparotomy, or even thoracotomy. Patients with nonlethal associated injuries who are hemodynamically stable should be diverted toward exclusion of aortic injury, and patients who are unstable require immediate direction toward life-saving operative intervention, bypassing time-consuming tests, in order to achieve the best chance of survival.

PREOPERATIVE IMAGING

After initial trauma evaluation, establishment of an airway, and control of ventilation and hemodynamics, a head CT should be obtained prior to any planned aortic operation in all patients with signs of an open or closed head injury. Relief of lesions occupying intracranial space takes priority over nonbleeding aortic injuries. Hemodynamically unstable patients with signs of exsanguinating hemorrhage should go directly to the operating room for control of hemorrhage, and TEE should be used to evaluate for aortic injury. Identification of blunt aortic injuries in hemodynamically stable patients should be done in the most efficient manner for a given institution, depending on availability of experienced imaging diagnosticians and imaging equipment, and should be coordinated with the evaluation of other life-threatening injuries. The usual scenario of the hemodynamically stable blunt trauma patient dictates leaving the emergency room to undergo head and abdominopelvic CT scan for identification of closed head injury and intra-abdominal injury. Patients with either an abnormal chest x-ray or a mechanism of injury that poses significant risk of aortic injury (e.g., falls greater than 3 m, motor vehicle crashes greater than 50 km/h, or pedestrians hit by automobiles) should undergo simultaneous helical chest CT at the time of head and/or abdominopelvic CT. In most institutions, aortography is now reserved for use in patients with equivocal helical CT or TEE results or in patients with complex aortic injuries that cannot be accurately defined by these other imaging techniques. Occasionally, thoracoscopy has been used to evaluate traumatic hemothoraces.[118] However, there is little role for thoracoscopy in the diagnosis of aortic rupture because, in experienced hands, the sensitivity and specificity of intraoperative TEE are so good.

In the preoperative period, patients with aortic injury should receive beta blockers and vasodilators for control of aortic wall tension and blood pressure.[3,60] Reduction of the change in pressure over the change in time ($\Delta P/\Delta t$) reduces the wall stress significantly.[119] These measures have been shown to reduce in-hospital aortic rupture rates without adversely affecting the outcome of other injuries.[3] These control measures should be employed both in patients going to the operating room and patients undergoing delayed aortic repair for the treatment of other life-threatening injuries.

TIMING OF OPERATION

Immediate thoracotomy and aortic repair are recommended in stable patients without the need for laparotomy, craniotomy, or pelvic stabilization once the diagnosis of aortic injury is made. Intracranial bleeding causing mass effect and thoracic, abdominal, pelvic, or retroperitoneal hemorrhage should all be addressed prior to thoracotomy for contained aortic injury.[62,120] Presentation of aortic disruption with aortic bleeding requires immediate surgery; however, this situation is rarely encountered as it is usually immediately fatal. Aortic injury should be monitored by TEE during surgical treatment of intracranial, thoracic, abdominal, or pelvic injuries. Treatment of injuries that are not life-threatening should be delayed until after definitive aortic repair. Hemodynamically unstable patients should be taken to the operating room immediately, prior to definitive testing. Laparotomy or even thoracotomy may be required to locate and control ongoing hemorrhage. Patients with instability secondary to associated trauma who require laparotomy or thoracotomy for damage control to establish hemodynamic stability may be better served by subsequent immediate transfer to the intensive care unit for further resuscitation, postponing definitive repair of aortic rupture until complete resuscitation and hemodynamic stability are achieved. Care should be taken during this stabilization period to avoid undue aortic wall stress and hypertension with maintenance of short-acting beta blockers.[3] Purposeful delay of definitive aortic repair may be a safe option when there is concomitant severe hepatic trauma that carries a significant risk of recurrent or ongoing hemorrhage.[121]

OPERATION

The technical issues of repairing aortic lacerations are straightforward. While no one method of repair of aortic transection has been proven superior, standards are being established. There remains considerable controversy surrounding the issue of spinal cord protection and which means of protection are optimal.[9,10,23,27,31,33,56,60,64,66,77,86,92,122–130] There remain two general perspectives: (1) "clamp-and-sew" techniques are sufficient alone, or (2) some form of lower body perfusion provides added spinal cord and visceral protection against the ischemia of the aortic cross-clamp. Regardless of the technical controversies, paraplegia occurs among these patients at an overall rate of approximately 10%.[9,10,31,33,77,131] Prospectively acquired data from multiple institutions demonstrate a marked reduction in paraplegia rates with the use of lower body perfusion techniques.[3,10,16,60]

Preparations Appropriate blood work including complete blood count, coagulation studies, electrolytes, urea nitrogen, and creatinine should be attained. Antihypertensive and beta-blockade therapy should be ongoing prior to induction of anesthesia. Single (right) lung ventilation is optimal and should be secured either by double-lumen endotracheal tube or single-lumen tube with left bronchial balloon blocker. After anesthetic induction, right femoral and right radial arterial lines should be placed for monitoring of upper and lower body perfusion. The left groin should be left alone for access for possible partial left heart bypass. Several large-bore intravenous catheters for infusion and a pulmonary arterial catheter should be placed for ongoing hemodynamic monitoring. A bladder catheter with temperature probe, peripheral arterial oxygen saturation monitor, and electrocardiogram should be placed for continuous monitoring. A nasogastric (NG) tube is inserted, the stomach emptied, and then the NG tube removed to allow insertion of a TEE probe. Subsequently, the patient is placed in the right lateral decubitus position with the table flexed and the hip rotated slightly leftward to facilitate left groin exposure. The patient's skin is prepped and draped from left shoulder to left knee. A cell-saver system is used for red blood cell salvage. Antifibrinolytic drugs (e.g., aprotinin, tranexamic acid, or ε-amino caproic acid) may offer a reduced incidence of blood transfusion requirements.[132]

Spinal cord protection Blood flow is supplied to the spinal cord by anterior and posterior spinal arteries that consist of anatomic vascular chains that run the length of the cord.[133] The anterior spinal artery supplies the anterior two thirds of the cord and is well developed in the upper thorax. Collateral arterial vessels also feed off of the left subclavian artery, and consequently its occlusion during repair may have added implications toward a heightened risk of spinal cord ischemia. In the lower thorax and upper abdomen the anterior spinal artery is less developed and relies on segmental branches from intercostal and lumbar arteries. The anterior artery is supplied by 7 to 10 unpaired anterior medullary branches that vary in location along the cord (Fig. 51-8). Usually at least two anterior medullary vessels supply the cervical cord, two or three supply the thoracic cord, and two supply the

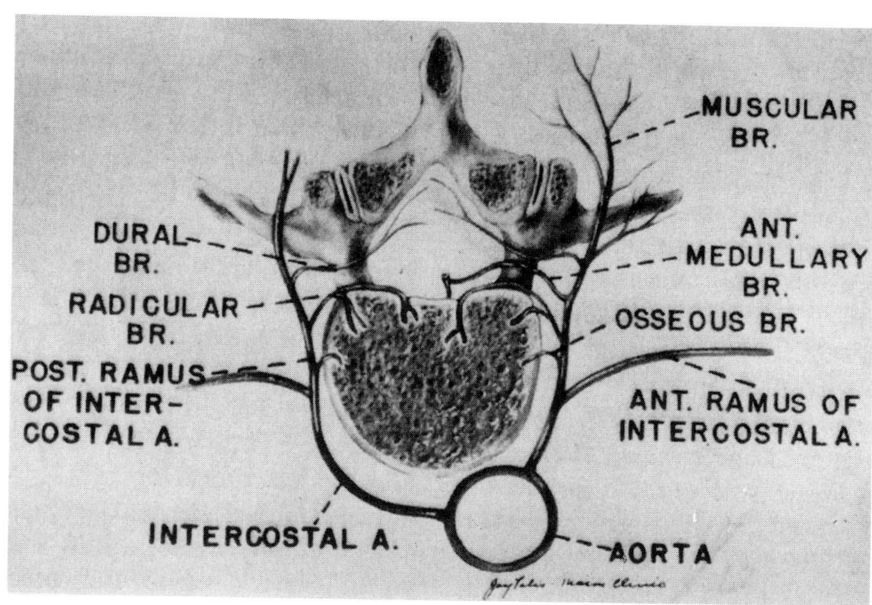

FIGURE 51–8 Cross-sectional diagram showing a medullary (radicular) arterial branch to the anterior spinal artery.

lumbar cord. At the level of the first lumbar vertebra (variations T8 to L4) the anterior spinal artery receives the arteria radicularis magna (or artery of Adamkiewicz), which for at least 25% of patients is essential for cord blood supply in this zone.[133,134]

Aortic cross-clamping near the aortic isthmus produces profound hypotension in the lower body and spinal cord below this region, and spinal cord injury is proportional to aortic cross-clamp time (Fig. 51-9).[135] Clamping the aorta above the takeoff of the left subclavian artery may increase the risk of paraplegia since there are collateral vessels fed by the internal thoracic, vertebral, and subscapular vessels, all emanating from the subclavian.[136] Paraplegia has occurred after only 9 minutes of aortic cross-clamping without extracorporeal perfusion of the lower body (J Bavaria, personal case).

Several adjuncts have been proposed to reduce the risk of paraplegia in cases of elective repair of thoracic or thoracoabdominal aneurysms, but many of these techniques are not practical in the trauma patient requiring repair of aortic transection. These include monitoring of somatosensory evoked potentials and lumbar cerebrospinal fluid drainage, both of which require added time and expertise in the preoperative setting that are often not available to trauma patients.[131,137–143] Hypothermia, while attractive as a means of spinal cord protection, is not practical in partial bypass

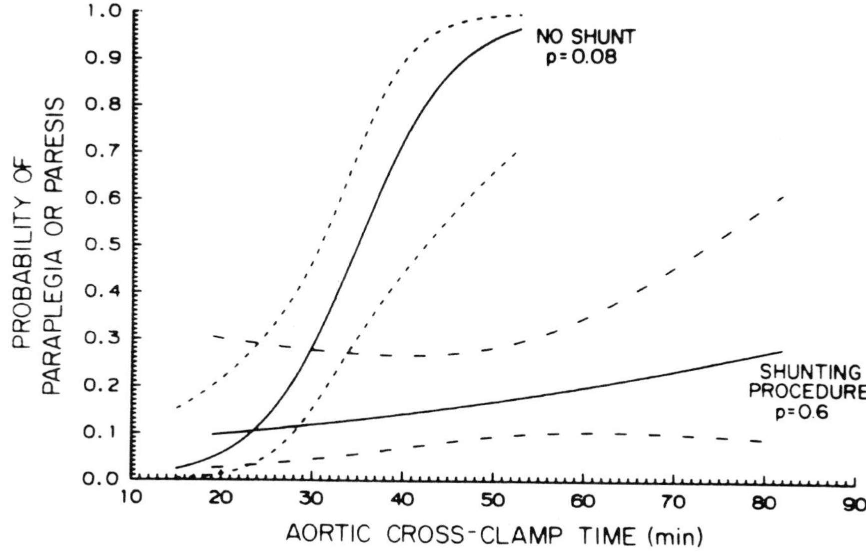

FIGURE 51–9 Probability of paraplegia in relation to aortic cross-clamp time with and without lower body perfusion in patients with traumatic aortic disruption at the isthmus. *(Reproduced with permission from Katz NM, Blackstone EH, Kirklin JW, Karp RB: Incremental risk factors for spinal cord injury following operation for acute traumatic aortic transection. J Thorac Cardiovasc Surg 1981; 81:669.)*

systems, which rely on the heart to perfuse the upper body. On rare occasions when aortic injury involves the aortic arch, hypothermic circulatory arrest techniques are required for repair and may actually offer added spinal cord protection.[144–147] Selective spinal cord hypothermia and perfusion have been studied in the laboratory, but to date these techniques have not been employed in humans.[148,149] Experience with theoretical neuroprotective pharmaceuticals like steroids, lidocaine, or magnesium has not been thoroughly studied in this patient population.

Based on the currently available data from the surgical community as a whole, it appears that cross-clamp times exceeding 30 minutes and utilization of the "clamp-and-sew" technique alone yield higher rates of paraplegia than techniques that include extracorporeal lower body perfusion. Certainly, some groups have had success with low paraplegia rates using exclusively simple cross-clamping technique,[9,23] but these results have not been reproducible throughout many institutions, and their results rely on short cross-clamp times (average 20 to 25 minutes). Recent data suggest that the paraplegia rate approaches zero when cross-clamp times are short (less than 30 minutes) and lower body perfusion techniques are employed.[10,125,131] At the University of Pennsylvania all patients undergoing repair of aortic transection receive some form of lower body perfusion during aortic cross-clamping. There have been no cases of paraplegia since this strategy was implemented in 1994 (over 40 patients; unpublished data).

Incisions A standard fourth interspace posterolateral thoracotomy with or without fifth rib removal or notching usually provides excellent exposure to the aortic isthmus and proximal descending aorta. The incision should be long enough to facilitate dissection of the descending aorta below the level of the inferior pulmonary vein and dissection of the arch of the aorta between the left common carotid and left subclavian arteries. Dissection near the isthmus or tear should be avoided until both proximal and distal aortic control are established. Depending on the stability of the patient, the decision of how to achieve lower body perfusion can be made prior to aortic exposure by gaining access to the left groin or after aortic exposure to facilitate left atrial to distal aortic bypass. The left groin is exposed in the standard fashion. The left common femoral artery is encircled with vessel loops, and the left femoral vein is exposed simply on its anterior surface because circumferential exposure may increase the incidence of deep venous thrombosis.

MANAGEMENT OF LOWER BODY CIRCULATION

Optimally, both right radial and femoral arterial catheters should be in place to allow for monitoring of upper and lower body perfusion. Both active and passive shunting systems have been successful with both full systemic heparinization and no heparinization.[10,23,25,27,86,122–124,126,127,129,137,150,151] Despite the theoretical risk of bleeding with heparinization in the trauma setting, most groups, including our own, that employ active partial left heart bypass techniques use full systemic heparinization and have not seen bleeding complications.[3,10] It is important to be well versed in the various lower body perfusion systems because distinct circumstances may require alterations in routine practice.

Simple aortic cross-clamping Simple aortic cross-clamping probably still has a role in the management of traumatic aortic rupture. The only advantage to this technique is its simplicity. In particular, it may be useful to the general, vascular, or trauma surgeon who is not experienced in the utilization of extracorporeal perfusion circuits or the cannulation of cardiac chambers or great vessels when thoracic surgical expertise is unavailable. It may also be useful in unstable patients who are actively bleeding from the aortic tear; in these patients there may be no time to employ a distal aortic perfusion system.

When aortic cross-clamp times are less than 25 to 30 minutes, low paraplegia rates have been achieved.[9,10,23] However, the average cross-clamp time reported in the literature is 41.0 minutes.[31] Many cases of aortic transection require more than 30 minutes to repair because of extravasated blood, fragility of the aorta, and difficulty in identifying local anatomy within a large hematoma. This is especially true if the tear extends proximally to involve the orifice of the left subclavian artery. These patients require clamping the aorta proximal to the left subclavian artery, which may increase the incidence of paraplegia in the absence of distal aortic perfusion.

Lower body perfusion systems The system used by any one group should be simply applied, reliable, and routine to that group. Distal perfusion pressure should be maintained at 60 to 70 mm Hg.[127] Full heparinization is relatively contraindicated in cases of intracranial hemorrhage and lung injury, but is otherwise safely used by many groups.[9,10,31,77,127,150,152] The least amount of heparin that can be used for a given circuit is probably best. Use of a Bio-Medicus pump with heparin-bonded tubing and active partial left heart bypass or use of a heparin-bonded passive shunt is an option that does not require systemic heparinization.[123,127,152] It is helpful to employ the use of a heat exchanger within extracorporeal circuits in order to maintain core temperatures above 35°C in those patients who cool quickly.

Partial left heart bypass This technique actively shunts blood from the left atrium to the lower body via either the distal thoracic aorta or left femoral artery.[127,150] Typically, a two-stage 20-20F cannula is placed into the left atrium through the left inferior pulmonary vein to provide inflow to the pump (Fig. 51-10). Arterial cannulation size is determined by body size and site of cannulation. We employ either a high-flow, atraumatic, aortic cannula for distal aortic

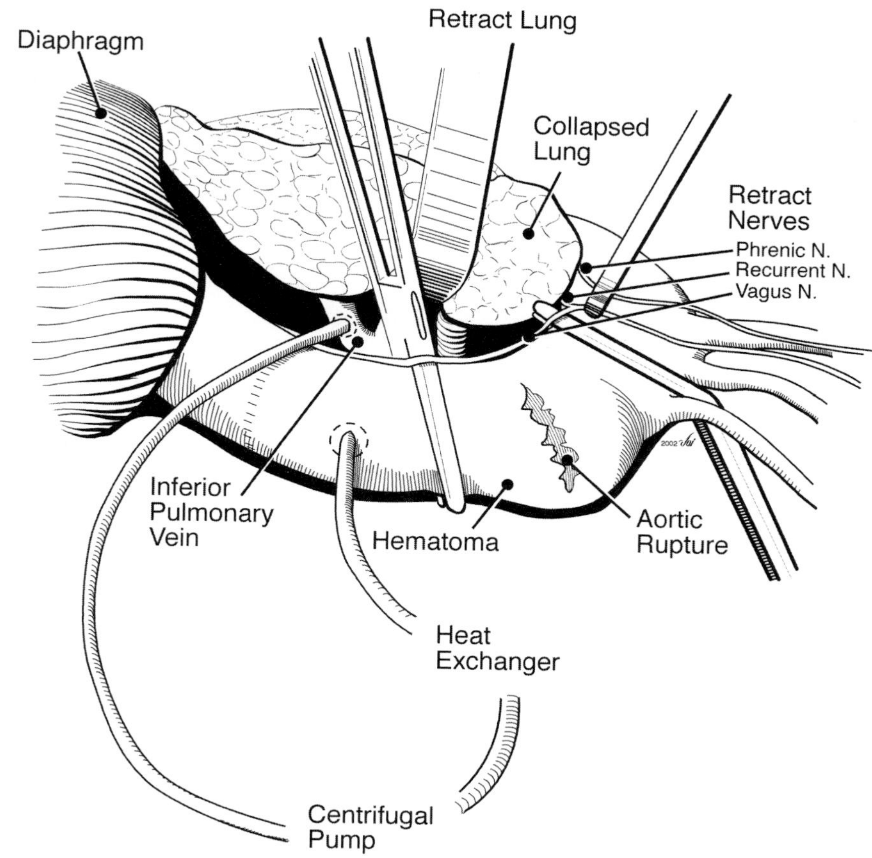

FIGURE 51–10 Diagram showing a typical setup for partial left heart bypass in a patient with aortic disruption at the isthmus.

cannulation or a 16F to 22F straight arterial cannula for femoral cannulation. Distal aortic cannulation has the advantage of convenience and speed. Partial left heart bypass serves several purposes:

1. Unloads the left heart and controls proximal hypertension at the time of cross-clamping
2. Maintains lower body perfusion
3. Allows rapid infusion of volume
4. Controls intravascular volume

The lower body is perfused at a flow rate of 2 to 3 L/min with lower body mean arterial pressure (MAP) of 60 to 70 mm Hg while maintaining an upper body MAP of 70 to 80 mm Hg. All field blood is returned to the circuit via a pump reservoir or is accumulated and returned by cell saver.

Ventricular arrhythmias pose a major risk since the native heart perfuses the upper body. Single-lung ventilation does not increase postoperative pulmonary problems after left heart bypass. If the system is used without systemic heparinization, heat exchangers and oxygenators should be removed from the circuit to minimize surface area and thrombotic risks, but in doing so great care must be taken to reduce heat losses and maintain near-normal temperatures.

Right atrial to femoral arterial bypass A long venous catheter (18F-22F) with multiple side holes is passed via the left common femoral vein into the right atrium using a guidewire technique. The left groin is exposed in the usual fashion, and the anterior wall of the common femoral vein is exposed as described above. A purse-string suture is placed within the vein, and the vein is cannulated. The femoral artery is cannulated. This bypass technique can be used with or without an oxygenator like partial left heart bypass, but it can also provide a complete cardiac output and full cardiopulmonary bypass. This becomes relevant if the aortic arch is involved in the aortic injury. When partial heart bypass is utilized, flows in the circuit are maintained at 2 to 3 L/min as in partial left heart bypass circuits. When neither an oxygenator nor a heat exchanger is used, no heparin is required as with left heart bypass.[153] In this case, the femoral arterial PaO_2 is approximately 40 mm Hg (saturation 45%-65%), which is adequate for tissue oxygen needs provided the hemoglobin concentration is maintained above 10 g/dL. The concern that perfusion of the lower body with this reduced blood oxygen saturation might increase the paraplegia rate has not been realized.[137]

Right atrial to femoral arterial bypass has the distinct advantage of allowing for establishment of partial or complete bypass prior to entering the chest. Additionally, this technique is preferred when there is concomitant right lung contusion in order to assure adequate tissue oxygenation during repair. Rarely, there may be a need to perform a proximal anastomosis under deep hypothermic circulatory arrest (HCA) because of an injury that involves the aortic arch, and right atrial cannulation provides an adequate amount of inflow to the pump to facilitate complete cardiopulmonary bypass while left atrial cannulation alone usually does not. Use of this technique should proceed with caution in a trauma patient and only after other associated injuries have been addressed to avoid bleeding complications. If HCA is required, it is essential to confirm the lack of aortic valvular insufficiency. When HCA is utilized within the left chest, the left ventricle should be vented via the left inferior pulmonary vein.

Passive proximal to distal aortic shunt (Gott shunt) Of predominantly historical interest, this technique shunts blood from the proximal aorta to the distal aorta with a tapered, heparin-coated polyvinyl tube.[123] The proximal end is placed in the ascending aorta, the arch of the aorta, or the left subclavian artery and the distal end is placed in the descending aorta or femoral artery. Ventricular cannulation had been used in the past, but it was abandoned due to a high rate of ventricular dysrhythmias, reduced shunt flows, and a higher rate of paraplegia.[25,123,124,151,154,155] The diameter of the shunt is obviously fixed, and therefore flow is passive, unmonitored, and dependent on a pressure gradient. Femoral arterial monitoring, as with all of these techniques, is recommended.[151] The Gott shunt is easy to use although it requires a more extensive dissection of either the aortic arch or ascending aorta. It does not offer the left ventricular unloading or loading advantage that partial bypass systems allow, and therefore blood pressure control is left to pharmacology alone.

INTRAOPERATIVE MANAGEMENT OF AORTIC DISRUPTION

The decisions about heparinization and method of lower body perfusion should be made prior to incision if feasible. It should be clear that if no heparin is planned, cannulation of vessels must be immediately followed by bypass to allow for immediate flow through the circuit to prevent thrombosis. The order of conduct for contained aortic disruptions should be to establish groin access first, if employing femoral bypass techniques, followed by chest incision and control of the proximal and distal aorta around the site of injury. If cannulation is planned in the chest, proximal and distal aortic control is established first. The left inferior pulmonary vein is dissected after establishing aortic control when planning partial left heart bypass. Excessive compression or traction of the lung should be avoided, particularly when dissecting out the aortic arch, as the pulmonary artery may be easily disrupted.

The mediastinal pleura is incised along the anterior surface of the proximal left subclavian artery. The subclavian artery is then encircled with a tape. The pleura overlying the distal aortic arch is incised lateral to the vagus nerve. Great care is taken to avoid injury to either the phrenic or vagus nerves as they pass over the aortic arch, which can be difficult since they are often obscured by the hematoma. They are reflected off the aorta with the overlying pleura and are retracted medially by attaching silk suture stays to the pleura just lateral to the vagus nerve. Loops around the nerves themselves should be avoided, because even stretch of these nerves will result in paresis. This reflection exposes the arch of the aorta between the left common carotid and left subclavian arteries, which is the point needed for proximal aortic control in most cases. Inferiorly, the vagus nerve and its branching left recurrent laryngeal nerve are reflected medially as well. This exposes the ligamentum arteriosum, which can be sharply divided. The aortic arch between the left carotid and subclavian artery superiorly and medial to the ligamentum inferiorly is encircled with a tape after establishing a plane between the posterior arch and the trachea using a combination of sharp and gentle finger dissection.

Distal aortic control is established at an adequate distance from the aortic injury to facilitate repair. The overlying pleura is incised, and the aorta encircled with a tape. The left inferior pulmonary vein is dissected out anteriorly. Opening the pericardium just anterior to the vein allows better exposure and a better site of pulmonary venous cannulation. Heparin, if employed, is given. We establish arterial cannulation first. Distal aortic purse-string sutures are fashioned below the distal clamp site, or the femoral artery is cannulated by Seldinger technique with serial dilatation to the desired cannula size. The inferior pulmonary vein is then cannulated with a 20-20F dual-stage catheter. The circuit for left heart bypass is connected. Lower body perfusion is initiated, and once systemic blood pressure is stabilized the left subclavian artery is clamped followed by the proximal aorta then the distal aorta. We prefer to clamp the proximal aorta between the left common carotid artery and the left subclavian artery because the tear frequently extends quite close to the ostium of the left subclavian artery. Upper and lower body pressures are stabilized with the bypass circuit to maintain upper body mean arterial pressures of 70 to 80 mm Hg and a lower body pressure of 60 to 70 mm Hg with flows of 2 to 3 L/min.

The periaortic hematoma is then entered, and the edges of the transected aorta identified. Usually the aorta is completely transected, and the edges are separated by 2 to 4 cm.[6,12] Less frequently the transection is only partial. Some authors advocate primary repair at this point,[25,156] but most surgeons place a short interposition graft after debridement of the torn edges.[9,10,23,26,33,81,124,126,128–130] Collagen-coated woven Dacron grafts or gelatin-impregnated grafts are used most commonly. Use of intraluminal prostheses has been abandoned by most groups.[157] Grafts are sewn using a running 3-0 or 4-0 polypropylene suture with the proximal anastomosis performed first, followed by the distal.

Generous amounts of adventitial tissue are included in each bite. Pledgeted reinforcing horizontal mattress sutures are placed intra- or extraluminally as necessary. Upon completion of the anastomoses, the distal clamp is removed first, followed by the proximal aortic, and finally the left subclavian arterial. The patient is then weaned off partial bypass. Heparin is reversed, and the bypass cannulae removed. Hemostasis is achieved, and the chest is closed in a standard fashion.

If the aorta is already ruptured with bleeding into the hemithorax, proximal aortic dissection between the left carotid and subclavian arteries is rapidly performed, and a cross-clamp quickly applied. The descending aorta is then clamped below the injury, and the hematoma opened. No attempt is made to establish lower body perfusion, but every attempt is made to maintain normal or slightly elevated mean arterial pressure during clamping. The aortic repair is done as expeditiously as possible in order to minimize clamp time. Repair sutures are placed accordingly after clamps are removed. Hemostasis is then achieved after continuity of the aorta is reestablished.

Previous left thoracotomy Emergency room thoracotomies are usually done in haste by inexperienced nonthoracic surgeons and are often placed at sites too low to effectively repair an aortic transection. Given this situation it is usually best to enter the chest through a fourth interspace thoracotomy even if this means creating a second intercostal incision. When a patient with a history of prior left thoracotomy presents with an aortic injury, the associated scarring offers both an advantage and disadvantage to the patient. The adhesions between the lung and mediastinum help contain the rupture and make it less likely to exsanguinate, but they also make the dissection considerably more difficult and time consuming. Optimally, dissection in these cases should be done prior to heparinization.

Extension of the tear into the left subclavian artery We recommend placing the proximal aortic clamp proximal to the left subclavian artery since most aortic ruptures tear close to it. This allows for an easier, more precise proximal anastomosis. The subclavian is controlled after encircling it with a tape just distal to its origin. Occasionally, the aortic tear will extend into the left subclavian orifice, and in this case the proximal clamp may have to partially or totally occlude the left common carotid. The left subclavian is then completely detached from the aorta, the proximal anastomosis completed, and the clamp then moved distally onto the graft. The left subclavian is then reattached to the aortic graft with an interposition graft after completing the distal aortic anastomosis. The left common carotid artery will usually tolerate occlusion for 10 to 15 minutes without sequelae. The left subclavian interposition graft is fashioned with an end-to-end anastomosis distally and an end-to-side anastomosis proximally.

Endoluminal stent grafts There are now reports of the use of endoluminal stent grafts in the setting of acute traumatic aortic disruption.[158,159] In each case reported, associated injuries were felt to render a prohibitive operative risk with conventional repair. Significant pulmonary contusions were cited most frequently. Currently, use of endoluminal stent grafts for aortic transection remains experimental. In the future, a defined role for their use may evolve, particularly in patients with prohibitive injuries, life-threatening comorbidities, or advanced age.

Nonisthmic Aortic/Arterial Lacerations

The incidence of acute rupture of the ascending aorta among motor vehicular or other trauma patients is not known as most of these patients do not survive beyond the site of the accident. However, there are reports of successful repairs of these injuries.[19,24,160] Most commonly the proximal ascending aorta at or just above the sinotubular junction is involved.[24] There are a few case reports of ascending aortic ruptures associated with the deployment of air bags.[19,20] Ascending aortic ruptures require full heparinization and cardiopulmonary bypass for repair. Therefore, these injuries should initially be managed with beta blockade and blood pressure control until a thorough evaluation of all other life-threatening injuries is completed. These injuries are approached through a median sternotomy. The survival among cases reported in the literature of those undergoing repair is about 85%.[24] They have been repaired either primarily or with an interposition graft. Rarely, a concomitant aortic valve replacement is required.[24]

Lacerations to the base of the innominate or left common carotid arteries should be approached through a median sternotomy and may require cardiopulmonary bypass depending on the degree of aortic involvement.[38] Extension of the incision into the right or left neck including detachment of the sternocleidomastoid from the sternum is usually helpful in obtaining adequate exposure. When the base of the left carotid or innominate artery is injured, the safest option is to oversew the base and create an interposition graft to the ascending aorta in an end-to-side fashion.[86,161,162] Injury to the base of the left subclavian artery can be approached either by sternotomy or left posterolateral thoracotomy, the latter of which typically provides better exposure.[161] Alternatively, when injuries extend out onto either the left or right subclavian arteries a thoracosternotomy, cervicosternotomy, or cervicosternothoracotomy "trap door" incision each provides good exposure depending on the level of the injury.[1] Finally, the transverse anterior thoracosternotomy "clam-shell" incision provides good exposure to the mediastinal structures and both hemithoraces when multiple injuries require repair.[1]

Aortic injuries of the descending aorta distal to the isthmus to the level of T8 should be approached through a posterolateral thoracotomy in the 4th, 5th, or 6th interspace depending on the level of injury. These types of aortic injuries from blunt trauma are rare. More commonly, this segment of aorta is injured by penetrating trauma. These patients rarely make it to the hospital alive. When the distal thoracoabdominal aorta is injured below T8, it should be approached by thoracoabdominal incision. This can be done either retroperitoneally or intraperitoneally. An intraperitoneal approach offers the advantage of allowing for abdominal exploration, but retraction of the abdominal contents with a thoracoabdominal incision and a violated peritoneum can be cumbersome. We use partial left heart bypass with left atrial to femoral arterial or distal aortic cannulation for all thoracoabdominal aortic procedures unless active bleeding precludes its setup, or there is an absolute contraindication to heparinization.

Associated Injuries

Life-threatening intracranial, thoracic, intra-abdominal, or retroperitoneal hemorrhage should be addressed prior to repair of aortic lacerations that are not bleeding.[60,62,163] Posterolateral thoracotomy should immediately follow laparotomy provided hemodynamic stability is achieved after control of intra-abdominal injury. Long bone fractures should be stabilized with only temporary splinting during preparation for thoracotomy. Exsanguinating pelvic fractures should be stabilized with external fixation and/or angiographic embolization prior to aortic repair.[77,164–166] Patients should be carefully monitored throughout these interventions with judicious fluid replacement, avoiding fluid overload and optimizing respiratory, circulatory, and renal function. Body temperature should be controlled to avoid hypothermia.

Postoperative Care

Postoperative care after aortic repair is similar to that given patients who have other major cardiothoracic surgery. Immediately following aortic repair in the operating room, patients should undergo flexible bronchoscopy for evacuation of bloody secretions to avoid plugging and atelectasis of the left lung. Vital signs, ventricular filling pressures, blood pressures, cardiac output, renal function, chest tube output, nasogastric drainage, body temperature, neurologic status, blood gases, and coagulation function are all monitored closely. Blood products are given as indicated. Chest x-rays are followed serially. Pulmonary toilet is extraordinarily important, and once clinically stable (usually on postoperative day one) an epidural catheter should be placed for narcotic and local anesthetic delivery if not placed preoperatively. This facilitates good pulmonary recovery. Antibiotics are given in a standard prophylactic fashion. Patients are extubated as soon as is clinically indicated. Chest tubes are removed when any air leak has stopped and drainage is less than 150 to 200 cc of serous fluid per day.

Complications

Complications after aortic repair occur at a rate of 40% to 50%.[10,25,27,33,86] Pneumonia is the most common complication and occurs at a rate of 17% to 34%.[10,25,27,33,86] Other complications include bacteremia, renal insufficiency, and paraplegia. Rates of frequency for several series are listed in Table 51-4.[10,25,27,33,86] Left vocal cord paralysis has been reported to occur at a rate of 4% to 14%, although recurrent nerve injuries are probably underreported. Late complications are rare in these patients. Aortobronchial fistula following repair of transection has been reported.[167,168]

TABLE 51–4 Major postoperative complications

	Schmidt[25] (n = 73)	Cowley[33] (n = 51)	Kodali[86] (n = 50)	AAST[10] (n = 207)
Paraplegia	5.4%	19.6%	10%	8.7%
Renal failure	9.6%	9.8%	4%	8.7%
Sepsis	13.7%	9.8%	—	—
ARDS/pneumonia	21.9%	17.7%	34%	33.0%
Left vocal cord paralysis	4.1%	13.7%	14%	4.3%
Left phrenic nerve palsy	1.4%	5.9%	—	—
Stroke	2.7%	—	4%	—
Reexploration for bleeding	1.4%	9.8%	4%	—
Pulmonary embolism	1.4%	3.9%	—	—
Deep vein thrombosis	2.7%	—	—	—
Empyema	—	—	—	1.9%
Wound infection	—	3.9%	—	—
Chylothorax	—	3.9%	—	—
Deaths	8.8%	43.1%	28%	14.0% (31.3%)*

*Twenty-nine deaths (14%) occurred among the 207 patients who presented in stable condition. An additional 46 patients presented either *in extremis* or with free rupture, and all of these patients died in the hospital. All told there were 86 deaths among 274 patients included in the AAST trial (31.3%).

TABLE 51–5 Incidence of postoperative paraplegia in relation to operative technique: meta-analysis

Operative technique	No. of patients	Paraplegia (%)	Clamp time (min.)
No shunt	443	19.2	31.8
Passive shunt	424	11.1	46.8
CPB*	490	2.4	47.8
Partial bypass†	71	1.4	39.5

*CPB, cardiopulmonary bypass with oxygenator and heparin.
†Partial bypass, partial left heart, or femoral vein to artery without systemic heparin.
Source: Reproduced with permission from von Oppell UO, Dunne TT, De Groot MK, Zilla P. Traumatic aortic rupture: twenty-year metaanalysis of mortality and risk of paraplegia. Ann Thorac Surg 1994; 58:585.

TABLE 51–6 Incidence of postoperative paraplegia in relation to operative technique: AAST prospective trial

Operative technique	No. of patients	Paraplegia (%)
Bypass	134	4.5
Gott shunt	4	0
Full bypass	22	4.5
Partial bypass	39	7.7
Centrifugal pump	69	2.9†
Clamp and sew	73	16.4*†

*$p < .004$, bypass vs. clamp and sew.
*†$p < .01$, centrifugal pump vs. clamp and sew.
Source: Reproduced with permission from Fabian TC, Richardson JD, Croce MA, et al: Prospective study of blunt aortic injury: Multicenter Trial of the American Association for the Surgery of Trauma. J Trauma 1997; 42:374.

Patients who survive an undiagnosed aortic injury may develop a chronic traumatic aortic aneurysm.[15,39–44,70–74] Among those patients with initial pseudoaneurysm formation, most develop progressive dilation with symptoms of pain referable to aneurysmal expansion. Other symptoms include dyspnea or cough secondary to compression of the left mainstem bronchus, hoarseness due to stretching of the recurrent nerve, hemoptysis, or dysphagia. These chronic traumatic aortic aneurysms, once discovered, should be repaired regardless of size unless there are contraindications due to age or comorbidity.

Results

The mortality rate of patients with aortic rupture who reach the hospital ranges from 7% to 55% depending on whether or not the injury is repaired.[9,10,23,31] Among hemodynamically stable patients undergoing planned thoracotomy and repair, the hospital mortality rate is 14% in the modern era.[10] The mortality rate of nonoperative patients with associated injuries precluding initial aortic repair was 55% in the AAST trial.[10] All patients who either presented *in extremis* or with free rupture died of aortic rupture. In his meta-analysis of 1492 patients, Von Opell reported an average of 7.8% of patients dying during aortic repair, and 13.5% dying in the postoperative period.[31]

Paraplegia or paraparesis occurred in an average of 9.9% of patients in the review by Von Opell.[31] However, paraplegia rates vary widely depending on the operative technique utilized with ranges of 0% to 20%.[9,10,23,31,33,64,86] Although several groups have reported very low paraplegia rates using the "clamp-and-sew" technique, these results have not been widely reproduced.[10,23] Alternatively, use of extracorporeal lower body perfusion systems has facilitated low rates of paraplegia.[10] At the University of Pennsylvania, since the practice of partial left heart bypass for all repairs of aortic transection was instituted in 1994 there have been no cases of paraplegia in a series of over 40 patients (unpublished data). It is also clear that increasing cross-clamp time, particularly beyond 30 minutes, increases the rate of paraplegia.[10,135] The preponderance of data suggests that the combination of partial left heart bypass for lower body perfusion with short (less than 30 minutes) cross-clamp time affords the lowest rate of paraplegia (Tables 51-5 and 51-6).[10,31]

NONAORTIC GREAT VESSEL INJURY

The majority of injuries to the great venous structures and the pulmonary arteries are a result of penetrating trauma. Blunt trauma to these structures is rare. The incidence of injury to the nonaortic great vessels among cases of penetrating thoracic trauma is not known, but the overall incidence of great vessel injury with thoracic gunshot wounds is approximately 5% and with stab wounds is 2%.[169] Patients with penetrating injuries to the thorax should all be managed utilizing standard ATLS protocol as outlined above. Wounds penetrating the thoracic "box" bordered between the midclavicular lines, the thoracic outlet, and xiphoid process should be explored operatively. Chest tubes should be inserted as a diagnostic and therapeutic measure, and a subxiphoid pericardial window performed to rule out hemopericardium. Patients with a high index of suspicion of mediastinal great vessel injury or with a confirmed hemopericardium should undergo sternotomy. Patients with central venous or pulmonary arterial rupture will decompensate from pericardial tamponade. Expeditious pericardial decompression will often provide enough stability to facilitate definitive repair. Exsanguination from a venous or pulmonary arterial injury into one of the hemithoraces requires immediate massive volume resuscitation and transfer to the operating room. Choice of incision should be made based on clinical suspicion of site of injury or objective data (arteriography, chest radiograph, or bleeding site). When site of injury is not clear, median sternotomy provides excellent access to the heart and great vessels, and it can be extended across a hemithorax or up the neck along either sternocleidomastoid to facilitate exposure of any vascular structure in the chest. Most venous injuries and pulmonary arterial injuries when localized and simple can be repaired without cardiopulmonary bypass. Large or complex venous, and particularly pulmonary arterial, injuries are often more easily repaired on full cardiopulmonary bypass with a decompressed heart. When repairing pulmonary venous injuries it is important to safeguard against air embolus, the result of which can be devastating. Therefore, complex pulmonary venous injury may require aortic cross-clamping with cardioplegia to prevent embolus to the brain.

REFERENCES

1. Reul GJ Jr, Beall AC Jr, Jordan GL Jr, Mattox KL: The early operative management of injuries to great vessels. *Surgery* 1973; 74:862.
2. Weaver FA, Suda RW, Stiles GM, Yellin AE: Injuries to the ascending aorta, aortic arch and great vessels. *Surg Gynecol Obstet* 1989; 169:27.
3. Fabian TC, Davis KA, Gavant ML, et al: Prospective study of blunt aortic injury: helical CT is diagnostic and antihypertensive therapy reduces rupture. *Ann Surg* 1998; 227:666.
4. Gavant ML, Flick P, Menke P, Gold RE: CT aortography of thoracic aortic rupture. *AJR Am J Roentgenol* 1996; 166:955.
5. Gavant ML: Helical CT grading of traumatic aortic injuries: impact on clinical guidelines for medical and surgical management. *Radiol Clin North Am* 1999; 37:553.
6. Parmley L, Mattingly T, Manion W: Nonpenetrating traumatic injury of the aorta. *Circulation* 1958; 17:1086.
7. Sailer S: Dissecting aneurysm of the aorta. *Arch Pathol* 1942; 23:704.
8. Williams JS, Graff JA, Uku JM, Steinig JP: Aortic injury in vehicular trauma. *Ann Thorac Surg* 1994; 57:726.
9. Razzouk AJ, Gundry SR, Wang N, et al: Repair of traumatic aortic rupture: a 25-year experience. *Arch Surg* 2000; 135:913.
10. Fabian TC, Richardson JD, Croce MA, et al: Prospective study of blunt aortic injury: Multicenter Trial of the American Association for the Surgery of Trauma. *J Trauma* 1997; 42:374.
11. Greendyke RM: Traumatic rupture of aorta; special reference to automobile accidents. *JAMA* 1966; 195:527.
12. Feczko JD, Lynch L, Pless JE, et al: An autopsy case review of 142 nonpenetrating (blunt) injuries of the aorta. *J Trauma* 1992; 33:846.
13. Dischinger P, Cowley R, Shankar B: The incidence of ruptured aorta among vehicular fatalities. *Proc Assoc Adv Automot Med Conf* 1988; 32:15.
14. Smith RS, Chang FC: Traumatic rupture of the aorta: still a lethal injury. *Am J Surg* 1986; 152:660.
15. Duhaylongsod FG, Glower DD, Wolfe WG: Acute traumatic aortic aneurysm: the Duke experience from 1970 to 1990. *J Vasc Surg* 1992; 15:331.
16. Demetriades D, Gomez H, Velmahos GC, et al: Routine helical computed tomographic evaluation of the mediastinum in high-risk blunt trauma patients. *Arch Surg* 1998; 133:1084.
17. Durham RM, Zuckerman D, Wolverson M, et al: Computed tomography as a screening exam in patients with suspected blunt aortic injury. *Ann Surg* 1994; 220:699.
18. Pillgram-Larsen J, Geiran O: [Air bags influence the pattern of injury in severe thoracic trauma]. *Tidsskr Nor Laegeforen* 1997; 117:2437.
19. Dunn JA, Williams MG: Occult ascending aortic rupture in the presence of an air bag. *Ann Thorac Surg* 1996; 62:577.
20. deGuzman BJ, Morgan AS, Pharr WF: Aortic transection following air-bag deployment. *N Engl J Med* 1997; 337:573.
21. Brown DK, Roe EJ, Henry TE: A fatality associated with the deployment of an automobile airbag. *J Trauma* 1995; 39:1204.
22. Pezzella AT: Blunt traumatic injury of the thoracic aorta following commercial airline crashes. *Tex Heart Inst J* 1996; 23:65.
23. Sweeney MS, Young DJ, Frazier OH, et al: Traumatic aortic transections: eight-year experience with the "clamp-sew" technique. *Ann Thorac Surg* 1997; 64:384.
24. Symbas PJ, Horsley WS, Symbas PN: Rupture of the ascending aorta caused by blunt trauma. *Ann Thorac Surg* 1998; 66:113.
25. Schmidt CA, Wood MN, Razzouk AJ, et al: Primary repair of traumatic aortic rupture: a preferred approach. *J Trauma* 1992; 32:588.
26. Hilgenberg AD, Logan DL, Akins CW, et al: Blunt injuries of the thoracic aorta. *Ann Thorac Surg* 1992; 53:233.
27. Kirsh MM, Behrendt DM, Orringer MB, et al: The treatment of acute traumatic rupture of the aorta: a 10-year experience. *Ann Surg* 1976; 184:308.
28. Sturm JT, Billiar TR, Dorsey JS, et al: Risk factors for survival following surgical treatment of traumatic aortic rupture. *Ann Thorac Surg* 1985; 39:418.
29. Arajarvi E, Santavirta S, Tolonen J: Aortic ruptures in seat belt wearers. *J Thorac Cardiovasc Surg* 1989; 98:355.
30. Rabinsky I, Sidhu GS, Wagner RB: Mid-descending aortic traumatic aneurysms. *Ann Thorac Surg* 1990; 50:155.
31. von Oppell UO, Dunne TT, De Groot MK, Zilla P: Traumatic aortic rupture: twenty-year meta-analysis of mortality and risk of paraplegia. *Ann Thorac Surg* 1994; 58:585.
32. Kieny R, Charpentier A: Traumatic lesions of the thoracic aorta: a report of 73 cases. *J Cardiovasc Surg* (Torino) 1991; 32:613.
33. Cowley RA, Turney SZ, Hankins JR, et al: Rupture of thoracic aorta caused by blunt trauma: a fifteen-year experience. *J Thorac Cardiovasc Surg* 1990; 100:652.
34. Katz S, Mullin R, Berger RL: Traumatic transection associated with retrograde dissection and rupture of the aorta: recognition and management. *Ann Thorac Surg* 1974; 17:273.
35. Strassman G: Traumatic rupture of the aorta. *Am Heart J* 1947; 33:508.
36. Butcher HJ: The elastic properties of the human aortic intima, media and adventitia: the initial effect of thromboendarterectomy. *Ann Surg* 1960; 1151:480.
37. Lundevall J: The mechanism of traumatic rupture of the aorta. *Acta Pathol Microbiol Scand* 1964; 62:34.
38. Pretre R, Chilcott M, Murith N, Panos A: Blunt injury to the supra-aortic arteries. *Br J Surg* 1997; 84:603.
39. Bennett DE, Cherry JK: The natural history of traumatic aneurysms of the aorta. *Surgery* 1967; 61:516.
40. Finkelmeier BA, Mentzer RM Jr, Kaiser DL, et al: Chronic traumatic thoracic aneurysm: influence of operative treatment on natural history: an analysis of reported cases, 1950–1980. *J Thorac Cardiovasc Surg* 1982; 84:257.
41. John LC, Hornick P, Edmondson SJ: Chronic traumatic aneurysm of the aorta: to resect or not, the role of exploration operation. *J Cardiovasc Surg* (Torino) 1992; 33:106.
42. McCollum CH, Graham JM, Noon GP, DeBakey ME: Chronic traumatic aneurysms of the thoracic aorta: an analysis of 50 patients. *J Trauma* 1979; 19:248.
43. Albuquerque FC, Krasna MJ, McLaughlin JS: Chronic, traumatic pseudoaneurysm of the ascending aorta. *Ann Thorac Surg* 1992; 54:980.
44. Prat A, Warembourg H Jr, Watel A, et al: Chronic traumatic aneurysms of the descending thoracic aorta (19 cases). *J Cardiovasc Surg* (Torino) 1986; 27:268.
45. Stapp J: Human tolerance to deceleration. *Am J Surg* 1957; 93:734.
46. Marsh C, Moore R: Deceleration trauma. *Am J Surg* 1957; 93:623.

47. Aldman B: Biodynamic studies on impact protection. *Acta Physiol Scand* 1962; 56(suppl):192.
48. Jackson FR, Berkas EM, Roberts VL: Traumatic aortic rupture after blunt trauma. *Dis Chest* 1968; 53:577.
49. Sevitt S: The mechanisms of traumatic rupture of the thoracic aorta. *Br J Surg* 1977; 64:166.
50. Sevitt S: Traumatic ruptures of the aorta: a clinico-pathological study. *Injury* 1977; 8:159.
51. Gotzen L, Flory PJ, Otte D: Biomechanics of aortic rupture at classical location in traffic accidents. *Thorac Cardiovasc Surg* 1980; 28:64.
52. Coermann R, Dotzauer G, Lange W, Voigt GE: The effects of the design of the steering assembly and the instrument panel on injuries (especially aortic rupture) sustained by car drivers in head-on collision. *J Trauma* 1972; 12:715.
53. Voigt GE, Wilfort K: Mechanisms of injuries to unrestrained drivers in head-on collisions, in *Proceedings of the 30th Stapp Car Crash Conference*. New York, New York Society of Automotive Engineers, 1969.
54. Crass JR, Cohen AM, Motta AO, et al: A proposed new mechanism of traumatic aortic rupture: the osseous pinch. *Radiology* 1990; 176:645.
55. Cohen AM, Crass JR, Thomas HA, et al: CT evidence for the "osseous pinch" mechanism of traumatic aortic injury. *AJR Am J Roentgenol* 1992; 159:271.
56. Cohen AM, Crass JR: Traumatic aortic injuries: current concepts. *Semin Ultrasound CT MR* 1993; 14:71.
57. Zehnder M: Delayed post-traumatic rupture of the aorta in a young healthy individual after closed injury: mechanical-etiological considerations. *Angiology* 1956; 7:252.
58. Oppenheim F: Gibt es eine spontanruptur der gesunden aorta und wie kommt sie zustande? *Muenchen Med Wochenschr* 1918; 65:1234.
59. Malhotra AK, Fabian TC, Croce MA, et al: Minimal aortic injury: a lesion associated with advancing diagnostic techniques. *J Trauma* 2001; 51:1042.
60. Nagy K, Fabian T, Rodman G, et al: Guidelines for the diagnosis and management of blunt aortic injury: an EAST Practice Management Guidelines Work Group. *J Trauma* 2000; 48:1128.
61. Fisher RG, Oria RA, Mattox KL, et al: Conservative management of aortic lacerations due to blunt trauma. *J Trauma* 1990; 30:1562.
62. Borman KR, Aurbakken CM, Weigelt JA: Treatment priorities in combined blunt abdominal and aortic trauma. *Am J Surg* 1982; 144:728.
63. Camp PC, Shackford SR: Outcome after blunt traumatic thoracic aortic laceration: identification of a high-risk cohort. Western Trauma Association Multicenter Study Group. *J Trauma* 1997; 43:413.
64. Akins CW, Buckley MJ, Daggett W, et al: Acute traumatic disruption of the thoracic aorta: a ten-year experience. *Ann Thorac Surg* 1981; 31:305.
65. Bodily K, Perry JF Jr, Strate RG, Fischer RP: The salvageability of patients with post-traumatic rupture of the descending thoracic aorta in a primary trauma center. *J Trauma* 1977; 17:754.
66. Camp PC Jr, Rogers FB, Shackford SR, et al: Blunt traumatic thoracic aortic lacerations in the elderly: an analysis of outcome. *J Trauma* 1994; 37:418.
67. Maggisano R, Nathens A, Alexandrova NA, et al: Traumatic rupture of the thoracic aorta: should one always operate immediately? *Ann Vasc Surg* 1995; 9:44.
68. Pezzella AT, Todd EP, Dillon ML, et al: Early diagnosis and individualized treatment of blunt thoracic aortic trauma. *Am Surg* 1978; 44:699.
69. Weimann S, Balogh D, Furtwangler W, et al: Graft replacement of post-traumatic thoracic aortic aneurysm: results without bypass or shunting. *Eur J Vasc Surg* 1992; 6:381.
70. Roques X, Bourdeaud'hui A, Collet D, et al: Traumatic rupture and aneurysm of the aortic isthmus: late results of repair by direct suture. *Ann Vasc Surg* 1989; 3:47.
71. Roques X: [Chronic post-traumatic aneurysms of the thoracic aorta]. *Rev Prat* 1991; 41:1789.
72. Becker HM, Ramirez J, Echave V, Heberer G: Traumatic aneurysms of the descending thoracic aorta. *Ann Vasc Surg* 1986; 1:196.
73. Russo P, Orszulak TA, Arnold PG, et al: Concomitant repair of a chronic traumatic aortic aneurysm with tracheal erosion. *Ann Thorac Surg* 1987; 43:559.
74. Heystraten FM, Rosenbusch G, Kingma LM, Lacquet LK: Chronic posttraumatic aneurysm of the thoracic aorta: surgically correctable occult threat. *AJR Am J Roentgenol* 1986; 146:303.
75. Clark DE, Zeiger MA, Wallace KL, et al: Blunt aortic trauma: signs of high risk. *J Trauma* 1990; 30:701.
76. Gundry SR, Williams S, Burney RE, et al: Indications for aortography in blunt thoracic trauma: a reassessment. *J Trauma* 1982; 22:664.
77. Kram HB, Appel PL, Wohlmuth DA, Shoemaker WC: Diagnosis of traumatic thoracic aortic rupture: a 10-year retrospective analysis. *Ann Thorac Surg* 1989; 47:282.
78. Sturm JT, Perry JF Jr, Olson FR, Cicero JJ: Significance of symptoms and signs in patients with traumatic aortic rupture. *Ann Emerg Med* 1984; 13:876.
79. Trachiotis GD, Sell JE, Pearson GD, et al: Traumatic thoracic aortic rupture in the pediatric patient. *Ann Thorac Surg* 1996; 62:724.
80. Vlahakes GJ, Warren RL: Traumatic rupture of the aorta. *N Engl J Med* 1995; 332:389.
81. Plume S, DeWeese JA: Traumatic rupture of the thoracic aorta. *Arch Surg* 1979; 114:240.
82. Kram HB, Wohlmuth DA, Appel PL, Shoemaker WC: Clinical and radiographic indications for aortography in blunt chest trauma. *J Vasc Surg* 1987; 6:168.
83. Goarin JP, Le Bret F, Riou B, et al: Early diagnosis of traumatic thoracic aortic rupture by transesophageal echocardiography. *Chest* 1993; 103:618.
84. Hengster P, Furtwangler W, Pernthaler H: Transesophageal echocardiography for the diagnosis of traumatic injury of the thoracic aorta. *J Thorac Cardiovasc Surg* 1994; 107:638.
85. Hartford JM, Fayer RL, Shaver TE, et al: Transection of the thoracic aorta: assessment of a trauma system. *Am J Surg* 1986; 151:224.
86. Kodali S, Jamieson WR, Leia-Stephens M, et al: Traumatic rupture of the thoracic aorta: a 20-year review, 1969–1989. *Circulation* 1991; 84:III40.
87. Cook AD, Klein JS, Rogers FB, et al: Chest radiographs of limited utility in the diagnosis of blunt traumatic aortic laceration. *J Trauma* 2001; 50:843.
88. Burney RE, Gundry SR, Mackenzie JR, et al: Chest roentgenograms in diagnosis of traumatic rupture of the aorta: observer variation in interpretation. *Chest* 1984; 85:605.
89. Cigarroa JE, Isselbacher EM, DeSanctis RW, Eagle KA: Diagnostic imaging in the evaluation of suspected aortic dissection: old standards and new directions. *N Engl J Med* 1993; 328:35.
90. Gundry SR, Burney RE, Mackenzie JR, et al: Assessment of mediastinal widening associated with traumatic rupture of the aorta. *J Trauma* 1983; 23:293.
91. Heystraten FM, Rosenbusch G, Kingma LM, et al: Chest radiography in acute traumatic rupture of the thoracic aorta. *Acta Radiol* 1988; 29:411.
92. Mattox KL: Fact and fiction about management of aortic transection. *Ann Thorac Surg* 1989; 48:1.

93. Parker MS, Matheson TL, Rao AV, et al: Making the transition: the role of helical CT in the evaluation of potentially acute thoracic aortic injuries. *AJR Am J Roentgenol* 2001; 176:1267.
94. Raptopoulos V, Sheiman RG, Phillips DA, et al: Traumatic aortic tear: screening with chest CT. *Radiology* 1992; 182:667.
95. Barker DE, Crabtree JD Jr, White JE, et al: Mediastinal evaluation utilizing the reverse Trendelenburg radiograph. *Am Surg* 1999; 65:484.
96. Agee CK, Metzler MH, Churchill RJ, Mitchell FL: Computed tomographic evaluation to exclude traumatic aortic disruption. *J Trauma* 1992; 33:876.
97. Gavant ML, Menke PG, Fabian T, et al: Blunt traumatic aortic rupture: detection with helical CT of the chest. *Radiology* 1995; 197:125.
98. Ishikawa T, Nakajima Y, Kaji T: The role of CT in traumatic rupture of the thoracic aorta and its proximal branches. *Semin Roentgenol* 1989; 24:38.
99. McLean TR, Olinger GN, Thorsen MK: Computed tomography in the evaluation of the aorta in patients sustaining blunt chest trauma. *J Trauma* 1991; 31:254.
100. Miller FB, Richardson JD, Thomas HA, et al: Role of CT in diagnosis of major arterial injury after blunt thoracic trauma. *Surgery* 1989; 106:596.
101. Mirvis SE, Shanmuganathan K, Miller BH, et al: Traumatic aortic injury: diagnosis with contrast-enhanced thoracic CT–five-year experience at a major trauma center. *Radiology* 1996; 200:413.
102. Mirvis SE, Shanmuganathan K, Buell J, Rodriguez A: Use of spiral computed tomography for the assessment of blunt trauma patients with potential aortic injury. *J Trauma* 1998; 45:922.
103. Morgan PW, Goodman LR, Aprahamian C, et al: Evaluation of traumatic aortic injury: does dynamic contrast-enhanced CT play a role? *Radiology* 1992; 182:661.
104. Pate JW, Minard G: Imaging of traumatic rupture of the aorta. *J Thorac Cardiovasc Surg* 1995; 109:190.
105. Richardson P, Mirvis SE, Scorpio R, Dunham CM: Value of CT in determining the need for angiography when findings of mediastinal hemorrhage on chest radiographs are equivocal. *AJR Am J Roentgenol* 1991; 156:273.
106. Wilson D, Voystock JF, Sariego J, Kerstein MD: Role of computed tomography scan in evaluating the widened mediastinum. *Am Surg* 1994; 60:421.
107. Vignon P, Boncoeur MP, Francois B, et al: Comparison of multiplane transesophageal echocardiography and contrast-enhanced helical CT in the diagnosis of blunt traumatic cardiovascular injuries. *Anesthesiology* 2001; 94:615.
108. Sturm JT, Hankins DG, Young G: Thoracic aortography following blunt chest trauma. *Am J Emerg Med* 1990; 8:92.
109. Smith MD, Cassidy JM, Souther S, et al: Transesophageal echocardiography in the diagnosis of traumatic rupture of the aorta. *N Engl J Med* 1995; 332:356.
110. Kearney PA, Smith DW, Johnson SB, et al: Use of transesophageal echocardiography in the evaluation of traumatic aortic injury. *J Trauma* 1993; 34:696.
111. Saletta S, Lederman E, Fein S, et al: Transesophageal echocardiography for the initial evaluation of the widened mediastinum in trauma patients. *J Trauma* 1995; 39:137.
112. LaBerge JM, Jeffrey RB: Aortic lacerations: fatal complications of thoracic aortography. *Radiology* 1987; 165:367.
113. Eddy AC, Nance DR, Goldman MA, et al: Rapid diagnosis of thoracic aortic transection using intravenous digital subtraction angiography. *Am J Surg* 1990; 159:500.
114. Nienaber CA, von Kodolitsch Y, Brockhoff CJ, et al: Comparison of conventional and transesophageal echocardiography with magnetic resonance imaging for anatomical mapping of thoracic aortic dissection: a dual noninvasive imaging study with anatomical and/or angiographic validation. *Int J Card Imaging* 1994; 10:1.
115. Goldstein SA, Lindsay J Jr, Vasan R: The diagnosis of thoracic aortic dissection by noninvasive imaging procedures. *N Engl J Med* 1993; 328:1637.
116. Hartnell G, Costello P: The diagnosis of thoracic aortic dissection by noninvasive imaging procedures. *N Engl J Med* 1993; 328:1637.
117. Nienaber CA, von Kodolitsch Y, Nicolas V, et al: The diagnosis of thoracic aortic dissection by noninvasive imaging procedures. *N Engl J Med* 1993; 328:1.
118. Feliciano DV, Rozycki GS: Advances in the diagnosis and treatment of thoracic trauma. *Surg Clin North Am* 1999; 79:1417.
119. Williams MJ, Low CJ, Wilkins GT, Stewart RA: Randomised comparison of the effects of nicardipine and esmolol on coronary artery wall stress: implications for the risk of plaque rupture. *Heart* 2000; 84:377.
120. Hanschen S, Snow NJ, Richardson JD: Thoracic aortic rupture in patients with multisystem injuries. *South Med J* 1982; 75:653.
121. Klena JW, Shweiki E, Woods EL, Indeck M: Purposeful delay in the repair of a traumatic rupture of the aorta with coexistent liver injury. *Ann Thorac Surg* 1998; 66:950.
122. Appelbaum A, Karp RB, Kirklin JW: Surgical treatment for closed thoracic aortic injuries. *J Thorac Cardiovasc Surg* 1976; 71:458.
123. Donahoo JS, Brawley RK, Gott VL: The heparin-coated vascular shunt for thoracic aortic and great vessel procedures: a ten-year experience. *Ann Thorac Surg* 1977; 23:507.
124. Merrill WH, Lee RB, Hammon JW Jr, et al: Surgical treatment of acute traumatic tear of the thoracic aorta. *Ann Surg* 1988; 207:699.
125. Pate JW, Gavant ML, Weiman DS, Fabian TC: Traumatic rupture of the aortic isthmus: program of selective management. *World J Surg* 1999; 23:59.
126. Stavens B, Hashim SW, Hammond GL, et al: Optimal methods of repair of descending thoracic aortic transection and aneurysms. *Am J Surg* 1983; 145:508.
127. Szwerc MF, Benckart DH, Lin JC, et al: Recent clinical experience with left heart bypass using a centrifugal pump for repair of traumatic aortic transection. *Ann Surg* 1999; 230:484.
128. Turney SZ, Attar S, Ayella R, et al: Traumatic rupture of the aorta: a five-year experience. *J Thorac Cardiovasc Surg* 1976; 72:727.
129. Zeiger MA, Clark DE, Morton JR: Reappraisal of surgical treatment of traumatic transection of the thoracic aorta. *J Cardiovasc Surg* (Torino) 1990; 31:607.
130. Wallenhaupt SL, Hudspeth AS, Mills SA, et al: Current treatment of traumatic aortic disruptions. *Am Surg* 1989; 55:316.
131. von Oppell UO, Dunne TT, De Groot KM, Zilla P: Spinal cord protection in the absence of collateral circulation: meta-analysis of mortality and paraplegia. *J Card Surg* 1994; 9:685.
132. Robinson J, Nawaz S, Beard JD: Randomized, multicentre, double-blind, placebo-controlled trial of the use of aprotinin in the repair of ruptured abdominal aortic aneurysm. On behalf of the Joint Vascular Research Group. *Br J Surg* 2000; 87:754.
133. Gillian L: The arterial blood supply of the human spinal cord. *J Comp Neurol* 1958; 110:75.
134. Adams H, Von Geertruyden H: Neurologic complications of aortic surgery. *Ann Surg* 1956; 144:574.
135. Katz NM, Blackstone EH, Kirklin JW, Karp RB: Incremental risk factors for spinal cord injury following operation for acute traumatic aortic transection. *J Thorac Cardiovasc Surg* 1981; 81:669.
136. Wadouh F, Arndt CF, Oppermann E, et al: The mechanism of spinal cord injury after simple and double aortic cross-clamping. *J Thorac Cardiovasc Surg* 1986; 92:121.
137. Grossi EA, Krieger KH, Cunningham JN Jr, et al: Venoarterial bypass: a technique for spinal cord protection. *J Thorac Cardiovasc Surg* 1985; 89:228.
138. Laschinger JC, Cunningham JN Jr, Catinella FP, et al: Detection and prevention of intraoperative spinal cord ischemia after cross-clamping of the thoracic aorta: use of somatosensory evoked potentials. *Surgery* 1982; 92:1109.

139. Laschinger JC, Cunningham JN Jr, Nathan IM, et al: Intraoperative identification of vessels critical to spinal cord blood supply—use of somatosensory evoked potentials. *Curr Surg* 1984; 41:107.
140. Laschinger JC, Cunningham JN Jr, Isom OW, et al: Definition of the safe lower limits of aortic resection during surgical procedures on the thoracoabdominal aorta: use of somatosensory evoked potentials. *J Am Coll Cardiol* 1983; 2:959.
141. Laschinger JC, Cunningham JN Jr, Nathan IM, et al: Experimental and clinical assessment of the adequacy of partial bypass in maintenance of spinal cord blood flow during operations on the thoracic aorta. *Ann Thorac Surg* 1983; 36:417.
142. Laschinger JC, Cunningham JN Jr, Cooper MM, et al: Prevention of ischemic spinal cord injury following aortic cross-clamping: use of corticosteroids. *Ann Thorac Surg* 1984; 38:500.
143. McCullough JL, Hollier LH, Nugent M: Paraplegia after thoracic aortic occlusion: influence of cerebrospinal fluid drainage: experimental and early clinical results. *J Vasc Surg* 1988; 7:153.
144. Kouchoukos NT, Wareing TH, Izumoto H, et al: Elective hypothermic cardiopulmonary bypass and circulatory arrest for spinal cord protection during operations on the thoracoabdominal aorta. *J Thorac Cardiovasc Surg* 1990; 99:659.
145. Kouchoukos NT, Masetti P, Rokkas CK, et al: Safety and efficacy of hypothermic cardiopulmonary bypass and circulatory arrest for operations on the descending thoracic and thoracoabdominal aorta. *Ann Thorac Surg* 2001; 72:699.
146. Kouchoukos NT, Rokkas CK: Hypothermic cardiopulmonary bypass for spinal cord protection: rationale and clinical results. *Ann Thorac Surg* 1999; 67:1940.
147. Rokkas CK, Kouchoukos NT: Profound hypothermia for spinal cord protection in operations on the descending thoracic and thoracoabdominal aorta. *Semin Thorac Cardiovasc Surg* 1998; 10:57.
148. Parrino PE, Kron IL, Ross SD, et al: Spinal cord protection during aortic cross-clamping using retrograde venous perfusion. *Ann Thorac Surg* 1999; 67:1589.
149. Parrino PE, Kron IL, Ross SD, et al: Retrograde venous perfusion with hypothermic saline and adenosine for protection of the ischemic spinal cord. *J Vasc Surg* 2000; 32:171.
150. Fullerton DA: Simplified technique for left heart bypass to repair aortic transection. *Ann Thorac Surg* 1993; 56:579.
151. Verdant A, Page A, Cossette R, et al: Surgery of the descending thoracic aorta: spinal cord protection with the Gott shunt. *Ann Thorac Surg* 1988; 46:147.
152. Hess PJ, Howe HR Jr., Robicsek F, et al: Traumatic tears of the thoracic aorta: improved results using the Bio-Medicus pump. *Ann Thorac Surg* 1989; 48:6.
153. Turney SZ: Blunt trauma of the thoracic aorta and its branches. *Semin Thorac Cardiovasc Surg* 1992; 4:209.
154. Pett SB Jr, Wernly JA, Akl BF: Observations on flow characteristics of passive external aortic shunts. *J Thorac Cardiovasc Surg* 1987; 93:447.
155. Marvasti MA, Meyer JA, Ford BE, Parker FB Jr: Spinal cord ischemia following operation for traumatic aortic transection. *Ann Thorac Surg* 1986; 42:425.
156. McBride LR, Tidik S, Stothert JC, et al: Primary repair of traumatic aortic disruption. *Ann Thorac Surg* 1987; 43:65.
157. Ablaza SG, Ghosh SC, Grana VP: Use of a ringed intraluminal graft in the surgical treatment of dissecting aneurysms of the thoracic aorta: a new technique. *J Thorac Cardiovasc Surg* 1978; 76:390.
158. Mattison R, Hamilton IN Jr, Ciraulo DL, Richart CM: Stent-graft repair of acute traumatic thoracic aortic transection with intentional occlusion of the left subclavian artery: case report. *J Trauma* 2001; 51:326.
159. Singh MJ, Rohrer MJ, Ghaleb M, Kim D: Endoluminal stent-graft repair of a thoracic aortic transection in a trauma patient with multiple injuries: case report. *J Trauma* 2001; 51:376.
160. Marzelle J, Nottin R, Dartevelle P, et al: Combined ascending aorta rupture and left main bronchus disruption from blunt chest trauma. *Ann Thorac Surg* 1989; 47:769.
161. Kirsh MM, Orringer MB, Behrendt DM, et al: Management of unusual traumatic ruptures of the aorta. *Surg Gynecol Obstet* 1978; 146:365.
162. Mattox KL, Wall MJR: Traumatic aneurysm of the thoracic aorta, in Najafi H (ed): *Chest Surgery Clinics of North America,* vol 2. Philadelphia, WB Saunders, 1992; p 413.
163. Hudson HM 2nd, Woodson J, Hirsch E: The management of traumatic aortic tear in the multiply-injured patient. *Ann Vasc Surg* 1991; 5:445.
164. Santini F, Gatti G, Cannarella A, Mazzucco A: Diagnosis and early surgical management of traumatic thoracic aortic disruption. *G Ital Cardiol* 1999; 29:1426.
165. Ochsner MG Jr, Hoffman AP, DiPasquale D, et al: Associated aortic rupture-pelvic fracture: an alert for orthopedic and general surgeons. *J Trauma* 1992; 33:429.
166. Ochsner MG Jr, Champion HR, Chambers RJ, Harviel JD: Pelvic fracture as an indicator of increased risk of thoracic aortic rupture. *J Trauma* 1989; 29:1376.
167. Kazerooni EA, Williams DM, Abrams GD, et al: Aortobronchial fistula 13 years following repair of aortic transection. *Chest* 1994; 106:1590.
168. Tsai FC, Lin PJ, Wu YC, Chang CH: Traumatic aortic arch transection with supracarinal tracheoesophageal fistula: case report. *J Trauma* 1999; 46:951.
169. Demetriades D: Penetrating injuries to the thoracic great vessels. *J Card Surg* 1997; 12:173.

Part **VI**

Surgery for Cardiac Arrhythmias

Chapter 52

Cardiologic Interventional Therapy for Atrial and Ventricular Arrhythmias

S. Dinakar Satti/Laurence M. Epstein

Cardiologic intervention for tachyarrhythmias has evolved from pharmacologic therapy to surgically based elimination of arrhythmogenic foci and circuits to transvenous catheter-based ablation procedures. It has dramatically changed the management of tachyarrhythmias. Catheter-based ablation has become the standard form of therapy for many tachyarrhythmias, surpassing pharmacologic and surgical methods.

This chapter will review the development of catheter-based ablation methods. It will focus on radiofrequency (RF) ablation, from the physics of RF energy as an ablation tool to clinical application to specific tachyarrhythmias. It will also review mapping techniques for localization of tachyarrhythmias to appropriately target the energy delivery. Lastly, future techniques and technologies will be discussed.

HISTORICAL EVOLUTION

Techniques for catheter-based ablation of tachyarrhythmias began with the development of methods for intracardiac recording of electrical signals. This led to the procedures for programmed stimulation of cardiac tissue for the induction and termination of tachyarrhythmias. In 1967, Durrer first described initiation and termination of tachycardia in a patient with WPW syndrome.[1] In 1969, the His bundle was first reproducibly recorded using a transvenous electrode catheter.[2] This led to a variety of tachyarrhythmias to be studied using intracardiac catheters. Catheters were used to identify mechanisms of tachycardia initiation and maintenance.

The idea emerged that critical regions of cardiac tissue were necessary for the initiation and propagation of tachyarrhythmias. If these regions could be interrupted, the tachyarrhythmia could then be clinically cured. Once catheter mapping could localize arrhythmogenic foci, surgical excision was explored. In 1968, such a surgical procedure for the elimination of an accessory pathway was first published.[3] This heralded an era of nonpharmacologic treatment of tachyarrhythmias.

Surgical Ablation

A variety of arrhythmogenic foci and circuits were successfully mapped and ablated using surgical techniques in the 1970s. Resection of an atrial focus was described in 1973 to cure atrial tachycardia.[4] Surgical ablation became more refined and precise as mapping techniques localized tachyarrhythmias with greater detail. With the elucidation of reentry circuits within the atrioventricular (AV) node, surgical dissection was performed to treat AV nodal reentrant tachycardia without causing AV block.[5]

Although surgical ablation was therapeutic for a variety of tachyarrhythmias, the morbidity and mortality associated with thoracotomy and open heart surgery limited its application. The risk of the procedure was not justified for most patients with tachyarrhythmias because they were not life threatening. Rather, ablation procedures were an option of last resort in highly symptomatic patients refractory to medical therapy. With these limitations of the surgical approach, catheter-based ablation procedures were explored.

Catheter Ablation

Once the His bundle could be recorded with consistency using catheters and thus localized, the idea evolved to using the catheter to delivery energy to cardiac tissue to achieve local tissue injury. In 1981 Scheinman et al reported the first catheter-based ablation procedure, describing the ablation of the His bundle in dogs.[6] This same group, in March of 1981, performed the first closed-chest ablation procedure in man. They described a patient with atrial fibrillation refractory to medical therapy. The patient was placed under general anesthesia and a catheter was advanced to the His bundle region. Using a standard external direct current (DC) defibrillator and by attaching one of the defibrillator pads to the intracardiac catheter, energy was delivered between the distal electrode of the catheter and a cutaneous grounding pad. A series of DC shocks were then delivered, achieving complete heart block.[7]

Induction of complete AV nodal blockage was then extended to the treatment of other supraventricular tachycardias (SVTs).[8] This necessitated the implantation of a pacemaker. As experienced was gained and specific catheters were developed, energy could be more precisely directed to target a variety of tachyarrhythmias, including ablation of accessory pathways, atrial tachycardia, single limb of AV nodal reentrant tachycardia, and ventricular tachycardia. Although DC shock ablation advanced the field of catheter-based ablation beyond surgical ablation, it had its own limitations. High-energy discharges resulted in the formation of a plasma ball at the distal electrode. Energy delivery was not titratable and lesions were patchy in nature. Cardiac rupture and perforation were associated risks with this procedure. In addition, since direct current energy stimulated skeletal muscle, general anesthesia was required for these procedures.

The development of the use of radiofrequency (RF) energy as an ablative energy source heralded a new era in the nonpharmacologic, nonsurgical treatment of tachyarrhythmias. RF energy had been used for decades by surgeons for surgical cutting and cautery and had a long history of safety and efficacy. Animal studies using RF energy were first described in 1987.[9] RF energy produces controlled lesions at the catheter tip over a period of 40 to 90 seconds. The improved safety and efficacy of RF catheter-based ablation procedures superseded the extensive and imprecise lesions created by DC shock ablation techniques.

BIOPHYSICS OF RADIOFREQUENCY ABLATION

Radiofrequency (RF) ablation involves the delivery of sinusoidal alternating current between the catheter tip at the endocardial surface and a large grounding pad on the skin. The current has a frequency of 350 to 700 kHz. The use of frequencies below 350 kHz results in direct skeletal and cardiac muscle stimulation. This results in perception of pain by the patient as well as induction of polymorphic tachyarrhythmias. The use of frequencies above 700 kHz results in loss of energy during transmission as well as a decrease in resistive heating. Limiting energy delivery to the range of 350 to 700 kHz makes the procedure relatively painless and eliminates the need for general anesthesia.

The principal method of tissue injury with RF delivery is thermal. As the RF energy passes through the tissue at the distal electrode of the ablation catheter, resistive heating produces coagulation necrosis. The lesions produced are well demarcated and are 5 to 6 mm wide by 2 to 3 mm deep when a standard catheter tip is used. No significant heating occurs at the tissue-grounding pad interface due to the large surface area of contact. To achieve irreversible tissue injury, a temperature of about 55°C to 58°C is required.[10] At temperatures above 100°C, plasma reaches the boiling point and coagulates on the catheter tip. Coagulum and desiccated tissue act as an insulating barrier to energy delivery, resulting in a rise in impedance and the prevention of tissue heating. If subendocardial tissue temperature exceeds 100°C, steam may be formed within the tissue, resulting in a rapid expansion and crater formation and an audible "pop." Such lesions can cause unpredictable injury, resulting in thromboembolic risk and rupture of thin-walled structures. Thus it is important to regulate the temperature of the catheter tissue interface either manually or automatically by regulating the energy delivered.

The morphology of the lesion formed by RF energy is distinct. There is a centralized region of necrosis with surrounding inflammation. As the lesion matures in a matter of weeks to months, the surrounding region of inflammation may progress to necrosis or inflammation may resolve without permanent damage. Thus it is critical to place RF lesions precisely. Tachyarrhythmias that initially disappear with RF delivery may recover if the lesion is peripheral to the site of the tachyarrhythmia and the temporary inflammation resolves. On the contrary, a lesion may extend as the border zone of inflammation becomes necrotic, resulting in unintentional injury to surrounding tissue.

RF lesion size is well suited for focal endocardial tachyarrhythmias. Tachyarrhythmias utilizing a reentrant circuit with a wide isthmus or localized deep in the myocardium may be more difficult to ablate. Advancements in catheter technology have improved the success rates of RF ablations. Primary of these was the inclusion of a thermistor or thermocouple within the ablation electrode to monitor catheter-tissue interface temperature. This allows the maximal energy delivery without the buildup of excessive temperature that results in coagulum and increases in impedance. Other advances have been the development of larger catheter tips, which increase the surface area, reducing current density and increasing cooling by surrounding blood pool. Irrigated catheters bathe the catheter tip internally or externally with a saline solution to cool the catheter-tissue interface, preventing coagulum formation and enhancing energy delivery. Catheters themselves have been designed to be steerable and allow precise positioning of the tip to the region of interest. Future advances in catheter technologies will be discussed later in the chapter.

ELECTROPHYSIOLOGY STUDY PROCEDURAL PROTOCOL

Catheter ablation of tachyarrhythmias is typically an elective procedure with the patients presenting on an outpatient basis. As it is an invasive procedure and thus carries some procedural risk, patients need to be thoroughly evaluated and informed regarding the procedure. Occasionally electrophysiology procedures are performed on an emergency basis in patients with recurrent or incessant hemodynamically significant arrhythmias.

Patient Screening

Patients are typically seen on a consultative basis. A complete history and physical examination are performed. An ECG at baseline and recordings of the tachyarrhythmia are crucial to planning the procedure. A patient may present to a physician's office or to an emergency room with the tachyarrhythmia, allowing the recording of a 12-lead ECG. A loop recorder is sometimes helpful to record tachyarrhythmias that are infrequent or of short duration. The recording of onset and termination of the tachyarrhythmia, either spontaneously, with vagal maneuvers, or with drugs, is also very helpful in determining the mechanism of the tachycardia.

Several adjunctive studies may be necessary to fully assess the patient. An echocardiogram is useful in evaluating for the presence of structural heart disease that will sway the differential diagnosis of an unknown tachyarrhythmia. A treadmill exercise stress test is useful in evaluating the relationship of catecholamine state in the induction of tachyarrhythmias. If clinical history indicates, right heart catheterization, stress testing with imaging, or coronary angiography may be performed to evaluate for volume status and coronary artery disease. This is useful to rule out ischemia in an atypical presentation and to assure that the patient will tolerate a prolonged period of supine posture, sustained tachycardias, and possible hypotension during the procedure.

Pharmacologic considerations include stopping all antiarrhythmic medications at least four half-lives prior to the procedure to allow for induction of tachyarrhythmias. In most cases, AV nodal blocking medications should also be stopped when the AV node may be involved in the reentrant circuit. Anticoagulation medications should also be stopped and, depending on the indication, the patient may be bridged for the procedure with subcutaneous low molecular heparin or admitted into the hospital for conversion to intravenous heparin. Because of the need for systemic anticoagulation for procedures that require left heart access, the menses cycle should be taken into consideration in timing the procedures in premenopausal women. Routine complete blood count, electrolyte status, and coagulation profile should be obtained. Additional laboratory tests that are sometimes useful are thyroid function tests in patients with history suggestive of hyperthyroid state and beta HCG serum levels in women of childbearing age.

Patients should present on the day of the procedure in a fasting state. Intravenous access is obtained for administration of conscious sedation and for emergency access. Procedures are typically performed using short-acting benzodiazepines and narcotics in combination. General anesthesia is rarely required. It may be used in patients with idiosyncratic reaction to benzodiazepines, those undergoing prolonged procedures, or in unstable patients, such as those undergoing ablation of ventricular tachycardia.

Patient Monitoring

Continuous monitoring is performed using 12-lead surface ECG, noninvasive or invasive blood pressure monitoring, continuous pulse oximetry, and capnography. An external defibrillator is available and attached to the patient with "hands-free" patches throughout the procedure. Intubation and resuscitation supplies should be readily available. Electrophysiological procedures are typically divided into diagnostic and ablative phases. The diagnostic phase involves obtaining venous access, passage of multiple catheters into the heart to record intracardiac electrograms, and induction and mapping of tachyarrhythmias. Once tachyarrhythmias are localized, ablation follows.

Diagnostic Electrophysiology Study

Diagnostic localization of tachyarrhythmias involves positioning catheters in strategic locations within the heart to obtain intracardiac recordings from all four chambers of the heart as well as from the His bundle. Venous access is typically obtained in the bilateral groins via the right and left femoral veins. Catheters of 4F to 6F in size are passed into the right atrium and right ventricle as well as positioned just across the tricuspid value to obtain His bundle recordings under fluoroscopic guidance. To obtain recordings of the left atrium and ventricle, a catheter is guided into the coronary sinus, which passes posteriorly in the atrioventricular groove and drains into the right atrium. Because of the angle of the entrance into the coronary sinus, cannulation is easier via the superior vena cava and thus typically venous access has been obtained from the right internal jugular, left subclavian, or left antecubital vein. However, steerable catheters allow for reliable access from the inferior approach and are now being used more frequently (Fig. 52-1).

Direct recordings of the left heart are sometimes necessary and accomplished either by trans-septal cannulation via the intra-atrial septum from the right atrium or via a retrograde approach from the femoral artery and across the aortic valve. Systemic anticoagulation with heparin is maintained during catheter manipulation in the left heart because of the risk of thromboembolic events due to platelet and thrombin aggregation on the catheters, coagulum formation with RF delivery, and fibrinolytic activation.

Once diagnostic catheters are positioned, programmed electrical stimulation is performed to induce and study the tachyarrhythmia. Sometimes modulation of the autonomic nervous system is required to induce tachyarrhythmias with the infusion of atropine or isoproterenol. As will be described later, there are specific pacing maneuvers to initiate and evaluate the mechanism of a variety of tachyarrhythmias. Once an optimal site for ablation is assessed, steerable ablation catheters are positioned at the target site. These catheters come with a variety of curvatures. Specifically shaped long vascular sheaths may also be used to direct catheters. Once RF energy is delivered to the target site, reinduction of the tachycardia is attempted.

At the end of the procedure, all catheters and sheaths are removed and manual pressure held to achieve hemostasis. If the patient was heparinized for the procedure, sheath removal is delayed until anticoagulation reverses. The patient is placed on bed rest for 4 or more hours. During this recovery, the patient is monitored for hemodynamical stability and recovery from sedation, and to assess for bleeding from puncture sites. The patient may be discharged to home the same day or be observed overnight in the hospital. Routine follow-up studies are not warranted unless to assess for a complication. Patients may be placed on 4 to 6 weeks of aspirin to reduce the risk of embolic events due to thrombus formation on ablated myocardium, especially those undergoing ablations in the left heart.

In referring patients for catheter ablation, it is important to weigh the risks and benefits of the procedure for the individual patient. Most tachyarrhythmias, although causing a variety of symptoms, are generally hemodynamically well

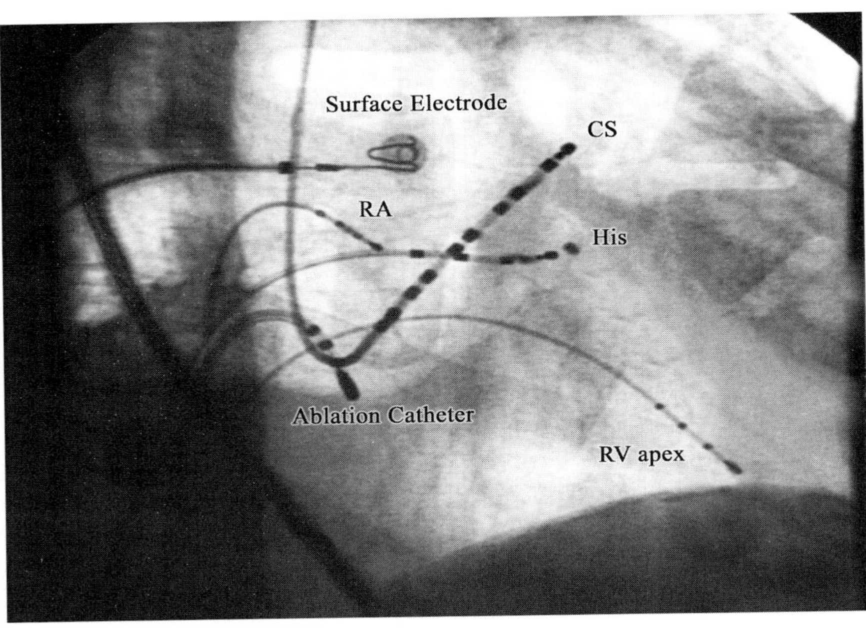

FIGURE 52–1 Radiograph in the right anterior oblique projections showing catheters positioned for a standard diagnostic electrophysiology procedure. Three nonsteerable diagnostic catheters are introduced from the inferior vena cava into the right heart. Two 4F catheters with 4 electrodes are positioned in the region of the right atrial appendage (RA) and right ventricular apex (RV apex). A 5F catheter with 6 electrodes is positioned across the tricuspid annulus to obtain a His bundle recording (His). A nonsteerable 6F catheter is introduced via the right internal jugular vein into the coronary sinus to obtain left atrial and ventricular recordings. Finally a deflectable 7F ablation catheter is positioned in the region of the low right atrium.

tolerated and are not life threatening. Thus an awareness of the potential complications of catheter ablation is necessary prior to referring a patient. Complications can be divided into those involving access, catheter manipulation within the heart, and ablation.

Access-related complications include pain, adverse drug reaction from anesthesia and sedation, infection, thrombophlebitis, and bleeding at the site of access. Associated with bleeding are hematoma or arteriovenous fistula formation. Arterial damage or dissection may also result. Systemic or pulmonary thromboembolism can occur, most seriously resulting in transient ischemic attack or stroke.

Complications associated with placement of intracardiac catheters can be more life threatening. These include trauma of a cardiac chamber or the coronary sinus resulting in myocardial infarction, perforation, hemopericardium, and cardiac tamponade. Programmed electrical stimulation can result in the induction of life-threatening tachyarrhythmias such as ventricular tachycardia or fibrillation. Catheter manipulation can also result in usually transient but sometimes permanent damage to valvular apparatus or to the conduction of the right or left bundles due to mechanical trauma.

RF delivery within cardiac structures carries with it its own set of risks. Inadvertent ablation of the normal conduction system could result in complete heart block requiring permanent pacing. Perforation of a cardiac chamber or vascular structure can also occur with RF delivery. Collateral damage to coronary circulation could result in myocardial infarction, heart failure, or cardiogenic shock. Phrenic nerve paralysis can occur. Ablation near the pulmonary veins within the left atrium can result in venous stenosis and pulmonary hypertension. Finally, new tachyarrhythmias can arise from the scar induced by RF ablation.

An 8-year prospective study of 3966 procedures found an overall complication rate of 3.1% for ablative and 1.1% for diagnostic procedures. Complications are more likely to occur in elderly patients and those with systemic disease.[11] No deaths were reported in this series and other studies have shown very low mortality rates directly attributable to the electrophysiology study. Body dosimetry studies have shown that the lifetime excess risk per 60 minutes of fluoroscopy exposure is 294 per million cases or 0.03% per patient. The risk is higher for obese patients and the lungs are the most susceptible organs.[12] Technology is evolving and advances will continue to improvethe safety and efficacy of this procedure.

DIAGNOSTIC ELECTROPHYSIOLOGY TECHNIQUES

A variety of techniques have been developed to elucidate the origin and mechanism of tachyarrhythmia propagation. These techniques are necessary to reveal targets for ablation. They involve pacing in a specific chamber at particular intervals to initiate a tachyarrhythmia, assess its response to pacing maneuvers, or terminate it. Thus some of these techniques involve pacing in sinus rhythm while others are performed during the tachyarrhythmia. Occasionally pharmacologic modulation of the autonomic nervous system is used in conjunction with pacing maneuvers.

Activation Mapping

Activation mapping is a technique of localizing focal tachycardias and accessory pathways. It involves positioning the mapping/ablation catheter during the tachyarrhythmia in such a way that activation at the catheter tip precedes any other intracardiac activation or corresponding surface P wave or QRS. The earliest site of activation during a focal tachycardia must by definition be the source of the tachycardia.

Accessory pathways can also be mapped using this technique by tracing the tricuspid and mitral annulus with the ablation catheter. The atrial insertion can be localized by determining the earliest site of retrograde atrial activation during atrioventricular reciprocating tachycardia or in sinus rhythm during ventricular pacing. The ventricular insertion can be localized in patients with preexcitation by determining the site of earliest ventricular activation during sinus rhythm.

Pace Mapping

Pace mapping is performed during sinus rhythm after obtaining a 12-lead surface ECG during tachycardia. By pacing at different sites and comparing the resulting paced ECG to the tachycardia ECG, the disparity can be assessed and the catheter can be repositioned until a perfect 12-lead match is obtained. These sites are then the targets for ablation. This technique is typically used for focal ventricular tachycardias, especially those of right ventricular outflow origin.

Mapping of local electrogram potentials requires recording an intracardiac signal from the structure targeted for ablation. For instance, to achieve complete heart block, the His bundle is the target and the ablation catheter is positioned such that the distal tip is recording a His bundle potential. Similarly for bundle branch reentry, the right bundle potential is used to target the right bundle to achieve right bundle branch block. Sometimes an accessory pathway potential can be recorded and used to localize a target for ablation.

Anatomic Mapping

Anatomic mapping is yet anther way to localize potential targets for ablation. This does not involve any electrical signal but instead uses fluoroscopy to localize anatomical landmarks for ablation. Catheters placed through the inferior vena cava into the coronary sinus and across the tricuspid valve delineate these structures. In typical atrial flutter that is dependent on the inferior vena cava and tricuspid annulus isthmus, these anatomical landmarks are used for the delivery of a line of lesions to prevent conduction across this isthmus. Bidirectional conduction block across this isthmus terminates flutter and prevents its reinitiation.

Entrainment Mapping

Entrainment mapping is a technique of localizing reentrant circuits for ablation. It involves positioning the catheter in a region thought to be involved in a reentrant tachycardia. This is confirmed by pacing during the tachycardia slightly faster than the tachycardia rate. If the pacing site is within the circuit, then activation should proceed orthodromically around the circuit resulting in an identical activation pattern. The resultant QRS or P wave should match that of the tachycardia. At the termination of the pacing the activation wavefront proceeds around the circuit. Therefore, if pacing was in the circuit, the first beat should be close to the cycle length of the tachycardia.

In clinical situations a combination of these mapping techniques is used to localize an arrhythmia for ablation. Usually an anatomical approach is used to find the general region and then more precise mapping used to specifically localize the focal arrhythmia or reentrant circuit.

Advanced Mapping Techniques

The success of ablation is very much dependent on localization of arrythmogenic foci and circuits. The previously mentioned mapping techniques are useful for arrhythmias that originate from specific anatomical locations or have characteristic endocardial electrograms. Conventional fluoroscopy and the use of a single roving mapping catheter have limited success in ablation of complex arrhythmias that may originate from sites without characteristic fluoroscopic landmarks or have variable electrograms as recorded from the catheter tip. Advanced mapping techniques have been developed as adjuncts to conventional methods to improve the efficacy of catheter ablation for arrhythmias that are transient, focal, or hemodynamically unstable and thus require rapid mapping.

Multielectrode "basket" catheters (Constellation, Boston Scientific Corp., Natick, MA) consist of eight collapsible arms at the distal end that deploy within a cardiac chamber to provide recordings from 64 electrodes. Multielectrode catheters allow acquisition of electrograms from multiple sites simultaneously to enable reconstruction of activation maps such that a single ectopic beat can be mapped online rapidly. Although these catheters are still fluoroscopically guided, multiple data points are acquired simultaneously, limiting procedure times, especially in patients with hemodynamically unstable arrhythmias.[13] The disadvantage of these catheters is the low spatial resolution (approximately 1 cm) due to the spacing between the electrodes and arms. As RF lesions are on the order of 0.5 cm in size, this limits the use of this technology to macro reentrant arrhythmias.

An electroanatomical mapping system (CARTO, Biosense, Diamond Bar, CA) uses a magnetic field to localize the mapping catheter tip in three-dimensional space. Three coils in a locator pad located beneath the patient's chest generate ultra-low-intensity magnetic fields in the form of a sphere that decays in strength. A sensor in the catheter tip measures the relative strength and hence the distance from each of the coils. This allows for the recording of the spatial and temporal location of the catheter. Electrodes at the catheter tip record local electrograms and this information is displayed on screen as a three-dimensional map of the local activation times relative to a reference catheter in a color-coded fashion. Data from multiple single mapping points acquired during tachycardia can be reconstructed to show animated sequences of arrhythymia propagation. Voltage maps can be obtained to delineate regions of scar and diseased myocardium.[14]

The advantages are that this system is nonfluoroscopic, and it allows for precise location of the catheter tip with a resolution of less than 1 mm. The catheter can be positioned independent of fluoroscopic landmarks. In addition, recordings of catheter position allow for the repositioning of the catheter to previously mapped sites of interest. A limitation of this mapping technique is that data acquisition is sequential and point to point. Construction of an activation sequence can be time consuming and difficult in nonsustained arrhythmias or those originating from multiple sites.[15]

A noncontact endocaridial mapping system (EnSite 3000, Endocardial Solutions, Inc, St Paul, MN) consists of a catheter with a woven braid of 64 insulated 0.003-mm-diameter wires with 0.025-mm breaks in insulation that serve as electrodes. Using a ring electrode on the shaft of the catheter as a reference, raw far field signals from the multielectrode array can be used to construct a virtual electrogram of the chamber of interest. A locator signal is also generated between the noncontact array and a standard mapping catheter to permit nonfluoroscopic localization of the catheter to regions of interest. The position of the roving catheter is acquired over time to construct a three-dimensional map of the endocardial surface. Landmarks can be tagged and labeled such as the His catheter or the coronary sinus.

Over 3360 virtual electrograms are simultaneously acquired by this system, allowing high-density maps to be acquired from a single beat. Thus this system is very useful for mapping in unstable or transient, nonsustained arrhythmias. It allows for nonfluoroscopic navigation of the mapping catheter, return to points of interest, and logging of ablation sites.[16]

Intracardiac echocardiography (ICE) has extended the principles of intravascular ultrasound (IVUS) for electrophysiological use.[17] In contrast to IVUS catheters, ICE catheters use lower-frequency (5.5-10 MHz) transducers to extend the imaging range. Newer ICE catheters are steerable and have Doppler capability (Acuson, Mountain View, CA), allowing for hemodynamic evaluation of intracardiac structures. For electrophysiological use, ICE catheters are useful for visualization of endocardial structures such as the fossa ovalis and guiding trans-septal catheterization. As the recognition of the importance of anatomy in the genesis of arrhythmias has grown, so has the importance of imaging. ICE catheters allow the accurate targeting of anatomical sites such as the crista terminalis and pulmonary vein ostia. They are useful for imaging diagnostic and ablation catheter positions and visualization of tissue contact for optimal ablation. Through visualization of pericardial effusions, rapid diagnosis of perforation and other complications is feasible.

CLINICAL APPLICATIONS

Using the techniques described above, a variety of tachyarrhythmias can be targeted for percutaneous catheter-based ablation, including both atrial and ventricular arrhythmias that are either focal or that utilize reentrant circuits.

Atrioventricular Nodal Reentrant Tachycardia

The most common supraventricular arrhythmia is atrioventricular nodal reentrant tachycardia (AVNRT). Of patients with supraventricular tachycardia, AVNRT represents up to 60% of cases that present to tertiary centers for electrophysiological studies. This tachycardia can present at any age although most patients that present for medical attention are in their 40s and the majority are female.[18,19] Advances in RF catheter ablation of this tachycardia has made it a first-line therapy for those symptomatic patients not wishing to take medications.[20]

This tachycardia has a reentrant mechanism utilizing two pathways within the AV nodal tissue. Controversy remains about whether atrial tissue is an integral part of the circuit. The pathways are the "slow pathway" and "fast pathway" based on their relative conduction velocities. The anatomical location of these pathways is variable but generally located within the triangle of Koch. Koch's triangle is bounded by the tricuspid annulus and the tendon of Todaro with the coronary sinus at the base. The apex of the triangle is the His bundle at the membranous septum where it passes through the central fibrous body. The anterior third of the triangle contains the compact AV node and the fast pathway, and the middle and posterior portion, near the coronary sinus os, contains the slow pathway (Fig. 52-2).[21] Recent studies suggest the left atrial extension of the AV node may be involved in the reentrant circuit.[22]

In the typical form of AVNRT, antegrade conduction from the atrium to the ventricle occurs over the slow pathway and

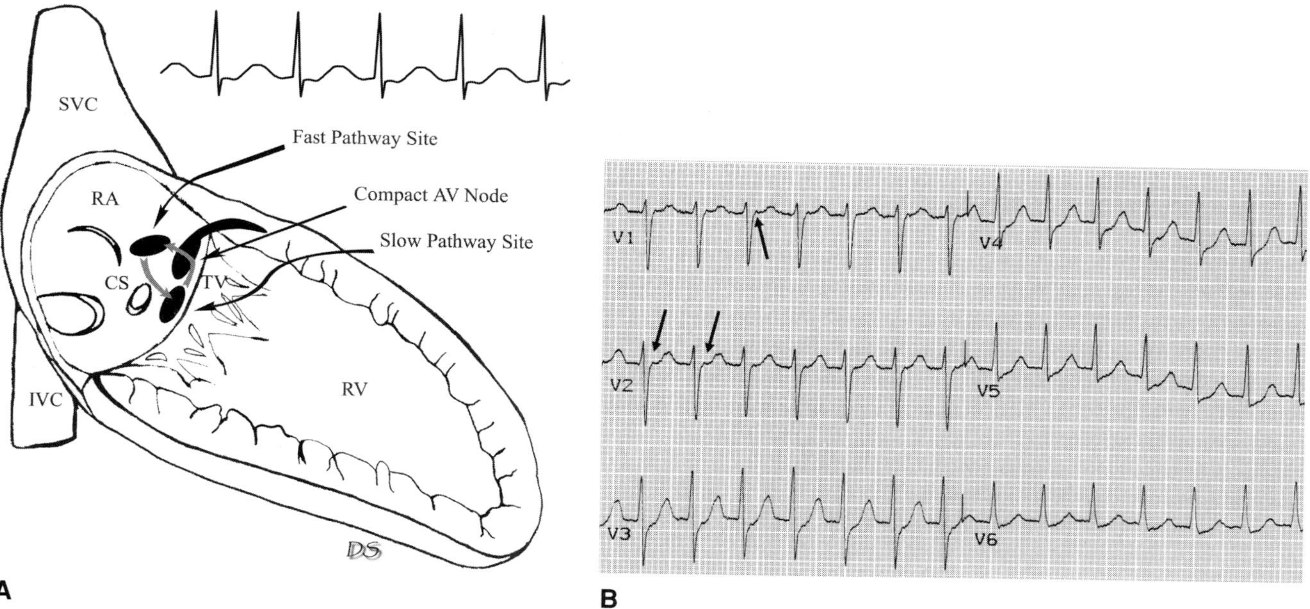

FIGURE 52–2 (A) Diagrammatic representation of typical atrioventricular nodal reentrant tachycardia. Surface ECG shows narrow complex tachycardia with no clear P waves. The reentrant circuit (gray arrows) consists of the posterior slow pathway region acting as the antegrade limb and the anterior fast pathway region acting as the retrograde limb. The slow pathway target site is located between the coronary sinus os (CS) and the tricuspid valve annulus (TV). SVC = superior vena cava; RA = right atrium; IVC = inferior vena cava; RV = right ventricle. (B) Surface ECG showing precordial leads in AVNRT. This demonstrates that the retrograde P waves are barely discernable in some leads. In V1, it forms a pseudo r′ wave (arrow). P waves are also visible in the terminal portions of QRS complexes in V2 and V3 but not in the lateral leads.

the retrograde conduction from the ventricle to the atrium occurs over the fast pathway. Since conduction in the retrograde direction is fast, the atria and ventricle are depolarized almost simultaneously. Thus the electrocardiographic feature of this tachycardia is P waves that are inscribed within the QRS and thus not seen or barely discernible at the termination of the QRS complex.[23]

In less then 10% of cases, the circuit is reversed. In atypical AVNRT, the antegrade limb occurs over the fast pathway and retrograde VA conduction occurs over the slow pathway. Thus the ECG of this tachycardia shows inverted P waves in the inferior leads denoting retrograde activation of the atria with short PR segment due to rapid antegrade conduction.

Ablation of either of these tachycardias involves disruption of the reentrant circuit. In the early days of catheter ablation therapy, highly symptomatic patients who had failed all medical therapy underwent complete atrioventricular junctional ablation utilizing DC current with the insertion of a permanent pacemaker. While this greatly improved these patients' quality of life, it made them pacemaker dependent. It was therefore not indicated for patients with less symptomatic arrhythmia.

Initial attempts to selectively eliminate AVNRT while leaving antegrade AV nodal conduction intact were performed with DC energy.[24] It was difficult to choose a specific target and in some patients the fast pathway and in others the slow pathway was ablated. With the advent of RF energy, more selective ablation could be performed. Early procedures utilizing RF energy targeted the fast pathway. While successful in up to 90% of patients, there was still a 5% to 10% incidence of inadvertent complete heart block.[25] In addition, ablation of the fast pathway left the patients with a prolonged PR interval. In some, this led to symptomatic atrial contraction during ventricular contraction (pseudopacemaker syndrome) especially during sinus tachycardia.

Subsequently it was found that the slow pathway could be successfully targeted in the posterior triangle of Koch.[26] Slow pathway ablation has a high degree of success with recurrence rate in the range of 2% to 7% with the complication of complete AV block occurring about 1% (range 0%-3%) of the time.[27] The 1992 NASPE self-reported survey on 3052 patients who underwent slow pathway ablation showed a success rate of 96% with complication rate of 0.96%,[28] and the 1998 NASPE survey reported a total of 1197 with a success rate of 96.1% and a complication rate of 1% incidence of AV block.[29]

Atrioventricular Reentrant Tachycardia

The next most common type of supraventricular tachycardia is atrioventricular reentrant tachycardia (AVRT). About 30% of supraventricular tachycardias are due to AVRT. This is a reentrant tachycardia utilizing the AV node and an accessory pathway. These accessory pathways are remnants of conductive tissue from embryonic development that span the normally electrically inert tricuspid and mitral valve annulus and provide an independent path of conduction outside of the AV node between the atria and the ventricles. The most common form of AVRT is part of the Wolf-Parkinson-White (WPW) syndrome of ventricular preexcitation and symptomatic arrhythmias. The most common accessory pathways connect the atrium to the ventricle. Other accessory pathways may connect the atria or AV node to the His-Purkinje system. In sinus rhythm, antegrade conduction over the accessory pathway results in preexcitation of the ventricles eccentric to the AV node and is manifested by a short PR segment and slurring of the onset of the QRS, the delta wave. Absence of these findings does not exclude an accessory pathway as the degree of preexcitation may vary or conduction may only occur in the retrograde direction (approximately 30% of accessory pathways).

Patients with WPW typically present with palpitations due to rapid heart rate. This may be the result of AVRT or due to any supraventricular tachycardia with resulting rapid atrioventricular conduction via the accessory pathway. Associated symptoms may be mild such as palpitations and shortness of breath or as severe as syncope and sudden death. Sudden death may be due to ventricular fibrillation resulting from the extremely rapid ventricular activation over the accessory pathway during atrial fibrillation in some patients.

Indications for ablation of accessory pathways include patients with symptomatic AVRT or those with atrial tachyarrhythmias with rapid ventricular conduction who fail or do not wish medical therapy. Relative indications for ablations include asymptomatic patients in high-risk professions, those with family history of sudden death, or those mentally distraught over their condition.[15]

In the typical or orthodromic form of AVRT, antegrade conduction from the atrium to the ventricle occurs over the AV node and retrograde conduction occurs over the accessory pathway. In this form of AVRT, the P wave in the tachycardia closely follows the preceding QRS complex with a long PR segment (Fig. 52-3). In the rare antidromic form of AVRT, antegrade conduction occurs over the accessory pathway with retrograde conduction over the AV node. This results in eccentric depolarization of the ventricle producing a wide complex tachycardia with retrograde P waves that can be easily mistaken for ventricular tachycardia with one-to-one VA conduction.

Patients with highly symptomatic WPW syndrome or asymptomatic patients in high-risk professions who had failed medical therapy were the initial population to undergo surgical interruption of accessory pathways. Although this procedure evolved with success rates near 100% and mortality rates of 1%,[30] it still involved a major surgical procedure. Catheter-based ablation of accessory pathways has success rates approaching surgical ablation with lower morbidity and mortality.

The first catheter ablation procedures were performed with direct current energy in patients with posteroseptal

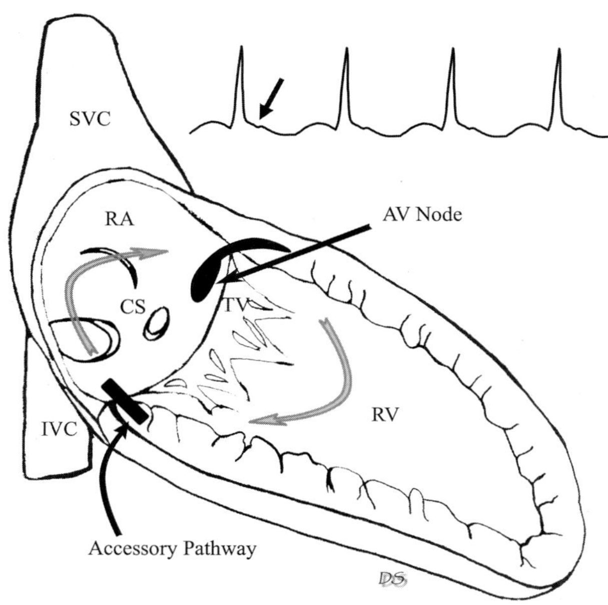

A

FIGURE 52–3 (A) Diagrammatic representation of atrioventricular reentrant tachycardia. This macro-reentrant circuit (gray arrows) utilizes the AV node and an accessory pathway (AP), in this case a right lateral pathway. In orthodromic AVRT, antegrade conduction occurs over the AV node and retrograde conduction occurs over the AP. Because of the conduction delay from the His-Purkinje system through the ventricular myocardium to reach the AP, retrograde P waves are discernable after the QRS complexes (arrow). In antidromic AVRT, the reentrant circuit is reversed and surface ECG shows P waves that closely precede the QRS complexes. SVC = superior vena cava; RA = right atrium; IVC = inferior vena cava; CS = coronary sinus, TV = tricuspid valve; RV = right ventricle. (B) Intracardiac recording of atrioventricular reentrant tachycardia with termination of eccentric conduction over the accessory pathway during RF ablation. The tracing at 50 mm per second speed shows four surface leads (V1, II, I, and a VF) and intracardiac recording from catheters: ablation (ABL), His distal, mid and proximal as well right ventricular apex (RVA). The first three beats of the tracing show evidence of eccentric conduction over an accessory pathway: short PR segment and delta wave. With onset of RF energy from the ablation catheter positioned in the region of shortest AV conduction, conduction becomes normal within two beats, with normalization of PR segment and loss of delta wave.

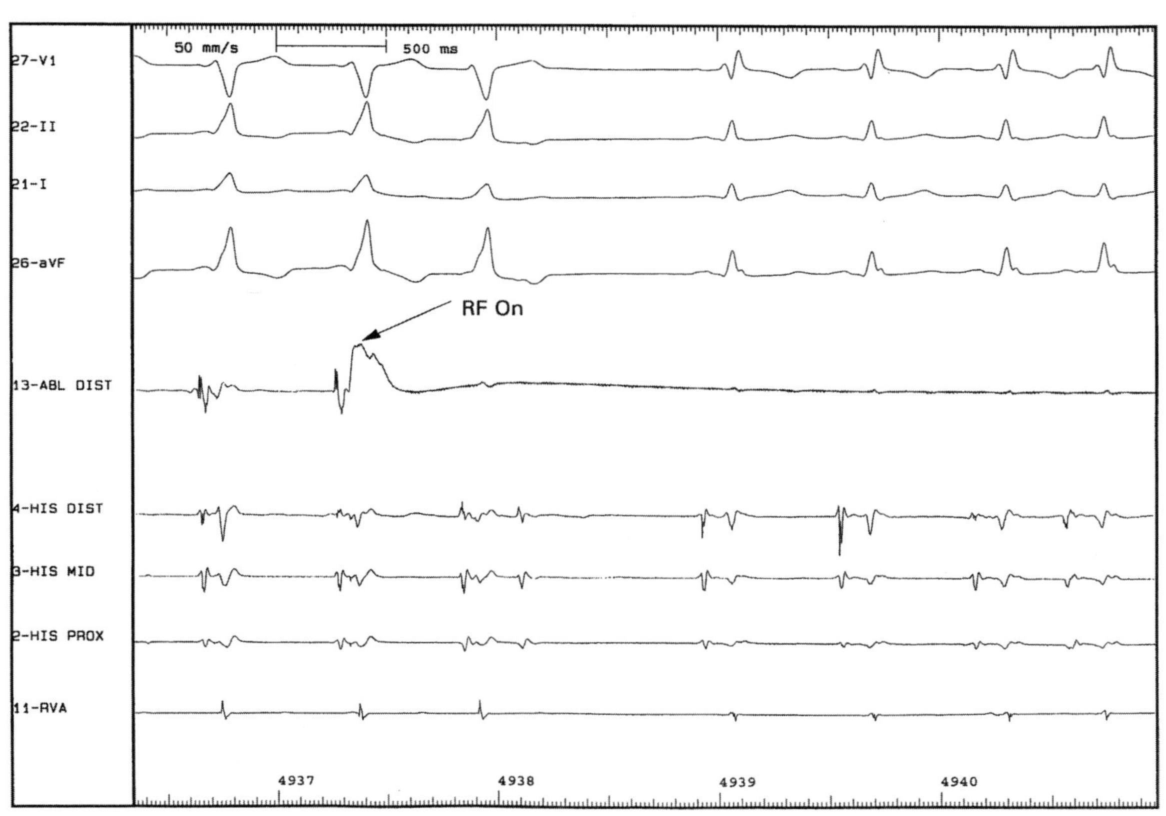

B

accessory pathways.[31] With the development of RF energy for ablation, accessory pathways in all locations could be treated.

Ablation of right-sided accessory pathways is performed by accessing the right heart via the femoral vein or occasionally via the antecubital, subclavian, or internal jugular veins. Left-sided accessory pathways are ablated via a trans-septal approach or via a retrograde approach from the femoral artery. The initial procedures to ablate left-sided accessory pathways were via a retrograde aortic approach. While successful in more than 95% of patients, there was a small risk of aortic valve perforation or dissection of a coronary artery.[32]

Most centers now perform ablation of left-sided accessory pathways via a trans-septal approach.

Rarely, left-sided accessory pathways can be ablated from within the coronary sinus if they are on the epicardial surface, which is unusual. Due to the more sloping architecture of the tricuspid annulus, it is more difficult to achieve a stable catheter position for right-sided pathways. While the use of long curved vascular sheaths may be helpful, the success rates for right free wall accessory pathways are lower then for other locations.

The major challenge that remains is the ablation of accessory pathways near the normal conduction system and those that are epicardial in location. Ablation of pathways that are anteroseptal and midseptal in location carries a high risk of causing complete heart block. It is hoped that newer ablative energies such as cryoablation may offer a safer alternative. Recently, elimination of epicardial accessory pathways via a pericardial approach has been attempted.[33]

Unusual accessory pathways include atriofasicular (Mahaim) pathways. These show decremental conduction and the atrial insertion is typically located in the right free wall. These can often be successfully ablated via an endocardial catheter approach.[34]

The 1998 NASPE prospective catheter ablation registry reported on 654 patients with a 94% success rate.[29] Success rates are lower (in the range of 84%-88%) for septal and right free wall pathways. Other pathways have success rates in the range of 90% to 95%.[35–37]

Complications associated with ablation of accessory pathways include those associated with all ablation procedures. The 1998 NASPE registry reports major complications of cardiac tamponade in 7 patients, pericarditis in 2 patients, and acute myocardial infarction, femoral artery pseudoaneurysm, AV block, and pneumothorax in 1 patient each. A specific complication associated with trans-septal catheterizations for left-sided pathways is persistent intra-atrial shunt. Although acute shunt may be present in up to 50% of patients, long-term sequelae and persistence beyond 3 weeks are rare.[38,39] Mortality rates are less than 1% and nonfatal complications are about 4%.

Atrial Tachycardia

Atrial tachycardias depend wholly on atrial tissue for initiation and maintenance of the tachycardia. Ectopic atrial tachycardia, sinoatrial nodal reentrant tachycardia, inappropriate sinus tachycardia, atrial flutter, and atrial fibrillation fall into this category. Atrial flutter and atrial fibrillation will be considered separately below. Focal atrial tachycardias, a less common type of supraventricular tachycardia, forms about 10% of all SVTs referred for electrophysiological studies. Multifocal atrial tachycardia is due to multiple foci of abnormal automaticity or triggered activity and is not amenable to catheter ablation.

Patients with atrial tachycardia present with palpitations and associated symptoms may include chest discomfort, shortness of breath, and dizziness. Symptoms most often are benign and not life threatening. These arrhythmias are more common in patients with structural heart disease. Indications for ablation include failure or intolerance of medical therapy. Rarely, incessant tachycardias can lead to cardiomyopathy. With ablation and control of heart rate, myocardial dysfunction can be reversed.[40,41]

Surface ECG features of atrial tachycardia include abnormal P-wave morphology or axes that are close to the following QRS complexes. Mapping and ablation of atrial tachycardias can be more difficult as they can originate from anywhere within the right or left atrium. But there are specific anatomical regions that have a high incidence of foci and these are primary targets. They include the crista terminalis, atrial appendages, valve annulus, and pulmonary ostia.[42] Intracardiac echocardiography has been used to localize these anatomic regions of interest. Mapping is facilitated by other techniques.

Activation mapping by means of a roving mapping catheter is used to localize a region of earliest activation. Successful targets for ablation usually have intracardiac activation 30 milliseconds or more prior to any surface P wave. Sometimes two catheters are used to triangulate a target by moving one catheter at a time toward sites of earlier activation. A caveat to this mapping technique is that an early right atrial activation site may in fact originate from the left atrium as the posterior septum of the right atrium overlies the left atrium.[43]

Other techniques that have aided focal ablation are the use of noncontact[44] and electroanatomical mapping systems. These newer mapping catheters have increased the success rate of ablation of focal tachycardias, especially in patients with altered atrial anatomy such as those with congenital anomalies and post–atrial surgery.[45]

Inappropriate sinus tachycardia and sinoatrial nodal reentry tachycardias occur more infrequently and experience with catheter ablation of these tachycardias is more limited. Inappropriate sinus tachycardia is also difficult to ablate due to the variability and diffuse location of sinoatrial tissue. Medical therapy is the preferred method of therapy and catheter ablation is attempted only after drug failure. Catheter ablation may result in complete loss of sinoatrial node function and resulting junctional rhythm, requiring insertion of a pacemaker. Even if resting heart rate is reduced with nodal modification, symptoms may continue with episodes of tachycardia. Sinoatrial nodal reentrant tachycardia is targeted for ablation using techniques similar to those used for other atrial tachycardias.

Success with ablation of atrial tachycardia is quite variable depending upon the location of the arrhythmogenic foci and the experience of the operator. The 1998 NASPE survey showed a success rate of 80% for right-sided versus 72% for left-sided versus 52% for septal foci in 216 cases of atrial tachycardia ablation.[29] Another large review examined the frequency of arrhythmias as a predictor of success. In 105 patients, the overall initial success rate was 77%, and 10% had recurrence over a 33-month follow-up period. There was an 88% success rate for paroxysmal form versus 71% for permanent and 41% for repetitive forms of atrial tachycardia.[46]

Atrial Flutter

Atrial flutter is a type of atrial tachycardia that utilizes a macro-reentrant circuit contained within the atria. A variety of natural and surgical barriers to conduction can create a reentrant circuit within the atria. Typical atrial flutter is due to a right atrial circuit, bound anteriorly by the tricuspid valve (TV) annulus. Posteriorly, it is confined by the superior vena cava, crista terminalis, inferior vena cava (IVC), eustachian ridge, and coronary sinus (CS) (Fig. 52-4).

In the typical and more common form of atrial flutter, the circuit transverses the right atrium in a counterclockwise manner in the frontal plane. In the inferior leads, the P waves are negative and have a "sawtooth" appearance. In V1, the P wave is usually upright and in V6 it is inverted. Clockwise flutter utilizes the same circuit but in a reversed manner. The ECG also shows a reversed pattern. In the inferior leads the P waves are upright, with inverted P waves in V1 and upright in V6. This surface ECG morphology is suggestive of the circuit but needs intracardiac confirmation.[47] These two forms of atrial flutter have been termed "isthmus dependent" due to the use of the IVC-tricuspid annular isthmus. Other types of atrial flutter are called "atypical."

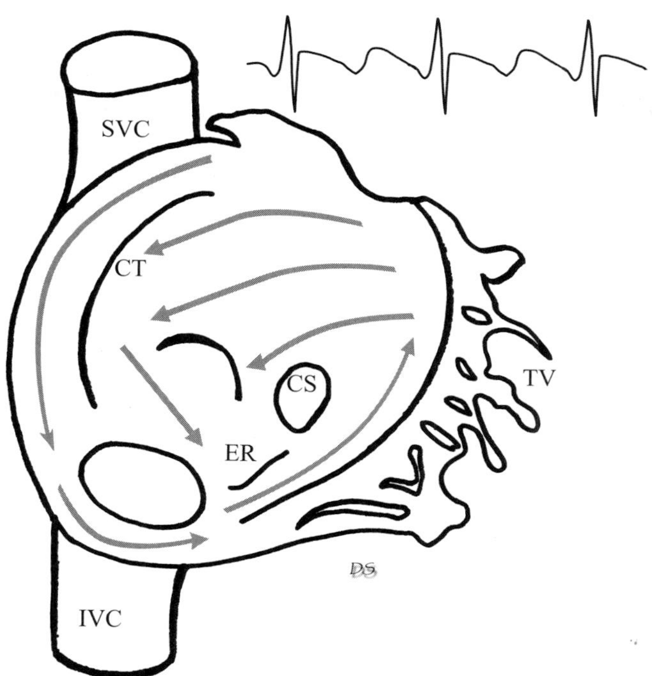

FIGURE 52–4 Diagrammatic representation of typical or counterclockwise right atrial flutter. Surface ECG shows large inverted P waves in the inferior leads. Lead III above shows 2:1 AV conduction with "sawtooth" flutter waves. The reentrant circuit (gray arrows) is confined to the right atrium by the tricuspid valve annulus (TV) and barriers to conduction within the right atrium. These include the superior vena cava (SVC), crista terminalis (CT), inferior vena cava (IVC), eustacian ridge (ER), and coronary sinus (CS). The isthmus between the IVC and TV is the preferred target for ablation.

A macro-reentrant circuit can be cured by lesions that transect the circuit between two anatomical barriers. In the case of isthmus-dependent flutter, the target for ablation is the isthmus between the IVC and TV. This is a relatively narrow target and easily reachable by ablation catheters introduced from the IVC. Success rates for ablation of this form of atrial flutter are high. Initial success rates are up to 90% with recurrence rates of 10% to 15%.[48] Given these results, ablation has become the first line of therapy for recurrent isthmus-dependent atrial flutter. In addition, studies have shown that the incidence of atrial fibrillation is markedly reduced in patients with atrial flutter treated with ablation as compared to medications.[49]

In some patients with atrial fibrillation, treatment with class IC antiarrhythmics or amiodarone results in the development of typical atrial flutter. A hybrid approach using ablation of the IVC-TV isthmus and continued use of the antiarrhythmic medication has been shown to be highly successful in reducing the incidence of atrial fibrillation.[50]

While the right atrial circuit described above is the most common, a variety of other circuits in the right and left atrium are possible. These are more common in patients with underlying heart disease. Although initially thought not to be amenable to ablative therapy, mapping and ablation of these arrhythmias are now routinely performed. However, the success rate are somewhat lower than that for typical isthmus-dependent atrial flutter. An electroanatomic map of a patient with left atrial flutter can be seen in Figure 52-5. Ablation in the isthmus between these scars resulted in termination of the flutter.

Surgical Scar–Related Atrial Arrhythmias

Incisional scars from prior cardiac surgery can be the substrate for reentrant atrial arrhythmias. The most common is an atypical atrial flutter related to a lateral right atrial incision. Mapping demonstrates a circuit circling the incision. Ablation from the end of the incision to either the superior vena cava or more commonly the inferior vena cava is often curative.[51]

It had been thought that there was conduction block between the donor and recipient atria in patients who have undergone heart transplantation. Recent reports have demonstrated reentrant arrhythmias due to donor-recipient atrial conduction. Mapping the connection between the atria can successfully ablate these arrhythmias.[52] Atrial arrhythmias

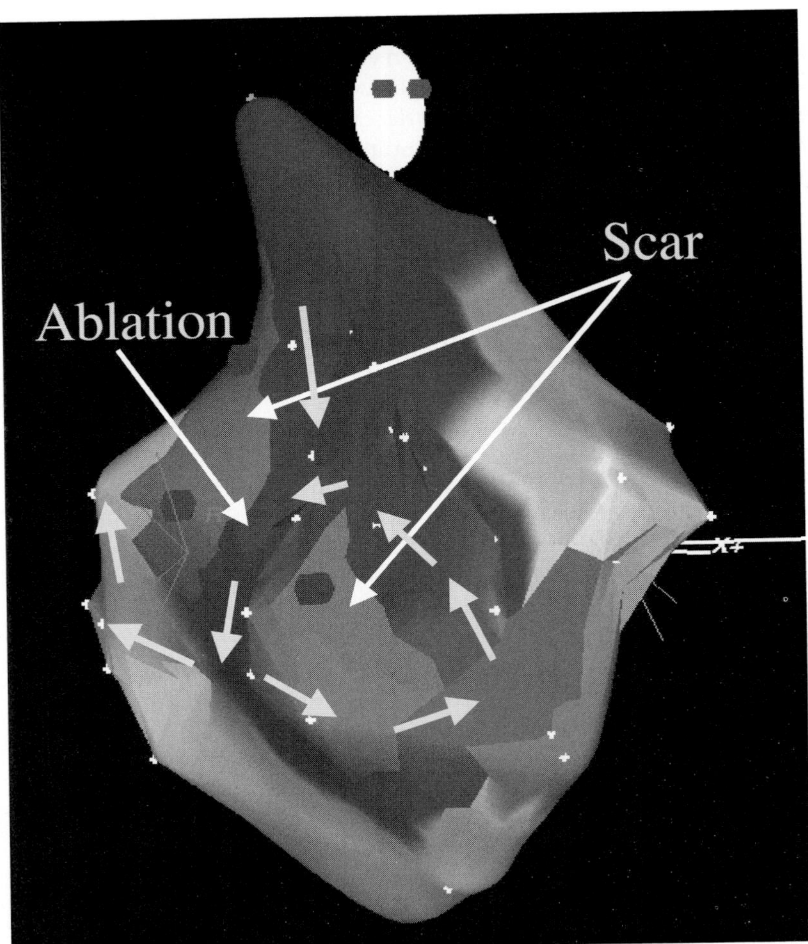

FIGURE 52–5 An electroanatomical map of a patient with left atrial flutter is shown in the RAO projection. Two large areas of scar can be seen in gray. Gradation in color shows activation sequence, with lighter being the earliest and darker being late in relation to a reference catheter, in this case positioned in the coronary sinus. The circulating wavefronts describe a figure-8 pattern around these two areas of scar but are confined by the narrow region (isthmus) between them. Ablation in the isthmus resulted in termination of the flutter.

have also been reported in a not insignificant number of patients who have undergone the surgical Maze procedure for atrial fibrillation. These treatment failures are most often due to reentrant circuits involving gaps in the Maze lesion or through alternative pathways such as the musculature surrounding the coronary sinus.[53] These arrhythmias can now be successfully mapped and ablated. Multipole noncontact and electroanatomical mapping systems are useful in improving success of these ablations. The principle of interrupting these circuits by placing lesions to connect conduction barriers remains the same.[54]

Atrial Fibrillation

Atrial fibrillation is another difficult to treat atrial tachycardia with variable targets for ablation. Atrial fibrillation is often symptomatic for patients due to irregular and/or rapid ventricular rates. Patients can also be completely asymptomatic and present with stroke or be diagnosed on routine examination. The prevalence of atrial fibrillation and the associated risk of stroke makes this arrhythmia a prime target for catheter-based ablation. Medical therapy for atrial fibrillation is of limited efficacy and can be associated with significant proarrhythmia in some patients. In addition, sustained rapid ventricular rates can lead to a tachycardia-related cardiomyopathy. When medical therapy aimed at maintaining sinus rhythm or blocking AV nodal conduction to slow ventricular response fails, ablation can be considered.

In the past, AV nodal or His ablation, with placement of a permanent pacemaker, was considered in patients with difficult to control ventricular rates and symptomatic palpitations. The advantages of the approach are the relative ease and speed at of the procedure. The downside is that it renders the patient pacemaker dependent. Success rates of this procedure are nearly 100%.[55] Complications of this procedure include the same complications as other ablation procedures. A unique complication associated with creation of complete heart block is bradycardia-related ventricular tachycardia (torsades de pointes). The incidence this complication is reduced with high-rate atrial pacing at 80 to 90 bpm for up to a month following ablation. In highly symptomatic patients, this approach to the treatment of atrial fibrillation has been associated with improvement in quality of life and left ventricular function, and with a reduction in hospitalizations.[56] With up to 3 years of follow-up, no long-term sequelae have been noted.[57] Patients with CHF and atrial fibrillation may particularly benefit from this approach. This population is at particular risk of proarrhythmia due to antiarrhythmic medications and has been shown to experience improved left ventricular function following this treatment.

Surgical experience with the Maze procedure to create lines of conduction block in the atrium has led the way for catheter-based ablation procedures to cure atrial fibrillation. Studies have attempted to replicate the success of the surgical procedure using a catheter-based approach. Atrial fibrillation consists of multiple reentrant circuits within the atrium, around the vena cava, pulmonary veins, and appendages, and around areas of functional block. Creation of multiple lines of block between these nonconducting structures prevents development of reentry.

A variety of catheter techniques have been employed including a “point-by-point” approach, a “drag” approach, and a multielectrode approach. Right atrial lesions alone were shown to be ineffective.[58] Attempts at left atrial or biatrial lesions have met with limited success due to the prolonged procedure times, high risk of complications, and limited efficacy.[59,60] There is also concern about reduced mechanical function of the atria following extensive ablation. This limits the hemodynamic benefit of the restored sinus rhythm.

As understanding of the mechanism of atrial fibrillation has evolved, attempts to block propagation of atrial fibrillatory circuits have been abandoned in favor of attempted ablation of the fibrillatory triggers. Data suggest that atrial fibrillation may in some cases be triggered by an organized supraventricular tachycardia. About 12% of patients with AVNRT or AVRT will develop symptomatic atrial fibrillation in 1 year of follow-up.[61] Thus ablation of the initiating trigger arrhythmia may prevent atrial fibrillation.

In a series of patients undergoing a left-sided catheter Maze procedure, it was discovered that rapidly firing foci arising from the musculature of the pulmonary veins were driving atrial fibrillation.[62] Ablation of these foci eliminated atrial fibrillation in some patients. This procedure has evolved to empiric electrical isolation of the pulmonary veins. One approach is the complete encircling of the pulmonary veins.[63] Another approach is segmental isolation of each vein by mapping the location of the connecting fibers. Electroanatomical mapping and intracardiac echocardiography have been employed to facilitate ablation. Data on the long-term efficacy and complications of this procedure are limited and it is still considered to be a procedure in evolution. In one series of 251 patients, the short-term success over 10.4 months of follow-up was 80%. There was an 85% success rate in those with paroxysmal and 68% success in those with permanent atrial fibrillation. There was a continued need for antiarrhythmic medications in some patients.[64]

A major complication of ablation within the pulmonary veins is focal pulmonary vein stenosis. In 102 patients undergoing pulmonary vein focal ablation, 39% with right upper vein ablation and 23% with left vein ablation developed focal pulmonary vein stenosis by transesophageal echocardiography 3 days after the procedure.[65] In this series, only 3 patients experienced symptoms of dyspnea on exertion and only 1 had mild increase in pulmonary pressure. Although most cases are asymptomatic, severe cases have been reported that progress to pulmonary hypertension and lung transplant. The ablation procedure is evolving in an attempt to prevent this complication. Changes have included limiting ablation to the vein ostia, limiting power, and using ultrasound imaging during ablation.

In some patients, triggering foci arise from outside the pulmonary veins. Reported sites have included the superior vena cava, ligament of Marshall, crista terminalis, posterior wall of the left atrium, tricuspid/mitral valve annulus, and limbus of the fossa ovalis. Pulmonary vein isolation failures in some cases may be due to the triggers from these alternative sites.

In patients with persistent and/or chronic atrial fibrillation, there may be a combination of triggers and substrate responsible. Successful ablation may require elimination of triggers combined with modification of substrate. The future role of focal ablation for atrial fibrillation will depend on advances in catheter technologies to improve efficacy, reduce procedure times, and reduce complications.

Ventricular Tachycardia

Ablation techniques can also target ventricular tachycardia (VT). Over 90% of life-threatening ventricular arrhythmias originate from myocardium with structural abnormalities. Regions of scarred or aneurysmal myocardium create channels for reentrant circuits. Initial successes with resection of ventricular arrhythmogenic foci and reentrant circuits surgically have led to advancements in catheter-based ablation techniques. Beginning with DC ablation, techniques have advanced with the use of radiofrequency ablation catheters and electroanatomical mapping systems. Despite these advances, ablation for VT in patients with coronary artery disease has a limited role. Given the life-threatening potential of VT in patients with structural heart disease, even a single recurrence can be disastrous. Therefore, implantable cardiac defibrillators have become the primary therapy. Indications for ablation in this population are failure of antiarrhythmic medication to suppress symptomatic, sustained monomorphic VT, or more often frequent shocks from an implanted defibrillator despite optimal medical therapy.[15]

There are several factors limiting the role of catheter ablation of ischemic VT. The hemodynamic instability of patients with coronary artery disease and depressed left ventricular function limits mapping during the tachycardia. A patient may have multiple reentrant circuits, not all of which are clinically significant. The VT reentrant circuits involve scarred myocardium or can be epicardial in locations that may be out of reach for radiofrequency energy to penetrate. Finally short-term success may be eclipsed by development of new ventricular tachycardias with further myocardial injury.

Success of ischemic VT ablation is variable due to the heterogeneity of the population. Reported studies have shown efficacy in the range of 60% to 90% using the criteria of reduced defibrillator shocks and decreased need for antiarrhythmic medications. Recurrence rate is as high as 40%. Recently, success has been reported with an approach employing "substrate mapping." This technique defines the potential arrhythmic substrate using electroanatomical voltage maps. Ablation is targeted to eliminate potential reentrant circuits. Complications are in the range of 2%, with concern for perforation and cardiac tamponade due to the thin, scarred ventricles that are the substrates for ablation and thromboembolic events in those undergoing extensive ablation.[66–68] One reason for failure of ischemic VT ablation is the deep or epicardial location of circuits. Catheter ablation has been directed at these epicardial circuits using a pericardial approach with some success.[69]

In patients with dilated cardiomyopathy and His-Purkinje system disease, sustained monomorphic VT can occur due to a macro-reentrant circuit using the bundle branches. Patients typically present with syncope or sudden death or can present with palpitations. The most common circuit is down the right bundle branch and up the left bundle branch resulting in a wide complex tachycardia with a left bundle branch block pattern. Treatment involves ablation of one of the fascicles involved in the reentrant circuit. The right bundle is most commonly targeted to interrupt the reentrant circuit. Long-term success is good for prevention of recurrent bundle branch reentry. Due to intrinsic conduction disease, patients may develop heart block. Patients may also develop other VTs due to other structural abnormalities, requiring further ablation, antiarrhythmic therapy, or defibrillator implantation.[70,71]

Other cardiac disorders can be associated with VT and are potential candidates for catheter ablation. This includes right ventricular dysplasia,[72] infiltrative disorders (sarcoid), and tumors. As in patients with atrial arrhythmias due to surgical incisions, patients with prior ventricular surgery can develop incision-related VT. This has occurred most often in patients who have undergone repair of congenital abnormalities such as tetrology of Fallot.

Ventricular tachycardia that presents in patients with no structural heart disease is termed idiopathic and represents up to 10% of all VTs that present to tertiary referral centers. Patients may be asymptomatic or present with palpitations, dizziness, or syncope. Idiopathic VT may be focal or a micro-reentrant circuit utilizing the Purkinje fibers.

Focal VT can originate from either the right or left ventricle. Right ventricular tachycardia typically originates from the outflow tract, on the septal or free wall sites. It has a typical left bundle branch morphology with leftward, inferior axis. This occurs more often in women than men, and patients typically present in their 30s to 50s. Idiopathic left ventricular tachycardia typically originates from the left posterior fascicle. It has a right bundle branch morphology with rightward, superior axis, and may be verapamil sensitive. It occurs more often in men. These VTs are localized by activation or pace mapping. Ablation is facilitated by the lack of other cardiac pathology and the presence of only one VT. Success rates for idiopathic VT are in the range of 70% to 90% with recurrence rates in the range of 15%. Complication rates are consistent with other ablative procedures.[73,74]

Cost-Effectiveness

Several studies have shown the cost-effectiveness of catheter ablation compared to medical therapy and surgical ablation. Catheter ablation has lower procedural costs than surgical ablation and reduces the need for further medical care and emergency room visits in comparison to drug therapy. A U.S. study comparing lifelong medical therapy versus catheter ablation for monthly episodes of supraventricular tachycardia showed a cost savings of $27,900 for ablation. There was also improvement in quality of life.[75] An Australian study compared 50 patients who underwent RF ablation to 20 who underwent surgical therapy and 12 who were treated medically. Costs over 20 years were estimated to be (in Australian dollars) $2911, $17,467, and $4959, respectively, for these groups.[76]

FUTURE DIRECTIONS

After the advent of steerable catheters, newer imaging techniques have been the most useful in directing the positioning of catheters to specific areas of interest within the heart. The techniques of nonfluoroscopic mapping discussed above have extended the efficacy of catheter-based ablation. Newer imaging techniques are in development that will continue to push the field of electrophysiology.

Imaging Technology

One novel technology in development is the use of magnetic resonance imaging (MRI) technology to visualize cardiac structures as well as catheter location with acquisition up to 10 frames per second. This would allow high-resolution three-dimensional mapping of the heart as well as localization of catheters in three-dimensional space in real time. A catheter has been developed that both acts as a receiver, allowing for visualization of its entire length by MRI, and functions as a traditional mapping and ablation catheter.[77]

Catheter Technology

Another area of active research is that of catheter design. A limit to tissue energy delivery with radiofrequency is the rise in temperature at the tissue-electrode interface leading to an impedance rise and limitation of energy delivery deep into the tissue. Coagulum begins to form at the catheter-tissue interface at temperatures above 100°C. This results in an increase in impedance and limits lesion size. This limitation in lesion size places some epicardial foci and arrhythmia circuits out of reach of endocardial ablations.

Cooling the ablation catheter tip with saline irrigation either through the catheter or external to the catheter prevents coagulum formation at the tissue interface. This prevents a rise in impedance and allows for more energy delivery deep into the tissue, resulting in deeper and larger lesions.[78] Catheters have been designed that are saline irrigated with infusion of saline through the catheter and then into the body through a porous tip. Catheters are also available that are completely contained, with recirculation of saline within the catheter.

Another method of increasing lesion size and depth also uses the principle of limiting coagulum size by increasing the electrode-tissue interface by increasing tip size. In vitro studies have shown that 8-mm catheter tips produced lesions that are twice as deep and four times larger than lesions produced by standard 4-mm tips.[79] Catheter tips of 12-mm size were also tried but this resulted in smaller lesions, perhaps due to poor tissue contact. A limitation of larger catheter tips is that the larger surface area makes it difficult to regulate power delivery and achieve even temperatures. High current densities develop at the edges of the electrode resulting in higher temperatures and coagulum formation. Larger lesions are particularly useful for higher successful rates for atrial flutter and ventricular tachycardia ablations that involve thicker myocardium. They also reduce procedure times and limit radiation exposure for patients.[80]

Hypothermia has been the preferred method of delivering linear lesions in surgical ablation. Cryoablation has been shown to be safe and effective. Cryothermal energy delivery via transvenous catheters is under development. This technique utilizes nitrogen or nitrogen oxide pressurized flow through a catheter tip nozzle. As the gas expands beyond the obstruction, there is a temperature drop to as much as −90°C. The blood pool forms an ice ball with resulting cooling of the underlying tissue. The advantages of cryoablation are that limited tissue cooling results in reversible injury causing transient conduction block. This allows for placement of test lesions, or "ice mapping," without causing permanent damage, reducing the chance of collateral damage. This may be especially true for high-risk ablations that are close to a normal conduction pathway. Once a successful safe site is localized, irreversible lesions can be placed by cooling further and freezing the tissue. Another advantage is that the resulting ice ball adheres the catheter tip to the myocardium, preventing catheter movement during lesion formation. This allows for ablation delivery during tachycardia when rapid heart movement may result in catheter movement.[81]

Alternative Energy Sources

Other energy sources for ablation are currently under development. These include laser, microwave, and ultrasound. The advantages of these systems are that direct tissue contact is not necessary for lesion formation. Theoretically, deeper and larger lesions could be formed with these energies. Ultrasound has the advantage of offering both imaging and ablation in a single catheter. Currently, catheter-based delivery systems for these energies are under development. The potential adverse effects of these systems remain the same as other ablation techniques such as proarrhythmic effects of lesions, inadvertent collateral damage, and perforation.[82] Energy delivery from a distance may someday allow noninvasive ablation of cardiac tissue.

CONCLUSION

The past 35 years have seen the development of intracardiac recording, programmed stimulation, and catheter ablation. The field of interventional electrophysiology is relatively young. Over the past two decades, great advances have been seen in the interventional management of atrial and ventricular tachyarrhythmias. Where the surgeons have gone with their scalpels, electrophysiologists have followed with their catheters. Transvenous RF ablation has become the standard of care for the treatment of many arrhythmias. These procedures have been proven to be safe and efficacious. Improved treatments for arrhythmias such as atrial fibrillation and ventricular tachycardias will come with further understanding of the mechanisms underlying these arrhythmias. Future advances in catheter design, energy delivery, and imaging techniques will continue to advance the field of electrophysiology.

REFERENCES

1. Durrer D, Schoo L, Schuilenburg RM, et al: The role of premature beats in the initiation and termination of supraventricular tachycardia with the WPW syndrome. *Ciruculation* 1967; 36:644.
2. Scherlag BJ, Lau SH, Helfant RH, et al: Catheter technique for recording His bundle activity in man. *Circulation* 1969; 39:13.
3. Cobb FR, Blumenschein SD, Sealy WC, et al: Successful surgical interruption of the bundle of Kent in a patient with Wolff-Parkinson-White syndrome. *Circulation* 1968; 38:1018.
4. Coumel P, Aigeperse J, Perrault MA, et al: Reperage et tentative d'exerese chirurgicale d'un foyer ectopique rebelled: evolution favorable. [Detection and attempted surgical exeresis of a left

auricular ectopic focus with refractory tachycardia: favorable outcome]. *Ann Cardiol Angeiol* 1973; 22:189.

5. Pritchett EL, Anderson RW, Benditt DG, et al: Reentry within the atrioventricular node: surgical cure with preservation of atrioventricular conduction. *Circulation* 1979; 60:440.
6. Gonzalez, R, Scheinman, MM, Margaretten, W, et al: Closed-chest electrode-catheter technique for His bundle ablation in dogs. *Am J Physiol* 1981; 24:H283.
7. Scheinman MM, Morady F, Hess DS, et al: Catheter-induced ablation of the atrioventricular junction to control refractory supraventricular arrhythmias. *JAMA* 1982; 248:851.
8. Gallagher JJ, Svenson RH, Kasel JH, et al: Catheter technique for closed-chest ablation of the atrioventricular conduction system. *N Engl J Med* 1982; 306:194.
9. Huang SK, Bharati S, Graham AR, et al: Closed chest catheter desiccation of the atrioventricular junction using radiofrequency energy—a new method of catheter ablation. *J Am Coll Cardiol* 1987; 9:349.
10. Nath S, Dimarco JP, Mounsey JP, et al: Correlation of temperature and pathophysiological effect during radiofrequency catheter ablation of the AV junction. *Circulation* 1995; 92:1188.
11. Chen SA, Chiang CE, Tai CT, et al: Complications of diagnostic electrophysiologic studies and radiofrequency catheter ablation in patients with tachyarrhythmias: an eight-year survey of 3,966 consecutive procedures in a tertiary referral center. *Am J Cardiol* 1996; 77:41.
12. Kovoor P, Ricciardello M, Collins L, et al: Risk to patients from radiation associated with radiofrequency ablation for supraventricular tachycardia. *Circulation* 1998; 98:1534.
13. Schalij MJ, van Rugge FP, Siezenga M, et al: Endocardial activation mapping of ventricular tachycardia in patients: first application of a 32-site bipolar mapping electrode catheter. *Circulation* 1998; 98:2168.
14. Gepstein L, Hayam G, Ben-Haim SA: A novel method for nonfluoroscopic catheter-based electroanatomical mapping of the heart: in vitro and in vivo accuracy results. *Circulation* 1997; 95:1611.
15. Hoffmann E, Reithmann C, Nimmermann P, et al: Clinical experience with electroanatomic mapping of ectopic atrial tachycardia. *Pacing Clin Electrophysiol* 2002; 25:49.
16. Gornick CC, Adler SW, Pederson B, et al: Validation of a new noncontact catheter system for electroanatomic mapping of left ventricular endocardium. *Circulation* 1999; 99:829.
17. Bruce CJ, Friedman PA: Intracardiac echocardiography. *Eur J Echocardiogr* 2001; 2:234.
18. Jazayeri MR, Hempe SL, Sra JS, et al: Selective transcatheter ablation of the fast and slow pathways using radiofrequency energy in patients with atrioventricular nodal reentrant tachycardia. *Circulation* 1992; 85:1318.
19. Akhtar M, Jazayeri MR, Sra J, et al: Atrioventricular nodal reentry: clinical, electrophysiological, and therapeutic considerations. *Circulation* 1993; 88:282.
20. ACC/AHA Task Force Report: Guidelines for clinical intracardiac electrophysiological and catheter ablation procedures: a report of the American College of Cardiology/American Heart Association Task Force on Practice Guidelines (Committee on Clinical Intracardiac Electrophysiologic and Catheter Ablation Procedures). Developed in collaboration with the North American Society of Pacing and Electrophysiology. *J Cardiovasc Electrophysiol* 1995; 6:652.
21. Doig JC, Saito J, Harris L, Downar E: Coronary sinus morphology in patients with atrioventricular junctional reentry tachycardia and other supraventricular tachyarrhythmias. *Circulation* 1995; 92:436.
22. Khalife K, Billette J, Medkour D, et al: Role of the compact node and its posterior extension in normal atrioventricular nodal conduction, refractory, and dual pathway properties. *J Cardiovasc Electrophysiol* 1999; 10:1439.
23. Kalbfleisch SJ, el-Atassi R, Calkins H, et al: Differentiation of paroxysmal narrow QRS complex tachycardias using the 12-lead electrocardiogram. *J Am Coll Cardiol* 1993; 21:85.
24. Epstein LM, Scheinman MM, Langberg JJ, et al: Percutaneous catheter modification of the atrioventricular node: a potential cure for atrioventricular nodal reentrant tachycardia. *Circulation* 1989; 80:757.
25. Hindricks G: Incidence of complete atrioventricular block following attempted radiofrequency catheter modification of the atrioventricular node in 880 patients. Results of the Multicenter European Radiofrequency Survey (MERFS): The Working Group on Arrhythmias of the European Society of Cardiology. *Eur Heart J* 1996; 17:82.
26. Kottkamp H, Hindricks G, Borggrefe M, et al: Radiofrequency catheter ablation of the anterosuperior and posteroinferior atrial approaches to the AV node for treatment of AV nodal reentrant tachycardia: techniques for selective ablation of "fast" and "slow" AV node pathways. *J Cardiovasc Electrophysiol* 1997; 8:451.
27. Kalbfleisch SJ, Strickberger SA, Williamson B, et al: Randomized comparison of anatomic and electrogram mapping approaches to ablation of the slow pathway of atrioventricular node reentrant tachycardia. *J Am Coll Cardiol* 1994; 23:716.
28. Scheinman MM: North American Society of Pacing and Electrophysiology (NASPE) survey on radiofrequency catheter ablation: implications for clinicians, third party insurers, and government regulatory agencies. *Pacing Clin Electrophysiol* 1992; 15:2228.
29. Scheinman MM, Huang S: The 1998 NASPE prospective catheter ablation registry. *Pacing Clin Electrophysiol* 2000; 23:1020.
30. Cox JL, Gallagher JJ, Cain ME: Experience with 118 consecutive patients undergoing operation for the Wolff-Parkinson-White syndrome. *J Thorac Cardiovasc Surg* 1985; 90:490.
31. Haissaguerre M, Montserrat P, Warin JF, et al: Catheter ablation of left posteroseptal accessory pathways and of long RP' tachycardias with a right endocardial approach. *Eur Heart J* 1991; 12:845.
32. Olsson A, Darpo B, Bergfeldt L, et al: Frequency and long term follow up of valvar insufficiency caused by retrograde aortic radiofrequency catheter ablation procedures. *Heart* 1999; 81:292.
33. Sapp J, Soejima K, Couper GS, et al: Electrophysiology and anatomic characterization of an epicardial accessory pathway. *J Cardiovasc Electrophysiol* 2001; 12:1411.
34. Okishige K, Goseki Y, Itoh A, et al: New electrophysiologic features and catheter ablation of atrioventricular and atriofascicular accessory pathways: evidence of decremental conduction and the anatomic structure of the Mahaim pathway. *J Cardiovasc Electrophysiol* 1998; 9:22.
35. Lesh MD, Van Hare GF, Schamp DJ, et al: Curative percutaneous catheter ablation using radiofrequency energy for accessory pathways in all locations: results in 100 consecutive patients. *J Am Coll Cardiol* 1992; 19:1303.
36. Jackman WM, Wang XZ, Friday KJ, et al: Catheter ablation of accessory atrioventricular pathways (Wolff-Parkinson-White syndrome) by radiofrequency current. *N Engl J Med* 1991; 324:1605.
37. Dagres N, Clague JR, Kottkamp H, et al: Radiofrequency catheter ablation of accessory pathways: outcome and use of antiarrhythmic drugs during follow-up. *Eur Heart J* 1999; 20:1826.
38. Fitchet A, Turkie W: Fitzpatrick accessory pathway transseptal approach to ablation of left-sided arrhythmias does not lead to persisting interatrial shunt: a transesophageal echocardiographic study. *Pacing Clin Electrophysiol* 1998; 21:2070.
39. Kessler DJ, Pirwitz MJ, Horton RP, et al: Intracardiac shunts resulting from transseptal catheterization for ablation of accessory pathways in otherwise normal hearts. *Am J Cardiol* 1998; 82:391.

40. Corey WA, Markel ML, Hoit BD, et al: Regression of a dilated cardiomyopathy after radiofrequency ablation of incessant supraventricular tachycardia. *Am Heart J* 1993; 126:1469.
41. Chiladakis JA, Vassilikos VP, Maounis TN, et al: Successful radiofrequency catheter ablation of automatic atrial tachycardia with regression of the cardiomyopathy picture. *Pacing Clin Electrophysiol* 1997; 20:953.
42. Callans DJ, Schwartzman D, Gottlieb CD, et al: Insights into the electrophysiology of atrial arrhythmias gained by the catheter ablation experience: "learning while burning, part II." *J Cardiovasc Electrophysiol* 1995; 6:229.
43. Tracy CM: Catheter ablation for patients with atrial tachycardia. *Cardiol Clin* 1997; 15:607.
44. Schmitt H, Weber S, Schwab JO, et al: Diagnosis and ablation of focal right atrial tachycardia using a new high-resolution, noncontact mapping system. *Am J Cardiol* 2001; 87:1017.
45. Reithmann C, Hoffmann E, Dorwarth U, et al: Electroanatomical mapping for visualization of atrial activation in patients with incisional atrial tachycardias. *Eur Heart J* 2001; 22:237.
46. Anguera I, Brugada J, Roba M, et al: Outcomes after radiofrequency catheter ablation of atrial tachycardia. *Am J Cardiol* 2001; 87:886.
47. Chen SA, Tai CT, Chiang CE, et al: Role of the surface electrocardiogram in the diagnosis of patients with supraventricular tachycardia. *Cardiol Clin* 1997; 15:539.
48. Fischer B, Jais P, Shah D, et al: Radiofrequency catheter ablation of common atrial flutter in 200 patients. *J Cardiovasc Electrophysiol* 1996; 7:1225.
49. Feld GK: New approaches for the management of atrial fibrillation: role of ablation of atrial flutter. *J Cardiovasc Electrophysiol* 1999; 10:1188.
50. Huang DT, Monahan KM, Zimetbaum P, et al: Hybrid pharmacologic and ablative therapy: a novel and effective approach for the management of atrial fibrillation. *J Cardiovasc Electrophysiol* 1998; 9:462.
51. Nakagawa H, Shah N, Matsudaira K, et al: Characterization of reentrant circuit in macroreentrant right atrial tachycardia after surgical repair of congenital heart disease: isolated channels between scars allow "focal" ablation. *Circulation* 2001; 103:699.
52. Strohmer B, Chen PS, Hwang C: Radiofrequency ablation of focal atrial tachycardia and atrioatrial conduction from recipient to donor after orthotopic heart transplantation. *J Cardiovasc Electrophysiol* 2000; 11:1165.
53. Ellenbogen KA, Hawthorne HR, Belz MK, et al: Late occurrence of incessant atrial tachycardia following the Maze procedure. *Pacing Clin Electrophysiol* 1995; 18:367.
54. Kalman JM, Olgin JE, Saxon LA, et al: Electrocardiographic and electrophysiologic characterization of atypical atrial flutter in man: use of activation and entrainment mapping and implications for catheter ablation. *J Cardiovasc Electrophysiol* 1997; 8:121.
55. Marshall HJ, Griffith MJ: Ablation of the atrioventricular junction: technique, acute and long-term results in 115 consecutive patients. *Europace* 1999; 1:26.
56. Kay GN, Ellenbogen KA, Giudici M, et al: The Ablate and Pace Trial: a prospective study of catheter ablation of the AV conduction system and permanent pacemaker implantation for treatment of atrial fibrillation. APT Investigators. *J Interv Card Electrophysiol* 1998; 2:121.
57. Ozcan C, Jahangir A, Friedman PA, et al: Long-term survival after ablation of the atrioventricular node and implantation of a permanent pacemaker in patients with atrial fibrillation. *N Engl J Med* 2001; 344:1043.
58. Jais P, Shah DC, Takahashi A, et al: Long-term follow-up after right atrial radiofrequency catheter treatment of paroxysmal atrial fibrillation. *Pacing Clin Electrophysiol* 1998; 21:2533.
59. Pappone C, Oreto G, Lamberti F, et al: Catheter ablation of paroxysmal atrial fibrillation using a 3D mapping system. *Circulation* 1999; 100:1203.
60. Zhou L, Keane D, Reed G, et al: Thromboembolic complications of cardiac radiofrequency catheter ablation: a review of the reported incidence, pathogenesis and current research directions. *J Cardiovasc Electrophysiol* 1999; 10:611.
61. Hamer ME, Wilkinson WE, Clair WK, et al: Incidence of symptomatic atrial fibrillation in patients with paroxysmal supraventricular tachycardia. *J Am Coll Cardiol* 1995; 25:984.
62. Haissaguerre M, Jais P, Shah DC, et al: Spontaneous initiation of atrial fibrillation by ectopic beats originating in the pulmonary veins. *N Engl J Med* 1998; 339:659.
63. Oral H, Knight BP, Tada H, et al: Pulmonary vein isolation for paroxysmal and persistent atrial fibrillation. *Circulation* 2002; 105:1077.
64. Pappone C, Oreto G, Rosanio S, et al: Atrial electroanatomic remodeling after circumferential radiofrequency pulmonary vein ablation: efficacy of an anatomic approach in a large cohort of patients with atrial fibrillation. *Circulation* 2001; 104:2539.
65. Yu WC, Hsu TL, Tai CT, et al: Acquired pulmonary vein stenosis after radiofrequency catheter ablation of paroxysmal atrial fibrillation. *J Cardiovasc Electrophysiol* 2001; 12:887.
66. Morady F, Harvey M, Kalbfleisch SJ, et al: Radiofrequency catheter ablation of ventricular tachycardia in patients with coronary artery disease. *Circulation* 1993; 87:363.
67. Stevenson WG, Khan H, Sager P, et al: Identification of the reentry circuit during catheter mapping and radiofrequency ablation of ventricular tachycardia late after myocardial infarction. *Circulation* 1993; 88:1647.
68. Gonska BD, Cao K, Schaumann A, et al: Catheter ablation of ventricular tachycardia in 136 patients with coronary artery disease: results and long-term follow-up. *J Am Coll Cardiol* 1994; 24:1506.
69. Sosa E, Scanavacca M, d'Avila A, et al: Nonsurgical transthoracic epicardial catheter ablation to treat recurrent ventricular tachycardia occurring late after myocardial infarction. *J Am Coll Cardiol* 2000; 35:1442.
70. Mehdirad AA, Keim S, Rist K, et al: Long-term clinical outcome of right bundle branch radiofrequency catheter ablation for treatment of bundle branch reentrant ventricular tachycardia. *Pacing Clin Electrophysiol* 1995; 18:2135.
71. Blanck Z, Dhala A, Deshpande S, et al: Bundle branch reentrant ventricular tachycardia: cumulative experience in 48 patients. *J Cardiovasc Electrophysiol* 1993; 4:253.
72. Marcus FI, Fontaine G: Arrhythmogenic right ventricular dysplasia/cardiomyopathy: a review. *Pacing Clin Electrophysiol* 1995; 18:1298.
73. Rodriguez LM, Smeets JL, Timmermans C, et al: Predictors for successful ablation of right- and left-sided idiopathic ventricular tachycardia. *Am J Cardiol* 1997; 79:309.
74. Wen MS, Taniguchi Y, Yeh SJ, et al: Determinants of tachycardia recurrences after radiofrequency ablation of idiopathic ventricular tachycardia. *Am J Cardiol* 1998; 81:500.
75. Cheng CH, Sanders GD, Hlatky MA, et al: Cost-effectiveness of radiofrequency ablation for supraventricular tachycardia. *Ann Intern Med* 2000; 133:864.
76. Weerasooriya HR, Murdock CJ, Harris AH, et al: The cost-effectiveness of treatment of supraventricular arrhythmias related to an accessory atrioventricular pathway: comparison of catheter ablation, surgical division and medical treatment. *Aust N Z J Med* 1994; 24:161.
77. Susil RC, Yeung CJ, Halperin HR, et al: Multifunctional interventional devices for MRI: a combined electrophysiology/MRI catheter. *Magn Reson Med* 2002; 47:594.

78. Demazumder D, Mirotznik MS, Schwartzman D: Biophysics of radiofrequency ablation using an irrigated electrode. *J Interv Card Electrophysiol* 2001; 5:377.
79. Langberg JJ, Gallagher M, Strickberger SA, et al: Temperature-guided radiofrequency catheter ablation with very large distal electrodes. *Circulation* 1993; 88:245.
80. Tsai CF, Tai CT, Yu WC, et al: Is 8-mm more effective than 4-mm tip electrode catheter for ablation of typical atrial flutter? *Circulation* 1999; 100:768.
81. Skanes AC, Dubuc M, Klein GJ, et al: Cryothermal ablation of the slow pathway for the elimination of atrioventricular nodal reentrant tachycardia. *Circulation* 2000; 102:2856.
82. Wang PJ, Homoud MK, Link MS, et al: Alternate energy sources for catheter ablation. *Curr Cardiol Rep* 1999; 1:165.

Chapter 53

Surgical Treatment of Supraventricular Tachyarrhythmias

James L. Cox

Supraventricular arrhythmias due to the Wolff-Parkinson-White (WPW) syndrome, AV node reentry, automatic atrial foci, and most forms of atrial flutter have essentially disappeared from the realm of the surgeon because of the phenomenal success of less invasive radiofrequency catheter ablation techniques. Thus, the numerous surgical procedures that were once in such vogue for the treatment of those arrhythmias are now of historical interest only. The only supraventricular arrhythmia of significance to the cardiac surgeon in 2002 is atrial fibrillation.

Atrial fibrillation is present in approximately 1% of the general population[1–5] and 6% of the population over the age of 65 years,[6–9] making it the most common of all sustained cardiac arrhythmias. According to the Health Care Finance Administration (HFCA), atrial fibrillation results in 1.4 million outpatient visits and 227,000 hospitalizations (50% as emergencies) in the United States annually.[10] The annual cost of atrial fibrillation to the federal budget is calculated by HFCA to be $6.6 billion, not including physician fees, outpatient expenses, medications, and non-Medicare patient expenses.[10]

Although atrial fibrillation is considered by many to be an innocuous arrhythmia, it is associated with significant morbidity and mortality due to its three detrimental sequelae: (1) an irregularly irregular heartbeat, which causes patient discomfort and anxiety; (2) loss of synchronous atrioventricular contraction, which compromises cardiac hemodynamics resulting in varying levels of congestive heart failure; and (3) stasis of blood flow in the left atrium, which increases the vulnerability to thromboembolism.

Optimal medical therapy of atrial fibrillation includes the use of drugs directed towards *rhythm* control, i.e., the conversion of atrial fibrillation to normal sinus rhythm. Unfortunately, these drugs frequently fail and the therapeutic goal shifts to *rate* control, i.e., slowing the ventricular response rate to atrial fibrillation. Although the ventricular response rate can usually be controlled medically, it is important to recognize the fact that the atria are still fibrillating and therefore all three of the detrimental sequelae associated with atrial fibrillation persist. Obviously, the hemodynamic compromise is not as great with a controlled ventricular response rate to atrial fibrillation but, just as obviously, cardiac hemodynamics are not restored to normal because of the absence of the atrial "kick." Thus pharmacologic therapy is less than optimal in a large number of patients with atrial fibrillation. Because medical therapy frequently fails to control atrial fibrillation, several surgical procedures were introduced in the 1980s to either ablate the arrhythmia or ameliorate its attendant detrimental sequelae.

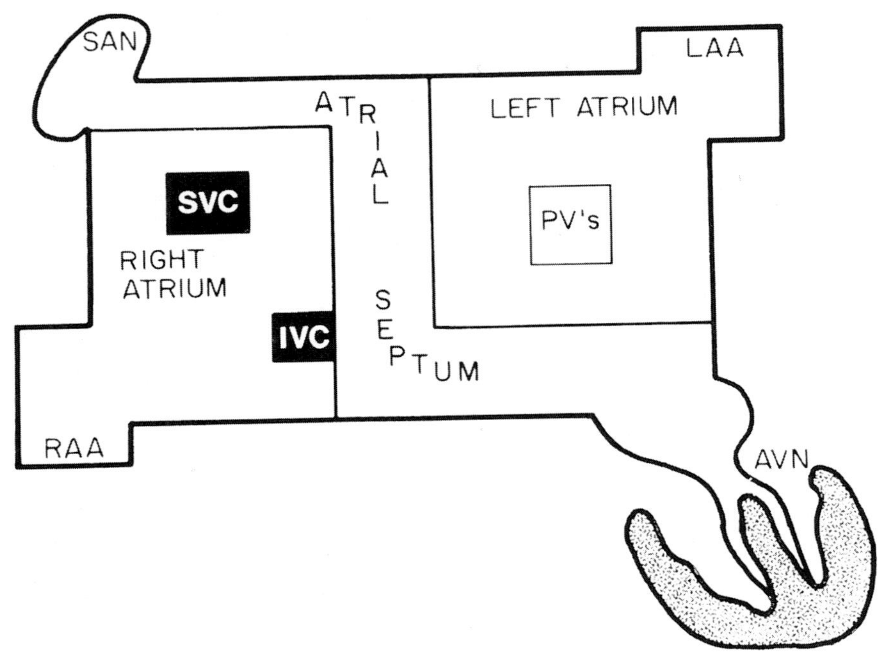

FIGURE 53–1 Schematic atrial anatomy. The atria are represented as a box with the left atrium and right atrium in the designated locations. The right atrium has two electrical "holes": the orifice of the superior vena cava (SVC) and the orifice of the inferior vena cava (IVC). It also has a right atrial appendage (RAA). The left atrium is contiguous with the pulmonary veins (PV's) and also has the left atrial appendage (LAA).

The atrial septum lies between the right and left atria. The sinoatrial node (SAN) is positioned at the top of the atrial septum, and the atrioventricular node (AVN) is at the bottom of the atrial septum, where conduction continues to the ventricles via the specialized conduction system.

EARLY SURGICAL PROCEDURES FOR ATRIAL FIBRILLATION

Even though the early procedures that were developed for the surgical treatment of atrial fibrillation are no longer employed, it is virtually impossible to understand the vagaries of treating atrial fibrillation in the operating theater without understanding the lessons of those initial efforts. Indeed, most of the failures of contemporary catheter and surgical techniques in ablating atrial fibrillation result from a lack of knowledge of the problems that were identified, elucidated, and solved in the early days of development of these surgical procedures. For purposes of clarity, the schema used to describe the results of all of these procedures is shown in Figure 53-1.

The Left Atrial Isolation Procedure

In 1980, we described the *left atrial isolation procedure* (Fig. 53-2),[11] which was capable of confining atrial fibrillation to the left atrium while leaving the remainder of the heart in normal sinus rhythm (Fig. 53-3). This procedure was successful in restoring a regular ventricular rhythm without the need for a permanent pacemaker, and, unexpectedly, it also restored normal cardiac hemodynamics. The reason for the latter is that the right atrium and right ventricle beat in synchrony following the procedure. This provides a normal right-sided cardiac output that is then delivered to the left side of the heart. Despite the fact that the left atrium is isolated, and therefore cannot beat in synchrony with the left ventricle, the left ventricle adapts instantaneously to the normal right-sided output and delivers a normal forward cardiac output (Fig. 53-4). Thus, the left atrial isolation procedure alleviates two of the three detrimental sequelae of atrial fibrillation, namely irregular heartbeat and compromised hemodynamics. Unfortunately, since the left atrium may continue to fibrillate, the vulnerability to systemic thromboembolism is unchanged following this procedure.

Catheter Ablation of the AV Node–His Bundle Complex

In 1982, Scheinman introduced *catheter fulguration of the His bundle* (Fig. 53-5) as a means of controlling the irregular cardiac rhythm associated with atrial fibrillation and other refractory supraventricular arrhythmias.[12] This procedure was also a type of isolation procedure in that it isolated the supraventricular arrhythmia to the atria and away from the ventricles. Catheter fulguration was eventually abandoned in favor of the less traumatic radiofrequency ablative techniques that are still in use today. Elective His bundle ablation necessitates the implantation of a permanent ventricular pacemaker, which restores a normal ventricular rhythm. However, the atria continue to fibrillate following His bundle ablation, and thus this technique alleviates only *one* of the detrimental sequelae of atrial fibrillation, the irregular heartbeat. The hemodynamic compromise due to loss of atrioventricular synchrony and the vulnerability to thromboembolism are unaffected by His bundle ablation.

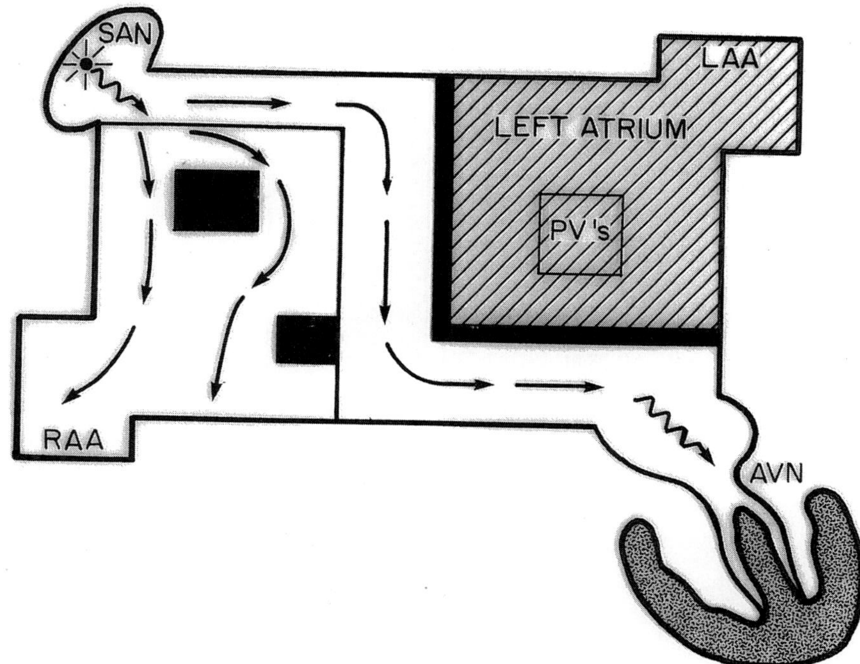

FIGURE 53–2 The left atrial isolation procedure confines all electrical activity in the left atrium, whether normal or abnormal, to the left atrium. This allows the normal cardiac impulse to originate in the sinoatrial node (SAN), conduct across the right atrium, and into the ventricles via the atrioventricular node (AVN). (Same schema as in Figure 53-1.)

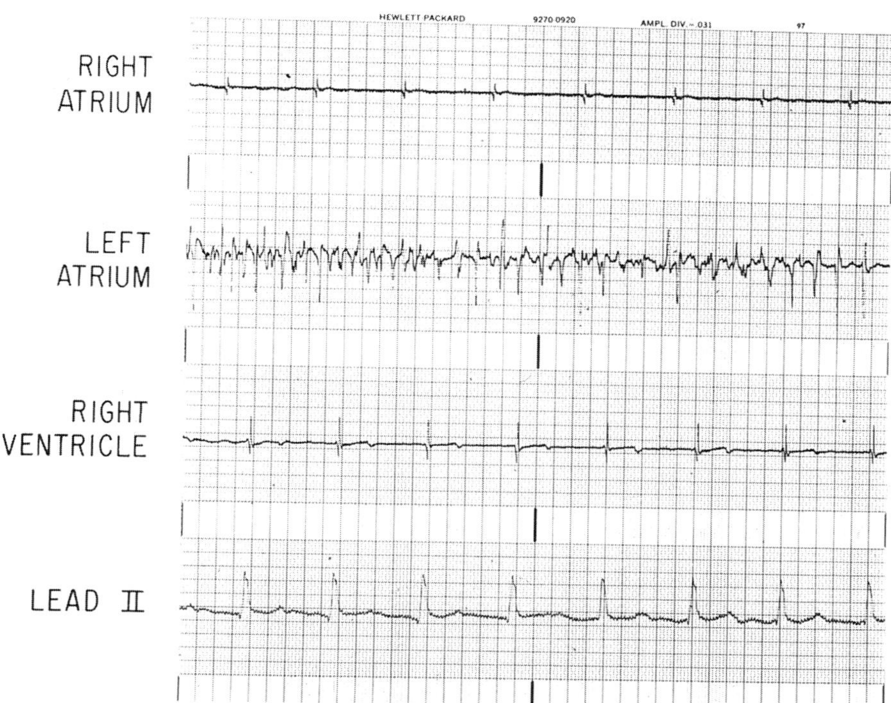

FIGURE 53–3 Following the left atrial isolation procedure, the left atrium may still fibrillate, but the atrial fibrillation is confined to the left atrium due to its electrical isolation from surgery. The remainder of the heart beats in a normal sinus rhythm. However, this may be difficult to discern on a standard ECG (for example, in lead II) because the size and morphology of the P wave is determined primarily by the electrical activity in the left atrium, not the right atrium. (*Reproduced with permission from Williams JM, Ungerleider RM, Lofland GK, Cox JL: Left atrial isolation: new technique for the treatment of supraventricular arrhythmias. J Thorac Cardiovasc Surg 1980; 80:373.*)

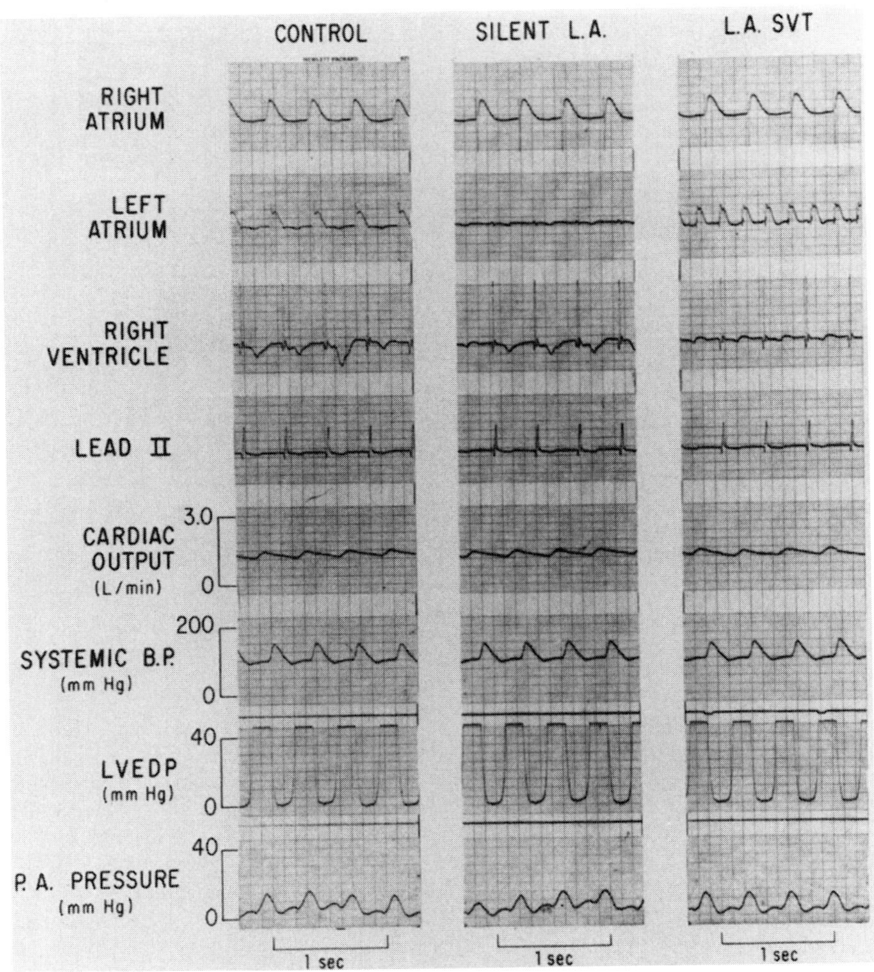

FIGURE 53–4 This example of one of several experiments documenting that as long as the right atrium is beating in synchrony with the right ventricle, the contractile function of the left atrium is irrelevant to forward cardiac output.

In the control panel, the right atrium is being paced first followed by pacing of the left atrium only 40 msec later, thus mimicking the normal activation sequence between the two atria during normal sinus rhythm. Both atria were contracting normally to visual inspection. Note the hemodynamic measurements at that time. The cardiac output (minus coronary artery blood flow) was being measured continuously by means of an electromagnetic flow probe positioned around the ascending aorta. The systemic blood pressure (B.P.), the left ventricular end-diastolic pressure (LVEDP), and the pulmonary artery (P.A.) pressure were all being measured simultaneously with three separate Millar high-fidelity catheters in appropriate positions.

Once the control measurements were recorded, the LA pacing wire was suddenly disconnected without changing anything else, resulting in an electrically silent LA (middle panel) and immediate loss of all LA contraction. Note that this caused no change in any of the measured pressures or in the forward cardiac output of the heart.

The left atrial wire was then connected to a rapid atrial pacemaker to mimick a left atrial tachycardia confined to the left atrium by the left atrial isolation procedure. Again, there were no changes in any of the measured pressures or in the forward cardiac output. (*Reproduced with permission from Williams JM, Ungerleider RM, Lofland GK, Cox JL: Left atrial isolation: new technique for the treatment of supraventricular arrhythmias. J Thorac Cardiovasc Surg 1980; 80:373.*)

The Corridor Procedure

In 1985, Guiraudon described the *corridor procedure* (Fig. 53-6) for the treatment of atrial fibrillation,[13] an open heart technique that isolated a strip of atrial septum (the "corridor") harboring both the SA node and the AV node, thereby allowing the SA node to drive the ventricles. This procedure corrected the irregular heartbeat associated with atrial fibrillation, but both atria either continued to fibrillate postoperatively or developed their own asynchronous intrinsic rhythm because they were both totally isolated from the septal "corridor." In addition, both atria were also isolated from their respective ventricles, thereby precluding the possibility of atrioventricular synchrony on either side of the heart. Therefore, neither the hemodynamic compromise nor the vulnerability to thromboembolism associated with atrial fibrillation was alleviated by the corridor procedure and it was soon abandoned.

The Atrial Transsection Procedure

All three of the surgical and/or catheter techniques developed up to that time had attempted to *isolate and confine* atrial fibrillation to a certain region of the atria so that its effects on the ventricles could be minimized. It was obvious that a much better approach would be to try to *ablate* the atrial fibrillation itself and thus restore the heart's normal sinus rhythm. Using our best canine model for atrial fibrillation,[14] the first ablative surgical procedure tried was a simple incision encompassing all of the orifices of the pulmonary veins to totally isolate them from the remainder of

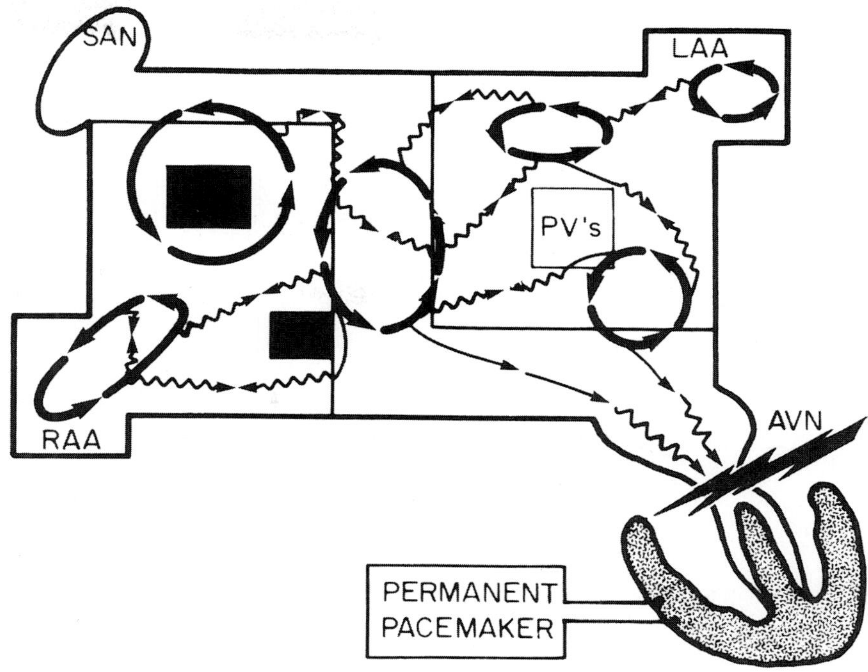

FIGURE 53–5 Catheter ablation of the AV node–His bundle complex for the treatment of atrial fibrillation simply confines the arrhythmia to the atria while dictating that a permanent ventricular pacemaker be inserted afterwards. The physiology of this procedure is the same whether the ablation is via the old fulguration technique introduced in 1981 or via the radiofrequency ablation catheters that are used today. (Same schema as in Figure 53-1.)

the heart (Fig. 53-7A).[15] Unfortunately, this incision had no effect whatsoever on the ability of the atria to fibrillate in any animal. This is particularly interesting in view of the subsequent demonstration of the importance of the pulmonary vein orifices in serving as the "initiating site" for paroxysmal atrial fibrillation.

The second series of experiments incorporated pulmonary vein isolation plus a lateral incision to the level of the mitral valve annulus and a medial incision to the interatrial septum (Fig. 53-7B). These incisions prevented the atria from fibrillating in every animal. However, once these left atrial and septal incisions were completed, the animals

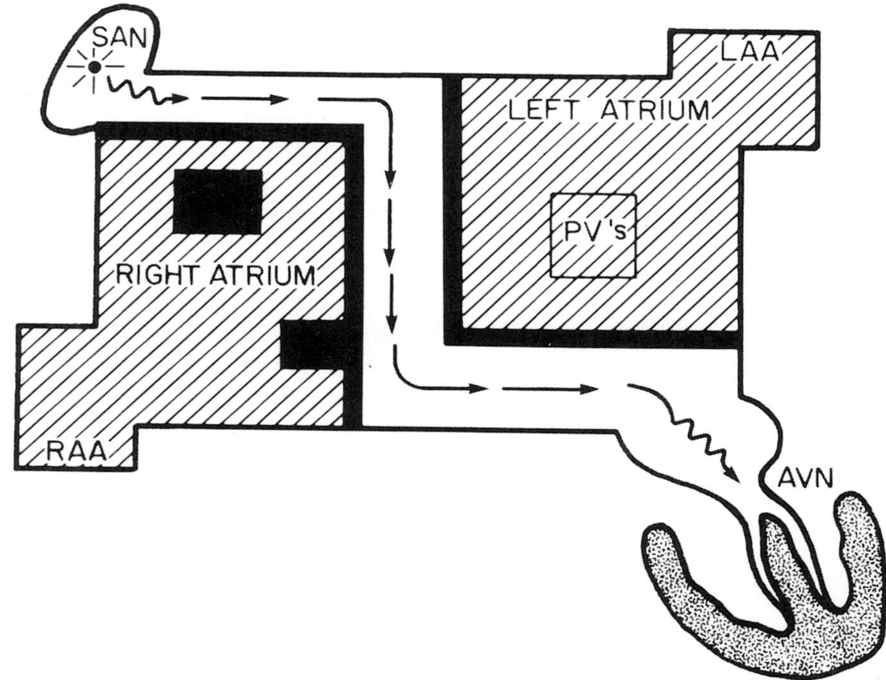

FIGURE 53–6 Guiraudon's corridor procedure resulted in the surgical isolation of both the right and left atria from their respective ventricles and allowed both to continue to fibrillate postoperatively. Since synchronous atrioventricular contraction was thereby precluded, the resultant physiology of this procedure was the same as that following catheter ablation of the His bundle and insertion of a rate-responsive pacemaker. The only potential advantage of the corridor procedure over catheter His bundle ablation was the lack of need for a permanent pacemaker. Unfortunately, a large number of these patients did in fact require permanent pacemakers postoperatively, probably because of devascularization of the sinoatrial node resulting in an iatrogenic sick sinus syndrome. Of course, the major disadvantage of the corridor procedure when comparing the two was that it was an open heart procedure. (Same schema as in Figure 53-1.)

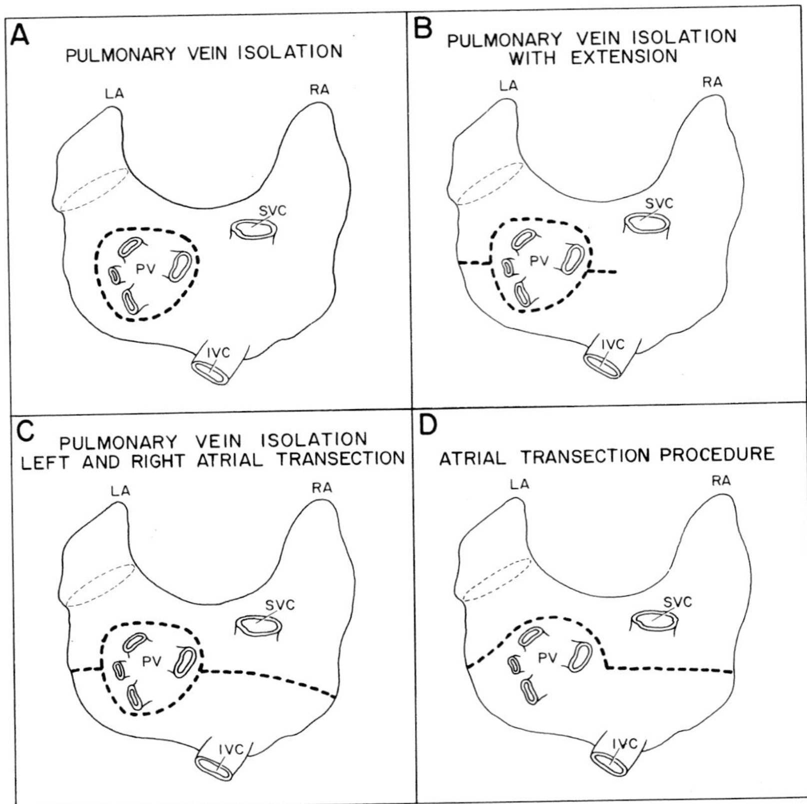

FIGURE 53–7 Various surgical procedures initially attempted in the experimental laboratory to ablate atrial fibrillation. See text for discussion. *(Reproduced with permission from Cox JL, Schuessler RB, D'Agostino HJ Jr, et al: The surgical treatment of atrial fibrillation, III: development of a definite surgical procedure. J Thorac Cardiovasc Surg 1991; 101:569.)*

immediately converted from atrial fibrillation to stable atrial flutter. Since we suspected that the atrial "flutter wave" was occurring in the right atrium, we simply extended the medial left atriotomy across the body of the left atrium between the superior vena cava (SVC) and inferior vena cava (IVC) posteriorly and down to the level of the right free-wall tricuspid valve annulus (Fig. 53-7C). We then worked backwards to see if we could eliminate a portion of the procedure and still cure atrial fibrillation in the animal model. We learned that, at least in this model, it was not necessary to encircle the pulmonary veins and therefore we were left with a single long incision across both atria and down into the septum (Fig. 53-7D). In the animal model we were employing, this so-called atrial transsection procedure invariably prevented the induction and maintenance of atrial fibrillation or atrial flutter in every animal.[15] Unfortunately, the procedure was effective but not curative in its clinical application and it became apparent that the surgical cure of atrial fibrillation would require a more complete understanding of the underlying electrophysiology of atrial fibrillation.

THE ANATOMICAL-ELECTROPHYSIOLOGICAL BASIS OF ATRIAL FIBRILLATION

Our experimental and clinical studies during the mid-1980s documented that there are three interacting components in atrial flutter and atrial fibrillation that determine the findings on the peripheral ECG and thus dictate the clinical diagnosis. These three components include: (1) macro-reentrant circuit(s), (2) passive atrial conduction in that portion of the atrium not involved in the macro-reentrant circuit, and (3) atrioventricular conduction (Figs. 53-8 and 53-9). The electrophysiological characteristics of these three components define a *spectrum* of atrial arrhythmias, extending from simple atrial flutter, through several types of transitional arrhythmias, to complex atrial fibrillation.[16]

In addition to elucidating the mechanism of atrial flutter and atrial fibrillation, these experimental and clinical electrophysiologic studies also documented that our initial hopes of obtaining computerized electrophysiological maps of atrial fibrillation and using them to guide the specific surgical technique, as we had done in other arrhythmias, was not feasible. Since the macro-reentrant circuits responsible for atrial flutter and atrial fibrillation are so fleeting in nature, it would be impossible to use activation maps to guide surgery even with on-line maps. As a result, we sought to develop a surgical technique that would be capable of interrupting *any and all* macro-reentrant circuits that might potentially develop in the atria, thereby precluding the ability of the atrium to flutter or fibrillate. In addition, it was recognized that the surgical incisions would have to be placed so that the SA node could resume activity postoperatively and "direct" the propagation of the sinus impulse throughout both atria.

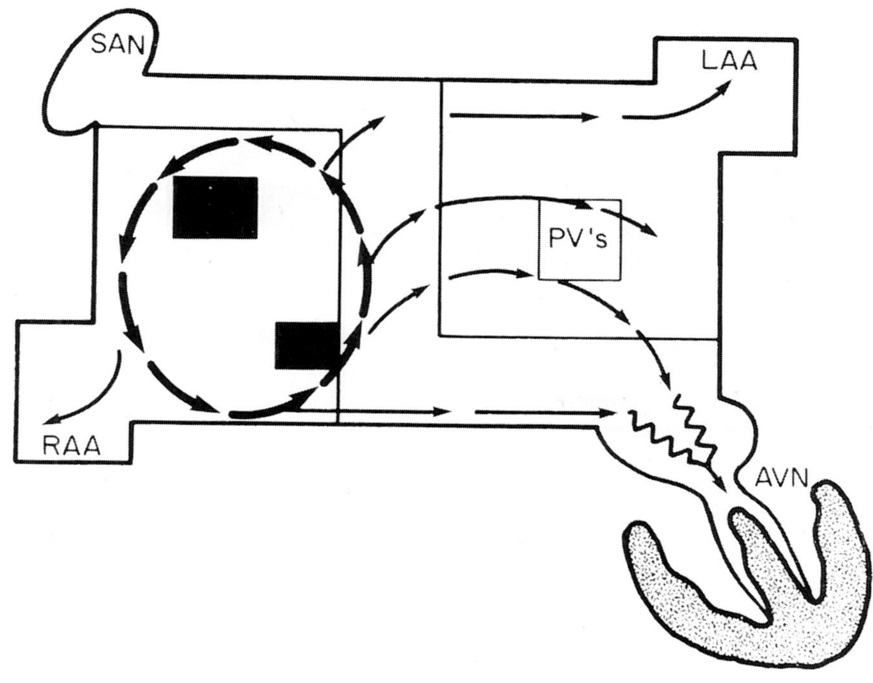

FIGURE 53–8 The three components of atrial flutter are the macro-reentrant circuit that is usually, but not always, located in the right atrium (the "flutter wave"); passive conduction to the rest of the atrial muscle; and conduction through the AV node where a 2:1 block occurs en route to the ventricles. The flutter wave drives all of the electrical activity in the heart, including both atria and both ventricles. In humans, it takes 200 msec for the electrical activity to complete one cycle around the flutter wave. This corresponds to 300 cycles per minute, which means that as long as the cycle length is stable and the passive atrial conduction is stable, both atria will beat regularly 300 times per minute. This gives rise to the "sawtooth" appearance of the P wave on the peripheral ECG during classic atrial flutter.

Because there is a 2:1 conduction block in the AV node, the ventricles are activated only 150 times per minute, but they activate in a very regular fashion in response to the consistent block of the stable atrial flutter wave. The combination of a regular P wave of 300 beats per minute and a regular ventricular response of 150 beats per minute on the standard ECG results in the clinical diagnosis of "atrial flutter." (Same schema as in Figure 53-1.) *(Reproduced with permission from Cox JL, Canavan TE, Schuessler RB, et al: The surgical treatment of atrial fibrillation, II: intraoperative electrophysiologic mapping and description of the electrophysiologic basis of atrial flutter and atrial fibrillation. J Thorac Cardiovasc Surg 1991; 101:406.)*

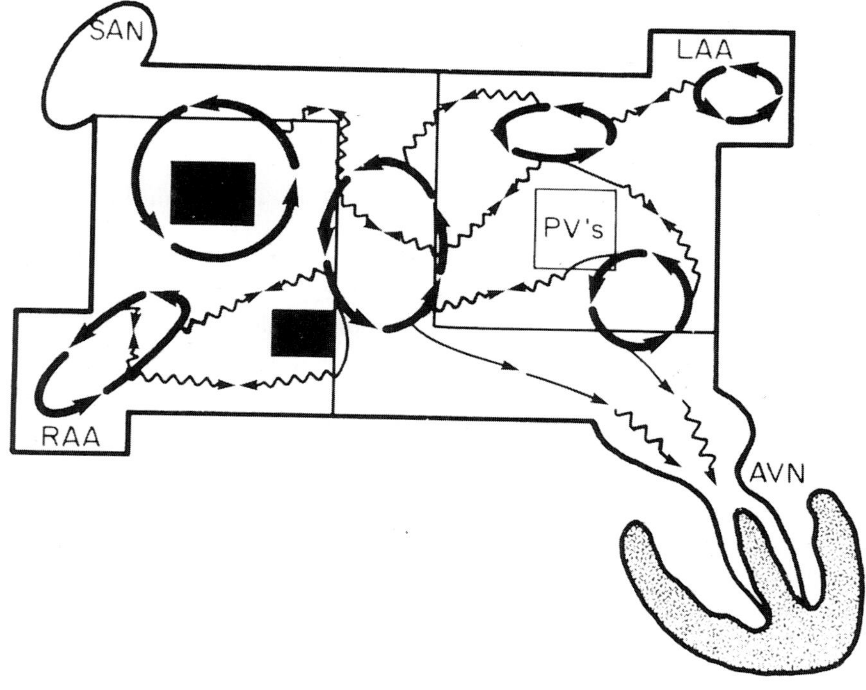

FIGURE 53–9 Atrial fibrillation may be induced by electrical stimuli in the pulmonary veins or elsewhere in the atria, or it may result from deterioration of a large atrial flutter wave. Regardless of its origin, once atrial fibrillation is established, it is characterized electrically by the presence of multiple macro-reentrant circuits in the atria. These reentrant circuits are usually smaller than the large single flutter wave that causes atrial flutter but they are still classified as macro-reentrant. Once atrial fibrillation is established, the electrical events are identical in paroxysmal (intermittent) atrial fibrillation and chronic (continuous) atrial fibrillation. (Same schema as in Figure 53-1.) *(Reproduced with permission from Cox JL, Canavan TE, Schuessler RB, et al: The surgical treatment of atrial fibrillation, II: intraoperative electrophysiologic mapping and description of the electrophysiologic basis of atrial flutter and atrial fibrillation. J Thorac Cardiovasc Surg 1991; 101:406.)*

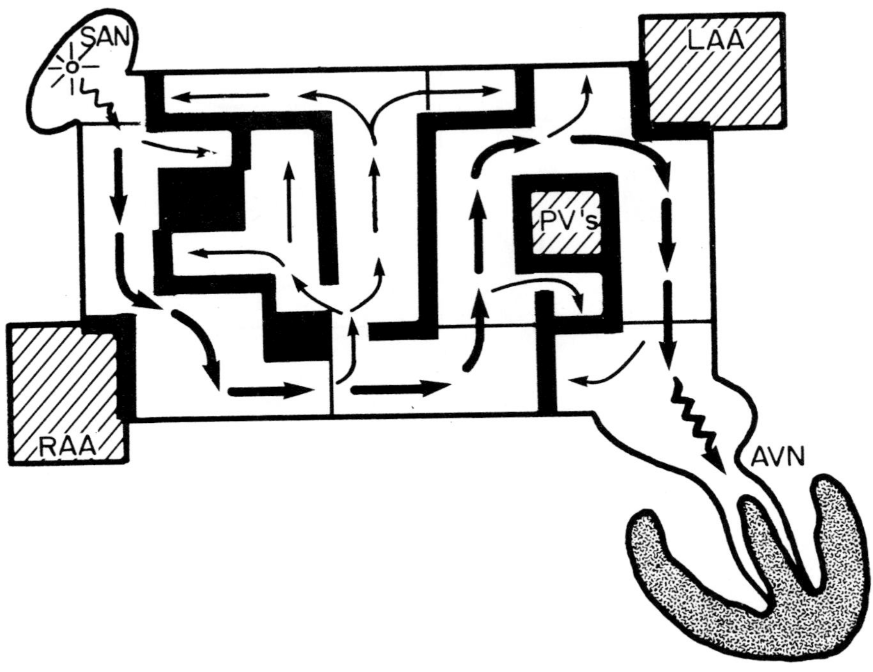

FIGURE 53–10 The Maze procedure is designed to preclude the ability of the atria to harbor any macro-reentrant circuits and therefore to preclude the ability of the atria to fibrillate. This could be accomplished by "bread-loafing" the heart, but the atria could not be activated by the SA node thereafter. Thus, the Maze procedure not only abolishes atrial fibrillation but is also designed to allow the SA node to take over atrial activation postoperatively and to allow the impulse generated in the SA node to activate all of the myocardium of both atria and then be conducted via the AV node into the ventricles. One way of accomplishing these goals is to create a set of lesions based on the concept of a maze with one site of entrance (the SA node) into the box (the atria) and one site of exit (the AV node) from the box, with one true route between the entrance and exit and multiple blind alleys along the way to provide activation to all areas of the atria. (Same schema as in Figure 53-1.) (*Reproduced with permission from Cox JL, Schuessler RB, D'Agostino HJ Jr, et al: The surgical treatment of atrial fibrillation, III: development of a definite surgical procedure. J Thorac Cardiovasc Surg 1991; 101:569.*)

This would allow all of the atrial myocardium to be activated postoperatively, resulting in preservation of atrial transport function, a prerequisite for the restoration of normal cardiac hemodynamics and the prevention of stasis of blood flow in the left atrium with the resultant potential for thromboembolism. The surgical procedure that was conceived to accomplish these goals is based on the concept of a maze[17] and, as a result, was named the "Maze procedure" (Fig. 53-10).

THE MAZE PROCEDURE

Surgical Technique

The original surgical technique, the Maze-I procedure (Fig. 53-11), [18] was modified to become the Maze-II procedure (Fig. 53-12) because of late chronotropic problems with the sinoatrial node and intra-atrial conduction delays that resulted in decreased left atrial contraction. However, the Maze-II procedure proved to be exceedingly difficult technically and as a result, it was modified again to become the Maze-III procedure (Fig. 53-13).[19,20] The Maze-III procedure soon became the surgical technique of choice for the treatment of medically refractory atrial flutter and atrial fibrillation. Most of the incisions originally performed as a part of the Maze-III procedure have been replaced by cryolesions so that the procedure can be performed by minimally invasive techniques.[21] In addition, the new minimally invasive technique avoids removal of the left atrial appendage. The orifice of the appendage is now cryoablated circumferentially and then closed from inside the left atrium.

Surgical Indications

The major indication for surgery is intolerance of the arrhythmia. In many respects, patients with paroxysmal atrial flutter/fibrillation are more symptomatic than those with chronic atrial fibrillation. Major symptoms in the paroxysmal group include dyspnea on exertion, easy fatigability, lethargy, malaise, and a general sense of impending doom during the periods of atrial flutter/fibrillation. The patients with chronic atrial fibrillation are usually better adapted to the sensation of an irregular heartbeat, but the majority of them complain of exercise limitations, dypsnea on exertion, and easy fatigability. In addition, they frequently express concern over the possibility of having a stroke. In fact, 19.5% of the patients in our series had experienced at least one episode of cerebral thromboembolism that resulted in significant temporary or permanent neurologic deficit. Finally, all patients who are considered for surgery must have failed the maximal drug therapy preoperatively.

Preoperative Electrophysiology Evaluation

For several years, a preoperative endocardial catheter electrophysiology study was required in all patients with atrial

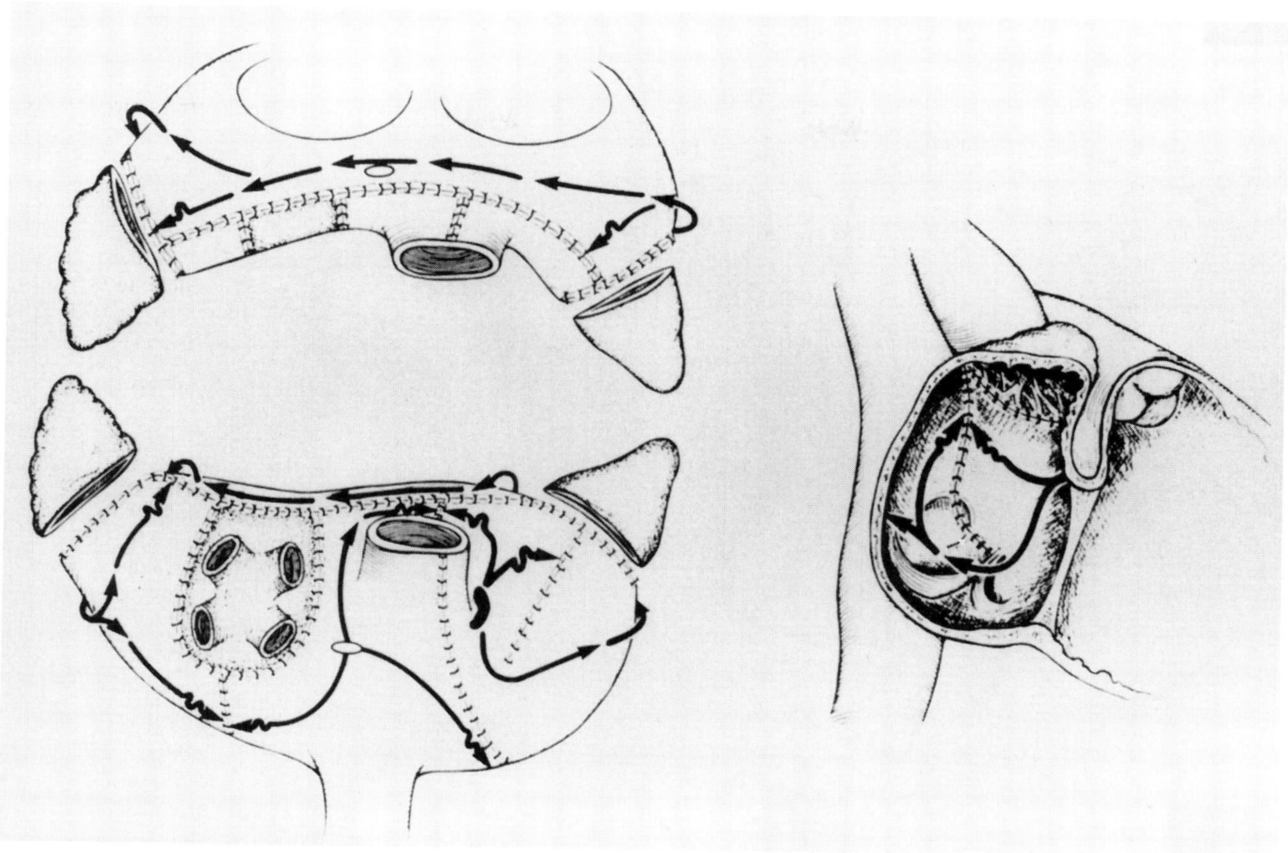

FIGURE 53–11 The Maze-I procedure. The lower left panel shows a posterior view of both atria. The left upper panel is drawn as if the atria had been cut in half with the front half flipped upwards. The incisions of the Maze-I procedure are shown and the heavy dark arrows represent the direction of propagation of a sinus beat away from the SA node following the procedure. The two atrial appendages are excised and the pulmonary veins are completely encircled.

The right panel is a cut-away view of the right atrium to show the position of the atrial septotomy and the direction of impulse propagation through the atrial septum in an anterior-to-posterior direction. Note that the septotomy is anterior to the orifice of the superior vena cava (SVC) and that there is a small atriotomy connecting the septotomy incision to the orifice of the SVC. (*Reproduced with permission from Cox JL, Jaquiss RD, Schuessler RB, Boineau JP: Modification of the Maze procedure for atrial flutter and atrial fibrillation, II: surgical technique of the Maze III procedure. J Thorac Cardiovasc Surg 1995; 110:485.*)

flutter and in patients with *paroxysmal* atrial fibrillation. The primary purpose of this study was to: (1) determine SA node function; (2) localize the site of the reentrant circuit in patients with atrial flutter; and (3) try to detect any underlying electrophysiological abnormality that might be triggering the atrial fibrillation, such as an automatic atrial focus, an accessory atrioventricular connection, or AV node reentry. These electrophysiological studies have proven to be a bit superfluous in today's environment and as a result we no longer require that a patient undergo a formal study prior to surgery. We have never thought it wise to try to perform electrophysiology studies in patients with *chronic* atrial fibrillation because the SA node cannot be evaluated without electrical cardioversion, which would introduce the risk of thromboembolism. We require all males over the age of 40 years to undergo an elective cardiac catheterization prior to surgery to rule out coronary artery disease.

Surgical Results

Between September 25, 1987, and April 16, 1992, 32 patients had the Maze-I procedure and 15 patients had the Maze-II procedure. For the reasons mentioned earlier, the Maze-III became the standard thereafter and by July 1, 2000, 308 patients had undergone the Maze-III procedure for the treatment of atrial flutter and/or atrial fibrillation.

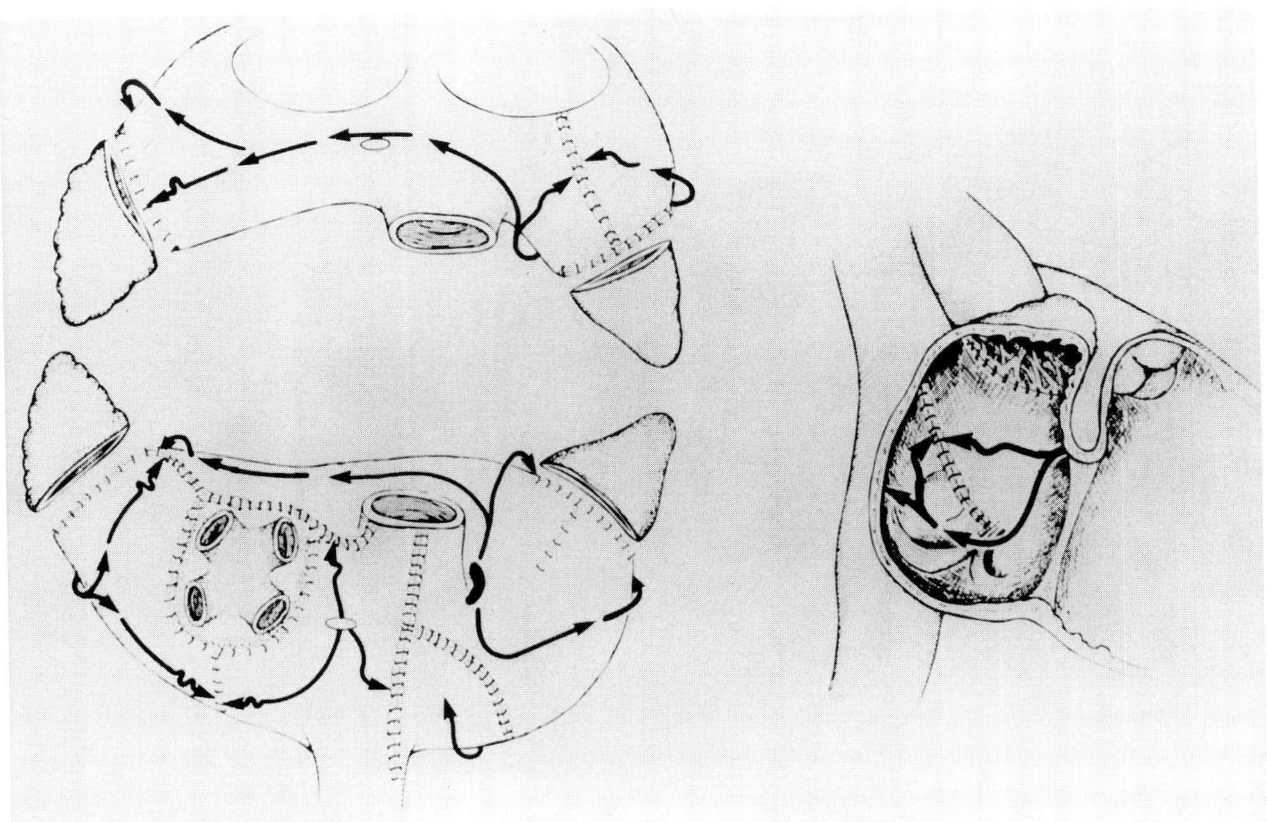

FIGURE 53–12 The Maze-II procedure. The small atriotomy located just anterior to the orifice of the SVC in the Maze-I procedure was later discovered to be traversing directly through the so-called "sinus tachycardia" region of the atrial pacemaker complex and as a result was responsible for the inability of patients to generate a normal chronotropic response to exercise or excitement following the Maze-I procedure. Moreover, the anterior location of the septotomy frequently interrupted or severely impeded interatrial conduction across the rapidly conducting Bachmann's bundle. This caused the left atrium to activate up to 150 msec after activation of the right atrium rather than the normal 40 msec. This delay in interatrial conduction resulted in the left atrium being activated nearly simultaneously with the left ventricle (AV interval of 150 msec.), i.e., when the mitral valve was closed. Thus, when this abnormal interatrial conduction delay occurred, it actually prevented the left atrium from contracting postoperatively.

For these two reasons, the culprit lesions of the Maze-I procedure were eliminated and the resultant modification is shown in this diagram. Unfortunately, the atrial septotomy in the Maze-II procedure was in the middle of the medial portion of the orifice of the SVC (right panel) and thus the left-sided exposure was limited, making the procedure extremely difficult to perform technically. As a result, it was further modified to become the Maze-III procedure. *(Reproduced with permission from Cox JL, Jaquiss RD, Schuessler RB, Boineau JP: Modification of the Maze procedure for atrial flutter and atrial fibrillation, II: surgical technique of the Maze III procedure. J Thorac Cardiovasc Surg 1995; 110:485.)*

PERIOPERATIVE RESULTS

The perioperative mortality rate (within 3 months following surgery) was 2.9% with the independent determinants of operative death being (1) preoperative congestive heart failure, (2) preoperative hypertension, and (3) performance of the Maze procedure concomitantly with a double valve replacement. The most common perioperative complication following the Maze procedure was postoperative arrhythmias, usually atrial flutter or atrial fibrillation, which occurred in 37% of patients. As described earlier, the Maze procedure was designed to interrupt the macro-reentrant circuits that must be able to form for the atria to fibrillate. The actual physical size of these circuits is determined by the duration of the refractory period at any given site in the atria (Figs. 53-14 and 53-15). Normally, atrial refractory periods

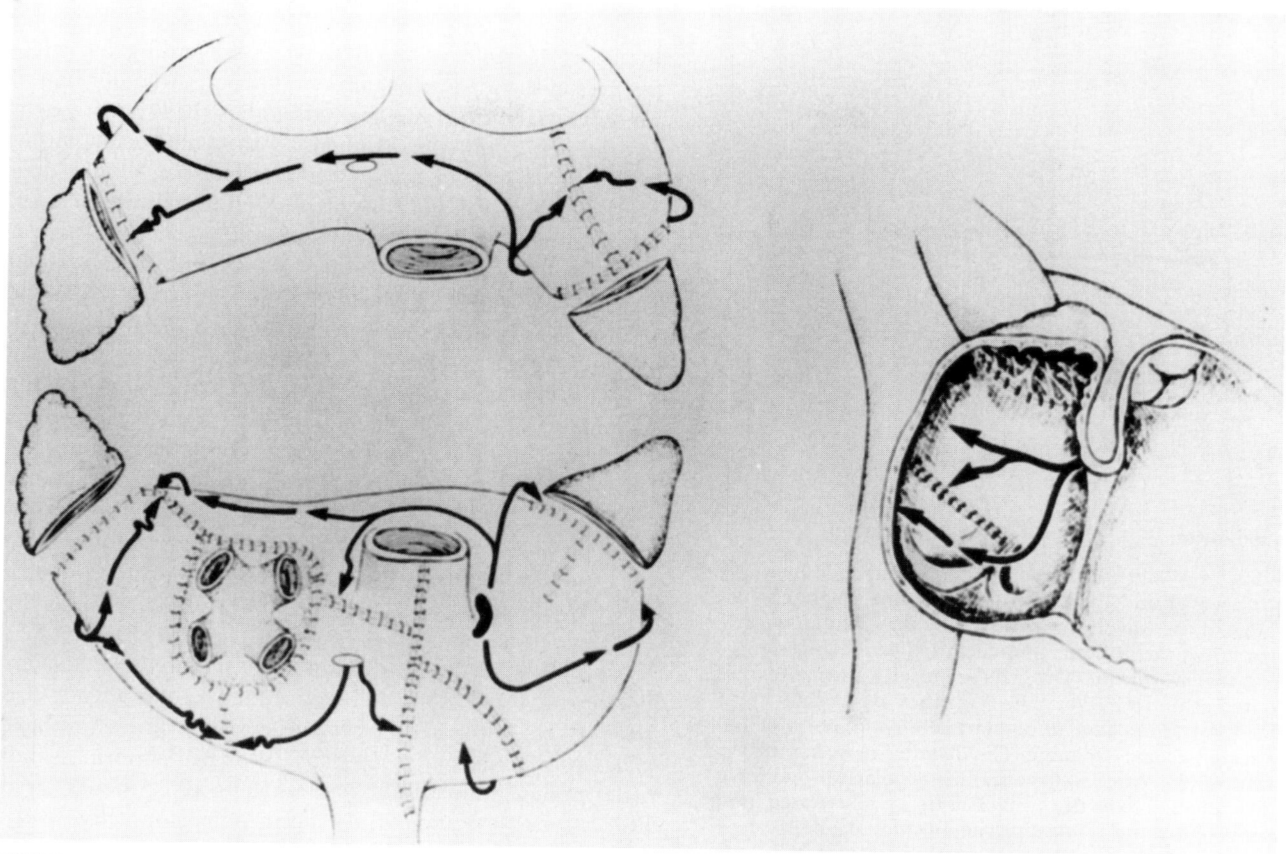

FIGURE 53–13 The Maze-III procedure. The atrial septotomy was moved to a position posterior to the orifice of the SVC without altering the concept of the Maze-II procedure. However, the Maze-III procedure is far easier to perform technically than the previous two iterations. This pattern of lesions has been used exclusively since April 1992. *(Reproduced with permission from Cox JL, Jaquiss RD, Schuessler RB, Boineau JP: Modification of the Maze procedure for atrial flutter and atrial fibrillation, II: surgical technique of the Maze III procedure. J Thorac Cardiovasc Surg 1995; 110:485.)*

are relatively long and as a result the macro-reentrant circuits are relatively large, i.e., over 6 to 7 cm in diameter. In this situation, the macro-reentrant circuits cannot form between the suture lines of the Maze procedure (Fig. 53-16A) and therefore the atrium cannot fibrillate. During the immediate postoperative period and until the atria heal from surgery, local refractory periods may be much shorter and thus the macro-reentrant circuits can be much smaller (Fig. 53-16B). As a result, it is possible to form macro-reentrant circuits between the suture lines of the Maze procedure and have postoperative atrial fibrillation even following the performance of a technically perfect operation.

Because there are critical relationships between the size of the macro-reentrant circuits, the distance between the Maze suture lines, and the effectiveness of the procedure in curing atrial fibrillation, the Maze procedure may fail when performed in extremely large atria. Since the pattern of incisions is always the same, even in the presence of normal long atrial refractory periods (and therefore of large macro-reentrant circuits), the distance between the incisions may be so great in large atria that the reentrant circuits can still form between them following the surgery. This is why the "cut-and-sew" technique is recommended for extremely large atria so that before the incisions are closed, atrial muscle can be resected to decrease the distance between the Maze suture lines.

A most gratifying result is the extremely low incidence (0.7%) of perioperative neurologic events that occur in association with performance of the Maze procedure (Fig. 53-17).[22] As noted, 20% of patients had suffered some type of significant thromboembolic event due to the atrial fibrillation preoperatively. Since these patients have early postperative atrial fibrillation as often as do other cardiac surgery patients, we believe that careful closure of the left atrial appendage during surgery most likely explains this apparent paradox.

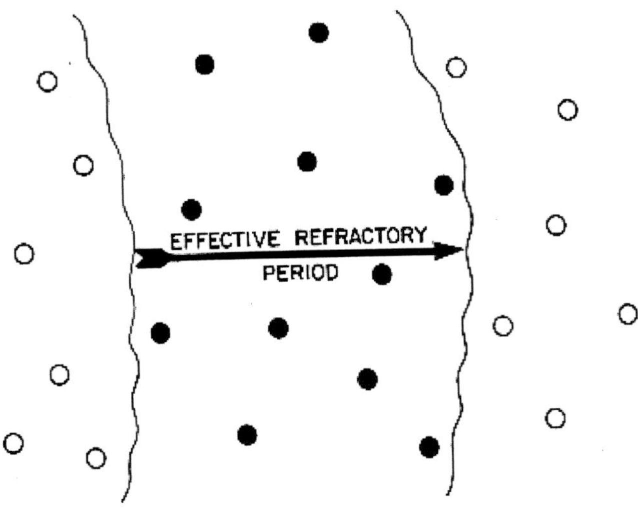

FIGURE 53–14 When atrial myocardium is activated by a propagating wavefront (from left to right in this diagram), the leading edge of the wavefront is caused by the simultaneous depolarization of the millions of myocardial cells lying along the edge of that wavefront. The cells are briefly incapable of being excited again (refractory) because they are already depolarized. A trailing edge of repolarization soon follows and the cells again become excitable. The distance between the depolarization wavefront and the trailing repolarization "wave" (sometimes referred to as the "wavelength") is illustrated as an arrow in this figure and represents the duration of the local refractory period in this region of the atrium. (*Reproduced with permission from Cox JL, Schuessler RB, Lappas DG, Boineau JP: An 8 1/2 year clinical experience with surgery for atrial fibrillation. Ann Surg 1996; 224:267.*)

LATE RESULTS

In reporting our own surgical results regarding the effectiveness of the Maze procedure in "curing" atrial fibrillation (and/or atrial flutter), we have adhered to the following definitions: *perioperative arrhythmias* are those that occur within 3 months of surgery, and *arrhythmia recurrence* is the documentation of a single episode of atrial flutter and/or atrial fibrillation more than 3 months after surgery.

Using these definitions, 98% of patients were cured of atrial fibrillation by the Maze procedure alone and half of the other 2% of patients were cured with a combination of surgery and postoperative drug therapy, an overall cure rate of 99%. Other groups that have adhered to the concept of the Maze procedure have attained similar results.[23–25] Groups that have chosen to modify the procedure by violating the basic concept of the Maze procedure have had poorer results.[26]

One of the major benefits of the Maze procedure is that it essentially abolishes the threat of stroke associated with atrial fibrillation.[27,28] The long-term stroke rate following the Maze procedure is 0.1% per year (Fig. 53-18).

Overall, 15% of our patients have required pacemakers postoperatively but virtually all of them either already had pacemakers implanted before surgery, were known to have sick sinus syndrome preoperatively, or had abnormal sinoatrial nodes "unmasked" by abolishing the patient's atrial fibrillation. Nevertheless, the need for postoperative pacemakers is higher in our own series than in most other series, probably because of the more extensive extracardiac dissection that we perform routinely in "preparing" the field

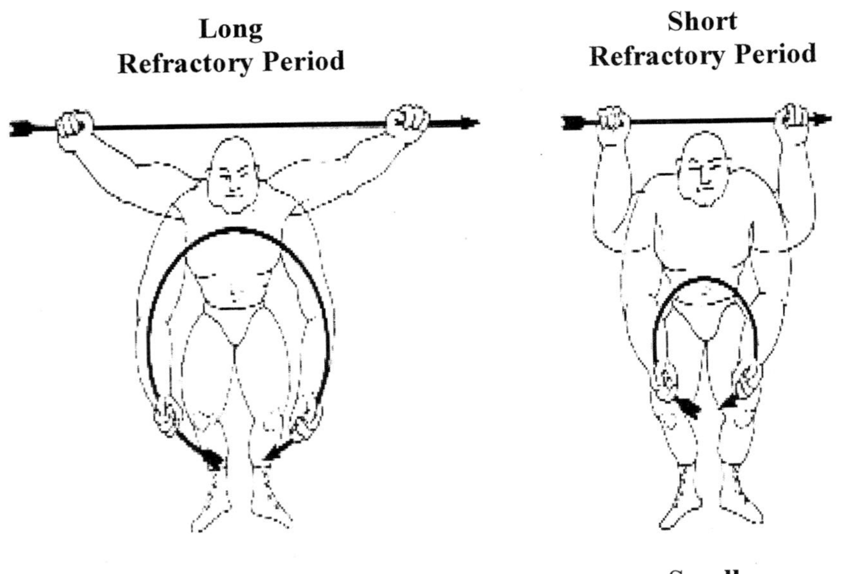

FIGURE 53–15 The length of the arrow in Figure 53-14 will determine the minimum size that a macro-reentrant circuit can be in that region of the atria. In other words, the duration of the local refractory period determines the lower limits of the size of the macro-reentrant circuit. In this illustrative diagram, if the arrow representing the duration of the local refractory period is bent so that its point almost, but not quite, touches its tail, this would represent the smallest size that a reentrant circuit can be in that region of the atrium. If the arrow is long, the reentrant circuit is large (left panel). If the arrow is shorter, the reentrant circuit can be smaller (right panel). (*Reproduced with permission from Cox JL, Schuessler RB, Lappas DG, Boineau JP: An 8 1/2 year clinical experience with surgery for atrial fibrillation. Ann Surg 1996; 224:267.*)

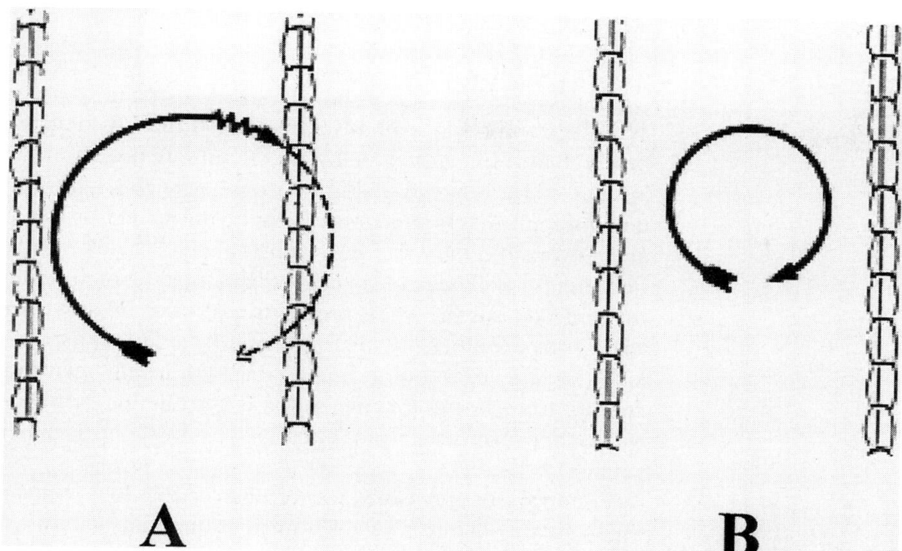

FIGURE 53–16 There is a critical relationship between the size of a local macro-reentrant circuit and the distance between the incisions (or other type of blocking lesions) of the Maze procedure. Under normal circumstances, even in diseased atria, the local refractory periods of the atria are relatively long and they are longer in the right atrium than in the left atrium. It is most fortuitous that the proximity of the incisions of the Maze procedure is such that they will prevent macro-reentry in the atrium in virtually all cases if the lesion pattern is placed correctly and if each and every lesion is transmural (A). There are two exceptions to this rule. Immediately postoperatively the refractory periods are shorter than normal for a few weeks, probably because of increased circulating catecholamines, atrial irritability, pericarditis, and other conditions associated with the surgery itself. As a result, smaller macro-reentrant circuits can form between the Maze incisions (B), a temporary phenomenon responsible for perioperative atrial fibrillation in over one third of patients having the Maze procedure. Fortunately, when the atria heal, the susceptiblility of the atria to fibrillation disappears because of the return of the refractory periods to their normal preoperative durations.

In the case of perioperative atrial fibrillation following the Maze procedure, the problem is that the reentrant circuits are too small. In extremely large atria, the Maze incisions may be too far apart to interrupt the normal-sized macro-reentrant circuits. Thus, it is absolutely essential to resect a portion of the atria when performing the Maze procedure in extremely large atria so that at the end of the procedure the size of both the right and left atria approaches normal. (*Reproduced with permission from Cox JL, Schuessler RB, Lappas DG, Boineau JP: An 8 1/2 year clinical experience with surgery for atrial fibrillation. Ann Surg 1996; 224:267.*)

for performance of the Maze procedure itself. This suspicion would seem to be confirmed by the fact that only 6% of our patients required pacemakers after undergoing the Maze procedure using minimally invasive techniques in which we perform very little extracardiac dissection.

In our series, all patients were documented to have both right atrial and left atrial transport function in the immediate postoperative period that contributed to forward cardiac output. On late follow-up evaluation, 98% of patients have continued to have right atrial transport function and 93% of patients with the Maze-III procedure have had documented left atrial function as well. Documentation of atrial transport function is difficult and for that reason we have used multiple tests in various combinations to arrive at these figures. These tests include transthoracic and transesophageal echocardiography, dynamic magnetic resonance imaging, and atrioventricular sequential pacing versus ventricular-only pacing with multiple determinations of cardiac output.

In 1996, we developed a minimally invasive Maze procedure that is performed through a 7-cm incision in the right anterior 4th intercostal space and utilizes cryosurgery rather than surgical incisions for the creation of the atrial lesions of the Maze procedure.[21] This newer, less invasive surgical approach has resulted in earlier extubation, shorter ICU stays, shorter hospitalizations, quicker recuperation and return to work, a decreased need for postoperative pacemakers (6% versus 17% following median sternotomy), and a decreased incidence of perioperative atrial fibrillation (22% versus 37% with median sternotomy).

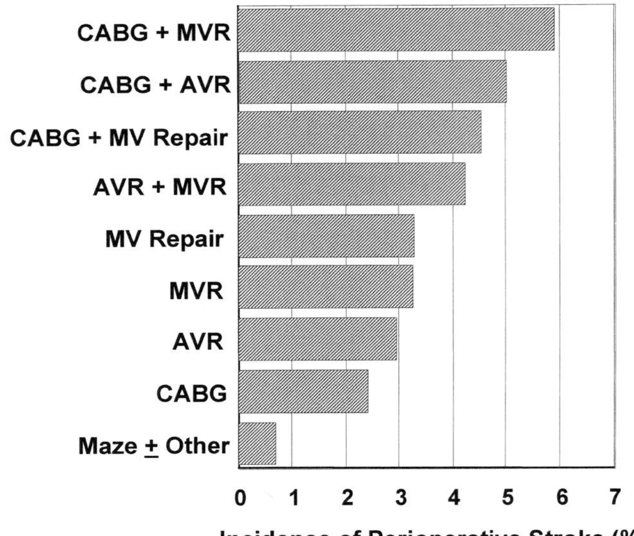

FIGURE 53–17 Relative percentages of patients undergoing cardiac surgery who experience either a minor or major cerebral thromboembolic event during the perioperative period. (CABG = coronary artery bypass grafting; MVR = mitral valve replacement; AVR = aortic valve replacement.) (Data from 1998 STS National Adult Surgery Database.)

CHANGING CONCEPTS OF THE ELECTROPHYSIOLOGY OF ATRIAL FIBRILLATION

The electrophysiology of atrial fibrillation described above, in which multiple macro-reentrant circuits are present in the atria, is relevant once atrial fibrillation has begun. Thus, the macro-reentrant circuits in the atria during atrial fibrillation are responsible only for the *maintenance* of atrial fibrillation, not for the *induction* of atrial fibrillation. Therefore, the real objective of the Maze procedure can best be described as creating atrial lesions that *preclude the ability of the atria to fibrillate* by preventing the possibility of macro-reentrant circuits from forming. The idea was that if the atria cannot harbor macro-reentrant circuits, then by definition they cannot fibrillate.

For a variety of reasons, we were never able to document the spontaneous onset of atrial fibrillation in any of our extensive experimental or clinical studies. However, in 1998, Haissaguerre et al published a seminal article documenting that atrial fibrillation is usually *induced* by stimulation from a site within the orifice of one or more of the pulmonary veins.[29] This article is at once one of the most important and yet one of the most poorly understood articles ever published in the electrophysiology literature. The findings were completely compatible with our earlier findings and in fact they completed the picture of the electrophysiology of atrial

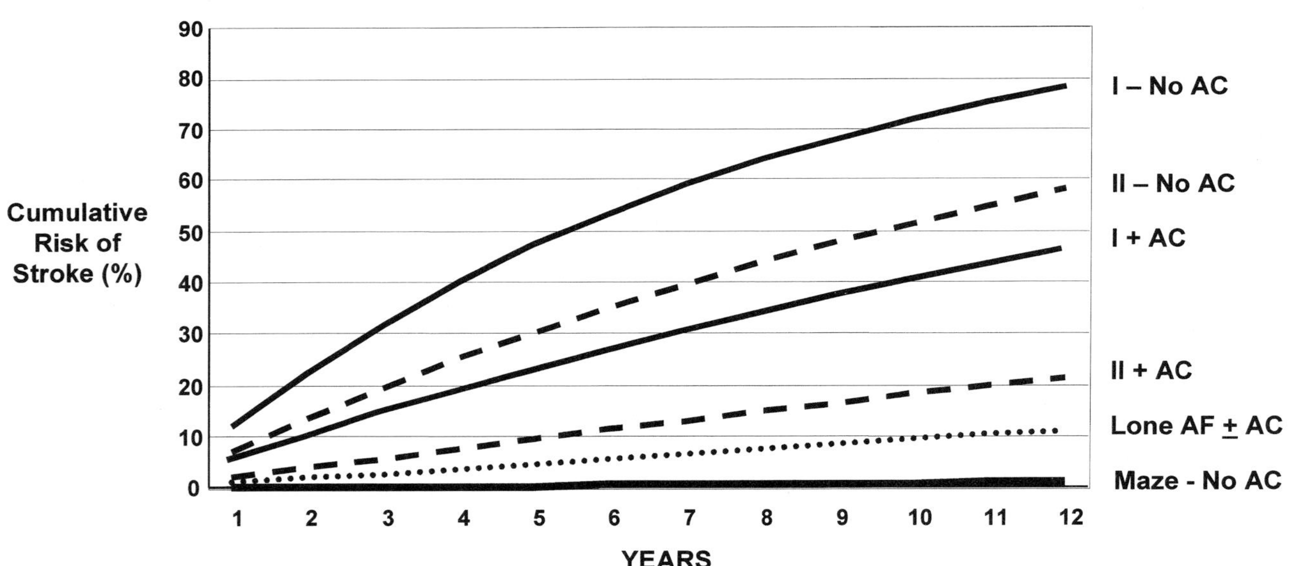

FIGURE 53–18 Group I risk factors that increase the likelihood of having a stroke and/or TIA due to atrial fibrillation include hypertension, old age, diabetes mellitus, ischemic heart disease, and congestive heart failure. (I = patients with group I risk factors plus a prior history of either a stroke or TIA due to atrial fibrillation; II = patients with group I risk factors for stroke due to atrial fibrillation; AC = anticoagulation; lone AF = atrial fibrillation in the absence of any other demonstrable heart disease.) (*Modified and reproduced with permission from Cox JL, Ad N, Palazzo T: Impact of the Maze procedure on the stroke rate in patients with atrial fibrillation. J Thorac Cardiovasc Surg 1999; 118:883.*)

fibrillation. The Hassaguirre article showed how atrial fibrillation is *induced* and our earlier work showed how atrial fibrillation is *maintained*. Unfortunately, the article was taken by many to mean that all that was needed to cure atrial fibrillation was to isolate the orifices of the pulmonary veins, a misconception that led to the development of our own first surgical procedure to ablate atrial fibrillation (see above). What resulted from the misinterpretation of this article was the development of a variety of surgical devices and procedures designed to encircle the pulmonary veins as the sole treatment for atrial fibrillation, an approach that has resulted in a predictable and unacceptable 30% failure rate.

This unfortunate misinterpretation of Hassaguirre's article ignores the fact that chronic (continuous) atrial fibrillation of 10 years duration or longer does not require any type of *induction* stimulus since the atria are always in atrial fibrillation. It also ignores the seminal work of Wijffels and Allessie, who showed that once the atria begin to fibrillate, they undergo a process of electrical "remodelling," in which the more they fibrillate, the more they will fibrillate in the future, or as those authors state, "Atrial fibrillation begets atrial fibrillation."[30,31] These established facts negate any importance of the pulmonary veins in *chronic* atrial fibrillation, which includes roughly one half of the patients who suffer from atrial fibrillation. Therefore, simple encirclement of the pulmonary veins is not a scientifically sound surgical approach to the treatment of chronic atrial fibrillation. On the other hand, pulmonary vein isolation for the treatment of paroxysmal atrial fibrillation is a reasonable procedure and can be expected to cure about 90% of patients with that specific type of atrial fibrillation. Thus, if surgeons are to treat atrial fibrillation effectively, it is extremely important that they understand the difference between the *induction* of atrial fibrillation and the *maintenance* of atrial fibrillation and the difference between *paroxysmal* (intermittent) and *chronic* (continuous) atrial fibrillation.

TECHNIQUES FOR ABLATING ATRIAL FIBRILLATION DURING MITRAL VALVE SURGERY

Following the phenomenal success of radiofrequency (RF) catheter ablation for the WPW syndrome, AV node reentry tachycardia, and other supraventricular arrhythmias in the 1990s,[32] clinical electrophysiologists began to apply it for the attempted treatment of atrial fibrillation.[33] Largely because of the availability of RF catheters and the initial reports of Hassaguirre's studies, surgeons began to use RF catheters intraoperatively in an effort to ablate atrial fibrillation in patients who were already undergoing surgery for mitral valve disease.[34] The major objective was no longer to create a Maze procedure but rather to encircle the pulmonary veins. Unfortunately, the RF lesions were frequently not transmural, thereby offering at best only a temporary barrier to electrical conduction and, in addition, pulmonary vein isolation was used in many patients with chronic atrial fibrillation. The 30% failure rate was thus predictable. Unfortunately, without really understanding the underlying electrophysiology of atrial fibrillation, several medical device companies have now developed products designed to do nothing more than encircle the pulmonary veins despite the fact that pulmonary vein encirclement, even when accomplished by completely transmural lesions, is effective in only 90% of 50% of the patients with atrial fibrillation. In actuality, pulmonary vein encirclement alone can occasionally ablate *chronic* atrial fibrillation if the isolated "cuff" of left atrium surrounding the pulmonary veins is so large that it inadvertently ablates all of the surrounding macro-reentrant circuits in the left atrium. The problem with this scenario is that so much of the left atrium is excluded by the isolated cuff that there may be not effective left atrial contraction postoperatively. Nevertheless, the overall atrial fibrillation ablation cure rate of 70% to 80% that is now being accomplished in some centers is certainly an improvement over simply ignoring the atrial fibrillation in patients undergoing mitral valve surgery as has been the practice in the past.

We continue to apply the complete Maze procedure in patients with atrial fibrillation who require mitral valve surgery, utilizing the cryosurgical rather than the "cut-and-sew" technique to avoid leaving suture lines in the posterior left atrium. The technique presently advocated adds only 20 minutes to the overall procedure and is, as it has always been, just as effective in patients with mitral valve disease as it is in patients without mitral valve or other cardiac disease.

REFERENCES

1. Savage DD, Garrison RJ, Castelli WP, et al: Prevalence of submitral (anular) calcium and its correlates in a general population-based sample (the Framingham study). *Am J Cardiol* 1983; 51: 1375.
2. Diamantopoulos EJ, Anthopoulos L, Nanas S, et al: Detection of arrhythmias in a representative sample of the Athens population. *Eur Heart J* 1987; 8(suppl D):17.
3. Onundarson PT, Thorgeirsson G, Jonmundsson E, et al: Chronic atrial fibrillation: epidemiologic features and 14 year follow-up: a case control study. *Eur Heart J* 1987; 8:521.
4. Hirosawa K, Sekiguchi M, Kasanuki H, et al: Natural history of atrial fibrillation. *Heart Vessels* 1987; 2(suppl):14.
5. Cameron A, Schwartz MJ, Kronmal RA, Kosinski AS: Prevalence and significance of atrial fibrillation in coronary artery disease (CASS Registry). *Am J Cardiol* 1988; 61:714.
6. Tammaro AE, Ronzoni D, Bonaccorso O, et al: Le aritmie nell'anziano. *Minerva Med* 1983; 74:1313.
7. Cobler JL, Williams ME, Greenland P: Thyrotoxicosis in institutionalized elderly patients with atrial fibrillation. *Arch Intern Med* 1984; 144:1758.
8. Martin A, Benbow LJ, Butrous GS, et al: Five-year follow-up of 101 elderly subjects by means of long-term ambulatory cardiac monitoring. *Eur Heart J* 1984; 5:592.
9. Treseder AS, Sastry BS, Thomas TP, et al: Atrial fibrillation and stroke in elderly hospitalized patients. *Age Aging* 1986; 15:89.

10. *Health Care Finance Administration Annual Report*, 1997.
11. Williams JM, Ungerleider RM, Lofland GK, Cox JL: Left atrial isolation: new technique for the treatment of supraventricular arrhythmias. *J Thorac Cardiovasc Surg* 1980; 80:373.
12. Scheinman MM, Morady F, Hess DS, Gonzalez R: Catheter-induced ablation of the atrioventricular junction to control refractory supraventricular arrhythmias. *JAMA* 1982; 248:851.
13. Guiraudon GM, Campbell CS, Jones DL, et al: Combined sinoatrial node atrio-ventricular node isolation: a surgical alternative to His bundle ablation in patients with atrial fibrillation. *Circulation* 1985; 72 (suppl 3):220.
14. Smith PK, Holman WL, Cox JL: Surgical treatment of supraventricular tachyarrhythmias. *Surg Clin North Am* 1985; 65:553.
15. Cox JL, Schuessler RB, D'Agostino HJ Jr, et al: The surgical treatment of atrial fibrillation, III: development of a definite surgical procedure. *J Thorac Cardiovasc Surg* 1991; 101:569.
16. Cox JL, Canavan TE, Schuessler RB, et al: The surgical treatment of atrial fibrillation, II: intraoperative electrophysiologic mapping and description of the electrophysiologic basis of atrial flutter and atrial fibrillation. *J Thorac Cardiovasc Surg* 1991; 101:406.
17. Cox JL, Schuessler RB, D'Agostino HJ Jr, et al: The surgical treatment of atrial fibrillation, III: development of a definite surgical procedure. *J Thorac Cardiovasc Surg* 1991; 101:569.
18. Cox JL: The surgical treatment of atrial fibrillation, IV: surgical technique. *J Thorac Cardiovasc Surg* 1991; 101:584.
19. Cox JL, Boineau JP, Schuessler RB, Lappas DG: Modification of the Maze procedure for atrial flutter and atrial fibrillation, I: rationale and surgical results. *J Thorac Cardiovasc Surg* 1995; 110:473.
20. Cox JL, Jaquiss RD, Schuessler RB, Boineau JP: Modification of the Maze procedure for atrial flutter and atrial fibrillation, II: surgical technique of the Maze III procedure. *J Thorac Cardiovasc Surg* 1995; 110:485.
21. Cox JL: The minimally invasive Maze-III procedure. *Oper Tech Thorac Cardiovasc Surg* 2000; 5:79.
22. Cox JL, Schuessler RB, Lappas DG, Boineau JP: An 8 1/2 year clinical experience with surgery for atrial fibrillation. *Ann Surg* 1996; 224:267.
23. McCarthy PM, Gillinov AM, Castle L, et al: The Cox-Maze procedure: the Cleveland Clinic experience. *Semin Thorac Cardiovasc Surg* 2000; 12:25.
24. Schaff HV, Dearani JA, Daly RC, et al: Cox-Maze procedure for atrial fibrillation: Mayo Clinic experience. *Semin Thorac Cardiovasc Surg* 2000; 12:30.
25. Arcidi JM, Doty DB, Millar RC: The Maze procedure: the LDS Hospital experience. *Semin Thorac Cardiovasc Surg* 2000; 12:38.
26. Kosakai Y: Treatment of atrial fibrillation using the Maze procedure: the Japanese experience. *Semin Thorac Cardiovasc Surg* 2000; 12:44.
27. Cox JL, Ad N, Palazzo T: Impact of the Maze procedure on the stroke rate in patients with atrial fibrillation. *J Thorac Cardiovasc Surg* 1999; 118:883.
28. Ad N, Cox JL: Stroke prevention as an indication for the maze procedure in the treatment of atrial fibrillation. *Semin Thorac Cardiovasc Surg* 2000; 12:56.
29. Haissaguerre M, Jais P, Shah DC, et al: Spontaneous initiation of atrial fibrillation by ectopic beats originating in the pulmonary veins. *N Engl J Med* 1998; 339:659.
30. Wifjjels MC, Kirchhof CJ, Dorland R, Allessie MA: Atrial fibrillation begets atrial fibrillation: a study in awake chronically instrumented goats. *Circulation* 1995; 92:1954.
31. Allessie MA, Dirchhof CJ, Konings KT: Unravelling the electrical mysteries of atrial fibrillation [review]. *Eur Heart J* 1996; 17(suppl C):2.
32. Jackman WM, Wang XZ, Friday KJ, et al: Catheter ablation of accessory atrioventricular pathways (Wolff-Parkinson-White syndrome) by radiofrequency current. *N Engl J Med* 1991; 324:1605.
33. Haissaguerre M, Gencel L, Fischer B, et al: Successful catheter ablation of atrial fibrillation. *J Cardiovasc Electrophysiol* 1994; 5:1045.
34. Melo J, Adragao PR, Neves J, et al: Electrosurgical treatment of atrial fibrillation with a new intraoperative radiofrequency ablation catheter. *Thorac Cardiovasc Surg* 1999; 47(suppl 3):370.

Chapter 54

Surgical Treatment of Ventricular Arrhythmias

Lynda L. Mickleborough

In the 1990s the number of patients referred for surgery for control of ventricular arrhythmias dramatically decreased. Alternative approaches gained in popularity, particularly implantable cardioverter-defibrillator (ICD) insertion and radiofrequency catheter ablation. I believe, however, that in selected patients with coronary artery disease, surgery still has an important role to play. This is particularly true in view of the recent resurgence of interest in left ventricular surgical remodelling or restoration as a potential treatment for congestive heart failure.[1] As ventricular arrhythmias are often a component of the clinical presentation in these cases, I think it is important at this time to review lessons learned from earlier experience with surgical ventricular tachycardia (VT) ablation.

In patients with ventricular arrhythmias due to coronary artery disease, ICD implantation has proven very effective for preventing sudden death. However, in such patients, electrical instability is only one manifestation of a complex problem. Other sequelae of coronary artery disease include the potential for recurrent ischemia and in many cases progressive heart failure related to poor left ventricular function and dilatation with or without mitral insufficiency. Optimal treatment in these patients would prevent further episodes of the arrhythmia, reverse ischemia, and restore left ventricular size, shape, and geometry towards normal. ICD insertion does not prevent recurrent arrhythmia episodes nor does it address ongoing ischemia or heart failure. A surgical procedure that can correct the underlying structural cardiac abnormality as much as possible may not only prevent arrhythmia recurrence but also offer additional improvements in quality of life as well as prolonged survival.

ROLE OF REVASCULARIZATION

In patients with coronary artery disease and ventricular arrhythmias, revascularization should be considered whenever possible to relieve symptoms of ischemia, to eliminate ischemia as a possible trigger for ventricular arrhythmias, and to improve prognosis.

In those with relatively good ventricular function who present with exercise-induced arrhythmias clearly associated with demonstrable ischemia, revascularization alone may be an effective treatment.[2–4] Following aortocoronary bypass grafting, repeat exercise testing and an electrophysiologic study (EPS) can be used to separate those who are noninducible and unlikely to have an arrhythmia recurrence from those still at risk in whom an ICD can be inserted as a staged procedure.

Most patients with coronary artery disease and clinical ventricular arrhythmias have dilated hearts and poor left ventricular function.[5] In these patients the arrhythmia is inducible by programmed stimulation and is due to reentry in a fixed anatomical substrate.

ANATOMICAL SUBSTRATE FOR VENTRICULAR ARRHYTHMIAS AND LESSONS LEARNED FROM MAPPING

Preoperative catheter mapping and intraoperative mapping using handheld roving electrodes or computerized multiple electrode arrays have been used to try to determine the arrhythmogenic site of origin in patients with ventricular tachycardia. Techniques involving handheld probes and sequential acquisition of data are time consuming and require a sustained monoform VT for appropriate analysis.[6,7] Endocardial mapping is performed through a ventriculotomy incision that often renders the tachycardia noninducible.[8–10] Such techniques therefore often provide incomplete mapping data, and ablation attempts relying on these data result in a higher inducibility rate at postoperative EPS and are associated with increased arrhythmias or sudden death during follow-up.[11,12]

Our group introduced a transatrial approach to mapping in the intact beating heart that has allowed us and others to obtain extensive mapping data in all patients within a relatively short period of time.[13] We used a multiple-balloon electrode array and a computer-generated flashing light display (Fig. 54-1), which demonstrates the endocardial activation sequence. Cox et al developed a different system for data analysis that allows rapid generation of serial potential distribution maps.[14] Whether the information derived is displayed as a series of color-coded isochrone maps, a real-time video light display of the activation sequence, or a dynamic color-coded potential map display is largely a matter of preference and availability.

After extensive mapping experience, three basic patterns of activation have been observed.[13] Based on our understanding of these patterns, ablation efforts have been directed not only towards the earliest site of activation, but also towards critical areas of the reentry circuit (Fig. 54-2). Results of mapping studies show that the substrate for inducible VT is usually located at the borderzone between viable myocardium and scar and corresponds to sheets of surviving muscle fibers mixed with areas of fibrosis.[15] In most cases at least part of the reentry circuit is subendocardial in location. In a small number of cases a mid myocardial circuit has been implicated.[16]

The majority of patients with coronary artery disease and poor left ventricular function who present with ventricular arrhythmias have an area of anteroapical scar (akinetic or

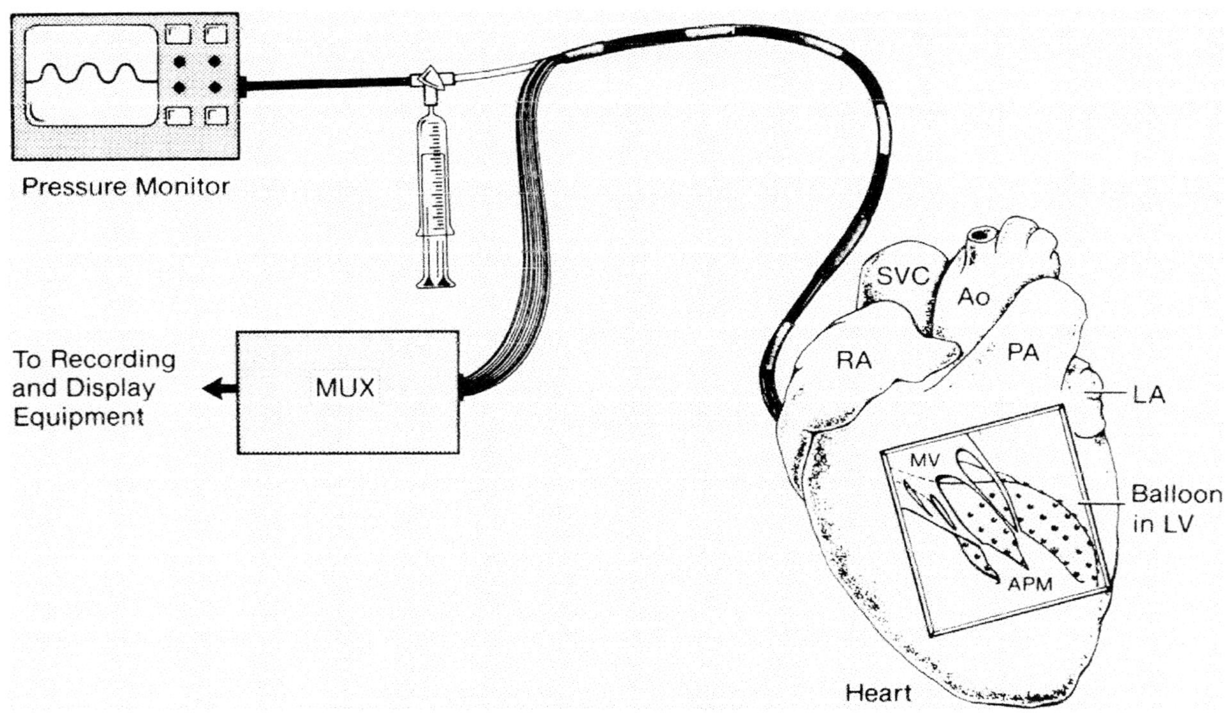

FIGURE 54–1 Diagram of transatrial approach to mapping. The balloon is inserted via a small left atrial incision and passed across the mitral valve. When positioned in the LV, it is inflated to achieve good electrode contact with the endocardium. Intraballoon pressure is monitored to prevent overinflation and possible subendocardial ischemia. (*Reproduced with permission* from Mickleborough LL: Surgery for ventricular arrhythmias following myocardial infarction, in David TE (ed): *Mechanical Complications of Myocardial Infarction*. Austin, TX, RG Landes Company, 1993; p 211.

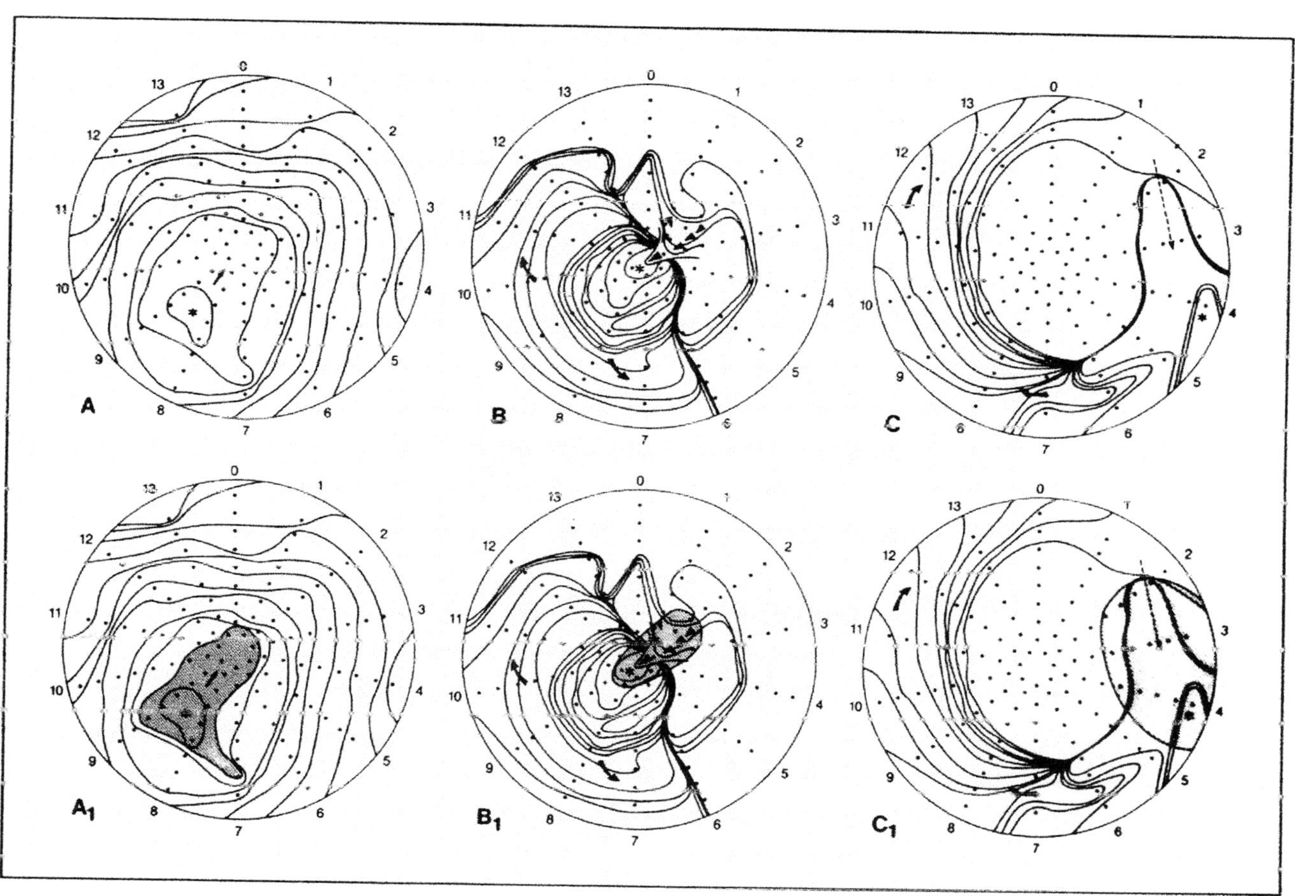

FIGURE 54–2 Patterns of activation observed with transatrial balloon mapping technique. (A) Monoregional. Endocardial activation radiates from well-defined focus indicated by asterisk. Shaded area (A1) corresponds to target area identified from video display. Surgical ablation techniques encompassed this region of interest. (B) Figure-of-8 pattern. Earliest site of endocardial activation indicated by asterisk lies to one side of two areas of block. Endocardial activity radiates in two directions around arcs of block in figure-of-8 pattern. An area of slow conduction can be identified between two areas of block that appears to lead up to site of earliest endocardial activation. We believe that this narrow corridor between two areas of block represents a reentry pathway. Target area as indicated by shading (B1) was chosen to include both presumed reentry pathway and earliest site of endocardial activity observed. (C) Circle (complete or incomplete). A large portion of myocardium is involved in sweeping circular front of activation. Earliest site of endocardial activation is indicated by asterisk. There is a spacial and temporal gap in upper right hand quadrant of circle and presumed pathway of reentry in this area is indicated by broken arrows. Shaded area (C1), which includes both presumed reentry circuit and earliest site of endocardial activation, indicates target area chosen for surgical ablation. (*Reproduced with permission from Mickleborough LL, Harris L, Downar E, et al: A new intraoperative approach for endocardial mapping of ventricular tachycardia. J Thorac Cardiovasc Surg 1988; 95:271.*)

dyskinetic), which often extends over the apex in cases of a wraparound left anterior descending (LAD) artery. In such patients mapping studies showed that the arrhythmogenic area almost always lies on the scarred septum.[11,17]

Because mapping is time consuming and requires specialized equipment and expertise, many centers have advocated a visually directed approach to VT ablation. Their approach is to resect areas of subendocardial scarring, and in cases of anteroapical infarcts such operations have been quite successful.[11,12,18,19] In less frequent cases of prior inferior myocardial infarction and a posterior aneurysm, results of VT ablation, even when guided by extensive mapping information, have been less successful.[11,20] Resection of endocardial scar and repair of the aneurysm may be hampered in this location by proximity of the posterior papillary muscle. Some centers have advocated resection and reimplantation of the papillary muscle or mitral valve replacement as a means of improving control of the arrhythmia, but such aggressive ablation procedures often result in decreased long-term survival[21] and in general results of VT surgery in cases of posterior aneurysm have been less satisfactory.

ABLATION TECHNIQUE FOR CONTROL OF VENTRICULAR TACHYCARDIA

Various techniques have been advocated for control of VT foci. All techniques involve destruction of tissue at the borderzone between scar and viable muscle and as such have potential negative effects on left ventricular structure and function. Some techniques such as encircling ventriculotomy have largely been abandoned because of their harmful effects on LV function.[22,23] In the late 1980s the most frequently used ablation techniques included endocardial excision (removal of visible endocardial scar) and cryoablation.[6,11,20,24] The depth of tissue injury achieved with cryoablation is critically dependent on the heat sink of the underlying tissue. Cryoablation using a 15-mm probe cooled to −60°C and applied for 2 minutes will result in depth of injury of only 2 to 3 mm in a well-perfused area of the heart but could result in much more extensive injury (6 mm or more) if applied in the heart under cold cardioplegia conditions. Other techniques for ablation that have been used at the time of surgery to control VT include direct shock ablation,[24] laser photoablation, or radiofrequency ablation.[25] In general, the more extensive the ablation procedure carried out, the less likely it is that inducible arrhythmias will appear on the postoperative EPS, but the more chance there is to have a negative effect on LV function or to damage surrounding structures including the papillary muscle apparatus. Such deleterious effects of the ablation procedure may have a negative effect on long-term survival.[26]

LEFT VENTRICULAR RECONSTRUCTION

In patients with coronary artery disease, ventricular arrhythmias, and poor left ventricular function, an important part of the surgical approach is to address poor LV function and associated mitral insufficiency in addition to revascularization and ablation of the arrhythmogenic focus. Following VT ablation in patients with akinetic or dyskinetic scar, LV reconstruction or remodelling should be undertaken to restore LV size and geometry towards normal.[24] We have advocated use of a modified linear closure technique that can be combined with septoplasty when there is significant aneurysmal involvement of the septum or when the septum has been thinned following extensive endocardial excision for control of VT.[27] Dor has popularized his approach utilizing an endoventricular patch plasty.[28] Both techniques have been associated with excellent results. The aim is to resect or exclude all nonfunctioning portions of the ventricle, thereby restoring ventricular cavity size and shape towards normal as much as possible. Potential benefits include decreased wall stress and decreased oxygen consumption in the surrounding myocardium as well as potential improvements in fiber orientation that may result in increased contractility.[27] Mechanical unloading with decreased stretch of remote ventricular wall may also help prevent recurrent arrhythmias.[29] Mitral regurgitation (MR) may be improved by LV remodelling, but intraoperative transesophageal echocardiography should be used to rule out residual MR for which additional valvuloplasty procedures may be indicated.

RESULTS OF SURGERY FOR VENTRICULAR ARRHYTHMIAS: COMPARISON WITH OTHER TREATMENT MODALITIES

In the 1980s results of surgery for control of ventricular tachycardia improved over time as experience was accumulated with various mapping and ablation techniques. Clearly, results achieved with respect to operative mortality, control of VT, and long-term survival will depend on many factors including patient selection, accuracy of mapping data if used, and type and extent of ablation technique employed. Most reported surgical series for control of VT include patients at high risk, i.e., those with extensive coronary artery disease, poor preoperative ejection fraction, and symptoms of congestive heart failure. By the late 1980s, average ejection fraction in most reported series ranged from 25% to 30%.[6,7,11,24] Operative mortality with map-directed or visually directed surgery was in the range of 2% to 10%.[7,11,24] Patients with a positive postoperative EPS were generally treated with either amiodarone or an ICD. Recurrence of clinical arrhythmias was low, ranging from 10% to 20%, and freedom from sudden death during follow-up was usually over 90%.[6,7,11,24] Long-term survival at 5 years was in the range of 70% to 80%. Factors associated with increased risk of surgery for control of VT included advanced age, decreased ejection fraction, and severe symptoms of congestive heart failure.[11,24,30–32] Decreased success of surgical VT ablation was reported in patients with an inferior infarct.[11] These results will be compared to results obtained with other treatment modalities.

Catheter ablation has been reported to successfully ablate the target VT in 82% of cases.[33] The procedural mortality is low (1.8%), but there is an 8% chance of major complications including stroke, transient ischemia attack, or tamponade.[34] Perhaps more importantly, when used in a patient population with a mean ejection fraction of 32% ± 11%, the 5-year survival following catheter ablation was only 49% with the recurrence rate of VT at 4 years of 72%.[33] Clearly, the results of catheter ablation are inferior to those achieved with surgical ablation in patients with coronary artery disease and poor LV function.

Thousands of ICDs have been employed in patients with coronary artery disease and ventricular arrhythmias. Most patients with an ICD do receive shocks, and if shocks are frequent they have a definite negative effect on quality of life.[35] It has recently been established in large randomized prospective trials in patients with prior VT or VF arrest (secondary prevention trials) that ICD treatment is superior to drug therapy including amiodarone with respect to prevention of sudden death and improving overall survival.[33] In these studies, survival benefit due to ICD increased with increasing patient risk, i.e., increasing age, decreasing ejection fraction, and increasing symptoms of heart failure. In the Antiarrhythmics Versus Implantable Defibrillators (AVID) series, the Canadian Implantable Defibrillator Study (CIDS) series, and the Cardiac Arrhythmic Suppression Trial (CAST) series, the mean ejection fraction was 30% to 45% and the average annual death rate ranged between 8% and 12%.[36,37] If the results in patients with an ejection fraction of less than 35%, which are comparable to surgical VT series, are analyzed, the 5-year survival rate was only 60%.[38] In the AVID registry the 3-year survival in patients with an ejection fraction less than 25% was only 55%.[39] Clearly, in patients with previous documented clinical ventricular arrhythmias and decreased ejection fraction, the 5-year survival following ICD implantation is less than that reported in patients with similar ejection fractions following surgical ablation for VT.

CURRENT RECOMMENDATIONS

Based on past experience and results reported with VT ablation surgery, we would currently recommend revascularization in patients with coronary artery disease, poor left ventricular function, and ventricular arrhythmias, if there is an area of anteroapical scarring (akinesis or dyskinesis) with no significant thinning of the wall.[40] If arrhythmias recur or are still inducible postoperatively, the patient should be treated with amiodarone or considered for an ICD.

We would recommend left ventricular remodelling in patients with coronary artery disease, poor left ventricular function, and ventricular arrhythmias, if the area of anteroapical scarring (akinesis or dyskinesis) corresponds to a region of significant thinning. At the time of surgery, the septum should be examined for scarring. We would recommend excision of all visible endocardial septal scar with cryoablation at the periphery of the excision as the strategy for control of VT.[27] A postoperative electrophysiologic study should be performed. If ventricular arrhythmias are still inducible, amiodarone therapy should be instituted. In our experience with this approach, ventricular arrhythmias have rarely been a problem during long-term follow-up and ICD use in our series has been low.[27] Further studies are needed to confirm effectiveness of this approach in patients with poor left ventricular function and dilated hearts. In such patients we believe symptoms of congestive heart failure, mitral insufficiency, and ventricular arrhythmias are all markers of advanced ischemic disease. Surgery should be undertaken early before progressive dilatation and adverse ventricular remodelling result, leaving transplantation as the only reasonable option.

REFERENCES

1. Cox JL: Ventricular shape and function in health and disease. *Semin Thorac Cardiovasc Surg* 2001; 13:297.
2. Berntsen RF, Gunnes P, Lie M, Rasmussen K: Surgical revascularization in the treatment of ventricular tachycardia and fibrillation exposed by exercise-induced ischemia. *Eur Heart J* 1993; 14:1297.
3. Lee JF, Folsom DL, Biblo LA, et al: Combined internal cardioverter-defibrillator implantation and myocardial revascularization for ischemic ventricular arrhythmias: optimal cost-effective strategy. *Cardiovasc Surg* 1995; 3:393.
4. Manolis AS, Rastegar H, Estes NAM: Effects of coronary artery bypass grafting on ventricular arrhythmias: results with electrophysiologic testing and long-term followup. *Pacing Clin Electrophysiol* 1993; 16:984.
5. Kleiman RB, Miller JM, Buxton AE, et al: Prognosis following sustained ventricular tachycardia occurring early after myocardial infarction. *Am J Cardiol* 1988; 62:528.
6. Geha AS, Elefteriades JA, Hsu J, Biblo L, et al: Strategies in the surgical treatment of malignant ventricular arrhythmias: an 8 year experience. *Ann Surg* 1992; 216:309.
7. Ostermeyer J, Borgraf M, Brighthart G, et al: Direct operations for the management of life-threatening ischemic ventricular tachycardia. *J Thorac Cardiovasc Surg* 1987; 94:848.
8. Krafchek J, Lawrie GM, Roberts R, et al: Surgical ablation of ventricular tachycardia: improved results with a map-directed regional approach. *Circulation* 1986; 73:1239.
9. DiMarco JP, Lerman BB, Kron IL, et al: Sustained ventricular tachyarrhythmias within two months of acute myocardial infarction: results of medical and surgical therapy in patients resuscitated from the initial episode. *J Am Coll Cardiol* 1985; 6:759.
10. Bolooki H, Palatianos GM, Zaman L, et al: Surgical management of postmyocardial infarction ventricular tachyarrhythmia by myocardial debulking, septal isolation and myocardial revascularization. *J Thorac Cardiovasc Surg* 1986; 92:716.
11. Lee R, Mitchell JD, Garan H, et al: Operation for recurrent ventricular tachycardia: predictors of short and long-term efficacy. *J Thorac Cardiovasc Surg* 1994; 107:732.
12. Fieguth HG, Trapp HG, Wallers T, et al: Surgical intervention in ischemic ventricular tachyarrhythmias: endocardial resection or implanted cardioverter-defibrillator. *Eur J Cardiothorac Surg* 1994; 8:400.
13. Mickleborough LL, Harris L, Downar, E et al: A new intraoperative approach for endocardial mapping of ventricular tachycardia. *J Thorac Cardiovasc Surg* 1988; 95:271.
14. Rokkas CK, Nittas T, Schuessler RB, et al: Human ventricular tachycardia: precise intraoperative localization with potential distribution mapping. *Ann Thorac Surg* 1994; 57:1628.
15. Downar E, Mickleborough LL, Harris L, Parson I: Endocardial mapping of ventricular tachycardia in the intact human ventricle: evidence for reentrant mechanisms. *J Am Coll Cardiol* 1988; 11:783.
16. Page PL, Cardinal R, Shenasa M, et al: Surgical treatment of ventricular tachycardia: regional cryoablation guided by computerized epicardial and endocardial mapping. *Circulation* 1989; 80 (suppl I):I124.
17. Mickleborough LL: Surgical management of left ventricular aneurysms. *Semin Thorac Cardiovasc Surg* 1995; 7:233.

18. Moran JM, Kehoe RF, Loeb JM, et al: Extended endocardial resection for the treatment of ventricular tachycardia and ventricular fibrillation. *Ann Thorac Surg* 1982; 34:538.
19. Landymore RW, Gardner MA, McIntyre AJ, Barker RA: Surgical intervention for drug-resistant ventricular tachycardia. *J Am Coll Cardiol* 1990; 16:37.
20. Hargrove WC, Miller JM, Vassallo JA, Josephson ME: Improved results in the operative management of ventricular tachycardia related to inferior wall infarction: importance of the annular isthmus. *J Thorac Cardiovasc Surg* 1986; 92:726.
21. Kron IL, DiMarco JP, Lerman BB, Nolan SP: Resection of scarred papillary muscles improves outcome after surgery for ventricular tachycardia. *Ann Surg* 1986; 203:685.
22. Guirudon G, Fontaine G, Frank R, et al: Encircling endocardial ventriculotomy: a new surgical treatment for life-threatening ventricular tachycardia resistant to medical treatment following myocardial infarction. *Ann Thorac Surg* 1978; 26:438.
23. Ungerleider RM, Holman WL, Calcagno D, et al: Encircling endocardial ventriculotomy for refactory ischemic ventricular tachycardia, III: effects on regional left ventricular function. *J Thorac Cardiovasc Surg* 1982; 83:857.
24. Mickleborough LL, Mizuno S, Downar E, Gray GC: Late results of operation for ventricular tachycardia. *Ann Thorac Surg* 1992; 54:832.
25. Selle JG, Svenson RH, Sealy WC, et al: Successful clinical laser ablation of ventricular tachycardia: a promising new therapeutic method. *Ann Thorac Surg* 1986; 42:380.
26. Frapier JM, Hubaut JJ, Pasquie JL, Chaptal PA: Large encircling cryoablation without mapping for ventricular tachycardia after anterior myocardial infarction: long-term outcome. *J Thorac Cardiovasc Surg* 1998; 116:578.
27. Mickleborough LL, Carson S, Ivanov J: Repair of dyskinetic or akinetic left ventricular aneurysm: results obtained with a modified linear closure. *J Thorac Cardiovasc Surg* 2001; 121:675.
28. Dor V, Saab M, Costa P, et al: Left ventricular aneurysm: a new surgical approach. *J Thorac Cardiovasc Surg* 1989; 37:11.
29. Franz MR, Cima R, Wang D, et al: Electrophysiological effects of myocardial stretch and mechanical determinants of stretch-activated arrhythmias. *Circulation* 1992; 86:968.
30. Bakker PFA, de Lange F, Hauer RNW, et al: Sequential map-guided endocardial resection for ventricular tachycardia improves outcome. *Eur J Cardiothorac Surg* 2001; 19:448.
31. Van Hemel NM, Kingma JH, Defauw JAM, Vermeulen FEE: Left ventricular wall motion score as a criterion for selecting patients for direct surgery in the treatment of post-infarction ventricular tachycardia. *Eur Heart J* 1989; 10:304.
32. Nath S, Haines DE, Kron IL, et al: Regional wall motion analysis predicts survival and functional outcome after subendocardial resection in patients with prior anterior myocardial infarction. *Circulation* 1993; 88:70.
33. O'Callaghan PA, Poloniecki J, Sosa-Suarez G, et al: Long-term clinical outcome of patients with prior myocardial infarction after palliative radiofrequency catheter ablation for frequent ventricular tachycardia. *Am J Cardiol* 2001; 87:975.
34. Hindricks G: The Multicentre European Radiofrequency Survey (MERFS): complications of radiofrequency catheter ablation of arrhythmias. The Multicentre European Radiofrequency Survey (MERFS) investigators of the Working Group on Arrhythmias of the European Society of Cardiology. *Eur Heart J* 1993; 14:1644.
35. Heller SS, Ormont MA, Lidagoster LC, et al: Psychosocial outcomes after ICD implantation: a current perspective. *Pacing Clin Electrophysiol* 1998; 127:978.
36. Sheldon R, Connolly S, Krahn A, et al: Identification of patients most likely to benefit from implantable cardioverter-defibrillator therapy: the Canadian implantable defibrillator study. *Circulation* 2000; 101:1660.
37. Sweeney MO, Ellison KE, Stevenson WG: Implantable cardioverter defibrillators in heart failure. *Cardiol Clin* 2001; 19:653.
38. Steinberg JS, Martins J, Safanandan S, et al: Antiarrhythmic drug use in the implantable defibrillator arm of the antiarrhythmics versus implantable defibrillators (AVID) study. *Am Heart J* 2001; 142:520.
39. Pinkski SL, Yao, Q, Epstein AE, et al: Determinants of outcome in patients with sustained ventricular tachyarrhythmias: the antiarrhythmics versus implantable defibrillators (AVID) study registry. *Am Heart J* 2000; 139:804.
40. Mickleborough LL, Carson S, Tamariz M, Ivanov J: Results of revascularization in patients with severe left ventricular dysfunction. *J Thorac Cardiovasc Surg* 2000; 119:550.

Chapter 55

Pacemakers and Automatic Defibrillators

Henry M. Spotnitz

Pacemaker and defibrillator management is increasingly complex and is the subject of comprehensive reviews.[1–3] A review of 2760 procedures at the Columbia-Presbyterian campus of New York Presbyterian Hospital revealed that 23% of pacemaker recipients and 5% of ICD recipients were octogenarians. The 80- to 90-year age group accounted for 22% of pacemaker generator replacements and 5% of ICD generator replacements. The incidence of pacemaker insertion in patients older than 75 was 2.6% in a recent survey of noninstitutionalized adults. Pacemaker efficacy and cost-effectiveness in the elderly are widely accepted,[4] but the appropriate role for ICD insertion in older patients is still evolving. Application of pacemaker and ICD technology is now feasible across the entire span of human age, and the spectrum of technology application continues to expand into pacing for heart failure and prophylactic applications of ICDs. Although arrhythmia control devices are increasingly the purview of the electrophysiologist, thoracic surgeons will continue to play an important role both as implanters and as a court of last resort for complex or complicated cases. This chapter is intended to provide an overview of practical information related to pacemaker and ICD insertion and management.

ANATOMY OF SURGICAL HEART BLOCK

The conduction system is vulnerable to injury during heart surgery. Complete heart block can occur as a result of suture placement during aortic, mitral, or tricuspid valve surgery, during closure of septal defects, or during myotomy for idiopathic hypertrophic subaortic stenosis (IHSS). The sites of these lesions are indicated schematically in Figure 55-1. Occlusion of the blood supply to the conduction system or incomplete myocardial protection can also result in surgical heart block.

PACEMAKERS

History

The early history of cardiac surgery was complicated by iatrogenic heart block, which was lethal. Transthoracic pacing was implemented with Zoll cutaneous electrodes.[5] Percutaneous endocardial pacing was described in 1959.[6] A "permanent" pacemaker using epicardial electrodes was described in 1960.[7] Pacemakers and implantation techniques have progressed rapidly since the 1960s, reflecting advances in bioengineering and technology. Persistent problems include lead durability, chronic inflammatory responses to pacemaker materials, infection, device size, programmer compatibility, and expense.

Device Description

A "permanent pacemaker" consists of pacing leads[8] and a pacemaker generator. The generator contains a battery, a telemetry antenna, and integrated circuits. The power source is generally lithium iodide, but rechargeable and nuclear batteries have been used. The integrated circuits include programmable microprocessors, oscillators, amplifiers, and sensing circuits.[9] The integrated circuits employ complementary metallic oxide semiconductor (CMOS) technology, which is subject to damage by ionizing radiation.[10] Current pacemakers store and can telemeter their internal status, the condition of their external connections, their programmed settings, and recent activity. Unfortunately, each device responds only to its own manufacturer's programmer.

International Pacemaker Code

The five-letter code in Table 55-1 describes pacemaker function.[11] Three letters are in common usage. The first letter is the chamber paced, and the second is the chamber sensed. The third letter describes the algorithm used to integrate pacing and sensing functions. Thus, fixed-rate ventricular and atrial pacemakers are VOO and AOO, respectively. Demand (rate-inhibited) pacers for the same chambers would be VVI and AAI. VDD refers to a pacemaker that paces the ventricle only but senses both the atrium and the ventricle.[12] DVI pacemakers involve atrial and ventricular pacing but

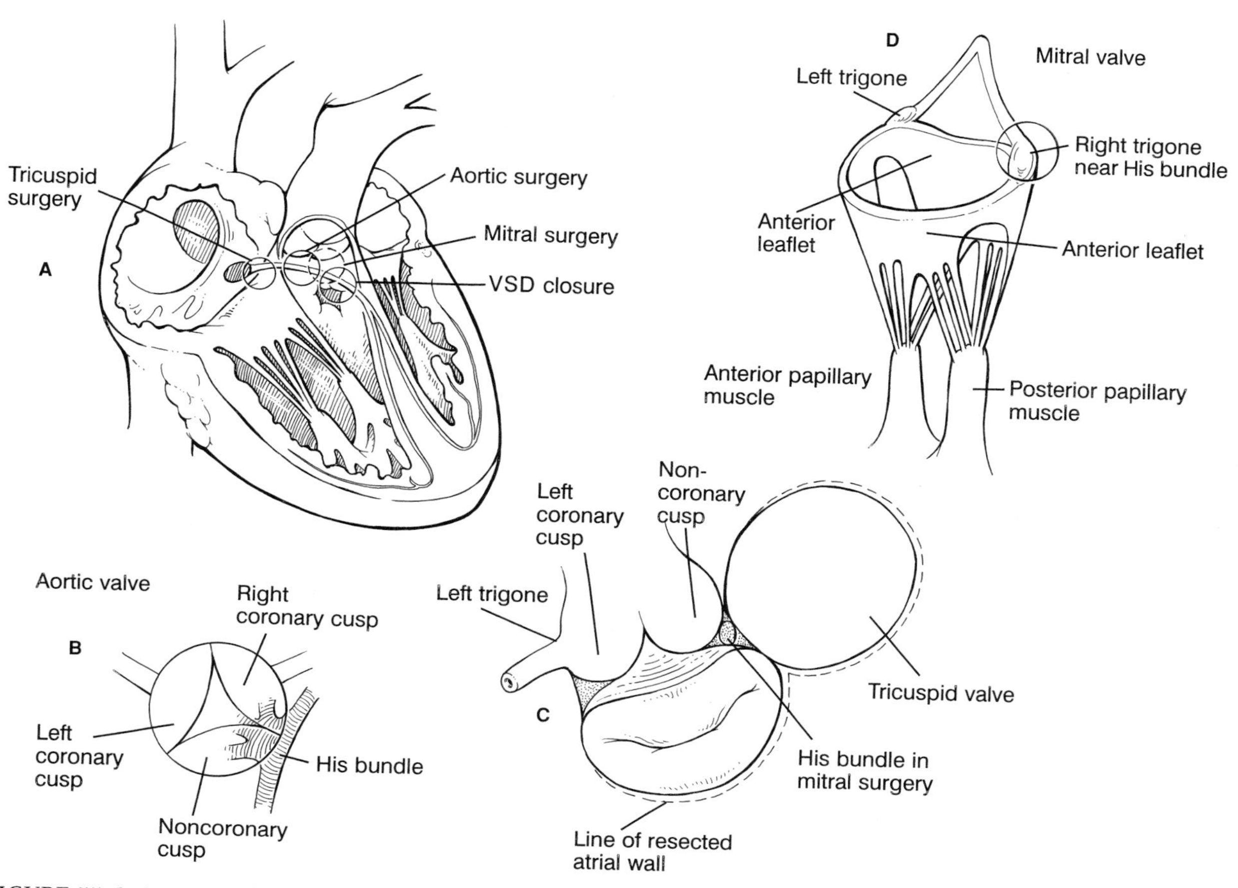

FIGURE 55–1 Anatomy of iatrogenic complete heart block. (A) The location of the His bundle and nearby cardiac structures is illustrated. Common sites of injury are indicated. (B) The His bundle lies within the ventricular septum, just below the commissure between the noncoronary and right coronary aortic cusps. (C) During mitral valve surgery, the His bundle is on the ventricular septum anteromedial to the posterior commissure and right fibrous trigone (see D).

only ventricular sensing. DDD is the most flexible of current designs.

Cellular Electrophysiology

Cellular membrane depolarization and repolarization provide a mechanism for automaticity of the cardiac chambers and the conduction system. In the resting state, the outer surface of the cell is positive, and the interior of the cell is negative. Applying a negative current to the outside of the cell theoretically produces a greater potential difference and would be expected to be more successful in depolarizing the cell than a positive current. Empirically, this is correct—unipolar pacing thresholds are lowest when the negative terminal (cathode) of a pacing system is connected to the heart and the positive terminal (anode) is connected to ground.[13] Electrogram amplitude is not substantially affected by polarity.

TABLE 55–1 International pacemaker code

I, chamber paced	II, chamber sensed	III, pacing algorithm
A	A	T
V	V	I
D	D	D
O	O	O
S	S	–

A = Atrium
V = Ventricle
D = Dual (both of the above)
O = None
S = Single

T = Triggered
I = Inhibited
D = Dual (both of the above)

Rhythm Disorders

INDICATIONS FOR PACEMAKER INSERTION

Concern about indiscriminate referral for pacemaker insertion led to Medicare guidelines (Table 55-2). Supporting documentation may be required for billing. Medicare divides indications into three categories: justified, never justified, and possibly justified. Symptomatic third-degree heart block

TABLE 55–2 Medicare guidelines for cardiac pacemaker implantation

Accepted, in symptomatic patients with chronic conditions
- Atrioventricular (AV) block
  - Complete (third-degree)
  - Incomplete (second-degree)
    - Mobitz I
    - Mobitz II
  - Incomplete with 2:1 or 3:1 block
- Sinus node dysfunction (symptomatic)
  - Sinus bradycardia, sinoatrial block, sinus arrest
  - Bradycardia-tachycardia syndrome

Controversial
- In symptomatic patients
  - Bifascicular/trifascicular intraventricular block
  - Hypersensitive carotid sinus syndrome
- In asymptomatic patients
  - Third-degree block
  - Mobitz II
  - Mobitz II AV block following myocardial infarction
  - Congenital AV block
  - Sinus bradycardia <45 bpm with long-term necessary drug therapy
  - Overdrive pacing for ventricular tachycardia

Not warranted
- Syncope of undetermined cause
- In asymptomatic patients
  - Sinus bradycardia, sinoatrial block, sinus arrest
  - Bundle branch blocks
  - Mobitz I

Source: Modified from AMA Council on Scientific Affairs: The use of cardiac pacemakers in medical practice. JAMA 1985; 254:1952.

or profound sinus bradycardia easily justifies pacemaker insertion if adequately documented. Sinus bradycardia with rates in the 50s may justify pacemaker insertion if symptoms can be causally related to the underlying bradyarrhythmia. Documentation often requires Holter monitoring. Medicare allows pacemakers in support of long-term necessary drug therapy for medical conditions such as supraventricular arrhythmias, ventricular tachycardia, hypertension, and angina. While novel indications for pacemaker therapy may be supported by clinical research, recognition of such advances by the FDA and insurance carriers is often slow. Electrophysiology (EP) study is often helpful in defining proper treatment.[14]

AV BLOCK

First-degree block refers to prolongation of the PR interval beyond 200 milliseconds. First-degree block at a low atrial rate may progress to Wenckebach as atrial rate is increased. Second-degree block involves incomplete dissociation of the atria and ventricles. This results in either progressive PR prolongation and dropped beats (Wenckebach, Mobitz I, usually AV nodal block) or frequently dropped beats without prior progression of the PR interval (Mobitz II, usually in the His-Purkinje system[15]). Third-degree block consists of complete atrioventricular dissociation, with the atrial rate usually exceeding the ventricular rate. Left and right bundle branch blocks and left anterior and posterior hemiblocks are partial conduction system blocks recognizable by electrocardiogram. The etiology of AV block includes ischemic heart disease, idiopathic fibrosis, cardiomyopathy, iatrogenic damage, AV node ablation, Lyme disease, bacterial endocarditis, lupus erythematosus, and congenital heart disease.

SINUS NODE DYSFUNCTION

Sinus node dysfunction that is producing symptoms warrants pacemaker insertion. Symptomatic bradycardia may be caused by administration of drugs required for treatment of ancillary conditions. Causes of sinus node dysfunction include coronary artery disease, cardiomyopathy, and reflex influences.

Reflex problems include carotid sinus hypersensitivity, vasovagal syncope, and oddities like micturation-induced and deglutition syncope.[16] Both cardioinhibitory (asystole >3 seconds) and vasodepressor (marked fall in blood pressure despite adequate heart rate) components of reflex-mediated syncope are recognized. Whether pacemaker insertion is indicated is determined by symptoms and clinical judgment based on the duration of asystole. Tilt table testing provides objective data. Current trends favor pacemaker insertion for asystolic intervals longer than 3 seconds; medical therapy is favored for vasodepressor syncope even with substantial sinus bradycardia.[17] Dual-chamber (DDD or VDD) pacing is favored for this population because of beneficial effects of AV synchrony on stroke volume and symptomatology.

Features of Permanent Pacing

AV SYNCHRONY AND SEQUENCE OF ACTIVATION

AV synchrony is important for maintenance of ventricular filling and stroke volume. In the normal heart, stroke volume is augmented 5% to 15% by AV synchrony compared with the asynchronous state.[18,19] Left ventricular hypertrophy, decreased diastolic compliance, and heart failure increase the quantitative importance of AV synchrony.[20] Apical pacing of the right ventricle disrupts the normal sequence of activation, because depolarization spreads slowly and progressively over the ventricular walls rather than spreading rapidly and symmetrically through the conduction system.

The hypothesis that abnormalities of the sequence of activation can impair mechanical performance of the left ventricle has been established experimentally, and recent developments have demonstrated clinical relevance. Thus, disruption of the activation sequence is believed to explain why the ventricular-aortic gradient in IHSS can be reduced in many patients by DDD pacing.[21–23] Further, some clinical studies suggest that RV outflow tract pacing may improve stroke volume when compared to apical pacing because of favorable effects on activation sequence.[24] Biventricular pacing with leads in the RV apex and coronary sinus in patients with advanced cardiomyopathy and an intraventricular conduction defect is believed to improve LV function by restoring simultaneous contraction of the septum and free wall, or "ventricular resynchronization."[25] Single-site, epicardial left ventricular pacing may provide similar benefits in some patients.

DUAL-CHAMBER PACING ALGORITHM

Programming of DDD pacemakers includes the lower rate, the upper rate, and the AV delay.[26] If the atrial rate lies between the upper and lower rate limits, the pacemaker will maintain a 1:1 response between the RA and RV without atrial pacing. If the atrial rate falls to the lower rate limit, the pacemaker adds atrial pacing at the lower rate limit. If the atrial rate is faster than the upper rate limit, the pacemaker maintains the ventricular rate at the upper rate limit, with loss of AV synchrony, resembling a Wenckebach effect.

The programmable AV delay is the allowable interval between atrial and ventricular contraction. Timing starts when an atrial electrogram or pacing stimulus is detected. If no ventricular depolarization is detected within the allowed interval, the ventricle is paced. When the atrium is paced, the physiologic P wave may occur as much as 100 milliseconds after the atrial pacing artifact. Thus, a longer AV delay is needed during atrial pacing than during atrial tracking, and these intervals are separately programmable.

Rate response to increased metabolic demand During high metabolic demand, cardiac output is potentiated physiologically by increased myocardial contractility, increased venous return, and increased heart rate. In patients with a normal sinus node rate response to exercise and complete AV block, dual-chamber pacemakers restore both AV synchrony and, by tracking the atrium, a normal rate response. With dual-chamber pacing and sinus node incompetence (no atrial rate increase with exercise) or with single-chamber ventricular pacing, alternative methods of assessing and compensating for metabolic demand are needed. Pacemakers with this capability are identified by the letter "R" (for "rate responsive") added to the three-letter pacemaker code. Body vibration[27] or respiratory rate[28] is commonly employed to estimate demand in commercial products. Other indicators under evaluation include body temperature,[29] venous oxygen saturation,[30] Q-T interval,[31] RV systolic pressure,[32] and RV stroke volume.[33] All proposed and implemented indicators can produce aberrant increases in heart rate.[34] For example, a pacemaker that senses body vibration may cause tachycardia during a bumpy car ride. Elderly patients with sedentary life styles are not likely to benefit substantially from rate-responsive pacing, and adverse effects can result from elevated heart rates in patients with evolving coronary disease.

CHOICE OF PACING TECHNIQUE

Enthusiasm for dual-chamber pacing is increasing. Paroxysmal atrial fibrillation is no longer a contraindication, because mode switching is available and sinus rhythm appears better maintained by atrial than ventricular pacing.[35] Similarly, dual-chamber pacing is now recommended for reflex-mediated syncope with cardioinhibitory features.[17] Whether the additional complexity of dual-chamber pacing is warranted in elderly patients who do not suffer from pacemaker syndrome is debatable. VVI or VVIR pacing is most appropriate for patients with bradycardia in chronic atrial fibrillation. AAIR is appropriate for cardiac allograft recipients with sinus arrest or sinus bradycardia.[36]

Pacemaker Technology

EPICARDIAL/ENDOCARDIAL LEADS

Epicardial leads have generally proven inferior to endocardial leads.[37,38] Lead fracture is an important cause. Small contact surfaces, associated with better pacing thresholds, have only recently been developed for epicardial systems.[8] Fibrosis and trauma associated with reoperations make epicardial pacing more difficult. Steroid eluting epicardial leads are now available.[8] Infected epicardial leads require a thoracotomy for lead removal. The epicardial approach is best reserved for congenital heart disease, patients with mechanical tricuspid valves, or unusual problems with venous access. Left ventricular pacing is more easily achieved with epicardial leads. At thoracotomy, the option of inserting endocardial leads through an atrial purse string is useful.[39] Minimal access approaches to LV lead insertion may prove valuable in patients requiring biventricular pacing.

For implantation of a DDD pacemaker during open heart surgery, a preferred scheme is indicated in Figure 55-2. Endocardial atrial and ventricular fixed-screw, positive fixation leads are introduced into the heart through small atrial punctures and passed to the appropriate cardiac chambers. They are fixed into position by axial rotation and tested. When a tricuspid prosthesis or ring is inserted, one option is to pass the leads between the sutures in the prosthetic ring and the valve annulus. A useful method for epicardial atrial application of endocardial pacing leads is illustrated in Figure 55-3. Additional epicardial approaches to the patient with limited venous access are described below.

UNIPOLAR/BIPOLAR

Bipolar lead designs include two conductors electrically separated by insulation. In unipolar systems, the patient's body is the ground for anodal conduction; leads containing only

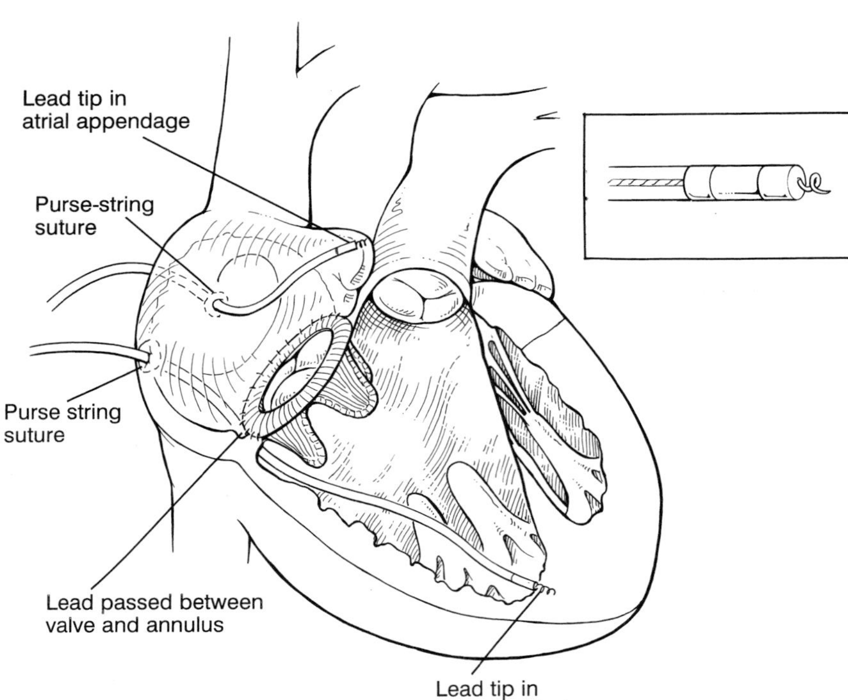

FIGURE 55–2 Endocardial pacing from epicardial approach during cardiac surgery. Purse-string sutures in atrium provide access; leads are advanced and screwed into position with aid of introducers or manual palpation. The ventricular lead is shown traversing the tricuspid plane between valve prosthesis and the annulus. Inset shows tip of endocardial screw-in lead.

a single conductor carry the negative current to the heart. Bipolar pacing systems are resistant to electrical noise (oversensing) and cause less adventitious pacing of the diaphragm or chest wall. These advantages are offset by the increased engineering complexity of two conductors in a single structure. Bipolar leads are subject to breakdown of insulation or conductors, which can severely compromise both sensing and pacing functions (Fig. 55-4).[8,40] Bipolar leads tend to be thicker, stiffer, and less easily maneuvered than unipolar leads. Flexibility facilitates J bends and loops (Fig. 55-5) and reduces the chance of perforation through the right ventricular apex. Recent bipolar leads have advanced insulation designs and are similar in diameter to unipolar leads (Fig. 55-6); handling characteristics have also improved. The long-term durability of these leads remains to be confirmed. The market for unipolar leads is contracting, and Oscor remains one of the few manufacturers producing a 6F unipolar screw-in lead suitable for use in infants and children.

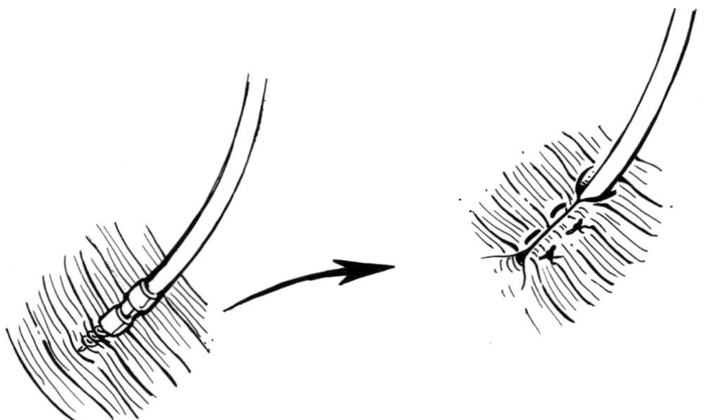

FIGURE 55–3 Permanent epicardial atrial pacing with an endocardial screw-in lead. The tip is screwed into the atrial myocardium, and atrial myocardium is then "Whitselled" over the electrode with 6-0 monofilament suture.

LEAD FIXATION

We prefer positive fixation techniques, particularly in locations with minimal trabeculation. Positive fixation involves a small wire spiral or "screw" at the tip of the lead (see Fig. 55-6). A fixed screw may be covered with soluble material to promote venous passage. Alternatives include a retractable screw (Bisping lead), which is extended or retracted by rotation of the pin at the lead tip. Axial clockwise rotation of these leads during fixation provides tactile feedback on the firmness and reproducibility of the fixation site. Lead impedance is an important clue to full extension of retractable screw designs.

Tined leads use miniature anchors in a variety of shapes and sizes that secure the lead tip by wedging between myocardial trabeculae (see Fig. 55-6). Tined leads require a larger introducer than screw-in leads and are not as secure in smooth-walled (as in corrected transposition of the great vessels) or massively dilated chambers. Tined leads are also less secure in atrial insertion. However, many physicians have reported excellent results with these leads.[41,42]

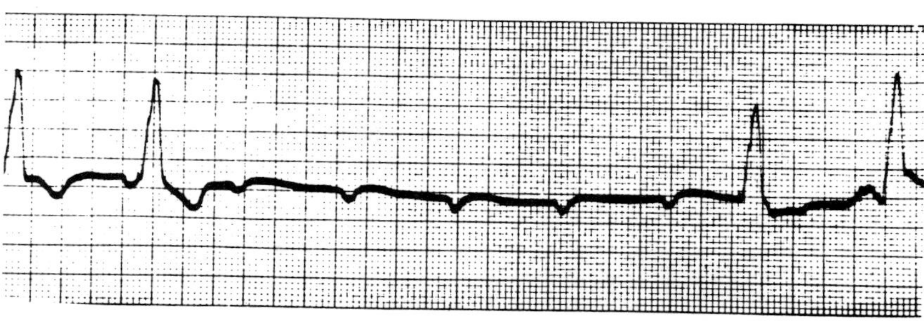

FIGURE 55–4 Telemetry from patient with third-degree heart block, no detectable escape rhythm, and malfunctioning bipolar VVI pacemaker. Patient was admitted with repeated presyncopal episodes. Differential diagnosis between oversensing and failure to capture was resolved when programming to VOO mode completely eliminated recurrent pauses. Patient underwent successful lead replacement and was discharged the next day. This is an example of a life-threatening effect of oversensing. This older model pacemaker was not capable of telemetry of electrograms to confirm the diagnosis (see Fig. 55-12).

TEMPORARY PACING

Acute bradycardia can be treated with transthoracic pacing, temporary endocardial pacing, or chronotropic drugs including atropine or isoproterenol. RV perforation has become less prevalent with current endocardial lead designs but must be borne in mind if hypotension develops acutely after removal of temporary wires.

Bradycardia after cardiac surgery is commonly treated with pacing via temporary atrial and ventricular epicardial wires. Problems include loss of RA or RV capture and loss of RA sensing. Competition between an atrial pacemaker and the patient's intrinsic rhythm can precipitate atrial fibrillation or atrial flutter. If atrial sensing is not adequate, pacing the atrium considerably faster than the intrinsic rate can reduce competition. Reversing polarity or inserting an independent ground wire in the skin under local anesthesia may alleviate problems with temporary epicardial pacing. The output of the external generator in volts or milliamps should be left at least twice as high as the threshold, measured daily. Improper ventricular sensing in critically ill patients is particularly hazardous, as pacing during the vulnerable period can precipitate ventricular tachycardia or fibrillation.

CARDIAC OUTPUT AND PACING RATE

For patients with hemodynamic compromise following cardiac surgery, pacing rate and AV delay can affect hemodynamics. Mean arterial pressure can be used to estimate cardiac output, if systemic resistance is constant. Rate and timing adjustments should be assessed over intervals of less than 20 seconds to minimize reflex effects. The settings producing the highest sustained mean arterial pressure should also produce the highest cardiac output. The addition of temporary LV wires adds pacing site (RV, LV, or both) and RV-LV delay to the variables affecting the hemodynamics of temporary pacing.

Pacemaker Insertion

ENVIRONMENT/ANESTHESIA

Recent trends suggest that pacemaker and ICD surgery can safely be performed in EP laboratories.[43] Whether the procedure takes place in the OR or EP lab, properly functioning equipment is essential. Infection control is critical[44]; operating room standards for air quality should be enforced. Pacemakers can be inserted in an EP laboratory by one skilled

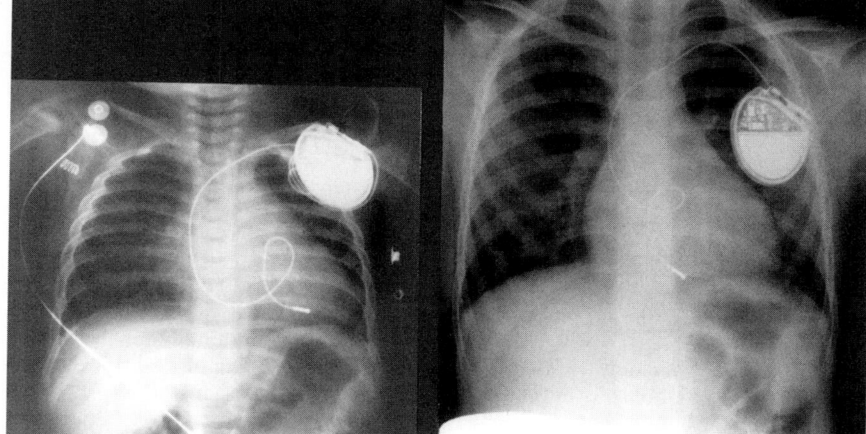

FIGURE 55–5 Tenacious fixation and flexibility of small-diameter, positive fixation leads is illustrated in these x-rays, demonstrating stability of transvenous pacing lead with intracardiac lead loop over four years of growth in a patient from age 1 (left) to age 5 (right).

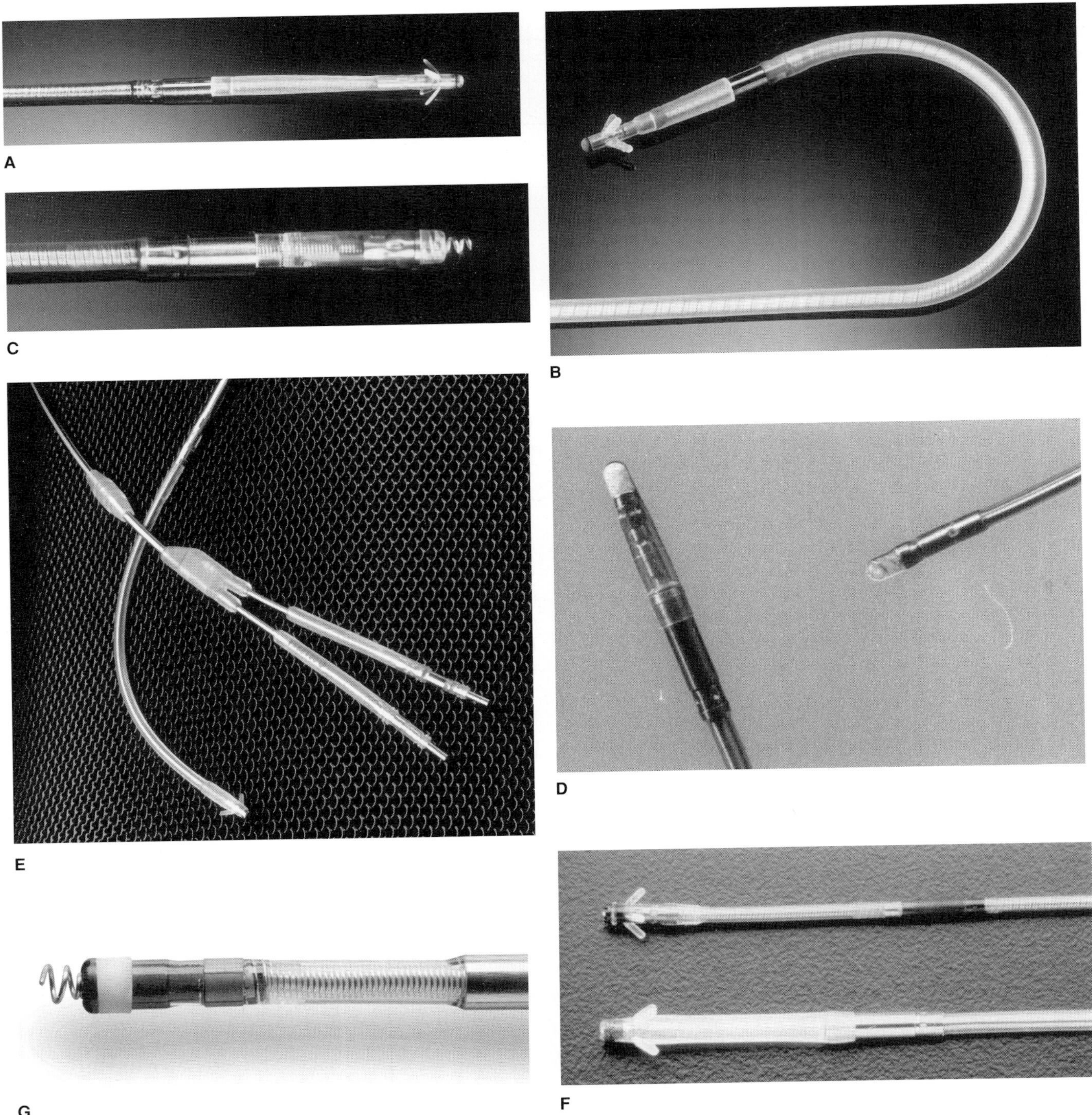

FIGURE 55–6 (A) Straight bipolar tined ventricular pacing lead with steroid-eluting tip. (B) J-shaped, bipolar tined atrial pacing lead with steroid-eluting tip. (C) Bisping bipolar ventricular pacing lead with retractable, screw-in tip. (D) Bipolar (left) and unipolar (right) pacing leads with fixed-screw tips. Soluble coating over tip, which quickly dissolves in the bloodstream, reduces chance of venous snagging during lead introduction. These leads can be used in atrial or ventricular position. The lead on the right was used by the author extensively for both atrial and ventricular transvenous pacing. (E) Single-pass lead for VDD pacing. (F) Current technology leads demonstrating progress in reduction of bipolar lead diameter. (G) Fixed-screw bipolar 7F lead with steroid-eluting white collar at lead tip. (*A-C, courtesy of Medtronic, Inc.; D-F, courtesy of Intermedics, Inc.; G, courtesy of Guidant Corp.*)

surgeon and one skilled circulating nurse. This is satisfactory until a problem like angina, transient ischemic attack, patient disorientation, or lidocaine toxicity arises. Also, certain patients are simply too unstable because of dementia, myocardial ischemia, heart failure, anxiety, or ventricular tachycardia to undergo pacemaker insertion without the presence of an anesthesiologist or an equivalent, full-time advocate. Vancomycin reactions (red man syndrome), pacing-induced ventricular fibrillation, air embolism, and Stokes-Adams attacks may occur, albeit rarely, requiring assistance of a skilled specialist. Intraoperative death can occur due to hemorrhage or myocardial infarction. Good clinical judgment about when an anesthesiologist is essential is an important issue. If English is not the patient's first language, a translator can also be helpful.

MONITORING

R-wave detection by an ECG monitor is inadequate for pacemaker insertion, because pacing artifacts that fail to capture may not be distinguished from those that do. Thus, subthreshold pacing can elicit regular beeping from the monitor in an asystolic patient. Oxygen saturation monitors are preferable in this application, as they beep only during blood flow. Palpation by an anesthesiologist or nurse of the temporal, facial, or radial artery pulse can be valuable for detecting asystole.

VENOUS ACCESS STRATEGY

Choices include which side will be employed and whether a cut-down or percutaneous venipuncture will be used. Cut-down approaches to the cephalic, subclavian, external jugular, and internal jugular system have been described.[45] Subclavian vein puncture has recently been modified[46] in an effort to reduce the frequency of subclavian crush (Fig. 55-7). Subclavian puncture is associated with an apparently unavoidable but low incidence of pneumo/hemothorax and major venous injury.

Access from below or even transhepatically is possible,[45,47] but the potential for venous thrombosis and pulmonary embolism are concerns. Right parasternal mediastinotomy has been advocated as a useful approach to the right atrium, using a Seldinger approach and small introducers through an atrial purse-string suture (Fig. 55-8).[39]

ANTIBIOTIC PROPHYLAXIS

Antibiotic prophylaxis is indicated before insertion of a prosthetic device.[44] We prefer cefazolin, 1 gram IV. We also irrigate the operative field with a portion of a solution of 1 gram of cefazolin in a liter of warm saline. Patients who have a valve prosthesis or who have a penicillin or cefazolin allergy receive vancomycin (500 mg) and gentamycin (1 mg/kg).

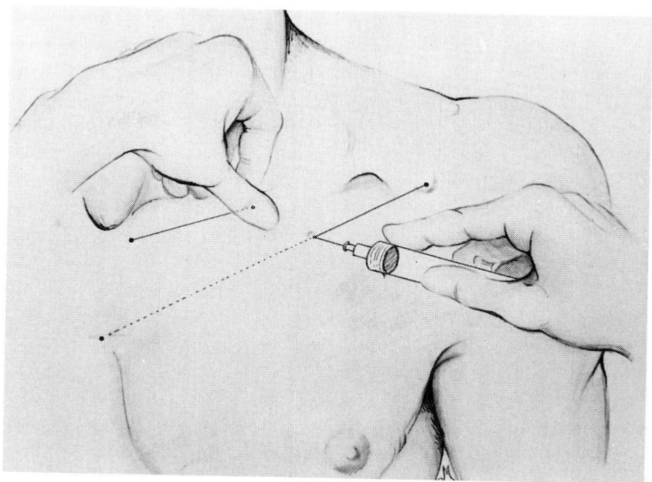

FIGURE 55–7 Landmarks for subclavian vein puncture.[40] Potential complications of this procedure include pneumothorax, hemothorax, and lead damage due to subclavian crush injury.

PACING SYSTEMS ANALYZER

Pacing thresholds and electrogram amplitudes are measured with a pacing systems analyzer. Electrogram characteristics and slew rate can be examined with many current analyzers, and electrogram telemetry is available from many current pacemakers. The analyzer must function properly, and should be serviced and tested periodically. The batteries must be checked and replaced when depleted. Any discrepancies between measurements by the analyzer and the pacemaker should be noted and related functions of the analyzer rechecked.

A skilled operator is needed to run the analyzer and record the results. Alternatively, the analyzer can be placed in a sterile bag and operated from the surgical field. Manufacturer's representatives, an increasing presence in the operating room and EP lab, are skilled in operation of these analyzers.

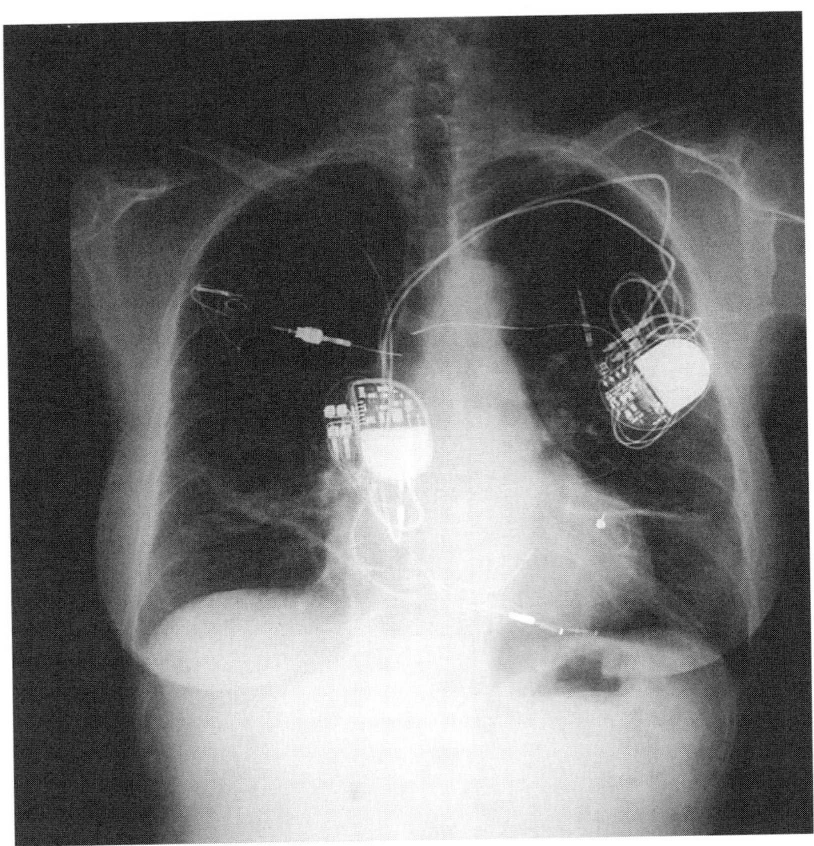

FIGURE 55–8 Female admitted from another hospital with very poor escape rhythm, bilateral venous obstruction, and severe exit block. A new pacing system was inserted through the right atrial appendage via right parasternal mediastotomy. Old pacemaker was programmed to backup mode and scheduled for removal at a later date.

CABLES

The cables connecting the analyzer to the leads are the patient's lifeline. Even with excellent quality control, defective cables may be delivered to the surgical field. Errors can also occur in connecting the cables to the analyzer, resulting in open or intermittent connections. A routine for testing the cables and the integrity of their connection to the analyzer is therefore recommended. After passing the cables from the operating table, pacing is initiated from the analyzer at maximum output. The alligator connectors are then briefly connected to the subcutaneous tissue. Impedance should be about 500 ohms, a current of 100 milliamperes at an output of 5 volts. No current flow and high impedance indicate an open circuit. The operation should not proceed until the problem is corrected, because the analyzer-cable circuit is defective. Connections to the analyzer should also be checked, since inadvertent reversal of polarity can make measured pacing thresholds inappropriately high. Many of these issues are resolved by disposable leads with polarized connectors.

FLUOROSCOPY

Fluoroscopy is essential for transvenous device implantation, and operating room personnel need to be familiar with the equipment. Distracting problems with image orientation, rebooting, timers, brakes, and locks can be avoided by a knowledgeable team. Sudden failure of fluoroscopy at a critical point happens to every pacemaker surgeon with a large enough clinical volume. If a backup unit is not available, the options include "blind" endocardial lead insertion, epicardial insertion, or postponement of the procedure. Overheating is an issue when fluoroscopy is prolonged, as may occur during biventricular pacemaker insertion. The use of low-dose and pulsed image options is desirable when prolonged use of the fluoroscope is planned.

SURGICAL APPROACH

Our preference is to approach the patient from the left. The fluoroscope is positioned carefully on the patient's right to allow visualization of the apex, right atrium, and deltopectoral groove. The right arm is extended to the right on an arm board. The drapes are suspended from IV poles. One pole is caudad to the arm board. Careful positioning allows the left clavicular region to be exposed while leaving the patient adequate light and air. After skin preparation, towels are aligned with the deltopectoral groove and clavicle to define the essential landmarks. The region of the incision and generator is infiltrated with 1% lidocaine to produce a field block. A 5- to 6-cm horizontal incision is created 4 cm beneath the clavicle, with the lateral extent of the incision just reaching the deltopectoral groove. This allows the generator to be positioned away from the deltopectoral groove and axilla, avoiding interference with motion of the left arm at the shoulder. An alternative incision directly over the deltopectoral groove facilitates exposure of the cephalic vein; this is particularly valuable in obese patients or elderly patients with atretic veins.

VENOUS ACCESS

When the deltopectoral groove has been exposed, additional anesthesia is infiltrated into lateral margin of the pectoralis and laterally into the deltoid. The dissection proceeds into the deltopectoral groove, following the lateral edge of the pectoralis, until the cephalic vein or another venous branch is exposed. Failure to find a vein may mean the incision is too far cephalad or caudad or not lateral enough. The incision can be deepened into the subpectoral fat, if necessary. If the vein is too small to pass a pacemaker lead, the curved end of the guidewire for a 7F introducer is passed centrally. The ability to manually stiffen and extend the curve by central manipulation of the tension in the guidewire is an important technical aid in tortuous veins. The method illustrated in Figure 55-9 can be used to enlarge the vein at the point of access. If the guidewire will not pass centrally,

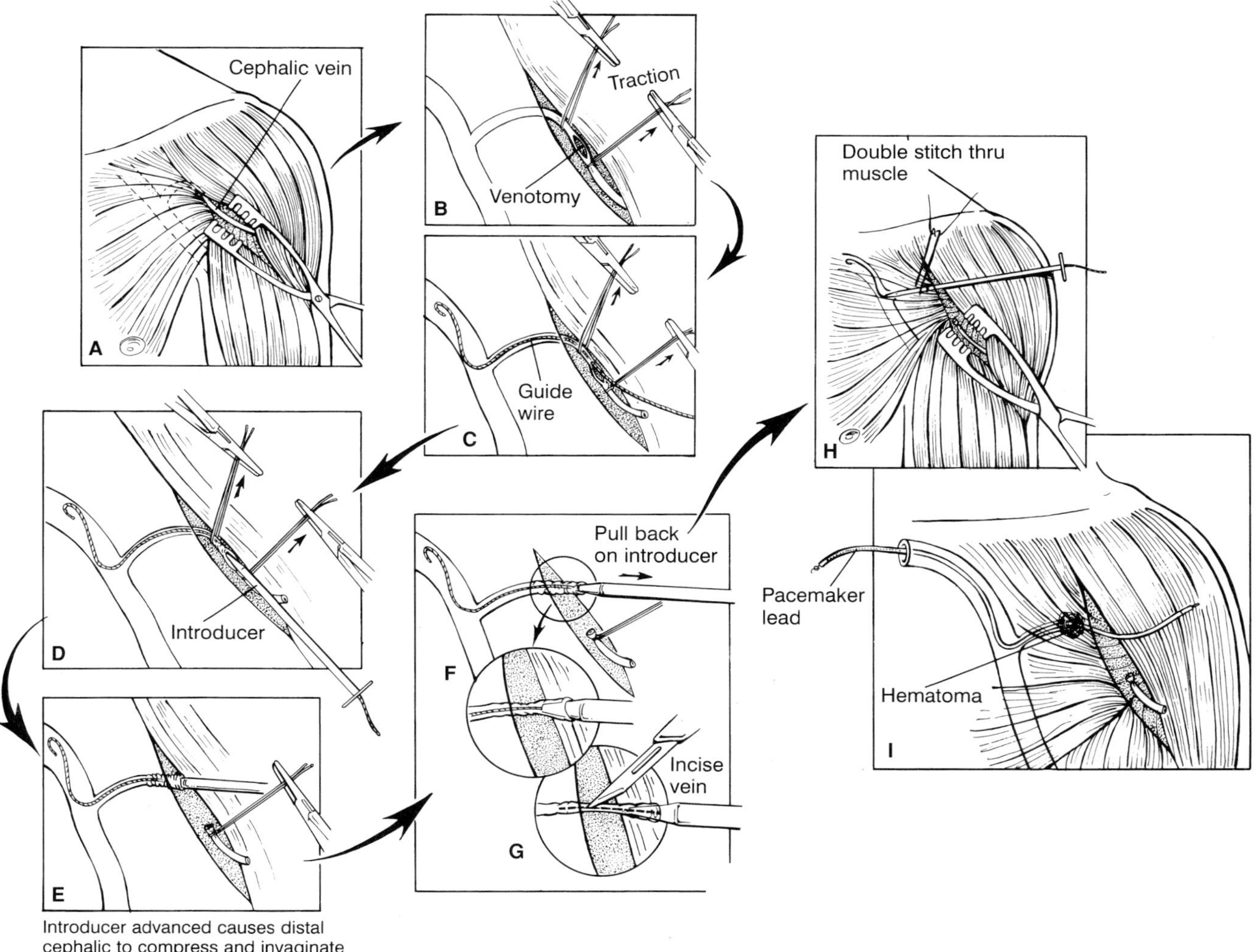

FIGURE 55–9 Cephalic cut-down approach to small veins that pass a guidewire but not an introducer to the central veins. Resistance results from entrapment of the introducer tip and invagination of the vein; the introducer can only be advanced by turning the vein outside-in. Fortunately, this entrapment can be put to good use. After the guidewire is advanced (C), a #16 Angiocath is passed over the guidewire to dilate the vein (not shown). This allows the introducer tip to enter the vein (D), but if the vein does not split, the introducer cannot be advanced (E). The impaled vein is exposed by gently withdrawing the introducer (F). The adherent, exposed segment of vein is then split longitudinally with a #11 blade (G). The procedure can be repeated, if necessary, to advance the introducer centrally. A purse-string suture approximates soft tissue around the path of the introducer to achieve hemostasis (H, I).

a #16 angiocath is advanced over the guidewire and used to inject a small amount of iodinated contrast to visualize the venous system fluoroscopically. If the cut-down approach must be abandoned, precise localization of the subclavian vein by venogram reduces the risk of subclavian puncture. If dual-chamber pacing is planned, the guidewire should be reinserted through the introducer before the introducer is stripped away. This provides venous access for the duration of the procedure.[48,49] A purse-string suture in the muscle usually provides adequate control of bleeding and allows stabilization of the lead(s).[50,51]

RV LEAD INSERTION

From the left side, a gentle spiral in the distal 10 cm of the stylet will guide the lead across the tricuspid valve to the RV. Ideally, the lead should first be advanced into the pulmonary artery outside the cardiac silhouette to confirm that it is not in the coronary sinus. For fixed-screw positive fixation leads, the stylet should be withdrawn 3 to 5 cm before screwing the lead into the myocardium with axial clockwise rotation. It is important to evaluate the reverse torque that develops as the lead is rotated; this torque is a guide to the security of fixation. We fix the lead with a sequence of three consecutive 360° clockwise rotations of the lead shaft and then release the torque. This fixation sequence is repeated as many times as is necessary, until the lead is secure, with substantial reverse torque after the first 360° rotation. No more than three complete axial rotations are employed in any sequence. A rare problem to avoid with screw-in leads is undetected ventricular perforation. The lead tip should be watched during the fixation process to look for sudden extra-anatomic movement. When the lead tip is fixed, the stylet should be withdrawn and thresholds tested. The patient is asked to hyperventilate and cough to confirm fixation. Ventricular pacing threshold should be less than 0.7 volt and R-wave amplitude should be more than 5 mv. For unipolar leads, impedance should be 400 to 1000 ohms, depending on lead design. There should be no diaphragmatic pacing at an output of 10 volts.

If the lead is dislodged by hyperventilation and coughing, or if thresholds are not adequate, the lead should be relocated. A positive fixation lead can be unscrewed by counterclockwise axial rotation until it floats free. Positive fixation leads can be secured almost anywhere along the margins of the RV silhouette (Fig. 55-10), including the RV outflow tract (Fig. 55-11).[52] In difficult cases, we have relocated these leads as many as 15 times. The geographic center of the silhouette is not a desirable location, as it can lead to entanglement of the lead in the chordae tendineae (see Fig. 55-10).

CS LEAD INSERTION

Left ventricular pacing via the coronary sinus (CS) will become increasingly popular if biventricular pacing for heart failure proves to have long-term benefit. Electrophysiologists

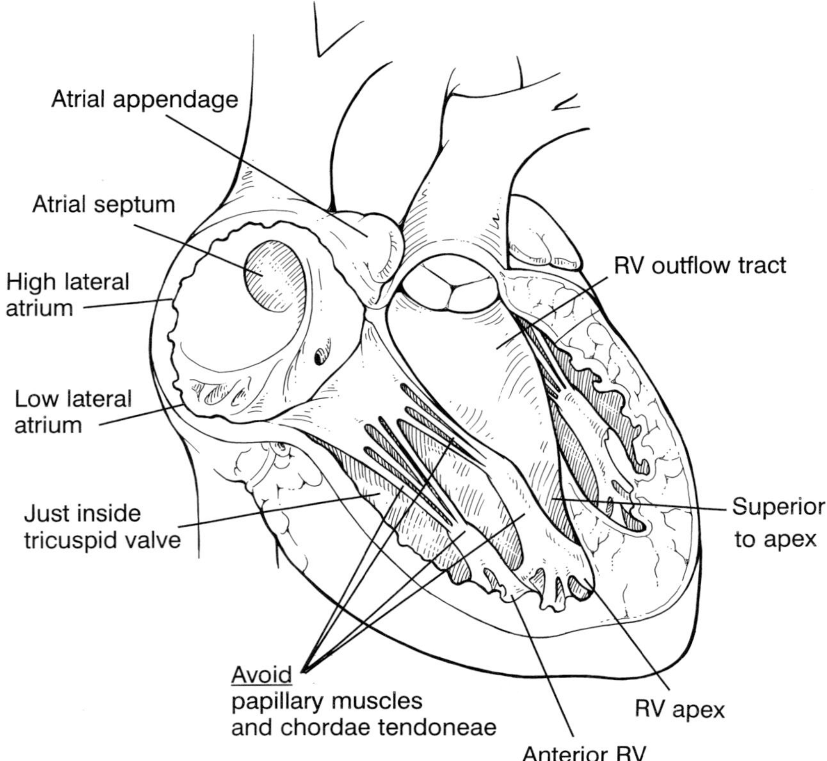

FIGURE 55–10 Useful sites for transvenous atrial and ventricular pacing using fixed-screw unipolar leads. The geographic center of the RV should be avoided; screwing leads into this location can result in lead entrapment in the chordae tendineae, which may necessitate lead abandonment.

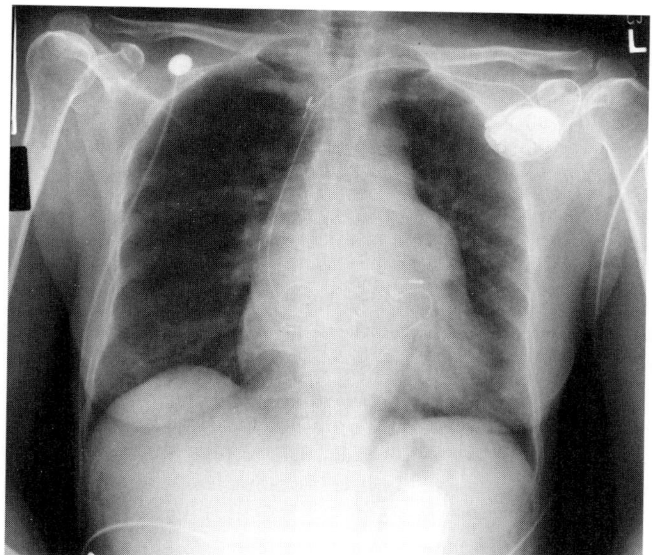

FIGURE 55–11 X-ray illustrates screw-in lead in the RV outflow tract of a patient with complete heart block after tricuspid valve replacement for Ebstein's anomaly. This location minimized lead motion and stress at the tricuspid annulus in this patient.

routinely place mapping leads in the CS and have many special tools for this, including steerable mapping catheters and biplane fluoroscopy. It appears that over-the-wire designs will be most successful, the key being entry to the CS with a guidewire. The CS is a posterior structure near the caudal aspect of the tricuspid valve (Fig. 55-12). Locating the CS in heart failure patients is difficult because the CS is angulated and distorted by enlargement of the RV and RA. Venography via special catheters can be advantageous. Transesophageal echo also is helpful in locating the os, but this requires general anesthesia. Patients with congestive heart failure are prone to ventricular tachycardia, making the application of R2 pads a reasonable precaution. Even experienced operators can take many hours to insert a CS catheter with present methods, but it is likely that technology in this area will improve for both endocardial and epicardial LV lead placement. We prefer to do the CS lead first via the cephalic approach, with RA and RV leads following via subclavian puncture if necessary. The difficulty of CS lead insertion in heart failure patients should not be underestimated; special training by an experienced preceptor is definitely worthwhile.

LENGTH ADJUSTMENT

Lead length should be adjusted between "too short," where a deep breath in the upright position results in lead displacement, and "too long," where a cough in the supine position may result in formation of a loop which effectively shortens the lead and pulls it out of the apex.

We ask patients to perform a maximal inspiration and expiration under fluoroscopy to aid in length adjustment. Vigorous coughing tests the security of lead tip fixation. Pacemaker syndrome can be detected immediately with VVI

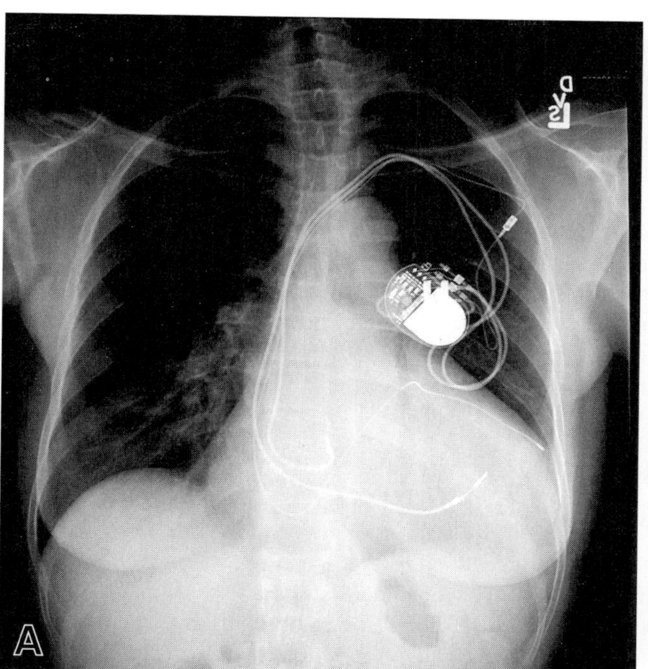

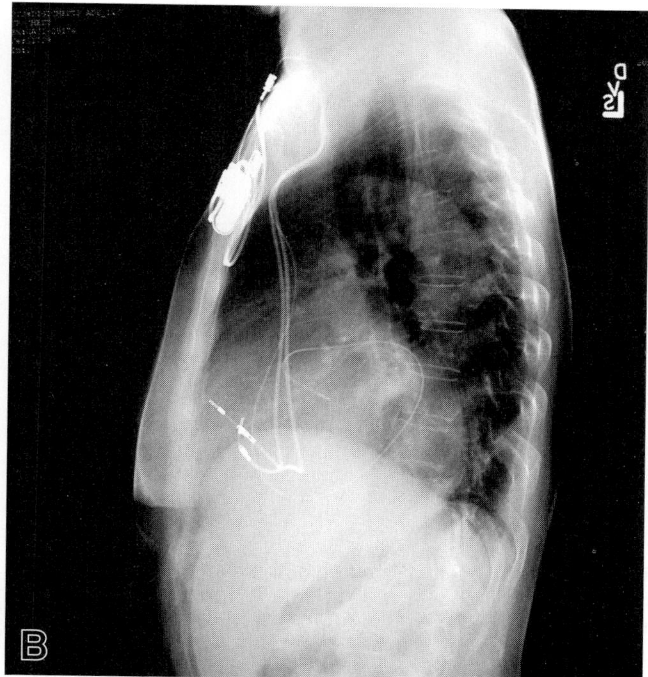

FIGURE 55–12 (A) Biventricular, dual-chamber pacemaker with endocardial leads in the RA, RV, and lateral branch of the coronary sinus (LV). This patient was relieved of dobutamine dependence by addition of LV lead. (B) Lateral x-ray of same patient. Posterior course of coronary sinus is apparent.

pacing in susceptible patients This valuable feedback is lost if the patient is too heavily sedated or cannot cooperate for other reasons.

ATRIAL LEAD INSERTION

For dual-chamber pacing, atrial lead is required. A "J" stylet shape is best for finding the atrial appendage from the left side.[51] An "S" shape is useful for passing a positive fixation lead to the right margin of the atrium near the junction of the right atrium and inferior vena cava (Figs. 55-10 and 55-13). P-wave amplitude is often better in this location than at other atrial sites. The atrial pacing threshold should be less than 2 volts. In the presence of complete heart block, it may be difficult to confirm atrial capture from the surface ECG. Pacing the atrium at 150 beats/min results in rapid motion of the lead tip, which is apparent fluoroscopically and can be used to determine atrial pacing threshold. This technique should only be used if the high atrial rate is not conducted to the ventricle. It is also possible that crosstalk from this atrial pacing can inhibit whatever temporary VVI pacing is supporting the patient, resulting in asystole.

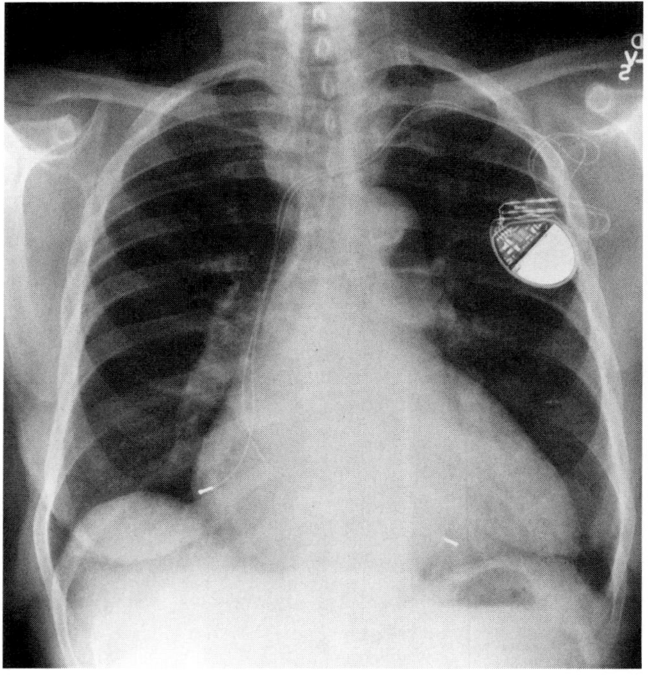

FIGURE 55–13 Dual-chamber pacemaker illustrates low, right lateral atrial lead placement. This location, particularly advantageous after obliteration of the atrial appendage at heart surgery, requires a positive fixation lead. P-wave amplitude in this location is often acceptable when other sites fail. If phrenic nerve stimulation is observed with 10-volt stimulation at 0.50-ms pulse width, however, the lead tip should be repositioned.

The P-wave electrogram is the Achilles heel of dual-chamber pacing. If atrial sensing is not satisfactory, a DDD pacemaker will not function properly. The P-wave amplitude should ideally be greater than 1.5 mv. Measurement of P-wave amplitude with unipolar leads can be confusing. Crosstalk or far-field sensing of ventricular depolarization from the atrial lead can occur, so that a 2-mv signal measured through a pacemaker analyzer from the atrium is not a P wave but a QRS complex. Simultaneous measurement and display of atrial and ventricular electrograms as well as the surface ECG can resolve this. An alternative solution involves programming the generator as a P-wave detector. The lower rate is set below the patient's intrinsic atrial rate, the AV delay is set shorter than the patient's PR interval, and atrial sensitivity is set at 2 mv. When the generator is connected to the atrial and ventricular leads, every P wave will be followed immediately by a ventricular pacing spike if P-wave amplitude is greater than 2 mv. The pacemaker must be reprogrammed to clinically appropriate settings at the conclusion of surgery. Telemetry of atrial and ventricular electrograms by pacemakers is a valuable source of EP data. For example, inability to pace the atrium or to measure atrial electrograms in the operating room may indicate low-amplitude atrial fibrillation or SVT; this may be invisible on the surface ECG but may be detectable as electrogram activity (Fig. 55-14A). Electrogram telemetry provides valuable confirmation of proper DDD pacing (Fig. 55-14B).

GENERATOR LOCATION

We utilize a watertight, two-layer skin closure for primary implants, three layers in some generator replacements. Cosmetic appearance is important to many patients, and in others technique is critical to optimize healing. Past injury to the chest wall or surgery/radiotherapy for breast cancer can present formidable technical problems. The use of bipolar systems facilitates generator placement behind the pectoralis. Diminutive generators are available, but battery life is reduced. Innovative locations for pacemaker generators include axillary, retromammary, intrathoracic, and preperitoneal sites. These approaches are rarely indicated with present generator designs.

Length of Stay After Pacemaker Implantation

AMBULATORY SURGERY

Early hospital discharge after pacemaker insertion is feasible in patients who have an adequate escape rhythm. Positive fixation leads are preferred. After monitoring and recovery from sedation, patients are ambulated and instructed in range of motion exercises for the shoulder. A chest x-ray is obtained to document lead position and rule out hemo/pneumothorax or pericardial enlargement.

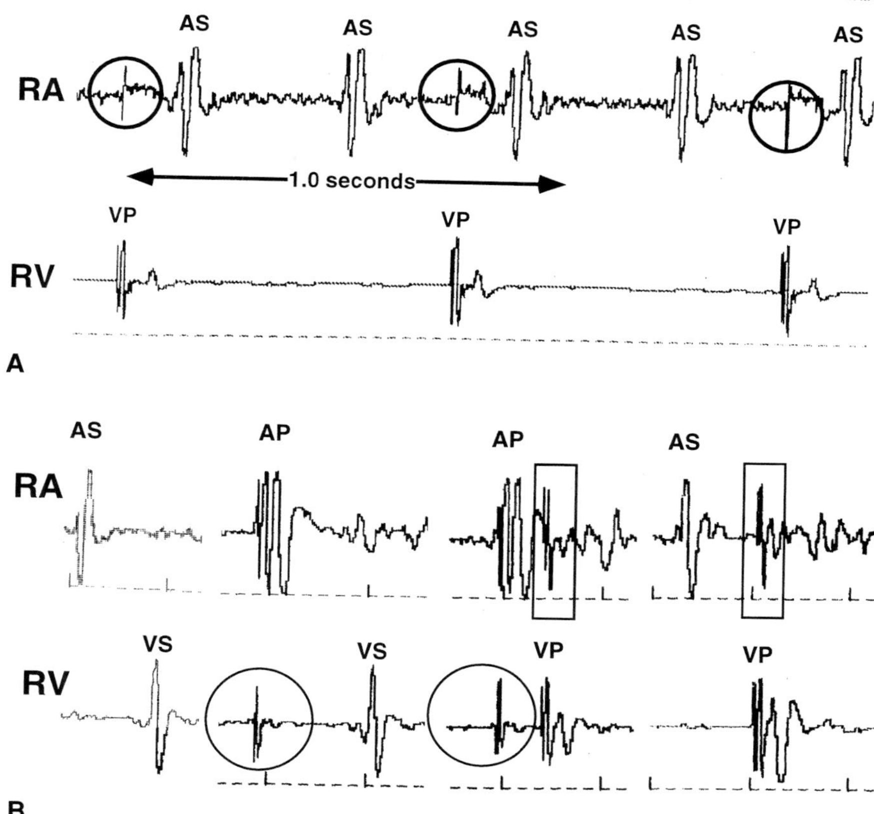

FIGURE 55–14 (A) RA and RV electrograms from a DDD pacemaker during supraventricular tachycardia (SVT). Regular atrial depolarizations appear (AS) at a rate of 160. The pacemaker paces the ventricle (VP) at 80, because alternate P waves fall inside the PVARP and are not detected. The circles illustrate far-field sensing of the RV pacing artifact in the RA lead. The SVT was not detected preoperatively, and, until this recording was obtained, the RA could not successfully be paced. After this electrogram was obtained, overdrive atrial pacing from the pacemaker converted the SVT to normal sinus rhythm, and normal pacemaker function was observed. (B) Atrial (upper, RA) and ventricular (lower, RV) electrograms illustrate unipolar DDD pacemaker function. The first cycle illustrates atrial sensing (AS) and ventricular sensing (VS) only. The second cycle illustrates atrial pacing (AP) and VS. The third cycle illustrates AP and ventricular pacing (VP). The last cycle from a different patient illustrates AS and VP, which provides atrial synchronous ventricular pacing in complete heart block. The circles demonstrate far-field sensing of RA pacing artifact in the RV lead. The rectangle illustrates far-field sensing of the RV pacing artifact in the RA lead.

PACEMAKER-DEPENDENT PATIENTS

Lead displacement can be caused by technical error, struggling of demented patients, and other factors. Since a small percentage of lead displacement is probably unavoidable,[41,42,53,54] patients who might suffer death or injury in the event of abrupt pacemaker failure should be observed in the hospital overnight on telemetry. However, lead displacement in our hands in ambulatory patients has not been more frequent than in hospitalized patients.

Pacemaker Generator Replacement

PLANNING

Fifteen percent of functioning pacemakers were replacements in a recent survey.[55] Complications of pacemaker generator replacement include infection, lead damage, connector problems, and asystole during the transition from the old generator to the new. Relatively minor conduction problems at the time of initial pacemaker implant may progress to severe pacemaker dependence by the time of generator replacement. Ambulatory surgery is usually appropriate. As a practical matter, we no longer reverse warfarin for pacemaker generator replacement, unless lead replacement is anticipated.[56] Patients with leads more than 10 years old should be carefully evaluated for pacemaker dysfunction prior to generator replacement; a Holter monitor should be obtained if lead dysfunction is suspected. Rising pacing threshold may indicate impending lead failure. Since unsuspected lead problems may be discovered during generator replacement, the option of lead replacement should be discussed with the patient in advance.

BACKUP PACING

Some practitioners insert a temporary transvenous pacing wire during pacemaker generator replacement, but this is rarely necessary. The output of the replacement unit must be high enough to match the pacing threshold of a chronically implanted lead. This is can be problematic if the generator is an older type with a fixed output of 5.4 volts. Lack of programmability prevents preoperative threshold testing, and the 5.4-volt output is considerably higher than nominal for most current generators. The standard approach with newer generators is to test the pacing threshold with a pacemaker analyzer and program the replacement to appropriate output before the unit is connected. Before disconnecting the old generator, be sure that the pacemaker analyzer, cables, and connections are intact and that personnel in the operating room are aware of where the cables run. Some place the analyzer in a sterile bag on the operative field. With many generators, an Allen wrench placed in the header establishes electrical continuity with the ventricular lead; the pacing threshold can then be established before disconnecting the old generator. The old generator should be kept within reach as a backup in case of trouble with the new generator, the analyzer, or the connectors.

LEAD SIZES

The three common sizes of lead connector for permanent pacing are 6 mm, 5 mm, and 3.5 mm (VS-1 or IS-1). Ideally, the new generator should be an exact match for the patient's lead size. A selection of step-up and step-down adapters should also be available. The contacts do not always line up correctly across VS-1 and IS-1 connectors, even though the connector diameter is the same. It is important to determine in advance whether connections can safely be made across the VS-1/IS-1 interface.

Postoperative Care

WOUND CARE

Patients are instructed to keep implant wounds dry until an office visit 7 to 10 days postoperatively. Any wound drainage at the postoperative visit is cultured, and prophylactic antibiotics are started until culture results are available. We have

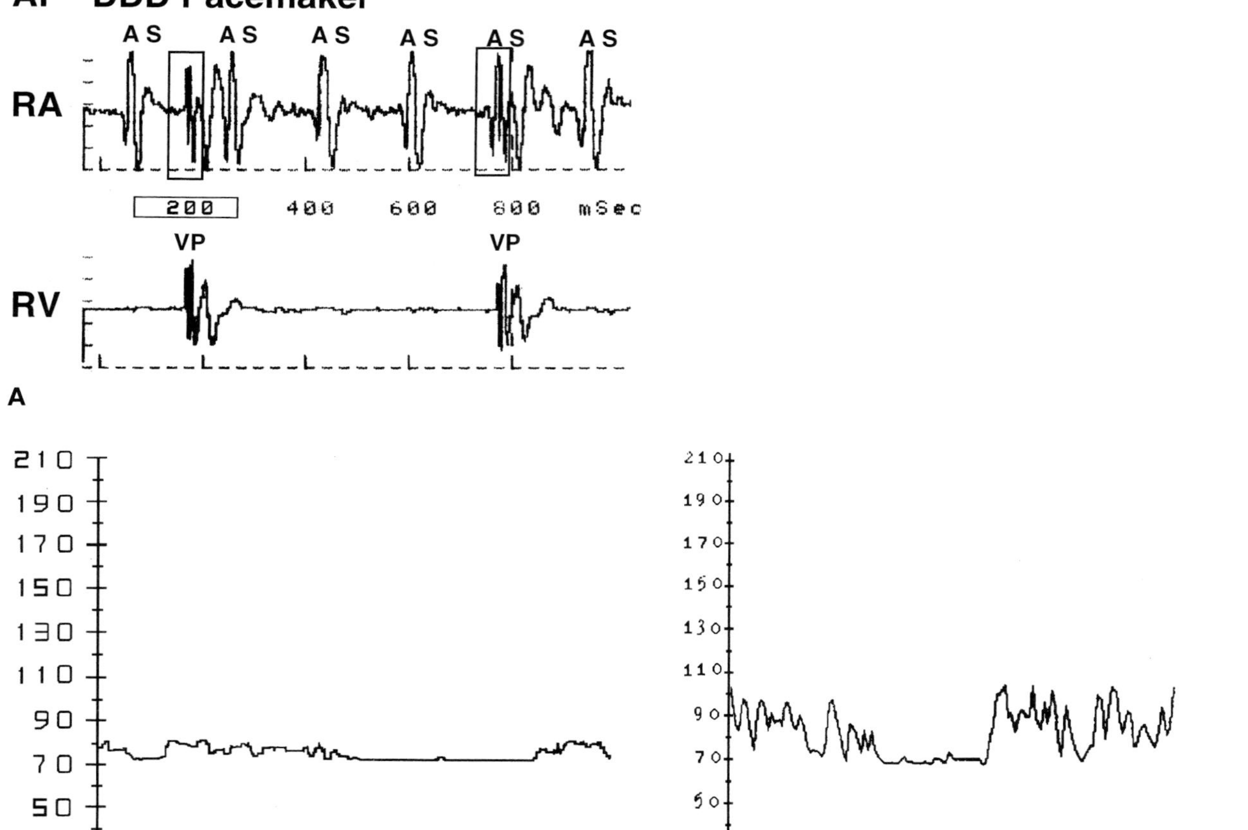

FIGURE 55–15 (A) Atrial (upper, RA) and ventricular (lower, RV) electrograms from a DDD pacemaker during atrial fibrillation (AF). The AF appears as rapid atrial depolarizations (AS). The upper rate limit and PVARP of the pacemaker determine the rate at which the pacemaker stimulates the ventricle (VP). (B,C) Average heart rate over 24 hours recorded by memory circuits in DDD pacemaker. The initial tracing (B) reveals sinus node incompetence, which developed during amiodarone therapy for paroxysmal atrial fibrillation. More normal rate variation resulted from activation of the rate-responsive feature of the generator (C), and the patient reported improved exercise tolerance.

abandoned aspiration of the rare postoperative hematoma in favor of close observation, unless infection is an issue or spontaneous drainage appears imminent.

ANTIBIOTIC PROPHYLAXIS

Routine use of prophylactic antibiotics before dental work and other invasive procedures in pacemaker or ICD recipients is not recommended under AHA/ACC guidelines. We recommend prophylaxis for 3 months after device insertion, allowing time for the pacing leads to become endothelialized.

Testing/Follow-up

OFFICE/CLINIC VERSUS TELEPHONE

Pacemakers require periodic testing to confirm sensing and pacing function and detect battery depletion. Current standards call for testing these functions at 1-to 3-month intervals. Whether follow-up should be done by transtelephonic monitoring, clinic, or office visits is in dispute.[57–59] Transtelephonic monitoring alleviates transportation issues for elderly patients, but some are too anxious or debilitated to manage the process. In addition to reducing patient travel and office resources, many commercial services provide emergency monitoring on a 24-hour basis, an important advantage in managing apprehensive or incapacitated patients.

PACEMAKER PROGRAMMING

Programming can be done in an office setting by trained, experienced personnel. In some situations, a manufacturer's representative may provide valuable help. Transtelephonic programming is not currently available.

DDD pacemaker programming allows adjustment of electrogram sensitivity as well as pacing stimulus amplitude/pulse width for both the atrium and ventricle. Lower rate, upper rate, atrioventricular delay, and refractory periods for atrial and ventricular sensing are programmable. Rate responsiveness, unipolar/bipolar configuration, and many other options are also adjustable noninvasively.

We initially program newly inserted pacemakers to stimulation amplitude and pulse width higher than nominal. At the initial office visit, pacing thresholds are retested and amplitude and pulse width are adjusted to nominal levels if pacing thresholds allow this. The use of high initial output is less important with steroid-eluting leads. Details of pacemaker programming have been described elsewhere.[59,60] Some current pacemakers are capable of automated threshold adjustment.

Programming allows most problems detected by transtelephonic or Holter monitoring to be corrected. The etiology of symptoms can often be elicited from real-time electrograms or stored data. Adjustments may include not only sensitivity or pacing output but also pacing mode for new onset atrial fibrillation[61] (Fig. 55-15A) or sinus node incompetence related to medication changes (Fig. 55-15B and C). Problems that may require reoperation include lead displacement, lead fracture (Fig. 55-16), insulation degradation, and exit block (Fig. 55-17).[53,54]

Pacemaker interrogation should include a printout of the initial settings, which can provide a valuable reference after an involved programming session. Telemetry should be examined to determine time-related variation in heart rate, percentage of beats sensed and paced, the quality of the electrograms, lead impedance, and battery voltage.

The pacing amplitude and pulse width are finely tuned at the 1-year follow-up visit. We generally provide at least 100%

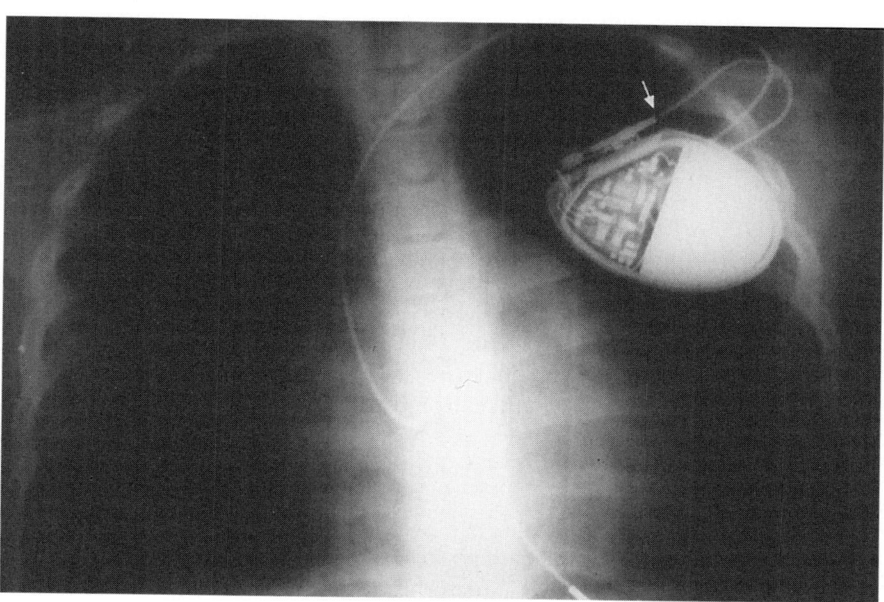

FIGURE 55–16 Unipolar lead fracture in a 3-year-old with complete heart block as revealed by x-ray. The patient underwent successful lead replacement.

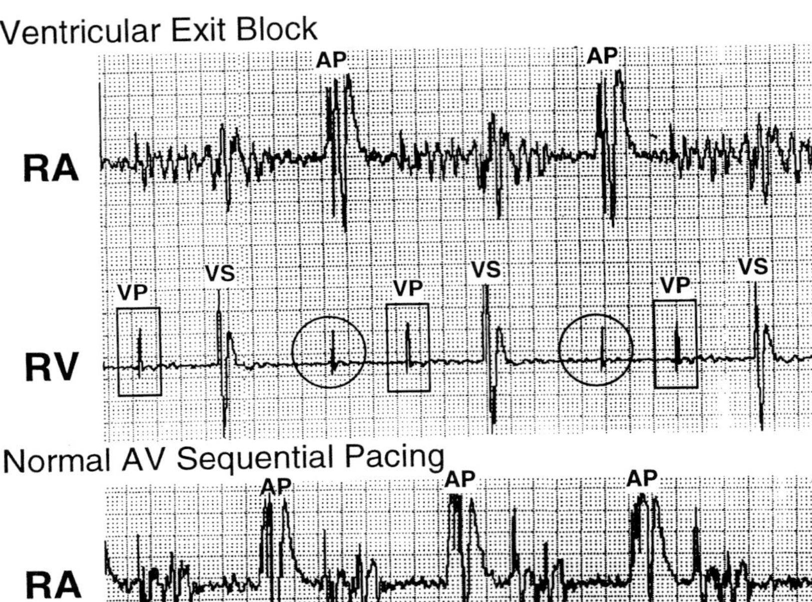

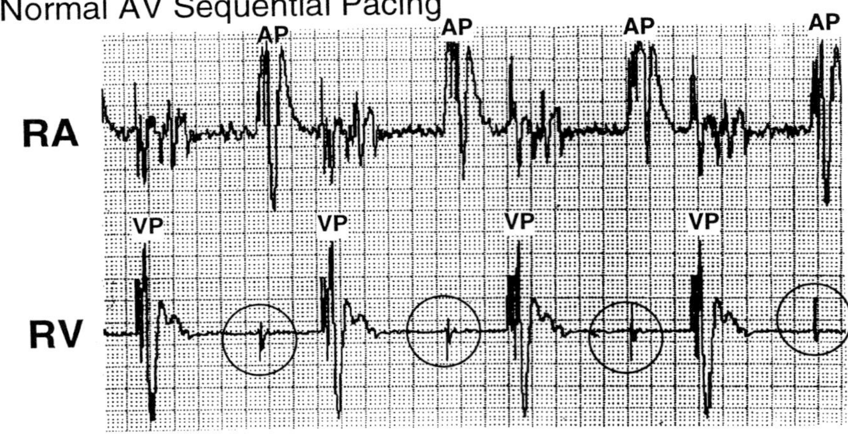

FIGURE 55–17 RA and RV electrograms illustrating RV exit block (above). This patient required atrial (AP) and ventricular (VP) pacing for sinus arrest and marked first-degree AV block. RV capture is restored after a programmed increase in RV pacing amplitude from 3.5 (top) to 5.4 volts (bottom). Ventricular capture increases the effective heart rate in this patient, because the late, conducted ventricular electrograms (VS) in the upper tracing are sensed by the pacemaker and used to begin a new cardiac timing cycle. The circles indicate far-field sensing of the RA pacing artifact in the RV lead.

safety margin on pulse width threshold. Pacing mode, rates, refractory periods, rate response, and delays are adjusted to optimize patient comfort and battery life. For example, some pacemakers allow programmed reduction of the lower rate at night, thereby eliminating unnecessary pacing during sleep. A very long AV delay will completely eliminate ventricular pacing in some patients with first-degree block.

Complications of Pacemaker Insertion

MORTALITY

Death is a rare complication of pacemaker insertion.[53,54,62] Lethal technical problems can include lead displacement, venous or cardiac perforation, air embolism, and ventricular tachycardia or fibrillation.[53,54] A review of 650 pacemaker insertions by the author between January 1984 and April 1993 revealed one perioperative death due to heart failure induced by general anesthesia in a child with congenital heart disease (Table 55-3).

INCIDENCE OF COMPLICATIONS

The incidence of early complications in one recent published series was 6.7%, with 4.9% requiring reoperation.[53] Reoperation in the author's series was required in 4.0% of 480 patients with long-term follow-up (Table 55-3). For patients over age 65, comparable figures were 6.1% and 4.4%, respectively.[54] Lead displacement, pneumothorax, and cardiac perforation were the commonest complications. The reported incidence of late complications was 7.2%.[53]

LEAD DISPLACEMENT

The incidence of endocardial lead displacement with early lead designs was greater than 10%.[54] With tined and positive fixation leads this has fallen to the range of 2%.[8,41,42,53,54,63–65] The overall incidence of this complication was 1.5% for both atrial and ventricular leads in all locations in a recent review (Table 55-3). Secure placement of pacemaker leads is a learned skill, and relevant technical issues have been described above. We have found that positive fixation leads can be applied in a variety of unusual locations with essentially no penalty in terms of lead displacement (Table 55-4).

MYOCARDIAL INFARCTION

Pacemaker insertion is often indicated as an adjunct to medical therapy of angina in patients with inoperable coronary

TABLE 55–3 Results of pacemaker implantation, Columbia-Presbyterian Medical Center 1984–93*

Surgical mortality	1/616 (general anesthesia related)
Mean follow-up	884±675 (SD) days (n = 480 patients, 679 leads)
Morbidity	19 reoperations (4.0% of 480)
	4 Infections (0.8%)
	7 Lead displacements (1.5%)
	4 Exit block (0.8%)
	4 Undersensing (0.8%)
	5 Suspected RV perforations
	2 Leads abandoned (chordal entrapment)
	41 Reprogrammed for dysfunction
	0 Hemothorax
	0 Pneumothorax
	1 Procedure abandoned for thoracotomy (newborn)
Characteristics at Generator Replacement (n = 40, 75±31 months after implant)	
Pacing threshold	1.3±0.5 v
	3.0±1.3 ma
R-wave amplitude	8.9±4.3 mv
Long-term DDD pacing	89% (1109±34 days folow-up)
Causes of DDD failure	8.4% Atrial fibrillation
	2.4% Lead dysfunction

*Models 479-01 and 435-02 unipolar, positive fixation leads, Intermedics, Inc.
Source: Spotnitz HM, Mason DP, Carter YM: Unpublished data.

artery disease. However, an increase in heart rate can be detrimental to the underlying coronary disease. Angina, myocardial infarction, or death can result from pacemaker-induced increases in heart rate of as little as 10 beats per minute.

HEMOPNEUMOTHORAX

Hemopneumothorax and pericardial tamponade can result from injury to the heart or to the arterial or venous system. Errors with the Seldinger technique can lead to such injuries. In patients over age 65, pneumothorax has been related to subclavian puncture.[54] In our experience with pacemaker insertion in more than 1000 patients by cephalic cut-down, hemopneumothorax has not occurred. In contrast, a recent review of 1088 consecutive implants by subclavian puncture revealed a 1.8% incidence of pneumothorax.[54] Deaths occur, albeit rarely, due to complications of subclavian puncture during pacemaker implantation.

TABLE 55–4 Lead stability in unusual locations, Columbia-Presbyterian Medical Center 1984–93*

Location	No.	Displaced
Coronary sinus (to LV)	2	0
Atrial conduit	1	0
RA of transplant	20	0
Lateral RA	27	1
RV outflow—single	22	0
RV outflow—paired (ICD recipients)	11 (×2)	0
Infants—looped leads (<1 y old)	7	0
Children—looped leads	42	2
Total	132	3 (2.3%)

*Models 479-01 and 435-02 unipolar, positive fixation leads, Intermedics, Inc.
Source: Spotnitz HM, Mason DP, Carter YM: Unpublished data.

PACEMAKER SYNDROME

Loss of AV synchrony produces symptoms related to contraction of the atria against closed AV valves and reflex effects. The resulting constellation of symptoms is known as pacemaker syndrome.[66] These symptoms are quite variable, but severely affected patients may refuse pacemaker magnet testing. Symptoms are relieved immediately by conversion from VVI to dual-chamber pacing.

LEAD ENTRAPMENT

Entanglement of a pacemaker lead in the chordae tendineae can lead to firm entrapment. Options under these circumstances include further escalation of force, application of lead extraction techniques,[67,68] or an open procedure. Our experience with this has involved 3 firmly entangled leads in 1000 lead implants. These leads were capped and abandoned rather than escalate the risk of the procedure. There were no untoward consequences of abandoning these leads. This experience taught us to avoid the anatomic center of the RV when implanting positive fixation leads. This problem has not recurred in more than 750 subsequent pacemaker implants.

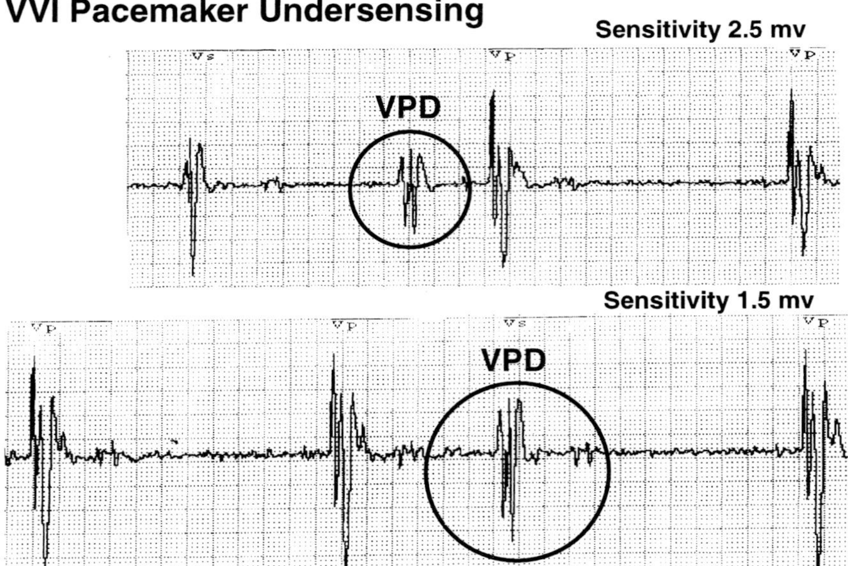

FIGURE 55–18 Undersensing of ventricular premature depolarizations (VPDs) illustrated in upper panel of electrograms obtained by telemetry from a VVI pacemaker. Effect of reprogramming is shown in lower panel; the amplitude of the electrograms increases and sensing is corrected after an increase in programmed sensitivity from 2.5 (top) to 1.5 mv (bottom).

INFECTION/EROSION

Pacemaker infection appears as frank sepsis, intermittent fever with vegetations or inflammation, purulence, and drainage at the pacemaker pocket. Established infection in implanted prosthetic devices can be suppressed but rarely eliminated by antibiotics. Antibiotic suppression may result in temporary resolution of signs of infection in a pacemaker or ICD pocket, but the problem usually recurs several months later.[69,70] Negative cultures from a pacemaker erosion may encourage the clinician to move the generator to a fresh, adjacent site, but the erosion usually recurs. Clinical resolution of recurrent device erosion in such individuals almost always requires removal of all hardware and insertion of a new device at a fresh site.[69,70] The incidence of erosions, infections, hematoma, and lead displacement early after pacemaker is increased by operator inexperience.[65]

PACEMAKER DYSFUNCTION

Mechanical defects in leads, lead displacement, or errors in connecting the lead and generator can cause pacemaker dysfunction. Most commonly, lead dysfunction represents scarring at the lead-myocardial interface, changes in myocardial properties due to tissue necrosis or drug effects, or a poor initial choice of lead position.

GENERATOR DYSFUNCTION

Electrical component failures are rare. Three pacemaker or ICD generator failures have required urgent device replacement over the past 10 years at our center. New pacemaker and lead designs may contain flaws that do not become apparent for many years.[8,71]

UNDERSENSING

This is failure to sense atrial or ventricular electrograms. The result is an atrial or ventricular pacing artifact that should have been inhibited by the preceding (unsensed) beat. In a dual-chamber pacemaker, undersensing may also cause failure to pace the ventricle after an atrial P wave. Undersensing can often be corrected by programming increased generator sensitivity, but this can also lead to oversensing. The latitude for reprogramming can be estimated by examining telemetered electrograms (Figs. 55-18 and 55-19).

OVERSENSING

Inappropriate pacemaker inhibition or triggering in unipolar systems may result from detection of myopotentials (muscular activity). This can occur without lead damage and may be correctable by reprogramming reduced pacemaker sensitivity. Oversensing in bipolar systems may indicate breakdown of lead insulation (see Fig. 55-4).

CROSSTALK AND FAR-FIELD SENSING

A deflection on the ventricular lead immediately after the atrial pacing artifact could be either ventricular premature contraction or far-field sensing of an atrial depolarization (see Fig. 55-17). Many pacemakers deal with this ambiguity by pacing the ventricle at a short (100-ms) AV delay. This short AV delay, known as "safety pacing," indicates that the pacemaker is detecting an ambiguous signal during the AV delay.[26]

Complexities of dual-chamber pacemaker programming involve blanking and refractory periods used to compensate for crosstalk or to prevent retrograde AV conduction from

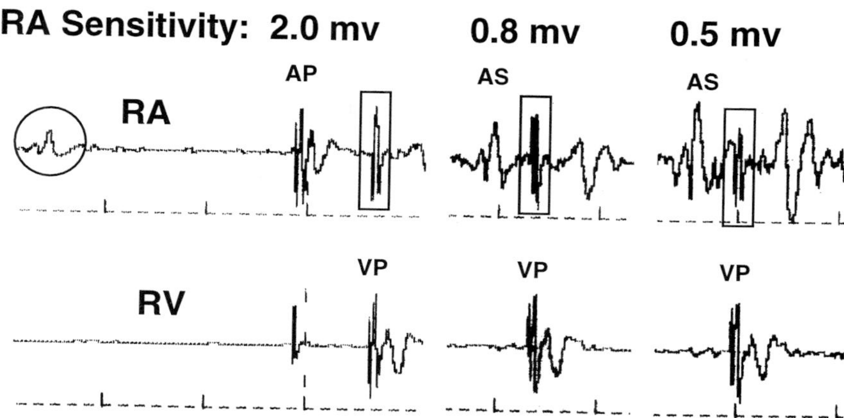

FIGURE 55–19 RA and RV electrograms telemetered from a DDD pacemaker during correction of atrial undersensing. The amplitude of the RA electrogram increases after atrial sensitivity is increased from 2.0 (left) to 0.8 mv (center) to 0.5 mv (right). The P-wave electrogram (circled) is not sensed at 2.0 mv, resulting in unnecessary atrial pacing (AP). Proper sensing is restored and the size of the electrogram increases (AS) as sensitivity is increased. VP indicates ventricular pacing. The rectangles in the RA tracing identify far-field sensing of the ventricular pacing artifact.

producing pacemaker-mediated tachycardia (see below). Crosstalk is ameliorated by bipolar lead systems.

EXIT BLOCK

This is a rising pacing threshold due to edema or scarring at the lead tip–myocardial interface. Pacing threshold is expected to increase over 7 to 14 days after lead insertion, and then stabilize at about six weeks. This phenomenon, which is related to inflammatory changes at the lead tip, is ameliorated by steroid-eluting leads.[8,72] Exit block may be corrected by programming increased amplitude or pulse width, but this shortens battery life. In unipolar systems, pacing of the chest wall and/or diaphragm may result from high generator output.

LEAD FRACTURE

Lead fracture, whether due to insulation or conductor breaks, is often demonstrable by chest x-ray (see Fig. 55-16). Lead impedance less than 300 ohms suggests an insulation break, while high lead impedance, more than 1000 ohms, may suggest conductor problems. High impedance also suggests incomplete extension of the fixation screw in Bisping leads. Office examination may detect impending lead fracture as electrical noise on telemetered electrograms when the patient hyperventilates, coughs, bends, or swing his arms. Oversensing related to body movement usually is an indication for lead replacement or repair.

At reoperation, dysfunctional leads can be capped or removed. Removal of chronically implanted leads is potentially hazardous and results in endothelial venous damage even when successful. Lead removal probably should be deferred unless infection or mechanical problems occur. The probability of lead fracture has been promoted historically by design errors, bipolar construction, certain forms of polyurethane insulation, and epicardial insertion.[59] Technical factors in fracture include tight ligatures applied to the lead without an anchoring sleeve, kinking, lead angulation, vigorous exercise programs, and "subclavian crush."[8,40,47]

SUBCLAVIAN CRUSH

This refers to entrapment of a pacemaker lead between the clavicle and first rib in the costoclavicular ligament. The lead is believed to be subjected to unusual stress during body movement, resulting in early lead failure. This problem pertains to leads implanted by percutaneous puncture of the subclavian vein and may be avoided through cephalic cut-down. Techniques to minimize this problem have been described.[8,40,47]

PACEMAKER-MEDIATED TACHYCARDIA

DDD pacemakers can inadvertently cause a reentrant arrhythmia, pacemaker-mediated tachycardia (PMT).[60] This involves retrograde conduction through the AV node, possibly triggered by a premature ventricular depolarization. If the pacemaker senses the resulting atrial depolarization and paces the ventricle, a recurring cycle is set up that could continue indefinitely at the upper rate limit of the pacemaker. This problem can be minimized by avoiding high upper rate limits in patients with retrograde conduction and by adjusting the postventricular atrial refractory period (PVARP) so that the pacemaker will ignore atrial depolarizations for 300 to 350 milliseconds after the QRS complex. Current pacemaker circuits also have built-in safeguards that attempt to break reentrant arrhythmias by periodic interruption of continuous high-rate pacing. In addition, pacemaker interrogation provides notification of high-rate pacing suspicious of PMT.

Innovations and Special Problems

PACEMAKER LEAD EXTRACTION

Indications for lead extraction include chronic infection or life-threatening mechanical defects.[73–75] Some recommend that any dysfunctional pacemaker lead be removed. Until recently, the techniques for extraction of a transvenous lead were external traction or thoracotomy/cardiotomy employing inflow occlusion or cardiopulmonary bypass. Chronically implanted leads may be densely fibrosed to the RV myocardium, vena cava, innominate, and subclavian veins.

Lead extraction has been advanced by techniques described by Byrd.[67,68] A carefully sized stylet is passed inside the central channel to the tip of the lead where it locks by uncoiling, allowing traction to be applied to the lead tip. A long plastic sheath slightly larger than the pacing lead is passed over the lead to the tip. Countertraction is applied to the myocardium with the sheath while traction is applied to the lead tip with the locking stylet (Fig. 55-20). Success with this technique has been greater than 90%, with a 3% chance of serious morbidity or death. Laser-based systems have also been used.[76] Technical details have been described.[67,68] Extraction of leads implanted for more than ten years is difficult and tedious.

ACCUFIX LEAD

An unusual form of lead fracture affects the Telectronics Accufix lead, a bipolar, Bisping type atrial screw-in lead.[73–75] A J shape was integrated into the design of this lead to direct the tip to the atrial appendage. A J-shaped retention wire was welded to the indifferent cathodal ring electrode near the tip and then was bonded to the lead body with polyurethane. This retention wire has proven susceptible to fracture, followed by extrusion. The extruded retention wire can resemble an open safety pin inside the right atrium (Fig. 55-21). Lead removal can be done with the Byrd technique employing Cook catheters (see Fig. 55-20), laser systems, or an open chest procedure.[67–69,76]

ATRIAL FIBRILLATION/MODE SWITCHING

Many DDD pacemaker recipients suffer from both sinus bradycardia and intermittent, paroxysmal atrial fibrillation

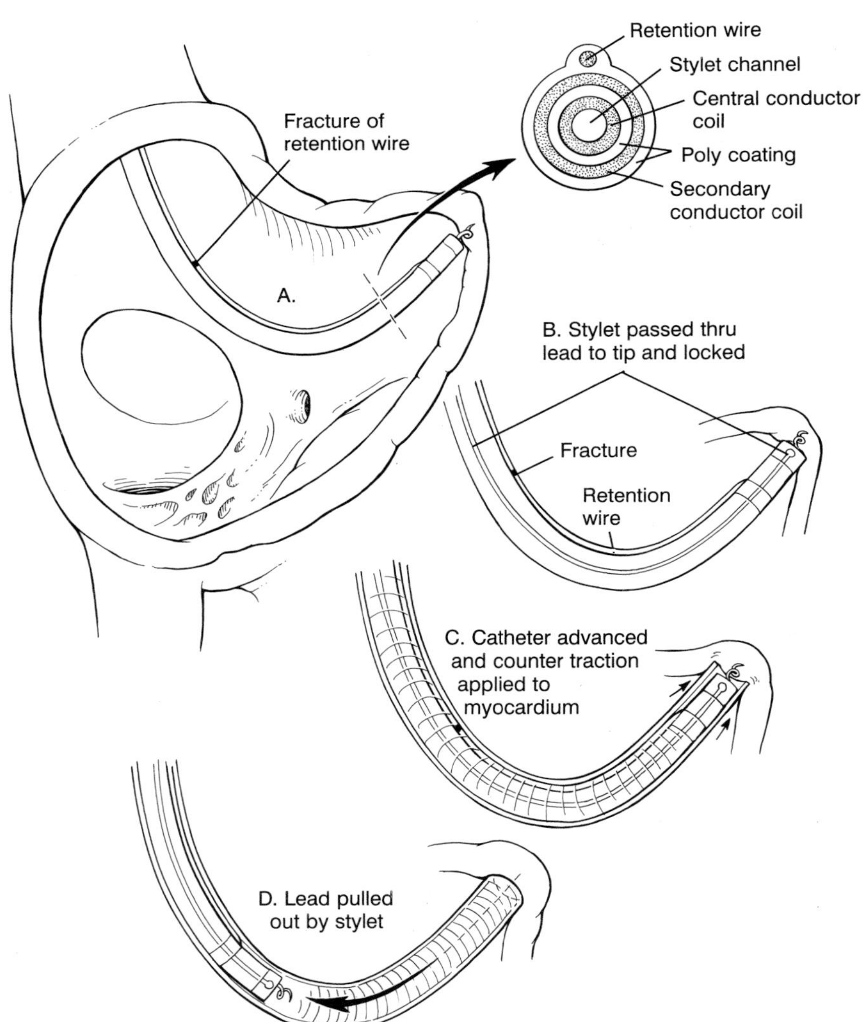

FIGURE 55–20 Byrd method of lead extraction using Cook catheters. Drawings illustrate successful removal or a Telectronics Accufix J lead with a fractured retention wire.

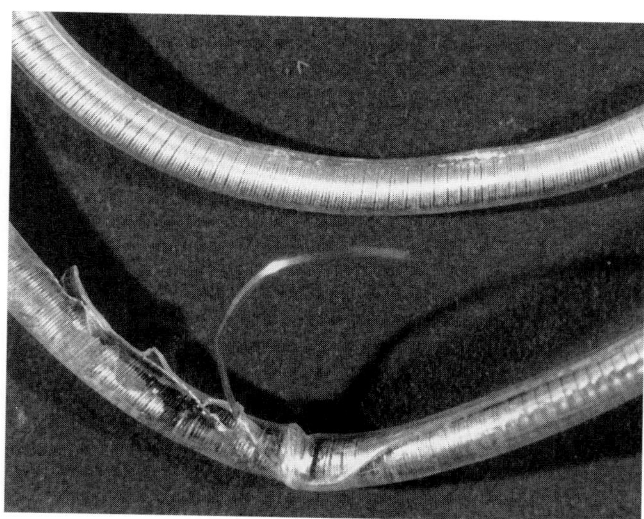

FIGURE 55–21 Telectronics Accufix atrial J leads removed for retention wire fracture. The region of the fracture appears relatively benign to gross inspection in the upper lead. In the lower example, the retention wire extruded during lead manipulations required for percutaneous extraction. The extruded wire is strong and sharp, creating a potential for injury.

(sick sinus syndrome). A standard DDD pacemaker responds to atrial fibrillation by pacing at the upper rate limit. While DDD pacing was initially felt to be contraindicated in atrial fibrillation, the current view is that atrial pacing may decrease the frequency of paroxysmal atrial fibrillation. Mode switching[77] achieves a useful compromise. Mode switching can be triggered by a programmed upper rate limit or by comparing the observed atrial rate to predictions based on the patient's activity level. If an atrial tachyarrhythmia is detected, the pacemaker switches to VVIR pacing until the atrial rate again appears appropriate. Management of atrial fibrillation in the elderly may involve less medications and interventions than in younger patients.[61]

DATABASE SUPPORT

Information to be maintained relative to pacemakers and ICDs includes information for billing and for generating operative notes, serial numbers of leads and generators, records of programming, management of follow-up visits/monitoring, and patient education. A large amount of data should be available at a moment's notice in the event of a query related to a device malfunction. For these purposes, a multiuser relational database, allowing simultaneous access by multiple users, is particularly valuable. A variety of commercial and homegrown software packages are helpful for this purpose.

GENERAL SURGERY AND PACEMAKERS

General surgery in the pacemaker-dependent patient presents a potentially serious problem.[78] Procedures like hip replacement that require unipolar cautery increase the chances of electromagnetic interference with pacemaker function. Preoperative evaluation is essential. The manufacturer and model of the pacemaker should be identified from the patient's pacemaker card, monitoring service, medical record, or x-ray appearance.[79,80] A programmer for the pacemaker should be obtained. The pacemaker's operating modes, programmed parameters, polarity, battery life, and lead characteristics should be determined. If the electrocardiogram reveals ventricular pacing of every beat, abrupt pacemaker failure during surgery must be considered, since electrocautery can result in pacemaker failure.[78] This is best determined by careful programmed reduction of pacing rate or output with ECG monitoring. Pacemaker dependence may increase during anesthesia because of withdrawal of sympathetic stimulation. If the patient is pacemaker dependent, backup pacing or chronotropic agents should be available during surgery. The pacemaker should be programmed to VOO, DOO, or VVT mode to prevent inhibition by electromagnetic interference.[78] Finally, a physician should be identified who agrees to deal with any pacemaker problems that develop in the operating room.

ELECTROCAUTERY

Manufacturers recommend that electrocautery should not be employed in pacemaker patients, because of the danger of electromagnetic interference (EMI) or pacemaker damage. If electrocautery must be used, unipolar cautery is far more likely to cause EMI than bipolar cautery. Unipolar pacemakers are also more susceptible to EMI than bipolar pacemakers. At a minimum, EMI from the electrocautery may be misinterpreted by pacemaker sensing circuits as a rapid heart rate, resulting in pacemaker inhibition. This inhibition reverses when the EMI stops. Cautery can also cause pacemaker reprogramming or reversion of the pacemaker to a "backup mode" or "magnet mode" (see below). Finally, electrocautery can cause complete and permanent loss of pacing, although this is rare.[78]

One approach to avoiding pacemaker inhibition by EMI is to program sensing off (VOO) and to increase rate to minimize competition with the intrinsic heart rate. However, competition with spontaneous beats can occur, including a risk of induction of atrial fibrillation or ventricular tachycardia in susceptible patients. In view of this, the pacemaker should be returned to an appropriate sensing mode as soon as possible after the completion of surgery.

MAGNET MODE

A permanent magnet placed over a pacemaker closes a magnetic reed switch and converts the pacemaker to "magnet mode." Magnet mode is not the same for all pacemakers. In some, a magnet initiates VOO mode, making the pacemaker

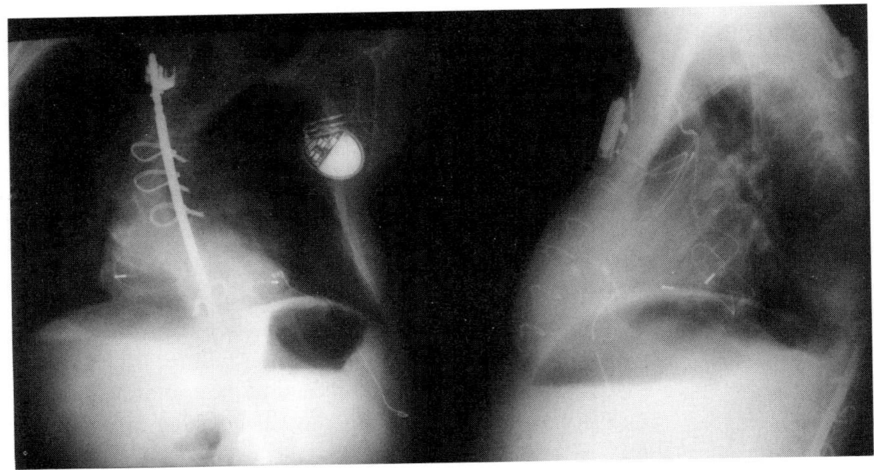

FIGURE 55–22 X-ray of dual-chamber pacing system illustrates successful ventricular pacing via the coronary sinus in a patient following the Fontan operation. This system functioned successfully for nearly 5 years and was replaced at the time of Fontan revision. An epicardial pacing wire, which failed due to exit block, is also illustrated.

insensitive to EMI. Other pacemakers will convert to VOO for a few beats and then revert to the underlying program. Most current generators perform a "threshold margin" test under the influence of a magnet; this investigates the adequacy of the pacing margin by decreasing the pulse width in a predictable pattern.

STEROID-ELUTING LEADS

A promising approach to the problem of fibrosis at the lead-myocardial interface involves incorporation of a pellet of dexamethasone at the lead tip. This improves early pacing thresholds, compared to conventional leads.[72] The long-term (>1 y) advantage of steroid-eluting leads remains to be defined.

ADULTS WITH CONGENITAL HEART DISEASE

Adults with congenital heart disease present special challenges. Pacemaker insertion in the presence of persistent left superior vena cava draining into the coronary sinus is more easily done from the right side, but can be done from the left, requiring a loop to get to the ventricle in some patients.[50,51] Preoperative echo-Doppler or angiographic studies may help define caval and coronary sinus anatomy. Persistent left superior vena cava may be associated with aberrant location of the subclavian vein, increasing the hazards of percutaneous subclavian vein puncture. High priority should be placed on the cephalic cut-down approach in patients with congenital heart disease.[50] Situs inversus and corrected transposition can be particularly confusing in the operating room if undetected prior to pacemaker insertion.

Positive fixation leads are particularly valuable in patients who need atrial pacing after a Mustard operation or a caval-pulmonary anastomosis. The smooth-walled "right" ventricle of corrected TGV also makes positive fixation leads advantageous.[50] In some adults who have undergone the Fontan operation, a small-diameter, positive fixation lead may be passed far enough distally in the coronary sinus to allow successful pacing of the right ventricle (Fig. 55-22). We have also found ventricular pacing via the coronary sinus advantageous in a patient with a mechanical valve in the tricuspid position.

PACING IN INFANTS AND CHILDREN

Transvenous pacing can be facilitated in this population by leaving an intracardiac loop to allow for growth (see Fig. 55-5). Unipolar, positive fixation leads are ideal for this purpose,[50,51] but other approaches have been described.[81] We prefer a cephalic vein cut-down with optical magnification if needed. A flexible guidewire is passed centrally and a 7F introducer is used to introduce the lead. A longitudinal split of the cephalic vein facilitates advancing the introducer (see Fig. 55-9). In very small infants, the external jugular vein at the thoracic inlet may be useful. Others prefer a subclavian vein puncture guided by a catheter introduced via the femoral vein.[81] Thoracotomy provides a third option for pacing in this group.[39] Our experience suggests that infants under 6 months of age are less than ideal candidates for transvenous pacing.

AV NODE ABLATION

AV node ablation controls ventricular rate in refractory atrial fibrillation but leads to permanent heart block. Conventionally, the AV node is ablated first. Temporary pacing supports heart rate until a permanent pacemaker is inserted. Ventricular escape rhythm is often poor in these patients, favoring positive fixation leads, overnight observation on telemetry, and high pacemaker output. Alternatively, the pacemaker can be inserted and allowed to heal prior to ablation, reducing the risk of lead displacement and avoiding the need for overnight hospitalization.

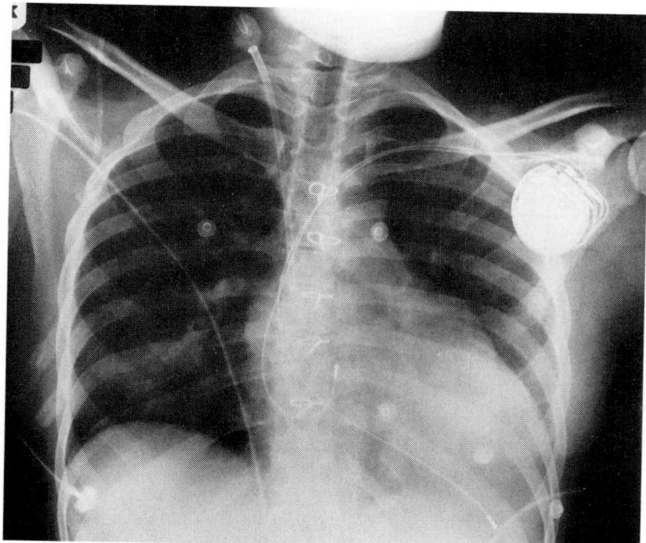

FIGURE 55–23 DDDR pacing system in cardiac allograft recipient illustrates shift of the atrial appendage toward the midline characteristic of these patients.

TRANSPLANT RECIPIENTS

The most common indication for pacemaker insertion in cardiac transplant recipients is sinus bradycardia or sinus arrest, which can be managed successfully by AAIR pacing.[36,82] In our experience, most patients outgrow the need for pacing within two years.[36,82] The surface ECG can be quite misleading and may suggest atrioventricular dissociation, because there are two sources of P waves: the atria of the donor and the atria of the recipient. Whether ventricular pacing is needed can be evaluated intraoperatively by pacing the atrium at a rate of 150. If a 1:1 response of the ventricle is observed, the AV node is essentially normal. The location of the atrial appendage is more medial than usual in these patients, and positive fixation leads are useful for secure lead positioning (Fig. 55-23).

ICD RECIPIENTS

Transvenous pacing in ICD recipients has stringent requirements for lead performance. Crosstalk between devices can result in inappropriate ICD shocks or failure of the ICD to detect and correct lethal ventricular arrhythmias. Although techniques have been described for simultaneous implantation of an independent pacemaker and an ICD in the same patient,[83] the currently preferred solution is use of ICDs with integrated DDD pacing capability.

LONG QT SYNDROME

This is a genetically determined repolarization abnormality that is associated with a high incidence of sudden death. Recommended therapy includes stellate ganglionectomy and/or adrenergic blockade.[84,85] In severe cases, pacing threshold may be too high for rapid ventricular pacing, and atrial pacing may be the only option.[84] ICD therapy is advocated in selected cases.[81]

IDIOPATHIC HYPERTROPHIC SUBAORTIC STENOSIS

Idiopathic hypertrophic subaortic stenosis (IHSS) or obstructive cardiomyopathy can cause LV outflow obstruction with angina and/or syncope. Permanent RV pacing at short AV intervals preexcites the right ventricle and decreases outflow gradients in some patients with IHSS (Fig. 55-24A and B).[21–23] A reduction in the incidence of sudden death has also been claimed with this approach in patients with a history of syncope, but an ICD may be indicated in selected patients.[84]

BIVENTRICULAR PACING

End-stage cardiomyopathy and heart failure tend to progress with advancing age. Advanced therapies like cardiac transplantation or left ventricular assist devices are appropriate for some patients, but biventricular pacing is widely applicable at a lower cost. Clinical trials have demonstrated modest subjective and objective improvement in patients with an ejection fraction less than 35% and a QRS duration greater than 120 milliseconds.[25,86] Marked clinical improvement is seen in some patients.

ATRIAL AND VENTRICULAR TACHYARRHYTHMIAS

Overdrive pacing techniques can be effective for VT, Wolff-Parkinson-White syndrome, or atrial flutter.[84] Implantable pacemaker-defibrillators are under development for atrial fibrillation. Antitachycardia ventricular pacing for VT has been integrated into implantable cardioverter-defibrillator (ICD) therapy.

Environmental Issues

ELECTROMAGNETIC INTERFERENCE

Electromagnetic interference (EMI) can be caused by electrocautery, cellular telephones, magnetic resonance imagers,[87] microwaves, diathermy, arc welders, powerful radar or radio transmitters, and theft detectors in department stores. Any defective, sparking electrical appliance or motor, electric razor, lawn mower, or electric light can be problematic. The importance of EMI is related to pacemaker dependence. Most pacemaker recipients are not pacemaker dependent, so that a brief period of pacemaker dysfunction will not result in loss of consciousness. Patients who are pacemaker dependent and work in electrically noisy environments may benefit from the added protection of bipolar pacing systems.

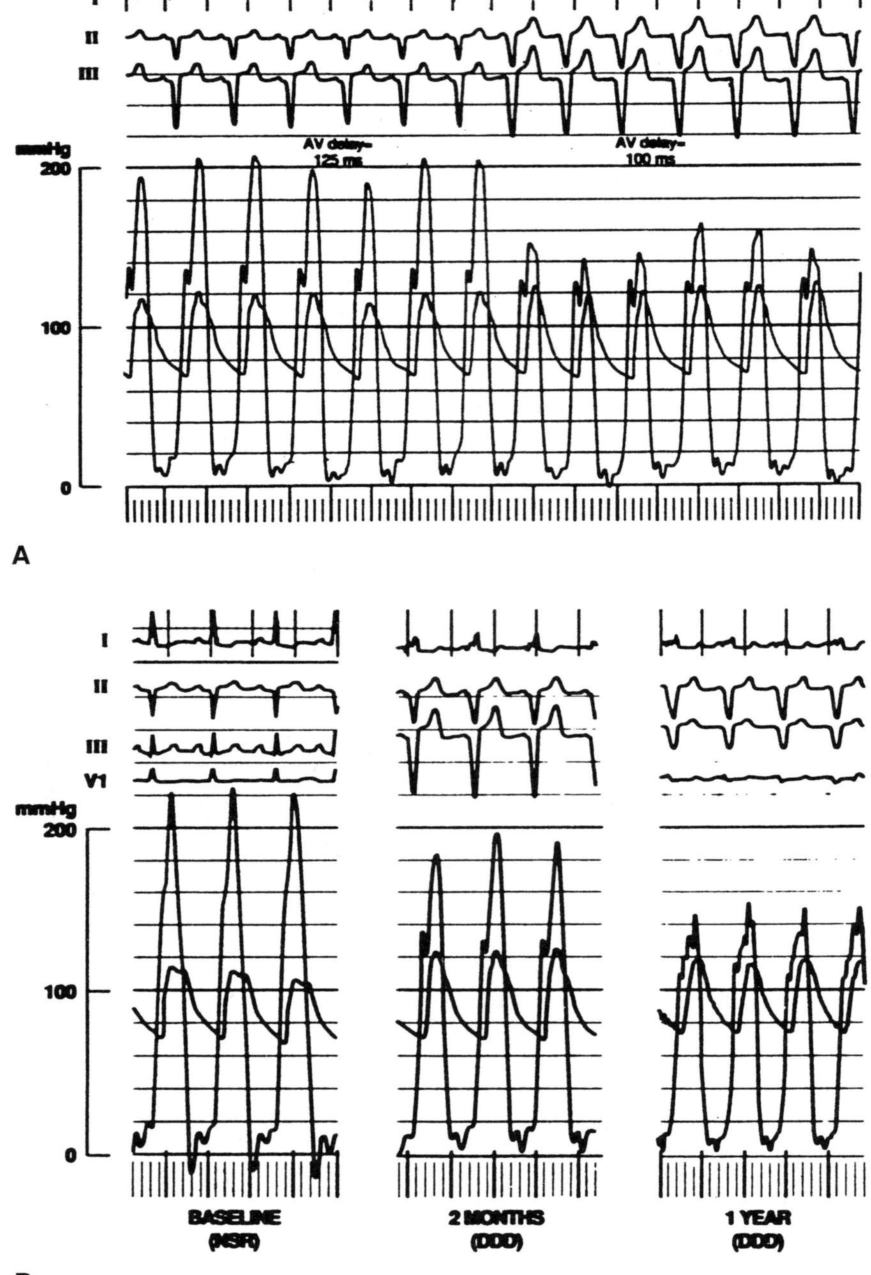

FIGURE 55–24 (A) Effect of reducing AV delay in DDD pacing from 125 ms (left tracings) to 100 ms (right tracings) on LV outflow tract gradient in IHSS. (B) Effect of time and DDD pacing on LV outflow tract gradient in IHSS. (*Reproduced with permission from Fananapazir L, Epstein ND, Curiel RV, et al: Long-term results of dual-chamber (DDD) pacing obstructive hypertrophic cardiomyopathy: evidence for progressive symptomatic and hemodynamic improvement and reduction of left ventricular hypertrophy. Circulation 1994; 90:2731.*)

Cellular telephones should be separated by several inches from pacemaker generators, preferably on the contralateral side.[88]

MECHANICAL INTERFERENCE

Lithotripsy, trauma, dental equipment, and even bumpy roads can affect pacemakers. Automobile accidents have caused pacemaker damage and disruption of pacemaker wounds.[89] Vibration in subways or automobiles causes inappropriately high heart rates in rate-responsive units. Patients with poor escape rhythms should be discouraged from exposure to deceleration injury, such as occurs in traditional contact sports as well as in basketball, handball, downhill skiing, surfing, diving, mountain climbing, and gymnastics. Participants in these activities should realize that abrupt pacemaker failure could occur in the event of lead displacement related to trauma.

RADIOACTIVITY

The integrated circuits of current pacemakers can be damaged by radiotherapy. If the pacemaker cannot be adequately shielded from the radiation field, it may be necessary to remove and replace it or move the pacing system to a remote site.

QUALITY OF LIFE

In contrast to ICD recipients, quality of life is not a major concern for most pacemaker recipients. While many clinics require periodic visits, the model of transtelephonic monitoring with office visits only for problems is highly acceptable to most patients. This latter system involves a preoperative visit, a 10-day postoperative visit, a 1-year visit to adjust output, and no additional visits unless functional problems or impending battery depletion are detected. Some recipients are never happy with their pacemaker because of body image problems, vague symptoms, or concern that life will be artificially prolonged. The value of generator replacement in patients with advanced debilitation has been a subject of ethical concerns.[90]

IMPLANTABLE CARDIOVERTER-DEFIBRILLATORS

More than 400,000 deaths in the United States each year are classified as sudden and likely to be caused by arrhythmias.[91] Michelle Mirowski conceptualized the implantable defibrillator in the late 1960s. He overcame numerous conceptual, engineering, and financial obstacles and participated in a successful clinical trial of his device in the early 1980s.[92] Today's implantable cardioverter-defibrillator (ICD) reflects dramatic and expensive growth in technology. The therapeutic efficacy of the ICD in survivors of sudden death is well established. Increasingly sophisticated clinical trials, clinical experience, and the passage of time only emphasize the survival advantages of the ICD over other modalities, including antiarrhythmic drugs and subendocardial resection. The ICD is associated with the lowest sudden death mortality (1%-2% annually) of any known form of therapy.[93–96] The ICD is expensive ($12,000-$20,000 for the generator; $2000-$8000 for the lead system), and is associated with discomfort and lifestyle issues. The role of prophylactic ICD insertion is under study.

Clinical trials, including Cardiac Arrest Study Hamburg (CASH), Antiarrhythmics Versus Implantable Defibrillators (AVID), Multicenter Unsustained Tachycardia Trial (MUSTT), Canadian Implantable Defibrillator Study (CIDS), and Multicenter Automatic Defibrillator Implantation Trial (MADIT), have demonstrated advantages for ICD therapy.[97–105] Only the CABG Patch Trial, which compared CABG to CABG + ICD, failed to demonstrate ICD benefits.[105] Trials now focus on prophylactic ICD insertion, its cost effectiveness, and formidable implied costs of widespread use of such therapy.

ICDs have been improved, with battery life increased beyond 5 years and broad programmability. Size and weight have been reduced to that of a large pacemaker. Lead systems have evolved from epicardial patches requiring thoracotomy to effective endocardial systems[93–96] potentiated by biphasic shocks[106] and "hot can" technology.[107] These advances make pectoral implant feasible and preferable for most patients. Implantation is increasingly done by electrophysiologists. Abdominal implantation is now reserved for special cases (Fig. 55-25A and B, Fig. 55-26). Diagnostic advances include downloadable real-time or stored electrograms.[108] VVI, DDD, and overdrive (shockless) antitachycardia pacing have been successfully integrated into ICDs.[109] Accelerated development has brought pressure on the Food and Drug Administration to rapidly approve new technology. When the U.S. Health Care Finance Administration refused in 1995 to allow Medicare reimbursement to support device development, ICD development shifted overseas.

Physiology

Ventricular tachycardia (VT) associated with ischemic cardiomyopathy is commonly a reentrant arrhythmia[110] that may be prevented by drugs, catheter ablation, or surgical maneuvers that alter the timing and electrical attributes of the reentrant circuit. Myocardial infarction creates areas of scarring and slow conduction needed for reentry. Other forms of VT and ventricular fibrillation (VF) involve aberrancies of automaticity related to acute myocardial ischemia, increased ventricular wall stress, and myopathic cellular injury. Some class I antiarrhythmics have been shown to increase postinfarction mortality,[111] possibly due to proarrhythmic effects.

Indications

A straightforward ICD candidate has suffered a documented cardiac arrest in the absence of acute myocardial infarction and has been proven unsuitable for antiarrhythmic drugs or surgical therapy, based on programmed electrical stimulation studies in the EP laboratory. However, many patients who suffer cardiac arrest do not have inducible VT at EP study, and many patients with a history of syncope and presyncope have inducible VT but no history of a clinical arrhythmia. Many antiarrhythmics have negative inotropic and proarrhythmic effects. Serial EP studies of drug efficacy have been discredited in clinical trials.[103] In mid-1996 the FDA approved an indication for prophylactic ICD insertion based on early termination of the MADIT trial.[102] If EP studies demonstrate inducible VT in patients with nonsustained VT and history of myocardial infarction, an ICD is indicated. MADIT II results support ICD insertion in all patients with

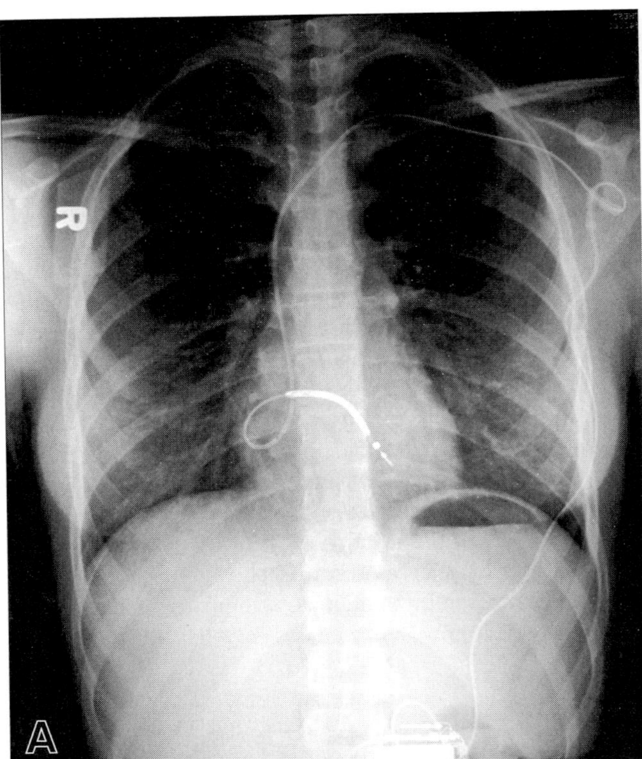

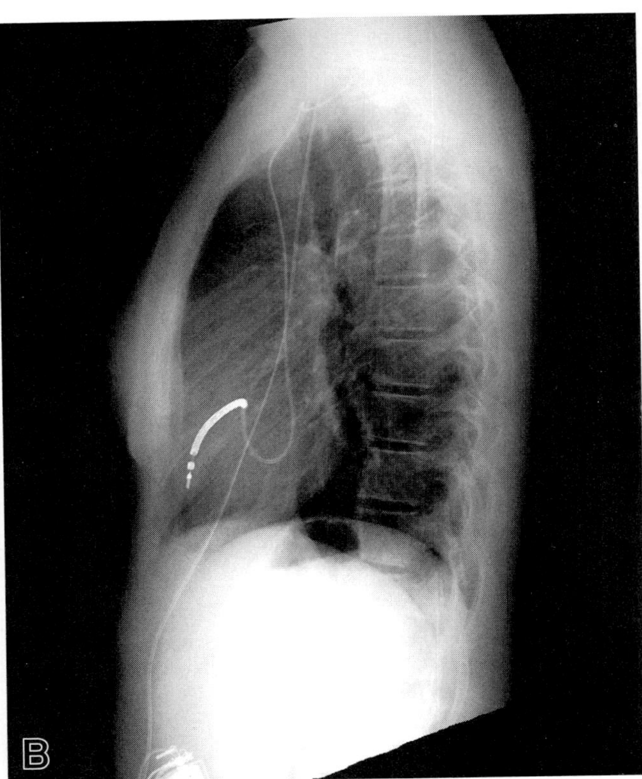

FIGURE 55–25 (A) ICD implant in 13-year-old female with long QT syndrome. X-rays reveal an intracardiac loop to allow for growth and a strain relief loop in the left shoulder. An intracardiac loop requires a screw-in ICD lead with only one defibrillation coil because the second coil is too stiff to loop. This implant was also done using a cosmetic technique including positioning the "hot can" generator in the posterior rectus sheath. (B) Lateral x-ray of same patient.

a history of myocardial infarctions and LV ejection fraction less than 30%.

Device Description

ICDs employ two lead systems (Fig. 55-27A and B), one for ventricular pacing/rate sensing and the other to deliver the defibrillation current. These systems are usually bipolar, but a unipolar ventricular lead paired with an "active can" delivers the defibrillation current in some designs. Algorithms intended to distinguish supraventricular arrhythmias from VT have fallen into disfavor, and rate alone is currently used to determine when a patient requires treatment, resulting in a substantial incidence of inappropriate therapy.[93,112] A bipolar atrial lead can be added for atrial pacing or differentiation of supraventricular arrhythmias from VT. Subcutaneous patch leads and arrays are available for patients with high defibrillation thresholds (DFTs). Leads come in standard lengths for pectoral implants and long lengths for abdominal implants. Positive fixation leads are available and preferred.

The ICD contains a high-energy battery (Fig. 55-27C) and a capacitor to step up the output voltage to 600 to 800 volts at 35 to 40 joules. Biphasic (positive and negative phases) shocks can reduce DFTs. The device includes integrated circuits and a telemetry antenna. A broad range of programmable diagnostic and therapeutic functions are supported.

Surgical Procedure

PATIENT PREPARATION

Most potential ICD recipients would be at high mortality/morbidity risk for any surgery. Therapy of ischemia, heart failure, and systemic illnesses should be optimized before ICD implantation. While the overall mortality in our program has been very low since we began ICD implants in 1983, we have found ischemia more lethal in our experience than ejection fraction below 15%. When ischemia is severe, a patient may be operable only with ancillary coronary artery bypass graft, percutaneous transluminal coronary angioplasty, intra-aortic balloon pump, or deferral of DFT measurement.

SURGICAL APPROACH

The epicardial approach[113,114] is now rarely useful, e.g., in patients who require ICD implantation during cardiac

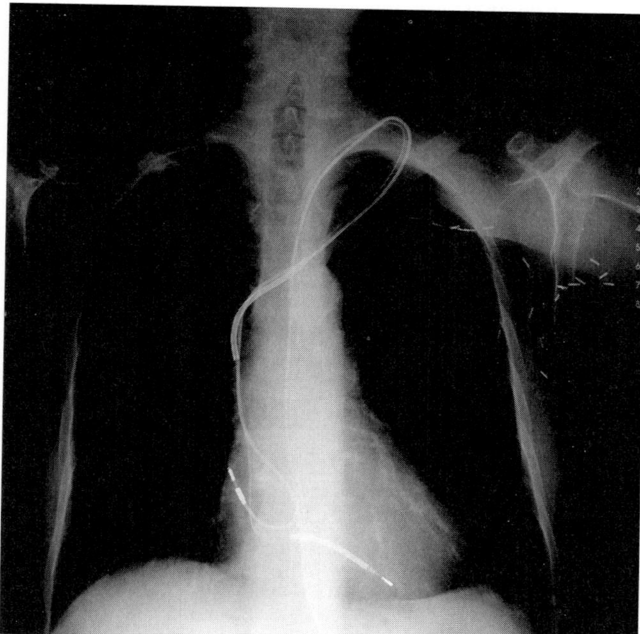

FIGURE 55–26 ICD/DDD pacemaker implant in female with ventricular tachycardia and previous bilateral radical mastectomies. Venous access was obtained via the external jugular vein. Positive fixation leads were tunneled vertically in the midline, which was the only location on the chest wall with adequate subcutaneous tissue. Generator was placed subcutanously in the abdomen. Cosmetic result was quite acceptable to the patient.

surgery. Even this has been discouraged since the CABG Patch Trial demonstrated increased infectious complications in ICD recipients.[107] Extrapericardial ICD patches cause less fibrotic reaction, less impairment of diastolic properties,[115,116] and less potential for graft impingement than intrapericardial leads. Biphasic waveforms, improved leads, high-output "hot can" generators, and ancillary subcutaneous patches and arrays contribute to a high rate of success for the endocardial approach.

MANUFACTURER'S REPRESENTATIVES

The complexity of current devices has legitimized the presence of manufacturer's representatives with electrophysiologists during ICD implants. This increases influence of the manufacturer on the selection of devices and techniques and warrants oversight.

TECHNIQUE

We prefer local anesthesia and unipolar cautery for ICD insertion. Positioning and draping is similar to that for pacemaker insertion with the addition of R2 electrodes over the right breast and beneath the left scapula. R2 electrodes should not be placed directly over the site of a possible subcutaneous ICD patch or array in the lateral axilla. This can result in serious equipment damage from arcing if external defibrillation is necessary.

The most difficult part of ICD insertion for the patient is the induction and reversal of VF. This can be managed with deep sedation by an experienced anesthesiologist, if only a few DFT measurements are expected, as in a generator replacement. When multiple shocks are required, endotracheal intubation gives better control. Intravenous vancomycin and gentamycin or aztreonam are used for perioperative antibiotic prophylaxis.

We prefer a cephalic vein cut-down via a 6-cm incision over the deltopectoral groove. If the vein is small, a guidewire is used to position an 9F introducer. A longitudinal slit in the cephalic vein may be helpful if the vein is too small for the introducer (see Fig. 55-9). The guidewire can be left in place if a multiple lead system is to be employed. Introducer kinking can lead to difficulty passing rough surfaced ICD leads through the introducer. This is awkward, and high central pressures can lead to bleeding until the introducer is out. Introducer kinking is avoided by aligning the introducer with the course of the cephalic vein before removing the obturator; this may require retracting the skin incision cephalad.

As the lead is advanced to the ventricle, VT or VF may be triggered. This is not disruptive if an external defibrillator is available, connected to disposable precharged R2 electrodes. It is important to advance the ventricular lead as far as possible to the apex and to find a secure location. We prefer positive fixation ICD leads for both the RA and RV. During measurement of DFTs, fluoroscopy should be used to check for lead displacement, particularly if external defibrillation is necessary. An intravenous infusion of norepinephrine is used when necessary to maintain systolic blood pressure. Transesophageal echocardiography is useful as a monitoring tool in anesthetized patients. We do not use Swan-Ganz catheters intraoperatively.

We currently position most ICD generators in the pectoral region. The left upper quadrant of the abdomen is reserved primarily for cosmetic insertions, which may include placing the generator in the posterior rectus sheath (see Fig. 55-25A). With general anesthesia or heavy sedation and local, a tunneler is passed from the abdomen to the subclavian incision. Extreme caution should be exercised with the tunneler; it must pass anterior to the costal margin. The lead is looped in the shoulder and firmly secured to minimize the possibility that a tug on the abdominal portion of the lead will displace the lead (see Fig. 55-25A). Hemostasis should be meticulously secured and antibiotic irrigation employed before a watertight closure.

DEFIBRILLATION THRESHOLD

The DFT is critical to ICD insertion and the point of maximum risk. Its measurement requires induction of VF. The DFT should be at least 10 joules less than the maximum

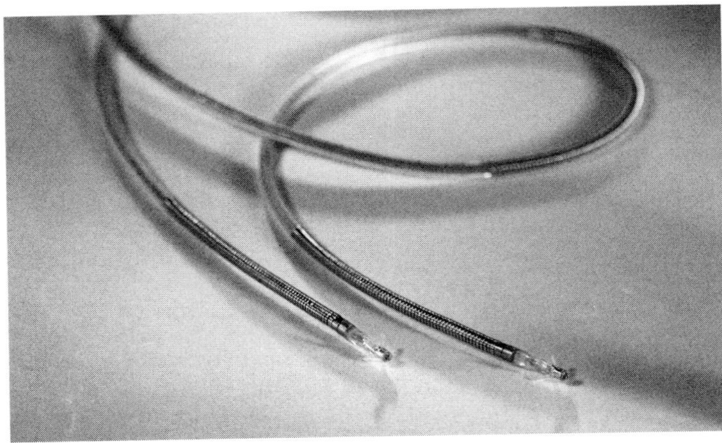

A

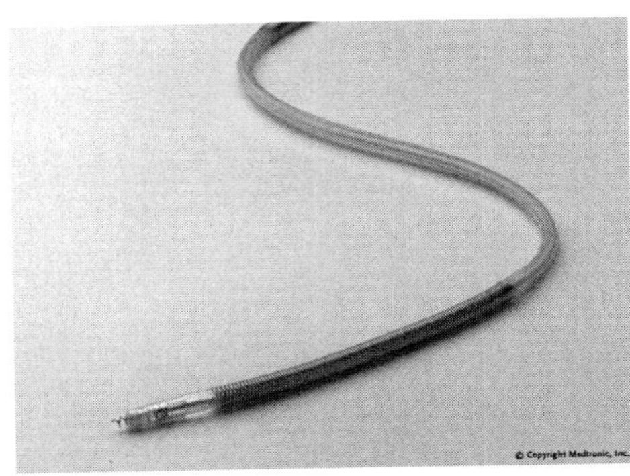

B

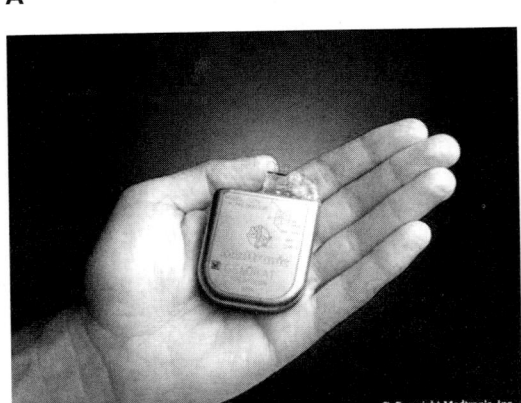

C

FIGURE 55–27 (A) Current generation ICD leads, tined. (B) Current generation ICD lead, retractable screw. (C) Current generation ICD. (*A, courtesy of Guidant Corp.; B, C, courtesy of Medtronic, Inc.*)

output of the ICD. If DFTs are too high with optimized endocardial leads, an axillary subcutaneous patch or array should help by distributing the defibrillation current over the lateral LV. High-output generators and reversal of shock polarity may also be helpful. DFT measurement can, rarely, depress LV function[102–104,117,118] and result in a low-output state. The mortality of ICD insertion with present techniques is on the order of 1%.[119] Complications include myocardial infarction, heart failure, lead displacement, infection, and venous occlusion.

REFRACTORY VF

A left-sided pneumothorax can result from errant subclavian puncture, a ruptured bleb, or technical error during subcutaneous array insertion. Pneumothorax, an effective insulator, dramatically raises DFTs and can cause refractory VF. This must be considered in the differential diagnosis of refractory VF, which includes myocardial ischemia, electromechanical dissociation, and poor distribution of the defibrillator shocks. Inability to defibrillate is an intraoperative emergency that may require open cardiac massage or cardiopulmonary bypass support until a solution can be found.

POSTOPERATIVE CARE

We recommend telemetry after ICD insertion if a postoperative EP test is planned. Postoperative EP testing may be deferred if intraoperative DFTs are low. If the EP test is deferred, pacing and sensing properties of the lead should be checked to confirm lead stability. Wherever patients with a fresh ICD system are located, telemetry and ready availability of a magnet are essential. Personnel must know how to use a magnet to inhibit ICD shocks that could be delivered inappropriately if the RV lead is displaced or a supraventricular arrhythmia develops. We prefer 24 hours of intravenous antibiotics followed by 5 days of ciprofloxacin to complete prophylaxis. A postoperative office visit is scheduled 7 to 14 days after discharge.

SURGICAL FOLLOW-UP

At the postoperative office visit, lead position, patient symptoms, and the surgical wound are assessed. If drainage is present, the wound is cultured and treated appropriately. For persistent sterile drainage, ciprofloxacin or Bactrim is administered for 10 days, and the patient is asked to keep the wound dry until it heals. Patients are referred for EP follow-up.

DEVICE FOLLOW-UP

ICDs require outpatient EP evaluation at 1- to 3-month intervals to cycle the capacitors, confirm battery life, test pacing thresholds, and download electrograms. The electrograms define aborted charging cycles and arrhythmias. Programming is adjusted accordingly. For patients reporting ICD shocks, telemetry downloads confirm proper function, detect inappropriate shocks, and demonstrate electrical noise and oversensing that may indicate a need for lead revisions.

Late Follow-up/Generator Replacement

BATTERY DEPLETION

ICD battery life is now typically more than 60 months. Infection, myocardial infarction, or death can complicate generator replacement. One reason for this is the progression of heart failure and/or coronary artery disease. Replacement is now commonly done under local anesthesia, with sedation during DFT measurement. DFT measurement may be deferred if the risk of the test appears greater than the risk of sudden death. Patients are usually discharged on the same day, unless the high-voltage lead is replaced.

LEAD DYSFUNCTION

The incidence of lead failure progresses with implant duration. Approximately 50% of ICD recipients require lead revision at 10 years of follow-up.[120–123] Problems include lead fracture, high DFTs, oversensing, undersensing, and exit block. The incidence of transvenous lead displacement is 7% and of fracture is 6% at 2-year follow-up.[123] Oversensing can be caused by insulation damage in the ICD pocket. Oversensing is usually corrected with a new transvenous rate sensing lead, preferably of the positive-fixation type. Outer insulation damage inside the defibrillator pocket may be repairable with silicone sleeves, silicone glue, and ligatures.[124]

Patch leads can fail due to conductor fracture or distortion by fibrosis. DFTs may increase with cardiac enlargement, which shifts the left ventricle leftward, away from the original lead system. Insertion of a new, transvenous defibrillator lead, a subcutaneous patch, and/or a high-output generator can correct high DFTs.

Additional Issues

BRIDGE TO TRANSPLANT

The benefits and liabilities of the ICD for treatment of VT/VF in patients who are candidates for cardiac allografting are under investigation.[125,126] Transvenous ICDs are likely to be advantageous in this group, but cost remains a concern.

QUALITY OF LIFE

Issues include the discomfort and distress of repeated shocks and mandatory outpatient visits. These are particularly trying for elderly patients and are an important part of the decision to implement ICD therapy. Dramatic progress has been made in reduction of ICD size, but ICDs remain bulky compared to current pacemakers. While many patients are elated to be rescued by their ICD from a malignant arrhythmia, others find their plight distressing.[127–129] Many ICD patients do not comply with recommended limitations on automobile driving. Fortunately, the rate of accidents in ICD recipients reportedly is low.[130]

COST-EFFECTIVENESS

ICD therapy is expensive, but the cost of VT/VF management in the absence of an ICD is also substantial. The incremental cost per year of life added has been estimated at $10,000 to $200,000.[131–133] Substantial reduction in the cost of ICD generators and leads is necessary before potential benefits of widespread implementation of ICD prophylaxis can be widely realized.

REFERENCES

1. Ellenbogen KA, Kay GN, Wilkoff BL (eds): *Clinical Cardiac Pacing and Defibrillation,* 2d ed. Philadelphia, WB Saunders, 2000.
2. Furman S, Hayes DL, Holmes DR Jr: *A Practice of Cardiac Pacing,* 3d ed. Mt. Kisco, NY, Futura, 1993.
3. Camm AJ, Lindemans FW: *Transvenous Defibrillation and Radiofrequency Ablation.* Armonk, NY, Futura, 1995.
4. Rosenheck S, Geist M, Weiss A, et al: Permanent cardiac pacing in octogenarians. *Am J Geriatr Cardiol* 1995; 4:42.
5. Zoll PM: Resuscitation of the heart in ventricular standstill by external electric stimulation. *N Engl J Med* 1952; 247:768.
6. Furman S, Schwedel JB: An intracardiac pacemaker for Stokes-Adams seizures. *N Engl J Med* 1959; 261:948.
7. Chardack WM, Gage AA, Greatbatch W: A transistorized self-contained, implantable pacemaker for the long-term correction of heart block. *Surgery* 1960; 48:643.
8. Mond HG: Engineering and clinical aspects of pacing leads, in Ellenbogen KA, Kay GN, Wilkoff BL (eds): *Clinical Cardiac Pacing and Defibrillation,* 2d ed. Philadelphia, WB Saunders, 2000; p 127.
9. Warren JA, Nelson JP: Pacemaker and ICD pulse generator circuitry, in Ellenbogen KA, Kay GN, Wilkoff BL (eds): *Clinical Cardiac Pacing and Defibrillation,* 2d ed. Philadelphia, WB Saunders, 2000; p 194.

10. Rodriguez F, Filimonov A, Henning A, et al: Radiation-induced effects in multiprogrammable pacemakers and implantable defibrillators. *Pacing Clin Electrophysiol* 1991; 14:2143.
11. Bernstein AD, Camm AJ, Fletcher R, et al: The NASPE/BPEG generic pacemaker code for antibradyarrhythmia and adaptive-rate pacing and antitachyarrhythmia devices. *Pacing Clin Electrophysiol* 1987; 10:794.
12. Wiegand UK, Potratz J, Bode F, et al: Cost-effectiveness of dual-chamber pacemaker therapy: does single lead VDD pacing reduce treatment costs of atrioventricular block? *Eur Heart J* 2001; 22:174.
13. Stokes KB, Kay GN: Artificial electrical cardiac stimulation, in Ellenbogen KA, Kay GN, Wilkoff BL (eds): *Clinical Cardiac Pacing and Defibrillation,* 2d ed. Philadelphia, WB Saunders, 2000; p 17.
14. Nelson SD, Kou WH, De Buitleir M, et al: Value of programmed ventricular stimulation in presumed carotid sinus syndrome. *Am J Cardiol* 1987; 60:1073.
15. Ellenbogen KA, de Guzman M, Kawanishi DT, et al: Pacing for acute and chronic atrioventricular conduction system disease, in Ellenbogen KA, Kay GN, Wilkoff BL (eds): *Clinical Cardiac Pacing and Defibrillation,* 2d ed. Philadelphia, WB Saunders, 2000; p 426.
16. Sheldon RS, Jaeger FJ: Carotid sinus hypersensitivity and neurally mediated syncope, in Ellenbogen KA, Kay GN, Wilkoff BL (eds): *Clinical Cardiac Pacing and Defibrillation,* 2d ed. Philadelphia, WB Saunders, 2000; p 455.
17. Sra JS, Jazayeri MR, Avitall B, et al: Comparison of cardiac pacing with drug therapy in the treatment of neurocardiogenic (vasovagal) syncope with bradycardia or asystole. *N Engl J Med* 1993; 328:1085.
18. Mitchell JH, Gilmore JP, Sarnoff SJ: The transport function of the atrium: factors influencing the relation between mean left atrial pressures and left ventricular end-diastolic pressure. *Am J Cardiol* 1962; 9:237.
19. Leclercq C, Gras D, Le Hellco A, et al: Hemodynamic importance of preserving the normal sequence of ventricular activation in permanent cardiac pacing. *Am Heart J* 1995; 129:1133.
20. Prech M, Grygier M, Mitkowski P, et al: Effect of restoration of AV synchrony on stroke volume, exercise capacity, and quality-of-life: can we predict the beneficial effect of a pacemaker upgrade? *Pacing Clin Electrophysiol* 2001; 24:302.
21. Fananapazir L, Cannon RO III, Tripodi D, et al: Impact of dual-chamber permanent pacing in patients with obstructive hypertrophic cardiomyopathy with symptoms refractory to verapamil and b-adrenergic blocker therapy. *Circulation* 1992; 85:2149.
22. Erwin JP 3rd, Nishimura RA, Lloyd MA, et al: Dual chamber pacing for patients with hypertrophic obstructive cardiomyopathy: a clinical perspective in 2000. *Mayo Clin Proc* 2000; 75:173.
23. Gadler F, Linde C, Daubert C, et al: Significant improvement of quality of life following atrioventricular synchronous pacing in patients with hypertrophic obstructive cardiomyopathy: data from 1 year of follow-up. PIC study group. Pacing in Cardiomyopathy. *Eur Heart J* 1999; 20:1044.
24. Karpawich PP, Mital S: Comparative left ventricular function following atrial, septal, and apical single chamber heart pacing in the young. *Pacing Clin Electrophysiol* 1997; 20:1983.
25. Leclercq C, Cazeau S, Ritter P, et al: A pilot experience with permanent biventricular pacing to treat advanced heart failure. *Am Heart J* 2000; 140:862.
26. Barold SS: Timing cycles and operational characteristics of pacemakers, in Ellenbogen KA, Kay GN, Wilkoff BL (eds): *Clinical Cardiac Pacing and Defibrillation,* 2d ed. Philadelphia, WB Saunders, 2000; p 727.
27. Lau CP, Butrous GS, Ward DE, et al: Comparison of exercise performance of six rate-adaptive right ventricular cardiac pacemakers. *Am J Cardiol* 1989; 63:833.
28. Kay GN, Bubien RS, Epstein AE, et al: Rate-modulated cardiac pacing based on transthoracic impedance measurements of minute ventilation: correlation with exercise gas exchange. *J Am Coll Cardiol* 1989; 14:1283.
29. Sellers TD, Fearnot NE, Smith HJ: Temperature controlled rate-adaptive pacing, in Ellenbogen KA, Kay GN, Wilkoff BL (eds): *Clinical Cardiac Pacing and Defibrillation,* 2d ed. Philadelphia, WB Saunders, 2000; p 219.
30. Kay GN, Bornzin GA: Rate-modulated pacing controlled by mixed venous oxygen saturation, in Ellenbogen KA, Kay GN, Wilkoff BL (eds): *Clinical Cardiac Pacing and Defibrillation,* 2d ed. Philadelphia, WB Saunders, 2000; p 212.
31. Connelly DT, Rickards AF: The evoked QT potential, in Ellenbogen KA, Kay GN, Wilkoff BL (eds): *Clinical Cardiac Pacing and Defibrillation,* 2d ed. Philadelphia, WB Saunders, 2000; p 250.
32. Yee R, Bennett TD: Rate-adaptive pacing controlled by dynamic right ventricular pressure (dp/dtmax), in Ellenbogen KA, Kay GN, Wilkoff BL (eds): *Clinical Cardiac Pacing and Defibrillation,* 2d ed. Philadelphia, WB Saunders, 2000; p 187.
33. Salo R, O'Donoghue S, Platia EV: The use of intracardiac impedance-based indicators to optimize pacing rate, in Ellenbogen KA, Kay GN, Wilkoff BL (eds): *Clinical Cardiac Pacing and Defibrillation,* 2d ed. Philadelphia, WB Saunders, 2000; p 234.
34. Furman S: Rate-modulated pacing. *Circulation* 1990; 82:1081.
35. Hesselson AB, Parsonnet B, Bernstein AD, et al: Deleterious effects of long-term single-chamber ventricular pacing in patients with sick sinus syndrome: the hidden benefits of dual-chamber pacing. *J Am Coll Cardiol* 1992; 15:1542.
36. Cooper MW, Smith CR, Rose EA, et al: Permanent transvenous pacing following orthotopic heart transplantation. *J Thorac Cardiovasc Surg* 1992; 104:812.
37. Cohen MI, Vetter VL, Wernovsky G, et al: Epicardial pacemaker implantation and follow-up in patients with a single ventricle after the Fontan operation. *J Thorac Cardiovasc Surg* 2001; 121:804.
38. Serwer GA, Dorostkar PC, LeRoy S, et al: Comparison of chronic thresholds between differing endocardial electrode types in children [abstract]. *Circulation* 1992; 86:I-43.
39. Hoyer MH, Beerman LB, Ettedgui JA, et al: Transatrial lead placement for endocardial pacing in children. *Ann Thorac Surg* 1994; 58:97.
40. Magney JE, Flynn DM, Parsons JA, et al: Anatomical mechanisms explaining damage to pacemaker leads, defibrillator leads, and failure of central venous catheters adjacent to the sternoclavicular joint. *Pacing Clin Electrophysiol* 1993; 16:445.
41. Mond H, Sloman G: The small tined pacemaker lead—absence of dislodgement. *Pacing Clin Electrophysiol* 1980; 3:171.
42. Mond HG, Hua W, Wang CC: Atrial pacing leads: the clinical contribution of steroid elution. *Pacing Clin Electrophysiol* 1995; 18:1601.
43. Garcia-Bolao I, Alegria E: Implantation of 500 consecutive cardiac pacemakers in the electrophysiology laboratory. *Acta Cardiol* 1999; 54:339.
44. Da Costa A, Kirkorian G, Cucherat M, et al: Antibiotic prophylaxis for permanent pacemaker implantation: a meta-analysis. *Circulation* 1998; 97:1796.
45. Belott PH, Reynolds DW: Permanent pacemaker and implantable cardioverter-defibrillator implantation, in Ellenbogen KA, Kay GN, Wilkoff BL (eds): *Clinical Cardiac Pacing and Defibrillation,* 2d ed. Philadelphia, WB Saunders, 2000; p 573.
46. Byrd CL: Recent developments in pacemaker implantation and lead retrieval. *Pacing Clin Electrophysiol* 1993; 16:1781.
47. Mathur G, Stables RH, Heaven D, et al: Permanent pacemaker implantation via the femoral vein: an alternative in cases with contraindications to the pectoral approach. *Europace* 2001; 3:56.
48. Ong LS, Barold S, Lederman M, et al: Cephalic vein guide wire technique for implantation of permanent pacemakers. *Am Heart J* 1987; 114:753.

49. Belott PH: A variation on the introducer technique for unlimited access to the subclavian vein. *Pacing Clin Electrophysiol* 1981; 4:43.
50. Spotnitz HM: Transvenous pacing in infants and children with congenital heart disease. *Ann Thorac Surg* 1990; 49:495.
51. Spotnitz HM: Transvenous pacemaker insertion in children under four years of age. American College of Surgeons Film Library, 1992.
52. Barin ES, Jones SM, Ward DE, et al: The right ventricular outflow tract as an alternative permanent pacing site: Long-term follow-up. *Pacing Clin Electrophysiol* 1991; 14:3.
53. Kiviniemi MS, Pirnes MA, Eranen HJ, et al: Complications related to permanent pacemaker therapy. *Pacing Clin Electrophysiol* 1999; 22:711.
54. Link MS, Estes NA 3rd, Griffin JJ, et al: Complications of dual-chamber pacemaker implantation in the elderly. Pacemaker Selection in the Elderly (PASE) Investigators. *J Interv Card Electrophysiol* 2:175, 1998.
55. Silverman BG, Gross TP, Kaczmarek RG, et al: The epidemiology of pacemaker implantation in the United States. *Public Health Rep* 1995; 110:42.
56. Goldstein DJ, Losquadro W, Spotnitz HM: Outpatient pacemaker procedures in orally anticoagulated patients. *Pacing Clin Electrophysiol* 1998; 21:1730.
57. Sweesy MW, Erickson SL, Crago JA, et al: Analysis of the effectiveness of in-office and transtelephonic follow-up in terms of pacemaker system complications. *Pacing Clin Electrophysiol* 1994; 17:2001.
58. Gessman LJ, Vielbig RE, Waspe LE, et al: Accuracy and clinical utility of transtelephonic pacemaker follow-up. *Pacing Clin Electrophysiol* 1995; 18:1032.
59. Schoenfeld MH: Follow-up of the paced patient, in Ellenbogen KA, Kay GN, Wilkoff BL (eds): *Clinical Cardiac Pacing and Defibrillation,* 2d ed. Philadelphia, WB Saunders, 2000; p 895.
60. Levine PA, Love CJ: Pacemaker diagnostics and evaluation of pacemaker malfunction, in Ellenbogen KA, Kay GN, Wilkoff BL (eds): *Clinical Cardiac Pacing and Defibrillation,* 2d ed. Philadelphia, WB Saunders, 2000; p 827.
61. Aronow WS: Management of the older person with atrial fibrillation. *J Am Geriatr Soc* 1999; 47:740.
62. Spotnitz HM, Mason DP, Carter YM: Application and performance of fixed helix unipolar pacemaker leads. Presented at the New York Society for Thoracic Surgery, May, 1994.
63. Brewster GM, Evans AL: Displacement of pacemaker leads-a 10-year survey. *Br Heart J* 1979; 42:266.
64. Perrins EJ, Sutton R, Kalebic B, et al: Modern atrial and ventricular leads for permanent cardiac pacing. *Br Heart J* 1981; 46:196.
65. Aggarwal RK, Connelly DT, Ray SG, et al: Early complications of permanent pacemaker implantation: no difference between dual and single chamber systems. *Br Heart J* 1995; 73:571.
66. Janosik DL, Ellenbogen KA: Basic physiology of cardiac pacing and pacemaker syndrome, in Ellenbogen KA, Kay GN, Wilkoff BL (eds): *Clinical Cardiac Pacing and Defibrillation,* 2d ed. Philadelphia, WB Saunders, 2000; p 333.
67. Smith HJ, Fearnot NE, Byrd CL, et al: Five-year experience with intravascular lead extraction. U.S. Lead Extraction Database. *Pacing Clin Electrophysiol* 1994; 17:2016.
68. Byrd CL: Management of implant complications, in Ellenbogen KA, Kay GN, Wilkoff BL (eds): *Clinical Cardiac Pacing and Defibrillation,* 2d ed. Philadelphia, WB Saunders, 2000; p 669.
69. Chua JD, Wilkoff BL, Lee I, et al: Diagnosis and management of infections involving implantable electrophysiologic cardiac devices. *Ann Intern Med* 2000; 133:604.
70. Molina JE: Undertreatment and overtreatment of patients with infected antiarrhythmic implantable devices. *Ann Thorac Surg* 1997; 63:504.
71. Furman S, Benedek ZM, Andrews CA, et al: Long-term follow-up of pacemaker lead systems: establishment of standards of quality. *Pacing Clin Electrophysiol* 1995; 18:271.
72. Mond H, Stokes KB: The electrode-tissue interface: the revolutionary role of steroid elution. *Pacing Clin Electrophysiol* 1992; 15:95.
73. Parsonnet V: The retention wire fix [editorial]. *Pacing Clin Electrophysiol* 1995; 18:955.
74. Brinker JA: Endocardial pacing leads: the good, the bad, and the ugly [editorial; comment]. *Pacing Clin Electrophysiol* 1995; 18:953.
75. Daoud EG, Kou W, Davidson T, et al: Evaluation and extraction of the Accufix atrial J lead. *Am Heart J* 1996; 131:266.
76. Epstein LM, Byrd CL, Wilkoff BL, et al: Initial experience with larger laser sheaths for the removal of transvenous pacemaker and implantable defibrillator leads. *Circulation* 1999; 100:516.
77. Ovsyshcher IE, Katz A, Bondy C: Initial experience with a new algorithm for automatic mode switching from DDDR to DDIR mode. *Pacing Clin Electrophysiol* 1994; 17:1908.
78. Madigan JD, Choudhri AF, Chen J, et al: Surgical management of the patient with an implanted cardiac device: implications of electromagnetic interference. *Ann Surg* 1999; 230:639.
79. Lloyd MA, Hayes DL: Pacemaker and implantable cardioverter-defibrillator radiography, in Ellenbogen KA, Kay GN, Wilkoff BL (eds): *Clinical Cardiac Pacing and Defibrillation,* 2d ed. Philadelphia, WB Saunders, 2000; p 710.
80. Morse D, Parsonnet V, Gessman L, et al (eds): *A Guide to Cardiac Pacemakers, Defibrillators, and Related Products.* Durham, NC, Droege Computing Services, Inc, 1996.
81. Serwer GA, Dorostkar PC, LeRoy SS: Pediatric pacing and defibrillator usage, in Ellenbogen KA, Kay GN, Wilkoff BL (eds): *Clinical Cardiac Pacing and Defibrillation,* 2d ed. Philadelphia, WB Saunders, 2000; p 953.
82. Raghavan C, Maloney JD, Nitta J, et al: Long-term follow-up of heart transplant recipients requiring permanent pacemakers. *J Heart Lung Transplant* 1995; 14:1081.
83. Spotnitz HM, Ott GY, Bigger JT Jr, et al: Methods of implantable cardioverter-defibrillator-pacemaker insertion to avoid interactions. *Ann Thorac Surg* 1992; 53:253.
84. Saksena S, Mehra R, Ellenbogen KA: Pacing for prevention of tachyarrhythmias, in Ellenbogen KA, Kay GN, Wilkoff BL (eds): *Clinical Cardiac Pacing and Defibrillation,* 2d ed. Philadelphia, WB Saunders, 2000; p 479.
85. Zareba W, Moss AJ: Long QT syndrome in children. *J Electrocardiol* 2001; 34(suppl):167.
86. Reuter S, Garrigue S, Bordachar P, et al: Intermediate-term results of biventricular pacing in heart failure: correlation between clinical and hemodynamic data. *Pacing Clin Electrophysiol* 2000; 23:1713.
87. Lauck G, von Smekal A, Wolke S, et al: Effects of nuclear magnetic resonance imaging on cardiac pacemakers. *Pacing Clin Electrophysiol* 1995; 18:1549.
88. Barbaro V, Bartolini P, Donato A, et al: Do European GSM mobile cellular phones pose a potential risk to pacemaker patients? *Pacing Clin Electrophysiol* 1995; 18:1218.
89. Brown KR, Carter W Jr, Lombardi GE: Blunt trauma-induced pacemaker failure. *Ann Emerg Med* 1991; 20:905.
90. Manganello TD: Disabling the pacemaker: the heart-rending decision every competent patient has a right to make. *Health Care Law Monthly,* 2000; Jan:3.
91. Weaver WE, Cobb LA, Hallstrom AP, et al: Factors influencing survival after out-of-hospital cardiac arrest. *J Am Coll Cardiol* 1986; 7:752.
92. Mirowski R, Reid PR, Mower MM, et al: Termination of malignant ventricular arrhythmia with an implantable automatic defibrillator in human beings. *N Engl J Med* 1980; 303:322.

93. Zipes DP, Roberts D: Results of the international study of the implantable pacemaker cardioverter-defibrillator: a comparison of epicardial and endocardial lead systems. *Circulation* 1995; 92:59.
94. Shahian DM, Williamson WA, Svensson LG, et al: Transvenous versus transthoracic cardioverter-defibrillator implantation. *J Thorac Cardiovasc* Surg 1995; 109:1066.
95. Fitzpatrick AP, Lesh MD, Epstein LM, et al: Electrophysiological laboratory, electrophysiologist-implanted, nonthoracotomy-implantable cardioverter/defibrillators. *Circulation* 1994; 89:2503.
96. Kim SG, Roth JA, Fisher JD, et al: Long-term outcomes and modes of death of patients treated with nonthoracotomy implantable defibrillators. *Am J Cardiol* 1995; 75:1229.
97. Moss AJ, Hall WJ, Cannom DS, et al: Improved survival with an implanted defibrillator in patients with coronary disease at high risk for ventricular arrhythmia. Multicenter Automatic Defibrillator Implantation Trial Investigators. *N Engl J Med* 1996; 335:1933.
98. The Antiarrhythmics Versus Implantable Defibrillators (AVID) Investigators: A comparison of antiarrhythmic drug therapy with implantable defibrillators in patients resuscitated from near-fatal ventricular arrhythmias. *N Engl J Med* 1997; 337:1576.
99. [No authors listed]: Causes of death in the Antiarrhythmics Versus Implantable Defibrillators (AVID) Trial. *J Am Coll Cardiol* 1999; 34:1552.
100. Hohnloser SH: Implantable devices versus antiarrhythmic drug therapy in recurrent ventricular tachycardia and ventricular fibrillation. *Am J Cardiol* 1999; 84:56R.
101. Klein H, Auricchio A, Reek S, et al: New primary prevention trials of sudden cardiac death in patients with left ventricular dysfunction: SCD-HEFT and MADIT-II. *Am J Cardiol* 1999; 83:91D.
102. Prystowsky EN, Nisam S: Prophylactic implantable cardioverter defibrillator trials: MUSTT, MADIT, and beyond. Multicenter Unsustained Tachycardia Trial. Multicenter Automatic Defibrillator Implantation Trial. *Am J Cardiol* 2000; 86:1214.
103. Klein HU, Reek S: The MUSTT study: evaluating testing and treatment. *J Interv Card Electrophysiol* 2000; 4(suppl 1):45.
104. Capucci A, Aschieri D, Villani GQ: The role of EP-guided therapy in ventricular arrhythmias: beta-blockers, sotalol, and ICD's. *J Interv Card Electrophysiol* 2000; 4(suppl 1):57.
105. Bigger JT Jr: Prophylactic use of implanted cardiac defibrillators in patients at high risk for ventricular arrhythmias after coronary-artery bypass graft surgery. Coronary Artery Bypass Graft (CABG) Patch Trial Investigators. *N Engl J Med* 1997; 337:1569.
106. Block M, Breithardt G: Optimizing defibrillation through improved waveforms. *Pacing Clin Electrophysiol* 1995; 18:526.
107. Libero L, Lozano IF, Bocchiardo M, et al: Comparison of defibrillation thresholds using monodirectional electrical vector versus bidirectional electrical vector. *Ital Heart J* 2001; 2:449.
108. Horton RP, Canby RC, Roman CA, et al: Diagnosis of ICD lead failure using continuous event marker recording. *Pacing Clin Electrophysiol* 1995; 18:1331.
109. Luceri RM: Initial clinical experience with a dual-chamber rate responsive implantable cardioverter defibrillator. *Pacing Clin Electrophysiol* 2000; 23:1986.
110. Boineau JP, Cox JL: Slow ventricular activation in acute myocardial infarction: a source of reentrant premature ventricular contractions. *Circulation* 1973; 49;702.
111. The Cardiac Arrhythmia Suppression Trial (CAST) Investigators: Preliminary report: effect of encainide and flecainide on mortality in a randomized trial of arrhythmia suppression after myocardial infarction. *N Engl J Med* 1989; 321:406.
112. Winkle RA, Mead RH, Ruder MA, et al: Long-term outcome with the automatic cardioverter-defibrillator. *J Am Coll Cardiol* 1989; 13:1353.
113. Spotnitz HM: Surgical approaches to ICD insertion, in Spotnitz HM (ed): *Research Frontiers in Implantable Defibrillator Surgery*. Austin, TX, RG Landes, 1992; p 23.
114. Watkins L Jr, Taylor E Jr: Surgical aspects of automatic implantable cardioverter-defibrillator implantation. *Pacing Clin Electrophysiol* 1991; 14:953.
115. Auteri JS, Jeevanandam V, Bielefeld MR, et al: effects of location of aicd patch electrodes on the left ventricular diastolic pressure-volume curve in pigs. *Ann Thorac Surg* 1991; 52:1052.
116. Barrington WW, Deligonul U, Easley AR, et al: Defibrillator patch electrode constriction: an underrecognized entity. *Ann Thorac Surg* 1995; 60:1112.
117. Spotnitz HM: Effects of ICD insertion on cardiac function, in Spotnitz HM (ed): *Research Frontiers in Implantable Defibrillator Surgery*. Austin, TX, RG Landes, 1992; p 98.
118. Park WM, Amirhamzeh MMR, Bielefeld MR, et al: Systolic arterial pressure recovery after ventricular fibrillation/flutter in humans. *Pacing Clin Electrophysiol* 1994; 17:1100.
119. Hauser RG, Kurschinski DT, McVeigh K, et al: Clinical results with nonthoracotomy ICD systems. *Pacing Clin Electrophysiol* 1993; 16:141.
120. Mattke S, Muller D, Markewitz A, et al: Failures of epicardial and transvenous leads for implantable cardioverter defibrillators. *Am Heart J* 1995; 130:1040.
121. Roelke M, O'Nunain, Osswald S, et al: Subclavian crush syndrome complicating transvenous cardioverter defibrillator systems. *Pacing Clin Electrophysiol* 1995; 18:973.
122. Argenziano M, Spotnitz HM, Goldstein DJ, et al: Longevity of lead systems in patients with implantable cardioverter-defibrillators. *Circulation* 1995; 102:II-397.
123. Jones GK, Bardy GH, Kudenchuk PJ, et al: Mechanical complications after implantation of multiple-lead nonthoracotomy defibrillator systems: implications for management and future systems design. *Am Heart J* 1995; 130:327.
124. Dean DA, Livelli FL Jr, Bigger JT Jr, et al: Safe repair of insulation defects in ICD leads [abstract]. *Pacing Clin Electrophysiol* 1996; 19:678.
125. Jeevanandam V, Bielefeld MR, Auteri JS, et al: The implantable defibrillator: an electronic bridge to cardiac transplantation. *Circulation* 1992; 86:II-276.
126. Bolling SF: Implantable cardioverter-defibrillators as a bridge to cardiac transplantation, in Spotnitz HM (ed): *Research Frontiers in Implantable Defibrillator Surgery*. Austin, TX, RG Landes, 1992; p 57.
127. May CD, Smith PR, Murdock CL, et al: The impact of implantable cardioverter defibrillator on quality-of-life. *Pacing Clin Electrophysiol* 1995; 18:1411.
128. Ahmad M, Bloomstein L, Roelke M, et al: Patients' attitudes toward implanted defibrillator shocks. *Pacing Clin Electrophysiol* 2000; 23:934.
129. Kohn CS, Petrucci RJ, Baessler C, et al: The effect of psychological intervention on patients' long-term adjustment to the ICD: a prospective study. *Pacing Clin Electrophysiol* 2000; 23:450.
130. Akiyama T, Powell JL, Mitchell LB, et al: Resumption of driving after life-threatening ventricular tachyarrhythmia. *N Engl J Med* 2001; 345:391.
131. Hoffmaster B: The ethics of setting limits on ICD therapy. *Can J Cardiol* 2000; 16:1313.
132. Stanton MS, Bell GK: Economic outcomes of implantable cardioverter-defibrillators. *Circulation* 2000; 101:1067.
133. O'Brien BJ, Connolly SJ, Goeree R, et al: Cost-effectiveness of the implantable cardioverter-defibrillator: results from the Canadian Implantable Defibrillator Study (CIDS). *Circulation* 2001; 103:1416.

Part VII

Other Cardiac Operations

Chapter 56

Adult Congenital Heart Disease

Hillel Laks/Daniel Marelli/Mark Plunkett/Jonah Odim/Jeff Myers

The steady rise in individuals who have survived congenital heart disease (with or without treatment) into adulthood is expected to create special cardiovascular issues that mandate strategic collaborative care protocols for this swelling subpopulation. If one neglects all patients born before 1990 and those not diagnosed in the first year, assuming stable mortality in early adulthood, nearly 760,000 adults will have congenital heart disease by 2020.[1,2]

Adults with congenital heart disease who are referred for surgery fall into three general categories: those without previous surgery, those with previous palliation, and those with complete physiological or anatomical repair returning for revision of their repair because of residual defects or sequelae from their repairs.[1,2]

In the current era, there is a trend toward surgical correction of congenital heart defects in the neonatal period or during infancy. This approach aims at minimizing the long-term consequences of congenital heart defects, such as myocardial dysfunction, endocarditis, and the hematologic and cerebral complications of cyanosis.[3–6]

There are, however, some patients who present as adults (particularly from underdeveloped countries) without previous surgery. More common lesions in this category include aortic valve disease, coarctation, pulmonary stenosis, atrial septal defect, and patent ductus arteriosus. Less commonly seen are tetralogy of Fallot, ventricular septal defect, Ebstein's anomaly, and coronary arteriovenous (AV) fistulae. Palliated adults are also unusual and include patients with systemic to pulmonary artery shunts, Glenn cavopulmonary shunts, and pulmonary artery bands. The largest group includes adults who present with residual lesions or sequelae from previous surgeries. These conditions may include patch leaks, recurrent valvular or ouflow tract stenoses, recurrent coarctation, pulmonary valve regurgitation, valve stenosis after tissue valve replacement or homograft insertion, or aneurysm formation in the pulmonary artery or aorta. Both primary repair and redo procedures are frequently complex and at increased risk from long-standing abnormal physiology and hemodynamics. Surgical care of the adult with congenital heart disease requires a multidisciplinary team experienced in pediatric and adult cardiology and cardiac surgery.

GENERAL MANAGEMENT

Preoperative Evaluation

The natural history of the congenital defect, the sequelae of previous surgical interventions, and the development of newly acquired cardiovascular disease mandate thorough evaluation during preoperative surgical planning. Long-standing cyanosis and pressure or volume overload may all result in right or left ventricular dysfunction and secondary valvular regurgitation that may require repair. Additionally, cyanosis and underperfusion of the lungs may cause the development of aortopulmonary collaterals that may require coil embolization prior to reoperation. Pulmonary vascular resistance is usually affected by long-standing excessive flow or by severe underperfusion and, in older patients, by ongoing pulmonary thromboembolism. Older patients may also develop coronary artery disease that requires concomitant revascularization.

Transthoracic or transesophageal echocardiography provides excellent information regarding the segmental and morphologic cardiac anatomy. Additionally, hemodynamic data can assist in evaluating valvular function, stenosis, and direction of shunting. In most complex cases, cardiac catheterization is required and pulmonary vascular resistance is calculated directly. Quantitative perfusion lung scans are useful to assess right- and left-sided blood flow. MR angiograms with three-dimensional reconstruction can provide excellent views of anatomy and are particularly helpful in preparation for redo coarctation procedures to delineate the aortic arch and descending aorta.

Procedures Requiring Reoperation

Redo median sternotomy can be hazardous and result in massive hemorrhage if thin-walled vascular structures are adherent to the posterior sternum. We obtain CT scans in select patients to view the retrosternal structures. In some patients, the femoral artery and vein are exposed prior to sternotomy. If the aorta, right atrium, or a conduit is adherent to the back of the sternum, cardiopulmonary bypass (CPB) may be initiated with femoral artery and vein cannulation using thin-walled cannulae. If the right atrium or right ventricle is entered inadvertently, an intracardiac defect such as ASD or VSD could result in catastrophic systemic air embolism. This complication can be avoided by instituting deep hypothermia with CPB, keeping the heart full, and discontinuing the cardiac dissection until the heart fibrillates. In the presence of aortic regurgitation, decompression of the left ventricle is accomplished by cannulating the left ventricular (LV) apex via a small submammary incision. Bleeding may be a problem during chest opening due to the presence of numerous large thin-walled vessels throughout the mediastinum that are commonly found in chronically cyanotic patients. Chronic cyanosis and polycythemia are associated with a coagulopathy due to platelet dysfunction. Chronic hepatic congestion affects the coagulation factors and exacerbates coagulopathy. The use of antifibrinolytic agents such as aprotinin, aminocaproic acid, or tranexamic acid is considered in high-risk patients except when circulatory arrest is used. Autologous blood donation (when not contraindicated) and the use of cell-saving devices are routine.

A polytetrafluoroethylene (Gore-Tex) pericardial substitute is used at closure for patients requiring later surgery, such as palliative procedures or after use of homografts or tissue valves. This membrane facilitates the dissection of reentry and the risk of injuring a retrosternal structure is markedly reduced.

Myocardial Protection

Right and left ventricular hypertrophy, dilatation, or dysfunction may be present. Noncoronary collateral flow is usually increased and bronchial flow can be torrential. Myocardial protection is therefore critical to the outcome of complex procedures. A left ventricular vent and deeper hypothermia to 24°C are required, and both antegrade and/or retrograde cardioplegia are given every 10 minutes. A purse string is placed around the coronary sinus to improve retrograde distribution.

Postoperative Care

The adult with congenital heart disease may present a far more complex postoperative course than the usual adult with acquired heart disease. Both right and left ventricular function may be compromised and require support. Both pulmonary and systemic vascular resistance may require manipulation. For this reason, right atrial (RA), pulmonary artery (PA), and left atrial (LA) pressure-monitoring lines are used when indicated. Left atrial lines are used rather than attempting to obtain PA wedge pressures because of the danger of PA rupture and possible discrepancy between PA diastolic pressures and LA pressure. Transesophageal echocardiography is required postoperatively to assess left and right ventricular function, to evaluate left- and right-sided valve function, and to look for shunts. Ventilator control to reduce P_{CO_2}, inhaled nitric oxide, and milrinone are useful to reduce pulmonary vascular resistance.

Associated Procedures

Many adults with congenital heart disease require corrective surgery after associated procedures. In particular, all patients above the age of 40 years require preoperative coronary angiography. Due to a history of shunts or increased chest wall collaterals from cyanosis, many patients have aortic insufficiency secondary to increased venous return to the systemic ventricle. Such patients should be considered for aortic valve repair.[7]

Other associated procedures often performed in adults with congenital heart disease include bicuspid aortic valve repair or replacement, mitral or tricuspid valve repair or replacement, and implantation of epicardial pacemaker leads and generator.[8–15]

Our preferred approach for epicardial pacemaker implantation is a subxyphoid approach. Atrial tissue is easily identified near the inferior vena cava in most patients. A ventricular site is usually identified on the diaphragmatic surface of the heart. We prefer nonpenetrating steroid-eluding leads that are sutured onto the epicardium. The pacemaker battery is placed in the preperitoneal position beneath the fascia or in the subcutaneous tissues of the left upper quadrant. Transvenous leads are generally contraindicated in the systemic circulation because of the risk of thromboembolism. This is of particular importance in patients with single ventricle physiology.

SPECIFIC CONGENITAL MALFORMATIONS

Atrial Septal Defects

ANATOMY

Atrial septal defects (ASD) of the secundum type are the most common lesions, but sinus venosus defects of both the superior and inferior vena caval types as well as ostium primum atrial septal defects are seen in adults (Fig. 56-1).

PHYSIOLOGY AND INDICATIONS FOR SURGERY

The amount of left-to-right atrial shunting is variable. In older patients, as right ventricular dysfunction and tricuspid regurgitation develop, the degree of left-to-right shunting

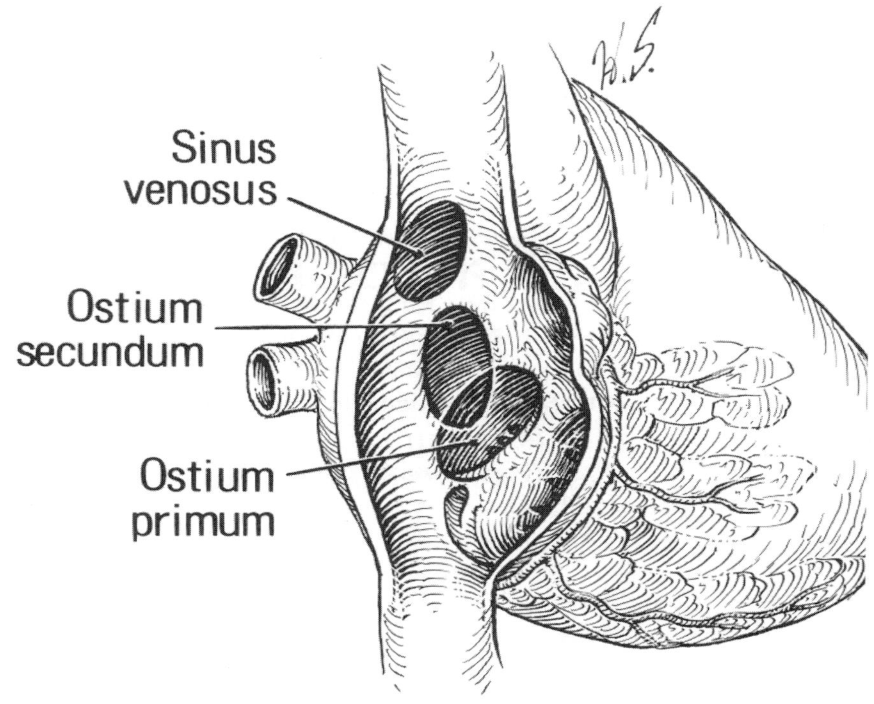

FIGURE 56–1 Diagram showing the locations of the most common types of atrial septal defects. Sinus venosus defects are close to the superior vena cava (SVC) to right atrial (RA) junction and are frequently associated with partial anomalous pulmonary venous drainage (not shown). The right superior pulmonary vein may drain directly into the SVC or at the junction of the SVC and RA.

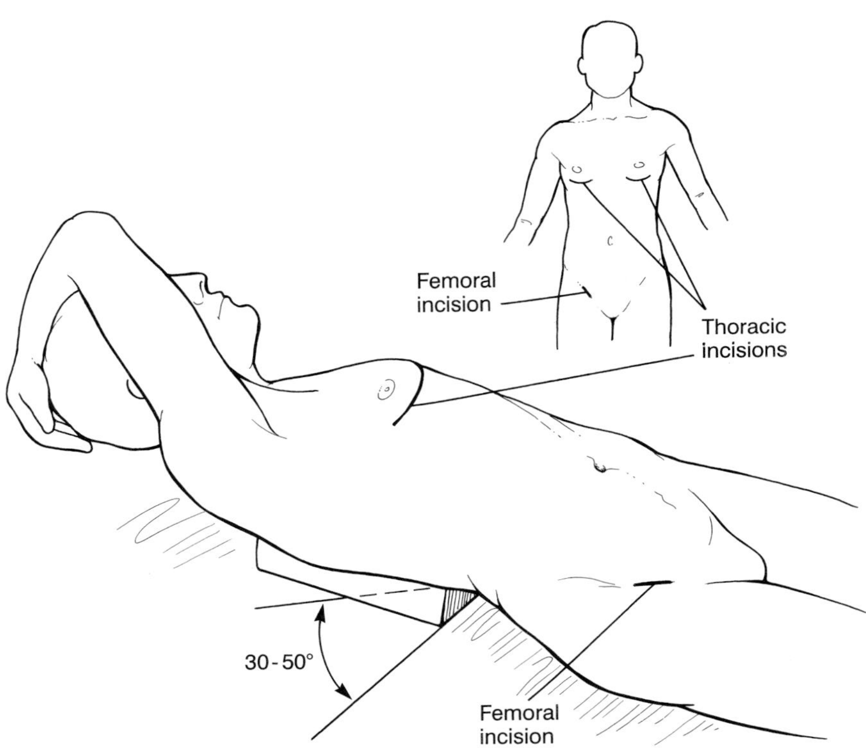

FIGURE 56–2 Patient position for minimally invasive right thoracotomy approach for repair of an atrial septal defect. A 5- to 7-cm incision is made in the submammary crease. An additional incision may be made in the groin crease for femoral artery cannulation.

may decrease. The left-to-right shunt may increase in other patients due to hypertension and reduced LV compliance. Although most patients with an ASD are asymptomatic through the second decade, by the third or fourth decade adults commonly develop atrial fibrillation or a reduction in exercise tolerance, and eventually heart failure.[16–22] It is preferable to close the defect when the diagnosis is made, before the development of these sequelae. As long as the Qp:Qs ratio (pulmonary flow to systemic flow) is greater than 1.5:1 and the calculated pulmonary vascular resistance (PVR) is less than 6 to 8 units/m^2(or Wood units/m^2), depending on systemic vascular resistance at the time of measurement, closure is usually indicated.

About 15% to 20% of children with an ASD eventually develop pulmonary vascular disease.[23–25] If it does not occur by the end of the second decade, it is very unlikely to occur. Pulmonary vascular disease eventually causes reversal of the shunt and development of hypoxia that may be intermittent and severe depending on right ventricular (RV) function and tricuspid regurgitation. Patients with a patent foramen ovale and systemic embolization are candidates for closure of the defect. In the past, patients with pulmonary vascular disease were considered inoperable and were candidates for eventual lung transplants and ASD closure. The use of long-term prostacyclin (Flolan) has allowed some patients to lower their pulmonary vascular resistance and develop a left-to-right shunt. We have successfully proceeded to ASD closure and continued prostacyclin therapy in some of these patients.

OPERATIVE PROCEDURE

The operation is performed using cardiopulmonary bypass and moderate hypothermia. For cosmetic purposes in young women, a submammary skin incision with median sternotomy is used. For the last 5 years we have used a small right anterolateral thoracotomy (Fig. 56-2). Superior and inferior vena cava cannulation is achieved directly through the thoracotomy incision using right-angled metallic-tipped cannulae. If aortic cannulation is difficult, femoral artery cannulation is used. The aorta is clamped and cold blood cardioplegia alternating with cold blood is run continuously to keep the left atrium and ventricle full to prevent air entry. The chest cavity is filled with CO_2throughout the procedure. The ASD is closed either primarily or with a pericardial patch. The right-sided pulmonary veins must all be identified, and if they are draining anomalously, they are baffled to the left side with a pericardial patch. It is also important to identify the inferior vena caval orifice so that it is not inadvertently baffled into the left atrium by sewing the patch to a well-developed eustachian valve. In adults, the redundant right atrial wall is excised and a regurgitant tricuspid valve (if present) is repaired with an annuloplasty. In patients with chronic atrial fibrillation, a Maze procedure is performed. The cleft in the mitral valve is routinely closed in the primum ASD, often combined with an annuloplasty. The suture line is placed on the tricuspid aspect of the defect and outside the conduction tissue, which is left beneath the patch. After closure of the defect and right atrium, extensive de-airing is performed prior to releasing the cross-clamp. This includes syringe and large-bore needles, de-airing of the left atrium, and venting of the aorta. Rarely, if air has entered the left ventricle during the procedure, a small submammary left-sided thoracotomy is made, and a small left ventricular apical vent is also inserted to assist in de-airing. The left ventricle is inspected with TEE for residual air prior to release of the cross-clamp.

Atrial septal defects are closed via a right minithoracotomy with a submammary skin incision. In most adults the aorta is cannulated in the chest. In some cases the femoral artery is cannulated. Carbon dioxide is infused into the chest cavity to reduce the risk of air embolism.

OUTCOMES

Long-term follow-up after repair of isolated ASDs is well documented.[26–29] When patients are operated on at or before 25 years of age, normal life expectancy is anticipated, but this may not be the outcome when patients are corrected after 25 years, when both right and left ventricular reserve are diminished following a long-standing ASD. However, patients with ASD closure after 40 years of age may still realize improvement of symptoms. At the University of Alabama, it was found that age and New York Heart Association (NYHA) class were fairly well correlated, thus suggesting that ASD closure is indicated when the defect is hemodynamically significant (Qp:Qs >1.5:1). Older age per se is not a risk factor for operative mortality.

Ostium primum defects are unusual in adults; however, survival similar to that of a large ASD is expected for partial AV canal defects with minimal valvular incompetence. There is also a group of previously operated patients that may present because of left AV valve malfunction following repair at an earlier age. These patients are often successfully treated with a re-repair of the mitral valve, particularly if a residual defect such as a cleft is present in the anterior leaflet. Some will require valve replacement.

Recently, keen interest in the use of intravascular devices to close ASDs has developed.[30,31] The Amplatzer device was recently approved by the FDA for clinical use. Follow-up of 5 to 7 years is now available showing good long-term results. This trend will grow as the Amplatzer and CardioSEAL devices are currently approved by the FDA for atrial septal defect closure. Long-term follow-up is pending. There is growing interest in the use of computer-assisted "robotic" closure of these defects. It is presently unclear what role this modality will play in future.

Ventricular Septal Defects

Unrestrictive ventricular septal defects (VSDs) are mostly associated with congestive heart failure in infancy, and are usually repaired in early childhood. Adult survival with an unrestrictive VSD can occur if there is concurrent pulmonary outflow obstruction that restricts pulmonary blood flow, or if the development of severe pulmonary vascular disease reduces or reverses the left-to-right shunt (Eisenmenger's syndrome). Restrictive VSDs are more commonly found in the adult and may be the result of a persistent small defect, partial spontaneous closure of a larger defect, or a residual patch leak following surgical repair.

ANATOMY

Most ventricular septal defects (VSDs) are categorized into four anatomical types. The *perimembranous* type is the most common. It is located under the septal leaflet of the tricuspid valve. The *subarterial* VSD is located in the supracristal area and may lie directly beneath the annulus of the pulmonary valve. Because of the proximity of the aortic annulus to such defects, the right cusp of the aortic valve may prolapse into the defect, reducing the effective orifice and limiting the shunt. Aortic regurgitation is frequently associated with this defect.[32] With surgical closure of a subarterial VSD, the aortic valve may require repair with suspension of the prolapsing valve leaflet (Fig. 56-3).

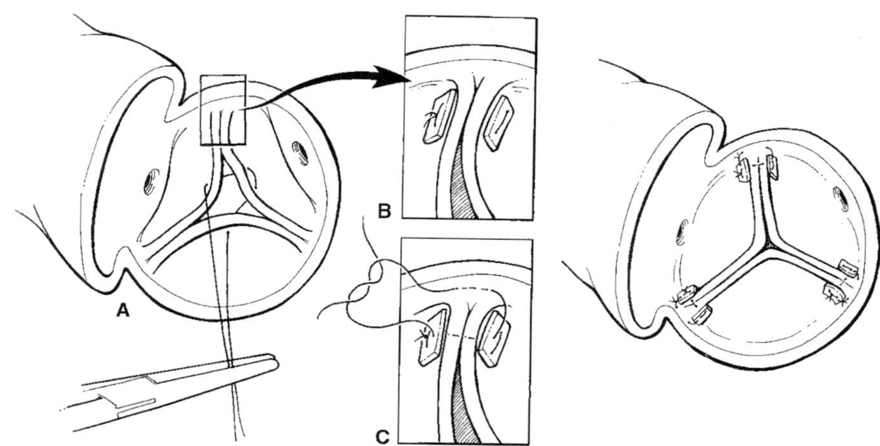

FIGURE 56–3 Technique of aortic valve repair using pericardial pledgetted sutures to resuspend redundant leaflets. Additional apposition can be achieved by adding sutures below the commissures or at the level of the annulus.

The *endocardial cushion* type of VSD is located in the inlet of the right ventricle and beneath the septal leaflet and posterior leaflet of the tricuspid valve. This VSD may have associated mitral valve defects such as cleft anterior leaflet and therefore require mitral valve repair at the time of surgery. The repair usually involves suture closure of the anterior leaflet cleft and reduction of the dilated annulus with annuloplasty. The *muscular* type of VSD may occur anywhere within the muscular ventricular septum. This type is unusual in adults, as it has a tendency to close spontaneously in the first years of life.[33]

PHYSIOLOGY

Use of the term *restrictive* implies a pressure gradient between the ventricles and a restriction to flow across the defect. The amount of left-to right shunting across the defect can be quantified by calculation of the Qp:Qs ratio. VSDs with left-to-right shunting that results in a Qp:Qs of less than 1.5:1 are usually not considered for repair, if there is no other associated pathology (e.g., aortic leaflet prolapse and insufficiency).

Double-chambered right ventricle is an obstruction in the mid-portion of the right ventricle that divides the chamber into two segments: a high-pressure lower chamber and a low-pressure upper chamber. The development of obstructive tissue in the right ventricle is a direct result of a restrictive VSD producing a "jet effect" that strikes adjacent myocardium and produces an area of fibromuscular proliferation. Right ventricular hypertrophy develops secondary to the obstruction and contributes to the progression of right ventricular hypertension. In many patients the VSD will eventually close, as the fibromuscular rim of tissue proliferates around and over the defect. In these patients, the VSD is often identified at the time of surgery with resection of the obstructing tissue in the right ventricle.

In patients with large unrestrictive VSDs, the probability of developing severe pulmonary vascular disease is about 50% by the third decade of life.[34,35] Consequently, patients eventually die of complications of Eisenmenger's syndrome if their VSDs remain unrepaired. These patients ultimately will become cyanotic as a result of right-to-left shunting, and the only surgical options available at that point are either heart-lung transplantation or lung transplantation with repair of the VSD. A pulmonary vascular resistance greater than 6 units/m^{2}is considered a high risk for isolated VSD closure. Preoperative long-term prostacyclin (Flolan) infusion may lower the pulmonary vascular resistance in some patients.

PREOPERATIVE EVALUATION

An adult patient with a VSD should be evaluated by chest radiograph, echocardiography, and possibly cardiac catheterization. A chest radiograph may show an enlarged right heart shadow and right ventricular hypertrophy. It may also reveal chronic changes in the pulmonary vasculature prompting further evaluation by catheterization. Transthoracic and transesophageal echocardiography are both useful in defining VSDs anatomically and identifying associated lesions.[36] An estimate of the pulmonary artery pressures may also be obtained. Right and left heart catheterization is useful to confirm the anatomical findings and to accurately measure the pulmonary vascular resistence and estimate the Qp:Qs. In patients more than 40 years old or in those with increased risk factors, coronary artery disease must also be excluded by angiography.

INDICATIONS FOR SURGERY

Adults with small restrictive VSDs who are asymptomatic often require no surgical intervention and should receive endocarditis prophylaxis as necessary. In general, if the Qp:Qs is greater than 1.5:1 and the calculated pulmonary vascular resistance is under 6 units/m^2, surgical closure of a VSD can be performed safely and is recommended. The development of a double-chambered right ventricle with outflow obstruction is also an indication for operative intervention. The occurrence of infective endocarditis in an adult with a restrictive VSD is a rare but compelling indication for repair of the defect. In adults with VSD and Eisenmenger's syndrome, heart-lung transplantation or lung transplantation with closure of the defect may be considered.

OPERATIVE PROCEDURE

Operative repair of VSDs is performed on cardiopulmonary bypass with moderate systemic hypothermia and blood cardioplegia for myocardial protection. Most adults with a perimembranous, inlet, and/or muscular VSD can have the defect repaired through the tricuspid valve annulus. If the edges of the defect are difficult to visualize due to multiple attachments of the septal leaflet to the edges of the defect, the septal leaflet may be incised at its base adjacent to the annulus, exposing the VSD under the septal leaflet. Subarterial VSDs may be approached through the pulmonary valve or the right ventricular outflow tract. The patch material for closure of VSDs may be synthetic (e.g., Gore-Tex, Dacron, etc.), or glutaraldehyde-treated autologous pericardium, which we have preferred for 10 years. Postoperatively, elevated pulmonary artery pressures may be treated with inhaled nitric oxide. Currently, transcatheter closure of VSDs remains experimental.[37,38]

OUTCOMES

Long-term follow-up is recommended to monitor pulmonary artery pressures in those adult patients with large VSDs that are repaired late in life.[39] This is achieved echocardiographically if there is a mild tricuspid regurgitation from which to calculate the RV pressure or by measuring the pulmonary-valve opening time. The pulmonary vascular resistance (PVR) may continue to rise after VSD closure, resulting in systemic or suprasystemic right ventricular pressures. This may eventually cause the onset of angina, right heart failure, or even sudden death.

At UCLA, we have repaired 52 VSDs in patients aged 16 to 67 years without mortality. In most patients, the VSD repair was combined with additional procedures such as aortic valve repair, pulmonary valve replacement, and tricuspid valve repair. Except in patients with congenitally corrected transposition, the incidence of complete heart block following VSD closure is approximately 1%. Overall, the long-term outcome for these patients has been excellent.

Patent Ductus Arteriosus

NATURAL HISTORY AND INDICATIONS FOR SURGERY

Isolated patent ductus arteriosus (PDA) may present with congestive heart failure by the third or fourth decade of life.[40] Occasionally, the ductus may become aneurysmal secondary to flow characteristics. The aortic end of the PDA is usually calcified in the older adult patient. A long-standing left-to-right shunt may lead to pulmonary vascular disease. Cumulative death rate in childhood is about 0.5% per year. This doubles to 1% by adulthood and increases to 2% to 4% by midlife. There is always a risk of endocarditis (regardless of the PDA size) that is dependent on the presence of abnormal flow. Adults with large PDAs may develop Eisenmenger's syndrome and the classic finding of differential cyanosis in the lower body. It is imperative to determine pulmonary vascular resistance and reactivity preoperatively. If the resistance is greater than 6 to 8 units/m^2, the ductus should not be closed, and the patient may be considered for lung or heart-lung transplantation.

OPERATIVE PROCEDURE

Surgical closure of a PDA is usually carried out via a small posterior thoracotomy. Thoracoscopic procedures are probably not appropriate for the adult because of the frequency of calcification and the greater risk of rupture while ligating the ductus.[41,42] In patients over 40 years of age, or in the presence of severe ductal calcification, consideration should be given to performing PDA ligation via a median sternotomy using cardiopulmonary bypass.[43,44] During cooling, the ductus is occluded by finger pressure on the PA and the branch pulmonary arteries are snared. This prevents steal from the descending aorta. The ductus is exposed via an incision in the PA. Using low flow, the ductus is closed on the PA side with horizontal pledgeted mattress sutures, or the PA defect is patched with glutaraldehyde-treated pericardium or a Gore-Tex patch.

Patients with Eisenmenger's syndrome may be candidates for either single or double lung transplantation combined with PDA closure or heart-lung transplantation if there is significant ventricular dysfunction and tricuspid valve regurgitation. Catheter closure using coils or other devices may be possible depending on the size and length of the ductus.[45–48]

Coarctation of the Aorta

ANATOMY

Aortic coarctation in adults usually presents with upper-body hypertension typically in the second or third decade of life.[49] Although these patients comprise a selected group who have survived free of complications beyond childhood, long-term complications include aneurysm formation of the aorta and aneurysmal dilatation of intercostal arteries, which may eventually rupture. This latter anomaly is important because the initial portion of these arteries should be occluded at the time of surgery if they appear disproportionately enlarged. Other complications include premature coronary artery disease, left ventricular hypertrophy, aortic dissection and rupture, endocarditis, and intracranial hemorrhage. The aorta distal to the coarctation site is frequently dilated and thin walled, and is prone to late aneurysm formation after repair. There is usually extensive collateral circulation in adults with coartcation. The source is mainly from branches of the subclavian artery and internal mammary arteries, and intercostal chest-wall circulation. Collateral flow *into* the descending aorta is dependent on enlarged intercostals at the level of the third and fourth ribs beyond the coarctation.

NATURAL HISTORY AND INDICATIONS FOR SURGERY

In adults with coarctation, congestive heart failure may develop from long-standing hypertension. Up to 40% of patients have an associated bicuspid aortic valve that also may become stenotic and/or incompetent.[9] If aortic coarctation is left untreated, 90% of patients eventually die by the age of 50 due to cardiac causes or stroke. The oldest patient in our series was 81 years old. Repair also may be required for patients who have had previous coarctation repairs with recurrence or for patients who have developed recurrence after previous balloon aortoplasty. Residual coarctation following repair in childhood is usually due to failure of growth of the anastomosis or technical factors such as a short subclavian flap aortoplasty. In patients who were initially treated with a patch, aneurysm formation may occur and require reoperation. Surgical repair is indicated when the gradient across the coarctation is greater than or equal to 30 mm Hg at rest.[50] If the gradient is less and the anatomical obstruction severe, an exercise test will reveal a more severe gradient, and repair is indicated.

PREOPERATIVE EVALUATION

Echocardiography is performed to evaluate the aortic valve, ventricular function and hypertrophy, and the aorta. In adults, magnetic resonance angiography with

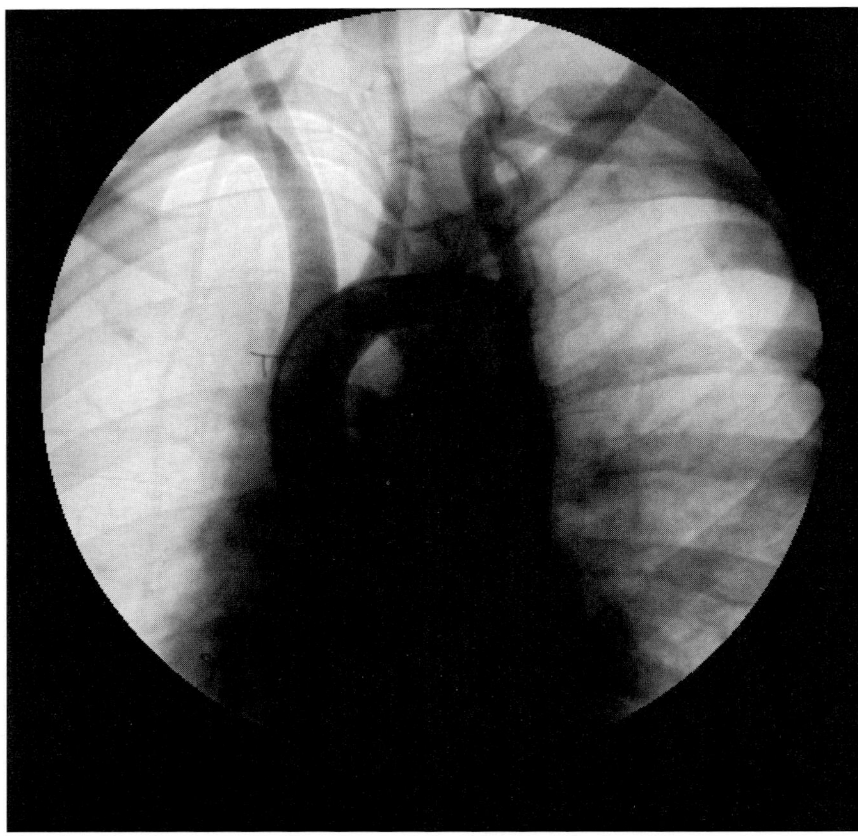

FIGURE 56–4 Angiogram of a 27-year-old patient who presented with residual coarctation after initial repair in which a 16-mm interposition graft was inserted. She presented with stenosis at the distal transverse arch and at the interposition graft with proximal hypertension. Repair using a left atrial to aortic bypass circuit involved repairing the distal arch and replacing the graft with a 20-mm Gore-Tex conduit and extended anastomosis.

three-dimensional computerized reconstruction to assess the transverse arch, isthmus, and descending aorta is often useful (Fig. 56-4).

OPERATIVE PROCEDURE

The preferred method is resection with extended end-to-end anastomosis (Fig. 56-5), although patch repair is used for reoperations or where the collaterals are particularly enlarged and difficult to mobilize.[49,51–53] Tube-graft interposition is used when indicated to relieve long segments of obstruction. Special precautions are taken to reduce the major risk of spinal cord ischemia. Arterial lines are placed in the upper and lower extremities for monitoring blood pressure during aortic clamping. The distal pressure should be maintained above 50 mm Hg throughout the procedure. Somatosensory evoked potentials (SSEPs) are monitored intraoperatively to aid in the decision to use extracorporeal circulation to help prevent spinal cord ischemia during aortic cross-clamping. In extensive reoperations or operations for aneurysms, the cerebrospinal fluid (CSF) pressure is monitored by catheter, and the fluid is allowed to drain if pressure exceeds 10 cm H_2O (essentially central venous pressure). The CSF pressure is monitored for 24 hours postoperatively. The goal is to optimize perioperative perfusion of the spinal cord by increasing the pressure gradient during and after aortic clamping.

The patient is placed on a temperature-regulated blanket and cooled to 33°C to 34°C. Cold saline is used to bathe the left chest cavity to aid in cooling, and the room is cooled. Positioning for the left thoracotomy is important in that one must prep and drape the groins to have access to the femoral arteries if left atrial-to-femoral artery (or descending aorta) bypass becomes necessary during the operation. One must carefully identify chest-wall collaterals, which can bleed massively and which must be ligated individually during the thoracotomy.

The aorta is mobilized extensively, and the ligamentum arteriosum is divided and oversewn. Large intercostal branches are identified and encircled in preparation for snaring. On induction of anesthesia, the patient is given 30 mg/kg of methylprednisolone sodium succinate and lidocaine 2mg/1kg IV, as well as 8 g of mannitol. The patient is anticoagulated with 1 mg/kg of heparin. The aorta is clamped when the rectal temperature is 34°C or below. Once the aorta is clamped proximally and distally, if the distal pressure is below 50 mm Hg, distal aortic bypass is instituted. The distal pressure is maintained above 60 mm Hg. This consists of left atrial-to-descending aortic bypass using a centrifugal pump. In more complex redo or aneurysm procedures, pulmonary artery to descending aortic bypass can be used with an oxygenator. Upper extremity pressure is maintained at about 120 mm Hg systolic. Once the aortic coarctation is resected,

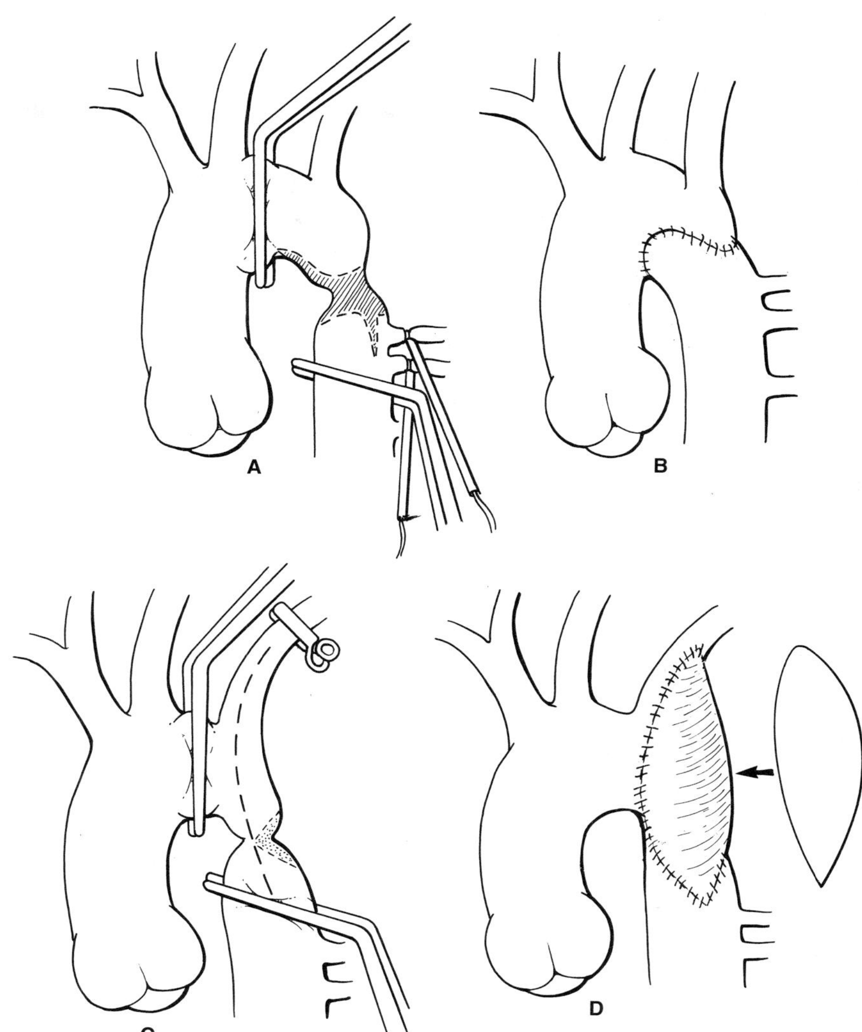

FIGURE 56–5 Resection of coarctation of the aorta. (A,B) With extended end-to-end anastomosis. (C,D) After excision of the coarctation site and reconstruction of the posterior wall by end-to-end anastomosis, a glutaraldehyde-treated autologous pericardial patch is used to enlarge the isthmus and the site of coarctation repair. The patch is measured to avoid excessive dilatation, which can result in late aneurysm formation.

reconstruction with a tube graft or end-to-end anastomosis is carried out with 4-0 polypropylene suture mounted on a small needle.

For patients undergoing reoperation for recurrent coarctation, mobilization of the aorta for end-to-end anastomosis may be difficult and cause excessive blood loss. In these patients, the aorta is clamped proximal to the left subclavian artery, and a glutaraldehyde-treated autologous pericardial patch may be used to enlarge the aorta from the base of the subclavian artery to the distal aorta. An excessively large patch should be avoided to prevent late aneurysm development.

There should be no gradient between upper and lower extremities upon release of the clamps. During closure, special care is taken to control intrathoracic bleeding and to check chest tube and pericostal suture sites.

Hypertension is controlled and is treated aggressively in the intensive care unit. Abdominal pain and distension may be present in 5% of patients postoperatively. Management is usually conservative. The patient is given nothing by mouth for at least 24 hours postoperatively until bowel sounds return.

In older patients who have a coarctation and also require coronary revascularization, we prefer a median sternotomy approach with cannulation of both the ascending aorta and the femoral artery. After completing the coronary revascularization, an adequately sized Dacron graft can be placed between the ascending aorta and the proximal abdominal aorta through the diaphragm. Another option to consider is a clamshell-type incision to access the descending thoracic aorta and the mediastinum simultaneously.

OUTCOMES

Outcome following repair is generally good, and follow-up may be assisted with transesophageal echocardiogram, computed tomographic (CT) scan, or magnetic resonance imaging (MRI). The latter is useful to detect aneurysm formation or recoarctation.[54,55] *Recoarctation* is defined as a gradient greater than 20 to 30 mm Hg at rest.. The possibility of coronary disease and systemic hypertension requires lifelong monitoring.

Catheter-based techniques are being used for both primary coarctations and recurrences.[56–58] Residual mild gradients are common after stenting primary coarctations and we therefore prefer surgical therapy.[49] For selected recurrent coarctations, stenting may be the preferred method provided that an excellent anatomical relief of the obstruction can be achieved.[59]

Tetralogy of Fallot

Tetralogy of Fallot (TOF) is the most common cyanotic heart defect in children, constituting approximately 10% of all congenital heart disease. It is, therefore, one of the most common cyanotic congenital heart defects found in adults. Successful repair of TOF in childhood has spanned almost four decades, with many of those patients now returning as adults for reoperation.[60–69] These patients constitute the majority of adults presenting for surgical intervention for TOF. There are also adults with TOF who underwent palliative procedures in childhood but never underwent complete repair of the defect.[70] Occasionally, a patient with a well-balanced TOF defect and adequate pulmonary stenosis to protect their pulmonary vasculature will reach adulthood without any operative intervention.

ANATOMY

TOF is classically defined by Fallot's four original pathologic findings: obstruction of the right ventricular outflow, ventricular septal defect, overriding aorta, and right ventricular hypertrophy. The defect is the result of an anterior displacement of the infundibular septum during development, resulting in obstruction to the right ventricular outflow and a malalignment ventricular septal defect. The aorta is displaced toward the ventricular septum resulting in an overriding position, and hypertrophy of the right ventricle is a direct consequence of the outflow obstruction. The obstruction to pulmonary blood flow is often at multiple levels, which may include subvalvular, valvular, and supravalvular stenosis. The pulmonary valve is frequently malformed or bicuspid and the annulus is often small. Hypoplasia of the pulmonary arteries may be present if the obstruction to pulmonary blood flow is severe, and there is often stenosis of the branch pulmonary arteries either primary or secondary to shunts. Aortopulmonary collaterals arising from the aorta may coexist, as is commonly found in patients having pulmonary atresia with ventricular septal defect. Occasionally, cyanotic adults will present with unrepaired TOF and severe pulmonary obstruction but adequate collateral pulmonary blood flow to allow survival beyond childhood.

PHYSIOLOGY

The pathophysiology of TOF results in restriction of pulmonary blood flow secondary to obstruction of right ventricular outflow and right-to-left shunting across the ventricular septal defect. The age at presentation and the degree of cyanosis vary directly with the degree of obstruction to pulmonary blood flow. Patients undergoing palliative shunt procedures in childhood to increase pulmonary blood flow may do quite well if the resulting oxygenation remains adequate with subsequent growth. These systemic-to-pulmonary shunts are often outgrown at an early age, requiring reintervention for additional palliation or more definitive repair. While currently the modified Blalock-Taussig shunt or central shunt is used for palliation in most patients, the Potts (ascending aorta-to-right pulmonary artery) and Waterston (descending aorta-to-left pulmonary artery) shunts were used in the past, and may be found in some adult patients.

INDICATIONS FOR SURGERY

Residual VSDs, residual or recurrent obstruction to pulmonary blood flow, and severe pulmonary insufficiency with progressive right ventricular dilatation and dysfunction are all indications to consider reoperation in adults who have undergone previous complete repair of TOF. Patients who have previously undergone right ventricle-to-pulmonary artery conduit placement often present later in life with conduit stenosis requiring replacement. Patients who have had TOF repair in late childhood may have other sequelae that may have an impact on late reoperative surgery. The long-term volume load from a large shunt may produce permanent left ventricular dysfunction. The pulmonary vascular resistance may be elevated. Mild or even moderate aortic valve regurgitation is not uncommon due to dilatation of the aorta and may require aortic valve repair or replacement.

Pulmonary valve regurgitation is very common after repair of TOF, since approximately 70% to 80% are repaired with a transannular patch. Even though exercise capacity may be decreased, the vast majority of patients tolerate this well unless they have an additional residual VSD or pulmonary artery stenosis. In addition, some patients, without these associated residual defects, will slowly develop right ventricular dilatation and severe tricuspid regurgitation. This may progress for over 20 years, and patients are currently presenting late as they become symptomatic from combined pulmonary and tricuspid valve regurgitation. In view of the risks of sudden death and the progressive nature of right ventricular dysfunction, surgical intervention is recommended.

Aneurysms of the right ventricular outflow tract may occur following the use of an excessively large transannular pericardial patch with the initial repair (Fig. 56-6). Such

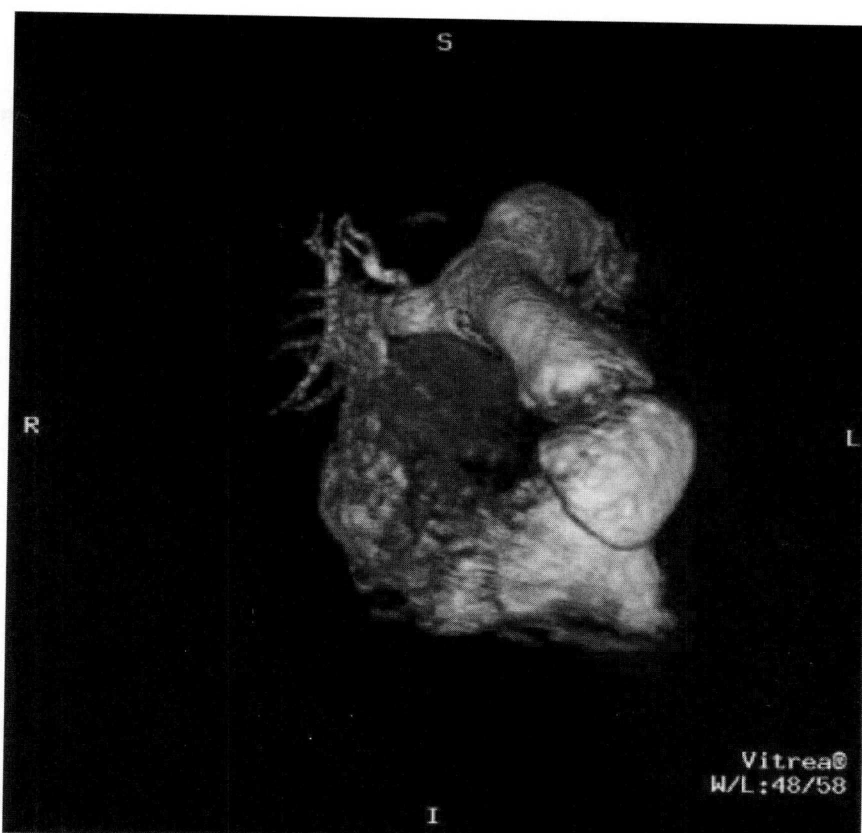

FIGURE 56–6 A three-dimensional magnetic resonance image documenting aneurysmal dilatation of the right ventricular outflow tract in a patient with previous repair of tetralogy of Fallot.

aneurysmal dilatation may progress, especially if there is associated right ventricular outflow tract obstruction.

Sudden death after TOF repair accounts for a significant number of late deaths. It usually occurs in patients who have had a right ventricular incision and have right ventricular dilatation combined with an elevated right ventricular pressure above 60 mm Hg.[71] All else being equal, a QRS duration of greater than 180 milliseconds is associated with an increased risk of sudden death and a progressive increase in QRS duration is considered a factor in deciding on reoperation.[72] Any ventricular arrhythmias should be evaluated by electrophysiological studies and focal pathways should be treated with catheter ablation. Pacemakers are required in less than 4% of patients late after TOF repair.[73] They may be indicated for sick sinus syndrome, the combination of right bundle branch block with left anterior hemiblock, or the late onset of complete heart block.

PREOPERATIVE EVALUATION

The preoperative evaluation in adults with TOF must take into consideration the patient's previous operative interventions. In addition to chest radiography and electrocardiography, transthoracic or transesophageal echocardiography has become the fundamental diagnostic tool in most of these patients. Angiography is indicated to define specific hemodynamics such as the pulmonary vascular resistance and to define the pulmonary artery anatomy. Aortic and selective injections are performed to look for aorta-pulmonary collaterals. The coronary anatomy must be known as 4% to 5% of TOF patients have an LAD arising from the right coronary artery, which can be injured by a transannular incision. Adults over age 40 and those with risk factors for early coronary artery disease should undergo coronary angiography to evaluate the need for concomitant coronary bypass. Magnetic resonance imaging with angiography (MRA) or computerized tomography (CT) scans with three-dimensional reconstruction have proven valuable for defining the anatomy. In all patients with TOF, there should be an evaluation of the size and patency of the pulmonary trunk and its branches, the size of the pulmonary annulus, the stenosis and/or competency of the pulmonary valve, the proximal coronary artery location, and the presence of systemic-to-pulmonary artery collaterals. If there is a right ventricle-to-pulmonary artery conduit or an aneurysmal transannular patch present, MRA or CT imaging studies should be used to evaluate the proximity of these structures to the sternum and to the midline site of the redo sternotomy. Preoperative electrophysiological studies may be indicated if significant arrhythmias are identified.

OPERATIVE PROCEDURE

In most adults with TOF, bicaval cannulation is used, and myocardial protection involves both antegrade and retrograde cold-blood cardioplegia followed by warm-blood cardioplegia and warm-blood reperfusion. Ventricular distension is avoided with venting of the left ventricle. Atrial septal defects should be sutured primarily or closed with a patch of native pericardium. Ventricular septal defects may be approached through the right atrium or through the right ventricular scar or outflow tract patch. A Gore-Tex or glutaraldehyde-treated pericardial patch may be used. The right ventricle is remodeled by resection of scar from the previous ventriculotomy and any aneurysmal tissue in the right ventricular outflow tract. The pulmonary valve is replaced, usually with an oversized porcine bioprosthetic valve seated below the native annulus in the right ventricular outflow tract (Fig. 56-7). A 27- or 29-mm porcine valve can usually be accommodated in all adults. A transannular hood of pericardium or Gore-Tex is used to cover the porcine valve and establish continuity to the pulmonary artery. Homografts are used to replace previously inserted conduits (Fig. 56-8). The pulmonary homograft lasts longer than the aortic homograft, but develops regurgitation earlier. The tricuspid valve can usually be repaired with an annuloplasty and rarely requires replacement. In some cases adherence of the septal leaflet to the VSD patch can be repaired by suturing it to the adjacent anterior and posterior leaflets.

Definitive procedures in adults may require takedown of previously placed shunts. Systemic-to-pulmonary artery type shunts should be controlled as soon as cardiopulmonary bypass is instituted. Takedown of a Waterston shunt is done from within the pericardium. The right pulmonary artery is mobilized. The aortic cannulation site for cardiopulmonary bypass is placed distally. When cardiopulmonary bypass is initiated, shunt flow is controlled with a clamp flush with the aorta, and the patient is cooled to 20°C. Cardioplegia is administered after aortic clamping. With the heart arrested and at low flow, the shunt clamp is released, and the anastomosis is excised from the aorta. This mobilizes the right pulmonary artery. The aorta is closed primarily. The incision in the right pulmonary artery is extended proximally and distally to relieve any stenoses. The right pulmonary artery is reconstructed with a pericardial or Gore-Tex patch. Takedown of a Potts anastomosis usually requires a period of low flow or circulatory arrest.[74] The shunt is occluded by pressure on the left pulmonary artery while blood is cooled to below 20°C. With the head down, the left pulmonary artery is incised and opened under low flow so that the opening to the aorta can be occluded with a Hegar dilator. Under low flow or circulatory arrest, the aortic side is closed primarily, and the pulmonary artery is repaired with a pericardial patch (Fig. 56-9). Takedown of a Blalock-Taussig shunt is usually achieved by dissection, ligation, and division of the shunt at the initiation of cardiopulmonary bypass.

OUTCOMES

Long-term results are well documented in patients who had complete repair of TOF in the late 1950s and early 1960s.[75–80] Actuarial survival ranges from 77% to 90% at

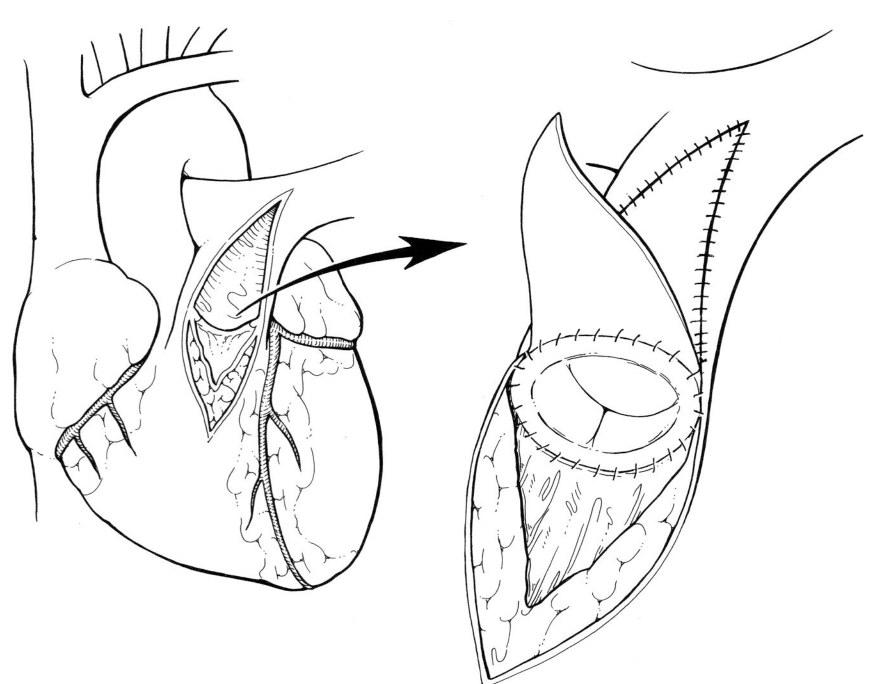

FIGURE 56–7 Pulmonary valve replacement with patch enlargement of the right ventricular outflow tract. The incision extends across the annulus and beyond the bifurcation to the left pulmonary artery. The outsized porcine valve (27 or 29 mm) is placed within the RV outflow tract to accommodate the larger size valve.

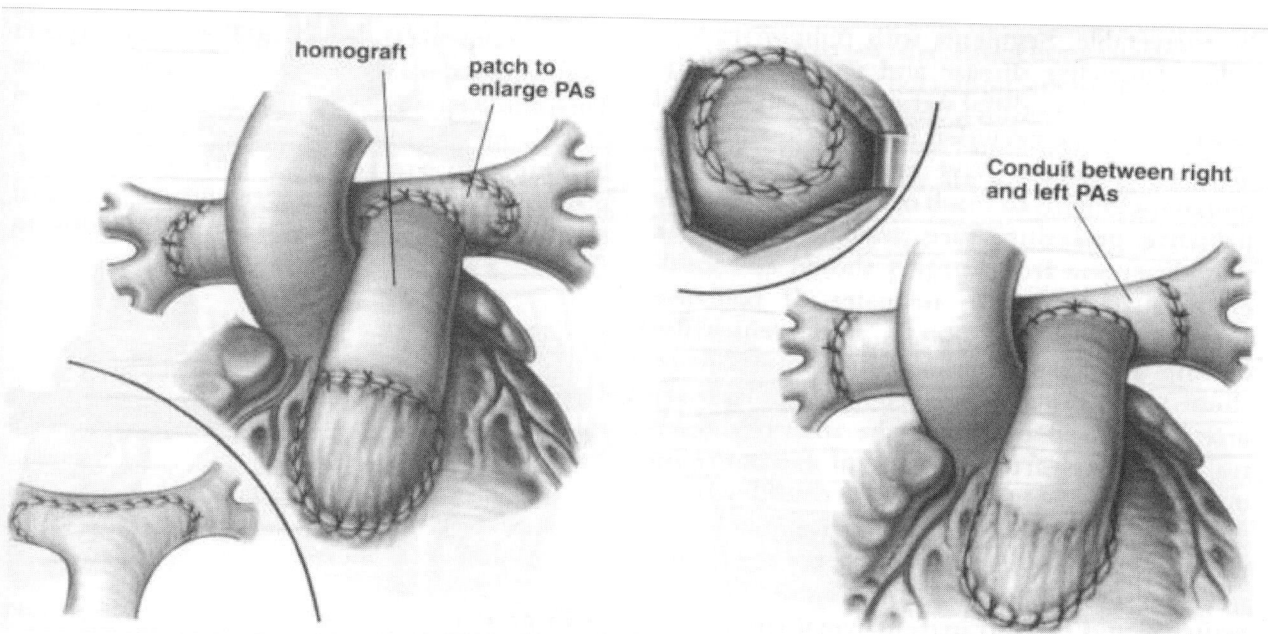

FIGURE 56–8 Homograft replacement of the right ventricular outflow tract with hood augmentation of the proximal anastomosis and patch enlargement of the branch pulmonary arteries. A reinforced Gore-Tex conduit may be placed behind the aorta to reestablish continuity between right and left pulmonary arteries.

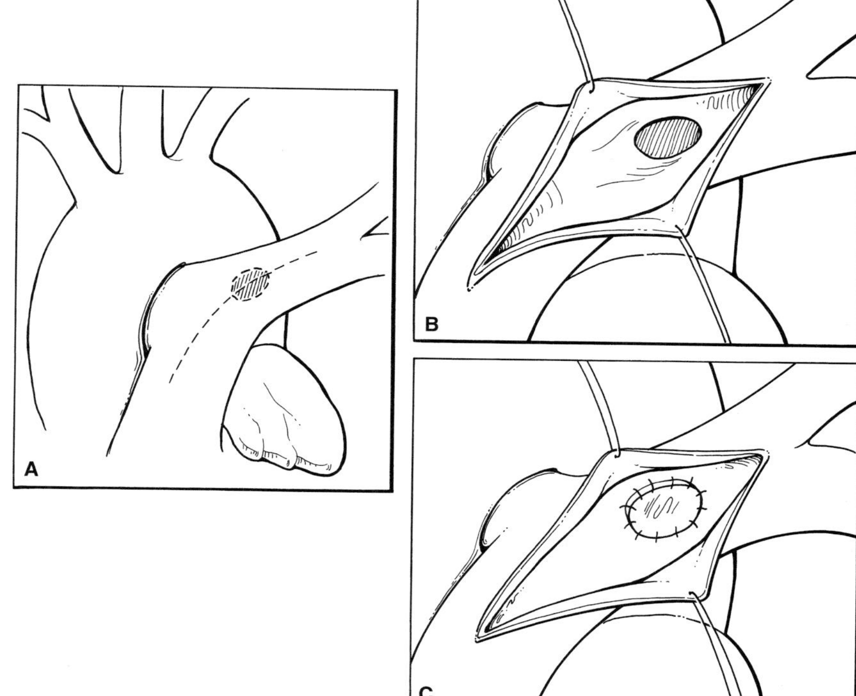

FIGURE 56–9 Patch repair of a Potts shunt anastomosis. The main and left pulmonary arteries are incised (A) to expose the opening (B) in the posterior proximal left pulmonary artery. The defect is closed with a pericardial or prosthetic patch (C).

between 20 and 30 years of follow-up. Late mortality from cardiac causes accounts for about two thirds of all late deaths. Between 40% and 60% of these are sudden and presumed to be due to arrhythmias or to heart block. Other causes include right ventricular outflow abnormalities (obstruction, pulmonary incompetence, aneurysm) and congestive heart failure partly related to residual VSDs, which are reported in 1% to 8% of all operated patients in these early series. Currently, residual VSDs are expected in less than 5% of repairs for TOF.

The results of primary repair of tetralogy in adults are very good. Presbitero et al reported an operative mortality of 2.8% in a series of 40 adults with TOF repairs.[75] There were two residual VSDs and two patients with residual RVOT obstruction. The results of reoperative surgery in adults with TOF are also generally good. Mortality ranges from 7% to 20%. Pome et al reported an actuarial survival of 87% for 22 patients at 20-year follow-up for this particular cohort.[68] Eighty-nine percent of patients were NYHA class I, and only 1 patient (5.5%) was in class III. Two women in this series experienced uncomplicated pregnancy. In the series from the Mayo Clinic reported by Uretzky et al, 5 patients (12%) had a second reoperation.[79]

At UCLA, we have operated on adults with TOF ranging in age from 16 to 65 years. Most had patch repairs of the ventricular septum, insertion of a right ventricular outflow patch, and pulmonary valve replacement. The oldest TOF patient underwent primary repair and coronary bypass grafting. There was no mortality or significant morbidity in this series.

Pulmonary Atresia with Ventricular Septal Defect and Major Aorta-to-Pulmonary Artery Collaterals

Patients with this complex lesion sometimes survive to adulthood without surgery because of adequate pulmonary blood flow from collaterals. Others have shunts or unifocalization procedures or complete repairs.[81–83]

ANATOMY

The true pulmonary arteries may be absent, hypoplastic, and continuous or discontinuous. The collaterals may be the dominant or only blood supply to the lung or supply only lesser areas of the lung. The VSD is subaortic and usually single. Depending on previous shunts, there may be stenoses in the proximal or distal pulmonary arteries. If repaired there may be a residual VSD, obstruction between RV and PA, and tricuspid valve regurgitation.

PHYSIOLOGY

In order to have arterial saturation of 75% to 84%, these patients with arterial and venous mixing have a left-to-right shunt of between 1:1 and 2:1. Therefore, they all have a variably volume overloaded circulation system. Because of high flow and elevated pressure, they may have developed increased pulmonary vascular resistance in the area of some of the collaterals. The volume overload results in reduced exercise tolerance. The aorta and aortic valve tend to dilate and 50% develop aortic valve regurgitation. Ventricular dilatation and dysfunction can also occur.

PREOPERATIVE EVALUATION

Echocardiography is used to exclude additional VSDs and to evaluate the aortic valve. Angiography is performed to delineate the collaterals and true pulmonary arteries as well as to evaluate transpulmonary gradient, which may be high if there was uncontrolled large collateral flow hypertension. Such elevated gradients may preclude complete repair. MR angiograms with three-dimensional reconstruction give detailed models of the anatomy.

INDICATIONS FOR SURGERY

Patients with inadequate pulmonary blood flow are limited due to cyanosis and may require unifocalization if they have an adequate bed for future repair. If they do not, they may be candidates for a palliative shunt. Patients with excessive pulmonary blood flow and failure can also be treated by unifocalization with reduction of the total flow. The size of the shunt to the unifocalization is crucial to adjust flow to the pulmonary vasculature. After unifocalization on one side (Fig. 56-10), the opposite side is unifocalized 6 months to 1 year later (Fig. 56-11), followed 6 months to 1 year later by a complete repair (Fig. 56-12).

Shunted patients should be repaired if they have an adequate size pulmonary bed, unless they are inoperable because of high pulmonary vascular resistance or poor ventricular function. A residual VSD should be closed in previously repaired patients if the left-to-right shunt is 1.5:1 or above. Conduit or valve obstruction is reoperated when there are symptoms, or if the RV pressure at rest is two thirds to three fourths of systemic pressure. If there is severe pulmonary valve regurgitation with RV dilatation or tricuspid regurgitation, reoperation should be undertaken.

STAGED SURGICAL REPAIR

The goal of surgical management of pulmonary atresia, ventricular septal defect, and multiple aorta-to-pulmonary collateral arteries is closing the ventricular septal defect and establishing continuity between the right ventricle and pulmonary artery. Ultimately, successful definitive repair requires an adequate pulmonary vascular bed, without which VSD closure and RV to PA continuity will lead to RV failure due to a prohibitively high pulmonary vascular resistance.

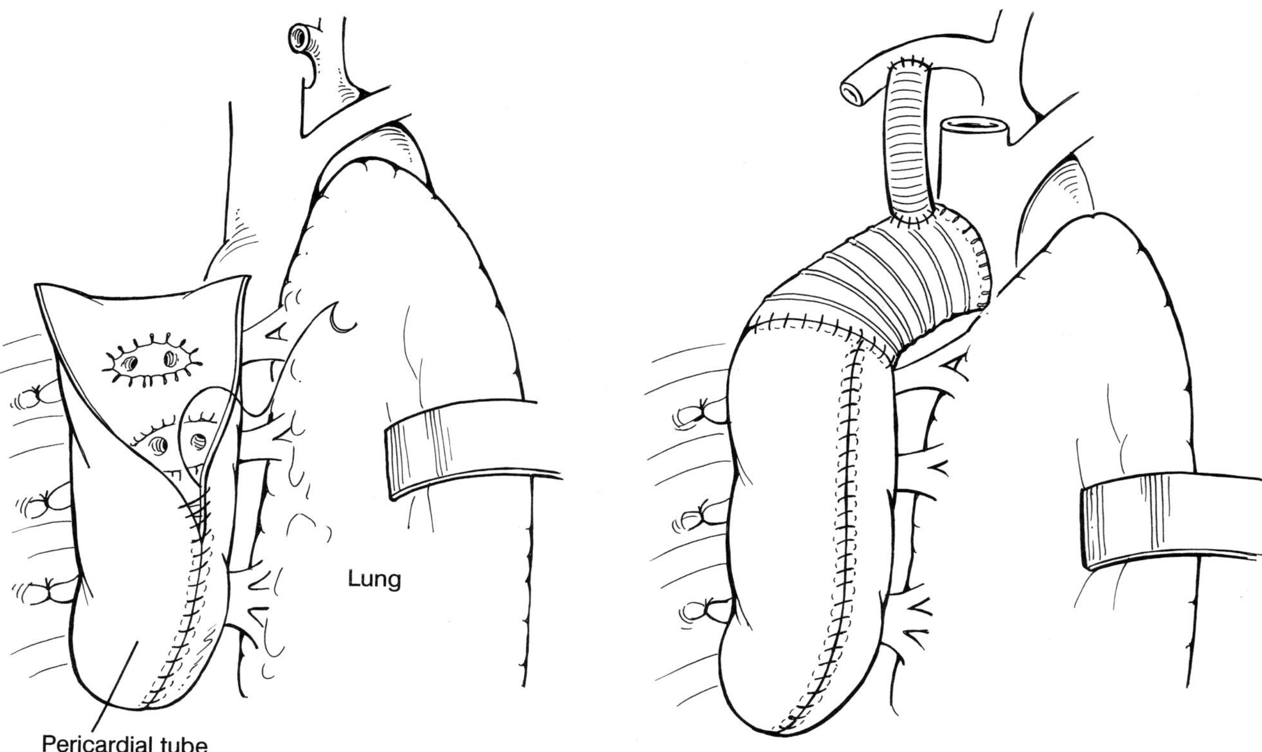

FIGURE 56–10 Unifocalization of the pulmonary artery blood supply to the right lung using a pericardial tube. Through a lateral thoracotomy a side-to-side anastomosis is created to each major collateral and an adjacent incision made in the autologous pericardium placed behind the lung. The pericardium is turned into a tube by suturing the edges and the collaterals are ligated proximal to the tube. The posteriorly lying tube is extended by a 16-mm Gore-Tex graft to the anterior mediastinum. A 6-mm Gore-Tex shunt is made between the subclavian artery and the 16-mm Gore-Tex extension.

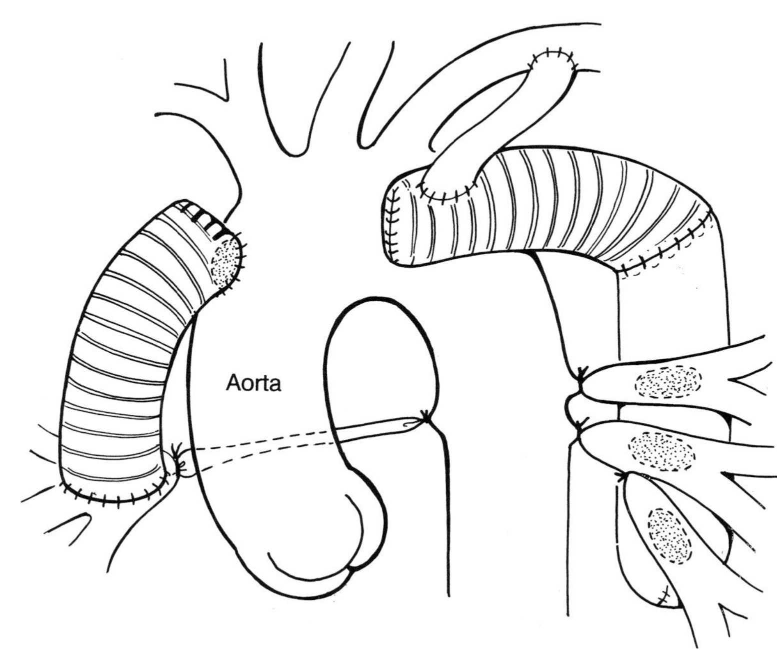

FIGURE 56–11 A 19 year-old patient who previously underwent left pericardial tube unifocalization to three collaterals at age 18 years. On the right side there was a single collateral to a large pulmonary artery supplying the entire right lung. Right-sided unifocalization was achieved by ligating the collateral and placing a 20-mm Gore-Tex graft from the right pulmonary artery to the ascending aorta creating a central restrictive anastomosis.

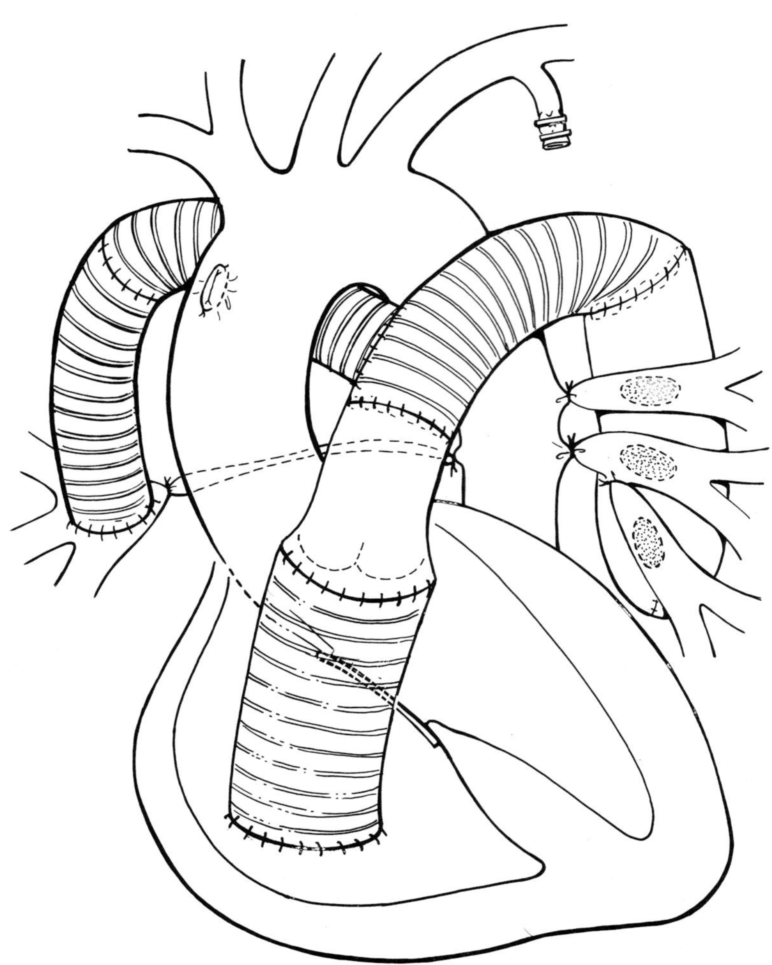

FIGURE 56–12 The complete repair performed 6 months after the right unifocalization shown in Figure 56-10. The ventricular septal defect was closed. An aortic homograft conduit was placed between the right ventricle and the left unifocalization. The right unifocalization was then connected to the homograft by a 16-mm reinforced Gore-Tex tube placed behind the aorta.

Thus, all efforts during the operative staging are designed to maximize the size, distribution, and normal flow of the pulmonary arteries while preserving myocardial function.

Early palliative procedures in patients with excessive or inadequate pulmonary blood flow are designed to create a balanced pulmonary blood flow and encourage growth of the true pulmonary arteries.

Unifocalization procedures join the multifocal sources of pulmonary flow (true pulmonary arteries and aorta-to-pulmonary artery collaterals) into a single source that can ultimately be accessed in the anterior mediastinum via median sternotomy. The unifocalization procedure is performed through a posterolateral thoracotomy incision. A double-lumen endotracheal tube is employed, when possible, for large children and adults. Single-lung ventilation of the contralateral lung, when tolerated, greatly facilitates exposure. We prefer autologous pericardial tube unifocalization of aortopulmonary collaterals and true pulmonary arteries.

Finally, definitive repair in this disorder entails patch closure of the anterior malaligned ventricular septal defect and establishment of continuity between the right ventricle and the pulmonary arteries. All systemic-to-pulmonary artery shunts, including redundant collaterals and surgically created shunts, have been previously occluded or are readily accessible from the anterior mediastinum for occlusion at the time of definitive biventricular repair. Measurement of the ratio of right ventricle to left ventricle systolic pressure allows intraoperative assessment of the repair. A ratio of 0.75 or less immediately after termination of cardiopulmonary bypass is acceptable, and the ratio can be expected to decrease in the first few days after operation. Higher ratios suggest inadequate pulmonary runoff, and will likely result in right ventricular failure. If the pressure on the right side is near systemic or suprasystemic, perforation of the ventricular septal defect patch may provide survival and reasonable palliation.

OUTCOMES

From 1983 through 2000, 105 children and adults have presented to our institution with pulmonary atresia, ventricular septal defect, and multiple aorta to pulmonary artery collaterals. All patients were subject to a strategy of staged repair. Sixty-four patients in this cohort underwent palliation in the newborn period at a median age of 1 week. Surgical palliation included systemic to pulmonary artery shunts, right ventricular outflow patches, and banding of aorta to pulmonary artery collaterals to reduce high pressure and flow. Interventional cardiac catheterization procedures were performed to promote growth of the pulmonary arteries as necessary.

Ninety-four patients underwent unifocalization at a median of 3.5 years (range, 6 months to 37 years). Fifty-eight (range, 1 to 34 years) of these 94 patients have proceeded to complete repair at a median of 7.2 years. Unifocalization was performed in 19 adults, and of this group, 8 patients have undergone uneventful complete repair. There was neither mortality nor important morbidity in this group. At a median follow-up of 60 months there were a total of 18 deaths for a 17% early and late mortality rate. Survival after initial palliation was 92%, after unifocalization, 91%, and after complete repair, 91%. There were 36 reoperations (12%) and 16 patients required catheter-based interventions after surgery. The mean right ventricle to left ventricle (RV/LV) pressure ratio was 0.46. Nearly all the survivors are asymptomatic and do not exhibit any signs of exercise intolerance.

Although there is some debate about whether a one-stage repair is preferable in neonates and children, patients presenting as adults, with or without prior palliation, may be excellent candidates for the staged approach described above. We prefer a staged approach to one-stage correction in adults whose predominant blood supply to the lungs is from collaterals. In adults with a predominant blood supply from the true pulmonary arteries a one-stage repair may be utilized. The strategy of staged repair for patients with tetralogy of Fallot with MAPCAs (Major Aorto-Pulmonary Collaterals) provides good functional results. The mortality rate and requirements for postoperative interventional cardiac catheterization with this approach are lower than published reports of single-stage repair.

As patients age and mature they will require reoperations to replace right ventricle to pulmonary artery homografts and degenerative bioprostheses in the pulmonary position. Long-standing pressure and volume load on the right ventricle will lead to tricuspid regurgitation and right atrial enlargement that may predispose some patients to atrial arrythmias.

Late Reoperations for Transposition of the Great Arteries

ANATOMY AND PHYSIOLOGY

D-transposition of the great arteries is characterized by atrioventricular concordance and associated ventriculoarterial discordance. Prior to the introduction of the arterial switch procedure in 1982, the Mustard and Senning procedures were the standard operations for d-transposition. In the Mustard procedure, a pericardial baffle was used to redirect the systemic and pulmonary venous return. In the Senning procedure, the atrial septum and wall were used for the baffle. This allowed the deoxygenated blood to be pumped to the pulmonary circulation and the oxygenated blood to be pumped to the systemic circulation. As a consequence of these operations, such patients have the morphologic right ventricle acting as the systemic ventricle, and the natural history of such anatomy is well documented. There is about 70% 80% survival at 20 years; 10% of patients have symptomatic right ventricular dysfunction, and about 60% have dysfunction that becomes evident at exercise testing. Additionally, atrial arrhythmias are common, and many patients are in junctional rhythm at 10 years of follow-up. With either procedure, baffle obstruction can lead to a high incidence of vena caval obstruction or pulmonary venous obstruction.[84,85]

PREOPERATIVE EVALUATION

Transthoracic or transesophageal echocardiography usually delineates the site of systemic or pulmonary venous obstruction, ventricular function, and valvular regurgitation. In some cases angiography is also required.

OPERATIVE PROCEDURE

Reoperation for obstruction of either systemic veins or pulmonary veins almost always can be accomplished by incision of the site of obstruction and patching using a pericardial patch when it is available. Usually, with repair of the caval part of the baffle, the functional left atrium is also enlarged.

For patients who present with right ventricular (RV) dysfunction and tricuspid valve regurgitation, the choice of therapy is more complex. If the major problem is tricuspid valve regurgitation in the presence of relatively well-preserved RV function, we prefer to repair or replace the tricuspid valve. The results of tricuspid valve repair or replacement in suitable patients are generally good. Care must be taken to avoid conduction tissue that is very vulnerable at the junction of the septal and anterior leaflets. If RV function is significantly depressed, the LV function and the left ventricular outflow tract (LVOT) and pulmonic valve are evaluated. If LV function is good and there is no fixed LVOT obstruction or pulmonic stenosis, the patient may be considered for LV preparation and the arterial switch procedure. Preparation of the LV requires PA banding to a pressure of 60% to 70% of systemic pressures initially and then delayed rebanding to systemic pressures. It should be noted that retraining the left ventricle in the mature heart is a longer process than in the neonate and that there is less margin for error when placing a band in a fully septated heart. Six months to a year may be required to achieve this and to obtain a normal LV wall thickness.

Once this is achieved, the arterial switch operation may be performed. The atrial baffle is removed, and a new atrial septum is constructed in the anatomic position (Fig. 56-13). In adults, LV preparation by successive tightening of a

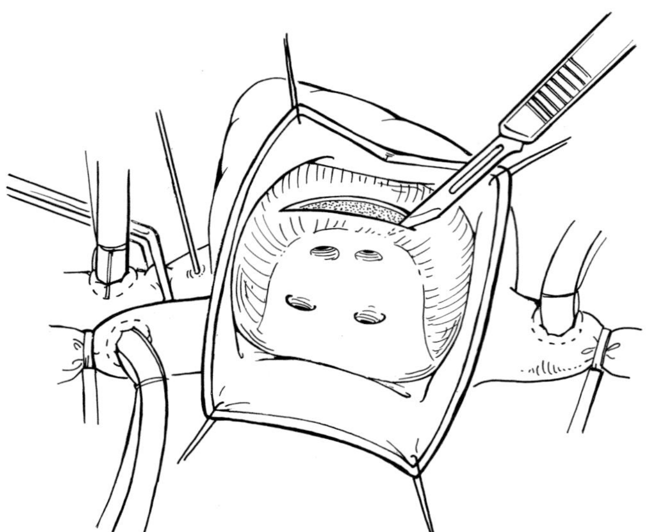

FIGURE 56–13 Takedown of a Mustard baffle. After opening the anatomic right (functional left) atrium, the four pulmonary veins surrounded on three sides by the Mustard baffle are visible. The illustrated incision enters the atrial chamber that receives systemic venous blood and when completed will expose both caval-atrial junctions and the four pulmonary veins entering a common atrial chamber. For venous return to the perfusion circuit, the superior and inferior vena cavae can be cannulated directly or via peripheral venous cannulas.

pulmonary artery band can be hazardous and ultimately unsuccessful with the onset of left ventricular failure. The outcomes from this approach have been quite variable and the overall experience is limited. If significant LV dysfunction or fixed LVOT obstruction is identified, the patient may be considered for heart transplantation.

RESULTS

The outcomes from reoperations in patients with previous Mustard and Senning procedures are quite good if the right ventricle is preserved as the systemic ventricle.[84–98] Generally adults are poor candidates for a staged conversion to an arterial switch procedure.[89,94] Results of cardiac transplantation in these patients has also been successful.

Single Ventricle

ANATOMY

This group includes many lesions characterized by the inability to create a two-ventricle repair. Examples include tricuspid atresia, mitral atresia, double-inlet left ventricle, and unbalanced AV canal.

PHYSIOLOGY

These patients have a mixed circulation with oxygenated and deoxygenated blood mixing in the single ventricle. Pulmonary blood flow is supplied either by the pulmonary artery (PA) or by a patent ductus or shunt. The PA may have pulmonary or subpulmonary stenosis or may have been surgically banded. In order to have an adequate arterial oxygen saturation of 80%, the pulmonary blood flow must be approximately 1.5 times the systemic flow, which results in the effects of volume overload on the ventricle and aorta.

INDICATIONS FOR SURGERY

Few patients with single ventricle survive to adulthood without surgical intervention. Patients may require intervention because of too much pulmonary blood flow, causing heart failure, or too little flow, causing cyanosis. Patients are stratified according to their pulmonary artery pressure, pulmonary vascular resistance (PVR), ventricular function, and anatomical complexity into low-, medium-, and high-risk candidates for a Fontan procedure. In medium- and high-risk patients with elevated PA pressure and PVR and impaired ventricular function, a bidirectional Glenn shunt is performed as a first stage to a Fontan procedure or as long-term palliation until a heart transplant may be indicated.

GLENN SHUNT

Physiology By connecting the end of the SVC to the superior aspect of the right PA, about one third of the systemic venous return is diverted to the lungs for oxygenation. This is a more efficient shunt than a systemic to PA shunt and does not cause a volume overload on the ventricle. It is therefore better tolerated in the presence of impaired ventricular function. Provided the SVC pressure is 18 mm Hg or less, the elevation in SVC pressure is well tolerated.

Operative procedure As shown in Figure 56-14, the Glenn shunt is performed without cardiopulmonary bypass in most patients by using an SVC to PA shunt. If additional procedures are required, such as the relief of subaortic obstruction, atrial septectomy, or AV valve repair, an open procedure on cardiopulmonary bypass is required. An additional source of pulmonary blood flow aims for a pulmonary to systemic blood flow ratio of 1 to 1.3 depending on the PVR. Either a banded pulmonary artery or a small systemic to PA shunt is used. The additional source of blood flow improves oxygenation at rest and with exercise and may prevent late arteriovenous fistula development in the lungs.

Outcomes The early mortality for an isolated Glenn shunt is low (1% to 4%), depending on factors such as the PVR and ventricular function.[99–102] Additional intracardiac procedures increase the risk. In the long term the Glenn shunt slowly loses its effectiveness due to the development of venous collaterals from the superior vena cava to the inferior vena cava.[99,101,102] These can be coil embolized by catheter technique. If there is no additional source of pulmonary

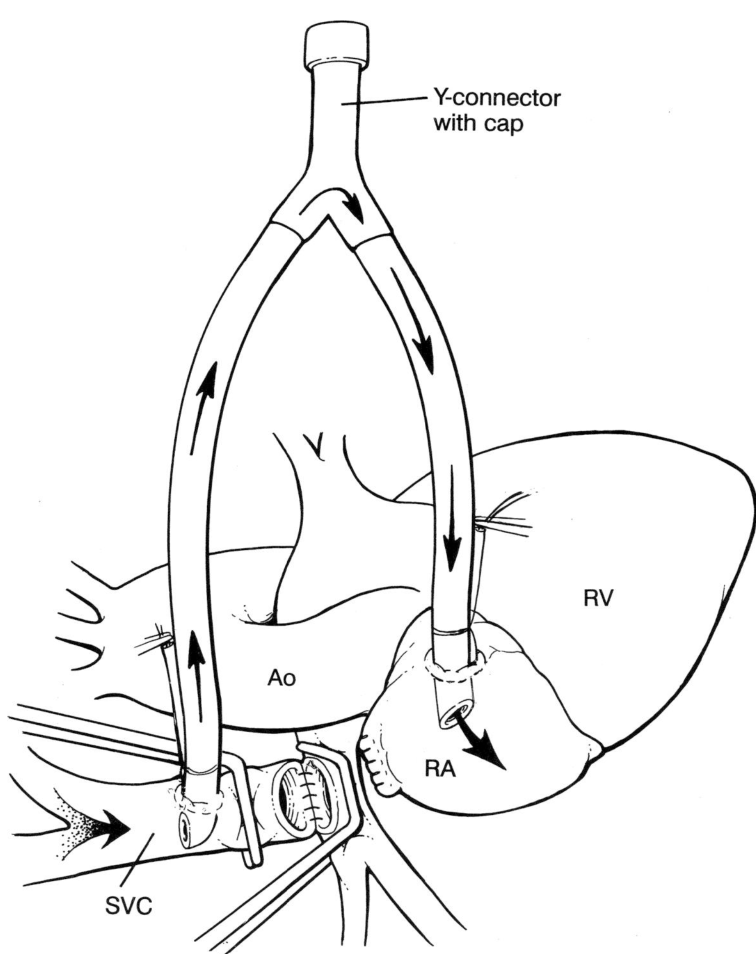

FIGURE 56–14 Creation of a bidirectional Glenn shunt (superior vena cava to right pulmonary artery) using an extracorporeal shunt (with systemic heparin) to maintain superior caval flow into the right atrium. A de-airing chamber and port are needed to prevent air entry into the heart.

blood flow, there is usually severe desaturation on exercise and systemic to PA collaterals develop over time. Intrapulmonary AV fistula can also develop in this situation, resulting in desaturation. In patients with no additional source of pulmonary blood flow and with severely impaired ventricular function, oxygenation can be improved with a controlled shunt by performing an axillary artery-to-vein fistula without thoracotomy.[103]

MODIFIED FONTAN PROCEDURE

Indications Because of the limited palliation provided by the Glenn shunt, patients who meet hemodynamic criteria are accepted for a Fontan procedure. The criteria include good ventricular function, ejection fraction 50% or higher, normal or close to normal PVR, PA pressure less than 20mm Hg, and no additional severe hemodynamic lesions that require prior attention, such as residual coarctation of the aorta, severe subaortic obstruction, or severe AV valve regurgitation. Generally, severe lesions should be addressed at the time of the Glenn shunt or before the Fontan procedure.

Operative procedure Many different types of connection have evolved to connect both SVC and IVC blood to the pulmonary arteries. The two most commonly performed operations are the lateral tunnel Fontan (Fig. 56-15) and the extracardiac Fontan (Fig. 56-16). The lateral tunnel has the advantage of not requiring warfarin anticoagulation in the majority of cases and a fenestration can be easily included in the procedure. The extracardiac Fontan can be done without arresting the heart and is therefore associated with excellent ventricular function. It requires warfarin anticoagulation for at least 1 year and possibly for life. Because of the extensive atrial suture lines, arrhythmias and sick sinus syndrome may be more common with the lateral tunnel Fontan, although they occur in the extracardiac group as well.

Outcomes The early mortality of the Fontan procedure in adults depends a great deal on selection of patients and the presence of risk factors. Reported series have an early mortality of 5%.[104] Fontan patients may be candidates for pacemakers (10%) and reoperations for valvular (5%) and obstructive problems, and may require transplantation for deteriorating

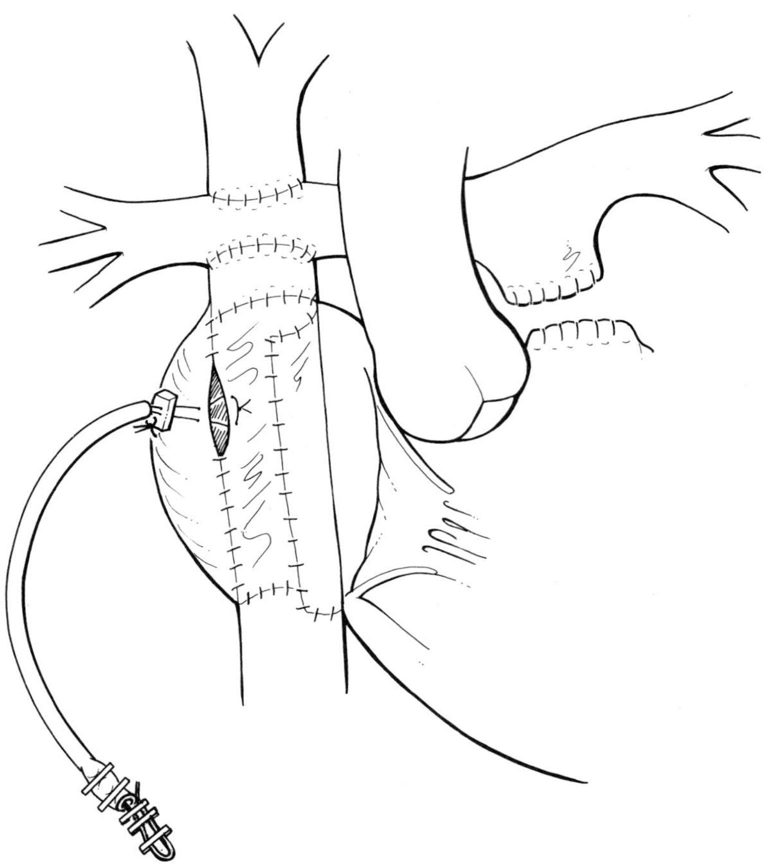

FIGURE 56–15 A lateral tunnel Fontan operation enlarges the right atrium and directs inferior caval flow into the right pulmonary artery using an end-to-side anastomosis to provide bidirectional flow into both pulmonary arteries. A snared purse-string suture adjusts the size of an atrial septal opening that is used to decompress caval pressures and to control the amount of right-to-left shunting.

ventricular function.[105] Protein-losing enteropathy can occur in 5% to 10% of patients.[104,106,107]

Late Reoperations After Modified and Classic Fontan Procedures

Patients who have had a right atrial to PA connection may develop massive right atrial enlargement.[104,106,107] This can eventually result in atrial arrhythmias, thrombus formation, and thromboembolism. Supraventricular arrhythmias as well as AV node dysfunction are not uncommon, and preoperative evaluation by an electrophysiologist is usually necessary. When the RA is enlarged, warfarin anticoagulation is indicated. Such patients are now considered for reoperation with conversion to either a lateral tunnel Fontan or to an extracardiac conduit with reduction of the enlarged RA and a right-sided Maze procedure.[108] If additional surgery is required for Fontan patients with an RA to PA connection, simultaneous conversion to a lateral tunnel is recommended if the RA is enlarged. If they do not meet the criteria, they could be candidates for a heart transplant.

The long-term results after modified Fontan procedures have shown that a significant number of patients require late reoperation. The highest incidence was for patients in whom a valved conduit was used.[109,110] Older age at operation remains a risk factor for late death after the Fontan procedure. Revision of the AV valve closure in double-inlet ventricles or repair of the AV valve in tricuspid atresia is needed in more than 5% of patients.

Protein-losing enteropathy (PLE) is sometimes difficult to diagnose. It occurs in about 10% of patients. It is characterized by a low serum albumin level, ascites, and peripheral edema with or without diarrhea. It may be associated with a mortality up to 20%.[104,105,107] This seems to occur more frequently in patients with heterotaxia or polysplenic syndromes, as well as in those with elevated pulmonary vascular resistance or abnormal systemic venous drainage. Some of these patients can be helped by transcatheter fenestration of the atrial septum. Conversion to a lateral tunnel or transplantation should be considered for these patients. If they do not meet criteria for a Fontan revision, they should be evaluated for transplantation.[111–118]

Ebstein's Anomaly

Ebstein's malformation is a rare congenital cardiac defect accounting for less than 1% of all congenital heart disease. The primary pathologic finding is an abnormal development of

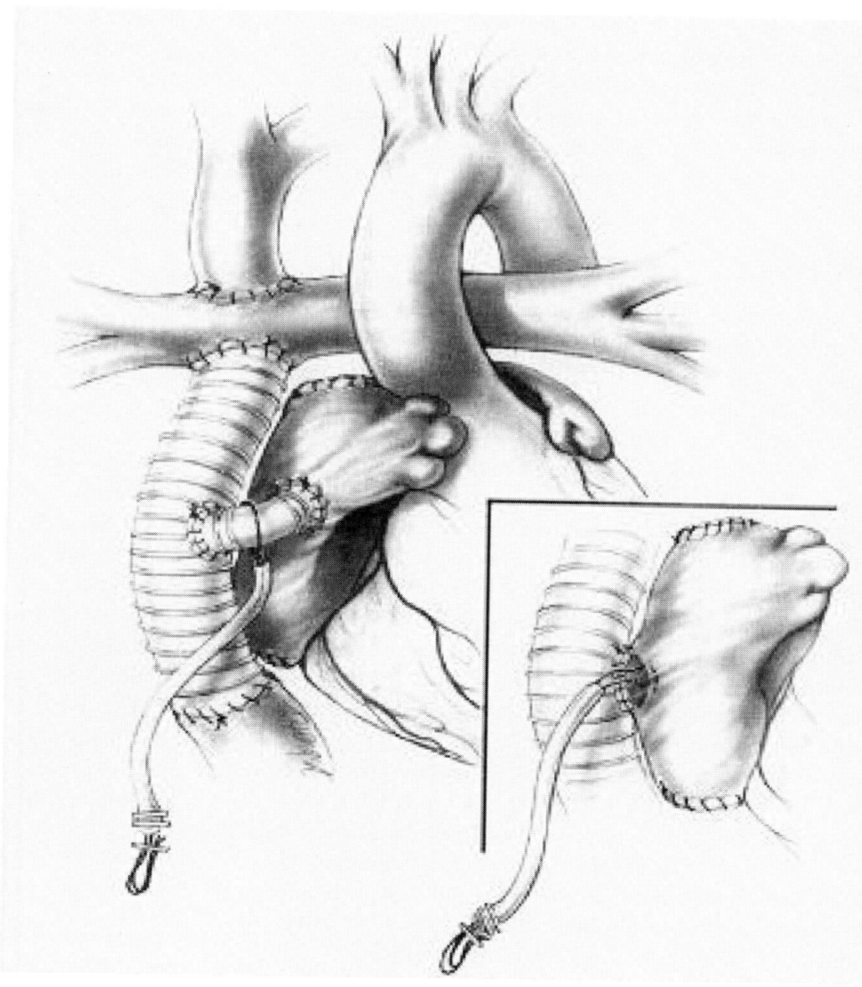

FIGURE 56–16 Extracardiac Fontan with adjustable conduit to atrial connection.

the tricuspid valve marked by a downward displacement of the septal and posterior leaflets into the cavity of the right ventricle. This defect is characterized by a remarkable morphologic variability and a broad spectrum of clinical presentations. Consequently, the diagnosis may be made in symptomatic newborn infants, in children, or in adults.[119,120] The degree of tricuspid regurgitation varies depending on the anatomic abnormality. If there is an atrial septal defect, patients may present with cyanosis. If the atrial septum is intact, they may present with cardiomegaly, right-sided heart failure, or arrhythmias. Those patients with atrial or ventricular arrhythmias may present with episodes of syncope, near syncope, or recurrent palpitations.

Paroxysmal supraventricular arrhythmias occur in 25% to 40% of patients and are most often found in teenagers or young adults.[121] Aberrant right atrial to RV tracts resulting in tachycardia (Wolff-Parkinson-White syndrome) occur in 10% to 18% of patients.[122] Sudden death due to ventricular arrhythmias may occur in as many as 5% to 7% of patients. Likewise, patients with mild manifestations of the Ebstein's malformation may present as late as the third or fourth decade of life with complaints of palpitations or mild exercise intolerance.[123,124] While some patients may reach advanced age without serious clinical manifestations, most will eventually develop significant symptoms.[125] The most common causes of death are congestive heart failure, severe hypoxia, and cardiac arrhythmias.[126]

ANATOMY

Ebstein's malformation is defined by a downward displacement of the annular attachments of the septal and posterior leaflets of the tricuspid valve into the inlet portion of the right ventricle.[127] This downward displacement of the leaflets reduces the distal chamber of the right ventricle, leaving part of the ventricle above the valve as an extension of the right atrium. The atrialized RV is variable in size and thickness, depending on the extent of downward displacement of the leaflets. The entire wall of the right ventricle, both above and below the tricuspid valve, is often thin, dilated, and dysfunctional. In most patients, annular dilatation and malformation of the leaflets result in moderate to severe insufficiency of the tricuspid valve. It usually occurs in the pulmonary right ventricle, but can occur in the systemic right ventricle in patients with corrected transposition of the great arteries. An atrial septal defect or patent foramen ovale is present in greater than 50% of patients, allowing predominantly right-to-left shunting at the atrial level.

PHYSIOLOGY

In patients with Ebstein's malformation, the tricuspid valve is incompetent, but the degree varies depending on the anatomical features. In addition, there is some degree of functional impairment of the right ventricle. The atrialized right ventricle moves paradoxically with right atrial and right ventricular contractions. The net effect is reduced forward blood flow through the right ventricle and pulmonary arteries. The impaired filling of the functional right ventricle and the incompetence of the tricuspid valve both result in systemic venous hypertension. The right atrium and the atrialized right ventricle become dilated, often to extreme degrees. In patients with atrial septal defects, right-to-left shunting occurs, resulting in cyanosis. Both atrial and ventricular arrhythmias may contribute to impaired right ventricular function.

Although the primary pathology involves the right ventricle, patients with Ebstein's malformation may also demonstrate abnormal left ventricular geometry and function. The severity of left ventricular dysfunction is associated with the degree of displacement of the tricuspid valve, the size and dysfunction of the right ventricle, and the severity of paradoxical motion of the interventricular septum.

PREOPERATIVE EVALUATION

On a chest radiograph, the right border of the heart in the area of the RA is enlarged and there may be massive cardiomegaly. Typically, the shadow of the great vessels is narrow due to a small aorta and main pulmonary artery. Right atrial and right ventricular enlargement produce a globular shape to the heart shadow. The apical region of the left ventricle may be elevated from the diaphragm, as seen in right ventricular enlargement. Pulmonary vascularity may range from normal to significantly decreased in the presence of an ASD. A cardiothoracic ratio greater than 0.65 has been shown to be a predictor of sudden death and is considered by some an indication for surgery.

Echocardiography has evolved as the primary diagnostic tool for patients with Ebstein's malformation. The preoperative echocardiogram is helpful in predicting the ability to repair the valve. Echocardiography can define the morphology of the tricuspid valve and the specific abnormalities of the leaflets. Of the greatest importance are the length and mobility of the anterior leaflet. In addition, the function, thickness, and size of the right and left ventricles can be assessed. Coexisting cardiac lesions can also be identified. Color flow Doppler allows a better assessment of tricuspid valve incompetence and the degree of shunting at the atrial level.[128] If echocardiography is inadequate, magnetic resonance angiography imaging with three-dimensional reconstruction is useful for diagnostic purposes. Cardiac catheterization should be avoided as it is usually unnecessary and can result in arrhythmias. Currently, cardiac catheterization is reserved for patients with associated cardiac defects, previous shunt placements, possible pulmonary artery stenosis, or possible coronary artery disease.

INDICATIONS FOR SURGERY

The indications for surgical intervention in patient with Ebstein's malformation include the following: functional New York Heart Association (NYHA) class III or IV symptoms; significant or progressive cyanosis; decline in exercise tolerance; severe cardiomegaly (cardiothoracic ratio greater than 0.65); associated cardiac anomalies (including right ventricular outflow tract obstruction); refractory atrial or ventricular arrhythmias; and a history of paradoxical embolus. With the improved outcomes and a greater ability to repair the valve, there is a trend to perform early repair in the presence of severe tricuspid regurgitation and atrial enlargement.

OPERATIVE PROCEDURE

The goals of surgical intervention in patients with Ebstein's malformation are to increase pulmonary blood flow, minimize tricuspid insufficiency, reduce or eliminate right-to-left shunting, optimize right ventricular function, and reduce or eliminate arrhythmias. Ideally, the tricuspid valve can be repaired, which may avoid valve replacement with a bioprosthetic valve and the need for future valve replacements. Patients with preoperative Wolff-Parkinson-White syndrome are treated by catheter ablation prior to the surgery.

If the anterior leaflet is adequate in size and is not extensively bound down by muscular attachments, repair is almost always possible. Two main techniques of repair have been described. Danielson was the first to demonstrate the ability to repair these valves and avoid replacement.[129] Repair includes plication of the atrialized RV back to the true annulus and an annuloplasty (Fig. 56-17).

Carpentier et al described a technique in which the atrialized right ventricle is plicated perpendicular to the valve annulus toward the apex of the heart.[130] The displaced leaflets are detached from the right ventricle at their base and attached to the true annulus (Fig. 56-18). We perform an annuloplasty using a glutaraldehyde-treated strip of pericardium. The redundant RA wall and appendage are excised, and the ASD is closed. In patients with a large preoperative right-to-left shunt and a thinned-out underdeveloped right ventricle,

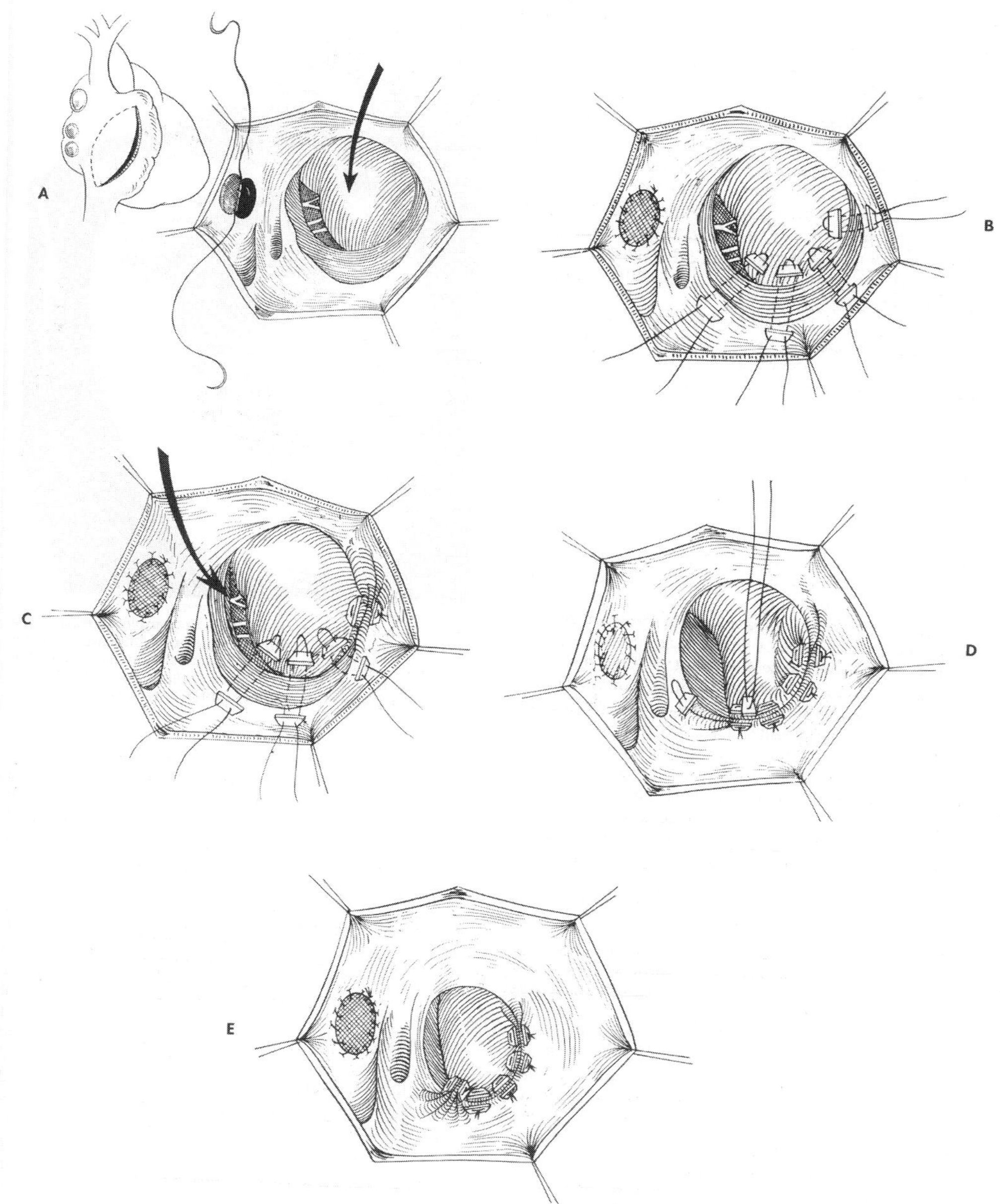

FIGURE 56–17 Danielson's repair of the tricuspid valve in Ebstein's anomaly.

a snare-controlled adjustable atrial septal defect may be used to allow continued controlled right-to-left shunting until the RV recovers. The ASD can then be closed using the snare, which is exposed under local anesthesia. In addition, electrophysiological mapping for localization of accessory pathways may be performed in patients with arrhythmias.

We prefer to use a porcine bioprosthetic valve. In the absence of atrial arrhythmias or severe atrial wall thickening, this allows anticoagulation with aspirin only. Generally, tissue valves are preferred in the tricuspid position because of the risk of thrombosis of a right-sided mechanical valve in a low-pressure setting.

The right atrial Maze procedure is a modification of the Maze procedure and has been used to treat atrial arrhythmias in patients with Ebstein's malformation. This procedure may reduce or eliminate atrial arrhythmias by preventing reentry conduction at the atrial level (Fig. 56-19).

OUTCOMES

Results of tricuspid valve repair continue to improve. Danielson and colleagues at the Mayo clinic currently have a surgical experience of more than 400 patients with Ebstein's malformation.[131] The data have recently been analyzed for

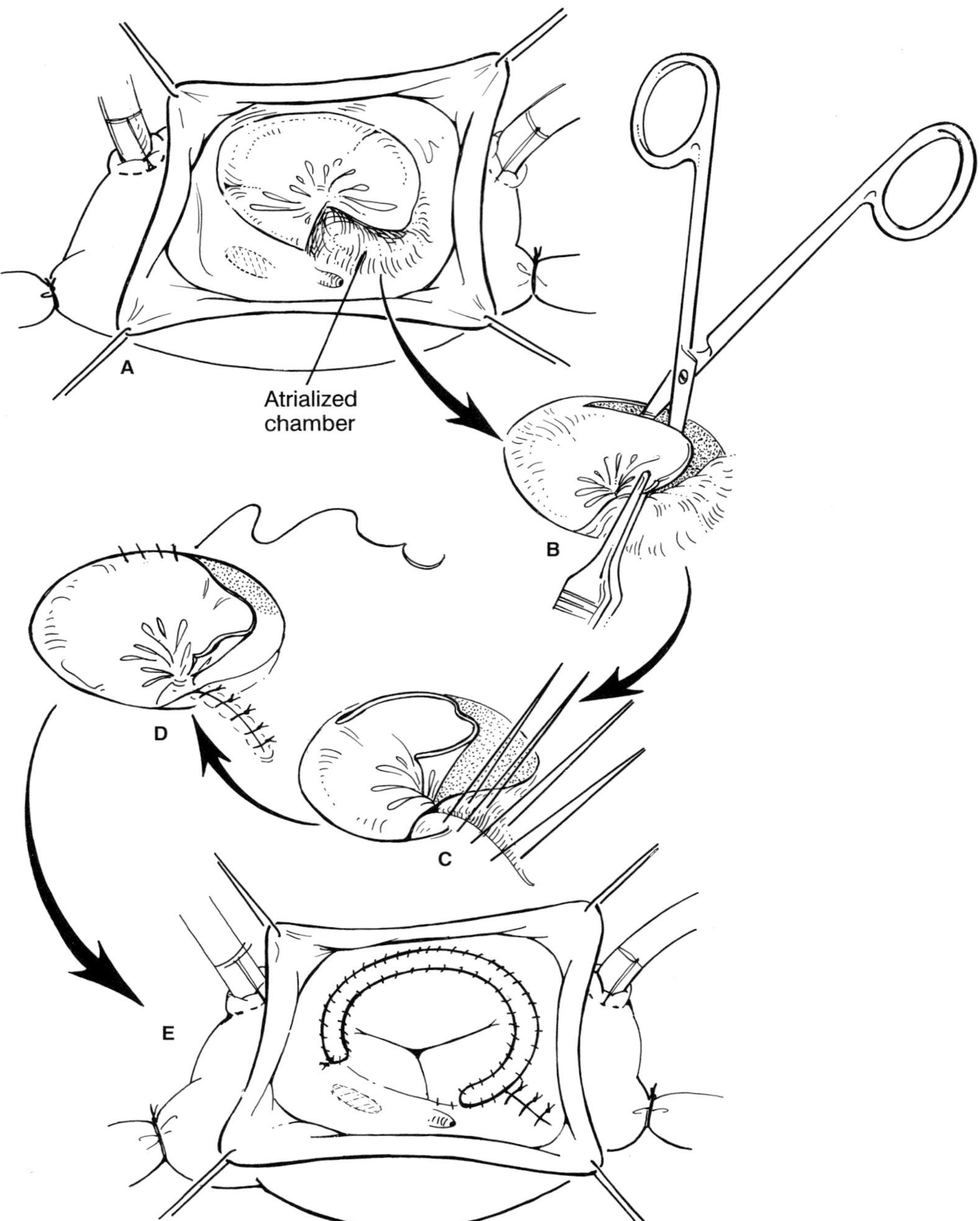

FIGURE 56–18 Carpentier's repair of the tricuspid valve in Ebstein's anomaly.

the first 312 patients undergoing surgical intervention from 1972 to 1996. The ages in this series range from 9 months to 71 years, with a mean age of 20.7 years. There were no neonates in this group. In 43% a tricuspid valve repair was successful, and in 53% a bioprosthesis was used to replace the tricuspid valve. Approximately 4% of patients underwent a Fontan reconstruction or other procedures. There were 20 hospital deaths (6.4% early mortality) in this series. Forty-four patients had accessory conduction pathways (Wolff-Parkinson-White syndrome) and underwent successful pathway ablation as part of their repair. Fifteen patients underwent right-sided Maze procedures for control of atrial dysrhythmias and 4 underwent ablation of the atrioventricular node for re-entry tachycardia. There were 24 late deaths (7.3%). Seventeen of the 135 patients (12.6%) who underwent valve repair required reoperation for valve regurgitation 1.5 to 18 years later (mean, 8.7 years). Eight bioprosthetic valves required replacement 1 to 16 years after implantation. Follow-up of those patients evaluated more than a year after operation determined that 93% were in NYHA functional

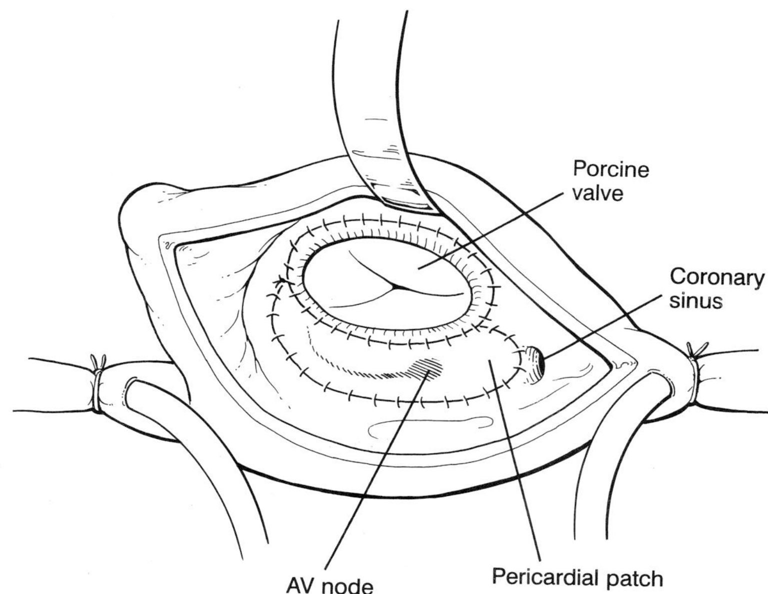

FIGURE 56–19 Injury to the conduction system may be avoided during tricuspid valve replacement by suturing a triangular patch of pericardium over the AV node and triangle of Koch.

class I or II. The addition of a right atrial Maze procedure to the repair is often successful in reducing or eliminating atrial arrhythmias. Furthermore, the durability of a porcine bioprosthesis for tricuspid valve replacement has been quite favorable.

Heart Transplantation

Adults with congenital heart disease may not be amenable to palliation or repair due to severe ventricular dysfunction or pulmonary vascular disease. They may be candidates for heart, lung, or heart-lung transplantation. In addition,

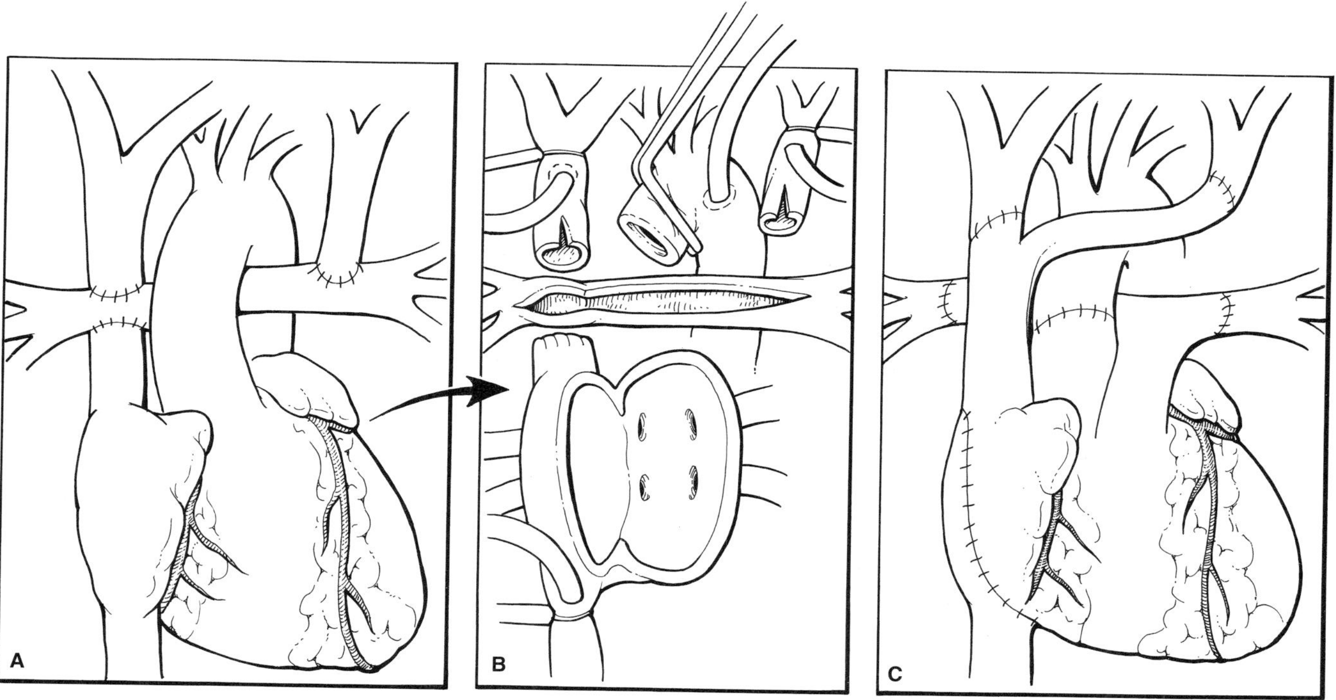

FIGURE 56–20 Heart transplantation after total cavopulmonary connection in a patient with bilateral superior vena cavae. The innominate vein from the donor is used to reconstruct the left superior vena cava. Alternatively (not shown), if the left superior vena cava is too short, a synthetic graft can be used to route the left superior vena cava blood along the coronary sinus of the donor heart into the recipient native inferior vena cava.

patients previously repaired may deteriorate and may have no other options.[132–147]

In symptomatic patients who are NYHA class III or IV and who have an acceptable pulmonary vascular resistance, heart transplantation is usually feasible. Anomalies of systemic and pulmonary venous return can be corrected. Deformities of the pulmonary artery can be repaired. This may require quite extensive repair, particularly in some patients after the Fontan procedure. Dextrocardia and transposition may be challenging, but with current reconstructive techniques, transplantation is almost always possible.[140–144,148,149]

PREOPERATIVE EVALUATION

General evaluation is as for all heart transplant recipients. Cardiopulmonary exercising testing, pulmonary, dental, and psychosocial evaluations are routine. Pulmonary vascular resistance must be carefully assessed; cut-off is at 4 to 6 Wood units or transpulmonary gradient of 12 to 14 mm Hg. Panel-reactive antibody screening is essential, as most patients have had previous surgery and blood transfusions. If these values are higher than 10%, then prospective cross-matching is preferable. Chest wall collaterals may increase left-sided return particularly after previous surgery, and therefore it is usual to oversize donors by 20%. Some larger aortopulmonary or veno-venous collaterals may be coil-embolized preoperatively.[150]

OPERATIVE PROCEDURE

It is important to anticipate the recipient's anatomy. For example, in tricuspid atresia d-transposition is common, and the aorta may be immediately behind the sternum. A CT scan is obtained preoperatively to assess the retrosternal structures. It may be necessary to institute bypass before opening the sternum. Aprotonin is used in all cases and it is important to plan correct timing for the arrival of the donor heart, since redo sternotomy in these patients is more complex than usual. Patients are cooled to 22°C to 24°C in order to minimize the pulmonary venous return, which can be torrential. This can warm the donor heart and, after the aortic anastamoses are completed, may wash out the preservation solution if the aortic root is not vented. A vent in the left atrium is therefore used. Anomalies in systemic or pulmonary venous return and the pulmonary arteries are reconstructed prior to bringing the donor heart onto the field. We apply intracardiac cooling to the left ventricle using a catheter passed through the left atrial anastamosis into the left ventricle apex. Generally, we prefer a bicaval anastamosis (Figs. 56-20 and 56-21).

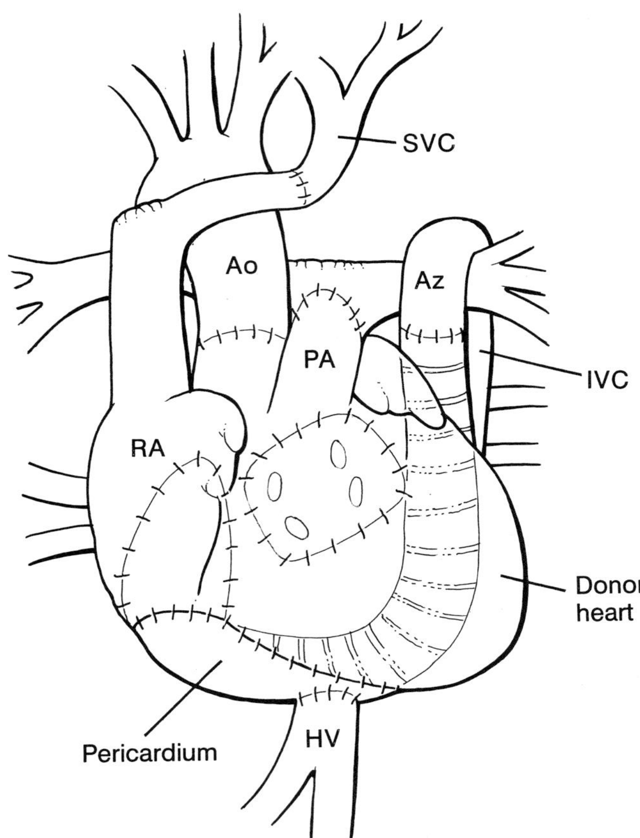

FIGURE 56–21 Heart transplant in a patient with dextrocardia, right-sided arch, and interrupted inferior vena cava with azygous continuity who previously had undergone a Fontan procedure.

OUTCOMES

Due to previous surgeries, anatomical complexity, borderline pulmonary vascular resistance, hepatic congestion, and other factors, these patients (particularly the Fontan patients) are at higher risk for transplantation. Over the last 18 years, 30 adults and adolescents with congenital heart disease have undergone transplantation at our institution. Close to 50% of the patients had single-ventricle physiology and on average all had at least two previous sternotomies. Age range was 13 to 49 years old. The early mortality for this high-risk group was 18%.

REFERENCES

1. Moodie D: Diagnosis and management of congenital heart disease in the adult. *Cardiol Rev* 2001; 9:276.
2. Brickner M, Hillis L, Lange R: Congenital heart disease in adults. *N Engl J Med* 2000; 324:256.
3. Perloff JK: *Congenital Heart Disease in Adults*. Philadelphia, WB Saunders, 1996; p 21.
4. Durack DT: Prevention of infective endocarditis. *N Engl J Med* 1995; 332:38.
5. Freed MD: Infective endocarditis in the adult with congenital heart disease. *Cardiol Clin* 1993; 11:589.
6. Perloff JK, Marelli AJ, Miner PD: Risk of stroke in adults with cyanotic congenital heart disease. *Circulation* 1993; 87:1954.

7. Rao V, Van Arsdell G, David T, et al: Aortic valve repair for adult congenital heart disease: a 22-year experience. *Circulation* 2000; 102:III40-3.
8. Overgaard C, Harrison D, Siu S, et al: Outcome of previous tricuspid valve operation and arrhythmias in adult patients with congenital heart disease. *Ann Thorac Surg* 1999; 68:2158.
9. Sabet H, Edwards W, Tazelaar H, Daly R: Congenitally bicuspid aortic valves: a surgical pathology study of 542 cases (1991 through 1996) and a literature review of 2,715 additional cases. *Mayo Clin Proc* 1999; 74:14.
10. Van Nooten GJ, Caes F, Tacymarrs Y, et al: Tricuspid valve replacement: postoperative and long-term results. *J Thorac Cardiovasc Surg* 1995; 110:672.
11. Milgalter E, Laks H: Use of a pericardial patch to bridge the conduction tissue during tricuspid valve replacement. *Ann Thorac Surg* 1991; 52:1337.
12. Kuckarczuk J, Cohen M, Rhodes L, et al: Epicardial atrial pacemaker lead placement after multiple cardiac operations. *Ann Thorac Surg* 2001; 71:2057.
13. Cohen M, Vetter V, Wernovsky G, et al: Epicardial pacemaker implantation and follow-up in patients with a single ventricle after the Fontan operation. *J Thorac Cardiovasc Surg* 2001; 121:804.
14. Ramesh V, Gaynor J, Shah M, et al: Comparison of left and right atrial epicardial pacing in patients with congenital heart disease. *Ann Thorac Surg* 1999; 68:2314.
15. Epstein M, Walsh E, Saul J, et al: Long-term performance of bipolar epicardial atrial pacing using an active fixation bipolar endocardial lead. *Pacing Clin Electrophysiol* 1998; 21:1098.
16. Donit A, Bonvicini M, Placci A, et al: Surgical treatment of secundum atrial septal defect in patients older than fifty years. *Ital Heart J* 2001; 2:428.
17. Jemielity M, Dyszkiewicz W, Paluszkiewicz L, et al: Do patients over forty years of age benefit from surgical closure of atrial septal defects? *Heart* 2001; 85:300.
18. Landzberg M: Closure of atrial septal defects in adult patients: justification of the "tipping point." *J Interven Cardiol* 2001; 14:267.
19. Moodie D, Sterba R: Long-term outcomes excellent for atrial septal defect repair in adults. *Cleve Clin J Med* 2000; 67:591.
20. Gatzoulis M, Redington A, Somerville J, Shore D: Should atrial septal defects in adults be closed? *Ann Thorac Surg* 1996; 61:657.
21. Oakley C: Closure of atrial septal defect in adult life. *Cardiologia* 1996; 41:31.
22. Perloff J: Surgical closure of atrial septal defect in adults. *N Engl J Med* 1995; 8:513.
23. Steele PM, Fuster V, Cohen M, et al: Isolated atrial septal defect with pulmonary vascular obstructive disease: long-term follow-up and prediction of outcome after surgical correction. *Circulation* 1987; 76:1037.
24. Campbell M: Natural history of atrial septal defect. *Br Heart J* 1970; 32:820.
25. Craig RJ, Selzer A: Natural history and prognosis of atrial septal defect. *Circulation* 1968; 37:805.
26. Kirklin JW, Barratt-Boyes BG: Atrial septal defect and partial anomalous pulmonary venous connection, in Kirklin JW, Barratt-Boyes BG (eds): *Cardiac Surgery*. New York, Churchill-Livingstone, 1993; p 620.
27. Kirklin JW, Barratt-Boyes BG: Atrioventricular canal defect, in Kirklin JW, Barratt-Boyes BG (eds): *Cardiac Surgery*. New York, Churchill-Livingstone, 1993; p 718.
28. Horvath KA, Burke RP, Collins JJ, Cohn LH: Surgical treatment of adult atrial septal defect: early and long-term results. *J Am Coll Cardiol* 1992; 20:1156.
29. Murphy JG, Gersh BJ, McGoon MD, et al: Long-term outcome after surgical repair of isolated atrial septal defect. *N Engl J Med* 1990; 323:1645.
30. Lloyd TR, Rao S, Beekman RH, et al: Atrial septal defect occlusion with the buttoned device (a multi-institutional U.S. trial). *Am J Cardiol* 1994; 73:286.
31. Rome JJ, Keane JF, Perry SB, et al: Double-umbrella closure of atrial defects. *Circulation* 1990; 82:751.
32. Rhodes LA, Keane JF, Keane JP, et al: Long follow-up (to 43 years) of ventricular septal defect with audible aortic regurgitation. *Am J Cardiol* 1990; 66:340.
33. Kirklin JW, Barratt-Boyes BG: Ventricular septal defect, in Kirklin JW, Barratt-Boyes BG (eds): *Cardiac Surgery*. New York, Churchill-Livingstone, 1993; p 800.
34. Ikawa S, Shimazaki Y, Nakano S, et al: Pulmonary vascular resistance during exercise late after repair of large ventricular septal defects: relation to age at the time of repair. *J Thorac Cardiovasc Surg* 1995; 109:1218.
35. Hornberger LK, Sahn DJ, Krabill KA, et al: Elucidation of the natural history of ventricular septal defects by serial Doppler color flow mapping studies. *J Am Coll Cardiol* 1989; 13:1111.
36. Rahko P: Doppler echocardiographic evaluation of ventricular septal defects in adults. *Echocardiography* 1993; 10:517.
37. O'Laughlin MP, Mullins CE: Transcatheter occlusion of ventricular septal defect. *Cathet Cardiovasc Diagn* 1989; 17:175.
38. Lock JE, Locherman JT, Jeane JF, et al: Transcatheter umbrella closure of congenital heart defects. *Circulation* 1987; 73:593.
39. Moller JH, Patton C, Varco RL, Lillehei W: Late results (30-35 years) after operative closure of isolated ventricular septal defect from 1954 to 1960. *Am J Cardiol* 1991; 68:1491.
40. Campbell M: Natural history of persistent ductus arteriosus. *Br Heart J* 1968; 30:4.
41. Ho A, Tan P, Yang M, et al: The use of multiplane transesophageal echocardiography to evaluate residual patent ductus arteriousus during video-assisted thoracoscopy in adults. *Surg Endosc* 1999; 13:975.
42. Schrader R, Kadel C, Cieslinski G, et al: Non-thoracotomy closure of persistent ductus arteriosus beyond age 60 years. *Am J Cardiol* 1993; 72:1319.
43. Yoshiyuki T, Matsumoto M, Sugita T: Optimal treatment for adult patent ductus arteriosus. *Ann Thorac Surg* 2001; 72:2186.
44. Toda R, Moriyama Y, Yamashita M, et al: Operation for adult patent ductus arteriosus using cardiopulmonary bypass. *Ann Thorac Surg* 2000; 70:1935.
45. Arora R: Patent ductus arteriosus: catheter closure in the adult patient. *J Interven Cardiol* 2001; 14:255-9.
46. Latson LA: Residual shunts after transcatheter closure of patent ductus arteriosus: a major concern or benign "techno-malady"? [editorial comment]. *Circulation* 1991; 84:2591.
47. Bridges ND, Perry SB, Parness I, et al: Transcatheter closure of a large patent ductus arteriosus with the clamshell septal umbrella. *J Am Coll Cardiol* 1991; 18:1297.
48. Hosking MCK, Benson LN, Musewe N, et al: Transcatheter occlusion of the persistently patent ductus arteriosus. *Circulation* 1991; 84:2313.
49. Bauer M, Alexi-Meskishvili V, Bauer U, et al: Benefits of surgical repair of coarctation of the aorta in patients older than fifty years. *Ann Thorac Surg* 2001; 72:2060.
50. Marx G: "Repaired" aortic coarctation in adults: not a "simple" congenital heart defect. *J Am Coll Cardiol* 2000; 35:1003.
51. Bouchart F, Dubar A, Tabley A, et al: Coarctation of the aorta in adults: surgical results and long-term follow-up. *Ann Thorac Surg* 2000; 70:1483.
52. Aris A, Subirana T, Ferres P, Torner-Soler M: Repair of aortic coarctation in patients more than fifty years of age. *Ann Thorac Surg* 1999; 67:1376.
53. Kirklin JW, Barratt-Boyes BG: Coarctation of the aorta and interrupted aortic arch, in Kirklin JW, Barratt-Boyes BG (eds): *Cardiac Surgery*. New York, Churchill-Livingstone, 1993; p 1263.

54. Cohen M, Fuster V, Steele PM, et al: Coarctation of the aorta: long-term follow-up and prediction of outcome after surgical correction. *Circulation* 1989; 80:840.
55. Presbitero P, Demarie D, Villani M, et al: Long term results (15-30 years) of surgical repair of aortic coarctation. *Br Heart J* 1987; 57:462.
56. Walhout R, Lekkerkerker J, Ernst S, et al: Angioplasty for coarctation in different aged patients. *Am Heart J* 2002; 144:180.
57. Rosenthal E: Stent implantation for aortic coarctation: the treatment of choice in adults? *J Am Coll Cardiol* 2001; 38:1524.
58. Hellenbrand WE, Allen HD, Golinko RJ, et al: Balloon angioplasty for aortic recoarctation: results of valvuloplasty and angioplasty of congenital anomalies registry. *Am J Cardiol* 1990; 65:793.
59. Harrison D, McLaughlin P, Lazzam C, et al: Endovascular stents in the management of coarctation of the aorta in the adolescent and adult: one year follow up. *Heart* 2001; 85:561.
60. Therrien J, Siu S, McLaughlin P, et al: Pulmonary valve replacement in adults late after repair of tetralogy of Fallot: are we operating too late? *J Am Coll Cardiol* 2000; 36:1670.
61. Oechslin E, Harrison D, Harris L, et al: Reoperation in adults with repair of tetralogy of Fallot: indications and outcomes. *J Thorac Cardiovasc Surg* 1999; 118:245.
62. Dittrich S, Vogel M, Dahnert I, et al: Surgical repair of tetralogy of Fallot in adults today. *Clin Cardiol* 1999; 22:460.
63. Rammohan M, Airan B, Bham A, et al: Total correction of tetralogy of Fallot in adults: surgical experience. *Int J Cardiol* 1998; 63:121.
64. Van der Weijden P, Baur L, Kool L, et al: Embolization as a treatment of life-threatening haemoptysis in an adult with tetralogy of Fallot with pulmonary atresia. *Int J Card Imaging* 1998; 14:123.
65. Nollert G, Fischlein T, Bouterwek S, et al: Long-term results of total repair of tetralogy of Fallot in adulthood: 35 years follow-up in 104 patients corrected at the age of 18 or older. *Thorac Cardiovasc Surg* 1997; 45:178.
66. Jonsson H, Ivert T, Jonasson R, et al: Work capacity and central hemodynamics thirteen to twenty-six years after repair of tetralogy of Fallot. *J Thorac Cardiovasc Surg* 1995; 110:416.
67. Rosenthal A: Adults with tetralogy of Fallot—repaired, yes: cured, no. *N Engl J Med* 1993; 9:655.
68. Pome G, Rossi C, Colucci V, et al: Late reoperations after repair of tetralogy of Fallot. *Eur J Cardiothorac Surg* 1992; 6:31.
69. Pacifico AD: Reoperations after repair of tetralogy of Fallot, in Stark J, Pacifico AD (eds): *Reoperations in Cardiac Surgery*. Berlin, Springer-Verlag, 1989; p 171.
70. Stewart S, Alexson C, Manning J: Long-term palliation with the classic Blalock-Taussig shunt. *J Thorac Cardiovasc Surg* 1988; 96:117.
71. Harrison D, Harris L, Siu S, et al: Sustained ventricular tachycardia in adult patients late after repair of tetralogy of Fallot. *J Am Coll Cardiol* 1997; 30:1368.
72. Cullen S, Celermajer DS, Franklin RCG, et al: Prognostic significance of ventricular arrhythmia after repair of tetralogy of Fallot: a 12-year prospective study. *J Am Coll Cardiol* 1994; 23:1151.
73. Garson A, Nihill MR, McNamara DG, Cooley DA: Status of the adult and adolescent after repair of tetralogy of Fallot. *Circulation* 1979; 59:1232.
74. Kirklin JW, Devloo RA: Hypothermic perfusion and circulatory arrest for surgical correction of tetralogy of Fallot with previously constructed Potts' anastomosis. *Dis Chest* 1961; 39:87.
75. Presbitero P, Demarie D, Aruta E, et al: Results of total correction of tetralogy of Fallot performed in adults. *Ann Thorac Surg* 1988; 46:297.
76. Zahka KG, Horneffer PJ, Rowe SA, et al: Long-term valvular function after total repair of tetralogy of Fallot: relation to ventricular arrhythmias. *Circulation* 1988; 78(suppl III):III-14.
77. Lillehei CW, Varco RL, Cohen M, et al: The first open heart corrections of tetralogy of Fallot: a twenty-six to thirty-one year follow-up of 106 patients. *Ann Surg* 1986; 204:490.
78. Deanfield JF, McKenna WJ, Presbitero P, et al: Ventricular arrhythmia in unrepaired and repaired tetralogy of Fallot: relation to age, timing of repair, and haemodynamic status. *Br Heart J* 1984; 52:77.
79. Uretzky G, Puga FJ, Danielson GK, et al: Reoperation after correction of tetralogy of Fallot. *Circulation* 1982; 66 (suppl I):I-202.
80. Fuster V, McGoon DC, Kennedy MA, et al: Long-term evaluation (twelve to twenty-two years) of open heart surgery for tetralogy of Fallot. *Am J Cardiol* 1980; 46:635.
81. Marelli A, Perloff J, Child J, Laks H: Pulmonary atresia with ventricular septal defect in adults. *Circulation* 1994; 89:243.
82. Reichenspurner H, Netz H, Uberfuhr P, et al: Heart-lung transplantation in a patient with pulmonary atresia and ventricular septal defect. *Ann Thorac Surg* 1994; 57:210.
83. Permut LC, Laks H: Surgical management of pulmonary atresia with ventricular septal defect and multiple aortopulmonary collaterals, in Karp RB, Laks H, Wechsler AS (eds): *Advances in Cardiac Surgery*. St. Louis, Mosby Year Book, 1999; p 75.
84. Webb GD, McLaughlin PR, Gow RM, et al: Transposition complexes. *Cardiol Clin* 1993; 11:651.
85. Turina M, Siebenmann R, Nussbaumer P, Senning A: Long-term outlook after atrial connection of transposition of great arteries. *J Thorac Cardiovasc Surg* 1988; 95:828.
86. Kirklin JW, Blackstone EH, Tchervenkov CI, et al: Clinical outcomes after the arterial switch operation for transposition of the great arteries. *Circulation* 1995; 109:289.
87. Hechter S, Webb G, Fredriksen P, et al: Cardiopulmonary exercise performance in adult survivors of the Mustard procedure. *Cardiol Young* 2001; 11:407.
88. Fredrikson P, Chen A, Veldtman G, et al: Exercise capacity in adult patients with congenitally corrected transposition of the great arteries. *Heart* 2001; 85:191.
89. Padalino M, Stellin G, Brawn W, et al: Arterial switch operation after left ventricular retraining in the adult. *Ann Thorac Surg* 2000; 70: 1753.
90. Cetta F, Bonilla J, Lichtenberg R, et al: Anatomic correction of dextrotransposition of the great arteries in a 36-year-old patient. *Mayo Clin Proc* 1997; 72:245.
91. Connelly M, Liu P, Williams W, et al: Congenitally corrected transposition of the great arteries in the adult: functional status and complications. *J Am Coll Cardiol* 1996; 27:1238.
92. Presbitero P, Somerville J, Rabajoli F, et al: Corrected transposition of the great arteries without associated defects in adult patients: clinical profile and follow up. *Br Heart J* 1995; 74:57.
93. Serraf A, Roux D, Lacour-Gayet F, et al: Reoperation after the arterial switch operation for transposition of the great arteries. *J Thorac Cardiovasc Surg* 1995; 110:892.
94. Cochrane AD, Karl TR, Mee RB: Staged conversion to arterial switch for late failure of the systemic right ventricle. *Ann Thorac Surg* 1993; 56:854.
95. Chang AC, Wernovsky G, Wessel DL, et al: Surgical management of late right ventricular failure after Mustard or Senning repair. *Circulation* 1992; 86(suppl II):II-140.
96. Stark J: Reoperations after Mustard and Senning operations, in Stark J, Pacifico AD (eds): *Reoperations in Cardiac Surgery*. Berlin, Springer-Verlag, 1989; p 187.
97. Peterson RJ, Franch RH, Fajman WA, Jones RH: Comparison of cardiac function in surgically corrected and congenitally corrected transposition of the great arteries. *J Thorac Cardiovasc Surg* 1988; 96:227.
98. Quaegebeur M, Rohmer J, Brom AG: Revival of the Senning operation in the treatment of transposition of the great arteries. *Thorax* 1977; 32:517.

99. Elizari A, Somerville J: Experience with the Glenn anastomosis in the adult with cyanotic congenital heart disease. *Cardiol Young* 1999; 9:257.
100. Bruckheimer E, Bulbul Z, Hellenbrand W, et al: Takedown of Glenn shunts in adults with congenital heart disease: technique and long-term follow-up. *J Thorac Cardiovasc Surg* 1997; 113:607.
101. Jonas RA: Indications and timing for the bidirectional Glenn shunt versus the fenestrated Fontan circulation. *J Thorac Cardiovasc Surg* 1994; 108:522.
102. Kopf GS, Laks H, Stansel HC, et al: Thirty-year follow-up of superior vena cava-pulmonary artery (Glenn) shunts. *J Thorac Cardiovasc Surg* 1990; 100:662.
103. Glenn WL, Fenn JE: Axillary arteriovenous fistula: a means of supplementing blood flow through a cava-pulmonary artery shunt. *Circulation* 1972; 46:1013.
104. Stamm C, Friehs I, Mayer J, et al: Long-term results of the lateral tunnel Fontan operation. *J Thorac Cardiovasc Surg* 2001; 121:28.
105. Harrison D, Liu P, Walters J, et al: Cardiopulmonary function in adult patients late after Fontan repair. *J Am Coll Cardiol* 1995; 26:1016.
106. Podzolkov V, Zaets S, Chiaureli M, et al: Comparative assessment of Fontan operation in modifications of atriopulmonary and total cavopulmonary anastomoses. *Eur J Cardiothorac Surg* 1997; 11:458.
107. Driscoll DJ, Offord KP, Feldt RH, et al: Five- to fifteen-year follow-up after Fontan operation. *Circulation* 1992; 85:469.
108. Deal BJ, Mavroudis C, Backer CC, et al: Comparison of anatomic isthmus block with the modified right atrial maze procedure for late atrial tachycardia in Fontan patients. *Circulation* 2002; 106:575.
109. Gentles T, Gauvreau K, Mayer J, et al: Functional outcome after the Fontan operation: factors influencing late morbidity. *J Thorac Cardiovasc Surg* 1997; 114:392.
110. Koutlas T, Harrison K, Bashore T, et al: Late conduit occlusion after modified Fontan procedure with classic Glenn shunt. *Ann Thorac Surg* 1996; 62:258.
111. Veldtman G, Nishimoto A, Siu S, et al: The Fontan procedure in adults. *Heart* 2001; 86:330.
112. Fredriksen P, Therrien J, Veldtman G, et al: Lung function and aerobic capacity in adults patients following modified Fontan procedure. *Heart* 2001; 85:295.
113. Dore A, Somerville J: Right atrioventricular extracardiac conduit as a Fontan modification: late results. *Ann Thorac Surg* 2000; 69:181.
114. Gates R, Laks H, Drinkwater D, et al: The Fontan procedure in adults. *Ann Thorac Surg* 1997; 63:1085.
115. Gelatt M, Hamilton RM, McCrindle BW, et al: Risk factors for atrial tachyarrhythmias after the Fontan operation. *J Am Coll Cardiol* 1994; 24:1735.
116. Kirklin JW, Barratt-Boyes BG: Tricuspid atresia and the Fontan operation, in Kirklin JW, Barratt-Boyes BG (eds): *Cardiac Surgery*. New York, Churchill-Livingstone, 1993; p 1055.
117. Giannico S, Corno A, Marino B, et al: Total extracardiac right heart bypass. *Circulation* 1992; 86(suppl II):II-110.
118. Laks H, Pearl JM, Haas GS, et al: Partial Fontan: advantages of an adjustable interatrial communication. *Ann Thorac Surg* 1991; 52:1084.
119. Celermajer DS, Bull C, Till JA, et al: Ebstein's anomaly: presentation and outcome from fetus to adult. *J Am Coll Cardiol* 1994; 23:170.
120. Kirklin JW, Barratt-Boyes BG: Ebstein's malformation, in Kirklin JW, Barratt-Boyes BG (eds): *Cardiac Surgery*. New York, Churchill-Livingstone, 1993; p 1105.
121. Hebe J: Ebstein's anomaly in adults. Arrhythmias: diagnosis and therapeutic approach. *Thorac Cardiovasc Surg* 2000; 48:214.
122. Pressley JC, Wharton JM, Tang ASL, et al: Effect of Ebstein's anomaly on short- and long-term outcome of surgically treated patients with Wolff-Parkinson-White syndrome. *Circulation* 1992; 86:1147.
123. Attie F, Rosas M, Rijlaarsdam M, et al: Analytical reviews of internal medicine, dermatology, neurology, pediatrics and psychiatry: the adult patient with Ebstein anomaly. *Medicine* (Baltimore) 2000; 79:27.
124. Saxena A, Fong LV, Tristam M, et al: Late noninvasive evaluation of cardiac performance in mildly symptomatic older patients with Ebstein's anomaly of tricuspid valve: role of radionuclide imaging. *J Am Coll Cardiol* 1991; 17:182.
125. Attie F, Rosas M, Rijlaarsdam M, et al: The adult patient with Ebstein anomaly. Outcome in 72 unoperated patients. *Medicine* (Baltimore) 2000; 79:27.
126. Gentles TL, Calder L, Clarkson PM, Neutze JM: Predictors of long-term survival with Ebstein's anomaly of the tricuspid valve. *Am J Cardiol* 1992; 69:377.
127. Frescura C, Angelini A, Daliento L, Thiene G: Morphological aspects of Ebstein's anomaly in adults. *Thorac Cardiovasc Surg* 2000; 48:203.
128. Oechslin E, Buchholz S, Jenni R: Ebstein's anomaly in adults: Doppler-echocardiographic evaluation. *Thorac Cardiovasc Surg* 2000; 48:209.
129. Mair DD, Seward JB, Driscoll DJ, Danielson GK: Surgical repair of Ebstein's anomaly: selection of patients and early and late operative results. *Circulation* 1985; 72:70.
130. Carpentier A, Chauvaud S, Mace L, et al: A new reconstructive operation for Ebstein's anomaly of the tricuspid valve. *J Thorac Cardiovasc Surg* 1988; 96:92.
131. Danielson, AHA newsletter.
132. Churgh R, Marelli D, Child J, et al: Heart transplantation in adolescents and adults with congenital heart disease. Presentation at the Annual Meeting of the American College of Cardiology, Atlanta, GA, March 2002.
133. Pigula F, Gandhi S, Ristich J, et al: Cardiopulmonary transplantation for congenital heart disease in the adult. *J Heart Lung Transplant* 2001; 20:297.
134. Stoica S, McNeil K, Perreas K, et al: Heart-lung transplantation for Eisenmenger syndrome: early and long-term results. *Ann Thorac Surg* 2001; 72:1887.
135. Lamour J, Addonizio L, Galantowicz M, et al: Outcome after orthotopic cardiac transplantation in adults with congenital heart disease. *Circulation* 1999; 100:II200.
136. Speziali G, Driscoll D, Danielson G, et al: Cardiac transplantation for end-stage congenital heart defects: the Mayo Clinic experience. Mayo Cardiothoracic Transplant team. *Mayo Clin Proc* 1998; 73:923.
137. Mendeloff E, Huddleston C: Lung transplantation and repair of complex congenital heart lesions in patients with pulmonary hypertension. *Semin Thorac Cardiovasc Surg* 1998; 10:144.
138. Fann J, Wilson M, Theodore J, Reitz B: Combined heart and single-lung transplantation in complex congenital heart disease. *Ann Thorac Surg* 1998; 65:823.
139. Carpentier A, Levy F, Mettauer B, et al: Successful sequential double lung transplantation and cardiac repair for aortopulmonary window: technical and functional advantages over heart-lung transplantation. *Transplant Proc* 1996; 28:2878.
140. Lupinetti F, Bolling S, Bove E, et al: Selective lung or heart-lung transplantation for pulmonary hypertension associated with congenital cardiac anomalies. *Ann Thorac Surg* 1994; 57:1545.
141. Bando K, Armitage JM, Paradis IL, et al: Indications for and results of single, bilateral, and heart-lung transplantation or pulmonary hypertension. *J Thorac Cardiovasc Surg* 1994; 108:1056.

142. Lupinetti FM, Bolling SF, Bove EL, et al: Selective lung or heart-lung transplantation for pulmonary hypertension associated with congenital cardiac anomalies. *Ann Thorac Surg* 1994; 57:1545.
143. Sarris GE, Smith JA, Shumway NE, et al: Long-term results of combined heart-lung transplantation: the Stanford experience. *J Heart Lung Transplant* 1994; 13:940.
144. Pearl JM, Laks H, Drinkwater DC: Cardiac transplantation following the modified Fontan procedure. *Transplant Sci* 1992; 2:1.
145. Spray TL, Mallory GB, Canter CE, et al: Pediatric lung transplantation for pulmonary hypertension and congenital heart disease. *Ann Thorac Surg* 1992; 54:216.
146. Madden B, Radley-Smith R, Hodson M, et al: Medium-term results of heart and lung transplantation. *J Heart Lung Transplant* 1992; 11:S241.
147. Mayer JE, Perry S, O'Brien P, et al: Orthotopic heart transplantation for complex congenital heart disease. *J Thorac Cardiovasc Surg* 1990; 99:484.
148. Rabago G, Copeland J, Rosapepe F, et al: Heart-lung transplantation in situs inversus. *Ann Thorac Surg* 1996; 62:296.
149. Carrel T, Neth J, Pasic M, et al: Should cardiac transplantation for congenital heart disease be delayed until adult age? *Eur J Cardiothorac Surg* 1995; 8:462.
150. Perry SB, Radtke W, Fellows KE, et al: Coil embolization to occlude aortopulmonary collateral vessels and shunts in patients with congenital heart disease. *J Am Coll Cardiol* 1989; 13:100.

Chapter 57

Pericardial Disease

Abeel A. Mangi/David F. Torchiana

The pericardium invests the heart like a cocoon; when incised and suspended from a chest retractor it nicely presents the heart for surgical correction. The surgical significance of the pericardium arises when cardiac filling is perturbed. When the limited space between the rigid pericardium and heart is acutely filled with blood or fluid, cardiac compression and tamponade may result. When inflammation and scarring cause the pericardium to shrink and densely adhere to the surface of the heart, constrictive pericarditis is the consequence. In this chapter, we will discuss pericardial anatomy and function and describe the conditions that commonly give rise to pericardial constriction and tamponade. The chapter includes steps for the diagnosis and therapy of these entities, the management of tamponade that occurs late after cardiac surgery, and the rationale for and against pericardial closure at the time of cardiac surgery.

ANATOMY AND FUNCTION

The pericardium serves two major functions: (1) to maintain the position of the heart within the mediastinum, and (2) to prevent cardiac distension by sudden volume overload. The position of the pericardium is maintained by loose attachments to the undersurface of the sternum and to the vertebral bodies, and by firm attachment to the central tendon of the diaphragm. The pericardium attaches to the ascending aorta, just inferior to the innominate vein, and attaches to the superior vena cava (SVC) several centimeters above the sinoatrial node. The pericardial reflection encompasses the superior and inferior pulmonary veins, and encircles the inferior vena cava (IVC), thereby making it possible for the surgeon to control the IVC from within the pericardium. The pericardial reflection attaches to the left atrium near the entrances of the pulmonary veins just above the atrioventricular groove (Fig. 57-1). The pericardium is perfused by the pericardiophrenic arteries that travel with the phrenic nerves, as well as by branches of the internal mammary arteries and feeder branches directly from the aorta. It is innervated by vagal fibers from the esophageal plexus, and the phrenic nerves course within it.

The pericardium is made up of two layers. The inner layer (visceral layer) of the pericardium is transparent, and is made up of a monolayer of mesothelial cells, making it essentially indistinguishable from the epicardium. Parietal pericardial lymphatic drainage is largely to the anterior and posterior

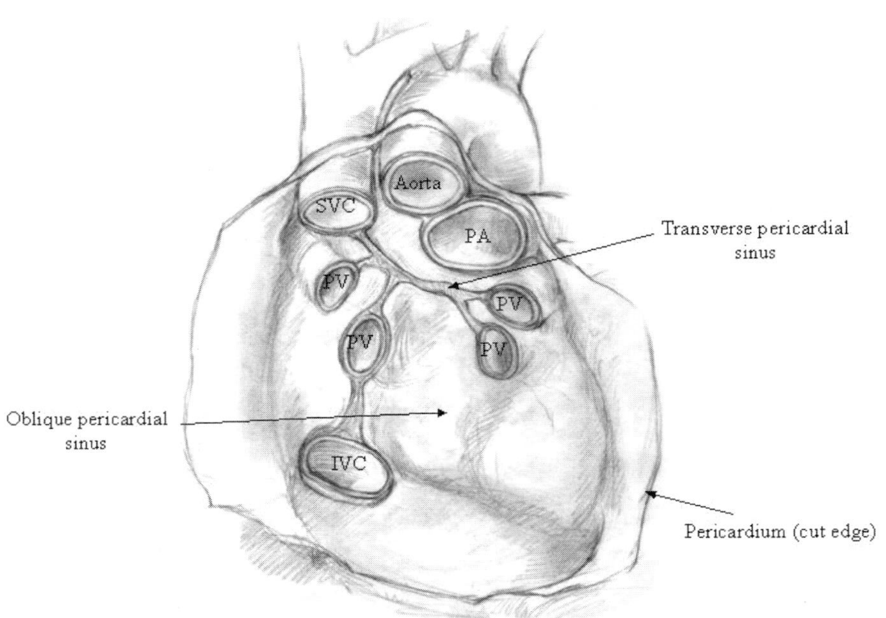

FIGURE 57–1 Pericardial attachments and reflections. PA = pulmonary artery; PV = pulmonary vein; IVC = inferior vena cava; SVC = superior vena cava.

mediastinal nodes, whereas visceral pericardial lymphatic drainage is via the tracheal and bronchial mediastinal lymph nodes.[1] The pericardial mesothelial cells contain dense microvilli that are $1\mu m$ wide and $3\mu m$ high,[2] ideal for facilitating fluid and ion exchange.[3]

The parietal layer is made up of elastin fibers interspersed amongst dense parallel bundles of collagen, which render this layer relatively noncompliant. Because the pericardium is stiffer than cardiac muscle, it tends to equalize the compliance of both chambers. By doing so, the pericardium contributes to the resting cavitary diastolic pressure of both ventricles, maximizing diastolic ventricular interaction.[4] An example of this phenomenon is the diminution of systemic arterial pressure during inspiration. Intrapericardial pressure tends to approximate pleural pressure, and varies with respiration. The negative intrathoracic pressure generated during inspiration augments right ventricular filling. The interventricular septum shifts towards the left to accommodate the increase in right ventricular volume. Because pericardial constraint does not allow equal filling of the left ventricle, the decrease in volume ejected by the systemic chamber results in a slight diminution of systemic arterial pressure during inspiration. This phenomenon is greatly magnified with an increase in intrapericardial pressure (for example, during acute filling of the pericardial space, or circulatory volume overload) resulting in production of the pulsus paradoxus.[5–7]

Normally, the volume of the pericardium exceeds that of the heart by about 10% to 20%.[8] The pericardium contains several sinuses and recesses that are not readily evident at the time of surgery or at postmortem examination (see Fig. 57-1). The largest (the transverse pericardial sinus) is the space between the ascending aorta and pulmonary artery bifurcation anteriorly, and the dome of the left atrium and SVC posteriorly. Such potential spaces allow the pericardium to expand and accommodate a limited volume load. Under normal conditions, the pericardium contains approximately 20 mL of fluid, which is an ultra-filtrate of plasma. This pericardial fluid serves to lubricate the junction of the beating heart with fixed structures.[9] The relative noncompliance of the pericardium results in a nonlinear relationship between intrapericardial volume and intrapericardial pressure. Although the pericardium may gradually expand to accommodate large volumes over time without appreciable increases in intrapericardial pressure, an acute volume overload may result in a large increase in intrapericardial pressure (Fig. 57-2). The pathophysiological sequelae of pericardial compliance and pericardial constraint are discussed below.

PATHOPHYSIOLOGY OF PERICARDIAL COMPRESSION

Tamponade

Tamponade is a state of circulatory decompensation that results from cardiac compression due to increased intrapericardial pressure. The clinical syndrome of tamponade varies widely, and is a reflection of the severity of hemodynamic impairment as well as the physiologic resilience of the host. Although hemorrhage is the most common etiology, pericardial diseases of almost any type can produce tamponade. It can be due to the accumulation of effusions, blood, clots, pus, or gas, or any combination of these. When pericardial filling commences, pericardial reserve volume (10-20 mL) is rapidly depleted. As fluid enters the pericardial space faster

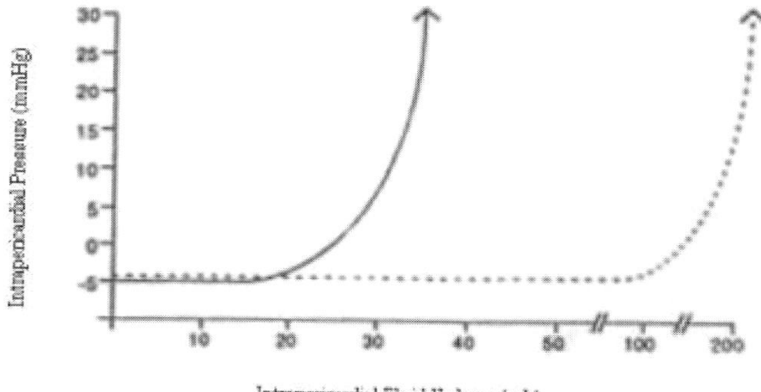

FIGURE 57–2 Relationship of intrapericardial volume and pressure. The pericardium of a healthy individual can accommodate 15 to 20 mL of fluid, with minimal increases in intrapericardial pressure. However, when the elastic limit of the pericardial space is acutely exceeded, small increases in intrapericardial volume will result in large increases in intrapericardial pressure (solid line). Intrapericardial volume and pressure are not linearly related. With gradual development of an effusion, the pericardial space can dilate considerably (dashed line). It may therefore accommodate a relatively large effusion without an appreciable increase in intrapericardial pressure. (*Modified with permission from Harken AH, Hammond GL, Edmunds LH Jr: Pericardial diseases, in Edmunds LH Jr (ed): Cardiac Surgery in the Adult. McGraw-Hill, New York, 1996; p 1303.*)

than the rate at which the parietal pericardium stretches, the noncompliant parietal pericardium prevents further expansion. At this point, pericardial volume can only increase by reducing cardiac chamber volumes. As a result, diastolic compliance is reduced equally in all chambers of the heart. This loss in compliance, coupled with the increase in intrapericardial pressures, means that higher pressures are required to fill the cardiac chambers, which may be partially achieved by parallel increases in systemic and pulmonary venous pressure by vasoconstriction.[10,11] Other compensatory mechanisms include tachycardia, time-dependent pericardial stretch, and blood volume expansion.[12] The latter two mechanisms are of little help in acute tamponade. The rapid accumulation of as little as 150 mL of fluid in the pericardial space (for example, after a penetrating cardiac wound) does not allow the parietal pericardium to develop any degree of compliance. In such a setting, the rapid accumulation of a relatively small volume of blood in the pericardial space can result in critical tamponade. On the other hand, the gradual accumulations of large pericardial effusions (over 1 L) can be compensated for in a more chronic setting such as inflammatory conditions. Distension of the pericardial space can be detected by chest roentgenogram (Fig. 57-3) or echocardiogram (Fig. 57-4).

Constriction

A wide range of disease processes can result in formation of a pericardial scar, the basic pathologic process behind constrictive pericarditis. The principal etiologies behind pericardial scar formation have changed over the last 25 years. The incidence of infectious etiologies (particularly tuberculosis) has declined, whereas the incidence of cases resulting from therapeutic irradiation of the mediastinum, cardiac surgery, and trauma (Fig. 57-5) has been increasing.[13] Constrictive pericarditis is important to recognize, because it is curable.

A

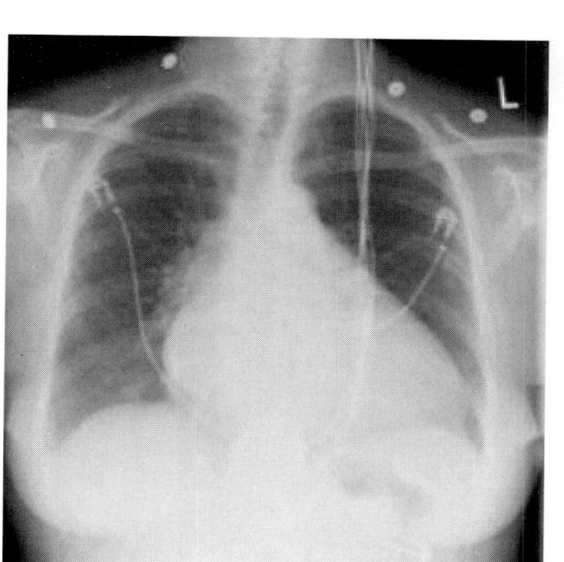

B

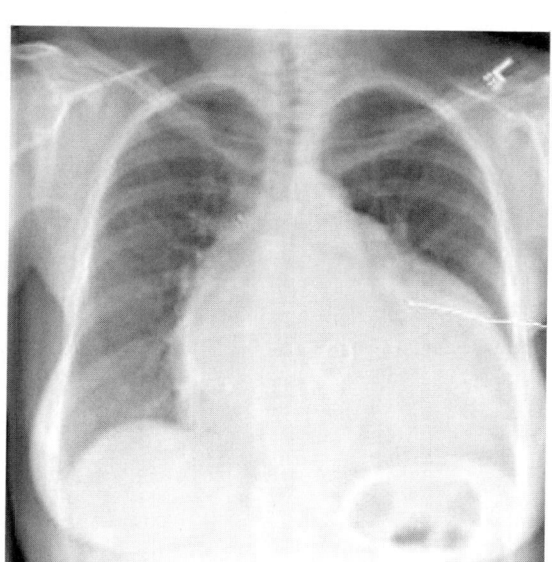

FIGURE 57–3 Enlarging pericardial effusion detected on chest x-ray. (A) At discharge; (B) on re-presentation, 3 weeks after discharge.

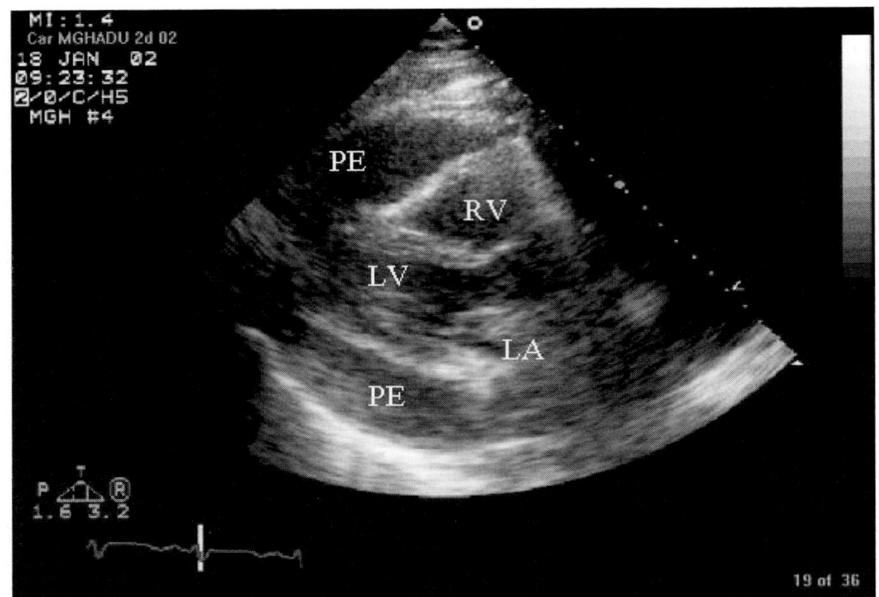

FIGURE 57–4 Large pericardial effusion detected on echocardiogram. LA = left atrium; LV = left ventricle; RV = right ventricle; PE = pericardial effusion.

Pericardial constriction exerts its pathophysiological effects by limiting cardiac filling. Unlike cardiac tamponade, in which cardiac filling is limited from the very beginning of diastole, constriction does not restrict filling in the earliest stages of diastole. As the ventricles fill, they are prevented from their normal distention as they encounter a stiff, contracted, and noncompliant pericardium. As a result, 70% to 80% of diastolic filling is forced to occur in the first 25% to 30% of diastole.[14] Although early diastolic filling pressures are normal (while the ventricle is free from the overlying stiff pericardium), later diastolic filling pressures are much higher. This sudden increase in diastolic pressure is reflected in the "dip and plateau" or "square-root" sign (Fig. 57-6), which occurs when ventricular pressures are measured

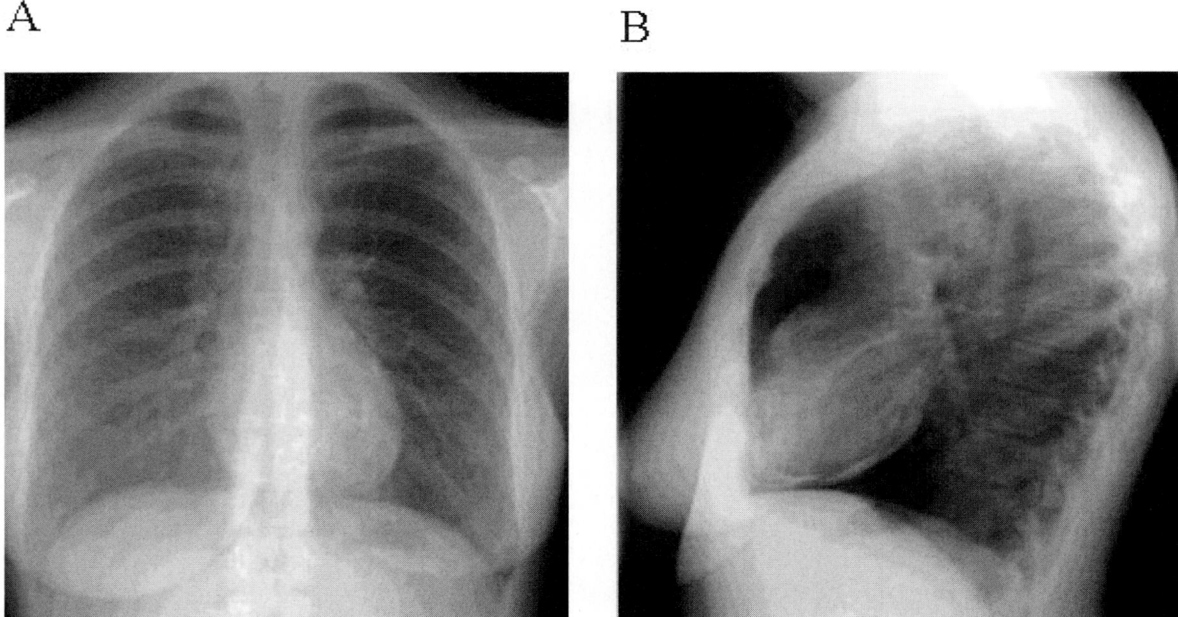

FIGURE 57–5 Pericardial calcification on PA (A) and lateral (B) chest x-ray in a young patient with a history of thoracic trauma.

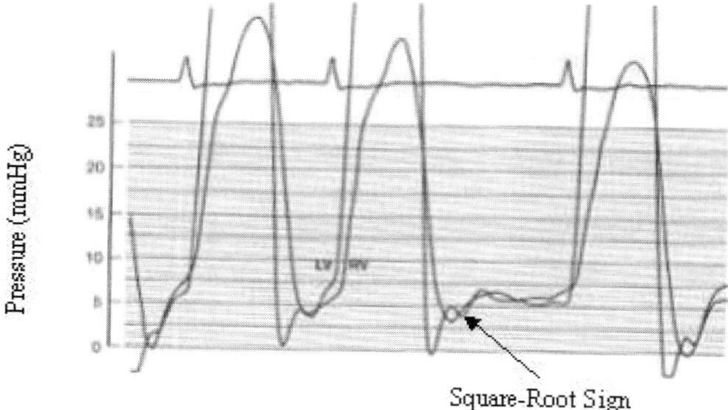

FIGURE 57–6 Square-root sign in right ventricular pressure tracing in constrictive pericarditis. (*Modified with permission from Spodick DH (ed): The Pericardium: A Comprehensive Textbook. Marcel Dekker, New York, 1997; p 4.*)

during cardiac catheterization. On this tracing, the gradual onset of diastolic filling is interrupted by an abrupt dip as the ventricles encounter the constrictive pericardium. The relaxing ventricles then spring back and reach the limit of the constrictive pericardium, generating a gentle rise in diastolic pressure that manifests itself as a plateau tracing. Similarly, right atrial pressure tracings reveal a deep *y* descent, which correlates to the nadir of the "square-root" sign. The clinical manifestation of this phenomenon is seen in the Kussmaul sign. Under normal circumstances, inspiration results in a 3- to 7-mm Hg drop in right atrial pressure. Venous flow from the neck veins therefore accelerates into the heart. The high pressure of pericardial constriction prevents the right atrium from accepting inspiratory acceleration of blood from the neck veins. As a result, neck veins become prominently distended during inspiration, a phenomenon referred to as Kussmaul's sign.[15]

These pathophysiological entities are all incorporated into the conventional diagnostic criteria for pericardial constriction at cardiac catheterization[16]:

1. *Equalization of pressures.* When pericardial compression is a dominant determinant of hemodynamic status, left and right ventricular end-diastolic pressures are within 5 mm Hg of each other. This classic criterion, however, has a sensitivity of only 60% and a specificity of only 38% for constrictive pericarditis.
2. *Elevation of mean atrial pressures.* Mean atrial pressure of over 10 mm Hg is suggestive of either cardiac tamponade or of pericardial constriction.
3. *Square-root sign.*
4. *Prominent* y *descent in right atrial pressure tracing.*
5. *Elevated right ventricular end-diastolic pressure.* Should be more than one third of right ventricular systolic pressure. This criterion has a sensitivity of 93% and a specificity of 57% for constrictive pericarditis.
6. *Left ventricular ejection fraction.* Must be above 40% for a diagnosis of pericardial constriction.

The low sensitivity and specificity of tests make the diagnosis of constrictive pericarditis a difficult one. It is important, however, to distinguish between constrictive pericarditis and other conditions such as restrictive cardiomyopathy because constrictive pericarditis is treatable. The diagnostic criteria for restrictive cardiomyopathy include:

1. Increased jugular venous pressure
2. Prominent *x* and *y* descents
3. A small or normal sized heart
4. Pulmonary congestion
5. Hepatic congestion
6. Absence of ventricular hypertrophy or dilatation
7. Depressed ventricular systolic function

Unfortunately, none of these tests are pathognomonic for restrictive cardiomyopathy. Although noninvasive tests such as echocardiography may qualitatively distinguish normal from thickened pericardium, and may reveal a depressed ejection fraction in the patient suffering from restrictive cardiomyopathy, they too, are not pathognomonic. Invasive hemodynamic monitoring can reveal nuanced differences between restrictive cardiomyopathy and constrictive pericarditis, such as decreased early diastolic filling in restrictive cardiomyopathy but not in pericardial constriction, and divergence in ventricular end-diastolic pressures in restrictive cardiomyopathy but convergence in pericardial constriction after fluid challenge.[17] Finally, endomyocardial biopsy may show pathologic change like amyloidosis or fibrosis in patients with restrictive cardiomyopathy, but be normal in the patient with pericardial constriction.[18]

The low sensitivity and specificity of these tests make it difficult to distinguish between constrictive pericarditis and other conditions such as restrictive cardiomyopathy. In an attempt to increase sensitivity and specificity of tests to diagnose constrictive pericarditis, Hurrell et al measured the respiratory variation of the gradient of left ventricular pressure to pulmonary capillary wedge pressure during the rapid filling of diastole. This was done to assess the dissociation of intrathoracic and intracardiac pressures that is seen in constrictive pericarditis. A difference of 5 mm Hg in the gradient between inspiratory and expiratory cycles had 93% sensitivity and 81% specificity for constrictive pericarditis. Furthermore, increased ventricular interdependence was assessed by comparing left ventricular systolic pressure and right ventricular systolic pressure during respiration. Although concordant increases in left ventricular systolic pressure and right ventricular systolic pressure are expected during inspiration, discordant pressures are encountered during inspiration in patients with constrictive pericarditis. This finding has 100% sensitivity and 95% specificity for constrictive pericarditis.[18]

CONGENITAL ABNORMALITIES

Most congenital abnormalities of the pericardium are discovered accidentally at cardiac surgery, on routine chest imaging, or while investigating unrelated problems.[19] They are rare, and less than 200 cases have been reported in the world literature.[20] The rarest of congenital pericardial abnormalities are pericardial bands that obstruct the superior vena cava. The most common are pericardial coelomic cysts.

Partial absence of the pericardium is the most common form of pericardial agenesis. It occurs in approximately 1 out of 14,000 births, and has a male preponderance.[20] It is usually associated with cardiac, pulmonary, or skeletal anomalies.[20] Most defects tend to occur on the left side, and are due to premature atrophy of the left common cardinal vein, or duct of Cuvier, which normally goes on to form a portion of the left superior intercostal vein. The right duct of Cuvier goes on to form the superior vena cava and ensures closure of the right pleuropericardial membrane.[21] Accordingly, right-sided defects tend to be lethal. While complete pericardial agenesis is of little clinical significance, unilateral absence is potentially problematic as it may accentuate cardiac mobility and allow the heart to be displaced into the pleural space with resulting incarceration[22] and tricuspid insufficiency.[21] The treatment for this lesion is pericardial resection, which may be accomplished thoracoscopically.[20] Alternatively, the pericardium can be replaced using patch material via thoracotomy. Both therapies appear to yield good outcomes.

Cysts can occur anywhere on the pericardium, but are found most often in the right costophrenic angle.[19] They do not communicate with the pericardial space, and contain a clear yellow fluid. They are typically unilocular, smooth, and less than 3 cm in diameter. Most remain clinically silent, and are discovered on routine chest imaging. Cysts have been associated with chest pain, dyspnea, cough, and arrhythmias probably owing to compression and inflammatory involvement of adjacent structures. They can also become secondarily infected.[23,24] Cysts are relatively easy to diagnose by echocardiography or CT imaging, and can be followed in asymptomatic patients. In symptomatic patients, cysts can be aspirated under radiologic guidance, or resected either via the thoracoscope or at thoracotomy.[25]

ACQUIRED ABNORMALITIES

A large number of factors can cause irritation of the pericardium, inducing the condition known as pericarditis (Table 57-1). The etiologies include myocardial infarction (Dressler's syndrome); drugs such as procainamide and hydralazine; viral, bacterial and fungal infections; metabolic (e.g., uremia) and autoimmune diseases (e.g., rheumatoid arthritis); neoplasms; trauma; and mechanical irritation at the time of surgery. The clinical syndrome in all these cases is similar, and includes pain, constitutional symptoms (such as weakness and malaise), fever (occasionally with rigors), and other symptoms such as cough or odynophagia. The pain is variably described as sharp, dull, aching, or pressure-like. It is generally acute in onset and precordial but can follow referred patterns similar to that of angina, such as to the arm, epigastrium, jaw, shoulder, or ridge of the trapezius. The pain is generally pleuritic, and exacerbated by inspiration, cough, or recumbency. These patients therefore like to sit up and lean forward for relief.

The cardinal sign of pericarditis is the pericardial rub. Echocardiogram may reveal fibrinous thickening of the pericardium with or without a small effusion. The electrocardiogram may range from normal, to nonspecific ST-segment deviations, to diffuse concave elevation of the ST segments without reciprocal depressions. This may be associated with PR-segment depression, and T-wave inversions in V_3 to V_6. It should be noted that arrhythmias and conduction abnormalities are not commonly seen in pericarditis, and are suggestive of an underlying cardiac abnormality if present.

After excluding other entities in the differential diagnosis, such as myocardial ischemia, pneumonia, chest wall pain, and pulmonary embolism, treatment should aim to relieve symptoms and eliminate etiologic agents. Nonsteroidal inflammatory drugs (NSAIDs) are the mainstay of treatment,[26] and may be supplemented with colchicine.[27] Further treatment must be tailored to address the specific etiologic agent, some of which are discussed in greater depth below.

Infectious Pericarditis

Microorganisms may invade the pericardial space from contiguous infections in the heart (e.g., endocarditis), lung, subdiaphragmatic space, or from the wound in postoperative patients. Patients with septicemia can also seed the pericardial space. This problem is more common in immunosuppressed patients.[28] Acute surgical intervention is required in the setting of purulent pericarditis, which may result in tamponade in a third of cases,[28] or in cases in which scarring results in pericardial constriction.

VIRAL PERICARDITIS

The cardiotropic viruses that cause myocarditis are the ones most likely to cause pericarditis as well. Pericardial inflammation is a result of immune complex deposition, direct viral attack, or both.[29] The clinical illness involves pain, friction rub, and typical changes on the electrocardiogram. Treatment is expectant, and symptoms generally resolve with 2 weeks. Surgical intervention is rarely required.

BACTERIAL (SUPPURATIVE) PERICARDITIS

Acute suppurative pericarditis is a life-threatening disease that has the potential to induce tamponade and septicemia.

TABLE 57–1 Acquired etiologies of acute pericarditis

INFECTIOUS
- **Bacterial**
  - Tuberculous (mycobacterial)
  - Suppurative (streptococcal, pneumococcal)
- **Viral**
  - Coxsackie
  - Influenza
  - HIV
  - Hepatitis A, B, C
  - Other
- **Fungal**
- **Parasitic**
- **Other**
  - Rickettsial
  - Spirochetal
  - *Spirillum*
  - *Mycoplasma*
  - Infectious mononucleosis
  - *Leptospira*
  - *Listeria*
  - Lymphograuloma venereum
  - Psittacosis

AUTOIMMUNE/VASCULITIDES
- **Rheumatoid arthritis**
- **Rheumatic fever**
- **Systemic lupus erythematosus**
- **Drug-induced lupus erythematosus**
- **Scleroderma**
- **Sjogrens syndrome**
- **Whipple's disease**
- **Mixed connective tissue disease**
- **Reiter's syndrome**
- **Ankylosing spondylitis**
- **Inflammatory bowel diseases**
  - Ulcerative colitis
  - Crohn's disease
- **Serum sickness**
- **Wegener's granulomatosis**
- **Giant cell arteritis**
- **Polymyositis**
- **Behçet's syndrome**
- **Familial Mediterranean fever**
- **Panmesenchymal syndrome**
- **Polyarteritis nodosa**
- **Churg-Strauss syndrome**
- **Thrombohemolytic-thrombocytopenic purpura**
- **Hypocomplementemic uremic vasculitis syndrome**
- **Leukoclastic vasculitis**
- **Other**

METABOLIC DISORDERS
- **Renal Failure**
  - Uremia in chronic or acute renal failure
  - "Dialysis" pericarditis
- **Myxedema**
  - Cholesterol pericarditis
- **Gout**
- **Scurvy**

DISEASE OF CONTIGUOUS STRUCTURES
- **Myocardial infarction/cardiac surgery**
  - Acute myocardial infarction
  - Post–myocardial infarction syndrome
  - Postpericardiotomy syndrome
  - Ventricular aneurysm
- **Aortic dissection**
- **Pleural and plumonary disease**
  - Pneumonia
  - Pulmonary embolism
  - Pleuritis
  - Malignancies of lung

NEOPLASTIC
- **Primary**
  - Mesothelioma
  - Sarcoma
  - Fibroma
- **Secondary**
  - Metastatic; carcinomas, sarcomas
  - Direct extension; bronchogenic, esophageal carcinomas
  - Hematogenous; lymphoma, leukemia

TRAUMA
- **Penetrating**
  - Stab wound or gunshot wound to the chest
- **Iatrogenic**
  - During diagnostic or therapeutic cardiac catheterization
  - During pacemaker insertion
- **Radiation pericarditis**

UNCERTAIN ETIOLOGIES AND PATHOGENESIS
- **Pericardial fat necrosis**
- **Loffler's syndrome**
- **Thalassemia**
- **Drug reactions**
  - Procainamide
  - Hydralazine
  - Others
- **Pancreatitis**
- **Sarcoidosis**
- **Fat embolism**
- **Bile fistula to pericardium**
- **Wissler syndrome**
- **"PIE" syndrome**
- **Stevens-Johnson syndrome**
- **Gaucher disease**
- **Diaphragmatic hernia**
- **Atrial septal defect**
- **Giant cell aortitis**
- **Takayasu syndrome**
- **Castleman disease**
- **Fabry disease**
- **Kawasaki disease**
- **Degos disease**
- **Histiocytosis X**
- **Campylodactyly-pleuritis-pericarditis syndrome**
- **Farmer's lung**
- **Idiopathic**

The most common organisms remain streptococcal, pneumococcal, and staphylococcal,[30] but the incidence of gram-negative infections such as *Escherichia coli, Salmonella,* and opportunistic infections is increasing. In adults, pneumopyopericardium is often due to fistula formation between a hollow viscus and the pericardium. However, invasion from contiguous foci, implantation at the time of surgery or trauma, mediastinitis, endocarditis, and subdiaphragmatic abscess can all induce this condition. The clinical course is acute and fulminant. The patient appears toxic and can have a high fever. Aggressive surgical drainage and antibiotic therapy are needed to avoid mortality, which is high.[28]

TUBERCULOUS PERICARDITIS

After decades of decrease, the incidence of tuberculous pericarditis has been increasing recently because of the rising numbers of immunocompromised patients, particularly those with HIV.[31] The pericardium is infected by hematogenous, lymphatic (from lung, bronchial, and mediastinal lymph nodes), peribronchial, or contiguous spread of tuberculosis. The classic pathologic stages of this entity include[32]:

1. Fibrinous exudation, with robust polymorphonuclear infiltration
2. Serous or serosanguinous effusions with a mainly lymphocytic exudation
3. Absorption of effusion, with organization of caseating granulomas, and pericardial thickening due to fibrin, collagen deposition, and fibrosis
4. Constrictive scarring, often with extensive calcification

Most often, the clinical course of this entity is insidious. Children and immunocompromised patients may, however, present with a more fulminant course, often demonstrating both constrictive and tamponade physiology.[30] The diagnosis is established by examining pericardial fluid for the presence of the mycobacterium. These patients require urgent institution of triple drug therapy. In addition certain groups advocate addition of aggressive surgical management in order to avoid development of chronic constrictive pericarditis.[33]

FUNGAL PERICARDITIS

Fungal pericarditis is an unusual entity and occurs predominantly in immunocompromised individuals, debilitated individuals, patients with severe burns, infants, and patients taking steroids. *Candida* and *Aspergillus* generate an insidious clinical picture, and may come to attention after the patient develops tamponade or constriction. Fungi such as *Histoplasma* that tend to be endemic to certain geographic areas may cause pericarditis in young, healthy, immunocompetent patients, and will often resolve within 2 weeks. There may be late sequelae such as constriction, but this is rare. Similarly, *Coccidioides* can also infect young healthy individuals, but will generally produce a more severe illness. Acute pericardial coccidiomycosis usually will accompany pneumonia from the same organism, with systemic adenopathy, osteomyelitis, or meningitis. The potential for chronic constriction is higher in this disease. These conditions all tend to resolve either spontaneously or after treatment with appropriate antifungal medical regimens. Surgical intervention is not usually required in the acute setting.

Metabolic Causes of Pericarditis

Pericarditis has been recognized to occur in the presence of renal failure, hypothyroidism, and autoimmune diseases (such as rheumatoid arthritis), in response to certain drugs (e.g., procainamide and hydralazine), and after mediastinal radiation.

UREMIC PERICARDITIS

Uremic pericarditis was first recognized by Bright in 1836.[34] Although it is recognized that nitrogen retention (blood urea nitrogen levels are generally greater than 60 mg/dL) is required for uremic pericarditis, the inciting agent is still unknown. The clinical profile is of a patient with chronic renal insufficiency who has symptoms of pain, fever, and a friction rub. There is usually a pericardial fluid collection, which can be exudative or transudative, and is usually hemorrhagic. The patient may be in tamponade; although the incidence of tamponade is decreasing due to the more widespread use of renal dialysis,[35,36] it remains the primary danger of this condition. Management of uremic pericarditis is controversial. Initial therapy includes NSAIDs and aggressive dialysis, and there is also a role for pericardiocentesis or drainage. The timing, however, remains uncertain.[37,38] Drainage has been advocated if a pericardial effusion persists despite 2 weeks of aggressive dialysis.[39] Any patient with hemodynamic compromise deserves immediate drainage.

DRUG-INDUCED PERICARDITIS

Procainamide (with or without associated lupus syndrome), hydralazine, methysergide, and emetine have all been associated with pericardial inflammation. Minoxidil has been associated with pericardial effusion.[40] The clinical presentation and guidelines for management in these settings are similar to those for other conditions. The inciting agent should be discontinued.

PERICARDITIS ASSOCIATED WITH RHEUMATOID ARTHRITIS

Pericarditis is common in patients with rheumatoid arthritis (RA). Approximately half of patients with RA have pericardial effusions, and almost half of all patients with RA have significant pericardial adhesions at autopsy.[41] The condition is encountered more often in patients with advanced RA, and is thought to be due to the higher rheumatoid factor titers. The deposition of immune complexes in the pericardium appears to be the inciting event behind the inflammatory response.[42] The clinical syndrome varies widely. The most common mode of presentation is a friction rub that lasts days to years with an asymptomatic effusion. The diagnosis is often compounded by the many clinical variants, and by intercurrent diseases such as viral pericarditis and drug-induced pericarditis. Treatment is required only in patients with symptomatic effusions. Constriction may occur late in RA patients. These patients should then be considered for pericardiectomy.

HYPOTHYROIDISM

Severe hypothyroidism produces large, clear, high-protein, high-cholesterol, and high-specific-gravity effusions in 5% to 30% of patients. The effusion may precede other signs of hypothyroidism.[43] These effusions are often asymptomatic and are recognized on chest roentgenogram. Clinical tamponade is rare because of the slow accumulation of fluid. However, acute exacerbation due to intercurrent acute pericarditis, hemorrhage, or cholesterol pericarditis can induce cardiac tamponade.[44]

Radiation Pericarditis

Radiation is the most common etiology of constrictive pericarditis in the United States.[45] This was first recognized in patients who received high-dose mantle radiation for Hodgkin's lymphoma in the 1960s and 1970s and later developed cardiac and pericardial diseases. Radiation induces acute pericarditis, pancarditis, and accelerated coronary artery disease in a dose-response fashion.[46,47] Cardiac surgery in these patients can be very challenging. Patients may present with a combination of pericardial constriction, restrictive cardiomyopathy, valvular heart disease, and a superimposed ischemic cardiomyopathy. In a large series from Stanford, over 20% of patients with "delayed pericarditis" went on to require surgical pericardiectomy.[48]

Neoplastic Pericarditis

Secondary neoplasms of the pericardium, that is, tumors that involve the pericardium by metastasis or by infiltration from adjoining structures, account for over 95% of pericardial neoplastic diseases. Rarely, primary pericardial tumors can also arise de novo, and paraneoplastic effusions can also occur that are in response to remote tumors.[49]

The most common secondary tumors involving the pericardium in males (including both metastasis and local extension) are carcinoma of the lung (31.7%), and esophagus (28.7%) and lymphoma (11.9%). In females, carcinoma of the lung (35.9%), lymphoma (17.0%), and carcinoma of the breast (7.5%) are most common.[50] Tumors of the lung, thymus, chest wall, or esophagus are more likely to involve the pericardium by direct spread. Lymphomas, Hodgkin's disease, leukemias, melanomas, and multiple myeloma can infiltrate the pericardium as well as the myocardium. Primary pericardial tumors are rare. Benign tumors are generally encountered in infancy or childhood. Malignant tumors such as mesotheliomas, sarcomas, and angiosarcomas are found in the third or fourth decade of life.[51]

In both primary and secondary tumor involvement, the clinical presentation is usually silent, and is associated with large pericardial effusions. Tamponade can result if hemorrhage occurs into a malignant effusion. Occasional tumors can induce constriction, due to neoplastic tissue, adhesions, or both. The role of the surgeon is limited to that of a diagnostician in most of these cases.[52] Large refractory and tamponading effusions may need to be drained. Pericardiocentesis has a very high failure rate. Subxiphoid drainage or percutaneous balloon pericardiotomy are transiently effective. A pericardioperitoneal shunt may be considered in children. While extensive resection and debulking is desirable in persistent or recurrent malignant pericardial constriction, it is transient without effective adjunctive chemotherapy and/or radiation therapy. In general, life expectancy after malignant pericardial involvement is less than 4 months.[53,54]

Traumatic Pericardial Disease

PENETRATING TRAUMA

Knives, bullets, needles, intracardiac instrumentation, and cardiac surgery are the most common causes of penetrating trauma to the pericardium.[55] Lacerating and penetrating objects like knives cause less physical damage than high-velocity projectiles like bullets. That being said, tamponade is more common in stab wounds than in gunshot wounds. The right ventricle is most commonly involved in anterior chest wounds. Because tamponade provides hemostasis and prevents exsanguination, patients in tamponade appear to have a better survival rate than patients with cardiac stab wounds not in tamponade.[56] The corollary of course, is that unless tamponade is released in a timely fashion, it can cause circulatory decompensation and death. Pericardiocentesis has no role in the management of penetrating wounds to the heart. Stable patients can be explored in the operating theater, but unstable patients should undergo thoracotomy in the emergency room.

BLUNT TRAUMA

Blunt injuries to the pericardium rarely occur in isolation. Trauma due to compression, blast, and deceleration will produce a spectrum of injuries, ranging from cardiac contusion to cardiac rupture, and pericardial laceration with herniation or luxation of the heart, which is a surgical emergency. The management of cardiac contusion and cardiac rupture are discussed elsewhere in this book. Here we will focus on pericardial laceration with cardiac herniation. These patients typically suffer deceleration injuries and are invariably hypotensive. They may initially respond to volume resuscitation. A pericardial rub may be the only physical finding, but is not specific for this entity. On chest imaging, free air may be seen in the pericardium, and the heart may be displaced. Intra-abdominal organs may have migrated into the pericardial sac. This is more likely to occur on the left. The immediate management consists of repositioning the patient so as to reduce the herniation. If the heart has herniated into the left pleural space, positioning the patient right-side down may reduce the herniation. Thoracotomy is required for definitive treatment and repair of associated injuries.[57–59]

Peridcarditis Associated with Myocardial Infarction/Dressler Syndrome

This entity is thought to occur in almost half of patients suffering a transmural myocardial infarction, but is discovered in far less.[60] Although chest pain is almost universally present, the pain of pericarditis can be distinguished from ischemic pain by its positional and pleuritic nature. The pain of pericarditis tends to start one week after myocardial infarction. A rub is present on auscultation. The electrocardiographic signs of pericarditis are obscured by those of infarction. Patients may develop a small pericardial effusion. Patients suffering from pericarditis appear to have a worse long-term prognosis than those without postinfarct pericarditis,[61] possibly because they tend to have larger infarctions as judged by enzyme release and degree of ST-segment elevation. The diagnosis is clinical, and is treated with aspirin and/or NSAIDs.

Cardiac Surgery and the Pericardium

POSTINFARCTION PERICARDITIS

Postinfarction pericarditis may be relevant to the surgeon. To the unwary it may masquerade as postinfarction angina and lead to a needless early operation after a myocardial infarction. Extensive fibrinous adhesions and murky gelatinous fluid may be present in the pericardial space and obscure epicardial vessels. When the pericardium is opened late in such a patient, the surgeon should expect dense pericardial adhesions.

POSTPERICARDIOTOMY SYNDROME

Pericardial friction rubs are almost universal after cardiac surgery, and some patients will develop Dressler's syndrome.[62] These patients will almost always respond to a course of NSAIDs, and may occasionally require a short course of corticosteroids. Despite these measures, pericardial effusions may develop in the later postoperative period.

LATE CARDIAC TAMPONADE

Early postoperative tamponade will usually be promptly detected because of a high level of vigilance and close hemodynamic monitoring. It is equally important for surgeons to be aware of the potential for late cardiac tamponade that usually presents after hospital discharge and often initially to a clinician other than the cardiac surgeon. This entity is a potentially lethal complication and occurs in between 0.5% and 6% of patients after heart surgery, almost exclusively in those taking warfarin. Late cardiac tamponade (that is, tamponade occurring more than 7 days after cardiac surgery) is more common in younger patients who have undergone cardiac valve surgery. Patients present on average within 3 weeks of surgery with elevated prothrombin times. They are generally very symptomatic, with declining exercise tolerance, dyspnea, and an inability to diurese, and sometimes hypotension. Although echocardiography will demonstrate a pericardial effusion, the typical echocardigraphic signs of tamponade are detected in only 30% of patients. The diagnosis is therefore a clinical one. Patients respond favorably to pericardiocentesis, and are able to safely resume anticoagulation.[63]

PERICARDIAL CLOSURE

Surgeons vary in their approach towards closing the pericardium after routine cardiac surgery. Redo sternotomy may be more hazardous when the right ventricle is adherent to the inner table of the sternum. Accordingly, it has been proposed that closing the pericardium at the time of the initial procedure will interpose a protective layer of tissue between the sternum and the heart and thereby reduce the risks of redo sternotomy. The value of this added protection against cardiac injury on sternal reentry is limited by the relative infrequency of reoperation and the low incidence of cardiac injury when the pericardium is left open. On the negative side, closing the pericardium can cause kinking of bypass grafts after coronary bypass surgery and may result in hemodynamic compromise due to cardiac compression. Rao et al demonstrated that pericardial closure at the time of cardiac surgery adversely affects postoperative hemodynamics.[64] In this study, the pericardial edges were marked with radiopaque markers and the pericardium was closed with a running suture, the ends of which were exteriorized. After obtaining a postoperative chest film that demonstrated pericardial approximation, a set of baseline hemodynamics were measured. The suture was then removed, another roentgenogram taken to demonstrate that the pericardial edges had become distracted, and then the

TABLE 57–2 Structural and hemodynamic changes after pericardial closure in patients undergoing elective isolated coronary artery bypass grafting

Parameters measured	Open pericardium	Closed pericardium	*p* value
Retrosternal space at 1 wk (cm)	13 ± 5	20 ± 7	.0003
Retrosternal space at 3 mo (cm)	7 ± 3	14 ± 7	.0001
CI L/min/m^2 1 h postoperation	3.1 ± 0.8	2.3 ± 0.6	.003
CI L/min/m^2 4 h postoperation	3.1 ± 0.9	2.7 ± 0.7	.156
CI L/min/m^2 8 h postoperation	3.0 ± 0.8	2.8 ± 0.5	.402
LVSWI g/m/m^2 1 h postoperation	72 ± 18	52 ± 13	.002
LVSWI g/m/m^2 4 h postoperation	68 ± 17	54 ± 8	.016
LVSWI g/m/m^2 8 h postoperation	62 ± 22	52 ± 10	.087

CI = cardiac index; LVSWI = left ventricular stroke work index.

hemodynamic measurements were repeated. Pericardial closure resulted in transient hemodynamic compromise in the first 8 hours after operation. Conversely, the retrosternal space was significantly larger both 1 week and 3 months after operation (Table 57-2). The risks and benefits of pericardial closure must therefore be weighed against its potential benefits if it is to be used in everyday clinical practice.

OPERATIONS

Mediastinal Reexploration

Standard management for the postoperative cardiac surgical patient involves leaving the pericardium open, and placing anterior and posterior mediastinal thoracostomy drains. Despite this, postoperative tamponade may occur. The typical clinical scenario is one in which chest tube output falls after a period of early postoperative bleeding, the patient develops tachycardia, narrowing of the pulse pressure, increase in right heart filling pressures, decrease in urine output, and a drop in the cardiac index. This setting is diagnostic of tamponade, and arrangements should be made for expedient mediastinal exploration. Echocardiography is not always helpful because the pericardial space is difficult to visualize in the immediate postoperative patient and thrombus is difficult to resolve. Subtle findings that have been reported include an inspiratory increase in right ventricular end-diastolic diameter and a reciprocal decrease in left ventricular diastolic diameter,[64] as well as an increase in early peak tricuspid flow velocity and reduction in flow across the mitral valve.[65,66]

Pericardiocentesis

Pericardiocentesis can be performed at the bedside under local anesthesia in a calm patient, but it is usually performed in the catheterization laboratory. Arterial and right heart catheterization monitoring are frequently used. After administration of 1% lidocaine to the skin and the deeper tissues of the left xiphocostal area, a 25-mL syringe is affixed to a three-way stopcock and then to an 18-gauge spinal needle. This pericardial needle is connected to an ECG "V" lead. Under ECG and fluoroscopic guidance, the needle is advanced from the left of the subxiphoid area aiming toward the left shoulder. A discrete pop may be felt as the needle enters the pericardial space. ST-segment elevation may be seen on the V lead tracing when the needle touches the epicardium. Under these circumstances, the needle is retracted slightly until ST-segment elevation disappears. Once the pericardial space is entered, a guidewire is introduced into the pericardial space through the needle. The needle is removed and a catheter is inserted in the pericardial sac over the guidewire. At our institution, a pigtail-shaped drainage catheter with an end and multiple side holes is used. Intrapericardial pressure is measured by attaching a pressure transducer system to the intrapericardial catheter. Pericardial fluid may then be removed. When appropriate, samples of pericardial fluid are sent for cell count, chemistry, cytology, cultures, and special stain studies to assist with the diagnosis of the etiology of the effusion. In the presence of pericardial tamponade, aspiration of fluid is continued until there is clear clinical and hemodynamic improvement. If blood is withdrawn, 5mL should be placed on a sponge to see if it clots. Clotting blood suggests that the needle has either inadvertently entered a cardiac chamber or caused epicardial injury. Defibrinated blood that has been present in the pericardial space for even a short time should not clot.[67] The catheter is frequently left in place to monitor pericardial fluid drainage. It is secured to the skin with 4-0 silk sutures and covered with a sterile dressing, and the patient is started on prophylactic antibiotics. The pericardial space is drained every 8 hours and the catheter flushed with heparinized solution and in general removed within the next 24 to 72 hours. Pneumothorax is a potential complication, and chest x-ray is mandatory after the procedure.

Pericardial Window

The purpose of partial pericardial resection (window) is to drain fluid into the pleural or peritoneal compartment in order to avoid the reaccumulation of pericardial fluid if the patient has failed prior pericardiocentesis. The procedure can be performed via thoracoscopy, anterior thoracotomy, or subxiphoid incision. General anesthetic is desirable, with the caveat that it may be poorly tolerated in patients with cardiac compression. When the pericardium is encountered, it should be incised. Fluid will invariably drain under pressure. The excised portion of pericardium should be as large as is feasible. Through an anterior thoracotomy, all accessible pericardium ventral to the phrenic nerve should be excised. The surgeon should remain mindful of the rare possibility of cardiac prolapse. Similarly, via the subxiphoid approach, as much diaphragmatic pericardium should be excised as is possible. Thoracostomy drainage catheters should be left within the pericardium.

Pericardial Stripping

Pericardial diseases that produce epicardial or pericardial inflammation (such as radiation or tuberculosis) can cause the pericardium to adhere to the epicardial surface, inducing chronic pericardial constriction. Because of dense adhesions and calcification that can penetrate into the myocardium, pericardial resection can be a technical challenge. The procedure is done via median sternotomy with the capability to go on full cardiopulmonary bypass.[18,33] Because of the additional complication of coagulopathy we do not use cardiopulmonary bypass routinely. Left anterior thoracotomy is preferred by some surgeons. The goal of the procedure is to release the ventricles from the densely adherent pericardial shell. The lack of a surgical plane can make this a very bloody operation, and attention must be paid to salvage and reinfusion of blood. Epicardial coronary vessels are at risk in this dissection and particular care must be taken dissecting in these regions. The pericardium should be excised from phrenic nerve to phrenic nerve, and also posteriorly, particularly around the entrance of the vena cavae and pulmonary veins to the pericardium. This complete resection should restore pressure-volume loops to their normal position.[68] The results vary with the etiology and severity of the disease. Operative mortality has been reported as high as 10% to 20%[69,70] and varies based on severity of heart failure, elevation of right atrial pressure, and comorbidities. Although surgery alleviates or improves symptoms in the vast majority of patients, long-term results are disappointing in patients over the age of 50 and in patients with radiation-induced constrictive pericarditis.[13,71]

ACKNOWLEDGMENTS

The authors would like to thank Marcia Williams for the preparation of Figure 57-1.

REFERENCES

1. Miller AJ, Pick R, Johnson PJ: The production of acute pericardial effusion: the effects of various degrees of interference with venous return and lymph drainage from the heart muscle in the dog. *Am J Cardiol* 1971; 28:463.
2. Ishihara T, Ferrans VJ, Jones M, et al: Histologic and ultrastructural features of normal human pericardium. *Am J Cardiol* 1980; 46:744.
3. Spodick DH: The normal and diseased pericardium: current concepts of pericardial physiology, diseases and treatment. *J Am Coll Cardiol* 1983; 1:240.
4. Hammond HK, White FC, Bhargava V, et al: Heart size and maximal cardiac output are limited by the pericardium. *Am J Physiol* 1992; 263:H1675.
5. Savitt MA, Tyson GS, Elbeery JR, et al: Physiology of cardiac tamponade and paradoxical pulse in conscious dogs. *Am J Physiol* 1993; 265:H1996.
6. Tyberg JV, Smith ER: Ventricular diastole and the role of the pericardium. *Hertz* 1990; 15:354.
7. Santamore WP, Dell'Italia LJ: Ventricular interdependence: significant left ventricular contributions to right ventricular systolic function. *Prog Cardiovasc Dis* 1990; 40:298.
8. Harken AH, Hammond GL, Edmunds LH Jr: Pericardial diseases, in Edmunds LH Jr (ed): *Cardiac Surgery in the Adult*. New York, McGraw-Hill, 1996; p 1303.
9. Spodick DH: Physiology of the normal pericardium: functions of the pericardium, in Spodick DH (ed): *The Pericardium: A Comprehensive Textbook*. New York, Marcel Dekker, 1997; p 15.
10. Spodick DH: Pathophysiology of cardiac tamponade. *Chest* 1998; 113:1372.
11. Spodick DH: Physiology of cardiac tamponade: functions of the pericardium, in Spodick DH (ed): *The Pericardium: A Comprehensive Textbook*. New York, Marcel Dekker, 1997; p 180.
12. Reddy PS, Curtiss EI, Uretsky BF: Spectrum of hemodynamic changes in cardiac tamponade. *Am J Cardiol* 1990; 66:1487.
13. Ling LH, Oh JK, Schaff HV, et al: Constrictive pericarditis in the modern era: evolving clinical spectrum and impact on outcome after pericardiectomy. *Circulation* 1999; 100:1380.
14. Myers RBH, Spodick DH: Constrictive pericarditis: clinical and pathophysiologic characteristics. *Am Heart J* 1999; 138:219.
15. Spodick DH: Constrictive pericarditis, in Spodick DH (ed): *The Pericardium: A Comprehensive Textbook*. New York, Marcel Dekker, 1997; p 214.
16. Aroney CN, Ruddy TD, Dighero H, et al: Differentiation of restrictive cardiomyopathy from pericardial constriction: assessment of diastolic function by radionuclide angiography. *J Am Coll Cardiol* 1989; 13:1007.
17. Bush CA, Stang JM, Wooley CF, et al: Occult constrictive pericardial disease: diagnosis by rapid volume expansion and correction by pericardiectomy. *Circulation* 1977; 56:924.
18. Hurrell DG, Nishimura RA, Higano ST, et al: Value of dynamic respiratory changes in left and right ventricular pressures for the diagnosis of constrictive pericarditis. *Circulation* 1996; 93:2007.
19. Spodick DH: Congenital abnormalities of the pericardium, in Spodick DH (ed): *The Pericardium: A Comprehensive Textbook*. New York, Marcel Dekker, 1997; p 65.
20. Risher WH, Rees AD, Ochsner JL, et al: Thoracoscopic resection of pericardium for symptomatic congenital pericardial defect. *Ann Thorac Surg* 1993; 56:1390.
21. VanSon JAM, Danielson GK, Callahan JA: Congenital absence of the pericardium: displacement of the heart associated with tricuspid insufficiency. *Ann Thorac Surg* 1993; 56:1405.
22. Saito R, Hotta F: Congenital pericardial defect associated with cardiac incarceration: case report. *Am Heart J* 1980; 100:866.

23. Barva GL, Magliani L, Bertoli D, et al: Complicated pericardial cyst: atypical anatomy and clinical course. *Clin Cardiol* 1998; 21:862.
24. Chopra PS, Duke DJ, Pellett JR, et al: Pericardial cyst with partial erosion of the right ventricular wall. *Ann Thorac Surg* 1991; 51:840.
25. Weder W, Klotz HP, Segesser LV, et al: Thoracoscopic resection of a pericardial cyst. *J Thorac Cardiovasc Surg* 1994; 107:313.
26. Ilan Y, Oren R, Ben-Chetrit E: Acute pericarditis: etiology, treatment, and prognosis: a study of 115 patients. *Jpn Heart J* 1991; 32:315.
27. Adler Y, Finkelstein Y, Guindo J, et al: Colchicine treatment for recurrent pericarditis: a decade of experience. *Circulation* 1998; 97:2183.
28. Rubin RH, Moellering RC: Clinical, microbiological and therapeutic aspects of purulent pericarditis. *Am Med J* 1975; 59:68.
29. Maisch B, Outzen H, Roth D, et al: Prognostic determinants in conventionally treated myocarditis and perimyocarditis—focus on antimyolemmal antibodies. *Eur Heart J* 1991; 12:81.
30. Spodick DH: Infectious pericarditis. in Spodick DH (ed): *The Pericardium: A Comprehensive Textbook*. New York, Marcel Dekker, 1997; p 260.
31. Fowler NO: Tuberculous pericarditis. *JAMA* 1991; 266:99.
32. Tirilomis T, Univerdoben S, von der Emde J: Pericardiectomy for chronic constrictive pericarditis: risks and outcome. *Eur J Thorac Cardiovasc Surg* 1994; 8:487.
33. Quale JM, Lipschik GY, Heurich AW: Management of tuberculous pericarditis. *Ann Thorac Surg* 1987; 43:653.
34. Bright R: Tabular view of the morbid appearance in 100 cases connected with albuminous urine: with observations. *Guys Hosp Rep* 1836; 1:380.
35. Spodick DH: Pericardial disease in systemic disease. *Cardiol Clin* 1990; 8:709.
36. Sever MS, Steinmuller DR, Hayes JM, et al: Pericarditis following renal transplantation. *Transplantation* 1991; 51:1229.
37. Lazarus JM: Pericardial effusion. *Arch Intern Med* 1984; 144:1317.
38. Leehey DJ, Daugirdas JT, Ing TS: Early drainage of pericardial effusions in patients with dialysis pericarditis. *Arch Intern Med* 1983; 143:1673.
39. Rustky EA, Rostard SG: Pericarditis in end stage renal disease: clinical characteristics and management. *Semin Dial* 1989; 2:25.
40. Oates JA, Wilkinson GR: Principles of drug therapy, in Isselbacher KJ, Braunwald E, Wilson JD, et al (eds): *Harrison's Principles of Internal Medicine*. New York, McGraw-Hill, 1994; p 409.
41. Turesson C, Lacobsson L, Bergstrom U: Extra-articular rheumatoid arthritis: prevalence and mortality. *Rheumatology* 1999; 38:668.
42. Gulati S, Kumar L: Cardiac tamponade as an initial manifestation of systemic lupus erythematosus in early childhood. *Ann Rheum Dis* 1992; 51:179.
43. Kabadi UM, Kumer SP: Pericardial effusion in primary hypothyroidism. *Am Heart J* 1990; 120:1393.
44. Bereket A, Yang TF, Dey S, et al: Cardiac decompensation due to massive pericardial effusion: a manifestation of hypothyroidism in children with Down's syndrome. *Clin Pediatr* 1994; 12:749.
45. Schiavone WA: The changing etiology of constrictive pericarditis in a large referral center. *Am J Cardiol* 1986; 58:373.
46. Stewart JR, Fajardo LF: Radiation induced heart disease: an update. *Prog Cardiovasc Dis* 1984; 27:173.
47. Fajardo LF: Radiation induced coronary artery disease. *Chest* 1977; 71:563.
48. Fajardo LF, Stewart JR: Radiation induced heart disease: human and experimental observations, in Bristow MR (ed): *Drug Induced Heart Disease*. Amsterdam, Elsevier, 1980; p 241.
49. Spodick DH: Neoplastic pericardial disease, in Spodick DH (ed): *The Pericardium: A Comprehensive Textbook*. New York, Marcel Dekker, 1997; p 301.
50. Lam KY, Dickens P, Chan AC: Tumors of the heart: a 20–year experience with a review of 12,485 consecutive autopsies. *Arch Pathol Lab Med* 1993; 117:1027.
51. Warren MH: Malignancies involving the pericardium. *Semin Thorac Cardiovas Surg* 2000; 12:119.
52. Bardales RH, Stanley MW, Schaefer RF, et al: Secondary pericardial malignancies: a critical appraisal of the role of cytology, pericardial biopsy, and DNA ploidy analysis. *Am J Pathol* 1996; 106:29.
53. Palacios IF, Tuzcu EM, Ziskind AA, et al: Percutaneous balloon pericardial window for patients with malignant pericardial effusions and tamponade. *Cathet Cardiovasc Diagn* 1991; 22:244.
54. Hazelrigg SR, Mack MJ, Landreneau RJ, et al: Thoracoscopic pericardiectomy for effusive pericardial disease. *Ann Thorac Surg* 1993; 56:792.
55. Asensio JA, Berne JD, Demetriades D, et al: One hundred five penetrating cardiac injures: a 2-year prospective evaluation. *J Trauma* 1998; 44:1073.
56. Sabers CJ, Levy NT, Bowen JM: A 33-year old man with chest pain and fever. *Mayo Clin Proc* 1999; 74:181.
57. Bitkover CY, Al-Khalili F, Ribeiro A, Liska J: Surviving resuscitation: successful repair of cardiac laceration. *Ann Thor Surg* 1996; 61:710.
58. Buckman RF, Buckman PD: Vertical deceleration trauma: principles of management. *Surg Clin North Am* 1991; 71:331.
59. Feghali NT, Prisant LM: Blunt myocardial injury. *Chest* 1995; 108:1673.
60. Spodick DH: Pericardial involvement in diseases of the heart and other contiguous structures, in Spodick DH (ed): *The Pericardium: A Comprehensive Textbook*. New York, Marcel Dekker, 1997; p 334.
61. Correale E, Maggioni AP, Romano S, et al: Comparison of frequency, diagnostic and prognostic significance of pericardial involvement in acute myocardial infarction treated with and without thrombolytics. *Am J Cardiol* 1993; 71:1377.
62. Miller RH, Horneffer PJ, Gardner TJ, et al: The epidemiology of the postpericardiotomy syndrome: a common complication of cardiac surgery. *Am Heart J* 1998; 116:1323.
63. Mangi AA, Palacios IF, Torchiana DF: Catheter pericardiocentesis for delayed tamponade after cardiac valve operation. *Ann Thorac Surg* 2002; 73:1479.
64. Rao W, Komeda M, Weisel RD, et al: Should the pericardium be closed routinely after heart operations? *Ann Thorac Surg* 1999; 67:484.
65. Gonzalez MS, Basnight MA, Appleton CP: Experimental cardiac tamponade: hemodynamic and Doppler echocardiographic reexamination of right and left heart ejection dynamics to the phase of respiration. *J Am Coll Cardiol* 1991; 18:243.
66. Appleton C, Hatle LK, Popp RL: Cardiac tamponade and pericardial effusion: respiratory variation in transvalvular flow velocities during experimental cardiac tamponade. *J Am Coll Cardiol* 1988; 11:1020.
67. Nkere UU, Whaawell SA, Thompson EM, et al: Changes in pericardial morphology and fibrinolytic activity during cardiopulmonary bypass. *J Thorac Cardiovasc Surg* 1993; 106:339.
68. Kuroda H, Sakaguchi M, Takano T, et al: Intraoperative monitoring of pressure-volume loops of the left ventricle in pericardiectomy for constrictive pericarditis. *J Thorac Cardiovasc Surg* 1996; 112:198.
69. McCaughan BC, Schaff HV, Piehler JM, et al: Early and late results of pericardiectomy for constrictive pericarditis. *J Thorac Cardiovasc Surg* 1985; 89:340.
70. Seifert FC, Miller DC, Oesterle SN, et al: Surgical treatment of constrictive pericarditis: analysis of outcome and diagnostic error. *Circulation* 72 (suppl II):II-264.
71. Ni Y, von Segesser LK, Turina M: Futility of pericardiectomy for postirradiation constrictive pericarditis. *Ann Thorac Surg* 1990; 149:445.

Chapter 58

Cardiac Neoplasms

Michael J. Reardon/W. Roy Smythe

Neoplasms of the heart can be divided into primary cardiac tumors arising in the heart and secondary cardiac tumors that have metastasized to the heart. Primary cardiac tumors can be further stratified into benign and malignant tumors. Secondary involvement of the heart is relatively uncommon; 10% to 20% of patients dying of disseminated cancer have metastatic involvement of the heart or pericardium.[1,2] Surgical resection is seldom possible or advisable for these tumors, and surgical intervention is usually limited to drainage of malignant pericardial effusions and/or diagnostic biopsies.

Primary tumors of the heart are uncommon but not rare. The incidence of primary cardiac neoplasm ranges between 0.17% and 0.19% in unselected autopsy series.[3–8] Approximately 75% of primary cardiac tumors are benign and 25% are malignant.[2,9] Approximately 50% of the benign tumors are myxomas, and about 75% of the malignant tumors are sarcomas.[2,9] The clinical incidence of these tumors is approximately 1 in 500 cardiac surgical cases and, with the exception of myxomas, most surgeons will encounter primary cardiac tumors rarely. The purpose of this chapter is to summarize useful information for the evaluation and management of patients with primary and secondary cardiac tumors and to provide a reference for additional study on these subjects.

HISTORICAL BACKGROUND

A primary cardiac neoplasm was first described by Realdo Colombo in 1559.[10,11] Alden Allen Burns of Edinburgh described cardiac neoplasm and suggested valvular obstruction by an atrial tumor in 1809.[12] A series of six atrial tumors, with characteristics we now recognize as myxoma, was published in 1845 by King.[13] In 1931, Yates reported nine cases of primary cardiac tumor and established a classification system similar to what we use today.[14] The first antemortem diagnosis of a cardiac tumor was made in 1934 when Barnes diagnosed a cardiac sarcoma using electrocardiography and biopsy of a metastatic lymph node.[15] In 1936 Beck successfully resected a teratoma external to the right ventricle[16] and Mauer removed a left ventricular lipoma in 1951.[17] Treatment of cardiac tumors was profoundly influenced by two events: the introduction of cardiopulmonary bypass in 1953 by John Gibbon, which allowed a safe and reproducible approach to the cardiac chambers, and the introduction of cardiac echocardiography, which allowed safe and noninvasive diagnosis of an intracardiac mass. The first echocardiographic diagnosis of an intracardiac tumor was made in 1959.[18] An intracardiac myxoma was diagnosed by angiography in 1952 by Goldberg, but attempts at surgical removal were unsuccessful.[13] A large right atrial myxoma was removed by Bhanson in 1952 using caval inflow occlusion but the patient expired 24 days later.[19] Crafoord in Sweden first successfully removed a left atrial myxoma in 1954 using cardiopulmonary bypass,[20] and Kay in Los Angeles first removed a left ventricular myxoma in 1959.[21] By 1964, 60 atrial myxomas had been removed successfully, with a steady increase due to increasing safety of cardiopulmonary bypass and increased use of echocardiography for detection.[22] Operations are currently routinely performed on the vast majority of patients with atrial myxoma with minimal mortality.[9,23–33] Primary malignant tumors, however, continue to represent a challenge.

CLASSIFICATION

Surgeons generally classify cardiac tumors as primary or secondary, as previously noted, and divide primary tumors into benign and malignant categories. However, the tissue of origin may influence clinical behavior, and an understanding of the pathologic classification of cardiac tumors is important. Pathologic classification is listed in Table 58-1. Mural thrombus is listed as a pseudotumor. Although not really a cardiac tumor, its presentation may clinically and pathologically mimic myxoma. Most mural thrombi are associated with underlying valvular disease, myocardial infarction or dysfunction, or atrial fibrillation.[32] Mural thrombi have also been noted in hypercoagulable syndromes, particularly antiphospolipid syndrome.[33] With increasing use of long-term central catheters, we have seen several right atrial masses that were difficult to tell from myxoma; these masses turned out to be mural thrombi on removal. Simple removal must be combined with addressing the underlying cause, and long-term anticoagulation is often needed.

Heterotopias and tumors of ectopic tissue include cystic tumors of the atrioventricular node consisting of multiple benign cysts in the region of the atrioventricular node, which can cause heart block or sudden death. Most are diagnosed at autopsy but biopsy diagnosis of atrioventricular nodal tumor has been reported.[34] Germ cell tumors of the heart are usually teratomas, occurring within the pericardial sac, but yolk sac tumors have been described in infants and children.[35–36] Ectopic thyroid tissue may occur within the myocardium and is referred to as "struma cordis." Right ventricular outflow track obstruction may be present, but most patients are asymptomatic.[37–38]

The majority of the remaining tumors arise in the mesenchymal, fat, fibrous, neural, or vascular cells of the heart, with myxoma representing a tumor of undetermined histogenesis. Primary cardiac lymphoma and mesothelioma and metastatic tumors to the heart represent the remaining pathologic categories that comprise the greater part of this chapter.

TABLE 58–1 Types of cardiac tumors by pathology

Pseudotumors
Mural thrombi
Heterotopias and tumors of ectopic tissue
Tumors of the atrioventricular nodal region
Teratoma
Ectopic thyroid
Tumors of mesenchymal tissue
Hamartoma of endocardial tissue
Papillary fibroelastoma
Hamartomas of cardiac muscle
Rhabdomyoma
Histiocytoid cardiomyopathy (Purkinje cell hamartoma)
Tumors and neoplasms of fat
Lipomatous hypertrophy, interarterial septum
Lipoma
Liposarcoma
Tumors and neoplasms of fibrous and myofibroblastic tissue
Fibroma
Inflammatory pseudotumor (inflammatory myofibroblastic tumor)
Sarcomas (malignant fibrous histiocytoma, fibrosarcoma, leiomyosarcoma)
Vascular tumors and neoplasms
Hemangioma
Epithelioid hemangioendothelioma
Angiosarcoma
Neoplasm of uncertain histogenesis
Myxoma
Neoplasms of neural tissue
Granular cell tumor
Schwannoma/neurofibroma
Paraganglioma
Malignant schwannoma/neurofibrosarcoma (rare)
Malignant lymphoma
Malignant mesothelioma
Metastatic tumors to the heart

PRIMARY BENIGN TUMORS

Myxoma

Myxoma comprises 50% of all benign cardiac tumors in adults but only 15% of such tumors in children. Occurrence during infancy is rare (Tables 58-2 and 58-3). A vast majority of myxomas occur sporadically and tend to be more common in women than men.[4,31] The peak incidence is between the third and sixth decades of life and 94% of tumors are solitary.[39] Approximately 75% occur in the left atrium.[31] The deoxyribonucleic acid (DNA) genotype of sporadic myxomas is normal in 80% of patients.[40] Tumors are

TABLE 58–2 Benign cardiac neoplasms in adults

Tumor	No.	Percentage
Myxoma	118	49
Lipoma	45	19
Papillary fibroelastoma	42	17
Hemangioma	11	5
A-V node mesothelioma	9	4
Fibroma	5	2
Teratoma	3	1
Granular cell tumor	3	1
Neurofibroma	2	<1
Lymphangioma	2	<1
Rhabdomyoma	1	<1
Total	241	100

Source: Reproduced with permission from McAllister HA Jr, Fenoglio JJ Jr: Tumors of the cardiovascular system, in Atlas of Tumor Pathology. Washington DC, Armed Forces Institute of Pathology; 1978, fas. 15.

unlikely to be associated with other abnormal conditions and have a low recurrence rate.[4,39]

About 5% of myxoma patients show a familial pattern of tumor development based on autosomal dominance inheritance.[41–42] These patients and 20% of those with sporadic myxoma have an abnormal DNA genotype chromosomal pattern.[40] In contrast to the "typical" sporadic myxoma profile of a middle-aged, frequently female, patient with a single left atrial myxoma, familial myxoma patients are more likely to be younger, equally likely to be male and female, and more often (22%) have multicentric tumors originating from either the atrium or ventricle.[43–48] Although familial myxomas have the same histology as sporadic tumors, familial myxoma has a higher recurrence rate after surgical resection (21%–67%).[44,49–50] Approximately 20% of familial patients have associated conditions such as adrenocortical nodule hyperplasia, Sertoli cell tumors of the testes, pituitary tumors, multiple myxoid breastfibroadenoma, cutaneous myomas, and facial or labial pigmented spots.[39,49]

TABLE 58–3 Benign cardiac neoplasms in children

	0-1 year old		1-15 years old	
Tumor	Number	Percentage	Number	Percentage
Rhabdomyoma	28	62	35	45.0
Teratoma	9	21	11	14.0
Fibroma	6	13	12	15.5
Hemangioma	1	2	4	5.0
A-V node mesothelioma	1	2	3	4.0
Myxoma	–	–	12	15.5
Neurofibroma	–	–	1	1.0
Total	45	100	78	100

Source: Reproduced with permission from McAllister HA Jr, Fenoglio JJ Jr: Tumors of the cardiovascular system, in Atlas of Tumor Pathology. Washington DC, Armed Forces Institute of Pathology, 1978; fas. 15.

These conditions are often described as "complex myxomas" within the group of familial myxoma.[40] A familial syndrome with autosomal X-linked inheritance characterized by primary pigmented nodular adrenocortical disease with hypercortisolism, cutaneous pigmentous lentigines, and cardiac myxoma is referred to as Carney's complex.[39,49]

PATHOLOGY

Myxomas occur in any chamber of the heart but have a special predilection for the left atrium, from which approximately 75% originate.[32] The next most frequent site is the right atrium, where 10%–20% are found. The remaining 6% to 8% are equally distributed between the left and right ventricle.[2] Both biatrial and multicentric tumors are more common in familial disease. Biatrial tumors probably arise from bidirectional growth of a tumor originating within the atrial septum.[51] Atrial myxomas generally arise from the interatrial septum at the border of the fossa ovalis but can originate anywhere within the atrium including the appendage (Figs. 58-1 and 58-2).[4] In addition, isolated reports confirm that myxomas arise from the cardiac valves, pulmonary artery and vein, and vena cava.[52–53] Right atrial myxomas are

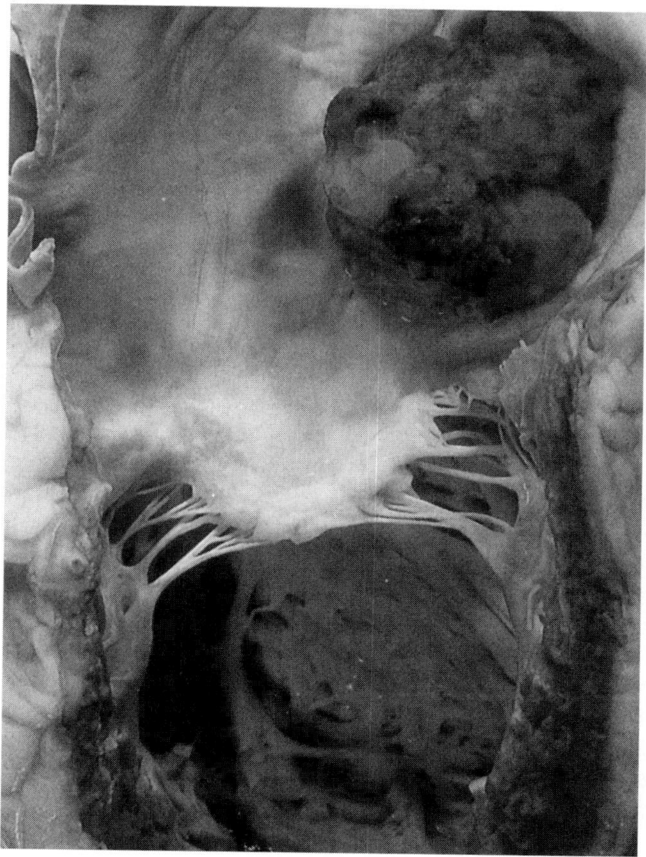

FIGURE 58–1 Left atrial myxoma obstructing the mitral orifice. *(Reproduced with permission from Hurst JW, et al: Atlas of the Heart. New York, McGraw-Hill, 1988.)*

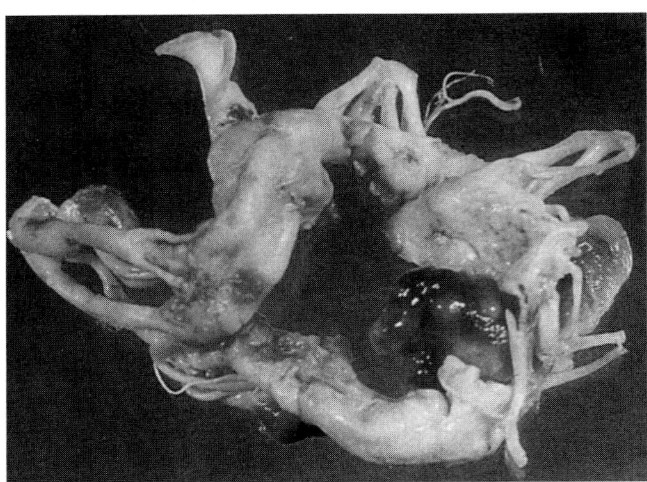

FIGURE 58–2 Left atrial myxoma arising from the posterior papillary muscle. (*Reproduced with permission from Hurst JW, et al: Atlas of the Heart. New York, McGraw-Hill, 1988.*)

more likely to have broad-based attachments than left atrial tumors; they also are more likely to be calcified[45–46] and thus visible on chest radiographs (Fig. 58-3). Ventricular myxomas occur more often in women and children and may be multicentric.[2,54] Right ventricular tumors typically arise from the free wall and left ventricular tumors tend to originate in the proximity of the posterior papillary muscle.

Grossly, about two thirds of myxomas are round or oval tumors with a smooth or slightly lobulated surface.[31] Most are polypoid, relatively compact, pedunculated, mobile, and not likely to fragment spontaneously.[2,4] Mobility depends on the length of the stalk, the extent of attachment to the heart, and the amount of collagen in the tumor.[4] Most tumors are pedunculated with a short broad base and although sessile forms occur they are unusual.[2,55] Less common villous or papillary myxomas are gelatinous and fragile and prone to fragmentation and embolization, occurring about one third of the time.[31,56] Myxomas are white, yellowish or brownish color, frequently covered with thrombus.[2] Focal areas of hemorrhage, cyst formation, or necrosis may be seen in cut section. The average size is about 5 cm in diameter but growth to 15 cm in diameter and larger has been reported.[4] Most myxoma tumors appear to grow rapidly, but growth rates vary and occasionally tumor growth arrests spontaneously.[4] Weights range from 8 to 175 g with a mean between 50 and 60 g.[8]

Histologically, myxomas are composed of polygonal shaped cells and capillary channels within an acid mucopolysaccharide matrix (Fig. 58-4).[4] The cells appear singularly or in small clusters throughout the matrix, and mitoses are rare.[57] The matrix also contains a smattering of smooth muscle cells, reticulocytes, collagen, elastin fibers, and a few blood cells. Cyst, areas of hemorrhage, and foci of extramedullary hematopoesis are present throughout the matrix.[49,56,58] Ten percent of the tumors have microscopic

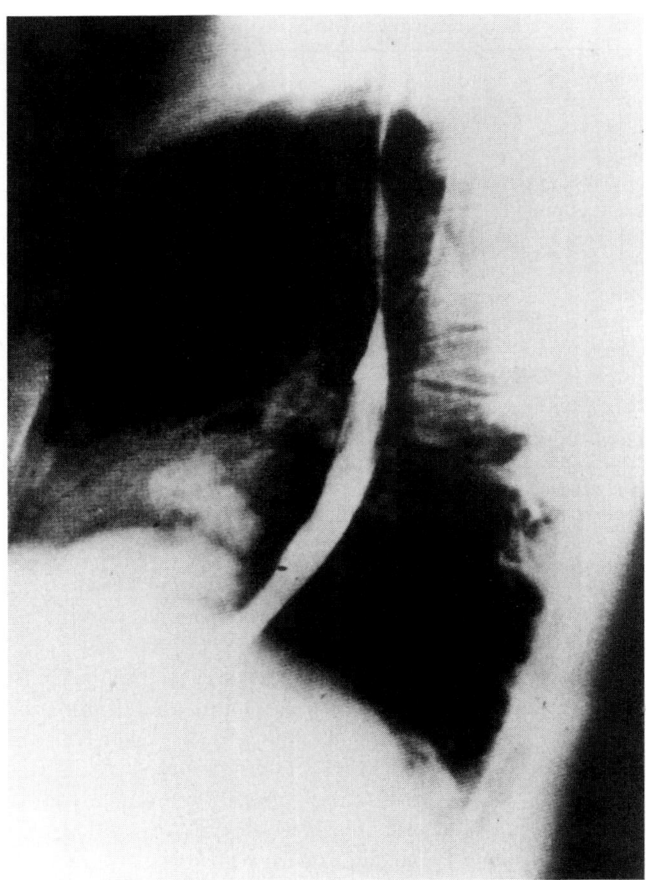

FIGURE 58–3 Calcified right atrial myxoma. (*Reproduced with permission from Hurst JW, et al: Atlas of the Heart. New York, McGraw-Hill, 1988.*)

deposits of calcium and metastatic bone deposits, and sometimes glandular-like structures.[49,56] The base of the tumor contains a large artery and veins that connect with the subendocardium but do not extend deeply beyond the subendocardium in most cases.[49] We have recently seen a myxoma that on coronary angiography had a large feeding vessel and was originally suspected of being a angiosarcoma, but on histology proved to be a typical benign myxoma. Myxomas tend to grow into the overlying cardiac cavity rather than into the surrounding myocardium. The tumor surface is covered by monolayer of polygonal cells with interspersed primitive blood vessels.

Myxomas arise from the endocardium and are considered derivative of the subendocardial multipotential mesenchymal cell,[59–60] although origin from endocardial nervous tissue has also been suggested.[61] The multipotential mesenchymal cells are thought to be embryonic cells left behind during septation of the heart, and are capable of differentiating into endothelial cells, smooth muscle cells, angioblasts, fibroblasts, myoblasts, and cartilage. This accounts for the occasional presence of hematopoietic tissue and bone in these tumors. There is no evidence that these tumors are of thrombotic origin as was formerly speculated.[62]

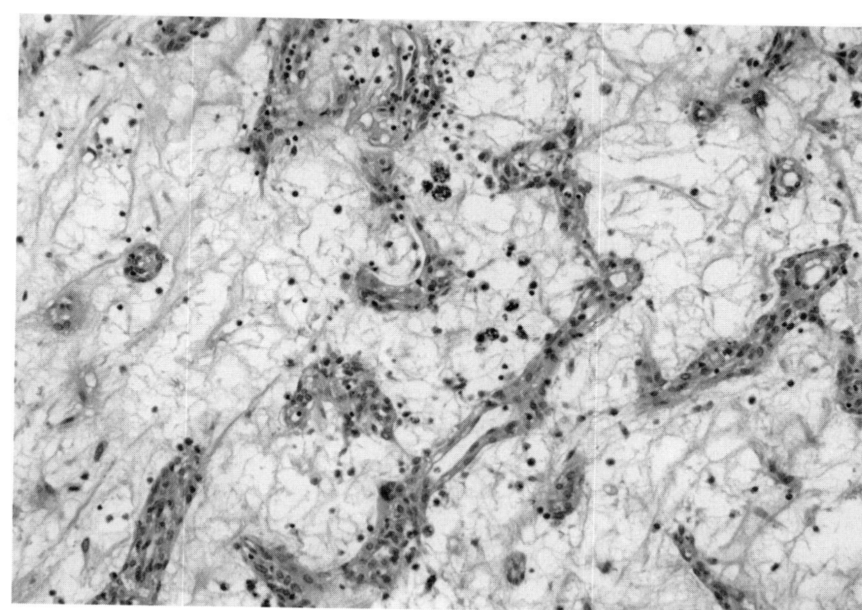

FIGURE 58–4 Typical microscopic appearance of atrial myxoma with nests of small stellate cells and blood vessels immersed in abundant accellular matrix rich in proteoglycams. These tumors often contain smooth muscle, areas of hemorrhage and calcification, hemosiderin-laden macrophages, and chronic inflammatory cells. Hematoxylin eosin X 200. (*Courtesy of Dr. G. G. Pietra.*)

Interestingly, myxomas have developed after cardiac trauma including repair of atrial septal defects and transseptal puncture for paracutaneous dilatation of the mitral valve.

CLINICAL PRESENTATION

The classic triad of myxoma clinical presentation is intracardiac obstruction with congestive heart failure (67%), signs of embolization (29%), systemic or constitutional symptoms of fever (19%) and weight loss or fatigue (17%), and immunologic manifestations of myalgia, weakness, and arthralgia (5%), with almost all patients presenting with one or more of these symptoms.[31] Cardiac rhythm disturbances and infection occur less frequently.

Constitutional symptoms Nearly all myxoma patients on careful questioning admit to a variety of constitutional symptoms that may include weight loss, fever, and lethargy. These complaints may be accompanied by laboratory abnormalities including leukocytosis, elevated erythrocyte levels and sedimentation rate, hemolytic anemia, thrombocytopenia, and elevated C-reactive protein. Immunoelectrophoresis may reveal abnormal immunoglobulin levels with increased circulating IgG.[63] These symptoms often suggest an inflammatory autoimmune disease and are unrelated to the location and size of the tumor.[4]

The recent discovery of elevated levels of interleukin-6 in patients with myxoma has been linked to a variety of associated conditions including lymphadenopathy, tumor metastasis, ventricular hypertrophy, and development of constitutional symptoms.[54,64–66] Other less frequent complaints include Raynaud's phenomenon, arthralgias, myalgias, erythematous rash, and clubbing of the digits.[4,67–68]

Possible etiologies of such varied complaints and symptoms include tumor embolization with secondary myalgias and arthralgias and elevated immunoglobulin response.[69] Circulating antibody tumor antigen complexes with complement activation may also play a role in the constitutional symptom complex.[70] More important, such symptom complexes tend to resolve following surgical resection of tumor.[58,71–72]

Obstruction Obstruction of blood flow in the heart is the most common cause of acute presenting symptoms. The nature of these symptoms is determined by which of the chambers is involved and the size of the tumor.

Myxomas in the left atrium tend to mimic mitral valvular heart disease. They produce dyspnea, which may be positional,[73] and other signs and symptoms of heart failure associated with elevated left atrial and pulmonary venous pressures. Clinically, mitral stenosis is often suspected and leads to echocardiography and diagnosis of myxoma. On occasion, large myxomas may interfere with mitral leaflet closure and produce mitral regurgitation, but this is uncommon.[4] Syncopal episodes occur in some patients and are thought to result from temporary occlusion of the mitral orifice.[46,73–75] Right atrial myxomas can produce a clinical picture of right heart failure with signs and symptoms of venous hypertension including hepatomegaly, ascites, and dependent edema. The tumor simulates tricuspid valve stenosis by partially obstructing the valve orifice.[46,73–75] If a patent foramen ovale is present, right to left atrial shunting may occur with central cyanosis, and paradoxal embolization has been reported.[74,76–77]

Large ventricular myxomas may mimic ventricular outflow obstruction. The left ventricular myxoma may produce the equivalent of subaortic or aortic valvular stenosis,[77–79] whereas right ventricular myxomas can simulate right ventricular outflow track or pulmonic valve obstruction.

Embolization Systemic embolization is the second most common mode of presentation for patients with myxoma. It occurs in 30% to 40% of patients.[2,4,46,73–74] Because the majority of myxomas are left-sided, approximately 50% of embolic episodes affect the central nervous system owing to both intracranial and extracranial vascular obstruction. The neurologic deficits following embolization range from transient to permanent but a high portion do not resolve.[80] Specific central nervous system consequences include intracranial aneurysms, seizures, hemiparesis, and brain necrosis.[81–84] Retinal artery embolization with visual loss has occurred in some patients.[85–86]

Embolic material for cardiac myxoma has been found in iliac and femoral arteries, causing acute lower extremity ischemia.[87–89] Other sites of tumor embolization include abdominal viscera and the renal and coronary arteries.[90] Histologic examination of surgically removed peripheral myxoma that has embolized provides the diagnosis of an otherwise unsuspected tumor.[46,91,92]

Right-sided myxomatous emboli usually do not cause clinical manifestations but do obstruct pulmonary arteries and cause pulmonary hypertension and even death from acute obstruction.[4,77]

Infection Infection arising in a myxoma is a rare complication and produces a clinical picture of infectious endocarditis,[91–95] and a variety of bacterial pathogens as well as fungus forms[93] have been isolated.[96] Infection increases the likelihood of systemic embolization[4] and infected myxoma warrants urgent surgical resection.

DIAGNOSIS

Clinical examination Findings at the time of clinical assessment of a patient with cardiac myxoma vary according to the size, location, and mobility of the tumor. Left atrial myxomas may produce auscultatory findings similar to mitral stenosis just as these tumors may mimic the symptoms of mitral disease. The well-described "tumor plop" is an early diagnostic sound heard and sometimes confused with a third heart sound. The diagnostic tumor plop occurs just after the opening snap of the mitral valve and is believed to be secondary to contact between the tumor and endocardial wall.[97–98] Of note, the murmur of cardiac myxoma may depend on its position and this may aid in the auscultatory diagnosis. Left atrial myxomas that cause partial obstruction of left ventricular filling may result in elevated pulmonary vascular pressures with augmentation of the pulmonary component of the second heart sound.[99]

Right atrial myxomas may produce the same auscultatory findings as left atrial myxomas with the exception that they are best heard along the lower right sternal border rather than the cardiac apex. These include both systolic and diastolic murmurs and a tumor plop. In addition, right atrial hypertension may produce a large A wave in the jugular venous pulse and when severe may mimic superior vena caval syndrome. Similarly, elevated right atrial pressure can lead to right-to-left shunting across the patent foramen ovale. This may produce polycythemia, cyanosis, and clubbing of the digits. Lower body manifestations of venous hypertension are hepatomegaly, ascites, and peripheral edema.

Chest radiograph and electrocardiogram The findings on chest roentgenogram, although not specific, may include generalized cardiomegaly, individual cardiac chamber enlargement, and pulmonary venous congestion. More specific occasional findings are density within the cardiac silhouette caused by calcification within the tumor (see Fig. 58-3). This finding occurs more often with right-sided myxomas;[4] however, the majority of our myxoma patients have normal chest roentgenograms.

Electrocardiographic findings Similar to plain film imaging, nonspecific abnormalities are noted, including chamber enlargements, cardiomegaly, bundle branch blocks, and axis deviation.[100] Fewer than 20% of patients have atrial fibrillation.[48] Evaluation of nonspecific electrocardiographic abnormalities occasionally leads to an incidental diagnosis of myxoma but, as with chest x-rays, most electrocardiograms are not helpful in establishing a diagnosis.

Echocardiography Cross-sectional echocardiography is the most useful test employed for the diagnosis and evaluation of myxoma. The sensitivity of 2-D echocardiography for myxoma is 100% and this imaging technique has largely supplanted angiocardiography.[101] However, coronary angiography usually is performed in patients over 40 years of age to rule out significant coronary arterial disease in a patient who has another indication for cardiac surgery. A transthoracic echocardiogram usually provides all the information for surgical resection, but transesophageal echocardiography (TEE) provides the best information concerning tumor size, location, mobility, and attachment.[102–103] Transesophageal echocardiograms detect tumors as small as 1–3 mm in diameter.[104] Our practice is to obtain a transesophageal echocardiogram in the operating room before commencing the operation (Fig. 58-5). We particularly evaluate the posterior left atrial wall, atrial septum, and right atrium, which often are not well displayed on transthoracic examination, to exclude the possibility of biatrial multiple tumors. Additionally, operative TEE assures a normal echocardiogram prior to leaving the operating room.

Computed tomography and magnetic resonance imaging Although myxomas have been identified using computed tomography (CT),[100,105] this modality is most useful in malignant tumors of the heart because of its ability to

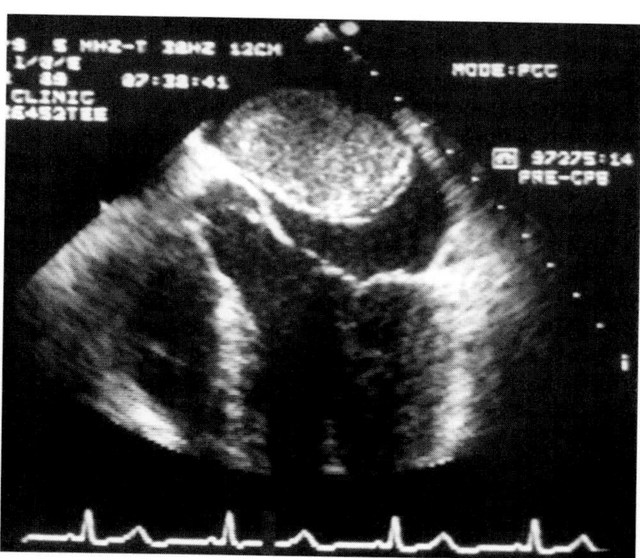

FIGURE 58–5 Transesophageal echocardiogram of large left atrial myxoma in patient presenting with symptoms of mitral valve disease. The tumor is attached to the interatrial septum above the normal mitral valve. (*Reproduced with permission from Hall RA, Anderson RP: Cardiac neoplasms, in Edmunds LH Jr: Cardiac Surgery in the Adult. New York, McGraw-Hill, 1997; p. 1350.*)

demonstrate myocardial invasion and tumor involvement of adjacent structures.[100] Similarly magnetic resonance imaging (MRI) has been employed in the diagnosis of myxomas and may yield a clear picture of tumor size, shape, and surface characteristics.[100,103,105–106] MRI is particularly useful in detecting intracardiac and pericardial extension and invasion of malignant secondary tumors, and is also useful in the evaluation of ventricular masses that occasionally turn out to be myxoma. Both CT and MRI detect tumors as small as 0.5 to 1.0 cm and provide information regarding the composition of the tumor.[4] Neither CT nor MRI is needed for atrial myxomas if an adequate echocardiogram is available because the information from these studies is not likely to alter surgical approach. The exception is the occasional right atrial myxoma that extends into one or both caval or tricuspid orifice. CT or MRI should be reserved for the situation in which the diagnosis or characterization of the tumor is unclear after complete echocardiographic evaluation.

SURGICAL MANAGEMENT

Surgical resection is the only effective therapeutic option for patients with cardiac myxoma and should not be delayed because death from obstruction to flow within the heart or embolization may occur in as many as 8% of patients awaiting operation.[107–108] Mediasternotomy approach with ascending aortic and bicaval cannulation is usually employed. Manipulation of the heart before initiation of cardiopulmonary bypass is minimized in deference to the known friability and embolic tendency of myxomas. For left atrial myxomas the vena cava are cannulated through the right atrial wall with the inferior cannula placed close and laterally to the inferior vena cava right atrial junction (Fig. 58-6). Caval snares are always used to allow opening of the right atrium, if necessary. If extensive exposure of the left atrium is needed, or a malignant left atrial tumor is suspected, we mobilize

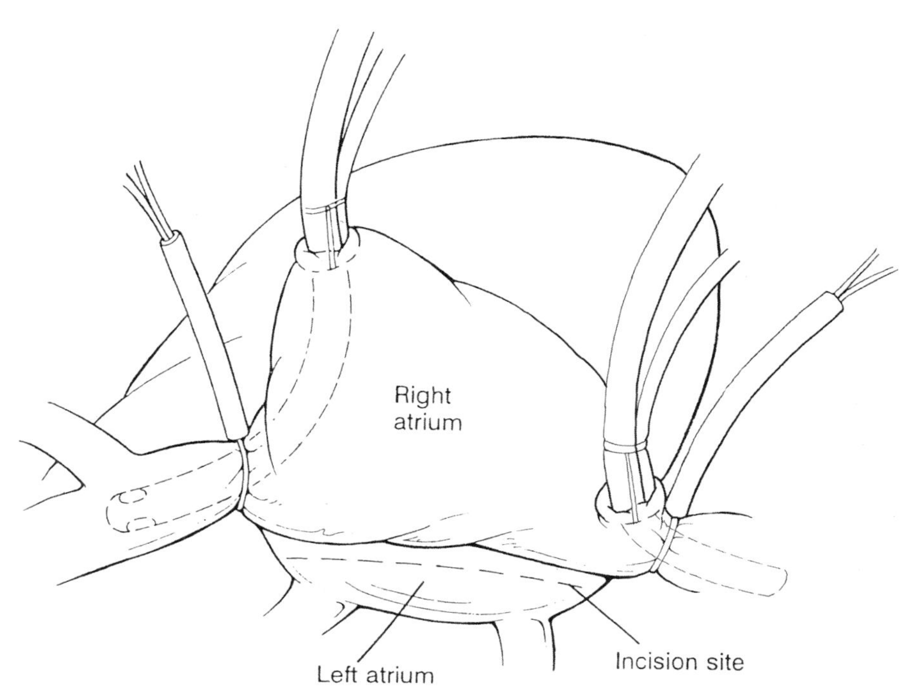

FIGURE 58–6 Standard venous cannulation for atrial myxomas and left arteriotomy site for left atrial myxoma.

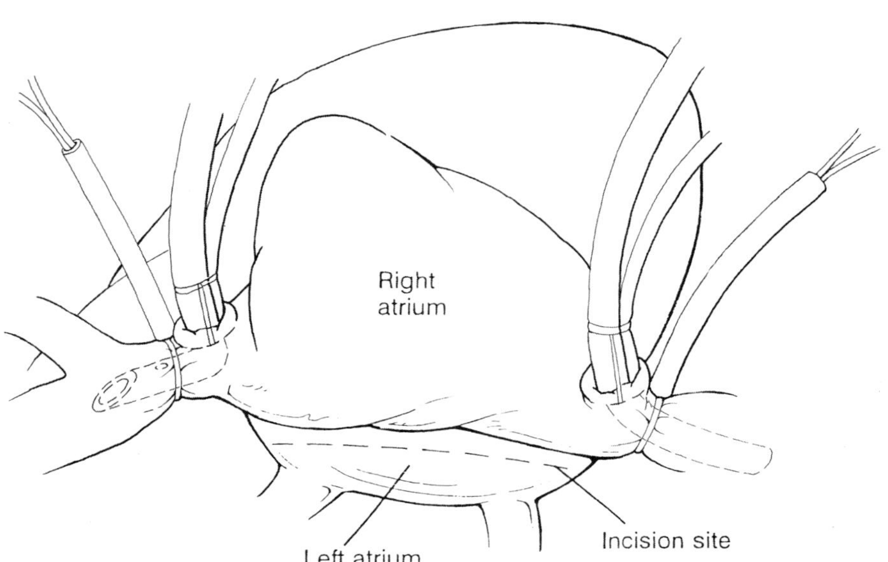

FIGURE 58–7 Superior vena cava cannula to allow increased right atrial exposure or division of superior vena cava for additional left atrial exposure.

and directly cannulate the superior vena cava, which allows it to be transected if necessary for additional exposure (Fig. 58-7). Body temperature is allowed to drift down but there is no attempt to induce systemic hypothermia unless the need for reduced perfusion flow is anticipated. Modern cardioplegic techniques yield a quiet operative field and protect the myocardium from ischemic injury during aortic cross-clamping. Cardiopulmonary bypass is started and the aorta is clamped prior to manipulation of the heart.

Exposure of left atrial myxomas is maximized by using several principles from mitral valve repair surgery. The surgeon desires the right side of the heart to rotate up and the left side of the heart to rotate down. Therefore, stay sutures are placed low on the pericardium on the right side

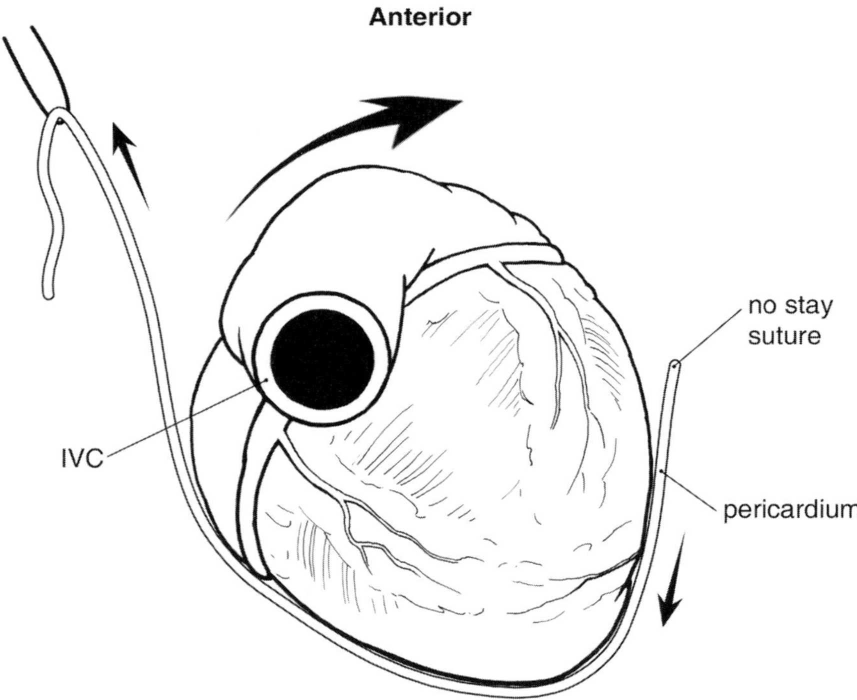

FIGURE 58–8 Rotation of the heart with pericardial stay sutures for left atrial exposure.

and no pericardial stay sutures on the left prior to placing the chest retractor. This rotates the heart for optimal exposure of both the right and, particularly, the left atrium (Fig. 58-8). For left atrial tumors the superior vena cava is extensively mobilized as is the inferior vena caval–right atrial junction, allowing increased mobility and exposing the left atrial cavity. Left atrial myxomas can be approached by an incision through the anterior wall of the left atrium anterior to the right pulmonary veins (Fig. 58-9). This incision can be extended behind both cava for greater exposure (Figs. 58-10 and 58-11). Exposure of large tumors attached to the interatrial septum and removal may be aided by a second incision parallel to the first in the right atrium going posterior to the superior vena caval cannula and anterior to the inferior vena caval cannula. This biatrial incision allows easy removal of tumor attached to the fossa ovalis with full thickness excision at the site of attachment and easy patch closure of the atrial septum if necessary.

Right atrial myxomas pose special venous cannulation problems and intraoperative echocardiography may be of benefit in allowing safe cannulation. Both vena cava may be cannulated directly. When low- or high-lying tumor pedicles preclude safe transatrial cannulation, cannulation of the jugular or femoral vein can provide venous drainage of the upper or lower body. In general, we can always cannulate the superior vena cava distal enough from the right atrium to allow adequate tumor resection, but occasionally femoral venous cannula drainage has been necessary for low-lying right atrial tumors encroaching on the inferior vena cava orifice. If the tumor is large or attached near both caval orifices, peripheral cannulation of both jugular and femoral vein may be used to initiate cardiopulmonary bypass and deep hypothermia. After the aorta is cross-clamped and the heart is arrested with antegrade cardioplegia, the right atrium may be opened widely for resection of the tumor and reconstruction of the atrium using pericardium or polyflorotetraethylene during a period of circulatory arrest if this is needed for a dry field. Resection of large or critically placed right atrial myxomas often requires careful preoperative planning, intraoperative transesophageal echocardiography, and special extracorporeal perfusion techniques to ensure complete removal of the tumor, protection of right atrial structures, and reconstruction of the atrium. Because myxomas rarely extend deep in the endocardium, it is not necessary to resect deeply around the conduction tissue. The tricuspid valve and the right atrium as well as the left atrium ventricle should be inspected carefully for multicentric tumors in patients with right atrial myxoma, with or without familial myxoma. However, in the age of pre- and intraoperative TEE, it is unusual to find additional tumors not seen on echocardiography.

Regardless of the surgical approach, the ideal resection encompasses the tumor and a portion of the cardiac wall or interatrial septum to which it is attached. Whether excision of full thickness wall is necessary or excision of only an endocardial attachment is sufficient to prevent recurrence is controversial. Our policy is to resect full thickness

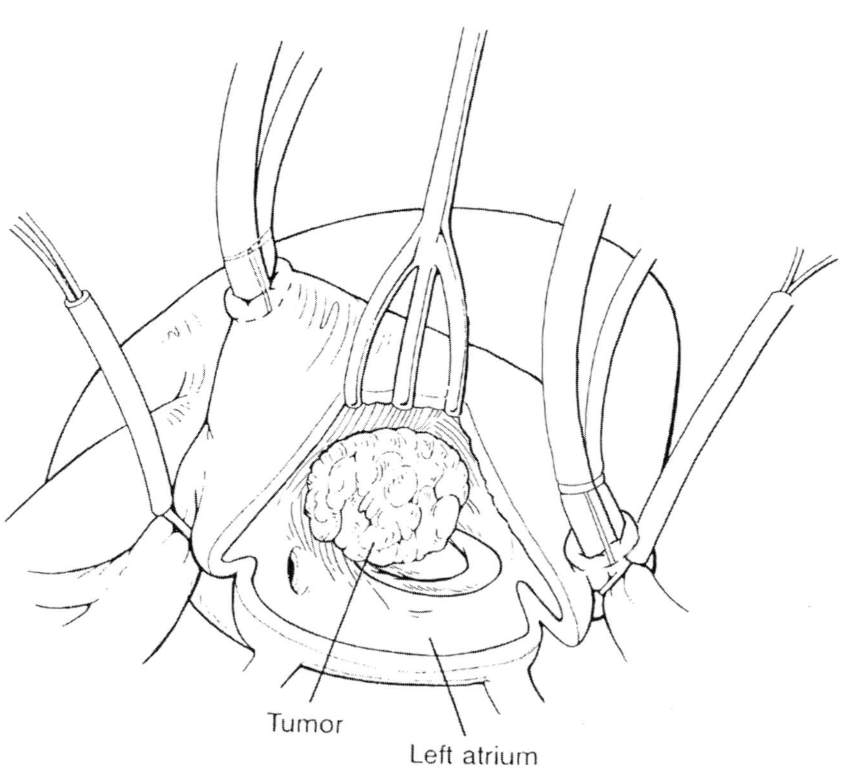

FIGURE 58–9 Left atriotomy and exposure of myxoma.

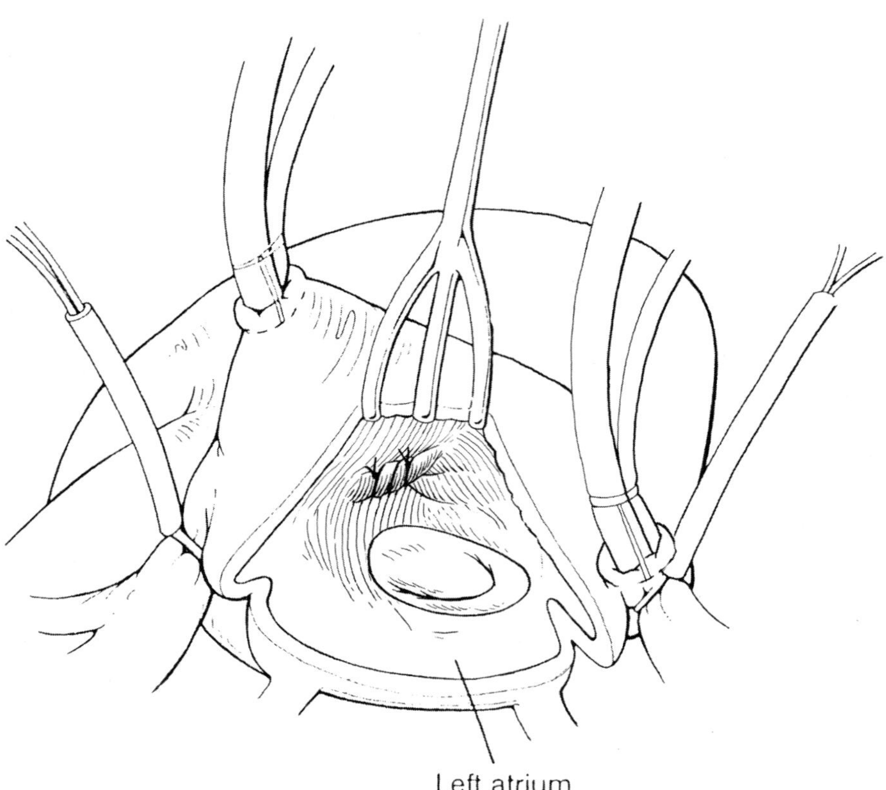

FIGURE 58–10 Repair of left atrial wall after removal of myxomas.

whenever possible. However, only partial thickness resection of the area of tumor attachment has been performed when anatomically necessary without a noted increase in recurrence rate.[109–110]

Ventricular myxomas usually are approached through the AV valve[111] or by detaching the anterior portion of the AV valve for exposure and resection and reattachment after resection (Fig. 58-12). Occasional small tumors in either outflow tract can be removed through the outflow valve.[111–112] If necessary, the tumor is excised through a direct incision into the ventricle, but this is unusual. It is not necessary to remove full thickness of the ventricular wall since no recurrences have been reported with partial thickness excisions. As with right atrial myxoma, the presence of ventricular myxoma prompts inspection for other tumors because of the high incidence of multiple tumors.

Every care should be taken to remove the tumor without fragmentation. Following tumor removal from the field, the area should be liberally irrigated, suctioned, and inspected for loose fragments. Whether blood removed from the field during tumor manipulation should be discarded or returned to the pump circuit is also controversial. There are rare instances of distant metastases from myxoma many years after tumor resection, and these reports raise the issue of potential intraoperative dissemination of tumor.[113–114] We use the cardiotomy suction during operation but use the wall suction during the brief time that the tumor is actually excised. We reason that macro tumor emboli entering the profusion circuit will be filtered out in the cardiotomy reservoir. Considering the growth of the tumor within the bloodstream, its friable character would seem to pose no greater threat for distant metastases during tumor removal than it did during tumor development. The low malignant potential of the vast majority of myxomas and the rarity of metastasis further support this policy of retaining rather than discarding blood and we believe most cases of metastatic implantation of myxoma represent a preoperative embolic event.

Minimally invasive approaches to surgical removal Minimally invasive approaches are being applied with increasing frequency in all areas of cardiac surgery and cardiac tumors are no exception. Experience is confined to benign tumors and is quite limited. Approaches have included right parasternal or partial sternotomy exposure with standard cardioplegic techniques,[115] right submammary incision with femoral-femoral bypass and non-clamped ventricular fibrillation,[116] and right submammary port-access method with antegrade cardioplegia and ascending aortic balloon occlusion.[117] Results in this limited number of selected patients have been good but more experience and longer follow-up are needed before this can be recommended as a standard approach.

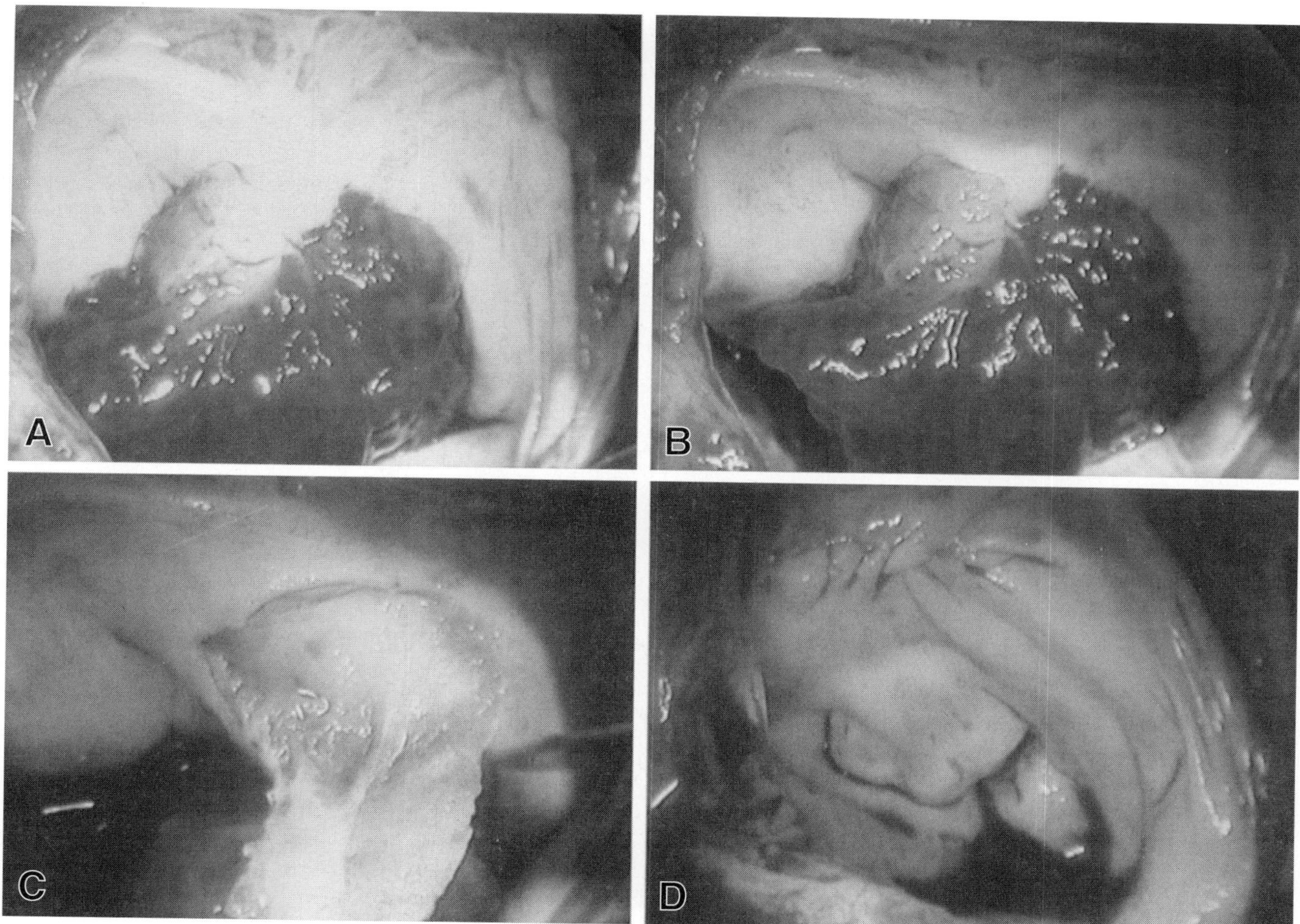

FIGURE 58–11 Photographs of left atrial mysoma removal and repair.

RESULTS

Removal of atrial myxomas carries an operative mortality rate of 5% or less.[31] A review of 202 resections indicates that operative mortality is related to advanced age or disability and comorbid conditions.[113] Excision of ventricular myxomas carries a higher risk (approximately 10%) but the experience is small. Our experience over the last 15 years with 85 myxomas shows no operative or hospital mortality.

Recurrence of nonfamilial sporadic myxoma is approximately 1% to 4%.[4,109–110] It probably is even lower in patients with a normal DNA genotype. Many large series report no recurrent tumors.[109,118–121] The 20% of patients with sporadic myxoma and abnormal DNA have a recurrence rate estimated between 12% and 40%.[4,62] The recurrence rate is highest in patients with familial complex myxomas, all of whom exhibit DNA mutation, and this is estimated to be about 22%.[4] Overall, recurrences are more common in younger patients. The disease-free interval averages about 4 years and can be as brief as 6 months.[109] Most recurrent myxomas occur within the heart, in the same or different cardiac chambers, and may be multiple.[29,46,122–123] Relationship of local recurrence to the adequacy of the original resection remains unsettled because sporadic tumors rarely recur even if full-thickness excision of the base is not done and because recurrent tumors often do not recur at the site of the original tumor.[109,124] Extracardiac recurrence after resection of tumor, presumably from embolization and subsequent tumor growth and local invasion, has been observed.[29,122–124] The biology of the tumor, dictated by gene expression rather than histology, may be the only reliable factor predicting recurrence. DNA testing of all patients with cardiac myxoma may prove to be the best predictor of the likelihood of recurrence.[125]

Uncertainty concerning the true malignant potential of myxomas has increased as reports that myxomas generally classified as "malignant" are found on subsequent review to be sarcomas with myxoid degeneration.[126] However, this issue also remains unsettled because of reports of metastatic growth of embolic myxoma fragments in the

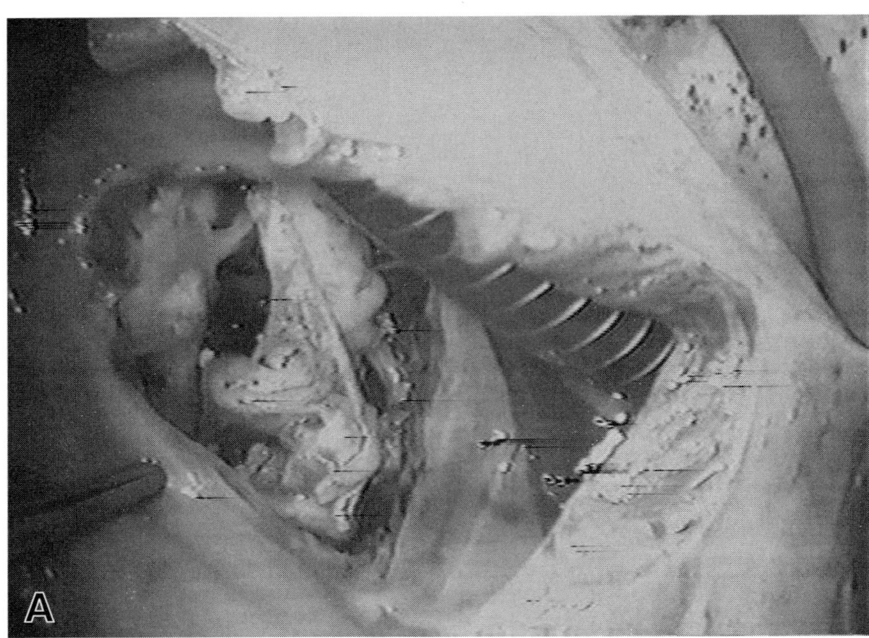

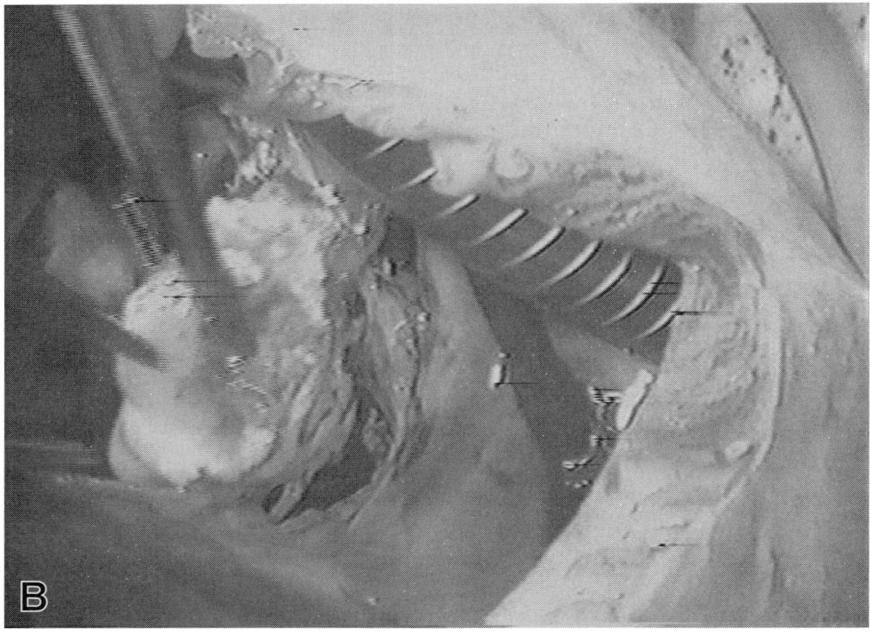

FIGURE 58–12 (A) Takedown of atrial ventricular valve for ventricular exposure. (B) Tumor exposure after valve takedown.

brain, arteries, soft tissue, and bones.[80,124,127–133] Symptomatic lesions of possible metastatic myxoma should be excised if possible.[80,127]

The extent to which patients should be subjected to long-term echocardiographic surveillance after myxoma resection is not standardized. It would seem prudent to closely follow patients who are treated initially for multicentric tumors, those whose tumors are removed from unusual locations in the heart, all tumors believed to have been incompletely resected, and tumors found to have an abnormal DNA genotype. Patients undergoing resection of tumors thought to be myxoma but with malignant characteristics at pathologic examination should have long-term, careful follow-up.

Other Benign Cardiac Tumors

As shown in Table 58-2, myxomas comprise approximately 41% of benign cardiac tumors, with three other tumors (lipoma, papillary fibroelastoma, and rhabdomyoma) together contributing a similar proportion. A variety of rarely encountered tumors accounts for the remainder.

LIPOMA

Lipomas are well-encapsulated tumors consisting of mature fat cells that may occur anywhere in the heart but also are found in the pericardium, subendocardium, subepicardium, or intra-atrial septum.[2] They may occur at any age and have no sex predilection. Lipomas are slow growing and may attain considerable size before producing obstructive or arrhythmic symptoms. Many are asymptomatic and are discovered incidentally on routine chest roentgenogram, echocardiogram, or at surgery or autopsy.[134,135] Subepicardial and parietal lipomas tend to compress the heart and may be associated with pericardial effusion. Subendocardial tumors may produce chamber obstruction. The right atrium and left ventricle are sites most often affected. Lipomas lying within the myocardium or septum can produce arrhythmias or conduction abnormalities.[136,137] Large tumors that produce severe symptoms should be resected. Smaller, asymptomatic tumors encountered unexpectedly during cardiac operation should be removed if excision can be performed without adding risk to the primary procedure. These tumors are not known to recur.

LIPOMATOUS HYPERTROPHY OF THE INTERATRIAL SEPTUM

Nonencapsulated hypertrophy of the fat within the atrial septum is known as lipomatous hypertrophy.[2] This abnormality is more common than cardiac lipoma and is usually encountered in elderly, obese, or female patients as an incidental finding during a variety of cardiac imaging procedures.[119] Various arrhythmias and conduction disturbances have been attributed to its presence.[120,137,138] The main problem is differentiation from a cardiac neoplasm when the lesion is discovered on echocardiography.[139] After the demonstration of a mass by echocardiography, the typical T1 and T2 signal intensity of fat on MRI can usually establish a diagnosis.[140,141] Arrhythmias or heart block are considered by some as an indication for resection, but data is lacking as to the long-term benefits from resection.[142]

PAPILLARY FIBROELASTOMA OF THE HEART VALVES

Papillary fibroelastomas are tumors that arise characteristically from the cardiac valves or adjacent endocardium.[143] Grossly, these tumors are described as resembling sea anemones with frond-like projections (Fig. 58-13). The AV and semilunar valves are affected with equal frequency. Papillary fibroelastomas were formerly thought to be innocuous because they were incidental findings at autopsy. It is now known that they are capable of producing obstruction of flow, particularly coronary ostial flow, and may embolize to the brain and produce stroke.[144–157] They are usually asymptomatic until a critical event occurs but now are found more often because of the more frequent use of echocardiography. Papillary fibroelastomas of the cardiac valve should be resected whenever diagnosed because of their known tendency to produce life-threatening complications. Valve repair rather than replacement should follow the resection of these benign tumors whenever technically feasible, using conservative margins of resection. Cytomegalovirus has been recovered in these tumors suggesting the possibility of viral induction of the tumor and chronic viral endocarditis.[152]

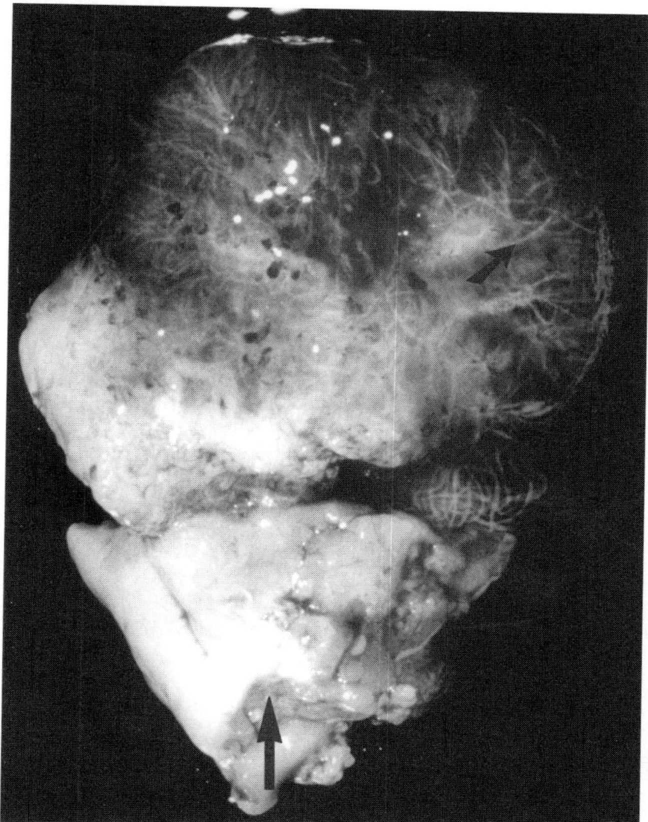

FIGURE 58–13 Papillary fibroelastoma of the tricuspid valve demonstrating delicate fronds.

RHABDOMYOMA

Rhabdomyoma is the most frequently occurring cardiac tumor in children. It usually presents during the first few days after birth. It is thought to be a myocardial hamartoma rather than a true neoplasm.[158] Although rhabdomyoma appears sporadically, it is associated strongly with tuberous sclerosis, a hereditary disorder characterized by hamartomas in various organs, epilepsy, mental deficiency, and sebaceous adenomas. Fifty percent of patients with tuberous sclerosis have rhabdomyoma but more than 50% of patients with rhabdomyoma have or will develop tuberous sclerosis.[159,160] The exceptional patient is one with a solitary, single rhabdomyoma who does not have or develop tuberous sclerosis.

Over 90% of rhabdomyomas are multiple and occur with approximate equal frequency in both ventricles.[161] The atrium is involved in fewer than 30% of patients. Pathologically, these tumors are firm, gray, and nodular and tend to project into the ventricular cavity. Micrographs show myocytes of twice normal size filled with glycogen and containing hyperchromatic nuclei and eosinophilic staining cytoplasmic granules.[2,162] Scattered bundles of myofibrils can be seen within cells by electron microscopy.[161]

The most common presentation is heart failure caused by tumor obstruction of cardiac chambers or valvular orifice flow. Clinical findings may mimic valvular or subvalvular stenosis. Arrhythmias, particularly ventricular tachycardia and sudden death, may be a presenting symptom.[162] Atrial tumors may produce atrial arrhythmias.[162] The diagnosis is suggested by clinical features of tuberous sclerosis and is made by echocardiography. Rarely, no intramyocardial tumor is found in a patient with ventricular arrhythmias and the site of rhabdomyoma is located by electrophysiologic study.[162]

Early operation is recommended in patients who do not have tuberous sclerosis before 1 year of age.[121] The tumor is usually removed easily in early infancy, and some can be enucleated.[121] Unfortunately, symptomatic tumors often are both multiple and extensive, particularly in patients with tuberous sclerosis who unfortunately have a dismal long-term outlook. In such circumstances, surgery offers little benefit.

FIBROMA

Fibromas are the second most common benign cardiac tumor, with over 83% occurring in children. These tumors are solitary, occur exclusively within the ventricle and the ventricular septum, and affect the sexes equally. Fewer than 100 tumors have been reported and most are diagnosed by age 2 years. These tumors are not associated with other disease, nor are they inherited. Fibromas are nonencapsulated, firm, nodular, gray-white tumors that can become bulky. They are composed of elongated fibroblasts in broad spiral bands and whirls mixed with collagen and elastin fibers. Calcium deposits or bone may occur within the tumor and occasionally are seen in roentgenography.

The majority of fibromas produce symptoms through chamber obstruction, interference with contraction, or arrhythmias. Depending on size and location, such a tumor may interfere with valve function, obstruct flow paths, or cause sudden death from conduction disturbances in up to 25% of patients.[121] Intracardiac calcification on chest roentgenograms suggests the diagnosis, which is confirmed by echocardiogram.

Surgical excision is successful in some patients, particularly if the tumor is localized, does not involve vital structures, and can be enucleated.[121,163–165] However, it is not always possible to completely remove the tumor and partial removal is only palliative although some patients have survived many years.[121,164] Operative mortality may be high in infants. Most cases are in adolescents and adults.[121,163,164] Successful, complete excision is curative.[163,164] Children with extensive fibromas have been treated by cardiac transplantation.[165,166]

MESOTHELIOMA OF THE AV NODE

Mesothelioma of the atrial ventricular node, also termed polycystic tumor, Purkinje tumor, or conduction tumor, was mentioned in the pathologic classification of tumors. It is a relatively small, multicystic tumor that arises in proximity to the atrial ventricular node and may extend upward into the interventricular septum and downward along the bundle of His.[2] Mesothelioma is associated with heart block, ventricular fibrillation,[167] and sudden death. Cardiac pacing alone does not prevent subsequent ventricular fibrillation. Surgical excision has been reported.[34]

PHEOCHROMOCYTOMA

Cardiac pheochromocytomas arise from chromaffin cells of the sympathetic nervous system and produce excess amounts of catecholamines, particularly norepinephrine. Approximately 90% of pheochromocytomas are in the adrenal glands. Fewer than 2% arise in the chest. Only 32 cardiac pheochromocytomas had been reported by 1991.[168] The tumor predominantly affects young and middle-aged adults with an equal distribution between the sexes. Approximately 60% occur in the roof of the left atrium. The remainder involve the interatrial septum or anterior surface of the heart. The tumor is reddish-brown, soft, lobular, and consists of nests of chromatin cells.

The patients usually present with symptoms of uncontrolled hypertension or are found to have elevated urinary catecholamines. The tumor is usually located by scintigraphy using 131-I-metaiodobenzylguanidine[169,170] and CT or MRI.[169,170] Cardiac catheterization with differential blood chamber sampling is sometimes necessary.[168] Because these tumors are vascular and may be near major coronary arteries, coronary arteriograms are advisable.

After the tumor is located, it should be removed, using cardiopulmonary bypass with cardioplegic arrest. Patients require preanesthetic alpha and beta blockade, and careful intraoperative and immediate postoperative monitoring. Most tumors are extremely vascular and uncontrollable operative hemorrhage has occurred.[170] Resection may require removal of the atrial and/or ventricular wall or a segment of a major coronary artery.[168] Explantation of the heart to allow resection of a large left atrial pheochromocytoma has been attempted (Fig. 58-14).[171] Transplantation has been performed for nonresectable tumor. Complete excision produces cure.[168–170]

HEMANGIOMA

Hemangiomas of the heart are rare tumors (24 clinical cases reported), affect all ages, and may occur anywhere within the heart.[172,173] These are vascular tumors composed of

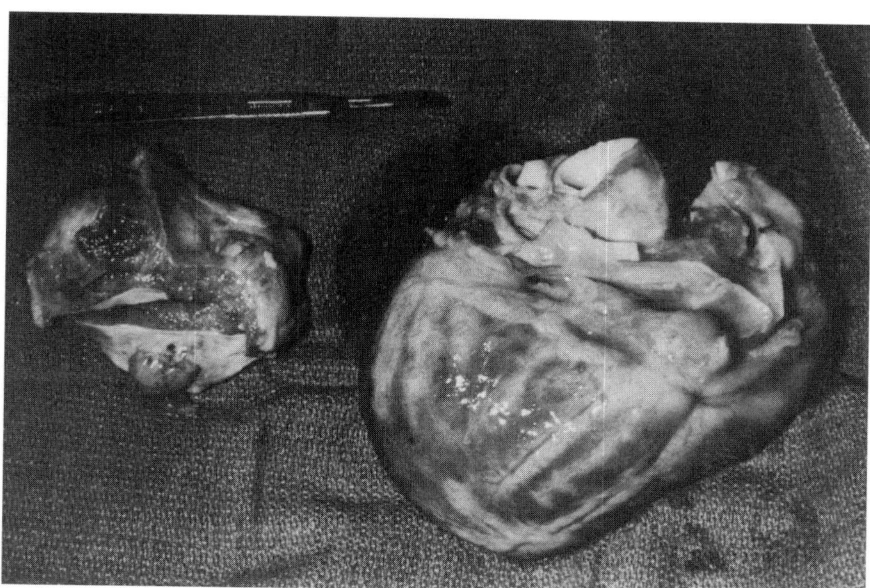

FIGURE 58–14 Excised left atrial pheochomocytoma and explanted heart prior to reimplantation.

capillaries or cavernous vascular channels. Patients usually develop dyspnea, occasional arrhythmias, or signs of right heart failure.[174] Diagnosis is difficult and chest roentgenography may be abnormal but is not specific. Echocardiography or cardiac catheterization usually but not always establishes a diagnosis of cardiac tumor by showing an intracavity filling defect.[175] CT and MRI should be done. Axial T_2-weighted MRI should show a high signal mass due to vascularity (Fig. 58-15).[176] Coronary angiography typically shows a tumor blush and maps the blood supply to the tumor.

The tumors can be resected in asymptomatic patients, and cardiopulmonary bypass is recommended. Meticulous ligation of feeding vessels is required to prevent postoperative residual arteriovenous fistulas or intracavity communications. Partial resections have produced long-term benefits.[172] Tumors rarely resolve spontaneously.[177]

TERATOMA

Cardiac teratoma is a rare tumor that usually presents in infants and young children but has occurred in adults.[178] About 80% of the tumors are benign and the remainder have microscopic or clinically malignant cells.[179] These tumors are discovered by echocardiography after a variety of symptoms lead to cardiac or mediastinal evaluation. There is little experience with surgical removal, which should be possible with modern imaging and surgical technology.

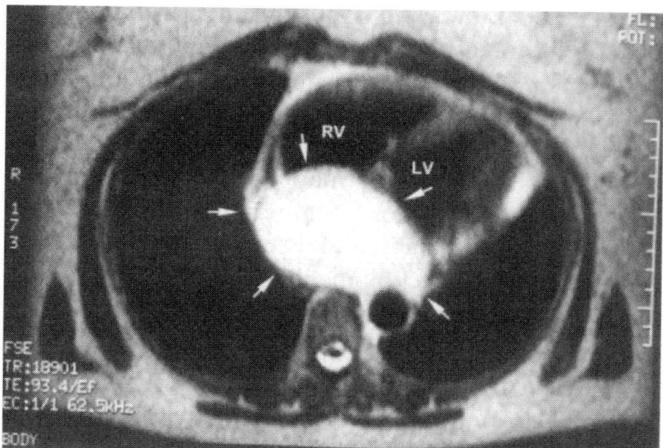

FIGURE 58–15 Axial T2-weighted magnetic resonance image showing high signal mass of left atrial hemangioma. *(Reproduced with permission from Lo JJ, Ramsay CN, Allen JW, et al: Left atrial cardiac hemangioma associated with shortness of breath and palpitations. Ann Thorac Surg 2002; 73:979.)*

PRIMARY MALIGNANT TUMORS

Primary cardiac malignancy is very uncommon, with only 21 surgically treated cases noted in a 25-year surgical experience from 1964–69, combining the experience of two large institutions, the Texas Heart Institute and the M.D. Anderson Cancer Center in Houston.[180] Even in busy centers, primary cardiac malignancy continues to challenge the diagnostic ability and surgical skills of thoracic surgeons. Approximately 25% of primary cardiac tumors are malignant and of these about 75% are sarcomas. McAllister's survey of cardiac tumors found the most common to be angiosarcomas (31%), rhabdomyosarcomas (21%), malignant mesotheliomas (15%), and fibrosarcomas (11%) (Table 58-4).[2]

Primary malignant cardiac tumors arise sporadically, showing no inherited linkage. Although they may span the entire age spectrum, they usually occur in adults over 40 years of age. The patients usually present with symptoms of congestive heart failure, pleuritic chest pain, malaise, anorexia, and weight loss.[178,181] The most common

TABLE 58–4 Primary malignant cardiac neoplasms in adults

Tumor	Number	Percentage
Angiosarcoma	39	33
Rhabdomyosarcoma	24	21
Mesothelioma	19	16
Fibrosarcoma	13	11
Lymphoma	7	6
Osteosarcoma	5	4
Thymoma	4	3
Neurogenic sarcoma	3	2
Leiomyosarcoma	1	<1
Liposarcoma	1	<1
Synovial sarcoma	1	<1
Total	117	100

Source: Reproduced with permission from McAllister HA Jr, Fenoglio JJ Jr: Tumors of the cardiovascular system, in Atlas of Tumor Pathology. Washington DC, Armed Forces Institute of Pathology, 1978; fas. 15.

symptom has been dyspnea (Table 58-5).[180] Some develop refractory arrhythmias, syncope, pericardial effusion, and tamponade.[180] The chest x-ray may be abnormal and even show a mass lesion, but the definite diagnosis is usually made with cardiac echocardiography.[182,183] We have seen angiosarcoma of the right heart that presented as multiple nodules on chest x-ray, and at thoracoscopy it was found to present multiple reddish lesions of the lung consistent with angiosarcoma. Subsequent cardiac echocardiography was used to confirm the diagnosis of a cardiac primary tumor. Right atrial lesions are more frequently malignant (usually angiosarcoma) than left-sided lesions (usually myxoma, but when malignant are often malignant fibrous histiocytoma). If malignancy is suspected, chest CT or MRI may suggest histology and provide detailed anatomy and help in staging and assessing resectability. The current status of positron emission tomography (PET) scans in evaluating these patients remains controversial. We perform cardiac catheterization on all patients over 40 years of age presenting with intracardiac masses, and on all patients with large right atrial masses. Malignancy may be suggested and coronary involvement suspected by tumor blush (Fig. 58-16). This is not pathognomonic as we have seen large feeding vessel and tumor blush in a histologically confirmed myxoma.

TABLE 58–5 Symptoms of primary malignant cardiac tumors

	Number	Percentage
Dyspnea	13/21	61.9
Chest pain	6/21	28
CHF	6/21	28
Palpitations	5/321	24
Fever	3/21	14
Myalgia	2/21	10

Source: Reproduced with permission from Murphy MC, Sweeney MS, Putnam JB Jr, et al: Surgical treatment of cardiac tumors: a 25-year experience. Ann Thorac Surg 1990; 49:612.

Unfortunately, primary cardiac malignancy may grow to a large size prior to detection and involve portions of the heart not amenable to resection. Some of these cases have been considered for transplantation and will be discussed later. Otherwise palliative medical therapy can be attempted with radiation therapy, although success in both symptom relief and longevity has been somewhat limited. Whether the tumor is primary or secondary, the decision to resect is based on tumor size and location and an absence of metastatic spread seen on complete evaluation. Unfortunately, the majority of primary cardiac malignancies that have been referred to our center were initially considered to be benign and incompletely resected at presentation. If malignancy is suspected or confirmed, and if the lesion appears anatomically resectable and there is no metastatic disease, then resection should be considered. If complete resection is possible, surgery provides better palliation and can possibly double survival.[183] After resection, we recommend adjuvant chemotherapy and believe this will slightly improve survival[179,183,184] and add to our ability to treat this desperate disease. Complete resection will depend on the location of the tumor, extent of involvement of the myocardium and/or fibrous skeleton of the heart, and histology.

Angiosarcoma

Angiosarcomas are two to three times more common in men than women and have a predilection for the right heart. Eighty percent arise in the right atrium.[181,185,186] These tumors tend to be bulky and aggressively invade adjacent structures, including the great veins, tricuspid valve, right ventricular free wall, interventricular septum, and right coronary artery (Fig. 58-17).[185] Obstruction and right heart failure are not uncommon. Pathologic examination of resected specimens demonstrates anastomosing vascular channels lined with typical anaplastic epithelial cells. Unfortunately, most of these tumors have spread by the time of presentation, usually to the lung, liver, and brain.[181] Without resection 90% of the patients are dead within 9 to 12 months after diagnosis despite radiation or chemotherapy.[32,187] We have found carefully selected patients without evidence of spread on metastatic evaluation who have undergone complete surgical resection with subsequent chemotherapy (Fig. 58-18). We have had no hospital mortality in this small group and the main problem remains metastasis rather than recurrence at the local site.

Malignant Fibrous Histiocytoma

Malignant fibrous histiocytoma (MFH) is the most common soft-tissue sarcoma in adults. Its occurrence as a cardiac primary malignancy has been relatively recently accepted as a

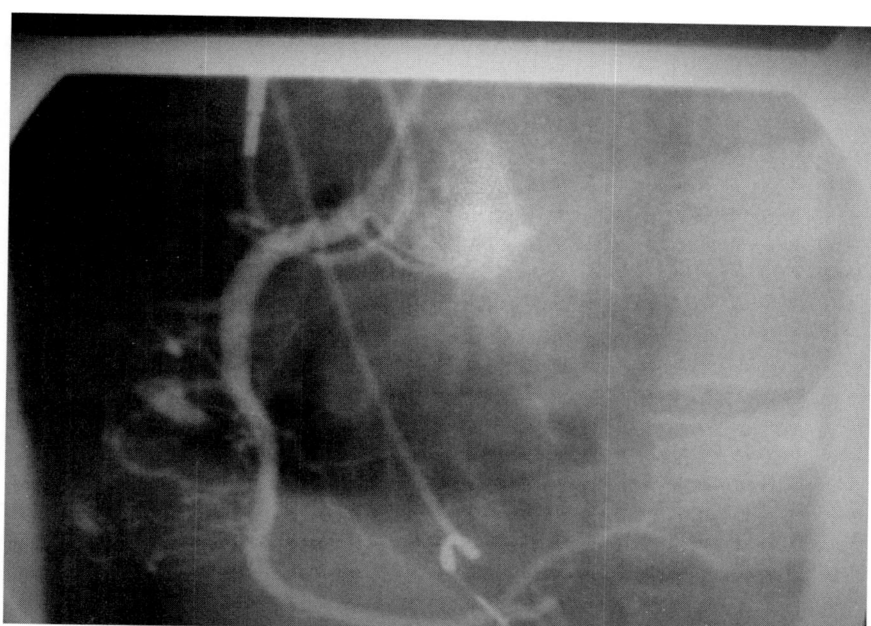

FIGURE 58–16 Tumor blush in right atrial sarcoma.

specific entity. It is characterized histologically by a mixture of spindle cells in a storiform pattern, polygonal cells resembling histiocytes, and malignant giant cells. The cell of origin is the fibroblast or histioblast.[182,188] It usually occurs in the left atrium and often mimics myxoma. In fact, every left atrial MFH referred to our institution has been previously incompletely resected when thought to represent a myxoma. The tendency to metastasize early is not as prominent as with angiosarcoma. Several reports exist with rapid symptomatic recurrence after incomplete resection despite chemotherapy. These patients often die of local cardiac disease prior to development of metastasis. We believe that if complete resection can be obtained (particularly if the malignant nature is recognized and complete resection can be done at the original operation) and adequate chemotherapy provided, we may improve the survival in this otherwise dismal disease. Our group believes incomplete resection is usually due to inadequate exposure of these broad-based tumors, which often extend to the anterior wall of the left atrium. Difficulty in exposing this posterior portion of the heart leads to inhibition

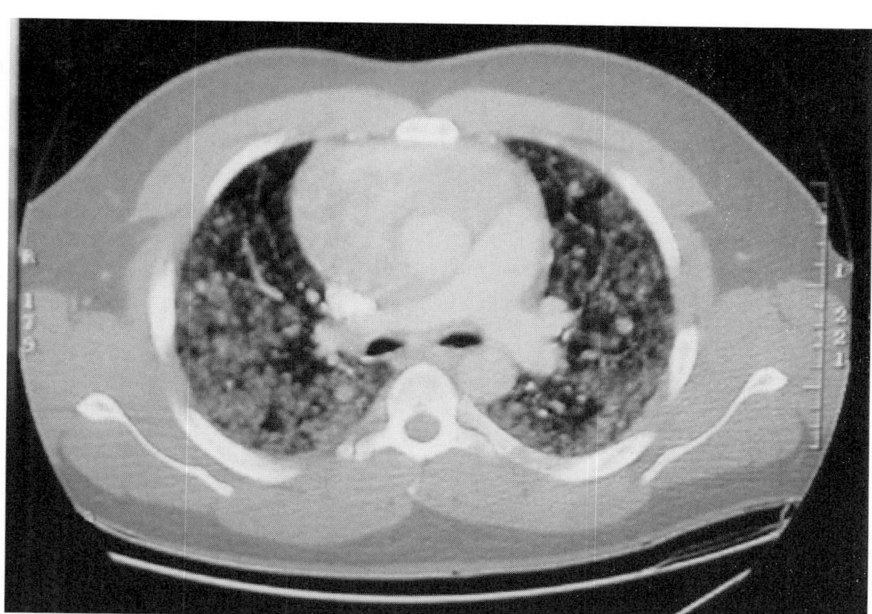

FIGURE 58–17 Angiosarcoma with extensive involvement of mediastinum.

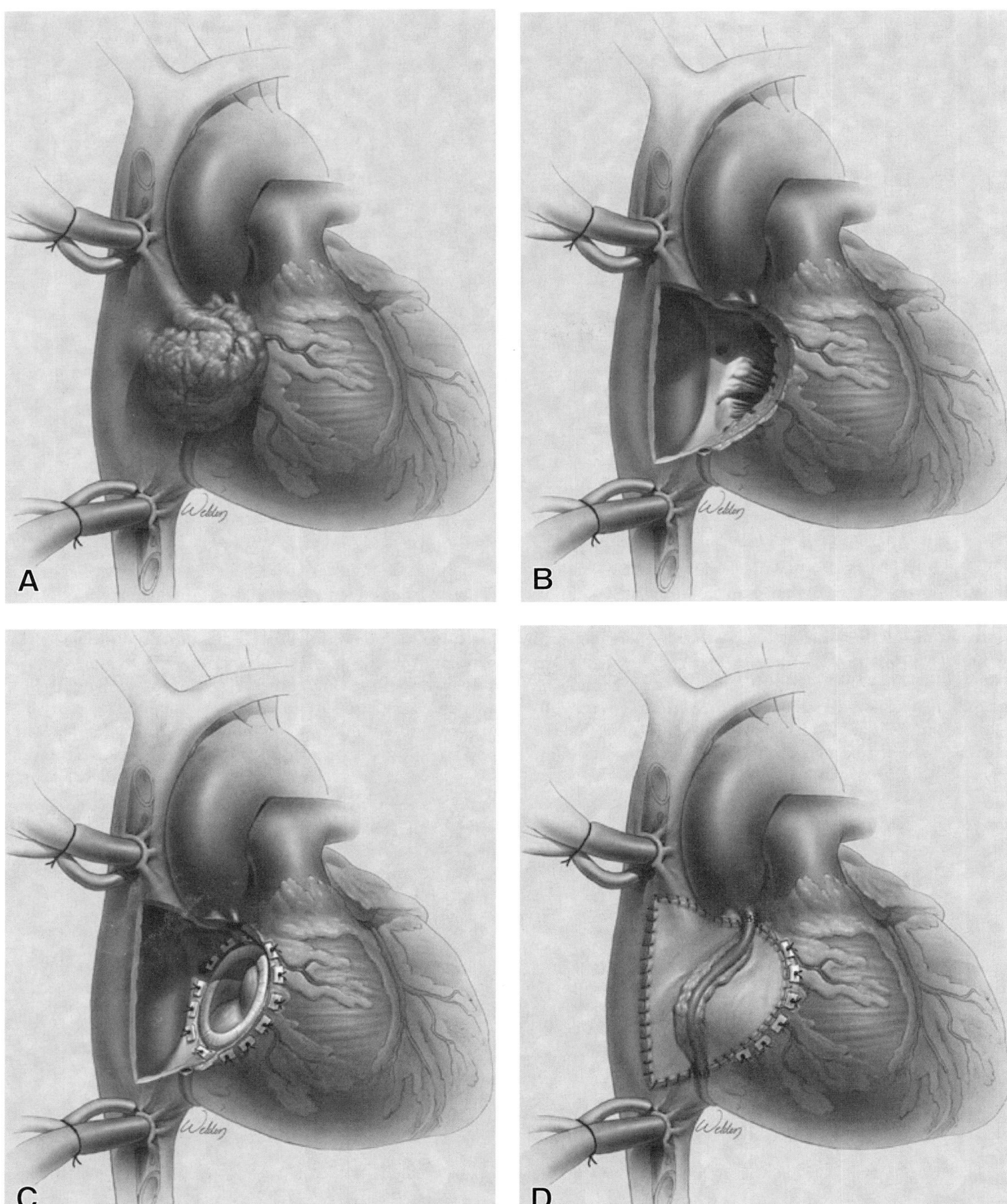

FIGURE 58–18 (A) Right atrial angiosarcoma involving right coronary artery and tricuspid valve. (B) Excision of tumor with right coronary artery and tricuspid valve. (C) Tricuspid valve replaced. (D) Completed repair using bovine pericardium. *(Copyright 2002, Baylor College of Medicine.)*

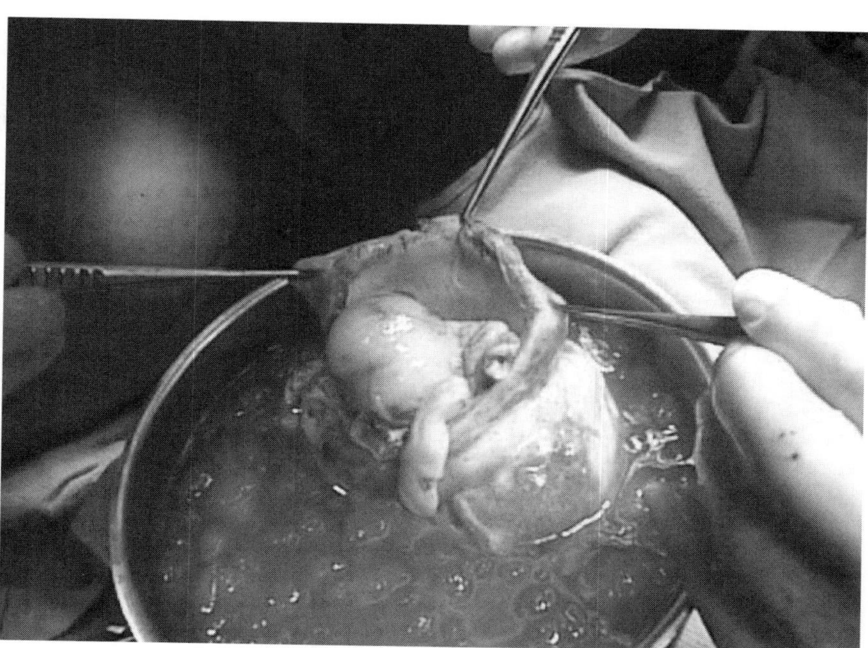

FIGURE 58–19 Ex vivo heart showing large sarcoma arising from the anterior left atrial wall.

of aggressive resection for clear margins, and makes reconstruction difficult. We believe that these difficulties can be overcome by excising the heart and inverting it so that the posterior left atrium is now an anterior structure. This allows excellent visualization for aggressive resection and reconstruction done ex vivo, after which the heart is reimplanted (Fig. 58-19). This was first attempted by Cooley in 1984 for a pheochromocytoma and, although technically accomplished, it was unsuccessful because of severe hemorrhage due to the vascular nature of the tumor.[178] Our program first attempted this approach for MFH in 1998 (Fig. 58-20).[188] We have performed six of these autotransplant procedures with no operative or hospital mortality. Three patients have died of metastatic disease without local recurrence and three are alive and disease-free 4 months to 3 years postoperatively. All were given adjuvant chemotherapy. This has proven to be an efficacious technique at local control with a low mortality in our hands, but metastasis is still common and strongly suggests that further improvements in survival will require more effective, biologically based systemic therapy.

Rhabdomyosarcoma

Rhabdomyosarcomas do not evolve from rhabdomyoma and occur equally in the sexes. The tumors are multicentric in 60% of patients and arise from either ventricle. These tumors frequently invade cardiac valves or interfere with valve function because of their intracavitary bulk. Microscopically, tumors cells demonstrate pleomorphic nuclei and spidery, wispy, streaming eosinophilic cytoplasm, usually in a muscle-like pattern (Fig. 58-21). The tumors are aggressive and may invade pericardium. Surgical excision of small tumors may be rational but local and distant metastasis and poor response to radiation or chemotherapy limit survival to less than 12 months in the majority of these patients.[163,178,179,183,189,190]

Other Sarcomas and Mesenchymal Origin Tumors

McAllister and Fenoglio found that malignant mesotheliomas arising from the heart or pericardium and not from the surrounding pleura were the third most common malignant cardiac tumors and that fibrosarcomas were fourth.[2] However, in the two decades since their work, clinicians have rarely encountered these tumors. This apparent decrease in incidence may be related to changes in histological criteria for classifying primary malignant neoplasm since their study.[5,172,179–184,190–192]

The histology of these tumors can be ambiguous and difficult. These neoplasms can resemble other sarcomas, and some might be deemed fibrous histiocytomas today. The behavior of these tumors is more important and, as with other cardiac sarcomas, resection of small tumors in the absence of known metastasis perhaps is justified but data is scarce.[32,180,183,190] This being said, it is important to rule out more diffuse thoracic involvement with mesothelioma before considering resection of an isolated cardiac or pericardial mesothelioma. A PET scan may be considered, and any suspicious pleural thickening or effusion should be carefully evaluated both radiographically and histologically.

Myosarcoma, liposarcoma, osteosarcoma, chondromyxosarcoma, plasmacytoma, and carcinosarcoma arising from the heart have all been reported,[121,192–195] but by the time diagnosis is made, only palliative therapy can usually be

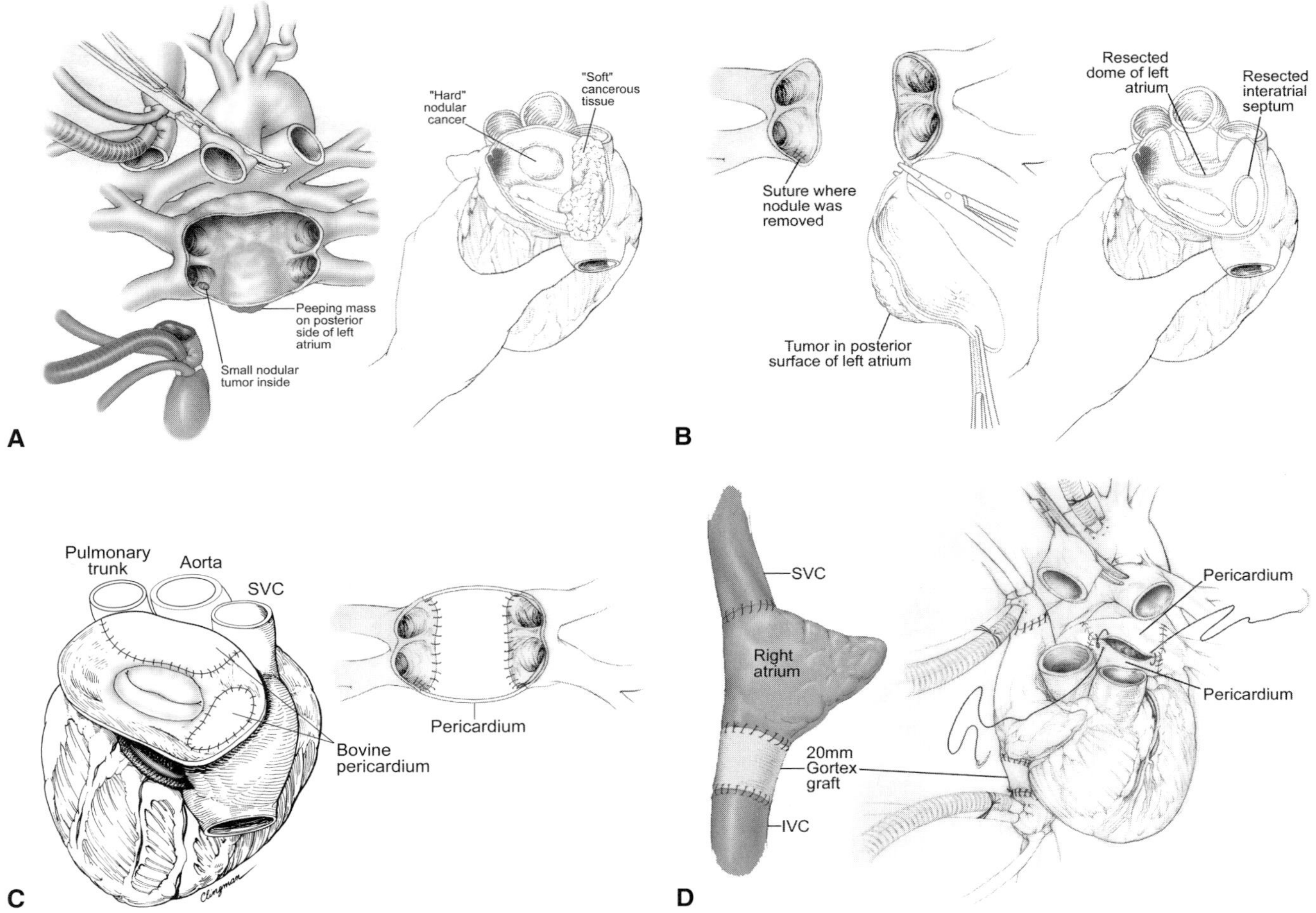

FIGURE 58–20 (A) Explanation of the heart for exposure of extensive left atrial sarcoma. (B) Resection of left atrial sarcoma. (C) Reconstruction of the heart with bovine pericardium after tumor resection. (D) Reimplantation of the heart using a 20-mm polytetrafluoroethylene graft between the inferior vena cava and right atrium.

offered and surgery is only occasionally indicated. Regardless of therapy, it is unusual for patients with these diagnoses to survive more than a year.

Lymphomas

Lymphomas may arise from the heart although it is rare.[196] Most of these tumors respond to radiation and chemotherapy. Even when complete resection is not possible, and incomplete resection is performed to relieve acute obstructive systems, radiation and chemotherapy have allowed for up to 3-year survival in selected patients.

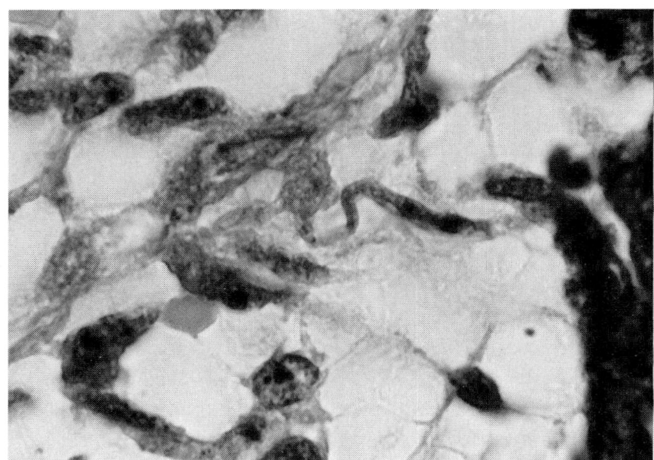

FIGURE 58–21 Representative microphotograph of rhabdomyosarcoma showing loosely elongated rhabdomyoblasts with distinct angulation of the muscle fibers and undifferentiated tumor cells with plump nuclei and prominent nucleoli. Masson's trichome X 800. (*Courtesy of Dr. G. G. Pietra.*)

Heart Transplantation

Malignant primary cardiac tumors may grow to a large size prior to detection. Additionally, extensive myocardial involvement or location affecting the fibrous skeleton of the heart may make complete resection impossible. Because complete resection yields better results than incomplete resection,[183] orthotopic cardiac transplantation has been considered as a treatment option in some cases. Reports of transplantation for a number of cardiac tumors including sarcoma,[197–199] pheochromocytoma,[200] lymphoma,[201] fibroma,[166] and myxoma[202] have appeared. However, the long-term results are uncertain because some patients die from recurrent metastatic disease despite transplantation.[200,201,203] As of 2000, 28 patients had been reported who had undergone orthotopic transplantation for primary cardiac tumors and, of these, 21 had malignant tumors.[203] The mean survival for patients with primary cardiac malignancy was 12 months. Although technically feasible in some cases, orthotopic transplantation is hindered by a scarcity of donor organs coupled with an extensive recipient list of patients without cancer. In addition, the large size of the tumor when diagnosed often necessitates rapid intervention for progressive congestive heart failure. Finally, the morbidity and mortality involved with immunosuppression as well as the unknown effect of immunosuppression on any remaining malignancy should be considered. For these reasons, orthotopic cardiac transplantation for primary cardiac tumor remains controversial and should be considered carefully on a case-by-case basis by experienced transplant and tumor boards. In most cases, orthotopic transplantation should be reserved for unresectable benign tumors, such as cardiac fibroma.

SECONDARY METASTATIC TUMORS

Approximately 10% of metastatic tumors eventually reach the heart or pericardium, and almost every type of malignant tumor has been known to do so.[2,5,9,204] Secondary neoplasms are 20 to 40 times more common than primary cardiac malignancies.[4,205] Up to 50% of patients with leukemia develop cardiac lesions.[5] Other cancers that commonly involve the heart include breast, lung, lymphoma, melanoma, and various sarcomas.[2,206,207] Metastasis involving the pericardium, epicardium, myocardium, and endocardium roughly follow that order of frequency[2,9] as well (Table 58-6).

TABLE 58–6 Metastatic cardiac disease

Tumor	Total (no.)	Cardiac (%)	Pericardial (%)
Leukemia	420	53.9	22.4
Melanoma	59	34.0	23.7
Lung ca	402	10.2	15.7
Sarcoma	207	9.2	9.2
Breast ca	289	8.3	11.8
Esophageal ca	65	7.7	7.7
Ovarian ca	115	5.7	7.0
Kidney ca	95	5.3	0.0
Gastric ca	308	3.6	3.2
Prostate ca	186	2.7	1.0
Colon ca	214	0.9	2.8
Lymphoma	75	–	14.6

Source: Reproduced with permission from Perry, MC: Cardiac metastasis, in Kapoor AS (ed): Cancer and the Heart. New York, Springer-Verlag Publishers, 1986.

The most common means of spread, particularly for melanoma, sarcoma, and bronchogenic carcinoma, is hematogenous, and ultimately via coronary arteries. In addition, metastasis can reach the heart through lymphatic channels, though direct extension from adjacent lung, breast, esophageal, and thymic tumors, and from the subdiaphragmatic vena cava. The pericardium most often is involved by direct extension of thoracic cancer; the heart is the target of hematologous and/or retrograde lymphatic metastasis.[5] Cardiac metastases rarely are solitary and nearly always produce multiple microscopic nests and discrete nodules of tumor cells (Fig. 58-22).[2,5,9] Cardiac metastases produce clinical symptoms in only about 10% of afflicted patients.[5,208,209] The most common symptom is pericardial effusion or cardiac tamponade. Occasionally patients develop refractory arrhythmias or congestive heart failure. Chest radiographs and electrocardiograms tend to show nonspecific changes but echocardiography is particularly useful for diagnosis of pericardial effusion, irregular pericardial thickening, or intracavity masses interfering with blood flow.

Surgical therapy is limited to relief of recurrent pericardial effusions or, occasionally, cardiac tamponade. In most instances, these patients have widespread disease with limited life expectancies. Surgical therapy is directed at providing symptomatic palliation with minimal patient discomfort and hospital stay. This is most readily accomplished via subxiphoid pericardiotomy, which can be accomplished under

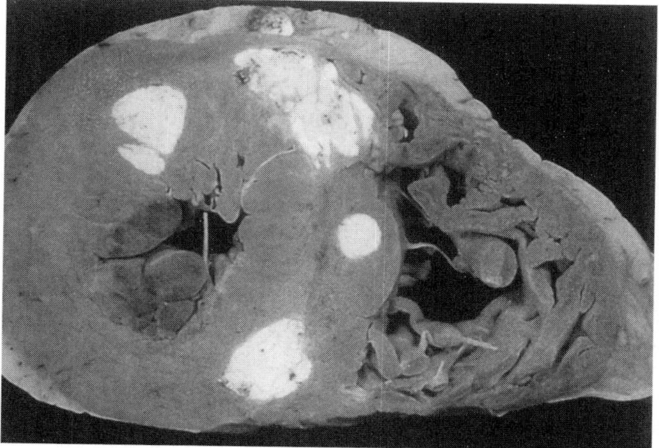

FIGURE 58–22 Hematogenous metastases within the myocardium of a patient with renal cell cancer. (*Reproduced with permission from Hurst JW, et al: Atlas of the Heart. New York, McGraw-Hill, 1988.*)

local anesthesia if necessary with reliable relief of symptoms, a recurrence rate of about 3%, and little mortality.[207] Alternatively, a large pericardial window in the left pleural space can be created using thoracoscopy, but we would recommend this only under unusual circumstances.[210] This can be accomplished with minimal patient discomfort, but does require general anesthesia with single-lung ventilation and may be poorly tolerated by patients with hemodynamic deterioration secondary to large effusions.

RIGHT ATRIAL EXTENSION OF SUBDIAPHRAGMATIC TUMORS

Abdominal and pelvic tumors on occasion may grow in a cephalad direction via the inferior vena cava to reach the right atrium. Subdiaphragmatic tumors are frequently renal carcinomas, although hepatic, adrenal, and uterine tumors have occasionally exhibited this behavior. Up to 10% of renal cell carcinomas invade the inferior vena cava, and nearly 40% of these reach the right atrium.[211] Radiation and chemotherapy are not effective in relieving the obstruction of blood flow. If the kidney can be fully removed as well as the tail of tumor thrombus, survival can approach 75% at 5 years.[121,213]

Renal cell tumors with atrial extension typically are resected with abdominal dissection to ensure resectability of the renal tumor. Initially we performed a concomitant median sternotomy and often used cardiopulmonary bypass with hypothermic circulatory arrest when treating these patients. However, we have changed our approach and now work closely with our liver transplant surgeons who have extensive experience in the area of the retrohepatic vena cava. We have found we can expose the vena cava up to the right atrium through an abdominal incision. With ligation of the arterial inflow, the tumor tail often shrinks below the diaphragm and, in almost all circumstances, this can be removed without the use of cardiopulmonary bypass. Occasionally veno-veno bypass as used in hepatic transplantation is necessary to occlude inflow through the inferior vena cava, but this is unusual. If the tumor is too extensive for that maneuver, then median sternotomy is performed and cardiopulmonary bypass with hypothermic circulatory arrest can be used to remove the tumor from the cardiac chambers down into the inferior vena cava. Perfusion can be restarted followed by removal of the rest of the tumor. Although it leads to adequate exposure, significant problems with coagulopathy are often apparent after cardiopulmonary bypass and profound hypothermia.

A 5-year survival rate of 75% has been achieved following nephrectomy with resection of right atrial tumor extension.[212,213] Other subdiaphragmatic tumors with atrial extension that have been resected successfully include hepatic and adrenal carcinoma as well gynecologic tumors.[214–218]

MOLECULAR AND BIOLOGIC-BASED DIAGNOSIS AND THERAPY FOR CARDIAC TUMORS

This is an exciting time for investigators involved in the search for novel therapies for tumors such as many of those discussed in this chapter. A "new biology" is being developed in laboratories around the world working in these areas, and this is supplanted by the knowledge that is being obtained from the concerted Human Genome Project and the subsequent development of proteomics.[219] It is incumbent upon the thoracic surgeon involved in the care of patients with cardiac tumors to have some degree of familiarity with the terms and promise of these advances because significant additional improvement in survival of many of these patients is unlikely to result from further advances in surgical technique.

Interestingly, many sarcomas demonstrate reproducible translocations that allow for the production of novel chimeric genes, which may code for a variety of fusion proteins. Many of these proteins have been found to engender cellular phenotypic malignant changes, resistance to apoptosis, and unfettered growth.[220] Although not associated with cardiac involvement, the fusion proteins EWS-FL11 and EWS-ERG are noted in Ewing's sarcoma. When full-length antisense oligonucleotide constructs are utilized to target the mRNA of these proteins, protein expression is downregulated, and an 8-fold increase in apoptosis sensitivity is noted.[211] These fusion proteins have been noted in some forms of rhabdomyosarcoma, and the most common is PAX3-FKHR. This oncoprotein combines components of two strong transcriptional activators, and may increase the production of the downstream anti-apoptotic protein bcl-xl. Antisense oligonucleotides directed at this oncoprotein mRNA have led to apoptosis in rhabdomyosarcoma cells.[221,222] Similarly, in our laboratory we have demonstrated that antisense oligonucleotides directed at the mRNA of the downstream anti-apoptotic protein bcl-xl in mesothelioma can induce apoptotic cellular death and engender chemosensitivity.[223] A similar translocation and fusion protein has been noted in fibrosarcoma. This translocation (t(12;15)(p13q25)) brings together genes from chromosomes 12 and 15, which combines a transcription factor with a tyrosine kinase receptor. The resultant fusion protein is a tyrosine kinase that has oncogenic potential.[224] Reproducible translocations and fusion proteins with downstream effectors of malignant behavior have not been described for angiosarcoma, but they are actively being sought. Antisense treatment has been maligned in the past due to problems with both delivery and stability of therapeutic constructs. However, sophisticated biochemical alteration of these molecules has improved stability, and two recent solid tumor trials utilizing antisense therapy for salvage have demonstrated positive results.[225,226] Additional methods of delivering antisense to tumor cells, including viral vector delivery, have been developed. Finally, in addition to antisense methods, small molecule inhibition of many of these fusion proteins should be possible.

Angiosarcoma is an obvious target for therapies based on antiangiogenesis. The weak antiangiogenic properties of interferon alpha are presumed to be the mechanism that accounts for responses to this agent in this tumor.[227] Multiple new antiangiogenic agents are being evaluated currently in phase I and II trials, and a number of noncardiac angiosarcoma patients have been treated at our institution on this basis. We have noted several to develop stabilized disease, but there are no definitive data yet published. Certainly, the use of these agents in these vascular origin tumors is theoretically attractive.

Viral vector-mediated gene therapy has been evaluated for various sarcomas in the preclinical setting. A number of potential targets exist for these sorts of therapies. Although p53 is not commonly mutated or absent, mdm-2 is often overexpressed in many sarcomas, including angiosarcoma. This gene is a known oncogene that is able to directly induce cellular transformation. Importantly, when overexpressed, it binds to and inhibits p53 activity, even though expression of p53 may appear normal. Overexpression of mdm-2 has also been associated with VEGF overproduction and angiogenesis.[227,228] Preclinical studies of adenoviral vector p53 transduction of sarcoma in SCID mice have demonstrated growth delay, tumor regression, and decreases in VEGF expression.[229] Many other targets for this approach, including the inhibition of Nf-kB expression utilizing an adenoviral dominant negative Ik-Bα construct and prodrug–mediated gene therapy utilizing a doxorubicin prodrug and adenoviral transfer of a metabolizing enzyme in sarcoma cells, have been shown to be effective.[230,231] Unfortunately, the application of viral-mediated gene therapy paradigms to this tumor suffer the same problems of targeting, transgene expression durability, and immune response that are problematic for the field in general.

In regard to molecular diagnosis, there are no reproducible familial patterns for development of most malignant tumors. However, familial cardiac myxoma, rhabdomyoma, and fibroma may exhibit reproducible genetic abnormalities that lend themselves to the development of genetic testing to identify individuals at risk. Familial myxoma syndrome, or Carney complex, has been associated with mutations in the 17q24 gene PRKAR1α that codes for the R1α regulatory subunit of cAMP-dependent protein kinase A (PKA).[232] Although not widely available, genetic diagnosis of this syndrome is now technically achievable.[233] Reproducible mutations in the TSC-1 and TSC-2 genes in patients with tuberous sclerosis and cardiac rhabdomyoma, as well as mutations in the PTC gene of patients with the Gorlin syndrome and cardiac fibroma have been noted.[234–236] It is hoped that in the near future we will be able to predict who is at particular risk for these and other cardiac tumors. This could allow for more intense surveillance, earlier detection, and a higher rate of surgical or multimodality cure for these patients.

REFERENCES

1. Smith C: Tumors of the heart. *Arch Pathol Lab Med* 1986; 110:371.
2. McAllister HA, Fenoglio JJ Jr: Tumors of the cardiovascular system, in *Atlas of Tumor Pathology,* series 2. Washington DC, Armed Forces Institute of Pathology, 1978.
3. Straus R, Merliss R: Primary tumors of the heart. *Arch Pathol* 1945; 39:74.
4. Reynen K: Cardiac myxomas. *N Engl J Med* 1995; 333:1610.
5. Fine G: Neoplasms of the pericardium and heart, in Gould SE (ed): *Pathology of the Heart and Blood Vessels.* Springfield IL, Charles C Thomas, 1968; p 851.
6. Nadas AD, Ellison RC: Cardiac tumors in infancy. *Am J Cardiol* 1968; 21:363.
7. Pollia JA, Gogol LJ: Some notes on malignancies of the heart. *Am J Cancer* 1936; 27:329.
8. Wold LE, Lie JT: Cardiac myxomas: a clinicopathologic profile. *Am J Pathol* 1980; 101:219
9. Silverman NA: Primary cardiac tumors. *Ann Surg* 1980; 91:127.
10. Columbus MR: *De Re Anatomica,* Liber XV. Venice, N Bevilacque, 1559; p 269.
11. Moes RJ, O'Malley CD: Realdo Columbo: on those things rarely found in anatomy. *Bull Hist Med* 1960; 34:508.
12. Burns A: *Observations of Some of the Most Frequent and Important Diseases of the Heart.* London, James Muirhead, 1809.
13. Goldberg HP, Glenn F, Dotter CT, et al: Myxoma of the left atrium: diagnosis made during life with operative and postmortem findings. *Circulation* 1952; 6:762.
14. Yater WM: tumors of the heart and pericardium: pathology, symptomatology, and report of nine cases. *Arch Intern Med* 1931; 48:267.
15. Barnes AR, Beaver DC, Snell AMP: Primary sarcoma of the heart: report of a case with electrocardiographic and pathological studies. *Am Heart J* 1934; 9:480.
16. Beck CS: An intrapericardial teratoma and tumor of the heart: both removed operatively. *Ann Surg* 1942; 116:161.
17. Mauer ER: Successful removal of tumor of the heart. *J Thorac Surg* 1952; 3:479.
18. Effert S, Domanig E: Diagnostik intraaurikularer Tumoren an grosser Thromben mit dem Ultraschall-Echoverfahren. *Dtsch Med Wochesch* 1959; 84:6.
19. Bahnson HT, Newman EV: Diagnosis and surgical removal of intracavitary myxoma of the right atrium. *Bull Johns Hopkins Hosp* 1953; 93:150.
20. Crafoord C: Panel discussion of late results of mitral commissurotomy, in Lam CR (ed): *Henry Ford Hospital International Symposium on Cardiovascular Surgery.* Philadelphia, WB Saunders, 1955; p 202.
21. Kay JH, Anderson RM, Meihaus J, et al: Surgical removal of an intracavity left ventricular myxoma. *Circulation* 1959; 20:881.
22. Malm JR, Bowman FO Jr, Henry HB: Left atrial myxoma associated with an ASD. *J Thorac Cardiovasc Surg* 1963; 45:490.
23. Attar S, Lee L, Singleton R, et al: Cardiac myxoma. *Ann Thorac Surg* 1980; 29:397.
24. Castenada AR, Varco RL: Tumors of the heart: surgical considerations. *Am J Cardiol* 1968; 21:357.
25. Collins HA, Collins IS: Clinical experience with cardiac myxoma. *Ann Thorac Surg* 1972; 13:450.

26. Donahoo JS, Weiss JL, Gardner TJ, et al: Current management of atrial myxomas with emphasis on a new diagnostic technique. *Ann Surg* 1979; 189:763.
27. Kabbani SS, Cooley DA: Atrial myxoma: surgical considerations. *J Thorac Cardiovasc Surg* 1973; 65:731.
28. Richardson JV, Brandt B 3rd, Doty DB, et al: Surgical treatment of atrial myxomas: early and late results of 11 operations and review of the literature. *Ann Thorac Surg* 1979; 28:354.
29. St. John Sutton MG, Mercier LA, Giuliani ER, et al: Atrial myxomas: a review of clinical experience in 40 patients. *Mayo Clin Proc* 1980; 55:371.
30. Dein JR, Frist WH, Stinson EB, et al: Primary cardiac neoplasms: early and late results of surgical treatment in 42 patients. *J Thorac Cardiovasc Surg* 1987; 93:502.
31. Pinede L, Duhaut P, Loire R: Clinical presentation of left atrial cardiac myxoma: a series of 112 consecutive cases. *Medicine* 2001; 80:159.
32. Waller R, Grider L, Rohr T, et al: Intracardiac thrombi: Frequency, location, etiology and, complications: a morphologic review, part I. *Clin Cardiol* 1995; 18:477.
33. Gertner E, Leatherman J: Intracardiac mural thrombus mimicking atrial myxoma in the antiphospholipid syndrome: *J Rheumatol* 1992; 19:1293.
34. Balasundaram S, Halees SA, Duran C: Mesothelioma of the atrioventricular node: first successful follow-up after excision. *Eur Heart J* 1992; 13:718.
35. Ali SZ, Susin M, Kahn E, Hajdu SI: Intracardiac teratoma in a child simulating an atrioventricular nodal tumor. *Pediatr Pathol* 1994; 14:913.
36. Swalwell CI: Benign intracardiac teratoma: a case of sudden death. *Arch Pathol Lab Med* 1993; 117:739.
37. Fujioka S, Takatsu Y, Tankawa H, et al: Intracardiac ectopic thyroid mass. *Chest* 1996; 110:1366.
38. Maillette S, Paquet E, Carrier L, et al: Asymptomatic heterotopic thyroid tumour in the right ventricular infundibulum. *Can J Cardiol* 1994; 10:37.
39. Carney JA: Differences between nonfamilial and familial cardiac myxoma. *Am J Surg Pathol* 1985; 64:53.
40. McCarthy PM, Schaff HV, Winkler HZ, et al: Deoxyribonucleic acid ploidy pattern of cardiac myxomas. *J Thorac Cardiovasc Surg* 1989; 98:1083.
41. Bortolotti U, Faggian G, Mazzucco A, et al: Right atrial myxoma originating from the inferior vena cava. *Ann Thorac Surg* 1990; 49:1000.
42. Kuroda H, Nitta K, Ashida Y, et al: Right atrial myxoma originating from the tricuspid valve. *J Thorac Cardiovasc Surg* 1995; 109:1249.
43. King YL, Dickens P, Chan ACL: Tumors of the heart. *Arch Pathol Lab Med* 1993; 117:1027.
44. Gelder HM, O'Brian DJ, Styles ED, et al: Familial cardiac myxoma. *Ann Thorac Surg* 1992; 53:419.
45. Kennedy P, Parry AJ, Parums D, et al: Myxoma of the aortic valve. *Ann Thorac Surg* 1995; 59:1221.
46. St. John Sutton MG, Mercier LA, Guiliana ER, et al: Atrial myxomas: a review of clinical experience in 40 patients. *Mayo Clin Proc* 1980; 55:371.
47. Burke AP, Virmani R: Cardiac myxoma: a clinicopathologic study. *Am J Clin Pathol* 1993; 100:671.
48. Peters MN, Hall RJ, Cooley DA, et al: The clinical syndrome of atrial myxoma. *JAMA* 1974; 230:695.
49. Carney JA, Hruska LS, Beauchamp GD, et al: Dominant inheritance of the complex of myxomas, spotty pigmentation, and endocrine overactivity. *Mayo Clin Proc* 1986;61:165.
50. Farrah MG: Familial cardiac myxoma: study of patients with myxoma. *Chest* 1994; 105:65.
51. Imperio J, Summels D, Krasnow N, et al: The distribution patterns of biatrial myxoma. *Ann Thorac Surg* 1980; 29:469.
52. McAllister HA: Primary tumors of the heart and pericardium. *Pathol Annu* 1979; 14:325.
53. Jones DR, Hill RC, Abbott AE Jr, et al: Unusual location of an atrial myxoma complicated by a secundum atrial septal defect. *Ann Thorac Surg* 1993; 55:1252.
54. Kuroki S, Naitoh K, Katoh O, et al: Increased interleukin-6 activity in cardiac myxoma with mediastinal lymphadenopathy. *Intern Med* 1992; 31:1207.
55. Reddy DJ, Rao TS, Venkaiah KR, et al: Congenital myxoma of the heart. *Indian J Pediatr* 1956; 23:210.
56. Prichard RW: Tumors of the heart: review of the subject and report of one hundred and fifty cases. *Arch Pathol* 1951; 51:98.
57. Merkow LP, Kooros MA, Macgovern G, et al: Ultrastructure of a cardiac myxoma. *Arch Pathol* 1969; 88:390.
58. Kaminsky ME, Ehlers KH, Engle MA, et al: Atrial myxoma mimicking a collagen disorder. *Chest* 1979; 75:93.
59. Lie JT: The identity and histogenesis of cardiac myxomas; a controversy put to rest. *Arch Pathol Lab Med* 1989; 113:724.
60. Ferrans VJ, Roberts WC: Structural features of cardiac myxomas: histology, histochemistry, and electron microscopy. *Hum Pathol* 1973; 4:111.
61. Krikler DM, Rode J, Davies MJ, et al: Atrial myxoma: a tumor in search of its origins. *Br Heart J* 1992; 67:89.
62. Dewald GW, Dahl RJ, Spurbeck HL, et al: Chromosomally abnormal clones and nonrandom telemetric translocations in cardiac myxomas. *Mayo Clin Proc* 1987; 62:558.
63. Glasser SP, Bedynek JL, Hall RJ, et al: Left atrial myxoma: report of a case including hemodynamic, surgical, and histologic characteristics. *Am J Med* 1971; 50:113.
64. Saji T, Yanagawa E, Matsuura H, et al: Increased serum interleukin-6 in cardiac myxoma. *Am Heart J* 1991; 122:579.
65. Seino Y, Ikeda U, Shimada K: Increased expression of interleukin-6 mRNA in cardiac myxomas. *Br Heart J* 1993; 69:565.
66. Senguin JR, Beigbeder JY, Hvass U, et al: Interleukin-6 production by cardiac myxoma may explain constitutional symptoms. *J Thorac Cardiovasc Surg* 1992; 103:599.
67. Skause B, Bava NO, Westfield TA: Atrial myxoma with Raynaud's phenomenon as the initial presenting symptom. *Acta Med Scand* 1959; 164:321.
68. Buchanan RC, Cairns JA, Krag G, et al: Left atrial myxoma mimicking vasculitis: echocardiographic diagnosis. *Can Med Assoc J* 1979; 120:1540.
69. Currey HLF, Matthew JA, Robinson J: Right atrial myxoma mimicking a rheumatic disorder. *Br Med J* 1967; 1:547.
70. Byrd WE, Matthew OP, Hunt RE: Left atrial myxoma presenting as a systemic vasculitis. *Arthritis Rheum* 1980; 23:240.
71. Huston KA, Combs JJ, Let JT, et al: Left atrial myxoma simulating peripheral vasculitis. *Mayo Clin Proc* 1978; 53:752.
72. Hattler BG, Fuchs JCA, Coson R, et al: Atrial myxomas: an evaluation of clinical and laboratory manifestations. *Ann Thorac Surg* 1970; 10:65.
73. Goodwin JF: The spectrum of cardiac tumors. *Am J Cardiol* 1968; 21:307.
74. Greenwood WF: Profile of atrial myxoma. *Am J Cardiol* 1968; 21:367.
75. Bulkley BH, Hutchins GM: Atrial myxomas: a fifty year review. *Am Heart J* 1979; 97:639.
76. Powers JC, Falkoff M, Heinle RA, et al: Familial cardiac myxoma: emphasis on unusual clinical manifestations. *J Thorac Cardiovasc Surg* 1979; 77:782.
77. Panidas IP, Kotler MN, Mintz GS, et al: Clinical and echocardiographic features of right atrial masses. *Am Heart J* 1984; 107:745.

78. Meller J, Teichholz LE, Pichard AD, et al: Left ventricular myxoma: echocardiographic diagnosis and review of the literature. *Am J Med* 1977; 63:81.
79. Rosenzweig A, Harrigan P, Popvic AD: Left ventricular myxoma simulating aortic stenosis. *Am Heart J* 1989; 117:962.
80. Desousa AL, Muller J, Campbell RL, et al: Atrial myxoma: a review of the neurological complications, metastases, and recurrences. *J Neurol Neurosurg Psychiatr* 1978; 41:1119.
81. Suzuki T, Nagai R, Yamazaki T, et al: Rapid growth of intracranial aneurysms secondary to cardiac myxoma. *Neurology* 1994; 44:570.
82. Chen HJ, Liou CW, Chen L: Metastatic atrial myxoma presenting as intracranial aneurysm with hemorrhage: case report. *Surg Neurol* 1993; 40:61.
83. Tonz M, Laske A, Carrel T, et al: Convulsions, hemiparesis and central retinal artery occlusion due to left atrial myxoma in a child. *Eur J Ped* 1992; 151:652.
84. Browne WT, Wijdicks EF, Parisi JE, et al: Fulminant brain necrosis from atrial myxoma showers. *Stroke* 1993; 24:1090.
85. Furlong BR, Verdile VP: Myxomatous embolization resulting in unilateral amaurosis. *Am J Emerg Med* 1995; 13:46.
86. Lewis JM: Multiple retinal occlusions from a left atrial myxoma. *Am J Ophthalmol* 1994; 117:674.
87. Eriksen UH, Baandrup U, Jensen BS: Total disruptions of left atrial myxoma causing cerebral attack and a saddle embolus in the iliac bifurcation. *Int J Cardiol* 1992; 35:127.
88. Zernivicky F, Kubis J, Vrtik L: Myxoma embolizing into both lower extremities. *Rozhledy V Chirurgii* 1994; 73:127.
89. Carter AB, Lowe K, Hill I: Cardiac myxomata and aortic saddle embolism. *Br Heart J* 1960; 22:502.
90. Hashimoto H, Tikahashi H, Fukiward Y, et al: Acute myocardial infarction due to coronary embolization from left atrial myxoma. *Jpn Circ J* 1993; 57:1016.
91. Kaplam LJ, Weiman DS, VanDecker W, et al: Infected biatrial myxoma: transesophageal echocardiography-guided surgical resection. *Ann Thorac Surg* 1994; 57:487.
92. ten Berg JM, Elbers HR, Defaux JJ, et al: Endocarditis of a left atrial myxoma. *Eur Heart J* 1992; 13:1592.
93. Joseph P, Himmerstein DU, Mahowald JM, Stullman WSL: Atrial myxoma infected with candida: first survival. *Chest* 1980; 78:340.
94. Rajpal RS, Leibsohn JA, Leikweg WG, et al: Infected left atrial myxoma with bacteremia simulating infective endocarditis. *Arch Intern Med* 1979; 139:1176.
95. Whitman MS, Rovito MA, Klions D, et al: Infected atrial myxoma: case report and review. *Clin Infect Dis* 1994; 18:657.
96. Quinn TJ, Codini MA, Harris AA: Infected cardiac myxoma. *Am J Cardiol* 1984; 53:381.
97. Bass NM, Sharratt GJP: Left atrial myxoma diagnoses by echocardiography with observation on tumor movement. *Br Heart J* 1973; 35:1332.
98. Martinez-Lopez JI: Sounds of the heart in diastole. *Am J Cardiol* 1974; 34:594.
99. Harvey WP: Clinical aspects of heart tumors. *Am J Cardiol* 1968; 21:328.
100. Case Records of the Massachusetts General Hospital, Weekly Clinicopathological Exercises: Case 14-1978. *N Engl J Med* 1978; 298:834.
101. Mundinger A, Gruber HP, Dinkel E, et al: Imaging cardiac mass lesions. *Radiol Med* 1992; 10:135.
102. Reeder GS, Khandheria BK, Senard JB, et al: Transesophageal echocardiographs and cardiac masses. *Mayo Clin Proc* 1991; 66:1101.
103. Ensberding R, Erbel DR, Kaspar W, et al: Diagnosis of heart tumors by transesophageal echocardiography. *Eur Heart J* 1993; 14:1223.
104. Samdarshi TE, Mahan EF 3rd, Nanda NC, et al: Transesophageal echocardiographic diagnosis of multicentric left ventricular myxomas mimicking a left atrial tumor. *J Thorac Cardiovasc Surg* 1992; 103:471.
105. Bleiweis MS, Georgiou D, Brungage BH: Detection of intracardiac masses by ultrafast computed tomography. *Am J Cardiac Imag* 1994; 8:63.
106. Sutton D, Al-Kutoubi MA, Lipkin DP: Left atrial myxoma diagnosed by computerized tomography. *Br J Radiol* 1982; 55:80.
107. Symbas PN, Hatcher CR Jr, Gravanis MB: Myxoma of the heart: clinical and experimental observations. *Ann Surg* 1976; 183:470.
108. Nkere UU, Pugsley WB: Time relationships in the diagnosis and treatment of left-atrial myxoma. *Thorac Cardiovasc Surg* 1993; 41:301.
109. McCarthy PM, Piehler JM, Schaff HV, et al: The significance of multiple, recurrent, and "complex" cardiac myxoma. *J Thorac Cardiovasc Surg* 1986; 91:389.
110. Dato GMA, Benedictus M, Dato AA, et al: Long-term follow-up of cardiac myxomas (7–31 years). *J Cardiovasc Surg* 1993; 34:141.
111. Bertolotti U, Mazzucco A, Valfre C, et al: Right ventricular myxoma: review of the literature and report of two patients. *Ann Thorac Surg* 1983; 33:277.
112. Gerbode F, Kerth WJ, Hill JD: Surgical management of tumors of the heart. *Surgery* 1967; 61:94.
113. Attum AA, Johnson GS, Masri Z, et al: Malignant clinical behavior of cardiac myxomas and "myxoid imitators." *Ann Thorac Surg* 1987; 44:217.
114. Read RC, White HJ, Murphy ML, et al: The malignant potentiality of left atrial myxoma. *J Thorac Cardiovasc Surg* 1974; 68:857.
115. Ravikumar E, Pawar N, Gnanamuthu R, et al: Minimal access approach for surgical management of cardiac tumors. *Ann Thorac Surg* 2000; 70:1077.
116. Ko PJ, Chang CH, Lin PJ, et al: Video-assisted minimal access in excision of left atrial myxoma. *Ann Thorac Surg* 1998; 66:1301.
117. Gulbins H, Reichenspurner H, Wintersperger BJ: Minimally invasive extirpation of a left-ventricular myxoma. *Thorac Cardiovasc Surg* 1999; 47:129.
118. Zingas AP, Carrera JD, Murray CA, et al: Lipoma of the myocardium. *J Comput Assist Tomogr* 1983; 7:1098.
119. Reyes CV, Jablokow VR: Lipomatous hypertrophy of the atrial septum: a report of 38 cases and review of the literature. *Am J Clin Pathol* 1979; 72:785.
120. McAllister HA: Primary tumors and cysts of the heart and pericardium, in Harvey WP (ed): *Current Problems in Cardiology*. Chicago, Year Book Medical, 1979.
121. Reece IJ, Cooley DA, Frazier OH, et al: Cardiac tumors: clinical spectrum and prognosis of lesions other than classic benign myxoma in 20 patients. *J Thorac Cardiovasc Surg* 1984; 88:439.
122. Markel ML, Armstrong WF, Waller BF, et al: Left atrial myxoma with multicentric recurrence and evidence of metastases. *Am Heart J* 1986; 111:409.
123. Hade Y, Takahashi T, Takenaka K, et al: Recurrent multiple myxomas. *Am Heart J* 1984; 107:1280.
124. Castells E, Ferran KV, Toledo MCO, et al: Cardiac myxomas: surgical treatment, long-term results and recurrence. *J Cardiovasc Surg* 1993; 34:49.
125. Seidman JD, Berman JJ, Hitchcock CL, et al: DNA analysis of cardiac myxomas: flow cytometry and image analysis. *Hum Pathol* 1991; 22:494.
126. Attum AA, Ogden LL, Lansing AM: Atrial myxoma: benign and malignant. *J Ky Med Assoc* 1984; 82:319.
127. Seo S, Warner TFCS, Colyer RA, et al: Metastasizing atrial myxoma. *Am J Surg Pathol* 1980; 4:391.
128. Hirsch BE, Sehkar L, Kamerer DB: Metastatic atrial myxoma to the temporal bone: case report. *Am J Otol* 1991; 12:207.

129. Kotani K, Matsuzawa Y, Funahashi T, et al: Left atrial myxoma metastasizing to the aorta, with intraluminal growth causing renovascular hypertension. *Cardiology* 1991; 78:72.
130. Diflo T, Cantelmo NL, Haudenschild DD, Watkins MT: Atrial myxoma with remote metastasis: case report and review of the literature. *Surgery* 1992; 111:352.
131. Hannah H, Eisemann G, Hiszvzynskyj R, et al: Invasive atrial myxoma: documentation of malignant potential of cardiac myxomas. *Am Heart J* 1982; 104:881.
132. Rankin LI, Desousa AL: Metastatic atrial myxoma presenting as intracranial mass. *Chest* 1978; 74:451.
133. Burton C, Johnston J: Multiple cerebral aneurysm and cardiac myxoma. *N Engl J Med* 1970; 282:35.
134. Harjola PR, Ala-Kulju K, Ketonen P: Epicardial lipoma. *Scand J Thorac Cardiovasc Surg* 1985; 19:181.
135. Arciniegas E, Hakimi M, Farooki ZQ, et al: Primary cardiac tumors in children. *J Thorac Cardiovasc Surg* 1980; 79:582.
136. Reyes LH, Rubio PA, Korompai FL, et al: Lipoma of the heart. *Int Surg* 1976; 61:179.
137. Voigt J, Agdal N: Lipomatous infiltration of the heart: an uncommon cause of sudden unexpected death in a young man. *Arch Pathol Lab Med* 1982; 106:497.
138. Isner J, Swan CS II, Mikus JP, et al: Lipomatous hypertrophy of the interatrial septum: in vivo diagnosis. *Circulation* 1982; 66:470.
139. Simons M, Cabin HS, Jaffe CC: Lipomatous hypertrophy of the atrial septum: diagnosis by combined echocardiography and computerized tomography. *Am J Cardiol* 1984; 54:465.
140. Basu S, Folliguet T, Anselmo M, et al: Lipomatous hypertrophy of the interatrial septum. *Cardiovasc Surg* 1994; 2:229.
141. Zeebregts CJAM, Hensens AG, Timmermans J, et al: Lipomatous hypertrophy of the interatrial septum: indication for surgery? *Eur J Cardiothorac Surg* 1997; 11:785.
142. Vander Salm TJ: Unusual primary tumors of the heart. *Semin Thorac Cardiovasc Surg* 2000; 2:89.
143. Edwards FH, Hale D, Cohen A, et al: Primary cardiac valve tumors. *Ann Thorac Surg* 1991; 52:1127.
144. Israel DH, Sherman W, Ambrose JA, et al: dynamic coronary ostial occlusion due to papillary fibroelastoma leading to myocardial ischemia and infarction. *Am J Cardiol* 1991; 67:104.
145. Grote J, Mugge A, Schfers HJ: Multiplane transesophageal echocardiography detection of a papillary fibroelastoma of the aortic valve causing myocardial infarction. *Eur Heart J* 1995; 16:426.
146. Gallas MT, Reardon MJ, Reardon PR, et al: Papillary fibroelastoma: a right atrial presentation. *Tex Heart Inst J* 1993; 20:293.
147. DiMattia DG, Assaghi A, Mangini A, et al: Mitral valve repair for anterior leaflet papillary fibroelastoma: two case descriptions and a literature review. *Eur J Cardiothorac Surg* 1999; 15:103.
148. Grinda JM, Couetil JP, Chauvaud S, et al: Cardiac valve papillary fibroelastoma: surgical excision for revealed or potential embolization. *J Thorac Cardiovasc Surg* 1999; 117:106.
149. Darvishian F, Farmer P: Papillary fibroelastoma of the heart: report of two cases and review of the literature. *Ann Clin Lab Sci* 2001; 31:291.
150. Shing M, Rubenson DS: Embolic stroke and cardiac papillary fibroelastoma. *Clin Cardiol* 2001; 24:346.
151. Shahian DM: Papillary fibroelastomas. *Semin Thorac Cardiovasc Surg* 2000; 12:101.
152. Grandmougin D, Fayad G, Moukassa D, et al: Cardiac valve papillary fibroelastomas: clinical, histological and immunohistochemical studies and a physiopathogenic hypothesis. *J Heart Valve Dis* 2000; 9:832.
153. Mazzucco A, Bortolotti U, Thiene G, et al: Left ventricular papillary fibroelastoma with coronary embolization. *Eur J Cardiothorac Surg* 1989; 3:471.
154. Topol EJ, Biern RO, Reitz BA: Cardiac papillary fibroelastoma and stroke: echocardiographic diagnosis and guide to excision. *Am J Med* 1986; 80:129.
155. McFadden PM, Lacy JR: Intracardiac papillary fibroelastoma: an occult cause of embolic neurologic deficit. *Ann Thorac Surg* 1987; 43:667.
156. Mann J, Parker DJ: Papillary fibroelastoma of the mitral valve: a rare cause of transient neurologic deficits. *Br Heart J* 1994; 71:6.
157. Ragni T, Grande AM, Cappuccio G, et al: Embolizing fibroelastoma of the aortic valve. *Cardiovasc Surg* 1994; 2:639.
158. Nicks R: Hamartoma of the right ventricle. *J Thorac Cardiovasc Surg* 1967; 47:762.
159. Bass JL, Breningstall GN, Swaiman DF: Echocardiographic incidence of cardiac rhabdomyoma in tuberous sclerosis. *Am J Cardiol* 1985; 55:1379.
160. Mehta AV: Rhabdomyoma and ventricular preexcitation syndrome: a report of two cases and review of the literature. *Am J Dis Child* 1993; 147:669.
161. Fenoglio JJ, McAllister HA, Ferrans VJ: Cardiac rhabdomyoma: a clinicopathologic and electron microscopic study. *Am J Cardiol* 1976; 38:241.
162. Garson A, Smith RT, Moak JP, et al: Incessant ventricular tachycardia in infants: myocardial hamartomas and surgical cure. *J Am Coll Cardiol* 1987; 10:619.
163. Burke AP, Rosado-de-Christenson M, Templeton PA, et al: Cardiac fibroma: clinicopathologic correlates and surgical treatment. *J Thorac Cardiovasc Surg* 1994; 108:862.
164. Yamaguchi M, Hosokawa Y, Ohashi H, et al: Cardiac fibroma: long term fate after excision. *J Thorac Cardiovasc Surg* 1992; 103:140.
165. Jamieson SA, Gaudiani VA, Reitz BA, et al: Operative treatment of an unresectable tumor on the left ventricle. *J Thorac Cardiovasc Surg* 1981; 81:797.
166. Valente M, Cocco P, Thiene G, et al: Cardiac fibroma and heart transplantation. *J Thorac Cardiovasc Surg* 1993; 106:1208.
167. Nishida K, Kaijima G, Nagayama T: Mesothelioma of the atrioventricular node. *Br Heart J* 1985; 53:468.
168. Jebara VA, Uva MS, Farge A, et al: Cardiac pheochromocytomas. *Ann Thorac Surg* 1991; 53:356.
169. Sisson JC, Shapiro B, Beiervaltes WH, et al: Locating pheochromocytomas by scintigraphy using 131-I-metaiodobenzylguanidine. *Cancer* 1984; 34:86.
170. Orringer MB, Sisson JC, Glazer G, et al: Surgical treatment of cardiac pheochromocytomas. *J Thorac Cardiovasc Surg* 1985; 89:753.
171. Cooley DA, Reardon MJ, Frazier OH, et al: Human cardiac explantation and autotransplantation: application in a patient with a large cardiac pheochromocytoma. *J Texas Heart Inst* 1985; 2:171.
172. Bizard C, Latremouille C, Jebara VA, et al: Cardiac hemangiomas. *Ann Thorac Surg* 1993; 56:390.
173. Grenadier E, Margulis T, Plauth WH, et al: Huge cavernous hemangioma of the heart: a completely evaluated case report and review of the literature. *Am Heart J* 1989; 117:479.
174. Soberman MS, Plauth WH, Winn KJ, et al: Hemangioma of the right ventricle causing outflow tract obstruction. *J Thorac Cardiovasc Surg* 1988; 96:307.
175. Weir I, Mills P, Lewis T: A case of left atrial hemangioma: echocardiographic, surgical, and morphologic features. *Br Heart J* 1987; 58:665.
176. Lo LJ, Ramsay CN, Allen JW, et al: Left atrial cardiac hemangioma associated with shortness of breath and palpitations. *Ann Thorac Surg* 2002; 73:979.
177. Palmer TC, Tresch DD, Bonchek LI: Spontaneous resolution of a large cavernous hemangioma of the heart. *Am J Cardiol* 1986; 58:184.

178. Thomas CR, Johnson GW, Stoddard MF, et al: Primary malignant cardiac tumors: update 1992. *Med Pediatr Oncol* 1992; 20:519.
179. Poole GV, Meredith JW, Breyer RH, et al: Surgical implications in malignant cardiac disease. *Ann Thorac Surg* 1983; 36:484.
180. Murphy MC, Sweeney MS, Putnam JB Jr., et al: Surgical treatment of cardiac tumors: a 25-year experience. *Ann Thorac Surg* 1990; 49:612.
181. Bear PA, Moodie DS: Malignant primary cardiac tumors: the Cleveland Clinic experience, 1956–1986. *Chest* 1987; 92:860.
182. Burke AP, Cowan D, Virmani R: Primary sarcomas of the heart. *Cancer* 1922; 69:387.
183. Putnam JB, Sweeney MS, Colon R, et al: Primary cardiac sarcomas. *Ann Thorac Surg* 1991; 51:906.
184. Janigan DT, Husain A, Robinson NA: Cardiac angiosarcomas: a review and case report. *Cancer* 1986; 57:852.
185. Rettmar K, Stierle U, Shiekhzadeh A, et al: Primary angiosarcoma of the heart: report of a case and review of the literature. *Jpn Heart J* 1993; 34:667.
186. Hermann MA, Shankerman RA, Edwards WD, et al: Primary cardiac angiosarcoma: a clinicopathologic study of six cases. *J Thorac Cardiovasc Surg* 1992; 102:655.
187. Wiske PS, Gillam LD, Blyden G, et al: Intracardiac tumor regression documented by two-dimensional echocardiography. *Am J Cardiol* 1986; 58:186.
188. Reardon MJ, DeFelice CA, Sheinbaum R, et al: Cardiac autotransplant for surgical treatment of a malignant neoplasm. *Ann Thorac Surg* 1999; 67:1793.
189. Nagata K, Irie K, Morimatsu M, et al: Rhabdomyosarcoma of the right ventricle. *Acta Pathol Jpn* 1982; 32:843.
190. Miralles A, Bracamonte MD, Soncul H, et al: Cardiac tumors: clinical experience and surgical results in 74 patients. *Ann Thorac Surg* 1991; 52:886.
191. Schwarz JE, Schwartz GP, Judson PL, et al: Complete resection of a primary cardiac rhabdomyosarcoma: case report, review of the literature and management recommendation. *Cardiovasc Issues (Bull Texas Heart Inst)* 1979; 6:413.
192. Winer HE, Kronzon I, Fox A, et al: Primary chrondromyxomosarcoma—clinical and echocardiographic manifestations: a case report. *J Thorac Cardiovasc Surg* 1977; 74:567.
193. Torsveit JF, Bennett WA, Hinchcliffe WA, et al: Primary plasmacytoma of the atrium: report of a case with successful surgical management. *J Thorac Cardiovasc Surg* 1977; 74:563.
194. Nzayinambabo K, Noel H, Brobet C: Primary cardiac liposarcoma simulating a left atrial myxoma. *J Thorac Cardiovasc Surg* 1985; 40:402.
195. Burke AP, Virmani R: Osteosarcomas of the heart. *Am J Surg Pathol* 1991; 15:289.
196. Takagi M, Kugimiya T, Fuii T, et al: Extensive surgery for primary malignant lymphoma of the heart. *J Cardiovasc Surg* 1992; 33:570.
197. Golstein DJ, Oz MC, Rose EA, et al: Experience with heart transplantation for cardiac tumors. *J Heart Lung Transplant* 1995; 14:382.
198. Baay P, Karwande SV, Kushner JP, et al: Successful treatment of a cardiac angiosarcoma with combined modality therapy. *J Heart Lung Transplant* 1994; 13:923.
199. Crespo MG, Pulpon LA, Pradas G, et al: Heart transplantation for cardiac angiosarcoma: should its indication be questioned? *J Heart Lung Transplant* 1993; 12:527.
200. Jeevanandam V, Oz MC, Shapiro B, et al: Surgical management of cardiac pheochromocytoma: resection versus transplantation. *Ann Surg* 1995; 221:415.
201. Yuh DD, Kubo SH, Francis GS, et al: Primary cardiac lymphoma treated with orthotopic heart transplantation: a case report. *J Heart Lung Transplant* 1994; 13:538.
202. Goldstein DJ, Oz MC, Michler RE: Radical excisional therapy and total cardiac transplantation for recurrent atrial myxoma. *Ann Thorac Surg* 1995; 60:1105.
203. Gowdamarajan A, Michler RE: Therapy for primary cardiac tumors: is there a role for heart transplantation? *Curr Opin Cardiol* 2000; 15:121.
204. Pillai R, Blauth C, Peckham M, et al: Intracardiac metastasis from malignant teratoma of the testis. *J Thorac Cardiovasc Surg* 1986; 92:118.
205. Hallahan ED, Vogelzang NJ, Borow KM, et al: Cardiac metastasis from soft-tissue sarcomas. *J Clin Oncol* 1986; 4:1662.
206. Skhvatsabaja LV: Secondary malignant lesions of the heart and pericardium in neoplastic disease. *Oncology* 1986; 43:103.
207. Press OW, Livingston R: Management of malignant pericardial effusion and tamponade. *JAMA* 1987; 257:1008.
208. Hanfling SM: Metastatic cancer to the heart: review of the literature and report of 127 cases. *Circulation* 1960; 2:474.
209. Weinberg BA, Conces DJ Jr, Waller BF: Cardiac manifestation of noncardiac tumors, part I: direct effects. *Clin Cardiol* 1989; 12:289.
210. Caccavale RJ, Newman J, Sisler GE, Lewis RH: Pericardial disease, in Kaiser LR, Daniel TM (eds): *Thorascopic Surgery*. Boston, Little, Brown, 1993; p 177.
211. Prager RL, Dean R, Turner B: Surgical approach to intracardial renal cell carcinoma. *Ann Thorac Surg* 1982; 33:74.
212. Vaislic CD, Puel P, Grondin P, et al: Cancer of the kidney invading the vena cava and heart: results after 11 years of treatment. *J Thorac Cardiovasc Surg* 1986; 91:604.
213. Shahian DM, Libertino JA, Sinman LN, et al: Resection of cavoatrial renal cell carcinoma employing total circulatory arrest. *Arch Surg* 1990; 125:727.
214. Fujisaki M, Kurihara E, Kikuchi K, et al: Hepatocellular carcinoma with tumor thrombus extending into the right atrium: report of a successful resection with the use of cardiopulmonary bypass. *Surgery* 1991; 109:214.
215. Theman TE: Resection of atriocaval adrenal carcinoma [letter]. *Ann Thorac Surg* 1990; 49:170.
216. Cooper MM, Guillem J, Dalton J, et al: Recurrent intravenous leiomyomatosis with cardiac extension. *Ann Thorac Surg* 1992; 53:139.
217. Vargas-Barron J, Keirns C, Barragan-Garcia R, et al: Intracardiac extension of malignant uterine tumors. *J Thorac Cardiovasc Surg* 1990; 99;1099.
218. Phillips MR, Bower TC, Orszulak TA, et al: Intracardiac extension of an intracaval sarcoma of endometrial origin. *Ann Thorac Surg* 1995; 59:742.
219. Gasparini G: Molecular-targeted anticancer therapy: challenges related to study design and choice of proper endpoints. *Cancer J* 2000; 6:117.
220. Tomescu O, Barr F: Chromosomal translocations in sarcomas: prospects for therapy. *Trends Mol Med* 2001; 7:554.
221. Marque CM: Transcriptional activation of the anti-apoptotic protein BCL-XL by the paired box transcription factors PAX3/FKHR. *Oncogene* 2000; 19:2921.
222. Bernasconi M, Remppis A, Fredericks WJ, et al: Induction of apoptosis in rhabdomyosarcoma cells through downregulation of PAX proteins. *Proc Natl Acad Sci U S A* 1996; 93:13164.
223. Smythe WR, Mohuiddin I, Ozvaran M, Cao X: Antisense therapy for malignant mesothelioma utilizing oligonucleotides targeting the bcl-xl gene product. *J Thorac Cardiovasc Surg* 2002; 123:1191.
224. Graadt van Roggen JF, Bovee JVMG, et al: Diagnostic and prognostic implications of the unfolding molecular biology of bone and soft tissue tumors. *J Clin Pathol* 1999; 52:481.
225. Waters JS, Webb A, Cunningham D, et al: Phase I clinical and pharmacokinetic study of bcl-2 antisense oligonucleotide therapy

in patients with non-Hodgkins lymphoma. *J Clin Oncol* 2000; 18:1812.

226. Jansen B, Wacheck V, Heere-Ress E, et al: Chemosensitization of malignant melanoma by BCL2 antisense therapy. *Lancet* 2000; 356:1728.
227. Momand J, Zambetti GP, Olson D, et al: The mdm-2 oncogene product forms a complex with the p53 protein and inhibits p53-mediated transactivation. *Cell* 1992; 69:1237.
228. Zietz C, Rossle M, Haas C, et al: MDM-2 oncoprotein overexpression, p53 gene mutation, and VEGF up-regulation in angiosarcomas. *Am J Pathol* 1998; 153:1425.
229. Milas M, Yu D, Lang A, et al: Adenovirus-mediated p53 gene therapy inhibits human sarcoma tumorigenecity. *Cancer Gene Ther* 2000; 7:422.
230. Feig BW, Lu X, Hunt KK, et al: Inhibition of the transcription factor nuclear factor kappa-B by adenoviral mediated expression of I kappa B alpha M results in tumor cell death. *Surgery* 1999; 126:399.
231. Mohuiddin IT, Cao X, Smythe WR: A novel gene therapy system utilizing an enzyme activated anthracycline prodrug and adenoviral transfer of the beta glucuronidase gene [abstract]. The International Gene Therapy of Cancer Meeting, San Diego CA, 2001.
232. Casey M, Vaughan CJ, He J, et al: Mutations in the protien kinase R1α regulatory subunit cause familial cardiac myxomas and Carney complex. *J Clin Invest* 2000; 106:R31.
233. Goldstein MM, Casey M, Carney JA, et al: Molecular genetic diagnosis of the familial myxoma syndrome (Carney complex). *Am J Med Genet* 1999; 86:62.
234. Van Siegenhorst M, de Hoogt R, Hermans C, et al: Identification of the tuberous sclerosis gene TSC1 on chromosome 9q34. *Science* 1997; 277:805.
235. The European Chromosome 16 Tuberous Sclerosis Consortium: Identification and characterization of the tuberous sclerosis gene on chromosome 16. *Cell* 1993; 75:1305.
236. Hahn H, Wicking C, Zaphiropoulos PG: Mutations of the human homolog of Drosophila patched in the nevoid basal cell carcinoma syndrome. *Cell* 1996; 85:841.

Part **VIII**

Cardiothoracic Transplantation and Chronic Circulatory Support

Chapter 59

Immunobiology of Heart and Heart-Lung Transplantation

Bartley P. Griffith/Robert S. Poston

The purpose of this chapter is to introduce the immune biology of heart and lung transplantation to the surgeon with the hope that it will provide a better understanding of the complex events that occur outside of the operating room and give the subsequent strategies of immunosuppression a clear rationale. This work differs from the more usual approach in the thoracic surgical textbook, which typically lists established classification systems utilized for diagnosing various grades of rejection and reiterates the results of various conventional immunosuppression therapies generally already well known to the reader. It has been a challenge to distill the more germane aspects of the molecular events surrounding the allogeneic response in a way that those events can be better understood by those heart and lung transplant surgeons not intimately involved in the field of immunology. It is hoped that transplant recipients will benefit if the fundamentals presented here can be understood and made useful by clinicians.

THE MAJOR HISTOCOMPATIBILITY COMPLEX

An allogeneic organ is one that is transferred from one individual to another of the same species but with a different genetic repertoire. A donor heart or lung is immunologically incompatible with the host tissues, and an immunologic reaction or alloresponse is directed against donor proteins or antigens located on the surface of the endothelial, mesenchymal, and epithelial cells of the allograft.

The major histocompatibility locus (MHC) is a complex of polymorphic genes whose glycoprotein MHC molecule products are expressed on the surface of cells. The protein products are the principal determinants of whether an organ is deemed self or nonself, and are the primary targets of the immune response to allografts. The MHC, also known as human leukocyte antigens (HLA), guide the development of T lymphocytes to have a low affinity to self and to use the reaction to self as a way in which foreign peptides are recognized (MHC restriction). The genes that express HLA are among the most variable (or have the largest number of polymorphisms) in the human genome.

Immune responses to organs with different HLA gene types define the alloresponse in humans. The HLA complex encodes class I HLA molecules A, B, and C, which present intracellular antigen to stimulate cytotoxic T lymphocytes expressing the cell surface receptor CD8 (Fig. 59-1). In

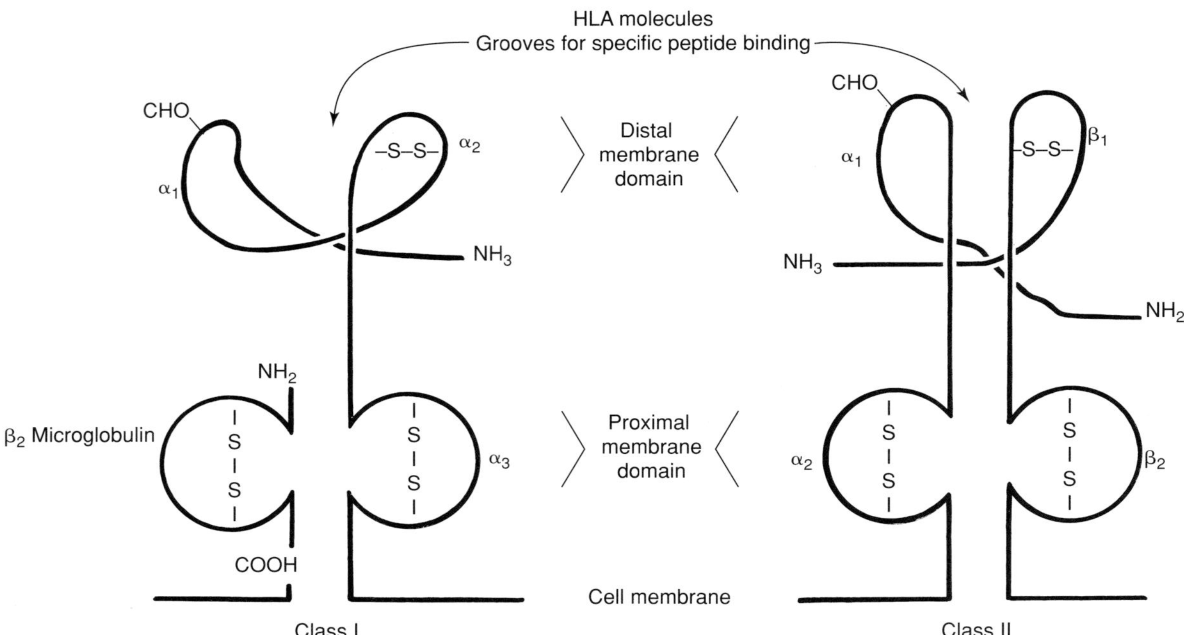

FIGURE 59–1 Class I and II HLA molecules are made up of polypeptide chains with intrachain disulfide bonds. The α_1 and α_2 distal domains of class I and α_1 and β_1 domains of class II make up the peptide binding site for alloantigen. *(Adapted with permission from Parham M, in Haber E (ed): Immunobiology of Transplantation Molecular Cardiovascular Medicines. New York, Scientific American Press, 1995.)*

addition, the HLA complex encodes HLA class II molecules DP, DQ, and DR, which are expressed on antigen-presenting cells that bind extracellular, foreign antigen that is recognized by the proinflammatory CD4-positive T lymphocytes.

At least 20 definable loci, or *alleles*, at HLA-A, 40 at HLA-B, and 10 at HLA-DR[1] have been identified that are inherited as a unit called the *haplotype*. With two possible alleles at each HLA-A, HLA-B, and HLA-DR loci, one maternal and one paternal, an antigen *mismatch* is possible for 0 through 6 antigens. Because of their proximity on chromosome 6, the alleles for HLA-C, HLA-DQ, and HLA-DP are predictably inherited as extended haplotypes with HLA-A, HLA-B, and HLA-DR in a defined donor population (i.e., linkage disequilibrium). Tissue compatibility for transplantation has traditionally required only HLA-A, HLA-B, and HLA-DR typing. Only in unusual cases, such as bone marrow transplant procedures that draw donors from a worldwide registry, have clinically important mismatches of these additional alleles been identified despite matching donor-recipient pairs for HLA-A, HLA-B, and HLA-DR.[2] Although either serology or DNA sequencing is used for typing, recent data suggest that a serologic (i.e., antigen) mismatch has a greater effect on outcome than a DNA (i.e. allele) mismatch.[3]

In heart and lung transplantation, several single-institution studies examining the effect of HLA matching on outcome have found an association between the degree of serologic HLA-DR matching and actuarial graft survival at 1, 5, and 10 years. In general, an association was not present for HLA-A and HLA-B matching. In fact, in a report from the Texas Heart Institute, Kerman et al reviewed 448 heart transplants[4] and found an inverse relationship between HLA-A and HLA-B mismatches and death from cardiac allograft vasculopathy.

Most studies draw from a system of random allocation of donor organs, resulting in less than 8% of closely matched donor-recipient pairs (i.e., 0, 1, or 2 mismatches). Given this low frequency, an adequate pool of closely matched pairs for comparison to recipients that are mismatched at multiple loci with the donor is made possible only by a multi-institutional study of significant size. Two cardiac transplantation registries have fulfilled this size requirement and verified the relationship between HLA matching and acute graft survival: the Collaborative Transplant Study,[5] with 8331 recipients, and the United Network for Organ Sharing/International Society for Heart-Lung Transplantation (UNOS/ISHLT) Registry[6] with 10,752. In the Collaborative Transplant Study, 128 patients (1.5%) with either 0 or 1 combined HLA-A, HLA-B, or HLA-DR mismatches were compared to those with 2 mismatches and 3 to 6 mismatches. Mean rates of survival at three years were a striking 83%, 76%, and 71%, respectively. Multifactorial regression analysis further established that HLA matching had a strong independent effect on graft survival, with the most pronounced effect at 6 months. While the timing might suggest a predominant role for acute rejection, only graft survival and not rejection rates were reported.

The UNOS/ISHLT Registry investigators also found a progressive reduction in risk for greater donor-recipient HLA matching. As opposed to the Collaborative Transplant Study, data obtained from this registry is derived from a database whose use is compulsory for all transplant centers in the United States and subject to auditing and verification. Follow-up in this patient population was found to be virtually complete. The primary benefit of matching appeared to be at the A and DR loci with no independent effect of matching of the B loci. However, these retrospective data, as with the previous study, were based on serologic methods of tissue typing that are less accurate than current recombinant techniques. Again, the effect of HLA matching was greatest at 6 months with the survival curves between matched and mismatched patients becoming parallel at later time points. Considering the results of these two registry studies in light of prior work,[7] HLA matching is unlikely to influence chronic graft rejection. Larger numbers of well-matched transplants studied at a prolonged follow-up are needed to investigate the influence of HLA matching on chronic rejection.

Data demonstrating the effect of HLA matching on outcomes in heart-lung and lung transplantation are sparse. In one study from the University of Pittsburgh, 74 single- and double-lung transplant recipients were analyzed, and a strong effect of HLA-DR matching on 6-month graft survival was evident (100% vs. 75% vs. 56% for 0, 1, and 2 DR mismatches, respectively).[8] Combining A, B, and DR mismatches showed 100% survival for 0 to 2 mismatches, 78% for 3 or 4, and 58% for 5 or 6. The Collaborative Transplant Study showed a trend toward improved survival for well-matched grafts in both heart-lung and lung recipients, but this did not reach statistical significance (1176 patients enrolled in the lung transplant group and 640 in the heart-lung group).[5] The UNOS/ISHLT registry data also showed a less impressive effect of matching on lung allograft outcome. A significant reduction in risk with any degree of HLA matching was seen but no progressive improvement with increasing levels of matching.

These data support the conclusion that HLA matching confers an important benefit after heart transplantation, and probably after heart-lung and lung transplantation. The conventional wisdom that deems prospective HLA matching to be logistically unfeasible in thoracic organ transplantation may be changing. The former requirement of HLA typing using serologic methods for donor splenic tissue retrieved during procurement did not provide sufficient time for prospective typing given that heart and lung allografts tolerate only 4 to 6 hours of ischemic time. This formidable restriction has been overcome by the use of PCR-based HLA typing on peripheral blood lymphocytes prior to the procurement procedure. Future advances in our current preservation methods such as the use of continuous, warm, sanguinous perfusion of the ex vivo cardiac allograft[9] will permit procurements from longer distances, a certain requirement of an organ allocation system that takes into consideration HLA matching.

Some groups have, in fact, reported impressive advances in achieving prospective HLA matching. One is the Harefield group, which recently reported that within their donor allocation zone, HLA typing was available before organ retrieval in 69% of cases performed in 1994. Based on outcome data from their institution, this group has focused on HLA-DR matching only and has seen an increase in prospective matching from 5% to 25% of transplants in a recent 1-year time period and a reduction in acute rejection in those matched. However, widespread adoption of cardiac HLA matching has been hindered by continued limitations. A benefit on early cardiac allograft survival was seen mainly for those with more than 3 antigen matches, an infrequent event (less than 8% of cases) in the current system of random allocation of donor organs. Increasing this frequency of close matches via prospective matching would require significantly prolonged ischemic and waiting list times for the donor organ and transplant candidate, respectively. Given current methods of organ preservation and the high recipient waiting list mortality, such a requirement would seem unacceptable in light of the modest impact on acute organ survival and lack of evidence supporting an effect on long-term graft outcome and chronic rejection.

ANTIGEN PROCESSING/AFFERENT RESPONSE

HLA class I and class II molecules are not uniformly expressed on the same cells. HLA expression is low at baseline in human donor hearts and lungs but can be found to stain prominently for both classes in response to inflammatory stimuli (Fig. 59-2). After transplantation, class I molecules present protein products produced from the endogenous breakdown of their own MHC protein to previously activated $CD8^+$ cytotoxic lymphocytes (CTL) (Fig. 59-3). Class I molecules are found on the surfaces of all cells except the erythrocyte, which incidentally protects a malarial red cell infection from $CD8^+$ cell surveillance. Class II expression is constitutively found on the professional *antigen-presenting cells* (APCs), dendritic cells, B lymphocytes, macrophages, and thymic epithelium, and induced on other cell types by cytokines like interferon (INF), also produced as part of the alloimmune response. Originating either from donor organ (i.e., passenger cells) or from the host, these APC internalize, process, and present shed fragments of donor MHC protein on class II molecules (see Fig. 59-3). The allogenic class II molecule and bound peptide exclusively react with a large number of $CD4^+$ T cells (perhaps 1%) in a process called the direct or allorestricted pathway.[10,11]

The direct recognition of a few allogenic donor class II and I MHC epitopes by host CD4 and CD8 cells soon draws other epitopes into the response as a result of a general upregulation of antigen processing and presentation.[12] This process,

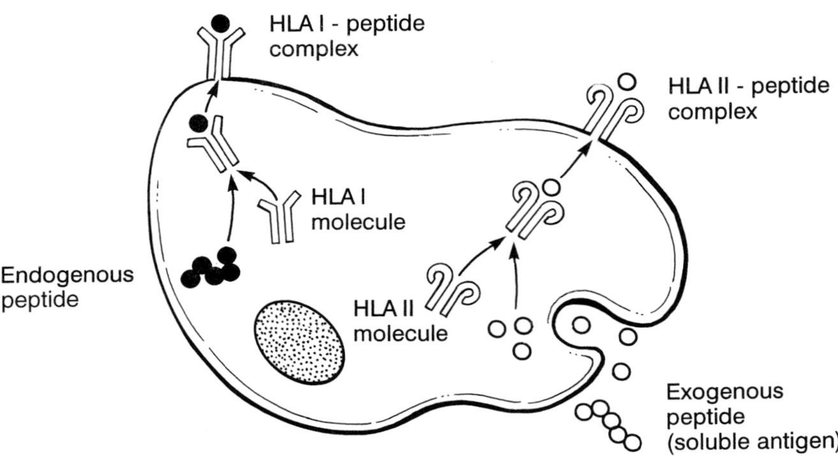

FIGURE 59–2 Donor antigen derives from either the endogenous pathway or exogenous path.

called epitope spreading, is a potent initiator of cell-mediated rejection when accompanied by costimulatory signals generated by the interaction of certain cell-surface proteins on antigen-presenting cells and T cells (Fig. 59-4). The indirect or self-restricted pathway is the physiological mechanism of T-cell immune recognition. In this pathway, host-derived APC process exogenous allo-MHC fragments and bind them to host class II and I MHC for presentation to host T cells. The exact role for the indirect alloresponse in transplantation is not well characterized, but it is believed to be a significant

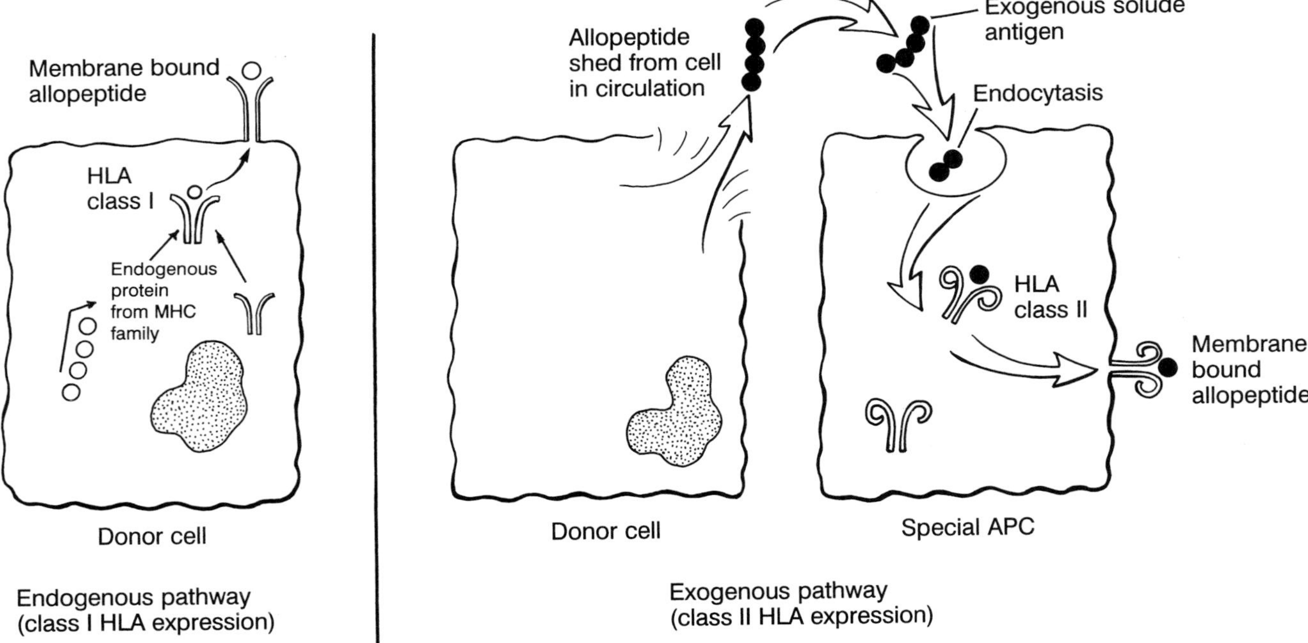

FIGURE 59–3 Generally HLA class I molecules bind protein fragments of donor MHC protein produced from endogenous cellular processes. Allopeptides from MHC donor cell membrane fragments are brought into special APCs that process and bind them to HLA class II molecules for presentation to host T cells.

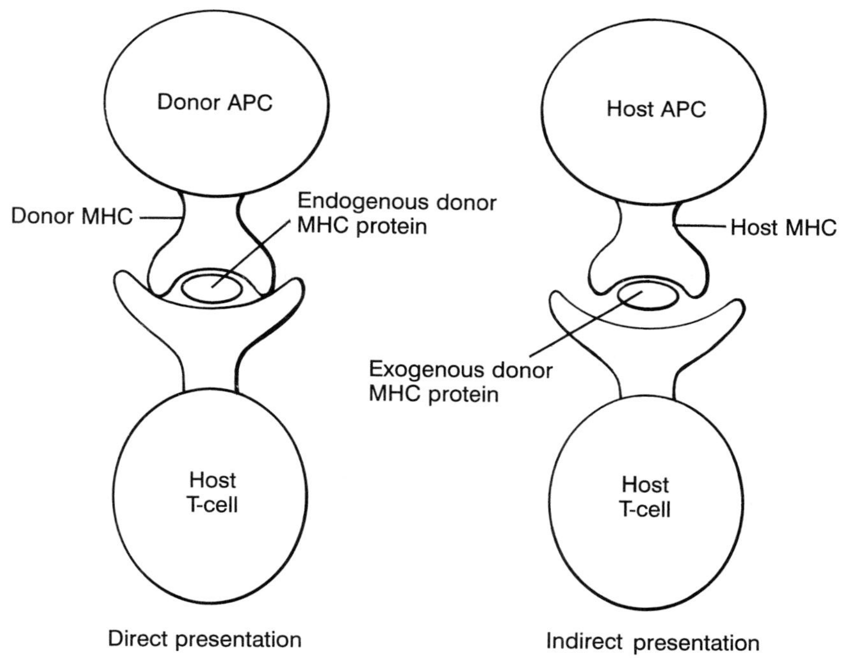

FIGURE 59–4 Host T lymphocytes can respond to alloantigens by the direct or indirect pathway. On direct presentation, donor cells bind endogenous MHC protein to donor MHC molecules (allorestricted). In the direct path, host cells respond to processed donor MHC peptide bound to host MHC (self-restricted). The direct pathway can stimulate many T cells and is responsible for most acute rejections, whereas fewer T cells respond to the small foreign peptide presented in host MHC molecule. The indirect pathway has been implicated as an important part of the late chronic rejection process when host APCs replace those of the donor within the allograft.

contributor to late and chronic rejection when donor APCs are eventually replaced by those of the host.[13] Its role in chronic rejection is supported by the observation that T cells from patients with chronically rejected renal, cardiac, and lung transplants show evidence of reactivity to indirectly, but not directly, presented donor HLA allopeptides.[14] Indirect alloresponses may be especially important in xenograft responses, in which recipient T cells and donor APC cannot make efficient contact with each other. On the other hand, indirect antigen presentation in the absence of costimulation has been proposed as one of the mechanisms of tolerance, which is thought to explain the immunosuppressive effects of blood transfusions. The direct and indirect pathways likely have differential sensitivities to immunosuppressive drugs.

CD4 cells elaborate various cytokines that amplify the generalized inflammatory response. Two different mature CD4 cells have been characterized: TH1 cells, which secrete cytokines INF and interleukin 2 (IL-2), and stimulate cellular immunity; and TH2 cells, which secrete interleukins 4 and 10, and stimulate B-lymphocytes to produce antibodies. Because TH1 cells and TH2 cells are known to mutually suppress each other's subsets, the TH2 cells have been implicated in tolerance against cell-mediated rejection.[15] While mechanisms are evolving, it appears that the TH1 cells arise in regional lymph nodes following class II presentation on macrophages and mature dendritic cells (DC). Mature DC are the most effective APC at activating naïve T cells because they express high levels of HLA, intercellular adhesion, and costimulatory molecules. TH2 cells arise from class II presentation by B lymphocytes or immature DC, cells that are capable of presenting antigen but that provide low levels of costimulation.[16]

Only mature DC provide the appropriate costimulatory signal for the conversion of naïve CD8 T cells to activated cytotoxic lymphocytes (CTL). In addition, this process typically requires exogenous IL-2 from CD4 "helper" T cells. A more stringent requirement for stimulation of $CD8^+$ versus $CD4^+$ T cells assures that CTL are formed only when evidence of their need is unambiguous.[1]

EFFERENT ALLORESPONSE

After recognizing a heart or lung allograft as foreign, the immune system unleashes cellular and humoral (antibody) attacks (Fig. 59-5). The efferent response usually begins when activated CD4 cells secrete various cytokines that drive the inflammatory response.[17] IL-2 increases the expression of IL-2R on CD4 cells, driving proliferation and further differentiation of CD4 cells. The activated CD4 cells secrete additional lymphokines, including INF, which with IL-2 stimulate the activated CTL cells to bind to the allograft cells presenting donor MHC protein molecules. The CTL proliferate and specifically kill the allotarget by at least two mechanisms.[18] In the presence of Ca^{2+}, the protein perforin polymerizes onto the target cell and causes 16 to 20 nm pores to open in the cell membrane, resulting in osmotic collapse. The other likely method is by stimulation of apoptosis or programmed cell death by interaction of the lymphocyte Fas ligand with the APO-1/Fas receptor of the target cell. Second messengers are elicited that activate endonucleases and proteases to cause fragmentation of DNA and T-cell dissolution. Tissues that appear to have an immune privilege, such as the testis, eye, brain, and some tumors, utilize this Fas/Fas-L apoptotic

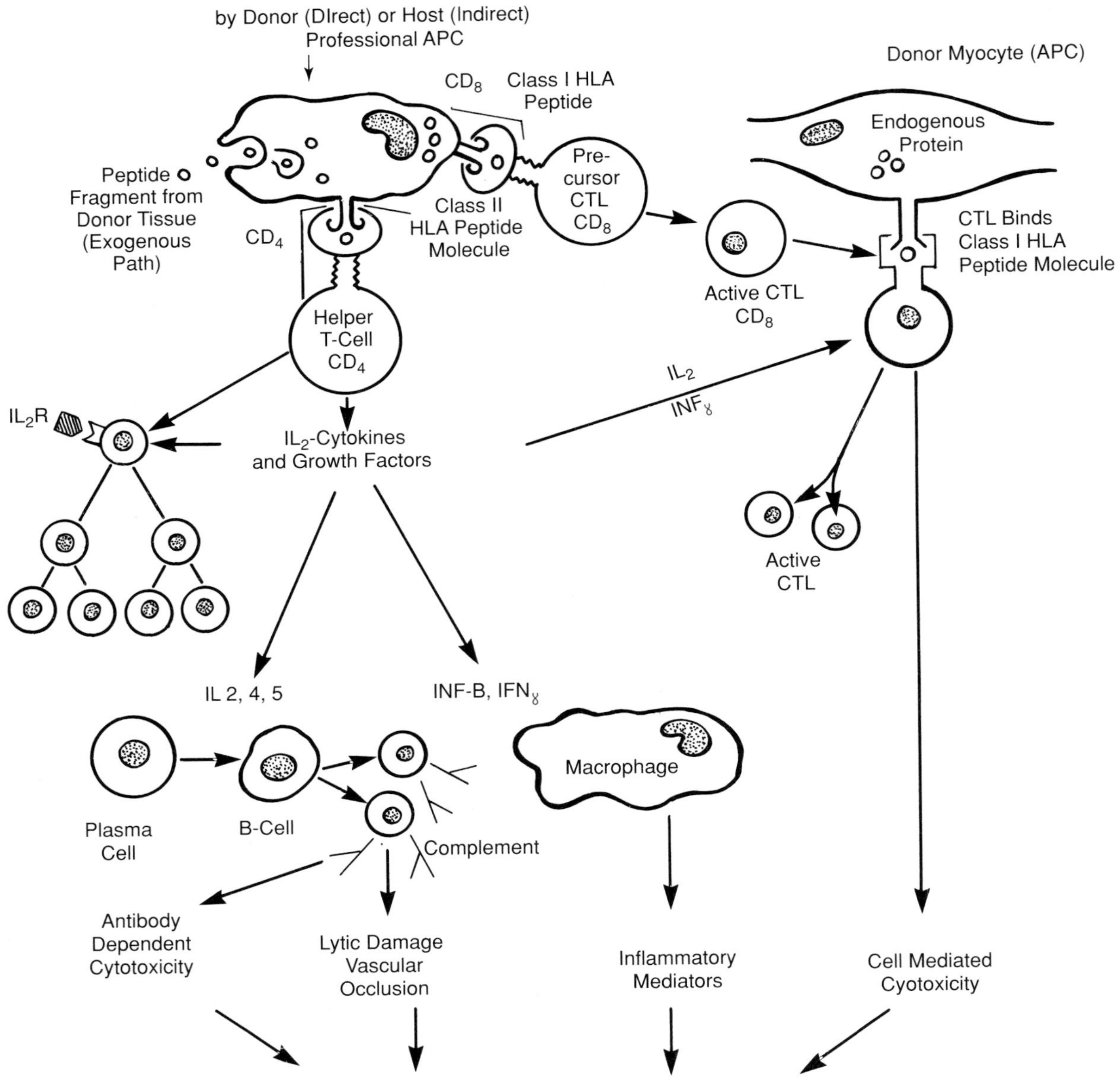

FIGURE 59–5 The alloresponse is a complicated cellular and humoral process that generally begins when a CD4 cell recognizes a class II donor HLA molecule peptide complex presented on a donor heart or lung APC (direct path) and a precursor CTL cell of CD8 lineage binds to a class I donor molecule. The CD4 proliferates and produces IL-2 that drives the process further. The activated CTL cells seek class I donor specific targets and are stimulated by IL-2 and INF to kill targets. These CTL CD8 cells are primarily responsible for destruction of the allograft. Antibodies are selectively produced by B cells and draw inflammatory cells to the targets by antibody-dependent cytotoxicity. The complement is also activated by the humoral arm and initiates lytic changes and thrombosis in the allograft. Other inflammatory cytokines attract polymorphonuclear cells into the response and TNF and INF mix to activate macrophages.

pathway to destroy autoreactive lymphocytes. This pathway is being exploited for the development of tolerance to allogenic tissues in experimental models.[19]

Graft ischemia and reperfusion provoke a nonspecific immune response involving neutrophils and macrophages. Through the production of cytokines such as INF and tumor necrosis factor (TNF), these cells upregulate costimulatory molecules and MHC class I and II, thereby enhancing immunogenicity and T-cell recruitment to the graft. Macrophages also release IL-1, which promotes a positive feedback cycle by driving IL-2 production by T cells. Through this mechanism, a significant bout of reperfusion injury (RI) has been shown clinically to increase the incidence of acute rejection.[20] In addition, by activating the coronary endothelium and initiating smooth muscle cell proliferation, RI has been hypothesized to be an important contributor to chronic allograft vasculopathy.[21] Inhibition of RI has been shown to reduce this vasculopathy both experimentally[22] and clinically.[23]

On the other hand, recent data suggest that host reparative responses may mitigate the immunogenic effects of RI. By analyzing female cardiac allografts transplanted into male recipients, Quaini et al documented the migration of host stem cells that matured into myocytes, endothelium, and capillaries in the donor hearts as soon as 4 days posttransplantation.[24] With the discovery of this capacity for rapid formation of an organ chimera with up to 20% mature host-derived tissue, it is hypothesized that RI may actually result in a reduction, rather than enhancement, of allograft immunogenicity. The overall effect of RI on the allograft likely depends on which pathway plays a greater role in any given donor-recipient pair, illustrating an important future area for investigation.

The humoral response begins as host and B cells are drawn into the alloresponse by the lymphokines and by their own class I and II cell receptor engagement with the donor cells. The activated B cells evolve into plasma cells that produce allospecific antibodies against the donor class I and II HLA molecules and engage the complement cascade.

T-CELL LYMPHOCYTE MATURATION AND ALLOACTIVATION

T cells form receptors (TCR) in the thymus that, similar to antibody, recognize specific peptide sequences. However, unlike antibody, the TCR cannot be released from the cell membrane and requires an association with five invariant polyproteins collectively called the *CD3 complex*. The TCR cannot recognize free antigen but is restricted by the HLA molecule with which it interacts. Genes responsible for the TCR randomly rearrange within the thymus to provide an astonishing array (10^{16}) of potential binding sites necessary for diversity. Immature T cells are selected to survive in the thymus based upon whether and how strongly their TCR binds the HLA class I and II molecules expressed on the thymic epithelium (Fig. 59-6). The importance of the thymus is illustrated when it fails to develop in DiGeorge's syndrome. This disease results in an increased risk for a wide range of opportunistic infections that is reversed by thymic transplantation.[25] It is believed that when T cells react too strongly or too weakly to HLA molecules in the thymus, they are negatively selected and die of apoptosis or DNA fragmentation to prevent the establishment of autoreactive clones and impotent cells. In fact, 95% of the thymocytes do not survive this selection.

T cells are said to be naive until they are exposed to specific antigens in the periphery. When the TCR expressed on a lymphocyte engages its specific membrane-bound MHC molecule on an APC, a series of reactions occur in the cell that result in a rise of intracellular calcium (Fig. 59-7). The Ca^{2+} influx results in the accumulation of calcineurin, which in turn removes a phosphate from nuclear factor for activating T cells (NFAT-P).[26] NFAT can then enter the nucleus, where it promotes transcription of the cytokine IL-2. IL-2 prompts the appearance of IL-2 receptors (IL-2R) on the surface of T cells with which it reacts, prompting proliferation and differentiation of the lymphocyte and enabling it to interact with B cells and cytotoxic T cells. While the TCR/CD3 dependent signal is necessary, it alone is not sufficient to activate quiescent T cells. Full activation requires a second or costimulatory signal provided by physical contact between various T-cell surface proteins known as integrins and their ligands on the APC surface.[27] The molecules on the surface of T cells that form an "immunological synapse" with costimulatory molecules on antigen-presenting cells include CD28, whose ligand is B7; CD154, which binds to CD40; CD2, the ligand for CD58 (LFA-3); and LFA-1, the ligand for ICAM-1. CD8 and CD4 also assist in the binding of the T cell to its MHC peptide of class I or class II specificity and modify the TCR signal (see Fig. 59-7). T cells that have been activated express CTLA-4, which may act as a competitive inhibitor of CD28, thereby blocking the generation of costimulatory signals.[28] Inhibition of costimulation using monoclonal antibodies against ICAM,[29] CD40L,[30] and CD28[31] has generated donor-specific tolerance in preclinical transplantation models. Stimulation of alloresponsive T cells in the absence of costimulation seems to be a central feature in this form of tolerance, because the addition of less specific immunosuppressive medications such as FK506 or corticosteroids inhibits its development. Other T-cell integrins combine with matrix molecules of the allograft that are exposed during inflammation, including fibronectin, lamenin, fibrinogen, and vitronectin. These sites link the immune response to the organizing framework of all tissues and provide a further evidence of the connection between early graft injury and chronic rejection. Another family of cell adhesion molecules called selectins has been identified on the endothelium and assists in the first contact of leukocytes, macrophages, and platelets with the donor organ by inducing a rolling, sticking,

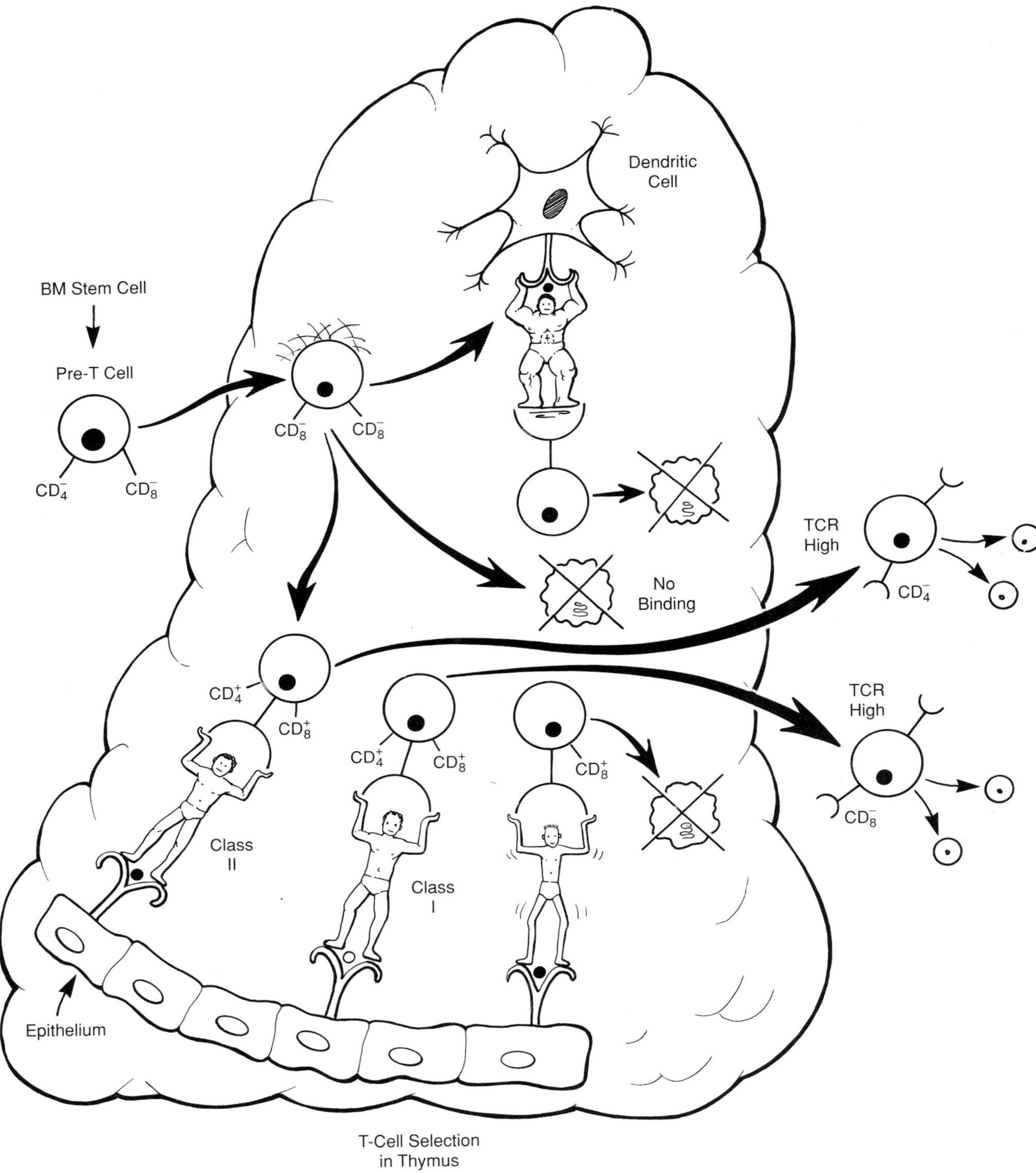

FIGURE 59–6 T cells enter the thymus from the bone marrow where they differentiate and assemble diverse TCRs that cause the cells to be pl or mi selected, based on their usefulness. Diversity is based on rearrangement of genes responsible for variable portions of the chains that form the TCR heterodimer. When the TCR is pl selected on a class I HLA molecule, CD8 will form part of the receptor complex, and when a class II molecule is involved, then CD4 will form.

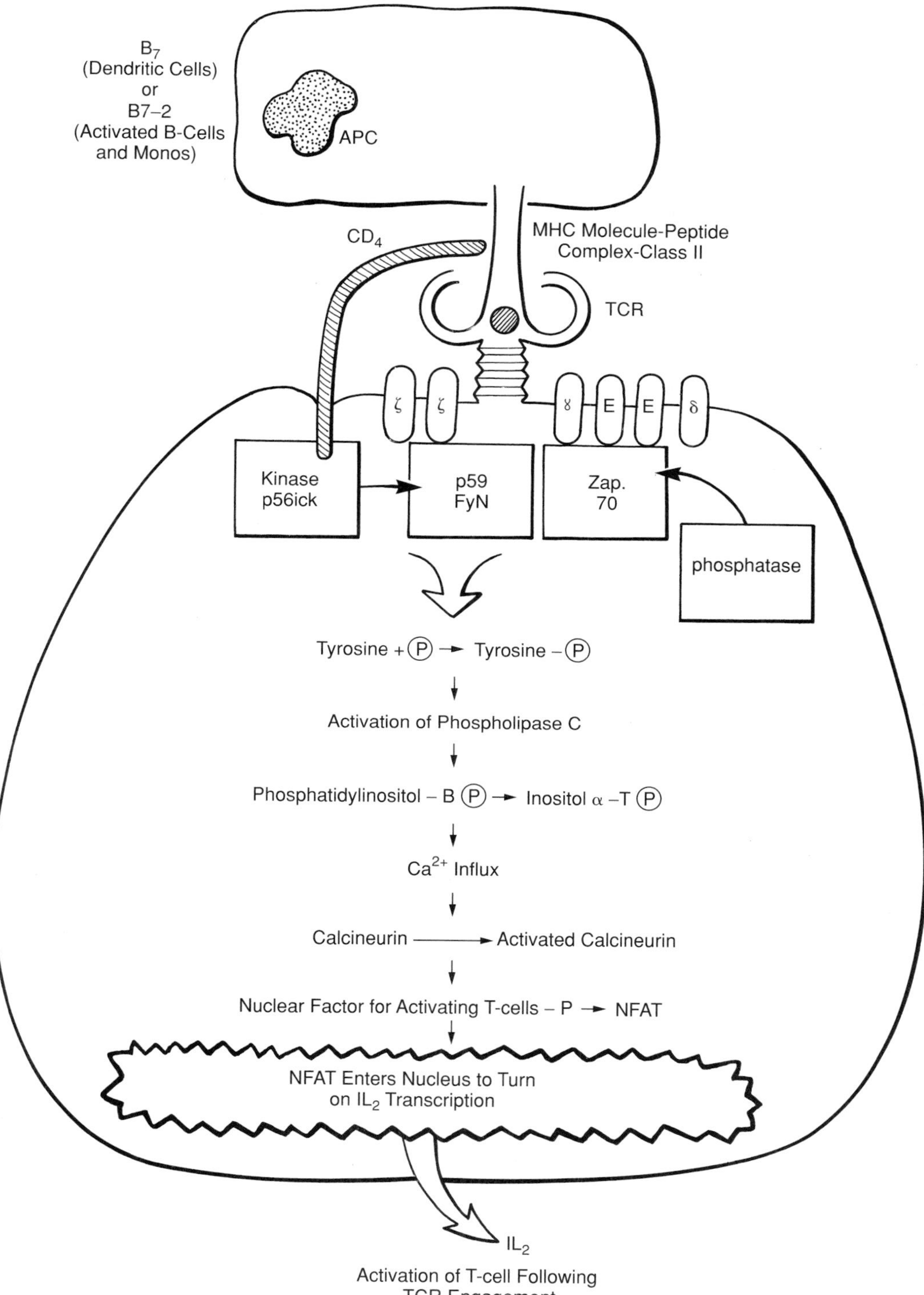

FIGURE 59–7 CD4 cells TCR has engaged its specific MHC class II molecule and bound allopeptide. The TCR complex initiates cytotoxic signal transduction that enables a Ca^{2+} influx activation of calcineurin nuclear factor for activating T cells, loses phosphate, and enters the nucleus to begin the promotor sequence to activate the IL-2 gene. (*Adapted with permission from Parham M, in Haber E (ed): Immunobiology of Transplantation Molecular Cardiovascular Medicines. New York, Scientific American Press, 1995.*)

and finally transepithelial migration. The selectins are upregulated by the inflammatory cytokines IL-1, INF, and TNF that are elaborated from immune cells during the alloresponse.

REJECTION OF HEART AND LUNGS

Hyperacute Rejection

Hyperacute rejection (HAR) is said to occur when edema, hemorrhage, and thrombosis are noted shortly following revascularization. This process involves preformed antibodies that immediately bind to and activate the endothelium, initiating the complement and coagulation cascades. These antibodies bind to oligosaccharide antigens of the ABO blood group and xenoreactive antigens that are similar to those found on numerous endemic bacteria, protozoa, and viruses. The cross-reactivity of antibodies directed against these endemic microbes is likely to be responsible for the preexisting natural antibodies that cause HAR after transplantation with either ABO-incompatible or xenogenic organs. Because the titer and avidity of preformed antibodies against the blood group antigens in newborn infants is low, ABO-incompatible cardiac allografts have shown greater success in these patients.[32] HAR also occurs from antibodies directed against nonself HLA antigens, especially in patients with a prior history of exposure to allogenic HLA through blood transfusions and pregnancies. Mechanical support with a ventricular assist device is also a strong risk factor for development of anti-HLA antibodies, which can be alleviated in part by the use of leukocyte-depleted, CMV-negative blood transfusions.[33]

Although anti–class I Ab are more destructive of the graft endothelial cells, class II HLA is induced on the graft vasculature during periods of inflammation and can also provoke HAR when bound by anti–class II Ab following allotransplantation. Although HAR can be treated by cobra venom factor to deplete complement,[34] it is best prevented during allotransplantation by avoiding blood group disparities and identifying preexisting antibodies to HLA antigens. This is accomplished by exposing candidate serum to panels of donor cells with most HLA types. If a patient is determined to react to more than 10% of the panel, specific pretransplant (i.e., prospective) crossmatching is recommended between lymphocytes from the proposed donor and candidate's serum.

Despite their high endothelial avidity, neither the pre- nor posttransplant presence of anti-HLA antibodies guarantees HAR. By using an aggressive perioperative regimen of plasmapheresis, IVIG, and cytoxan, patients have successfully avoided HAR after transplantation despite a positive prospective crossmatch.[35] Anti–donor HLA antibodies have developed in some after transplant despite a negative prospective crossmatch. Titers may rise as early as 3 to 4 days after transplant, which implies a secondary antibody response with undetectable levels of preformed anti-HLA antibodies despite prior exposure. Although a process known as accelerated, acellular rejection occurs in a few, the induction of a protective phenotype (e.g. bcl-x_L, bcl-2, and A20) inhibits endothelial activation and prevents vascular injury in the vast majority.[36]

Acute Rejection

Acute rejection involves both cellular and humoral immunity and is most common within weeks to months after transplantation. Although late acute episodes can occur, they often do so in the setting of a change in the balance of immunosuppression versus host immunity. A decrease in the blood level of immunosuppressant either by prescription drug interaction or by an upregulation in alloreactivity owing to viral infection can cause a late allorejection. Myocardial and pulmonary cytolysis on endomyocardial or pulmonary biopsy is the finding that supports a higher rejection grade (Table 59-1). Nonimmunological modalities, including measurement of hemodynamic parameters, radionuclide scanning, and magnetic resonance imaging have shown good

TABLE 59–1 New International Society of Heart and Lung Transplantation morphologic grading of acute rejection

Heart		Lung	
Grade 1A	Focal aggregates of perivascular activated lymphocytes; rarely interstitial foci	Grade 1	Minimal perivascular and interstitial mononuclear infiltrates*
Grade 1B	Diffuse but sparse interstitial foci; activated lymphocytes	Grade 2	Mild perivascular and interstitial mononuclear infiltrates*
Grade 2	One focus of perimyocytic-activated lymphocytes with myocyte damage	Grade 3	Moderate perivascular and interstitial mononuclear infiltrates*
Grade 3A	Multifocal areas of myocyte damage caused by activated lymphocytes and eosinophils	Grade 4	Severe perivascular and interstitial mononuclear infiltrates*
Grade 3B	Borderline severe rejection		
Grade 4	Diffuse mixed (eosinophils, often neutrophils) infiltrate with vasculitis, hemorrhage, and myocyte necrosis		

*Without lymphocytic bronchitis or bronchiolitis.

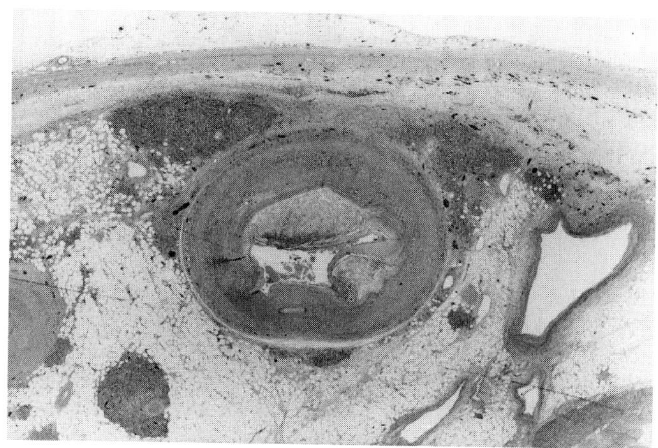

FIGURE 59–8 Obliterative arteriopathy, or chronic allograft vasculopathy (CAV), results in concentric narrowing of the epicardial coronary arteries and their large intramyocardial branches. This section was taken from an explanted cardiac allograft resected at the time of retransplantation for chronic rejection. Note the fibrointimal hyperplasia, and adventitial and mural inflammation.

correlation with established high-grade rejections but have not demonstrated sufficient predictive value to be included in routine clinical management.

Acute vascular rejection has been primarily used after cardiac transplantation to refer to depositions of immunoglobulin and complement within the walls of the coronary artery.[37] Although it has been proposed that this is a common form of acute rejection that can lead to allograft ischemia and dysfunction, many believe that the deposits are nonspecific and more related to endothelial injury from ischemia. In addition, enhanced perioperative immunosuppression such as the mouse anti-CD3 antibody, OKT3, can protract the healing phase of ischemic myocardial injury and confuse the histologic diagnosis of ischemic injury versus acute rejection.[38] Although some physicians advocate aggressive therapy when there is a suspicion, most will not treat with increased immunotherapy unless there is significant allograft dysfunction.

Chronic Rejection of the Heart

Although chronic, persistent cell-mediated rejection causes progressive myocardial fibrosis and dysfunction, the term chronic allograft vasculopathy (AV) takes into consideration the role of multiple nonimmune factors in the etiology of this process. AV has a prevalence of at least 60% within 5 years of transplantation.[39] This obstructive process can progress to near-complete occlusion of the epicardial coronary arteries causing micro- and macroinfarction (Figs. 59-8 and 59-9) and is the leading cause of death after the first year following cardiac transplantation. The histologic findings differ from those seen in typical atherosclerosis with a uniform pattern of near-luminal occlusion by neointimal proliferation, and fewer early accumulations of extracellular lipid. Infiltrates of T cells that encircle the entire vessel are characteristic.[40] The concentric nature of the lesion has led to emergence of intravascular ultrasound (IVUS) as the optimal method for clinical detection of AV.[41] Endothelial cells generally remain intact but are known to be dysfunctional based on a paradoxical constrictive response to acetylcholine.[42]

AV has been linked to multiple potential etiologies but the most important clinical explanation has not emerged. Earlier belief that AV might be solely due to an arterial injury that occurs during cardiac harvest and implantation is not tenable as animal models of syngeneic transplants do not develop the lesion. However, events around the procurement

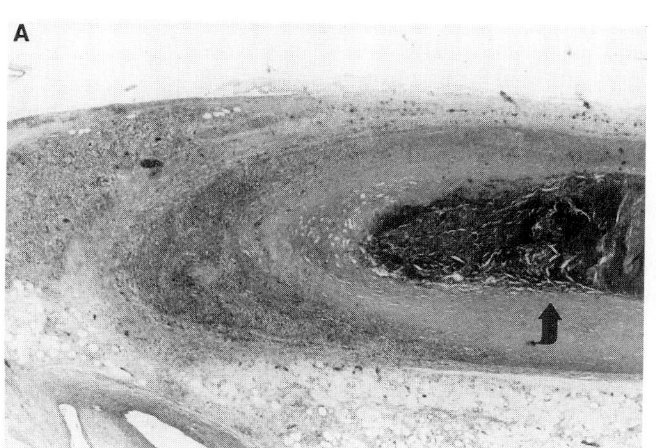

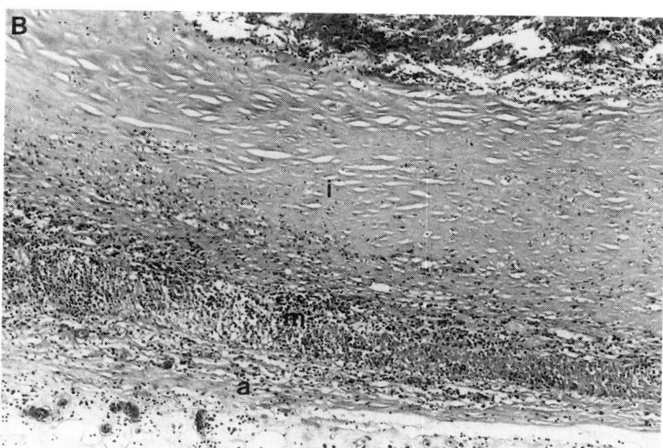

FIGURE 59–9 (A) Predisposition to thrombosis is a complication of chronic allograft vasculopathy (CAV). In this photomicrograph, an artery already narrowed by CAV shows a complicating thrombus (arrow). (B) A higher magnification of the artery shown in *A* illustrates the adventitial (a), medial (m), and intimal (i) mononuclear inflammation, which is more prevalent and severe in CAV than in atherosclerosis seen in the general population.

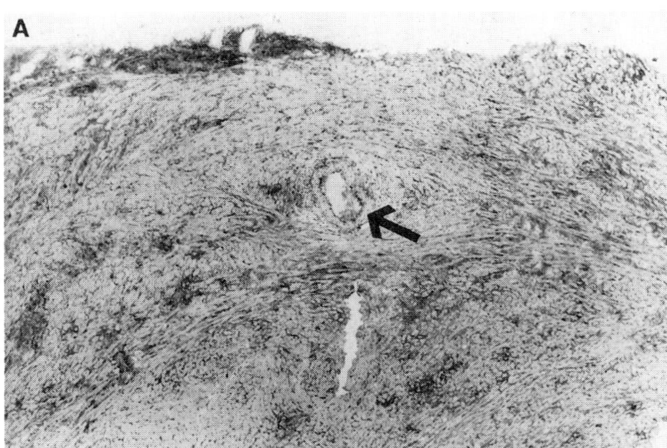

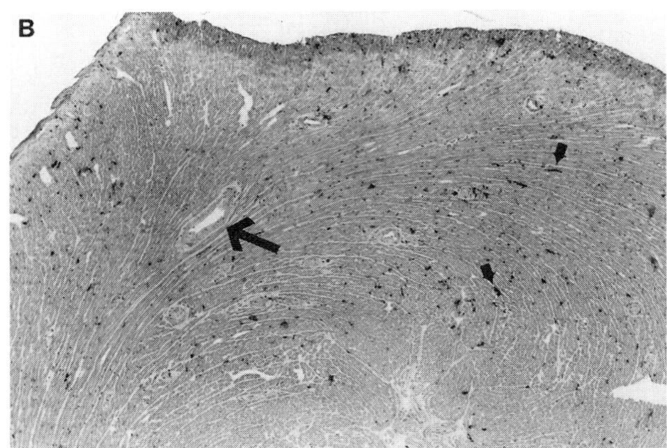

FIGURE 59–10 (A) Experimental animal models of chronic allograft vasculopathy suggest that tolerance induction via the introduction of hematolymphoid chimerism can prevent chronic class II antigens on the microvasculature and large intramyocardial coronary arteries, which show early changes of chronic allograft vasculopathy (arrow). (B) In contrast, staining for donor MHC class II antigens in a cardiac allograft that is resistant to chronic rejection shows staining only in the interstitial hematolymphoid cells (small arrows), whereas the arteries are normal appearing (large arrows).

process that result in early endothelial activation and dysfunction have demonstrated a convincing correlation with the development of experimental[43] and clinical AV.[44] It has been difficult to correlate any of the usual risk factors for natural atherosclerosis including hypertension, pretransplant hyperlipidemia, history of smoking, or prior atherosclerosis with an increased risk of AV. However, aggressive treatment of posttransplantation hyperlipidemia with pravastatin was shown to reduce the incidence of AV in a randomized, placebo-controlled clinical trial, using both IVUS and angiography.[45] Some studies have suggested that cytomegalovirus (CMV) infection might prompt the atherosclerotic process and, although there appears to be some association, it has been clearly demonstrated that cytomegalic infection is not required for the process to occur and the association may be more an association than cause and effect.[46,47] Antidonor cellular[48,49] and humoral[50–52] immune responses are associated with clinical AV lesions, but these processes might equally well be a marker for high risk as opposed to a direct cause of chronic rejection. Despite a significant improvement in the 1-year half-life of allografts in the modern cyclosporin era of improved immunosuppression, AV has remained refractory.[53] Increased expression of ICAM-1 and other adhesion molecules in AV lesions[54–56] point to the role of a smoldering, nonspecific immune response in the chronic rejection process as documented in development and activation of nontransplant atherosclerosis.[57]

Our current limited pathophysiologic understanding of this relentless process is based largely on small animal models. By systematically isolating possible etiologic factors, these models have provided significant insight into the basic science of the vasculopathy process in cardiac allografts. However, out of logistical necessity, the surrogate pathologic lesion occurs much earlier than the typical changes of chronic rejection in clinical patients. Thus, the pathogenesis of the process being studied experimentally is almost certainly not the same as that occurring clinically. Indeed, many of the commonly used rodent models demonstrate suppression of AV lesion formation with standard immunosuppression such as cyclosporin,[58] a finding that significantly limits clinical relevance (Fig. 59-10).

Murase et al. have investigated pathogenic mechanisms of AV using MHC class I–mismatched miniature swine.[59] This more clinically relevant large animal model supports the findings of most rodent models and suggests that there is an immune-mediated injury that initiates changes in the arterial wall. The artery then follows a "response to injury" pathway common to other forms of arteriosclerosis, prompting physical changes and relocation of smooth muscle cells from the media to a neointima. In addition, there is evidence that host stem cells deposit in the vessel wall and contribute to this neointimal formation.[60] Irrespective of the cell of origin, neointimal formation is accelerated with growth factors, TNF and IFN elaborated from the endothelium, and CD4 cells. Macrophages are recruited and contribute cytokines and growth factors that promote the proliferation and synthesis of matrix by vascular smooth muscle cells.

Treatment strategies will remain elusive unless more complete control of the alloresponse can be maintained by the newer xenobiotics and monoclonal antibodies or induction of tolerance. Clinicians are anxious to explore the potential for new xenobiotics that have demonstrated striking reduction in experimental AV based on their suppression of the smooth muscle response to the growth factors.[58]

Chronic Rejection of Lung Allografts

The lung allograft, too, appears to be affected by a chronic process that limits the long-term usefulness of the organ. This chronic attrition can affect 30% to 50% of recipients

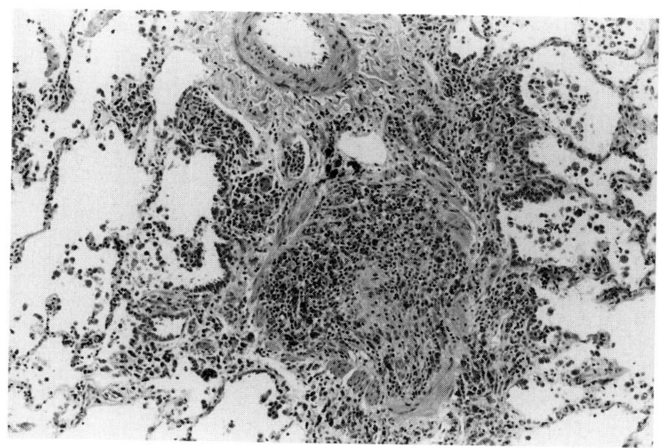

FIGURE 59–11 **Bronchiolitis obliterans. A small bronchiole has its lumen completely obliterated by dense scar tissue and mononuclear inflammatory cells.**

within 3 years of pulmonary transplantation and 60% to 70% of patients who survive for 5 years.[61] In the majority of patients, the problem is difficult to resolve once it develops, and the mortality rate at 3 years after diagnosis is 40% or higher. The term used to describe this chronic loss of function, obliterative bronchiolitis (OB), comes from the histologic findings of obliteration and fibrotic scarring of the terminal bronchioles (Fig. 59-11).[62] However, the clinical diagnosis is rarely based on histology given the low sensitivity of transbronchial biopsy.[63] The lesions of OB involve the lung in a nonuniform manner and biopsy is performed mostly to rule out other causes of graft dysfunction such as acute rejection, infection, and airway complications. Because symptoms are nonspecific, the most sensitive test for early detection of OB is a fall in forced expiratory flow between 25% and 75% of the FVC (FEF 25-75).[64] The term "bronchiolitis obliterans syndrome" (BOS) was formulated to describe chronic allograft dysfunction in the absence of confirming histology by a progressive decline in FEV1, deemed a more reliable and reproducible pulmonary function test.[65] BOS grades 0 to 3 are assigned according to the percentage of FEV1 to best postoperative baseline value obtained. Bronchial wall thickening, distention of distal airways with air trapping, and frequent association of secondary acute infection have been detected on high-resolution chest CT scanning and are proposed as helpful in making the diagnosis.[66]

The histologic changes provide insight into the etiology of the process, including potential therapy. As in cardiac AV, OB appears to be the end result of an exaggerated injury response to the interplay between allogenic, ischemic, and viral etiologies. The lungs and airways appear to be quite susceptible to ischemia-reperfusion injury. Possible reasons include a propensity for ischemic damage of the delicate alveolar-capillary unit, difficulty in lung preservation given a static column of air in the graft, postoperative pulmonary hypertension due to a hypertrophic right ventricle, and the lack of a direct arterial supply to the bronchus after transplant. It has been proposed that ischemia to the bronchial epithelium causes an exaggerated and chronic inflammatory response resulting in airway scarring. Although animal models have demonstrated a connection, ischemic time has not been convincingly shown to be an independent clinical risk factor for long-term graft failure.[67] However, clinical success has been achieved against chronic rejection in renal transplantation with the perioperative use of the free radical scavenger, superoxide dismutase[23]; the availability of a proven strategy for inhibiting RI in lung transplants with inhaled nitric oxide and pentoxifylline[68] warrants further follow-up to investigate a long-term effect on OB.

The transplanted lung is unique amongst solid organ transplants in that it is exposed to the outside world. As a result, these lungs are particularly susceptible to the immunomodulary effects of respiratory viruses. By serving as an adjuvant for the cellular immune response or by a direct cytopathic effect on the airway, respiratory viruses such as CMV, respiratory syncytial virus, adenovirus, influenza, and parainfluenza infection have all been implicated as risk factors for BOS.[69] CMV infection, in particular, has a potent effect on donor-specific and nonspecific immune responses. An increase in INF and MHC class II antigen expression has been noted in bronchoalveolar lavage (BAL) cells during infections with CMV.[70] Most transplant centers believe in an association between CMV infection and BOS, although a precise relationship is far from uniformly accepted.

Although other facilitating factors certainly exist, several lines of clinical evidence support the alloresponse as a more important force behind the development of OB than cardiac AV (Figs. 59-12 and 59-13). First, acute rejection has consistently been found to be the leading risk factor for the eventual development of OB.[71] In particular, OB develops in the setting of indirect alloimmune[72] and alloantibody[73] responses to HLA-A mismatches and is occasionally stabilized by augmented immunosuppression (Fig. 59-13).[74,75]

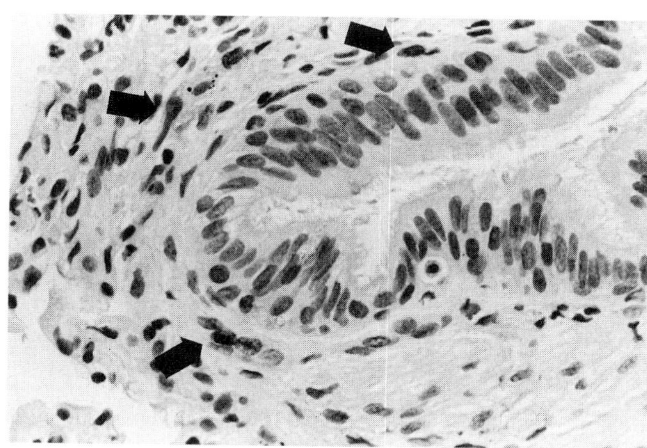

FIGURE 59–12 **Bronchiolitis obliterans. Stains for S100 protein decorate antigen-processing dendritic cells (arrows) present in increased numbers in the airways of lung allografts experiencing rejection.**

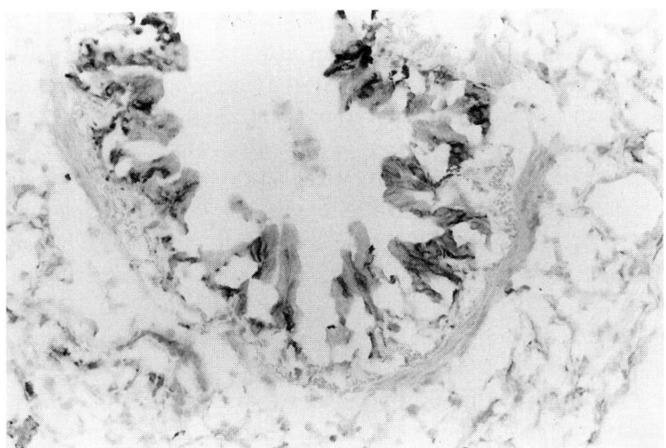

FIGURE 59–13 Bronchiolitis obliterans. Chronic airway rejection is characterized by increased expression of HLA class II antigens, especially HLA-DR (shown here) on respiratory epithelial cells.

Second, an identical form of OB can occur in bone marrow transplant recipients with graft-versus-host disease following the recognition of the host lungs by the grafted alloreactive T cells.[76] Third, cells from bronchial lavages of OB patients have demonstrated TH1 cytokine mRNA profiles (IL-1, IL-2, IL-6 and IFN).[77] Finally, in the Pittsburgh study of microchimerism, it appeared that those patients with OB had less evidence of microchimerism in blood, lymph nodes, and skin, which follows the general concept of less immune reactivity for those patients with a generalized chimeric state.[78]

The currently available experimental models of OB have provided insight into the human condition and new avenues for investigation. However, the lack of a large animal model significantly limits their relevance. Attempts to model OB in nonhuman primate lung allografts have resulted in either acute rejection or normal lung tissue depending on the level of immunosuppression used. Subcutaneous and intraabdominal tracheal implants in rodents, but not nonhuman primates, develop close approximations of the pathologic lesions of OB at 1 and 2 months.[79,80] As in cardiac AV, the dissimilarity of the pathophysiology of these lesions prevents conclusions that have direct clinical relevance, especially regarding treatment. At present, the focus is on the newer immune drugs that might reduce not only the initial allogeneic response but also the secondary effects that result in mesenchymal cell recruitment for luminal scarring.

NEW IMMUNOSUPPRESSIVE DRUGS

The improved outlook for transplant recipients has followed the introduction of xenobiotic immunosuppressants, that is, those drugs produced by organic synthesis or microorganisms that suppress the immune system. Between 1960 and 1985 only steroids, azathioprine (AZA), and cyclosporin (CsA) had been adopted for use in clinical transplantation. These agents have been more recently joined by polyclonal and monoclonal anti–T-cell antibodies. In the last few years, progress in the molecular understanding of the alloresponse has made new discoveries possible and allowed agents to be classified by mechanism of molecular action (Fig. 59-14 and Table 59-2).

Corticosteroids

Transplant physicians have recognized the benefits of corticosteroids from the very early days of clinical transplantation. These molecules have protean effects that, like any steroid, are mediated through intracellular receptors that alter gene transcription. The predominant anti-inflammatory effects of glucocorticoids such as the blockade of NFKB-induced transcription of inflammatory cytokines and adhesion molecules derive from the inhibition of gene transcription. On the other hand, the metabolic side effects such as muscle wasting and diabetes derive from positive transcriptional effects.[81] This concept of differing mechanisms of action has prompted investigations to develop corticosteriod analogues that bind to intracellular receptors to promote the inflammatory effects without the metabolic effects.

Glucocorticoids have been found to induce apoptosis in malignant T cells[82] and are therefore an especially appropriate choice of sole immunosuppression in the setting of posttransplant lymphoproliferative disorder. Outside of this subgroup, however, recent advances in the development of tolerance protocols have suggested that steroid use blocks certain immune signaling pathways necessary to induce donor-specific anergy or suppressor cells.[30] In addition, steroid weaning reduces the tendency towards diabetes and dyslipidemia, which may decrease the incidence of AV.[83]

Cytokine Synthesis Inhibitors

Cyclosporin (CsA) inhibits the gene activation necessary for IL-2 production. To accomplish this, CsA inhibits the function of a Ca^{2+} activated calcineurin phosphatase when bound to its cytoplasmic receptor.[84] This prevents the activation and nuclear translocation of the nuclear factor for activation of T cells (NFAT), precluding its engagement with the promoter sequence of the IL-2 gene. Blockade of the Ca^{2+} calcineurin phosphatase complex also inhibits the production of nitric oxide synthetase, a potential mechanism by which CsA seems to promote AV in animal models.[85]

Originally oil-based, CsA has been replaced by a novel microemulsion formula, Neoral, which has significantly improved its bioavailability and reduced pharmacokinetic variability between patients. Approximately 30% of heart transplant recipients develop nephrotoxicity, the primary toxicity of CsA, which appears to be mediated by the inhibition of prostaglandin metabolites. However, the prostaglandin

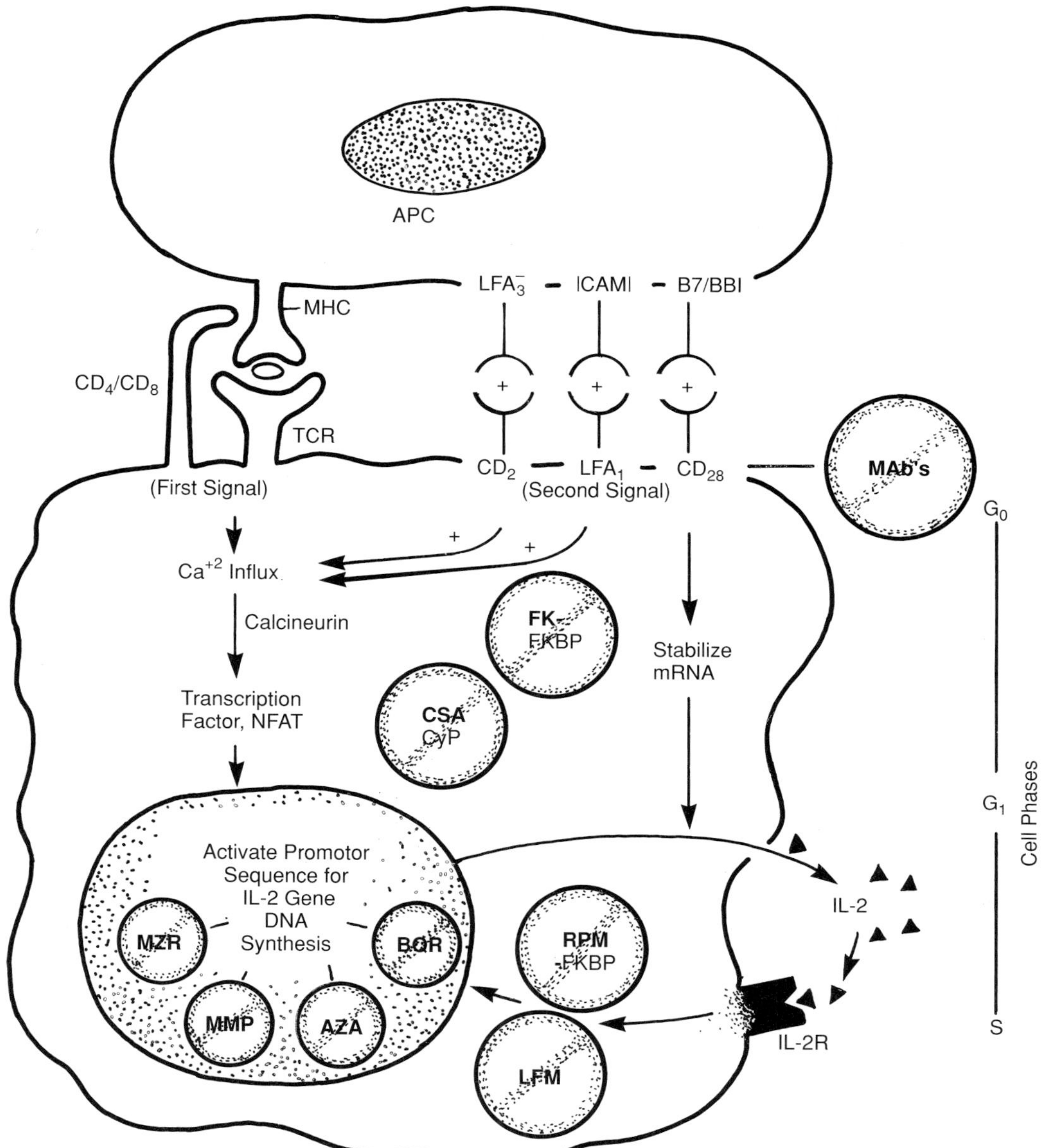

FIGURE 59–14 Immunosuppressants available to clinicians are directed toward inhibiting T-cell activation at various steps and by varied mechanisms, including interference with TCR complex (OKT3 Mab) and other surface ligands (anti–ICAM-1, anti-CD2, others); Ca^{2+}-dependent (CsA, FK) signal transduction; inhibition of cytokine IL-2 action in promoting cellular proliferation (RPM, LFM); and inhibition of purine (AZA, MZR, MMP) or pyrimidine synthesis BQR.

analogue misoprostol has afforded little clinical benefit.[86] In two recent series of heart transplant patients, calcineurin inhibition was the sole indication for metachronous kidney transplantation.[87,88] CsA-induced alterations in cell phenotype explain other side effects such as hypertension and dyslipidemia.[89,90]

CsA was widely embraced as the central component for effective multidrug immunosuppression until FK506 (tacrolimus) was introduced to patients in Pittsburgh in 1988. Tacrolimus combines with a different cytosolic protein than CsA (FK binding protein) but complexes with the same Ca^{2+} activated calcineurin to prevent the activation of NFAT.[76] Tacrolimus has proven to be at least as effective in heart transplant patients[91] and possibly better in lung transplant patients.[92] It has found particular success following a switch from CsA-based immunosuppression when faced with a refractory acute rejection of the heart or lung[93] or bronchiolitis obliterans.[74] Given a mechanism of action

TABLE 59–2 Compendium of immunosuppressants

Drug	Proposed mechanism	Status
Cytokine synthesis		
Cyclosporine A	Inhibits SER/THR phosphatase	FDA approved
Tacrolimus (FK 506)	Inhibits SER/THR phosphatase	FDA approved
Growth factor inhibitor		
Rapamycin	Unclear	FDA approved
Leflunomide (LFM)	Inhibits tyrosine kinase	In clinical trials
DNA synthesis inhibitor		
Azathioprine (AZA)	Inhibits PRPP amidotransferase (purine)	FDA approved
Methotrexate	Inhibits dihydrofolate reductase	FDA approved
Mycophenolate (MFF)	Inhibits IMP dehydrogenase (purine)	FDA approved
Mizoribine (MZR)	Inhibits IMP dehydrogenase (purine)	In clinical trials
Brequinar (BQR)	Inhibits DHO dehydrogenase (pyrimidine)	On hold
Receptor antagonists		
Antithymocyte globulin (equine or rabbit)	Kills T cells or alters traffic	FDA approved
Anti-CD3 (OKT3)	Kills CD3+ cells or alters traffic	FDA approved
Anti-IL-2 receptor	Kills IL-2R+ or alters traffic	In phase III clinical trials
DAB486-IL-2	Kills CD25+ cells or alters traffic	In clinical trials
Anti-LFA-1	Inhibits intercellular adhesion	In clinical trials
Anti-ICAM-I	Inhibits intercellular adhesion	In clinical trials
OKT4A	Induces CD4+ cell anergy	In clinical trials
IL-1 receptor antagonist	Inhibits IL-1 receptor	In clinical trials
Soluble HLA	Inhibits antigen presentation	Preclinical
Deoxyspergualin	Inhibits antigen presentation	In clinical trials
Cytokine inhibitors		
Anti-IL-6	Neutralizes IL-6	In clinical trials
Anti-TNF	Neutralizes TNF	In clinical trials
Soluble IL-1 receptor	Neutralizes IL-1	In clinical trials
IL-10	Inhibits cytokine synthesis	Preclinical

Source: Adapted with permission from Przepiorka D: Rational use of new immunosuppressive agents, in Recent Developments in Transplantation Medicine. Glenview, IL, Physicians & Scientists, 1994.

similar to that of CsA, the reason for the improved effectiveness of tacrolimus in refractory rejection likely relates to more predictable pharmacokinetics.[94] Therefore, ongoing clinical trials comparing tacrolimus with Neoral are of great interest with regard to efficacy but are not likely to change the improved side effect profile already demonstrated with tacrolimus in multicenter trials.[91] Compared to recipients receiving CsA, tacrolimus was found to be associated with less facial disfigurement, hirsutism, hypertension, and hyperlipidemia but equal nephrotoxicity, and was perhaps associated with greater neurotoxic and diabetogenic effects.

Inhibitors of DNA Synthesis

Antimetabolites are immunosuppressive because they inhibit the synthesis of nucleotides necessary for DNA's rapidly dividing cells. The classic antimetabolite has been azathioprine (AZA), which inhibits purine synthesis and therefore DNA and RNA synthesis throughout all dividing cells. Mycophenolate mofetil (MMF) appears to be more selective for T and B cells than AZA[95] based on its ability to block the activity of enzyme inosine monophosphate dehydrogenase, and therefore the synthesis of purines in the de novo pathway. Unlike other parenchymal and peripheral blood cells, T cells and B cells cannot use the salvage pathway and depend solely on the de novo pathway for purine synthesis. Compared to AZA, randomized clinical trials have shown a reduction in acute rejection events and antibody production with MMF in both heart[96] and lung[97] transplant patients. The reduction in chronic graft loss that has been demonstrated with the use of MMF versus AZA in renal transplantation has not yet been confirmed in cardiothoracic transplants. Neutropenia has not been a limiting factor as it has been with AZA.

Brequinar sodium (BQR) is a new addition to the antimetabolite group.[98] Unlike MMF, its action appears to be directed against dihydroorotate dehydrogenase (DHODH), an enzyme in the pathway leading to synthesis of pyrimidines. The rationale for use of BQR is similar to that for MMF, given that activated immune cells are relatively more dependent on de novo synthesis of pyrimidine's effects than nonimmune cells, although unlike for purines, a salvage pathway does exist. As a result, BQR appears to be less selective for immune cells. Another DHODH inhibitor, leflunomide, has demonstrated a much more favorable therapeutic window although a profound weight loss has been seen in animal and human trials.[99] Leflunomide depletes ATP-dependent enzymes, which inhibits the glycosylation of adhesion molecules, providing another possible mechanism of immunosuppression.[100] Clinical utility of both BQR and leflunomide has been limited by myelotoxicity and GI effects; planned clinical trials have been stopped.

IL-2 Signal Transduction Inhibitor

Rapamycin (sirolimus; RPM) is structurally similar to tacrolimus and binds with FK binding protein (FKBP) but surprisingly does not inhibit the calcium-activated calcineurin.[94] Instead, RPM acts at a point downstream from the cytokine inhibitors and upstream from the antiproliferative agents. In alloreactive T cells, stimulation of the IL-2 receptor leads to clonal proliferation following initiation of the cell cycle and conversion from the resting (G_0) to proliferative (G_1/S) state. The RPM/FKBP complex binds the so-called "target of rapamycin," a lipid kinase,[101] and prevents the signaling between IL-2 receptor activation and cell-cycle initiation. Because of theoretical concerns of competition for FK binding protein, sirolimus was combined initially with CsA[102] but recent clinical trials in renal transplantation have actually demonstrated greater success when combined with FK506.[103] In vitro studies have demonstrated that RPM also induces cell cycle arrest in B cells and smooth muscle cells.[104] This smooth muscle cell antiproliferative effect is thought responsible for the arrest of AV in both small[60] and large[105] animal experimental models, and for the clinical prevention of restenosis after using RPM-coated intracoronary stents.[106] In preliminary randomized studies, the use of RPM instead of AZA following heart transplantation has resulted in reduced AV by IVUS evaluation at 6 months[107] and 1 year.[108] Sirolimus is not nephroxic but it may enhance the renal toxic effects of calcineurin inhibitors[103]; its main toxicity is hyperlipidemia.

Combinations of these drugs that act at the level of cytokine production, the proliferative response to cytokines, and/or the signaling between the two have demonstrated additive immunosuppressive effects.[109] This will not only effectively reduce the alloresponse but also potentially do so with lower doses of each.

Inhibition of T- and B-Cell Maturation

Deoxyspergualin (DSG) does not inhibit the synthesis or actions of cytokine but has been shown to inhibit the maturation of T and B cells and APC.[110] Clinical trials that were conducted in high-risk renal allograft recipients were stopped due to a high incidence of leukopenia.

Receptor Antagonists and Monoclonal Antibodies

Polyclonal anti–T-cell preparations (ATG) have been developed that recognize T-cell surface structures and kill these targets by inducing F_C-receptor–mediated cell lysis or by complement-dependent cell lysis. In the mid-1980s, the murine anti–human CD3 monoclonal antibody (OKT3) was developed that recognizes the epsilon protein of the CD3 complex on all T cells. When used as induction agents in thoracic transplantation, ATG and OKT3 have been found only to delay the onset of acute rejection at the expense of a profound, uncontrolled immunosuppression that increases the risk for opportunistic infections and malignancy.[111] Furthermore, their main toxicity, the cytokine release syndrome, is tolerated particularly poorly in heart and lung transplant recipients. As a result, their current use is limited in most centers for the treatment of refractory acute rejection and as a calcineurin-inhibitor sparing agent in those with prolonged postoperative renal dysfunction.

The development of a humanized monoclonal antibody (mAb) against the IL-2 receptor provided the opportunity for a more selective targeting of activated T cells, the only cells that express this receptor. In a small (55 heart transplant recipients), randomized, clinical trial, induction therapy using this mAb, dacluzimab, reduced the frequency and severity of acute rejection events over the study period. In addition, there were essentially no side effects and no increased risk of infections or malignancy.[112] Pilot studies using mAb against the cell adhesion molecules LFA-1[113] or ICAM-1[114] showed promise in preventing reperfusion injury but variable success against acute rejection. The combination of the two, which was synergistic against acute rejection in rodent models, has not been tried clinically. Also awaiting clinical trial is a strategy which inhibits T-cell costimulation such as the anti–CD154 mAb or CTLA-4 Ig which have produced tolerance in the nonhuman primate model.[30] Other monoclonal antibodies that are in various stages of clinical development may have a specific role in therapy, but hopes for a magic bullet likely will not be realized, as the immune response is far from simple and is based on redundancy by way of alternative pathways. A combination of various mAb would likely be the best protocol to address this redundancy. Unfortunately, no preclinical or clinical trials using a combination strategy have been performed in large part due to financial conflicts between the different pharmaceutical companies that own the rights to these agents.

TOLERANCE

While immunosuppressive agents have permitted the replacement of heart and lungs to become realities, their toxic side effects and inability to prevent more chronic forms of rejection have driven the search for alternative strategies. Experimental models have suggested that the induction of tolerance is the most effective way to prevent chronic rejection.[115] Indeed, the absence of AV or OB has been considered to be the best clinical end point for the evaluation of successful tolerance induction in future trials by the National Heart, Lung and Blood Institute Heart and Lung Tolerance

Working Group.[116] While a myriad of protocols have induced tolerance in small animals, only a few have been reproduced in swine or nonhuman primate transplant models. The list of studies relevant to thoracic surgery shrinks further when considering the elusiveness of translating tolerance protocols from one organ to the other. In addition, there is a general belief that induction of tolerance in thoracic organs is more difficult than for other organs such as the liver or kidney.[117] To date, only three protocols have induced prolonged survival of cardiac allografts in large animals without immunosuppression (none in lung allografts): (1) the induction of mixed chimerism which is thought to work through central tolerance; (2) the use of costimulatory blockade to induce peripheral tolerance; and (3) the cotransplantation of heart and kidney allografts, which works by unknown mechanisms.[117]

By introducing allogenic bone marrow cells into newborn mice, Billingham et al induced a mixed chimeric state that was the first demonstration of allograft tolerance in 1953.[118] A recent analysis of renal transplant recipients from sibling donors has shown this type of tolerance to occur towards noninherited maternal HLA due to prior in utero exposure to this foreign antigen.[119] In these mixed chimeras, bone marrow–derived elements of both host and donor appear in the thymus and present ligands for negative selection of newly developing T cells that are either donor or host reactive.[120] This induces clonal deletion, one of the most reliable approaches to achieving long-term donor-specific tolerance. In an adult organism, creation of a mixed chimera requires the infusion of donor hematopoietic cells along with a conditioning regimen to enhance engraftment. Conditioning using antilymphocyte serum has been attempted but has produced little[121] to no[122] evidence of durable hematopoietic cell engraftment and minimal impact on allograft survival. The most common method used in preclinical and clinical trials has been the use of a toxic dose of total lymphoid irradiation (TLI), similar to that used to treat Hodgkin disease.[123] The use of a nonmyeloablative conditioning regimen of CD3 monoclonal Ab bound to the diphtheria immunotoxic instead of TLI has enabled the induction of stable mixed chimerism using donor stem cells with significantly less toxicity. Subsequent transplantation resulted in long-term tolerance in the swine model despite a minor-antigen mismatched histocompatibility barrier. Recently, the use of pleuripotent embryonic stem cells has allowed the development of mixed chimerism and tolerance without conditioning in rodents.[124] These preliminary results have not yet been reproduced in large animal models.

It has been observed that in heart[125] and lung[126] transtplant recipients enjoying long-term survival, donor-type lymphoid and dendritic cells migrate from the graft and establish themselves in the unconditioned recipient's periphery.[127] In this case, donor cells exist at levels less than cytometric detection in the periphery of solid organ transplant recipients (1 in 10^5 cells as detected by polymerase chain reaction techniques) with a kinetics and patchy distribution that resemble a spreading infection. In lung transplant recipients, this microchimerism has been associated with donor-specific hyporeactivity and lower incidence of OB.[128]

The observation that microchimerism is a common event after heart and lung transplantation and associated with long-term graft acceptance has stimulated attempts to augment microchimerism with perioperative bone marrow transfusion. Pham et al have provided proof of the principle that induced microchimerism influences acute and chronic rejection in clinical heart[129] and lung[130] transplantation without producing GVHD. However, a causal relationship between microchimerism and a decrease in target events such as rejection or graft survival was not established. The association between microchimerism and graft survival is inconsistent with the identification of both long-term survivors who do not have it and patients with multiple episodes of rejection who do.[131] Furthermore, only mixed chimerism, and not microchimerism, has been shown in animal models to induce systemic, stable allograft-specific tolerance.[132]

The second mechanism for the induction and maintenance of tolerance that occurs following costimulatory blockade is anergy, also known as peripheral tolerance.[133] The two-signal model of T-cell activation holds that an alloresponse to the interaction of the T-cell receptor with its antigen requires a second signal prompted by the other molecular participants of the immunologic synapse. Engagement of the T-cell receptor without these signals induces anergy or a lack of T-cell proliferation on antigen stimulation. The advantage of this mechanism is achieved by exposing T cells to alloantigen under the umbrella of mAb blocking costimulatory molecules such as CD28,[31] LFA-1, or CD2 ligand. The period of immunosuppression lasts only as long as the mAb are at therapeutic levels in the host. As the mAb clear, the immune competence returns to all antigens other than those to which tolerance had been induced.

It has long been recognized that passenger leukocytes, that is, cells derived from the organ transplant most commonly dendritic in nature, can escape the organ and accumulate in peripheral host lymphoid tissues. It is possible that donor-derived immature passenger dendritic cells mediate a form of anergy by indirect and direct presentation of alloantigen with limited secondary signals necessary for T-cell proliferation. Kidney transplants are thought to have enhanced numbers of these cells as the proposed mechanism of their immunosuppressive effect on cardiac allograft rejection.

XENOTRANSPLANTATION

Animal-to-human transplantation, known as xenotransplantation, has been proposed to alleviate the critical shortage of human donor organs. Approximately 30% of the patients waiting for hearts and lungs will die without receiving a transplant. In 1964, 4 years before the first human allotransplant,

Hardy attempted to replace a 68-year-old man's failing heart with one obtained from a chimpanzee.[134] Since then, there have been only six additional attempts of xenotransplantation reported using pig, sheep, baboon, or chimpanzee donors.[135–138] These cases, although unsuccessful, have provided insight and promise to the field. In 1984, Bailey et al placed an ABO-incompatible baboon heart into a child with a hypoplastic left heart syndrome. Baby Faye, as the child was known, made remarkable progress for 20 days when rather suddenly the xenograft stopped functioning. Examination of the heart gave evidence consistent with a humoral rejection, perhaps related to the blood group incompatibility.

Although nonhuman primates provide concordant organs for cross-species transplantation, phylogenetically disparate or discordant donor organs from pigs are favored for several reasons. First, broad use of the relatively rare and sentient primates is unlikely to gain societal acceptance. Second, retroviruses from pigs are much less likely than those from nonhuman primates to transmit disease to humans.[139] Finally, the short gestation, time to maturation, and large litters of pigs relative to primates simplifies their breeding and improves their candidacy for germ-line gene therapy. Accordingly, the porcine heart has been the focus of most of the experimental work in heart and lung xenotransplantation and was the most recent clinical xenograft reported for use in cardiac transplantation in 1992.[138]

Xenograft Hyperacute Rejection

The first major obstacle to discordant cross-species transplantation is generally believed to be the process described as hyperacute rejection (HAR). Hyperacute rejection is mediated largely by preformed xenoreactive antibodies and the relative incompatibility of discordant xenograft complement regulatory proteins (e.g., decay accelerating factor) with the human complement system. The primary human xenoreactive antibodies that initiate HAR against discordant pig hearts are specific for the blood group carbohydrate Gal (1-3 Gal), an antigen not present in concordant nonhuman primates.[140] Utilizing the classical pathway, the binding of xenoreactive antibodies to the pig endothelium leads to the unregulated activation of complement due to inadequate function of swine counter-regulatory proteins for human complement. The resulting uncontrolled deposition of the terminal complement complexes (C5b67) on the swine endothelial cells disrupts the endothelial cell barrier function as they retract and generate intracellular gaps (type 1 activation). Platelets then are attracted to exposed extracellular matrix and release vasoactive substances, including thromboxane A2, that stimulate vasoconstriction. The procoagulant state is intensified because of the loss of heparin sulfate proteoglycans from their surface.

These findings have led White, Pedor, and Platt to develop swine that are transgenic for human DAF and CD-59. By overexpressing human DAF and CD-59, these transgenic organs successfully avert hyperacute rejection following pig to primate renal, heart and lung transplantation.[141–143] The temporary, pretransplant depletion of complement using cobra venom[34] and anti-Gal antibodies using any of several different methods have provided further success against HAR.[144] Evidence exists that if HAR and AVR can be prevented initially, then the xenograft may "accommodate" in a manner in which it becomes resistant to future exposure to human antibody and complement.[36,145] This is thought to be mediated by increased expression of antiapoptotic genes and inhibition of NFKB transcriptional activation in the xenograft endothelium. The enhancement of this pathway would serve obvious benefits in xenotransplantation. However, the greatest potential for a significant advance has been achieved by the recent creation of Gal-1,3 galactosyl transferase knockout pigs.

Acute Vascular Xenograft Reaction

Despite prevention of HAR by either disrupting antibody binding or by depletion or inhibition of complement, xenografts are subjected to a process named acute vascular rejection (AVR).[145] Although the histologic picture of AVR with its hemorrhage and thrombosis is very characteristic of HAR, it appears to be a distinct process not dependent on complement nor appearing in concordant transplant combinations. The pathophysiology begins with naturally occurring anti–pig antibodies binding to the endothelial surface. This leads to levels of complement activation through the membrane attack complex (MAC) that are below lytic levels but that lead to the induction of IL-1, which mediates other changes on the surface of the endothelial cell that, by and large, create a strongly procoagulant state (type 2 activation). These changes include the induction of procoagulant tissue factor, release of plasminogen activator inhibitor, decrease in tissue plasminogen activator, and a loss in thrombomodulin activity. Thrombomodulin is expressed on the surface of vascular endothelial cells and reduces thrombotic process by thrombin-dependent activation of protein C, which in turn degrades the procoagulant cofactor's factors Va and VIIIa. It has been noted also that E-selectin, responsible for leukocyte rolling on the endothelium, is also upregulated during AVR.

Cell-Mediated Xenograft Rejection

Although cell-mediated rejection has not been studied extensively in the xenograft model because of difficulties in overcoming HAR and AVR, recent investigations have suggested that xenografts have increased susceptibility to cell-mediated injury and also to attack by NK cells.[146] NK cells normally are inhibited by class I MHC receptors, yet when added to xenograft tissue culture, NK cells have been demonstrated to cause cytotoxicity and phenotypic changes in a disruptive endothelial cell monolayer consistent with retraction and gap formation typical of the activated endothelium described in HAR.[147,148] It was hoped that thymic selection, which permits T lymphocytes to recognize allogeneic cells directly, might be less effective in producing T lymphocytes that might recognize the porcine xenogenic cells. However, it has been determined that human T cells can recognize porcine cells directly through MHC class II antigen.[149]

Significant progress has been made with the discordant porcine-to-primate model. However, an impact on human transplantation awaits additional studies that promote a further understanding of the effects of the inhibition of early HAR, methods to persistently reduce AVR, and finally a way of dealing with an enhanced cell-mediated rejection. It is likely that a combination of immunosuppressants, transgenic animals, and even tolerance-induction protocols may provide a suitable therapeutic cocktail. Chief clinical investigators in the field of xenotransplantation have stressed the need to look for intermediate end points as means of understanding processes, since the long-term goal of routinely successful discordant xenografting will require solving multiple complex processes. It is likely then that well-prepared surgical groups will soon initiate bridge trials in which short-term survival of the xenograft might be predicted, and information gained will be invaluable to the science.

REFERENCES

1. Parham P: *The Immune System*. New York, Garland Publishing, 2000.
2. Petersdorf EW, Longton GM, Anasetti C, et al: Definition of HLA-DQ as a transplantation antigen. *Proc Natl Acad Sci U S A* 1996; 93:15358.
3. Petersdorf EW, Hansen JA, Martin PJ, et al: Major-histocompatibility-complex class I alleles and antigens in hematopoietic-cell transplantation. *N Engl J Med* 2001; 345:1794.
4. Kerman RH, Kimball P, Scheinen S, et al: The relationship among donor-recipients HLA mismatches, rejection, and death from coronary artery disease in cardiac transplant recipients. *Transplantation* 1994; 57:884.
5. Opelz G, Wujciak T: The influence of HLA compatibility on graft survival after heart transplantation: the Collaborative Transplant Study. *N Engl J Med* 1994; 330:816.
6. Hosenpud JD, Edwards EB, Lin H-M, Daily OP: Influence of HLA matching on thoracic transplant outcomes: an analysis from the UNOS/ISHLT* Thoracic Registry. *Circulation* 1996; 94:170.
7. Hornick P, Smith J, Pomerance A, et al: Influence of acute rejection episodes, HLA matching, and donor/recipient phenotype on the development of "early" transplant-associated coronary artery disease. *Circulation* 1997; 96(suppl):II-148.
8. Iwaki Y, Yuichi Y, Griffith B: The HLA matching effect in lung transplantation. *Transplantation* 1993; 56:1528.
9. Hassanein WH, Zellos L, Tyrrell TA, et al: Continuous perfusion of donor hearts in the beating state extends preservation time and improves recovery of function. *J Thorac Cardiovasc Surg* 1998; 116:821.
10. Fischer Lindahl K, Wilson DB: Histocompatibility antigen-activated cytotoxic T lymphocytes, II: estimates of frequency and specificity of precursors. *J Exp Med* 1977; 145:508.
11. Teh HS, Harley E, Phillips RA, Miller RG: Quantitative studies on the precursors of cytotoxic lymphocytes, I: characterization of a clonal assay and determination of the size of clones derived from single precursors. *J Immunol* 1977; 118:1049.
12. Vanderlugt CJ, Miller SD: Epitope spreading. *Curr Opin Immunol* 1996; 8:831.
13. Lee RS, Yamada K, Houser SL, et al: Indirect recognition of allopeptides promotes the development of cardiac allograft vasculopathy. *Proc Natl Acad Sci U S A* 2001; 98:3276.
14. Hornick PI, Mason PD, Baker RJ, et al: Significant frequencies of T cells with indirect anti-donor specificity in heart graft recipients with chronic rejection. *Circulation* 2000; 101:2405.
15. Sayegh MH, Akalin E, Hancock WW, et al: CD28–B7 blockade after alloantigenic challenge in vivo inhibits Th1 cytokines but spares Th2. *J Exp Med* 1995; 181:1869.
16. Stumbles, PA, Thomas JA, Pimm CL, et al: Resting respiratory tract dendritic cells preferentially stimulate T helper cell type 2 (Th2) responses and require obligatory cytokine signals for induction of Th1 immunity. *J Exp Med* 1998; 188:2019.
17. Binah O: Immune effector mechanisms in heart transplant rejection. *Cardiovasc Res* 1994; 28:1748.
18. Podack ER: Functional significance of two cytolytic pathways of cytotoxic T lymphocytes. *J Leukoc Biol* 1995; 57:548.
19. Green DR, Ferguson TA: The role of Fas ligand in immune privilege. *Nat Rev Mol Cell Biol* 2001; 2:917.
20. Foerster A, Abdelnoor M, Geiran O, et al: Morbidity risk factors in human cardiac transplantation: histoincompatibility and protracted graft ischemia entail high risk of rejection and infection. *Scand J Thorac Cardiovasc Surg* 1992; 26:169.
21. Day JD, Rayburn BK, Gaudin PB, et al: Cardiac allograft vasculopathy: the central pathogenetic role of ischemia-induced endothelial cell injury. *J Heart Lung Transplant* 1995; 14:S142.
22. Poston RS, Ennen M, Pollard J, et al: *Ex vivo* gene therapy prevents chronic graft vascular disease in cardiac allografts. *J Thor Cardiovasc Surg* 1998; 116:128.
23. Land W, Zweler JL: Prevention of reperfusion-induced, free radical-mediated acute endothelial injury by superoxide dismutase as an effective tool to delay/prevent chronic renal allograft failure: a review. *Transplant Proc* 1997; 29:2567.
24. Quaini F, Urbanek K, Beltrami AP, et al: Chimerism of the transplanted heart. *N Engl J Med* 2002; 346:5.
25. Markert ML, Boeck A, Hale LP, et al: Transplantation of thymus tissue in complete DiGeorge syndrome. *N Engl J Med* 1999; 341:1180.
26. Jain J, McCaffrey PG, Miner Z, et al: The T cell transcription factor NFAT is a substrate for calcineurin and interacts with *Fos* and *Jun*. *Nature* 1993; 365:352.
27. Jenkins MK, Johnson JG: Molecules involved in T cell costimulation. *Curr Opin Immunol* 1993; 5:361.
28. Lenschow DJ, Walunas TL, Bluestone JA: CD28/B7 system of T cell costimulation. *Annu Rev Immunol* 1996; 14:233.
29. Isobe M, Yagita H, Okumura K, Ihara A: Specific acceptance of cardiac allograft after treatment with antibodies to ICAM-1 and LFA-1. *Science* 1992; 255:1125.
30. Kirk AD, Burkly LC, Batty DS, et al: Treatment with humanized monoclonal antibody against CD154 prevents acute renal allograft rejection in nonhuman primates. *Nat Med* 1999; 5:686.
31. Larsen CP, Elwood ET, Alexander DZ, et al: Long-term acceptance of skin and cardiac allografts after blocking CD40 and CD28 pathways. *Nature* 1996; 381:434.
32. West LJ, Pollock-Barziv SM, Dipchand AI, et al: ABO-incompatible heart transplantation in infants. *N Engl J Med* 2001; 344:793.
33. Massad MG, Cook DJ, Schmitt SK, et al: Factors influencing HLA sensitization in implantable LVAD recipients. *Ann Thorac Surg* 1997; 64:1120.
34. Auchincloss H Jr: Xenogeneic transplantation: a review. *Transplantation* 1988; 46:1.

35. Pisani BA, Mullen GM, Malinowska K, et al: Plasmapheresis with intravenous immunoglobulin G is effective in patients with elevated panel reactive antibody prior to cardiac transplantation. *J Heart Lung Transplant* 1999; 18:701.
36. Bach FH, Ferran C, Hechenleitner P, et al: Accommodation of vascularized xenografts: expression of "protective genes" by donor endothelial cells in a host Th2 cytokine environment. *Nature Med* 1997; 3:196.
37. Hammond EH, Yowell RL, Nunoda S, et al: Vascular (humoral) rejection in heart transplantation: pathologic observations and clinical implications. *J Heart Lung Transplant* 1989; 8:430.
38. Fyfe B, Loh E, Winters GL, et al: Heart transplantation-associated perioperative ischemic myocardial injury: morphological features and clinical significance. *Circulation* 1996; 93:1133.
39. Pierson RN, III, Miller GG: Late graft failure: lessons from clinical and experimental thoracic organ transplantation. *Graft* 2000; 3:88.
40. Billingham ME: Cardiac transplant atherosclerosis. *Transplant Proc* 1987; 19:19.
41. Lim TT, Liang DH, Botas J, et al: Role of compensatory enlargement and shrinkage in transplant coronary artery disease: serial intravascular ultrasound study. *Circulation* 1997; 95:855.
42. Hollenberg SM, Klein LW, Parrillo JE, et al: Coronary endothelial dysfunction after heart transplantation predicts allograft vasculopathy and cardiac death. *Circulation* 2001; 104:3091.
43. Poston RS, Billingham ME, Hoyt EG, et al: Effects of increased ICAM-1 on reperfusion injury and chronic graft vascular disease. *Ann Thor Surg* 1997; 64:1004.
44. Davis SF, Yeung AC, Meredith IT, et al: Early endothelial dysfunction predicts the development of transplant coronary artery disease at 1 year posttransplant. *Circulation* 1996; 93:457.
45. Kobashigawa JA, Katznelson S, Laks H, et al: Effect of pravastatin on outcomes after cardiac transplantation. *N Engl J Med* 1995; 333:621.
46. Grattan MT, Moreno-Cabral CE, Starnes VA, et al: Cytomegalovirus infection is associated with cardiac allograft rejection and atherosclerosis. *JAMA* 1989; 261:3561.
47. Everett JP, Hershberger RE, Norman DJ, et al: Prolonged cytomegalovirus infection with viremia is associated with development of cardiac allograft vasculopathy. *J Heart Lung Transplant* 1992; 11:S133.
48. Salomon RN, Hughes CCW, Schoen FJ, et al: Human coronary transplantation-associated arteriosclerosis: evidence for a chronic immune reaction to activated graft endothelial cells. *Am J Pathol* 1991; 138:791.
49. Hruban RH, Beschorner WE, Baumgartner WA, et al: Accelerated arteriosclerosis in heart transplant recipients is associated with a T-lymphocyte-mediated endothelialitis. *Am J Pathol* 1990; 137:871.
50. Rose ML: Role of antibody and indirect antigen presentation in transplant associated coronary artery vasculopathy. *J Heart Lung Transpant* 1996; 15:342.
51. Rose EA, Smith CR, Petrossian GA, et al: Humoral immune responses after cardiac transplantation: correlation with fatal rejection and graft atherosclerosis. *Surgery* 1989; 106:203.
52. Reed EF, Hong B, Ho E, et al: Monitoring of soluble HLA alloantigens and anti-HLA antibodies identifies heart allograft recipients at risk of transplant-associated coronary artery disease. *Transplantation* 1996; 61:566.
53. Cecka JM, Terasaki PI (eds): *Clinical Transplants 1995*. Los Angeles, UCLA Tissue Typing Laboratory, 1995.
54. Briscoe DM, Schoen FJ, Rice GE, et al: Induced expression of endothelial-leukocyte adhesion molecules in human cardiac allografts. *Transplantation* 1991; 51:537.
55. Taylor PM, Rose ML, Yacoub MH, et al: Induction of vascular adhesion molecules during rejection of human cardiac allografts. *Transplantation* 1992; 54:541.
56. Qiao JH, Ruan XM, Trento A, et al: Expression of cell adhesion molecules in human cardiac allograft rejection. *J Heart Lung Transplant* 1992; 11:920.
57. McKechnie RS, Rubenfire M: The role of inflammation and infection in coronary artery disease: a clinical perspective. *Curr J Rev* 2002; 11:32.
58. Poston RS, Billingham M, Hoyt EG, et al: Rapamycin reverses chronic graft vascular disease in a novel cardiac allograft model. *Circulation* 1999; 100:67.
59. Madsen JC, Yamada K, Allen JS, et al. Transplantation tolerance prevents cardiac allograft vasculopathy in major histocompatility complex in class I-disparate swine. *Transplantation* 1998; 63:304.
60. Saiura A, Sata M, Hirata Y, et al: Circulating smooth muscle progenitor cells contribute to atherosclerosis. *Nat Med* 2001; 7:382.
61. Heng D, Sharples LD, McNeil K, et al: Bronchiolitis obliterans syndrome: incidence, natural history, prognosis, and risk factors. *J Heart Lung Transplant* 1998; 17:1255.
62. Yousem SA, Berry GJ, Brunt EM, et al: A working formulation for the standardization of nomenclature in the diagnosis of heart and lung rejection: Lung Rejection Study Group. *J Heart Lung Transplant* 1990; 9:593.
63. Chamberlain D, Maurer J, Chaparro C, et al: Evaluation of transbronchial lung biopsy specimens in the diagnosis of bronchiolitis obliterans after lung transplantation. *J Heart Lung Transplant* 1994; 13:963
64. Nathan SD, Ross DJ, Belman MJ, et al: Bronchiolitis obliterans in single-lung transplant recipients [see comments]. *Chest* 1995; 107:967.
65. Cooper JD, Billingham M, Egan T, et al: A working formulation for the standardization of nomenclature and for clinical staging of chronic dysfunction in lung allografts. *J Heart Lung Transplant* 1993; 12:713.
66. Worthy SA, Park CS, Kim JS, et al: Bronchiolitis obliterans after lung transplantation: high-resolution CT findings in 15 patients. *AJR Am J Roentgenol* 1997; 169:673.
67. Meyer DM, Bennett LE, Novick RJ, Hosenpud JD: Effect of donor age and ischemic time on intermediate survival and morbidity after lung transplantation. *Chest* 2000; 118:1255.
68. Thabut G, Brugiere O, Leseche G, et al: Preventive effect of inhaled nitric oxide and pentoxifylline on ischemia/reperfusion injury after lung transplantation. *Transplantation* 2001; 71:1295.
69. Palmer SM Jr, Henshaw NG, Howell DN, et al: Community respiratory viral infections in adult lung transplant recipients. *Chest* 1998; 113:944.
70. Zeevi A, Dauber JH, Yousem SA, et al: Immunologic alterations in chronic lung rejection, in Senib H (ed): *Immunology of the Lung Allograft*. Montreal, CA, Lands Med Publisher, 1995; p 75.
71. Bando K, Paradis IL, Similo S, et al: Obliterative bronchiolitis after lung and heart-lung transplantation: an analysis of risk factors and management. *J Thorac Cardiovasc Surg* 1995, 109:49.
72. SivaSai SR, K Smith MA, Poindexter NJ, et al: Indirect recognition of donor HLA class I peptides in lung transplant recipients with bronchiolitis obliterans syndrome. *Transplantation* 1999; 67:1094.
73. Sundaresan S, Mohanakumar T, Smith MA, et al: HLA-A locus mismatches and development of antibodies to HLA after lung transplantation correlate with the development of bronchiolitis obliterans syndrome. *Transplantation* 1998; 65:648.
74. Ross DJ, Lewis MI, Kramer M, et al: FK 506 "rescue" immunosuppression for obliterative bronchiolitis after lung transplantation. *Chest* 1997; 112:1175.
75. Ross DJ, Jordan SC, Nathan SD, et al: Delayed development of obliterative bronchiolitis syndrome with OKT_3 after unilateral lung transplantation: a plea for multicenter immunosuppressive trials. *Chest* 1996; 109:870.

76. Mathew P, Bozeman P, Krance RA, et al: Bronchiolitis obliterans organizing pneumonia (BOOP) in children after allogeneic bone marrow transplantation. *Bone Marrow Transplant* 1994; 13:221.
77. Whitehead BF, Stoehr, C, Wu JC, et al: Cytokine gene expression in human lung transplant recipients. *Transplantation* 1993; 56:956.
78. Keenan R, Zeevi A, Banan R, Griffith B: Microchimerism is associated with a lower incidence of chronic rejection after lung transplantation. *J Heart Lung Transplant* 1994; 13:533.
79. Hertz MI, Jessurun J, King MB, et al: Reproduction of the obliterative bronchiolitis lesion after heterotopic transplantation of mouse airways. *Am J Pathol* 1993; 142:1945.
80. Huang XH, Reichenspurner H, Shorthouse R, et al: Heterotopic tracheal allograft transplantation: a new model to study the molecular events causing obliterative airway disease (OAD) in rats. *J Heart Lung Transplant* 1995; 14:S49.
81. Newton R: Molecular mechanisms of glucocorticoid action: what is important? *Thorax* 2000; 55:603.
82. Ramdas J, Hasday JD: Glucocorticoid-induced apoptosis and regulation of NF-kappaB activity in human leukemic T cells. *Endocrinology* 1998; 139:3813.
83. Baran DA, Segura L, Kushwaha S, et al: Tacrolimus monotherapy in adult cardiac transplant recipients: intermediate-term results. *J Heart Lung Transplant* 2001; 20:59.
84. Clipstone NA, Crabtree GR: Calcineurin is a key signaling enzyme in T lymphocyte activation and the target of immunosuppressive drugs cyclosporin A and FK 506. *Ann NY Acad Sci* 1993; 696:20.
85. Sudhir K, MacGregor JS, DeMarco T, et al: Cyclosporine impairs release of endothelium-derived relaxing factors in epicardial and resistance coronary arteries. *Circulation* 1994; 90:3018.
86. Boers M, Bensen WG, Ludwin D, et al: Cyclosporine nephrotoxicity in rheumatoid arthritis: no effect of short term misoprostol treatment. *J Rheumatol* 1992; 19:534.
87. Poston R, McCurry K, Griffith B: Kidney transplantation following heart transplantation: effects on cardiac outcome. *J Heart Lung Transplant* 2002; 21:102.
88. Coopersmith CM, Brennan DC, Miller B, et al: Renal transplantation following previous heart, liver, and lung transplantation: an 8–year single-center experience. *Surgery* 2001; 130:457.
89. Wu J, Zhu H, Patel SB: CsA-induced dyslipoproteinemia is associated with selective activation of SREBP-2. *Am Physiol Soc* 1999; 277:E1087.
90. Ventura HO, Malik FS, Mehra MR, et al: Mechanisms of hypertension and the role of CsA. *Curr Opin Cardiol* 1997; 12:375.
91. Taylor DO, Barr ML, Radovancevic B, et al: A randomised, multicenter comparison of TAC and CsA immunosuppressive regimens in cardiac transplantation: decreased hyperlipidemia and hypertension with TAC. *J Heart Lung Transplant* 1999; 18:336.
92. Treede H, Klepetko W, Reichenspurner H, et al: Tacrolimus versus cyclosporine after lung transplantation: a prospective, open, randomized two-center trial comparing two different immunosuppressive protocols. *J Heart Lung Transplant* 2001; 20:511.
93. Onsager DR, Canver CC, Jahania MS, et al: Efficacy of tacrolimus in the treatment of refractory rejection in heart and lung transplant recipients. *J Heart Lung Transplant* 1999; 18:448.
94. Fruman D, Burakoff SJ, Biarer BE: Molecular actions of cyclosporin A, FK 506 and rapamycin, in Thompson AW, Starzl TE (eds): *Immunosuppressive Drugs: Developments in Anti-Rejection Therapy*. London, Edward Arnold, 1994; p 15.
95. Allison A, Eugui EM: Mycophenolate mofetil (RS-61443): mode of action and effects on graft rejection, in Thompson AW, Starzl TE (eds): *Immunosuppressive Drugs: Developments in Anti-Rejection Therapy*. London, Edward Arnold, 1994; p 144.
96. Kobashigawa J, Miller L, Renlund D, et al: A randomized active-controlled trial of mycophenolate mofetil in heart transplant recipients. Mycophenolate Mofetil Investigators. *Transplantation* 1998; 66:507.
97. Corris P, Glanville A, McNeil K, et al: One year analysis of an ongoing international randomized study of mycophenolate mofetil (MMF) vs azathioprine (AZA) in lung transplantation. *J Heart Lung Transplant* 2001; 20:149.
98. Murphy MM, Morris RE: Brequinar sodium is a highly potent antimetabolite immunosuppressant that suppresses heart allograft rejection. *Med Sci Res* 1991; 19:835.
99. Smolen JS, Kalden JR, Scott DL, et al: Efficacy and safety of leflunomide compared with placebo and sulphasalazine in active rheumatoid arthritis: a double-blind, randomised, multicentre trial. *Lancet* 1999; 353:259.
100. Breedveld FC, Dayer J-M: Leflunomide: mode of action in the treatment of rheumatoid arthritis. *Ann Rheum Dis* 2000; 59:841.
101. Kuntz J, Henriquez R, Schneider U, et al: Target of rapamycin in yeast TOR2, as an essential phosphatidylinositol kinase homolog required for G1 progression. *Cell* 1993; 73:585.
102. Halloran PF: Immunosuppressive agents in clinical trials in transplantation. *Am J Med Sci* 1997; 313:283.
103. McAlister VC, Gao Z, Peltekian K, et al: Sirolimus-tacrolimus combination immuno-suppression. *Lancet* 2000; 355:376.
104. Gregory CR, Huang X, Pratt RE, et al: Treatment with rapamycin and mycophenolic acid reduces arterial intimal thickening after balloon catheter injury and allows endothelial replacement. *Transplantation* 1995; 59:655.
105. Ikonen TS, Gummert JF, Hayase M, et al: Sirolimus (rapamycin) halts and reverses progression of allograft vascular disease in non-human primates. *Transplantation* 2000; 70:969.
106. Morice M-C, Serruys PW, Sousa JE, et al: A randomized comparison of a sirolimus-eluting stent with a standard stent for coronary revascularization. *N Engl J Med* 2002; 346:1773.
107. Keogh A: Progression of graft vessel disease in cardiac allograft recipients is significantly reduced by sirolimus immunotherapy: 6-month results from a phase 2, open-label study [abstract #431]. *Am J Transpl* 2002; 2(suppl 3):246.
108. Tuzcu EM, Schoenhagen P, Starling RC, et al: Impact of everolimus on allograft vasculopathy: the SDZ RAD/heart intravascular ultrasound study. *J Heart Lung Transplant* 2002; 21:68.
109. Hausen B, Gummert J, Berry GJ, et al: Prevention of acute allograft rejection in nonhuman primate lung transplant recipients: induction with chimeric anti-interleukin-2 receptor monoclonal antibody improves the tolerability and potentiates the immunosuppressive activity of a regimen using low doses of both microemulsion cyclosporine and 40–O-(2–hydroxyethyl)-rapamycin. *Transplantation* 2000; 69:488.
110. Kerr P, Nikotic-Patterson DJ, Lan HY, et al: Deoxyspergualin suppresses local macrophage proliferation in rat renal allograft rejection. *Transplantation* 1994; 58:596.
111. Johnson MR, Mullen GM, O'Sullivan EJ, et al: Risk/benefit ratio of perioperative OKT3 in cardiac transplantation. *Am J Cardiol* 1994; 74:261.
112. Beniaminovitz A, Itescu S, Lietz K, et al: Prevention of rejection in cardiac transplantation by blockade of the interleukin-2 receptor with a monoclonal antibody. *N Engl J Med* 2000; 342:613.
113. Hourmant M, Bedrossian J, Durand D, et al: A randomized multicenter trial comparing leukocyte function-associated antigen-1 monoclonal antibody with rabbit antithymocyte globulin as induction treatment in first kidney transplantations. *Transplantation* 1996; 62:1565.
114. Haug CE, Colvin RB, Delmonico FL, et al: A phase I trial of immunosuppression with anti-ICAM-1 (CD54) mAb in renal allograft recipients. *Transplantation* 1993; 55:766.
115. Womer KL, Lee RS, Madsen JC, Sayegh M: Tolerance and chronic rejection. *Philos Trans R Soc Lond B Biol Sci* 2001; 356:727.

116. Massicot-Fisher J, Noel P, Madsen J: Recommendations of the National Heart, Lung And Blood Institute Heart And Lung Tolerance Working Group. *Transplantation* 2001; 72:1467.
117. Madsen JC, Yamada K, Allan JS, et al: Transplantation tolerance prevents cardiac allograft vasculopathy in major histocompatibility complex class I–disparate miniature swine. *Transplantation* 1998; 65:304.
118. Billingham RE, Brent L, Medawar PB: Actively acquired tolerance to foreign cells. *Nature* 1953; 172:606.
119. Burlingham WJ, Grailer AP, Heisey DM, et al: The effect of tolerance to noninherited maternal HLA antigens on the survival of renal transplants from sibling donors. *N Engl J Med* 1998; 339:1657.
120. Blackman M, Kappler JW, Marrack P: The role of the T cell receptor in positive and negative selection of developing T cells. *Science* 1990; 248:1335.
121. Barber WH, Mankin JA, Laskow DA, et al: Long-term results of a controlled prospective study with transfusion of donor specific bone marrow in 57 cadaveric renal allograft recipients. *Transplantation* 1991; 51:70.
122. Monaco AP, Clark AW, Wood ML, et al: Possible active enhancement of a human cadaver renal allograft with anti-lymphocyte serum (ALS) and donor bone marrow: case report of an initial attempt. *Surgery* 1976; 79:384.
123. Kahn DR, Hong R, Greenberg AJ, et al: Total lymphatic irradiation and bone marrow in human heart transplantation. *Ann Thorac Surg* 1984; 38:169.
124. Fandrich F, Lin X, Chai GX, et al: Preimplantation-stage stem cells induce long-term allogeneic graft acceptance without supplementary host conditioning. *Nat Med* 2002; 82:171.
125. Masaki Y, Hirasawa S, Okuyama G, et al: Microchimerism and heart allograft acceptance. *Transplant Proc* 1995; 27:148.
126. Kubit V, Sonmez-Alpan E, Zeevi A, et al: Mixed allogeneic chimerism in lung allograft recipients. *Hum Pathol* 1994; 25:408.
127. Starzl TE, Demetris AJ, Murase N, et al: Cell migration, chimerism, and graft acceptance. *Lancet* 1992; 339:1579.
128. Keenan RJ, Zeevi A, Banas E, et al: Microchimerism is associated with a lower incidence of chronic rejection after lung transplantation. *J Heart Lung Transplant* 1994; 13(suppl):S32.
129. Pham SM, Rao AS, Zeevi A, et al: A clinical trial combining donor bone marrow infusion and heart transplantation: intermediate-term results. *J Thorac Cardiovasc Surg* 2000; 119:673.
130. Pham SM, Rao AS, Zeevi A, et al: Effects of donor bone marrow infusion in clinical lung transplantation. *Ann Thorac Surg* 2000; 69:345.
131. Schlitt HJ, Hundroeser K, Hisanaga M, et al: Patterns of donor-type microchimerism after heart transplantation. *Lancet* 1994; 343:1469.
132. Li H, Kaufman CL, Ildstad ST, et al: Allogeneic chimerism induces donor-specific tolerance to simultaneous islet allografts in nonobese diabetic mice. *Surgery* 1995; 118:192.
133. Ramsdell F, Lantz T, Faulkes BJ: A non-deletional mechanism of thymic self tolerance. *Science* 1989; 246:1038.
134. Hardy JD, Chavez CM, Kurrus FD, et al: Heart transplantation in man. *JAMA* 1964; 188:1132.
135. Cooley DA, Hallman GL, Bloodwell RD, et al: Human heart transplantation: experience with 12 cases. *Am J Cardiol* 1968; 22:804.
136. Barnard CN, Wolpitz A, Losman JG: Heterotopic cardiac transplantation with a xenograft for assistance of the left heart in cardiogenic shock after cardiopulmonary bypass. *S Afr Med J* 1977; 52:1035.
137. Bailey LL, Nehlsen-Cannarella SL, Concepcion W, et al: Baboon-to-human cardiac xenotransplantation in a neonate. *JAMA* 1985; 254:3321.
138. Czaplicki J, Blonska B, Religa Z: The lack of hyperacute xenogeneic heart transplant rejection in a human [letter]. *J Heart Lung Transplant* 1992; 11:393.
139. Paradis K, Langford G, Long Z, et al. Search for cross-species transmission of porcine endogenous retrovirus in patients treated with living pig tissue [see comments]. *Science* 1999; 285:1236.
140. Jozaisse DH: Mammalian glycosyltransferases: genomic organization and protein structure. *Glycobiology* 1992; 2:271.
141. Cozzi E, Bhatti F, Schmoeckel M, et al: Long-term survival of nonhuman primates receiving life-supporting transgenic porcine kidney xenografts. *Transplantation* 2000; 70:15.
142. White DJG, Braidley P, Dunning J, et al: Hearts from pigs transgenic for human DAF are not hyperacutely rejected when xenografted to primates. Plenary Presentation at the Third International Congress for Xenotransplantation, Boston, MA, September 27–October 1, 1995.
143. Lau CL, Daggett WC, Yeatman MF, et al: The role of antibodies in dysfunction of pig-to-baboon pulmonary transplants. *J Thorac Cardiovasc Surg* 2000; 120:29.
144. Kozlowski T, Ierino FL, Lambrigts D, et al: Depletion of anti-Gal(alpha)1-3Gal antibody in baboons by specific alpha-Gal immunoaffinity columns. *Xenotransplantation* 1998; 5:122.
145. Parker W, Saadi S, Lin SS, et al: Transplantation of discordant xenografts: a challenge revisited. *Immunol Today* 1996; 17:373.
146. Murray AG, Khodadoust MM, Pober JS, et al: Porcine aortic endothelial cells activate human T cells: direct presentation of MHC antigens and costimulation by ligands for human CD2 and CD28. *Immunity* 1994; 1:57.
147. Lanier LL, Phillips JH: Inhibitory MHC class I receptors on NK cells and T cells. *Immunol Today* 1996; 17:86.
148. Inverardi L, Samaja M, Motterlini R, et al: Early recognition of a discordant xenogeneic organ by human circulating lymphocytes. *J Immunol* 1992; 149:1416.
149. Yamada K, Sachs DH, DerSimonian H: Human anti-porcine xenogeneic T cell response; evidence for allelic specificity of mixed leukocyte reaction and for both direct and indirect pathways of recognition. *J Immunol* 1995; 155:5249.

Chapter 60

Heart Transplantation

Brian T. Bethea/David D. Yuh/John V. Conte/William A. Baumgartner

Cardiac transplantation has emerged as the therapeutic procedure of choice for patients with end-stage heart failure. Tremendous advances in the fields of immunosuppression, rejection, and infection have transformed what was once considered an experimental intervention into a routine treatment readily available worldwide. Today, the success of cardiac transplantation is no longer measured by patient survival alone, but also by the quality of life attained by the transplant recipient.

HISTORY OF HEART TRANSPLANTATION

The birth of cardiac transplantation can be traced back to the innovative French surgeon Alexis Carrel who performed the first heterotopic canine heart transplant with Charles Guthrie in 1905.[1,2] Twenty years later, the concept of cardiac allograft rejection was proposed by Frank Mann at the Mayo Clinic to explain the eventual failure of heterotopic canine allografts.[3] He described the rejection process as a biological incompatibility between donor and recipient manifested by an impressive leukocytic infiltration of the rejecting myocardium. In 1946, Vladimir Demikhov of the Soviet Union successfully implanted the first intrathoracic heterotopic heart allograft.[4] He later demonstrated that heart-lung and isolated lung transplantation were also technically feasible. The use of moderate hypothermia, cardiopulmonary bypass, and an atrial cuff anastomotic technique permitted Norman Shumway and Richard Lower at Stanford University to surmount the formidable barriers of orthotopic heart transplantation using a canine model in 1960 (Fig. 60-1).[5] The first human cardiac transplant was a chimpanzee xenograft performed at the University of Mississippi by James Hardy in 1964.[6] Although the procedure using Shumway's technique was technically satisfactory, the primate heart was unable to maintain the recipient's circulatory load and the patient succumbed several hours postoperatively. Despite great skepticism that cardiac transplantation would ever be successfully performed in humans, South African Christiaan Barnard surprised the world when he performed the first human-to-human heart transplant on December 3, 1967.[7]

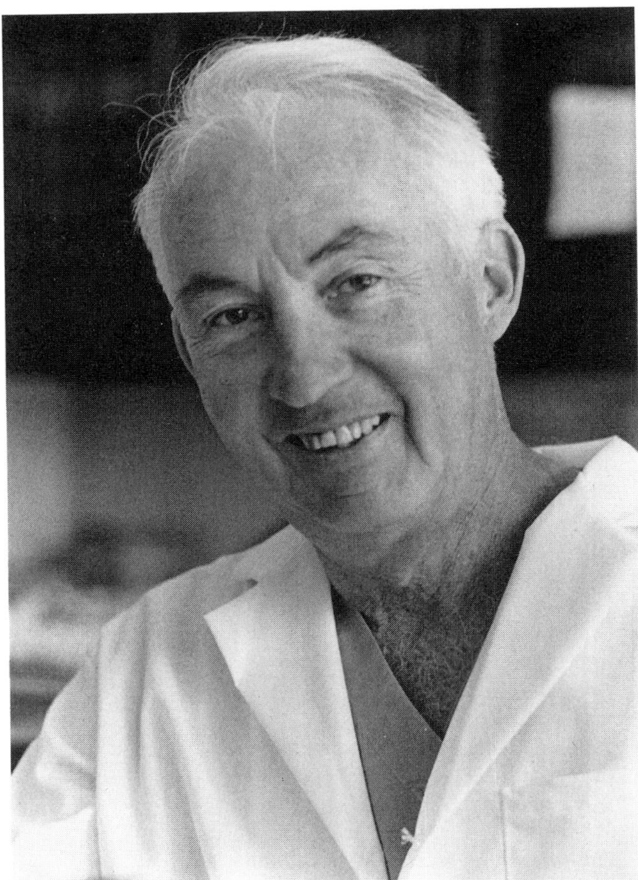

FIGURE 60–1 Norman Shumway.

Over the next several years, poor early clinical results led to a moratorium on heart transplantation, with only the most dedicated centers continuing experimental and clinical work in the field. The pioneering efforts of Shumway and his colleagues at Stanford eventually paved the way for the reemergence of cardiac transplantation in the late 1970s. The introduction of transvenous endomyocardial biopsy by Philip Caves in 1973 finally provided a reliable means for monitoring allograft rejection.[8] The advent of the immunosuppressive agent cyclosporine dramatically increased patient survival and marked the beginning of the modern era of successful cardiac transplantation in 1981.[9] Heart transplantation is now a widely accepted therapeutic option for end-stage cardiac failure; however, the annual number of transplants in the United States (approximately 2200 per year) has remained relatively constant because of limited donor organ availability.[10]

THE CARDIAC TRANSPLANT RECIPIENT

Recipient Selection

The evaluation of patients with end-stage heart disease and the selection of potential candidates for cardiac

TABLE 60–1 Recipient selection for heart transplantation

Indications	Eligibility criteria
1. Systolic heart failure (as defined by ejection fraction <35%) Inclusive etiology Ischemic Dilated Valvular Hypertensive Other Excluded etiology Amyloid HIV Cardiac sarcoma 2. Ischemic heart disease with intractable angina Not amenable to coronary artery bypass graft or percutaneous revascularization Ineffective maximal tolerated medical therapy Not a candidate for direct myocardial revascularization or transmyocardial revascularization procedure. Unsuccessful myocardial revascularization 3. Intractable arrhythmia Uncontrolled with pacing cardioverter defibrillator Not amenable to electrophysiology-guided single or combination medical therapy Not a candidate for ablative therapy 4. Hypertrophic cardiomyopathy Class IV symptoms persist despite interventional therapies Alcohol injection Myotomy and myomectomy Mitral valve replacement Maximal medical therapy Pacemaker therapy 5. Congenital heart disease in which severe fixed pulmonary hypertension is not a complication	Age 55-65 (center-specific) Healthy apart from heart disease Compliant with medical advice Psychosocially stable, supportive family or companions **Absolute contraindications** Age>70 Fixed pulmonary hypertension (unresponsive to pharmacologic intervention) Pulmonary vascular resistance >5 Wood units Transpulmonary gradient >15 mm/Hg Systemic illness that will limit survival despite transplant Neoplasm other than skin cancer HIV/AIDS (CDC definition of CD4 count of <200 cells /mm^3) SLE or sarcoid that has multisystem involvement and is currently active Any systemic process with a high probability of recurrence in the transplanted heart Irreversible renal or hepatic dysfunction **Potential contraindications** Chronic obstructive pulmonary disease Peripheral vascular or cerebrovascular disease Peptic ulcer disease Insulin-dependent diabetes mellitus with end-organ damage Past malignancy Recent and unresolved pulmonary infarction Current or recent diverticulitis Other systemic illness likely to limit survival or rehabilitation Cachexia Active alcohol or drug abuse History of noncompliance or psychiatric illness likely to interfere with long-term compliance Absence of psychosocial support

transplantation is undertaken by a multidisciplinary committee to ensure an equitable, objective, and medically justified allocation of the limited donor organs to patients with the greatest chance of postoperative survival and rehabilitation. Because of the current excellent results of transplantation and improved immunosuppression, eligibility criteria have been significantly expanded, contributing to the escalating donor shortage, complicating the selection process, and perhaps jeopardizing the results of future procedures. Indications and potential contraindications for cardiac transplantation are outlined in Table 60-1.[10] These inclusion and exclusion criteria vary somewhat among transplantation centers. The basic objective of the selection process is to identify those relatively healthy patients with end-stage cardiac disease refractory to medical therapies who possess the potential to resume a normal active life and maintain compliance with a rigorous medical regimen after cardiac transplantation. Accumulating transplant experience will facilitate optimal donor organ allocation through improved risk stratification of potential recipients and prediction of successful outcomes for cardiac transplantation.

ETIOLOGY OF END-STAGE CARDIAC FAILURE

Determination of the etiology and potential reversibility of end-stage cardiac failure is critical for the selection of transplant candidates. The vast majority of patients are referred with New York Heart Association (NYHA) class III or IV symptoms caused by ischemic heart disease or idiopathic dilated cardiomyopathy.[11] The spectrum of known causes of dilated cardiomyopathy include infectious (viral), inflammatory, toxic, metabolic, and familial etiologies.[12] Infrequent indications for transplantation include intractable angina, refractory malignant ventricular arrhythmias, allograft occlusive coronary artery disease, and cardiac failure caused by valvular or congenital heart disease. The perception of the irreversibility of advanced cardiac failure is changing with the growing popularity of tailored medical therapy, high-risk revascularization procedures, and newer antiarrhythmic pharmacologic agents and devices.

EVALUATION OF THE POTENTIAL CARDIAC RECIPIENT

The initial evaluation involves a comprehensive history and physical examination, chest roentgenogram, routine hematologic and biochemical laboratories, a limited panel of infectious disease serologies, and an exercise test with maximal oxygen consumption (V_{O_2}) measurements. Although the majority of referred patients have already undergone right heart cardiac catheterization and coronary angiography, the former study is repeated at the transplantation center before listing and at routine intervals thereafter to rule out irreversible pulmonary hypertension. Cine coronary angiography should be reviewed to confirm the inoperability of coronary artery lesions in ischemic cardiomyopathy. Endomyocardial biopsy should be performed on all patients with nonischemic cardiomyopathies symptomatic for less than 6 months to assist in therapeutic decision making. The complete routine preoperative evaluation in patients selected for transplantation includes thyroid function studies, fasting and postprandial blood sugar, creatinine clearance, lipoprotein electrophoresis, viral titers, fungal serologies, 12-lead electrocardiogram, Holter monitor, echocardiogram, pulmonary function tests, panel reactive antibody screen, and HLA typing. Abdominal ultrasound, carotid and lower extremity Doppler flow studies, esophagogastroduodenoscopy, and screening studies for malignancy are indicated in selected patients.

INDICATIONS FOR CARDIAC TRANSPLANTATION

Cardiac transplantation is reserved for a select group of patients with end-stage heart disease not amenable to optimal medical therapy or other surgical procedures (such as revascularization, balloon angioplasty, or catheter ablation techniques).[13] Prognosis for 1-year survival without transplantation should be less than 50%. Prediction of patient survival involves considerable subjective clinical judgment by the transplant committee, as no reliable objective prognostic criteria are currently available. Low ejection fraction (<20%), reduced serum sodium (<135 mEq/dL), high pulmonary capillary wedge pressure (>25 mm Hg), elevated plasma norepinephrine (>600 pg/mL), increased cardiothoracic ratio, and reduced maximal V_{O_2} (<10 mL/kg/min) have all been proposed as predictors of poor prognosis and potential indications for transplantation in patients receiving optimal medical therapy.[14–20] A V_{O_2} value between 10 and 15 mL/kg/min may be an indication if a steady decline has been noted. Reduced left ventricular ejection fraction and low maximal oxygen consumption are the strongest independent predictors of survival.[24]

CONTRAINDICATIONS FOR CARDIAC TRANSPLANTATION

Age is one of the most controversial exclusionary criteria for transplantation. The upper age limit for recipients is determined by each center, but emphasis is placed on the patient's physiologic rather than chronologic age.[21] Survival and quality of life in carefully selected older patients is comparable to that of younger recipients.[22] Although the elderly have a greater potential of occult systemic disease that may complicate their postoperative course, they have fewer rejection episodes than younger patients.[23]

Elevated pulmonary vascular resistance (PVR) is one of the few absolute contraindications for orthotopic cardiac transplantation. A fixed PVR greater than 6 Wood units or a transpulmonary gradient greater than 15 mm Hg are criteria for rejection of a candidate.[24–27] Preoperative assessment of these patients should include evaluation of the reversibility of the pulmonary hypertension with vasodilators (oxygen, milrinone, sodium nitroprusside, or prostaglandin E1) in the cardiac catheterization laboratory. If this hemodynamic maneuver does not reduce PVR by 50%, a trial of parenteral inotropes or vasodilators is initiated and after 48 to 72 hours repeat catheterization is performed. A fixed elevated PVR is defined as one that cannot be significantly reduced with the aforementioned interventions and predicts fatal graft right heart failure in the immediate postoperative period.[28–29] These patients may be candidates for heterotopic heart or heart-lung transplantation.[30–31] For a recipient with moderate pulmonary hypertension (3-6 Wood units), a larger donor heart often is selected to provide additional right ventricular reserve.

Transplantation in patients with diabetes mellitus is contraindicated only in the presence of significant end-organ damage (diabetic nephropathy, retinopathy, or neuropathy).[32–33] Control of blood sugar is possible with the reduction (or elimination) of corticosteriods in the cyclosporine era.[34–36] Active infection (including human immunodeficiency virus), irreversible renal or hepatic dysfunction, significant chronic lung disease, severe noncardiac arteriosclerotic vascular disease, and malignancy are generally considered contraindications for transplantation. Poor nutritional status as manifested by cachexia increases risk of infection and may limit early postoperative rehabilitation.

The ultimate success of transplantation is intimately dependent on the psychosocial stability and compliance of the recipient.[36] The rigorous postoperative regimen of multidrug therapy, frequent clinic visits, and routine endomyocardial biopsies demands commitment on the part of the patient. A history of psychiatric illness, substance abuse, or previous noncompliance (particularly with medical therapy for end-stage heart failure) may be sufficient cause to reject the candidacy of a patient.[37–39] Lack of supportive family members or companions is an additional relative contraindication.

Management of the Potential Cardiac Recipient

TAILORED MEDICAL THERAPY FOR END-STAGE CARDIAC FAILURE

Pharmacologic advances in the treatment of heart failure have clearly led to improvements in both quality of life and long-term outcomes. Conventional outpatient management of congestive heart failure includes angiotensin-converting enzyme (ACE) inhibitors, beta blockers, and diuretics (especially spironolactone).[40–47] Patients with moderate to severe congestive heart failure have shown improved survival with drug therapy.[41–43]

PHARMACOLOGIC BRIDGE TO TRANSPLANTATION

Critically compromised patients require admission to the intensive care unit for intravenous inotropic therapy. Milrinone, dobutamine, and dopamine are the agents of choice.[44–45] Placement of an intra-aortic balloon pump (IABP) also may be necessary in heart failure refractory to initial pharmacologic measures. Patients with continued pulmonary congestion or global hypoperfusion despite maximal pharmacologic and IABP therapies have been shown to improve with placement of mechanical devices as bridges to transplantation.[46–49]

MECHANICAL BRIDGE TO TRANSPLANTATION

The increased success of cardiac transplantation in conjunction with the static number of available organs has created a need for mechanical assist devices as a bridge to transplantation.[50] Ventricular assist devices (VAD) or total artificial hearts (TAH) may be indicated in potential cardiac recipients who remain unstable after 24 to 48 hours of maximal pharmacologic support (Table 60-2).[51–57] Since these devices are rarely weaned, however, it is imperative that the patient's candidacy for transplantation be scrutinized prior to placement of a VAD or TAH. Patient selection for a mechanical device is a complex, evolving field closely followed by the U.S. Food and Drug Administration.[58] Recent data shows that approximately 70% of patients are successfully bridged to transplantation and the actuarial survival is 80% at one year.[59] Most large series suggest an improvement in survival because the devices allow patients to be rehabilitated while on the device.[47,60] Initial results from the Randomized Evaluation of Mechanical Assistance for the Treatment of Congestive Heart Failure (REMATCH) study indicate that patients with devices have improved survival and quality of life at 1 year compared to medical therapy and may prove to be an acceptable long term option in those patients who are not candidates for cardiac transplantation.[61]

TABLE 60–2 Recipient selection criteria for ventricular assist device

Accepted as candidate for cardiac transplantation
Absence of coagulopathy or gastrointestinal hemorrhage
Ventricular failure (CI <1.8 L/min/m^2, left atrial pressure >25 mmHg, systolic blood pressure <90 mmHg), despite:
Corrected metabolism (temperature, acid-base, electrolytes)
Adequate preload, appropriate afterload reduction
Maximal inotropic support
Intra-aortic balloon pump assistance

LIFE-THREATENING VENTRICULAR ARRHYTHMIAS

Symptomatic ventricular tachycardia or fibrillation and a history of sudden cardiac death (SCD) are indications for placement of an automatic implantable cardioverter-defibrillator (AICD), long-term amiodarone therapy, or occasionally radiofrequency catheter ablation.[62–63] SCD is the most common cause of death in patients awaiting heart transplantation and is most common within the first 3 months after referral for transplantation.[64–65] Several studies have shown that implantation of a defibrillator improved survival in patients with either a history of or inducible ventricular tachycardia or fibrillation.[66–67]

Recipient Prioritization for Transplantation

The prioritization of appropriate recipients for transplantation is based on survival and quality of life expected to be gained in comparison to maximal medical and surgical alternatives.[68] Organ allocation is based on recipient priority status (IA, IB, or II), duration on the waiting list, and geographic distance between donor and potential recipient. Highest priority is given to local status IA patients possessing the earliest listing dates. The recipient status criteria established by the United Network for Organ Sharing (UNOS) in 1999 are outlined in Table 60-3. In 1999, of the patients who received cardiac transplants, 34% of recipients were in status IA, 37% were in status IB, and only 26% were in status II.[69] Furthermore, the cardiac transplant waiting list has more than doubled over the last 10 years and, in 1999, more than 39% of the waiting list was comprised of patients who have been listed for more than 2 years.[69] Patients considered for transplantation should be examined at least every 3 months for reevaluation of recipient status. Yearly right heart catheterization is indicated for all candidates on the waiting list, and in selected cases, for patients rejected because of pulmonary hypertension. Presently, there is no established method to de-list patients who have stabilized on medical therapy without loss of their previously accrued waiting time.

TABLE 60–3 Current recipient status criteria of the United Network for Organ Sharing (UNOS)*

Status IA

Patient requires mechanical circulatory assistance with one or more of the following devices:
- Total artificial heart
- Left and/or right ventricular assist device implanted for 30 days or less
- Intra-aortic balloon pump
- Extracorporeal membrane oxygenator (ECMO)

Mechanical circulatory support for more than 30 days with significant device-related complications

Mechanical ventilation

Continuous infusion of high-dose inotrope(s) in addition to continuous hemodynamic monitoring of left ventricular filling pressures

Life expectancy without transplant is less than 7 days

Status IB

Patient has at least one of the following devices or therapies in place:
- Left and/or right ventricular assist device implanted for more than 30 days
- Continuous infusion of intravenous inotropes

Status II

All other waiting patients who do not meet Status IA or IB criteria

*UNOS Executive Order, August, 1999.

THE CARDIAC DONOR

Donor Availability

The availability of donor organs remains the major limiting factor to heart transplantation. The number of heart transplants performed in the United States has declined over the past 10 years but appears to have leveled at approximately 2200 per year. Interestingly, likely due to improved preoperative care, the death rate for patients on the waiting list for a cardiac allograft declined to an all time low of 172.4 per 1000 patients in 1999.[69] The Uniform Anatomic Gift Act of 1968 states that all competent individuals over the age of 18 (may) donate all or part of their bodies and established the current voluntary basis of organ donation practiced in the United States.[70] To accommodate the increasing demand for organs, the original stringent criteria for donor eligibility have been relaxed and educational campaigns have increased awareness of the need for a larger donor pool. Interestingly, several reports indicate that the most important reason for the organ shortage is not the indifference of the public, but rather a failure of health care providers to discuss the option of organ donation with families of dying patients.[71] In 1986, the Required Request Law, which required hospitals to request permission from next of kin to harvest organs, was passed to encourage physician compliance in the donor request process.[72] Several European countries have implemented controversial "presumed consent" legislation whereby organ procurement may automatically proceed in brain-dead individuals if wishes to the contrary are not expressed by the patient prior to death.[73] Even in the presence of documentation of the patient's wishes to donate, consent for organ donation in the United States usually is verified with the family. The adoption of presumed consent legislation, the use of anencephalic newborns as donors, and financial incentives for the donor family have all stimulated considerable controversy.[74–75] Future reforms will be molded by the evolving public attitude towards transplantation and will likely focus on continued public and physician education as well as enforcement and expansion of required request legislation.[76]

Allocation of Donor Organs

In an effort to increase organ donation and to coordinate an equitable allocation of allografts, Congress passed the National Organ Transplant Act in 1984.[77] This act resulted in the drafting of the aforementioned Required Request Law as well as the awarding of a federal contract to the United Network of Organ Sharing (UNOS) for the development of a national organ procurement and allocation network.[78] Eleven regions were created that are locally managed by transplant coordinators of individual organ procurement organizations (OPOs).

Brain Death

Establishment of criteria for brain death was imperative with the advent of heart transplantation so that the organ could be procured while still functioning to minimize ischemic injury. After early attempts to define brain death by the Harvard Committee, the University of Minnesota, and the National Institutes of Health, the Uniform Brain Death Act (1978) and later the Uniform Determination of Death Act (1980) were passed to provide national guidelines for state legislators to adopt.[79–82] The basic criteria used for the diagnosis of brain death include loss of cortical function, apnea, absence of brain stem reflexes, and irreversibility over a 12 to 24 hour observation period. Furthermore, any potentially reversible cause for the patient's neurologic status, including metabolic disturbances, pharmacologic agents, and hypothermia must be ruled out.[83–84] The vast majority of donors are victims of blunt head trauma (motor vehicle accident), penetrating head trauma (gunshot wound), or cerebrovascular accident. The diagnosis of brain death can be made by clinically established criteria by the patient's physician. However, if uncertainty exists or the observation period must be abbreviated because of patient instability, ancillary confirmatory tests should be performed for uncertainty or declining clinical status of the donor and include electroencephalogram, cerebral angiography, or radionuclide cortical blood flow studies.[85] Declaration of brain death and confirmation of written informed consent must be documented in the patient's chart.

TABLE 60–4 **Donor selection for heart transplantation**

Suggested criteria for cardiac donor
- Age <55
- Absence of the following:
  - Prolonged cardiac arrest
  - Prolonged severe hypotension
  - Preexisting cardiac disease
  - Intracardiac drug injection
  - Severe chest trauma with evidence of cardiac injury
  - Septicemia
  - Extracerebral malignancy
  - Positive serologies for human immunodeficiency virus, hepatitis B, or hepatitis C
  - Hemodynamic stability without high-dose inotropic support (<20 μg/kg/min dopamine)

Cardiac donor evaluation
- Past medical history and physical examination
- Electrocardiogram
- Chest roentgenogram
- Arterial blood gases
- Laboratory tests (ABO, HIV, HBV, HCV)
- Cardiology consultation (echocardiogram, and in selected cases, coronary angiogram)

Donor Selection

Once a brain-dead individual has been identified as a potential cardiac donor, the patient undergoes a rigorous three-phase screening regimen. The primary screening is undertaken by the organ procurement agency. Information regarding the patient's age, height, weight, gender, ABO blood type, hospital course, cause of death, and routine laboratory data including CMV, HIV, HBV, and HCV serologies are collected. Cardiac surgeons or cardiologists perform the secondary screening, which involves further investigation in search of potential contraindications (Table 60-4), determination of the hemodynamic support necessary to sustain the donor, and review of the electrocardiogram, chest roentgenogram, arterial blood gas, and echocardiogram. Although adverse donor criteria may be reported, a team is often dispatched to the hospital to evaluate the donor onsite. Echocardiography is performed in the United States but not in Europe. While echocardiography has been extremely useful for detection of wall motion abnormalities and unsuspected congenital heart lesions, pulmonary catheters are used to determine cardiac output because of inaccuracies of echocardiography.[80] Coronary angiography is indicated in the presence of advanced donor age (male donors >45 years of age, female donors >50 years of age) or risk factors for atherosclerotic coronary artery disease (tobacco abuse, diabetes, significant family history). The final and often most important screening of the donor occurs intraoperatively at the time of organ procurement by the cardiac surgical team. Direct visualization of the heart is performed for evidence of ventricular or valvular dysfunction, previous infarction, or myocardial contusion secondary to closed-chest compressions or blunt chest trauma. The coronary arterial tree is palpated for gross calcifications indicative of atheromatous disease. If direct examination of the heart is unremarkable, the recipient hospital is notified and the procurement surgeons proceed with donor cardiectomy, usually in conjunction with multiorgan procurement.

In light of continued attempts to liberalize the criteria for donor eligibility,[86] the screening process continues to evolve and intensify to predict early allograft failure because of latent cardiac disease. Currently, several studies have been evaluating the routine use of angiography in potential cardiac donors in an effort to increase the number of available organs.[87] Considerable experimental work is still necessary for the development of a simple, reproducible test for detecting cardiac allograft injury prior to explantation.

Management of the Cardiac Donor

Medical management of cardiac donors, an integral part of organ preservation, is complicated by the complex physiological phenomenon of brain death and the need to coordinate procurement with other organ donor teams. Optimal care requires that the donor be treated as any other intensive care unit patient with invasive hemodynamic monitoring, ventilatory support, and meticulous attention to intravascular volume status and electrolytes (Table 60-5).[88]

TABLE 60–5 **Management of the cardiac donor**

- Continuous monitoring with intra-arterial catheter, central venous or Swan-Ganz catheter, telemetry, pulse oximetry, and urinary catheter
- Cardiovascular goals: mean arterial pressure 80-90 mm Hg, central venous pressure 5-12 mm Hg
- Volume resuscitation: initial bolus of 1-2 L of lactated Ringer's, followed by maintenance rate of 100 mL/h plus previous hour's urine output
- Hypotension: inotropic support (dopamine) and/or vasopressor support (phenylephrine)
- Hypertension: afterload reduction (sodium nitroprusside, esmolol)
- Thermoregulation goal: 34°C-36°C utilizing warming blankets and lights, warm intravenous fluids, warm inspired air
- Fluid and electrolyte balance goals: Urine output >100 mL/h, normal serum electrolyte levels
  - Diabetes insipidus: volume replacement, vasopressin (0.8-1.0 U/h)
  - Oliguria: fluid boluses, diuretics (furosemide, mannitol)
  - Correct electrolyte disturbances
- Ventilatory support managed by serial arterial blood gases
- Blood transfusions for hemoglobin <10 gm/dL
- Hormonal therapy: triiodothyronine (T3), cortisol, insulin

Continuous monitoring of arterial pressure, central venous pressure, and urinary output is mandatory. As the number of marginal donors increases with the acceptance of more lenient eligibility criteria, some transplant centers have established mobile intensive care teams that are dispatched to ensure appropriate management of these highly labile patients.[89] Hemodynamic instability in the donor may result from vasomotor dysfunction, hypovolemia, hypothermia, and dysrhythmias. Increased intracranial pressure may lead to massive sympathetic discharge with elevated levels of circulating endogenous catecholamines. The resultant episodes of systemic hypertension and coronary vasospasm place the allograft at significant risk of ischemic injury.[90] Rapid afterload reduction may be achieved with sodium nitroprusside, whereas volatile anesthetics assist in reducing the intensity of sympathetic bursts. To minimize cerebral edema prior to the declaration of brain death, potential donors have been intravascularly volume depleted via strict fluid restriction and osmotic diuresis. Aggressive volume resuscitation is sometimes necessary and may require use of a Swan-Ganz catheter.[91] Fluid overload, however, should be avoided to prevent postoperative allograft dysfunction caused by chamber distention and myocardial edema. Blood transfusions are indicated to optimize oxygen delivery if the hemoglobin falls below 10 g/dL. Mean arterial pressure should be maintained between 80 and 90 mm Hg. If fluid resuscitation is inadequate to restore blood pressure in the hypotensive donor, a dopamine infusion is initiated for inotropic support.[92–93] Vasopressors are occasionally indicated for hypotension caused by loss of systemic vasomotor tone. Prolonged administration of high-dose catecholamine therapy (dopamine >10–15 μg/kg/min) has been associated with poor cardiac function in the posttransplant period because of depletion of myocardial norepinephrine stores.[94–95] Traditionally, these patients were rejected for use as cardiac donors, but high-dose inotropic support is no longer an absolute contraindication for donation.[96] Maintenance of normal temperatures, electrolyte levels, osmolarity, acid-base balance, and oxygenation is critical for optimal donor management. Common electrolyte disturbances include hypernatremia, hypokalemia, hypomagnesemia, and hypophosphatemia.[97] Central diabetes insipidus develops in more than 50% of donors because of pituitary dysfunction, and massive diuresis complicates fluid and electrolyte management.[98] A low-dose aqueous vasopressin (Pitressin) infusion is initiated at 0.8 to 1.0 U/h and titrated to keep urinary output at approximately 100 to 200 mL/h.[99] Alternatively, vasopressin may be administered periodically subcutaneously or intramuscularly (10 U every 4 hours). Standard ventilator management with diligent endotracheal suctioning is essential in these vulnerable patients.[100]

Broad-spectrum antibiotic therapy with a cephalosporin is initiated following collection of blood, urine, and tracheal aspirate for culture. Brain death is associated with the depletion of a variety of hormones, including free triiodothyronine (T3), cortisol, and insulin.[101–102] Donor pretreatment with hormone replacement therapy has proven to be beneficial.[103–105]

Donor Heart Procurement

A median sternotomy is performed and the pericardium incised longitudinally. The heart is inspected and palpated for evidence of cardiac disease or injury. The superior and inferior vena cava and azygous vein are circumferentially mobilized and encircled with ties. The aorta is dissected from the pulmonary artery and isolated with umbilical tape. To facilitate access to the epigastrium by the liver procurement team, the cardiac team often then temporarily retires from the operating room table or assists with retraction. Once preparation for liver, pancreas, lung, and kidney explantation is completed, the patient is administered 30,000 U of heparin intravenously. The azygous vein and superior vena cava are doubly ligated (or stapled) and divided distal to the azygous vein leaving a long segment of superior vena cava (Fig. 60-2). The inferior vena cava is clamped at the level of the diaphragm (if the abdominal IVC is vented) and then divided proximal to the clamp to permit efflux of the cardioplegia. Additional venting is achieved with transection of

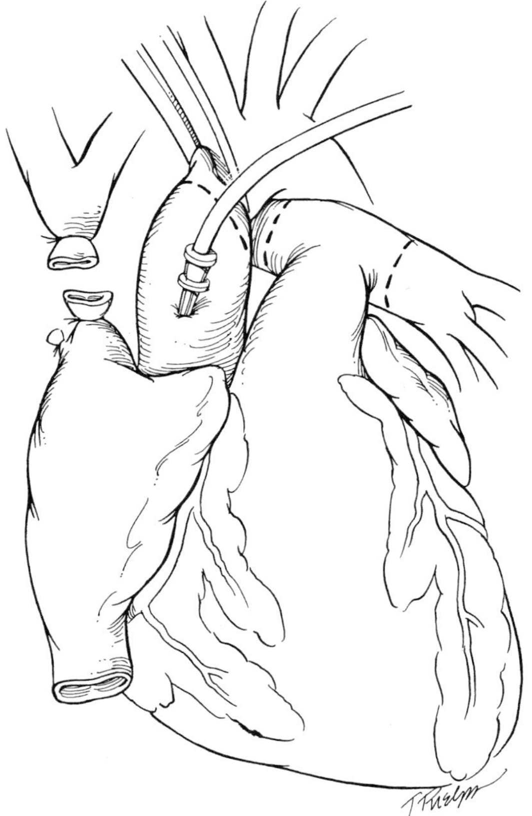

FIGURE 60–2 Donor cardiectomy.

the right superior pulmonary vein. The aortic cross-clamp is applied at the takeoff of the innominate artery and the heart is arrested with a single flush (500 mL) of cardioplegic solution infused through a 14-gauge needle inserted proximal to the cross-clamp. Rapid cooling of the heart is achieved with copious amounts of cold saline and cold saline slush poured into the pericardial well. Following the delivery of cardioplegia, cardiectomy proceeds as the apex of the heart is elevated cephalad and any remaining intact pulmonary veins are divided. This maneuver is appropriately modified to retain adequate left atrial cuffs for both lungs and the heart if the lungs also are being procured. While applying caudal traction to the heart with the nondominant hand, the ascending aorta is transected proximal to the innominate artery and the pulmonary arteries are divided distal to bifurcation (again, modification is necessary if the lungs are being procured). More generous segments of the great vessels and superior vena cava may be required for recipients with congenital heart disease.

Once the explantation is complete, the allograft is examined for evidence of a patent foramen ovale, which should be closed at that time, or any valvular anomalies. The allograft is then placed in a sterile container for transport back to the recipient hospital.

Organ Preservation

Current clinical graft preservation techniques generally permit a safe ischemic period of 4 to 6 hours. The donor heart is vulnerable to injury at all stages of the transplantation procedure. Factors contributing to the severity of postoperative myocardial dysfunction include insults associated with suboptimal donor management, hypothermia, ischemia-reperfusion injury, and depletion of energy stores. A single flush of a cardioplegic or preservative solution followed by static hypothermic storage is the preferred preservation method by most transplant centers.[130] Despite two decades of investigation, no single preservation regimen has demonstrated consistent, clinically significant superior myocardial protection when used within the current safe limits of ischemia.[106] Controversy abounds in the literature regarding optimal storage temperature, composition of cardioplegic and storage solutions, techniques of solution delivery, additives, and reperfusion modification. Hypothermia remains the cornerstone of organ preservation. The ideal storage temperature is unknown, but most institutions aim for temperatures between 4°C and 10°C.[107] Crystalloid solutions of widely different compositions are available and the debate over them speaks for the fact that no ideal solution currently exists. Depending on their ionic composition, solutions are classified as intracellular or extracellular.[108–110] Intracellular solutions, characterized by moderate to high concentrations of potassium and low concentrations of sodium, purportedly reduce hypothermia-induced cellular edema by mimicking the intracellular milieu. Commonly used examples of these solutions include University of Wisconsin, Euro-Collins, and in Europe, Bretschneider (HTK) solutions. Extracellular solutions, characterized by low to moderate potassium and high sodium concentrations, avoid the theoretical potential for cellular damage and increased vascular resistance associated with hyperkalemic solutions. Stanford, Hopkins, and St. Thomas Hospital solutions are representative extracellular cardioplegic solutions. Although a plethora of pharmacologic additives have been included in cardioplegic storage solutions, the greatest potential for future routine use may lie with impermeants, substrates, and antioxidants. Currently used impermeants (mannitol, lactobionate, raffinose, and histidine) counteract intracellular osmotic pressure to reduce hypothermia-induced cellular edema in the allograft. The preservation of myocardial high-energy phosphates during ischemia (to prevent contracture bands) and their rapid regeneration at reperfusion (to fuel the newly contracting heart) are the primary objectives for the use of substrate-enhanced media. Adenosine, L-pyruvate, and L-glutamate have been studied most intensely.[111] Recognizing that oxygen-derived free radicals and neutrophils likely are critical mediators of myocardial reperfusion injury, considerable investigative effort has been undertaken to modify the untoward effects of ischemia-reperfusion with antioxidant additives including allopurinol, glutathione, superoxide dismutase, catalase, mannitol, and histidine. A variety of pharmacologic and mechanical strategies for leukocyte inhibition and depletion are also being explored.[112–113] Potential benefits of continuous perfusion preservation techniques are currently overshadowed by exacerbation of extracellular cardiac edema and logistical problems inherent to a complex perfusion apparatus.[114] Experimental low-pressure (microperfusion) and intermittent flush techniques theoretically provide sufficient oxygen and substrates for basal metabolic demands without causing significant edema.[115] Continued research will be necessary to resolve these ongoing debates over the various aspects of cardiac allograft preservation, since the heart transplant registry continues to report that 20% of perioperative deaths are caused by cardiac dysfunction.

Donor-Recipient Matching

Criteria for matching potential recipients with the appropriate donor are based primarily on ABO blood group compatibility and patient size. ABO barriers should not be crossed in heart transplantation, as incompatibility frequently results in fatal hyperacute rejection. Donor weight should be within 30% of recipient weight except in pediatric patients, where closer size matching is required. In cases of elevated pulmonary vascular resistance in the recipient (>6 Wood units), a larger donor is preferred to reduce the risk of right ventricular failure in the early postoperative period. A random panel of pooled lymphocytes representing the major histocompatibility antigens in the community is used to screen the recipient for anti–human lymphocyte antigen (HLA) antibodies that may also mediate hyperacute rejection. If the percentage (or panel) of reactive antibody (PRA) is greater than 10% to 15%, indicating recipient presensitization to alloantigen, a prospective negative T-cell crossmatch between the recipient and donor sera is mandatory prior to transplantation.[116–117] A positive crossmatch is an absolute contraindication to transplantation. A crossmatch is always performed retrospectively, even if the PRA is absent or low. Retrospective studies have also demonstrated that better matching at the HLA-DR locus results in fewer episodes of rejection and infection with an overall improved survival.[118] Because of current allocation criteria and limits on ischemic time of the cardiac allograft, prospective HLA matching is not possible logistically.

Hyperacute Rejection

Hyperacute rejection results from preformed, donor-specific antibodies in the recipient.[119] ABO blood group and panel reactive antibody screening have made this condition a rare complication. The onset of hyperacute rejection occurs within minutes to several hours after transplantation and the results are catastrophic. Gross inspection reveals a mottled or dark red, flaccid allograft,[120] and histologic examination confirms the characteristic global interstitial hemorrhage and edema without lymphocytic infiltrate. Immunofluorescence techniques reveal deposits of immunoglobulins and complement on the vascular endothelium.[121] No treatment is effective except retransplantation, and even this aggressive strategy frequently is unsuccessful.

OPERATIVE TECHNIQUES IN HEART TRANSPLANTATION

Orthotopic cardiac transplantation, the surgical technique of choice, involves the replacement of part (or occasionally all) of the recipient's heart with a healthy donor allograft. Heterotopic cardiac transplantation, the piggy-backing of an allograft onto the patient's heart, is rarely performed today. It may be indicated if orthotopic transplantation is not possible because of elevated pulmonary vascular resistance or when a donor heart is too small to sustain the recipient.[122–123] Even in these selected cases, results are not equivalent to orthotopic transplant.[124]

Orthotopic Heart Transplantation

ANESTHETIC MANAGEMENT

Once the organ procurement team has confirmed the acceptability of the donor allograft at time of operation, recipient induction may commence. High-dose narcotics (e.g., fentanyl) usually are employed for induction and maintenance anesthesia.[125–126] In light of the poor ventricular function of the recipient, all anesthetic agents should be titrated carefully with inotropic and vasoactive agents readily accessible for the rapid management of induction-induced hypotension. Inhaled agents may be added if necessary, but their potential myocardial depressant effects limit widespread use in this patient population. Prior to skin incision, some centers initiate aprotinin or aminocaproic acid therapy to minimize perioperative blood loss.[127]

OPERATIVE PREPARATION OF THE RECIPIENT

The surgical technique of orthotopic cardiac transplantation has changed little from the original description reported by Shumway and Lower.[5] Following median sternotomy and vertical pericardiotomy, the patient is heparinized and prepared for cardiopulmonary bypass. Bicaval venous cannulation and distal ascending aortic cannulation just proximal to the origin of the innominate artery is optimal. Umbilical tape snares are passed around the superior and inferior vena cava. Bypass is initiated, the patient is cooled to 28°C, caval snares are tightened, and the ascending aorta is cross-clamped. The great vessels are transected above the semilunar commissures, whereas the atria are incised along the atrioventricular grooves leaving cuffs for allograft implantation. Removal of the atrial appendages reduces the risk of postoperative thrombus formation.[128] Following cardiectomy, the proximal 1 to 2 cm of aorta and pulmonary artery are separated from one another with electrocautery, taking care to avoid injuring the right pulmonary artery. Continuous aspiration of pulmonary venous return from bronchial

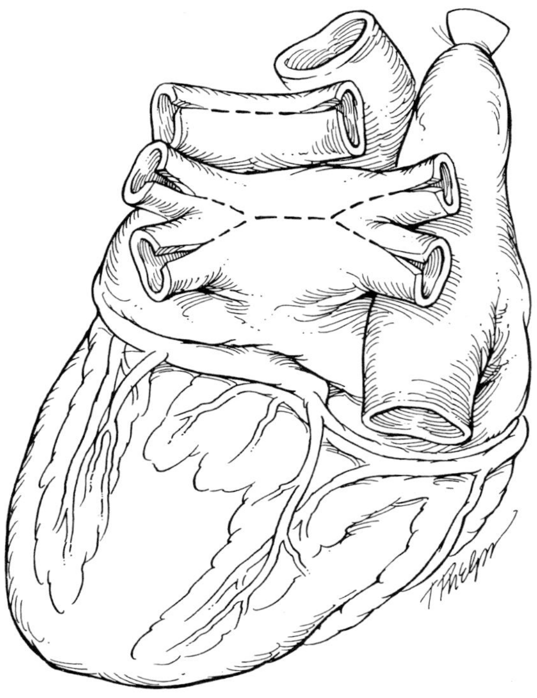

FIGURE 60–3 Donor allograft preparation for orthotopic heart transplantation. Pulmonary vein orifices joined to form left atrial cuff.

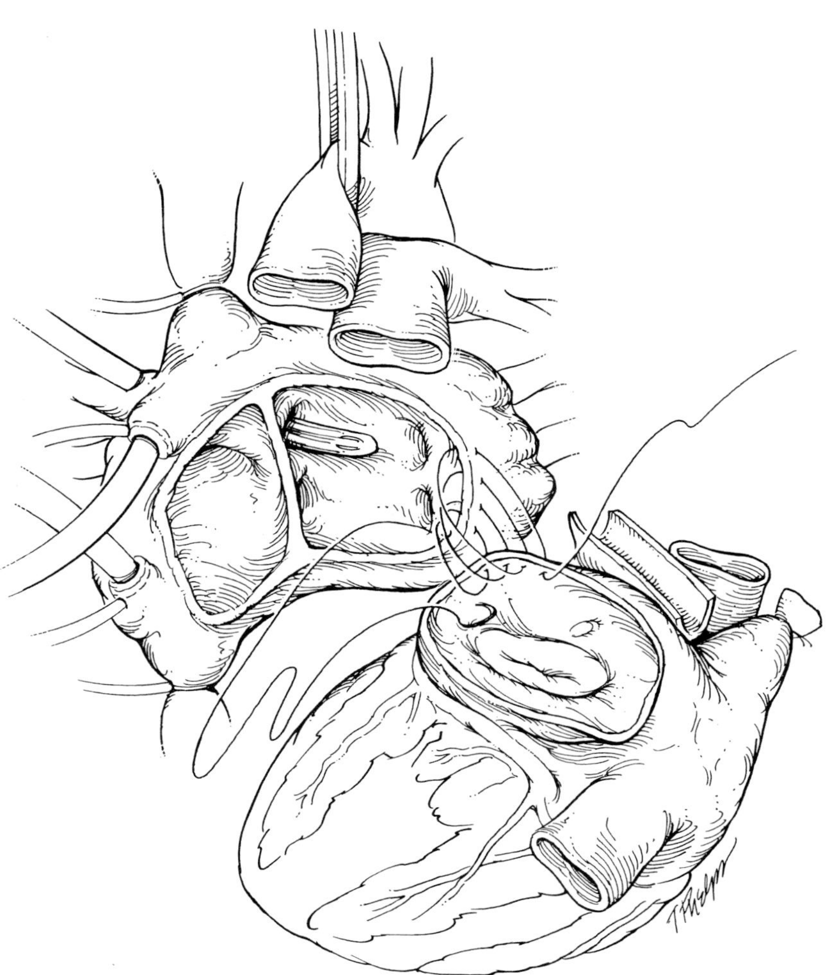

FIGURE 60–4 Implantation of allograft. First suture is placed at the level of the left superior pulmonary vein.

collaterals is achieved by insertion of a vent into the left atrial remnant, either directly or via the right superior pulmonary vein.

Timing of donor and recipient cardiectomies is critical to minimize allograft ischemic time and recipient bypass time. Frequent communication between the procurement and transplant teams permits optimal coordination of the procedures. Ideally, the recipient cardiectomy is completed just prior to the arrival of the cardiac allograft.[129]

IMPLANTATION

The donor heart is removed from the transport cooler and placed in a basin of cold saline. If not previously performed, preparation of the donor heart is accomplished. Electrocautery and sharp dissection are used to separate the aorta and pulmonary artery. The left atrium is incised by connecting the pulmonary vein orifices and excess atrial tissue is trimmed forming a circular cuff tailored to the size of the recipient left atrial remnant (Fig. 60-3). Implantation begins with placement of a double-armed 3-0 Prolene through the recipient left atrial cuff at the level of the left superior pulmonary vein and then through the donor left atrial cuff near the base of the atrial appendage (Fig. 60-4). The allograft is lowered into the recipient mediastinum atop a cold sponge to insulate it from direct thermal transfer from adjacent thoracic structures. The suture is continued in a running fashion caudally and then medially to the inferior aspect of the interatrial septum (Fig. 60-5). Upon completion of the posterior left atrial suture line, continuous topical cold saline irrigation of the pericardial well is initiated, and the patient is oriented in a left side down–head up position to allow drainage of the saline away from the operative field and maximal cold saline exposure of the left and right ventricles. The second arm of the suture is run along the roof of the left atrium and down the interatrial septum. It is important to continually assess size discrepancy between donor and recipient atria so that appropriate plication of excess tissue may be performed. The left atrium is filled with saline and the two arms of suture are tied together on the outside of the heart. Some centers introduce a line into the left atrial appendage for continuous endocardial cooling of the allograft (50-75 mL/min) and evacuation of intracardiac air.

Once the left atrial anastomosis is complete, a curvilinear incision is made from the inferior vena caval orifice toward

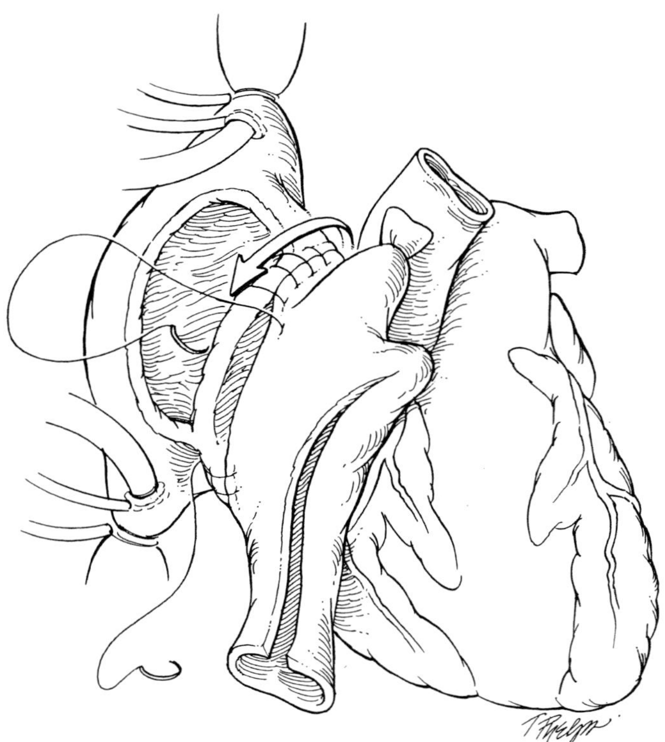

FIGURE 60–5 Implantation of allograft (continued). Left atrial anastomosis.

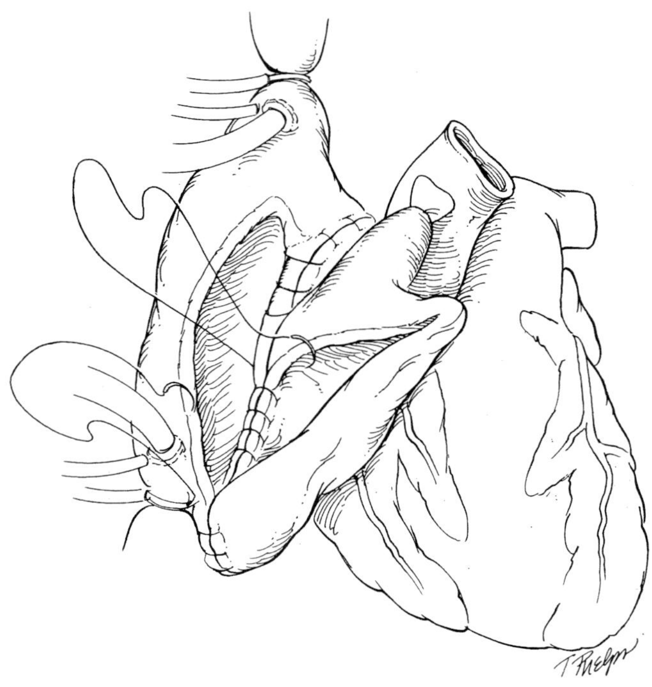

FIGURE 60–6 Implantation of allograft (continued). Right atrial anastomosis.

the right atrial appendage of the allograft. This modification in the right atriotomy initially introduced by Barnard reduces the risk of injury to the sinoatrial node and accounts for the preservation of sinus rhythm observed in most recipients.[130] The tricuspid apparatus and interatrial septum are inspected. Recipients are predisposed to increased right-sided heart pressures in the early postoperative period owing to preexisting pulmonary hypertension and volume overload. Both conditions are poorly tolerated by the recovering right ventricle. To avoid refractory arterial desaturation associated with right-to-left shunting, patent foramen ovale are oversewn.[131] The right atrial anastomosis is performed in a running fashion similar to the left with the initial anchor suture placed either at the most superior or inferior aspect of the interatrial septum so that the ends of the suture meet in the middle of the anterolateral wall (Fig. 60-6).

The end-to-end pulmonary artery anastomosis is next performed using a 4-0 Prolene suture beginning with the posterior wall from inside of the vessel and then completing the anterior wall from the outside. It is crucial that the pulmonary artery ends be trimmed to eliminate any redundancy in the vessel that might cause kinking.[132] Rewarming is initiated at this time. Finally, the aortic anastomosis is performed using a technique similar to the pulmonary artery except that some redundancy is desirable in the aorta as it facilitates visualization of the posterior suture line (Fig. 60-7). Rewarming is usually begun prior to the aortic anastomosis,

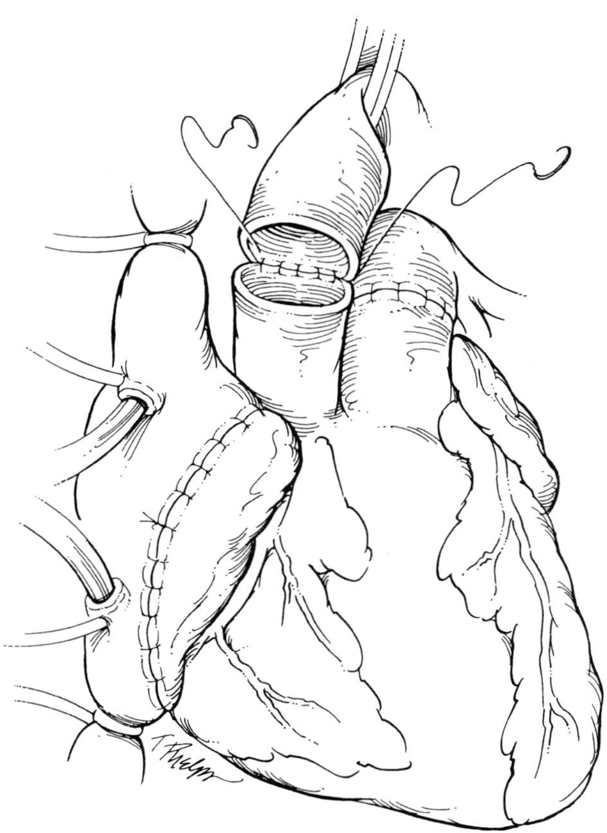

FIGURE 60–7 Implantation of allograft (continued). Aortic anastomosis.

which is performed in a standard end-to-end fashion. Routine de-airing techniques are then employed.[133] Cold saline lavage is discontinued, lidocaine (100-200 mg IV) is administered, and the aortic cross-clamp is removed. Half of patients require electrical defibrillation. A needle vent is inserted in the ascending aorta for final de-airing with the patient in steep Trendelenburg. Suture lines are carefully inspected for hemostasis. Inotrope infusion is initiated and titrated to achieve a heart rate between 90 and 110 bpm.[134] The patient is weaned from cardiopulmonary bypass and the cannulae are removed. Temporary epicardial pacing wires are placed in the donor right atrium and ventricle. Following insertion of mediastinal and pleural tubes, the median sternotomy is closed in standard fashion.

ALTERNATIVE TECHNIQUES FOR ORTHOTOPIC HEART TRANSPLANTATION

Two alternative techniques for orthotopic heart transplantation have been gaining popularity over the past several years. Total heart transplantation involves complete excision of the recipient heart with bicaval end-to-end anastomoses and bilateral pulmonary venous anastomoses.[135–137] The Wythenshawe bicaval technique is performed in a similar fashion except that the recipient left atrium is prepared as a single cuff with all four pulmonary vein orifices (Fig. 60-8).[138] Although these procedures are more technically difficult than standard orthotopic transplantation, series using these techniques have reported shorter hospital stays and reduced postoperative dependence on diuretics, in addition to lower incidences of atrial dysrhythmias, conduction disturbances, mitral and tricuspid valve incompetence, and right ventricular failure.[138–140] Furthermore, a recently completed randomized study comparing bi-atrial versus bicaval transplant showed an improved twelve month survival in the bicaval group.[141] Long term outcomes and additional randomized studies evaluating these alternative techniques are still needed.

RECIPIENTS WITH CONGENITAL ANOMALIES

Unlike children and infants, transplantation in adults with previous palliative procedures for congenital anomalies is uncommon. It is critical that a generous donor cardiectomy be performed so that sufficient tissue is available for optimal reconstruction. There are a variety of anomaly-specific implantation techniques.[142–144]

Heterotopic Heart Transplantation

Pulmonary hypertension and right heart failure has remained one of the leading causes of death in cardiac transplantation. This has led to an interest in heterotopic heart tranplantation. Currently, heterotopic heart transplants are indicated in patients with irreversible pulmonary hypertension or significant donor-recipient size mismatch.

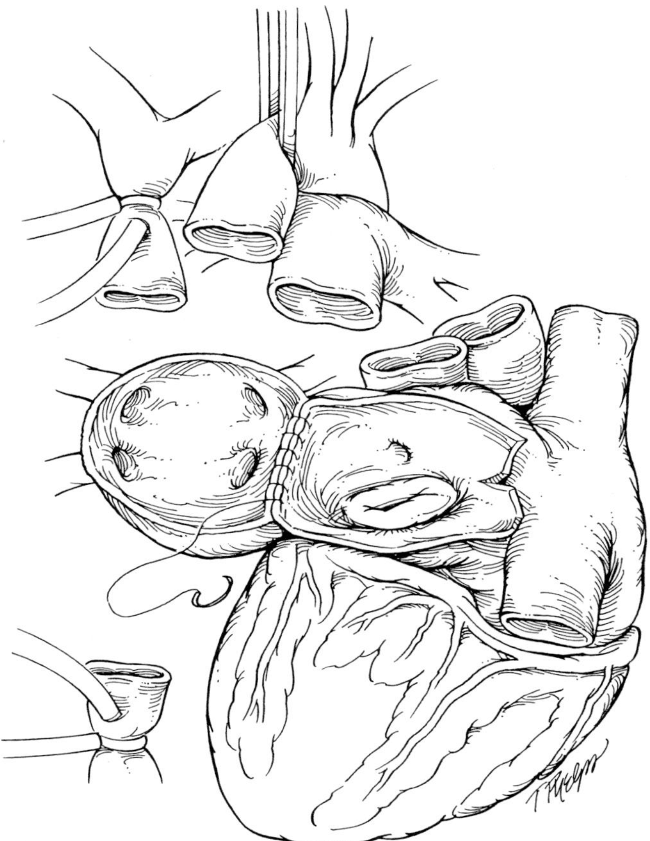

FIGURE 60–8 Bicaval heart transplantation.

DONOR ALLOGRAFT PREPARATION

Like the cardiectomy for patients with congenital disease, the maximal length of aorta, superior vena cava, and pulmonary arteries is procured. The inferior vena cava and the right pulmonary veins are oversewn, and a common left pulmonary vein orifice is created (Fig. 60-9). A linear incision is made along the long axis of the posterior right atrium extending 3 to 4 cm into the superior vena cava.

IMPLANTATION

The details of the technique are well described in the literature[145–147] and are beyond the scope of this chapter. Briefly, the sequence of anastomoses is as follows: donor left pulmonary vein orifice to recipient left atrium, donor superior vena cava-right atrial orifice to recipient right atrium, end-to-side aortic-aortic anastomosis, and finally an end-to-side anastomosis joining the pulmonary arteries of donor and recipient (Fig. 60-10). By employing this technique, the strengths of both the native and transplanted heart are utilized. The conserved recipient's right ventricle provides the necessary assistance to the transplanted heart to overcome significant pulmonary hypertension.

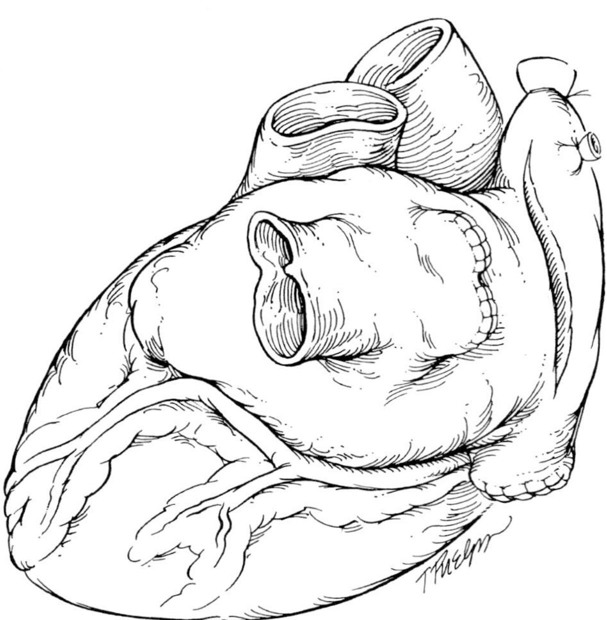

FIGURE 60–9 Donor allograft preparation for heterotopic heart transplantation.

Domino Donor Procedure

Of historical interest, the Domino donor procedure was used to avoid wasting relatively healthy hearts from selected heart-lung transplant recipients. These organs were transplanted into a different recipient using standard orthotopic or heterotopic techniques.[148–149]

POSTOPERATIVE MANAGEMENT

Hemodynamic Management

HEART ALLOGRAFT PHYSIOLOGY

The intact heart is innervated by antagonistic sympathetic and parasympathetic fibers of the autonomic nervous system. Transplantation necessitates transection of these fibers, yielding a denervated heart with altered physiology. Devoid of autonomic input, the sinoatrial (SA) node of the transplanted heart fires at its increased intrinsic resting rate of 90 to 110 bpm.[150–151] The allograft relies on distant noncardiac sites as its source for catecholamines; thus, its response to stress (e.g., hypovolemia, hypoxia, anemia) is somewhat delayed until circulating catecholamines can exert their positive chronotropic effect on the heart.[152–154] Careful examination of the electrocardiogram occasionally may reveal a distinct P wave originating from the innervated atrial remnant of the recipient, and an increase in its rate may be used as an early indicator of stress. The absence of a normal reflex tachycardia in response to venous pooling accounts for the frequency of orthostatic hypotension in transplant patients.

Denervation alters the heart's response to therapeutic interventions that act directly through the cardiac autonomic nervous system. Carotid sinus massage, Valsalva maneuver, and atropine have no effect on sinoatrial node firing or atrioventricular conduction.[150] Because of depletion of myocardial catecholamine stores associated with prolonged inotropic support of the donor, the allograft often requires high doses of catecholamines.

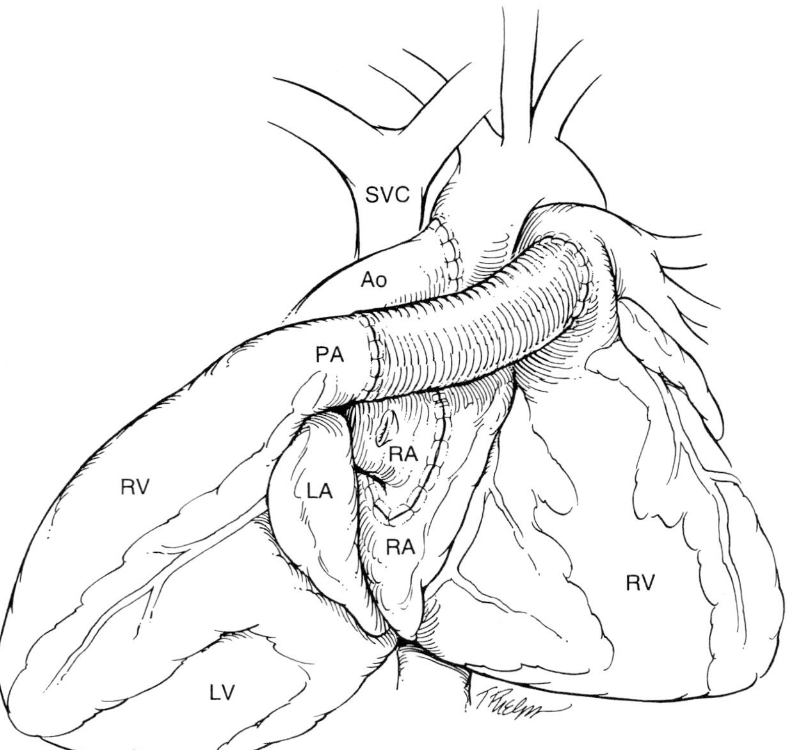

FIGURE 60–10 Heterotopic heart transplantation.

ROUTINE HEMODYNAMIC MANAGEMENT

Donor myocardial performance is transiently depressed in the immediate postoperative period. Allograft injury associated with donor hemodynamic instability and the hypothermic, ischemic insult of preservation contribute to the reduced ventricular compliance and contractility characteristics of the newly transplanted heart.[155–157] Abnormal atrial dynamics owing to the midatrial anastomosis exacerbate the reduction in ventricular diastolic loading. An infusion of epinephrine or dobutamine is initiated routinely in the operating room to provide temporary inotropic support.[157–159] Restoration of normal myocardial function usually permits the cautious weaning of inotropic support within 2 to 4 days.[160]

EARLY ALLOGRAFT FAILURE

Early cardiac failure accounts for up to 25% of perioperative deaths of transplant recipients.[160–162] The cause may be multifactorial, but the most important etiologies are pulmonary hypertension, ischemic injury during preservation, and acute rejection. Mechanical support with an intra-aortic balloon pump or ventricular assist device is indicated in cases refractory to pharmacologic interventions.[163] Retransplantation in this setting is associated with very high mortality.[164–165]

Chronic left ventricular failure frequently is associated with elevated pulmonary vascular resistance, and the unprepared donor right ventricle may be unable to overcome this increased afterload. Although recipients are screened to ensure that those with irreversible pulmonary hypertension are not considered for transplantation, right heart failure remains a leading cause of early mortality.[166–168] Initial management involves employing pulmonary vasodilators such as inhaled nitric oxide, nitroglycerin, or sodium nitroprusside. Pulmonary hypertension refractory to these vasodilators will often respond to prostaglandin E_1 (PGE_1).[169–171] Inhalation nitric oxide is considered the standard at several institutions. Intra-aortic or pulmonary artery balloon counterpulsation and right ventricular assist devices have been utilized in patients unresponsive to medical therapy.[172]

DYSRHYTHMIAS

Sinus or junctional bradycardia occurs in more than half of transplant recipients.[173] The primary risk factor for sinus node dysfunction is prolonged organ ischemia. Adequate heart rate is achieved with inotropic drug infusions and/or temporary epicardial pacing. Most bradyarrhythmias resolve over 1 to 2 weeks, although recovery may be further delayed in patients who received preoperative amiodarone therapy.[174] Theophylline has been effective in patients with bradyarrhythmias and has decreased the need for permanent pacemakers in this patient population.[175–176] Ventricular arrhythmias, primarily premature ventricular beats (PVCs) and nonsustained ventricular tachycardia, have been reported in up to 60% of recipients when monitored continuously.[177–179] Atrial fibrillation-flutter is treated with digoxin, but at a higher dose than used in the setting of an innervated heart.[180] Arrhythmias occasionally are markers for acute rejection.

SYSTEMIC HYPERTENSION

Mean arterial pressures greater than 80 mm Hg should be treated to prevent unnecessary afterload stress on the allograft. In the early postoperative period, intravenous sodium nitroprusside or nitroglycerin is administered.[181–182] Nitroglycerin is associated with less pulmonary shunting because of a relative preservation of the pulmonary hypoxic vasoconstrictor reflex.[183] If hypertension persists, an oral antihypertensive can be added to permit weaning of the parenteral agents.

Respiratory Management

The respiratory management of the cardiac transplant recipient utilizes the same protocols used following routine cardiac surgery.

Renal Function

Preoperative renal insufficiency owing to chronic heart failure and the nephrotoxic effects of cyclosporine places the recipient at increased risk of renal insufficiency. Acute cyclosporine-induced renal insufficiency usually will resolve with the reduction in cyclosporine dose. Patients at risk for renal failure initially may receive cyclosporine as a continuous intravenous infusion to eliminate the wide fluctuations in levels associated with oral dosing. Furthermore, concurrent administration of mannitol with cyclosporine may reduce its nephrotoxicity. Alternatively, some centers administer a cytolytic agent in the immediate postoperative period and delay the initiation of cyclosporine therapy.

Intermediate Care Unit and Convalescent Ward

The increasing risk of nosocomial infections with resistant organisms has led to shorter hospital stays for cardiac transplant recipients. Most patients are discharged 7 to 14 days following transplantation.[184] Patient education is performed by the cardiac nursing staff. Topics include medications (regimens and potential side effects), diet, exercise (routines and restrictions), and infection recognition.

Outpatient Follow-up

Close follow-up by an experienced transplant team is the cornerstone for successful long-term survival after cardiac transplantation. This comprehensive team facilitates the early detection of rejection, opportunistic infections, patient

TABLE 60–6 Complications associated with immunosuppressive agents

Agent	Side effect or toxicity
Corticosteroids	Water and salt retention (weight gain, hypertension), glucose intolerance, peptic and esophageal ulceration, osteoporosis, cushingoid appearance, cataracts, hypercholesterolemia, hyperlipidemia, impotence, aseptic necrosis, myopathy, psychosis, poor wound healing, easy bruising
Azathioprine	Bone marrow suppression (leukopenia, anemia, thrombocytopenia), pancreatitis, hepatitis, gastrointestinal (GI) distress (nausea, vomiting, abdominal pain, diarrhea), cholestatic jaundice, alopecia
Cyclosporine	Nephrotoxicity, hypertension, hepatotoxicity, neurotoxicity (seizures, tremor), gingival hyperplasia, hypertrichosis, hyperuricemia, pericardial effusion
Polyclonal antibodies*	Fever and chills, serum sickness, thrombocytopenia, GI distress, anemia, leukopenia, arthralgias, rash, alopecia
OKT3	Fever and chills, GI distress, leukopenia, serum sickness, bronchospasm, pulmonary edema, hypotension (peripheral vasodilatation), rash, headache
Methotrexate	Leukopenia, ulcerative stomatitis, GI distress
Cyclophosphamide	Leukopenia, hemorrhagic cystitis

*ATS/ATG = Antithymocyte sera/globulin, ALG = Antilymphocyte globulin.

noncompliance, and adverse sequelae of immunosuppression. Clinic visits routinely are scheduled concurrently with endomyocardial biopsies and include physical examination, a variety of laboratory studies, chest roentgenogram, and electrocardiogram.

IMMUNOSUPPRESSIVE THERAPY

An organism's ability to distinguish self from nonself is critical for its survival in a hostile environment. In transplantation, the recipient's host defense mechanisms recognize the human leukocyte antigens (HLA) on allograft cells as being nonself and, if permitted, will respond to eradicate the foreign cells.[185] The ultimate goal of immunosuppressive therapy is the selective modulation of the recipient's immune response to prevent rejection, while concurrently sparing immune defenses against infections or neoplasia and minimizing the toxicity associated with immunosuppressive agents (Table 60-6).

Pharmacologic Immunosuppressive Strategies

Immunosuppression following transplantation consists of an early induction phase followed by a long-term maintenance phase. This basic strategy essentially is universal, although the choice of immunosuppressive agents, dosages, and combination protocols vary among transplantation centers.[186] Since the tendency for allograft rejection is greatest in the early postoperative period, the most intense immunosuppression is administered during this induction phase. Most programs employ a triple immunosuppressive regimen while some centers also provide additional induction prophylaxis with potent polyclonal antibodies, and OKT3 or IL-2 blockers. After several months, immunosuppression and rejection surveillance are gradually reduced to chronic maintenance phase levels and frequencies.

Currently, most centers use triple drug therapy consisting of cyclosporine, steroids, and mycophenolate mofentil or azathioprine.[187] The use of a multidrug regimen permits adequate immunosuppression with reduced doses of individual agents to minimize their toxicity. The immunosuppressive regimen currently used at the Johns Hopkins Hospital is outlined in Table 60-7.

The use of cyclosporine has allowed for steroid-free maintenance immunosuppression, thus avoiding the multiple untoward sequelae associated with chronic corticosteroid therapy immunosuppression.[188–189] The timing of steroid withdrawal varies as some clinicians discontinue prednisone

TABLE 60–7 Immunosuppressive regimen for heart transplantation at the Johns Hopkins Hospital

Preoperative preparation
- Cyclosporine: 4-10 mg/kg PO (dosage based on serum creatinine)

Intraoperative management
- Methylprednisolone: 500 mg IV (after administration of protamine)

Immediate postoperative therapy
- Methylprednisolone: 125 mg/kg IV for 3 doses
- Prednisone: 1 mg/kg PO Qd tapered to 0.4 mg/kg by 2 wks
- Cyclosporine: 0.5 mg/kg/day IV until taking PO then 5-10 mg/kg/day PO

Postoperative maintenance therapy
- Prednisone: 0.2 mg/kg PO Qd
- Mycophenolate mofetil: 1 g PO/IV B.I.D.
- Cyclosporine: 5 mg/kg PO Qd (dose adjusted to maintain serum levels between 200-350 ng/mL)*

*CycloTrac SP ^{125}I RIA Kit, INCSTAR, Stillwater, MN.

within several weeks of transplantation,[188,190–191] whereas others delay the taper until 6 to 12 months posttransplantation.[189,192–193] Recently, it has been suggested that the majority of patients can be completely tapered off steroids without an increased incidence of rejection.[194] Attempts at corticosteroid withdrawal in patients with history of rejection, however, have usually been unsuccessful.[195]

Individual Immunosuppressive Agents

CORTICOSTEROIDS

Corticosteroids have played an integral role in immunosuppression since the beginning of cardiac transplantation. These nonselective agents influence essentially all limbs of the immune response.[196–198] Currently, methylprednisolone is used during induction, and prednisone is usually part of maintenance immunosuppressive regimens. Corticosteroids are also the first-line therapy for acute rejection in most centers. The numerous untoward sequelae associated with long-term corticosteroid therapy have driven clinicians to significantly reduce doses of or even eliminate these drugs from maintenance regimens.[199]

CYCLOSPORINE

Cyclosporine (cyclosporin A), a cyclic undecapeptide fungal metabolite,[200] inhibits the production of the lymphokine interleukin-2 (IL-2) by helper T-lymphocytes, attenuating cytotoxic T-lymphocyte proliferation.[201] By sparing macrophages, neutrophils, suppressor T lymphocytes, and some B lymphocytes, cyclosporine provides more selective immunosuppression compared to azathioprine and corticosteroids.[202,203] It has also permitted the reduction in corticosteroid doses in maintenance immunosuppression.[204,205] Indeed, the improved survival of cardiac recipients in the cyclosporine era is primarily secondary to a reduction in infection-related mortality likely associated with a relative preservation of host defense against microbials. Although the introduction of cyclosporine has not altered the incidence of acute rejection, it has dramatically attenuated the severity and associated morbidity of rejection episodes.[206] Doses of cyclosporine are adjusted to achieve trough serum levels between 150 and 300 ng/mL.[207–208] The low therapeutic index of cyclosporine and the wide variation in individual pharmacokinetics mandate close monitoring of levels to maximize immunosuppression while minimizing nephrotoxicity.[209–211] In light of the frequency of cyclosporine drug interactions, the initiation or discontinuation of drugs should prompt frequent measurements of levels. For patients who develop renal insufficiency, cyclosporine may be administered temporarily as a continuous infusion to reduce wide fluctuations in serum levels. Neoral, the preferred formulation, has been shown to have more predictable intestinal absorption and improved pharmacokinetics compared with the original formulation.[212–213] Nephrotoxicity and hypertension are the primary complications associated with cyclosporine.[214]

TACROLIMUS

Tacrolimus or FK506 is derived from the fungus *Streptomyces* and is an alternative to cyclosporine. Like cyclosporine, FK506 ihibits calcineurin and thus decreases the formation of IL-2.[215] Similarly, the side effect profile of FK106 also resembles cyclosporine. Furthermore, several recent studies have compared FK506 to cyclosporine and report similar survival and rejection rates and a possible improvement in the side effect profile.[216] Furthermore, recent studies have found FK506 to be most effective in reversing recalcitrant rejection.[217] This has prompted some institutions that use cyclosporine to employ FK506 as a "rescue" agent.

MYCOPHENOLATE MOFETIL

The mechanism of action of mycophenolate mofetil (MMF, or CellCept) involves lymphocyte-specific inhibition of de novo purine synthesis and has largely replaced azathioprine.[218] In randomized trials comparing MMF to azathioprine, the MMF groups had decreased mortality, while maintaining similar rejection rates.[218] MMF currently provides the most promise for the induction of allograft-specific unresponsiveness.[219]

AZATHIOPRINE

An imidazole derivative from 6-mercaptopurine, azathioprine inhibits antigen-stimulated proliferation of lymphocytes.[220] Dosage adjustments are made to maintain the leukocyte count between 4000 and 5000/mm^3. Azathioprine causes a dose-related bone marrow suppression that can be profound if administered concurrently with allopurinol.[221]

SIROLIMUS

Sirolimus, or rapamycin, is another antibiotic derived from *Streptomyces*. Rapamycin, however, inhibits the action (not the transcription) of IL-2 (and IL-4)-driven proliferation of T-lymphocytes instead of blocking IL-2 production.[222] Clinical trials are ongoing to evaluate the efficacy and toxicity of rapamycin.[223] Several studies have indicated that rapamycin is effective in cases of refractory rejection.[224–225]

POLYCLONAL ANTIBODIES

Polyclonal antibodies (antithymocyte, antilymphocyte) are produced by animals following immunization with human lymphocytes. By attaching to circulating lymphocytes and thus promoting cytolysis or opsonization by the reticuloendothelial system, these antibodies can decrease the level of circulating T cells to less than 10% of normal. The precise mechanism by which polyclonal antibodies provide their immunosuppressive effect is still under investigation. Antithymocyte globulin (ATG) and sera (ATS) have been used as part of induction therapy protocols and for rescue therapy for acute rejection refractory to corticosteroids.[226–227] Use in the immediate postoperative period permits a reduction in early corticosteroid doses and a delay in initiating cyclosporine therapy in the patient at risk of perioperative renal failure.[228–229]

OKT3

OKT3 is a murine monoclonal antibody that binds and modulates the CD3 receptor site on cytotoxic T lymphocytes interfering with antigen recognition and preventing cellular proliferation.[230–231] Like polyclonal preparations, administration of OKT3 can also eliminate almost all circulating T lymphocytes, though its monoclonal specificity prevents it from having a cytolytic effect on other circulating cells.[232] Monitoring of T3 subpopulation cell counts can be used to determine adequacy of therapy. While it has been used for induction therapy, OKT3 has demonstrated its greatest benefit on rescue therapy.[233–236] Thirty percent of patients develop antibodies against OKT3, but few patients develop high enough titers to preclude reuse of the drug in the future.[237–238] Studies comparing efficacy of OKT3 and ATG have yielded conflicting results.[239–240] Controversy exists concerning the long-term side effects of both monoclonal and polyclonal antibody therapy (i.e., increased risk of viral infections and malignancy).

Nonpharmacologic Immunosuppressive Strategies

TOTAL LYMPHOID IRRADIATION (TLI)

Fractionated delivery of radiation to lymphatic tissues using an inverted Y-mantle field provides several weeks of generalized, nonspecific immunosuppression. Experimental indications for TLI include recurrent rejection unresponsive to pharmacologic intervention and treatment-limiting toxicity associated with standard immunosuppressive agents.[241–243] Because of the potential for life-threatening bone marrow suppression, azathioprine is discontinued during TLI therapy.

PHOTOPHERESIS

Peripheral mononuclear blood cells are obtained via leukopheresis from recipients who have received a photoactivatable agent (e.g., 8-methoxypsoralen). Following ex vivo activation with ultraviolet A light, the mononuclear cells are reinfused into the recipient where they have a suppressor effect on T lymphocytes (mechanism unclear). Preliminary studies have demonstrated that this nontoxic immunomodulating technique can reverse acute rejection (including recalcitrant cases).[244–245]

APHERESIS

Apheresis procedures (e.g., therapeutic plasma exchange) permit the removal of circulating antibodies and cytokines. In the future, selective immunoabsorption filtration techniques may allow the reduction of antibodies and HLA antigens in sensitized patients as well as the removal of specific cellular subsets. Controversy exists regarding current indications for the use of apheresis.

ACUTE REJECTION

Cardiac allograft rejection is the normal host response to cells recognized as nonself. The vast majority of cases are mediated by the cellular limb of the immune response through an elegant cascade of events involving macrophages, cytokines, and T lymphocytes. Humoral-mediated rejection (also called vascular rejection) is less common. More than 80% of episodes of acute rejection occur in the first 3 months after transplantation, and most recipients will have at least one episode of rejection during this period.[246–247] The highest risk factors are female gender, human leukocyte antigen (HLA) mismatches, and allografts from younger or female donors.[248] Although 80% to 96% of episodes can be reversed with corticosteroid therapy alone,[249–251] rejection is still a major cause of morbidity in cardiac recipients.[252–253]

Diagnosis of Acute Rejection

In the era before cyclosporine, the classic clinical manifestations of acute rejection included low-grade fever, malaise, leukocytosis, pericardial friction rub, supraventricular arrhythmias, low cardiac output, reduced exercise tolerance, and signs of congestive heart failure. In the cyclosporine era, however, most episodes of rejection are characteristically insidious and patients can remain asymptomatic even with late stages of rejection. Thus, routine surveillance studies for early detection are crucial to minimize cumulative injury to the allograft.

Right ventricular endomyocardial biopsy remains the gold standard for the diagnosis of acute rejection.[254–255] The most frequently utilized technique for orthotopic allografts is a percutaneous approach through the right internal jugular vein.[256–257] Interventricular septal specimens are fixed in formalin for permanent section although frozen sections occasionally are performed if urgent diagnosis is necessary. Hemodynamic parameters may also be obtained with a pulmonary artery catheter. Complications are infrequent (1%-2%), but include venous hematoma, carotid puncture,

TABLE 60–8 ISHLT standard cardiac biopsy grading system*

Grade		Histologic findings
0	No rejection	No lymphocytic infiltration
1A	Focal, mild	Focal infiltrate without necrosis
1B	Diffuse, mild	Diffuse infiltrate without necrosis
2	Focal, moderate	One focus of aggressive infiltration and/or focal myocyte damage
3A	Multifocal, moderate rejection	Multifocal aggressive infiltration and/or myocyte damage
3B	Diffuse, borderline severe rejection	Diffuse inflammatory infiltration with myocyte necrosis
4	Severe rejection	Diffuse aggressive, WBC infiltration with myocyte necrosis; edema, hemorrhage, or vasculitis

ISHLT = International Society of Heart and Lung Transplantation.

Source: Adapted from Billingham ME, et al: A working formulation for the standardization of nomenclature in the diagnosis of heart and lung rejection: Heart rejection study group. J Heart Lung Transplant 1990; 9:587.

pneumothorax, arrhythmias, heart block, and right ventricular perforation. The exact schedule for endomyocardial biopsies varies among institutions but reflects the greater risk of rejection during the first 6 months following transplantation. Biopsies are initially performed every 7 to 10 days in the early postoperative period and eventually tapered to 3- to 6-month intervals after the first year. Suspicion of rejection warrants additional biopsies.

The pattern and density of lymphocyte infiltration in addition to the presence or absence of myocyte necrosis in the endomyocardial biopsy determine the severity grade of cellular rejection (Table 60-8).[258] Interpretation of histology may be complicated by the lymphocyte infiltration and perimyocytic fibrosis associated with cyclosporine therapy.[259–260] Inflammatory infiltrates associated with organ preservation injury or infection may also mimic rejection.[261] Etiologies of biopsy-negative allograft dysfunction include focal rejection, accelerated coronary artery disease, and occasionally, vascular (humoral-mediated) rejection.

Noninvasive studies for the diagnosis of acute rejection have been unreliable. Electrocardiographic voltage summation and E-rosette assay techniques were useful adjuncts in the early cardiac transplant experience[262]; however, they currently are of no value in patients receiving cyclosporine.[263] More recent attempts with signal-averaged electrocardiography,[264–265] echocardiography,[266–267] magnetic resonance imaging,[268] technetium ventriculography,[269] and a variety of immunologic markers[270–271] have not provided sufficient sensitivity to warrant widespread use.[272]

Treatment of Acute Rejection

Corticosteroids are the cornerstone for antirejection therapy. The treatment of choice for any rejection episode occurring during the first 1 to 3 postoperative months or for an episode considered to be severe is a short course (3 days) of intravenous methylprednisolone (1000 mg/d). Virtually all other episodes are initially treated with increased doses of oral prednisone (100 mg/d) followed by a taper to baseline over several weeks.[273] Although not yet universally accepted, many centers successfully reduce the doses of these corticosteroids with reversal rates of rejection similar to traditional dosing.[274]

Repeat endomyocardial biopsy should be performed 7 to 10 days after the cessation of antirejection therapy to assess adequacy of treatment. If the biopsy does not show significant improvement, a second trial of pulse-steroid therapy is recommended; if rejection has progressed (or if the patient becomes hemodynamically unstable), rescue therapy is indicated.

Rescue protocols for recurring or refractory rejection include methylprednisolone plus OKT3 polyclonal antibody therapy (ATS, ATG, ALG), or methotrexate.[275–277] Methotrexate has been particularly successful in eradicating chronic low-grade rejection. Clinical studies using FK-506, rapamycin, and mycophenolate mofetil have also shown to be effective and further trials are ongoing. Total lymphoid irradiation and photopheresis also demonstrate success in some cases of refractory rejection. Cardiac retransplantation is the ultimate therapeutic option for patients who do not respond to the aforementioned interventions. However, the results of retransplantation for rejection are dismal and, in most centers, it is no longer performed for this indication.

Except in the occasional case of rejection associated with significant symptoms or hemodynamic instability, the decision to treat acute rejection is complex. The risk of infection associated with increased immunosuppression must be carefully weighed against the potential sequelae of untreated rejection. Asymptomatic mild rejection (grade 1) is usually not treated but is monitored with repeat endomyocardial biopsies, because only 20% to 40% of mild cases progress to moderate rejection.[278–279] On the other hand, presence of myocyte necrosis (grades 3B and 4) represents a definite threat to allograft viability and is a universally accepted indication for therapy. Management of moderate rejection (grade 3A) is controversial and requires consideration of multiple variables.[280–281] Regardless of the biopsy results, allograft dysfunction is an indication for hospitalization, antirejection therapy, and, if severe, invasive hemodynamic monitoring and inotropic support. Interestingly, biopsy results of up to 60% of patients presenting with hemodynamically significant rejection reveal only mild or moderate rejection.[282]

Acute Vascular Rejection

Vascular rejection is mediated by the humoral limb of the immune response.[283–285] There is growing interest in antibody-mediated mechanisms of acute rejection particularly in patients with a history of treatment with cytolytic agents, an elevated panel of reactive antibodies, or multiparity.[286–287] Unlike cellular rejection, hemodynamic instability often necessitating inotropic support is common in cases of vascular rejection.[288] Diagnosis requires evidence of endothelial cell swelling on light microscopy and immunoglobulin-complement deposition by immunofluorescence techniques.[289–290] Aggressive treatment of patients with allograft dysfunction consists of plasmapheresis, high-dose corticosteroids, heparin, IgG and cyclophosphamide.[291–293] Despite these interventions, symptomatic acute vascular rejection is associated with a high mortality.[294] Repeated episodes of acute vascular rejection or chronic low-grade vascular rejection are believed to play a dominant role in the development of allograft coronary artery disease.[295–297]

INFECTIOUS COMPLICATIONS IN HEART TRANSPLANTATION

Infection is a leading cause of morbidity and mortality in the cardiac transplant population.[298–299] Impaired host defense secondary to chronic immunosuppression is the primary predisposing factor for the increased susceptibility to microbial pathogens. The introduction of cyclosporine (CsA), coincident with a more aggressive approach to diagnosis and treatment, has resulted in a dramatic reduction in the frequency and severity of transplant-related infections over the past decade.[300–302] Patients are at greatest risk of life-threatening infections in the first 3 months after transplantation and following increases in immunosuppression for acute rejection episodes or retransplantation.[298,303]

Organisms and Timing of Infections

The source of posttransplant infection may be exogenous (nosocomial, latent infection in the donor organ, and community-acquired) or endogenous (reactivation of a latent recipient infection). Table 60-9 illustrates the most common organisms causing infections in the cardiac recipient. The types of infections often follow a predictable temporal sequence following transplantation.[304–305] During the first postoperative month, nosocomial bacterial pathogens common to any patient undergoing surgery and requiring intensive care unit admission account for the majority of early infections.[306] Opportunistic pathogens (e.g., microorganisms that almost never cause severe illness in healthy

TABLE 60–9 Infections in cardiac transplant recipients

Early infections (first month)
Pneumonia
Gram-negative bacilli (GNB)
Mediastinitis and sternal wound infections
Staphylococcus epidermidis
Staphylococcus aureus
GNB
Catheter-associated bacteremia
S. epidermidis
S. aureus
GNB
Candida albicans
Urinary tract infections
GNB
Enterococcus
C. albicans
Mucocutaneous infections
Herpes simplex virus (HSV)
Candida sp.
Late infections (after first month)
Pneumonia
Diffuse interstitial pneumonia
Pneumocystis carinii
Cytomegalovirus (CMV)*
HSV
Lobar or nodular (± cavitary) pneumonia
Cryptococcus
Aspergillus
Bacteria (community-acquired, nosocomial)
Nocardia asteroides
Mycobacterium sp.
Central nervous system infections
Abscess or meningoencephalitis
Aspergillus
*Toxoplasma gondii**
Meningitis
Cryptococcus
Listeria
Gastrointestinal (GI) infections
Esophagitis
Candida albicans
HSV
Diarrhea or lower GI hemorrhage
Aspergillus
Candida sp.
Cutaneous infections
Vesicular lesions
HSV
Varicella-zoster
Nodular or ulcerating lesions
Nocardia
Candida (disseminated)
Atypical *Mycobacterium* sp.
Cryptococcus

*Known donor-transmitted pathogens.

individuals with normal cellular immunity) are responsible for the majority of infections between 1 and 6 months.[307] Thereafter, infections in the immunosuppressed recipient are caused by a mixture of community-acquired bacterial and opportunistic organisms.[308–309] Major infections are rare after the first year in the absence of recurrent acute rejection episodes.

Preventive Measures and Prophylaxis against Infection

PREOPERATIVE SCREENING

Prevention of postoperative infection begins with pretransplant screening of the donor and recipient.[310] Current suggested guidelines are outlined in Table 60-10. Potential donors or recipients with active systemic infection or positive serologies for human immunodeficiency virus (HIV) or hepatitis B virus (HBV) are not candidates for transplantation.[311] Controversy exists regarding cardiac transplantation in patients seropositive for hepatitis C virus (HCV).[312–313] Recipient prophylaxis is indicated for donors seropositive for cytomegalovirus (CMV) or *Toxoplasma gondii* if the recipient is seronegative.[314–315]

TABLE 60–10 Guidelines for routine screening and prophylaxis of infections in heart transplantation

Preoperative screening
Donor
Clinical assessment
Serologic studies (HIV, HBV, HCV, CMV, *Toxoplasma gondii*)
Recipient
History and physical examination
Serologic studies (HIV, HBV, HCV, CMV, *Toxoplasma gondii*, herpes simplex virus, varicella-zoster virus, Epstein-Barr virus, endemic fungi)
PPD (tuberculin) skin test
Urine culture
Stool for ova and parasites (*Strongyloides stercoralis*; center-specific)
Antimicrobial prophylaxis
Perioperative
First-generation cephalosporin (or vancomycin)
Postoperative
Trimethoprim-sulfamethoxazole or pentamidine (for *Pneumocystis carinii*)
Nystatin or clotrimazole (for *Candida* species)
Ganciclovir followed by acyclovir once discharged (for all patients except CMV-negative recipient and donor)
Acyclovir (for herpes simplex and zoster; routine use is controversial)
Standard endocarditis prophylaxis
Postoperative immunizations
Pneumococcal (booster every 5-7 years)
Influenza A (yearly; center-specific)

PERIOPERATIVE INFECTION PREVENTION

A first-generation cephalosporin, or vancomycin for patients with beta-lactam allergy, should be initiated prior to induction of anesthesia and continued for 48 hours following transplantation.[316] Although transplant recipients are still admitted to a private room, elaborate protective isolation procedures are no longer used.[317] Meticulous handwashing and a concerted effort to decrease the risk of infection have been shown to be effective prophylaxis.[318] Patients requiring prolonged intubation for ventilatory support may benefit from selective oropharyngeal and bowel decontamination.[319]

POSTOPERATIVE ANTIMICROBIAL PROPHYLAXIS

Trimethoprim-sulfamethoxazole (TMP/SMX) or aerosolized pentamidine (if TMP/SMX not tolerated) provide effective prophylaxis against *Pneumocystis carinii* pneumonia.[320–321] TMP/SMX also reduces the incidence of *Toxoplasma gondii, Listeria, Legionella,* and possibly *Nocardia* infections. Nystatin or clotrimazole is routinely given to prevent mucocutaneous candidiasis.[322] The frequency and severity of recurrences of herpes simplex and varicella-zoster infections can be reduced with low-dose oral acyclovir although routine prophylaxis is not universally accepted.[323] Standard endocarditis antibiotic prophylaxis is indicated prior to bacteremia-producing procedures. Recipients with a positive PPD skin test should be considered for prophylactic isoniazid (rifampin) therapy.[324]

POSTOPERATIVE IMMUNIZATIONS

Recommended postoperative vaccinations are listed in Table 60-10.[325–326] Live, attenuated virus vaccines should be avoided in the immunocompromised transplant patient. Immunization for influenza A virus is controversial as this pathogen is not responsible for significant morbidity in cardiac transplantation.[327] Exposure to measles, varicella, tetanus, or hepatitis B by a nonimmunized recipient often warrants specific immunoglobulin therapy (e.g., varicella-zoster immune globulin, VZIG).[328]

Donor-Transmitted Infection

CMV, *Toxoplasma gondii*, HBV, HCV, and HIV may be transmitted to the recipient via the donor allograft.[329–330] Ideally, recipients seronegative (SN) for CMV or *Toxoplasma* would receive appropriately SN organs to prevent the development of a life-threatening primary infection postoperatively.[331] However, due to the improvement in CMV prophylaxis and treatment, CMV serologic matching is no longer performed. Currently, the most effective prophylaxis for CMV is intravenous ganciclovir for 1 to 2 weeks followed by oral dosing for 3 months.[332]

Specific Organisms Causing Infection Following Heart Transplantation

BACTERIA

Gram-negative bacilli are the most common cause of bacterial infectious complications following heart transplantation. Furthermore, *Escherichia coli* and *Pseudomonas aeruginosa* are the most prevalent organisms and usually cause urinary tract infections and pneumonias respectively.[333] *Staphylococcus* species have been shown to cause the majority of gram-positive related infections.

VIRUS

CMV remains the most common causative pathogen in patients following cardiac transplantation.[334] Infections develop secondary to donor transmission, reactivation of latent recipient infection, or reinfection of a CMV-seropositive patient with a different viral strain.[335] Mortality from serious CMV infections has been dramatically reduced with ganciclovir. The reduction in leukocytes associated with CMV infection predisposes the patient to superinfection with other pathogens (e.g., CMV, *Pneumocystis carinii* pneumonia).[336] Although not a cure for herpes simplex or zoster viruses, acyclovir can reduce recurrences and the discomfort associated with the vesicular lesions. Epstein-Barr virus infection may be associated with posttransplant lymphoproliferative disorders in immunocompromised hosts.[337]

FUNGUS

Mucocutaneous candidiasis is common and usually can be treated with topical antifungal agents (nystatin or clotrimazole). Fluconazole is indicated for candidiasis refractory to this therapy or involving the esophagus.[338] *Aspergillus* causes a serious pneumonia in 5% to 10% of recipients during the first 3 months after transplantation and requires intravenous amphotericin B (or oral itraconazole).[339] Dissemination of *Aspergillus* to the central nervous system is almost uniformly fatal.[340]

PROTOZOA

Pneumocystis carinii is the most common cause of late pneumonia.[341] Since the organism resides in the alveoli, bronchoalveolar lavage usually is necessary for diagnosis. TMP/SMX or pentamidine are the agents of choice for treatment of this protozoa.[316–317] In addition to donor transmission, *Toxoplasma gondii* infection may be acquired from undercooked meat and cat feces. It usually causes CNS infections and is effectively treated with pyrimethamine and sulfonamides for 6 months.[342]

CHRONIC COMPLICATIONS FOLLOWING HEART TRANSPLANTATION

Allograft Coronary Artery Disease

Long-term survival of cardiac transplant recipients is primarily limited by the development of allograft coronary artery disease (ACAD), the leading cause of death after the first posttransplantation year.[343–345] Angiographically detectable ACAD is reported in approximately 50% of patients by 5 years after transplantation. The etiology of this allograft vasculopathy is multifactorial and involves both immunologic and nonimmunologic components. Recently, it has been shown that immune-related risk factors appear to be more significant in the development of ACAD.[346–348] Likewise, many nonimmune-associated related risks have been implicated in ACAD including increased donor age, hyperlipidemia, and CMV infection.[349–352] These immune and nonimmune risk factors lead to unique coronary pathology characterized by diffuse, concentric intimal proliferation with infiltration by smooth muscle cells and macrophages leading to narrowing along the entire length of the vessel.[353–354] Furthermore, collateral vessels are notably absent. ACAD may begin within several weeks posttransplantation and insidiously progress at an accelerated rate to complete obliteration of the coronary lumen with allograft failure secondary to ischemia.[355]

The clinical diagnosis of ACAD is difficult and complicated by allograft denervation resulting in silent myocardial ischemia. Ventricular arrhythmias, congestive heart failure, and sudden death are commonly the initial presentation of significant ACAD. Noninvasive screening tests (e.g., thallium scintigraphy) are unreliable in transplant recipients.[356] Annual coronary angiogram is the current gold standard for ACAD surveillance. However, due to the previously mentioned pathological changes, it underestimates the extent of disease and is insensitive to early atherosclerotic lesions.[357] This has led to growing interest in intravascular ultrasound (IVUS) devices.

IVUS is better equipped to provide important quantitative information regarding vessel wall morphology and the degree of intimal thickening.[358–359] Some centers have begun to use IVUS for the early detection of ACAD; however, concerns have been raised concerning its ability to assess more long-term lesions.[360] Currently, the only definitive treatment for advanced ACAD is retransplantation due to the diffuse and distal nature of ACAD. Based on this lack of effective treatment options, an emphasis has been placed on prevention of ACAD. Currently, prophylactic management focuses on empiric risk factor modification (dietary and pharmacologic reduction of serum cholesterol, cessation of smoking, hypertension control, etc.). Several studies have demonstrated a decrease in ACAD in patients treated with a calcium channel blocker or HMG-CoA reductase inhibitors.[348,361]

Renal Dysfunction

Irreversible interstitial fibrosis caused by cyclosporine nephrotoxicity is chiefly responsible for the chronic renal dysfunction observed in cardiac transplant recipients.[362–363] Its pathogenesis is unclear but is believed to be secondary to afferent arteriolar vasoconstriction with secondary ischemia.[364–365] Direct tubular toxicity also may play a contributory role.[366] Most renal injury occurs during the first 6 months following transplantation concurrent with the highest levels of cyclosporine. Little additional decline in renal function occurs after 1 year.[367] Frequent monitoring of cyclosporine levels and avoidance of intravascular volume depletion are important preventive measures.[368] Approximately 3% to10% of patients develop end-stage renal failure requiring dialysis or renal transplantation.[369]

Hypertension

Moderate to severe systemic hypertension afflicts 50% to 90% of cardiac transplant recipients and is a difficult problem to manage.[370] Peripheral vasoconstriction in combination with fluid retention seem to play the greatest role. Although the exact mechanisms are unclear, it likely involves a combination of cyclosporine-induced tubular nephrotoxicity and vasoconstriction of renal and systemic arterioles mediated by sympathetic neural activation.[371–373] No single class of antihypertensive agents has proven uniformly effective, and treatment of this refractory hypertension remains empiric and difficult.

Malignancy

Chronic immunosuppression is associated with an increased incidence of malignancy.[374–375] The estimated risk of carcinoma in transplant recipients is almost 100-fold greater than in the general population.[376] Lymphoproliferative disorders[377–378] and carcinoma of the skin[379] are the most common malignancies found in heart transplant recipients. Attenuation of T-lymphocyte control over Epstein-Barr virus (EBV)–stimulated B-lymphocyte proliferation appears to be the primary mechanism for the development of lymphoproliferative disorders.[380–382] The risk of these malignancies is increased further following monoclonal and polyclonal antibody therapy.[383] Unlike lymphomas in nontransplant patients, these lymphoproliferative disorders demonstrate a predilection for unusual extranodal locations (e.g., lung, bowel, and brain).[384] Treatment options in transplantation include a reduction in immunosuppression and high-dose acyclovir (to attenuate EBV replication) in addition to conventional therapies for carcinoma (chemotherapy, radiation therapy, and surgical resection).[385–387] Despite these efforts, mortality remains high.

Other Chronic Complications

Hyperlipidemia eventually develops in the majority of recipients and is managed with dietary restrictions, exercise, and lipid-lowering agents.[388] Other complications that commonly contribute to posttransplant morbidity include osteoporosis,[389] avascular necrosis of weight-bearing joints,[390] obesity,[391] and cholelithiasis.[392–393]

CARDIAC RETRANSPLANTATION

Retransplantation accounts for fewer than 3% of the cardiac transplants currently performed.[10] Primary indications for retransplantation are allograft coronary artery disease and refractory acute rejection.[394–395] The operative technique and immunosuppressive regimen are similar to those employed for the initial transplantation.[396] Despite reduced mortality in the cyclosporine era, actuarial survival remains markedly reduced following retransplantation if performed within 6 months of the initial procedure or in the setting of acute rejection.[395,397] A recently completed study showed that the survival rate for cardiac retransplantation at 1 year was 55%.[396]

Interestingly, however, recent data from the International Society for Heart and Lung Transplantation (ISHLT) shows that if retransplantation occurs 2 years after the initial transplant procedure, the 1-year survival rate markedly improves but remains approximately 4% to 6% below that of primary cardiac transplantation.[10]

RESULTS OF HEART TRANSPLANTATION

Operative (i.e., 30-day) mortality for cardiac transplantation ranges from 5% to 10%.[398] Primary graft failure is the most frequent cause of early death. Overall 1-year survival is approximately 80% with a 4% mortality per year for subsequent years.[10] Infection and rejection account for the majority of deaths in the first 6 months; thereafter, accelerated coronary artery disease eventually claims the lives of most recipients. Risk factors associated with increased mortality include ventilator dependence, previous cardiac transplantation, preoperative ventricular assist device or balloon pump, recipient age greater than 65 years, female gender (donor or recipient), and donor age greater than 50 years.[10]

Studies examining the health-related quality of life (HRQOL) in patients following cardiac transplantation demonstrate that most experience a HRQOL that approaches that of the normal population.[399–400] Although cardiac reserve is reduced, exercise tolerance is improved dramatically compared to preoperative level, and recipients usually can enjoy an active lifestyle.[401] Nevertheless, because of concerns about future disability, recipients often encounter significant problems with postoperative employment and health insurance coverage particularly if over 50 years of age.[402]

FUTURE

As a result of a series of unprecedented advances over the past drecade, the clinical outcome of heart transplantation has dramatically improved. Although cardiac replacement remains the best therapeutic option for patients with end-stage heart failure, a number of challenges await future investigators to further improve survival and reduce transplant-related morbidity.

A major factor limiting long-term survival of recipients is allograft rejection and the untoward effects of immunosuppression. Development of reliable, noninvasive diagnostic studies will permit more frequent evaluations for the early detection of rejection and for monitoring the effectiveness of therapy. Ultimately, this will allow more precise control of immunosuppression, and in turn a reduction in cumulative allograft injury and infectious complications.

Immunosuppressive strategists will continue their efforts to establish specific unresponsiveness to antigens of transplanted organs in hopes of preserving much of the recipient's immune responses. Novel immunosuppressive agents and techniques are under continuous investigation for this purpose. Alternatively, donor organs may be made less susceptible to immunologic attack through genetic engineering techniques by altering the expression of cell membrane-bound molecules. This approach is being currently utilized in the pursuit of clinically applicable xenotransplant sources.

Xenografts eventually may be an additional source of donor organs, although extended xenograft survival remains an elusive goal. Complicating this alternative are unresolved ethical issues concerning transgenic experimentation and the potential for transmission of veterinary pathogens to an immunosuppressed recipient.

Future improvements in organ preservation permitting extension of the storage interval will have several benefits. In addition to a modest increase in the donor pool, extension of storage times would permit better allocation of organs with respect to donor-recipient immunologic matching. There is growing evidence that human lymphocyte antigen (HLA) matching may be important for long-term graft function through attenuation of chronic rejection. Reducing the ischemic injury may also result in an attenuation of transplant coronary artery disease.

Finally, mechanical assist devices are being used more frequently in patients with end-stage heart failure and may prove to be the best solution for the current organ shortage. Assist devices are being currently used both as a bridge to transplantation and a destination therapy. The Randomized Evaluation of Mechanical Assistance for the Treatment of Congestive Heart Failure (REMATCH) study demonstrated a survival benefit in heart failure patients in which assist devices were utilized versus all other forms of treatment for heart failure.[61] It appears that as the technology of assist devices continues to improve, it is only a matter of time before they become a long-term solution for patients with severe congestive heart failure.

Clearly, in light of the advancements witnessed over recent years, solutions to many of the aforementioned obstacles in cardiac transplantation are within reach in the foreseeable future. Further research into these solutions will require dedicated resources and financial investments from government agencies, foundations, and interested organizations.

REFERENCES

1. Carrel A, Guthrie CC: The transplantation of veins and organs. *Am Med* 1905; 10:1101.
2. Carrel A: The surgery of blood vessels. *Johns Hopkins Hosp Bull* 1907; 18:18.
3. Mann FC, Priestly JT, Markowitz J, et al: Transplantation of the intact mammalian heart. *Arch Surg* 1993; 26:219.
4. Demikhov VP: *Experimental Transplantation of Vital Organs*. Haigh B. (trans). New York, Consultants' Bureau, 1962.
5. Lower RR, Shumway NE: Studies on the orthotopic homotransplantation of the canine heart. *Surg Forum* 1960; 11:18.
6. Hardy JD, Chavez CM, Kurrus FD, et al: Heart transplantation in man. *JAMA* 1964; 188:114.
7. Barnard CN: A human cardiac transplant: an interim report of a successful operation performed at Groote Schuur Hospital, Capetown. *S Afr Med J* 1967; 41:1271.
8. Caves PK, Stinson EB, Billingham ME, et al: Percutaneous endomyocardial biopsy in human heart recipients. *Ann Thorac Surg* 1973; 16:325.
9. Oyer PE, Stinson EB, Jamieson SA, et al: Cyclosporin A in cardiac allografting: a preliminary experience. *Transplant Proc* 1983; 15:1247.
10. Steinman TI, Becker BN, Frost AE, et al: Guidelines for the referral and management of patients eligible for solid organ transplantation. *Transplantation* 2001; 71:1189.
11. Hosenpud JD, Leah BE, Keck BM, et al: The Registry of the International Society for Heart and Lung Transplantation: Eighteenth Official Report—2001. *J Heart Lung Transplant* 2001; 20:805.
12. Stevenson LW, Perloff JK: The dilated cardiomyopathies: clinical aspects. *Cardiol Clin* 1988; 6:187.
13. Ad Hoc Committee for Cardiothoracic Surgical Practice Guidelines: transplantation (heart, lung, heart-lung) and heart assist devices: I. *Ann Thorac Surg* 1994; 58:903.
14. Stevenson LW, Tillisch JH, Hamilton M, et al: Importance of hemodynamic response to therapy in predicting survival with ejection fraction <20 percent secondary to ischemic or nonischemic dilated cardiomyopathy. *Am J Cardiol* 1990; 66:1348.
15. Lee WH, Packer M: Prognostic importance of serum sodium concentration and its modification by converting enzyme inhibition in patients with severe heart failure. *Circulation* 1986; 73:257.
16. Mancini DM, Eisen H, Kussmaul W, et al: Value of peak exercise oxygen consumption for optimal timing of cardiac transplantation in ambulatory patients with heart failure. *Circulation* 1991; 83:778.
17. Unverferth DV, Magorien RD, Moeschberger ML, et al: Factors influencing the one-year mortality of dilated cardiomyopathy. *Am J Cardiol* 1984; 54:147.

18. Cohn JN, Levine TB, Olivari MT, et al: Plasma norepinephrine as a guide to prognosis in patients with chronic congestive heart failure. *N Engl J Med* 1984; 311:819.
19. Keogh AM, Baron DW, Hickie JB: Prognostic guides in patients with idiopathic or ischemic dilated cardiomyopathy assessed for cardiac transplantation. *Am J Cardiol* 1990; 65:903.
20. Cohn JN, Johnson GR, Shabetai R, et al: Ejection fraction, peak exercise oxygen consumption, cardiothoracic ratio, ventricular arrhythmias, and plasma norepinephrine as determinants of prognosis in heart failure. *Circulation* 1993; 87(suppl):VI-5.
21. Miller LW, Pennington DG, Kanter K, et al: Heart transplantation in patients over 55 years of age. *J Heart Transplant* 1986; 5:367.
22. Laks H, Marelli D, Odim J, et al: Heart transplantation in the young and elderly. *Heart Failure Rev* 2001; 6:221.
23. Frazier OH, Radovancevic B, Abou-Awdi N, et al: Cardiac transplantation in patients over 60 years of age. *Ann Thorac Surg* 1997; 64:1866.
24. Myers J, Gullestad L, Vagelos R, et al: Clinical, hemodynamic and cardiopulmonary exercise test determinants of survival in patients referred for evaluation of heart failure. *Ann Intern Med* 1998; 129:286.
25. Erickson KW, Costanzo-Nordin MR, O'Sullivan EJ, et al: Influence of preoperative transpulmonary gradient on late mortality after orthotopic heart transplantation. *J Heart Transplant* 1990; 9:526.
26. Kormos RL, Thompson M, Hardesty RL, et al: Utility of preoperative right heart catheterization data as a predictor of survival after heart transplantation. *J Heart Transplant* 1986; 5:391.
27. Kirklin JK, Naftel DC, Kirklin JW, et al: Pulmonary vascular resistance and the risk of heart transplantation. *J Heart Transplant* 1988; 7:331.
28. Addonizio LJ, Gersony WM, Robbins RC, et al: Elevated pulmonary vascular resistance and cardiac transplantation. *Circulation* 1987; 76(suppl V):52.
29. Stinson EB, Griepp RB, Schroeder JS, et al: Hemodynamic observations one and two years after cardiac transplantation in man. *Circulation* 1972; 45:1183.
30. Griepp RB, Stinson EB, Dong EJ, et al: Determinants of operative risk in human heart transplantation. *Am J Surg* 1971; 122:192.
31. Losman JG, Barnard CN: Heterotopic heart transplantation: a valid alternative to orthotopic transplantation: results, advantages, and disadvantages. *J Surg Res* 1982; 32:297.
32. Desruennes M, Muneretto C, Gandjbakhch I, et al: Heterotopic heart transplantation: current status in 1988. *J Heart Transplant* 1989; 8:479.
33. Munoz E, Lonquist J, Radovancevic B, et al: Long-term results in diabetic patients undergoing cardiac transplantation. *J Heart Transplant* 1991; 10:189.
34. Rhenman MJ, Rhenman B, Icenogle T, et al: Diabetes and heart transplantation. *J Heart Transplant* 1988; 7:356.
35. Renlund DG, O'Connell JB, Gilbert EM, et al: Feasibility of discontinuation of corticosteroid maintenance therapy in heart transplantation. *J Heart Transplant* 1987; 6:71.
36. Szentpetery S, Richardson J, Hanrahan J, et al: Cardiac transplantation without oral steroids: the McGuire VA Hospital experience [abstract]. *J Heart Transplant* 1989; 8:103.
37. Mai FM, McKenzie FN, Kostuk WJ, et al: Psychiatric aspects of heart transplantation: preoperative evaluation and postoperative sequela. *Br Med J* 1986; 292:311.
38. Holland C, Hagan M, Volkman K, et al: Substance abuse: does this warrant exclusion for transplant? [abstract]. *J Heart Transplant* 1988; 7:70.
39. Hanrahan JS, Taylor DO, Eberly C, et al: Cardiac allograft survival reformed substance abusers [abstract]. *J Heart Lung Transplant* 1991; 1:158.
40. Bristow MR, O'Connell JB, Gilbert EM, et al: Dose response of chronic beta blocker treatment in heart failure from either idiopathic dilated or ischemic cardiomyopathy. *Circulation* 1994; 89:1632.
41. Packer M, Coats AJ, Fowler MB, et al: Effect of carvedilol on survival in severed chronic heart failure. *N Engl J Med* 2001; 344: 1651.
42. The SOLVD Investigators: Effect of enalapril on survival in patients with reduced left ventricular ejection fractions and congestive heart failure. *N Engl J Med* 1991; 325:293.
43. Pitt B, Zannad F, Remme WJ, et al: The effect of spironolactone on morbidity and mortality in patients with severe heart failure. *N Engl J Med* 1999; 341:709.
44. Leier CV, Binkley PF: Parenteral inotropic support for advanced congestive heart failure. *Prog Cardiovasc Dis* 1998; 41: 207.
45. Canver CC, Chandra J: Milrinone for long term pharmacologic support of status I heart transplant candidates. *Ann Thorac Surg* 2000; 69:1823.
46. Bank AJ, Mir SH, Nguyen DQ, et al: Effects of left ventricular assist devices on outcomes in patients undergoing heart transplantation. *Ann Thorac Surg* 2000; 69:1369.
47. Morales DLS, Catanese KA, Helman DN, et al: Six year experience of caring for forty-four patients with left ventricular assist device at home: safe, economical, necessary. *J Thorac Cardiovasc Surg* 2000; 119:251.
48. Hardesty RL, Griffith BP, Trento A, et al: Mortally ill patients and excellent survival following cardiac transplantation. *Ann Thorac Surg* 1986; 41:126.
49. Peric M, Frazier OH, Macris M, et al: Intra-aortic balloon pump as a bridge to transplantation [abstract]. *J Heart Transplant* 1986; 5:380.
50. Slaughter MS, Ward HB: Heart failure in the elderly. *Clin Geriatr Med* 2000;16:3.
51. Hodgson JM, Aja M, Sorkin RP: Intermittent ambulatory dobutamine infusions for patients awaiting cardiac transplantation. *Am J Cardiol* 1984; 53:375.
52. Miller LW: Ambulatory inotropic therapy as a bridge to cardiac transplantation. *J Am Coll Cardiol* 1987; 9:89A.
53. Dies F: Intermittent dobutamine in ambulatory patients with chronic cardiac failure. *Circulation* 1986; 74(suppl):II-39.
54. Leier CV, Huss RN, Lewis RP, et al: Drug-induced conditioning in congestive heart failure. *Circulation* 1982; 65:1382.
55. Unverferth DV, Magorien RD, Lewis RP, et al: Long-term benefit of dobutamine in patients with congestive cardiomyopathy. *Am Heart J* 1980; 100:622.
56. Pennington DG, McBride LR, Kanter KR, et al: Bridging to heart transplantation with circulatory support devices. *J Heart Transplant* 1989; 8:116.
57. Miller LW: Mechanical assist devices in intensive cardiac care. *Am Heart J* 1991; 121:1887.
58. Pennington DG, Joyce LD, Pae WE Jr, et al: Patient selection [panel discussion]. *Ann Thorac Surg* 1989; 47:77.
59. Birovljev S, Radovancevic B, Burnell BL, et al: Heart transplantation after mechanical circulatory support: four years experience. *J Heart Lung Transplant* 1992; 11:240.
60. Pennington DG, Oaks TE, Lohmann DP: Permanent ventricular assist device support versus cardiac transplantation. *Ann Thorac Surg* 1999; 68:729.
61. Rose EA, Gelijns AC, Moskowitz AJ, et al: Long-term use of a left ventricular assist device for end-stage heart failure. *N Engl J Med* 2001; 345:1435.
62. Bolling S, Deeb GM, Morady F, et al: Automatic internal cardioverter defibrillator: a bridge to heart transplantation. *J Heart Lung Transplant* 1991; 10:562.

63. Jeevanandam V, Bielefeld M, Auteri J, et al: The implantable defibillator: an electronic bridge to cardiac transplantation.*Circulation* 1992; 86(suppl):II-276.
64. Stevenson WG, Stevenson LW, Weiss J, et al: Programmed ventricular stimulation in severe heart failure: high, short-term risk of sudden death despite noninducibility. *Am Heart J* 1988; 116:1447.
65. Auricchio A, Stellbrink C, Block M, et al: Effect of pacing chamber and atrioventricular delay on acute systolic function of pace patients with congestive heart failure. *Circulation* 1999; 99:2993.
66. Moss AJ, Hall WJ, Cannom DS, et al: Improved survival with an implanted defibrillator in patients with coronary disease at high risk for ventricular arrhythmia. *N Engl J Med* 1996; 335:1933.
67. Buxton AE, Lee KL, Fisher JD, et al: A randomized study of the prevention of sudden death in patients with coronary artery disease. *N Engl J Med* 1999; 341:1882.
68. Deng MC: Cardiac transplantation. *Heart* 2002; 87:177.
69. *UNOS 2000 Annual Report*. http://www.unos.org.
70. Sadler AM, Sadler BL, Statson EB: The Uniform Anatomical Gift Act. *JAMA* 1968; 206:2501.
71. The Hastings Center: *A Report on the Project on Organ Transplantation: Ethical, Legal and Policy Issues Pertaining to Solid Organ Procurement*. Hastings-on-Hudson, NY, October, 1985.
72. Omnibus Budget Reconciliation Act of 1986, Public Law 99–509.
73. Stuart FP: Need, supply and legal issues related to organ transplantation in the United States. *Transplant Proc* 1984; 16:87.
74. Miller M: A proposed solution to the present organ donation crisis based on a hard look at the past. *Circulation* 1987; 75:20.
75. Arras JD, Shinnar S: Anencephalic newborns as organ donors: a critique. *JAMA* 1988; 259:2284.
76. *Legislative Update: Transplant Action*. Alexandria, VA, American Council on Transplantation, Jan–Feb 1987; p 3.
77. *National Task Force on Organ Transplantation: Final Report*. Rockville, MD, Office of Organ Transplantation, Health Resources, and Services Administration, 1986.
78. *Minutes of the Task Force on Organ Transplantation*. United States Department of Health and Human Services, Office of Organ Transplantation. Rockville, MD, November 18, 1985.
79. Report of Ad Hoc Committee of the Harvard Medical School to Examine the Definition of Brain Death: a definition of irreversible coma. *JAMA* 1968; 205:337.
80. Mohandas A, Chou SN: Brain death: a clinical and pathological study. *J Neurosurg* 1971; 35:211.
81. Walker AE: The neurosurgeon's responsibility for organ procurement. *J Neurosurg* 1976; 44:1.
82. Uniform Brain Death Act, approved at Annual Conference of National Conference of Commissioners on Uniform State Laws, Washington, DC, July 28–August 4, 1978.
83. Jennett B: The donor doctors dilemma: observations on the recognition and management of brain death. *J Med Ethics* 1975; 1:63.
84. Pallis C: ABS of brain stem death. Pitfalls and safeguards. *Br Med J* 1982; 285:1720.
85. Goodman JM, Mishkin FS, Dyken M: Determination of brain death by isotope angiography. *JAMA* 1969; 209:1869.
86. Guerraty A, Wechsler AS: Defining the limits of suitability of cardiac allografts. *Ann Thorac Surg* 1990; 50:1.
87. Hauptman PJ, O'Connor KJ, Wolf RE, et al: Angiography in cardiac donors. *J Am Coll Cardiol* 2001; 37:1252.
88. Baumgartner WA, Reitz BA, Oyer PE, et al: Cardiac homotranplantation. *Curr Probl Surg* 1979; 16:17.
89. Wheeldon DR, Potter CD, Oduro A, et al: Transplantation of marginal donor organs [abstract]. *J Heart Lung Transplant* 1994; 13.
90. Frilman NF, Jeffers WA: Effect of progressive sympathectomy on hypertension produced by increased intracranial pressure. *Am J Physiol* 1940; 128:662.
91. Slapak M: The immediate care of potential donors for cadaveric organ transplantation. *Anaesthesia* 1978; 33:700.
92. Frist WH, Fanning WJ: Donor management and matching. *Cardiol Clin* 1990; 8:55.
93. Raferty AT, Johnson RWG: Dopamine pretreatment in unstable kidney donors. *BMJ* 1979; 1:522.
94. Rose AG, Novitzky D, Cooper DK: Myocardial and pulmonary histopathologic changes. *Transplant Proc* 1988; 20(suppl 7):29.
95. Szakals JE, Mehlman B: Pathologic changes induced by L-norepinephrine. *Am J Cardiol* 1960; 5:619.
96. Sweeney MS, Lammermeier DE, Frazier OH, et al: Extension of donor criteria in cardiac transplantation: surgical risk versus supply-side economics. *Ann Thorac Surg* 1990; 50:7.
97. Lentz RD, Brown DM, Kjellstrand CM: Treatment of severe hypophosphatemia. *Ann Intern Med* 1978; 89:941.
98. Harms J, Isemer FE, Kolenda H: Hormonal alteration and pituitary function during course of brain stem death in potential organ donors. *Transplant Proc* 1991; 23:2614.
99. Davis FD: Coordination of cardiac transplantation: patient processing and donor organ procurement. *Circulation* 1987; 75:29.
100. Salter DR, Dyke CM, Fabian JA: Cardiopulmonary dysfunction after brain death, in Fabian JA(ed): *Anesthesia for Organ Transplantation*. Philadelphia, JB Lippincott, 1992; p 81.
101. Montero JA, Mallol J, Alvarez, et al: Biochemical hypothyroidism and myocardial damage in organ donors: are they related? *Transplant Proc* 1988; 20:746.
102. Novitzky D, Cooper DKC, Reichart B: Hemodynamic and metabolic responses to hormonal therapy in brain dead potential organ donors. *Transplantation* 1987; 43:852.
103. Gifford RPM, Weaver AS, Burg JE, et al: Thyroid hormone levels in heart and kidney cadaver donors. *J Heart Transplant* 1986; 5:249.
104. Novitzky D, Wicomb WN, Cooper DKC, et al: Improved cardiac function following hormonal therapy in brain dead pigs: relevance to organ donation. *Cryobiology* 1987; 24:1.
105. Novitzky D, Cooper DKC, Zuhdi N: The physiological management of cardiac transplant donors and recipients using triiodothyronine. *Transplant Proc* 1988; 20:803.
106. Schaal SF, Sugimoto T, Wallace AG, et al: Effects of digitalis on the functional refractory period of the AV node: studies in awake dogs with and without cardiac denervation.*Cardiovasc Res* 1968; 2:356.
107. Keon KJ, Hendry PJ, Taichman GC, et al: Cardiac transplantation: the ideal myocardial temperature for graft transport. *Ann Thorac Surg* 1988; 46:337.
108. Fremes SE, Li RK, Weisel RD, et al: Prolonged hypothermic cardiac storage with University of Wisconsin solution. *J Thorac Cardiovasc Surg* 1991; 102:666.
109. Human PA, Holl J, Vosloo S, et al: Extended cardiopulmonary preservation: University of Wisconsin solution versus Bretschneider's cardioplegic solution. *Ann Thorac Surg* 1993; 55:1123.
110. Demertzis S, Wippermann J, Schaper J, et al: University of Wisconsin versus St. Thomas' Hospital solution for human donor heart preservation. *Ann Thorac Surg* 1993; 55:1131.
111. Segel LD, Follette DM, Contino JP, et al: Importance of substrate enhancement for long-term heart preservation. *J Heart Lung Transplant* 1993; 12:613.
112. Zehr KJ, Herskowitz A, Lee P, et al: Neutrophil adhesion inhibition prolongs survival of cardiac allografts with hyperacute rejection. *J Heart Lung Transplant* 1993; 12:837.
113. Pillai R, Bando K, Schueler S, et al: Leukocyte depletion results in excellent heart-lung function after 12 hours of storage. *Ann Thorac Surg* 1990; 50:211.
114. Wicomb WN, Cooper DKC, Barnard CN: Twenty-four hour preservation of the pig heart by a portable hypothermic perfusion system. *Transplantation* 1982; 34:246.

115. Ferrera R, Marcsek P, Larese A, et al: Comparison of continuous microperfusion and cold storage for pig heart preservation. *J Heart Lung Transplant* 1993; 12:463.
116. Braun WE: Laboratory and clinical management of the highly sensitized organ transplant recipient. *Hum Immunol* 1989; 26:245.
117. Loh E, Bergin JD, Couper GS, et al: Role of panel-reactive antibody crossreactivity in predicting survival after orthotopic heart transplantation. *J Heart Lung Transplant* 1994; 13:194.
118. Jarcho J, Naftel DC, Shroyer JK, et al: Influence of HLA mismatch on rejection after heart transplantation: a multiinstitutional study. *J Heart Lung Transplant* 1994; 13:583.
119. Trento A, Hardesty RL, Griffith BP, et al: Role of the antibody to vascular endothelial cells in hyperacute rejection in patients undergoing cardiac transplantation. *J Cardiovasc Surg* 1988; 95:37.
120. Weil R, Clarke DR, Iwaki Y, et al: Hyperacute rejection of transplanted human heart. *Transplantation* 1981; 32:71.
121. Forbes RDC, Guttman RD: Evidence for complement-induced endothelial injury *in vivo*: A comparative ultrastructural tracer study in a controlled model of hyperacute rate cardiac allograft rejection. *Am J Pathol* 1982; 106:378.
122. Losman JG, Campbell CD, Replogle RL: The advantages of heterotopic cardiac transplantation: critical review of initial results. *Heart Transplant* 1981; 1:53.
123. Nakatani T, Frazier OH, Lammermeier DE, et al: Heterotopic heart transplantation: a reliable option for a select group of high-risk patients. *J Heart Transplant* 1989; 8:40.
124. Cooper DKC, Novitzky D, Becerra E, et al: Are there indications for heterotopic heart transplantation in 1986? *Thorac Cardiovasc Surg* 1986; 34:300.
125. Wynands JE, Wong P, Whalley DG, et al: Oxygen-fentanyl anesthesia in patients with poor left ventricular function. *Anesth Analg* 1983; 62:476.
126. Hensley FA, Martin DE, Larach DR, et al: Anesthetic management for cardiac transplantation in North America—1986 survey. *J Cardiothorac Anesth* 1987; 1:429.
127. Royston D: Aprotinin therapy in heart and heart-lung transplantation. *J Heart Lung Transplant* 1993; 12:19.
128. Ross D: Report of a heart transplant operation. *Am J Cardiol* 1968; 22:838.
129. Yacoub M, Mankad P, Ledingham S: Donor procurement and surgical techniques for cardiac transplantation. *Semin Thorac Cardiovasc Surg* 1990; 2:153.
130. Barnard CN: What have we learned about heart transplants. *J Thorac Cardiovasc Surg* 1968; 56:457.
131. Schulman LL, Smith CR, Drusin R, et al: Patent foramen ovale complicating heart transplantation. *Chest* 1987; 92:569.
132. Baumgartner WA, Reitz BA, Achuff SC: Operative techniques utilized in heart transplantations, in Achuff SC (ed): *Heart and Heart-Lung Transplantation*. Philadelphia, WB Saunders, 1990.
133. Cabrol C, Gandjbakhch I, Pavie A, et al: Heart and heart-lung transplantation: techniques and safeguards. *J Heart Transplant* 1984; 3:110.
134. Stinson EB, Caves PK, Griepp RB, et al: Hemodynamic observation in the early period after human heart transplantation. *J Thorac Cardiovasc Surg* 1975; 69:264.
135. Blanche C, Valenza M, Aleksic I, et al: Technical considerations of a new technique for orthotopic heart transplantation. *J Cardiovasc Surg* 1994; 35:283.
136. Couetil JP, Mihaileanu S, Lavergne T, et al: Total excision of the recipient atria (TERA) in orthotopic heart transplantation (OHT) as a new clinical procedure: technical consideration and early results. *J Heart Lung Transplant* 1991; 10:101.
137. Dreyfus G, Jebara V, Mihaileanu S, et al: Total orthotopic heart transplantation: an alternative to the standard technique. *Ann Thorac Surg* 1991; 52:1181.
138. Sarsam MA, Campbell CS, Yonan NA, et al: An alternative surgical technique in orthotopic cardiac transplantation. *J Cardiovasc Surg* 1993; 8:344.
139. Gamel AE, Yonan NA, Grant S, et al: Orthotopic cardiac transplantation: a comparison of standard and bicaval Wythenshawe techniques. *J Thorac Cardiovasc Surg* 1995; 109:721.
140. Deleuze PH, Benvenuti C, Mazzucotelli JP, et al: Orthotopic cardiac transplantation with direct caval anastomosis: is it the optimal procedure? *J Thorac Cardiovasc Surg* 1995; 109:731.
141. Aziz T, Burgess M, Khafagy R, et al: Bicaval and standard techniques in orthotopic heart transplantation: medium-term experience in cardiac performance and survival. *J Thorac Cardiovasc Surg* 1999; 118:115.
142. Bailey LL: Heart transplantation techniques in complex congenital heart disease. *J Heart Lung Transplant* 1993; 12:S168.
143. Allard M, Assaad A, Bailey LL, et al: Session IV: surgical techniques in pediatric heart transplantation. *J Heart Lung Transplant* 1996; 10:808.
144. Reitz BA, Jamieson SA, Gaudiani VA, et al: Method for cardiac transplantation in corrected transposition of the great arteries. *J Thorac Cardiovasc Surg* 1982; 23:29.
145. Frazier OH, Okereke OUJ, Cooley DA, et al: Heterotopic heart transplantation in three patients at the Texas Heart Institute. *Tex Heart Inst J* 1985; 12:221.
146. Novitzky D, Cooper DKC, Barnard CN: The surgical technique of heterotopic heart transplantation. *Ann Thorac Surg* 1983; 36:476.
147. Ridley PD, Khaghani A, Musumeci F, et al: Heterotopic heart transplantation and recipient heart operation in ischemic heart disease. *Ann Thorac Surg* 1992; 54:333.
148. Baumgartner WA, Traill TA, Cameron DE, et al: Unique aspects of heart and lung transplantation exhibited in the "domino-donor" operation. *JAMA* 1989; 261:3121.
149. Oaks TE, Aravot D, Dennis C, et al: Domino heart transplantation: the Papworth experience. *J Heart Lung Transplant* 1994; 13:433.
150. Stinson EB, Schroeder JS, Griepp RB, et al: Observations on the behavior of recipient atria after cardiac transplantation in man. *Am J Cardiol* 1972; 30:615.
151. Urelsky BF: Physiology of the transplanted heart. *Cardiovasc Clin* 1990; 20:23.
152. Fowles RE, Reitz BA, Ream AK, Kaplan J: Drug actions in a transplanted or artificial heart, in Kaplan J (ed): *Cardiac Anesthesia*. New York, Grune & Stratton, 1983.
153. Griepp RB, et al: Hemodynamic performance of the transplanted human heart. *Surgery* 1971; 70:88.
154. Pope SE, et al: Exercise response of the denervated heart in long-term cardiac transplant recipients. *Am J Cardiol* 1980; 46:213.
155. Tischler MD, Lee RT, Plappert T, et al: Serial assessment of left ventricular function and mass after orthotopic heart transplantation: a four-year longitudinal study. *J Am Coll Cardiol* 1992; 19:60.
156. Stinson EB, Griepp RB, Bieber CP, et al: Hemodynamic observations after orthotopic transplantation of the canine heart. *J Thorac Cardiovasc Surg* 1972; 63:344.
157. Stinson EB, Caves PK, Griepp RB, et al: The transplanted heart in the postoperative period. *Surg Forum* 1983; 24:189.
158. Sonnenblick EH, Frishman WH, LeJemtel TH: Dobutamine: a new synthetic cardioactive sympathetic amine. *N Engl J Med* 1979; 300:17.
159. Cannon DS, Rider AK, Stinson EB, et al: Electrophysiological studies in the denervated transplanted heart, II: response to norepinephrine, isoproterenol and propranolol. *Am J Cardiol* 1975; 36:859.
160. Bourge RC, Naftel DC, Costanzo-Nordin MR, et al: Pretransplantation risk factors for death after heart transplantation: a multiinstitutional study. *J Heart Lung Transplant* 1993; 12:549.

161. Costanzo-Nordin MR, Heroux AL, Radvany R, et al: Role of humoral immunity in acute cardiac allograft dysfunction. *J Heart Lung Transplant* 1993; 12:S143.
162. Reemtsma K, Hardy MA, Drusin RE, et al: Cardiac transplantation: changing patterns in evaluation and treatment. *Ann Surg* 1985; 202:418.
163. Kanter KR, Pennington DG, McBride LR, et al: Mechanical circulatory assistance after heart transplantation. *J Heart Transplant* 1987; 6:150.
164. Dein JR, Oyer PE, Stinson ER, et al: Cardiac retransplantation in the cyclosporine era. *Ann Thorac Surg* 1989; 48:350.
165. Karwande SV, Ensley RD, Renlund DG, et al: Cardiac retransplantation: a viable option? *Ann Thorac Surg* 1992; 54:840.
166. Baumgartner WA, Reitz BA, Oyer PE, et al: Cardiac transplantation. *Curr Probl Surg* 1979; 16:6.
167. Murali S, Urelsky BF, Armitage JM, et al: Utility of prostaglandin E_1 in the pretransplantation evaluation of heart failure patients with significant pulmonary hypertension. *J Heart Lung Transplant* 1992; 11:716.
168. Kirklin JK, Naftel DC, McGiffin DC, et al: Analysis of morbid events and risk factors for death after cardiac transplantation. *J Am Coll Cardiol* 1988; 11:917.
169. D'Ambra MN, LaRaia PJ, Philbin DM, et al: Prostaglandin E_1: a new therapy for refractory right heart failure and pulmonary hypertension after mitral valve replacement. *J Thorac Cardiovasc Surg* 1985; 89:567.
170. Armitage JM, Hardy RL, Griffith BP: Prostaglandin E_1: an effective treatment of right heart failure after orthotopic heart transplantation. *J Heart Transplant* 1987; 6:348.
171. Esmore DS, Spratt PM, Branch JM, et al: Right ventricular assist and prostacyclin infusion for allograft failure in the presence of high pulmonary vascular resistance. *J Heart Transplant* 1990; 9:136.
172. Odom NJ, Richens D, Glenville BE, et al: Successful use of mechanical assist device for right ventricular failure after orthotopic heart transplantation. *J Heart Transplant* 1990; 9:652.
173. Jacquet L, Ziady G, Stein K, et al: Cardiac rhythm disturbances early after orthotopic heart transplantation. *J Am Coll Cardiol* 1990; 16:832.
174. Cameron DE, Augustine SM, Gardner TJ, et al: Preoperative amiodarone therapy causes graft bradycardia following orthotopic heart transplantation. *J Heart Transplant* 1988; 7:67.
175. Redmond JM, Zehr K, Gillinov MA, et al: Use of theophylline for treatment of prolonged sinus node dysfunction in human orthotopic heart transplantation [abstract]. *J Heart Lung Transplant* 1992; 11:203.
176. Bertolet BD, Eagle DA, Conti JB, et al: Bradycardia after heart transplantation: reversal with theophylline. *J Am Coll Cardiol* 1996; 28:396.
177. Corcos T, Tamburino C, Leger P, et al: Early and late hemodynamic evaluation after cardiac transplantation. *J Am Coll Cardiol* 1988; 1:264.
178. Romhilt DW, Doyle M, Sagar KB, et al: Prevalence and significance of arrhythmias in long term survivors of cardiac transplantation. *Circulation* 1982; 66(suppl 1):219.
179. Little RE, Kay GN, Epstein AE, et al: Arrhythmias after orthotopic cardiac transplantation: Prevalence and determinants during initial hospitalization and late follow-up. *Circulation* 1989; 80:III-140.
180. Goodman DJ, Rossen RM, Cannon DS, et al: Effect of digoxin on atrioventricular conduction: studies in patients with and without cardiac autonomic innervation. *Circulation* 1975; 51:251.
181. Flaherty JT, Magee PA, Gardner TL, et al: Comparison of intravenous nitroglycerin and sodium nitroprusside for treatment of acute hypertension developing after coronary artery bypass surgery. *Circulation* 1982; 65:1072.
182. Bixler TJ, Gardner TJ, Donahoo JS, et al: Improved myocardial performance in postoperative cardiac surgical patients with sodium nitroprusside. *Ann Thorac Surg* 1978; 25:444.
183. Hill NS, Antman EM, Green LH, et al: Intravenous nitroglycerin: a review of pharmacology, indications, therapeutic effects and complications. *Chest* 1981; 79:69.
184. Holt C, Fandrich R, Leonard L, et al: Nursing strategy to allow early discharge after cardiac transplantation: is it safe? *J Heart Transplant* 1990; 9:84.
185. Bach FH, Sachs DH: Transplantation immunology. *N Engl J Med* 1987; 317:489.
186. Evans R, Manninen DL, Dong FB, et al: Immunosuppressive therapy as a determinant of transplantation outcomes. *Transplantation* 1993; 55:1297.
187. Ranjit J, Rajasinghe HA, Chen JM, et al: Long-term outcomes after cardiac transplantation: an experience based on different eras of immunosuppressive therapy. *Ann Thorac Surg* 2001; 72:440.
188. Price GD, Olsen SL, Taylor DO, et al: Corticosteroid-free maintenance immunosuppression after heart transplantation: feasibility and beneficial effects. *J Heart Lung Transplant* 1992; 11:403.
189. Miller LW, Wolford T, McBride LR, et al: Successful withdrawal of corticosteroids in heart transplantation. *J Heart Lung Transplant* 1992; 11:431.
190. Keogh A, Macdonald P, Mundy J, et al: Five-year follow-up of a randomized double-drug versus triple-drug therapy immunosuppressive trial after heart transplantation. *J Heart Lung Transplant* 1992; 11:550.
191. Katz M, Barnhardt G, Szentpetery S, et al: Are steroids essential for successful maintenance of immunosuppression in heart transplant patients? *J Heart Lung Transplant* 1987; 6:293.
192. Kobashigawa JA, Stevenson LW, Brownfield ED, et al: Initial success of steroid weaning late after heart transplantation. *J Heart Lung Transplant* 1992; 11:428.
193. Olivari MT, Jessen ME, Baldwin BJ, et al: Triple-drug immunosuppression with steroid discontinuation by six months after heart transplantation. *J Heart Lung Transplant* 1995; 14:127.
194. Oaks TE, Wannenberg T, Close SA, et al: Steroid-free maintenance immunosuppression after heart transplantation. *Ann Thorac Surg* 2001; 72:102.
195. Miller LW, Wolford T, McBride LR, et al: Successful withdrawal of corticosteroids in heart transplantation. *J Heart Transplant* 1992; 11:431.
196. Chan GLC, Gruber SA, Skjei KL, et al: Principles of immunosuppression. *Crit Care Clin* 1990; 6:841.
197. Woodley SL, Renlund DG, O'Connell JB, et al: Immunosuppression following cardiac transplantation. *Cardiol Clin* 1990; 8:83.
198. Lan NC, Karin M, Nguyen T, et al: Mechanisms of glucocorticoid hormone action. *J Steroid Biochem* 1984; 20:77.
199. Livi U, Luciani GB, Boffa GM, et al: Clinical results of steroid-free induction immunosuppression after heart transplantation. *Ann Thorac Surg* 1993; 55:1160.
200. Borel JF, White DJG: The history of cyclosporin A and its significance, in White DJG (ed): *Cyclosporin A: Proceedings of an International Conference on Cyclosporin A*. New York, Elsevier Biomedical, 1982.
201. Hess AD, Tutschka PJ: Effect of cyclosporin A on human lymphocytic responses in vivo. *J Immunol* 1980; 124:2601.
202. Cohen DJ, Loertscher R, Rubin MF, et al: Cyclosporine: a new immunosuppressive agent for organ transplantation. *Ann Intern Med* 1984; 101:667.
203. Borel JF: Immunological properties of cyclosporin A. *J Heart Transplant* 1982; 1:237.

204. Griffith BP, et al: Cardiac transplantation with cyclosporin A and prednisone. *Ann Surg* 1982; 196:324.
205. Griffith BP, et al: Powerful but limited immunosuppression for cardiac transplantation with cyclosporine and low-dose steroid. *J Thorac Cardiovasc Surg* 1984; 87:35.
206. Merion RM, White DJG, Calne RY: Early renal rejection episodes are less aggressive with cyclosporin A immunosuppression. *Transplant Proc* 1983; 15:2172.
207. Hausen B, Demertzis S, Rohde R, et al: Low-dose cyclosporine therapy in triple-drug immunosuppression for heart transplant recipients. *Ann Thorac Surg* 1994; 58:999.
208. Valantine HA: Long-term management and results in heart transplant recipients. *Cardiol Clin* 1990; 8:141.
209. Kahan BD, Ried M, Newberger J: Pharmacokinetics of cyclosporine in human renal transplantation. *Transplant Proc* 1983; 15:446.
210. Keown PA, Stiller CR, Sinclair NR, et al: The clinical relevance of cyclosporine blood vessels as measures by radioimmunoassay. *Transplant Proc* 1983; 15(suppl I):I-2438.
211. Lemaire M, Fahr A, Maurer G: Pharmacokinetics of cyclosporin: inter and intra-individual variations and metabolic pathways. *Transplant Proc* 1990; 22:1110.
212. Holt DW: The pharmacokinetics of Sandimmune Neoral—a new oral formulation of cyclosporin. The Third International Congress on Cyclosporin, Seville, Spain, 1994; p 128.
213. Neumayer HH, Faber L, Haller P, et al: Conversion of Sandimmune to Sandimmune Neoral: experience in 300 patients after renal transplantation. The Third International Congress on Cyclosporin, Seville, Spain, 1994; p 131.
214. Myers BD, et al: Cyclosporine-associated chronic nephropathy. *N Engl J Med* 1984; 311:699.
215. Cotts WG, Johnson MR: The challenge of rejection and cardiac allograft vasculopathy. *Heart Failure Rev* 2001; 6:227.
216. Taylor DO, Barr ML, et al: A randomized, multicenter comparison of tacrolimus and cyclosporine immunosuppressive regimens in cardiac transplantation: decreased hyperlipidemia and hypertension with tacrolimus. *J Heart Lung Transplant* 1999; 18:336.
217. Meiser BM, Fuchs UA, Schmidt D, et al: Single center randomized trial comparing tacrolimus (FK 506) and cyclosporine in the prevention of acute myocardial rejection. *J Heart Lung Transplant* 1998; 17:782.
218. Koegh A, Bourge R, Costanzo M, et al.: Three year results of the double-blinded randomized multicenter trial of mycophenolate Mofetil in heart transplant patients. *J Heart Lung Transplant* 1999; 18:53. title.
219. Taylor DO, Ensley D, Olsen SL, et al: Mycophenolate Mofetil (RS-61443): Preclinical, clinical and three year experience in heart transplantation. *J Heart Lung Transplant* 1994; 13:571.
220. Elion GB: Pharmacologic and physical agents: immunosuppressive agents. *Transplant Proc* 1978; 9:975.
221. McCormack JJ, Johns DG, Chabner B: Purine antimetabolites, in Chabner B (ed): *Pharmacologic Principles of Cancer Treatment*. Philadelphia, WB Saunders, 1982; p 213.
222. Jain A, Khanna A, Molmenti E, et al: Immunosuppressive therapy. *Surg Clin North Am* 1999; 79:1.
223. Haddad H, MacNeil DM, Howlett J, et al: Sirolimus, a new potent immunosuppressant agent for refractory cardiac transplantation rejection: two case reports. *Can J Cardiol* 2000; 16:221.
224. Snell GI, Levvey BJ, Chin W, et al: Rescue therapy: A role for sirolimus in lung and heart transplant recipients. *Transplant Proc* 2001; 33:1084.
225. Radovancevic B, El-Sabrout R, Thomas C, et al: Rapamycin reduces rejection in heart transplant recipients. *Transplant Proc* 2001; 33:3221.
226. Griepp RB, Stinson EB, Dong EJ, et al: The use of antithymocyte globulin in human heart transplantation. *Circulation* 1972; 45(suppl 2):147.
227. Szenpetery S, Mohanakumar T, Barnhart G, et al: Beneficial effects of prophylactic use of rabbit antihuman thymocyte globulin in heart transplant recipients innumosuppressed with cyclosporine. *J Heart Transplant* 1986; 5:365.
228. Carey JA, Frist WH: Use of polyclonal antilymphocytic preparations for prophylaxis in heart transplantation. *J Heart Transplant* 1990; 9:297.
229. Kawaguchi A, Szenpetery S, Mohanakumar T, et al: Effects of prophylactic rabbit antithymocyte globulin in cardiac allograft recipients treated with cyclosprorine. *J Heart Transplant* 1987; 6:214.
230. Kung PC, Goldstein G, Reinherz EL, et al: Monoclonal antibodies defining distinctive human T cell surface antigens. *Science* 1979; 206:347.
231. Reinherz EL, Meuer S, Fitzgerald KA, et al: Antigen recognition by human T lymphocytes is linked to surface expression of the T3 molecular complex. *Cell* 1982; 30:735.
232. Jaffers GJ, et al: The human immune response to murine OKT3 monoclonal antibody. *Transplant Proc* 1983; 15:646.
233. Haverty TP, Sanders M, Sheahan M: OKT3 treatment of cardiac allograft rejection. *J Heart Lung Transplant* 1993; 12:591.
234. Frist WH, Gerhardt EB, Merrill WH, et al: Therapy of refractory, recurrent heart rejection with multiple courses of OKT3. *J Heart Transplant* 1990; 9:724.
235. Gilbert EM, Dewitt CW, Eiswirth CC, et al: Treatment of refractory cardiac allograft rejection with OKT3 monoclonal antibody. *Am J Med* 1987; 82:202.
236. Normann DJ: The clinical role of OKT3. *Cardiol Clin* 1990; 8:97.
237. Norman DJ, Shield CF, Henell KR, et al: Effectiveness of a second course of OKT3 monoclonal anti-T cell antibody for treatment of renal allograft rejection. *Transplantation* 1988; 46:52.
238. First MR, Schroeder TJ, Hurtubise PE, et al: Successful retreatment of allograft rejection with OKT3. *Transplantation* 1989; 47:88.
239. Renlund DG, O'Connell JB, Gilbert EM, et al: A prospective comparison of murine monoclonal CD-3 (OKT3) antibody-based and equine antithymocyte globulin-based rejection prophylaxis in cardiac transplantation. *Transplantation* 1989; 47:599.
240. Kormos RL, Armitage JM, Dummer S, et al: Optimal perioperative immunosuppression in cardiac transplantation using rabbit antithymocyte globulin. *Transplantation* 1990; 49:306.
241. Rubin RH: Prevention and treatment of cytomegalovirus disease in heart transplant patients. *J Heart Lung Transplant* 2000; 19:731.
242. Frist WH, Winterland AW, Gerhardt EB, et al: Total lymphoid irradiation in heart transplantation: adjunctive treatment for recurrent rejection. *Ann Thorac Surg* 1989; 48:863.
243. Salter MM, Kirklin JK, Bourge RC, et al: Total lymphoid irradiation in the treatment of early or recurrent heart rejection. *J Heart Lung Transplant* 1992; 11:902.
244. Wieland M, Randels MJ, Strauss RG, et al: Photopheresis: a promising therapy for intractable cardiac allograft rejection. *J Clin Apheresis* 1992; 7:42.
245. Barr ML, Meisner BM, Eise HJ, et al: Photopheresis for the prevention of rejection in cardiac transplantation. *N Engl J Med* 1998; 339:1744.
246. Baumgartner WA, Reitz BA, Oyer PE, et al: Cardiac homotransplantation. *Curr Probl Surg* 1979; 16:1.
247. Hunt SA, Stinson EB: Cardiac transplantation. *Annu Rev Med* 1981; 32:213.
248. Opelz G, Reichert B, Mollner H, et al: Preliminary results of the collaborative heart transplant study, in Reichert B (ed): *Recent Advances in Cardiovascular Surgery*. Heidelberg, Springer-Verlag, 1989.
249. Hosenpud JD, Norman DJ, Pantely GA, et al: Low dose oral prednisone in the treatment of acute cardiac allograft rejection not

associated with hemodynamic compromise. *J Heart Lung Transplant* 1990; 9:292.

250. Miller LW: Treatment of cardiac allograft rejection with intervenous corticosteriods. *J Heart Transplant* 1990; 9:283.
251. Wahlers TH, Heublein B, Lowes D, et al: Treatment of rejection following cardiac transplantation: what dosage of pulsed steroids is necessary? *J Heart Transplant* 1989; 8:96.
252. Cooper DKC, Boyde ST, Lanza RP, et al: Factors influencing survival following heart transplantation. *J Heart Transplant* 1983; 3:86.
253. Sharples LD, Caine N, Mullins P, et al: Risk factor analysis for the major hazards following heart transplantation—rejection, infection, and coronary occlusive disease. *Transplantation* 1991; 52:244.
254. Billingham ME: Diagnosis of cardiac rejection by endomyocardial biopsy. *Heart Transplant* 1980; 1:25.
255. Gokel JM, Reichart B, Strauck E: Human cardiac transplantation—evaluation of morphological changes in serial endomyocardial biopsies. *Path Res Pract* 1985; 178:354.
256. Caves PK, Coltart J, Billingham ME, et al: Transvenous endomyocardial biopsy—application of a method for diagnosing heart disease. *Postgrad Med J* 1975; 51:286.
257. Pierard L, ElAllaf D, D'Orio V, et al: Two-dimensional echocardiographic guiding of endomyocardial biopsy. *Chest* 1984; 85:759.
258. Billingham ME, Cary NRB, Hammond ME, et al: A working formulation for the standardization of nomenclature in the diagnosis of heart and lung rejection: Heart rejection study group. *J Heart Lung Transplant* 1990; 9:587.
259. Karch SB, Billingham ME: Cyclosporine induced myocardial fibrosis: a unique controlled case report. *Heart Transplant* 1985; 4:210.
260. Cohen RG, Hoyte EG, Billingham ME, et al: Myocardial fibrosis due to cyclosporine in rat heterotopic heart transplantation. *Heart Transplant* 1984; 3:355.
261. Billingham ME: Cardiac transplantation, in Sale GE (ed): *The Pathology of Organ Transplantation*. Stoneham, MA, Butterworth-Heinemann, 1990; p 133.
262. Lower RR, Dong E, Glazener FS: Electrocardiogram of dogs with heart homografts. *Circulation* 1966; 33:455.
263. Cooper DK, Charles RG, Rose AG, et al: Does the electrocardiogram detect early acute heart rejection? *J Heart Transplant* 1985; 4:546.
264. Warnecke H, Schuler S, Goetze HJ, et al: Non-invasive monitoring of cardiac allograft rejection by intramyocardial electrogram recordings. *Circulation* 1986; 76(suppl III):72.
265. Keren A, Gillis AM, Freedman RA, et al: Heart transplant rejection monitored by signal-average electrocardiography in patients receiving cyclosporine. *Circulation* 1984; 70(suppl I): I-124.
266. Hsu DT, Spotritz HM: Echocardiographic diagnosis of cardiac allograft rejection. *Prog Cardiovasc Dis* 1990; 33:149.
267. Desruennes M, Corocos T, Cabrol A, et al: Doppler echocardiography for the diagnosis of acute cardiac allograft rejection. *J Am Coll Cardiol* 1988; 12:63.
268. Revel D, Chapelon C, Mathieu D, et al: Magnetic resonance imaging of human orthotopic heart transplantation correlation with endomyocardial biopsy. *J Heart Transplant* 1989; 8:139.
269. Addonizio LJ: Detection of cardiac allograft rejection using radionuclide techniques. *Prog Cardiovasc Dis* 1990; 33:73.
270. Hanson CA, Bolling SF, Stoolman LM, et al: Cytoimmunologic monitoring and heart transplantation. *J Heart Transplant* 1988; 7:424.
271. Jutte NHPM, Daane R, Bemd JMG, et al: Cytoimmunologic monitoring to detect rejection after heart transplantation. *Transplant Proc* 1989; 21:2519.
272. Carrier M: Noninvasive assessment of cardiac transplant rejection: a critical look at the approach to acute rejection. *Can J Surg* 1991; 34:569.
273. Michler RE, Smith CR, Drusin RE, et al: Reversal of cardiac transplant rejection without massive immunosuppression. *Circulation* 1986; 74(suppl III):68.
274. Cochrane PJ, Cavarocchi NC, Jessup M, et al: Moderate acute rejections (MRx) in cardiac transplantation (CTx): a comparison of treatment with oral vs. intravenous steroids. *Circulation* 1988; 78:II-251.
275. Carrier M, Jenicek M, Pelletier LC: Value of monoclonal antibody OKT3 in solid organ transplantation: a meta-analysis. *Transplant Proc* 1992; 24:2586.
276. Olsen SL, O'Connell JB, Bristow MR, et al: Methotrexate as an adjunct in the treatment of persistent mild cardiac allograft rejection. *Transplantation* 1990; 50:773.
277. Bourge RC, Kirklin JK, Williams CW, et al: Methotrexate pulse therapy in the treatment of recurrent acute heart rejection. *J Heart Lung Transplant* 1992; 11:1116.
278. Laufer G, Lackovics A, Wollenek G, et al: The progression of mild acute cardiac rejection evaluated by risk factor analysis. *Transplantation* 1991; 51:184.
279. Lloveras JJ, Escourrou G, Delisle MG, et al: Evolution of untreated mild rejection in heart transplant recipients. *J Heart Lung Transplant* 1992; 11:751.
280. McGoon MD, Fronty RP: Techniques of immunosuppression after cardiac transplantation. *Mayo Clin Proc* 1992; 67:586.
281. Hutter JA, Wallwork J, English TAH: Management of rejection in heart transplant recipients: does moderate rejection always require treatment? *J Heart Transplant* 1990; 9:87.
282. Kobashigawa JA, Kirklin JK, Naftel DC, et al: Pretransplantation risk factors for acute rejection after heart transplantation: a multi-institutional study. *J Heart Lung Transplant* 1993; 12:355.
283. Yowell RL, Hammond EH, Bristow MR, et al: Acute vascular rejection involving the major coronary arteries of a cardiac allograft. *J Heart Transplant* 1988; 7:191.
284. Miller LW, Wesp A, Jennison SH, et al: Vascular rejection in heart transplant recipients. *J Heart Lung Transplant* 1993; 12:S147.
285. Jambroes G, Borleffs JC, Slootweg PJ, et al: Acute humoral rejection after heart transplantation. *Transplantation* 1988; 46:603.
286. Hammond EH, Wittwer CT, Greenwood J, et al: Relationship of OKT3 sensitization and vascular rejection in cardiac transplant patients receiving OKT3 rejection prophylaxis. *Transplantation* 1990; 50:776.
287. Normann SJ, Salomon DR, Leelachaikul P, et al: Acute vascular rejection of the coronary arteries in human heart transplantation: pathology and correlations with immunosuppression and cytomegalovirus infection. *J Heart Lung Transplant* 1991; 10:674.
288. Ensley RD, Hammond EH, Renlund DG, et al: Clinical manifestations of vascular rejection in cardiac transplantation. *Transplant Proc* 1991; 23:1130.
289. Herskowitz A, Soule LM, Ueda K, et al: Arteriolar vasculitis on endomyocardial biopsy: a histologic predictor of poor outcome in cyclosporine-treated heart transplant recipients. *J Heart Transplant* 1987; 6:127.
290. Hammond EH, Yowell RL, Nunoda S, et al: Vascular (humoral) rejection in heart transplantation: pathologic observations and clinical implications. *J Heart Transplant* 1989; 8:430.
291. Partanen J, Nieminen MS, Krogerus L, et al: Heart transplant recipients treated with plasmapheresis. *J Heart Lung Transplant* 1992; 11:301.
292. Olsen SL, Wagoner LE, Taylor DO, et al: Treatment of vascular rejection in the 1990s: the Utah experience. *Circulation* 1992; 86:2500.
293. Ratkovec RM, Hammond EH, O'Connell JB, et al: Outcome of cardiac transplant recipients with a donor specific crossmatch—

preliminary results with plasmapheresis. *Transplantation* 1992; 54:651.

294. Olsen SL, Wagoner LE, Hammond EH, et al: Vascular rejection in heart transplantation: clinical correlation, treatment options, and future considerations. *J Heart Lung Transplant* 1993; 12:S135.
295. Hammond EH, Yowell RL, Price GD, et al: Vascular rejection and its relationship to allograft coronary artery disease. *J Heart Lung Transplant* 1992; 11:S111.
296. Hammond EH, Ensley RD, Yowell RL, et al: Vascular rejection of human cardiac allografts and the role of humoral immunity in chronic allograft rejection. *Transplant Proc* 1991; 23:26.
297. Rose AG, Pepino P, Barr ML, et al: Relation of HLA antibodies and graft atherosclerosis in human cardiac allograft recipients. *J Heart Lung Transplant* 1992; 11:S120.
298. Miller LW, Naftel DC, Bourge RC, et al: Infection after heart transplantation: a multiinstitutional study. *J Heart Lung Transplant* 1994; 13:381.
299. Petri WA Jr: Infections in heart transplant recipients. *Clin Infect Dis* 1994; 18:141.
300. Dresdale AR, Drusin RE, Lamb J, et al: Reduced infection in cardiac transplant recipients. *Circulation* 1985; 72(suppl II):237.
301. Hofflin JM, Potasam J, Baldwin JC, et al: Infectious complications in heart transplant recipients receiving cyclosporine and corticosteroids. *Ann Intern Med* 1987; 106:209.
302. Andreone PA, Olivari MT, Elick B, et al: Reduction of infectious complications following heart transplantation with triple-drug immunotherapy. *J Heart Transplant* 1986; 5:13.
303. Mason JW, Stinson EB, Hunt SA, et al: Infections after cardiac transplantation: relation to rejection therapy. *Ann Intern Med* 1976; 85:69.
304. Rubin RH, Cosimi AB: Infection in the immunocompromised host, in Simmons RL, Howard RJ (eds): *Surgical Infectious Disease*. New York, Appleton-Century-Crofts, 1982; p 1101.
305. Rubin RH, Wolfson JS, Cosimi AB, et al: Infection in the renal transplant recipient. *Am J Med* 1981; 70:405.
306. Gentry LO, Zeluff BJ: Diagnosis and treatment of infection in cardiac transplant patients. *Surg Clin North Am* 1986; 66:459.
307. Hosenpud JD, Herschberger RE, Pantely GA, et al: Late infection in cardiac allograft recipient: profiles, incidence and outcome. *J Heart Transplant* 1987; 10:80.
308. Dummer SJ: Infectious complications of transplantation. *Cardiovasc Clin* 1990; 20:163.
309. Garibaldi R: Infections in organ transplant recipients. *Infect Control* 1983; 4:460.
310. Gottesdiener KM: Transplanted infections: donor-to-host transmission with the allograft. *Ann Intern Med* 1989; 110:1001.
311. Love KR, Emery RW, Pritzker MR (eds): Nonbacterial infections in thoracic transplantation, in Vandersalm TJ (ed): *State of the Art Reviews: Cardiac Surgery*. Philadelphia, PA, Hanley & Belfus, 1988; p 647.
312. Lake K, Milfred T, Reutzel J, et al: Practices of cardiothoracic transplant centers regarding hepatitis Cpl candidates and donors—A follow-up survey [abstract]. *J Heart Lung Transplant* 1995; 14:S70.
313. Pereira BJG, Milford EL, Kirkman RL: Transmission of hepatitis C virus organ transplantation. *N Engl J Med* 1991; 325:454.
314. Snydman DR, Werner BG, Heinze-Lacey B, et al: Use of cytomegalovirus immune globulin to prevent cytomegalovirus disease in renal transplant recipients. *N Engl J Med* 1987; 317:1049.
315. Holliman RE, Johnson JD, Adams S, et al: Toxoplasmosis and heart transplantation. *J Heart Transplant* 1991; 10:608.
316. Kaiser AB: Antimicrobial prophylaxis in surgery. *N Engl J Med* 1986; 315:1129.
317. Walsh TR, Gyttendorf J, Dummer S, et al: The value of protective isolation procedures in cardiac allograft recipients. *Ann Thorac Surg* 1989; 47:539.
318. Wade JC, Schimpff SC: Epidemiology and prevention of infection in the compromised host, in Rubin RH, Young LS (eds): *Clinical Approach to Infection in the Compromised Host*, 2d ed. New York, Plenum, 1988; p 5.
319. Pugin J, Auckenthaler R, Lew DP, et al: Oropharyngeal decontamination decreases incidence of ventilator-associated pneumonia: a randomized, placebo-controlled, double-blind clinical trial. *JAMA* 1991; 264:2704.
320. Hughes WT, Rivera GK, Schell MJ, et al: Successful intermittent chemoprophylaxis for *Pneumocystis carinii* pneumonitis. *N Engl J Med* 1987; 316:1627.
321. Jules-Elysee KM, Stover DE, Zaman MB, et al: Aerosolized pentamidine: effect on diagnosis and presentation of *Pneumocystis carinii* pneumonia. *Ann Intern Med* 1990; 112:750.
322. Gombert ME, duBouchet L, Aulcino TM, et al: A comparative trial of clotrimazole troches and oral nystatin suspension in recipients of renal transplants: use in prophylaxis of oropharyngeal candidiasis. *JAMA* 1987; 258:2553.
323. Seale L, Jones CJ, Kathpalia S, et al: Prevention of herpes virus infections in renal allograft recipients by low-dose oral acyclovir. *JAMA* 1985; 254:3435.
324. The use of preventive therapy for tuberculous infection in the United States. Recommendations of the Advisory Committee for Elimination of Tuberculosis. *MMWR* 1990; 39:9.
325. Houston SH, Glossa JS, Fisher A, et al: Immunization of solid organ transplant candidates and recipients. *Infect Dis Newsl* 1993; 12:86.
326. Health and Public Policy Committee, American College of Physicians: Pneumococcal vaccine. *Ann Intern Med* 1986; 104:118.
327. Kobashigawa JA, Stevenson LW, Moriguchi J: Influenza vaccine does not cause rejection after cardiac transplantation [abstract]. *J Am Coll Cardiol* 1990; 15:225.
328. Varicella-zoster immune globulin for the preventation of chickenpox. *MMWR* 1984; 33:84.
329. Luft BJ, Naot Y, Araujo FG, et al: Primary and reactivated toxoplasma infection in patients with cardiac transplantation. *Ann Intern Med* 1983; 99:27.
330. Ho M, Suwannsirikul S, Dowling JN, et al: The transplanted kidney as a source of cytomegalovirus infection. *N Engl J Med* 1975; 293:1109.
331. Wreghitt T: Cytomegalovirus infections in heart-lung transplant recipients. *J Antimicrob Chem* 1989; 49(suppl E):60.
332. Mergan T, Renlund D, Keay S, et al: A multicenter, randomized, double-blind, placebo controlled study of CMV prophylaxis with intravenous ganciclovir (DHPG) in cardiac transplantation [abstract]. *J Heart Lung Transplant* 1991; 10:175.
333. Montoya JG, Giraldo LF, Efron B, et al: Infectious complications among 620 consecutive heart transplant patients at Stanford university medical center. *Clin Infect Dis* 2001; 33:629.
334. Kirklin JK, Naftel DC, Levine TB, et al: Cytomegalovirus after heart transplantation: risk factors for infection and death: a multiinstitutional study. The Cardiac Transplant Research Database group. *J Heart Lung Transplant* 1994; 13:394.
335. Chou S: Acquisition of donor strains of cytomegalovirus by renal transplant recipients. *N Engl J Med* 1986; 314:1418.
336. Rand KH, Pollard RB, Merigan TC: Increased pulmonary superinfections in cardiac transplant patients undergoing primary cytomegalovirus infection. *N Engl J Med* 1978; 298:951.
337. Dummer JS, Bound L, Singh G, et al: Epstein-Barr virus-induced lymphoma in a cardiac transplant patient. *Am J Med* 1984; 77:179.
338. Samonis G, Rolston K, Karl C: Prophylaxis of oropharyngeal candidiasis with fluconazole. *Rev Infect Dis* 1990; 12(suppl 3):S369.
339. Denning DW, Tucker RM, Hanson LH, et al: Treatment of invasive aspergillosis with itraconazole. *Am J Med* 1989; 86:791.

340. Hummel M, Thalmann U, Jautzke G, et al: Fungal infections following heart transplantation. *Mycoses* 1992; 35:23.
341. Montgomery JR, Barett FF, Williams TW Jr: Infectious complications in cardiac transplant patients. *Transplant Proc* 1973; 5:1239.
342. Carey RM, Kimball AC, Armstrong D, et al: Toxoplasma: clinical experiences in a cancer hospital. *Am J Med* 1973; 54:30.
343. Urelsky BF, Murali S, Reddy PS, et al: Development of coronary artery disease in cardiac transplant patients receiving immunosuppressive therapy with cyclosporine and prednisone. *Circulation* 1987; 76:827.
344. Bieber CP, Hunt SA, Schwinn DA, et al: Complications in long-term survivors of cardiac transplantation. *Transplant Proc* 1981; 8:20783.
345. Mullins PA, Cary NR, Sharples LD, et al: Coronary occlusive disease and late graft failure after cardiac transplantation. *Br Heart J* 1992; 68:260.
346. Kobashigwa J: What is the optimal prophylaxis for treatment of cardiac allograft vasculopathy. *Curr Control Trials Cardiovasc Med* 2000; 1:166.
347. Day JD, Rayburn BK, Gaudin PB, et al: Cardiac allograft vasculopathy: the central pathogenic role of ischemia-induced endothelial cell injury. *J Heart Lung Transplant* 1995; 14:S142.
348. Rose EA, Pepino P, Barr ML, et al: Relation of HLA antibodies and graft atherosclerosis in human cardiac allograft recipients. *J Heart Lung Transplant* 1992; 11:S120.
349. Fields BL, Hoffman RM, Berkoff HA: Assessment of the impact of recipient age and organ ischemic time on heart transplant mortality. *Transplant Proc* 1988; 20:1035.
350. Johnson MR: Transplant coronary disease: non-immunologic risk factors. *J Heart Lung Transplant* 1992; 11:S124.
351. Winters GL, Kendall TJ, Radio SJ, et al: Posttransplant obesity and hyperlipidemia: major predictors of severity of coronary arteriopathy in failed human heart allografts. *J Heart Lung Transplant* 1990; 9:364.
352. Grattan MT, Moreno-Cabral CE, Starnes VA, et al: Cytomegalovirus infection is associated with cardiac allograft rejection and atherosclerosis. *JAMA* 1989; 261:3561.
353. Johnson DE, Gao SZ, Schroeder JS, et al: The spectrum of coronary artery pathologic findings in human cardiac allografts. *J Heart Transplant* 1989; 8:349.
354. Billingham ME: Cardiac transplant atherosclerosis. *Transplant Proc* 1987; 19(suppl 5):19.
355. St. Goar FG, Pinto FJ, Alderman EL, et al: Detection of coronary atherosclerosis in young adult hearts using intravascular ultrasound. *Circulation* 1992; 86:756.
356. Smart FW, Ballantyne CM, Farmer JA, et al: Insensitivity of non-invasive tests to detect coronary artery vasculopathy after heart transplant. *Am J Cardiol* 1991; 67:243.
357. Johnson DE, Alderman EL, Schroeder JS, et al: Transplant coronary artery disease: histopathologic correlations with angiographic morphology. *J Am Coll Cardiol* 1991; 17:449.
358. St. Goar FG, Pinto FJ, Alderman EL, et al: Intravascular ultrasound imaging of angiographically normal coronary arteries: an in vivo comparison with quantitative angiography. *J Am Coll Cardiol* 1991; 18:952.
359. Anderson TJ, Meredith IT, Uehata A, et al: Functional significance of initimal thickening as detected by intravascular ultrasound early and late after cardiac transplantation. *Circulation* 1993; 88:1093.
360. Mehra MR, Ventura HO, Stapleton DD, et al: The prognostic significance of intimal proliferation in cardiac allograft vasculopathy: a paradigm shift. *J Heart Lung Transplant* 1995;14:S207.
361. Wenke K, Meiser B, Thiery J, et al: Simvistatin reduces graft vessel disease and mortality after heart transplantation: a 4 year randomized trial. *Circulation* 1997; 96:1398.
362. Myers BD, Sibley R, Newton L, et al: The long-term course of cyclosporine-associated chronic nephropathy. *Kidney Inst* 1988; 33:590.
363. Myers BD: Cyclosporine nephrotoxicity. *N Engl J Med* 1986; 30:964.
364. Kahan BD: Cyclosporine nephrotoxicity: pathogenesis, prophylaxis, therapy and prognosis. *Am J Kidney Dis* 1986; 8:323.
365. Myers BD, Newton L: Cyclosporine-induced chronic nephropathy: an obliterative microvascular renal injury. *J Am Soc Nephrol* 1991; 2(suppl 1):S45.
366. Kahan BD: Cyclosporine. *N Engl J Med* 1989; 321:1725.
367. Miller LW, Pennington DG, McBride LR: Long-term effects of cyclosporine in cardiac transplantation. *Transplant Proc* 1990; 22(suppl 1):15.
368. Moyer TP, Post GR, Sterioff S, et al: Cyclosporine nephrotoxicity is minimized by adjusting dosage on the basis of drug concentration in blood. *Mayo Clin Proc* 1988; 63:241.
369. Greenberg A, Thompson ME, Griffith BJ, et al: Cyclosporine nephrotoxicity in cardiac allograft patients: a seven year follow-up. *Transplantation* 1990; 50:589.
370. Andreassen AK, Hartmann A, Offstad J, et al: Hypertension prophylaxis with omega-3 fatty acids in heart transplant recipients. *J Am Coll Cardiol* 1997; 29:1324.
371. Schacter M: Cyclosporine A and hypertension. *J Hypertens* 1988; 6:511.
372. Starling RC, Cody RJ: Cardiac transplant hypertension. *Am J Cardiol* 1990; 65:106.
373. Mark AL: Cyclosporine, sympathetic activity, and hypertension. *N Engl J Med* 1990; 323:748.
374. Cole W: The increase in immunosuppression and its role in the development of malignant lesions. *J Surg Oncol* 1985; 30:139.
375. Penn I: Cancers complicating organ transplantation. *N Engl J Med* 1990; 323:1767.
376. Penn I: Cancers following cyclosporine therapy. *Transplantation* 1987; 43:32.
377. Armitage JM, Kormos RL, Stuart RS, et al: Posttransplant lymphoproliferative disease in thoracic organ transplant patients: ten years of cyclosporine-based immunosuppression. *J Heart Lung Transplant* 1991; 10:877.
378. Randhawa PS, Yousem SA, Paradis IL, et al: The clinical spectrum, pathology, and clonal analysis of Epstein-Barr virus-associated lymphoproliferative disorders in heart-lung transplant recipients. *Am J Clin Pathol* 1989; 92:177.
379. Krikorian JG, Anderson JL, Bieber CP, et al: Malignant neoplasms following cardiac transplantation. *JAMA* 1978; 240:639.
380. Nalesnik MA, Makowka L, Starzl TE: The diagnosis and treatment of posttransplant lymphoproliferative disorders. *Curr Probl Surg* 1988; 25:371.
381. Hanto DW, Sakamoto K, Purtilo DT, et al: The Epstein-Barr virus in the pathogenesis of posttransplant lymphoproliferative disorders. *Surgery* 1981; 90:204.
382. Klein G, Purtillo DT: Summary: symposium on Epstein-Barr virus-induced lymphoproliferative diseases in immunodeficient patients. *Cancer Res* 1981; 41:4302.
383. Swinnen LJ, O'Sullivan EJ, Johnson MR, et al: OKT3 therapy is associated with an increased incidence of lymphoproliferative disorder following cardiac transplantation. *N Engl J Med* 1990; 323:1723.
384. Weintraub J, Warnke RA: Lymphoma in cardiac allograft recipients: clinical and histological features and immunological phenotype. *Transplantation* 1981; 33:347.
385. Penn I: Cancers after cyclosporine therapy. *Transplant Proc* 1988; 20:276.
386. Hanto DW, Binkenbach M, Frizzera G, et al: Confirmation of the heterogeneity of posttransplant Epstein-Barr virus-associated

B cell proliferations by immunoglobular gene management analysis. *Transplantation* 1989; 47:458.

387. Sullivan JL, Medveczky P, Forman SJ, et al: Epstein-Barr virus induced lymphoproliferation: implications for antiviral chemotherapy. *N Engl J Med* 1984; 311:1163.
388. Keogh A, Simons L, Spratt P, et al: Hyperlipidemia after heart transplantation. *J Heart Transplant* 1988; 7:171.
389. Lee AH, Mull RL, Keenan GF, et al: Osteoporosis and bone morbidity in cardiac transplant recipients. *Am J Med* 1994; 96:35.
390. Ibels LS, Alfrey AC, Huffer WE, et al: Aseptic necrosis of bone after renal transplantation: experience in 194 transplant recipients and review of the literature. *Medicine (Baltimore)* 1978; 57:25.
391. Hagan ME, Holland CS, Herrick CM, et al: Amelioration of weight gain after heart transplantation by corticosteroid-free maintenance immunosuppression. *J Heart Transplant* 1990; 9:382.
392. Spes CH, Angermann CE, Beyer RW, et al: Increased evidence for cholelithiasis in heart transplant recipients receiving cyclosporine therapy. *J Heart Transplant* 1990; 9:404.
393. Augustine SM, Yeo CJ, Buchman TG, et al: Gastrointestinal complications in heart and in heart-lung transplant patients. *J Heart Lung Transplant* 1991; 10:547.
394. Michler RE, McLaughlin MJ, Chen JM, et al: Clinical experience with cardiac retransplantation. *J Thorac Cardiovasc Surg* 1993; 106:622.
395. Schroeder JS, Hunt SA, Alderman EL, et al: Retransplantation for severe accelerated coronary vascular disease in heart transplant [abstract]. *J Am Coll Cardiol* 1987; 9:29A.
396. Srivastava R, Keck BM, Bennett LE, et al: The result of cardiac retransplantation: an analysis of the joint international society of heart lung transplantation/united network for organ sharing thoracic registry. *Transplantation* 2000; 4:606.
397. DeBoer J, Cohen B, Thorogood J, et al: Results of acute heart retransplantation. *Lancet* 1991; 337:1158.
398. Sarris GE, Moore KA, Schroeder JS, et al: Cardiac transplantation: the Stanford experience in the cyclosporine era. *J Thorac Cardiovasc Surg* 1994; 108:240.
399. Fisher DC, Lake KD, Reutzel TJ, et al: Changes in health-related quality of life and depression in heart transplant recipients. *J Heart Lung Transplant* 1995; 14:373.
400. Rosenblum DS, Rosen ML, Pine ZM, et al: Health status and quality of life following cardiac transplantation. *Arch Physiol Med Rehabil* 1993; 74:490.
401. Kavanagh T, Yacoub MH, Mertens DJ, et al: Cardiorespiratory responses to exercise training after orthotopic cardiac transplantation. *Circulation* 1988; 77:162.
402. Paris W, Woodbury A, Thompson S, et al: Returning to work after heart transplantation. *J Heart Lung Transplant* 1993; 12:46.

Chapter 61

Heart-Lung and Lung Transplantation

Leora B. Balsam/David D. Yuh/Robert C. Robbins/Bruce A. Reitz

The birth and evolution of thoracic organ transplantation have occurred over the past 60 years. With the development of improved operative techniques, organ preservation techniques, and immunosuppressive regimens, combined heart-lung and isolated lung transplantation have emerged as lifesaving procedures for patients with end-stage cardiopulmonary or pulmonary disease. To date, 2861 combined heart-lung transplants, 7204 single lung transplants, and 5420 bilateral lung transplants have been performed worldwide.[1] While the number of heart-lung transplants performed annually has declined in recent years, the number of single and bilateral lung transplantation procedures remains stable. Clinical progress in thoracic organ transplantation has been considerable, yet significant barriers that limit the scope of these procedures still remain. These include donor organ shortage, limited preservation techniques, graft rejection, and infectious complications. This chapter summarizes the state of the art in combined heart-lung and isolated lung transplantation.

HISTORICAL BACKGROUND

History of Heart-Lung Transplantation

Long before the first successful human heart-lung transplants were reported, thoracic organ transplantation flourished in the laboratory. In the 1940s, Demikhov developed the first successful method of en bloc heart-lung transplantation in dogs. In his series of 67 dogs, the longest survivor lived for 6 days postoperatively.[2] These remarkable studies

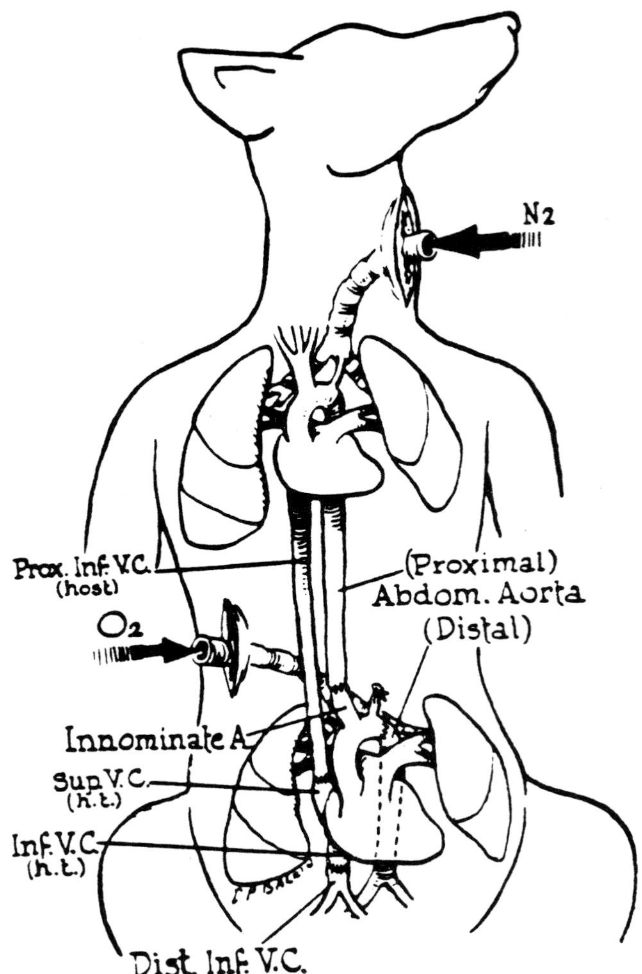

FIGURE 61–1 Heterotopic heart-lung transplantation in canines as reported by Marcus et al in 1953. (*Reproduced with permission from Marcus E, Wong SNT, Luisada AA: Homologous heart grafts. Arch Surg 1953; 66:179. Copyright ©1953, American Medical Association.*)

demonstrated the technical feasibility of heart and lung replacement, yet remained largely unknown in the West until the 1960s. In 1953, Marcus and colleagues at the Chicago Medical School described a technique for heterotopic heart-lung grafting to the abdominal aorta and inferior vena cava in dogs (Fig. 61-1).[3] Later studies in the 1960s and early 1970s examined the physiological effect of total denervation on heart and lung function. Discouraging studies by Webb and Howard in 1957 showed failure to resume normal spontaneous respiration following heart-lung replacement in dogs.[4] This physiologic phenomenon was confirmed by several other groups doing research in dogs, including Lower et al in 1961.[5] Fortunately, later studies in primates by Haglin,[6] Nakae,[7] Castaneda,[8,9] and their colleagues showed that unlike dogs, primates resume a normal respiratory pattern following complete denervation with cardiopulmonary replacement. The 1970s saw the development of improved immunosuppressive medications, particularly cyclosporine, which prevented rejection of primate heart-lung allografts after transplantation. A Stanford series showed survival for well over 5 years after heart-lung allografting in primates.[10] In the 1980s, Reitz et al reported a modification to the standard technique of heart-lung replacement, using a retained portion of the right atrium for a single inflow anastomosis instead of separate caval anastomoses (Fig. 61-2).[11] This technique preserved the donor sinoatrial node and eliminated the potential for caval anastomotic stenosis. These studies laid the groundwork for a clinical trial of heart-lung transplantation at Stanford University. On March 9, 1981, Reitz et al performed the first successful human heart-lung transplant in a 45-year-old woman with end-stage primary pulmonary hypertension.[12]

History of Lung Transplantation

Experimental lung transplantation developed in parallel with heart-lung transplantation. In 1949, Henry Metras described important technical concepts, including preservation of the left atrial cuff for the pulmonary venous anastomoses and reimplantation of an aortic patch containing the origin of the bronchial arteries to prevent bronchial dehiscence.[13] Airway dehiscence was a major obstacle in experimental lung transplantation, and he proposed that preservation of the bronchial arterial supply was critical to airway healing. Unfortunately, this technique was technically cumbersome and never gained widespread popularity. In the 1960s, Blumenstock et al advocated transection of the transplant bronchus close to the lung parenchyma to prevent ischemic bronchial necrosis.[14] Additional surgical modifications were developed to prevent bronchial anastomotic complications, including telescoping of the bronchial anastomosis, described by Veith in 1969,[15] and coverage of the anastomosis with an omental pedicle flap, described by the Toronto group in 1982.[16] Corticosteroids were found to be another contributor to poor bronchial healing,[17] so with the introduction of cyclosporine immunosuppression in the 1970s, the stage was set for successful clinical lung transplantation.

The first human lung transplant was described in 1963 by Hardy et al at the University of Mississippi.[18] The patient, a 58-year-old man with lung cancer, survived 18 days postoperatively. Over the next two decades, nearly 40 lung transplants were performed without long-term success. In 1986, the Toronto Lung Transplant Group reported the first series of successful single lung transplants with long-term survival.[19] Improved immunosuppression, along with careful recipient and donor selection, were pivotal to their success. For patients with bilateral lung disease, en-bloc double lung replacement was introduced by Patterson in 1988.[20] This technique was later replaced by sequential bilateral lung transplantation, described by Pasque et al in 1990.[21]

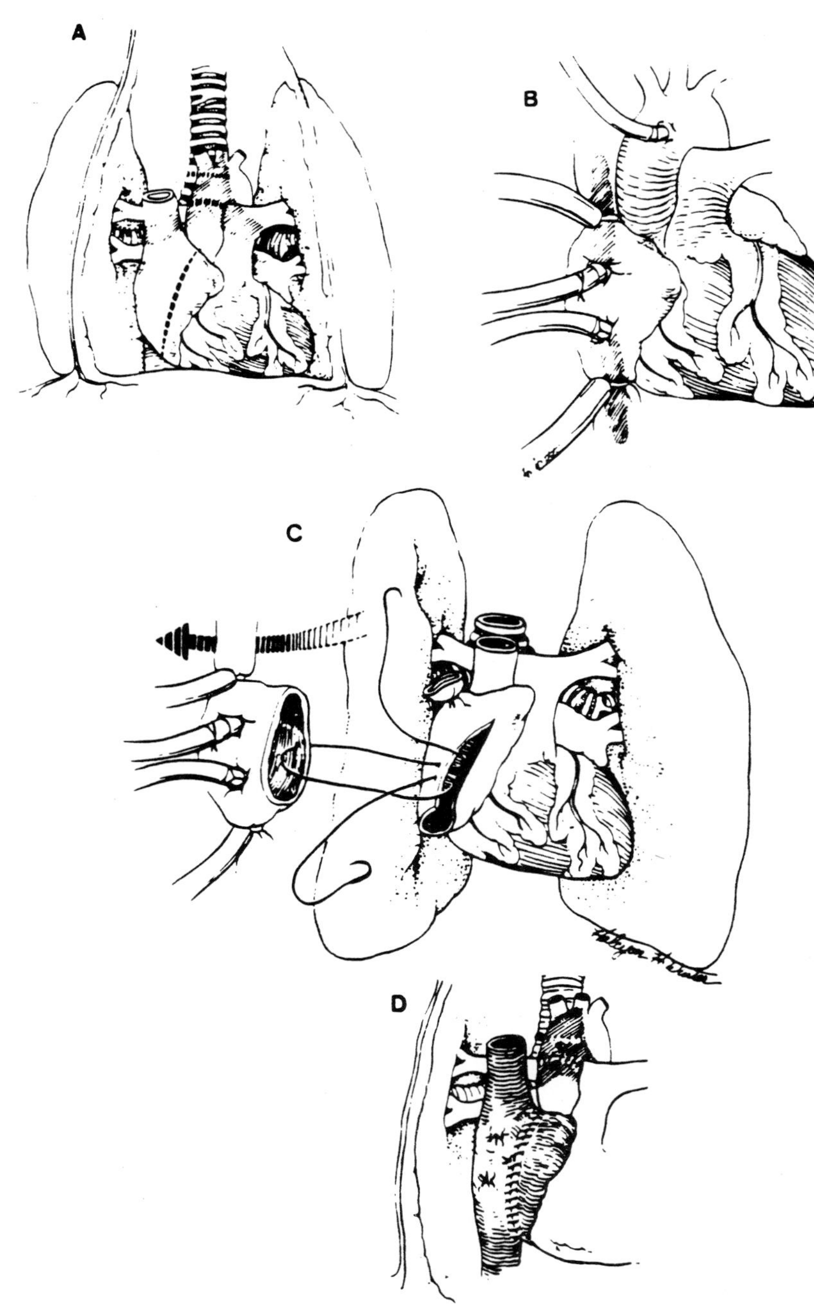

FIGURE 61–2 Simplified technique for heart-lung transplantation as described by Reitz et al in 1981. (A) Native heart-lung bloc dissection with preservation of phrenic nerves on pedicles and lines of transection along the right atrium, aorta, and trachea. (B) Cannula configuration for recipient cardiopulmonary bypass with venous cannulas placed in the lower right atrium and arterial cannula in the ascending aorta. (C) Inflow (right atrial) anastomosis. The graft right atrial cuff is constructed by ligating the superior vena cava and opening the right atrium from the inferior vena caval orifice toward the appendage. Note that the right lung is passed behind the vena cava and right phrenic nerve pedicle. (D) Completed transplantation with right atrial, aortic, and tracheal anastomoses shown. (*From Reitz BA, Pennock JL, Shumway NE: Simplified operative method for heart and lung transplantation. J Surg Res 1981; 31:1. Reproduced with permission from Academic Press, Inc.*)

More recent operative innovations include living lobar transplantation, an alternative to cadaveric bilateral lung transplantation.

INDICATIONS AND EVALUATION FOR HEART-LUNG AND LUNG TRANSPLANTATION

Indications for Heart-Lung Transplantation

When heart-lung transplantation was introduced in 1982, it provided a lifesaving therapeutic option for patients with end-stage cardiopulmonary disease and end-stage septic lung disease. Since that time, the techniques of single and double lung transplantation have improved considerably, and the indications for combined heart-lung replacement have become fewer. Moreover, donor organ distribution algorithms, which appropriately distribute donor hearts to critical heart recipients, have also limited the availability of heart-lung blocs.

Heart-lung transplant volumes peaked in the late 1990s; in 2001, only 104 operations were performed worldwide.[1] The most common indications include congenital heart

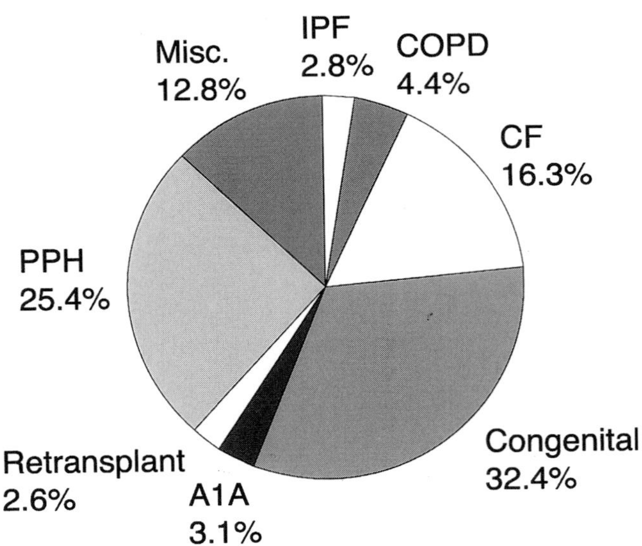

FIGURE 61–3 Indications for heart-lung transplantation. A1A = α_1 antitrypsin deficiency; CF = cystic fibrosis; COPD = chronic obstructive pulmonary disease; IPF = idiopathic pulmonary fibrosis; Misc = miscellaneous; PPH = primary pulmonary hypertension. (*Adapted from Hosenpud JD, Bennett LE, Keck BM, et al: The Registry of the International Society for Heart and Lung Transplantation: Eighteenth Official Report—2001. J Heart Lung Transplant 2001; 20:805 with permission from Elsevier Science.*)

disease with Eisenmenger's syndrome, primary pulmonary hypertension, and cystic fibrosis. The diagnostic profile of heart-lung transplant recipients reported to the Registry of the International Society for Heart and Lung Transplantation (ISHLT) is shown in Figure 61-3.

Congenital heart disease (atrial and ventricular septal defects, patent ductus arteriosus) with secondary pulmonary hypertension (Eisenmenger's syndrome) is the most frequent indication, found in over one third of the patients. Other complex congenital heart defects have also been treated successfully with heart-lung transplantation, including univentricular heart with pulmonary atresia, truncus arteriosus, and hypoplastic left heart syndrome.

The data regarding the long-term survival benefit of heart-lung transplantation in patients with Eisenmenger's syndrome remains unclear.[22] Some data suggests that pulmonary hypertension in these patients has a more favorable prognosis than other types of pulmonary hypertension. There is clear evidence, however, that quality of life is improved by transplantation.[23] In patients with simpler cardiac defects, repair of the cardiac defect combined with single or bilateral lung transplantation is another option.

Primary pulmonary hypertension with right-sided heart failure is the second most common diagnosis in heart-lung transplant recipients. Nearly one quarter of patients in the ISHLT registry carry this diagnosis. Recently, there has been a shift toward single and bilateral lung transplantation in this population.[24] The shift in paradigm is based on the finding that right heart function often recovers after normalization of pulmonary pressures with lung transplantation. However, in patients with severe right-sided heart failure and primary pulmonary hypertension, heart-lung transplantation is clearly the operation of choice.

The balance of heart-lung transplants are performed for a variety of cardiac and pulmonary diseases. These include cystic fibrosis and other septic lung diseases, severe coronary artery disease with intercurrent end-stage lung disease, and primary parenchymal lung disease with severe right-sided heart failure (e.g., idiopathic pulmonary fibrosis, lymphangioleiomyomatosis, sarcoidosis, and desquamative interstitial pneumonitis).

Septic lung disease was historically a significant indication for heart-lung transplantation. The domino procedure, which emerged in the late 1980s, took explanted hearts from these patients and offered them to a second recipient in need of heart transplantation.[25–27] While studies have shown equivalent survival in recipients of domino heart grafts, currently the domino procedure is rarely performed. Instead, bilateral lung transplantation has become the procedure of choice for end-stage septic lung disease.[28,29] It avoids the pitfalls of cardiac denervation and graft coronary artery disease that characterize heart-lung transplantation.

Indications for Lung Transplantation

In recent years, the number of lung transplant procedures performed annually has reached a plateau. Worldwide, 1412 lung transplants were performed in 2000. Nearly half were single lung transplants and the remainder were bilateral lung transplants. A small number of living lobar transplants are also being performed annually.[1]

The primary indications for single lung transplantation are emphysema and pulmonary fibrosis (Fig. 61-4A). Patients with emphysema comprise nearly one half of single lung transplant recipients. In some cases, hyperinflation of the native emphysematous lung may lead to compressive atelectasis and restriction of the donor lung. This may result in a significant ventilation/perfusion mismatch. In such cases, native lung volume reduction can be used to preserve allograft function.[30] Some evidence exists that late allograft function may be superior in emphysema patients treated with bilateral rather than single lung transplantation;[31] however, given the donor organ shortage, single lung transplantation remains the preferred therapeutic option.

The principal indications for bilateral lung transplantation are septic lung disease, emphysema, primary pulmonary hypertension, and pulmonary fibrosis (Fig. 61-4B).[30] While single lung transplantation may be performed for emphysema, primary pulmonary hypertension, and pulmonary fibrosis, it is not an option for septic lung disease. In these patients, bilateral sepsis mandates removal of both native lungs. Primary pulmonary hypertension has been treated

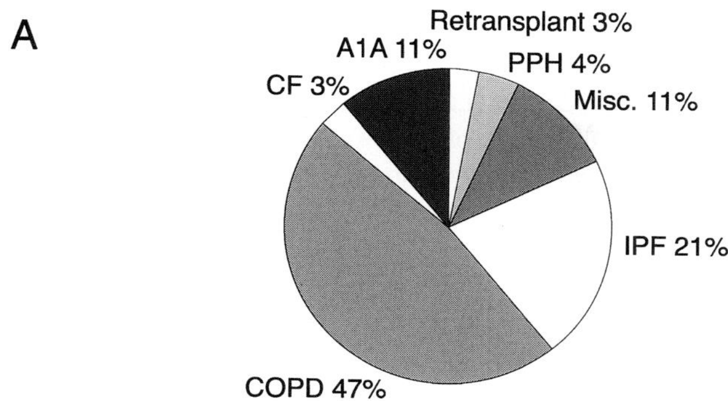

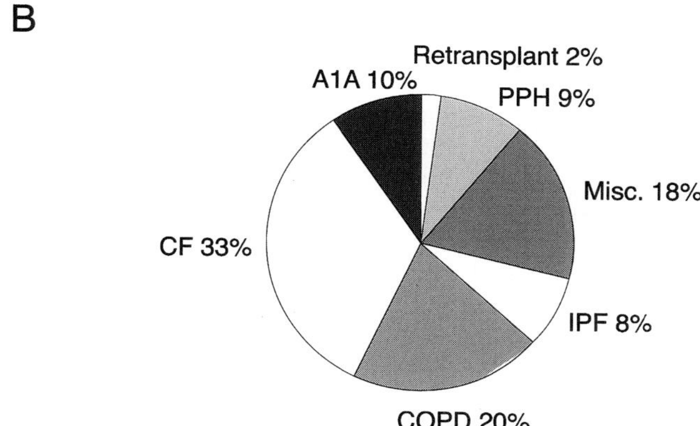

FIGURE 61–4 Indications for single (A) and bilateral (B) lung transplantation. A1A = α_1 antitrypsin deficiency; CF = cystic fibrosis; COPD = chronic obstructive pulmonary disease; IPF = idiopathic pulmonary fibrosis; Misc = miscellaneous; PPH = primary pulmonary hypertension. *(Adapted from Hosenpud JD, Bennett LE, Keck BM, et al: The Registry of the International Society for Heart and Lung Transplantation: Eighteenth Official Report—2001. J Heart Lung Transplant 2001; 20:805 with permission from Elsevier Science.)*

with both bilateral and single lung transplants, though most advocate bilateral lung transplantation. There is evidence that the effects of bronchiolitis obliterans on long-term survivors are better tolerated in recipients of bilateral lung transplants. However, in a single-center retrospective study of 58 patients undergoing either single lung or bilateral lung transplantation for pulmonary hypertension, Gammie et al found equivalent survival at 1 and 4 years.[24] While they advocate the preferential application of single lung transplantation in this patient group, this indication will remain controversial until larger clinical trials are reported.

Less than 3% of all single and bilateral lung transplants are retransplantations.[1] Overall, survival is poorer compared to first-time transplantation, though certain subsets of patients perform better than others. The Pulmonary Retransplant Registry has collected data from 230 patients at over 40 centers and has found that 1-year survival of ambulatory, nonventilated patients undergoing retransplantation after 1991 is in fact comparable to first-time transplants.[32]

Finally, lobar transplantation is another option for end-stage lung disease. Living lobar transplantation was developed by Starnes et al, and has its greatest application in children with cystic fibrosis. The left lower lobe and right lower lobe from two donors are transplanted into the recipient. The procedure is most applicable to children and adults of small stature. Results in children have been superior to cadaveric transplants in terms of long-term survival and freedom from bronchiolitis obliterans syndrome. In adults, results have been comparable to cadaveric transplants.[33–35]

Recipient Selection Criteria

The primary objective in recipient evaluation is to select individuals with progressively disabling cardiopulmonary or pulmonary disease who still possess the capacity for full rehabilitation after transplantation. It is notable that early attempts in the history of thoracic transplantation were thwarted by selection of critically ill recipients, and it was not until the development of strict recipient selection criteria that heart-lung and lung transplantation were met with success.

Candidates should have a life expectancy of less than 18 to 24 months despite the use of appropriate medical or alternative surgical strategies. On average, waiting times can be from 6 to 36 months. Unfortunately, mortality while on the waiting list remains nearly 20% for both lung and heart-lung transplant candidates. Therefore, it is imperative that recipients be identified as early as possible within the "transplant window."[36]

Disabling symptoms prompting consideration for transplantation typically include dyspnea, cyanosis, syncope, and hemoptysis. Most recipients for heart-lung transplantation also fall within New York Heart Association functional classes III or IV.[37] Potential recipients are identified by their local primary physicians and referred to transplantation centers for further evaluation. This includes a complete history, physical exam, laboratory tests, specialized studies, and a psychosocial evaluation.

Among most heart-lung transplant programs, the upper recipient age limit is 50 years. For bilateral lung transplantation, the upper limit is 55 years, and for single lung transplantation, it is 60 years. These values represent a relaxation of previous age limits, reflecting the ongoing evolution in recipient selection criteria. Unfortunately, with the expansion of recipient eligibility, the problem of donor organ shortage is further exacerbated.

There are well-established contraindications to lung and heart-lung transplantation (Table 61-1). Significant multisystem disease is a contraindication, though occasionally multiorgan transplants have been performed. Renal dysfunction, active malignancy, infection with HIV, hepatitis B antigen positivity, hepatitis C infection with biopsy-proven liver disease, and infection with panresistant respiratory flora are

TABLE 61–1 Recipient contraindications to heart-lung and lung transplantation

Age >50 (heart-lung), >55 (bilateral lung), >60 (single lung)
Significant systemic or multisystem disease (e.g., peripheral or cerebrovascular disease, portal hypertension, poorly controlled diabetes mellitus)
Significant irreversible hepatic or renal dysfunction (e.g., bilirubin >3.0 mg/dL, creatinine clearance <50 mg/mL/min)
Active malignancy
Corticosteroid therapy (>10 mg/day)
Panresistant respiratory flora
Cachexia or obesity (<70% or >130% ideal body weight)
Current cigarette smoking
Psychiatric illness or history of medical noncompliance
Drug or alcohol abuse
Previous cardiothoracic surgery (considered on a case-by-case basis)
Severe osteoporosis
Prolonged mechanical ventilation
HIV
HBsAg positivity
Hepatitis C infection with biopsy-proven liver disease

absolute contraindications. Relative contraindications include active extrapulmonary infection, symptomatic osteoporosis, recent history of active peptic ulcer disease, cachexia or obesity, drug or alcohol abuse, and psychiatric illness or history of medical noncompliance. Cigarette smokers must quit smoking and remain abstinent for several months before transplantation. Patients with previous histories of thoracic surgery are evaluated on a case-by-case basis. In patients requiring systemic corticosteroids, tapering to the lowest tolerable level, preferably below 10 mg/day, is critical to prevent airway healing complications. Finally, mechanical ventilation is generally considered a contraindication to transplantation; repeated studies have shown that these patients have significantly worse immediate and long-term survival after transplantation.[38] In addition to meeting these criteria, a stable and supportive socioeconomic environment is an important criterion.

TABLE 61–2 Typical laboratory tests and studies obtained during recipient evaluation for heart-lung and lung transplantation

Suitability for transplantation (phase I)
Required laboratory tests and studies
- CBC with differential, platelet, and reticulocyte count
- Blood type and antibody screen (ABO, Rh)
- Prothrombin and activated partial thromboplastin time (PT, PTT)
- Bleeding time
- Immunology panel (FANA, RF)
- Electrolytes, including Mg^{2+}
- CK with isoenzymes
- Serum protein electrophoresis
- Urinalysis
- Viral serologies
  - Compromised host panel (cytomegalovirus, adenovirus, varicella-zoster, herpes simplex, Epstein-Barr virus)
  - Hepatitis A, B, and C antibodies, hepatitis B surface antigen (HBsAg)
  - Cytomegalovirus (quantitative antibodies and IgM)
  - Human immunodeficiency virus
- Electrocardiogram
- Chest x-ray

Studies obtained as indicated
- Echocardiogram with bubble study
- MUGA for right and left ventricular ejection fraction
- Cardiac catheterization with coronary angiogram
- Thoracic CT scan
- Quantitative ventilation-perfusion scans
- Carotid duplex
- Mammogram
- Colonoscopy
- Sputum for Gram stain, AFB smear, KOH, and routine bacterial, mycobacterial, and fungal cultures

Required for listing (phase II)
HLA and DR typing
Transplant antibody
Quantitative immunoglobulins
Histoplasma, Coccidiodes, and *Toxoplasma* titers
PPD
Pulmonary function tests with arterial blood gases
12-hour urine collection for creatinine clearance and total protein
Urine viral culture

Clinical and Laboratory Criteria for Listing

Tests required for transplant listing are reviewed in Table 61-2. Diagnostic studies that are particularly useful in evaluating potential recipients include full pulmonary function tests, an exercise performance test, electrocardiogram, echocardiogram, 24-hour creatinine clearance, and liver function tests.

Certain patient populations may be held to additional requirements. For example, cystic fibrosis recipients should have an otolaryngologic evaluation before being placed on an active waiting list. Most of these patients will require endoscopic maxillary antrostomies for sinus access and monthly antibiotic irrigation. This measure, designed to decrease the bacterial load of the upper respiratory tract,[39] has decreased the incidence of serious posttransplant bacterial infections in this group of patients. Previous smokers must undergo screening to exclude smoking-related illnesses such as peripheral vascular disease and malignancy. A negative sputum cytology, thoracic computed tomographic (CT) scan, bronchoscopy, otolaryngologic evaluation, and carotid duplex scan are required. In addition, left heart catheterization and coronary angiography are performed in previous smokers considered for transplantation.

Patients deemed suitable for transplantation during the initial evaluation are subjected to a final phase of testing (see Table 61-2). If accepted by the transplant review committee, they are listed on the national transplant registry on the basis of clinical urgency, time on the waiting list, ABO blood group, and thoracic cage dimensions. Most transplant centers will require patients to reside within several hours of the center by automobile or air charter.

ABO compatibilities are strictly adhered to, because isolated cases of hyperacute rejection have been reported in transplants performed across ABO barriers. Donor-to-recipient lung volume matching is based on the vertical (apex to diaphragm along the midclavicular line) and transverse (level of diaphragmatic dome) radiologic dimensions on chest x-ray, as well as body weight, height, and chest circumference. In practice, matching donor and recipient height seems to be the most reproducible method for selecting the appropriate donor lung size, and the dimensions of the donor lungs should not be greater than 4 cm over those in the recipient. It is possible, however, to downsize donor lungs by lobectomy if needed.

In a series of 82 heart-lung transplants at Papworth Hospital, Tamm et al recorded recipient lung volumes after transplantation and compared them to preoperative and predicted volumes to evaluate the influence of donor lung size and recipient underlying disease.[40] The investigators demonstrated that by 1 year after surgery, total lung capacity (TLC) and dynamic lung volume returned to values predicted by the patient's sex, age, and height. They proposed that the simplest method of matching donor lung size to that of the recipient is to use their respective predicted TLC values. Moreover, they concluded that the recipient's predicted lung volumes should be attained by 1 year after transplantation, and that failure to do so suggests possible complications within the transplanted lungs.

In contrast to renal transplantation, HLA matching is not a criteria for thoracic organ allocation. Because only short ischemic times are tolerated by lung and heart-lung blocs, it is not possible to perform this tissue typing preoperatively.[41] However, several retrospective studies have been performed to look at the influence of HLA matching on long-term graft survival and the development of obliterative bronchiolitis. Wisser et al examined the relationship between HLA matching and long-term survival in 78 lung transplant recipients.[42] They found improved graft survival with matching at the HLA-B locus. In a retrospective study of 74 lung transplant patients, Iwaki et al also correlated improved graft survival with matching at the HLA-B and HLA-DR loci.[43] Harjula et al at Stanford evaluated the relationship between HLA matching and outcome in heart-lung transplantation.[44] Among 40 heart-lung transplant recipients evaluated, they found a significant increase in graded obliterative bronchiolitis with total mismatch at the HLA-A locus. These studies all suggest that there is a relationship between HLA matching and long-term graft function.

Once an appropriate donor-recipient pairing is made, the recipient is screened for preformed antibodies against a panel of random donors. A percent reactive antibody (PRA) level greater than 25 prompts a prospective specific crossmatch between the donor and recipient. A positive crossmatch indicates the presence of anti–donor circulating antibodies in the recipient that would likely lead to hyperacute rejection of the donor organ. In the event of a positive crossmatch, the donor organ cannot be accepted for that recipient.

RECIPIENT MANAGEMENT AFTER LISTING

It is extremely important that a candidate's medical condition be optimized prior to heart-lung and lung transplantation. Standard medical measures should be aggressively employed by the patient's local physician, and the patient should have routine follow-up at the transplant center.

Supplemental oxygen is recommended for any patient exhibiting arterial hypoxemia, defined as either an arterial oxygen saturation less than 90% or an arterial P_{O_2} less than 60 mm Hg at rest, during exertion, or while asleep.

For patients with heart failure, standard therapeutic measures are applied, including dietary restrictions, diuretics, and vasodilators. Dietary water and salt restriction as well as diuretic therapy facilitate intravascular fluid management. However, particular care must be exercised when using loop diuretics in patients with underlying pulmonary disease; this class of potent diuretics results in a metabolic alkalosis that depresses the effectiveness of carbon dioxide as a stimulus for breathing. Vasodilators result in afterload reduction, and have been proven to effectively improve functional capacity and prolong survival in patients suffering from severe cardiac failure.[45] Commonly used vasodilators include nitrates, hydralazine, and angiotensin-converting enzyme inhibitors.

Despite the clinical heterogeneity among patients with primary pulmonary hypertension, conventional medical therapy targets the sequelae of the pulmonary vascular derangements associated with this disease process. Supplemental oxygen therapy is recommended to eliminate the stimulus for hypoxic pulmonary vasoconstriction and secondary erythropoiesis, thus lessening the burden placed on the right side of the heart and diminishing the likelihood of cardiac arrhythmias. Pulmonary vasodilator therapy is important in the treatment of primary pulmonary hypertension, and includes the use of calcium channel blockers and continuous prostacyclin infusions.[46] Because most standard vasodilators have potent systemic effects, careful dosing and follow-up is essential. Approximately 20% of patients with primary pulmonary hypertension will respond to calcium channel blockers, and this favorable response can usually be predicted by the response to short-acting vasodilators during cardiac catheterization, but response to the acute vasodilator challenge does not always predict the response to long-term prostacyclin infusion.

Interstitial lung disease in patients awaiting transplantation results from a wide variety of diffuse inflammatory processes, such as sarcoidosis, asbestosis, and collagen-vascular diseases. Increases in pulmonary vascular resistance leading to right-sided heart failure are thought to result from interstitial inflammatory infiltrates that entrap and eventually destroy septal arterioles, reducing the distensibility of the remaining pulmonary vessels.[47] This process, coupled with closure of peripheral bronchioles, results in arterial hypoxemia, which further aggravates pulmonary hypertension. Corticosteroids are the mainstay of treatment in this class of diseases. The adverse effects of steroids on airway healing are well established,[17,48] and mandate significant dose reductions in anticipation of heart-lung and isolated lung transplantation.

The multisystem manifestations of cystic fibrosis, particularly chronic bronchopulmonary infection, malabsorption, malnutrition, and diabetes mellitus, pose difficult management problems and require aggressive chest physiotherapy, antibiotics, enteral or parenteral nutritional supplementation, and tight serum glucose control.[49]

Certain underlying diagnoses are associated with increased rates of pulmonary and systemic thrombosis and embolization. These include dilated cardiomyopathy, congestive heart failure, and primary pulmonary hypertension,[47] and most centers recommend routine prophylactic anticoagulation with heparin, warfarin, or antiplatelet agents.

ORGAN PROCUREMENT AND PRESERVATION

Donor Selection

Standard criteria have been established for donor selection (Table 61-3).[50,51] Donors must have sustained irreversible brain death, but due to the susceptibility of the lungs to edema and infection, particularly in the setting of brain death and trauma, suitable heart-lung and lung blocs are more difficult to obtain than other organs. Less than 20% of organ donors possess lungs suitable for transplantation.

Initial donor evaluation consists of a directed history and physical examination, chest x-ray, 12-lead ECG, arterial blood gases, and serologic screening [including human immunodeficiency virus (HIV), hepatitis B surface antigen, hepatitis C antibodies, herpes simplex virus (HSV), cytomegalovirus (CMV), *Toxoplasma*, RPR]. A donor age younger than 50 is preferred. The chest x-ray should be clear and the arterial Po_2 should exceed 140 mm Hg on an Fio_2 of 40% and 300 mm Hg on an Fio_2 of 100%. Lung compliance can be estimated by measuring peak inspiratory pressures, which should be less than 30 cm H_2O. Bronchoscopy should ensure the absence of purulent secretions or signs of aspiration. For combined heart-lung donors, echocardiographic evidence of normal cardiac function and the absence of a significant cardiac history and significant coronary atherosclerosis must be established. Coronary angiography may also be indicated in donors with cardiac risk factors. Finally, direct inspection and palpation of the heart and lungs at explantation is an essential part of the donor evaluation process.

TABLE 61–3 Heart-lung and lung donor selection criteria

Age <40 (heart-lung), <50 (lung)
Smoking history less than 20 pack-years
Arterial Po_2 of 140 mm Hg on an Fio_2 of 40% or 300 mm Hg on an Fio_2 of 100%
Normal chest x-ray
Sputum free of bacteria, fungus, or significant numbers of white blood cells on Gram and fungal staining
Bronchoscopy showing absence of purulent secretions or signs of aspiration
Absence of thoracic trauma
HIV negative

Absolute contraindications to lung and heart-lung donation include prolonged cardiac arrest, arterial hypoxemia, active malignancy (excluding basal cell and squamous cell carcinoma of the skin), and positive HIV status. For heart-lung donation, severe coronary or structural heart disease and prior myocardial infarction are additional contraindications. Relative contraindications to both lung and heart-lung donation include thoracic trauma, sepsis, significant smoking history, prolonged severe hypotension (i.e., less than 60 mm Hg for more than 6 hours), HBsAg or hepatitis C antibodies, multiple resuscitations, and a prolonged high inotropic requirement (e.g., dopamine in excess of 15 μg/kg/min for 24 hours). It is important to rule out correctable metabolic or physiological causes of cardiac rhythm disturbances and electrocardiographic anomalies (e.g., brain herniation, hypothermia, and hypokalemia).

The last decade has seen a trend toward liberalization of standard donor selection criteria. This strategy, which was initiated in response to the donor organ shortage, has been employed at a large number of transplant centers.[52–54] Donors up to age 60 have been used in thoracic transplantation, with good long-term graft survival. However, recent reports from the ISHLT document worse outcomes in recipients of lung allografts from donors over age 55 who had ischemic times longer than 6 to 8 hours.[55] In this group of recipients, long-term survival is impaired and the risk of developing bronchiolitis obliterans is increased. A limitation on smoking history is another criterion that has been liberalized. Conventional guidelines limit smoking history to less than 20 pack years, but modified criteria have allowed for a more extensive smoking history, assuming there is no evidence of COPD or other lung disease on screening tests. Other extended criteria include use of lungs from donors whose sputum Gram stain shows presence of bacteria; in these cases, treatment with antimicrobials is initiated in the donor and continued posttransplantation in the recipient. In general, the presence of fungus in donor sputum samples is a contraindication to donation. Some groups have accepted donors with small pulmonary infiltrates on chest x-ray, though clinical correlation is necessary. Others have selectively used donor lungs in patients with Pa_{O_2} less than 300 mm Hg on Fi_{O_2} of 100%.

Gabbay et al in Australia have adopted an aggressive approach to donor management and "organ resuscitation."[54] By manipulating donors with antibiotic therapy, chest physiotherapy, careful fluid management, ventilator adjustments, and bronchial toilet, 34% of donors with an initial Pa_{O_2} less than 300 mm Hg on Fi_{O_2} of 100% had a rise in their Pa_{O_2} and became acceptable donors.

Areas of investigation in the field of donor organ procurement include the use of non–heart-beating donors. In 2001, Steen et al reported on the transplantation of lungs from a non–heart-beating donor into a 54-year-old woman with COPD.[56] The functional result has been good during the first 5 months of follow-up. However, ethical, logistic, and scientific questions remain on the use of non–heart-beating donors, and this strategy is far from being widely applicable.

Donor Management

The overriding goal in managing the thoracic organ donor is the maintenance of hemodynamic stability and pulmonary function. Patients suffering from acute brain injury are often hemodynamically unstable due to neurogenic shock, excessive fluid losses, and bradycardia. Donor lungs are prone to neurogenic pulmonary edema, aspiration, nosocomial infection, and contusion. Continuous arterial and central venous pressure monitoring, judicious fluid resuscitation, vasopressors, and inotropes are usually required.

Meticulous fluid management prevents intraoperative blood pressure instability and minimizes the need for inotropes and vasopressors that stress the myocardium. Intravascular volume replacement should be given to maintain the central venous pressure between 5 and 8 mm Hg, though fluids should not be administered at rates far in excess of hourly urine output. In general, crystalloid fluid boluses are to be avoided. Diabetes insipidus is common in organ donors and requires the use of intravenous vasopressin (0.8 to 1.0 unit/h) to reduce excessive urine losses.

To maintain adequate perfusion pressures, dopamine is the standard inotropic agent used, although alpha agonists (e.g., phenylephrine) are often appropriate. Blood transfusions should be used sparingly to maintain the hemoglobin concentration around 10g/dL to ensure adequate myocardial oxygen delivery. CMV-negative and leukocyte-filtered blood should be used whenever possible. Hypothermia should be avoided because it predisposes to ventricular arrhythmias and metabolic acidosis.

With regard to mechanical ventilation, Fi_{O_2} values in excess of 40%, especially 100% oxygen "challenges," should be avoided, since these oxygen levels may be toxic to the denervated lung. Ventilator settings should include positive end-expiratory pressures (PEEP) between 3 and 5 cm H_2O to prevent atelectasis.

Donor Operation

The donor operation is performed via a median sternotomy (Fig. 61-5A). After the sternum is divided, a standard chest retractor is placed, and both pleural spaces are opened immediately with inspection of the lungs and pleural spaces, particularly in cases of trauma. The lungs are briefly deflated, and the pulmonary ligaments are divided inferiorly using electrocautery. After completely excising the thymic remnant, the pericardium is opened vertically and laterally on the diaphragm and cradled during dissection of the great vessels and trachea. The ascending aorta, pulmonary artery, and venae cavae are dissected. Umbilical tapes are placed around the ascending aorta and venae cavae (Fig. 61-5B). The pericardium overlying the trachea is incised vertically, and the trachea is encircled with an umbilical tape between the aorta and superior vena cava at the highest point possible and at least four rings above the carina (Fig. 61-5B). The entire anterior pericardium is excised back to each hilum (Fig. 61-5C).

Approximately 15 minutes prior to applying the aortic cross-clamp, prostaglandin E_1 (PGE_1) is infused intravenously, initially at a rate of 20 ng/kg/min, followed by incremental increases of 10 ng/kg/min to a target rate of 100 ng/kg/min (Fig. 61-5D). During PGE_1 infusion, the mean arterial blood pressure should be maintained at or above 55 mm Hg. Ventilation is continued with an Fi_{O_2} of 40% and a PEEP of 3 to 5 cm H_2O. The donor is heparinized. The superior vena cava is ligated and a straight Potts clamp is placed across the inferior vena cava. After the heart is allowed to empty, the aortic cross-clamp is applied, and 10 mL/kg of cold crystalloid cardioplegia, commonly the Stanford formulation, is rapidly infused into the aortic root. The inferior vena cava is incised, and the left atrial appendage is amputated to avoid cardiac distention. While the antegrade cardioplegia is being delivered, pulmonoplegia is rapidly flushed into the main pulmonary artery at a rate of 15 mL/kg/min for 4 minutes. Ice-cold saline or Physiosol solution (Abbott Laboratories, North Chicago, IL) is immediately poured over the heart and lungs. During the cardioplegic and pulmonoplegic infusions, ventilation is maintained with half-normal tidal volumes of room air. Upon completion of the plegic infusions and topical cold application, all solutions are aspirated from the thoracic cavity and the lungs are fully deflated.

For combined heart-lung blocs, the bloc is dissected free from the esophagus commencing at the level of the diaphragm and continuing cephalad to the level of the carina. Dissection is kept close to the esophagus, and care is taken to avoid injury to the trachea, lung, or great vessels. The posterior hilar attachments are divided. The lungs are inflated to a full normal tidal volume, and the trachea is

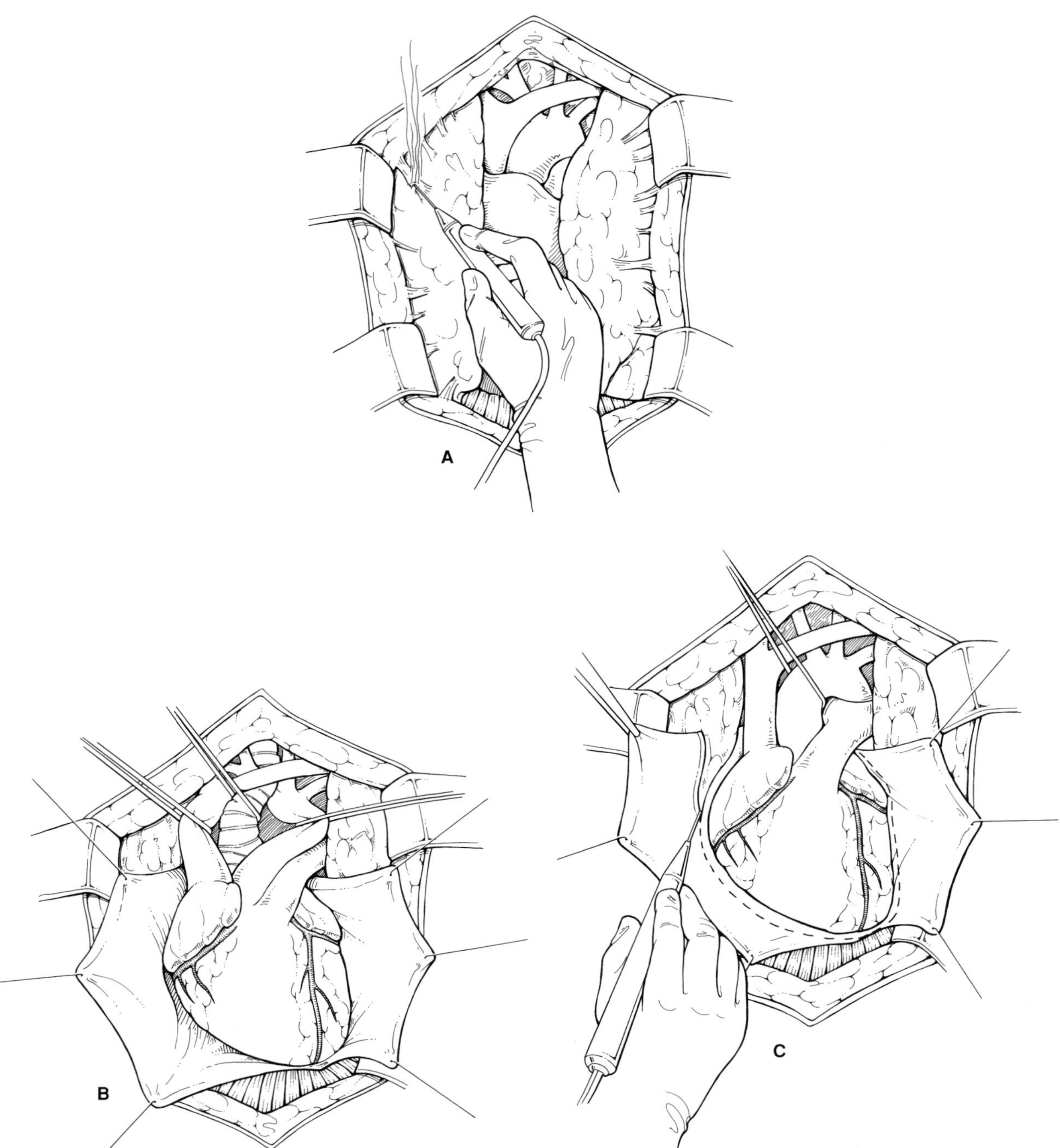

FIGURE 61–5 Donor operation for heart-lung transplantation. (A) Through a median sternotomy, adhesions are lysed and the pulmonary ligaments are divided inferiorly. (B) The pericardium is opened and cradled followed by dissection of the ascending aorta, venae cavae, pulmonary artery, and trachea. (C) The entire anterior pericardium is excised back to each hilum.

stapled at the highest point possible with a TA-55 stapler (U.S. Surgical, Norwalk, CT), at least four rings above the carina (Fig. 61-5E). The trachea is then divided above the staple line, and the entire heart-lung bloc is removed from the chest.

For separate heart and lung blocs, the donor operation is modified slightly, allowing for in situ separation of the heart from the lungs. After delivery of plegic solutions, the great vessels are divided. The heart is reflected anteriorly and a left atriotomy is performed, leaving a 2-cm cuff of atrium around

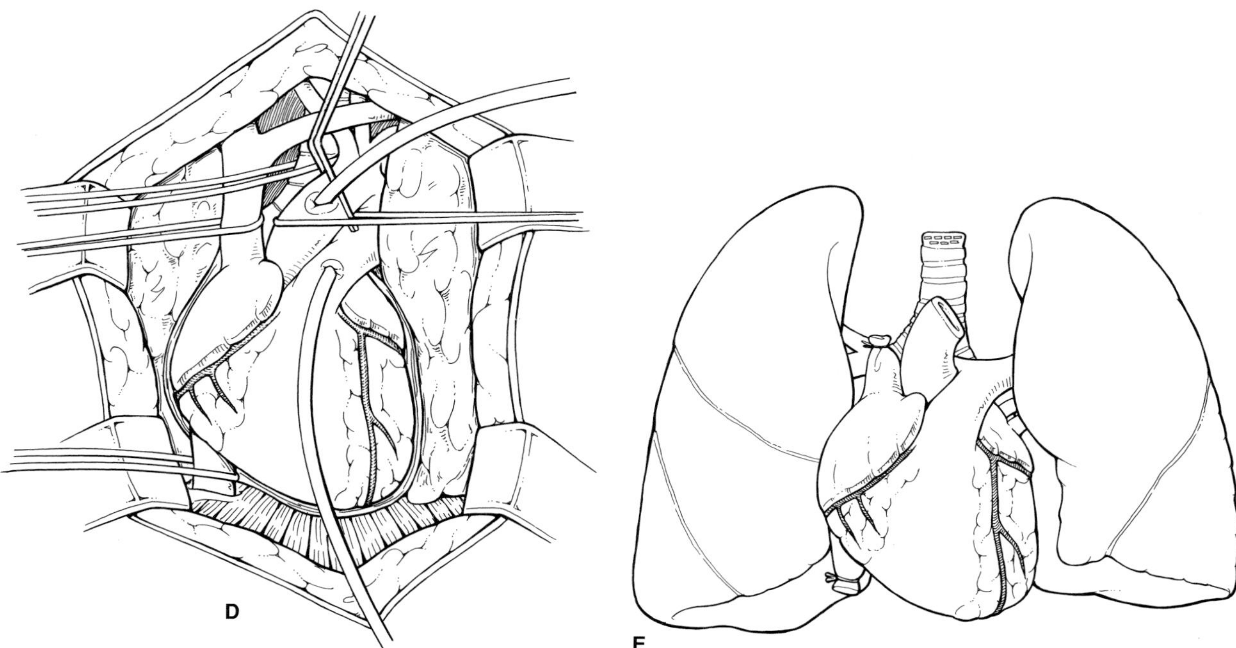

FIGURE 61–5 *(Continued)* (D) Cardioplegia and pulmonoplegia are infused simultaneously into the aorta and main pulmonary artery after aortic cross-clamping. Application of topical cold Physiosol follows immediately. (E) The venae cavae and aorta are divided, and the heart-lung bloc is dissected free from the esophagus and posterior hilar attachments. After the trachea is stapled and divided at the highest point possible, the entire heart-lung bloc is removed from the chest.

the pulmonary vein orifices. Once this division is complete, the heart is removed from the chest. The lung bloc is then dissected free along the pre-esophageal plane above the level of the carina. The lungs are inflated and the trachea is stapled at the highest possible point. If needed, the bilateral lung bloc can be further separated into left and right lung blocs. The left atrial cuff containing the orifices of the pulmonary veins is divided in half vertically. The left and right pulmonary arteries are divided at their junction. Finally, the left mainstem bronchus is stapled near its junction with the trachea.

Once removed from the donor, grafts are wrapped in sterile gauze pads and immersed in ice-cold saline at 2°C to 4°C in several sterile plastic bags placed within a sterile plastic container. This, in turn, is placed in an ice-filled chest and transported to the transplant center.

Organ Preservation and Transport

On-site lung procurement was considered essential between 1981 and 1984 due to inadequate lung preservation techniques.[57] Since then, active research and clinical experience have produced several different preservation protocols that have permitted distant procurement. Most centers currently tolerate a maximum of 6 to 8 hours of ischemia in lung and heart-lung allografts. This practice is supported by several studies, including independent retrospective studies from the University of Pittsburgh[58] and the University of Virginia[59] that showed comparable long-term survival and rates of acute rejection and bronchiolitis obliterans among recipients of grafts with over 6 hours of ischemia compared with those with less than 4 or with 4 to 6 hours of ischemia. In animal studies, reports of successful transplantation of lung allografts with cold ischemia times up to 18 hours have been reported. However, it is believed that beyond a certain threshold, organ ischemia will likely lead to primary graft failure and/or impaired long-term function.

The overriding principle in preservation is to minimize injury to the allograft from ischemia and reperfusion.[60] Ischemia-reperfusion injury is mediated by reactive oxygen species, which disrupt the homeostatic mechanisms in myocyte and endothelial cells. As receptors for leukocyte adhesion molecules are upregulated and leukocyte chemotactic factors are released, an inflammatory response ensues, leading to cellular injury. Several approaches to minimizing ischemia-reperfusion injury have developed, and these include donor pretreatment, development of specialized preservation solutions, and recipient treatments.

Hypothermia is considered by many to be the most important method of organ preservation. It works by reducing the tissue's metabolic demand by up to 99%. In a small number of centers, hypothermic preservation includes donor core cooling on CPB. Universally, hypothermia is employed during explantation, storage, and implantation. During explantation, organs are flushed with cold plegic solutions (between 0°C to 10 °C, depending on the institution and solution employed). They are stored at 0°C to 10°C, and during implantation, they are covered with gauze soaked in saline slush or recipients are cooled through CPB. The optimal temperature for flush and storage of organs remains unknown, but common practice is to rely on ice bath temperature for convenience.

Heart-lung and lung blocs are typically preserved with a cold pulmonary artery flush in conjunction with standard crystalloid cardioplegic arrest. A variety of crystalloid flush solutions are used worldwide, and they can be divided into two categories based on their electrolyte compositions: intracellular and extracellular. Intracellular solutions contain moderate to high concentrations of potassium and little calcium and sodium; Euro-Collins, University of Wisconsin (UW), and Cardiosol are examples. Extracellular solutions contain high concentrations of sodium and low to moderate concentrations of potassium; low-potassium dextran solution is an example. While Euro-Collins is the most frequently used preservation solution, data comparing the merits of the various solutions is sparse and for now inconclusive.

Prostaglandins are commonly used for donor pretreatment and as an additive in pulmonary flush solutions. PGE_1, a vasodilator, is given to counteract reflex pulmonary vasoconstriction resulting from the cold flush and to permit uniform distribution of the perfusate throughout the lung. Experimental studies also suggest that PGE_1 treatment may minimize reperfusion injury through its anti-inflammatory properties.[61]

Another commonly used donor pretreatment strategy is steroid treatment. Experimental evidence suggests that donor lymphocytes may play a role in ischemic lung graft injury, so methylprednisolone is given intravenously to the donor to inactivate them.

Experimental studies suggest that lung graft function is improved when the explanted organ is inflated, when 100% oxygen is used for inflation, and when the lung is transported at 10°C.[62] Research in the field of lung preservation has recently focused on the role of various flush and storage solution additives, such as antioxidants, which may act as free radical scavengers. Other additives that have been shown to decrease reperfusion injury in research models include nitric oxide donors and phosphodiesterase inhibitors. Additional areas of research interest include the development of leukocyte depletion strategies, examining the role of gene therapy in modifying donor organ susceptibility to ischemia-reperfusion injury, and the development of colloid-based perfusates.

These preservation techniques, coupled with streamlined donor and recipient protocols, have permitted procurements as far as 1000 miles from the transplant center. Extensive communication and coordination must be maintained between the organ procurement agency, donor and recipient operative teams, medical centers, and abdominal procurement teams.

RECIPIENT OPERATION

The recipient operation in heart-lung and lung transplantation proceeds in two phases. The first is excision of the native organ(s) and the second is implantation of the allograft. Cardiopulmonary bypass is mandatory in heart-lung transplantation and occasional in single and bilateral lung transplantation. At all times, it should be available as standby. At Stanford, we have favored the use of CPB during bilateral lung transplantation for a variety of reasons. There is improved exposure of the hilar strutures, which is particularly helpful in patients with dense adhesions and bronchial collaterals. CPB allows for early pneumonectomies without hemodynamic or respiratory instability, and the ischemic time of the second lung is substantially reduced when compared to off-CPB bilateral lung transplants. Its use also prevents overperfusion of the first lung graft with the entire cardiac output. In patients with suppurative lung disease, the use of CPB facilitates careful washout of the distal trachea and proximal bronchi to prevent contamination of the first implanted lung. Others prefer to avoid CPB, as it may be associated with increased blood loss, transfusion needs, and reperfusion injury. More detailed experimental and clinical studies are needed to resolve these questions, but in the meanwhile, each recipient should be evaluated individually in deciding if CPB is needed.

Anesthetic monitoring includes arterial pressure monitoring, pulse oximetry, continuous electrocardiography, pulmonary artery catheter monitoring, temperature monitoring, and urine output monitoring. The use of double-lumen endotracheal tubes is particularly helpful, allowing for single lung ventilation during certain portions of the dissection. Large bore intravenous lines are placed for volume infusion. Transesophageal echocardiography is often performed during the procedure.

Heart-Lung Transplantation

The recipient is positioned supine on the operating table. The chest is entered through a median sternotomy, a sternal retractor is placed, and both pleural spaces are opened anteriorly from the level of the diaphragm to the level of the great vessels (Fig. 61-6A). Any pleural adhesions are divided using electrocautery. In patients in whom dense pleural adhesions are anticipated, such as those with previous thoracotomies or cystic fibrosis, a bilateral "clamshell" thoracotomy is performed. Combined with the use of perioperative antifibrinolytic therapy (e.g., aprotinin) and an argon beam coagulator, this approach improves exposure and facilitates both lysis of adhesions and hemostasis.

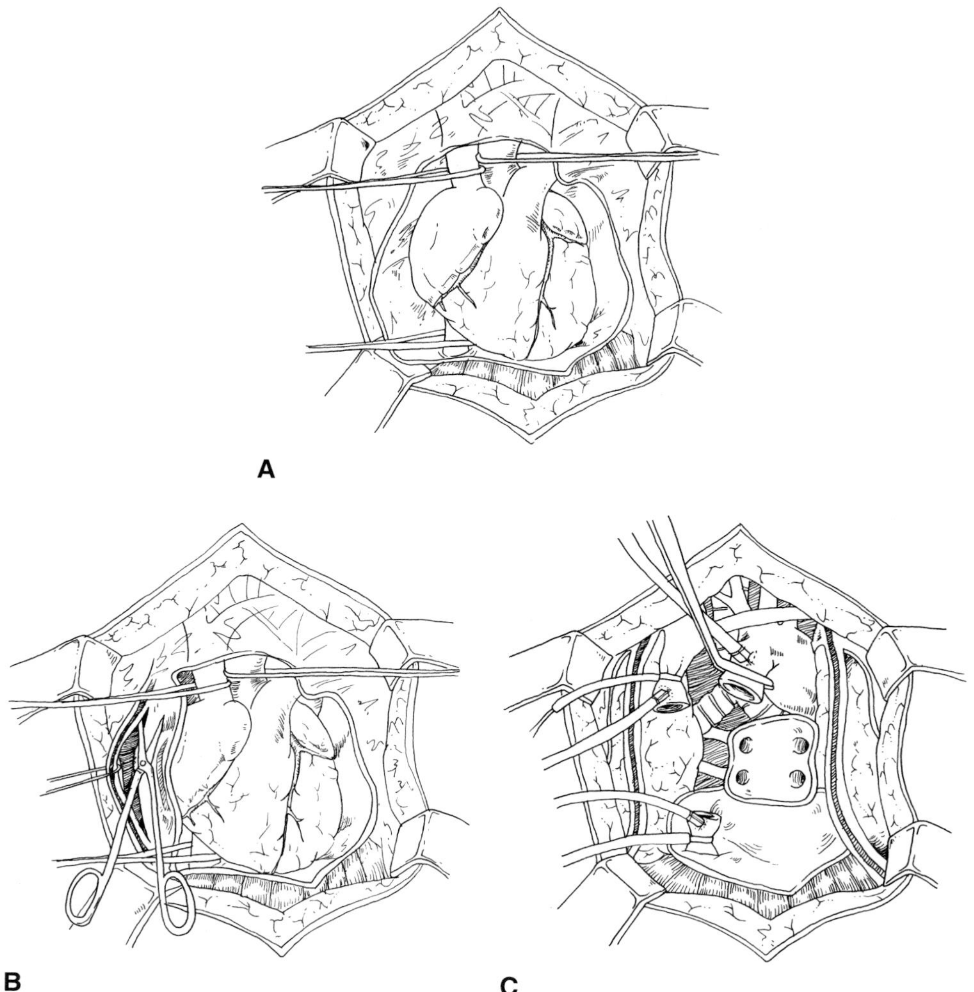

FIGURE 61–6 Recipient operation for heart-lung transplantation. (A) Through a median sternotomy, the anterior pericardium is partially removed and the ascending aorta and both venae cavae are dissected and encircled with tapes. (B) The right phrenic nerve is carefully separated from the right hilum, providing a space for inserting the right lung of the graft. (C) Cannulation for cardiopulmonary bypass consists of a cannula in the high ascending aorta and separate vena caval cannulas. Once on bypass, the native heart is excised in a manner similar to that for standard cardiac explantation.

The anterior pericardium is excised, while lateral segments are preserved to support the heart and protect the phrenic nerves. A 3-cm border of the pericardium should be left both anteriorly and posteriorly to each phrenic nerve extending from the level of the diaphragm to the level of the great vessels (Fig. 61-6B).

After fully heparinizing the recipient, the ascending aorta is cannulated near the base of the innominate artery, and the venae cavae are individually cannulated laterally and snared. Cardiopulmonary bypass with systemic cooling to 28°C to 30°C is instituted, and the heart is excised at the midatrial level. The aorta is divided just above the aortic valve, and the pulmonary artery is divided at its bifurcation (Fig. 61-6C). The left atrial remnant is then divided vertically at a point halfway between the right and left pulmonary veins.

The posterior edge of the left atrial and pulmonary venous remnant is developed in a manner that allows the left inferior and superior pulmonary veins to be displaced over into the left chest. Following division of the pulmonary ligament, the left lung is moved into the field, allowing full dissection of the posterior aspect of the left hilum, being careful to avoid the vagus nerve posteriorly. Once this is completed, the left main pulmonary artery is divided (Fig. 61-6D), and the left main bronchus is stapled with a TA-30 stapler and divided. The same technique of hilar dissection and division is repeated on the right side (Fig. 61-6E), and both lungs are removed from the chest.

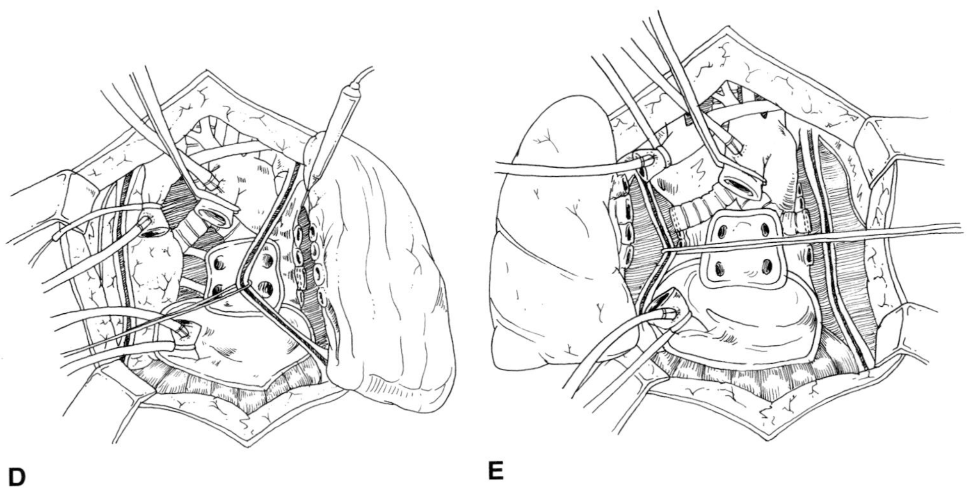

FIGURE 61–6 *(Continued)* (D,E) Left and right pneumonectomies are performed by dividing the respective inferior pulmonary ligament, pulmonary artery and veins, and mainstem bronchus.

The native main pulmonary artery remnant is removed, leaving a portion of the pulmonary artery intact adjacent to the underside of the aorta near the ligamentum arteriosum to preserve the left recurrent laryngeal nerve. Attention is then turned to preparing the distal trachea for anastomosis. The stapled ends of the right and left bronchi are grasped and dissection is carried up to the level of the distal trachea. Bronchial vessels are individually identified and carefully ligated. Patients with congenital heart disease and pulmonary atresia or severe cyanosis secondary to Eisenmenger's syndrome may have large mediastinal bronchial collaterals that must be meticulously ligated. Perfect hemostasis is necessary in this area of the dissection, because it is obscured once graft implantation is completed. Once absolute hemostasis is achieved, the trachea is divided at the carina with a no. 15 blade. The chest is now prepared to receive the heart-lung graft.

The donor heart-lung bloc is removed from its transport container and prepared by irrigating, aspirating, and culturing the tracheobronchial tree and by trimming the trachea to leave one cartilaginous ring above the carina. The heart-lung graft is then lowered into the chest, passing the right lung beneath the right phrenic nerve pedicle. The left lung is then gently manipulated under the left phrenic nerve pedicle (Fig. 61-6F). The tracheal anastomosis is performed using continuous 3-0 polypropylene suture (Fig. 61-6G). The posterior membranous portion of the anastomosis is performed first, followed by completion of the anastomosis anteriorly. The lungs are then ventilated with room air at half-normal tidal volumes to inflate the lungs and reduce atelectasis. Topical cooling with a continuous infusion of cold Physiosol into both thoraces is begun. To augment endomyocardial cooling and to exclude air from the graft, a third cold "bubble-free" line is placed directly into the left atrial appendage.

Next, the bicaval venous anastomosis is performed. The recipient inferior vena cava is anastomosed to the donor inferior vena cava-right atrial junction with a continuous 4-0 polypropylene suture. At this point the patient is rewarmed toward 37°C, and the superior vena caval and aortic anastomoses are performed end-to-end with continuous 4-0 polypropylene sutures (Fig. 61-6H). After the ascending aorta and pulmonary artery are cleared of air, the aortic cross-clamp and caval tapes are removed. The left atrial catheter is removed, and the atrium is allowed to drain. The amputated left atrial stump is oversewn, and the pulmonoplegia infusion site on the pulmonary artery is closed. The heart is defibrillated, and the patient is gradually weaned from cardiopulmonary bypass in the standard fashion. Methylprednisolone (500 mg) is administered to the recipient following heparin reversal with protamine sulfate.

PEEP at 3 to 5 cm H_2O and an FiO_2 of 40% are maintained. As in cardiac transplantation, isoproterenol (0.005 to 0.01 μg/kg/min) is usually initiated on graft reperfusion to increase the heart rate to about 100 to 110 bpm and to lower pulmonary vascular resistance. Temporary right atrial and ventricular pacing wires are placed. Right and left pleural chest tubes (right angle) are placed along each diaphragm, as well as one mediastinal tube. The chest is closed in the standard fashion. Finally, the double-lumen endotracheal tube is exchanged for a single-lumen tube and the tracheal anastomosis is checked endoscopically before transporting the patient to the intensive care unit.

Lick et al at the University of Texas and the University of Arizona have recently described an interesting alternative to the standard technique in which the pulmonary hila are placed anterior to the phrenic nerves and direct caval anastomoses are used whenever feasible.[63] This modification obviates extensive dissection of the phrenic nerves and posterior

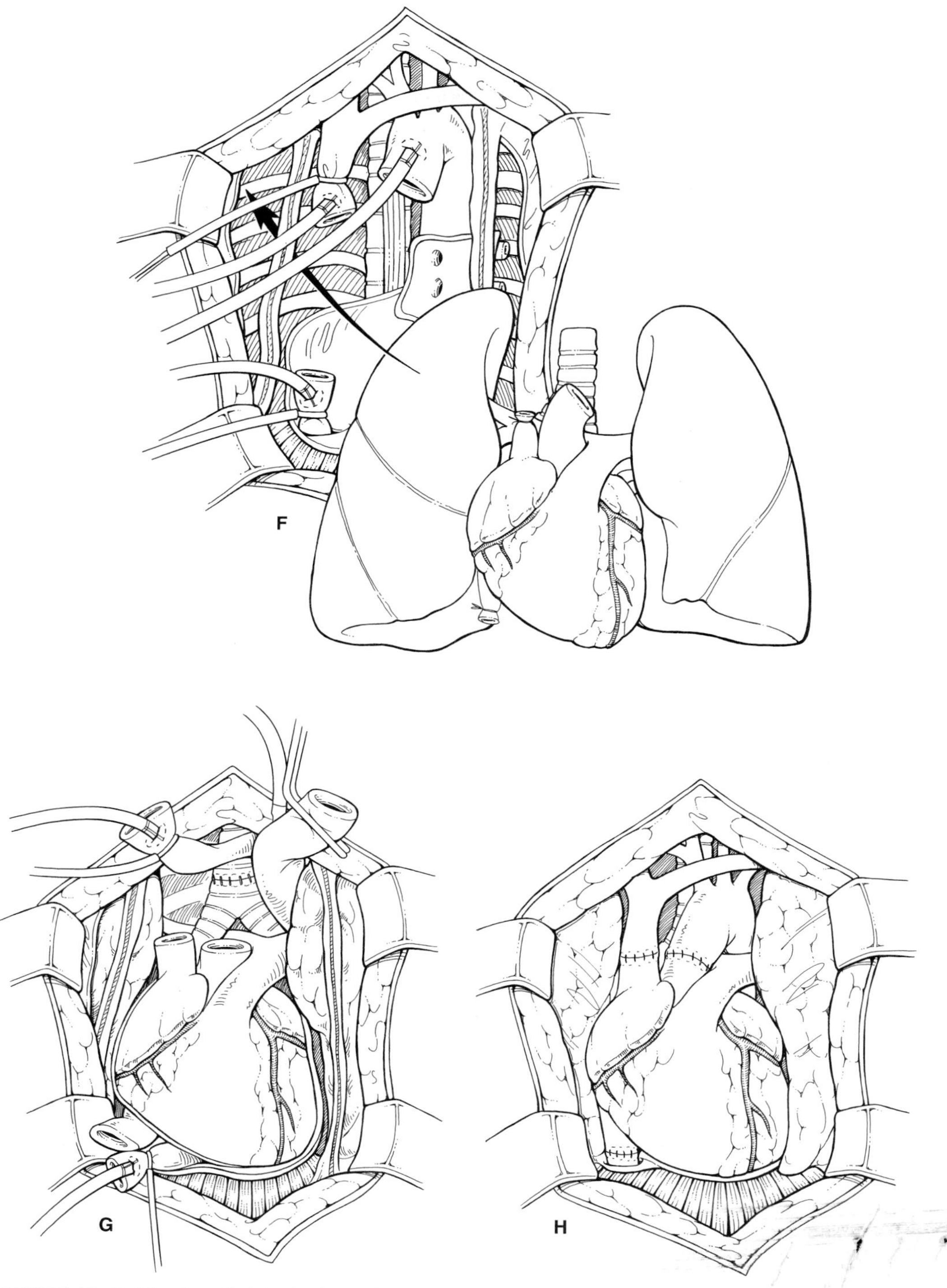

FIGURE 61–6 *(Continued)* (F) The heart-lung graft is moved into the chest, beginning with passage of the right lung underneath the right phrenic nerve pedicle, followed by manipulation of the left lung beneath the left phrenic nerve pedicle. (G) The tracheal anastomosis is performed with a continuous 3-0 polypropylene suture. (H) The caval and aortic anastomoses are performed with a continuous 4-0 polypropylene suture.

mediastinum, decreasing the likelihood of phrenic and vagus nerve injury. Furthermore, the posterior mediastinum can be inspected more easily for bleeding after implantation by rotating the heart-lung bloc anteriorly and medially while still on bypass.

Single Lung Transplantation

If possible, the lung with the least function determined by preoperative ventilation-perfusion scan is selected for replacement. The patient is placed in a standard thoracotomy position, with access to the groin should CPB be needed. A posterior lateral thoracotomy is made at the level of the fourth or fifth intercostal space. Adhesions are lysed and the hilar dissection is performed. The pulmonary artery, the superior and inferior pulmonary veins, and the mainstem bronchus are isolated. A trial occlusion of the pulmonary artery is used to determine whether the procedure will be tolerated without CPB. If it is tolerated, the pulmonary artery is ligated and divided distal to the upper lobe branch. The pulmonary veins are also ligated and divided. The mainstem bronchus is stapled and divided, and the native lung is explanted.

The donor lung is removed from its transport container and prepared for implantation. The donor bronchus is opened and secretions are aspirated and cultured. The bronchus is trimmed, leaving two cartilaginous rings proximal to the orifice of the upper lobe. Any remaining pericardial and lymphatic tissue is removed, and the left atrial cuff is trimmed as needed. The donor lung is then placed in the recipient's chest and covered with saline slush and iced laparotomy pads.

The sequence of anastomoses is a matter of preference, though most perform the deepest anastomosis (the bronchial anastomosis) first and then proceed to the more superficial ones. The bronchial anastomosis is fashioned with 4-0 polypropylene suture. We favor a continuous suture technique; alternatively, the membranous portion can be sewn with interrupted suture. Alternatively, the entire anastomosis can be sewn with a running suture. Variations on the end-to-end bronchial anastomosis include the use of a telescoping technique, in which the donor bronchus is intussuscepted into the recipient bronchus, and the placement of an omental pedicle flap around the anastomosis. These techniques were developed to prevent bronchial anastomotic dehiscence but are now rarely performed.

Once the bronchial anastomosis is complete, attention is then turned to making the pulmonary venous anastomosis. A side-biting clamp is applied to the left atrium to include the pulmonary veins. The recipient pulmonary vein stumps are opened and the intervening atrial tissue is cut. This creates a cuff that is anastomosed to the donor atrial remnant using continuous 4-0 polypropylene suture; this suture is not tied down until reperfusion. Donor and recipient pulmonary arteries are anastomosed with 5-0 polypropylene suture. Upon graft inflation, kinking can occur if the arteries are left too long, so they must be carefully trimmed to an appropriate length before fashioning the anastomosis. The pulmonary artery anastomosis is de-aired. The lung is inflated, and the pulmonary artery clamp is temporarily released to allow flushing of air through the atrial suture line, and the left atrial clamp is removed to allow retrograde de-airing of the atrial anastomosis. The pulmonary venous anastomosis is then secured.

After hemostasis is ensured, apical and basal chest tubes are inserted. The ribs are reapproximated and the chest is closed in a standard fashion. The double-lumen endotracheal tube is exchanged for a single-lumen tube and bronchoscopy is performed to evaluate the bronchial anastomosis.

Bilateral Lung Transplantation

Bilateral lung transplantation is performed as sequential single lung transplants. The patient is positioned supine and a bilateral anterior thoracosternotomy (clamshell) incision is made at the level of the fourth intercostal space. The lung with the least amount of function (as determined by a preoperative ventilation-perfusion scan) is removed first and replaced with an allograft as described for single lung transplantation above. Once ventilation and perfusion are established in the first allograft, the second native lung is explanted and the second allograft is implanted. Bilateral chest tubes are placed and the chest is closed. Bronchoscopy is performed to evaluate the bronchial anastomoses.

Many centers use CPB routinely during bilateral lung transplantation. It allows for improved exposure, shorter graft ischemic times, controlled reperfusion, and the use of leukocyte-depleting filters. Because the risk of bleeding may be increased with CPB, strategies have been developed to minimize the chance of hemorrhage. These include the routine use of aprotinin and heparin-coated CPB circuits, as well as the availability of an argon beam coagulator.

POSTOPERATIVE MANAGEMENT

Heart-Lung and Lung Graft Physiology

Interesting corollaries to the clinical benefits of heart-lung and isolated lung transplantation are the structural and functional aspects of the transplanted heart-lung or lung bloc (Table 61-4).

Denervation of the lungs results in diminished cough reflex as well as impaired mucociliary clearance mechanisms. This predisposes recipients to pulmonary infections and necessitates aggressive postoperative pulmonary toilet.[64] Moreover, ischemia and reperfusion injury in the transplanted lung, along with disrupted pulmonary lymphatics, can result in increased vascular permeability and

TABLE 61–4 Structural and functional aspects of the transplanted heart-lung and lung allograft

Heart-lung only
- Denervation from sympathetic and parasympathetic cardiac plexus
- Higher resting heart rate
- Absence of respiratory sinus arrhythmia and carotid reflex bradycardia
- Increased chronotropic and inotropic sensitivity to circulating catecholamines
- Slower initial rise in heart rate in response to exercise or stress
- Normal coronary flow reserve in the absence of rejection

Heart-lung and isolated lung
- Increased pulmonary vascular permeability and interstitial edema (early)
- Disrupted pulmonary lymphatics
- Diminished cough reflex
- Impaired mucociliary airway clearance mechanisms
- Hypoxic pulmonary vasoconstriction intact

varying degrees of interstitial edema. For the heart-lung recipients, denervation of the cardiac allograft leads to additional physiologic characteristics. The denervated heart has lost its sympathetic and parasympathetic autonomic regulation; therefore recipients of heart-lung grafts do not have normal autonomic regulation of heart rate, contractility, or coronary artery caliber. The resting heart rate is generally higher due to the absence of vagal tone. Respiratory sinus arrhythmia and carotid reflex bradycardia are absent. Interestingly, the denervated heart develops an increased sensitivity to catecholamines; this is due to an increase in beta-adrenergic receptor density and a loss of norepinephrine uptake in postganglionic sympathetic neurons.[65,66] This augmented sensitivity plays an important role in maintaining an adequate cardiac response to exercise and stress. During exercise, the recipient experiences a steady but delayed increase in heart rate, primarily due to a rise in circulating catecholamines. This initial rise in heart rate is subsequently accompanied by an immediate increase in filling pressures resulting from augmented venous return. These changes lead to an augmentation of stroke volume and cardiac output sufficient to sustain an increase in activity. The ability of the coronary circulation to dilate and increase blood flow in response to increased myocardial oxygen demand is normal in cardiac transplant recipients and would likewise be expected to be so in recipients of heart-lung grafts. Conversely, graft coronary vasodilator reserve is abnormal in the presence of rejection, hypertrophy, or regional wall abnormalities.

Clinical Management in the Early Postoperative Period

The acute postoperative management for heart-lung and isolated lung graft recipients centers around careful fluid and ventilatory management. Simply put, the primary objective in the immediate postoperative period is to maintain adequate perfusion and gas exchange in the recipient while minimizing intravenous fluid administration, cardiac work, and barotrauma.

Upon completion of the transplant, the patient is transported to the intensive care unit (ICU), where cardiac rhythm and arterial and central venous pressures are monitored. Strict isolation precautions, previously enforced to reduce the incidence of infection in these immunosuppressed patients, are no longer required; simple handwashing is now considered sufficient.

Approximately 10% to 20% of heart-lung graft recipients experience some degree of transient sinus node dysfunction in the immediate perioperative period, often manifested as sinus bradycardia, which usually resolves within a week. The use of bicaval venous anastomoses has been reported to lower the incidence of sinus node dysfunction and improve tricuspid valve function.[67] Because cardiac output is primarily rate dependent after heart-lung transplantation, the heart rate should be maintained between 90 and 110 bpm during the first few postoperative days using temporary pacing or isoproterenol (0.005–0.01 μg/kg/min) as needed. Although rarely seen, persistent sinus node dysfunction and bradycardia may require a permanent transvenous pacemaker. The systolic blood pressure should be maintained between 90 and 110 mm Hg using afterload reduction in the form of nitroglycerin or nitroprusside if necessary. Renal-dose dopamine (3–5 μg/kg/min) is used frequently to augment renal blood flow and urine output. The adequacy of cardiac output is indicated by warm extremities and a urine output great than 0.5 mL/kg/hr without diuretics. Cardiac function generally returns to normal within 3 to 4 days, at which time parenteral inotropes and vasodilators can be weaned.

In the heart-lung graft recipient, several factors may contribute to some form of depressed global myocardial performance in the acute postoperative setting. The myocardium is potentially subject to prolonged ischemia, inadequate preservation, or catecholamine depletion prior to implantation. Hypovolemia, cardiac tamponade, sepsis, and bradycardia may also be contributory and should be treated expeditiously if they are present. A Swan-Ganz pulmonary artery catheter should be used in cases of persistently abnormal hemodynamics.

Ventilatory management is a key element in the postoperative management of both heart-lung and isolated lung graft recipients. Barotrauma and high airway pressures that might compromise bronchial mucosal flow should be avoided. Lower tidal volumes and flow rates may be necessary to limit peak airway pressures to less than 40 cm H_2O. Upon arrival to the ICU, an anteroposterior chest x-ray is obtained, and the ventilator is typically set to an F_{IO_2} of 50%, tidal volume of 10 to 15 mL/kg, an assist-control rate of 10 to 14 breaths per minute, and PEEP of 3 to 5 cm H_2O. These settings are adjusted every 30 minutes to achieve an arterial P_{O_2} greater than 75 mm Hg on an F_{IO_2} of 40%, an arterial carbon

TABLE 61–5 Typical immunosuppression protocol for heart-lung and lung transplant recipients

Immunosuppressant	Early postoperative period	Late postoperative period
Cyclosporine	5-10 mg/kg/d orally[a,b] (PO) or 0.05-0.1 mg/kg/h IV	3-6 mg/kg/d PO[c]
Methylprednisolone	500 mg IV after reperfusion followed by 125 mg IV every 8 hours for 3 doses	None
Prednisone	0.6 mg/kg/d PO starting on day 15	0.1-0.2 mg/kg/d PO
Azathioprine	2 mg/kg/d PO[a]	1-2 mg/kg/d PO[d]
RATG	2.5 mg/kg/d IV on days 1, 2, 3, 5, and 7	

[a]Intravenous dose only if preoperative serum creatinine >1.5 mg/dL.
[b]Maintain trough serum concentration between 150-250 ng/mL.
[c]Maintain trough serum concentration between 100-150 ng/mL.
[d]Maintain white blood cell count greater than 4000/mm^3.

dioxide pressure (Pa_{CO_2}) between 30 and 40 mm Hg, and a pH between 7.35 and 7.45. Pulmonary toilet with endotracheal suctioning is an effective means of reducing mucous plugging and atelectasis. Ventilatory weaning is initiated after the patient is deemed stable, awake, and alert. Usually, weaning is accomplished through successive decrements in intermittent mandatory ventilation rate followed by a trial of continuous positive airway pressure. Once ventilatory mechanics and arterial blood gases are deemed acceptable, the patient is extubated. This usually occurs within the first 24 hours after transplantation. Subsequent pulmonary care consists of vigorous diuresis, supplemental oxygen for several days, continued aggressive pulmonary toilet and incentive spirometry, and serial chest x-rays.

A diffuse interstitial infiltrate is often found on early postoperative chest x-rays. Previously referred to as a *reimplantation response,* this finding is better defined as graft edema due to inadequate preservation, reperfusion injury, or early rejection.[68] It appears that the degree of pulmonary edema is inversely related to the quality of preservation. Judicious administration of fluid and loop diuretics is required to maintain fluid balance and minimize this pulmonary edema.

Early lung graft dysfunction manifested by persistent marginal gas exchange without evidence of infection or rejection occurs in less than 15% of transplants.[69] This primary graft failure is often the result of ischemia-reperfusion injury and is manifested histologically by diffuse alveolar damage. Of course, technical causes of graft failure, such as pulmonary venous anastomotic stenosis or thrombosis, must always be considered. In cases of persistent severe pulmonary graft dysfunction refractory to mechanical ventilatory maneuvers, extracorporeal membrane oxygenation (ECMO)[70] and inhaled nitric oxide[71] have been used successfully to stabilize gas exchange in several patients. In others, urgent retransplantation has been performed.

Expedient removal of vascular lines has been shown to reduce the incidence of line sepsis. Pleural and mediastinal chest tubes are removed when drainage has fallen to less than 25 mL/h. For heart-lung graft recipients, pacing wires are removed between 7 and 10 days after transplantation, provided that pacing is not required. After several days, barring significant complications, the patient is transferred from the ICU to a standard cardiothoracic surgical ward for the remainder of the hospital stay.

Immunosuppressive Management: Early and Late Postoperative Regimens

For heart-lung and lung graft recipients, immunosuppression begins intraoperatively and is continued for the patient's lifetime. The conventional triple-drug combination consists of cyclosporine, azathioprine, and prednisone. Initially, high doses of these drugs are given, and they are later tapered for chronic administration. A typical dosing protocol employed at Stanford University Hospital is outlined in Table 61-5. Cyclosporine is initiated in the early postoperative period, initially intravenously (0.05-0.1 mg/kg/h) and subsequently orally when oral intake is well established (5-10 mg/kg/d in two divided doses). Dosing is titrated to maintain a trough serum concentration between 150 and 250 ng/mL in the first few weeks after transplantation and from 100 to 150 ng/mL thereafter. Azathioprine is administered intravenously at 4 mg/kg preoperatively and subsequently maintained at approximately 2 to 3 mg/kg/d. Azathioprine dosages are adjusted to maintain the white blood cell count greater than 4000 cells/mm^3. Methylprednisolone is administered intraoperatively at graft reperfusion (500 mg intravenously) and then continued for the first 24 hours at 125 mg intravenously every 8 hours. Steroids are then suspended for 2 weeks, based on experimental and clinical evidence that they impede bronchial anastomotic healing. After 2 weeks, prednisone is started at a daily oral dose of 0.6 mg/kg and gradually tapered over the next 3 to 4 weeks to 0.1 to 0.2 mg/kg/d.

The conventional triple-drug combination of cyclosporine, azathioprine, and prednisone is modified at some centers. Tacrolimus (FK506) and mycophenolate mofetil are two drugs that have been used widely in kidney and liver transplantation; experience with use of these drugs in heart-lung and lung transplant recipients is limited. One promising study by Keenan et al compared triple therapy with tacrolimus, azathioprine, and steroids to triple therapy with cyclosporine, azathioprine, and steroids.[72] Among the 133 lung allograft recipients studied, they found decreased acute rejection episodes and increased freedom from obliterative bronchiolitis at 2 years in the tacrolimus/azathioprine/steroid group. Reichenspurner et al also found lower acute rejection rates and comparable infection rates in lung transplant recipients treated with tacrolimus-based immunotherapy rather than cyclosporine.[73] Larger studies and longer follow-up periods will be needed before conventional immunosuppressive regimens are modified.

Many centers have added prophylactic induction therapy to the standard triple-drug regimen. This includes the use of OKT3, antithymocyte globulin (RATG and ATGAM), and daclizumab. OKT3 is a murine monoclonal antibody preparation that recognizes the CD3 antigen of human T cells. RATG and ATGAM are polyclonal anti–T cell antibody preparations. Daclizumab is a monoclonal antibody preparation that blocks IL-2-dependent activation of human T cells by binding to their IL-2 receptors. Use of these agents may reduce the rate of acute pulmonary rejection, but may also predispose to infection. Several retrospective and prospective studies have compared the efficacy of all or some of these induction agents. Palmer et al found a decreased incidence of acute rejection in lung transplant recipients receiving RATG induction and conventional triple-drug therapy when compared to patients receiving triple-drug therapy alone.[74] Barlow et al found that the incidence of acute pulmonary rejection was significantly lower in recipients induced with RATG compared with those induced with OKT3; in addition, there was a trend toward decreased infection rate in the RATG group when compared to the OKT3 cohort.[75] Brock et al performed a prospective nonrandomized trial comparing OKT3, ATGAM, and daclizumab as induction agents in 87 lung allograft recipients.[76] Among all groups, they found comparable freedom from acute rejection and bronchiolitis obliterans syndrome and comparable long-term survival. However, daclizumab was associated with a lower rate of infections. Unfortunately, the follow-up for the daclizumab cohort was only 7 months, whereas the other cohorts were followed for 2 years. Long-term follow-up will be important in ascertaining which induction therapy is optimal in heart-lung and lung allograft recipients. Moreover, because of the increased risk of infection with some agents and an association with increased risk of development of posttransplant lymphoproliferative disorder, induction agents should be used with caution.

Judicious doses of immunosuppressives are usually well tolerated by patients; however, each is associated with side effects. Cyclosporine is commonly associated with nephrotoxicity, hypertension, hepatotoxicity, hirsutism, and an increased incidence of lymphoma. The primary toxicity of azathioprine is generalized bone marrow depression, which manifests as leukopenia, anemia, and thrombocytopenia. Steroids are associated with a myriad of side effects, including the development of cushingoid features, hypertension, diabetes, osteoporosis, and peptic ulcer disease. Initial doses of OKT3 and antithymocyte globulin can be associated with a "cytokine release syndrome"; significant hypotension, bronchospasm, and fever can result. Therefore, patients receiving these induction agents are premedicated with acetominophen, antihistamines, and corticosteroids, and are monitored closely. Interestingly, daclizumab is not associated with the cytokine release syndrome.

Infection Prophylaxis

Antiviral and antifungal prophylaxis are important components of postoperative management in heart-lung and lung transplant recipients. Cytomegalovirus prophylaxis (CMV) with ganciclovir is employed by many centers in any CMV-positive recipient and in any CMV-negative recipient receiving an allograft from a CMV-positive donor. Ganciclovir is typically given for a several week course, and can be associated with leukopenia. Some patients may require G-CSF if their white blood cell count falls below 4000. Fungal prophylaxis against mucosal *Candida* infection includes use of daily nystatin swish and swallow. *Pneumocystis carinii* prophylaxis consists of trimethoprim-sulfamethoxazole or aerosolized pentamidine. In the immediate postoperative period, *Aspergillus* colonization is inhibited by the use of aerosolized amphotericin B. For *Toxoplasma*-negative recipients of grafts from *Toxoplasma*-positive patients, pyrimethamine prophylaxis is maintained for the first 6 months after transplantation.

Graft Surveillance: Patient Follow-Up Schedule

Routine clinical follow-up for heart-lung and lung allograft recipients is required to monitor graft function and modify immunosuppressive regimens. Regular surveillance protocols have been developed to monitor graft function, and these typically consist of serial pulmonary function tests, arterial blood gases, and bronchoscopic evaluation at 2 weeks, 4 to 6 weeks, 12 weeks, and 6 months after transplantation, and yearly thereafter. Transbronchial biopsies are obtained from each transplanted lung, and lavage specimens are submitted for staining (i.e., Gram, fungal, acid-fast bacillus, and silver), culture, and cytology. Surveillance endomyocardial biopsies are performed at 3 months and then annually in heart-lung graft recipients.

In addition to routine surveillance, follow-up is often needed to address changes in clinical status. Complications related to transplantation are many, and these must be addressed carefully and expediently to prevent long-term graft failure.

POSTOPERATIVE COMPLICATIONS

Early morbidity and mortality after heart-lung and lung transplantation (within 30 days of operation or before initial discharge from hospital) are most commonly caused

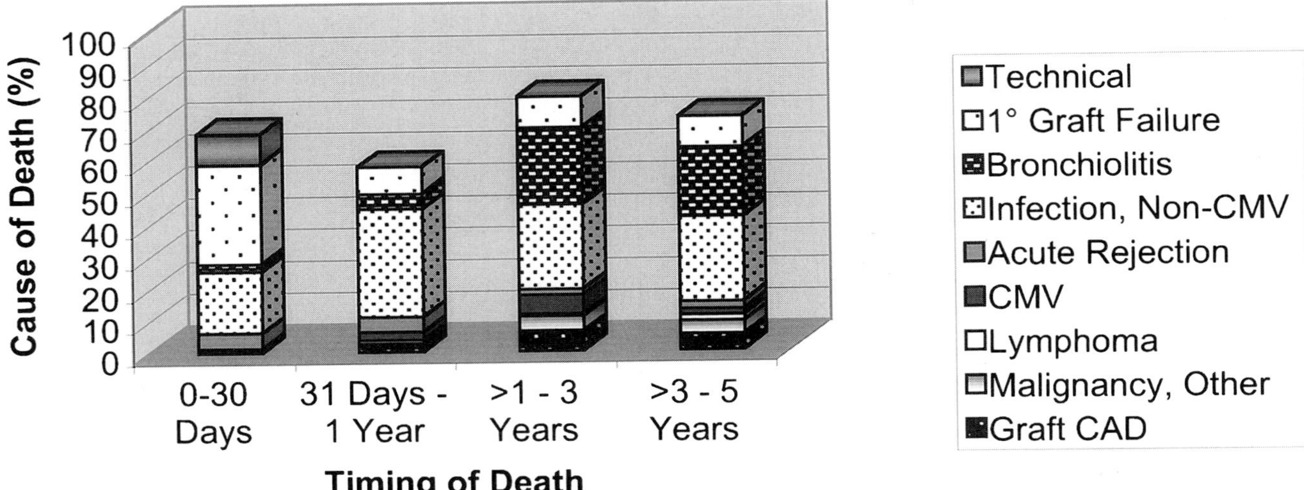

FIGURE 61–7 Causes of death at various periods after heart-lung transplantation. (*Adapted from Hosenpud JD, Bennett LE, Keck BM, et al: The Registry of the International Society for Heart and Lung Transplantation: Eighteenth Official Report—2001. J Heart Lung Transplant 2001; 20:805 with permission from Elsevier Science.*)

by primary graft failure or infection. Late mortality is most commonly caused by obliterative bronchiolitis or infection.[1] Causes of death at various time points after transplantation have been compiled by the ISHLT and are presented in Figures 61-7 and 61-8.

Hemorrhage

Perioperative hemorrhage is an infrequent but significant cause of early death in heart-lung and lung transplantation. Much of this stems from operating in the midst of dense adhesions from previous operations or the inflammatory response to chronic lung infection. As mentioned previously, meticulous attention to hemostasis is mandatory, and all available means should be used to achieve a dry field on completing the operation.

Hyperacute Rejection

ABO matching of donor and recipient has decreased the rate of hyperacute rejection. This complication, which is almost universally fatal, is mediated by preformed antibodies in the recipient that recognize antigens on the donor vascular endothelium. This humoral immune response results in activation of inflammatory and coagulation cascades, and results in extensive thrombosis of graft vessels and subsequent graft failure.[68] To reduce the incidence of hyperacute rejection, a

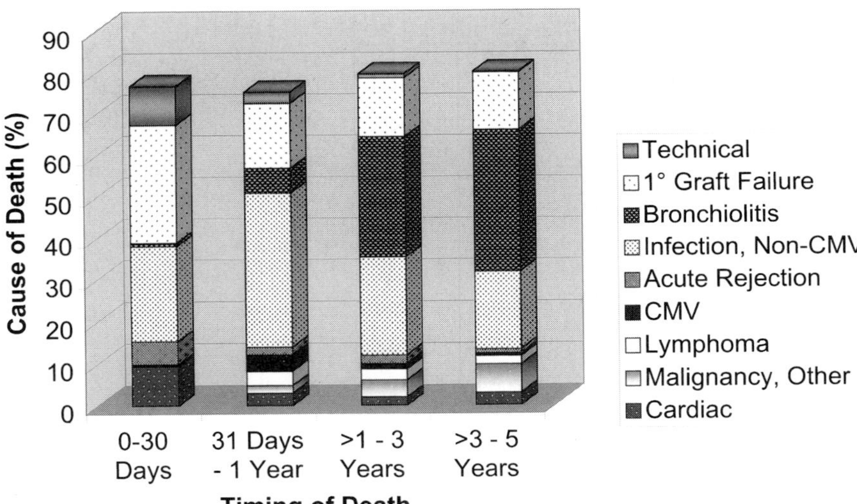

FIGURE 61–8 Causes of death at various periods after isolated lung transplantation. (*Adapted from Hosenpud JD, Bennett LE, Keck BM, et al: The Registry of the International Society for Heart and Lung Transplantation: Eighteenth Official Report—2001. J Heart Lung Transplant 2001; 20:805 with permission from Elsevier Science.*)

prospective crossmatch should be performed in recipients with a PRA greater than 25%.

Early Graft Dysfunction and Primary Graft Failure

Graft dysfunction in the first few days after transplantation is common. It has often been referred to as the "reimplantation response" and is manifested by abnormal lung function, pulmonary edema, and pulmonary infiltrates on chest x-ray. This phenomenon is thought to be linked to ischemia and reperfusion. It may also be related to allograft contusion, inadequate preservation, or use of cardiopulmonary bypass during transplantation. While most cases are mild and resolve with supportive care, some progress to primary graft failure. The rates of primary graft failure following lung and heart-lung transplantation are reported between 10% and 15%; treatment may include the use of ECMO and inhaled nitric oxide (NO). Unfortunately, primary graft failure is associated with a mortality of over 60%.[69]

Acute Rejection

As in cardiac transplantation, the majority of acute rejection episodes occur within the first year after transplant. From 1981 through 1994 at Stanford University, acute lung rejection (either isolated or simultaneous with heart rejection) occurred in more than 67% of heart-lung patients within the first year.[77] Similar rates of acute rejection have been reported among isolated lung transplant recipients. Despite its prevalence, death is very rarely a direct consequence of acute rejection. It is recognized, however, that the number and severity of acute rejection episodes is a risk factor for the ultimate development of obliterative bronchiolitis.

In the early posttransplant period, the diagnosis of acute rejection is often based on clinical parameters. Symptoms and signs of rejection include fever, dyspnea, impaired gas exchange manifested by a decrease in arterial Po_2, a diminished forced expiratory volume during 1 second (FEV_1, a measure of airway flow), a fall in vital capacity (VC), and the development of a characteristic bilateral interstitial infiltrate on chest x-ray (Fig. 61-9A). After the first postoperative month, the chest x-ray is frequently normal during episodes of acute rejection, placing greater emphasis on other clinical parameters of rejection.

Based on clinical findings, it is often difficult to distinguish between the diagnosis of acute lung rejection and pulmonary infection. It is of paramount importance to distinguish between the two before initiating therapy. Fiberoptic bronchoscopy with transbronchial parenchymal lung biopsy and bronchoalveolar lavage is the "gold standard" in the diagnosis of acute lung rejection and pulmonary infection. At least five biopsy specimens are taken from the lung allografts, along with bronchoalveolar lavage, which is evaluated for cytology, microbial staining, and culture.[78] In

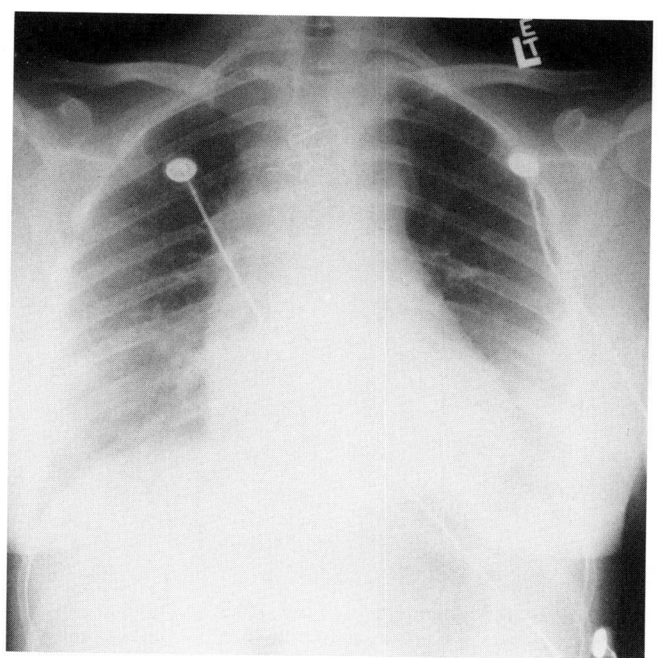

A

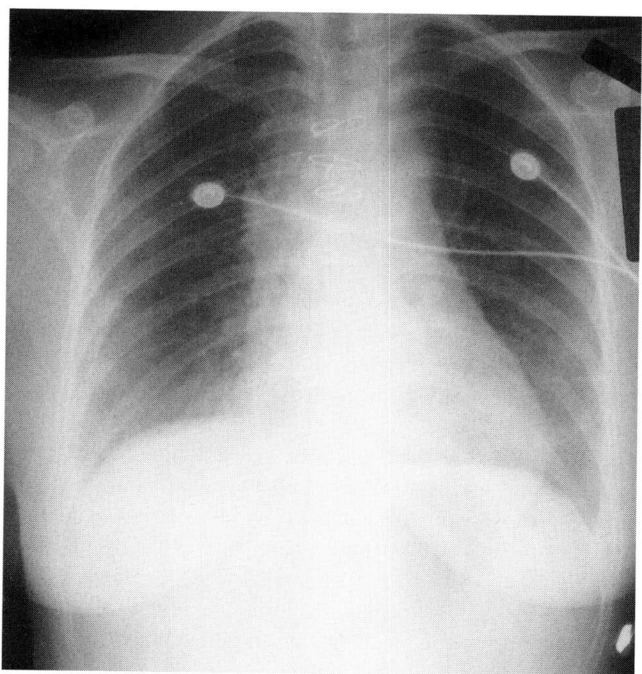

B

FIGURE 61–9 Acute and resolving lung rejection. (A) Chest radiograph illustrates bilateral infiltrates characteristic of acute pulmonary rejection. (B) Follow-up radiograph after pulsed methylprednisolone treatment of acute rejection demonstrating resolution of infiltrates.

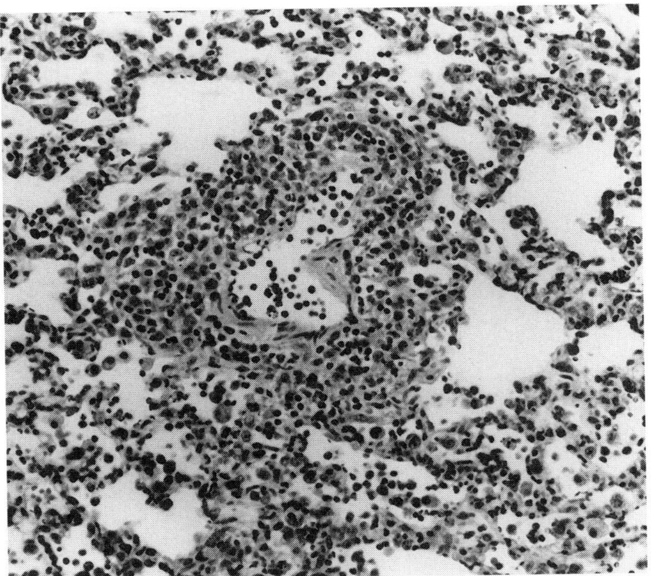

FIGURE 61–10 Moderate acute lung rejection. Moderate rejection is characterized by perivascular mononuclear cell infiltrates with extension into the adjacent alveolar septa (H&E stain; X 200).

TABLE 61–6 Grading system for acute lung rejection

Grade	Histologic appearance (transbronchial biopsy)
0	No significant inflammation; normal specimen
1	Small, infrequent perivascular infiltrates with or without bronchiolar lymphocytic infiltrates
2	Larger, more frequent perivascular lymphocytic infiltrates with or without moderate bronchiolar lymphocytic inflammation; occasional neutrophils and eosinophils
3	Extension of infiltrates into alveolar septa and alveolar spaces with or without bronchiolar mucosal ulceration

addition to performing bronchoscopy with transbronchial biopsy in response to changes in clinical status and graft performance, most centers maintain a schedule of surveillance biopsies for lung and heart-lung allograft recipients. Interestingly, occult rejection or infection is found on transbronchial biopsy specimens of 17% to 25% of asymptomatic heart-lung and lung allograft recipients undergoing surveillance bronchoscopy. For patients undergoing bronchoscopy for clinical indications, 50% to 72% of biopsy specimens have shown evidence of rejection or infection. In most cases, positive biopsies directly guide successful treatment of rejection or infection.[79,80]

Acute lung rejection is characterized histologically by lymphocytic perivascular infiltrates (Fig. 61-10). A histologic grading scheme for acute lung rejection was developed by Clelland and Colin[81] and is presented in Table 61-6; a similar scheme was also developed by the Lung Rejection Study Group.[78]

In heart-lung transplantation, experimental and clinical evidence suggests that pulmonary and cardiac rejections occur independently of each other. Higenbottam et al at Papworth Hospital reported a surprisingly low diagnostic yield from routine endomyocardial biopsies in heart-lung recipients compared with functional or histologic tests of pulmonary rejection. The authors advanced that, because of this, transbronchial biopsy eliminates the need for routine endomyocardial biopsies in heart-lung transplant recipients.[82] These findings were confirmed by Sibley et al at Stanford University, who demonstrate a discordance between findings on endomyocardial biopsy and transbronchial biopsy during episodes of acute rejection; endomyocardial biopsies are most often normal despite findings of pulmonary rejection on transbronchial biopsy.[80] Combined, these results have led to modifications in surveillance biopsy programs. At Stanford, surveillance endomyocardial biopsies have been abandoned in patients in whom transbronchial biopsies can be performed reliably.

As in cardiac transplantation, efforts are being made to develop noninvasive ways of diagnosing early acute lung rejection. Loubeyre et al at the Hôpital Cardiovasculaire et Pneumologique report an association between "ground-glass" density areas seen on high-resolution computed tomography (HRCT) and histologically diagnosed acute lung rejection in heart-lung transplant recipients.[83] They found that ground-glass opacities on HRCT had a sensitivity of 65% for detecting lung rejection and a specificity of 85% for detecting an acute lung complication.

Treatment strategies for rejection involve augmentation of immunosuppression. At most institutions, the timing and severity of rejection episodes dictate therapy. A typical algorithm is shown in Figure 61-11. Rejection episodes that are graded moderate or severe are treated with a "steroid pulse" (intravenous methylprednisolone 500-1000 mg/d for 3 consecutive days), followed by augmentation of the oral prednisone maintenance dose to 0.6 mg/kg/d. This maintenance dose is then tapered to 0.2 mg/kg/d over 3 to 4 weeks. Clinical and radiographic improvement (see Fig. 61-9B) following steroid therapy is often rapid and dramatic and is considered confirmatory of rejection. Mild episodes are treated initially with an increased oral prednisone dose, followed by a gradual taper over 3 to 4 weeks. Transbronchial biopsies are repeated 10 to 14 days following antirejection therapy to assess efficacy. Recurrent rejection episodes may be treated by a second steroid pulse and taper. Acute rejection refractory to steroid therapy may be treated with antilymphocyte preparations. Alternatively, primary immunosuppression may be switched from cyclosporine-based therapy to tacrolimus-based therapy. Finally, in especially difficult persistent cases of rejection, total lymphoid irradiation (TLI) may be useful.[84]

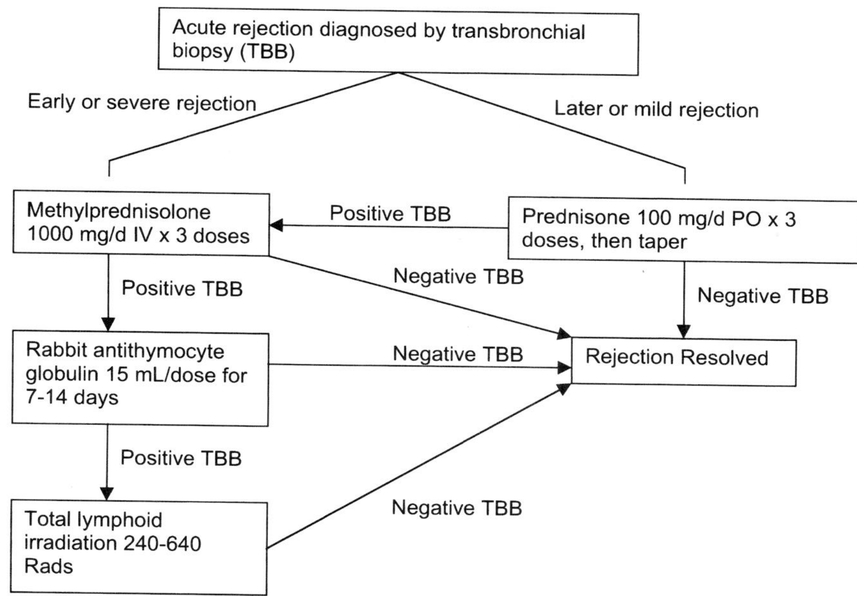

FIGURE 61–11 Typical algorithm for treating acute rejection in heart-lung and lung transplant recipients.

Chronic Rejection

Chronic lung allograft rejection poses the greatest limitation to the long-term benefits of lung and heart-lung transplantation. Chronic lung rejection most commonly presents as obliterative bronchiolitis (OB). It was first noted as a pulmonary corollary to chronic cardiac rejection (cardiac graft atherosclerosis) in recipients of heart-lung transplants.[85] Later, obliterative bronchiolitis was shown to occur in recipients of isolated lung transplants as well. The onset of OB typically occurs after the first 6 months to 1 year after transplantation. Its incidence increases steadily thereafter. Recent data demonstrate that 70% of heart-lung and lung graft recipients are diagnosed with OB by the fifth postoperative year.[86]

Transbronchial biopsies are the "gold standard" for diagnosing OB. The sensitivity of transbronchial biopsy for detecting OB has been reported between 17% and 87%.[80,87] The diagnostic yield of the biopsy procedure is related to the number of specimens taken, and current recommendations are that at least 5 specimens be taken from each transplanted lung. Clearly, OB is a patchy process and therefore a large number of samples will be falsely negative.

OB is a histologic diagnosis and is characterized by dense eosinophilic submucosal scar tissue that partially or totally obliterates the lumen of small (2 mm) airways, specifically the terminal and respiratory bronchioles (Fig. 61-12). The physiologic consequences are decreased arterial P_{O_2}, FEV_1, FEF_{25-75} [forced expiratory flow at 25% to 75% (midrange) of lung volumes], and FEF_{50}/FVC (ratio of FEF_{50} to forced vital capacity). A characteristic "bowing" of the expiratory limb of the flow-volume loop has also been associated with OB. Clinical symptoms may be nonspecific, and include cough and dyspnea with or without exertion. The term *bronchiolitis obliterans syndrome* (BOS) was developed to refer to patients who have clinical manifestations of obliterative bronchiolitis with or without proven histologic characteristics. A standardized working formulation for the clinical staging of BOS was established by the ISHLT and is based on the ratio of the current FEV_1 to the best posttransplant FEV_1. Patients with a decline of 20% or greater in their FEV_1 (in the absence of infection or other process) are diagnosed with BOS, irrespective of pathologic evidence of obliterative bronchiolitis (Table 61-7).[88]

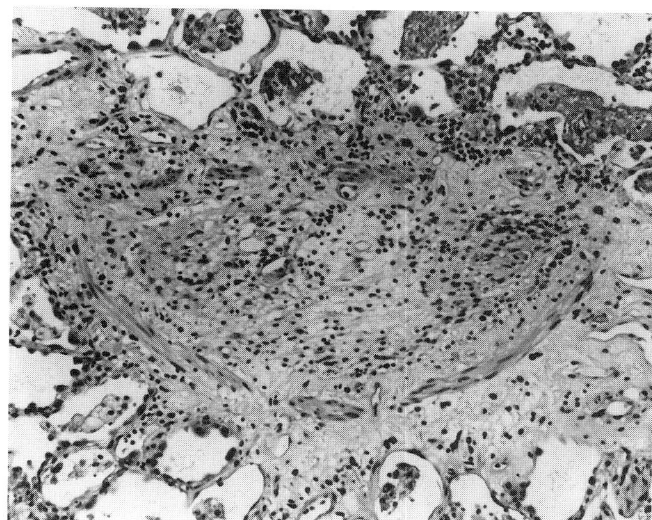

FIGURE 61–12 Bronchiolitis obliterans. Chronic airway rejection is characterized by luminal narrowing or replacement by dense eosinophilic collagenous scar tissue. Inflammatory cells may be seen in this case (H&E stain; X 150).

TABLE 61–7 Working formulation for bronchiolitis obliterans syndrome

$0_{a\ or\ b}$	No significant abnormality: FEV_1 80% of baseline
$1_{a\ or\ b}$	Mild bronchiolitis obliterans syndrome: FEV_1 66%-80% of baseline
$2_{a\ or\ b}$	Moderate bronchiolitis obliterans syndrome: FEV_1 51%-65% of baseline
$3_{a\ or\ b}$	Severe bronchiolitis obliterans syndrome: FEV_1 50% of baseline

a = without pathologic evidence of obliterative bronchiolitis; b = with pathologic evidence of obliterative bronchiolitis.

Valentine and the Stanford group have reported that measurements of small airway function (i.e., FEF_{25-75}, FEF_{50}/FVC) are more sensitive indicators of BOS than the FEV_1 in heart-lung and bilateral lung transplant recipients.[86] An FEF_{50}/FVC persistently below 0.7 for 6 consecutive weeks was selected as the most sensitive predictor of OB. Approximately 50% of heart-lung and bilateral lung recipients with biopsy-proven OB developed a fall in their FEF_{50}/FVC nearly 4 months prior to fulfilling the ISHLT working group criteria for BOS.

With regard to the etiologies of OB, experimental and clinical evidence points to injury of the bronchial epithelium by one or more mechanisms. These include infection (particularly CMV), chronic inflammation stemming from impaired mucociliary clearance, and immunologic mechanisms.[68] These insults result in airway epithelial damage and a subsequent exaggerated healing response. Along with this injury, there is increased expression of major histocompatibility class II antigens in the bronchial epithelium. In a recent meta-analysis, Sharples et al[89] found that acute rejection is a risk factor for later development of OB. In keeping with this finding is the association between BOS and decreased levels of immunosuppression (as may occur with noncompliance). Lymphocytic bronchitis and bronchiolitis were also closely associated with development of OB. CMV pneumonitis, other pulmonary infections, and HLA mismatching have been linked to the development of OB in small retrospective studies. Novick et al recently reported on the relationship between OB, donor age, and graft ischemic times.[55] Using data from the ISHLT registry, they found a higher rate of OB at 3 years in recipients of grafts from donors over 55 who were also subjected to 6 to 8 hours of ischemia.

The current management of OB hinges on prevention, close surveillance, and immediate therapeutic intervention when patients are symptomatic or when asymptomatic physiologic changes occur. Patients are encouraged to perform incentive spirometry to prevent microatelectasis of lungs deprived of native innervation, bronchial circulation, and normal mucociliary clearance mechanisms. Moreover, all recipients are instructed to contact their transplant center or primary physician when respiratory tract symptoms develop so that pulmonary function tests can be performed. Any alteration in FEF_{25-75}or FEF_{50}/FVC or specific changes in the flow-volume loop are an indication for bronchoscopy with bronchoalveolar lavage and transbronchial biopsy, especially in the absence of infectious bronchitis or pulmonary edema.

Augmentation of immunosuppression is the mainstay of therapy for BOS. The prednisone dose is increased to 0.6 to 1.0 mg/kg/d and slowly tapered to 0.2 mg/kg/d while concomitantly optimizing cyclosporine and azathioprine dosing. Ganciclovir is reinstituted during treatment for those patients at risk of reactivation CMV infection, and antimicrobial therapy is directed against any organisms isolated from bronchoalveolar lavage. Follow-up pulmonary function tests are performed. Pulmonary function can be stabilized in most patients, but significant improvement is uncommon. Unfortunately, relapse rates are greater than 50% and progressive pulmonary failure or infection due to increased immunosuppression are the most common causes of death in lung transplant patients after the second year. Among 89 heart-lung and 13 bilateral lung recipients who underwent transplantation at Stanford University between 1981 and 1995, a 5-year survival rate of 49% among recipients diagnosed with OB (n = 59) was noted compared to 74% among recipients without OB (n = 43). The 1-, 3-, 5-, 8-, and 10-year actuarial survival rates following the diagnosis of OB were 74%, 50%, 43%, 23%, and 11%, respectively, with a median survival of 3 years following diagnosis.

Retransplantation is the only option for terminal respiratory failure secondary to OB. While survival for patients undergoing retransplantation for OB is better than for those undergoing retransplantation for other reasons, it is still worse than survival of first-time transplant recipients. Among heart-lung recipients with OB, Adams et al at Harefield Hospital noted worse survival rates if combined heart-lung replacement, as opposed to isolated lung replacement, is performed on retransplantation.[90] They also noted that the absence of preformed antibodies, retransplantation at least 18 months after the original transplantation, and negative preoperative sputum cultures were associated with improved survival after retransplantation. Novick et al recently reported results from the Pulmonary Retransplant Registry.[32] They reviewed survival rates in 237 patients who underwent pulmonary retransplantation between 1985 and 1996. At 1, 2, and 3 years after retransplantation, survival was 47%, 40%, and 33%, respectively. Survival was higher in nonventilated ambulatory patients and their freedom from OB was comparable to first-time transplant recipients. The authors conclude that pulmonary retransplantation should be performed only in carefully selected recipients who have a reasonable likelihood of long-term survival.

Accelerated graft coronary artery disease (CAD) or graft atherosclerosis is another major obstacle to long-term survival in heart-lung transplant recipients. Significant graft CAD resulting in diminished coronary artery blood flow may lead to arrhythmias, myocardial infarction, sudden death, or

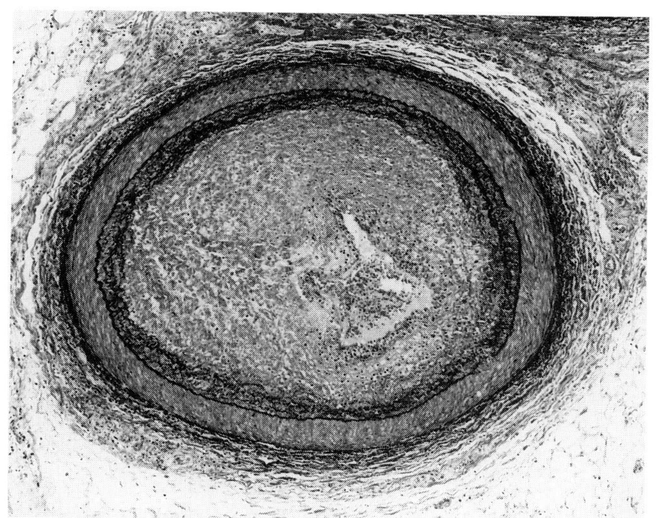

FIGURE 61–13 Cardiac graft atherosclerosis. Complete luminal obliteration by a concentric fibrointimal proliferation was observed at postmortem in this heart-lung transplant patient (Elastin von Gieson stain; X 60).

impaired left ventricular function with congestive heart failure. Classic angina due to myocardial ischemia is usually not noted in transplant recipients because the cardiac graft has been denervated. Multiple etiologies for graft CAD have been proposed, but they all focus on chronic, immunologically mediated damage to the coronary vascular endothelium. In fact, elevated levels of antiendothelial antibodies have been correlated with graft CAD. Unlike coronary artery occlusive disease in the native heart, which tends to be more focal in nature, transplant atherosclerosis represents a more diffuse vascular narrowing extending symmetrically into distal branches. Histologically, transplant arteriopathy is characterized by concentric intimal proliferation with smooth muscle hyperplasia (Fig. 61-13).

Coronary angiograms are performed on a yearly basis to identify recipients with accelerated CAD. Because graft CAD manifests as diffuse coronary intimal thickening, intracoronary ultrasound has been advanced as a more sensitive means to detect graft atherosclerosis due to its ability to assess vascular wall morphology in addition to luminal diameter. Interestingly, graft CAD occurs at a reduced incidence in heart-lung recipients compared with the cardiac transplantation population.[91] In a retrospective survey at Stanford, 89% of heart-lung recipients were free from graft CAD at 5 years compared with 73% of heart transplant recipients. Clinically observed risk factors for developing this condition in heart transplant recipients include donor age greater than 35 years, incompatibility at the HLA-A1, A2, and DR loci, hypertriglyceridemia (serum concentration greater than 280 mg/dL), frequent acute rejection episodes, and documented recipient CMV infection. It is not clear whether these risk factors can be extended to the heart-lung transplant population.

Percutaneous transluminal coronary angioplasty and coronary artery bypass grafting have been used to treat discrete proximal lesions in some cases of graft CAD; however, the only definitive therapy for diffuse disease is retransplantation. Effective prevention of graft CAD will rely on development of improved immunosuppression, recipient tolerance induction, improved CMV prophylaxis, and inhibition of vascular intimal proliferation.

Airway Complications

Improvements in surgical technique and posttransplant management have resulted in a relatively low incidence of airway complications after heart-lung and lung transplantation. Kshettry et al at the University of Minnesota report an airway complication rate of 15% in lung transplant recipients.[92] The avoidance of perioperative steroids has long been considered important in preventing airway complications; however, recent experimental and clinical evidence suggests that the detrimental effect of steroids may be overestimated.[93] The most common airway complications are partial anastomotic dehiscence and stricture. Such complications are usually diagnosed by bronchoscopy. Airway dehiscence is treated by reoperation or close observation and supportive care. Strictures are treated by balloon or bougie dilatation, often with stent placement.

Infection

Bacterial, viral, and fungal infections are leading causes of morbidity and mortality in both heart-lung and lung transplant recipients. The rate of infection is higher in this transplant group than in other solid organ transplant recipients; this may be related to the lung allograft's direct exposure to airway colonization and aspiration, as well as its impaired cough reflex and mucociliary clearance. The risk of infection and infection-related death peaks in the first few months after transplantation and declines to a low persistent rate thereafter. Between 1981 and 1994 at Stanford, only 20% of heart-lung transplant recipients were free from infection 3 months after transplantation. In a retrospective analysis of 200 episodes of serious infections occurring in 73 heart-lung recipients at Stanford between 1981 and 1990, Kramer et al[94] found that bacterial infections accounted for half of all infections; fungal infections accounted for 14%; and CMV was the most common viral agent, comprising 15% of viral infections and occurring primarily in the second month after transplantation. Other viral infections (i.e., herpes simplex, adenovirus, and respiratory syncitial virus) were less common. Five percent of infections were attributed to *Pneumocystis carinii,* typically occurring 4 to 6 months after transplantation, and 2% were due to *Nocardia,* generally appearing after the first year. There was no significant difference in the incidence of infections between patients receiving triple-drug or double-drug (cyclosporine and prednisone) immunosuppression. Infectious mortality comprised 40% of all deaths.

Posttransplant infections can be classified broadly into those that occur early or late after transplantation. Early infections, occurring in the first month after transplantation, are commonly bacterial (especially gram-negative bacilli) and manifest as pneumonia, mediastinitis, catheter sepsis, and urinary tract and skin infections. In the late posttransplant period, opportunistic viral, fungal, and protozoan pathogens become more prevalent. The lungs, central nervous system, gastrointestinal tract, and skin are the usual sites of invasion.

Bacterial infections, particularly caused by gram-negative bacteria, predominate during the early postoperative period. Between 75% and 97% of bronchial washings obtained from donor lungs before organ retrieval culture at least one organism.[95] Posttransplant invasive infections frequently are caused by organisms cultured from the donor. Conversely, bacterial infections developing in patients with septic lung disease, particularly cystic fibrosis, most commonly originate from the recipient's airways and sinuses. Treatment of bacterial infections generally involves characterization of the infective agent (e.g., cultures, antibiotic sensitivities), source control (e.g., catheter removal, debridement), and appropriate antibiotic regimens.

CMV infection presents either as a primary infection or as reactivation of a latent infection; it occurs most often at 1 to 3 months after transplantation. By definition, primary infection results when a previously seronegative recipient is infected though contact with tissue or blood from a seropositive individual. The donor organ itself is thought to be the most common vector of primary CMV infections. Reactivation infection occurs when a recipient who is seropositive prior to transplant develops clinical CMV infection during immunosuppressive therapy. Seropositive recipients are also subject to infection by new strains of CMV.

Clinically, CMV infection has protean manifestations, including leukopenia with fever, pneumonia, gastroenteritis, hepatitis, and retinitis. CMV pneumonitis is the most lethal of these, with a 13% mortality rate, while retinitis is the most refractory to treatment. Diagnosis of CMV infection is made by direct culture of the virus from blood, urine, or tissue specimens, by a 4-fold increase in antibody titers from baseline, or by the characteristic histologic changes (i.e., markedly enlarged cells and nuclei containing basophilic inclusion bodies). Most cases respond to ganciclovir and hyperimmune globulin.

The significance of CMV as an infective agent becomes clear when one realizes that it is implicated as a trigger for accelerated graft CAD[96] and OB,[89] as well as an inhibitor of cell-mediated immunity. CMV-negative donors comprise less than 20% of the donor organ pool and, because of organ scarcity, most transplant centers perform transplants across CMV serologic barriers using ganciclovir and/or hyperimmune globulin prophylactic protocols in CMV-positive donors and/or recipients. A recent study by Valantine et al in 80 heart-lung and lung transplant recipients found that the combined use of ganciclovir and hyperimmune globulin was superior to ganciclovir alone as prophylaxis for CMV; moreover, the ganciclovir/hyperimmune globulin cohort had longer survival at 3 years and greater freedom from obliterative bronchiolitis.[97]

Invasive fungal infections peak in frequency between 10 days and 2 months after transplantation. Treatment consists of fluconazole, itraconazole, or amphotericin B. Reichenspurner et al have reported that the actuarial incidence and linearized rate of fungal infections after heart, heart-lung, and lung transplants performed at Stanford University were significantly reduced in recipients who received inhaled amphotericin prophylaxis.[98]

Pneumocystis carinii pneumonia has been prevented effectively in lung and heart-lung transplant patients since the institution of prophylaxis with oral trimethoprim-sulfamethoxazole or inhalational pentamidine for sulfa-allergic patients.

Infection prophylaxis in heart-lung and lung recipients is comprised of vaccinations, perioperative broad-spectrum antibiotics, and long-term prophylactic antibiotics.

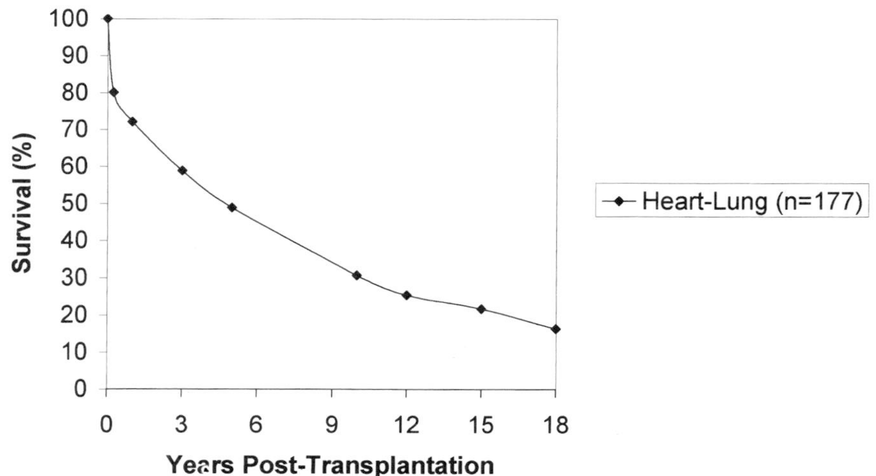

FIGURE 61–14 Survival for Stanford heart-lung transplantation, 1981 through 2002.

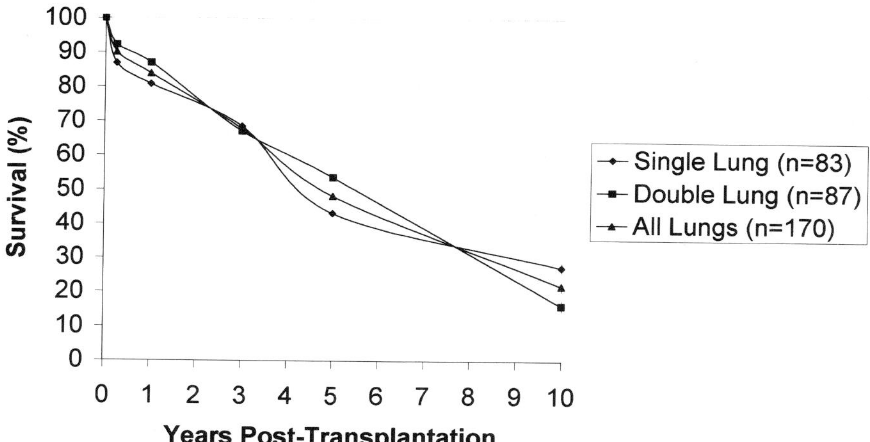

FIGURE 61–15 Survival for Stanford lung transplantation, 1989 through 2002.

Pretransplant inoculations with pneumococcal and hepatitis B vaccines, as well as DPT boosters, are recommended. Perioperative antibiotic regimens vary widely between transplant centers; however, first-generation cephalosporins (e.g., cefazolin) or vancomycin are commonly used. Long-term prophylaxis typically includes nystatin mouthwash, trimethoprim-sulfamethoxazole, aerosolized amphotericin B, and antivirals such as acyclovir or ganciclovir.

Neoplasm

The incidence of neoplasia is higher in transplant recipients than in the general population.[99] Undoubtedly, this is due to chronic immunosuppression. Recipients are predisposed to a variety of tumors, including skin cancer, B-cell lymphoproliferative disorders, carcinoma in situ of the cervix, carcinoma of the vulva and anus, and Kaposi's sarcoma. On average, tumors appear approximately 5 years after transplantation.[1]

The incidence of B-cell lymphoproliferative disorders in transplant patients is a staggering 350 times greater than that seen in the normal age-matched population. Posttransplant lymphoproliferative disorder (PTLD) has been reported in 6% of lung transplant recipients.[100] PTLD most commonly occurs within the first year after transplantation, and has been associated with Epstein-Barr virus infection. Treatment consists of reduction in immunosuppression and administration of an antiviral agent such as acyclovir or ganciclovir, with a response rate of 30% to 40%.

LONG-TERM RESULTS IN HEART-LUNG AND LUNG TRANSPLANTATION

The Stanford long-term survival for heart-lung and lung transplant recipients is shown in Figures 61-14 and 61-15 respectively. Similar results are recorded in the ISHLT registry (Figs. 61-16 and 61-17). At Stanford, 1-, 5-, 10-, and 15-year survival after heart-lung transplantation are 72%, 49%, 31%, and 22% respectively. Lung transplantation survival at 1-, 5-, and 10-years posttransplantation are 84%, 48%, and 22% respectively. Most recipients are able to resume active lifestyles without supplemental oxygen and demonstrate significant increases in posttransplant exercise capacity. Pulmonary function measured by spirometry and arterial blood gases is markedly improved within several months after transplantation, with a normalization of ventilation and gas exchange after 1 to 2 years.[101]

CONCLUSION

The evolution of heart-lung and lung transplantation from rudimentary laboratory experimentation to its current prominence as an accepted therapy for end-stage cardiopulmonary disease is a product of ingenuity, perseverance, skill, and courage. Many debilitated patients, both adult

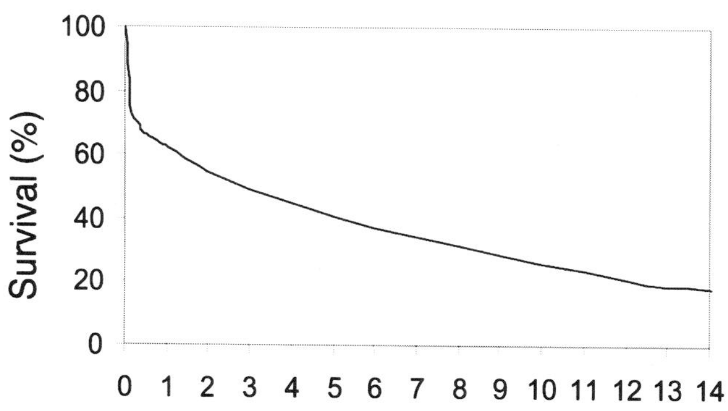

FIGURE 61–16 Actuarial survival for heart-lung transplantation, 1982 through 2000. (*Data from Hosenpud JD, Bennett LE, Keck BM, et al: The Registry of the International Society for Heart and Lung Transplantation: Eighteenth Official Report—2001. J Heart Lung Transplant 2001; 20:805 with permission from Elsevier Science.*)

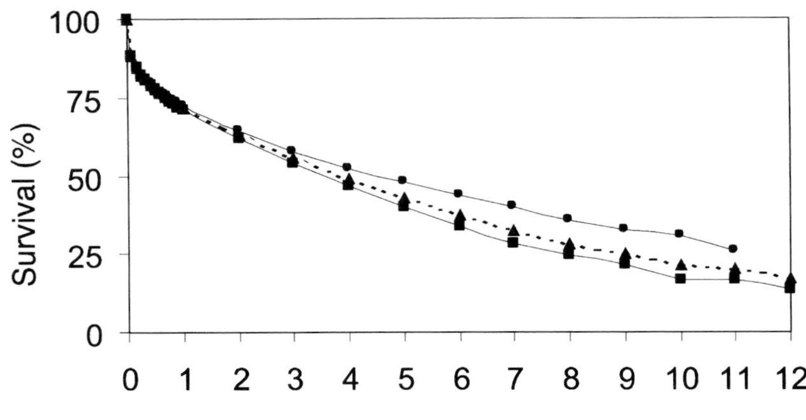

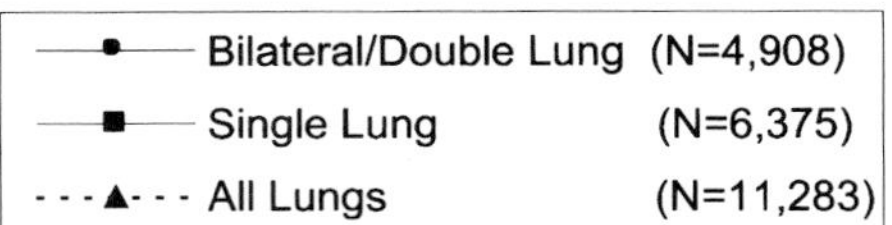

FIGURE 61–17 Actuarial survival after isolated lung transplantation, 1983 through 2000. (*Data from Hosenpud JD, Bennett LE, Keck BM, et al: The Registry of the International Society for Heart and Lung Transplantation: Eighteenth Official Report—2001. J Heart Lung Transplant 2001; 20:805 with permission from Elsevier Science.*)

and pediatric, now have an opportunity to resume full and active lifestyles after heart-lung and lung transplantation. Nevertheless, significant hurdles have yet to be overcome, particularly graft rejection, infection, and a limited donor pool. Important advances on the horizon include cross-species transplantation, improved immunosuppression, the induction of immunologic tolerance to foreign tissue, and improved organ preservation techniques.

REFERENCES

1. Hosenpud JD, Bennett LE, Keck BM, et al: The Registry of the International Society for Heart and Lung Transplantation: Eighteenth Official Report—2001. *J Heart Lung Transplant* 2001; 20:805.
2. Demikhov VP: *Experimental Transplantation of Vital Organs*. New York, Consultants Bureau, 1962.
3. Marcus E, Wong SNT, Luisada AA: Homologous heart grafts: transplantation of the heart in dogs. *Surg Forum* 1951; 2:212.
4. Webb WR, Howard HS: Cardiopulmonary transplantation. *Surg Forum* 1957; 8:313.
5. Lower RR, Stofer RC, Hurley EJ, et al: Complete homograft replacement of the heart and both lungs. *Surgery* 1961; 50:842.
6. Haglin J, Telander RL, Muzzall RE, et al: Comparison of lung autotransplantation in the primate and dog. *Surg Forum* 1963; 14:196.
7. Nakae S, Webb WR, Theodorides T, et al: Respiratory function following cardiopulmonary denervation in dog, cat, and monkey. *Surg Gynecol Obstet* 1967; 125:1285.
8. Castaneda AR, Arnar O, Schmidt-Habelmann P, et al: Cardiopulmonary autotransplantation in primates. *J Cardiovasc Surg (Torino)* 1972; 13:523.
9. Castaneda AR, Zamora R, Schmidt-Habelmann P, et al: Cardiopulmonary autotransplantation in primates (baboons): late functional results. *Surgery* 1972; 72:1064.
10. Reitz BA, Burton NA, Jamieson SW, et al: Heart and lung transplantation: autotransplantation and allotransplantation in primates with extended survival. *J Thorac Cardiovasc Surg* 1980; 80:360.
11. Reitz BA, Pennock JL, Shumway NE: Simplified operative method for heart and lung transplantation. *J Surg Res* 1981; 31:1.
12. Reitz BA, Wallwork JL, Hunt SA, et al: Heart-lung transplantation: successful therapy for patients with pulmonary vascular disease. *N Engl J Med* 1982; 306:557.
13. Metras H: Preliminary note on lung transplants in dogs. *Compte Rendue Acad Sci* 1950; 231:1176.
14. Blumenstock DA, Kahn DR: Replantation and transplantation of the canine lung. *J Surg Res* 1961; 1:40.
15. Veith FJ, Richards K: Improved technic for canine lung transplantation. *Ann Surg* 1970; 171:553.
16. Lima O, Goldberg M, Peters WJ, et al: Bronchial omentopexy in canine lung transplantation. *J Thorac Cardiovasc Surg* 1982; 83:418.
17. Lima O, Cooper JD, Peters WJ, et al: Effects of methylprednisolone and azathioprine on bronchial healing following lung autotransplantation. *J Thorac Cardiovasc Surg* 1981; 82:211.
18. Hardy JD, Webb WR, Dalton ML, et al: Lung homotransplantation in man: report of the initial case. *JAMA* 1963; 186:1065.
19. Unilateral lung transplantation for pulmonary fibrosis. Toronto Lung Transplant Group. *N Engl J Med* 1986; 314:1140.
20. Patterson GA, Cooper JD, Goldman B, et al: Technique of successful clinical double-lung transplantation. *Ann Thorac Surg* 1988; 45:626.
21. Pasque MK, Cooper JD, Kaiser LR, et al: Improved technique for bilateral lung transplantation: rationale and initial clinical experience. *Ann Thorac Surg* 1990; 49:785.
22. De Meester J, Smits JM, Persijn GG, et al: Listing for lung transplantation: life expectancy and transplant effect, stratified by type of end-stage lung disease, the Eurotransplant experience. *J Heart Lung Transplant* 2001; 20:518.
23. Stoica SC, McNeil KD, Perreas K, et al: Heart-lung transplantation for Eisenmenger syndrome: early and long-term results. *Ann Thorac Surg* 2001; 72:1887.
24. Gammie JS, Keenan RJ, Pham SM, et al: Single- versus double-lung transplantation for pulmonary hypertension. *J Thorac Cardiovasc Surg* 1998; 115:397.

25. Oaks TE, Aravot D, Dennis C, et al: Domino heart transplantation: the Papworth experience. *J Heart Lung Transplant* 1994; 13:433.
26. Yacoub MH, Banner NR, Khaghani A, et al: Heart-lung transplantation for cystic fibrosis and subsequent domino heart transplantation. *J Heart Transplant* 1990; 9:459.
27. Kells CM, Marshall S, Kramer M, et al: Cardiac function after domino-donor heart transplantation. *Am J Cardiol* 1992; 69:113.
28. Barlow CW, Robbins RC, Moon MR, et al: Heart-lung versus double-lung transplantation for suppurative lung disease. *J Thorac Cardiovasc Surg* 2000; 119:466.
29. Egan TM, Detterbeck FC, Mill MR, et al: Improved results of lung transplantation for patients with cystic fibrosis. *J Thorac Cardiovasc Surg* 1995; 109:224.
30. Patterson GA: Indications: unilateral, bilateral, heart-lung, and lobar transplant procedures. *Clin Chest Med* 1997; 18:225.
31. Sundaresan RS, Shiraishi Y, Trulock EP, et al: Single or bilateral lung transplantation for emphysema? *J Thorac Cardiovasc Surg* 1996; 112:1485.
32. Novick RJ, Stitt LW, Al Kattan K, et al: Pulmonary retransplantation: predictors of graft function and survival in 230 patients. Pulmonary Retransplant Registry. *Ann Thorac Surg* 1998; 65:227.
33. Barr ML, Schenkel FA, Cohen RG, et al: Recipient and donor outcomes in living related and unrelated lobar transplantation. *Transplant Proc* 1998; 30:2261.
34. Starnes VA, Woo MS, MacLaughlin EF, et al: Comparison of outcomes between living donor and cadaveric lung transplantation in children. *Ann Thorac Surg* 1999; 68:2279.
35. Barr ML, Baker CJ, Schenkel FA, et al: Living donor lung transplantation: selection, technique, and outcome. *Transplant Proc* 2001; 33:3527.
36. Maurer JR: Patient selection for lung transplantation. *JAMA* 2001; 286:2720.
37. Marshall SE, Kramer MR, Lewiston NJ, et al: Selection and evaluation of recipients for heart-lung and lung transplantation. *Chest* 1990; 98:1488.
38. Hosenpud JD, Bennett LE, Keck BM, et al: The Registry of the International Society for Heart and Lung Transplantation: Seventeenth Official Report—2000. *J Heart Lung Transplant* 2000; 19:909.
39. Umetsu DT, Moss RB, King VV, et al: Sinus disease in patients with severe cystic fibrosis: relation to pulmonary exacerbation. *Lancet* 1990; 335:1077.
40. Tamm M, Higenbottam TW, Dennis CM, et al: Donor and recipient predicted lung volume and lung size after heart-lung transplantation. *Am J Respir Crit Care Med* 1994; 150:403.
41. Hosenpud JD, Edwards EB, Lin HM, et al: Influence of HLA matching on thoracic transplant outcomes: an analysis from the UNOS/ISHLT Thoracic Registry. *Circulation* 1996; 94:170.
42. Wisser W, Wekerle T, Zlabinger G, et al: Influence of human leukocyte antigen matching on long-term outcome after lung transplantation. *J Heart Lung Transplant* 1996; 15:1209.
43. Iwaki Y, Yoshida Y, Griffith B: The HLA matching effect in lung transplantation. *Transplantation* 1993; 56:1528.
44. Harjula AL, Baldwin JC, Glanville AR, et al: Human leukocyte antigen compatibility in heart-lung transplantation. *J Heart Transplant* 1987; 6:162.
45. Cohn JN, Archibald DG, Ziesche S, et al: Effect of vasodilator therapy on mortality in chronic congestive heart failure. Results of a Veterans Administration Cooperative Study. *N Engl J Med* 1986; 314:1547.
46. McLaughlin VV, Rich S: Pulmonary hypertension—advances in medical and surgical interventions. *J Heart Lung Transplant* 1998; 17:739.
47. Palevsky HI, Fishman AP: Chronic cor pulmonale: etiology and management. *JAMA* 1990; 263:2347.
48. Goldberg M, Lima O, Morgan E, et al: A comparison between cyclosporin A and methylprednisolone plus azathioprine on bronchial healing following canine lung autotransplantation. *J Thorac Cardiovasc Surg* 1983; 85:821.
49. Madden BP, Kamalvand K, Chan CM, et al: The medical management of patients with cystic fibrosis following heart-lung transplantation. *Eur Respir J* 1993; 6:965.
50. International guidelines for the selection of lung transplant candidates. The American Society for Transplant Physicians (ASTP)/American Thoracic Society (ATS)/European Respiratory Society (ERS)/International Society for Heart and Lung Transplantation (ISHLT). *Am J Respir Crit Care Med* 1998; 158:335.
51. Frost AE: Donor criteria and evaluation. *Clin Chest Med* 1997; 18:231.
52. Shumway SJ, Hertz MI, Petty MG, et al: Liberalization of donor criteria in lung and heart-lung transplantation. *Ann Thorac Surg* 1994; 57:92.
53. Bhorade SM, Vigneswaran W, McCabe MA, et al: Liberalization of donor criteria may expand the donor pool without adverse consequence in lung transplantation. *J Heart Lung Transplant* 2000; 19:1199.
54. Gabbay E, Williams TJ, Griffiths AP, et al: Maximizing the utilization of donor organs offered for lung transplantation. *Am J Respir Crit Care Med* 1999; 160:265.
55. Novick RJ, Bennett LE, Meyer DM, et al: Influence of graft ischemic time and donor age on survival after lung transplantation. *J Heart Lung Transplant* 1999; 18:425.
56. Steen S, Sjoberg T, Pierre L, et al: Transplantation of lungs from a non-heart-beating donor. *Lancet* 2001; 357:825.
57. Hardesty RL, Griffith BP: Procurement for combined heart-lung transplantation: bilateral thoracotomy with sternal transection, cardiopulmonary bypass, and profound hypothermia. *J Thorac Cardiovasc Surg* 1985; 89:795.
58. Gammie JS, Stukus DR, Pham SM, et al: Effect of ischemic time on survival in clinical lung transplantation. *Ann Thorac Surg* 1999; 68:2015.
59. Fiser SM, Kron IL, Long SM, et al: Influence of graft ischemia time on outcomes following lung transplantation. *J Heart Lung Transplant* 2001; 20:1291.
60. Conte JV, Baumgartner WA: Overview and future practice patterns in cardiac and pulmonary preservation. *J Card Surg* 2000; 15:91.
61. Novick RJ, Reid KR, Denning L, et al: Prolonged preservation of canine lung allografts: the role of prostaglandins. *Ann Thorac Surg* 1991; 51:853.
62. Kirk AJ, Colquhoun IW, Dark JH: Lung preservation: a review of current practice and future directions. *Ann Thorac Surg* 1993; 56:990.
63. Lick SD, Copeland JG, Rosado LJ, et al: Simplified technique of heart-lung transplantation. *Ann Thorac Surg* 1995; 59:1592.
64. Dummer JS, Montero CG, Griffith BP, et al: Infections in heart-lung transplant recipients. *J Heart Lung Transplant* 1986; 41:725.
65. Lurie KG, Bristow MR, Reitz BA: Increased beta-adrenergic receptor density in an experimental model of cardiac transplantation. *J Thorac Cardiovasc Surg* 1983; 86:195.
66. Vatner DE, Lavallee M, Amano J, et al: Mechanisms of supersensitivity to sympathomimetic amines in the chronically denervated heart of the conscious dog. *Circ Res* 1985; 57:55.
67. Kendall SW, Ciulli F, Mullins PA, et al: Total orthotopic heart transplantation: an alternative to the standard technique. *Ann Thorac Surg* 1992; 54:187.
68. DeMeo DL, Ginns LC: Clinical status of lung transplantation. *Transplantation* 2001; 72:1713.
69. Christie JD, Bavaria JE, Palevsky HI, et al: Primary graft failure following lung transplantation. *Chest* 1998; 114:51.

70. Slaughter MS, Nielsen K, Bolman RM 3rd: Extracorporeal membrane oxygenation after lung or heart-lung transplantation. *ASAIO J* 1993; 39:M453.
71. Adatia I, Lillehei C, Arnold JH, et al: Inhaled nitric oxide in the treatment of postoperative graft dysfunction after lung transplantation. *Ann Thorac Surg* 1994; 57:1311.
72. Keenan RJ, Konishi H, Kawai A, et al: Clinical trial of tacrolimus versus cyclosporine in lung transplantation. *Ann Thorac Surg* 1995; 60:580.
73. Reichenspurner H, Kur F, Treede H, et al: Optimization of the immunosuppressive protocol after lung transplantation. *Transplantation* 1999; 68:67.
74. Palmer SM, Miralles AP, Lawrence CM, et al: Rabbit antithymocyte globulin decreases acute rejection after lung transplantation: results of a randomized, prospective study. *Chest* 1999; 116:127.
75. Barlow CW, Moon MR, Green GR, et al: Rabbit antithymocyte globulin versus OKT3 induction therapy after heart-lung and lung transplantation: effect on survival, rejection, infection, and obliterative bronchiolitis. *Transpl Int* 2001; 14:234.
76. Brock MV, Borja MC, Ferber L, et al: Induction therapy in lung transplantation: a prospective, controlled clinical trial comparing OKT3, anti-thymocyte globulin, and daclizumab. *J Heart Lung Transplant* 2001; 20:1282.
77. Sarris GE, Smith JA, Shumway NE, et al: Long-term results of combined heart-lung transplantation: the Stanford experience. *J Heart Lung Transplant* 1994; 13:940.
78. Yousem SA, Berry GJ, Brunt EM, et al: A working formulation for the standardization of nomenclature in the diagnosis of heart and lung rejection: Lung Rejection Study Group. The International Society for Heart Transplantation. *J Heart Transplant* 1990; 9:593.
79. Guilinger RA, Paradis IL, Dauber JH, et al: The importance of bronchoscopy with transbronchial biopsy and bronchoalveolar lavage in the management of lung transplant recipients. *Am J Respir Crit Care Med* 1995; 152:2037.
80. Sibley RK, Berry GJ, Tazelaar HD, et al: The role of transbronchial biopsies in the management of lung transplant recipients. *J Heart Lung Transplant* 1993; 12:308.
81. Clelland CA, Higenbottam TW, Stewart S, et al: The histological changes in transbronchial biopsy after treatment of acute lung rejection in heart-lung transplants. *J Pathol* 1990; 161:105.
82. Higenbottam T, Hutter JA, Stewart S, et al: Transbronchial biopsy has eliminated the need for endomyocardial biopsy in heart-lung recipients. *J Heart Transplant* 1988; 7:435.
83. Loubeyre P, Revel D, Delignette A, et al: High-resolution computed tomographic findings associated with histologically diagnosed acute lung rejection in heart-lung transplant recipients. *Chest* 1995; 107:132.
84. Valentine VG, Robbins RC, Wehner JH, et al: Total lymphoid irradiation for refractory acute rejection in heart-lung and lung allografts. *Chest* 1996; 109:1184.
85. Burke CM, Theodore J, Dawkins KD, et al: Post-transplant obliterative bronchiolitis and other late lung sequelae in human heart-lung transplantation. *Chest* 1984; 86:824.
86. Valentine VG, Robbins RC, Berry GJ, et al: Actuarial survival of heart-lung and bilateral sequential lung transplant recipients with obliterative bronchiolitis. *J Heart Lung Transplant* 1996; 15:371.
87. Chamberlain D, Maurer J, Chaparro C, et al: Evaluation of transbronchial lung biopsy specimens in the diagnosis of bronchiolitis obliterans after lung transplantation. *J Heart Lung Transplant* 1994; 13:963.
88. Cooper JD, Billingham M, Egan T, et al: A working formulation for the standardization of nomenclature and for clinical staging of chronic dysfunction in lung allografts. International Society for Heart and Lung Transplantation. *J Heart Lung Transplant* 1993; 12:713.
89. Sharples LD, McNeil K, Stewart S, et al: Risk factors for bronchiolitis obliterans: a systematic review of recent publications. *J Heart Lung Transplant* 2002; 21:271.
90. Adams DH, Cochrane AD, Khaghani A, et al: Retransplantation in heart-lung recipients with obliterative bronchiolitis. *J Thorac Cardiovasc Surg* 1994; 107:450.
91. Sarris GE, Moore KA, Schroeder JS, et al: Cardiac transplantation: the Stanford experience in the cyclosporine era. *J Thorac Cardiovasc Surg* 1994; 108:240.
92. Kshettry VR, Kroshus TJ, Hertz MI, et al: Early and late airway complications after lung transplantation: incidence and management. *Ann Thorac Surg* 1997; 63:1576.
93. Colquhoun IW, Gascoigne AD, Au J, et al: Airway complications after pulmonary transplantation. *Ann Thorac Surg* 1994; 57:141.
94. Kramer MR, Marshall SE, Starnes VA, et al: Infectious complications in heart-lung transplantation: analysis of 200 episodes. *Arch Intern Med* 1993; 153:2010.
95. Davis RD Jr, Pasque MK: Pulmonary transplantation. *Ann Surg* 1995; 221:14.
96. Grattan MT, Moreno-Cabral CE, Starnes VA, et al: Cytomegalovirus infection is associated with cardiac allograft rejection and atherosclerosis. *JAMA* 1989; 261:3561.
97. Valantine HA, Luikart H, Doyle R, et al: Impact of cytomegalovirus hyperimmune globulin on outcome after cardiothoracic transplantation: a comparative study of combined prophylaxis with CMV hyperimmune globulin plus ganciclovir versus ganciclovir alone. *Transplantation* 2001; 72:1647.
98. Reichenspurner H, Gamburg P, Yun K, et al: Inhaled amphotericin B prophylaxis significantly reduces the number of fungal infections after heart, lung, and heart-lung transplantation [abstract]. International Society for Heart and Lung Transplantation 16th Annual Meeting and Scientific Sessions, New York, 1996.
99. Penn I: Incidence and treatment of neoplasia after transplantation. *J Heart Lung Transplant* 1993; 12:S328.
100. Paranjothi S, Yusen RD, Kraus MD, et al: Lymphoproliferative disease after lung transplantation: comparison of presentation and outcome of early and late cases. *J Heart Lung Transplant* 2001; 20:1054.
101. Theodore J, Morris AJ, Burke CM, et al: Cardiopulmonary function at maximum tolerable constant work rate exercise following human heart-lung transplantation. *Chest* 1987; 92:433.

Chapter 62

Long-Term Mechanical Circulatory Support

Eugene L. Kukuy/Mehmet C. Oz/Yoshifumi Naka

HISTORY

Heart failure accounts for approximately 250,000 deaths in America each year.[1] Hundreds of thousands of additional patients experience debilitating symptoms despite maximal medical management. About 50% of patients with chronic heart failure will die within 1 year and about 70% within 5 years. Even though heart transplantation has been an effective treatment, the number of donors is limited to about 2300 annually and thousands of people die awaiting heart transplantation.[2] Man has long sought to find a mechanical means to support the failing heart, and since the mid-1980s this dream has become a reality. More recently, as the results have improved, the indications for the use of these devices have broadened.

In 1953, Gibbon introduced cardiopulmonary bypass and revolutionized the practice of heart surgery.[3] The bypass machine not only started a new era in heart surgery, but also showed that a mechanical device could replace the function of the heart. Spencer in 1959 showed that circulatory support could be used to assist the failing heart.[4]

DeBakey was the first to successfully use an implantable mechanical assist device in 1963 to aid a failing heart. Cooley followed this in 1969 with the first implantable device used as a bridge to transplantation.[5] Subsequently, in the 1970s and early 1980s, further research on these devices was undertaken with the help of government sponsorship, and on several occasions circulatory assist devices were used successfully as a bridge to transplantation.

In 1982, DeVries implanted a total artificial heart (Jarvik-7) into a patient in a much-publicized case. The patient died 112 days after implantation.[6] Several subsequent patients in the 1980s received the total artificial heart and many were thus bridged to transplantation. However, these devices were plagued by thromboembolic and infectious complications, and by the end of the 1980s the enthusiasm for the use of a total artificial heart was waning. During the same time, heart transplantation surged with the new use of cyclosporine and focus was turned to devices that could "bridge" the failing heart to transplantation.[7,8]

The last two decades saw the renaissance of the ventricular assist device as a bridge to transplantation. More recently the use of these devices has been expanded to include bridge to recovery and permanent long-term heart support/replacement. At the same time, the total artificial heart and new smaller devices have emerged as options in the treatment of heart failure.

In this chapter, we will review the major left ventricular assist systems (LVAS) and devices (LVAD) subdivided into categories that include: implantable tethered pulsatile devices, paracorporeal pulsatile devices, rotary axial flow pumps, totally implantable pulsatile devices, centrifugal devices, and the total artificial heart. We will also talk about patient selection, operative technique, postoperative care, and complications. The three end points of treatment will be discussed: bridge to transplantation, bridge to recovery, and destination therapy.

SYSTEMS

Implantable Pulsatile Devices

HEARTMATE

The HeartMate LVAD (Thoratec Corporation, Pleasanton, CA) was designed in 1975 (Fig. 62-1).[9] The system was originally a pneumatic vented system that required a large

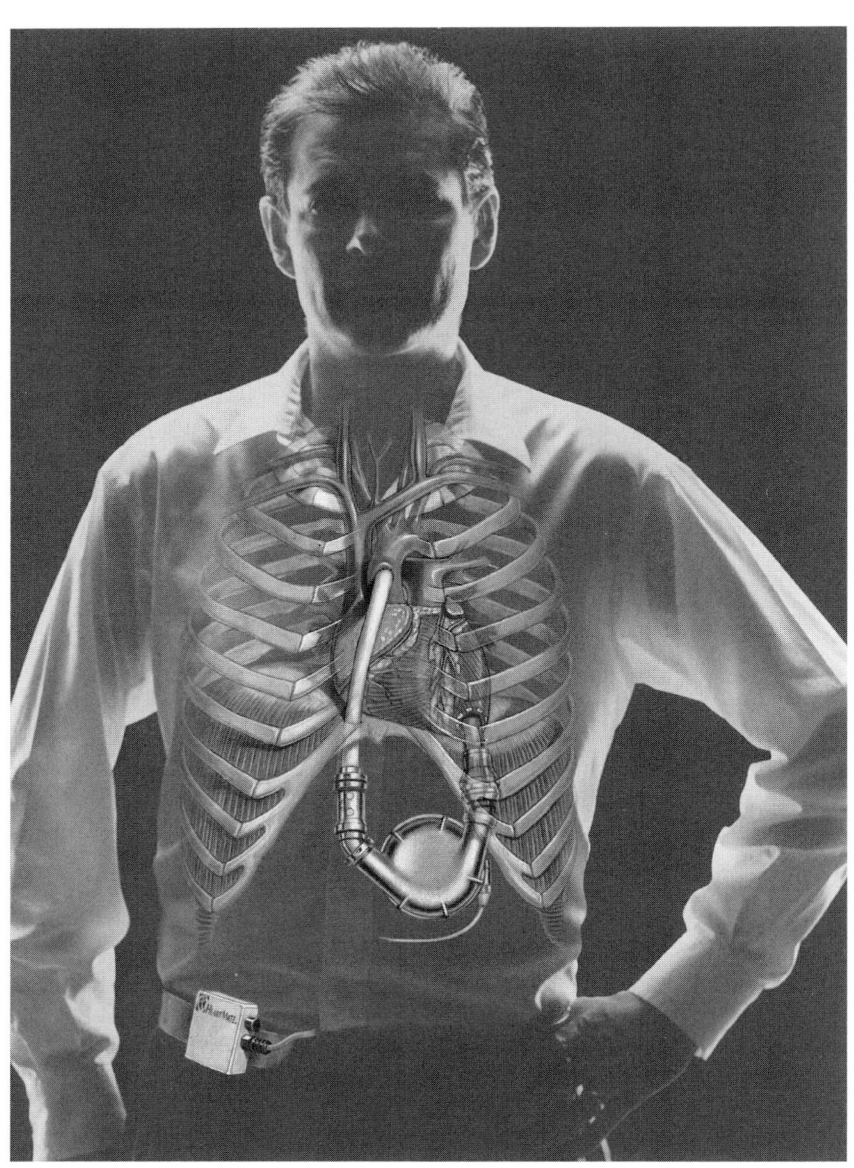

FIGURE 62–1 HeartMate left ventricular assist device. (*Reproduced with the permission of Thoratec Corp., Pleasanton, CA.*)

cumbersome console that did not allow patients much mobility outside the hospital. Since 1986, this system has proven to be effective as a long-term support device with the end goal of heart transplantation. The system underwent years of development and in 1991 a clinical trial of an electric vented (VE) model was begun.[10] This electric system allowed a greater amount of mobility with portable battery units carried in a holster. Since then, both models have shown a 60% to 70% rate of survival to transplantation.[11–13] The worldwide average implant duration is 80 to 100 days, and maximum duration on support has exceeded 2 years.[13] The probability of device failure has been shown to be 35% at 2 years.[14]

The device is made of a titanium alloy external housing with inflow and outflow tracts that utilize porcine xenograft valves (25 mm). The unique characteristic of the device is its internal blood-contacting surface, which is made on one side of textured titanium and on the other of textured polyurethane. This textured surface encourages the deposition of a fibrin-cellular matrix that forms a pseudoneointima. The formation of this surface greatly reduces the need for anticoagulation because thrombus formation is greatly reduced.[13] Patients with these devices take aspirin (primarily as an anti-inflammatory, not as an anticoagulant) as their only anticoagulation with a subsequent low rate of thromboembolic complications (7%).[12,13,15] The device has a pumping capacity in excess of 10 L/min and a stroke volume of 83 mL. The pulsatile flow is created using a pusher plate system.[13] The device is operated in either a fixed-rate or automatic mode. In automatic mode, the pump senses when the chamber is full and activates the pusher plate. The pump is inserted into the left upper quadrant of the abdomen either pre- or intraperitoneally. The driveline, consisting of an air vent and power cables, is tunneled and brought out of the skin in the right upper quadrant. Small battery units, worn in a harness, are connected to the cables. Battery life is between 4 and 6 hours depending on activity level.[13] In case of an emergency, a portable hand pump can be used to activate the device. The patient's body size is an important factor in allowing device placement. The size of the device requires patients to have a body surface area of more than 1.5 m^2. This device was used in the Randomized Evaluation of Mechanical Assistance for the Treatment of Congestive Heart Failure (REMATCH) trial to compare medical and circulatory assist device treatments for end-stage heart failure. Patients with this device showed better results than the medically treated group (see later section on destination therapy).

NOVACOR

The Novacor (World Heart Corp., Ottawa, ON, Canada) left ventricular assist system (LVAS) was developed by Peer Portner in collaboration with Stanford University and was first used in 1984 in a successful bridge to transplant application (Fig. 62-2).[16] Initially designed as a totally implantable system for long-term support, it has evolved through a console-based controller system to a wearable controller that has been available since 1993. This system has proven to be reliable, with about 60% to 70% of patients surviving to transplantation.[16–18] The worldwide median time of LVAS support using this system is 100 days with the device lasting as long as 1512 days.[16,17] The company currently claims a 3-year pump reliability of greater than 90%.[19]

The pump works using dual pusher plates that compress a polyurethane sac; 21-mm bioprosthetic valves are used in both inflow and outflow tracts. Stroke volume reaches 70 mL. Similar to the HeartMate device, the pump is placed in the left upper abdominal quadrant, anterior to the posterior rectus sheath. The inflow tract is connected to the left ventricle, and the outflow tract to the ascending aorta. The percutaneous lead is brought out in the right lower quadrant of the abdomen and connected to a controller worn on a belt system. Unlike the HeartMate system, patients require anticoagulation with warfarin to avoid embolic events. Currently the Investigation of Non-Transplant-Eligible Patients Who Are Inotrope Dependent (INTREPID) trial is underway to evaluate the use of this device as a long-term alternative to transplantation.

Paracorporeal Pulsatile Devices

Numerous Pierce-Donachy type pumps are available, such as Thoratec, Medos, German Heart, and Toyobo Heart. We will discuss here the most utilized device, the Thoratec VAD.

THORATEC

The Thoratec VAD (Thoratec Laboratories Corp., Pleasanton, CA) is another reliable and often used system for ventricular support (Fig. 62-3). Unlike the previously mentioned Novacor and HeartMate, Thoratec is a paracorporeal system that can be applied for univentricular or biventricular support. Since the actual pump chamber is outside of the body, this device can be used on patients with small body size who would not meet the size criteria to house a HeartMate or Novacor system. However, a paracorporeal system limits mobility and presents an obstacle for patients in a long-term setting. William Pierce and James Donachy of Pennsylvania State University designed the pump. In 1984 the first Thoratec system was used as a successful bridge to transplantation. The system received FDA approval for bridging to transplantation in 1995 and for postcardiotomy support in 1998.[20]

The pump consists of a prosthetic ventricle with 65-mL stroke volume and cannulas for ventricular or atrial inflow and arterial outflow. Currently a large pneumatic drive console is available and a smaller briefcase-sized power driver

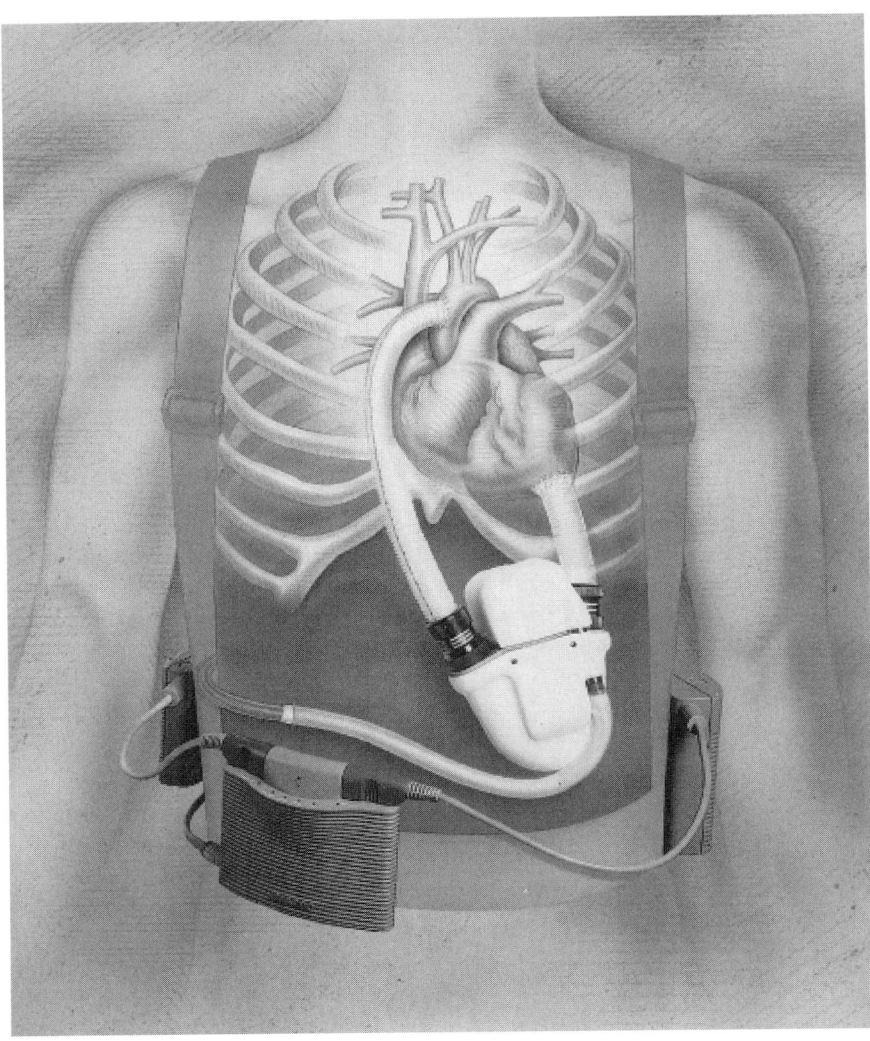

FIGURE 62–2 Novacor left ventricular assist system. (*Courtesy of World Heart Corp., Ottawa, ON.*)

unit is in trial.[20] Pneumatic drivers provide alternating air pressure to fill and empty the blood pump. The pump flow rate ranges from 1.3 to 7.2 L/min.[20] The smallest patient receiving the device was a 7-year-old child weighing 17 kg with a BSA of $0.7m^2$. Inflow cannula placement can occur in an atrial or ventricular position. Ventricular cannula placement is better for left side support as it allows for greater flow rates than the atrial cannulation. Anticoagulation is similar to that used for patients with mechanical valves, with warfarin as a typical therapy.[20]

The device has been used in over 1000 patients for uni- and biventricular support for both bridge to transplantation and postcardiotomy recovery. Survival to transplantation has been in the 60% to 80% range depending on which ventricle was supported.[20,21] The great benefit of this system is its versatility. It is easy to place with less surgical dissection, can be used for different sized patients, can be attached to either the atrium or ventricle, and can be used for right and left support. However, its paracorporeal location limits its use as a long-term device.

Rotary Axial Flow Pumps

Continuous blood flow in circulatory support is a concept as old as the heart-lung machine of the 1950s. Researchers realized that axial pumps had the advantage of smaller size, less power consumption, minimal moving parts, and no valves. Early research focused on problems of hemolysis and questionable problems with long-term nonpulsatile blood flow. Numerous experiments with different pumps were carried out throughout the 1960s, 1970s, and 1980s. However, it is the MicroMed-DeBakey VAD, the HeartMate II, and the Jarvik 2000 pumps that have lately shown most promise in the clinical setting.[22]

MICROMED-DEBAKEY

The MicroMed-DeBakey VAD (Houston, TX) was initially developed in the 1980s as a collaboration between Dr. George Noon and Dr. Michael DeBakey of Baylor College of Medicine and engineers from NASA (Fig. 62-4).

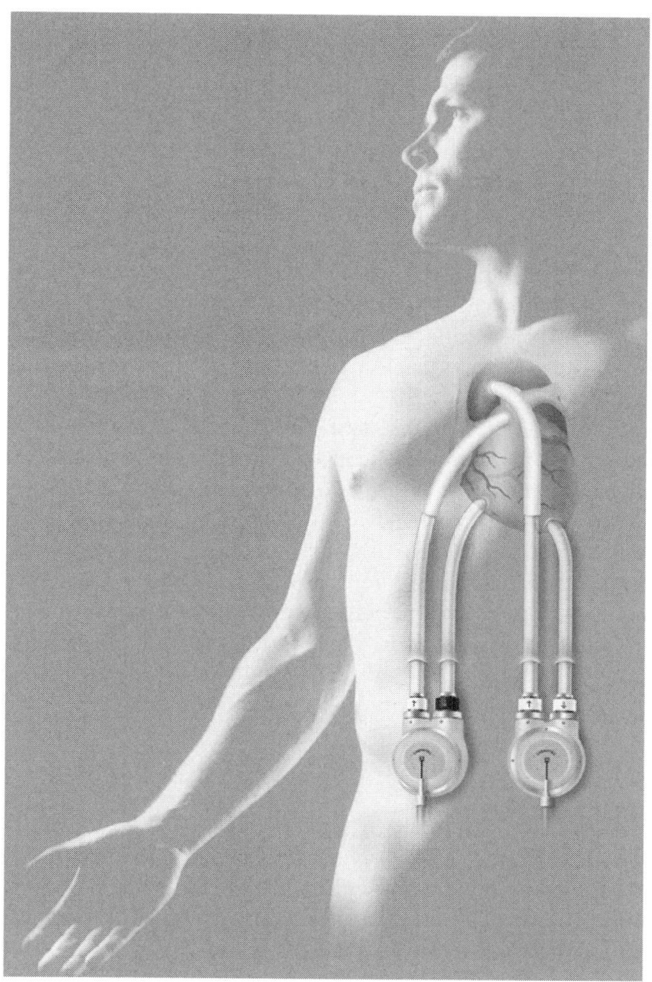

FIGURE 62–3 Thoratec ventricular assist device. (*Reproduced with the permission of Thoratec Corp., Pleasanton, CA.*)

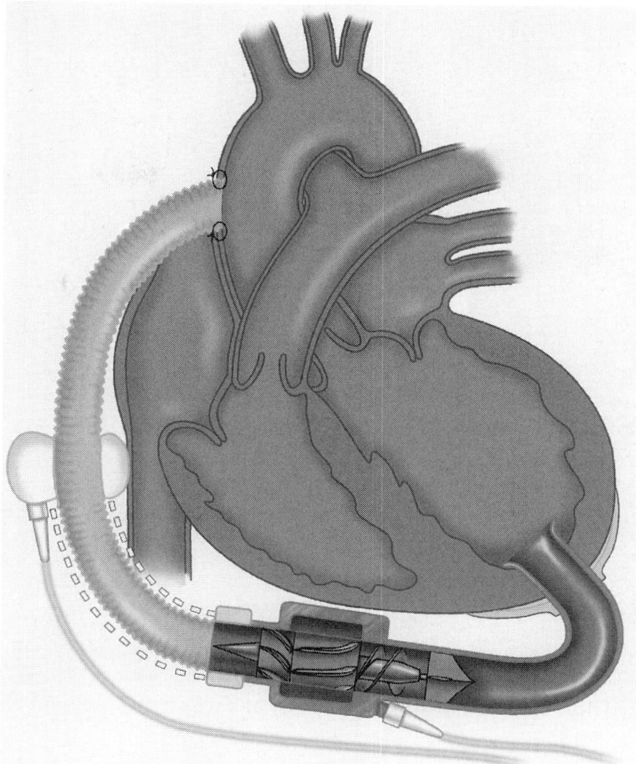

FIGURE 62–4 MicroMed-DeBakey ventricular assist device. (*Courtesy of MicroMed Technology Inc., Houston, TX.*)

MicroMed Technology, Inc., received the license for this technology in 1996 and has continued to develop this device for clinical use.[23] The first clinical use of the device was in Europe in November of 1998 with subsequent trials starting in United States in June of 2000.[23,24]

The pump unit is 1.2 inches in diameter, 3 inches long, and weighs 95 grams. It is made of titanium casing with an impeller/inducer capable of pumping 10 L/min. The rest of the pump consists of a titanium inflow cannula, a flow meter, a Dacron outflow graft (Sulzer Inc., Austin, TX), and a percutaneous cable connected to a wearable battery/control console.[23] The inflow cannula is inserted into the left ventricular apex, the pump is placed into a small abdominal pocket, and the outflow graft is anastomosed to the ascending or descending aorta. Patients are chronically anticoagulated with warfarin.[23,25] A pump index of 2.0 to 2.5 L/min/m^2 or higher is recommended and the pump is started at 7500 rpm and then adjusted. Average pump flow is 3.9 to 5.4 L/min. The flow is volume and preload related. High rpm with inadequate preload can cause suction and ventricular collapse, but this problem is not typically seen.[23,25] The flow is not nonpulsatile but is low pulsatile due to the recovering ventricle and change in ventricular volume. Increase in rpm leads to diminished pulses. No consistent significant clinical hemolysis based on plasma-free hemoglobin has been reported. Lactate dehydrogenase, however, is consistently elevated.[24,26]

In the clinical trial in Europe, the device was tested as a bridge to cardiac transplantation. The trial lasted from November 1998 to March 2001 with 78 patients enrolling in 12 centers. The U.S. trial was begun in June 2000 with 18 patients implanted as of this writing. The total number of worldwide implants is 140. Average time on pump is 79 days with 11 patients surviving longer than 111 days on pump. Longest duration with the pump has been greater than 1 year.[25] The probability of 30-day survival is 81%. Out of the initial 32 patients receiving the device, 11 were transplanted and 10 died on support. Death was the result of multiorgan failure but could not be related to device performance as there was no difference in pump index between survivors and nonsurvivors.[23] The major complication was late bleeding and was apparently related to the level of anticoagulation, which has since been decreased to a target International Normalized Ratio (INR) of 2.0–2.5.[23] Follow-up of patients with

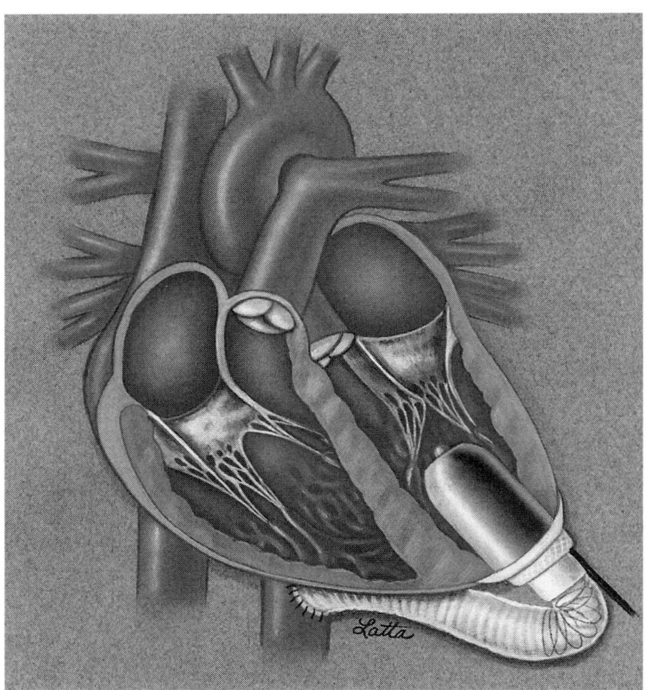

FIGURE 62–5 Jarvik 2000. (*Courtesy of Texas Heart Institute.*)

the device has shown improved exercise tolerance and ability to go home with the device while awaiting transplantation.[27]

JARVIK 2000

The Jarvik 2000 (Jarvik Heart, Inc., New York, NY) is another extensively developed axial-flow pump initially developed by Dr. Jarvik (Fig. 62-5). The pump underwent animal testing at the Texas Heart Institute and Columbia-Presbyterian Medical Center from 1991 to 1999.[28] Clinical patient trials to evaluate the device as a bridge to heart transplantation started in April 2000 at the Texas Heart Institute and shortly thereafter in Oxford, United Kingdom. The Oxford protocol included patients who were not transplant candidates and who received the device as destination therapy.[29]

The titanium pump measures 2.5 cm in diameter, displaces 25 mL, and weighs 90 grams. The rotor includes titanium impeller blades and is held in place by two ceramic bearings. The impeller rotates at 8,000 to 12,000 rpm producing a flow rate of 7 L/min. Unlike the DeBakey VAD or the HeartMate II pump, the pump is positioned inside the ventricle with the outflow graft extended to the descending aorta. The pump can operate in fixed rate or variable mode and has a manual rate adjustment capability for times of increased activity. Three different control and energy systems are currently under investigation. A percutaneous model that, like most other LVAD systems, has a power lead that exits the patient's skin; a fully implantable model that uses the transcutaneous energy transfer system (TETS), which is still in development; and a modified percutaneous system that uses a titanium pedestal screwed into the skull with a connector piercing the skin and attaching to the external cable. The fixed skull implantation provides a low level of repeated trauma and minimizes the risk of infection seen with percutaneous systems due to high vascularity of the scalp; however, a risk of subsequent intracranial bleeding exists. Clinical implantations of the skull pedestal are currently used in Britain.[29,30] Unlike the other systems, which require a sternotomy, the Jarvik 2000 is implanted through a left thoracotomy incision. Similar to other systems, the pump provides a low pulsatile flow with a narrowing of pulse pressure at higher speeds.[29]

Required anticoagulation is reported to be minimal with some patients taking warfarin while others showing no clot formation with only aspirin. No significant hemolysis is observed between 8,000 and 12,000 rpm. The small size of the device allows patients with small body surface areas to be treated, and the manual control with the ability to increase the pump rate allows patients to control pump output during exercise as shown in the Oxford experience. Patients receiving destination therapy in the United Kingdom have also been discharged from the hospital on the device.[30]

HEARTMATE II

The HeartMate II LVAD (Thoratec Corp., Pleasanton, CA), like the two previously mentioned pumps, is an axial flow pump that had its origin in the early 1990s with a collaboration between Nimbus Company and the University of Pittsburgh (Fig. 62-6). After many years of animal experiments and development, the device was first implanted in July 2000 in a patient in Israel. Six other patients have received the device in Europe and the company is currently starting a European and U.S. study involving 20 patients in multiple centers.[31]

Similar to the other pumps, this is an axial-flow rotary LVAD made of titanium with a rotor capable of producing flow rates greater than 10 L/min at rpms greater than 10,000. Like the DeBakey VAD, the inflow cannula is joined to the apex of the left ventricle, with the outflow graft connected to the ascending aorta. Like the other axial-flow pumps, there is a risk of generating negative intraventricular pressure and collapsing the ventricle. As a result, inflow cannula positioning and ventricular preload are important. The intraventricular portion of the inflow tract has been elongated and as a result tends to stent open the middle of the ventricle, thus improving reliability of continuous flow throughout the cardiac cycle.[31] Anticoagulation is at present required to keep INR between 1.5 and 2.5. The pump is small (124 mL) and is inserted preperitoneally or within the abdominal musculature. Power and control are supplied by a percutaneous lead that is attached to a system driver that can be connected to a power base unit or to rechargeable batteries and worn in a

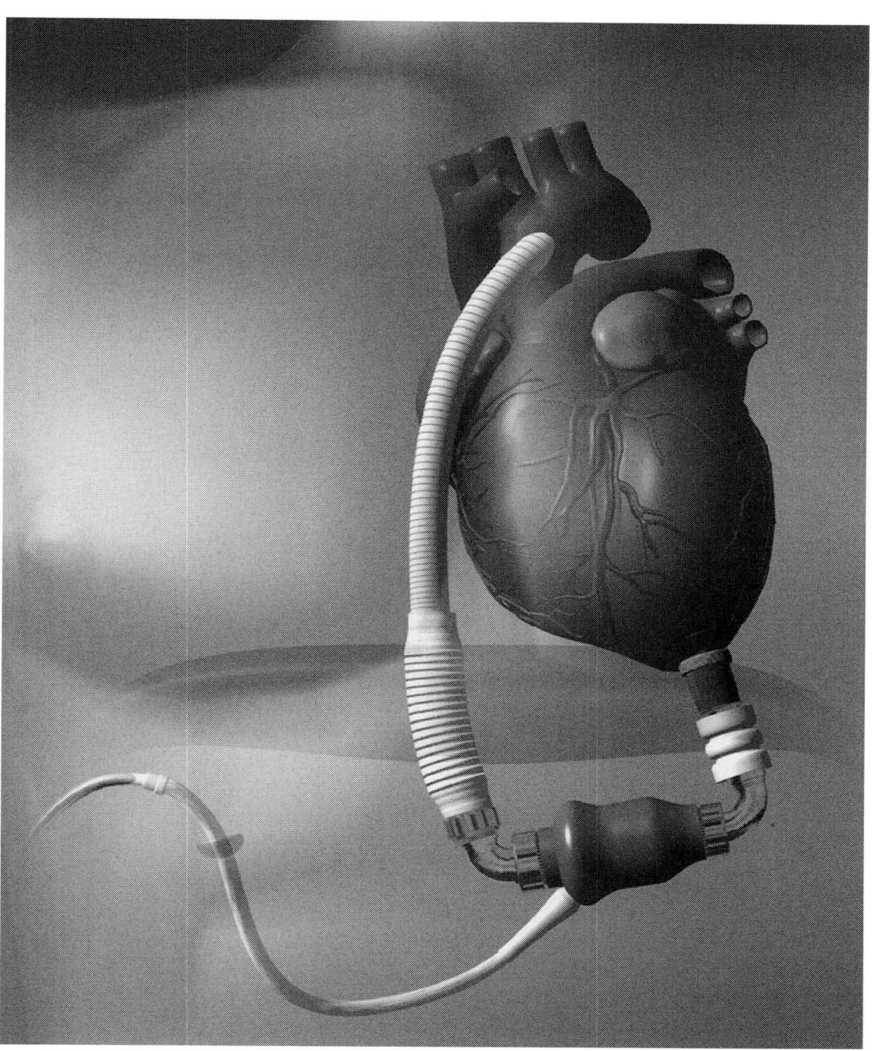

FIGURE 62–6 HeartMate II left ventricular assist device. (*Reproduced with the permission of Thoratec Corp., Pleasanton, CA.*)

manner similar to the pulsatile HeartMate LVAD. The system can be operated in manual or auto mode with the auto mode preferred for everyday use.[31] Currently research is underway to develop and test a totally implantable system using TETS coil to deliver power to the system.[32] This pump is a promising system and with the upcoming trials more results are expected in the near future.

Totally Implantable Pulsatile Devices

As our experience with long-term devices improves and the future of destination therapy draws near, completely implantable devices become increasingly important. Two design issues with total implantable systems involve energy transfer and volume displacement. Several models are currently under investigation, including the current Arrow LionHeart LVD-2000 designed with collaboration between Pennsylvania State University and Arrow International (Reading, PA).

ARROW LIONHEART LVD-2000

The Arrow LionHeart LVD-2000 is the first system designed specifically with destination support in mind. It is a completely implantable system with a transcutaneous energy transmission system (TETS) and a compliance chamber, which allows for complete implantation with no percutaneous lines or connections. The pump is made of a titanium casing with pumping activated by a pusher plate. Unidirectional blood flow is maintained via two Delrin disk monostrut valves (27-mm inlet; 25-mm outlet). The inflow and outflow tracts are positioned in the ventricular apex and aorta respectively. Maximum pump flow is 8 L/min with stroke volume of 64 mL.[33] The controller is housed in a titanium casing that also houses rechargeable batteries. The control system is dependent on continual monitoring of end-diastolic volume, and thus the patient's physiologic demands control the filling volume of the pump.[33] The compliance chamber consists of a circular polymer sac and an attached subcutaneous port infusion system. This compliance chamber loses gas through the polymer and requires replenishment of gas once a month.[34] Recharging of the battery is accomplished through a transcutaneous system with a wand overlying the skin over the recharging coil. The patient may be completely disconnected from the external power supply for a short period of time and rely on internal back-up batteries. The internal coil must be positioned under the skin so as to allow no more than 1 cm of tissue thickness between the coil and skin surface.[33,34]

The LionHeart underwent initial studies in Europe using 5 centers with 20 patients receiving the device. A U.S. clinical trial has begun with FDA approval for a phase I clinical human trial.[34]

Total Artificial Heart

CARDIOWEST

Mechanical left ventricular support is adequate for the majority of heart failure patients. However, a subgroup of patients requires biventricular support and complete replacement of native heart function. The total artificial heart (TAH) has been under development for decades. In 1982 a Jarvik-7 TAH was used in a much publicized case.[6] The CardioWest Total Artificial Heart (CardioWest Technologies, Inc., Tucson, AZ) is a device derived from the Jarvik pump and subsequently modified into the Symbion Jarvik-70 TAH and finally the CardioWest C-70 TAH. Since its inception, the device has been implanted in over 300 people worldwide, and since an FDA-approved study was begun in 1993, the device has been successfully used in over 150 patients as a bridge to transplantation.[35] The pneumatic device is implanted into the chest cavity of critically ill patients with a minimal body surface area of 1.7 m^2. The prosthetic ventricles of the device replace the patient's native ventricles and connections are made to the patient's great vessels and atrial cuffs. The patients require chronic anticoagulation. Those who are eligible to receive the device must have large chests with 10-cm anteroposterior diameter at T10. The overall survival of patients on the device has been as high as 83% with a low postoperative stroke rate of 0.6 events/patient-year. Serious infection has occurred in approximately 20% of patients, and the mean duration of device support until transplantation has been 84 days. The CardioWest pump should be considered in a patient with biventricular failure and a large chest cavity. The lack of a small portable controller does limit ambulation on this device.[35,36]

ABIOCOR

Another device showing much promise is the AbioCor (ABIOMED Inc, Danvers, MA) totally implantable artificial heart (Fig. 62-7). The pump is an electrohydraulically

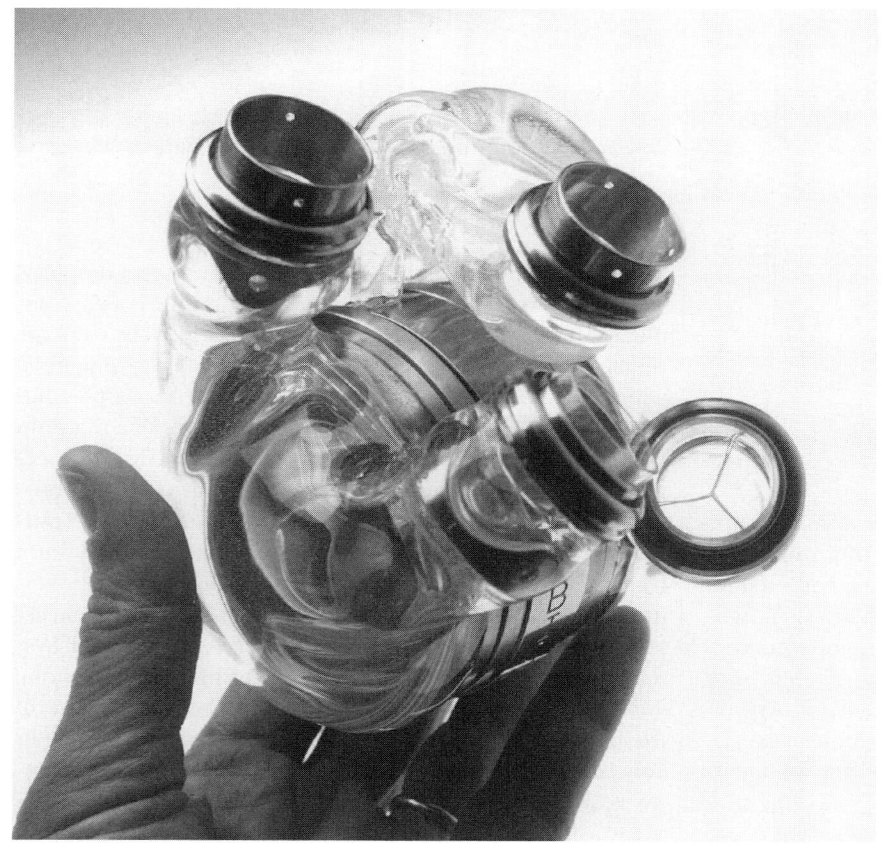

FIGURE 62–7 AbioCor totally implantable artificial heart. (*Courtesy of ABIOMED Inc., Danvers, MA.*)

actuated device implanted in the pericardial space after excision of the native heart. The pump chambers are sutured to atrial tissue and great vessels by textured Dacron atrial cuffs and grafts. Two polyurethane blood pump chambers with a 60-mL stroke volume produce 8 L/min of flow. The pump is connected to internal components including controller, battery, and transcutaneous energy transfer (TET) coil.[37] The patients require chronic anticoagulation after implantation to prevent thromboembolic events.

After extensive animal testing starting in 1998 at the University of Louisville and the Texas Heart Institute, the device received FDA approval for a multicenter limited human testing trial involving patients requiring total heart support who did not qualify for heart transplantation. The first patient received the heart on July 2, 2001, and was kept alive for almost 5 months on the device. His death was a result of anticoagulation complications and was not device related.[38] This early experience will heighten awareness of the significance of right heart failure during left ventricular support.

PATIENT AND DEVICE SELECTION

As LVAD technology improves so does the desire to apply this technology to an ever growing population. However, patients receiving this therapy still experience a large risk of morbidity and mortality. In order to minimize this risk, both the technology and the patient selection need to improve.

Patient Selection

The HeartMate and the Novacor LVAD systems have been tested for years and have a greater than 70% rate of survival to transplantation.[11–13,16–18] One of the most important aspects of device implantation is patient selection. Heart failure in some form (chronic congestive, idiopathic dilated, acute postcardiotomy, or other) must be present. Signs of failure such as pulmonary capillary wedge pressure higher than 20 mm Hg, cardiac index less than 2.0 L/min/m^2, or systolic blood pressure below 80 mm Hg despite best medical management should be present.[11] Columbia University and the Cleveland Clinic Foundation devised a scoring system in 1995 to predict which patients would have a successful outcome after LVAD implantation.[39] However, as the technology evolved, it widened and extended the use of these devices and the Columbia score was revised to better reflect the current LVAD-eligible population.[40] The previous score utilized 10 factors found to be significant for mortality using univariate analysis with a score higher than 5 corresponding to more than a 33% risk of postimplantation death.[39] The revised score was based on 130 patients receiving vented electric HeartMate devices from 1996 to 2001 (Table 62-1). Univariate and multivariate analyses were performed to determine operative mortality.

The new preoperative risk factors predicting mortality by univariate analysis are: previous LVAD/RVAD, acute MI, postcardiotomy, central venous pressure (CVP) greater than 16 mm Hg, prothrombin time (PT) greater than 16 seconds, preoperative ventilation, redo surgery, coronary artery disease, and dilated cardiomyopathy. Interestingly, preoperative renal insufficiency was not found to impact survival in the new scoring system, unlike the old system. This is likely due to aggressive treatment of renal insufficiency with ultrafiltration and hemodialysis. A stepwise linear regression model identified a ventilated patient and a previous LVAD as independent predictors of mortality following device insertion.[42] After multivariate analysis the 5 new factors included in the scoring system were: ventilated patients (score of 4), redo surgery (score of 2), previous LVAD inserted (score of 2), CVP higher than 16 mm Hg (score of 1), and PT higher than 16 seconds (score of 1). A score higher than 5 corresponds with a 47% mortality, compared with 9% mortality for a score lower than 5. The positive and negative predictive value of this scoring system is 79% and 70% respectively.[40]

TABLE 62–1 Scoring systems for prediction of successful outcome after LVAD implantation

Variable	Points
Original system	
Urine output <30cc/h	3
Ventilated	2
CVP >16 mm Hg	2
PT >16 sec	2
Redo surgery	1
Revised system	
Ventilated	4
Redo surgery	2
Previous LVAD	2
CVP >16 mm Hg	1
PT >16 sec	1

The urgency of device placement has also been shown to play a factor in survival. In a study by Deng et al, patients receiving emergent LVADs had a lower survival to transplantation rate than those receiving devices urgently or those who did not need devices. However, electively implanted LVAD patients with no subsequent transplantation had better survival than medically treated heart failure patients who also did not get transplanted. This occurred despite the fact that the LVAD recipients were a sicker group of patients.[41]

Device Selection

Once we decide that the patient will receive an assist device, the next step is to select the right device for the patient. As mentioned previously, numerous reliable devices are available, and many more will be available in the near future. However, not all of the devices are ideal for every situation. First, the decision needs to be made about the goals for the patient. Will it be short-term or long-term heart recovery? Is it bridge to transplantation or destination therapy? What is the size of the patient, and what size device will they tolerate? Does the patient need biventricular or only left-sided support? A paracorporeal system such as the Thoratec system can be used for short- and medium-term support of less than 6 months as well as for right-sided support. The implantable systems such as the Novacor and Thoratec VADs can be used for medium-term, long-term, and destination therapy and have become the workhorses in this field. However, these devices support only the left side and require a minimum body size greater than 1.5 m^2. For smaller patients an axial-flow pump such as the DeBakey VAD, Jarvik 2000, or HeartMate II would be ideal; however, a Thoratec system can also be used until the other devices become fully approved. For destination therapy and biventricular support, the AbioCor TAH may become the system of choice. Biventricular support can be considered in patients with high central venous pressures (CVP), increased pulmonary vascular resistance, multiple organ dysfunction, or severe malignant arrhythmias refractory to medical therapy.[42] It is important to tailor the device to the patient and not the patient to the device.

SURGICAL TECHNIQUE

The techniques for implantation of these multiple devices are varied. We will briefly describe the placement of the HeartMate LVAD. The patient is prepared for open heart cardiopulmonary bypass surgery as usual. The sternum is opened and prior to heparinization a pre-peritoneal LVAD pocket is created in the abdominal left upper quadrant through an extension of the midline sternotomy incision. Once the pocket is created, the heart is cannulated for bypass. The device is primed and brought into the field. The LVAD driveline is passed through its tract and out of the skin in the right upper quadrant of the abdomen. If the patient's hemodynamic status allows, we prefer to do off-pump aortic anastomosis first with the use of a side-biting clamp to minimize bypass time. After full heparinization, we measure the length of the graft. Once the graft is measured and trimmed, a side-biting aortic clamp is applied and an elipticolongitudinal aortotomy is created. The graft is sewn into place using 4-0 Prolene sutures. To prevent bleeding, BioGlue (CryoLife Inc., Kennesaw, GA) is generously applied over the entire anastomosis line. Bypass is instituted and aortic pressure is lowered prior to releasing the aortic side clamp to minimize the bleeding associated with high pressure. Hemostasis is confirmed immediately after releasing the clamp. A circular core bored out of the apex of the left ventricle allows for placement of the inflow cannula. Sutures are placed circumferentially around the cored opening and passed through the inflow cannula Teflon ring. Once all the sutures are placed, the cannula is brought down to the ventricle and all the sutures are tied. The inflow cannula is secured to the LVAD body and additional BioGlue is used to reinforce the anastomosis. The pump is manually primed and vented through the outflow tract as the patient is weaned from bypass with the pump on. Chest tubes are placed in the pleural cavities and drains are placed in the mediastinum and in the LVAD pocket. After hemostasis is achieved, the chest and upper abdomen are closed in the standard fashion.

POSTOPERATIVE CARE

After LVAD implantation patients are moved to the intensive care unit on a ventilator. Extra care needs to be taken to ensure that the right heart is well supported, and as a result milrinone and inhaled nitric oxide (iNO) therapy are now routinely used in the immediate postoperative period.[12] If excessive bleeding is encountered in the operating room, the chest may be packed and left open upon transfer to the intensive care unit. The patient is then brought back to the operating room after the coagulopathy is corrected for irrigation and chest closure. In the intensive care unit, the patient is weaned from NO and extubated once pulmonary artery pressures are in the normal range. With no further sign of active bleeding, the drains and chest tubes are removed. Anticoagulation with aspirin is used for patients with all devices. Additional anticoagulation with warfarin is used for patients receiving the Thoratec and Novacor, as well as the axial-flow devices. Physical therapy and nutrition are addressed early. The LVAD recipient discharge program was instituted in 1993 by the FDA. Since then, numerous centers have reported selective patients who are sent home to live with their devices while awaiting transplantation or as destination therapy. The FDA program created numerous functional and clinical discharge criteria. General criteria include physical rehabilitation, echocardiographic evidence of marginal heart function (to keep the patient alive until manual pumping can be instituted in case the device fails), and a training course in use and care of the device. Once these criteria are met, patients undergo a gradual program with longer trips outside the hospital and finally discharge with weekly returns.[11,43]

COMPLICATIONS

Six common complications occur after VAD implantation. We will review these in context of the three most common pumps used: Thoratec, HeartMate, and Novacor.

Bleeding

Postoperative bleeding occurs frequently after device placement. Normal postoperative bleeding is made excessive by preoperative heart failure leading to hepatic dysfunction, need for anticoagulation, coagulopathy caused by human-device interaction, extensive surgical dissection, and prolonged cardiopulmonary bypass time. Excessive perioperative bleeding occurs between 20% and 50% of the time in all three devices. This rate, however, has decreased as the experience with the devices has grown.[42,44] Coagulation parameters as well as complete blood count must be monitored closely and products replaced as necessary. Death due to bleeding has been reported in the range of 0% to 15% for the three devices.[16,44] Reexploration for bleeding is also common and at times can be planned. If excessive bleeding is noted at the time of chest closure, the chest can be left open, packed, and the patient taken to the ICU for resuscitation. The chest is closed once coagulation is normalized.

Infection

Infection is another serious complication affecting long-term mechanical circulatory support patients. There is some controversy and lack of definitions regarding what constitutes the various subgroups of device infection. LVAD infection can manifest as driveline, pocket, blood, or device endocarditis. At times it can be difficult to decide if a pocket infection is present or exactly where the offending organism is harbored in an LVAD-supported patient with positive blood cultures and multiple catheters and intravenous lines. In addition to device infections, the patients are susceptible to the standard common infections seen in critically ill patients such as pneumonia, line sepsis, and urinary tract infections. The reported infection rates in these patients range from 12% to 55%.[42,45] Pocket infection rates have been reported to be 11% to 24% for the HeartMate and Novacor systems with the driveline infection rates even higher and in the range of 18% to 30% for the two devices.[42,44] There is much variability in this data since definitions for these infections have not been standardized and in many cases clinical presentation is not clear cut. Sepsis accounts for 21% to 25% of LVAD deaths and occurs in 11% to 26% of patients.[14,16,42,44] Infection, however, is not a contraindication to transplantation in this population and transplantation can successfully be accomplished.[46]

The interaction between device and human that occurs after VAD implantation is a topic of much interest. It is well established that B-cell hyperreactivity in LVAD patients leads to the development of antibodies to HLA class I or II antigens with subsequent high panel reactive antibody (PRA) results. Several studies from Columbia University have also pointed to immune system activation with T-cell dysfunction, apoptosis, and elevation in CD-95 levels in patients after LVAD implantation. In comparison to medically managed patients, LVAD patients were also found to have lower T-cell proliferative responses after activation.[47,48] This immunologic dysfunction may play a key role in the high infection rates seen in patients with long-term circulatory assist devices. More work is needed in this area to further define the causes of this phenomenon.

Thromboembolism

Thromboembolism is a major concern in any patient with mechanical circulatory support due to blood-device interface. The prevalence of embolism varies depending on the system used and varies from 7% to 47%, with the majority occurring in cerebral distribution in the 25% range.[42,44] The HeartMate device has the lowest thromboembolic rate, reported to be as low as 7.4%.[42] This is likely due to its unique textured blood-interface surface, which promotes a formation of neointima with subsequent low thrombus formation despite minimal anticoagulation with aspirin. All other pumps require warfarin as well as antiplatelet agents for anticoagulation to prevent this complication. In addition to device-surface interaction, thrombus formation can occur due to turbulent flow in any one of the conduits or in the device itself.

Mechanical Failure

Mechanical failure is a complication on the decline. Constant modifications of pump design result in more reliable systems. The failure can occur in multiple places in the device itself or in the controller. The rate of failure is 10% or less including the long-term studies with device duration longer than 1 year.[14,44] Device failure, however, does not always result in patient death. In many cases ample time or reserve is available to replace the device or the controller.

Right Heart Failure

Patients must be observed for signs of right ventricular failure from the time before device implantation until the early postoperative period. The clinician must keep right heart function in mind when evaluating a patient for LVAD placement. In most cases, the unloading and support of the left ventricle will help the right side. However, a rise in central venous pressure with a decrease in device flow and an empty left ventricle signals right ventricular failure. Inhaled nitric oxide is useful in this situation; however, at times an RVAD needs to be implanted. The incidence of right heart failure is above 10%, and 20% of patients are on prolonged inotropic support due to right heart failure. Right heart failure is also associated with high transfusion rate and increased rate of end-organ failure. The number of days in the intensive care unit and the mortality rate are also increased in the right heart failure patients.[49]

Multiorgan Failure

Multiorgan failure is another frequent complication in this population. Due to a significant amount of preoperative end-organ dysfunction and comorbid conditions, some of these patients do not fully recover after device implantation. In many situations multiorgan failure is the end result of a long cascade of complications including sepsis, bleeding, and other events. At other times it may be the result of significant preoperative multiorgan dysfunction that gets worse after the insult of surgery. In all these scenarios it can account for 11% to 29% of deaths with the device.[44]

BRIDGE TO VENTRICULAR RECOVERY/ REMODELING

There is increasing evidence that hemodynamic unloading of the ventricle can reverse and in some cases normalize several aspects of a failing heart's structure and function. Consistent data show that LVAD support provides both pressure and volume unloading of the left ventricle.[50,51] LVADs have been shown to cause a reversal of ventricular chamber enlargement, reduction of left ventricular mass, regression of myocyte hypertrophy, increased contractile properties of myocytes, and normalization of gene expression encoding for proteins involved in calcium metabolism in the failing heart.[50,52] Clinical experience has shown that in some patients LVAD support may lead to improvement of pump function of sufficient magnitude to allow explantation of the device without transplantation.[51,53,54] These findings have led to the idea of using LVADs as a bridge to recovery. Reports of heart failure recovery leading to explantation of the device date back to 1991.[55] Since the mid-1990s an increasing amount of work has been done in this field. Some of the studies were done using the HeartMate LVAD system in which a flow limiter was used to decrease LVAD flow and assess potential candidates for device explantation, using exercise testing, echocardiography, and max V_{O_2}. Other centers have used rate weaning and dobutamine stress studies in combination with cardiac echocardiography to select patients who may tolerate the removal of device. As of now, this "recovery" has been shown to occur in a limited number of patients. Additional work is currently being done in this area under the LVAD Working Group (LWG) multicenter study in an attempt to better classify who will benefit from this form of therapy and what parameters are to be used to wean the patient off the LVAD.[56] Specific and unique pharmacotherapy may also prove to be beneficial in this patient population with the resulting treatment formula being a combination of device implantation and pharmacologic manipulation. Yacoub has previously published work showing the benefit of this combined treatment with medications such as clenbuterol.[57] At present this form of therapy is not the standard of care.

DESTINATION THERAPY

Due to the constant shortage of available donor organs, the large group of patients who would benefit from circulatory assistance, and the positive results from the use of current LVADs as long-term support, a multicenter trial was conducted to evaluate the use of a LVAD as a permanent device in the treatment of heart failure. The REMATCH Study was undertaken in 1998 and included 129 patients in 20 centers. The Thoratec HeartMate vented electrical LVAD was used as the tested device. Eligible patients were adults with end-stage heart failure and contraindications for transplantation. The patients in the study were randomly assigned to receive either an LVAD or optimal medical therapy. The study used death as the primary end point and included a number of secondary end points to assess quality of life, complications, and hospitalizations. The study ended in July 2001 once a predetermined number of deaths occurred. Sixty-eight percent of patients received LVADs and 61% received only medical management. The two groups were similar in baseline characteristics. There was a reduction of 48% in the risk of death in the group treated with LVADs as compared to the medically treated group. Quality of life measurements were also better in the LVAD-treated groups. In the adverse events category, patients with devices were more than twice as likely to have an adverse event. Patients with LVADs had a higher median number of days spent in and out of the hospital.[14]

The INTREPID trial is another similar study currently under way and near completion. This study involves the Novacor LVAS, which has been shown to work without failure an average of 4 years in 12 patients.[58] The results of this study may further reconfirm the LVAD as an alternative to transplantation and a good tool in the fight against heart failure.

FUTURE

Long-term mechanical circulatory support is at a point of intense research and development. The potential of these devices not only as a bridge to transplantation but also as destination therapy is being shown in clinical trials. A number of devices are currently under development and will soon reach clinical application.

HeartSaver LVAD

The HeartSaver LVAD (World Heart Corporation, Ottawa, ON, Canada) is designed as a totally implantable LVAD system using TET coil for transcutaneous energy transfer. Similar to other LVADs, the inflow cannula is inserted into the apex of the left ventricle with the outflow going to the ascending aorta. The pump has an attached volume displacement chamber and as an entire unit is implanted into the left thoracic cavity. The preclinical work with the device is being done at the University of Ottawa Heart Institute and numerous animal studies have shown promise.[59]

Thoratec Intracorporeal VAD

The Thoratec Intracorporeal VAD (Thoratec Laboratories Corp., Pleasanton, CA) is being designed by the same firm that developed the paracorporeal device. The intracorporeal system is the same size as the external system but is cased in a titanium alloy housing and will be implantable. The advantages of this system will be its use as implantable right ventricular support, and its small size, reliability, and proven and extensively tested technology based on the currently used Thoratec system. It will be targeted toward patients who would benefit from long-term support and the benefits of an implanted device.[60]

Novacor II

Novacor II (World Heart Corp., Ottawa, ON, Canada) is a concept heart created by a company with extensive LVAD experience. It will be a totally implantable pump for definitive treatment of heart failure. Its unique dual-chamber, four-valve pump requires no volume compensator. The pusher plate is suspended and magnetically driven thus providing for a system with few moving parts. The two chambers fill alternately creating pulsatile flow. The system also uses transcutaneous energy transfer technology to supply power. It is currently in preclinical testing.[18]

Centrifugal Pumps

Years after the invention of centrifugal pumps, researchers in several centers are looking into these pumps as next-generation implantable circulatory assist devices. The HeartQuest System (MedQuest Products Inc., Salt Lake City, UT) is one such pump built on the maglev (magnetic levitation) concept, which allows for frictionless pumping, low thrombogenicity, minimal noise and vibration, and durability due to lack of metal to metal contact. These pumps have been tested in animals with promising results.[61] The VentrAssist (Micromedical Industries, Ltd., Chatswood, NSW, Australia) is another promising centrifugal pump currently undergoing animal testing. It has been implanted in animals without cardiopulmonary bypass. The centrifugal pump is hydrodynamically suspended resulting in no wear, no hemolysis, and no need for anticoagulation.[62] Another centrifugal pump in the making is the HeartMate III from the Thoratec Corporation, which created the HeartMate I and II. This pump is their third-generation pump powered by a magnetically levitated centrifugal impeller. It is about one third the size of the HeartMate I pump and is about 3 times the volume of HeartMate II.[63,64] Another unique pump, the Terumo DuraHeart LVAS (Terumo Cardiovascular Systems, Ann Arbor, MI) incorporates a unique centrifugal pump with a magnetically levitated impeller. The pump provides contact-free rotation of the impeller without material wear and tear and therefore is one of the most durable blood pumps. More than 50 animal experiments have been conducted with the longest thrombus-free operation up to 864 days. The first human clinical study is expected to begin in 2002. The Kriton VAD (Kriton Medical Inc., Miramar, FL) is also a small centrifugal pulsatile pump now in long-term animal studies. The pump's displaced volume is 48 and the pump is capable of pumping 15 L/min in a pulsatile fashion. Since the pump's bearings are magnetically suspended, the pump should last for years with minimal wear.[65] All of these centrifugal pumps share the common advantage of ease of operation and dependability with few moving parts. Within the next few years we will see further advancement of mechanical circulatory support as these next devices come into clinical use.

Long-term mechanical circulatory support has become a tool for the treatment of congestive heart failure. In the years to come, further understanding of heart failure, myocardial recovery, and immunology and further device modifications will lead to improved outcomes and greater utilization of this treatment option. FDA approval of this new technology as treatment for heart failure is a critical step in the future of this field.

REFERENCES

1. DeRose JJ, Argenziano M, Sun BC, et al: Implantable left ventricular assist devices – An evolving long-term cardiac replacement therapy. *Ann Surg* 1997; 226:461.
2. DeBakey ME: The odyssey of the artificial heart. *Artif Organs* 2000; 24:405.
3. Gibbon JH: Application of a mechanical heart and lung apparatus to cardiac surgery. *Minn Med* 1954; 37:171.
4. Spencer FC, Eiseman B, Trinkle JK, et al: Assisted circulation for cardiac failure following intracardiac surgery with cardiorespiratory bypass. *J Thorac Cardiovasc Surg* 1959; 49:56.
5. Frazier OH: Long-term mechanical circulatory support, in Edmunds LH Jr (ed): *Cardiac Surgery in the Adult*. New York, McGraw-Hill, 1995; p 1477.
6. DeVries WC, Anderson JL, Joyce LD, et al: Clinical use of the total artificial heart. *N Engl J Med* 1984; 310:273.
7. Pierce WS: Permanent heart substitution: better solutions lie ahead. *JAMA* 1988; 259:891.
8. Lawrie GM: Permanent implantation of the Jarvik-7 total artificial heart: a clinical perspective. *JAMA* 1988; 259:892.
9. Poirier VL: Heartmate VE LVAS improvements. Oral presentation at the International Society for Heart and Lung Transplantation 3d Fall Education Meeting: Mechanical Cardiac Support and Replacement II, Anaheim, CA, Nov. 9–10, 2001.
10. Frazier OH: First use of an untethered, vented electric left ventricular assist device for long-term support. *Circulation* 1994; 89:2908.
11. DeRose JJ, Umana JP, Argenziano M, et al: Implantable left ventricular assist devices provide an excellent outpatient bridge to transplantation and recovery. *J Am Coll Cardiol* 1997; 30:1773.
12. Sun BC, Catanese KA, Spanier TB, et al: 100 Long-term implantable left ventricular assist devices: the Columbia Presbyterian interim experience. *Ann Thorac Surg* 1999; 68:688.
13. Poirier VL: Worldwide experience with the TCI HeartMate system: issues and future perspective. *Thorac Cardiovasc Surg* 1999; 49(suppl):316.

14. Rose EA, Gelijns AC, Moskowitz AJ, et al: Long-term use of a left ventricular assist device for end-stage heart failure. *N Engl J Med* 2001; 345:1435.
15. McCarthy PM, Smedira NO, Vargo RL, et al: One hundred patients with the HeartMate left ventricular assist device: evolving concepts and technology. *J Thorac Cardiovasc Surg* 1998; 155:904.
16. Deng MC, Loebe M, El-Banayosy A, et al: Mechanical circulatory support for advanced heart failure: effect of patient selection on outcome. *Circulation* 2001; 103:231.
17. Portner PM: Permanent mechanical circulatory assistance, in Baumgartner WA, Reitz B, Kasper E, Theodore J (eds): *Heart and Lung Transplantation,* 2d ed. Philadelphia, WB Saunders, 2002; p 531.
18. Robbins RC, Kown MH, Portner PM, et al: The totally implantable Novacor left ventricular assist system. *Ann Thorac Surg* 2001; 71:S162.
19. Portner P: Novacor LVAS. Oral presentation at the International Society for Heart and Lung Transplantation 3d Fall Education Meeting: Mechanical Cardiac Support and Replacement II, Anaheim, CA, Nov. 9–10, 2001.
20. Farrar DJ: The Thoratec ventricular assist device: a paracorporeal pump for treating acute and chronic heart failure. *Semin Thorac Cardiovasc Surg* 2000; 12:243.
21. El-Banayosy A, Korfer R, Arusoglu L, et al: Bridging to cardiac transplantation with the Thoratec ventricular assist device. *Thorac Cardiovasc Surg* 1999; 47(suppl):307.
22. Olsen DB: The history of continuous-flow blood pumps. *Artif Organs* 2000; 24:401.
23. Noon GP, Morley DL, Irwin S, et al: Clinical experience with the MicroMed DeBakey ventricular assist device. *Ann Thorac Surg* 2001; 71:S133.
24. Wieselthaler GM, Schima H, Hiesmayr M, et al: First clinical experience with the DeBakey VAD continuous-axial-flow pump for bridge to transplantation. *Circulation* 2000; 101:356.
25. Noon GP: MicroMed-DeBakey VAD. Oral presentation at the International Society for Heart and Lung Transplantation 3d Fall Education Meeting: Mechanical Cardiac Support and Replacement II, Anaheim, CA, Nov. 9–10, 2001.
26. Agati S, Bruschi G, Russo C, et al: First successful Italian clinical experience with DeBakey VAD. *J Heart Lung Transplant* 2001; 20:914.
27. Wieselthaler GM, Schima H, Dworschak M, et al: First experience with outpatient care of patients with implanted axial flow pumps. *Artif Organs* 2001; 25:331.
28. Kaplon RJ, Oz MC, Kwiatkowski PA, et al: Miniature axial flow pump for ventricular assistance in children and small adults. *J Thorac Cardiovasc Surg* 1996; 111:13.
29. Frazier OH, Myers TJ, Jarvik RK, et al: Research and development of an implantable, axial-flow left ventricular assist device: the Jarvik 2000 Heart. *Ann Thorac Surg* 2001; 71:S125.
30. Westaby S, Banning AP, Jarvik R, et al: First permanent implant of the Jarvik 2000 Heart. *Lancet* 2000; 356:900.
31. Griffith BP, Kormos RL, Borovetz HS, et al: HeartMate II left ventricular assist system: from concept to first clinical use. *Ann Thorac Surg* 2001; 71:S116.
32. Burke DJ, Burke E, Parsaie F, et al: The HeartMate II: design and development of a fully sealed axial flow left ventricular assist system. *Artif Organs* 2001; 25:380.
33. Mehta SM, Pae WE, Rosenberg G, et al: The LionHeart LVD-2000: a completely implanted left ventricular assist device for chronic circulatory support. *Ann Thorac Surg* 2001; 71:S156.
34. Pae WE: LionHeart LVD. Oral presentation at the International Society for Heart and Lung Transplantation 3d Fall Education Meeting: Mechanical Cardiac Support and Replacement II, Anaheim, CA, Nov. 9–10, 2001.
35. Copeland JG: Mechanical assist device; my choice: the CardioWest total artificial heart. *Transplant Proc* 2000; 32:1523.
36. Copeland JG, Smith RG, Arabia FA, et al: Comparison of the CardioWest total artificial heart, the Novacor left ventricular assist system and the Thoratec ventricular assist system in bridge to transplantation. *Ann Thorac Surg* 2001; 71(suppl):S92-7.
37. Dowling RD, Etoch SW, Stevens KA, et al: Current status of the AbioCor implantable replacement heart. *Ann Thorac Surg* 2001; 71:S147.
38. SoRelle R: First AbioCor trial patient dies. *Circulation* 2001; 104:E9050.
39. Oz MC, Goldstein DJ, Pepino P, et al: Screening scale predicts patients successfully receiving long-term implantable left ventricular assist devices. *Circulation* 1995; 92:169.
40. Rao V, Oz MC, Flannery MA, et al: Revised screening scale to predict survival following left ventricular assist device insertion. *J Thorac Cardiovasc Surg (in press).*
41. Deng MC, Weyand M, Hammel D, et al: Selection and management of ventricular assist device patients: the Muenster experience. *J Heart Lung Transplant* 2000; 19:77.
42. El-Banayosy A, Korfer R, Arusoglu L, et al: Device and patient management in a bridge-to-transplant setting. *Ann Thorac Surg* 2001; 71:S98.
43. El-Banayosy A, Fey O, Sarnowski P, et al: Midterm follow-up of patients discharged from hospital under left ventricular assistance. *J Heart Lung Transplant* 2001; 20:53.
44. Minami K, El-Banayosy A, Sezai A, et al: Morbidity and outcome after mechanical ventricular support using Thoratec, Novacor, and HeartMate for bridging to heart transplantation. *Artif Organs* 2000; 24:421.
45. El Banayosy A, Minami K, Arusoglu L, et al: Long-term mechanical circulatory support. *Thorac Cardiovasc Surg* 1997; 45:127.
46. Oz MC, Argenziano M, Catanese KA, et al: Bridge experience with long-term implantable left ventricular assist devices: are they an alternative to transplantation? *Circulation* 1997; 95:1844.
47. Ankersmit HJ, Tugulea S, Spanier T, et al: Activation-induced T-cell death and immune dysfunction after implantation of left-ventricular assist device. *Lancet* 1999; 354:550.
48. Ankersmit HJ, Edwards NM, Schuster M, et al: Quantitative changes in T-cell populations after left ventricular assist device implantation: relationship to T-cell apoptosis and soluble CD95. *Circulation* 1999; 100(19 suppl):II211.
49. Kavarana MN, Pessin-Minsley MS, Urtecho J, et al: Right ventricular dysfunction and organ failure in left ventricular assist device recipients: a continuing problem. *Ann Thorac Surg* 2002; 73:745.
50. Burkhoff D, Holmes JW, Madigan J, et al: Left ventricular assist device-induced reverse ventricular remodeling. *Prog Cardiovasc Dis* 2000; 43:19.
51. Young JB: Healing the heart with ventricular assist device therapy: mechanisms of cardiac recovery. *Ann Thorac Surg* 2001; 71(suppl 1):S210.
52. Zafeiridis A, Jeevanandam V, Houser SR, et al: Regression of cellular hypertrophy after left ventricular assist device support. *Circulation* 1998; 98:656.
53. Mancini DM, Beniaminovitz A, Levin H, et al: Low incidence of myocardial recovery after left ventricular assist device implantation in patients with chronic heart failure. *Circulation* 1998; 98: 2383.
54. Nakatani T, Sasako Y, Kobayashi J, et al: Recovery of cardiac function by long-term left ventricular support in patients with end-stage cardiomyopathy. *ASAIO J* 1998; 44:M516.
55. Holman WL, Bourge RC, Kirklin JK: Case report: circulatory support for 70 days with resolution of acute heart failure. *J Thorac Cardiovasc Surg* 1991; 102:932.

56. Maybaum S: Strategies to assess recoverability. Oral presentation at the International Society for Heart and Lung Transplantation 3d Fall Education Meeting: Mechanical Cardiac Support and Replacement II, Anaheim, CA, Nov. 9–10, 2001.
57. Yacoub MH: A novel strategy to maximize the efficacy of left ventricular assist devices as a bridge to recovery. *Eur Heart J* 2001; 22:534.
58. Pasque MK: INTREPID trial. Oral presentation at the International Society for Heart and Lung Transplantation 3d Fall Education Meeting: Mechanical Cardiac Support and Replacement II, Nov. 9–10, 2001.
59. Hendry PJ, Mussivand TV, Masters RG, et al: The HeartSaver left ventricular assist device: an update. *Ann Thorac Surg* 2001; 71:S166.
60. Farrar D: Thoratec. Oral presentation at the International Society for Heart and Lung Transplantation 3d Fall Education Meeting: Mechanical Cardiac Support and Replacement II, Anaheim, CA, Nov. 9–10, 2001.
61. Khanwilkar P: Heart Quest System. Oral presentation at the International Society for Heart and Lung Transplantation 3d Fall Education Meeting: Mechanical Cardiac Support and Replacement II, Anaheim, CA, Nov. 9–10, 2001.
62. Woodard J: VentrAssist Pump. Oral presentation at the International Society for Heart and Lung Transplantation 3d Fall Education Meeting: Mechanical Cardiac Support and Replacement II, Anaheim, CA, Nov. 9–10, 2001.
63. Maher TR, Butler KC, Poirier VL, et al: HeartMate left ventricular assist devices: A multigeneration of implanted blood pumps. *Artif Organs* 2001; 25:422.
64. Loree HM, Bourque K, Gernes DB, et al: The HeartMate III: design and in vivo studies of a Maglev centrifugal left ventricular assist device. *Artif Organs* 2001; 25:386.
65. Boyce SW, Crevensten G, Fine RB: An anatomically compatible, wearless, reliable, and nonthrombogenic centrifugal blood pump. *Ann Thorac Surg* 2001; 71(suppl):S190.

Chapter 63

Total Artificial Heart

O. H. Frazier/Nyma A. Shah/Timothy J. Myers

Cardiovascular disease (CVD) is the leading cause of morbidity and mortality in the United States and a significant public health problem in most industrialized nations. Since 1900, CVD has been the leading cause of death in the United States every year except 1918.[1] In 1999, it caused 958,775 American deaths. At the same time, the number of people with CVD, especially its advanced forms, is increasing. There are several reasons for this. First, while there is still no cure for CVD, palliative therapy has improved to the point that more people are surviving past their initial episodes of CVD to live on with some form of the disease. Second, the average age of the U.S. population is rising as the "baby boom" generation ages.

An increasingly prevalent form of advanced CVD is congestive heart failure (CHF). Today, almost 4.8 million Americans (approximately 2.3 million men and 2.4 million women) are living with CHF.[2] Its etiology can be ischemic, idiopathic, or viral. More than $36 billion is spent each year on the care of CHF patients, and many therapeutic advances have been made. Nevertheless, between 1979 and 1999, the incidence of CHF increased by 145%. Each year, CHF directly causes 30,000 to 40,000 deaths and indirectly contributes to another 250,000. Large as the problem is now, its magnitude is expected to worsen as more cardiac patients are able to survive and live longer with their disease and thus increase their chances of developing end-stage CHF.

At present, treatment of advanced CHF takes three forms: medical therapy, surgical therapy, and cardiac replacement.[3] Medical therapy (e.g., intravenous inotropes and vasodilators) relieves symptoms by reducing cardiac load and increasing myocardial contractility. However, while advances in medical therapy have helped improve quality of life for those with heart failure, mortality remains unaffected. Surgical therapy (e.g., aortocoronary bypass, transmyocardial laser revascularization, valve replacement or repair) relieves symptoms of ischemia and valvular dysfunction, but in most cases does not stop the underlying disease process from progressing until death. When conventional medical and surgical therapies for CHF are exhausted, cardiac replacement (i.e., heart transplantation or implantation of an artificial heart) may in some cases become the only therapeutic alternative.

Heart transplantation has evolved into a suitable treatment for advanced CHF. However, it has severe limitations related to patient selection, organ procurement and distribution, and cost-effectiveness. About 2500 patients with end-stage heart failure receive heart transplants each year in the United States. However, about 4000 patients are on the active heart transplant waiting list at any given time, and as many as 40,000 more are potential candidates for heart transplantation.[4,5] Heart transplantation for the relatively young (<40 years old) is not very promising because the life expectancy of a donor heart recipient is about 10 years on average and 20 years at most. In 2001, 458 patients on the active waiting list died while awaiting a donor heart. Heart transplantation is also associated with continuous, lifelong, expensive medical therapy.

To help overcome these limitations, engineers and physicians have continued efforts begun over 4 decades ago to develop systems for providing either temporary or permanent mechanical circulatory support (MCS). Originally, such systems were intended to support patients indefinitely because other forms of heart replacement did not appear to be feasible. Temporary MCS has been shown to be a suitable option for some CHF patients who are awaiting heart transplants[6,7] and for others who are not transplant candidates but need support for indefinite periods of time.[8] In recent clinical studies, myocardial function improved sufficiently in some cases to allow removal of the MCS device and avoid heart transplantation.[9,10] Nevertheless, in light of the shortcomings of medical therapy, surgical therapy, and heart transplantation, efforts have continued to develop a total artificial heart (TAH) that would not only save the lives of critically ill CHF patients but also allow them to resume relatively normal lifestyles. Here, we review the historical development and current status of TAH technology.

EARLY DEVELOPMENT AND EXPERIENCE

In 1812, LeGallois first proposed the idea of supporting a failing heart with either a permanent or temporary device.[11] In the 1930s, Lindbergh and Carrel discussed and planned an artificial heart.[12] Throughout the 1940s, researchers including Dennis and Gibbon were developing a machine that would bypass the circulation of the heart and lungs to allow open heart surgery. The modern era of MCS began in 1951 when Dennis first used a heart-lung machine to sustain the circulation while the heart was opened to repair an atrial septal defect.[13] Two years later, Gibbon repeated this procedure.[14] However, high mortality in the first few cases led both Dennis and Gibbon to abandon the use of their heart-lung machines. In 1954, Lillehei began to use cross-circulation (human-to-human perfusion) as a means to support heart and lung function during congenital heart defect repair.[15] However, because of the controversy engendered by Lillehei's procedure in using human donors and putting two individuals at risk of death, researchers continued efforts to develop a machine that would allow open heart surgery.

By 1955, Kirklin at the Mayo Clinic had refined the Mayo-Gibbon machine and the techniques that allowed open heart surgery.[16] Likewise, DeWall and Lillehei had developed their machine that also allowed for safe open heart operations.[17] By 1960, Kirklin and Lillehei in Minneapolis and DeBakey and Cooley in Houston had perfected their machines and techniques to the point where heart surgery was becoming routine in Minnesota and Texas. The early developmental work on the use of mechanical circulatory systems by Dennis, Lillehei, DeWall, Gibbon, and Kirklin allowed for many new cardiac operations, including coronary artery bypass, heart transplantation, valve repair, and implantation of the total artificial heart. After refinements of the heart-lung machines, Debakey and Cooley began to develop many of the surgical techniques that eventually made open heart surgery routine around the world.

In 1957, Akutsu and Kolff became the first to implant a TAH in vivo.[18] Inserted into the chest of a dog, the pump adequately maintained the circulation for approximately 90 minutes. However, Akutsu and Kolff never applied their TAH technology clinically. In 1964, the National Heart Institute established the Artificial Heart Program to promote the development of the TAH and other cardiac assist devices. In the early 1960s, DeBakey and researchers at Baylor College of Medicine in Houston began developing a TAH. In 1963, DeBakey implanted the first clinical left ventricular assist device (LVAD) into a 42-year-old patient.[19] The pump functioned well, but the patient died of pulmonary complications after 4 days of support. In 1967, DeBakey implanted an LVAD into a 37-year-old who presented with symptoms of CHF including easy fatigability and severe dyspnea on slight exertion. This patient also had history of rheumatic heart disease since age 18 and closed mitral valvulotomy at age 25. The intention was to use the LVAD until sufficient myocardial recovery could be gained. The LVAD supported the patient's circulation for 10 days and was then electively removed. The patient was discharged from the hospital on postoperative day 29 and later resumed normal activity. On follow-up at 18 months after LVAD removal, the patient remained free of CHF symptoms, and a chest x-ray showed a significant reduction in cardiac size.

FIRST TOTAL ARTIFICIAL HEART

The first implantation of a TAH into a human was done by Cooley on April 4, 1969, in a 47-year-old man who could not be weaned from cardiopulmonary bypass (CPB) following left ventricular aneurysmectomy.[20] The intent was to support the patient until a donor heart could be found. The TAH (Fig. 63-1), designed by Liotta, was a pneumatically powered, double-chambered pump with Dacron-lined right and left inflow cuffs and outflow grafts. Wada-Cutter hingeless valves controlled the direction of blood flow through the pump. The TAH itself was connected to a large external power unit, which unfortunately severely restricted patient mobility. The TAH performed adequately for 64 hours until transplantation. The donor heart also functioned well, but the patient died of pseudomonal pneumonia 32 hours after transplantation. Though the Liotta device performed as designed, it was never used clinically again. Nevertheless, this case clearly demonstrated that a TAH could be safely and effectively used in a human as a bridge to transplantation.

AKUTSU-III TOTAL ARTIFICIAL HEART

The second implantation of a TAH in a human was also done by Cooley. On July 23, 1981, Cooley implanted the Akutsu-III TAH into a critically ill 26-year-old man who suffered heart failure after undergoing coronary artery bypass surgery for severe arteriosclerosis. Unable to be weaned from CPB after surgery, the patient was fitted with the TAH in a final effort to sustain his life. The Akutsu-III TAH (Fig. 63-2) consisted of two pneumatically powered, double-chambered pumps featuring reciprocating hemispherical diaphragms.[21] CPB was discontinued 90 minutes after implantation. The

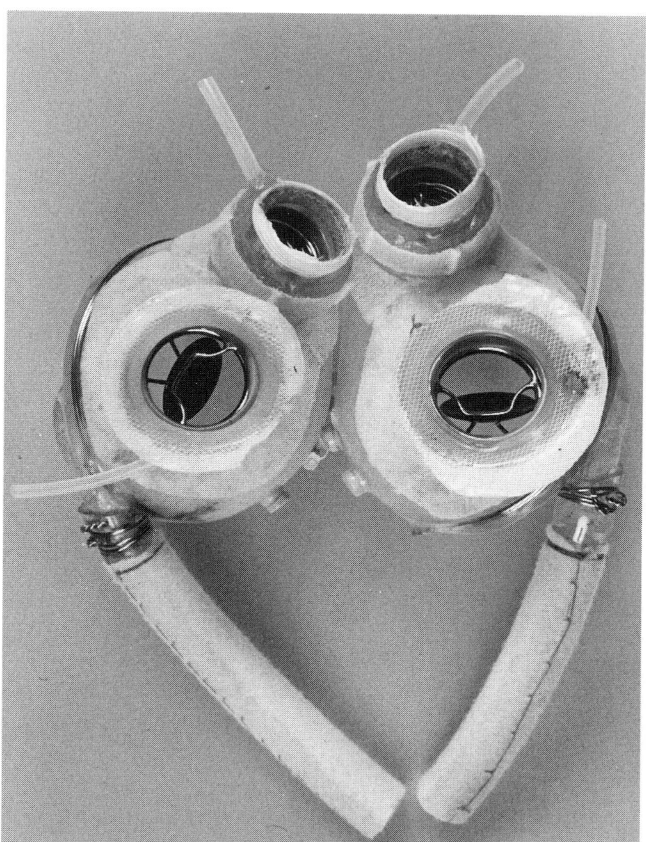

FIGURE 63–1 The Liotta total artificial heart, the first TAH implanted in a human.

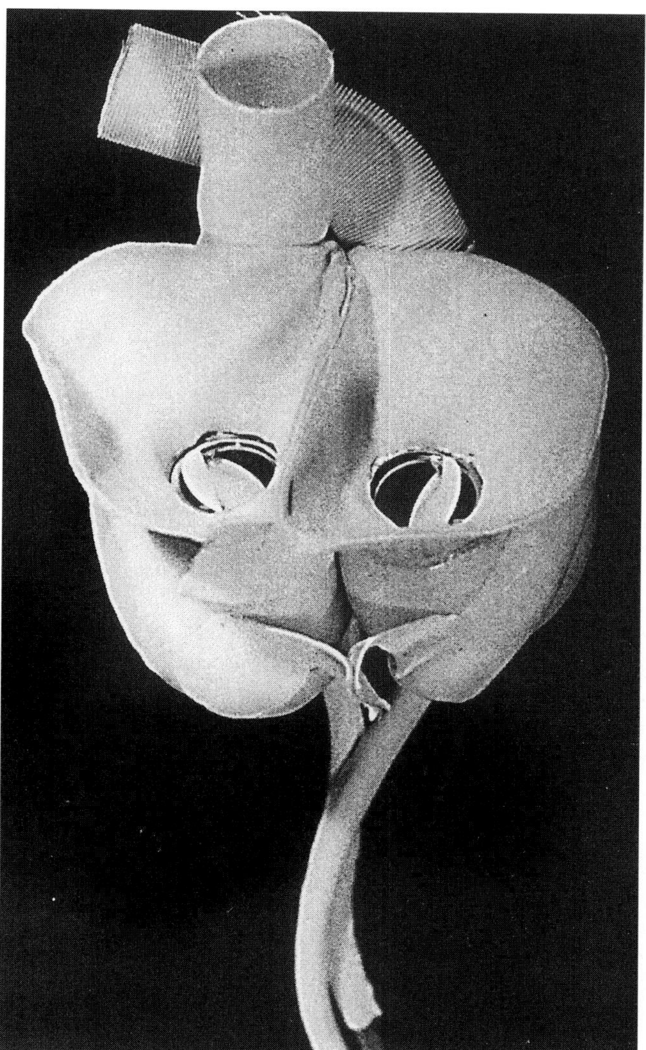

FIGURE 63–2 The Akutsu-III total artificial heart, the second TAH implanted in a human.

TAH provided excellent hemodynamics and supported the patient in stable condition for a total of 55 hours until a suitable donor heart was found. The patient finally received a transplant but died of infectious, renal, and pulmonary complications 10 days later. Despite the fatal outcome, this case demonstrated that the TAH could adequately sustain a patient for several days, with no evidence of hemolysis or thromboembolism, until heart transplantation.

JARVIK-7 TOTAL ARTIFICIAL HEART

In the late 1970s, Kolff and his team at the University of Utah developed the Jarvik-7 TAH. In 1982, DeVries became the first to permanently implant a TAH when he implanted a Jarvik-7 into a dying patient.[22] The Jarvik-7 TAH (Fig. 63-3) was a pneumatically powered, biventricular pulsatile device that replaced the heart.[23,24] The pumps were connected to their respective native atria by synthetic cuffs and connectors. Each pump had chambers for air and blood separated by a smooth flexible polyurethane diaphragm. The inflow and outflow conduits contained Medtronic-Hall tilting disk valves. The filling of the pumps was aided by vacuum. Pneumatic drivelines, brought out through the chest wall to connect with an external console, shuttled air to the pumps during systole, thereby causing collapse of the pump sac and blood ejection. Pump rate, drive pressure, and systolic duration were monitored and optimized from the external console. The Jarvik-7 had a stroke volume of 70 mL and a normal cardiac output of 6 to 8 L/min (maximum, 15 L/min).

In the initial clinical experience with the Jarvik-7 TAH, a total of 5 patients were permanently supported for periods ranging from 10 days to 620 days. The TAH was able to adequately support circulation, but its large drive console and frequent medical complications limited patient activity. Four patients were able to make brief trips out of the hospital and to see family and friends. Long-term outcomes, however, were poor. Patients supported by the Jarvik-7 for longer periods suffered several complications, including thromboembolism, stroke, infection, and multiorgan failure.

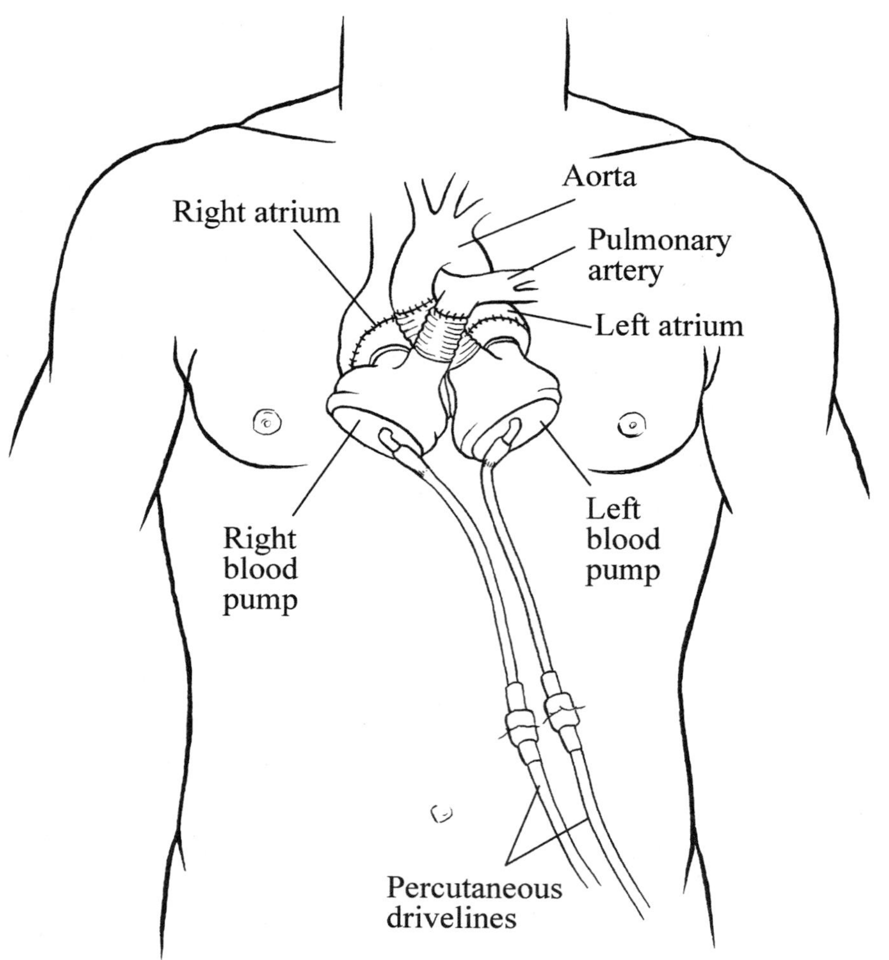

FIGURE 63–3 The CardioWest total artificial heart (CardioWest Technologies Inc., Tucson, AZ), formerly the Jarvik-7 and Symbion TAH.

Despite these mixed results, in 1985 the Jarvik-7 (renamed the Symbion) TAH entered clinical trials as a bridge to transplantation. In 1986, Copeland reported the first successful use of this device for this indication.[25] Between 1985 and 1991, approximately 170 patients were supported with the Symbion TAH as a bridge to transplantation.[26] Sixty-six percent underwent successful heart transplantation, a rate similar to those in bridge-to-transplantation studies of left ventricular assist devices. Sepsis and multiorgan failure were the primary causes of death during TAH support.

Although the bridge-to-transplantation study demonstrated that the Jarvik-7 (Symbion) TAH was clinically effective, the U.S. Food and Drug Administration withdrew the device's investigational device exemption (IDE) for clinical use in January 1991 because of inadequate compliance with FDA regulations.[27] In January 1993, the IDE was restored to what was now called the CardioWest TAH, which differed little from the original Jarvik-7. The CardioWest TAH has since been used successfully in the United States, Canada, and France. Worldwide, 63% of CardioWest-supported patients eventually undergo successful heart transplantation and 92% of those are eventually discharged to home. In the United States, the rates are even better (93% and 96%, respectively).

ABIOCOR TOTAL ARTIFICIAL HEART

On July 2, 2001, as part of an FDA-sponsored clinical trial, surgeons at Jewish Hospital in Louisville, Kentucky, performed the first implantation of the AbioCor TAH in a 59-year-old man suffering from end-stage CHF.[28] The AbioCor totally implantable replacement heart is a self-contained electrohydraulic TAH (Fig. 63-4) that has been developed and tested by ABIOMED, Inc. (Danvers, MA) and the Texas Heart Institute, with the support of the National Heart, Lung, and Blood Institute (NHLBI).[29,30] It is designed to sustain the circulation and extend the lives of patients with end-stage heart failure who have suffered irreversible left and right ventricular failure, for whom surgery or medical therapy is inadequate, and who would otherwise soon die (Table 63-1). The AbioCor is the first TAH to be used

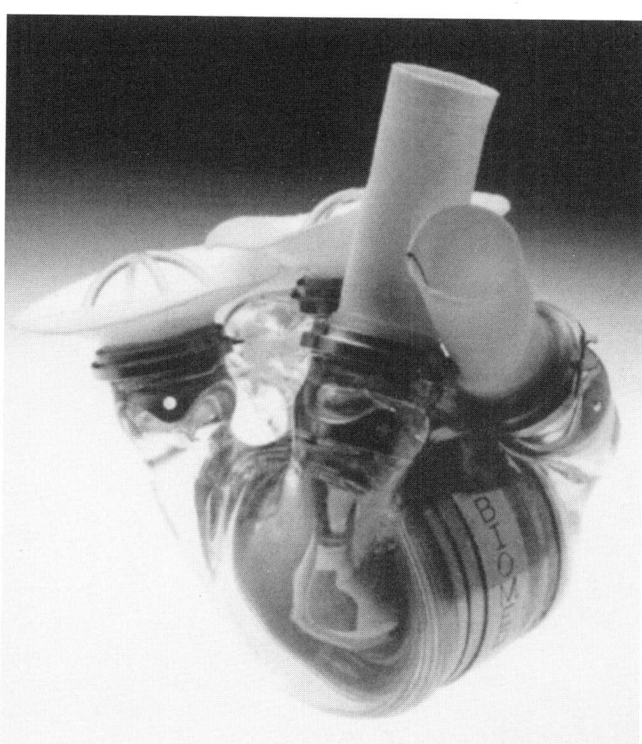

FIGURE 63–4 The AbioCor total artifical heart (ABIOMED, Inc., Danvers, MA).

clinically that is fully implantable and communicates to external hardware without penetrating the skin. The device utilizes a transcutaneous energy transfer (TET) system and a radiofrequency communication (RF Comm) system that allows it to be powered and controlled by signals transmitted across intact skin. A unique feature of the AbioCor is a right-left flow balancing mechanism that eliminates the need for an external vent or internal compliance chamber.[31]

The internal components of the AbioCor system consist of a thoracic unit, internal TET coil, controller, and battery.[32] The thoracic unit (pump) weighs about 2 pounds and consists of 2 artificial ventricles, 4 valves, and an innovative motor-driven hydraulic pumping system (Fig. 63-5). The pump's motor rotates at 6000 to 8000 rpm, which allows sufficient hydraulic fluid pressure to compress the diaphragm around the blood chamber and eject blood. A miniaturized electronics package implanted in the patient's abdomen monitors and controls the pump rate, right-left balance, and motor speed. An internal rechargeable battery, also implanted within the abdomen, provides emergency or backup power. The internal battery is continually recharged via the TET system and can provide up to 30 minutes of tether-free operation.

The AbioCor's external components include a computer console, an external TET coil, and external battery packs. The external computer communicates via the RF Comm system with the abdominally implanted controller, which controls the pump. The external TET coil provides power to the pump from the console or from the external battery packs. The external battery packs can power the AbioCor TAH for 2 to 4 hours.

Since its first implantation, the AbioCor has been implanted 6 more times at several institutions (Table 63-2). As of this writing, 1 patients continues to be supported at 474 days. Four of the 6 patients survived beyond the 60-day study end point, which is twice their predicted life expectancy. Four patients became ambulatory and were able to leave the hospital for short periods. Quality of life improved in 4 patients.

TABLE 63–1 Inclusion/exclusion criteria for FDA-sponsored clinical trial of AbioCor total artificial heart

Criteria
Inclusion criteria
End-stage heart failure
>70% probability of death within 30 days
Ineligibility for a heart transplant
No other surgical or medical treatment options
Biventricular failure
Exclusion criteria
Significant potential for reversibility of heart failure
Chronic dialysis
Recent cerebrovascular accident (CVA)
Irreversible liver failure
Blood dyscrasia

COMPLICATIONS

Use of a TAH is associated with serious complications. The most frequent complications are infection, severe postoperative bleeding, and thromboembolism.[33–36] Potentially serious but less frequent complications are renal, hepatic, pulmonary, and neurologic dysfunction, and complications due to technical problems.[33,37] Complicating factors include patient selection, device size, implantation timing and location, the need for extensive surgery at implantation, and the reliability of support equipment.

Life-threatening infections have been the most important complication for patients being supported permanently by a TAH.[38] In the Jarvik-7 experience, all patients supported for many months developed serious infections that eventually contributed to their deaths.[22,39] Patients supported by a TAH for shorter periods while awaiting heart transplantation had infection rates of 30% to 40%.[34–38] During the 1980s, driveline and mediastinal infections in TAH-supported patients were frequent and severe, regardless of the duration of support. However, in the more recent bridge-to-transplantation experience with the CardioWest TAH, the infection rate was no more than 20%.[40,41]

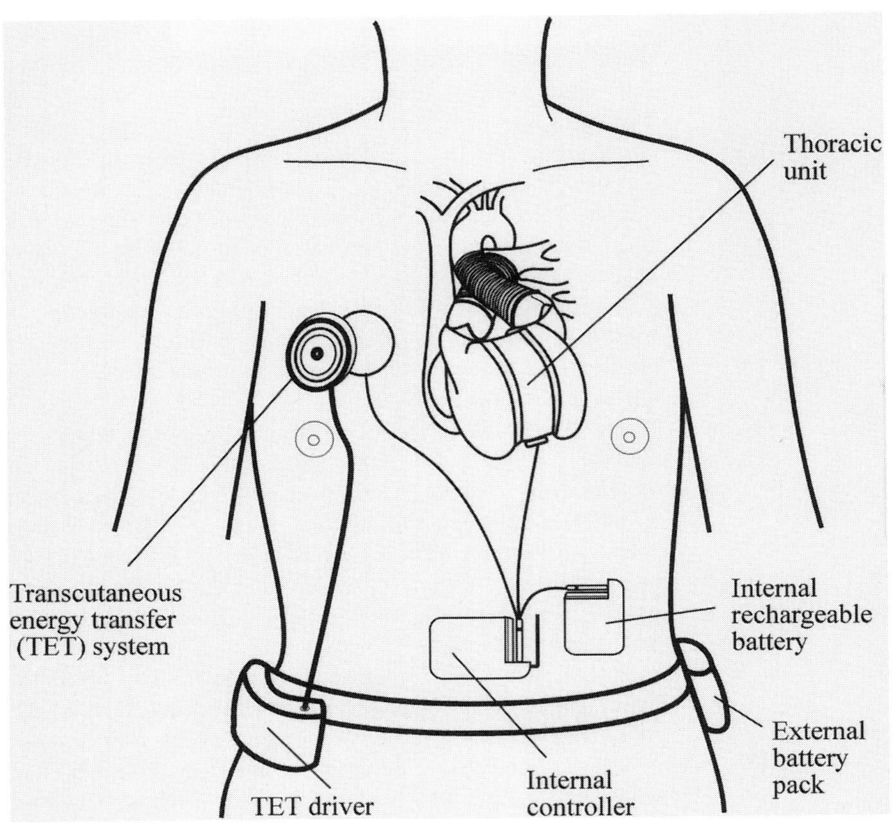

FIGURE 63–5 The AbioCor system is designed to increase or decrease its pump rate in response to the body's needs. The AbioCor also includes an active monitoring system that provides detailed performance feedback and alarms in the event of irregularities.

Patients supported with a TAH, regardless of the intended use, are very susceptible to infection. Predisposing factors include the tissue trauma of the surgery; contamination of the implanted device; depressed immune defenses; a large foreign material surface area; and use of the drivelines, tubes, catheters, and other devices that are necessary for the care of these patients. Infections can occur at any point during TAH support. Once an internal component of the TAH system is infectiously colonized, treatment is difficult and often ineffective. Infections are more likely to occur in the early postoperative period, especially in the most critically ill patients, due to device contamination during the course of their care and to postoperative bleeding resulting from intensive care procedures and exposure during reoperation. Meticulous care and numerous infection prevention measures are vital in all TAH patients.

Postoperative bleeding is a frequent and serious complication of TAH implantation. It generally occurs in 40% to 50% of TAH or ventricular assist device recipients.[33] In the more recent CardioWest experience, the rate was approximately 25%. Contributing factors include severe CHF and associated hepatic dysfunction, the extensive surgery and lengthy CPB time required for implantation, and the necessity for postoperative anticoagulation therapy. Severe CHF often leads to hepatic dysfunction and subsequent derangement of the coagulation system. Patients with severe CHF are often receiving continuous preoperative anticoagulant or antiplatelet therapy, the effects of which are often difficult to reverse before TAH implantation. The extensive surgery and lengthy CPB time required for implantation can lead to severe depletion of clotting factors. The necessity for postoperative anticoagulation therapy requires that a proper balance be established between preventing thrombosis and allowing blood to clot, through the careful management of hemostasis and anticoagulant therapy.

Thrombosis within the TAH is of particular concern. Five of the first 6 Jarvik-7 recipients suffered thromboembolic events. However, the frequency of thromboembolism has decreased significantly since that initial experience and is now an estimated 10% to 15%.[33,34,42] Preventive measures are primarily targeted at precisely monitoring the thrombotic and fibrinolytic systems, maintaining sufficient flow through the device to avoid stasis, and providing adequate anticoagulation and antiplatelet therapy. Generally, heparin and warfarin are used as antithrombotic therapy to achieve a prothrombin time, activated thromboplastin time, or international normalized ratio 2 to 3 times greater than the baseline or normal value. Aspirin or dipyridamole or both are also used.

There is a complex though poorly understood interrelationship between infection, bleeding, and thromboembolism. Thrombus formation may lead to the development of infection, and bacterial colonization may lead to thrombus formation. Bacteria are often seen in thrombi found in

TABLE 63–2 Summary of initial clinical experience with AbioCor total artificial heart*

Patient	Implantation date	No. days supported	Age (y)	Institution/city	Outcome
1	July 2, 2001	151	59	Jewish Hospital, Louisville, KY	Died
2	September 13, 2001	474	70	Jewish Hospital, Louisville, KY	Alive
3	September 26, 2001	142	68	THI/St. Luke's Episcopal Hospital, Houston, TX	Died
4	October 17, 2001	56	74	UCLA, Los Angeles, CA	Died
5	November 5, 2001	294	51	MCP Hahnemann University Hospital, Philadelphia, PA	Died
6	November 27, 2001	1	79	THI/St. Luke's Episcopal Hospital, Houston, TX	Died
7	April 9, 2002	1	61	Jewish Hospital, Louisville, KY	Died

*As of December 31, 2002.

cardiovascular devices.[43] Bacteria embedded in a thrombus are protected from circulating antibiotics and leukocytes. Bacteria, endotoxins, and inflammatory cells may contribute to thrombus formation by their effect on platelet aggregation.[44] Bacterial endotoxins can cause platelet aggregation, endothelial injury, and increased endothelial thromboplastin activity. Excessive bleeding most often results in reoperation, which increases the patient's exposure to contamination. Also, blood transfusions and intravascular monitoring for these critically ill patients are more extensive and result in frequent exposure to the external environment. Infection, bleeding, and thromboembolism can contribute individually and collectively to the development of multiorgan failure, one of the most frequent causes of death in TAH recipients.

Other important problems and issues related to TAH implantation are device malfunction, poor fit or size mismatch between TAH and patient, social and ethical issues, mobility, and nutrition. Device malfunction leading to catastrophic failure of the TAH or ventricular assist device is rare. Most technical issues have involved external components and have been readily resolved. Fit and size mismatch remain a problem. All TAH models used to date have been relatively large and only fit adequately into patients with a body surface area greater than 1.7 m^2. Because the cost of TAH technology is fairly high and most candidates for TAH implantation are in their sixth to seventh decade of life, many question whether society should bear the cost of developing this technology. Until recently, the external components of the TAH equipment have been large and cumbersome, thus limiting patient mobility, exercise, and rehabilitation. More recent designs of the TAH allow for much more mobility.

COMMENT

Since the 1950s, when the heart-lung bypass machine was developed, many advances have been made in the surgical treatment of CVD. Many surgical procedures considered impossible just 40 years ago are today considered routine. A classic example is heart transplantation. However, TAH technology has not evolved at the same pace. Though the first human heart transplantation and first human TAH implantation occurred within 2 years of each other, TAH implantation is still neither routine nor widely available. However, two TAHs are undergoing clinical trials at present in the United States. The CardioWest (formerly the Jarvik-7) TAH is more widely used but still has not yet received FDA market approval, though it may be approved for use as a bridge to transplantation in the near future. The AbioCor TAH is still in the early stages of its FDA-sponsored feasibility study and is likely years away from approval as an alternative to heart transplantation. However, should its unique TET system and flow-balancing mechanism prove to be reliable for extended periods of time, the AbioCor may become a widely used alternative to heart transplantation for those patients who have no other treatment options.

There are many obstacles to overcome before any TAH is widely accepted. Infection, bleeding, thromboembolism, and biocompatibility issues are serious problems that affect nearly all implantable cardiovascular devices including TAHs. Improved biomaterials, better prevention, and more effective antibiotic and anticoagulant medications may help overcome these problems. Acceptance by the public, by some critics in the health professions, and by third-party payers may be slow. Quality in manufacturing is needed to ensure reliability of TAH components. Addressing these problems will help bring the TAH more quickly into routine clinical use.

REFERENCES

1. American Heart Association: *2002 Heart and Stroke Statistical Update*. Available at http://www.americanheart.org. Accessed April 2002.
2. Congestive heart failure in the United States: a new epidemic [data fact sheet]. Bethesda (MD), National Heart Lung and Blood Institute, National Institutes of Health, September 1996.
3. Frazier OH, Myers TJ: Surgical therapy for severe heart failure [review]. *Curr Probl Cardiol* 1998; 23:721.
4. United Network for Organ Sharing: *Critical Data: U.S. Facts about Transplantation*. Available at http://www.unos.org. Accessed April 2002.
5. Kottke TE, Pesch DG, Frye RL: The potential contribution of cardiac replacement to the control of cardiovascular disease: a population-based estimate. *Arch Surg* 1990; 125:1148.
6. Frazier OH, Rose EA, McCarthy PM, et al: Improved mortality and rehabilitation of transplant candidates treated with a long-term implantable left ventricular assist system. *Ann Surg* 1995; 222:327.
7. Frazier OH, Rose EA, Oz MC, et al: Multicenter clinical evaluation of the HeartMate vented electric left ventricular assist system in patients awaiting heart transplantation. *J Thorac Cardiovasc Surg* 2001; 122:1186.
8. Rose EA, Gelijns AC, Moskowitz AJ, et al: Long-term mechanical left ventricular assistance for end-stage heart failure. *N Engl J Med* 2001; 345:1435.
9. Mueller J, Weng Y, Dandel M: Long-term results of weaning from LVAD: it does work. *ASAIO J* 1999; 45:153.
10. Frazier OH, Myers TJ: Left ventricular assist system as a bridge to myocardial recovery. *Ann Thorac Surg* 1999; 68(2 suppl):734.
11. LeGallois CJJ: *Experience on the Principle of Life*. Philadelphia, Thomas, 1813. Translation of LeGallois CJJ, *Experience sur la principe de la vie*. Paris, 1812.
12. Miller GW: *King of Hearts: The True Story of the Maverick Who Pioneered Open Heart Surgery*. New York, Random House, 2000; p 12.
13. Dennis C: A heart-lung machine for open-heart operations: how it came about. *Trans Am Soc Artif Intern Organs* 1989; 35:767.
14. Gibbon JH: Application of a heart and lung apparatus to cardiac surgery. *Minn Med* 1954; 37:171.
15. Lillehei CW, Cohen M, Warden HE, Varco RL: The direct-vision intracardiac correction of congenital anomalies by controlled cross circulation. *Surgery* 1955; 38:11.
16. Kirklin JW, DuShane JW, Patrick RT, et al: Intracardiac surgery with the aid of a mechanical pump-oxygenator system (Gibbon type): report of eight cases. *Mayo Clin Proc* 1955; 30:201.
17. Lillehei CW, DeWall RA, Read R, et al: Direct-vision intracardiac surgery in man using a simple, disposable artificial oxygenator. *Dis Chest* 1956; 29:1.
18. Akutsu T, Kolff WJ: Permanent substitute for valves and hearts. *Trans Am Soc Artif Intern Organs* 1958; 4:230.
19. DeBakey ME: Left ventricular bypass for cardiac assistance: clinical experience. *Am J Cardiol* 1971; 27:3.
20. Cooley DA, Liotta D, Hallman GL, et al: Orthotopic cardiac prosthesis for two-staged cardiac replacement. *Am J Cardiol* 1969; 24:723.
21. Frazier OH, Akutsu T, Cooley DA: Total artificial heart (TAH) utilization in man. *Trans Am Soc Artif Intern Organs* 1982; 23:534.
22. DeVries WC: The permanent artificial heart: four case reports. *JAMA* 1988; 259:849.
23. DeVries WC, Anderson JL, Joyce LD, et al: Clinical use of the total artificial heart. *N Engl J Med* 1984; 310:273.
24. DeVries WC: Surgical technique for implantation of the Jarvik-7-100 total artificial heart. *JAMA* 1988; 259:875.
25. Copeland CG, Smith RG, Icenogle TB, Ott RA: Early experience with the total artificial heart as a bridge to cardiac transplantation. *Surg Clin North Am* 1988; 68:621.
26. Johnson KE, Prieto M, Joyce LD, et al: Summary of the clinical use of the Symbion total artificial heart: a registry report. *Ann Surg* 1995; 222:327.
27. Copeland JG: Current status and future directions for a total artificial heart with a past. *Artif Organs* 1998; 22:998.
28. SoRelle R: Cardiovascular news: totally contained AbioCor artificial heart implanted July 3, 2001. *Circulation* 2001; 104:E9005.
29. Kung RTV, Yu LS, Ochs BD, et al: Progress in the development of the ABIOMED total artificial heart. *ASAIO J* 1995; 41:M245.
30. Parnis SM, Yu LS, Ochs BD, et al: Chronic in vivo evaluation of an electrohydraulic total artificial heart. *ASAIO J* 1994; 40:M489. .
31. Kung RTV, Yu LS, Ochs BD, et al: An artificial hydraulic shunt in a total artificial heart: a balance mechanism for the bronchial shunt. *ASAIO J* 1993; 39:M213.
32. Yu LS, Finnegan M, Vaughan S, et al: A compact and noise-free electrohydraulic total artificial heart. *ASAIO J* 1993; 39:M386.
33. Quaini E, Pavie A, Chieco S, Mambrito B: The Concerted Action "Heart" European registry on clinical application of mechanical circulatory support systems: bridge to transplant. The Registry Scientific Committee. *Eur J Cardiothorac Surg* 1997; 11:182.
34. Mehta SM, Aufiero TX, Pae WE Jr, et al: Combined Registry For The Clinical Use Of Mechanical Ventricular Assist Pumps and the Total Artificial Heart in Conjunction with Heart Transplantation: Sixth Official Report—1994. *J Heart Lung Transplant* 1995; 14:585.
35. Myers TJ, Khan T, Frazier OH: Infectious complications associated with ventricular assist systems. *ASAIO J* 2000; 46:S28.
36. Conger JL, Inman RW, Tamez D, et al: Infection and thrombosis in total artificial heart technology: past and future challenges—a historical review. *ASAIO J* 2000; 46:S22.
37. Arabia FA, Copeland JG, Smith RG, et al: International experience with the CardioWest total artificial heart as a bridge to heart transplantation. *Eur J Cardiothorac Surg* 1997; 11(suppl):S5.
38. Gristina AG, Dobbins JJ, Giammara B, et al: Biomaterial-centered sepsis and the total artificial heart: microbial adhesion versus tissue integration. *JAMA* 1988; 259:870.
39. Joyce LD, DeVries WC, Hastings WL, et al: Response of the human body to the first permanent implant of the Jarvik-7 total artificial heart. *Trans Am Soc Artif Intern Organs* 1983; 29:81.
40. Copeland JG, Pavie A, Duveau D, et al: Bridge to transplantation with the CardioWest total artificial heart: the international experience 1993 to 1995. *J Heart Lung Transplant* 1995; 15:94.
41. Copeland JG 3rd, Smith RG, Arabia FA, et al: Comparison of the CardioWest total artificial heart, the Novacor left ventricular assist system, and the Thoratec ventricular assist system in bridge to transplantation. *Ann Thorac Surg* 2001; 71(3 suppl):S92.
42. Copeland JG, Smith RG, Arabia FA, et al: The CardioWest total artificial heart as a bridge to transplantation. *Semin Thorac Cardiovasc Surg* 2000; 12:238.
43. Chiang BY, Burns GL, Pantalos GM, et al: Microbially infected thrombus in animals with total artificial hearts. *Trans Am Soc Artif Intern Organs* 1991; 37:M256.
44. Didisheim P, Olsen DB, Farrar DJ, et al: Infections and thromboembolism with implantable cardiovascular devices. *Trans Am Soc Artif Intern Organs* 1989; 35:54.

Chapter 64

Nontransplant Surgical Options for Heart Failure

Vinay Badhwar/Steven F. Bolling

Congestive heart failure (CHF) has become a major worldwide public health problem. In our ever-aging population, medical advances that have extended our average life expectancy have also left more people living with chronic cardiac disease than ever before. In the United States alone, there are nearly 4.9 million suffering with heart failure; yet of the 500,000 new patients diagnosed each year, less than 3000 are offered transplantation due to limitations of age, comorbid conditions, and donor availability. Despite the significant improvements with medical management, CHF patients are repeatedly readmitted for inpatient care and the vast majority will die within 3 years of diagnosis.[1]

The successful and reproducible long-term results with orthotopic heart transplantation (OHT) have made it the treatment of choice for patients with medically refractory end-stage heart failure.[2] Unfortunately, the obvious limitations to OHT include the need for immunosuppression and the severe shortage of donor organs. This past decade has seen the annual number of transplants performed worldwide plateau at less than 4000.[3] This lack of donor availability has thus necessitated a rigorous selection criteria be applied to potential recipients in order to optimize the utility of these precious organs, indicated only for patients with end-stage cardiomyopathy in whom all other modes of therapy have been exhausted. Access to OHT has thus been restricted to those without comorbid medical conditions and relatively restricted to those younger than age 65. This leaves the vast majority of CHF patients seeking other options.

Despite the technologic strides being made towards total implantability, the role for mechanical support presently remains primarily as a bridge to transplantation or for temporary support. Though there have been a number of clearly successful cases of ventricular assist device (VAD) use as a bridge to recovery, its long-term efficacy for this purpose or its use as a long-term therapy for chronic heart failure remains to be fully evaluated by multicenter clinical trials.[4–9] Though assist device technology may be on the verge of being implemented as a destination therapy for CHF, its current primary indication as a bridge to transplantation results in the restriction of its use to patients fulfilling candidacy for OHT. These confines, and the high cost associated with these devices, have yet to make the VAD an unrestricted surgical solution for the management of most CHF patients.

This clinical dilemma has provided the impetus for surgeons to develop new alternatives for the treatment of heart failure. As OHT and VAD use is more stringently applied, techniques to restore myocardial perfusion, eliminate valvular regurgitation, and restore ventricular geometry have emerged as the first-line surgical approach to heart failure. In response to the growing need for the proficient application and critical appraisal of the expanding menu of surgical options, the new subspecialty of heart failure surgery has emerged. The following will briefly review established nontransplant surgical modalities for heart failure such as coronary revascularization, geometric mitral reconstruction, and geometric ventricular reconstruction. Alternative options such as partial left ventriculectomy and cardiomyoplasty as well as some innovative devices currently being evaluated for clinical application will also be discussed.

CORONARY REVASCULARIZATION

We have known for nearly 20 years that revascularizing patients with left ventricular dysfunction can result in upwards of a 25% improvement in long-term survival.[10,11] Early enthusiasm was tempered by reports of high operative mortality in patients with a low ejection fraction (EF). Since then, as success with the medical and surgical management of heart failure and transplantation grew, so did the interest in applying this experience to patients with ischemic cardiomyopathy. Successful revascularization can now be performed on patients with an EF less than 30% with hospital mortalities as low as 5%.[12–14]

The premise behind the improvements in EF, long-term survival, and quality of life of these patients following coronary artery bypass grafting (CABG) is believed to be due to postoperative myocyte recruitment. Restoration of perfusion resuscitates dormant viable myocardium and serves to protect the previously functioning portions of the ventricle from further ischemic insults, arrhythmias, and infarction.

In order to minimize morbidity, a multidisciplinary approach to the preoperative management of heart failure is essential. Patients ideally suited for CABG are those who are medically optimized, with or without angina, who have good distal coronary targets, functional hibernating myocardium identified preoperatively, and no evidence of right ventricular dysfunction.[15] As experience in managing these patients increases, many surgeons have operated on patients with ejection fractions less than 10%, those requiring reoperation, and those with moderate elevations in pulmonary artery pressure. Nevertheless, patients with clear documentation of poor right ventricular EF, clinical right-sided congestive symptoms, or fixed pulmonary hypertension above 60 mm Hg systolic should be approached cautiously, because these patients may in fact be better suited for transplantation.

The process of preoperative investigation should coincide with optimizing the patient's medical management. This should entail an aggressive regimen of diuretic and vasodilator therapy to minimize ventricular afterload and normalize the patient's circulating volume. For patients with severe heart failure, a brief period of inotropic therapy for ventricular resuscitation may be necessary to optimize their medical management. Inability to be weaned from this support is often indicative of severe myocardial injury and poor overall prognosis with any surgical therapy other than mechanical ventricular assistance or transplantation.

Preoperative investigations should begin with transthoracic echocardiography to grossly evaluate ventricular function and identify any underlying valvular pathology. Baseline screening physiological studies of oxygen consumption, pulmonary function, and cardiopulmonary endurance are recommended. Identification of reversible ischemia by means of a nuclear study can be helpful; however, for patients with angina, many centers will proceed directly to coronary angiography. Though angina may be indicative of living ventricular muscle, perhaps the most important correlate of successful surgical recovery is the quantification of myocardial viability. Not only is a determination of myocardial contractile reserve essential to ensure that the patient can be safely separated from cardiopulmonary bypass (CPB), but this information is predictive of ventricular recovery and long-term survival after operation. Though thallium-201 perfusion scans may distinguish myocytes with membrane integrity from scar, PET scanning and dobutamine stress echocardiography permit the preoperative identification of myocardial viability and the prediction of postoperative function.[16–18]

The fundamental premise behind a successful operation is to attain an expeditiously performed and yet complete revascularization. As the failing myocardium is particularly intolerant to further episodes of ischemia, careful consideration should be given to the quality of the distal vessels and the ease with which good anastomoses can be achieved. Operative time expended grafting small or extensively diseased vessels, or performing additional techniques such as endarterectomy, may be counterproductive. Since the price to pay for incomplete revascularization or transient ischemia may be severe, off-pump techniques may not be ideally suited for these patients unless performed flawlessly.

Multiple groups have been uniformly successful in demonstrating improvements in survival, ventricular function, and functional status with coronary revascularization in patients with ischemic cardiomyopathy with ejection fractions less than 25%.[19–21] The 5-year survival with transplantation ranges from 62% to 82%, whereas with medical therapy alone, it is less than 20%. Most series report survival following CABG for ischemic cardiomyopathy ranging from 85% to 88% at 1 year, 75% to 82% at 2 years, 68% to 80% at 3 years, and 60% to 80% at 5 years. Operative mortality has been reported from 3% to 12%, with the main predictor of increased risk being urgency of operation. When compared to medical therapy, revascularized patients have significant improvements in quality of life. Most series consistently report considerable enhancements in patient mobility, peak oxygen consumption, and functional status. The average preoperative NYHA class of 3.5 reportedly drops to 1.5 after revascularization. Postoperatively, there are substantial reductions in readmissions for CHF and many patients return to work.

It is encouraging to note that the long-term survival of CHF patients following CABG is equivalent to transplantation in many series. The superior survival of CABG over transplant in the first 2 years postoperatively may be due to early attrition from rejection or infection in the latter group. Although there has been little reported on patients with ejection fractions under 10%, from the above data, one could infer that these patients would have a similarly better outcome than their nonrevascularized counterparts. As experience with heart failure surgery expands, refinements in preoperative and operative management of CABG patients will no doubt be reflected in the uniformity of future long-term results.

GEOMETRIC MITRAL RECONSTRUCTION

Functional mitral regurgitation (MR) is a significant complication of end-stage cardiomyopathy and it may affect almost all heart failure patients as a preterminal or terminal event. Its presence in these patients is associated with progressive ventricular dilatation, an escalation of CHF symptomatology, and significant reductions in long-term survival estimated between only 6 and 24 months.[22]

A firm understanding of the functional anatomy of the mitral valve is fundamental to the management of MR in heart failure. The mitral valve apparatus consists of the annulus, leaflets, chordae tendineae, and papillary muscles as well as the entire LV. Thus the maintenance of chordal, annular, and subvalvular continuity is essential for the preservation of mitral geometric relationships and overall ventricular function. As the ventricle fails, the progressive dilatation of the LV gives rise to MR, which begets more MR and further ventricular dilatation (Fig. 64-1). With postinfarction remodeling and lateral wall dysfunction, similar processes combine to result in ischemic mitral regurgitation (Fig. 64-2). Left uncorrected, the end result of progressive MR and global ventricular remodeling is similar regardless of the etiology of cardiomyopathy. Incomplete leaflet coaptation, loss of the zone of coaptation, and regurgitation develop secondary to alterations in the annular-ventricular apparatus and ventricular geometry.[23,24] Thus, reconstruction of this geometric abnormality serves to not only restore valvular competency but also improve ventricular function.[25–29]

Historically, the surgical approach to MR was mitral valve replacement, yet little was understood of the interdependence of ventricular function and annulus-papillary muscle continuity.[30] Consequently, patients with low EF who underwent mitral valve replacement with removal of the subvalvular apparatus had prohibitively high mortality rates.[31] In an attempt to explain these outcomes, the concept of a beneficial "pop-off" effect of mitral regurgitation was conceived. This idea erroneously proposed that mitral incompetence provided a low-pressure relief during systolic ejection from the failing ventricle, and that removal of this effect through mitral replacement was responsible for deterioration of ventricular function. Consequently, mitral valve replacement in patients with heart failure was discouraged. More recent studies documenting the importance of maintaining subvalvular integrity to preserve postoperative LV function have led to surgical techniques that have been applicable to

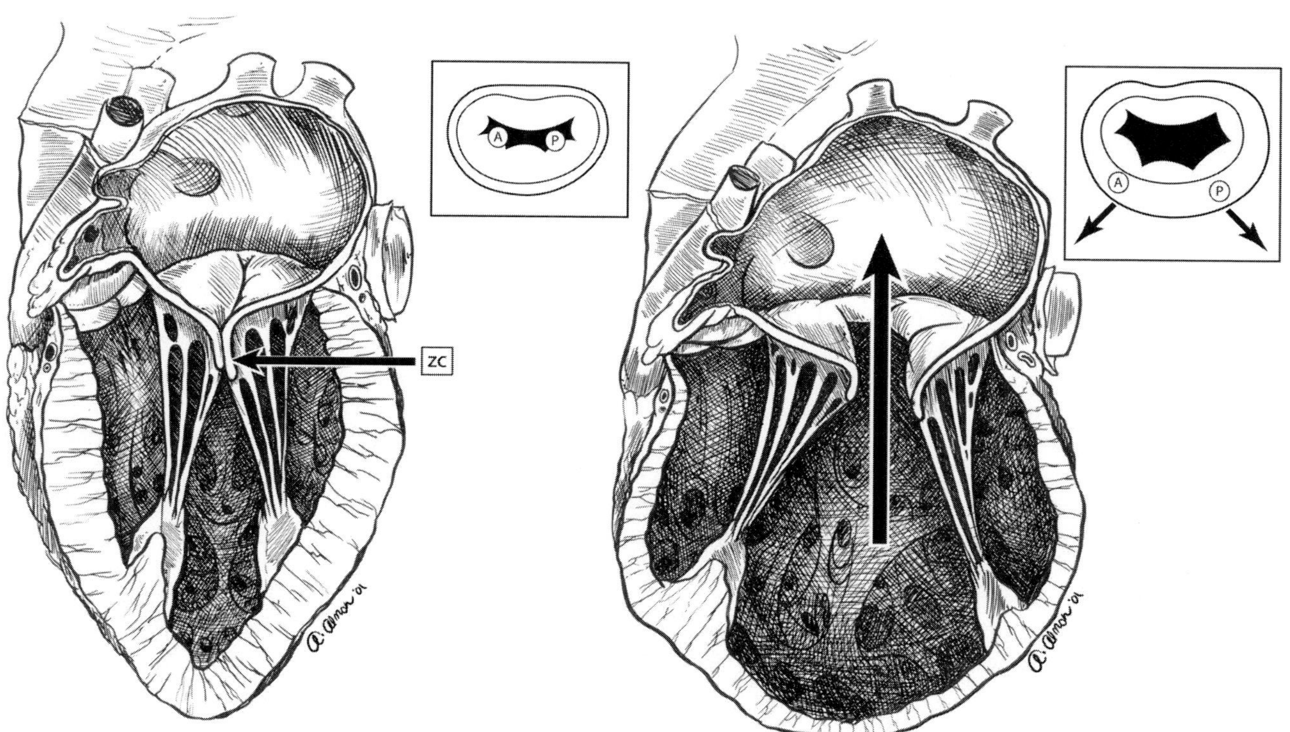

FIGURE 64–1 Note the geometric changes that occur from the normal to the failing LV. With the ventricular and annular dilatation of heart failure, the mitral leaflets cannot adequately cover the enlarged mitral orifice. Geometric mitral regurgitation results from a combination of annular dilatation, papillary muscle displacement, increased leaflet tethering forces, and weakened leaflet closing forces.

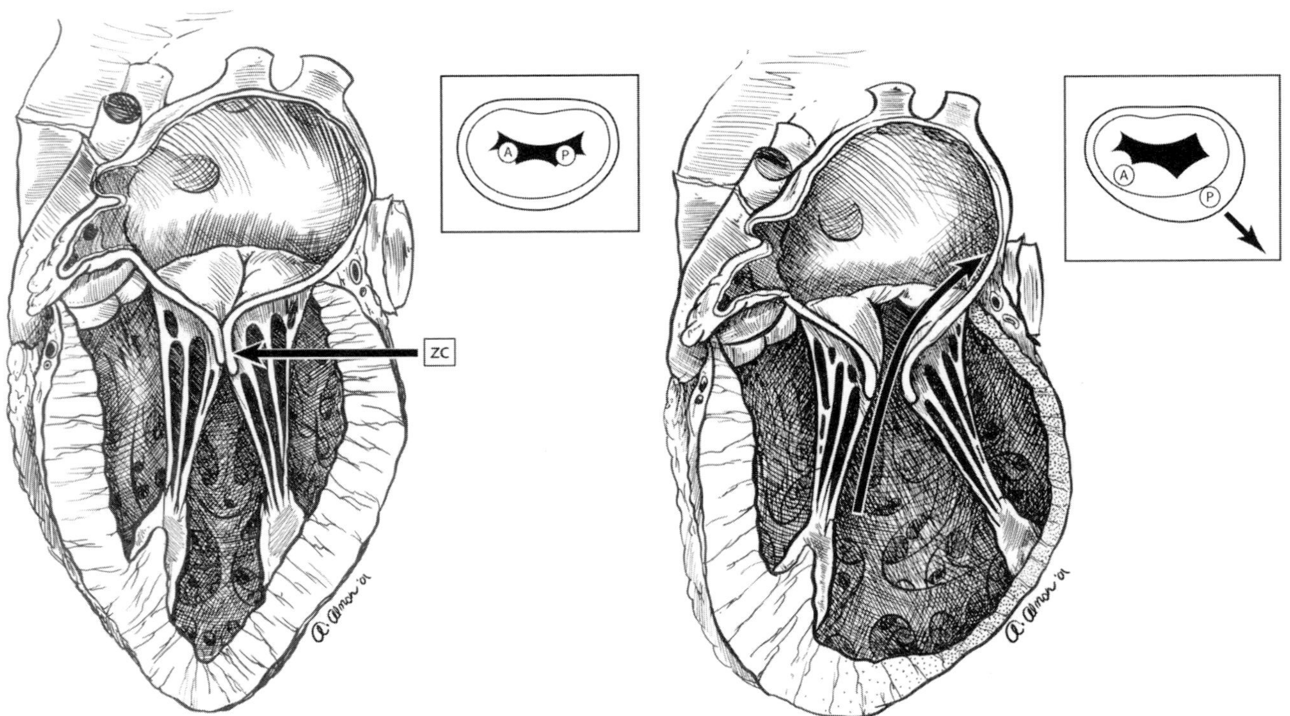

FIGURE 64–2 Note the structural changes that occur from the normal to the ischemic LV. With ischemic damage and thinning of the ventricular wall, there is lateral tethering and displacement of the papillary muscle resulting in an eccentric jet of mitral regurgitation. This illustrates the concept that ischemic mitral regurgitation results from "lateral wall dysfunction" that, if left untreated, will progress to global LV dysfunction and severe heart failure.

patients with heart failure.[32] Accordingly, preservation of the mitral valve apparatus in mitral surgery has been demonstrated to enhance ventricular geometry, decrease wall stress, and improve systolic and diastolic function.[33] Therefore, maintenance of chordal, annular, and subvalvular continuity is essential for the preservation of optimal mitral geometry and overall ventricular function. Furthermore, preservation of both the leaflet integrity as well as the dynamic function of the mitral apparatus with mitral repair has unmistakable functional benefits.

In treating heart failure patients, the most significant determinant of leaflet coaptation and MR is the diameter of the mitral valve annulus. The left ventricular dimension is of less importance in functional MR, as the lengths of the chordae and papillary muscles are similar in myopathic hearts regardless of the presence of MR. Observations with medically managed patients with severe heart failure and MR reveal that decreasing filling pressure and systemic vascular resistance lead to reductions in the dynamic MR associated with their heart failure.[34] This is attributed to a reduction in mitral orifice area relating to decreased LV volume and decreased annular distension. This complex relationship between mitral annular area and leaflet coaptation may thus explain why an undersized "valvular" repair may help a "ventricular" problem. This restoration of the mitral apparatus and ventricle forms the premise behind geometric mitral reconstruction (GMR) for the treatment of heart failure.

At the University of Michigan, over 150 patients with end-stage cardiomyopathy and refractory severe MR have undergone mitral valve repair with an undersized flexible annuloplasty ring (Fig. 64-3). All patients were in NYHA class III or IV heart failure despite receiving maximal medical therapy. Patients had severe preoperative LV dysfunction as defined by an EF under 25%, with a mean of 14%. On immediate postoperative echocardiograms, the mean transmitral gradient has been 3 ± 1 mm Hg (range 2-6 mm Hg). The overall operative mortality has been under 5%. There were 730-day mortalities: 1 from a cerebrovascular accident, 2 from CHF, 3 from multisystem organ failure, and only 1 intraoperative death, which resulted from right ventricular failure. Five patients have required intra-aortic balloon counterpulsation, yet mechanical LV assistance has not been necessary in any patient. The duration of follow-up of these patients has been between 2 and 83 months, with a mean of 45 months. There have been 27 late deaths: 12 from sudden ventricular arrhythmias, 9 from progression of CHF but without MR, 3 related to complications from other operative procedures, 2 that progressed to transplantation, and 1 suicide. The

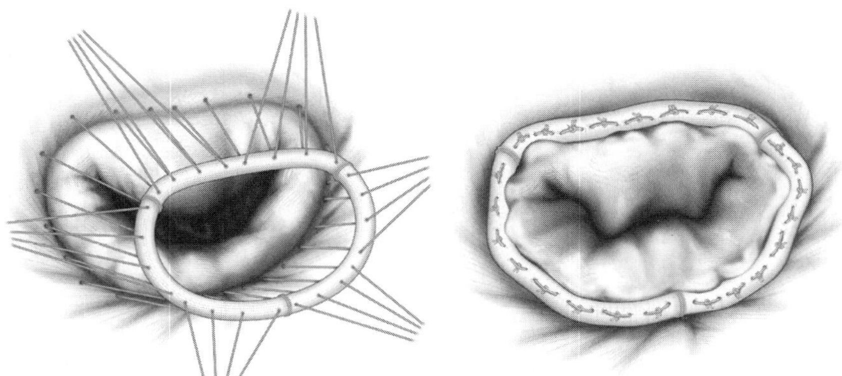

FIGURE 64–3 Geometric mitral reconstruction for heart failure. Successful augmentation of the zone of coaptation and prevention of recurrent MR can be achieved with placement of an undersized circumferential annuloplasty ring performed with multiple annular sutures.

1-, 2-, 3-, and 5-year actuarial survivals following GMR are 82%, 71%, 68%, and 57% respectively.

At 24-month assessment, mean EF increased to 26% and all patients were in NYHA class I or II. NYHA symptom scores were reduced from 3.2 ± 0.2 preoperatively to 1.8 ± 0.4 postoperatively. These improvements paralleled subjective functional improvements reported by all patients. Echocardiographically, there were marked improvements in regurgitant fraction, end-diastolic volume, cardiac output, and sphericity index (Table 64-1). Although significant undersizing of the mitral annulus was employed to overcorrect for the zone of coaptation (Fig. 64-4), no systolic anterior motion (SAM) of the anterior leaflet or mitral stenosis was noted in these patients.

The technique of undersizing in mitral reconstruction avoids SAM in these myopathic patients likely due to widening of the aorto-mitral angle in these hearts with increased LV size. Furthermore, acute remodeling of the base of the heart with this reparative technique may also reestablish the somewhat normal geometry and ellipsoid shape the LV. As evidenced by the decreased sphericity index and LV volumes seen in these patients, the geometric restoration from mitral reconstruction not only effectively corrects MR but also achieves surgical unloading of the ventricle.

Recently, several centers have reported consistent findings following GMR.[28,35–38] With outcomes equating to transplant while avoiding immunosuppression, this straightforward reparative operation performed in conjunction with medical management may be offered to all patients with MR and cardiomyopathy as a first-line therapy.

GEOMETRIC VENTRICULAR RECONSTRUCTION

Myocardial revascularization and GMR reliably improve ventricular function. However, further surgical techniques have been developed that attempt to augment LV function through a reduction of end-diastolic wall tension following the principles of the law of LaPlace. Since ventricular wall tension is directly proportional to LV radius and pressure and inversely proportional to wall thickness, any intervention to optimize this relationship would be beneficial. As heart failure progresses, so does the progressive thinning and dilatation of the LV thus leading to increasing wall stress and further dilatation. This remodeling process may result in regional LV dysfunction, as occurs following segmental myocardial infarction, or global LV dysfunction, which may arise from either ischemic or nonischemic etiologies. The concept of reducing wall stress through the surgical restoration of LV cavity size and geometry remains the guiding principle behind many innovative techniques including those developed for the isolation of LV aneurysms and nonfunctioning ventricular segments.

After an acute myocardial infarction, the noncontractile myocardium undergoes thinning and fibrous replacement often following the segmental distribution of the arterial occlusion. This nonfunctional LV segment may remain akinetic or transform into a dyskinetic aneurysm depending on factors such as age and regional collateral circulation. Though such postinfarct pathologic remodeling may occur in any area of the heart, the most common clinically relevant region that manifests is the anteroapical segment of the LV. The

TABLE 64–1 Matched preoperative and postoperative echocardiographic data at 24 months following mitral reconstruction for heart failure

Echocardiographic parameter	Preoperative	Postoperative (24 months)	*p* value
End-diastolic volume (mL)	281 ± 86	206 ± 88	<.001
Ejection fraction (%)	16 ± 5	26 ± 8	.008
Regurgitant fraction (%)	70 ± 12	13 ± 10	<.001
Cardiac output (L/min)	3.1 ± 1.0	5.2 ± 0.8	.001
Sphericity index (D/L)	0.82 ± 0.10	0.74 ± 0.07	.005

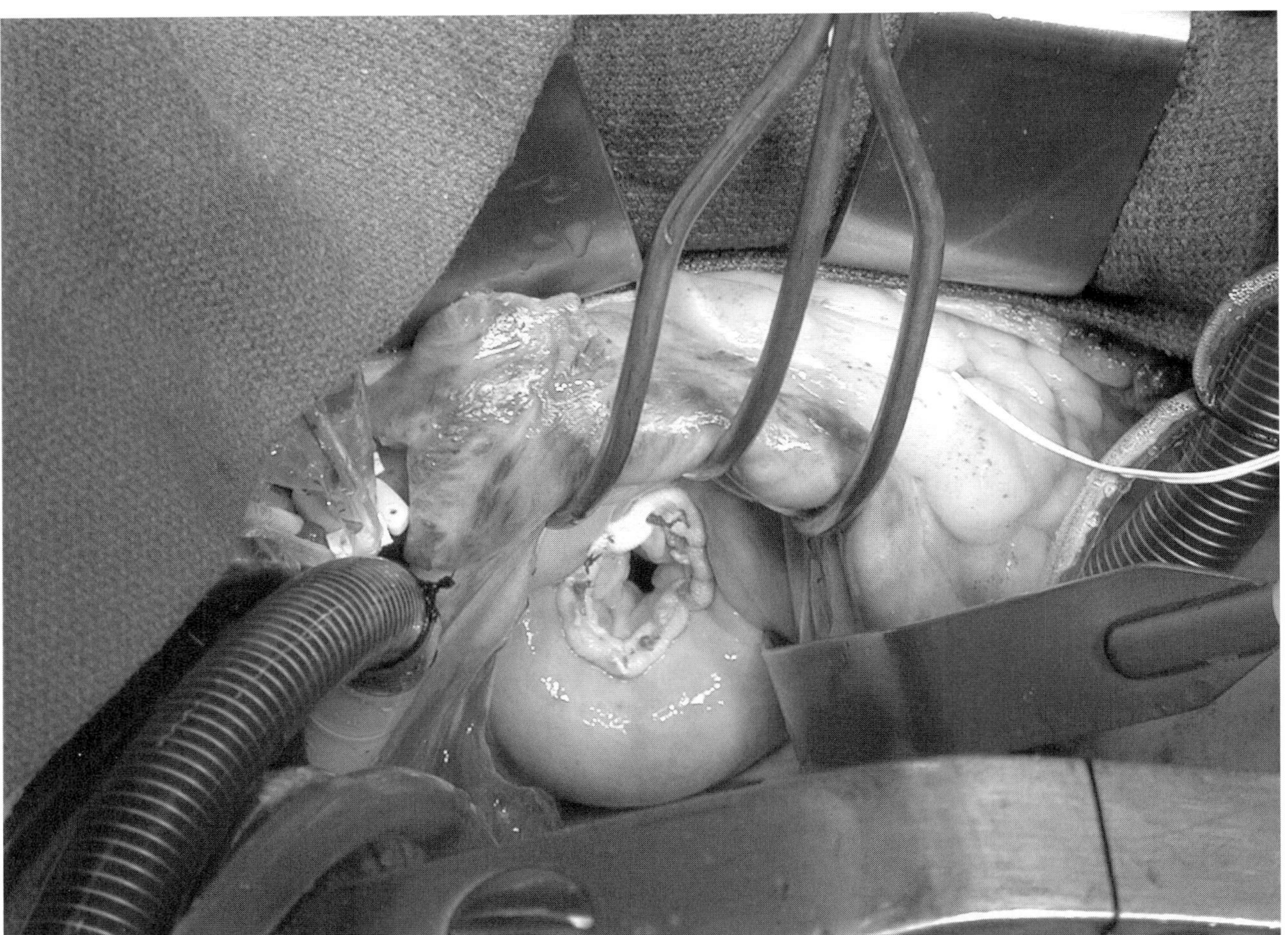

FIGURE 64–4 Technique of geometric mitral reconstruction. Bicaval cannulation, approaching the mitral valve through the interatrial groove, and the use of a self-retaining retractor greatly enhances exposure. Multiple circumferential annular sutures are placed followed by the implantation of an undersized flexible ring. Note the reduced size of the annulus after successful reconstruction.

resulting loss of contractile function in the affected segment results in global increases in LV wall tension and myocardial oxygen consumption in turn leading to compensatory LV dilatation in accordance with the law of LaPlace. These geometric ventricular changes may also result in loss of the zone of coaptation and MR following infarction, as discussed earlier. Moreover, when a dyskinetic region expands and becomes aneurysmal, cardiac work is further increased due to the paradoxical systolic motion of the thinned segment. These pathological alterations often result in CHF. The principle of surgical restoration of LV geometry involves the isolation of these nonfunctional areas and a subsequent reduction in LV volumes. This concept has been clearly illustrated by Dor and others, who have revealed significant improvement in heart failure after endoventricular patch exclusion of dyskinetic or akinetic ventricular segments.[39–42]

The preoperative selection and preparation for LV reconstruction should follow the identical medical optimization discussed earlier. In addition to viability assessment, echocardiography, and contrast ventriculography, cardiac MRI and LV-gated nuclear imaging have proved valuable tools for pre- and postoperative volume estimation and anatomic assessment of the LV wall and septum. The pre- and intraoperative decision on when to perform LV reconstruction should be based on the function, viability, and thinning of the segment as well as the location of viability-targeted concomitant coronary grafting. Benefits obtained from repairing dyskinetic thin aneurysmal defects are well established.[40,43] More recently, however, preliminary reports have revealed encouraging results with endoventricular repair of nondilated akinetic segments when combined with CABG. These findings have spawned the multicenter Surgical Treatment of Ischemic Heart Failure (STICH) trial to evaluate its long-term functional benefit.

The operative principles of LV reconstruction involve optimal myocardial preservation, septal exclusion of the nonfunctioning segment with an endoventricular patch, and closure of the excluded ventricular myocardium. To improve

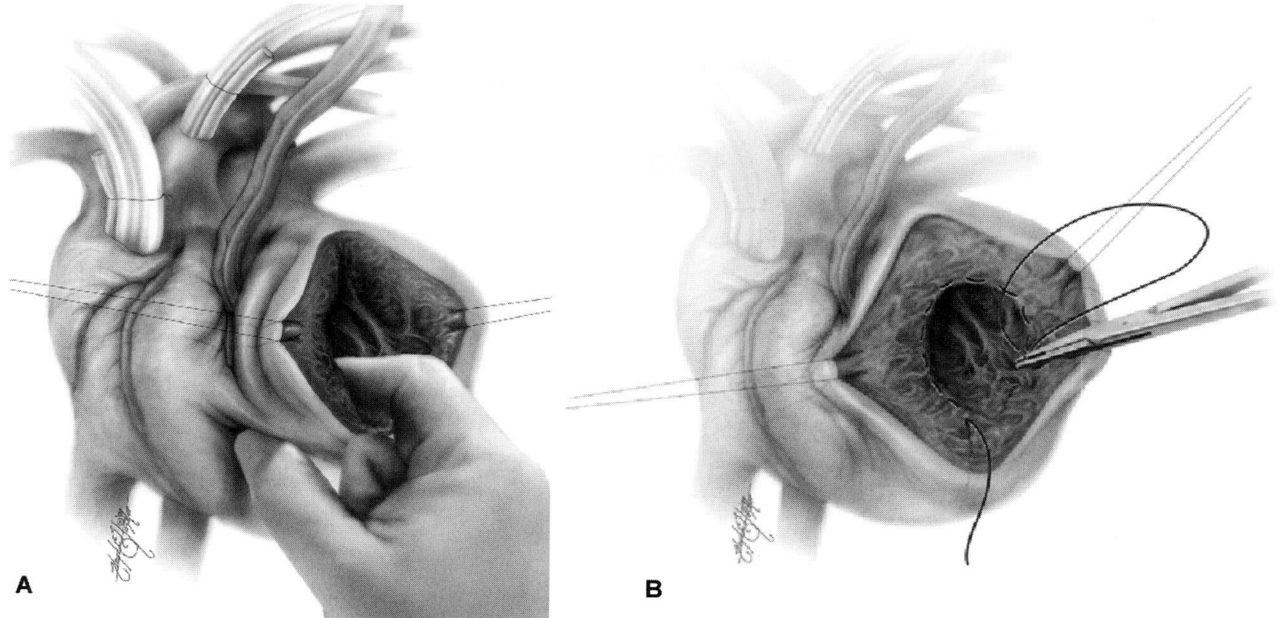

FIGURE 64–5 (A) Left ventricular reconstruction on the beating heart decompressed on CPB. Palpation assists in identification of the demarcation zone between functioning and nonfunctioning myocardium. (B) Placement of a circumferential monofilament suture at the level of demarcation between functional and nonfunctional myocardium permits reduction of the ventricular opening in preparation for placement of a bovine pericardial patch. Patch closure is performed with either a running or interrupted technique and the covering myocardium is reapproximated with the aid of strips of bovine pericardium or felt.

the visual and tactile identification of the nonfunctioning segment, the ventricular repair is often performed on the perfused beating unvented heart decompressed with CPB. Entry should be at least 1 to 2 cm to the left of the anterior descending coronary artery to avoid the septum. The thinned segment often will pucker when the LV is decompressed, thus marking the initial access point. A point knife is used to gain entry to permit complete decompression and endocardial visualization under direct vision as the incision is further developed. This allows for the safe removal of any LV thrombus if present, as well as for the visual and tactile identification of the septum and demarcation zone between functioning and nonfunctioning myocardium (Fig. 64-5A). A circumferential monofilament suture or "Fontan stitch" is then placed within this zone and tied as advocated by Dor (Figure 64-5B). The resulting reduced size of the defect is then patched with bovine pericardium and the residual myocardial defect is buttressed closed with strips of bovine pericardium or felt. Though concomitant GMR and CABG can be performed before or after LV reconstruction, it is often advocated before so as to allow for improved myocardial recovery and reperfusion following removal of the aortic cross-clamp.

Results from LV reconstruction have been favorable and consistent between groups regardless if endoventricular circular patch plasty or a modified linear patch closure technique is utilized. Significant reductions in left ventricular end-systolic volume index and improvements in EF, NYHA class, and long-term survival have resulted. It is being regularly performed with hospital mortalities of under 8% and with a 12-month freedom from readmission for CHF of over 80%.[40–45] Therefore, geometric left ventricular reconstruction by endoventricular exclusion of nonfunctional segments should be placed alongside high-risk CABG and GMR as a first-line surgical option for heart failure.

PARTIAL LEFT VENTRICULECTOMY

Batista has furthered the concept of surgical ventricular remodeling to optimize wall tension in dilated ventricles with the contention that all mammalian hearts should share the same mass-diameter ratio regardless of size. He proposes that all hearts not complying with this relationship should have a segment of the LV wall excised in order to diminish mural tension and improve myocardial oxygen consumption in accordance with the law of LaPlace.[46,47] This interesting concept was initially presented as a case report of a 34-year-old patient who underwent a partial left ventriculectomy (PLV) that reportedly increased the EF from 17% to 44% at 2 months postoperatively. Batista performed over 150 such procedures predominantly on patients with Chagas disease and dilated cardiomyopathy. Though this experience stimulated much interest, unfortunately no meaningful follow-up data or statistical analyses has ever been made available from this series.

To further evaluate the potential benefits of PLV, the Cleveland Clinic performed 62 such cases on patients with idiopathic dilated cardiomyopathy awaiting transplant. The ventriculectomy involved resection of the lateral wall of the LV in the circumflex coronary artery distribution to the base of the papillary muscles with closure between two strips of felt or bovine pericardium. This was one of the largest North American series, reporting a 3.5% operative mortality with 7 late deaths and a 1-year actuarial survival of 82%. However, of the total 62 patients, 24 (39%) were considered short-term treatment failures: 11 required LVAD support, 6 were listed for transplantation again, and 7 non-LVAD patients died.[48] Moreover, a further 30% attrition rate at 2 years following PLV has been reported.[49,50] These results may be superior to no surgical treatment but they fall short of those obtained by other surgical options for heart failure. As a result, PLV has fallen into disfavor in North America. However, in the Asian-Pacific region, where transplantation is not widely available, efforts by Suma et al to improve selection criteria and introduce echo-guided surgical decision making have resulted in PLV persisting as a viable option for heart failure in this part of the world.[51]

In attempting to elucidate the mechanism behind the relative success of PLV, it is quite interesting to note that over 95% of the cases performed in the Cleveland Clinic experience also involved a mitral reconstruction. Therefore, it becomes difficult to discern the role mitral repair plays in the overall utility of PLV, since patients undergoing mitral reconstruction alone also attain normalization of the LV mass to volume ratio, but without the excision of viable myocardium.[26] Furthermore, experimental models of heart failure have revealed that correction of the MR alone permits LV remodeling that may be rapid and complete with resulting regurgitant fractions of less than 30%.[52]

Though the concept of instantly remodeling the LV through PLV is mechanically appealing, discarding functioning myocardium is not. Patients with ischemic cardiomyopathy with a dyskinetic aneurysmal segment have undergone successful remodeling with an endoventricular patch repair. Patients with dilated cardiomyopathy and MR have undergone mitral reconstruction thereby altering the angulation of the base of the heart and promoting favorable LV geometry and remodeling. Thus at this time, when similar if not superior results can be obtained by methods that preserve myocardial integrity, the application of PLV to patients with end-stage heart failure should be approached with an element of caution.

DYNAMIC CARDIOMYOPLASTY

Another alternative method to surgically optimize LaPlace's law is dynamic cardiomyoplasty (DCMP). This procedure is conceptually based upon imparting the contractile and supportive forces of the patient's own skeletal muscle for purposes of cardiac assistance and the reduction of myocardial wall stress. It is accomplished by wrapping the latissimus dorsi muscle (LDM) around the failing heart and, by means of an implantable cardiomyostimulator, stimulating the muscle to contract in synchrony with cardiac systole. DCMP has been proposed as an alternative to transplant or LVAD. It has the obvious advantages of total implantability; it avoids the power constraints and thromboembolic risks experienced with mechanical assist devices; and the LDM with its single neurovascular pedicle can be easily utilized with no loss of shoulder function.

Prior to using skeletal muscle as a power source, the concerns of fatigability and performance loss with altered geometry must be addressed. The biological principles governing the plausibility of biomechanical assistance center on three main concepts: transformation, conformation, and burst stimulation.

Skeletal muscle is comprised of variable amounts of oxidative slow-twitch type I fibers and glycolytic fast-twitch type II fibers. Early work with cross-innervation of muscle preparations noted that certain fiber types could be altered through neural stimulation.[53] It was further noted that mixed type I and II fatigue-prone fibers could be morphologically converted into totally type II fatigue-resistant muscle with repeated low frequency electrical stimulation.[54] This ability to phenotypically and histologically alter fiber composition and confer fatigue resistance to skeletal muscle is known as transformation.

All muscle, skeletal or myocardial, responds to strain following the principles of a Frank-Starling functional curve.[55] In determining the ideal stretch or orientation of the muscle wrap for optimal performance, it has been observed that within weeks after DCMP the LDM adapts by altering its geometric shape to conform to the epicardial surface; this phenomenon persists even after the native heart is removed. This morphologic ability of skeletal muscle to delete or add sarcomeres to restore optimal resting tension and performance is known as conformation.[56,57]

Unlike the all-or-none contractile syncytium found in myocardium, skeletal muscle performance is a reflection of the recruitment of individual motor units. A single electrical impulse stimulates only a few motor units and results in only a twitch. By studying the application of a burst of stimuli in the form of a pulse train, it was deemed possible to induce a summation of twitches into a graded full contractile response.[58] This technique of burst stimulation forms the basis of the design of the cardiomyostimulator used for DCMP.

For optimal results, indications for DCMP include patients with NYHA class III symptoms, EF greater than 20%, and maximal oxygen consumption (V_{O_2}) higher than 15 mL/kg/min.[59] Since adhesions may increase the technical difficulty and risk to these fragile patients, caution should be exercised when considering those with previous cardiac or thoracic procedures. Clinical experience has revealed a higher risk in patients with high pulmonary vascular resistance, V_{O_2} less than 10 mL/kg/min, poor EF, and NYHA class IV heart failure.[60]

As with other surgical approaches to heart failure, the preoperative preparation of the patient should be optimized. As the goal is to perform the operation off pump, anesthesia must be carefully induced with double-lumen endotracheal intubation and a primed CPB circuit; a perfusionist should be on standby. In the right lateral decubitus position, the left LDM is atraumatically dissected with preservation of its thoracodorsal pedicle. The graft is detached from its ligamentous humeral insertion, two intramuscular leads are placed along its proximal margin, and the graft is placed into the left chest through a window in the second interspace created by a segmental resection of the third rib. The ligamentous proximal portion of the LDM is fixed to the periosteum of the second rib and the wound is closed. The patient is repositioned, a median sternotomy is performed, and the left pleura is opened to retrieve the LDM. Two epicardial sensing electrodes are secured on the RV for LDM synchronization. Using minimal manipulation, the LDM is slid posteriorly where it is anchored to the posterior pericardial reflection. It is then folded from posterior to anterior as the edges are sutured together to form the completed cardiomyoplasty. The leads are then tunneled to a subcutaneously implanted cardiomyostimulator prior to sternal closure. Postoperatively, afterload reduction is reinstituted while avoiding high-dose vasoconstrictors due to the tenuous LDM blood supply, and care must be taken with intravenous infusions to avoid volume overload. The LDM is left unstimulated for a 14-day period of vascular delay, which is followed by a graded 8-week protocol of stimulation to induce LDM transformation and attain optimal burst capacity for cardiac assistance.[61]

Starting in 1985, Medtronic Inc. began coordinating a multicenter FDA trial to evaluate the cardiomyostimulator. In effect, the rigorous evaluation of this device uniquely subjected DCMP to the scientific analysis of a multiphase prospective trial. Phase I set out to assess the selection criteria for the procedure and safety of the stimulator. From July 1985 to April 1991, data from 118 patients revealed that patients with NYHA class IV failure and an EF less than 20% had a prohibitive mortality, but those with class III had an acceptable outcome and enjoyed a mean reduction of 1.6 functional classes at 3 months.[59] With this refined selection criteria, the phase II trial set out to assess the efficacy of DCMP. From May 1991 to September 1993, data from 68 patients in refractory NYHA class III failure of mixed etiology revealed that DCMP could be performed with a mortality of 12% and result in an average EF increase of 15%. Over 85% of these patients had an improvement in their functional status and quality of life. This prompted a phase III randomized controlled trial to definitively assess the benefits of DCMP.[62]

Starting in 1994, the Cardiomyoplasty-Skeletal Muscle Assist Randomized Trial (C-SMART) was established to assess if DCMP has a benefit over conventional medical therapy for heart failure. The sample size calculation required to reach this conclusion was determined to be 400 patients. Unfortunately after 4 years, only slightly over 100 patients were enrolled in this North American trial. This illustrated the unique adversity C-SMART faced, as recruitment appeared impeded by slow physician referral that showed the "too well/too sick" phenomenon. Projecting that it would take over 9 years to complete the trial and surmising a lack of enthusiasm for DCMP, Medtronic decided to withdraw their device. At that time, over 54 patients had undergone DCMP with only a single mortality (1.9%).[62] When attempting to ascertain its efficacy as a therapy for heart failure, pooled observations after DCMP reveal a paucity of positive quantitative hemodynamic data yet, paradoxically, patients report over 30% functional improvement when compared to medical therapy alone.[63,64]

Though DCMP is now only rarely performed in North America, the recently available LD Pace myostimulator out of Russia has allowed this procedure to continue to be an available in that country as well as throughout various centers in Europe, Asia, and the Caribbean.

Investigations into the mechanisms of DCMP, which continue today, have generated spin-offs in the fields of myoblast transplantation and remodeling surgery. As the initial vision of simple systolic assist did not sufficiently explain why unstimulated DCMP patients showed benefit, further studies revealed that the wrap actually contributes to significant reductions in myocardial wall stress.[65,66] In effect, this conceptually protects myocytes from overt functional stresses and thereby prevents the adaptive progressive dilatation of heart failure. Working in favor of the law of LaPlace, this girdling effect of DCMP was seen with unstimulated adynamic cardiomyoplasty. Furthermore, original experiments comparing adynamic cardiomyoplasty to synthetic material revealed that this beneficial girdling effect even occurs when a passive constraint of prosthetic mesh fabric is applied to the ventricles.[67] These findings of girdling and myocardial sparing provide a potential explanation for the reverse remodeling seen with DCMP, and they have spawned the development of novel biomedical devices currently under clinical investigation.

EMERGING BIOMEDICAL DEVICES FOR HEART FAILURE

The Acorn Cardiac Support Device (ACSD; Acorn Medical, Minneapolis, MN) is a polyester mesh fabric that attempts to reduce ventricular wall stress by providing external support. Much like DCMP, the ACSD is placed around the ventricles from posterior to anterior, using stay sutures, as well as an anterior fabric seam for snug tailoring to the patient's heart (Fig. 64-6). Taking advantage of the girdling effect, the purpose of this device is to passively support the failing ventricles and prevent further dilatation. Preclinical data have shown decreased LV volumes and improvements in regional

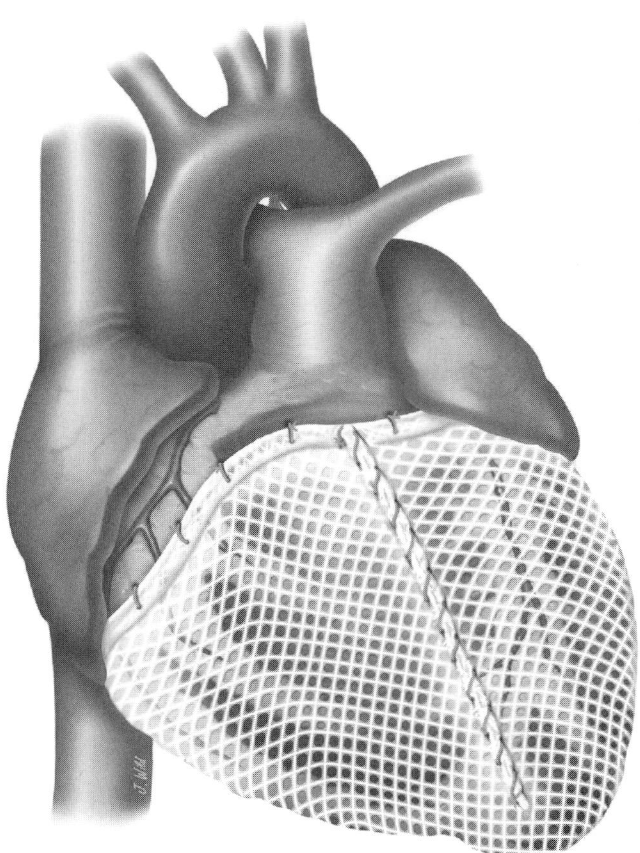

FIGURE 64–6 The Acorn Cardiac Support Device.

wall motion, EF, and other functional parameters without any evidence of constrictive physiology.[68,69] Histologic animal studies have also demonstrated decreased myocyte hypertrophy and interstitial fibrosis, as well as improvements in several biochemical markers of failure.[70,71] A phase I-II clinical trial is underway to assess the safety and the early remodeling ability of the ACSD when used on heart failure patients with or without concomitant cardiac procedures. Preliminary experience reveals that the ACSD is easily applied, and may even be performed without the necessity of cardiopulmonary bypass.

The Myocor Myosplint (Myocor Medical, St. Paul, MN) is a second device developed to reduce ventricular wall stress by directly altering cardiac geometry. Working on the premise of optimizing the law of LaPlace, it involves the placement of transventricular tension bands through the RV and LV walls that have the unique ability to be individually tightened in order to achieve a 20% reduction in wall stress. Preclinical animal data have shown improvements in end-diastolic volume, end-systolic volume, and EF. These experiments reveal the Myocor device becomes readily incorporated within a fibrous capsule that has been free of thrombus formation. A phase I clinical trial is under way to assess device safety in patients prior to cardiectomy at the time of transplant. Preliminary data reveal that the device can be readily deployed without harm to other cardiac structures. Further chronic studies are required to address the efficacy of this unique device.

CONCLUSIONS

As surgical therapies for heart failure rapidly evolve, the need for their critical appraisal is essential so that they may be offered to the growing population of CHF patients in a prompt yet effective manner. Transplantation continues to offer selected patients reliable long-term survival in a reproducible fashion, and it thus remains as a gold standard surgical therapy for heart failure. Though in time we may see mechanical assist devices play a more prevalent role in myocardial recovery or destination therapy, currently their main utility is as a bridge to transplantation. With the growing disparity between donor availability and heart failure patients, experience is mounting with effective nontransplant surgical solutions.

The results of the more conventional techniques of CABG, geometric mitral reconstruction, and ventricular reconstruction when combined with the optimal medical management of heart failure may now be on a par with transplantation. Therefore, these modalities now form the new first-line surgical therapy for heart failure when applicable. Patients with primary ischemic cardiomyopathy with favorable anatomy may be effectively managed with revascularization alone or in combination with LV reconstruction. Myopathic patients with MR, regardless of etiology, may be effectively managed with mitral reconstruction. With the superior results of these approaches, the use of other techniques such as PLV and DCMP should be reserved as viable alternative surgical options for heart failure. The prudent and effective application of the growing menu of surgical strategies for heart failure enables the scarcely available donor hearts be efficiently used for patients with truly no other surgical or medical alternatives. Along with the utility of emerging biomedical devices, each of these unique modalities has enhanced the clinically effective armamentarium of the modern surgeon treating patients with heart failure.

REFERENCES

1. Tavazzi L: Epidemiology of dilated cardiomyopathy: a still undetermined entity. *Eur Heart J* 1997; 18:4.
2. Hunt SA: Current status of cardiac transplantation. *JAMA* 1998; 280:1692.
3. Hosenpud JD, Bennett LE, Keck BM, et al: The Registry of the International Society for Heart and Lung Transplantation: Fifteenth Official Report—1998. *J Heart Lung Transplant* 1998; 17:656.
4. Rose EA, Moskowitz AJ, Packer M, et al: The REMATCH trial: rationale, design, and end points. Randomized Evaluation of Mechanical Assistance for the Treatment of Congestive Heart Failure. *Ann Thorac Surg* 1999; 67:723.

5. Stevenson LW, Kormos RL: Mechanical cardiac support 2000: current applications and future trial design. *Circulation* 2001; 103:337.
6. Westaby S, Banning AP, Jarvik R, et al: First permanent implant of the Jarvik 2000 Heart. *Lancet* 2000; 356:900.
7. Dipla K, Mattiello JA, Jeevanandam V, et al: Myocyte recovery after mechanical circulatory support in humans with end-stage heart failure. *Circulation* 1998; 97:2316.
8. Kumpati GS, McCarthy PM, Hoercher KJ: Left ventricular assist device bridge to recovery: a review of the current status. *Ann Thorac Surg* 2001; 71:S103.
9. Deng Mario C, Loebe M, El-Banayosy A, et al: Mechanical circulatory support for advanced heart failure: effect of patient selection on outcome. *Circulation* 2001; 103:231.
10. CASS Principle Investigators. Coronary Artery Surgery Study (CASS): A randomized trial of coronary artery bypass surgery: survival data. *Circulation* 1983; 68:939.
11. European Coronary Surgery Study Group. Long-term results of prospective randomized study or coronary artery bypass surgery in stable angina pectoris. *Lancet* 1982; 2:1173.
12. Elefteriades JA, Tolis G Jr, Levi E, et al: Coronary artery bypass grafting in severe left ventricular dysfunction: excellent survival with improved ejection fraction and functional state. *J Am Coll Cardiol* 1993; 22:1411.
13. Samady H, Elefteriades JA, Abbot B, et al: Failure to improve left ventricular function after coronary revascularization for ischemic cardiomyopathy is not associated with worse outcome. *Circulation* 1999; 100:1298.
14. Kim RW, Ugurlu BS, Tereb DA, et al: Effect of left ventricular volume on results of coronary artery bypass grafting. *Am J Cardiol* 2000; 86:1261.
15. Louie HW, Laks H, Milgalter E, et al: Ischemic cardiomyopathy: criteria for coronary revascularization and cardiac transplantation. *Circulation* 1991; 84(suppl III):III290.
16. Di Carli MF, Maddahi J, Roshsar S, et al: Long-term survival of patients with coronary artery disease and left ventricular dysfunction: implications for the role of myocardial viability assessment in management decisions. *J Thorac Cardiovasc Surg* 1998; 116:997.
17. Marwick TH, Zuchowski C, Lauer MS, et al: Functional status and quality of life in patients with heart failure undergoing coronary bypass surgery after assessment of myocardial viability. *J Am Coll Cardiol* 1999; 33:750.
18. Senior R, Kaul S, Lahiri A: Myocardial viability on echocardiography predicts long-term survival after revascularization in patients with ischemic congestive heart failure. *J Am Coll Cardiol* 1999; 33:1848.
19. Elefteriades JA, Morales DLS, Gradel C, et al: Results of coronary artery bypass grafting by a single surgeon in patients with left ventricular ejection fractions <30%. *Am J Cardiol* 1997; 79:1573.
20. Mickelborough LL, Maruyama H, Takagi Y, et al: Results of revascularization in patients with poor left ventricular function. *Circulation* 1995; 92(suppl II):II73.
21. Kaul TK, Agnihotri A, Fields B, et al: Coronary artery bypass grafting in patients with an ejection fraction of twenty percent or less. *J Thorac Cardiovasc Surg* 1996; 111:1001.
22. Blondheim DS, Jacobs LE, Kotler MN, et al: Dilated cardiomyopathy with mitral regurgitation: decreased survival despite a low frequency of left ventricular thrombus. *Am Heart J* 1991; 122(3 pt 1):763.
23. Boltwood CM, Tei C, Wong M, Shah PM: Quantitative echocardiography of the mitral complex in dilated cardiomyopathy: the mechanism of functional mitral regurgitation. *Circulation* 1983; 68:498.
24. Kono T, Sabbah HN, Rosman H, et al: Left ventricular shape is the primary determinant of functional mitral regurgitation in heart failure. *J Am Coll Cardiol* 1992; 20:1594.
25. Bolling SF, Deeb GM, Brunsting LA, et al: Early outcome of mitral valve reconstruction in patients with end-stage cardiomyopathy. *J Thorac Cardiovasc Surg* 1995; 109:676.
26. Bach DS, Bolling SF: Improvement following correction of secondary mitral regurgitation in end-stage cardiomyopathy with mitral annuloplasty. *Am J Cardiol* 1996; 78:966.
27. Bolling SF, Pagani FD, Deeb GM, et al: Intermediate-term outcome of mitral reconstruction in cardiomyopathy. *J Thorac Cardiovasc Surg* 1998; 115:381.
28. Chen FY, Adams DH, Aranki SF, et al: Mitral valve repair in cardiomyopathy. *Circulation* 1998; 98:II-124.
29. Badhwar V, Bolling SF: Mitral valve surgery in the patient with left ventricular dysfunction. *Semin Thorac Cardiovasc Surg* 2002; 14:133.
30. Pitarys CJ II, Forman MB, Panayiotou H, et al: Long-term effects of excision of the mitral apparatus on global and regional ventricular function in humans. *J Am Coll Cardiol* 1990; 15:557.
31. Phillips HR, Levine FH, Carter JE, et al: Mitral valve replacement for isolated mitral regurgitation: analysis of clinical course and late postoperative left ventricular ejection fraction. *Am J Cardiol* 1981; 48:647.
32. David TE, Uden DE, Strauss HD: The importance of the mitral apparatus in left ventriuclar function after correction of mitral regurgitation. *Circulation* 1983; 68(3 pt 2):II76.
33. Sarris GE, Cahill PD, Hansen DE, et al: Restoration of left ventricular systolic performance after reattachment of the mitral chordae tendineae: the importance of valvular-ventricular interaction. *J Thorac Cardiovasc Surg* 1988; 95:969.
34. Rosario LB, Stevenson LW, Solomon SD, et al: The mechanism of decrease in dynamic mitral regurgitation during heart failure treatment: importance of reduction in the regurgitant orifice size. *J Am Coll Cardiol* 1998; 32:1819.
35. Bishay ES, McCarthy PM, Cosgrove DM, et al: Mitral valve surgery in patients with severe left ventricular dysfunction. *Eur J Cardiothorac Surg* 2000; 17:213.
36. Calafiore AM, Gallina S, Di Mauro M, et al: Mitral valve procedure in dilated cardiomyopathy: repair or replacement? *Ann Thorac Surg* 2001; 71:1146.
37. Bitran D, Merin O, Klutstein MW, et al: Mitral valve repair in severe cardiomyopathy. *J Card Surg* 2001; 16:79.
38. Radovanovic N, Mihajlovic B, Selestiansky J, et al: Reductive annuloplasty of double orifices in patients with primary dilated cardiomyopathy. *Ann Thorac Surg* 2002; 73:751.
39. Di Donato M, Sabatier M, Montiglio F, et al: Outcome of left ventricular aneurysmectomy with patch repair in patients with severely depressed pump function. *Am J Cardiol* 1995; 76:557.
40. Dor V, Sabatier M, Montiglio F, et al: Endoventricular patch reconstruction in large ischemic wall-motion abnormalities. *J Card Surg* 1999; 14:46.
41. Mickleborough LL, Carson S, Ivanov J: Repair of dyskinetic or akinetic left ventricular aneurysm: results obtained with modified linear closure. *J Thorac Cardiovasc Surg* 2001; 121:675.
42. Athanasuleas CL, Stanley AWH Jr, Buckberg GD, et al: Surgical anterior ventricular endocardial restoration (SAVER) in the dilated remodeled ventricle after anterior myocardial infarction. *J Am Coll Cardiol* 2001; 37:1199.
43. Dor V, Di Donato M, Sabatier M, et al: Left ventricle reconstruction by endoventricular circular patch plasty repair: a 17-year experience. *Semin Thorac Cardiovasc Surg* 2001; 13:435.
44. Athanasuleas CL, Stanley AW, Buckberg GD: Restoration of contractile function in the enlarged left ventricle by exclusion of remodeled akinetic anterior segment: surgical strategy, myocardial protection, and angiographic results. *J Card Surg* 1998; 13:418.
45. Dor V, Sabatier M, Di Donato M, et al: Efficacy of endoventricular patch plasty in large postinfarction akinetic scar and severe left

ventricular dysfunction: comparison with a series of large dyskinetic scars. *J Thorac Cardiovasc Surg* 1998; 116:50.
46. Batista RJ, Santos JL, Takeshita N, et al: Partial left ventriculectomy to improve LV function in end-stage heart disease. *J Card Surg* 1996; 11:96.
47. Batista R: Partial left ventriculectomy—the Batista procedure. *Eur J Cardiothorac Surg* 1999; 15(suppl 1):S12.
48. McCarthy JF, McCarthy PM, Starling RC, et al: Partial left ventriculectomy and mitral valve repair for end-stage CHF. *Eur J Cardiothorac Surg* 1998; 13:337.
49. Stolf NA, Moreira LF, Bocchi EA, et al: Determinants of midterm outcome of partial left ventriculectomy in dilated cardiomyopathy. *Ann Thorac Surg* 1999; 67:1541.
50. Kawaguchi AT, Bergsland J, Ishibashi-Ueda H, et al: Partial left ventriculectomy in patients with dilated failing ventricle. *J Card Surg* 1998; 13:335.
51. Isomura T, Suma H, Horii T, et al: Partial left ventriculectomy, ventriculoplasty or valvular surgery for idiopathic dilated cardiomyopathy—the role of intra-operative echocardiography. *Eur J Cardiothorac Surg* 2000; 17:239.
52. Nagatsu M, Ishihara K, Zile MR, et al: The effects of complete versus incomplete mitral valve repair in experimental MR. *J Thorac Cardiovasc Surg* 1994; 107:416.
53. Buller AJ, Eccles JC, Eccles RM: Interactions between motorneurons and muscles in respect of the characteristic speeds of their responses. *J Physiol* 1960; 150:417.
54. Salmons S, Sreter FA: Significance of impulse activity in the transformation of skeletal muscle type. *Nature* 1976; 263:30.
55. Kochamba G, Chiu RCJ: The physiologic characteristics of transformed skeletal muscle for cardiac assist. *Trans Am Soc Artif Organs* 1987; 33:404.
56. Tardieu C, Tabary JC, Tardieu G, et al: Adaptation of sarcomere numbers to the length imposed on muscle. *Adv Physiol Sci* 1981; 24:29.
57. Gealow KK, Solien EE, Bianco RW, et al: Conformational adaptation of muscle: implications in cardiomyoplasty and skeletal muscle ventricles. *Ann Thorac Surg* 1993; 56:520.
58. Drinkwater DC, Chiu RCJ, Modry D, et al: Cardiac assist and myocardial repair with synchronously stimulated skeletal muscle. *Surg Forum* 1980, 31:271.
59. Furnary AP, Jessup M, Moreira LFP: Multicenter trial of dynamic cardiomyoplasty for chronic heart failure. *J Am Coll Cardiol* 1996; 28:1175.
60. Carpentier A, Chachques JC, Acar C, et al: Dynamic cardiomyoplasty at seven years. *J Thorac Cardiovasc Surg* 1993; 106:42.
61. Li CM, Chiu RCJ: The mechanisms and optimization of programming, in Brachman J, Stephenson LW (eds): *Current Clinical Practices in Dynamic Cardiomyoplasty*. New York, Futura, 1997; p 1.
62. Badhwar V, Francischelli D, Chiu RCJ: Dynamic cardiomyoplasty, in Masters RG (ed): *Surgical Options for the Treatment of Heart Failure*. Dordrecht, The Netherlands, Kluwer, 1999; p 137.
63. Orghetti-Mario SA, Romano W, Bocchi EA, et al: Quality of life after cardiomyoplasty. *J Heart Lung Transplant* 1994; 13:271.
64. Tasdemir O, Kucukaksu SD, Vural KM, et al: A comparison of the early and midterm results after dynamic cardiomyoplasty in patients with ischemic or idiopathic cardiomyopathy. *J Thorac Cardiovasc Surg* 1997; 113:73.
65. Chen F, Aklog L, deGuzman B, et al: New techniques measure decreased transmural myocardial pressure in cardiomyoplasty. *Ann Thorac Surg* 1995; 60:1678.
66. Oh JH, Badhwar V, Chiu RCJ: Mechanisms of dynamic cardiomyoplasty: current concepts. *J Card Surg* 1996; 11:194.
67. Oh JH, Badhwar V, Mott BD, et al: The effects of prosthetic cardiac binding and adynamic cardiomyoplasty in a model of dilated cardiomyopathy. *J Thorac Cardiovasc Surg* 1998; 116:148.
68. Sabbah HN, Chaudry PA, Kleber F, et al: Passive mechanical containment of progressive left ventricular dilation: a surgical approach to the treatment of heart failure. *J Heart Failure* 2000; 6:115.
69. Power JM, Raman J, Dornom A, et al: Passive ventricular constraint amends the course of heart failure: a study in an ovine model of dilated cardiomyopathy. *Cardiovasc Res* 1999; 44:549.
70. Chaudhry PA, Mishima T, Sharov VG, et al: Passive epicardial containment prevents ventricular remodeling in heart failure. *Ann Thorac Surg* 2000; 70:1275.
71. Konertz WF, Shapland JE, Hotz H, et al: Passive containment and reverse remodeling by a novel textile cardiac support device. *Circulation* 2001; 104(suppl I):1270.

Chapter 65

Tissue Engineering for Cardiac Surgery

Fraser W. H. Sutherland/John E. Mayer, Jr.

Tissue engineering is a term that embraces the many processes involved in trying to recreate organs in the laboratory. The impetus for this work derives from the need to replace tissues that have either been lost to disease/trauma or that failed to develop properly during embryogenesis. Although a relatively new term, the underlying concept is a natural scientific progression from the ability to culture cells in vitro, the development of biodegradable materials for use in surgery, the widespread acceptance of orthotopic transplantation by the medical community, and stark realization of the many problems that attend organ transplantation today. The potential demand for replacement tissues is high and in the last decade many biotechnology companies have entered this space, chasing forward multiples that are truly astounding. The total market for tissue engineering by 2006 has been estimated at $80 billion. Nevertheless, except in a few specific areas, tissue engineering remains in its infancy.

This chapter summarizes some of the progress that has been made in tissue engineering research as it relates to cardiac surgery and will seek to identify areas within the specialty where it is likely to have most impact. Even within this one specialty there are many different pathologies, and tissue engineering does not hold equal promise for all. Nevertheless, there are some areas where one might anticipate that tissue engineering solutions may have a profound impact on future surgical practice.

Tissue engineering is driven by the quest to restore function. It follows that in the creation of first-generation products, emphasis should be placed on their functional behavior in vivo rather than on esoteric parameters such as detailed tissue microstructure and elaborate histologic comparisons with normal tissues. At a very superficial level, it is clear that the heart has parts that function *actively*, such as the muscle and conduction pathways, and parts whose function is largely *passive* in response to intravascular flow and pressures created by the former elements. Historically, it has been possible to replace those parts of the heart that passively provide function, such as the cardiac valves and great arteries, baffles within the chambers of the heart, and patches to close defects between adjacent chambers with wholly synthetic elements. The results of these techniques have largely been very successful and hampered only by the interaction of body fluids with the surface of materials[1,2] or cavitation in the flow of blood through rigid moving parts.[3,4] With the possible exception of pacemakers, attempts to mimic actively functioning elements of the heart such as the myocardium have either failed or remain outside of wide clinical practice. There are still many problems to be overcome in respect of ventricular assist devices and artificial hearts.[5–7] So too it is anticipated that in the creation of tissue-engineered elements for the cardiovascular system, heart valves, conduits, and baffles/patches are likely to be somewhat easier to develop than a segment of graftable, coordinated, and contracting muscle.

Tissue engineering holds one further promise that has peculiar significance to the pediatric population: the potential to create replacement materials that can grow or at least increase in size with the increase in size and attendant physiological demands on blood flow of the developing child.[8] Although there remains no absolutely clear evidence to support the growth hypothesis, it is this anticipation that forms the cornerstone of research efforts in the field of tissue-engineered heart valves.

THE CREATION OF HEART VALVES AND SIMPLE CONDUITS

It is natural that tissue engineering research should focus first on the pulmonary circulation where existing solutions are unsatisfactory,[9,10] and lower physiological pressures make this environment much more forgiving to the developing technology. The intention is then to translate these findings into valves and conduits for the systemic circulation that have the potential to benefit adult patients suffering from acquired valvular heart disease and ischemic heart disease. In a multidisciplinary collaborative effort that has come to characterize tissue engineering research in general, work at Children's Hospital, Boston, in conjunction with the Brigham and Women's Hospital and the Massachusetts Institute of Technology has focused on the optimizing the cell source, mechanisms for cell delivery, and scaffold design as they relate to the tissue engineering of heart valves.

A considerable effort has been placed on selecting the optimal cell source for tissue engineering applications. In brief, the choice may be broadly categorized into stem cells or pleuripotent cells that exhibit the potential to differentiate into multiple cell types and fully committed or differentiated cells. The choice is further segmented between autologous and allogeneic cells, and between the anatomical source of those cells, i.e., from the proposed tissue that is to be fabricated or from anatomically distinct elements. The ultimate choice will likely reflect, however, a complex interplay between what is favored in terms of basic cell biology, what tissues are available for harvest in the individual patient, and what is clinically acceptable to both patient and physician.

In the field of heart valves, considerable early success was achieved using immature myofibroblasts and endothelial cells derived from systemic arteries.[11–13] These cells were chosen by virtue of their anatomical location within the arterial limb of the cardiovascular system and their known ability to synthesize structural extracellular elements such as collagen. The prospect of harvesting segments of artery from an otherwise normal peripheral circulation presents a somewhat unattractive solution clinically, however, and led to the search for alternative cell sources. A comparison of myofibroblasts from the wall of the ascending aorta with those from discarded segments of saphenous vein revealed that the latter cells exhibit superior collagen formation and mechanical strength when cultured on biodegradable polyurethane scaffolds.[14] Enhanced collagen formation may be a two-edged sword. The rapid formation of new tissue in the early culture period could give rise to uncontrolled proliferation and synthesis of matrix elements, similar to the development of intimal hyperplasia when venous grafts are introduced into the arterial circulation. Mature cells may, furthermore, present a problem of senescence in long-term culture, which typically spans many weeks. Techniques are currently being explored to increase the replicative lifespan of human vascular cells while maintaining their differentiated phenotype and capability of synthesizing extracellular matrix in vitro.

The search for a more attractive source of cells has stimulated interest in the use of stem cells for tissue engineering. The latter may be isolated from a variety of tissues including skeletal muscle,[15] adipose tissue,[16] bone marrow,[17] and peripheral blood.[18] The latter study demonstrated that endothelial progenitor cells may be isolated from peripheral blood, expanded in vitro, and delivered onto decellularized allografts. These grafts remained functional for up to 130 days as carotid interposition grafts in sheep. The feasibility of using stem cells derived from the bone marrow of sheep to create semilunar valves has also been demonstrated by our own group both in vitro and in vivo (unpublished data).

One final cell strategy is *not* to provide cells at all, but to allow grafts to "repopulate" in vivo from the host.[19] In one study, porcine or sheep heart valves were decellularized and implanted as pulmonary or aortic valve replacements in sheep. Recellularization was evaluated histologically after intervals of between 3 and 11 months with cell phenotypes identified using specific antibodies. The heart valves showed progressive recellularization, with cell density and distribution at 11 months approaching that of native valve leaflets and localization of smooth muscle actin positive cells at the ventricularis/spongiosa interface. Of course this strategy is only applicable to grafts that are capable of functioning in the circulation as scaffolds alone, which is currently not the case with synthetic biodegradable scaffolds.

Cell Delivery Methodologies

A reliable method for delivering cells to polymer scaffolds in vitro is fundamental to the development of tissue-engineered structures. In early tissue engineering methodologies developed in our laboratory, valves were made on an individual basis by delivering cells in a concentrated paste onto scaffolds held in an open dish. These constructs were then left for an arbitrary period of time for cell attachment before being immersed in cell culture medium.[13,20] There were a number of theoretical problems intrinsic to this technique. First, it is very difficult to obtain an even distribution of cells over complex surfaces such as that of a semilunar heart valve scaffold; second, there is the potential for cell death through depletion of metabolites and accumulation of metabolic waste products in this extremely concentrated paste during the time allowed for cell attachment. An alternative technique is to deliver cells from suspension by immersing the entire scaffold within that suspension. However, in a static system, cells that do not immediately encounter the scaffold tend to deposit onto the base of the container and are effectively lost. It therefore becomes necessary to develop a mechanism for continual resuspension of unattached cells. Shaker and spinner flasks have been used in the past for this purpose.[21] However, the physical forces created by such violent movements have the disadvantage of tending to disrupt nascent cell-polymer interactions. We compared the efficacy of two rotating systems as vehicles for cell delivery to our cardiovascular scaffolds, a rotating wall vessel (RWV, Synthecon Inc., TX), originally developed by NASA scientists to study the behavior of cells under conditions of microgravity, and a system of rotating individual sealed tubes (RIST). Scaffolds were fabricated from polyglycolic acid mesh dip-coated in poly-4-hydrobutyrate according to a method developed previously[13] and placed in each of the cell culture systems. Cell-scaffold constructs were assayed for DNA content as a surrogate for cell number after 5 days. Total DNA per conduit was $226 \pm 7\mu g$ for conduits seeded in the RIST and $396 \pm 18\mu g$ for conduits in the RWV, suggesting that the RWV culture system provides a superior environment to the RIST for delivering cells onto polymer scaffolds. In this system, scaffolds are placed in the annular space between a cylindrical outer wall and a central core membrane; the entire assembly is placed in an incubator with atmosphere enriched with 5% CO_2 maintained at 37°C. This maintains a relatively constant physiological milieu protecting constructs from fluctuating temperature, pH, and mechanical forces disruptive to cell attachment. Indeed, the RWV has also seen wider application within tissue engineering, specifically to mature small pieces of PGA mesh seeded with chondrocytes.[22] Such constructs exhibited far superior tissue formation to those grown in static culture or to the mixer flasks alluded to above.[23] It has further been shown that cell delivery systems that utilize rotation favor the uniform distribution of cells over polymer scaffolds and by corollary the uniform formation of tissue on valves engineered in vitro (FWH Sutherland and TE Perry, unpublished data). Work is currently underway to devise a system that combines the benefits of gas exchange afforded by the RWV with a scaffold-enclosing membrane that restricts the movement of cells to the vicinity of the scaffold yet allows free movement of media, nutrients and dissolved gases with the much larger volume of the RWV. At the time of writing we are seeking to overcome technical difficulties related to the selecting a membrane of suitable pore size for this purpose.

In summary, the ability to deliver cells to cardiovascular scaffolds in a uniform and predictable manner will permit the generation of groups of scaffolds with identical numbers of cells. This is a prerequisite to the design of experiments to interrogate subsequent steps in the tissue engineering process. Ongoing research in this area is essential in order to facilitate scale-up and commercial application of tissue engineering for the benefit of patients.

Optimal Scaffold Design

A fundamental difference in the various tissue engineering strategies that have been adopted in the cardiovascular field centers on the choice of scaffold. The options fall broadly between the use of decellularized tissues or wholly synthetic matrices. Until recently, a significant advantage of decellularized grafts has been their established and appropriate geometry for valves and the density of extracellular material contained therein, which contributes significantly to the short-term integrity of small vessel conduits[18] or heart valves.[24] Tissue-engineered grafts made in this manner and using a variety of cell types have proved functional following implantation in animal models.[18] However, the disadvantages of decellularized grafts include the relative shortage of available homografts and immunogenecity problems that may arise from the use of decellularized xenogeneic tissues. Perhaps more importantly, the density of residual extracellular matrix that proves attractive from a structural point of view prevents the penetration of seeded cells into the interstices of the matrix. Furthermore, given the complex and ill-understood interaction between the cytoskeleton and extracellular matrix in normal tissues, it may be naïve to expect cells seeded onto decellularized tissues to assume those same relationships with foreign matrix elements.

One further scaffold that deserves mention is small intestinal submucosa (SIS). Grafts of SIS are prepared by removing the serosal layer, inverting the material, and removing the surface mucosa. The remaining submucosa and stratum compactum constitute the graft material.[25] SIS is an acellular structure that elicits relatively little cross-species immunogenicity.[26] In these respects, SIS represents the ideal naturally occurring material and preliminary studies have suggested that it may provide a very favorable substrate for tissue regeneration. Indeed, SIS has been implanted, as a substitute patch, into a variety of anatomical locations including the ureter,[27] dura,[28] and small bowel itself.[29] Each study has demonstrated regeneration of host tissue without histologic evidence of sensitization or graft rejection. SIS has also recently been sutured into a tubular form and implanted as an interposition graft into the carotid artery of dogs. Mechanical properties, over time, appear to approach those of the native carotid artery, angiograms show uniform flow without dilatation at two months, and the luminal surface of explanted grafts appears white, shiny, and glistening.[30] These encouraging results prompted interest in the use of this material for the fabrication of a substitute heart valve. Unfortunately, a major stumbling block remains in how to fabricate the highly complex, multiply curved, surface geometry of a heart valve and accompanying root from *flat* sheets of tissue. This is a problem that has faced heart valve manufacturers for many years. One could certainly draw upon traditional methods of heart valve assembly that, for example, utilize Elgiloy stents. However, this approach would seem to offer little or no advantage over the well-proven, stented, pericardial valves in use today.

Biodegradable polymers that have thus far been used for tissue engineering applications are mainly based on materials already in clinical use. In the group of macromolecules of natural origin collagen, alginate, agarose, hyaluronic acid derivatives, chitosan, and fibrin glue have been used as scaffolds. Man-made polymers such as polyglycolide (PGA), polylactides (PLLA, PDLA), poly(caprolactone) (PCL), and poly(dioxanone) (PDS) have also been studied. More recently, the fabrication of biodegradable elastomers has broadened the biomechanical possibilities of available scaffolds even further. Appropriate selection of a scaffold material in terms of its mechanical properties and degradation characteristics must be matched to each specific tissue engineering application.

Nonwoven textiles manufactured from these materials have proved to be particularly well suited to tissue engineering applications because they can be made highly porous and exhibit extensive interporous connections that allow cells to penetrate and adhere to fibers through the full thickness of the scaffold. Furthermore, the fibers are not stretched taught as in a woven material, and therefore the material exhibits a degree of "give" that, it is hoped, should not restrict subsequent growth of the nascent tissue. From an engineering perspective, the Young's modulus is larger for nonwovens than for equivalent textiles made using a weave, and it is possible, at least in principle, to match the change in modulus of the nonwoven mesh as the polymer degrades over time with the requirement for growth imposed by the pediatric application.

Polyglycolic acid, PGA, was introduced into clinical practice as a biodegradable suture material and marketed under the trade name Dexon (U.S. Surgical, Norwalk, CT). It has since been adopted by many research groups as a scaffold for a variety of potential tissue engineering applications.[31] The ability to extrude PGA into fibers permits it to be fabricated into nonwoven sheets with an open structure. Pore size has been shown to be important in the choice of scaffold for tissue engineering liver for a variety of cell types including hepatocytes.[32] An open pore structure is thought to facilitate both cell delivery and subsequent cell proliferation by allowing free access to suspended cells, free diffusion of nutrients and dissolved gases, and removal of waste products of metabolism. These spatial properties combined with a consistent and rapid loss of polymer mass relative to other biodegradable materials make PGA an attractive choice for tissue engineering.

Biodegradable scaffolds for tissue engineering heart valves have been assembled from flat sheets of nonwoven PGA fibers, impregnated with the thermoplastic polymer poly-4-hydroxybutyrate (P4HB). These flat sheets were then assembled into a trileaflet structure by a series of two or more wraps around a cylindrical mandrel. Seams were heat welded at a temperature above the melting point of the P4HB to provide a tube-like, trileaflet-valved conduit.[13]

Despite promising early results using the PGA/P4HB composite, ongoing studies experienced a number of problems with the use of this particular scaffold material. Specifically, because of the rapid hydrolysis of PGA, there was a tendency for collapse of the cell-polymer construct during culture in vitro. A further, unfavorable, characteristic of PGA is that its tensile strength decays far more rapidly than the decay in its residual mass. At the time of implantation, the strength of the construct was highly dependent on the degree of new tissue growth and spontaneous rupture of the conduit wall occurred not infrequently at the time of implantation. One further but related problem was tearing of the grafts at the suture line during implantation. It appeared that most, if not all, of these problems were attributable to loss in tensile strength of the nonwoven mesh over time, itself a reflection of changes in the tensile properties of the individual fibers. Based on these problems we formally set out a number of criteria required of the scaffold at different time points in the tissue engineering process. It was clear that first and foremost we require a *template* in the geometry of a normal heart valve to which cells will attach at the time of cell delivery; second, we required a *mechanical support* for the cell-template construct that would maintain the structural integrity during culture, implantation, and into the short- to mid-term postoperative period; and finally, a *skeleton* was required onto which sutures could be anchored at the time of implantation and the resultant forces distributed through the whole body of the graft. We perceived that these requirements could be served by a composite nonwoven mesh incorporating the rapidly degrading PGA fibers to provide the geometric template with the much more slowly degrading PLLA fibers to provide the structural support and anchorage for the suture lines.

Poly L-lactic acid, PLLA, the α-methyl–substituted form of PGA, was initially developed for the biodegradable suture market but failed to become popular in that capacity. The polymer hydrolyzes at a much slower rate than PGA, which is made from the unsubstituted glycolide monomer. The initial tensile strength of PLLA is, however, less than that of PGA or many of the other biodegradable sutures such as PDS, vicryl, or silk, making it less suitable as an absorbable suture material. Studies in vivo conducted on rats have shown the breaking force of PLLA to diminish by 20% during the first 2 weeks but to remain relatively constant for up to 4 weeks thereafter when used for fascial closure. Suture material in this study appeared intact at 28 weeks but had largely disappeared by 52 weeks.[33] In a separate study, 8-0 PLLA fibers were found to retain 70% to 100% of their strength over a 12-week period of in vitro degradation. The more sustained tensile properties of PLLA have already led to its use in orthopedic applications where fixation with biodegradable miniplates and screws avoids the need for subsequent removal. Comparison of PGA and PLLA miniscrews implanted into the calvarium of sheep showed fragmentation and hydrolysis of PGA at 4 to 6 weeks and total absorption by 12 weeks. In contrast, PLLA miniscrews retained their integrity and holding power at 26 weeks but had mostly resorbed by 2 years.[34] PLLA materials are now being investigated for use in a range of biodegradable applications including urethral and cardiovascular stents[35] where the rapid loss of tensile properties exhibited by PGA might permit early restenosis or closure.

Stress-strain data have been collected for combinations of PGA/PLLA in nonwoven meshes using uniaxial tests of tensile strength and found to be highly suited to a role in the wall of tissue-engineered heart valves on the pulmonary side of the circulation. Further mechanical studies are underway, in conjunction with Dr. Michael Sacks' laboratory for soft tissue biomechanics at the University of Pittsburgh, to optimize the flexural behavior of this nonwoven textile for the valve leaflets.

The next problem has been to develop a means of assembling scaffolds from sheets of nonwoven textiles that recapitulate the surface geometry of the native pulmonary valve and trunk. On the surface of it this would appear to be a perfectly straightforward task. However, the necessity of fabricating such a structure from a nonwoven material required the development of some novel textile technologies. We have developed a means of fitting flat sheets of mesh over molds with multiple axes of curvature. This is achieved by needle punching around the periphery of the mold using custom-cut felting needles. The needle-punching process permits adjoining layers of nonwoven textiles to be united without evidence of layering in the final product.[36] While these technologies have been developed for use with the PGA/PLLA mesh described above, the methods remain broadly applicable to a wide range of nonwoven textiles in the fabrication of a variety of anatomical elements. In essence, these techniques permit the fabrication of a structure comprising the multiply curved surfaces of three symmetrical valve leaflets and their respective sinuses of Valsalva. This mode of assembly creates a wholly symmetrical and unitary structure with no sutures or residual evidence of lamination.

The role of computational models with respect to heart valves presents a much less complex problem than presented below for the development of soft tissues. Nevertheless, models have proved useful in predicting and optimizing the geometry of valves. The role of computational fluid dynamics, important as it is to the design and characterization of flow through prosthetic mechanical valves, assumes much less importance to the tissue-engineered valve in which one seeks to mimic nature in terms of geometry and viscoelastic properties of the valve leaflets over time. Even with very stiff leaflets it is unlikely that the normal function of flexible tissue-engineered valve leaflets will generate microcavitation in the flow of blood between them.

As to the future, there are a number of emerging technologies that have the potential to provide scaffolds with the desired geometry, porosity, and connectivity between pores for tissue engineering applications. Specifically, advanced manufacturing technologies known as rapid prototyping or solid freeform fabrication are under investigation. In essence, rapid prototyping (RP) is the process of creating a three-dimensional (3-D) object through repetitive deposition of material in 2-D layers from a computer-aided design (CAD) virtual model of the object using a slicing algorithm.[37] Although RP has been available for a decade now and data on the geometry of anatomical elements has been widely available from MRI or CT images of normal human subjects for even longer, conventional RP techniques do not have sufficient resolution to fabricate scaffolds with the porosity and extensive interporous connections considered necessary for tissue engineering and which are currently available from textile technologies.

One further perspective on the future of scaffolds for tissue engineering in general will be the ability to deliver cytokines locally to developing tissues through advances in the field of drug delivery in conjunction with existing human recombinant technologies. This has already proved possible in the engineering of regenerative elements for orthopedic surgery by the provision of bone morphogenic proteins (BMPs) from poly-D,L-lactic acid-p-dioxanone-polyethylene glycol block coplymer (PLA-DX-PEG), a synthetic biodegradable polymer used to tissue engineer bone.[38] As yet these techniques have not been applied widely to the engineering of soft tissues, however.

It is clear that the success of tissue-engineered grafts in cardiac surgery will be intimately related to the properties of the underlying scaffold. Despite the promise of emerging technologies, it is likely that a plethora of first-generation products utilizing existing polymers and established technologies will emerge over the next decade.

Evaluation of Tissue-Engineered Heart Valves in Vivo

Tissue-engineered valve leaflets and valves proper have been evaluated in a series of experiments spanning several years and many design and tissue culture iterations.[11,13,39,40] Most recently, we have undertaken a detailed evaluation of the hemodynamic performance of tissue-engineered valves acutely in the sheep model. Valves grown over many weeks in culture (Fig. 65-1) exhibit the histology shown in Figure 65-2 with dense tissue formation on inner and outer surfaces and relatively less tissue in the depth of the structure. Following implantation (Fig. 65-3), valve gradients are typically found to be less than 5 mm Hg with only trivial regurgitation in the resting state. Through the use of echocardiography, the valve leaflets are seen to open symmetrically into their respective sinuses, creating an effective orifice area that is typically in the region of 2.0 to 2.5 cm^2 for a 21-mm valve at 5 L/min cardiac output. Echocardiography has furthermore enabled a detailed analysis of the shape and morphology of various components of the valve throughout the cardiac cycle. Figure 65-4 demonstrates the curvaceous outline of the valve sinus and the smooth continuity that exists between the sinus and the valve leaflets. Close inspection of the leaflets in the commissural regions in late systole (Fig. 65-5) shows an absence of the reverse bending that has been the cause of stress-related tears in

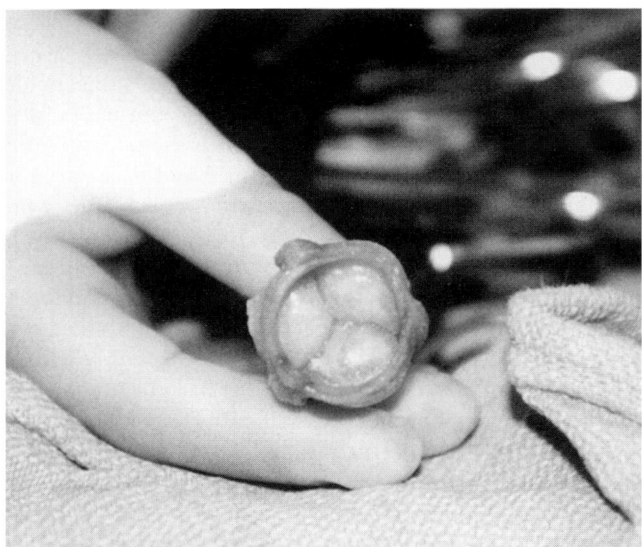

FIGURE 65–1 The tissue-engineered substitute pulmonary valve viewed from below prior to implantation.

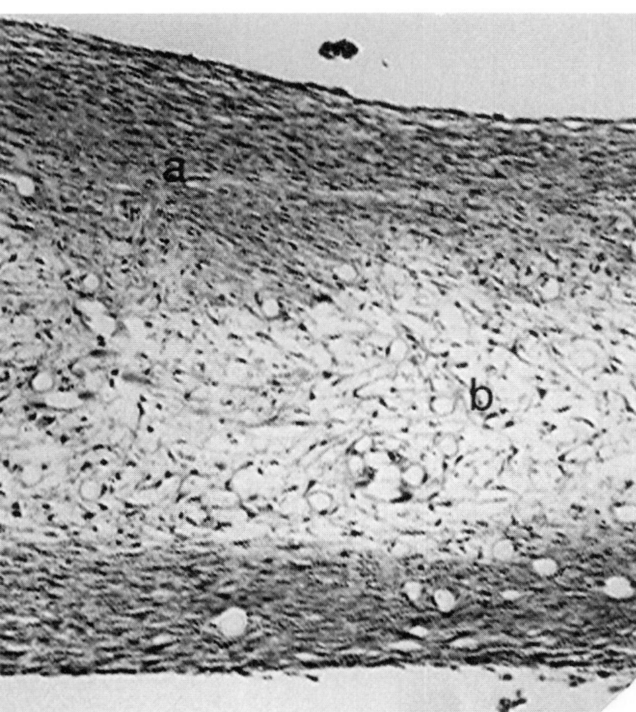

FIGURE 65–2 Histology of the tissue-engineered substitute pulmonary valve showing dense surface tissue formation (a) and relatively fewer cells deep in the wall of the construct (b). H.& E. ×100.

explanted bioprostheses. Stress sharing between the valve leaflet and its respective sinus together with the absence of reverse bending are expected to have a significant impact on the longevity of tissue-engineered valves just as they have for classical biologic prostheses.

The results from these short-term studies are indeed very encouraging. However, it is too early to say what the long-term fate of tissue-engineered grafts will be in terms of their function and ability to increase in size, as required by our pediatric patients.

THE CREATION OF HEART MUSCLE SUBSTITUTES

In regard to heart muscle, the central problem facing physicians is that adult myocardium lacks the ability to regenerate. Tissue engineering of heart muscle is principally aimed at improving the outlook for patients who have lost the function of substantial portions of their left ventricular wall because of ischemic heart disease. Conceivably a variety of other smaller patient groups may also potentially benefit from these advances.

Approaches to the tissue engineering of myocardium have many similarities to those that address the fabrication of substitute heart valves, as outlined above. One principal difference, however, is the notion of using the scar itself as a scaffold. The idea that a scar may be repopulated with functional cells has emerged over the last decade and stimulated many research groups to look for a suitable cell type. A variety of cell types have indeed been injected into myocardium under different experimental conditions. While transformed cell lines appear intuitively very attractive, the risk of uncontrolled cellular proliferation is real. For example, primary myoblasts engineered to contain vascular endothelial growth factor (VEGF) and injected into myocardium in one study resulted in the formation of hemangiomas and the appearance of VEGF in the circulation.[41] Until recently, however, most studies have concentrated on the use of fetal cardiomyocytes or satellite cells from skeletal muscle.

Cultured fetal cardiomyocytes, in particular, have been extensively investigated.[42–48] Fetal cardiomyocytes have been shown to survive after implantation into host myocardium.[49,50] Furthermore, the functional benefits of cardiomyocyte injection have been demonstrated in two well-established models of myocardial infarction created by cryonecrosis[43] and coronary artery ligation.[48] These cells have then been shown to form gap junctions with those of the recipient myocardium.[42] The hope is that connections such as these should permit the transplanted cells to beat in synchrony with the recipient myocardium.

In contrast to fetal cardiomyocytes, satellite cells within skeletal muscle are morphologically undifferentiated cells that lie dormant between the plasma membrane and basal lamina. With appropriate stimuli, these cells will proliferate and differentiate into new skeletal muscle fibers.[51] The hypothesis that satellite cells might be able to undergo "milieu-dependent" differentiation into cardiac myocytes was first put forward by Chiu et al in 1995.[52] They began by

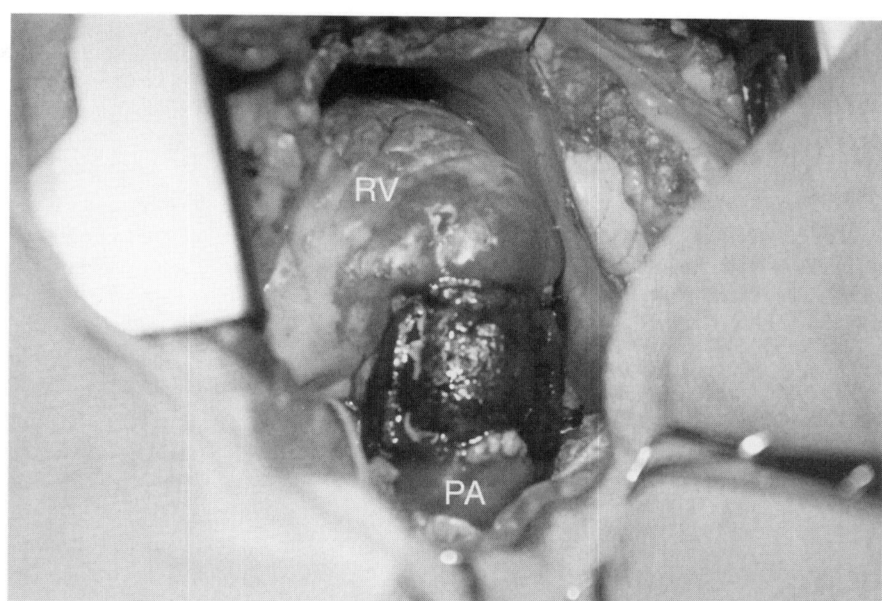

FIGURE 65–3 The tissue-engineered substitute pulmonary valve interposed within the main pulmonary artery as seen through a right fourth space thoracotomy. RV = right ventricle; PA = pulmonary artery.

implanting autologous satellite cells isolated from skeletal muscle into canine myocardium in a cryoinjury model and were able to demonstrate the presence of striated muscle fibers at the implant sites. These cells showed morphologic characteristics of cardiac myofibrils such as the centrally located nuclei and the presence of intercalated disks. They later confirmed the feasibility of satellite cell differentiation into muscle fibers after implantation into the myocardium of isogenic rats using the cell marker 4',6-diamidino-2-phenylindone, which binds to DNA and to the protein tubulin to form a fluorescent complex.[51] There are obvious advantages to using autologous donor myoblasts in preference to fetal tissues. Ethical and regulatory issues abound in the area of human fetal cells. Furthermore, cells transplanted

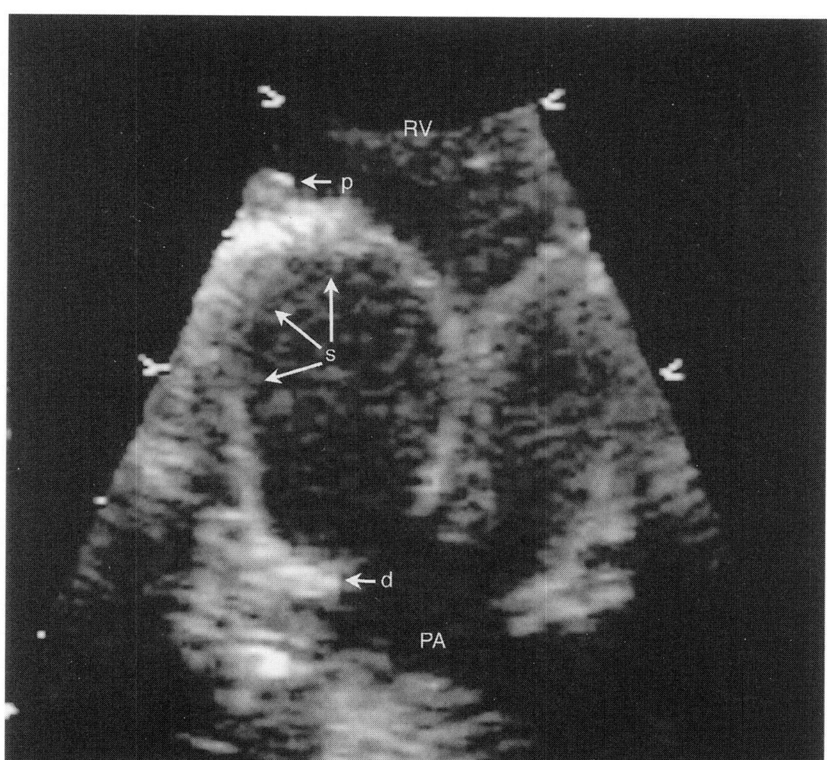

FIGURE 65–4 Long axis echocardiogram of the substitute pulmonary valve in diastole showing proximal (p) and distal (d) suture lines and smooth continuity between the sinus (s) and the valve leaflet. RV = right ventricle; PA = pulmonary artery.

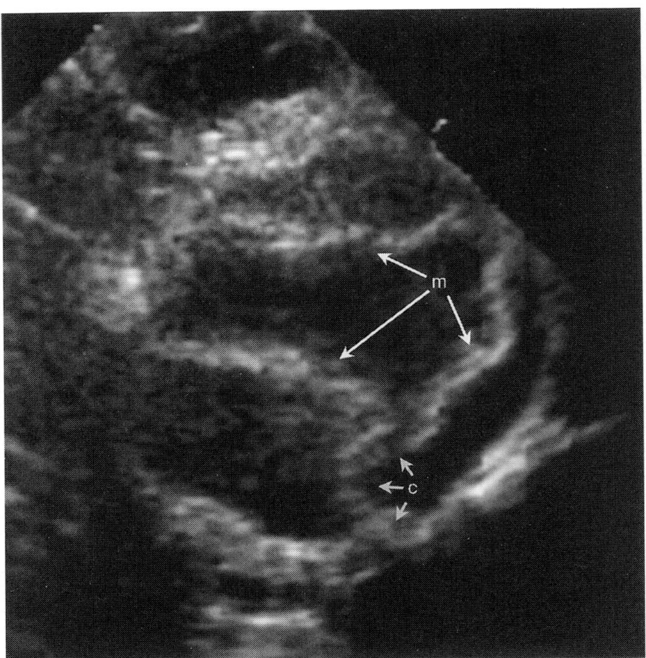

FIGURE 65–5 Short axis echocardiogram of substitute pulmonary valve in late systole showing the leaflet free margins (m) and absence of reverse bending at the commissures (c).

into potential adult patients would, by necessity, be allogeneic, raising the possibility of rejection.

Scorsin et al compared the use of cellular transplantation of fetal cardiomyocytes with that of neonatal skeletal myoblasts and uninjected controls in rats. Their model used coronary artery ligation to create a zone of myocardial infarction. Functional assessment was made by 2-D echocardiography. In this study, they were able to demonstrate a decrease in LV function following coronary artery ligation, as anticipated. However, a significant improvement was seen in the calculated ejection fraction of injured hearts that had been injected with both fetal cardiomyocyte and skeletal myoblast groups 1 month earlier. Although the sample size was quite small, there was no difference demonstrable between the two experimental groups. This and other studies have opened the door to the future possibility of "cellular cardiomyoplasty" by removing the requirement for fetal tissues.

These studies also led some groups to take a closer look at the myocardium itself. Although the lack of regenerative capacity of adult myocardium would appear to preclude its use as a potential cell source, some researchers have questioned this traditional dogma. Indeed, atrial cardiomyocytes may be cultured in the presence of fetal calf serum and resemble immature cardiomyocytes, more so even than ventricular cardiomyocytes, which may also be cultured in vitro.[53] Atrial cardiomyocytes are of course clinically quite accessible by endomyocardial biopsy. The Toronto group has transplanted cardiomyocytes cultured from the left atrial appendage of adult rats and expanded in vitro into a transmural scar created 3 weeks earlier at the time of cell harvest. Five weeks later ventricular function, evaluated after explantation in a Langendorff preparation, showed systolic and developed pressures as well as maximal rates of myocardial contraction and relaxation significantly better in the transplanted group than controls. Histologically, the cultured cells were shown to have survived within the scar tissue, even in the absence of an apparent blood supply. The area occupied by the LV scar was smaller and its thickness greater than that of controls and LV chamber volume was furthermore noted to be smaller in the transplanted group.

Although the future prospects of cardiomyocyte transplantation or "cellular cardiomyoplasty" are intriguing, especially for patients with established scar formation who are not expected to benefit from coronary revascularization, the mechanism of action remains elusive. A criticism of early experimental models that used cryoinjury alone was a failure of the model to wholly reflect the occlusive pathology that characterizes ischemic heart disease. Nevertheless, the demonstration of these same functional improvements in hearts in which the model for injury has been created by coronary artery ligation has perplexed cardiac surgeons. One would anticipate that the survival of cells implanted deep within myocardial scar tissue would necessitate rapid and thorough revascularization. However, there appears to be little evidence of neovascularization in these studies. Indeed, the functional benefits may not be related to any ongoing cellular functionality but follow simply from changes to the physical characteristics of the scar itself. These and many other questions need to be addressed before this technique finds its way to the clinic.

More generally, the survival of cells that are deeply embedded within cell-polymer constructs raises the question of how to provide for the rapid and thorough revascularization of tissue-engineered elements. One approach to this problem has been through the delivery of angiogenic molecules from the underlying polymer scaffolds. The delivery of specific growth factors, or plasmid DNA encoding the factors, with defined doses and rates at the site where blood vessel growth is desired may now be possible. Such systems will likely have significant utility in the engineering of large tissue volumes and may indeed provide novel, model systems for studying human angiogenesis in vivo.[54]

The more traditional approach to tissue engineering, trying to create of a segment of cardiac muscle from its constituent elements in vitro, would seem to present a much more complex problem than that of creating a functional heart valve. While a heart valve functions largely passively in response to pressure changes in adjacent cardiac chambers and great arteries, cardiac muscle must assume an active role in its function. A noncontractile patch is destined to suffer from paradoxical motion if interposed into the ventricular free wall, a point well illustrated by transmural scars arising from earlier myocardial infarction. In essence, individual cells are required to contract and to do so in a coordinated manner in synchrony with the recipient myocardium. The creation of a contractile element is thus the core of the problem. Furthermore, it would appear that, at least intuitively, the final product will require a blood supply and that cells must be assembled in such a way that the integrity of the structure is maintained in the face of significant intraventricular pressures and shortening of tissue-engineered elements that allows them to contribute meaningfully to contraction of the structure as a whole. This equates to the building of a very complex system and one for which armchair (qualitative) thinking is wholly inadequate. For this reason, it is thought that modeling, through the use of computers, may provide a useful tool. Indeed, the results of modeling very complex systems are frequently counterintuitive.[55]

The amount of biological data currently available that relates to the heart and generated by new technologies is truly overwhelming. There is, already, rich data available in the literature on the three-dimensional geometry of the heart as a whole. Anatomically detailed models of the heart include fiber orientations and sheet structure that permit one to reconstruct the electrical and mechanical behavior of the organ. Furthermore, accurate cellular models have also become highly sophisticated. Models exist for the electromechanical function of all of the main types of cardiac myocyte; in many cases there are multiple models for a given cell type. Connecting these two levels, an accurate reconstruction of the depolarization waveform has been beautifully demonstrated across a virtual framework of the heart. Extensions of this work by incorporation of the ventricular model into a virtual torso have enabled computers to simulate the conducting properties of different tissues and reconstruct the ECG chest and limb leads.[56] Despite, the complex anatomy and lack of symmetry in most soft tissues, a special computational challenge, material properties of the native heart and its ventricular mechanics have also been modeled during the early filling phase of diastole by coupling finite elasticity theory with finite element analysis.[57] These examples serve to illustrate the potential power that in silico biology has to offer tissue engineering.

By way of example, in one potential iteration, anatomically detailed models of the coronary circulation, developed to study the effects of transmural pressure on blood flow, could be rapid prototyped and serve as the scaffold onto which various myocardial elements could be assembled. This model could be connected to existing models of cellular function or new models of specific cell types, such as skeletal myoblasts that are envisaged as potential cell sources, to predict the electrical behavior of the construct. Further connections with models that describe the material properties of those cells and the underlying scaffold over time might be able to predict the ventricular mechanics of potential tissue substitutes even before they have been formed.

In contrast to models of individual cellular functions, which typically run on PCs, this kind of work that uses integrative elements from several models requires massive computing power and program codes, such as CMISS developed at the University of Auckland as part of the Cardiome project, to enable such models to communicate freely with one another. The true prospects for regenerative medicine in the future will likely be closely tied to the development of new supercomputers and to the continued sophistication of mathematical models that describe nature.

We must anticipate that there will be many experimental iterations between now and the clinical reality of tissue engineering. Nevertheless, the mere prospect of being able to fashion substitute elements for the cardiovascular system in the laboratory provides a healthy stimulus for ongoing research in this area.

REFERENCES

1. Bolz A, Schaldach M: Haemocompatibility optimisation of implants by hybrid structuring. *Med Biol Eng Comput* 1993; 31 (suppl): S123.
2. Bruck SD: The effect of the physiological environment on the mechanical properties of biomaterials in cardiovascular applications. *Biomater Med Devices Artif Organs* 1978; 6:341.
3. Chandran KB, Aluri S: Mechanical valve closing dynamics: relationship between velocity of closing, pressure transients, and cavitation initiation. *Ann Biomed Eng* 1997; 25:926.
4. Bachmann C, Kini V, Deutsch S, et al: Mechanisms of cavitation and the formation of stable bubbles on the Bjork-Shiley Monostrut prosthetic heart valve. *J Heart Valve Dis* 2002; 11:105.
5. Nose Y: Is a totally implantable artificial heart realistic? *Artif Organs* 1992; 16:19.
6. Arabia FA, Copeland JG, Smith RG, et al: International experience with the CardioWest total artificial heart as a bridge to heart transplantation. *Eur J Cardiothorac Surg* 1997; 11(suppl):S5.
7. Copeland JG 3rd, Smith RG, Arabia FA, et al: Comparison of the CardioWest total artificial heart, the Novacor left ventricular assist system and the Thoratec ventricular assist system in bridge to transplantation. *Ann Thorac Surg* 2001; 71(3 suppl):S92.
8. Mayer JE Jr: Uses of homograft conduits for right ventricle to pulmonary artery connections in the neonatal period. *Semin Thorac Cardiovasc Surg* 1995; 7:130.
9. Stark J, Bull C, Stajevic M, et al: Fate of subpulmonary homograft conduits: determinants of late homograft failure. *J Thorac Cardiovasc Surg* 1998; 115:506.
10. Forbess JM, Shah AS, St Louis JD, et al: Cryopreserved homografts in the pulmonary position: determinants of durability. *Ann Thorac Surg* 2001; 71:54.
11. Shinoka T, Breuer CK, Tanel RE, et al: Tissue engineering heart valves: valve leaflet replacement study in a lamb model. *Ann Thorac Surg* 1995; 60(6 suppl):S513.
12. Sodian R, Hoerstrup SP, Sperling JS, et al: Tissue engineering of heart valves: in vitro experiences. *Ann Thorac Surg* 2000; 70:140.
13. Hoerstrup SP, Sodian R, Daebritz S, et al: Functional living trileaflet heart valves grown in vitro. *Circulation* 2000; 102(suppl 3):III44.
14. Schnell AM, Hoerstrup SP, Zund G, et al: Optimal cell source for cardiovascular tissue engineering: venous vs. aortic human myofibroblasts. *Thorac Cardiovasc Surg* 2001; 49:221.
15. Deasy BM, Jankowski RJ, Huard J: Muscle-derived stem cells: characterization and potential for cell-mediated therapy. *Blood Cells Mol Dis* 2001; 27:924.
16. Zuk PA, Zhu M, Mizuno H, et al: Multilineage cells from human adipose tissue: implications for cell- based therapies. *Tissue Eng* 2001; 7:211.

17. Perry TE, Kaushal S, Sutherland FWH, et al: Bone marrow as a cell source for tissue engineering heart valves. *Ann Thorac Surg (in press)*.
18. Kaushal S, Amiel GE, Guleserian KJ, et al: Functional small-diameter neovessels created using endothelial progenitor cells expanded ex vivo. *Nat Med* 2001; 7:1035.
19. Elkins RC, Goldstein S, Hewitt CW, et al: Recellularization of heart valve grafts by a process of adaptive remodeling. *Semin Thorac Cardiovasc Surg* 2001; 13(suppl 1):87.
20. Shinoka T, Breuer CK, Tanel RE, et al: Tissue engineering heart valves: valve leaflet replacement study in a lamb model. *Ann Thorac Surg* 1995; 60(6 suppl):S513.
21. Kim BS, Putnam AJ, Kulik TJ, Mooney DJ: Optimizing seeding and culture methods to engineer smooth muscle tissue on biodegradable polymer matrices. *Biotechnol Bioeng* 1998; 57:46.
22. Freed LE, Vunjak-Novakovic G, Langer R: Cultivation of cell-polymer cartilage implants in bioreactors. *J Cell Biochem* 1993; 51:257.
23. Vunjak-Novakovic G, Martin I, Obradovic B, et al: Bioreactor cultivation conditions modulate the composition and mechanical properties of tissue-engineered cartilage. *J Orthop Res* 1999; 17:130.
24. Steinhoff G, Stock U, Karim N, et al: Tissue engineering of pulmonary heart valves on allogenic acellular matrix conduits: in vivo restoration of valve tissue. *Circulation* 2000; 102(suppl 3):III50.
25. Marshall SE, Tweedt SM, Greene CH, et al: An alternative to synthetic aortic grafts using jejunum. *J Invest Surg* 2000; 13:333.
26. Allman AJ, McPherson TB, Badylak SF, et al: Xenogeneic extracellular matrix grafts elicit a TH2-restricted immune response. *Transplantation* 2001; 71:1631.
27. Jaffe JS, Ginsberg PC, Yanoshak SJ, et al: Ureteral segment replacement using a circumferential small-intestinal submucosa xenogenic graft. *J Invest Surg* 2001; 14:259.
28. Cobb MA, Badylak SF, Janas W, et al: Porcine small intestinal submucosa as a dural substitute. *Surg Neurol* 1999; 51:99.
29. Chen MK, Badylak SF: Small bowel tissue engineering using small intestinal submucosa as a scaffold. *J Surg Res* 2001; 99:352.
30. Roeder R, Wolfe J, Lianakis N, et al: Compliance, elastic modulus, and burst pressure of small-intestine submucosa (SIS), small-diameter vascular grafts. *J Biomed Mater Res* 1999; 47:65.
31. Saxena AK, Marler J, Benvenuto M, et al: Skeletal muscle tissue engineering using isolated myoblasts on synthetic biodegradable polymers: preliminary studies. *Tissue Eng* 1999; 5:525.
32. Ranucci CS, Moghe PV: Polymer substrate topography actively regulates the multicellular organization and liver-specific functions of cultured hepatocytes. *Tissue Eng* 1999; 5:407.
33. Heino A, Naukkarinen A, Kulju T, et al: Characteristics of poly(L-) lactic acid suture applied to fascial closure in rats. *J Biomed Mater Res* 1996; 30:187.
34. Peltoniemi HH, Hallikainen D, Toivonen T, et al: SR-PLLA and SR-PGA miniscrews: biodegradation and tissue reactions in the calvarium and dura mater. *J Craniomaxillofac Surg* 1999; 27:42.
35. Talja M, Valimaa T, Tammela T, et al: Bioabsorbable and biodegradable stents in urology. *J Endourol* 1997; 11:391.
36. Sutherland FWH, Perry TE, Masuda Y, et al: Method of assembly of semi-lunar heart valve scaffold having non-woven mesh structure and total symmetry between three leaflet/sinus units. Presented at the 2002 Prosthetic Valve Workshop, Hilton Head, SC, March 7, 2002.
37. Hutmacher DW: Scaffold design and fabrication technologies for engineering tissues—state of the art and future perspectives. *J Biomater Sci Polym Ed* 2001; 12:107.
38. Saito N, Okada T, Horiuchi H, et al: A biodegradable polymer as a cytokine delivery system for inducing bone formation. *Nat Biotechnol* 2001; 19:332.
39. Stock UA, Nagashima M, Khalil PN, et al: Tissue-engineered valved conduits in the pulmonary circulation. *J Thorac Cardiovasc Surg* 2000; 119:732.
40. Sodian R, Hoerstrup SP, Sperling JS, et al: Early in vivo experience with tissue-engineered trileaflet heart valves. *Circulation* 2000; 102(suppl 3):III-22.
41. Springer ML, Chen AS, Kraft PE, et al: VEGF gene delivery to muscle: potential role for vasculogenesis in adults. *Mol Cell* 1998; 2:549.
42. Soonpaa MH, Koh GY, Klug MG, Field LJ: Formation of nascent intercalated disks between grafted fetal cardiomyocytes and host myocardium. *Science* 1994; 264:98.
43. Li RK, Jia ZQ, Weisel RD, et al: Cardiomyocyte transplantation improves heart function. *Ann Thorac Surg* 1996; 62:654.
44. Li RK, Mickle DA, Weisel RD, et al: Natural history of fetal rat cardiomyocytes transplanted into adult rat myocardial scar tissue. *Circulation* 1997; 96(suppl):II-86.
45. Van MC Jr, Claycomb WC, Delcarpio JB, et al: Myoblast transplantation in the porcine model: a potential technique for myocardial repair. *J Thorac Cardiovasc Surg* 1995; 110:1442.
46. Scorsin M, Marotte F, Sabri A, et al: Can grafted cardiomyocytes colonize peri-infarct myocardial areas? *Circulation* 1996; 94(suppl):II337.
47. Leor J, Patterson M, Quinones MJ, et al: Transplantation of fetal myocardial tissue into the infarcted myocardium of rat: a potential method for repair of infarcted myocardium? *Circulation* 1996; 94(suppl):II332.
48. Scorsin M, Hagege AA, Marotte F, et al: Does transplantation of cardiomyocytes improve function of infarcted myocardium? *Circulation* 1997; 96(suppl):II-93.
49. Connold AL, Frischknecht R, Dimitrakos M, Vrbova G: The survival of embryonic cardiomyocytes transplanted into damaged host rat myocardium. *J Muscle Res Cell Motil* 1997; 18:63.
50. Koh GY, Soonpaa MH, Klug MG, et al: Stable fetal cardiomyocyte grafts in the hearts of dystrophic mice and dogs. *J Clin Invest* 1995; 96:2034.
51. Dorfman J, Duong M, Zibaitis A, et al: Myocardial tissue engineering with autologous myoblast implantation. *J Thorac Cardiovasc Surg* 1998; 116:744.
52. Chiu RC, Zibaitis A, Kao RL: Cellular cardiomyoplasty: myocardial regeneration with satellite cell implantation. *Ann Thorac Surg* 1995; 60:12.
53. Benardeau A, Hatem SN, Rucker-Martin C, et al: Primary culture of human atrial myocytes is associated with the appearance of structural and functional characteristics of immature myocardium. *J Mol Cell Cardiol* 1997; 29:1307.
54. Bouhadir KH, Mooney DJ: Promoting angiogenesis in engineered tissues. *J Drug Target* 2001; 9:397.
55. Noble D: Modeling the heart—from genes to cells to the whole organ. *Science* 2002; 295:1678.
56. Bradley CP, Pullan AJ, Hunter PJ: Geometric modeling of the human torso using cubic hermite elements. *Ann Biomed Eng* 1997; 25:96.
57. Nash MP, Hunter PJ: Computational mechanics of the heart. *J Elasticity* 2000; 61:113.

Index

Page numbers followed by an *f* indicate figures; numbers followed by a *t* indicate tables.